ANESTHESIA
BIOLOGIC FOUNDATIONS

ANESTHESIA
BIOLOGIC FOUNDATIONS

Edited by

Tony L. Yaksh, PhD

Professor and Vice Chairman for Research
Department of Anesthesiology
University of California, San Diego
La Jolla, California

Carl Lynch III, MD, PhD

Professor
Department of Anesthesiology
University of Virginia Health Sciences Center
Charlottesville, Virginia

Warren M. Zapol, MD

Reginald Jenney Professor of Anesthesia
Harvard Medical School
Anesthetist-in-Chief
Massachusetts General Hospital
Boston, Massachusetts

Mervyn Maze, MB, ChB, FRCP

Professor and Research Director
Department of Anesthesia
Stanford University School of Medicine
Stanford, California

Julien F. Biebuyck, MB, DPhil

Eric A. Walker Professor and Chair
Department of Anesthesia
Associate Dean for Academic Affairs
The Pennsylvania State University College of Medicine
Hershey, Pennsylvania

Lawrence J. Saidman, MD

Department of Anesthesia
Stanford University School of Medicine
Stanford, California

Lippincott - Raven
PUBLISHERS
Philadelphia • New York

Acquisitions Editor: R. Craig Percy
Developmental Editor: Anne Snyder
Manufacturing Manager: Tim Reynolds
Production Manager: Larry Bernstein
Production Editor: Pamela Blamey
Cover Designer: Joseph DePinho
Indexer: Kathy Unger
Compositor: Lippincott–Raven Electronic Production
Printer: Courier-Kendallville

Printed in the United States of America

9 8 7 6 5 4 3 2 1

Library of Congress Cataloging-in-Publication Data

Anesthesia : biologic foundations / edited by Tony L. Yaksh ... [et al.].
p. cm.
Includes bibliographical references and index.
ISBN 0-397-58742-2
1. Anesthetics—Mechanism of action. 2. Anesthetics—Physiological effect. 3. Anesthesia—Physiological aspects
I. Yaksh, T. L. (Tony L.), 1944–
[DNLM: 1. Anesthesia—methods. 2. Anesthetics—metabolism. 3. Pain—therapy. WO 200 A5787 1997]
RD85.5.A54 1997
617.9′6—dc21
DNLM/DLC
for Library of Congress 97-23913
CIP

To future scientific researchers in anesthesiology and pain medicine, and the impact of the knowledge they will create on the future of clinical practice.

A portion of the proceeds from the sales of this book will be donated by the Editors and the Publisher to the Foundation for Anesthesia Education and Research (FAER).

CONTENTS

Color plates appear after p. 764.

CONTRIBUTORS

Stephen E. Abram, MD
Professor
Department of Anesthesiology
University of New Mexico
School of Medicine
Surge Building
2701 Frontier Street
Albequerque, New Mexico
87131-5216

Steven J. Allen, MD
Professor
Department of Anesthesiology
The University of Texas-Houston
Medical School
6431 Fannin, MSB 5.020
Houston, Texas 77030

Robert S. Aronstam, PhD
Scientific Director and Senior Scientist
Guthrie Research Institute
One Guthrie Square
Sayre, Pennsylvania 18840

Flemming W. Bach, MD
Department of Neurology
The National University Hospital
University of Copenhagen
Blegdamsvej 9
Dk-2100 Copenhagen
Denmark

Helen A. Baghdoyan, PhD
Department of Anesthesia
The Pennsylvania State University
College of Medicine
500 University Drive
Hershey, Pennsylvania 17033

Lawrence J. Baudendistel, MD, PhD
Professor and Chairman
Department of Anesthesiology
St. Louis University
Health Sciences Center
3635 Vista Avenue at Grand Boulevard
PO Box 15250
St. Louis, Missouri 63110-0250

Karen J. Berkley, PhD
Program in Neuroscience
Florida State University
Tallahassee, Florida 32306-1051

Julien F. Biebuyck, MB, DPhil
Eric A. Walker Professor and Chair
Department of Anesthesia
Associate Dean for Academic Affairs
The Pennsylvania State University College of Medicine
500 University Drive
Hershey, Pennsylvania 17033

Thomas J.J. Blanck, MD, PhD
Professor of Anesthesiology and
Physiology and Biophysics
Cornell University Medical College
Director of Anesthesiology
The Hospital for Special Surgery
535 East 70th Street
New York, New York 10021

Zeljko J. Bosnjak, PhD
Professor
Departments of Anesthesiology
and Physiology
The Medical College of Wisconsin
8701 Watertown Plank Road
Milwaukee, Wisconsin 53226

Geoffrey M. Bove, DC, PhD
Research Fellow in Anesthesia
Beth Israel Hospital
and Harvard Medical School
330 Brookline Avenue, Dana 719
Boston, Massachusetts 02215

William G. Brose, MD
Associate Professor
Department of Anesthesiology
Stanford University
S-268 300 Pasteur Drive
Stanford, California 94305

Kay Brune MD
Institut Fur Experimentelle
und Klinische Pharmakologie
und Toxikologie
Universitat of Erlangen-Nurnberg
Erlangen, Germany

Ann Buttermann, MD, PhD
Assistant Professor
Department of Anesthesiology
University of Minnesota Hospitals
and Clinics
420 Delaware Street, SE
Box 294 Mayo Building
Minneapolis, Minnesota 55455

Nigel A. Calcutt, PhD
Assistant Professor
Department of Pathology
University of California, San Diego
9500 Gilman Drive
La Jolla, California 92093-0612

James N. Campbell, MD
Professor
Department of Neurosurgery
The Johns Hopkins Hospital
600 N. Wolfe Street, Meyer 5-109
Baltimore, Maryland 21287-7509

Berit X. Carlson, PhD
Department of Pharmacology
UCLA School of Medicine
Los Angeles, California 90024

Susan M. Carlton, PhD
Professor
Marine Biomedical Institute
University of Texas Medical Branch
301 University Boulevard
Galveston, Texas 7555-1069

Daniel B. Carr
Saltonstall Professor of Pain Research
Departments of Anesthesia and Medicine
New England Medical Center
Box 298
750 Washington Street
Boston, Massachusetts 02111

Sandra R. Chaplan, MD
Department of Anesthesiology
University of California, San Diego
9500 Gilman Drive
La Jolla, California 92093

Victoria Chapman, PhD
Department of Pharmacology
University College London
Gower Street
London
England WC1 6BT

Randall C. Cork, MD
Professor and Chair
Department of Anesthesiology
Louisiana State University Medical Center
1501 Kings Highway
Shreveport, Louisiana 71130-3932

Lawrence J. Couture, MA
Department of Psychology
University of Arizona
Tucson, Arizona 85721

A. D. Craig, PhD
Senior Staff Scientist
Division of Neurobiology
Barrow Neurological Institute
350 West Thomas Road
Phoenix, Arizona 85013

Carl E. Creutz, PhD
Department of Pharmacology
University of Virginia
Box 448 Jordan Hall
Charlottesville, Virginia 22908

Thomas E. Dahms, PhD
Associate Professor of Anesthesiology
Department of Anesthesiology
St. Louis University Medical School
3635 Vista Avenue at Grand Boulevard
PO Box 15250
St. Louis, Missouri 63110-0250

Cynthia K. Damer, PhD
Department of Pharmacology
Health Sciences Center
Box 448
Charlottesville, Virginia 22908

Anthony H. Dickenson, BSc, PhD
Professor of Neuropharmacology
Department of Pharmacology
University College London
Gower Street
London
England WC1 6BT

James P. Dilger, PhD
Associate Professor of Anesthesiology
Departments of Anesthesiology, Physiology, and Biophysics
University at Stony Brook
Stony Brook, New York 11794-8480

Raymond A. Dionne, DOS, PhD
Pain & Neurocensory Mechanism Branch
National Institute of Dental Research
10 Center Drive, Building 10
Bethesda, Maryland 20892-1258

Marek K. Dobke, MD, DSc
Associate Professor of Surgery
Chief, Section of Plastic and Reconstructive Surgery
University of Medicine and Dentistry of New Jersey
New Jersey Medical School
90 Bergen Street, Suite 7200
Newark, New Jersey 07103-2499

Karen B. Domino, MD
Associate Professor of Anesthesiology
University of Washington
School of Medicine
Department of Anesthesiology
Box 356540
Seattle, Washington 98195

J. O. Dostrovsky, PhD
Professor
Department of Physiology
University of Toronto
Medical Sciences Building
Toronto, Ontario
Canada M5S 1A8

Robert E. Drake, PhD
Department of Anesthesiology
The University of Texas-Houston Medical School
6431 Fannin, MSB 5.020
Houston, Texas 77030

Andy Dray, PhD
ASTRA Research Centre Montreal
7171 Frederick Banting Street
Ville St-Laurent, Quebec
Canada H4S 1Z9

Marcel E. Durieux, MD
Assistant Professor of Anesthesiology, Pharmacology, and Neurological Science
Department of Anesthesiology
University of Virginia HSC
P.O. Box 10010
Charlottesville, Virginia 22906-0010

Thomas J. Ebert, MD, PhD
Professor of Anesthesiology/Adjunct Professor of Physiology
Department of Anesthesiology and Physiology
Medical College at Wisconsin
8701 Watertown Plank Road
Milwaukee, Wisconsin 53226

Roderic G. Eckenhoff, MD
Associate Professor
Departments of Anesthesia and Physiology
University of Pennsylvania Health System
Philadelphia, Pennsylvania 19104-4283

James C. Eisenach, MD
Professor and Chair for Anesthesia Research
Bowman Gray School of Medicine
Winston-Salem, North Carolina 27157-1009

Kathyn J. Elliott, MD
Assistant Professor of Neurology
Cornell University Medical College
1275 York Avenue
New York, New York 10021

Leonard Firestone, MD
Professor and Chair
Department of Anesthesiology and Critical Care Medicine
University of Pittsburgh
A1305 Scaife Hall
Pittsburgh, Pennsylvania 15261

Susan Firestone, MD
Associate Professor of Anesthesiology
Department of Anesthesiology and Critical Care Medicine
Children's Hospital of Pittsburgh
3705 5th Avenue
Pittsburgh, Pennsylvania 15213-2583

Joanna Floros, PhD
Departments of Cellular and Molecular Biology, and Pediatrics
The Pennsylvania State University College of Medicine
500 University Drive
Hershey, Pennsylvania 17033

Robert D. Foreman, PhD
Professor and Chair
George Lynn Cross Research Professor
Department of Physiology
University of Oklahoma Health Sciences Center
940 S. L. Young Boulevard
Oklahoma City, Oklahoma 73104

Stuart A. Forman, MD, PhD
Assistant Professor in Anesthesia
Department of Anaesthesia and Critical Care
Massachusetts General Hospital
Blossom Street
Boston, Massachusetts 02114

Mary G. Garry, PhD
Instructor
Department of Anesthesiology and Pain Management
The University of Texas Southwestern Medical Center
5323 Harry Hines Boulevard
Dallas, Texas 75235-9068

Dorothee Gaumann, MD
Privat Dozent-University of Geneva
Department of Anesthesiology
Regional Hospital Thun
Kruakennausstr. 12
Thun
Switzerland

Torsten Gordh, MD, PhD
Department of Anaesthesiology
and Intensive Care
Uppsala University Hospital
S-751 85 Uppsala
Sweden

Sharon M. Gordon, DDS, MPH
Research Associate
Department of Pain Management and Neurosensory Mechanism Branch
National Institute of Dental Research
9000 Rockville Pike, Building 10, Room 1N-103
Bethesda, Maryland 20892

Brent A. Graham, MD
Assistant Professor
Department of Anesthesia and Critical Care Medicine
University of Chicago
5841 S. Maryland Avenue
Chicago, Illinois 60637

Patrice G. Guyenet, PhD
Professor of Pharmacology
Department of Pharmacology
University of Virginia Health Sciences Center
Box 448, Jordan Hall, 5th Floor
1300 Jefferson Park Avenue
Charlottesville, Virginia 22908

Tim G. Hales, PhD
Assistant Professor of Anesthesiology
Department of Anesthesiology
University of California, Los Angeles
Los Angeles, California 90095-1778

Donna L. Hammond, PhD
Associate Professor
Department of Anesthesia and Critical Care
University of Chicago
5841 S. Maryland Avenue, M/C 4028
Chicago, Illinois 60637

Kenneth M. Hargreaves, DDS, PhD
Professor
Department of Endodontics
University of Texas Health Sciences Center
at San Antonio
7703 Floyd Curl Drive
San Antonio, Texas, 78284-7906

Goran Hedenstierna, MD, PhD
Professor in Clinical Physiology
Department of Clinical Physiology
University Hospital
Uppsala
Sweden

Mary M. Heinricher, PhD
Associate Professor
Division of Neurosurgery, L472
Oregon Health Sciences University
3181 S.W. Sam Jackson Park Road
Portland, Oregon 97201

Hugh C. Hemmings, Jr, MD, PhD
Associate Professor of Anesthesiology and Pharmacology
Director of Research
Department of Anesthesiology
Box 50, LC-203
Cornell Medical Center
525 East 68th Street
New York, New York 10021

Dean Hess, PhD, RRT
Assistant Professor of Anesthesia
Harvard Medical School
Assistant Director of Respiratory Care
Massachusetts General Hospital
Ellison 401
55 Fruit Street
Boston, Massachusetts 02114

J. Allan Hobson, MD
Professor of Psychiatry
Department of Psychiatry
Harvard Medical School
74 Fenwood Road
Boston, Massachusetts 02115

Francis A. Hopp, Jr., MSEE
Biomedical Engineer
Department of Anesthesiology
The Medical College of Wisconsin
5000 W. National Avenue
Milwaukee, Wisconsin 53295

William E. Hurford, MD
Assistant Professor of Anesthesia
Harvard Medical School
Associate Anesthetist
Massachusetts General Hospital
55 Fruit Street
Boston, Massachusetts 02114

Paul A. Iaizzo, PhD
Associate Professor
Departments of Anesthesiology and Physiology
University of Minnesota
Box 294
420 Delaware Street SE
Minneapolis, Minnesota 55455

Jonas S. Johansson, MD, PhD
Assistant Professor
Departments of Anesthesia, Biochemistry,
and Biophysics, and the Johnson Foundation
University of Pennsylvania Medical Center
3400 Spruce Street
Philadelphia, Pennsylvania 19104

Roger A. Johns, MD
Professor
Department of Anesthesiology
University of Virginia Health Sciences Center
P.O. Box 10010
1 Hospital Drive
Charlottesville, Virginia 22906-0010

Rosemary C. Jones, PhD
Associate Professor of Pathology in Anesthesia
Harvard Medical School
Department of Anesthesia
Massachusetts General Hospital
149 Thirteenth Street, Room 3416
Charlestown, Massachusetts 02129

Judy R. Kersten, MD
Assistant Professor of Anesthesiology
Department of Anesthesiology
Medical College of Wisconsin
8701 Watertown Plank Road
Milwaukee, Wisconsin 53226

John F. Kihlstrom, MD
Professor
Department of Psychology
University of California, Berkeley
Tolman Hall
Berkeley, California 94720

Jeffrey R. Kirsch, MD
Associate Professor
Director Resident Education
Department of Anesthesiology and
Critical Care Medicine
The Johns Hopkins Hospital
Blalock 1412
600 North Wolfe Street
Baltimore, Maryland 21287-4963

Paul R. Knight, MD, PhD
Professor and Chairman
Department of Anesthesiology
State University of New York
Hamlin House, 2nd Floor
100 High Street
Buffalo, New York 14203

Jens D. Kristensen, MD
Department of Anaesthesiology
and Intensive Care
University Hospital
S-751 85 Uppsala
Sweden

Wai-Meng Kwok, PhD
Department of Anesthesiology
Medical College of Wisconsin
8701 Watertown Plank Road
Milwaukee, Wisconsin 53226

David Langleben, MD
Associate Professor of Medicine
McGill University
Division of Cardiology
Sir Mortimer B. Davis Jewish General Hospital
3755 Chemin de la Cote Ste. Catherine
Montreal, Quebec H3T 1E2
Canada

Ryan E. Lesh, MD
Assistant Professor
Department of Anesthesiology
Instructor
Department of Molecular Physiology
and Biological Physics
University of Virginia
1300 Jefferson Park Avenue
Charlottesville, Virginia 22908

Martin K. Lotz, MD
Head
Division of Arthritis Research
Department of Molecular and
Experimental Medicine
The Scripps Research Institute
10550 North Torrey Pines Road, SBR7
La Jolla, California 92093-0663

R. Lydic, PhD
Professor of Anesthesia, Cellular and
Molecular Physiology
Department of Anesthesia
The Pennsylvania State University
College of Medicine
500 University Drive
Hershey, Pennsylvania 17033

Carl Lynch III, MD, PhD
Professor of Anesthesiology
Department of Anesthesiology
University of Virginia Health Sciences Center
P.O. Box 10010
Charlottesville, Virginia 22908

M. Bruce MacIver, MSc, PhD
Assistant Professor of Neurophysiology
Department of Anesthesia
Stanford University School of Medicine
Room 5284A, SUMC
300 Pasteur Drive
Stanford, California 94305-5117

Rayaz A. Malik, BSc, MSc, MBChB, PhD, MRCP
Lecturer in Medicine
Department of Medicine
Manchester Royal Infirmary
Oxford Road
Manchester
United Kingdom

Mervyn Maze MB, ChB, FRCP
Professor and Research Director
Department of Anesthesia
Stanford University and Anesthesiology Service
Palo Alto VA Health Care System
Anesthesiology Service (112A)
3801 Miranda Avenue
Palo Alto, California 94304

John S. McDonald, MD
Professor and Chairman of Anesthesiology
Department of Anesthesia
Ohio State University Hospital
410 W. 10th Avenue, N-429
Columbus, Ohio 433210

Richard A. Meyer, MS
Professor of Neurosurgery and of
Biomedical Engineering
Department of Neurosurgery
Johns Hopkins University School of Medicine
600 N. Wolfe Street
Baltimore, Maryland 20223

Keith W. Miller, MD
Mallinckropt Professor of Pharmacology
Department of Anesthesia
Massachusetts General Hospital
White 4, Room 430
32 Fruit Street
Boston, Massachusetts 02114

J. Randall Moorman, MD
Associate Professor
Department of Medicine and Physiology
University of Virginia Health Sciences Center
Box 6012, MR4 Building
300 Park Place
Charlottesville, Virginia 22908

Michael A. Moskowitz, MD
Professor of Neurology
Massachusetts General Hospital and
Harvard Medical School
149 13th Street, CNY 6403
Charlestown, Massachusetts 02129

Robert R. Myers, PhD
Professor of Anesthesiology
Professor of Pathology (Neuropathology)
Department of Anesthesiology
University of California, San Diego
9500 Gilman Drive
La Jolla, California 92093-0629

Therese C. O'Connor
FFARCSI
Consultant Anesthetist
Cavan/Monaghan Hospital Group
Loughanelton
Calry
Sligo
Ireland

Richard W. Olsen, PhD
Professor
Department of Molecular and Medical Pharmacology
UCLA School of Medicine, CHS 23-120
10833 Le Conte Avenue
Los Angeles, California 90095-1735

Patricia F. Osgood, PhD
Assistant Professor
Department of Anesthesia
Harvard Medical School
P.O. Box 146
Kearsarge, New Hampshire 03847

Paul S. Pagel, MD, PhD
Associate Professor of Anesthesiology
Department of Anesthesiology
Medical College of Wisconsin
MEB–Room 462C
8701 Watertown Plank Rd
Milwaukee, Wisconsin 53226

Joseph J. Pancrazio, PhD
Research Assistant Professor
Departments of Anesthesiology and Biomedical Engineering
University of Virgina Health Sciences Center
Box 238
Charlottesville, Virginia 22908

Leonardo Paroli MD, PhD
Department of Anesthesiology
New York Hospital Cornell Medical Center
525 East 68th Street
New York, New York 10021

Robert W. Peoples, PhD
Laboratory of Molecular and Cellular Neurobiology
National Institute on Alcohol Abuse and Alcoholism
National Institutes of Health
12501 Washington Avenue
Rockville, MD 20852

David S. Phelps, PhD
Associate Professor of Pediatrics
Department of Pediatrics
Pennsylvania State University
College of Medicine
500 University Drive
Hershey, Pennsylvania 17033

Pamela A. Pierce, MD, PhD
Assistant Professor in Residence
Department of Anesthesiology
University of California, San Francisco
513 Parnaisus Avenue, Box 0464, Rm 5455
San Francisco, California 94143-0648

Russell K. Portenoy, MD
Chairman
Department of Pain Medicine and Palliative Care
Beth Israel Medical Center
First Avenue at 16th Street
New York, New York 10003

Donald D. Price, PhD
Professor and Director of Research
Department of Anesthesiology
Medical College of Virginia
P.O. Box 980337, MCV Station
Richmond, Virginia 23298-0337

Douglas E. Raines, MD
Assistant Professor in Anesthesia
Department of Anesthesia
Harvard Medical School
Massachusetts General Hospital
55 Fruit Street
Boston, Massachusetts 02114

Srinivasa N. Raja, MD
Associate Professor
Department of Anesthesiology and
Critical Care Medicine
The Johns Hopkins Hospital, Osler 304
600 N. Wolfe Street
Baltimore, Maryland 21287-5354

Andrea Rapkin, MD
Associate Professor of Obstetrics and Gynecology
Department of Obstetrics and Gynecology
UCLA School of Medicine
10833 LeConte Avenue, Rm 22-177 CH5
Los Angeles, California 90095-1740

Natalia Luzina Rasgon, MD, PhD
Assistant Clinical Professor
Department of Ob/Gyn
Clinical Instructor
Department of Psychiatry
UCLA School of Medicine
Neuro-Psychiatric Institute
760 Westwood Plaza, Room C8-532
Los Angeles, California 90024

Hans Ulrich Rothen, MD, PhD
Institute for Anesthesiology and Intensive Care
University Hospital
Bern, CH-3010
Switzerland

Michael C. Rowbotham, MD
Departments of Neurology and Anesthesia
University of California, San Francisco
P.O. Box 1635
San Francisco, California 94143-1635

Debra A. Schwinn, MD
Associate Professor of Anesthesiology,
Pharmacology, and Surgery
Department of Anesthesiology
Duke University Medical Center
Box 3094
Durham, North Carolina 27710

Jeanne L. Seagard, PhD
Professor of Anesthesiology
Department of Anesthesiology
The Medical College of Wisconsin
VA Medical Center
Anesthesiology Research Service 151
5000 W. National Avenue
Milwaukee, Wisconsin 53295

Virginia Seybold, PhD
Professor
Department of Cell Biology and
Neuroanatomy
University of Minnesota
4-144 Jackson Hall
321 Church Street SE
Minneapolis, Minnesota 55455

Brendan S. Silbert, MBBS, FANZCA
Department of Anaesthesia
St. Vincent's Hospital
Melbourne
Australia

S. H. Sindrup, MD, PhD
Department of Clinical Pharmacology
Odense University
Institute of Medical Biology
Winslowparken 19
DK-5000 Odense C
Denmark

Claudia L. Sommer, MD
Neurologische Universitatsklinik
Josef-Schneider-Str 11
97080 Wurzburg
Germany

Linda S. Sorkin, PhD
Associate Professor in Residence
of Anesthesiology
Department of Anesthesiology
University of California San Diego
9500 Gilman Drive
La Jolla, California 92093-0818

Louise C. Stanfa, PhD
Research Fellow
Department of Pharmacology
University College London
Gower Street
London WC1 6BT
England

Thomas A. Stekiel, MD
Assistant Professor
Department of Anesthesiology
Medical College of Wisconsin
8701 Watertown Plank Road
Milwaukee, Wisconsin 53226

William J. Stekiel, PhD
Professor
Department of Physiology
Medical College of Wisconsin
8701 Watertown Plank Road
Milwaukee, Wisconsin 53226-0509

Ruth L. Stornetta, PhD
Research Assistant Professor
Department of Pharmacology
University of Virginia
1300 Jefferson Park Avenue
Rm 5024 Jordan Hall
Charlottesville, Virginia 22908

Gary R. Strichartz, PhD, AM
Professor of Anesthesia
(Pharmacology)
Department of Anesthesia
Brigham and Women's Hospital
Anesthesia Research Laboratories
75 Francis Street
Boston, Massachusetts 02116

James Q. Swift, DDS
Associate Professor and Director
Division of Oral and Maxillofacial Surgery
University of Minnesota
7-174 Moos Tower
515 Delaware Street SE
Minneapolis, Minnesota 55455-0329

Darrell L. Tanelian, MD, PhD
Associate Professor
Department of Anesthesiology and Pain Management
The University of Texas Southwestern Medical Center
5323 Harry Hines Boulevard
Dallas, Texas 75235-9068

Kirk Taylor, MD
Clinical Instructor
Department of Neurology
Pain Clinical Research Center
University of California, San Francisco
San Francisco, California 94115

John A. Temp, MD
Assistant Professor
Department of Anesthesiology
School of Medicine and Dentistry
University of Rochester
601 Elmwood Avenue
Rochester, New York 14642

Richard J. Traystman, PhD
Distinguished Research Professor
Vice Chair for Research
Director, A/CCM Laboratories
Department of Anesthesiology and
Critical Care Medicine
The Johns Hopkins Medical Institutions
600 North Wolfe Street (Blalock 1408)
Baltimore, Maryland 21287-4961

Robert L. Trelstad, MD
Professor and Chairman
Department of Pathology
Robert Wood Johnson Medical School
New Brunswick, New Jersey 08903-0019

Yvonne Vulliemoz, PhD
Senior Research Scientist in Anesthesiology
College of Physicians and Surgeons
Columbia University
Department of Anesthesiology, P&S Box 46
Columbia University
630 West 168th Street
New York, New York 10032

Anne M. Wallace, MD
Assistant Clinical Professor of Surgery
Department of Plastic Surgery
University of California, San Diego
200 West Arbor Drive
La Jolla, California 92103-8890

Mark S. Wallace, MD
Assistant Clinical Professor
Department of Anesthesiology
University of California, San Diego
200 West Arbor Drive
San Diego, California 92103-8770

Denham S. Ward, MD, PhD
Professor and Chairman
Department of Anesthesiology
School of Dentistry and Medicine
University of Rochester
601 Elmwood Avenue, Box 604
Rochester, New York 14642

David C. Warltier, MD, PhD
Professor of Anesthesiology, Pharmacology, and Cardiology
Department of Anesthesiology
Medical College of Wisconsin
8701 Watertown Plank Road
Milwaukee, Wisconsin 53226

David O. Warner, MD
Associate Professor of Anesthesiology
Department of Anesthesiology
Mayo Clinic
200 First Street SW
Rochester, Minnesota 55905

W. David Watkins, MS, PhD, MD
Professor of Anesthesiology/Critical Care Medicine
Departments of Anesthesiology/Critical Care Medicine
University of Pittsburgh
A-1305 Scaife Hall
Pittsburgh, Pennsylvania 15261

Forrest F. Weight, MD
Chief
Laboratory of Molecular and Cellular Neurobiology
National Institute on Alcohol Abuse and Alcoholism
National Institutes of Health
Bethesda, Maryland 20892-8205

George L. Wilcox, PhD
Professor
Department of Pharmacology
University of Minnesota
3-249 Millard Hall
Minneapolis, Minnesota 55455

Frederick Wolfe, MD
Clinical Professor of Internal Medicine
and Family and Community Medicine
University of Kansas-Wichita
1035 N. Emporia, Suite 230
Wichita, Kansas 67214

Yan Xu, PhD
Assistant Professor
Departments of Anesthesiology and Critical Care
Medicine, and of Pharmacology
University of Pittsburgh
W-1358 Biomedical Science Tower
Pittsburgh, Pennsylvania 15261

Fang Xu, PhD
Department of Anesthesiology
The Hospital for Special Surgery
535 East 70th Street
New York, New York 10021

Tony L. Yaksh, PhD
Professor and Vice Chairman for Research
Department of Anesthesiology
University of California, San Diego
9500 Gilman Drive
La Jolla, California 92093-0818

Warren M. Zapol, MD
Reginald Jenney Professor of Anesthesia
Harvard Medical School
Anesthetist-in-Chief
Massachusetts General Hospital
Boston, Massachusetts 02114

PREFACE

Anesthesiology has progressed through several stages in the past 150 years. The first, beginning in the 1840s, was best characterized by the observation by Morton, Wells and others that unconsciousness and at times unresponsiveness were reliably caused by administration of one of several vapors—any of which could also cause death if given in too great a concentration. Truly this discovery of anesthesia represents one of medicine's great achievements since, for the first time, surgery could be performed without patients suffering the agony of surgically related pain. For nearly the next half-century, the principal advances consisted of improvements in anesthesia-related apparatus and in the development of a small cadre of individuals specializing in administration of anesthetics. This stage also represented a period of consolidation of the not-yet-developed clinical specialty, which was necessary before progress leading to an understanding of the mechanisms underlying anesthesia could occur. As an aside, imagine what it must have been like to administer anesthetics in this period at the latter half of the 19th century. Precise doses of inhaled drugs were not known; supplemental oxygen was not routinely administered; monitoring of vital signs was not practiced; only inhaled anesthetics and local anesthetics were available; patients breathed spontaneously; often the least-trained individuals (usually not physicians) were administering the anesthesia; resuscitation techniques were crude at best; intravenous therapy was not yet commonly used; and transfusion science had not yet been developed.

The next era of our specialty occurred over the first third of the 20th century and paralleled the development of new knowledge in areas of basic science related to anesthesiology. Developments included new drugs and new classes of drugs, the characterization of altered physiology related to the surgical state, availability of anesthetic-related equipment permitting precise administration of anesthetic gases and supplemental oxygen, the possiblity of transfusions (although for a number of reasons they were not terribly practical), the use of tracheal intubation, and the advancement of surgical science apace with that of other medical specialties. At the same time, anesthesia practitioners still understood little of the science behind why they did what they did, and thus flexibility and variations of care based on logic rather than empiricism were nearly impossible. Further, there were few individuals committed to developing the science of the specialty, virtually no Departments of Anesthesia existed, and in addition, only a few physicians were committed to the specialty to the exclusion of other aspects of medical practice.

The middle third of the 20th century brought with it many changes that assisted in a rapid increase in the size and impact of the specialty, providing conditions propitious for achieving a more detailed and scientifically accurate description of the mechanisms underlying the anesthetized state. First was the formation of the American Society of Anesthesiologists (ASA) and the American Board of Anesthesiology (ABA). These organizations provided an organized voice for political and economic issues of concern to anesthesiologists (ASA) as well as a way to credentialed anesthesiologists (ABA) on a plane similar to that of other specialties. Second, the World War II and the need for expert anesthesia care necessitated by war-associated injuries resulted in an increase in the number of physicians receiving at least some training in anesthesia. Third was the establishment in many medical schools of Departments of Anesthesiology, and the exposure of medical students to the specialty. Fourth, the specialty was increasingly attracting individuals interested in and capable of performing quality clinical and laboratory research. This coincided with and was perhaps in part driven by a massive expansion in biomedical research funding by Congress, administered by the National Institutes of Health (NIH). The result was a number of medical school Departments of Anesthesia with substantial NIH-supported research budgets. The fifth major change was the development of techniques useful for studying the physiologic consequences and pharmacologic effects of anesthetics as well as the physiologic impact of the surgical experience, for use in the operating room as well as in the laboratory. This research in turn lead to an understanding of and the ability to better treat acute respiratory failure, shock, and other states of circulatory decompensation, as well as the physical principles defining pharmacokinetics related to anesthetics and other drugs administered to the anesthetized patient. Lastly, there was the recruitment by departments of anesthesiology of talented PHDs who, in addition to performing their own anesthesia-related research, created an environment suitable for other anesthesiologists to do the same. This resulted in the close relationship between basic and clinical researchers that enabled complex physiologic and biochemical as well as clinically related research issues to be studied.

In the latter third of the 20th century remarkable advances have occurred in all areas of science. Of particular importance to our specialty is the increased understanding of how the nervous system functions on both a cellular and subcellular basis. New tools such as MRI and PET scanning are now available to noninvasively probe where and perhaps how anesthetics act. Molecular biologic techniques, including gene knockouts, permit the most detailed investigations of the processes affected by the drugs we administer. Taken together, these latter tools are beginning to provide answers to the century-and-a-half old question of how and where anesthetics act to produce their effects.

Thus, the stage was set for this book.

In the late 1980s, a number of university-based anesthesiologists were asked by Mary Rogers from Raven Press to consider organizing a multiauthored textbook describing what was then known regarding the biology underlying anesthesia. The basis for such a comprehensive approach to a clinical specialty had been established by Raven Press with their Scientific Foundation series that included the Lung and the Heart and Cardiovascular System. Although it was acknowledged that such an approach was needed in anesthesia, several years elapsed before the composition of the editorial board could be finalized, and several additional years passed before the organization and final content of this textbook could be agreed upon. In the meantime, Raven Press had become Lippincott–Raven and Mary Rogers had become President of the new company.

The book is broadly divided into two sections—Cell Biology of Anesthetic Action and Anesthetic Effects Upon Physiological Integrated Systems. The first section is comprised of chapters describing basic processes underlying the most fundamental activities that regulate cell function, as well as chapters detailing laboratory techniques available to study these processes. The integrated systems covered in Section Two describe the biology involved in a number of the behavioral states including sleep, consciousness, memory and recall, as well as an in-depth analysis of the physiology and pharmacology of pain and a variety of painful states, the cardiovascular system, and the respiratory system (with special emphasis on the effects of anesthetics).

This textbook is intended for use by basic researchers both within and out of the field of anesthesiology as well as for anesthesiologists interested in the "why" of what they do. Anesthetics are powerful agents that remain incompletely understood and often misused. Thus we hope that this textbook will be available as a reference within all libraries in which information on the broad science of anesthetics and anesthesia is needed.

We thank the large number of contributors and our publisher who have helped produce this first textbook attempting to consider the totality of the biologic foundations of anesthesia. As with all such efforts, some areas are treated more completely than others, and if we have erred, it is because of our wish to comprehensively examine areas of anesthesia-related science not available elsewhere within the covers of a single anesthesiology text.

Tony L. Yaksh, PhD
Julien Biebuyck, MB, DPhil
Carl Lynch III, MD, PhD
Mervyn Maze, MB, ChB, FRCP
Lawrence J. Saidman, MD
Warren M. Zapol, MD

ACKNOWLEDGMENTS

To the scientists whose laboratory and clinical investigations have enriched the specialty of anesthesiology and those clinicians who have boldly applied the results of these investigations to the benefit of their patients.

ANESTHESIA
BIOLOGIC FOUNDATIONS

I

CELL BIOLOGY OF ANESTHETIC ACTION

A

CONTROL OF CELL SIGNALING

Anesthesia: Biologic Foundations, edited by
Tony L. Yaksh et al. Lippincott–Raven Publishers,
Philadelphia © 1997.

CHAPTER 1

THE INTERACTIONS OF GENERAL ANESTHETICS WITH MEMBRANES

STUART A. FORMAN, DOUGLAS E. RAINES,
AND KEITH W. MILLER

Despite our rapidly increasing knowledge of the cellular processes underlying neuronal excitability, we do not yet understand the molecular and cellular mechanisms underlying consciousness, pain perception, memory formation, and other higher brain functions (see Chap. 26). The suppression of these brain functions by general anesthetics demonstrates a unique nonspecific pharmacology. While our ability to determine how general anesthetics act may ultimately depend on defining mechanisms underlying important brain functions, a great deal is known about anesthetic actions on various molecular components that are involved in neuronal excitability. Indeed, when viewed from a historical perspective, hypotheses of general anesthetic mechanisms reflect the development of evermore sophisticated models of neuronal function. In this introductory chapter we review the development of models of general anesthetic action with particular emphasis on the cell membrane and its role as a modulator of excitability.

THE UNIQUE PHARMACOLOGY OF GENERAL ANESTHETICS: PHENOMENOLOGY

The major feature that distinguishes general anesthetics from other drug classes is the extraordinary diversity of chemical structures that possess general anesthetic activity. These range from simple gases such as xenon and nitrous oxide to the more familiar alcohols and halogenated hydrocarbons and also include complex organic structures such as barbiturates and steroids (Fig. 1) (63). A characteristic of most potent anesthetics is their *lipophilicity*, a property that may be expressed as the partition coefficient for the drug between an oily solvent (frequently olive oil or octanol) and another standard state (partial pressure in air or concentration in aqueous solution). High lipophilicity is generally accompanied by high *hydrophobicity* (very low solubility in water) and the two terms are often used interchangeably. Indeed, it has been known since the turn of the century that anesthetic potency correlates strongly with the oil/gas partition coefficient (C_{oil}/C_{aq}) over many orders of magnitude of potency (the *Meyer-Overton rule*; Fig. 2) (72).

The discussion that follows enumerates a number of other features of anesthetic pharmacology, in addition to hydrophobicity, in experimental animals that provide hints as to the nature of the general anesthetic site and experimental guidelines for assessing various hypotheses of general anesthetic action.

First, there is no pharmacologic antagonist for general anesthesia. This is consistent with the nonspecificity suggested by the Meyer-Overton rule and implies that an effector site is not involved.

Second, when the actions of a homologous series of compounds, such as the n-alcohols, are assessed, they generally show smoothly increasing anesthetic potencies as methylene groups are added, such that

$$\mathrm{ECS(n,50)\ /\ ECS(n+1,50)} \approx 3,$$

where n is the number of carbons in the methylene chain and EC_{50} is the half effect concentration of a given action of anesthetics. This is fully consistent with the change in hydrophobicity measured with each additional methylene. However, as the chain length increases, there comes a point where addition of another methylene fails to increase anesthetic potency or actually causes a loss of anesthetic activity despite increased hydrophobicity (Fig. 3). This phenomenon is known as *anesthetic cutoff* and occurs between $n = 12$ and 13 for the normal alkanol series.

A third phenomenon associated with anesthetics is *pressure reversal*. Experimental animals anesthetized at atmospheric pressure will awaken if the hydrostatic pressure of the experimental chamber is increased, then return to the anesthetized state as the chamber is decompressed. A related observation concerns the anesthetic effects of the inert gases. Although, helium is often used to transmit pressure and demonstrate pressure reversal in mammals, it does have an anesthetic effect of its own because it causes less pressure reversal than hydrostatic pressure (22). Argon, by contrast, is a full general anesthetic.

Fourth, the general anesthetics have very small safety margins; typically, concentrations double those required for surgery produce undesirable side effects. This suggests that

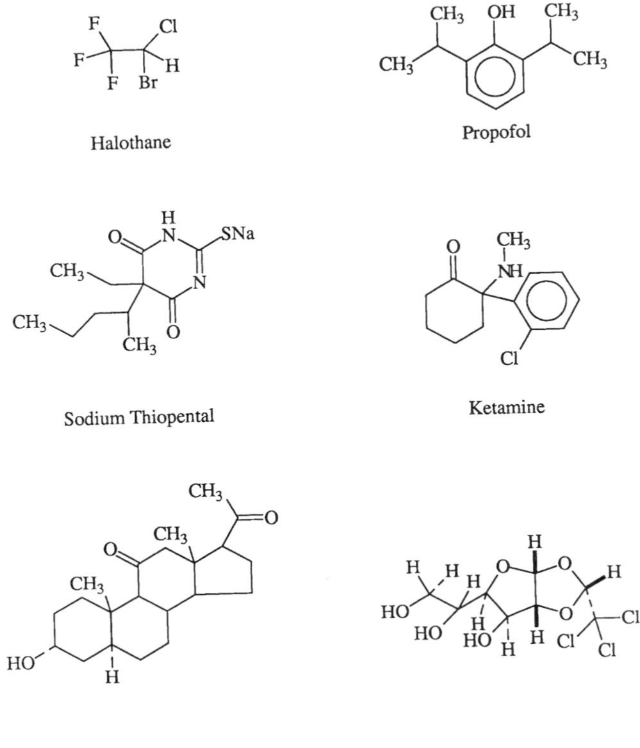

Figure 1. The structures of some general anesthetics. (From ref. 39, with permission.)

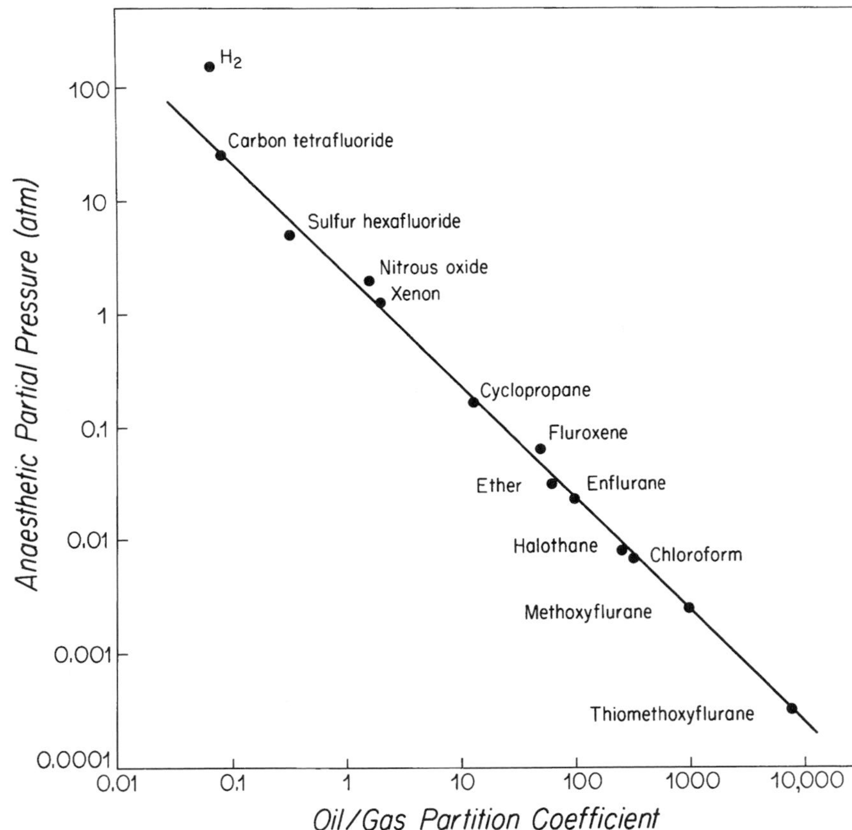

Figure 2. Anesthetic potency correlates with oil solubility. Anesthetic partial pressure in mammals (minimum alveolar concentration, MAC) correlates over a 74,300-fold range of potency with the olive oil/gas partition coefficient at 37°C. The linearity of the Log-Log plot means that the product of the anesthetic partial pressure and the oil/gas partition coefficient is a constant, equivalent to a concentration in oil of ~0.1 M on average. Hydrogen deviates from the correlation because of the pressure reversal effect. (From ref. 90, with permission.)

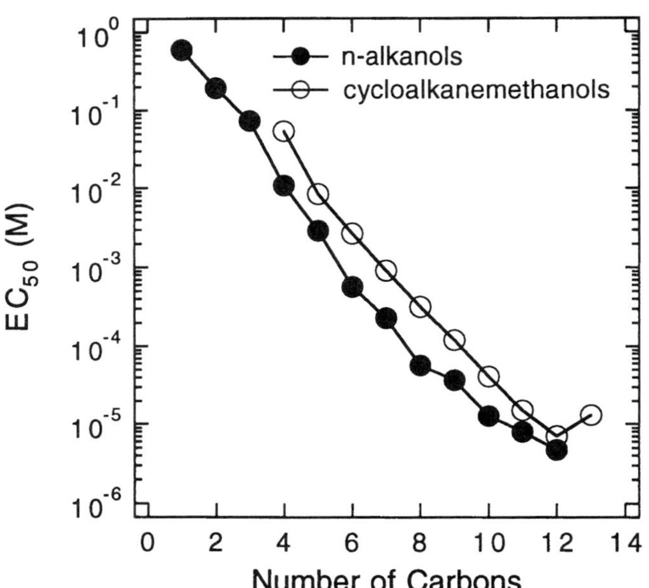

Figure 3. The anesthetic potency of members of both the normal alkanol series and a series of cyclic analogues of normal alkanols called cycloalkanemethanols increases logarithmically with the addition of successive carbons (2,74). However, tridecanol (n-alkanol with 13 carbons) and cyclotetradecanemethanol (cycloalkanemethanol with 15 carbons) do not induce anesthesia even when present as saturated aqueous solutions.

there may be secondary sites of action in the nervous system with very similar affinity for general anesthetics as the sites in the central nervous system that produce general anesthesia per se.

Fifth, the potency of a given general anesthetic varies little across many species, which suggests that the structures involved in anesthesia are conserved.

Recently, two additional features of anesthetic pharmacology have come to light that appear to be exceptions to the Meyer-Overton rule. Stereoselectivity is not predicted by this rule, and it has long been thought that only anesthetic steroids and barbiturates were the exception. However, Lysko et al. (55) have demonstrated a less than twofold degree of stereoselectivity for a halogenated ether (isoflurane) in mammals, but a study employing a much larger cohort of tadpoles failed to find any stereoselectivity (26). Other experiments have demonstrated that a set of hydrophobic halogenated volatile compounds that are predicted to be anesthetics are either much less potent than predicted or are completely devoid of anesthetic activity (45).

CELL MEMBRANES

Hydrophobic Sites for Hydrophobic Drugs

Neuronal cell membranes have long been the focus of research into anesthetic mechanisms because of two important concepts. First, while no specific structure within the central nervous system has been identified as a target for anesthetics, they generally depress the excitability of neurons and it is believed that cell membranes contain the mechanisms that underlie electrical excitability. More specifically, when compared to axonal action potential propagation, synaptic transmission between neurons is much more sensitive to anesthetics (48). Second, the cell membrane is hydrophobic; thus, it is predicted that anesthetics will concentrate in membranes. Indeed, the concept of hydrophobicity as a force in biology has historically linked studies of membrane structure to anesthetic actions. Overton, who helped establish the importance of hydrophobicity in anesthetic action, was one of the first to propose that cell membranes were composed of lipids (72).

The Hydrophobic Effect

The hydrophobic effect is the thermodynamic force that underlies the formation of both lipid bilayers and the structure of proteins in the membrane (89). The hydrophobic effect originates in the unfavorable entropic effects of packing water molecules around nonpolar hydrocarbon solutes. The dynamic structure of pure water is determined by intermolecular hydrogen bonds. When any nonpolar molecule becomes solvated in water, the water is forced to pack around the solute in an ordered way (in order to avoid breaking hydrogen bonds), reducing the entropy (ΔS) of the water. Since a reduction in entropy translates to an increase in Gibbs free energy ($\Delta G = \Delta H - T\Delta S$, where ΔH is the change in enthalpy and T is the absolute temperature), this entropy change is unfavorable and increases in proportion to the surface area of the solute (35). The forces between these nonpolar solutes and water are not strong enough to provide a compensatory enthalpy change (ΔH), and therefore the free energy of transfer from a nonpolar to a polar environment is positive (unfavorable). In contrast, ions and polar solutes also order water around them in a different way by interacting with the water molecules through strong charge-dipole, dipole-dipole, or hydrogen-bonding interactions. Such strong interactions are reflected in large enthalpic terms that more than compensate for the unfavorable entropy change caused by electrostriction of water, and thus these solutes have a negative Gibbs free energy of solvation.

The formation of lipid bilayers can be readily understood when the underlying forces are appreciated. Phospholipids are amphiphilic, with nonpolar acyl chains as well as charged and polar moieties in their head groups and ester regions (Fig. 4). To minimize the nonpolar surface area in contact with water, the acyl chains (which also have favorable van der Waals interactions with each other) tend to aggregate and are separated from the water phase by the hydrophilic head groups. Thus, the overall free energy of the water/lipid mixture is minimized. Similar arguments apply to soluble proteins, which tend to fold in such a way that their hydrophobic amino acid residues are placed inside the structure and hidden from water. The extramembranous regions of membrane proteins behave similarly, but in their lipid bilayer-associated regions they must present hydrophobic amino acid residues to the acyl chains of the lipids.

Membrane Structure and Function

Our present concept of cell membrane structure has developed from simple beginnings to the complex models of today. Overton's lipid layer model was modified to one of a lipid bilayer with a hydrophobic core and relatively hydrophilic head groups in contact with water on either side (38). Danielli (18) added protein to the membrane model; since at that time proteins were felt to be mostly water-soluble, they pictured the membrane as a sandwich with the lipid bilayer between two layers of protein. Current views of membrane structure date to the "fluid mosaic model" of Nicholson (82) (Fig. 4), in which proteins are embedded in a lipid matrix. The fluid mosaic model has undergone much revision, with the addition of molecular details about the structures and functions of lipids and proteins, as well as the important interactions between these two membrane components. This knowledge allows us to identify hydrophobic regions that are potential sites for general anesthetic action.

Membrane Lipids

The fundamental role of the cell membrane is to separate the cytoplasm from the extracellular environment, enabling active processes to set up gradients of ions and nutrients across this diffusion barrier. Membrane lipids also provide an environment in which both intrinsic membrane proteins and membrane-associated proteins can function (more below). However, to view lipids only as a passive matrix is an oversimplification. Lipids play important roles in cell adhesion and growth, phagocytosis, and exocytosis. Specific lipid species also play a role in the regulation of both membrane protein activity and other cellular functions; for example, phosphatidylinositol turnover regulates intracellular calcium and the activity of protein kinase C (PKC; see Chapter 7).

The composition and structure of lipid bilayers have been studied for many years, but the functional significance of many bilayer structures is unknown. Cell membranes may contain up to 100 different lipid species; while some of these have known functions, the importance of the others is unknown.

Lipid/water mixtures form a variety of structures depending on the shape of the specific lipid molecules (Fig. 5) (16). A number of these phases have been invoked in theories of anesthetic action and are reviewed below. First, the *lamellar liquid crystalline phase* (L_α) is a bilayer structure in which individual phospholipids diffuse freely in the plane of the bilayer but not at right angles to it. The acyl chains in the bilayer core are quite

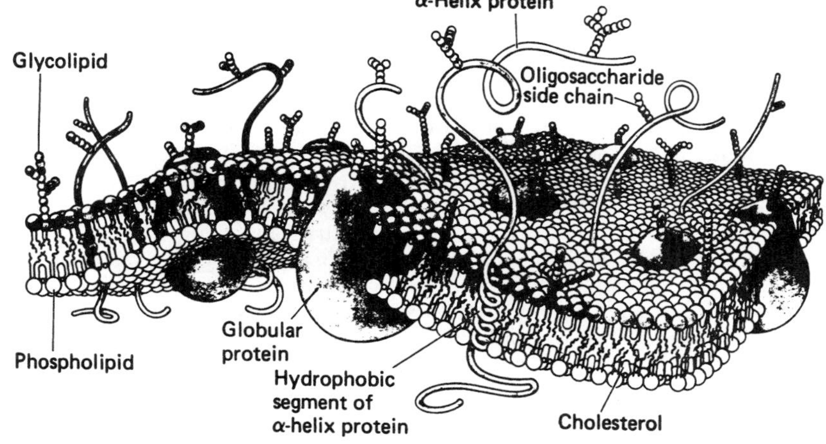

Figure 4. Cartoon illustrating the fundamentals of membrane structure. A section of plasma membrane consisting of a lipid bilayer, composed of various phospholipids, in which cholesterol and intrinsic membrane proteins are embedded. The polar head groups of the phospholipids (represented by balls) face the aqueous phase on both sides of the bilayer, while the hydrocarbon chains form the interior of the bilayer. The cytoplasmic side of this membrane faces down. Various intrinsic membrane proteins are shown with their hydrophobic sequences passing through the bilayer. Not shown are extrinsic, or membrane-associated, proteins attached to this surface (see text). (From ref. 9, with permission.)

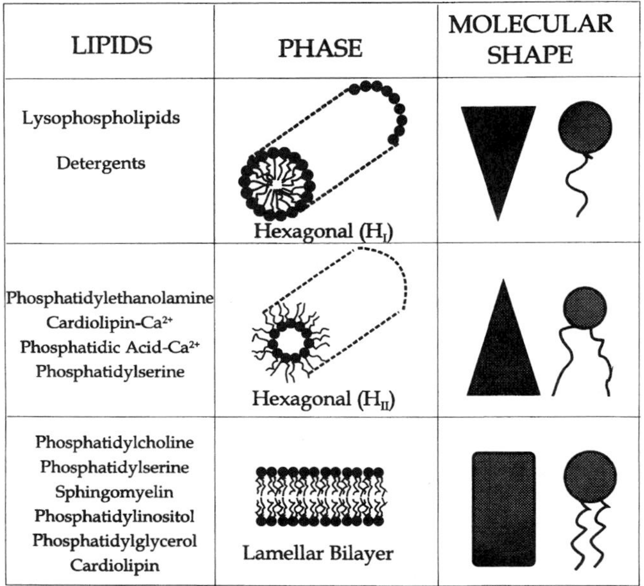

Figure 5. Phases and molecular shapes for some common membrane lipids. (From ref. 36.)

mobile and can take up many conformations. Second, the *lamellar gel phase* (L_β) is formed when bilayers in the liquid crystalline phases are cooled and freeze into a solid state. There are several different solid structures, L_β being the most common. The individual phospholipid molecules exhibit no lateral motion and the acyl chains are fully extended (all *trans*) perpendicular to the bilayer plane, causing a closer packing of molecules in the bilayer surface and an increase in bilayer thickness relative to the liquid crystalline phase. Both lamellar structures are preferred by cylindrically shaped lipid species such as phosphatidylcholine, phosphatidylserine, phosphatidylinositol, sphingomyelin, and cholesterol. Third, unlike the lamellar phase which has a plane of symmetry, the *hexagonal I phase* (H_I) has an axis of symmetry and forms cylindrical structures with polar head groups on the outside in contact with water. This phase is preferred by lipids with large polar head groups that have an inverted cone shape such as lysophospholipids. Fourth, *the hexagonal II phase* (H_{II}) is a similar cylindrical form, but with polar head groups facing inward toward a cylinder of water. Cone-shaped lipids with small head groups, such as phosphatidylethanolamine, and/or with large, difficult to pack, acyl chains, for example with *cis*-unsaturated bonds, favor this phase (Fig. 5).

Lipids within bilayers may be distributed nonhomogeneously in two ways—across the plane of the bilayer (asymmetry) or within the plane (lateral domains). Glycolipids are found only on the outer membrane leaflet. The red cell membrane has phosphatidylserine and phosphatidylethanolamine primarily in the cytoplasmic leaflet, while phosphatidylcholine and sphingomyelin are concentrated in the outer leaflet (95). Lateral heterogeneity in cell membranes is usually associated with different protein species and functions (44). A straightforward example is the different lipid compositions of the apical and basolateral surfaces of epithelial cells. Concentrations of specific membrane protein species, such as occurs in purple membrane patches containing bacteriorhodopsin in *Halobacterium halobium* are enriched in lipids that associate with these proteins. Similar domains are thought to exist within synapses, where proteins involved in cell to cell communication are concentrated. In protein-free bilayers, there is also evidence of discrete lipid domains with different structures on the bilayer surface (61). "Lipidic particles" observed in binary lipid mixtures where one lipid forms bilayers and the other prefers the hexagonal II phase are thought to represent such microdomain structures (17). While such structures have been proposed to facilitate membrane fusion or stabilize membrane regions with high curvature, evidence supporting these roles in cells is absent.

Physical Properties of Bilayers and Membranes

The physical properties of membranes are dependent on composition and environmental factors. Two important concepts in the biophysics of membranes are *fluidity*, which is essentially the inverse of viscosity and a measure of the mobility of molecules within the bilayer, and *order*, which is a measure of the degree to which the acyl chains are extended parallel to each other and orthogonal to the plane of the bilayer. Often these two parameters parallel one another and the terms have often been used interchangeably, although this is strictly incorrect. A number of techniques, including fluorescence relaxation measurements, electron spin, or paramagnetic resonance (ESR or EPR; see Chap. 28), and nuclear magnetic resonance (NMR) use reporter probes incorporated into membranes to assess these parameters. The lamellar gel phase lacks fluidity and is nearly perfectly ordered. The liquid crystalline phase is fluid but its viscosity is much higher than that of isotropic fluids. Furthermore, it exhibits different degrees of fluidity at different depths in the bilayer. Near the membrane surface, where head groups are tightly packed, mobility is low but increases at the ends of the acyl chains near the middle of the bilayer. The fluidity of membranes may be an important factor in the function of intrinsic membrane proteins (see below). Indirect evidence for this concept comes from studies of bacteria, which actively alter the composition of their membrane lipids in order to maintain constant fluidity in the face of changing environmental conditions such as temperature and pressure. *Escherichia coli* grown at low temperatures incorporate a higher fraction of unsaturated fatty acids into membrane lipids to counter the decrease in fluidity that the cool environment induces (79). Analogously, a barophilic bacterium (NPT3) increases its unsaturated fatty acid composition to oppose increased membrane order induced by high hydrostatic pressures (19).

The most common method for studying phase transitions between lamellar gel and liquid crystalline phases is the use of differential scanning calorimetry (DSC) to measure the heat absorbed or released as the phase transition occurs. The temperature at which such transitions occur can be altered by changes in pH, ionic strength, and pressure. DSC demonstrates that lipid mixtures of even closely related species often do not mix ideally, leading to separation of microdomains with distinct phase transition characteristics. Transitions in mixtures containing negatively charged lipids are strongly influenced by Ca^{2+} concentration, which causes clustering of the anionic head groups into distinct domains. The effect of sterols such as cholesterol is to broaden the transition range between gel and crystalline phases. In the liquid crystalline state, cholesterol tends to take up empty space between acyl chains, limiting their mobility and causing a more ordered bilayer. In the highly ordered gel phase, cholesterol interferes with the close packing of acyl chains, reducing bilayer order. Thus, cholesterol promotes a bilayer structure somewhere between gel and crystalline (56).

Membrane Proteins: General Structure and Function

Many of the chapters of this book detail specific information about different classes of membrane proteins and their interactions with anesthetics. Here we introduce some of the broad concepts of membrane protein structure, emphasizing interactions with membrane lipids. It is important at the outset to realize that membrane proteins are very difficult to crystallize and that so few structures are known that general rules are based on little hard data.

The proteins on a cell's surface are essential for biochemical activity and determine many of the cell's characteristics. Membrane proteins act as transporters for a cell's nutrients and wastes; they also act as molecular receptors and sensors, triggering intracellular activities. Membrane proteins transduce energy, using light or chemical potential to move ions and nutrients across membranes or using ion gradients to induce chemical catalysis. Ion pumps and ion channels are membrane proteins that determine the dynamic electrical activity of cells, the sine qua non of neurons.

Membrane proteins are broadly classified into two groups depending on how readily they can be separated from membranes. *Intrinsic* membrane proteins cannot be purified without solubilizing membranes because they contain domains that pass through the membrane (transmembrane domains); most excitable proteins and ion pumps belong to this class. *Extrinsic,* or membrane-associated, proteins copurify with membranes, but are easily separated from them by procedures such as ionic strength or pH changes. In general, these associated proteins are weakly bound by electrostatic or hydrophobic forces to either lipids or intrinsic membrane proteins. Cytoskeletal proteins, which help maintain a cell's shape and facilitate interactions between cytoplasmic organelles and the cell membrane, are membrane-associated proteins.

Transmembrane domains of intrinsic proteins are predicted to consist of continuous sections of hydrophobic amino acids that are long enough to cross the bilayer, although shorter sections that dip into the bilayer are possible. Based on the few structures available (15), these transmembrane domains apparently take on one of two structures—an α-helix or a β-sheet.

The α-helical structure allows the amino acid backbone to internally hydrogen bond, while exposing the hydrophobic side chains to the lipid core of the membrane. Thus, the thermodynamic requirement of minimizing interactions between polar and nonpolar molecular structures is fulfilled. Each helical turn takes 3.6 amino acids and the helix rises 1.5 Å per residue (5.4 Å rise per turn); therefore, some 22 amino acids are required to cross a typical 35 Å width bilayer structure.

The other secondary structure motif is the β-sheet in which the backbone hydrogen bonds are satisfied between adjacent strands. It rises 3.5 Å per amino acid residue, so some nine residues will cross the bilayer. However, if the interstrand hydrogen bonds are staggered by one residue the β-sheet takes on a tilt of 60° relative to the plane of the bilayer and 18 hydrophobic amino acids are required in a transmembrane sheet (59).

With the advent of genetic techniques, there is now a great deal known about the amino acid sequences (primary structure) of membrane proteins, and it is common for investigators to use side-chain hydrophobicity profiles to predict transmembrane domains (47). Stretches of 22 hydrophobic amino acids indicate transmembrane regions but not necessarily their structure. In bacterial rhodopsin, a member of the G-protein–associated family, hydropathy analysis suggests there are seven transmembrane regions and structural studies have shown that there are seven transmembrane α-helices arranged nearly parallel to each other and at right angles to the plane of the bilayer. In the bacterial protein porin, where hydropathy analysis reveals no continuous stretches of hydrophobic amino acids, there is a continuous "bracelet" of β-sheet arranged at 60° relative to the plane of the bilayer (called a β-barrel) exposed to the bilayer on the one side and to the aqueous channel on the other (15,47). Thus, based on the little data available, hydropathy analysis has so far proved reasonably reliable.

Indirect approaches to transmembrane protein topology utilizing glycosylation analysis, chemical modification techniques, antibodies, and high-resolution micrographic methods are beginning to provide additional data to refine structural models. Membrane proteins contain cytoplasmic and extracellular domains that form important interactive and functional structures. Glycosylation is exclusively extracellular, and membrane receptors are formed by extracytoplasmic protein regions. Cytoplasmic domains of intrinsic membrane proteins function as regulatory sites or enzymes, ion binding sites, and cytoplasmic protein binding sites. Such studies have recently led to a revision of the structure of the glycine receptor that had been inferred from hydropathy analysis (99).

In addition to their obvious roles as anchors in the membrane, transmembrane sequences of amino acids are thought to form important functional components of some membrane proteins, such as the ion channels. There is convincing evidence that α-helices from multiple subunits combine to form the transmembrane ion channel of the nicotinic acetylcholine receptor (nAcChoR) (12), but it remains controversial whether the channel helices are separated from the bilayer by more helices or by a β-barrel structure.

Membrane proteins are often assembled from multiple subunits that are independently encoded in the cell genome, but little is known about the nature of the interactions between subunits that govern assembly of functional proteins. Most models of intrinsic membrane proteins suggest that α-helices make extensive contacts with other helices, excluding lipids from the inside of the protein; however, some workers have emphasized the role of interstitial lipids trapped within the protein's structure and exchanging only slowly, or not at all, with the bulk lipids (80).

Lipid-Protein Interactions

When lipids containing a covalently bound spin label are added at low concentration into membranes, their electron spin resonance spectra (see Chap. 28), which are sensitive to small differences in mobility, resolve a population of lipids whose mobility is restricted compared to the lipid bilayer (24,58,97). This restricted component results from the interaction of lipids with membrane proteins. These so-called boundary or annular lipids typically have rotational correlation times some 10 to 100 times longer than lipids not directly in contact with proteins (bulk lipids) (75). They are not "fixed" to the protein but exchange with the bulk lipids once every 10 to 100 nanoseconds.

When a protein is purified and inserted (reconstituted) into bilayers of known lipid composition, it is possible to estimate the number of lipid molecules directly surrounding the protein as well as the distribution of lipids between annular and bulk membrane environments, a measure of a lipid's affinity for a protein. In general, the number of lipid molecules that surround a membrane protein increases with the protein's size. This is not surprising since the intramembranous surface area of a membrane protein is expected to roughly correlate with its molecular weight.

The functions of some membrane proteins, including gated ion channels, appear to be dependent on the physicochemical properties of the lipids immediately surrounding the protein or upon more specific lipid-protein interactions (10,27,37,88). The role of lipid-protein interactions in modulating membrane protein function can be examined by modifying the lipid composition of the membrane bilayer and then determining whether the activity of a protein embedded in that bilayer changes. However, an important limitation of this approach is that since even a subtle alteration in the membrane composition may alter many physicochemical properties of the lipid bilayer, it may be difficult to precisely define the relevant lipid-protein interactions.

Some Representative Membrane Proteins

In this chapter we have chosen to present a few membrane proteins in some detail. The action of general anesthetics on these proteins will be discussed in a later section. The basis of our choice is twofold. First, structural details are known about only a few proteins that happen to be available in sufficient quantity to allow such studies; none of these comes from the central nervous system. Second, we have chosen proteins that are representatives of superfamilies of proteins. The existence of these superfamilies offsets the technical limitations referred to above and allows one to extrapolate to other members of the family that may be of interest.

The Nicotinic Acetylcholine Receptor Lipid-protein interactions have been extensively studied in nAcChoR membranes. The structure of this receptor is reviewed by Taylor and Dilger in Chaps. 15 and 16, respectively (Fig. 6). Early ESR studies used native membrane preparations in which the molar ratio of lipid:protein is high, in the range of 500–1000:1 (34). Thus, only a small portion of the lipid in such samples is at the lipid-protein interface, resulting in a relatively small annular lipid ESR spectral component. With the development of affinity purification and reconstitution techniques, it became possible to precisely control the lipid composition of the membrane, to adjust the lipid/protein ratio, and to remove nonreceptor protein components (60). Approximately 50 (annular) lipid molecules surround each nAcChoR (23). If the lipid/protein molar ratio is reduced below 45:1, activity is reduced (40). This activity can be recovered by simply increasing the lipid content of the bilayers. However, if the lipid/protein molar ratio is reduced to 20:1, activity is irreversibly lost, presumably due to protein unfolding.

The distribution of lipids between annular and bulk environments is not random in nAcChoR membranes but is dependent on the identity of the lipid head group. In general, the spin-labeled cholesterol analogue androstanol and negatively charged phospholipids and fatty acids exhibit a high affinity for the lipid-protein interface (23,75). This selectivity reflects both electrostatic and steric interactions between the nAcChoR and the lipid bilayer.

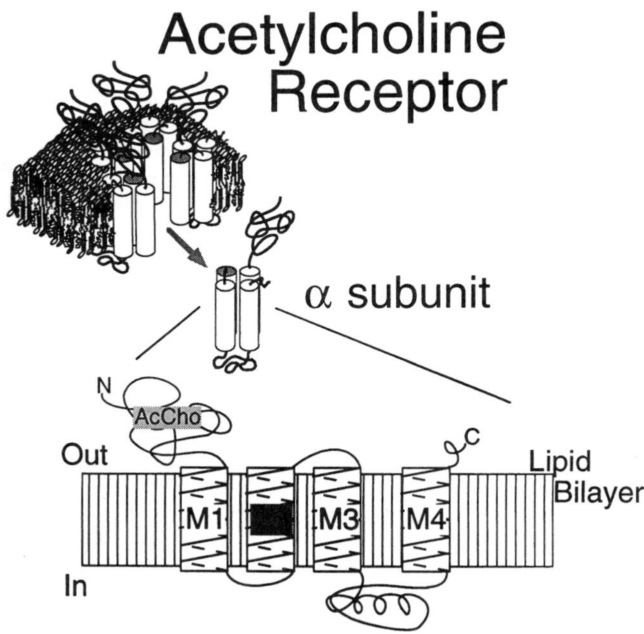

Figure 6. Schematic of the nAcChoR, a representative ligand gated ion channel. The receptor is an oligomer (*upper diagram*) of five highly homologous subunits of which two are identical (α subunits, which bind acetylcholine) and three (β, δ, γ) are distinct. The subunits are arranged in a centro-symmetric manner around a central funnel that contains the ion channel. In this figure, one α subunit is pulled forward of the oligomer to reveal this funnel. As shown in the *lower diagram,* each subunit has four hydrophobic transmembrane domains. The M2 domain lines the pore and the top of this helix is shaded in the upper two diagrams.

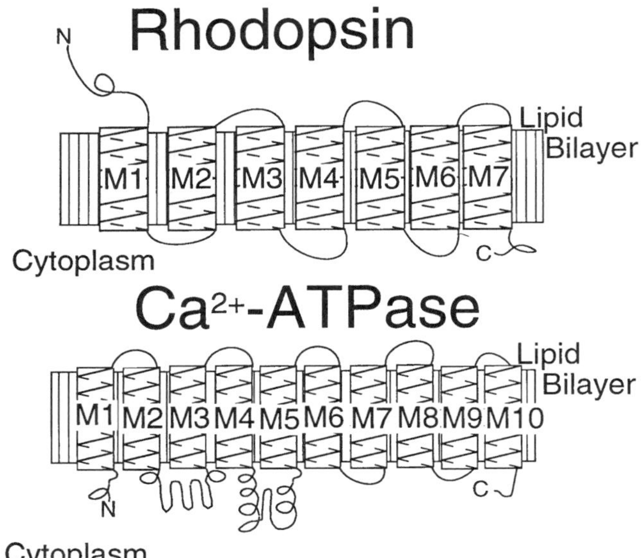

Figure 7. Schematic of a second messenger receptor and an ion pump. The upper schematic shows the structure of rhodopsin, which is the best-characterized member of a seven transmembrane helix superfamily that includes most of the ligand-activated second messenger receptors. The lower schematic shows Ca-ATPase, a member of the ten transmembrane helix superfamily of membrane transporters.

The selectivity of certain lipids for the lipid-protein interface of the nAcChoR may have important structural and functional implications. Fourier transform infrared studies suggest that the secondary structure of the nAcChoR depends on cholesterol and negatively charged phospholipids (3,28). Cholesterol increases the α-helical content while phosphatidic acid increases the β-sheet content of the receptor. In addition, these lipids are required for normal channel gating function and modulate desensitization kinetics (87). A correlation has been detected between the membrane order parameter and ion channel activity (27). Based on these findings, it has been proposed that an optimal membrane fluidity window exists such that if the membrane fluidity is above or below this range, receptor activity is reduced. More recently, however, it has been suggested that specific interactions between annular lipids and the receptor at the lipid-protein interface are more important than bulk membrane properties in determining receptor function (88).

Sarcoplasmic Reticulum Ca-ATPase The calcium–adenosine triphosphatase (Ca-ATPase) enzyme is responsible for Ca^{2+} transport within muscle cells and accounts for approximately 80% of the total protein content of sarcoplasmic reticulum membranes (Fig. 7). Studies using both delipidated and reconstituted Ca-ATPase indicate that 20 to 30 lipid molecules surround the enzyme (85,91). As with the nAcChoR, a minimum number of lipid molecules per protein is needed to preserve full activity. This number is approximately equal to the number of lipid molecules that surround each protein. In contrast to the nAcChoR, however, there is only a small degree of selectivity at the lipid-protein interface for negatively charged lipids.

The activity of the Ca-ATPase is dependent on the physicochemical properties of the lipid bilayer. For example, reconstitution studies reveal that the enzyme's activity is dependent on the thickness of the lipid bilayer. Activity is greatest when the enzyme is reconstituted into bilayers of lipids that have a chain length of 18 carbons, the average chain length of phospholipids in biologic membranes, but less active when in membranes whose lipids are longer or shorter than 18 carbons (14). Presumably, mismatch between the length of the membrane's hydrophobic acyl chains and the nonpolar transmembrane regions of the enzyme alters its function. The activity of the Ca-ATPase also varies with the head group of the lipid forming the bilayer, with phosphatidylcholine supporting activity the best. Enzyme activity has also been correlated with membrane fluidity as well as protein mobility, although the underlying mechanism that accounts for these correlations is not known with certainty (84). One possibility is that the lipid bilayer composition modulates protein function by altering the aggregation state of the protein; protein dimers exhibit the greatest activity, while monomers are less active, and aggregates larger than dimers are even less active (5). This hypothesis is supported by the observation that the induction of protein aggregation by melitin reduces both protein mobility and activity while anesthetics have the opposite effect (see below) (57,96).

Rhodopsin Rhodopsin is a G-protein–coupled receptor that is the major protein component of rod outer segment disk membranes (Fig. 7). Absorption of a photon by the retina induces a series of very rapid conformational transitions in rhodopsin, followed by a slower conformational change from the meta I state to the meta II state, which causes G-protein activation. The states are identified by their unique absorption spectrograms, and the quasi-equilibrium between the meta I and meta II states that exists on the millisecond time scale (meta II/meta I ratio equals K_{eq}) has been used as a measure of rhodopsin activity (70).

Approximately 40% of the lipids in rod outer segment disk membranes are motionally restricted. The mobilities of these motionally restricted lipids are on the order of tenfold lower than the mobilities of lipids not in direct contact with the protein. This tenfold difference is similar to that found in both nAcChoR and Ca-ATPase membranes. However, by reconstituting rhodopsin into bilayers of different lipid composition, it has become apparent that the molecular properties of the lipids are not the major determinates of protein photochemical function in contrast to the strong selectivity of nAcChoR and the weak lipid selectivity for the Ca-ATPase.

However, the average or bulk properties of the bilayer do appear to modulate rhodopsin function (69). Straume and Litman (86) suggest that a property they refer to as the acyl chain packing free volume, quantified by a parameter, f_v, modulates K_{eq}. They propose that f_v is a measure of the overall ability of a bilayer to accommodate integral membrane protein conformational changes. Since the meta II state has a larger volume than the meta I state, the meta I–meta II equilibrium is predicted to shift toward meta II (K_{eq} increases) when f_v increases. Thus, increasing f_v either by raising the temperature of the bilayer or by decreasing its cholesterol content causes equivalent increases in K_{eq} (69,70). The slope derived from a plot of f_v versus K_{eq} is a measure of the bilayer's ability to use the increase in acyl chain packing free volume to accommodate the transition to the meta II state and is referred to by Mitchell et al. (69,70) as a "permissiveness index." These studies indicate that the permissiveness index is larger for membranes composed of unsaturated lipids than saturated ones. Thus, increasing f_v leads to a larger increase in K_{eq} when rhodopsin is reconstituted into polyunsaturated lipids than when it is reconstituted into lipids with greater degrees of saturation.

The value of K_{eq} also increases when rhodopsin is reconstituted into mixed lipid bilayers containing increasing quantities of lipids that by themselves would form the H_{II} phase (10). It has been suggested that the latent tendency to form the nonbilayer phase provides an additional driving force that shifts the conformational equilibrium toward the meta II state leading to greater activity (37).

MECHANISMS OF ANESTHESIA

At the beginning of this chapter, we introduced the general reasons why conserved hydrophobic regions of membranes, particularly those at synapses, are considered likely targets for anesthetics. Based on this and our current concepts of membrane structure, we can broadly define several likely locations of membrane-anesthetic interactions (Fig. 8) that form the basis of various hypotheses of general anesthetic action. The first hypothesis considers the membrane lipids as the target for anesthetics, the second considers that anesthetics interact directly with membrane proteins, and the third that anesthetics act, directly or indirectly, at the interface between the lipid interior of the bilayer and the hydrophobic structures of intrinsic membrane proteins. Fourth, the possibility that protein-protein interactions within the bilayer (i.e., protein aggregation) may be involved in anesthetic action must be considered. The next section of this chapter considers these possible sites of general anesthetic action in turn. Then, to examine the evidence for the role of proteins or lipid-protein interactions in general anesthetic action, the action of anesthetics on selected specific membrane protein targets is considered.

Before outlining specific mechanistic models, it is important to assess some of the underlying assumptions common to all of them. The central assumption, which has been called the "unitary hypothesis," was first espoused by Claude Bernard in 1875. In essence, the unitary hypothesis states that all general anesthetics act by the same mechanism at the same molecular site(s). Arguments about the suitability of this assumption center around whether one wishes to emphasize the commonality of actions or the differences between drugs. That so diverse a group of drugs (Fig. 1) all induce similar changes in the behavior of animals and the function of some subcellular components is remarkable. This observation makes the unitary hypothesis both elegant and attractive, and it continues to provide a philosophical underpinning for research. On the other hand, the differences between actions of different anesthetics provide important clues as to the sites where these drugs act. Whether such different actions are intrinsic to the drugs' anesthetic activity or simply an additional drug action unrelated to

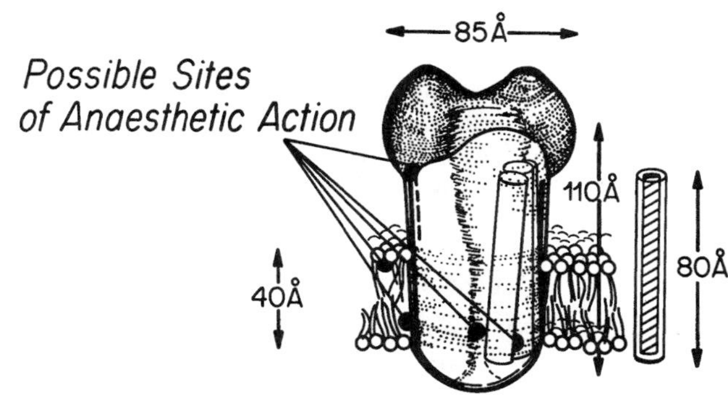

Figure 8. Possible locations of general anesthesia sites in membranes. A three-dimensional model of a ligand-gated ion channel in its lipid bilayer based on the AcChoR. The protein is about 11 nm long, perpendicular to the plain of the lipid bilayer, which is 4 nm thick (1 nm is 10Å). Nearly half the protein projects well out into the extracellular space (*top*) and the binding sites for acetylcholine are thought to be at the top of the protein. Cylinders indicate α-helices, which are probably packed perpendicular to the plane of the bilayer. *Filled circles* indicate possible sites of anesthetic action in the lipid bilayer: the lipid-protein interface, the intramembranous region of the protein, a short hydrophobic cylinder lining the channel or a hydrophobic cleft in the extramembranous region of the protein. The amino acid composition of all the protein hydrophobic regions is highly conserved. (From ref. 42, with permission.)

anesthesia is often impossible to determine. We know too little about the mechanisms underlying consciousness, pain sensation, and memory to establish a universally accepted definition of the anesthetized state—if indeed it is a single state.

Anesthetic Interactions with Membrane Lipids

Lipid Solubility Hypothesis

Hans Meyer summarized his theory of anesthesia by stating that "narcosis commences when any chemically indifferent substance attains a certain molar concentration in the lipoids of the cell." This statement can be expressed mathematically as:

$$EC_{50} \times \lambda = CS(m,50) = E_{50}$$

where EC_{50} is the aqueous concentration of anesthetic that anesthetizes half of a population of test animals, λ is the membrane/buffer partition coefficient, CS(m,50) is the membrane concentration of the anesthetic at the EC_{50} (equal to about 25–50 mmol/l in lipid bilayers), and E_{50} represents the change associated with any functional process when it is half maximally affected, for example, anesthesia of half a group of animals (63).

The lipid solubility hypothesis is remarkably successful at correlating the potency of the majority of general anesthetics with their lipid solubility, but it fails to account for a number of the pharmacologic features outlined at the beginning of this chapter. A number of hydrophobic molecules that are chemically similar to known anesthetics are much less potent than their lipid/membrane partition coefficients predict, or they may actually antagonize anesthetics (45). The solubility hypothesis fails to explain pressure reversal, since pressure does not sufficiently alter lipid solubility. The cutoff effect was once thought to be due to aqueous solubility limitations, which prevented the lipid concentration of very hydrophobic drugs from reaching the necessary concentration range for action. However, recent studies demonstrate that nonanesthetic alcohols can achieve the necessary membrane concentration (32). These shortcomings, together with the need to define a mechanism by which the general anesthetics produce their action once they are in the bilayer, led to the formulation of a number of hypotheses that focused on specific lipid properties that anesthetics perturb. These are briefly reviewed in the following sections.

Lipid Perturbation Hypotheses

The proliferation of membrane theories of general anesthetic action, occurring mainly in the 1970s, can be formally categorized by extending the Meyer-Overton equation to include terms both for the perturbation of lipid structure by general anesthetics in the bilayer and for the resultant of this perturbation on membrane protein function (39). Thus, one may write

$$E_{50} = CS(m,50) \times P_1 \times T_P$$

where P_1 reflects the change in lipid properties per mole of anesthetic in the bilayer, and T_P reflects the alteration in membrane protein function or structure that results from the change in lipid properties (39,63). Much is known about the lipid perturbation term, but our current knowledge of lipid-protein interactions is so rudimentary that no clear principles have emerged. In the sections immediately following we discuss models that deal solely with the lipid perturbation term. In a later section we consider the rather preliminary evidence for the involvement of lipid-protein interactions in general anesthetic action.

Membrane Expansion Pressure reversal of anesthesia suggests that anesthetics may act by altering the volume of their site of action. The *critical volume hypothesis* states that anesthesia occurs when a hydrophobic membrane phase expands beyond a critical point, and this expansion in turn causes dysfunction of membrane proteins. At physiologic anesthetic concentrations, model bilayers expand 0.2% to 0.6% (43). This degree of expansion is close to that predicted from in vivo pressure reversal data (39,66). The volume change in the bilayer is anisotropic. Because the acyl chains are disordered there is no increase in thickness; consequently, the largest change caused by anesthetics is an increase in membrane surface area. While pressure reversal is implicitly explained by the critical volume hypothesis, it fails to adequately explain the cutoff (11). On the other hand, the pharmacology of the inert gases is elegantly predicted by the critical volume hypothesis (22).

Phase Transitions Another biophysical feature of membranes that may be perturbed by anesthetics is their phase state. The *lateral phase transition hypothesis* suggests that lipid microdomains surrounding membrane proteins undergo a crystalline to gel phase transition due to changes in the shape of the protein (93). Anesthetics therefore inhibit protein function by eliminating the gel phase lipids. While anesthetics have been shown to alter the transition temperature for crystalline to gel phase in bilayers, the pressure required to reverse this effect is an order of magnitude smaller than that required to reverse anesthesia. Although overt phase transitions are unlikely to occur in synaptic membranes because of their complex lipid composition, the tendency of some lipids within these membranes to form other phases may be important (see, for example, the section on rhodopsin, above).

Lipid Fluidity and Order When anesthetics dissolve in lipid bilayers, they decrease the measured order parameter. The lipid fluidity hypothesis assumes that this physical property of lipids is critical for function of synaptic membrane proteins, such as ion channels. Indeed this kind of modulation is observed for Na/K ATPase, where a 6% increase in order parameter decreases function tenfold (81). In cholesterol-containing model membranes, there is a good correlation between the ability of anesthetics to disorder lipids and their activity. In addition, the anesthetic activity (or lack thereof) of halogenated ethers correlates with their inability to fluidize membranes (62). The stereoselective anesthetic actions of cannabinols also correlate with their membrane fluidizing potencies (49), but the smaller stereoselective effects of isoflurane enantiomers do not (33). In *Torpedo* postsynaptic membranes, a cutoff for n-alcohols for membrane disordering is observed at about the same chain length as the cutoff for anesthesia in tadpoles (65). Pressure is predicted to oppose the fluidizing effects of anesthetics, and this has been observed experimentally (13).

Critique of Lipid Hypotheses

The unitary lipid theories account for the potencies of a wide range of anesthetics. By incorporating specific lipid perturbations, features such as anesthetic cutoff and pressure reversal can also be explained. Experimental evidence best supports a lipid fluidity or disorder model; however, all the lipid hypotheses fail to satisfy the requirements of a working model in several important ways. First, none of these hypotheses easily accounts for the stereoselectivity of isoflurane, but then this stereoselectivity is not well established and is at best rather modest. In addition, it is the ester region of phospholipids that are chiral and the question of isoflurane's interaction with such regions has not been examined. Second, the membrane changes induced by clinical concentrations of anesthetics are quite small and difficult to measure. Indeed, membrane changes of the same magnitude are caused by a temperature increase of less than 1°C, which does not cause anesthesia in experimental animals. While anesthetic and temperature perturbations are not thermodynamically equivalent (heat is sensed by the whole system, general anesthetics mainly by the bilayer), this fact suggests that the observed membrane perturbations may not be linked to anesthesia. Finally, all the lipid hypotheses explicitly state that anesthetics ultimately affect membrane protein function, without specifying at the molecular level how such lipid perturbations cause protein function to change. For the present, a serious barrier to testing this extension of the lipid theories is the fact that the proteins at the heart of general anesthetic action have not been identified. A similar problem faces those theories that invoke direct protein-anesthetic interactions. Nonetheless, since sufficient targets exist where general anesthetics exert effects at or near clinical levels, work seeking to establish general principles is able to proceed. Aspects of this work are presented in the succeeding sections, and later chapters provide more details (31,39).

Anesthetic Interactions with Membrane Proteins

While it has been known for many decades that certain general anesthetics bind to soluble proteins and that they tend to do so without altering the conformations of those proteins (at least at clinical concentrations) (see Chapter 2), technical difficulties have prevented testing the hypothesis that general anesthetics bind directly to excitable membrane proteins in the central nervous system. These difficulties stem from two sources. First, and most important, their high lipid solubility and their low expected affinity for putative binding sites make general anesthetics the most challenging of all pharmacologic ligands to study by classical radioligand binding techniques (see Chapter 25). Second, if general anesthetics do bind to membrane proteins they would be expected to exert their actions allosterically. This means that they will bind to the different conformational states exhibited by such proteins with different affinities. It is most likely that general anesthetics will bind with highest affinity to the active state of a membrane protein, yet such a state is often only present for a few milliseconds. In this section we consider how these difficulties may be overcome and briefly illustrate the progress achieved with examples.

The difficulties that face classical radioligand binding techniques may be illustrated by a simple calculation (63). If a general anesthetic with a membrane/buffer partition coefficient of 10 binds to a single site on each γ-aminobutyric acid (GABA) receptor in the brain with a dissociation constant of 200 μM, then one can calculate that for every molecule bound to the receptor there will be several hundred thousand associated with membrane lipid. Thus, the one molecule we are interested in will be undetectable against the background binding. Can this problem be overcome by increasing the affinity of the general anesthetic? Insofar as any theory conforms to the empirical Meyer-Overton rule, we must expect that all general anesthetics will exhibit a simple relationship between lipid solubility and binding site affinity. Thus, searching for a higher affinity general anesthetic in order to increase the ratio of protein- to lipid-associated general anesthetic will probably not lead to success. Two further strategies to solve this problem are available.

First, one might seek to purify, or at least to concentrate, the protein of interest in order to increase the ratio of general anesthetic binding sites to lipid. This would require purifications of the order of 10- to 100,000-fold, and these are difficult to achieve. In some specialized tissues nature has already performed this trick for us. For example, in the electroplax of *Torpedo*, an electric fish, the nAcChoR concentration is so high that it has proved possible to study the binding of radiolabeled barbiturates to the receptor (21). In the future it may prove possible to exploit expression systems to produce high concentrations of other proteins in the plasma membrane and extend the applicability of such measurements to a wider range of proteins.

Second, one might attempt a filtration assay with the object of quickly washing away much of the lipid-associated general anesthetic before the protein-bound general anesthetic can dissociate. However, a ligand bound with an affinity in the micromolar range will be expected to dissociate almost as rapidly as that dissolved in the lipid, so this strategy is of limited utility unless the ligand can be detained on the protein in some way. One strategy for doing so involves covalent binding. This method is limited to general anesthetics that can be induced to react while bound to the protein. For example, when halothane is exposed to ultraviolet light the bromine-carbon bond is broken and the reactive species generated can combine with the protein. To date this method has been applied to both brain and *Torpedo* synaptic membranes. Evidence for protein binding has been found, but this binding seems rather unselective (see Chapter 2). It is therefore evident that this technique suffers from many of the limitations of the normal binding assay because even lipids are labeled. However, this limitation can be overcome if the covalently labeled membranes are digested into their components. An interesting example of how far this technique can be pushed is provided by the classical photolabel TID (3-trifluoromethyl-3-(m-iodophenyl) diazirine), which has recently been shown to be a general anesthetic (50). Covalent photoincorporation of the radio iodinated derivative of this agent into nAcChoR-containing membranes occurs at many sites but three types of region predominate. The first of these is the lipid bilayer, a component that can be discarded by purifying the protein on gels. The second of these is the lipid-protein interface, where TID binds in a nondisplaceable manner to most of the amino acid residues exposed to the lipid. The third is the hydrophobic lining of the channel where a single TID binds in a displaceable fashion. The detection of this single site against the background of nondisplaceable binding to the rest of the receptor is only possible if the receptor is digested with proteases into several fragments that are then separated on gels (98). By extending this technique to include amino acid sequencing, it is possible to detect the actual residues to which the agent has bound. However, this extra information is bought at a high price because sequencing requires milligrams of protein; thus, once again we have a powerful method that will be of limited utility until efficient expression systems are devised (7).

In addition to the direct approaches above, several less direct approaches offer useful solutions to the nonspecific binding problem. The oldest involves finding a high affinity nonanesthetic radioligand whose site is allosterically modulated when the general anesthetic occupies its own separate site. Often this allosteric ligand will be the agonist itself. For example, the action of barbiturates on [^{3}H]acetylcholine binding provided the first clue that there was a barbiturate binding site on the AcChoR (21). In other cases the allosteric ligand used to detect the effect of anesthetics may itself bind to a relatively uncharacterized site. For example, the GABA receptor radiolabeled ligand, t-butylbicyclophosphorothionate, binds to the picrotoxin (convulsant) site. Barbiturates allosterically modulate this site, suggesting that they occupy another allosteric site (92; see also Chapter 18).

We now turn to the problem of general anesthetic binding to transient conformational states. Because these states may exist for only a few milliseconds, the only way to directly detect such binding is to "catch" the protein in this conformational state. One way to do so is by rapidly freezing the protein-anesthetic complex while it is in the transient active state. A general anesthetic such as halothane or TID could then be photoactivated and permanently bound to the trapped transiently available anesthetic site. This direct approach has not yet been exploited. Instead, it is common to infer the existence of anesthetic sites on transient states by studying function with techniques of high time resolution. These studies variously involve single-channel kinetic studies, inhibition of brief macroscopic currents, additivity between inhibitory anesthetics to test for mutually exclusive occupation of a single site, and site-directed mutagenesis to probe the location of sites. Examples of such approaches appear below and in later chapters of this book.

Anesthetic Effects on Lipid-Protein Interactions

The hypothesis that general anesthetics act by perturbing interactions between neuronal membrane proteins and their lipid environment has been investigated by a number of methods. As mentioned above, photolabeling shows general anesthetics to be present in the lipid-protein interface, but this does not prove they have a functional role there. Electron paramagnetic resonance studies with spin-labeled lipids provide another approach. A third approach is to reconstitute proteins into bilayers whose lipid composition can be precisely controlled. It has been found in several instances that the action of general anesthetics is modulated by the composition of the lipid surrounding the protein in question.

Because the underlying principles governing lipid-protein interaction are poorly understood, we consider some specific examples as part of the sections that follow.

Anesthetic Interactions with Some Representative Membrane Proteins

The Nicotinic Acetylcholine Receptor

General anesthetics have several actions on the nAcChoR, which are reviewed in detail elsewhere (64; see Chap. 14). The two actions with which we concern ourselves here are desensitization and channel inhibition.

At relatively high concentrations, general anesthetics shift the conformational equilibrium of nAcChoR from the resting state toward the inactive, desensitized state with very steep concentration-response curves. The potency with which anesthetics induce this conformational change correlates with both their lipid solubility and their ability to fluidize neuronal membranes (25). Anesthetic-induced desensitization of the nAcChoR can be reversed by applying pressure (8). Consequently, this receptor provides a promising model for studying the actions of general anesthetics on neuronal membrane proteins. General anesthetics reduce the affinity of spin-labeled lipids for the lipid-protein interface of native nAcChoR membranes (34). This effect occurs at the high anesthetic concentrations required to shift the nAcChoR to the desensitized state. This seemed to support the theory that anesthetics modify the receptor's conformational equilibrium by altering interactions between the nAcChoR and membrane lipids. However, subsequent studies using nAcChoR reconstituted into pure dioleoylphosphatidylcholine (DOPC) failed to detect any anesthetic-induced changes at the lipid-protein interface (1). The reason for the discrepancy between studies using receptors in native membranes and receptors reconstituted into pure DOPC is not known with certainty. However, if anesthetics act by perturbing specific lipid-nAcChoR interactions, then the anesthetic sensitivity of the nAcChoR should be sensitive to the lipid composition of the membrane. Preliminary studies do suggest that when the nAcChoR is reconstituted into pure DOPC, it becomes relatively insensitive to the actions of general anesthetics (76). This is not an artifact of reconstitution because when such receptors are re-reconstituted into bilayers that contain cholesterol and negatively charged lipids, sensitivity to general anesthetics is restored.

Photolabeling studies show that halothane labels all five subunits of the nAcChoR as well as the phospholipids in nAcChoR membranes (see Chap. 2). The precise nAcChoR sites that are photolabeled by halothane are not yet known, but the lipid-protein interface with its abundance of hydrophobic amino acids is a likely location. TID, one of the most potent general anesthetics known with an EC_{50} of 610 nM (50), photolabels the lipid-protein interface of the nAcChoR extensively (7). Thus, there is little doubt that general anesthetics access the lipid-protein interface.

At clinically relevant concentrations, general anesthetics neither alter the degree of desensitization nor have marked effects on bulk lipid properties or lipid-protein interfacial lipid mobility (25,34), but they do increase the apparent rate of agonist-induced desensitization (77). The mechanism is unknown, but it might involve the perturbation of specific interactions between the nAcChoR and its annular membrane lipids or direct anesthetic-protein interactions.

In contrast to the nonspecific pharmacology of desensitization, channel inhibition is much more selective. Some common agents, such as ethanol and ethylcarbamate (urethane), do not inhibit channel opening, which would seem to rule out a lipid mechanism. Here we concentrate on those agents that do inhibit the channel. Kinetic (see Chapter 14) and pharmacologic (29) studies suggest that inhibitory anesthetics may block the open channel by binding directly to it after activation by the agonist (called open channel block). Anesthetics may bind within the ion channel and thereby directly obstruct the lumen, or alternatively they may bind elsewhere and inhibit in an allosteric manner. The hypothesis that anesthetics bind to a specific site is consistent with the slopes of inhibition curves, which often have Hill coefficients of 1, but a more secure proof of the existence of such a site depends on kinetic work that established that two anesthetic alcohols, octanol and heptanol, mutually excluded each other from occupying an inhibitory site. This alcohol site is distinct from the local anesthetic site where local anesthetics block the channel. Ethanol, which does not block the channel, does not interact with the octanol site (100).

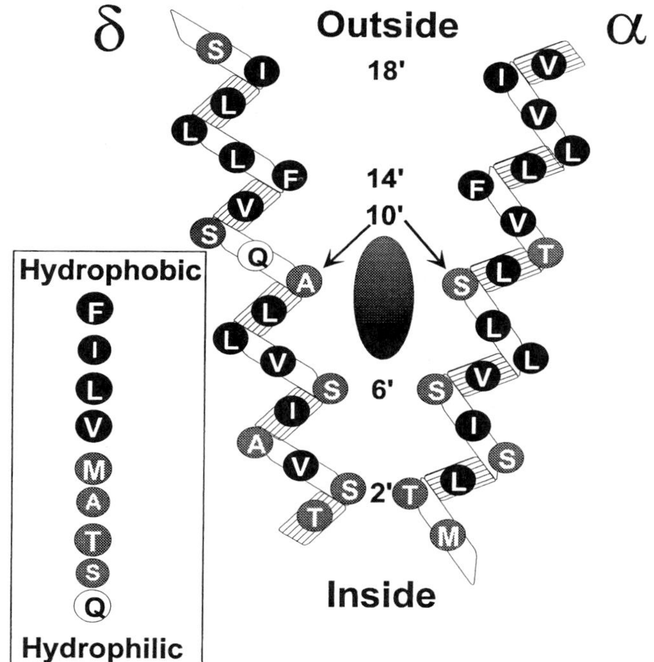

Figure 9. Model of the nicotinic receptor's ion channel site for general anesthetics. Transmembrane domains (M2) for three (two αs and one δ) of the five subunits ($\alpha_2\beta\gamma\delta$) that combine to form a functional receptor/ion channel unit are depicted as α-helices (see Figs. 6 and 8). The amino acid residues are labeled with single-letter codes, and the numbering scheme (1′ through 20′) indicates the aligned residue number starting at the cytoplasmic end of the M2 domains. A hydrophobic blocking molecule is depicted in the center of the channel model. Site-directed mutagenesis experiments indicate that the hydrophobicity of the amino acid residues at the 10′ level in the channel are major determinants of the receptorís sensitivity to block by general anesthetics (see text) (30). A three-tone gray scale is employed to depict the relative hydrophobicity of the amino acid residues found in the M2 domains shown (see inset for scale). Note that largely hydrophobic amino acids are present both above and below the 10′ level in the wild-type channel. These hydrophobic protein regions may allow ions to pass through the channel, but bind to general anesthetics, which then prevent ion movement.

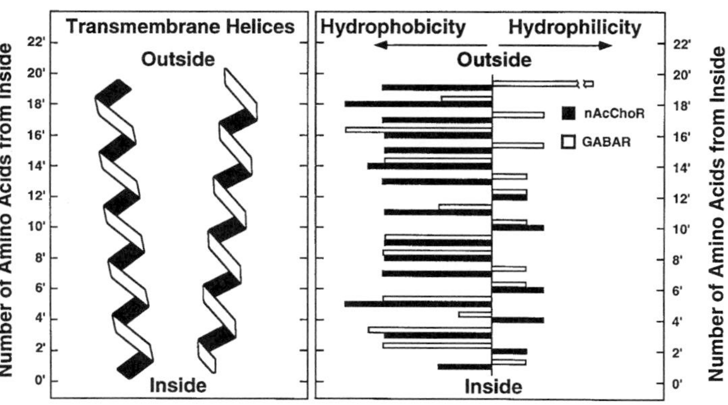

Figure 10. The channel lining helices (M2 domains) of the acetylcholine receptor compared to those of the GABA receptor. In the GABA receptor, the two turns of the α-helix at the outer end of the M2 region are not continuously hydrophobic as they are in the acetylcholine receptor. The relative hydrophobicity of the individual amino acid residues are displayed as a bar chart in the *right panel.* Their position corresponds to their vertical distribution along the M2 helices lining the channel, which are diagrammed in the *left panel.* The helices shown in the *right panel* are the rat muscle acetylcholine receptor's α subunit, and the rat central nervous system GABA receptor's α1 subunit. The other subunits of each receptor are highly homologous in each case with the ones shown.

The presence of a functional inhibitory site for general anesthetics in the nAcChoR ion channel has recently been confirmed (30). Using site-directed mutagenesis of cloned nAcChoR subunits, serines, threonines, and alanines near the middle of the channel-forming M2 domains (10′ level; see Fig. 9 for model) were replaced with more hydrophobic amino acids, such as phenylalanine and isoleucine, to increase the interaction energy between drug and site. When these mutated receptors were expressed in cells, their sensitivity to blockade by general anesthetics was dramatically increased. Similar mutations at the 6′ level did not change the channel sensitivity to anesthetics, suggesting that the site is closer to 10′ than to 6′ in the channel. Furthermore, the kinetic mechanism of inhibition in these studies is consistent with a predominantly open-channel block mechanism for both the wild-type and mutant receptors. The location of this site is explored in Fig. 9. The polar ring at the 10′ position is near to the midpoint of the putative channel. Above these serines lies a cylinder lined with hydrophobic amino acid residues (14′ to 18′). Presumably this nonpolar lining is designed to allow the ions to pass through the channel without hindrance. However, it might have the opposite effect on general anesthetics and provide an inhibitory binding site for them.

The above hypothesis predicts that only members of the superfamily that have this hydrophobic patch at the outer end of their channel should undergo channel inhibition by general anesthetics. The GABA receptor is not inhibited by general anesthetics, so it provides a test of this hypothesis (see Chaps. 11 and 18). The M2 domains of the GABA and the nAcChoR receptors are compared in Fig. 10. The subunit sequences of each of these channel lining helices is so highly conserved for each receptor that we only need to examine one subunit of each to make the comparison. The outer part of the nAcChoR channel has a stretch of seven contiguous hydrophobic amino acids (six are shown), enough to make two whole turns of the helix, but this hydrophobic cylinder is missing in GABA receptors where in the same region hydrophobic amino acids alternate with hydrophilic ones. Thus, the hypothesis holds but further tests will be needed, for example, with the $5HT_3$ receptor.

The situation is probably more complex than suggested above, however. Isoflurane has effects on closed as well as open nAcChoR channels (20). The inhibitory potency of halothane on nAcChoRs expressed in oocytes decreases when the membrane concentration of cholesterol is increased by equilibrating with cholesterol-containing liposomes (51). That mutations in the lipid-protein interface alter the channel closing rate also suggests a role for that site in channel kinetics (52). Indeed, it may be that channel opening is so concerted that the whole nAcChoR complex must be considered, and that a complete description of general anesthetic–induced inhibition of acetylcholine-gated channels may involve more than one mechanism.

Sarcoplasmic Reticulum Ca-ATPase The effects of halothane and hexanol on sarcoplasmic reticulum Ca-ATPase activity are complex, and seemingly contradictory results have been reported by several groups (6,54,71). However, by studying the effects of halothane on the enzyme's activity as well as on protein regional mobility and lipid fluidity at various temperatures, Karon and Thomas (41) seem to have resolved many of these discrepancies (Fig. 11). They concluded that at low temperatures, activity is largely dependent on the aggregation state of the enzyme; dimers exhibit the highest activities, monomers have intermediate activities, and tetramers and higher order oligomers have the lowest activities. At low temperatures the addition of halothane increases activity by dissociating large aggregates into more active dimers and monomers. Similarly, increasing the temperature of sarcoplasmic reticulum membranes dissociates large aggregates leading to an increase in Ca-ATPase activity. At higher temperatures, where little of the enzyme is in the form of tetramers or higher order oligomers, the effect of halothane on Ca-ATPase activity is biphasic. At low concentrations, halothane increases sarcoplasmic reticulum Ca-ATPase activity (perhaps due to an increase in lipid fluidity), while at high concentrations halothane inhibits activity by converting the more active dimers into the less active monomers.

The changes in aggregation state of the sarcoplasmic reticulum Ca-ATPase are not insubstantial over the clinical concentration range, and this suggests that modulation of protein-protein interactions should be given serious attention as one mechanism by which general anesthetics might act. For example, alteration of subunit-subunit interactions in oligomeric proteins might have significant implications for ligand-gated ion channels (which include the nAcChoR, GABA, and glutamate receptors), which are all believed to be oligomeric proteins, although in their case such alterations are unlikely to lead to disaggregation.

The role of lipids in modulating the aggregation state of this enzyme is less clear. Studies with spin-labeled lipids suggest that

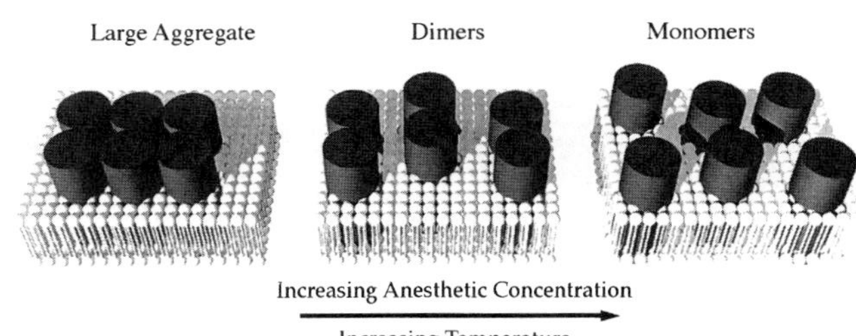

Figure 11. The activity of the Ca-ATPase is dependent on its aggregation state. At low temperature (i.e., 0°C), much of the enzyme is present as large aggregates that exhibit low activity (5). If a general anesthetic is added or the temperature increased, the relative proportion of enzyme present as high activity dimers and intermediate activity monomers increases while that of large aggregates decreases (41).

anesthetics act by selectively fluidizing and reducing the number of the annular lipids surrounding the enzyme (4,53). However, changes in annular lipid properties are smaller than those in the aggregation state and are generally detected only at concentrations that far exceed those required to induce anesthesia. Kutchai et al. (46) found that at an aqueous hexanol concentration of 10 mM (which is more than 10 times the anesthesia EC_{50} for tadpoles), the effect of hexanol on the fluidity of annular lipids and their affinity for the enzyme were on the order of a few percent.

Rhodopsin Spectroscopic studies of rhodopsin conformational states indicate that ethanol shifts the conformational equilibrium between the meta I and meta II states of rhodopsin toward the meta II state (increases K_{eq}) (67). The concentration range over which ethanol shifts the meta I–meta II equilibrium generally corresponds to the range that increases the acyl chain packing free volume. In addition, rhodopsin's sensitivity to ethanol is dependent on the composition of the lipid acyl chains in a manner that is generally predicted by the bilayer's permissivity index (see above). For example, increasing lipid polyunsaturation enhanced the potency of ethanol. These findings are consistent with a mechanism in which ethanol alters lipid packing. A recent preliminary report indicates that butanol and hexanol also increase K_{eq}, although the efficacy with which these alcohols shift the meta I–meta II equilibrium decreases with increasing chain length from ethanol to hexanol (68). The addition of octanol to rhodopsin-containing membranes actually decreases K_{eq}. Although the effect of these alcohols on f_v have not been reported, such a study would test the hypothesis that f_v plays an important modulatory role in determining K_{eq}.

Other Protein Systems The ability of the lipids surrounding a protein to modulate the action of general anesthetics appears to be a general phenomenon that occurs in a wide variety of proteins, including the oligomeric four transmembrane ligand gated ion channels, the seven transmembrane second messenger receptors, the voltage gated ion selective channels, and an extrinsic, or membrane-associated protein, protein kinase C.

Thus, Rehberg, et al. (78) characterized the actions of pentobarbital on the channel kinetics of sodium channels that had been incorporated into phospholipid bilayers containing varying mole fractions of cholesterol. Increasing the amount of cholesterol in the bilayer did not alter the properties of the sodium channel, but it elevated the IC_{50} for pentobarbital-mediated inhibition of the channel. This IC_{50} doubled between 0 and 17 mole percent cholesterol but did not change at higher concentrations; remarkably, over half the change occurred by 3.7 mole percent cholesterol, the lowest concentration examined. This suggests that cholesterol plays a more direct role than would be inferred from lipid properties alone. On the other hand, it is interesting to note that pentobarbital orders phosphatidylcholine bilayers below 10 mole percent cholesterol but disorders them at higher cholesterol contents (73).

Protein kinase C (PKC; see Chap. 7) modulates neuronal signal transduction by phosphorylating membrane proteins. It exists in soluble and membrane-associated conformations. In the absence of lipids, anesthetics can inhibit the protamine sulfate activation of PKC with potencies that correlate with their lipid solubilities, suggesting there is a hydrophobic site for general anesthetics on the protein (83). Although lipids are not required for inhibition, they exert a modulatory action. For example, increasing acyl chain unsaturation enhances general anesthetic potency (compare rhodopsin). These observations suggest that both general anesthetics and phospholipids interact as allosteric modulators of PKC.

CONCLUSION

The unique pharmacology of the general anesthetics is well accounted for by the Meyer-Overton rule and its derivative lipid perturbation theories. However, these theories have yet to yield a satisfactory mechanism for general anesthetic action. Hydrophobic protein sites also exist in soluble proteins and in some cases may be occupied at clinical concentrations and obey the Meyer-Overton rule, but to date no one site has been found to account for the diversity of general anesthetic structures. Thus, the specificity of protein binding sites implies that there are several mechanisms of anesthesia and several proteins sites, where different anesthetics act (94).

The traditional physicochemical approach has now yielded to much more detailed studies of selected membrane proteins. Such studies are aimed at deriving the mechanism of general anesthetic action on a single structure, leaving the question of its relationship to general anesthesia for another day. The results of this line of research have been surprising. Rather than simplifying the problem, it appears to be a general rule that general anesthetics act in a multitude of ways even when a single target is considered. The unitary hypothesis is an immediate victim of these studies, unless one takes the position that all the structures studied to date are irrelevant to anesthesia and the true site for general anesthetics still lies beyond our ken.

Although it is too early to draw definitive conclusions, a number of features of the mode of action of general anesthetics on membrane proteins have begun to emerge. Where there is clear evidence for protein-anesthetic interactions, the sites exhibit structural selectivity, implying that other classes of general anesthetics may exert their actions at other sites either on the same protein or elsewhere. The first inklings of the location of a site for some general anesthetics in the channel of the acetylcholine receptor lead to testable predictions on why a related ligand gated channel, the GABA receptor, is not inhibited. On the other hand, it is difficult to rule out a role for lipids in the action of general anesthetics on membrane proteins because the dependence of their kinetics on their membrane environment is so poorly understood. It does seem to be a general rule that the lipids interacting with both extrinsic and intrinsic membrane proteins are able to modulate the potency and/or the efficacy of general anesthetic action.

Overall, it is emerging that the membrane targets of general anesthetics studied to date have highly allosteric structures. The different conformations in which they can exist have different affinities for both general anesthetics and lipids. Thus, a complete description of the mechanisms involved in anesthetic action on membrane proteins requires that they be considered in their membrane environment. Although this complexity means that molecular mechanisms are only now beginning to emerge, it is clear that research has passed beyond the "black box" stage and that new advances are to be expected. New experimental techniques are now capable both of resolving the mechanisms by which general anesthetics act and of locating their target sites. These techniques include rapid-perfusion electrophysiology, site-directed mutagenesis, reconstitution of purified proteins into membranes of defined lipid composition, and photolabeling. The combination of rapid-perfusion electrophysiology with site-directed mutagenesis can now be applied to any known channel and should displace more classical approaches. Biophysical techniques are limited in their applicability, but only until advances in expression systems make many more membrane proteins available in the quantities required. We are thus about to enter a golden age during which our understanding of the molecular mechanisms by which general anesthetics act will advance to the point at which one may expect significant benefits to patient care.

REFERENCES

1. Abadji VC, Raines DE, Watts A, Miller KW. The effect of general anesthetics on the dynamics of phosphatidylcholine-acetylcholine receptor interactions in reconstituted vesicles. *Biochim Biophys Acta* 1993;1147:143–153.

2. Alifimoff JK, Firestone LL, Miller KW. Anaesthetic potencies of primary alkanols: implications for the molecular dimensions of the anaesthetic site. *Br J Pharmacol* 1989;96:9–16.
3. Bhushan A, McNamee MG. Correlation of phospholipid structure with functional effects on the nicotinic acetylcholine receptor. A modulatory role for phosphatidic acid. *Biophys J* 1993;64:716–723.
4. Bigelow DJ, Thomas DD. Rotational dynamics of lipid and the Ca-ATPase in sarcoplasmic reticulum. The molecular basis of activation by diethyl ether. *J Biol Chem* 1987;262:13449–13456.
5. Birmachu W, Thomas DD. Rotational dynamics of the Ca-ATPase in sarcoplasmic reticulum studied by time-resolved phosphorescence anisotropy. *Biochemistry* 1990;29:3904–3914.
6. Blanck TJ, Peterson CV, Baroody B, Tegazzin V, Lou J. Halothane, enflurane, and isoflurane stimulate calcium leakage from rabbit sarcoplasmic reticulum. *Anesthesiology* 1992;76:813–821.
7. Blanton MP, Cohen JB. Mapping the lipid-exposed regions in the Torpedo californica nicotinic acetylcholine receptor. *Biochemistry* 1992;31:3738–3750.
8. Braswell LM, Miller KW, Sauter JF. Pressure reversal of the action of octanol on postsynaptic membranes from Torpedo. *Br J Pharmacol* 1984;83:305–311.
9. Bretscher MS. The molecules of the cell membrane. *Sci Am* 1985;253:100–108.
10. Brown MF. Modulation of rhodopsin function by properties of the membrane bilayer. *Chem Phys Lipids* 1994;73:159–180.
11. Bull MH, Brailsford JD, Bull BS. Erythrocyte membrane expansion due to the volatile anesthetics, the 1-alkanols, and benzyl alcohol. *Anesthesiology* 1982;57:399–403.
12. Changeux JP, Galzi JL, Devillers TA, Bertrand D. The functional architecture of the acetylcholine nicotinic receptor explored by affinity labelling and site-directed mutagenesis. *Q Rev Biophys* 1992;25:395–432.
13. Chin JH, Trudell JR, Cohen EN. The compression-ordering and solubility-disordering effects of high pressure gases on phospholipid bilayers. *Life Sci* 1976;18:489–497.
14. Cornea RL, Thomas DD. Effects of membrane thickness on the molecular dynamics and enzymatic activity of reconstituted Ca-ATPase. *Biochemistry* 1994;33:2912–2920.
15. Cowan SW, Schirmer T, Rummel G, et al. Crystal structures explain functional properties of two *E. coli* porins. *Nature* 1992; 358:727–733.
16. Cullis PR, deKruiff B, Hope MJ, et al. Structural properties of lipids and their functional roles in biological membranes. In: Aloia RC, ed. *Membrane fluidity in biology*. New York: Academic Press, 1983;39–81.
17. Cullis PR, Hope MJ, Tilcock CPS. Structural properties of phospholipids in the rat liver inner mitochondrial membrane: A 31-P-NMR Study. *Biochim Biophys Acta* 1986;600:625–635.
18. Danielli JF, H D. A contribution to the theory of permeability of thin films. *J Cell Comp Physiol* 1935;5:495–508.
19. DeLong EF, Yayanos AA. Adaptation of the membrane lipids of a deep-sea bacterium to changes in hydrostatic pressure. *Science* 1985;228:1101–1103.
20. Dilger JP, Brett RS, Lesko LA. Effects of isoflurane on acetylcholine receptor channels. 1. Single-channel currents. *Mol Pharmacol* 1992;41:127–133.
21. Dodson BA, Braswell LM, Miller KW. Barbiturates bind to an allosteric regulatory site on nicotinic acetylcholine receptor-rich membranes. *Mol Pharmacol* 1987;32:119–126.
22. Dodson BA, Furmaniuk ZJ, Miller KW. The physiological effects of hydrostatic pressure are not equivalent to those of helium pressure on Rana pipiens. *J Physiol* 1985;362:233–244.
23. Ellena JF, Blazing MA, McNamee MG. Lipid-protein interactions in reconstituted membranes containing acetylcholine receptor. *Biochemistry* 1983;22:5523–5535.
24. Esmann M, Marsh D. Spin-label studies on the origin of the specificity of lipid-protein interactions in Na+,K+-ATPase membranes from Squalus acanthias. *Biochemistry* 1985;24:3572–3578.
25. Firestone LL, Alifimoff JK, Miller KW. Does general anesthetic-induced desensitization of the Torpedo acetylcholine receptor correlate with lipid disordering? *Mol Pharmacol* 1994;46:508–515.
26. Firestone S, Ferguson C, Firestone L. Isoflurane's optical isomers are equipotent in Rana pipiens tadpoles. *Anesthesiology* 1992;77: A758.
27. Fong TM, McNamee MG. Correlation between acetylcholine receptor function and structural properties of membranes. *Biochemistry* 1986;25:830–840.
28. Fong TM, McNamee MG. Stabilization of acetylcholine receptor secondary structure by cholesterol and negatively charged phospholipids in membranes. *Biochemistry* 1987;26:3871–3880.
29. Forman SA, Miller KW. Molecular sites of anesthetic action in postsynaptic nicotinic membranes. *Trends Pharmacol Sci* 1989;10: 447–452.
30. Forman SA, Miller KW, Yellen G. A discrete site for general anesthetics on a postsynaptic receptor. *Mol Pharmacol* 1995;(in press).
31. Franks NP, Lieb WR. Molecular mechanisms of general anaesthesia. *Nature* 1982;300:487–493.
32. Franks NP, Lieb WR. Partitioning of long-chain alcohols into lipid bilayers: implications for mechanisms of general anesthesia. *Proc Natl Acad Sci USA* 1986;83:5116–5120.
33. Franks NP, Lieb WR. Molecular and cellular mechanisms of general anaesthesia. *Nature* 1994;367:607–614.
34. Fraser DM, Louro SR, Horvaath LI, Miller KW, Watts A. A study of the effect of general anesthetics on lipid-protein interactions in acetylcholine receptor enriched membranes from Torpedo nobiliana using nitroxide spin-labels. *Biochemistry* 1990;29:2664–2669.
35. Frommel C. The apolar surface area of amino acids and its empirical correlation with hydrophobic free energy. *J Theoret Biol* 1984; 111:247–260.
36. Gennis RB. *Biomembranes: molecular structure and function*. New York: Springer-Verlag, 1989.
37. Gibson NJ, Brown MF. Lipid headgroup and acyl chain composition modulate the MI-MII equilibrium of rhodopsin in recombinant membranes. *Biochemistry* 1993;32:2438–2454.
38. Gorter E, Grendel F. On biomolecular layers of lipid on the chromacytes of the blood. *J Exp Med* 1895;41:439–443.
39. Janoff AS, Miller KW. A critical assessment of the lipid theories of general anaesthetic action. In: Chapman D, ed. *Biological membranes*. London: Academic Press, 1982;417–469.
40. Jones OT, Eubanks JH, Earnest JP, McNamee MG. A minimum number of lipids are required to support the functional properties of the nicotinic acetylcholine receptor. *Biochemistry* 1988;27: 3733–3742.
41. Karon BS, Thomas DD. Molecular mechanism of Ca-ATPase activation by halothane in sarcoplasmic reticulum. *Biochemistry* 1993; 32:7503–7511.
42. Kistler J, Stroud RM, Klymkowsky MW, Lalancette RA, Fairclough RH. Structure and function of an acetylcholine receptor. *Biophys J* 1982;37:371–383.
43. Kita Y, Bennett LJ, Miller KW. The partial molar volumes of anesthetics in lipid bilayers. *Biochim Biophys Acta* 1981;647:130–139.
44. Klausner RD, Kleinfeld AM, Hoover RL, Karnovsky MJ. Lipid domains in membranes. Evidence derived from structural perturbations induced by free fatty acids and lifetime heterogeneity analysis. *J Biol Chem* 1980;255:1286–1295.
45. Koblin DD, Chortkoff BS, Laster MJ, Eger EI, Halsey MJ, Ionescu P. Polyhalogenated and perfluorinated compounds that disobey the Meyer-Overton hypothesis. *Anesth Anal* 1994;79:1043–1048.
46. Kutchai H, Mahaney JE, Geddis LM, Thomas DD. Hexanol and lidocaine affect the oligomeric state of the Ca-ATPase of sarcoplasmic reticulum. *Biochemistry* 1994;33:13208–13222.
47. Kyte J, Doolittle RF. A simple method for displaying the hydropathic character of a protein. *J Mol Biol* 1982;157:105–132.
48. Larabee MG, Posternak J. Selective action of anesthetics on synapses and axons in mammalian sympathetic ganglia. *J Neurophysiol* 1952;15:91–114.
49. Lawrence DK, Gill EW. Structurally specific effects of some steroid anesthetics on spin-labeled liposomes. *Mol Pharmacol* 1975;11: 280–286.
50. Leal SM, Evers AS. The photolabeling reagent 3-trifluoromethyl-3-(m-iodophenyl) diazirine (TID) is a potent general anesthetic in tadpoles. *Anesthesiology* 1994;81:A897.
51. Lechleiter J, Wells M, Gruener R. Halothane-induced changes in acetylcholine receptor kinetics are attenuated by cholesterol. *Biochim Biophys Acta* 1986;856:640–645.
52. Lee YH, Li L, Lasalde J, Rojas L, McNamee M, Ortiz-Miranda SI, Pappone P. Mutations in the M4 domain of Torpedo californica acetylcholine receptor dramatically alter ion channel function. *Biophys J* 1994;66:646–653.
53. Lopes CMB, Louro SRW. The effects of n-alkanols on the lipid/protein interface of Ca-ATPase of sarcoplasmic reticulum vesicles. *Biochim Biophys Acta* 1991; 1070:467–473.
54. Louis CF, Zualkernan K, Roghair T, Mickelson JR. The effects of volatile anesthetics on calcium regulation by malignant hyperthermia-susceptible sarcoplasmic reticulum. *Anesthesiology* 1992; 77:114–125.

55. Lysko GS, Robinson JL, Casto R, Ferrone RA. The stereospecific effects of isoflurane isomers in vivo. *Eur J Pharmacol* 1994;263:25–29.
56. Mabrey S, Mateo PL, Sturtevant JM. High-sensitivity calorimetric study of mixtures of cholesterol with dimyristoyl and dipalmitoylphosphatidylcholines. *Biochemistry* 1978;17:2464–2468.
57. Mahaney JE, Kleinschmidt J, Marsh D, Thomas DD. Effects of melittin on lipid-protein interactions in sarcoplasmic reticulum membranes. *Biophys J* 1992;63:1513–1522.
58. Marsh D. ESR spin label studies of lipid-protein interactions. In: Watts A, DePont JM, eds. *Progress in protein-lipid interactions.* Amsterdam, New York, Oxford: Elsevier, 1985;143–172.
59. Marsh D. The nature of the lipid-protein interface and the influence of protein structure on protein-lipid interactions. In: Watts A, ed. *Protein-lipid interactions.* Oxford: Elsevier, 1993;41–66.
60. McNamee MG, Ochoa EL. Reconstitution of acetylcholine receptor function in model membranes. *Neuroscience* 1982;7: 2305–2319.
61. Melchoir DL. Lipid domains in fluid membranes: a quick-freeze differential scanning calorimetry study. *Science* 1986;234:1577–1580.
62. Mihic SJ, McQuilkin SJ, II EIE, Ionescu P, Harris RA. Potentiation of γ-aminobutyric acid type A receptor-mediated chloride currents by novel halogenated compounds correlates with their abilities to induce general anesthesia. *Mol Pharmacol* 1994;46:851–857.
63. Miller KW. The nature of the site of general anesthesia. *Int Rev Neurobiol* 1985;27:1–61.
64. Miller KW, Braswell LM, Firestone LL, Dodson BA, Forman SA. General anesthetics act both specifically and nonspecifically on acetylcholine receptors. In: Roth SH, Miller KW, eds. *Molecular and cellular mechanisms of anesthetics.* New York: Plenum, 1986; 125–138.
65. Miller KW, Firestone LL, Alifimoff JK, Streicher P. Nonanesthetic alcohols dissolve in synaptic membranes without perturbing their lipids. *Proc Natl Acad Sci USA* 1989;86:1084–1087.
66. Miller KW, Paton WD, Smith RA, Smith EB. The pressure reversal of general anesthesia and the critical volume hypothesis. *Mol Pharmacol* 1973;9:131–143.
67. Mitchell DC, Litman BJ. Effect of ethanol on metarhodopsin II formation is potentiated by phospholipid polyunsaturation. *Biochemistry* 1994;33:12752–12756.
68. Mitchell DC, Litman J. The effects of alcohols on receptor activation is potentiated by phospholipid polysaturation. *Alcoholism Clin Exp Res* 1995;19:60A.
69. Mitchell DC, Straume M, Litman BJ. Role of sn-1-saturated, sn-2-polyunsaturated phospholipids in control of membrane receptor conformational equilibrium: effects of cholesterol and acyl chain unsaturation on the metarhodopsin I in equilibrium with metarhodopsin II equilibrium. *Biochemistry* 1992;31:662–670.
70. Mitchell DC, Straume M, Miller JL, Litman BJ. Modulation of metarhodopsin formation by cholesterol-induced ordering of bilayer lipids. *Biochemistry* 1990;29:9143–9149.
71. Nelson TE, Sweo T. Ca2+ uptake and Ca2+ release by skeletal muscle sarcoplasmic reticulum: differing sensitivity to inhalational anesthetics. *Anesthesiology* 1988;69:571–577.
72. Overton E. Uber die somotischen eigenshaften der lebenden pflanzen und tierzelle. *Vjsch Naturf Ges Zurich* 1895;40:159–201.
73. Pang KY, Miller KW. Cholesterol modulates the effects of membrane perturbers in phospholipid vesicles and biomembranes. *Biochim Biophys Acta* 1978;511:1–9.
74. Raines DE, Korten SE, Hill AG, Miller KW. Anesthetic cutoff in cycloalkanemethanols. A test of current theories. *Anesthesiology* 1993;78:918–927.
75. Raines DE, Miller KW. The role of charge in lipid selectivity for the nicotinic acetylcholine receptor. *Biophys J* 1993;64:632–641.
76. Raines DE, Rankin SE, Miller KW. Isofluraneís actions on the nicotinic acetylcholine receptor are dependent upon the composition of the lipid bilayer. *Anesthesiology* 1994;81:A884.
77. Raines DE, Rankin SE, Miller KW. General anesthetics modify the kinetics of nicotinic acetylcholine receptor desensitization at clinically relevant concentrations. *Anesthesiology* 1995;82:276–287.
78. Rehberg B, Urban BW, Duch DS. The membrane cholesterol modulates anesthetic actions on a human brain ion channel. *Anesthesiology* 1995;82:749–758.
79. Rock CO, Cronan JE. Lipid metabolism in procaryotes. In: Vance DE, Vance JE, eds. *Biochemistry of lipids and membranes.* Menlo Park, CA: Benjamin/Cummings, 1985;73–115.
80. Simmonds AC, East JM, Jones OT, Rooney EK, McWhirter J, Lee AG. Annular and non-annular binding sites on the (Ca2+ + Mg2+)-ATPase. *Biochim Biophys Acta* 1982;693:398–406.
81. Sinensky M, Pinkerton F, Sutherland E, Simon FR. Rate limitation of (Na+ + K+)-stimulated adenosinetriphosphatase by membrane acyl chain ordering. *Proc Natl Acad Sci USA* 1979;76:4893–4897.
82. Singer SJ, Nicholson GL. The fluid mosaic model of the structure of cell membranes. *Science* 1972;175:720–731.
83. Slater SJ, Cox KJ, Lombardi VJ, Ho C, Kelly MB, Rubin E, Stubbs CD. Inhibition of protein kinase C by alcohols and anaesthetics. *Nature* 1993;364:82–84.
84. Squier TC, Bigelow DJ, Thomas DD. Lipid fluidity directly modulates the overall protein rotational mobility of the Ca-ATPase in sarcoplasmic reticulum. *J Biol Chem* 1988;263:9178–9186.
85. Squier TC, Thomas DD. Selective detection of the rotational dynamics of the protein-associated lipid hydrocarbon chains in sarcoplasmic reticulum membranes. *Biophys J* 1989;56:735–748.
86. Straume M, Litman BJ. Influence of cholesterol on equilibrium and dynamic bilayer structure of unsaturated acyl chain phosphatidylcholine vesicles as determined from higher order analysis of fluorescence anisotropy decay. *Biochemistry* 1987;26:5121–5126.
87. Sunshine C, McNamee MG. Lipid modulation of nicotinic acetylcholine receptor function: the role of neutral and negatively charged lipids. *Biochim Biophys Acta* 1992;1108:240–246.
88. Sunshine C, McNamee MG. Lipid modulation of nicotinic acetylcholine receptor function: the role of membrane lipid composition and fluidity. *Biochim Biophys Acta* 1994;1191:59–64.
89. Tanford C. *The hydrophobic effect: formation of micelles and biological membranes.* New York: Wiley, 1980.
90. Tanifuji Y, Eger Ed, Terrell RC. Some characteristics of an exceptionally potent inhaled anesthetic: thiomethoxyflurane. *Anesth Analg* 1977;56:387–390.
91. Thomas DD, Bigelow DJ, Squier TC, Hidalgo C. Rotational dynamics of protein and boundary lipid in sarcoplasmic reticulum membrane. *Biophys J* 1982;37:217–225.
92. Ticku MK, Rastogi SK. Barbiturate-sensitive sites in the benzodiazepine-GABA receptor-ionophore complex. In: Roth SH, Miller KW, eds. *Molecular and cellular mechanisms of anesthetics.* New York: Plenum, 1986;179–188.
93. Trudell JR. A unitary theory of anesthesia based on lateral phase separations in nerve membranes. *Anesthesiology* 1977;46:5–10.
94. Urban BW. Modifications of excitable membranes by volatile and gaseous anesthetics. In: Covino BG, Fozzard HA, Rehder L, Strichartz G, eds. *Effects of anesthesia.* Bethesda, MD: American Physiological Society, 1985;13–28.
95. Verkliej AJ, Zwaal RFA, Roelofsen B, Comfurius P, Kastelijn D, Van Deenen LLM. The asymmetric distribution of phospholipids in the human red cell membrane. *Biochim Biophys Acta* 1973;323:178–193.
96. Voss J, Birmachu W, Hussey DM, Thomas DD. Effects of melittin on molecular dynamics and Ca-ATPase activity in sarcoplasmic reticulum membranes: time-resolved optical anisotropy. *Biochemistry* 1991;30:7498–7506.
97. Watts A, Marsh D. Saturation transfer ESR studies of molecular motion in phosphatidylglycerol bilayers in the gel phase: effects of pretransitions and pH titration. *Biochim Biophys Acta* 1981;642: 231–241.
98. White BH, Howard S, Cohen SG, Cohen JB. The hydrophobic photoreagent 3-(trifluoromethyl)-3-m-(125I iodophenyl) diazirine is a novel noncompetitive antagonist of the nicotinic acetylcholine receptor. *J Biol Chem* 1991;266:21595–21607.
99. Wo ZG, Oswald RE. Unraveling the modular design of glutamate-gated ion channels. *Trends Neurosci* 1995;18:161–168.
100. Wood SC, Tonner PH, de Armendi AJ, Bugge B, Miller KW. Channel inhibition by alkanols occurs at a binding site on the nicotinic acetylcholine receptor. *Mol Pharmacol* 1995;47:121–130.

Anesthesia: Biologic Foundations, edited by
Tony L. Yaksh et al. Lippincott–Raven Publishers,
Philadelphia © 1997.

CHAPTER 2

INHALATIONAL ANESTHETIC INTERACTIONS WITH PROTEINS

RODERIC G. ECKENHOFF AND JONAS S. JOHANSSON

There is little doubt that anesthetics can directly interact with and alter the function of a variety of proteins. The nature of these interactions is less clear, but at a minimum must involve binding and some subsequent conformational or dynamic change in the protein target. This chapter presents and discusses some of the evidence for such interactions, with the intent of demonstrating the plausibility of a direct functional effect. Because of the large number of compounds that can produce the behavioral state termed "anesthesia," we will restrict our focus to the inhalational anesthetics, including those with vapor pressures higher than atmospheric at room temperature, such as xenon and nitrous oxide. Further, most of this chapter focuses on soluble proteins, because the binding and structural investigations have been more productive, and are not confounded by the presence of lipid. This is not to suggest, however, that these proteins mediate important components of anesthetic action; there seems to be consensus that membrane proteins serve this role (51,61,103). Rather, the information derived from the soluble proteins will allow an unambiguous definition of binding character and energetics, and the local and global conformational consequences of anesthetic binding, which almost certainly share features of relevance to the more complex membrane proteins. We intend this chapter to be used as a companion to those that follow, to aid in the interpretation of the behavioral, cellular, and receptor level investigations that form the bulk of this volume.

HISTORY

The idea that inhalational anesthetics might interact directly with protein dates back to the latter half of the nineteenth century. Claude Bernard (8) suggested that diethyl ether and chloroform caused a reversible coagulation of the "albuminoid" cell contents, and that this caused anesthesia. Somewhat later, Moore and Roaf (95,96) reported that chloroform and diethyl ether were more soluble in serum or hemoglobin solutions than in water or saline, suggesting binding interactions. They went on to propose that the uptake of anesthetics by "proteoid" rather than by "lipoid" components was responsible for the production of anesthesia. Countering this idea was the independent work of Overton and Meyer at about the same time, which demonstrated the now-famous correlation of anesthetic potency with olive oil solubility, suggesting that anesthetics work by interacting with the lipid components of the cell (92).

In 1915 Harvey (62) reported that n-alkanols, diethyl ether, and chloroform reversibly depressed the luminescence of certain marine bacteria, and that inhibitory potency correlated with n-alkanol length. This early work spawned a whole series of more recent investigations with purified light-emitting proteins, to be discussed later, with the goal of demonstrating and characterizing direct anesthetic-protein interactions.

That the small anesthetic molecules might cause a change in protein structure was proposed by Östergren (100), based on observations of anesthetic effects on the mitotic spindle. He postulated that general anesthetics such as the n-alkanols, nitrous oxide, chloroform, and trichloroethylene exert their effects on the lipophilic portion of proteins, finally reconciling the observations of Overton and Meyer with those of protein target proponents. The interaction of anesthetics with the hydrophobic domains was hypothesized to lead to decreased flexibility of the protein (100), a fairly precocious proposal.

The description of the structure of the cell membrane (120), when combined with the observations of Overton and Meyer, led the field of anesthetic mechanisms research into the lipid bilayer, which unfortunately has produced much ambiguity. It appears that many investigators have now returned their attention to protein, but with an improved appreciation of the importance of hydrophobic forces to protein structure and function. Further, the functional inseparability of lipid and protein in the cell membrane is now better understood, and thus provides a rich environment for reconciliation of the lipid and protein proponents.

As new protein systems are described and their function determined, it is inevitable that someone will add an anesthetic and examine the consequences. What follows is a distillation of some of this work, and that of our own laboratory, in an attempt to concisely describe the essential interactions of anesthetics and proteins.

ANESTHETIC BINDING TO PROTEIN

Equilibrium Kinetics

For any compound to have a direct effect on protein function, it must first bind in some way. Traditionally, anesthetics have been thought to partition into, and not necessarily to "bind" to, biologic macromolecules. However, the distinction is largely semantic, and the confusion over this issue results from the fact that only marginal binding forces are involved. While many pharmacologic principles probably remain valid (e.g., some kind of binding must occur for functional consequence), it is necessary to adjust one's view as to the meaning of high and low affinity, and specific and nonspecific binding in the context of these very weak ligands. For example, it is possible that what would traditionally be termed nonspecific binding is functionally very important in the case of the membrane proteins, given the relatively high concentration of ligand in at least part of the protein's solvent (lipid). Also, as we shall see, the discrete, saturable binding sites found in some soluble proteins, in general, appear to have only modest functional consequences.

The binding of an anesthetic *(A)* to a protein target *(P)* can be described as follows:

$$A + P \underset{k_{-1}}{\overset{k_1}{\rightleftarrows}} AP \qquad [1]$$

with forward and reverse rate constants k_1 and k_{-1}, respectively. The dissociation constant of this interaction, K_d, is defined by:

$$K_d = \frac{k_{-1}}{k_1} = \frac{[A][P]}{[A \cdot P]} \qquad [2]$$

The dissociation constant is important because it reflects the strength (duration) of an interaction, and in general, the stronger the interaction, the more probable a structural and functional consequence. If we propose that anesthesia is produced by anesthetic binding to a limited number of sites, then it is reasonable to assume that the aqueous median effective concentration (EC_{50}) approximates the K_d, which, for most inhalational anesthetics, is in the high-micromolar range (50). If we also assume that the forward rate constant is diffusion controlled (10^9 M^{-1} sec^{-1}), then a dissociation rate constant k_{-1} of about 0.25 to 1.0 · 10^6 sec^{-1} can be calculated, implying that binding sites are occupied for lifetimes on the order of 1 to 4 μsec, confirming the predicted weak binding interactions for these small molecules. Compare this to lifetimes of many minutes for more familiar ligands like the catecholamines or the peptide hormones, which bind to their receptors with dissociation constants of 2 to 10 nM (22).

Because of the difficulty of directly measuring rate constants, the K_d is usually estimated from equilibrium binding studies with radiolabeled ligands. However, even these studies have been challenging for the inhalational anesthetics because of the difficulty of reliably separating the free from bound states with such rapidly dissociating compounds. At least three methods, however, have been used to estimate the K_d for inhalational anesthetic-protein interactions. First, simple partitioning between the gas phase and a solution of protein, as compared to buffer alone, can be used to estimate that amount bound by the protein (32,33). The separation of specific from nonspecific binding is problematic with this approach, however, but can be occasionally approximated by measuring partitioning into the denatured protein, such as occurs with a low pH solution of albumin to produce the "E" or extended form (16), or with the protein denatured in a high concentration of guanidinium chloride. This requires sufficient structural knowledge to ensure that the binding domain is removed by the denaturing conditions. Using this approach to measure nonspecific binding, bovine serum albumin has been shown to bind isoflurane and halothane with K_d values of 1.4 mM and 1.3 mM, respectively (32,33). Very similar estimates of the halothane K_d for binding to bovine serum albumin have been obtained with ^{19}F–nuclear magnetic resonance (NMR) (33) and tryptophan fluorescence quenching (72). A somewhat lower estimate of the halothane K_d (0.4 mM) was obtained with direct photoaffinity labeling (34). However, all of these K_d estimates are well within an order of magnitude, and therefore comparable when considering the overall energetics of the binding interactions. It is also important to note, however, that all of these affinity estimates for the anesthetic binding to albumin are higher than the clinical EC_{50} values for the same drugs, and therefore the bovine albumin binding site(s) may not accurately reflect the character of the site(s) responsible for "anesthesia." It should be emphasized, however, that EC_{50} and K_d need only be similar if one assumes that anesthesia is produced by interactions at one site or a very few similar sites. This seems unlikely when considering the remarkably steep dose-response curves for anesthesia, and the widely varied targets for anesthetics covered in the remainder of this volume.

The ^{19}F-NMR measurements have also allowed an estimation of the average lifetime ($1/k_{-1}$) of a bound anesthetic molecule, which for isoflurane was about 250 μsec, or about two orders of magnitude longer than estimated above (32). This discrepancy probably results from the use of a diffusion-controlled rate constant for k_1. Although all molecules in solution undergo collisions, it should not be surprising that few diffusional encounters between ligand and protein will result in binding. The actual binding site(s) on the protein surface, or the pathway to an interior binding domain, is expected to comprise only a small fraction of the protein surface area, and therefore the fraction of collisions resulting in binding should be smaller. Further, normal protein dynamics may limit the duration that an access route to an interior binding domain is "open," which will clearly have an effect on k_1. Therefore, using the experimentally derived K_d and k_{-1} values, k_1 can be estimated to be about 3•10^6 M^{-1} sec^{-1}, or almost three orders of magnitude slower than expected for a diffusion-controlled process. This is comparable with the binding rate constants of 10^4 to 10^7 M^{-1} sec^{-1} observed for other ligand-receptor interactions (56,121). Such kinetic evidence is consistent with a limited number of discrete anesthetic binding sites in soluble proteins, rather than simple nonspecific surface (interfacial) binding as proposed by some investigators (131).

Thermodynamics

The magnitude of the dissociation constant allows calculation of the Gibbs free energy change ($\Delta G°$) associated with anesthetic binding to protein.

$$\Delta G° = RT \ln K_d \qquad [3]$$

where R is the gas constant and T is the absolute temperature, under molar standard state at pH7. The Gibbs free energy change corresponds to the work involved in the binding step of ligand to receptor, and is negative if binding occurs spontaneously at the temperature and pressure of the experiment. The magnitude of the Gibbs free energy difference between the free and bound states determines the stability of the interaction. Analysis of anesthetic binding as a function of temperature allows estimation of the enthalpy ($\Delta H°$) and entropy ($\Delta S°$) changes associated with binding, from the Gibbs-Helmholtz equation:

$$\Delta G° = \Delta H - T\Delta S° \qquad [4]$$

Combining equations [3] and [4] yields the integrated van't Hoff equation:

$$\ln K_d = \frac{\Delta H°}{RT} - \frac{\Delta S°}{R} \qquad [5]$$

A plot of $\ln K_d$ as a function of T^{-1} then allows calculation of $\Delta H°$ and $\Delta S°$ from the slope ($\Delta H°/R$) and intercept ($\Delta S°/R$), respectively, assuming that the changes in enthalpy and entropy are constant over the temperature range examined. Although the majority of the biochemical data on ligand binding has been obtained using such van't Hoff plots, more recently investigators have used titration calorimetry, allowing direct measurement of the enthalpy change associated with ligand binding to protein (70),

Thermodynamic analysis can provide clues to the types of interactions associated with binding (107,126). For example, while the formation of a complex between an anesthetic molecule and a protein target implies that there is an increase in the order of the system (a negative change in entropy), the more important entropic event is thought to occur in the bulk water due to removal of the structured water (more extensively hydrogen bonded) surrounding the hydrated anesthetic molecules (hydrophobic hydration) (97). Therefore, the net entropic change associated with the hydrophobic effect is positive. In addition, if the hydrophobic anesthetic binding site of a protein is normally hydrated or exposed to water, then the displacement of these more structured water molecules will also contribute a positive entropic component (such as occurs in when dichloroethane binds to insulin—see below). Enthalpic contributions to hydrophobic binding or partitioning tend to be minimal, but if there are electrostatic contributions (e.g., van der Waals and/or hydrogen bonding—see below), the binding is more favorable and is therefore associated with a decrease in enthalpy (i.e., a decrease in heat content, or an exothermic process), suggesting an increase in stability of the system.

Thermodynamic analyses of anesthetic-protein interactions have, to date, been limited to only a few systems. Using a light-emitting enzyme purified from fireflies, Dickinson et al. (26)

reported that the interaction between inhalational anesthetics and firefly luciferase was characterized by negative enthalpic contributions at 20°C, implying that heat was released when anesthetics bind to this protein. This is consistent with earlier work by Ueda and Kamaya (130), and, as suggested above, is different than expected for simple hydrophobic partitioning, which should have a less negative enthalpic change (122) .

Studies of the temperature dependence of halothane binding to bovine serum albumin in our laboratory, using both tryptophan fluorescence quenching and photoaffinity labeling, reveal that the apparent K_d decreases as the temperature is reduced, giving the van't Hoff plot shown in Fig. 1. This analysis yields a ΔH° of –1.9 kcal mol^{-1} and a ΔS° of +6.0 cal $mol^{-1}K^{-1}$, quantitatively similar to the values for the halothane-luciferase interaction (26). In addition, a manometric analysis of xenon binding to myoglobin demonstrated a primarily enthalpic-driven process with a ΔG° of –2.9 kcal mol^{-1} at 25°C (43). Thus, it is possible that protein-anesthetic interactions are characterized by a negative enthalpic change, implying a significant electrostatic contribution, but the relevance of this characteristic to anesthetic action must wait for more such studies in many different protein systems.

The thermodynamics of anesthetic binding to membrane-bound protein could be very different because the target is partitioned between two solvents—water and lipid. For example, inhalational anesthetic inhibition of the erythrocyte Ca^{2+}–adenosine triphosphatase (ATPase) (78) demonstrates a higher IC_{50} at 25°C as compared to physiologic temperature, implying a more positive ΔH° as compared with anesthetic interactions with the soluble proteins mentioned above, and more consistent with the classical view of the hydrophobic effect. Although speculative, this may reflect the greater role of hydrophobicity and a lesser role for an electrostatic contribution to anesthetic interactions with membrane proteins, possibly pointing toward the lipid-protein interface of such proteins as a functional binding domain. While consistent with studies trying to localize the inhalational anesthetic binding sites in such proteins (see below), it clearly points toward the need for more work on the thermal dependence of anesthetic effects in membrane systems.

Binding Forces

Hydrophobic Effect

The hydrophobic effect is classically thought to result from the strong attraction of water molecules for each other, and the energetic cost of forcing these strongly hydrogen-bonded molecules into a cagelike structure (clathration shell) to form a cavity, or void, for the hydrophobic molecule (124). While this energetic cost can be overcome by the strong electrostatic interactions between charged species (like ions) and the relatively high partial charges of water, the weakly polar molecules characteristic of those with anesthetic properties have only feeble interactions with water, and are therefore forced into macromolecular domains of low hydration, e.g., hydrophobic regions. This movement of the anesthetic compound from the bulk water into a hydrophobic domain should therefore be a favorable entropic event, consistent with the albumin data cited above and a multitude of partitioning studies between organic solvents and water at 25°C (3,124). While confirming an inability of the hydrocarbon molecule to form any energetically important attractive (electrostatic) interactions with water molecules, it also suggests that mutual attraction of hydrocarbon molecules through van der Waals interactions is not an important contributor to "de-solvation."

More recently, however, this view of the energetic contributions to the hydrophobic effect has been questioned (104,105). The controversy relates to whether these nonpolar molecules leave water because the structure of water excludes them, or because they are able to make more favorable interactions with a less polar environment. In support of the latter interpretation is that partitioning of hydrophobic molecules between water and nonpolar solvent is much more favorable than the partitioning of the same molecule between water and the vapor phase, where van der Waals interactions are essentially absent (111).

Despite the possibility of an electrostatic attraction (see below), the strong correlation between oil solubility and anesthetic potency (Meyer-Overton rule) suggests that the hydrophobic effect is important in creating productive anesthetic-macromolecule interactions in some relevant targets. Indeed, the few studies that have examined the structural features of anesthetic binding sites in soluble proteins (see below) reveal internal cavities lined by hydrophobic amino acids. This preference for hydrophobic protein domains was unambiguously demonstrated by an examination of the interactions between halothane and a simple homopolymer, poly-(L-lysine), with photoaffinity labeling and fluorescence spectroscopy (74). When the butylamino side chains of lysine were charged (pH = 7), and circular dichroism spectroscopy showed the homopolymer to be in a random-coil configuration, only low and nonspecific halothane binding was observed. However, when the pH was raised above the pK_a of the ε-amino group (pH = 10.2), these side chains no longer repel each other and the secondary structure spontaneously changes to that of an α-helix. In an attempt to reduce this now-hydrophobic surface area, the long helices (>200 residues) fold to produce interhelix hydrophobic domains, demonstrated by a large increase in fluorescence yield and a blue-shift of the hydrophobic fluorescent probe, 8-anilino-1-naphthalene-sulfonate (ANS). Under these conditions, photoaffinity labeling of the lysine residues was substantially increased, and acquired a saturable character (Fig. 2). We have also found that ornithine polymers, with a side chain similar to lysine except one methylene group shorter, bind halothane less well, and that inclusion of bulky aromatics in such polymers increases the binding of halothane. Such results suggest that anesthetic binding is controlled in part by interhelical side chain packing as well as by the hydrophobic effect.

Crystallographic and NMR data indicate that native protein side chains tend to fit together in a complementary fashion with a packing density (the ratio of the summed atomic volumes to the total molecular volume) comparable to that of organic crystals (109). Defects in this tight packing are found in the majority of proteins whose structures have been determined at high resolution. The term *cavity* refers to such a packing defect in the protein tertiary structure, which may or may not normally be occupied by water molecules. These cavities are present in

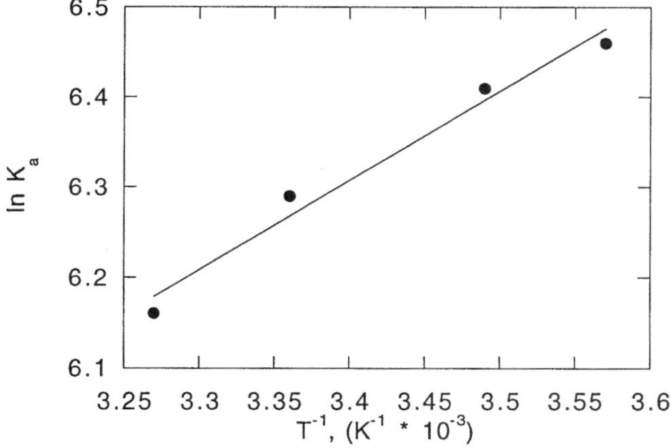

Figure 1. The dependence of the affinity of bovine serum albumin (5 μM) for halothane at pH 7 in phosphate buffer as a function of temperature. Data points are the means of three separate experiments. Buffer pH varied by only ±0.2 units over this temperature range.

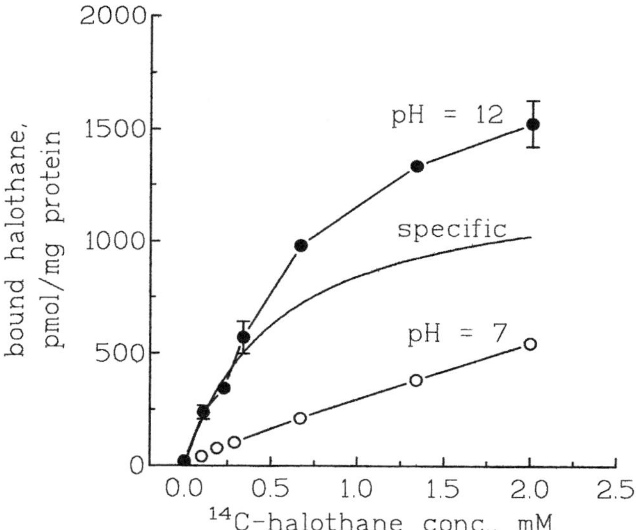

Figure 2. Direct photoaffinity labeling of poly-(L-lysine) (PLL) (approx. 200 residues) at pH 7 and 12. Circular dichroism spectra (not shown) demonstrated only random coil character at pH 7, and predominately α-helix at pH 12. Halothane labeling of PLL is substantially increased under alkaline conditions, and acquires a saturable character as shown from the curve fitted to the specific binding data (pH12-pH7), implying the creation of a suitable hydrophobic domain for halothane immobilization (binding).

monomeric proteins (68,108) and also occur at protein-protein interfaces (67). Richards and Lim (110) have postulated that while the presence of cavities is energetically costly (secondary to the loss of van der Waals contacts), they have evolved in order to allow the conformational changes required for protein function. This was recently confirmed in the case of λ repressor, where site-directed mutations produced an increase in packing density and stability (to thermal unfolding), but a decrease in function (82).

While the structure or cavity volume distribution in high pH lysine homopolymers is not clear, x-ray crystallography has shown that cavity volume and shape in natural proteins can vary substantially (67,68,108), and in some cases is large enough to accommodate even bulky anesthetic molecules like methoxyflurane (2,2-dichloro-1,1-difluoroethyl methyl ether) (0.144 nm^3). In myoglobin and hemoglobin, for example (see below), numerous packing defects exist with volumes on the order of 0.03 to 0.18 nm^3 (108,128), which can accommodate anesthetic molecules up to cyclopropane or dichloromethane in size (99). Clearly, the shape and preexisting occupancy of these cavities is also relevant to the binding of anesthetic molecules, demonstrated by the lack of halothane binding to hemoglobin or myoglobin, using either photoaffinity labeling (Eckenhoff, *unpublished observations*) or tryptophan fluorescence quenching (72), despite the fact that suitable volume cavities exist in these proteins. Consistent with these binding results are the minimal effects that halothane has on myoglobin and hemoglobin structure or function (137), whereas the smaller dichloromethane produces an important allosteric antisickling effect on hemoglobin (116). Such cavity volume considerations may be responsible for the well-known "cutoff" effect (44), whereby anesthetic potency is abruptly lost as the homologous series of either n-alkanes or n-alkanols is ascended. While once thought to reflect a cutoff with respect to lipid solubility, it is now appreciated that bilayer partitioning continues to increase as one ascends the series (23).

Electrostatic Interactions

The original Meyer-Overton rule was based on the solubility of anesthetics in olive oil, an uncertain mixture of various lipids (57,63). A somewhat better correlation has been found for n-octanol than for aliphatic solvents (47), demonstrating the possible importance of a polar component at the anesthetic site of action. Further, an improved correlation of potency with solubility in lecithin also suggests the importance of amphipathic and polar components to the interaction of macromolecules with these formally uncharged anesthetic molecules (57,123). Such weak electrostatic interactions can be conveniently divided into those due to hydrogen bonding and those due to van der Waals interactions. It is important to recognize, however, that such interactions represent more of a continuum than distinct entities, and thus some overlap in our discussion will be apparent. We also consider stereoselectivity here, because the weak electrostatic interactions that define anesthetic binding, when spatially distributed in a cavity, confer differential binding selectivity for enantiomers.

Hydrogen Bonding This relatively strong noncovalent bond arises when two electronegative atoms share (usually asymmetrically) the same hydrogen atom. Such hydrogen bonds play a central role in protein structure, stability, and function (45,119), and underlie the structure and properties of water. The electronegative atoms at either end of the hydrogen bond are generally oxygen and nitrogen in biologic macromolecules. Other atoms or structures that may serve as hydrogen bond donors include sulfur and carbon atoms (14,136), while the π-electrons of aromatic rings (80) and possibly the electronegative halogens may serve as hydrogen bond acceptors (135).

It is now clear that inhalational anesthetics possessing a single or few hydrogen atoms in addition to the halogens are more potent than the perhalogenated analogues (38,58). Also, there is a reasonably good correlation between anesthetic potency in tadpoles (9), and possibly for firefly luciferase inhibition, with the relative ability to donate this proton in a hydrogen bond (4). The ability of a compound like halothane to accept a hydrogen bond is probably limited, although this may be important in the case of ether compounds, like isoflurane and methoxyflurane (5). Indeed, the presumed ability of the halogenated ethers to hydrogen bond is reflected in their increased aqueous phase solubility compared to similar-sized alkanes. Experimental evidence supporting the ability of inhalational anesthetics to form hydrogen bonds comes primarily from infrared spectroscopic studies. DiPaolo and Sandorfy (28,29), for example, found that halothane decreased the association between well hydrogen-bonded solutions such as *N*-methylpivalamide and 2,6-diisopropylphenol. Perfluorinated molecules, on the other hand, did not influence these systems, but the presence of heavier halogens like chlorine, bromine, and iodine had a progressively greater hydrogen bond weakening effect. Further, both of the chlorine atoms of 1,2-dichloroethane have been shown crystallographically to interact with the indole NH groups of two tryptophan residues and the aromatic hydrogens of two phenylalanine residues in the active site of haloalkane dehalogenase (135). The chlorine-nitrogen bond length of about 0.32 to 0.36 nm, and chlorine-carbon bond lengths of 0.36 nm, however, are longer than the typical hydrogen bonds of water (0.28 nm), suggesting a relatively weak interaction. Indeed, the K_m for dichloroethane dehalogenation by this enzyme is about 0.7 to 1.1 mM. Somewhat lower K_m values of about 0.2 mM were obtained for halothane metabolism and adduct formation by liver microsomes, suggesting slightly stronger binding forces of this pentahalogenated ethane to a catalytic site on one of the cytochrome P450 enzymes (53). This latter example is complex, however, since higher concentrations of halothane inhibit its own metabolism (83), so the apparent K_m may not accurately reflect the catalytic site K_d.

Although it is possible that weak hydrogen bonds could occur between the halogens and an "acidic" proton on a protein target, as suggested above, a hydrogen bond between a haloalkane, or haloether proton, and a target electron donor sites is also plausible. Accordingly, proton NMR studies have provided evidence for hydrogen bonding between halothane and chloroform protons and electron donors such as ethers, amines, and carbonyl groups (11,88). The dimerization of gramicidin monomers in a phospholipid bilayer, essential for channel formation and driven by hydrogen bonding in the membrane hydrocarbon core, is also impeded by halothane and other inhalational anesthetics (13). Although these gramicidin results did not allow assignment of the interacting groups, they are consistent with the premise that hydrogen bonding is important to the anesthetic-target interaction.

The ability of these small molecules to donate a hydrogen bond, however, may not be consistent across the entire range of inhalational anesthetics. In recent molecular dynamic simulations of halothane in water, Scharf (University of Pennsylvania, *personal communication*, 1995) was unable to demonstrate an association of the sole proton of halothane with the water oxygen atom, except at distances over 0.27 nm (total carbon-oxygen distance of 0.38 nm). If this represents a form of weak hydrogen bond, it is unlikely to be strong enough to compete with the much stronger water-water or macromolecular structural hydrogen bonds. Finally, at least in the case of halothane, it also suggests that the ability to donate a proton is unlikely to play a significant role in binding interactions with a target site.

van der Waals Interactions This category of interatomic forces includes the stabilizing forces known as hydrophobic bonding, confusing because of overlap with the hydrophobic effect. All such stabilizing forces are ultimately derived from Coulomb's law of attraction between unlike charges. Given the chemical composition, structure and the lack of formal charge on the inhalational anesthetics, it is clear that van der Waals forces must play an important role in the stabilizing energetics that determine binding to a protein. The attractive van der Waals forces include dipole-dipole, induced dipole-dipole, and London (or dispersion) interactions. Induced dipole-dipole interactions result from the distortion of an atom's electron cloud (polarization) in the presence of a strong dipole moment (such as in a protein cavity lined by polar residues). Polarizability is a function of atomic mass, and thus is more prominent with the larger halogens often included on the inhalational anesthetics. Accordingly, it is interesting to note that for a given structure, both anesthetic potency and degree of metabolism are progressively increased as heavier halogens are substituted (60,125), suggesting that this van der Waals force may be important in producing functional binding interactions. London interactions between molecules arise from the normal transient fluctuations in the charge distribution symmetry of the electron clouds of two neighboring molecules. The energy of all these van der Waals interactions varies as a function of $1/[\text{distance}]^6$, rendering these forces significant only at very close range. Xenon binding to myoglobin is an example of binding that occurs entirely through van der Waals interactions, but limited to induced dipole-dipole and London-type interactions. On the other hand, the clinically used anesthetics have a permanent (but small) dipole moment, allowing all three forces to potentially act in the stabilization of binding interactions.

Stereoselectivity

One of the determinants of specific binding to a protein target has to do with the spatial arrangements of the important interactive groups in the binding cavity or pocket. Such relationships may produce chirality of ligand binding, and thereby stereoselective alterations in function. The small size, low-affinity, and probable small electrostatic interactive potential of the inhalational anesthetics suggest that chiral selectivity should be small. Indeed, Pfeiffer's (102) rule suggests that, based on the average required dose (mass) of a drug, the inhalational anesthetics should demonstrate almost no stereoselectivity. Thus, two in vivo studies have found the (+) isomer of isoflurane (1-chloro-2,2,2-trifluoroethyl difluoromethyl ether) to be only twice as potent as the (–) isomer (59,84), and in vitro, several studies have shown approximately the same magnitude of difference using various models like activation of a potassium channel in the pond snail *L. stagnalis* (49), binding to serum albumin (34), and γ-aminobutyric acid ($GABA_A$) chloride channel potentiation (106). The enantiomers of the even simpler compound, halothane, have been found to have slightly different immobilizing potency in specific mutants of the nematode *C. elegans* (117), and a two- to threefold difference in metabolism in vivo as detected by trifluoroacetylated liver proteins (87), but no differences in anesthetic potency in mammals has yet been reported. There are at least three important caveats of these observations. First, modest stereoselectivity for the action of inhalational anesthetics has now been observed in many reductionist systems, limiting the usefulness of this approach in searching for a single important site of action. Second, even the less potent isomer has behavioral effects that include anesthesia, suggesting that distinction at the molecular level might be difficult unless, again, one proposes a single site of action for these compounds. Third, because stereoselectivity suggests spatial constraints to binding in a cavity, it seems unlikely that the many diverse structures producing anesthesia could all satisfy these constraints, again implying multiple sites of action. While the initial goal of such studies was to unambiguously demonstrate that interactions with protein (as opposed to lipid) were responsible for anesthetic action, the result has been somewhat less definitive because of the possibility of lipid-based chirality. To address this, Dickinson et al. (27) reported that the isoflurane enantiomers partition equally into bilayers of phosphatidylcholine, phosphatidic acid, and cholesterol, and lower phase transition temperatures equally (49). However, it remains plausible that other lipid components of biologic membranes not yet examined may contribute to stereoselective anesthetic partitioning or function. In summary, then, the low degree of selectivity is predicted for ligands with such limited interactive capability, and does point toward chiral sites of interaction, which include protein.

Location and Character of Anesthetic Binding Sites

The determination of the location of anesthetic binding sites in protein is important because it predicts the interactions that produce binding and may also provide clues for the structural consequences of binding. Further, it should allow optimization of anesthetic structure, something that has not been possible to date. Such location and structural information can be provided by a number of different approaches, from kinetic studies to x-ray crystallography. We very briefly present and discuss each of the approaches, as it is important to realize their individual strengths and limitations.

Functional and Equilibrium Binding Assays

The most common approach is to first ask whether the binding site overlaps with a native substrate or ligand site, or whether it is located elsewhere on the protein (allosteric). This information may be provided by examining the concentration dependence of the anesthetic effect on some functional assay, or an equilibrium (radioligand) binding assay for some previously established ligand. From double reciprocal plots, the process can be classified as competitive, noncompetitive, or some combination. Competitive kinetics are typically interpreted as binding at the same or overlapping sites in the protein. There are numerous examples of this approach, ranging from soluble proteins, such as adenylate kinase (112), firefly, and bacterial luciferases (6,48), to membrane bound proteins, such as the ligand-gated ion channels or catecholamine transporters (41,94). In firefly luciferase, the double reciprocal plot suggests competitive kinetics with the native substrate luciferin and indicates that two halothane molecules fit in the luciferin binding pocket on the protein (48). This is consistent with the approximate molecular volumes of these two ligands.

On the other hand, apparent competitive kinetics in the case of anesthetics and fatty acid binding by bovine serum albumin has now been shown to be largely an allosteric effect, since recent halothane photoaffinity labeling (unpublished observations) and tryptophan fluorescence quenching studies (72) have demonstrated that saturable binding of halothane is to different binding regions (domains IA and IIA) of this protein than what is thought to be the high-affinity fatty acid binding domain (IIIA) (see below). Also, competitive kinetics in the case of halothane's effect on serotonin transport and cocaine binding were shown by other methods to represent allosterism (35,85,86). Therefore, competitive kinetics can be mimicked by anesthetic binding to a site that is distinct from the native ligand or substrate site, sometimes termed "allosteric competition" (90), and thus using only these functional approaches may lead to ambiguity with respect to the actual location or character of the anesthetic binding site.

This functional/kinetic approach is even more difficult to interpret for the membrane bound proteins because of the dramatic functional influence of the lipid component. A modification of the equilibrium binding approach that more directly addresses the issue of the site is to determine whether both the native ligand and the anesthetic can protect the same site from alkylation by a compound such as n-ethylmaleimide (75). Unfortunately, it is not yet clear whether such nonequilibrium protection assays are valid when the kinetics for the ligand and anesthetic are very different, as they typically are (see above).

Reporter Groups

A potentially powerful approach to determining the location of an anesthetic binding site, and one to which we will return when considering alterations to protein structure, is the use of reporter groups on the protein target, or on the anesthetic itself. It is important to recognize that such groups typically provide information on the character of their immediate environment, and that more than one reason could explain this change in environment.

^{19}F-NMR Spectroscopy The volatile general anesthetics that are currently in clinical use (e.g., halothane, isoflurane, and desflurane) are heavily fluorinated in order to decrease metabolism and flammability. Since organofluorine compounds are not normally present in biologic systems, the naturally occurring ^{19}F isotope (which has a nucleus with a nonzero spin) has been used as a probe for NMR spectroscopy with little background noise. We have discussed the use of this approach to define kinetics above, but it can also be used to define features of the anesthetic environment in whole animals, tissue, and phospholipid vesicle systems. Trudell and Hubbell (129) used ^{19}F-NMR to show that halothane rapidly equilibrated between water and the entire thickness of the bilayer of model membranes composed of egg phosphatidylcholine. Wyrwicz et al. (139) found multiple environments for halothane in rabbit sciatic nerve, but only a single environment in intact rabbit brain (140). Of interest is the fact that the single anesthetic environment in brain was characterized as being hydrophobic with some polar component, based on the fluorine chemical shift. The most recent example of this approach examined the distribution of sevoflurane in the rat head in vivo, and concluded that there were two distinct environments for this anesthetic, similar to environments defined by several other investigators, and that the more confined environment correlated better with the onset and offset of behavioral anesthesia than the less confined environment (141). While the nature of these NMR environments remains unclear and may be difficult to characterize further with this approach, one reasonable possibility is that the confined environment represents that fraction of anesthetic molecules bound to macromolecules, perhaps proteins, and the less confined environment is that in water and perhaps lipid.

Proton NMR Spectroscopy This technique examines the environment of hydrogen atoms in, for example, macromolecules. Because of the large number of protons in biologic systems, one-dimensional NMR spectra are characterized by fairly broad resonances, due to overlap from the many chemically identical protons in slightly different environments. One-dimensional proton NMR spectroscopy has been used to examine the effect of halothane and methoxyflurane on human hemoglobin structure (7). Clinical concentrations of these anesthetics caused reversible changes in two peaks in the portion of the spectrum that reported on aromatic and histidine resonances. This was interpreted to be due to localized pK_a changes brought on by alterations in the dielectric constant of the environment of these residues, probably because of conformational changes. These results were confirmed by another study, which also reported perturbations in the aliphatic regions of the spectrum following the addition of halothane (10).

More recently, two-dimensional (and now three- and four-dimensional) proton- and heteronuclear NMR spectroscopy has been applied to solving the structure of smaller (15 to 25 kd) proteins (20). Although these approaches have not yet been used to study anesthetic-protein interactions, they are anticipated to provide much useful information as to location and character of anesthetic binding domains, and also the structural consequences.

Fluorescence Spectroscopy This method allows the study of biomolecular systems under conditions of thermodynamic equilibrium, as well as the rapid kinetics associated with dynamic changes in protein structure. Most proteins contain fluorescent aromatic residues, such as phenylalanine, tyrosine, and tryptophan. Of these, tryptophan is the least common, but has the highest quantum yield. The rarity can be advantageous, however, since the observed fluorescence signal results from few amino acids, which may have known positions in the protein. For example, bovine serum albumin contains two tryptophans, one of which is conserved and is in a well-characterized binding cavity for small charged aromatic molecules, such as warfarin or triiodobenzoic acid (64). Binding of an anesthetic in this site, provided it contains a heavy halogen like bromine or chlorine, will quench the fluorescence signal. This can then serve as a marker for the location of the ligand in the protein matrix, since heavy atom quenching occurs only at short range (~0.5 nm). The analysis can be extended to examine the thermodynamics and kinetics of binding as mentioned above. It is important, however, to realize that alterations in the structure of a protein by binding of the anesthetic at a remote site could change the environment of the tryptophan sufficiently to produce charge transfer interactions with neighboring residues that also quench the fluorescence signal. Thus, it is necessary to have some independent means of ruling out significant structural changes on binding of the ligand, in order to conclude that binding occurs in the vicinity of the fluorescent group. In the case of albumin, photoaffinity labeling confirmed that halothane was binding in the immediate vicinity of the tryptophans, and circular dichroism (CD) spectroscopy demonstrated a lack of change in the secondary structure (72). On the other hand, the two tryptophan residues in myoglobin are apparently in a smaller cavity, or one lacking a suitable access pathway, since halothane failed to quench the fluorescence in any reasonable concentrations and, as stated previously, is also unable to bind saturably by photoaffinity labeling.

This approach will be less definitive in proteins containing several tryptophan residues, since they will all contribute to the steady-state fluorescence signal, and determination of those tryptophan residues whose fluorescence is altered by anesthetic binding is problematic. Some information, however, could be obtained if the multiple tryptophans were in similar domains, such as the transmembrane sequences of membrane proteins. It may also be feasible to dissect out interactions with individual tryptophan residues using fluorescence lifetime measurements.

Fluorescence Lifetime Analysis This method permits study of the dynamic interactions in the vicinity of the fluorescent groups and also to classify the mechanism of the quenching interaction as static versus collisional (37). Collisional quenching results from the random diffusional encounters between quencher and fluorophore as might occur between halothane and indole (for example) in a suitable organic solvent. The measured lifetime of the fluorophore, under these conditions, will be inversely proportional to the halothane concentration. On the other hand, a static interaction occurs when a complex is formed between the fluorophore and quencher (or between the fluorescent group in a protein and a bound quencher). Under these conditions, no change in the fluorescence lifetime is observed as the quencher concentration is increased. This is because the quencher molecule is already present in the vicinity of the fluorophore at the moment of excitation, and therefore causes instantaneous fluorescence quenching. This type of behavior has been observed for the quenching of the tryptophan fluorescence of a four-helix bundle protein by halothane, demonstrating that binding to the protein has occurred (73).

Fluorescence Anisotropy This technique is used to study the rotational diffusion of the protein as a whole (relatively slow), and also the dynamics of individual tryptophan residues (relatively fast) within the protein (71). Tryptophan residues in proteins experience considerable mobility about the C_α-C_β bond, limited only by the structural barriers imposed by the macromolecular framework. Fluorescence anisotropy measurements may prove useful for detecting changes in local protein dynamics and conformation that result from anesthetic binding. To date, this approach has not been used to study anesthetic-protein interactions; however, Vanderkooi et al. (134) showed that general anesthetics depolarize the fluorescence of the hydrophobic probe 1-phenyl-6-phenylhexatriene (DPH), indicating an increase in the fluidity of biologic membranes.

Electron Paramagnetic Resonance (EPR) Spectroscopy Specific labels with environment-sensitive spectra can be attached to proteins and lipids. The use of nitroxide spin labels covalently incorporated into macromolecular structures allows determination of the local viscosity, topology, and dielectric features of the environment (81,93). Such probes have been used to characterize the effect of anesthetics on lipid bilayer fluidity (46). The effect of general anesthetics on the properties of spin labeled membrane proteins has also received some attention. For example, the extracellular domain of the anion-exchange protein in human erythrocytes has been labeled with bis(sulfo-N-succinimidyl)doxyl-2-spiro-5'-azlate (21) and the rotational mobility of the probe was reversibly increased by diethyl ether. Although this could have represented a localized structural change due to direct anesthetic binding to protein, it was interpreted as probably being due to changes in surrounding lipid bilayer order. These probes have also been used to examine the effects of general anesthetics on the interactions of the nicotinic acetylcholine receptor (nAChR) with neighboring lipid molecules in the bilayer (1). Isoflurane and hexanol were unable to displace boundary lipids from their association with the receptor. Enhancement of protein side chain mobility by ethanol, as detected by spectral changes in a covalently attached maleimide spin-label to selected cysteine residues on the nAChR, has also been reported (2). Further studies with carefully positioned EPR probes should allow further insight into the influence of anesthetics on target dynamics, but not necessarily the binding locations.

Direct Photoaffinity Labeling

A recently described approach in use in our laboratory is halothane direct photoaffinity labeling (34,40). The rapid kinetics of halothane equilibrium binding can be converted to a stable covalent bond by first cleaving the C-Br bond of halothane with UV light to produce a reactive chlorotrifluoroethyl (CTFE) radical, which then covalently attaches to adjacent residues in its bound environment, probably through a two-step process. Unless confined, the CTFE radical recombines with the free bromine radical to reform halothane, as suggested by the low loss of halothane from UV-irradiated aqueous systems, as compared to ethanolic systems (*unpublished observations*). The adduct location can be tracked by including a radioactive atom, such as ^{14}C on the trifluoromethyl carbon, or ^{3}H on the 1-carbon, or by monitoring regional protein mass with mass spectrometry. The use of this approach has permitted the mapping of halothane binding sites in soluble proteins, such as serum albumin. Two specific binding sites are identified in bovine serum albumin (BSA), and these correspond roughly to the location of the two tryptophans in BSA, in agreement with the tryptophan quenching studies. In accordance with the rapid kinetics and relatively small size (compared to triiodobenzoic acid) of the parent molecule, halothane, the label is found bound to several amino acid residues in this cavity (Trp214-Arg219). Despite clear competition between fatty acids and halothane (32,34) for binding to BSA, the photolabeled residues do not coincide with the presumed fatty acid binding domains (16), indicating allosteric communication between these sites. The dissimilarity of fatty acid and halothane binding sites is consistent with the low affinity (K_d >5 mM) interactions of other fatty acid binding proteins and halothane (42).

Photoaffinity labeling has allowed the initial assignment of halothane binding domains in membrane proteins as well. The halothane binding domains in a ligand-gated ion channel, the nicotinic acetylcholine receptor (nAChR), was determined in membranes from *Torpedo nobiliana* (36). Photoaffinity labeling with approximately 0.5 mM free halothane concentration and subsequent affinity purification of the receptor revealed each subunit of the nAChR to be specifically labeled to a similar degree. On digesting the α-subunit with V8 protease (endoprotease Glu-C), greater than 90% of the label was found in the fragments known to contain the four putative transmembrane sequences, but it is not yet clear if the probable channel lining helix (M2) is labeled by halothane. Thus, results in this member of the ligand-gated ion channel family suggest that there are multiple halothane (anesthetic) binding sites. Most are specific, and the majority are found in the transmembrane domain in a distribution that is different from lipid distribution. Such data hints of the importance of these functionally crucial transmembrane regions (lipid-protein or interhelical interfaces) for anesthetic binding and possibly action. Other evidence has accumulated to implicate the lipid-protein interface of membrane proteins as a favored binding site for anesthetic-like molecules (52,76,98).

Crystallographic Approaches

X-Ray Diffraction This approach requires the formation of suitable three-dimensional crystals of similarly oriented protein molecules to allow amplification of the diffracted x-rays. Such crystals are often difficult to produce [human serum albumin (HSA), for example, required crystallization in microgravity], have until recently been limited to the soluble proteins, and may not reflect the native structure of a protein in the biologically relevant aqueous state (133). Further, the assumptions and algorithms for reducing the electron density map to a three-dimensional structure involve a degree of subjectivity so that not every detail of the structure is necessarily accurate (77). Nevertheless, x-ray crystal structures are considered the gold standard for comparison at this point, and have resulted in substantial insights into protein structure/function relationships, and protein-ligand interactions (39).

The binding of xenon to crystals of myoglobin has characterized the anesthetic-protein interaction at the highest resolution. Using 2.5 atm of xenon and x-ray diffraction analysis of sperm whale myoglobin, this weak anesthetic was noted to bind through van der Waals interactions at a single site equidistant from the proximal histidine and one of the pyrrole rings of the heme moiety (114). Interestingly, cyclopropane and dichloromethane were found to bind to metmyoglobin in the same site (99,115). While this site is in the interior of myoglobin, there is no obvious access pathway from the solvent to this proximal heme region. Molecular dynamic simulations have resolved this problem by revealing transient structural fluctuations away from the average crystal structure, resulting in the opening of pathways for ligand entry and exit (24,128). These fluctuations caused a 3% to 4% change in overall volume, and created small cavities with lifetimes on the order of 1 to 20 psec. As many as four binding sites for xenon in myoglobin could be demonstrated on raising the xenon pressure to 7 atm (127). As pointed out by Miller et al. (91), however, the relative affinities of xenon and cyclopropane for myoglobin are not consistent with their relative anesthetic potency, suggesting that this site may not adequately represent the character of the "anesthetic" binding site. Nevertheless, this work is important in that it has demonstrated the concept of the binding of weak ligands to the hydrophobic interior of soluble proteins in the vicinity of aromatic structures, the recruitment of binding sites, as well as the dynamic nature of these sites and access routes.

Xenon binding to hemoglobin has also been studied with x-ray diffraction analysis (113), and demonstrates a single binding site on each of the α and β chains. Interestingly, these sites are not equivalent to the myoglobin sites, but are instead located more peripherally. The residues with which xenon makes contact at both sites in hemoglobin are valine, leucine, and phenylalanine. Likewise, dichloromethane was found to bind to hemoglobin at three to four distinct sites, each of which lies in an interior hydrophobic site close to aromatic residues such as Trp14α or Phe71β, or at the interface between the hemoglobin subunits near Tyr145 (116).

Dichloroethane binding to both bacterial haloalkane dehalogenase (135) and insulin (55) has also been analyzed with x-ray diffraction. In the former, the dihaloalkane is the native substrate from which the microorganism derives energy. As shown in Fig. 3, the dihaloalkane binds in an interior hydrophobic site with electrostatic contacts to two tryptophan and two phenylalanine residues and an aspartate residue. This site also binds and dehalogenates smaller haloalkanes such as methyl chloride and ethyl chloride, but with lower apparent K_m values, suggesting the importance of the two additional electrostatic contacts on the 2-carbon halogen, or loss of van der Waals contacts. The insulin cavity, on the other hand, is lined by serine, valine, glutamate, and tyrosine, and is sufficiently small and sterically hindered to prohibit binding of the *trans*-conformation of dichloroethane. In addition, all of the clinically used haloalkane anesthetics are too large to bind in this insulin cavity, and those that are much smaller, like dichloromethane, also bind poorly. Interestingly, the insulin cavity contains structured water molecules, some of which are displaced on haloalkane binding, suggesting an additional entropic contribution to the binding interaction. Sufficient structural resolution has not been achieved in other protein-anesthetic systems to determine whether this is a general feature of anesthetic binding.

The only x-ray diffraction data that incorporate a clinically important haloalkane anesthetic are those of halothane binding to adenylate kinase (112). Halothane was shown to inhibit this enzyme with a K_i of 2.5 mM, at low-adenosine monophosphate (AMP) concentration (100 μM), suggesting a competitive interaction (see above). Crystals soaked in "saturated" solutions of halothane showed localization of the halothane molecule in a discrete interhelical niche, lined by the hydrophobic residues valine, leucine, and isoleucine, but also by the more polar residues tyrosine, arginine, and glutamine (101). Such a site satisfies the suggestions made above that an anesthetic site, while necessarily hydrophobic, should also have some polar (aromatic?) character. Confirming the kinetic results, this site was also identified as that involved in AMP

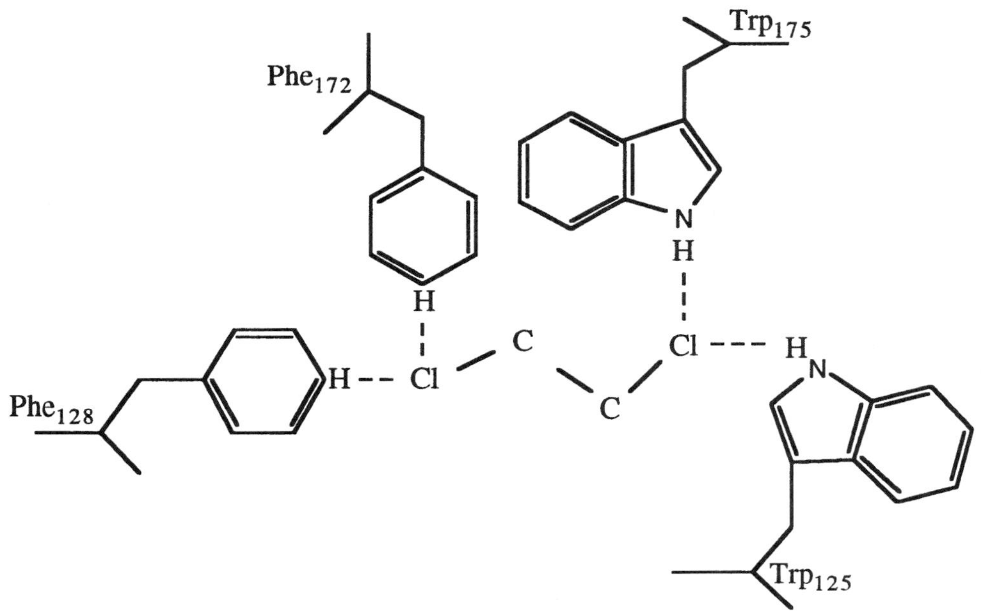

Figure 3. Binding of the substrate 1,2-dichloroethane to the active site of dehaloalkane dehalogenase from *X. autotrophicus*. One of the chlorine atoms electrostatically interacts with the ring nitrogen protons of Trp 125 and 175, while the other chlorine interacts with the side chains (probably peripheral ring protons) of Phe 128 and 172. (Adapted from ref. 135.)

binding. While of low resolution (0.6 nm), this study confirms many of our impressions of what the character of an anesthetic binding site should be and brings clear evidence of competitive interactions. Interestingly, there was no evidence for a structural consequence to adenylate kinase as a result of halothane binding. More such studies at higher resolution should allow further refinement of our concepts of anesthetic-protein interactions.

Although x-ray diffraction studies of membrane proteins have been difficult, some progress has been made with novel crystallographic approaches using short chain detergents or monoclonal antibody fragments (25,69), or with highly ordered natural membrane proteins such as bacteriorhodopsin (98). In the latter case, low-resolution difference analysis of electron density maps with and without diiodomethane found the anesthetic to be located in the lipid-filled center of the naturally occurring protein trimers, suggesting lipid-protein interfacial binding.

Electron Diffraction A related technique that may prove useful for studying anesthetic interactions with the membrane proteins at high resolution is electron cryomicroscopy (19,31). The advantage is that the structure of proteins that form thin two-dimensional crystals, such as several membrane proteins under native conditions, can be analyzed at up to 0.35-nm resolution. This technique was used to define the structure of bacteriorhodopsin at high resolution (65). In addition, Unwin (132) has used this approach to show that binding of acetylcholine to the *T. marmorata* nAChR results in allosteric conformational changes in the α-helices that line the pore of this ligand-gated ion channel. The paucity of suitable crystals and low-resolution inherent to this approach, however, may limit its usefulness in defining the presumably more subtle influences of the inhalational anesthetics.

Neutron Diffraction Because neutron scattering is unrelated to the atomic number, it is possible to locate hydrogens that typically constitute half of the total number of atoms in a protein (79). In addition, neutron diffraction provides higher resolution maps than x-ray diffraction, providing more precise structural detail. In relation to anesthetics, this approach has only been used to study interactions with lipid bilayers. For example, Franks and Lieb (47) found that cyclopropane at one atmosphere had no detectable effect on the gross structure of model lipid bilayers, and White et al. (138) showed that hexane localized to the center of dioleoyl lecithin bilayers. While potentially very useful, the difficulty and expense of neutron diffraction experiments will undoubtedly limit the application of this technology to protein-anesthetic studies.

Infrared Spectroscopy This form of spectroscopy has the advantage of rapid time resolution (10^{-13} sec), allowing discrimination of environments not possible with NMR. Caughey and coworkers (30,54) have used infrared spectroscopy to characterize the binding environment of nitrous oxide in a variety of protein targets. They examined the shift in the wave number position of a specific antisymmetric stretch frequency (υ_3) of N_2O close to 2230 cm^{-1}, which reflects the polarity of the environment. Two distinct sites for N_2O were found in HSA and BSA (30,63). One is near a benzene-like structure, and the other is in an alkane-like environment, consistent with the general features of anesthetic binding sites identified above. Although currently limited to nitrous oxide, this approach should be useful for examining the interactions of other anesthetics with proteins because the low-energy photons can probe the weak associations characteristic of these compounds.

Binding Site Character Summary At present there is clearly a limited data base from which to generalize the structural features of an anesthetic binding site in a protein target. However, the available information indicates that the binding site for inhalational anesthetics has an appropriate cavity volume, shape, and hydrophobic character—all of which may in part be contributed by the bulky hydrophobic side chains such as leucine, isoleucine, tryptophan, and phenylalanine. In addition, the site has some polar character, which stabilizes the binding interaction, and which could also be contributed by the aromatic side chains, and by residues such as histidine, arginine, and glutamate. Discrete binding sites are less apparent in membrane proteins; available evidence suggests multiple binding sites at the lipid-protein, and protein-protein interfaces. Figure 4 illustrates potential electrostatic interactions between aromatic rings and haloalkane/haloether anesthetics.

STRUCTURAL CONSEQUENCES OF ANESTHETIC BINDING

Structural and conformational changes to proteins as a result of anesthetic binding have been difficult to demonstrate. This is not unreasonable when one considers the primitive state of

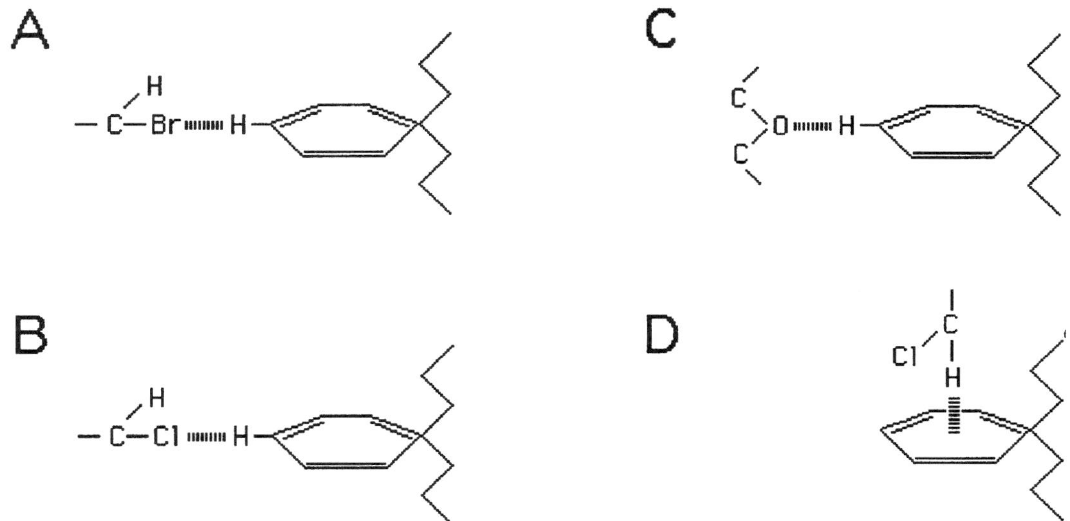

Figure 4. Potential electrostatic interactions between aromatic rings (shown here by a benzene side chain, i.e., Phe) and anesthetics. **A,B:** A C-H X hydrogen bonding between either bromine or chlorine atoms of the anesthetic and the aromatic ring protons. **C:** A more conventional hydrogen bond between an ether oxygen (such as on diethyl ether or isoflurane) and the aromatic proton. **D:** An electrostatic interaction between an "acidic" proton on an anesthetic an the π-electrons of the aromatic ring.

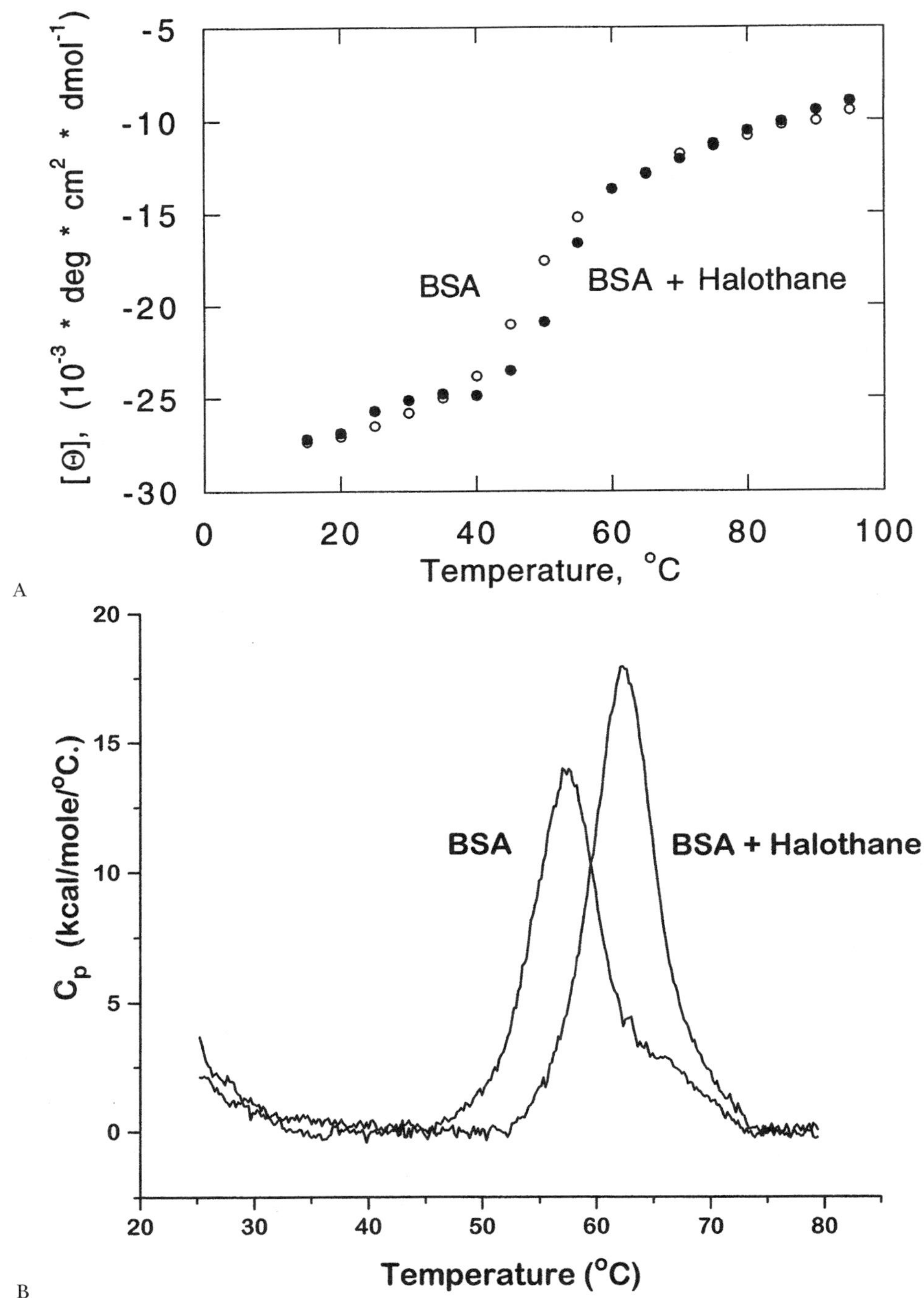

Figure 5. Soluble protein stabilization by an inhalational anesthetic. **A:** A thermal denaturing circular dichroism scan of serum albumin in the presence of 1.5 M guanidinium chloride with *(closed circles)* and without *(open circles)* 5 mM halothane, with clear evidence of stabilization of α-helical character (negative ellipticity at 222 nm). **B:** Shows data from differential scanning microcalorimetry experiments of 15 mM albumin, clearly showing stabilization of the folded structure in the presence of 3 mM halothane (PA Liebman, University of Pennsylvania, *unpublished observations*, 1996).

our ability to discern changes in protein structure, and the fact that the functional effects of anesthetics in vivo are well tolerated and generally reversible. The tools for defining protein structure at high resolution are only just now becoming widely used to define protein/ligand interactions, and the most easily characterized proteins are the small soluble ones that anesthetics appear to influence minimally or not at all. Further, the recently described creative approaches for crystallizing membrane proteins, using short chain detergents or monoclonal antibody fragments (25,69) to allow x-ray diffraction analysis, may well limit the ability to study ligand interactions.

Nevertheless, the fact that inhalational anesthetics bind to and alter protein function dictates that a change in protein structure or dynamics must be occurring. One example of this is the multiple effects that halothane has on the binding of ligands by serum albumin. Halothane has been shown to compete with warfarin binding (15), but also to increase the binding of other drugs, such as the barbiturates and benzodiazepines

(12), and to alter the chirality of bilirubin binding (89). These clearly cannot all be competitive effects, especially since the binding domains for halothane are now known to be distinct (see above). The changes to membrane protein function cannot yet be unambiguously assigned to protein (see Chap. 1 by Forman et al.), but if due to a direct effect on protein, little evidence has emerged to point to anesthetic competition at agonist sites; the interaction is likely to be allosteric in nature, through subtle alterations in stability or conformation. We will briefly discuss the potential impact of anesthetic binding to each aspect of protein structure, but again, substantial overlap between these areas must exist.

Secondary Structure

The few hydrogen atoms on potent inhalational anesthetics are thought to be relatively "acid" in character, meaning that they possess a relative positive charge due to the electron withdrawing effect of the halogens. An extension of the proposition that anesthetic binding forces may be contributed by an atypical hydrogen bond (see above) is that the hydrogen bonding ability (donor or acceptor) may be sufficiently strong to disrupt or reduce the stability of peptide hydrogen bonds. This "competitive" hydrogen bonding could have widespread effects on protein structure through destabilization of secondary structure, which is principally formed by intrapeptide hydrogen bonds. As stated above, such widespread influences have been difficult to demonstrate. Ueda's group (17,118) reported a slight shift from α-helix to β-sheet for poly-(L-lysine) in the presence of anesthetics, using Fourier transform infrared ratio (FTIR) and CD spectroscopy, but in more recent experiments with the same homopolymer, we were unable to observe any significant change in secondary structure with up to 12 mM halothane (74). Also, no change was observed in the secondary structure of albumin as measured by CD spectroscopy in the presence of 12 mM halothane (almost 2 orders of magnitude greater than clinical EC_{50}), even though significant binding is observed (72). In fact, recent studies in our laboratory suggest that the secondary structure of bovine serum albumin is actually stabilized in the presence of halothane (see Fig. 5A).

Tertiary Structure

Most approaches to protein tertiary structure are even more indirect. As mentioned above, the alteration in ligand binding in the presence of anesthetics is most likely due to subtle alterations in tertiary structure. In at least one case, anesthetic-induced alterations in the tertiary structure of proteins could be observed by electron microscopy. The exposure of crayfish axonal microtubules to 5 mM halothane produced a dramatic change in filament organization, such that a completely different structure, the macrotubule, was reversibly created (66). As suggested above, x-ray crystallography has only revealed subtle local changes in protein structure after anesthetic binding (xenon, cyclopropane, dichloromethane). In addition, Gursky et al. (55) found that the binding of 1,2-dichloroethane to insulin crystals results in displacement of sulfate ions from distant sites on the protein, apparently through allosteric conformational changes.

Occupancy of these internal cavities may have little effect on the average global structure (as represented by crystallography) of proteins, but could have a more marked effect on the protein dynamics that are essential in many cases for protein function. It seems likely that if the anesthetic binding step is characterized by a negative enthalpy, the tertiary, folded state of the protein may actually be more stable than the unbound protein. For example, this could be revealed in some cases by thermal unfolding. Preliminary data from our laboratory has suggested (Fig. 5B) that bovine serum albumin is rendered more stable to thermal unfolding in the presence of 3 mM halothane. Other investigators, on the other hand, have suggested that the enzyme firefly luciferase is actually destabilized by ethanol, also based on differential scanning calorimetry (18). While such differences may relate to the choice of anesthetic (alcohol versus alkane), or the target itself (luciferase has an unusually low thermal transition temperature), such discrepancies point toward the need for more such studies.

FUNCTIONAL CONSEQUENCES OF ANESTHETIC BINDING

The final consequence of anesthetic binding and the resulting structural changes is a functional effect. Whether or not a functional result occurs is presumably dependent on whether a suitable cavity exists in the protein in question and how crucial this cavity is to protein function. In some cases, this binding site will overlap with that of some other ligand, and therefore directly influence function in a competitive fashion. In others, the vacancy of the cavity will be important for protein dynamics (110), so its occupancy may slow or prevent normal dynamics and function. In still others, occupancy of some cavity may have no functional effect whatsoever.

Throughout this chapter, we have been alluding to the well-documented functional effects of the inhalational anesthetics, and aside for these few examples, will go into no more detail. The remainder of this volume deals exhaustively with the functional influences of this interesting set of compounds at a variety of levels, from the receptor to the intact organism.

CONCLUSIONS

The fundamental interactions of the inhalational anesthetics with proteins have been considered in some detail, using specific examples where appropriate to illustrate these interactions. It is clear that these low-affinity molecules with rapid kinetics can specifically bind to discrete sites in protein, and some general features of these sites are beginning to emerge. The structural consequences of anesthetic binding, however, are still vague at best. The remaining challenges are to define which interactions produce anesthetic binding, what the attributes of an optimal anesthetic binding site are, and finally, how the occupancy of these pockets, patches, or cavities result in the subtle alteration to protein conformation and dynamics that confound their function and ultimately produce the behavioral response that we term "anesthesia." One reasonable (but generic) hypothesis at this point would be that occupancy of protein cavities, formed by folding or interfacial (protein-protein or lipid-protein) contacts, increases van der Waals contacts and electrostatic attractions, thereby stabilizing the target and preventing or slowing the dynamics necessary for function. Implicit in this hypothesis is that the average protein structure may be altered little by anesthetic binding, and thus testing will require a multifaceted approach that crosses traditional disciplinary lines.

REFERENCES

1. Abadji VC, Raines DE, Watts A, Miller KW. The effect of general anesthetics on the dynamics of phosphatidylcholine-acetylcholine receptor interactions in reconstituted vesicles. *Biochim Biophys Acta* 1993;1147:143–153.
2. Abadji VC, Raines DE, Dalton LA, Miller KW. Lipid-protein interactions and protein dynamics in vesicles containing the nicotinic acetylcholine receptor: a study with ethanol. *Biochim Biophys Acta* 1994;1194:25–34.
3. Abraham MH, Whiting GS, Fuchs R, Chambers EJ. Thermodynamics of solute transfer from water to hexadecane. *J Chem Soc Perkin Trans* 1990;2:291–300.

4. Abraham MH, Lieb WR, Franks NP. Role of hydrogen bonding in general anesthesia. *J Pharm Sci* 1991;80:719–724.
5. Abraham MH. Scales of solute hydrogen-bonding: their construction and application to physicochemical and biochemical processes. *Chem Soc Rev* 1993;22:73–83.
6. Adey G, Wardley-Smith B, White D. Mechanism of inhibition of bacterial luciferase by anaesthetics. *Life Sci* 1975;17:1849–1854.
7. Barker RW, Brown FF, Drake R, Halsey MJ, Richards RE. Nuclear magnetic resonance studies of anaesthetic interactions with haemoglobin. *Br J Anaesth* 1975;47:25–29.
8. Bernard CM. *Leçons sur les anesthésiques et sur l'asphyxie.* Paris: Libraire J.-B. Ballière et Fils, 1875.
9. Brockerhoff H, Brockerhoff S, Box LL. Mechanism of anesthesia: the potency of four derivatives of octane corresponds to their hydrogen bonding capacity. *Lipids* 1986;21:405–408.
10. Brown FF, Halsey MJ, Richards RE. Halothane interactions with haemoglobin. *Proc R Soc Lond B* 1976;193:387–411.
11. Brown JM, Chaloner PA. Strong amide-halothane hydrogen-bonding observed by nuclear magnetic resonance. *Can J Chem* 1977;55: 3380–3383.
12. Büch HP, Altmeyer P, Büch U. Thiopental binding to human serum albumin in the presence of halothane. *Acta Anaesthesiol Scand* 1990;34:35–40.
13. Buchet R, Sandorfy C, Trapane TL, Urry DW. Infrared spectroscopic studies on gramicidin ion channels: relation to the mechanisms of anesthesia. *Biochim Biophys Acta* 1985;821:8–16.
14. Burley SK, Petsko GA. Weakly polar interactions in proteins. *Adv Protein Chem* 1988;39:125–189.
15. Calvo R, Aguilera L, Suárez E, Rodriguez-Sasiaín JM. Displacement of warfarin from human serum albumin by halothane anaesthesia. *Acta Anaesthesiol Scand* 1989;33:575–577.
16. Carter DC, Ho JX. Structure of serum albumin. *Adv Protein Chem* 1994;45:153–203.
17. Chiou J-S, Tatara T, Sawamura S, Kaminoh Y, Kamaya H, Shibata A, Ueda I. The α-helix to β-sheet transition in poly (L-lysine): effects of anesthetics and high pressure. *Biochim Biophys Acta* 1992; 1119:211–217.
18. Chiou J-S, Ueda I. Ethanol unfolds firefly luciferase while competitive inhibitors antagonize unfolding: DSC and FTIR analyses. *J Pharm Biomed Analysis* 1994;12:969–975.
19. Chiu W. What does electron cryomicroscopy provide that X-ray crystallography and NMR spectroscopy cannot? *Annu Rev Biophys Biomol Struct* 1993;22:233–255.
20. Clore GM, Gronenborn AM. Two-, three-, and four-dimensional NMR methods for obtaining larger and more precise three-dimensional structures of proteins in solution. *Annu Rev Biophys Biophys Chem* 1991;20:29–63.
21. Cobb CE, Juliao S, Balasubramanian K, Staros JV, Beth AH. Effects of diethyl ether on membrane lipid ordering and on rotational dynamics of the anion exchange protein in intact human erythrocytes: correlations with anion exchange function. *Biochemistry* 1990;29:10799–10806.
22. Cooper JR, Bloom FE, Roth RH. *The biochemical basis of neuropharmacology,* 4th ed. New York: Oxford University Press, 1982;73.
23. Curatola G, Lenaz G, Zolese G. Anesthetic-membrane interactions: effects on membrane structure and function. In: Aloia RC, Curtain CC, Gordon LM, eds. *Drug and anesthetic effects on membrane structure and function.* New York: Wiley-Liss, 1991;35–70.
24. Daggett V, Levitt M. Realistic simulations of native-protein dynamics in solution and beyond. *Annu Rev Biophys Biomol Struct* 1993;22: 353–380.
25. Deisenhofer J, Michel H. High-resolution structures of photosynthetic reaction centers. *Annu Rev Biophys Biophys Chem* 1991;20: 247–266.
26. Dickinson R, Franks NP, Lieb WR. Thermodynamics of anesthetic/protein interactions. *Biophys J* 1993;64:1264–1271.
27. Dickinson R, Franks NP, Lieb WR. Can the stereoselective effects of the anesthetic isoflurane be accounted for by lipid solubility? *Biophys J* 1994;66:2019–2023.
28. DiPaolo T, Sandorfy C. Hydrogen bond breaking potency of fluorocarbon anesthetics. *J Med Chem* 1974;17:809–814.
29. DiPaolo T, Sandorfy C. Fluorocarbon anaesthetics break hydrogen bonds. *Nature* 1974;252:471–472.
30. Dong A, Huang P, Zhao XJ, Sampath V, Caughey WS. Characterization of sites occupied by the anesthetic nitrous oxide within proteins by infrared spectroscopy. *J Biol Chem* 1994;269:23911–23917.
31. Dorset DL. Structural electron crystallography. New York: *Plenum Press,* 1995;405–427.
32. Dubois BW, Evers AS. ^{19}F-NMR spin-spin relaxation (T_2) method for characterizing anesthetic binding to proteins: analysis of isoflurane binding to albumin. *Biochemistry* 1992;31:7069–7076.
33. Dubois BW, Cherian SF, Evers AS. Volatile anesthetics compete for common binding sites on bovine serum albumin: a ^{19}F-NMR study. *Proc Natl Acad Sci USA* 1993;90:6478–6482.
34. Eckenhoff RG, Shuman H. Halothane binding to soluble proteins determined by photoaffinity labeling. *Anesthesiology* 1993;79:96–106.
35. Eckenhoff RG, Fagan D. Inhalation anaesthetic competition at high-affinity cocaine binding sites in rat brain synaptosomes. *Br J Anaesth* 1994;73:820–825.
36. Eckenhoff RG. An inhalational anesthetic binding domain in the nicotinic acetylcholine receptor. *Proc Natl Acad Sci USA* 1996; 93:2807–2810.
37. Eftink MR. Fluorescence quenching: theory and applications. In: Lakowicz JR, eds. Topics in fluorescence spectroscopy, vol 2: principles. New York: *Plenum Press,* 1991;53–126.
38. Eger EI, Liu J, Koblin DD, Laster MJ, Taheri S, Halsey MJ, Ionescu P, Chortkoff BS, Hudlicky T. Molecular properties of the "ideal" inhaled anesthetic: studies of fluorinated methanes, ethanes, propanes, and butanes. *Anesth Analg* 1994;79:245–251.
39. Eisenberg D, Hill CP. Protein crystallography: more surprises ahead. *TIBS* 1989;14:260–264.
40. El-Maghrabi EA, Eckenhoff RG, Shuman H. Saturable binding of halothane to rat brain synaptosomes. *Proc Natl Acad Sci USA* 1992; 89:4329–4332.
41. El-Maghrabi EA, Eckenhoff RG. Inhibition of dopamine transport in rat brain synaptosomes by volatile anesthetics. *Anesthesiology* 1993;78:750–756.
42. Evers AS, Dubois BW, Burris KE. Saturable binding of volatile anesthetics to proteins studied by ^{19}F-NMR spectroscopy and photoaffinity labeling. *Prog Anesth Mechanism* 1995;3:151–157.
43. Ewing GJ, Maestas S. The thermodynamics of absorption of xenon by myoglobin. *J Physiol Chem* 1970;74:2341–2344.
44. Ferguson J. The use of chemical potentials as indices of toxicity. *Proc R Soc Lond B* 1939;127:387–404.
45. Fersht AR, Shi J-P, Knill-Jones J, Lowe DM, Wilkinson AJ, Blow DM, Brick P, Carter P, Waye MMY, Winter G. Hydrogen bonding and biological specificity analysed by protein engineering. *Nature* 1985;314:235–238.
46. Firestone LL, Alifimoff JK, Miller KW. Does general anesthetic-induced desensitization of the *Torpedo* acetylcholine receptor correlate with lipid disordering? *Mol Pharmacol* 1994;46:508–515.
47. Franks NP, Lieb WR. Where do general anesthetics act? *Nature* 1978;274:339–342.
48. Franks NP, Lieb WR. Do general anaesthetics act by competitive binding to specific receptors? *Nature* 1984;310:599–601.
49. Franks NP, Lieb WR. Stereospecific effects of inhalational general anesthetic optical isomers on nerve ion channels. *Science* 1991; 254:427–430.
50. Franks NP, Lieb WR. Selective actions of volatile general anaesthetics at molecular and cellular levels. *Br J Anaesth* 1993;71:65–76.
51. Franks NP, Lieb WR. Molecular and cellular mechanisms of general anaesthesia. *Nature* 1994;367:607–614.
52. Fraser DM, Louro SRW, Horváth LI, Miller KW, Watts A. A study of the effect of general anesthetics on lipid-protein interactions in acetylcholine receptor enriched membranes from *Torpedo nobiliana* using nitroxide spin-labels. *Biochemistry* 1990;29:2664–2669.
53. Gandolfi AJ, White RD, Sipes IG, Pohl LR. Bioactivation and covalent binding of halothane *in vitro:* studies with [^{3}H]- and [^{14}C]halothane. *J Pharmacol Exp Ther* 1980;214:721–725.
54. Gorga JC, Hazzard JH, Caughey WS. Determination of anesthetic molecule environments by infrared spectroscopy. *Arch Biochem Biophys* 1985;240:734–746.
55. Gursky O, Fontano E, Bhyravbhatla B, Caspar DLD. Stereospecific dihaloalkane binding in a pH-sensitive cavity in cubic insulin crystals. *Proc Natl Acad Sci USA* 1994;91:12388–12392.
56. Gutfreund H. Reflections on the kinetics of substrate binding. *Biophys Chem* 1987;26:117–121.
57. Halsey MJ. Molecular interactions of anaesthetics with biological membranes. *Gen Pharmacol* 1992;23:1013–1016.
58. Hansch C, Vittoria A, Silipo C, Jow PYC. Partition coefficients and the structure-activity relationship of the anesthetic gases. *J Med Chem* 1975;18:546–548.

59. Harris B, Moody E, Skolnick P. Isoflurane anesthesia is stereoselective. *Eur J Pharmacol* 1992;217:215–216.
60. Harris JW, Jones JP, Martin JL, LaRosa AC, Olson MJ, Pohl LR, Anders MW. Pentahaloethane-based chlorofluorocarbon substitutes and halothane: correlation of in vivo hepatic protein trifluoroacetylation and urinary trifluoroacetic acid excretion with calculated enthalpies of activation. *Chem Res Toxicol* 1992;5: 720–725.
61. Harris RA, Mihic SJ, Dildy-Mayfield JE, Machu TK. Actions of anesthetics on ligand-gated ion channels: role of receptor subunit composition. *FASEB J* 1995;9:1454–1462.
62. Harvey EN. The effect of certain organic and inorganic substances upon light production by luminous bacteria. *Biol Bull* 1915;29:308–311.
63. Hazzard JH, Gorga JC, Caughey WS. Determination of anesthetic molecule environments by infrared spectroscopy. *Arch Biochem Biophys* 1985;240:747–756.
64. He XM, Carter DC. Atomic structure and chemistry of human serum albumin. *Nature* 1992;358:209–215.
65. Henderson R, Baldwin JM, Ceska TA, Zemlin F, Beckmann E, Downing KH. Model of the structure of bacteriorhodopsin based on high-resolution electron cryomicroscopy. *J Mol Biol* 1990;213: 899–929.
66. Hinkley RE. Microtubule-macrotubule transformation induced by volatile anesthetics. *J Ultrastruct Res* 1976;57:237–250.
67. Hubbard SJ, Argos P. Cavities and packing at protein interfaces. *Protein Sci* 1994;3:2194–2206.
68. Hubbard SJ, Gross K-H, Argos P. Intramolecular cavities in globular proteins. *Protein Eng* 1994;7:613–626.
69. Iwata S, Ostermeier C, Ludwig B, Michel H. Structure at 2.8 Å resolution of cytochrome C oxidase from *Paracoccus denitrificans*. *Nature* 1995;376:660–669.
70. Jakoby MG, Covey DF, Cistola DP. Localization of tolbutamide binding sites on human serum albumin using titration calorimetry and heteronuclear 2-D NMR. *Biochemistry* 1995;34:8780–8787.
71. Jameson DM, Sawyer WH. Fluorescence anisotropy applied to biomolecular interactions. *Methods Enzymol* 1995;246:283–300.
72. Johansson JS, Eckenhoff RG, Dutton PL. Binding of halothane to serum albumin demonstrated using tryptophan fluorescence. *Anesthesiology* 1995;83:316–324.
73. Johansson JS, Rabanal F, Dutton PL. Halothane binds to the hydrophobic interior of a four-helix bundle protein. *Anesthesiology* 1995;83:A1258.
74. Johansson JS, Eckenhoff RG. Minimum structural requirement for an inhalational anesthetic binding site on a protein target. *Biochim Biophys Acta* 1996;1290:63–68.
75. Johnson KM, Bergmann JS, Kozikowski AP. Cocaine and dopamine differentially protect [^{3}H] mazindol binding sites from alkylation by N-ethylmaleimide. *Eur J Pharmacol* 1992;227: 411–415.
76. Jørgensen K, Ipsen JH, Mouritsen OG, Zuckermann MJ. The effect of anaesthetics on the dynamic heterogeneity of lipid membranes. *Chem Phys Lipids* 1993;65:205–216.
77. Kleywegt GJ, Jones TA. Where freedom is given, liberties are taken. *Structure* 1995;3:535–540.
78. Kosk-Kosicka D. Plasma membrane Ca^{2+}-ATPase as a target for volatile anesthetics. *Adv Pharmacol* 1994;31:313–322.
79. Kossiakoff AA. The application of neutron crystallography to the study of dynamic and hydration properties of proteins. *Annu Rev Biochem* 1985;54:1195–1227.
80. Levitt M, Perutz MF. Aromatic rings act as hydrogen bond acceptors. *J Mol Biol* 1988;201:751–754.
81. Likhtenshtein GI. *Biophysical labeling methods in molecular biology.* Cambridge: Cambridge University Press, 1993;1–44.
82. Lim WA, Hodel A, Sauer RT, Richards FM. The crystal *structure* of a mutant protein with altered but improved hydrophobic core packing. *Proc Natl Acad Sci USA* 1994;91:423–427.
83. Lind RC, Gandolfi AJ. Concentration-dependent inhibition of halothane biotransformation in the guinea pig. *Drug Metab Dispos* 1993;21:386–389.
84. Lysko GS, Robinson JL, Casto R, Ferrone RA. The stereospecific effects of isoflurane isomers in vivo. *Eur J Pharmacol* 1994;263: 25–29.
85. Martin DC, Adams RJ, Introna RPSI. Halothane inhibits 5-hydroxytryptamine uptake by synaptosomes from rat brain. *Neuropharmacology* 1990;29:9–16.
86. Martin DC, Introna RP, Aronstam RS. Inhibition of neuronal 5-HT uptake by ketamine, but not halothane, involves disruption of substrate recognition by the transporter. *Neurosci Lett* 1990;112: 99–103.
87. Martin JL, Meinwald J, Radford P, Liu Z, Graf MLM, Pohl LR. Stereoselective metabolism of halothane enantiomers to trifluoroacetylated liver proteins. *Drug Metab Rev* 1995;27:179–189.
88. Martire DE, Sheridan JP, King JW, O'Donnell. Thermodynamics of molecular association. 9. An NMR study of hydrogen bonding of $CHCl_3$ and $CHBr_3$ in Di-*n*-octyl ether, Di-*n*-octyl thioether, and Di-*n*-octylmethylamine. *J Am Chem Soc* 1976;98:3101–3106.
89. McDonagh AF, Pu YM, Lightner DA. Effect of volatile anesthetics on the circular dichroism of bilirubin bound to human serum albumin. *Experientia* 1992;48:246–248.
90. Miles JL, Morey E, Crain F, Gross S, San Julian J, Canady WJ. Inhibition of α-chymotrypsin by diethyl ether and certain alcohols: a new type of competitive inhibition. *J Biol Chem* 1962;237: 1319–1322.
91. Miller KW, Paton WDM, Smith EB, Smith RA. Physicochemical approaches to the mode of action of general anesthetics. *Anesthesiology* 1972;36:339–351.
92. Miller KW. Molecular mechanisms by which general anaesthetics act. In: Feldman SA, Paton W, Scurr C, eds. *Mechanisms of drugs in anaesthesia.* Boston: Hodder & Stoughton, 1993;191–200.
93. Millhauser GL, Fiori WR, Miick SM. Electron spin labels. *Methods Enzymol* 1995;246:589–610.
94. Moody EJ, Harris BD, Skolnick P. Stereospecific actions of the inhalation anesthetic isoflurane at the $GABA_A$ receptor complex. *Brain Res* 1993;615:101–106, 1993.
95. Moore B, Roaf HE. On certain physical and chemical properties of solutions of chloroform in water, saline, serum, and haemoglobin. A contribution to the chemistry of anaesthesia. *Proc R Soc Lond* 1904;73:382–412.
96. Moore B, Roaf HE. On certain physical and chemical properties of solutions of chloroform and other anaesthetics. A contribution to the chemistry of anaesthesia. *Proc R Soc Lond* 1905;B77: 86–102.
97. Muller N. Search for a realistic view of hydrophobic effects. *Acc Chem Res* 1990;23:23–28.
98. Nakagawa T, Hamanaka T, Nishimura S, Uruga T, Kito Y. The specific binding site of the volatile anesthetic diiodomethane to purple membrane by X-ray diffraction. *J Mol Biol* 1994;238:297–301.
99. Nunes AC, Schoenborn BP. Dichloromethane and myoglobin function. *Mol Pharmacol* 1973;9:835–839.
100. Östergren G. Colchicine mitosis, chromosome contraction, narcosis and protein chain folding. *Hereditas* 1944;30:429–467.
101. Pai EF, Sachsenheimer W, Schirmer RH, Schulz GE. Substrate positions and induced-fit in crystalline adenylate kinase. *J Mol Biol* 1977;114:37–45.
102. Pfeiffer CC. Optical isomerism and pharmacological action, a generalization. *Science* 1956;124:29–31.
103. Pocock G, Richards CD. Cellular mechanisms in general anaesthesia. *Br J Anaesth* 1991;66:116–128.
104. Privalov PL, Gill SJ. Stability of protein *structure* and hydrophobic interaction. *Adv Protein Chem* 1988;39:191–234.
105. Privalov PL, Gill SJ. The hydrophobic effect: a reappraisal. *Pure Appl Chem* 1989;61:1097–1104.
106. Quinlan JJ, Firestone S, Firestone LL. Isoflurane's enhancement of chloride flux through rat brain γ-aminobutyric acid type A receptors is stereoselective. *Anesthesiology* 1995;83:611–615.
107. Raffa RB, Porreca F. Thermodynamic analysis of the drug-receptor interaction. *Life Sci* 1989;44:245–258.
108. Rashin AA, Iofin M, Honig B. Internal cavities and buried waters in globular proteins. *Biochemistry* 1986;25:3619–3625.
109. Richards FM. Areas, volumes, packing, and protein structure. *Annu Rev Biophys Bioeng* 1977;6:151–176.
110. Richards FM, Lim WA. An analysis of packing in the protein folding problem. *Q Rev Biophys* 1994;26:423–498.
111. Rose GD, Wolfenden R. Hydrogen bonding, hydrophobicity, packing, and protein folding. *Annu Rev Biophys Biomol Struct* 1993; 22:381–415.
112. Sachsenheimer W, Pai EF, Schulz GE, Schirmer RH. Halothane binds in the adenine-specific niche of crystalline adenylate kinase. *FEBS Lett* 1977;79:310–312.
113. Schoenborn BP. Binding of xenon to horse haemoglobin. *Nature* 1965;208:760–762.

114. Schoenborn BP, Watson HC, Kendrew JC. Binding of xenon to sperm whale myoglobin. *Nature* 1965;207:28–30.
115. Schoenborn BP. Binding of cyclopropane to sperm whale myoglobin. *Nature* 1967;214:1120–1122.
116. Schoenborn BP. Dichloromethane as an antisickling agent in sickle cell hemoglobin. *Proc Natl Acad Sci USA* 1976;73:4195–4199.
117. Sedensky MM, Cascorbi HF, Meinwald J, Radford P, Morgan PG. Genetic differences affecting the potency of stereoisomers of halothane. *Proc Natl Acad Sci USA* 1994;91:10054–10058.
118. Shibata A, Morita K, Yamashita T, Kamaya H, Ueda I. Anesthetic-protein interaction: effects of volatile anesthetics on the secondary structure of poly (L-lysine). *J Pharm Sci* 1991;80:1037–1041.
119. Shirley BA, Stanssens P, Hahn U, Pace CN. Contribution of hydrogen bonding to the conformational stability of ribonuclease T1. *Biochemistry* 1992;31:725–732.
120. Singer SJ, Nicolson GL. The fluid mosaic model of the structure of cell membranes. *Science* 1972;175:720–731.
121. Sklar LA. Real-time spectroscopic analysis of ligand-receptor dynamics. *Annu Rev Biophys Biophys Chem* 1987;16:479–506.
122. Smith RA, Porter EG, Miller KW. The solubility of anesthetic gases in lipid bilayers. *Biochim Biophys Acta* 1981;645:327–338.
123. Taheri S, Halsey MJ, Liu J, Eger EI, Koblin DD, Laster MJ. What solvent best represents the site of action of inhaled anesthetics in humans, rats, and dogs? *Anesth Analg* 1991;72:627–634.
124. Tanford C. *The hydrophobic effect: formation of micelles and biological membranes.* New York: John Wiley, 1973.
125. Targ AG, Yasuda N, Eger EI, Huang G, Vernice GG, Terrell RC, Koblin DD. Halogenation and anesthetic potency. *Anesth Analg* 1989;68:599–602.
126. Testa B, Jenner P, Kilpatrick GJ, El Tayar N, van de Waterbeemd H, Marsden CD. Do thermodynamic studies provide information on both the binding to and the activation of dopaminergic and other receptors? *Biochem Pharmacol* 1987;36:4041–4046.
127. Tilton RF, Kuntz ID, Petsko GA. Cavities in proteins: structure of a metmyoglobin-xenon complex solved to 1.9 Å. *Biochemistry* 1984; 23:2849–2857.
128. Tilton RF, Singh UC, Kuntz ID, Kollman PA. Protein-ligand dynamics. A 96 picosecond simulation of a myoglobin-xenon complex. *J Mol Biol* 1988;199:195–211.
129. Trudell JR, Hubbell WL. Localization of molecular halothane in phospholipid bilayer model nerve membranes. *Anesthesiology* 1976; 44:202–205.
130. Ueda I, Kamaya H. Kinetic and thermodynamic aspects of the mechanism of general anesthesia in a model system of firefly luminescence *in vitro*. *Anesthesiology* 1973;38:425–436.
131. Ueda I. Interfacial effects of anesthetics on membrane fluidity. In: Aloia RC, Curtain CC, Gordon LM, eds. *Drug and anesthetic effects on membrane structure and function.* New York: Wiley-Liss, 1991;15–33.
132. Unwin N. Acetylcholine receptor channel imaged in the open state. *Nature* 1995;373:37–43.
133. Urbanova M, Dukor RK, Pancoska P, Gupta VP, Keiderling TA. Comparison of α-lactalbumin and lysozyme using vibrational circular dichroism. Evidence for a difference in crystal and solution *structures*. *Biochemistry* 1991;30:10479–10485.
134. Vanderkooi JM, Landesberg R, Selick H, McDonald GG. Interaction of general anesthetics with phospholipid vesicles and biological membranes. *Biochim Biophys Acta* 1977;464:1–16.
135. Verschueren KHG, Seljée F, Rozeboom HJ, Kalk KH, Dijkstra BW. Crystallographic analysis of the catalytic mechanism of haloalkane dehalogenase. *Nature* 1993;363:693–698.
136. Viguera AR, Serrano L. Side-chain interactions between sulfur-containing amino acids and phenylalanine in α-helices. *Biochemistry* 1995;34:8771–8779.
137. Weiskopf RB, Nishimura M, Severinghaus JW. The absence of an effect of halothane on blood hemoglobin O_2 equilibrium *in vitro*. *Anesthesiology* 1971;35:579–581.
138. White SH, King GI, Cain JE. Location of hexane in lipid bilayers determined by neutron diffraction. *Nature* 1981;290:161–163.
139. Wyrwicz AM, Li Y, Scofield JC, Burt CT. Multiple environments of fluorinated anesthetics in intact tissues observed with ^{19}F-NMR spectroscopy. *FEBS Lett* 1983;162:334–338.
140. Wyrwicz AM, Pszenny MH, Schofield JC, Tillman PC, Gordon RE, Martin PA. Noninvasive observations of fluorinated anesthetics in rabbit brain by fluorine 19 nuclear magnetic resonance. *Science* 1983;222:428–430.
141. Xu Y, Tang P, Zhang W, Firestone L, Winter P. ^{19}F-NMR imaging and spectroscopy of sevoflurane uptake, distribution, and elimination in rat brain. *Anesthesiology* 1995;83:766–774.

Anesthesia: Biologic Foundations, edited by
Tony L. Yaksh et al. Lippincott–Raven Publishers,
Philadelphia © 1997.

CHAPTER 3

BASIC CONCEPTS OF MOLECULAR BIOLOGY

MARCEL E. DURIEUX AND DEBRA A. SCHWINN

As will be obvious to anyone who follows the biomedical literature, an ever increasing fraction of the new information in the biologic sciences derives from the application of molecular biology techniques. To a large extent this is a result of the shift in application of these techniques from the interesting, but relatively narrow, field of gene cloning, to a wide range of approaches used to probe a variety of cellular processes, including gene function, expression, and regulation, as well as protein function. While, therefore, much molecular biology work performed currently attempts to answer questions not primarily related to the genome (questions such as determining the presence of a specific receptor in a specific cell type or defining the catalytic site of an enzyme), our understanding of gene structure and function has also expanded considerably with the application of these techniques. Not only do we understand the information flow from DNA to RNA to protein in much greater detail than ever before, but completely new areas of study have developed, molecular evolution being an example.

This chapter provides a brief introduction to basic molecular biology concepts. We cover primarily the conceptual background necessary for understanding the techniques of molecular biology described in Chapter 22, placing particular emphasis on the regulation of the genetic system. To place this information in practical perspective, we provide brief overviews of some ways in which our knowledge of the genome and its functioning can be put to clinical use.

THE BUILDING BLOCKS

This section summarizes briefly the essential molecular biology of the genome and its expression: the flow of information from DNA to RNA to protein. For readers interested in a more in-depth description of our current understanding of this complex information-processing system, several excellent standard texts on this subject are available (1,3).

DNA

The business of the genome is information management. The massive amounts of information encoding the building instructions for all proteins needed by all cells in the body during all of the stages of life must be stored compactly, yet be easily accessible, and must not only be copied faithfully during the innumerable cell divisions that take place in the organism between conception and death, but also passed on to subsequent generations. The task of acting as the mass storage medium for our genetic database has been assigned to the nucleic acid DNA (deoxyribonucleic acid). Thus, each normal human diploid cell holds two copies of each of 24 chromosomes, each chromosome consisting of a single, huge DNA molecule packaged in a covering of histone proteins.

DNA exists in long strands of alternating sugar residues (deoxyribose) linked together by phosphodiester bonds (Fig. 1A). As the phosphate moiety links the 3′ carbon atom of one sugar to the 5′ carbon of the next, the sugar-phosphate backbone is polar: one end of the molecule has a free 3′ hydrogen (the 3′ end), whereas the other end has a phosphorylated 5′ carbon (the 5′ end). Attached to each sugar residue is a base (see Fig. 1B), which is either a purine (adenine, A, or guanine, G) or a pyrimidine (cytosine, C, or thymine, T). Base and sugar together form a nucleotide. In the mature DNA molecule two of these strands are wound together in an antiparallel fashion (i.e., with one strand running 5′ to 3′ and the other 3′ to 5′) to form a double helix (Fig. 2). As Watson and Crick surmised correctly in 1953, in such a DNA helix the sugar-phosphate backbone is located on the outside, and the bases point inward, with bases from each strand pairing in an exact complementary fashion: each A pairs with a T, with two hydrogen bonds, and each C pairs with a G, with three hydrogen bonds (Fig. 1B).

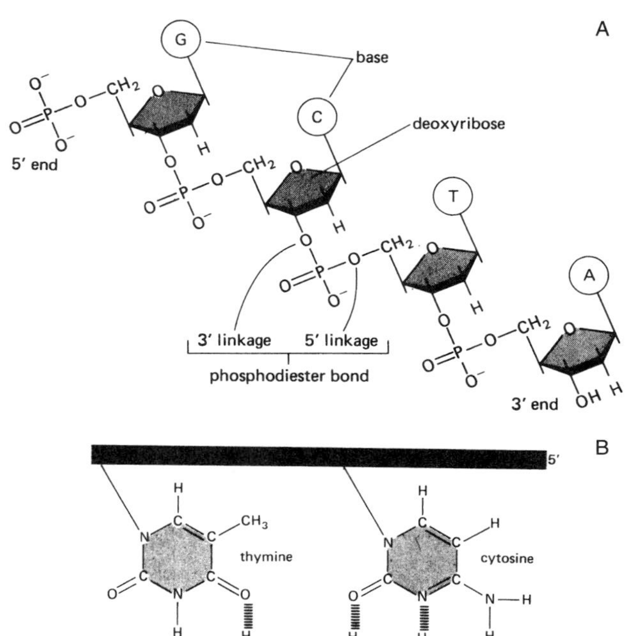

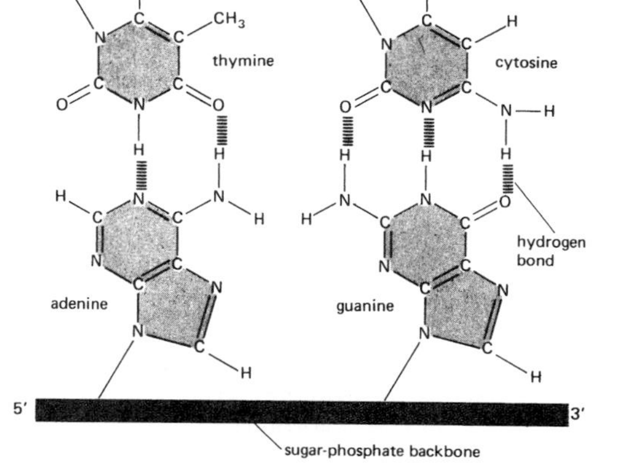

Figure 1. Molecular structure of DNA. **A:** The sugar-phosphate backbone of a DNA molecule. Deoxyribose groups are linked together through phosphodiester bonds, forming the backbone, whereas bases (G, C, T, A) attached to the sugar carry the genetic information. As the phosphodiester bond is asymmetrical, each DNA molecule has polarity: one end (the 5′ end) carries a free phosphate group, whereas the other end (the 3′ end) carries a free hydroxyl group on the sugar. **B:** Bases in DNA. Four bases carry the genetic information in DNA: the purines adenine and guanine, and the pyrimidines cytosine and thymine. During base pairing, a purine always pairs with a pyrimidine and vice versa. Base pairs are held together by hydrogen bonds. Thus, there are no covalent links between the two strands of a DNA molecule. AT pairs have two hydrogen bonds and GC pairs three, making the latter base pair stronger.

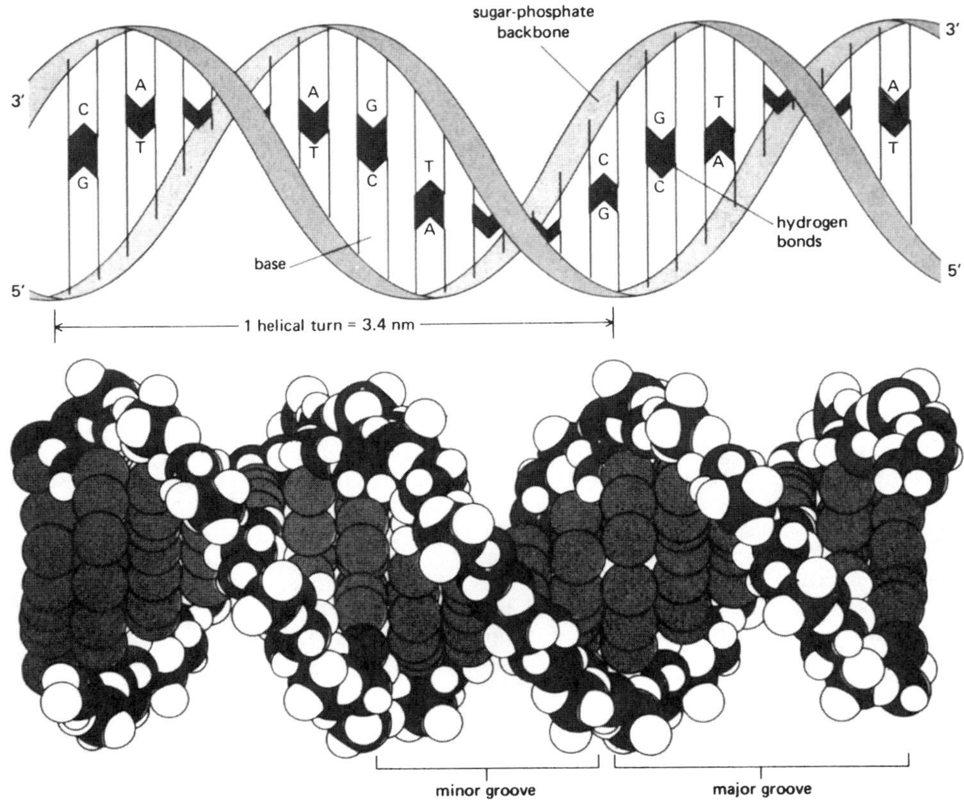

Figure 2. The double helix. *Top:* diagrammatic representation. *Bottom:* space-filling model. The double-stranded DNA molecule is twisted into a right-handed helix, making one turn every 3.4 nm. The sugar-phosphate backbone occupies the outside of the helix, and the bases are located on the inside. This topography results in the presence of two grooves, the major and the minor, running along the helix. The presence of these grooves is of importance to allow proteins access to the bases inside the helix.

The strict base-pairing means that the two strands hold essentially the same information. However, in each protein-coding region of DNA only the information on one of the two strands, the sense strand, can be translated into protein. The complementary strand is named the antisense strand. Each strand can act as a template for the construction of the other, and this mechanism is of the utmost importance for the accurate replication of DNA during cell division. During DNA replication the two strands are separated by breaking the hydrogen bonds between the bases, and a complex polyenzyme, DNA polymerase, assembles a new complementary strand on each of the old single strands (Fig. 3), beginning at an area called the origin of replication and advancing along the chromosome. It is important to realize that only double-stranded DNA can serve as a template for this enzyme. Built into the polymerase is an error correction function that proofreads newly incorporated nucleotides and minimizes the error rate to a remarkably low 10^{-9}: a single error in each billion replicated base pairs. As the human genome consists of 3×10^9 base pairs, complete duplication of chromosomal material in a cell would result in only three misincorporated bases. The efficacy of storage of information in DNA is extremely high. An average mammalian genome of 6×10^9 base pairs can be packed in a cube 1.9 μm on each side. In contrast, a book containing 6×10^9 letters would be more than a million pages in length (1).

RNA

Although DNA is our current genetic storage medium, it was not always the genetic material on this earth. Current understanding of the development of life on the planet assumes that the first life forms, which developed about four billion years ago, consisted of the nucleic acid RNA (ribonucleic acid) only. RNA is different from DNA in two ways: (a) the sugar moiety is ribose, rather than deoxyribose, and (b) the base uracil (U, see Fig. 4) substitutes for T. RNA is found generally as a single-stranded molecule, although complementary regions in a single RNA strand can fold back on themselves and base pair. As a primordial life form RNA acted not only as a storage medium for genetic information, but also as a catalyst directing its own

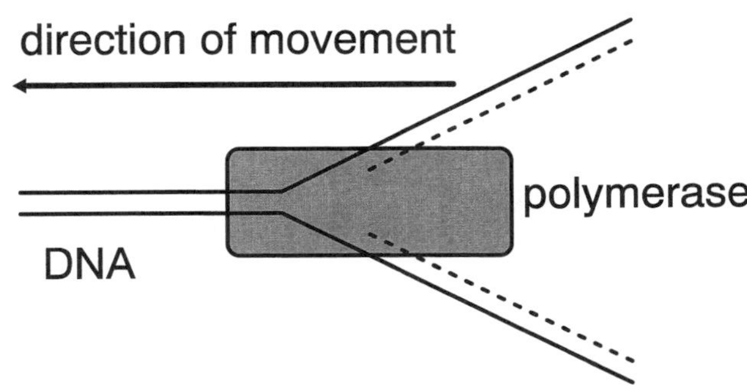

Figure 3. DNA replication. To replicate DNA, the helix must be untwisted and the two strands must be separated. Each strand is then used as a template for the construction of a complementary one. This highly simplified picture shows the DNA polymerase complex, which performs all these functions, moving along a DNA molecule, leaving behind it the duplicated DNA.

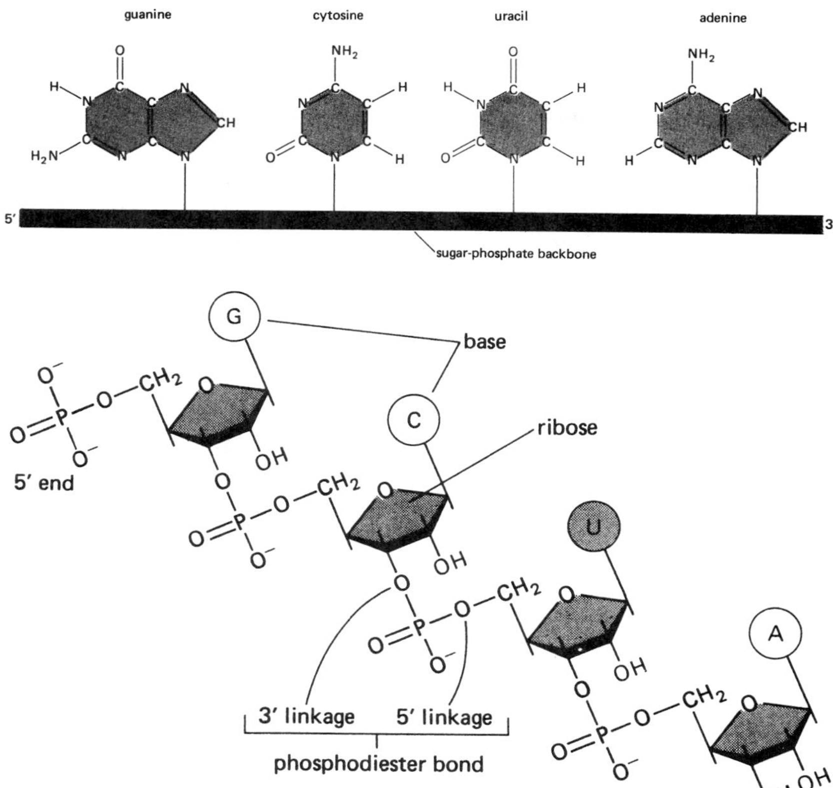

Figure 4. Molecular structure of RNA. **A:** The sugar-phosphate backbone of RNA is different from that of DNA in that the sugar ribose, rather than deoxyribose, is present. The extra hydroxyl group makes RNA a less stable molecule. **B:** The bases of RNA. In RNA molecules, the pyrimidine uracil replaces thymidine.

replication. No separate polymerase was involved, and this RNA therefore was a self-replicating unit. Once this ability for self-replication existed, natural selection could begin to play its role. Although RNA can thus act as an "enzyme" (some RNA molecules in present-day organisms still act in a catalytic role, e.g., by cutting pieces out of themselves, and, as noted in the section on antisense therapy, ribozymes are considered as a novel form of gene therapy), it was only with the much more versatile polypeptides that modern cells could develop. The first polypeptides must have been assembled by RNA catalysts using RNA templates, and, indeed, the high RNA content of ribosomes, the organelles where proteins are constructed, is a remnant of this original translation system. As cells developed, RNA yielded its role as a storage medium to DNA, which is less susceptible to hydrolysis due to the absence of a hydroxyl group at the 2′ position. The molecule that began life has retained only a few specialized positions in protein synthesis. It acts as a constituent of ribosomes (ribosomal RNA or rRNA) and spliceosomes (see below), as the molecule carrying a selected piece of genomic information to the ribosomes for translation into protein (messenger RNA or mRNA), and as an adapter bringing in amino acids from the cytosol to be linked to a growing amino acid chain (transfer RNA or tRNA).

INFORMATION TRANSFER

Transcription

The process by which a piece of genomic information in the nucleus is selected and copied into RNA for transfer to the cytoplasm and translation into a polypeptide is called DNA transcription. Transcription is performed by multisubunit enzymes called RNA polymerases. In eukaryotes different polymerases exist, one for each of the types of RNA mentioned in the previous section; prokaryotes and viruses (such as the bacteriophages) use only a single type.

The first step of the transcription process is the recognition by RNA polymerase of a specific DNA sequence, just in front of the DNA to be transcribed. This area, the promoter, determines which strand of DNA is to be used as a template for transcription. As DNA can only be transcribed in one direction (5′ to 3′) the promoter determines completely which DNA sequence will be copied. Many promoter sequences have been analyzed as to their ability to bind RNA polymerase, and a consensus sequence has been determined for "strong" promoters (i.e., promoters with high binding ability and resulting high levels of transcribed RNA). In eukaryotes, two short sequences, one so-called TATA box approximately 30 nucleotides, and a GC-rich area and CCAAT sequence 50 to 100 nucleotides upstream from the start of transcription, appear to be essential for effective initiation of transcription.

Once transcription is initiated, the polymerase moves 5′ to 3′ along the DNA. It unwinds temporarily the double helix, and uses one strand as a template for the construction of a single-stranded RNA molecule. Behind, the DNA helix is reformed. This process continues until a transcription stop signal is reached. The stop sequence consists of two short areas of DNA complementary to each other, followed by a run of T residues. Presumably the two resulting complementary regions in the synthesized RNA molecule will fold upon themselves and base pair, leaving only relatively unstable base pairing between the run of T and U to hold the DNA and the newly formed RNA together. This area will then spontaneously come apart, ending transcription. Although the definition has become less clear as we learn more about the function of the genome, the term *gene* has usually been applied to a sequence of DNA encoding a polypeptide, beginning with the promoter and associated regulatory regions, and ending at the transcription stop signal.

RNA Processing

Whereas prokaryotic RNA, synthesized as described, is ready for transfer to ribosomes and translation into protein, eukaryotic RNA undergoes a number of specific modifications before it is transported from the nucleus. First, both the 5′ and the 3′ end of the RNA molecule are altered. At the 5′ end, a methylated guanine nucleotide is linked to the RNA molecule through a triphosphate bridge. This is known as capping, and it is important for the efficient initiation of protein translation. The 3′ end is cleaved 10 to 30 nucleotides upstream (i.e., 5′) from a polyadenylation sequence (AAUAAA), and a string of 100 to 200 A residues is added (Fig. 5). This poly-A tail probably plays a role in preventing degradation of the RNA in the cytoplasm. Still more complex processing is required before the RNA transcript is ready for translation. For reasons unclear, eukaryotic genes frequently contain, within the area that encodes a protein (the coding region), sequences of noncoding DNA (Fig. 5). These areas are called introns, whereas the coding regions are called exons. Introns are removed from the transcribed RNA in a process called splicing, by enzyme complexes called spliceosomes. These consist of both RNA (a remnant of primordial RNA life) and protein, and recognize subtle sequences on the intron-exon boundaries. Frequently, multiple introns have to be removed, and, at times, alternative splicing allows the generation of different mRNAs from a single primary RNA transcript (see below). After processing, the mRNA is coated with small protein and ribonucleoprotein particles that help to package it efficiently, and is subsequently transported out of the nucleus to the cytoplasm. It should be recognized that even after this processing the mRNA still consists of more than just the sequence encoding a protein. Both on the 5′ and on the 3′ side of the protein-coding area are variably large noncoding regions.

PROTEIN EXPRESSION

Translation

Once in the cytoplasm, the mRNA is ready to be translated into a polypeptide chain. For this translation to take place, the four nucleotide types in the RNA must be able to encode the 20 amino acid types used to construct proteins. The coding scheme is a straightforward one, with a group of three nucleotides (a codon) representing a single amino acid. This genetic code (Table 1) is virtually the same for all organisms, indicating that it evolved early in evolution.

The initial step in translation is binding of the mRNA to a ribosome. The 5′ cap, added after RNA transcription, is the recognition site for this initial contact. Next, the ribosome slides along the RNA in a 5′ to 3′ direction until it recognizes

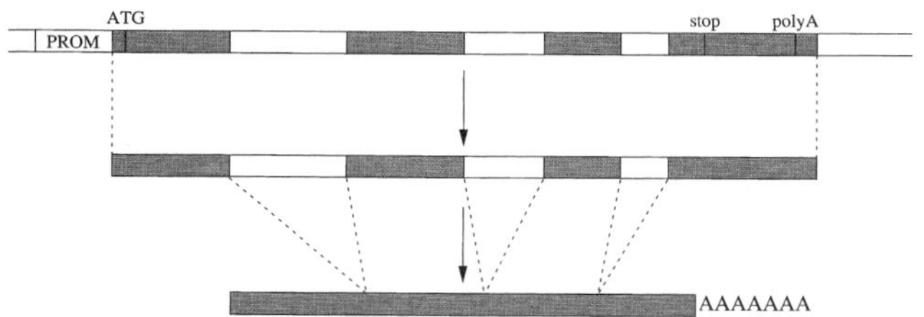

Figure 5. RNA processing. This hypothetical gene contains three exons (coding regions, *dark*) interrupted by two introns (noncoding regions, *light*). In front of the first exon is the promoter region. The start signal for translation (the initiator ATG), however, is downstream of the transcription initiation site. Similarly, the stop codon is followed by noncoding region. A poly-A addition site is present just in front of the transcriptional termination signal. After the primary RNA transcript has been made, it is modified in several ways: introns are removed, the RNA is cleaved at the poly-A addition site, and a poly-A tail is added.

Table 1. THE GENETIC CODE*

	Second position				
First position	**U**	**C**	**A**	**G**	**Third position**
U	Phe	Ser	Tyr	Cys	U
	Phe	Ser	Tyr	Cys	C
	Leu	Ser	Stop	Stop	A
	Leu	Set	Stop	Trp	G
C	Leu	Pro	His	Arg	U
	Leu	Pro	His	Arg	C
	Leu	Pro	Gln	Arg	A
	Leu	Pro	Gln	Arg	G
A	Ile	Thr	Asn	Ser	U
	Ile	Thr	Asn	Ser	C
	Ile	Thr	Lys	Arg	A
	Met	Thr	Lys	Arg	G
G	Val	Ala	Asp	Gly	U
	Val	Ala	Asp	Gly	C
	Val	Ala	Glu	Gly	A
	Val	Ala	Glu	Gly	G

*Each amino acid is encoded by three bases (a codon). Most amino acids are encoded by several codons, i.e., the genetic code is degenerate. Generally, the degeneracy is in the third base of the codon. Note the three elongation termination or stop codons.

the initiation codon (AUG) on the mRNA, at which point translation begins. As AUG encodes a methionine, all newly translated proteins begin with this amino acid. The actual translation of the genetic code is performed by tRNA molecules. These display a triplet of nucleotides (an anticodon) on one side, where it can base pair with complementary sequence on the mRNA, and on the other side bind to a single amino acid of a specific kind, which can then be added to the growing polypeptide chain (Fig. 6). There are tRNAs in the cytoplasm for each of the possible codons in the genetic code. As with DNA replication, the translation process involves several error-correcting mechanisms. Translation ends when a termination codon (stop codon) is reached (Table 1), which leads to release of the polypeptide chain from the ribosome.

Posttranslational Modifications

Most proteins are modified to a greater or lesser extent after their production. Often, the initial methionine is removed. Signal peptides are present on proteins designated for the plasma membrane, and after appropriate folding of the protein these are removed. Further modifications include selective attachment of sugar groups on sections of proteins exposed to the extracellular space (glycosylation) and the attachment of fatty acid moieties that help anchor the proteins in the membrane (e.g., palmytoylation). In addition, covalent disulfide bonds (frequently between two cysteine residues) are formed in some proteins and result in a more rigid conformation, a process that may be important in functionality. Together, such changes in protein structure are referred to as posttranslational modifications.

Protein Structure

The goal of everything we have described thus far about the flow of information from DNA to RNA to protein is, of course, the creation of a protein that is able to perform a specific function in the cell. At this point in our description, however, we are left with a linear chain of amino acids, as yet devoid of function. This level of protein structure is called the primary structure. We now delineate briefly how this polypeptide is organized into successive levels of protein structure. It is indicative of the enormous

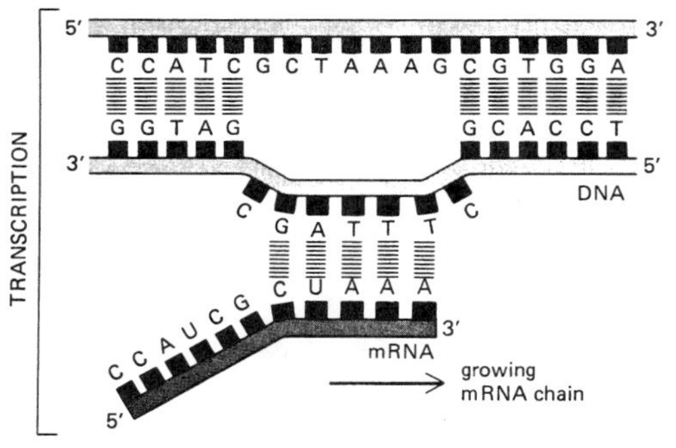

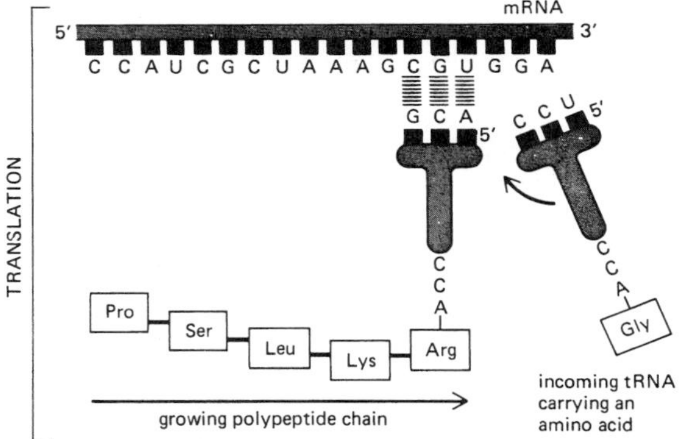

Figure 6. Protein synthesis. A: A nmRNA molecule is transcribed from genomic *DNA*. B: The information in the mRNA is translated into a polypeptide sequence. Each amino acid is encoded by a group of three bases (a codon). Although the construction of polypeptides takes place on ribosomes, the actual translation is performed by a subclass of RNA, named tRNA. A tRNA molecule can carry a specific amino acid on one side, linked to a CCA sequence. On the other side it contains an anti-codon: a three-base sequence complementary with a codon for the specific amino acid carried. Translation consists of sequential matching of tRNA anti-codons to codons on the mRNA, followed by linking together of the amino acids carried by the tRNAs into a polypeptide chain.

step in versatility from nucleotides to amino acids that out of relatively simple linear polypeptide chains the enormous variety of cellular proteins with all their varied functions—from the strength of collagen, to the high ion selectivity of channels, to the myriad catalytic surfaces of enzymes—can be generated. One of the most remarkable features of this whole system is that all the information necessary to convert this string of amino acids to a functional protein is contained in the sequence of the amino acids themselves. The chemical bonds along the polypeptide chain allow a large degree of rotational freedom, and as a result the newly synthesized chain will assume a large number of random conformations. Some of these conformations will be more stable than others and thus will be preferred, and eventually the protein will assume a single, most stable conformation. This conformation is to a large extent determined by the distribution of polar and nonpolar residues. For cytoplasmic proteins, the most stable conformation is that where the polar residues are in contact with the aqueous cell interior, and nonpolar side chains are sequestered in the interior of the protein, where they interact with each other but where water is excluded. The optimal conformation obtained is stabilized by interactions between amino acid side chains, in the form of hydrogen bonds, and sometimes by covalent links such as disulfide bonds between two cysteine residues. The result is a protein folded in a precisely defined conformation, namely the functional one. This level of protein structure is called the secondary structure.

When the secondary structure of many proteins became known, it was obvious that there are recurrent themes in the folding patterns. Two particularly common features are helices and sheets. Protein helices are stabilized by interactions between residues in neighboring turns, and are commonly seen as lipid bilayer-spanning components of membrane proteins, as well as in many other polypeptides. Sheets are often found in the interior of proteins, and are formed by an extended polypeptide chain folding back upon itself, with stabilization accomplished by interaction between neighboring stretches. But recurrent themes occur on higher levels as well. It is now known that many proteins consist of a number of functional domains stitched together. These functional domains themselves show high levels of similarity between various proteins, and current thinking supposes that these domains used to be the original functional units, which later, by duplication and gene recombination, were used in more complex, multidomain proteins with more complex functions.

On an even higher level of organization, many proteins consist of several polypeptide chains held together by noncovalent interactions. An example is the hemoglobin molecule, which is built up of four subunits (two α and two β units in adult hemoglobin) surrounding a central heme moiety. This level of protein organization is called tertiary structure.

REGULATION OF GENE EXPRESSION

Earlier we mentioned promoter strength as one of the determinants controlling whether or not a particular segment of DNA is transcribed and translated into protein. It will be obvious, however, that this is only a very elementary form of control of gene expression, and that much more sophisticated regulatory systems are necessary for proper functioning of cell and organism. Although each cell in the body holds a copy of the full genome, each cell type expresses only its own set of genes—or, stated more exactly, it is a specific cell type only because it expresses a particular set of genes. Complex regulatory systems control this selective gene expression, making possible such differences in structure and function as exist between muscle cells and neurons. But even in a single cell, gene expression is constantly regulated. The levels of enzymes, receptors, and structural elements are continuously adapted to the changing environment. Liver cells that increase their metabolic systems when exposed to drugs such as barbiturates and muscle cells that change the number and type of nicotinic acetylcholine receptors in the absence of nerve stimulation are just two examples. We still have a rather limited understanding of these regulatory mechanisms, but patterns are beginning to emerge. Much progress in our understanding of the functioning of the genome will likely come from new discoveries in the area of the regulation of gene expression. For this reason we provide an overview of the current ideas in this area. Due to space limitations, however, we can review only a few well-studied examples.

Regulatory systems can be divided as to the location of control; most of the regulation of gene expression takes place at the level of transcription, but examples exist for regulation on virtually all levels between DNA and protein.

Transcriptional Regulation

Control of gene expression at the level of DNA transcription is the most efficient form of regulation, as no metabolic energy is wasted on the creation of intermediates that are later discarded. A variety of mechanisms are known to act at this level, whereas undoubtedly others await discovery. We highlight only some of the more common ones, beginning with those active in prokaryotes, and advancing to the most common—but less understood—eukaryotic control systems.

Regulatory Proteins

A very common regulatory system, found in prokaryotes as well as eukaryotes, employs regulatory DNA-binding proteins that are able to either repress or enhance DNA transcription. In prokaryotes these systems often take the form of operons.

Operons are groups of genes in adjacent locations that are regulated together under the control of a single regulating region. An example is the lactose (or lac) operon in *Escherichia coli,* which consists of three genes encoding enzymes involved in lactose metabolism: β-galactosidase, lactose permease, and thiogalactosidase (Fig. 7). Expression of these enzymes is regulated by a feedback loop involving the amount of lactose present in the cell. A regulatory gene located in a different location of the genome expresses a constant amount of regulatory protein, in this instance a repressor protein. Such constant-rate production is called constitutive synthesis, and is determined by the strength of the promoter of the regulatory gene. The repressor protein recognizes and binds reversibly to an area (the operator) between the lactose operon promoter and the three genes, and thereby inhibits transcription of the genes. However, if lactose (called the inducer) is present in the bacterial cell, it combines with the repressor protein. The resulting repressor-inducer complex can no longer bind to the operator, and as a result the lactose-metabolizing genes are transcribed from the operon promoter. When their protein products metabolize the lactose present, free repressor protein will again be available to bind to the operator. Thus, a constant balance is maintained between the amount of substrate and the amount of metabolizing enzymes in the cell.

The lactose operon, described by Jaques Monod and François Jacob, was the first discovery of a feedback regulator of gene expression. Since then, many similar systems have been described. The lac operon is an example of negative regulation: a bound repressor protein prevents gene transcription. In the lac operon the inducer removes the repressor from the operator, but other systems exist where the inducer in contrast allows the repressor to bind to DNA. Examples include the synthesizing machinery for various amino acids. These genes are switched off by the presence of the amino acid (the inducer) in the environment. In contrast to these forms of negative regulation, some operons use positive regulation, where bound protein (called an activator) enhances transcription. Again, the inducer can either function to remove the activator or to allow it to bind to the DNA.

The genes encoding repressors and activators are examples of *trans*-acting control elements; these can regulate gene expression even when not in close proximity to the gene regulated. In contrast, promoters are examples of *cis*-acting control elements; they only affect genes immediately downstream.

In prokaryotes regulatory DNA-binding proteins are probably the main regulators of gene expression, but they perform many important functions in eukaryotes as well. In fact, whereas prokaryotic RNA polymerase interacts directly with the DNA sequence of the promoter, eukaryotic polymerase requires the presence of regulatory proteins for initiation of transcription. As an example, the TATA box (see above), which forms part of the eukaryotic promoter system, needs to combine with a regulatory factor, the TATA factor, before it is recognized by polymerase.

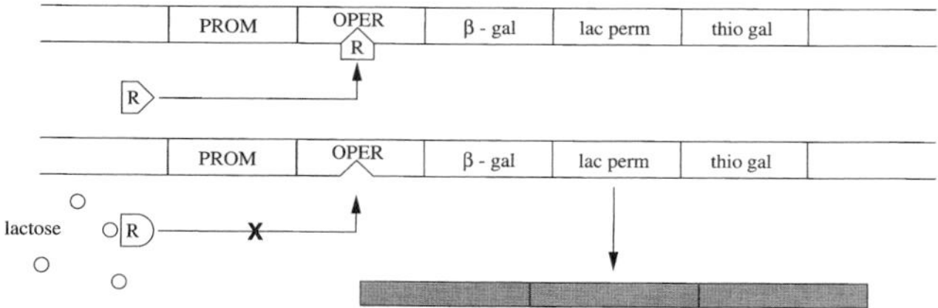

Figure 7. The lactose operon. A regulatory gene produces constitutively a repressor protein (R), which is able to bind to the operator (OPER) and prevent transcriptions of the structural genes β-galactosidase (β-gal), lactose permease (lac perm), and thiogalactosidase (thio gal). In the presence of inducer (lactose) the inducer-repressor complex does not bind to the operator and the structural genes can be transcribed from the promoter (PROM).

Eukaryotic systems are also more complex, in that apart from promoter and operator regions the regulatory domain of a gene usually includes an additional cis-acting element, the enhancer. Enhancers are similar to operators in being DNA domains where regulatory proteins bind, but there are some major differences between the two. First, enhancers are located much farther away from the gene regulated, often up to thousands of nucleotides upstream (or sometimes downstream). Second, it does not seem to matter what direction the enhancer sequence has, i.e., it regulates expression of the gene just as well when reversed in the DNA strand. Although many details of enhancer function are as yet unclear, it is thought that many function by looping back the DNA between promoter and enhancer, thus allowing protein bound to the enhancer to contact the polymerase on the promoter. Protein regulation of gene expression in eukaryotes can be extraordinarily complex. As an example, the β-globin gene in the chick has an upstream enhancer region with binding sites for at least seven proteins, and another enhancer downstream with an additional six binding sites, with each of these proteins having variable activating or repressing effects (making, incidentally, the term *enhancer* a misnomer). Another indication of the complexity of these systems is our gradual realization that many of the dramatic changes during development and cellular differentiation result from changes in gene expression controlled by regulatory proteins.

A particularly important group of protein regulators are the steroid receptors. Members of this family of regulatory proteins (including, among others, the glucocorticoid, mineralocorticoid, estrogen, progesterone, and thyroid hormone receptors) all include a hormone-binding domain and a DNA-binding domain, and for some a transcription-activating domain has been located as well. When a steroid hormone enters the cell and binds to its receptor, the receptor becomes activated and is able to bind to specific sequences of DNA, so-called glucocorticoid-responsive elements (GREs), thereby regulating gene expression. The presence of a GRE in front of a cloned gene indicates that it is probably regulated by steroid hormones. Cyclic adenosine monophosphate (cAMP) is another example of a signaling molecule that regulates gene expression by activating a regulatory protein. Other regulators are activated or inactivated by changes in phosphorylation or by binding to an accessory protein.

Heterochromatin

In addition to regulation by DNA-binding proteins eukaryotic organisms have other means of transcriptional control of gene expression. The presence of histone proteins around the DNA makes the task of DNA transcription more complex, as these proteins need to be removed before the polymerase can have access to its template. However, with nature's usual efficiency this system has evolved into a regulatory system as well. By changing the conformation of DNA into a more condensed form named heterochromatin, the information in the DNA is made physically inaccessible. Heterochromatin is not only inaccessible for transcription, but also occupies less space in the nucleus. Two forms exist, constitutive and facultative heterochromatin. The constitutive form contains short repeated sequences of DNA, is located at the centromeres, and is of obscure function. Facultative heterochromatin contains genes that are excluded from transcription. In embryonic cells only a small part of the genome is in this form, whereas in more specialized cells progressively more genes are packaged this way.

An extreme example of heterochromatin is the condensation of a complete chromosome. This takes place with one of the X chromosomes in females. Whereas male animals only have one X chromosome, females have two. Supposedly, the presence of two functioning X chromosomes would have detrimental effects on the organism, so one of them is condensed into a clump of heterochromatin, called a Barr body. Barr body formation takes place in the embryo, and is inherited as the cell divides, through mechanisms that are as yet unclear. During the formation of germ cells the condensed X chromosome is reactivated, indicating that no structural damage to the DNA has occurred.

It must be appreciated that the condensation of DNA into heterochromatin is the result of a regulatory process, rather than a regulatory process itself. At the moment, we know very little about how the genes that are no longer needed are selected and induced to condense. A hint as to the mechanism may come from the observation that in yeast cells "silencer" DNA sequences exist that block expression in regions of DNA thousands of nucleotides downstream.

DNA Methylation

One important issue in the study of gene regulation is the question how regulatory decisions are transmitted during cell division. The development of a liver cell is accomplished by selectively turning on and off a large number of genes, and these decisions need to be passed on to the daughter cells if these are to remain liver cells as well. Several specific examples of "molecular switches" that could accomplish this function have been described. However, a common system that undoubtedly plays a role in reinforcing these decisions is the covalent modification of DNA. In vertebrates the C in the sequence CG is often methylated, as is the C in the GC sequence on the opposite strand. This methylation has no effect on base pairing, and is easily maintained during DNA replication by a methylating enzyme that only methylates a C when the C on the opposite strand is already methylated (Fig. 8). Thus, methylated C's remain methylated in offspring, and unmethylated C's do not become methylated. The finding that inactive genes are generally heavily methylated and active genes are not supplies a potential explanation as to how decisions about gene activity are propagated during rounds of cell division. Methylation is thought to be a signal for other regulatory systems indicating that a gene is not to be expressed.

Posttranscriptional Regulation

As stated earlier, transcriptional control of gene expression is the most economical mode of regulation. Nonetheless, examples exist of regulation at virtually every step between DNA and protein. Here we will discuss only two important sites of control, both prominent in higher organisms: alternative splicing and differences in mRNA stability.

Alternative Splicing

As mentioned above, in many eukaryotic genes the coding areas (exons) are interrupted by, often much larger, noncoding regions called introns. After transcription the introns are spliced out and the exons are stitched together to form the mRNA. Although introns do not occur in prokaryotes, it should not be concluded that the development of introns and splicing is of recent evolutionary origin. In contrast, it is assumed that these are very ancient processes, but that bacteria have lost their introns in order to streamline their genomes to the maximum extent possible.

In many eukaryotic genes several splicing possibilities exist. In the case of such alternative splicing, a single primary transcript can give rise to several mRNA species, i.e., different forms of protein can be derived from the same gene. Usually, alternative splicing is accomplished by skipping an exon during splicing. As a result, the process generally results in closely related proteins.

Alternative splicing does not occur at random but is regulated, although the mechanisms of regulation are not understood. Sometimes, particular splice forms are preferentially expressed in different tissues. Examples also exist of different splice products being expressed at different stages of development. A well-known example is differential splicing of antibodies produced in B cells, where a membrane-bound form, including a hydrophobic transmembrane domain, is produced during the initial stages of development, and a secreted form, with the hydrophobic domain replaced by a hydrophilic one, is produced later. Alternative splicing can even act as a molecular switch, as when one splice product is completely inactive and only a change in splicing allows a gene to be expressed as functional protein.

mRNA Stability

After splicing has produced a mature mRNA and it has been transported to the cytoplasm, expression of the protein can still

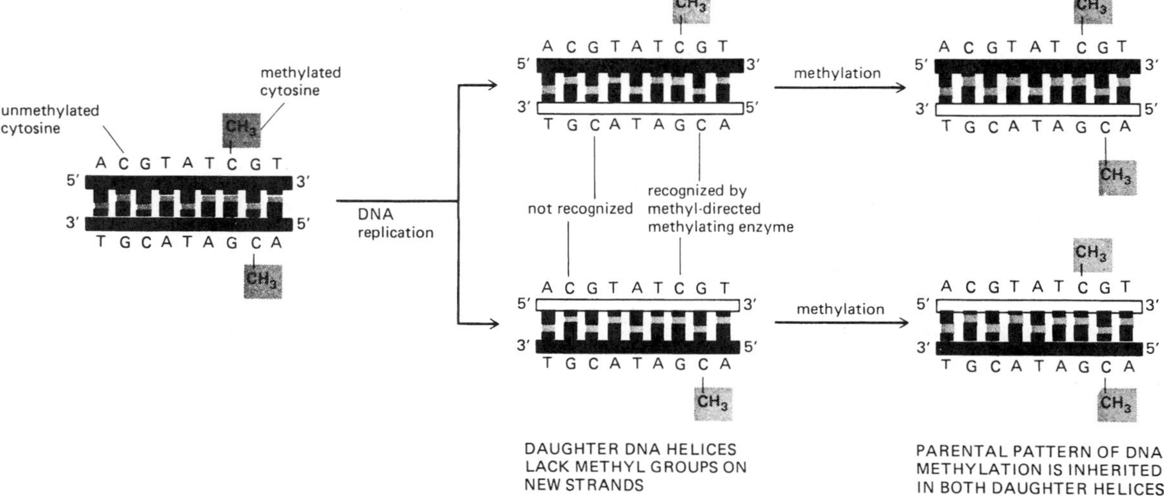

Figure 8. DNA methylation. In vertebrate DNA a large fraction of the cytosine bases in the sequence CG are methylated. Because of the existence of a methyl-directed methylating enzyme, once a pattern of DNA methylation is established each site of methylation is inherited in the progeny DNA.

be regulated by modifying the life span of the mRNA. Generally, eukaryotic mRNAs are more stable than their prokaryotic counterparts, with half-lives measured in hours, as compared to minutes in bacteria. Yet there are significant differences in stability between various mRNAs. Particularly those coding for regulatory proteins such as growth factors are often unstable. This type of instability is built into the 3′ untranslated region.

In addition, mRNA half-life can be regulated by extracellular signals. A well-known example is the regulation of transferrin mRNA by iron levels, but steroids also have significant effects on the stability of mRNA from several genes. A very interesting example is the mRNA for histone protein, whose stability depends on the cell cycle; during DNA synthesis half-life is about one hour, whereas in other stages it decreases to several minutes.

Oncogenes

Often, advances in our knowledge of biologic systems have come from the detailed study of aberrations in these systems. In the case of the regulation of gene expression, much information has been obtained from cases of regulation gone awry, in particular cancer. Although human cancer is a molecularly highly complex disease, simpler types of neoplasia, especially those caused by retroviruses, have helped pinpoint a number of genes of importance in the regulation of cell proliferation.

Retroviruses are RNA viruses, whose genome, after introduction into the host cell, is copied into DNA and inserted in the host chromosome. Many retroviruses cause tumors when infecting specific hosts, and their small genomes made them attractive, although controversial (see Chap. 26), models for study. It was found that those retroviruses causing cancer do so not because of an inherent ability of their genes, but because they carry a mutated gene picked up from a previous host. In other words, the gene causing cancer is originally not a viral gene at all. Such mutated genes are called oncogenes, and the nonmutated host genes they derive from are called proto-oncogenes. Transformation of the host cell arises when the oncogene is inserted into the host cell genome and begins to act as the proto-oncogene—with the difference that the mutation causes it to be overly active. There can be other reasons for this high activity apart from the mutation: often it is due to high levels of expression, either by gene duplication, by an unhappy location close to a strong enhancer, or by any number of other mechanisms.

If expression of an oncogene leads to uncontrolled proliferation, it is likely that the proto-oncogene it derives from is involved in the regulation of proliferation. For this reason much effort has been put in a search for proto-oncogenes, and more than 50 have been discovered thus far. Two findings are of interest. First, the same oncogenes are found repeatedly. This suggests that there may not be many more than about 50 proto-oncogenes, and if that is true, proliferation might be regulated by a relatively small number of genes. Second, the functions of proto-oncogenes fall into a relatively small number of categories. About half of them have domains indicating a protein kinase activity. This indicates that protein phosphorylation plays an essential role in the regulation of cellular proliferation. The remainder have roles in growth-signaling systems; examples exist of growth factors, growth factor receptors, cytoplasmic G proteins, and several classes of transcription regulating proteins. One hopes that study particularly of the latter oncogenes, such as *jun* and *fos,* will lead to a better understanding of the mechanisms of gene regulation.

Gene Regulation and Human Disease

Cancer is not the only human disease resulting from irregularities in gene regulation. As is well known, many diseases have a strong genetic component, although genetic predisposition to a disease may not necessarily lead to disease until such regulatory abnormalities become apparent and the abnormally regulated gene is expressed. Oncogenes, discussed in the previous section, are one example of aberrant gene regulation. What causes derepression or activation of oncogenes remains a mystery but is being investigated actively by several laboratories. Another way gene regulation may be altered in human disease is through increased or decreased expression of normal transmembrane receptors or other cellular proteins. For example, renin is important in the control of blood pressure. Upregulation of the renin gene in mice, using molecular techniques, has been demonstrated to increase renin production and ultimately increase blood pressure. As described above, regulatory elements in the 5′ untranslated regions of many genes are affected by circulating second messengers and drugs such as cAMP, steroids, thyroid hormone, and many other molecules. Once we begin to understand how these elements can be activated (or inappropriately fail to be dampened) then we can begin to understand and treat many human diseases. Perhaps we can even begin to decrease the use of terms such as *idiopathic* in describing many diseases.

In addition to a better understanding of the underlying mechanisms of disease, our knowledge of the details of gene expression will allow the development of novel genetic therapies. In the next section we give, as an extended example of the possibilities and problems of such approaches, an overview of one that appears likely to find its place in the clinic within the next years, namely antisense therapy.

ANTISENSE THERAPY

The molecular cloning of a variety of cellular genes has made possible the study of a new therapeutic modality: selective interference with protein expression. Conventional cancer chemotherapy in particular suffers significantly from its lack of selectivity. Compounds disrupting the flow of information from gene to protein act on all messages expressed, and a relative selective effect on cancer cells results only from the generally higher growth rate and consequent higher protein production of cancer cells as compared with their normal counterparts. In contrast to generally acting chemotherapeutic drugs, knowledge of the DNA sequence of a gene makes it possible to target specifically its protein product through a process named antisense translation arrest.

If oligonucleotides, 15 to 30 nucleotides in length and complementary to the mRNA encoding the protein to be blocked, are introduced into a cell, they will anneal with the mRNA present in the cytoplasm. The resulting double-stranded RNA-DNA hybrid does not act well as a template on ribosomes. First, the presence of the second strand interferes with binding at the ribosome, and in addition there is competitive inhibition between the annealed antisense DNA and the tRNA anticodon that uses the mRNA as a template. As a result of these effects, expression of the protein encoded by the mRNA is decreased. In addition, many cells contain significant amounts of an RNA degrading enzyme, RNAse H, that specifically cuts the RNA component of DNA-RNA hybrids. The hybrids resulting from antisense oligonucleotide annealing are a substrate for this enzyme, which will thus destroy the mRNA for the targeted protein.

The idea of antisense therapy, which was already voiced as far back as 1967, could not be studied seriously until it became possible to make oligonucleotides of the required length (which determines specificity) and until the genes to be targeted had been cloned. Once serious attempts were made to inhibit protein expression in this way, several problems surfaced, not all of which have yet been solved to satisfaction.

First, it rapidly became apparent that normal, phosphodiester-linked DNA oligonucleotides were degraded rather quickly in cells. A number of DNAses exist that either cut these short DNA sequences (endonucleotides) or degrade them from one of the ends (exonucleotides). To circumvent this problem and to obtain the stability needed for adequate suppression of protein translation, a variety of backbone modifications have been made in an attempt to make the compounds less susceptible to DNAse. The most successful thus far are the phosphorothioate compounds, where one of the nonbridging oxygens on the phosphate is replaced by a sulfur atom. One of the difficulties inherent in this substitution is that a chiral center is created at each phosphorus, with poorly defined effects on the enzymes interacting with DNA. An interesting alternative to circumvent this is to use α-oligonucleotides, where the base on the backbone is transposed from the natural β position to the α position. These compounds, which form parallel rather than antiparallel helices, are resistant to nucleases, but unfortunately do not create, when bound to mRNA, a substrate for RNAse H. More research on backbone substitutions is needed to determine fully the impact of modifications on mRNA binding and degradation. As an example, the presence of a sulfur, rather than an oxygen atom, decreases the binding affinity between the oligonucleotide and its target mRNA. The effects of chirality have not been defined completely, and it should be known if it is worth the effort to eliminate chirality by double substitutions on the phosphorus. One way to circumvent some of the difficulties resulting from substitution is to alternate substituted bonds with regular phosphodiester bonds in a certain, optimal arrangement. This approach might decrease some of the difficulties, but at the same time also decrease some of the advantages of substitutions.

A second area that needs to be defined in more detail before antisense therapy can be used clinically is the confusing results of what is called, in a rather cumbersome manner, non–sequence-specific effects, i.e., effects of oligonucleotides that cannot be attributed to complementary mRNA annealing. Sometimes these effects can be pronounced. Production of the human immunodeficiency virus (HIV) p24 gag protein, encoded by the *rev* gene, which is essential for viral reproduction, was shown to be inhibited by an antisense 28mer (i.e., an oligonucleotide consisting of 28 nucleotides, the "mer" being derived from "polymer"), but HIV replication is inhibited with similar effectiveness by oligonucleotides of almost any composition, even homopolymers of cytidine and adenosine! These non–sequence-specific effects are thought to be brought about by activities on a variety of other cellular components, most of which have not been defined clearly.

A third issue is the introduction of antisense oligonucleotides into the target cells. At first thought it seems remarkable that large, charged compounds like DNA would be taken up by cells at all. However, it has been shown that many cell types have DNA-binding proteins present in the cell membrane, and that binding of DNA to these proteins leads to internalization of both protein and DNA. Presumably the complex will be present in intracellular vesicles at that point. It is unclear how the DNA is released from the binding protein and the vesicle, and how it reaches its mRNA target in the cytoplasm. Novel methods of enhancing oligonucleotide uptake are being investigated. These include administration of the DNA in the presence of cationic lipid, adding a cholesteryl moiety to the oligonucleotide in an attempt to secure internalization through the low-density lipoprotein receptor, and other approaches to force uptake through existing receptor systems.

Another question being studied is where in the mRNA transcript the antisense oligonucleotide should be targeted. The variables involved have not been defined clearly. Generally, antisense oligonucleotides have been produced against the initiation region or against the 5′ cap. Targeting of a splice site also seems to be effective, as is disruption of regions with presumed three-dimensional structure. Correct targeting might well be of major influence in the final effect of the antisense therapy.

Where can antisense therapy be applied? At present, the two most promising areas appear to be the suppression of tumor growth and the inhibition of viral replication. As discussed earlier in this chapter, many tumors are caused by the presence and expression of oncogenes. Many of these have been cloned and form adequate targets for antisense therapy. Most studies thus far have been performed in vitro, particularly on leukemic cell lines, and show much promise for the future. Although the issue of non–sequence-specific effects confuses some of the results, many experiments have demonstrated the ability of directed antisense oligonucleotides to inhibit tumorous growth of cells and to induce differentiation. In studies of viral suppression much effort has been directed toward HIV. In p24 gag, the protein product of the *rev* gene, an appropriate target for inhibition of HIV has been found. This protein is essential for viral replication and, in contrast to much of the HIV genome, is highly conserved. As mentioned earlier, studies in this area are also plagued by non–sequence-specific effects, but progress is being made.

There seems to be little doubt that antisense therapy will be a viable therapeutic option for selected disorders. One purely technical issue that needs to be resolved is how to generate large amounts of oligonucleotides at acceptable cost. At the same time, related methods are being studied that could lead to novel applications. As an example, it has been shown that oligonucleotides can be targeted directly to genomic DNA, in which case a triple helix results that is unavailable for transcription. The advantage is that only the (usually) single copy of the gene needs to be inhibited, rather than all or most of the mRNA message transcribed from it. Other approaches considered include DNA minihelices that anneal to and inactivate transcription factors, and the development of catalytic RNA molecules, ribozymes, that selective anneal and then cut their targets. Interestingly enough, this latter approach would bring us back to the method by which, billions of years ago, life began.

An up-to-date review on the subject of antisense therapy is available for the interested reader (2).

CLONING A GENE

In this section we describe how our knowledge of gene structure and expression, summarized above, can be applied in order to obtain even more detailed knowledge of the genome. Here only concepts will be discussed, while technical matters are detailed in Chapter 22.

What Is Cloning and Why Clone a Gene?

Since purifying proteins can be a long and sometimes difficult process, it is often useful to produce a protein to be studied in vitro using molecular techniques. It is important to note at this point that it is far easier to manipulate DNA than it is to manipulate proteins. Thus, when one wishes to study protein function, one can first make changes in the nucleotide sequence of DNA encoding the protein, and this DNA can be translated into a new synthetic protein; properties of this new protein can then be compared with the naturally occurring protein in order to gain insight into regions important in protein function. However, to manipulate the DNA encoding a protein, it is necessary first to find the gene that encodes the protein as well as to establish expression systems that will enable the production of synthetic protein.

The word *cloning* refers to the process of isolating the gene encoding a specific protein from the rest of the genome. Two sources of DNA are used commonly to clone a gene. The first is chromosomal DNA. Since every cell in the body contains a full complement of chromosomes, any cell can be used to isolate every gene in the body from chromosomal DNA. However, since usually a gene is only present once at the level of the chromosome, isolating a single gene from genomic DNA is like finding a needle in a haystack. When the gene of interest encodes a protein known to be present in high concentrations in a certain cell type or tissue, then an enriched pool of DNA containing many copies of the gene of interest can be created artificially from mRNA extracted from the cells or tissue. This is done by taking advantage of an enzyme called reverse transcriptase, which generates DNA from RNA; DNA created in this manner from cellular mRNA is called complementary DNA (cDNA). A third scheme used to clone a gene is to isolate RNA samples from several sources and inject them into systems such as oocytes, where functional protein is made directly from injected RNA. If the protein serves an identifiable function (such as mediating ion currents in the case of a channel protein, binding ligands in the case of a receptor protein, or activating an enzyme which activity can be assayed), then the function can be used as a marker for the presence of the desired RNA. This process is called expression cloning. In this section, we review briefly several classic cloning techniques.

DNA Probes and Restriction Enzymes

Once a source of DNA is found, it is necessary to have a probe for the gene to be cloned, in order to identify it among the other DNA. In the early days of molecular biology, proteins of interest were purified to homogeneity and enzymatically degraded into small polypeptides that could be sequenced with an amino acid analyzer. Once polypeptide sequences of 10 to 15 amino acids were known, an oligonucleotide that could conceivably encode the polypeptide fragment was designed using tables that predict which triplet of nucleotides should encode the amino acid. Although there is some redundancy in the genetic code (i.e., more than one nucleotide triplet encodes a given amino acid), knowledge about the relative frequency of codon usage frequently enables a fairly accurate "best guess" primer to be synthesized. Once the oligonucleotide probe is synthesized and labeled (usually by incorporating radioactive atoms), it can anneal to and thereby identify the corresponding DNA. It is used much as a magnet would be used to find a needle in a haystack—a difficult but not impossible task.

Since a labeled probe will hybridize to the corresponding DNA fragment under the correct conditions, the researcher can determine which fragment of DNA to isolate in order to find the gene of interest. However, since chromosomal DNA is very long, it is necessary to cut the DNA into smaller fragments, one of which will contain the area of interest, before it can be analyzed. Bacteria contain so-called restriction enzymes that cut very specific sequences of DNA. More than 100 of these enzymes have been isolated that cut DNA in different locations (due to their nucleotide specificity). Hence, the molecular biologist can cut chromosomal DNA (or cDNA) into small fragments. The nucleotide sequence of the DNA fragment to which the probe has annealed can then be determined to see if the entire gene has been isolated and from the nucleotide sequence the putative protein sequence can be derived using the genetic code. If the entire gene is not present, then another restriction enzyme "digest" can be performed to isolate a slightly larger DNA fragment that might contain the entire gene of interest. Once this is accomplished, the gene has been cloned. However, further manipulations of the DNA are required so that it can be expressed conveniently in cells or used to generate large quantities of RNA. This process is called subcloning and frequently involves a special form of DNA called plasmids.

Plasmids and Selection

Plasmids are relatively small pieces of circular DNA. Many plasmids have been engineered to contain a region of DNA (called a polylinker) with a sequence that can be cut by several restriction enzymes. In addition to containing several sites for restriction enzyme digestion, plasmids often also contain an antibiotic resistance gene and promoter regions. Many plasmids with different promoter regions, different antibiotic resistance genes, or other convenient genes (such as the luciferase gene to be used as a marker) are available commercially; the choice of plasmid depends on the experiment to be performed. A gene subcloned into a plasmid can be manipulated, expressed, and modified with relative ease. To insert the cloned gene into a plasmid, the gene of interest is cut with restriction enzymes that correspond to the ones present in the polylinker of a desired plasmid and then inserted into the plasmid at the corresponding sites, creating a new plasmid that now contains the gene of interest.

The beauty of subcloning a gene into a plasmid is that the plasmid can be inserted into *E. coli* bacteria. Every time the bacteria divide, the plasmid is replicated, doubling the concentration of the cloned gene. In addition, by adding antibiotic to the growth media, only those bacteria containing the plasmid DNA will survive (since the plasmid contains an antibiotic resistance gene in addition to the cloned gene). This process is called selection. Since bacteria replicate thousands of times over several hours, large quantities of bacteria can be grown easily in the laboratory (frequently overnight while the researcher sleeps). Large quantities of plasmid DNA can be isolated by rupturing the bacteria and quickly purifying the DNA. The entire cloned gene can be cut out of the plasmid at this point using restriction enzymes, or plasmid DNA can be used to generate RNA probes, using the plasmid promoter, to perform mutagenesis experiments (changing nucleotide sequences and creating various synthetic DNA and proteins), or for expression in cells.

Clonal Expression Cell Systems

Cells expressing specific proteins are valuable in many kinds of experiments. Hence, the creation of a cell line expressing a single type of protein (i.e., membrane receptor, channel protein, or cytoplasmic enzyme) is very helpful for the study of the protein. Plasmid DNA can be inserted into the cell's DNA so that the cell will begin to manufacture the given protein where it previously did not. Assuming the cell has all of the proper second messenger machinery, many studies of protein function can now be accomplished. Such protein expression can be transient or stable. Transient expression refers to the situation where a protein is manufactured by the cells for a short time span, whereas stably expressing cell lines continue to express the protein over many months or years. There is a difference in preparation technique as well. Stably expressing cell lines have to be tested carefully one by one until a single population of cells is found with appropriate protein concentrations. Every cell in this selected population will express the protein of interest. On the other hand, transiently expressing cells have the gene randomly incorporated (roughly 10% of the cell population take up very large concentrations of plasmid DNA and make protein); these cells are therefore not a homogeneous population and cannot be perpetuated indefinitely as can stable cell lines.

MOLECULAR TECHNIQUES IN CLINICAL STUDIES—POSSIBILITIES AND PITFALLS

Molecular biology techniques are now so common that they can be adapted easily for use in clinical studies. In fact, many assays can be purchased in the form of complete kits, with instructions, reagents, and a toll-free telephone number for assistance included. Clinical studies using molecular techniques can have a wide variety of goals, ranging from the determination of changes in mRNA levels during acute interventions such as cardiopulmonary bypass, surgery, and different disease states, to trials of genetically altered (corrected) genes for diseases such as cystic fibrosis. Molecular techniques are also used frequently to answer mechanistic questions. For example, by investigating the impact of organ ischemia (for example in the liver) on expression of mRNAs encoding for various proteins (such as tumor necrosis factor), possible mechanisms for resulting organ injury can be determined. Molecular techniques are now becoming increasingly common diagnostic tools for diseases such as hemophilia, cystic fibrosis, and malignant hyperthermia. By identifying the existence of a detrimental DNA abnormality, early diagnosis and therapy can be instituted for genetic diseases. This type of diagnostic testing will become increasingly important for routine preoperative screening for various diseases in the future.

It is important to note at this point that although molecular information can be accumulated rather easily, correct interpretation of resulting data is essential and requires in-depth knowledge of the limitations of the molecular biology techniques used. For example, many clinical studies rely on rapid amplification of small segments of DNA from patient samples (frequently blood or tissue samples) using a technique called the polymerase chain reaction (PCR, a technique explained in detail in Chapter 22). PCR technology enables a single copy of DNA to be amplified several million times. Therefore, large quantities of DNA are available within hours for genetic testing or for quantitation of DNA or RNA present in tissues. PCR results, however, are prone to interpretation errors. In genetic testing such as the identification of sickle cell disease, the abnormality is present in the genomic DNA and therefore amplification of this DNA by PCR is a useful and appropriate technique. However, if RNA levels are to be studied, it is important to remember that all tissue samples contain both genomic DNA as well as RNA. RNA is amplified by converting it to cDNA using the enzyme reverse transcriptase prior to PCR amplification. However, since traces of genomic DNA may be amplified as well as the cDNA, it is critical to treat each sample with an enzyme called DNAse to eradicate any genomic DNA prior to making cDNA from RNA. Simply using PCR techniques in clinical studies without being aware of this caveat can easily result in erroneous conclusions. Hence, molecular-based clinical studies should always provide appropriate controls to ensure that they have been performed correctly.

CONCLUSION

Molecular biology has ushered in an exciting era for medicine. These tools are now readily available for both clinical and basic science studies. Imagine the potential value of simple genetic blood tests available the night before surgery to determine if your patient is susceptible to malignant hyperthermia or has pseudocholinesterase deficiency. While such tests are not available yet, they are not inconceivable in the future. Understanding proteins (be they new receptor subtypes, targets of anesthetic action, or enzyme systems harnessed to new medical therapies) at the molecular level will greatly facilitate the development of new drugs for our use in the perioperative period. In addition, molecular biology tools are rapidly unlocking the mechanisms of many diseases. This may enable us to intervene more appropriately when such patients are stressed during surgery. Few things can compare to molecular biology in terms of the rapidity of change that these techniques have brought at all levels of medicine. For further information regarding details of molecular biology techniques, see Chapter 22.

REFERENCES

1. Alberts B, Bray D, Lewis J, Raff M, Roberts K, Watson JD. *Molecular biology of the cell,* 2nd ed. New York: Garland, 1989.
2. Stein CA, Cheng Y-C. Antisense oligonucleotides as therapeutic agents—is the bullet really magical? *Science* 1993;261:1004–1012.
3. Watson JD, Gilman M, Witkowski J, Zoller M. *Recombinant DNA,* 2nd ed. New York: W.H. Freeman, 1992.

Anesthesia: Biologic Foundations, edited by
Tony L. Yaksh et al. Lippincott–Raven Publishers,
Philadelphia © 1997.

CHAPTER 4

G-PROTEIN SYSTEMS

ROBERT S. ARONSTAM

G proteins comprise a large family of regulatory proteins that are involved in both intracellular and intercellular signal transduction processes (25,76). G proteins are molecular switches whose activities are determined by their interaction with guanine nucleotides, hence their name. G proteins cycle between an inactive, guanosine diphosphate (GDP)-bound form and an active guanosine triphosphate (GTP)-bound form. This cycling may be regulated by a guanine nucleotide exchange factor (GEF) on the one hand, and a guanosine triphosphatase (GTPase) activating factor (GAF) on the other (Fig. 1).

G proteins can be divided into two groups: the heterotrimeric, membrane-bound proteins prominent in synaptic signal transduction, and smaller (20–30 kd), monomeric G proteins involved in regulating a number of intracellular processes. This chapter discusses the heterotrimeric proteins because of the central importance of synaptic function in anesthesia. General anesthesia involves a global depression of synaptic transmission processes, the same processes that are globally mediated by heterotrimeric G proteins.

HISTORY

The discovery of G proteins arose from the study of hormonal control of adenylate cyclase activity (12,40). In 1971 Martin Rodbell and coworkers (68,69) demonstrated that GTP regulates receptor control of adenylate cyclase. Rodbell et al. postulated a three-step signal transduction pathway in cell membranes encompassing an outwardly directed receptor, a GTP-sensitive intermediary, and an inwardly directed effector (i.e., adenylate cyclase). This theory was supported by the demonstration that guanine nucleotide regulation of hormonal control of adenylate cyclase was mediated by a protein subunit that was distinct from either the receptor or the enzyme (62). The molecular nature of the pathway came into clearer focus with Cassel and Selinger's (17) demonstration that GTP hydrolysis was associated with hormone stimulation of adenylate cyclase.

Transducin (G_t), which activates a cyclic guanosine monophosphate (cGMP)-specific phosphodiesterase in response to the activation of the opsins, was the first G protein characterized that was not involved in the regulation of adenylate cyclase. Transducin was partially purified and its subunit nature determined in 1979 (26). In a remarkable series of experiments, Alfred Gilman and his coworkers fused cells deficient in G proteins with wild-type cells (56,81). The consequent regeneration of hormonal control of adenylate cyclase activity was exploited to detect and subsequently purify G proteins (56,81). Additional G proteins were identified and purified over the next several years. In 1985 the primary amino acid sequences of G-protein α subunits were reported (28,42,51,84,93). To date, the presence of about 17 G_α genes has been reported (91). In 1994 Rodbell and Gilman were awarded the Nobel Prize in Physiology and Medicine for their work on G proteins.

G-PROTEIN STRUCTURE

The G proteins involved in synaptic signal transduction are heterotrimeric proteins comprised of α, β, and γ subunits (Figs. 2 and 3). Within the α subunit resides the binding site for guanine nucleotides, a GTPase catalytic activity, amino acid residues that are substrates for adenosine diphosphate (ADP)-ribosylation by bacterial toxins (cholera and pertussis

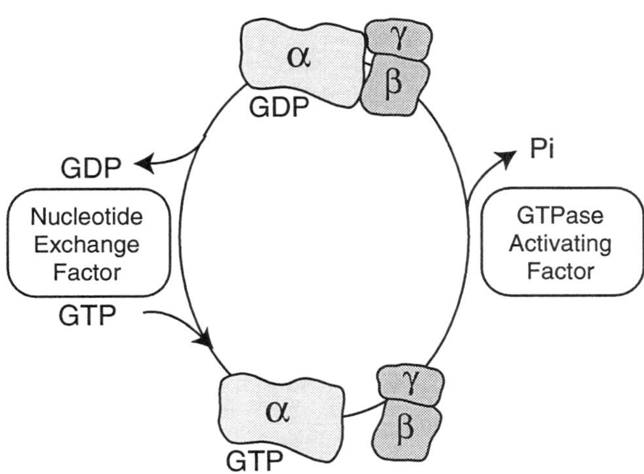

Figure 1. Basic G-protein cycle. The G protein alternates between an inactive, trimeric form in which GDP occupies the nucleotide binding site on the α subunit and an active, dissociated form in which GTP occupies the nucleotide binding site. Switching between the two states is controlled by nucleotide exchange and GTPase-activating factors. In the heterotrimeric G proteins subserving synaptic signal transduction, receptors function as the nucleotide exchange factor while at least certain effector structures can act as GTPase-activating factors.

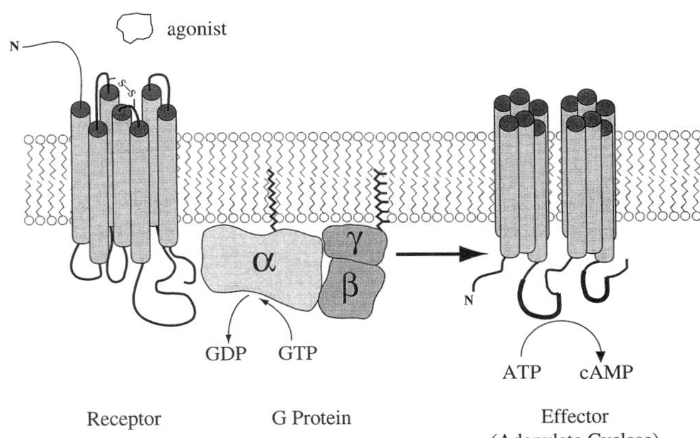

FIG. 2. General scheme for G-protein mediation of synaptic signal transduction. A hormonal or neurotransmitter/neuromodulator messenger binds to an intrinsic membrane receptor. This is usually a member of the superfamily of synaptic receptors that incorporate seven transmembrane spanning domains. Activation of this receptor induces an interaction ("coupling") to a heterotrimeric G protein. This interaction involves the third intracellular protein loop and C terminal chain of the receptor and the C terminal region of the G protein α subunit. This interaction catalyzes the release of GDP from the α subunit and the subsequent binding of GTP. This allows the dissociated G-protein subunits to affect the activity of effector structures. In this example, the effector is adenylate cyclase, which converts ATP to the second messenger cAMP.

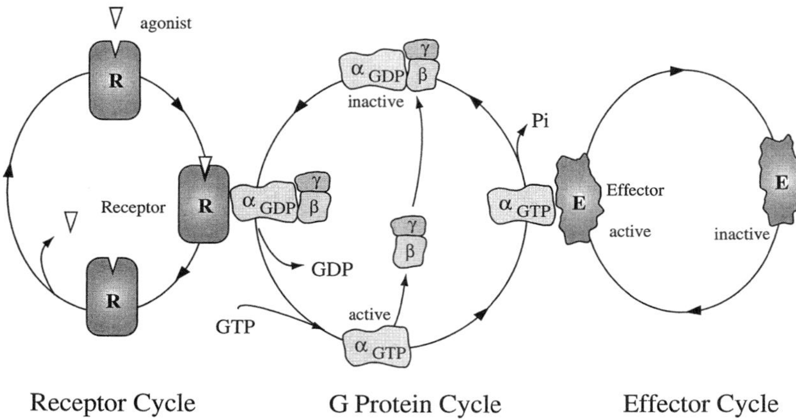

Figure 3. Interacting receptor, G protein, and effector cycles in synaptic transmission. The G-protein cycle involves the cycling of G proteins between an inactive, GDP-bound, trimeric form and an active, GTP-bound dissociated form *(center circular pathway)*. The rate-limiting step in this cycling is the release of GDP from the α subunit. This step is accelerated by G-protein interaction with an activated neurotransmitter/hormonal/sensory receptor *(left circular pathway)*. The termination of G-protein stimulation of the messenger-producing effector molecule (E, typically an enzyme or ion channel) may be accelerated by the interaction with the effector molecule itself (11). Thus, G-protein stimulation is a self-limiting process that is under the control of membrane receptors. Synaptic signaling through G proteins can be viewed as three interacting cycles, with a G-protein cycle bridging an externally oriented receptor cycle and an internally oriented effector cycle.

toxins), and sites involved in interactions with both receptors and effector mechanisms. Thus, most attention has focused on the α subunit. The βγ subunit complex demonstrates less variability and was originally thought to play a supportive role, especially in G-protein association with the membrane. However, it has become clear that β and γ subunits show selectivity for the signal transduction system, and the βγ dimer itself regulates the activity of numerous effector mechanisms.

α Subunit

The α subunit is comprised of a polypeptide of molecular weight 40,000–46,000. Molecular cloning has revealed the presence of at least 17 α subunit genes, although alternate RNA splicing results in additional isoforms (e.g., the four species of $G_{\alpha s}$). Most G-protein α subunits are tightly associated with the cytosolic face of the plasma membrane, even though amino acid analysis indicates an absence of membrane-spanning domains (Fig. 2). One source of this association is an anchoring effect of the βγ subunits; α subunits do not associate with phospholipid vesicles unless βγ is present (79). A second source of this association may be covalent modification of the protein α subunit with fatty acids. In several members of the G_i family (including G_o and G_i), myristic acid (n-tetradecanoic acid) is cotranslationally attached to the Gly2 residue of the α subunit via a stable amide bond after removal of Met1. The α subunits of transducin (G_t) are modified with a variety of different fatty acids. These N-terminal additions may be responsible for hydrophobic interactions of α subunits with the membrane lipid bilayer, the βγ subunit, or perhaps other membrane-bound structures. However, not all α subunits display this modification, even though all are membrane associated. Monoclonal antibodies to N-terminal fragments (49) and proteolytic removal of an N-terminal peptide (22) also disrupt α subunit association with βγ subunits and release a soluble α subunit fragment, emphasizing the importance of the N-terminal region in membrane association.

In contrast, the C terminal domain of the α subunit appears to play an important role in interactions with receptor and effector structures. Pertussis toxin catalyzes the ADP-ribosylation of a cysteine moiety located four residues from the C terminal of the α subunits of certain G proteins in the G_i family, including $G_{i1\text{-}3}$, G_{oA+B}, and G_{t1+2}. As a consequence of this modification, G proteins are functionally uncoupled from the receptors (33,58). Antibodies to the C-terminal sequence, chimeric replacement of the C terminus, and mutational alteration of the C terminal (not necessarily including the C-terminal cysteine) also alter α subunit interactions with receptors and effectors (47,59,82).

The guanine nucleotide binding domain of the α subunit has been deduced from similarities with the structure of crystallized small GTP binding proteins. Five highly conserved domains (G1-G5) involved in this binding have been delineated and the amino moieties involved in the catalytic activity have been identified (15). The catalytic activity of the α subunit is lost upon ADP-ribosylation of Arg201 of G_s and G_{olf} by cholera toxin. This results is a constitutitively active subunit and persistent stimulation of the associated effector.

The βγ Dimer

The β (35–36 kd) and γ (8–9 kd) subunits remain closely associated with each other and appear to function as a unit. Four β subunit genes have been cloned, β1–β4. β1, β2, and β4 have a 90% amino acid identity to each other, while β3 has an 80% amino acid identity to the other subunits. Six γ subunit genes have been cloned and sequenced. Amino acid identity of the γ chains ranges from 30% to 76% (91).

βγ dimers are tightly associated with the membrane and require detergent for extraction, even though amino acid analysis does not reveal a highly hydrophobic character or the presence of membrane-spanning domains. One source of this hydrophobic character is the posttranslational addition of a long-chain isoprenyl group to the C-terminus of the γ subunit. The isoprenyl group is attached to the cysteine in the terminal CAAX sequence (where C is cysteine, A is an aliphatic residue, and X is any amino acid). The AAX residues are then enzymatically removed and the terminal cysteine is carboxymethylated. Different isoprenyl groups are attached to different γ subunits. For example, a farnesyl moiety is attached to the γ1 subunit that is associated with rod photoreceptors, while a 20 carbon geranylgeranyl moiety is attached to the γ2 subunit that is prominent in brain. When isoprenylation of γ subunits is blocked, an inactive and soluble form of the βγ dimer is produced.

Several functions have been ascribed to the βγ dimer: (a) promoting the association of α_{GDP} with the receptor, (b) decreasing nucleotide dissociation from α_{GDP}, thereby decreasing inadvertent signal transduction through the G-protein cycle (30), (c) anchoring the G protein to the cytosolic surface of the membrane, and (d) direct roles in activating or inhibiting signal transduction pathways (Table 1). The expression of specific β and γ subunits shows regional, tissue, and developmental selectivity, emphasizing their active role in signal transduction. Moreover, β subunits display specificity for the receptor species. Thus, muscarinic and somatostatin receptors that inhibit Ca^{2+} channels in GH_3 cells are coupled to β1 and β3, but not β2 and β4, subunits (36). Details on the specificity of βγ subunits for the different signal transduction pathways are rapidly emerging, and it is becoming abundantly evident that

Table 1. ACTIVITIES OF G-PROTEIN SUBUNITS

Activity	Stimulation	Inhibition	References
Adenylate cyclase	α_s, $\beta\gamma$, α_{olf}	α_{i1-3}, α_o, α_z, $\beta\gamma$	86
Calcium channels (N-type)	α_s	α_{oA}, α_{oB}, α_s, $\beta\gamma$	31,95
Phospholipase C	α_q, α_{11}, α_{14}, α_{15}, α_{16}, $\beta\gamma$		61
cGMP phosphodiester	$\alpha_{t1\ (rods)}$, $\alpha_{t1\ (cones)}$		83
Potassium channels	α_{i3}, $\beta\gamma$	$\alpha_{q/11}$	19,43,66
Phospholipase A_2	$\beta\gamma$		8,35

A number of less well established activities have also been described. References are generally to review articles.

$\beta\gamma$ subunits are as important as α subunits in regulating the activity of cellular effector mechanisms.

THE G-PROTEIN CYCLE

A generally accepted model for G-protein activity is outlined in Fig. 3 (25). In the resting state, the G protein exists in its trimeric form with GDP occupying the nucleotide binding site on the α subunit. Activation of G proteins involves the release of GDP and rapid binding of GTP (to the α subunit). The binding of GTP induces (a) the dissociation of receptor and G protein and (b) the dissociation of the G protein into its α and $\beta\gamma$ subunits. The α_{GTP} (and possibly $\beta\gamma$) complex then interacts with various effector entities (e.g., enzymes, ion channels), stimulating or inhibiting their activity. The activity of the α_{GTP} complex is terminated by hydrolysis of GTP by an intrinsic enzymatic activity. In the GDP-bound state, the α subunit reassociates with $\beta\gamma$ subunits and is subject to reactivation. The association of G proteins and receptors has consequences for the receptor's binding properties: Receptors coupled to G proteins have a higher affinity for receptor agonists than receptors not coupled to G proteins. Thus, inclusion of guanine nucleotides in in vitro binding assays lowers agonist affinity by effectively dissociating receptor–G-protein complexes. This guanine nucleotide-sensitivity of agonist binding is frequently used as an indication of receptor–G-protein interactions.

There are two critical control points in the G-protein cycle, the release of GDP from the α subunit and the hydrolysis of GTP catalyzed by the α subunit (85). The lifetime of the α_{GTP} complex is several seconds, but the basal rate of GDP dissociation from the α subunit is even slower. Thus, in the resting condition most of the G protein is in the inactive, GDP-bound state. GDP release is catalyzed by an interaction with an activated neurotransmitter, sensory, or hormonal receptor: The binding of an agonist to a receptor induces a conformational change in the receptor that promotes its association with the G-protein trimer. As a consequence of its association with the activated receptor, there is a conformational change in the α subunit, and GDP is released. This release is the crucial step in signal transduction through G proteins.

The second control point is in the hydrolysis of GTP, which terminates Gα regulation of the effector. This turnover is normally quite low. In the small signaling G proteins such as Ras, GTP hydrolysis requires the action of a GTP activating protein (GAP). Berstein et al. (11) demonstrated that an effector (in this case, phospholipase C) can stimulate G-protein–GTPase activity. Thus, effectors can mediate the fast physiologic deactivation of G-protein–mediated signaling, and represent a self-limiting mechanism. Another possibility is that the α subunit incorporates a GAP-like domain within its primary structure (15).

The arrestins comprise a class of proteins that modulate the activation of G-protein–coupled receptors by disrupting receptor–G-protein coupling (27,44). Receptor desensitization mediated by arrestins involves at least two steps: (a) agonist activation of the receptor stimulates phosphorylation of the receptor by receptor kinases; (b) arrestins bind to phosphorylated forms of the receptors, thereby depressing receptor–G-protein coupling, and thus receptor-mediated signaling. Multiple forms of both receptor kinases and arrestins have been described, each with a unique, and not generally exclusive, selectivity for the receptor species. This multiplies even further the possibilities for cellular control of signal transduction activity.

G-PROTEIN FAMILIES AND ACTIVITIES

The existence of four families of G proteins has been inferred from the amino acid homology of the α subunit: G_s, G_i, G_q, and G_{12} (Fig. 4) (76,91). The most highly conserved regions of the α subunits are the domains involved in nucleotide binding and GTP hydrolysis; presumably the more variable regions are involved in interactions with the different receptor and effector structures. The most firmly established activities of the different G-protein subunits are summarized in Table 1.

G_s family α subunits are substrates for ADP-ribosylation catalyzed by cholera toxin and mediate stimulation of adenylate cyclase. $G_{\alpha s}$ is expressed in a wide variety of tissues, while $G_{\alpha olf}$ is prominent in the olfactory neuroepithelium and central nervous system.

The G_i family comprises at least nine α subunits, most of which are susceptible to ADP-ribosylation catalyzed by pertussis toxin. These G proteins are widely expressed, but are especially prominent in the central nervous system and heart. $G_{\alpha i}$ and $G_{\alpha o}$ are the most widely expressed G-protein α subunits in the brain, and may be the source of $\beta\gamma$ subunits that play direct roles in modulating signal transduction processes. $G_{\alpha z}$ has less homology to the other α subunits in this family; $G_{\alpha z}$ is expressed in neural tissues and inhibits adenylate cyclase, but apparently it is not a substrate for ADP-ribosylation by pertussis toxin. The transducins, $G_{\alpha t\text{-}1}$ and $G_{\alpha t\text{-}2}$, are expressed in retinal rod and cone cells, respectively, while $G_{\alpha gust}$ expression is restricted to the tongue, where it probably plays a role in the transduction of taste stimuli (50). G_i family proteins are involved in the inhibition of adenylate cyclase ($G_{\alpha i}$), and the inhibition of calcium ($G_{\alpha o}$) and potassium channels ($G_{\alpha i}$) (Table 1).

The G_q family of G proteins contains α subunits that are involved in the stimulation of the B-isoforms of phospholipase C, thereby producing the second messengers IP_3 and diacylglycerol that, in turn, increase intracellular Ca^{2+} and protein kinase C activities (Table 1). Gq proteins are not substrates for ADP-ribosylation by bacterial toxins. Certain G_q proteins (G_q and G_{11}) are widely expressed, while others are restricted to specific tissues and cell lines (G_{14}, G_{15}, and G_{16}; Fig. 4). G_{15} and G_{16} are only expressed in certain hematopoietic cells (1,92).

The G_{12} family is comprised of the pertussis toxin-insensitive and widely expressed proteins G_{12} and G_{13}. Specific physiologic functions have not been linked to these proteins (57).

The heterotrimeric G proteins show structural and functional similarities to the low-molecular-weight GTP-binding proteins (LMWGs), such as Ras, Rho, Rab, and Rac (90). LMWGs are involved in signaling processes underlying cell

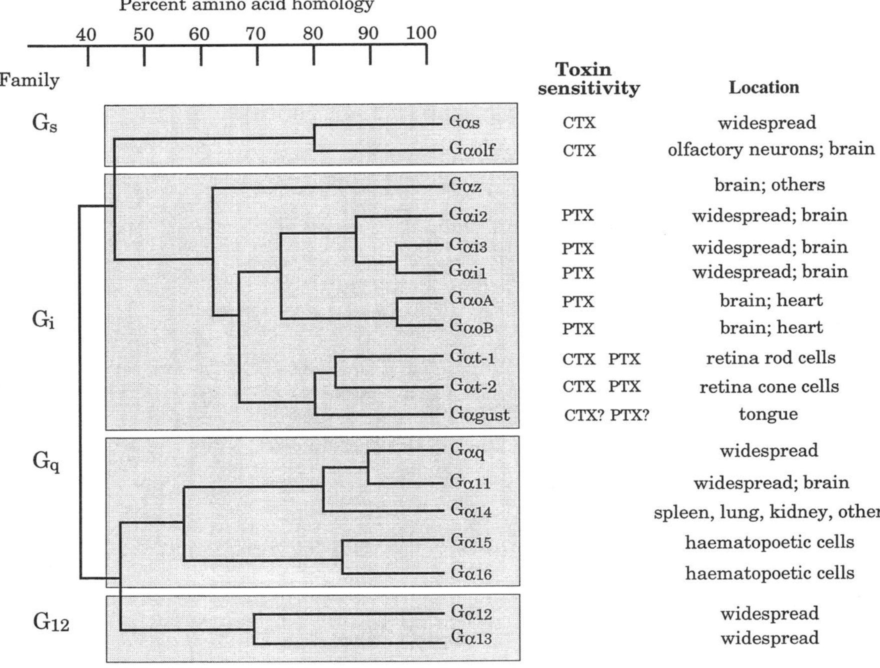

Figure 4. G-protein α subunits: structural and evolutionary relationships, biochemical actions and tissue distribution. Eighteen α subunits are listed, although alternate splicing accounts for a number of variants with similar properties (e.g., 4 α_s and 2 α_o subunits). Four families of G proteins can be distinguished on the basis of amino acid homology, G_s, G_i, G_q, and G_{12} (76,91). These proteins differ in the selectivity for receptor protein and effectors and in the tissue distribution.

growth and differentiation, cytoskeletal regulation, vesicular trafficking, enzyme regulation, and protein synthesis. Like the heterotrimer G proteins, the LMWGs are molecular switches that are active when complexed with GTP. Moreover, their activity is regulated by guanine nucleotide exchange factors and GTPase activating proteins, corresponding to G-protein control by receptor and effector molecules. In both classes of molecules, the hydrolysis of the high-energy phosphate bond of GTP is used as a switching signal rather than a source of energy to drive reactions. The α subunits of heterotrimer G proteins share structural homology with the LMWGs in the domains involved in nucleotide binding and hydrolysis (15,34).

G-PROTEIN TOOLS

G-protein research has benefited from the development of specific probes for G-protein function:

1. Certain bacterial toxins catalyze the ADP-ribosylation of α subunit amino acids. Cholera toxin transfers ADP-ribose from NAD to a cysteine residue in the α subunits of G_s and G_t (54). This cysteine is located in a region (G2) (15) that is highly conserved among the α subunits and that probably participates in guanine nucleotide binding and hydrolysis. As a consequence of this modification, GTPase activity is suppressed and the G protein is locked into its activating mode (16). As noted above, pertussis toxin ADP-ribosylates a C terminal cysteine in G proteins in the G_i family (with the exception of G_z), thereby disrupting receptor–G-protein coupling. These toxins have been widely used in physiologic studies to establish whether G_α or G_i family proteins are involved in specific signaling pathways. The extent of endogenous ADP-ribosylation of G proteins, and the role it plays in the physiologic control of G-protein activity, are unsettled issues.
2. Immunologic probes in the form of antibodies to defined segments of the various G proteins have proven useful in the detection and quantitation of the different G proteins (78). However, not all G-protein antibodies inactivate G-protein function. Moreover, due to the high degree of homology between G proteins, it is not yet possible to discriminate all subunits using these probes.
3. Sodium fluoride reacts with aluminum to form fluoroaluminates such as AlF_4^-. AlF_4^- binds to the γ-phosphate position of the nucleotide binding site on the α subunit next to GDP, thereby mimicking GTP occupancy of the site and eliciting the conformational changes associated with G-protein activation. The result is a hydrolysis-resistant activation of the G protein (29,80).
4. GTP analogues, such as 5′-guanylylimidodiphosphate and guanosine 5′-O-(3-thiotriphosphate), may replace GTP and support G-protein activation. Since they are resistant to hydrolysis, their use results in persistent activation. These agents have been widely used in both physiologic studies and binding assays to determine whether actions are mediated by G-protein transducers, or whether specific receptors are coupled to G proteins.

G PROTEINS AND ANESTHESIA

General anesthetics abolish sensation and produce unconsciousness by depressing certain functions of the central nervous system in a reversible manner. It has been recognized for at least 90 years that anesthetics preferentially affect the chemical transmission between neurons, rather than axonal conductance or the electrical activity of neurons (39,77). Complex effects of anesthetics on both excitatory and inhibitory synaptic transmission have been described (18,37,64,67).

The molecular mechanisms underlying anesthesia are poorly understood. General anesthetics include a disparate set of compounds, including inert gases, halogenated hydrocarbons, and ethers. Most theories of anesthesia have focused on the physicochemical properties of the drugs, and in particular the strong correlation between anesthetic potency and lipid solubility (52,60). For example, it has been suggested that anesthetics insert into the lipid bilayer of nerve membranes, thereby altering fluidity, phase transitions, membrane dimensions, or ionic permeability (71). However, the physical changes caused by anesthetics (at clinical concentrations) can be quite small, and are often in opposing directions (e.g., membrane fluidity may be either increased or decreased by anesthetic agents that are clinically equipotent). Franks and Lieb (23,24) have presented evidence that direct actions of anesthetics on specific proteins may underlie anesthetic action.

Thus, current information indicates that (a) anesthesia primarily involves a reversible disruption of synaptic communication between neurons in the central nervous system, and (b) anesthesia is likely to involve specific interactions with hydrophobic domains of particularly sensitive proteins, presumably those proteins involved in the synaptic processes that are disrupted by the anesthetic.

In view of their strategic locations and critical functions in intercellular communication, receptors, G proteins, and effectors are all logical candidates for targets of anesthetic action. However, general anesthetics have not been found to be particularly potent disrupters of receptor function, at least as indicated by ligand binding activity, except at very high concentrations. The literature dealing with anesthetic effects on effector mechanisms is extensive, complex, and often contradictory. Moreover, it is important to note that it has not always been possible to distinguish anesthetic effects on receptors and effector mechanisms from anesthetic effects on intermediary transducer proteins. For instance, certain drug and physical effects on synaptic transmission that had been previously ascribed to receptors or effectors we now know to reflect actions on G proteins. Some information indicating an action of liquid volatile general anesthetics on G-protein activity has been reported and is summarized below. A few commentaries addressing possible roles of G proteins in anesthetic actions have been published (6,38,48,94).

VOLATILE GENERAL ANESTHETICS AND G-PROTEIN–RECEPTOR INTERACTIONS

The potency of volatile anesthetics is affected by activation or inhibition of a number of G-protein–coupled receptors, including the α_2-adrenergic receptor (73), the dopamine receptor (74), and opiate receptors (94).

Puil and El-Beheiry (64) found that the postsynaptic depolarizations caused by acetylcholine, glutamate, *N*-methyl-d-aspartate (NMDA) and γ-aminobutyric acid (GABA) in rat cortical slices were depressed by the volatile anesthetics isoflurane and halothane. The excitation induced by acetylcholine was the most sensitive to inhibition by the anesthetics; isoflurane depressed acetylcholine response with an EC_{50} of less than 1 minimum alveolar concentration (MAC). Thus, inhibition of muscarinic transmission would be expected during routine anesthetic administration.

The muscarinic acetylcholine receptor has been one of the most extensively studied receptors of the G-protein–coupled receptor superfamily. Central cholinergic systems are involved in several processes (memory, attention, arousal) that are disrupted by anesthetics. Moreover, cholinergic pathways project diffusely to brain areas that are selectively depressed by anesthetics. Therefore, it is reasonable to question whether a disruption of cholinergic transmission contributes to the development of at least certain aspects of the anesthetic state.

[^{3}H]*N*-methylscopolamine ([^{3}H]MS) binding to muscarinic receptors in membranes prepared from rat brainstem or cerebral cortex was increased after equilibration of the tissue with halothane (5). Saturation binding experiments indicated that halothane increased [^{3}H]MS binding affinity 67%. Halothane had no effect on the rate constant of association, but decreased the rate constant of dissociation. Similar results were obtained with other volatile general anesthetics.

Information on the status of receptor–G-protein interactions is provided by the binding properties of the receptor ligands. The affinity of the receptors for their ligand is affected by whether or not the receptor is coupled to a G protein. In many systems, this coupling is revealed as a higher affinity for agonists when the receptor is coupled to its associated G protein (Fig. 3). This "agonist affinity" effect is readily monitored in vitro.

Examples of the guanine nucleotide effect on agonist binding to a variety of G-protein-coupled receptors are provided in Fig. 5. In each case, the binding of a tritiated agonist to the receptor was measured in the presence of varying concentrations of 5′-guanylylimidodiphosphate (Gpp(NH)p), a stable analogue of GTP. As

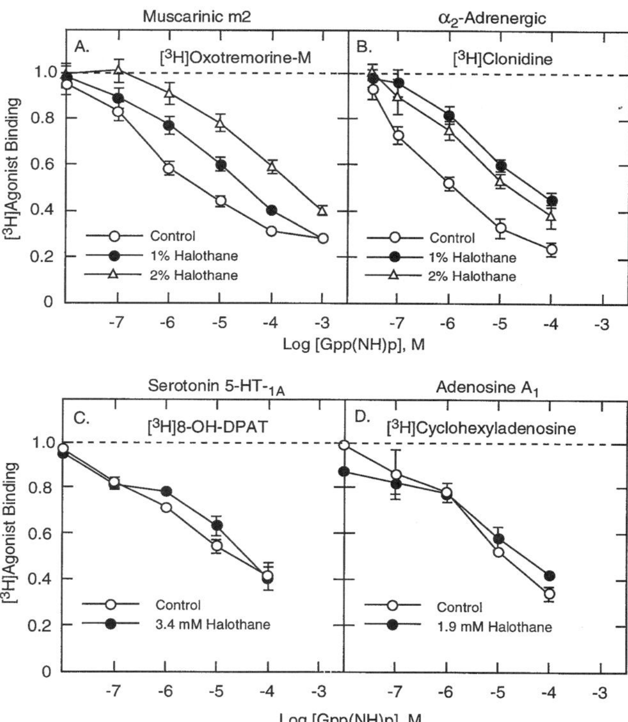

Figure 5. Influence of halothane on receptor–G-protein coupling of a variety of neurotransmitter receptors coupled to pertussis toxin–sensitive G proteins (especially G_i and G_o). The radiolabeled agonist/receptor combinations were as follows: (1) [^{3}H]oxotremorine-M and m_2-muscarinic receptors from rat atrium **(A)**, (2) [^{3}H]clonidine and α_2-adrenergic receptors in rat cerebral cortex **(B)**, (3) [^{3}H]8-hydroxy-dipropylaminotetralin ([^{3}H]8-OH-DPAT) and serotonin 5-HT_{1A} receptors from rat hippocampus **(C)**, and (4) [^{3}H]cyclohexyladenosine and adenosine-A_1 receptors from rat forebrain **(D)**. Binding was measured by filtration after an incubation at room temperature. In the presence of Gpp(NH)p, a stable analogue of GTP, [^{3}H]agonist binding decreased. This decrease reflects uncoupling of receptor and G protein: receptor–G protein complexes have a higher affinity for agonists than uncoupled receptors. Halothane decreased the sensitivity of m_2-muscarinic and α_2-adrenergic receptors to Gpp(NH)p. Although apparently coupled to the same G proteins, 5-HT_{1A} and A_1-receptors were not affected by halothane. At the same concentrations, halothane decreased muscarinic stimulation of G-protein–GTPase activity (see Fig. 6), but not muscarinic stimulation of guanine nucleotide binding. These findings indicate that halothane disrupts m_2-muscarinic and α_2-adrenergic receptor–G-protein cycles, perhaps by preventing GDP release from the α subunit or by stabilizing receptor–G-protein complexes by some other means. Binding is expressed as fraction of total specific binding measured in the absence of guanine nucleotide. (Data are from refs. 10 and 46, and Aronstam et al., *unpublished data.*)

the concentration of Gpp(NH)p increased, [^{3}H]agonist binding decreased. This reflects a guanine nucleotide-induced decrease in agonist affinity; in the presence of guanine nucleotide the receptor and G-protein complexes dissociate and the receptor assumes a conformation characterized by low affinity for agonists (low affinity [^{3}H]agonist binding would not be detected in the experiments depicted in Fig. 5). In the presence of halothane, the ability of Gpp(NH)p to decrease agonist binding to m_2-muscarinic receptors from rat atrium and α_2-adrenergic receptors from rat brain was depressed; higher concentrations of Gpp(NH)p were required to depress [^{3}H]agonist binding (10). This ability to disrupt muscarinic receptor–G proteins was a general phenomenon shared by all liquid volatile anesthetics examined, including halothane, isoflurane, enflurane, chloroform, and diethyl ether (2,4).

Note, however, that not all receptors examined displayed a sensitivity to guanine nucleotides (Fig. 5). Thus, the Gpp(NH)p sensitivity of [^{3}H]agonist binding to 5-HT_{1A} receptors from rat hippocampus and adenosine A_1 receptors from rat forebrain was not affected by high concentrations of halothane (46). These findings are all the more unexpected since each of the receptors depicted in Fig. 5 is coupled via a pertussis toxin–sensitive G_i protein to an inhibition of adenylate cyclase activity. Thus, the source of this differential sensitivity is not clear, but appears to reside in the receptor itself.

The suppression of the guanine nucleotide effect on agonist binding suggests a stabilization of receptor–G-protein complexes. Possible explanations for this effect include (a) an inhibition of GDP dissociation from the α subunit, (b) an inhibition of GTP binding to the α subunit, and (c) a failure of the receptor–G-protein complex to dissociate in the face of GTP binding. These possibilities require separate evaluation of each step of the G-protein cycle (Fig. 3). One such study is summarized in Fig. 6 (Aronstam, Dennison and Martin, *unpublished data*). Acetylcholine stimulation of G-protein–GTPase activity was monitored in membranes isolated from rat atrium as an indication of turnover of the G-protein cycle. Acetylcholine activation of cardiac M2-muscarinic receptors caused an increase in low K_M GTPase activity; activity increased by up to 90% with an EC_{50} of ≈ 3 μM (Fig. 6). This increase was completely blocked by 10 μM atropine. Halothane decreased basal GTPase activity measured in the absence of acetylcholine slightly (5–10%), but completely eliminated acetylcholine stimulation of G-protein–GTPase activity with an IC_{50} of ≈ 0.3 mM, a concentration well within anesthetic ranges expected to be achieved during routine clinical use. While this provides powerful evidence for anesthetic disruption of muscarinic signaling in this tissue, the precise site of the inhibition has yet to be determined.

The functional significance of these effects is indicated by anesthetic inhibition of muscarinic control of (a) Ca^{2+} responses in *Xenopus* oocytes expressing muscarinic receptors (21,41), and (b) forskolin- and isoproterenol-stimulated adenylate cyclase activity (3,55). In the latter studies, anesthetics did not affect basal effector activity or isoproterenol-stimulation of adenylate cyclase. Isoproterenol stimulation of adenylate cyclase is mediated by G_s, again indicating that not all receptor–G-protein interactions are affected by volatile anesthetics. In contrast, Sanuki et al. (72) found that sevoflurane depressed stimulation of cAMP production by isoproterenol and GTP-γ-S, but not forskolin, in rat myocardial membranes. Moreover, sevoflurane also affected ligand binding in a manner that suggested anesthetic actions on both the receptor and receptor–G-protein coupling.

Bohm et al. (13,14) found that halothane increased isoprenaline-, NaF-, cholera toxin-, and Gpp(NH)p-stimulated adenylate cyclase in human myocardial membranes. Forskolin stimulation of cyclase activity was not affected, and halothane's action was eliminated by treatment with pertussis toxin. Pertussis toxin alone increased adenylate cyclase activity 40%, presumably due to a release from a tonic inhibitory control exercised by $G_{i\alpha}$. The magnitude of halothane's effect was greater in tissue from failing human heart, which had a greater content of Gi, leading to the suggestion that halothane's actions reflected an impairment of $G_{i\alpha}$ function.

Puig et al. (63) found that pertussis toxin decreased the ability of halothane to depress electrically induced contractions of guinea pig ileum, and concluded that the contractile effects of halothane involved a pertussis toxin–sensitive G protein.

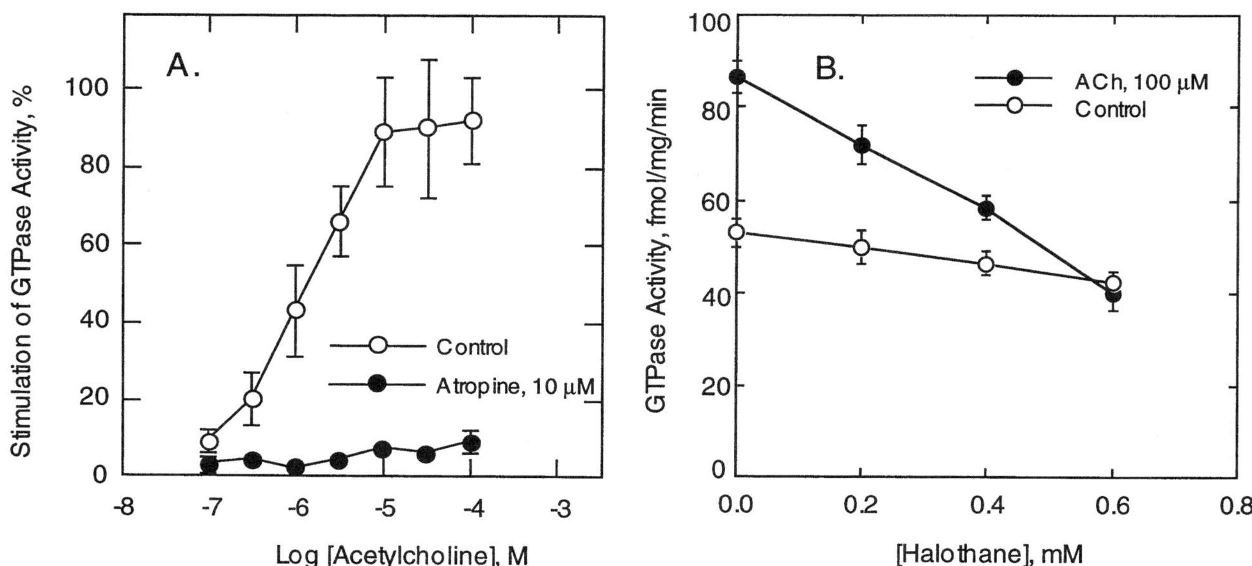

Figure 6. Influence of halothane on muscarinic receptor–stimulated G-protein–GTPase activity in rat atrium. Acetylcholine stimulated low K_M GTPase activity in atrial membranes (m_2-muscarinic receptors) by up to 90% with an EC_{50} of ≈ 3 μM **(A)**. GTPase activity was measured after incubation of 10 μg atrial membrane protein at 37°C for 10 minutes. Acetylcholine stimulation of GTPase activity was completely blocked by 10 μM atropine. Halothane inhibited acetylcholine-stimulated activity (without affecting basal GTPase activity) with an IC_{50} of less than 0.4 mM **(B)**.)Data are from Aronstam and Dennison, *unpublished.*)

However, a number of authors have reported results that are not consistent with the notion of anesthetic disruption of receptor–G-protein interactions. For example, Seifen et al. (75) found that halothane, isoflurane, and enflurane did not affect the inotropic and chronotropic effects of norepinephrine and acetylcholine in isolated guinea pig atria. Similarly, Morimoto et al. (53) found that treatment with pertussis toxin did not affect halothane relaxation of airway smooth muscle precontracted with acetylcholine, and concluded that halothane did not affect pertussis toxin–sensitive G proteins.

Vulliemoz et al. (89) found that halothane decreased the cAMP and increased the cGMP content of mouse ventricular myocardium. Atropine had no effect on these anesthetic actions, indicating that they were not mediated by muscarinic receptors. Pertussis toxin, however, eliminated halothane's increase in cGMP (88). Vulliemoz (87) also found that, while both halothane and acetylcholine decreased the contractile force of rat heart left papillary muscle and atrium, pretreatment with pertussis toxin selectively abolished the myocardial depressant effect of muscarinic agonists without affecting the depression caused by halothane. These results indicate that volatile anesthetic depression of the myocardium does not involve a functional, pertussis toxin–sensitive G protein, but rather a pathway that is distinct from that utilized by muscarinic agonists.

A few studies have raised the possibility that volatile anesthetics modulate the signaling mediated by the pertussis toxin–insensitive G proteins of the G_q family. Lin et al. (41) found that enflurane inhibited the ion channels activated by phosphatidylinositol-linked acetylcholine (M1) and serotonin receptors expressed in *Xenopus* oocytes. Enflurane suppressed the currents activated by injected guanine nucleotide, but not inositol triphosphate, indicating a selective effect on G-protein activity. Rooney et al. (70) reported that halothane activated phospholipase C activity in turkey erythrocyte membranes; this activation required guanine nucleotide. The authors suggested that anesthetics modify the responsiveness of this system to receptor agonists.

It is interesting, although not surprising, that anesthetics and ethanol have many of the same effects on G-protein–mediated signal transduction processes. Several studies have implicated guanine nucleotide–dependent transducer proteins (G proteins) in the actions of ethanol. Ethanol increases the activation of adenylate cyclase by G_s (45,65). Hoffman and Tabakoff (32) proposed that ethanol selectively enhances the rate of activation of G_s (an action that is normally catalyzed by an interaction with receptors), as well as the interaction of $G_{\alpha s}$ with guanine nucleotides. Bauché et al. (9) have presented evidence that ethanol also disrupts G_i-mediated control of adenylate cyclase in rat brain, and Charness et al. (20) have demonstrated differential regulation by ethanol of the expression of both $G_{i\alpha}$ and $G_{s\alpha}$ in several neuronal cell lines.

We have demonstrated that ethanol diminishes the guanine nucleotide sensitivity of agonist binding to muscarinic receptors at concentrations as low as 25 mM (7). This effect was seen in both carbamylcholine/[^{3}H]*N*-methylscopolamine competition curves and in direct measurements of high-affinity [^{3}H]oxotremorine-M binding. At the same concentrations, ethanol depressed muscarinic stimulation of G-protein–GTPase activity and GTP binding to striatal membranes, two measures of G-protein cycle activity (Aronstam et al., *unpublished data*).

SUMMARY

Anesthetics globally depress synaptic transmission in the central nervous system. Insofar as signaling at the majority of neurotransmitter receptor is mediated by transducer G proteins, G-protein systems are a logical site of action for anesthetic action. Interference with receptor–G-protein coupling has been demonstrated in certain systems but not in others. Variable direct effects of anesthetics on both receptors or effector structures have also been reported, although certain of these effects may reflect actions on G-protein–receptor or G-protein–effector interactions. The existence of multiple receptor subtypes, G proteins (α and $\beta\gamma$ subunits), and effector structures is likely to underlie some of this variability. The situation calls for a more complete analysis of anesthetic action on each transmitter system, as well as on the partial reactions of the G-protein cycle.

ACKNOWLEDGMENTS

The preparation of this chapter was supported by PHS grants GM-46408 and NS-25296, the Department of the Army grant number DAMD17-94-J-4011, and the Research Service of the Veterans Administration.

REFERENCES

1. Amatruda TT, Steele DA, Slepak VZ, Simon MI. $G_{\alpha 16}$, a G protein α subunit specifically expressed in hematopoietic cells. *Proc Natl Acad Sci USA* 1991;88:5587–5591.
2. Anthony BL, Dennison RL, Aronstam RS. Disruption of muscarinic receptor-G protein coupling is a general property of liquid volatile anesthetics. *Neurosci Lett* 1989;99:191–196.
3. Anthony BL, Dennison RL, Aronstam RS. Influence of volatile anesthetics on muscarinic regulation of adenylate cyclase activity. *Biochem Pharmacol* 1990;40:376–379.
4. Anthony BL, Dennison RL, Narayanan TK, Aronstam RS. Diethyl ether effects on muscarinic acetylcholine receptor complexes in rat brainstem. *Biochem Pharmacol* 1988;37:4041–4046.
5. Aronstam RS, Anthony BL, Dennison RL. Halothane effects on muscarinic acetylcholine receptor complexes in rat brain. *Biochem Pharmacol* 1986;35:667–672.
6. Aronstam RA, Dennison RL. Anesthetic effects on muscarinic signal; transduction. *Int Anesth Clin* 1989;27:265–272.
7. Aronstam RS, Dennison RL, Martin DC, Ravindra R. Ethanol disruption of muscarinic acetylcholine receptor-G protein interactions in rat brainstem revealed by ligand binding measurements. *Neurosci Res Commun* 1993;12:175–182.
8. Axelrod J. Phospholipase A_2 and G proteins. *Trends Neurosci* 1995; 18:64–65.
9. Bauché F, Bourdeaux-Jaubert AM, Giudicelli Y, Nordmann R. Ethanol alters the adenosine receptor-*Ni*-mediated adenylate cyclase inhibitory response in rat brain cortex in vitro. *FEBS Lett* 1987;219:296–300.
10. Baumgartner MK, Dennison RL, Narayanan TK, Aronstam RS. Halothane disruption of α_2-adrenergic receptor-mediated inhibition of adenylate cyclase and receptor G-protein coupling in rat brain. *Biochem Pharmacol* 1990;39:223–225.
11. Berstein G, Blank JL, Jhon D-Y, Exton JH, Rhee SG, Ross EM. Phospholipase C-b1 is a GTPase-activating protein for $G_{q/11}$, its physiologic regulator. *Cell* 1992;70:411–418.
12. Birnbaumer L. On the origins and present state of the art of G protein research. *J Receptor Res* 1991;11:577–585.
13. Bohm M, Schmidt U, Gierschick P, Schwinger RH, Bohm S, Erdmann E. Sensitization of adenylate cyclase by halothane in human myocardium and S49 lymphoma wild-type and *cyc-* cells: evidence for inactivation of the inhibitory G protein G_{ia}. *Mol Pharmacol* 1994;45:380–389.
14. Bohm M, Schmidt U, Schwinger RH, Bohm S, Erdmann E. Effects of halothane on β-adrenoceptors and M-cholinoceptors in human myocardium: radioligand binding and functional studies. *J Cardiovasc Pharmacol* 1993;21:296–304.
15. Bourne HR, Sanders DA, McCormick F. The GTPase superfamily: conserved structure and molecular mechanism. *Nature* 1991;349: 117–127.
16. Cassel D, Selinger Z. Mechanism of adenylate cyclase activation by cholera toxin: inhibition of GTP hydrolysis at the regulatory site. *Proc Natl Acad Sci USA* 1977;74:3307–3311.
17. Cassel D, Selinger Z. Catecholamine-stimulated GTPase activity in turkey erythrocyte membranes. *Biochim Biophys Acta* 1978;252: 538–551.
18. Catchlove RFH, Krnjevic K, Maretic H. Similarity between effects of

general anesthetics and dinitrophenol on cortical neurones. *Can J Physiol Pharmacol* 1972;50:1111–1114.
19. Caulfield, MP, Jones S, Vallis Y, Buckley NJ, Kim GD, Milligan G, Brown DA. Muscarinic M-current inhibition via $G_{\alpha q/11}$ and α-adrenoceptor inhibition of Ca^{2+} current via $G_{\alpha o}$ in rat sympathetic neurones. *J Physiol* 1994;477:415–422.
20. Charness ME, Querimit LA, Henteleff M. Ethanol differentially regulates G proteins in neural cells. *Biochem Biophys Res Commun* 1988;155:138–143.
21. Durieux ME, Salafranca MN. Halothane inhibits signaling through m1 muscarinic receptors expresses in *Xenopus* oocytes. *Anesthesiology* 1993;79:A734.
22. Eide B, Giershick P, Milligan G, Mullaney I, Unson C, Goldsmith P, Spiegel A. GTP-binding proteins in brain and neutrophil are tethered to the plasma membrane via their amino termini. *Biochem Biophys Res Commun* 1987;148:1398–1405.
23. Franks NP, Lieb WR. Molecular mechanisms of general anaesthesia. *Nature* 1982;300:487–493.
24. Franks NP, Lieb WR. Mapping of general anaesthetic target sites provides a molecular basis for cutoff effects. *Nature* 1985;316: 349–351.
25. Gilman AG. G proteins: transducers of receptor-generated signals. *Annu Rev Biochem* 1987;56:615–649.
26. Godchaux W, Zimmerman WF. Membrane-dependent guanine nucleotide binding and GTPase activities of soluble protein from bovine rod cell outer segments. *J Biol Chem* 1979;254:7874–7884.
27. Gurevich VV, Dion SB, Onorato JJ, Ptasiewnski J, Kim CM, Sterne-Marr R, Hosey MM, Benovic JL. Arrestin interactions with G protein-coupled receptors: direct binding studies of wild type and mutant arrestins with rhodopsin, β_2-adrenergic, and m2 muscarinic cholinergic receptors. *J Biol Chem* 1995;270:720–731.
28. Harris BA, Robishaw JD, Mumby SM, Gilman AG. Molecular cloning of complementary DNA for the alpha subunit of the G protein that stimulates adenylate cyclase. *Science* 1985;229:1274–1277.
29. Haug A, Shi B, Vitorello V. Aluminum interaction with phosphoinositide-associated signal transduction. *Arch Toxicol* 1994;68:1–7.
30. Higashijima T, Ferguson KM, Sternweis PC, Smigel MD, Gilman AG. Effects of Mg^{2+} and the beta gamma-subunit complex on the interactions of guanine nucleotides with G proteins. *J Biol Chem* 1987;262:762–766.
31. Hille B. Modulation of ion-channel function by G-protein-coupled receptors. *Trends Neurosci* 1994;17:531–536.
32. Hoffman PL, Tabakoff B. Ethanol and guanine nucleotide binding proteins: a selective interaction. *FASEB J* 1990;4:2612–2622.
33. Huff RM, Neer EJ. Subunit interactions of native and ADP-ribosylated alpha 39 and alpha 41, two guanine nucleotide-binding proteins from bovine cerebral cortex. *J Biol Chem* 1986;261:1105–1110.
34. Kaziro Y, Itoh H, Nakafuku M. Organization of genes coding for G protein α subunits in higher and lower eukaryotes. In: Iyengar R, Birnbaumer L, eds. *G proteins.* San Diego: Academic Press, 1990; 63–80.
35. Kim D, Lewis DL, Graziadei L, Neer EJ, Bar-Sagi D, Clapham DE. G-protein βγ-subunits activate the cardiac muscarinic K^+ channel via phospholipase A2. *Nature* 1989;337:557–560.
36. Kleuss C, Hescheler J, Ewel C, Rosenthal W, Schultz G, Wittig B. Assignment of G-protein subtypes to specific receptors inducing inhibition of calcium currents. *Nature* 1992;358:424–426.
37. Krnjevic K, Phillis JW. Acetylcholine-sensitive cells in the cerebral cortex. *J Physiol Lond* 1963;166:296–327.
38. Lambert DG. Signal transduction: G proteins and second messengers. *Br J Anaesth* 1993;71:86–95.
39. Larrabee MG, Posternak JM. Selective action of anesthetics on synapses and axons in mammalian sympathetic ganglia. *J Neurophysiol* 1952;15:91–114.
40. Lefkowitz RJ. Rodbell and Gilman win 1994 Nobel prize for physiology and medicine. *Trends Pharmacol Sci* 1994;15:442–444.
41. Lin LH, Leonard S, Harris A. Enflurane inhibits the function of mouse and human brain phosphatidylinositol-linked acetylcholine and serotonin receptors expressed in *Xenopus* oocytes. *Mol Pharmacol* 1993;43:941–948.
42. Lochrie MA, Hurley JB, Simon MI. Sequence of the α subunit of photoreceptor G protein: homologies between transducin, ras and elongation factors. *Proc Natl Acad Sci USA* 1985;82:96–99.
43. Logothetis De, Kurachi Y, Galper J, Neer EJ, Clapham DE. The βγ subunits of GTP-binding proteins activate the muscarinic K^+ channel in heart. *Nature* 1987;325:321–326.
44. Lohse MJ, Andexinger S, Pitcher J, Trukawinski S, Codina J, Faure J-P, Caron MG, Lefkowitz RJ. Receptor specific desensitization with purified proteins: Kinase dependence and receptor specificity of β-arrestin and arrestin in the β_2-adrenergic receptor and rhodopsin systems. *J Biol Chem* 1992;267:8558–8564.
45. Luthin GR, Tabakoff B. Activation of adenylate cyclase by alcohol requires the nucleotide-binding protein. *J Pharmacol Exp Ther* 1984; 228:579–587.
46. Martin DC, Dennison RL, Introna RPS, Aronstam RS. Influence of halothane on the interactions of $serotonin_{1A}$ and $adenosine_{A1}$ receptors with G proteins in rat brain membranes. *Biochem Pharmacol* 1991;42:1313–1316.
47. Masters SB, Sullivan KA, Miller RT, Beiderman B, Lopez NG, Ramachandran J, Bourne HR. Carboxyl terminal domain of Gsa specifies coupling of receptors to stimulation of adenylyl cyclase. *Science* 1988;241:448–451.
48. Maze, M. Transmembrane signalling and the Holy Grail of anesthesia. *Anesthesiology* 1990;72:959–961.
49. Mazzoni MR, Hamm HE. Effect of monoclonal antibody binding on alpha-beta gamma subunit interactions in the rod outer segment G protein, Gt. *Biochemistry* 1989;28:9873–9880.
50. McLaughlin SK, McKinnon PJ, Margolskee RF. Gustducin is a taste-cell-specific G protein closely related to the transducins. *Nature* 1992;357:563–569.
51. Medynski DC, Sullivan K, Smith D, Van Dop C, Chang FH, Fung BK, Seeburg PH, Bourne HR. Amino acid sequence of the alpha subunit of transducin deduced from the cDNA sequence. *Proc Natl Acad Sci USA* 1985;82:4311–4315.
52. Meyer HH. Zur Theorie Alkoholnarkose I Mitt Welche Eigenschaft der Anesthetika bedingt ihre narkotische Wirkung? *Arch Exp Pathol Pharmacol* 1899;42:109.
53. Morimoto N, Yamamoto K, Jones KA, Warner DO. Halothane and pertussis toxin-sensitive G proteins in airway smooth muscle. *Anesth Analg* 1994;78:328–334.
54. Moss J, Vaughan M. Participation of guanine nucleotide-binding protein cascade in activation of adenylyl cyclase by cholera toxin (choleragen). In: Iyengar R, Birnbaumer L, eds. *G proteins.* San Diego: Academic Press, 1990;179–200.
55. Narayanan TK, Confer RA, Dennison RL, Anthony BL, Aronstam RS. Halothane attenuation of muscarinic inhibition of adenylate cyclase in rat heart. *Biochem Pharmacol* 1988;37:1219–1223.
56. Northup JK, Sternweis PC, Smigel MD, Schleifer LS, Ross EM, Gilman AG. Purification of the regulatory component of adenylate cyclase. *Proc Natl Acad Sci USA* 1980;77:6516–6520.
57. Offermanns S, Schultz G. What are the functions of the pertussis toxin-insensitive G proteins G_{12}, G_{13} and G_z? *Mol Cell Endocrinol* 1994;100:71–74.
58. Okajima F, Katada T, Ui M. Coupling of the guanine nucleotide regulatory protein to chemotactic peptide receptors in neutrophil membranes and its uncoupling by islet-activating protein, pertussis toxin. A possible role of the toxin substrate in Ca^{2+}-mobilizing receptor-mediated signal transduction. *J Biol Chem* 1985;260: 6761–6768.
59. Osawa S, Dhanasekaran N, Woon CW, Johnson GL. $G_{\alpha i}$-$G_{\alpha s}$ chimeras define the function of a chain domains in control of G protein activation and βγ subunit complex interactions. *Cell* 1990; 63:697–706.
60. Overton E. *Studien uber die Narkose zugleich ein Beitrag zur allgemeinen Pharmakologie.* Jena: G Fisher, 1901.
61. Park, D, Jhon DY, Kriz R, Knopf J, Rhee SG. Cloning, sequencing, expression and G_q-independent activation of phospholipase C-β2. *J Biol Chem* 1992;267:16048–16055.
62. Pfeuffer T, Helmreich EJM. Activation of pigeon erythrocyte membrane adenylate cyclase by guanylnucleotide analogs and separation of nucleotide binding protein. *J Biol Chem* 1975;250:867–876.
63. Puig MM, Turndorf H, Warner W. Effect of pertussis toxin on the interaction of azepexole and halothane. *J Pharmacol Exp Ther* 1990; 252:1156–1159.
64. Puil E, El-Beheiry. Anaesthetic suppression of transmitter actions in neocortex. *Br J Pharmacol* 1990;101:61–66.
65. Rabin RA, Molinoff PB. Multiple sites of action of ethanol on adenylate cyclase. *J Pharmacol Exp Ther* 1983;227:551–556.
66. Reuveny E, Slesinger PA, Inglese J, Morales JM, Iñiguez-Lluhi JA, Lefkowitz RJ, Bourne HR, Jan YN, Jan LY. Activation of the cloned muscarinic potassium channel by G protein βγ subunits. *Nature* 1994;370:143–146.

67. Richards CD. Action of general anesthetics on synaptic transmission in the CNS. *Br J Anaesthesiol* 1983;55:201–207.
68. Rodbell M, Birnbaumer L, Pohl SL, Krans HMJ. The glucagon-sensitive adenyl cyclase system in plasma membranes of rat liver. V. An obligatory role of guanyl nucleotides in glucagon action. *J Biol Chem* 1971;246:1877–1812.
69. Rodbell M, Krans HMJ, Pohl SL, Birnbaumer L. The glucagon-sensitive adenyl cyclase system in plasma membranes of rat liver. IV. Binding of glucagon: Effect of guanyl nucleotides. *J Biol Chem* 1971; 246:1872–1876.
70. Rooney TA, Hager R, Stubbs CD, Thomas AP. Halothane regulates G-protein-dependent phospholipase C activity in turkey erythrocyte membranes. *J Biol Chem* 1993;268:15550–15556.
71. Roth SH. Physical mechanisms of anesthesia. *Annu Rev Pharmacol Toxicol* 1979;19:159–178.
72. Sanuki M, Yuge O, Kawamoto M, Fuji K, Azuma T. Sevoflurane inhibited β-adrenoceptor-G protein bindings in myocardial membrane in rats. *Anesth Analg* 1994;79:466–471.
73. Savola MK, MacIver MB, Doze VA, Kendig JJ, Maze M. The α_2-adrenoceptor agonist dexmedetomidine increases the apparent potency of the volatile anesthetic isoflurane in rats in vivo and in hippocampal slice in vitro. *Brain Res* 1991;548:23–28.
74. Segal IS, Walton JK, Irwin I, DeLanney LE, Ricaurte GA, Langston JW, Maze M. Modulating role of dopamine on anesthetic requirements. *Eur J Pharmacol* 1990;186:9–15.
75. Seifen AB, Kennedy RH, Seifen E. Effects of volatile anesthetics on response to norepinephrine and acetylcholine in guinea pig atria. *Anesth Analg* 1991;73:304–309.
76. Simon MI, Strathmann MP, Gautam N. Diversity of G proteins in signal transduction. *Science* 1991;252:802–808.
77. Sowton SCM, Sherrington CS. On the relative effects of chloroform upon the heart and other muscular organs. *Br Med J* 1905;2: 181.
78. Spiegel AM. Immunologic probes for heterotrimeric GTP-binding proteins. In: Iyengar R, Birnbaumer L, eds. *G proteins.* San Diego: Academic Press, 1990;115–143.
79. Sternweis PC. The purified α subunits of Go and Gi from bovine brain require βγ for association with phospholipid vesicles. *J Biol Chem* 1986;261:631–637.
80. Sternweis PC, Gilman AG. Aluminum: a requirement for activation of the regulatory component of adenylate cyclase by fluoride. *Proc Natl Acad Sci USA* 1982;79:4888–4891.
81. Sternweis PC, Northup JK, Smigel MD, Gilman AG. The regulatory component of adenylate cyclase. *J Biol Chem* 1981;256:11517–11526.
82. Sullivan KA, Miller RT, Masters SB, Beiderman B, Heideman W, Bourne HR. Identification of receptor contact site involved in receptor-G protein coupling. *Nature* 1987;330:758–760.
83. Stryer L. Cyclic GMP cascade of vision. *Annu Rev Neurosci* 1986;9: 87–119.
84. Tanabe T, Nukada T, Nishikawa Y, Sugimoto K, Suzuki H, Takahashi H, Noda M, Haga T, Ichiyama A, Kangawa K, Minamoto N, Matsuo H, Numa S. Primary structure of the alpha-subunit of transducin and its relationship to *ras* proteins. *Nature* 1985;315:242–245.
85. Tang W-J, Iñiguez-Lluhi JA, Mumby S, Gilman AG. Regulation of mammalian adenylyl cyclases by G-protein α and βγ subunits. *Cold Spring Harb Symp Quant Biol* 1992;57:135–144.
86. Taussig R, Gilman AG. Mammalian membrane-bound adenylyl cyclases. *J Biol Chem* 1995;270:1–4.
87. Vulliemoz Y. The myocardial depressant effect of volatile anesthetics does not involve arachidonic acid metabolites or pertussis toxin-sensitive G proteins. *Eur J Pharmacol* 1990;203:345–351.
88. Vulliemoz Y, Verosky M. Halothane interaction with guanine nucleotide binding proteins in mouse heart. *Anesthesiology* 1988;69: 876–880.
89. Vulliemoz Y, Verosky M, Triner L. Effect of halothane on myocardial cyclic AMP and cyclic GMP content of mice. *J Pharmacol Exp Ther* 1986;236:181–186.
90. Wagner ACC, Williams JA. Low molecular weight GTP-binding proteins: molecular switches regulating diverse cellular functions. *Am J Physiol* 1994;266:G1–G14.
91. Watson S, Arkinsall S. *The G-protein linked receptor facts book.* San Diego: Academic Press, 1994.
92. Wilkie TM, Scherle PA, Strathmann MP, Slepak VZ, Simon MI. Characterization of G-protein alpha subunits in the Gq class: expression in murine tissues and in stromal and hematopoietic cell lines. *Proc Natl Acad Sci USA* 1991;88:10049–10053.
93. Yatsunami K, Khorana HG. GTPase of bovine rod outer segments: the amino acid sequence of the α subunit as derived from the cDNA sequence. *Proc Natl Acad Sci USA* 1985;82:4316–4320.
94. Yost CS. G proteins: basic characteristics and clinical potential for the practice of anesthesia. *Anesth Analg* 1993;77:822–834.
95. Zhu Y, Ikeda SR. VIP inhibits N-type Ca^{2+} channels of sympathetic neurons via a pertussis toxin-insensitive but cholera toxin-sensitive pathway. *Neuron* 1994;13:657–669.

Anesthesia: Biologic Foundations, edited by
Tony L. Yaksh et al. Lippincott–Raven Publishers,
Philadelphia © 1997.

CHAPTER 5

G PROTEIN–COUPLED RECEPTORS

MERVYN MAZE AND ANN BUTTERMANN

G protein-coupled receptors (GPCRs) recognize and process multiple external (e.g., photons of light, odorant, and taste molecules) and internal (e.g., catecholamines, acetylcholine, neurokinins) signals. The activated GPCRs couple to a wide variety of G proteins, which in turn alter the activity of several effector mechanisms (31) (Table 1). Despite the diverse ligands that bind to these receptors and the diverse cellular events that they produce, there is a high degree of sequence homology (approximately 20%) in the receptors themselves. The conservation of the primary structure among GPCRs permitted isolation of new cDNA and genomic clones by cross-hybridization (see Chap. 22) and the polymerase chain reaction (PCR) methods. A recent estimate suggests that there are more than 400 GPCRs that have been isolated and cloned (2). Among the GPCRs that are particularly important for anesthesiologists are all the receptors involved in transducing the function of the autonomic nervous system, receptors for transducing the action of opiate narcotics, adenosine compounds, serotonin compounds, and α_2-adrenergic agonists. This chapter addresses the structure, function, and regulation of this important class of proteins.

STRUCTURE

Several predictive techniques have been developed to derive secondary structures of proteins from their amino acid sequence. Among these is the analysis of hydrophobicity of the different regions, which can be quantified easily (29) (Fig. 1). Such analysis of GPCRs has shown that they are characterized by seven hydrophobic domains, each composed of 20 to 30 amino acids, of sufficient length to span the lipid bilayer (Fig. 1). These putative transmembrane domains exhibit more homology across the GPCRs than the intervening hydrophilic loops, which are exposed intra- and extracellularly.

Detailed comparison of the GPCRs reveals that they share a number of conserved residues in the transmembrane domains. The strictly conserved residues probably play an essential role in maintaining the structure of the protein, while those residues conserved only among major classes of receptors may determine their unique functional properties (1). The amino-terminus of the polypeptide is extracellular and contains probable sites for N-linked glycosylation, while the carboxy terminus is intracellular. The glycosylation sites on the amino terminus are variable and are not found on analogous α_2-adrenergic receptor subtypes in either humans (52) or rats (53). On the carboxy terminus there are consensus sequences for phosphorylation, which are important for functional regulation (see below).

The tertiary structure of GPCRs has proven insoluble because of the difficulty in extracting large amounts of pure protein from the natural membranes for crystallography studies. In the absence of biophysical analysis, structural models have been devised, based largely on the folding pattern of the ancient retinal-linked visual pigment bacteriorhodopsin (24). This proton pump is found in large amounts in naturally occurring lattices within the purple membrane of *Halobacterium halobium.* Although bacteriorhodopsin is not coupled to G proteins, it is similar to the opsin family (e.g., rhodopsin) since both have a covalently linked retinal chromophore that undergoes photoisomerization to initiate either proton pump action (in the case of bacteriorhodopsin) or signal transduction (in the case of rhodopsin). The first structural studies of bacteriorhodopsin utilized electron diffraction to determine the orientation of the transmembrane regions (24). Using this method investigators showed that bacteriorhodopsin has seven α-helices arranged in a bundle perpendicular to the plane of the lipid bilayer (50) (Fig. 2). This characteristic feature of seven transmembrane helices is used as a scaffold for molecular modeling of the GPCRs. Subsequently, a higher resolution structural study, to a level of 3.5Å, was achieved with electron cryomicroscopy resolution. This method refined the orientation of the helices and the position of the chromophore on the protein (23). Yet, there is less than 10% sequence homology between bacteriorhodopsin and eukaryotic GPCRs, except in models in which the sequence ordering of the helices is permitted to vary (35). Therefore, it has proven difficult to precisely identify the ends of the helices and the beginnings of the more variable hydrophilic loop regions, except where charged and polar residues signal the change from the membrane-buried portion to the hydrophilic loop structure. Another method by which one can predict where the α-helix exits the membrane involves detection of a region in the lipid-facing side of the helix that has no charged residues in any of the available sequences (11). The point at which charged residues can be accommodated on this face of the helix indicates the point at which the external face reaches a polar, extramembrane environment.

Mammalian visual pigments (the opsin family) were the first GPCRs for which sequence data were obtained (21). These proteins, which also are retinal bound, have been the only GPCR for which structural information (but only to a 9Å level) is available because large quantities are present in the retina; therefore, it is relatively easy to purify and examine the protein in its membranous state using small-angle x-ray diffraction, circular dichroism, polarized infrared spectroscopy, and Raman spectroscopy (41). From the projection maps derived using these techniques (Fig. 3), four peaks have been resolved, probably corresponding to helices IV, V, VI, and VII, which are approximately perpendicular to the membrane. A further arc-shaped feature appears to be the density created from three tilted helices (helices I, II, and III) that overlap in the projection maps.

Perhaps the most widely cited structural model of GPCRs is the Baldwin model, based on the structural details that emerged from bovine rhodopsin data (3). The sequential arrangement of the helices in this model of rhodopsin is based on the fact that in one or more of the GPCRs, each of the interhelical hydrophilic loops is too short to permit any other arrangement. Thus, each helix is thought to be next to those closest to it in the amino acid sequence. The rotation of each of the helices in Baldwin's model is based on the theory that conserved, hydrophilic residues are likely to face inward toward the other transmembrane domains. This theory has been bolstered by a plethora of site-directed mutagenesis data (4) that show that the important residues for binding and activation are on the inner face of the helix. A pivotal but until recently untested

Table 1. SELECTED G PROTEIN–COUPLED SYSTEMS[a]

Ligand	Receptor	Subtypes	G protein	Effector mechanism	Second messenger effects
Catecholamines	β-adrenergic	(3)	→G_s→	↑AC activity	↑cAMP protein phosphorylation
Norepinephrine	α_1-adrenergic	(3)	→G_q→	↑PLC activity	↑IP_3, DAG Ca release
Epinephrine	α_2-adrenergic	(3)	→G_i→	↓AC, ↓Ca, and ↑K channel	↓cAMP hyperpolarization, ↓[Ca],
Dopamine	$D_{1,5}$	(5)	→G_s→	↑AC activity	↑cAMP protein phosphorylation
	$D_{2,3,4}$		→G_i→	↓AC, ↑K channel	↓cAMP, hyperpolarization
Acetylcholine	$M_{2,4}$	(5)	→$G_{i,o}$→	↓AC, ↑K channel	↓cAMP, hyperpolarization
(muscarinic)[b]			→G_q→	↑PLC activity, ↑AC activity	↑IP_3, DAG Ca release
Serotonin (5-HT)[b]	5-$HT_{1A,1B,1D}$	(8)	→G_i→	↓AC activity and ↑K channel	↓cAMP, hyperpolarization
	5-$HT_{2,1c}$		→G_q→	↑PLC activity	↑IP_3, DAG Ca release
	5-HT_4		→G_s→	↑AC activity	↑cAMP protein phosphorylation
Histamine	H1	(3)	→$G_?$→	↑PLC activity	↑IP_3, DAG Ca release
	H2		→G_s→	↑AC activity	↑cAMP protein phosphorylation
ATP (P2 purinergic)[b]	P_{2y}	(?1)	→G_q→	↑PLC activity	↑IP_3, DAG Ca release
Adenosine					
(P1 purinergic)	$A_{1,3}$	(4)	→G_i→	↓AC activity and ↑K channel	↓cAMP hyperpolarization
	$A2_{a,b}$		→G_s→	↑AC activity	↑cAMP protein phosphorylation
γ-aminobutyric acid[b]	$GABA_B$	(1)	→G_i→	↓AC, ↓Ca, and ↑K channel	↓cAMP hyperpolarization, ↓[Ca],
Opioid	μ, σ, δ	(≥3)	→$G_{o,i}$→	↓Ca and ↑K channel	↓cAMP hyperpolarization, ↓[Ca],
Somatostatin	SST	(?1)	→G_i→	↓AC, ↓Ca, and ↑K channel	↓cAMP hyperpolarization, ↓[Ca],
Cannabinoid		(?1)	→G_i→	↓AC activity	↓cAMP
Bombesin (GRP)		(?1)	→G_q→	↑PLC activity	↑IP_3, DAG Ca release
Bradykinin	$B_{1,2,3}$	(3)	→G_q→	↑PLC activity	↑IP_3, DAG Ca release
Vasopressin,	$V_{1A,\ 1B}$OT	(4)	→G_q→	↑PLC activity	↑IP_3, DAG Ca release
oxytocin	V_2		→G_s→	↑AC activity	↑cAMP protein phosphorylation
Angiotensin II	AT1	(2)	→$G_{i,q}$→	↑PLC activity, ↓AC activity	↑IP_3, DAG ↓cAMP Ca release
Prostanoid	D, E_2, prostacyclin	(?5)	→G_s→	↑AC activity	↑cAMP protein phosphorylation
	$E_{1,3}$ F, thromboxane		→$G_{i,q}$→	↑PLC activity, ↓AC activity	↑IP_3, DAG Ca release
Leukotriene	LT	(?3)	→G_q→	↑PLC activity	↑IP_3, DAG Ca release
PAF		(?1)	→G_q→	↑PLC activity	↑IP_3, DAG Ca release
Endothelin	ET_A, ET_B	(≥2)	→G_q→	↑PLC, PLA_2 activity	↑IP_3, DAG, AA Ca release
Tachykinins[c]	$NK_{1,2,3}$	(3)	→G_q→	↑PLC activity	↑IP_3, DAG Ca release
Chemotactic factors	C5a, fMLP, lgE	(≥4)	→$G_{i,q}$→	↑PLC activity	↑IP_3, DAG Ca release
Neuropeptides	NPY, neurotensin	(2)	→$G_{i,q}$→	↑PLC activity, ↓AC activity	↑IP_3, DAG, ↓cAMP Ca release
Anterior pituitary glycopeptide hormones	Thyrotropin (TSH), LH/CG; FSH	(3)	→G_s→	↑AC activity	↑cAMP protein phosphorylation
Hypothalamic releasing factors	GnRF, TRF	(?3)	→G_i→	↑PLC activity	↑IP_3, DAG Ca release
	CRF		→G_s→	↑AC activity	↑cAMP protein phosphorylation
CCK and gastrin	$CCK_{A,B}$	(2)	→G_q→	↑PLC activity	↑IP_3, DAG Ca release
Thrombin	Thrombin	(?1)	→$G_{i,?q}$→	↓AC activity, ↑PLC activity	↓cAMP, ↑IP_3, DAG
Light	Rhodopsin	(2)	→G_t→	↑phosphodiesterase activity	↓cGMP closed cation channel
Taste	Taste receptors	(?)	→G_g→	?↑phosphodiesterase activity	?↓cAMP closed cation channel
Odorant molecules	Odorant receptor	(?100s)	→G_{olf}→	↑AC activity	↑cAMP open cation channel
Glutamate	$mGIR_{1\alpha,\beta,\gamma,5}$	(8)	→$G_{q,s}$→	↑PLD activity, ↑AC activity	↑ DAG, ↑cAMP Ca release
(metabotropic)[b,d]	$mGIR_{2,3,4,6}$		→G_i→	↓AC, ↓Ca, and ↑K channel	↓cAMP, hyperpolarization, ↓[Ca],
Peptide hormones[d]	VIP, secretin, calcitonin parathyroid hormone, glucagon, PACAP		→G_s→	↑AC activity	↑cAMP protein phosphorylation

AA, arachidonic acid metabolites; AC, adenylate cyclase; cAMP, cyclic 3′ 5′-adenosine monophosphate; CCK, cholecystokinin; DAG, diacyglycerol; fMLP, N-formyl-Met-Leu-Phe; GRP, gastrin-releasing peptide; IP_3, inositol 1,4,5-trisphosphate; PACAP, pituitary adenylyl cyclase–activating polypeptide; PAI, platelet-activating factor; PDE, phosphodiesterase; PL, phospholipase (A_2, C, or D); VIP, vasoactive intestinal peptide.

[a]The ligands and receptors listed represent a partial list of those clearly identified as mediated by G proteins. The receptors listed are those that have been either cloned or clearly defined as G-protein linked using pertussis toxin or nonhydrolyzable guanosine triphosphate analogues. In the latter case, receptor sybtypes have been defined by pharmacologic agents.

[b]Acetycholine (ACh), serotonin, glutamate, γ-aminobutyric acid, and adenosine triphosphate (ATP) have both ligand-gated channel receptors in addition to these G protein–linked receptors. The nicotinic ligand-gated channel is typically excitatory. The 5-HT_4 and ATP ligand-gated receptors are nonspecific (typically excitatory) ion channels. Glutamate activates *N*-methyl-D-aspartate (NMDA) receptors, which permits depolarizing cation entry. Like $GABA_B$ (G protein linked), the $GABA_A$ (ligand-gated) receptors are also inhibitory.

[c]Tachykinins include substance P, substance K, neurokinin B (neuromedin K).

[d]While sharing the apparent seven hydrophobic domain transmembrane structure, the metabotrobic glutamate and peptide hormone receptors share no apparent homology with the other G protein–linked receptors and appear to represent separate families.

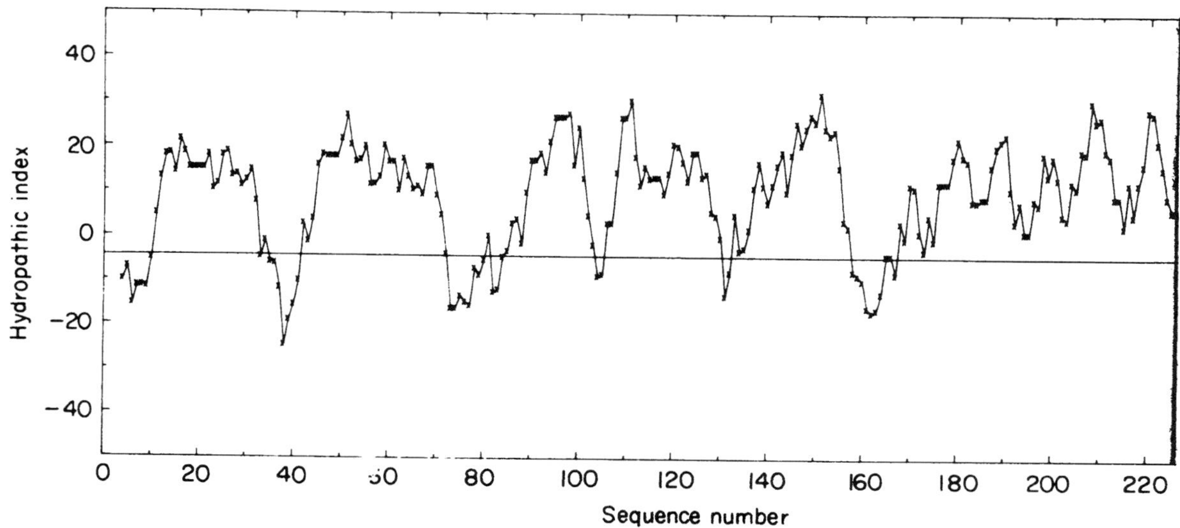

Figure 1. Kyte-Doolittle hydropathy plot of bacteriorhodopsin. Using a moving segment approach, the protein has been progressively evaluated for the hydophilicity and hydrophobicity of its residue side chains. The portions of the sequence that are located on the hydrophobic side of the midpoint line are located within the lipid bilayer. (From ref. 29, with permission.)

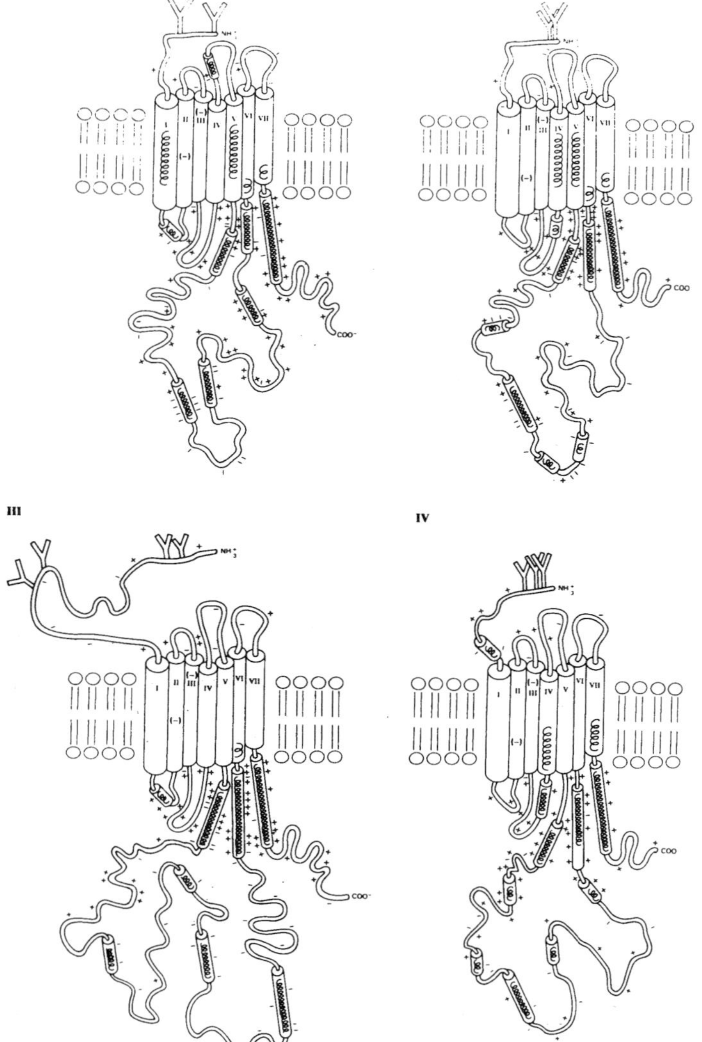

Figure 2. Models of the rat muscarinic receptors M_1 (I), M_2 (II), M_3 (III), and M_4 (IV). (From ref. 50, with permission.)

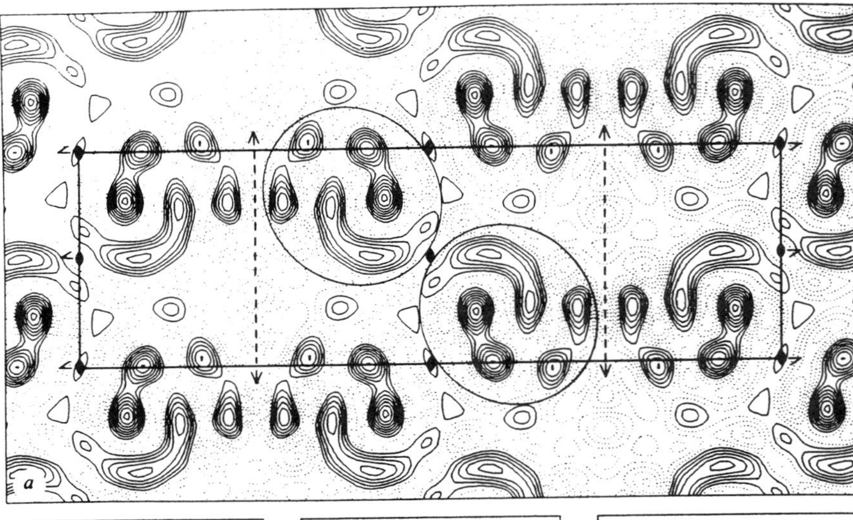

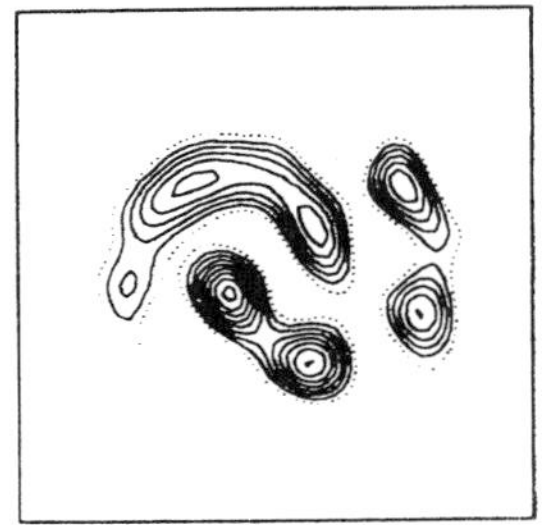

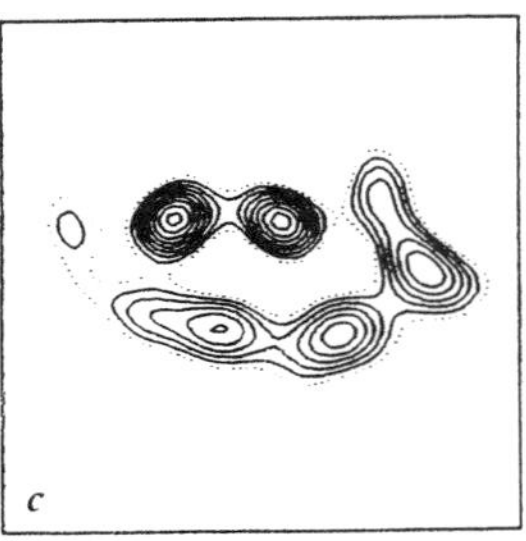

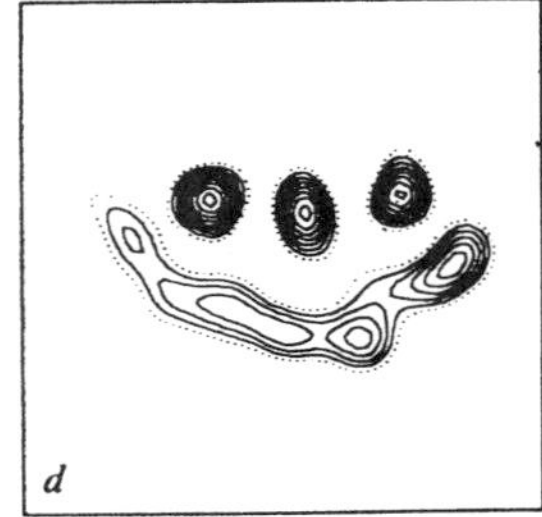

Figure 3. Projection density maps of rhodopsin at 9 Å resolution. **A:** Calculated from merged and corrected image amplitudes and phases obtained from 13 independent crystalline areas. **B–D:** The density for a single rhodopsin molecule with negative contours omitted and the zero contour represented by a *dotted line.* (From ref. 41, with permission.)

feature of the model is the orientation of the bundle of helices in a clockwise direction when viewed from the inside of the cell. This prediction has now been borne out by recent experiments (34). Structural information regarding the hydrophilic loops is totally lacking, however.

STRUCTURE FUNCTION RELATIONSHIPS

Keeping in mind that receptors of this GPCR superfamily bind different ligands and interact with different G proteins, the following set of general principles governs how ligands are bound, how agonists activate a receptor, and how receptors interact with G proteins.

Binding of Ligands to GPCR

Experiments designed to demonstrate which sites in the receptor structure contribute to its ligand-binding properties often involve site-directed mutagenesis. For antagonists, changes in binding affinity after site-directed mutagenesis usually are due to alterations in the ligand-binding pocket while changes in binding affinity for agonists can involve both alterations in the ligand-binding pocket as well as alterations in the equilibrium between the high- and low-affinity states of the receptor (38). A rule of thumb from site-directed mutagenesis studies suggests that small ligands bind in a pocket located in the extracellular half of the transmembrane domain formed by the helical bundle. Also, nearly all the sites that have been identified as modulating ligand binding lie in the lower two thirds of the membrane and point inward toward the other helices. With the exception of helix I, all helices appear to contribute to the ligand-binding site with strong involvement of helices III, V, VI, and VII and a smaller contribution from IV and II (4).

Rhodopsin contains a retinal chromophore covalently attached via a Schiff base formed between the aldehyde group of retinal and the ε-amino group in the side chain of Lys296 in helix VII of rhodopsin (26). On exposure to photons of light, the covalently bound retinal undergoes a conversion from the 9-*cis* to the all-*trans* conformation. In this manner the bound light-activated retinal can be considered the agonist. It is buried in rhodopsin at a depth of 22Å into the membrane bilayer (48).

For catecholamines (and most of the other ligands), the membrane-spanning domains are critical since binding of neither agonists nor antagonists is affected following deletion of the extracellular and cytoplasmic loops of the β-adrenoceptor (9). Furthermore, there is now physical evidence obtained with the fluorescent ligand carazolol (antagonist at the β-adrenergic receptor) that the binding site is within the membrane and is more than 11Å from the surface (49).

Pharmacophore analysis of biogenic amines (32) demonstrates that the basic amine moiety is the source of much of the binding energy of these compounds. An acidic group in the binding pocket provides a counterion for the protonated amine of the ligand. This salt bridge can provide up to 10 kcal/mol of binding energy within an essentially hydrophobic environment. The β-hydroxyl group of epinephrine and norepinephrine is important for stereoselective binding of agonists and antagonists to the receptor, requiring a hydrogen bond donor or acceptor in the binding site to interact with this moiety. Also, the hydroxyl groups on the catechol ring are essential for full agonist responsiveness, and require a pair of hydrogen donors or acceptors in the receptor that can interact with the catechol hydroxyl groups. Furthermore, some type of aromatic side chain needs to interact with the phenyl ring of the phenylethylamines. From a series of site-directed mutagenesis studies, Strader et al. (47) demonstrated that the critical residues responsible for adrenergic agonist binding involves aspartic acid^{113} on transmembrane domain (TMD) III (for the protonated amine), and the serine^{204} and serine^{207} on TMD V (for the hydroxyl groups on the catechol ring) (Fig. 4). However, it is noteworthy that serine^{204} does not exist for certain α-adrenergic receptors (51). Because of the

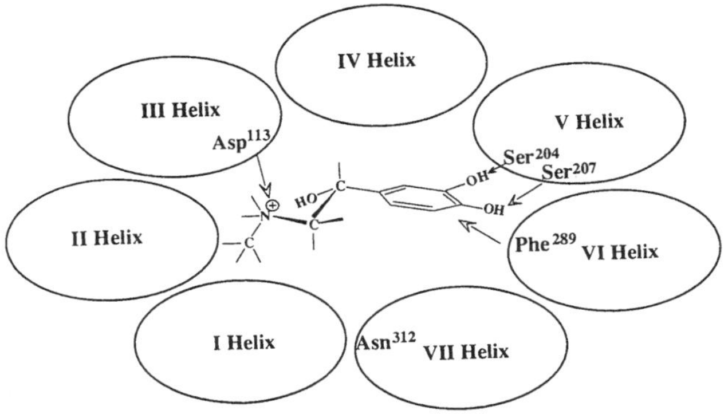

Figure 4. Model proposed for the interaction of epinephrine with the adrenergic receptor. The amino nitrogen interacts with the Asp[113] in the third hydrophobic segment and the two catechol hydroxyls form hydrogen bonds with Ser[204] and Ser[207] in the fifth hydrophobic segment.

homology of the transmembrane domains among the GPCRs, one would expect a certain pattern of conservation of key binding residues across the family of receptors. This has proven to be the case.

Binding of peptide ligands differs somewhat from the monoamine ligands because of the wide range of size, from tripeptides such as thyrotropin-releasing hormone (TRH) to glucagon, a 20 amino acid ligand. Given the larger surface area of these ligands, it is probable that extracellular domains are also involved (13). Three residues in TMD II (Asn[85], Asn[89], and Tyr[92]) and Tyr[287] in TMD VII are involved in the binding of all neurokinin peptides (14).

Activation of G Proteins

Mutant receptors demonstrating constitutive activity (activity not requiring occupation by the agonist) have provided insight into the sites in the GPCR that are required for activation of the G proteins. The most important domains for activation of G proteins appear to be the intracellular areas, including the intracellular end of TMD III, the cytoplasmic loop between TMDs V and VI, and the carboxy-terminal region near TMD VII (27).

Synthetic sequences that correspond to naturally occurring sequences have been shown to block the interaction with some G proteins (8) or to directly stimulate different G proteins (46). Recently, investigators have examined naturally occurring constitutively active receptors. These mutant receptors are thought to be responsible for the pathogenesis of some endocrine disease states (12,36).

Asp[79] in TMD II is one of the most highly conserved residues throughout the GPCR family. Substitution with alanine decreases agonist efficacy with no change in antagonist binding consistent with a role for this residue in promoting receptor activation (47). A disulfide bridge between the cysteine at the extracellular end of TMD II and a cysteine in the extracellular loop between TMDs IV and V occurs in more than 90% of GPCRs. Apparently, its role is to stabilize the active form of the receptor. There appear to be particular sequence patterns governing the association with the various G proteins (37). Thus, coupling to a G protein responsible for a particular effect on an intracellular signaling pathway requires a specific structure in the cytoplasmic loops and carboxy terminus of the GPCR. Inhibition of adenylate cyclase by activation of G_i requires a long third cytoplasmic loop and a short carboxy terminus; stimulation of phosphoinositide hydrolysis via G_q requires a short third cytoplasmic loop and a long carboxy terminus; and stimulation of adenylate cyclase via G_s requires a long carboxy terminus with many serine and threonine residues. However, there is a great deal of promiscuity, since a single receptor subtype is capable of activating several different G proteins in the same cell.

A knowledge of the basis of receptor action mandates an understanding of the conformational changes that allow the binding of a ligand to TMDs of the receptor to affect protein-protein interaction at the intracellular surfaces. To study this dynamic process one needs nonstatic methods such as fluorescence and nuclear magnetic resonance (NMR). A critical issue to be resolved is whether the conformational states induced by agonists, inverse agonists (sometimes referred to as negative antagonists), and true antagonists (also referred to as neutral antagonists) are different. (The manner by which the receptor transmits its signal to the G protein is covered in the Aronstam Chap. 4.)

FUNCTIONAL REGULATION OF GPCRs

For most GPCRs, agonist stimulation is followed by desensitization, in which there is a reduction in effector stimulation over time despite the continued presence of the stimulus. The molecular components of the effector signaling pathway are plastic and can be regulated dynamically at several different levels including gene transcription, posttranscription, and posttranslation (16) (Fig. 5). The receptor is but one component of the pathway at which regulation can occur. Receptor expression is regulated at the level of the gene, the messenger RNA (mRNA), and the protein through various transcriptional and postsynthetic mechanisms.

Regulation of GPCRs is divided into two distinct time frames. In the short-term, posttranslational modifications (especially alterations in the phosphorylation state) alter the function of the receptor with no alteration in its steady-state concentration. The most well-studied GPCR in this regard is the β adrenoceptor. Following prolonged exposure of the receptor to agonist, the receptor is phosphorylated (43). One of the kinases responsible is the β-adrenoceptor kinase (BARK), an adenosine 3',5'-cyclic monophosphate (cAMP)-independent cytosolic enzyme (5) that is activated when the receptor is occupied by the agonist. The phosphorylation sites are at the C terminus (10). The phosphorylated receptor is functionally uncoupled from the G protein and is therefore less capable of activating the effector mechanism (44). A different type of phosphorylation and uncoupling occurs when receptors are exposed to a lower level of agonist, in which case the kinase responsible appears to be cAMP-dependent protein kinase (22). In the case of muscarinic receptors (and probably adrenoceptors too), agonist occupation activates receptor phosphorylation via the coupling of the βγ dimer of the G protein to appropriate kinases (20).

Longer-term regulation involves transcriptional activation, posttranscriptional effects, and posttranslational regulation of the turnover of the receptor. Transcriptional activation is measured by nuclear run-in transcription assays (15). Posttranscriptional effects are due to changes in mRNA stability and are assessed by determining the mRNA half-life (19). Longer term (>4 hours) agonist challenges of cells results in a sustained downregulation (<50%) of steady-state β_2-adrenergic receptor mRNA levels by destabilization (19). This destabilization involves both cAMP-dependent and -independent processes (18). Glucocorticoids, acting at a 5′ noncoding region of the β_2-adrenergic receptor gene, cause an upregulation of receptor expression through an increase in the steady-state mRNA levels (7).

Persistent activation of adenylyl cyclase induces desensitization of the stimulatory G protein pathways, but also increases responsiveness to inhibitory ligands by increasing the expression of inhibitory receptors (39). This appears to be due to the presence of cAMP-responsive elements in the 5′ promoter

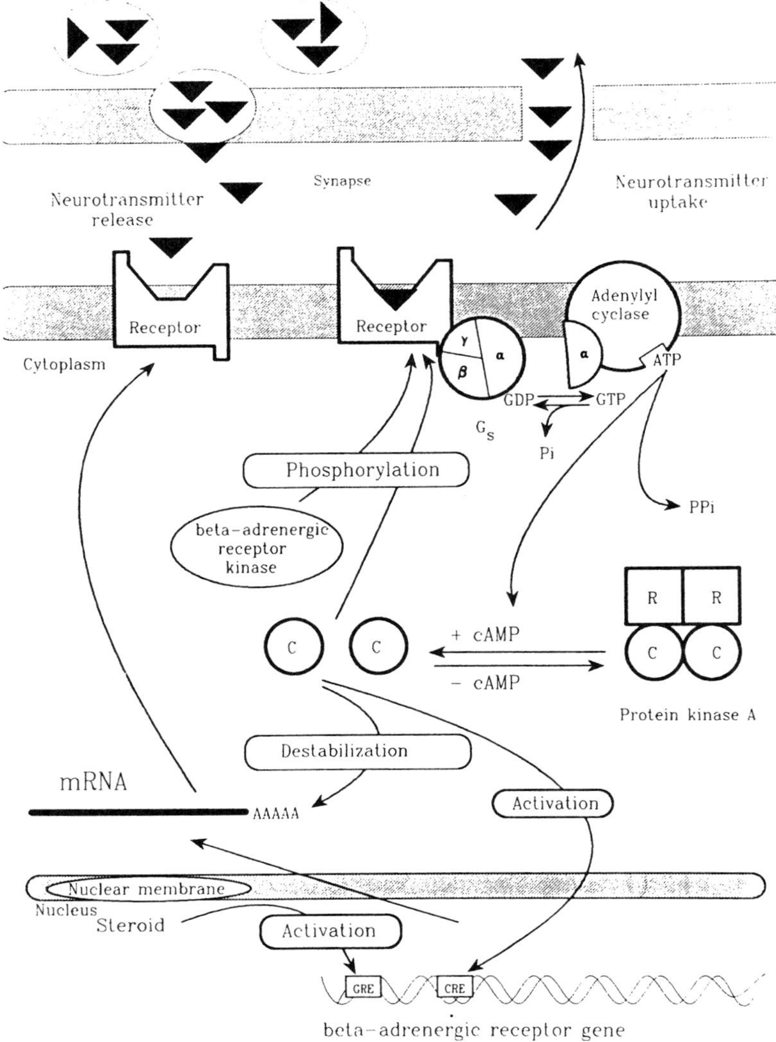

Figure 5. Agonist regulation of G protein–coupled receptor mRNA: transcriptional, posttranscriptional, and posttranslational controls. Agonist regulation of β-adrenergic receptors is divided into two distinct phases. In the early phase (up to 4 hours of stimulation) uptake of the neurotransmitter and phosphorylation of the receptor play central roles in attenuating the response to catecholamines. An early, transient, agonist-induced increase in the transcription rate (after 1 hour of stimulation) of the β-adrenergic receptor gene increases receptor mRNA levels. In the late phase of agonist regulation (more than 4 hours of stimulation), the rate of transcription of the receptor gene is unaffected by the agonist. Agonist-induced downregulation of receptor reflects downregulation of receptor mRNA by the destabilization of the mRNA. CRE, cAMP-responsive element; GRE, glucocorticoid responsive element; G_s, the stimulatory G protein coupled to adenylyl cyclase; Ppi and Pi, inorganic phosphate; R and C, regulatory and catalytic subunits of cAMP-dependent protein kinase, respectively. (From ref. 16, with permission.)

region of the α_{2A} adrenergic receptor gene. Thus, receptors responding through multiple G protein–linked pathways integrate information and cross-regulate each other (17).

MOLECULAR MODELING

A three-dimensional molecular model is not an end itself but a starting point, since it is likely to be wrong in detail, especially those models that are based on the experimentally derived structure of a closely related homologue. The model must be predictive and lend itself to experimental testing of the new predictions. In "homology modeling" the sequence of the protein being modeled (the "unknown") is aligned with the structure of at least one protein (the "known") with which it is believed to share a common three-dimensional fold. The latter is used as a template on which the model of the "unknown" is constructed. The final model is thus totally dependent on the accuracy of the alignment of the sequence of the unknown protein with the template structure. However, the results of such approaches provide useful information that is open to empirical testing and can be used to suggest new experiments. Loop regions connecting the individual helices are omitted because of the difficulty in predicting the conformation of these loops. This is not a limitation for modeling ligand binding and activation sites since these loops are uninvolved.

The only spatial information on structure of GPCRs is derived from bacteriorhodopsin and rhodopsin. When these structural data are compared at a 9Å resolution, the projection footprints of the helical arrangements differ in the following respects (Fig. 6). TMD III is relatively buried in rhodopsin, especially on the intracellular side of the membrane, while it is more exposed to the lipid environment in bacteriorhodopsin.

The arrangement of the helices in the bundle appear different because of differences in the helical axes. For bacteriorhodopsin TMDs II, III, and IV are perpendicular to the membrane while V, VI, VII, and I are tilted. For rhodopsin the assignment of the helices in less certain, but it appears that IV, V, VI, and VII are perpendicular while I, II, and III slope. The distance between the extracellular ends of helices III and V need to be quite close in GPCRs such as rhodopsin because of the disulfide bridge between the conserved cysteine at the extracellular end of TMD III and the cysteine positioned in the second extracellular loop close to the extracellular end of TMD V. The extracellular ends of helices II and V are relatively far apart for bacteriorhodopsin. The binding sites for the catecholamines to the conserved aspartic acid on TMD III and to the conserved serines on TMD V cannot be easily accomplished for bacteriorhopdopsin because TMD IV is interpolated at this level between TMDs III and V in the helical bundle. However, these differences may be mitigated by a tilt rotation of the projections through 15° around an axis, perpendicular to the membrane. Such a tilting may be necessary to normalize for the extreme differences in the crystallization condition (25). Finally, there is a good likelihood that the helical packing will be different because of the different positions of conserved proline residues that induce bending. In the bacteriorhodopsin family there are conserved prolines in II, III, and VI, while in the GPCRs there are conserved prolines in IV, V, VI, and VII. Also, the proline residues in helix VI are on the opposite side of the helix.

Therefore, there is a fair modicum of uncertainty introduced when bacteriorhodopsin is used as a template for molecular models of GPCRs. The assumptions remain to be rigorously tested experimentally.

AGONISTS, ANTAGONISTS, AND INVERSE AGONISTS

The cornerstone of classical receptor theory is the occupancy-response relationship in which the magnitude of the response obtained is directly proportional to the number of receptors occupied by ligand. A corollary of this statement is that the agonist-unoccupied receptor is in an unactivated state. However, recent data utilizing a transgenic mouse with an overexpressed, constitutively active β_2-adrenergic receptor in the heart forces one to reexamine these precepts (6) since it appears that the unoccupied receptors exist in an active form.

In the basal state, transgenic animals' hearts behaved similarly to control animals that were being maximally stimulated

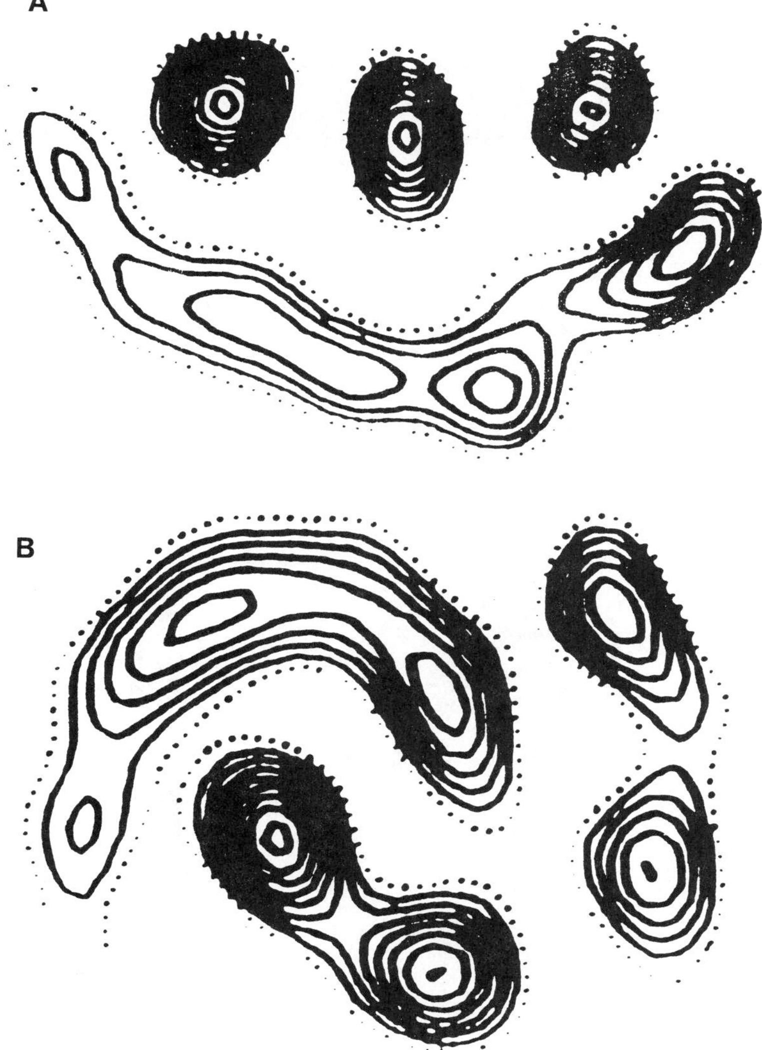

Figure 6. Experimental projection density maps for **(A)** bacteriorhodopsin and **(B)** bovine rhodopsin. (From ref. 25, with permission.)

with isoproterenol. To rule out the possibility that there was a "high endogenous tone" from overproduction of endogenous agonists, the transgenic animals were given reserpine to deplete cardiac stores of catecholamines. Even in this catecholamine-depleted state, the hearts behaved as if they were maximally stimulated with isoproterenol.

To satisfy these data, a new model has been proposed in which receptors exist in an equilibrium between two allosterically different conformations: an active and an inactive state (6) (Fig. 7). Spontaneous isomerization occurs between these two receptor forms, and only the active form can interact productively with a G protein to couple to the effector mechanisms. In this model, agonists do not activate receptors; rather, their agonist activity is a consequence of disturbing the equilibrium to favor the active receptor state. Inverse agonists will tend to pull the equilibrium in the opposite direction. Competitive ìneutralî antagonists do not disturb the equilibrium because they have equal affinity for both receptor states and can ìblockî the effect of both agonists and inverse agonists.

Higher levels of receptor expression are expected to increase basal activity as more copies of the activated receptor will be present stochastically at any one time. Also, mutant receptors can have their equilibrium shifted to the active state, providing a physiologic basis for the mutation-induced activated state that have been reported for adrenergic receptors (38,40). The characteristics of inverse agonists will be especially apparent in systems that express relatively high receptor levels or activate mutant G protein–coupled receptors (33). Therefore, a concept that had only been alluded to before from computer simulations can now be appreciated in an in vivo setting (6). Inverse agonists may be particularly use-

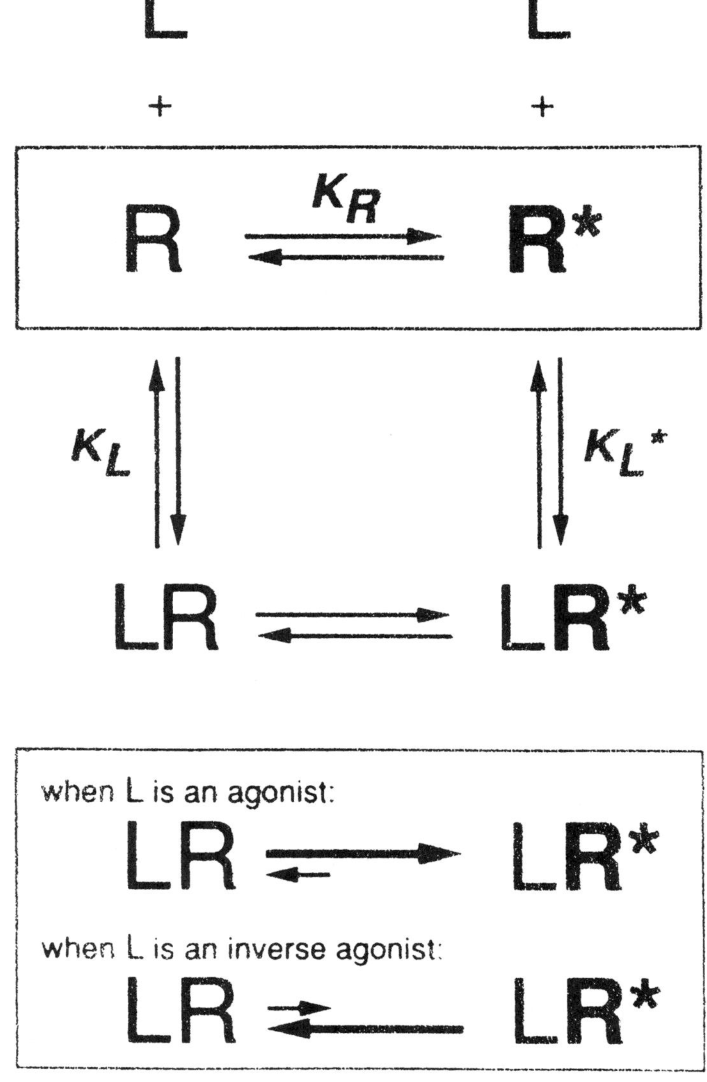

Figure 7. The two-state model of receptor activation depicting the receptor existing in inactive (R) and active (R*) conformations; L, ligand; K_R, the equilibrium constant for the distribution of receptor between R and R* in the absence of the ligand; K_L and K_{L*}, the dissociation equilibrium constants for ligand at the two receptor states. These equilibria are defined as follows: $K_R = [R]/[R^*]$; $K_L = [R][L]/[LR]$; $K_{L*} = [R^*][L]/[LR^*]$; and the total receptor population $([R]_{TOT})=[R] + [R^*] + [LR] + [LR^*]$. Using these equations a relationship can be derived between the concentrations of the agonist ([L]) and the concentration of the receptors in the active form ([R]+[LR*]), which is expressed as the fraction of the total receptor concentration $(f_{R*})=(K_{L*} + [L])/K_L.(1 + K_R) + (1 + K_RK_{L*}/K_L)[L]$. The interactions between two ligands can be modeled by including the additional equilibrium equations, $K_B = [R][B]/[BR]$; $K_{B*} = [R^*][B]/[BR^*]$, and extending the distribution equation. (From ref. 6, with permission.)

ful therapeutic agents to negate constitutive activity that is seen in certain disease states. In addition, inverse agonists may be useful in disease states in which there has been inappropriate expression or overexpression of receptors. The dopamine D_4 receptor has been shown to be present in very high levels in brain tissue obtained at necropsy of patients with schizophrenia. An inverse agonist for this particular receptor subtype may prove to be effective therapy for this intractable disease.

TOOLS FOR INVESTIGATING FUNCTION OF G PROTEIN–COUPLED RECEPTORS

Continuous Expression

The overexpression of receptors in permanent cell lines provides a unique source of receptor protein for detailed biochemical and structural studies. To this end one can use plasmid vectors containing selectable markers for the expression of the receptors of interest. The permanent expression of specific receptors provides a pure population of human receptors for drug development and testing, a substantial improvement over the use of animal tissues.

Binding Assays

Data on chemical interactions with GPCRs can be obtained by competitive binding assays.

Functional Assays

These assays are based on measuring discrete biologic responses following application of chemicals of interest to isolated tissue or cells in culture. Cloning and expression of GPCRs has resulted in demand for rapid functional assays usually involving a reporter system. In such a system accumulation of the second messenger reduces the transcription of a gene coding for a reporter protein. Typically, the reporter proteins are enzymes whose activity can be measured by the conversion of a substrate to an easily detectable product. Recently, a new approach has been advocated that uses chromatophores or skin cells that regulate color (30).

Chimeric Receptors

Chimeric receptors are formed between two related GPCRs by splicing together complementary helical regions from two receptors. By moving the splice junction to different positions in the receptor sequence one can obtain information as to which helical domains are the most critical for binding of specific ligands. This strategy locates general regions that can then be further characterized by specific point mutations in those regions (28). However, structural effects can make these mutants difficult to interpret, since formation of a fully active chimeric receptor requires that all the interhelical contacts responsible for tertiary structure of the receptor be maintained in the chimeric protein. Chimeric receptors frequently display a reduced binding affinity or decreased level of expression that probably signifies a disruption of the tertiary structure of the receptor. Further information must be obtained by single amino acid substitutions that may be less likely to cause an overall disruption of the structure of the protein.

Site-Directed Mutagenesis

Two different types of mutants can be constructed, namely, deletion mutations in which large stretches of nucleotides encoding specific amino acids are removed from the gene sequence for deletion mutants, whereas only a single nucleotide, which converts one amino acid to another, is used for point mutants. In theory, deletion mutations can provide information as to the importance of a defined receptor domain. However, in practice, interpretation of the results from deletion mutations can be difficult if the mutation alters receptor processing or membrane insertion. For this reason, the information obtained from point mutations may be of greatest utility in elucidating important functional domains of a receptor.

ANESTHETIC EFFECTS ON G PROTEIN–COUPLED RECEPTORS

Studies addressing the effects of anesthetic agents on G protein–coupled receptors is covered in Chap. 4 by Aronstam.

REFERENCES

1. Attwood TK, Eliopoulos EE, Findlay JBC. Multiple sequence alignment of protein families showing low sequence homology: a methodological approach using database pattern-matching discriminators for G-protein-linked receptors. *Gene* 1991;98:153–159.
2. Attwood TK, Findlay JBC. Design of a discriminating fingerprint for G-protein-coupled receptors. *Protein Engineer* 1993;6:167–176.
3. Baldwin JM. The probable arrangement of the helices in G protein-coupled receptors *EMBO* 1993;12:1693–1703.
4. Baldwin JM. Structure and function of receptors coupled to G proteins. *Curr Opinion Cell Biol* 1994;6:180–190.
5. Benovic JL, Mayor F, Staniszewski C, Lefkowitz RJ, Caron MG. Purification and characterization of the beta-adrenergic receptor kinase *J Biol Chem* 1987;262:9026–9032.
6. Bond RA, Leff P, Johnson TD, et al. Physiologic effects of inverse agonists in transgenic mice with myocardial overexpression of the β_2 adrenergic receptor. *Nature* 1995;374:272–276.
7. Collins S, Caron MG, Lefkowitz RJ. β2-Adrenergic receptors in hamster smooth muscle cells are transcriptionally regulated by glucocorticoids. *J Biol Chem* 1988;263:9067–9070.
8. Dalman HM, Neubig RR. Two peptides from the α_{2A}-adrenergic receptor alter receptor G protein coupling by distinct mechanisms. *J Biol Chem* 1991;266:11025–11029.
9. Dixon RAF, Sigal IS, Rands E, et al. Ligand binding to the beta-adrenergic receptor involves its rhodopsin-like core. *Nature* 1987; 326:73–77.
10. Dohlman HG, Bouvier M, Benovic JL, Caron MG, Lefkowitz RJ. The multiple membrane spanning topography of the beta 2-adrenergic receptor. Localization of the sites of binding, glycosylation, and regulatory phosphorylation by limited proteolysis. *J Biol Chem* 1987;262:14282–14288.
11. Donnelly D, Cogdell RJ. Predicting the point at which transmembrane helices protrude form the bilayer: a model of the antenna complexes from photosynthetic bacteria. *Protein Engineer* 1993;6: 629–635.
12. Dryja TP, Berson EL, Rao VT, Oprian DD. Heterozygous missense mutation in the rhodopsin gene as a cause of congenital night blindness. *Nature Genet* 1993;4:280–283.
13. Fong TM, Huang RRC, Strader CD. Localization of agonist and antagonist binding domains of the human neurokinin-1 receptor. *J Biol Chem* 1992;267:25664–25667.
14. Fong TM, Yu H, Huang RRC, Strader CD. The extracellular domain of the neurokinin-1 receptor is required for high affinity binding of peptides. *Biochemistry* 1992;31:11806–11811.
15. Greenberg ME, Ziff EB. Stimulation of 3T3 cells induces transcription of the c-fos proto-oncogene. *Nature* 1984;311:433–438.
16. Hadcock JR, Malbon CC. Regulation of receptor expression by agonists: transcription and post-translational control. *Trends Neurosci* 1991;14:242–247.
17. Hadcock JR, Malbon CC. Agonist regulation of gene expression of adrenergic receptors and G proteins. *J Neurochem* 1993;60:1–9.
18. Hadcock JR, Ros M, Malbon CC. Agonist regulation of b-adrenergic receptor mRNA: analysis in S 49 mouse lymphoma mutants. *J Biol Chem* 1989;264:13956–13961.
19. Hadcock JR, Wang H-Y, Malbon CC. Agonist-induced destabilization of β-adrenergic receptor mRNA. Attenuation of glucocorticoid-

induced up-regulation of β-adrenergic receptors. *J Biol Chem* 1989; 264:19928–19933.

20. Haga T, Haga K, Kameyama K, Nakata H. Phosphorylation of muscarinic receptors: regulation by G proteins. *Life Sci* 1993;52:421–428.
21. Hargrave PA, McDowell JH, Curtis DR, et al. The structure of bovine rhodopsin. *Biophys Structure Mech* 1983;9:235–244.
22. Hausdorff WP, Bouvier M, O'Dowd BF, et al. Phosphorylation sites on two domains of the beta 2-adrenergic receptor are involved in distinct pathways of receptor desensitization *J Biol Chem* 1989;264: 12657–12665.
23. Henderson R, Baldwin JM, Ceska TA, et al. Model for the structure of bacteriorhodopsin based on high-resolution electron microscopy. *J Mol Biol* 1990;213:899–929.
24. Henderson R, Unwin PNT. Three-dimensional model of purple membrane obtained by electron microscopy. *Nature* 1975;257:28–32.
25. Hoflack J, Trumpp-Kallmeyer S, Hibert M. Re-evaluation of bacteriorhodopsin as a model for G protein-coupled receptors. *Trends Pharmacol Sci* 1994;15:7–9.
26. Khorana HG. Rhodopsin, photoreceptor of the rod cell. An emerging pattern for structure and function. *J Biol Chem* 1992;267:1–4.
27. Kjelsberg MA, Cotecchia S, Ostrowski J, Caron MG, Lefkowitz RJ. Constitutive activation of the α1β-adrenergic receptor by all amino acid substitutions at a single site. Evidence for a region which constrains receptor activation. *J Biol Chem* 1992;267:1430–1433.
28. Kobilka BK, Kobilka TS, Daniel K, et al. Chimeric alpha 2-, beta 2-adrenergic receptors: delineation of domains involved in effector coupling and ligand binding specificity. *Science* 1988;240:1310–1316.
29. Kyte J, Doolittle RFA. A simple method for displaying the hydropathic character of a protein. *J Mol Biol* 1982;157:105–132.
30. Lerner M. Tools for investigating the functional interactions between ligands and G-protein coupled receptors. *Trends Neurosci* 1994; 17:142–146.
31. Lynch CL III, Jaeger JM. The G protein cell signaling system. *Adv Anesth* 1994;11:65–112.
32. Main BG, Tucker H. Recent advances in beta-adrenergic blocking agents *Prog Med Chem* 1985;22:122–164.
33. Milligan G, Bond RA, Lee M. Inverse agonism: pharmacological curiosity or potential therapeutic strategy? *Trends Pharmacol Sci* 1995; 16:10–13.
34. Mizobe T, Maze M, Lam V, Suryanarayana S, Kobilka B. Arrangement of transmembrane domains in adrenergic receptors: similarity to bacteriorhodopsin. *J Biol Chem* 1996;271:2387–2389.
35. Pardo L, Ballesteros JA, Osman R, Weinstein H. On the use of the transmembrane domain of bacteriorhodopsin as a template for modeling the three-dimensional structure of guanine nucleotide-binding regulatory protein-coupled receptors *Proc Natl Acad Sci USA* 1992;89:4009–4912.
36. Parma J, Duprez L, VanSande J, et al. Somatic mutation in the thyrotropin receptor gene cause hyperfunctioning thyroid adenomas. *Nature* 1993;365:649–651.
37. Raymond JR, Hnatowich M, Caron MG, Lefkowitz RJ. Structure-function relationships of G-protein-coupled receptors. In: Moss J, Vaughan ASM, eds. *ADP-ribosylating toxins and G proteins: insights into signal transduction.* Washington: American Society for Microbiology, 1990;163–188.
38. Ren Q, Kurose H, Lefkowitz RJ, Cotecchia S. Constitutively active mutants of the α_2-adrenergic receptor. *J Biol Chem* 1993;268: 16483–16487.
39. Sakaue M, Hoffman BB. cAMP regulates transcription of the α_{2A} adrenergic receptor gene in HT-29 cells. *J Biol Chem* 1991;266: 5743–5740.
40. Samama P, Cotecchia S, Costa T, Lefkowitz FJ. A mutation-induced activated state of the beta 2-adrenergic receptor. Extending the ternary complex model. *J Biol Chem* 1993;268:4635–4636.
41. Schertler GF, Villa C, Henderson R. Projection structure of rhodopsin. *Nature* 1993;362:770–772.
42. Shenker A, Laue L, Kosugi S, et al. A constitutively activating mutation of the luteinizing hormone receptor gene in familial male precocious puberty. *Nature* 1993;365:652–656.
43. Sibley DR, Lefkowitz RJ. Identification of residues required for ligand binding to the beta-adrenergic receptor. *Nature* 1987;317: 124–129.
44. Sibley DR, Strasser RH, Benovic JL, Daniel K, Lefkowitz RJ. Phosphorylation/dephosphorylation of the beta-adrenergic receptor regulates its functional coupling to adenylate cyclase and subcellular distribution *Proc Natl Acad Sci USA* 1986;83:9408–9412.
45. Strader CD, Candelore MR, Hill WS, Sigal IS, Dixon RAF. Identification of two serine residues involved in agonist activation of the beta-adrenergic receptor. *J Biol Chem* 1989;264:13572–13578.
46. Strader CD, Fong TM, Tota MR, Underwood D. Structure and function of G protein-coupled receptors. *Annu Rev Biochem* 1994;63: 101–132.
47. Strader CD, Sigal IS, Register RB, et al. Identification of residues required for ligand binding to the beta-adrenergic receptor. *Proc Natl Acad Sci USA* 1987;84:4384–4388.
48. Thomas DD, Stryer L. Transverse location of the retinal chromophore of rhodopsin in rod outer segment disc membranes. *J Mol Biol* 1982;154:145–157.
49. Tota M, Strader CD. Characterization of the binding domain of the beta-adrenergic receptor with the fluorescent antagonist carazolol. Evidence for a buried ligand binding site. *J Biol Chem* 1990;265: 16891–16897.
50. Venter JC, Fraser CM, Kerlavage AR, Buck MA. Molecular biology of adrenergic and muscarinic cholinergic receptors. *Biochem Pharmacol* 1989;38:1197–1208.
51. Wang CD, Buck MA, Fraser CM. Site-directed mutagenesis of alpha 2A-adrenergic receptors: identification of amino acids involved in ligand binding and receptor activation by agonists. *Mol Pharmacol* 1991;40:168–179.
52. Weinshank RL, ZgombickJM, Macchi M, Adham N, Lichtblau H, Branchek TA, Hartig PR. Cloning, expression, and pharmacological characterization of a human alpha2B-adrenergic receptor. *Mol Pharmacol* 1990;38:681–688.
53. Zeng DW, Harrison JK, D'Angelo DD, Barber CM, Tucker AL, Lee Z, Lynch KR. Molecular characterization of a rat alpha 2B-adrenergic receptor. *Proc Natl Acad Sci USA* 1990;87:3102–3106.

Anesthesia: Biologic Foundations, edited by
Tony L. Yaksh et al. Lippincott–Raven Publishers,
Philadelphia © 1997.

CHAPTER 6

ADENYLATE CYCLASE

YVONNE VULLIEMOZ

HISTORY—FROM SUTHERLAND TO RODBELL AND BEYOND

The discovery by Earl W. Sutherland and his collaborators in 1957 of adenosine 3′,5′-cyclic monophosphate (cAMP) as an intracellular mediator of hormone action started a new era in cellular biology. This discovery, for which Sutherland received the Nobel Prize in Medicine in 1971, is at the origin of our understanding of signal transduction.

Cyclic AMP was first isolated from the liver during a study of the mechanisms of epinephrine and glucagon glycogenolytic activity. In their earlier studies Sutherland and collaborators had found that the hormone stimulation was due in part to activation of glycogen phosphorylase. If phosphorylase activation by the hormones could be shown easily in intact cells or in whole tissue homogenates, it was lost when a particulate fraction was removed from the preparation by centrifugation and was restored upon addition of the particulate fraction. Quoting from the summary of the paper by Rall, Sutherland and Berthet (60): "It has been possible to show that the response of the homogenates to the hormones occurred in two stages. In the first stage, a particulate fraction of homogenates produced a heat-stable factor in the presence of the hormones; in the second stage, this factor stimulated the formation of [active] liver phosphorylase in the supernatant fractions of the homogenates in which the hormones themselves were inactive." This heat-stable factor was then shown to be cAMP (Fig. 1). At about the same time, cAMP was prepared and isolated chemically by a group of chemists (13). This was a fortunate coincidence, because chemical synthesis could provide large quantities of the compound, which greatly facilitated the development and understanding of the wide role of cAMP in biologic functions (62). The enzymatic activity that catalyzes the formation of cAMP from adenosine triphosphate (ATP) and can be stimulated by hormones was named adenylate cyclase. It was also found that tissue extracts contain cAMP-inactivating enzymes, cAMP phosphodiesterases, which convert cAMP to 5′AMP (Fig. 2). Sutherland had observed that phosphorylase activation by the hormone was a phosphorylation reaction. It was shown later that cAMP activates a specific protein kinase, named protein kinase A, and that this enzyme mediates not only the glycogenolytic action of cAMP, but most of the cAMP-mediated cellular functions (Fig. 3) (39).

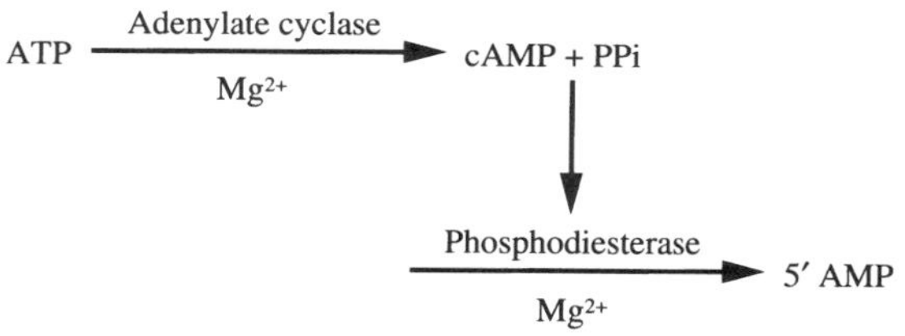

ATP —Adenylate cyclase, Mg^{2+}→ cAMP + PPi

cAMP + PPi —Phosphodiesterase, Mg^{2+}→ 5′ AMP

Figure 2. cAMP synthesis and degradation.

The unraveling of the sequence of events leading to the hormone-induced breakdown of glycogen was very important for many reasons. The concept of a hormone, the extracellular messenger, acting at the outside of the cell membrane and initiating a series of events leading to the formation of an intracellular messenger, called by Sutherland the second messenger, which by phosphorylation of an enzyme promotes the functional change, was new. It became obvious very soon that it represented a general mode of action of many hormones and transmitters and has opened the search for other intracellular mediators, of which guanosine 3′,5′-cyclic monophosphate (cGMP), inositol 1,4,5-triphosphate, and nitric oxide are the best known. Last, but not least, Sutherland demonstrated, against the credo of that time, that intact cells were not required to study hormone effects and that hormones could be studied in broken cell preparations, allowing a more precise analysis of their action.

At that time it was thought that the adenylate cyclase system was composed of two subunits, a regulatory subunit at the extracellular side of the cell membrane that contains the hormone binding sites, and a catalytic subunit at the intracellular side of the membrane. In the following years Rodbell and collaborators observed that guanosine triphosphate (GTP) plays an obligatory role in the activation of adenylate cyclase by the hormone and that the actions of hormones and GTP were interdependent (63). They inferred from their studies that the adenylate cyclase system was a multimeric enzyme complex

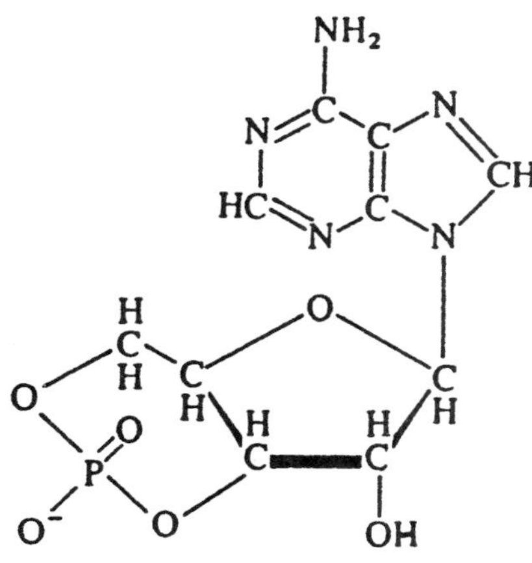

Figure 1. Structural formula of cAMP.

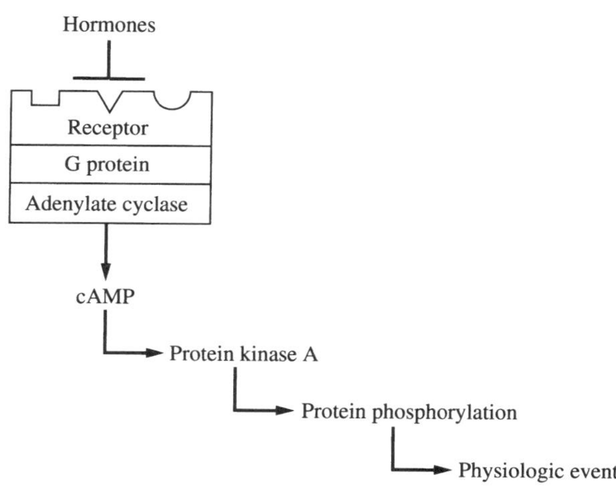

Figure 3. The cAMP cascade.

composed of at least three components: a hormone discriminator (receptor), a transducer (a GTP regulatory protein), and an amplifier (adenylate cyclase itself) (64). This pioneer work led to the identification in the mid-1970s of a guanine nucleotide-binding protein (G protein), separate from the adenylate cyclase and receptor proteins (54). When purified forms of β-adrenoceptor, G protein, and adenylate cyclase were combined in phospholipid vesicles, hormone-dependent synthesis of cAMP could be demonstrated. This confirmed Rodbell's insightful proposal that the adenylate cyclase system consists of three components, the G protein being the transducer that couples the receptor to the effector. This reconstituted system also proved that no additional protein component is required for the transfer of the hormonal signal. This very simple system is quite efficient. The binding of one molecule of a β-adrenergic agonist to its receptor can catalyze the formation of 1000 molecules of cAMP, a 10^3 amplification of the signal (45). Today over 30 receptors that are coupled to adenylate cyclase have been identified, but the β-adrenoceptor pathway, which has been the first and most fully characterized, has remained the model for signal transduction via G protein.

Since physiologic functions mediated by these receptors depend in great part on the specific interactions between the three protein components of the hormonally regulated adenylate cyclase system, it is essential to identify their structures and their sites of interaction and of regulation. Over the past 10 years an explosion of new information has been derived from purification and from isolation and characterization of the genes that encode these proteins. Gilman and collaborators have greatly contributed to this endeavor. For their work Rodbell and Gilman received the Nobel Prize in Medicine in 1994.

GENERAL ANESTHETICS AND SIGNAL TRANSDUCTION

General anesthetics alter central and peripheral functions mediated by hormones and transmitters; however, little is known about the cellular mechanism(s) underlying these effects. There is accumulating evidence that the cell membrane is the site of action of general anesthetics and that the anesthetics alter cell communication by disturbing synaptic transmission and postsynaptic signal transduction (61,68). At anesthetic concentrations they probably act by binding directly to hydrophobic pockets of selective membrane proteins, causing small changes in protein conformation (20). Thus the cAMP system, which serves as intracellular mediator in the transduction of the signal from a class of receptors that regulates central and peripheral autonomic functions, is a potential target for the action of anesthetics. While the preceding chapters have dealt with the receptors and G proteins, this chapter is about the enzyme that catalyzes cAMP synthesis, adenylate cyclase, and the effect of general anesthetics on the enzyme activity. The reader is also referred to recent review articles on this topic (31,40,43,73,79).

ADENYLATE CYCLASE

There are different classes of adenylate cyclase. This review is concerned with the mammalian membrane-bound enzymes that are coupled to hormone receptors by a G protein.

Adenylate Cyclase Isozymes

The mammalian adenylate cyclases are a family of thermolabile membrane-bound glycoproteins found in extremely small amounts in the cell (0.001–0.01% of total membrane protein, compared to brain G proteins, which represent 1–2%). The existence of multiple forms of the enzyme was suggested by the results of the early biochemical studies that showed that the characteristics of the enzyme differ from tissue to tissue. In brain and in heart, for example, the adenylate cyclase response to hormonal stimulation was the same, but the response to calcium was different. Because of the low amount of the enzyme and of the instability of the protein during purification, detailed characterization of these enzymes has been difficult and lagged behind that of the receptors and G proteins until Pfeuffer and Metzger (55), using the new affinity chromatography technique, succeeded in purifying myocardial adenylate cyclase 2000-fold. The enzyme can now be purified to homogeneity. Preparation of antibodies raised against purified bovine brain adenylate cyclase provided the first direct evidence for the existence of two distinct adenylate cyclases in brain tissue (48). It was subsequently cloned and sequenced, and arbitrarily designated type I. Using probes based on type I sequence, five additional cDNA (type II to VI) have been cloned from different tissues and species, sequenced, and expressed in various cells (3,18,23,29,37,56,74). Two cDNA from human brain, localized on different chromosomes, have been cloned and partly sequenced. One of them shows similarities with type II, the other is a distinct species (53,70). Corresponding cDNA sequences for these two types, tentatively designated VII and VIII, have been identified in mouse S49 lymphoma cells and rat tissues, respectively (42). Yet another type has been found, which is widely distributed in human tissues (25). It is possible that more adenylate cyclase isoforms will be found in the future, since the messages for the known types could only be detected in some tissues in which adenylate cyclase plays an important physiologic role. Adenylate cyclase type I to VI are proteins consisting of 1098 to 1166 amino acids with a molecular weight of 110 to 180 kDa.

Structure

All types of adenylate cyclase share the same topology: a cytoplasmic amino terminal of varying length followed by two large alternating sets of hydrophobic and hydrophilic domains (Fig. 4) (31,41,73). The two large hydrophilic domains are cytoplasmic and each contain one region of about 250 amino acids with a very similar sequence (50–92% identity). These regions, which are highly conserved, also show a high degree of homology with other nonmammalian enzyme, as well as with guanylate cyclases. The C terminal of the molecule is part of the second cytoplasmic domain. Each of the hydrophobic domains contains six transmembrane spanning elements with 1 to 4 putative N-glycosylation sites exposed to the extracellular milieu. The amino acid sequence of these domains differs significantly among the adenylate cyclases and the degree of divergence varies between adenylate cyclases. While type I and III share the lower degree of homology with the others, there is some similarity between type

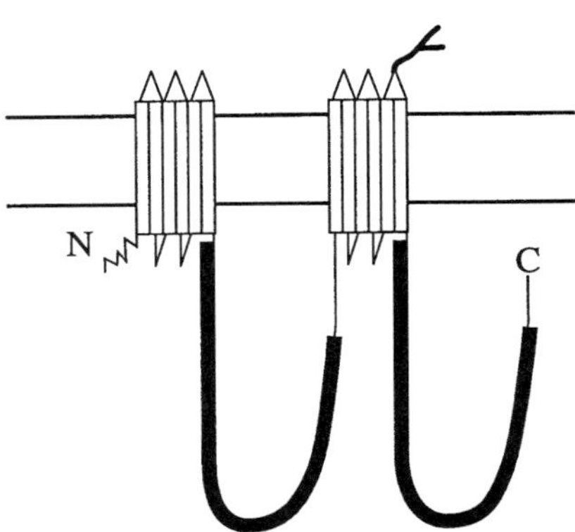

Figure 4. Adenylate cyclase structure. *Bold lines* indicate regions of amino acid sequence homology.

II and IV and between type V and VI, the latter showing the highest sequence homology.

Tissue Distribution

The tissue distribution of the different adenylate cyclases also varies and more than one type has been identified in a single cell or tissue, although with widely different frequencies among tissues (Table 1) (3,18,23,37,42,49,90). Type I is expressed in brain with high levels in neurons of selected regions; type II is also found in brain as well as in lungs and kidney; type III is predominantly in olfactory neurons; type IV in many peripheral tissues, including the heart, and in the CNS; type V is very selective for the heart and specific brain regions, e.g., striatum; type VI is widely distributed among tissues in small amounts. This selective distribution of adenylate cyclases has permitted some speculations about the physiologic function of the different isozymes. Type I, which is highly expressed in areas of the brain implicated with learning and memory, is also expressed in the *Drosophila* fly, where it has been associated with the ability of the fly to learn and remember some simple tasks, suggesting that type I is important for acquisition and storage of information (44,90).

Regulation

Purification and cloning of the adenylate cyclase isozymes have permitted a detailed analysis of their characteristics. As could be expected from the high degree of structural diversity, each adenylate cyclase has its own regulatory properties.

Substrate

All types I–VI use the same substrate, ATP complexed with a divalent metal magnesium or manganese (Mg/Mn.ATP). In addition a free metal is a requisite cofactor, increasing the maximum capacity (V_{max}) of the enzyme. Various observations suggest that the regions within the two hydrophilic domains that share a high degree of homology are important for catalytic activity. Each has a putative nucleotide binding site and share similarity with the region in guanylate cyclase that encode the catalytic site. Mutations in these regions compromise catalytic activity. However, both hydrophilic domains must be expressed together for catalytic activity, suggesting that each has its own nucleotide binding properties and that an interaction between the two sites is necessary for catalysis (37,73). An inhibitory site, called "P-site," has been identified on adenylate cyclase; it binds adenosine and analogues and interacts allosterically with the substrate binding site. Based on the results of kinetic studies on the inhibition of adenylate cyclase by adenosine, it has been proposed that one cytoplasmic domain contains the substrate binding site, the other the "P-site" (34,40,73). This proposition is interesting in view of the fact that so far the physiologic role of the P-site has remained elusive.

Forskolin

This diterpene, known for its hypotensive properties, is a potent activator of adenylate cyclase (67). It interacts directly with the enzyme, presumably at a site within the hydrophobic domains. Although the physiologic role of this site is not clear, stimulation of adenylate cyclase by forskolin and G_s, the G protein that stimulates adenylate cyclase, is synergistic, indicating an interaction between the two sites (23,72). In addition forskolin has been used extensively as a tool to test adenylate cyclase activity independently of G protein.

G Protein Subunits

The regulation of adenylate cyclase by G proteins has been extensively studied and the mechanism by which hormones activate G proteins has been reviewed in details in the previous chapter. In brief, adenylate cyclase is bidirectionally regulated by stimulatory and inhibitory receptors that are coupled to the enzyme by a specific G protein, G_s and G_i, respectively. G proteins are heterotrimeric proteins consisting of three subunits, α, β, and γ. Binding of an agonist to its receptor promotes the activation of a G protein by catalyzing the exchange of tightly bound GDP on the α subunit for GTP. This is followed by the dissociation of the inactive heterotrimeric G protein into $\beta\gamma$ and GTP.Gα. GTP.Gα carries the hormonal signal to adenylate cyclase by directly interacting with the enzyme. In contrast the role of the $\beta\gamma$ subunits in adenylate cyclase regulation has remained uncertain until recently (24,51).

Because G_s stimulation of all membrane-bound mammalian adenylate cyclases is mediated by the α subunit of G_s, the role of $G_i\alpha$ in adenylate cyclase inhibition by G_i has been more difficult to assess. The results of recent studies indicate that subtypes of purified activated $G_i\alpha$ do inhibit adenylate cyclase (75,88). In membranes from Sf9 cells expressing adenylate cyclase I, II, III, V, and VI the inhibition was dependent on the type of adenylate cyclase, types V and VI being most sensitive, type II the least, and on the nature of the activator (75,77). As to the site of interaction of the α subunits with adenylate cyclase, site-specific mutagenesis has suggested some putative regions of the cytosolic domains at the interface close to the transmembrane domains (75,77) Competition studies with type V indicate that $G_s\alpha$ and $G_i\alpha$ bind to distinct sites of the enzyme (77).

It was considered for a long time that the major role of the $\beta\gamma$ subunits was to modulate the activation of $G_s\alpha$ (24,51). Inhibition of adenylate cyclase by $\beta\gamma$ was thought to be indirect, due to their capacity to associate with and thereby deactivate $G_s\alpha$. Katada et al. (36) in 1987 proposed that the $\beta\gamma$ subunit may also inhibit adenylate cyclase by a mechanism independent of the α subunit. The results of recent studies with purified preparations

Table 1. PROPERTIES OF MEMBRANE-BOUND MAMMALIAN ADENYLATE CYCLASE ISOZYMES

	Regulator								
Type	$G_s\alpha$	$G_i\alpha$	$G\beta\gamma$	Calcium	Forskolin	P-site inhibitor	PKC	PKA	Tissue distribution
I	+	-	-	+(CaM)[b]	+	-	+	-	CNS (selected brain regions)
II	+	-	+[a]	0	+	-	+	NA[c]	CNS (diffuse) olfactory neuron, lungs
III	+	-	0	+(CaM)[a]	+	-	+	NA[c]	Olfactory neuron
IV	+	NA	+[a]	0	+	-	+	0	CNS and peripheral tissue (diffuse)
V	+	-	0	-	+	-	+	-	Heart, brain (selected regions)
VI	+	-	0	-	+	-	+	-	Heart, brain, kidney, other tissues (diffuse)

PKA, protein kinase A; PKC, protein kinase C; NA, not available; +, stimulation; -, inhibition; 0, no effect; CaM, calmodulin dependent.
[a]In the presence of activated α_s.
[b]Synergistic with GTP $G_s\alpha$.
[c]PKA phosphorylation site has been predicted, but effect on adenylate cyclase has not been reported.

of adenylate cyclase or with membranes of cells expressing a specific type of adenylate cyclase indicate that $\beta\gamma$ subunits do interact directly with adenylate cyclase (28,72,76,82). Furthermore, mutational experiments have tentatively assigned the site for activation of adenylate cyclase by $\beta\gamma$ to the carboxyl terminal in the second hydrophilic domain, a site different from that of $G_s\alpha$. Their effect depends not only on the type, but also on the activation state of the enzyme. The $\beta\gamma$ subunits have essentially no effect on unstimulated adenylate cyclase. They will, however, stimulate types II and IV when the enzyme is simultaneously activated by $G_s\alpha$, but inhibit type I. In contrast types III, V, and VI are unaffected by the $\beta\gamma$ subunits (Table 1). Their capacity to stimulate or inhibit adenylate cyclase is similar and independent of the subtype of $\beta\gamma$. The apparent affinity of individual $\beta\gamma$s for adenylate cyclase, however, varies and these differences appear to be dictated by the identity of the γ subunit. The concentration of $\beta\gamma$ required to activate or inhibit adenylate cyclase activity is significantly greater than that of $G_s\alpha$ and it is considered that G_i and G_o, which are much more abundant in the cell than G_s, at least in brain, are the source of $\beta\gamma$. This implies that adenylate cyclase receives signals not only from G_s- or G_i-linked receptors, but also from receptors linked to other G proteins (Fig. 5). How α and $\beta\gamma$ subunits can influence adenylate cyclase activity is demonstrated in a study by Bourne and collaborators (17). In transfected cells expressing adenylate cyclase II, activation of α_2-adrenoceptors that are negatively coupled to adenylate cyclase via the inhibitory G protein G_i will either decrease or increase cAMP accumulation depending on the state of adenylate cyclase activation by $G_s\alpha$. $G_i\alpha$ will inhibit adenylate cyclase when $G_s\alpha$ is not in an active state. In the presence of an activated $G_s\alpha$, the $\beta\gamma$ released upon activation of the inhibitory receptor will potentiate the $G_s\alpha$ stimulation of adenylate cyclase, overcoming the $G_i\alpha$-mediated inhibition (Fig. 5). This requires in vivo that the signal transmitted from G_i by $\beta\gamma$ coincides with that transmitted by $G_s\alpha$, since $\beta\gamma$ by itself has no effect.

Calcium

As observed in early studies with nonpurified preparations, the adenylate cyclase response to calcium varies greatly. Calcium can be stimulatory (types I and III), inhibitory (types V and VI), or have no effect (types II and IV) (Table 1) (3,18,23,29,37,74). The stimulation of types I and III by calcium is dependent on calmodulin, a well-conserved calcium-binding protein, first identified in brain, where it is found in high concentrations. Calmodulin has no known intrinsic activity, but it modulates the activity of numerous enzymes. In its active calcium-bound form, calmodulin forms a reversible complex with adenylate cyclase (Fig. 6). Calcium, not calmodulin, is the rate-limiting factor in the enzyme activation (10). Recently a hydrophobic site that binds calmodulin at nanomolar concentrations has been identified in a region of adenylate cyclase type I that protrudes in the cytosol from the sixth putative transmembrane domain (84).

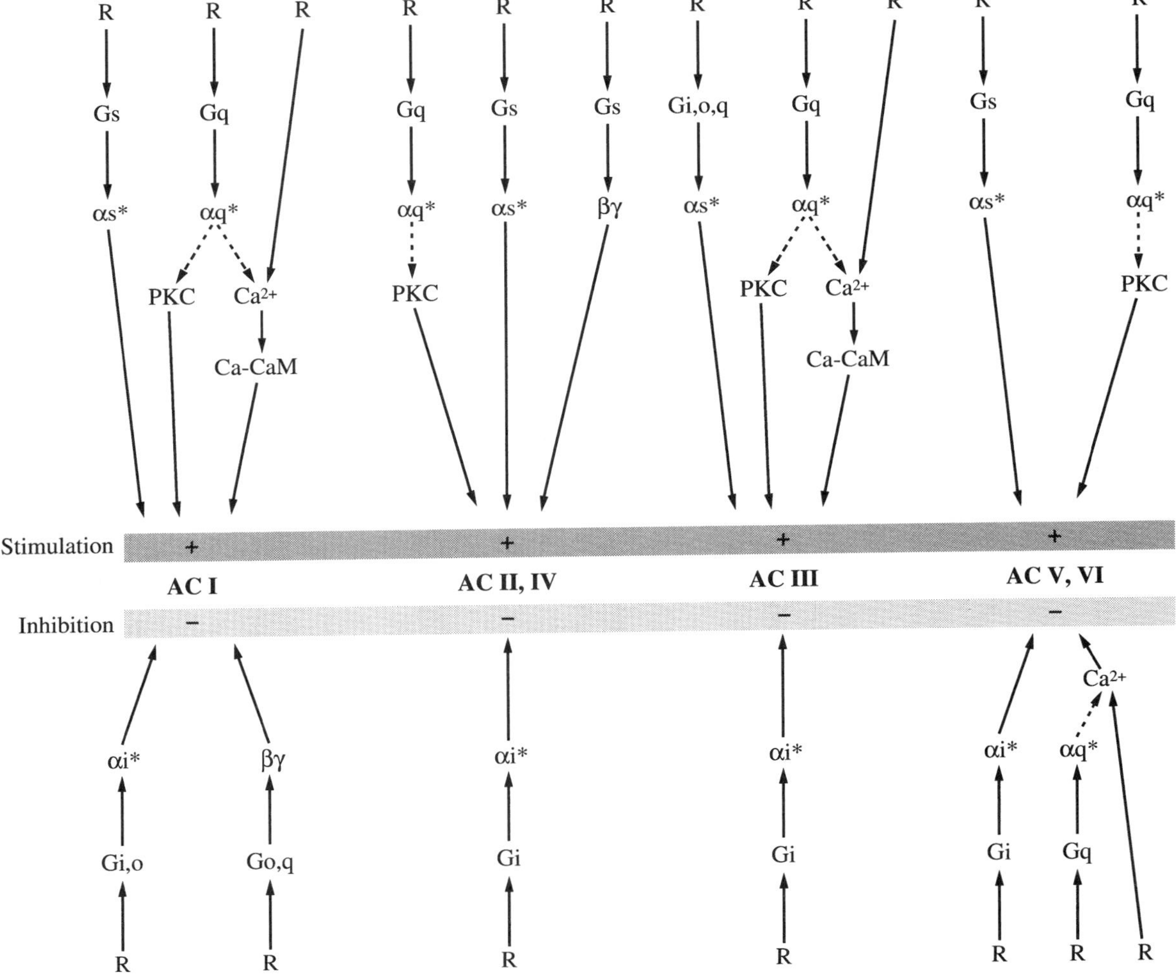

Figure 5. Pathways of regulation of adenylate cyclase (AC) isozymes. +, stimulation; -, inhibition; PKC, protein kinase C; Ca-CaM, calcium-activated calmodulin; *, activated subunit; —>, direct interaction; - - - - >, indirect modulation; αq*, activates phospholipase C, which in turn produces inositol triphosphate, which releases calcium from intracellular stores, and diacylglycerol, which activates PKC. (Modified from ref. 77.)

$$4\ Ca^{2+} + \underset{\text{Inactive}}{(CaM)} \longrightarrow \underset{\text{Active}}{(Ca_4^{2+} \bullet CaM)} + AC \longrightarrow (Ca_4^{2+} \bullet CaM) \bullet AC$$

Figure 6. Activation of adenylate cyclase by calcium-calmodulin. AC, adenylate cyclase; CaM, calmodulin.

The sensitivity of types I and III to stimulation by calcium and calmodulin differs. Type III is 100 times less sensitive than type I. In addition type III is stimulated by calcium-calmodulin only when the enzyme is already activated, while type I is stimulated in the absence of other activators and calmodulin acts synergistically with forskolin and GTP derivatives (11,74). This indicates that type I can be stimulated indirectly by receptors not coupled to G_s (Fig. 5).

Inhibition by calcium, on the other hand, does not require calmodulin. The results of kinetic studies indicate two calcium inhibitory sites, of high and low affinity. At the high affinity site calcium inhibits adenylate cyclase at the same submicromolar range of concentrations that stimulate the enzyme. The magnitude of inhibition is often greater than that elicited by G_i coupled receptors and is additive to their effect. In contrast, at the low affinity site calcium most likely competes with magnesium ions for an allosteric divalent ion binding site. This inhibition, observed at submillimolar concentrations, is not subtype specific, but is displayed by all adenylate cyclases regardless of their response to calcium at the submicromolar range (12,14,18).

Calcium represents an intracellular messenger through which adenylate cyclase can receive external signals from multiple receptor pathways: receptors coupled to G_s, G_o, or G_q, and receptors not coupled to a G protein (Fig. 5). Activation of G_s coupled receptors, e.g., the β-adrenoceptor, will increase intracellular calcium by stimulation of the adenylate cyclase–cAMP pathway and by directly opening dihydropyridine-sensitive voltage-gated calcium channels in the cell membrane. Activation of G_o coupled receptors, e.g., α_2-adrenoceptors, opiate, or neuropeptide Y receptors, will close voltage-gated calcium channels. Activation of G_q coupled receptors, e.g., α_1-adrenoceptors or M_1- and M_3-muscarinic receptors, will stimulate phospholipase C, which produces two second messengers, inositol triphosphate and diacylglycerol. Inositol triphosphate facilitates the release of calcium from intracellular stores into the cytosol (8). Activation of receptors that are an integral part of a specific ion channel complex and that transmit the signal independently of G proteins, e.g., γ-aminobutyric acid (GABA) A or *N*-methyl-D-aspartate (NMDA) receptors, will increase intracellular calcium by depolarizing the cell membrane and opening the calcium ion channels (83).

Regulation of adenylate cyclase by calcium may be of major significance in the heart, which contains predominantly types V and VI. These isozymes are stimulated by $G_s\alpha$ and inhibited by $G_i\alpha$ and calcium (Fig. 5). In the heart calcium can be elevated by the increase in cAMP induced by activation of receptors that are coupled to adenylate cyclase by G_s, e.g., β-adrenoceptor. The inhibition of adenylate cyclase caused by the elevated calcium provides a negative feedback control on the hormonal stimulus. Thus an increase in transient calcium induced by cAMP will reduce the cAMP signal by inhibiting its synthesis; as a consequence calcium will fall, allowing cAMP to rise again. It has been proposed that these oscillations between calcium and cAMP may in part control cardiac rhythmicity and contractility (15).

Protein Kinases

In addition to regulation by G proteins and calcium, adenylate cyclase, like the receptors and G proteins, can be modulated by phosphorylation, either by protein kinase C or protein kinase A (57,92). In a variety of cells, phorbol esters, which are potent activators of protein kinase C, produce stimulation or inhibition of cAMP synthesis (33,46). Evidence has been provided that adenylate cyclase can be phosphorylated and stimulated by activation of protein kinase C (38,93). In a recent study purified protein kinase C isozymes α and ξ phosphorylated purified type V adenylate cyclase and activated the enzyme in an isoform specific manner. Phosphopeptide mapping of the adenylate cyclase molecule showed that the pattern and the degree of phosphorylation by the two isoforms were different (38). In addition, adenylate cyclases types I to VI appear to have different sensitivities for protein kinase C (32,46). Protein kinase C is activated by diacylglycerol, a second messenger produced by stimulation of receptors coupled to phospholipase C by G_q. This is yet another route through which adenylate cyclase can receive signals from receptors not coupled to G_s or G_i. Thus, signals through receptors coupled to G_q can modulate the enzyme activity in three ways: by calcium, protein kinase C phosphorylation, and βγ subunits (Fig. 5). This means that type I adenylate cyclase can be simultaneously activated by both intracellular messengers produced by phospholipase C activation, inositol triphosphate and diacylglycerol, and this could provide for a powerful stimulus independent of G_s. On the other hand, protein kinase C greatly increases the basal activity of type II and the βγ subunits of G_q may further enhance G_s stimulation of the enzyme. Indeed, in neuronal cells the increase in cAMP induced by a β-adrenergic agonist is significantly enhanced by simultaneous treatment with activators of protein kinase C (71).

Protein kinase A has also been shown to phosphorylate the purified adenylate cyclase. When reconstituted in phospholipid vesicles with purified G_s the response of the phosphorylated adenylate cyclase to a GTP analogue was greatly diminished (92). Analysis of the homologous regions of the cytoplasmic domains proposed to encode the catalytic site of adenylate cyclase types V and VI show that both types have a conserved putative protein kinase A phosphorylation site at the end of the first cytoplasmic domain near transmembrane span 7. This site was not conserved in any other type of adenylate cyclase. Types I, II, and III have one or two putative sites at another location of the cytoplasmic domains, while type IV has none (56). Direct phosphorylation of adenylate cyclase by protein kinase A may be partly responsible for the heterologous desensitization of glucagon-induced adenylate cyclase activity in hepatocytes, which contain types V and VI adenylate cyclase (57). It is well documented that cAMP-dependent phosphorylation of hormone receptors by protein kinase A is one of the mechanisms of the diminished adenylate cyclase responsiveness that occurs in heterologous desensitization. Phosphorylation of adenylate cyclase by protein kinase A may be another level of regulation of the adenylate cyclase system in the presence of persistent stimulus.

Ever since the discovery of cAMP, investigators have remained puzzled by the intriguing question, namely, how can a ubiquitous molecule provide for the selective regulation of so many diverse cellular functions? Part of the answer can be found in the presence of adenylate cyclase isozymes, in the diversity of their regulation by endogenous factors and of their distribution within and between cells and tissues. The identification of many isoforms of membrane-bound adenylate cyclase in mammalian tissues has been surprising, since the function of adenylate cyclase in all cells is to synthesize cAMP and for a long time the major site of regulation of cAMP formation was assigned to the receptor and the G protein. Adenylate cyclases are regulated not only by signals from receptors coupled to the enzyme by G_s or G_i, but also by receptors coupled to other G proteins or independent of G proteins. At least nine putative independent but interacting regulatory sites can be found on the adenylate cyclase molecule. The putative catalytic region is very well conserved in all cyclases from bacteria to human. All isoforms are stimulated by the α subunit of G_s, but there is a type-specific, bidirectional regulation by G_i and other G proteins, e.g., G_o, G_q. The effect can be a direct effect of the subunit α or $\beta\gamma$, or secondary to the G protein–mediated modulation of an endogenous factor, calcium, or a protein, such as protein kinase A or C. In most instances the regulatory factors have a more pronounced effect when adenylate cyclase is stimulated by $G_s\alpha$. This may suggest that in vivo G_s maintains adenylate cyclase under a certain tone, which is modulated by signals from other receptors. Thus, one single adenylate cyclase can integrate separate interactive signals from the same or different receptors. The final response will depend on the temporal convergence of the signals, the properties, the relative amounts and the activation state of the adenylate cyclases present in a given cell. One can visualize a wide network of cell- and tissue-specific pathways formed by the interaction of different isoforms of adenylate cyclase, G subunits, and protein kinases to control cAMP synthesis. It is this complexity in adenylate cyclase regulation that can account in part for the selective response of the cell to cAMP, but it does not stop at the level of cAMP formation. The cAMP level in the cell is determined not only by its rate of synthesis, but also by its rate of degradation by phosphodiesterases. Phosphodiesterases belong to a large family of isozymes with a tissue-specific distribution pattern. These isozymes are also differently regulated by endogenous factors, e.g., calcium-CaM, cGMP, protein kinases (5). These enzymes, therefore, will not only terminate the action of cAMP, but also provide another mean of regulation of cAMP level, affecting the length and magnitude of the signal and the cross-talk between the adenylate cyclase and other pathways. The last selection will depend on the protein kinase A isoforms and their substrates, which determine the functional state of the cell (39). One can now start to understand how defects or mutations at any step along the cAMP cascade can lead to pathologic states.

Furthermore, identification of the structural divergences between the particular isozyme(s) present in individual cells and of the sequences essential for adenylate cyclase activity and regulation will permit the development of new therapeutic agents that will specifically alter the activity of one isozyme linked to a particular function. Such effector-selective drugs should be more specific than the current receptor-selective drugs and thereby have fewer side effects.

General Anesthetics and Adenylate Cyclase

There is a small body of literature spanning over 20 years that describes the interaction of general anesthetics, mainly volatile anesthetics, with the cAMP system in various tissues and species in in vivo and in vitro preparations. Since hormones and transmitters regulate the synthesis of cAMP, the effect of the anesthetics has been studied mainly on adenylate cyclase using tissue homogenates or membrane preparations as the source of enzyme. Even though the adenylate cyclase response to volatile anesthetics varies greatly between tissues and preparations and is often inconsistent, the results of these studies reveal some characteristics of the action of volatile anesthetics on adenylate cyclase. Within a clinically relevant range of concentrations the changes in adenylate cyclase were dose dependent and reversible, suggesting that the effect of the anesthetics is not due to a nonspecific disruption of the membrane bilayer. Most studies have examined the effects of halothane, but enflurane, isoflurane, sevoflurane and diethyl ether, where tested, produced similar qualitative changes in adenylate cyclase activity.

Volatile anesthetics have been reported to increase non-stimulated adenylate cyclase in vitro in various brain preparations, cerebral cortex, cerebellum and caudate nucleus, and in preparations from peripheral tissues, vascular, bronchial or uterine smooth muscle, platelets, and liver lymphocytes. The anesthetics further increased the adenylate cyclase response to hormones, transmitters, and autacoids that activate adenylate cyclase via receptors coupled to G_s, e.g., catecholamines, dopamine, glucagon, and prostaglandins, as well as to compounds that activate G_s, GTP and derivatives, or cholera toxin and sodium fluoride, which maintain G_s in an active state (6,19,65,69,80,81,85,87,89,91). In contrast, in myocardial homogenates from healthy animals from different species halothane 1 to 3 vol% or sevoflurane inhibited the adenylate cyclase response to β-adrenergic agonists or to GTP derivatives (21,26,66). In human ventricle and atrial membrane preparations from patients with terminal heart failure, however, halothane 2 vol% further increased basal as well as adenylate cyclase stimulated by isoproterenol, GTP, or cholera toxin, but not by forskolin (9). In preparations from cerebral cortex and normal and failing heart, halothane also diminished hormonal or GTP-induced inhibition of adenylate cyclase, an effect mediated by G_i (1,4,9). The effect of the anesthetics does not appear to be dependent on calcium and/or calmodulin (22,81).

The differences observed in the adenylate cyclase response to volatile anesthetics appear to be tissue related and may reflect the tissue dependent distribution of the adenylate cyclase isozymes. As described earlier in this chapter, the heart contains high amounts of types V and VI, while the brain contains predominantly type I, and the properties of types V and VI are very different from those of type I (Table 1). In addition, the qualitative difference between the healthy rat heart and the human failing heart is probably not due to species differences, since the properties of the adenylate cyclase isozymes do not vary from species to species (42), but it may reflect pathologic changes in the components of the adenylate cyclase system or in the regulatory factors. Indeed, as mentioned above, alterations in all three components of the β-adrenergic–adenylate cyclase system, receptor, G protein, and adenylate cyclase have been reported in the failing human heart and in a dog model of heart failure (27,30).

Volatile anesthetics alter adenylate cyclase activity independently of the type of stimulatory or inhibitory receptor regulating adenylate cyclase and modify the capability of the G protein to activate adenylate cyclase, suggesting that volatile anesthetics alter the enzyme activity by an action at the level of the G protein. This is in agreement with the observation that volatile anesthetics do not change the properties of the hormone receptor, but affect the coupling between the receptor and the G protein (2). Since the effect of volatile anesthetics is noncompetitive with hormones and GTP, it is possible, in view of the evidence that anesthetics interact at hydrophobic sites of membrane proteins, that the anesthetics induce conformational changes in the G protein, thereby altering the accessibility or availability of the G protein to its substrate GTP or/and to adenylate cyclase itself. This hypothesis is supported by the observation that detergents, which also partition into membranes, can selectively modulate the activation state of G proteins in a tissue selective pattern, an effect that is related to their concentration and chemical structure (50).

Another important class of anesthetics that also regulate adenylate cyclase activity are those that bind to specific membrane receptors that are coupled to adenylate cyclase by G_i. These include the opioids and the α_2-adrenergic agonists. The characteristics of these receptor pathways have been dealt with in a preceding chapter. However, it is interesting to note the synergistic effect observed experimentally and/or clinically between volatile anesthetics and opiates or α_2-adrenergic agonists. The mechanism of their interaction is still unknown, but there are indications that the anesthetic may interact with these receptor pathways at the level of the G protein (59; Vulliemoz, *unpublished data*).

There are very few reports of the interaction of other general anesthetics with the cAMP system. Anesthetic barbiturates and ketamine also appear to interfere selectively with the G protein–mediated activation of the enzyme. In rat brain synaptosomal membranes, barbiturates prevent G_s activation of adenylate cyclase, but do not affect G_i interaction with the enzyme (7,16,52).

At this time there is only circumstantial evidence that G proteins are a target for the action of anesthetics, and it is not clear whether the anesthetics interact selectively with any G protein. Future studies in reconstituted systems with purified isoforms of the three components of the cAMP system, receptor, G protein subunits, and adenylate cyclase will permit the identification of the site(s) of action of the anesthetics in the adenylate cyclase system.

As presented in other chapters of this book, general anesthetics also interact with receptors that are coupled to effectors other than adenylate cyclase, but that indirectly influence adenylate cyclase as well as cAMP phosphodiesterase. Furthermore, anesthetics modulate the release of transmitters, such as catecholamines, an effect that will influence the activation of receptors that modulate adenylate cyclase. To evaluate the overall effect of the anesthetic on cAMP in vivo, tissue cAMP level has been determined after exposure of an animal to a clinically relevant concentration of anesthetic (7,35,47,86). In most studies the change in cAMP level was qualitatively similar to that observed in vitro and in the direction expected from the functional change induced by the anesthetic. In mice exposed to 1.2 vol% halothane, for example, myocardial cAMP was decreased by about 50%, an effect that was prevented by pretreatment of the mice with propranolol, but was not affected by atropine (86). These data corroborate those obtained in vitro indicating that the anesthetic antagonizes the β-adrenoceptor–adenylate cyclase pathway and lend support to the hypothesis that the decreased positive inotropic effect of catecholamines induced by halothane is related to the anesthetic-induced changes in adenylate cyclase activity.

In addition, the results of a few studies suggest that anesthetics can also affect functions mediated by cAMP at a step distal to cAMP formation (58,78). Thus, evidence has been slowly accumulating supporting the hypothesis that general anesthetics alter signal transduction, but there is still much to learn. An important question is what defines the selectivity of their action. It has been proposed that halothane may modulate phosphorylation reactions. Since phosphorylation-dephosphorylation reactions are a primary mean of regulating key proteins in signal transduction cascades, this is an attractive unifying hypothesis that has not yet been investigated.

REFERENCES

1. Anthony BL, Dennison RL, Aronstam RS. Influence of volatile anesthetics on muscarinic regulation of adenylate cyclase activity. *Biochem Pharmacol* 1990;40:376–379.
2. Aronstam RS, Dennison RL. Anesthetic effects on muscarinic signal transduction. *Int Anesth Clin* 1989;27:265–272.
3. Bakalyar HA, Reed RR. Identification of a specialized adenylyl cyclase that may mediate odorant detection. *Science* 1990;250: 1403–1406.
4. Baumgartner MK, Dennis RL Jr, Narayanan TK, Aronstam RS. Halothane disruption of α_2-adrenergic receptor-mediated inhibition of adenylate cyclase and receptor G-protein coupling in rat brain. *Biochem Pharmacol* 1990;39:223–225.
5. Beavo JA. Multiple isozymes of cyclic nucleotide phosphodiesterase. *Adv Second Messenger and Phosphoprotein Res* 1988;22:1–38.
6. Bernstein KJ, Verosky M, Triner L. Effect of halothane on rat liver adenylate cyclase. *Anesth Analg* 1985;64:531–537.
7. Biebuyck JF, Dedrick DF, Scherer YD. Brain cyclic AMP and putative transmitter amino acids during anesthesia. In: Fink RB, ed. *Molecular Mechanisms of Anesthesia.* New York: Raven Press, 1975;1: 451–470.
8. Birnbaumer L, Abramowitz J, Brown AM. Receptor-effector coupling by G proteins. *Biochim Biophys Acta* 1990;1031:163–224.
9. Böhm M, Schmidt U, Gierschik P, Schwinger RHG, Böhm S, Erdmann E. Sensitization of adenylate cyclase by halothane in human myocardium and S49 lymphoma wild-type and cyc$^-$ cells: evidence for inactivation of the inhibitory G protein $G_{i\alpha}$. *Mol Pharmcol* 1994;45:380–389.
10. Cheung WY, Storm DR. Calmodulin regulation of cyclic AMP metabolism. In: Nathanson JA, Kebabian JW, eds. *Cyclic Nucleotides I.* New York: Springer-Verlag, 1982;301–323.
11. Choi EJ, Xia Z, Storm DR. Stimulation of the type III olfactory adenylyl cyclase by calcium and calmodulin. *Biochemistry* 1992;31: 6492–6498.
12. Colvin RA, Oibo JA, Allen RA. Calcium inhibition of cardiac adenylyl cyclase. Evidence for two distinct sites of inhibition. *Cell Calcium* 1991;12:19–27.
13. Cook WH, Lipkin D, Markham R. The formation of a cyclic dianhydrodiadenylic acid by the alkaline degradation of adenosine-5′-triphosphoric acid. *J Am Chem Soc* 1957;79:3607–3608.
14. Cooper DMF. Inhibition of adenylate cyclase by Ca^{2+}. *Biochem J Lett* 1991;278:903–904.
15. Cooper DMF, Brooker G. Ca^{+2}-inhibited adenylyl cyclase in cardiac tissue. *TIPS* 1993;14:34–36.
16. Dan'ura T, Kurokawa T, Yamashita A, Higashi K, Ishibashi S. Inhibition of brain adenylate cyclase by barbiturates through the effect on the interaction between guanine nucleotide-binding stimulatory regulatory protein and catalitic unit. *J Pharmacobiodyn* 1987; 10:98–103.
17. Federman AD, Conklin BR, Schrader KA, Reed RR, Bourne HR. Hormonal stimulation of adenylyl cyclase through G_i protein βγ subunit. *Nature* 1992;356:159–161s.
18. Feinstein PG, Schrader KA, Bakalyar HA, et al. Molecular cloning and characterization of a Ca^{2+}/calmodulin-insensitive adenylyl cyclase from rat brain. *Proc Natl Acad Sci USA* 1991;88:10173–10177.
19. Ferrero E, Ferrero ME, Marni A, et al. In vitro effects of halothane on lymphocytes. *Eur J Anaesth* 1986;3:321–330.
20. Franks NP, Lieb WR. Molecular and cellular mechanisms of general anesthesia. *Nature* 1994;367:607–614.
21. Gangat Y, Vulliemoz Y, Verosky M, Danilo P, Bernstein K, Triner L. Action of halothane on myocardial adenylate cyclase of rat and cat. *Proc Soc Exp Biol Med* 1979,160:154–159.
22. Gangat Y, Bernstein K, Vulliemoz Y, Verosky M, Triner L. Halothane- and butyrophenone-induced alterations of myocardial adenylate cyclase activity. In: Fink RB, ed. *Molecular Mechanisms of Anesthesia (Progress in Anesthesiology).* New York: Raven Press, 1980; 2:417–422.
23. Gao B, Gilman AG. Cloning and expression of a widely distributed (type IV) adenylyl cyclase. *Proc Natl Acad Sci USA* 1991;88: 10178–10182.
24. Gilman AG. G proteins: transducers of receptor-generated signals. *Annu Rev Biochem* 1987;56:615–649.
25. Hellevuo K, Yoshimura M, Kao M, Hoffman PL, Cooper DMF, Tabakoff B. A novel adenylyl cyclase sequence cloned from the human erythroleukemia cell line. *Biochem Biophys Res Comm* 1993; 192:311–318.
26. Hirota K, Ito Y, Kuze S, Momose Y. Effects of halothane on electrophysiologic properties and cyclic adenosine 3′,5′-monophosphate content in isolated guinea pig hearts. *Anesth Analg* 1992,74:564–569.
27. Homcy CJ, Vatner SF, Vatner DE. Beta-adrenergic receptor regulation in the heart in pathophysiological states: abnormal adrenergic responsiveness in cardiac disease. *Annu Rev Physiol* 1991;53:137–159.
28. Iniguez-Lluhi JA, Simon MI, Robishaw JD, Gilman AG. G protein βγ subunits synthesized in Sf9 cells. *J Biol Chem* 1992;267:23409–23417.
29. Ishikawa Y, Katsushika S, Chen L, et al. Isolation and characterization of a novel cardiac adenylylcyclase cDNA. *J Biol Chem* 1992;267: 13553–13557.
30. Ishikawa Y, Sorota S, Kiuchi K, et al. Downregulation of adenylylcyclase types V and VI mRNA levels in pacing-induced heart failure in dogs. *J Clin Invest* 1994;93:2224–2229.
31. Iyengar R. Molecular and functional diversity of mammalian G_s-stimulated adenylyl cyclases. *FASEB J* 1993;7:768–775.
32. Jacobowitz O, Chen J, Premont RT, Iyengar R. Stimulation of specific types of G_s-stimulated adenylyl cyclase by phorbol ester treatment. *J Biol Chem* 1993;268:3829–3832.
33. Jacobowitz O, Iyengar R. Phorbol ester-induced stimulation and phosphorylation of adenylyl cyclase 2. *Proc Natl Acad Sci USA* 1994;91:10630–10634.
34. Johnson RA, Shoshani I. Kinetics of "P"-site-mediated inhibition of

adenylyl cyclase and the requirements of substrate. *J Biol Chem* 1990;265:11595–11600.
35. Kant GJ, Muller TW, Leno RH, Meyerhoff JL. In vivo effects of pentobarbital and halothane anesthesia on levels of adenosine 3′,5′-monophosphate and guanosine 3′,5′-monophosphate in rat brain regions and pituitary. *Biochem Pharmacol* 1980;29:1891–1896.
36. Katada T, Katsukabe K, Oinuma M, Ui M. A novel mechanism for the inhibition of adenylate cyclase via inhibitory GTP binding proteins. *J Biol Chem* 1987;262:11897–11900.
37. Katsushika S, Chen L, Kawabe JI, Nilakantan R, Halnon NJ, Homcy CJ, Ishikawa Y. Cloning and characterization of a sixth adenylyl cyclase isoform: types V and VI constitute a subgroup within the mammalian adenylyl cyclase family. *Proc Natl Acad Sci USA* 1992;89: 8774–8778.
38. Kawabe J, Iwami G, Ebina T, et al. Differential activation of adenylyl cyclase by protein kinase C isoenzymes. *J Biol Chem* 1994;269: 16554–16558.
39. Krebs EG. Role of the cyclic AMP-dependent protein kinase in signal transduction. *JAMA* 1989;262:1815–1818.
40. Krupinski J. The adenylyl cyclase family. *Mol Cell Biochem* 1991;104: 73–79.
41. Krupinski J, Coussen F, Bakalyar HA, et al. Adenylyl cyclase amino acid sequence: possible channel- or transporter-like structure. *Science* 1989;244:1558–1564.
42. Krupinski J, Lehman TC, Frankenfield CD, Zwaagstra JC, Watson PA. Molecular diversity in the adenylylcyclase family. *J Biol Chem* 1992;267:24858–24862.
43. Lambert DG. Signal transduction: G proteins and second messengers. *Br J Anaesth* 1993;71:86–95.
44. Levin LR, Han PL, Hwang PM, Feinstein PG, Davis RL, Reed RR. The Drosophila learning and memory gene rutabaga encodes a Ca^{2+}/calmodulin-responsive adenylyl cyclase. *Cell* 1992;68: 479–489.
45. Levitzki A. From epinephrine to cyclic AMP. *Science* 1988;241: 800–806.
46. Lustig KD, Conklin BR, Herzmark P, Taussig R, Bourne HR. Type II adenylyl cyclase integrates coincident signals from G_s, G_i, and G_q. *J Biol Chem* 1993;268:13900–13905.
47. MacMurdo SD, Nemoto EM, Nikki, P, Frankenberry MJ. Brain cyclic AMP and possible mechanisms of cerebrovascular dilation by anesthetics in rats. *Anesthesiology* 1981;55:435–438.
48. Mollner S, Pfeuffer T. Two different adenylyl cyclases in brain distinguished by monoclonal antibodies. *Eur J Biochem* 1988;171: 265–271.
49. Mons N, Cooper DMF. Selective expression of one Ca^{2+}-inhibitable adenylyl cyclase in dopaminergically innervated rat brain regions. *Mol Brain Res* 1994;22:236–244.
50. Morris SA, Horn EM, Hawley T, Manning D, Bilezikian JP. The influence of detergents on the availability of pertussis toxin substrates. *Arch Biochem Biophys* 1991;290:1–7.
51. Neer EJ, Clapham DE. Roles of G protein subunits in transmembrane signalling. *Nature* 1988;333:129–134.
52. Okuda C, Miyazaki M, Kuriyama K. Alterations in cerebral β-adrenergic receptor-adenylate cyclase system induced by halothane, ketamine and ethanol. *Neurochem Int* 1984;6:237–244.
53. Parma J, Stengel D, Gannage MH, et al. Sequence of a human brain adenylyl cyclase partial cDNA. *Biochem Biophys Res Commun* 1991;179:455–462.
54. Pfeuffer T, Helmreich EJM. Activation of pigeon erythrocyte membrane adenylate cyclase by guanyl nucleotide analogues and separation of a nucleotide binding protein. *J Biol Chem* 1975; 250: 867–876.
55. Pfeuffer T, Metzger H. 7-O-Hemisuccinyl-deacetyl forskolin-sepharose: a novel affinity support for purification of adenylyl cyclase. *FEBS Lett* 1982;369–375.
56. Premont RT, Chen J, Ma HW, Ponnapalli M, Iyengar R. Two members of a widely expressed subfamily of hormone-stimulated adenylyl cyclases. *Proc Natl Acad Sci USA* 1992;89:9809–9813.
57. Premont RT, Jacobowitz O, Iyengar R. Lowered responsiveness of the catalyst of adenylyl cyclase to stimulation by G_s in heterologous desensitization: a role for adenosine 3′,5′-monophosphate-dependent phosphorylation. *Endocrinology* 1992;131:2774–2784.
58. Prokocimer PG, Maze M, Vickery RG, Kraemer FB, Gandjei R, Hoffman BB. Mechanism of halothane-induced inhibition of isoproterenol-stimulated lipolysis in isolated rat adipocytes. *Mol Pharmacol* 1988;33:338–343.
59. Puig MM, Turndorf H, Warner W. Effect of pertussis toxin on the interaction of azepexole and halothane. *J Pharmacol Exp Ther* 1990; 252:1156–1159.
60. Rall TW, Sutherland EW, Berthet J. The relationship of epinephrine and glucagon to liver phosphorylase. *J Biol Chem* 1957;224: 463–475.
61. Richards CD. Actions of general anesthetics on synaptic transmission in the CNS. *Br J Anaesth* 1983;55:201–207.
62. Robison GA, Butcher RW, Sutherland EW. *Cyclic AMP.* New York: Academic Press, 1971.
63. Rodbell M, Birnbaumer L, Pohl SL, Krans HMJ. The glucagon-sensitive adenyl cyclase system in plasma membrane of rat liver. *J Biol Chem* 1971; 246:1877–1882.
64. Rodbell M, Lin MC, Salomon Y, et al. Role of adenine and guanine nucleotides in the activity and response of adenylate cyclase systems to hormones: evidence for multisite transition states. *Adv Cyclic Nucleotide Res* 1975;5:3–29.
65. Rosenberg H, Pohl S. Stimulation of rat liver adenylate cyclase by halothane. *Life Sci* 1975;17:431–434.
66. Sanuki M, Yuge O, Kawamoto M, Fujii K, Azuma T. Sevoflurane inhibited β-adrenoceptor–G protein bindings in myocardial membrane in rats. *Anesth Analg* 1994;79:466–471.
67. Seamon KB, Daly JW. Forskolin: its biological and chemical properties. *Adv Cyclic Nucleotide Protein Phosphoryl Res* 1986;20:1–150.
68. Seeman P. The membrane action of anaesthetics and tranquillizers. *Pharmacol Rev* 1972;24:583–655.
69. Sprague DH, Yang JD, Ngai SH. Effects of isoflurane and halothane on contractility and the cyclic 3′,5′-adenosine monophosphate system in the rat aorta. *Anesthesiology* 1974;40:162–167.
70. Stengel D, Parma J, Gannage MH, Roeckel N, Mattei MG, Barouki R, Hanoune J. Different chromosomal localization of two adenylyl cyclase genes expressed in human brain. *Hum Genet* 1992;90: 126–130.
71. Sugden D, Klein DC. Activators of protein kinase C act at a postreceptor site to amplify cyclic AMP production in rat pinealocytes. *J Neurochem* 1988;50:149–155.
72. Tang WJ, Gilman AG. Type-specific regulation of adenylyl cyclase by G protein βγ subunits. *Science* 1991;254:1500–1503.
73. Tang WJ, Gilman AG. Adenylyl cyclases. *Cell* 1992;70:869–972.
74. Tang WJ, Krupinski J, Gilman AG. Expression and characterization of calmodulin-activated (type I) adenylylcyclase. *J Biol Chem* 1991; 266:8595–8603.
75. Taussig R, Iniguez-Lluhi JA, Gilman AG. Inhibition of adenylyl cyclase by $G_i\alpha$. *Science* 1993;261:218–221.
76. Taussig R, Quarmby, Gilman AG. Regulation of purified type I and type II adenylyl cyclases by G protein βγ subunits. *J Biol Chem* 1993; 268:9–12.
77. Taussig R, Tang WJ, Helper JR, Gilman AG. Distinct patterns of bidirectional regulation of mammalian adenylyl cyclases. *J Biol Chem* 1994;269:6093–610.
78. Thurston TA, Glusman S. Halothane myocardial depression: interactions with the adenylate cyclase system. *Anesth Analg* 1993;7: 63–68.
79. Towler SC, Evers AS. Anesthesia and chemical second messenger generation in the adrenergic nervous system. *Int Anesthesiol Clin* 1989;27:234–247.
80. Triner L, Vulliemoz Y, Verosky M. The action of halothane on adenylate cyclase. *Mol Pharmacol* 1977;13:976–979.
81. Triner L, Vulliemoz Y, Woo SY, Verosky M. Halothane effect on cAMP generation and hydrolysis in rat brain. *Eur J Pharmacol* 1980; 66:73–80.
82. Ueda N, Tang WJ. Conditional regulation of adenylyl cyclases by G-protein βγ-subunits. *Biochem Soc Trans* 1993;21:1132–1138.
83. Unwin N. Neurotransmitter action: opening of ligand-gated ion channel. *Cell/Neuron* 1993;72(suppl):31–41.
84. Vorherr T, Knöpfel L, Hofmann F, Mollner S, Pfeuffer T, Carafoli E. The calmodulin binding domain of nitric oxide synthase and adenylyl cyclase. *Biochemistry* 1993;32:6081–6088.
85. Vulliemoz Y, Verosky M, Triner L. The cyclic adenosine 3′,5′-monophosphate system in bronchial tissue. In: Stephens NL, ed. *The Biochemistry of Smooth Muscle.* Baltimore: University Press, 1977; 293–314.
86. Vulliemoz Y, Verosky M, Triner L. Effect of halothane on myocardial cyclic AMP and cyclic GMP content of mice. *J Pharmacol Exp Ther* 1986;236:181–186.
87. Walter F, Vulliemoz Y, Verosky M, Triner L. The action of halothane on the cyclic 3′,5′-adenosine monophosphate enzyme system in human platelets. *Anesth Analg* 1980;59:856–861.

88. Wong YH, Federman A, Pace AM, Zachary I, et al. Mutant α subunits of G_{i2} inhibit cyclic AMP accumulation. *Nature* 1991;351:63–65.
89. Woo SY, Verosky M, Vulliemoz Y, Triner L. Dopamine-sensitive adenylate cyclase activity in the rat caudate nucleus during exposure to halothane and enflurane. *Anesthesiology* 1979;51:27–33.
90. Xia Z, Refsdal CD, Merchant KM, Dorsa DM, Storm D. Distribution of mRNA for the calmodulin-sensitive adenylate cyclase in rat brain: expression in areas associated with learning and memory. *Neuron* 1991;6:431–443.
91. Yang JC, Triner L, Vulliemoz Y. Effects of halothane on the cyclic 3′,5′-adenosine monophosphate system in the rat uterine muscle. *Anesthesiology* 1973;38:244–250.
92. Yoshimasa T, Bouvier M, Benovic JL, Amlaiky N, Lefkowitz RJ, Caron MG. Regulation of the adenylate cyclase signalling pathway: potential role for the phosphorylation of the catalytic unit by protein kinase A and protein kinase C. In: Chretien M, Mckerns KW, eds. *Molecular Biology of Brain and Endocrine Peptidergic Systems.* New York: Plenum Press, 1988;123–139.
93. Yoshimasa T, Sibley DR, Bouvier M, Lefkowitz RJ, Caron MG. Cross-talk between cellular signalling pathways suggested by phorbol-ester-induced adenylate cyclase phosphorylation. *Nature* 1987;327:67–70.

Anesthesia: Biologic Foundations, edited by
Tony L. Yaksh et al. Lippincott–Raven Publishers,
Philadelphia © 1997.

CHAPTER 7

PROTEIN KINASE C

SUSAN FIRESTONE AND LEONARD FIRESTONE

Protein kinase C (PKC) was first identified in 1977 by Nishizuka's group (36,62) as a histone protein kinase activated not by a cyclic nucleotide, but rather by the combined effects of calcium ion, phospholipid, and diacylglycerol (DAG; Fig. 1) or phorbol ester. This led to the understanding that PKC acts as the intracellular effector for G protein–linked cell surface receptors, including muscarinic cholinergeric, serotonin (5-HT), and α_1-adrenergic types, whose activation generates that array of second messengers. A prodigious amount of investigation has now established PKC's central role in signal transduction in cell types as diverse as neurons, T cells, and endocrine acinar cells, and in biologic processes such as development (53), memory (5), and carcinogenesis (6). This central role is the basis for speculation that the heterogeneous tissue responses of anesthetics can be accounted for, at least in part, by effects on PKC.

To date, virtually all anesthesia research relating to PKC has focused on the CNS enzyme. This chapter discusses PKC's physiologic role in the nervous system. PKC is particularly abundant in the nervous system, and has been implicated in many key neuronal functions, and even diseases such as Alzheimer's (13), Parkinson's (45), and Huntington's (29). For example, activation of PKC is associated with modulation of ion channels (reviewed in 58) including the γ-aminobutyric acid $GABA_A$ receptor (42), receptor desensitization (35), and enhancement of neurotransmitter release (56). Given this broad array, it is clear that the PKC pathway can readily modulate the efficacy of synaptic transmission at virtually all sites in the nervous system. Coupled with the well-known effects of general anesthetics on synaptic transmission, this formed the basis for our initial interest in CNS-derived PKC as a putative anesthetic target (21,24).

MOLECULAR HETEROGENEITY AND MECHANISM OF ACTIVATION

Early work with nerve and other tissue revealed that agonist-induced G-protein activation enhanced DAG production in membranes, as a consequence of immediate hydrolysis of inositol phospholipid (PIP_2; Fig. 1) by phospholipase C (PLC) (46), and a slower hydrolysis of membrane phospholipid (e.g., phosphatidylserine [PS]) by phospholipase D (PLD) with further dephosphorylation to DAG (19). The production of DAG parallels the formation of inositol 1,3,4-trisphosphate (IP_3), which in turn gives rise, through a receptor-mediated mechanism, to the release of Ca^{2+} from intracellular membrane stores. Release of another second messenger, arachidonic acid (AA), often

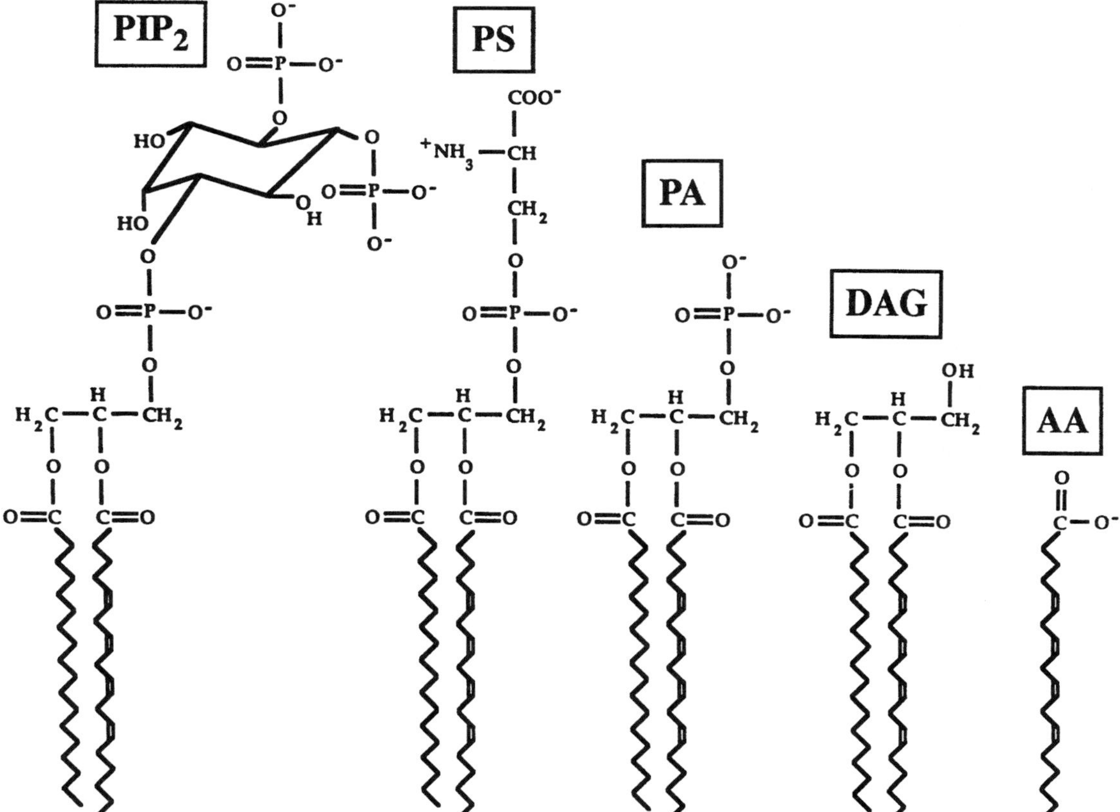

Figure 1. Lipids involved in the activation of protein kinase C. Abbreviations are specified in the text.

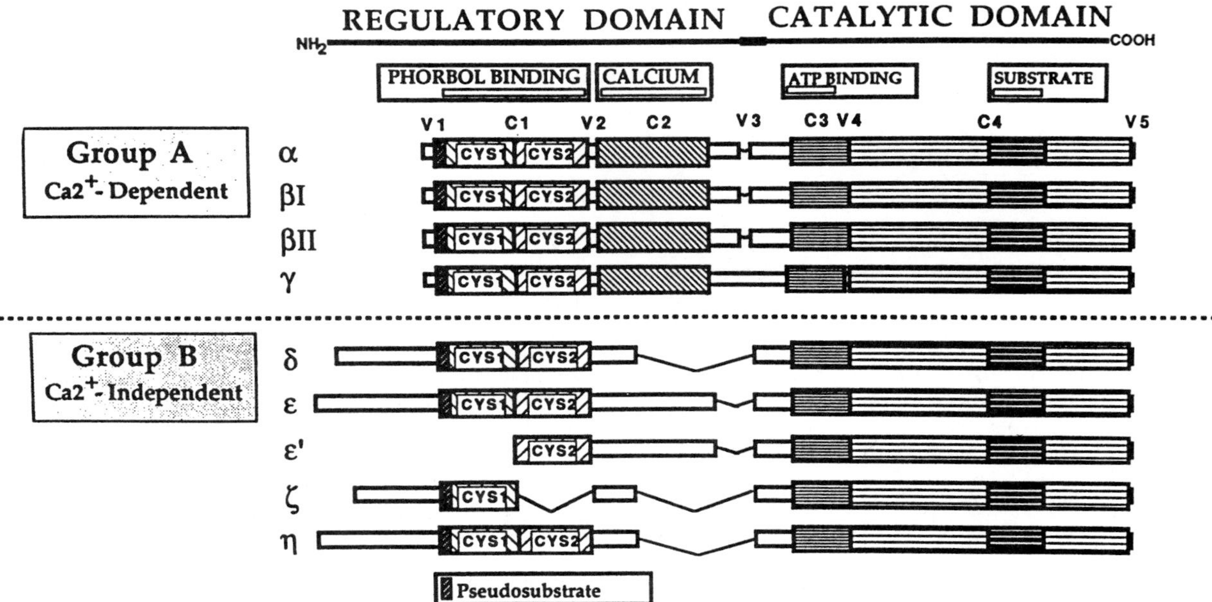

Figure 2. Domain structure of the PKC family of isozymes. C1–C5 are conserved regions; V1–V5 are variable regions. Areas of shared homology are highlighted. The regulatory domain contains the phorbol and Ca^{2+} interaction sites; the catalytic domain contains the substrate and ATP recognition sites. (From ref. 11, with permission.)

accompanies activation of PLC and PLD as well, through phospholipase A_2-catalyzed hydrolysis.

To date, ten isoforms (α, β1, βII, γ, δ, ε, η, θ, ς, and λ) have been identified in mammalian tissues, differing in their cofactor dependence, intracellular localization, and tissue expression. This makes the PKC family the largest serine/threonine-specific kinase subfamily known, rivaling even the expansive *src*-related tyrosine-specific kinase family. The first four isoforms identified, α, β1, βII, and γ (47), are activated by DAG and Ca^{2+}, with further enhancement by free fatty acids (FFA) and

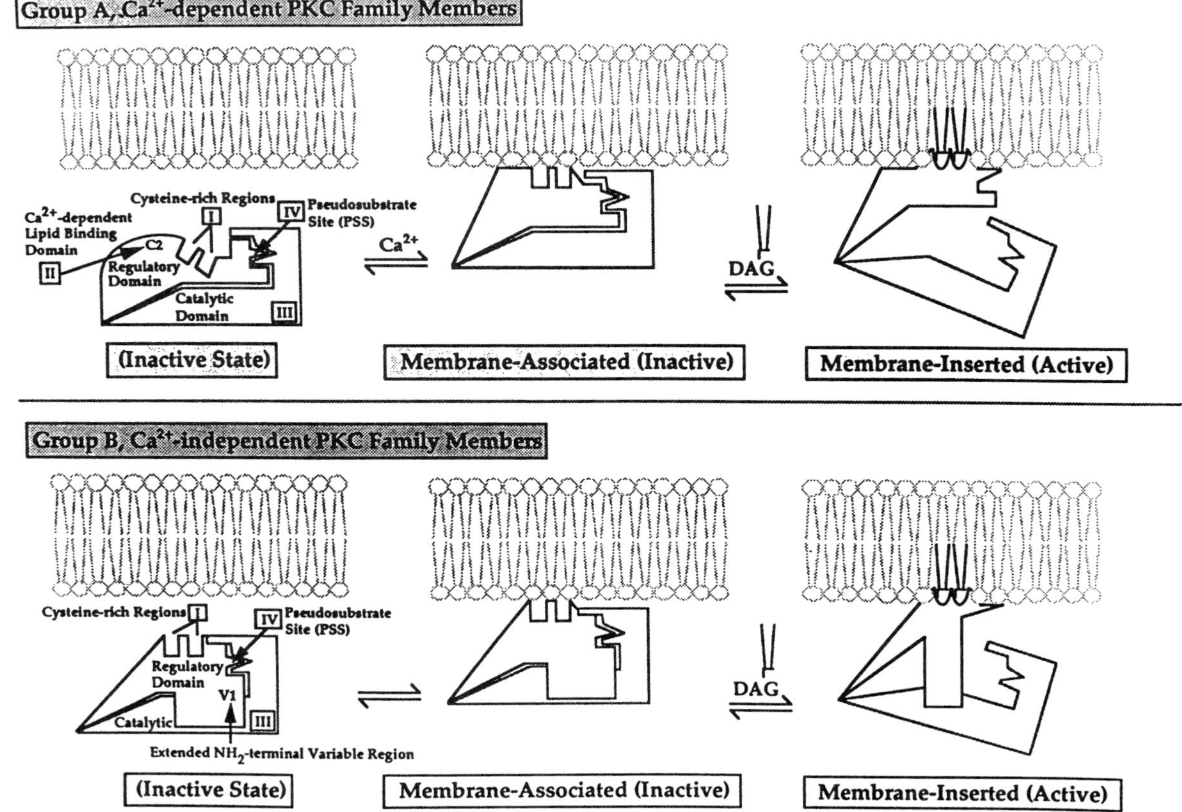

Figure 3. Activation mechanism for the PKC family of enzymes. *Top*: Activation of the Ca^{2+}-dependent isozymes. *Bottom*: Activation of the Ca^{2+}-independent isozymes. (From ref. 11, with permission.)

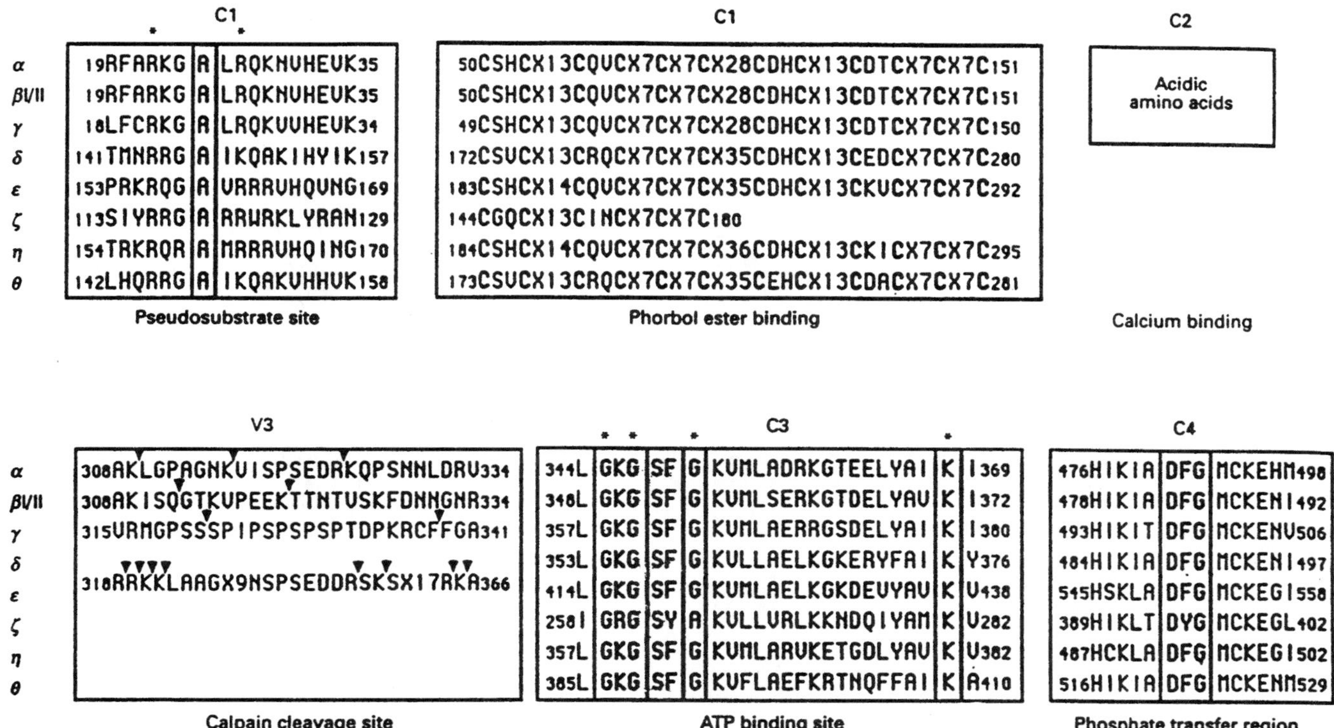

Figure 4. Sequence motifs of PKC isoenzymes. Sequences are taken from human, rat, and mouse isoforms. *Asterisks* indicate conserved amino acids; *arrowhead,* the calpain I and II, or tryptic cleavage sites. Longer stretches of nonhomologous amino acids within the conserved sequences are marked with X followed by the number of amino acids not depicted. (From ref. 34, with permission.)

lysophosphatidylcholine, and have four regions of conserved sequence (C1–C4; Fig. 2) and five regions of variable sequence (V1–V5). The cysteine-rich sequence repeat in C1 is essential for phorbol ester binding, while C2 is related to Ca^{2+} sensitivity (although in the presence of DAG and FFA, basal levels of Ca^{2+} are sufficient for maximal activation). The enzyme's catalytic site is within C3, while C4 is required for substrate recognition. A generic activation mechanism for this group of isozymes is represented in Fig. 3 (Group A); briefly, activation involves transient elevation in intracellular Ca^{2+}, followed by translocation of the enzyme to the membrane (via Ca^{2+}-dependent interaction with membrane lipids at lipid interaction site II). The membrane-associated, inactive form is then activated following DAG-induced insertion of the cysteine-rich regions (lipid interaction site I) into the membrane bilayer. During the insertion process, a conformational isomerization dislocates the intrinsic pseudosubstrate (see Fig. 2) from the substrate site, yielding an active enzyme. Biochemical and physical aspects of lipid activation of PKC have been reviewed (11).

The next four isoforms, δ, ε, η, and θ, sometimes known as nPKCs, are missing C2 and therefore not Ca^{2+} dependent, but do require PS and DAG for activation (51,52) (Fig. 3, Group B). These may be the effectors for growth factor receptors, ultimately controlling the cell cycle via the nucleus (3). The δ and ε isoforms are found in brain; ε has been localized to nerve terminals. Figure 3 (Group B) illustrates the activation mechanism for nPKCs, where elevation of intracellular Ca^{2+} is not necessary to permit membrane translocation; activation otherwise proceeds as in the Ca^{2+}-dependent isoforms. Note that in the figure, the regulatory domain still contacts the catalytic domain in the Ca^{2+}-independent isoforms; this represents the finding in nPKCs that substrate preference of the catalytic domain can still be modulated even after activation of the kinase.

The final two isoforms, ς and λ, known as the aPKCs, lack the C2 region and have only one cysteine-rich region. They are unaffected by DAG, phorbol esters, and Ca^{2+}, but are activated by PS. The physiologic stimulus that activates the aPKC isoforms is still unknown, although they are ubiquitous in tissues.

Partial genomic clones have been isolated only for the human PKC-β and human and rat PKC-γ genes (12,54); thus, little is known about the DNA sequence or genomic organization of mammalian PKC genes. It has been demonstrated that the βI and βII isoforms are generated by alternative splicing of a common primary transcript. In contrast, there is detailed amino acid sequence information available; similarities in the critical functional domains are presented in Fig. 4.

DIFFERENTIAL EXPRESSION IN THE NERVOUS SYSTEM

The cellular distribution of the predominant isoforms found in the nervous system are represented in Table 1. These and the ς isoform have been identified in the spinal cord and brain by Western and Northern blot analysis, as well as by in situ hybridization. Differential distribution has been revealed by immunohistochemical analysis using isoform-specific antibodies (64). For example, the γ isoform seems to be expressed exclusively in the brain and spinal cord, mainly in excitatory and inhibitory amino acidergic neurons, such as hippocampal pyramidal and granule cells, cerebellar Purkinje cells, cortical pyramidal cells, and thalamic neurons. In developing rats, γ is virtually absent at birth but progressively increases for several weeks postnatally; the same is true for βII. In contrast, the βI isoform is already significantly expressed (mainly in the brain stem) at birth, and continues to increase thereafter. βII is localized primarily in amino acidergic neurons; ε is expressed principally in nerve terminals in the forebrain, spinal cord, and primary sensory neurons. Interestingly, in the striatum and substantia nigra, expression of each of the four members of the Ca^{2+}-dependent group is confined to a different neuron with a

Table 1. CELLULAR DISTRIBUTION OF COMMON PROTEIN KINASE C ISOFORMS IN MAMMALIAN BRAIN

	α	βI	βII	γ	ε
Neocortex	Round cell (I) Pyramidal cell (III) Nonpyramidal (IV–VI)	Horizontal cell (I) Nonpyramidal (II–VI, GABA)	Pyramidal cell (II, III, V)	Pyramidal cell (II, V, VI)	Nerve terminal
Hippocampal formation	Pyramidal cell (CA1–CA3) Interneuron	–	Pyramidal cell (CA1)	Pyramidal cell (CA1–CA3) Granule cell (DG)	Pyramidal cell (CA3) Mossy fiber Schaffer collateral Perforant pathway
Stratum	ACh neuron	GABA neuron (intrinsic)	GABA neuron (projecting)	Medium-sized cell (projecting)	Nerve terminal
Substantia nigra	Dopamine neuron (pars compacta)	Nondopamine (pars reticulata)	GABA terminal	Nerve terminal	Nerve terminal
Cerebellar cortex	Climbing fiber Basket cell Stellate cell	Mossy fiber Basket cell Stellate cell	Parallel fiber	Purkinje cell Basket cell Stellate cell Golgi cell	Parallel fiber
Deep nuclei cerebellar	–	–	Purkinje cell terminal	–	–

From ref. 63.

specific neurotransmitter (71); in contrast, glutaminergic neurons in the hippocampus contain multiple PKC isoforms. The α, βII, and γ isoforms are present in pyramidal cells; α and γ in granule cells.

The subcellular distribution in neurons is also heterogeneous: γ is localized mostly presynaptically, in the cytoplasm near ribosomes and the outer membranes of cell organelles. (The exception is in the terminals of Purkinje cells.) The α isoform is usually in the periphery of perikarya but has also been found near nuclei. The significance of such subcellular distribution patterns is not yet known, but may provide important clues regarding their respective roles in short- and long-term neuromodulation.

ROLE OF PKC IN NEUROMODULATION

The principal mechanism by which PKC influences excitability is by modification of membrane ion channels (35,58). Arguably the most important among these are voltage-dependent calcium channels, since they have major influence over neuronal firing patterns, the morphology of action potentials, and the quantity of neurotransmitter released by a neuron. The bag cell neurons of the invertebrate *Aplysia* have been extensively studied for kinase-linked modulation of calcium channels (15). Inhibitors of PKC can block the progressive increase in the amplitude of bag cell action potentials typically observed during evoked discharge (16), without affecting the pattern of firing. Microinjection of PKC, or application of PKC activators, reproduces the enhancement. In bag cell neurons, the mechanism by which calcium currents are enhanced by PKC involves unmasking a new species of voltage-dependent calcium channel in the plasma membrane (61).

Calcium channels from vertebrate cells are also modulated by PKC (reviewed in 39). For example, in rat dorsal root ganglion (DRG) neurons, PKC activators result in inhibition of calcium currents mediated by T- and N-type channels. In contrast, in hippocampal neurons, N-type calcium currents are reduced without effects on L- or T-types. In these and many other examples, inhibition may occur by one of three general mechanisms illustrated in Fig. 5. Activation of PKC may selectively affect one or more calcium (or other) channel type, possibly by direct phosphorylation. Alternatively, PKC may produce a more generalized effect by phosphorylation of enzymes or guanosine triphosphate (GTP)-binding proteins that are components of second messenger pathways that, in turn, influence the activity of channels. In addition, PKC activators may have a nonspecific pharmacologic action on channels based on binding site homology, unrelated to their effects on the activation of PKC.

Other mammalian neuronal channels known to be affected by activation of PKC include calcium-activated K^+ channels from CA1 hippocampal pyramidal neurons (18); M-current K^+ channels in sympathetic ganglia (10); delayed-rectifier K^+ channels in acutely dissociated hippocampal neurons (17); brain GABA-gated Cl^- channels expressed in ooctyes (38); and, voltage-dependent Na^+ channels (VDSC) (59). In $GABA_A$-gated channels, site-directed mutagenesis of the Ser-410 residue in the β_2 subtype, and the Ser-327 residue in the γ_{2S} subtype, was used to demonstrate that phosphorylation of these residues by a phorbol-stimulated kinase was responsible for inhibition of function (38). With a similar strategy, a phosphorylation site was identified in the intracellular loop of VDSCs between putative membrane-spanning domains III and IV of the α subunit, which is required for modulation by PKC.

The ultimate effect of PKC-mediated channel modulation is likely to be a change in the efficacy of synaptic transmission. For example, in cerebellum, through desensitization of postsynaptic glutamate receptors, phorbol esters enhance coactivation of climbing fiber and parallel fiber input to Purkinje cells, leading to long-term depression (LTD) of the parallel fiber input. PKC inhibitors prevent the LTD response (37,41). In contrast, in dentate gyrus and the CA1 region of the hippocampus (4), PKC activation is associated with long-term potentiation (LTP), which is the persistent enhancement of synaptic efficacy due to a Ca^{2+}-dependent phosphorylation (33,43). Because the γ isoform is localized on the postsynaptic side of the glutaminergic synapse related to LTP or LTD, this PKC isoform is the most likely candidate for mediating these events.

PKC's influence on neurotransmitter release would also be expected to affect neuronal network activity. Ca^{2+}-dependent release of neurotransmitter evoked by chemical or electrical depolarization is usually potentiated by PKC activators (reviewed in 63; see also 56). This has been demonstrated in cerebellar Purkinje cells (where the γ isoform is involved in GABA release), substantia nigra (where the βII isoform is located in the terminals of GABAergic neurons), and striatum

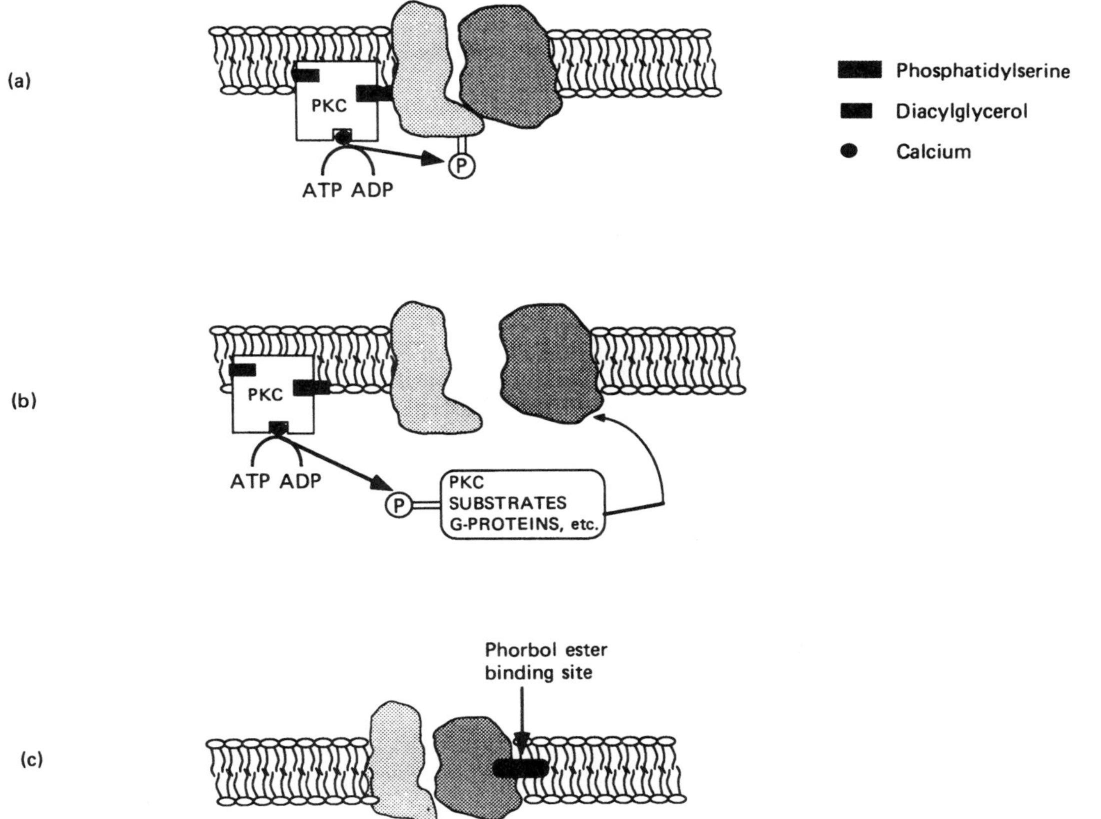

Figure 5. Mechanisms of ion channel modulation by PKC activators. **a:** Direct phosphorylation of the channel. **b:** Indirect modulation of channel activity by alterations in the phosphorylation state of other proteins such as components of second messenger pathways. **c:** Direct block of channel activity by PKC activators. (From ref. 39, with permission.)

(where the α isoform colocalizes with choline acetyltransferase in striatal neurons). Presynaptic proteins thought to be involved in transmitter release are also known to be PKC substrates; these include GAP-43 (14) and dephosphin (56). The α and βII isoforms, localized presynaptically in hippocampus, may be responsible for their phosphorylation.

In 1993 a strain of mice with complete deletion of the gene encoding the γ isoform of PKC was generated using the gene targeting method (2). These animals were tested for their ability to carry out hippocampal-dependent spatial and contextual learning. This was based on prior findings correlating hippocampal PKC with performance in learning tasks (7,50), and that an increase in γ in the hippocampus is observed with spatial learning (68). These mutant mice were noted to have an abnormal gait, resembling cerebellum-lesioned animals, consistent with the γ isoform's high level of expression in cerebellar Purkinje cells (47). Performance in the hidden-platform Morris water maze task, a test for spatial as well as contextual learning that requires the hippocampus, indicated mild deficits in both of these forms of learning. In separate experiments (1), it was shown that LTP in the CA1 hippocampal region of the PKC-γ–deficient mice was abnormal; it could rarely be induced after conventional high-frequency stimulation (tetanus), although apparently normal LTP was observed if the tetanus was preceded by a low-frequency stimulation. In contrast, ordinary synaptic transmission was normal, as was induction of LTD. The results of observations made upon administration to PKC-γ–deficient mice of intoxicating levels of alcohol are discussed in the next section.

These experiments amply illustrate the great utility of the gene targeting method for elucidating the physiologic role of each PKC isoform; analogous experiments are no doubt under way for some or all of the other isoforms.

ANESTHETIC EFFECTS ON PROTEIN KINASE C

The tumor-promoting phorbol esters activate PKC by specifically binding to its DAG interaction site (40). Using a ^{3}H-phorbol dibutyrate (PDBu) and membrane-bound PKC from rat brain, Firestone and Firestone assessed the ability of a homologous series of *n*-alkanols (21) and several structurally heterogeneous general anesthetics, including halothane, thiopental, etomidate, and ethanol (24), to affect activator binding. At physiologic concentrations, all agents significantly inhibited PDBu binding in a reversible, concentration-dependent fashion (Fig. 6), with potencies that paralleled lipophilicity. At high concentrations, binding was completely but reversibly inhibited; however, the maximal number of (noninteracting) PDBu sites was unchanged by exposure to anesthetics. Similarly, anesthetics such as halothane, diethylether, and ethanol were found to inhibit the enzymatic activity of crudely purified soluble PKC (27; Table 2), using a ^{32}P-incorporation assay adapted from the procedure of Bell et al. (8). Although the efficiency of ^{32}P-incorporation depended to some degree on the identity of the protein substrate (histone III*S* > myosin light chain kinase > troponin), clinically relevant concentrations of these anesthetics still inhibited phosphorylation of all three substrates (26). In 1993 confirmatory findings of PKC inhibition by *n*-alkanols (Fig. 7), halothane, and enflurane were reported (60), using crudely purified PKC from rat brain activated both in a lipid-free assay by protamine sulfate (36), as well as with lipid vesicles

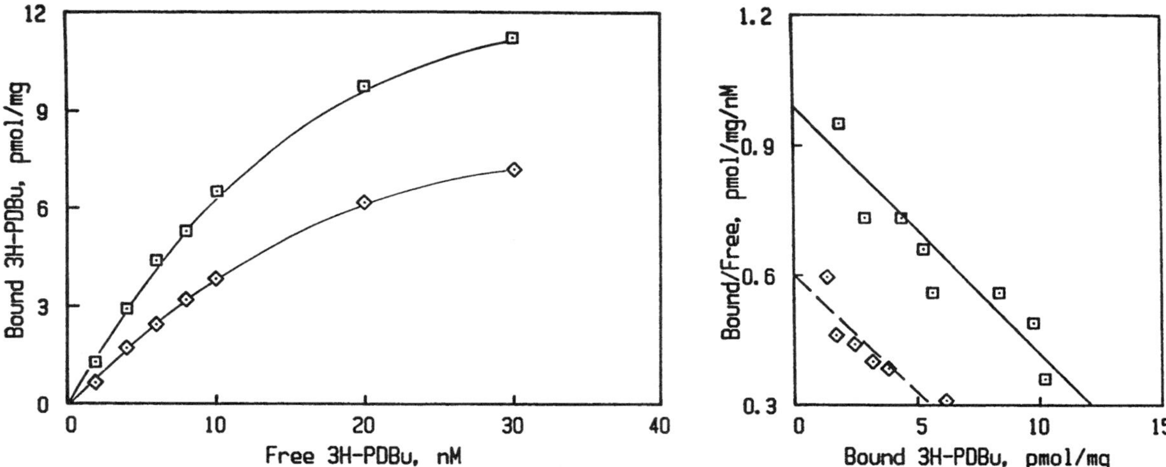

Figure 6. Effect of ethanol on phorbol dibutyrate (PDBu) association with PKC. *Left:* Binding in the presence of ethanol 100 mM (diamonds) is compared to that of controls *(squares)*. Membrane fragments and cytosol containing PKC, purified from rat whole brain homogenates, were incubated to equilibrium (40 min, 20ºC), and bound ^{3}H-PDBu was separated from free by ultracentrifugation. Nonspecific binding, determined in the presence of 1 μM unlabeled PDBu, amounted to <10% of total binding and was subtracted to yield specifically bound ^{3}H-PDBu. Gas chromatography was used to monitor for ethanol losses due to evaporation. Data are fit to functions using an iterative, nonlinear least squares routine. *Right:* Scatchard analysis of these same data; the parallel leftward shift in the presence of ethanol indicates that there is a decrease in PKC sites (X-intercept) rather than a change in apparent affinity (−1/slope). (Firestone and Firestone, unpublished results.)

and the DAG analogue 12-O-tetradecanoylphorbol-13-acetate (TPA) (8). The degree of ethanol-induced inhibition was found to be lipid dependent such that PS-eggPC > PS-POPC > PS, but inhibition by these mixtures did not parallel their "fluidity" as reflected by diphenylhexatriene rotational mobility.

In apparent conflict, other groups have reported that anesthetics *enhance* PKC activity. For example, Tsuchiya et al. (67) observed that ^{32}P incorporation into both histone III*S* and cerebral cytoplasmic proteins by rat cerebral PKC was strongly enhanced by 10 to 30 mM (!) halothane, and modestly enhanced by similar concentrations of isoflurane and enflurane. The PKC employed was purified on diethylaminoethyl (DEAE) cellulose and Superose columns, and reaction mixtures included 300 μM Ca^{2+}, 100 μM phospholipid, 5 μM diolein, and 100 μM TPA as in Boni and Rando (9). Hemmings and Adamo (30,73) found that halothane and propofol also stimulated phosphorylation by partially purified rat forebrain PKC, depending on the lipid mixture and substrate (Table 3). Specifically, stimulation was marked when lipid vesicles contained PC, PS, and DAG, and the substrate was histone H1; much less stimulation occurred with PS/DAG, or when protamine or poly(lysine, serine) peptides were used as substrates. Stimulation was absent with PS/DAG/Triton X-100 micelles, with all three artificial substrates, and when activation was induced by AA or oleic acid. Substitution of PDBu for DAG in the lipid vesicles did not interfere with anesthetic-induced activation, and since the activity of the PKC's catalytic fragment was unaffected by halothane, it was concluded that the anesthetics acted through the lipid-binding regulatory domain. Further biochemical characterization of anesthetic-induced activation (31) revealed that these same agents increased V_{max} without affecting the K_m for phosphorylation of histone H1, and increased PKC's sensitivity to activation by PS, DAG, and Ca^{2+} (Table 4). Because anesthetics affected all of these activators, and increased the IC_{50} value for sphingosine, a regulatory domain-specific PKC inhibitor, these data were taken as further

Table 2. EFFECT OF ANESTHETICS ON THE ENZYMATIC ACTIVITY OF PKC[a]

Agent	Concentration (mM)	Activity (pmol/min/10 λ eluate)	% Control Activity[b]
Control	0	8.1–8.5	100
Ethanol	90	6.2	82
	180	4.8	63
	400	3.1	41
Halothane	0.6	4.4	52
Diethylether	20	5.1	63
	40	4.4	54

[a]PKC was released from rat brain homogenates by Ca^{2+} chelator treatment, purified by DEAE-Sephacel, then eluted by ionic gradient. PKC concentration was determined under conditions of saturating ^{3}H-PDBu as in Fig. 6. Reaction mixtures consisted of aliquots of dilute enzyme, lipid (phosphatidylserine-DAG) dispersion, calcium/magnesium chloride (final Ca^{2+} 20 μM; Mg^{2+} 10 mM), substrate protein (histone III*S*) and general anesthetic diluted in buffer. After equilibration (at 30°C), reactions were initiated by addition of 10 μM (final concentration) γ-^{32}P-ATP, allowed to incubate for 2.5 minutes (period of linear activity), then quenched with excess iced 25% trichloroacetate. Following filtration through GF/C glass fiber (Whatman), filters were dried and counted in scintillation cocktail, and ^{32}P incorporation corrected for other kinase activities determined in the absence of added lipids. General anesthetic concentrations were confirmed by gas chromatography.

[b]% Control activity = (Activity with GAs/Activity without GAs) × 100%. (Firestone and Firestone, unpublished results.)

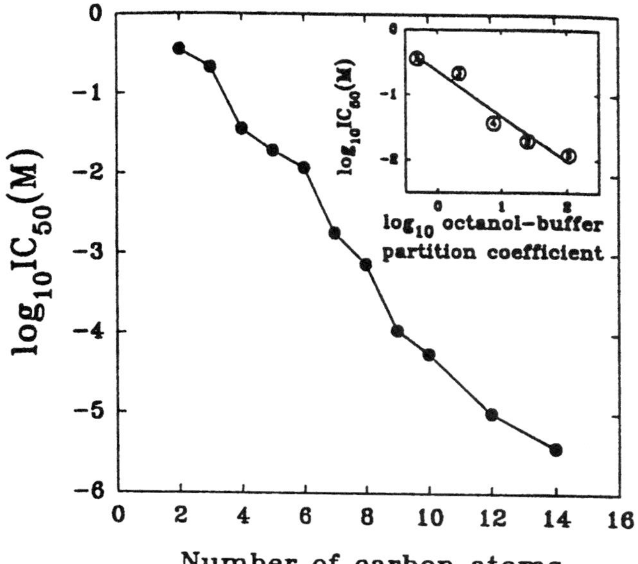

Figure 7. The dependence of PKC inhibition potency (IC_{50}) on methylene carbon chain length of a homologous series of *n*-alkanols. IC_{50} values were calculated from PKC activities determined over a range of alcohol concentrations. *Inset:* Potency of inhibition by alcohols as a function of the buffer-octanol partition coefficients. (From ref. 60, with permission.)

support that anesthetics stabilize PKC's active conformation, probably through interactions with the regulatory domain.

Because the concentrations of the agents employed by Tshuchiya et al. (67) exceeded their reported saturated solubilities in buffer [i.e., halothane, 17 mM; isoflurane, 15 mM; enflurane, 15 mM (20)], it is possible that conflicting results are explained by partial enzyme denaturation after exposure to undissolved anesthetic droplets in reaction mixtures. By analogy with site-directed mutagenesis (55) and proteolytic (calpain or trypsin) cleavage studies (57), the result of selective denaturation of the regulatory domain might be constitutively enhanced activity. It should also be mentioned that the effective concentrations for activation of PKC reported by Hemmings et al. (30,31) exceeded clinical half-effect concentrations by at least three- and fivefold (halothane and propofol), respectively.

Whatever the findings in vitro, the physiologically relevant effects of anesthetics on PKC can only be revealed by observations in living systems, such as intact cultured cells and animals. Using neutrophils as a model, Tshuchiya et al. (66) assayed the effects of halothane on superoxide generation ex vivo following stimulation by a phorbol ester. Halothane enhanced superoxide generation, as reflected by the reduction of cytochrome C and monitored spectrophotometrically, with the half-effect concentration described as 0.3 mM and the maximal effect as 1.0 mM; stimulation could be completely blocked by H-7, a PKC inhibitor. Similarly, Tas and Koschel (65) studied the effects of halothane, enflurane, isoflurane, and methoxyflurane on phorbol ester-enhanced norepinephrine release from rat pheochromocytoma PC12 cells. These cells share many properties with adrenergic neurons, including high-affinity catecholamine uptake and storage, and release after depolarization or nicotinic stimulation. ^{3}H-norepinephrine release from PC12 cells, known to be enhanced synergistically by PKC and Ca^{2+}, was stimulated by therapeutic concentrations of volatile agents, with effective concentrations paralleling their clinical potencies. Separate studies in which cells were loaded with the Ca^{2+}-sensitive fluorescent dye Fura-2 revealed anesthetic dose-dependent increases in cytoplasmic Ca^{2+} levels, leading to the conclusion that stimulation of PKC-mediated neurotransmitter release in PC12 cells by anesthetics is mediated by a rise in Ca_i^{2+}. The mechanism(s) involved in this rise, which might include diminished uptake of Ca^{2+} into intracellular storage sites, decreased Ca^{2+} efflux from cells, enhanced cellular influx, or even production of IP_3 with receptor-mediated release from intracellular stores, was not determined.

Messing et al. (44) reported that 2- to 8-day exposure to intoxicating concentrations of ethanol upregulated PKC activity in both PC12 and NG108-15 neuroblastoma-glioma cells. Cellular PKC increased, particularly the δ and ε isoforms (Fig. 8), and was associated with an increase in PKC-mediated phosphoryla-

Table 3. EFFECTS OF HALOTHANE 2.4 VOL% ON PROTEIN KINASE C ACTIVITY[a]

		PKC Activity[b]								
		Histone H1			Protamine			Poly (Lys, Ser)		
		Halothane			Halothane			Halothane		
Lipid Cofactors	Ca^{2+}	−	+	Ratio[c] (%)	−	+	Ratio (%)	−	+	Ratio (%)
None	-	1.69 ± 0.12	1.92 ± 0.62	114	63.2 ± 7.8	52.5 ± 10††	83.0	9.95 ± 1.54	9.18 ± 1.66	92.3
PS/DG dispersion[d]	-	20.4 ± 4.4	26.7 ± 4.6**	131	1.39 ± 9.8	140 ± 21	101	9.54 ± 1.81	9.50 ± 2.19	99.6
	+	32.2 ± 3.0	46.0 ± 5.6**	143	92.2 ± 6.5	82.0 ± 12††	88.9	7.54 ± 2.02	7.79 ± 0.95	103
PC/PS/DG vesicles[e]	-	3.90 ± 0.48	4.88 ± 0.54**	125	74.0 ± 6.8	101 ± 15††	136	10.8 ± 2.2	12.4 ± 2.0††	115
	+	16.7 ± 2.6	35.2 ± 10.4**	211	91.5 ± 10	92.8 ± 23	101	11.2 ± 2.5	10.8 ± 2.0	96.4
PS/DG Triton X-100	-	5.55 ± 0.89	7.39 ± 1.76	133	173 ± 22	182 ± 25	106	69.3 ± 10.2	68.6 ± 13.0	99.3
Mixed micelles[f]	+	51.6 ± 7.0	57.0 ± 4.8	110	198 ± 22	160 ± 14	108	52.6 ± 8.8	52.3 ± 9.1	99.4

[a]Qualitatively similar results were obtained for propofol 240 μM.

[b]PKC activity was assayed at 30°C using 0.25 μg/ml [for histone H1 and poly(Lys, Ser)] or 0.05 μg/ml (for protamine) purified PKC. Values for protamine assays have been normalized to an enzyme concentration of 0.25 μg/ml to allow direct comparison to other substrates. Data are mean ± SD; $n = 5$. Each experiment included duplicate assays of each experimental condition in the absence or presence of 2.4 vol% halothane. Differences between means were analyzed by the two-tailed ± test.

[c]Values are expressed as percentage of PKC activity in the presence of halothane normalized to activity in the absence of anesthetic.

[d]Assayed by the method of Taki et al. (62).

[e]Assayed by the method of Boni and Rando (9).

[f]Assayed by the method of Hannun Y, Loomis C, Bell RM. Activation of protein kinase C by Triton X-100 mixed micelles containing diacylglycerol and phosphatidylserine. *J Biol Chem,* 1985;260:10039–10043.

**$p < .02$; ††$p < .05$.

Adapted from ref. 30.

Table 4. BIOCHEMICAL EFFECTS OF HALOTHANE 2.4 VOL% AND PROPOFOL 200 μM ON PROTEIN KINASE C ACTIVITY

		PKC activity[a]			
		Halothane		Propofol	
Variable	*n*	–	+	–	+
K_m (mg/mL histone H1)	2	0.14	0.14	0.11	0.10
V_{max} (μmol·min^{-1}·mg^{-1})	2	0.46	0.73	0.27	0.48
Phosphatidylserine EC_{50} (mol%)	3	18 ± 2.5	11 ± 0.6†	18 ± 1.9	11 ± 1.2‡
Diacylglycerol EC_{50} (mol %)	3	1.6 ± 0.3	0.87 ± 0.2†	2.5 ± 0.3	1.2 ± 0.4‡
Ca^{2+} EC_{50} (free Ca^{2+}, μM)	3	4.5 ± 1.0	2.8 ± 0.4†	2.8 ± 0.7	1.9 ± 0.2†
Sphingosine IC_{50} (μM)	3	20 ± 1.5	26 ± 0.6‡	24 ± 4.8	34 ± 4.8†

[a]Protein kinase C (PKC) activity was determined at 30°C in the absence or presence of halothane (2.4 vol% determined by gas chromatography) or propofol [200 μM with 5% (vol/vol) ethanol present as a vehicle; controls contained 5% (vol/vol) ethanol]. K_m and V_{max} values were determined by Michaelis-Menton analysis. EC_{50} and IC_{50} values were determined by a graded concentration-response analysis. Values are presented as mean ± SD. Statistical significance was assessed by Student's unpaired two-tailed *t*-test.

†p <.05; ‡p <.01 (versus control value without anesthetic).

Adapted from ref. 31.

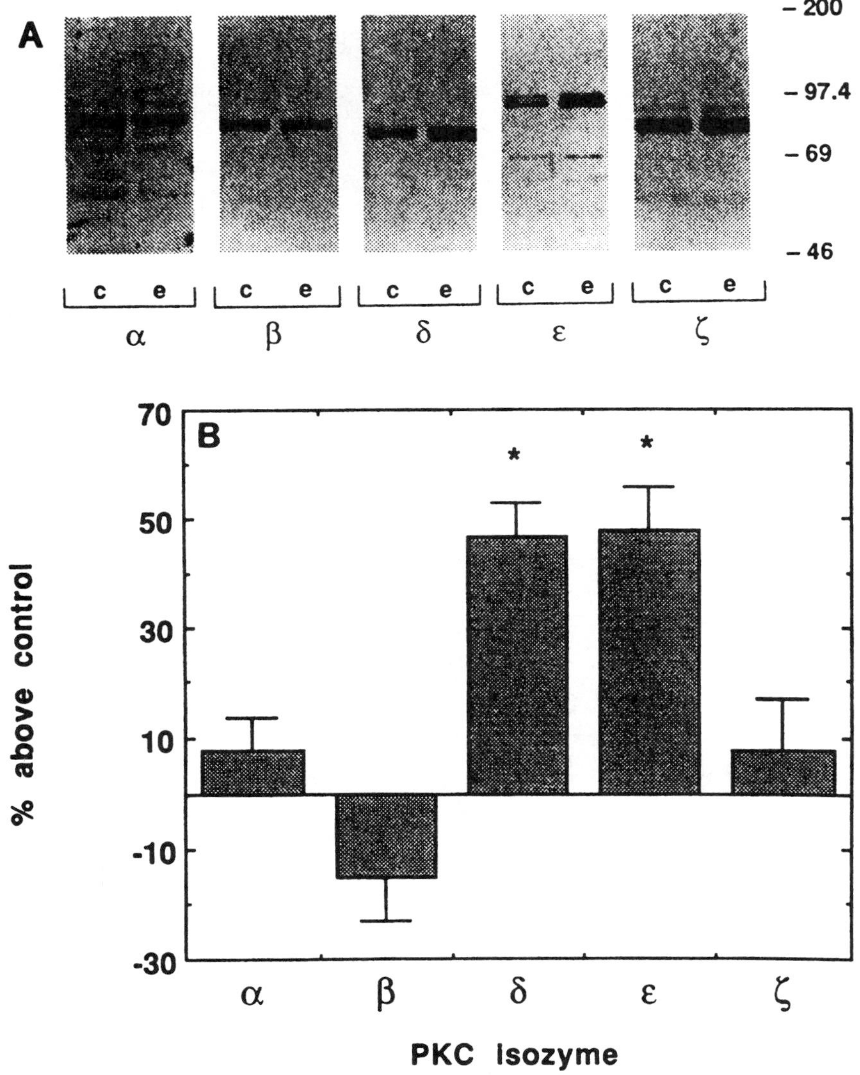

Figure 8. PKC immunoreactivity in ethanol-treated cells. *Top:* Representative blots from PC12 cells cultured without (c) or with (e) 100 mM ethanol for 6 days. Cells were lysed in SDS and proteins were separated by SDS-polyacrylamine gel electrophoresis,transferred to nitrocellulose paper, and analyzed for immunoreactivity with antibodies against PKC isoenzymes. *Bottom:* Values of isozymes expressed as mean ± SE; *asterisks* indicate significant increases. (From ref. 44, with permission.)

TABLE 5. COMPARISON OF *n*-ALKANOL EC50S IN STAUROSPORINE-TREATED AND CONTROL GROUPS[a]

		Control			+Staurosporine			
Agent	Experiment no.	EC_{50} (mM)	SE	*n*	EC_{50}(mM)	SE	*n*	*p*
Ethanol	1	126	19	25	80	12	25	
	2	200	36	55	117	13	25	
	3	152	13	50	87	11	25	
	4	125	19	25				
	Pooled	170	11	155	95	6.0	75	<.001
Butanol	1	12	0.9	50	4.0	1.2	25	
	2	12	0.8	25	5.6	1.8	50	
	Pooled	12	0.7	75	4.6	1.4	75	<.001
Octanol	1	59 μM	5.9	60	35	6.1	25	
	2	45 μM	6.7	60	35	3.5	50	
	3	53 μM	6.3	50				
	4	60 μM	10	25				
	Pooled	59 μM	4.0	195	35	3.0	75	<.001

[a]Loss-of-righting reflex responses to ethanol (50–350 mM) in *Rana pipiens* tadpoles preincubated for 90 min with staurosporine 1 μM (confirmed by UV spectroscopy) were compared to those of untreated controls. Data from each separate experiment were fit to logistic equations yielding slopes, EC_{50}s and errors; experiments were performed two to four times, pooled, and refit. *n* Represents total tadpoles in each experiment; *p* refers to the probability of a difference from controls at least as large as the observed difference under the assumption that the true difference is 0.

From ref. 25.

tion. In vitro, ethanol 200 mM reportedly failed to affect the crudely purified brain enzyme. In contrast, in a mixed micelle assay using pure recombinant PKC-α and -γ isolated from SF9 cells after baculoviral expression, Firestone and Firestone (23) observed that this same concentration of ethanol inhibits activity of these pure brain-specific isoforms by some 50%. Interestingly, in *Rana pipiens* tadpoles, the PKC inhibitor staurosporine decreases ethanol's median effective concentration for loss-of-righting reflex by virtually the same percent (Table 5) (25). Qualitatively similar results were obtained in analogous experiments in tadpoles with staurosporine, halothane, and diethylether (22).

Alcohol responses have also been assayed in mice with complete deletion of the gene encoding for PKC-γ (28), to assess the role of this brain-specific isoform in ethanol sensitivity. The mutation eliminated the expression of PKC-γ, without altering the levels of the α, βI, or βII isoforms, and although modest impairments in learning, memory, and gait were detectable (2), null mutant mice were otherwise normal in appearance.

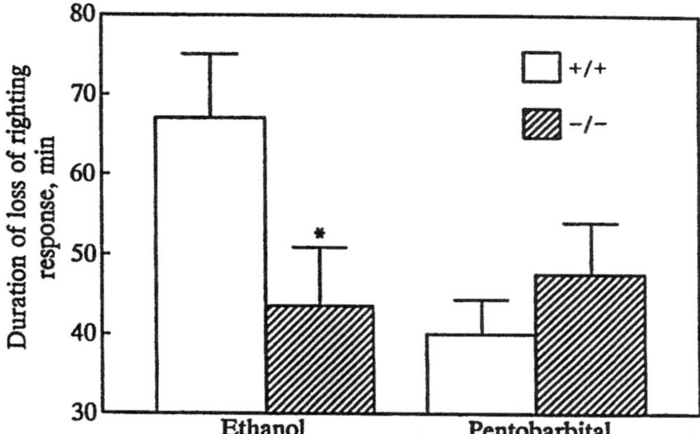

Figure 9. Behavioral effects of ethanol or pentobarbital in wild-type (+/+, *open bars)* and PKC-γ null mutant (-/-, *hatched bars)* mice. Sensitivity to ethanol and pentobarbital was measured by the duration of the loss-of-righting reflex; ethanol (3.5 g/kg) or pentobarbital (62 mg/kg) was administered by i.p. injection. Each value is the mean ± SEM. The *asterisk* indicates that mutant mice are less sensitive to ethanol; $p < .05$. (From ref. 28, with permission.)

Ethanol sensitivity was significantly reduced in the mutant mice when tested by loss-of-righting reflex (Fig. 9), although flunitrazepam and pentobarbital responses were unaffected. That removal of PKC-γ should block the behavioral effects of ethanol is consistent with results from $GABA_A$ receptor subtype expression studies, where ethanol's enhancement of GABA-gated currents specific for the γ_{2L} spice-variant depends on PKC-mediated phosphorylation at the γ_{2L} splice insert's PKC consensus sequence (69). The responses of PKC-γ null mutants to volatile and other general anesthetics, an obvious and important experiment, has yet to be reported.

PKC AND PAIN

Although relatively little information is currently available on whether PKC activation modulates pain pathways, the presence of PKC in spinal cord (Table 2) and its widespread distribution in pain-processing areas of the brain suggest this possibility. PKC is an intracellular effector for the inflammatory pain mediator, bradykinin (32). Opiate receptors are coupled to a variety of ion channels (48), as well as to G proteins (49); the latter may couple opiate receptors to PLC, the enzyme that initiates PKC's activation cascade. Glutamate- and GABA-activated channels have also been localized to pain networks, and their sensitivity to PKC-mediated phosphorylation has already been mentioned. Hammond's group has recently demonstrated that the $GABA_A$ antagonists bicuculline and picrotoxin, antagonize the suppression of noxious-evoked movement produced by halothane (72). Considering that potent and selective modulators of PKC activity have now been developed (70), important new therapeutic strategies for pain are likely to come from this work.

ACKNOWLEDGMENTS

The authors gratefully acknowledge the support of BRS grant RR05416 from the National Institutes of Health; the Department of Anesthesiology and Critical Care Medicine, University of Pittsburgh; and Dr. Peter M. Winter.

REFERENCES

1. Abeliovich A, Paylor R, Chen C, Kim JJ, Wehner JM, Tonegawa S. PKCγ mutant mice exhibit mild deficits in spatial and contextual learning. *Cell* 1993;75:1263–1271.

2. Abeliovich A, Cehn C, Goad Y, Silva AJ, Stevens CF, Tonegawa S. Modified hippocampal long-term potentiation in PKCγ-mutant mice. *Cell* 1993;75:1253–1262.
3. Ahn NG, Weiel JE, Chan CP, Krebs EG. Identification of multiple epidermal growth factor-stimulated protein serine/threonine kinases from Swiss 3T3 cells. *J Biol Chem* 1990;265:11487–11494.
4. Aniksztejn L, Otani S, Ben-Ari Y. Quisqualate metabotropic receptors modulate NMDA currents and facilitate induction of long-term potentiation through protein kinase C. *Eur J Neurosci* 1992;4: 500–505.
5. Alkon DL. Memory storage and neuronal systems. *Sci Am* 1989;261:42–50.
6. Ashendel CL. The phorbol ester receptor: a phospholipid-regulated kinase. *Biochim Biophys Acta* 1985;822:219–242.
7. Bank B, LoTurco JJ, Alkon DL. Learning-induced activation of protein kinase C: a molecular memory trace. *Mol Neurobiol* 1989;3:55–70.
8. Bell RM, Hannun Y, Loomis C. Mixed micellar assay of protein kinase C. *Methods Enzymol* 1986;124:353–359.
9. Boni LT Rando RR. The nature of protein kinase C activation by physically defined phospholipid vesicles and diacylglycerol. *J Biol Chem* 1985;260:10819–10825.
10. Brown DA, Marrion NV, Smart TG. On the transduction mechanism for muscarine induced inhibition of M-current in cultured rat sympathetic neurones. *J Physiol (Lond)* 1989;413:468–488.
11. Burns DJ, Bell RM. Lipid regulation of protein kinase C. In: Lester DS, Epand RM, eds. *Protein kinase C: current concepts and future perspectives.* New York: E. Horwood, 1992;25–40.
12. Chen K-H, Widen S, Wilson SG, Huang K-P. Characterization of the 5'-flanking region of the rat protein kinase C γ gene. *J Biol Chem* 1990;265:19961–19965.
13. Cole G, Dobkins KR, Hansen LA. Decreased levels of protein kinase C in Alzheimer brain. *Brain Res* 1988;452:165–170.
14. Coggins PJ, Zweirs H. B-50(GAP-43): Biochemistry and functional neurochemistry of a neuron-specific phosphorylation. *J Neurochem* 1991;56:1095–1106.
15. Conn PJ, Kaczmarek LK. A model for the study of the molecular mechanisms involved in the control of prolonged animal behaviors. *Mol Neurobiol* 1989;3:237–273.
16. Conn PJ, Strong JA, Kaczmarek LK. Inhibitors of protein kinase C prevent enhancement of calcium current and action potentials in peptidergic neurons of Aplysia. *J Neurosci* 1988;9:480–487.
17. Doerner D, Pitler TA, Alger BE. Protein kinase C activators block specific calcium and potassium current components in isolated hippocampal neurons. *J Neurosci* 1988;8:4069–4078.
18. Dutar P, Nicoll RA. Classification of muscarinic responses in hippocampus in terms of receptor subtypes and second-messenger systems: electrophysiological studies in vitro. *J Neurosci* 1988;8: 4214–4224.
19. Exton JH. Signaling through phosphatidylcholine breakdown. *J Biol Chem* 1990;265:1–4.
20. Firestone L, Miller JC, Miller KW. Tables of physical and pharmacological properties of anesthetics. In: Roth SH, Miller KW, eds. *Molecular and cellular mechanisms of anesthetics.* New York: Plenum Medical, 1986;455–470.
21. Firestone S, Firestone L. Anesthetic alcohols modulate membrane-bound protein kinase C function. *FASEB J* 1988;2:A1381.
22. Firestone S, Firestone L, Ferguson C, Blanck D. Staurosporine, a protein kinase inhibitor, decreases the general anesthetic requirement in *Rana pipiens* tadpoles. *Anesth Analg* 1993;77:1026–1030.
23. Firestone S, Firestone LL. Differential effects of general anesthetics on protein kinase C isoforms α and γ. *Anesth Analg* 1995;80:S125.
24. Firestone S, Firestone L. Protein kinase C is a target for general anesthetics. *Anesthesiology* 1989;71:A255.
25. Firestone S, Firestone L. Staurosporine, a protein kinase inhibitor, increases the intoxicating potencies of ethanol and other *n*-alkanols in *Rana pipiens* tadpoles. *Alcoholism Clin Exp Res* 1995;19: 416–419.
26. Firestone S, Gray K, Firestone LL. General anesthetic effects on protein kinase C are substrate-dependent. *Anesthesiology* 1991;75:A1042.
27. Firestone S, Gray K, Firestone LL. General anesthetics and ethanol inhibit enzymatic activity of CNS-derived protein kinase C. *Anesthesiology* 1990;73:A706.
28. Harris RA, McQuilkin SJ, Paylor R, Abeliovich A, Tonegawa S, Wehner JM. Mutant mice lacking the gamma isoform of protein kinase C show decreased behavioral actions of ethanol and altered function of gamma-aminobutyrate type A receptors. *Proc Natl Acad Sci USA* 1995;92:3658–3662.
29. Hashimoto T, Kitamura N, Saito N. The loss of βII-protein kinase C in the striatum from patients with Huntington's disease. *Brain Res* 1992;585:303–306.
30. Hemmings HC, Adamo AI. Effects of halothane and propofol on purified brain protein kinase C activation. *Anesthesiology* 1994;81: 147–155.
31. Hemmings HC, Adamo AIB, Hoffman MM. Biochemical characterization of the stimulatory effects of halothane and propofol on purified brain protein kinase C. *Anesth Analg* 1995;81:1216–1222.
32. Higashida H, Brown DA. Two polyphosphatidylinositide metabolites control two K^+ currents in a neuronal cell. *Nature* 1986;323:333–335..
33. Hu G-Y, Hvalby O, Walaas SI. Protein kinase C injection into hippocampal pyramidal cells elicits features of long term potentiation. *Nature* 1987;328:426–429.
34. Hug H, Sarre TF. Protein kinase C isoenzymes: divergence in signal transduction? *Biochem J* 1993;291:329–343.
35. Huganir RL, Greengard P. Regulation of neurotransmitter receptor desensitization by protein phosphorylation. *Neuron* 1990;5:555–567.
36. Inoue M, Kishimoto A, Takai Y, Nishizuka Y. Studies on a cyclic nucleotide-independent protein kinase and its proenzyme in mammalian tissues II. *J Biol Chem* 1977;252:7610–7616.
37. Ito M. Long term depression. *Annu Rev Neurosci* 1989;12:85–102.
38. Kellenberger S, Malherbe P, Sigel E. Function of the $\alpha_1\beta_2\gamma_{2S}$ γ-aminobutyric acid type A receptor is modulated by protein kinase C via multiple phosphorylation sites. *J Biol Chem* 1992;267:25660–25663.
39. Knox RJ, Kaczmarek LK. Regulation of neuronal ion channels by protein kinase C. In: Lester DS, Epand RM, eds. *Protein kinase C: current concepts and future perspectives.* New York: E. Horwood, 1992; 274–296.
40. Konig B, Dinitto PA, Blumberg PM. Stoichiometric binding of diacylglycerol to the phorol ester receptor. *J Cell Physiol* 1985;29:37–43.
41. Linden DJ, Conner JA. Participation of postsynaptic PKC in cerebellar long-term depression in culture. *Science* 1991;254:1656–1659.
42. Macdonald RL, Olsen RW. $GABA_A$ receptor channels. *Annu Rev Neurosci* 1994;17:569–602.
43. Malinow R, Schulman H, Tsien RW. Inhibition of postsynaptic PKC or CaMKII blocks induction but not expression of LTP. *Science* 1989;245:862–866.
44. Messing RO, Petersen PJ, Henrich CJ. Chronic ethanol exposure increases levels of protein kinase C δ and ε and protein kinase C-mediated phosphorylation in cultured neural cells. *J Biol Chem* 1991;266:23428–23432.
45. Nishino N, Kitamura N, Nakai T. Phorbol ester binding sites in human brain: characterization, regional distribution, age-correlation, and alterations in Parkinson's disease. *J Mol Neurosci* 1989;1:9–26.
46. Nishizuka, Y. The role of protein kinase C in cell surface signal transduction and tumour promotion. *Nature* 1984;308:693–698.
47. Nishizuka Y. The molecular heterogeneity of protein kinase C and implications for cellular regulation. *Nature* 1988;334:661–665.
48. North RA. Opioid receptor types and membrane ion channels. *Trends Neurosci* 1986;9:114–117.
49. North RA, Williams JT, Suprenant A, Christie M. Mu and delta receptors belong to a family of receptors that are coupled to potassium channels. *Proc Natl Acad Sci USA* 1987;84:5487–5491.
50. Olds JL, Alkon DL. A role for protein kinase C in associative learning. *New Biol* 1991;3:27–35.
51. Ono Y, Fujii T, Igarashi K. Phorbol ester binding to protein kinase C requires a cysteine-rich zinc-finger like sequence. *Proc Natl Acad Sci USA* 1989;86:4868–4871.
52. Ono Y, Fujii T, Ogita K. The structure, expression, and properties of additional members of the protein kinase C family. *J Biol Chem* 1988;263:6927–6932.
53. Otte AP, Kramer IM, Durston AJ. Protein kinase C and regulation of the local competence of *Xenopus* ectoderm. *Science* 1991;251: 570–573.
54. Parker PJ. Protein kinase C: a structurally related family of enzymes. In: Lester DS, Epand RM, eds. *Protein kinase C: current concepts and future perspectives.* New York: E. Horwood, 1992;3–24.
55. Pears CJ, Kour G, House C, Kemp BE, Parker PJ. Mutagenesis of the pseudosubstrate site of protein kinase C leads to activation. *Eur J Biochem* 1990;194:89–94.
56. Robinson PJ. The role of protein kinase C and its neuronal substrates dephosphin B-50, and MARCKS in neurotransmitter release. *Mol Neurobiol* 1992;5:87–130.
57. Schaap D, Hsuan J, Totty N, Parker PJ. Proteolytic activation of protein kinase C-ε. *Eur J Biochem* 1990;191:431–435.
58. Shearman MS, Sekiguchi K, Nishizuka Y. Modulation of ion chan-

nel activity: a key function of the protein kinase C enzyme family. *Pharmacol Rev* 1989;41:211–237.
59. Sigel E, Baur R. Activation of protein kinase C differentially modulates neuronal Na^+, Ca^{++}, and $GABA_A$-type channels. *Proc Natl Acad Sci USA* 1988;85:6192–6196.
60. Slater SJ, Cox KJA, Lombardi JV, Ho C, Kelly MB, Rubin E, Stubbs CD. Inhibition of protein kinase C by alcohols and anesthetics. *Nature* 1993;364:82–84.
61. Strong JA, Fox AP, Tsien RW, Kaczmarek LK. Stimulation of protein kinase C recruits convert calcium channels in *Aplysia* bag cell neurons. *Nature* 1987;325:714–717.
62. Takai Y, Kishimoto A, Inoue M, Nishizuka Y. Studies on a cyclic nucleotide-independent protein kinase and its proenzyme in mammalian tissue I. Purification and characterization of an active enzyme from bovine cerebellum. *J Biol Chem* 1977;252:7603–7609.
63. Tanaka C, Nishizuka Y. The protein kinase C family for neuronal signaling. *Annu Rev Neurosci* 1994;17:551–567.
64. Tanaka C, Saito N. Localization of subspecies of protein kinase C in the mammalian central nervous system. *Neurochem Int* 1992;21: 499–512.
65. Tas PWL, Koschel K. Volatile anesthetics stimulate the phorbol ester evoked neurotransmitter release from PC12 cells through an increase of the cytoplasmic Ca^{++} ion concentration. *Biochim Biophys Acta* 1991;1091:401–404.
66. Tsuchiya M, Okimasu E, Ueda W, Hirakawa, Utsumi K. Halothane, an inhalation anesthetic, activates protein kinase C and superoxide generation by neutrophils. *FEBS Lett* 1988;242: 101–105.
67. Tshuchiya M, Tomoda M, Ueda W, Hirakawa M. Halothane enhances the phosphorylation of H1 histone and rat brain cytoplasmic proteins by protein kinase C. *Life Sci* 1990;46:819–825.
68. Van der Zee EA, Compaan JC, de Boer M, Luiten PGM. Changes in PKCg immunoreactivity in mouse hippocampus induced by spatial discrimination learning. *J Neurosci* 1992;12:4808–4815.
69. Wafford KA, Whiting PJ. Ethanol potentiation of $GABA_A$ receptors requires phosphorylation of the alternatively spliced variant of the gamma 2 subunit. *FEBS Lett* 1992;313:113–117.
70. Wilkinson SE, Hallam TJ. Protein kinase C: is its pivotal role in cellular activation overstated? *Trends Pharmacol Sci* 1994;15:53–57.
71. Yoshihara C, Saito N, Taniyama K, Tanaka C. Differential localization of four subspecies of protein kinase C in the rat striatum and substantia nigra. *J Neurosci* 1991;11:690–700.
72. Mason P, Owens CA, Hammond DL. Antagonism of the antinocifensive action of halothane by intrathecal administration of $GABA_A$ receptor antagonists. *Anesthesiology* 1996;84:1205–1214.
73. Hemmings HC, Adama AIB. Activation of endogenous protein kinase C by halothane in synaptosomes. *Anesthesiology* 1996;84: 652–662.

Anesthesia: Biologic Foundations, edited by Tony L. Yaksh et al. Lippincott–Raven Publishers, Philadelphia © 1997.

CHAPTER 8

ARACHIDONATE METABOLITE SIGNALING

LAWRENCE J. BAUDENDISTEL, THOMAS E. DAHMS, AND W. DAVID WATKINS

The ability of cells to respond to, and interact with, their environment is a fundamental property and a decisive determinant of survival. Further, the capacity of cells to work in concert provides the flexibility and subtle gradations in cooperative responses that are requisite for and characterize homeostatic control. To assure adequacy of response in the face of diverse stimuli, complex biochemical processes of information integration through intra- and intercellular signal transmission have been developed. In this regard, phospholipid metabolism has been increasingly recognized for its importance in cell signaling. A variety of hormones, neurotransmitters, and other cellular mediators exert their action through phospholipid-related messenger systems (11,118,152).

The principle of a phospholipid-mediated messenger system rests in the signal-mediated hydrolysis of phospholipids within cellular membranes. The importance of the cell membrane in this type of lipidic signaling system is paramount. It not only maintains receptor mechanisms but also serves as the reservoir of lipid mediator precursors for the transmission of receptor-associated information that ultimately activates specific processes within the cell.

Arachidonic acid and its oxygenated metabolites were the first phospholipid-derived messengers identified. This system remains the most important and encompasses the most diverse set of lipidic messenger molecules coupling cellular responses to various stimuli and in mediating cell-to-cell interactions at several levels (paracrine, autocrine, and juxtacrine) of biologic organization (263). A distinct feature of this signaling system is the ability to contain the responses to biologic stimuli in close proximity to the activation site leading to efficient and specific cell signaling.

This chapter focuses on the role of arachidonic acid metabolites in cell signaling both as ligands and as intracellular messengers. Pertinent information regarding the biosynthesis and control of these compounds has been presented in order to better understand the pivotal role of arachidonate and its metabolites as a lipidic messenger system. Selected biologic activities and physiologic implications are presented for eicosanoids as intracellular signals since ligand responses have been widely reviewed elsewhere.

THE ARACHIDONIC ACID CASCADE

Prostaglandins, leukotrienes, and epoxides are families of oxygenated 20 carbon fatty acids that possess profound biologic activities and play key regulatory roles in cell and organ physiology. Collectively referred to as eicosanoids (41), these compounds are not stored in tissues, as are many hormones and neurotransmitters, but are synthesized via the activity of specific enzymes immediately prior to their intracellular and/or extracellular release. In the adult, these compounds generally do not circulate in blood in effective concentrations (endocrines), but act locally (paracrines) or near (juxtacrines) their sites of production.

A number of polyunsaturated fatty acids such as linoleic, linolenic, and docosahexaenoic acids are substrates for the oxygenases involved in the synthesis of eicosanoids. However, because of its abundant presence esterified to hormonally sensitive glycerolipid pools, arachidonic acid is the predominant fatty acid precursor to this integrated system of phospholipid intracellular signal molecules, so much so, that the biosynthetic pathways leading to the production of eicosanoids are referred to as the arachidonic acid (AA) cascade (Fig. 1). The known pathways for oxidative metabolism of AA leading to the formation of eicosanoids are generally classified as resulting from one of three main enzymatic pathways. Oxidation of AA via the cyclooxygenase (COX) pathway generates a labile endoperoxide from which a series of products including the prostaglandins (PGs) and thromboxanes (TXs) are derived; oxidation by various lipoxygenases (LOX) yields metabolites that include the leukotrienes (LTs), lipoxins (LXs), and hepoxilins (HX); finally, a family of cytochrome P450 monooxygenases catalyze the biotransformation of AA to a variety of metabolites including epoxides and a series of fatty acid alcohols.

Eicosanoids are widely distributed phylogenetically and are formed by virtually every mammalian tissue that has been examined. Even though all cells (except nonnucleated erythrocytes) are capable of producing eicosanoids, differentiation results in each cell type producing its own characteristic pattern of metabolites. Some cell types are distinguished by the predominant products they synthesize (Table 1). The ultimate fate of AA depends on the complement of enzymes present and their relative abundance (227). In a similar manner, the biologic activity of a specific eicosanoid will vary among constituent cell types of an organ as well as from organ to organ in any given species and can differ markedly from species to species. Even the stage of development or the phase of a biologic cycle can elicit profound alterations in the synthesis of and responses to individual eicosanoids (142,167,190,197). Table 2 lists some of the well-substantiated, prominent biologic actions of eicosanoids in various tissues and organs.

EICOSANOID SYNTHESIS

Arachidonic Acid Release

Hydrolysis of esterified AA from cellular glycerophospholipids (Fig. 2) is the first and rate-limiting step in response to extracellular stimuli in the pathways leading to eicosanoid production. Physical stimuli as disparate as sheer force on vascular endothelium (122,129) or tissue ischemia (112) can lead to the nonspecific release of fatty acids from phospholipid stores. Activation of diverse classes of cell surface receptors of many cell types elicit selective AA release from membrane phospholipids (48,80,118,128,181). Agonists to these receptors take the form of hormones, neurotransmitters, growth factors, and cytokines including thyrotropin-releasing hormone (120), bradykinin (80), serotonin (64), glutamate (3), angiotensin II, antidiuretic hormone, fibroblast-derived growth factor (60), platelet-derived growth factor (14), epidermal growth factor (209), and the interferons (99,196). Agonist-receptor interaction results in the activation of one or more cellular, calcium-dependent phospholipases. This enzyme activity results in a relatively selective, discrete release of AA via two pathways (Fig. 3). Activated phospholipase A_2 (PLA_2) catalyzes the hydrolysis of phosphatidylcholine (and, to a lesser extent, phosphatidylethanolamine and

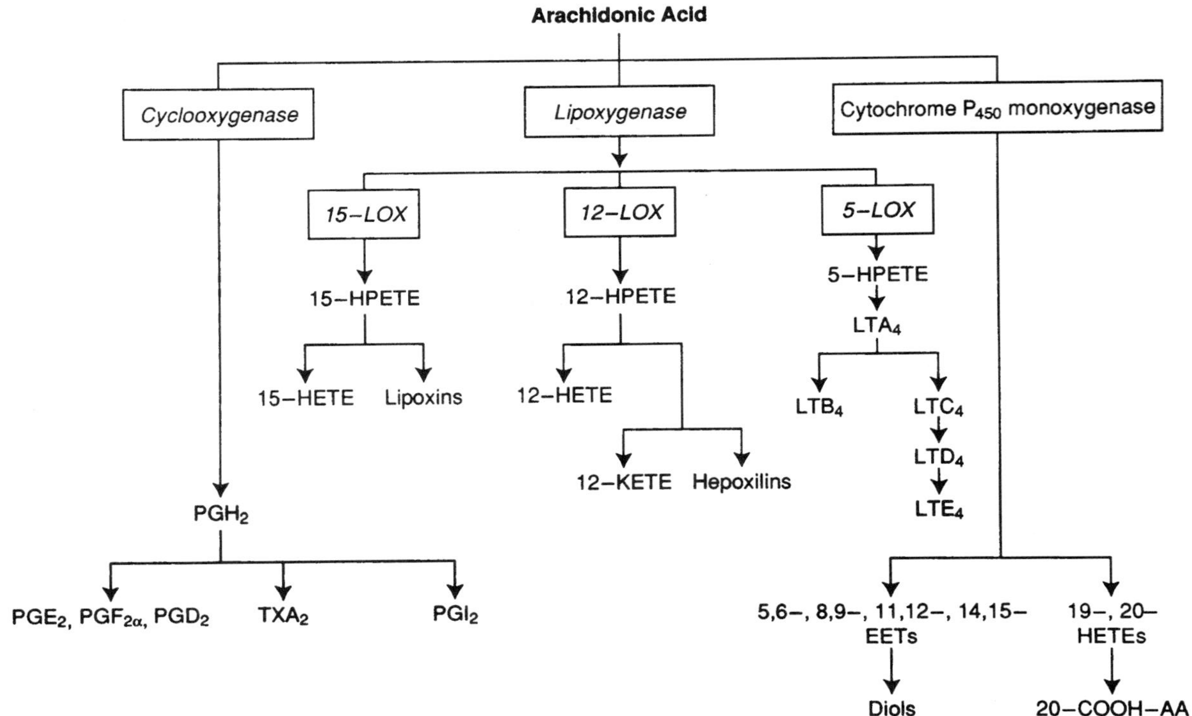

Figure 1. Arachidonic acid cascade: biochemical pathways involved in the generation of prostaglandins, leukotrienes, and epoxides. The rate-limiting step in this cascade is the mobilization of arachidonic acid from membrane phospholipids. Free arachidonic acid can be oxygenated by three principal routes: cyclooxygenase, lipoxygenase, and cytochrome P450 monooxygenase. Each pathway consists of a distinct biosynthetic sequence and enzymatic mechanisms. The immediate products of these pathways: prostaglandin endoperoxide, hydroperoxyeicosatetraenoic acid, and epoxyeicosatrienoic acid may act as mediators in and of themselves or may be further transformed into other bioactive metabolites depending on the enzyme complement of the tissue or cell type under consideration. LOX, lipoxygenase; PG, prostaglandin, followed by a class [D, E, F, H, I] and a subclass [subclass 2] designation; LT, leukotriene, followed by a class [A, B, C, D, E] and a subclass designation [subclass 4]; PGI_2, prostacyclin; TXA_2, thromboxane A_2; HPETE, hydroperoxyeicosatetraenoic acids; HETE, hydroxyeicosatetraenoic acid; KETE, ketoeicosatetraenoic acid; EET (epoxide), epoxyeicosatrienoic acid; Diols, dihydroxyeicosatetraenoic acid; 20-COOH-AA, 20-eicosatetraenedioic acid.

phosphatidylinositol) at the sn-2 position, yielding free AA and lysophospholipid (146,245). The second pathway involves phosphatidylinositol that is cleaved at the phosphate ester bond by phospholipase C (PLC) producing diacylglycerol, which is subsequently broken down by diacyl- and monoacylglycerol lipases yielding free AA and glycerol. Quantitatively, an arachidonoyl-specific PLA_2 is most important in regard to substrate mobilization leading to eicosanoid formation in most cells (48,181).

Phospholipase A_2 is directly regulated through guanine nucleotide-binding (G) proteins so that the production of AA can be an independent receptor-activated event. The mechanism for G-protein activation of PLA_2 appears to be direct cou-

Table 1. PREDOMINANT EICOSANOID[a] PRODUCTS OF SPECIFIC TISSUE AND/OR CELL TYPES

	Biosynthetic pathway		
Cell/tissue type	COX	LOX	P450
Corneal epithelium	PGE_2(83)		12(R)-HETE(46,217,218)
Large vessel endothelial cells	PGI_2[b](89,117)	5- & 15-HETE(89)	
Microvessel endothelial cells	PGE_2(82)		
Platelets	TXA_2(97)		
Eosinophils		LTC_4(106,255)	
Mast cells	PGD_2(174)		
Neutrophils		LTB_4(16)	
Thick ascending limb of the loop of Henle	PGE_2(67)		20-HETE[b](27,49,67)
Renal collecting tubule cells	PGE_2(43,128)		
Uterine endometrium	$PGF_{2\alpha}$(116)		
Testes	$PGF_{2\alpha}$(205)	12-HPETE(205)	

[a]Eicosanoids listed were measured in amounts approximately 2 to 10 times greater than other products generated within the same pathway.
[b]Predominant product within and across pathways.
COX, cyclooxygenase; LOX, lipoxygenase; P450, cytochrome P450 monooxygenase; PG, prostaglandin: PGD_2, PGE_2, $PGF_{2\alpha}$; PGI_2, prostacyclin; TXA_2, thromboxane A_2; LT, leukotriene: LTB_4, LTC_4; HPETE, hydroperoxyeicosatetraenoic acids; HETE, hydroxyeicosatetraenoic acid.

Table 2. PARTIAL LIST OF PROMINENT BIOLOGIC ACTIVITIES OF SELECTED EICOSANOIDS

Eicosanoid	Biologic activities
PGD_2	Systemic vasodilatation (1,250), pulmonary vasoconstriction (126,250), bronchoconstriction and airway hyperreactivity (72,126,147), sleep induction (101,186)
PGE_2	Bronchodilatation (70,149), vasodilatation (30), diuresis (237), natriuresis (42,103), hyperalgesia (66), hyperthermia (160,236), cytoprotection (130,256), and gastric antisecretory actions (31,241), promotes arousal (101)
$PGF_{2\alpha}$	Bronchoconstriction (183), vasoconstriction (147,223), luteolysis (167,190)
PGI_2	Vasodilatation (30), platelet antiaggregation (261), hyperalgesia (66), stimulates renin release (2,75)
TXA_2	Bronchoconstriction (72,76), vasoconstriction (22,226), promotes platelet activation and aggregation (238,261)
LTB_4	Leukocyte chemotaxis and adhesion to endothelial cells (44,71), promotes neutrophil-dependent increase in microvascular permeability (13,20)
LTC_4,D_4,E_4 (SRS-A)	Bronchoconstriction (21,76,221,253), vasoconstriction (7,224,246), increase in vascular permeability (44,239,248), augments bronchial mucous secretion (155), decreased myocardial contractility and coronary blood flow (90,141)
LTC_4	Opening of cardiac atrial K^+ channel (125,133), stimulates secretion of luteinizing hormone releasing hormone (81,213) and luteinizing hormone (113,124,213), prolonged depolarization of cerebellar Purkinje fibers (188,189)
LXA_4	Chemokinesis (36,138), bronchoconstriction (38,45,139), arteriolar vasodilatation without permeability (23,45,105), activation of protein kinase C (100,220), inhibition of natural killer cells (201,202)
LXB_4	Bronchoconstriction (45,139), inhibition of natural killer cells (201,202)
12-HPETE	Vasoconstriction, increases neuronal K^+ channel conductance (195,249)
12-HETE	Renal vasoconstriction (148), natriuresis (59,200), inhibition of renin secretion (2,108,200), stimulates migration of vascular smooth muscle cells (175)
5,6-EET	Vasodilatation (26,199), secretion of growth hormone (233), luteinizing hormone (232), somatostatin (121), and prolactin (28)
14,15-EET	Platelet antiaggregation (198,153)

PG, prostaglandins: PGD_2, PGE_2, $PGF_{2\alpha}$; PGI_2, prostacyclin; TXA_2, thromboxane A_2; LT, leukotrienes: LTB_4, LTC_4, LTD_4, LTE_4; SRS-A, slow releasing substance of anaphylaxis; LXA_4 (lipoxin A_4): 5,6,15-trihydroxyeicosatetraenoic acid; LXB_4 (lipoxin B_4): 5,14,15-trihydroxyeicosatetraenoic acid; HPETE, hydroperoxyeicosatetraenoic acids; HETE, hydroxyeicosatetraenoic acid; EET (epoxide), epoxyeicosatrienoic acid.

pling of the two proteins (Fig. 3), resulting in a reduction in the enzyme's requirement for free calcium (177). This mechanism is similar to that described for G-protein activation of PLC (225). The linking of heteromeric G proteins to PLA_2 activation is probably through the α subunit, although the β-γ subunits may be the GTP-binding transducer protein component responsible for phospholipase A_2 regulation in several cell types (6).

Although Ca^{2+}-independent forms of PLA_2 exist, most PLA_2s require Ca^{2+} for full activity. Following receptor activation, elevation in cytosolic Ca^{2+} mediates (facilitates) the translocation of PLA_2 from the cytosol to the membrane, thus promoting the juxtaposition of the enzyme to its phospholipid substrate as well as to competent G proteins (29,35). However, there are indications that increasing cytosolic Ca^{2+}, in and of itself, does not ensure increased PLA_2 activity in intact cells, with the possible exception of vascular endothelium. The lack of specificity of Ca^{2+} precludes its use as the exclusive regulator of PLA_2 (i.e., consider the consequences in muscle cells and neurons if PLA_2 were activated every time the Ca^{2+} increased). In addition, studies suggest that hormonally stimulated calcium flux is insufficient in itself to induce activation of PLA_2 (12,41). However, calcium-mobilizing ligands such as dopamine (194), norepinephrine (65), adenosine (58), and acetylcholine that do not directly participate in AA release can facilitate its liberation.

In certain tissues, receptor-dependent activation of PLA_2 appears to require the activity of a serine protein kinase (144) in addition to Ca^{2+} and an activated G protein. One protein kinase capable of phosphorylating PLA_2 has been identified as mitogen-activated protein (MAP), which in turn may be activated by PKC-dependent protein phosphorylation (145). Protein kinase C (PKC) also enhances the Ca^{2+} sensitivity of PLA_2. There are probably a number of specific PLA_2-activating proteins residing in different cell types.

PLA_2-independent mechanisms also participate in the regulation of AA levels. For example, the intracellular concentration of unesterified "free" AA is maintained at low concentrations primarily as a result of the sequential actions of arachidonoyl–coenzyme A (CoA) synthetase and arachidonoyl-phospholipid transferase that promote the rapid reincorporation of unesterified arachidonate into membrane phospholipids (Fig. 3) (33). In this regard, mobilization of AA can involve perturbation of the reacylation pathway (118) that has been shown to be regulated by protein kinase C (78). Intracellular AA levels are also influenced by the extent of its provision via the uptake of low-density lipoproteins (LDLs) by the LDL receptor pathway (95).

Cyclooxygenase Products

In prostanoid-forming cells, biotransformation of free AA to the endoperoxide PGH_2 is mediated by the enzyme cyclooxygenase (COX), alternately known as prostaglandin endoperoxide synthase (PGG/H synthase) (51,208). Integral to the endoplasmic reticulum, COX catalyzes two reactions: (a) the addition of molecular oxygen to AA at the C-9, C-11, and C-15 positions to form the cyclic endoperoxide prostaglandin G_2 (PGG_2) (cyclooxygenase activity); and (b) reduction of the C-15 peroxide of PGG_2 to a hydroxyl group to yield PGH_2 (peroxidase activity) (184,187). The endoperoxides PGG_2 and PGH_2 are unstable (half-life of approximately 4 minutes), biologically

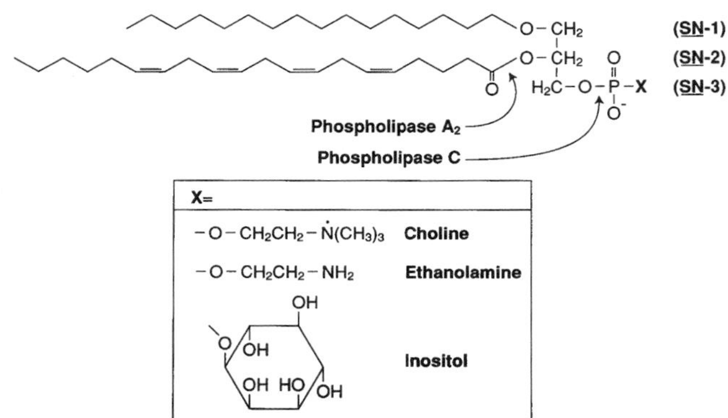

Figure 2. Major molecular species of arachidonate-containing phospholipids involved in transmembrane signaling. In eukaryotic membranes glycerol-based phospholipids predominate. Glycerol serves as a spine coupling a hydrophobic domain consisting of two long chain fatty acids esterified at the sn-l position (usually a saturated fatty acid) and the sn-2 position (usually an unsaturated fatty acid) and a hydrophilic domain consisting of a polar moiety attached to a primary hydroxyl of glycerol by either a glycosidic or a phosphodiester linkage. Fatty acyl groups are most commonly of 16, 18, or 20 carbons with 0 to 4 double bonds. Sites of hydrolysis of the major pathways, where activation leads to arachidonic acid release, are indicated by *arrows*. PLA_2 hydrolyzes the 2-acyl ester. PLC cleaves the glycerol-phosphate bond. PLA_2, phospholipase type A_2; PLC, phospholipase type C; sn, standard numbering (systems are shown beside the glycerolphospholipid moiety for substituents on the glycerol backbone); X, corresponds to the polar head group: choline, ethanolamine, or inositol.

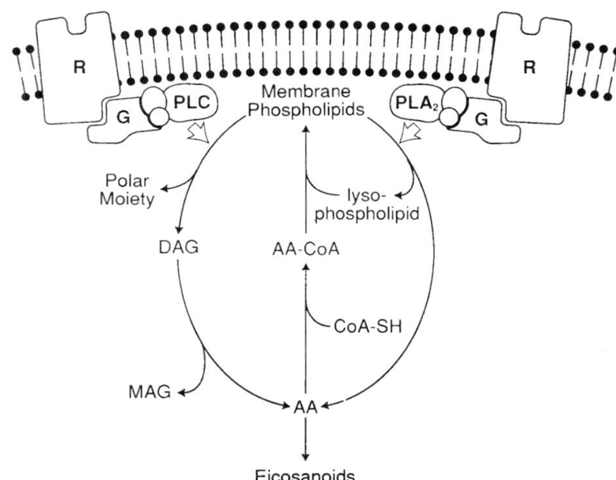

Figure 3. The steps in the sequence leading to receptor-phospholipase coupling that results in arachidonic acid mobilization. PLA_2 assumes a key role in eicosanoid production because it acts on the sn-2 position of the glycerol backbone of phospholipid pools to cleave arachidonate. As shown, AA can be produced by both PLA_2 and PLC pathways, however the predominant pathway is via PLA_2. Control of PLA_2 activity has important implications for the control of eicosanoid production. AA, arachidonic acid; DAG, 1,2-diacylglycerol; MAG, monoacylglycerol; AA-CoA, arachidonoyl-coenzyme A; G, GTP-binding protein complex; R, membrane receptor; PLA_2, phospholipase type A_2; PLC, phospholipase type C.

active intermediates that can effectively aggregate platelets and contract smooth muscle. PGH_2 subsequently serves as a substrate for tissue-specific enzymes (isomerases, synthases, and reductases) that ultimately form a variety of biologically active products depending on the tissue or cell under consideration (Fig. 4). Cells that generate prostaglandins typically synthesize one or two major products, a reflection of the enzyme(s) constitutively present that metabolize PGH_2. For example, in endothelial cells from large arteries, synthases convert PGH_2 principally to PGI_2 (50,117), in platelets, to TXA_2 (89), while PGE_2 is the major cyclooxygenase product of macrophages and collecting tubule cells (3,117), and $PGF_2\alpha$ is the product of uterine endometrium (116).

Cyclooxygenase activity is specifically inhibited by aspirin and nonsteroidal anti-inflammatory drugs (169,247). Aspirin-induced acetylation leads to irreversible cyclooxygenase inhibition (229), and enzyme synthesis is required prior to the generation of additional prostanoid. However, in cells that are incapable of supporting protein synthesis (i.e., platelets) new cells must be formed. Indomethacin and meclofenamate also cause irreversible inactivation of cyclooxygenase activity but without covalent modification of the enzyme (209,235). Other nonsteroidal, anti-inflammatory drugs, such as ibuprofen, are reversible enzyme inhibitors that are competitive inhibitors of arachidonate binding (209).

Eicosanoid synthesis is regulated at several stages throughout the COX pathway. In addition to the acute regulation of AA substrate mobilization, COX activity is controlled by free-radical-dependent mechanisms. The reduction of PGG_2 generates a reactive oxygen singlet that can promote the rearrangement of COX to an inactive enzyme species. This "suicide" inactivation occurs approximately once in every 1200 turnovers and may be a mechanism to limit PG biosynthesis (123,157). Various reducing cosubstrates can increase the number of turnover cycles of COX prior to deactivation. Reduced glutathione has been shown to increase the synthesis of PGE_2 through activation of its isomerase. Thromboxane synthase is readily inhibited by lipid hydroperoxides, which can be reversed by free radical scavengers.

The quantity of COX protein is influenced in various cells and organ systems by steroids (9,116), growth factors (9,104, 253), and tumor promoters (86). Several tiers of control (49, 230) exist at this level, the importance of which depend on the cell type and/or stage of differentiation of the tissue. Developmental control is exemplified by the induction of COX in ovarian follicles. On exposure to a rising concentration of circulating luteinizing hormone, the levels of COX mRNA, protein, and enzyme activity, previously unmeasurable, increase dramatically. At another level of control, constitutive levels of COX activity may be variably regulated. Human vascular endothelial cells normally express COX at constitutively high levels. Humoral stimulation of these cells results in a further increase in enzyme activity and gene transcription (49). Induction of COX gene expression has been shown to be relatively rapid with increases in COX activity and mRNA levels occurring within several hours (44). Although information concerning the enzymes that catalyze the metabolism of PGH_2 is limited compared to COX, evidence suggests the levels of PGH_2 metabolizing enzymes are regulated in concert with that of COX by growth factors and hormones (254).

Cyclooxygenase has recently been proposed to have two forms: a constitutive form (COX1, steroid insensitive) and an inducible form (COX2, steroid sensitive) (159,204,212). This concept reconciles the earlier findings that corticosteroids did not alter COX activity with the more recent reports that dexamethasone alters the production of prostaglandins by a wide variety of cell types following challenge with inflammatory agents. This distinction in types of COX has been proposed to explain the ability of glucocorticoids to primarily inhibit COX activity after injection of inflammatory agents. For example, endotoxin injection in animals leads to a more severe response in adrenalectomized animals; the reaction to endotoxin can be reversed by injection of steroids or COX inhibitors. Masferrer et al. (158) reported an increase in inducible COX in macrophages but not in kidney cells by LPS. In adrenalectomized animals without endogenous corticosterone, the COX2 enzyme became more highly induced, resulting in increased production of prostaglandins and a more severe

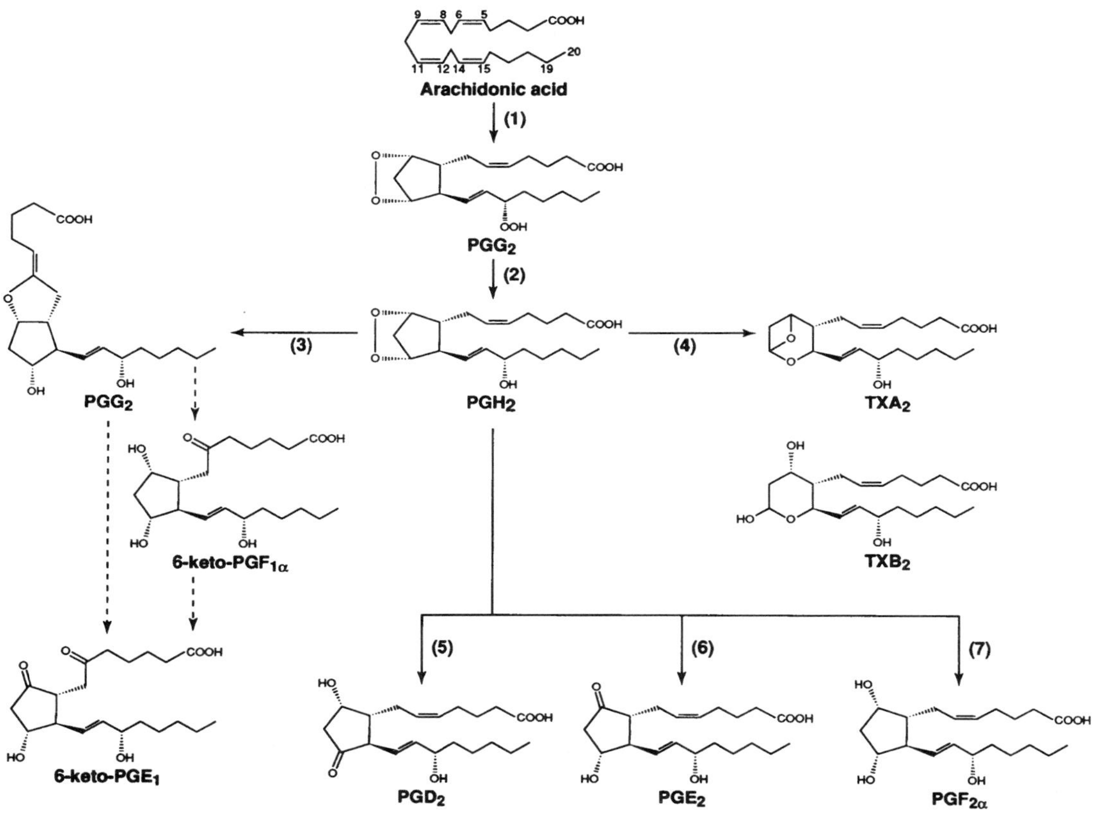

Figure 4. Pathways leading to the formation of the primary prostanoids. PG, prostaglandins: PGD_2, PGE_2, $PGF_{2\alpha}$; PGI_2, prostacyclin; TXA_2, thromboxane A_2. Enzyme nomenclature: 1, PGG/H synthase (cyclooxygenase); 2, PGG/H synthase (hydroperoxidase); 3, prostacyclin synthase; 4, thromboxane synthase; 5, PGD synthase (PGH-D isomerase); 6, PGE synthase (PGH-E isomerase); 7, PGF synthase (PGF reductase). Broken lines indicate nonenzymic processes.

response to the LPS. This points to possible control over the potentially injurious extracellular prostanoid release during inflammation if selective inhibitors can be found for the induced (steroid-sensitive) form of COX. In this regard, nonsteroidal anti-inflammatory drugs have been shown to be relatively selective inhibitors of either COX-1 or COX-2 in a range of animal models of disease (168).

Lipoxygenase Products

An alternate oxidation pathway of arachidonic acid is through the action of lipoxygenase (LOX) enzymes that generate leukotrienes and related mono-, di-, and trihydroxy fatty acids (Fig. 5). Three mammalian lipoxygenases differ in their specificity for inserting molecular oxygen into either the 5, 12, or 15 position of AA, producing the corresponding hydroperoxyeicosatetraenoic acid (i.e., 5-, 12-, or 15-HPETEs). Not all tissues possess the same spectrum of LOX enzymes. Different HPETEs are formed in different tissues and thus their distribution is tissue specific. For example, blood platelets possess only 12-LOX, and therefore the exclusive product of the human platelet is 12-HPETE (17,182). In contrast, the human neutrophil makes predominantly 5-HPETE (15), but 15-LOX activity is also present (87,178). The distribution of LOX enzymes is also a function of species variation. Although HPETEs are essential intermediates in LOX pathways, they also possess a diversity of important biologic properties. These include the regulation of eicosanoid synthesis, electrolyte flux, the release of histamine, the regulation of oocyte maturation, and the release of a number of reproductive hormones.

The HPETEs are unstable intermediates and are further metabolized by a variety of enzymes. Most importantly, HPETEs can be reduced by peroxidases to their corresponding hydroxyeicosatetraenoic acid (i.e., 5-, 12-, or 15-HETEs). A number of potentially important actions have been attributed to the HETEs. These include effects on prostaglandin formation and regulation, intracellular calcium concentration, cell proliferation, and regulation of phospholipase activity and hormone secretion (Table 2). Catalyzed molecular rearrangement can also transform 12-HPETE to hydroxyeicosatrienoic acids called hepoxilins. 15-LOX is detected in developing red cells (203), in eosinophils (244), and in airway epithelial cells (107,115) as well as in leukocytes. Metabolites generated from 15-lipoxygenation of arachidonic acid include 15-HETE, dihydroxy acids (e.g., 8,15-diHETE), and trihydroxy acids called lipoxins (215). Lipoxins may also result from sequential action of 5-, 12-, or 15-LOX. Products of 15-LOX have been detected in human bronchoalveolar lavage (137,172) and may contribute to airway inflammation (127,219).

Because of the biologic activity profiles of its products, which include the leukotrienes, the 5-lipoxygenase pathway has been the focus of considerable experimental attention. The enzymatic activities of 5-LOX catalyzes the first two steps of leukotriene biosynthesis (110,199,244). First, molecular oxygen is inserted in position five to produce the intermediate 5-hydroperoxyeicosatetraenoic acid (5-HPETE), and second, a dehydrase step converts 5-HPETE to the unstable triene epoxide leukotriene A_4 (LTA_4). Two enzymatic pathways have been described in the subsequent metabolism of LTA_4. LTA_4 can be converted to LTB_4 (5,12-diHETE) by the specific enzyme LTA_4 hydrolase (77,166). This enzyme is suicide-deactivated by its substrate, which can lead to the accumulation of LTA_4 in cells and subsequent transfer to other cells for enzymatic transformation (161). LTB_4 is the most potent chemoattractant for leukocytes and causes adherence

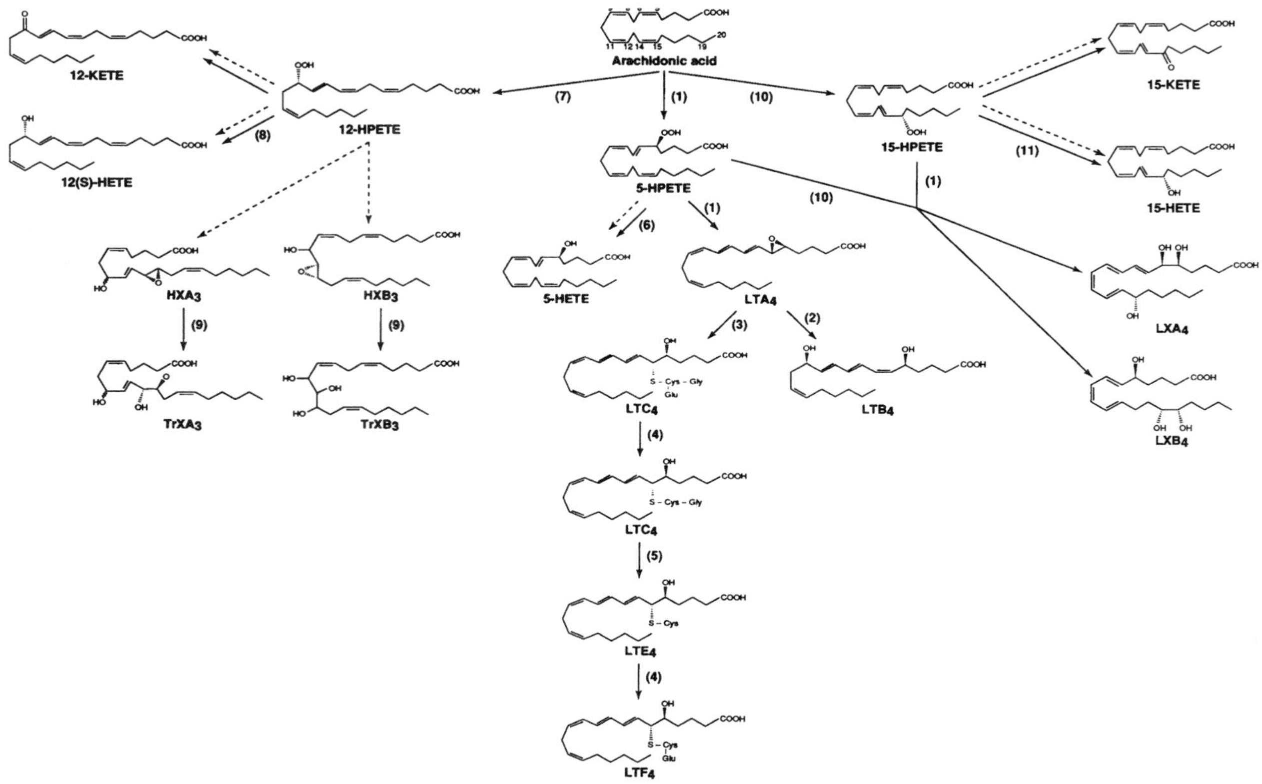

Figure 5. Alternate lipoxygenase pathways of arachidonic acid metabolism. LT, leukotrienes: LTB_4, LTC_4, LTD_4, LTE_4, LTF_4; HPETE, hydroperoxyeicosatetraenoic acids; HETE, hydroxyeicosatetraenoic acid; KETE, ketoeicosatetraenoic acid; LXA_4 (Lipoxin A_4): 5,6,15-trihydroxyeicosatetraenoic acid; LXB_4 (Lipoxin B_4): 5,14,15-trihydroxyeicosatetraenoic acid; HxA_3, (Hepoxilin A_3), 8-hydroxy-11,12-epoxyeicosatrienoic acid; HxB_3 (Hepoxilin B_3), 10-hydroxy-11,12-epoxyeicosatrienoic acid; $TrXA_3$ (Trioxilin A_3), 8,11,12-trihydroxyepoxyeicosatrienoic acid; $TrXB_3$ (Trioxilin B_3), 10,11,12-trihydroxyepoxyeicosatrienoic acid. Enzyme nomenclature: 1, 5-lipoxygenase; 2, LTA_4 hydrolase; 3, LTC_4 synthase (glutathione S-transferase); 4, gamma-glutamyltranspeptidase; 5, dipeptidase; 6, peroxidase; 7, 12-lipoxygenase; 8, glutathione peroxidase; 9, epoxide hydrolase; 10, 15-lipoxygenase; 11, peroxidase. *Broken lines* indicate nonenzymic processes or an unknown process (i.e., unknown enzyme).

and chemotaxis of leukocytes at nanomolar concentrations (71). Alternately, LTA_4 may be conjugated with glutathione to form LTC_4 by glutathione S-transferase (98). This enzyme is present in those cells that convert AA to peptidoleukotrienes (leukotrienes containing peptides or amino acids at C-6) including the mast cell, basophils, eosinophils, and monocytes.

LTC_4 can be subsequently cleaved of glutamic acid by γ-glutamyl transpeptidase to produce LTD_4, which is the major peptidoleukotriene in a number of tissues. Removal of glycine from LTD_4 by specific membrane-bound dipeptidases (98) yields LTE_4 with concomitant loss in activity (215). The exact peptidoleukotriene(s) observed in a tissue or cell type is a function of its complement and activity of ancillary enzymes such as γ-glutamyl transpeptidase and LTD-dipeptidase.

LTC_4, LTD_4, and LTE_4 are important mediators of human bronchial asthma and allergic diseases and comprise the major active elements of the slow-reacting substances of anaphylaxis (SRS-A). They are also potent vasoconstrictors in a variety of vascular beds including the coronary and cerebral circulations. In comparison, LTB_4 possesses potent chemotactic, chemokinetic, and neutrophil aggregation properties. In addition, LTB_4 induces vascular permeability changes and modulation of pain responses, implicating this leukotriene as a significant mediator in a number of inflammatory conditions. Recent evidence suggests a possible role for LTB_4 in myocardial infarction (79).

Regulation of 5-LOX is complex and implies its eminence in the management of the effects of, and responses to, the leukotrienes. The efficient generation of leukotrienes depends not only on substrate availability (free arachidonate) as with COX products, but also on the activation of 5-LOX. 5-LOX appears to be the only Ca^{2+}-dependent enzyme within this pathway and this activation is dose dependent (105). In the unstimulated cell, 5-LOX is localized to the cytosol. Stimulation leading to Ca^{2+} mobilization results in a rapid burst of leukotriene synthesis that is associated with a Ca^{2+}-dependent translocation of 5-LOX to a membrane site (211,257). Five lipoxygenase-activating protein (FLAP), a transmembrane protein, has been shown to facilitate the binding of 5-LOX to the plasma membrane (52,165). Synthesis of 5-LOX products are inhibited in intact cells by MK886 (84), which prevents and reverses the membrane association of 5-LOX and its activation (210). Thus, a complex of 5-LOX, FLAP, and possibly other proteins form at the cell membrane upon activation of the cell. 5-LOX is also prone to inactivation by peroxides, high levels of superoxide, and possibly hydroxyl radicals. Following cell stimulation, glutathione S-transferase activation does not appear responsible for enhanced production of LTC_4.

Cytochrome P450 Products

A number of cell/tissue types can oxidatively metabolize AA via cytochrome P450–dependent monooxygenase pathways. Epoxidation of AA generates a series of epoxyeicosatrienoic acids (EETs) that subsequently can be hydrolyzed by epoxide hydrolase to the corresponding dihydroxyeicosatrienoic acids (DHETs) (Fig. 6). Twenty- and 19-hydroxyeicosatetraenoic acids (HETEs) are formed by ω- and ω-1 hydroxylation. 20-HETE can be further metabolized to 1,20-eicosatetraenedioic acid (20-COOH-AA). AA metabolites from this pathway may play important roles in vascular reactivity and in Na^+/K^+ transport functions in kidney and corneal epithelium (169). Other products have been shown to possess activities including the capability to liberate luteinizing hormone, prolactin, and somatostatin from brain tissue (185). The exact roles of cytochrome P450–mediated AA metabolites remain to be precisely defined.

MECHANISMS OF EICOSANOID ACTIONS

Eicosanoids behave somewhat differently than other mediators in that, in addition to their intracellular functions, they can also pass through the plasma membrane to bind to specific receptors on neighboring cells and tissues (231). That is, communication between cells, cell types, and/or tissues occur through the action of eicosanoids. Eicosanoids were considered by many to be principally primary messengers regulating cell functions through the alteration of cyclic nucleotide levels. Recent evidence, however, suggests that eicosanoids act both as intracellular second messengers as well as intercellular local mediators. As second messenger molecules, they propagate the primary message by regulating ion fluxes, Ca^{2+} mobilization, and the activity of intracellular enzymes. As local mediators or primary messengers, these compounds are released from the cell of origin and elicit cellular responses in neighboring cells by binding to high-affinity membrane receptors. In the latter case eicosanoids function to coordinate the effects of the primary stimulus that initially provoked eicosanoid synthesis and release.

Transmembrane signal transduction is the process by which extracellular information (encoded in the form of hormones, growth factors, and neurotransmitters) is decoded into an intracellular physiologic response. The decoding process begins with the binding of an agonist (hormone, growth factor) to a plasma membrane receptor on a responsive cell, resulting in activation of the receptor and propagation of the signal leading to an intracellular effect.

Intercellular Signaling: Eicosanoids as Primary Messages

The proposition that eicosanoids are local hormones that act near their site of generation (228,230) was based on observations that infused eicosanoids failed to survive a single pass through the circulation. Support of this concept has been strengthened by the observation that under normal physiologic conditions the plasma concentrations of eicosanoids are less than that required to elicit most biologic responses, approximately 10^{-9} M (34,56,68), the fetal circulation not withstanding. A reasonable conclusion, therefore, is that eicosanoids must exert their effect proximate to their site of synthesis and before dilution in the circulation. Furthermore, unlike typical circulating hormones, eicosanoids are not stored nor is eicosanoid synthesis restricted to a central endocrine organ, but rather occur in virtually all organs, tissues, and cell types (15,227).

Current evidence supports the concept that all eicosanoid actions (in the role of primary ligands) are mediated through specific membrane receptors that are coupled to effector enzymes via guanine nucleotide (GTP)-binding regulatory proteins, or G proteins, which transmit signals into the cell interior (Fig. 7). In general, three membrane-bound constituents comprise this signal transduction system—receptors, effectors, and G proteins, which transduce the information from activated receptors to effectors. When activated by ligands coupling with their receptors, distinct heterotrimeric G-protein complexes

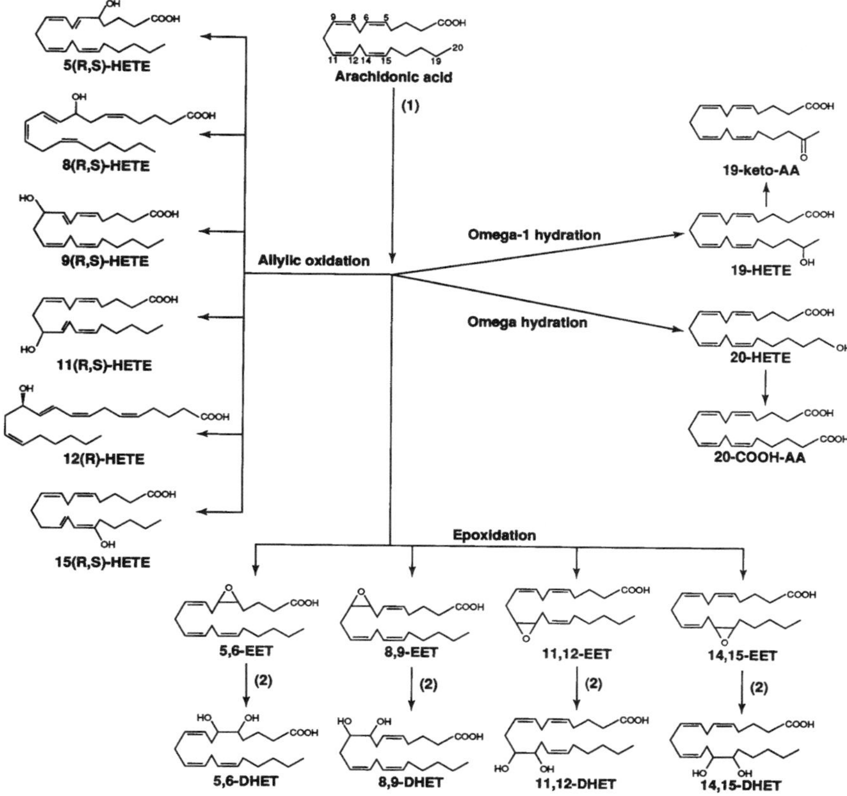

Figure 6. Arachidonic acid metabolism via the three types of oxidative reactions (epoxidation, allylic oxidation, omega hydroxylation) catalyzed by the cytochrome P450 system. HETE, hydroxyeicosatetraenoic acid; EET (epoxide), epoxyeicosatrienoic acid; DHET, (Diols), dihydroxyeicosatetraenoic acid; 20-COOH-AA, 20-eicosatetraenedioic acid. Enzyme nomenclature: 1, Cytochrome P450 monooxygenases; 2, epoxide hydrolases.

induce changes in the concentrations of second messengers or intracellular ions (Table 3).

Eicosanoids mediate a remarkable diversity of physiologic responses. Multiplicity of receptor subtypes specific for each eicosanoid with each receptor coupled to a different G-protein complex mediating a different effector system may explain some of the diversity. Thus, relative to the number of primary messengers (PGs, TXs, LTs, etc.), there is a significantly greater number of distinct receptors that mediate their effects. This is illustrated by the existence of at least two types of PGH_2/TXA_2 receptors (150,151), and two types of PGI_2/PGE_1 receptors (4). Three receptor subtypes have been proposed for PGE_2 (114). Multiple receptor subtypes have also been demonstrated for LTD_4 (69,131) and for LTB_4 (88,91). As yet, no receptor has been identified that selectively recognizes LTE_4. In some tissues LTE_4 has been shown to bind to LTD_4 receptors (32,171).

Signal transduction GTP-binding or G proteins form a group of plasma membrane-associated heterotrimers that function as signaling intermediates between the cell surface receptors and the intracellular effector-second messenger systems. G proteins are comprised of α, β, and γ subunits. The α subunit is the principal signal transducer. Approximately 16 G proteins have been identified based upon α subunit genes. However, the number of distinct G proteins is higher as a result of subunit isoforms. The extent to which a specific receptor uses a particular G protein varies as a function of cell type and differentiations (39). Besides modulating effector activity, G proteins are able to regulate the functional state of the receptors; GTP-dependent dissociation of the G protein from the receptor induces its transition from the high- to the low-affinity state for the hormone.

Terminal effector functions regulated by these receptors number approximately 15 to 30. The spectrum of effectors and the second messenger(s) they generate include adenyl cyclase (cAMP), phospholipase A_2 (AA), phospholipase C (IP_3, DAG, Ca^{2+}), and various ion membrane channels (Ca^{2+}, K^+, Na^+, H^+). It should be noted that modulation of the cell's membrane

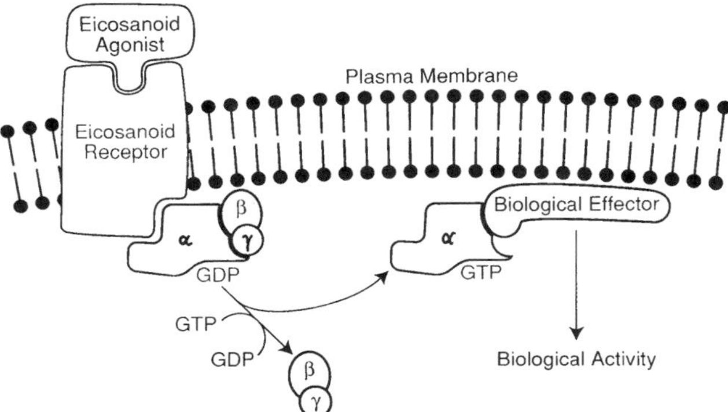

Figure 7. Schematic of the G-protein–coupled sequence shown to be involved in transmembrane signal transduction following eicosanoid-receptor interaction. Eicosanoid receptors are coupled to a family of regulatory GTP-binding proteins (G proteins) that have been shown to modulate the activity of a spectrum of intracellular effector systems. The more common effectors include adenyl cyclase, polyphosphoinositide-specific phospholipase C, phospholipase A_2, and ion channels. The binding of eicosanoid to its receptor provokes an exchange of GTP for GDP at the nucleotide-binding site of the coupled G protein. This GTP-binding induces the heterotrimeric G protein to dissociate to the α:GTP subunit and a β:subunit complex. Now free, the α:GTP subunits interact with and induce a functional state transition in the effector(s) (e.g., ion channels or PLA_2). Hydrolysis of the bound GTP to GDP, catalyzed by the α subunits, results in dissociation of α:GDP from the effector and its reassociation with β: complex. G proteins also regulate the functional state of receptors. GTP-dependent dissociation of the G protein from the receptor induces a transition from a high-affinity to a low-affinity state for the ligand.

potential through the modulation of ion channels is in itself a critical regulator of cellular function.

Generally, second messenger molecules stimulate the activity of specific protein kinase(s), which in turn phosphorylate and regulate the activity of protein substrates, which include enzymes, membrane ion channels and pumps, and structural proteins. Some of these substrates may be other kinases, which may themselves be positively or negatively regulated by phosphorylation (135,193). Second messengers can activate protein phosphatases directly and can also activate indirectly through phosphorylation of phosphatase inhibitors. In some cases second messengers function without the participation of enzyme intermediates by binding directly to a membrane ion channel or to closely applied regulatory proteins, thereby changing the functional state of the channel (73).

As primary messengers, eicosanoids generate a characteristic physiologic response by triggering one of several principal signal transduction pathways including the phosphatidylinositol-dependent PLC pathway and the adenyl cyclase–cAMP pathway. The latter pathway is considered to have two branches: one resulting in increased cAMP and the other down-modulating cAMP. These systems are referred to as "pathways" because of the cascade of events that is initiated by binding agonist to its receptor.

The best-characterized receptor/G protein/effector coupling system is that which regulates adenyl cyclase activity. In the platelet, for example, receptor binding by PGI_2 activates the membrane-bound enzyme adenyl cyclase. This enzyme catalyzes the synthesis of the second messenger cAMP from adenosine triphosphate (ATP) on the cytoplasmic side of the plasma membrane, and the resultant increase in intracellular cAMP mediates most of the activities of PGI_2. The PGI_2 receptor is coupled to adenyl cyclase by the guanine nucleotide binding protein, G_s, which is characteristic of cyclase stimulatory receptors. Increased cellular cAMP concentration, in turn, activates cAMP-dependent protein kinase (protein kinase A), stimulating the cellular changes peculiar to cAMP elevation in the cell in question.

Eicosanoids also activate the phosphatidylinositol-dependent PLC pathway. Platelet activation by TXA_2 is associated with activation, via a G protein, of the enzyme phospholipase C. PLC stimulates the hydrolysis of membrane glycerophospholipids such as phosphatidylinositol 4,5-bisphosphate (PIP_2) with the production of two second messengers: inositol 1,4,5-triphosphate (IP_3) and 1,2 diacylglycerol (DAG). IP_3 provokes an increase in intracellular Ca^{2+} by mobilizing stores from an endoplasmic reticular-storage site (19) and/or stimulating transport across the plasma membrane. DAG activates protein kinase C (PKC) in various tissues (47). PKC is responsible for the phosphorylation (and activation) of certain proteins. This cascade leads to platelet aggregation and secretion. In addition to the activation of PLC, the binding of eicosanoids to some membrane receptors also activates PLA_2, which results in the liberation of AA. Alternatively, AA may be generated from inositol phospholipids through the consecutive actions of PLC and DAG-lipase. Elevated AA exerts its effect either by functioning as a second messenger through the direct stimulation of PKC or as substrate for the generation of eicosanoids. In this regard, the PGF_2 receptor may couple to both PLC and PLA_2, whereas PGE_2 can stimulate both enzyme pathways independently through different receptor isotypes.

Intracellular Signaling: Eicosanoids as Second Messengers

In addition to their intercellular signaling roles, eicosanoids exhibit characteristics attributed to intracellular modulators and messengers within their cells of origin. A modulator performs briefly and reversibly at a specific location to modify or fine-tune the attributes of a signal. A second messenger has the

Table 3. SIGNAL TRANSDUCTION MECHANISMS DEMONSTRATING THE INVOLVEMENT OF SIMILAR G-PROTEIN–COUPLED MESSENGER SYSTEMS IN A VARIETY OF CELL TYPES

Receptor	Coupling protein	Regulated effector system	Second messenger	Cell type and/or organ
PGD_2	G_s	↑ AC	cAMP	
	G_{plc}	PI-PLC	IP_3, DAG, Ca^{2+}	Osteoblastis cells (243)
PGE_2[a]	G_s	↑ AC	cAMP	CCD (180,234)
	G_i	↓ AC	cAMP	CCD (234,242,251), adrenal medulla (179,260)
	G_{plc}	PI-PLC	IP_3, DAG, Ca^{2+}	CCD (102,234), adrenal medulla (179,260)
	$G_?$	ROC	Cl^-	Rabbit parietal cells (214)
$PGF2_\alpha$	G_{plc}	PI-PLC	IP_3, DAG, Ca^{2+}	Luteal cells (142,207), 3T3-fibroblasts (176)
	G_{pla}	PLA_2	LOX products	Platelets (19,47), endothelial cells (114)
PGI_2[b]	G_s	↑ AC	cAMP	Platelets (5,57,140)
	G_i	↓ AC	cAMP	Hepatocytes (163)
TXA_2	$G_?$	PI-PLC	IP_3, DAG, Ca^{2+}	Platelets (10,19,47), Vascular SM (53,252)
LTB_4	G_{plc}	PI-PLC	IP_3, DAG, Ca^{2+}	Neutrophils, monocytes (206)
LTD_4	G_{plc}	PI-PLC	IP_3, DAG, Ca^{2+}	Lung (40,170), airway SM (111)
	$G_?$	ROC	Ca^{2+}	Monocyte (222)

[a]Distinct receptors on the same- and/or on different-cell types can mediate the effects of PGE_2: as in the present example, CDD (234).

[b]PGI_2 and PGE_1 may act at distinct receptor, but in some tissues (i.e., platelets) they mediate their effects by interacting with the same receptor protein (5,57,180).

PG, prostaglandins: PGD_2, PGE_2, $PGF_{2\alpha}$; PGI_2, prostacyclin; TXA_2, thromboxane A_2; LT, leukotrienes: LTB_4, LTD_4; G, GTP-binding protein: G_s, activates AC; G_i, inhibits AC; G_{plc}, activates PLC; G_{pla}, activates PLA_2; $G_?$, of unknown type; AC, adenyl cyclase; , Stimulation; , inhibition (downregulate); PI-PLC, phosphatidylinositol-dependent PLC; ROC, receptor operated channel; cAMP, 3′,5′-cyclic adenosine monophosphate; IP_3, inositol 1,4,5-triphosphate; DAG, 1,2-diacylglycerol; LOX, lipoxygenase; CCD, cortical collecting ducts; SM, smooth muscle.

following characteristics: its concentration is altered in response to the primary ligand, mechanisms must exist for its removal to allow for rapid signal termination, and its effect on cellular processes must correlate with the physiologic effects of the primary signal. Over the last several years evidence has accumulated suggesting that eicosanoids, functioning as intracellular second messengers, play significant roles in the regulation of ion channels, cytoskeletal structure, and Na^+/K^+ adenosine triphosphatase (ATPase) activity.

Regulation of Ion Channels, Ion Gradients, and Secretion

Evidence gleaned from a number of studies suggests that hormone and neurotransmitter secretion (18,73,135) as well as the functional state of membrane ion channels (8,154,173) may be modulated by AA metabolites. For example, there is a growing body of evidence that products of 12-LOX metabolism function as second messengers in *Aplysia* sensory neurons (195). 12-HPETE has been shown to mimic the inhibitory effect (increased K^+ conductance, membrane hyperpolarization) of FMRFamide, which increases the open time of S-type K^+ channels (Fig. 8) (249). It appears that the effect of FMRFamide is mediated directly by 12-HPETE or possibly a metabolite (i.e., hepoxillin A_3, 12-KETE).

That LOX products may act as intracellular messengers is also supported by patch-clamp studies on guinea pig atrial cells (133). In these studies, 5-LOX products, possibly LTC_4, activate a class of muscarinic K^+ channels ($I_{K.ACh}$) that are modulated by acetylcholine. These data suggest that following agonist binding to α_1-adrenergic receptors, activation of $I_{K.ACh}$ results from G-protein–mediated stimulation of PLA_2, mobilization of AA, and the synthesis of LOX metabolites (125,133). LOX products have also been implicated in the stimulation of luteinizing hormone secretion from anterior pituitary (192), and through modulation of ion currents may participate in certain forms of long-term potentiation in the hippocampus (62,109,164). Thus, these data support the proposition that AA metabolites, in general, and LOX products, in particular, play widespread roles as intracellular messengers.

Many of the metabolites of arachidonic acid can contract smooth muscle presumably by altering membrane potentials and increasing intracellular calcium in the myocytes. The physiologic mechanisms linking extracellular eicosanoids (primary messengers) and contraction for specific eicosanoids (i.e., TXA_2) have been characterized in some systems. There are several reports of intracellular eicosanoids altering ion channel activity, which could lead to increased contractile activity. These results are summarized in Table 4 and demonstrate a primary role for 5-LOX products in this endeavor. In all cases COX products had no effect on any of these ion channels. These LOX products have satisfied the necessary criteria to be classified as second messengers. The sequence of events usually involves the binding of an agonist to its receptor leading to activation of

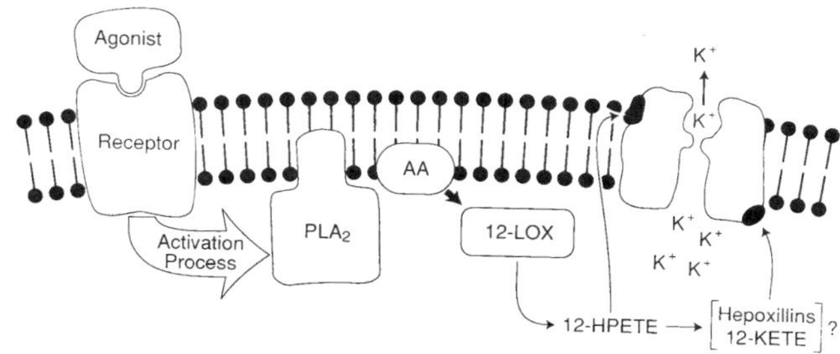

Figure 8. Example of eicosanoid second messenger pathway regulation of ion conductance: modulation of S type K^+ channel by 12-lipoxygenase products. Binding of agonist to its specific receptor activates a receptor-linked G protein that in turn activates phospholipase A_2 to hydrolyze membrane glycerophospholipids to free arachidonate, which becomes available for oxidation by 12-lipoxygenase (12-LOX). Produced through the 12-LOX pathway, 12-HPETE interacts with a channel protein through proposed receptors located either on the exterior surface of the cell or on the interior of the cell membrane. This receptor can interact with 12-HPETE originating from the same cell in which it was produced or from adjacent cells. Evidence exists suggesting that the cytochrome P450 system, which is known to convert HPETE to epoxyhydroxy and trihydroxy fatty acids, plays an important role in S-K channel regulation. In the present system, metabolite(s) of 12-HPETE (Hepoxillin A_3 or 12-KETE) may be specific ligands for the internal receptor.

Table 4. INTRACELLULAR EFFECTS OF EICOSANOIDS ON ION CHANNELS

Ion channel	Cell type	Mediator	Action
Ca^{2+}, voltage insensitive, plasma membrane	Human carcinoma	LTC_4	Activation of Ca^{2+}-dependent K^+ channels: membrane hyperpolarization (192)
	Murine embryonic carcinoma		
Na^+	Xenopus renal tubular cells	12-HPETE, LTD_4	Activation: ↑ Na^+ uptake (25)
K^+, muscarinic	Guinea pig myocytes	LTA_4, LTC_4	Activation (133)
K^+, muscarinic	Neonatal rat myocytes	12-HETE, LTB_4, C_4, D_4	Activation (125)
Cl^-	Bovine chromaffin cells	LTs	Activation (54)
K^+, Cl^-	Ehrlich tumor cells	LTD_4	Activation (134)

LT, leukotrienes: LTB_4, LTC_4, LTD_4, LTE_4; HPETE, hydroperoxyeicosatetraenoic acids; HETE, hydroxyeicosatetraenoic acid.

PLA_2 through the coupling of this enzyme with a G protein. Then, the mobilization of arachidonic acid by PLA_2 within the cell results in the production of the LOX messengers. In some cell types G-protein activity is not essential for the function of this second messenger system; in cardiac tissue, K^+ channels were activated by products of arachidonic acid without G-protein involvement (125).

The maintenance of cellular ion gradients is fundamental to the homeostasis of virtually all cells and depends on the activity of Na^+/K^+-ATPase. Although various metabolic pathways participate in the regulation of Na^+/K^+-ATPase (216,240,262), recent studies have identified intracellular second messenger effects of eicosanoids in regulating this enzyme. A cytochrome P450 (epoxygenase) product has been demonstrated to inhibit microsomal Na^+/K^+-ATPase activity in cells derived from rabbit kidney medullary thick ascending limb (162). Eicosanoids have also been shown to modulate Na^+/K^+-ATPase activity in brain tissue (74).

Modulation of the Cytoskeleton

One of the fundamental self-regulatory functions of cells is to maintain cell shape, which is accomplished by the maintenance of the cytoskeletal proteins. The major cytoskeletal protein is actin, which, when in the filamentous form (F-actin), determines the shape of the cell and provides the potential for shape change in response to agonists of both intracellular and extracellular origin. Downey et al. (55) recently presented evidence suggesting that leukotriene B_4 can control the assembly/polymerization of F-actin in polymorphonuclear (PMN) leukocytes, which in turn results in PMNs being less deformable. PMNs that are stiff have more difficulty in passing through small capillaries resulting in prolonged contact of PMNs with endothelial cells in any given tissue. Increased intracellular calcium levels induced by addition of the ionophore A23187 resulted in actin assembly in human neutrophils. This actin assembly was completely inhibited by the LTB_4 receptor antagonist LY-223982, implying that LTB_4 was essential for actin assembly. The proposed mechanism of action of the ionophore involves the increase in intracellular Ca^{2+}, which activates/facilitates phospholipase A_2, releasing AA that is converted to LTB_4 in the PMNs. The LTB_4 effect was proposed to be on the GTP-binding proteins necessary for F-actin formation.

The role of leukotrienes in actin assembly reported by Downey et al. (55) has also been reported in several diverse cell lines by Peppelenbosch et al. (191). In HeLa (human leukemia), A431 (squamous carcinoma), and Rat-1 (embryonic fibroblasts) cells, epidermal growth factor results in cell shape change—movement from flat toward spherical. This shape change was demonstrated to be accompanied by a corresponding increase in F-actin in a time-dependent manner. These authors provided greater detail regarding the involvement of the intermediate steps involved in this process. The mechanism proposed by Peppelenbosch et al. and Downey et al. indicates that F-actin formation may be dependent on phospholipase A_2 activity, releasing AA, and the activity of 5-LOX producing sulfido-peptidoleukotrienes (Fig. 9). The data on the activity of the LTC_4, LTD_4, and LTE_4 were obtained both by use of the specific inhibitor of 5-LOX (FLAP inhibitor MK-886) and by the addition of LTs to these cells in culture. In addition, these authors reported that prostaglandins resulted in the depolymerization of actin. It appears that metabolites of AA can play an important role in the maintenance of cell morphology.

Modulation of Endothelial Barrier Function

Contraction of the assembled F-actin in confluent monolayers of endothelial cells results in the separation of the junctions between endothelial cells without detachment of these cells from the substratum (259). This contraction of the F-actin in endothelial cells has been shown to be due to the activation of myosin light chain kinase (258). Addition of leukotrienes to endothelial cells also results in separation of endothelial cells, which is assumed to be due to contraction of F-actin. If the scheme in Fig. 9 is applicable to endothelial cells, then LTs not only increase the formation of F-actin into an array of stress fibers but also result in the contraction of these fibers pulling

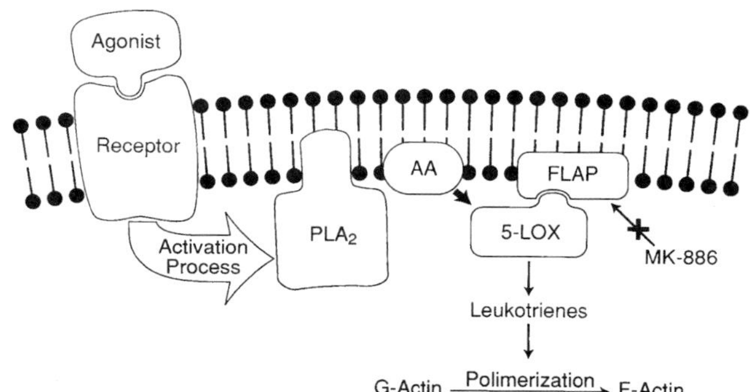

Figure 9. Proposed involvement of leukotrienes in changes in cytoskeletal proteins leading to changes in cell morphology. Binding of agonist to its cell surface receptor provokes an activation process that stimulates receptor-coupled PLA_2 activity. As a consequence of the enhanced activity of PLA_2, unesterified AA is liberated from membrane glycerophospholipids and becomes available for oxidation by 5-lipoxygenase (5-LOX). The 5-lipoxygenase pathway metabolizes AA to leukotrienes, which serve as second messengers effecting cortical actin polymerization. The exact mechanism by which leukotrienes, as second messengers, regulate actin reorganization has not been identified. Unlike cyclooxygenase, 5-LOX requires activation in addition to substrate (AA) mobilization. Activation of 5-LOX takes place concomitantly with its Ca^{2+}-dependent translocation from the cytoplasm to plasma membrane and binding to the transmembrane protein 5-lipoxygenase-activating protein (FLAP). Occupation of FLAP binding sites by the 5-LOX inhibitor MK-886 blocks the formation of leukotrienes and also prevents cytoskeletal changes.

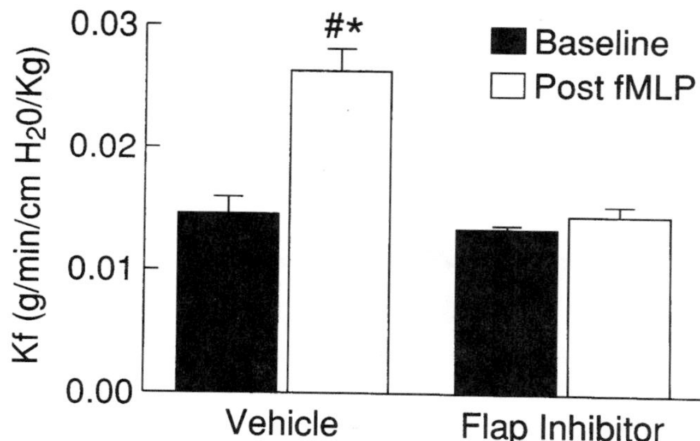

Figure 10. Effect of inhibition of 5-LOX on endothelial permeability following neutrophil-mediated oxidant injury. Pulmonary microvascular fluid filtration coefficient (K_f) at baseline *(solid bars)* and 30 minutes after the addition of 10^{-6} M FMLP *(open bars)*. Rabbit polymorphonuclear leukocytes (PMNs) (1×10^9) were added to the perfusate 30 minutes before baseline measurements were obtained. Five minutes after the addition of the PMNs either vehicle or the FLAP inhibitor MK-886 were added to the perfusate reservoir of the corresponding animal group. *Significant difference from baseline; #significant difference from corresponding group (p <.05).

the cells apart. This contraction of endothelial cells would result in an increase in pericellular permeability.

Addition of LTs to isolated perfused rat lungs has been demonstrated to result in an increase in microvascular permeability (248). Further, addition or increased production of free radicals results in leukotriene production that increases edema formation in isolated perfused rabbit lungs (61). Stimulation of PMNs with the bacterial product N-formyl-L-methionyl-L-leucyl-L-phenylalanine (FMLP) in isolated perfused rabbit lungs results in an increase in permeability and increase in the production of sulfido-peptidoleukotrienes (239). In these investigations when 1×10^9 PMNs were added to the perfusate, FMLP addition resulted in a significant increase in permeability as determined by the filtration coefficient (K_f) (Fig. 10). Addition of FMLP alone did not increase microvascular permeability (K_f). Wet-to-dry weight ratio was also significantly increased with PMNs + FMLP compared with FMLP only.

Perfusate LT levels were measured before and 30 min after adding FMLP (Table 5). LT levels were not increased when PMNs alone were added to the preparation. When FMLP was added to lungs primed with 1×10^9 PMNs, LT levels were markedly increased. Pretreatment with MK-886 attenuated the increase in LTs. MK-886 blocked the FMLP-induced increase in K_f. These data suggested that cysteinyl LT production has an important role in the development of edema caused by FMLP stimulation of PMNs. Further, manipulation of the normal intracellular action of leukotrienes on actin polymerization and contraction by addition of LTs or by stimulation of the LT production by neutrophil-endothelial cell combinations results in increased permeability due to shape change in the endothelial cells.

The source of LTs in these experiments is complex, because although PMNs are the likely source, their lack of glutathione S-transferase precludes the production of cysteinyl LTs. In contrast endothelial cells lack 5-LOX while containing the requisite enzymes to generate cysteinyl LTs. Thus, Grimminger et al. (94) reported that the calcium ionophore A23187 stimulated PMNs to produce LTA_4. Endothelial cells stimulated with A23187 have been shown to be unable to convert arachidonic acid to detectable levels of LTA_4-derived products, including the biologically active metabolites LTB_4 and LTC_4. However, when A23187-stimulated neutrophils were coincubated with endothelial cells, a significant increase in LTC_4 levels were detected over neutrophils alone. The glutathione required for the conversion of LTA_4 to LTC_4 has been shown to be endothelial glutathione, demonstrating one potential mechanism for the synthesis of LTC_4 in the pulmonary circulation (63). The results of the coincubation experiments have been supported by those in isolated blood-free perfused rabbit lungs (92), which have investigated the fate of intravascularly administered LTA_4. Pulmonary artery injection of LTA_4 resulted in the rapid appearance of LTC_4, -D_4, and -E_4, as well as LTB_4, in the recirculating perfusate. These results indicate that pulmonary vascular or perivascular tissue rapidly converts intraluminally available LTA_4 to both cysteinyl LT and LTB_4 in the absence of PMNs, platelets, erythrocytes, and other circulating cells. Therefore, the PMNs stimulated by FMLP in our experiment may have released LTA_4, which could have been converted to LTC_4, -D_4, and -E_4 by the rabbit lung tissue (Fig. 11). The present data support a role for cell-cell interactions via transcellular synthesis of eicosanoids and exemplify the potential contribution of such biosynthetic collaborations to eicosanoid formation in vivo.

REFERENCES

1. Alving K, Matran R, Lundberg JM. The possible role of prostaglandin D_2 in the long-lasting airways vasodilatation induced by allergen in the sensitized pig. *Acta Physiol Scand* 1991;143:93–103.
2. Antonipillai I. 12-Lipoxygenase products are potent inhibitors of prostacyclin-induced renin release. *Proc Soc Exp Biol Med* 1990;194: 224–230.
3. Aramori I, Nakanishi S. Signal transduction and pharmacological characteristics of a metabotropic glutamate receptor, mGluR1, in transfected CHO cells. *Neuron* 1992;8:757–765.
4. Ashby B. Kinetic evidence indicating separate stimulatory and inhibitory prostaglandin receptors on platelet membranes. *J Cyclic Nucleotide Protein Phosphoryl Res* 1986;11:291–300.
5. Ashly B. Model of prostaglandin-regulated cyclic AMP metabolism in intact platelets: examination of time-dependent effects on

Table 5. EFFECT OF FLAP INHIBITOR (MK-886) ON FMLP-INDUCED INCREASES IN PERFUSATE SULFIDOPEPTIDOLEUKOTRIENE DEMONSTRATING THE KEY ROLE OF FLAP IN THE 5-LOX PATHWAY

		Baseline			Experimental		
Group	n	LTC_4	LTD_4	LTE_4	LTC_4	LTD_4	LTE_4
Vehicle	6	5.5 ± 1.6	3.4 ± 1.6	5.9 ± 3.4	234.0 ± 56.0*	85.4 ± 9.1*	239.4 ± 52.0*
MK-886	6	2.9 ± 206	1.8 ± 0.9	1.7 ± 1.0	6.9 ± 2.2	11.7 ± 5.6	14.3 ± 4.9

Values are mean ± SE in pg/ml. Leukotriene (LT) C_4, LTD_4, LTE_4 perfusate levels were measured at baseline and 30 minutes after FMLP administration (experimental). Rabbit polymorphonuclear leukocytes (PMNs) (1×10^9) were added to the perfusate 30 minutes before baseline measurements were obtained. Five minutes after the addition of the PMNs either vehicle or the FLAP inhibitor MK-886 were added to the perfusate reservoir of the corresponding animal group. Perfusate concentrations of individual leukotrienes were assayed by radioimmunoassay following high-performance liquid chromatography separation. *Significant difference from corresponding baseline value (p <.05).

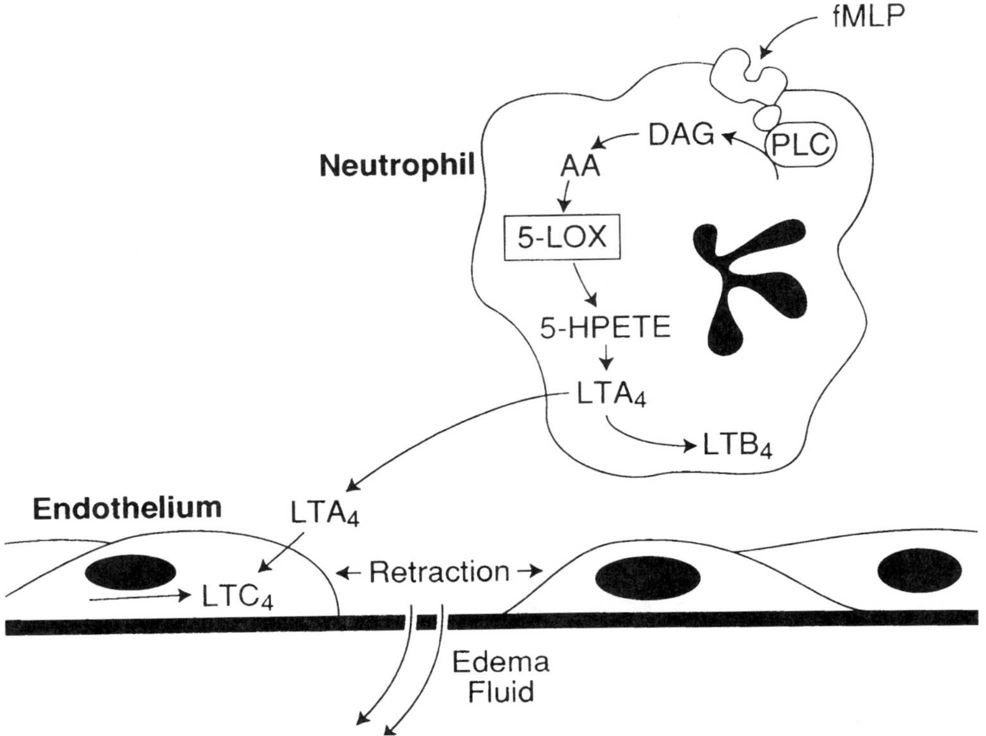

Figure 11. Model of proposed mechanism underlying FMLP stimulated PMN-induced increase in pulmonary microvascular permeability: transcellular metabolism of LTA_4. Binding of the bacterial product FMLP to its specific neutrophil membrane receptor results in receptor-mediated, G-protein–linked activation of and hydrolysis of glycerophospholipids by phospholipase C(189). Liberated AA is metabolized to the unstable intermediate LTA_4 in considerable amounts. PMNs do not generate peptidoleukotrienes because of their constitutive lack of glutathione-S-transferase. Endothelial cells do not contain 5-lipoxygenase and thus are unable to synthesize LTA_4 from AA. LTA_4 is released in the immediate vicinity of the neutrophils, which, when sequestered within the microvasculature, results in the transfer of LTA_4 to vascular endothelium with glutathione-S-transferase activity. The leukotrienes that are generated within the endothelial cells serve as second messengers effecting cortical actin polymerization, endothelial cell retraction, and permeability.

adenylate cyclase and phosphodiesterase activities. *Mol Pharmacol* 1990;36:866–873.
6. Axelrod J, Burch RM, Jelsema CL. Receptor-mediated activation of phospholipase A_2 via GTP-binding proteins: arachidonic acid and its metabolites as second messengers. *Trends Neurosci* 1988;11: 117–123.
7. Badr KF. Sepsis associated renal vasoconstriction: potential targets for future therapy. *Am J Kidney Dis* 1992;20:207–213.
8. Bahls FH, Richmond JE, Smith WL, Haydon PG. A lipoxygenase pathway of arachidonic acid metabolism mediates FMRFamide activation of a potassium current in an identified neuron of Helisoma. *Neurosci Lett* 1992;138:165–168.
9. Bailey JM, Muza B, Hla T, Salata K. Restoration of prostacyclin synthase in vascular smooth muscle cells after aspirin treatment: regulation by epidermal growth factor. *J Lipid Res* 1985;26:54–61.
10. Baldassare JJ, Tarver AP, Henderson PA, Mackin WM, Sahagan B, Fisher GJ. Reconstitution of thromboxane A_2 receptor-stimulated phosphoinositide hydrolysis in isolated platelet membranes: involvement of phosphoinositide-specific phospholipase C-beta and GTP-binding protein Gq. *Biochem J* 1993;291:235–240.
11. Berridge JM. Inositol triphosphate and diacylglycerol: two interacting second messengers. *Annu Rev Biochem* 1987;56:159–193.
12. Bicknell R, Vallee BL. Angiogenin stimulates endothelial cell prostacyclin secretion by activation of phospholipase A_2. *Proc Natl Acad Sci USA* 1989;86:1573–1577.
13. Bjork J, Hedqvist P, Arfors KE. Increase in vascular permeability induced by leukotriene B_4 and the role of polymorphonuclear leukocytes. *Inflammation* 1982;6:189–200.
14. Bonventre JV, Weber, PC, Gronich JH. PAF and PDGF increase cytosolic [Ca^{++}] and phospholipase activity in mesangial cells. *Am J Physiol* 1988;254:F87–94.
15. Borgeat P. Prostaglandins and related lipids. In: Willis AL, ed. *Handbook of eicosanoids.* Boca Raton, FL: CRC Press, 1987;1: 193–211.
16. Borgeat P, Samuelsson B. Arachidonic acid metabolism in polymorphonuclear leukocytes: effects of ionophore A23187. *Proc Natl Acad Sci USA* 1979;76:2148–2152.
17. Borgeat P, Samuelsson B. Metabolisms of arachidonic acid in polymorphonuclear leukocytes. *J Biol Chem* 1979;254:7865–7869.
18. Bourdeau A, Souberbielle J-C, Bonnet P, Herviaux P, Sachs C, Lieberherr, M. Phospholipase-A_2 action and arachidonic acid metabolism in calcium-meditated parathyroid hormone secretion. *Endocrinology* 1992;130:1339–1344.
19. Brass LF, Shaller CC, Belmonte J. Inositol 1,4,5-triphosphate-induced granule secretion in platelets. *J Clin Invest* 1987;79: 1269–1275.
20. Bray MA, Cunningham FM, Ford-Hutchinson AW, Smith MJH. Leukotriene B_4: a mediator of vascular permeability. *Br J Pharmacol* 1981;72:483–486.
21. Buckner CK, Krell RD, Laravuso RB, Coursin DB, Bernstein PR, Will JA. Pharmacological evidence that human intralobar airways do not contain different receptors that mediate contractions to leukotriene C_4 and leukotriene D_4. *J Pharmacol Exp Ther* 1986;237: 558–562.
22. Bunting S, Buchanan LV, Holzgrefe HH, Fitzpatrick FA. Pharmacology of synthetic thromboxane A_2. *Adv Prostaglandins Thromboxane Leukotriene Res* 1987;17A:192–198.
23. Busija DW, Armstead W, Leffler CW, Mirro R. Lipoxins A_4 and B_4 dilate cerebral arterioles of newborn pigs. *Am J Physiol* 1989;256: H468–471.
24. Busija DW, Khreis I, Chen J. Prostanoids promote pial arteriolar dilatation and mask constriction to oxytocin in piglets. *Am J Physiol* 1993;264:H1023–H1027.
25. Cantiello HF, Patenaude CR, Codina J, Birnbaumer L, Ausiello DA. $G\alpha$ i-3 regulates epithelial Na^+ channels by activation of phospholipase A^2 and lipoxygenase pathways. *J Biol Chem* 1990;265: 21624–21628.
26. Carroll MA, Balazy M, Margiotta P, Falck JR, McGiff, JC. Renal

vasodilator activity of 5, 6-epoxyeicosatrienoic acid depends upon conversion by cyclooxygenase and release of prostaglandins. *J Biol Chem* 1993;268:12260–12266.
27. Carroll MA, Sala A, Dunn CE, McGiff JC, Murphy RC. Structural identification of cytochrome P450-dependent arachidonate metabolites formed by rabbit medullary thick ascending limb cells. *J Biol Chem* 1991;266:12306–12312.
28. Cashman JR, Snowdowne KW. Prolactin secretion in anterior pituitary cells: effect of eicosanoids. *Eicosanoids* 1992;5:153–161.
29. Channon JY, Leslie CC. A calcium-dependent mechanism for associating a soluble arachidonoyl-hydrolyzing phospholipase A_2 with membrane in the macrophage cell line RAW 264.7. *J Biol Chem* 1990;265:5409–5413.
30. Chatziantoniou C, Arendshorst WJ. Vascular interactions of prostaglandins with thromboxane in kidneys of rats developing hypertension. *Am J Physiol* 1993;265:F250–256.
31. Chen MCY, Amirian DA, Toomey M, Sanders MJ, Soll AH. Prostanoid inhibition of canine parietal cells: mediation by the inhibitory guanosine triphosphate-binding protein of adenylate cyclase. *Gastroenterology* 1988;94:1121–1129.
32. Cheng JB, Townley RG. Evidence for a similar receptor site for binding of [3H]-leukotriene E_4 and [3H]-leukotriene D_4 to the guinea-pig crude lung membrane. *Biochem Biophys Res Commun* 1984;122:949–954.
33. Chilton FH, Hadley JS, Murphy RC. Incorporation of arachidonic acid into l-acyl-2-lyso-*sn*-glycero-3-phosphocholine of the human neutrophil. *Biochim Biophys Acta* 1987;917:48–56.
34. Christ-Hazelhof E, Nugteren DH. Prostacyclin is not a circulating hormone. *Prostaglandins* 1981;22:739–746.
35. Clark JD, Lin L-L, Kriz RW, et al. A novel arachidonic acid-selective cytosolic PLA_2 contains a Ca^{++}-dependent translocation domain with homology to PKC and GAP. *Cell* 1991;65:1043–1051.
36. Colgan SP, Serhan CN, Parkos CA, Delp-Archer C, Madara JL. Lipoxin A_4 modulates transmigration of human neutrophils across intestinal epithelial monolayers. *J Clin Invest* 1993;92:75–82.
37. Corey EJ, Niwa H, Falck JR, Mioskowski C, Arai Y, Marfat A. Recent studies on the chemical synthesis of eicosanoids. *Adv Prostaglandin Thromboxane Leukotriene Res* 1980;6:19–25.
38. Cristol JP, Sirois P. Comparative activity of leukotriene D_4, 5, 6-dihydroxy-eicosatetraenoic acid and lipoxin A on guinea pig lung parenchyma and ileum smooth muscle. *Res Commun Chem Pathol Pharmacol* 1988;59:423–426.
39. Crooke ST, Mong S, Sarau HM, Winkler JD, Vegesna VK. Mechanisms of regulation of receptors and signal transduction pathways for the peptidyl leukotrienes. *Ann N Y Acad Sci* 1988;524:153–161.
40. Crooke S, Monia BP, Chiang MY, Bennett CF. Leukotriene receptors and mechanisms of signal transduction. *Ann N Y Acad Sci* 1991; 629:120–124.
41. Crouch MF, Lapetina EG. No direct correlation between Ca^{++} mobilization and dissociation of G_i during platelet phospholipase A_2 activation. *Biochem Biophys Res Commun* 1988;153:21–30.
42. Culpepper RM, Andreoli TE. Interactions among prostaglandin E_2, antidiuretic hormone, and cyclic adenosine monophosphate in modulating Cl^- absorption in single mouse medullary thick ascending limbs of Henle. *J Clin Invest* 1983;71:1588–1601.
43. Currie MG, Needleman P. Renal arachidonic acid metabolism. *Annu Rev Physiol* 1984;46:327–341.
44. Dahlen SE, Bjork J, Hedqvist P, et al. Leukotrienes promote plasma leakage and leukocyte adhesion in postcapillary venules: in vivo effects with relevance to the acute inflammatory response. *Proc Natl Acad Sci USA* 1981;78:3887–3891.
45. Dahlen SE, Raud J, Serhan CN, Bjork J, Samuelsson B. Biological activities of lipoxin A include lung strip contraction and dilation of arterioles in vivo. *Acta Physiol Scand* 1987;130:643–647.
46. Davies KL, Dunn MW, Schwartzman ML. Hormonal stimulation of 12(R)-HETE, a cytochrome P450 arachidonic acid metabolite in the rabbit cornea. *Curr Eye Res* 1990;9:661–667.
47. de Chaffoy de Courcelles D, Roevens P, Van Belle H, Kennis L, Somers Y, DeClerck F. The role of endogenously formed diacylglycerol in the propagation and termination of platelet activation. A biochemical and functional analysis using the novel diacylglycerol kinase inhibitor R59 949. *J Biol Chem* 1989;264:3274–3285.
48. Dennis EA. Regulation of eicosanoid production: role of phospholipases and inhibitors. *Biotechnology* 1985;5:1294–1300.
49. DeWitt DL. Prostaglandin endoperoxide synthase: regulation of enzyme expression. *Biochim Biophys Acta* 1991;1083:121–134.
50. DeWitt DL, Day JS, Sonnenburg WK, Smith WL. Concentrations of prostaglandin endoperoxide synthase and prostaglandin I_2 synthase in the endothelium and smooth muscle of bovine aorta. *J Clin Invest* 1983;72:1882–1888.
51. DeWitt DL, Rollins TE, Day JS, Gauger JA, Smith WL. Orientation of the active site and antigenic determinants of prostaglandin endoperoxide synthase in the endoplasmic reticulum. *J Biol Chem* 1981;256:10375–10382.
52. Dixon RAF, Diehl RE, Opas E, et al. Requirement of a 5-lipoxygenase-activating protein for leukotriene synthesis. *Nature* 1990;343: 282–284.
53. Dorn GW, Becker MW. Thromboxane A_2 stimulated signal transduction in vascular smooth muscle. *J Pharmacol Exp Ther* 1993;265 (1):447–456.
54. Doroshenko P. Second messengers mediating the activation of chloride current by intracellular GTPγs in bovine chromaffin cells. *J Physiol* 1991;436:725–738.
55. Downey GP, Takai A, Zamel R, Grinstein S, Chan CK. Okadaic acid-induced actin assembly in neutrophils: role of protein phosphatases. *J Cell Physiol* 1993;155:505–519.
56. Dunn MJ, Liard JF, Dray F. Basal and stimulated rates of renal secretion and excretion of prostaglandins E_2, Fα, and 13, 14-dihydro-15-keto Fα in the dog. *Kidney Int* 1978;13:36–43.
57. Dutta-Roy AK, Sinha AK. Purification and properties of prostaglandin E_1/prostacyclin receptor of human blood platelets. *J Biol Chem* 1987;262:12685–12691.
58. El-Etr M, Marin P, Tence M, et al. 2-Chloroadenosine potentiates the α_1-adrenergic activation of phospholipase C through a mechanism involving arachidonic acid and glutamate in striatal astrocytes. *J Neurosci* 1992;4:1363–1369.
59. Escalante B, Erlij D, Falck JR, McGiff JC. Effect of cytochrome P450 arachidonate metabolites on ion transport in rabbit kidney loop of Henle. *Science* 1991;251(4995):799–802.
60. Fafeur V, Jiang ZP, Bohlen P. Signal transduction by bFGF, but not TGFb1, involves arachidonic acid metabolism in endothelial cells. *J Cell Physiol* 1991;149:277–283.
61. Farrukh IS, Michael JR, Peters SP, et al. The role of cyclooxygenase and lipoxygenase mediators in oxidant-induced lung injury. *Am Rev Respir Dis* 1988;137:1343–1349.
62. Fazeli MS. Synaptic plasticity: on the trail of the retrograde messenger. *Trends Neurosci* 1992;15:115–117.
63. Feinmark SJ, Cannon PJ. Endothelial cell leukotriene C_4 synthesis results from intercellular transfer of leukotriene A_4 synthesized polymorphonuclear leukocytes. *J Biol Chem* 1986;261:16466–16472.
64. Felder CC, Kanterman RY, Ma AL, Axelrod J. Serotonin stimulates phospholipase A_2 and the release of arachidonic acid in hippocampal neurons by a type 2 serotonin receptor that is independent of inositolphospholipid hydrolysis. *Proc Natl Acad Sci USA* 1990;87:2187–2191.
65. Felder CC, Williams HL, Axelrod J. A transduction pathway associated with receptors coupled to the inhibitory guanine nucleotide binding protein Gi that amplifies ATP-mediated arachidonic acid release. *Proc Natl Acad Sci USA* 1991;88:6477–6480.
66. Ferreira SH, Nakamura M, Abreu-Castro MS. The hyperalgesic effects of prostacyclin and PGE_2. *Prostaglandins* 1978;16:31–37.
67. Ferreri N, Schwartzman M, Abraham N, Chander P, McGiff J. Arachidonic acid metabolism in a cell suspension isolated from rabbit renal outer medulla. *J Pharmacol Exp Ther* 1984;231:441–448.
68. FitzGerald GA, Brash AR, Falardeau P, Oates JA. Estimated rate of prostacyclin secretion into the circulation of normal man. *J Clin Invest* 1981;68:1272–1275.
69. Fleisch JH, Rinkema LE, Baker SR. Evidence for multiple leukotriene D_4 receptors in smooth muscle. *Life Sci* 1982;31: 577–581.
70. Folkerts G, Engels F, Nijkamp FP. Endotoxin-induced hyperreactivity of the guinea-pig isolated trachea coincides with decreased prostaglandin E2 production by the epithelial layer. *Br J Pharmacol* 1989;96:388–394.
71. Ford-Hutchinson AW, Bray MA, Doig MV, Shipley ME, Smith MJH. Leukotriene B, a potent chemokinetic and aggregating substance released from polymorphonuclear leukocytes. *Nature* 1980;186:264–265.
72. Francis HP, Greenham SJ, Patel UP, Thompson AM, Gardiner PJ. BAY U3405 an antagonist of thromboxane A_2- and prostaglandin D_2-induced bronchoconstriction in the guinea-pig. *Br J Pharmacol* 1991;104:596–602.
73. Freeman EJ, Damron DS, Terrian DM, Dorman RV. 12-Lipoxygenase products attenuate the glutamate release and Ca^{2+} accumulation evoked by depolarization of hippocampal mossy fiber nerve endings. *J Neurochem* 1991;56:1079–1082.

74. Freeman EJ, Terrian DM, Dorman RV. Presynaptic facilitation of glutamate release from isolated hippocampal mossy fiber nerve endings by arachidonic acid. *Neurochem Res* 1990;15:743–750.
75. Freeman RH, Davis JO, Villarreal D. Role of renal prostaglandins in the control of renin release. *Circ Res* 1984;54:1–9.
76. Fujimura M, Ogawa H, Saito M, Sakamoto S, Miyake Y, Matsuda T. Inhibitory effect of inhalation of a thromboxane synthetase inhibitor on bronchoconstriction induced by aerosolized leukotriene C_4 and thromboxane A_2 analogue in anesthetized guinea pigs. *Allergy* 1991;46:534–539.
77. Funk CD, Radmark O, Fu JY, et al. Molecular cloning and amino acid sequence of leukotriene A_4 hydrolase. *Proc Natl Acad Sci USA* 1987;84:6677–6681.
78. Fuse I, Iwanaga T, Tai HH. Phorbol ester, 1, 2-diacylglycerol, and collagen induce inhibition of arachidonic acid incorporation into phospholipids in human platelets. *J Biol Chem* 1989;264:3890–3895.
79. Gapinski DM, Mallett BE, Froelich LL, Jackson WT. Benzophenone dicarboxylic acid antagonists of leukotriene B_4. 1. Structure-activity relationships of the benzophenone nucleus. *J Med Chem* 1990;33:2798–2807.
80. Garcia-Perez A, Smith WL. Apical-basolateral membrane asymmetry in canine cortical collecting tubule cells. Bradykinin, arginine vasopressin, prostaglandin E_2 interrelationships. *J Clin Invest* 1984;74:63–74.
81. Gerozissis K, Rougot C, Dray F. Leukotriene C_4 is a potent stimulator of LHRH secretion. *Eur J Pharmacol* 1986;121:159–160.
82. Gerritsen ME, Cheli CD. Arachidonic acid and prostaglandin endoperoxide metabolism in isolated rabbit and coronary microvessels and isolated and cultivated coronary microvessel endothelial cells. *J Clin Invest* 1983;72(5):1658–1671.
83. Gerritsen ME, Rimarachin J, Perry CA, Weinstein BI. Arachidonic acid metabolism by cultured bovine corneal endothelial cells. *Invest Ophthalmol Vis Sci* 1989;30(4):698–705.
84. Gillard JA, Ford-Hutchinson AW, Chan C, et al. L-663, 536 (MK-886) (3-[1-(4-chlorobenzyl)-3-t-butyl-thio-5-isopropylindol -2-yl]-2,2-dimethylpropanoic acid), a novel, orally active leukotriene biosynthesis inhibitor. *Can J Physiol Pharmacol* 1989;67:456–464.
85. Glasgow WC, Afshari CA, Barrett JC, Eling TE. Modulation of the epidermal growth factor mitogenic response by metabolites of linoleic and arachidonic acid in Syrian hamster embryo fibroblasts. Differential effects in tumor suppressor gene (+) and (−) phenotypes. *J Biol Chem* 1992;267:10771–10779.
86. Goerig M, Habenicht AJ, Heitz R, et al. sn-1, 2-Diacylglycerols and phorbol diesters stimulate thromboxane synthesis by de novo synthesis of prostaglandin H synthase in human promyelocytic leukemia cells. *J Clin Invest* 1987;79:903–911.
87. Goetzl EJ, Sun FF. Generation of unique monohydroxy-eicosatetraenoic acids from arachidonic acid by human neutrophils. *J Exp Med* 1979;150:406–411.
88. Goldman DW, Goetzl EJ. Heterogeneity of human polymorphonuclear leukocyte receptors for leukotriene B_4. Identification of a subset of high affinity receptors that transduce the chemotactic response. *J Exp Med* 1984;159:1027–1041.
89. Goldsmith JC, Needleman SW. A comparison study of thromboxane and prostacyclin release from ex vivo and cultured bovine vascular endothelium. *Prostaglandins* 1982;24:173–178.
90. Goldstein RE. Involvement of leukocytes and leukotrienes in ischemic dysfunction of the coronary microcirculation. *Eur Heart J* 1990;11:B16–B26.
91. Gorman RR, Ruppel PL, Lin AH. Evidence for leukotriene B_4 receptors in human neutrophils. *Adv Prostaglandin Thromboxane Leukotriene Res* 1985;15:661–665.
92. Grimminger F, Becker G, Seeger W. High yield enzymatic conversion of intravascular leukotriene A_4 in blood-free perfused lungs. *J Immunol* 1988;141:2431–2436.
93. Grimminger F, Kreusler B, Schneider U, Becker G, Seeger W. Influence of microvascular adherence on neutrophil leukotriene generation. Evidence for cooperative eicosanoid synthesis. *J Immunol* 1990;144:1866–1872.
94. Grimminger F, Menger M, Becker G, Seeger W. Potentiation of leukotriene production following sequestration of neutrophils in isolated lungs: indirect evidence for intercellular leukotriene A_4 transfer. *Blood* 1988;72:1687–1692.
95. Habenicht AJ, Salbach P, Goerig M, et al. The LDL receptor pathway delivers arachidonic acid for eicosanoid formation in cells stimulated by platelet-derived growth factor. *Nature* 1990;345: 634–636.
96. Haines KA, Weissmann G. Protein I of *N. gonorrhoeae* shows that phosphatidate from phosphatidylcholine via phospholipase C is an intracellular messenger in neutrophil activation by chemoattractants. *Adv Prostaglandin Thromboxane Leukotriene Res* 1990;21: 545–552.
97. Hamberg M, Svensson J, Samuelsson B. Thromboxanes: a new group of biologically active compounds derived from prostaglandin endoperoxides. *Proc Natl Acad Sci USA* 1975;72:2994–2998.
98. Hammarstrom S, Orning L, Bernstrom K, Gustafsson B, Norin E, Kaijser L. Metabolism of leukotriene C_4 in rats and humans. *Adv Prostaglandin Thromboxane Leukotriene Res* 1985;15:185–188.
99. Hannigan GE, Williams BR. Signal transduction by interferon-α through arachidonic acid metabolism. *Science* 1991;251:204–207.
100. Hansson A, Serhan CN, Haeggstrom J, Ingelman-Sundberg M, Samuelsson B. Activation of protein kinase C by lipoxin A and other eicosanoids. Intracellular action of oxygenation products of arachidonic acid. *Biochem Biophys Res Commun* 1986;134:1215–1222.
101. Hayaishi O, Matsumura H, Onoe H, Koyama Y, Watanabe Y. Sleep-wake regulation by PGD_2 and PGE_2. *Adv Prostaglandin Thromboxane Leukotriene Res* 1990;21:723–726.
102. Hebert RL, Jacobson HR, Breyer MD. PGE_2 inhibits AVP-induced water flow in cortical collecting ducts by protein kinase C activation. *Am J Physiol* 1990;259:F318–325.
103. Hebert S, Andreoli TE. Control of NaCl transport in the thick ascending limb. *Am J Physiol* 1984;246:F745–F756.
104. Hedin L, Gaddy-Kurten D, Kurten R, DeWitt DL, Smith WL, Richards JS. Prostaglandin endoperoxide synthase in rat ovarian follicles: content, cellular distribution, and evidence for hormonal induction preceding ovulation. *Endocrinology* 1987;121:722–731.
105. Hedqvist P, Raud J, Palmertz U, Haeggstrom J, Nicolaou KC, Dahlen SE. Lipoxin A_4 inhibits leukotriene B_4-induced inflammation in the hamster cheek pouch. *Acta Physiol Scand* 1989;137: 571–572.
106. Henderson WR, Harley JB, Fauci AS. Arachidonic acid metabolism in normal and hypereosinophilic syndrome human eosinophils: generation of leukotrienes B_4, C_4, D_4 and 15-lipoxygenase products. *Immunology* 1984;51:679–686.
107. Henke D, Danilowicz RM, Curtis JF, Boucher RC, Eling TE. Metabolism of arachidonic acid by human nasal and bronchial epithelial cells. *Arch Biochem Biophys* 1988;267:426–436.
108. Henrich WL, Falck JR, Campbell WB. Inhibition of renin secretion from rat renal cortical slices by (R)-12-HETE. *Am J Physiol* 1992;263:F665–670.
109. Herroro I, Niras-Portugal MT, Sanchez-Prieto JS. Positive feedback of glutamate exocytosis by metabotropic presynaptic receptor stimulation. *Nature* 1992;360:163–166.
110. Hogaboom GK, Cook M, Newton JF, et al. Purification, characterization, and structural properties of a single protein from rat basophilic leukemia (RBL-1) cells possessing 5-lipoxygenase and leukotriene A_4 synthetase activities. *Mol Pharmacol* 1986;30:510–519.
111. Howard S, Chan-Yeung M, Martin L, Phaneuf S, Salari H. Polyphosphoinositide hydrolysis and protein kinase C activation in guinea pig tracheal smooth muscle cells in culture by leukotriene D_4 involve a pertussis toxin sensitive G-protein. *Eur J Pharmacol* 1992;227(2):123–129.
112. Hsueh W, Isakson PC, Needleman P. Hormone selective lipase activation in the isolated rabbit heart. *Prostaglandins* 1977;13: 1073–1091.
113. Hulting AL, Lindgren JA, Hokfelt T, et al. Leukotriene C_4 as a mediator of luteinizing hormone release from rat anterior pituitary cells. *Proc Natl Acad Sci USA* 1985;82:3834–3838.
114. Hunt JA, Keen M. Mechanism of thromboxane receptor activation of phospholipase A_2 in endothelial cells. *Biochem Soc Trans* 1991;19(2):99S.
115. Hunter JA, Finkbeiner WE, Nadel JA, Goetzl EJ, Holtzman MJ. Predominant generation of 15-lipoxygenase metabolites of arachidonic acid by epithelial cells from human trachea. *Proc Natl Acad Sci USA* 1985;82:4633–4637.
116. Huslig RL, Fogwell RL, Smith WL. The prostaglandin forming cyclooxygenase of ovine uterus: relationship to luteal function. *Biol Reprod* 1979;21:589–600.
117. Ingerman-Wojenski C, Silver MJ, Smith JB, Macarak E. Bovine endothelial cells in culture produce thromboxane as well as prostacyclin. *J Clin Invest* 1981;67:1292–1296.
118. Irvine RF. How is the level of free arachidonic acid controlled in mammalian cells? *Biochem J* 1982;204:3–16.
119. Johnson HG, McNee ML, Sun FF. 15-Hydroxyeicosatetraenoic

acid is a potent inflammatory mediator and agonist of canine tracheal mucus secretion. *Am Rev Respir Dis* 1985;31:917–922.
120. Judd AM, MacLeod RM. Thyrotropin-releasing hormone and lysine-bradykinin stimulate arachidonate liberation from rat anterior pituitary cells through different mechanisms. *Endocrinology* 1992;131:1251–1260.
121. Junier MP, Dray F, Blair I, Capdevila J, Dishman E, Falck JR, Ojeda SR. Epoxygenase products of arachidonic acid are endogenous constituents of the hypothalamus involved in D_2 receptor-mediated, dopamine-induced release of somatostatin. *Endocrinology* 1990;126:1534–1540.
122. Karwatowska-Prokopczuk E, Ciabbattoni G, Wennmalm A. Effects of hydrodynamic forces on coronary production of prostacyclin and purines. *Am J Physiol* 1989; 256:H1532–H1538.
123. Kent RS, Diedrich SL, Whorton AR. Regulation of vascular prostaglandin synthesis by metabolites of arachidonic acid in perfused rabbit aorta. *J Clin Invest* 1983;72:455–465.
124. Kiesel L, Przylipiak AF, Habenicht AJ, Przylipiak MS, Runnebaum B. Production of leukotrienes in gonadotropin-releasing hormone-stimulated pituitary cells: potential role in luteinizing hormone release. *Proc Natl Acad Sci USA* 1991;88:8801–8805.
125. Kim D, Lewis DL, Graziadei L, Neer EJ, Bar-Sagi D, Clapham DE. G-protein, $\beta\gamma$-subunits activate the cardiac muscarinic K^+-channel via phospholipase A_2. *Nature* 1989;337:557–560.
126. King LS, Fukushima M, Banerjee M, Kang KH, Newman JH, Biaggioni I. Pulmonary vascular effects of prostaglandin D_2, but not its systemic vascular or airway effects, are mediated through thromboxane receptor activation. *Circ Res* 1991;68(2):352–358.
127. Kirsch CM, Sigal E, Djokic TD, Graf PD, Nadel JA. An in vivo chemotaxis assay in the dog trachea: evidence for chemotactic activity of 8,15-diHETE. *J Appl Physiol* 1988;64:1792–1795.
128. Kirschenbaum MA, Lowe AG, Trizna W, Fine LG. Regulation of vasopressin action by prostaglandins. Evidence for prostaglandin synthesis in the rabbit cortical collecting tubule. *J Clin Invest* 1982; 70:1193–1204.
129. Kollter A, Sun D, Kaley G. Role of shear stress and endothelial prostaglandins in flow- and viscosity-induced dilation of arterioles in vitro. *Circ Res* 1993;72(6):1276–1284.
130. Konda Y, Nishisaki H, Nakano O, et al. Prostaglandin protects isolated guinea pig chief cells against ethanol injury via an increase in diacylglycerol. *J Clin Invest* 1990; 86:1897–1903.
131. Krell RD, Tsai BS, Berdoulay A, Barone M, Giles RE. Heterogeneity of leukotriene receptors in guinea-pig trachea. *Prostaglandins* 1983;25:171–178.
132. Kujubu DA, Fletcher BS, Varnum BC, Lim RW, Herschman HR. TIS10, a phorbol ester tumor promoter-inducible mRNA from Swiss 3T3 cells, encodes a novel prostaglandin synthase/cyclooxygenase homologue. *J Biol Chem* 1991;266:12866–12872.
133. Kurachi Y, Ito H, Sugimoto T, Shimizu T, Miki I, Ui M. Arachidonic acid metabolites as intracellular modulators of the G-protein-gated cardiac K^+ channel. *Nature* 1989;337:555–557.
134. Lambert IH. Leukotriene D_4 induced cell shrinkage in Ehrlich ascites tumor cells. *J Membr Biol* 1989;108(2):165–176.
135. Landt M, Easom RA, Colca JR, et al. Parallel effects of arachidonic acid on insulin secretion, calmodulin-dependent protein kinase activity and protein kinase C. Activity in pancreatic islets. *Cell Calcium* 1992;13:163–172.
136. Lang J, Boulay F, Guodong L, Wollheim CB. Conserved transducer coupling but different effector linkage upon expression of the myeloid fMet-Leu-Phe receptor in insulin secreting cells. *EMBO J* 1993;12:2671–2679.
137. Lee TH, Crea AEG, Gant V, et al. Identification of lipoxin A_4 and its relationship to the sulfidopeptide leukotrienes C_4, D_4 and E_4 in the bronchoalveolar lavage fluids obtained from patients with selected pulmonary diseases. *Am Rev Respir Dis* 1990;141: 1453–1458.
138. Lee TH, Horton CE, Kyan-Aung U, Haskard D, Crea AE, Spur BW. Lipoxin A_4 and lipoxin B_4 inhibit chemotactic responses of human neutrophils stimulated by leukotriene B_4 and n-formyl-methionyl-leucyl-l-phenylalanine. *Clin Sci* 1989;77:195–203.
139. Lefer AM, Stahl GL, Lefer DJ, et al. Lipoxins A_4 and B_4: comparison of eicosanoids having bronchoconstrictor and vasodilator actions but lacking platelet aggregatory activity. *Proc Natl Acad Sci USA* 1988;85:8340–8344.
140. Lerea KM, Glomset JA. Agents that elevate the concentration of cAMP in platelets inhibit the formation of a NaDodSO4-resistant complex between thrombin and a 4O-kDa protein. *Proc Natl Acad Sci USA* 1987;84:5620–5624.
141. Letts LG, Piper PJ. The actions of leukotrienes C_4 and D_4 on guinea-pig isolated hearts. *Br J Pharmacol* 1982;76:169–176.
142. Leung PCK, Minegishi T, Ma F, Shou F, Ho Yuen B. Induction of polyphosphoinositide breakdown in rat corpus luteum by prostaglandin $F_{2\alpha}$. *Endocrinology* 1986;119:12–18.
143. Levine JD, Lam D, Taiwo YO, Donatoni P, Goetzl EJ. Hyperalgesic properties of 15-lipoxygenase products of arachidonic acid. *Proc Natl Acad Sci USA* 1986;83:5331–5334.
144. Lin LL, Lin AY, Knopf JL. Cytosolic phospholipase A_2 is coupled to hormonally regulated release of arachidonic acid. *Proc Natl Acad Sci USA* 1992;89:6147–6151.
145. Lin LL, Wartmann M, Lin AY, Knopf JL, Seth A, Davis R. $cPLA_2$ is phosphorylated and activated by MAP kinase. *Cell* 1993;72: 269–278.
146. Lister MD, Deems RA, Watanabe Y, Ulevitch R, Dennis EA. *J Biol Chem* 1988;263:7506–7513.
147. Liu MC, Bleecker ER, Lichtenstein LM, et al. Evidence for elevated levels of histamine, prostaglandin D_2, and other bronchoconstricting prostaglandins in the airways of subjects with mild asthma. *Am Rev Respir Dis* 1990;142:126–132.
148. Ma YH, Harder DR, Clark JE, Roman RJ. Effects of 12-HETE on isolated dog renal arcuate arteries. *Am J Physiol* 1991;261:H451–456.
149. Madison JM, Jones CA, Sankary RM. Brown JK. Differential effects of prostaglandin E_2 on contractions of airway smooth muscle. *J Appl Physiol* 1989;66(3):1397–1407.
150. Mais DE, DeHoll D, Sightler H, Halushka P. Different pharmacologic activities for 13 azapinane thromboxane A_2 analogs in platelets and blood vessels. *Eur J Pharmacol* 1988;148:309–315.
151. Mais D, Dunlap C, Hamanaka N, Halushka P. Further studies on the effects of epimers of 13-azapinanethromboxane A_2 antagonists on platelets and veins. *Eur J Pharmacol* 1985;111:125–128.
152. Majerus PW, Connolly TM, Deckmyn H, et al. The metabolism of phosphoinositide-derived messenger molecules. *Science* 1986;234: 1519–1526.
153. Malcolm KC, Fitzpatrick FA. Epoxyeicosatrienoic acids inhibit Ca^{++} entry into platelets stimulated by thapsigargin and thrombin. *J Biol Chem* 1992;267:19854–19858.
154. Margalit A, Livne AA. Lipoxygenase product controls the regulatory volume decrease of human platelets. *Platelets* 1991;2:207–214.
155. Marom Z, Shelhamer JH, Bach MK, Morton DR, Kaliner M. Slow reacting substances, leukotrienes C_4 and D_4 increase the release of mucous from human airway in vitro. *Am Rev Respir Dis* 1982;126: 449–451.
156. Marom A, Shelhamer JH, Sun F, Kaliner M. Human airway monohydroxyeico-satetraenoic acid generation and mucus release. *J Clin Invest* 1983;72:122–127.
157. Marshall PJ, Kulmacz RJ, Lands WEM. Constraints of prostaglandin biosynthesis in tissues. *J Biol Chem* 1987;262:3510–3517.
158. Masferrer JL, Seibert K, Zweifel B, Needleman P. Endogenous glucocorticoids regulate an inducible cyclooxygenase enzyme. *Proc Natl Acad Sci USA* 1992;89(9):3917–3921.
159. Masferrer JL, Zweifel BS, Seibert K, Needleman P. Selective regulation of cellular cyclooxygenase by dexamethasone and endotoxin in mice. *J Clin Invest* 1990;86(4):1375–1379.
160. Matsumura K, Watanabe Y, Onoe H, Hayaishi O. High density of prostaglandin E_2 binding sites in the anterior wall of the third ventricle: a possible site of hyperthermic action. *Brain Res* 1990;533: 147–151.
161. McGee J, Fitzpatrick FA. Enzymatic hydration of leukotriene A_4: purification and characterization of a novel epoxide hydrolase from human erythrocytes. *J Biol Chem* 1985;260:12832–12837.
162. McGiff JC. Cytochrome P-450 metabolism of arachidonic acid. *Annu Rev Pharmacol Toxicol* 1991;31:339–369.
163. Melien O, Winsnes R, Refsnes M, Gladhaug IP, Christoffersen T. Pertussis toxin abolishes the inhibitory effects of prostaglandins E_1, E_2, I_2 and $F_{2\alpha}$ on hormone-induced cAMP accumulation in cultured hepatocytes. *Eur J Biochem* 1988;172:293–297.
164. Miller B, Sarantis M, Traynellis SF, Attwell D. Potentiation of NMDA receptor currents by arachidonic acid. *Nature* 1992;355: 722–725.
165. Miller DK, Gillard JW, Vickers PJ, et al. Identification and isolation of a membrane protein necessary for leukotriene production. *Nature* 1990;343:278–281.
166. Minami M, Ohno S, Kawasaki H, et al. Molecular cloning of a cDNA coding for human leukotriene A_4 hydrolase. Complete pri-

mary structure of an enzyme involved in eicosanoid synthesis. *J Biol Chem* 1987;262:13873–13876.

167. Mitchell DE, Lei ZM, Rao CV. The enzymes in cyclooxygenase and lipoxygenase pathways of arachidonic acid metabolism in human corpora lutea: dependence on luteal phase, cellular and subcellular distribution. *Prostaglandins Leukot Essent Fatty Acids* 1991;43: 1–12.
168. Mitchell JA, Akarasereenont P, Thiemermann C, Flower RJ, Vane JR. Selectivity of nonsteroidal antiinflammatory drugs as inhibitors of constitutive and inducible cyclooxygenase. *Proc Natl Acad Sci USA* 1993;90:11693–11697.
169. Mizuno K, Yamamoto S, Lands WE. Effects of non-steroidal anti-inflammatory drugs on fatty acid cyclooxygenase and prostaglandin hydroperoxidase activities. *Prostaglandins* 1982;23:743–757.
170. Mong S, Miller J, Wu H, Crooke S. Leukotriene D_4 receptor-mediated hydrolysis of phosphoinositide and mobilization of calcium in sheep tracheal smooth muscle cells. *J Pharmacol Exp Ther* 1988; 244:508–515.
171. Mong S, Scott MO, Lewis MA, et al. Leukotriene E_4 binds specifically to LTD_4 receptors in guinea pig lung membranes. *Eur J Pharmacol* 1985;109:183–192.
172. Murray JJ, Brash AR. Rabbit reticulocyte lipoxygenase catalyzes specific 12(s) and 15(S) oxygenation of arachidonoylphosphatidylcholine. *Arch Biochem Biophys* 1988;263:514–523.
173. Nakajima T, Sugimoto T, Kurachi Y. Platelet-activation factor activates cardiac G_K via arachidonic acid metabolites. *FEBS Lett* 1991; 289:239–243.
174. Nakamura T, Fonteh AN, Hubbard WC, et al. Arachidonic acid metabolism during antigen and ionophore activation of the mouse bone marrow derived mast cell. *Biochim Biophys Acta* 1991; 1085:191–200.
175. Nakao J, Ooyama T, Ito H, Chang W, Murota S. Comparative effect of lipoxygenase products of arachidonic acid on rat aortic smooth muscle cell migration. *Atherosclerosis* 1982;44:339–342.
176. Nakao A, Watanabe T, Taniguchi S, Nakamura M, Honda Z, Shimizu T, Kurokawa K. Characterization of prostaglandin F_2 α receptor of mouse 3T3 fibroblasts and its functional expression in Xenopus laevis oocytes. *J Cell Physiol* 1993;155(2):257–264.
177. Nakashima S, Nagata KI, Ueeda K, Nozawa Y. Stimulation of arachidonic acid release by guanine nucleotide in saponin-permeabilized neutrophils: evidence for involvement of GTP-binding protein in phospholipase A_2 activation. *Arch Biochim Biophys* 1988; 261:375–383.
178. Narumiya S, Salmon JA, Cottee FH, Weatherley BC, Flower RJ. Arachidonic acid 15-lipoxygenase from rabbit peritoneal polymorphonuclear leukocytes. Partial purification and properties. *J Biol Chem* 1981;256:9583–9592.
179. Negishi M, Ito S, Hayaishi O. Prostaglandin E receptors in bovine adrenal medulla are coupled to adenylate cyclase via Gi and to phosphoinositide metabolism in a pertussis toxin-insensitive manner. *J Biol Chem* 1989;264:3916–3923.
180. Negishi M, Sugimoto Y, Hayashi Y, et al. Functional interaction of prostaglandin E receptor EP3 subtype with guanine nucleotide-binding proteins, showing low-affinity ligand binding. *Biochim Biophys Acta* 1993;1175(3):343–350.
181. Neufeld EJ, Majerus PW. Arachidonate release and phosphatidic acid turnover in stimulated human platelets. *J Biol Chem* 1983;258: 2461–2467.
182. Nugteren DH. Arachidonic acid 12-lipoxygenase from bovine platelets. *Methods Enzymol* 1982;86:49–54.
183. O'Byrne PM, Aizawa H, Bethel RA, Chung KF, Nadel JA, Holtzman MJ. Prostaglandin $F_{2\alpha}$ increases responsiveness of pulmonary airways in dogs. *Prostaglandins* 1984;28:537–543.
184. Ohki S, Ogino N, Yamamoto S, Hayaishi O. Prostaglandin hydroperoxidase, an integral part of prostaglandin endoperoxide synthetase from bovine vesicular gland microsomes. *J Biol Chem* 1979;254:829–836.
185. Oliw EH, Guengenrich FP, Oates JA. Oxygenation of arachidonic acid by hepatic monooxygenases. Isolation and metabolism of four epoxide intermediates. *J Biol Chem* 1982;257:3771–3781.
186. Onoe H, Ueno R, Fujita I, Nishino H, Oomura Y, Hayaishi O. Prostaglandin D_2, a cerebral sleep-inducing substance in monkeys. *Proc Natl Acad Sci USA* 1988;85:4082–4086.
187. Pagels WR, Sachs RJ, Marnett LJ, DeWitt DL, Day JS, Smith WL. Immunochemical evidence for the involvement of prostaglandin H synthase in hydroperoxide-dependent oxidations by ram seminal vesicle microsomes. *J Biol Chem* 1983;258:6517–6523.
188. Palmer MR, Matheus R, Hoffer BJ, Murphy RC. Electrophysiological response of cerebellar purkinje neurons to leukotriene D_4 and B_4. *J Pharmacol Exp Ther* 1981;219:91–96.
189. Palmer MR, Mathews R, Murphy RC, Hoffer BJ. Leukotriene C elicits a prolonged excitation of cerebellar Purkinje neurons. *Neurosci Lett* 1980;18:173–180.
190. Patton PE, Stouffer RL. Current understanding of the corpus luteum in women and nonhuman primates. *Clin Obstet Gynecol* 1991;34:127–143.
191. Peppelenbosch MP, Tertoolen LG, Hage WJ, deLaat SW. Epidermal growth factor-induced actin remodeling is regulated by 5-lipoxygenase and cyclooxygenase products. *Cell* 1993;74(3): 565–575.
192. Peppelenbosch MP, Tertoolen LGJ, Hertog J, deLaat SW. Epidermal growth factor activates calcium channels by phospholipase A_2/5-lipoxygenase-mediated leukotriene C_4 production. *Cell* 1992; 69:295–303.
193. Piomelli D, Greengard P. Lipoxygenase metabolites of arachidonic acid in neuronal transmembrane signalling. *Trends Pharmacol Sci* 1990;11:367–373.
194. Piomelli D, Pilon C, Giros B, Sokoloff P, Martres MP, Schwartz JC. Dopamine activation of the arachidonic acid cascade as a basis for D_1/D_2 receptor synergism. *Nature* 1991;353:164–167.
195. Piomelli D, Volterra A, Dale N, Siegelbaum A, Kandel ER, Schwartz JH, Belardetti F. Lipoxygenase metabolites of arachidonic acid as second messengers for presynaptic inhibition of aplysia sensory cells. *Nature* 1987;328:38–43.
196. Ponzoni M, Montaldo PG, Cornaglia-Ferraris P. Stimulation of receptor-coupled phospholipase A_2 by interferon-γ. *FEBS Lett* 1992;310:17–21.
197. Priddy AR, Killick SR, Elstein M, et al. Ovarian follicular fluid eicosanoid concentrations during the preovulatory period in humans. *Prostaglandins* 1989;38:197–202.
198. Proctor KG, Capdevila JH, Falck JR, Fitzpatrick FA, Mullane KM, McGiff JC. Cardiovascular and renal actions of cytochrome P-450 metabolites of arachidonic acid. *Blood Vessels* 1989;26:53–64.
199. Proctor KG, Falck JR, Capdevila J. Intestinal vasodilation by epoxyeicosatrienoic acids: arachidonic acid metabolites produced by a cytochrome P450 monooxygenase. *Circ Res* 1987;60:50–59.
200. Quilley CP, McGiff JC. Isomers of 12-hydroxy-5,8,10,14-eicosatetraenoic acid reduce renin activity and increase water and electrolyte excretion. *J Pharmacol Exp Ther* 1990;254:774–780.
201. Ramstedt U, Ng J, Wigzell H, Serhan CN, Samuelsson B. Action of novel eicosanoids lipoxin A and B on human natural killer cell cytotoxicity: effects on intracellular cAMP and target cell binding. *J Immunol* 1985;135:3434–3438.
202. Ramstedt U, Serhan CN, Nicolaou KC, Webber SE, Wigzell H, Samuelsson B. Lipoxin A-induced inhibition of human natural killer cell cytotoxicity: studies on stereospecificity of inhibition and mode of action. *J Immunol* 1987;138:266–270.
203. Rapoport SM, Schewe T, Wiesner R, et al. The lipoxygenase of reticulocytes. Purification, characterization and biological dynamics of the lipoxygenase; its identity with the respiratory inhibitors of the reticulocyte. *Eur J Biochem* 1979;96:545–561.
204. Raz A, Wyche A, Fu J, Seibert K, Needleman P. Regulation of prostanoids synthesis in human fibroblasts and human blood monocytes by interleukin-1, endotoxin, and glucocorticoids. *Adv Prostaglandin Thromboxane Leukotriene Res* 1990;20:22–27.
205. Reddy GP, Prasad M, Sailesh S, Kumar YV, Reddanna P. The production of arachidonic acid metabolites in rat testis. *Prostaglandins* 1992;44(6):497–507.
206. Rediske J, Morrissey MM, Jarvis M. Human monocytes respond to leukotriene B_4 with a transient increase in cytosolic calcium. *Cell Immunol* 1993;147(2):438–445.
207. Rodway MR, Baimbridge KG, Ho Yuen B, Leung PCK. Effect of prostaglandin $F_{2\alpha}$ on cytosolic free calcium ion concentrations in rat luteal cells. *Endocrinology* 1991;129:889–895.
208. Rollins TE, Smith WL. Subcellular localization of prostaglandin-forming cyclooxygenase in Swiss mouse 3T3 fibroblasts by electron microscopic immunocytochemistry. *J Biol Chem* 1980;255: 4872–4875.
209. Rome LH, Lands WE. Structural requirements for time-dependent inhibition of prostaglandin biosynthesis by anti-inflammatory drugs. *Proc Natl Acad Sci USA* 1975;72:4863–4865.
210. Rouzer CA, Ford-Hutchinson AW, Morton HE, Gillard JW. MK886, a potent and specific leukotriene biosynthesis inhibitor blocks and reverses the membrane association of 5-lipoxygenase

in ionophore-challenged leukocytes. *J Biol Chem* 1990;265: 1436–1442.
211. Rouzer CA, Kargman S. Translocation of 5-lipoxygenase to the membrane in human leukocytes challenged with ionophore A23187. *J Biol Chem* 1988;263:10980–10988.
212. Rouzer CA, Matsumoto T, Samuelsson B. Single protein from human leukocytes possesses 5-lipoxygenase and leukotriene A_4 synthase activities. *Proc Natl Acad Sci USA* 1986;83:857–861.
213. Saadi M, Gerozissis K, Rougeot C, Minary P, Dray F. Leukotriene C_4-induced release of LHRH into the hypophyseal portal blood and of LH into the peripheral blood. *Life Sci* 1990;46:1857–1865.
214. Sakai H, Takeguchi N. Small-conductance Cl^- channels in rabbit parietal cells activated by prostaglandin E_2 and inhibited by GTPγS. *J Physiol* 1993;461:201–212.
215. Samuelsson B, Dahlen SE, Lindgren JA, Rouzer CA, Serhan CH. Leukotrienes and lipoxins: structures, biosynthesis, and biological effects. *Science* 1987;237:1171–1176.
216. Satoh T, Cohen HT, Katz AI. Intracellular signaling in the regulation of renal Na-K-ATPase. II. Role of cyclic AMP and phospholipase A_2. *J Clin Invest* 1992;89:1496–1500.
217. Schwartzman ML, Abraham NG, Masferrer IL Dunn WW, McGiff JC. Cytochrome P450 dependent metabolism of arachidonic acid in bovine corneal epithelium. *Biochem Biophys Res Commun* 1985; 132:343–351.
218. Schwartzman ML, Balazy M, Masferrer J, Abraham NG, McGiff JC, Murphy RC. 12(R)-hydroxyeicosatetraenoic acid: a cytochrome-P450-dependent arachidonate metabolite that inhibits Na^+, K^+-ATPase in the cornea. *Proc Natl Acad Sci USA* 1987;84:8125–8129.
219. Shak S, Perez HD, Goldstein IM. A novel dioxygenation product of arachidonic acid possesses potent chemotactic activity for human polymorphonuclear leukocytes. *J Biol Chem* 1983;258:14948–14953.
220. Shearman MS, Naor Z, Sekiguchi K, Kishimoto A, Nishizuka Y. Selective activation of the γ-subspecies of protein kinase C from bovine cerebellum by arachidonic acid and its lipoxygenase metabolites. *FEBS Lett* 1989;243:177–182.
221. Sjolander A, Gronroos E, Hammarstrom S, Andersson T. Leukotriene D_4 and E_4 induce transmembrane signaling in human epithelial cells. *J Biol Chem* 1990;265:20976–20981.
222. Skoglund G, Claesson HE. Intracellular mechanisms involved in keukotriene C_4-stimulated adhesion of U-937 cells. *Cell Signal* 1991;3(5):399–404.
223. Skoner DP, Page R, Asman B, Gillen L, Fireman P. Plasma elevations of histamine and a prostaglandin metabolite in acute asthma. *Am Rev Respir Dis* 1988;137:1009–1014.
224. Smedegard G, Hedqvist P, Dahlen SE, Revenas B, Hammarstrom S, Samuelsson B. Leukotriene C_4 affects pulmonary and cardiovascular dynamics in monkey. *Nature* 1982;295:327–329.
225. Smith CD, Cox CC, Snyderman R. Receptor-coupled activation of phosphoinositide-specific phospholipase C by an N protein. *Science* 1986;232:97–100.
226. Smith JB, Yanagisawa A, Zipkin R, Lefer AM. Constriction of cat coronary arteries by synthetic thromboxane A_2 and its antagonism. *Prostaglandins* 1987;33:777–781.
227. Smith WL. Prostaglandins and related compounds. In: Willis AL, ed. *Handbook of eicosanoids.* Boca Raton, FL: CRC Press, 1987;1: 175–184.
228. Smith, WL. The eicosanoids and their biochemical mechanisms of action. *Biochem J* 1989;259:315–324.
229. Smith WL, Lands WE. Stimulation and blockade of prostaglandin biosynthesis. *J Biol Chem* 1971;246:6700–6702.
230. Smith WL, Marnett LJ, DeWitt DL. Prostaglandin and thromboxane biosynthesis. *Pharmacol Ther* 1991;49:153–179.
231. Smith WL, Watanabe T, Umegaki K, et al. General biochemical mechanisms for prostaglandin action. Direct coupling of prostanoid receptors to guanine nucleotide regulatory protein. *Adv Prostaglandin Thromboxane Leukotriene Res* 1987;17:463–466.
232. Snyder GD, Capdevila J, Chacos N, Manna S, Falck JR. Action of luteinizing hormone-releasing hormone: involvement of novel arachidonic acid metabolites. *Proc Natl Acad Sci USA* 1983;80: 3504–3507.
233. Snyder GD, Yadagiri P, Falck JR. Effect of epoxyeicosatrienoic acids on growth hormone release from somatotrophs. *Am J Physiol* 1989;256:E221–E226.
234. Sonnenburg WK, Smith WL. Regulation of cyclic AMP metabolism in rabbit cortical collecting tubule cells by prostaglandins. *J Biol Chem* 1988;263:6155–6160.
235. Stanford N, Roth GJ, Shen TY, Majerus PW. Lack of covalent modification of prostaglandin synthetase (cyclo-oxygenase) by indomethacin. *Prostaglandins* 1977;13:669–675.
236. Stitt JT. Differential sensitivity in the sites of fever production by prostaglandin E1 within the hypothalamus of the rat. *J Physiol* 1991;432:99–110.
237. Stokes JL. Modulation of vasopressin-induced water permeability of the cortical collecting tubule by endogenous and exogenous prostaglandins. *Miner Electrolyte Metab* 1985;11:240–248.
238. Takahara K, Murray R, Fitzgerald GA, Fitzgerald DJ. The response to thromboxane A_2 analogues in human platelets. Discrimination of two binding sites linked to distinct effector systems. *J Biol Chem* 1990;265(12):6836–6844.
239. Tanaka H, Bradley JD, Baudendistel LJ, Dahms TE. Mechanisms of increased pulmonary microvascular permeability induced by FMLP in isolated rabbit lungs. *J Appl Physiol* 1992;73(5):2074–2082.
240. Taub MD, Wang Y, Yang IS, Fiorella P, Lee SM. Regulation of the Na, K-ATPase activity of Madin-Darby canine kidney cells in defined medium by prostaglandin E_1 and 8-bromocyclic AMP. *J Cell Physiol* 1992;151:337–346.
241. Thomas FJ, Koss MA, Hogan DL, Isenberg JI. Enprostil, a synthetic prostaglandin E_2 analogue, inhibits meal-stimulated gastric acid secretion and gastrin release in patients with duodenal ulcer. *Am J Med* 1986;81:44–49.
242. Torikai S, Kurokawa K. Effect of prostaglandin E_2 on vasopressin dependent cell cAMP in isolated segments. *Am J Physiol* 1983;245: F58–66.
243. Tsushita K, Kozawa O, Tokuda H, Oiso Y, Saito H. Proliferative effect of PGD_2 on osteoblast-like cells; independent activation of pertussis toxin-sensitive GTP-binding protein from PGE_2 or $PGF_{2\alpha}$. *Prostaglandins Leukot Essent Fatty Acids* 1992;45(4):267–274.
244. Turk J, Mass RL, Brash AR, Roberts LJ, II, Oates JA. Arachidonic acid 15-lipoxygenase products from human eosinophils. *J Biol Chem* 1982;257:7068–7076.
245. Ulevitch RJ, Watanabe Y, Sano M, Lister MD, Deems RA, Dennis EA. Solubilization, purification, and characterization of a membrane-bound phospholipase A_2 from the P388D1 macrophage-like cell line. *J Biol Chem* 1988;263:3079–3085.
246. Uski TK, Hogestatt ED. Effects of various cyclooxygenase and lipoxygenase metabolites on guinea-pig cerebral arteries. *Gen Pharmacol* 1992;23:109–113.
247. Van Der Ouderaa FJ, Buytenhek M, Nugteren DH, Van Dorp DA. Acetylation of prostaglandin endoperoxide synthetase with acetylsalicylic acid. *Eur J Biochem* 1980;109:1–8.
248. Voelkel NF, Morganroth M, Stenmark K, Feddersen OC, Murphy RC, Reeves JT. Leukotrienes in the lung circulation: actions and interactions. *Prog Clin Biol Res* 1983;136:141–153.
249. Volterra A. Arachidonic acid metabolites as mediators of synaptic modulation. *Cell Biol Int Rep* 1989;13:1189–1199.
250. Wasserman MA, Ducharme DW, Griffin RL, DeGraaf GL, Robinson FG. Bronchopulmonary and cardiovascular effects of prostaglandin D_2 in the dog. *Prostaglandins* 1977;13:255–269.
251. Watanabe T, Umegaki K, Smith WL. Association of a solubilized prostaglandin E_2 receptor from renal medulla with a pertussis toxin reactive guanine nucleotide regulatory protein. *J Biol Chem* 1986;261:13430–13439.
252. Watanabe T, Yatomi Y, Sunaga S, et al. Characterization of prostaglandin and thromoboxane receptors expressed on a megakaryoblastic leukemia cell line, MEG-01s. *Blood* 1991;78(9):2328–2336.
253. Weiss JW, Drazen JM, Coles N, et al. Bronchoconstrictor effects of leukotriene C in humans. *Science* 1982;216:196–198.
254. Weksler BB. Regulation of cyclooxygenase activity in human vascular tissue. *Adv Prostaglandin Thromboxane Leukotriene Res* 1987; 17A:238–243.
255. Weller PF, Lee CW, Foster DW, Corey EJ, Austen KF, Lewis RA. Generation and metabolism of 5 lipoxygenase pathway leukotrienes by human eosinophils: predominant production of leukotriene C_4. *Proc Natl Acad Sci USA* 1983;80:7626–7630.
256. Wilson DE. Role of prostaglandins in gastroduodenal mucosal protection. *J Clin Gastroenterol* 1991;13:S65–S71.
257. Wong A, Hwang SM, Cook MN, Hogaboom GK, Crooke ST. Interactions of 5-lipoxygenase with membranes: studies on the association of soluble enzyme with membranes and alterations in enzyme activity. *Biochemistry* 1988;27:6763–6769.
258. Wysolmerski RB, Lagunoff D. Involvement of myosin light-chain kinase in endothelial cell retraction. *Proc Natl Acad Sci USA* 1990; 87(1):16–20.
259. Wysolmerski RB, Lagunoff D. Regulation of permeabilized

endothelial cell retraction by myosin phosphorylation. *Am J Physiol* 1991;261(1 Pt 1):C32–40.

260. Yokohama H, Tanaka T, Ito S, Negishi M, Hayashi H, Hayaishi O. Prostaglandin E receptor enhancement of catecholamine release may be mediated by phosphoinositide metabolism in bovine adrenal chromaffin cells. *J Biol Chem* 1988;263:1119–1122.
261. Yun JC, Ohman KP, Gill JR Jr, Keiser H. Effects of prostaglandins, cAMP, and changes in cytosolic calcium on platelet aggregation induced by a thromboxane A_2 mimic. *Can J Physiol Pharmacol* 1991; 69(5):599–604.
262. Zeidel ML, Brady HR, Kohan DE. Interleukin-1 inhibition of Na^+/K^+ ATPase in inner medullary collecting duct: role of PGE_2. *Am J Physiol* 1991;261:F1013–F1016.
263. Zimmerman GA, Lorant DE, McIntyre TM, Prescott SM. Juxtacrine intercellular signaling: another way to do it. *Am J Respir Cell Mol Biol* 1993;9:573–577.

Anesthesia: Biologic Foundations, edited by Tony L. Yaksh et al. Lippincott–Raven Publishers, Philadelphia © 1997.

CHAPTER 9

INTRACELLULAR Ca^{2+} REGULATION

RYAN E. LESH AND CARL LYNCH III

Ca^{2+} plays a ubiquitous and critical role in cell function. Alteration of the normally low (~0.1 μM) free intracellular [Ca^{2+}] ([Ca^{2+}]$_i$) is the most common system employed by eukaryotic cells to initiate and control cell behavior. The level of [Ca^{2+}]$_i$ regulates a myriad of cellular enzyme systems that carry out the "work" of any particular cell line. Unlike Na^+, which is segregated outside the cell with a 10- to 20-fold gradient, Ca^{2+} is maintained with a much higher gradient (10,000-fold) across the cell membrane. Also unlike Na^+, Ca^{2+} is selectively sequestered and maintained with a similarly high gradient in membrane-bound organelles within the cell. Because of its critical role in maintaining so many aspects of cell function, the Ca^{2+} fluxes across the cell surface and intracellular membranes are under exquisite control by ion channels, pumps, and exchangers.

As suggested by early studies of Ca^{2+} injection (123), it became evident in the 1960s that Ca^{2+} was the mediator of myofibrillar activation (65). The demonstration of the abundant pool of Ca^{2+} within internal muscle membrane systems (the sarcoplasmic reticulum, SR), combined with A. V. Hill's demonstration that skeletal muscle activation of tension is too rapid to be mediated by diffusion from the extracellular surface (129,130), defined the critical role of the SR in skeletal muscle for excitation-contraction (EC) coupling in striated muscle. While SR Ca^{2+} release has served as a paradigm and model for intracellular Ca^{2+} release, it has become obvious that internal stores of Ca^{2+} play critical roles in the activation of numerous cell types by mechanisms that are distinct but possibly related to EC coupling.

The regulation of intracellular [Ca^{2+}] can be divided into (a) nonmembrane Ca^{2+}-binding proteins and processes, and (b) membrane-delimited Ca^{2+} storage sites. The latter systems have distinct transmembrane proteins that are responsible for accumulation and release. While control of [Ca^{2+}]$_i$ by regulation of Ca^{2+} entry, release, reuptake, and elimination is of critical importance, Ca^{2+}-binding proteins present within the cell also provide another form of [Ca^{2+}]$_i$ regulation.

PROCESSES CONTROLLED BY INTRACELLULAR Ca^{2+} CONCENTRATIONS

Ca^{2+} is a universal second messenger, activating a variety of different processes in cells depending on their specialization. Table 1 lists a variety of cell types whose major function is mediated by alteration in cell [Ca^{2+}]. A notable feature of Ca^{2+} is its activation of nitric oxide synthesis, which acts as an intra- and intercellular messenger, frequently activating intracellular processes that counteract processes activated by Ca^{2+}. In addition to activating major cell-specific functions (contraction, secretion, etc.), Ca^{2+} plays a critical role in regulating cell replication, modulating transcription, and controlling the rate of mitochondrial respiration.

DISTRIBUTION AND COMPARTMENTATION OF INTRACELLULAR Ca^{2+}

Cytosomal Ca^{2+}-Binding Proteins

Cytosolic Ca^{2+}-binding proteins, along with other cellular mechanisms of Ca^{2+} homeostasis, participate in the dynamic control of cytosolic free Ca^{2+} concentrations. In addition to the anatomical compartmentalization of intracellular Ca^{2+} within the endoplasmic reticulum (ER)/SR network and the mitochondria (which probably buffer Ca^{2+} only under certain pathologic conditions), as well as the membrane-bound Ca^{2+} pumps and channels that contribute to intracellular Ca^{2+} regulation, all cells contain cytosolic Ca^{2+}-binding proteins that bind ionized Ca^{2+} with high affinity (kd 1–1000 nM). The three-dimensional structure of many Ca^{2+}-binding proteins has now been determined, and a partial list of some important proteins and their physical characteristics appears in Table 2. Protein crystal structures have revealed homologies among many of these molecules and have allowed their classification into groups that may also represent common genetic origins. In

Table 1. CELL-SPECIFIC Ca^{2+}-REGULATED PROCESSES

Ca regulated processes	Cell type	Protein
Electrophysiologic		
Depolarization	Certain muscle and neuronal cells	Voltage-gated Ca channels
Repolarization	Neurons, smooth muscle	Ca^{2+}-activated K and Cl channels
Movement		
Contraction, smooth muscle and platelets	Various smooth muscle	Myosin light chain kinase (CaM)
Contraction, striated muscle	Skeletal muscle, myocardium	Troponin
Regulation of cell shape	Various cell lines	Spectrin, actin
Secretion		
Vesicle release	Neurons	Synapsin
Secretion	Endocrine	
Degranulation	Platelets, mast cells	
Biochemical synthesis		
Nitric oxide synthesis	Neurons, endothelium	Neuronal and endothelial NOS (CaM)
Peroxide synthesis	Polymorphonuclear leukocytes	
Cytokine release	Lymphocytes	

CaM, calmodulin acts regulator.

Table 2. SELECTED CALCIUM-BINDING PROTEINS

Helix-loop-helix motif calcium-binding proteins (EF-hand)
- Calmodulin (kd ~$10^{-5}/10^{-6}$)
- Troponin C (kd ~$10^{-5}/10^{-7}$)
- Parvalbumin (kd ~$10^{-8}/10^{-9}$)
- Myosin Light Chains:
  - Essential
  - Regulatory
- S-100 (kd ~10^{-3} to 10^{-5}, depending on intracellular [cation])(76)
- Sarcoplasmic Ca^{2+}-binding protein(127)

Nonhelix-loop-helix motif calcium-binding proteins
- Protein kinase C (257) (multiple Ca^{2+}-sensitive isoforms with different Ca^{2+}-binding affinities)
- Annexins (phospholipid and Ca^{2+} concentrations (54) determine K_d's for Ca^{2+} binding)
- Gelsolin

Modified from ref. 331.

addition to structural characteristics, these proteins may also be characterized by functional criteria: (a) proteins that buffer Ca^{2+}; (b) molecules that are conformationally activated upon binding Ca^{2+}; and (c) proteins in which bound Ca^{2+} directly participates in enzymatic catalysis (224).

The structure of many cytosolic Ca^{2+}-binding proteins has now been determined using physical methods such as x-ray crystallography and nuclear magnetic resonance (NMR) spectroscopy in conjunction with circular dichroism measurements and knowledge of the protein's primary sequence. Ca^{2+}-binding proteins can be divided into two broad categories based upon their structures: EF-hand-containing proteins and those that have a non-EF-hand Ca^{2+}-binding pocket. The term *EF-hand* was originally coined by Kretsinger and colleagues to describe the helix-loop-helix (HLH) Ca^{2+}-binding motif found in carp parvalbumin (244). Since their solution of this crystal structure, numerous other proteins have been found that contain HLH-binding motifs as defined by Kretsinger's (178) criteria. The classic EF-hand motif is a 12-amino-acid loop flanked by two orthogonal α-helices, and in many HLH proteins EF-hands occur in pairs of adjacent domains (256). Ca^{2+} is bound in the loop of the EF-hand–binding motif, although some HLH proteins contain EF-hands that appear not to bind Ca^{2+} (or Mg^{2+}) under physiologic conditions. Ca^{2+} is coordinated in these metal-protein complexes exclusively by oxygen atoms; most coordinating oxygens are contributed by polypeptide backbone carbonyl oxygens, the side chains of aspartate, asparagine, glutamine, and glutamate residues in the loop, or, in a few instances, by the oxygen of a water molecule (224). While it appears that the number of oxygen ligands in the coordinating sphere can vary from 4 to 12, most proteins have between 6 and 8 (224). Analysis of the known EF-hand protein structures together with the sequences of genes encoding these proteins has led to the theory that EF-hand proteins evolved from a common ancestral gene (256).

The specificity and affinity of Ca^{2+}-binding proteins for a Ca^{2+} ligand are determined by complex relationships between the amino acid sequence and geometry of the metal-binding domain. Physical factors including the presence of other ions (particularly Mg^{2+}), temperature, ionic strength, pH, and the concentration of the binding proteins themselves also affect the specificity and affinity of ligand binding both in vitro and in vivo (196). At rest, the cytosolic concentration of free Mg^{2+} (~0.5 mM) is several orders of magnitude greater than the resting concentration of free Ca^{2+} (~100 nM); K^+ and Na^+ concentrations are even higher. To function biologically as a Ca^{2+} buffer or as a Ca^{2+}-activated enzyme, the protein must selectively bind Ca^{2+}. Many metal-binding domains of HLH proteins are geometrically optimal for Ca^{2+} binding: hydrated Mg^{2+} ions are smaller than Ca^{2+}, which leads to an unfavorable binding enthalpy; for Na^+ and K^+, the large ionic radius to charge ratio is unfavorable for binding. Studies of several metal-binding proteins reveal that the binding free energies (ΔG) are generally determined by entropic changes (ΔS) as water is lost from the hydration sphere of the metal ion (196). Despite these thermodynamic considerations, however, there are conditions in the resting cell where some of the divalent metal-binding sites will be occupied by Mg^{2+}. With cell stimulation and a rise in the cytosolic free Ca^{2+} concentration, many of these metal-binding sites will be occupied by Ca^{2+} (72). However, for a low-affinity Ca^{2+}-binding site (which has bound Mg^{2+} in the unstimulated state) to buffer cytosolic Ca^{2+}, Ca^{2+} must exchange with Mg^{2+}, and the kinetics of Ca^{2+}-Mg^{2+} exchange will determine the protein's contribution to Ca^{2+} buffering rather than the absolute levels of free Ca^{2+} (72, 297). Parvalbumin, for example, has Ca^{2+}-binding sites that are occupied by Mg^{2+}; the rate of Mg^{2+} dissociation from these binding sites is sufficiently slow that, unless there is a very protracted Ca^{2+} transient, these binding sites will have no significant Ca^{2+}-buffering effect. For this reason, the biologic implications of measured cytosolic Ca^{2+} and Mg^{2+}-binding affinities are further complicated by our recent understanding of the regional inhomogeneities in cytosolic $[Ca^{2+}]_i$ when cells are stimulated. The presence of high Ca^{2+} microdomains (see below) around plasma membrane Ca^{2+} channels and activated SR/ER Ca^{2+}-release channels, as well as cytosolic Ca^{2+} oscillations, make static Ca^{2+}-binding equilibria difficult to interpret in the context of an activated cell. While the ubiquitous EF-hand Ca^{2+}-binding proteins are most prominent and best understood, these generalizations extend to other Ca^{2+}-binding proteins such as calsequestrin, a major Ca^{2+}-binding protein in the lumen of the sarcoplasmic reticulum, and the annexins, a major class of extracellular Ca^{2+}-binding proteins.

Buffering by Parvalbumin

The parvalbumins are a family of monomeric, acidic Ca^{2+}-binding proteins (pI ~4.25) with a molecular weight of ~12 kd. They were first described in fast-twitch skeletal muscles of poikilotherms, but have since been shown to exist in the skeletal muscles and brain of various vertebrate classes. They are hypothesized to serve only a Ca^{2+} buffering function in all of these tissues. Parvalbumins are virtually absent from cardiac or smooth muscle. Crystal structures of several parvalbumins have been resolved with ~1.6 to 1.9 Å resolution, and these proteins assume a globular shape described geometrically as a prolate ellipsoid (331). Generally, they contain two high-affinity EF-hand metal-binding sites (kd 0.1–^{4} × 10^{-6} mol/L) that, in the resting cell, are occupied by Mg^{2+} ions (124,331). The physiologic role of parvalbumin during contraction of skeletal muscle has been debated, since (as discussed above) the Mg^{2+} off-rate is sufficiently slow that it probably serves no practical Ca^{2+}-buffering function during the initial Ca^{2+} rise in stimulated muscle. It may, however, bind Ca^{2+} that dissociates from troponin C and provide a sink for Ca^{2+} removal during relaxation of the muscle fiber.

Parvalbumin, in addition to calretinin and calbindin (also HLH Ca^{2+}-binding proteins) is present in the vertebrate CNS in characteristic subpopulations of cells, making them markers for certain cell types (8,13). Altered expression of some of these Ca^{2+}-binding proteins has been the subject of intense investigation in neurodegenerative disorders, particularly those in which abnormal neuronal Ca^{2+} homeostasis is thought to play a role (125). The distribution of similar Ca^{2+}-binding proteins in the rat spinal cord has also suggested that they may play a role in nociception and dorsal column sensory pathways (295). In light of the importance of intracellular Ca^{2+} levels in neuronal functions, such as neurotransmitter release, the concentrations of Ca^{2+}-binding proteins may prove, with further investigation, to be essential for normal neurologic function. In vitro (cell culture) and in vivo (transgenic animal) systems for altering expression of the Ca^{2+}-binding proteins in both glial and neuronal cells will help to elucidate the functional role of these proteins in a number of disease states (125).

Calmodulin-Signaling via a Ca^{2+}-Binding Protein

Calmodulin is a small acidic protein (pI ~4.2) with a molecular weight of ~16.5 kd that was originally shown to activate a bovine brain adenosine 3′,5′-cyclic monophosphate (cAMP) phosphodiesterase. Like troponin C (with which it shares ~60% sequence homology), calmodulin belongs to the superfamily of EF-hand proteins and contains two pair of metal-binding sites that appear to bind Ca^{2+} cooperatively and sequentially (Fig. 1A) (168). Ca^{2+} binding induces a conformational change in the protein structure that allows for Ca^{2+}-calmodulin's interaction with a variety of effector molecules (168,369). Other metals can complex with and activate calmodulin. Lanthanides (Tb^{3+}, Nd^{3+}, and Pr^{3+}) bind to calmodulin with a higher affinity than Ca^{2+}; Mn^{2+}, Sr^{2+}, Zn^{2+}, and Co^{2+} bind with a lower affinity to calmodulin, yet all yield biologically active complexes when bound (168).

Calmodulin, unlike the parvalbumins, acts as a Ca^{2+}-activated switch for a growing number of intracellular enzymes. Ca^{2+}-calmodulin, the active complex, is known to regulate smooth muscle contraction by binding to and activating myosin light chain kinase (MLCK). This complex also plays a role in the activation of a family of Ca^{2+}-calmodulin–activated protein kinases (CaM-kinases), the phosphatase calcineurin, and a host of other enzymes. The binding domain for calmodulin on MLCK is a region near the C-terminus (termed M13) that appears to form a 17 residue helix. In this interaction, the connecting helix of the "dumbbell"-shaped calmodulin molecule bends around the helix of the target protein (Fig. 1B) (276), apparently thereby modulating its activity. In addition to its cytosolic location, calmodulin has been localized in the nuclei of cells using biochemical and immunohistochemical techniques. Nuclear calmodulin has been implicated in Ca^{2+}-sensitive processes such as DNA replication, repair, and possibly gene expression (12,106). Calmodulin's function as an enzyme cofactor appears to be ubiquitous, by virtue of its presence in nearly every eukaryotic cell type.

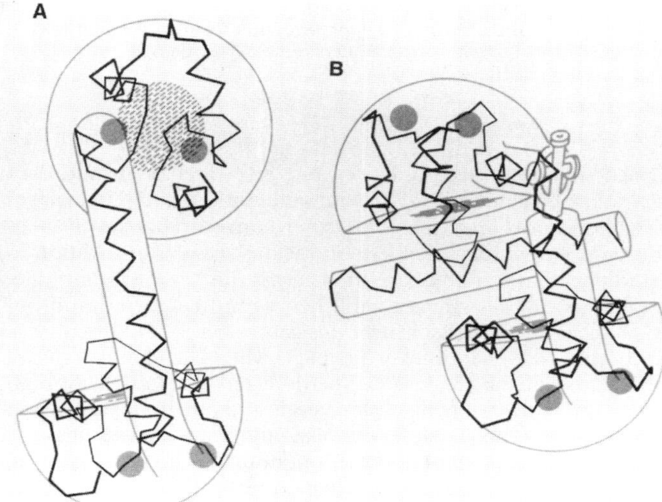

Figure 1. The structure of $(Ca^{2+})_4$-calmodulin and its proposed interaction with M13 peptide. M13 represents the CaM-binding domain of myosin light chain kinase. **(A)** An α-carbon tracing of the 3 Å resolution CaM structure currently being refined. The C terminus is uppermost; coordinated Ca^{2+} is indicated by *shaded circles*. The *gray outline* superimposed on the α-carbon tracing illustrates how the structure can be approximated by two hemispheres joined by a cylinder. *Stippled areas* on the hemispheres indicate the positions of hydrophobic clefts. **(B)** The proposed calmodulin-M13 complex. The two lobes of CaM enfold the M13 helix, with hydrophobic surfaces of M13 (not indicated) mated to the hydrophobic clefts of CaM. As represented in the figure, a bend in the central helix of CaM is analogous to a universal joint; it allows the two lobes to adopt a wide range of relative positions. (Reprinted with permission from ref. 276.)

Both local and volatile anesthetics have been shown to affect the Ca^{2+}-binding properties of calmodulin, although many of these studies have shown this effect indirectly (266). Recent publications by Blanck's group (23,192) demonstrate that halothane and isoflurane induce biphasic changes in the Kd of Ca^{2+} for calmodulin; however, they were unable to show a similar effect in the closely related HLH protein troponin C in its isolated state. While these few studies suggest that local and volatile anesthetics may alter the Ca^{2+} affinity for Ca^{2+}-binding proteins, none to date has unambiguously demonstrated a clear physiologic effect at pharmacologically relevant concentrations of anesthetic. Anesthetics are known to have effects on intracellular Ca^{2+} homeostasis; however, the available data suggest that their effects on the Ca^{2+}-binding proteins are small.

Mitochondrial Ca^{2+} Buffering

Alternative sites of intracellular Ca^{2+} storage and release have been proposed in addition to the intracellular reticular membrane network discussed below. Mitochondrial membranes possess the capability to sequester Ca^{2+} through an electrogenic Ca^{2+} uniporter; however, in smooth muscle, the threshold for Ca^{2+} accumulation exceeds the physiologic concentrations of free cytoplasmic Ca^{2+} (~1 mM), even during maximal contraction (26). Studies employing electron probe x-ray microanalysis in vascular smooth muscle have shown that, under physiologic conditions of EC coupling, the mitochondria play no significant role in Ca^{2+} uptake and release (26). Evidence now exists to suggest that, in some cells, the threshold for mitochondrial Ca^{2+} uptake may be lower than that estimated by the electron probe in smooth muscle. In rat adrenal chromaffin cells, there appears to be significant mitochondrial accumulation of Ca^{2+} when intracellular Ca^{2+} rises above ~400 nM, as measured with fluorescence photometry (128). Whether mitochondrial Ca^{2+} accumulation is important for sequestering Ca^{2+} under conditions of pathologically elevated cytosolic Ca^{2+}, seen for example under conditions of ischemia, remains to be established.

Mitochondrial Maintenance of Ca^{2+} Gradient

Mitochondria generate adenosine triphosphate (ATP) by employing the cytochrome cascade and flow of protons down a large electrochemical gradient, the inside of the mitochondria being strongly electronegative (−140 mV) relative to the cytoplasm. As a consequence of this large gradient, Ca^{2+} exists at a slightly higher concentration in the mitochondria (approximately 200 nm) compared to one-half or one-quarter that concentration in the bulk cytoplasm. The intramitochondrial Ca^{2+} concentration is regulated by a Ca^{2+}-proton exchanger that permits relatively rapid equilibration between the intramitochondrial space and the cytoplasm (113). As a consequence, when the cell cytosol becomes more acidic, Ca^{2+} in the mitochondria may rise. As Ca^{2+} in the cytoplasm rises it likewise builds up in the mitochondria, decreasing the proton gradient and inhibiting ATP synthesis. For other ions, water is carried into osmotic neutrality, resulting in mitochondrial swelling. Up to a point, water loading of the mitochondrion with Ca^{2+} accumulation is reversible; however, at some point the combined Ca^{2+} overload and swelling results in irreversible disruption of the mitochondria. Although the role of the mitochondria in regulating Ca^{2+} at very rapid rates (<10 msec) is highly unlikely, recent evidence suggests that the mitochondria can provide relatively rapid buffering (50–500 msec level) and can alter the Ca^{2+} gradients that may activate regenerative Ca^{2+} release (Ca^{2+} waves) within the cell (155). Likewise, the mitochondria may also alter Ca^{2+} transients elicited by electrical or receptor-mediated stimulation.

At high concentrations, anesthetics may alter mitochondrial metabolism (121,252), but the changes as assessed by cardiac reduced nicotinamide adenine dinucleotide (NADH) fluorometry of clinical concentrations are small enough (<10%) to suggest that effects are modest (167). Furthermore, earlier studies do not rule out the possibility that alterations in intracellular Ca^{2+} by the anesthetics may have been responsible in part for modulating the function of Ca^{2+}-sensitive dehydrogenase enzymes within the mitochondria (31,222,223).

Microdomains and Inhomogeneities of Intracellular [Ca^{2+}]

Researchers have long recognized the second-messenger function of Ca^{2+} as well as the importance of changes that occur in cellular Ca^{2+} concentrations that modulate cell function; likewise, it has become increasingly evident that spatial inhomogeneities of Ca^{2+} concentration exist within the cell so that various regions of the cell see different concentrations. Consequently, different processes and Ca^{2+}-controlled pathways within the cell may be differentially regulated by inhomogeneities of [Ca^{2+}] due to Ca^{2+} transients within the cell.

Concentration gradients exist at various levels within the cell and depend on the rate of Ca^{2+} flux through specific point sources (sarcolemmal or reticular membrane channels) and on the concentration of binding sites (membrane, phospholipids, as well as membrane and soluble Ca^{2+}-binding proteins), both of which interact to create varying gradients of Ca^{2+} concentration. Use of fluorometric dyes has been helpful in permitting visualization of the gradients extant in a variety of cell types, particularly in myocytes, neurons and their dendritic processes, and epithelial cells. While visualizations of gradients at the micron level are possible (67), Ca^{2+} gradients at the nanometer level have been defined by theoretical analysis (19,328) and substantiated by electrophysiologic experimentation (145).

Membrane Domains

When ions enter through a channel, the mouth of the intracellular pore represents a point source where a high concentration of Ca^{2+} exists. After the channel opens, 10 to 500 μM [Ca^{2+}] rapidly accumulates near the pore mouth. This Ca^{2+} provides feedback regulation of channel function by binding near the channel. High concentrations (>10 mM) of rapidly acting buffers such as BAPTA are necessary to bind Ca^{2+} in sufficient quantity to prevent the local [Ca^{2+}] elevation that normally causes Ca^{2+} channel inactivation. Ca^{2+} diffuses from the entry site to the surrounding cytoplasm and becomes bound by proteins and phospholipids in the membrane as well as by soluble proteins. While buffering in the vicinity (5–10 nm) is difficult to achieve, entering Ca^{2+} binds to cytoplasmic Ca^{2+}-binding proteins at greater distances (>10 nm), thereby reducing the free Ca^{2+}; the [Ca^{2+}] gradient declines steeply from the intramembranous surface (Fig. 2). In neurons, it can be demonstrated that, upon stimulation, the increased [Ca^{2+}] is restricted to a subneurolemmal space 1 to 3 μm in thickness (67). This very steep decrease in concentration is highly dependent on the buffering ability within the cytoplasm. While a decreasing concentration gradient exists from the inner pore mouth, both calculations (19) and macroscopic measurements (18) suggest that with sufficient activity, Ca^{2+} depletion can occur in the interstitial fluid near the external pore mouth as Ca^{2+} enters the cell. With ongoing depolarization, as one might anticipate during a cardiac action potential, a small gradient may be established between the interstitial fluid and the external pore mouth as well as between the internal pore mouth and the bulk cytoplasmic fluid.

Ca^{2+} "Sparks" and Waves

Membrane-delimited spaces, such as those between the transverse- or t-tubule and the SR membrane, may represent spaces in which accumulation and higher concentrations of Ca^{2+} may be achieved (277). Such membrane-delimited spaces may be important to permit higher concentrations of Ca^{2+} to develop, which may then gate intracellular Ca^{2+}. In addition to gradients that can be established across the plasma membrane, gradients can clearly be established within cells. Activation of Ca^{2+}-release channels in myocytes can result in a high concentration of Ca^{2+} that quickly dissipates when the channel closes; this transient Ca^{2+} release can be detected as a "spark" of high Ca^{2+} concentration typically located in the junctional SR. When Ca^{2+} release is activated by depolarization, a massive release of Ca^{2+} is uniformly generated throughout the cell. In contrast, when myocytes become overloaded with Ca^{2+}, spontaneous release of Ca^{2+} may be sufficient to activate ongoing release that can sweep through the cell as a wave of Ca^{2+}. Such waves of Ca^{2+} release have also been reported in other tissues, such as oocytes. In many of these, the process appears to be mediated by IP_3-gated Ca^{2+} channels, which have a component of Ca^{2+} dependence (see below). This Ca^{2+} released from the endoplasmic reticulum engenders the release of Ca^{2+} by its binding to adjacent IP_3 channels. Such waves of Ca^{2+} can be modulated by alterations within the Ca^{2+} store as well as by manipulation of IP_3 receptors. In addition, it has recently been noted that alteration in mitochondrial function can alter the waves of Ca^{2+} and their frequency, suggesting that mitochondrial buffering of Ca^{2+} may interact with the IP_3-gated channels in altering Ca^{2+} domains (155,296).

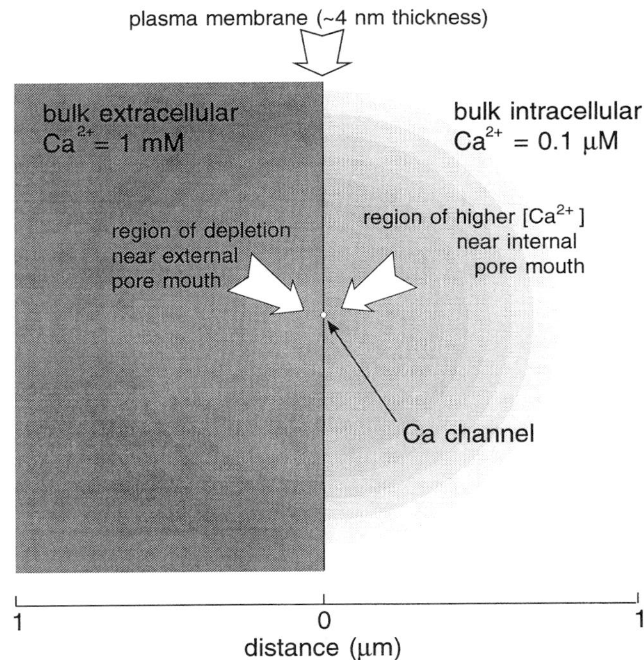

Figure 2. Graphic representation of the Ca^{2+} gradients surrounding an open Ca^{2+} channel. When the channel opens, there is depletion of the surrounding extracellular fluid by the Ca^{2+} ions entering the membrane. The entering Ca^{2+} then creates a gradient of high to low concentration into the myoplasm, which has a far lower bulk concentration. At the surface of the extracellular membrane there may be a slight increase in Ca^{2+} concentration due to binding to phospholipids and proteins as well as the slightly higher concentration due to the negative surface charge on the extracellular membrane (Guoy-Chapman effect). In addition, gradients within the cell may be altered by localized binding of Ca^{2+} to buffered proteins as well as membrane uptake systems. Nevertheless, gradients are calculated to extend for a significant distance into the myoplasm. This representation assumes a channel conductance of 25 picoSiemans and a current of N picoamps.

THE RETICULAR NETWORK—STORAGE SITE FOR INTRACELLULAR Ca^{2+}

The requirement for intracellular Ca^{2+} stores was evident from the time of A. V. Hill (129), whose calculations of Ca^{2+} diffusion indicated that skeletal muscle fiber activation by Ca^{2+} diffusion from the extracellular membrane could not explain the rapidity of activation. It required development of the electron microscope to clearly delineate the netlike internal membrane system (the sarcoplasmic reticulum) surrounding the 0.5 to 2 μm diameter myofibrils within striated muscle fibers.

Both excitable and nonexcitable cells contain an elaborate, interconnecting labyrinth of membranous tubules and fenestrated sheets called the endoplasmic reticulum (ER). This cytoplasmic organelle is the site for ribosome docking and protein synthesis (ER with ribosomes attached is termed "rough" ER, versus "smooth" ER), lipid synthesis, drug metabolism, and protein modification and transport. The ER also plays an important role in intracellular Ca^{2+} homeostasis, not only for muscle cells and neurons, but also for nonexcitable cells such as hepatocytes and endothelial cells (322). The endoplasmic reticulum of nonmuscle cells and the sarcoplasmic reticulum of muscle, which is generally regarded to be a specialized endoplasmic reticulum, both contain ATP-driven Ca^{2+} pumps, intraluminal Ca^{2+}-binding proteins, and tightly regulated Ca^{2+}-release channels that subserve the rapid sequestration, storage, and release of Ca^{2+} ions, respectively. In this section, the morphology of the ER/SR network and its function in Ca^{2+} homeostasis is reviewed. The term *endoplasmic reticulum* is used to refer to the Ca^{2+}-sequestering membranous network in nonmuscle cells, and *sarcoplasmic reticulum* refers to this specialized network in muscle.

Basic Functional Organization

Most mammalian cells possess internal membrane systems. The perinuclear membrane is composed of two lipid membrane layers enclosing a thin lumen. This membrane system that envelops the nuclear genetic machinery appears to be contiguous with a far more extensive, widely distributed cytosolic membrane network. This latter extensive internal membrane system, the endoplasmic reticulum (ER), serves a variety of functions. One major form incorporates ribosomes that gives it a rough appearance on electron micrographs (hence, rough ER), and is a major location of protein synthesis within the cell. This form typically assumes a smoother, multilayered structure (the Golgi apparatus) that is involved in packaging the synthesized proteins into vesicle. Another major form of the ER is smooth, and assumes various conformations and locations within the cell depending on the type of cell. Smooth ER is typically involved in regulation of Ca^{2+} within the cell, the Ca^{2+} in turn serving as a regulatory switch for a variety of processes.

Sarcoplasmic Reticulum

The structure and function of the SR/ER network have been extensively characterized in muscle, beginning with the early studies of Porter and Palade (285). In both skeletal and cardiac muscle, this organelle is a cytoplasmic "reticulum" of tubules that is discontinuous with the sarcolemma, but continuous with the outer nuclear envelope (326). The morphology of the SR in both cardiac and skeletal muscle is similar, and its general organization around the myofibrils can be seen schematically in Fig. 3. Two distinct regions of the SR in striated muscle have been characterized: (a) the longitudinal SR, which envelopes the contractile filaments in the A-band region, which has a high concentration of membrane-bound Ca^{2+} ATPases; and (b) the junctional SR, or "terminal cisterns" (TC), which are the specialized regions of the SR most closely apposed to the sarcolemma—either at the transverse- or t-tubules (near the Z-lines or the A-I interface depending on the muscle type and species) or at the peripheral sarcoplasmic reticulum (326). Electron-dense structures, originally termed "SR feet," span the ~150 Å separation between the TC and the sarcolemmal invaginations (91); these are now known to be the ryanodine-binding Ca^{2+}-release channels in both skeletal and cardiac muscle. The longitudinal SR, with its high concentration of Ca^{2+} adenosine triphosphatases (ATPases), is the predominant site of Ca^{2+} reuptake during muscle relaxation, while the terminal cisternae, which contain the highest concentration of ryanodine receptors in the SR membrane, are the site of activator Ca^{2+} release (81). Corbular SR, found predominantly in cardiac muscle, is an extrajunctional SR that makes no peripheral cou-

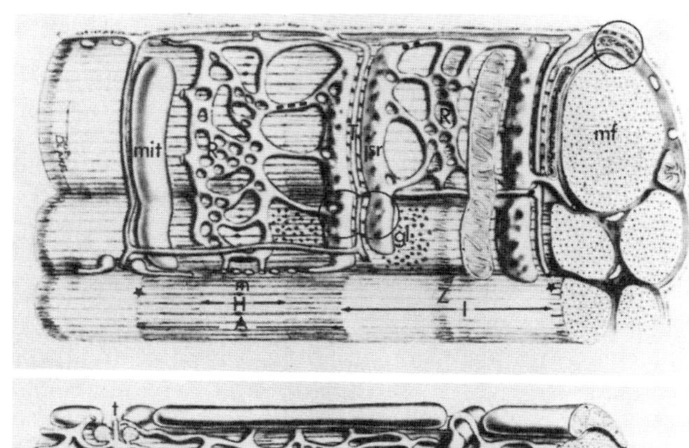

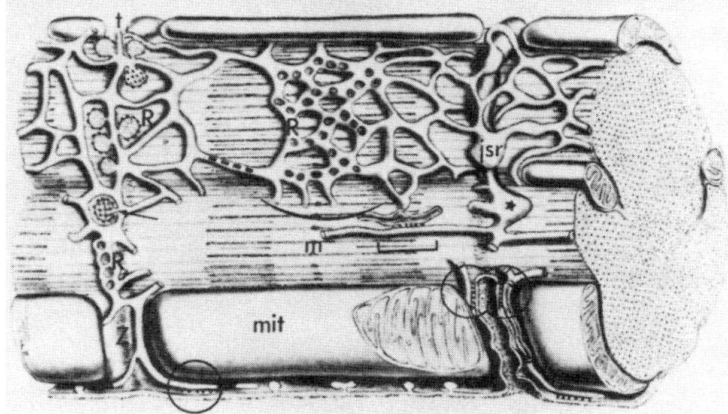

Figure 3. Relationships between sarcoplasmic reticulum (SR) and myofibrils in skeletal muscle (**A**) and mammalian cardiac muscle (**B**). Free SR is all the SR except junctional SR (jsr; terminal cisternae). Junctional SR forms peripheral couplings *(circles)* and interior couplings *(double circles)* with plasma membrane of cell surfaces and transverse tubules, respectively. Two couplings make a triad *(double circles)*; one coupling makes a dyad (*single circles* and jsr with underlying transverse tubule). Junctional SR has processes that make quasi-contact with transverse tubules. Free SR is differentiated into two retes (R) at M and Z lines, respectively. Z rete includes Z tubule, which is a tubule of SR in mammalian cardiac muscle that is found on most Z lines as if attached to it. Retes have many fenestrations that are also seen in junctional SR of skeletal muscle. M rete is connected to junctional SR via longitudinal tubules *(broken line)*; in skeletal muscle general region of transition between longitudinal tubules and junctional SR is called intermediate cisternae (*dots* in A). Corbular SR (*arrows* in B) is a specialization of SR in the region of Z rete and is found especially where the transverse tubules are absent—such as in mammalian atrial muscle, in fibers of the conduction system. Corbular SR has only one connection with free SR in contrast to extended junctional SR, which has two or more. Corbular SR often occurs in clusters, contains electron-dense granular material, and has processes on its surface. In skeletal muscle (A) transverse tubules (T) are small in diameter as compared with those in cardiac muscle and are situated at either A-I junction *(stars)* or at Z lines (Z). In mammalian cardiac muscle they are at Z lines. Transverse tubules form interior couplings with junctional SR. Transverse tubules in cardiac muscle are very polymorphous in size and shape with bulbous outpouchings in many places (*star* in B). The fuzzy coat over the plasma membrane, the laminar coat, extends into transverse tubules of cardiac but apparently not of skeletal muscle. mit, mitochondria; gl glycogen; m, M line; A, A band; I, I band; H, H band; Z, Z line. (Adapted with permission from ref. 28.)

pling to the sarcolemma; however, the junctional face membrane of corbular SR contains ryanodine receptors (154,325). The activation of corbular SR Ca^{2+}-release channels and its function in excitation-contraction coupling remain unknown at this time.

The SR in smooth muscle is distributed more randomly throughout the cell, forming an elaborate, interconnected labyrinth of tubules and stacks of fenestrated sheets that occupy between 2% and 9% of the cytoplasmic volume (Fig. 4) (61,265). As in other cell types, the smooth muscle SR is continuous with the outer leaflet of the nuclear membrane, and it is often found closely apposed to mitochondrial outer membranes (265). Unlike the case with striated muscle, no histologic characteristics of smooth muscle SR allow it to be characterized as "longitudinal" or "junctional" SR. Arbitrarily, however, SR tubules located within a distance of three caveolae widths from the sarcolemma have been termed "peripheral" SR, whereas the remaining SR is termed "central" SR. A careful study employing morphometry has characterized the different percentages of central and peripheral SR in different types of tonic and phasic smooth muscles: tonic smooth muscles, such as aorta and main pulmonary artery, contain greater central SR than phasic smooth muscles like vas deferens and ileum (61,265). Peripheral SR occasionally closely approaches the plasma membrane of the cell where it makes peripheral couplings; electron micrographs reveal electron-dense objects spanning the distance between the sarcolemma and the SR, suggestive of the "SR feet" seen in striated muscle, which are known to be the ryanodine receptor–Ca^{2+}-release channels (91). Identification of these ~100 Å objects and their role in excitation-contraction coupling, however, await further study.

The geometry of the SR in cardiac and skeletal, as well as in smooth muscle, reflects its role in excitation-contraction (EC) coupling. In skeletal and cardiac myofibers, the functional unit that subserves EC coupling is the triad. As a wave of membrane depolarization sweeps across the sarcolemma and into discrete invaginations of the membrane (called t-tubules), rows of SR terminal cysternae on either side of the t-tubules release Ca^{2+} in response either to the membrane depolarization, directly, as in skeletal muscle, or to the influx of extracellular Ca^{2+} through L-type Ca^{2+} channels, as in cardiac muscle (81). The specialized apposition of two SR terminal cisternae (TC) and a t-tubule defines a "triad" (Fig. 3). In both skeletal and cardiac muscle, the rapid release of Ca^{2+} from the SR is, in part, dependent on the close apposition of the surface membrane with the underlying Ca^{2+} storage organelle. In smooth muscle, the release of Ca^{2+} from the SR is in response either to agonist binding at the cell surface (pharmacomechanical coupling) or to membrane depolarization (electromechanical coupling) (323). While the exact mechanisms that subserve electromechanical coupling in smooth muscle are somewhat controversial, the events that couple agonist binding to intracellular Ca^{2+} release are better understood. It is generally agreed that agonists, such as phenylephrine or acetylcholine, bind to their receptors and activate G-protein–mediated production of 1,4,5-inositol trisphosphate (IP_3); in turn, IP_3 binds to its receptor on the surface of the SR and induces the release of Ca^{2+}, which initiates contraction (323). Interestingly, a recent study of IP_3 receptors in the SR of both tonic and phasic smooth muscle indicates no subcompartmentalization of the IP_3 receptor or calsequestrin, indicating that the entire SR in smooth muscle is able to participate in agonist-induced EC coupling (Fig. 4) (265), unlike the localization of Ca^{2+}-release channels to the TC in skeletal and cardiac muscles.

The lumen of the SR/ER in muscle and nonmuscle cells contains Ca^{2+}-binding proteins that enhance the capacity for Ca^{2+} accumulation. Calsequestrin, a high-capacity, low-affinity Ca^{2+}-binding protein, is the major luminal Ca^{2+}-buffering protein in the SR of cardiac and skeletal muscle, and it is present in both the longitudinal SR and terminal cysternae (213). Calsequestrin binds large amounts of Ca^{2+} (40–50 mol Ca^{2+}/mol protein) with a relatively low affinity (kd ~1 mM) after it has been transported into the SR lumen by the SR-Ca^{2+}-ATPase (212). The C-terminus of calsequestrin contains a large number of acidic amino acid residues, which are thought to be the sites of Ca^{2+} binding. The predominant SR Ca^{2+}-buffering protein in smooth muscle has been more difficult to identify; however, recent studies have identified the "calsequestrin-like" proteins in smooth muscle and nonmuscle cells to be calreticulin (34,242). Calreticulin has been identified as a major luminal Ca^{2+}-binding protein in both hepatocytes and smooth muscle cells (241). Similar to calsequestrin, it is a high-capacity, low-affinity Ca^{2+}-binding protein

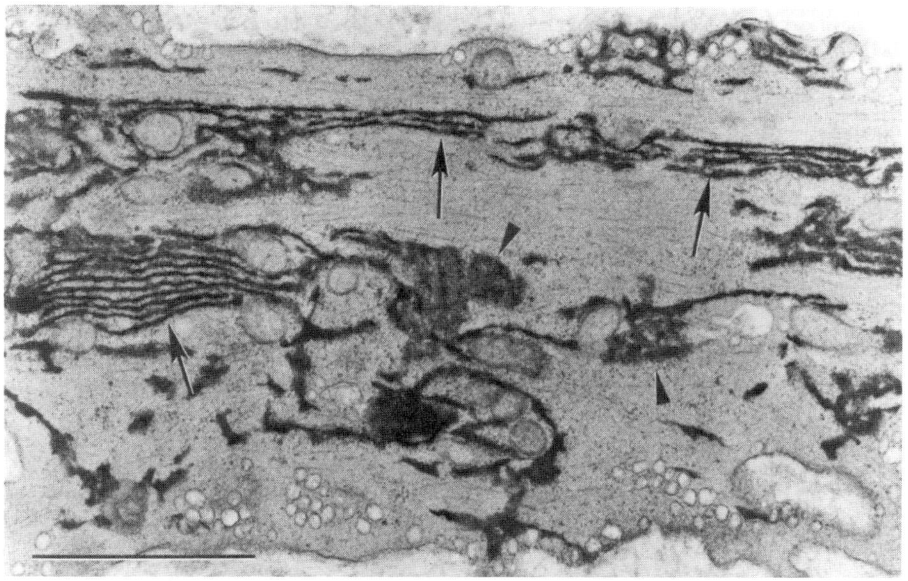

Figure 4. Osmium ferricyanide-stained section of main pulmonary artery. Stacks of sarcoplasmic reticulum can be easily recognized *(arrows)* in the central region of the cell. *Arrowheads* denote possible fenestrated stacks or tubules of SR viewed en face. SR tubules can also be seen in close apposition to mitochondria and close to the plasma membrane. Scale bar—1μm. (Reprinted with permission from ref. 265.)

that binds ~25 mol Ca^{2+}/mol protein with a K_d of ~250 mM; however, it contains one high-affinity binding site (K_d ~1 mM) and can also bind Zn^{2+} with high capacity (~14 mol/mol protein) and low affinity (242). The amino acid sequence of calreticulin from several species has recently been obtained from DNA cloning studies, and analysis of the sequence indicates no EF-hand consensus sequences. Calreticulin contains an ER-retention signal "KDEL," which is known to signal retention of newly synthesized peptides in the ER, which supports the immunohistochemical and biochemical data that localize the protein to the ER/SR lumen. Several other Ca^{2+}-binding proteins are found in the lumen of the SR in both cardiac and skeletal muscle as well as smooth muscle: sarcolumenin, endoplasmin (Grp96), T3BP/PDI, and HCP (242). The physiologic importance of these proteins in maintaining the luminal Ca^{2+} buffering capacity of the SR/ER, however, is not known at present.

Neurons also have an ER that participates in the control of intracellular Ca^{2+} concentrations. Early experiments identified an ATP-dependent Ca^{2+}-sequestering function of the axoplasm that was independent of mitochondrial function (240). This nonmitochondrial Ca^{2+} storage site was associated with the microsomal fraction of cell homogenates and later identified as the ER. Similar to the ER/SR network in muscle, the ER in neurons is a membranous labyrinth of cisterns; some studies show stacks of these cisterns that are contiguous with the nuclear envelope and encircle the outer membrane of the mitochondria. Like muscle SR, this network of membranes contains a Ca^{2+}-ATPase that concentrates Ca^{2+} within the lumen of the organelle, luminal Ca^{2+} buffering proteins, and both ryanodine-sensitive and IP_3-sensitive Ca^{2+}-release channels. Additionally, the existence of an extra-ER/SR Ca^{2+} storage site called the "calciosome" has been proposed. The ontogeny of this proposed organelle is unknown, and the direct evidence supporting its existence is not abundant. A description of this structure and hypotheses regarding its function can be found in a review by Rossier and Putney (300).

The regulation of intraluminal Ca^{2+} concentrations in the ER/SR network has recently become an area of intense research interest. The description of plasmalemmal Ca^{2+} entry gated by depletion of intracellular Ca^{2+} stores has been termed "capacitative entry" of Ca^{2+} (288). Several Ca^{2+}-selective, voltage-independent Ca^{2+} channels have been described that, although having a low conductance relative to the voltage-gated L-type channels, can be activated by depletion of intracellular Ca^{2+} stores (49). The most extensively studied has been termed I_{CRAC}, or the "Ca^{2+}-release activated channel" current (49,77). Signaling mechanisms that communicate the depletion of intracellular Ca^{2+} to plasma membrane Ca^{2+}-conductance channels are, at present, poorly understood.

The definition of SR accumulation and Ca^{2+} release was greatly enhanced by the fact that these membrane systems reformed into functional vesicles after muscles were homogenized. Although uptake characteristics of the Ca^{2+}-ATPase were intensively explored implying these preparations (see Chapter 20), the ability of loaded SR vesicles to also release Ca^{2+} provides an insight into the release pathway.

MECHANISMS OF INTRACELLULAR Ca^{2+} RELEASE

To activate rapid processes such as contraction, specific protein channels exist for the release of Ca^{2+} from the SR/ER lumen into the cytoplasm. Two classes of very large tetrameric channels located on the internal membrane systems constitute an important feature in muscle; these are also common in a variety of other cells. The first class of channels has been termed ryanodine (Ry) receptors, based on their high affinity for the plant alkaloid ryanodine, which permitted their isolation and the subsequent cloning of the genetic substrate for three different isoforms (53,226). While the Ry receptor is gated by Ca^{2+} and/or the L-type Ca channel (skeletal muscle subunit α_{1S}), a somewhat smaller but structurally similar class of Ca^{2+}-release channels is the ligand-gated inositol-1,4,5-trisphosphate receptors (IP_3 receptor). These two classes of Ca^{2+}-releasing channels are widely distributed in various tissues of the muscular, neural, endothelial, vascular, and immunologic systems (53,226). As a general rule, Ry receptors are present in those systems that require very rapid (<10 msec) activation (e.g., skeletal and cardiac muscle, and certain neurons), while IP_3 receptors appear to have a more prominent functional role in tissues whose response time is slower (≥0.2 sec). These systems frequently overlap and interact within single cell types, although in the nervous system the two release systems seem to be largely separate and distinctly distributed (309).

The Ryanodine (Ry) Receptor Ca^{2+}-Release Channels

The protein responsible for rapid release of activating Ca^{2+} was first described in structural studies of skeletal muscle, the tissue in which it is the most prominent both functionally and anatomically. High-resolution electron micrographs of skeletal muscle identified regularly spaced, electron-dense structures between the tubular surface membrane invaginations of muscle fibers (the t-tubules) and the sarcoplasmic reticulum (SR). These structures, termed "SR feet" in their initial description, juxtapose and appear to hold together the t-tubules and SR membrane (91). It was not until the discovery of a toxin that acts specifically on these proteins that researchers proposed they mediate Ca^{2+} release. In this case, the toxin was ryanodine, an insecticide derived from the vine *Ryanodinia.* Ryanodine markedly alters EC coupling in vertebrate striated muscle, causing contracture of skeletal muscle and severe contractile depression in myocardium (152,160,338). When radiolabeled, [^{3}H]ryanodine was found to bind with extremely high affinity to SR membranes isolated from the junction of the SR and t-tubules (junctional SR [JSR]), in both skeletal (144,147,181) and cardiac muscle (6,146,180,195,294). Studies from a variety of laboratories determined that the SR feet present at the junction of the SR with the t-tubule were the receptors for ryanodine (144,146,147,279,282), and that these receptors had the capability to act as highly conductive Ca^{2+}-activated and Ca^{2+}-selective channels (137,181,305,306,317,319).

Structure

The large size of the Ry receptor Ca^{2+}-release channel (RyR/CaRC) has permitted detailed analysis of its structure. Initial studies of isolated junctional SR yielded a protein with a very high estimated molecular weight (>450 kd) (82,282), which was subsequently documented by isolating the genetic material encoding the protein (219,342,381). Both molecular biologic techniques and detailed optical studies of the isolated channel complex have proven useful, the former having permitted cloning of the genes for this class of intracellular channels.

Tertiary Structure Each RyR/CaRC is a homotetramer, composed of four 450-kd monomers arranged with a rosette or quatrefoil symmetry (53,226,359) (Fig. 5). Each monomer is thought to have a transmembrane domain, which extends through the SR membrane into its lumen, and a very prominent cytoplasmic domain on the N-terminus. It is the large cytoplasmic domains that occupy the space between the nearly adjacent SR and t-tubular membranes and that appear in electron micrographs as the electron dense SR feet. Optical image analysis of the isolated tetrameric complex reveals a protein structure with numerous and variably oriented indentations and clefts, in addition to an apparent central channel (292,293). The cytoplasmic domains may contain internal channels and binding sites for associated proteins (see below),

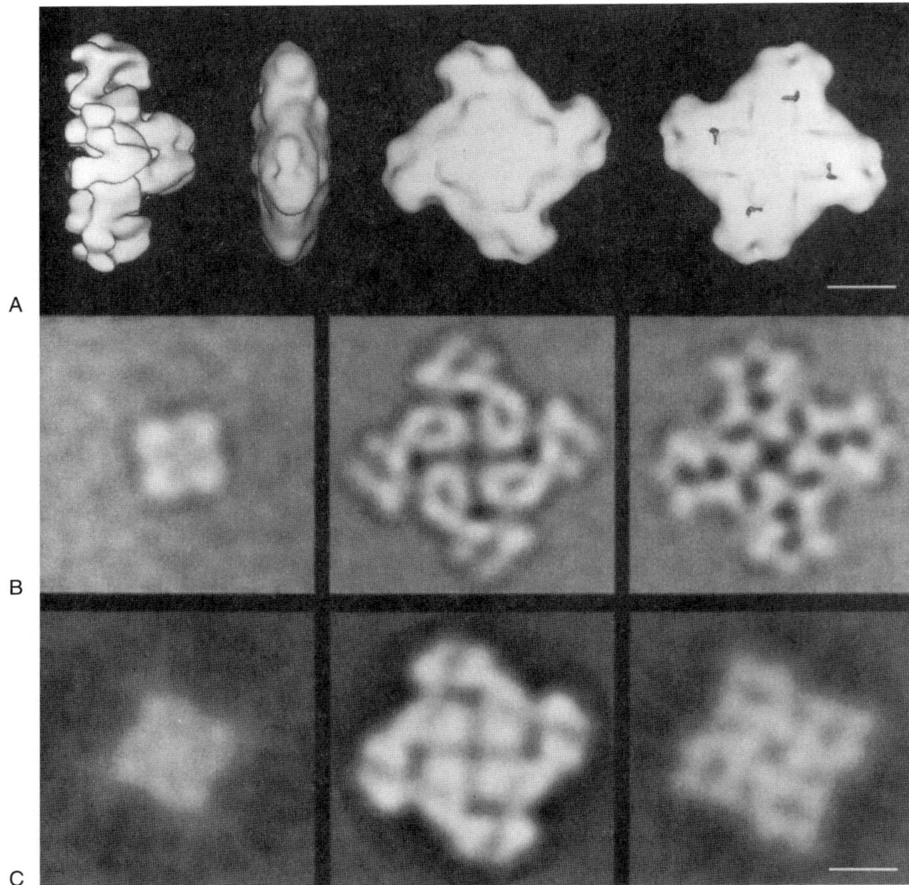

Figure 5. Three-dimensional reconstructions of the skeletal muscle ryanodine receptor (RyR1) determined from negatively stained and frozen-hydrated CRCs. **(A)** Surface representations of frozen-hydrated *(left image)* and negatively stained *(second image)* CRC in the side view. Views of the negatively stained CRC in SR- and cytoplasmic-facing views are shown in the third and fourth images from the left. The reconstruction from a negatively stained specimen is from Wagenknecht et al.(359), but has been refined with projection onto convex sets (POCS). **(B,C)** Z-sections at selected levels from reconstructions of negatively stained (C) and frozen-hydrated (B) CRC. The three sections are at comparable z-coordinates in the two reconstructions. (Reproduced with permission from ref. 292.)

as well as sites for chemical species that regulate or alter channel gating such as Ca^{2+}, ATP, anthraquinones, and a wide variety of different drugs.

Sequence and Distribution of Three Isoforms After isolation and purification of Ry receptors from the junctional SR of rabbit, cleavage peptides of the very large protein were generated, their sequence determined, and synthetic oligodeoxynucleotide probes were made based on the predicted nucleotide sequence. These probes were then used to screen cDNA library (complementary DNA derived from muscle mRNA), which encoded a very large protein of over 5000 amino acids (219,342,381). Sequence analysis of the encoded protein suggests a modest number of hydrophobic regions consistent with distinct transmembrane spanning regions (postulated as either four [342] or 12 [381]) located near the carboxy terminus (Fig. 6, lower two lines). A very large hydrophilic region is consistent with the enormous cytoplasmic structure observed microscopically (25, 91,92). Subsequently, the cDNA sequence was defined for a distinct cardiac form of the channel subunit (RYR2, cRyR, Ry_2 receptor), which is somewhat smaller (4968–4976 amino acids, depending on the variant) than the Ry_1 receptor, to which it bears a 66% sequence identity (269). A distinct subunit has also been defined from brain mRNA (RYR3, Ry_3 receptor) (119), which was also partially described in mink lung epithelium (105). The mRNA for the Ry_3 receptor encodes a protein of almost comparable size (4872 amino acids) to Ry_1 and Ry_2 receptors and bears 67% and 70% homology with those isoforms, respectively. Since each monomer is composed of ~5000 amino acids, over twice the size of the α_1-subunit of the L-type plasmalemmal Ca channel, the total weight of the ion conductive, tetrameric RyR-CaRC complex is ~2 million daltons, one of the largest known protein complexes.

The Ry_1 receptor (RyR1, sRyR) is present primarily in skeletal muscle. It has also been detected in cerebellar Purkinje cells (179), where it is also the dominant isoform, and a trace is present in myocardium and aortic smooth muscle (219). The mRNA of a considerably truncated form of this protein has also been isolated in brain (343). This smaller message encodes only 565 amino acids (13% of full isoform) at the carboxy terminus, which leaves the four postulated hydrophobic transmembrane domains intact as well as binding sites for Ca^{2+} and ATP. The Ry_2 receptor (cardiac isoform) is also found prominently in brain and is present in a variety of other tissues (96–98,179,226). The Ry_3 isoform is present in brain (predominantly hippocampal CA1, striated and dorsal thalamus [97]) and smooth muscle (119). All three Ry receptors appear to be expressed in vascular smooth muscle (263). It is not known whether heterotetramers form in such tissues, perhaps generating release channels with properties distinct from those of the homotetramers.

Common Biophysical Characteristics

The skeletal and cardiac forms of the Ry receptor have been the most widely studied with respect to ionic conductance, gating, and modulation. Incorporation of junctional SR membrane into artificial membrane bilayers demonstrated a very highly conductive channel that transmits cations at very high rates (10,133,194,195,302,303,305,317–320,368). When vesicles are formed from heavy SR following tissue homogenization, they typically form with the lumen of the vesicle equivalent to the lumen of the native SR, and the external vesicle surface is exposed to what would correspond to the cytoplasmic milieu. Isolation of such uniformly similar vesicles not only has permitted studies of Ca^{2+} uptake by this Ca^{2+} ATPase (SERCA), but has also permitted elucidation of the Ca^{2+}-release pathway in those vesicles that retain Ry receptor (142,166,227,228). While studies in isolated SR vesicles have provided considerable insight into activation and blockade of Ca^{2+} release by various compounds

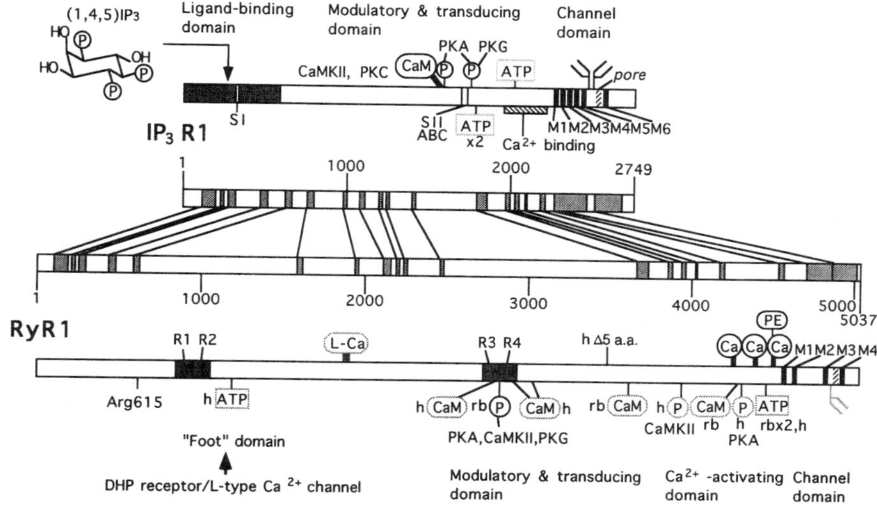

Figure 6. Structural comparison between the intracellular Ca^{2+}-release channels, IP_3R1 and RyR1. The IP_3R1 *(upper two lines)* consists of 2,749 amino acids (SI^-/SII^+ splicing subtype) in the mouse (99) and rat (237) and 2,695 amino acids (SI^+/SII^+) in the human (371). The following sites and regions are shown: splicing segments SI (residues 318–332) and SII (SII-ABC, where A, B, and C represent subsegments) (255); ligand-binding domain with a *dotted box* (IP_3-binding site, N-terminal 650 amino acids); modulatory and transducing domain, including CaM (CaM-binding site; M. Kobayashi et al., *unpublished data*), PKA (Ser_{1588} and Ser_{1755}, for PKA phosphorylation), PKG (Ser_{1755} for PKG phosphorylation), ATP (potential ATP-binding sites) (79), and Ca^{2+} binding with a *shaded horizontal bar* (Ca^{2+}-binding sites, residues 1,961–2,219) (236). The channel domain (six *solid vertical bars;* six putative MSDs [M1–M6] between residues 2,276 and 2,2589 in the mouse) includes two N-glycosylation sites (two branched bars, Asn_{2475} and Asn_{2503}) (234) and one putative "pore"-forming sequence (*shaded vertical bar,* residues 2,530–2,552) between M5 and M6 (234). CaMKII and PKC phosphorylation sites are not identified. The RyR1 *(lower two lines)* from rabbit skeletal muscle (5,037 amino acids) (342) is five amino acids longer (hΔ5a.a., residues 3,481–3,485) than the RyR1 from the human skeletal muscle (5,032 amino acids) (381). Most of the receptor molecule is the cytoplasmic region composed of the putative "foot" domain and the modulatory and transducing domain containing the following regions and sites: four long repeats in two doublets, R1–R2 (residues 841–954, 955–1,068) and R3–R4 (residues 2,725–2,844, 2,845–2,958); L-Ca, putative low-affinity Ca^{2+}-binding sites (residues 1,872–1,923) in the human; ATP, putative ATP-binding sites (residues 4,449–4,454 and 4,452–4,457 in the rabbit, 1,194–1,199 and 4,447–4,452 in the human); CaM, putative CaM-binding sites; rb-P-PKA, CaMKII, PKG, Ser_{2846} of the rabbit RyR1 phosphorylated by PKA, CaMKII, and PKG (336); h-P-PKA, potential PKA phosphorylation site (Thr_{4317}) in the human; and h-P-CaMKII, potential CaMKII phosphorylation site (Ser_{3944}) in the human. The Ca^{2+}-activation domain consists of three high-affinity Ca^{2+}-binding sites (Ca^{2+}; residues 4,253–4,264, 4,407–4,416, and 4,489–4,499) (44) and Pro-Glu repeat (PE; residues 4,489–4,499) (45). The channel domain contains a putative N-glycosylation site (*branched bar;* residue 4,864 in the rabbit), four putative MSDs (M1–M4; *solid vertical bars;* between residues 4,564 and 4,937 in the rabbit), and a putative "pore"-forming sequence *(shaded bar).* Note that functional sites that have not yet been experimentally determined are encircled by *dotted lines.* The *middle two lines* represent the regions *(dotted boxes)* in which identical amino acid sequences are clustered in the IP_3R1 and RyR1 (99). DHP, dihydropyridine. (Reprinted with permission from ref. 98.)

(38,39,270–272,358), additional insight has been gained when such vesicles have been incorporated into artificial membrane bilayers, which permits study of their activity as single-ion transmitting channels (10,95,317–320,368).

Channel Gating The major physiologic regulator of the Ry receptor appears to be Ca^{2+} itself, an effect that can be demonstrated in skinned muscle fibers (75,327), isolated vesicles (142,166,227,228), and by using bilayer techniques (48,117, 306,317). The amino acid sequences in all three isoforms appear to contain multiple Ca^{2+}-binding sites, of which the most clearly identified are those in Ry_1 receptor (43–45). When isolated SR vesicles are added to a chamber on one side of an artificial bilayer, vesicle incorporation usually occurs with the cytoplasmic face facing the *cis* chamber, while the luminal face is the *trans* chamber. For both skeletal and cardiac muscle, opening of single channels can be observed as brief, discrete currents of highly variable duration (<1 to >100 msec) (303,317). Ionic constituents on either surface can be manipulated to determine their effect on gating and conductance characteristics of the channels. A prominent feature of the CaRCs is the increased probability of opening (P_o), which occurs when the [Ca^{2+}] in the *cis* chamber (cytoplasmic face) is increased from 0.1 μM to 1 to 10 μM concentrations (144,181, 317). Channel opening, as well as ryanodine binding, is enhanced when [Ca^{2+}] achieves ~0.3 μM in the vicinity of the cytoplasmic domain, with peak activity appearing at ~5 to 20 μM (48,117,233,282). The open- and closed-state durations suggest that the channels exist in many distinct states, with at least two closed and two open states when activated by Ca^{2+} and/or ATP (317). In single-channel bilayer studies, CaRCs derived from either cardiac (canine) or skeletal muscle (rabbit), the Ca^{2+} activation site had a K_d of 1 to 2 μM with a Hill coefficient of ~1 (48,117). By utilizing flash photolysis of caged Ca^{2+} near CaRCs incorporated into lipid bilayers, Györke et al. (117) sought also to determine how quickly Ca^{2+} entering cells near release channels could activate opening. The time constant for either cardiac or skeletal muscle channels opening was ~1 msec, sufficiently rapid to explain physiologic muscle activation. Based on sequence-specific antibody studies, the modulatory Ca^{2+}-binding site appears to be located in regions near the transmembrane domains, one of the regions containing a proline-glutamate multiple repeat region (44,45).

It is the open CaRC to which ryanodine binds with a high affinity, with K_d of 5 to 50 nM depending on the isoform and the conditions. There appears to be one high-affinity site for ryanodine on the intact tetramer; with the solubilization and disaggregation of the tetramer into the 500-kd proteins, ryanodine affinity is lost. Ryanodine binding causes the CaRC to be locked into an open state, with a conductance of approximately 40% of the normal open value (144,251,306). When such modulatory binding occurs in intact skeletal muscle fibers, the Ca^{2+} loss from the SR causes a contracture; in cardiac myocytes, the Ca^{2+} lost from the SR is eliminated and results in decreased contractions (152,337,338). Ry binding at low concentrations (10–100 nM) can be used to define open channels (47), in which the gating and activation of both skeletal and cardiac muscle CaRC by Ca^{2+} (47,281) and a variety of other activating compounds (1,47,134,135,278,281,376,380) including anesthetics (52,207) has been extensively investigated using the activation of ryanodine binding as an assay of channel opening. However, ryanodine binding to the receptor is complex at higher [Ry], since the intact tetramer has four probable binding sites that appear to demonstrate negative cooperativity (211,283,379), and that are able to modulate the conductance and gating state of the channel. The presence of higher [Ry] of ≥100 μM and binding to low-affinity sites is associated with blockade of Ca^{2+} release and closure of the channel (32,47).

The mechanism of Ca^{2+} activation of the CaRC appears to be a self-regulating and adaptive response. As assessed by a variety of methods (flux studies, ryanodine binding, single channel) the skeletal muscle Ry_1 receptor typically shows decreased channel opening and ryanodine binding when Ca^{2+} is increased beyond 10 to 50 μM (48,117). In contrast, the cardiac Ry_2 receptor appears to show less inhibition as [Ca^{2+}] is increased. With a sustained increase in [Ca^{2+}], the increased P_o decays and the channel opening decreases over a few seconds (115). Luminal Ca^{2+} also appears to influence the behavior of the Ca^{2+}-release channel. No binding sites have been identified on the rather minuscule portion of the molecule that exists in the area adjacent to the SR lumen. It may be that sufficiently high luminal concentrations and random channel openings may permit leakage of Ca^{2+}, which could increase the local cytoplasmic concentration sufficiently to influence channel gating.

The inactivation of Ry receptors by Ca^{2+} can be described by a single Ca^{2+}-binding site with a K_d of ~400 μM as assessed by single-channel opening or [^3H] Ry binding (45,233,282). Carbodiimide derivatization of Ry_1 receptors results in the loss of the ability of mM concentrations of Ca^{2+} (as well as Mg^{2+} and ruthenium red) to inhibit Ca^{2+} release from vesicles, suggesting this low-affinity Ca^{2+}-binding site is distinct from the higher affinity Ca^{2+}-binding site that activates channel opening (220). Mg^{2+} at millimolar concentrations appears to compete for the Ca^{2+} site present in the cytoplasmic face of the channel and inhibit Ca^{2+}-mediated activation in the channel (166,228,254,317), although at higher concentrations it may also compete and substitute as the permeant ion.

In the absence of other activating agents, however, Ca^{2+} does not usually increase the P_o beyond 0.4. When various second messengers such as ATP are added, opening can be synergistically enhanced in combination with Ca^{2+}, so that channels may remain open continuously ($P_o = 1.0$) (317). ATP by itself, as well as other agents (sulmazole, milrinone, doxorubicin; see Table 3), have been shown to activate Ry_1 receptors (316) and in combination with Ca^{2+}, ATP elicits a synergistic response (317). In contrast, calmodulin when bound with Ca^{2+} appears to cause inhibition of channel opening (320) and could be responsible in part for feedback pathways that shut down the channel once release has taken place. An additional physiologic regulator, in addition to ATP, may be the nucleotide derivative cyclic adenosine diphosphate (ADP) ribose (cADPR) that also appears to cause activation of the channel (187,230,247), although this has not been proven uniformly true (94,314), and its physiologic role in situ remains uncertain.

In addition to Ca^{2+}, a variety of drugs induce activation of the Ry receptors and Ca^{2+} release from the SR. Caffeine and other methylxanthines have long been employed as agents that activate SR Ca^{2+} release, and they are well documented to activate Ry binding and channel opening (53). Such Ca^{2+} release is typically "quantal" in nature, that is, Ca^{2+} flux from SR vesicles occurs, whereby there is dynamic adaptation and increment detection (59). By this process, Ca^{2+} release is dynamically slowed following the initial activation by a drug, but residual Ca^{2+} can be released by an increased concentration of the agonist. Such behavior is demonstrable for a variety of compounds known to activate the Ry receptor such as caffeine, doxorubicin, and sulmazole (59). Such an adaptive release process for such a wide variety of compounds suggests that the effect is an intrinsic characteristic of the channel-gating process. The effect can be observed not only for Ry receptors from rabbit skeletal muscle, but also those from crayfish skeletal (116) and rat cardiac muscle (373). As listed in Table 3, a wide variety of chemically distinct compounds have also been found to activate Ca-release channels. Volatile anesthetics have been found to activate such channels, although activity varies depending on the chemical structure (see below).

Protons also have a modulating action on Ry function and Ca^{2+} release. With increasing pH above 6.0, ryanodine binding by Ry receptors increases, reaching a peak value at 7.1, and subsequently declining as pH is increased beyond 8.0 (380). Although channel opening is inhibited by acidic pH, as pH is increased above 7.1 activity continues to increase, consistent with a titratable site with a pK of 7.2 (208,304), suggesting that ryanodine binding and channel activity may not correlate in alkaline medium. Likewise, the alkaline-induced enhancement of Ca^{2+} release from SR can be partially inhibited by Ry receptor blockade with ruthenium red (60). However, proton modulation of channel-opening probability demonstrates hysteresis, that is, greater acidosis is required to block channels that are opening, and a higher pH is required to open channels blocked by increased [H^+] (209). Whether or not these effects of pH are mediated by direct competition of protons for the Ca^{2+} activation or inactivation binding sites is uncertain. Blockade of Ca^{2+} release and its retention in the SR in setting of intracellular acidosis has clear beneficial effects in decreasing further energy expenditure.

Conductance The opening of the Ca^{2+}-release channels is remarkable for the very high conductance observed, with single-channel conductances for Ca^{2+} in the range of 75 to 100 pS equivalent to >10,000 Ca^{2+} per msec when 50 to 60 mM Ca^{2+} is present on the luminal (*trans* chamber) side of the channel (303,315,317,318). Single-channel conductance does not appear to be affected by the type of agonist used to activate the channel. Ba^{2+} appears to have a slightly higher conductance than Ca^{2+}, while Mg^{2+} is also conducted by the channel at a rate of about 40% to 70% of that seen with Ca^{2+}(368). Monovalent ions appear to have an even higher conductance through the channel, with Cs^+ having a conductance of 400 pS. Approximately 4% of channels exhibit subconductance states of one half to three quarters of the peak levels. When CaRCs have been isolated from SR and chromatographically purified, their incorporation into bilayers shows the high conductance channels seen with heavy SR (368). Unlike the native SR channel, purified Ry receptor channels display far more prominent variable conductance levels with openings of both 110 and 50 pS. When different monovalent cations are studied, Cs^+, Na^+, and K^+ show similar high unit conductances of 400 to 500 pS, again with multiple conductance states being present.

As with the L-type Ca channel, divalent ion and especially Ca^{2+} selectivity arises from tighter binding of the divalent ion as it passes through the channel. The pore itself appears to have ample dimensions and is of sufficient magnitude to permit small organic cations (156,319) and sugar molecules to pass (157). The resulting estimated cross-sectional area of 38 Å^2 (53) is similar to that of the acetylcholine channel (64), and is sufficient for some water molecules that hydrate permeating cations to be retained as they pass through the channel. The

Table 3. AGENTS THAT AFFECT RYANODINE RECEPTORS

Agent	Effective concentration	Ca^{2+} release	Ryanodine binding	Single channel	Tissue
Anthraquinones (doxorubicin)	1–300 μM	Activated	Activated	Activated	Skeletal, cardiac
Polyamines					
Protamine	1 μg/ml	Activated	ND	ND	Skeletal
Putrescine, spermidine	1–100 mM	ND	Activated	ND	Skeletal
Spermine	1–100 mM	Activated	Activated	ND	Skeletal
Local anesthetics					
Lidocaine	0.1–15 mM	ND	Activated	ND	Skeletal, brain
Procaine	1–20 mM	Inactivated	Inhibited	Inhibited	Skeletal
Tetracaine	0.01–2 mM	Inactivated	Inhibited	Inhibited	Skeletal, cardiac, brain, liver
Volatile anesthetics					
Enflurane	2% vol	ND	?Activated	Activated	Cardiac
Halothane	1.55%, 2% vol	Activated	Activated	Activated	Cardiac
Isoflurane	2%, 2.5% vol	?Activated	NE	NE	Cardiac
Fatty acid derivatives					
Long-chain acyl CoA	50 μM	Activated	ND	ND	Skeletal
Arachidonic acid	1–50 μM	Activated	ND	ND	Skeletal, cardiac
Acyl carnitines		Activated	ND	ND	Skeletal
Palmitoyl carnitine	50 μM	Activated	Activated	Activated	Skeletal
Sphingosine	1–100 μM	Activated	Inhibited	ND	Skeletal
	30–50 μM	Inactivated	Inhibited	ND	Skeletal
Stearic acid	0.1–10 μM	Activated	ND	ND	Skeletal
	16–32 μM				
Toxins					
Bulthotus venom	0.1–500 μg/ml	ND	Activated	Activated	Skeletal, cardiac, brain
Imperatoxin A	1–1,000 nM	ND	Activated	Activated	Skeletal
Imperatoxin I	1–1,000 nM	ND	Inhibited	Inhibited	Skeletal, cardiac
Bastadins	0.5–20 μm	Activated	Activated		Skeletal
Methylxanthines(caffeine, theophylline)	1–20 mM	Activated	Activated	Activated	Skeletal, cardiac
Alkylphenols					
4-Alkylphenol	10–25 nmol/mg	Activated	ND	ND	Skeletal
Chlorocresol	0.1–100 μM	Activated	ND	ND	Skeletal
Cyclic ADP ribose	1–17 μM	Activated	NE	NE	Skeletal
	1–2 μM	NE	Inhibited	NE	Cardiac
	1–2 μM	Activated	Activated	Activated	Skeletal
Dantrolene, azumolene	23 nM	Inhibited	NE	*	Skeletal
Perchlorate	8–100 mM	Activated	Activated	Activated	Skeletal, cardiac
Ruthenium red	0.001–20 μM	Inactivated	Inhibited	Inhibited	Skeletal, Cardiac
PDE inhibitors					
Milrinone	100 μM–2 mM	ND	Activated	Activated	Cardiac
Sulmazole	0.1–10 μM	ND	Activated	Activated	Cardiac
Oxidizing agents					
Rose bengal	1–200 μM	Inactivated	Inhibited	Activated	Skeletal

PDE, phosphodiasterase; NE, no effect; ND, not determined; *, activates at ≤10 μM, inhibits at higher concentrations.
Adapted from ref. 53.

channel can be represented by multiple cation binding sites arranged in single file (319). Monovalent ions presumably bind less tightly and pass through more rapidly, while when Ca^{2+} is present it binds more tightly to a central region of the pore (351,352). As a consequence, the added presence of Ca^{2+} decreases the conductance of monovalent ions.

Associated Proteins

In addition to the large tetrameric CaRC complex, additional protein components that have been defined in the junctional SR appear to be intimately involved in modulation and function of the channels in releasing Ca^{2+} from the SR. Their association is shown schematically in Fig. 7 for skeletal muscle, in which most studies have been performed.

FKBP12: When the Ry_1 receptor purified by continuous sucrose density gradient centrifugation is digested with endoprotease, sequence analysis of 30 of the 31 proteolytic peptide fragments is generated from the 5037 amino acid Ry_1 receptor monomer (217). One exogenous peptide fragment (KC7), which copurifies with Ry_1 receptor, is unrelated by sequence analysis and has recently been shown to be identical to the major cytoplasmic immunophilin of human T-cells, *FKBP12* (FK506-binding protein–12 kd) (151). FKBP12 is a 12-kd protein that belongs to a growing class of cytosolic proteins first identified in human T-cells. FKBPs are *cis-trans* proline isomerases with important functions in regulating nuclear DNA transcription and signal transduction pathways essential to immune function. However, one FKBP12 is associated with each RyR subunit, four being present with each complete Ca^{2+}-release complex. Micromolar concentrations of the immunosuppressant FK506 promote dissociation of FKBP12 from SR membrane preparations and reduce the rates of active Ca^{2+} accumulation in SR vesicles, suggesting that the FKBP12/Ry_1 receptor heterocomplex stabilizes the closed conformation of the Ca^{2+}-release channels (350). Binding of FK506 by FKBP12 also increases RyR open time and relieves the inactivation caused by high cytoplasmic levels of Ca^{2+} (3), reinforcing the modulatory role of FKBP12 on SR Ca^{2+} channel function. A recently defined class of macrocyclic alkaloids isolated from the marine sponge *Ianthella basta* and known as bastadins mediate activation of the Ry_1 receptor via FKBP12 (210). Unlike FK506, bastadins do not induce dissociation of FKBP12 from Ry_1 receptors, but instead markedly alter the FKBP12-Ry_1 interaction, resulting in a marked (~50-fold) increase in channel mean open

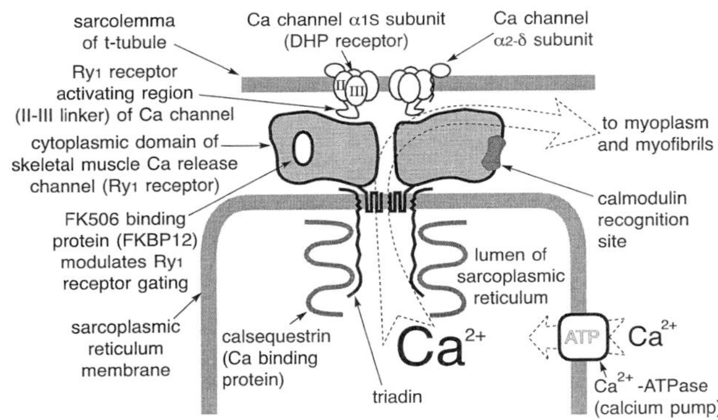

Figure 7. The major components of the excitation-contraction pathway of skeletal muscle shown schematically. The major feature is the Ca^{2+}-release channel of the junctional sarcoplasmic reticulum (JSR). A voltage-dependent conformation change in the skeletal muscle Ca channel (DHP receptor, α_{1S} subunit) is transmitted to the Ca-release channel (Ry_1 receptor) through the protein segment linking motifs II and III, which activates its opening. Other Ry_1 receptors have no associated DHP receptors and are activated by a rise in local [Ca^{2+}] (Ca^{2+}-induced Ca^{2+} release). The large cytoplasmic domain ("foot process") has multiple-binding sites for ATP, Ca^{2+}, Mg^{2+}, and a variety of drugs including volatile anesthetics. The FK-binding protein (FKBP12) binds to Ry_1 receptor and modulates its gating. Triadin is a protein closely associated with JSR that appears to regulate Ca^{2+} release from the SR lumen, possibly by transmitting the release signal to calsequestrin, an acidic protein with many sites that bind Ca^{2+} with low affinity. (Reprinted from ref. 280.)

time with no change in unitary conductance. Intact BC3H1 cells and isolated skeletal SR vesicles suggest that, through their actions on FKBP12, bastadins modulate the ratio of ryanodine-insensitive "leak" states to ryanodine-sensitive channel states in the SR membrane. The incidence of subconductance states is reduced when purified FKBP12 protein is added to expressed recombinant Ry_1 receptors, but normal (rapid) gating behavior is not completely restored (29). In addition, the Ry_1 receptor expressed in these cells also shares characteristics similar to Ry_1 receptor found in SR membranes, including recognition by native RyR1 antibodies, the binding of [^{3}H]ryanodine, and formation of an ion channel in bilayers (29). However, the channel-gating kinetics are greatly altered in bilayer studies, exhibiting numerous channel conductances and subconductances that are not evident in channels studied in fused native SR vesicles.

Triadin is a 95-kd glycoprotein isolated from junctional SR (36) and cloned by Campbell's group (170). It appears to associate with the Ry_1 receptor and may play a structural role in coupling L-type Ca^{2+} channels of the t-tubule membrane with the SR Ca^{2+}-release channel. Using a fluorescent coumarin maleimide (CPM), a small number of highly reactive sulfhydryl moieties that reside on both RyR1 and triadin proteins have been identified, which appear to be essential for normal channel function (198). Close association of Ry_1 receptor and triadin is evident from coimmunoprecipitation of CPM-labeled proteins from detergent-solubilized SR membranes. Either anti-Ry_1 antibodies or antitriadin monoclonal antibodies coprecipitate both fluorescently tagged Ry_1 receptor and triadin protein and specific high-affinity [^{3}H]ryanodine-binding sites (114). Even in the absence of dihydropyridine (DHP) receptors in dysgenic mice, triadin and Ry_1 are able to aggregate and form clusters (86). The presence of the sulfhydryl moietics may be responsible for the ability of silver (Ag^+) and other heavy metal ions that react with sulfhydryl groups to alter SR vesicle Ca^{2+} retention (287).

Calsequestrin (Ca^{2+}-binding protein) is a highly acidic protein of 45 kd isolated from the SR, which appears to reside in the SR lumen (215). This protein has a high proportion of acidic amino acids that provide for a low-affinity, high-capacity binding of Ca^{2+}. Ikemoto et al. (141) have shown that activation of Ry_1 receptors by ligands elicits a signal in the junctional face membrane, which is transmitted to calsequestrin. This signal appears to be important to release of bound Ca^{2+} within the SR lumen. In support, intraluminal SR Ca^{2+} has been shown to be an important factor in Ry_1 receptor function; furthermore, triadin may functionally relate calsequestrin to Ry_1 receptor (114). Although first identified in skeletal muscle (215), a cardiac distinct isoform has also been defined (35). In addition, a 106-kd protein has also been identified as distinct from the others and may be involved in Ry receptor regulation.

Cellular Control of RyReceptor Function

In addition to such modulation by associated proteins and simple intracellular mediators, phosphorylation of Ry receptors can modulate the gating and response of the release channel (361). Numerous amino acid sequences on Ry receptors exist near serines and threonines that make them candidates for phosphorylation by protein kinase C (PKC), cAMP-dependent kinase (PKA), CaM kinase II, and others (Fig. 6, lower two lines). β-Adrenergic stimulation of mammalian skeletal muscle enhances release of activator Ca^{2+}, a process that has been attributed to phosphorylation of the release channel, presumably by PKA (33). In contrast, in isolated SR preparations, phosphorylation attributed to CaM kinase II was suggested as a mechanism for inactivation (361). However, comparative studies of cardiac and skeletal Ry receptors have suggested that skeletal muscle Ry_1 receptor is not a prominent substrate for CaM kinase II or PKA (330,370). The cardiac Ry receptor appears to readily phosphorylated by CaM kinase II and PKA (330,370,374). Phosphorylation has measurable physiologic effects; when Ca^{2+} is released by photolysis in the proximity of channels in permeabilized myocardium, Ca^{2+} release is enhanced, even though Ca^{2+} stores are no greater, suggesting that the release pathway is enhanced (275). Obviously, since phosphorylation can augment Ry receptor channel function, phosphorylase activity may provide a negative modulatory mechanism.

The Skeletal Muscle Ca^{2+}-Release Channel

When extracellular Ca^{2+} is removed from the medium perfusing myocardium, either in the absence or presence of repetitive depolarizations and contractile activity, contractions will cease. This requirement for extracellular Ca^{2+} to activate contractions in the myocardium is not present in skeletal muscle. When Ca^{2+} is removed from the extracellular fluid, even for a sustained period, a contraction or contracture can be elicited if no prior activity has occurred (9,110). Consequently, Ca^{2+} does not appear to be required for EC coupling in skeletal muscle. However, removal of Ca^{2+} does appear to result in depletion of a pool of Ca^{2+}, which somehow contributes to EC coupling (110), perhaps being bound to the DHP receptor or to the intracellular membrane.

EC Coupling and the Dihydropyridine (DHP) Receptor Evidence for activation of Ry_1 receptor by the α_{1S} L-type Ca^{2+} channel subunit has been discovered using dysgenic mice, animals that die at birth because their skeletal muscles are nonfunctional and that lack the DHP receptor (169). In an extensive series of studies, Beam and coworkers (2,169,345) have found that EC coupling can be restored by introducing α_{1S} cDNA into the dysgenic mouse muscle. A somewhat truncated form of the α_{1S} is present in skeletal muscle; this form is also is effective in restoring EC coupling (15). Interestingly, the cardiac L-type Ca channel (a_{1C}) is also able to restore EC coupling in skeletal muscle; unlike the skeletal muscle Ca channel, however, it requires extracellular Ca^{2+} (346). Recent work employing chimeric Ca channels, which include the components of either the skeletal or cardiac-type muscle, has demonstrated clearly that the 2-3 cytoplasmic linker appears to be involved in coupling to and activation of the Ry_1 receptor (344), as shown in Fig. 7. Specific peptide regions have been identified, one of which seems to serve as an activator and the other as an inhibitor of Ca^{2+} release from isolated SR vesicles containing Ry_1 receptors (68). In addition to its functional defect, skeletal muscle of dysgenic mice lacking DHP receptors (α_{1S} subunit) show a marked decrease in clustering of Ry receptors during development; replacement of DHP receptor gene into dysgenic mouse muscle restores the organized structure (86,340). When mice are mutated to generate a strain lacking Ry_1 receptors, the SR feet and EC coupling are absent (341). Surprisingly, the formation of t-tubular/SR junctions still occurs in the absence of Ry_1 receptors, emphasizing role of other proteins in providing the developmental organization to this complex membrane structure. During the period in which researchers were defining the structure of the JSR, electrophysiologic measurements disclosed an intramembranous charge movement in voltage-clamped skeletal muscle that was closely associated with tension development and Ca^{2+} release (41,307). It was proposed that this charge movement somehow gated the Ca^{2+} flux from the SR that activated the myofibrils. The charge movement could be eliminated by interventions that disrupted the t-tubule–surface membrane connection, and it was assumed to be located in the t-tubule membrane (40,41). Subsequently, DHP receptors, sarcolemmal L-type Ca channels (α_{1S}), were isolated from t-tubules (27,55). Notably, the myocytes of dysgenic mice that lack the α_{1S} DHP receptor also lack the gating charge (15).

Freeze-fracture electron microscopic studies of the t-tubule/junctional SR region demonstrate a clear square configuration of surface membrane particles (termed tetrad) that appear to be DHP receptor Ca channels. In a roughly alternating pattern, each tetrad was aligned with a larger SR foot process or Ry receptor present on the SR membrane (25,92). Consequently, about half the Ry receptors have no associated DHP receptor tetrad (92). Since each Ry receptor (four monomers) binds a single Ry and each DHP receptor tetrad binds four DHP molecules, this feature has been employed to explore the stoichiometric relationships in muscle membrane. Typically, a binding ratio of the radiolabeled ligands is 2 DHP:1 Ry, a ratio consistent with one DHP tetrad for every two Ry receptors (20,216). However, in rat and rabbit skeletal muscle the ratio is lower, with less than one DHP bound per Ry, suggesting that there is an even greater excess of Ry receptors (5,216). Although they were initially defined by their presence as the SR feet between the t-tubule and junctional SR, it is now clear that Ry receptors are also located at a distance from the triad (63). Obviously, these "excess" Ryl receptors, some located at considerable distance from DHP receptors, cannot be activated by the DHP receptors; instead, they are most likely activated by the rise in cytoplasmic Ca^{2+}, Ca^{2+}-induced Ca^{2+} release (CICR), a process prominent in myocardium (see below). Recently, two components of Ca^{2+} release in skeletal muscle have been identified, with a fast component that desensitizes or is lost with the absence of extracellular Ca^{2+} (7). Nevertheless, the close association of Ry_1 receptors and a portion of DHP receptors in skeletal muscle heavy SR is emphasized by the fact that following homogenization, the proteins cosediment upon centrifugation (221). Thus, a dual Ca^{2+}-release pathway is present in skeletal muscle, with both CICR and direct RyR activation. In vascular smooth muscle and cerebellar Purkinje cells, other cells where Ry_1 is expressed, it is unclear whether DHP receptors (specifically α_{1S}) directly couple depolarization to Ry_1, or whether only Ca^{2+} entry is present to activate their opening.

Malignant Hyperthermia The genetic disease termed malignant hyperthermia (MH) is a hypermetabolic state resulting from the activation of skeletal muscle due to increased sarcoplasmic Ca^{2+} concentration, usually caused by volatile anesthetics and succinylcholine. When left untreated, or in the ongoing presence of anesthetics, the massive metabolic requirement caused by contractures in all the skeletal muscles of the body severely strains the capacity of the cardiovascular system. A combined metabolic and respiratory acidosis secondary to the massive production of CO_2 occurs as the skeletal muscle attempts to generate enough ATP to meet the ongoing metabolic requirement. The increases in sarcoplasmic Ca^{2+} are typically associated with contracture formation, but this is not uniformly the case, since certain forms of MH appear even when tension development is not massively activated (111). Anesthetic-inducible MH is observed in humans and pigs, the latter serving as a model for human disease (111); the disease has also been described recently in dogs (260).

Tests employing ion-selective microelectrodes have detected increased resting levels of sarcoplasmic Ca^{2+} in skeletal muscle from MH susceptible (MHS) individuals and animals (199,200). In the presence of anesthetics, particularly halothane, massive elevations in Ca^{2+} occur in the sarcoplasm, an effect not seen in MH nonsusceptible (MHN) tissue (201). This anesthetic-induced increase in Ca^{2+} serves in part as the basis for the in vitro contracture test (IVCT) in which small cut segments of skeletal muscle (2–3 cm in length) are exposed to halothane, which causes a contracture to develop (30). In nonsusceptible muscle, concentrations of 4% halothane are required to elicit even small contractures, while concentrations as small as 0.5% may be sufficient to induce contracture in MHS muscle (229). Likewise in MHS muscle, caffeine causes contraction at concentrations 4 to 10 times lower than in normal muscle. The behavior of such muscle in vitro has served as the basis for diagnosis of MHS in both humans and pigs. In spite of efforts at standardization of the IVCT (74,183), since the muscle specimens will inevitably vary in length, damage, and handling, all of which may influence contractile behavior (78,83,101), some variation in test sensitivity seems inevitable.

THE MH MUTATION IN SWINE When exposed to volatile anesthetics and/or muscle depolarization by succinylcholine, MHS swine show massive whole-body contracture and rigor. These swine can also be induced to enter a hypermetabolic state by stress alone, leading to the diagnosis of "porcine stress syndrome" (261). Although MH can be detected in a variety of breeds of pigs, the effect appears to be mediated by a specific gene defect that is identical across all breeds and occurs in the RyR_1 gene on chromosome 6 (95). The defect is the substitution of thymine for cytosine at nucleic acid 1843, resulting in the substitution of cysteine for an argenine at amino acid 615 within the large cytoplasmic domain of the channel protein. Swine that are homozygous for this gene demonstrate MH, while the heterozygous animals show far less profound behavior. For example, stress alone is insufficient to cause the syndrome; however, expression of a mildly hypermetabolic state may occur under certain circumstances (103).

The MHS mutation does not alter ionic selectivity (312), while the single-channel conductance of porcine Ry_1 receptor is only modestly increased (80), if at all (262,310,312). However, the alteration causes a variety of important functional changes in the SR and Ry_1 receptor: (a) the luminal $[Ca^{2+}]$ of the SR before activation of release is decreased in MHS (258, 268); (b) under mildly stimulating conditions, the MHS Ry_1 receptor binds more ryanodine to the high-affinity site (235), consistent with a higher fraction of open channels, although the mutated receptor appears to have lower K_d (310); (c) the $[Ca^{2+}]_i$ required to inhibit channel opening is significantly higher for MHS Ry_1 (80,310), so that channels will continue to open at $[Ca^{2+}]_i$, which would inhibit the normal channel; and (d) the Ry_1 receptor channel demonstrates increased open times (80,262,310). The channels appear to be more sensitive to voltage activation, since smaller K^+ depolarizations are required to activate contractures in MHS muscle (100,102); whether the effect is mediated via the DHP receptor or Ca^{2+}-induced Ca^{2+} release is not known. The close linkage between the DHP receptor and Ry_1 receptor is emphasized in that not only is the behavior of the mutated Ry_1 receptor altered, but also it affects the DHP binding of the associated DHP receptor (73).

These changes in Ry_1 channel function apparently result in the elevated resting $[Ca^{2+}]_i$ (200), but result in no major effects in muscle in the absence of stress or anesthetics. However, halothane at subclinical concentrations (≥10 μM, equivalent to ≥0.05% inspired) increases the mean open time of MHS channels, as well as their conductance, while normal channels are unaltered (262). It is this further enhancement of channel Ca^{2+} release that leads to increasing myoplasmic $[Ca^{2+}]$, and ultimately to contractures and an MH episode. Such anesthetic effects when combined with enhanced response to depolarization (e.g., succinylcholine administration) are presumably responsible for the rapid and severe MH episodes that occur with combined succinylcholine/halothane administration. Anesthetic actions are also transmitted from the Ry_1 receptor to the DHP receptor, which demonstrates decreased DHP binding (204). Halothane has served as the prototypical triggering agent for MH episodes and Ry_1 channel studies. Desflurane and isoflurane appear in vivo to be slightly less potent triggers (363), but their efficacy compared to halothane in activating mutated Ry_1 channels is not known. Ryanodine binding to isolated skeletal muscle SR from normal swine is enhanced by isoflurane and halothane, but curiously not by enflurane (52). While anesthetics may enhance channel opening of the MHS Ry receptor, other factors appear to contribute to the occurrence of the MH episode in a positive feedback manner. The muscle activation caused by the uncontrolled increase in $[Ca^{2+}]_i$ would be expected to induce a metabolic acidosis that would inhibit Ry_1 receptor opening. Instead the MH mutated Ry_1 stays open under more acidic conditions (205,311), permitting ongoing Ca^{2+} release and further aggravating the metabolic stress.

Ry_1 receptors isolated from heterozygous animals show an array of gating behaviors that suggest the formation of heterotrimers (313). The presence of one or more MHS Ry monomer appears sufficient to induce abnormal behavior, with heterotetramers showing closed times and gating that is distinct from the MHS and normal homotetramers (313).

A number of additional changes can be observed in MHS swine that, at first, do not appear to be directly related to this RyR_1 defect alone; for example, altered IP_3 concentration are observed (84,87). It is likely that the elevated resting $[Ca^{2+}]_i$ can induce additional changes in muscle that cause the secondary effects observed. While the RyR_1 gene is expressed in other tissues, it is unclear what disorder if any may result from the gene defect in these tissues. For example, little or no Ry_1 may be expressed in cardiac muscle (186,219,381), and whether the presence of MHS Ry_1 receptors in myocardium can account for the electrophysiologic changes observed in this tissue isolated from MHS pigs (prolonged AP) (298) is not known. Likewise, whether neuronally expressed Ry_1 receptors explain early changes in brain electrical activity remains to be determined (173).

HUMAN MH: LINKAGE WITH THE RY_1 RECEPTOR GENE Although both the porcine and human forms are triggered by anesthetics, and the porcine form served as a model for the human disease, differences have been clearly apparent. While the porcine form of MH has a recessive inheritance, human MH appears to have more dominant inheritance, although variable expression of the MH syndrome contributes to the diagnostic dilemma (225). The vagaries of the clinical triggering, with early therapeutic interventions, frequently prevent definitive diagnosis. Contractures observed with other myopathies (138,188,243) or rigidity of specific muscle groups such as the masseter muscle (185,197) has further complicated exact definition of the disease. Diagnosis is based on the IVCT of specimens of human muscle (usually quadriceps femoris); small specimens of muscle fibers removed from MH susceptible (MHS) patients enter a contracture (sustained continuous tension in the absence of electrical stimulus) with either halothane or caffeine exposure, an effect seen only at far higher concentrations than those required for contracture of non-MH muscle (30). In spite of the fact that the study is performed with cut skeletal muscle fibers, which may show variable "sealing" of their membrane and restoration of normal function (78,189), the IVCT test has proved to have rather high selectivity and excellent sensitivity (182), although false-negative results have been reported (150). The necessity for removal of tissue and the inaccuracies of such a bioassay have increased the desire for a genetic test (193).

The abnormality in Ca^{2+} handling by human skeletal muscle has been documented by a number of methods. Activation of Ca^{2+} release from isolated MHS human SR by ≤1 μM Ca^{2+}, but not in normal SR, was initially documented (71). Subsequent reports demonstrated increased resting $[Ca^{2+}]_i$ in MHS muscle (199), and enhanced CICR in skinned human muscle fibers (161). Once the Ry_1 mutation responsible for the porcine form of MH was identified, its presence in the human syndrome was also determined. Clear linkage of clinical MH or a positive biopsy could be made with the location of the RYR1 gene on the long limb of chromosome 19, specifically 19 r13.1. Although clear linkage is apparent, only 1 in 35 (109) and 1 in 62 (132) families specifically demonstrated the comparable mutation, that is, Arg 614 to Cys. However, a number of additional mutations of the human RyR1 have been described that are linked to MH susceptibility (Table 4), some of which are also coincident with central core disease (289,290,378), a muscle disease previously associated with MH susceptibility (90). In contrast to studies in swine, isolated SR from five patients demonstrated an increased sensitivity to Ca^{2+} activation of ryanodine binding (355). Likewise in single-channel studies, only certain patients showed altered behavior in response to halothane stimulation, suggesting that distinct pathogenic forms may be present in the isolated Ry_1 channels (259). Detailed examination of the IVCT results (including twitch potentiation) in 47 patients from four separate families suggests that genetic factors influence the positive responses, resulting in distinctive patterns of response (354). Additional genetic studies have clearly shown that for perhaps half of individuals with MHS, the disease is not linked to the RYR1 gene, or even to chromosome 19 (14,153). Clearly, volatile anesthetic-induced leakage of Ca^{2+} must be mediated by mutations in other muscle regulatory proteins, or proteins involved in muscle activation. The associated triadic proteins represent possible sites in which mutations might alter muscle Ca^{2+} regulation. In one case, there is apparent linkage to the DHP receptor α_2-δ subunit (143), suggesting that some alteration is transmitted to the a_1 subunit, which in turn alters the control of Ca^{2+} release.

DANTROLENE The hydantoin derivative dantrolene and its more nitro-substituted analogue azumolene have been long recognized to decrease skeletal muscle contractile force (58,69,

Table 4. RY_1 RECEPTOR MUTATIONS ASSOCIATED WITH MALIGNANT HYPERTHERMIA OR CENTRAL CORE DISEASE

Amino acid substitution	Nucleotide substitution	Association	Reference
$Arg^{163} \rightarrow Cys$	C487 → T	MH, CCD	289
$Gly^{248} \rightarrow Arg$	G742 → A	MH	108
$Gly^{341} \rightarrow Arg$	G1021 → A	MH	291
$Ile^{403} \rightarrow Met$	C1209 → G	MH, CCD	289
$Tyr^{522} \rightarrow Ser$	A1565 → C	MH, CCD	290
$Arg^{614} \rightarrow Cys$	C1840→ T	MH	109
$Gly^{2433} \rightarrow Arg$	G7297 → A	MH	164, 284
$Arg^{2433} \rightarrow His$	G7301 → A	MH, CCD	378

Adapted from ref. 214.

70,118,177,191) in a process involving inhibition of Ca^{2+} release from the SR (118,246,357). The agent clearly inhibits the Ca^{2+}-induced release of Ca^{2+} from the SR (268). By virtue of its potent action in blocking Ca^{2+} release, this agent proved to prevent MH in swine (111,112,122) and has now become a mainstay in the therapy of human MH, both to prevent episodes as well as to relax and reverse hypermetabolic episodes once they are started (85,111,174). The increased resting level of $[Ca^{2+}]_i$ in MH muscle can be reduced by dantrolene (202,203), while the explosive rise in $[Ca^{2+}]_i$ increases observed following triggering agents are also inhibited by this agent (201). Recently, a distinct dantrolene binding site with a K_d of ~280 nM has been isolated from the junctional SR of skeletal muscle (274). However, this dantrolene-binding site appears to be associated with proteins smaller than the Ry_1 itself, suggesting that dantrolene may mediate its actions via one of the associated triadic proteins (273). While dantrolene has clear actions in depressing Ca^{2+} release at >100 nM, lower concentrations (<10 nM) appear to activate Ry_1 receptor channel opening, suggesting that it binds to a high-affinity site yielding biphasic actions (375).

The effect of decreasing the Ca^{2+} release has actions in other tissues as well. In neurons, dantrolene prevents injury mediated by excess glutamate stimulation (88,89,190), while it also is able to depress long-term potentiation, suggesting a role for intracellular Ca^{2+} stores in this process (267).

The Cardiac Ca^{2+}-Release Channel

In contrast to skeletal muscle, in which a large fraction of Ry_1 receptor activation is via the DHP receptor, a fundamental feature of cardiac excitation-contraction coupling is Ca^{2+}-induced Ca^{2+} release (CIRC), in which Ca^{2+} entry activates Ry_2 receptors to open, resulting in Ca^{2+} flux into the myocardium. Considering the proximity of L-type Ca channels at the junctional SR membrane, one would expect that once Ca^{2+} release was initiated by a small amount of entering Ca^{2+}, a positive feedback loop would develop and all the Ry_2 receptors at a t-tubule-SR coupling would activate an explosion of Ca^{2+} release from the junctional SR. Remarkably, this does not occur because the cardiac Ry_2 receptor shows a graded response to Ca^{2+} entry. In cardiac tissues, small "sparks" of release can be observed that appear to be self-limited openings of a single or a few release channels; it does not spread to involve the entire junctional region (46). Part of the explanation may be the geometry of the junctional cleft (329), as well as buffering of the increased $[Ca^{2+}]$ by binding to membrane phospholipids (277,286,362). A major contribution to this muting of positive feedback may be the apparent accommodation to Ca^{2+} activation observed with its persistent presence (115). Following a rise in Ca^{2+} near the receptor, activity immediately (~1 msec) increases and then slowly declines until a subsequent increase in Ca^{2+} elicits a subsequent marked increase in channel opening, which again declines. While such adaptation can occur with a time constant of over 1 sec, in the presence of physiologic concentrations of Mg^{2+} (0.3–1 mM) adaptation and inactivation occur faster (200 msec) (356). In addition, phosphorylation by PKA of Ry_2 receptors, as expected during β-adrenergic stimulation, has important modulating actions. While the initial probability of opening is increased, adaptation and decline of opening is also accelerated (356). While initial Ca^{2+} release would be enhanced, the rapid decay of channel opening permits a shorter systolic release period before relaxation, and more rapid availability of channels for the next contraction.

The volatile anesthetics have dramatic and distinct actions on cardiac Ry receptors. It has long been recognized that volatile anesthetics decrease the Ca^{2+} available for release from the SR (332–334). Halothane clearly depletes SR Ca^{2+} (158,159, 175,366,367), with similar effects demonstrable for enflurane (158,159,364,365). In contrast, isoflurane had less or no action in this regard in most direct or indirect studies evaluating SR Ca^{2+} stores (176,365). Evidence for the specific effect of halothane on Ry receptors is that its release of myocardial SR Ca^{2+} could be inhibited by Ry receptor blockade with ruthenium red (126); in addition, specific Ry binding by cardiac Ry receptors is enhanced by halothane and enflurane (52,207). While halothane clearly increases the number of high-affinity sites (open channels), isoflurane has no such action (207). In a study of single channels incorporated into bilayers, halothane and enflurane, but not isoflurane, clearly activated cardiac Ry receptor channels (51). Consequently, the cardiac Ry receptor shows a striking specificity for volatile anesthetic binding and activation, an action that may explain the greater myocardial depressant action of halothane. While a few studies have suggested that isoflurane may decrease the cardiac SR Ca^{2+} store (158,332), however, this action may be a nonspecific effect, since it occurs in SR membrane lacking functional Ry receptors and derived from either skeletal (24) or cardiac tissue (93).

Other Ion Channels in the Recticular Membrane

The rapid efflux of Ca^{2+} from the SR lumen would create a large negative charge, retarding further efflux, unless that efflux were balanced by an equivalent charge movement in the opposite direction. Influx of K^+ into and/or Cl^- efflux from the SR lumen is able to provide the balancing charge movement. The SR has a high conductance (230 pS) single-ion site K^+ channel, investigated as a model channel for study of ion permeation (184,239), which can permit the balancing charge movement necessary to permit rapid Ca^{2+} efflux from the SR. The chloride channel has been found when SR membrane has been incorporated into bilayers (301,347). It has a moderate conductance (70 pS in 250 mM Cl^-), and appears to be activated by PKA-mediated phosphorylation and inhibited by the Ca^{2+}-calmodulin complex (162,163); it could thereby be an additional mechanism by which SR function can be controlled. In addition, an anion channel has been described in the SR of skeletal muscle that appears to permit translocation of Ca^{2+} as an ion pair with Cl^-, which may provide an alternate pathway for Ca^{2+} efflux into the myoplasm (335).

The IP_3 Receptor/Ca^{2+}-Release Channels

Like its relative the ryanodine receptor, the inositol 1,4,5-trisphosphate receptor (IP_3 receptor) is a tetrameric structure of considerable molecular mass (~1 Md) (107) and is one of the largest known cellular protein complexes. In contrast to the DHP receptor-gated RyR in skeletal muscle (Ry_1) and the Ca^{2+}-gated Ry receptor of cardiac muscle (Ry_2, the site of Ca^{2+}-induced Ca^{2+} release [75]), the IP_3 receptor is a Ca^{2+}-release channel that is activated upon binding the triply phosphated hexose sugar, inositol *myo*-inositol 1,4,5-trisphosphate (IP_3), which initiates the flux of Ca^{2+} from internal stores (81). The release of intracellular Ca^{2+} from its ER stores through the IP_3 receptor, and the subsequent activation of a variety of processes, is characteristic of cells that respond to neurotransmitters, hormones, and growth factors (17). The SR/ER membranes of many cell types contain both IP_3 receptors and the Ry receptors; however, the physiologic relationship and functional interaction between both Ca^{2+}-mediated and IP_3-mediated Ca^{2+} release channels in the same or contiguous internal membrane system of a single-cell type is, at present, unclear.

General and Molecular Structure

The IP_3-receptor family is a group of closely related, IP_3-gated, intracellular cation channels. One receptor is a tetrameric complex composed of large ligand-binding domains (one on each subunit) and four transmembrane domains that coalesce to form a membrane channel, having an overall structure similar to that of the Ry receptor (Fig. 6, upper two lines). Individual subunit masses differ depending on whether they are predicted from cDNA sequence (~330 kd) (99,237) or estimated from their migration in SDS-polyacrylamide gels (~260 kd) (37,339). The three known IP_3 receptor isoforms are primarily thought to be homotetramers of different gene products (IP_3R-1, IP_3R-2, and IP_3R-3), which share approximately 60% to 70% amino acid sequence homology (97). Heterotetrameric combinations of the different IP_3R gene products have recently been described; however, in studies of Chinese hamster ovary cells (CHO-K1), which express abundant quantities of all three isoforms and in native rat hepatocytes, where IP_3R-1 and IP_3R-2 are both highly expressed (245). Since the first IP_3R subunit was cloned from cerebellar Purkinje neurons (99), at least six IP_3R splice variants have also been identified using polymerase chain reaction (PCR) techniques (56,79,97). The sequences and locations of variable insert regions suggest that IP_3 receptors derived by alternative splicing may account for some observed differences in ligand-binding affinity, and alternative splicing may subserve some role in the regulation of channel function (56,79).

Most eukaryotic cells express IP_3 receptors in the membranes of their SR/ER (16,17); they are frequently present throughout the internal membrane systems, being represented not only on the smooth ER, but also on the rough ER, the nuclear envelope, and on membranes juxtaposed to mitochondria (Figs. 4 and 8) (98). However, the relative abundance and pattern of isoform expression is tissue specific (299). The brain expresses large quantities of all three IP_3R isoforms, although certain isoforms appear to be characteristic in specific CNS regions; the cerebellum, for example, expresses largely IP_3R-2s. Hepatocytes, however, contain only IP_3R-1 and IP_3R-2 (245). T-lymphocytes contain predominantly the IP_3R-1 (120,218), vascular endothelium contains IP_3R-2, while type IP_3R-3 is found in certain lymphoma and hematopoietic cell lines (372). Several reports also indicate that IP_3 receptors are expressed at low levels in cardiac muscle (IP_3R mRNA levels are approximately 50-fold lower in heart than the cardiac RyR), although it remains to be determined whether these receptors transduce a Ca^{2+} signal (165,248). Smooth muscle cells contain numerous IP_3R-1 in their SR/ER network (37,218); these receptors are of central importance in transducing agonist-induced contraction (pharmacomechanical coupling) in smooth muscle (171,324). Skeletal muscle fibers contain IP_3R mRNA; however, expression of primarily IP_3R-1 is most prominent in slow oxidative (type I) and fast oxidative-glycolytic (type IIA) fibers, as opposed to fast glycolytic fibers (type IIB) fibers (249). However, their functional role in EC coupling remains uncertain.

Each IP_3 receptor subunit can be divided into three distinct functional domains, as originally described by Mignery and Südhof (238). The N-terminal ~650 amino acids of each receptor subunit encode the IP_3-binding domain. This region is ~70% conserved among all IP_3 receptor subtypes in humans (372). The midportion of the receptor contains consensus sequences for phosphorylation by various protein kinases (PKA, PKG, PKC, CamKII) and a site for autophosphorylation (Fig. 6, upper two lines), although the presence of these regulatory sites varies between IP_3 receptor isoforms (98). In addition, this "regulatory" region contains binding sites for Ca^{2+} and nucleotides, which modulate the receptor's channel function. Hydropathy analysis of the IP_3 receptor carboxy terminus reveals six putative transmembrane-spanning segments (labeled M1 through M6) that are thought to comprise a hydrophobic domain, which in the tetrameric complex combine to form the cation pore. Supporting this view are the conserved distribution of negatively charged amino acids in this segment of the molecule, and recent data that show a monoclonal antibody generated to a 12 amino acid, C-terminal epitope (residues 2648–2749 of the mouse cerebellar IP_3 receptor) decreased Ca^{2+} flux through IP_3 receptors of cerebellar microsomes in response to IP_3. Interestingly, this antibody also increased the affinity of the IP_3 receptor for IP_3: K_d decreased with antibody binding from 43 ± 12 nM to 25 ± 4 nM (253). Several isoforms of the IP_3 receptor also contain one or two potential N-glycosylation sites in the C-terminal region. These hydrophobic C-terminal segments are more conserved among the different IP_3 receptor isoforms and among species than other regions of the molecule. While each of the four IP_3 receptor subunits is thought to contribute a portion of the cation channel, gating and regulation is mediated by the N-terminal IP_3-binding region and the central "regulatory" sequence.

The macromolecular structure of the IP_3 receptor has been investigated using electron microscopy and computer-assisted three-dimensional image reconstruction. Like the Ry receptor, the IP_3 receptor isoform isolated from smooth muscle displays a fourfold "pinwheel" symmetry with a prominent central pore, which is thought to be the cation channel. Electron micrographs of purified, negatively stained, membrane-associated receptors show the smooth muscle IP_3 receptor has dimensions of ~250 × 250 Å (37).

Regulation of IP_3 Receptor Function by IP_3

Binding of inositol 1,4,5-trisphosphate (IP_3) IP_3 to the cytoplasmic N-terminal IP_3-binding domain of the receptor monomers induces opening of the channel, and is the major physiologic activator ligand for the various IP_3 receptor isoforms. Extracellular hormones or growth factors bind to their cell surface receptors and activate phospholipase C, either through a G-protein (e.g., acetylcholine, 5-HT, angiotensin-II, odorants, bradykinin, etc.) or a tyrosine kinase-linked receptor, for example, platelet-derived growth factor (PDGF) or epidermal growth factor (EGF). Phospholipase C is a family of enzymes that are activated in response to the binding of ligands to either het-

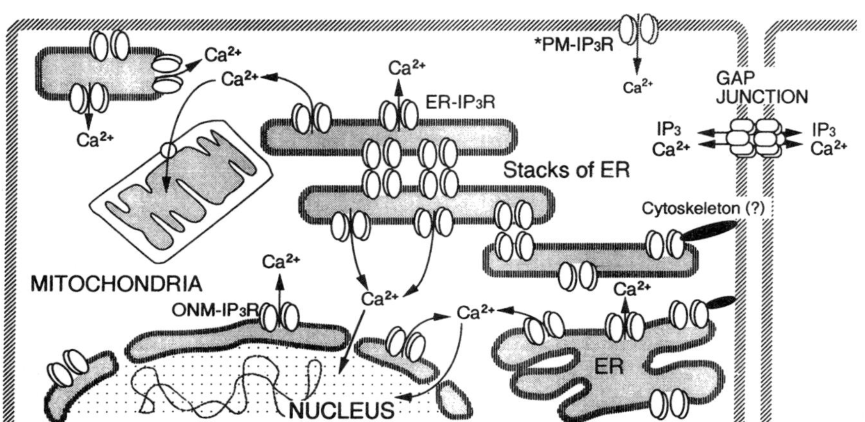

Figure 8. Local IP_3R-mediated Ca^{2+} signaling. IP_3R is subcellularly localized in Ca^{2+} pools, such as the smooth ER, rough ER, and its outer nuclear membrane (ONM). IP_3R-Ca^{2+} pools (or the IP_3R itself) appear to interact with the cytoskeleton (see text). In the Purkinje cells of the cerebellum, IP_3R immunoreactivity was observed especially on the stacked cisternae and subplasmalemmal cisternae. In the space interposed between adjacent cisternae, it appears that IP_3R apposed on individual stacks face each other head to head as perpendicular bridges. Cytoplasmic Ca^{2+} signals mediated by IP_3Rs appear to be transported into mitochondria and nuclei as well. Moreover, IP_3 and Ca^{2+} signals appear to be intracellularly propagated via gap junctions. Putative IP_3Rs on the PM are also indicated by *dotted symbols.* (Reprinted with permission from ref. 98.)

erotrimeric G-protein–linked receptors (which activate PLC-β1) or tyrosine kinase-linked receptors (which activate PLC-γ1); these two parallel signal transduction pathways thus converge upon the activation of different PLC isoforms (16). Phosphatidylinositol 4,5-bisphosphate (PIP_2), the IP_3 precursor, is a normal lipid component of the plasma membrane that is enzymatically converted (by activated PLC) to IP_3 and diacylglycerol (DAG). DAG binds to some isoforms of protein kinase C (PKC) to activate this enzyme and a parallel limb of the signal transduction cascade (see Chapter 7) (264). Among the large number of effector molecules PKC can phosphorylate is IP_3 receptor itself, providing additional modulation and control of cellular responses to hormone or growth factor stimulation.

IP_3 diffuses from the surface membrane to the IP_3 receptor on the ER/SR, binds with high affinity (kd ~18 nM) to the IP_3-binding domain on the IP_3 receptor subunits, and causes release of stored Ca^{2+}. Kinetic studies indicate that opening of the IP_3 receptor calcium channel requires a minimum of three bound IP_3 molecules. The binding of IP_3 to its receptor sites has been shown to be highly cooperative in rat basophilic leukemia cells—the Hill coefficient over a range of IP_3 from 2 to 40 nm was ~2.7 (231). The onset kinetics of IP_3-induced Ca^{2+} increases were also found to be highly cooperative in cultured HL-60 granulocytes, with Hill coefficients of between 4 and 12 (308). In contrast, others have described noncooperative behavior of the channel, which may reflect the methods of study (22). The major differences among ligand-gated ion channels studied to date are the off-rates for the ligand and the equilibrium dissociation constants. These characteristics imply that the IP_3 receptor channel is slow, kinetically, when compared to other ligand-gated channels such as the nicotinic acetylcholine receptor. The higher affinity binding sites, and the slower off-rate constants may be favorable, energetically, since signal transduction events can be accomplished with smaller concentrations of ligand (IP_3) (232). Like Ry receptors response to Ca^{2+} and other agonists, IP_3 receptors also show adaptation to the ongoing presence of IP_3, demonstrating a decreasing activity and Ca^{2+} flux with continued stimulation (50).

IP_3 is rapidly metabolized by either phosphorylation (IP_3 3-kinase) or by dephosphorylation (IP_3 5-phosphatase) (for review see ref. 62). Either reaction limits the duration of the IP_3 effect and generates IP_3 metabolites, which may also have effects on calcium homeostasis, apart from the IP_3 receptor. Irvine and Moor (149) have hypothesized that inositol 1,3,4,5-tetrakisphosphate (IP_4) may, in sea urchin oocytes, gate Ca^{2+} channels in the plasma membrane and/or stimulate the refilling of IP_3-dependent calcium stores by extracellular Ca^{2+}. Data from mouse lachrymal cells support these observations; however, the activation of a plasma membrane Ca^{2+} channel by IP_4 may require the synergistic effect of IP_3. Further evidence for the role of IP_4 in stimulating plasma membrane Ca^{2+} influx has been found in endothelial cells where 1,3,4,5-IP_4 stimulates a plasma membrane Ca^{2+} channel (206). The specific effect of IP_4 on extracellular Ca^{2+} entry would suggest a specific IP_4 receptor protein in the plasma membrane. Several groups have identified IP_4- and IP_6-binding proteins from rat brain homogenates that may be Ca^{2+} channels, suggesting that the production of IP_4 and its subsequent binding to a "receptor" may aid in the refilling of depleted internal calcium stores (148,349). Additional kinases have been found in rat brain homogenates that can phosphorylate (1,3,4,6) IP_4 to IP_5 and, possibly, IP_6; however, the physiologic function of these phosphorylated myoinositols remains unclear.

IP_3 Receptor Regulation by Ca^{2+} and Other Species

In addition to IP_3, other regulators of Ca^{2+} release have also been described for the various IP_3 receptors. Most notably and like their structural homologs the Ry receptors, IP_3 receptors can be modulated in a complex way by Ca^{2+} (both cytosolic and ER-luminal) and nucleotides (17,66,348). The IP_3 receptor in brain is negatively regulated by Ca^{2+}, an effect that requires the calcium-binding protein, calmedin (57,353). In tissues such as vas deferens, where Ca^{2+} ions have been shown to have less of a regulatory effect, the addition of exogenous calmedin to membrane preparations of IP_3 receptor changes the IP_3-binding affinity (79,250), suggesting a pivotal role for calmedin in Ca^{2+} regulation of the IP_3 receptor in this tissue. Ca^{2+} exerts a biphasic, dose-dependent regulation of the IP_3 receptor in saponin-permeabilized taenia caeci (smooth muscle); $[Ca^{2+}]_i$ less than 300 nM enhanced Ca^{2+} flux through the IP_3 receptor when stimulated by IP_3 (139). $[Ca^{2+}]_i$ greater than 300 nM inhibited the IP_3R channel activity, giving rise to the idea that Ca^{2+} is able to modulate or regulate IP_3R channel function at both high and low concentrations. The amount of calmedin in taenia caeci was not measured in this study, however, and its requirement for such Ca^{2+} regulation is not clear. The inhibition of IP_3 receptor channel function by rising levels of Ca^{2+} has been proposed to generate the spatiotemporal dynamic of intracellular Ca^{2+}, or "calcium waves" (4,321); however, the cellular mechanisms of calcium wave generation and their physiologic function are far from clear at this time. The responsiveness of the receptor, the size of the cell, as well as the extent and exact structure of the membrane system probably determines the pattern of Ca^{2+} release that can be observed.

Adenosine triphosphate (ATP) appears to enhance the frequency of IP_3 receptor channel opening in the presence of IP_3; however, adenine nucleotides in the absence of IP_3 are insufficient to cause IP_3 receptor activation. At concentrations above 4 mM, ATP decreased activity of the IP_3 receptor, and this effect is thought to result from competition with IP_3 at the IP_3-binding site. Other factors such as intracellular pH and Mg^{2+} concentrations have also been thought to modify IP_3 receptor channel function (21).

Heparin, a polysulfated glycosaminoglycan (polyanionic), has been shown to antagonize IP_3 binding to its receptor. The importance of IP_3-induced Ca^{2+} release in contraction of smooth muscle has been demonstrated directly (324) and also by demonstrating that cystosolic heparin, by binding to the IP_3 receptor, could selectively block agonist-induced contraction in permeabilized smooth muscle (171,172). The specificity of heparin binding to the IP_3 receptor has also been seen in liver, cultured smooth muscle cells, and a variety of other cell types (104,131). While heparin's antagonism of IP_3 binding to its receptor has been used as an indicator of IP_3 receptor-mediated effects, the selectivity of this effect for the IP_3 receptor has also been questioned. It appears that heparin can also *activate* Ca^{2+} release from the Ry receptor in a Ca^{2+}-dependent way, making it a less selective antagonist than once thought. However, the Ca^{2+}-dependence of heparin's Ry receptor activation probably limits the general observation of its effect, since the threshold $[Ca^{2+}]$ appears to be greater than 100 nM (66).

As with Ry receptor, not only is IP_3 receptor regulated by Ca^{2+} and nucleotides, but phosphorylation of the IP_3 receptor by protein kinase A (in response to a rise in cytosolic cyclic AMP) shifts the dose-response curve for Ca^{2+} regulation of IP_3 receptor channel function (reviewed in ref. 98). In addition, the activity of phosphatases may provide an additional level of control to modulate channel activity and rate of Ca^{2+} release.

With regard to anesthetic interactions with the IP_3 receptor, few studies have been performed to elucidate any specific interaction. Halothane, isoflurane, and octanol have been found to deplete the IP_3-releasable pool of Ca^{2+} in clonal pituitary (GH3) cells, but whether activation of the IP_3 receptor is involved, as is the case for the Ry receptor, is not known (136).

Diseases of the IP_3 Regulation

There are, presently, no known diseases that result from mutations of the IP_3 receptor, equivalent to the RyR mutations that cause malignant hyperthermia. However, IP_3 metabolism is thought to be altered in Lowe's oculocerebrorenal syndrome

(11). This rare, X-linked recessive disorder is characterized by cataracts, renal tubular dysfunction and severe cognitive deficits (42). A novel gene (named OCRL-1) that shares ~70% homology with the human inositol polyphosphate-5-phosphatase has been cloned; mRNA transcripts of OCRL-1 are absent from some patients affected by Lowe's syndrome or abnormally sized in others (11). More recent work has shown that a baculovirus-expressed cDNA construct encoding a partial sequence of the OCRL gene catalyzes a reaction similar to the platelet 5-phosphatase II. The affinity of this recombinant OCRL protein was greatest for PIP_2, which suggests that the endogenous OCRL gene product may function as a lipid phosphatase that regulates membrane levels of phosphatidylinositol 4,5-bisphosphate—the membrane precursor of IP_3 (377). Such studies have led to the speculation that the progressive deterioration seen in patients with Lowe's syndrome may result from altered PIP_2 metabolism and resultant errors in inositol phosphate signaling; however, the exact biochemical basis for the disease remains unknown.

Interaction of Ca^{2+}-Release Stores

It is clear that many cell types contain both the IP_3-gated channel and the ryanodine-receptor Ca^{2+}-release channel. Both immunohistochemical techniques and functional Ca^{2+}-release experiments have demonstrated the coexistence of both proteins in the same cell. Cerebellar Purkinje cells, for example, contain a large number of both IP_3-receptor epitopes and ryanodine-receptor epitopes in their internal membrane system (360) as seen by immunofluorescent labeling. Smooth muscle also contains both a ryanodine-receptor-gated Ca^{2+} store and an IP_3-receptor-gated Ca^{2+} store. In smooth muscle, these channels have been thought to release functionally different internal Ca^{2+} reserves; however, studies were done in detergent-permeabilized preparations of smooth muscle under conditions that can vesiculate the SR and possibly lead to artifactual compartmentalization of the Ca^{2+} (139,140).

While the coexpression of different Ca^{2+}-release channels in the SR/ER membranes of many cells is no longer in question, the functional role for both channels is not yet clear. Studies, such as those discussed above, have pointed to a functional compartmentalization; however, there are no data that conclusively support anatomical compartmentalization of the SR/ER network or suggest separate Ca^{2+} stores are subserved by either the IP_3 or ryanodine-sensitive Ca^{2+}-release channels. It is possible that Ca^{2+} release through the IP_3 receptor serves to modulate the Ca^{2+}-release function of the ryanodine-sensitive Ca^{2+}-release channel, as previously discussed, and vice versa. The coexistence of both IP_3 and Ry receptors in neuronal cells also suggests that there is a role for both receptors in brain, although no gating mechanisms are distinct for the two Ca^{2+}-release channels. Recent evidence showing complex intracellular Ca^{2+} wave formation may result from the presence of two separate pathways for intracellular Ca^{2+} release and by the inherent Ca^{2+}-sensitivity of the release channel proteins themselves (4); however, a physiologic function for complex regenerative Ca^{2+} wave phenomena is unclear.

Future work on the regulation of intracellular Ca^{2+} release will be required to answer a number of important questions. The mechanism of the signaling interaction between the DHP receptor and the skeletal muscle ryanodine receptor needs to be elucidated. While this has been attributed to a "direct" interaction, further research is required to characterize the nature of the signaling. The exact role for ryanodine receptors in tissues, such as smooth muscle, endothelium, brain, and in the corbular SR of cardiac muscle, where the RyRs are not directly apposed to DHP receptors, is most likely gated by increases in local Ca^{2+} "domains"; however, the specific functions subserved by these receptors is unclear. Finally, the integration of intracellular Ca^{2+}-release responses, modulation of IP_3 and Ry receptor responses by intracellular messengers or phosphorylation, and the coordinated refilling of intracellular Ca^{2+} stores are not well understood. Given the critical importance of cytosolic free Ca^{2+} in most cells, further understanding of Ca^{2+} regulation will shed light on disease states as diverse as malignant hyperthermia and Ca^{2+} overload in states of ischemia and reperfusion.

ANESTHETIC INTERACTIONS CA^{2+} REGULATION

In addition to the Ry receptors, anesthetics alter a variety of specific Ca^{2+} pathways (see Chapters 13 and 20). While actions on specific transport proteins have been emphasized, it is important to recognize that anesthetic effects may be due to more "nonspecific" effects. Anesthetics have been found to enhance Ca^{2+} leakage from membrane stores that do not contain release proteins (24,93), suggesting that other membrane proteins or the lipids bilayer itself may be altered so that more Ca^{2+} will travel down its enormous electrochemical gradient. In analyzing the action of any anesthetic on Ca^{2+} regulation and the subsequent cellular effects, it is important to recognize that the observed change in $[Ca^{2+}]_i$ (or the consequent cellular action) is the net effect of such nonspecific actions, as well as specific effects on transport pathways across both the plasma membrane and the intracellular membranes, and protein binding. Two questions must be addressed. First, what is the particular cellular compartment of interest and which subcellular processes are present? Such a cellular compartment may have both by structural boundaries (e.g., membranes) and functional restrictions (e.g., diffusion), as well as being defined by the balance of the Ca^{2+} transport processes (Ca^{2+} entry vs. release of intracellular stores; Ca^{2+} removal by Na-Ca exchange vs. Ca^{2+}-ATPases). Second, how does the anesthetic in question alter the various subcellular processes that are present regulating Ca^{2+}? For example, if an anesthetic blocks Ca^{2+} entry by voltage-gated channels, but also inhibits Ca^{2+} elimination from the cell, the net effect could be relatively neutral. If a process responds to both Ca^{2+} entering the cell as well as that which is released from an intracellular store, biphasic effects may result. If anesthetic action causes leakage or activates release from the intracellular store, but also blocks Ca^{2+} entry, $[Ca]_i^{2+}$ may transiently rise above normal until the store is depleted, and subsequently remain below normal since the decreased Ca^{2+} entry prevents replenishing the stores. Such an action seems to occur with halothane in the myocardium. Considering major roles in cell function played by Ca^{2+}, and the major alteration in behavior caused by anesthetics, it is not surprising that these agents alter important aspects of Ca^{2+} regulation. While analysis of anesthetic actions on various subcellular components is useful, a combined model of anesthetic actions on the various components of Ca^{2+} handling is required to explain the integrated response within the whole tissue.

REFERENCES

1. Abramson JI, Buck E, Salama G, Casida JE, Pessah IN. Mechanism of anthraquinone-induced calcium release from skeletal muscle sarcoplasmic reticulum. *J Biol Chem* 1988;263:18750–18758.
2. Adams BR, Tanabe T, Mikami A, Numa S, Beam KG. Intramembrane charge movement restored in dysgenic skeletal muscle by injection of dihydropyridine receptor cDNAs. *Nature* 1990;346:569–572.
3. Ahern GP, Junankar PR, Dulhunty AF. Single channel activity of the ryanodine receptor calcium release channel is modulated by FK-506. *FEBS Lett* 1994;352:369–374.
4. Amundson J, Clapham D. Calcium waves. *Curr Opin Neurobiol* 1993;3:375–382.
5. Anderson K, Cohn AH, Meissner G. High affinity [^{3}H]PN200-110 and [^{3}H]ryanodine binding to rabbit and frog skeletal muscle. *Am J Physiol* 1994;266:C462–C466.
6. Anderson K, Lai FA, Liu Q, Rousseau E, Erickson HP, Meissner G. Structural and functional characterization of the purified cardiac

ryanodine receptor-Ca^{2+} release channel complex. *J Biol Chem* 1989;264:1329–1335.
7. Anderson K, Meissner G. T-tubule depolarization-induced SR Ca^{2+} release is controlled by dihydropyridine receptor- and Ca^{2+}-dependent mechanisms in cell homogenates from rabbit skeletal muscle. *J Gen Physiol* 1995;105:363–384.
8. Andressen C, Blümcke I, Celio MR. Calcium-binding proteins: selective markers of nerve cells. *Cell Tissue Res* 1993;271:181–208.
9. Armstrong CM, Bezanilla FM, Horowicz P. Twitches in the presence of ethylene-glycol-bis(β-amino-ethyl ether)-*N,N'*-tetraacetic acid. *Biochim Biophys Acta* 1972;267:605–608.
10. Ashley RH, Williams AJ. Divalent cation activation and inhibition of single calcium release channels from sheep cardiac sarcoplasmic reticulum. *J Gen Physiol* 1990;95:981–1005.
11. Attree O, Olivos IM, Okabe I, et al. The Lowe's oculocerebrorenal syndrome gene encodes a protein highly homologous to inositol polyphosphate-5-phosphatase. *Nature* 1992;358:239–242.
12. Bachs O, Agell N, Carafoli E. Calcium and calmodulin function in the cell nucleus. *Biochim Biophys Acta* 1992;1113:259–270.
13. Baimbridge KG, Celio MR, Pogers JH. Calcium-binding proteins in the nervous system. *Trends Neurosci* 1992;15:303–308.
14. Ball SP, Johnson KJ. The genetics of malignant hyperthermia. *J Med Genet* 1993;30:89–93.
15. Beam KG, Adams BA, Niidome T, Numa S, Tanabe T. Function of a truncated dihydropyridine receptor as both voltage sensor and calcium channel. *Nature* 1992;360:169–171.
16. Berridge MJ. Inositol trisphosphate and calcium signalling. *Nature* 1993;361:315–325.
17. Berridge MJ, Irvine RF. Inositol triphosphate, a novel second messenger in cellular signal transduction. *Nature* 1984;312:315–321.
18. Bers DM, MacLeod KT. Cumulative depletions of extracellular calcium in rabbit ventricular muscle monitored with calcium-selective microelectrodes. *Circ Res* 1986;58:769–782.
19. Bers DM, Peskoff A. Diffusion around a cardiac calcium channel and the role of surface bound calcium. *Biophys J* 1991;59:703–721.
20. Bers DM, Stiffel VM. Ratio of ryanodine and dihydropyridine receptors in cardiac and skeletal muscle and implications for excitation-contraction coupling. *Am J Physiol* 1993; 264:C1587–C2600.
21. Bezprozvanny I, Ehrlich BE. ATP modulates the function of inositol 1,4,5-triphosphate-gated channels at two sites. *Neuron* 1993;10: 1175–1184.
22. Bezprozvanny I, Watras J, Ehrlich BE. Bell-shaped calcium-response curves of $Ins(1,4,5)P_3$- and calcium-gated channels from endoplasmic reticulum of cerebellum. *Nature* 1991;351:751–754.
23. Blanck TJJ, Chiancone E, Salviati G, et al. Halothane does not alter Ca^{2+} affinity of troponin C. *Anesthesiology* 1992;76:100–105.
24. Blanck TJJ, Peterson CV, Baroody B, Tegazzin V, Lou J. Halothane, enflurane, and isoflurane stimulate calcium leakage from rabbit sarcoplasmic reticulum. *Anesthesiology* 1992;76:813–821.
25. Block BA, Imagawa T, Campbell KP, Franzini-Armstrong C. Structural evidence for direct interaction between the molecular components of the transverse tubule/sarcoplasmic reticulum junction in skeletal muscle. *J Cell Biol* 1988;107:2587–2600.
26. Bond M, Shuman H, Somlyo AP, Somlyo AV. Total cytoplasmic calcium in relaxed and maximally contracted rabbit portal vein smooth muscle. *J Physiol* 1984;357:185–201.
27. Borsotto M, Barhanin J, Norman RI, Lazdunski M. Purification of the dihydropyridine receptor of the voltage-dependent Ca^{2+} channel from skeletal muscle transverse tubules using (+) [^{3}H]PN 200–110. *Biochem Biophys Res Commun* 1984;122:1357–1366.
28. Bossen E, Sommer JR, Waugh RA. Comparative stereology of the SR of the mouse and finch left ventricle. *Tissue Cell* 1978;10: 773–784.
29. Brillantes A-MB, Ondrias K, Scott A, et al. Stabilization of calcium release channel (ryanodine receptor) function by FK506-binding protein. *Cell* 1994;77:513–523.
30. Britt BA, Frodis W, Scott E, Clements M-J, Endrenyi L. Comparison of the caffeine skinned fibre tension (CSFT) test with the caffeine-halothane contracture (CHC) test in the diagnosis of malignant hyperthermia. *Can Anaesth Soc J* 1982;6:550–562.
31. Brown GC. Control of respiration and ATP synthesis in mammalian mitochondria and cells. *Biochem J* 1992;284:1–13.
32. Buck E, Zimanyi, Abramson JJ, Pessah IN. Ryanodine stabilized multiple conformational states of the skeletal muscle calcium release channel. *J Biol Chem* 1992;267:23560–23567.
33. Cairns SP, Dulhunty AF. β-Adrenergic potentiation of E-C coupling increases force in rat skeletal muscle. *Muscle Nerve* 1993;16: 1317–1325.
34. Cala SE, Scott BT, Jones LR. Intralumenal sarcoplasmic reticulum Ca^{2+}-binding proteins. *Semin Cell Biol* 1990;1:265–275.
35. Campbell KP, MacLennan DH, Jorgensen AO, Mintzer MC. Purification and characterization of calsequestrin from canine cardiac sarcoplasmic reticulum and identification of the 53,000 dalton glycoprotein. *J Biol Chem* 1983;258:1197–1204.
36. Caswell AH, Brandt NR, Brunschwig J-P, Purkerson S. Localization and partial characterization of the oligomeric disulfide-linked molecular weight 95,000 protein (triadin) which binds the ryanodine and dihydropyridine receptors in skeletal muscle triadic vesicles. *Biochemistry* 1991;30:7507–7513.
37. Chadwick CC, Saito A, Fleischer S. Isolation and characterization of the inositol trisphosphate receptor from smooth muscle. *Proc Natl Acad Sci USA* 1990;87:2132–2136.
38. Chamberlain BK, Volpe P, Fleischer S. Calcium-induced calcium release from purified sarcoplasmic reticulum vesicles. General characteristics. *J Biol Chem* 1984;259:7540–7546.
39. Chamberlain BK, Volpe P, Fleischer S. Inhibition of calcium-induced Ca^{++} release from purified cardiac sarcoplasmic reticulum vesicles. *J Biol Chem* 1984;259:7547–7553.
40. Chandler WK, Rakowski RF, Schneider MF. Effects of glycerol treatment and maintained depolarization on charge movement in skeletal muscle. *J Physiol* 1976;254:285–316.
41. Chandler WK, Rakowski RF, Schneider MF. A non-linear voltage dependent charge movement in frog skeletal muscle. *J Physiol* 1976;254:245–283.
42. Charnas LR, Bernardini I, Rader D, Hoeg JM, Gahl WA. Clinical and laboratory findings in the oculocerebrorenal syndrome of Lowe, with special reference to growth and renal function. *N Engl J Med* 1991;324:1318–1325.
43. Chen SRW, MacLennan DH. Identification of calmodulin, Ca^{2+} and ruthenium red binding domains in the Ca^{2+} release channel (ryanodine receptor) of rabbit skeletal muscle sarcoplasmic reticulum. *J Biol Chem* 1994;269:22698–22704.
44. Chen SRW, Zhang L, MacLennan DH. Characterization of a Ca^{2+} binding and regulatory site in the Ca^{2+} release channel (ryanodine receptor) of rabbit skeletal muscle sarcoplasmic reticulum. *J Biol Chem* 1992;267:22318–23326.
45. Chen SRW, Zhang L, MacLennan DH. Antibodies as probes for Ca^{2+} activation sites in the Ca^{2+} release channel (ryanodine receptor) of rabbit skeletal muscle sarcoplasmic reticulum. *J Biol Chem* 1993;268:13414–13421.
46. Cheng H, Lederer WJ, Cannell MB. Calcium sparks: Elementary events underlying excitation-contraction coupling in heart muscle. *Science* 1993;262:740–744.
47. Chu A, Díaz-Muñoz M, Hawkes MJ, Brush K, Hamilton SL. Ryanodine as a probe for the functional state of the skeletal muscle sarcoplasmic reticulum calcium release channel. *Mol Pharmacol* 1990; 37:735–741.
48. Chu A, Fill M, Stefani E, Entman ML. Cytoplasmic Ca^{2+} does not inhibit the cardiac muscle sarcoplasmic reticulum ryanodine receptor channel, although Ca^{2+}-induced Ca^{2+} inactivation of Ca^{2+} release is observed native vesicles. *J Membr Biol* 1993;135:49–59.
49. Clapham DE. Calcium signaling. *Cell* 1995;80:259–268.
50. Combettes L, Hannaert-Merah Z, Coquil J-F, et al. Rapid filtration studies of the effect of cytosolic Ca^{2+} on inositol 1,4,5-trisphosphate-induced $^{45}Ca^{2+}$ release from cerebellar microsomes. *J Biol Chem* 1994;269:17561–17571.
51. Connelly TJ, Coronado R. Activation of the Ca^{2+} release channel of cardiac sarcoplasmic reticulum by volatile anesthetics. *Anesthesiology* 1994;81:459–469.
52. Connelly TJ, Hayek R-E, Rusy BF, Coronado R. Volatile anesthetics selectively alter [^{3}H]ryanodine binding to skeletal and cardiac ryanodine receptors. *Biochem Biophys Res Commun* 1992;186:595–600.
53. Coronado R, Morrissette M, Sukhareva M, Vaughn DM. Structure and function of ryanodine receptors. *Am J Physiol* 1994;266: C1485–C1504.
54. Creutz CE. The annexins and exocytosis. *Science* 1992;258:924–931.
55. Curtis BM, Catterall WA. Purification of the calcium antagonist receptor of the voltage-sensitive calcium channel from skeletal muscle transverse tubules. *Biochemistry* 1984;23:2113–2119.
56. Danoff SK, Ferris CD, Donath C, et al. Inositol 1,4,5-trisphosphate receptors: distinct neuronal and nonneuronal forms derived by alternative splicing differ in phosphorylation. *Proc Natl Acad Sci USA* 1991;88:2951–2955.
57. Danoff SK, Supattapone S, Snyder SH. Characterization of a membrane protein from brain mediating the inhibition of inositol 1,4,5-trisphosphate receptor binding. *Biochem J* 1988;254:701–705.

58. Dershwitz M, Sréter FA. Azumolene reverses episodes of malignant hyperthermia in susceptible swine. *Anesth Analg* 1990;70: 253–255.
59. Dettbarn C, Györke S, Palade P. Many agonists induce "quantal" Ca2+ release or adaptive behavior in muscle ryanodine receptors. *Mol Pharmacol* 1994;46:502–507.
60. Dettbarn C, Palade P. Effect of alkaline pH on sarcoplasmic reticulum Ca^{2+} release and Ca^{2+} uptake. *J Biol Chem* 1991;266:8993–9001.
61. Devine CE, Somylo AV, Somylo AP. Sarcoplasmic reticulum and excitation-contraction coupling in mammalian smooth muscle cells. *J Cell Biol* 1972;52:690–718.
62. Downes CP. Inositol phosphates: a family of signal molecules. *Trends Neurosci* 1988;11:336–339.
63. Dulhunty AF, Junankar PR, Stanhope C. Extra-junctional ryanodine receptors in the terminal cisternae of mammalian skeletal muscle fibres. *Proc R Soc Lond B* 1992;247:69–75.
64. Dwyer TM, Adams DJ, Hille B. The permeability of the endplate channel to organic cations in frog skeletal muscle. *J Gen Physiol* 1980;75:469–492.
65. Ebashi S, Endo M. Calcium ions and muscle contraction. *Prog Biophys Mol Biol* 1968;18:123–183.
66. Ehrlich BE, Kaftan E, Bezprozvannaya S, Bezprozvanny I. The pharmacology of intracellular Ca^{2+}-release channels. *Trends Pharmacol Sci* 1994;15:145–149.
67. Eilers J, Callewaert G, Armstrong C, Konnerth A. Calcium signaling in a narrow somatic submembrane shell during synaptic activity in cerebellar Purkinje neurons. *Proc Natl Acad Sci USA* 1995;92: 10272–10276.
68. El-Hayek R, Antoniu B, Wang J, Hamilton SL, Ikemoto N. Identification of calcium release-triggering and blocking regions of the II-III loop of the skeletal muscle dihydropyridine receptor. *J Biol Chem* 1995;270:22116–22118.
69. Ellis KO, Butterfield JL, Wessels FL, Carpenter JF. A comparison of skeletal, cardiac, and smooth muscle actions of dantrolene sodium-a skeletal muscle relaxant. *Arch Int Pharmacodyn* 1976;224: 118–132.
70. Ellis KO, Wessels FL, Carpenter JF. Effects of intravenous dantrolene sodium on respiratory and cardiovascular functions. *J Pharm Sci* 1976;65:1359–1364.
71. Endo M, Yagi S, Ishizuka T, Horiuti K, Koga Y, Amaha K. Changes in Ca-induced Ca release mechanism in the sarcoplasmic reticulum of the muscle from a patient with malignant hyperthermia. *Biomed Res* 1983;4:83–92.
72. England PJ. Intracellular calcium receptor mechanisms. *Br Med Bull* 1986;42:375–383.
73. Ervasti JM, Claessens MT, Mickelson JR, Louis CF. Altered transverse tubule dihydropyridine receptor binding in malignant hyperthermia. *J Biol Chem* 1989;264:2711–2717.
74. European Malignant Hyperpyrexia Group. A protocol for the investigation of malignant hyperpyrexia (MH) susceptibility. *Br J Anaesth* 1984;56:1267–1269.
75. Fabiato A. Calcium-induced release of calcium from the cardiac sarcoplasmic reticulum. *Am J Physiol* 1983;245:C1–C14.
76. Fano G, Biocca S, Fulle S, Mariggio MA, Belia S, Calissano P. The S-100: a protein family in search of a function. *Prog Neurobiol* 1995; 46:71–82.
77. Fasolato C, Innocenti B, Pozzan T. Receptor-activated Ca^{2+} how many mechanisms for how many channels? *Trends Pharmacol Sci* 1994;15:77–83.
78. Faulkner JA, Clafin DR, McCully KK, Jones DA. Contractile properties of bundles of fiber segments from skeletal muscles. *Am J Physiol* 1982;243:C66–C73.
79. Ferris CD, Snyder SH. Inositol 1,4,5-trisphosphate-activated calcium channels. *Annu Rev Physiol* 1992;54:469–488.
80. Fill M, Coronado R, Mickelson JR, et al. Abnormal ryanodine receptor channels in malignant hyperthermia. *Biophys J* 1990;57: 471–476.
81. Fleischer S, Inui M. Biochemistry and biophysics of excitation-contraction coupling. *Annu Rev Biophys Biophys Chem* 1989;8:333–364.
82. Fleischer S, Ogunbunmi EM, Dixon MC, Fleer EAM. Localization of Ca2+ release channels with ryanodine in junctional terminal cisternae of sarcoplasmic reticulum of fast skeletal muscle. *Proc Natl Acad Sci USA* 1985;82:7256–7259.
83. Fletcher JE, Conti PA, Rosenberg H. Comparison of North American and European malignant hyperthermia group halothane contracture testing protocols in swine. *Acta Anaesthesiol Scand* 1991;35: 483–487.
84. Fletcher JE, Erwin K, Karan SM, Rosenberg H. Elevated IP_3 in malignant hyperthermia (MH) muscle results from increase phospholipase C (PLC) activity (abstract). *Anesthesiology* 1995;83:A729.
85. Flewellen EH, Nelson TE, Jones WP, Arens JF, Wagner DL. Dantrolene dose response in awake man: implications for management of malignant hyperthermia. *Anesthesiology* 1983;59:275–280.
86. Flucher BE, Andrews SB, Fleischer S, Marks AR, Caswell A, Powell JA. Triad formation: organization and function of the sarcoplasmic reticulum calcium release channel and triadin in normal and dysgenic mice. *J Cell Biol* 1993;123:1161–1174.
87. Foster PS, Gessini E, Claudianos C, Hopkinson KC, Denborough MA. Inositol 1,4,5-triphosphate deficiency and malignant hyperpyrexia in swine. *Lancet* 1989;2(8655):124–127.
88. Frandsen A, Schousboe A. Dantrolene prevents glutamate cytotoxicity and Ca^{2+} release from intracellular stores in cultured cerebral cortical neurons. *J Neurochem* 1991;56:1075–1078.
89. Frandsen A, Schousboe A. Mobilization of dantrolene-sensitive intracellular calcium pools is involved in the cytotoxicity induced by quisqualate and *N*-methyl-D-aspartate but not by 2-amino-3-(3-hydroxy-5-methylisoxazol-4-yl)propionate and kainate in cultured cerebral cortical neurons. *Proc Natl Acad Sci USA* 1992;89: 2590–2594.
90. Frank JP, Harati Y, Butler IJ, Nelson TE, Scott CI. Central core disease and malignant hyperthermia syndrome. *Ann Neurol* 1979;7: 11–17.
91. Franzini-Armstrong C. Studies of the triad. I. Structure of the junction in frog twitch fibers. *J Cell Biol* 1970;47:488–499.
92. Franzini-Armstrong C, Kish JW. Alternate disposition of tetrads in peripheral couplings of skeletal muscle. *J Muscle Res Cell Motil* 1995;16:319–324.
93. Frazer MJ, Lynch C, III. Halothane and isoflurane effects on Ca^{2+} fluxes of isolated myocardial sarcoplasmic reticulum. *Anesthesiology* 1992;77:316–323.
94. Fruen BR, Mickelson JR, Shomer NH, Velez P, Louis CF. Cyclic ADP-ribose does not affect cardiac or skeletal muscle ryanodine receptors. *FEBS Lett* 1994;352:123–126.
95. Fujii J, Otsu K, Zorzato F, et al. Identification of a mutation in porcine ryanodine receptor associated with malignant hyperthermia. *Science* 1991;253:448–451.
96. Furuichi T, Furutama D, Hakamata Y, Nakai J, Takeshima H, Mikoshiba K. Multiple types of ryanodine receptor/Ca^{2+} release channels are differentially expressed in rabbit brain. *J Neurosci* 1994;14:4794–4805.
97. Furuichi T, Kohda K, Miyawaki A, Mikoshiba K. Intracellular channels. *Curr Opin Neurobiol* 1994;4:294–303.
98. Furuichi T, Mikoshiba K. Inositol 1,4,5-trisphosphate receptor-mediated Ca^{2+} signalling in brain. *J Neurochem* 1995;64:953–960.
99. Furuichi T, Yoshikawa S, Miyawaki A, Kentaroh W, Maeda N, Mikoshiba K. Primary structure and functional expression of the inositol 1,4,5-triposphate-binding protein P_{400}. *Nature* 1989;342: 32–38.
100. Gallant EM, Donaldson SK. Skeletal muscle excitation-contraction coupling. II. Plasmalemmal voltage control of intact bundle contractile properties in normal and malignant hyperthermic muscle. *Pflugers Arch* 1989;414:24–30.
101. Gallant EM, Fletcher TF, Goettl VM, Rempel WE. Porcine malignant hyperthermia: cell injury enhances halothane sensitivity of muscle biopsies. *Muscle Nerve* 1986;9:174–184.
102. Gallant EM, Gronert GA, Taylor SR. Cellular membrane potential and contracture threshold in mammalian skeletal muscle susceptible to malignant hyperthermia. *Neurosci Lett* 1982;28:181–186.
103. Gallant EM, Mickelson JR, Raggow BD, Donaldson SK, Louis CF, Rempel WE. Halothane-sensitivity gene and muscle contractile properties in malignant hyperthermia. *Am J Physiol* 1989;257: C781–C786.
104. Ghosh TK, Eis PA, Mullaney JM, Ebert CL, Gill DL. Competitive, reversible, and potent antagonism of inositol 1,4,5-triphosphate-activated calcium release by heparin. *J Biol Chem* 1988;263: 11075–11079.
105. Giannini G, Clementi E, Ceci R, Marziali G, Sorrentino V. Expression of a ryanodine receptor-Ca^{2+} channel that is regulated by TGF-β. *Science* 1992;257:91–94.
106. Gilchrist JSC, Czubryt MP, Pierce GN. Calcium and calcium-binding proteins in the nucleus. *Mol Cell Biochem* 1994;135:79–88.
107. Gill DL. Receptor kinships revealed. *Nature* 1989;342:16–18.
108. Gillard EF, Otsu K, Fujii J, et al. Polymorphisms and deduced amino acid substitutions in the coding sequence of the ryanodine receptor (RYR1) gene in individuals with malignant hyperthermia. *Genomics* 1992;13:1247–1254.

109. Gillard EF, Otsu K, Fujii J, et al. A substitution of cysteine for arginine 614 in the ryanodine receptor is potentially causative of human malignant hyperthermia. *Genomics* 1991;11:751–755.
110. Graf F, Schatzmann HH. Some effects of removal of external calcium on pig striated muscle. *J Physiol* 1984;349:1–13.
111. Gronert GA. Malignant hyperthermia. *Anesthesiology* 1980;53: 395–423.
112. Gronert GA, Milde JH, Theye RA. Dantrolene in porcine malignant hyperthermia. *Anesthesiology* 1976;44:488–495.
113. Gunter TE, Pfeiffer DL. Mechanisms by which mitochondria transport calcium. *Am J Physiol* 1990;258:C755–C786.
114. Guo W, Campbell KP. Association of triadin with the ryanodine receptor and calsequestrin in the lumen of the sarcoplasmic reticulum. *J Biol Chem* 1995;270:9027–9030.
115. Györke S, Fill M. Ryanodine receptor adaptation: control mechanism of Ca^{2+}-induced Ca^{2+} release in heart. *Science* 1993;260: 807–809.
116. Györke S, Palade P. Ca^{2+}-dependent negative control mechanism for Ca^{2+}-induced Ca^{2+} release in crayfish muscle. *J Physiol* 1994;476: 315–322.
117. Györke S, Vélez P, Suárez-Isla B, Fill M. Activation of single cardiac and skeletal ryanodine receptor channels by flash photolysis of caged Ca^{2+}. *Biophys J* 1994;66:1879–1886.
118. Hainaut K, Desmedt JE. Effect of dantrolene sodium on calcium movements in single muscle fibers. *Nature* 1974;252:728–730.
119. Hakamata Y, Nakai J, Takeshima H, Imoto K. Primary structure and distribution of a novel ryanodine receptor/calcium release channel from rabbit brain. *FEBS Lett* 1992;312:229–235.
120. Harnick DJ, Jayaraman T, Ma Y, Mulieri P, Go LO, Marks AR. The human type 1 inositol 1,4,5-trisphosphate receptor from T lymphocytes. *J Biol Chem* 1995;270:2833–2840.
121. Harris RA, Farmer B, Kim KC, Jenkins P. Action of halothane upon mitochondrial respiration. *Arch Biochem Biophys* 1971;142: 435–444.
122. Harrison GG. Control of the malignant hyperpyrexic syndrome in MHS swine by dantrolene sodium. *Br J Anaesth* 1975;47:62–75.
123. Heilbrunn LV, Wiercinski FJ. The action of various cations ion muscle protoplasm. *J Cell Comp Physiol* 1947;29:15–32.
124. Heizmann CW. Parvalbumin, an intracellular calcium-binding protein;distribution, properties and possible roles in mammalian cells. *Experientia* 1984;40:910–921.
125. Heizmann CW, Braun K. Changes in Ca^{2+}-binding proteins in human neurodegenerative disorders. *Trends Neurosci* 1992;15: 259–264.
126. Herland JS, Julian FJ, Stephenson DG. Halothane increases Ca^{2+} efflux via Ca^{2+} channels of sarcoplasmic reticulum in chemically skinned rat myocardium. *J Physiol* 1990;426:1–18.
127. Hermann A, Cox JA. Sarcoplasmic calcium-binding protein. *Comp Biochem Physiol* 1995;111B:337–345.
128. Herrington J, Park YB, Babcock DF, Hille B. Dominant role of mitochondria in calcium clearance from rat adrenal chromaffin cells (Abstract). *Biophys J* 1995;68:A230.
129. Hill AV. On the time required for diffusion and its relation to processes in muscle. *Proc R Soc Lond B* 1948;135:446–453.
130. Hill AV. The abrupt transition from rest to activity in muscle. *Proc R Soc Lond B* 1949;136:399–420.
131. Hill TD, Berggren P-O, Boynton AL. Heparin inhibits inositol trisphosphate-induced calcium release from permeabilized rat liver cells. *Biochem Biophys Res Commun* 1987;149:897–901.
132. Hogan K, Couch F, Powers PA, Gregg RG. A cysteine-for-arginine substitution (R614C) in the human skeletal muscle calcium release channel cosegregates with malignant hyperthermia. *Anesth Analg* 1992;75:441–448.
133. Holmberg SRM, Williams AJ. The cardiac sarcoplasmic reticulum calcium-release channel: modulation of ryanodine binding and single-channel activity. *Biochim Biophys Acta* 1990;1022:187–193.
134. Holmberg SRM, Williams AJ. Patterns of interaction between anthraquinone drugs and the calcium-release channel from cardiac sarcoplasmic reticulum. *Circ Res* 1990;67:272–283.
135. Holmberg SRM, Williams AJ. Phosphodiesterase inhibitors and the cardiac sarcoplasmic reticulum calcium release channel: differential effects of milrinone and enoximone. *Cardiovasc Res* 1991;25: 537–545.
136. Hossain MD, Evers AE. Volatile anesthetic-induced efflux of calcium from IP_3-gated stores in clonal (GH_3) pituitary cells. *Anesthesiology* 1994;80:1379–1389.
137. Hymel L, Inui M, Fleischer S, Schindler H. Purified ryanodine receptor of skeletal muscle sarcoplasmic reticulum forms Ca^{2+}-activated oligomeric Ca^{2+} channels in planar bilayers. *Proc Natl Acad Sci USA* 1988;85:441–445.
138. Iaizzo PA, Lehmann-Horn F. Anesthetic complications in muscle disorders. *Anesthesiology* 1995;82:1093–1096.
139. Iino M. Biphasic Ca^{2+} dependence of inositol 1,4,5-triphosphate-induced Ca release in smooth muscle cells of the guinea pig teania caeci. *J Gen Physiol* 1990;95:1103–1122.
140. Iino M, Kobayashi T, Endo M. Use of ryanodine for functional removal of the calcium store in smooth muscle cells of the guinea pig. *Biochem Biophys Res Commun* 1988;152:417–422.
141. Ikemoto N, Antoniu B, Kang J-J, Mészáros LG, Ronjat M. Intravesicular calcium transient during calcium release from sarcoplasmic reticulum. *Biochemistry* 1991;30:5230–5237.
142. Ikemoto N, Antoniu B, Mézáros LG. Rapid flow chemical quench studies of calcium release from isolated sarcoplasmic reticulum. *J Biol Chem* 1983;260:14096–14100.
143. Iles DE, Lehmann-Horn F, Scherer SW, et al. Localization of the gene encoding the α_2/δ-subunits of the L-type voltage-dependent calcium channel to chromosome 7q and analysis of the segregation of flanking markers in malignant hyperthermia susceptible families. *Hum Mol Genet* 1994;3:969–975.
144. Imagawa T, Smith JS, Coronado R, Campbell KP. Purified ryanodine receptor from skeletal muscle sarcoplasmic reticulum is the Ca^{2+}-permeable pore of the calcium release channel. *J Biol Chem* 1987;262:16636–16643.
145. Imredy JP, Yue DT. Submicroscopic Ca^{2+} diffusion mediates inhibitory coupling between individual Ca^{2+} channels. *Neuron* 1992;9:197–207.
146. Inui M, Saito A, Fleischer S. Isolation of the ryanodine receptor from cardiac sarcoplasmic reticulum and identity with the feet structures. *J Biol Chem* 1987;262:15643–15648.
147. Inui M, Saito A, Fleischer S. Purification of the ryanodine receptor and identity with feet structures of junctional terminal cisternae of sarcoplasmic reticulum from fast skeletal muscle. *J Biol Chem* 1987;262:1740–1747.
148. Irvine RF. Inositol phosphates and Ca^{2+} entry: toward a proliferation or a simplification? *FASEB J* 1992;6:3085–3090.
149. Irvine RF, Moor RM. Microinjection of inositol 1,3,4,5-tetrakisphosphate activates sea urchin eggs by a mechanism dependent on external Ca^{2+}. *Biochem J* 1986;240:917–920.
150. Isaacs HI, Badenhorst M. False negative results with muscle caffeine halothane contracture testing for malignant hyperthermia. *Anesthesiology* 1993;79:5–9.
151. Jayaraman T, Brillantes A, Timerman A, et al. FK506 binding protein associated with the calcium release channel (ryanodine receptor). *J Biol Chem* 1992;267:9474–9477.
152. Jenden DJ, Fairhurst AS. The pharmacology of ryanodine. *Pharmacol Rev* 1969;21:1–25.
153. Johnson K. Malignant hyperthermia hots up! *Hum Mol Genet* 1993; 2:849.
154. Jorgenson AO, Shen AC-Y, Arnold W, McPherson PS, Campbell KP. The Ca^{2+} release channel/ryanodine receptor is localized in junctional and corbular sarcoplasmic reticulum in cardiac muscle. *J Cell Biol* 1993;120:969–980.
155. Jouaville LS, Ichas F, Holmuhamedov EL, Camacho P, Lechleiter JD. Synchronization of calcium waves by mitochondrial substrates in *Xenopus laevis* oocytes. *Nature* 1995;377:438–441.
156. Kasai M, Kawasaki T. Effects of ryanodine on permeability of choline and glucose through calcium channels in sarcoplasmic reticulum vesicles. *Biochem J* 1993;113:327–333.
157. Kasai M, Kawasaki T, Yamamoto K. Permeation of neutral molecules through calcium channel in sarcoplasmic reticulum vesicles. *Biochem J* 1992;112:197–203.
158. Katsuoka M, Kobayashi K, Ohnishi T. Volatile anesthetics decrease calcium content of isolated myocytes. *Anesthesiology* 1989;70: 954–960.
159. Katsuoka M, Ohnishi ST. Inhalation anaesthetics decrease calcium content of cardiac sarcoplasmic reticulum. *Br J Anaesth* 1989;62: 669–673.
160. Katz NL, Ingenito A, Procita L. Ryanodine-induced contractile failure of skeletal muscle. *J Pharmacol Exp Ther* 1970;171:242–248.
161. Kawana Y, IIno M, Horiuti K, et al. Acceleration in calcium-induced calcium release in the biopsied muscle fibers from patients with malignant hyperthermia. *Biomed Res* 1992;13: 287–292.
162. Kawano S, Kiraoka M. Protein kinase A-activated chloride channel is inhibited by the Ca^{2+}-calmodulin complex in cardiac sarcoplasmic reticulum. *Circ Res* 1993;73:751–757.

163. Kawano S, Nakamura F, Tanaka T, Kiraoka M. Cardiac sarcoplasmic reticulum chloride channels regulated by protein kinase A. *Circ Res* 1992;71:585–589.
164. Keating KE, Quane KA, Manning BM, et al. Detection of a novel RYR1 mutation in four malignant hyperthermia pedigrees. *Hum Mol Genet* 1994;3:1855–1856.
165. Kijima Y, Saito A, Jetton TL, Magnuson MA, Fleischer S. Different intracellular localization of inositol 1,4,5-triphosphate and ryanodine receptors in cardiomyocytes. *J Biol Chem* 1993;268:3499–3506.
166. Kirino Y, Osakabe M, Shimizu H. Ca^{2+}-induced Ca^{2+} release from fragmented sarcoplasmic reticulum: Ca^{2+}-dependent passive efflux. *J Biochem(Tokyo)* 1983;94:1111–1118.
167. Kissin I, Aultman DF, Smith LR. Effects of volatile anesthetics on myocardial oxidation-reduction status assessed by NADH fluorometry. *Anesthesiology* 1983;59:447–452.
168. Klee CB, Vanamo TC. Calmodulin. In: Anfinsen CB, Edsall JT, Richards FM, eds. *Advances in protein chemistry*, vol 35. New York: Academic Press, 1982;213–321.
169. Knudson CM, Chaudhari N, Sharp AH, Powell JA, Beam KG, Campbell KP. Specific absence of the a1 subunit of the dihydropyridine receptor in mice with muscular dysgenesis. *J Biol Chem* 1989;264:1345–1348.
170. Knudson CM, Stang KK, Jorgensen AO, Campbell KP. Biochemical characterization and ultrastructural localization of a major junctional sarcoplasmic reticulum glycoprotein (triadin). *J Biol Chem* 1993;268:12637–12645.
171. Kobayashi S, Kitazawa T, Somlyo AV, Somlyo AP. Cytosolic heparin inhibits muscarinic and α-adrenergic Ca^{2+} release in smooth muscle. *J Biol Chem* 1989;264:17997–18004.
172. Kobayashi S, Somlyo AV, Somlyo AP. Heparin inhibits the inositol 1,4,5-trisphosphate-dependent, but not the independent, calcium release induced by guanine nucleotide in vascular smooth muscle. *Biochem Biophys Res Commun* 1988;153:625–631.
173. Kochs E, Hoffman WE, Roewer N, Schulte Am Esch J. Alterations in brain electrical activity may indicate the onset of of malignant hyperthermia in swine. *Anesthesiology* 1993;73:1236–1242.
174. Kolb ME, Horne ML, Martz R. Dantrolene in human malignant hyperthermia—a multicenter trial. *Anesthesiology* 1982;56:254–262.
175. Komai H, Rusy BF. Effect of halothane on rested-state and potentiated state contraction in rabbit papillary muscle relationship to negative inotropic effect. *Anesth Analg* 1982;61:403–409.
176. Komai H, Rusy BF. Negative inotropic effects of isoflurane and halothane in rabbit papillary muscles. *Anesth Analg* 1987;66:29–33.
177. Kotsias BA, Muchnik S. Reversible effect of dantrolene sodium on twitch tension of rat skeletal muscle. *Arch Neurol* 1978;35:234–236.
178. Kretsinger RH. Structure and evolution of calcium-modulated proteins. *CRC Critical Reviews in Biochemistry* 1980;8:119–174.
179. Kuwajima G, Futatsugi A, Ninobe M, Nakanishi S, Mikoshiba K. Two types of ryanodine receptors in mouse brain: skeletal muscle type exclusively in Purkinje cells and cardiac muscle type in various neurons. *Neuron* 1992;9:1133–1142.
180. Lai FA, Anderson K, Rousseau E, Liu Q-Y, Meissner G. Evidence for a Ca^{2+} channel within the ryanodine receptor complex from cardiac sarcoplasmic reticulum. *Biochem Biophys Res Commun* 1988;151: 441–449.
181. Lai FA, Erickson LP, Rousseau E, Liu Q-Y, Meissner G. Purification and reconstitution of the calcium release channel from skeletal muscle. *Nature* 1988;331:315–319.
182. Larach MG. Should we use muscle biopsy to diagnose malignant hyperthermia susceptibility. *Anesthesiology* 1993;79:1–4.
183. Larach MG, North American Malignant Hyperthermia Group. Standardization of the caffeine halothane muscle contracture test. *Anesth Analg* 1989;69:511–515.
184. Latorre R, Miller C. Conduction and selectivity in potassium channels. *J Membr Biol* 1983;71:11–30.
185. Leary NP, Ellis FR. Masseteric muscle spasm as a normal response to suxamethonium. *Br J Anaesth* 1990;64:488–492.
186. Ledbetter MW, Preiner JK, Louis CF, Mickelson JR. Tissue distribution of ryanodine receptor isoforms and alleles determined by reverse transcription polymerase chain reaction. *J Biol Chem* 1994; 269:31544–31551.
187. Lee HC, Aarhus R, Graeff RM. Sensitization of calcium-induced calcium release by cyclic ADP-ribose and calmodulin. *J Biol Chem* 1995;270:9060–9066.
188. Lehmann-Horn F, Iaizzo PA. Are myotonias and periodic paralyses associated with susceptibility to malignant hyperthermia. *Br J Anaesth* 1990;65:692–697.
189. Lehmann-Horn F, Iaizzo PA. Resealed fiber segments for the study of the pathophysiology of human skeletal muscle. *Muscle Nerve* 1990;13:222–231.
190. Lei SZ, Zhang D, Abele AE, Lipton SA. Blockade of NMDA receptor-mediated mobilization of intracellular Ca^{2+} prevents neurotoxicity. *Brain Res* 1992;598:196–202.
191. Leslie GC, Part NJ. Effects of dantrolene sodium on twitch contractions of intrafusal and extrafusal muscle in rat. *J Physiol* 1980; 301:776–778.
192. Levin A, Blanck TJJ. Halothane and isoflurane alter the Ca^{2+} binding properties of calmodulin. *Anesthesiology* 1995;83:120–126.
193. Levitt RC. Prospects for the diagnosis of malignant hyperthermia susceptibility using molecular genetic approaches. *Anesthesiology* 1992;76:1039–1048.
194. Lindsay ARG, Manning SD, Williams AJ. Monovalent cation conductance in the ryanodine receptor-channel of sheep cardiac muscle sarcoplasmic reticulum. *J Physiol* 1991;439:463–480.
195. Lindsay ARG, Williams AJ. Functional characterisation of the ryanodine receptor purified from sheep cardiac muscle sarcoplasmic reticulum. *Biochim Biophys Acta* 1991;1064:89–102.
196. Linse S, Forsén S. Determinants that govern high-affinity calcium binding. In: Means AR, Greengard P, Nairn AC, Shenolikar S, eds. *Advances in second messenger and phosphoprotein research*, vol 30. New York: Raven Press, 1995;89–151.
197. Littleford JA, Patel LR, Bose D, Cameron CB, McKillop C. Masseter muscle spasm in children: implications of continuing the triggering anesthetic. *Anesth Analg* 1991;72:151–160.
198. Liu G, Pessah IN. Molecular interaction between ryanodine receptor and glycoprotein triadin involves redox cycling of functionally important hyperreactive sulfhydryls. *J Biol Chem* 1994;269:33028–33034.
199. López J, Alamo L, Caputo C, Wikinski J, Ledezma D. Intracellular ionized calcium concentration in muscles from humans with malignant hyperthermia. *Muscle Nerve* 1985;8:355–358.
200. López JR, Alamo LA, Jones DE, et al. $[Ca^{2+}]_i$ in muscles of malignant hyperthermia susceptible pigs determined in vivo with Ca^{2+} selective microelectrodes. *Muscle Nerve* 1986;9:85–86.
201. López JR, Allen PD, Alamo L, Jones D, Sreter F. Myoplasmic free $[Ca^{2+}]$ during a malignant hyperthermia episode in swine. *Muscle Nerve* 1988;11:82–88.
202. López JR, Allen PD, Alamo L, Ryan JF, Jones DE, Sreter F. Dantrolene prevents the malignant hyperthermic syndrome by reducing free intracellular calcium concentration in skeletal muscle of susceptible swine. *Cell Calcium* 1987;8:385–396.
203. López JR, Medina P, Alamo L. Dantrolene sodium is able to reduce the resting ionic $[Ca^{2+}]_i$ in muscle from humans with malignant hyperthermia. *Muscle Nerve* 1987;10:77–79.
204. Louis CF, Roghair T, Mickelson JR. Volatile anesthetics inhibit dihydropyridine binding to malignant hyperthermia-susceptible and normal pig skeletal muscle membranes. *Anesthesiology* 1994; 80:618–624.
205. Louis CF, Zualkernan K, Roghair T, Mickelson JR. The effects of volatile anesthetics on calcium regulation by malignant hyperthermia-susceptible sarcoplasmic reticulum. *Anesthesiology* 1992; 77:114–125.
206. Lückhoff A, Clapham DE. Inositol 1,3,4,5-tetrakisphosphate activates an endothelial Ca^{2+}-permeable channel. *Nature* 1992;355: 356–358.
207. Lynch C, III, Frazer MJ. Anesthetic alteration of ryanodine binding by cardiac calcium release channels. *Biochim Biophys Acta* 1994; 1194:109–117.
208. Ma J, Fill M, Knudson M, Campbell KP, Coronado R. Ryanodine receptor of skeletal muscle is a gap junction-type channel. *Science* 1988;242:99–102.
209. Ma J, Zhao J. Highly cooperative and hysteretic response of the skeletal muscle ryanodine receptor to changes in proton concentration. *Biophys J* 1994;67:626–633.
210. Mack MM, Molinski TF, Buck ED, Pessah IN. Novel modulators of skeletal muscle FKBP12/calcium channel complex from *Ianthella basta*. *J Biol Chem* 1994;269:23236–23249.
211. Mack MM, Zimanyi I, Pessah IN. Discrimination of multiple binding sites for antagonists of the calcium release channel complex of skeletal and cardiac sarcoplasmic reticulum. *J Pharmacol Exp Ther* 1992;262:1028–1037.
212. MacLennan DH. Molecular tools to elucuidate problems in excitation-contraction coupling. *Biophys J* 1990;58:1355–1365.
213. MacLennan DH, Campbell KP, Reithmeier RAF. *Calsequestrin. Calcium and cell function,* vol 4. New York: Academic Press, 1983.

214. MacLennan DH, Phillips MS. The role of skeletal muscle ryanodine receptor (RYR1) gene in malignant hyperthermia and central core disease. In: Dawson DC, Frizzell RA, eds. *Ion channels and genetic diseases.* Society of General Physiologists Series, vol 50. New York: Rockefeller University Press, 1995;89–100.
215. MacLennan DH, Wong PTS. Isolation of a calcium-sequestering protein from sarcoplasmic reticulum. *Proc Natl Acad Sci USA* 1971; 68:1213–1235.
216. Margath A, Damiani E, Tobaldin G. Ratio of dihydropyridine to ryanodine receptors in mammalian and frog twitch muscles in relation to the mechanical hypothesis of excitation-contraction coupling. *Biochem Biophys Res Commun* 1993;197:1303–1311.
217. Marks A, Fleischer S, Tempst P. Surface topography analysis of the ryanodine receptor/junctional channel complex based on proteolysis sensitivity mapping. *J Biol Chem* 1990;265:13143–13149.
218. Marks AR. The calcium channels expressed in vascular smooth muscle. *Circulation* 1992;86(6 suppl):III61–III67.
219. Marks AR, Tempst P, Hwang KS, et al. Molecular cloning and characterization of the ryanodine receptor/junctional channel complex cDNA from skeletal muscle sarcoplasmic reticulum. *Proc Natl Acad Sci USA* 1989;86:8683–8687.
220. Martinez-Azorin F, Gomez-Fernandez JC, Fernandez-Belda F. Limited carbodiimide derivatization modifies some functional properties of the sarcoplasmic reticulum Ca^{2+} release channel. *Biochemistry* 1993;32:8553–8559.
221. Marty I, Robert M, Villaz M, et al. Biochemical evidence for a complex involving dihydropyridine receptor and ryanodine receptor in triad junctions of skeletal muscle. *Proc Natl Acad Sci USA* 1994;91:2270–2274.
222. McCormack JG, Denton RM. Role of Ca^{2+} ions in the regulation of intramitochondrial metabolism in rat heart. Evidence from studies with isolated mitochondria that adrenalin activates the pyruvate and 2-oxyglutarate dehydrogenase complexes by increasing the intramitochondrial concentration of Ca^{2+}. *Biochem J* 1990; 218:235–247.
223. McCormack JG, Halestrap AP, Denton RM. Role of calcium ions in regulation of mammalian intramitochondrial metabolism. *Physiol Rev* 1990;70:391–425.
224. McPhalen CA, Strynadka NCJ, James MNG. Calcium-binding sites in proteins: a structural perspective. *Adv Protein Chem* 1991;42: 77–144.
225. McPherson E, Taylor Jr CA. The genetics of malignant hyperthermia: evidence for heterogeneity. *Am J Med Genetics* 1982;11:273–285.
226. McPherson PS, Campbell KP. The ryanodine receptor/Ca^{2+} release channel. *J Biol Chem* 1993;268:13765–13768.
227. Meissner G. Adenine nucleotide stimulation of Ca^{2+}-induced Ca^{2+} release in sarcoplasmic reticulum. *J Biol Chem* 1984;259:2365–2374.
228. Meissner G, Darling E, Eveleth J. Kinetics of rapid Ca^{2+} release by sarcoplasmic reticulum. Effects of Ca^{2+}, Mg^{2+}, and adenine nucleotides. *Biochemistry* 1986;25:236–244.
229. Melton AT, Martucci RW, Kien ND, Gronert GA. Malignant hyperthermia in humans—standardization of contracture testing protocol. *Anesth Analg* 1989;69:437–443.
230. Mészáros LG, Bak J, Chu A. Cyclic ADP-ribose as an endogenous regulator of the non-skeletal type ryanodine receptor Ca^{2+} channel. *Nature* 1993;364:76–79.
231. Meyer T, Holowka D, Stryer L. Highly cooperative opening of calcium channels by inositol 1,4,5-trisphosphate. *Science* 1988;240: 653–656.
232. Meyer T, Wensel T, Stryer L. Kinetics of channel opening by inositol 1,4,5-trisphosphate. *Biochemistry* 1990;29:32–37.
233. Michalek M, Dupraz P, Shoshan-Rarmatz V. Ryanodine binding to sarcoplasmic reticulum membrane;comparison between cardiac and skeletal muscle. *Biochim Biophys Acta* 1988;939:587–594.
234. Michikawa T, Hamanaka H, Otsu H, et al. Transmembrane topology and sites of N-glycosylation of inositol 1,4,5-triphosphate receptor. *J Biol Chem* 1994;269:9184–9189.
235. Mickelson JR, Gallant EM, Litterer LA, Johnson KM, Rempel WE, Louis CF. Abnormal sarcoplasmic reticulum ryanodine receptor in malignant hyperthermia. *J Biol Chem* 1988;263: 9310–9315.
236. Mignery GA, Johnson PA, Südhof TC. Mechanism of Ca^{2+} inhibition of inositol 1,4,5-triphosphate ($InsP_3$) binding to the cerebellar $InsP_3$ receptor. *J Biol Chem* 1992;267:7450–7455.
237. Mignery GA, Newton CL, Archer BT, III, Südhof TC. Structure and expression of the rat inositol 1,4,5-triphosphate receptor. *J Biol Chem* 1990;265:12679–12685.
238. Mignery GA, Südhof TC. The ligand binding site and transduction mechanism in the inositol-1,4,5-triphosphate receptor. *EMBO J* 1990;9:3893–3898.
239. Miller C. Voltage-gated cation conductance channel from fragmented sarcoplasmic reticulum: steady state electrical properties. *J Membr Biol* 1978;40:1–23.
240. Miller RJ. The control of neuronal Ca^{2+} homeostasis. *Prog Neurobiol* 1991;37:255–285.
241. Milner RE, Baksh S, Shemanko C, et al. Calreticulin, and not calsequestrin, is the major calcium binding protein of smooth muscle sarcoplasmic reticulum and liver endoplasmic reticulum. *J Biol Chem* 1991;266:7155–7165.
242. Milner RE, Famulski KS, Michalak M. Calcium binding proteins in the sarcoplasmic/endoplasmic reticulum of muscle and nonmuscle cells. *Mol Cell Biochem* 1992;112:1–13.
243. Mitchell MM, Ali HH, Savarese JJ. Myotonia and neuromuscular blocking agents. *Anesthesiology* 1978;49:44–48.
244. Moews PC, Kretsinger RH. Refinement of the structure of carp muscle calcium-binding parvalbumin by model building and difference fourier analysis. *J Mol Biol* 1975;91:201ff.
245. Monkawa T, Miyawaki A, Sugiyama T, et al. Heterotetrameric complex formation of inositol 1,4,5-trisphosphate receptor subunits. *J Biol Chem* 1995;270:14700–14704.
246. Morgan KG, Bryant SH. The mechanism of action of dantrolene sodium. *J Pharmacol Exp Ther* 1977;201:138–147.
247. Morrissette J, Heisermann G, Cleary J, Ruoho A, Coronado R. Cyclic ADP-ribose induced Ca^{2+} release in rabbit skeletal muscle sarcoplasmic reticulum. *FEBS Lett* 1993;330:270–274.
248. Moschella MC, Marks AR. Inositol 1,4,5-trisphosphate receptor expression in cardiac myocytes. *J Cell Biol* 1993;120:1137–1146.
249. Moschella MC, Marks AR. Inositol 1,4,5-trisphosphate receptor in skeletal muscle: differential expression in myofibres. *J Muscle Res Cell Motil* 1995;16:390–400.
250. Mourey RJ, Verma A, Supattapone S, Snyder SH. Purification and characterization of the inositol 1,4,5-trisphosphate receptor protein from rat vas deferens. *Biochem J* 1990;272:383–389.
251. Nagasaki K, Fleischer S. Ryanodine sensitivity of the calcium release channel of sarcoplasmic reticulum. *Cell Calcium* 1988;9:1–7.
252. Nahrwold ML, Cohen PJ. The effects of forane and fluroxene on mitochondrial respiration. *Anesthesiology* 1973;38:437–444.
253. Nakade S, Maeda N, Mikoshiba K. Involvement of the *C*-terminus of the inositol 1,4,5-trisphosphate receptor in Ca^{2+} release analyzed using region-specific monoclonal antibodies. *Biochem J* 1991; 277:125–131.
254. Nakagaki K, Kasai M. Fast release of calcium from fragmented sarcoplasmic reticulum: steady-state electrical properties. *J Biochem (Tokyo)* 1983;94:1101–1108.
255. Nakagawa T, Okano H, Furuichi T, Aruga J, Mikoshiba K. The subtypes of inositol 1,4,5-triphosphate receptors are expressed in a tissue-specific and developmentally specific manner. *Proc Natl Acad Sci USA* 1991;88:6244–6248.
256. Nakayama S, Kretsinger RH. Evolution of the EF-Hand family of proteins. *Annu Rev Biophys Struct* 1994;23:473–507.
257. Nelsestuen GL, Bazzi MD. Activation and regulation of protein kinase C enzymes. *J Bioenerg Biomem* 1991;23:43–61.
258. Nelson TE. Abnormality in calcium release from skeletal sarcoplasma reticulum of pigs susceptible to malignant hyperthermia. *J Clin Invest* 1983;72:862–870.
259. Nelson TE. Halothane effect on calcium release channel from human malignant hyperthermia skeletal muscle. *Biophys J* 1991;59: 85a.
260. Nelson TE. Malignant hyperthermia in dogs. *J Am Vet Med Assoc* 1991;198:989–994.
261. Nelson TE, Jones EW, Hendrickson RL. Porcine malignant hyperthermia: observations on the occurrence of pale, soft exudative musculature among susceptible pigs. *Am J Vet Res* 1974;35:347–350.
262. Nelson TE, Lin M. Abnormal function of porcine malignant hyperthermia calcium release channel in the absence and presence of halothane. *Cell Physiol Biochem* 1995;5:10–22.
263. Neylon CB, Richards SM, Larsen MA, Agrotis A, Bobik A. Multiple types of ryanodine receptor/Ca2+ release channels are expressed in vascular smooth muscle. *Biochem Biophys Res Commun* 1995; 215:814–821.
264. Nishizuka Y. Protein kinases 5: protein kinase C and lipid signalling for sustained cellular responses. *FASEB J* 1995;9:484–496.
265. Nixon GF, Mignery GA, Somlyo AV. Immunogold localization of inositol 1,4,5-triphosphate receptors and characterization of ultra-

structural features of the sarcoplasmic reticulum in phasic and smooth muscle. *J Muscle Res Cell Motil* 1994;15:682–700.
266. Nosaka S, Kamaya H, Ueda I, Wong KC. Smooth muscle contraction and local anesthetics: calmodulin-dependent myosin light-chain kinase. *Anesth Analg* 1989;69:504–510.
267. Obenaus A, Mody I, Baimbridge KG. Dantrolene-Na (Dantrium) blocks induction of long-term potentiation in hippocampal slices. *Neurosci Lett* 1989;98:172–178.
268. Ohnishi ST, Taylor S, Gronert GA. Calcium-induced Ca^{2+} release from sarcoplasmic reticulum of pigs susceptible to malignant hyperthermia. The effects of halothane and dantrolene. *FEBS Lett* 1983;161:103–107.
269. Otsu K, Willard HF, Khanna VK, Zorzato F, Green NM, MacLennan DH. Molecular cloning of cDNA encoding of the Ca^{2+} release channel (ryanodine receptor) of rabbit cardiac muscle sarcoplasmic reticulum. *J Biol Chem* 1990;265:13472–13483.
270. Palade P. Drug-induced Ca^{2+} release from isolated sarcoplasmic reticulum: I. use of pyrophosphate to study caffeine-induced Ca^{2+} release. *J Biol Chem* 1987;262:6135–6141.
271. Palade P. Drug-induced Ca^{2+} release from isolated sarcoplasmic reticulum: II. releases involving Ca^{2+} induced Ca^{2+} release channel. *J Biol Chem* 1987;262:6142–6148.
272. Palade P. Drug-induced Ca^{2+} release from isolated sarcoplasmic reticulum: III. block of Ca^{2+} induced Ca^{2+} by organic polyamines. *J Biol Chem* 1987;262:6149–6154.
273. Palnitkar SS, Parness J. Partial purification of the dantrolene receptor from skeletal muscle: non-identity with the ryanodine receptor (abstract). *Anesthesiology* 1995;83:A729.
274. Parness J, Palnitkar SS. Identification of dantrolene binding sites in porcine skeletal muscle sarcoplasmic reticulum. *J Biol Chem* 1995;270:18465–18472.
275. Patel JR, Coronado R, Moss RL. Cardiac sarcoplasmic reticulum phosphorylation increases Ca^{2+} release induced by flash photolysis of Nitr-5. *Circ Res* 1995;77:943–949.
276. Persechini A, Moncrief ND, Kretsinger RH. The EF-hand family of calcium-modulated proteins. *Trends Neurosci* 1989;12:462–467.
277. Peskoff A, Post JA, Langer GA. Sarcolemmal calcium binding sites in heart: II. Mathematical model for diffusion of calcium release from the sarcoplasmic reticulum into the diadic region. *J Membr Biol* 1992;129:59–69.
278. Pessah IN, Durie EM, Schiedt MJ, Zimanyi I. Anthraquinone-sensitized Ca^{2+} release channel from rat cardiac sarcoplasmic reticulum: possible receptor-mediated mechanism of doxorubicin cardiomyopathy. *Mol Pharmacol* 1990;37:503–514.
279. Pessah IN, Francini AO, Scales DJ, Waterhouse AL, Casida JE. Calcium-ryanodine receptor complex. Solubilization and partial characterization from skeletal muscle junctional sarcoplasmic reticulum vesicles. *J Biol Chem* 1986;261:8643–8648.
280. Pessah IN, Lynch C, III, Gronert GA. The complex pharmacology of malignant hyperthermia (Editorial). *Anesthesiology* 1996;84: 1275–1279.
281. Pessah IN, Stambuk RA, Casida JE. Ca^{2+}-activated ryanodine binding: mechanisms of sensitivity and intensity modulation by Mg^{2+}, caffeine and adenine nucleotides. *Mol Pharmacol* 1987;31:232–238.
282. Pessah IN, Waterhouse AL, Casida JE. The calcium-ryanodine receptor complex of skeletal and cardiac muscle. *Biochem Biophys Res Commun* 1985;128:449–456.
283. Pessah IN, Zimanyi I. Characterization of multiple [^{3}H]ryanodine binding sites on the Ca^{2+} release channel of the sarcoplasmic reticulum from skeletal and cardiac muscle: evidence for a sequential mechanism in ryanodine action. *Mol Pharmacol* 1991; 39:679–689.
284. Phillips MS, Khanna VK, De Leaon S, Frodis W, Britt BA, MacLennan DH. The substitution of Arg for Gly2433 in the human skeletal muscle ryanodine receptor is associated with malignant hyperthermia. *Hum Mol Genet* 1994;3:2181–2186.
285. Porter KR, Palade GE. Studies on the Endoplasmic Reticulum III: Its Form and Distribution in Striated Muscle Cells. *J Biophys Biochem Cytol* 1957;3:269–299.
286. Post JA, Langer GA. Sarcolemmal calcium binding sites in heart: I. Molecular origin in "gas dissected" sarcolemma. *J Membr Biol* 1992;129:49–57.
287. Prabhu SD, Salama G. The heavy metal ions Ag^+ and Hg^{2+} trigger calcium release from cardiac sarcoplasmic reticulum. *Arch Biochem Biophys* 1990;277:47–55.
288. Putney JW. Capacitative Calcium Entry Revisited. 1990;11: 611–624.
289. Quane KA, Healy JMS, Keating KE, et al. Mutations in the ryanodine receptor gene in central core disease and malignant hyperthermia. *Nature Genet* 1993;5:51–55.
290. Quane KA, Keating KE, Healy JM, et al. Mutation of the RYR1 gene in malignant hyperthermia: detection of a novel Tyr to Ser mutation in a pedigre with associated central cores. *Genomics* 1994;23:236–239.
291. Quane KA, Keating KE, Manning BM, et al. Detection of a novel common mutation in the ryanodine receptor gene in malignant hyperthermia: implications for diagnosis and heterogeneity studies. *Hum Mol Genet* 1994;3:471–476.
292. Radermacher M, Rao V, Grassucci R, et al. Cryo-electron microscopy and three-dimensional reconstruction of the calcium release channel/ryanodine receptor from skeletal muscle. *J Cell Biol* 1994;127: 411–423.
293. Radermacher M, Wagenknecht T, Grassucci R, et al. Cryo-EM of the native structure of the calcium release channel/ryanodine receptor from sarcoplasmic reticulum. *Biophys J* 1992;61:936–940.
294. Rardon DP, Cefali DC, Mitchell RD, Seiler SM, Jones LR. High molecular weight proteins purified from cardiac junctional sarcoplasmic reticulum vesicles are ryanodine-sensitive calcium channels. *Circ Res* 1989;64:779–789.
295. Ren K, Ruda MA. A comparative study of the calcium-binding proteins calbindin-D28K, calretinin, calmodulin and parvalbumin in the rat spinal cord. *Brain Res Rev* 1994;19:163–179.
296. Rizzuto B, Brini M, Murgia M, Pozzan T. Microdomains with high Ca^{2+} close to IP_3-sensitive channels that are sensed by neighboring mitochondria. *Science* 1995;262:744–747.
297. Robertson SP, Johnson DJ, Potter JD. The time-course of Ca2+ exchange with calmodulin, troponin, parvalbumin, and myosin in response to transient increases in Ca2+. *Biophys J* 1981;34:559–569.
298. Roewer N, Dziadzka A, Greim CA, Kraas E, Schulte am Esch J. Cardiovascular and metabolic responses to anesthetic-induced malignant hyperthermia in swine. *Anesthesiology* 1995;83:141–159.
299. Ross CA, Danoff SK, Schell MJ, Snyder SH, Ullrich A. Three additional inositol 1,4,5-trisphosphate receptors: molecular cloning and differential localization in brain and peripheral tissues. *Proc Natl Acad Sci USA* 1992;89:4265–4269.
300. Rossier MF, Putney JW, Jr. The identity of the calcium-storing, inositol 1,4,5-trisphosphate-sensitive organelle in non-muscle cells: calciosome, endoplasmic reticulum...or both? *Trends Neurosci* 1991;14:310–314.
301. Rousseau E. Single chloride-selective channel from cardiac sarcoplasmic reticulum studied in planar bilayers. *J Membr Biol* 1989; 110:39–47.
302. Rousseau E, Chabot H, Beaudry C, Muller B. Reconstitution and regulation of cation-selective channels from cardiac sarcoplasmic reticulum. *Mol Cell Biochem* 1992;114:109–117.
303. Rousseau E, Meissner G. Single cardiac sarcoplasmic reticulum Ca^{2+}-release channel: activation by caffeine. *Am J Physiol* 1989;256: H328–H333.
304. Rousseau E, Pinkos J. pH modulates conductance and gating behavior of single calcium release channels. *Pflugers Arch* 1990;415: 645–647.
305. Rousseau E, Smith JS, Henderson JS, Meissner G. Single channel and $^{45}Ca^{2+}$flux measurements of the cardiac sarcoplasmic reticulum calcium channel. *Biophys J* 1986;50:1009–1014.
306. Rousseau E, Smith JS, Meissner G. Ryanodine modifies conductance and gating behavior of single Ca^{2+} release channel. *Am J Physiol* 1987;253:C364–C368.
307. Schneider M, Chandler W. Voltage dependent charge movement in skeletal muscle: a possible step in excitation-contraction coupling. *Nature* 1973;242:244–246.
308. Schrenzel J, Demaurex N, Foti M, et al. Highly cooperative Ca^{2+} elevations in response to Ins(1,4,5)P_3 microperfusion through a patch-clamp pipette. *Biophys J* 1995;69:2378–2391.
309. Sharp AH, McPherson PS, Dawson TM, Aoki C, Campbell KP, Snyder SH. Differential immunohistochemical localization of inositol 1,4,5-triphosphate and ryanodine-sensitive Ca^{2+} release channels in rat brain. *J Neurosci* 1993;13:3051–3063.
310. Shomer NH, Louis CF, Fill M, Litterer LA, Mickelson JR. Reconstitution of abnormalities in the malignant hyperthermia-susceptible pig ryanodine receptor. *Am J Physiol* 1993;264:C125–C135.
311. Shomer NH, Mickelson JR, Louis CF. Caffeine stimulation of malignant hyperthermia-susceptible sarcoplasmic reticulum Ca^{2+} release channel. *Am J Physiol* 1994;267:C1253–C1261.
312. Shomer NH, Mickelson JR, Louis CF. Ion selectivity of porcine

skeletal muscle Ca^{2+} release channels is unaffected by the Arg615 to Cys615 mutation. *Biophys J* 1994;67:641–646.
313. Shomer NH, Mickelson JR, Louis CF. Ca^{2+} release channels of pigs heterozygous for malignant hyperthermia. *Muscle Nerve* 1995;18: 1167–1176.
314. Sitsapesan R, McGarry SJ, Williams AJ. Cyclic ADP-ribose competes with ATP for the adenine nucleotide binding site on the cardiac ryanodine receptor Ca^{2+}-release channel. *Circ Res* 1994;75: 596–600.
315. Small DL, Monette R, Mealing G, Buchan AM, Morley P. Neuroprotective effects of ω-Aga-IVA against *in vitro* ischaemia in the rat hippocampal slice. *NeuroReport* 1995;6:1617–1620.
316. Smith JS, Coronado R, Meissner G. Sarcoplasmic reticulum contains adenine nucleotide-activated channels. *Nature* 1985;316: 446–449.
317. Smith JS, Coronado R, Meissner G. Single channel measurements of the calcium release channel from skeletal muscle sarcoplasmic reticulum. *J Gen Physiol* 1986;88:573–588.
318. Smith JS, Coronado R, Meissner G. Single-channel calcium and barium currents of large and small conductance from sarcoplasmic reticulum. *Biophys J* 1986;50:921–928.
319. Smith JS, Imagawa T, Ma J, Fill M, Campbell KP, Coronado R. Purified ryanodine receptor from rabbit skeletal muscle is the calcium-release channel of sarcoplasmic reticulum. *J Gen Physiol* 1988;92:1–26.
320. Smith JS, Rousseau E, Meissner G. Calmodulin modulation of single sarcoplasmic reticulum Ca^{2+}-release channels from cardiac and skeletal muscle. *Circ Res* 1989;64:352–359.
321. Sneyd J, Keizer J, Sanderson MJ. Mechanisms of calcium oscillations and waves: a quantitative analysis. *FASEB J* 1995;9:1463–1472.
322. Somlyo AP. Cellular site of calcium regulation. *Nature* 1984; 309:516–517.
323. Somlyo AP, Somlyo AV. Smooth Muscle structure and function. In: Fozzard HA, Haber E, Katz AM, Morgan HE, eds. *The heart and cardiovascular system.* New York: Raven Press, 1991;1295–1324.
324. Somlyo AV, Bond M, Somlyo AP, Scarpa A. Inositol trisphosphate-induced calcium release and contraction in vascular smooth muscle. *Proc Natl Acad Sci USA* 1985;82:5231–5235.
325. Sommer JR. Comparative anatomy: in praise of a powerful approach to elucidate mechanisms translating cardiac excitation into purposeful contraction. *J Mol Cell Cardiol* 1995;27:19–35.
326. Sommer JR, Johnson EA. *Ultrastructure of cardiac muscle. Handbook of physiology:* the cardiovascular system, vol 1. Baltimore: Williams & Wilkins, 1979.
327. Stephenson EW. Activation of fast skeletal muscle: contributions of studies on skinned fibers. *Am J Physiol* 1981;240:C1–C9.
328. Stern MD. Buffering of calcium in the vicinity of a channel pore. *Cell Calcium* 1992;13:183–192.
329. Stern MD. Theory of excitation-contraction coupling in cardiac muscle. *Biophys J* 1992;63:497–517.
330. Strand MA, Louis CF, Mickelson JR. Phosphorylation of the porcine skeletal and cardiac muscle sarcoplasmic reticulum ryanodine receptor. *Biochim Biophys Acta* 1993;1175:319–326.
331. Strynadka NCJ, James MNG. Crystal structures of the helix-loop-helix calcium-binding proteins. *Annu Rev Biochem* 1989;58:951–59.
332. Su JY, Bell JG. Intracellular mechanism of action of isoflurane and halothane on striated muscle of the rabbit. *Anesth Analg* 1986;65: 457–462.
333. Su JY, Kerrick WGL. Effects of halothane on caffeine-induced tension transients in functionally skinned myocardial fibers. *Pflugers Arch* 1979;380:29–34.
334. Su JY, Kerrick WGL. Effects of enflurane on functionally skinned myocardial fibers from rabbits. *Anesthesiology* 1980;52:385–389.
335. Sukhareva M, Morrissette J, Coronado R. Mechanism of chloride-dependent release of Ca^{2+} in the sarcoplasmic reticulum of rabbit skeletal muscle. *Biophys J* 1994;67:751–765.
336. Suko J, Maurer-Fogy I, Plank B, et al. Phosphorylation of serine 2843 in ryanodine receptor-calcium release channel of skeletal muscle by cAMP-, and CaM-dependent protein kinase. *Biochim Biophys Acta* 1993;1175:193–206.
337. Sutko JL, Willerson JT. Ryanodine alteration of the contractile state of rat ventricular myocardium. *Circ Res* 1980;46:332–343.
338. Sutko JL, Willerson JT, Templeton GH, Jones LR, Besch HR Jr. Ryanodine: its alterations of cat papillary muscle contractile state and responsiveness to inotropic interventions and a suggested mechanism of action. *J Pharmacol Exp Ther* 1979;209:37–47.
339. Suttapone S, Worley PF, Baraban JM, Snyder S. Solubilization, purification and characterization of an inositol triphosphate receptor. *J Biol Chem* 1988;263:1530–1534.
340. Takekura H, Bennet L, Tanabe T, Beam KG, Franzini-Armstrong C. Restoration of junctional tetrads in dysgenic myotubes by dihydropyridine receptor cDNA. *Biophys J* 1994;67:793–803.
341. Takekura H, Nishi M, Noda T, Takeshima H, Franzini-Armstrong C. Abnormal junctions between surface membrane and sarcoplasmic reticulum in skeletal muscle with a mutation targeted to the ryanodine receptor. *Proc Natl Acad Sci USA* 1995;92:3381–3385.
342. Takeshima H, Nishimura S, Matsumoto T, et al. Primary structure and expression from complementary DNA of skeletal muscle ryanodine receptor. *Nature* 1989;339:439–445.
343. Takeshima H, Nishimura S, Nishi M, Ikeda M, Sugimoto T. A brain-specific transcript from the 3′-terminal region of the skeletal muscle ryanodine receptor gene. *FEBS Lett* 1993;322:105–110.
344. Tanabe T, Beam KG, Adams BA, Niidome T, Numa S. Regions of the skeletal muscle dihydropyridine receptor critical for excitation-contraction coupling. *Nature* 1990;346:567–569.
345. Tanabe T, Beam KG, Powell JA, Numa S. Restoration of excitation-contraction coupling and slow calcium current in dysgenic mice by dihydropyridine receptor complementary DNA. *Nature* 1988; 336:134–139.
346. Tanabe T, Mikami A, Numa S, Beam KG. Cardiac-type excitation-contraction coupling in dysgenic skeletal muscle injected with cardiac dihydropyridine receptor. *Nature* 1990;344:451–453.
347. Tanifuji M, Sokabe M, Kassai M. An anion channel of sarcoplasmic reticulum incorporated into planar bilayers: single channel properties. *J Membr Biol* 1987;99:103–111.
348. Taylor CW, Marshall CB. Calcium and inositol 1,4,5-trisphosphate receptors: a complex relationship. *Trends Biochem Sci* 1992;17: 403–493.
349. Theibert AB, Estevez VA, Mourey RJ, et al. Photoaffinity labeling and characterization of isolated inositol 1,3,4,5-tetrakisphosphate- and inositol hexakisphosphate-binding proteins. *J Biol Chem* 1992;267:9071–9079.
350. Timerman AP, Ogunbumni E, Freund E, Wiederrecht G, Marks AR, Fleischer S. The calcium release channel of sarcoplasmic reticulum is modulated by FK506-binding protein. *J Biol Chem* 1993;268:22992–22999.
351. Tinker A, Lindsay ARG, Williams AJ. A model for ionic conduction in the ryanodine receptor channel of sheep cardiac muscle sarcoplasmic reticulum. *J Gen Physiol* 1992;100:495–517.
352. Tinker A, Williams AJ. Divalent cation conduction in the ryanodine receptor channel of sheep cardiac muscle sarcoplasmic reticulum. *J Gen Physiol* 1992;100:479–493.
353. Tsien RW, Tsien RY. Calcium channels, stores, and oscillations. *Annu Rev Cell Biol* 1990;6:715–760.
354. Urwyler A, Censier K, Kaufmann MA, Drewe J. Genetic effects on the variability of the halothane and caffeine muscle contracture tests. *Anesthesiology* 1994;80:1287–1295.
355. Valdivia HH, Hogan K, Coronado R. Altered binding site for Ca^{2+} in the ryanodine receptor of human malignant hyperthermia. *Am J Physiol* 1991;261:C237–C245.
356. Valdivia HH, Kaplan JH, Ellis-Davies GHR, Lederer WJ. Rapid adaptation of cardiac ryanodine receptors: modulation by Mg^{2+} and phosphorylation. *Science* 1995;267:1997–2000.
357. Van Winkle WB. Calcium release from skeletal muscle sarcoplasmic reticulum: site of action of dantrolene sodium? *Science* 1976; 193:1130–1131.
358. Volpe P, Palade P, Costello B, Mietchell RD, Fleischer S. Spontaneous calcium release from sarcoplasmic reticulum. Effect of local anesthetics. *J Biol Chem* 1983;258:12434–12442.
359. Wagenknecht T, Grassucci R, Frank J, Saito A, Inui M, Fleischer S. Three-dimensional architecture of the calcium channel/foot structure of sarcoplasmic reticulum. *Nature* 1989;338:167–170.
360. Walton PD, Airey JA, Sutko JL, et al. Ryanodine and inositol triphosphate receptors coexists in avian cerebellar Purkinje neurons. *J Cell Biol* 1991;113:1145–1157.
361. Wang J, Best P. Inactivation of the sarcoplasmic reticulum calcium channel by protein kinase. *Nature* 1992;359:739–743.
362. Wang S-Y, Peskoff A, Langer GA. Inner sarcolemmal leaflet Ca^{2+} binding: its role in cardiac Na/Ca exchange. *Biophys J* 1996;70: 2266–2274.
363. Wedel DJ, Gammel SA, Milde JH, Iaizzo PA. Delayed onset of malignant hyperthermia induced by isoflurane and desflurane compared with halothane in susceptible swine. *Anesthesiology* 1993; 78:1138–1144.

364. Wheeler DM, Katz A, Rice RT. Effects of volatile anesthetics on cardiac sarcoplasmic reticulum as determined in intact cells. In: Blanck TJJ, Wheeler DM, eds. *Mechanisms of anesthetic action in skeletal, cardiac and smooth muscle.* New York: Plenum Press, 1991;143–154.
365. Wheeler DM, Katz A, Rice RT, Hansford RG. Volatile anesthetic effects on sarcoplasmic reticulum Ca content and sarcolemmal Ca flux in isolated rat cardiac cell suspensions. *Anesthesiology* 1994;80: 372–382.
366. Wheeler DM, Rice RT, Hansford RG, Lakatta EG. The effect of halothane on the free intracellular calcium concentration of isolated rat heart cells. *Anesthesiology* 1988;69:578–583.
367. Wheeler DM, Rice RT, Lakatta EG. The action of halothane on spontaneous contractile waves and stimulated contractions in isolated rat and dog heart cells. *Anesthesiology* 1990;72:911–920.
368. Williams AJ. Ion conduction and discrimination in the sarcoplasmic reticulum ryanodine receptor/calcium-release channel. *J Muscle Res Cell Motil* 1992;13:7–26.
369. Williams RJP. Calcium and calmodulin. *Cell Calcium* 1992;13:355–362.
370. Witcher DR, Kovacs RJ, Schulman H, Cefali DC, Jones LR. Unique phosphorylation site on the cardiac ryanodine receptor regulates calcium channel activity. *J Biol Chem* 1991;266:11114–11152.
371. Yamada N, Makino Y, Clark RA, et al. Human inositol 1,4,5-triphosphate type 1 receptor, $InsP_3R1$: structure, function, regulation of expression and chromosomal localization. *Biochem J* 1994; 302:781–890.
372. Yamamoto-Hino M, Sugiyama T, Hikichi K, et al. Cloning and characterization of human type 2 and type 3 inositol 1,4,5-trisphosphate receptors. *Receptors Channels* 1994;2:9–22.
373. Yasui K, Palade P, Györke S. Negative control mechanism with features of adaptation controls Ca^{2+} release in cardiac myocytes. *Biophys J* 1994;67:457–460.
374. Yoshida A, Takahashi M, Imagawa T, Shigekawa M, Takisawa H, Nakamura T. Phosphorylation of ryanodine receptors during β-adrenergic stimulation. *J Biochem(Tokyo)* 1992;111:186–190.
375. Zapata-Sudo G, Nelson TE, Sudo RT. Dantrolene paradox: activation of calcium channel and muscle contracture by dantrolene binding to a high affinity site. *Anesthesiology* 1995;83:A349.
376. Zarka A, Shoshan-Barmatz V. The interaction of spermine with the ryanodine receptor from skeletal muscle. *Biochim Biophys Acta* 1992;1108:13–20.
377. Zhang X, Jefferson AB, Auethavekiat V, Majerus PW. The protein deficient in Lowe syndrome is a phosphatidylinositol-4,5-biphosphate 5-phosphatase. *Proc Natl Acad Sci USA* 1995;92:4853–4856.
378. Zhang Y, Chen HS, Khanna VK, et al. A mutation in the human ryanodine receptor gene associated with central core disease. *Nature Genetics* 1993;5:46–50.
379. Zimányi I, Buck E, Abramson JJ, Mack MM, Pessah IN. Ryanodine induces persistent inactivation of the Ca^{2+} release channel from skeletal muscle sarcoplasmic reticulum. *Mol Pharmacol* 1992;42: 1049–1057.
380. Zimanyi I, Pessah IN. Comparison of [^{3}H]ryanodine receptors and Ca^{2+} release from rat cardiac and rabbit skeletal muscle sarcoplasmic reticulum. *J Pharmacol Exp Ther* 1991;256:938–946.
381. Zorzato F, Fujii J, Otsu K, et al. Molecular cloning of cDNA encoding human and rabbit forms of the Ca^{2+} release channel (ryanodine receptor) of skeletal muscle sarcoplasmic reticulum. *J Biol Chem* 1990;265:2244–2256.

Anesthesia: Biologic Foundations, edited by Tony L. Yaksh et al. Lippincott–Raven Publishers, Philadelphia © 1997.

CHAPTER 10

THE NITRIC OXIDE–GUANYLYL CYCLASE SIGNALING PATHWAY

ROGER A. JOHNS

Nitric oxide (NO) is a novel cell signaling molecule whose identity and broad physiologic importance were discovered recently as a result of converging research in vascular biology, immunology, and neuroscience. In vascular biology, a labile but unidentified vasodilating factor released from endothelium was reported in 1980 as the mediator of acetylcholine-induced vasodilation and given the name endothelium-derived relaxing factor (EDRF) (53). EDRF was subsequently found to be the common mediator for a wide array of endogenous and exogenous vasodilators (50,52), and was demonstrated to activate soluble guanylyl cyclase in vascular smooth muscle following its release from endothelium (76,128,153). Prior to this time, nitric oxide had been recognized as the mechanism by which nitrovasodilators could activate soluble guanylyl cyclase and cause vasodilation, but an in vivo activator of soluble guanylyl cyclase was unknown (198). EDRF was not recognized as nitric oxide until a symposium in 1986 when it was suggested by Furchgott and Vanhoutte (52) that this labile vasodilator had many pharmacologic properties similar to nitric oxide. It was then demonstrated that endothelial cells were capable of producing nitric oxide (25) and that the source of NO was the amino acid L-arginine (143). In parallel but unrelated research in immunology, nitric oxide was recognized as a mediator of the cytotoxic effects of macrophages (137). Activation of macrophages by endotoxin and cytokines resulted in a large increase in NO production coincident with bactericidal and tumoricidal action. These actions were prevented by inhibition of NO synthesis. Subsequently, neuroscientists recognized that NO was the mediator of excitatory amino acid and acetylcholine stimulated increases in guanosine 3',5'-cyclic monophosphate (cGMP) in neuronal tissue (57). In fact, an isoform of nitric oxide synthase (NOS), the enzyme responsible for producing NO, was first isolated and cloned from brain tissue (11).

Synthesized from L-arginine by a family of NO synthase(s), NO is now recognized as a novel cell messenger implicated in wide-ranging physiologic and pathophysiologic actions in the cardiovascular, immune, and nervous systems (128). In blood vessels, EDRF/NO is produced by endothelium where it is a primary determinant of resting vascular tone through basal release and causes vasodilation when synthesized in response to a wide range of vasodilator agents (51,212). It also inhibits platelet aggregation and adhesion, and it may play a major role in disease states such as atherosclerosis and hypertension, cerebral and coronary vasospasm, and ischemia-reperfusion injury (80,128). In the immune system, it is an effector mechanism for macrophage-induced cytotoxicity (109), and its overproduction is an important mediator of the septic shock syndrome. In neuronal tissue, EDRF/NO appears to subserve multiple functions (13). It is present in several specific neuronal pathways and is known to mediate the *N*-methyl-D-aspartate (NMDA) and acetylcholine receptor-stimulated increases in neuronal cGMP (12,57–59,127). NO has been implicated in long-term potentiation in the CA1 region of the hippocampus (9,13,141), thus mediating an important step in learning and memory. NO is the potential agent responsible for NMDA-mediated cytotoxicity (33) and is the mediator of nonadrenergic, noncholinergic neurotransmission (18,61,191). Recent studies have suggested a role for NO in mediating central nociceptive pathways (117,118) and a possible involvement in mechanisms of anesthesia (84). The L-arginine to NO pathway is being explored as a physiologic mediator in multiple other cell and tissue types where it is present, including bronchial epithelium, renal tubular and juxtaglomerular cells, hepatocytes and Kupffer cells, the pituitary, the ovary, and the adrenal medulla (125,127).

This chapter reviews the biochemistry and cell and molecular biology involved in the NO-guanylyl cyclase signaling system and the evidence for and importance of anesthetic interaction with this pathway.

BIOCHEMISTRY, MOLECULAR BIOLOGY, AND REGULATION OF NO SYNTHESIS

Three major NO synthase isoforms have been described (Table 1) (128,186). Two require calcium and calmodulin binding for activation and are constitutively expressed (i.e., normally present) in neurons and in endothelium. As such, these enzymes have been found to be part of a common pathway of cell communication. These constitutive enzymes are activated by a rise in cytosolic free Ca^{2+} ($[Ca^{2+}]_i$) and subsequent binding of Ca^{2+} to calmodulin. In neural tissue, the enzyme is in a soluble form in the cytosol. In endothelium it is bound to the membrane by myristoylation, in which the lipid moiety myristic acid is conjugated with an amino acid residue, providing a lipophilic anchor in the bilayer (120). The third isoform is only expressed following induction by cytokines or microbial products such as endotoxin (lipopolysaccharide) and participates in host defense, mediating many of the cytotoxic actions of macrophages. This inducible isoform has calmodulin tightly bound as a subunit (33,70) and produces NO continuously and in large amounts without a calcium requirement. The cytokine-induced isoform may also participate in pathophysiology associated with cytokine overproduction, such as in sepsis (21,128,149). While this inducible form of the enzyme is present in the macrophage under basal conditions, it is not normally found in the endothelial cell or vascular smooth muscle. Indeed, many cell types appear capable of expressing inducible NOS following exposure to the appropriate cytokines. Unlike the constitutive form, the induced form is present in vascular tissues only following induction by cytokines (21,137,149). In endotoxin-induced sepsis, the inducible NOS is prominent in endothelium and vascular smooth muscle, accounting for excessive NO production, leading to sepsis-related hypotension and possibly contributing to cytotoxicity (89,119,177,184).

In contrast to their differences in location, expression, and function, the NO synthase isoforms appear to be biochemically similar. The inducible and constitutive NO synthases are active as homodimers with dimeric molecular weight of 130 kd (inducible) and 150 kd (constitutive) (11,178). Both are members of a rare class of proteins that contain both the riboflavin-containing nucleotides flavin adenine dinucleotide (FAD) and flavin mononucleotide (FMN) as prosthetic groups (178,205), and share homology with the cytochrome P450 reductase class

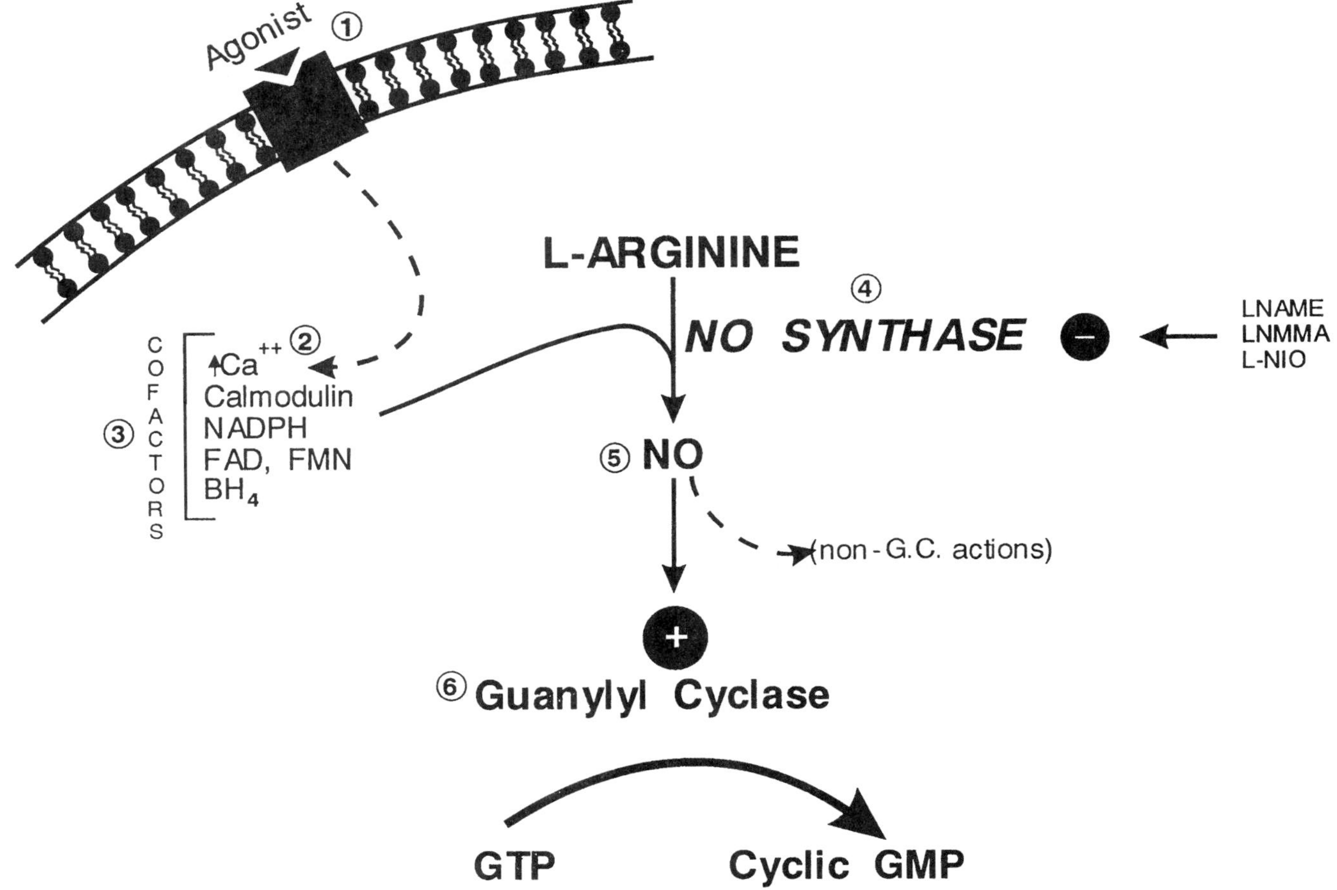

Figure 1. The nitric oxide (NO) signaling pathway. In the brain and endothelium, NO is produced from L-arginine by similar constitutive enzymes called NO synthase(s). These enzymes are activated by the binding of calcium and calmodulin, often in response to agonist-receptor interaction leading to increased intracellular calcium. They are homologous to P450 reductase enzymes, having recognition sites for reduced nicotinamide adenine dinucleotide phosphate (NADPH), flavin adenine dinucleotide (FAD), and flavin mononucleotide (FMN). Tetrahydrobiopterin (BH4) is another cofactor. In addition to L-arginine, two O_2 molecules are involved as substrates, one being incorporated into NO and the other into the stable by-product of the reaction, L-citrulline. After its production, NO binds to the heme moiety of guanylyl cyclase (GC), which catalyzes the production of cyclic 3' ,5-guanosine monophosphate (cGMP) from guanosine triphosphate (GTP). Specific analogues of L-arginine, including nitro-L-arginine methylester (LNAME), monomethyl-L-arginine (LNMMA) and N-imino-L-ornithine (L-NIO) are competitive inhibitors of NO synthase. The numbers 1 to 6 represent potential sites of biochemical regulation and of inhalational anesthetic interaction as discussed in the text. (Modified from ref. 81, with permission.)

of proteins (11,201) typically involved in oxidation-reduction reaction pathways. The constitutive brain enzyme, the constitutive endothelial cell enzyme, and the cytokine-induced macrophage enzyme have been sequenced and cloned (11,78,107,144,178,205). The deduced amino acid sequence of the endothelial cell NO synthase reveals 57% and 50% homology with the brain and macrophage enzymes, respectively (178). In addition, the endothelial cell NO synthase contains a unique N-myristoylation consensus sequence not shared by the brain and macrophage enzymes that is responsible for its membrane localization (19). Previous work indicated that this membrane myristoylation is controlled by protein kinase C (PKC)-mediated phosphorylation, leading to removal of the enzyme from the membrane and a decrease in activity (120). However, a recent report demonstrates that palmitoylation is responsible for the removal of the enzyme from the membrane (20,161), and that phosphorylation through PKC only occurs once the enzyme is cytosolic, resulting in a decrease in NOS activity (161). The primary sequences of these enzymes demonstrate that the monomers are composed of an oxygenase and reductase domain (11,201). The combination of these two domains on one protein makes this family of enzymes a unique class of P450 enzyme. In addition to flavins, both isoforms contain bound tetrahydrobiopterin, a proton-transferring component, and a recently recognized heme moiety (46,71,72,178,201). The NOS enzymes are functional only as homodimers, each monomer containing a heme moiety. Stoichiometric quantities of tetrahydrobiopterin appear to play a critical role in maintaining the dimeric form of the enzyme (46).

These NO synthases are termed mixed function monooxygenases that utilize reduced nicotinamide adenine dinucleotide phosphate (NADPH) to oxidize L-arginine in a stepwise manner to form NO and citrulline as primary products (11,119,201). NADPH serves as the electron donor and oxygen is the electron acceptor. It is now recognized that the initial step in NO synthesis is an NADPH- and oxygen-dependent hydroxylation of arginine that forms N-hydroxyarginine. Enzymatic conversion of the intermediate N-hydroxyarginine to NO and citrulline also utilizes NADPH and O_2 (92,124). One molecule of O_2 is incorporated into NO and one into L-citrulline in a process involving five electron reductions (156,175). It is proposed that NADPH passes electrons through the flavins which

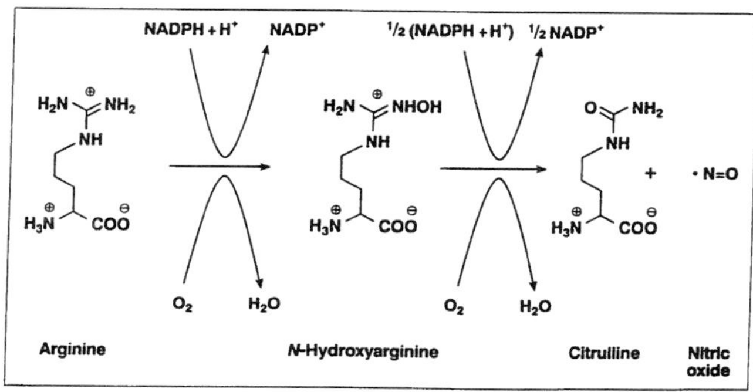

Figure 2. The reaction catalyzed by nitric oxide synthase. (From ref. 147.)

subsequently reduce the iron in heme to its ferrous form, which can then bind oxygen and oxidize the substrate L-arginine (92). Limiting the availability of substrate molecular oxygen is the likely mechanism by which hypoxia inhibits NO synthase activation and EDRF/NO dependent vasodilation (156).

All forms of the enzyme can be specifically and competitively inhibited (Table 2) by analogues of L-arginine, in which a substitution is made at one of the guanidino nitrogen atoms (155). These include N^G-monomethyl L-arginine (LNMMA), N^G-L-arginine methyl ester (LNAME), and N-imino-L-ornithine (L-NIO) (85,128). While these L-arginine analogues are effective inhibitors of both the constitutive and inducible forms of NO synthase, aminoguanidine has been reported to be highly selective for the inducible isoform (123). These inhibitors are proving to be of enormous benefit in elucidating the physiologic and pathophysiologic roles of the NO pathway. Agents that inhibit protoporphyrin heme-based enzymes are under active investigation as NOS inhibitors. In particular, a number of indazole derivatives have been shown to be effective NOS inhibitors through interaction at the heme moiety (129). In addition to direct interaction with NOS, there are a number of other potential sites at which NO signaling can be inhibited. Diphenyleneiodonium and other aromatic iodonium compounds that irreversibly inhibit nucleotide-requiring flavoproteins inhibit both inducible and constitutive NO synthases at nanomolar concentrations (137). Agents that inhibit or compete with NO synthase cofactors have also been employed. These include calmodulin inhibitors, flavoprotein binders, and agents that deplete tetrahydrobiopterin (128). The interaction of carbon monoxide with the heme of NO synthase also results in inactivation of the enzyme (201). In situations where NO synthase is activated by receptor-mediated increases in cytosolic calcium, such as neuronal NMDA receptors, specific receptor antagonists are highly indirect inhibitors of NO production.

In addition to inhibition of the pathway through interference with NO synthase activity, NO itself can be inactivated following its production (Table 3). It binds avidly to hemoglobin and other hemoproteins and also interacts with superoxide to form peroxynitrate (6). The regulation of cellular superoxide dismutase activity and subsequent superoxide levels has been suggested as a potentially physiologic regulatory mechanism (95). The rapid binding and inactivation of NO by hemoglobin in the pulmonary vessels is responsible for the selective pulmonary vasodilation effect of inhaled NO (160).

Interference with NO activation of guanylyl cyclase is another means of blocking NO action. This has most commonly been accomplished with methylene blue; however, one must be cautious in using this agent, as its avid role as an electron acceptor makes it very nonspecific (66). Indeed, it has recently been reported that methylene blue exerts much of its action by inhibiting NO synthase in addition to guanylyl cyclase (112).

GUANYLYL CYCLASE AND CGMP

Following its production, the primary biologic function of NO is the activation of soluble guanylyl cyclase to increase the cGMP content of several tissues, including vascular smooth muscle and brain (76,153). It does so by binding to the heme moiety of soluble guanylyl cyclase, resulting in movement of the heme away from the protein and causing a conformational change leading to increased catalytic activity (175). Cyclic GMP then serves as the "second messenger" for carrying out many of the actions of NO. There are two major forms of guanylyl cyclase, particulate (membrane bound) and soluble (cytosolic). The soluble form is that which is activated by nitric oxide, while the particulate form is activated only by atrial natriuretic peptides (Fig. 3). The guanylyl cyclases are structurally and functionally distinct from adenyl cyclase, which is activated by β-adrenergic agents to catalyze adenosine 3',5'-cyclic monophosphate (cAMP) production from adenosine triphosphate (ATP).

The particulate (membrane associated) guanylyl cyclase is a single protein containing an intracellular catalytic domain and an extracellular ligand-binding domain, which are adjoined by a single transmembrane spanning portion. The ligand-binding component is present on the cell surface, serving as the receptor for atrial natriuretic peptides (175). Four mammalian membrane receptor guanylyl cyclases have been cloned and characterized (175). Atrial natriuretic peptide receptor type A (ANPR-A) is prevalent in brain and vasculature and is activated by both brain and atrial natriuretic peptides (BNP, ANP) (55,209). Atrial natriuretic peptide receptor type B (ANPR-B) is activated selectively by atrial natriuretic peptide type C

Table 1. COMPARISON OF NITRIC OXIDE SYNTHASE ISOFORMS

	Endothelium	Brain	Macrophage
Regulation	Constitutive, agonist activated	Constitutive, agonist activated	Inducible, no for activation
Calcium dependent	CA^{2+}, CaM activation	Ca^{2+}, CaM activation	CaM tightly bound, no Ca^{2+} requirement
Membrane vs cytosol	Particulate	Soluble	Soluble
Substrates	L-arginine, O_2	L-arginine, O_2	L-arginine, O_2
Cofactors	FAD, FMN, NADPH, BH4, Heme, CaM, Ca^{2+}	FAD, FMN, NADPH, BH4, Heme, CaM, Ca^{2+}	FAD, FMN, NADPH, BH4, Heme
Homology	——	57% homology to EC	57% homology to EC
Molecular size	135 kd	155 kd	150 kd
Amount NO produced	pmoles NO produced	pmoles NO produced	nmoles NO produced

Ca2+, calcium; CaM, calmodulin; FAD, flavin adenine dinucleotide; FMN, flavin adenine mononucleotide; BH4, tetrahydroborpterin; NADPH, nicotinamole adenine dinucleotide phosphate; EC, endothelial cell nitric oxide sythase.

Table 2. STRATEGIES OF NITRIC OXIDE SYNTHASE INHIBITION

- Agonist-receptor inhibition
- Interaction with arginine binding site
  - L-NAME, L-NMA, L-NIO, etc.
- Heme ligands
  - indazoles, hydrazines, nitric oxide
- Interference with BH4 binding, biosynthesis
- Calcium-calmodulin antagonists
- Transcriptional and translational regulation

L-NAME = L-nitro arginine methyl ester; L-NMA = monomethyl L-arginine, L-NIO = L-imino ornithine

(CNP) (209). A third membrane receptor guanylyl cyclase is the intestinal receptor for *Escherichia coli* heat-stable enterotoxin, which is activated by the recently discovered endogenous intestinal peptide, guanylin (175). Human retinal guanylyl cyclase is a fourth membrane receptor cyclase that has been cloned and sequenced, but for which an endogenous ligand has not yet been found (55). The physiologic function of these particulate guanylyl cyclase isoforms is still being defined. The natriuretic peptides ANP, BNP, and CNP stimulate vasodilation, natriuresis, and diuresis, inhibit aldosterone synthesis (55,27), as well as hasten relaxation and increase compliance of the myocardium (28). While ANP and BNP are widely distributed, CNP appears specific to brain or neuronal tissue and has been proposed to be a neurotransmitter (209). The guanylin and enterotoxin activated cyclase controls cGMP-mediated salt and fluid transport in the intestine while the role of the retinal particulate gyanylyl cyclase remains unknown (175). (For detailed review of particulate guanylyl cyclases, see refs. 27,55,175,209.)

Nitric oxide–stimulated increases in cGMP are mediated by NO activation of the soluble guanylyl cyclase(s) and are unrelated to the particulate guanylyl cyclases. Soluble guanylyl cyclase(s) are a family of heterodimers consisting of a 70-kd protein (α subunit) and an 82-kd protein (β subunit) (91,136,198), each containing a heme of the ferroprotoporphyrin IX family (175,198). In addition to iron, copper is another transition metal contained in the enzyme, although its function is unknown (198). Multiple α and β subunits have been demonstrated including α and β from rat and bovine lung, rat kidney β and human fetal α (91,101,136,175,198). The extent of variation in subunits is not yet well investigated, and it is likely that additional isoforms will be discovered. What is clear, however, is that the coexpression of both α and β subunits is essential for enzyme activity (91,175).

NO activates soluble guanylyl cyclase by binding to the heme moiety resulting in dislocation of the heme-iron moiety and a subsequent conformational change in the protein permitting access to the catalytic site (175). NO is clearly the most effective and potent activator of soluble guanylyl cyclase. Both carbon monoxide (CO) and hydroxyl radical have been proposed as additional physiologic activators of soluble guanylyl cyclase, but they appear to be less important and their role remains undefined (175).

The physiologic functions of cGMP are diverse, as described above, and as reviewed in detail elsewhere (13,50,51,53,80,96, 128,137,175,198). There are three known classes of receptor proteins through which these actions of cGMP are mediated. These include cGMP-dependent protein kinases, cyclic nucleotide-binding phosphodiesterases, and ion channel proteins that directly bind cGMP and are regulated by such action.

Cyclic GMP kinases phosphorylate specific serine and threonine residues in proteins and exist in two distinct classes (101). The most widely distributed cGMP kinase is type I, a homodimer, which is isolated from the soluble fraction of tissues as a mixture of two isoforms, type Ia and type Ib. Type II cGMP kinase is a monomer and is less well described. Cyclic GMP kinases are most abundant in smooth muscle, platelets and cerebellum as well as cardiac myocytes and neutrophils (101). Little if any is found in skeletal muscle, hepatocytes, vascular endothelial cells or renal tubular epithelium, suggesting that cGMP kinase does not mediate all of the effects of cGMP (101). Thus, cGMP may have limited function in some tissues or may act through a kinase-unrelated mechanism. Cyclic GMP kinase does mediate a cGMP-induced decrease in $[Ca^{2+}]_i$ in vascular smooth muscle, although the mechanism by which it acts is not clearly understood. One effect is the stimulation of smooth muscle Ca^{2+}–adenosine triphosphatase (ATPase), which would lead to stimulation of uptake of Ca^{2+} into the sarcoplasmic reticulum and extrusion from the plasmalemma (100,101). Phospholamban, a sarcoplasmic reticulum Ca^{2+}-ATPase regulatory protein, is phosphorylated by cGMP kinase (89,120,151,170). Cyclic GMP kinase is also capable of phosphorylating the inositol 1,4,5-phosphate receptor leading to decreased Ca^{2+} release from the sarcoplasmic reticulum (100,101). Cyclic GMP activation of K^+ channels in smooth muscle leads to hyperpolarization of the smooth muscle cell membrane and a reduction in $[Ca^{2+}]_i$ (26,46,190,201), but whether this involves protein kinase phosphorylation of the receptor or other mechanisms remains unclear (24,56,60,85,92,116,124,155,175,202). Cyclic GMP has also been found to activate Na^+/Ca^{2+} exchange of cultured vascular smooth muscle cells (54), which would decrease the intracellular Ca^{2+} store available for release. Cyclic GMP has also been proposed to decrease smooth muscle $[Ca^{2+}]_i$ by inhibition of G protein function (73,76,99,112) and inhibition of phospholipase C activation (154). In platelets, cGMP reduces $[Ca^{2+}]_i$ by an effect on phospholipase C. In neutrophils, cGMP mediates agonist-induced increases in motility (chemotaxis) and degranulation through protein kinase phosphorylation of vimentin, an intermediate filament cytoskeleton protein, independent of Ca^{2+} (149,204).

The ability of cGMP to directly gate ion channels represents another major mode of cGMP action, particularly important to the role of the NO–guanylyl cyclase pathway in the nervous system. This function of cGMP has been primarily characterized in the vertebrate photoreceptor (31,88,118,122,154,204). In the absence of light, cGMP binds to and opens a nonspecific cation channel, which causes a depolarization of rod outer segment membrane through the influx of Na^+ and Ca^{2+} ions into the cell. The subunit of the cGMP gated ion channel is a 63-kd protein that has been cloned, sequenced, and shown to have

Table 3. TARGETS OF NITRIC OXIDE ACTION

Activation of DNA binding factors
  NF-κβ (induce TNF, IL-1)
  CREB (induce c-*fos*, c-*jun*)
  Sox R (induce sox S)
Activation of RNA binding factors
  IRE-BP (suppression of ferritin translation)
Activation of enzymes
  Soluble guanylyl cyclase
  Cyclooxygenase
Inactivation of enzymes
  Cis aconitase, NADH ubiquinone oxidoreductase, succinate ubiquinone reductase, GAPDH, ribonucleotide reductase, NO synthase
Mutation of DNA
  Deamination
  Oxidation
  Cross-linking
Generalized inactivation of oxidoreductants
  O2–: peroxynitrite, nitrite
  Thiols: s-nitrosothiols

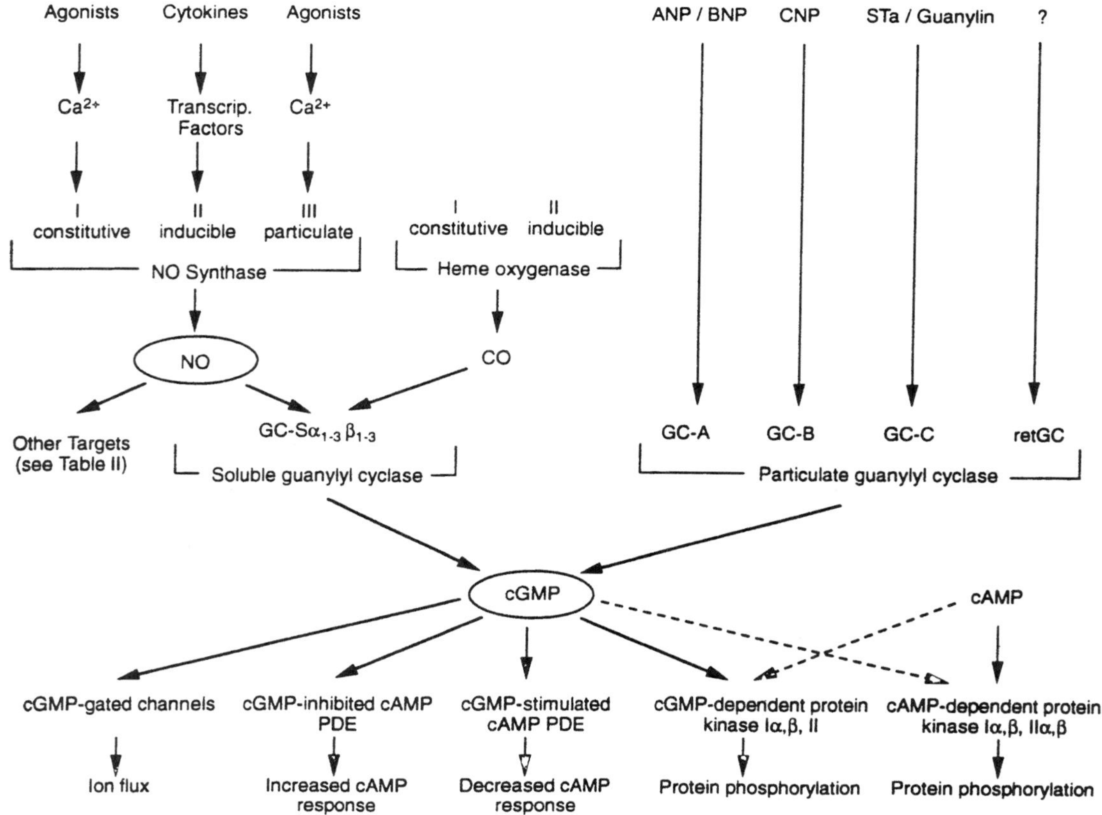

Figure 10-3. Model of the signal transduction pathways leading to cGMP synthesis and subsequent actions. Specific pathways are discussed in detail in the text. (Modified from ref. 175, with permission.)

six probable membrane-spanning regions. By analogy with the voltage-gated K^+ channel (31,88,154,204), to which it is similar in structure, four subunits combine to form a homotetramid with a central pore. This cation channel has an relatively low affinity for cGMP, which plays a critical role in phototransduction; when cGMP dissociates from the receptor, and is hydrolyzed by its phosphodiesterase, the channel rapidly closes, providing the essential decrease in membrane conductance (101). A similar cGMP gated receptor/channel composed of 76-kd subunits is present in olfactory epithelium (87). The renal epithelium has also been reported to have a cGMP regulated, amiloride-sensitive cation channel that has been suggested to regulate diuretic-sensitive Na^+ and Cl^- transport in renal tubular cells (99,112).

The third known class of receptor proteins for cGMP is the family of cGMP-binding phosphodiesterases (PDE) (101). By altering the activity of PDEs, changes in the levels of intracellular cyclic nucleotides are induced that result in changes in protein phosphorylation and other signaling events (101). Cyclic GMP binds to two PDEs as an allosteric effector (100,101). These include the cGMP-stimulated PDE and the cGMP-binding, cGMP-specific PDE. Another PDE, the high-affinity cAMP-specific PDE is widely distributed in vertebrate tissues and occurs as two isoforms, one of which is inhibited by cGMP and one of which is unaffected (100,101). By binding to and inhibiting this latter PDE, cGMP causes an increase in cellular cAMP. The inhibition of this latter PDE by cGMP is responsible for the cGMP-mediated potentiation of cAMP-activated Ca^{2+} current in mammalian ventricular myocytes (142).

While these three classes of receptor-binding proteins for cGMP are now recognized, it is clear that our understanding of the interconnected intracellular mechanisms by which cGMP acts is still very limited. The discovery of the important physiologic functions of signaling molecules such as NO and the natriuretic peptides has brought new interest to investigation of mechanisms of cGMP action.

NONGUANYLYL CYCLASE ACTIONS OF NO

NO, a reactive free radical, has also been reported to have other, non–cGMP-mediated actions. It has been shown to activate adenosine diphosphate (ADP) ribosyltransferase (16), and to inhibit a number of enzymes including mitochondrial aconitase, electron transport chain complexes I and II, ribonucleotide reductase (69,94,113), and protein kinase C (62). These protein/enzyme interactions of NO have been suggested to be a result of its ability to form complexes with both heme and non-heme iron proteins (114). Recently, White and Marletta (201) have demonstrated that both the inducible and constitutive NO synthases contain a heme moiety. We have recently reported the feedback inhibition of NO synthase by NO, a potentially important mechanism for regulation of this signaling pathway (157,158). The binding of NO to the heme of NO synthase would be a likely mechanism of this observed inhibition.

NO also interacts avidly with reactive oxygen species resulting in its rapid inactivation (126,131). It combines with superoxide radical to form peroxynitrite (6) and with oxygen to form nitrite, nitrate, and nitric acid (6,49). This explains the ability of high oxygen concentrations to inhibit EDRF/NO (156,164) and superoxide dismutase to markedly prolong its biologic half-life (156,163,164). This is a potential mechanism of anesthetic inactivation of NO, as inhalational anesthetics have been shown to generate oxygen-derived radicals that would avidly combine with NO (180,207).

NO has recently been shown to play an important role in gene regulation. It is capable of activating several DNA and RNA binding factors and has also been shown capable of DNA mutation through deamination, oxidation, and cross-linking (135,137,139).

BIOCHEMICAL REGULATION OF NO SIGNALING PATHWAY

The NO signaling pathway is biochemically regulated at multiple sites (Table 4). An understanding of the regulation of NO signaling will form a basis for understanding the likely sites of inhalational anesthetic inhibition of NO signaling. Potential sites of regulation are indicated in Fig. 1 and include (a) receptor activation and signal transduction; (b) calcium availability; (c) availability of other cofactors; (d) direct effects on NO synthase, including phosphorylation and feedback inhibition; (e) interactions with nitric oxide itself; and (f) interactions with guanylyl cyclase and cGMP. In addition, recent cloning and analysis of the promoter regions of human endothelial NO synthase and of mouse macrophage–inducible NO synthase have revealed multiple potential mechanisms of molecular regulation of NO synthase expression.

The requisite activation of constitutive NO synthase by increases in cytosolic calcium (104,121,145,165,168,182,183) provides one of the most significant modes of regulation of NO production. The calcium dependence of the activation of NO synthase and production of NO has been studied extensively in the endothelial cell (104,183). Endothelium-dependent responses are enhanced by the calcium ionophore A23187 and attenuated or abolished by the removal of extracellular calcium (182). While the removal of extracellular calcium consistently causes inhibition of EDRF-dependent responses (145), however, calcium entry blockers do not inhibit endothelium-dependent relaxations in all vessels studied (121,183). Both extracellular influx of calcium and release of calcium from intracellular stores are involved in EDRF release from endothelial cells. In the absence of extracellular calcium, bradykinin-stimulated endothelial cells release EDRF in an attenuated and transient manner (182). An increase in endothelial cell $[Ca^{2+}]_i$ has been shown to accompany the release of EDRF in response to a wide variety of endothelium-dependent dilators including histamine, bradykinin, ATP, melittin, thrombin, and norepinephrine (23,29,35,36,45,83, 111,115,165,183,197), implicating receptor-mediated release of intracellular Ca^{2+} stores as the initial step in the production NO. This increase in $[Ca^{2+}]_i$ associated with EDRF release correlates with an increase in the concentration of endothelial cell inositol 1,4,5-trisphosphate (IP_3) (79,82,102,168), while inhibition of phospholipase C by gentamicin, thus blocking IP_3 production, prevents EDRF release from cultured endothelial cells (34).

Several calcium-stimulating endothelial cell receptor and signaling pathways have been related to EDRF/NO production. An increase in $[Ca^{2+}]_i$ leads to Ca-calmodulin activation of NO synthase (1,22,38,41,63,93,150,171,172) as discussed above. There are multiple mechanisms by which $[Ca^{2+}]_i$ may be increased in the endothelial cell. Agonist binding to a receptor may lead to opening of receptor-operated calcium channels present in the plasma membrane (1,30,63,68,168,173,174,189), that is, channels that open when intracellular $Ca^{2+}{}_i$ stores are depleted. Alternatively, receptor-mediated G-protein activation of phospholipase C can lead to the cleavage of phosphatidylinositol 4,5-bisphosphate generating IP_3 and diacylglycerol (DAG) (38,48,150). IP_3 releases Ca^{2+} from intracellular stores (38,48,150), while DAG activates protein kinase C (see below). While not definitively demonstrated in the endothelial cell, it is also possible that inositol 1,3,4,5-tetrakisphosphate (IP_4) can stimulate receptor-operated channels allowing entry of Ca^{2+} (77). Both a Ca^{2+} leak channel, dependent on the electrochemical gradient for Ca^{2+}, as well as internal Na^+-dependent calcium entry (Na^+-Ca^{2+} exchange) have been proposed but not well demonstrated (1,150,203). While there are reports of voltage-operated calcium channels in endothelial cells, the overwhelming evidence suggests that L-type voltage-operated channels are not present (61). Thus, the well-documented action of anesthetics on these channels is unlikely to influence endothelium cell function. The presence of other potential operated channels remains controversial. The rate of Ca^{2+} entry can be modulated by the resting membrane potential that may be regulated by two types of K channels (1): (a) inwardly rectifying K channels activated upon hyperpolarization or shear stress, and (b) a calcium-activated K channel activated upon depolarization that may function to repolarize the agonist-stimulated endothelial cell (22,41,171,172). By maintaining a more negative membrane potential, these K channels increase the electrochemical gradient for Ca^{2+} entry, and blockade of the channels decreases Ca^{2+} entry. ATP sensitive K channels have also been demonstrated in endothelial cells (22,150).

Phosphorylation is another likely regulatory mechanism for NO synthase. Study of the NO synthase amino acid sequence reveals recognition sites for protein phosphorylation in addition to sites for NADPH, FAD, FMN and calmodulin (10,11,176). Indeed, NO synthase has recently been reported to be stoichiometrically phosphorylated by cAMP-dependent protein kinase, protein kinase C, and calcium/calmodulin-dependent protein kinase (10,17,135,137), each kinase phosphorylating a different serine in the amino acid sequence of the enzyme. The phosphorylation by protein kinase C resulted in a marked inhibition of the enzyme. Previous work indicated that this membrane myristoylation is controlled by PKC-mediated phosphorylation, leading to removal of the enzyme from the membrane and a decrease in activity (120). However, a recent report demonstrates that palmitoylation is responsible for the removal of the enzyme from the membrane (20,161), and that phosphorylation through PKC only occurs once the enzyme is cytosolic, resulting in a decrease in NOS activity (161).

As mentioned, the receptor-mediated activation of phospholipase C (PLC), in conjunction with initiating the inositol phosphate cascade, produces diacylglycerol (DAG), which leads to protein kinase C activation. The DAG response to receptor stimulation in endothelial cells has two components. An initial peak correlates with PLC- mediated inositol 1,4,5-trisphosphate release. A secondary, sustained release of DAG may be related to the action of other lipases (1). DAG, through activation of protein kinase C, may play an important physiologic role in modulating endothelial cell responsiveness to vasoactive agents (34). Activation of protein kinase C by phorbol esters has been shown by several investigators to inhibit EDRF production stimulated by receptor-mediated agents but not in response to the calcium ionophore A23187 (98,200). This is consistent with known protein kinase C inactivation of receptor GTP binding proteins involved in PLC activation, a negative feedback pathway observed in other cell types.

Table 4. BIOCHEMICAL REGULATION OF NITRIC OXIDE AND NITRIC OXIDE SYTHASE

Receptor activation
Calcium/calmodulin
Cofactor availability
Substrate availability
Phosphorylation
NO feedback inhibition
Product metabolism
NO + O_2, O_2-produces NO2, NO3, HOON-, etc.
L-citrulline recycled to L-arginine
Cyclic GMP

The mechanisms of Ca^{2+} sequestration by endoplasmic reticulum (ER) are poorly defined in endothelial cells, although an ER Ca^{2+}-ATPase isoform is responsible for intracellular Ca^{2+} accumulation. Two recent papers suggest the histochemical (97) and functional (210) presence of a ryanodine receptor in endothelium. Thus, the ryanodine receptor would be an obvious site for investigation of anesthetic effects on endothelial cell signaling based on inhalational anesthetic interactions at this site in myocytes (187,106,108).

MOLECULAR REGULATION OF NOS ISOFORMS

While the promoter structures of the NOS isoforms are established, there is yet only limited information on the processes that regulate these genes. The molecular regulation of NOS is now under active investigation and three recent publications present the analysis and cloning of the promoter regions for the constitutive human endothelial NOS, the inducible murine macrophage NOS, and the constitutive human neuronal NOS genes (67,105,110,206). The endothelial NOS gene is tumor-associated transplantation antigen (TATA)-less and exhibits proximal promoter elements consistent with a constitutively expressed gene, namely, Sp1 and GATA motifs. The 5'-flanking region contains AP-1, AP-2, NF-1, heavy metal, acute phase response, shear stress, estrogen recognition sites, and sterol-regulatory *cis*-elements (110). The latter four elements are consistent with pharmacologic studies implicating NOS in reperfusion injury and in the vascular remodeling of hypertension and atherosclerosis. The role of these elements in pathophysiologic states, however, is just beginning to be investigated. Thus far, shear stress (140), chronic exercise (179), and estrogen (74,199) have been shown to upregulate endothelial NOS messenger RNA (mRNA) and protein, while tumor necrosis factor-α increases endothelial NOS mRNA turnover (208). The macrophage-inducible NOS, in contrast to the endothelial constitutive enzyme, contains a TATA box preceding its mRNA initiation site and at least 22 elements homologous to consensus sequences for the binding of transcription factors related to cytokines or bacterial products (206). Maximal expression depends on two discrete regulatory regions upstream of the TATA box. Region I contains LPS-related response elements, including a binding site for interleukin-6 and for NF-κB. Region II contains binding motifs for interferon α-related transcription factors and is probably responsible for the interferon α-mediated regulation of LPS-induced NOS. The cooperative interaction of these two regions explains, at the level of transcription, how interferon α and LPS act together to maximally induce the macrophage NOS gene and how interferon α augments the inflammatory response to LPS (105). Transforming growth factor β (TGFβ forms 1, 2, and 3) regulates inducible NOS at multiple sites. It decreases translation, enhances mRNA breakdown, and increases degradation of the NOS protein once produced (137–139). The structural organization of the human neuronal NOS gene has recently been reported (67). There is a major transcription initiation site 28 nucleotides downstream from a TATA box. Analysis of the 5 -flanking regions revealed potential *cis*-acting DNA elements: AP-2, TEF-1/MCBF, CREB/ATF/*c-fos*, NRF-1, Ets, NF-1, and NF-κB-like sequences. Multiple alleles were evident in normal individuals indicating allelic mRNA sequence variation. Analysis of variant human neuronal NOS cDNAs demonstrated structural mRNA diversity due to alternative splicing.

EVIDENCE FOR INHALATIONAL ANESTHETIC INTERACTION WITH NO SIGNALING IN THE VASCULATURE

Several studies have examined the role of the endothelium in mediating the vascular responses of anesthetics or the effects of anesthetics on endothelium-dependent responses. Blaise et al. (7) have demonstrated that isoflurane impairs the contractile response of canine coronary arteries induced by phenylephrine in an endothelium-dependent manner, and they proposed that this might be due to isoflurane-induced release of EDRF. Consistent with these observations, in a report by Greenblatt et al. (65), the microsphere technique was used to measure tissue-specific blood flow, suggesting indirectly that isoflurane may stimulate EDRF/NO production in certain vascular beds. Several laboratories have provided strong direct evidence, however, that anesthetics are not capable of stimulating EDRF release (14,43,44). Rather, inhalational anesthetics appear to be potent inhibitors of EDRF-dependent vascular relaxation at clinically relevant doses. Muldoon et al. (132) have demonstrated that halothane inhibits endothelium-dependent vasodilation in response to the receptor-mediated agonists, acetylcholine and bradykinin. Stone and Johns (185) previously reported that a small vasoconstricting response observed with low concentrations of isoflurane, enflurane, and halothane requires an intact endothelium and may be due to the inhibition of EDRF production or action.

Recently, Uggeri et al. (195) have more directly and definitively demonstrated that these three volatile anesthetics can inhibit both receptor and non–receptor-mediated EDRF/NO-dependent vasodilation. Halothane, enflurane, and isoflurane inhibited the endothelium-dependent vasodilation induced by muscarinic (MI) receptor activation by methacholine as well as that by the receptor-independent calcium ionophore A23187, but the anesthetics had no effect on the endothelium-independent vasodilation induced by sodium nitroprusside (SNP). While this study demonstrated that anesthetic inhibition of EDRF/NO vasodilation occurred distal to receptor activation of the endothelial cell, it did not rule out an additional effect on receptor mechanisms as was suggested by Muldoon et al. (132), and that has been demonstrated in other cell types (2,4,15,37,96,195). Toda et al. (134,193) have recently reported that both isoflurane and halothane inhibited acetylcholine-induced endothelium-dependent relaxation of rat aorta and simultaneously prevented acetylcholine-induced increases in cGMP). Consistent with the work by Uggeri et al., isoflurane was more potent than halothane in this regard. Unlike Uggeri et al., however, these investigators did not demonstrate an inhibition of A23187-induced vasodilation. One explanation for the apparent anesthetic stimulation of NO synthase in vivo but not in isolated preparations has been suggested by Crystal et al. (32), who demonstrated that NO release by isoflurane in intact coronary vessels is due to flow-dependent (shear stress related) NO release resulting from direct coronary smooth muscle vasodilation by isoflurane, independent of the NO pathway.

In the studies by Muldoon et al. (132) and by Uggeri et al. (185) of inhalational anesthetic inhibition of EDRF-dependent vasodilation, it was shown that this inhibition was due to an effect on the production, release, or transport of EDRF, and independent of any effect on guanylyl cyclase activation in the vascular smooth muscle. The evidence for this was that nitroglycerin (TNG) or SNP-induced relaxation, which is mediated by a direct activation of vascular smooth muscle soluble guanylyl cyclase following its breakdown to NO, was not affected by any of the anesthetics. A recent study, also by the Muldoon laboratory, however, suggests that vasodilation induced by TNG is inhibited by halothane, and that halothane inhibits vasodilation and cGMP accumulation in response to NO. It is implied that halothane might act to inhibit NO-dependent vasodilation through inhibition of guanylyl cyclase (133). This action appears specific for halothane, however, as isoflurane did not inhibit NO vasodilation (Muldoon, *personal communication*). Thus, it is not clear from isolated vascular ring studies whether inhalational anesthetics are capable of interfering with NO signaling through an action in vascular smooth muscle involving guanylyl cyclase.

Blaise et al. (8) have studied the site of anesthetic interaction with NO signaling using a superfusion-bioassay technique for nitric oxide production in which buffer passes through a column of endothelial cells and subsequently onto an endothelium-denuded vascular ring, the relaxation of which serves as a bioassay for EDRF/NO. These studies demonstrate that halothane does not interfere with endothelial cell release of EDRF/NO or its action on vascular smooth muscle guanylyl cyclase. These data suggest that halothane may modify EDRF/NO half-life or its activated redox form (8).

A recent report on the vascular actions of sevoflurane demonstrated that sevoflurane selectively impaired EDRF-dependent relaxation induced by acetylcholine, bradykinin, and the calcium ionophore A23187, and that this effect was partially reversed by superoxide dismutase (207). These authors demonstrated with electron paramagnetic resonance spectroscopy techniques that sevoflurane generated the superoxide free radical and suggested superoxide inactivation of NO as a possible mechanism of sevoflurane's inhibition of EDRF-dependent vasodilation. Subsequent work has failed to confirm this and suggests that sevoflurane acts by limiting Ca^{2+} availability (5).

POTENTIAL AND LIKELY SITES FOR ANESTHETIC INTERACTION WITH NO SIGNALING

There are multiple sites at which inhalational anesthetics may potentially inhibit EDRF/NO production or release based on the known mechanisms of EDRF/NO synthesis and action, and on the observed effects of these anesthetics in endothelial cells, neurons, and other cell types. Likely sites of interaction are indicated in Fig. 1 by circled numbers that correlate with the discussion below.

1 and 2: Receptor Activation and Cytosolic Calcium Availability

As inhalational anesthetics have been shown to have profound and specific effects on calcium homeostasis in other cell types (167) (see Chap. 9), an effect of inhalational anesthetics on calcium availability is a highly likely site of anesthetic interaction with EDRF/NO generation. As discussed above, inhalational anesthetics have been shown to impair receptor activation (2,4,15,37,96,132,195). Anthony et al. (2), Dennison et al. (37), and Aronstam et al. (4) have investigated the mechanisms of inhalational anesthetic inhibition of muscarinic acetylcholine receptors in rat brain. They found both an increase in antagonist, but not agonist-binding affinity, caused by a decrease in the rate of dissociation, and a decrease in the guanine nucleotide sensitivity of agonist binding. These effects were common to halothane, enflurane, isoflurane, diethyl ether, and chloroform, suggesting that interference with muscarinic receptor–G protein interactions is a common property of volatile anesthetics and may represent a general mechanism for the disruption of signal transmission between cells during anesthesia. Puil et al. (148), studying calcium transients in response to NMDA receptor activation in rat hippocampal neurons, observed that both isoflurane and halothane inhibited the calcium response to glutamate. While anesthetic inhibition of muscarinic receptor (or other receptor) activation may be a component of the mechanism by which anesthetics inhibit EDRF/NO production in response to those specific agonists, receptor activation is not likely to be the major or only site of anesthetic inhibition of NO signaling, as we have demonstrated significant anesthetic inhibition of calcium ionophore (A23187)-stimulated EDRF/NO production that bypasses receptor effects (195).

Inhalational anesthetics have also been shown to affect calcium homeostasis in endothelial cells. Uhl et al. (196), using fluorescent dye studies, have shown that halothane modestly decreased basal intracellular calcium and impaired the ATP-stimulated calcium transient in endothelial cells. Loeb et al. (103), using the fluorescent Ca^{2+} indicator dye FURA-2, have reported that both halothane and isoflurane enhance basal Ca^{2+} concentrations, and that halothane significantly inhibited the calcium transient evoked by bradykinin. Tsuchida et al. (194), studying endothelium-denuded rat aorta, found a decrease in cytosolic calcium that correlated with halothane and isoflurane-induced vasodilation. The most established actions of inhalational anesthetics on cytosolic Ca^{2+} concentration in other cell types have been through an effect on calcium movement into the cell, either by changing Ca^{2+} influx through receptor- or voltage-activated membrane Ca^{2+} channels, or by altering Ca^{2+} release from or uptake into the sarcoplasmic reticulum (90,167,188).

EDRF/NO activity may be attenuated by an interaction with the phospholipase C–inositol phosphate pathway in the endothelial cell. Indeed, halothane has been shown to inhibit stimulated phosphatidylinositol 4,5-bisphosphate hydrolysis in RBL-2H3 cells (162). Sill et al. (181) have demonstrated that halothane inhibits serotonin-stimulated phosphatidylinositol 4,5-bisphosphate hydrolysis in vascular smooth muscle and that isoflurane inhibits acetylcholine stimulated phosphatidylinositol-4,5-bisphosphate hydrolysis in coronary smooth muscle. In preliminary studies, they demonstrated that halothane does not inhibit phorbol-12,13-dibutyrate–stimulated protein kinase C action in vascular smooth muscle, suggesting that an effect through diacylglycerol is unlikely (181). Other recent work suggests that inhalational anesthetics do inhibit protein kinase C (see Chap. 7). Thus, inhalational anesthetics are clearly capable of decreasing Ca^{2+} availability for NO synthase activation and may do so by altering calcium entry through the plasma membrane, Ca^{2+} release from or reuptake into intracellular stores, or through inhibiting phospholipase C and altering IP_3-mediated calcium release.

3: Availability of Other Cofactors for NO Synthase

Halothane may interact with and inhibit calmodulin, perhaps by interacting with hydrophobic sites on the protein (169). Halothane potentiation of the antitumor activity of interferon is suggested to be mediated through inhibition of calmodulin. It was shown that halothane clearly mimicked specific calmodulin blocking agents (166). Excess calmodulin has been shown to reverse the activating effects of halothane on sarcoplasmic reticulum calcium release in skeletal muscle, suggesting that this action of halothane may be partially mediated through an inhibition of calmodulin (171).

4: Direct Interactions with NO Synthase

Inhalational anesthetics have been shown to bind competitively to specific hydrophobic regions of proteins (39). For example, halothane, methoxyflurane, and chloroform caused a 50% inhibition of luciferase activity (47). There appears to be a specific anesthetic-binding pocket on this enzyme, the hydrophobicity of which (and therefore anesthetic sensitivity of luciferase activity) is modulated by ATP (130). In the endothelial cell, NO synthase is 80% to 90% membrane associated (46,146), providing an additional potential mechanism for anesthetic interaction. Inhalational anesthetics could directly impair endothelial NO synthase activity through interaction with a hydrophobic site on the enzyme or by altering the fluidity or structure of enzyme-associated membrane. While an initial report implicated a direct interaction of inhalational anesthetics with NO synthase (192), a recent study suggests that this does not occur (159). Extensive study of the effects of isoflurane, halothane, and enflurane on purified and homogenate preparations of endothelial and neuronal NOS have failed to demonstrate any inhibition of NOS activity (159).

5: Inactivation of NO

It is also possible that inhalational anesthetics may inactivate NO following its production either via a direct interaction, or indirectly by enhancing free radical activity within the endothelial cell leading to the inactivation of EDRF by superoxide (see above discussion regarding sevoflurane) (96,127,180,195,207). Shayevitz et al. (180) have shown that halothane and isoflurane increase the sensitivity of rat pulmonary artery endothelial cells to injury by oxygen metabolites by inhibiting processes involved in intracellular antioxidant defenses. Anesthetic mediated increases in oxygen radicals within endothelial cells would clearly be a means of inactivating NO. The recent report by Blaise et al. (8) suggests that halothane either modifies the half-life of EDRF/NO or its activated redox form. Recently, by studying the effects of anesthetics on NO activation of guanylyl cyclase in cultured vascular smooth muscle and by studying the effects of anesthetics on NO activation of isolated soluble guanylyl cyclase and observing no significant effect, it has effectively been demonstrated, however, that inactivation of NO following its production is an unlikely mechanism for anesthetic inhibition of the NO pathway (86,211).

6: Inhibition of Guanylyl Cyclase

Muldoon et al. (133) have recently suggested that, in contrast to their original work, halothane may inhibit endothelium-dependent vasodilation through direct inhibition of soluble guanylyl cyclase. They suggest that halothane may interact with the heme moiety of guanylyl cyclase, as it has previously been shown to interact with the heme of a cytochrome P450. While work in vascular rings would suggest this is not the major site of anesthetic inhibition of NO signaling, an additional action on guanylyl cyclase cannot be ruled out by such studies. Eskinder et al. (40) studied the effects of halothane on the activity of isolated soluble and particulate guanylyl cyclases. While halothane had no effect on the soluble cyclase (which is involved in vasodilation by EDRF/NO), it significantly stimulated the activity of the particulate guanylyl cyclase (normally stimulated by atrial natriuretic peptide and some bacterial toxins but not involved in EDRF/NO dependent vasodilation). Recent work in our laboratory (86,211), studying the effects of inhalational anesthetics on both soluble and particulate guanylyl cyclase activity in cultured endothelial and vascular smooth muscle cells as well as in soluble and particulate guanylyl cyclase enzymes purified from brain, demonstrates that both halothane and isoflurane at 1% to 5% concentrations have no stimulatory or inhibitory effect on soluble or particulate guanylyl cyclase.

IMPORTANCE OF ANESTHETIC INTERACTION WITH NO SIGNALING

An understanding of the mechanisms of the observed inhibitory interactions of inhalational anesthetics with NO signaling and their potential stimulation of this pathway under certain conditions is clearly of tremendous clinical importance, given the widespread role of this pathway in the physiology and pathophysiology of multiple systems (13,80,125,128,137), the extensive use of these anesthetics, and their potent hemodynamic and central nervous system effects. NO actions have been most studied in the vasculature, the site at which anesthetics have clearly been shown to inhibit NO-dependent vasodilation. The pathway for NO production is present in all vascular beds, large and small vessels, and in a wide range of species (13,64,80,96,128). EDRF/NO is a potent endogenous vasodilator and an inhibitor of platelet aggregation and adhesion (128). Its activity is impaired in hypertension and atherosclerosis (128), and its absence due to endothelial damage may play a role in cerebral and coronary vasospasm (80). It is a mediator of flow-dependent vasodilation (75), and a modulator of the hypoxic pulmonary vasoconstrictor response (3). Endothelial cell damage and impairment of EDRF/NO production may also contribute to acute and chronic pulmonary hypertension, and EDRF/NO may be responsible for the low resting tone of the pulmonary vasculature (42). Inhaled exogenous NO is a potent, selective, and clinically useful pulmonary vasodilator (49,160). The central nervous system functions of NO are just beginning to be explored, but it is clear that NO mediates excitatory amino acid receptor stimulation of neuronal cGMP (11–13,57–59,80,109,127), that it mediates nonadrenergic, noncholinergic neurotransmission through which it may control peristalsis of the gastrointestinal tract, and also mediates relaxation of the corpora cavernosae of the penis (61,18,152,191). NO is also a mediator in synaptic plasticity such as its role in long-term potentiation (9,141). We have recently demonstrated that inhibitors of NO synthase decrease the threshold (MAC) for halothane and isoflurane anesthesia in the rat, suggesting an exciting new role for the NO signaling pathway in modulating consciousness and a possible involvement in the central mechanisms of anesthetic action (84).

ACKNOWLEDGMENT

This work is supported in part by National Institutes of Health Grants HL39706 and GM49111.

REFERENCES

1. Adams DJ, Barakeh J, Laskey R, van Breemen C. Ion channels and regulation of intracellular calcium in vascular endothelial cells. *FASEB J* 1989;3:2389–2400.
2. Anthony BL, Dennison RL, Aronstam RS. Disruption of muscarinic receptor-G protein coupling is a general property of liquid volatile anesthetics. *Neurosci Lett* 1989;99:191–196.
3. Archer SL, Tolins JP, Raij L, Weir EK. Hypoxic pulmonary vasoconstriction is enhanced by inhibition of the synthesis of an endothelium derived relaxing factor. *Biochem Biophys Res Commun* 1989;164:1198–1205.
4. Aronstam RS, Anthony BL, Dennison RL. Halothane effects on muscarinic acetylcholine receptor complexes in rat brain. *Biochem Pharmacol* 1986;35:667–672.
5. Az-ma T, Fujii K, Yuge O. Inhibitory effect of sevoflurane on nitric oxide release from cultured endothelial cells. *Eur J Pharmacol Mol Pharmacol* 1995;289:33–39.
6. Beckman JS, Beckman TW, Chen J, et al. Apparent hydroxyl radical production by peroxynitrite: implications for endothelial injury from nitric oxide and superoxide. *Proc Natl Acad Sci USA* 1990;87:1620–1624.
7. Blaise G, Sill JC, Nugent M, et al. Isoflurane causes endothelium-dependent inhibition of contractile responses of canine coronary arteries. *Anesthesiology* 1987;67:513–517.
8. Blaise G, To Q, Parent M, et al. Does halothane interfere with the release, action, or stability of endothelium-derived relaxing factor/nitric oxide? *Anesthesiology* 1994;80:417–426.
9. Bohme GA, Bon C, Stutzmann JM, et al. Possible involvement of nitric oxide in long-term potentiation. *Eur J Pharmacol* 1991;199: 379–381.
10. Bredt DS, Ferris C, Snyder SH. Nitric oxide synthase regulatory sites. *J Biol Chem* 1992;267:10976–10981.
11. Bredt DS, Hwang PM, Glatt CE, et al. Cloned and expressed nitric oxide synthase structurally resembles cytochrome P-450 reductase. *Nature* 1991;351:714–718.
12. Bredt DS, Snyder SH. Nitric oxide mediates glutamate linked enhancement of cGMP levels in the cerebellum. *Proc Natl Acad Sci USA* 1989;86:9030–9033.
13. Bredt DS, Snyder SH. Nitric oxide, a novel neuronal messenger. *Neuron* 1992;8:3–11.
14. Brendel J, Johns RA. Isoflurane does not vasodilate rat thoracic

aortic rings by endothelium-derived relaxing factor or other cyclic GMP-mediated mechanisms. *Anesthesiology* 1990;77:126–131.
15. Brett RS, Dilger JP, Yland KF. Isoflurane causes flickering of the acetylcholine receptor channel: Observations using patch clamp. *Anesthesiology* 1988;69:157–160.
16. Bruce B, Lapetina EG. Activation of a cytosolic ADP-ribosyltransferase by nitric oxide-generating agents. *J Biol Chem* 1989;264: 8455–8458.
17. Brune B, Lapetina EG. Phosphorylation of nitric oxide synthase by protein kinase A. *Biochem Biophys Res Commun* 1991;181: 921–926.
18. Bult H, Boeckxstaens GE, Pelckmans PA, et al. Nitric oxide as an inhibitory non-adrenergic non-cholinergic neurotransmitter. *Nature* 1990;345:346–347.
19. Busconi L, Michel T. Endothelial nitric oxide synthase. N-terminal myristoylation determines subcellular localization. *J Biol Chem* 1993;268:8410–8413.
20. Busconi L, Michel T. Recombinant endothelial nitric oxide synthase: Post-translational modifications in a baculovirus expression system. *Mol Pharmacol* 1995;47:655–659.
21. Busse R, Mulsch A. Induction of nitric oxide synthase by cytokines in vascular smooth muscle cells. *FEBS* 1990;275:87–90.
22. Cannell MB, Sage SO. Bradykinin-evoked changes in cytosolic calciumand membrane currents in cultured bovine pulmonary artery endothelial cells. *J Physiol* 1989;419:555–568.
23. Chand N, Altura BM. Acetylcholine and bradykinin relax intrapulmonary arteries by acting on endothelial cells: role in lung vascular diseases. *Science* 1981;213:1376–1379.
24. Chen GF, Cheung DW. Characterization of acetylcholine-induced membrane hyperpolarization in endothelial cells. *Circ Res* 1992; 70:257–263.
25. Chen WZ, Palmer RMJ, Moncada S. The effects of nitric oxide on the isolated perfused rabbit heart. *Br J Pharmacol* 1988;92: 643(abstr).
26. Chen XL, Rembold CM. Cyclic nucleotide-dependent regulation of Mn^{2+} influx, $[Ca^{2+}]_i$, and arterial smooth muscle relaxation. *Am J Physiol* 1992;C468:C4731992.
27. Chrisman TD, Schulz S, Garbers DL. Guanylyl cyclases: Ligands and functions. *Cold Spring Harbor Symp Quant Biol* 1992;57:155–162.
28. Clemo HF, Feher JJ, Baumgarten CM. Modulation of rabbit ventricular cell volume and $Na^+/K^+/2Cl^-$ cotransport by cGMP and atrial natriuretic factor. *J Gen Physiol* 1992;100:89–114.
29. Cocks TH, Angus JA. Endothelium-dependent relaxation of coronary arteries by noradrenaline and serotonin. *Nature* 1983;305: 627–630.
30. Coldeu-Stanfield M, Schilling WP, Ritchie AK, et al. Bradykinin-induced increases in cytosolic calcium and ionic channels in cultured bovine aortic endothelial cells. *Circ Res* 1987;61:632–640.
31. Cook NJ, Hanke W, Kaupp UB. Identification, purification, and functional reconstitution of the cyclic GMP-dependent channel from rod photoreceptors. *Proc Natl Acad Sci USA* 1987;84:585-589.
32. Crystal GJ, Kim SJ, Salem MR, Khoury E. Role of nitric oxide in isoflurane-induced coronary vasodilation. *Anesthesiology* 1992;77: A681.
33. Dawson VL, Dawson TM, London ED, et al. Nitric oxide mediates glutamate neurotoxicity in primary cortical culture. *Proc Natl Acad Sci USA* 1991;88:6368–6371.
34. de Nucci G, Gryglewski RJ, Warner TD, Vane JR. Receptor-mediated release of endothelium-derived relaxing factor and prostacyclin from bovine aortic endothelial cells is coupled. *Proc Natl Acad Sci USA* 1988;85:2334–2338.
35. DeMey JG, Claeys M, Vanhoutte PM. Endothelium-dependent inhibitory effects of acetylcholine, adenosine triphosphate-thrombin and arachidonic acid in the canine femoral artery. *J Pharmacol Exp Ther* 1982;222:166–173.
36. DeMey JG, Vanhoutte PM. Role of the intima in cholinergic and purinergic relaxation of isolated canine femoral arteries. *J Physiol (Lond)* 1981;316:347–355.
37. Dennison RL, Anthony BL, Narayanan TK, Aronstam RS. Effects of halothane on high affinity agonist binding and guanine nucleotide sensitivity of muscarinic acetylcholine receptors from brainstem of rat. *Neuropharmacology* 1987;26:1201–1205.
38. Dolor RJ, Hurwitz LM, Mirza Z, et al. Regulation of extracellular calcium entry in endothelial cells: role of intracellular calcium pool. *Am J Physiol* 1992;262:C171–C181.
39. Dubois BW, Cherian SF, Evers AS. Volatile anesthetics compete for common binding sites on bovine serum albumin: $A^{19}F$-NMR study. *Proc Natl Acad Sci USA* 1993;90:6478–6482.
40. Eskinder H, Hillard CJ, Flynn N, et al. Role of guanylate cyclase-cGMP systems in halothane-induced vasodilation in canine cerebral arteries. *Anesthesiology* 1992;77:482–487.
41. Fichtner H, Frobe U, Busse R, Kohlhardt M. Single nonselective cation channels and Ca^{2+}-activated K- channels in aortic endothelial cells. *J Membr Biol* 1987;98:125–133.
42. Fineman JR, Chang R, Soifer SJ. EDRF inhibition augments pulmonary hypertension in intact newborn lambs. *Am J Physiol Heart Circ Physiol* 1992;262:H1365–H1371.
43. Flynn N, Bosnjak ZJ, Kampine JP. Isoflurane effect on isolated canine cerebral vascular segments is not endothelium-dependent. *Anesthesiology* 1990;73:A5771990.
44. Flynn N, Bosnjak ZJ, Warltier DC, Kampine JP. Endothelium dependent relaxation in canine coronary collateral vessels. *Anesthesiology* 1990;73:A590.
45. Forstermann U, Neufang B. Endothelium-dependent vasodilation by melittin are lipoxygenase products involved. *Am J Physiol* 1985; 249:H14–H19.
46. Forstermann U, Pollock JS, Schmidt HHHW, et al. Calmodulin-dependent endothelium-derived relaxing factor/nitric oxide synthase activity is present in the particulate and cytosolic fractions of bovine aortic ECs. *Proc Natl Acad Sci USA* 1991;88:1788–1792.
47. Franks NP, Lieb WR. Do general anesthetics act by competitive binding to specific receptors? *Nature* 1987;310:599–601.
48. Freay A, Johns A, Adams DJ, Ryan US, van Breemen C. Bradykinin and inositol 1,4,5-trisphosphate-stimulated calcium release from intracellular stores in cultured bovine endothelial cells. *Pflugers Arch* 1989;414:377–384.
49. Frostell C, Fratacci MD, Wain JC, et al. Inhaled nitric oxide: selective pulmonary vasodilator reversing hypoxic pulmonary vasoconstriction. *Circulation* 1991;83:2038–2047.
50. Furchgott RF. Role of endothelium in responses of vascular smooth muscle. *Circ Res* 1983;53:557–573.
51. Furchgott RF. The role of endothelium in the responses of vascular smooth muscle to drugs. *Annu Rev Pharmacol Toxicol* 1984;24: 175–197.
52. Furchgott RF, Vanhoutte PM. Endothelium-derived relaxing and contracting factors. *FASEB J* 1989;3:2007–2018.
53. Furchgott RF, Zawadzki JV. The obligatory role of endothelial cells in the relaxation of arterial smooth muscle by acetylcholine. *Nature* 1980;288:373–376.
54. Furukawa K-I, Ohshima N, Tawada-Iwata Y, Shigekawa M. Cyclic GMP stimulates Na^+/Ca^{2+} exchange in vascular smooth muscle cells in primary culture. *J Biol Chem* 1991;266:12337–12341.
55. Garbers DL. Guanylyl cyclase receptors and their ligands. *Adv Second Messenger Phosphoprotein Res* 1993;28:91–95.
56. Garland CJ, McPherson GA. Evidence that nitric oxide does not mediate the hyperpolarization and relaxation to acetylcholine in the rat small mesenteric artery. *Br J Pharmacol* 1992;105:429–435.
57. Garthwaite J, Charles SL, Chess Williams R. Endothelium-derived relaxing factor release on activation of NMDA receptors suggests role as intercellular messenger in the brain. *Nature* 1988;336: 385–388.
58. Garthwaite J, Garthwaite G, Palmer RM, Moncada S. NMDA receptor activation induces nitric oxide synthesis from arginine in rat brain slices. *Eur J Pharmacol* 1989;172:413–416.
59. Garthwaite J, Southam E, Anderton M. A kainate receptor linked to nitric oxide synthesis from arginine. *J Neurochem* 1989;53: 1952–1954.
60. Geiger J, Nolte C, Butt E, et al. Role of cGMP and cGMP-dependent protein kinase in nitrovasodilator inhibition of agonist-evoked calcium elevation in human platelets. *Proc Natl Acad Sci USA* 1992;89:1031–1035.
61. Gillespie JS, Liu X, Martin W. The effects of L-arginine and NG-monomethyl L-arginine on the response of the rat anococcygeus muscle to NANC nerve stimulation. *Br J Pharmacol* 1989;98: 1080–1082.
62. Gopalakrishna R, Chen ZH, Gundimeda U. Nitric oxide and nitric oxide-generating agents induce a reversible inactivation of protein kinase C activity and phorbol ester binding. *J Biol Chem* 1993; 268:27180–27185.
63. Graier WF, Schmidt K, Kukovetz WR. Activation of G protein evokes Ca^{2+} influx in endothelial cells without correlation to inositol phosphates. *J Cardiovasc Pharmacol* 1991;17:S71–S78.
64. Graser T, Leisner H, Vedernikov YP, Tiedt H. The action of acetyl-

choline on isolated coronary arteries of different species. *Cor Vasa* 1987;29:70–80.

65. Greenblatt EP, Loeb AL, Longnecker DE. Influences of halothane and isoflurane on endothelium-dependent circulatory control in vivo. *Anesthesiology* 1991;75:A531.
66. Griffith TM, Edwards DH, Lewis MJ, Newby AC. The nature of endothelium-derived vascular relaxant factor. *Nature* 1984;308: 645–647.
67. Hall AV, Antoniou H, Wang Y, et al. Structural organization of the human neuronal nitric oxide synthase gene (NOS1). *J Biol Chem* 1994;269(52):33082–33090.
68. Hallam TJ, Pearson JD. Exogenous ATP raises cytoplasmic free calcium in fura-2 loaded piglet aortic endothelial cells. *FEBS Lett* 1986;207:95–99.
69. Harbrecht BG, Stadler J, Billiar TR, et al. Inhibition of glutathione metabolism decreases hepatocyte nitric oxide synthesis. *FASEB J* 1991;5:A371–ABS# 4364.
70. Hearn JC, Xie Q, Calaycay J, et al. Calmodulin is a subunit of nitric oxide synthase from macrophages. *J Exp Med* 1992;176: 599–604.
71. Hevel JM, Marletta MA. Macrophage nitric oxide synthase: Relationship between enzyme-bound tetrahydrobiopterin and synthase activity. *Biochemistry* 1992;31:7160–7165.
72. Hevel JM, Marletta MA. Macrophage nitric oxide synthase: Tetrahydrobiopterin decreases the NADPH stoichiometry. *Adv Exp Med Biol* 1993;338:285–288.
73. Hirata M, Kohse KP, Chang C-H, et al. Mechanism of cyclic GMP inhibition of inositol phosphate formation in rat aorta segments and cultured bovine aortic smooth muscle cells. *J Biol Chem* 1990; 265:1268–1273.
74. Hishikawa K, Nakaki T, Marumo T, et al. Up-regulation of nitric oxide synthase by estradiol in human aortic endothelial cells. *FEBS Lett* 1995;360:291–293.
75. Holtz J, Forstermann U, Pohl U, et al. Flow-dependent-endothelium-mediated dilation of epicardial coronary arteries in conscious dogs. effects of cyclooxygenase inhibition. *J Cardiovasc Pharmacol* 1984;6:1161–1169.
76. Holzmann S. Endothelium-induced relaxation by acetylcholine associated with larger rises in cyclic GMP in coronary arterial strips. *J Cyc Nucleotide Res* 1982;8:409–419.
77. Irvine RF, Moore RM. Micro-injection of inositol 1,3,4,5-tetrakisphosphate activates sea urchin eggs by a mechanism dependent on external Ca^{2+}. *Biochem J* 1986;240:917–920.
78. Janssens SP, Shimouchi A, Quertermous T, et al. Cloning and expression of a cDNA encoding human endothelium-derived relaxing factor/nitric oxide synthase. *J Biol Chem* 1992;267: 14519–14522.
79. Johns A, Freay AD, Adams DJ, et al. Role of calcium in the activation of endothelial cells. *J Cardiovasc Pharmacol* 1988;12: S119–S123.
80. Johns RA. Endothelium-derived relaxing factor: Basic review and clinical implications. *J Cardiothorac Vasc Anesth* 1991;5:69–79.
81. Johns RA. Endothelium, anesthetics, and vascular control. *Anesthesiology* 1993;79:1381–1391.
82. Johns RA, Izzo NJ, Milner PJ, et al. Use of cultured cells to study the relationship between arachidonic acid and endothelium-derived relaxing factor. *Am J Med Sci* 1988;295:287–292.
83. Johns RA, Linden JM, Peach MJ. Endothelium-dependent relaxation and cyclic GMP accumulation in rabbit pulmonary artery are selectively impaired by hypoxia. *Circ Res* 1989;65:1508–1515.
84. Johns RA, Moscicki JC, DiFazio CA. Nitric oxide synthase inhibitor dose-dependently and reversibly reduces the threshold for halothane anesthesia: A role for nitric oxide in mediating consciousness. *Anesthesiology* 1992;77:779–784.
85. Johns RA, Peach MJ, Linden JM, Tichotsky A. NG-monomethyl-L-arginine causes specific, dose-dependent inhibition of cyclic GMP accumulation in cocultures of bovine pulmonary endothelium and rat VSM through an action specific to the endothelium. *Circ Res* 1990;67:979–985.
86. Johns RA, Tichotsky A, Muro M, et al. Halothane and isoflurane inhibit EDRF-dependent cyclic GMP accumulation in endothelial cell-vascular smooth muscle co-cultures independent of an effect on guanylyl cyclase activation. *Anesthesiology* 1995;83: 823–834.
87. Kaupp UB. The cyclic nucleotide-gated channels of vertebrate photoreceptors and olfactory epithelium. *Trends Neurosci* 1991; 14:150–157.
88. Kaupp UB, Niidome T, Tanabe T, et al. Primary structure and functional expression from complementary DNA of the rod photoreceptor cyclic GMP-gated channel. *Nature* 1989;342:762–766.
89. Kilbourn RG, Griffith OW. Overproduction of nitric oxide in cytokine-mediated and septic shock. *J Natl Cancer Inst* 1992;84: 827–831.
90. Klip A, Britt BA, Elliott ME, et al. Changes in cytoplasmic free calcium caused by halothane. Role of the plasma membrane and intracellular Ca^{2+} stores. *Biochem Cell Biol* 1986;64:1181–1189.
91. Koesling D, Bohme E, Shultz G. Guanylyl cyclases, a growing family of signal-transducing enzymes. *FASEB J* 1991;5:2785–2791.
92. Kwon NS, Nathan CF, Gilker C, et al. L-citrulline production from L-arginine by macrophage nitric oxide synthase. *J Biol Chem* 1990;265:13442–13445.
93. Lambert TL, Kent RS, Whorton AR. Bradykinin stimulation of inositol polyphosphate production in porcine aortic endothelial cells. *J Biol Chem* 1986;261:15288–15293.
94. Lancaster JE, Hibbs JB. EPR demonstration of iron-nitrosyl complex formation by cytotoxic activated macrophages. *Proc Natl Acad Sci USA* 1990;87:1223–1227.
95. Langenstroer P, Pieper GM. Regulation of spontaneous EDRF release in diabetic rat aorta by oxygen free radicals. *Am J Physiol Heart Circ Physiol* 1992;263:H257–H265.
96. Lechlecter J, Greuner R. Halothane shortens acetylcholine receptor channel kinetics without affecting conductance. *Proc Natl Acad Sci USA* 1989;81:2929–2933.
97. Lesh RE, Marks AR, Somlyo AV, et al. Anti-ryanodine receptor antibody binding sites in vascular and endocardial endothelium. *Circ Res* 1993;72:481–488.
98. Lewis MJ, Henderson AH. A phorbol ester inhibits the release of endothelium-derived relaxing factor. *Eur J Pharmacol* 1987;137: 167–171.
99. Light DB, Corbin JD, Stanton BA. Dual ion-channel regulation by cyclic GMP and cyclic GMP-dependent protein kinase. *Nature* 1990;344:336–339.
100. Lincoln TM. Cyclic GMP and mechanisms of vasodilation. *Pharmacol Ther* 1989;41:479–502.
101. Lincoln TM, Cornwell TL. Intracellular cyclic GMP receptor proteins. *FASEB J* 1993;7:328–338.
102. Loeb AL, Izzo NJ, Johnson RM, et al. Endothelium-derived relaxing factor release associated with increased endothelial cell inositol trisphosphate and intracellular calcium. *Am J Cardiol* 1988; 62:36G–40G.
103. Loeb AL, Longnecker DE, Williamson JR. Alteration of calcium mobilization in endothelial cells by volatile anesthetics. *Biochem Pharmacol* 1993;45:1137–1142.
104. Long CJ, Stone TW. The release of endothelium-derived relaxant factor is calcium dependent. *Blood Vessels* 1985;22:205–208.
105. Lowenstein CJ, Alley EW, Raval P, et al. Macrophage nitric oxide synthase gene: Two upstream regions mediate induction by interferon gamma and lipopolysaccharide. *Proc Natl Acad Sci USA* 1993;90:9730–9734.
106. Lynch C. Differential depression of myocardial contractility by halothane and isoflurane in vitro. *Anesthesiology* 1986;64: 620–631.
107. Lyons CR, Orloff GJ, Cunningham JM. Molecular cloning and functional expression of an inducible nitric oxide synthase from a murine macrophage cell line. *J Biol Chem* 1992;267:6370–6374.
108. Malinconico ST, McCarl RL. Effect of halothane on cardiac sarcoplasmic reticulum Ca^{2+}-ATPase at low calcium concentrations. *Mol Pharmacol* 1982;22:8–10.
109. Marletta MA, Yoon PS, Yengar R, et al. Macrophage oxidation of L-arginine to nitrite and nitrate: Nitric oxide is an intermediate. *Biochem J* 1988;27:8706–8711.
110. Marsden PA, Heng HHQ, Scherer SW, et al. Structure and chromosomal localization of the human constitutive endothelial nitric oxide synthase gene. *J Biol Chem* 1993;268:17478–17488.
111. Martin W, Villani G, Jothianandan D, Furchgott R. Selective blockade of endothelium-dependent and glyceryl trinitrate-induced relaxation by hemoglobin and by methylene blue in the rabbit aorta. *J Pharmacol Exp Ther* 1985;232:703–716.
112. Mayer B, Brunner F, Schmidt K. Inhibition of nitric oxide synthesis by methylene blue. *Biochem Pharmacol* 1993;45:367–374.
113. Mayer B, Heinzel B, Klatt P, et al. Nitric oxide synthase-catalyzed activation of oxygen and reduction of cytochromes: Reaction mechanisms and possible physiological implications. *J Cardiovasc Pharmacol* 1992;20(suppl 12):S54–S56.

114. McDonald CC, Philips WO, Mower HF. An electron spin resonance study of some complexes of iron, nitric oxide, and amionic ligands. *J Am Chem Soc* 1965;87:3319–3326.65.
115. McMurtry IF, Morris KG. Platelet-activating factor causes pulmonary vasodilation in the rat. *Am Rev Respir Dis* 1986;134: 757–762.
116. Meisheri KD, Cipkus-Dubray LA, Hosner JM, Khan SA. Nicorandil-induced vasorelaxation: functional evidence for K- channel-dependent and cyclic GMP-dependent components in a single vascular preparation. *J Cardiovasc Pharmacol* 1991;17:903–912.
117. Meller ST, Dykstra C, Gebhart GF. Production of endogenous nitric oxide and activation of soluble guanylate cyclase are required for N-methyl-D-aspartate-produced facilitation of the nociceptive tail-flick reflex. *Eur J Pharmacol* 1992;214:93–96.
118. Meller ST, Pechman PS, Gebhart GF, Maves TJ. Nitric oxide mediates the thermal hyperalgesia produced in a model of neuropathic pain in the rat. *Neuroscience* 1992;50:7–10.
119. Meyer J, Traber LD, Nelson S, et al. Reversal of hyperdynamic response to continuous endotoxin administration by inhibition of NO synthesis. *J Appl Physiol* 1992;73:324–328.
120. Michel T, Li GK, Busconi L. Phosphorylation and subcellular translocation of endothelial nitric oxide synthase. *Proc Natl Acad Sci USA* 1993;90:6252–6256.
121. Miller RC, Schoeffter P, Stoclet JC. Insensitivity of calcium-dependent endothelial stimulation in rat isolated aorta to the calcium entry blocker-flunarizine. *Br J Pharmacol* 1985;85:481–487.
122. Miller WH. Physiological effects of cyclic GMP in the vertebrate retinal rod outer segment. *Adv Cyclic Nucleotide Res* 1983;15: 495–511.
123. Misko TP, Moore WM, Kasten TP, et al. Selective inhibition of the inducible nitric oxide synthase by aminoguanidine. *Eur J Pharmacol* 1993;233:119–125.
124. Moncada S. The L-arginine: nitric oxide pathway. *Acta Physiol Scand* 1992;145:201–227.
125. Moncada S, Higgs EA. Endogenous nitric oxide: physiology, pathology and clinical relevance. *Eur J Clin Invest* 1991;21: 361–374.
126. Moncada S, Palmer RM, Gryglewski RJ. Mechanism of action of some inhibitors of endothelium-derived relaxing factor. *Proc Natl Acad Sci USA* 1986;83:9164–9168.
127. Moncada S, Palmer RMJ, Higgs EA. Nitric oxide: Physiology, pathophysiology, and pharmacology. *Pharmacol Rev* 1991;43: 109–142.
128. Moncada S, Palmer RM. Nitric oxide: physiology, pathophysiology, and pharmacology. *Pharmacol Rev* 1991;43:109–142.
129. Moore PK, Babbedge RC, Wallace P, et al. 7-nitro indazole, an inhibitor of nitric oxide synthase, exhibits anti-nociceptive activity in the mouse without increasing blood pressure. *Br J Pharmacol* 1993;108:296–297.
130. Moss GWJ, Franks NP, Lieb WR. Modulation of the general anesthetic sensitivity of a protein: A transition between two forms of firefly luciferase. *Proc Natl Acad Sci USA* 1991;88:134–138.
131. Mugge A, Elwell JH, Peterson TE, Harrison DG. Release of intact endothelium-derived relaxing factor depends on endothelial superoxide dismutase activity. *Am J Physiol (Cell Physiol)* 1991;260: C219–C225.
132. Muldoon SM, Hart JL, Bowen KA, Freas W. Attenuation of endothelium-mediated vasodilation by halothane. *Anesthesiology* 1988;68:31–37.
133. Muldoon SM, Jing M, Freas W, et al. Proposed mechanism for the attenuation of endothelial induced relaxation by volatile anesthetics. *Anesthesiology* 1992;77:A687.
134. Nakamura K, Hatano Y, Toda H, Mori K. Isoflurane inhibits endothelium-dependent relaxation and cyclic GMP formation in rat aorta. *Anesthesiology* 1991;75:A530.
135. Nakane M, Mitchell J, Forstermann U, Murad F. Phosphorylation by calcium calmodulin-dependent protein kinase II and protein kinase C modulates the activity of nitric oxide synthase. *Biochem Biophys Res Commun* 1991;180:1396–1402.
136. Nakane M, Saheki S, Kuno T, et al. Molecular cloning of a 70 kilodalton subunit of soluble guanylate cyclase from rat lung. *Biochem Biophys Res Commun* 1987;157:1138–1147.
137. Nathan C. Nitric oxide as a secretory product of mammalian cells. *FASEB J* 1992;6:3051–3064.
138. Nathan C, Xie Q. Regulation of biosynthesis of nitric oxide. *J Biol Chem* 1994;269:13725–13728.
139. Nathan C, Xie Q. Nitric oxide synthases: Roles, tolls, and controls. *Cell* 1994;78:915–918.
140. Nishida K, Harrison DG, Navas JP, et al. Molecular cloning and characterization of the constitutive bovine aortic endothelial cell nitric oxide synthase. *J Clin Invest* 1992;90:2092–2096.
141. Son H, Hawkins RD, Martin K, Kiebler M, Huang PL, Fishman MC, Kandel ER. Long-term potentiation is reduced in mice that are doubly mutant in endothelial and neuronal nitric oxide synthase. *Cell* 1996;87:1015–1023.
142. Ono K, Trautwein W. Potentiation by cyclic GMP of beta-adrenergic effect on Ca^{2+} current in guinea-pig ventricular cells. *J Physiol* 1991;443:387–404.
143. Palmer RM, Ashton DS, Moncada S. Vascular endothelial cells synthesize nitric oxide from L-arginine. *Nature* 1988;333:664–666.
144. Palmer RMJ, Moncada S. A novel citrulline-forming enzyme implicated in the formation of NO by vascular endothelial cells. *Biochem Biophys Res Commun* 1989;58:348–352.
145. Peach MJ, Singer HA, Izzo NJ, Loeb AL. Role of calcium in endothelium-dependent relaxation of arterial smooth muscle. *Am J Cardiol* 1987;59:35A–43A.
146. Pollock JS, Forstermann U, Mitchell JA, et al. Purification and characterization of particulate endothelium-derived relaxing factor synthase from cultured and native bovine aortic endothelial cells. *Proc Natl Acad Sci USA* 1991;88:10480–10484.
147. Prince RC, Gunson DE. Rising interest in nitric oxide synthase. *Trends Biochem Sci* 1993;18:35–36.
148. Puil E, El-Beheiry H, Baimbridge KG. Anesthetic effects on glutamate-stimulated increase in intraneuronal calcium. *J Pharm Exp* 1990;255:955–961.
149. Radomski MW, Palmer RML, Moncada S. Glucocorticoids inhibit the expression of an inducible, but not the constitutive, nitric oxide synthase in vascular ECs. *Proc Natl Acad Sci USA* 1990;87: 10043–10047.
150. Rae JL, Dewey J, Cooper K, Gates P. A non-selective cation channel in rabbit corneal endothelium activated by internal calcium and inhibited by internal ATP. *Exp Eye Res* 1990;50:373–384.
151. Raeymaekers L, Hofmann F, Casteels R. Cyclic GMP-dependent protein kinase phosphorylates phospholamban in isolated sarcoplasmic reticulum from cardiac and smooth muscle. *Biochem J* 1988;252:269–273.
152. Raifer J, Aronson WJ, Bush PA, et al. Nitric oxide as a mediator of relaxation of the corpus cavernosum in response to noradrenergic, noncholinergic neurotransmission. *N Engl J Med* 1992;326:90–94.
153. Rapoport R, Murad F. Endothelium-dependent and nitrovasodilator-induced relaxation of vascular smooth muscle: Role of cyclic GMP. *J Cyclic Nucleotide Prot Phos Res* 1983;9:281–296.
154. Rapoport RM. Cyclic guanosine monophosphate inhibition of contraction may be mediated through inhibition of phosphatidylinositol hydrolysis in rat aorta. *Circ Res* 1986;58:407–410.
155. Rees D, Palmer RMJ, Hodson HF, Moncada S. A specific inhibitor of nitric oxide formation from L-arginine attenuates endothelium-dependent relaxation. *Br J Pharmacol* 1989;96:418–424.
156. Rengasamy A, Johns RA. Characterization of EDRF/NO synthase from bovine cerebellum and mechanism of modulation by high and low oxygen tensions. *J Pharmacol Exp Ther* 1991;259:310–316.
157. Rengasamy A, Johns RA. Feedback inhibition of EDRF/NO synthase. *FASEB J* 1992;6:A2257.
158. Rengasamy A, Johns RA. Regulation of nitric oxide synthase by nitric oxide. *Mol Pharmacol* 1993;44:124–128.
159. Rengasamy A, Ravichandran LV, Reikersdorfer CG, Johns RA. Inhalational Anesthetics do not Alter Nitric Oxide Synthase Activity. *J Pharmacol Exp Ther* 1995;273:599–604.
160. Rich GF, Roos CM, Anderson SM, et al. Inhaled nitric oxide: Dose-response and the effects of blood in the isolated rat lung. *J Appl Physiol* 1993;75:1278–1284.
161. Robinson LJ, Busconi L, Michel T. Agonist-modulated palmitoylation of endothelial nitric oxide synthase. *J Biol Chem* 1995;270: 995–998.
162. Robinson-White A. Mechanisms of action of anesthetics on inositol phospholipid hydrolysis in vascular endothelial cells and rat basophilic leukemia cells in tissue culture. In: Blanck TJJ, Wheeler DM, eds. *Mechanisms of anesthetic action in skeletal, cardiac and smooth muscle.* New York: Plenum Press, 1991;271–287.
163. Rubanyi GM, Kauser K, Gräser T. Effect of cilazapril and indomethacin on endothelial dysfunction in the aortas of spontaneously hypertensive rats. *J Cardiovasc Pharmacol* 1993;22(suppl 5): S23–S30.
164. Rubanyi GM, Vanhoutte PM. Superoxide anions and hyperoxia inactivate endothelium-derived relaxing factor. *Am J Physiol* 1986; 250:H822–H827.

165. Rubanyi GM, Vanhoutte PM. Calcium and activation of the release of endothelium-derived relaxing factor. *Ann NY Acad Sci* 1988;522:226–233.
166. Rudnick S, Stevenson GW, Hall SC, et al. Halothane potentiates antitumor activity of gamma-interferon and mimics calmodulin-blocking agents. *Anesthesiology* 1991;74:115–119.
167. Rusy BF, Komai H. Anesthetic depression of myocardial contractility: A review of possible mechanisms. *Anesthesiology* 1987;67: 745–766.
168. Ryan US, Avdonin PV, Posin EY, et al. Influence of vasoactive agents on cytoplasmic free calcium in vascular endothelial cells. *J Appl Physiol* 1988;65:2221–2227.
169. Salviati G, Ceoldo S, Fachechi-Cassano G, Betto R. Ca release from skeletal muscle SR: Effects of volatile anesthetics. In: Blanck TJJ, Wheeler DM, eds. *Mechanisms of anesthetic action in skeletal, cardiac, and smooth muscle.* New York: Plenum Press, 1991;31–41.
170. Sarcevic B, Brookes V, Martin TJ, et al. Atrial natriuretic peptide-dependent phosphorylation of smooth muscle cell particulate fraction proteins is mediated by cGMP-dependent protein kinase. *J Biol Chem* 1989;264:20648–20654.
171. Sauve R, Chahine M, Tremblay J, Hamet P. Single-channel analysis of the electrical response of bovine aortic endothelial cells to bradykinin stimulation: contribution of a Ca^{2+}-dependent K^+ channel. *J Hypertens* 1990;8:S193–S201.
172. Schilling WP. Effect of membrane potential on cytosolic calcium of bovine aortic endothelial cells. *Am J Physiol (Heart Circ Physiol* 26) 1989;257:H778–H784.
173. Schilling WP, Rajan L, Strobl-Jager E. Characterization of the bradykinin-stimulated calcium influx pathway of cultured vascular endothelial cells. *J Biol Chem* 1989;264:12838–12848.
174. Schilling WP, Ritchie AK, Navarro LT, Eskin SG. Bradykinin-stimulated calcium influx in cultured bovine aortic endothelial cells. *Am J Physiol* 1988;255:H219–H227.
175. Schmidt HHHW, Lohmann SM, Walter U. The nitric oxide and cGMP signal transduction system: Regulation and mechanism of action. *Biochim Biophys Acta Mol Cell Res* 1993;1178:153–175.
176. Schmidt HHHW, Pollock JS, Nakane M, et al. Ca^{2+}/calmodulin-regulated nitric oxide synthases. *Cell Calcium* 1992;13:427–434.
177. Schott CA, Gray GA, Stoclet J-C. Dependence of endotoxin-induced vascular hyporeactivity on extracellular L-arginine. *Br J Pharmacol* 1993;108:38–43.
178. Sessa WC, Harrison JK, Barber CM, et al. Molecular cloning and expression of a cDNA encoding endothelial cell nitric oxide synthase. *J Biol Chem* 1992;267:15274–15276.
179. Sessa WC, Pritchard K, Seyedi N, et al. Chronic exercise in dogs increases coronary vascular nitric oxide production and endothelial cell nitric oxide synthase gene expression. *Circ Res* 1994;74: 349–353.
180. Shayevitz JR, Varani J, Ward PA, Knight PR. Halothane and isoflurane increase pulmonary artery endothelial cell sensitivity to oxidant-mediated injury. *Anesthesiology* 1991;74:1067–1077.
181. Sill JC, Nelson OR, Uhl C. Isoflurane-, halothane- and agonist-evoked responses in pig coronary arteries and vascular smooth muscle cells. In: Blanck TJJ, Wheeler DM, eds. *Mechanisms of anesthetic action in skeletal, cardiac, and smooth muscle.* New York: Plenum Press, 1991;257–269.
182. Singer HA, Peach MJ. Calcium- and endothelial-mediated vascular smooth muscle relaxation in rabbit aorta. *Hypertension* 1982;4: 19–25.
183. Singer HA, Peach MJ. Endothelium-dependent relaxation of rabbit aorta. I-Relaxation stimulated by arachidonic acid. *J Pharmacol Exp Ther* 1983;226:790–795.
184. Smith REA, Radomski MW, Moncada S. Nitric oxide mediates the vascular actions of cytokines in septic shock. *Eur J Clin Invest* 1992; 22:438–439.
185. Stone DJ, Johns RA. Endothelium-dependent effects of halothane, enflurane, and isoflurane on isolated rat aortic vascular rings. *Anesthesiology* 1989;71:126–132.
186. Stuehr DJ, Kwon NS, Gross SS, et al. Synthesis of nitrogen oxides from L-arginine by macrophage cytosol: Requirement for inducible and constitutive components. *Biochem Biophys Res Commun* 1989;161:420–426.
187. Su JY, Kerrick WGL. Effect of halothane on caffeine-induced tenison transients in functional skinned myocardial fibers. *Pflugers Arch* 1979;380:29–34.79.
188. Su JY, Zhang CC. Intracellular mechanisms of halothane's effect on isolated aortic strips of the rabbit. *Anesthesiology* 1989;71: 409–417.
189. Takata S, Fukase M, Takagi Y, et al. Rapid Ca^{2+} refilling system of intracellular store(s) in human vascular endothelial cells. *Biochem Biophys Res Commun* 1990;167:933–940.
190. Thornbury KD, Ward SM, Dalziel HH, et al. Nitric oxide and nitrosocysteine mimic nonadrenergic, noncholinergic hyperpolarization in canine proximal colon. *Am J Physiol* 1991;261: G553–G557.
191. Tittrup A, Svane D, Forman A. Nitric oxide mediating NANC inhibition in opossum lower esophageal sphincter. *Am J Physiol* 1991; 260:G385–G389.
192. Tobin JR, Martin LD, Breslow MJ, Traystman RJ. Selective anesthetic inhibition of brain nitric oxide synthase. *Anesthesiology* 1994; 81:1264–1269.
193. Toda H, Nakamura K, Hatano Y, et al. Halothane and isoflurane inhibit endothelium-dependent relaxation elicited by acetylcholine. *Anesth Analg* 1992;75:198–203.
194. Tsuchida H, Notsuki E, Yamakage M, et al. Inhibitory effect of halothane and isoflurane on cytosolic Ca^{2+} increase and contraction in vascular smooth muscle of rat aorta. *Anesthesiology* 1991;75:A531.
195. Uggeri MJ, Proctor GJ, Johns RA. Halothane, enflurane, and isoflurane attenuate both receptor- and non-receptor-mediated EDRF production in rat thoracic aorta. *Anesthesiology* 1992;76: 1012–1017.
196. Uhl C, Sill JC, Nelson R, et al. Isoflurane and halothane and responses of cultured pig coronary artery endothelial cells. *Anesthesiology* 1990;73:A621.
197. VandeVoorde J, Lausen I. Role of endothelium in the vasodilator response of rat thoracic aorta to histamine. *Eur J Pharmacol* 1983; 87:113–120.
198. Waldman SA, Murad F. Cyclic GMP synthesis and function. *Pharm Rev* 1987;39:163–196.
199. Weiner CP, Lizasoain I, Baylis SA, et al. Induction of calcium-dependent nitric oxide synthases by sex hormones. *Proc Natl Acad Sci USA* 1994;91:5212–5216.
200. Weinheimer G, Wagner B, Osswald H. Interference of phorbolesters with endothelium-dependent vascular smooth muscle relaxation. *Eur J Pharmacol* 1986;130:319–322.
201. White KA, Marletta MA. Nitric oxide synthase is a cytochrome P-450 type hemoprotein. *Biochemistry* 1992;31:6627–6631.
202. Williams DL, Katz GM, Roy-Contancin L, Reuben JP. Guanosine 5'-monophosphate modulates gating of high-conductance Ca^{2+}-activated K- channels in vascular smooth muscle cells. *Proc Natl Acad Sci USA* 1988;85:9360–9364.
203. Winquist RJ, Bunting PB, Schofield TL. Blockade of endothelium-dependent relaxation by the amiloride analog dichlorobenzamil. possible role of Na^+/Ca^{2+} exchange in the release of endothelium-derived relaxant factor. *J Pharmacol Exp Ther* 1985;235:644–650.
204. Wyatt TA, Lincoln TM, Pryzwansky KB. Vimentin is transiently colocalized with and phosphorylated by cyclic GMP-dependent protein kinase in formyl-peptide stimulated neutrophils. *J Biol Chem* 1991;266:21274–21280.
205. Xie QE, Cho HJ, Calaycay J, et al. Cloning and characterization of inducible nitric oxide synthase from mouse macrophages. *Science* 1992;256:225–228.
206. Xie Q, Cho HJ, Calaycay J, et al. Cloning and characterization of inducible nitric oxide synthase from mouse macrophages. *Science* 1992;256:225–228.
207. Yoshida K, Okabe E. Selective impairment of endothelium-dependent relaxation by sevoflurane: Oxygen free radicals participation. *Anesthesiology* 1992;76:440–447.
208. Yoshizumi M, Perrella MA, Burnett JC Jr, Lee M-E. Tumor necrosis factor downregulates an endothelial nitric oxide synthase mRNA by shortening its half-life. *Circ Res* 1993;73:205–209.
209. Yuen PST, Garbers DL. Guanylyl cyclase-linked receptors. *Annu Rev Neurosci* 1992;15:193–225.
210. Ziegelstein RC, Spurgeon HA, Pili R, et al. A functional ryanodine-sensitive intracellular Ca^{2+} store is present in vascular endothelial cells. *Circ Res* 1994;1–156.
211. Zuo Z, Johns RA. Halothane, enflurane and isoflurane do not affect the basal or agonist-stimulated activity of partially isolated soluble and particulate guanylyl cyclases of rat brain. *Anesthesiology* 1995;83:395–404.
212. Zwiller J, Ciesielski Treska J, Ulrich G, et al. Activation of brain guanylate cyclase by phospholipase A2. *J Neurochem* 1982;6–858.

Anesthesia: Biologic Foundations, edited by Tony L. Yaksh et al. Lippincott–Raven Publishers, Philadelphia © 1997.

CHAPTER 11

SODIUM CHANNELS

J. RANDALL MOORMAN

The object of anesthesia is to curtail sensation and as little else as possible. An ideally direct approach would be to prevent action potentials in sensory nerves. Since action potentials in sensory neurons are initiated by the opening of voltage-dependent Na channels, it is no wonder that Na channel blockers have been used so successfully as targets for anesthetic agents. The strategy, however, is not without flaws. Just as sensory neurons rely on Na channels to work, so do all other neurons, not to mention muscle cells in skeletal muscle and the heart. The most desirable kind of anesthetic, which would interact with Na channels of sensory nerves but no other kinds, has not been found.

Happily, the exploding knowledge field of molecular electrophysiology may lead to just such an agent. At the molecular level, Na channels in nerve, muscle, and heart differ sufficiently that selective interventions appear to be feasible goals. Our purpose is to map the territory of molecular studies of Na channels, for here clinically significant advances will eventually be made. The chapter emphasizes molecular studies, and especially emphasizes studies of cloned, expressed Na channel molecules. The chapter has several sections. The first discusses studies of Na channel physiology and concludes with a list of Na channel behaviors. The second explores recent studies of cloned, expressed Na channels that have sought to ascribe function to pieces of the structure. Later sections highlight studies of Na channels in human diseases, and their developmental regulation. A recurring motif is the difference among Na channel molecules of different tissues. Unfortunately, a great deal of important information is omitted for lack of space, and the reader is referred to many excellent reviews (38–40,45,61,62,84,88,106,122,146,220,222,230).

HETEROGENEITY OF NA CHANNELS

Na channels from nerve, muscle, and heart have distinct biochemical, electrophysiologic, and pharmacologic differences. Moreover, multiple Na channel types are present within the same tissue, and the balance of power shifts among the types depending on developmental stage, innervation (in skeletal muscle), presence of blocking drugs, activation of protein kinases, and probably countless other factors. The response, then, of an organ to an Na channel blocking agent may vary dramatically according to internal and external conditions, most of them unknown to the clinician.

Biochemical differences first become evident when Na channel proteins are purified. In brain and muscle, Na channels are an assembly of subunits (117). The largest, the α subunit, is itself sufficient when expressed in *Xenopus* oocytes to form a perfectly functional channel, replete with characteristic voltage-dependence, ion selectivity, and toxin binding (85,174). Indeed, eel electroplax (162), chick heart (143), and some brain preparations (58) of purified Na channels show the α subunit alone, and the purified eel a subunit can be functionally reconstituted in phospholipid vesicles (197,198). Smaller β subunits are present in brain, which has two, and in muscle, which has one or two (16,34). One kind of noncovalently bound β subunit, called β_1, is apparently common to both, and is both necessary for functional reconstitution (224,225) and strongly modulatory (when expressed in *Xenopus* oocytes). The other brain channel subunit, called β_2, is linked by disulfide bonds, and is apparently not critical for channel function.

There are more subtle biochemical differences evident when the amino acid sequences of cloned Na channel proteins are compared. Brain Na channels are 85% to 90% homologous to each other and about 60% homologous to eel. It is likely, moreover, that each of brain channel types I, II, and III are encoded by different genes. Similarly, the two genes from flies are as homologous to each other as to the mammalian genes, suggesting that gene duplication occurred early in evolution.

Electrophysiologic differences are evident from studies of Na currents in different tissues. Kinetic analyses have been used to distinguish several populations of Na channels in different tissues, or in the same tissue in different stages of development. For example, Kirsch and Brown (127) demonstrated large differences in the behavior of Na channels from brain and heart when studied under identical conditions. These differences are important in shaping action potentials and may help explain differences in local anesthetic effects in different tissues.

Finally, there are important *pharmacologic differences* among Na channels. The most important distinctions can be made by testing the sensitivity to the specific Na channel blocker tetrodotoxin (TTX). For example, cardiac Na channels are much less sensitive to block by TTX than are nerve Na channels (24,65). Cardiac Na channels, on the other hand, are two to three orders of magnitude more sensitive to the local anesthetic compound lidocaine than are neuronal Na channels, and skeletal muscle Na channels have intermediate sensitivity. This may be due in part to the presence of a lidocaine binding site on the extracellular face of cardiac Na channels that is not present in nerve Na channels. This is suggested by the finding that a permanently charged lidocaine analogue blocks cardiac Na channels from both the extracellular and intracellular side (4,18), but it blocks neuronal and skeletal muscle Na channels only from the inside (104,221,236). The existence of such a site is extremely important, as the rationale of Na channel block as therapy for cardiac arrhythmias rests on the difference between cardiac and nerve Na channels in binding local anesthetics. At doses used clinically, local anesthetics should block cardiac Na channels but not brain Na channels. This strategy is not perfect, as central nervous system side effects of antiarrhythmic drugs are common. Moreover, currently available antiarrhythmic drugs are not useful for long-term therapy (35). In addition, cardiac Na channels are less sensitive to scorpion toxins and more sensitive to sea anemone toxin than Na channels from nerve (36,251).

These heterogeneities should permit targeting of specific populations of Na channels with specific drugs.

ASPECTS OF NA CHANNEL PHYSIOLOGY

Gating

Gating is the opening and closing of channels. In their pioneering works Hodgkin and Huxley (107–110) delivered depolarizing voltage steps to squid axon and observed Na currents that increased quickly to a maximum, then decayed rather more slowly. They gave the name *activation* to the process that increased current, and the name *inactivation* to the decay of current. They envisioned two working parts of the channel molecule—an activation gate (termed *m*) that opened to initiate current, and a separate inactivation gate (termed *h*) that closed thereafter, despite a persistent depolarizing stimulus. The whole process is complete in a few milliseconds. The relatively rapid inactivation of Na channels is one of their most important functional characteristics. Without it, excitable cells would be unable to generate the rapid trains of action potentials necessary for neuronal and muscular function.

Na channel activation gating is extremely sensitive to membrane potential. Over the range of potentials where some, but not all, Na channels open, the proportion of Na channels opening at a given test potential increases tenfold every 9 to 10 mV. Thus, the voltage range between threshold and the point at which nearly all the channels are open is only about 30 mV or so. Inactivation gating, on the other hand, is not very strongly voltage-dependent, and is considered to derive any apparent voltage-dependence from its association with the process of activation gating—put simply, a channel must open before it can close. This turns out to be less than completely true, as channel transitions from closed to inactivated states can take place without channel opening (137).

Experimentally, two kinds of current recordings can be made. *Macroscopic* currents (denoted *I*) are measured in whole cell recordings, and represent the sum of all the currents through individual channel molecules. They are smooth waveforms. *Microscopic* currents (denoted *i*) are measured in single-channel recordings using patch clamp technology. They are abrupt events, and represent currents through the individual channel molecules themselves. Single-channel analysis consists of measuring the statistical properties of the unitary events, and begins with measuring the times when the channel opens and closes.

Two important points should be made. First, at any test potential, the sum of a large number of single-channel records should be the same as the whole cell current. Second, many different patterns of single-channel events can sum to be identical whole-cell currents. Thus, analysis of macroscopic currents does not definitively elucidate the single-channel characteristics.

The fast-peaking, more slowly decaying waveforms led Hodgkin and Huxley to hypothesize that Na channels activated quickly, then inactivated slowly. This hypothesis is testable directly in single-channel recordings. Here, the process of activation is gauged by the time between the initiation of the voltage step and the appearance of the first unitary current event. This measure is the first latency, or waiting time. The inactivation process is gauged by the average time that the channel stays open, the mean open time. Customarily, these averages can be estimated from a histographic representation of the observed waiting or open times. These histograms have the appearance of exponential decay processes and are fit to single or sums of exponential functions where the exponential factors are the averages of the populations.

Thus, when Aldrich et al. (2,3) began to examine single Na channels in neuronal cells, they might have expected to see channels opening at the very beginning of the voltage step, remaining open for variable periods with a mean of a few milliseconds (the decay time constant of whole-cell Na currents). Instead, they saw quite the opposite. Although Na channels opened soon after the start of the voltage step, they did not open instantly. The latency to first opening, in fact, varied over several milliseconds. The channels, on the other hand, closed or inactivated very quickly after opening. This led to a fundamentally new idea of how Na channels worked—rather than fast activation and slow inactivation, the reverse is true. The terms *fast* and *slow* are entirely relative, as even the longest waiting times are on the order of just a few milliseconds.

This gating scheme is not observed in all kinds of Na channels, however. In particular, cardiac and skeletal muscle Na channels have distinctly different kinds of inactivation gating. Macroscopic cardiac Na currents decay more slowly than in neuronal preparations, and they decay in two phases—one quite rapid, like neuronal Na channels, and the other severalfold slower (24,65). At the single-channel level, the difference lies in the ability for these Na channels to reopen after initially closing (136), a process not allowed in the Aldrich et al. model. Indeed, some traces show dozens of reopenings, as if the process of inactivation had failed altogether. These prolonged bursts of prolonged openings of Na channels in skeletal muscle (180) and cardiac muscle (87,120,136,179) are a feature we call *slow inactivation gating*. These differences are apparent in brain and heart cells studied under identical experimental conditions (127). Excision of membrane patches from cells can lead to marked increases in the proportion of sweeps showing slow inactivation gating (127,170) and Kohlhardt (129) has presented evidence that this may be due to the presence of fluoride ion in the bath solution. Records of channel activity during cardiac action potentials confirms that Na channel openings occur during the plateau (142). The importance of this persistent Na current in cardiac physiology is evident—the late current contributes, along with Ca currents, to the characteristic prolongation of the cardiac action potential that allows protracted entry of Ca. Grant's group (257) have described another kind of noninactivating Na channels in heart cells. These channels are active at diastolic, hyperpolarized potentials and may contribute to total Na current near threshold. They are distinct from bursting channels, which are initiated by depolarization and quickly terminated by hyperpolarization. For the most part, neuronal Na channels do not display slow inactivation gating.

There are other situations where fast inactivation fails, and studies in these areas have led to an idea of what the inactivation gate must look like. First, Armstrong et al. (8) found that treatment of the cytoplasmic surface of squid axon with pronase, a mixture of proteolytic enzymes, led to persistent Na currents. There was no effect of pronase added extracellularly. This finding led to a number of speculations about structural basis of the inactivation process. First, it must involve a protein, since pronase attacks only peptides. Second, the peptide must be intracellular, as extracellular pronase had no effect. Third, since copious washing with nonproteolytic solutions did not affect inactivation, the peptide must be bound to or part of the membrane-bound ion channel itself. Fourth, this part of the protein must contain several positive charges, as pronase attacks peptides at lysines and arginines, which are positively charged. These kinds of speculations led to investigation of a specific part of the cloned Na channel, as described below. Fast inactivation also fails after treatment with a number of other enzymes, chemicals, and toxins, after excision of patches. It has proven a useful maneuver to study Na channel with fast inactivation removed, especially in studying features of drug interactions with open channels.

Gating currents are small membrane currents that flow outward at the beginning of depolarizing steps before ionic currents themselves begin (6,7). Their presence was predicted by Hodgkin and Huxley (108) as the manifestation of a direct effect on the membrane electrical field on the charge-bearing channel proteins themselves. If the voltage step is short, another gating current of equal magnitude and opposite direction can be seen when the membrane is repolarized. If, however, the depolarizing voltage step has much duration, the gating current at the end of the pulse is smaller than that at the beginning. This phenomenon is called "charge immobilization" and, importantly, has the same time course as Na channel inactivation (7) and is prevented by the agents that prevent inactivation (126). The molecular interpretation is that gating current represents the outward twisting of a charged segment of the channel protein in response to membrane depolarization. As described below, such segments of the channel molecule have been identified. Detailed models of this molecular motion have been proposed—the "sliding helix" (37), "helical screw" (95), and "propagating helix" (94) models. For short pulses, no other conformational change occurs, and the removal of the depolarizing stimulus results in the relaxation of the charged segments to their original position. After short times, however, a conformational change occurs that prohibits the easy return of the charged segments, and thus gating charge is immobilized. This second conformation also closes the pore, and ionic current ceases—this is what we have been calling inactivation gating. There may be more than one kinetic component of gating currents (121), and very highly resolved studies of gating current indicate that it, like the ionic currents that follow, is discrete in nature (47). Three "shots" of gating charge, each consisting of about two elemental charges, move per channel.

Modulation by Phosphorylation

Modulation of ion channels by phosphorylation has long been a well-established concept for cardiac Ca channels. It has only more recently become apparent that phosphorylation is an important means of regulating Na channels as well. The effects of phosphorylation have been studied in brain, in heart, and in skeletal muscle Na channels, both in native channels and in channels expressed from cDNA clones. The most important findings are (a) the single phosphorylation site in the III–IV linker is phosphorylated by at least two kinases—protein kinase C (PKC) and human myotonin protein kinase (HMPK), the product of the gene that is abnormal in myotonic muscular dystrophy; (b) the effect of one kinase may depend on the prior activity of other kinases; and (c) Na channel phosphorylation may affect local anesthetic efficacy.

Biochemically, purified rat brain Na channels are substrates for PKC and adenosine 3',5'-cyclic monophosphate (cAMP)-dependent protein kinase (PKA) (200,201). Both phosphorylate at multiple sites, and at some common sites in the channel protein (141). Functional modulation of Na channels by phosphorylation has been studied in cardiac and neuronal channels. In cell-attached patches of heart cells, angiotensin II increases the amplitude and changes the inactivation gating pattern of single Na channels (20,164,172). Since angiotensin II activates PKC, this result has been attributed to phosphorylation of the channel protein. The picture is made unclear by the different effects of 1-oleoyl-2-acetyl-*sn*-glycerol (OAG) (20), a membrane-permeant diacylglycerol analogue that should activate PKC directly. In brain channels, the effect of phosphorylation by PKC is to reduce current (177), and the phosphorylation site is in the III–IV linker (241). Likewise, currents through rat brain type IIA Na channels expressed in *Xenopus* oocytes are reduced by maneuvers that activate PKC (54,144).

The effect on cardiac Na channels of activation of PKA is pronounced, but whether the current increases or decreases or changes inactivation properties is controversial. Schubert and coworkers (211) showed that activation of β-adrenergic receptors by isoproterenol reduced the amplitude of whole-cell currents, shifted their steady-state inactivation to more hyperpolarized potentials, and reduced the probability of opening of single channels. Similarly, Ono and coworkers (178), using perforated patches (a patch-clamp technique that does not disrupt the intracellular milieu), showed that isoproterenol and a membrane-permeant cAMP analogue shifted conductance steady-state inactivation to more negative potentials. A role for PKA was suggested by the ability of a protein kinase inhibitor to block the cAMP effect. Kirstein and coworkers (128) used loose patch clamp—a similar technique—to show that sympathetic stimulation of heart cells by isoproterenol not only shifted steady-state inactivation parameters to more negative potentials, but also increased the maximum available Na conductance. Thus, Na currents elicited from normal holding potentials *increased,* but currents elicited from depolarized holding potentials *decreased* compared with control conditions. Shibata's group (154) showed that the effect of isoproterenol was to increase cardiac Na current amplitude and shift activation kinetics to more hyperpolarized potentials, an effect that was mollified by acetylcholine binding to muscarinic receptors (155). To some extent, these differences might be explained by differences in experimental preparations. For example, Gintant and Liu (82) showed that the effects of β-adrenergic stimulation in heart were different when measured in tissue than when measured in isolated cells. Whatever the details, there is likely to be not only physiologic but also developmental relevance of phosphorylation of Na channels by PKA, as Zhang and coworkers (254) found a similar effect of both development and sympathetic innervation on Na channels of neonatal cardiac myocytes.

The effect of the catalytic subunit of PKA plus adenosine triphosphate (ATP) on Na channels in excised patches of neurons is to reduce current by increasing the number of traces without channel openings (140). In brain channels expressed in *Xenopus* oocytes, on the other hand, results are inconsistent. In one study, activation of β-adrenergic receptors or application of a membrane permeant cAMP analogue increased rat brain IIA current amplitude (214). In another study published at the same time, the opposite result was observed—injection of cAMP or the catalytic subunit of PKA or bath application of forskolin reduced currents (80). Both groups studied the effect of phosphatases, again with opposite results.

Recently, we have speculated that the human illness myotonic muscular dystrophy (DM) may be due in part to abnormal regulation of muscle Na channels by phosphorylation (167). The gene that is abnormal in DM has sequence homology to PKA and to PKC, leading to the hypothesis that it was itself a serine-threonine protein kinase, and to its name—human myotonin protein kinase (HMPK) (10,22,71,148). Coexpression of HMPK with rat skeletal muscle Na channels in *Xenopus* oocytes reduced the amplitude of Na currents and accelerated current decay. The consequence of an abnormal amount of HMPK would be altered muscle cell excitability, consistent with the clinical finding of myotonia in myotonic dystrophy (31).

Clinical ramifications of this modulation of Na channels are potentially very important. Cummins and coworkers (51) showed that anoxia and metabolic inhibition shifted steady-state inactivation gating to more negative potentials in human neocortical pyramidal neurons, possibly underlying the decrease in excitability seen in similarly treated tissue slices. In guinea pig ventricular myocytes, on the other hand, metabolic inhibition by 2,4-dinitrophenol or iodoacetate did not have significant effects on the voltage dependence of Na channel gating (161). Perhaps most importantly, the effect of lidocaine to block cardiac Na channels is reversed by isoproterenol (138). This may underlie the clinical phenomenon of exercise-induced cardiac arrhythmias despite antiarrhythmic therapy, and relates directly to the problems of Na channel blockade as a means to treat patients with arrhythmias (90).

There is strong evidence for direct effects of G proteins in cardiac and brain Na channels. In cardiac channels, G_s appears to mediate the effect, which is inhibitory (211). In brain channels, on the other hand, a pertussis toxin–sensitive G_i is the effector, and serves to increase current amplitude (46,147). In both systems, the voltage dependence of the inactivation process is affected.

Nongating effects of phosphorylation are also important. Innervation of cardiac myocytes by sympathetic neurons alters the voltage dependence of Na channel gating, an effect mediated by the β-adrenergic receptor (254). Hypoxia increases the Na current density in cells of rat carotid body, an effect mimicked by a membrane-permeant cAMP analogue (219). Signal transduction pathways initiated by neuronal growth factor (NGF) lead to increased levels of Na channel expression, an effect that requires activation of PKA (53,124). Fibroblast growth factor (FGF), on the other hand, increases Na channel expression using a non-PKA pathway. Similarly, a PKA-deficient cell line had severalfold higher Na current amplitudes, at least partially explained by a higher number of channels as estimated by radiolabeled STX binding (140). Most interestingly, studies of PKA-deficient pheochromocytoma cells show that both NGF and FGF still lead to increases in Na channel messenger RNA (mRNA) level but not to increased protein levels (83). This suggests a role for PKA in the stability of the nascent channel peptide.

Effects of Local Anesthetics

Local anesthetic (LA) agents stop sensation by blocking conduction of nerve impulses, an effect achieved by blocking Na channels. Despite a wealth of clinical and experimental data, many major issues of the exact mechanism of this effect are entirely unresolved. The most important clinical issue is selectivity—as we note above, the object of anesthesia is to stop sensation but not function. Thus, nerve Na channels are the targets, not muscle channels. This difficult area has been recently reviewed (26,90,220).

Local anesthetics are tertiary amines. At physiologic pH, they exist in charged and neutral forms, both of which block Na channels. Lidocaine, the most commonly used local anesthetic agent, has a pK of about 7.9, and therefore has a neutral/charged form ratio of about 3:1 at pH 7.4. Although both permanently charged (QX compounds, pK >10) and neutral (benzocaine, pK <3) local anesthetics can block Na channels, the mechanisms are thought to differ. Charged forms should be restricted to the aqueous pore of the ion channel and cause block by physical occlusion. Logically, channels would have to be open and allow the drug in before block could be established. Uncharged forms, on the other hand, might interact with the channel from a site within the lipid membrane. They would not necessarily be restricted in their access to the channel by its gating history. Prevailing conditions within the aqueous pore might well allow interconversion between charged and uncharged forms once bound to the channel—thus, an uncharged molecule might find easy entry to the channel binding site, acquire charge there, and preclude an easy exit. In addition to charge, the size (48,49), shape (50), and lipid solubility (23) of the local anesthetic molecule play a critical role in blocking characteristics.

Earlier investigations of the mechanisms of LA block of Na channels exploited measurements of macroscopic Na currents or of dV/dt_{max}, the maximum rate of rise of the action potential. Two visions emerged. The first, called the *modulated receptor* theory, was proposed by Hille and coworkers (104,212) and by Hondegehm and Katzung (112,113). It states that the affinity of the Na channel for binding lidocaine depends on the conformational state of the Na channel protein. The inactivated form was felt to be most avid, the open state next-most avid, and the closed or resting state the least avid. In other words, hyperpolarized Na channels bound less drug than depolarized ones. Moreover, the drug-bound inactivation gate was postulated to display abnormal kinetics. The major experimental finding was a shift of steady-state inactivation parameters to more hyperpolarized potentials in the presence of lidocaine. The second vision, called the *guarded/trapped receptor* model, was proposed by Starmer and coworkers (215–218). In this view, the affinity of the channel protein stays constant regardless of the kinetic state. Rather, the drug is allowed to access the binding site only at specific times. Specifically, the channel must be open for the charged form to find and to bind to the binding site, and the drug is trapped there by the inactivation gate. The fundamental observation that both models address is a shift in steady-state inactivation gating to more negative potentials. That is to say, fewer channels are available for opening at any given resting potential. This might be because drug binds more avidly to the inactivated state (the affinity of the receptor is *modulated* by its gating state). Alternatively, it might be because the drug binding site is available only after the activation gate opens (the receptor is *guarded* by the gate), and the inactivation gate must be open for the drug to exit (the drug is *trapped* by the gate).

Binding studies favor the idea of a higher affinity state when channels are inactivated (103). These studies, however, require the presence of batrachotoxin, tetrodotoxin, and aconitine. The structural integrity of the channel molecule may be altered by these toxins (191,235). Moreover, the membrane potential in binding studies is not known. Depolarization would inactivate most of the channels, biasing the results. Although a clear distinction between hypotheses has not been achieved in voltage clamp studies, a recent study by Hanck and coworkers (96) has provided a new perspective. They demonstrated that cardiac Na channels continued to gate in the presence of local anesthetics, and that the gating kinetics differed from control. Specifically, they demonstrated reduced voltage dependence of gating charge movement in the presence of drug, as if the voltage sensor itself were altered in the presence of drug. These findings uphold one of the tenets of the modulated receptor hypothesis, that local anesthetics cause Na channels to gate with different kinetics.

Studies have suggested that the local anesthetic binding site interacted with the inactivation mechanism. For example, a recent study of cardiac Na channels in which fast inactivation was removed by papain, a permanently charged local anesthetic, had two different effects (81). First, the closed times between openings became prolonged, a finding that may be attributed to inactivation gating. Second, the current amplitude of individual openings was reduced, an effect attributable to binding of the agent within the pore. Moreover, as described below, the modulated receptor hypothesis for local anesthetic block of Na channels is predicated on the idea that the inactivated channel conformation favors binding of local anesthetics. From the study of Na channel gating currents comes other evidence that local anesthetics interact with the inactivation gate. The important observation is that local anesthetics produce charge immobilization just like inactivation gating does. Gating current is altered in amplitude and kinetics by local anesthetics that are neutral (209) and charged (28), and the charged form shows phasic block as well. As described below, recent molecular experiments bear out this association.

Other studies have suggested that local anesthetics bind in or near the pore. An early finding in the study of the antiarrhythmic properties of local anesthetics was that blockade increased with stronger and more frequent depolarization (221). This property, which is called phasic block (26) or frequency-dependent block, and which has the appealing feature of predicting maximum antiarrhythmic activity during tachycardia, is taken to mean that channels must open before they can be blocked. Phasic block is voltage dependent—it is enhanced by depolarization and mitigated by hyperpolarization—and it is pH dependent—it is favored at low pH (240). The accumulating block would logically be due to the charged form of the agent, as the neutral form has continuous access to the channel through the lipid membrane. According to the modulated-receptor hypothesis, the activated channel has more affinity for the agent than the resting state (though less than the inactivated state). According to the guarded receptor hypothesis, the receptor is not accessible until the channel opens, though the affinity of the receptor itself does not change.

Single-channel recordings should tell us a lot about the molecular mechanism of phasic block. One possible mechanism of channel block is interference of the drug molecule with the pore through which ions flow. This "open-channel block" is characterized in single-channel recordings by rapid flickering of the current. Another possibility is that the drug-burdened channel cannot open, or opens less readily. This "closed state" block would be manifest as an increase in the number of traces without channel activity. Perplexingly, single-channel recordings of Na channels in the presence of local anesthetics have revealed both kinds of results, and they differ among agents that ought to be the same.

Ordinarily, the open time of a Na channel is so short that it would not be possible to show a convincing reduction due to flickering block. Hence, it is a common strategy first to remove fast inactivation gating with one of the treatments noted above. Kohlhardt and coworkers (131), for example, studied cardiac Na channels where fast inactivation was removed by a chemical, the diphenylpiperazinylindole derivative DPI 201-106. This results in prolonged bursts of long openings and simplifies the kinetic analysis, but also allows the possibility that the structures underlying the usual interaction of the agent with the channel molecule were modified. Flickering block is then evident in recordings of Na channels treated with quinidine, propafenone, or procainamide, but, interestingly, *not* evident when lidocaine is present (21,130). Instead, the effect of lidocaine is to decrease the number of sweeps with channel activity. This has been interpreted as meaning that lidocaine, unlike other local anesthetics, blocks Na current by interacting with the channel when it is closed. What could this mean? Perhaps these two distinct kinds of effects of antiarrhythmic local anesthetic agents demonstrate a multiplicity of local anesthetic binding sites within the channel molecule. One site would be in the open pore, produce flickering block, and not bind lidocaine. Another would favor closed states and be accessible to different local anesthetics. In support of this, Zamponi and French (253) found that diethylamide, which is analogous to the hydrophilic end of the lidocaine molecule, induced a rapid channel block, manifest as a reduction in i, while phenol, which is analogous to the ring at the other end of lidocaine, induced long closures.

Is there really more than one binding site? A single binding site is suggested by the observation that one LA can competitively displace another. This has been exploited clinically in the treatment of patients overdosed with amitryptilene and propoxyphene with phenytoin and lidocaine. The strategy is to replace a LA with slow kinetics with one that has faster kinetics (239). Conversely, multiple binding sites are suggested by Yue (252), who found that QX-314, a permanently charged lidocaine analogue that should produce blocking phenomena specific to the charged form of lidocaine, in fact had two kinds of effects. First, the amplitude of unitary currents was reduced, as if the drug entered and exited the channel too quickly for the individual blocking events to be resolved. Second, there were relatively prolonged closures, as if the drug entered the channel, blocked it, and there reposed for a few milliseconds. In this study, any confounding effects of inactivation gating had been removed by exposing the channel to papain. Thus, in even this simplified experimental approach the matter appears to be quite complex. Likewise, Grant's group (14) found that amitryptilene produced phasic block of cardiac Na currents in a fundamentally different way than either lidocaine or diphenylhydantoin, suggesting more than one binding site may be involved in generating phasic block.

To confuse matters further, the effect of lidocaine on mean channel open time in different studies have not been consistent. Nilius and coworkers (171) and McDonald and coworkers (159) found a reduction in open times, but Grant and coworkers (86) and Benz and Kohlhardt (21) did not. In the latter two studies, traces with slow inactivation gating were clearly present in the presence of lidocaine, arguing further against the idea of open channel block. These studies, which enjoy the advantage of examining unmodified channels, suggest that phasic block involves closed as well as open states of the channel. Overall, McDonald and coworkers found intermediate results. In their study, phasic block by lidocaine did not require channel openings during the conditioning pulses, arguing at least partially that interactions of the drug molecule with open channels were not required. Disopyramide, on the other hand, clearly decreased mean channel open time (91). This suggests that it interacts with Na channels in a manner fundamentally different than lidocaine, a suggestion further strengthened by the observation that extracellular Na ions appear to displace disopyramide but not lidocaine (15). Thus, single-channel studies have yet to agree on the molecular details of the mechanism of phasic block by lidocaine.

Ionic block and pH potentiation of block of Na channels by local anesthetics also suggest they bind within the pore. The effect of reduced extracellular pH is to reduce Na current and shift gating to more positive potentials. Woodhull (246) analyzed this phenomenon in nerve and made two important observations. First, the block was half-complete at pH 5.4, suggesting that protons titrated a site such as a carboxylic acid. Second, the block was voltage-dependent; specifically, the reduction of currents at very strong depolarization was less proportionate than block at weaker depolarization. This suggested that the proton-binding site lay within the membrane electric field. Woodhull developed a mathematical model to fit the data that suggested that the proton binding site was about a fourth of the way into the pore from the outside. On the other hand, others have suggested a multiplicity of proton binding sites in the pore (55,168), and at least one alternative view is that protons bind outside the pore and alter activation gating (29) or surface charge (255). While controversy persists, the majority opinion is that protons bind to a site within the Na channel pore.

There is a clear-cut but complex relationship between use-dependent block by local anesthetics and extracellular pH. Extracellular protons dramatically increase the depth and tenacity of use-dependent block (89,105,212). To some extent, this may be explained by the increasing fraction of drug present in the charged form, which is responsible for use-dependent block. Lipid solubility also plays a role (23), to the extent that a neutral but poorly lipid soluble local anesthetic shows prominent use-dependence (44). Some of the kinetic details are not fully explained by physicochemical properties of the drugs, and we have suggested that the drug molecule has a different pK once it has bound to the channel (166). This concept has had a mixed reception (44,50,169).

The effect of extracellular pH is likely to be clinically important. In animals, acidemia results in enhanced effect of lidocaine to reduce impulse conduction velocity (111). In tissue preparations, low pH delays recovery from lidocaine-induced depression of Na currents in nerve (105) and of maximum upstroke velocity of cardiac action potentials, a rough measure of Na current (89). Since ischemic and infarcted myocardium is more acidotic than normal myocardium, local anesthetics used as antiarrhythmic agents during myocardial ischemia and infarction should prevent arrhythmias without interfering with impulse propagation through normal myocardium.

Although nearly all studies of the effects of local anesthetics on Na channels are confined to acute applications of drugs, it should be remembered that chronic therapy has other, additional effects. Prolonged treatment of rat cardiac muscle with the type I antiarrhythmic drug mexilitene increases both mRNA and protein levels of Na channels (56). Interestingly, the effect is mimicked by the Ca channel antagonist verapamil and opposed by a Ca ionophore, suggesting that the mechanism involved intracellular Ca^{2+}. Moreover, the effect of lidocaine differs greatly in the adult compared to the neonate (247).

Effects of General Anesthetics

Where Na channel block by local anesthetics has drawn a great deal of attention, the effects of general anesthetic agents are less well characterized. The lipid solubility of these agents, moreover, makes interpretation of the results more problematic. That is, while direct interactions of general anesthetic agents with ion channel proteins is certainly possible and likely, the agents' effect of generalized membrane perturbation may affect channel function in ways that are not well delineated (194).

In squid axon Na currents, Haydon and Urban studied the effects of aliphatic hydrocarbons (98), inhalation anesthetics (99), alcohols and other nonionic surface-active compounds (100), and hydrocarbons and carbon tetrachloride (101). Generally, all shared the effect of reversible depression of Na current amplitudes. Using a Hodgkin-Huxley model, they could demonstrate alterations of steady-state activation and inactivation parameters, time constants of activation and inactivation, and the maximum Na conductance. These global effects argue against the kind of specific, single residue-to-drug kind of interaction that is the current model for channel-local anesthetic interaction. Membrane capacitance, moreover, was significantly decreased by some (but not all) of the agents, in keeping with the idea that some of the effects on the ion channels were mediated through generalized membrane effects.

In preparations of human brain Na channels reconstituted in planar lipid bilayers, Urban and coworkers have studied the effects of pentobarbital (67,68,193), ketamine (70), and propofol (69). In these more resolved studies, the actions of all three agents was found to be a reduction in channel opening probability and a shift of activation to more negative potentials. To begin to address the all-important question of specific protein interaction versus generalized membrane effect, Rehberg and coworkers (194) used the same experimental system to test the effect of adding the membrane structural lipid cholesterol. They found that cholesterol mollified the effect of pentobarbital, adding credence to the idea that at least some of the Na channel blocking effect of anesthesia is mediated by the membrane and not by a protein-drug interaction.

As yet, there are no studies of general anesthetic agents in which a drug effect can be mollified by point mutations of the channel protein. Without doubt, these kinds of experiments will help determine the relative roles of generalized membrane effects and specific channel-drug interactions in producing Na channel block.

In summary, Na channels have a limited repertoire:

- they open in response to depolarization of the membrane
- prior to channel opening, a charged segment of the channel moves within the membrane
- they close after opening, perhaps utilizing an intracellular, charged part of the peptide
- they are modulated by phosphorylation
- they bind and are blocked by local anesthetics.

STRUCTURE AND FUNCTION OF THE NA CHANNEL

Molecular Structure (Fig. 1)

Na channel molecules consist of about 2000 amino acids grouped into four homologous domains of 40% to 50% homology. Each domain has six putative membrane-spanning segments, based on predictions from hydrophobicity plots. Evidence supporting this overall structure has been supplied by Barchi, Cohen, and coworkers (258), who have used Na channel antibodies to evaluate channel topology. They have found that the beginning of the amino terminus interacts with the end of the carboxyl terminus. Thus, domains I and IV are adjacent, as expected from the intuitive model in which the protein domains encircle a potential aqueous pore. The domains are joined by cytoplasmic linkers. Generally, the transmembrane segments are better conserved than the cytoplasmic linkers, with the exception of the linker between domains III and IV, which is very highly conserved. This structure is preserved from fly (202) to eel (175) to rat (173), and from nerve (11,119,125, 173) to skeletal muscle (123,231) to heart muscle (73,74,195). In fact, the homology of any one domain in any two species is considerably higher than the homology between any two domains within the same species.

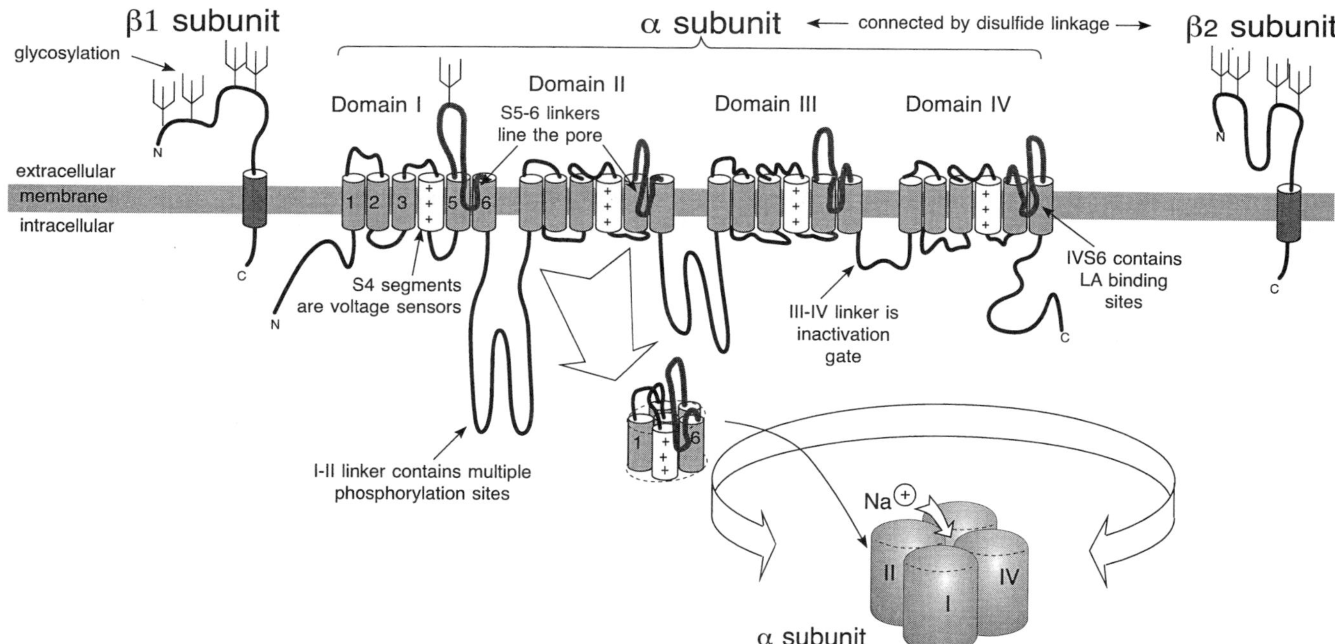

Figure 1. Structural model of the Na channel based on amino acid sequence analysis. The α subunit is composed of a sequence of approximately 2000 amino acids in which 24 hydrophobic regions are hypothesized to form α-helical transmembrane segments (indicated by the small cylinders). As shown for domain II, the six transmembrane segments (S1 to S6) coalesce to form four domains (I to IV). The four domains gather as indicated to form a tetrameric structure with a central pore through which the ions pass. Also shown in the figure are the β_1 and β_2 subunits that occur with the α subunit, modulating channel gating.

Structure-Function Relationships

Several influential molecular models of Na channel structure based on its amino acid sequence have been proposed (93,95,173). Testing of predictions of these models continues to provide new and exciting insights into the details of ion channel function, but are time- and labor-intensive. The studies mandate point mutagenesis of a large molecule, successful expression, and electrophysiologic studies often employing patch clamp technology. An important and gratifying finding is that single amino acids in well-conserved sequences can determine phenotypic differences. For instance, single point mutations can drastically alter ion selectivity, inactivation gating, toxin and divalent binding, and conductance. Thus, these kinds of studies can lead to impressive strides in understanding.

S4 Segments are Voltage Sensors (Fig. 2)

The most unusual feature of the amino acid sequence of Na channels is the presence of positively charged residues in the fourth transmembrane segment of all four domains. This energetically unfavorable situation—indeed, the first structural model placed them outside the membrane (175)—is present in all voltage-gated channels, including K and Ca channels, and must serve an important teleologic function. The charged residues are spaced three apart—if the segment is an α helix, the charges would be aligned nearly vertically. If they indeed move during channel activation, they would provide a structural basis for gating current—the so-called "sliding helix" and "propagating helix" models described above. Tamkun's group (78) has described an Na channel in human heart and uterus

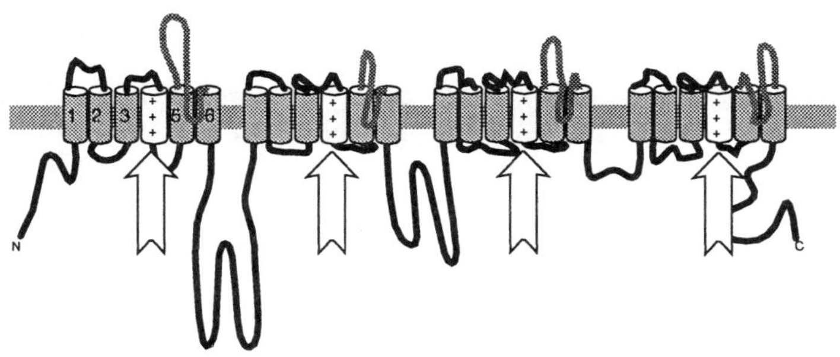

S4 mutations alter voltage-sensitivity

I	VSAL**R**TF**R**VL**R**AL**K**TISVIPGL**K**TIV
II	LSVL**R**SF**R**LL**R**VF**K**LA**K**SWPTLNMLI
III	LGAI**K**SL**R**TL**R**AL**R**PL**R**ALS**R**FEGM**R**
IV	PTLF**R**VI**R**LA**R**IG**R**IL**R**LI**K**GA**K**GI**R**

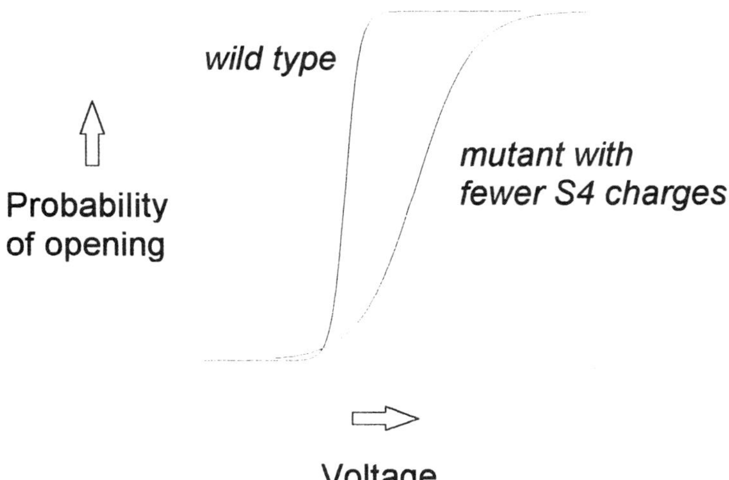

Figure 2. Positively charged residues in the S4 segments allow voltage-dependent Na channel activation. The amino acid sequence for the highly conserved S4 segments in the four domains are shown. The highlighted residues are positively charged Arg (R) and Lys (K), and occur in every third position throughout the domains. The idealized lines below are plots of channel activation as a function of membrane potential. Normally, activation of Na channels occurs over a very narrow range of voltage. Mutant channels with their voltage sensors partially disarmed by neutralization of one or more of the positive charges in the S4 segments require larger voltages for all channels to become fully activated.

in which some of the charged residues are histidine (His, H) instead of arginine (Arg, R) or lysine (Lys, K), pointing to a significant departure from the highly conserved structure of the other cloned Na channels.

Important mutagenesis experiments by Stühmer, Numa, and coworkers (223) established a major role for these residues as the voltage-sensing mechanism of the rat brain type II Na channel. The experimental strategy was to use recombinant DNA technology to replace, one by one, the positively charged Lys or Arg with chemically similar but electrically neutral glycine (Gln, G). Voltage clamp recordings of large patches containing many channels were analyzed using the Hodgkin-Huxley model, and the effect of each mutation on activation gating parameters was described. Ordinarily, Na channels are extremely sensitive to changes in membrane potential near their threshold for opening. The experimental results showed that this degree of sensitivity was modulated by positively charged residues in the S4 segments. Specifically, reducing the positive charges by 1, 2, or 3 perceptibly reduced the voltage sensitivity of activation gating, measured as the steepness of a Boltzmann distribution fit to a plot of proportion of channels open as a function of test potential. This major work was the first fulfillment of the promise that the marriage of molecular biology to cellular electrophysiology would lead to a new era of mechanistic insight into the workings of ion channels.

S4 segments contribute to Na channel function in other ways. For example, mutations of the S4 segment in domain IV cause the human illness paramyotonia congenita. Horn's group (42) investigated the single-channel gating kinetics of these mutants, and found more effects on inactivation gating than on activation gating, suggesting that the S4 segments may play an important role in coupling activation to inactivation. Nearby leucines in the S4-5 segment of Na channels play an important role in voltage-dependent activation as well (11). In addition, a fundamental structural role for the S4 segments has been suggested for the entire superfamily of ion channels (118).

III–IV Linker Modulates Inactivation Gating (Fig. 3)

In the same work that examined the role of S4 segments, Stühmer, Numa, and coworkers (223) tested the idea that the III–IV linker was the inactivation gate. This was a most reasonable conjecture, as it fulfilled the prediction of Armstrong et al. (8) that the inactivation gate was intracellular and was positively charged. Moreover, Catterall's group (233,234) had just reported that an antibody to this region effectively removed inactivation from Na channels in rat skeletal myoballs. Stühmer and coworkers transected the cDNA in the proximal III–IV linker, and coinjected mRNAs encoding the two fragments. Amazingly, Na currents appeared, demonstrating that the two fragments, one with three domains and the other with one, found and joined one another to form functional channels. The currents, though, had greatly impaired inactivation. This was the first demonstration that the III–IV linker played a role in Na channel inactivation.

A striking feature of the amino acid sequence in this linker is the presence of multiple positively charged residues. One early idea was that these charges served to close the inactivation gate, and that neutralization of them would remove fast inactivation. In fact, exactly the opposite occurs. Point mutations in the very slowly inactivating rat brain type III Na channel (119) that replaced groups of nearby Lys with Asn led to currents that decayed more quickly at the whole-cell level, and single-channel recordings showed the mechanism was a reduction in burst duration (163). Instructively, one of the mutations led to whole-cell currents that were identical to the wild type, but greatly different at the single-channel level where offsetting changes in activation and inactivation kinetics could be detected. In the faster-inactivating type II rat brain Na channel, neutralization of these charged residues had no discernible effect on macroscopic current decay (182). The critical residues in the III–IV linker turned out to be an innocuous-looking trio of hydrophobic residues—isoleucine (Ile, I), phenylalanine (Phe, F), methionine (Met, M)—in the amino end, near domain III (142, 182,242). Substitution of a single Phe with Gln removes fast inactivation nearly completely. This was confirmed with the elegant experimental strategy of using a synthetic peptide containing this sequence to restore fast inactivation to slowly inactivating mutant Na channels (57). The mechanism is not known, but the current notion is that these residues serve as a latch that attaches to a receptor elsewhere in the channel. Interestingly, the same mutation in heart Na channels has less profound effects, suggesting that the receptor for the IFM amino acid sequence may be different in the two channels (97).

Interestingly, the III–IV linker is relatively inaccessible to protease (258), suggesting it lies close to or within the membrane.

Inactivation is modulated by other parts of the channel protein. Chimeras of the rat skeletal muscle Na channel isoforms SkM1 and SkM2 in which domain I was exchanged had intermediate rates of channel inactivation (43), and Tomaselli and coworkers (227) have identified a residue in the pore region of domain IV that greatly influences current activation and decay.

Region Linking S5 to S6 Contributes to the Pore (Figs. 4 and 5)

Early models of Na channel structure differed on the position of the long, apparently extracellular region linking the S5 and S6 segments of the four domains. Where Numa and coworkers (175) initially envisioned this to lie outside the cell, Guy and Seetharamulu (95) thought the hydrophobic nature sufficient to position at least the midportion near or in the membrane. They gave the names SS1 and SS2 to the nearby parts of the sequence that most likely to approach and then exit the membrane. Indeed, point mutations in this area have strong effects on channel properties usually ascribed to the channel pore.

The first evidence came from Stühmer, Numa, and coworkers (176,188,226), who found that the S5-6 segment in domain I modulated both the binding of TTX, a pore blocker, and the single-channel conductance . Specifically, they found that mutation of either of two well-conserved negatively charged amino acids (E387 and D384) rendered brain type II channels almost insensitive to TTX, and reduced *i* by several orders of magnitude without altering gating current (Fig. 4). They reasoned that these residues must therefore be in or near the aqueous pore of the channel that forms the pathway for ion conductance. Similarly, well-conserved negatively charged residues are found in domain II (Fig. 4). These observations led to a systematic study of negatively charged residues in this region for all four domains (226). They found that mutations of any of eight amino acids had the combined effects of reducing toxin sensitivity and single-channel conductance. The eight amino acids were precisely distributed: two were in each of the four SS2 regions, and the pairs were exactly aligned among the four domains. Mutations of a number of other, nearby charged and uncharged residues had no effect, and no mutation affected gating kinetics. The results suggested that there are two rings of negative charges just inside the outer mouth of the channel that dictate toxin binding and single-channel conductance. Reducing the net negative charge here invariably reduced *both* toxin binding and conductance. Other mutations in this study showed dissociation of toxin binding and conductance—for instance, two mutations that increased the negative charge reduced toxin binding but did not affect conductance. A third nearby negative residue plays a smaller role in toxin binding (132). The picture emerges of negative charges that collect Na ions for transit through the pore and bind the large, positively charged TTX and STX molecules.

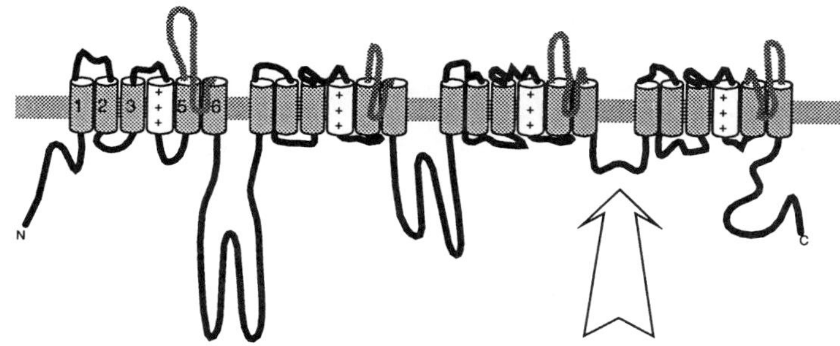

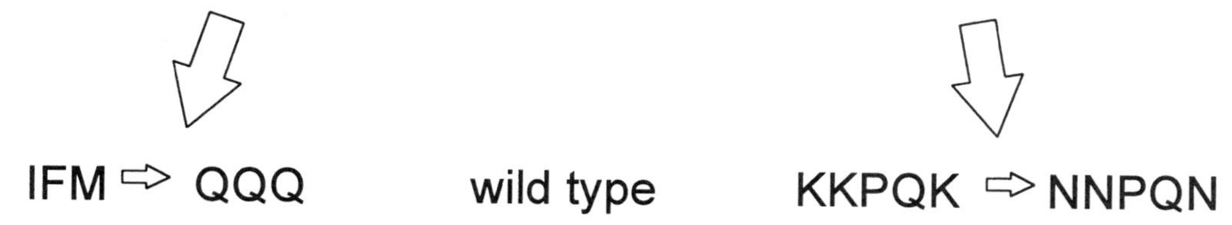

Figure 3. The III–IV linker is part or all of the Na channel inactivation gate. The 53 amino acid sequence, which is nearly completely conserved, is shown above.

Further evidence came in studies aiming to elucidate the molecular determinants of an interesting phenotypic difference of brain and skeletal muscle Na channels compared to cardiac Na channels (13,204). Divalent cations such as Ca, Zn, and Cd block some types of Na channels (9,66,192,208), but only those that are insensitive to TTX. Where brain and skeletal muscle channels are sensitive to TTX but not to Cd, cardiac channels have the opposite phenotype. Other studies had shown that sulfhydryl alkylating agents modified block by both toxin and Cd, suggesting that cysteine (Cys, C) residues might be involved in the binding site (Fig. 4, domain I). Two groups found a Cys that occurs in cardiac but not brain or skeletal muscle channels. This was a likely site, as Cys, with its sulfhydryl moiety, avidly binds Cd. In skeletal muscle channels, this residue was Tyr. Both groups found that the TTX/Cd binding profile was carried by Cys at this site, one group by mutating cardiac channels, the other by mutating skeletal muscle channels. Likewise, the different toxin sensitivities of rat skeletal muscle Na channel isoforms SkM1 and SkM2 can be explained by the presence of a Cys in this position in the TTX-resistant SkM2 channel (43).

The same area houses the selectivity filter (Fig. 5). Ca channels have much the same overall organization as Na channels, but the selectivity is vastly different. Stühmer, Numa, and coworkers aligned the S5-6 regions of domains III and IV of brain Ca and Na channels, and saw two strikingly conserved negatively charged glutamic acid (Glu, E) residues in Ca channels where Na channels had equally well-conserved positive Lys and neutral alanine (Ala, A) residues. They made three mutant Na channels—Lys to Glu in domain III (K1422E), Ala to Glu in domain IV (A1714E), and the double mutant. The mutant channels had clear differences in Na selectivity (102). As far as phenotypic changes following point mutations go, this is the most stunning.

Sixth Transmembrane Segment of the Fourth Domain (IVS6) Binds Local Anesthetics and Interacts with the Inactivation Mechanism

In systematic set of mutagenesis experiments, Catterall's group (189) has recently made two important observations on the role of IVS6 in brain Na channel function. Motivated by their findings that this region was responsible for binding phenylalkylamines in Ca channels, they made Na channel mutants in which each residue in this segment was changed, one by one, to Ala. They identified several mutants that were insensitive to block by etidocaine, a more lipophilic lidocaine derivative, and some other mutants that were more sensitive (189). Both tonic and phasic block were affected. Further studies of these and related mutant Na channels should shed a great deal of light on the mechanisms of local anesthetic block of Na channels.

In related experiments, they found that mutant channels in which three consecutive hydrophobic residues—valine (Val, V), Ile, and leucine (Leu, L) at positions 1774 to 1776—were all changed to Ala displayed almost no fast inactivation (160). Records of single mutant channels revealed two abnormalities of inactivation. First, reopenings were more frequent than in control, suggesting that the inactivated conformation was not stable. Second, the mean channel open time was prolonged, suggesting that access to the inactivated state was partially prohibited. Such global impairment of the inactivation process suggests a crucial role of this region, and Catterall and coworkers have proposed that it forms the binding site of the Ile-Phe-Met segment of the III–IV linker.

Given the importance of this region in binding, permeation, and selectivity in Na, Ca, and K channels, Catterall and coworkers have proposed that the S6 segment forms part or all of the intracellular mouth of channel pores.

Phosphorylation Sites are on Intracellular Linkers (Fig. 6)

The primary amino acid sequences allow distinction of two groups of Na channel molecules based on the size and features of the poorly conserved cytoplasmic linker between domains I and II. Brain Na channels have a long linker with five consensus sites for phosphorylation by PKA. Muscle Na channels, on the other hand, have a 200+ amino acid deletion in this linker and lose all five sites. This leads to the prediction that skeletal muscle Na channels would not be phosphorylated by PKA.

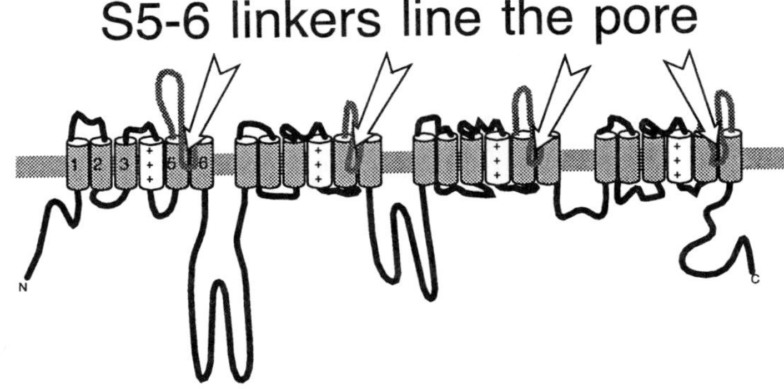

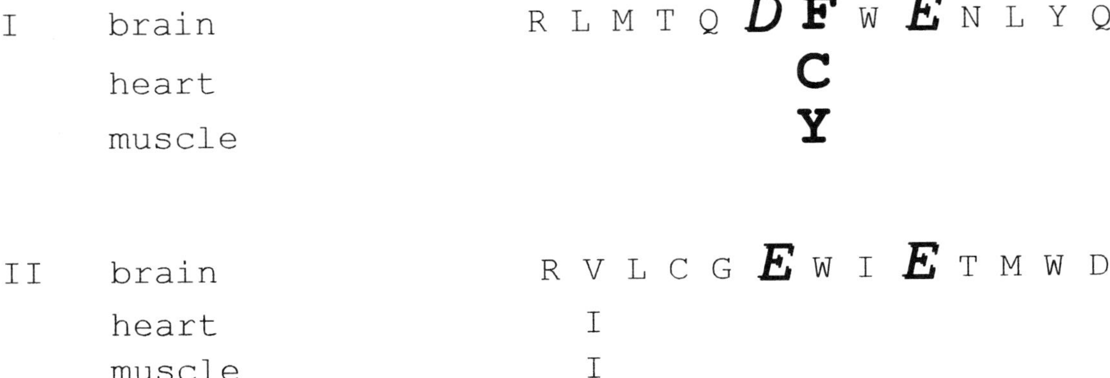

Figure 4. Small differences in the pore region, which is formed by the S5-6 linkers, are important. The amino acid sequences of this region from domains I and II are shown. Missing residues are either identical or conservative substitutions. In domain I, neutralization of the highlighted negatively charged Asp (D) or Glu (E) sites does away with block by TTX and greatly reduces the single-channel conductance. The other highlighted site (F in brain, C in heart, and Y in skeletal muscle) determines the differences in TTX and Cd sensitivity between heart and skeletal muscle Na channels. In domain II, there are other well-conserved negatively charged residues.

This, however, is not the case. Yang and Barchi (248) showed that the purified rat muscle α–subunit was readily phosphorylated by PKA, and that the site was likely to be in the I–II linker or in domain II. Although the total amount of incorporated phosphate was severalfold less than in brain—consistent with the loss of at least several phosphorylation sites—the rate of muscle Na channel phosphorylation was comparable to that in brain. One study of skeletal muscle Na channels expressed in *Xenopus* oocytes showed no effect of maneuvers that increase intracellular cAMP (214).

The Na channel from eel electroplax, like the skeletal muscle Na channel, has a short I–II linker with few phosphorylation sites. Agnew's group (59,60) has nonetheless shown biochemical and electrophysiologic evidence that this channel is regulated by phosphorylation by PKA at sites in the amino and carboxyl termini as well as a single site in the I–II linker. Here, the effect is to reduce current amplitude.

The effect of PKC activation has been determined at the molecular level. In skeletal muscle Na channels, activation of PKC by OAG leads first to slowed inactivation and then to reduced peak current amplitude. A specific peptide inhibitor of PKC prevented the OAG effect (256). In Chinese hamster ovary (CHO) cells transfected with a plasmid encoding wild-type and mutated type IIA brain Na channels, activation of PKC led to reduction of wild type current but not in a mutation that disables the potential phosphorylation site in the III–IV linker (S1506A) (241). In the same way, this site must be a serine (Ser, S) for HMPK to exert its effect (167). Most interestingly, this site must be phosphorylated in order for PKA to exert functional effects (141). This convergent regulation of the Na channel by multiple protein kinases places it in the role of an integrator of inputs into the central nervous system. The same work presented the important finding that replacement of a phosphorylation site with a negatively charged residue mimicked the effect of phosphorylation, simultaneously showing that the effects of phosphorylation are electrostatic and showing an important strategy for mutagenesis studies in the future. At the level of single-channel analysis of RNA-injected *Xenopus* oocytes, the mechanism is reduced channel activation kinetics (210).

Subunits

Auxiliary subunits are important to the function of Na, K, and Ca channels, as recent studies make clear (117). Although expression of α subunits alone is sufficient to induce currents in *Xenopus* oocytes, coexpression of β subunits usually has profound effects to restore normal gating parameters.

Although biochemical purification of sodium channels had long shown that smaller subunits copurified with the large a subunit and were important in toxin binding, cloning of the first β subunit came only recently (116). The β_1 subunit from rat brain

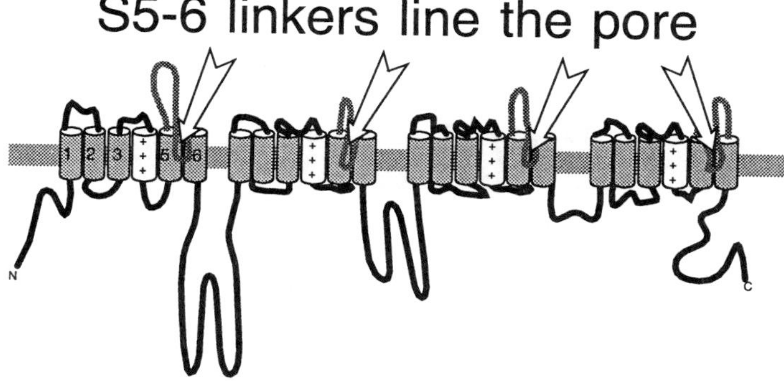


```
all Na channels      Q V A T F K G W M D I M Y
brain Ca channel     T V S T G E G W P Q E L K

brain Na channel     Q I T T S A G W D G L L A
brain Ca channel     R S A T G E A W H   N T M L
```

Figure 5. Other small differences in the pore region allow distinction between Na and Ca ions. The amino acid sequences of this region in the Na and Ca channels are shown. The highlighted site is the negatively charged Glu (E) in both domains of Ca channels, but the positively charged Lys (K) or neutral Ala (A) in Na channels. Substitution of E in the aligned site of Na channels results in Ca selectivity. The highlighted Asp (D) in Na channels, like the conserved negatively charged residues in domains I and II, plays a role in TTX block and in channel conductance.

proves to be a relatively small 218 amino acids and has a single putative transmembrane domain. Where α subunits vary at least perceptibly across tissues and species, the b_1 subunit is essentially identical wherever it is found (149,229). The functional effect of coexpressing the β_1 subunit with a subunits in *Xenopus* oocytes is to enhance the element of fast inactivation and to shift steady-state inactivation gating parameters to more negative potentials (19,32,116,181). To a large extent, the effect of the β_1 subunit may explain the observation that coinjection of low-molecular-weight (MW) brain RNA with a brain Na channel a subunit RNA induced currents with more rapid inactivation properties (256), and that Na channels expressed in mammalian cell lines have faster inactivation kinetics than when expressed in *Xenopus* oocytes (41,232,243). Although the β_1 subunit modifies brain and the µ1 or SkM1 muscle Na channel, it does not affect cardiac or SkM2 channels (249). Interestingly, Na currents induced by cardiac mRNA (134,228) or by mRNA encoding the cloned cardiac Na channel (73,205) inactivate quickly. In addition, β_1 subunit mRNA levels followed those of µ1 or SkM1 muscle Na channels but not of SkM2 channels. Most interestingly, the β_1 subunit maps to a locus on the mouse chromosome 7 associated with neuromuscular disorders, suggesting a role for the β subunits in disease processes (229).

NA CHANNELS IN HUMAN DISEASES

Importantly, human muscle diseases have been linked to Na channel mutations. For instance, paramyotonia congenita may result from a Leu to Arg mutation in IVS3 (186), an Arg to Cys or His at the extracellular end of IVS4 (184), or Gly to Val, or Thr to Met in the proximal III–IV linker (157). Hyperkalemic periodic paralysis is associated with a Thr to Met mutation at the intracellular end of IIS5 (185) or a Met to Val in IVS6 (196). An atypical myotonia congenita maps to the skeletal muscle Na channel locus (187). Other Na channel mutations lead to other, intermediate phenotypes (158). No mechanism has been ascribed for certain in these diseases, but the effect of the hyperkalemic periodic paralysis mutations is to shift the threshold for activation to more negative potentials, allowing channels to open near the resting potential (52), and to allow repetitive channel openings during a depolarizing stimulus, as if the process of inactivation had failed (30,33,139). Extracellular $[K^+]$ thus has the effect of modulating Na channel inactivation gating in muscle cells of patients with hyperkalemic periodic paralysis (30). Interestingly, extracellular $[K^+]$ diminishes Na current in cardiac ventricle (but not atrium), a potential mechanism for cardiac arrhythmias during ischemia and infarction (245).

Slow inactivation of normal muscle Na channels, including cardiac muscle, is observed only very rarely (reviewed in 165). This pattern is accentuated in channels expressed in *Xenopus* oocytes by α subunits alone (133,165,256) and relieved by coexpression of the β subunit (116). Interestingly, this pattern was observed in cell-attached patches of muscle cells from patients with myotonic muscular dystrophy (63), myotonia congenita (115), and generalized recessive myotonia (64). As subtle as the finding seems, mathematical models show that the increased late Na current would lead to myotonia or paralysis (31).

The genetic abnormality in myotonic muscular dystrophy, the most common myotonic disease and the most common

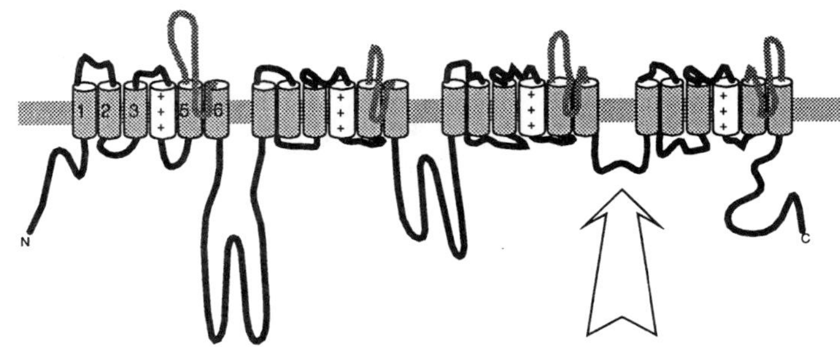

The III-IV linker is the inactivation gate

KKKFGGQD**IFM**TEEQKKYYNAMKKLG*S*KKPQKPIPRPANK

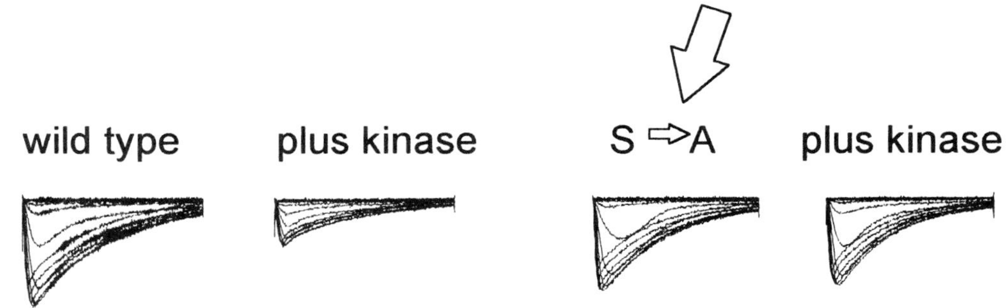

Figure 6. A phosphorylation site (*S*, italicized) in the III–IV linker allows channel modulation. *Below* are macroscopic recordings from four oocytes: The first is expressing the wild-type skeletal muscle Na channel alone. The second is coexpressing human myotonin protein kinase, a serine/threonin kinase; the effect of coexpression is to reduce current amplitude. The third current is from an oocyte expressing a mutant skeletal muscle Na channel in which the phosphorylation site has been inactivated by Ser to Ala mutation. The fourth current shows that coexpression of the kinase has no effect on the amplitude of currents through mutant channels, strongly implying that the kinase exerts its effect by phosphorylation of the III–IV linker site.

muscular dystrophy in adults, lies not in a Na channel, but rather in a molecule with structural similarities to protein kinases. As discussed above, studies of Na currents in *Xenopus* oocytes expressing both skeletal muscle Na channels and the myotonic dystrophy gene product show modulation of current amplitudes and kinetics.

DEVELOPMENTAL ASPECTS

Both functional and molecular studies have demonstrated developmental regulation of Na channel number and type. Many cell types have phenotypically distinct Na currents at different phases of development. Neonatal rat myotubes have both TTX-sensitive and TTX-resistant Na channels, where adult muscle has only the TTX-sensitive isoform, which also had a larger conductance (237). In dorsal root ganglion cells, the cohort of Na channel types depends on the size and class of neuron (27). Huguenard and coworkers (114) showed that TTX-sensitive Na channels develop slow gating as they mature. Barres and coworkers (17) found that Na channels from glial precursor cells have fast gating, but those from glial cells 6 to 7 days after birth have slow gating. In a human neuroblastoma cell line, undifferentiated cells display both TTX-insensitive and TTX-sensitive Na currents. After differentiation, the TTX-sensitive population increases in number, but the TTX-insensitive population stays the same (238).

Brain, heart, and skeletal muscle all express multiple Na channel genes. In mammalian skeletal muscle, for example, at least seven different Na channel RNAs can be distinguished (207). Genes encoding neuronal Na channels appear to be clustered near one another on chromosome 2 of mouse and human (Table 1). Genes encoding skeletal and cardiac muscle Na channel isoforms, on the other hand, appear on chromosomes 3 and 17 as well.

Alternative splicing appears to be a regulatory mechanism. The rat brain type II channel has two isoforms that differ in but a single amino acid—Asp versus Asn—at position 209. Type II predominates at birth and then declines (203). The mutation causes a large shift in the voltage dependence of activation (11). The rat brain type III channel also has two isoforms that differ in a single amino acid—Asp versus Ser—in domain I (92). One isoform is expressed preferentially in neonate, and the other in adult. The functional consequences of the mutation have not been explored.

In skeletal muscle, regulation of gene expression can explain developmental changes in the channel phenotype of Na currents. Early in development, the currents are resistant to TTX, but later are TTX sensitive. The SkM2 isoform is preferentially expressed in the embryo and decreases over the first month postpartum: SkM1 is expressed at low levels at birth and then rises. Expression of the two channel types is regulated independently by innervation (250). In normal innervated muscle, only SkM1 is found. After denervation, SkM1 mRNA levels fall, then rebound to normal, and SkM2 mRNA levels rise to very high levels before stabilizing. Interestingly, denervation by botulinum toxin leads to higher SkM2 mRNA levels than denervation by axotomy. Kallen's group (213) has identified positive- and negative-transcriptional regulator elements of the SkM2 gene.

Table 1. SODIUM CHANNELS

Tissue	Species	Name	Comments	Reference
	Jellyfish		Lowest organism with Na-action potentials	5
	Squid		Shortest known, at 1522 amino acids	206
			1784 amino acids	199
	Fly		One is at the *para* locus	145,190,202
Electroplax	Eel		Not expressed at all in oocytes	175
Brain	Rat	I	Not expressed sufficiently in oocytes	173
		II	The best studied	173
		IIA	Splice variant of II—rightward shift in gating explained by S4 mutation	11,12
		III	Very slow gating	119,125
	Human	HBA, HBB	Both map to chromosome 2 (band 2q23–24.3)	1,150
		HBSC I,II	Same chromosomal location	146
		SCN3A	Also chromosome 2 (2q24–31); analogous to rat brain III	151
		SCN6A	Also chromosome 2 (2q21–23)	75
Glia		Na-G	Also chromosome 2	72,183
Skeletal muscle	Rat	μ1; rSkM1	Innervated muscle; sensitive to TTX, μ-CTX	231
		rSkM2	Developing or denervated muscle; insensitive to TTX, μ-CTX; identical to RH1	123
	Human	hSkM1	Product of the SCN4A gene on chromosome 17	76,79
Heart	Rat	RH1	Identical to rSkM2	195
		hNav2.1	His replaces several positive charges in S4 segments; also in uterus	74
	Human	hH1	TTX insensitive; *i* twice that of RH1; product of the SCN5A gene on chromosome 3, band 3p21	73,77

Regulation of expression of brain Na channels has been reviewed by Mandel (152,153). Type I expression is low in brain and spinal cord at birth, and the levels rise together. The highest expression was found in caudate nucleus, hippocampus, striatum, thalamus, and cerebellum (25). Type II is expressed equally in brain and spinal cord at birth. Subsequently, levels rise in brain and fall in spinal cord. It is the most abundant at all stages in rat brain (25). Type III is also expressed equally in brain and spinal cord at birth; levels subsequently fall in brain and disappear from spinal cord. In mouse brain, type I and III channels are on cell bodies, and type II channels are on axons where their level decreases with myelination (244). Thus, a defect in myelination leads to overexpression of Na channels, and the mice have a characteristic phenotype—they shiver. Mandel and coworkers (135,156) have identified a genetic silencer element that allows, through cell-specific binding proteins, patterned expression of Na channels in the nervous system.

WHAT IS THE GOOD OF MOLECULAR STUDIES OF NA CHANNELS?

It is fair to ask why so much effort is going into characterizing Na channels and other ion channels at the molecular level. Although we know that cardiac arrhythmias, which must certainly be related to ion channel pathophysiology, are among the commonest means of death in this country, and although we know an ever-increasing amount about the molecular mechanisms of ion channels, we have not the first idea how these two things are related. There is not a single therapeutic strategy at this time that is based on anything other than empiricism. In fact, our best antiarrhythmic drugs—all of which block Na channels—have now been shown to be harmful to patients with coronary disease and ventricular arrhythmias (35), the people most in need of antiarrhythmic drugs. Instead, the attention of the medical community has turned, not unreasonably, to devices such as the automatic implantable cardioverter-defibrillator and to potentially curable interventional procedures such as radiofrequency catheter ablation.

Does this mean that the molecular knowledge is wasted? Perhaps it is simply too early to ask for practical results. The current investigation is at so highly resolved a level that thousands of bits of information will have to be presented before meaningful synthesis can be attempted and a coherent drug development program begun.

ACKNOWLEDGMENTS

Studies in the author's laboratory have been supported by the National Institutes of Health and MDA. I am grateful to Al George, Gus Grant, and Gordon Tomaselli for correcting and enhancing sections of the chapter.

REFERENCES

1. Ahmed CM, Ware DH, Lee SC, et al. Primary structure, chromosomal localization, and functional expression of a voltage-gated sodium channel from human brain. *Proc Natl Acad Sci USA* 1992; 89:8220–8224.
2. Aldrich RW, Corey DP, Stevens CF. A reinterpretation of mammalian sodium channel gating based on single channel recording. *Nature* 1983;306:436–441.
3. Aldrich RW, Stevens CF. Voltage-dependent gating of single sodium channels from mammalian neuroblastoma cells. *J Neurosci* 1987;7:418–431.
4. Alpert LA, Fozzard HA, Hanck DA, Makielski JC. Is there a second external lidocaine binding site on mammalian cardiac cells? *Am J Physiol* 1989;257:H79–H84.
5. Anderson PA, Holman MA, Greenberg RM. Deduced amino acid sequence of a putative sodium channel from the scyphozoan jellyfish *Cyanea capillata*. *Proc Natl Acad Sci USA* 1993;90:7419–7423.
6. Armstrong CM, Bezanilla F. Charge movement associated with the opening and closing of the activation gates of the Na channels. *J Gen Physiol* 1974;63:533–552.
7. Armstrong CM, Bezanilla F. Inactivation of the sodium channel. *J Gen Physiol* 1977;70:567–590.
8. Armstrong CM, Bezanilla F, Rojas E. Destruction of sodium conductance inactivation in squid axons perfused with pronase. *J Gen Physiol* 1973;62:375–391.
9. Armstrong CM, Cota G. Calcium ion as a cofactor in Na channel gating. *Proc Natl Acad Sci USA* 1991;88:6528–6531.
10. Aslanidis C, Jansen G, Amemiya C, et al. Cloning of the essential myotonic dystrophy region and mapping of the putative defect. *Nature* 1992;355:548–551.
11. Auld VJ, Goldin AL, Krafte DS, Catterall WA, Lester HA, Davidson

N, Dunn RJ. A neutral amino acid change in segment IIS4 dramatically alters the gating properties of the voltage-dependent sodium channel. *Proc Natl Acad Sci USA* 1990;87:323–327.
12. Auld VJ, Goldin AL, Krafte DS, et al. A rat brain Na⁺ channel α subunit with novel gating properties. *Neuron* 1988;1:449–461.
13. Backx PH, Yue DT, Lawrence JH, Marban E, Tomaselli GF. Molecular localization of an ion-binding site within the pore of mammalian sodium channels. *Science* 1992;257:248–251.
14. Barber MJ, Starmer CF, Grant AO. Blockade of cardiac sodium channels by amitriptyline and diphenylhydantoin. Evidence for two use-dependent binding sites. *Circ Res* 1991;69:677–696.
15. Barber MJ, Wendt DJ, Starmer CF, Grant AO. Blockade of cardiac sodium channels. Competition between the permeant ion and antiarrhythmic drugs. *J Clin Invest* 1992;90:368–381.
16. Barchi RL. Protein components of the purified sodium channel from rat skeletal muscle sarcolemma. *J Neurochem* 1983;40:1377–1385.
17. Barres BA, Chun LLY, Corey DP. Glial and neuronal forms of the voltage-dependent sodium channel: characteristics and cell-type distribution. *Neuron* 1989;2:1375–1388.
18. Baumgarten CM, Makielski JC, Fozzard HA. External site for local anesthetic block of cardiac Na⁺ channels. *J Mol Cell Cardiol* 1991;23:85–93.
19. Bennett PBJ, Makita N, George ALJ. A molecular basis for gating mode transitions in human skeletal muscle Na⁺ channels. *FEBS Lett* 1993;326:21–24.
20. Benz I, Herzig JW, Kohlhardt M. Opposite effects of angiotensin II and the protein kinase C activator OAG on cardiac Na⁺ channels. *J Membr Biol* 1992;130:183–190.
21. Benz I, Kohlhardt M. Differential response of DPI-modified cardiac Na⁺ channels to antiarrhythmic drugs; no flicker blockade by lidocaine. *J Membr Biol* 1992;126:257–263.
22. Brook JD, McCurrach ME, Harley HG, et al. Molecular basis of myotonic dystrophy: expansion of a trinucleotide (CTG) repeat at the 3′ end of a transcript encoding a protein kinase family member. *Cell* 1992;68:799–808.
23. Broughton A, Grant AO, Starmer CF, Klinger JK, Stambler BS, Strauss HC. Lipid solubility modulates pH potentiation of local anesthetic block of Vmax reactivation in guinea pig myocardium. *Circ Res* 1984;55:513–523.
24. Brown AM, Lee KS, Powell T. Sodium current in single rat heart muscle cells. *J Physiol* 1981;318:479–500.
25. Brysch W, Creutzfeldt OD, Luno K, Schlingensiepen R, Schlingensiepen KH. Regional and temporal expression of sodium channel messenger RNAs in the rat brain during development. *Exp Brain Res* 1991;86:562–567.
26. Butterworth JF, Strichartz GR. Molecular mechanisms of local anesthesia: a review. *Anesthesiology* 1990;72:711–734.
27. Caffrey JM, Eng DL, Black JA, Waxman SG, Kocsis JD. Three types of sodium channels in adult rat dorsal root ganglion neurons. *Brain Res* 1992;592:283–297.
28. Cahalan MD, Almers W. Interactions between quaternary lidocaine, the sodium channel gates, and tetrodotoxin. *Biophys J* 1979;27:39–56.
29. Campbell DT. Do protons block Na⁺ channels by binding to a site outside the pore? *Nature* 1982;298:165–167.
30. Cannon SC, Brown RH, Corey DP. A sodium channel defect in hyperkalemic periodic paralysis: potassium-induced failure of inactivation. *Neuron* 1991;6:619–626.
31. Cannon SC, Brown RH, Corey DP. Theoretical reconstruction of myotonia and paralysis caused by incomplete inactivation of sodium channels. *Biophys J* 1993;65:270–288.
32. Cannon SC, McClatchey AI, Gusella JF. Modification of the Na⁺ current conducted by the rat skeletal muscle α subunit by coexpression with a human brain b subunit. *Pflugers Arch* 1993;423:155–157.
33. Cannon SC, Strittmatter SM. Functional expression of sodium channel mutations identified in families with periodic paralysis. *Neuron* 1993;10:317–326.
34. Casadei JM, Gordon RD, Barchi RL. Immunoaffinity isolation of Na⁺ channels from rat skeletal muscle. *J Biol Chem* 1986;261:4318–4323.
35. CAST Investigators. Preliminary report: effect of encainide and flecainide on mortality in a randomized trial of arrhythmia suppression after myocardial infarction. *N Engl J Med* 1989;321:406–412.
36. Catterall WA. Neurotoxins that act on voltage-sensitive sodium channels in excitable membranes. *Annu Rev Pharmacol Toxicol* 1980;20:15–43.
37. Catterall WA. Voltage-dependent gating of sodium channels: correlating structure and function. *Trends Neurosci* 1986;9:7–10.
38. Catterall WA. Structure and function of voltage-sensitive ion channels. *Science* 1988;242:50–61.
39. Catterall WA. Cellular and molecular biology of voltage-gated sodium channels. *Physiol Rev* 1992;72:S15–48.
40. Catterall WA, Gonoi T, Costa M. Sodium channels in neural cells: molecular properties and analysis of mutants. In: *Anonymous current topics in membranes and transport.* Academic Press, 1985; 79–100.
41. Chahine M, Bennett PB, George AL Jr, Horn R. Functional expression and properties of the human skeletal muscle sodium channel. *Pflugers Arch Eur J Physiol* 1994;427:136–142.
42. Chahine M, George ALJ, Zhou M, Ji S, Sun W, Barchi RL, Horn R. Sodium channel mutations in paramyotonia congenita uncouple inactivation from activation. *Neuron* 1994;12:281–294.
43. Chen LQ, Chahine M, Kallen RG, Barchi RL, Horn R. Chimeric study of sodium channels from rat skeletal and cardiac muscle. *FEBS Letters* 1992;309:253–257.
44. Chernoff DM, Strichartz GR. Tonic and phasic block of neuronal sodium currents by 5-hydroxyhexano-2′,6′-xyide, a neural lidocaine homologue. *J Gen Physiol* 1989;93:1075–1090.
45. Cohen SA, Barchi R. Voltage-dependent sodium channels. *Int Rev Cytol* 1993;137C:55–103.
46. Cohen-Armon M, Sokolovsky M, Dascal N. Modulation of the voltage-dependent sodium channel by agents affecting G-proteins: a study in *Xenopus* oocytes injected with brain RNA. *Brain Res* 1989;4966:197–203.
47. Conti F, Stühmer W. Quantal charge redistributions accompanying the structural transitions of sodium channels. *Eur Biophys J* 1989;17:53–59.
48. Courtney KR. Structure-activity relations for frequency-dependent sodium channel block in nerve by local anesthetics. *J Pharmacol Exp Ther* 1980;213:114–119.
49. Courtney KR. Size-dependent kinetics associated with drug block of sodium current. *Biophys. J.* 1984;45:42–44.
50. Courtney KR. Sodium channel blockers: the size/solubility hypothesis revisited. *Mol Pharmacol* 1990;37:855–859.
51. Cummins TR, Jiang C, Haddad GG. Human neocortical excitability is decreased during anoxia via sodium channel modulation. *J Clin Invest* 1993;91:608–615.
52. Cummins TR, Zhou J, Sigworth FJ, Ukomadu C, Stephan M, Ptacek LJ, Agnew WS. Functional consequences of a Na⁺ channel mutation causing hyperkalemic periodic paralysis. *Neuron* 1993;10:667–678.
53. D'Arcangelo G, Paradiso K, Shepherd D, Brehm P, Halegoua S. Neuronal growth factor regulation of two different sodium channel types through distinct signal transduction pathways. *J Cell Biol* 1993;122:915–921.
54. Dascal N, Lotan H. Activation of protein kinase C alters voltage dependence of a Na⁺ channel. *Neuron* 1991;6:165–175.
55. Daumas P, Andersen OS. Proton block of rat brain sodium channels. Evidence for two proton binding sites and multiple occupancy. *J Gen Physiol* 1993;101:27–43.
56. Duff HJ, Offord J, West J, Catterall WA. Class I and IV antiarrhythmic drugs and cytosolic calcium regulate mRNA encoding the sodium channel alpha subunit in rat cardiac muscle. *Mol Pharmacol* 1992;42:570–574.
57. Eaholtz G, Scheuer T, Catterall WA. Restoration of inactivation and block of open sodium channels by an inactivation gate peptide. *Neuron* 1994;12:1041–1048.
58. Elmer LW, O'Brien BJ, Nutter TJ, Angelides KJ. Physicochemical characterization of the α-peptide of the sodium channel from rat brain. *Biochemistry* 1985;24:8128–8137.
59. Emerick MC, Agnew WS. Identification of phosphorylation sites for adenosine 3′,5′-cyclic phosphate dependent protein kinase on the voltage-sensitive sodium channel from electrophorus electricus. *Biochemistry* 1989;28:8367–8380.
60. Emerick MC, Shenkel S, Agnew WS. Regulation of the eel electroplax Na channel and phosphorylation of residues on amino- and carboxyl-terminal domains by cAMP-dependent protein kinase. *Biochemistry* 1993;32:9435–9444.
61. Fozzard HA, Hanck DS. Sodium channels. In: Fozzard HA, et al., eds. *The heart and cardiovascular system.* New York: Raven Press, 1992;1091–1119.

62. Fozzard HA, January CT, Makielski JC. New studies of the excitatory sodium current in heart muscle. *Circ Res* 1985;56:475–485.
63. Franke C, Hatt H, Iaizzo PA, Lehmann-Horn F. Characteristics of Na^+ and Cl^- conductance in resealed muscle fibre segments from patients with myotonic dystrophy. *J Physiol* 1990;425:391–405.
64. Franke C, Iaizzo PA, Hatt H, Spittelmeister W, Ricker K, Lehmann-Horn F. Altered Na^+ channel activity and reduced Cl^- conductance cause hyperexcitability in recessive generalized myotonia (Becker). *Muscle Nerve* 1991;14:762–770.
65. Freeman LC, Kass RS. Expression of a minimal K^+ channel protein in mammalian cells and immunolocalization in guinea pig heart. *Circ Res* 1993;73:968–973.
66. French RJ, Worley JF 3rd, Wonderlin WE, Kularatna AS, Krueger BK. Ion permeation, divalent ion block, and chemical modification of single sodium channels. Description by single- and double-occupancy rate-theory models. *J Gen Physiol* 1994;103:447–470.
67. Frenkel C, Duch DS, Recio-Pinto E, Urban BW. Pentobarbital suppresses human brain sodium channels. *Mol Brain Res* 1989;6: 211–216.
68. Frenkel C, Duch DS, Urban BW. Molecular actions of pentobarbital isomers on sodium channels from human brain cortex. *Anesthesiology* 1990;72:640–649.
69. Frenkel C, Urban BW. Human brain sodium channels as one of the molecular target sites for the new intravenous anaesthetic propofol (2,6-diisopropylphenol). *Eur J Pharmacol* 1991;208:75–79.
70. Frenkel C, Urban BW. Molecular actions of racemic ketamine on human CNS sodium channels. *Br J Anaesth* 1992;69:292–297.
71. Fu Y, Pizzuti A, Fenwick RG, et al. An unstable triplet repeat in a gene related to myotonic muscular dystrophy. *Science* 1992;255: 1256–1258.
72. Gautron S, Dos Santos G, Pinto-Henrique D, Koulakoff A, Gros F, Berwald-Netter Y. The glial voltage-gated sodium channel: cell- and tissue-specific mRNA expression. *Proc Natl Acad Sci USA* 1992; 89:7272–7276.
73. Gellens ME, George ALJ, Chen LQ, Chahine M, Horn R, Barchi RL, Kallen RG. Primary structure and functional expression of the human cardiac tetrodotoxin-insensitive voltage-dependent sodium channel. *Proc Natl Acad Sci USA* 1992;89:554–558.
74. George AL, Knittle TJ, Tamkun MM. Molecular cloning of an atypical voltage-gated sodium channel expressed in human heart and uterus: evidence for a distinct gene family. *Proc Natl Acad Sci USA* 1992;89:4893–4897.
75. George AL, Knops JF, Han J, Finley WH, Knittle TJ, Tamkun MM, Brown GB. Assignment of a human voltage-dependent sodium channel α-subunit gene (SCN6A) to 2q21–q23. *Genomics* 1994;19: 395–397.
76. George AL, Komisarof J, Kallen RG, Barchi R. Primary structure of the adult human skeletal muscle voltage-dependent sodium channel. *Ann Neurol* 1992;31:131–137.
77. George AL, Varkony TA, Drabkin HA, et al. Assignment of the human heart tetrodotoxin-resistant voltage-gated Na channel a-subunit gene (SCN5A) to band 3p21. *Cytogenet Cell Genet* 1995;68: 67–70.
78. George AL Jr, Knittle TJ, Tamkun MM. Molecular cloning of an atypical voltage-gated sodium channel expressed in human heart and uterus: evidence for a distinct gene family. *Proc Natl Acad Sci USA* 1992;89:4893–4897.
79. George ALJ, Iyer GS, Kleinfield R, Kallen RG, Barchi RL. Genomic organization of the human skeletal muscle sodium channel gene. *Genomics* 1993;15:598–606.
80. Gershon E, Weigl L, Lotan I, Schreibmayer W, Dascal N. Protein kinase A reduces voltage-dependent Na^+ current in *Xenopus* oocytes. *J Neurosci* 1992;12:3743–3752.
81. Gingrich KJ, Beardsley D, Yue DT. Ultra-deep blockade of Na^+ channels by a quaternary ammonium ion: catalysis by a transition-intermediate state? *J Physiol* 1993;471:319–341.
82. Gintant GA, Liu DW. Beta-adrenergic modulation of fast inward sodium current in canine myocardium. Syncytial preparations versus isolated myocytes. *Circ Res* 1992;70:844–850.
83. Ginty DD, Fanger GR, Wagner JA, Maue RA. The activity of cAMP-dependent protein kinase is required at a posttranslational level for induction of voltage-dependent sodium channels by peptide growth factors in PC12 cells. *J Cell Biol* 1992;116:1465–1473.
84. Goldin AL. Accessory subunits and sodium channel inactivation. *Curr Opin Neurobiol* 1993;3:272–277.
85. Goldin AL, Snutch T, L¸bbert H, et al. Messenger RNA coding for only the a subunit of the rat brain Na channel is sufficient for expression of functional channels in *Xenopus* oocytes. *Proc Natl Acad Sci USA* 1986;83:7503–7507.
86. Grant AO, Dietz MA, Gilliam, I, Starmer CF. Blockade of cardiac sodium channels by lidocaine: single-channel analysis. *Circ Res* 1989;65:1247–1262.
87. Grant AO, Starmer CF. Mechanisms of closure of cardiac sodium channels in rabbit ventricular myocytes: single-channel analysis. *Circ Res* 1987;60:897–913.
88. Grant AO, Starmer CF, Strauss HC. Antiarrhythmic drug action: blockade of the inward sodium current. *Circ Res* 1984;55:427–439.
89. Grant AO, Strauss LJ, Wallace AG, Strauss HC. The influence of pH on the electrophysiological effects of lidocaine in guinea pig ventricular myocardium. *Circ Res* 1980;47:542–550.
90. Grant AO, Wendt DJ. Block and modulation of cardiac Na^+ channels by antiarrhythmic drugs, neurotransmitters and hormones. *Trends Pharmacol Sci* 1992;13:352–358.
91. Grant AO, Wendt DJ, Zilberter Y, Starmer CF. Kinetics of interaction of disopyramide with the cardiac sodium channel: fast dissociation from open channels at normal rest potentials. *J Membr Biol* 1993;136:199–214.
92. Gustafson TA, Clevinger EC, O'Neill TJ, Yarowsky PJ, Krueger BK. Mutually exclusive exon splicing of type III brain sodium channel alpha subunit RNA generates developmentally regulated isoforms in rat brain. *J Biol Chem* 1993;268:18648–18653.
93. Guy HR. A model relating the structure of the sodium channel to its function. In: Agnew WS, Claudio T, Sigworth F, eds. *Current topics in membranes and transport*. F. Academic Press, 1988;289–308.
94. Guy HR, Conti F. *Trends Neurosci* 1990;13:201–206.
95. Guy HR, Seetharamulu P. Molecular model of the action potential sodium channel. *Proc Natl Acad Sci USA* 1986;83:508–512.
96. Hanck DA, Makielski JC, Sheets MF. Kinetic effects of quarternary lidocaine block of cardiac sodium channels: a gating current study. *J Gen Physiol* 1994;103:19–43.
97. Hartmann HA, Tiedeman AA, Chen SF, Brown AM, Kirsch GE. Effects of III–IV linker mutations on human heart Na^+ channel inactivation gating. *Circ Res* 1994;75:114–122.
98. Haydon DA, Requena J, Urban BW. Some effects of aliphatic hydrocarbons on the electrical capacity and ionic currents of the squid giant axon membrane. *J Physiol* 1980;309:229–245.
99. Haydon DA, Urban BW. The effects of some inhalation anaesthetics on the sodium current of the squid giant axon. *J Physiol* 1983;341:429–439.
100. Haydon DA, Urban BW. The action of alcohols and other non-ionic surface active substances on the sodium current of the squid giant axon. *J Physiol* 1983;341:411–427.
101. Haydon DA, Urban BW. The action of hydrocarbons and carbon tetrachloride on the sodium current of the squid giant axon. *J Physiol* 1983;338:435–450.
102. Heinemann SH, Terlau H, Stuhmer W, Imoto K, Numa S. Calcium channel characteristics conferred on the sodium channel by single mutations. *Nature* 1992;356:441–443.
103. Hill RJ, Duff HJ, Sheldon RS. Class I antiarrhythmic drug receptor: biochemical evidence for state-dependent interaction with quinidine and lidocaine. *Mol Pharmacol* 1989;366:150–159.
104. Hille B. Local anesthetics: hydrophilic and hydrophobic pathways for the drug-receptor reaction. *J Gen Physiol* 1977;69:497–515.
105. Hille B. The pH-dependent rate of action of local anesthetics on the node of Ranvier. *J Gen Physiol* 1977;69:475–496.
106. Hille B. *Ionic channels of excitable membranes*. Sunderland, MA: Sinauer, 1992.
107. Hodgkin AL, Huxley AF. The dual effect of membrane potential on sodium conductance in the giant axon of *Loligo*. *J Physiol* 1952; 116:497–506.
108. Hodgkin AL, Huxley AF. A quantitative description of membrane current and its application to conduction and excitation in nerve. *J Physiol* 1952;117:500–544.
109. Hodgkin AL, Huxley AF. The components of membrane conductance in the giant axon of *Loligo*. *J Physiol* 1952;116:473–496.
110. Hodgkin AL, Huxley AF. Currents carried by sodium and potassium ions through the membrane of the giant axon of *Loligo*. *J Physiol* 1952;116:449–472.
111. Hondeghem LM. Effects of lidocaine phenytoin and quinidine on ischemic canine of hypoxic cells. *J Electrocardiol* 1976;9:203–209.
112. Hondeghem LM, Katzung BG. Time-and voltage-dependent interactions of antiarrhythmic drugs with cardiac sodium channels. *Biochim Biophys Acta* 1977;472:373–398.
113. Hondeghem LM, Katzung BG. Antiarrhythmic agents: the modu-

lated receptor mechanism of action of sodium and calcium channel-blocking drugs. *Annu Rev Pharmacol Toxicol* 1984;24:387–423.
114. Huguenard JR, Hamill OP, Prince DA. Developmental changes in Na^+ conductances in rat neocortical neurons: appearance of a slowly inactivating component. *J Neurophysiol* 1988;59(3):778–795.
115. Iaizzo PA, Franke C, Hatt H, Spittelmeister W, Ricker K, Rudel R, Lehmann-Horn F. Altered sodium channel behaviour causes myotonia in dominantly inherited myotonia congenita. *Neuromusc Disord* 1991;1:47–53.
116. Isom LL, De Jongh KS, Patton DE, et al. Primary structure and functional expression of the b1 subunit of the rat brain sodium channel. *Science* 1992;256:839–842.
117. Isom LL, DeJongh KS, Catterall WA. Auxiliary subunits of voltage-gated ion channels. *Neuron* 1994;12:1183–1194.
118. Jan LY, Jan YN. A superfamily of ion channels. *Nature* 1990;345: 672.
119. Joho RH, Moorman JR, VanDongen AMJ, Kirsch GE, Silberberg H, Schuster G, Brown AM. Toxin and kinetic profile of rat brain type III Na^+ channels expressed in *Xenopus* oocytes. *Mol Brain Res* 1990;7:105
120. Josephson IR, Sperelakis N. Tetrodotoxin differentially blocks peak and steady-state sodium channel currents in early embryonic chick ventricular myocytes. *Pflugers Arch* 1989;414:354–359.
121. Josephson IR, Sperelakis N. Kinetic and steady-state properties of Na^+ channel and Ca^{2+} channel charge movements in ventricular myocytes of embryonic chick heart. *J Gen Physiol* 1992;100: 195–216.
122. Kallen RG, Cohen SA, Barchi RL. Structure, function and expression of voltage-dependent sodium channels. *Mol Neurobiol* 1993;7: 383–428.
123. Kallen RG, Sheng Z, Yang J, Chen L, Rogart RB, Barchi RL. Primary structure and expression of a sodium channel characteristic of denervated and immature rat skeletal muscle. *Neuron* 1990;4: 233–242.
124. Kalman D, Wong B, Horvai AE, Cline MJ, O'Lague PH. Nerve growth factor acts through cAMP-dependent protein kinase to increase the number of sodium channels in PC12 cells. *Neuron* 1990;4:355–366.
125. Kayano T, Noda M, Flockerzi V, Takahashi H, Numa S. Primary structure of rat brain sodium channel III deduced from the cDNA sequence. *FEBS Lett* 1988;228:187–194.
26. Keynes RD. Voltage-gated ion channels in the nerve membrane. *Proc R Soc Lond [Biol]* 1983;220:1–30.
127. Kirsch GE, Brown AM. Kinetic properties of single sodium channels in rat heart and rat brain. *J Gen Physiol* 1989;93:85–99.
128. Kirstein M, Eickhorn R, Langenfeld H, Kochsiek K, Antoni H. Influence of beta-adrenergic stimulation on the fast sodium current in the intact rat papillary muscle. *Basic Res Cardiol* 1991;86: 441–448.
129. Kohlhardt M. Gating properties of cardiac Na^+ channels in cell-free conditions. *J Membr Biol* 1991;122:11–21.
130. Kohlhardt M, Fichtner H. Block of single cardiac Na^+ channels by antiarrhythmic drugs: the effect of amiodarone, propafenone, and diprafenone. *J Membr Biol* 1988;102:105–119.
131. Kohlhardt M, Fichtner H, Frobe U, Herzig JW. On the mechanism of drug-induced blockade of Na^+ currents: interaction of antiarrhythmic compounds with DPI-modified single cardiac Na^+ channels. *Circ Res* 1989;64:867–881.
132. Kontis KJ, Goldin AL. Site-directed mutagenesis of the putative pore region of the rat IIA sodium channel. *Mol Pharmacol* 1993;43: 635–644.
133. Krafte DS, Goldin AL, Auld VJ, Dunn RJ, Davidson N, Lester HA. Inactivation of cloned Na channels expressed in *Xenopus* oocytes. *J Gen Physiol* 1990;96:689–706.
134. Krafte DS, Volberg WA, Dillon K, Ezrin AM. Expression of cardiac Na channels with appropriate physiological and pharmacological properties in *Xenopus* oocytes. *Proc Natl Acad Sci USA* 1991;88: 4071–4074.
135. Kraner SD, Chong JA, Tsay HJ, Mandel G. Silencing the type II sodium channel gene: a model for neural-specific gene regulation. *Neuron* 1992;9:37–44.
136. Kunze DL, Lacerda AE, Wilson DL, Brown AM. Cardiac Na currents and the inactivating, reopening, and waiting properties of single cardiac Na channels. *J Gen Physiol* 1985;86:691–719.
137. Lawrence JH, Yue DT, Rose WC, Marban E. Sodium channel inactivation from resting states in guinea-pig ventricular myocytes. *J Physiol* 1991;443:629–650.
138. Lee HC, Matsuda JJ, Reynertson SI, Martins JB, Shibata EF. Reversal of lidocaine effects on sodium currents by isoproterenol in rabbit hearts and heart cells. *J Clin Invest* 1993;91:693–701.
139. Lehmann-Horn F, Iaizzo PA, Hatt H, Franke C. Altered gating and conductance of Na^+ channels in hyperkalemic periodic paralysis. *Pflugers Archiv Eur J Physiol* 1991;418:297–299.
140. Li M, West JW, Lai Y, Scheuer T, Catterall WA. Functional modulation of brain sodium channels by cAMP-dependent phosphorylation. *Neuron* 1992;8:1151–1159.
141. Li M, West JW, Numann R, Murphy BJ, Scheuer T, Catterall WA. Convergent regulation of sodium channels by protein kinase C and cAMP-dependent protein kinase. *Science* 1993;261:1439–1442.
142. Liu YM, DeFelice LJ, Mazzanti M. Na channels that remain open throughout the cardiac action potential plateau. *Biophys J* 1992;63: 654–662.
143. Lombet A, Lazdunski M. Characterization, solubilization, affinity labeling and purification of the cardiac Na^+ channel using *Tityus* toxin gamma. *Eur J Biochem* 1984;141:651–660.
144. Lotan I, Dascal N, Naor Z, Boton R. Modulation of vertebrate brain Na^+ and K^+ channels by subtypes of protein kinase C. *FEBS Lett* 1990;267:25–28.
145. Loughney K, Kreber R, Ganetsky B. Molecular analysis of the *para* locus, a sodium channel gene in *Drosophila*. *Cell* 1989;58: 1143–1154.
146. Lu CM, Han J, Rado TA, Brown GB. Differential expression of two sodium channel subtypes in human brain. *FEBS Lett* 1992;303: 53–58.
147. Ma JY, Li M, Catterall WA, Scheuer T. Modulation of brain Na^+ channels by a G-protein-coupled pathway. *Proc Natl Acad Sci USA* 1994;91:12351–12355.
148. Mahadevan M, Tsilfidis C, Sabourin L, et al. Myotonic dystrophy mutation: an unstable CTG repeat in the 3′ untranslated region of the gene. *Science* 1992;255:1253–1255.
149. Makita N, Bennett PBJ, George ALJ. Voltage-gated Na^+ channel β_1 subunit mRNA expressed in adult human skeletal muscle, heart, and brain is encoded by a single gene. *J Biol Chem* 1994;269: 7571–7578.
150. Malo D, Schurr E, Dorfman J, Canfield V, Levenson R, Gros P. Three brain sodium channel α-subunit genes are clustered on the proximal segment of mouse chromosome 2. *Genomics* 1991;10: 666–672.
151. Malo MS, Srivastava K, Andresen JM, Chen X, Korenberg JR, Ingram VM. Targeted gene walking by low stringency polymerase chain reaction: assignment of a putative human brain sodium channel gene (SCN3A) to chromosome 2q24–31. *Proc Natl Acad Sci USA* 1994;91:2975–2979.
152. Mandel G. Tissue-specific expression of the voltage-sensitive sodium channel. *J Membr Biol* 1992;125:193–205.
153. Mandel G. Sodium channel regulation in the nervous system: how the action potential keeps in shape. *Curr Opin Neurobiol* 1993;3: 278–282.
154. Matsuda JJ, Lee H, Shibata EF. Enhancement of rabbit cardiac sodium channels by beta-adrenergic stimulation. *Circ Res* 1992;70: 199–207.
155. Matsuda JJ, Lee HC, Shibata EF. Acetylcholine reversal of isoproterenol-stimulated sodium currents in rabbit ventricular myocytes. *Circ Res* 1993;72:517–525.
156. Maue RA, Kraner SD, Goodman RH, Mandel G. Neuron-specific expression of the rat brain type II sodium channel gene is directed by upstream regulatory elements. *Neuron* 1990;4: 223–231.
157. McClatchey A, Van den Bergh P, Pericak-Vance M, et al. Temperature-sensitive mutations in the III-IV cytoplasmic loop region of the skeletal muscle sodium channel gene in paramyotonia congenita. *Cell* 1992;68:769–774.
158. McClatchey AI, McKenna-Yasek D, Cros D, et al. Novel mutations in families with unusual and variable disorders of the skeletal muscle sodium channel. *Nature Genet* 1992;2:148–152.
159. McDonald TV, Courtney KR, Clusin WT. Use-dependent block of single sodium channels by lidocaine in guinea pig ventricular myocytes. *Biophys J* 1989;55:1261–1266.
160. McPhee JC, Ragsdale DS, Scheuer T, Catterall WA. A mutation in segment IVS6 disrupts fast inactivation of sodium channels. *Proc Natl Acad Sci USA* 1994;91:12346–12350.
161. Mejia-Alvarez R, Marban E. Mechanism of the increase in intracellular sodium during metabolic inhibition: direct evidence against mediation by voltage-dependent sodium channels. *J Mol Cell Cardiol* 1992;24:1307–1320.
162. Miller JA, Agnew WS, Levinson SR. Principal glycopeptide of the

tetrodotoxin/saxitoxin binding protein from *Electrophorus electricus:* isolation and partial chemical and physical characterization. *Biochemistry* 1983;22:462–470.
163. Moorman JR, Kirsch GE, Brown AM, Joho RH. Changes in sodium channel gating produced by point mutations in a cytoplasmic linker. *Science* 1990;250:688–691.
164. Moorman JR, Kirsch GE, Lacerda AE, Brown AM. Angiotensin II modulates cardiac sodium channels in neonatal rat. *Circ Res* 1989; 65:1804
165. Moorman JR, Kirsch GE, VanDongen AMJ, Joho RH, Brown AM. Fast and slow gating of sodium channels encoded by a single mRNA. *Neuron* 1990;4:243–252.
166. Moorman JR, Yee R, Bjornsson T, Starmer CF, Grant AO, Strauss HC. pKa does not predict pH potentiation of sodium channel blockade by lidocaine and W6211 in guinea pig ventricular myocardium. *J Pharmacol Exp Ther* 1986;238:159–166.
167. Mounsey JP, Xu P, John JE, Horne LT, Gilbert J, Roses AD, Moorman JR. Modulation of skeletal muscle sodium channels by human myotonin protein kinase. *J Clin Invest* 1995;95:2379–2384.
168. Mozhayeva GN, Naumov AP, Neguoyaev YA. Evidence for existence of two acid groups controlling the conductance of sodium channel. *Biochim Biophys Acta* 1981;643:251–255.
169. Nettleton J, Wang GK. pH-dependent binding of local anesthetics in single batrachotoxin-activated Na$^+$ channels. *Biophys J* 1990;58: 95–106.
170. Nilius B. Modal gating behavior of cardiac sodium channels in cell-free membrane patches. *Biophys J* 1988;52:857–862.
171. Nilius B, Benndorf K, Markwardt F. Effects of lidocaine on single cardiac sodium channels. *J Mol Cell Cardiol* 1987;19:865–874.
172. Nilius B, Tytgat J, Albitz R. Modulation of cardiac Na channels by angiotensin II. *Biochim Biophys Acta* 1989;1014:259–262.
173. Noda M, Ikeda T, Kayano T, et al. Existence of distinct sodium channel messenger RNAs in rat brain. *Nature* 1986;320:188–192.
174. Noda M, Ikeda T, Suzuki H, Takeshima H, Takahashi T, Kuno M, Numa S. Expression of functional sodium channels from cloned cDNA. *Nature* 1986;322:826–828.
175. Noda M, Shimuzu S, Tanabe T, et al. Primary structure of *Electrophorus electricus* sodium channel deduced from cDNA sequence. *Nature* 1984;312:121–127.
176. Noda M, Suzuki H, Numa S, Stühmer W. A single point mutation confers tetrodotoxin and saxitoxin insensitivity on the sodium channel II. *FEBS Lett* 1989;259:213–216.
177. Numann R, Catterall WA, Scheuer T. Functional modulation of brain sodium channels by protein kinase C phosphorylation. *Science* 1991;254:115–118.
178. Ono K, Fozzard HA, Hanck DA. Mechanism of cAMP-dependent modulation of cardiac sodium channel current kinetics. *Circ Res* 1993;72:807–815.
179. Patlak JB, Ortiz M. Slow currents through single sodium channels of the adult rat heart. *J Gen Physiol* 1985;86:89–104.
180. Patlak JB, Ortiz M. Two modes of gating during late Na$^+$ channel currents in frog sartorius muscle. *J Gen Physiol* 1986;87:305–326.
181. Patton DE, Isom LL, Catterall WA, Goldin AL. The adult rat brain beta 1 subunit modifies activation and inactivation gating of multiple sodium channel alpha subunits. *J Biol Chem* 1994;269: 17649–17655.
182. Patton DE, West JW, Catterall WA, Goldin AL. Amino acid residues required for fast Na(+)-channel inactivation: charge neutralizations and deletions in the III-IV linker. *Proc Natl Acad Sci USA* 1992;89:10905–10909.
183. Potts JF, Regan MR, Rochelle JM, Seldin MF, Agnew WS. A glial-specific voltage-sensitive Na channel gene maps close to clustered genes for neuronal isoforms on mouse chromosome 2. *Biochem Biophys Res Commun* 1993;197:100–107.
184. Ptacek LJ, George AL, Barchi R, Griggs RC, Riggs JE, Robertson M, Leppert MF. Mutations in an S4 segment of the adult skeletal muscle sodium channel cause paramyotonia congenita. *Neuron* 1992;8:891–897.
185. Ptacek LJ, George AL, Griggs RC, et al. Identification of a mutation in the gene causing hyperkalemic periodic paralysis. *Cell* 1991;67:1021–1027.
186. Ptacek LJ, Guow L, Kwiecinski H, et al. Sodium channel mutations in paramyotonia congenita and hyperkalemic periodic paralysis. *Ann Neurol* 1993;33:300–307.
187. Ptacek LJ, Tawil R, Griggs RC, Storvick D, Leppert M. Linkage of atypical myotonia congenita to a sodium channel locus. *Neurology* 1992;42:431–433.
188. Pusch M, Noda M, Stühmer W, Numa S, Conti F. Single point mutations of the sodium channel drastically reduce the pore permeability without preventing its gating. *Eur Biophys J* 1991;20: 127–133.
189. Ragsdale DS, McPhee JC, Scheuer T, Catterall WA. Molecular determinants of state-dependent block of Na$^+$ channels by local anesthetics. *Science* 1994;265:1724–1728.
190. Ramaswami M, Tanouye MA. Two sodium channel genes in *Drosophila:* implications for channel diversity. *Proc Natl Acad Sci USA* 1989;86:2079–2082.
191. Rando TA, Strichartz GR. Saxitoxin blocks batrachotoxin-modified sodium channels in the node of Ranvier in a voltage-dependent manner. *Biophys J* 1986;49:785–794.
192. Ravindran A, Schild L, Moczydlowski E. Divalent cation selectivity for external block of voltage-dependent Na$^+$ channels prolonged by batrachotoxin. Zn2+ induces discrete substates in cardiac Na$^+$ channels. *J Gen Physiol* 1991;97:89–115.
193. Rehberg B, Duch DS, Urban BW. The voltage-dependent action of pentobarbital on batrachotoxin-modified human brain sodium channels. *Biochim Biophys Acta* 1994;1194:215–222.
194. Rehberg B, Urban BW, Duch DS. The membrane lipid cholesterol modulates anesthetic actions on a human brain ion channel. *Anesthesiology* 1995;82:749–758.
195. Rogart RB, Cribbs LL, Muglia LK, Kephart DD, Kaiser MW. Molecular cloning of a putative tetrodotoxin-resistant rat heart Na$^+$ channel isoform. *Proc Natl Acad Sci USA* 1989;86:8170–8174.
196. Rojas CV, Wang J, Schwartz LS, Hoffman E, Powell B, Brown RA. Met to Val mutation in the skeletal muscle Na$^+$ channel α-subunit in hyperkalemic periodic paralysis. *Nature* 1991;354: 387–389.
197. Rosenberg RL, Tomiko SA, Agnew WS. Single-channel properties of the reconstituted voltage-regulated Na channel isolated from the electroplax of *Electrophorus electricus. Proc Natl Acad Sci USA* 1984;81:5594–5598.
198. Rosenberg RL, Tomiko SA, Agnew WS. Reconstitution of neurotoxin-modulated ion transport by the voltage-regulated sodium channel isolated from the electroplax of *Electrophorus electricus. Proc Natl Acad Sci USA* 1984;81:1239–1243.
199. Rosenthal JJ, Gilly WF. Amino acid sequence of a putative sodium channel expressed in the giant axon of the squid *Loligo opalescens. Proc Natl Acad Sci USA* 1993;90:10026–10030.
200. Rossie S, Catterall WA. Phosphorylation of the a subunit of rat brain sodium channels by cAMP-dependent protein kinase at a new site containing Ser^{686} and Ser^{687}. *J Biol Chem* 1989;264: 14220–14224.
201. Rossie S, Gordon D, Catterall WA. Identification of an intracellular domain of the sodium channel having multiple cAMP-dependent phosphorylation sites. *J Biol Chem* 1987;262:17530–17535.
202. Salkoff L, Butler A, Wei A, et al. Genomic organization and deduced amino acid sequence of a putative sodium channel gene in *Drosophila. Science* 1987;237:744–749.
203. Sarao R, Gupta SK, Auld VJ, Dunn RJ. Developmentally regulated alternative RNA splicing of rat brain sodium channel mRNAs. *Nucleic Acids Res* 1991;19:5673–5679.
204. Satin J, Kyle JW, Chen M, Bell P, Cribbs LL, Fozzard HA, Rogart RB. A mutant of TTX-resistant cardiac sodium channels with TTX-sensitive properties. *Science* 1992;256:1202–1205.
205. Satin J, Kyle JW, Chen M, Rogart RB, Fozzard HA. The cloned cardiac Na channel α-subunit expressed in *Xenopus* oocytes show gating and blocking properties of native channels. *J Membr Biol* 1992;130:11–22.
206. Sato C, Matsumoto G. Primary structure of squid sodium channel deduced from the complementary DNA sequence. *Biochem Biophys Res Commun* 1992;186:61–68.
207. Schaller KL, Krzemien DM, McKenna NM, Caldwell JH. Alternatively spliced sodium channel transcripts in brain and muscle. *J Neurosci* 1992;12:1370–1381.
208. Schild L, Ravindran A, Moczydlowski E. Zn2(+)-induced subconductance events in cardiac Na$^+$ channels prolonged by batrachotoxin. Current-voltage behavior and single-channel kinetics. *J Gen Physiol* 1991;97:117–142.
209. Schneider MF, Dubois J. Effects of benzocaine on the kinetics of normal and batrachotoxin-modified Na channels in frog node of Ranvier. *Biophys J* 1986;50:523–530.
210. Schreibmayer W, Dascal N, Lotan I, Wallner M, Weigl L. Molecular mechanism of protein kinase C modulation of sodium channel alpha-subunits expressed in *Xenopus* oocytes. *FEBS Lett* 1991;291: 341–344.

211. Schubert B, VanDongen AMJ, Kirsch GE, Brown AM. β-adrenergic inhibition of cardiac sodium channels by dual G-protein pathways. *Science* 1989;245:516–519.
212. Schwarz W, Palade PT, Hille B. Local anesthetics: effect of pH on use-dependent block of sodium channels in frog muscle. *Biophys J* 1977;20:343–368.
213. Sheng ZH, Zhang H, Barchi RL, Kallen RG. Molecular cloning and functional analysis of the promoter of rat skeletal muscle voltage-sensitive sodium channel subtype 2 (rSkM2): evidence for muscle-specific nuclear protein binding to the core promoter. *DNA Cell Biol* 1994;13:9–23.
214. Smith RD, Goldin AL. Protein kinase A phosphorylation enhances sodium channel currents in *Xenopus* oocytes. *Am J Physiol* 1992;263:C660–C666.
215. Starmer CF, Courtney KR. Modeling ion channel blockade at guarded binding sites: application to tertiary drugs. *Am J Physiol* 1986;251:H848–H856.
216. Starmer CF, Grant AO. Phasic ion channel blockade. A kinetic model and parameter estimation procedure. *Mol Pharmacol* 1985; 28:348–356.
217. Starmer CF, Grant AO, Strauss HC. Mechanisms of use-dependent block of sodium channels in excitable membranes by local anesthetics. *Biophys J* 1984;46:15–27.
218. Starmer CF, Nesterenko VV, Undrovinas AI, Grant AO, Rosenshtraukh LV. Lidocaine blockade of continuously and transiently accessible sites in cardiac sodium channels. *J Mol Cell Cardiol* 1991; 23(suppl 1):73–83.
219. Stea A, Jackson A, Nurse CA. Hypoxia and N6,02′-dibutyryladenosine 3′,5′-cyclic monophosphate, but not nerve growth factor, induce Na^+ channels and hypertrophy in chromaffin-like arterial chemoreceptors. *Proc Natl Acad Sci USA* 1992;89: 9469–9473.
220. Strauss HC. Mechanisms of local anesthetic interaction with the sodium channel. In: Rosen MR, Janse MJ, Wit AL, eds. *Cardiac electrophysiology: a textbook.* Mount Kisco, NY: Futura 1990;995–1012.
221. Strichartz GR. The inhibition of sodium currents in myelinated nerve by quaternary derivatives of lidocaine. *J Gen Physiol* 1973;62: 37–57.
222. Stühmer W. Structure-function studies of voltage-gated ion channels. *Annu Rev Biophys Biophys Chem* 1991;20:65–78.
223. Stühmer W, Conti F, Suzuki H, et al. Structural parts involved in activation and inactivation of the sodium channel. *Nature* 1989; 339:597–603.
224. Talvenheimo JA, Tamkun MM, Catterall WA. Reconstitution of neurotoxin-stimulated sodium transport by the voltage-sensitive sodium channel purified from rat brain. *J Biol Chem* 1982;257: 11868–11871.
225. Tamkun MM, Talvenheimo JA, Catterall WA. The sodium channel from rat brain—reconstitution of neurotoxin-activated ion flux and scorpion toxin binding from purified components. *J Biol Chem* 1984;259:1676–2688.
226. Terlau H, Heinemman SH, Stühmer W, Pusch M, Conti F, Imoto K, Numa S. Mapping the site of block by tetrodotoxin and saxitoxin of sodium channel II. *FEBS Lett* 1991;293:93–96.
227. Tomaselli GF, Chiamvimonvat N, Nuss HB, et al. A mutation in the pore of the sodium channel alters gating. *Biophys J* 1995;68: 1814–1827.
228. Tomaselli GF, Feldman AM, Yellen G, Marban E. Human cardiac sodium channels expressed in *Xenopus* oocytes. *Am J Physiol* 1990; 258:H903–H906.
229. Tong J, Potts JF, Rochelle JM, Seldin MF, Agnew WS. A single β1 subunit mapped to mouse chromosome 7 may be a common component of Na channel isoforms from brain, skeletal muscle and heart. *Biochem Biophys Res Commun* 1993;195:679–685.
230. Trimmer JS, Agnew WS. Molecular diversity of voltage-sensitive Na channels. *Annu Rev Physiol* 1989;51:401–418.
231. Trimmer JS, Cooperman SS, Tomiko SA, et al. Primary structure and functional expression of a mammalian skeletal muscle sodium channel. *Neuron* 1989;3:33–49.
232. Ukomadu C, Zhou J, Sigworth FJ, Agnew WS. mI Na^+ channels expressed transiently in human embryonic kidney cells: biochemical and biophysical properties. *Neuron* 1992;8:663–676.
233. Vassilev PM, Scheuer T, Catterall WA. Identification of an intracellular peptide segment involved in sodium channel inactivation. *Science* 1988;241:1658–1661.
234. Vassilev PM, Scheuer T, Catterall WA. Inhibition of inactivation of single sodium channels by a site-directed antibody. *Proc Natl Acad Sci USA* 1989;86:8147–8151.
235. Wang GK. Binding affinity and stereoselectivity of local anesthetics in single batrachotoxin-activated Na^+ channels. *J Gen Physiol* 1990;96:1105–1127.
236. Wang GK, Simon R, Wang SY. Quaternary ammonium compounds as structural probes of single batrachotoxin-activated Na^+ channels. *J Gen Physiol* 1991;98:1005–1024.
237. Weiss RE, Horn R. Functional differences between two classes of sodium channels in developing rat skeletal muscle. *Science* 1986; 233:361–364.
238. Weiss RE, Sidell N. Sodium currents during differentiation in a human neuroblastoma cell line. *J Gen Physiol* 1991;97:521–539.
239. Wendt DJ, Starmer CF, Grant AO. Kinetics of interaction of the lidocaine metabolite glycylxylidide with the cardiac sodium channel. Additive blockade with lidocaine. *Circ Res* 1992;70:1254–1273.
240. Wendt DJ, Starmer CF, Grant AO. pH dependence of kinetics and steady-state block of cardiac sodium channels by lidocaine. *Am J Physiol* 1993;264:H1588–98.
241. West JW, Numann R, Murphey BJ, Scheuer T, Catterall WA. A phosphorylation site in the Na^+ channel required for modulation by protein kinase C. *Science* 1991;254:866–868.
242. West JW, Patton DE, Scheuer T, Wang Y, Goldin AL, Catterall WA. A cluster of hydrophobic amino acid residues required for fast Na(+)-channel inactivation. *Proc Natl Acad Sci USA* 1992;89: 10910–10914.
243. West JW, Scheuer T, Maechler L, Catterall WA. Efficient expression of rat brain type IIA Na^+ channel alpha subunits in a somatic cell line. *Neuron* 1992;8:59–70.
244. Westenbroek RE, Noebels JL, Catterall WA. Elevated expression of type II Na^+ channels in hypomyelinated axons of shiverer mouse brain. *J Neurosci* 1992;12:2259–2267.
245. Whalley DW, Wendt DJ, Starmer CF, Rudy Y, Grant AO. Voltage-independent effects of extracellular K^+ on the Na^+ current and phase 0 of the action potential in isolated cardiac myocytes. *Circ Res* 1994;75:491–502.
246. Woodhull AM. Ionic blockage of sodium channels in nerve. *J Gen Physiol* 1973;61:687–708.
247. Xu YQ, Pickoff AS, Clarkson CW. Developmental changes in the effects of lidocaine on sodium channels in rat cardiac myocytes. *J Pharmacol Exp Ther* 1992;262:670–676.
248. Yang J, Barchi R. Phosphorylation of the rat skeletal muscle sodium channel by cyclic AMP-dependent protein kinase. *J Neurochem* 1990;54:954–962.
249. Yang JS, Bennett PB, Makita N, George AL, Barchi RL. Expression of the sodium channel b_1 subunit in rat skeletal muscle is selectively associated with the tetrodotoxin-sensitive a subunit isoform. *Neuron* 1993;11:915–922.
250. Yang JS, Sladky JT, Kallen RG, Barchi RL. TTX-sensitive and TTX-insensitive sodium channel mRNA transcripts are independently regulated in adult skeletal muscle after denervation. *Neuron* 1991; 7:421–427.
251. Yatani A, Kirsch GE, Posani LD, Brown AM. Effects of new world scorpion toxins on single-channel and whole-cell cardiac sodium currents. *Am J Physiol* 1988;254:H443–H451.
252. Yue DT. Bridging the gap between anomalous sodium channel molecules and aberrant physiology. *Biophys J* 1993;65:13–14.
253. Zamponi GW, French RJ. Dissecting lidocaine action: diethylamide and phenol mimic separate modes of lidocaine block of sodium channels from heart and skeletal muscle. *Biophys J* 1993; 65:2335–2347.
254. Zhang JF, Robinson RB, Siegelbaum SA. Sympathetic neurons mediate developmental change in cardiac sodium channel gating through long-term neurotransmitter action. *Neuron* 1992;9:97–103.
255. Zhang JF, Siegelbaum SA. Effects of external protons on single cardiac sodium channels from guinea pig ventricular myocytes. *J Gen Physiol* 1991;98:1065–1083.
256. Numann R, Hauschka SD, Catterall WA, Scheuer T. Modulation of skeletal muscle sodium channels in a satellite cell line by protein kinase C. *J Neurosci* 1994;14:4226–4236.

Anesthesia: Biologic Foundations, edited by Tony L. Yaksh et al. Lippincott–Raven Publishers, Philadelphia © 1997.

CHAPTER 12

VOLTAGE-GATED CALCIUM CHANNELS

CARL LYNCH III

Increases in intracellular Ca^{2+} concentration ($[Ca^{2+}]_i$) serve to activate a variety of critical cellular processes that require a rapid response between the initiating signal and the consequent response, including muscle contraction, synaptic transmission, secretion, and membrane excitability. While the change in $[Ca^{2+}]_i$ is frequently augmented or amplified by release from intracellular Ca^{2+} stores, it is the voltage-gated Ca^{2+}-selective ion channels (VGCC) that are primarily responsible for regulating the alterations in $[Ca^{2+}]_i$ in many tissues. Furthermore, microdomains of Ca^{2+} exist within cells, and changes in $[Ca^{2+}]_i$ just inside the plasma membrane (87) may be of particular importance in providing graded local control of ion channel gating, fusion of neurotransmitter vesicles with the membrane, as well as gating of intracellular Ca^{2+} stores. Combined electrophysiologic and molecular biologic investigations have provided a detailed understanding of these VGCC and their regulation by membrane potentials, membrane proteins, and cellular second messengers.

THE Ca^{2+} CHANNEL SUBTYPES

Evidence for Ca^{2+} influx into cells via a pathway distinct from other ions was first evident in invertebrate tissue (97,127). While it was known that a wide variety of processes were mediated by entry of extracellular Ca^{2+} in vertebrates, e.g., secretion (80,81), it was in the myocardium that distinct ionic currents carried by Ca^{2+} were most clearly defined (301). The inhibition of these distinct Ca^{2+} currents by a variety of pharmacologic agents such as verapamil and nifedipine permitted definitive separation from the prominent inward, fast Na^+ current (103, 190), ultimately leading to the labeling of the responsible membrane proteins (400). At the same time, certain processes—most notably synaptic transmission—were shown to be unaltered by these early "calcium channel blockers," and researchers postulated the existence of multiple Ca channel subtypes. Subsequent studies defined Ca^{2+} entry into cells via different Ca^{2+} specific channels based on a number of criteria. First, distinct biophysical characteristics were identified; second, the discovery of toxins as well as additional drugs made possible the blockade of specific components of Ca^{2+} currents; finally, application of molecular biologic techniques permitted isolation of the various distinct proteins that constitute Ca channel subunits.

Biophysical Criteria for Separation

Delineation of the various Ca channels was initiated by the separation of the currents according to biophysical criteria. Such separation was employed because no specific toxins or agents were initially available to distinguish the Ca channel types. In the mid-1980s, a number of laboratories identified inward currents carried by divalent cations that had distinctive biophysical behavior (47,98,259,266). First, the channels differed in their *voltage threshold* for opening, that is, the degree of depolarization required to open the channel was a distinguishing trait. Second, the *single channel conductance* varied among the different Ca channels, that is, the number of ions passed per second, typically measured in picoSiemans (pS), which is 600 univalent ions/msec for a 100 mV potential driving force. Furthermore, the channels varied in their selectivity, with some channels passing certain ions faster than others. Third, the channels differed in their *kinetic properties,* the rate at which they opened and then inactivated in response to the transmembrane voltage. Such differences could be detected in both the whole cell currents (as the activation and inactivation rates) as well as the single channel recordings (open time duration and bursting). In general, these three characteristics dramatically affect the number of ions that enter or exit a cell when activated.

The presence of multiple Ca channels had been suggested by work in cultured neurons (102,246), but the existence of distinct Ca^{2+} currents in whole cells and through single channels was clarified in vertebrate sensory neurons (Fig. 1), where a "fast" inactivating current was seen with small depolarizations (to ~-40 mV) and a larger, kinetically slower current was evident with greater depolarizations (to +10 mV) (47,98). Single channel Ca^{2+} currents were initially described in cultured myocytes (52,304), and two forms of Ca^{2+} currents were subsequently examined in isolated cardiac myocytes (240,259). With modest (20 to 30 mV) depolarizations from more negative membrane potentials (-80 mV, typical of resting myocytes), there was a rapidly inactivating or transient (T-type) Ca^{2+} current similar to that observed in neurons. This current, which was activated at lower voltages (hence low-voltage-activated [LVA]), also exhibited a lower single channel conductance (~7–9 pS) than the currents activated at higher (more positive) voltages and showed equivalent ionic conductance for Ca^{2+} and Ba^{2+}.

The bulk of the Ca^{2+} current in myocytes was found to be carried by a channel with the following characteristics: (a) activation with depolarizations positive to -30 mV (hence the term high-voltage activated [HVA]); (b) single channel conductances of about 20 to 25 pS in 10 mM Ca^{2+}, 2.5 to 3 times greater than the T-type channel; and (c) repeated channel openings that persisted throughout a sustained depolarization (hence long-lasting, or L-type) (259). Ba^{2+} was transported even more rapidly than Ca^{2+}, as demonstrated by a higher single channel conductance and increased whole cell current with Ba^{2+} in place of Ca^{2+}. When Ba^{2+} is the charge-carrying ion in L-type VGCC, the channel shows modest inactivation; however, when Ca^{2+} is present, inactivation is more rapid and profound (86,141). Another prominent feature of L-type channels is their labile nature due to the rapid loss of activity in a cell-free environment (e.g., when a patch of membrane is pulled away from the cell for study) (52). Nevertheless, this L-type Ca channel has been the most widely studied Ca channel type for a variety of reasons. It is present in large amounts in heart and vascular smooth muscle (VSM), which has made it readily available for study in isolated myocytes and demonstrates its critical role in these tissues. It is also blocked with high specificity by a variety of drugs (the dihydropyridines, the phenylalkylamines, the benzothiazepines), which has permitted labeling and high-affinity binding studies.

In dorsal root ganglion (DRG) neurons from the rat, a second type of HVA Ca channel was detected that was activated with large depolarizations from very negative membrane potentials (-70 mV) and that was termed N-type (266). This channel

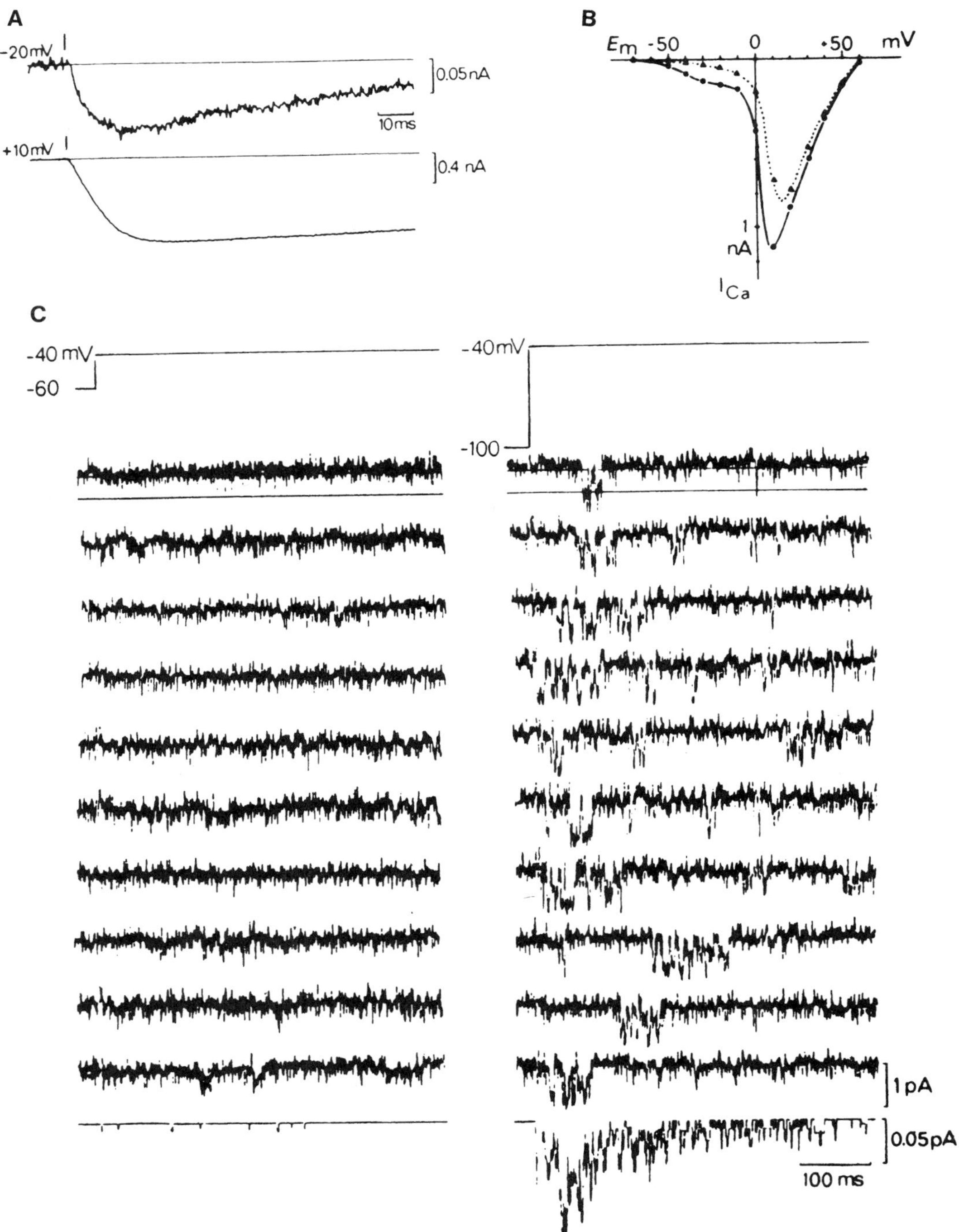

Figure 1. Activation of whole cell **(A)** and single channel Ca^{2+} currents **(C)** of chick dorsal root ganglion cells studied at 12°C in solution containing (in mM): 120 choline-Cl, 20 $CaCl_2$, 2 $MgCl_2$, 10 HEPES-CsOH (pH 7.2) plus 3 μM tetrodotoxin to block fully any inward Na^+ current. **A:** Appearance of an inactivating low-voltage-activated (LVA) Ca^{2+} current of the whole cell during a step to −20 mV from −90 mV membrane potential *(upper trace)*. Both turn-on and inactivation of this current are faster than those observed for the larger high-voltage-activated (HVA) current seen during a depolarizing step to +10 mV (lower trace), also from −90 mV. **B:** Peak current–voltage relationship of whole cell inward currents for depolarizations from −90 mV *(continuous line)*; the "shoulder" of current at −50 to −10 mV represents the peak LVA current, such as the upper trace in A. With depolarizations from −60 mV, the LVA current is largely inactivated and the current–voltage relation *(dotted line)* defines peak HVA currents. **C:** Single channel Ca^{2+} currents from an outside-out patch appear *(right)* during successive depolarizing steps to −40 mV from a holding potential of −100 mV from an initial −60 mV *(left)*. Lines in the upper current traces give the detection level for computing openings with the level (3.5 times background r.m.s. determined from event-free intervals). A second level near baseline at a similar distance from the average amplitude served to define closures. Sample averages of computed events are given in the *bottom traces*. Each sample contained 21 recordings. Recordings with the inactivated channel *(left)* are shown for comparison. The pipette solution contained (in mM): 100 CsCl, 16 tetraethylammonium-Cl, 1.6 $MgCl_2$, 0.2 $CaCl_2$, 5 EGTA, 7 glucose, 10 HEPES-NaOH at pH 7.2. (From ref. 47, with permission.)

proved resistant to the classic L-type Ca channel blockers, showed substantial inactivation (which was initially suggested to be a distinguishing feature from L-type channels), and exhibited an intermediate unitary channel conductance (14 to 16 pS) between that of L- and T-type channels (107). Figure 2 shows the initial description of the three distinct single channel currents through T-, L-, and N-type channels in DRG cells (266). It has subsequently become clear from studies of mammalian sympathetic neurons, which have predominantly N-type channels, that these channels do not fully inactivate and can have a large persistent current depending on various modulatory influences (287). An additional distinction was the ability of hyperpolarization to increase a component of inactivating N-type channel current, a feature not seen with L-type VGCC (287).

In the large and prominent Purkinje neuron of the cerebellum, a noninactivating current was observed that was not blocked by the classic L-type Ca channel blockers, yet its behavior was clearly distinct from the N-type channel (213). This channel was termed the P-type, and its definition in part rested on its specific blockade by certain spider toxins, which were found to have little effect on the previously defined T-, N-, and L-type channels.

Drug and Toxin Sensitivities

Biochemical isolation of the first VGCC (L-type) was possible because of its affinity for and modulation (inhibition or activation) by the dihydropyridine (DHP) class of synthetic "Ca channel blockers" (nifedipine, nicardipine, nitrendipine, etc.) (390,400). A variety of other synthetic drug classes have been described that also depressed the VGCC of the cardiovascular system (103,297,390) (see below), and refinement of drug properties within these various classes remains an important thrust of the pharmaceutical industry.

Since the presence of prominent DHP-resistant, HVA Ca^{2+} currents suggested the existence of additional types of Ca channels (299), numerous naturally occurring substances have been and are being evaluated and exploited to characterize other VGCC. An array of peptide toxins was discovered and isolated from various species of the Pacific cone snail *Conus*, which employ their poisons to paralyze and capture fish (270). A peripheral neural toxin derived from *C. geographus*, denoted ω-conotoxin-GVIA (Ctx-GVIA) was found to irreversibly block the N-type channel (5,228,287). In addition, a toxin isolated from *C. magus*, ω-Ctx-MVIIC (270,271), was found to block another component of HVA Ca current insensitive to both DHPs and ω-Ctx-GVIA; this additional HVA current is prominent in cerebellar granule cells and has been termed Q-type (298). Prior to the isolation of ω-Ctx-MVIIC, another group of extremely potent toxins was isolated from the venom of the funnel web spider. Both a relatively low-molecular-weight (200 to 400 kd) acylpolyamine molecule (213) and a 48 amino acid peptide synthesized by the spider (239) have proved to have a high affinity for the P-type VGCC associated with Purkinje cells. A drawback of these toxins is that their specificity is sometimes imperfect. For example, certain drugs and toxins such as Aga-IIIA react with more that one channel type (238).

Nevertheless, the discovery of these naturally occurring toxins in addition to the synthetic Ca channel blocking drugs provided the biochemical tools to more clearly define specific channels types, which in turn correspond to specific membrane proteins that are products of distinct genes. Included in Table 1 are the classes of VGCC now recognized based on their biophysical and pharmacologic behavior. Isolation and cloning of the genetic material that encodes various Ca channels has provided a molecular biologic basis for separation of the various channels.

Molecular Biologic Isolation of Ca Channel Types

In addition to the myocardial Ca^{2+} currents, DHP-sensitive Ca^{2+} currents were also identified in skeletal muscle cells. While

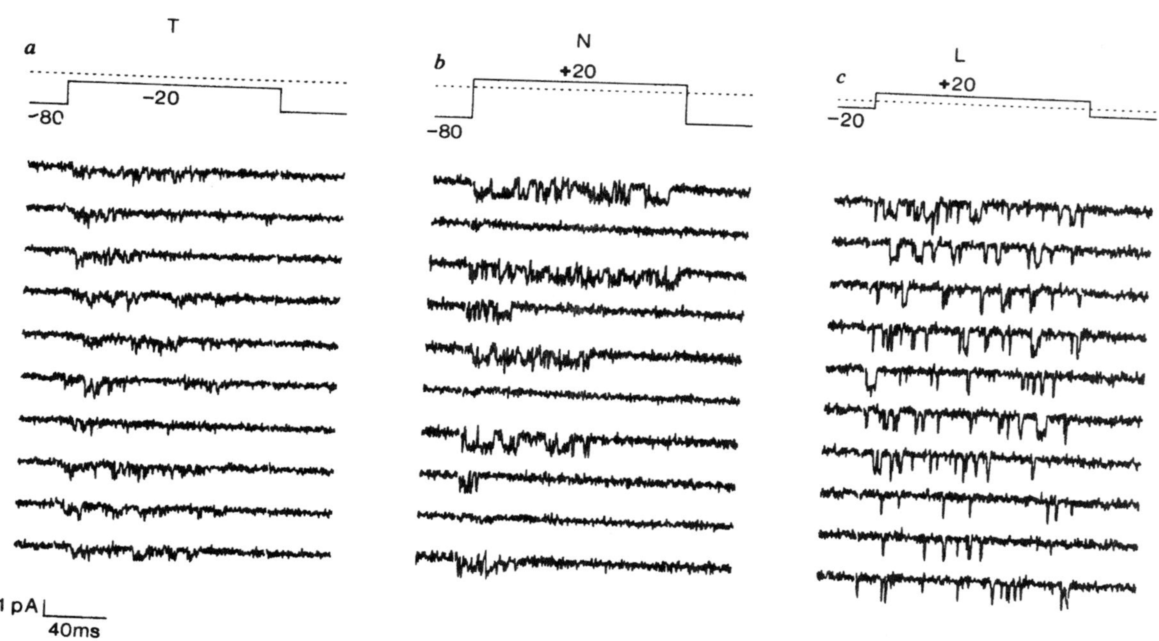

Figure 2. Three types of unitary Ca channel activity seen in cell-attached patch recordings with 110 mM Ba^{2+} as the charge carrier in cultured chick dorsal root ganglion cells. **a:** Transient or T-type single channel currents with low-voltage activation (LVA). **b:** Neither T- nor L-type, hence N-type unitary channel currents. **c:** Large, long-lasting or L-type unitary channel currents. Within each panel traces are consecutive. Current signals were filtered at 1 kHz and sampled at 5 kHz. Each of the three channel types may occur in isolation and in all possible combinations, while the number of channels under the patch pipette varied considerably from one to many. (From ref. 266, with permission.)

Table 1. MAJOR CLASSES OF Ca CHANNELS

Functional class	Sites of expression	Drug/toxin sensitivity (μm)	Single channel conductance (pS)[a]	Inactivation kinetics	α_1 Subunit consensus name
L-type (HVA)	Skeletal muscle, BC3H1 cells	0.01–0.10 Dihydropyridine, (insensitive to < μM ω-Ctx-GVIA, ω-Aga-IVA, FTX)	25–30	Ca dependent and voltage dependent	α_{1S}
	Heart				$\alpha_{1C\text{-a}}$
	Smooth muscle, lung				$\alpha_{1C\text{-b}}$
	Brain				$\alpha_{1C\text{-c}}$
	Brain, pancreas, HIT cells, GH3 cells, PC 12 cells				α_{1D}
N-type (HVA)	Brain, peripheral neurons, PC12 cells	0.1–0.5 ω-Ctx-GVIA >0.10 ω-Ctx-MVIIC	14	Moderate (requires β1 subunit)	α_{1B}
Q-type (HVA)	Brain, kidney, cerebellar granule cells	0.15 ω-Ctx-MVIIC 0.2 ω-Aga-IVA	20	Moderate	α_{1A}
P-type (HVA)	Neuronal (esp. cerebellar Purkinje cells), mammalian neuromuscular junction	0.002 ω-Aga-IVA, ? FTX, >1 ω-Ctx-MVIIC	15	Modest	α_{1A}
R-type (HVA)	Brain	Resistant to most toxins? ω-Aga-IA	14?	Rapid	α_{1E}
T-type (LVA)	Many tissues, modest amount	100 ω-Aga-IVA, 100 ω-Aga-IA	7–9	Very rapid	?

[a]Conductance estimates are based on high $[Ba^{2+}]$ (≥ 100 mM) rather than physiologic $[Ca^{2+}]$.

these Ca^{2+} currents activated very slowly and did not appear to contribute to excitation-contraction (EC) coupling in skeletal muscle (312,330), the transverse tubules of skeletal muscle, which invaginate into each muscle fiber and carry the depolarization into the interior of the fiber, were found to be a rich source of the skeletal muscle Ca channels that bind DHPs (hence the term *DHP receptors*). From the initial biochemical isolation and partial characterization of isolated Ca channels from skeletal muscle, skeletal muscle VGCC were found to be composed of a number of distinct subunits that were ultimately separated and defined as α_1, α_2, β, δ, and γ (50,104,373,374, 398). Employing its high affinity for DHPs, the 165-kd α_1 polypeptide was isolated and purified, making possible the enzymatic preparation of protein fragments and determination of their amino acid sequence. Sequences of the DNA encoding each segment were then prepared and ultimately used to isolate the cellular mRNA, which encoded the full 1873 amino acid sequence of the skeletal muscle DHP receptor (382). The amino acid sequence of the DHP receptor revealed a pattern of hydrophobic and basic amino acids that was very similar (55% amino acid sequence homology) to that previously defined for the α subunit of the Na channel (262).

α_1 Subunit

The proposed and now generally accepted structure for the major pore-forming subunit (α_1) of all VGCC is one in which there are four major domains (I to IV) surrounding a central pore. Each domain (or motif) is formed from six hydrophobic transmembrane α-helical segments, designated S1 to S6 (Fig. 3) (51,278,382). This four hexahelical domain structure was initially surmised for the Na channel, with which the L-type VGCC shares such striking homology (262). The similarity in structure may explain, in part, the fact that a number of drugs show only partial specificity. For example, both the phenylalkylamines and the DHPs can block Na channels as well as Ca channels, although at higher concentrations (15,114,429), while phenytoin and local anesthetics can block Ca as well as Na channels (321,322). Two prominent features of the α_1 subunit are shared with the Na channel. One is the presence of multiple positively charged residues in the fourth α-helix (S4) of each domain, a feature also seen in K channels. This region is thought to be the "voltage sensor" that responds to changes in membrane potential and is responsible for the conformational change within the protein that opens the pore permitting ions to flow. The second feature is a larger span of amino acids on the extracellular face of the channel between the fifth and sixth helix of each of the four domains (P-loop). These four P-loops are thought to fold back into the pore, forming binding sites for the ions passing through the channel and contributing to ion selectivity.

Following the initial isolation of the skeletal muscle α_1 subunit (α_{1S}, also termed CaCh1 and CACN1), comparable subunits were cloned based on the assumption that the primary amino acid sequence would be similar (Table 2) Based on sequence homologies, two additional closely related DHP-binding L-type Ca channels clones were isolated, each possessing 60% to 70% amino acid sequence identity with the α_{1S} subunit (233,280). The region of greatest identity (>90%) is in the postulated hydrophobic, α-helical transmembrane spanning region. The messenger RNA (mRNA) encoding these α_1 subunits predicts a size ~15% larger than the α_{1S} subunit, but shows some variation in structure due to the presence of splice variants generated during mRNA transcription. One L-type channel clone subtype was isolated from cardiac, smooth muscle, and brain tissue (now termed α_{1C}) and encoded a protein of 2200 (25,189,233,280,329,345,346). The other L-type clone was most prominent in endocrine (pancreatic) tissue (α_{1D}) and was of similar size (59,280,334), although a form with an abbreviated carboxy terminus has been described (159).

Based on cDNA isolated from rat brain, subunits for five distinct VGCC were discovered and initially designated rbA, rbB, rbC, rbD, rbE (343). Whereas rbC and rbD have been identified as subunits associated with L-type (DHP-sensitive) VGCC, three additional α_1 subunits show less homology and are more distantly related to the α_{1S} subunit, showing only 30% to 40% sequence identity with L-type α_1 subunits. The first of the neuronal α_1 subunits studied in detail (designated as B-I, now α_{1A}) was found to be somewhat larger than the L-type α_1 subunits, with different open reading frames resulting from splice variants encoding proteins of 2212 to 2424 amino acids (247,356).

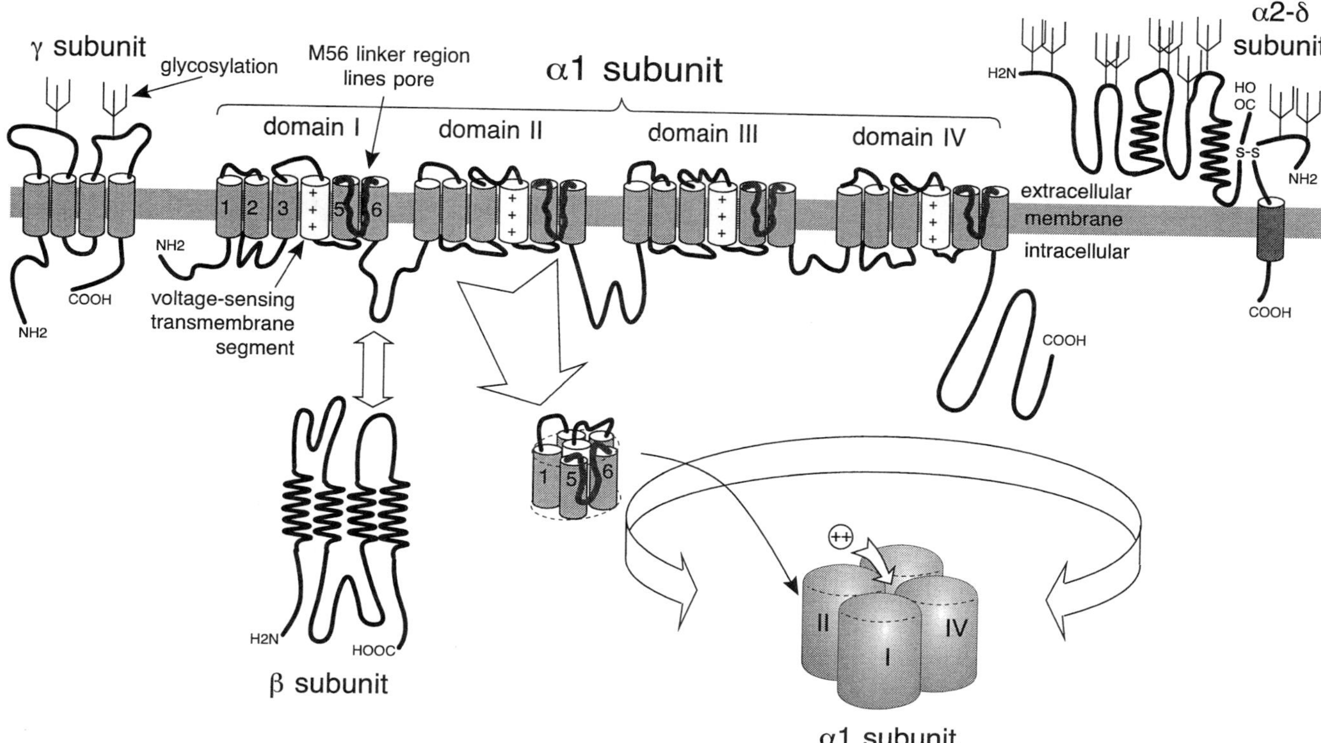

Figure 3. Structural model of the L-type Ca channel based on amino acid sequence analysis. The α_1 subunit is composed of 2171 amino acids in which 24 hydrophobic regions are hypothesized to form α helical transmembrane segments (as indicated by the small cylinders) (233). As shown for domain II, the six transmembrane segments (S1–S6) coalesce to form four domains (I–IV). The four domains gather as indicated to form a tetrameric structure with a central pore through which the ions pass. The pore itself appears to be lined by the extracellular-linking segment between helix spans 5 and 6, which is thought to fold back into the pore so that the polar or negatively charged sites become available for binding by ions as they pass through the channel. The fourth transmembrane segment (S4) of each domain contains a number of positively charged amino acids (typically arginine) that can respond to the membrane voltage field, acting as a "voltage sensor" and inducing a conformational change that will permit ions to flow through the central pore (261). Also shown in the figure are the other subunits that occur with the α_1 subunit. The β subunit, which appears to adjoin an intracellular aspect of the α_1 subunit appears to enhance channel opening and activation. The α_2-δ subunit also appears to modulate channel voltage responses, while the role of the γ subunit is unclear. (Adapted from various sources including refs. 51 and 170.)

When expressed in *Xenopus* oocytes, the α_{1A} subunit from rabbit acted as a divalent ion channel and proved to be insensitive to both dihydropyridines and ω-Ctx. While it showed marked inactivation uncharacteristic of the P-type channel, it demonstrated some sensitivity to the spider venoms (247). The similar subunit clone isolated from rat brain (rbA), like the rabbit B-I subunit, showed a high density of expression in the cerebellum expected for P-type channels (356). The two other neuronal α_1 subunits were subsequently described in greater detail. The rbB clone (now α_{1B}) splice variants encoded a protein of 2237-2339 amino acids, which when expressed was found to be sensitive to ω-Ctx and thus appeared to be the genetic material responsible for the N-type α_1 subunit (63,85, 109,417). The third neuronal α_1 subunit clone, initially designated B-II (rabbit) or rbE (rat), and subsequently termed α_{1E}, encodes a protein of 2178 to 2259 amino acids, depending on transcriptional splicing (258,349,419). When expressed, this α_1 subunit lacks DHP sensitivity and corresponds to neuronal channels that are insensitive to the other specific toxins and drugs (258,349,419).

Certain features are common for all six α_1 subunit clones (Fig. 4). First, splice variants exist for most of these Ca^{2+} pore subunits; that is, insertions of different series of amino acids occur at various points in the sequence. In addition to the splice variants, there may also be deletion of certain amino acid segments when these channels are expressed in different tissues. Second, tissue-specific expression of the splice variants of the α_{1C} channel seems to occur; the $\alpha_{1C\text{-}a}$ subtype is expressed primarily in heart, the $\alpha_{1C\text{-}b}$ is prominent in the vasculature, and the $\alpha_{1C\text{-}c}$ is most evident in neurons (279). Although some splice variant-tissue correlation exists, it is by no means exclusive. The neuronal α_1 subunits also show splice variants; however, the functional significance and tissue distribution has not been well clarified. A noteworthy feature distinguishing the predominantly neuronal α_{1A}, α_{1B}, and α_{1E} subunits from the DHP-binding channels is the far longer (by approximately 300 amino acids) cytoplasmic-linking segment present between domains II and III. Considering the important role played by the neuronal VGCC in vesicular release of neurotransmitters, this region may be likewise important in those processes (see below). All of the α_1 subunits also have multiple amino acid residues (serines, threonines) on the cytoplasmic regions that can be phosphorylated by the various protein kinases (adenosine 3',5'-cyclic monophosphate [cAMP]-dependent, guanosine 3',5'-cyclic monophosphate [cGMP]-dependent, and protein kinase C). Phosphorylation of these sites, and possibly sites on the β subunit, appears to be critical in modulating channel gating.

Table 2. CLONED SUBUNITS OF MAMMALIAN VOLTAGE-GATED Ca CHANNELS (26,279,399)

Subunit	Consensus	Cloned gene product —other names	Chromosome (human)	Splice variants	Primary tissue
α_1 (channel subunit)	α_{1S}	CaCh1, α_{1skm}, CACN1	1q32	1 (2[a])	Skeletal muscle
	$\alpha_{1C\text{-}a}$	CaCh2a, CaCh2-II			Heart
	$\alpha_{1C\text{-}b}$	CaCh2b, CaCh2-II, CACN2	12p13.3	3 (a,b,c)	Vascular, fibroblast, lung
	$\alpha_{1C\text{-}c}$	rbC, CaCh2-III			Neuronal
	α_{1D}	rbD, CaCh3, CACN4	3p14.3	4	Endocrine, neuronal
	α_{1A}	BI, CaCh4, rbA, CACN3	ND	4	Neuronal
	α_{1B}	BIII, rbB, CaCh5	ND	2	Neuronal
	α_{1E}	BII, CaCh6, rbE	ND		Neuronal
α_2-δ (extracellular)			7q21-22	5 (a–e)	
β (intracellular)	β_{1a}	β_{1M}			Skeletal muscle
	β_{1b}	β_{1B2}, β_2	17q21-22	4 (a–d)	Brain, heart
	β_{1c}	β_{1B1}			Brain, heart
	β_2	β_3	ND	4 (a–d)	
	β_3		12q13	2 (a,b)	Brain, heart, aorta
	β_4		ND	2 (a,b)	Brain
γ			17q24	1	Skeletal muscle only

[a]Posttranslational variants.
ND, not determined.

Whereas the rbE α_1 subunit (α_{1E}) was initially thought to be an LVA channel, possibly the T-type (349), that is no longer considered likely. A clone has yet to be expressed that convincingly shows the characteristics of the rapidly inactivating T-type channel.

α_2-δ Subunit

Subsequent cloning of the α_2 subunit indicated that the α_2 and the δ subunits were actually a single-gene product linked by a cysteine residue (418). The α_2 subunit proved to be a large (170 kd), highly glycosylated protein that bound with high affinity to wheat germ gluten affinity columns. In fact, it was binding of this protein with the still attached α_1 subunit that initially permitted isolation of the DHP receptor (279). Subsequent microsequencing permitted isolation of the full-length rabbit skeletal muscle α_2 cDNA, which proved to encode a protein of 1106 amino acids (91). Purification and sequencing of the δ peptide(s) showed that it was included in the DNA sequence for the isolated α_2 subunit (66). The α_2-δ subunit is synthesized as a propeptide that is cleaved near the carboxyl terminus between the two alanine residues at positions 934 and 935 after formation of a covalent disulfide linkage between cysteine residues of the α_2 and δ fragments (66). Although the α_2 subunit was initially hypothesized to contain transmembrane regions, it has been shown that the α_2 subunit is located entirely outside the cell (37,170) and is anchored in the membrane only by the δ subunit, which has a single transmembrane domain. In many ways the α_2-δ subunit, with its highly glycosylated extracellular domain, is similar to the β subunit of the Na channel. The prominence and glycosylation of the α_2 extracellularly (Fig. 3) may account for the apparent ability of the α_2 subunit to elicit autoimmunologic responses under some circumstances (248).

Functionally, α_2-δ appears to enhance the expression of α_1, especially in the presence of other accessory subunits such as β (see below). This has suggested to some investigators that the α_2-δ may play a role in determining the spatial distribution of Ca^+ channels. Two isoforms of the α_2-δ appear to be present, depending on the insertion or deletion of a particular exon (418). Subunits associated with the α_1 subunits are indicated schematically in Fig. 3. Coexpression of the α_2-δ subunit with an α_1 subunit may augment the currents observed (233,341); however, the effect is not so great as that observed with β subunits (see below).

β Subunit

Following its biochemical isolation as a Ca channel subunit of approximately 55 kd, the β subunit was subsequently fragmented, and oligonucleotide primers were generated that permitted determination of the underlying genetic code and amino acid sequence. The first of the four β subunits described proved to be composed of 524 amino acids, with a structure suggesting at least four major α-helical domains (310). These helical domains are not highly hydrophobic and, unlike the α_1 subunit, do not appear to represent transmembrane domains. This is consistent with the biochemical evidence suggesting that the β subunit is not membrane bound. Multiple splice variants of the subunits have been defined (277,292). The failure to observe the initially described β subunit in all tissues suggested that other isoforms existed, which was subsequently demonstrated by other workers (48,277,292,294). Of the four β subunit genes, the β_1 and β_2 appear to be expressed in at least four different splice variants, which appear to be somewhat tissue specific in their distribution (279,292) (Table 2).

The β subunits have multiple sites for phosphorylation by protein kinases, although how such phosphorylation modifies gating behavior of the channel complex is not well understood. The β subunits appear to have considerable role in modulating the behavior of the α_1 subunit gating. It was noted in the initial expression studies that the coexpression of the β subunit with the α_1 subunit resulted in a marked increase in the amount of current seen in oocytes or other cells compared with expression of the α_1 subunits (247,409). The presence of the β_3 subunit, for example, markedly increased the currents observed with α_{1C} (cardiac L-type) VGCC (48). In addition, there was a shift in the activation voltage to higher potentials, as well as an increased rate of activation and an enhanced degree of inactivation (48). The β subunit appears to enhance coupling between the voltage-dependent conformational change in the α_1 subunit and the rate of ion flux (260). Expression experiments in oocytes show that while the gating charge movement of the VGCC, which reflects the conformational change in the α_1 subunit, is the same in the presence of an expressed β subunit, the amount of current increases by over fourfold (255). Furthermore, the presence of the β subunit with α_{1C} subunits also mediates greater voltage-dependent facilitation of the channel; that is, prior depolarization causes a greater enhancement of the channel when the β_1 subunit (35).

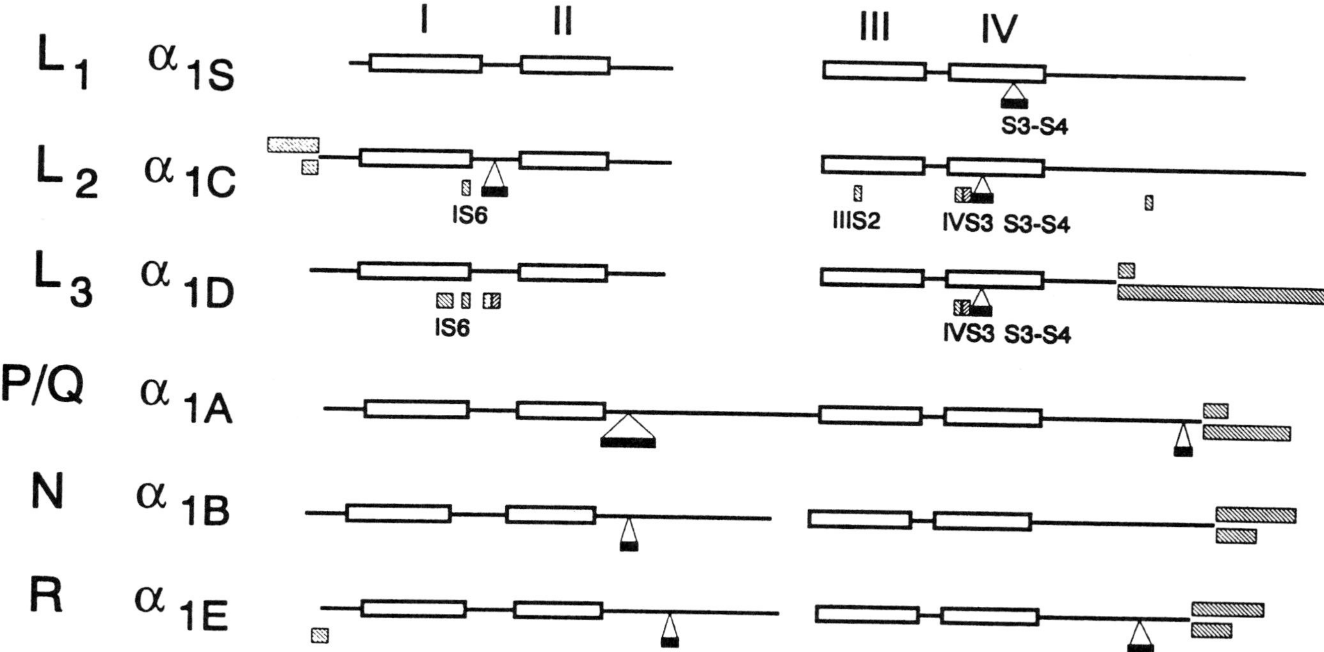

Figure 4. Gene structure of Ca channel α_1 subunits that are approximately 7,000 to 8,000 base pairs in length. L_1, L_2, L_3, P/Q, N, and R represent the channel designations for the indicated α_1 subunit genes. The regions encoding the four motifs (I–IV), each composed of six transmembrane segments, are indicated by the *open boxes.* Alternative splicing of exons is indicated by the *hatched boxes,* while insertions/deletions of >10 amino acids are indicated by the *thick line.* (From ref. 279, with permission.)

Enhancement of current by β subunits has also been noted for the α_{1A} subunit and can be mediated by the β_{1B}, β_{2A}, β_3, and β_4 subunits, with the β_{1B} and the β_4 subunits having the most profound effect (68). Likewise, enhancement of the α_{1B} subunit has also been observed by coexpression with the β_{1B} subunit (357). The α_2 subunit by itself has no effect; however, when expressed with the β_{1B}, α_2 appears to cause additional enhancement of current. For the α_{1A} and α_{1B} subunits, coexpression of the β_3 subunits abolishes the ability of G proteins to inhibit currents through these two channels (307).

The sites of interaction between the β and α_1 subunits have been well defined by Campbell's group (293). The β_1 subunit appears to bind to a site on the cytoplasmic linker between domains I and II of the α_{1S}, $\alpha_{1C\text{-}a}$, and the α_{1A} subunits. Sequence analysis identified a conserved motif of amino acids (Gln-Gln-X-Glu-X-X-Leu-X-Gly-Tyr-X-X-Trp-Ile-X-X-X-Glu) that is located 24 amino acids from the S6 transmembrane helix of domain 1. The complementary region of the β subunit appears to be a region in the central portion of the subunit straddled by two domains containing α-helices. Modification of the β_{1B} subunit by point mutations in this region resulted in the abolition of binding to the α_{1A} subunit and the loss of enhancement of currents when the α_1 subunits are expressed in oocytes (68). The K_D for the region of the α_1 subunit for the β subunit is approximately 5 nM, with the β_4 and β_{2A} subunits showing even greater affinity, and the β_3 subunit showing less affinity. Phosphorylation sites for protein kinase C are also located in the binding region of the β subunit.

γ Subunit

The γ subunit was first isolated biochemically as a 32-kd subunit of the skeletal muscle DHP receptor. The subunit clone was found to encode a 222 amino acid protein with four hydrophobic α-helical domains, which are thought to span the membrane (169). Analysis of various tissues for mRNA demonstrated that this subunit is expressed exclusively in skeletal muscle. The role the γ subunit plays in regulating the DHP receptors in skeletal muscle is unclear; however, it does not enhance the current of coexpressed α_{1S} subunits (409). It may play a particular role in excitation-contraction coupling.

In summary, the following general observations regarding the VGCC may be made: (a) The α_1 subunit is an ~2000 amino acid protein that forms the voltage-gated pore region of the VGCC. (b) The function of the α_1 subunit is modulated by the other subunits. (c) Splice variants of the α_1 subunit create VGCC subtypes ($\alpha_{1C\text{-}a}$, $\alpha_{1C\text{-}b}$, $\alpha_{1C\text{-}c}$), which may impart differing pharmacologic and physiologic characteristics of the channel.

L-TYPE Ca CHANNELS

In part because of its distinctive binding of DHPs, its plentiful expression in skeletal muscle and cardiac myocytes, and its importance in cardiovascular function, the L-type Ca channel has been the most widely studied Ca channel. In skeletal muscle, in which it acts as the voltage-sensor controlling Ca^{2+} release, this distinctive Ca channel was the first to be isolated and to have its subunits cloned and its amino acid sequence defined. Electrophysiologic methods, especially in combination with molecular biologic manipulation of the structure, have permitted determination of the sites and mechanisms of ion permeation, Ca^{2+} release channel activation, and drug binding. The L-type channels have served as models both for the biophysical mechanism of ion passage through the channel as well as for characterization of its gating and modulation, providing a useful standard for comparison with the other VGCC.

While a variety of drugs and physiologic regulators affect VGCC behavior, a primary determinant of channel behavior is Ca^{2+} itself, which modulates and directs channel function at several levels. The concentration of extracellular Ca^{2+} ($[Ca^{2+}]_o$) dramatically influences the rate of ion passage channel because Ca^{2+} binds within the pore. Intracellular Ca^{2+} ($[Ca^{2+}]_i$) markedly accelerates inactivation of L-type channels, and by binding to various regulatory enzymes inside the cell Ca^{2+} may modulate channel function.

Ion Permeation

Since no carrier molecule model could explain the high ionic conductances observed, a pore-like structure was surmised for ion channels even prior to the definition of their structure and the description of single channel currents. Nevertheless, an ion channel may still be viewed as an enzyme that facilitates the transport of ions through the hydrophobic barrier created by the membrane bilayer. The actual transit of the ion through the pore is a complicated biochemical process in which ions transiently bind to sites in the ion channel as they pass from one side of the membrane to the other. The acidic amino acid residues (glutamate, aspartate) can present their carboxyl side chains as a negatively charged site with which cations may electrostatically interact. Such binding sites are critical in providing a decreased energy state for the ion once surrounding waters of hydration are removed (187). For example, the passage of Ba^{2+} through the L-type channel can be described by simple saturable enzyme kinetics in which the maximum reaction rate V_{max} is defined by the maximal rate of ion flux through the channel (i.e., the single channel conductance, γ). When $[Ba^{2+}]_o$ is > 100 mM the γ_{max} is 24 pS. That concentration at which half of the maximum γ is observed defines the dissociation constant K_D for Ba^{2+} (4.7 mM) (185). As with enzymes, competitive ions can bind tightly to these sites and prevent passage of other ions. Because of the more complex electron orbital structure of the transition metal ions (Cd^{2+}, Ni^{2+}, Zn^{2+}, Fe^{2+}) and certain rare earth metal ions (La^{3+}, Nd^{+2}, Gd^{2+}, Yb^{2+}) and the stronger coordination bonds they may form with organic acid residues, these ions typically block ion channels at relatively low concentrations (1 to 100 μM) (200, 201).

Pore Structure and Selectivity

In the absence of extracellular Ca^{2+}, the L-type VGCC permits rapid passage of monovalent ions (Li^+, Na^+, K^+, Cs^+), producing very large currents (141,196) that far exceed those in the presence of Ca^{2+}. However, the presence of even sub-μM $[Ca^{2+}]_o$ markedly decreases the rate of monovalent ion passage through the channel (141), suggesting that the channel's selectivity for Ca^{2+} can be attributed to the ion's ability to bind within the channel. Because of its higher affinity, Ca^{2+} traverses the channel slowly and at the same time prevents the rapid flux of other ions, thereby reducing the conductance through the channel. In the presence of Ca^{2+}, extreme depolarization to highly positive potentials (>+90mV) yields large outward currents, suggesting that the "blocking" action of Ca^{2+} can be reduced by outward monovalent currents (198,199,205). Likewise, Ba^{2+} is highly permeant through L-type channels, with a single conductance over twice that of Ca^{2+}; that is, at equivalent concentrations, twice as many Ba^{2+} as Ca^{2+} can pass through the channel (187). The greater permeability Ba^{2+} than Ca^{2+} is one of the criteria for separating L- from T-type channels. However, when equal fractions of Ba^{2+} and Ca^{2+} are present in the extracellular bathing solution (e.g., 5 and 5 mM), rather than the current appearing as an average of the two it is lower than expected, similar to that with the 5 mM Ca^{2+} alone (the "anomalous mole fraction" effect). This effect can even be observed in single channels (108). Surprisingly, in the absence of Ca^{2+} the L-type channel permits the passage of such large organic cations as tri- and even tetramethylammonium, as well as hydrazinium, methyl-, amino-, and unsubstantiated guanidium (227). Such studies suggest that the L-type channel is a large pore with a diameter of 0.5 to 0.55 nm (5 to 5.5 Å), which could permit the passage of a Ca^{2+} with a single water of hydration. The pore size is larger than that of the voltage-dependent Na or K channels (143,144), leading to the conclusion that high selectivity is achieved by selective binding of Ca^{2+} rather than by rejection of monovalent ions (227).

Positing a scheme similar to enzyme models, Kostyuk et al. (193) proposed an allosteric binding for Ca^{2+} at the extracellular surface of the channel as well as a site within the pore that is responsible for the block of monovalent ion currents. An alternative scheme proposed by Hess and Tsien (141) and McCleskey and Almers (227) involved a pore model that had multiple sites for ion binding. Low-affinity ion binding sites within the pore permit the rapid passage of monovalent ions such as Na^+ or Li^+ when Ca^{2+} is absent. In the absence of Ca^{2+}, Na^+ has a conductance almost tenfold greater than that of Ca^{2+} (187). In the absence of other ions, low $[Ca^{2+}]_o$ (<100 μM) results in one intrapore site binding Ca^{2+} with a slow rate of ion flux. However, when Ca^{2+} concentrations are elevated (>100 μM), both sites may be bound by Ca^{2+} and the electrostatic repulsion between the closely bound ions is sufficient to destabilize them. The entry of another Ca^{2+} into the pore generates sufficient electrostatic repulsion to cause ions to move through the channel and generate far greater I_{Ca}. When competing ions are present Ca^{2+} is prevented from binding to both sites, and its slow transit reduces conductance. However, as predicted from double-ion binding site models (43), a sufficient increase in Ba^{2+} ion concentrations prevents Ca^{2+} binding since Ba^{2+} occupies the sites with a lower affinity; thus, higher currents are permitted (108). When the membrane is markedly hyperpolarized, Ca^{2+} affinity is decreased and conductance of the ions is also less inhibited.

Sophisticated electrophysiologic studies using various charge carriers and different ionic concentrations on either side of the membrane have permitted a detailed characterization of the channel. Employing the ability of Ca^{2+} to block the influx of monovalent ions, Kuo and Hess (196) found that the access to the Ca^{2+} binding site was in fact diffusion limited, as if the extracellular mouth of the pore were extremely wide and the binding site for Ca^{2+} very near the extracellular surface (196,198). Subsequent studies more fully characterized the ability of monovalent ions from the intracellular or extracellular side of the channel to displace Ca^{2+} and enhance flow, and suggest that the Ca channel has a "long pore" with low-affinity cation binding sites to which at least two ions may reside (199). Likewise, experiments in which aqueous diffusion is decreased by glycerol to increase the viscosity are consistent with a long pore (199) and also demonstrate the asymmetry in the channel mouth on the external and internal sides (196) (Fig. 5).

Site-directed mutagenesis of the channel combined with electrophysiologic studies has suggested a structure that is clearly compatible with measured ionic permeability. A critical glutamate residue is located in each of four the P-loops (also termed the SS1-SS2 region) of all of the Ca channel types (133,180,384,427). The presence of four glutamate residues in the pore-lining segments of the channel (P-loop) fit well with the hypothesis that Ca^{2+} selectivity is achieved by two high-affinity Ca^{2+} binding sites within the channels. In the P-loops from domains II and IV, glutamate residues are located close to the pore mouth and may provide an initial binding site. In domains I and III, glutamate residues slightly deeper in the pore may bind Ca^{2+} and provide an inner site (Figs. 3 and 6). With low (<0.1 mM) Ca^{2+} concentrations, both sites (all four glutamates) may form a single high-affinity binding site permitting little current. When $[Ca^{2+}]_o$ is increased >1 mM the pairs of glutamates may form separate, lower-affinity binding sites that permit greater current. The importance of the glutamate residues is emphasized by the site-directed mutagenesis of the Na channel, in which three of the equivalent amino acids of the SS1-SS2 regions are alanine or other uncharged residues (132,317). If one of the Na channel nonglutamate amino acids are mutated to glutamates, Ca^{2+} selectivity increases; if two of the Na chan-

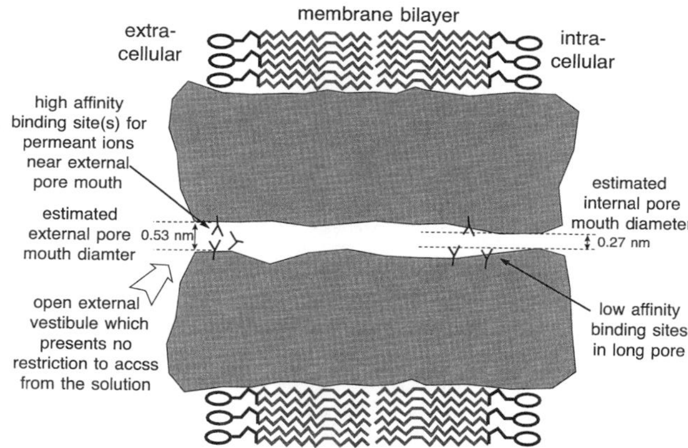

Figure 5. A longitudinal schematic of the L-type channel based on electrophysiologic investigations. The α_1 subunit pore is shown without other associated subunits. The high-affinity binding site for Ca^{2+} is not subject to voltage dependence and appears to be present very close to the external pore mouth of the channel. Furthermore, diffusion to this site is not limited and there is no evidence of a pore suppressant, so there appears to be ready access from the extracellular medium. In contrast, a long pore exists from the intracellular side that has low-affinity binding sites for a variety of ions. Based on ionic permeability in the presence of glycerol, the effective pore diameter appears to be approximately 0.53 nM at its external pore mouth and 0.27 nM at its internal pore mouth. (Based on data from refs. 196–199.)

nel residues become glutamates (for a total of three) then the Na channel shows ion selectivity similar to Ca channels.

Effects of H⁺ and Mg²⁺

Two major ionic species that provide physiologic modulation on VGCC are Mg^{2+} and H^+. It has long been recognized that acidosis inhibits Ca^{2+} currents (402), an action that may contribute to physiologic regulation of vascular tone and myocardial contractility. Detailed studies have clarified the distinctive action of variation in $[H^+]$ from the physiologically normal range, both at intra- and extracellular locations (185,186). Intracellularly, acidosis decreases the probability of channel opening and reopening, while conductance and open time are unaltered (186). The result is a decrease in peak current and an even greater decrease in late current. Such actions can decrease the activity of Ca^{2+}-modulated cell processes (e.g., contractility) and energy utilization. In contrast, excess extracellular protons differ in their action. For a given divalent ion concentration, lower pH decreases the single channel conductance (γ). The observed effect is compatible with a scheme in which two protons transiently bind to and block the anionic sites in the pore to which divalent cations bind in their passage through the channel (185). The resulting decreased rate of passage leads to lower γ. However, by increasing the divalent ion concentration, the same γ_{max} (24 pS) can be achieved at pH 6.4 or 8.4 , since the greater divalent ion concentration can compete with proton for binding sites in the pore.

Mg^{2+} is a physiologically important ion that has been employed clinically to modulate the entry of Ca^{2+} into cells, being used to decrease uterine smooth muscle tone, inhibit neural hyperexcitability, and treat cardiac arrhythmias. Increases in $[Mg^{2+}]_o$ from 1.2 to 9.6 or 16.8 mM decreased $I_{Ca,L}$ by 45% to 65% (72,422). Although Mg^{2+} competes poorly with Ca^{2+} for the high-affinity external site of the channel, at high enough external concentrations it may displace Ca^{2+} in the channel. Because Mg^{2+} is poorly permeant through the "long pore" of the channel, a decrease in $I_{Ca,L}$ results (197). While in this light it may be considered a physiologic Ca channel blocker, its elevation decreases Ca^{2+} via multiple effects. Normally, the $[Ca^{2+}]$ at the cell membrane surface increased above that in bulk solution ($[Ca^{2+}]_o$) because Ca^{2+} is attracted to the negative surface charge of the external membrane bilayer and membrane proteins. By competing with Ca^{2+}, Mg^{2+} "dilutes" the $[Ca^{2+}]$ at the membrane surface and also decreases the external charge surface (249). The dilutional effect could also contribute to decreased $I_{Ca,L}$. In addition, a shift in the voltage dependence of the L-type channel to more positive membrane potentials is also observed (72), similar to that described for Na channels (130) and consistent with a neutralization of the negative-surface charge. Such a shift might decrease Ca^{2+} entry into cells that are partially depolarized and near the threshold of L-type channel activation. A high free intracellular $[Mg^{2+}]$ of 5 to 10 mM inhibits $I_{Ca,L}$ (2,131,197), an effect compatible with a model in which Mg^{2+} cannot readily pass through the long pore of the channel (197). It seems unlikely that significant blocking actions at relevant physiologic free intracellular $[Mg^{2+}]$ (<1 mM) can occur.

In summary, the VGCC pore has a high-affinity Ca^{2+} site at the external surface composed of four glutamate residues and from which a long pore leads intracellularly. While early models of the channel assumed that it is a relatively inert structure that interacts with the permeant ions and presents a relatively

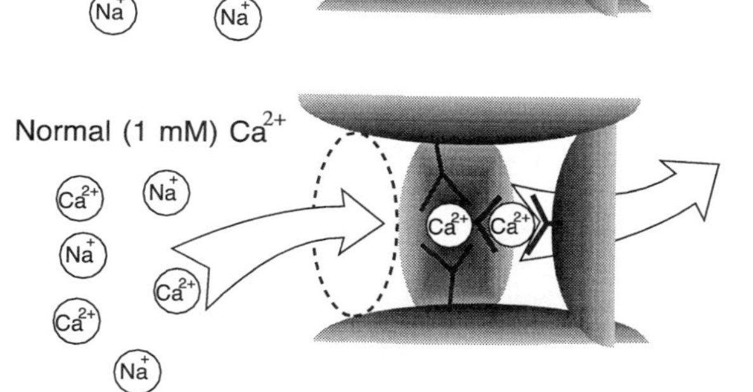

Figure 6. Ion permeation through the L-type Ca channel with binding to carboxyl moieties on glutamate residues located on the P-loops of each domain. These sites are located near the external channel mouth. **A:** With sub-µM external Ca^{2+}, monovalent ions such as Na^+ can readily pass through the channel due to their low affinity for the glutamate residues, and the relative absence of Ca^{2+} that binds with high affinity. **B:** With low-extracellular $[Ca^{2+}]$, Ca^{2+} binds to the four residues, the channel is largely occluded, and has a low conductance. **C:** When extracellular $[Ca^{2+}]$ is increased (~1 mM), the four glutamates may be occupied by two Ca^{2+}, which is inherently less stable due to mutual repulsion. Approach of another Ca^{2+} results in transfer through the channel and a far greater conductance.

uniform energy barrier, it is clear that the entire structure is dynamic and interactive. When Ca^{2+} occupies the binding site, other aspects of the conformation of the channel are altered significantly. For example, protons can bind more tightly to certain sites (286). If a glutamate residue at the Ca^{2+} selectivity site is genetically altered, the binding of DHPs is also changed (283).

Channel Gating and Modulation

The voltage-dependent gating of calcium channels is thought to be due to the S4 segments in each domain that contain multiple positively charged arginine residues. The regions of high-charge density are postulated to serve as voltage sensors, similar to their role in other voltage-gated ion channels. When the membrane depolarizes and the membrane potential becomes more positive, the positively charged S4 segments will shift outward with a resulting conformational change in the α_1 subunit that permits ions to permeate through the pore of the molecule. L-type channels and the other high-voltage-activated channels require a depolarization more positive than -40 mV in order to cause channel opening. The movement of the charged components of the channel in response to alterations in the transmembrane potential can be detected as a "gating current" (22,101,171,339), first described for Na channels (6). The probability of channel opening with depolarization increases exponentially and saturates at approximately +10 mV. Because the channel does not open immediately upon charge movement, it is suggested that there are a number of closed states (protein conformations) through which the channel must pass before the pore opens to become accessible for ion flux. While charge movement (or dipole movement) within the protein occurs during the early conformational changes, the lack of voltage dependence of the open durations and the fact that channel opening can be induced without charge movement suggests that the final conformational change to the open state does not involve a charge movement within the molecule (125,158). The coupling between the charge movement (of the S4 transmembrane segments within each domain) and activation of current appears to be strongly influenced by the specific amino acid sequence in domain I (379), specifically the S3 transmembrane segment and S3-S4 linker (251).

While Ca^{2+} plays a prominent role in regulating ion permeation, it is also a very important regulator of channel gating and channel opening. Considering its importance in intracellular processes, it is not surprising that Ca^{2+} plays a role in regulating its own entry into the cell. The clustering of Ca channels, which has been observed by anatomic studies (135) and suggested by electrophysiologic studies (69,164), may lead to a higher level $[Ca^{2+}]$ at the inner membrane surface than that which occurs with isolated Ca channels, which can in turn modulate channel function.

Ca Channel Inactivation—Voltage and Ca^{2+} Dependent

Following activation of the channel there is a gradual voltage-dependent inactivation; however, the rate of inactivation may be extremely variable, ranging from almost negligible to profound depending on the magnitude of depolarization and the permeant ion. In the absence of Ca^{2+} as the charge carrying ion, this voltage-dependent inactivation is relatively modest, resulting in a 20% to 40% decrease in channel currents over 100 msec (122), but inactivation increases markedly when Ca^{2+} is present (Fig. 7) (67,437).

When Ca^{2+} is the permeant ion, inactivation occurs more rapidly and the probability of channel opening is diminished with increasing duration of depolarization (121,437). Single channel studies document the requirement for channel opening and movement of Ca^{2+} through the channel (in the absence of internal Ca^{2+}) to mediate the process (165,437). A variety of studies have documented the influence of accumulating Ca^{2+} immediately inside the membrane on its intracellular surface (14,121,123,164). Somewhat less inactivation of L-type Ca^{2+} currents ($I_{Ca,L}$) is observed with profound buffering of the intracellular medium (Fig. 7), so that there is minimal accumulation of free Ca^{2+}, although Ca^{2+}-dependent inactivation is not eliminated (23,113,121). In contrast, if Ca^{2+} is released at the intracellular surface, either by photorelease of caged Ca^{2+} (14,123) or by release of intracellular stores (336), Ca^{2+} current inactivation is enhanced. The presence of Ca^{2+} at the intracellular surface appears to shift the channel into a state with a mode of gating in which the probability of opening is very low. Since the process is not altered by inhibition of phosphatases or by calmodulin, it appears to be mediated by a direct action of Ca^{2+} on the channel, presumably at the immediate intracellular surface (165).

Consistent with a site on the channel itself, Yue and collaborators (67) have identified a Ca^{2+} binding site on the proximal carboxy terminus of the α_{1C} subunit, within 19 amino acids of the IVS6 transmembrane helix. The 35 amino acid Ca^{2+} binding site meets the criteria for an "EF hand" Ca^{2+} binding region

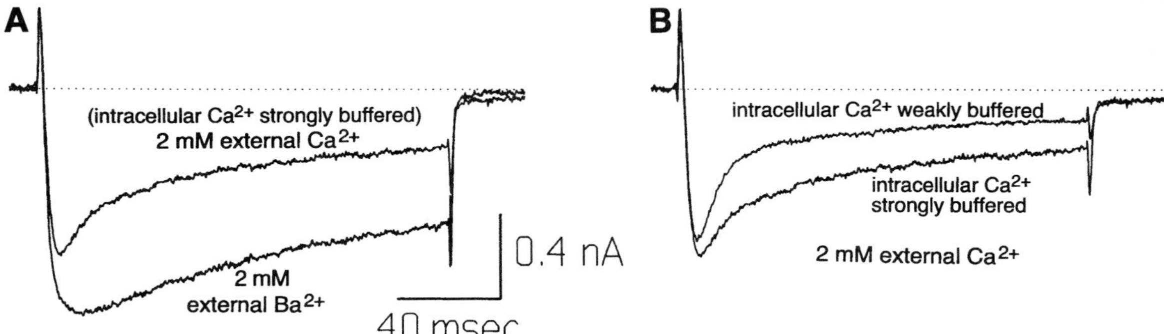

Figure 7. Ca^{2+} currents through L-type Ca channels ($I_{Ca,L}$) in guinea pig ventricular myocytes, demonstrating Ca^{2+}-dependent inactivation. Inward current is downward deflection. Whole cell Ca^{2+} currents observed in response to a depolarization from -80 to 0 mV (corrected for capacitance and leakage currents). Na^+ and K^+ currents were blocked by 10 µM tetrodotoxin and by 20 mM TEA^+/120 mM Cs^+, respectively. **A:** Currents observed in 2 mM external Ca^{2+} and subsequently with substitution of 2 mM Ba^{2+} for 2 mM Ca^{2+} in the same cell. In spite of strongly buffered intracellular Ca^{2+} with 10 mM ethyleneglycoltetraacetic acid (EGTA) ($[Ca^{2+}]_i < 0.05$ µM), the $I_{Ca,L}$ shows lower peak amplitude and greater inactivation when compared $I_{Ba,L}$. **B:** More rapid rate of inactivation of $I_{Ca,L}$ when myoplasmic Ca^{2+} is weakly buffered with 0.5 mM EGTA in the pipette vs. more strongly buffered with 10 mM EGTA (same cell as shown in A). (Courtesy of J.J. Pancrazio, unpublished results.)

characteristic of calmodulin, parvalbumin, and a wide variety of Ca^{2+} binding proteins. When this α_{1C} amino acid segment is substituted for the native carboxy terminus of the α_{1E} subunit, which shows no Ca^{2+}-dependent inactivation, then Ca^{2+}-dependent activation becomes apparent for the α_{1E} subunit. Likewise, the α_{1E} carboxy terminus substituted on the α_{1C} subunit eliminates Ca^{2+}-dependent inactivation. However, when the distal portion of the α_{1E} carboxy terminus is eliminated, Ca^{2+}-dependent inactivation persists (67,440). The $[Ca^{2+}]_i$ required may actually be quite high, since in steady-state experiments ≥600 μM Ca^{2+} is required to decrease channel opening when Ba^{2+} is used as the permeant ion (147). Theoretical analyses estimate such high concentrations at the inner pore mouth with entering Ca^{2+} (360).

Channel Modulation by Ca^{2+}

In addition to its action in inhibiting channel activity, Ca^{2+} entry also potentiates its own channel opening. In the setting of steady-state elevations in $[Ca^{2+}]_i$ in guinea pig myocytes, employing Ba^{2+} as the charge carrier in the patch electrode only, activation of increased channel opening has been demonstrated for $[Ca^{2+}]_i$ in the range of 180 to 500 μM (147). In addition, the photorelease of Ca^{2+} in cells also increases Ca^{2+} current (14,120). In both smooth muscle cells (225) as well as ventricular myocytes (436), the stimulation or frequency-dependent enhancement of current appears to be mediated by calmodulin-dependent protein kinase II (CaM KII). The rise in $[Ca^{2+}]_i$ in the immediate vicinity of the inner channel mouth presumably results in Ca^{2+}-bound calmodulin activating the kinase, which in turn phosphorylates the channel and results in increased activity. The presence of Ca channel clustering would enhance the rate at which $[Ca^{2+}]_i$ accumulates locally to activate CaMK II, and thereby increase the Ca channel potentiation (69,224).

Phosphorylation Sites and Gating Modes

Another major feature of L-type Ca^{2+} channels is their marked enhancement by neurotransmitters. The most prominent increases (up to a threefold increase) occur with β-adrenergic activation (302,303) and other interventions that activate cAMP-dependent protein kinase (PKA) (352). $I_{Ca,L}$ can be increased when cAMP is increased directly (174,254) or when its synthesis is increased by activated adenylyl cyclases with guanosine triphosphate (GTP)-bound stimulatory G proteins (G_s) or forskolin (352). Direct application of the PKA catalytic subunit (39,272) is also effective. When PKA is inactivated, the enhancement of $I_{Ca,L}$ by β-adrenergic stimulation is about 10% of that when PKA is active (173). Nevertheless, a direct association with (129) and modest activation of L-type channels by G_s acting alone has been described (430,431), but this feature is disputed and may not be of major consequence (20). The time course of β-adrenergic stimulation, requiring 1 to 2 sec to begin and 20 to 30 sec to become maximum at 34°C, is consistent with a more slowly mediated, multistep process such as the cascade that activates PKA. Also when PKA is inhibited, enhancement by β-adrenergic stimulation is reduced from 160% to 17% (173). Although L-type VGCC in some cell lines must be phosphorylated in order to open (9), this does not appear to be an absolute necessity since a modest fraction of channels open under conditions strongly favoring dephosphorylation (173). The importance of channel phosphorylation has also been demonstrated by dephosphorylation with oximes, which act as chemical phosphatases and markedly decrease the observed $I_{Ca,L}$ (4,54).

Numerous amino acid residues that can be phosphorylated by various protein kinases have been demonstrated on both the α_1 subunit and the β subunit. While the β subunit can be phosphorylated, phosphorylation of the α_{1C} subunit expressed alone is sufficient to demonstrate enhanced current (333). Furthermore, the facilitation of $I_{Ca,L}$ by previous depolarizations also appears to be mediated by a voltage activated, state-dependent phosphorylation (332,435). While suggesting that the other VGCC subunits are not required for this enhancement, phosphorylation of the β subunit may be involved since α_1 subunits expressed in isolation do not always show enhanced currents (154). One major site of phosphorylation appears to be on the α_1 carboxyl terminus attached to domain IV, since there appears to be PKA phosphorylation in this region that is exclusively associated with enhanced currents (435). When myocytes are subjected to intracellular trypsin treatment, Ca^{2+} currents can be markedly increased (139), and the effect is not additive with β-adrenergic stimulation. Likewise, if the carboxyl terminus is reduced in length by 300 amino acids using site-directed mutations, $I_{Ca,L}$ is likewise markedly enhanced (408). Phosphorylation sites are clearly located in this region of the channel, and like phosphorylation, loss of the carboxyl terminus appears to increase the probability of channel opening (408).

Whereas phosphorylation by PKA has been stated to increase the number of functional channels (21,303,352), the increased $I_{Ca,L}$ actually results from a number of changes in channel protein function (Table 3). Phosphorylation increases the fraction of channels available at any given time for opening (20,438), or rather increases their probability of opening (40,173,174,438). A second major mechanism that contributes to the increase in inward Ca^{2+} current has been described as a change in gating "mode," an effect first described for the DHP agonist Bay K 8644 (140,265). Phosphorylation by PKA shifts the channel from mode 0 (no opening) or mode 1 (brief openings) to mode 2, so that not only is probability of opening increased, but the channel remains open for a more sustained period (40,438). Instead of brief openings lasting less than 0.5 msec, openings are extended to an average of ~8 msec in length (Fig. 8). The appearance of the long-duration mode 2 openings appears to require a higher PKA activity, although it is not clear if this represents a separate phosphorylation site from that which increases opening probability. Such mode 2 gating can also be induced by prolonged depolarizations, although the mechanism is likewise unclear (158,285). It is noteworthy that the potentiation of channel activity by PKA activation was not fully additive with increased $[Ca^{2+}]_i$ (147) or by preceding depolarizations (21), suggesting that the pathways share at least in part a common final phosphorylation pathway. While these two gating modes have been formally recognized, other less-defined modes may also exist, emphasizing the complexity of the channel protein conformational response to membrane voltage fields, which constitutes channel gating. In addition, there is a negative shift in the voltage dependence so that the channels open with a smaller depolarization. Examination of the effects of β-adrenergic stimulation on the gating charge movements associated with I_{Ca} indicates that there is no increase in the amount of charge movement (171), suggesting that no greater number of channels are undergoing a charge movement. However, the charge movement occurs at more negative potentials, consistent with the negative shift in $I_{Ca,L}$ voltage dependence, while the rate of charge movement is also accelerated. Consequently, the increase in $I_{Ca,L}$ must result from more effective coupling of the charge movement within the channel to channel opening; that is, the protein conformational change from closed to open occurs more readily following charge movement, and the channels have an increased open time.

Drug Actions and Binding Sites

The association of contractile inhibition by certain antianginal and antihypertensive agents with their inhibition of Ca^{2+} entry into the myocardium and vascular smooth muscle was first defined by Fleckenstein and coworkers (103,191). The L-type VGCC was found to be a receptor not only for DHPs, but for a variety of drugs that inhibit or alter Ca^{2+} flux. Since that

Table 3. MECHANISMS OF INCREASED $I_{Ca,L}$ BY PROTEIN KINASE A PHOSPHORYLATION

Observation	Interpretation	Reference
Increased number of functional channels, i.e., increased probability of channel opening	Shift from mode 0 to mode 1 gating	21,40,173,174
Increased duration of opening	Channel shifts to mode 2 gating in which open times are greatly prolonged	40,438
Charge movement and channel opening at lower (more negative) membrane potentials	Channel activation threshold is more negative	171
Decreased rate of inactivation	?Shift to mode 2	21

time it has become clear that the L-type calcium channel has a rich molecular pharmacology, with a variety of receptors for various agents. Increased understanding of the interaction of the various drugs with the channel arose from a convergence of biochemical, electrophysiologic, and molecular biologic techniques (51,112,315,390). Distinct, yet interactive, binding sites have been clearly documented on the L-type Ca channel for DHPs, the phenylalkylamines (PAAs), and the benzothiazepines (BTZs), represented by nifedipine, verapamil, and diltiazem, respectively (351). Additional distinct sites for other drug classes are also being defined (182,183,350). The major classes of drugs active on L-type VGCCs and their interactions are listed in Table 4.

Dihydropyridines

As previously noted, the high affinity of the L-VGCC for the DHP class of drugs permitted its isolation and cloning. Isolated membranes containing L-VGCC have a specific K_D of <1 nM, while in many of the initial electrophysiologic studies concentrations approximately 100 times greater were required to cause

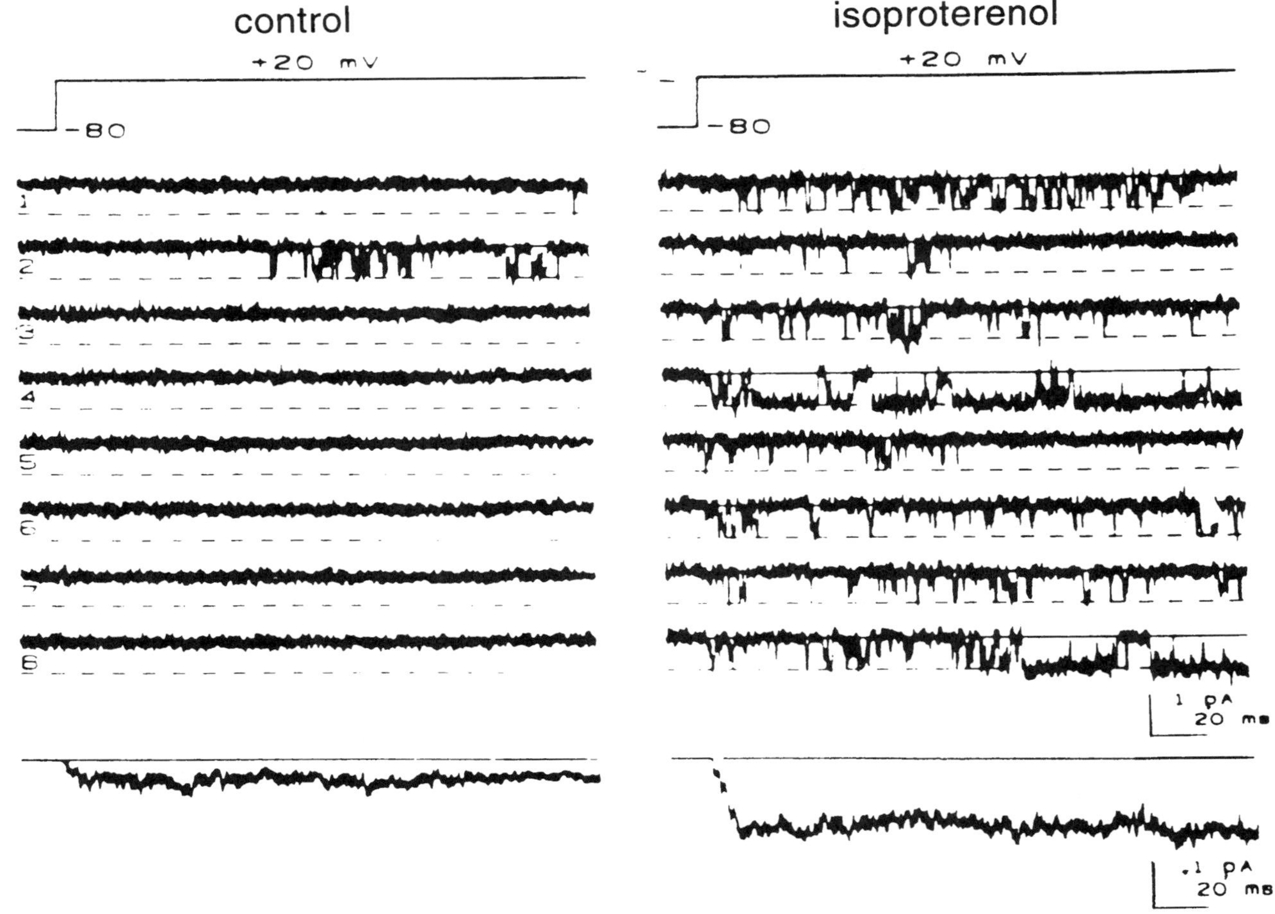

Figure 8. Ca^{2+} currents through unitary L-type channels ($I_{Ca,L}$) in guinea pig ventricular myocytes, demonstrating short- or long-opening modes of gating. Inward current is a downward deflection. Single channel recordings of single L-type channel from a patch of myocyte membrane containing two channels that was depolarized from -80 to +20 mV (*dashed line* represents single open-channel current). The lowest tracing in each panel shows the average response from 200 to 300 sweeps. **Left:** Normal brief openings (mode 1) or absent responses (mode 0). **Right:** Longer-sustained channel openings typical of mode 2 gating observed with β-adrenergic stimulation. (From ref. 438, with permission.)

Table 4. CLASSES OF L-TYPE Ca CHANNEL ANTAGONISTS

Drug class	Typical agents	Effective concentration	Drug binding site	Comments
Dihydropyridine (DHPs)	Nifedipine, nicardipine, amlodipine, nitrendipine	1–50 nM (voltage dependent)	External pore mouth on α_1 subunit, at P-loop junction with S6 in domains III and IV	Agonist properties of certain agents Binding enhanced by BTZs Binding enhanced by Ca^{2+}, decreased by transition metal cations (Cd^{2+}, Ni^{2+}, Co^{2+}) and La^{3+}
Phenylalkylamines (PAAs)	Verapamil, D600	10–100 nM	On intracellular aspect of S6 of domain IV	Binding enhanced by Ca^{2+}, decreased by transition metal cations
Benzothiazepines (BTZs)				
Benzazepinones Benzylisoquinoline alkaloids	Diltiazen (MII conformation) SQ32,910, SQ32,428 Tetrandrine, daurocine	10–100 nM	Near DHP site	Binding increased by Ca^{2+}, inhibited by transition metal cations Binding decreased by PAAs and DHPs Site may also bind desinethoxyverapamil
Others				
Diphenylbutylpiperidines (DPBPs)—antipsychotic neuroleptics, D_{2-4} receptor antagonists	Fluspirilene, pimozide, penfluridol, clopimozide	10–200 nM (voltage dependent)	? External pore	In contrast to the above: Binding inhibited by Ca^{2+}, activated by transition metal cations such as Cd^{2+}, Ni^{2+}, Mn^{2+} and by La^{3+} Mutual inhibition of binding with DHPs, PAAs, and BTZs Also inhibit T-, P-, N- and R-type VGCC
Benzhydrydryl piperiazines	Cinnarizine, flunarizine	~1 µM	Low affinity	
Pyrazines	Aryl and alkyl derivatives, Amiloride	1–10 µM	Within pore?	Inhibit binding of all of the above
Indolizinsulfones	Fantofarone	5–400 nM		

a 50% decrease in current. One explanation for this behavior appears to be due to voltage-dependent binding of DHPs by the channel. When cells are maintained in a partially depolarized state, the blockade of $I_{Ca,L}$ by DHP antagonists is far greater (17,314), leading to the suggestion that DHPs have a far higher affinity for the inactivated state of the channel. The affinity of the channel for radio labeled DHPs is increased by depolarization (323), while the blockade of I_{Ca} observed with partial depolarization (resting potential of -20 or -10 mV) is much greater than with normally polarized cells (17). This effect may explain in part the greater action of DHPs on vascular smooth muscle in which the resting potential is 20 to 40 mV more positive than the values of -80 mV and below typically observed in myocardium. Unlike verapamil, the DHPs do not appear to require repetitive depolarizations and channel opening. A mere shift in the population of channels to the inactivated state is sufficient to markedly decrease $I_{Ca,L}$ (314). Phosphorylation appears to enhance the action of DHP agonists (e.g., Bay K 8644), suggesting that the action of PKA modulates the pharmacologic behavior of the channel (389). If these agents bind more readily to channels that have opened and inactivated, the increased likelihood of channel opening caused by phosphorylation might be expected to increase drug binding.

An extracellular binding site was suggested by electrophysiologic studies demonstrating that charged DHPs, which cannot cross the membrane, have no effect on Ca^{2+} currents when perfused intracellularly (178). The exact binding site(s) for DHPs on the channel protein have been elucidated employing photolabile chemical groups attached to the main portion of the molecule by Catterall and colleagues (51,253,363,364). Photoaffinity DHP analogues bind to domains III and IV of the Ca^{2+} channels, at similar locations where the H5 pore-lining amino acids join the S6 transmembrane helix on the extracellular surface, that is, a site at the immediate extracellular pore mouth (Fig. 9). However, recent data suggest that more distant sites can influence DHP binding. The smooth muscle α_{1C} variant ($\alpha_{1C\text{-}b}$) shows greater voltage-dependent depression of current by DHP antagonists than does that of cardiac muscle (410,432), suggesting that such structural variation may influence drug actions. Splice variations between $\alpha_{1C\text{-}a}$ and $\alpha_{1C\text{-}b}$ occur in a number of portions of the subunit (I–II linker, as well as the IS6, IIIS2, and IVS3 transmembrane helices) that are somewhat distant from the DHP binding site. Experiments employing site-directed mutagenesis suggest that the region that determines the difference in voltage dependence resides in the IIIS2 transmembrane region (347). Alteration in this portion of the subunit is able to modify binding of the DHP at its site near the external pore mouth.

Of considerable interest is the fact that certain DHP analogues that are Ca channel agonists or stimulators, such as BayK 8644 and (+) (S) 202-791, cause the channel to shift into a state in which it remains open for a more sustained period, or into mode 2 gating (140,192,265), thereby markedly increasing the total $I_{Ca,L}$. While the binding of inhibitory DHPs to an external site of the inactivated channel tends to lock it in this state, binding of DHPs also appears to alter the rate at which conformational rearrangements take place that result in ion permeation. The gating charge associated with the L-type VGCC is also altered by DHPs; however, the actions are not correlated with the effects on $I_{Ca,L}$ (101,124). To elucidate these actions, Hadley and Lederer (125) made use of the fact that DHPs are photolabile and, while bound to their active site, they can be degraded to an inactive form by high-intensity light (313). When blocked channels are illuminated, there are two stages of recovery that can be explained by DHP binding to two states. As noted, DHPs bind with high affinity to the inactivated state, which is most prominent at depolarized potentials, and prevent the transition back to the closed state (from which channels can open). DHP binding to the channel also modulates the final (non–voltage-dependent) transition between the closed and open state; inhibitory DHPs slow the transition while stimulatory DHPs promote the transition to the open state. The fact that DHP stereoisomers may have opposite actions is interesting in this regard (192).

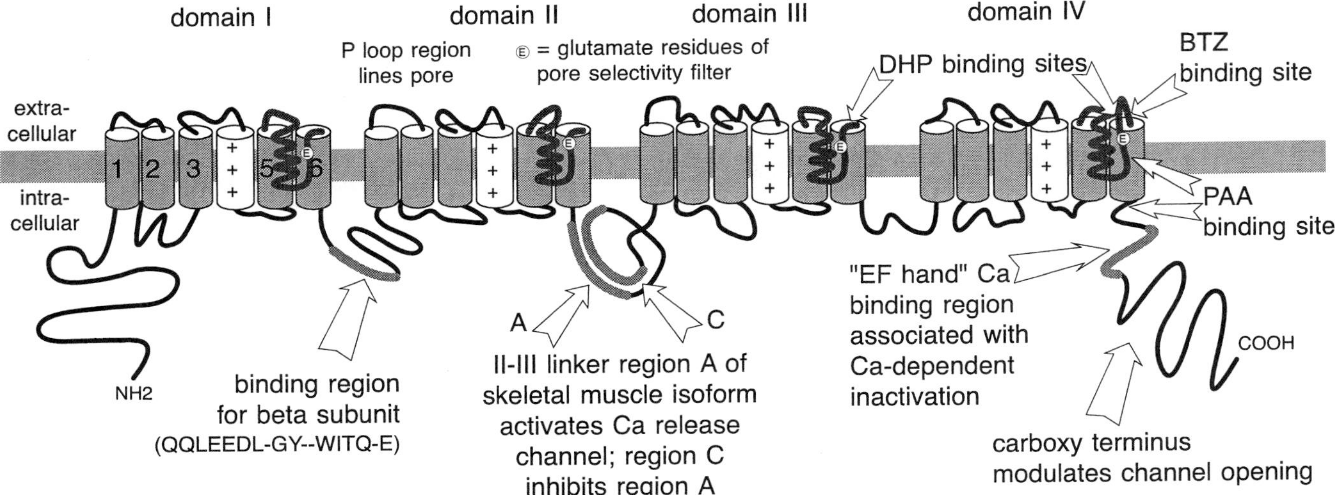

Figure 9. Identified sites of activity on the α_1 subunit of L-type Ca channels (α_{1S}, α_{1C}, α_{1D}). Dihydropyridines (DHPs, e.g., nifedipine) and benzothiazepines (BTZs, e.g., diltiazem) bind to extracellular sites on the L-type channels, while phenylalkylamines (PAA, e.g., verapamil) bind at the intracellular aspect of the channel. Specific sites are also associated with β subunit binding, activation (by α_{1S} only) of the Ca release channel (ryanodine receptor), and phosphorylation.

Phenylalkylamines (PAA)

In contrast to the DHPs, the PAAs such as verapamil are effective only when applied internally and have no effect on external applications (184,202). Photoaffinity-labeled PAAs bind to domain IV, where the S6 segment joins the amino end of the Ca channel protein (Fig. 9). It is also noteworthy that unlike the DHPs, the PAAs show a distinct frequency-dependent blockade of Ca^{2+} current (206,396), suggesting that the channel must pass through an open configuration before the PAAs have access to their binding site. Evidence from molecular biologic studies of the channel suggest that PAAs bind within the pore. When three critical amino acids (Tyr^{1463}, Ala^{1467}, Ile^{1470}) located in the IVS6 transmembrane helix are altered, sensitivity to the PAA compound (-)D888 decreases by over 100-fold to resemble that of the N-type VGCC (151). Mutations of the individual amino acids causes a partial loss of PAA sensitivity. The frequency-dependent VGCC blockade by PAAs is similar in behavior to that of the local anesthetics with regard to the Na channel. Similarly, local anesthetics possess binding sites in the IVS6 transmembrane segment of Na channel that are homologous to these PAA binding sites in the L-type Ca channel (295).

Benzothiazepines (BTZs)

The binding site for the BTZs is clearly distinct from those for PAAs and DHP, yet alters the L-type VGCC by enhancing the binding of the DHPs while decreasing binding of the PAAs (172,390). The BTZ site requires a specific conformation of the diltiazem molecule, similar to that of the closely related benzazepinones, which also bind to the site (181). Attempts to localize the binding site have demonstrated that quaternary BTZ analogues are only active with the extracellular application (363), while a photo-activatable BTZ analogue binds to α_{1S} sites near the IV P loop (406). In addition to BTZs and benzazepinones, a family derived from Chinese medicinal herb *Stefania tetrandra*, *bis*-benzoisoquinolines, also appears to bind the L-type VGCC at the BTZ site (172,182). Although a variety of drugs of this class (e.g., tetrandrine, daurocine) appear to compete with diltiazem for the site, these various agents have distinct actions on DHP and PAA binding, which can differ from those of the BTZs themselves.

Diphenylbutylpiperidines (DPBPs) and Other Agents

An additional class of VGCC modulating drugs are the DPBPs (e.g., fluspirilene, pimozide, clopimozide, penfluridol), a group of agents widely employed as antipsychotic agents that bear a modest resemblance to the PAAs (two or more aromatic rings linked by an 8- to 10-atom hydrocarbon-amine chain). These agents inhibit binding of DHPs, PAAs, and BTZs (172), while themselves depressing I_{Ca} in a voltage-dependent fashion (94,110). Although initially thought to bind at the PAA site (115), the complex interaction with the other L-type VGCC blockers suggests that this drug class has a distinct receptor site on the α_1 subunit (172,183). However, unlike the other agents, DPBPs are rather promiscuous in their Ca channel effects and depress T- (94,95), N-, and P-type VGCC (311) as well, although their affinity for the latter seems lower than that for the L-type channel.

A variety of other drug classes have also been defined that block L-VGCC with varying degrees of specificity, such as the indolizinsufones (fantofarone, SR33805), benzhydrylpiperazines (e.g., cinnarizine, flunnarizine), and pyrazines (e.g., amiloride and its derivatives) (181,350,363). Although altered binding of the more specific DHPs and PAAs can be seen with these agents, they are characterized by difficulty in defining specific binding sites as well as by a lack of specificity. Cinnarizine and flunnarizine are noteworthy for their blockade of a wide variety of VGCC, while amiloride blocks T-type channels as well as the Na^+/H^+ antiport.

While gating, permeation, and drug binding have been discussed individually, it is clear that these various characteristics interact intimately to generate the variable behavior observed in the context of channel protein structure.

Skeletal Muscle L-Type Channels

Excitation-Contraction Coupling

Although it was clear for a number of years that entry of extracellular Ca^{2+} was not required for excitation-contraction (EC) coupling in skeletal muscle (7), it likewise became clear that skeletal muscle possessed a robust, albeit slowly developing, $I_{Ca,L}$ (312,353). While the skeletal muscle $I_{Ca,L}$ was far too slow to initiate contraction by triggering Ca^{2+} release from the sarcoplasmic reticulum (SR) of the muscle, a charge movement within the membrane (i.e., charge movement in the absence of ion flux and due to movement of a dipole through the electrical field) had been identified by Schneider and Chandler (53,326), the size and appearance of which correlated closely with Ca^{2+} mobilization and contraction. Ultimately, it became clear that the charge movement as well as the Ca^{2+} current was inhibited by DHPs (305,330). An elegant series of experiments by Beam and colleagues (16,188,376,380,381) using a strain of dysgenic mice that lack the α_{1S} subunit has been particularly revealing. The major α_1 subunit of the L-type Ca channel of skeletal muscle (α_{1S}) is a particularly specialized type subtype, possessing a specific intracellular region of the linking domains II and III that is critical for EC coupling. Substitution of the equivalent linker region from the α_{1C} cannot restore EC coupling in mice, although the entry of Ca^{2+} via this channel can activate a slower cardiac form of EC coupling. Membrane protein particles evident on the T-tubular membrane, and of a structure appropriate for Ca channels, are closely aligned with the Ca release channel (ryanodine receptor, RYR1) of the SR (30). The picture that has subsequently emerged agrees with the much earlier proposal of a direct linkage between a "voltage sensor" and a SR Ca^{2+} release pathway (53). Membrane depolarization causes a measurable intramembranous charge movement due to the voltage-dependent rearrangement in α_{1S}. The molecular rearrangement must in turn alter the conformation of the II–III linking region, which is critical to activating RYR1 to open and release Ca^{2+} (380). A 20 amino acid segment (Thr^{671}–Leu^{690}) of the II–III linker next to the IIS6 transmembrane segment has been found to activate RYR1 to release Ca^{2+}, while a more central 36 amino acid segment (Glu^{724}–Pro^{760}) of the II–III linker apparently binds to the activating segment, thereby inhibiting its RYR1 activating capability (88). The depolarization must cause uncoupling of the two regions of the II–III linker, so that the activating segment can interact with RYR1. The role of the other skeletal muscle Ca channel subunits is unclear; the skeletal muscle specific γ subunit may play a role. One form of malignant hyperthermia appears related to an abnormality in the α_2-δ subunit (163), suggesting that this largely extracellular subunit can somehow influence coupling to the Ca^{2+} release pathway.

While volatile anesthetics have been shown to inhibit $I_{Ca,L}$, no systematic study has been carried out to determine if these agents interfere with coupling between the α_{1S} coupling regions and the Ca release channel (ryanodine receptor). Certainly, no obvious interference is apparent at relevant clinical concentrations. One possibility is that anesthetic activation of the Ca release channel by anesthetics, particularly halothane (61,257), may offset the inhibitory action on skeletal muscle L-type Ca channels.

Cardiac L-Type Channels

Splice Variants and Their Distribution

Although the α_{1C} subunit was first defined in cardiac muscle and is the predominant form there, both the mRNA transcripts as well as the channel subunits are present in a wide variety of tissues. This channel is alternatively spliced in at least six regions and has at least three major splice variants (a, b, c) (25,26,280). Two splice variants that differ in the IVS3 transmembrane region may be present in the same tissue (280), and the splice variant expressed may vary during myocardial development (73,154). As noted previously, the differing splice variants may also differ in their sensitivity to DHPs (410). In addition to its presence in cardiac tissue, one major site of expression is in vascular smooth muscle (VSM) in which the $\alpha_{1C\text{-}b}$ splice variant is expressed (24). In VSM, the L-type VGCC represents the major pathway for voltage-dependent Ca^{2+} influx (202,226). This pathway is highly sensitive to the membrane potential established by the K^+ conductances, which may represent a major mechanism controlling Ca^{2+} entry (256). This channel is also widely distributed in neurons and constitutes the predominant form of DHP-sensitive channel present in brain (135). A longer and a shorter splice variant of the neuronal α_{1C} are expressed, and while both forms can be phosphorylated by PKC, CaM K II, and cGMP-dependent kinase, only the longer form is a substrate for PKA. Such differential expression may be important in differential modulation of responses to stimulation.

Anesthetic Effects on the Cardiac L-Type Channels

The initial studies suggesting that volatile anesthetics block I_{Ca} were based on slow action potential experiments in papillary muscles (216–219), although prior to that halothane had been shown to decrease uptake of $^{45}Ca^{2+}$ into isolated atria (290). Subsequent voltage clamp studies in isolated myocytes from a variety of species have confirmed the depression of isolated $I_{Ca,L}$ by volatile anesthetics (34,149,150,162,387,388). Depression is typically in the range of 20% to 30% for 1 minimal alveolar concentration of anesthetic and is observed in isolated cerebral vascular myocytes as well (42). In addition to decreasing the peak $I_{Ca,L}$, the anesthetics typically increase the rate of inactivation, whether Ca^{2+} or Ba^{2+} is the charge carrier (273). When single channel currents are examined, both halothane (273) and enflurane (372) have been found to decrease the probability of opening, decrease the open channel lifetime, and increase the closed duration (Fig. 10).

Such electrophysiologic evidence is supplemented by biochemical evidence that volatile anesthetics can alter L-type channel function in myocardium. The volatile anesthetics decreased the amount of DHP binding to isolated cardiac sarcolemmal membranes (27,83,153,252,325), while halothane was notable for decreasing affinity for DHP in some studies (83,252). Halothane was also found to decrease the binding of the verapamil analogue D600 (152). Because these agents typically bind more strongly to channels in the inactivated state, decreased binding would be consistent with fewer channels having passing from closed to open to inactivated. It is interesting that in models of ischemic injury in both heart (82,204) and brain (153), halothane appears to "protect" the L-type VGCC as assessed by binding of DHP. The mechanism(s) by which anesthetics alter the function of these channels remains the object of investigation, since it is unclear whether the effects are mediated by direct binding to the channel protein(s) via the membrane lipid or by alteration in secondary modulatory actions such as phosphorylation.

In addition to the volatile anesthetics, thiopental and methohexital also inhibit $I_{Ca,L}$ and may contribute to their cardiodepressant actions (162,274,426). These action are observed with concentrations in the higher clinical range, particularly when protein binding is considered (276). Likewise, propofol decreases the lifetime of the L-type VGCC open channel and decreases the probability of opening (372), but the 100 μM concentration is well beyond the concentration of free drug present clinically (276).

Endocrine L-Type Channels

The α_{1D}-DHP-sensitive channel is prominent in pituitary and insulin-secreting β-islet cells, but is also expressed widely in brain where two isoforms are present (135). One of those isoforms is missing a major carboxy terminus, the absence of which has been shown to markedly enhance the currents present in α_{1C}-type channels (135). It is unclear whether the absence of this terminus contributes to the behavior of the L-type channels observed in certain endocrine tissues. Pituitary cells have a large L-type channel component that appears to regulate release of hormones such as prolactin, growth hor-

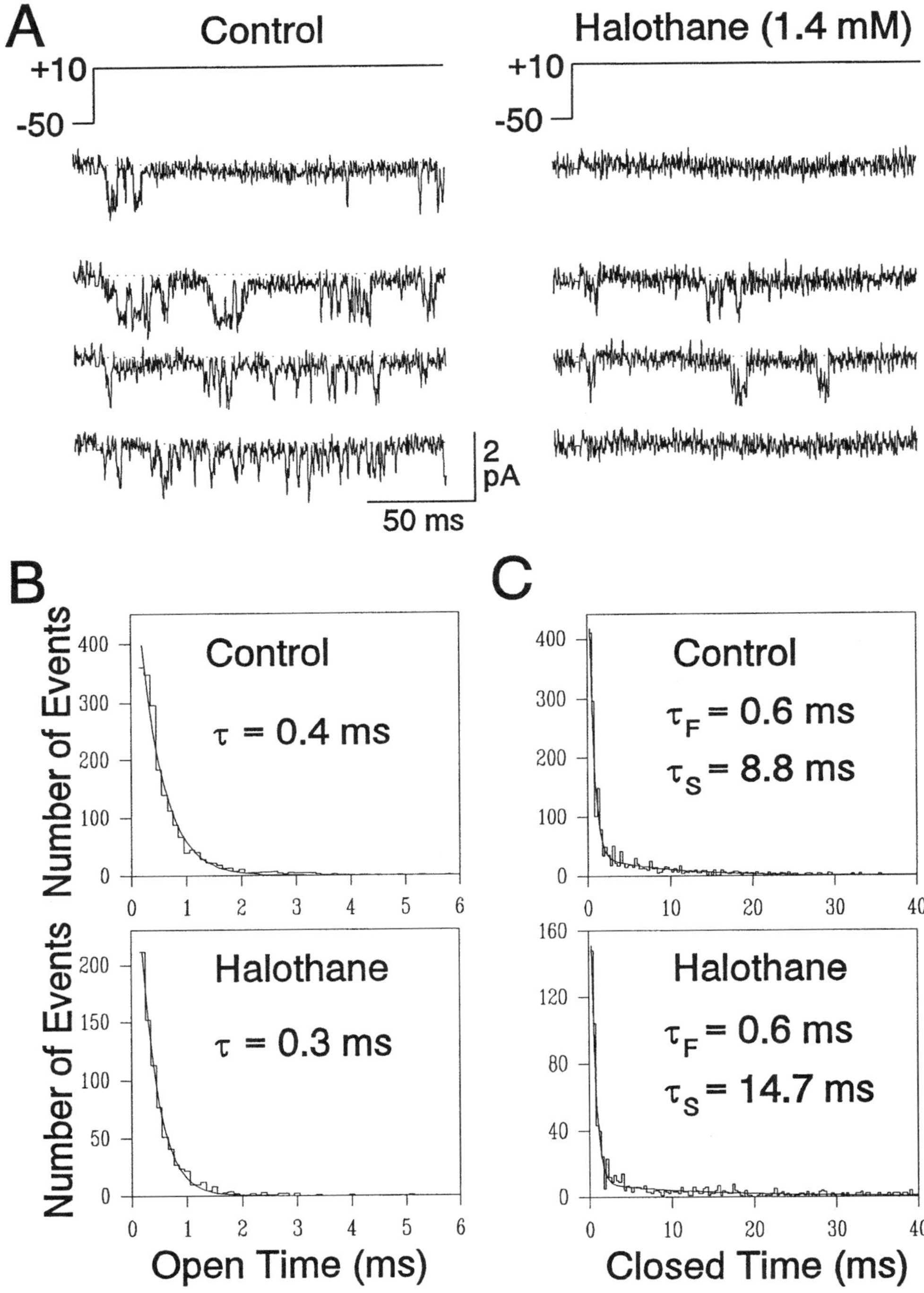

Figure 10. Halothane depresses the frequency and duration of L-type Ca channel opening. Isolated guinea pig ventricular myocytes were bathed in a solution containing (in mM): 120 K^- aspartate, 20 KCl, 2 EGTA, 10 HEPES, pH 7.4 with KOH, to effectively zero the resting membrane potential. The patch pipettes contained (in mM): 120 $BaCl_2$, 10 HEPES, 1 EGTA, pH 7.4 with 1M CsOH. Unitary Ca channel currents were filtered at 1 kHz with a four-pole low-pass Bessel filter and digitized at 10 kHz. Voltage pulses 200 msec in duration in groups of 64 episodes were applied at a rate of 0.5 Hz with a total of 256 sweeps collected for each experimental condition. Leak and capacitative currents were subtracted by fitting a null sweep, i.e., a record with no observable opening, with the sum of three exponential decay functions and subtracting the fitted result from each data trace. **A:** Four consecutive sweeps evoked by voltage steps from −50 mV to +10 mV from the same membrane patch with a single Ca channel under control conditions after application of 1.4 mM halothane. The *downward deflections* signify channel opening and the *dotted lines* indicate the zero current level. **B:** Comparison of open time distributions before and after application of halothane. **C:** Comparison of closed time distributions before and after administration of 1.4 mM halothane (equivalent to 2.2% at 22°C), a high concentration used to accentuate effects. Halothane decreased mean channel open time, equal to τ_O, and increased the time constant of the slow closed state component, t_{CS}, with no effect on the time constant of the fast closed state component, τ_{CF} (273).

mone, and luteinizing hormone (LH) . For example, in GH3 cells, inward Ca^{2+} flux can be observed with very modest depolarizations (244), although it is not clear if the distinctive behavior may be related to the particular splice variant of the α_{1D} channel that is present.

In insulin-secreting β islet cells, there is characteristic bursting behavior that is sustained over several seconds (62). There is modest voltage-dependent inactivation in Ca^{2+} currents over this period (318,320). Although N-type channels are present in at least some preparations of β cells, it is the sustained noninactivating L-type current during depolarizations that is responsible for actual release of insulin (319). The entry of Ca^{2+} into such cells is localized near the secretory granules, around which L-type channels appear to be clustered (31).

THE NEURONAL CA CHANNELS

Although DHP application to neurons typically caused a modest reduction in current (10–30%), there was clearly a large I_{Ca} component resistant to the effects of DHPs, suggesting that additional varieties of VGCC were present. The subsequent cloning of three α_1 subunits from brain, which were sensitive to various toxins and were far less homologous with the skeletal and cardiac channels, correlated with the presence of DHP-resistant channels. In certain highly homologous regions there are subtle distinctions between the DHP-sensitive and -insensitive classes. For example, in the highly conserved β subunit binding the I–II linker region, in which all six VGCC channels have 9 of 18 amino acids in common, the three L-type channels (α_{1S}, α_{1C}, α_{1D}) have 14 of 18 common amino acids, while the three neuronal α_1 subunits (α_{1A}, α_{1B}, α_{1E}) have 15 of 18 in common (Figs. 9 and 11) (279). However, the major feature that differs between the two families of α_1 subunits is the size of the intracellular linking region between domains II and III. In the neuronal α_1 subunits, this region is typically 200 amino acids longer.

The N-Type Channel

Structure and Distribution

The N-type channel, defined from biophysical characteristics and by sensitivity to ω-conotoxin, is now unequivocally associated with the neuronal VGCC α_{1B} subunit clone, variously named BIII, rbB, and CaCh5. Overlapping segments of cDNA for rbB-I were used to determine the complete amino acid sequence for the Ca channel α_1 subunit, which when expressed was found to be sensitive to ω-conotoxin (GVIA) (85). A human ω-conotoxin–sensitive channel α_{1B} subunit has also been described, with the isolated cDNA suggesting two forms: α_{1B-1} with 2339 amino acids (~262 kd) and α_{1B-2} with 2237 amino acids (~252 kd) (417). These distinctively spliced gene products may correlate with the two distinct forms isolated for class β N-type calcium channel; a smaller form has a shortened carboxy terminus (134,412). While both forms are phosphorylated by PKA, PKC, and cyclic GMP-modulated protein kinase, only the longer form is phosphorylated by CaM kinase II (134). Since CaM KII will be sensitive to $[Ca^{2+}]_i$, there exists a pathway for Ca^{2+} entry (via voltage- or ligand-gated channels) to provide feedback regulation (positive or negative) of Ca^{2+} entry via one of the N-type channel subtypes.

Employing site-directed mutagenesis of this α_{1B} subunit, the large hydrophilic cytoplasmic segment linking domains II and III has been found to possess an 87 amino acid sequence that binds to the neurotransmitter vesicle-associated protein syntaxin (338). This protein is located in the active zone membrane of synaptic nerve endings where vesicle release occurs. Since synaptic vesicles appear docked near these regions, this channel-synaptic protein linkage is strategically located to mediate exocytosis. Most studies suggest that Ca^{2+} entry is required for transmitter release (12,74), and there is little evidence to suggest that voltage-dependent conformational change is directly linked to initiate membrane fusion by itself.

N-type VGCC are prominent in neurons of the peripheral sympathetic nervous system (299). In the brain these N-type VGCC appear to be located on the presynaptic terminals and dendrites of various neurons, consistent with an important role in synaptic function in sympathetic neurons. In other cell lines they may contribute a smaller amount to the total I_{Ca} (89,167,298,397).

Modulation and Regulation

Regulation of synaptic transmission by inhibition of presynaptic release processes is widely recognized as a means of neural modulation. Presynaptic Ca^{2+} entry can be decreased indirectly by decreasing the excitability (ease of depolarization), or directly by depression of Ca channels, and a variety of neuromodulators act by both mechanisms. By enhancing K^+ conductance, the resulting hyperpolarization at the synaptic terminal inhibits depolarizations and repetitive firing, which in turn reduces Ca^{2+} entry and consequently decreases neurotransmitter release (155). By inhibiting presynaptic Ca channels, activation of trans-

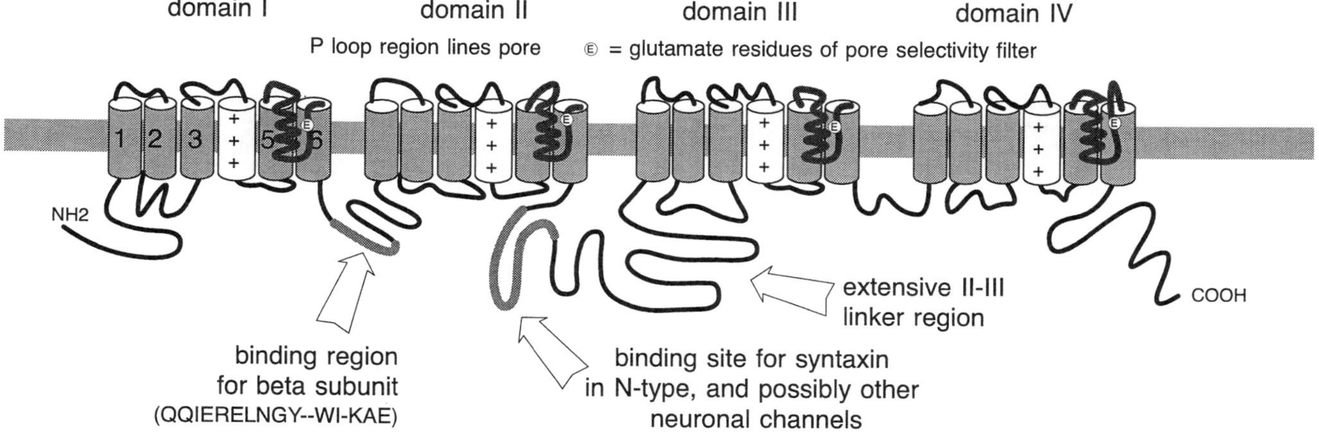

Figure 11. Identified sites of activity on the α_1 subunit of neuronal Ca channels (α_{1A}, α_{1B}, α_{1E}). On the large II–III linker of the N-type channel there is a 87 amino acid region with a helix-loop-helix protein binding motif that selectively binds syntaxin, a membrane-bound protein that regulates docking of small neurotransmitter vesicles. The P-loops possess glutamate in homologous locations to those in the L-type channels.

mitter release is depressed. Similar to the activation of K channels (38,264,392), inhibition of N-type channels is seen with activation of a variety of receptors (Table 5): opioid receptors (116, 138,156,243,335,337,392,416), α_2-adrenergic (328,337), $GABA_B$ (78), somatostatin (probably SS_2) (161), neuropeptide Y (NPY) (96), and muscarinic receptors (405). Such inhibition represents a major mechanism of modulation of Ca^{2+} and consequent neurotransmitter release. Based on the sensitivity to pertussis toxin (PTX), the receptor-mediated depression of neuronal I_{Ca} was linked to activation of $G_i\alpha$ or $G_o\alpha$ protein subunits, which are ADP-ribosylated by the PTX (78,138,405). The receptor-mediated inhibition can be mimicked by cell treatment with GTP-γS, the nonhydrolyzable analogue of GTP (78,138,405). When combined with the G protein α subunit, GTP-γS causes ongoing interaction with the channel receptor.

A variety of studies have now clearly identified $G_o\alpha$ as the major species responsible for the inhibition of N-type channels. Initially, replacement of $G_o\alpha$ as opposed to $G_i\alpha$ was found to be far more effective in restoring the ability of the opiate analogue DADLE to depress I_{Ca} in neurons (96,138). More recent studies have more clearly delineated the effect as being on ω-Ctx-sensitive N-type channels . When the $G_o\alpha$ subunit is eliminated by antibodies injected into cells (230,231), or when $G_o\alpha$ is eliminated by injection of antisense nucleotides that prevent its synthesis (44), the inhibitory effects of neurotransmitters (i.e., norepinephrine, GABA) are diminished. Additional studies indicate that $G_o\alpha$ may compete for the binding site of the β subunit on the N-type channel (45). These findings suggest that binding of the $G_o\alpha$ instead of the β subunit to the α_1 VGCC subunit results in the profound changes in gating of the channel itself, consistent with the observation that β subunits typically accelerate activation of currents and shift them to lower voltages. Coexpression of the β_3 subunit with α_{1B} (also α_{1A}) VGCC subunits is actually able to prevent inhibition mediated by G protein pathways (307).

Recent studies have suggested that even in the absence of receptor-mediated $G_o\alpha$ action, a tonic inhibition may be present in certain cells (160,176,177). Considering that $G_o\alpha$ exists in extremely high concentrations in brain, constituting up to 1% of brain protein (361), it is perhaps not surprising that some tonic effect may be present even in the absence of receptor-mediated activation of $G_o\alpha$. Although $G_{oA}\alpha$ is the typical inhibitory protein, somatostatin appears to mediate its action via one of the $G_i\alpha$ subtypes (or possibly $G_{oB}\alpha$) (386). K channel activation has been found to be mediated by the βγ G protein subunit (268). While initial evidence suggested no such interaction in neuronal VGCC (138), more recent studies suggest that the βγ subunit might mediate a steady-state inactivation of N-type channels (75).

The interaction of the activated $G_o\alpha$ with the N-type channel causes two prominent changes: a marked slowing in the rate of activation of the $I_{Ca,N}$, so that early inward Ca^{2+} is markedly reduced; and a shift in the voltage dependence of N-type channels to much more positive potentials, so that a greater depolarization is required for opening (78,93,289). N-type VGCC exhibit at least three gating modes (low, medium, and high) that differ in levels of channel activity (70). When the G proteins bind to the N-type channel, they appear to shift the probability of opening (P_o) of the channel from a prevalence of the high P_o mode, to the medium and low P_o modes (71)—from a "willing" to a "reluctant" mode (19). The channel can be described by a model in which up to four $G_o\alpha$ subunits can bind to the channel, shifting the voltage dependence of each of the voltage sensing regions (33). Previously, G protein had been found to alter the conductance behavior of N-type channels by decreasing the single channel current carried by Ba^{2+}, while leaving the ionic flux carried by Ca^{2+} or Cs^+ relatively unaltered (195). Thus, the conformational change induced by the G protein binding appears to influence the selectivity pathway.

The block is also voltage dependent in the sense that a depolarizing prepulse disrupts the inhibition caused by $G_o\alpha$ activation (93,289); the longer and the larger the depolarization, the greater the effect (33,160). With depolarizing prepulses, it is as if the channel conformational change decreases the affinity for the G proteins, so that the channel becomes available for opening with subsequent depolarizations. It seems possible that trains of impulses can physiologically duplicate this action and overcome such neurotransmitter inhibition.

In addition to the depolarizing prepulses, G protein–dependent inhibition can be overcome by other interventions. Nitric oxide (NO), via activation of guanylate cyclase and increase of cGMP, is also able to overcome the inhibition mediated by nor-

Table 5. MODULATORS OF N-TYPE Ca CHANNEL

Agonists	Receptor	Mechanism	Comment	Reference
Norepinephrine, clonidine	α_2	$G_o\alpha$	Slowing of activation	75,92,105,211,230, 288,289,366,369
Dexmetotomidine		$G_i\beta\delta \rightarrow$ PLC $\rightarrow$ PKC?	? Steady-state inhibition	
Opioids, endorphins:				138,243,263,
DAMGO	μ	$G_o\alpha$		335,416
Dynorphin A	κ	$G_o\alpha$		116,118,243
LHRH		$G_o\alpha$	PKC modulated	29,33,93,369
GABA, baclofen	$GABA_B$	$G_o\alpha$	PKC modulated	44,75,76,78,369
Somatostatin	SS_2	$G_i\alpha$?	Possibly $G_{oB}\alpha$	161,386
Adenosine, 2-chloro-adenosine	A_1	$G_o\alpha$	PKC modulated	77,220,242,369
Dopamine	D_2	?		179,222
Acetylcholine	M_1	$G_o\alpha$	PKC modulated	92,288,369,405
Neuropeptide Y	NPY	$G_o\alpha$		96,288
Substance P		$G_o\alpha$		29,92
Glutamate	mGluR	$G_o\alpha$	Strongly PKC modulated	370,371
Cortisol	GR	$G_o\alpha$ or $G_i\alpha$	Strongly PKC modulated	100
Bradykinin	BK1	?G_q	PKC activation	32,386

$G_i\alpha$, α subunit of inhibitory G protein; $G_o\alpha$, α subunit of "other" G protein, prominent in brain; PTX, pertussis toxin; PKC, protein kinase C; GR, glucocorticoid receptor.

epinephrine (57,58). In the absence of active inhibition, NO is able to modestly enhance I_{Ca}, presumably because a small, persistent G protein–mediated inhibition is ongoing (58). It is unclear whether activation of cGMP-dependent kinase results in modification of G protein inhibition. PKC activation is also able to reverse the inhibition of I_{Ca} in neurons by muscarinic, α_2-adrenergic, $GABA_B$, adenosine, or glutamate stimulation (369,371). PKC activation can enhance N-type channels (428), apparently reversing the tonic inhibition of N-type channels that appears to be G protein mediated (369). Since both the G protein subunits as well a the α_{1B} VGCC subunit can be phosphorylated, either (or both) may be a site of action. When expressed α_{1B} subunits are studied, PKC activation by phorbol esters can increase the current by 30% to 40%; however, coexpression with the β subunit (in this case β_{1b}) is required (358). The cytoplasmic I–II linker also plays a critical role. The complexity of the situation is emphasized by the fact that PKC enhancement exceeds the effect removing G protein inhibition. In addition, under certain settings PKC activation has been found to decrease N-type Ca^{2+} currents depending on the cell type (207).

Anesthetic Effects

While the predominantly L-type VGCC of cardiovascular tissues have been well documented to be depressed by volatile anesthetics, depression of N-type VGCC of hippocampal pyramidal cells is also depressed by isoflurane (Fig. 12). The peak ω-Ctx-sensitive current was diminished by ~35% and sustained current by 68% in solutions equilibrated with 2 MAC anesthetic (at 22°C) (365). In contrast, the HVA currents in rat sensory neurons, of which the majority are N-type, were found to be modestly sensitive (depressed by 20%) by 0.5 mM halothane at 22°C (equivalent to equilibration with 0.75% gas phase) (377). In adrenal chromaffin cells, which show a mixed population of Ca channels, the volatile anesthetics show more modest depression, with values in solution equivalent to greater than 3% gas phase required to cause >40% depression (55,275).

The intravenous anesthetic agents also appear to depress neuronal Ca^{2+} currents. Anesthetic concentrations, as opposed to anticonvulsant levels, of barbiturates depress Ca^{2+}-dependent APs (142) and VGCC currents (411) induced in cultured neurons. When investigated at very high concentrations (500

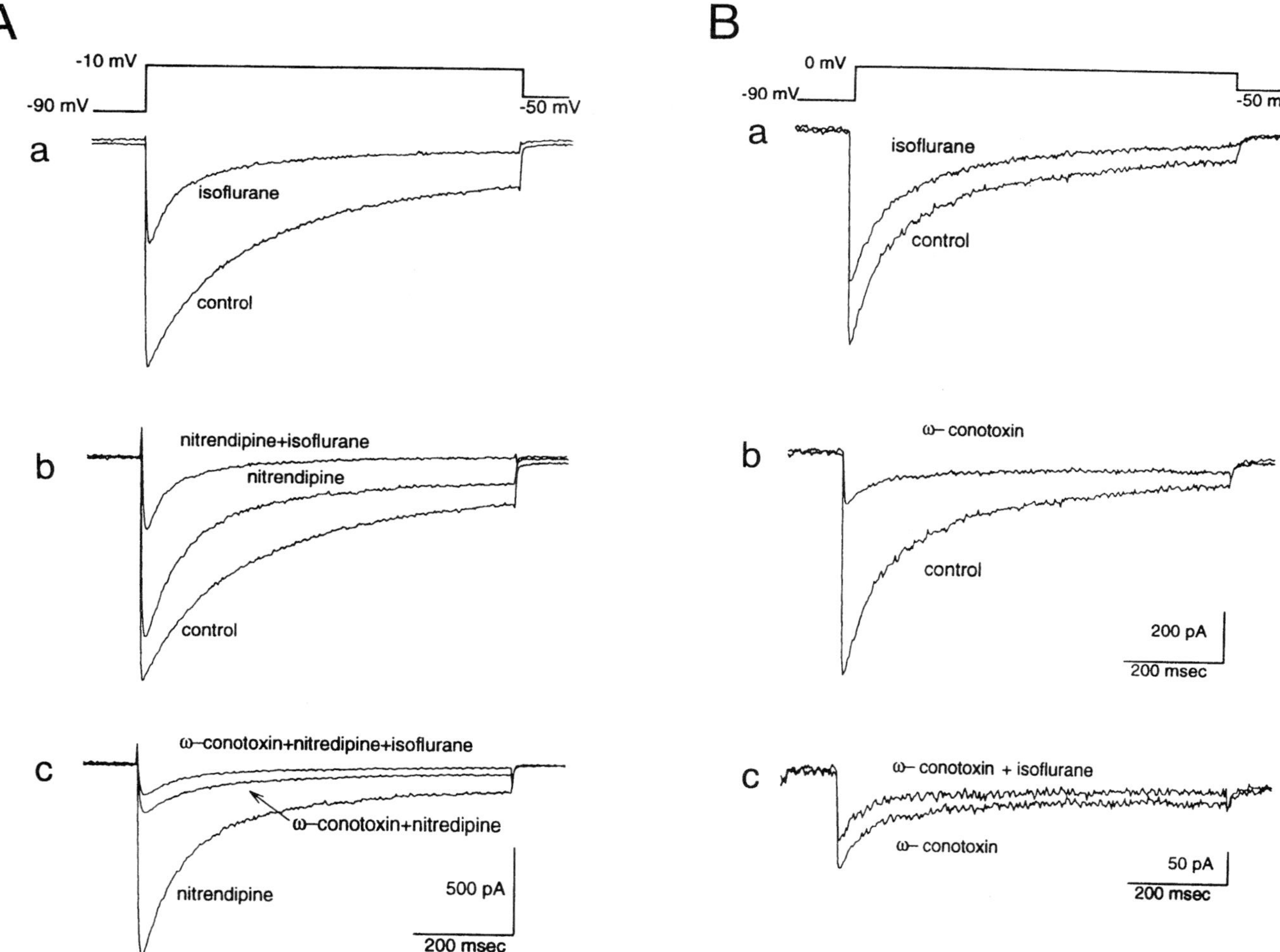

Figure 12. Isoflurane inhibition of Ca^{2+} currents in the presence and absence of L-type and N-type Ca channel blockade by nitrendipine and ω-Ctx-GVIA, respectively. **A:** Isoflurane (2.5%) was applied by puffer pipette and currents were measured in 5 mM Ca^{2+}. (a) Isoflurane (2.5%) inhibits the high-voltage-activated current resulting from a depolarization from -90 to -10 mV. (b) The same cell before and after a supramaximal concentration of 10 μM nitrendipine was added to block L-type Ca channels, leaving other Ca channels. (c) The same cell with 0.5 ω-Ctx-GVIA was added to also eliminate N-type channels (this cell had no T-type Ca^{2+} current). **B:** Isoflurane inhibition of Ca^{2+} current in the presence and absence of 0.5 μM ω-Ctx-GVIA (ω-Ctx). (a) Isoflurane inhibition of Ca^{2+} current in the absence of ω-Ctx. (b) Inhibition of most of the Ca^{2+} current in this cell with ω-Ctx. (c) Inhibition of the ω-Ctx–resistant current with isoflurane. Isoflurane (2.5%) was applied from a pressure pipette. (From ref. 365, with permission.)

μM), pentobarbital decreased N-type currents by speeding the rate of inactivation and increasing the fraction of inactivated channels (shifting the voltage dependence of inactivation to more negative potentials (117). When rat RNA is expressed in *Xenopus* oocytes, the resulting inward Ba^{2+} current is highly sensitive to ω-Ctx-GVIA. This largely N-type current is blocked by high clinical concentrations (IC_{50} ~250 μM for secobarbital, amobarbital and phenobarbital) of barbiturates (119). In hippocampal CA1 neurons, *R*(-)-pentobarbital inhibited I_{Ca} in a voltage-dependent manner with an IC_{50} of 3.5 μM, well within the clinical range, while a much higher concentration of phenobarbital (IC_{50} = 72 μM) and L(+)-pentobarbital (>1 mM) were required for an equivalent action (99). In PC12 cells, which have a mixed population of VGCC, I_{Ca} as well as Ca^{2+} entry and catecholamine release were depressed by methohexital (IC_{50} = 110 to 150 μM) at concentrations about three to four times the clinical levels of free drug (55). Concentrations of etomidate (IC_{50} = 230 μM) required for significant reduction of I_{Ca} were well beyond the clinical range (55). In contrast, propofol (300 μM) at over 100 times the clinical levels had minimal effects on ω-Ctx-G_{VIA} sensitive channels (269).

The α_{1A} Subunit: P- and Q-Type Ca Channels

The first brain VGCC cloned and expressed was initially termed BI (247). In addition to having a similar overall structure, it also shared with the L-type VGCC the presence of glutamate residues on each of the P-loops (SS2) that line the pore. Mutational replacement of the glutamates of domains III or IV resulted in the expected decrease in divalent ion selectivity and altered blockage by Cd^{2+} (180). The most perplexing feature of the α_{1A} (BI) subunit is the convergence of toxityping and molecular biologic methods that suggests that this VGCC is responsible for Ca channels with two different toxin sensitivities.

P-Type Channels

After the description of the highly selective blockade on N- and L-type HVA Ca channels, the persistence of DHP- and ω-Ctx-resistant I_{Ca} in a variety of neurons became evident, especially for the I_{Ca} in Purkinje cells from mammalian and avian cerebellum (213,299). In contrast to a rapidly inactivating $I_{Ca,T}$ activated at lower (<-50 mV) membrane potentials, the observed HVA current frequently demonstrated minimal inactivation and was blocked by a polyamine toxin (FTX) from the funnel web spider (213). Of interest and consistent with a role in central neuronal function, when half the lethal dose of FTX is injected into mice, animals entered a state similar to deep sleep (213). This channel was termed P-type by Llinás and coworkers (213) for its predominance in Purkinje cells, where it exhibits distinctive kinetic behavior and pharmacologic sensitivity. This channel was found to be exquisitely sensitive to nM concentrations of a 48 amino acid peptide toxin from *Agelenopsis aperta* (funnel web spider) termed Aga-IVA toxin (235,239). While profoundly blocking the I_{Ca} in Purkinje cells, Aga-IVA is ineffective on L-, N-, and T-type channels. An interesting characteristic of the blockade by Aga-IVA is that it is reversed by a profound positive prepulse (e.g., +100 mV), suggesting that the voltage-dependent conformation of the channel can modulate toxin binding. Using antibody labeling techniques, P-type channels have been localized to the molecular layer of the cerebellar cortex of the rat, particularly at Purkinje cell dendritic spines and bifurcations (145). While labeling was light in the neocortex, strong labeling was also present in the olfactory bulb, inferior olive, fourth ventricular floor, habelula, and trapezoid nucleus.

Complementary DNA derived from rabbit brain was first employed to generate a VGCC common in the central nervous system, and the clone was initially designated BI (247). The homologous α_1 subunit was subsequently isolated from rat brain as rbA (344), and is now termed class A (α_{1A}). This clone was initially speculated to be the channel observed in Purkinje cells (P-type) and sensitive to the toxin Aga-IVA (247). When the mRNA of the α_{1A} channel subunit has been mapped by in situ hybridization with antisense RNA, this subunit transcript was found to be extremely prominent in the cerebellar Purkinje cells (359). Surprisingly, when the α_{1A} channel subunit clone is expressed in oocytes, it shows only modest sensitivity to Aga-IVA, and moderate inactivation (359). It is likely that the apparent lack of sensitivity of isolated α_{1A} subunits to Aga-IVA results from posttranslational modulation, the presence of other subunits, or alternative splicing of the gene. In fact, when expressed with different β subunits or combinations of subunits, this clone shows marked variation in current kinetics (Fig. 13) (359).

In addition to the Purkinje cells, the transcripts for the α_{1A} subunit have been found to be prominent in the dentate gyrus, the hippocampus (CA1, CA2, CA3 fields), the olfactory bulb (mitral cell layer), and cerebral cortical layers II to VI, regions that have not necessarily proven particularly rich in Aga-IVA–sensitive (P-type) channels (359). Melanotrophic neuroendocrine cells of the intermediate pituitary also possess an inward Ca^{2+} current that is blocked by FTX (420).

Modulation and Regulation The effects of $GABA_B$ receptor activation on P-type VGCC currents are very similar to those previously described for N-type. Application of GABA or baclofen decreases the rate of activation of current as well as a steady-state reduction in current, effects that are in part reversed by stronger depolarizations (236). Like the effect on N-type channels, the effect is augmented by processes that enhance G protein activation. In contrast to the inhibition by GABA, adenosine potentiates P-type channels in CA1 hippocampal neurons, an effect mediated by A2b receptors and subsequent activation of the adenylyl cyclase cascade (242). When α_{1A} VGCC subunits are expressed in oocytes, PKC causes little enhancement of current unless the domain I–II cytoplasmic linker from α_{1B} (N-type) subunits has been substituted in the channel protein sequence and a β subunit is present (358).

Anesthetic Effects Employing a model of cerebellar Purkinje neurons that had predominantly P-type Ca channels, Hall et al. (128) found modest reductions caused by 0.2 mM halothane. However, by assuming that the volatile anesthetic MAC was reduced at the lower temperatures at which the experiments were conducted, they studied concentrations that are not comparable to the gas phase partial pressure employed at normothermia.

Q-Type Channels

Electrophysiologic and toxinologic evaluation of the α_{1A} subunit channel when expressed in oocytes showed it to be sensitive (<15 nM) to the toxin ω-Ctx-MVIIC. This sensitivity stands in contrast to the P-type VGCC, which requires far higher concentrations of ω-CTx-MVIIC to be blocked (316) and that is far more sensitive to Aga-IVA (359). These rapidly inactivating, Ctx-MVIIC-sensitive VGCCs with this latter behavior have been dubbed Q-type channels (439), although they have also been termed O-type channels based on an earlier biochemical evaluation (1). Although the currents through isolated, expressed α_{1A} subunits show modest inactivation, when combined with various β subunits inactivation can be slowed by β_{2a} subunits (359), or markedly enhanced by β_{1b} or β_3 subunits (316,359). Figure 13 shows the differing patterns of I_{Ca} observed in oocytes with the α_{1A} subunit, depending on the type β subunit expressed with α_{1A}. These results also suggest that it is possible for the α_{1A} subunit to behave kinetically represent like the Q- or the P-type channel depending on the β subunit present.

The importance of the Q-type VGCCs in modulating Ca^{2+} entry into neuronal tissue has been documented in isolated brain synaptosomes (1,36). Furthermore, blockade of Ca^{2+} entry via this channel has been shown to inhibit catecholamine release in bovine chromaffin cells (214) and glutamate release

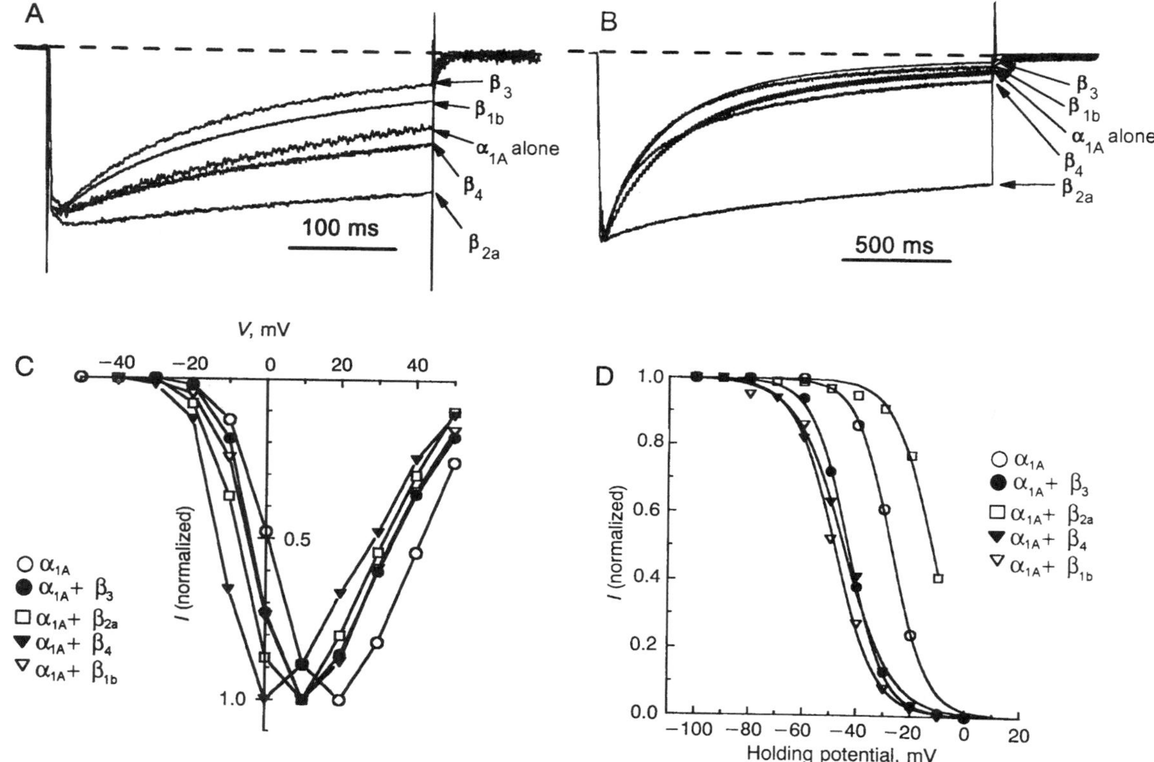

Figure 13. Effects of β-subunit coexpression on α_{1A}-current properties. **A:** Superimposed normalized current traces show differential inactivation rates of α_{1A} coexpressed with different β subunits over a 400-msec test pulse (applied voltage step from -100 mV to +10mV). **B:** Inactivation of α_{1A} currents with expression of different β subunits over a 2-sec test pulse (-100 to 10 mV). All oocytes were injected with BAPTA (2–5 mM estimated final concentration) to buffer internal Ca^{2+}. **C:** Normalized current-voltage relation of whole cell currents for α_{1A} alone, α_{1A} + β_{1b}, α_{1A} +β_{2a}, α_{1A} + β_3, and α_{1A} + β_4, where depolarizations were made from a holding potential of -100mV. **D:** Voltage dependence of inactivation for α_{1A} subunit coexpressed with β_{1b}, β_{2a}, β_3, or β_4 subunit. Oocytes were held at each holding potential for 20 sec prior to a test pulse to +10 mV. (From ref. 359, with permission.)

by hippocampal CA3 cells as assessed by depression of excitatory postsynaptic potentials (EPSPs) in CA1 cells (414). In the latter case, these channels appeared to be inhibited by activation of muscarinic, metabotropic glutamate (mGlu), adenosine, and $GABA_B$ receptors, similar to reports for N-type channels. Activation of PKC markedly augmented channel function and suppressed the receptor-mediated inhibition (288). As observed for the N-type channels in certain cell lines, modulation of Q-type channels may also exercise considerable control of neurotransmitter release.

R-Type Channels (α_{1E} Subunit)

In a number of studies of neuronal I_{Ca} (or I_{Ba}) in the presence of DHP blocking agents combined with toxins (w-Ctx (GVIA), MVIIC, Aga-IVA), an inactivating HVA current persists that is blocked by Cd^{2+} (299,439). This residual current displaying toxin-resistance has been termed R-type. One prominent feature of this current is its inactivating behavior, which makes it distinct from P-type channels. When studied in cerebellar granule cells, this DHP- and toxin-resistant current shows a slightly higher conductance for Ba^{2+} versus Ca^{2+}, and is sensitive to blockade by Cd^{2+} (IC_{50} = 1.2 μM) and Ni^{2+} (IC_{50} = 66 μM) (298,439).

Although there is electrophysiologic evidence for a channel possessing none of the characteristics of the L-, N-, P-, or Q-types, molecular physiologic techniques have isolated a class of mammalian brain mRNA encoding a typical α_1 sequence (termed BII in rabbit [258] and rbE-II in rat [349]). This VGCC subunit clone, now termed the α_{1E}, has a counterpart in marine rays termed doe-1, which has 76% amino acid identity (90). When expressed in oocytes, the resulting channel has a conductance of 14 pS, less than that reported for L- and N-type under comparable conditions (327); it also shows distinct inactivation and is resistant to blockade by DHPs, ω-Ctx (GVIA), and ω-Aga-IVA. Although certain characteristics of the current resulting from expression of the α_{1E} subunit are shared with T-type LVA currents, its pharmacology and biophysical behavior are sufficiently distinct to suggest that it is responsible for the R-type current. Four alternatively spliced variants of α_{1E} exist, with variations in the carboxy terminus as well as in the II–III cytoplasmic linker region (279,419). Since the latter region has been shown to play a prominent role in coupling to cellular events in other classes of VGCC, this may represent a site at which cell/tissue specific expression yields physiologically relevant consequences.

In situ hybridization of the α_{1E} mRNA has permitted localization of this VGCC with in the brain. The α_{1E} mRNA in rat brain is most prominent in hippocampus (pyramidal cells and granule cells of the dentate gyrus), the hypothalamus (supraoptic and tuberal regions), and the thalamus (the intralaminar, parafascicular, and reticular nuclei) (349). The subunit transcript is also present in medial habenula, substantia nigra pars compacta, dorsal raphe, pontine nuclei, inferior olive, and solitary tract nucleus. Although a specific R-type toxin has not yet been identified, its toxin resistance and distinct kinetics have permitted its functional localization in neurons. Within neurons, this channel has been localized by electrophysiologic methods to the dendrites of isolated pyramidal neurons (221). While no specific pharmacologic tool to specifically inhibit R-type channels has been defined, such DHP- and multi-toxin-resistant current in hippocampal neurons can be eliminated by the DPBP fluspirilene (30 μM) (311). When expressed α_{1E} subunits are studied, PKC activation by phorbol esters can increase the current by 30% to 40%, similar to that seen with α_{1B} subunits; however, coexpression with the β subunit is required (358).

Since this VGCC lacks a specific blocker, anesthetic alterations have not been clearly delineated. However, in hippocampal neurons, the residual, inactivating current present after application of both nitrendipine and ω-Ctx shows 44% inhibition of peak current and 71% inhibition of sustained current by 2.5% isoflurane (see Fig. 12).

Functions of Ca Channels in Neurons

As assessed by electrophysiologic experiments using toxins to eliminate the various currents, the distributions of the different Ca channels in neurons from various locations in the central and peripheral nervous system are listed in Table 6. While the L-type channels frequently account for 25% to 30% of Ca^{2+} current observed, the bulk of neuronal Ca^{2+} current is carried by the N-, P/Q-, and R-type VGCC. While there are clearly exceptions in the central nervous system, such as the Purkinje cell with its very high predominance of P-type channels, one-quarter to one-fifth of the channels observed are frequently of the N-type, P/Q-type, and R-type.

Ca Channels and Synaptic Release

The role of Ca^{2+} in mediating stimulus-secretion coupling has been appreciated for decades (79,81). In cells that secrete peptides, such as endocrine cells, L-type VGCCs contribute to the exocytotic process and are prominent in mediating secretion (210,319,362). However, the lack of a role for L-type channels in synaptic processes and fast neurotransmitter release (acetylcholine, glutamate, glycine, norepinephrine) is well established (65,250,284,296,306,367). Studies in isolated synaptosomes have documented the important role of the neuronal Ca^{2+} channels (N- and P/Q-) in mediating the rise in Ca (239, 306,385,403) and activating vesicle-mediated release (391). In mixed synaptosomes, glutamate release seems to be most sensitive to blockade of P-channels by ω-Aga-IVA (391), while the rise in Ca^{2+} activated by K^+ depolarization is likewise markedly inhibited by P-type channel blockade (385).

When assessed electrophysiologically, the VGCC mediating Ca^{2+} influx and the subsequent transmitter release varies depending on the neuronal preparation (56,106,245,284,300, 375,414). Using the polyamine FTX to block P-type channels, a prominent depression of presynaptic I_{Ca} and excitatory postsynaptic responses (EPSCs) at the mammalian neuromuscular junction was observed, an effect not seen with ω-Ctx-GVIA (395). P-type channels appear to play a prominent role in neurotransmitter release as assessed by blockade with Aga-IVA in many central neurons, particularly in the cerebellum (245, 300). The evoked release of inhibitory neurotransmitter from cerebellar cells is markedly inhibited by ω-Aga-IVA, and is less altered by N-type Ca channel blockade (375). Mossy fiber transmission in the hippocampus (49) as well as climbing fiber transmission to Purkinje fibers in the cerebellum (300) are unaffected by nifedipine, partially blocked by ω-Ctx-GVIA, and virtually abolished by 1 μM ω-Aga-IVA. In thalamic neurons, saturating ω-Ctx-GVIA depressed I_{Ca} and EPSCs by only 32% (284). Blockade by 200 nM ω-Aga-IVA of P-type in channels has also been shown to increase the tolerance of hippocampal CA1 pyramidal neurons in the rat to an ischemic insult, preserving function and preventing cell death (342). In many of the studies documenting P-type channel effects, ω-Aga-IVA concentrations of ≥200 nM have frequently been used (49,245,300,342,375), which may have inhibitory effects upon Q-type channels (298). Consequently, Wheeler et al. (414) have suggested that in hippocampal cells, neurotransmission in mediated by N- and Q-type currents. Likewise, in chromaffin cells, Q-type, in addition to L-type channels, appear to dominate control of secretion (214).

Table 6. FUNCTIONAL DISTRIBUTIONS OF DIFFERENT HVA NEURONAL Ca^{2+} CURRENTS

	Approximate Percent of VGCC type					
Neuronal type	L-type[a] (DHP sensitive)	N-type (ω-Ctx sensitive)	P-type (Aga-IVA sensitive)	Q-type	R-type	Reference
CENTRAL NERVOUS SYSTEM						
Substantia nigra	36	27	25	4	8	167
Ventromedial hypothal.	30	32	26	5	9	167
Tuberomammillary	12	43	35	3	6	167
Nuc. tractus solitarius	36	29	12	7	16	167
Hippocampal CA1 cells	38	27	13	9	13	167
	30	24		⇐ 51[b] ⇒		299
Cerebellar Purkinje cells	2	9	89	0	0	167
	8	7	92[b]	—	—	299
Cerebellar granule cells	15	20	11	35	19	298
Dentate gyrus granule cells	39	21	≤20	?	≤20	89
Visual cortex	31	41		⇐ 38[b] ⇒		299
Hypoglossal motoneurons	6	33	50[c]			397
Spinal cord	30	52		⇐ 33[b] ⇒		299
	18	35	45			234
PERIPHERAL NEURONS						
Dorsal root ganglion	31	54		⇐ 31[b] ⇒		299
Sympathetic ganglion	18	85		⇐ 10[b] ⇒		299

Failure to include T-type and overlap of sensitivities means that total % may exceed or fall below 100%.
[a]No classification of DHP-sensitive channels to α_{1C} or α_{1D}.
[b]Indicates percent of current DHP and ω-Ctx-resistance with no subclassification to P-, Q- or R-type.
[c]May include some Q-type current.
From refs. 89,167,234,298,299,397.

In central neurons, a component of neurotransmitter release appears to be contributed by N-type VGCC, since treatment with ω-Ctx-GVIA also inhibits release (203,375,423). Typically, the inhibitory postsynaptic potentials in hippocampus are inhibited by ω-Ctx more than the excitatory postsynaptic potentials, which appear somewhat more resistant (157,291,375). In synaptic transmission between CA3 and CA1 neurons, N-type and Q-type channels appear to play a predominant role (414). In a study of the granule cell synapse to Purkinje cells in the cerebellum, the P-type VGCC appeared to be most contributory to transmitter release as assessed by excitatory postsynaptic potentials (237). However, sensitivity to N-type channel blockade by ω-Ctx-GVIA indicated that multiple types of currents contribute synergistically to control release of neurotransmitter.

There are certain types of cells in which N-type channels appear to predominate in regulating transmitter release, such as in sympathetic neurons (148,281). Recordings of Ca^{2+} currents are possible in cholinergic presynaptic nerve terminals from ciliary ganglia, and in this setting the presynaptic current (355) and the postsynaptic response (354) is blockable by ω-Ctx-GVIA. The prominent role of N-type VGCC in mediating synaptic release processes is consistent with biochemical evidence that, at least for N-type channels, there is a strong association with the vesicle-release proteins syntaxin, synaptotagmin, and neurexin (208, 209,267,434). This combined association has been dubbed a "synaptosecretosome" (267), although the interaction between the various units is unclear. As noted previously, a syntaxin binding site has been demonstrated on the N-type channel (338). Considering the prominent role of P-type channel in synaptic release, a similar binding site on the large cytoplasmic II–III linker domain would be anticipated, although in P-type channels this region shares only a 38% sequence homology with the N-type channel (338).

Anesthetic Effects How much anesthetic inhibition of VGCCs might contribute to a decrease in neurotransmitter release and communication between central neurons is not yet defined. Although miniature end-plate postsynaptic potentials are unchanged by thiopental and pentobarbital, these agents can decrease neurotransmitter release by spinal motorneurons (407), while pentobarbital at anesthetic levels depresses Ca^{2+}-dependent action potentials (142). Both thiopental and halothane in vivo have been found to decrease the probability of transmitter release from spinal motorneurons, attributable to a presynaptic site of action (194). Isoflurane in hippocampal neurons (241) and halothane in rat spinal neurons (378) dose-dependently decreased synaptic transmission, attributed to depression of presynaptic release. In isolated synaptosomes, volatile anesthetics can be shown to depress both the $[Ca^{2+}]_i$ transients and neurotransmitter release (232,324). One study has attributed the anesthetic effect to possible actions on Na channels, observing little effect attributable to anesthetic-induced VGCC effects (324). However, a similar study identified close parallels between the decreases in intrasynaptosomal $[Ca^{2+}]$ and glutamate release, which could be induced by either isoflurane, halothane, or enflurane, or by reducing $[Ca^{2+}]$ in the medium (232). In contrast, halothane and isoflurane have been found not to inhibit the release of the inhibitory neurotransmitter GABA from rat striatal synaptosomes, although decreased release could be achieved by thiopental (0.01–1 mM) and by N-type channel blockade by ω-conotoxin (203). When Ca^{2+} transients are assessed in intact cultured neurons, isoflurane, halothane, enflurane, as well as methohexital can depress the depolarization induced rise in Ca^{2+} (28). Since this effect is not observed with nimodipine, neuronal VGCC are implicated in the observed depression.

Postsynaptic Ca Channels

It is also important to note the subcellular distribution of the channels in neurons. The neuronal channels typically appear to be more prominent at pre- and postsynaptic locations, in contrast to the cell soma. For example, the N-type Ca channel appears to be localized predominantly on dendrites, as assessed by antipeptide antibody staining (412). Both dendritic shafts and postsynaptic structures upon the dendrites were found to be labeled. In the dentate gyrus, the mossy fibers of granule cells were heavily labeled at their large terminals, indicating the high density of N-type VGCC in this region. The cell bodies of pyramidal cells in the cerebral cortex, as well as the Purkinje cells and other cell bodies, were typically labeled at a very low level.

When assessed by electrophysiologic techniques, hippocampal CA1 pyramidal neurons show prominent evidence of a 17 pS channel, which is neither N, P, nor Q type, and appears to represent the α_{1E} subunit on the dendritic shafts. Such neurons demonstrated evidence of all of the major types of Ca channels on the neuronal soma, although the dominant types appear to be the N and L type (221).

Neuronal L-Type Channels

The endocrine L-type channel (α_{1D}) accounts for only about 20% of neuronal L-type channels; they appear to be uniformly distributed in the cell soma and in proximal dendrites (135). A specific splice variant of α_{1C} channels as assessed by antibodies binding assays accounts for the large majority (80%) of neuronal L-type VGCC. In addition, the α_{1C} subunit channels are distributed in clusters within the cell soma, particularly near proximal dendrites (135), with little presence on the dendrites themselves. Although neurotransmitter release is not coupled to L-type channels, such channel may contribute to neuronal function in other ways. In ciliary ganglion neurons, blockade of N-type channels does not inhibit activation of Ca^{2+}-activated K current ($I_{K(Ca)}$), while L-type VGCC blockade did decrease $I_{K(Ca)}$ (421). In contrast, in sympathetic neurons, N-type VGCC blockade clearly decreased $I_{K(Ca)}$. The L-type VGCC also seem to be important in directing and regulating the growth cones and neurite outgrowth from neurons during development (11,308). The clustering of the L-type channels causes a Ca^{2+} "hotspot" in the cell, regions of locally elevated $[Ca^{2+}]_i$ that activate protein synthesis and development of growth cones (340). Likewise, the presence of L-type channels may modulate neurotransmitter-related enzyme expression, since the effects can be modulated by DHP antagonists and agonists (401). The expression of L-type VGCC can also be altered depending on the growth medium, for example, depending on whether normal or elevated concentrations of K^+ are present (298).

T-TYPE CA CHANNELS

The particular gene responsible for the α-subunit of T-type VGCCs has not yet been identified. The rapidly inactivating behavior of the α_{1E} subunit is consistent with $I_{Ca,T}$; however, when α_{1E} is expressed in oocytes it activates at less negative potentials than is typical of T-type channels, and shows somewhat slower activation behavior. The activation of T-type channels with modest depolarizations (hence the designation low-voltage activated [LVA]), the distinctive rapid inactivation of currents, and the modest single channel conductance permitted their early identification as a distinct type of Ca^{2+} current (8,47,259). While it has not been possible to employ immunocytochemical techniques to permit tissue localization of T-type channels as employed for other Ca channels, the distinct biophysical characteristics of the T-type channel have been used to demonstrate its wide distribution. It has been studied in detail in dorsal root ganglion cells (215,282,377), Purkinje cells (175), thalamic (348,368) and hippocampal (425) neurons, pituitary cells (8,136,223), ventricular (240,259,393) and atrial (18) myocytes, and smooth muscle cells (3,84,111). An additional feature is the slow deactivation, that is, the slow rate of closing upon returning to the resting potential that permitted its early definition in pituitary cells (223). Unlike L-type channels, T-type VGCCs do not "run down" with whole cell perfusion and do not appear to require phosphorylation to be active (136,223). It is also of interest that removal of sialic acid from the exterior of the sarcolemma with neuraminidase markedly increased $I_{Ca,T}$ in cardiac myocytes, while $I_{Ca,L}$ was unaffected (433).

The distinctive low conductance of these channels has permitted identification, but has sometimes limited studies of their microscopic gating behavior. Typically, following a brief pause after depolarization, these channels show bursts of opening, and the open probability correlates with that observed from the average of the ensemble currents (84). The time to the first opening also correlates strongly with the time constant of activation, decreasing markedly with depolarization. The channel inactivates rapidly (time constant ~20 msec) once activated, with little voltage dependence, and recovery has a fast (200 msec) and slow (1–2 sec) components . Sustained depolarizations of greater than 4 sec positive to -70 mV are required for half of the channels to be inactivated. Another feature of the T-type channel observed with single channel recording is the presence of a subconductance state, although its relevance is unclear (84).

As in other Ca channels, Ca^{2+} inhibits passage of monovalent ions through the T-type channel (K_D = 1.8 μM). The blockade is voltage dependent, however, which is best accounted for by a single, centrally located Ca^{2+} binding site (215). The ion binding sites within the pore are also distinct from the other VGCCs in that they are sensitive to blockade by 100 to 200 μM Ni^{2+} (13,107,175), relatively resistant to blockade by Cd^{2+} (136,175), and show no enhanced conductance in the presence of Ba^{2+} (98,136). However, the LVA channels of rat clonal pituitary GH3 cells (136) and lateral geniculate cells (64) appear relatively more resistant to blockade by Ni^{2+}. Whereas inhibition by Ni^{2+} characterizes the expressed α_{1E} subunit, its depression by Cd^{2+} is atypical for T-type channels. Furthermore, expressed α_{1E} subunits have a single channel conductance of 14 pS, almost twice that of T-type VGCC (327).

Physiologic Role and Modulation

The relatively high probability of opening and modest inactivation rates at membrane potentials of -60 to -40 mV permit T-type channels to play a prominent role in pacemaking behavior of various cells. Current through these channels is the major source of Ca^{2+} entry during subthreshold depolarizations (13). Activation at these lower voltages contributes to depolarization, which ultimately reaches threshold and leads to an action potential. T-type currents are present in cardiac pacemaking tissues (126,166) and in cardiac Purkinje fibers (146). Ni^{2+}, at concentrations sufficient for T-type channel blockade, slows the diastolic depolarization of sinoatrial and AV nodal tissue (126,166). Likewise, these channels appear to play a prominent role in the pacemaking and the spontaneous action potential bursting behavior of thalamic neurons (368,415). In neurons of the lateral geniculate nucleus, depolarizations of greater than 30 mV/sec are necessary to permit activation of $I_{Ca,T}$ in a fashion that can contribute to depolarization or AP generation (64). The distinctive slow steady-state inactivation and rapid recovery from fast inactivation may permit the channel to contribute depolarizing currents around threshold, yet show more profound inactivation with bursts of spiking activity. Although the most prominent role of T-type channels appears to be in pacemaking, it also plays a role in secretory activity in certain cells. In adrenal glomerulosa cells, steroidogenesis and aldosterone secretion is activated by elevations in [Ca^{2+}] (46). Blockade of L-type channels shows modest effects on Ca^{2+} influx in these cells (226), while blockade of T-type VGCC by tetrandrine (212) also inhibits steroidogenesis (309).

T-type VGCCs appear to be specifically regulated during development in a number of tissues. These channels are present in embryonic tissue (13,229), but decline markedly during embryonic growth, at least in motor neurons (229). T-type VGCCs show variable presence in the cells bodies of neurons in later development, maintaining prominence in the dendritic arborizations as the neurons mature (221). Developmental changes in neurons contrast with myocardium, in which $I_{Ca,T}$ density increases as the cells mature (413). This increased $I_{Ca,T}$ may be mediated by growth hormone (424).

T-type VGCC appear to be modulated by G proteins, as assessed by GTPγS activation of G protein α subunits (and release βγ subunits), or by stimulation of $GABA_B$ receptors. With low levels of stimulation there is activation, but high stimulation levels result in depression of $I_{Ca,T}$ (331). Activation of adrenal glomerulosa cells by angiotensin II results in activation of $I_{Ca,T}$ (60). However, specific activation of AT_2 receptors in another cell line, which typically decreases cGMP within cells, can in contrast decrease $I_{Ca,T}$ (41).

Pharmacologic Behavior

Unlike other Ca channels, no high-affinity drug or toxin that is highly specific for T-type channels has been described. The effects of the classic L-type VGCC blockers is variable; while PAAs and diltiazem typically possess IC_{50} values above 40 μM, DHPs have an IC_{50} ranging from 0.7 to 50 μM, depending on the tissue studied (136). Such varied responses make it possible that currents blocked by ≥10 μM DHPs and attributed to L-type currents may have included some component of $I_{Ca,T}$. Amiloride (10–100 μM) has been proposed as a specific blocker of T-type channels (383,394); however, relatively high concentrations are required for certain LVA Ca^{2+} currents (136). Valproic acid, a commonly used antiseizure medication, has been demonstrated to be a specific inhibitor of T-type channels (10), which may contribute to its antiepileptic activity. Although tetrandrine binds to the BTZ site on L-type VGCC, in neuroblastoma cells it has an even lower EC_{50} for inhibition of $I_{Ca,T}$ (9 μM) compared to its EC_{50} for $I_{Ca,L}$ (~30 μM) (212). The DPBP class of antipsychotics (94,95) as well as the flunarizine class of compounds have been shown to block T-type channels (404); however, their blockade of other channels suggests that they too lack specificity. A diphenylmethylpiperazine (U-92032) has been found to be a potent and selective T-type Ca channel antagonist, which appears to have the ability to protect neurons from ischemic injury at least as effectively as flunarizine (168). Clearly, the role of T-type channels in mediating

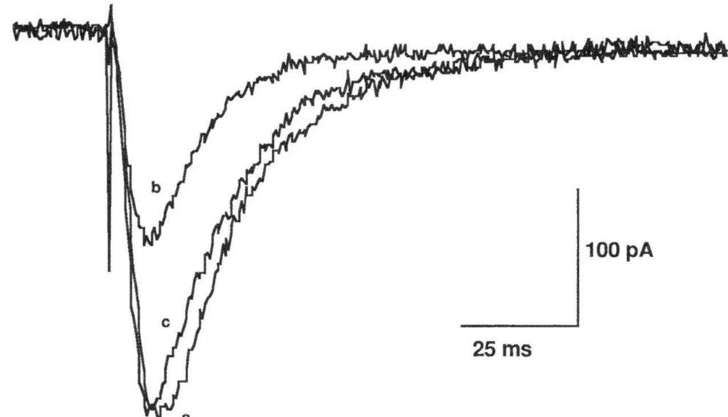

Figure 14. Effects of isoflurane on T-type Ca^{2+} currents recorded from a C-type thyroid cell line (calcitonin secreting). Currents observed were elicited under whole cell patch clamp, with a holding potential of –80 mV and a depolarization to –30 mV. a: control; b: 2.5% isoflurane; c: recovery from isoflurane. (Data courtesy of T.S. McDowell and J. J. Pancrazio.)

Table 7. CELLULAR FUNCTION OF VGCC

VGCC type	α_1 Subunit classification	Tissue location	Subcellular site	Function	Mechanism
	α_{1S}	Skeletal muscle	T-tubules, especially at junctional SR	Excitation-contraction coupling	Direct coupling to ryanodine receptors to activate SR Ca^{2+} release
	$\alpha_{1C\text{-}a}$	Heart	Surface and t-tubular sarcolemma	Excitation-contraction coupling	Ca^{2+} entry opens ryanodine receptors to release stored Ca^{2+} (CIRC)
L-type (HVA)	$\alpha_{1C\text{-}b}$	Smooth muscle	Surface membrane	Excitation-contraction coupling	Ca^{2+} binds to calmodulin and activates MLCK and contractile cascade; some CICR may be present
	$\alpha_{1C\text{-}c}$	Brain, neurons	Cell soma and axon hillock	?Modulation of neuronal growth	Ca^{2+} entry activates various cell growth pathways
	α_{1D}	Pancreas, endocrine tissues, brain	Soma and larger dendrites of neurons	Endocrine cell excitation-secretion coupling	Ca^{2+} entry activates release of endocrine peptides
N-type (HVA)	α_{1B}	Brain, peripheral neurons	Presynaptic and dendrites	Excitation-secretion coupling, modulation of cell growth	Mediated in part via synaptotagmin binding site? Ca^{2+} entry mobilizes vesicles
Q-type (HVA)	α_{1A}	Brain, kidney	Presynaptic	Excitation-secretion coupling	Mediated in part via synaptotagmin binding site? Ca^{2+} entry mobilizes vesicles
P-type (HVA)	α_{1A}	Neuronal	Presynaptic and dendrites	Excitation-secretion coupling, neuromuscular junction and centrally	Mediated in part via synaptotagmin binding site? Ca^{2+} entry mobilizes vesicles
R-type (HVA)	α_{1E}	Brain	Neuronal soma and dendrites		
T-type (LVA)	?	Cardiovascular and neuronal tissues	? surface membrane	Pacemaking, gradual depolarization leading to single or multiple APs	Ca^{2+} entry depolarizes cell to threshold for other channels

HVA, high-voltage-activated; LVA, low-voltage-activated; SR, sarcoplasmic reticulum; AP, action potential; CICR, Ca^{2+}-induced Ca^{2+} release.

ischemic damage would be of interest due to their widespread presence in a variety of neuronal tissues.

Anesthetic Effects

Anesthetics can have relatively profound effects on $I_{Ca,T}$. In rat sensory neurons, T-type currents had an EC_{50} of ~100 μM (equivalent to ~0.15% halothane gas phase) (377). In hippocampal pyramidal neurons, 2.5% isoflurane depressed $I_{Ca,T}$ by ~75% (365). Likewise, in calcitonin-secreting thyroid C cells, in which large component of the current is T-type, there is marked depression by isoflurane, halothane, enflurane, and sevoflurane (Fig. 14). In contrast, Herrington et al. (137) observed far more modest effects of anesthetics on $I_{Ca,T}$ in GH3 cells. Whether such blockade of T-type channels by anesthetics might contribute to the anesthetic state, perhaps by altering spontaneous potentials in thalamic neurons, or alter physiologic regulations by interfering with certain secretory effects remains unproven. Propofol (300 μM) caused an 80% depression of LVA VGCCs in chick sensory neurons, but whether any significant effect occurs at clinical concentrations of free (non-protein bound) drug is uncertain (269). In mouse dorsal root ganglion cells, pentobarbital was without effect on LVA Ca^{2+} currents (117).

CONCLUSIONS

The various VGCC types, their primary α_1 subunit, and their function in the various tissues in which they appear are summarized in Table 7. While Ca^{2+} entry via VGCC plays a critical role in the function of various cells, in some tissues these ubiquitous membrane proteins link membrane depolarization directly to cellular processes. Of the three major types of dihydropyridine-sensitive channels (L-type), the skeletal muscle type is an intrinsic component of excitation-contraction coupling. In other muscle tissue and endocrine cells, Ca^{2+} influx is mediated by these channels and plays a prominent activating role. Of the four major types of neuronal VGCC, at least three forms appear to couple depolarization to vesicle release of neurotransmitters, in part directly. Considering the critical activating and regulating role played by Ca^{2+} in so many tissues, it is not surprising that Ca^{2+} entry via these channels is carefully modulated. The VGCCs exhibit marked intrinsic modulation by Ca^{2+} itself, with regard to permeation, inactivation, and indirect modulation of channel opening. Extrinsic modulation of VGCCs by various neuroendocrine mediators in order to regulate signal transmission and the degree of cell activation is widely evident in various tissues. Since Ca^{2+} entry represents depolarizing current, VGCCs can also serve a role by mediating depolarization, especially pacemaking; the T-type VGCC appears to play a prominent role in this regard.

ACKNOWLEDGMENTS

The author thanks Joseph J. Pancrazio for invaluable discussion and sharing unpublished data, and Anna Hall Evans for excellent editorial assistance. The author's research has been funded by NIH grant GM-31144.

REFERENCES

1. Adams ME, Myers RA, Imperial JS, Olivera BM. Toxityping rat brain calcium channels with ω-toxins from spider and cone snail venoms. *Biochemistry* 1993;32:12566–12570.
2. Agus ZS, Kelepouris E, Dukes I, Morad M. Cytosolic magnesium modulates calcium channel activity in mammalian ventricular cells. *Am J Physiol* 1989;256:C452–C455.
3. Akaike N, Kanaide H, Kuga T, Nakamura M, Sadoshima J, Tomoike H. Low-voltage-activated calcium current in rat aorta smooth muscle cells in primary culture. *J Physiol* 1989;416:141–160.
4. Allen TJA, Chapman RA. The effect of a chemical phosphatase on single calcium channels and the inactivation of whole-cell calcium current from isolated guinea-pig ventricular myocytes. *Pflugers Arch* 1995;430:68–80.
5. Aosaki T, Kasai H. Characterization of two kinds of high-voltage-

activated Ca-channel currents in chick sensory neurons. Differential sensitivity to dihydropyridines and omega-conotoxin GVIA. *Pflugers Arch* 1989;414:150–156.
6. Armstrong CM, Bezanilla F. Currents related to the movement of gating particles of the sodium channel. *Nature* 1973;242:459–461.
7. Armstrong CM, Bezanilla FM, Horowicz P. Twitches in the presence of ethylene-glycol-bis(β-amino-ethyl ether)-*N,N'*-tetraacetic acid. *Biochim Biophys Acta* 1972;267:605–608.
8. Armstrong CM, Matteson DR. Two distinct populations of calcum channels in a clonal line of pituitary cells. *Science* 1985;227:65–67.
9. Armstrong D, Eckert R. Voltage-activated calcium channels that must be phosphorylated to respond to membrane depolarization. *Proc Natl Acad Sci USA* 1987;84:2518–2522.
10. Ashcroft FM, Kelly RP, Smith PA. Two types of Ca channel in rat pancreatic β cells. *Pflugers Arch* 1990; 415:504–506.
11. Audesirk G, Audesirk T, Ferguson C, et al. L-type calcium channels may regulate neurite initiation in cultured chick embryo brain neurons and N1E-115 neuroblastoma cells. *Dev Brain Res* 1990; 55:109–120.
12. Augustine GJ, Charlton MP, Smith SJ. Calcium action in synaptic transmitter action. *Annu Rev Neurosci* 1987;10:633–653.
13. Barish ME. Voltage-gated calcium currents in cultured embryonic *Xenopus* spinal neurones. *J Physiol* 1991;444:523–543.
14. Bates SE, Gurney AM. Ca^{2+}-dependent block and potentiation of L-type calcium current in guinea-pig ventricular myocytes. *J Physiol* 1993;466:345–365.
15. Bayer R, Kalusche D, Kaufmann R, Mannhold R. Inotropic and electrophysiological actions of verapamil and D600 in mammalian myocardium. III. Effects of optical isomers on transmembrane action potentials. *Naunyn Schmiedebergs Arch Pharmacol* 1975;290: 87–97.
16. Beam KG, Adams BA, Niidome T, Numa S, Tanabe T. Function of a truncated dihydropyridine receptor as both voltage sensor and calcium channel. *Nature* 1992;360:169–171.
17. Bean BP. Nitrendipine block of cardiac calcium channels: high-affinity to the inactivated state. *Proc Natl Acad Sci USA* 1984;81: 6388–6392.
18. Bean BP. Two kinds of calcium channels in canine atrial cells: differences in kinetics, selectivity, and pharmacology. *J Gen Physiol* 1985;86:1–31.
19. Bean BP. Neurotransmitter inhibition of neuronal calcium currents by changes in channel voltage dependence. *Nature* 1989;340: 153–156.
20. Bean BP. β-Adrenergic modulation of cardiac calcium channel gating. In: Spooner PM, Brown AM, Catterall WA, Kaczorowski GJ, Strauss HC, eds. *Ion channels in the cardiovascular system.* Armonk, NY: Futura, 1994;237–252.
21. Bean BP, Nowycky MC, Tsien RW. β-Adrenergic modulation of calcium channels in frog ventricular heart cells. *Nature* 1984;307: 371–375.
22. Bean BP, Rios E. Nonlinear charge movement in mammalian cardiac ventricular cells. *J Gen Physiol* 1989;94:65–93.
23. Bechem M, Pott L. Removal of Ca current inactivation in dialysed guinea-pig atrial cardioballs by Ca chelators. *Pflugers Arch* 1985; 404:10–20.
24. Biel M, Hullin R, Freunder S, et al. Tissue-specific expression of high-voltage-activated dihydropyridine-sensitive L-type calcium channels. *Eur J Biochem* 1991;200:81–88.
25. Biel M, Ruth P, Bosse E, et al. Primary structure and functional expression of a high voltage activated calcium channel from rabbit lung. *FEBS Lett* 1990; 269:409–412.
26. Birnbaumer L, Campbell KP, Catterall WA, et al. The naming of voltage-gated calcium channels. *Neuron* 1994;13:505–506.
27. Blanck TJJ, Runge S, Stevenson RL. Halothane decreases calcium channel antagonist binding to cardiac membranes. *Anesth Analg* 1988;67:1032–1035.
28. Bleakman D, Jones MV, Harrison NL. The effects of four general anesthetics on intracellular $[Ca^{2+}]$ in cultured rat hippocampal neurons. *Neuropharmacology* 1995;34:541–551.
29. Bley KR, Tsien RW. Inhibition of Ca^{2+} and K^+ channels in sympathetic neurons by neuropeptides and other ganglionic transmitters. *Neuron* 1990; 2:379–391.
30. Block BA, Imagawa T, Campbell KP, Franzini-Armstrong C. Structural evidence for direct interaction between the molecular components of the transverse tubule/sarcoplasmic reticulum junction in skeletal muscle. *J Cell Biol* 1988;107:2587–2600.
31. Bokvist K, Eliasson L, Ammala C, Renstrom E, Rorsman P. Co-localization of L-type Ca channels and insulin-containing secretory granules and its significance for the initiation of exocytosis in mouse pancreatic β cells. *EMBO J* 1995;14:50–57.
32. Boland LM, Allen AC, Dingledine R. Inhibition by bradykinin of voltage-activated barium current in a rat dorsal root ganglion cell line: role of protein kinase C. *J Neurosci* 1991;11:1140–1149.
33. Boland LM, Bean BP. Modulation of N-type calcium channels in bullfrog sympathetic neurons by luteinizing hormone-releasing hormone: kinetics and voltage dependence. *J Neurosci* 1993;13: 516–533.
34. Bosnjak ZJ, Supan FD, Rusch NJ. The effects of halothane, enflurane and isoflurane on calcium currents in isolated canine ventricular cells. *Anesthesiology* 1991;74:340–345.
35. Bourinet E, Charnet P, Tomlinson WJ, Stea A, Snutch TP, Nargeot J. Voltage-dependent facilitation of a neuronal α_{1C} L-type calcium channel. *EMBO J* 1994;13:5032–5039.
36. Bowman D, Alexander S, Lodge D. Pharmacological characterisation of the calcium channels coupled to the plateau phase of KCl-induced intracellular free Ca^{2+} elevation in chicken and rat synaptosomes. *Neuropharmacology* 1993;32:1195–1202.
37. Brickley K, Campbell V, Berrow N, et al. Use of site-directed antibodies to probe the topography of the α_2 subunit of voltage-gated Ca channels. *FEBS Lett* 1995;364:129–133.
38. Brown DA. G-proteins and potassium currents in neurons. *Annu Rev Physiol* 1990; 52:215–242.
39. Brum G, Flockerzi V, Hofmann F, Osterrieder W, Trautwein W. Injection of catalytic subunit of cAMP-dependent protein kinase into isolated cardiac myocytes. *Pflugers Arch* 1983;398:147–154.
40. Brum G, Osterrieder W, Trautwein W. β-adrenergic increase in the calcium conductance of cardiac myocytes studied with the patch clamp. *Pflugers Arch* 1984;401:111–118.
41. Buisson B, Bottari SP, de Gasparo M, Gallo-Payet N, Payet MD. The angiotensin AT_2 receptor modulates T-type calcium current in non-differentiated NG108-15 cells. *FEBS Lett* 1992;309:161–164.
42. Buljubasic N, Rusch NJ, Marijic J, Kampine JP, Bosnjak ZJ. Effects of halothane and isoflurane on calcium and potassium channel currents in canine coronary arterial cells. *Anesthesiology* 1992;76: 990–998.
43. Campbell DL, Rasmusson RL, Strauss HL. Theoretical study of the voltage and concentration dependence of the anomalous mole fraction effect in single calcium channels. New insights into the characterization of multi-ion channels. *Biophys J* 1988;54: 945–954.
44. Campbell V, Berrow N, Dolphin AC. $GABA_B$ receptor modulation of Ca^{2+} currents in rat sensory neurones by the G protein G_o: antisense oligonucleotide studies. *J Physiol* 1993;470:1–11.
45. Campbell V, Berrow NS, Fitzgerald EM, Brickley K, Dolphin AC. Inhibition of the interaction of G protein G_o with calcium channel β subunit in rat neurons. *J Physiol* 1995;485:365–372.
46. Capponi AM, Rossier MF, Davies E, Vallotton MB. Calcium stimulates steroidogenesis in permeabilized bovine adrenal cortical cells. *J Biol Chem* 1988;263:16113–16117.
47. Carbone E, Lux HD. A low voltage-activated, fully inactivating Ca channel in vertebrate sensory neurones. *Nature* 1984;310:501–502.
48. Castellano A, Wei X, Birnbaumer L, Perez-Reyes E. Cloning and expression of a third calcium channel β subunit. *J Biol Chem* 1993; 268:3450–3455.
49. Castillo PE, Weisskopf MG, Nicoll RA. The role of Ca channels in hippocampal mossy fiber synaptic transmission and long-term potentiation. *Neuron* 1994;12:261–269.
50. Catterall WA, Seagar MJ, Takahashi M. Molecular properties of dihydropyridine-sensitive calcium channels in skeletal muscle. *J Biol Chem* 1988;263:3535–3538.
51. Catterall WA, Striessnig J. Receptor sites for Ca channel antagonists. *Trends Pharmacol Sci* 1992;13:256–262.
52. Cavalie A, Ochi R, Pelzer D, Trautwein W. Elementary currents through Ca channels in guinea pig myocytes. *Pflugers Arch* 1983; 398:284–297.
53. Chandler WK, Rakowski RF, Schneider MF. A non-linear voltage dependent charge movement in frog skeletal muscle. *J Physiol* 1976;254:245–283.
54. Chapman RA. The effect of oximes on the dihydropyridine-sensitive Ca current of isolated guinea-pig ventricular myocytes. *Pflugers Arch* 1993;422:325–331.
55. Charlesworthy P, Pocock G, Richards CD. Calcium channel currents in bovine adrenal chromaffin cells and their modulation by anaesthetic agents. *J Physiol* 1994;481:543–553.

56. Charlton MP, Augustine GJ. Classification of presynaptic calcium channels at the squid giant synapse: neither T-, L- nor N-type. *Brain Res* 1990; 525:133–139.
57. Chen C, Schofield GG. Nitric oxide modulates Ca channel currents in rat sympathetic neurons. *Eur J Pharmacol* 1993;243:83–86.
58. Chen C, Schofield GG. Nitric oxide donors enhanced Ca^{2+} currents and blocked noradrenaline-induced Ca^{2+} current inhibition in rat sympathetic neurons. *J Physiol* 1995;482:521–531.
59. Chin H, Kozak CA, Kim H-L, Mock B, McBride OW. A brain L-type calcium channel α_1 subunit gene (CCHL1A2) maps to mouse chromosome 14 and human chromosome 3. *Genomics* 1991;11:914–919.
60. Cohen CJ, McCarthy RT, Barrett PQ, Rasmussen H. Calcium channels in adrenal glomerulosa cells: potassium and angiotensin II increase T-type current. *Proc Natl Acad Sci USA* 1988;85:2412–2416.
61. Connelly TJ, Coronado R. Activation of the Ca^{2+} release channel of cardiac sarcoplasmic reticulum by volatile anesthetics. *Anesthesiology* 1994;81:459–469.
62. Cook DL, Satin LS, Hopkins WF. Pancreatic β cells are bursting, but how? *Trends Neurosci* 1991;14:411–414.
63. Coppola T, Waldmann R, Borsotto M, et al. Molecular cloning of an N-type calcium channel α_1 subunit: evidence for isoforms, brain distribution, and chromosomal localization. *FEBS Lett* 1994;338:1–5.
64. Crunelli V, Lightowler S, Pollard CE. A T-type Ca^{2+} current underlies low-threshold Ca^{2+} potentials in cells of the cat and rat lateral geniculate nucleus. *J Physiol* 1989;413:543–561.
65. Daniell LC, Barr EM, Leslie SW. $^{45}Ca^{2+}$ uptake into rat whole brain synaptosomes unaltered by dihydropyridine calcium antagonists. *J Neurochem* 1983;41:1455–1459.
66. De Jongh KS, Warner C, Catterall WA. Subunits of purified calcium channels: alpha 2 and delta are encoded by the same gene. *J Biol Chem* 1990;265:14738–14741.
67. de Leon M, Wang Y, Jones L, et al. Essential Ca^{2+}-binding motif for Ca^{2+}-sensitive inactivation of Ca channels. *Science* 1995;270: 1502–1506.
68. De Waard M, Pragnell M, Campbell KP. Ca channel regulation by a conserved β subunit domain. *Neuron* 1994;13:495–503.
69. DeFelice LJ. Molecular and biophysical view of the Ca channel: a hypothesis regarding oligomeric structure, channel clustering, and macroscopic current. *J Membr Biol* 1993;133:191–202.
70. Delcour AH, Lipscombe D, Tsien RW. Multiple mosed of N-type calcium channel activity distinguished by differences in gating kinetics. *J Neurosci* 1993;13:181–194.
71. Delcour AH, Tsien RW. Altered prevalence of gating modes in neurotransmitter inhibition of N-type calcium channels. *Science* 1993;259:980–984.
72. Dichtl A, Vierling W. Inhibition by magnesium of calcium inward current in heart ventricular muscle. *Eur J Pharmacol* 1991;204: 243–248.
73. Diebold RJ, Koch WJ, Ellinor PT, et al. Mutually exclusive exon splicing of the cardiac calcium channel α_1 subunit gene generates developmentally regulated isoforms in the rat heart. *Proc Natl Acad Sci USA* 1992;89:1497–1501.
74. Dingledine R, Somjen G. Calcium dependence of synaptic transmission in the hippocampal slice. *Brain Res* 1981;207:218–222.
75. Diversé-Peirluissi M, Goldsmith PK, Dunlap K. Transmitter-mediated inhibition of N-type calcium channels in sensory neurons involves multiple GTP-binding proteins and subunits. *Neuron* 1995;14:191–200.
76. Dolphin AC. G protein modulation of calcium currents in neurons. *Annu Rev Physiol* 1990; 52:243–255.
77. Dolphin AC, Forda SR, Scott RH. Calcium-dependent currents in cultured rat dorsal root ganglion neurones are inhibited by an adenosine analogue. *J Physiol* 1986;373:47–61.
78. Dolphin AC, Scott RH. Calcium channel currents and their inhibition by (-)-baclofen in rat sensory neurones: modulation by their guanine nucleotides. *J Physiol* 1987;386:1–17.
79. Douglas WW, Poisner AM. Calcium movement in the neurohypophysis of the rat and its relation to the release of vasopressin. *J Physiol* 1964;172:19–30.
80. Douglas WW, Poisner AM. Stimulus-secretion coupling in a neurosecretory organ: the role of calcium in the release of vasopressin from the neurohypophysis. *J Physiol* 1964;172:1–18.
81. Douglas WW, Rubin RP. The role of calcium in the secretory response of the adrenal medulla to acetylcholine. *J Physiol* 1961; 159:40–57.
82. Drenger B, Ginosar Y, Chandra M, Reches A, Gozal Y. Halothane modifies ischemia-associated injury to the voltage-sensitive calcium channels in canine heart sarcolemma. *Anesthesiology* 1994;81: 221–228.
83. Drenger B, Quigg M, Blanck TJJ. Volatile anesthetics depress calcium channel blocker binding to bovine cardiac sarcolemma. *Anesthesiology* 1991;74:155–165.
84. Droogmans G, Nilius B. Kinetic properties of the cardiac T-type calcium channel in the guinea-pig. *J Physiol* 1989;419:627–650.
85. Dubel SJ, Starr TVB, Hell J, et al. Molecular cloning of the α-1 subunit of an ω-conotoxin-sensitive calcium channel. *Proc Natl Acad Sci USA* 1992;89:5058–5062.
86. Eckert R, Chad JE. Inactivation of Ca channels. *Prog Biophys Mol Biol* 1984;44:215–267.
87. Eilers J, Callewaert G, Armstrong C, Konnerth A. Calcium signaling in a narrow somatic submembrane shell during synaptic activity in cerebellar Purkinje neurons. *Proc Natl Acad Sci USA* 1995;92: 10272–10276.
88. El-Hayek R, Antoniu B, Wang J, Hamilton SL, Ikemoto N. Identification of calcium release-triggering and blocking regions of the II-III loop of the skeletal muscle dihydropyridine receptor. *J Biol Chem* 1995;270:22116–22118.
89. Eliot LS, Johnston D. Multiple components of calcium current in acutely dissociated dentate gyrus granule neurons. *J Neurophysiol* 1994;72:762–777.
90. Ellinor PT, Zhang J-F, Randall AD, et al. Functional expression of a rapidly inactivating neuronal calcium channel. *Proc Natl Acad Sci USA* 1993;363:455–458.
91. Ellis SB, Williams ME, Ways NR, et al. Sequence and expression of mRNAs encoding the α_1 and α_2 subunits of a DHP-sensitive calcium channel. *Science* 1988;241:1661–1664.
92. Elmslie KS. Calcium current modulation in frog sympathetic neurones: multiple neurotransmitters and G proteins. *J Physiol* 1992; 451:229–246.
93. Elmslie KS, Zhou W, Jones SW. LHRH and GTP-g-S modify calcium current activation in bullfrog sympathetic neurons. *Neuron* 1990; 5:75–80.
94. Enyeart JJ, Biagi BA, Day RN, Sheu S, Maurer RA. Blockade of low and high threshold Ca channels by diphenylbutylpiperidine antipsychotics linked to inhibition of prolactin gene expression. *J Biol Chem* 1990; 265:16373–16379.
95. Enyeart JJ, Biagi BA, Mlinar B. Preferential block of T-type calcium channels by neuroleptics in neural crest-derived rat and human C cell lines. *Mol Pharmacol* 1992;42:364–372.
96. Ewald DA, Sternweis PC, Miler RJ. Guanine nucleotide-binding protein G_o-induced coupling of neuropeptide Y receptors to Ca channels in sensory neurons. *Proc Natl Acad Sci USA* 1988;85: 3633–3637.
97. Fatt P, Katz B. The electrical properties of crustacean muscle fibers. *J Physiol* 1953;120:171–204.
98. Fedulova SA, Kostyuk PG, Veselovsky NS. Two types of calcium channels in the somatic membrane of new-born rat dorsal root ganglion neurones. *J Physiol* 1985;359:431–446.
99. Ffrench-Mullen JM, Barker JL, Rogawski MA. Calcium current block by (+)-pentobarbital, phenobarbital, and CHEB but not (+)-pentobarbital in acutely isolated hippocampal CA1 neurons: comparison with effects on GABA-activated Cl- current. *J Neurosci* 1993; 13:3211–3221.
100. Ffrench-Mullen JMH. Cortisol inhibition of calcium currents in guinea pig hippocampal CA1 neurons via G-protein-coupled activation of protein kinase C. *J Neurosci* 1995;15:903–911.
101. Field AC, Hill C, Lamb GD. Asymmetric charge movement and calcium currents in ventricular myocytes of neonatal rat. *J Physiol* 1988;406:277–297.
102. Fishman MC, Spector I. Potassium current suppression by quinidine reveals additional calcium currents in neuroblastoma cells. *Proc Natl Acad Sci USA* 1981;78:5245–5249.
103. Fleckenstein A. Specific pharmacology of calcium in myocardium, cardiac pacemakers, and vascular smooth muscle. *Annu Rev Pharmacol Toxicol* 1977;17:149–166.
104. Flockerzi V, Oeken H-J, Hofmann F. Purification of a functional receptor for calcium-channel blockers from rabbit skeletal-muscle microsomes. *Eur J Biochem* 1986;161:217–224.
105. Forscher P, Oxford GS, Schultz D. Noradrenaline modulates calcium channels in avian dorsal ganglion cells through tight receptor-channel coupling. *J Physiol* 1986;379:131–144.
106. Fossier P, Baux G, Tauc L. N- and P-type Ca channels are involved

in acetylcholine release at a neuroneuronal synapse: only the N-type channel is the target of neuromodulators. *Proc Natl Acad Sci USA* 1994;91:4771–4775.

107. Fox AP, Nowycky MC, Tsien RW. Kinetic and pharmacological properties distinguishing three types of calcium currents in chick sensory neurons. *J Physiol* 1987;394:149–172.
108. Friel DD, Tsien RW. Voltage-gated calcium channels: direct observation of the anomalous mole fraction effect at the single-channel level. *Proc Natl Acad Sci USA* 1989;86:5207–5211.
109. Fujita Y, Mynlieff M, Dirken RT, et al. Primary structure and functional expression of the omega-conotoxin-sensitive N-type channel from rabbit brain. *Neuron* 1993;10:585–598.
110. Galizzi J-P, Fosset M, Romay G, Laduron P, Lazdunski M. Neuroleptics of the diphenylbutylpiperidine series are potent calcium channel inhibitors. *Proc Natl Acad Sci USA* 1986;83:7513–7517.
111. Ganitkevich VY, Isenberg G. Stimulation-induced potentiation of T-type Ca channel currents in myocytes from guinea-pig coronary artery. *J Physiol* 1991;443:703–725.
112. Garcia ML, King VF, Siegl PKS, Reuben JP, Kaczorowski GJ. Binding of Ca^{2+} entry blockers to cardiac sarcolemmal membrane vesicles. *J Biol Chem* 1986;261:8146–8157.
113. Giannattasio B, Jones SW, Scarpa A. Calcium currents in the A7r5 smooth muscle-derived cell line. Calcium-dependent and voltage-dependent inactivation. *J Gen Physiol* 1991;98:987–1003.
114. Gilliam FR, III, Rivas PA, Wendt DJ, Starmer CF, Grant AO. Extracellular pH modulates block of both sodium and calcium channels by nicardipine. *Am J Physiol* 1990; 259:H1178–H1184.
115. Gould RJ, Murphy KMM, Reynolds IJ, Snyder SH. Antischizophrenic drugs of the diphenylbutylpiperidine type act as calcium channel antagonists. *Proc Natl Acad Sci USA* 1983;80:5122–5125.
116. Gross RA, Macdonald RL. Dynorphin A selectively reduces a large transient (N-type) calcium current of mouse dorsal root ganglion neurons in culture. *Proc Natl Acad Sci USA* 1987;84:5469–5473.
117. Gross RA, MacDonald RL. Differential actions of pentobarbitone on calcium current components of mouse sensory neurones in culture. *J Physiol* 1988;405:187–203.
118. Gross RA, Moises HC, Uhler MD, Macdonald RL. Dynorphin A and cAMP-dependent protein kinase independently regulate neuronal calcium currents. *Proc Natl Acad Sci USA* 1990; 87:7025–7029.
119. Gundersen CB, Umbach JA, Swartz BE. Barbiturates depress currents through human brain calcium channels studies in *Xenopus* oocytes. *J Pharmacol Exp Therap* 1988;247:824–248.
120. Gurney AM, Charnet P, Pye JM, Nargeot J. Augmentation of cardiac calcium current by flash photolysis of intracellular caged-Ca^{2+} molecules. *Nature* 1989;341:65–68.
121. Haack JA, Rosenberg RL. Calcium-dependent inactivation of L-type channels in planar lipid bilayers. *Biophys J* 1994;86:1051–1060.
122. Hadley RW, Hume JR. An intrinsic potential-dependent inactivation mechanism associated with calcium channels in guinea-pig myocytes. *J Physiol* 1987;389:205–222.
123. Hadley RW, Lederer WJ. Ca^{2+} and voltage inactivate Ca channels in guinea-pig ventricular myocytes through independent mechanisms. *J Physiol* 1991;444:257–268.
124. Hadley RW, Lederer WJ. Comparison of the effects of BAY K 8644 on cardiac Ca^{2+} current and Ca channel gating current. *Am J Physiol* 1992;262:H472–H477.
125. Hadley RW, Lederer WJ. Nifedipine inhibits movement of cardiac calcium channels through late, but not early, gating transitions. *Am J Physiol* 1995;269:H1784–H1790.
126. Hagiwara N, Irisawa H, Kameyama M. Contribution of two types of calcium currents to the pacemaker potentials of rabbit sinoatrial node cells. *J Physiol* 1988;395:233–253.
127. Hagiwara S, Byerly L. Calcium channel. *Annu Rev Neurosci* 1981;4:69–125.
128. Hall AC, Lieb WR, Franks NP. Insensitivity of P-type calcium channels to inhalational and intravenous general anesthetics. *Anesthesiology* 1994;81:117–123.
129. Hamilton SL, Codin J, Hawkes MJ, et al. Evidence for direct interaction of $G_s\alpha$ with the Ca channel of skeletal muscle. *J Biol Chem* 1991;266:19528–19535.
130. Hanck DA, Sheets MF. Extracellular divalent and trivalent cation effects on sodium current kinetics in single canine cardiac Purkinje cells. *J Physiol* 1992;454:267–298.
131. Hartzell HC, White RE. Effects of magnesium on inactivation of the voltage-gated calcium current in cardiac myocytes. *J Gen Physiol* 1989;94:745–749.
132. Heinemann SH, Schlief T, Mori Y, Imoto K. Molecular pore structure of voltage-gated sodium and calcium channels. *Braz J Med Bio Res* 1994;27:2781–2802.
133. Heinemann SH, Terlau H, Stuhmer W, Imoto K, Numa S. Calcium channel characteristics conferred on the sodium channel by single mutations. *Nature* 1992;356:441–443.
134. Hell JW, Appleyard SM, Yokoyama CT, Warner C, Catterall WA. Differential phosphorylation of two size forms of the N-type calcium channel a1 subunit which have different COOH termini. *J Biol Chem* 1994;269:7390–7396.
135. Hell JW, Westenbroek RE, Warner C, et al. Identification and differential subcellular localization of the neuronal class C and class δ L-type calcium channel α1 subunits. *J Cell Biol* 1993;123:949–962.
136. Herrington J, Lingle CJ. Kinetic and pharmacological properties of low-voltage-activated Ca^{2+} current in rat clonal (GH_3) pituitary cells. *J Neurophysiol* 1992;68:213–232.
137. Herrington J, Stern RC, Evers AS, Lingle CJ. Halothane inhibits two components of calcium current in clonal (GH_3) pituitary cells. *J Neurosci* 1991;11:2226–2240.
138. Hescheler J, Rosenthal W, Trautwein W, Schultz G. The GTP-binding protein, G_o, regulates neuronal calcium channels. *Nature* 1987;325:445–447.
139. Hescheler J, Trautwein W. Modification of L-type calcium current by intracellularly applied trypsin in guinea-pig ventricular myocytes. *J Physiol* 1988;404:259–274.
140. Hess P, Lansman JB, Tsien RW. Different modes of Ca channel gating behaviour favoured by dihydropyridine Ca agonists and antagonists. *Nature* 1984;311:538–544.
141. Hess P, Tsien RW. Mechanism of ion permeation through calcium channels. *Nature* 1984;309:453–456.
142. Heyer EJ, Macdonald RL. Barbiturate reduction of calcium-dependent action potentials: correlation with anesthetic action. *Brain Res* 1982;236:157–171.
143. Hille B. The permeability of the sodium channel to organic cations in myelinated nerve. *J Gen Physiol* 1971;58:599–619.
144. Hille B. Potassium channels in myelinated nerve: selective permeability to small cations. *J Gen Physiol* 1973;61:669–686.
145. Hillman D, Chen S, Aung TT, Cherksey B, Sugimori M, Llinás RR. Localization of P-type calcium channels in the central nervous system. *Proc Natl Acad Sci USA* 1991;88:7076–7080.
146. Hirano Y, Fozzard HA, January CT. Inactivation properties of T-type calcium current in canine cardiac Purkinje cells. *Biophys J* 1989;56:1007–1016.
147. Hirano Y, Hiraoka M. Dual modulation of unitary L-type Ca channel currents by $[Ca^{2+}]_i$ in fura-2–loaded guinea-pig ventricular myocytes. *J Physiol* 1994;480:449–463.
148. Hirning LD, Fox AP, McClesky EW, et al. Dominant role of N-type Ca channels in evoked release of norepinephrine from sympathetic neurons. *Science* 1988;239:57–60.
149. Hirota K, Ito Y, Masuda A, Momose Y. Effects of halothane on membrane potentials and membrane ionic currents in single bullfrog atrial myocytes. *Acta Anaesthesiol Scand* 1988;32:333–338.
150. Hirota K, Ito Y, Masuda A, Momose Y. Effects of halothane on membrane ionic currents in guinea pig atrial and ventricular myocytes. *Acta Anaesthesiol Scand* 1989;33:239–244.
151. Hockerman GH, Johnson BD, Scheuer T, Catterall WA. Molecular determinants of high affinity phenylalkylamine block of L-type calcium channels. *J Biol Chem* 1995;270:22119–22122.
152. Hoehner P, Quigg M, Blanck T. Halothane depresses D600 binding to bovine heart sarcolemma. *Anesthesiology* 1991;75:1019–1024.
153. Hoehner PJ, Blanck TJJ, Roy R, Rosenthal RE, Fiskum G. Alteration of voltage-dependent calcium channels in canine brain during global ischemia and reperfusion. *J Cereb Blood Flow Metab* 1992;12:418–424.
154. Hofmann F, Biel M, Bosse E, Flockerzi V, Ruth P, Welling A. Functional expression of cardiac and smooth muscle calcium channels. In: Spooner PM, Brown AM, Catterall WA, Kaczorowski GJ, Strauss HC, eds. *Ion channels in the cardiovascular system.* Armonk, NY: Futura, 1994;369–381.
155. Holz GG, IV, Kream RM, Spiegel A, Dunlap K. G proteins couple α-adrenergic and $GABA_B$ receptors to inhibition of peptide secretion from peripheral sensory neurons. *Neuroscience* 1989;9:657–666.
156. Holz GG, IV, Rane SG, Dunlap K. GTP-binding proteins mediate transmitter inhibition of voltage-dependent calcium channels. *Nature* 1986;319:670–672.
157. Horne AL, Kemp JA. The effect of ω-conotoxin GVIA on synaptic

transmission within the nucleus accumbens and hippocampus of the rat *in vitro*. *Br J Pharmacol* 1991;103:1733–1739.
158. Hoshi T, Smith SJ. Large depolarization induces long openings of voltage-dependent calcium channels in adrenal chromaffin cells. *J Neurosci* 1987;7:571–580.
159. Hui A, Ellinor PT, Krizanova O, Wang J-J, Diebold RJ, Schwartz A. Molecular cloning of multiple subtypes of a novel rat brain isoform of the α_1 subunit of the voltage-dependent calcium channel. *Neuron* 1991;7:35–44.
160. Ikeda SR. Double-pulse calcium channel current facilitation in adult rat sympathetic neurones. *J Physiol* 1991;439:181–214.
161. Ikeda SR, Schofield GG. Somatostatin blocks a calcium current in rat sympathetic ganglion neurones. *J Physiol* 1989;409:221–240.
162. Ikemoto Y, Yatani A, Arimura H, Yoshitake J. Reduction of the slow inward current of isolated rat ventricular cells by thiamylal and halothane. *Acta Anaesthesiol Scand* 1985;29:583–586.
163. Iles DE, Lehmann-Horn F, Scherer SW, et al. Localization of the gene encoding the α_2/δ-subunits of the L-type voltage-dependent calcium channel to chromosome 7q and analysis of the segregation of flanking markers in malignant hyperthermia susceptible families. *Hum Mol Genet* 1994;3:969–975.
164. Imredy JP, Yue DT. Submicroscopic Ca^{2+} diffusion mediates inhibitory coupling between individual Ca channels. *Neuron* 1992; 9:197–207.
165. Imredy JP, Yue DT. Mechanism of Ca^{2+}-sensitive inactivation of L-type Ca channels. *Neuron* 1994;12:1301–1318.
166. Irisawa H, Brown HF, Giles W. Cardiac pacemaking in the sinoatrial node. *Physiol Rev* 1993;73:197–227.
167. Ishibashi H, Rhee JS, Akaike N. Regional difference of high voltage-activated Ca channels in rat CNS neurones. *Neuroreport* 1995; 6:1621–1624.
168. Ito C, Im WB, Takagi H, et al. U-92032, a T-type Ca channel blocker and antioxidant, reduces neuronal ischemic injuries. *Eur J Pharmacol* 1994;257:203–210.
169. Jay SD, Ellis SB, McCue AF, et al. Primary structure of the γ subunit of the DHP-sensitive calcium channel from skeletal muscle. *Science* 1990; 248:490–492.
170. Jay SD, Sharp AH, Kahl SD, Vedvick TS, Harpold MM, Campbell KP. Structural characterization of the dihydropyridine-sensitive calcium channel α-2 subunit and the associated δ peptides. *J Biol Chem* 1991;266:3287–3293.
171. Josephson IR, Sperelakis N. Phosphorylation shifts the time-dependence of cardiac Ca^{++} channel gating currents. *Biophys J* 1991;60:491–497.
172. Kaczorowski GJ, Slaughter RS, Garcia ML. Strategies to discover novel ion channel modulators. In: Spooner PM, Brown AM, Catterall WA, Kaczorowski GJ, Strauss HC, eds. *Ion channels in the cardiovascular system.* Armonk, NY: Futura, 1994;463–488.
173. Kameyama M, hescheler J, Hofmann F, Trautwein W. Modulation of Ca current during the phosphorylation cycle in the guinea pig heart. *Pflugers Arch* 1986;407:123–128.
174. Kameyama M, Hofmann F, Trautwein W. On the mechanism of β-adrenergic regulation of the Ca channel in the guinea-pig heart. *Pflugers Arch* 1985;405:285–293.
175. Kaneda M, Wakamori M, Ito C, Akaike N. Low-threshold calcium current in isolated Purkinje cell bodies of rat cerebellum. *J Neurophysiol* 1990; 63:1046–1051.
176. Kasai H. Tonic inhibition and rebound facilitation of a neuronal calcium channels by a GTP-binding protein. *Proc Natl Acad Sci USA* 1991;88:8855–8859.
177. Kasai H. Voltage- and time-dependent inhibition of neuronal calcium channels by a GTP-binding protein in a mammalian cell line. *J Physiol* 1992;448:189–209.
178. Kass RS, Arena JP, Chin S. Block of L-type calcium channels by charged dihydropyridines. Sensitivity to side of application and calcium. *J Gen Physiol* 1991;98:63–75.
179. Keja JA, Stoof JC, Kits KS. Dopamine D_2 receptor stimulation differentially affects voltage-activated calcium channels in rat pituitary melanotropic cells. *J Physiol* 1992;451:409–435.
180. Kim M-S, Morii T, Sun L-X, Imoto K, Mori Y. Structural determinants of ion selectivity in brain calcium channel. *FEBS Lett* 1993; 318:145–148.
181. Kimball SD, Barrish JC, Hunt JT, Floyd DM, Gougoutas JZ, Lau WF. The design of new calcium antagonists. In: Spooner PM, Brown AM, Catterall WA, Kaczorowski GJ, Strauss HC, eds. *Ion channels in the cardiovascular system.* Armonk, NY: Futura, 1994; 489–508.
182. King VF, Garcia ML, Himmel D, et al. Interaction of tetrandrine with slowly inactivating calcium channels. Characterization of calcium channel modulation by an alkaloid of Chinese medicinal herb origin. *J Biol Chem* 1987;263:2238–2244.
183. King VF, Garcia ML, Shevell JL, Slaughter RS, Kaczorowski GJ. Substituted diphenylpiperidines bind to a unique high affinity site on the L-type calcium channel. Evidence for a fourth site in the cardiac calcium entry blocker complex. *J Biol Chem* 1989;264: 5633–5641.
184. Klöckner U, Isenberg G. Myocytes isolated from porcine coronary arteries: reduction of currents through L-type Ca-channels by verapamil-type Ca-antagonists. *J Physiol Pharmacol* 1991;42:163–179.
185. Klöckner U, Isenberg G. Calcium channel current of vascular smooth muscle cells: extracellular protons modulate gating and single channel conductance. *J Gen Physiol* 1994;103:665–678.
186. Klöckner U, Isenberg G. Intracellular pH modulates the availability of vascular L-type Ca channels. *J Gen Physiol* 1994;103:647–663.
187. Klöckner U, Schiefer A, Isenberg G. L-type Ca-channels: similar Q_{10} of Ca- , Ba- and Na-conductance points to the importance of ion-channel interaction. *Pflugers Arch* 1990; 115:638–641.
188. Knudson CM, Chaudhari N, Sharp AH, Powell JA, Beam KG, Campbell KP. Specific absence of the a1 subunit of the dihydropyridine receptor in mice with muscular dysgenesis. *J Biol Chem* 1989;264:1345–1348.
189. Koch WJ, Ellinor PT, Schwartz A. cDNA cloning of a dihydropyridine-sensitive calcium channel from rat aorta. Evidence for the existence of alternatively spliced forms. *J Biol Chem* 1990; 265: 17786–17791.
190. Kohlhardt M, Bauer B, Krause H, Fleckenstein A. Differentiation of the transmembrane Na and Ca channels in mammalian myocardial fibres by the use of specific inhibitors. *Pflugers Arch* 1972;335:309–322.
191. Kohlhardt M, Bauer B, Krause H, Fleckenstein A. Selective inhibition of the transmembrane Ca conductivity of mammalian myocardial fibres. *Pflugers Arch* 1973;338:115–123.
192. Kokubun S, Prod'hom B, Becker C, Porzig H, Reuter H. Studies on Ca channels in intact cardiac cells: voltage-dependent effects and cooperative interactions of dihydropyridine enantiomers. *Mol Pharmacol* 1986;30:571–184.
193. Kostyuk PG, Mironov SL, Shuba YM. Two ion-selecting filters in the calcium channel of the somatic membrane of mollusc neurons. *J Membr Biol* 1983;76:83–93.
194. Kullmann DM, Martin RL, Redman SJ. Reduction by general anaesthetics of group Ia excitatory postsynaptic potentials and currents in the cat spinal cord. *J Physiol* 1989;412:277–296.
195. Kuo C-C, Bean BP. G-protein modulation of ion permeation through N-type calcium channels. *Nature* 1993;365:258–262.
196. Kuo C-C, Hess P. A functional view of the entrances of L-type Ca^{2+}channels: estimates of the size and surface potential at the pore mouths. *Neuron* 1992;9:515–526.
197. Kuo C-C, Hess P. Block of the L-type Ca channel pore by external and internal Mg^{2+} in rat phaeochromocytoma cells. *J Physiol* 1993; 466:683–706.
198. Kuo C-C, Hess P. Characterization of the high-affinity Ca^{2+} binding sites in the L-type Ca channel pore in rat phaeochromocytoma cells. *J Physiol* 1993;466:657–682.
199. Kuo C-C, Hess P. Ion permeation through the L-type Ca channel in rat phaeochromocytoma cells: two sets of ion binding sites in the pore. *J Physiol* 1993;466:629–655.
200. Lansman JB. Blockade of current through single calcium channels by trivalent lanthanide cations. *J Gen Physiol* 1990; 95:679–696.
201. Lansman JB, Hess P, Tsein RW. Blockade of current through single calcium channels by Cd^{2+}, Mg^{2+}, and Ca^{2+}. Voltage and concentration dependence of calcium entry into the pore. *J Gen Physiol* 1986;88:321–347.
202. Leblanc N, Hume JR. δ 600 Block of L-type Ca channel in vascular smooth muscle cells: comparison with permanently charged derivative, δ 890. *Am J Physiol* 1989;257:C689–C695.
203. Lecharny J-B, Salord F, Henzel D, Desmonts J-M, Mantz J. Effects of thiopental, halothane and isoflurane on the calcium-dependent and -independent release of GABA from striatal synaptosomes in the rat. *Brain Res* 1995;670:308–312.
204. Lee DL, Zhang J, Blanck TJJ. The effects of halothane on voltage-dependent calcium channels in isolated Langenforff-perfused rat heart. *Anesthesiology* 1994;81:1212–1219.
205. Lee KS, Tsien RW. Reversal of current through calcium channels in dialysed single heart cells. *Nature* 1982;297:498–503.

206. Lee KS, Tsien RW. Mechanism of calcium channel blockade by verapamil, D600, diltiazem and nitrendipine in single dialysed heart cells. *Nature* 1983;302:790–794.
207. Leighton C, Mathie A, Dolphin AC. Modulation by phosphorylation and neuro-transmitters of voltage-dependent calcium channel currents in cultured rat cerebellar granule neurons. *J Physiol* 1994;477:89P-90P.
208. Lévêque C, El Far O, Martin-Moutot N, et al. Purification of the N-type calcium channel associated with syntaxin and synaptotagmin. *J Biol Chem* 1994;269:6306–6312.
209. Lévêque C, Hoshino T, David P, et al. The synaptic vesicle protein synaptotagmin associates with calcium channels and is a putative Lambert-Eaton myasthenic syndrome antigen. *Proc Natl Acad Sci USA* 1992;89:3625–3629.
210. Li G, Hidaka H, Wollheim CB. Inhibition of voltage-gated Ca channels and insulin secretion in HIT cells by the Ca^{2+}/calmodulin-dependent protein kinase II inhibitor KN-62: comparison with antagonists of calmodulin and L-type Ca channels. *Mol Pharmacol* 1992;42:489–498.
211. Lipscombe D, Kongsamut S, Tsien RW. a-Adrenergic inhibition of sympathetic neurotransmitter release mediated by modulation of N-type calcium-channel gating. *Nature* 1989;340:639–642.
212. Liu QY, Karpinski E, Rao MR, Pang PKT. Tetrandrine: a novel calcium channel antagonist inhibits type I calcium channels in neuroblastoma cells. *Neuropharmacology* 1991;30:1325–1331.
213. Llinás R, Sugimori M, Lin JW, Cherksey B. Blocking and isolation of a calcium channel from neurons in mammals and cephalopods utilizing a toxin fraction (FTX) from funnel-web spider poison. *Proc Natl Acad Sci USA* 1989;86:1689–1693.
214. López MG, Villarroya M, Baldomero L, et al. Q- and L-type Ca channels dominate the control of secretion in bovine chromaffin cells. *FEBS Lett* 1994;349:331–337.
215. Lux HD, Carbone E, Zucker H. Na^+ currents through low-voltage activated Ca channels of chick sensory neurons: block by external Ca^{2+} and Mg^{2+}. *J Physiol* 1990; 430:159–188.
216. Lynch C III. Differential depression of myocardial contractility by halothane and isoflurane *in vitro*. *Anesthesiology* 1986;64: 620–631.
217. Lynch C III. Effects of halothane and isoflurane on isolated human ventricular myocardium. *Anesthesiology* 1988;68:429–432.
218. Lynch C III, Vogel S, Pratila MG, Sperelakis N. Enflurane depression of myocardial slow action potentials. *J Pharmacol Exp Ther* 1982;222:405–409.
219. Lynch C III, Vogel S, Sperelakis N. Halothane depression of myocardial slow action potentials. *Anesthesiology* 1981;55:360–368.
220. MacDonald RL, Skerritt JH, Werz MA. Adenosine agonists reduce voltage-dependent calcium conductance of mouse sensory neurones in cell culture. *J Physiol* 1986;370:75–90.
221. Magee JC, Johnston D. Characterization of single voltage-gated Na^+ and Ca channels in apical dendrites of rat CA1 pyramidal neurons. *J Physiol* 1995;487:67–90.
222. Marchetti C, Carbone E, Lux HD. Effects of dopamine and noradrenaline on Ca channels of cultured sensory and sympathetic neurons of chick. *Pflugers Arch* 1986;406:104–111.
223. Matteson DR, Armstrong CM. Properties of two types of calcium channels in clonal pituitary cells. *J Gen Physiol* 1986;87:161–182.
224. Mazzanti M, DeFelice LJ, Liu Y-M. Gating of L-type Ca channels in embryonic chick ventricle cells: dependence on voltage, current and channel density. *J Physiol* 1991;443:307–334.
225. McCarron JG, McGoeown JG, Reardon S, Ikebe M, Fay FS, Walsh JV, Jr. Calcium-dependent enhancement of calcium current in smooth muscle by calmodulin-dependent protein kinase II. *Nature* 1992;357:74–77.
226. McCarthy RT, Fry HK. Nitrendipine block of calcium channel currents in vascular smooth muscle and adrenal glomerulosa cells. *J Cardiovasc Pharmacol* 1988;12(suppl 4):S98–S101.
227. McCleskey EW, Almers W. The Ca channel in skeletal muscle is a large pore. *Proc Natl Acad Sci USA* 1985;82:7149–7153.
228. McCleskey EW, Fox AP, Feldman DH, Cruz LJ, Olivera BM, Tsien RW. ω-Conotoxin: direct and persistent blockade of specific types of calcium channels in neurons but not muscle. *Proc Natl Acad Sci USA* 1987;84:4327–4331.
229. McCobb DP, Best PM, Beam KG. Development alters the expression of calcium currents in chick limb motoneurons. *Neuron* 1989; 2:1633–1643.
230. McFadzean I, Mullaney I, Brown DA, Mulligan G. Antibodies to the GTP binding protein, G_o, antagonize noradrenaline-induced calcium current inhibition in NG108–15 hybrid cells. *Neuron* 1989; 3:177–182.
231. Menon-Johansson AS, Berrow N, Dolphin AC. G_O traduces $GABA_B$-receptor modulation of N-type calcium channels in cultured dorsal root ganglion neurons. *Pflugers Arch* 1993;425: 335–343.
232. Miao N, Frazer MJ, Lynch C, III. Volatile anesthetic depress Ca^{2+} transients and glutamate release in isolated cerebral synaptosomes. *Anesthesiology* 1995;83:593–603.
233. Mikami A, Imoto K, Tanabe T, et al. Primary structure and functional expression of the cardiac dihydropyridine-sensitive calcium channel. *Nature* 1989;340:230–233.
234. Mintz IM, Adams ME, Bean BP. P-type calcium channels in rat central and peripheral neurons. *Neuron* 1992;9:85–95.
235. Mintz IM, Bean BP. Block of calcium channels in rat neurons by synthetic ω-Aga-IVA. *Neuropharmacology* 1993;32:1161–1170.
236. Mintz IM, Bean BP. $GABA_B$ receptor inhibition of P-type Ca channels in central neurons. *Neuron* 1993;10:889–898.
237. Mintz IM, Sabatini BL, Regehr WG. Calcium control of transmitter release at a cerebellar synapse. *Neuron* 1995;15:675–688.
238. Mintz IM, Venema VJ, Adams ME, Bean BP. Inhibition of N- and L-type Ca channels by the spider venom toxin omega-Aga-IIIA. *Proc Natl Acad Sci USA* 1991;88:6628–6631.
239. Mintz IM, Venema VJ, Swiderek KM, Lee TD, Bean BP, Adams ME. P-type calcium channels blocked by the spider toxin ω-Aga-IVA. *Nature* 1992;353:827–829.
240. Mitra R, Morad M. Two types of Ca^{2+} in guinea pig ventricular myocytes. *Proc Natl Acad Sci USA* 1986;83:5340–5344.
241. Miu P, Puil E. Isoflurane-induced impairment of synaptic transmission in hippocampal neurons. *Exp Brain Res* 1989;75:354–360.
242. Mogul DJ, Adams ME, Fox AP. Differential activation of adenosine receptors decreases N-type but potentiates P-type Ca^{2+} current in hippocampal CA3 neurons. *Neuron* 1993;10:327–334.
243. Moises HC, Rusin KI, Macdonald RL. μ- and κ-Opioid receptors selectively reduce the same transient components of high-threshold calcium current in rat dorsal root ganglion sensory neurons. *J Neurosci* 1994;14:5903–5916.
244. Mollard P, Theler J-M, Guérineau N, Vacher P, Chiavaroli C, Schlegel W. Cytosolic Ca^{2+} of excitable pituitary cells at resting potentials is controlled by steady state Ca^{2+} currents sensitive to dihydropyridines. *J Biol Chem* 1994;269:25158–25164.
245. Momiyama A, Takahashi T. Calcium channels responsible for potassium-induced transmitter release at rat cerebellar synapses. *J Physiol* 1994;476:197–202.
246. Moolenaar WH, Spector I. Ionic currents in cultured mouse neuroblastoma cells under voltage-clamp conditions. *J Physiol* 1978; 278:265–286.
247. Mori Y, Friedrich T, Kim M-S, et al. Primary structure and functional expression from a complementary DNA of a brain calcium channel. *Nature* 1991;350:398–402.
248. Morton ME, Cassidy TN, Froehner SC, Gilmour BP, Laurens RL. α_1 and α_2 Ca channel subunit expression in human neuronal and small cell carcinoma cells. *FASEB J* 1994;8:884–888.
249. Muller RU, Finkelstein A. The electrostatic basis of Mg^{++} inhibition of transmitter release. *Proc Natl Acad Sci USA* 1974;71: 923–926.
250. Nachshen DA, Blaustein MP. Influx of calcium, strontium, and barium in presynaptic nerve endings. *J Gen Physiol* 1982;79: 1065–1087.
251. Nakai J, Adams B, Imoto K, Beam KG. Critical roles of the S3 segment and S3–S4 linker of repeat I in activation of L-type calcium channels. *Proc Natl Acad Sci USA* 1994;91:1014–1018.
252. Nakao S, Hirat H, Kagawa Y. Effects of volatile anesthetics on cardiac calcium channels. *Acta Anaesthesiol Scand* 1989;33:326–330.
253. Nakayama H, Taki M, Striessnig J, Glossmann H, Catterall WA, Kanaoka Q. Identification of 1,4–dihydropyridine binding regions within the α1 subunit of skeletal muscle Ca channels by photoaffinity labeling with diazepine. *Proc Natl Acad Sci USA* 1991;88: 9203–9207.
254. Nargeot J, Nerbonne J, Engels J, Lester HA. The time course of the increase in the myocardial slow inward current after a photochemically generated concentration jump of intracellular cAMP. *Proc Natl Acad Sci USA* 1983;80:2395–2399.
255. Neely A, Wei X, Olcese R, Birnbaumer L, Stefani E. Potentiation by the β subunit of the ratio of the ionic current to the charge movement in the cardiac calcium channel. *Science* 1993;262: 575–578.

256. Nelson MT, Patlak JB, Worley JF, Standen NB. Calcium channels, potassium channels, and voltage dependence of arterial smooth muscle tone. *Am J Physiol* 1990; 259:C3–C18.
257. Nelson TE, Lin M. Abnormal function of porcine malignant hyperthermia calcium release channel in the absence and presence of halothane. *Cell Physiol Biochem* 1995;5:10–22.
258. Niidome T, Kin M-S, Friedrich T, Mori Y. Molecular cloning and characterization of a novel calcium channel from rabbit brain. *FEBS Lett* 1992;308:7–13.
259. Nilius B, Hess P, Lansman JB, Tsien RW. A novel type of cardiac calcium channel in ventricular cells. *Nature* 1985;316:443–446.
260. Nishimura S, Takeshima H, Hofmann F, Flockerzi V, Imoto K. Requirement of the calcium channel β subunit for functional conformation. *FEBS Lett* 1993;324:283–286.
261. Noda M, Ikeda T, Kayano T, et al. Existence of distinct sodium channel messenger RNAs in rat brain. *Nature* 1986;320:188–192.
262. Noda M, Shimizu S, Tanabe T, et al. Primary structure of *Electrophorus electricus* sodium channel deduced from cDNA sequence. *Nature* 1984;312:121–126.
263. Nomura K, Reuveny E, Narahashi T. Opioid inhibition and desensitization of calcium channel currents in rat dorsal root ganglion neurons. *J Pharmacol Exp Ther* 1994;270:466–474.
264. North RA, Williams JT, Surprenant A, Christie MJ. μ and δ Receptors belong to a family of receptors that are coupled to potassium channels. *Proc Natl Acad Sci USA* 1987;84:5487–5491.
265. Nowycky MC, Fox AP, Tsien RW. Long-opening mode of gating of neuronal calcium channels and its promotion by the dihydropyridine calcium agonist Bay K 8644. *Proc Natl Acad Sci USA* 1985;82: 2178–2182.
266. Nowycky MC, Fox AP, Tsien RW. Three types of neuronal calcium channels with different calcium agonist sensitivity. *Nature* 1985; 316:440–443.
267. O'Connor VM, Shamotienko O, Grishin E, Betz H. On the structure of the "synaptosecretosome": evidence for a neurexin/synaptotagmin/syntaxin/Ca channel complex. *FEBS Lett* 1993;326: 255–260.
268. Oh U, Ho Y-K, Kim D. Modulation of the serotonin-activated K^+ channel by G protein subunits and nucleotides in rat hippocampal neurons. *J Membr Biol* 1995;147:241–253.
269. Olcese R, Usai C, Maestrone E, Nobile M. The general anesthetic propofol inhibits transmembrane calcium current in chick sensory neurons. *Anesth Analg* 1994;78:955–960.
270. Olivera BM, Gray WR, Seikus R, et al. Peptide neurotoxins from fish-hunting cone snails. *Science* 1985;230:1338–1343.
271. Olivera BM, Miljanich GP, Ramachandran J, Adams ME. Calcium channel diversity and neurotransmitter release: the ω-conotoxins and ω-agatoxins. *Annu Rev Biochem* 1994;63:823–867.
272. Osterrieder W, Brum G, Hescheler J, Trautwein W, Hofmann F, Flockersi V. Injection of subunits of cyclic AMP-dependent kinase into cardiac myocytes modulates Ca^{2+} current. *Nature* 1982;298: 576–578.
273. Pancrazio JJ. Halothane and isoflurane preferentially depress a component of calcium channel current which undergoes slow inactivation. *J Physiol* 1996;494:91–103.
274. Pancrazio JJ, Frazer MJ, Lynch C III. Barbiturate anesthetics depress the resting K^+ conductance of myocardium. *J Pharmacol Exp Ther* 1993;265:358–365.
275. Pancrazio JJ, Park WK, Lynch C III. Inhalational anesthetic actions on voltage-gated ion currents of bovine chromaffin cells. *Mol Pharmacol* 1993;43:783–794.
276. Park WK, Lynch C III. Propofol and thiopental depression of myocardial contractility—a comparative study of mechanical and electrophysiologic effects in isolated guinea pig ventricular muscle. *Anesth Analg* 1992;74:395–405.
277. Perez-Reyes E, Castellano A, Kim HS, et al. Cloning and expression of a cardiac/brain beta subunit of the L-type calcium channel. *J Biol Chem* 1992;267:1792–1797.
278. Perez-Reyes E, Kim HS, Lacerda AE, et al. Induction of calcium currents by the expression of the α_1-subunit of the dihydropyridine receptor from skeletal muscle. *Nature* 1989;340:233–236.
279. Perez-Reyes E, Schneider T. Calcium channels: structure, function and classification. *Drug Dev Res* 1994;33:295–318.
280. Perez-Reyes E, Wei X, Castellano A, Birnbaumer L. Molecular diversity of L-type calcium channels—evidence for alternative splicing of the transcripts of three non-allelic genes. *J Biol Chem* 1990; 265:20430–20436.
281. Perney TM, Hirning LD, Leeman SE, Miller RJ. Multiple calcium channels mediate neurotransmitter release from peripheral neurons. *Proc Natl Acad Sci USA* 1986;83:6656–6659.
282. Petersen M, LaMotte RH. Relationships between capsaicin sensitivity of mammalian sensory neurons, cell size and type of voltage gated Ca-currents. *Brain Res* 1991;561:20–26.
283. Peterson BZ, Catterall WA. Calcium binding in the pore of L-type calcium channels modulates high affinity dihydropyridine binding. *J Biol Chem* 1995;270:18201–18204.
284. Pfreiger FW, Veselovsky NS, Gottmann K, Lux HD. Pharmacological characterization of calcium currents and synaptic transmission between thalamic neurons in vitro. *J Neurosci* 1992;12: 4347–4357.
285. Pietrobon D, Hess P. Novel mechanism of voltage-dependent gating in L-type calcium channels. *Nature* 1990; 346:651–655.
286. Pietrobon D, Prod'hom B, Hess P. Conformational changes associated with ion permeation in L-type calcium channels. *Nature* 1988;333:373–376.
287. Plummer MR, Logothetis DE, Hess P. Elementary properties and pharmacological sensitivities of calcium channels in mammalian peripheral neurons. *Neuron* 1989;2:1453–1463.
288. Plummer MR, Rittenhouse A, Kanevsky M, Hess P. Neurotransmitter modulation of calcium channels in rat sympathetic neurons. *J Neurosci* 1991;11:2339–2348.
289. Pollo A, Lovallo M, Sher E, Carbone E. Voltage-dependent noradrenergic modulation of ω-conotoxin-sensitive Ca channels in human neuroblastoma IMR32 cells. *Pflugers Arch* 1992;422:75–83.
290. Porsius AJ, van Zwieten PA. Influence of halothane on calcium movements in isolated heart muscle and in isolated plasma membranes. *Arch Int Pharmacodyn* 1975;218:29–39.
291. Potier B, Dutar P, Lamour Y. Different effects of ω-conotoxin GVIA at excitatory and inhibitory synapses in rat CA1 hippocampal neurons. *Brain Res* 1993;616:236–241.
292. Powers PA, Liu S, Hogan K, Gregg RG. Skeletal muscle and brain isoforms of a β subunit of human voltage-dependent calcium channels are encoded by a single gene. *J Biol Chem* 1992;267: 22967–22972.
293. Pragnell M, De Waard M, Mori Y, Tanabe T, Snutch T, Campbell K. Calcium channel β subunit binds to a conserved motif in the I-II cytoplasmic linker of the α_1-subunit. *Nature* 1994;368:67–70.
294. Pragnell M, Sakamoto J, Jay SD, Campbell KP. Cloning and tissue-specific expression of the brain calcium channel β-subunit. *FEBS Lett* 1991;291:253–258.
295. Ragsdale DS, McPhee JC, Scheuer T, Catterall WA. Molecular determinants of state-dependent block of Na^+ channels by local anesthetics. *Science* 1994;265:1724–1728.
296. Rampe D, Janis RA, Triggle DJ. Bay K 8644, a 1,4–dihydropyridine Ca channel activator: dissociation of binding and functional effects of brain synaptosomes. *J Neurochem* 1984;43:1688–1691.
297. Rampe D, Triggle DJ. New ligands for L-type Ca channels. *Trends Pharmacol Sci* 1990;11:112–115.
298. Randall A, Tsien RW. Pharmacological dissection of multiple types of Ca channel currents in rat cerebellar granule neurons. *J Neurosci* 1995;15:2995–3012.
299. Regan LJ, Sah DWY, Bean BP. Ca channels in rat central and peripheral neurons: high-threshold current resistant to dihydropyridine blockers and ω-conotoxin. *Neuron* 1991;6:269–280.
300. Regehr WG, Mintz IM. Participation of multiple calcium channel types in transmission at single climbing fiber to Purkinje cell synapses. *Neuron* 1994;12:605–613.
301. Reuter H. The dependence of slow inward current in Purkinje fibers on the extracellular calcium concentration. *J Physiol* 1967; 192:479–492.
302. Reuter H. Calcium channels modulation by neurotransmitters, enzymes and drugs. *Nature* 1983;301:569–574.
303. Reuter H, Scholz H. The regulation of the calcium conductance of cardiac muscle by adrenaline. *J Physiol* 1977;264:49–62.
304. Reuter H, Stevens CF, Tsien RW, Yellen G. Properties of single calcium channels in cardiac cell culture. *Nature* 1982;297:501–504.
305. Rios E, Brum G. Involvement of dihydropyridine receptors in excitation-contraction coupling in skeletal muscle. *Nature* 1987; 325:717–720.
306. Rivier J, Galyean R, Gray WR, et al. Neuronal calcium channel inhibitors: synthesis of ω-conotoxin GVIA and effect on ^{45}Ca uptake by synaptosomes. *J Biol Chem* 1987;262:1194–1198.
307. Roche JP, Anantharam V, Treistman SN. Abolition of G protein inhibition of α_{1A} and α_{1B} calcium channels by co-expression of the β_3 subunit. *FEBS Lett* 1995;371:43–46.

308. Rogers M, Hendry I. Involvement of dihydropyridine-sensitive calcium channels in nerve growth factor-dependent neurite outgrowth by sympathetic neurons. *J Neurosci Res* 1990; 26:447–454.
309. Rossier MF, Python CP, Capponi AM, Schlegel W, Kwan CY, Vallotton MB. Blocking T-type calcium channels with tetrandrine inhibits steroidogenesis in bovine adrenal glomerulosa cells. *Endocrinology* 1993;132:1035–1043.
310. Ruth P, Röhrkasten A, Biel M, et al. Primary structure of the β subunit of the DHP-sensitive calicum channel from skeletal muscle. *Science* 1989;245:1115–1118.
311. Sah DWY, Bean BP. Inhibition of P-type and N-type calcium channels by dopamine receptor antagonists. *Mol Pharmacol* 1994;45: 84–92.
312. Sanchez JA, Stefani E. Inward calcium current in twitch muscle fibres of the frog. *J Physiol* 1978;283:197–209.
313. Sanguinetti MC, Kass RS. Photoalteration of calcium channel blockade in the cardiac Purkinje fiber. *Biophys J* 1984;45:873–880.
314. Sanguinetti MC, Kass RS. Voltage-dependent block of calcium channel current in the calf cardiac Purkinje fiber by dihydropyridine calcium channel antagonists. *Circ Res* 1984;55:336–348.
315. Sanguinetti MC, Krafte DS, Kass RS. Voltage-dependent modulation of Ca channel current in heart cells by BAY K 8644. *J Gen Physiol* 1986;88:369–392.
316. Sather WA, Tanabe T, Zhang J-F, Mori Y, Adams ME, Tsien RW. Distinctive biophysical and pharmacological properties of class A (BI) calcium channel α_1 subunits. *Neuron* 1993;11:291–303.
317. Sather WA, Yang J, Tsien RW. Structural basis of ion channel permeation and selectivity. *Cur Opin Neurobiol* 1994;4:313–323.
318. Satin LS, Cook DL. Calcium current inactivation in insulin-secreting cells is mediated by calcium influx and membrane depolarization. *Pflugers Arch* 1989;414:1–10.
319. Satin LS, Tavalin SJ, Kinard TA, Teague J. Contribution of L-type and non-L-type calcium channels to voltage-gated calcium current and glucose-dependent insulin secretion in HIT-T15 cells. *Endocrinology* 1995;136:4589–4601.
320. Satin LS, Tavalin SJ, Smolen PD. Inactivation of HIT cell Ca^{2+} current by a simulated burst of Ca^{2+} activation potentials. *Biophys J* 1994;66:141–148.
321. Scamps F, Undrovinas A, Vassort G. Inhibition of I_{Ca} in single frog cardiac cells by quinidine, flecainide, ethmozin, and ethacizin. *Am J Physiol* 1989;25:C549–C559.
322. Scheuer T, Kass RS. Phenytoin reduces calcium current in the cardiac Purkinje fiber. *Circ Res* 1983;53:16–23.
323. Schilling WP, Drews JA. Voltage-sensitive nitrendipine binding in an isolated cardiac sarcolemma preparation. *J Biol Chem* 1985;261: 2750–2758.
324. Schlame M, Hemmings HC, Jr. Inhibition by volatile anesthetics of endogenous glutamate release from synaptosomes by a presynaptic mechanism. *Anesthesiology* 1995;82:1406–1416.
325. Schmidt U, Schwinger RHG, Böhm S, et al. Evidence for an interaction of halothane with the L-type Ca channel in human myocardium. *Anesthesiology* 1993;79:332–339.
326. Schneider M, Chandler W. Voltage dependent charge movement in skeletal muscle: a possible step in excitation-contraction coupling. *Nature* 1973;242:244–246.
327. Schneider T, Wei X, Olcese R, et al. Molecular analysis and functional expression of the human type E α_1 subunit. *Receptors Channels* 1994;2:255–270.
328. Schofield GG. Norepinephrine inhibits a Ca^{2+} current in rat sympathetic neurons via a G-protein. *Eur J Pharmacol* 1991;207: 195–207.
329. Schultz D, Mikala G, Yatani A, et al. Cloning, chromosomal localization, and functional expression of the α_1 subunit of the L-type voltage-dependent calcium channel from normal human heart. *Proc Natl Acad Sci USA* 1993;90:6228–6232.
330. Schwartz LM, McCleskey EW, Almers W. Dihydropyridine receptors in muscle are voltage-dependent but most are not functional calcium channels. *Nature* 1985;314:747–750.
331. Scott RH, Wootton JF, Dolphin AC. Modulation of neuronal T-type calcium channel currents by photoactivation of intracellular guanosine 5'-*o*(3–thio) triphosphate. *Neuroscience* 1990; 38:285–294.
332. Sculptoreanu A, Figourov A, de Groat WC. Voltage-dependent potentiation of neuronal L-type calcium channels due to state-dependent phosphorylation. *Am J Physiol* 1993;269:C725–C732.
333. Sculptoreanu A, Scheuer T, Catterall WA. Voltage-dependent potentiation of L-type Ca channels due to phosphorylation by cAMP-dependent protein kinase. *Nature* 1993;364:240–243.
334. Seino S, Chen L, Seino M, et al. Cloning of the α_1 subunit of a voltage-dependent calcium channel expressed in pancreatic β cells. *Proc Natl Acad Sci USA* 1992;89:584–588.
335. Seward E, Hammond C, Henderson G. μ-Opioid-receptor-mediated inhibition of the N-type calcium-channel current. *Proc R Soc Lond B* 1991;244:129–135.
336. Sham JSK, Cleeman L, Morad M. Functional coupling of Ca channels and ryanodine receptors in cardiac myocytes. *Proc Natl Acad Sci USA* 1995;92:121–125.
337. Shen K-Z, Surprenant A. Noradrenaline, somatostatin and opioids inhibit activity of single HVA/N-type calcium channels in excised neuronal membranes. *Pflugers Arch* 1991;418:614–616.
338. Sheng Z-H, Rettig J, Takahashi M, Catterall WA. Identification of a syntaxin-binding site on N-type calcium channels. *Neuron* 1994; 13:1303–1313.
339. Shirokov R, Levis R, Shirokova N, Rios E. Two classes of gating current from L-type Ca channels in guinea pig ventricular myocytes. *J Gen Physiol* 1992;99:863–895.
340. Silver RA, Lamb AG, Bolsover SR. Calcium hotspots caused by L-channel clustering promote morphological changes in neuronal growth cones. *Nature* 1990; 343:751–754.
341. Singer D, Biel M, Lotan I, Flockerzi V, Hofmann F, Dascal N. The roles of the subunits in the function of the calcium channel. *Science* 1991;253:1553–1557.
342. Small DL, Monette R, Mealing G, Buchan AM, Morley P. Neuroprotective effects of ω-Aga-IVA against *in vitro* ischaemia in the rat hippocampal slice. *NeuroReport* 1995;6:1617–1620.
343. Snutch TP, Leonard JP, Gilbert MM, Lester HA, Davidson N. Rat brain expresses a heterogeneous family of calcium channels. *Proc Natl Acad Sci USA* 1990; 87:3391–3395.
344. Snutch TP, Reiner PB. Ca channels: diversity of form and function. *Curr Opin Neurobiol* 1992;2:247–253.
345. Snutch TP, Tomlinson WJ, Leonard JP, Gilbert MM. Distinct calcium channels are generated by alternative splicing and are differentially expressed in the mammalian CNS. *Neuron* 1991;7: 45–57.
346. Soldatov NM. Molecular diversity of L-type Ca channel transcripts in human fibroblasts. *Proc Natl Acad Sci USA* 1992;89:4628–4632.
347. Soldatov NM, Bouron A, Reuter H. Different voltage-dependent inhibition by dihydropyridines of human Ca channel splice variants. *J Biol Chem* 1995;270:10540–10543.
348. Soltesz I, Lightowler S, Leresche N, Jassik-Gerschenfeld D, Pollard CE, Crunelli V. Two inward currents and the transformation of low-frequency oscillations of rat and cat thalamocortical cells. *J Physiol* 1991;441:175–197.
349. Soong TW, Stea A, Hodson CD, Dubel SJ, Vincent SR, Snutch TP. Structure and functional expression of a member of the low voltage-activated calcium channel family. *Science* 1993;260:1133–1136.
350. Spedding M, Kenny B, Chatelain P. New drug binding sites in Ca channels. *Trends Pharmacol Sci* 1995;16:139–142.
351. Spedding M, Paoletti R. Classification of calcium channels and the sites of action of drugs modifying channel function. *Pharmacol Rev* 1992;44:363–376.
352. Sperelakis N. Phosphorylation hypothesis of the myocardial slow channel and control of Ca^{++} influx. In: Zipes DP, Jaliffe J, eds. *Cardiac electrophysiology and arrhythmias.* New York: Grune & Stratton, 1985;123–135.
353. Stanfield PR. A calcium dependent inward current in frog skeletal muscle fibres. *Pflugers Arch* 1977;368:267–270.
354. Stanley EF, Atrakchi AH. Calcium currents recorded from a vertebrate presynaptic nerve terminal are resistant to the dihydropyridine nifedipine. *Proc Natl Acad Sci USA* 1990; 87:9683–9687.
355. Stanley EF, Goping G. Characterization of a calcium current in a vertebrate cholinergic presynaptic nerve terminal. *J Neurosci* 1991; 11:985–993.
356. Starr TVB, Prystay W, Snutch TP. Primary structure of a calcium channel that is highly expressed in the rat cerebellum. *Proc Natl Acad Sci USA* 1991;88:5621–5625.
357. Stea A, Dubel SJ, Pragnell M, Leonard JP, Campbell KP, Snutch TP. A β-subunit normalizes the electrophysiologic properties of a cloned N-type Ca channel α_1-subunit. *Neuropharmacology* 1993;32: 1103–1116.
358. Stea A, Soong TW, Snutch TP. Determinants of PKC-dependent modulation of a family of neuronal calcium channels. *Neuron* 1995;15:929–940.
359. Stea A, Tomlinson J, Soong TW, et al. Localization and functional properties of a rat brain α_{1A} calcium channel reflect similarities to

neuronal Q- and P-type channels. *Proc Natl Acad Sci USA* 1994;91: 10576–10580.
360. Stern MD. Buffering of calcium in the vicinity of a channel pore. *Cell Calcium* 1992;13:183–192.
361. Sternweis PC, Robishaw JD. Isolation of two proteins with high affinity for guanine nucleotides from membranes of bovine brain. *J Biol Chem* 1984;259:13806–13813.
362. Stojilkovic S, Iida T, Virmani MA, Izumi S, Rijas E, Catt KJ. Dependence of hormone secretion on activation-inactivation kinetics of voltage-sensitive Ca channels in pituitary gonadotrophs. *Proc Natl Acad Sci USA* 1990; 87:8855–8859.
363. Striessnig J, Hering S, Berger W, Catterall WA, Glossman H. Calcium antagonist binding domains of L-type calcium channels. In: Spooner PM, Brown AM, Catterall WA, Kaczorowski GJ, Strauss HC, eds. *Ion channels in the cardiovascular system.* Armonk, NY: Futura, 1994;441–458.
364. Striessnig J, Murphy BJ, Catterall WA. Dihydropyridine receptor of L-type Ca channels: identification of binding domains for [^{3}H](+)-PN200-110 and [^{3}H]azidopine within the alpha 1 subunit. *Proc Natl Acad Sci USA* 1992;88:10769–10773.
365. Study RE. Isoflurane inhibits multiple voltage-gated calcium currents in hippocampal pyramidal neurons. *Anesthesiology* 1994;81: 104–116.
366. Surprenant A, Shen K-Z, North RA, Tatsumi H. Inhibition of calcium currents by noradrenaline, somatostatin and opioids in guinea-pig submucosal neurones. *J Physiol* 1990; 431:585–608.
367. Suszkiw JB, O'Leary ME, Murawsky MM, Wang T. Presynaptic calcium channels in rat cortical synaptosomes: fast-kinetics of phasic calcium influx, channel inactivation, and relationship to nitrendipine receptors. *J Neurosci* 1986;6:1349–1357.
368. Suzuki S, Rogawski MA. T-type calcium channels mediate the transition between tonic and phasic firing in thalamic neurons. *Proc Natl Acad Sci USA* 1989;86:7228–7232.
369. Swartz KJ. Modulation of Ca channels by protein kinase C in rat central and peripheral neurons: disruption of G protein-mediated inhibition. *Neuron* 1993;11:305–320.
370. Swartz KJ, Bean BP. Inhibition of calcium channels in rat CA3 pyramidal cells by metabotropic glutamate receptor. *J Neurosci* 1993;12:4358–4371.
371. Swartz KJ, Merritt A, Bean BP, Lovinger DM. Protein kinase C modulates glutamate receptor inhibition of Ca channels and synaptic transmission. *Nature* 1993;361:165–168.
372. Takahashi H, Puttick RM, Terrar DA. The effects of propofol and enflurane on single calcium channel currents of guinea-pig isolated ventricular myocytes. *Br J Pharmacol* 1994;111:1147–1153.
373. Takahashi M, Catterall WA. Identification of an α subunit of dihydropyridine-sensitive brain calcium channels. *Science* 1987;236: 88–91.
374. Takahashi M, Seager MJ, Jones JF, Reber BFX, Catterall WA. Subunit structure of dihydropyridine-sensitive calcium channels from skeletal muscle. *Proc Natl Acad Sci USA* 1987;84:5478–5482.
375. Takahashi T, Momiyama A. Different types of calcium channels mediate central synaptic transmission. *Nature* 1993;366:156–158.
376. Takekura H, Bennet L, Tanabe T, Beam KG, Franzini-Armstrong C. Restoration of junctional tetrads in dysgenic myotubes by dihydropyridine receptor cDNA. *Biophys J* 1994;67:793–803.
377. Takenoshita M, Steinbach JH. Halothane blocks low-voltage-activated calcium current in rat sensory neurons. *J Neurosci* 1991;11: 1404–1412.
378. Takenoshita M, Takahashi T. Mechanisms of halothane action on synaptic transmission in motoneurons of the newborn rat spinal cord in vitro. *Brain Res* 1987;402:303–310.
379. Tanabe T, Adams BA, Numa S, Beam KG. Repeat I of the dihydropyridine receptor is critical in determining calcium channel activation kinetics. *Nature* 1991;352:800–803.
380. Tanabe T, Beam KG, Adams BA, Niidome T, Numa S. Regions of the skeletal muscle dihydropyridine receptor critical for excitation-contraction coupling. *Nature* 1990; 346:567–569.
381. Tanabe T, Beam KG, Powell JA, Numa S. Restoration of excitation-contraction coupling and slow calcium current in dysgenic mice by dihydropyridine receptor complementary DNA. *Nature* 1988; 336:134–139.
382. Tanabe T, Takeshima H, Mikami A, et al. Primary structure of the receptor for calcium channel blockers from skeletal muscle. *Nature* 1987;328:313–318.
383. Tang CM, Presser F, Morad M. Amiloride selectively blocks the low threshold (T) calcium channel. *Science* 1988;240:213–215.
384. Tang S, Mikala G, Bahinski A, Yatani A, Varadi G, Schwartz A. Molecular localization of ion selectivity sites within the pore of a human L-type cardiac calcium channel. *J Biol Chem* 1993;268: 13026–13029.
385. Tareilus E, Schoch J, Adams M, Breer H. Analysis of rapid calicum signals in synaptosomes. *Neurochem Int* 1993;23:331–341.
386. Taussig R, Sanchez S, Rifo M, Gilman AG, Belardetti F. Inhibition of the ω-conotoxin-sensitive calcium current by distinct G proteins. *Neuron* 1992;8:799–809.
387. Terrar DA, Victory JGG. Effects of halothane on membrane currents associated with contraction in single myocytes isolated from guinea-pig ventricle. *Br J Pharmacol* 1988;94:500–508.
388. Terrar DA, Victory JGG. Isoflurane depresses membrane currents associated with contractions in myocytes isolated from guinea-pig ventricle. *Anesthesiology* 1988;69:742–749.
389. Tiaho F, S R, Lory P, Nerbonne JM, Nargeot J. Cyclic-AMP-dependent phosphorylation modulates the stereospecific activation of cardiac Ca channels by Bay K 8644. *Pflugers Arch* 1990; 417:58–66.
390. Triggle DJ. Calcium, calcium channels, and calcium channel antagonists. *Can J Physiol Pharmacol* 1989;68:1474–1481.
391. Turner TJ, Adams ME, Dunlap K. Calcium channels coupled to glutamate release identified by omega-Aga-IVA. *Science* 1992;258: 310–313.
392. Twitchell WA, Rane SG. Opioid peptide modulation of Ca^{2+}-dependent K^+ and voltage-activated Ca^{2+} currents in bovine adrenal chromaffin cells. *Neuron* 1993;10:701–709.
393. Tytgat J, Vereecke J, Carmeliet E. A combined study of sodium current and T-type calcium current in isolated cardiac cells. *Pflugers Arch* 1990; 417:142–147.
394. Tytgat J, Vereecke J, Carmeliet E. Mechanism of cardiac T-type Ca channel blockade by amiloride. *J Pharmacol Exp Ther* 1990; 252: 546–551.
395. Uchitel OD, Protti DA, Sanchez V, Cherksey BD, Sugimori M, Llinás R. P-type voltage-dependent calcium channel mediates presynaptic calcium influx and transmitter release in mammalian synapses. *Proc Natl Acad Sci USA* 1992;89:3330–3333.
396. Uehara A, Hume JR. Interactions of organic calcium channel antagonists with calcium channels in single frog atrial cells. *J Gen Physiol* 1985;85:621–647.
397. Umemiya M, Berger AJ. Properties and function of low- and high-voltage-activated Ca channels in hypoglossal motoneurons. *J Neurosci* 1994;14:5652–5660.
398. Vaghy PL, McKenna E, Itagaki K, Schwartz A. Resolution of the identity of the Ca^{2+}-antagonist receptor in skeletal muscle. *Trends Pharmacol Sci* 1988;9:398–402.
399. Varadi G, Mori Y, Mikala G, Schwartz A. Molecular determinants of Ca channel function and drug action. *Trends Pharmacol Sci* 1995; 16:43–49.
400. Vetner JC, Fraser CM, Schaber JS, Jung CY, Bolger G, Triggle DJ. Molecular properties of the slow inward channel—molecular weight determinations by radiation inactivation and covalent affinity labeling. *J Biol Chem* 1983;258:9344–9348.
401. Vidal S, Raynaud B, Weber MJ. The role of Ca channels of the L-type in neurotransmitter plasticity of cultured sympathetic neurons. *Brain Res* 1989;6:187–196.
402. Vogel S, Sperelakis N. Blockade of myocardial slow inward current at low pH. *Am J Physiol* 1977;233:C99–C103.
403. Wang G, Lemos JR. Effects of funnel web spider toxin on Ca^{2+} currents in neurophysical terminals. *Brain Res* 1994;663:215–222.
404. Wang R, Karpinski E, Wu L, Pang PKT. Flunarizine selectively blocks transient calcium currents in N1E-115 cells. *J Pharmacol Exp Ther* 1990; 254:1006–1011.
405. Wanke E, Ferroni A, Malgaroli A, Ambrosini A, Pozzan T, Meldolesi J. Activation of a muscarinic receptor selectively inhibits a rapidly inactivated Ca^{2+} current in rat sympathetic neurons. *Proc Natl Acad Sci USA* 1987;84:4313–4317.
406. Watanabe T, Kalasz H, Yabana H, et al. Azidobutyryl clentiazem, a new photoactivatable diltiazem analog, labels benzothiazepine binding sites in the α_1 subunit of the skeletal muscle calcium channel. *FEBS Lett* 1993;334:261–264.
407. Weakly JN. Effect of barbiturates on 'quantal' synaptic transmission in spinal motorneurones. *J Physiol* 1969;204:63–77.
408. Wei X, Neely A, Lacerda AE, et al. Modification of Ca channel activity by deletions at the carboxyl terminus of the cardiac α_1 subunit. *J Biol Chem* 1994;269:1635–1640.
409. Wei X, Perez-Reyes E, Lacerda AE, Schuster G, Brown AM, Birnbaumer L. Heterologous regulation of the cardiac Ca channel α_1

subunit by skeletal muscle β and γ subunits. *J Biol Chem* 1991;266: 21943–21947.

410. Welling A, Kwan YW, Bosse E, Flockerzi V, Hofmann F, Kass RS. Subunit-dependent modulation of recombinant L-type calcium channels. *Circ Res* 1993;73:974–980.
411. Werz MA, Macdonald RL. Barbiturates decrease voltage-dependent calcium conductance of mouse neurons in dissociated cell culture. *Mol Pharmacol* 1985;28:269–277.
412. Westenbroek R, Hell J, Warner C, Dubel S, Snutch T, Catterall W. Biochemical properties and subcellular distribution of an N-type calcium channel alpha 1 subunit. *Neuron* 1992;9:1099–1115.
413. Wetzel GT, Chen F, Klitzner TS. L- and T-type calcium channels in acutely isolated neonatal and adult cardiac myocytes. *Pediatr Res* 1991;30:89–94.
414. Wheeler DB, Randall A, Tsien RW. Roles of N-type and Q-type Ca channels in supporting hippocampal synaptic transmission. *Science* 1994;264:107–111.
415. White G, Lovinger DM, Weight FF. Transient low-threshold Ca^{2+} current triggers burst firing through afterdepolarizing potential in adult mammalian neurons. *Proc Natl Acad Sci USA* 1989;86: 6802–6806.
416. Wilding TJ, Womack MD, McCleskey EW. Fast, local signal transduction between the m opioid receptor and Ca channels. *J Neurosci* 1995;15:4124–4132.
417. Williams ME, Brust PF, Feldman DH, et al. Structure and functional expression of an ω-conotoxin-sensitive human N-type calcium channel. *Science* 1992;257:389–395.
418. Williams ME, Feldman DH, McCue AF, et al. Structure and functional expression of α_1, α_2, and β subunits of a novel human neuronal calcium channel subtype. *Neuron* 1992;8:71–84.
419. Williams ME, Marubio LM, Deal CR, et al. Structure and functional characterization of neuronal alpha 1E calcium channel subtypes. *J Biol Chem* 1994;269:22347–22357.
420. Williams PJ, Pitman QJ, MacVicar BA. Blockade by funnel web toxin of a calcium current in the intermediate pituitary of the rat. *Neurosci Lett* 1993;157:171–174.
421. Wisgirda ME, Dryer SE. Functional dependence of Ca^{2+}-activated K^+ current on L- and N-type Ca channels: differences between chicken sympathetic and parasympathetic neurons suggest different regulatory mechanisms. *Proc Natl Acad Sci USA* 1994;91: 2858–2862.
422. Wu J, Lipsius SL. Effects of extracellular Mg^{2+} on T- and L-type Ca^{2+} currents in single atrial myocytes. *Am J Physiol* 1990; 259: H1842–H1850.
423. Wu L-G, Saggau P. Pharmacological identification to two types of presynaptic voltage-dependent calcium channels at CA3–CA1 synapses of the hippocampus. *J Neurosci* 1994;14:5613–5622.
424. Xu XP, Best PM. Increase in calcium current from adult rats with growth hormone-secreting tumors. *Proc Natl Acad Sci USA* 1990; 87:4655–4659.
425. Yaari Y, Hamon B, Lux HD. Development of two types of calcium channels in cultured mammalian hippocampal neurons. *Science* 1987;235:680–682.
426. Yamakage M, Hirschman CA, Croxton TL. Inhibitory effects of thiopental, ketamine, and propofol on voltage-dependent Ca channels in porcine tracheal smooth muscle cells. *Anesthesiology* 1995;83:1274–1282.
427. Yang J, Ellinor PT, Sather WA, Zhang J-F, Tsien RW. Molecular determinants of Ca^{2+} selectivity and ion permeation in L-type Ca channels. *Nature* 1993;366:158–161.
428. Yang J, Tsien RW. Enhancement of N- and L-type calcium currents by protein kinase C in frog sympathetic neurons. *Neuron* 1993;10:127–136.
429. Yatani A, Brown AM. The calcium channel blocker nitrendipine blocks sodium channels in neonatal rat cardiac myocytes. *Circ Res* 1985;56:868–875.
430. Yatani A, Brown AM. Rapid β-adrenergic modulation of cardiac calcium channel currents by a fast G protein pathway. *Science* 1989;245:71–74.
431. Yatani A, Codina J, Imoto Y, Reeves JP, Birnbaumer L, Brown AM. A G protein directly regulates mammalian cardiac calcium channels. *Science* 1987;238:1288–1292.
432. Yatani A, Seidel CL, Allen J, Brown AM. Whole-cell and single-channel calcium currents of isolated cells from saphenous vein. *Circ Res* 1987;60:523–533.
433. Yee HF Jr, Weiss JN, Langer GA. Neuraminidase selectively enhances transient Ca2+ current in cardiac myocytes. *Am J Physiol* 1989;256:C1267–C1272.
434. Yoshida A, Oho C, Omori A, Kuwahara R, Ito T, Takahashi M. HPC-1 is associated with synaptotagmin and ω-conotoxin receptor. *J Biol Chem* 1992;267:24925–24928.
435. Yoshida A, Takahashi M, Nishimura S, Takeshima H, Kokubun S. Cyclic AMP-dependent phosphorylation and regulation of the cardiac dihydropyridine-sensitive Ca channel. *FEBS Lett* 1992;309: 343–349.
436. Yuan W, Bers DM. Ca-dependent facilitation of cardiac Ca current is due to Ca-calmodulin-dependent protein kinase. *Am J Physiol* 1994;267:H982–H993.
437. Yue DT, Backx PH, Imredy JP. Calcium-sensitive inactivation in the gating of single calcium channels. *Science* 1990; 250:1735–1738.
438. Yue DT, Herzig S, Marban E. β-Adrenergic stimulation of calcium channels occurs by potentiation of high-activity gating modes. *Proc Natl Acad Sci USA* 1990; 87:753–757.
439. Zhang J-F, Randall AD, Ellinor PT, et al. Distinctive pharmacology and kinetics of cloned neuronal Ca channels and their possible counterparts in mammalian CNS neurons. *Neuropharmacology* 1993;32:1075–1088.
440. Zong S, Zhou J, Tanabe T. Molecular determinants of calcium-dependent inactivation in cardiac L-type calcium channels. *Biochem Biophys Res Commun* 1994;201:1117–1123.

Anesthesia: Biologic Foundations, edited by Tony L. Yaksh et al. Lippincott–Raven Publishers, Philadelphia © 1997.

CHAPTER 13

POTASSIUM CHANNELS

ZELJKO J. BOSNJAK, WAI-MENG KWOK, AND JOSEPH J. PANCRAZIO

OVERALL ROLE

As modern patch-clamp and molecular biologic techniques have been applied to different cell types and tissue, our understanding of K channels has steadily grown. It is now clear that K channels constitute the most diverse and prevalent group of ion channels. Their diversity is not strictly due to differences between cell types such as differing requirements for bioelectrical behavior, since various types of K channels can often be found in the same cell. By nature of their selectivity for K^+ ions and the strong chemical gradient for K^+ ions, which exists across many cell membranes, e.g., intracellular $[K^+] \sim 140$ mM and extracellular $[K^+] \sim 4$ to 5 mM, the opening of any of the K channels leads to a hyperpolarization and/or maintenance of the membrane at negative potentials. Despite the somewhat misleading names attached to some K channel types (e.g., the "inward rectifier"), all K channels pass outward current over a physiologic range of membrane potentials and K^+ concentrations in excitable cells. As long as the K^+ concentrations remain intact, K channels can be viewed as membrane stabilizers whose roles in excitable cells may include maintenance of the resting membrane potential, repolarization after an action potential, reduction of the frequency of spikes during repetitive firing, or even termination of firing after a period of marked activity. To perform these various functions, nature has provided a diversity of K-channel types that differ in their voltage-dependence, kinetics, and Ca^{2+}/ligand sensitivity. This chapter surveys the classes of K channels relevant to excitable cells with a special emphasis on the known molecular characteristics of these channel types, and reviews the effects of anesthetics on K channels from cardiac, smooth muscle, and neuronal tissue types.

DIVERSITY

From extensive studies in *Drosophila,* several mechanisms that contribute to the extreme diversity of K-channel proteins have been identified at the genomic, molecular, and posttranslational levels (12). The genomic level diversity can result from multiplicity of the genes that code for K-channel proteins and from alternative splicing of those genes. On the other hand, at the molecular level diversity can result from differences in the subunits of different types of K channels. At the posttranslational level, there are differences in the ways in which diverse subunits are assembled in the cell membrane along with differences in posttranslational glycosylation and phosphorylation. Furthermore, it is not yet known whether there are endogenous modulators of K-channel activity in addition to the neurotransmitters and the relevant G proteins, which may contribute to the variety of K-channel properties in different tissues (12).

CHARACTERISTICS

K channels represent the largest and most diverse group of any ion channel family that has been identified in cells of the animal and plant kingdoms. The wide range of K channels include some channels that are activated or modulated by second messengers such as Ca^{2+}, adenosine triphosphate (ATP), inositol 1,4,5-triphosphate, and G proteins, while others are activated by changes in membrane potential (170). In addition, other K channels such as the inward rectifier appear voltage dependent because their pores are blocked in a voltage-dependent manner by certain cations (230) or polyamines (108, 219), while other channels appear to be intrinsically sensitive to voltage so that changes of membrane potential induce specific conformational changes leading to channel openings. Many of these voltage-gated K channels differ in the range over which membrane potential changes elicit channel activation and in the rates of transition between the open and various closed states of the channel. Activation of voltage-gated K channels is thought to result from a voltage-driven conformational change that opens a transmembrane pore through the protein (58). Depolarization of the membrane exerts an electric force on voltage sensors in the channel that contain the charged residues of the channel located within the transmembrane electric field.

Previous work supports the view that the K channel is a multi-ion single file pore that selects primarily for K^+ (274). Even though Na^+ is smaller than K^+ in its nonhydrated form, K channels permit K^+ ions to pass through the pore 10,000 times more readily than Na^+ ions (170). This type of selectivity is achieved with little or no compromise in the rate of K^+ flux since more than 1,000,000 K^+ ions can permeate the pores of certain K channels in one second (244,402). It is likely that K channels have multiple K^+-binding sites within the pore and either some or all of these sites can discriminate between K^+ and Na^+ resulting in a high affinity for K^+. Because the narrowest part of the K channel pore is probably about 3 Å wide, K^+ ions must occupy certain binding sites to achieve high selectivity while passing through the pore in a single file (148,170). To allow for this selectivity and high flow, it is likely that unique structural contributions exist for K^+ ions including filter dimensions, electrical site field strength, and the strength of ion-water interactions (400). An additional factor that might contribute to the high-flow rates might be multi-ion repulsion within the K channel pore (213). It has been proposed that ions other than K^+ would remain destabilized and unable to compensate for the strong dehydration as the channel narrows to approximately 3 Å (148). These types of factors that are selecting for and against certain ions essentially leave the K channel like many other channels—imperfectly selective, since at least three other ions can permeate K channels including Tl^+, NH_4^+, and Rb^+ (274). Other ions known to block certain K channels, such as Ba^{2+}, may bind tightly to sites in the channel pore.

MOLECULAR BIOLOGY OF POTASSIUM CHANNELS

Given the extensive work clarifying the structure-function relationships of K channels, it is important to highlight some of the key studies in this rapidly growing field. The different structural classes are depicted in the cartoon in Fig. 1, which include voltage-gated K channels, Ca^{2+}-dependent "BK_{Ca}" K channels, inwardly rectifying K channels, *ether-à-go-go* (eag), and minK, each of which will be discussed in detail.

Flies and Ether: Identification of Voltage-Gated K-Channel Clones

Anesthesiologists can take pride, however small, in the knowledge that the anesthetic ether has played an important

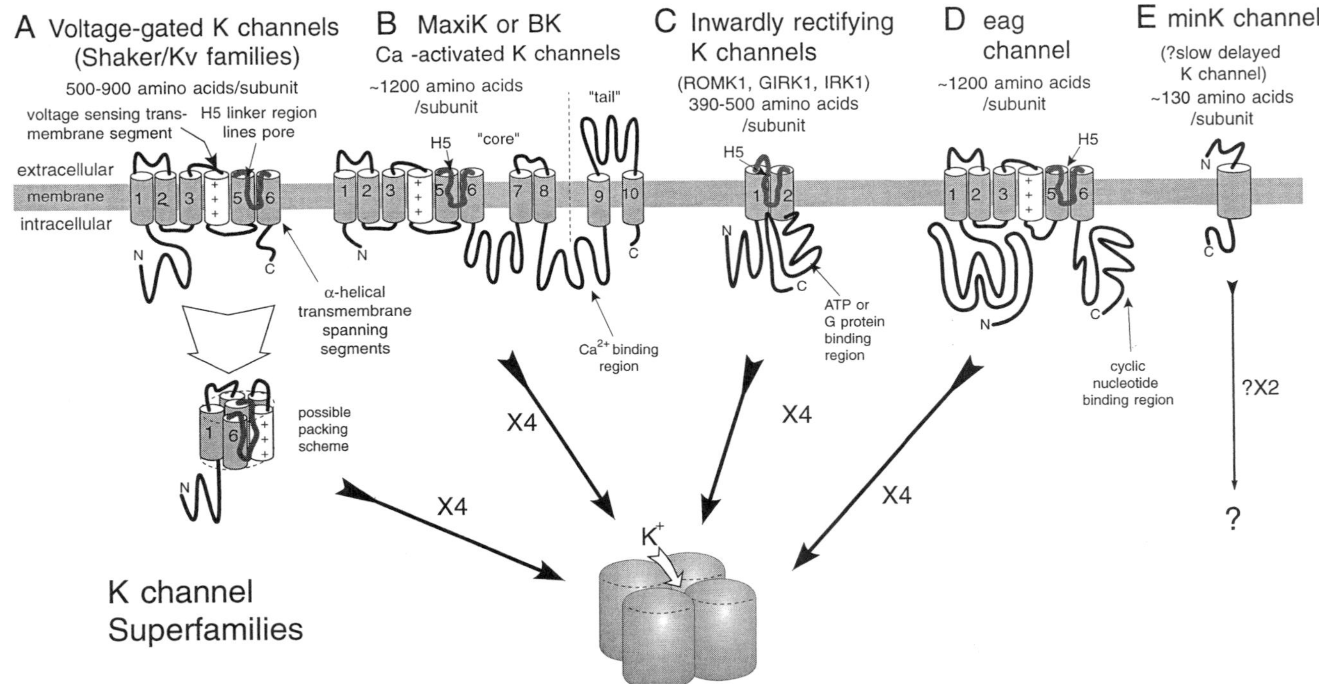

Figure 1. Structure of identified K channels. **(A)** Voltage-gated K channels typified by *Shaker* and related Kv subfamily of channels. **(B)** "BKCa" Ca^{2+}-dependent K channels, also referred to as *slo*. **(C)** Inwardly rectifying K channels that include IRK, ROMK, and GIRK. **(D)** Ether-à-go-go *(eag)*, which shares homology with both the Kv subfamily and the cyclic nucleotide gated ion channels. **(E)** MinK, a protein that underlies the slow delayed outward K current in cardiac cells. With the exception of minK, each of these channel types exhibits a hydrophilic loop, H5, which is thought to contribute to the ion-conducting pore and is separated by two transmembrane α-helices. Although there is substantial evidence that the Kv subfamily forms functional K channels as homo- or heterotetramers, the subunit stoichiometry of the other K channels is, at present, speculative.

role in the molecular biologic study of K channels. The recognition that a peculiar leg-shaking behavior was triggered by exposure to ether in a particular strain of fruit flies, *Drosophila melanogaster*, opened the door to K-channel cloning. Voltage-clamp analysis of muscle and neuronal cells isolated from *Drosophila* with the *Shaker* mutation revealed an altered or missing transient outward (A-type) K current (311,399). In 1987 efforts by several groups resulted in the preparation of cDNAs from the region of the *Shaker* gene defect (21,176,280). Examination of the hydropathy plot from the ~600 amino acid long peptide encoded by the cDNA indicated the presence of six membrane spanning segments with similarities to the motif used by the α subunit of the Na channel (94,170,244,247,290, 291,356). Fig. 1A illustrates the major structural components of this gene product including the six α-helical transmembrane segments, S1 to S6, which are composed largely of hydrophobic amino acid residues and the S5 to S6 loop, called the H5 segment, which is composed of mostly charged residues. In addition, the fourth membrane spanning segment, S4, has an arrangement of a positively charged residue every third position that is highly conserved among other voltage-dependent channels (356) and thought to be important for sensitivity to voltage (94,170,291). In addition, the loop linking the S1 and S2 segments has been experimentally confirmed to be located extracellularly (324). As is true for Na and Ca channels, the H5 loop appears to fold back to contribute to the "P region," which is thought to participate to the formation of the ion conduction pore. Note, however, that recent evidence implicates the S4 to S5 loop (333) as well as the S6 segment (220) as part of the pore region. Although the Na and Ca channel α subunits, each with a molecular weight of ~260 kD, have four homologous domains as shown in Fig. 1A, the *Shaker* peptide has only a single domain with a molecular weight of ~70 kD. These findings led to the proposal that the *Shaker* gene product assembles as a tetramer to form a voltage-dependent K channel (356). Voltage-clamp measurements from *Xenopus* oocytes injected with mRNA generated from the *Shaker* cDNA indeed produced an A-type K channel (167,359). The evidence that the *Shaker* peptide forms a tetramer, although strongly suspected based on comparisons with Na and Ca channels, was provided by MacKinnon (225) based on the kinetics of charybdotoxin binding, and more recently by Li et al. (214) using electron microscopy revealing a square like appearance of the purified *Shaker* protein (Fig. 2).

The molecular basis of tetraethylammonium (TEA) sensitivity of voltage-gated K channels appears to involve a tyrosine at the carboxyl terminal end of the P region (403). Internal TEA blocks voltage-gated K channels by interacting with a second site on the inner surface of the pore. 4-aminopyridine (4-AP) appears to block many of the voltage-gated K channels with variable potency. The 4-AP-binding site appears to be formed from the association of the amino terminal end of S5 and carboxyl terminal end of S6, which are both thought to lie in the inner vestibule of the channel pore (185).

The voltage dependence of *Shaker* K channels resides mainly in the transitions between several closed states prior to channel opening (189,338,405). The transition from the last closed state to the open state of the channel has been shown to be voltage-independent for *Shaker* K channels (405). Therefore, part of the channel molecule functions as a voltage sensor and is capable of detecting and responding to changes of membrane potential. The voltage sensor itself is expected to reside in the hydrophobic interior of the membrane (10,148). Voltage-clamp studies of expressed channels in oocytes has shown that the gating charge of the *Shaker* K channel is approximately +4 (358). Therefore, channel activation is associated with the

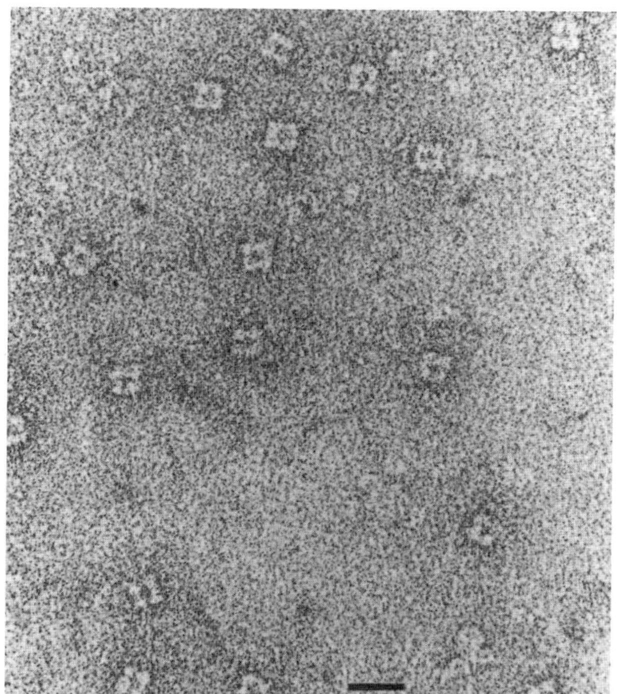

Figure 2. Electron microscopic images of *Shaker* K channels expressed in insect Sf9 cells revealing the striking fourfold symmetry, resulting in a square-shaped appearance. The *bar* corresponds to a length of 150 Å. (Reprinted with permission from ref. 214.)

translocation of about 4 positive charges in the direction from the cytoplasmic side to the extracellular side of the membrane.

Examination of *Drosophila* led to the identification of other genes similar to *Shaker: Shal, Shab,* and *Shaw,* when expressed in *Xenopus* oocytes and measured electrophysiologically, exhibit progressively less inactivation as shown in Fig. 3 (387). There is considerable diversity in the length of the carboxyl and amino terminal regions of the K channel polypeptides. For instance, the *Shaker*-related channels all have longer amino termini than carboxyl termini, while, overall, *Shab*-related proteins have the longest amino terminus. With the polypeptide sequences known, the molecular basis of inactivation exhibited by the *Shaker* and *Shaker*-related K channels was shown to be due to several mechanisms, two of which are illustrated in Fig. 4. First, like the "ball-and-chain" model initially proposed to explain rapid inactivation of voltage-dependent Na channels (10,11), the α subunits of those A-type K channels possess an inactivating region in the amino terminus sequence that blocks the pore from the cytoplasmic side upon membrane depolarization (156,406). Deletion of the amino terminal from the *Shaker* channel removes rapid inactivation (156), while addition of an amino terminal peptide to the inner surface of this channel restores inactivation (406). For this amino-terminal (N-type) inactivation, the inactivating domain consists of approximately 20 amino acids and binds to the channel mouth, perhaps at the S4 to S5 loop (163). Mutations in the intracellular loop linking S4 and S5 segments of the *Shaker* channel alter inactivation kinetics, suggesting that this region maybe indeed the receptor for amino terminal segment (164). Internal application of TEA produces a slower N-type inactivation in the *Shaker* channel probably by competing for a common binding site (60). Therefore, it has been suggested that the receptor for the fast inactivation segment must lie close to the cytoplasmic mouth of the ion conducting pathway. If this site is occupied by the ball, the gating charges within the voltage sensor may be immobilized and prevented from returning to its original position (27). Based on the time course of internally perfused hydrolytic enzyme action, it appears that rapidly inactivating K channels can have a total of four segments, one from each α subunit, each of which behave independently (127). Second, there is strong evidence for a role for the β subunit in inactivation. At least in some of the *Shaker*-related family of channels, the ~70 kD α subunits can form a tight association with a ~39-kD β subunit (281). As shown in Fig. 5, coexpression of the Kvβ1 with α subunits exhibiting two extremes in the rate of inactivation, RCK1 and RCK4 (Kv1.1 and Kv1.4, respectively, Table 1),

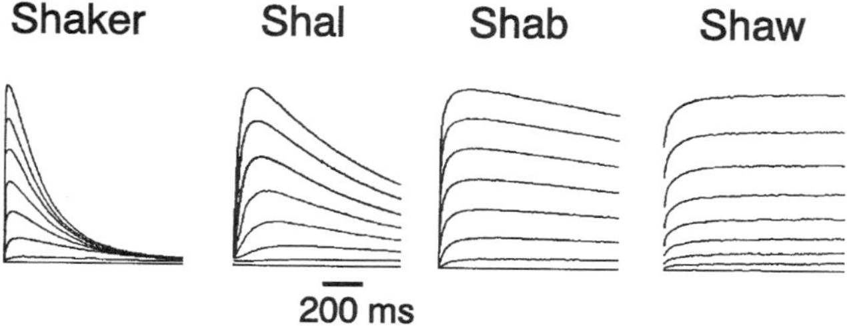

Figure 3. Measurement of voltage-gated K currents in *Xenopus* oocytes injected with cRNAs from *Shaker, Shal, Shab,* and *Shaw.* Test potentials 1 second in duration from −80 mV to +20 mV in 10-mV increments were applied from a holding potential of −90 mV. Note that the measurements from *Shaker* and *Shal* were made at 11°C, whereas those from *Shab* and *Shaw* were performed at 23°C. (Reprinted with permission from ref. 387.)

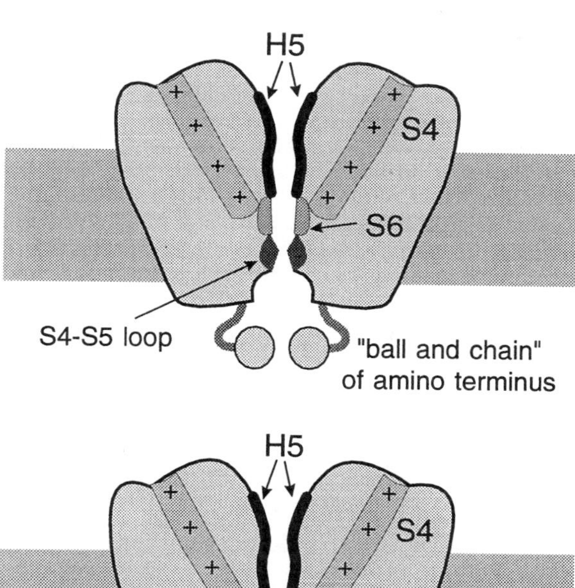

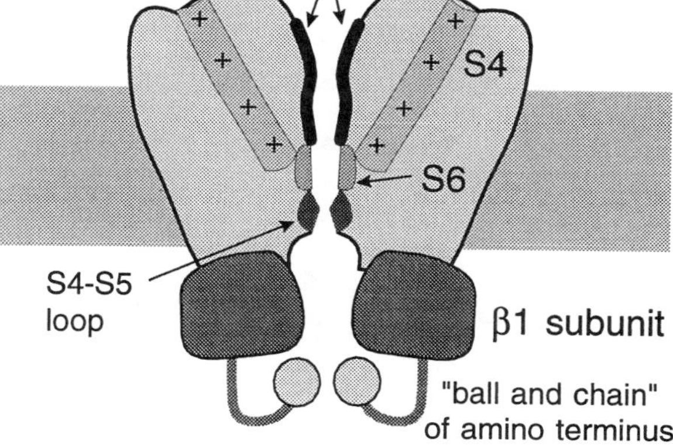

Figure 4. Side-view model of structural characteristics of *Shaker*-related voltage-dependent K channels. The S4 segment features a pattern of positively charged residues thought to serve as a voltage sensor, whereas the H5 loop, S4 to S5 loop, and the S6 segments contribute to the formation of the ion selective pore. Two types of amino-terminal or N-type inactivation are depicted by the inclusion of "ball-and-chain" assemblies from the amino terminus of the α subunits, as observed with Kv1.1, or from the β subunit, specifically Kvβ1. (Adapted from ref. 333.)

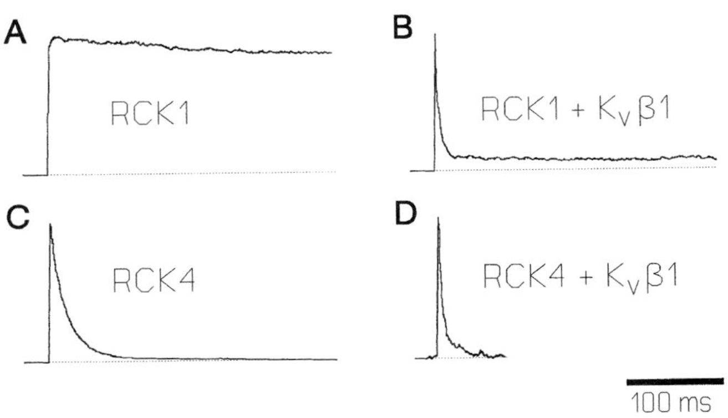

Figure 5. Coexpression of Kvβ1 with the slowly and rapidly inactivating α subunits, RCK1 (Kv1.1) and RCK4 (Kv1.4), respectively, results in even faster inactivation. Expression of Kvβ1 in the absence of α subunits fails to produce any outward current. Outward K currents were recorded from injected *Xenopus* oocytes using the cell-attached patch-clamp configuration. (Reprinted with permission from ref. 298.)

resulted in profound enhancements in the rate of decay of each (298). Sequence alignment of the N-terminal regions from Kvβ1 and α subunits that show rapid inactivation revealed structural similarity, suggesting that the Kvβ1 subunit can provide a ball-and-chain assembly (298). While Kvβ3, which is most abundantly expressed in the aorta and left ventricle, promotes inactivation of Kv1.4, it does not alter Kv1.1 gating (252). Note, however, that the promotion of inactivation should not be considered a general property of K channel β subunits, since Kvβ2 has poor homology with Kvβ1 and Kvβ3 over the section of the amino-terminal critical for inactivation (298). Channel blockade by TEA can distinguish N-type inactivation from another mechanism of inactivation, core or C-type, which has a time constant of seconds and appears to be a function of an extracellular domain (60,128). Whereas internally perfused TEA blocks N-type inactivation, possibly through a simple competition for the blocking site, externally administered TEA blocks C-type inactivation, perhaps also by competition where the C-type inactivation gate cannot swing shut with the TEA "foot in the door."

The availability of the *Shaker* clones paved the way for the identification of the first mammalian K-channel clones by screening the *Shaker* cDNA against mouse brain cDNA libraries (236,344). The original *Shaker* gene from *Drosophila* gave rise to five alternative spliced variants (317), four of which produced identifiable phenotypes (358) when expressed heterologously in *Xenopus* oocytes. Different names were given to these clones that reflected the tissue source, and as a consequence identical cDNAs often have different names. Further complicating this confusion is that significant differences in tissue distribution may occur between closely related genes (160). As one might expect, the growing interest and productivity in K channel cloning led to a situation where several laboratories cloned the same K channel gene, but gave it different names. To alleviate confusion, a standardized nomenclature has been adopted (59) where K channel genes can be designated in the form Kvn.m (Table 1). *Kv* indicates that a voltage-gated K channel is encoded by the gene, *n* designates the *Drosophila* subfamily to which the clone is most homologous such that Kv1, Kv2, Kv3, and Kv4 correspond to *Shaker, Shab, Shaw,* and *Shal* subfamilies, respectively. The second number, *m*, indicates the order in which the clone was identified. How similar are gene products within a subfamily and how different are the subfamilies? Regardless of species, sequence homology of 60% or more is typical of members within a subfamily, whereas homology of less than 40% distinguishes one subfamily from another (310).

In spite of the seemingly extensive variation afforded by these multiple genes in the formation of homomeric channels, K channels can also form as heterotetramers. Coexpression of *Shaker*-related clones in oocytes yielded evidence for the formation of heterotetrameric K channels (163), suggesting an even larger degree of K channel diversity. This hypothesis has been verified in native cells and tissue with the use of specific antibodies directed against *Shaker*-like polypeptides (318,382). In fact, Kv1.4 and Kv1.2 appear to coassemble in the rat brain to form the presynaptic A-type K channel that exhibits properties common to both gene products (326). Heteropolymerization, does not appear to occur between α subunits from different subfamilies (74). For example Kv1.4 and Kv4.2, appear to be strongly influenced by the amino terminal (209), specifically a region called the T1 assembly domain (325).

Table 1. NOMENCLATURE FOR VOLTAGE-DEPENDENT K CHANNELS

Drosophila subfamily	Standardized nomenclature	Rat pseudonym(s)	Human pseudonym(s)	Human genome nomenclature
ShI (*Shaker*)	Kv1.1	RCK1, RBK1, RMK1, RK1	HBK1, HuK1	KCNA1
Kv1	Kv1.2	RCK5, BK2, RK2, NGK1	HBK5, HuKIV	KCNA2
	Kv1.3	RCK3, RGK3, KV3	HPCN, HuKIII	KCNA3
	Kv1.4	RCK4, RHK1, RK3	HBK4, HK1, hPCN2, HuKII	KCNA4
	Kv1.5	RCK7, KV1, RK4	hPCN1, HK2	KCNA5
	Kv1.6	RCK2, KV2	HBK2	KCNA6
	Kv1.7		HaK6	KCNA7
	Kv1.8	RCK9		KCNA8
ShII (*Shab*)	Kv2.1	DRK1	DHK1, h-DRK1	KCNB1
Kv2	Kv2.2	cdrk		KCNB2
ShIII (*Shaw*)	Kv3.1	KV4, Raw2, Raw2a, KShIIIB	KCN1, NGK2-KV4	KCNC1
Kv3	Kv3.2	RkShIIIA, KV3.2b, KV3.2c, Raw1	KCN2, KShIIIA	KCNC2
	Kv3.3		KCN3	KCNC3
	Kv3.4	Raw3	KCN4, KShIIIC	KCNC4
ShIV (*Shal*)	Kv4.1	RShal	–	KCND1
Kv4	Kv4.2	RK5	–	KCND2
	Kv4.3		–	KCND3
?	aKv5.1*	?	?	?

Adapted largely from (77,290,300,354,389).

*aKv5.1 encodes a new subfamily of noninactivating, voltage-dependent K channel in Aplysia, which, unlike Kv1 through Kv4, can contribute to the resting potential (408).

"Maxi-BK" Ca^{2+}-Dependent K Channels

Another *Drosophila* mutation, *Slowpoke (slo),* permitted access to the genes encoding large-conductance, "BK_{Ca}" or "maxi," Ca^{2+}-activated K channels. Fruit flies with the *slo* mutation, which can be paralyzed with a protocol involving sudden temperature changes, fail to express a Ca^{2+}-dependent K current during voltage clamp investigation of dorsal longitudinal flight muscle (97). Genomic and cDNA clones from the *slo* locus were isolated and sequenced, indicating that the predicted gene product shared some resemblance with a number of regions of the *Shaker* family of K channels (18). The greatest similarity between the *slo* and *Shaker* polypeptides occurs over the H5 segment thought to line the pore (18). As shown in Fig. 1B, the *slo* polypeptide has the six transmembrane domains with a highly conserved S4 segment. However, the *slo* polypeptide is much longer, including ~850 amino acids between the S6 domain and the carboxyl terminus (183), and incorporating four additional hydrophobic segments, S7 to S10, which may span the membrane (51). Expression of the mRNAs constructed from the *slo* cDNA results in functional BK_{Ca} channels, while alternative splicing can result in extensive diversity (4). A mammalian homologue of the *Drosophila slo (dSlo)* clone, called *mSlo,* was isolated from mouse brain and skeletal muscle showing a 60% sequence homology of the amino acid sequence between the two polypeptide gene products (51). Evidence exists for differential roles for the core, comprised of the residues from the amino terminus through the S8 transmembrane region, and the tail, which contains the remaining residues. Whereas the core appears to determine the single-channel properties such as voltage-dependence, permeation, and kinetics, the tail influences Ca^{2+} sensitivity (388). Nine isoforms of *slo* have recently been cloned from human brain that are 92% similar to *mSlo* in protein sequence and are generated by alternative RNA splicing. These variants arise from separate but adjacent splice sites located within the tail region, resulting in differing Ca^{2+} sensitivity among the isoforms (370).

Immunoprecipitation experiments using [^{125}]I-charybdotoxin as a marker during purification of the BK_{Ca} channel in bovine smooth muscle revealed a heavily glycosylated 32-kD a protein (β subunit) that appeared in a 1:1 stoichiometry with the larger 62-kd α subunit (119,187). The β subunit consists of two possible transmembrane domains, a large extracellular domain, two short amino and carboxyl terminal domains, and a putative protein kinase A (PKA) phosphorylation site at the amino terminal (187). Recent work indicates that coexpression of the β subunit with the α subunit results in a BK_{Ca} channel that is much more sensitive to Ca^{2+} and voltage than the channels composed of the α subunit alone. Furthermore, expression of the β subunit has been shown to confer pharmacologic sensitivity to the BK channel. Dehydrosoysaponin-1 at a concentration that increases BK-channel probability of opening (P_o) by 50-fold in native smooth muscle channels (240) was without action in the absence of the β subunit while very effective when both α and β subunits were coexpressed (241).

The Ca^{2+}-dependent K-channel group does include at least two other functional channel types beyond BK_{Ca} channels: an intermediate "IK_{Ca}" and small conductance "SK_{Ca}" (205). While there is presently no information about the molecular structure of IK_{Ca} channels, Sokol and colleagues (337) have sequenced the protein binding to the bee venom apamin, a specific blocker of SK_{Ca} channels. The resulting sequence reveals four putative membrane spanning segments and a Ca^{2+}-binding domain, with similarities to the "EF hand" motif used by calmodulin. However, the sequence shows no significant homology with any known voltage or ligand-dependent channel and it remains to be shown that this protein forms a functional channel when expressed (337).

Missing a Few Segments: Inwardly Rectifying K Channels

While the *Shaker* family and the *slo* classes of K channels are characterized by the six transmembrane segment domains, the inwardly rectifying K channels have a strikingly different architecture. ROMK1 and IRK1, cloned from the outer medulla of rat kidney (151) and from a mouse macrophage cell line (194), respectively, encode polypeptides with only two transmembrane segments, M1 and M2, with an apparent H5 region. This region bears some resemblance to the S5 and S6 segments with the pore-forming segment (Fig. 1C). Expression of IRK1 and ROMK1 in *Xenopus* oocytes revealed that the IRK1 K channel exhibits a far more prominent inward rectification than ROMK1 K channel (151), attributable to differential sensitivity to intracellular Mg^{2+} or endogenous polyamines (108,219) that are largely conveyed by a different residue at a particular sequence location (393). Although IRK1 and ROMK1 differ in terms of single-channel conductance, exchange of the H5 region, which is thought to be a major determinant of pore properties, failed to affect K^+ conductance (349). Instead, the substitution of the carboxyl terminal region imparts Mg^{2+} sensitivity and K^+ conductance from IRK1 to ROMK1 (349), suggesting that this region governs pore function in these channels. Two other members of the IRK family, IRK2 (350) and IRK3 (253), have the greatest level of expression in the rat brain. Another member of the IRK family has been recently cloned from the human hippocampus, HIR, which is characterized by a relatively small unitary channel conductance of 13 pS, significantly lower than the 20 to 40 pS typically observed with other inwardly rectifying K channels recorded under similar conditions (287). In addition, a subunit of the G-protein–linked muscarinic K channel, GIRK1, which was cloned from rat heart, possesses the same fundamental architecture as the other members of the IRK subfamily (195). Coexpression of GIRK1 with $G_{\beta\gamma}$, but not G_α, results in a high probability of channel opening, which is consistent with a primary role for the βγ subunits in muscarinic K channel activation (299). It appears that a segment of the carboxyl terminus approximately 100 amino acids in length and exhibiting strong homology to β-adrenergic-receptor-kinase (βARK1) may serve as the $G_{\beta\gamma}$-binding domain for GIRK1 (332). It has recently been shown that in cardiac tissue GIRK1 coimmunoprecipitates with another protein, CIR, which is homologous to other members of the inwardly rectifying K channel family (192). Coexpression of CIR with GIRK1 results in a significant increase in G protein activated inwardly rectifying K current with properties quite similar to those observed for the ACh-activated K current, $I_{K(ACh)}$, suggesting that these K_{ACh} channels are the result of heteropolymerization (192). Whereas the IRK subfamily appears most often expressed in excitable tissue, ROMK1, along with splice variants ROMK2 and ROMK3, have been identified in tissue typically viewed as nonexcitable where the primary roles of these channels may be to maintain the membrane potential and mediate K^+ ion secretion (151,410). The subunit stoichiometry is presently uncertain for the inwardly rectifying K channels; however, it has been speculated that this family forms functional channels with tetrameric assembly (171).

Another member of the inwardly rectifying K channel family may prove to be the ATP-sensitive K channel (K_{ATP}), which has been reported to possess the hallmark structural features of this class, i.e., two membrane spanning domains separated by a putative H5 region (17). Recent work has raised significant doubts that the K_{ATP} channel protein complex has been truly identified (192). Instead, it may be that the polypeptide cloned previously by Ashford and colleagues (17) constitutes a subunit of K_{ATP} (192), where the sulfonylurea receptor might be part of a separate molecule (207).

eag Channels: A Missing Link?

Another structural class of K channels was determined using the *Drosophila* mutant *ether-à-go-go (eag)*, which exhibits a particular leg-shaking phenotype. The *eag* mutant shows spontaneous, repetitive firing of action potentials at larval neuromuscular junctions (118), which was attributed to an altered K conductance (409). As shown in Fig. 1D, the polypeptide encoded by the *eag* gene is structurally similar to the Kv family, featuring six α-helical membrane spanning segments and a pore region (170). But the *eag* polypeptide also shares significant homology with the cyclic nucleotide-gated ion channels, particularly at a cytoplasmic region beyond S6 (132,323,385). Interestingly, *eag* channels are permeable to both Ca^{2+} and K^+ ions, open with depolarization like Kv channels, and are upregulated by adenosine 3′,5′-cyclic monophosphate (cAMP) (47). These observations have led to the suggestion that *eag* channels may be an evolutionary "missing link" between cyclic nucleotide gated channels and the Kv family (47,169). An entire family of *eag*-related genes has been identified in mammals (386); however, little is known about their distribution and function. Recent evidence has implicated *HERG*, a human homologue of *eag*, as a major subunit of $I_{Kr(V)}$ (312,368). Mutations to *HERG* may be the molecular basis of long QT syndrome, an inherited disorder that is associated with torsades de pointes (78). Unlike some of the *eag* variants (47), *HERG* is unresponsive to cyclic nucleotides (312) and exhibits extremely rapid inactivation to account for its apparent inwardly rectifying nature (368). Since $I_{Kr(V)}$, which is a component of the delayed rectifier K current in cardiac tissue, may constitute an important target for class III antiarrhythmics (314), knowledge of the molecular structure of *HERG* may have profound implications for the rational design of antiarrhythmic agents.

MinK: K Channel or Transporter?

Although substantial strides have been made to understand the structure-function relations of the inwardly rectifying and Kv classes of K channels, minK remains somewhat enigmatic. An apparently isolated channel protein, minK, or I_{sK} consists of only ~130 amino acids and a single putative α-helical transmembrane domain (Fig. 1E) and was initially identified in rat kidney (353), heart (109), and uterus (292). It is difficult to imagine how this single hydrophobic membrane spanning domain might form a K-selective channel, unless the amino or carboxyl termini can contribute to pore formation. This possibility seems unlikely since extensive deletions to the amino and carboxyl regions have little or no effect on minK function (352). In fact, the lack of sequence homology of minK with other K channels, particularly the absence of an H5 segment, and the inability to measure single-channel currents led to the suggestion that minK might operate as a carrier rather than a channel, or that it might be a regulator of an endogenous, ordinarily silent K channel in *Xenopus* oocytes (31). The findings that the current carried by minK (a) shows voltage-dependent gating and pharmacologic similarities with delayed rectifiers in intact preparations (139), (b) exhibits altered cation selectivity and block by TEA with point mutations to the membrane spanning region (126), and (c) can be expressed in a mammalian cell line (112) have been used to support the argument that minK forms a K channel. Thus, voltage-gated K currents are carried by at least two structurally diverse classes of proteins, the Kv family of channels and minK. Like the inwardly rectifying K channels, it is unclear how many minK subunits must combine to form functional channels; however, preliminary data suggest that only two monomers may be sufficient (383). The absence of single-channel records may be due to the extremely low conductance on minK channels, recently estimated with noise analysis techniques to be less than 1 fA (401), which is on the same order of magnitude as a transporter (148). Regardless of whether minK functions in the membrane as a channel or transporter, there is now evidence that the slow component of K current in cardiac cells, a major determinant of action potential duration, is mediated by minK (112,373).

TYPES OF POTASSIUM CHANNELS: FUNCTION AND PHARMACOLOGY

In this section, a number of K-channel classes are presented that are distinguished on a functional and pharmacologic basis. Designations such as "delayed rectifier" refers to a broad group of functionally similar K currents rather than a particular class of channel proteins.

Voltage-Sensitive K Channels

Voltage-sensitive K currents are subdivided into several groups as shown in Table 2.

Delayed Rectifier Current—$I_{K(V)}$

The most well-known example of IK(V) is that from the squid giant axon initially described in detail by the remarkable efforts of Hodgkin and Huxley (152,153). After a delay, which varies in duration depending on the particular channel protein, this K current activates to repolarize a membrane during excitation, thus providing the outwardly rectifying characteristics of the membrane (154). As demonstrated in a variety of neuronal tissue and cell types, $I_{K(V)}$ activates upon depolarization with sigmoid kinetics (305) and exhibits slow time-dependent inactivation (2,96,116,319). Delayed rectifier (K_V) channels typically range from 5 to 20 pS in neuronal tissue (305). While most excitable membranes express at least one type of $I_{K(V)}$, some membranes contain even more. For example, at a single node of Ranvier in frog, there are at least three components of K current—fast, intermediate, and slow—distinguished on differential voltage-dependence of activation and pharmacologic criteria, which appeared to represent distinct K channel types (91,92). While the fast channels, which have a conductance of 55 pS, fall under a different functional category of K channel, i.e., the transient outward K channel class, the slow and intermediate channels are considered members of the K_V class and exhibit a single-channel conductance of 33 and 10 pS in symmetrical K^+ solution, respectively (307).

The K_V channels of smooth muscle cells, which have a dominant role in membrane repolarization and are responsible for slow wave activity, have been investigated in several tissue types (23,50,271). In rabbit portal vein, the K_V channel opens in response to depolarizing potentials above −40 mV, and at the single-channel level, the conductance was found to be approximately 5 to 7 pS (23,376). $I_{K(V)}$ in these cells is blocked by externally applied 4-AP while relatively insensitive to TEA.

The K_V channels of cardiac tissue require special attention since there is not only marked diversity between cell types, e.g., atrial versus ventricular versus pacemaker tissue, but also among different species. Clearly, issues of diversity are of critical importance for the choice of appropriate animal models of cardiac function in the study of pharmacologic agents, which include class III antiarrhythmics and anesthetics. There are at least three distinct types of $I_{K(V)}$ that have been identified in isolated cardiac cells based on differences in rate of activation, rectification properties, and pharmacology (125,238,263,315). These types include slowly activating outward rectifying current, $I_{Ks(V)}$, a rapidly activating inwardly rectifying current, $I_{Kr(V)}$, and a rapidly activating outwardly rectifying current, I_{RAK}. As mentioned earlier, minK appears to be responsible for $I_{Ks(V)}$ (112,373), while *HERG* may underlie the pore-forming subunit of $I_{Kr(V)}$ (312,368). In addition, Boyle and Nerbonne (39) identified a voltage-dependent, ultrarapid activating, noninactivating K current in rat atrial myocytes that is distinct from I_{Kr} called I_{RAK}, which appears to be encoded by Kv1.5

Table 2. K CHANNELS—THE RANGE OF SINGLE-CHANNEL CONDUCTANCE, γ, VALUES ARE GIVEN BELOW FOR EACH FUNCTIONAL CHANNEL CATEGORY ALONG WITH A BRIEF LIST OF COMMON BLOCKERS/INHIBITORS

Channel type	γ (pS)	Characteristics	Typical blockers
Voltage sensitive			
Delayed rectifier—K_V	5–33	Activated by depolarization above –45 mV with some delay; little or no inactivation (τ 0.1–10 sec)	TEA, 4-AP (weak), Cs^+, Ba^{2+}
Transient outward, A-type—K_A	15–55	Activated by modest depolarizations; rapid inactivation (τ 10–100 ms) and marked steady-state inactivation	4-AP (potent), TEA (weak), dendrotoxins
Inwardly rectifying			
Inward (anomalous) rectifier—K_{IR}	13–40	Inward rectification depends on intracellular Mg^{2+} and/or polyamines; conductance depends on extracellular [K^+]	TEA, Cs^+ (potent), Na^+, Ba^{2+}
ACh-sensitive—K_{ACh}	40–45	Directly activated by the βγ subunits of the G_i GTP-binding protein	Cs^+, Ba^{2+}
Neurotransmitter-activated, G-protein linked	30–70	Receptors for serotonin, opiates, and $GABA_B$ agonists to GIRK channels	Cs^+, Ba^{2+}
ATP-sensitive—K_{ATP}	30–260	Intracellular ATP reduces channel opening; intracellular ADP, pH, and Na may also modulate channel opening	Tolbutamide, glibenclamide, TEA (weak), Ba^{2+}, Cd^{2+}
Ca^{2+}-dependent			
High conductance—BK_{Ca}	150–300	Increased intracellular Ca^{2+} shifts the voltage for activation to more negative potentials	TEA (submillimolar), charybdotoxin
Small conductance—SK_{Ca}	<50	Voltage-insensitive; Ca^{2+} sensitivity of SK_{Ca}>BK_{Ca} at negative potentials	Apamin, TEA (weak)
Intermediate conductance—IK_{Ca}	50–150	Unclear at this time	Charybdotoxin, Cs^+, TEA
Other K specific			
M current—K_M	10–15	Time and voltage-dependent, activated above –60 mV; protein kinase C activation decreases activity	TEA (weak), Ba^{2+}, substance P
Na^+-activated—K_{Na}	170–210	Activated by an increase in intracellular Na^+ >20 mM	TEA, 4-AP

(107,334,335). I_{RAK} is expressed in adult human ventricle (76) and to a greater extent in human atria (301). While neither $I_{Kr(V)}$ nor $I_{Ks(V)}$ has been reported in human ventricle, both have been identified in human atrial myocytes (381).

In guinea pig myocytes, which express only $I_{Ks(V)}$ and $I_{Kr(V)}$, fully activated $I_{Ks(V)}$ evoked by step potentials is about 11-fold greater than $I_{Kr(V)}$ (315). While it might appear that $I_{Ks(V)}$ is the primary current responsible for repolarization in these cells, full activation of $I_{Ks(V)}$ requires many seconds while $I_{Kr(V)}$ activates very fast. During the time course of a normal action potential, these two currents activate to nearly equivalent magnitudes (314) and, therefore, both may substantially influence repolarization. At the single-channel level, the channels underlying $I_{Kr(V)}$ exhibit a conductance of 13 pS in symmetrical K^+ solution (375), whereas efforts to resolve single channels underlying $I_{Ks(V)}$ have met with failure (378). $I_{Kr(V)}$ and $I_{Ks(V)}$ were initially distinguished on the basis of activation and deactivation kinetics as well as differential pharmacologic sensitivity (314). $I_{Kr(V)}$ is specifically blocked by La^{3+} and certain class III antiarrhythmic agents including d-sotalol, E-4031, and dofetilide (174,313,314). The kinetics of this current are similar to an $I_{K(V)}$ present in the atrial node (327), and recently identified in rabbit ventricular myocytes, where an E-4031–sensitive $I_{Kr(V)}$ appears to be the only type of $I_{K(V)}$ present (375). In addition, the distribution of $I_{Ks(V)}$ and $I_{Ks(V)}$ may be influenced by the location of a myocyte within the ventricle: epicardial, midmyocardial, or endocardial (217). Midmyocardial canine ventricular myocytes have a distinctive phase-3 repolarization that may be in part due to a significantly smaller contribution of $I_{Ks(V)}$ to repolarization than in other myocytes from the canine ventricle (217). $I_{Ks(V)}$ appears to be modulated by a number of factors including intracellular Ca^{2+} (360–362), protein kinase C (PKC) (360–363,379,380), and PKA (379,380). Interestingly, whole-cell $I_{K(V)}$ is increased by the β-adrenergic agonist isoproterenol during blockade of phosphorylation pathways (113). These findings argue that guanine nucleotides and β-adrenergic receptor activation can enhance $I_{K(V)}$ by phosphorylation-independent pathway and, therefore, suggest the existence of direct coupling of the β-adrenergic receptor to a cardiac K_V channel via a membrane-delimited G- protein pathway.

Transient Outward Current—$I_{K(A)}$

The transient outward "A-type" K current, $I_{K(A)}$, which activates in response to small depolarizations from the resting potential followed by marked inactivation, was originally described independently by Neher (260) and Connor and Stevens (66) using molluscan neurons. Modeling work in molluscan neurons, which exhibit repetitive firing, demonstrated a role for $I_{K(A)}$ in mediating the duration of the interspike interval (67). Subsequent work identified $I_{K(A)}$ in mammalian central neurons (131) from the hippocampus (64,320,407), spinal cord (320), and nerve terminals of the posterior pituitary (28). The classic $I_{K(A)}$ exhibits profound steady-state inactivation that is nearly complete at −40 mV, sensitivity to millimolar concentrations of 4-AP (302,305), and a single-channel conductance ranging from 15 to 55 pS (28,71,179,307). Note, however, that there are a number of transient K currents that activate at more depolarized potentials and inactivate more slowly than the classic $I_{K(A)}$ (305). This observation is entirely consistent with the molecular biologic findings that K_V and K_A channels comprise a larger family of related proteins (148), as discussed earlier.

In cardiac cells, $I_{K(A)}$ is also referred to as I_{to} and is largely responsible for early phase-one repolarization of the cardiac action potential in certain species/tissues (124,256,369). There appear to be several transient outward currents that are variably expressed in different cardiac tissues (72,173,329,330) that are sensitive to the K channel blockers 4-AP (93,122,183,196, 216) and internally applied quaternary ammonium ions (180).

A prominent feature of the Purkinje fiber action potential is the phase-one repolarization. Although the $I_{K(A)}$ is present in all Purkinje fibers, its exact character seems to be species dependent. While the cow and calf Purkinje fibers clearly demonstrate a Ca^{2+}-activated current that has a very high single-channel conductance (52,330), in the sheep conduction system, $I_{K(A)}$ appears to be Ca^{2+}-independent (52,72).

A transient outward current has been demonstrated in the pacemaker tissue of the rabbit sinoatrial node. Although it contributes to repolarization, it differs from other $I_{K(A)}$ in being somewhat less selective for K^+ (257). Transient outward currents also have been documented in atrial muscle from a variety of tissues. The most prominent is the Ca^{2+}-independent form of these currents, which is largely responsible for the dramatically abbreviated plateau of the atrial action potentials (63,99).

The expression of $I_{K(A)}$ in ventricular myocytes varies with species. For instance, it is the major repolarizing current in rat (93,174), but absent in guinea pig (363). $I_{K(A)}$ appears to be the predominant repolarization current in human ventricle (374, 390), and has pharmacologic properties and kinetics most consistent with a heterotetrameric channels encoded by both Kv1.2 and Kv1.4 (301). Like $I_{Ks(V)}$, there appears to be a differential transmural distribution of $I_{K(A)}$ in rabbit ventricular myocytes (196). Close to the epicardial surface, ventricular cells, like Purkinje fibers, have shorter APs and a phase-one repolarization distinct from endocardial cells (111,123,184). Moreover, 4-AP eliminates the phase-one repolarization in the epicardial action potential and increases action potential duration, but has minimal effect on endocardial action potential duration.

Inwardly Rectifying K Channels

Inward (Anomalous) Rectifier K Channel—K_{IR}

Discovered by Katz (181)in skeletal muscle, inwardly rectifying K (K_{IR}) channels carry large inward current at potentials negative to the K equilibrium potential (E_K) and somewhat smaller current at potentials positive to E_K (Table 2). This property was termed "anomalous rectification" because the K conductance increases with hyperpolarization and decreases with depolarization, an action opposite to that of the delayed rectifier K current. Depending on the potential applied and transmembrane ion concentrations, many ion channels pass ions equally well in either direction. Although K_{IR} readily permits K^+ ions to traverse the membrane with the membrane potential near E_K, during the positive electrical potentials obtained during excitation, K_{IR} channels become far less permissive to the flow of K^+ ions. This rectification appears to be due to the voltage-dependent blockade of K_{IR} by intracellular Mg^{2+} (165,230,232,372) or endogenous polyamines such as spermine (108,219). In cardiac tissue, K_{IR} channels are expressed prominently in atrial and ventricular, but are absent in pacemaker cells (121,159,264). K_{IR} channels carry the current that generates the resting potential and modulates the final phase of repolarization of the cardiac action potential (161,223,328). Hyperpolarization of a cardiac myocyte results in an inward $I_{K(IR)}$ that activates rapidly and then appears to inactivate slowly, largely due to voltage-dependent block of K_{IR} channels by external Na^+ (29).

At the single-channel level, the conductance of K_{IR} channels is proportional to the square root of the extracellular K^+ concentration (178,286,309), which accounts for the observed whole-cell conductance increase in response to elevated extracellular K^+ (81,309). In symmetrical K^+ solutions, K_{IR} conductance is 27 to 32 pS at room temperature (159,309) reaching approximately 40 pS at 30 to 37°C in guinea pig myocytes (166,175,198) and human myocytes (190,316). Whereas many ionic channels exhibit brief open times that may average 1 to 10 ms, K_{IR} channels show comparatively long open times that average 150 to 220 ms in guinea pig myocytes (159,309) and 32 ms in human ventricular myocytes (190). The presence of three subconductance states for the K_{IR} channel at ¼, ½, and ¾ the main conductance has been reported, an observation that suggests that the main conductance may be the result of the simultaneous opening of four conducting subunits (234, 309). Expression of subconductance states may depend on the concentration of intracellular Mg^{2+} and other blocking ions or molecules. Increasing intracellular Mg^{2+} results in a rise in the probability of entry of K_{IR} channels into one of two subconductance states (229,231). In contrast to the four conducting subunits suggested above (234,309), work by Matsuda and colleagues (229,231) suggests that K_{IR} is triple-barreled with three conducting subunits. Future efforts with cloned inwardly rectifying K channels may clarify this issue.

Several lines of evidence indicate that adrenergic agonists can modulate K_{IR} channel activity. Isoproterenol, possibly via a novel adrenergic receptor subtype, causes an increase in $I_{K(IR)}$ inactivation and a shift of the current-voltage relationship toward more depolarized potentials in cardiac Purkinje cells (367). In contrast, β-adrenergic stimulation in spinal cord astrocytes results in a reduction in $I_{K(IR)}$ (304). In rabbit ventricular myocytes, both inward and outward components of $I_{K(IR)}$ were suppressed by α_1-adrenergic stimulation via a pertussis toxin-insensitive pathway (106) probably involving membrane-associated guanosine triphosphatase (GTPase) activity (40).

Acetylcholine-Sensitive K Channel—K_{ACh}

The G_i family of proteins is not limited to inhibition of adenylyl cyclase but includes linking the atrial myocardial cell muscarinic cholinergic receptor to the activation of the K_{ACh} channel (43). Acetylcholine (ACh) shortens the action potential and hyperpolarizes the resting membrane potential in a variety of cardiac tissues from many species (56,138,218,267). These actions of ACh are due to an increase in K conductance in the atrium (24), sinoatrial, and AV nodal tissues (265,308). Although it was initially thought that ACh modulated K_{IR} channels, it has been thoroughly demonstrated that there are marked differences between $I_{K(IR)}$ and $I_{K(ACh)}$ (143,144). While an agonist-induced increase in $I_{K(ACh)}$ occurs after a delay, implicating participation of a second messenger pathway (137,267), it was subsequently demonstrated that muscarinic activation of $I_{K(ACh)}$ does not involve diffusible cytoplasmic factors (336,348). Experimental evidence provided support that a membrane-bound G protein couples the muscarinic receptors to K_{ACh} channels (348). K_{ACh} channels can be persistently activated by application of hydrolysis resistant guanosine triphosphate (GTP) analogues, if Mg^{2+} and GTP are present at the intracellular surface, even after pertussis toxin uncouples the channel from the ACh receptor (42). Furthermore, K_{ACh} channels do not absolutely require a muscarinic agonist for channel opening, as these channels contribute substantially to the resting K^+ conductance in unstimulated myocytes (175).

Single K_{ACh} channels are readily distinguished from K_{IR} channels by their higher unitary conductance of approximately 43 pS in symmetrical K^+ solution and brief open times that average 1 to 2 ms among several mammalian species including human (175,190,316). Most recently, the most significant progress in the study of K_{ACh} channels has been made in the field of molecular biology. It is now clear that the G-protein βγ subunits, rather than the α subunit, have the major role in the activation of GIRK1, a subunit of the K_{ACh} channel (299). Furthermore, K_{ACh} may be a heterotetramer encoded by both GIRK1 and CIR (192).

Neurotransmitter-Activated, G-Protein–Linked K Channels

In central neurons, several neurotransmitters appear to upregulate one or more G-protein–linked inwardly rectifying K (GIRK) channels. Opiates (5,130,243,395,397), α_2-agonists (61, 254,347), gamma-aminobutyric acid ($GABA_B$) agonists (61,272, 293), and serotonin (8,9,272,284,293) have been shown to increase neuronal K^+ conductance via an inwardly rectifying, pertussis toxin–sensitive pathway. There is evidence that in some neurons multiple receptors may converge on the same GIRK channel. For example, $GABA_B$ and serotonin activate a similar K^+ conductance in a nonadditive manner in hippocampal neurons (9,272) while α_2-agonists and opiate appear to both activate a common GIRK channel in the rat locus coeuleus (5). However, single-channel measurements indicate that $GABA_B$ and serotonin appear to potentiate different channels; K channels opened by $GABA_B$ agonists had a larger conductance, 67 pS versus 36 pS, and longer average open times, 2.9 ms versus 0.7 ms, than the K channels activated by serotonin (293). Further work will be necessary to clarify this issue.

ATP-Sensitive Potassium Channel—K_{ATP}

K_{ATP} channels, which exhibit some inwardly rectifying characteristics, are present in various tissues such as heart muscle (266), the pancreas (129), skeletal muscle, smooth muscle (341), and the central nervous system (15) (Table 2). The single-channel conductance of the K_{ATP} channel varies greatly among different tissues (84): 80 pS in cardiac muscle (22); 44 pS in skeletal muscle (339); 30 pS (250,377), 135 pS (261), and 258 pS (221) in smooth muscle; up to 64 pS in pancreatic β cells (13); and up to 150 pS in neurons (15). In the pancreatic β cells, the K_{ATP} channels have a key role in glucose-induced insulin secretion (288). Inhibition of K_{ATP} channels by ATP can be achieved by nonhydrolyzable ATP analogues that are equally effective in blocking the channel (85,288). Moreover, other nucleotides such adenosine diphosphate (ADP), GTP, and guanosine diphosphate (GDP) also inhibit the K_{ATP} channel, although with lower efficacy and at higher concentrations than ATP (339). It appears that under physiologic conditions the ratio of intracellular ATP/ADP is probably the important variable in K_{ATP} channel regulation (84,288).

Activation of this channel in the presence of intracellular ATP depletion, which can occur during hypoxia (79,82) or ischemic insult as a result of reduced aerobic energy yield (100), might play a protective role by abbreviating electrical activity and subsequent voltage-gated Ca^{2+} influx. In many cases, changes in ATP concentration itself may not be the major regulator of the ATP-sensitive K channel. It could very well be that ATP may bind to the channel to set a low background probability of opening against which other substances act to modulate channel activity. For instance, in cardiac muscle ADP may be an important coregulator along with other substances that could modulate K_{ATP} channel activity by altering the sensitivity of the channel to ATP (340). It is now recognized that K_{ATP} constitutes a family of at least five different types (14) that vary not only in their sensitivity to Ca^{2+} and ATP, but also in their selectivity of K^+ over other ions and their susceptibility to pharmacologic modulation (95). An important modulator of K_{ATP} appears to be intracellular pH (191). While K_{ATP} channel activity increases with decreasing pH over the range of 7.6 to 6, a further reduction in intracellular pH results in a decrease in channel activity (191).

Many endogenous vasodilating factors modulate K_{ATP} channels in smooth muscle cells. These endogenous vasodilating factors include the calcitonin gene related peptide (CGRP), endothelial factors, β-adrenergic agonists, and adenosine. A common mode of action among CGRP (294) and β-adrenergic agonists (186,248) and perhaps other vasodilating agents is the activation of adenylyl cyclase, which results in the increase of intracellular cAMP levels. Several studies have shown that the vasodilatory action of adenosine appears to be mediated by K_{ATP} channels (80,242), which may involve a G-protein pathway (80). In rabbit arterial smooth muscle, the effect of CGRP on K_{ATP} channels was mimicked by stimulation of adenylyl cyclase with forskolin and by increased intracellular cAMP (294). Furthermore, the effect of CGRP on K_{ATP} channels was blocked by inhibition of cAMP. However, there is a report that in arterioles isolated from hamster cheek pouch, glibenclamide inhibited vasodilation induced by adenosine and isoproterenol, but not by forskolin and membrane-permeable cAMP, suggesting that adenosine and isoproterenol may activate K_{ATP} channels through a pathway not involving cAMP (168).

Several investigations have provided evidence for the activation of K_{ATP} channels as a mechanism of arterial smooth muscle relaxation induced by the endothelium-derived relaxing factor (EDRF), presumably nitric oxide (162,275) and/or the endothelium-derived hyperpolarizing factor. Endothelium-dependent relaxation induced by hyperpolarization of the smooth muscle cell membrane potential was reported to be blocked by K_{ATP} channel inhibitors (41). One recent study has demonstrated direct activation of vascular smooth muscle cell K_{ATP} channels by nitric oxide (249).

Compounds categorized as potassium channel openers target the K_{ATP} channel. In smooth muscle cells, glibenclamide markedly inhibits K_{ATP} channel activity (341). K-channel openers such as pinacidil, nicorandil, and cromakalim, which are known vasodilating compounds, primarily act on K_{ATP} channels (105,150,268,351,357). Nonspecific blockers of K channels, such as 4-AP and Ba^{2+}, also block K_{ATP} channel activity (69,295), whereas external TEA blocks with low affinity (K_d >7 mM) (83). Furthermore, externally applied Cd^{2+}, a blocker of the L-type Ca channel, and Zn^{2+} have also been shown to inhibit K_{ATP} channel activity (199). Note, however, that studies have also shown that K^+ channels other than the K_{ATP} channel are also activated by some K-channel openers. For example, cromakalim activation of a large-conductance Ca^{2+}-activated K channel (BK_{Ca}) has been reported in rabbit aorta (53,120), while a related K_{ATP} channel agonist lemakalim increases the activity of a subset of BK_{Ca} channels in hippocampal neurons (384). At least in smooth muscle, vasodilating actions of the potassium channel openers appear to involve primarily K_{ATP} channels, since the effects of the agonists are readily reversed by glibenclamide (65,396,398).

Ca^{2+}-Dependent K Channels

Ca^{2+}-dependent K channels are found in many different cell types and are involved in a variety of cellular functions (149). Ca^{2+}-dependent K currents have been identified in a number of cell types under whole-cell conditions by elevation of intracellular Ca^{2+} with the use of an ionophore (Fig. 6) or activation of voltage-gated Ca^{2+} entry (228). Underlying whole-cell current records, Ca^{2+}-dependent K channels can be subdivided into three primary groups based on their conductance in symmetrical K^+ solutions (Table 2) (239,273): (a) "maxi" or "big" conductance K channels (BK_{Ca}) more than 150 pS; (b) small conductance K channels (SK_{Ca}) of less than 50 pS; and (c) intermediate conductance K channels (IK_{Ca}) of approximately 50 to 150 pS.

High-Conductance Potassium Channels—BK_{Ca}

The BK_{Ca} channel has been the subject of numerous biophysical studies that have explored the complex dependence of voltage and Ca^{2+} in the gating of these channels (149,239). Regardless of this wealth of information, the functional significance of BK_{Ca} channels is not completely understood (205). In excitable cells, BK_{Ca} channels have been implicated in action potential repolarization in neuroendocrine cells (202,277), neurons (46,75,237), and smooth muscle (54,157). In addition, activation of BK_{Ca} channels contributes to the fast afterhyperpolarization (AHP) phase in hippocampal neurons (200) and sympathetic neurons (285). Reconstitution experiments with rat brain BK_{Ca} channels demonstrated channel types I and II that differed in terms of charybdotoxin sensitivity, gating kinetics, and sensitivity to PKA (296,297). Such differences are not surprising given the number of BK_{Ca} splice variants possible, as described earlier (4,370).

At the single-channel level, the BK_{Ca} channels can be described by one or two open states and two to four closed states (25,55,157,239). Subconductance states have also been reported, indicative of more open states (279). Despite their large unitary conductance, BK_{Ca} channels demonstrate an

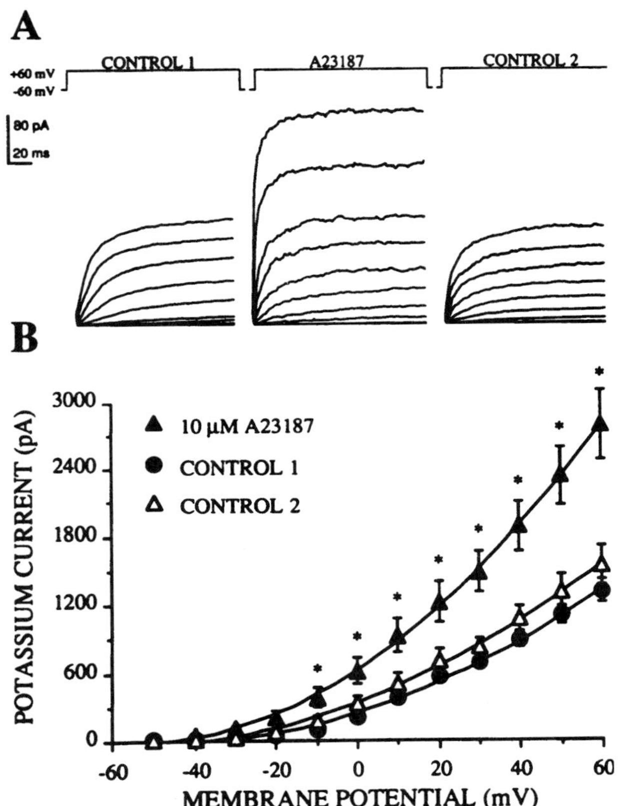

Figure 6. Whole-cell Ca^{2+}-activated K current. In many smooth muscle cell types, the major outward current in response to membrane depolarization is carried by the Ca^{2+}-activated K channels (23,25,49,235,343). Effects of 10 µM A23187 (Ca^{2+} ionophore) on the whole-cell K current are demonstrated on a single coronary smooth muscle cell depolarized from −60 up to +60 mV. **(A)** Current tracings shown before (control 1), during (A23187), and after (control 2) exposure to A23187. **(B)** Summary of changes in current amplitude plotted against membrane potential. (Reprinted with permission from ref. 49.)

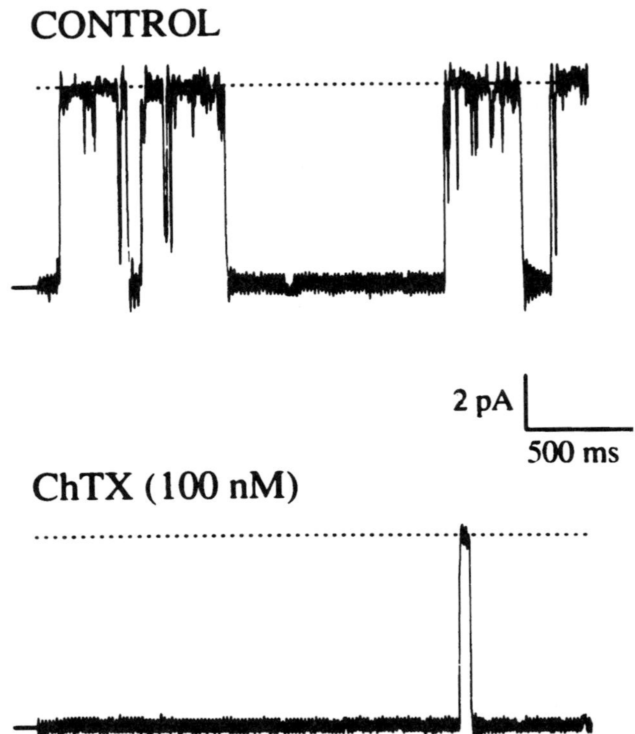

Figure 7. Effects of 100 nM charybdotoxin on K channel activity. Recordings from an inside-out patch held at a membrane potential of +60 mV are shown. The continuous rule at the beginning of current tracings represents the closed channel state, while the broken rule represents an open channel state. Recordings were made in symmetrical 145 mM K^+. The intracellular Ca^{2+} concentration was 10^{-7} M. (Reprinted with permission from ref. 49.)

extremely high degree of ionic selectivity (30). Although Na^+ ions are unable to pass through the BK_{Ca} channels, Na^+ ions block these channels when present on the cytosolic side of the membrane (149,404).

Several toxins purified from scorpion venom that are structurally related to charybdotoxin (Fig. 7) are specific to K channels as described in detail recently (245). For example, charybdotoxin inhibits BK_{Ca} channel activity (70,226,246), whereas noxiustoxin appears to block K channels of the Kv family (245, 251). Although it was originally thought that charybdotoxin is specific for BK_{Ca} channels, subsequent work has shown that several other K channels are also inhibited by charybdotoxin (149). Iberiotoxin may prove to be most specific of the scorpion toxins for BK_{Ca} channels (117). In addition, submillimolar concentrations of TEA ions can block the channel from the outside of the membrane, whereas higher concentrations are required for blockade when TEA is applied to the cytoplasmic side of the membrane (158). Several neuromuscular blocking agents have been shown to inhibit BK_{Ca} channels. Decamethonium induces a "flickery" blockade of the channel with an IC_{50} of approximately 120 µM, while hexamethonium exerts a similar effect with lower affinity: IC_{50} ~4 mM (73). Other factors that modulate these channels, either directly or via phosphorylation, include norepinephrine, histamine, acetylcholine, angiotensin II, endothelin, nitroglycerin, nitric oxide, guanosine monophosphate (GMP), and cGMP (365,366,394). Regulation of BK_{Ca} channels can be achieved via second messengers, protein kinase A (104,197,206,331,391,392), and/or protein kinase C (7,149,205).

Phosphorylation can play an important role in the modulation of BK_{Ca} channels. Studies from aortic smooth muscle have shown that extracellularly applied isoproterenol and forskolin increased P_o (306). Results from studies on myometrial BK_{Ca} channels incorporated into bilayers also provided evidence for regulation via a membrane-delimited G-protein pathway (364). It has been reported that phosphorylation by exogenous PKA can lead to a downregulation of BK_{Ca} channel activity in ovine pituitary gonadotrophs (331) and GH_4C_1 rat pituitary tumor cells (391,392) and an upregulation of BK_{Ca} channel activity in *Helix* neurons (104), mouse lacrimal cells (206), and tracheal myocytes (197). Reinhart and colleagues (297) have identified two types of BK_{Ca} channels in rat brain that differ in their response to exogenous PKA. Interestingly, evidence exists for a closely associated endogenous protein kinase that can upregulate BK_{Ca} channel activity (62). Excised patch experiments using gastric smooth muscle cells (208) and cloned *Drosophila Slo (dSlo)* BK_{Ca} channels expressed in oocytes (101) have confirmed this observation. Furthermore, evidence suggests that not only does an endogenous protein kinase associate with BK_{Ca} channels, but also an endogenous phosphatase, probably similar to protein phosphatase-1 (208).

Small Conductance K Channels—SK_{Ca}

SK_{Ca} channels lack the voltage dependence in gating that BK_{Ca} channels exhibit, while being far more sensitive to Ca^{2+} than BK_{Ca} channels (239). Consequently, SK_{Ca} channels are well suited for influencing excitability near the resting potential. SK_{Ca} channels underlie the slow AHP observed in hippocampal neurons (200,201), neuroendocrine cells (202), skeletal muscle cells (303), and sympathetic neurons (285), but not guinea pig olfactory neurons (68). SK_{Ca} channels have been suggested to influence the duration and frequency of action potentials in rat adrenal chromaffin cells (258,282). Whereas BK_{Ca} channels appear to require localized, high Ca^{2+} concentrations associated with Ca^{2+} influx for activation (211), there is evidence to support a role for the release of Ca^{2+} from intracellular stores as a physiologic modulator of SK_{Ca} (146,259,270,371). Apamin, a bee venom polypeptide composed of 18 amino acids (133), is a specific inhibitor of SK_{Ca} channels (30).

Intermediate Conductance K Channels—IK_{Ca}

IK_{Ca} channels appear to have slightly greater sensitivity for Ca^{2+} as compared to the BK_{Ca} channels, but not to the same degree as SK_{Ca} channels (239). While TEA blocks IK_{Ca} channels of rat brain at low concentrations (296), it has no effect on the channels in rabbit portal vein (149). In addition, charybdotoxin inhibits some IK_{Ca} channels (296). With regard to modulation, application of PKA causes an approximate fourfold increase in activity of rat brain IK_{Ca} channels (104). Further studies will be required to better distinguish the function and pharmacology of IK_{Ca} channels from BK_{Ca} and SK_{Ca} channels.

Other K-Specific Channels

Na^+-Activated K channels—K_{Na}

K_{Na} channels have been described in a variety of excitable cells including cardiac myocytes (177) and central neurons (19, 90,134) (Table 2). K_{Na} channels measured in inside-out patches have a unitary conductance of ranging from 170 to 210 pS in isotonic K^+ with many subconductance states, are voltage independent, are insensitive to Ca^{2+} or ATP, and require at least 20 mM Na^+ to become active (88,90,134,177). The physiologic function of K_{Na} channels has been difficult to ascertain in part because K_{Na}-channel activation typically requires Na^+ concentrations considerably higher than those that would be expected in the cytosol. Since the normal intracellular Na^+ concentrations in excitable cells is less than 10 mM, K_{Na} channels would not be expected to become active (89). However, comparison of K_{Na} channels measured under cell-attached and excised patch inside-out recording modes has provided evidence that either internal Na^+ concentration can reach very high levels near the membrane, possibly due to transient accumulation of Na^+ that enters via Na channels. Alternatively, a soluble cytoplasmic factor that is lost during patch excision may be critical for K_{Na}-channel functioning in quail sensory neurons (135). In cardiac cells, it has been proposed that ischemia and hypoxia can result in increases in the intracellular Na^+ concentration, due to cessation of Na^+ pump activity, which would make it possible for K_{Na} channels to contribute to the shortening of the action potential (177). Consistent with this view, it has been shown that inhibition of Na^+/K^+-ATPase by cardiac glycosides causes activation of K_{Na} channels in guinea pig ventricular myocytes (222). Therefore, K_{Na} channels might indeed play a role in the responses of cardiac myocytes to ischemia and hypoxia as well as in digitalis toxicity.

Muscarinic Receptor–Sensitive K Channels—K_M

In neuronal cells, the M-current ($I_{K(M)}$), in the absence of neurotransmitters, activates with depolarization and exhibits no inactivation. ACh acting at the muscarinic receptor and certain peptide hormones, such as luteinizing hormone–releasing hormone, substance P, and bradykinin, inhibit K_M channels, resulting in increased neuronal excitability (3,44,45,172). K_M channels exhibit two open conductance states of 10 and 15 pS (227) in isotonic K^+ solution and are insensitive to 4-AP and Cs^+ (44). ACh-mediated inhibition of K_M channels requires a pertussis toxin–insensitive G protein (289) and diffusible messenger (322), perhaps cyclic adenosine diphosphatase ribose (147), which serves as a second messenger similar to IP_3 (115). Muscarinic receptor activation reduces K_M channel activity through a selective inhibition of a gating mode associated with a high probability of opening (227).

ANESTHETIC EFFECTS ON POTASSIUM CHANNELS

Cardiac K Channels

To date, there are only a limited number of studies investigating the effects of anesthetics on cardiac K channels. Preliminary results have shown that halothane, isoflurane, and enflurane all have inhibitory effects on $I_{K(V)}$ in canine cardiac Purkinje cells (346). More recently, an investigation of the effects of intravenous anesthetics on $I_{K(V)}$ in mammalian ventricular myocytes showed that ketamine (20) has no effect on this current while propofol has a depressant effect. The general anesthetics heptanol, octanol, and halothane suppress $I_{K(V)}$ (262). Preliminary results from our laboratory (Kwok and Bosnjak) also show that guinea pig ventricular $I_{K(V)}$ is partially suppressed by halothane (Fig. 8).

Intravenous anesthetics showed differential effects on the cardiac $I_{K(IR)}$ current (20). Ketamine decreased $I_{K(IR)}$ amplitude, while propofol and methohexital had no effect on this current. In addition, heptanol, octanol, and halothane also suppress cardiac $I_{K(IR)}$ (262). Pancrazio and colleagues (276), utilizing the whole-cell patch-clamp technique, have examined the effect of thiopental on $I_{K(IR)}$ in frog atrial and guinea pig ventricular myocytes. Thiopental (30 μM) reduced the magnitude of $I_{K(IR)}$ by approximately 50%. Preliminary results from our laboratory (Kwok and Bosnjak) have shown that the ventricular $I_{K(IR)}$ is partially inhibited by halothane, sevoflurane, and isoflurane (Fig.

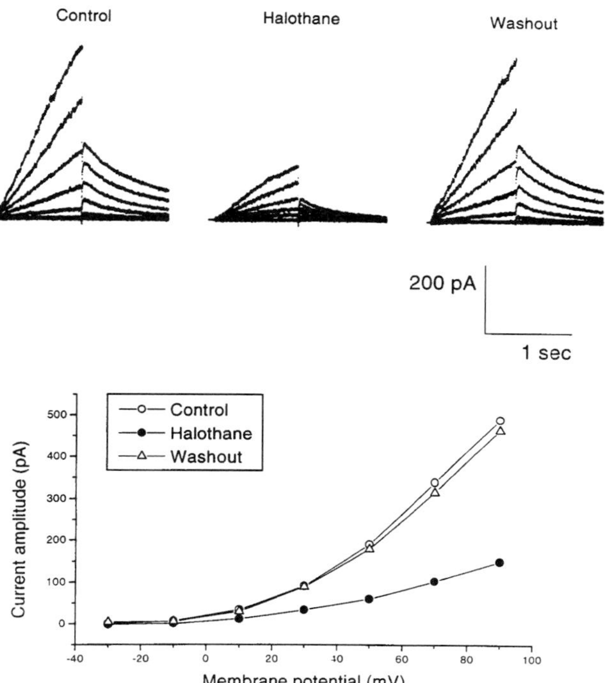

Figure 8. Effects of halothane on the whole-cell delayed rectifier K current $I_{K(V)} = I_{Ks(V)} + I_{Kr(V)}$ in guinea pig cardiac ventricular myocytes. **Top:** Effect of halothane (1 mM) on $I_{K(V)}$ under whole-cell conditions. Currents were measured during 1-second test pulses from −30 mV to +90 mV in steps of 20 mV and returned to the holding potential set at −40 mV. In the presence of halothane, current amplitude is substantially decreased. The inhibitory effect of halothane is readily reversible. **Bottom:** Effect of halothane on the $I_{K(V)}$ at various membrane potentials. Current amplitude was measured at the end of the 1-second test pulse to +90 mV.

9). Experiments on $I_{K(IR)}$ at the single-channel level suggest possible interactions between forskolin and halothane (Fig. 10). Single-channel activity was obtained from a cell-attached membrane patch using a guinea pig ventricular myocyte under control conditions, exposure to a high level of halothane (1.2 mM in solution), in 5 μM forskolin, and in the presence of both halothane and forskolin. Halothane decreased both mean open time (MOT) and P_o, while forskolin dramatically increased P_o with a slight increase in MOT. In the presence of both forskolin and halothane, P_o was increased compared to control; however, it was less than with forskolin alone. Neither halothane nor forskolin altered K^+ conductance. The overall blockade of $I_{K(IR)}$ is likely to lead to slight action potential prolongation and, more importantly, to a decrease in time-to-threshold for the action potential generation (276). These actions can increase the excitability of the myocardium and potentially lead to a greater likelihood of cardiac arrhythmias.

Preliminary results from the guinea pig atrial cells illustrate the inhibitory effects of halothane on the K_{ACh} channel (Fig. 11). Single-channel activity was obtained from a cell-attached membrane patch under control conditions, during exposure to a high level of halothane (1.2 mM), with 0.1 μM ACh (in pipette), and in the presence of both ACh and halothane. Whereas ACh increased both MOT and P_o, halothane had an opposite effect. In the presence of both halothane and ACh, MOT increased without an alteration in the P_o.

Smooth Muscle K Channels

Although several investigations have reported that inhalational anesthetics cause vasodilation in specific vascular beds, the modulatory mechanism of volatile anesthetics on the electrical properties of vascular smooth muscle is largely unknown (34,136). While it has been shown that anesthetics depress Ca channels in smooth muscle (48,50) as in cardiac tissue (32–38), studies examining anesthetic action on the K channels in smooth muscle are, at the present time, limited. Nevertheless, a 4-AP-sensitive $I_{K(V)}$, which has been identified in canine coronary and rabbit pulmonary arterial cells (50,271), is reversibly suppressed by clinically relevant concentrations of halothane (0.75% and 1.5%; 0.4 mM and 0.8 mM in solution) and isoflurane (2.6%; 1.0 mM in solution) (Figs. 12 and 13) (50). The depressant effects of halothane were less marked on $I_{K(V)}$ than on the L-type Ca current also found in these smooth muscle cells (48,50). Furthermore, at equianesthetic concentrations, $I_{K(V)}$ suppression by halothane was significantly greater than that by isoflurane. Similarly, in canine cerebral arterial muscle cells, a 4-AP-sensitive $I_{K(V)}$ was characterized and also found to be reversibly suppressed by halothane in a concentration-dependent manner (102).

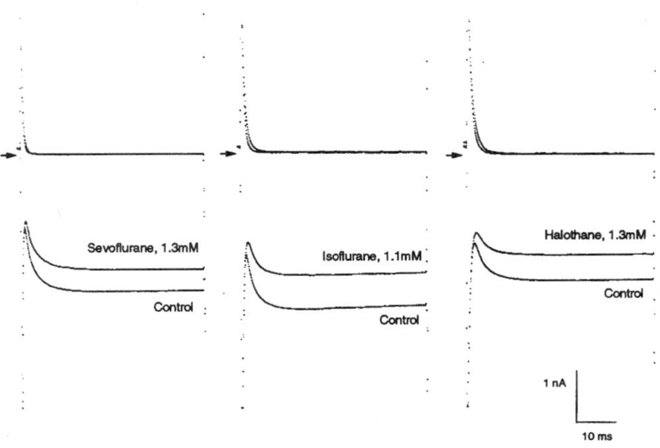

Figure 9. Effects of anesthetics on the cardiac inward rectifier K current, $I_{K(IR)}$, from guinea pig ventricular myocytes. Whole-cell current traces were measured during a 50 ms test pulse to −110 and 0 mV from a holding potential of −40 mV. The inhibitory effects of sevoflurane, isoflurane, and halothane on $I_{K(IR)}$ current amplitude are shown.

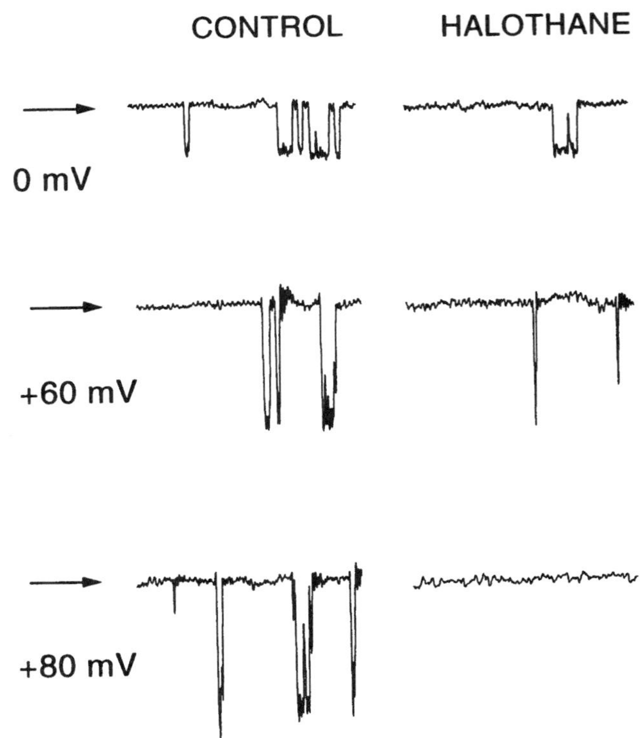

Figure 10. Effects of halothane on $I_{K(IR)}$ at the single-channel level. Single-channel activity obtained from a cell-attached membrane patch from guinea pig ventricular myocyte. Downward deflections indicate channel openings (inward current); *arrows* show zero current levels. Potentials indicated are pipette potentials. Recordings were obtained under control conditions and exposure to 1.2 mM halothane. Halothane decreased both mean open time and probability of opening; however, it did not alter K conductance.

Studies on the effects of anesthetics on K channels in smooth muscle have mainly concentrated on the BK_{Ca} channels. As shown in Fig. 14, isoflurane depresses a Ca^{2+}-activated K current in canine cerebral arterial cells (48). Several investigations at the single-channel level have directly demonstrated inhibitory effects of volatile anesthetics on BK_{Ca} channels (102,155,278,279). In cerebrovascular smooth muscle cells isolated from rat, halothane was shown to decrease open probability of the BK_{Ca} channel in a concentration-dependent manner without altering the single-channel conductance (155). The change in P_o was attributed to a decrease in MOT and an increase in the mean closed time of the channel. Likewise, single-channel studies revealed that halothane (102) and isoflurane (48) decreased event frequency, the MOT, and P_o of BK_{Ca} channels in canine cerebral arterial muscle cells. At the mechanistic level, the reduction in P_o by halothane was found to be dependent on the cytoplasmic Ca^{2+} concentration, such that the blocking effect of halothane diminishes at higher Ca^{2+} concentrations (155), a finding that is consistent with earlier work (279). These results, combined with other studies that have shown that the Ca^{2+}-binding sites on the BK_{Ca} channel probably lie within the intramembrane domain of the channel (188,205), suggest that halothane interacts with the BK_{Ca} channel protein from within the lipid bilayer. A potential site of action may involve a lipophilic domain of the channel that is important for Ca^{2+} sensitivity such as the tail region (388). At the present time, there are no documented reports on anesthetic effects on the SK_{Ca} or IK_{Ca} channels.

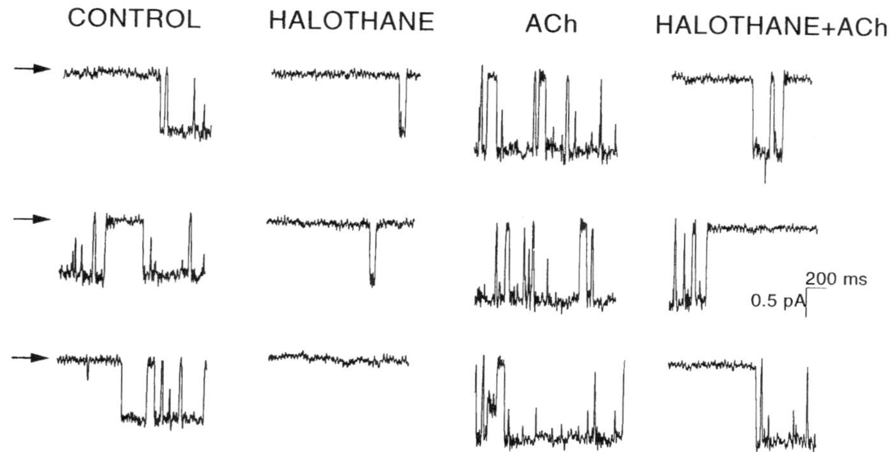

Figure 11. Effect of halothane on acetylcholine-sensitive K (K_{ACh}) channel. Single-channel activity obtained from a cell-attached membrane patch from guinea pig atrial cell. Downward deflections indicate channel openings (inward current); *arrows* indicate zero current levels. The membrane patch was held at a pipette potential of 0 mV with extracellular K^+ = 4.7 mM. Recordings were obtained under control conditions, during exposure to 1.2 mM halothane, in 0.1 μM ACh (in the pipette solution), and in the presence of both ACh and halothane. Halothane decreased both mean open time (MOT) and probability of opening (P_o), while ACh increased MOT and P_o. In the presence of both halothane and ACh, MOT increased without altering P_o.

Due to their functional importance in smooth muscle relaxation, the K_{ATP} channel could be a reasonable target for anesthetic effects. Although there are currently no reports of the direct effects of anesthetic on K_{ATP} channel activity in smooth muscle cells, an investigation has provided pharmacologic evidence that isoflurane might open K_{ATP} channels in vascular smooth muscle (57). Likewise, functional studies from isolated ring segments of rat coronary resistance vessels and porcine coronary arteries showed that glibenclamide, but not TEA, attenuated halothane-induced vasodilation (203,204). Halothane treatment of the rat coronary rings did not allow further relaxation by the K_{ATP} channel opener cromakalim (203), consistent with the view that halothane opens K_{ATP} channels. Interestingly, the glibenclamide attenuation of halothane-induced relaxation was dependent on the underlying vascular tone. For coronary arteries constricted with endothelin-1, an endothelial-derived vasoconstrictor peptide, glibenclamide, inhibited the halothane-induced vasodilation, whereas for methacholine or by high-extracellular K^+-induced constriction, glibenclamide had no effect on the relaxation caused by halothane (204). These results suggest that mechanisms other than K_{ATP} channel activation may be involved in anesthetic action on smooth muscle vasodilation. Moreover, monitoring direct anesthetic effects on the K_{ATP} channel will also need to be established using biophysical methodologies such as the patch clamp technique.

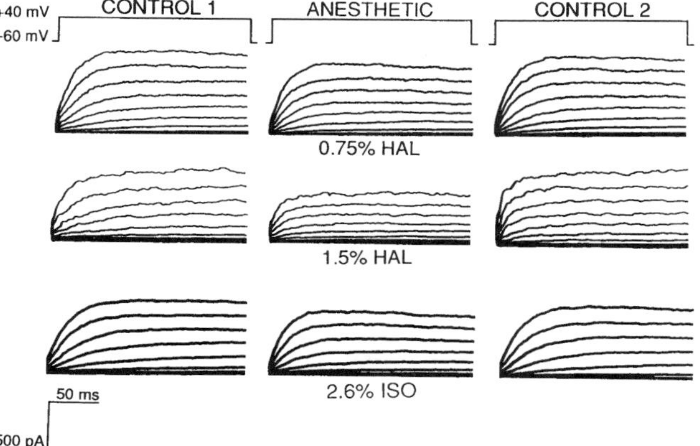

Figure 12. Effects of halothane and isoflurane on $I_{K(V)}$ from coronary arterial smooth muscle cells. Current tracings shown during control (control 1), in the presence of 0.75 and 1.5% halothane (0.4 and 0.8 mM in solution) and 2.6% isoflurane (1.0 mM in solution), and during washout of halothane and isoflurane (control 2). $I_{K(V)}$ were elicited by progressive 10 mV test pulses from −60 to +40 mV. (Reprinted with permission from ref. 50.)

Neuronal K Channels

During surgical anesthesia, there has been interest in the use of α_2-agonists that selectively bind to α_2-adrenoreceptors in the locus ceruleus to produce their pharmacologic action (98). While α_2-adrenoceptor activation is associated with a reduction of N-type Ca current and a subsequent depression of neurotransmitter release (215), a number of studies have shown that α_2-agonists also increase neuronal K^+ conductance (103,210,254, 347), an effect that appears to be shared with μ and δ opioid receptors (5,269). This K^+ conductance augmentation depends on a pertussis toxin–sensitive pathway (210,347), which implicates the GIRK family of K channels that are found throughout the brain (212). In support of a clinical role for this pathway, Doze and colleagues (87) reported that the analgesic effect of the α_2-agonist dexmedetomidine, through a pathway independent of $GABA_A$ receptors, can be suppressed by pertussis toxin or the 4-AP. While it is well known that opioids reduce inhalational anesthetic requirements for surgery, it appears that α_2-agonists share this property (1,182,233). These observations are consistent with the notion that there may be common site(s) of action, perhaps K channels or a regulator thereof, between α_2-agonists, opioids and inhalational anesthetics.

The fact that the opening of K channels leads to "membrane stabilization" has made these channels an attractive hypothetical site for inhalational anesthetic action. Indeed, the exciting finding that relevant concentrations of halothane activate a novel K^+ conductance in snail neurons, resulting in a hyperpolarization (110), led to speculation that a homologue of these anesthetic-sensitive K channels might exist in mammalian systems to contribute to the development of the anesthetic state. Although no such homologue has been definitively identified, there is some evidence of anesthetic-induced decreases in excitability in identified central neurons that may be due to an augmentation of K^+ conductance (26,345). Use of intracellular recording tech-

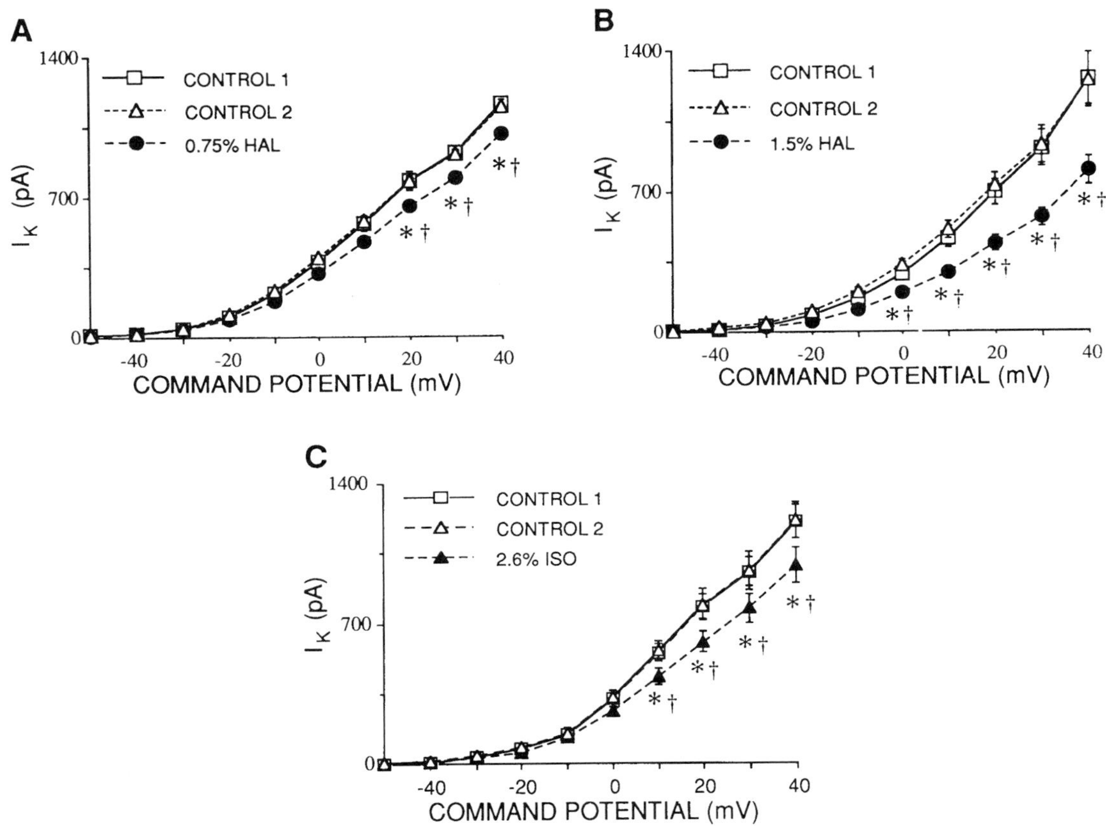

Figure 13. The current-voltage relationship for $I_{K(V)}$ from coronary arterial smooth muscle cells under control conditions and in the presence of halothane (**A** and **B**) and isoflurane (**C**). Halothane and isoflurane depressed current amplitude in a concentration-dependent manner. *p <.05 versus control 1 and control 2 (washout). (Reprinted with permission from ref. 50.)

niques revealed a concentration-dependent increase in a K conductance in guinea pig thalamic neurons with application of halothane (Fig. 15) that can be suppressed with K-channel antagonists Ba^{2+} and 4-AP (345). This anesthetic-sensitive K current appears to be active at or near the resting potential similar to the inwardly rectifying K channels. Although the activity of K_{ATP} channels may be increased by isoflurane in smooth muscle (57), it is unlikely that this type of inwardly rectifying K channel is involved in the development of the anesthetic state at the level of the central nervous system (412). These minimum alveolar concentration (MAC) studies cannot completely eliminate the involvement of K_{ATP} channels, since ATP-modulated K channels of ventral medial hypothalamic neurons are unaffected by either cromakalin or pinacidil (321) while suppressed by tolbutamide, a sulfonylurea inhibitor of K_{ATP} channels (16). Characterization of the anesthetic-sensitive K^+ conductance in thalamic neurons and motoneurons must await further experimentation. Alternatively, it has been proposed that anesthetics activate neuronal Ca^{2+}-dependent K^+ conductance by increasing the intracellular Ca^{2+} concentration, leading to reduced neuronal excitability (193,255). However, the experimental data suggest that mechanisms involving activation of Ca^{2+}-dependent K channels are unlikely.

Excitatory effects of inhalational anesthetics on neuronal tissue are not uncommon. Transient excitation of the squid axon by general anesthetics (141), including halothane, appears to be due to a reduction of a resting K^+ conductance component that is carried by channels distinct from $I_{K(V)}$ (140). Utilizing isolated crayfish stretch receptors, MacIver and Roth (224) showed that a large number of anesthetic agents, including halothane, produce biphasic responses, that is, excitation at low concentrations and depression at higher levels. Most of the voltage-clamp studies of intact neuronal or neuroendocrine cells or preparations have reported a slight blockade of $I_{K(V)}$ over the clinically relevant range of anesthetic concentrations. Halothane at concentrations of 6.4 mM and 3 mM are required to diminish by 50% $I_{K(V)}$ from the squid giant axon (142) and GH3 clonal pituitary cells (145), respectively.

Several studies have shown that neuronal Ca^{2+}-activated K channels are suppressed by the inhalational anesthetics. ^{86}Rb flux through Ca^{2+}-activated K channels of rat glioma C6 cells is diminished by halothane with an IC_{50} of ~1% at 36°C (~0.2 mM in solution) (355). Halothane has been reported to depress the fast and slow AHPs of hippocampal neurons at concentrations where no impairment of voltage-activated Ca^{2+} entry was observed (114,283). The fast AHP is mediated by BK_{Ca} channels, whereas the slow AHP is due to SK_{Ca} (201). Since the suppression of this fast AHP phase can increase hippocampal epileptiform burst duration (6), it is not surprising that the incidence and duration of spontaneous firing of hippocampal neurons is escalated with low concentrations of halothane or isoflurane (114), which is consistent with the view that the inhalational anesthetics inhibit hippocampal BK_{Ca} and, possibly, SK_{Ca} channel activity. Detailed electrophysiologic measurements of anesthetic effects have been made using bovine adrenal chromaffin cells, which are considered a classic model of neuronal electrophysiology and secretion. These cells express two types of K_V channels and BK_{Ca} channels (228). The anesthetics exerted only minor effects on the total delayed rectifier K current, as shown in Fig. 16A; however, BK_{Ca} channel P_o was markedly depressed (Fig. 16B). Although the mechanism of anesthetic action at the level of single BK_{Ca} channels may involve a reduction in the long-duration channel open time in smooth muscle (102), for neuroendocrine BK_{Ca} channels

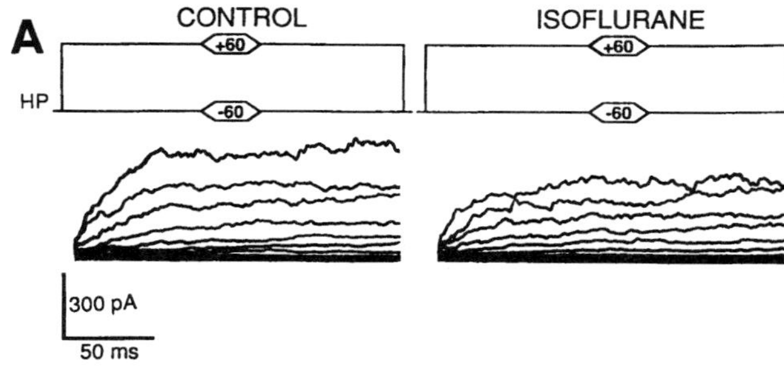

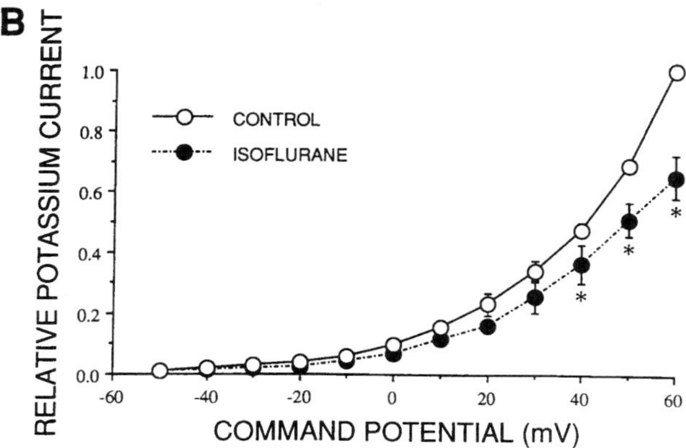

Figure 14. (A) Effect of 2.6% isoflurane (1.0 mM in solution at room temperature) on Ca^{2+}-activated K current from canine cerebral arterial smooth muscle cells elicited by progressive 10-mV test pulses from −60 to +60 mV. (B) The current-voltage relationship for peak whole-cell current under control conditions and in the presence of isoflurane. Isoflurane significantly depressed peak outward current only at the most positive voltages examined. (Reprinted with permission from ref. 48.)

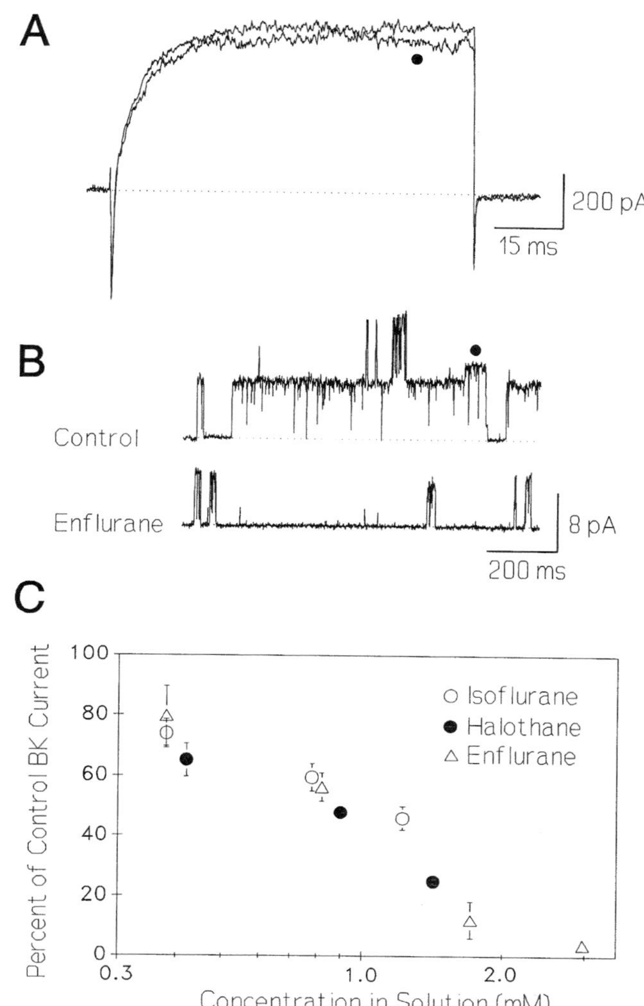

Figure 16. Effect of inhalational anesthetics on delayed rectifier K current and BK_{Ca} channel activity from bovine adrenal chromaffin cells. (A) Whole-cell patch-clamp recording under Ca^{2+}-free conditions to isolate the delayed rectifier K current elicited by a voltage step to +30 mV from a holding potential of −80 mV. (For details, see ref. 279.) Control outward current and after application of 1.5% halothane (0.9 mM in solution) denoted by *solid circle.* The *dotted line* indicates zero transmembrane current. (B) Excised inside-out membrane patch containing three BK_{Ca} channels in the presence of ~900 nM free Ca^{2+} at the cytoplasmic side and voltage-clamped to +30 mV. (For details, see ref. 278.) In the presence of 3.5% enflurane (1.7 mM in solution), the probability of channel opening was dramatically diminished with no change in the open channel amplitude. The *dotted line* indicates zero transmembrane current. Occasional subconductance state of BK_{Ca} channel denoted by *solid circle.* (C) Comparative concentration-dependent blockade of BK_{Ca} current by halothane, isoflurane, and enflurane.

volatile anesthetics (278,279), as well as ketamine (86), appear to decrease the likelihood of occupying a long-duration open state. Examination of the concentration-dependent blockade of BK_{Ca} channel current by halothane, isoflurane, and enflurane suggests that there is little difference between the anesthetics in the potency (Fig. 16C). The fact that higher vapor pressures of enflurane are necessary for anesthesia may create conditions where there is an increased likelihood for seizure activity (342), perhaps largely due to the concurrent blockade of neuronal BK_{Ca} channels.

Cloned K Channels

To date, there is a single brief study reporting the effect of an inhalational anesthetic on cloned K channels. Given that such studies offer the possibility of identifying channel domains that may serve as "anesthetic receptors," it will undoubtedly be the topic of future work. Four *Shaker*-related clones and minK, which were expressed in *Xenopus* oocytes, resulted in K currents that were all depressed with application of halothane (411). As shown in Fig. 17, two of these clones, *Shal*II and minK, were relatively sensitive to the halothane with IC_{50} values near 1% (~0.8 mM in solution at room temperature). In an effort to identify possible anesthetic sites of action a "minimal minK" (min^2K) was constructed with extensive deletions to the amino and carboxyl regions, which do not alter minK function. Interestingly, there was no difference in the efficacy of halothane between minK and min^2K, suggesting that the site(s) of anes-

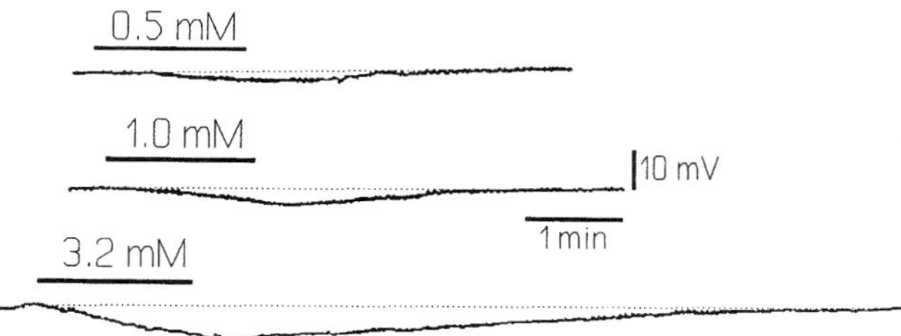

Figure 15. Halothane-induced hyperpolarization in parafasicular thalamic neurons from guinea pig recorded using standard glass microelectrode techniques. Halothane was applied to the same neuron for durations denoted by the *solid bars.* The baseline resting membrane potential of the neuron shown was −61 mV. (Reprinted with permission from ref. 345.)

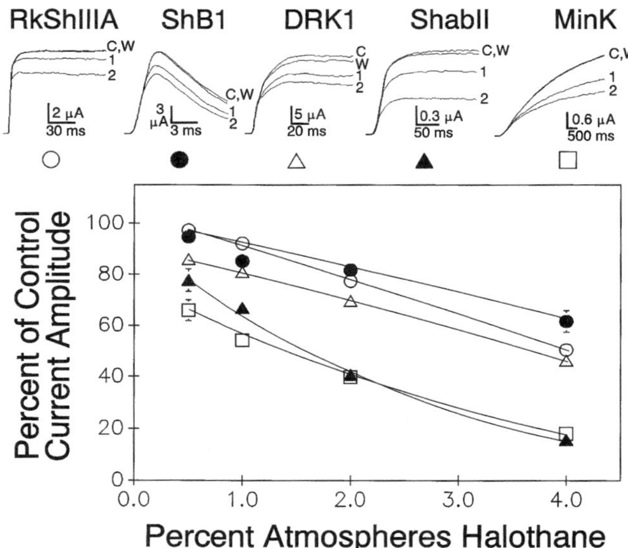

Figure 17. Comparative effects of the inhalational anesthetic halothane on cloned K channels. K currents were measured from *Xenopus* oocytes injected with cRNA encoding various K channels from the Kv subfamily and minK. (Reprinted with permission from ref. 411.)

thetic action for this protein is probably located on the transmembrane segment (411).

REFERENCES

1. Aantaa R, Kanto J, Scheinin M, Kallio A, Scheinin H. Dexmedetomidine, an α_2-adrenoceptor agonist, reduces anesthetic requirements for patients undergoing minor gynecologic surgery. *Anesthesiology* 1990;73:230–235.
2. Adams PR, Brown DA, Constanti A. M-currents and other currents in bullfrog sympathetic neurons. *J Physiol (Lond)* 1982;330: 537–572.
3. Adams PR, Brown DA, Constanti A. Pharmacological inhibition of the M-current. *J Physiol (Lond)* 1982;332:223–262.
4. Adelman JP, Shen K-Z, Kavanaugh MP, et al. Calcium-activated potassium channels expressed from cloned complementary DNAs. *Neuron* 1992;9:209–216.
5. Aghajanian GK, Wang Y-Y. Common alpha-2 and opiate effector mechanisms in the rat locus coeruleus: intracellular studies in brain slices. *Neuropharmacology* 1987;26:789–800.
6. Alger BE, Williamson A. A transient calcium-dependent potassium component of the epileptiform burst after hyperpolarization in rat hippocampus. *J Physiol (Lond)* 1988;399:191–205.
7. Alkon D, Kubota M, Neary J, Naito S, Coulter D, Rasmussen H. C-kinase activation prolongs Ca^{2+}-dependent inactivation of K^+ currents. *Biochem Biophys Res Commun* 1986;134:1245–1253.
8. Andrade R, Malenka RC, Nicoll RA. A G protein couples serotonin and $GABA_B$ receptors to the same channel in hippocampus. *Science* 1986;234:1261–1265.
9. Andrade R, Nicoll RA. Pharmacologically distinct actions of serotonin on single pyramidal neurons of the rat hippocampus recorded in vitro. *J Physiol (Lond)* 1987;394:99–124.
10. Armstrong CM. Sodium channels and gating currents. Physiol Rev 1981;61:644–683.
11. Armstrong CM, Bezanilla F. Inactivation of the sodium channel. II. Gating current experiments. *J Gen Physiol* 1977;70:567–590.
12. Aronson JK. Potassium channels in nervous tissue. *Biochem Pharmacol* 1992;43:11–14.
13. Ashcroft FM, Kakei M. ATP-sensitive K^+ channels in rat pancreatic beta-cells: modulation by ATP and Mg^{2+} ions. *J Physiol (Lond)* 1989; 416:349–367.
14. Ashcroft SJ, Ashcroft FM. Properties and functions of ATP-sensitive K-channels. *Cell Signal* 1990;2:197–214.
15. Ashford MLJ, Boden PR, Treherne JM. Glucose-induced excitation of hypothalamic neurones is mediated by ATP-sensitive K^+ channels. *Pflugers Arch* 1990;415:479–483.
16. Ashford MLJ, Boden PR, Treherne JM. Tolbutamide excites rat glucoreceptive ventromedial hypothalamic neurones by indirect inhibition of ATP-K^+ channels. *Br J Pharmacol* 1990;101:531–540.
17. Ashford MLJ, Bond CT, Blair TA, Adelman JP. Cloning and functional expression of a rat heart K_{ATP} channel. *Nature* 1994;370: 456–459.
18. Atkinson NS, Robertson GA, Ganetzky B. A component of calcium-activated potassium channels encoded by *Drosophila slo* locus. *Science* 1991;253:551–555.
19. Bader CR, Bernheim L, Bertrand D. Sodium-activated potassium current in cultured avian neurones. *Nature* 1985;317:540–542.
20. Baum VC. Distinctive effects of three intravenous anesthetics on the inward rectifier (I_{K1}) and the delayed rectifier (I_K) potassium currents in myocardium: implications for the mechanism of action. *Anesth Analg* 1993;76:18–23.
21. Baumann A, Krah-Jentgens I, Müller-Holtkamp F, et al. Molecular organization of the maternal effect region of the *Shaker* complex of Drosophila: characterization of an I_A channel transcript with homology to vertebrate Na^+ channel. *EMBO J* 1987;6:3419–3429.
22. Bechem M, Glitsch HG, Pott L. Properties of an inward rectifying K channel in the membrane of guinea-pig atrial cardioballs. *Pflugers Arch* 1983;399:186–193.
23. Beech DJ, Bolton TB. Two components of potassium current activated by depolarization of single smooth muscle cells from the rabbit portal vein. *J Physiol (Lond)* 1989;418:293–309.
24. Belardinelli L, Isenberg G. Isolated atrial myocytes: adenosine and acetylcholine increase potassium conductance. *Am J Physiol* 1983; 244:H734–H737.
25. Benham CD, Bolton TB, Lang RJ, Takewaki T. Calcium-activated potassium channels in single smooth muscle cells of rabbit jejunum and guinea-pig mesenteric artery. *J Physiol (Lond)* 1986; 371:45–67.
26. Berg-Johnsen J, Langmoen IA. Mechanisms concerned in the direct effect of isoflurane on rat hippocampal and human neocortical neurons. *Brain Res* 1990;507:28–34.
27. Bezanilla F, Perozo E, Papazian DM, Stefani E. Molecular basis of gating charge immobilization in Shaker potassium channels. *Science* 1991;254:679–683.
28. Bielefeldt K, Rotter JL, Jackson MB. Three potassium channels in rat posterior pituitary nerve terminals. *J Physiol (Lond)* 1992;458: 41–67.
29. Biermans G, Vereecke J, Carmeliet E. The mechanism of the inactivation of the inward-rectifying K current during hyperpolarizing steps in guinea-pig ventricular myocytes. *Pflugers Arch* 1987;410: 604–613.
30. Blatz AL, Magleby KL. Single apamin-blocked Ca-activated K^+ channels of small conductance in cultured rat skeletal muscle. *Nature* 1986;323:718–720.
31. Blumenthal E M, Kaczmarek LK. The minK potassium channel exists in functional and nonfunctional forms when expressed in the plasma membrane of Xenopus oocytes. *J Neurosci* 1994;14: 3097–3105.
32. Bosnjak ZJ. Cardiac effects of anesthetics. *Adv Exp Med Biol* 1991; 301:91–96.
33. Bosnjak ZJ. Effects of volatile anesthetics on the intracellular calcium transient and calcium current in cardiac muscle cells. *Adv Exp Med Biol* 1991;301:97–107.
34. Bosnjak ZJ. Ion channels in vascular smooth muscle. Physiology and pharmacology. *Anesthesiology* 1993;79:1392–1401.
35. Bosnjak ZJ, Aggarwal A, Turner LA, Kampine JM, Kampine JP. Differential effects of halothane, enflurane, and isoflurane on Ca^{2+} transients and papillary muscle tension in guinea pigs. *Anesthesiology* 1992;76:123–131.
36. Bosnjak ZJ, Kampine JP. Effects of halothane on transmembrane potentials, Ca^{2+} transients, and papillary muscle tension in the cat. *Am J Physiol* 1986;251:H374–H381.
37. Bosnjak ZJ, Kampine JP. Effects of halothane, enflurane, and isoflurane on the SA node. *Anesthesiology* 1983;58:314–321.
38. Bosnjak, ZJ, Supan FD, Rusch NJ. The effects of halothane, enflurane, and isoflurane on calcium current in isolated canine ventricular cells. *Anesthesiology* 1991;74:340–345.
39. Boyle WA, Nerbonne JM. A novel type of depolarization-activated K^- current in isolated adult rat atrial myocytes. *Am J Physiol* 1991; 260:H1236–H1247.
40. Braun AP, Walsh MP, Clark RB, Giles WR. α_1-adrenergic effects on

potassium currents and membrane GTPase in single rabbit cardiac cells. In: Spooner PM, Brown AM, eds. *Ion channels in the cardiovascular system: function and dysfunction.* New York: Futura, 1994; 221–236.

41. Brayden JE. Membrane hyperpolarization is a mechanism of endothelium-dependent cerebral vasodilation. *Am J Physiol* 1990; 259:H668–H673.
42. Breitwieser GE, Szabo G. Mechanism of muscarinic receptor-induced K^+ channel activation as revealed by hydrolysis-resistant GTP analogues. *J Gen Physiol* 1988;91:469–493.
43. Brown AM. A cellular logic for G-protein-coupled ion channel pathways. *FASEB J* 1991;5:2175–2179.
44. Brown DA. M-currents: an update. *Trends Neurosci* 1988;11:294–299.
45. Brown DA, Adams PR. Muscarinic suppression of a novel voltage-sensitive K^+ current in a vertebrate neurone. *Nature* 1980;283: 673–676.
46. Brown DA, Constanti A, Adams PR. Ca-activated potassium current in vertebrate sympathetic neurones. *Cell Calcium* 1983;4:407–420.
47. Brüggemann A, Pardo LA, Stühmer W, Pongs O. Ether-à-go-go encodes a voltage-gated channel permeable to K^+ and Ca^{2+} and modulated by cAMP. *Nature* 1993;365:445–448.
48. Buljubasic N, Flynn NM, Marijic J, Rusch NJ, Kampine JP, Bosnjak ZJ. Effects of isoflurane on K^+ and Ca^{2+} conductance in isolated smooth muscle cells of canine cerebral arteries. *Anesth Analg* 1992;75:590–596.
49. Buljubasic N, Marijic J, Kampine JP, Bosnjak ZJ. Calcium-sensitive potassium current in isolated canine coronary smooth muscle cells. *Can J Physiol Pharmacol* 1994;72:189–198.
50. Buljubasic N, Rusch NJ, Marijic J, Kampine JP, Bosnjak ZJ. Effects of halothane and isoflurane on calcium and potassium channel currents in canine coronary arterial cells. *Anesthesiology* 1992;76: 990–998.
51. Butler A, Tsunoda S, McCobb DP, Wei A, Salkoff L. mSlo, a complex mouse gene encoding "maxi" calcium-activated potassium channels. *Science* 1993;261:221–224.
52. Callewaert G, Vereecke J, Carmeliet E. Existence of calcium-dependent potassium channel in the membrane of cow cardiac Purkinje cells. *Pflugers Archiv* 1986;406:424–426.
53. Carl A, Bowen S, Gelband CH, Sanders KM, Hume JR. Cromakalim and lemakalim activate Ca^{2+}-dependent K^+ channels in canine colon. *Pflugers Arch* 1992;421:67–76.
54. Carl A, Frey BW, Ward SM, Sanders KM, Kenyon JL. Inhibition of slow-wave repolarization and Ca^{2+}-activated K^+ channels by quaternary ammonium ions. *Am J Physiol* 1993;264:C625–C631.
55. Carl A, Sanders KM. Ca^{2+}-activated K channels of canine colonic myocytes. *Am J Physiol* 1989;257:C470–C480.
56. Carmeliet E, Mubagwa K. Characterization of the acetylcholine-induced potassium current in rabbit Purkinje fibres. *J Physiol (Lond)* 1986;371:219–237.
57. Cason BA, Shubayev I, Hickey RF. Blockade of adenosine triphosphate-sensitive potassium channels eliminates isoflurane-induced coronary artery vasodilation. *Anesthesiology* 1994;81:1245–1255.
58. Catterall WA. Structure and function of voltage-gated ion channels. *Trends Neurosci* 1993;16:500–506.
59. Chandy KG. Simplified gene nomenclature. *Nature* 1991;352:26.
60. Choi KL, Aldrich RW, Yellen G. Tetraethyl ammonium blockade distinguishes two inactivation mechanisms in voltage-gated K^+ channels. *Proc Natl Acad Sci USA* 1991;88:5092–5095.
61. Christie MJ, North RA. Agonists at μ-opioid, M_2-muscarinic and $GABA_B$ receptors increase the same potassium conductance in rat lateral parabrachial neurones. *Br J Pharmacol* 1988;95:896–902.
62. Chung S, Reinhart PH, Martin BL, Brautigan D, Levitan IB. Protein kinase activity closely associated with reconstituted calcium-activated potassium channel. *Science* 1991;253:560–562.
63. Clark RB, Giles WR, Imaizumi Y. Properties of the transient outward currents in rabbit atrial cells. *J Physiol (Lond)* 1988;405: 147–168.
64. Cobbett P, Legendre P, Mason WT. Characterization of three types of potassium current in cultured neurones of rat supraoptic nucleus area. *J Physiol (Lond)* 1989;410:443–462.
65. Coldwell MC, Howlett DR. Specificity of action of the novel antihypertensive agent, BRL 34915, as a potassium channel activator. Comparison with Nicorandil. *Biochem Pharmacol* 1987;36:3663–3669.
66. Connor JA, Stevens CF. Voltage clamp studies of a transient outward membrane current in gastropod neural somata. *J Physiol (Lond)* 1971;213:21–30.
67. Connor JA, Stevens CF. Prediction of the repetitive firing behaviour from voltage clamp data on an isolated neurone soma. *J Physiol (Lond)* 1971;213:31–53.
68. Constanti A, Simm J. Calcium-dependent potassium conductance in guinea pig olfactory cortex in vitro. *J Physiol (Lond)* 1987;387: 173–194.
69. Cook DL, Hales CN. Intracellular ATP directly blocks K^+ channels in pancreatic B-cells. *Nature* 1984;311:271–273.
70. Cook NS. The pharmacology of potassium channels and their therapeutic potential. *Trends Pharmacol Sci* 1988;9:21–28.
71. Cooper E, Shrier A. Single-channel analysis of fast transient potassium currents from rat nodose neurons. *J Physiol (Lond)* 1985;369: 199–208.
72. Coraboeuf E, Carmeliet E. Existence of two transient outward currents in sheep Purkinje fibres. *Pflugers Arch* 1982;392:352–359.
73. Coronado R, Miller C. Decamethonium and hexamethonium block K^+ channels of sarcoplasmic reticulum. *Nature* 1980;288: 495–497.
74. Covarrubias M, Wei A, Salkoff L. Shaker, Shal, Shab, and Shaw express independent K^+ current systems. *Neuron* 1991;7:763–773.
75. Crest M, Gola M. Large conductance Ca^{2+}-activated K^+ channels are involved in both spike shaping and firing regulation in Helix neurones. *J Physiol (Lond)* 1993;465:265–287.
76. Crumb WJ Jr, Wible B, Arnold DJ, Payne JP, Brown AM. Blockade of multiple human cardiac potassium currents by the antihistamine terfenadine: possible mechanism for terfenadine-associated cardiotoxicity. *Mol Pharmacol* 1995;47:181–190.
77. Curran ME, Landes GM, Keating MT. Molecular cloning, characterization, and genomic localization of human potassium channel gene. *Genomics* 1992;12:729–737.
78. Curran ME, Splawski I, Timothy KW, Vincent GM, Green ED, Keating MT. A molecular basis for cardiac arrhythmia: HERG mutations cause long QT syndrome. *Cell* 1995;80:795–803.
79. Dart C, Standen NB. Activation of ATP-dependent K^+ channels by hypoxia in smooth muscle cells isolated from the pig coronary artery. *J Physiol (Lond)* 1995;483:29–39.
80. Dart C, Standen NB. Adenosine-activated potassium current in smooth muscle cells isolated from the pig coronary artery. *J Physiol (Lond)* 1993;471:767–786.
81. Daut J. The passive electrical properties of guinea pig ventricular muscle as examined with a voltage-clamp technique. *J Physiol (Lond)* 1982;330:221–242.
82. Daut J, Maier-Rudolph W, von Beckerath N, Mehrke G, Gunther K, Goedel-Meinen L. Hypoxic dilation of coronary arteries is mediated by ATP-sensitive potassium channels. *Science* 1990;247: 1341–1344.
83. Davies NW, Spruce AE, Standen NB, Stanfield PR. Multiple blocking mechanisms of ATP-sensitive potassium channels of frog skeletal muscle by tetraethylammonium ions. *J Physiol (Lond)* 1989; 413:31–48.
84. de Weille JR. Modulation of ATP sensitive potassium channels. *Cardiovasc Res* 1992;26:1017–1020.
85. de Weille JR, Lazdunski M. Regulation of the ATP-sensitive potassium channel. *Ion Channels* 1990;2:205–222.
86. Denson DD, Duchatelle P, Eaton DC. The effect of racemic ketamine on the large conductance Ca^{2+}-activated potassium (BK) channels in GH_3 cells. *Brain Res* 1994;638:61–68.
87. Doze VA, Chen B-X, Tinkleberg JA, Segal IS, Maze M. Pertussis toxin and 4-aminopyridine differentially affect the hypnotic-anesthetic action of dexmedetomidine and pentobarbital. *Anesthesiology* 1990;73:304–307.
88. Dryer SE. Na^+-activated K^+ channels and voltage-evoked ionic currents in brain stem and parasympathetic neurones of the chick. *J Physiol (Lond)* 1991;435:513–532.
89. Dryer SE. Na^+-activated K^+ channels: a new family of large-conductance ion channels. *Trends Neurosci* 1994;17:155–160.
90. Dryer SE, Fujii JT, Martin AR. A Na^+-activated K^+ current in cultured brain stem neurones from chicks. *J Physiol (Lond)* 1989;410: 283–296.
91. Dubois JM. Evidence for the existence of three types of potassium channels in the frog Ranvier node membrane. *J Physiol (Lond)* 1981;318:297–316.
92. Dubois JM. Potassium currents in the frog node of Ranvier. *Prog Biophys Mol Biol* 1983;42:1–20.
93. Dukes ID, Morad M. The transient K^+ current in rat ventricular myocytes: evaluation of its Ca^{2+} and Na^+ dependence. *J Physiol (Lond)* 1991;435:395–420.

94. Durell SR, Guy HR. Atomic scale structure and functional models of voltage-gated potassium channels. *Biophys J* 1992;62:238–247.
95. Edwards G, Weston AH. The pharmacology of ATP-sensitive potassium channels. *Annu Rev Pharmacol Toxicol* 1993;33:597–637.
96. Ehrenstein G, Gilbert DL. Slow changes in the potassium permeability in the squid giant axon. *Biophys J* 1966;6:553–566.
97. Elkins T, Ganetzky B, Wu C-F. A *Drosophila* mutation that eliminates a calcium-dependent potassium current. *Proc Natl Acad Sci USA* 1986;83:8415–8419.
98. Engelman E, Lipszye M, Gilbart E, Van der Linden P, Bellens B, Van Romphey A, de Rood M. Effects of clonidine on anesthetic drug requirements and hemodynaic response during aortic surgery. *Anesthesiology* 1989;71:178–187.
99. Escande D, Coulombe A, Faivre JF, Deroubaix E, Coraboeuf E. Two types of transient outward currents in adult human atrial cells. *Am J Physiol* 1987;252:H142–H148.
100. Escande D, Henry P. Potassium channels as pharmacological targets in cardiovascular medicine. *Eur Heart J* 1993;14:2–9.
101. Esguerra M, Wang J, Foster CD, Adelman JP, North RA, Levitan IB. Cloned Ca^{2+}-dependent K^+ channel modulated by functionally associated protein kinase. *Science* 1994;369:563–565.
102. Eskinder H, Gebremedhin D, Lee JG, Rusch NJ, Supan FD, Kampine JP, Bosnjak ZJ. Halothane and isoflurane decrease the open state probability of K^+ channels in dog cerebral arterial muscle cells. *Anesthesiology* 1995;82:479–490.
103. Evans RJ, Surprenant A. Effects of phospholipase A_2 inhibitors on coupling of α_2-adrenoceptors to inwardly rectifying potassium currents in guinea pig submucosal neurones. *Br J Pharmacol* 1993;10:591–596.
104. Ewald D, Williams A, Levitan I. Modulation of single Ca^{2+}-dependent K^+-channel activity by protein phosphorylation. *Nature* 1985;315:503–506.
105. Fan Z, Nakayama K, Hiraoka M. Pinacidil activates the ATP-sensitive K^+ channel in inside-out and cell-attached patch membranes of guinea-pig ventricular myocytes. *Pflugers Arch* 1990;415:387–394.
106. Fedida D, Braun AP, Giles WR. Alpha$_1$-adrenoceptors reduce background K^+ current in rabbit ventricular myocytes. *J Physiol (Lond)* 1991;441:673–684.
107. Fedida D, Wible B, Wang Z, Fermini B, Faust F, Nattel S, Brown AM. Identity of a novel delayed rectifier current from human heart with a cloned K^+ channel current. *Circ Res* 73: 210–216, 1993.
108. Ficker E, Taglialatela M, Wible BA, Henley CM, Brown AM. Spermine and spermidine as gating molecules for inward rectifier K^+ channels. *Science* 1994;266:1068–1072.
109. Folander K, Smith JS, Antanavage J, Bennett C, Stein RB, Swanson R. Cloning and expression of the delayed-rectifier I_{sK} channel from neonatal rat heart and diethylstilbestrol-primed rat uterus. *Proc Natl Acad Sci USA* 1990;87:2975–2979.
110. Franks NP, Lieb WR. Volatile general anesthetics activate a novel neuronal K^+ current. *Nature* 1988;333:662–664.
111. Franz MR, Bargheer K, Rafflenbeul W, Haverich A, Lichtlen PR. Monophasic action potential mapping in human subjects with normal electrocardiograms: direct evidence for the genesis of the T wave. *Circulation* 1987;75:379–386.
112. Freeman LC, Kass RS. Expression of a minimal K^+ channel protein in mammalian cells and immunolocalization in guinea pig heart. *Circ Res* 1993;73:968–973.
113. Freeman LC, Kwok W-M, Kass RS. Phosphorylation-independent regulation of cardiac I_K by guanine nucleotides and isoproterenol. *Am J Physiol* 1992;262:H1298–H1302.
114. Fujiwara N, Higashi H, Nishi S, Shimoji K, Sugita S, Yoshimura M. Changes in spontaneous firing patterns of rat hippocampal neurones induced by volatile anaesthetics. *J Physiol (Lond)* 1988;402: 155–175.
115. Galione A, White A, Willmont N, Turner M, Potter BVL, Watson SP. cGMP mobilizes intracellular Ca^{2+} in sea urchin eggs by stimulating cyclic ADP-ribose synthesis. *Nature* 1993;365:456–459.
116. Galvan M, Sedlmeir C. Outward currents in voltage-clamped rat sympathetic neurones. *J Physiol (Lond)* 1984;356:115–133.
117. Galvez A, Gimenez-Gallego G, Reuben JP, Roy-Contancin L, Feigenbaum P, Kaczorowski GJ, Garcia ML. Purification and characterization of a unique, potent, peptidyl probe for the high conductance calcium-activated potassium channel from venom of the scorpion *Buthus tamulus*. *J Biol Chem* 1990;265:11083–11090.
118. Ganetzky B, Wu C. Neurogenetics of membrane excitability in *Drosophila*. *Annu Rev Gen* 1986;20:13–44.
119. Garcia-Calvo M, Knaus H-G, McManus OB, Giangiacomo KM, Kaczorowski GJ, Garcia ML. Purification and reconstitution of the high-conductance, calcium-activated potassium channel from tracheal smooth muscle. *J Biol Chem* 1994;269:676–682.
120. Gelband CH, Lodge NJ, Van Breemen C. A Ca^{2+}-activated K^+ channel from rabbit aorta: modulation by cromakalim. *Eur J Pharmacol* 1989;167:201–210.
121. Giles WR, Imaizumi Y. Comparison of potassium currents in rabbit atrial and ventricular cells. *J Physiol (Lond)* 1988;405:123–145.
122. Giles WR, van Ginneken AC. A transient outward current in isolated cells from the crista terminalis of rabbit heart. *J Physiol (Lond)* 1985;368:243–264.
123. Gilmour Jr RF, Zipes DP. Different electrophysiological responses of canine endocardium and epicardium to combined hyperkalemia, hypoxia, and acidosis. *Circ Res* 1980;46:814–825.
124. Gintant GA, Cohen IS, Datyner NB, Kline RP. Time-dependent outward currents in the heart. In: Fozzard HA, Haber E, Jennings RB, Kate AM, Morgan HE, eds. *The heart and cardiovascular system.* New York: Raven Press, 1992;1121–1169.
125. Gintant GA, Datyner NB, Cohen IS. Gating of delayed rectification in acutely isolated canine cardiac Purkinje myocytes. *Biophys J* 1985;48:1059–1064.
126. Goldstein SAN, Miller C. Site-specific mutations in a minimal voltage-dependent K^+ channel alter ion selectivity and open-channel block. *Neuron* 1991;7:403–408.
127. Gomez-Lagunas F, Armstrong CM. Inactivation in ShakerB K^+ channels: a test for the number of inactivating particles on each channel. *Biophys J* 1995;68:89–95.
128. Grissmer S, Cahalan M. TEA prevents inactivation while blocking open K^+ channels in human T-lymphocytes. *Biophys J* 1989;55: 203–206.
129. Gross GJ, Auchampach JA. Role of ATP dependent potassium channels in myocardial ischaemia. *Cardiovasc Res* 1992;26: 1011–1016.
130. Grudt TJ, Williams JT. κ-opioid receptors also increase potassium conductance. *Proc Natl Acad Sci USA* 1993;90:11429–11432.
131. Gustafsson B, Galvan M, Grafe P, Wigstrom H. A transient outward current in a mammalian central neurone blocked by 4-aminopyridine. *Nature* 1982;299:252–254.
132. Guy HR, Durell SR, Warmke J, Drysdale R, Ganetzky B. Similarities in amino-acid sequences of Drosophila eag and cyclic nucleotide-gated channels. *Science* 1991;254:730.
133. Habermann E. Bee and wasp venoms. *Science* 1972;177:314–322.
134. Haimann C, Bernheim L, Bertrand D, Bader CR. Potassium current activated by intracellular sodium in quail trigeminal ganglion neurons. *J Gen Physiol* 1990;95:961–980.
135. Haimann C, Magistretti J, Pozzi B. Sodium-activated potassium current in sensory neurons: a comparison of cell-attached and cell-free single-channel activities. *Pflugers Arch* 1992;422:287–294.
136. Harder DR, Gradall K, Madden JA, Kampine JP. Cellular actions of halothane on cat cerebral arterial muscle. *Stroke* 1985;16: 680–683.
137. Hartzell HC. Adenosine receptors in frog sinus venosus: slow inhibitory potentials produced by adenosine compounds and acetylcholine. *J Physiol (Lond)* 1979;293:23–49.
138. Hartzell HC, Simmons MA. Comparison of effects of acetylcholine on calcium and potassium currents in frog atrium and ventricle. *J Physiol (Lond)* 1987;389:411–422.
139. Hausdorff SF, Goldstein SAN, Rushin EE, Miller C. Functional characterization of a minimal K^+ channel expressed from a synthetic gene. *Biochemistry* 1991;30:3341–3346.
140. Haydon DA, Requena J, Simon AJB. The potassium conductance of the resting squid axon and its blockage by clinical concentrations of general anesthetics. *J Physiol (Lond)* 1988;402:363–374.
141. Haydon DA, Simon AJB. Excitation of the giant squid axon by general anesthetics. *J Physiol (Lond)* 1988;402:375–389.
142. Haydon DA, Urban BW. The actions of some general anaesthetics on the potassium current of the squid giant axon. *J Physiol (Lond)* 1986;373:311–327.
143. Heidbuchel H, Vereecke J, Carmeliet E. The electrophysiological effects of acetylcholine in single human atrial cells. *J Mol Cell Cardiol* 1987;19:1207–1219.
144. Heidbuchel H, Vereecke J, Carmeliet E. Three different potassium channels in human atrium. Contribution to the basal potassium conductance. *Circ Res* 1990;66:1277–1286.
145. Herrington J, Stern RC, Evers AS, Lingle CJ. Halothane inhibits two components of calcium current in clonal (GH_3) pituitary cells. *J Neurosci* 1991;11:2226–2240.

146. Higashida H, Brown DA. Ca^{2+}-dependent K^+ channels in neuroblastoma hybrid cells activated by intracellular inositol triphosphate and extracellular bradykinin. *FEBS Lett* 1988;238:395–400.
147. Higashdi H, Robbins J, Egorova A, Noda M, Taketo M, Ishizaka N, Takasawa S, Okamoto H, Brown DA. Nicotinamide-adenine dinucleotide regulates muscarinic receptor-coupled K^+ (M) channels in rodent NG108-15 cells. *J Physiol (Lond)* 1995;482:317–323.
148. Hille B. *Ionic channels of excitable membranes.* Sunderland, MA: Sinauer Associates, 1992.
149. Hinrichsen RD. *Calcium-dependent potassium channels.* Austin: R.G. Landes, 1993.
150. Hiraoka M, Fan Z. Activation of ATP-sensitive outward K^+ current by nicorandil (2-nicotinamidoethyl nitrate) in isolated ventricular myocytes. *J Pharmacol Exp Ther* 1988;250:278–285.
151. Ho K, Nichols CG, Lederer WJ, Lytton J, Vassilev PM, Kanazirska MV, Hebert SC. Cloning and expression of an inwardly rectifying ATP-regulated potassium channel. *Nature* 1993;362:31–38.
152. Hodgkin AL, Huxley AF. Currents carried by sodium and potassium ions through the membrane of the giant axon of *Loligo. J Physiol (Lond)* 1952;116:449–472.
153. Hodgkin AL, Huxley AF. A quantitative description of membrane current and its application to conduction and excitation in nerve. *J Physiol (Lond)* 1952;117:500–544.
154. Hodgkin AL, Huxley AF, Katz B. Ionic currents underlying activity in the giant axon of the squid. *Arch Sci Physiol* 1949;3:129–150.
155. Hong Y, Puil E, Mathers DA. Effect of halothane on large-conductance calcium-dependent potassium channels in cerebrovascular smooth muscle cells of the rat. *Anesthesiology* 1994;81: 649–656.
156. Hoshi T, Zagotta WN, Aldrich RW. Biophysical and molecular mechanisms of Shaker potassium channel inactivation. *Science* 1990;250:533–538.
157. Hu SL, Yamamoto Y, Kao CY. The Ca^{2+}-activated K^+ channel and its functional roles in smooth muscle cells of guinea pig taenia coli. *J Gen Physiol* 1989;94:833–847.
158. Hu SL, Yamamoto Y, Kao CY. Permeation, selectivity, and blockade of the Ca^{2+}-activated potassium channel of the guinea pig taenia coli myocyte. *J Gen Physiol* 1989;94:849–862.
159. Hume JR, Uehara A. Ionic basis of the different action potential configurations of single guinea-pig atrial and ventricular myocytes. *J Physiol (Lond)* 1985;368:525–544.
160. Hwang PM, Glatt CE, Bredt DS, Yellen G, Snyder SH. A novel K^+ channel with unique localizations in mammalian brain: molecular cloning and characterization. *Neuron* 1992;8:473–481.
161. Ibarra J, Morley GE, Delmar M. Dynamics of the inward rectifier K^+ current during the action potential of guinea pig ventricular myocytes. *Biophys J* 1991;60:1534–1539.
162. Ignarro LJ, Buga GM, Wood KS, Byrns RE, Chaudhuri G. Endothelium-derived relaxing factor produced and released from artery and vein is nitric oxide. *Proc Natl Acad Sci USA* 1987; 84:9265–9269.
163. Isacoff EY, Jan YN, Jan LY. Evidence for the formation of heteromultimeric potassium channels in Xenopus oocytes. *Nature* 1990; 345:530–534.
164. Isacoff EY, Jan YN, Jan LY. Putative receptor for the cytoplasmic inactivation gate in the Shaker K^+ channel. *Nature* 1991;353:86–90.
165. Ishihara K, Mitsuiye T, Noma A, Takano M. The Mg^{2+} block and intrinsic gating underlying inward rectification of the K^+ current in guinea-pig cardiac myocytes. *J Physiol (Lond)* 1989;419:297–320.
166. Ito H, Vereecke J, Carmeliet E. Intracellular protons inhibit inward rectifier K^+ channel of guinea pig ventricular cell membrane. *Pflugers Arch* 1992;422: 280–286.
167. Iverson LE, Tamouge MA, Lester HA, Davidson N, Rudy B. A-type potassium channels expressed *Shaker* locus cDNA. *Proc Natl Acad Sci USA* 1988;85:5723–5727.
168. Jackson WF. Arteriolar tone is determined by activity of ATP-sensitive potassium channels. *Am J Physiol* 1993;265:H1797–H1803.
169. Jan LY, Jan YN. A superfamily of ion channels. *Nature* 1990;345: 672.
170. Jan LY, Jan YN. Structural elements involved in specific K^+ channel functions. *Annu Rev Physiol* 1992;54:537–555.
171. Jan LY, Jan YN. Potassium channels and their evolving gates. *Nature* 1994;371:119–122, 1994.
172. Jones S, Brown DA, Milligan GM, Willer E, Buckley NJ, Caulfield MP. Bradykinin excites rat sympathetic neurons by inhibition of M current through a mechanism involving B2 receptors and $G\alpha q/11$. *Neuron* 1995;14:399–405.
173. Josephson IR, Sanchez-Chapula J, Brown AM. Early outward current in rat single ventricular cells. *Circ Res* 1984;54:157–162.
174. Jurkiewicz NK, Sanguinetti MC. Rate-dependent prolongation of cardiac action potentials by a methanesulfonanilide class III antiarrhythmic agent. *Circ Res* 1993;72:75–83.
175. Kaibara M, Nakajima T, Irisawa H, Giles WR. Regulation of spontaneous opening of muscarinic K^+ channels in rabbit atrium. *J Physiol (Lond)* 1991;433:589–613.
176. Kamb A, Iverson LE, Tanouye MA. Molecular characterization of Shaker, a Drosophila gene that encodes a potassium channel. *Cell* 1987;50:405–413.
177. Kameyama M, Kakei M, Sato R, Shibasaki T, Matsuda H, Irisawa H. Intracellular Na^+ activates a K^+ channel in mammalian cardiac cells. *Nature* 1984;309:354–356.
178. Kameyama M, Kiyosue T, Soejima M. Single channel analysis of the inward rectifier K current in rabbit ventricular cells. *Jpn J Physiol* 1983;33:1039–1056.
179. Kasai H, Kameyama D, Yamaguchi K, Fukuda J. Single transient K channels in mammalian sensory neurons. *Biophys J* 1986;49: 1243–1247.
180. Kass RS, Scheuer T, Malloy KJ. Block of outward current in cardiac Purkinje fibres by injection of quaternary ammonium ions. *J Gen Physiol* 1982;79:1041–1063.
181. Katz B. Les constantes electriques de la membrane du muscle. *Arch Sci Physiol*1949;3:285–300.
182. Kaukinen S, Pyykko K. The potentiation of halothane anesthesia by clonidine. *Acta Anaesthesiol Scand* 1979;23:1007–1111.
183. Kenyon JL, Gibbons WR. 4-Aminopyridine and the early outward current of sheep cardiac Purkinje fibres. *J Gen Physiol* 1979;73: 139–157.
184. Kimura S, Bassett AL, Kohya T, Kozlovskis PL, Myerburg RJ. Simultaneous recording of action potentials from endocardium and epicardium during ischemia in the isolated cat ventricle: relation of temporal electrophysiologic heterogeneities to arrhythmias. *Circulation* 1986;74:401–409.
185. Kirsch GE, Drewe JA. Gating-dependent mechanism of 4-aminopyridine block in two related potassium channels. *J Gen Physiol* 1993;102:797–816.
186. Kitazono T, Faraci FM, Heistad DD. Effect of norepinephrine on rat basilar artery in vivo. *Am J Physiol* 1993;264:H178–H182.
187. Knaus H-G, Eberhart A, Glossman H, Munujos P, Kaczorowski GJ, Garcia ML. Pharmacology and structure of high conductance calcium-activated potassium channels. *Cell Signal* 1994;6:861–870.
188. Kolb HA. Potassium channels in excitable and non-excitable cells. *Rev Physiol Biochem Pharmacol* 1990;115:51–91.
189. Koren G, Liman ER, Logothetis DE, Nadal-Ginard B, Hess P. Gating mechanism of a cloned potassium channel expressed in frog oocytes and mammalian cells. *Neuron* 1990;4:39–51.
190. Koumi S-I, Wasserstrom JA. Acetylcholine-sensitive muscarinic K^+ channels in mammalian ventricular myocytes. *Am J Physiol* 1994; 266:H1812–H1821.
191. Koyano T, Kakei M, Nakashima H, Yoshinaga M, Matsuoka T, Tanaka H. ATP-regulated K^+ channels are modulated by intracellular H^+ in guinea-pig ventricular cells. *J Physiol (Lond)* 1993;463: 747–766.
192. Krapivinsky G, Gordon EA, Wickman K, Velimirovic B, Krapivinsky L, Clapham DE. The G-protein-gated atrial K^+ channel I_{KACh} is a heteromutimer of two inwardly rectifying K^+ channel proteins. *Nature* 1995;374:135–141.
193. Krnjevic K. Cellular and synaptic effects of general anesthetics. In: Roth SH, Miller KW, eds. *Molecular and cellular mechanisms of anesthetics.* New York: Plenum Press, 1986;3–16.
194. Kubo Y, Baldwin TJ, Jan YN, Jan LY. Primary structure and functional expression of a mouse inward rectifier potassium channel. *Nature* 1993;362:127–133.
195. Kubo Y, Reuveng E, Slesinger PA, Jan YN, Jan LY. Primary structure and functional expression of a rat G-protein-coupled muscarinic potassium channel. *Nature* 1993;364:802–806.
196. Kukushkin NI, Gainullin RZ, Sosunov EA. Transient outward current and rate dependence of action potential duration in rabbit cardiac ventricular muscle. *Pflugers Arch* 1983;399:87–92.
197. Kume H, Takai A, Tokuno H, Tomita T. Regulation of Ca^{2+}-dependent K^+-channel activity in tracheal myocytes by phosphorylation. *Nature* 1989;341:152–154.
198. Kurachi Y. Voltage-dependent activation of the inward-rectifier potassium channel in the ventricular cell membrane of guinea-pig heart. *J Physiol (Lond)* 1985;366:365–385.

199. Kwok W-M, Kass RS. Block of cardiac ATP-sensitive K^+ channels by external divalent cations is modulated by intracellular ATP. Evidence for allosteric regulation of the channel protein. *J Gen Physiol* 1993;102:693–712.
200. Lancaster B, Nicoll RA. Properties of two calcium-activated hyperpolarizations in rat hippocampal neurones. *J Physiol (Lond)* 1987; 389:187–203.
201. Lancaster B, Nicoll RA, Perkel DJ. Calcium activates two types of potassium channels in rat hippocampal neurons in culture. *J Neurosci* 1991;11:23–30.
202. Lang DG, Ritchie AK. Tetraethylammonium blockade of apamin-sensitive and insensitive Ca^{2+}-activated K^+ channels in a pituitary cell line. *J Physiol (Lond)* 1990;425:117–132.
203. Larach DR, Schuler HG. Potassium channel blockade and halothane vasodilation in conducting and resistance coronary arteries. *J Pharmacol Exp Ther* 1993;267:72–81.
204. Larach DR, Schuler HG, Zangari KA, McCann RL. Potassium channel opening and coronary vasodilation by halothane. In: Bosnjak ZJ, Kampine JP, eds. *Advances in pharmacology. Anesthesia and cardiovascular disease.* San Diego: Academic Press, 1994; 253–267.
205. Latorre R, Oberhauser A, Labarca P, Alvarez O. Varieties of calcium-activated potassium channels. *Annu Rev Physiol* 1989;51: 385–399.
206. Lechleiter JD, Dartt DA, Brehm P. Vasoactive intestinal peptide activates Ca^{2+}-dependent K^+ channels through a cAMP pathway in mouse lacrimal cells. *Neuron* 1988;1:227–235.
208. Lee M-Y, Bang HW, Lim I-J, Uhm D-Y, Rhee S-D. Modulation of large conductance calcium-activated K^+ channel by membrane delimited protein kinase and phosphatase activities. *Pflugers Arch* 1994;429:150–152.
207. Lee K, Ozanne SE, Hales CN, Ashford MLJ. Mg^{2+}-dependent inhibition of K_{ATP} by sulphonylureas in CRI-G1 insulin-secreting cells. *Br J Pharmacol* 1994;111:632–640.
209. Lee TE, Philipson LH, Kuznetsov A, Nelson DJ. Structural determinant for assembly of mammalian K^+ channels. *Biophys J* 1994;66: 667–673.
210. Lefkowitz RJ, Caron MG. Molecular and regulatory properties of adrenergic receptors. *Rec Prog Hormone Res* 1987;43:469–497.
211. Leinders T, Vijverberg HPM. Ca^{2+} dependence of small Ca^{2+}-activated K^+ channels in cultured N1E-115 neuroblastoma cells. *Pflugers Arch* 1992;422:223–232.
212. Lesage F, Duprat F, Fink M, Guillemare E, Coppola T, Lazdunski M, Hugnot J-P. Cloning evidence for a family of inward rectifier and G-protein coupled K^+ channels in the brain. *FEBS Lett* 1994; 353:37–42.
213. Lester HA. Strategies for studying permeation at voltage-gated ion channels. *Annu Rev Physiol* 1991;53:477–496.
214. Li M, Unwin N, Stauffer KA, Jan YN, Jan LY. Images of purified Shaker potassium channels. *Curr Biol* 1994;4:110–115.
215. Lipscombe D, Kongsamut S, Tsien RW. α-adrenergic inhibition of sympathetic neurotransmitter release mediated by modulation of N-type calcium-channel gating. *Nature* 1989;340:639–642.
216. Litovsky SH, Antzelevitch C. Transient outward current prominent in canine ventricular epicardium but not endocardium. *Circ Res* 1988;62:116–126.
217. Liu D-W, Antzelevitch C. Characteristics of the delayed rectifier current (I_{Kr} and I_{Ks}) in canine ventricular epicardial, midmyocardial, and endocardial myocytes—a weaker I_{Ks} contributes to the longer action potential of the M cell. *Circ Res* 1995;76:351–365.
218. Loffelholz K, Pappano AJ. The parasympathetic neuroeffector junction of the heart. *Pharmacol Rev* 1985;37:1–24.
219. Lopatin AN, Makhina EN, Nichols CG. Potassium channel block by cytoplasmic polyamines as the mechanism of intrinsic rectification. *Nature* 1994;372:366–369.
220. Lopez GA, Jan YN, Jan LY. Evidence that the S6 segment of the Shaker voltage-gated K^+ channel comprises part of the pore. *Nature* 1994;367:179–182.
221. Lorenz JN, Schnermann J, Brosius FC, Briggs JP, Furspan PB. Intracellular ATP can regulate afferent arteriolar tone via ATP-sensitive K^+ channels in the rabbit. *J Clin Invest* 1992;90:733–740.
222. Luk HN, Carmeliet E. Na^+ activated K^+ current in cardiac cells: rectification, open probability, block and role in digitalis toxicity. *Pflugers Arch* 1990;416:766–768.
223. Luo C, Rudy Y. A model of the ventricular cardiac action potential: depolarization, repolarization, and their interaction. *Circ Res* 1991;68:1501–1526.
224. MacIver MB, Roth SH. Anesthetics produce differential actions on the discharge activity of a single neuron. *Eur J Pharmacol* 1987;139: 43–52.
225. MacKinnon R. Determination of the subunit stoichiometry of a voltage-activated potassium channel. *Nature* 1991;350:232–235.
226. MacKinnon R, Miller C. Mechanism of charybdotoxin block of the high-conductance Ca^{2+}-activated K^+ channel. *J Gen Physiol* 1988;91:335–349.
227. Marrion NV. Selective reduction of one mode of M-channel gating by muscarine in sympathetic neurons. *Neuron* 1993;11:77–84.
228. Marty A, Neher E. Potassium channels in cultured bovine adrenal chromaffin cells. *J Physiol (Lond)* 1985;367:117–141.
229. Matsuda H. Open-state substructure of inwardly rectifying potassium channels revealed by magnesium block in guinea pig heart cells. *J Physiol (Lond)* 1988;397:237–258.
230. Matsuda H. Magnesium gating of the inwardly rectifying K^+ channel. *Annu Rev Physiol* 1991;53:289–298.
231. Matsuda H, Matsuura H, Noma A. Triple-barrel structure of inwardly rectifying K^+ channels revealed by Cs^+ and Rb^+ block inguineal pig heart cells. *J Physiol (Lond)* 1989;413:139–157.
232. Matsuda H, Saigusa A, Irisawa H. Ohmic conductance through the inwardly rectifying K channel and blocking by internal Mg^{2+}. *Nature* 1987;325:156–159.
233. Maze M, Vickery RG, Merlone SC, Gaba DM. Anesthetic and hemodynamic effects of $alpha_2$-adrenergic agonist, azepexole, in isoflurane-anesthetized dogs. *Anesthesiology* 1988;68:689–694.
234. Mazzanti M, DiFrancesco D. Intracellular Ca modulates K-inward rectification in cardiac myocytes. *Pflugers Arch* 1989;413:322–324.
235. McCann JD, Welsh MJ. Neuroleptics antagonize a calcium-activated potassium channel in airway smooth muscle. *J Gen Physiol* 1987;89:339–352.
236. McCormack T, Vega-Saenz de Miera EC, Rudy B. Molecular cloning of a member of a third class of Shaker-family K^+ channel genes in mammals. *Proc Natl Acad Sci USA* 1990;87:5227–5231.
237. McDermott AB, Weight FF. Action potential repolarization may involve a transient, Ca^{2+}-sensitive outward current in a vertebrate neuron. *Nature* 1982;300:185–188.
238. McDonald TF, Trautwein W. The potassium current underlying delayed rectification in cat ventricular muscle. *J Physiol (Lond)* 1978;274:217–246.
239. McManus OB. Calcium-activated potassium channels: regulation by calcium. *J Bioenerg Biomembr* 1991;23:537–560.
240. McManus OB, Harris GH, Giangiacomo KM, et al. An activator of calcium-dependent potassium channels isolated from a medicinal herb. *Biochemistry* 1993;32:6128–6133.
241. McManus OB, Helms LMH, Pallanck L, Ganetzky B, Swanson R, Leonard RL. Functional role of the β subunit of high conductance calcium-activated potassium channels. *Neuron* 1995;645–650.
242. Merkel LA, Lappe RW, Rivera LM, Cox BF, Perrone MH. Demonstration of vasorelaxant activity with an A1-selective adenosine agonist in porcine coronary artery: involvement of potassium channels. *J Pharmacol Exp Ther* 1992;260:437–443.
243. Mihara S, North RA. Opioids increase potassium conductance in submucous neurones of guinea pig caecum by activating δ-receptors. *Br J Pharmacol* 1986;88:315–322.
244. Miller C. Diffusion-controlled binding of a peptide neurotoxin to its K^+ channel receptor. *Biochemistry* 1990;29:5320–5325.
245. Miller C. The charybdotoxin family of K^+ channel-blocking peptides. *Neuron* 1995;15:5–10.
246. Miller C, Moczydlowski E, Latorre R, Phillips M. Charybdotoxin, a protein inhibitor of single Ca^{2+}-activated K^+ channels from mammalian skeletal muscle. *Nature* 1985;313:316–318.
247. Miller RJ. Glucose-regulated potassium channels are sweet news for neurobiologists. *Trends Neurosci* 1990;13:197–199.
248. Miyoshi H, Nakaya Y. Activation of ATP-sensitive K^+ channels by cyclic AMP-dependent protein kinase in cultured smooth muscle cells of porcine coronary artery. *Biochem Biophys Res Commun* 1993; 193:240–247.
249. Miyoshi H, Nakaya Y, Moritoki H. Nonendothelial-derived nitric oxide activates the ATP-sensitive K^+ channel of vascular smooth muscle cells. *FEBS Lett* 1994;345:47–49.
250. Miyoshi Y, Nakaya Y, Wakatsuki T, Nakaya S, Fujino K, Saito K, Inoue I. Endothelin blocks ATP-sensitive K^+ channels and depolarizes smooth muscle cells of porcine coronary artery. *Circ Res* 1992;70:612–616.
251. Moczydlowski E, Lucchesi K, Ravindran A. An emerging pharmacology of peptide toxins targeted against potassium channels. *J Membr Biol* 1988;105:95–111.

252. Morales MJ, Castellino RC, Crews AL, Rasmusson RL, Strauss HC. A novel b subunit increases rate of inactivation of specific voltage-gated potassium channel a subunits. *J Biol Chem* 1995;270: 6272–6277.
253. Morishige K, Takahashi N, Jahangir A, Yamada M, Koyama H, Zanelli JS, Kurachi Y. Molecular cloning and functional expression of a novel brain-specific inward rectifier potassium channel. *FEBS Lett* 1994;346:251–256.
254. Morita K, North RA. Clonidine activates membrane potassium conductance in myenteric neurones. *Br J Pharmacol* 1981;74: 419–428.
255. Morris ME. General anesthetics and intracellular free calcium ions. In: Roth SH, Miller KW, eds. *Molecular and cellular mechanisms of anesthetics*. New York: Plenum Press, 1986;65–74.
256. Murray KT, Fahrig SA, Deal KK, Po SS, Hu NN, Snyders DJ, Tamkun MM, Bennett PB. Modulation of an inactivating human cardiac K^+ channel by protein kinase C. *Circ Res* 1994;75:999–1005.
257. Nakayama T, Irisawa H. Transient outward current carried by potassium and sodium in quiescent atrioventricular node cells of rabbit. *Circ Res* 1985;57:65–73.
258. Neely A, Lingle CJ. Two components of calcium-activated potassium current in rat adrenal chromaffin cells. *J Physiol (Lond)* 1992; 453:97–131.
259. Neely A, Lingle CJ. Effects of muscarine on single rat adrenal chromaffin cells. *J Physiol (Lond)* 1992;453:133–166.
260. Neher E. Two transient current components during voltage clamp in snail neurons. *J Gen Physiol* 1971;61:385–399.
261. Nelson MT, Huang Y, Brayden JE, Hescheler J, Standen NB. Arterial dilations in response to calcitonin gene-related peptide involve activation of K^+ channels. *Nature* 1990;344:770–773.
262. Niggli E, Rüdisüli A, Maurer P, Weingart R. Effects of general anesthetics on current flow across membranes in guinea pig myocytes. *Am J Physiol* 1989;256:C273–C281.
263. Noble D, Tsien RW. Outward membrane currents activated in the plateau range of potentials in cardiac Purkinje fibres. *J Physiol (Lond)* 1969;200:205–231.
264. Noda A, Nakayama T, Kurachi Y, Irisawa H. Resting K conductances in pacemaker and non-pacemaker heart cells of the rabbit. *Jpn J Physiol* 1984;34:245–254.
265. Noda A, Trautwein W. Relaxation of the ACh-induced potassium current in the rabbit sinoatrial node cell. *Pflugers Arch* 1978;377: 193–200.
266. Noma A. ATP-regulated K^+ channels in cardiac muscle. *Nature* 1983;305:147–148.
267. Noma A. Chemical-receptor dependent potassium channels in cardiac muscle. In:Noble D, Powell T, eds. *Electrophysiology of single cardiac cells*. Orlando: Academic Press, 1987;223–246.
268. Noma A, Takano M. The ATP-sensitive K^+ channel. *Jpn J Physiol* 1991;41:177–187.
269. North RA, Williams JT, Surprenant A, MacDonald JC. μ and δ Receptors belong to a family of receptors that are coupled to potassium channels. *Proc Natl Acad Sci USA* 1987;84:5487–5491.
270. Oakes SG, Iaizzo PA, Richelson E, Powis G. Histamine-induced intracellular free Ca^{2+}, inositol phosphates and electrical changes in murine N1E-115 neuroblastoma cells. *J Pharmacol Exp Ther* 1988;247:114–121.
271. Okabe K, Kitamura K, Kuriyama H. Features of 4-aminopyridine sensitive outward current observed in single smooth muscle cells from the rabbit pulmonary artery. *Pflugers Arch* 1987;409:561–568.
272. Okuhara DY, Beck SG. 5-HT_{1A} receptor linked to inward-rectifying potassium current in hippocampal CA3 pyramidal cells. *J Neurophysiol* 1994;71:2161–2167.
273. Pallotta BS, Blatz AL, Magleby KL. Recording from calcium-activated potassium channels. In Rudy B, Iverson LE, eds. *Methods in enzymology, vol 207, ion channels*. San Diego: Academic Press, 1992; 194–207.
274. Pallotta BS, Wagoner PK. Voltage-dependent potassium channels since Hodgkin and Huxley. *Physiol Rev* 1992;72:S49–S67.
275. Palmer RMJ, Ferrige AG, Moncada S. Nitric oxide release accounts for the biological activity of endothelium-derived relaxing factor. *Nature* 1987;327:524–526.
276. Pancrazio JJ, Frazer MJ, Lynch III C. Barbiturate anesthetics depress the resting K^+ conductance of myocardium. *J Pharmacol Exp Ther* 1993;265:358–365.
277. Pancrazio JJ, Johnson PA, Lynch III C. A major role for calcium-dependent potassium current in action potential repolarization in adrenal chromaffin cells. *Brain Res* 1994;668:246–251.
278. Pancrazio JJ, Park WK, Lynch III C. Effects of enflurane on voltage-gated membrane currents of bovine adrenal chromaffin cells. *Neurosci Lett* 1992;146:147–151.
279. Pancrazio JJ, Park WK, Lynch III C. Inhalational anesthetic actions on voltage-gated ion currents of bovine chromaffin cells. *Mol Pharmacol* 1993;43:783–794.
280. Papazian DM, Schwarz TL, Tempel BL, Jan YN, Jan LY. Cloning of genomic and complementary DNA from Shaker, a putative potassium channel gene from Drosophila. *Science* 1987;237:749–753.
281. Parcej DN, Scott VES, Dolly JO. Oligomeric properties of α-dendrotoxin-sensitive potassium ion channels purified from bovine brain. *Biochemistry* 1992;31:11084–11088.
282. Park YB. Ion selectivity and gating of small conductance Ca^{2+}-activated K^+ channels in cultured rat adrenal chromaffin cells. *J Physiol (Lond)* 1994;481:555–570.
283. Pearce RA. Halothane blocks the afterhyperpolarization but not calcium spike in hippocampal CA1 neurons. *FASEB J* 1991;74: A867.
284. Penington NJ, Kelly JS, Fox AP. Whole-cell recordings of inwardly rectifying K^+ currents activated by 5-HT_{1A} receptors on dorsal raphe neurones of the adult rat. *J Physiol (Lond)* 1993;469:387–405.
285. Pennefather P, Lancaster B, Adams PR, Nicoll RA. Two distinct Ca-dependent K currents in bullfrog sympathetic ganglion cells. *Proc Natl Acad Sci USA* 1985;82:3040–3044.
286. Perier F, Coulter KL, Radeke CM, Vandenberg CA. Expression of an inwardly rectifying potassium channel in Xenopus oocytes. *J Neurochem* 1992;59:1971–1974.
287. Perier F, Radeke CM, Vandenberg CA. Primary structure and characterization of a small-conductance inwardly rectifying potassium channel from human hippocampus. *Proc Natl Acad Sci USA* 1994;91:6240–6244.
288. Petersen OH, Dunne MJ. Regulation of K^+ channels plays a crucial role in the control of insulin secretion. *Pflugers Arch* 1989;414: S115–S120.
289. Pfaffinger PJ. Muscarine and t-LHRH suppress M-current by activating an IAP-insensitive G-protein. *J Neurosci* 1988;8:3343–3353.
290. Pongs O. Molecular biology of voltage-dependent potassium channels. *Physiol Rev* 1992;72:S69–S88.
291. Pongs O. Structural basis of voltage-gated K^+ channel pharmacology. *Trends Pharmacol Sci* 1992;13:359–365.
292. Pragnell M, Snay KJ, Trimmer JS, MacLusky NJ, Naftolin F, Kaczmarek LK, Boyle MB. Estrogen induction of a small, putative K^+ channel mRNA in rat uterus. *Neuron* 1990;4:807–812.
293. Premkumar LS, Gage PW. Potassium channels activated by $GABA_B$ agonists and serotonin in cultured hippocampal neurons. *J Neurophysiol* 1994;71:2570–2575.
294. Quayle JM, Bonev AD, Brayden JE, Nelson MT. Calcitonin gene-related peptide activated ATP-sensitive K^+ currents in rabbit arterial smooth muscle via protein kinase A. *J Physiol (Lond)* 1994;475:9–13.
295. Quayle JM, Standen NB, Stanfield PR. The voltage-dependent block of ATP-sensitive potassium channels of frog skeletal muscle by caesium and barium ions. *J Physiol (Lond)* 1988;405:677–697.
296. Reinhart PH, Chung S, Levitan IB. A family of calcium-dependent potassium channels from rat brain. *Neuron* 1989;2:1031–1041.
297. Reinhart PH, Chung S, Martin BL, Brautigan DL, Levitan IB. Modulation of calcium-activated potassium channels from rat brain by protein kinase A and phosphatase 2A. *J Neurosci* 1991;11: 1627–1635.
298. Rettig J, Heinemann SH, Wunder F, Lorra C, Parcej DN, Dolly JO, Pongs O. Inactivation properties of voltage-gated K^+ channels altered by presence of β-subunit. *Nature* 1994;369:289–294.
299. Reuveny E, Slesinger PA, Inglese J, et al. Activation of the cloned muscarinic potassium channel by G protein βγ subunits. *Nature* 1994;370:143–146.
300. Ried T, Rudy B, Vega-Saenz de Miera E, Lau D, Ward DC, Sen K. Localization of a highly conserved human potassium channel gene (NGK2-KCNCl) to chromosome 11p15. *Genomics* 1993;15: 405–411.
301. Roberds SL, Knoth KM, Po S, et al. Molecular biology of the voltage-gated potassium channels of the cardiovascular system. *J Cardiovasc Electrophysiol* 1993;4:68–80.
302. Rogawski MA. The A-current: how ubiquitous a feature of excitable cells is it? *Trends Neurosci* 1985;5:214–219.
303. Romey G, Lazdunski M. The coexistence in rat muscle cells of two distinct classes of Ca^{2+}-dependent K^+ channels with different pharmacological properties and different physiological functions. *Biochem Biophys Res Commun* 1984;118:669–674.

304. Roy ML, Sontheimer H. β-adrenergic modulation of glial inwardly rectifying potassium channels. *J Neurochem* 1995;64:1576–1584.
305. Rudy B. Diversity and ubiquity of K channels. *Neuroscience* 1988;25: 729–749.
306. Sadoshima J, Akaike N, Kanaide H, Nakamura M. Cyclic AMP modulates Ca-activated K channel in cultured smooth muscle cells of rat aortas. *Am J Physiol* 1988;255:H754–H759.
307. Safronov BV, Kampe K, Vogel W. Single voltage-dependent potassium channels in rat peripheral nerve membrane. *J Physiol (Lond)* 1993;460:675–691.
308. Sakmann B, Noma A, Trautwein W. Acetylcholine activation of single muscarinic K^+ channels in isolated pacemaker cells of the mammalian heart. *Nature* 1983;303:250–253.
309. Sakmann B, Trube G. Conductance properties of single inwardly rectifying potassium channels in ventricular cells from guinea-pig heart. *J Physiol (Lond)* 1984;347:641–657.
310. Salkoff L, Baker K, Baker A, Covarrubias M, Pak MD, Wei A. An essential "set" of K^+ channels conserved in flies, mice and humans. *Trends Neurosci* 1992;15:161–166.
311. Salkoff L, Wyman R. Genetic modification of potassium channels in Drosophila Shaker mutants. *Nature* 1981;293:228–230.
312. Sanguinetti MC, Jiang C, Curran ME, Keating MT. A mechanistic link between an inherited and an acquired cardiac arrhythmia: *HERG* encodes the I_{Kr} potassium channel. *Cell* 1995;81:299–307.
313. Sanguinetti MC, Jurkiewicz NK. Lanthanum blocks a specific component of I_K and screens membrane surface charge in cardiac cells. *Am J Physiol* 1990;28:H1881–H1889.
314. Sanguinetti MC, Jurkiewicz NK. Two components of cardiac delayed rectifier K^+ current. Differential sensitivity to block by class III antiarrhythmic agents. *J Gen Physiol* 1990;96:195–215.
315. Sanguinetti MC, Jurkiewicz NK. Delayed rectifier potassium channels of cardiac muscle. In: Spooner PM, Brown AM, eds. *Ion channels in the cardiovascular system: function and dysfunction.* New York: Futura, 1994;121–143.
316. Sato R, Hisatome I, Wasserstrom JA, Arentzen CE, Singer DH. Acetylcholine-sensitive potassium channels in human atrial myocytes. *Am J Physiol* 1990;259:H1730–H1735.
317. Schwarz TL, Tempel BL, Papazian DM, Jan YN, Jan LY. Multiple potassium-channel components are produced by alternative splicing at the Shaker locus in Drosophila. *Nature* 1988;331:137–142.
318. Scott VES, Muniz ZM, Sewing S, Lichtinghagen R, Parcej DN, Pongs O, Dolly JO. Antibodies specific for distinct Kv subunits unveil a heterooligomeric basis for subtypes of alpha-dendrotoxin-sensitive K^+ channels in bovine brain. *Biochemistry* 1994;33:1617–1623.
319. Segal M, Barker JL. Rat hippocampal neurones in culture: potassium conductances. *J Neurophysiol* 1984;51:1409–1433.
320. Segal M, Rogawski MA, Barker JL. A transient potassium conductance regulates the excitability of cultured hippocampal and spinal neurons. *J Neurosci* 1984;4:604–609.
321. Sellers AJ, Boden PR, Ashford MLJ. Lack of effect of potassium channel openers on ATP-modulated potassium channels recorded from rat ventromedial hypothalamic neurones. *Br J Pharmacol* 1992;107:1068–1074.
322. Selyanko AA, Stanfeld CE, Brown DA. Closure of potassium M-channels by muscarinic acetylcholine-receptor stimulants requires a diffusible messenger. *Proc R Soc Lond B* 1992;250:119–125.
323. Shabb JB, Corbin JD. Cyclic nucleotide-binding domains in proteins having diverse functions. *J Biol Chem* 1992;267:5723–5726.
324. Shen NV, Chen X, Boyer MM, Pfaffinger PJ. Deletion analysis of K^+ channel assembly. *Neuron* 1993;11:67–76.
325. Shen NV, Pfaffinger PJ. Molecular recognition and assembly sequences involved in the subfamily-specific assembly of voltage-gated K^+ channel subunit proteins. *Neuron* 1995;14:625–633.
326. Sheng M, Liao YI, Jan YN, Jan LY. Presynaptic A-current based on heteromultimeric K^+ channels detected in vivo. *Nature* 1993;365: 72–75.
327. Shibasaki T. Conductance and kinetics of delayed rectifier potassium channels in nodal cells of the rabbit heart. *J Physiol (Lond)* 1987;387:227–250.
328. Shimoni Y, Clark RB, Giles WR. Role of an inwardly rectifying potassium current in rabbit ventricular action potential. *J Physiol (Lond)* 1992;448:709–727.
329. Siegelbaum SA, Tsien RW. Calcium-activated transient outward current in calf Purkinje fibres. *Nature* 1980;299:485–506.
330. Siegelbaum SA, Tsien RW, Kass RS. Role of intracellular calcium in the transient outward current of calf Purkinje fibres. *J Physiol (Lond)* 1977;269:611–613.
331. Sikdar SK, McIntosh RP, Mason WT. Differential modulation of Ca^{2+}-activated K^+ channels in ovine pituitary gonadotrophs by GnRH, Ca^{2+} and cyclic AMP. *Brain Res* 1989;496:113–123.
332. Slesinger PA, Huang CL, Reuveny E, Jan YN, Jan LY. Identification of the cytoplasmic structures involved in the activation of the muscarinic potassium channel (GIRK1) by Gβγ subunits. *Biophys J* 1995;68:A362.
333. Slesinger PA, Jan YN, Jan LY. The S4-S5 loop contributes to the ion selective pore of potassium channels. *Neuron* 1993;11:739–749.
334. Snyders DJ, Tamkun MM, Bennett PB. A rapidly activating and slowly inactivating potassium channel cloned from human heart. Functional analysis after stable mammalian cell culture expression. *J Gen Physiol* 1993;101:513–543.
335. Snyders J, Knoth KM, Roberds SL, Tamkun MM. Time-, voltage-, and state-dependent block by quinidine of a cloned human cardiac potassium channel. *Mol Pharmacol* 1992;41:322–330.
336. Soejima M, Noma A. Mode of regulation of the ACh-sensitive K-channel by the muscarinic receptor in rabbit atrial cells. *Pflugers Arch* 1984;400:424–431.
337. Sokol PT, Hu W, Yi L, Toral J, Chandra M, Ziai MR. Cloning of an apamin binding protein of vascular smooth muscle. *J Protein Chem* 1994;13:117–128.
338. Solc, CK, Aldrich RA. Gating of single non-Shaker A-type potassium channels in larval Drosophila neurons. *J Gen Physiol* 1990;96: 135–165.
339. Spruce AE, Standen NB, Stanfield PR. Studies of the unitary properties of adenosine-5 -triphosphate-regulated potassium channels of frog skeletal muscle. *J Physiol (Lond)* 1987;382:213–236.
340. Standen NB. The G. L. Brown Lecture. Potassium channels, metabolism and muscle. *Exp Physiol* 1992;77:1–25.
341. Standen NB, Quayle JM, Davies NW, Brayden JE, Huang Y, Nelson MT. Hyperpolarizing vasodilators activate ATP-sensitive K^+ channels in arterial smooth muscle. *Science* 1989;245:177–180.
342. Stevens JE, Fujinaga M, Oshima E, Mori K. The biphasic pattern of the convulsive property of enflurane in cats. *Br J Anaesth* 1984; 56:395–403.
343. Stuenkel EL. Single potassium channels recorded from vascular smooth muscle cells. *Am J Physiol* 1989;257:H760–H769.
344. Stühmer W, Ruppersberg P, Schröter KH, et al. Molecular basis and functional diversity of voltage-gated potassium channels in mammalian brain. *EMBO J* 1989;8:3235–3244.
345. Sugiyama K, Muteki T, Shimoji K. Halothane-induced hyperpolarization and depression of postsynaptic potentials of guinea pig thalamic neurons in vitro. *Brain Res* 1992;576:97–103.
346. Supan FD, Buljubasic N, Eskinder H, Kampine JP, Bosnjak ZJ. Effects of halothane, isoflurane and enflurane on K^+ current in canine cardiac Purkinje cells. *Anesth Analg* 1991;72:S286.
347. Surprenant A, North RA. Mechanism of synaptic inhibition by noradrenaline acting at α_2-adrenoceptors. *Proc R Soc Biol* 1988; 234:85–114.
348. Szabo G, Otero AS. G protein mediated regulation of K^+ channels in heart. *Annu Rev Physiol* 1990;52:293–305.
349. Taglilatela M, Wible BA, Caporaso R, Brown AM. Specification of pore properties by the carboxyl terminus of inwardly rectifying K^+ channels. *Science* 1994;264:844–847.
350. Takahashi N, Morishige K-I, Jahangir A, Yamada M, Findlay I, Koyama H, Kurachi Y. Molecular cloning and functional expression of cDNA encoding a second class of inward rectifier potassium channels in the mouse brain. *J Biol Chem* 1994;269: 23274–23279.
351. Takano M, Noma A. Selective modulation of the ATP-sensitive K^+ channel by nicorandil in guinea-pig cardiac cell membrane. *Naunyn Schmiedebergs Arch Pharmacol* 1990; 342:592–597.
352. Takumi T, Moriyoshi K, Aramori I, et al. Alteration of channel activities and gating by mutations of slow I-SK potassium channel. *J Biol Chem* 1991;266:22192–22198.
353. Takumi T, Ohkubo H, Nakanishi S. Cloning of a membrane protein that induces a slow voltage-gated potassium current. *Science* 1988;242:1042–1045.
354. Tamkun MM, Knoth KM, Walbridge JA, Kroemer H, Roden DM, Glover DM. Molecular cloning and characterization of two voltage-gated K^+ channel cDNAs from human ventricle. *FASEB J* 1991; 5:331–337.
355. Tas PW, Kress HG, Koschel K. Volatile anesthetics inhibit the ion flux through Ca^{2+}-activated K^+ channels of rat glioma C6 cells. *Biochim Biophys Acta* 1989;983:264–268.
356. Tempel BL, Papazian DM, Schwartz TL, Jan YN, Jan LY. Sequence

of a probable potassium channel component encoded at *Shaker* locus of Drosophila. *Science* 1987;237:770–775.
357. Thuringer D, Escande D. Apparent competition between ATP and the potassium channel opener RP 49356 on ATP-sensitive K+ channels of cardiac myocytes. *Mol Pharmacol* 1989;36:897–902.
358. Timpe LC, Jan YN, Jan LY. Four cDNA clones from the Shaker locus of Drosophila induce kinetically distinct A-type potassium currents in Xenopus oocytes. *Neuron* 1988;1:659–667.
359. Timpe LC, Schwartz TL, Tempel BL, Papazian DM, Jan YN, Jan LY. Expression of functional potassium channels from *Shaker* cDNA in *Xenopus* oocytes. *Nature* 1988;331:143–145.
360. Tohse N. Calcium-sensitive delayed rectifier potassium current in guinea pig ventricular cells. *Am J Physiol* 1990;258:H1200–H1207.
361. Tohse N, Kameyama M, Irisawa H. Intracellular Ca^{2+} and protein kinase C modulate K^+ current in guinea pig heart cells. *Am J Physiol* 1987;22:H1321–H1324.
362. Tohse N, Kameyama M, Sekiguchi K, Shearman MS, Kanno M. Protein kinase C activation enhances the delayed rectifier potassium current in guinea-pig heart cells. *J Mol Cell Cardiol* 1990;22: 725–734.
363. Tohse N, Nakaya H, Kanno M. Alpha$_1$-adrenoceptor stimulation enhances the delayed rectifier K^+ current of guinea pig ventricular cells through the activation of protein kinase C. *Circ Res* 1992; 71:1441–1446.
364. Toro L, Ramos-Franco J, Stefani E. GTP-dependent regulation of myometrial KCa channels incorporated into lipid bilayers. *J Gen Physiol* 1990;96:373–394.
365. Toro L, Stefani E. Calcium-activated K^+ channels: metabolic regulation. *J Bioenerg Biomembr* 1991;23:561–576.
366. Toro L, Vaca L, Stefani E. Calcium-activated potassium channels from coronary smooth muscle reconstituted in lipid bilayers. *Am J Physiol* 1991;260:H1779–H1789.
367. Tromba C, Cohen IS. A novel action of isoproterenol to inactivate a cardiac K^+ current is not blocked by beta and alpha adrenergic blockers. *Biophys J* 1990;58:791–795.
368. Trudeau MC, Warmke JW, Ganetzky B, Robertson GA. HERG, a human inward rectifier in voltage-gated potassium channel family. *Science* 1995;269:92–95.
369. Tseng GN, Hoffman BF. Two components of transient outward current in canine ventricular myocytes. *Circ Res* 1989;64:633–647.
370. Tseng-Crank J, Foster CD, Krause JD, Mertz R, Godinot N, DiChiara TJ, Reinhart PH. Cloning, expression and distribution of functionally distinct Ca^{2+}-activated K^+ channel isoforms from human brain. *Neuron* 1994;13:1315–1330.
371. Uceda G, Artalejo AR, Lopez MG, Abad F, Neher E, Garcia AG. Ca^{2+}-activated K^+ channels modulate muscarinic secretion in cat chromaffin cells. *J Physiol (Lond)* 1992;454:213–230.
372. Vandenberg CA. Inward rectification of a potassium channel in cardiac ventricular cells depends on internal magnesium ions. *Proc Natl Acad Sci USA* 1987;84:2560–2564.
373. Varnum MD, Busch AE, Bond CT, Maylie J, Adelman JP. The min K channel underlies the cardiac potassium current IKs and mediates species-specific responses to protein kinase C. *Proc Natl Acad Sci USA* 1993;90:11528–11532.
374. Varró A, Nanasi PP, Lathrop DA. Potassium currents in isolated human atrial and ventricular cardiocytes. *Acta Physiol Scand* 1993; 149:133–142.
375. Veldkamp MW, van Ginneken AC, Bouman LN. Single delayed rectifier channels in the membrane of rabbit ventricular myocytes. *Circ Res* 1993;72:865–878.
376. Volk KA, Shibata EF. Single delayed rectifier potassium channels from rabbit coronary artery myocytes. *Am J Physiol* 1993;264: H1146–H1153.
377. Wakatsuki T, Nakaya Y, Inoue I. Vasopressin modulates K(+)-channel activities of cultured smooth muscle cells from porcine coronary artery. *Am J Physiol* 1992;263:H491–H496.
378. Walsh KB, Arena JP, Kwok W-M, Freeman L, Kass RS. Delayed-rectifier potassium channel activity in isolated membrane patches of guinea pig ventricular myocytes. *Am J Physiol* 1991;260:H1390–H1393.
379. Walsh KB, Begenisich TB, Kass RS. β-adrenergic modulation in the heart: independent regulation of K and Ca channels. *Pflugers Arch* 1988;411:232–234.
380. Walsh KB, Kass RS. Regulation of a heart potassium channel by protein kinase A and C. *Science* 1988;242:67–69.
381. Wang Z, Fermini B, Nattel S. Rapid and slow components of delayed rectifier current in human atrial myocytes. *Cardiovasc Res* 1994;28:1540–1546.
382. Wang H, Kunkel DD, Martin TM, Schwartkroin PA, Tempel BL. Heteromultimeric K^+ channels in terminal and juxtaparanodal regions of neurons. *Nature* 1993;365:75–79.
383. Wang K-W, Goldstein SAN. Subunit composition of minK potassium channels. *Neuron* 1995;14:1303–1309.
384. Wann KT, Richards CD. Properties of single calcium-activated potassium channels of large conductance in rat hippocampal neurons in culture. *Eur J Neurosci* 1994;6:607–617.
385. Warmke JW, Drysdale R, Ganetzky B. A distinct potassium channel polypeptide encoded by the Drosophila eag locus. *Science* 1991; 252:1560–1562.
386. Warmke JW, Ganetzky B. A family of potassium channel genes related to *eag* in *Drosophila* and mammals. *Proc Natl Acad Sci USA* 1994;91:3438–3442.
387. Wei A, Covarrubias M, Butler A, Baker K, Pak M, Salkoff L. K^+ current diversity is produced by an extended gene family conserved in *Drosophila* and mouse. *Science* 1990;248:599–604.
388. Wei A, Solaro C, Lingle C, Salkoff L. Calcium sensitivity of BK-type K_{Ca} channels determined by a separable domain. *Neuron* 1994;13: 671–681.
389. Weiser M, Vega-Saenz de Miera E, Kentros C, et al. Differential expression of *Shaw*-related K^+ channels in the rat central nervous system. *J Neurosci* 1994;14:949–972.
390. Wettwer E, Amos G, Gath J, Zerkowski H-R, Reidemeister J-C, Ravens U. Transient outward current in human and rat ventricular myocytes. *Cardiovasc Res* 1993;27:1662–1669.
391. White RE, Lee AB, Shcherbatko AD, Lincoln TM, Schonbrunn A, Armstrong DL. Potassium channel stimulation by natriuretic peptides through cGMP-dependent dephosphorylation. *Nature* 1993; 361:263–266.
392. White RE, Schonbrunn A, Armstrong DL. Somatostatin stimulates Ca^{2+}-activated K^+ channels through protein dephosphorylation. *Nature* 1991;351:570–573.
393. Wible BA, Taglialatela M, Ficker E, Brown AM. Gating of inwardly rectifying K^+ channels localized to a single negatively charged residue. *Nature* 1994;371:246–249.
394. Williams Jr D, Katz GM, Roy-Contancin L, Reuben JP. Guanosine 5 -monophosphate modulates gating of high-conductance Ca^{2+}-activated K^+ channels in vascular smooth muscle cells. *Proc Natl Acad Sci USA* 1988;85:9360–9364.
395. Williams JT, North RA. Opiate-receptor interactions on single locus coeruleus neurones. *Br J Pharmacol* 1984;26:489–497.
396. Wilson C. Inhibition by sulphonylureas of vasorelaxation induced by K^+ channel activators in vitro. *J Auton Pharmacol* 1989;9:71–78.
397. Wimpey TL, Chavkin C. Opioids activate both an inward rectifier and novel voltage-gated potassium conductance in the hippocampal formation. *Neuron* 1991;6:281–289.
398. Winquist RJ, Heaney LA, Wallace AA, Baskin EP, Stein RB, Garcia ML, Kaczorowski GJ. Glyburide blocks the relaxation response to BRL 34915 (Cromakalim), minoxidil sulfate and diazoxide in vascular smooth muscle. *J Pharmacol Exp Ther* 1989;248:149–156.
399. Wu C-F, Haugland FN. Voltage-clamp analysis of membrane currents in larval muscle fibres of *Drosophila:* alteration of potassium currents in *Shaker* mutants. *J Neurosci* 1985;5:2626–2640.
400. Wu J. Microscopic model for selective permeation in ion channels. *Biophys J* 1991;60:238–251.
401. Yang Y, Sigworth FJ. The conductance of minK 'channels' is very small. *Biophys J* 1995;68:A22.
402. Yellen G. Permeation in potassium channels: implications for channel structure. *Annu Rev Biophys Chem* 1987;16:227–246.
403. Yellen G, Jurman ME, Abramson T, MacKinnon R. Mutations affecting internal TEA blockade identify the probable pore-forming region of a K^+ channel. *Science* 1991;251:939–942.
404. Yellen G, Sodickson D, Chen TY, Jurman ME. An engineered cysteine in the external mouth of a K^+ channel allows inactivation to be modulated by metal binding. *Biophys J* 1994;66:1068–1075.
405. Zagotta WN, Aldrich RW. Voltage-dependent gating of Shaker A-type potassium channels in Drosophila muscle. *J Gen Physiol* 1990; 95:29–60.
406. Zagotta WN, Hoshi T, Aldrich RW. Restoration of inactivation in mutants of Shaker potassium channels by a peptide derived from ShB. *Science* 1990;250:568–571.
407. Zbicz KL, Weight FF. Transient voltage and calcium-dependent outward currents in hippocampal CA3 pyramidal neurons. *J Neurophysiol* 1985;53:1038–1058.

408. Zhao B, Rassendren F, Kaang B-K, Furukawa Y, Kubo T, Kandel E. A resting new class of noninactivating K^+ channels from Aplysia capable of contributing to the resting potential and firing patterns of neurons. *Neuron* 1994;13:1205–1213.
409. Zhong Y, Wu C-F. Alteration of four identified K^+ currents in *Drosophila* muscle by mutations in eag. *Science* 1991;252:1562–1564.
410. Zhou H, Tate SS, Palmer LG. Primary structure and functional properties of an epithelial K channel. *Am J Physiol* 1994;266: C809–C824.
411. Zorn L, Kulkarni R, Anantharam V, Bayley H, Treistman SN. Halothane acts on many potassium channels including a minimal potassium channel. *Neurosci Lett* 1993;161:81–84.
412. Zucker JR. ATP-sensitive potassium channels do not alter MAC for isoflurane in rats. *Anesthesiology* 1992;76:560–563.

Anesthesia: Biologic Foundations, edited by Tony L. Yaksh et al. Lippincott–Raven Publishers, Philadelphia © 1997.

CHAPTER 14

STRUCTURE AND FUNCTION OF THE NICOTINIC ACETYLCHOLINE RECEPTOR

JAMES P. DILGER

The nicotinic acetylcholine receptor (AChR) protein is an ionotropic ligand-gated ion channel, that is, a single protein containing both the ligand-binding sites and the transmembrane ion channel. Nicotinic AChRs are found on muscle cells at the neuromuscular junction and on neurons in both the peripheral and central nervous systems. The muscle-type and neuronal-type AChRs are highly homologous, but not identical. Considerably more is known about the detailed structure and function of the muscle type of AChR than the neuronal type. Similarly, the neuromuscular synapse is better understood than any other synapse. Nevertheless, there are still significant gaps in our knowledge about the AChR and neuromuscular transmission.

The AChR mediates rapid synaptic transmission by increasing the conductance of the postsynaptic cell in response to ACh. High speed is achieved because the receptor and ion channel are parts of a single protein molecule. Consider synaptic transmission at the neuromuscular junction. The time between ACh release from the motor neuron and the opening of the ion channel in the muscle cell is about 0.2 ms. During this time, ACh diffuses about 0.05 μm across the synaptic cleft, spreads laterally over an area of about 0.1 μm^2, binds to the AChR, and induces the channel to undergo a conformational change from a closed (nonconducting) state to an open (conducting) state. The channels remain open for an average of 1 ms. After channel closure, ACh dissociates from the receptor and is hydrolyzed by acetylcholinesterase (AChE) within 0.2 ms. The synapse is then ready to transmit another signal from nerve to muscle.

The open AChR channel is a pathway for sodium ions to enter and depolarize the muscle cell. This depolarization persists for a few milliseconds. If the depolarization reaches the excitation threshold, the muscle cell fires an action potential. The action potential propagates along the muscle fiber and ultimately results in muscle contraction.

The importance of the nicotinic AChR to anesthesiologists is fourfold. First, it is the site of action of the muscle relaxant drugs used to paralyze patients during surgery. Second, some general anesthetics themselves affect the muscle-type AChR. Third, neuronal AChRs in autonomic ganglia may be affected by drugs used by anesthesiologists. Fourth, the roles of neuronal AChRs in the cerebral cortex, hypothalamus, hippocampus, and other areas of the central nervous system are largely unknown but may be important in many brain functions.

Several recent reviews of the structure and function of the nicotinic AChR are available (20,32,51,76).

ANATOMY OF THE NEUROMUSCULAR JUNCTION

Synapses contain many highly specialized structures that work together to allow chemical communication between cells (37). Some of these are identified in the drawing of the neuromuscular junction (NMJ) shown in Fig. 1. The terminal of the presynaptic cell (a motor neuron at the NMJ) lies in a depression on the surface of the postsynaptic cell (a skeletal muscle cell at the NMJ). The nerve terminal is filled with 50 nm diameter synaptic vesicles that contain the neurotransmitter (10,000 molecules of ACh^+ at the NMJ with ATP^{3-} as the counterion). Some vesicles are concentrated around active zones that are aligned opposite to junctional folds on the surface of the muscle cell. During synaptic transmission, the entry of calcium into the nerve terminal causes vesicles in the active zone to fuse with the nerve cell membrane and release ACh. Larger, dense core vesicles contain neuropeptides that, when secreted, may affect the development of the muscle cell. Many mitochondria reside in the presynaptic neuron to fuel the high level of transport and synthesis activity that takes place.

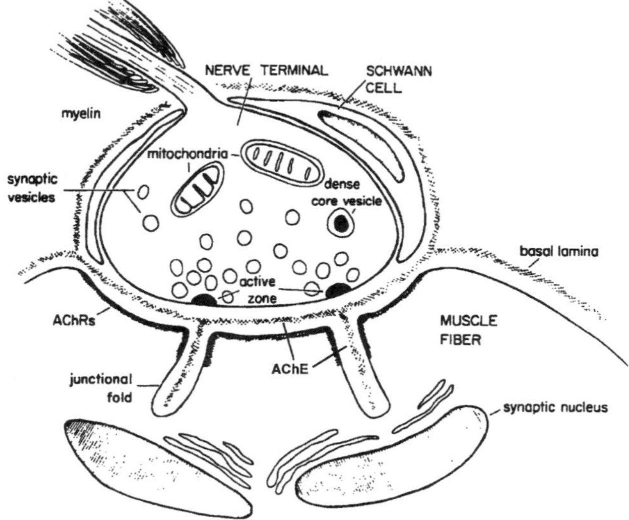

Figure 1. The anatomy of the neuromuscular junction. Some of the structures in the presynaptic nerve terminal, synaptic cleft and postsynaptic muscle cell are illustrated. See text for details. (From ref. 37, used with permission.)

The presynaptic and postsynaptic cells are separated by a 50-nm wide synaptic gap. A network of connective tissue, the basal lamina, extends through the synaptic cleft and into the junctional folds of the muscle cell. The synaptic basal lamina is continuous with the basal lamina that surrounds the entire muscle cell and the one that surrounds the Schwann cells. AChE (at a density of ≈1,000 sites/μm^2) is associated with the synaptic basal lamina where it is used to rapidly hydrolyze free ACh. The basal lamina also contains enzymes that help in the development and maintenance of the NMJ.

The surface of the postsynaptic membrane is dimpled to accommodate the nerve terminal and is wrinkled with 1-μm deep junctional folds. The AChRs are densely packed (>10,000/μm^2) at the tops and halfway down the folds. The density of AChRs in the muscle cell membrane decreases steeply with distance from the junction; at 15 μm from the junction, the density is <20/μm^2 (29). The muscle cell also contains synaptic nuclei dedicated to the synthesis of AChR and other proteins.

The synapse contains many molecular components not shown in Fig. 1. On the presynaptic side there are voltage-gated Ca^{2+} channels, proteins that help synaptic vesicles dock close to the active zones, a Na^+-choline$^+$ cotransport protein to recycle choline from the synapse, choline acetyltransferase to synthesize ACh from choline and acetylcoenzyme A, a mechanism for concentrating ACh into vesicles, a mechanism for endocytosis of vesicle membrane, and nicotinic AChRs, whose function is uncertain. The fate of the ATP^{3-} anions released from synaptic vesicles along with ACh^+ is also unclear (74); nature would certainly not waste such a precious energy resource. On the postsynaptic side there are voltage-gated Na^+ channels that initiate the muscle action potential and a host of proteins that participate in clustering of AChRs.

STRUCTURE OF THE ACETYLCHOLINE RECEPTOR

The muscle AChR channel has been, and remains today, the ion channel protein for which the most detailed structural information is available. The receptor was biochemically isolated in 1970 (13) and the subunit composition was determined four years later (96). The complete primary structure of the subunits was known by 1982 (4). This led to proposals for the folding of the subunits within the membrane (64). The tertiary and quaternary structure of the AChR is now being revealed by high resolution electron microscopy. This is made possible by the large, tubular crystalline arrays of AChRs that can be isolated from the electric organ of *Torpedo* rays. The most detailed structure determinations to date are those of the closed channel at 9 Å resolution (87; Fig. 2A; also see Fig. 4A) and the open channel (obtained by freezing the preparation within 5 ms of adding ACh), also at 9 Å resolution (88; see Fig. 5).

The nicotinic AChR has a molecular weight of 270 kd (calculated from the amino acid sequence) and is composed of five subunits arranged around a central pore (Fig. 2). The muscle-type AChR is composed of one of two possible subunit combinations: (a) ααβγδ—found in embryonic muscle, in nonsynaptic (extrajunctional) regions of adult muscle, and in the electric organ of rays (e.g., *Torpedo*) and eels; and (b) ααβεδ—found at the synapse of adult muscle. (The differences between the two types of muscle AChRs are discussed in later sections.) Functional channels composed of α+β+γ-subunits (ααβγγ) or α+β+δ-subunits (ααβδδ) have been expressed in vitro (44,48), but it is thought that these combinations do not occur significantly in vivo. There is more diversity in the subunit composition of neuronal AChRs. So far, genes for eight different α-subunits (α2–α9) and three different β-subunits (β2–β4) have been identified (76). At least six different combinations of these subunits form functional channels composed of two α- and three β-subunits. In addition, five α7-, α8-, or α9-subunits aggregate to form homo-oligomeric channels (68). The most common AChR isoform found in CNS neurons is the combination of α4 and β2. There are also some neuronal AChRs that are permeable to chloride rather than cations (47). The structure of these channels has not yet been determined. However, the homo-oligomeric α7 neuronal receptor can be converted to an anionic channel by mutation of three amino acid residues within the M2 region (31).

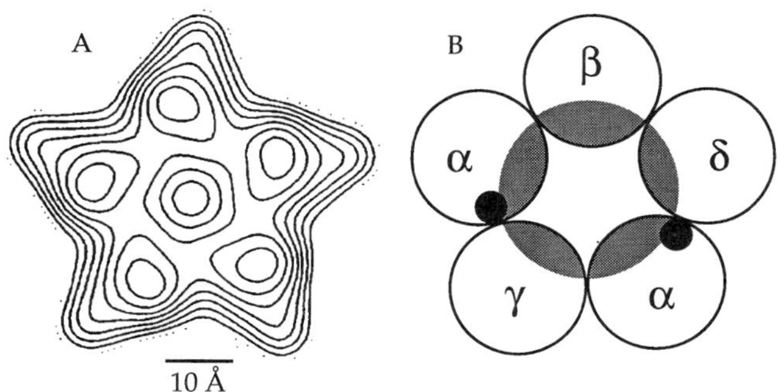

Figure 2. Top view of the AChR. **(A)** Electron density map constructed from high-resolution electron microscopy of AChRs from the electric organ of *Torpedo*. The degree of fivefold symmetry is exaggerated in this image because of the averaging techniques used. (From ref. 87, used with permission.) **(B)** Drawing of the subunit arrangement of AChRs from *Torpedo*. Extrajunctional and embryonic AChRs have the same subunit arrangement, adult junctional AChRs have an ε-subunit instead of a γ-subunit. The *black circles* represent the ACh-binding sites on the two α-subunits. The *shaded regions* are the M2 transmembrane regions that line the pore of the channel.

There is an additional protein, a 43-kd peripheral protein, that is associated with the cytoplasmic side of the AChR (Fig. 3). It is a distinct protein from the AChR but we mention it in this section only because it is seen on the high-resolution structural maps (Fig. 4A). The 43-kd protein is weakly bound to the β-subunit with a 1:1 stoichiometry. It appears to have no functional significance for the AChR, but is likely to be involved in aggregating the receptors into clusters at a synapse (72).

Each subunit contains between 440 and 500 amino acid residues: (α<β≈ε<γ≈δ). The sequence for the α-subunit from the human muscle AChR is shown in Fig. 3. A comparison of the human α-subunit with the α-subunit of other animals reveals a high degree of homology among mammals (20 differences between human and mouse) but more variation between human and *Torpedo* (89 differences). There is a fair amount of sequence similarity among subunits. Each subunit has four regions that contain highly conserved sequences of 19 to 27 amino acids, many of which are hydrophobic. These regions (denoted as M1, M2, M3, and M4; Fig. 3) span the membrane. They were originally thought to have an α-helical conformation, but recent data indicate that while M2 and M4 may have a mixture of α-helix and beta sheet structure, M1 and M3 may be mostly beta sheet (40). Also, the possibility of additional membrane spanning regions cannot be entirely discounted yet.

The first 200 amino acids of the N-terminus of each subunit form the large synaptic portion of the AChR (Fig. 4). Near the center of this sequence, each subunit has a similar series of 15 amino acids bounded by cysteines (the *large box* in Fig. 3). The significance of this region is unknown; however, it is one of several glycosylation sites found on the extracellular side of the protein. The β-, δ-, γ-, and ε-subunits each have two to five additional glycosylation sites.

The physiologic neurotransmitter ACh (see Fig. 15) is a hydrolyzable ester of acetic acid with choline and is positively charged at the quaternary nitrogen of the choline. The α-subunit of the AChR contains the primary part of the ligand-binding region. Specific aromatic amino acids (tyrosines and tryptophans) and two cysteines are known to participate in ACh binding (*squares* in Fig. 3). These three separate areas probably fold to form a binding pocket for ACh on the synaptic side of the AChR. A putative binding pocket has been identified in the high-resolution structure of the AChR (87). This binding site is 30 to 35 Å above the synaptic surface of the membrane (87,89). Because the AChR has two α-subunits, there are two ACh-binding sites. Although the primary structures of the two α-subunits are identical, the two binding sites have distinct binding affinities for ACh (79) and other ligands (63). This implies that ACh binding involves other subunits either directly (ACh makes contact with the neighboring subunit) or indirectly (the neighboring subunit affects the structure of the α-subunit). Ligand binding is influenced by both the δ- and γ-subunits, so the binding sites are considered to be at the α–δ and α–γ interfaces (denoted by *filled circles* in Figs. 2B and 4B).

The ligand-binding site is also the site at which α-bungarotoxin, a peptide toxin from snake venom, binds. (Naturally, α-bungarotoxin does not bind to the AChRs of either snake or mongoose [5]). Because α-bungarotoxin binding is specific

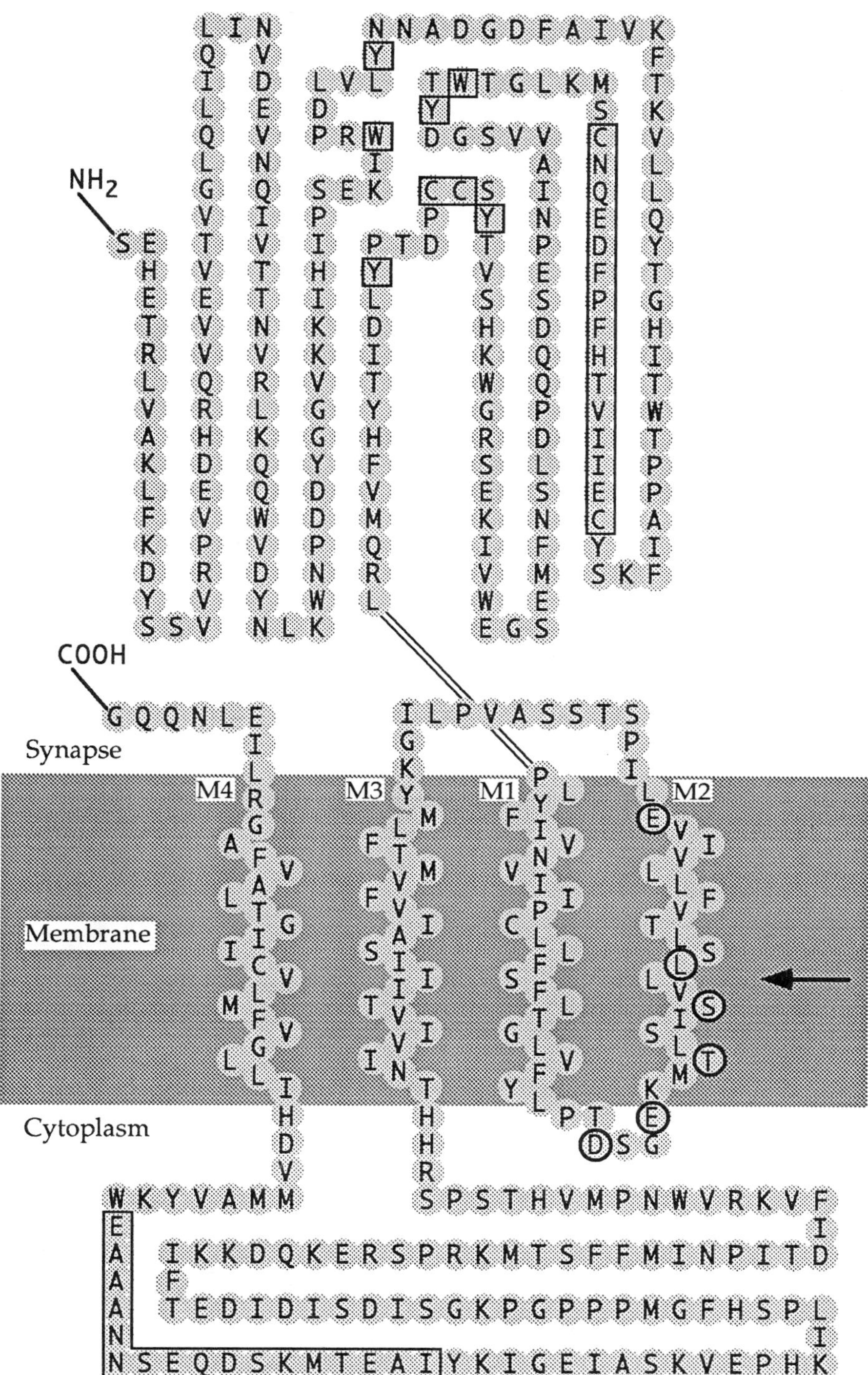

Figure 3. The amino acid sequence and proposed topology of the α-subunit from human muscle AChR (15). The four transmembrane regions are labeled M1 to M4. The six *circled* amino acids in the M2 region are conserved in all subunits and form negatively charged rings in the pore of the channel. The *arrow* denotes the point at which the M2 region is kinked and may be involved in channel gating. The residues outlined by *squares* are important in the binding of ACh. The large region bounded by cysteines is highly conserved in all subunits but its function is not yet known. The residues *outlined* in the *lower left corner* are important for subunit assembly.

and irreversible, it is an ideal tool for identification and purification of the muscle-type AChR.

The M2 transmembrane region of each of the five subunits of the AChR (Fig. 3) lines the pore of the channel. When the M2 regions of all five subunits are aligned, six rings of negatively charged amino acids can be identified (*circled residues* in Fig. 3). The threonine ring near the cytoplasmic end of the pore may form the narrowest part of the pore and determine the maximum size of permeable ions (16,28,90). The roles of the other negatively charged rings include selectivity for cations over anions and the relative permeability of different cations (16). The rings might also act to align permeable

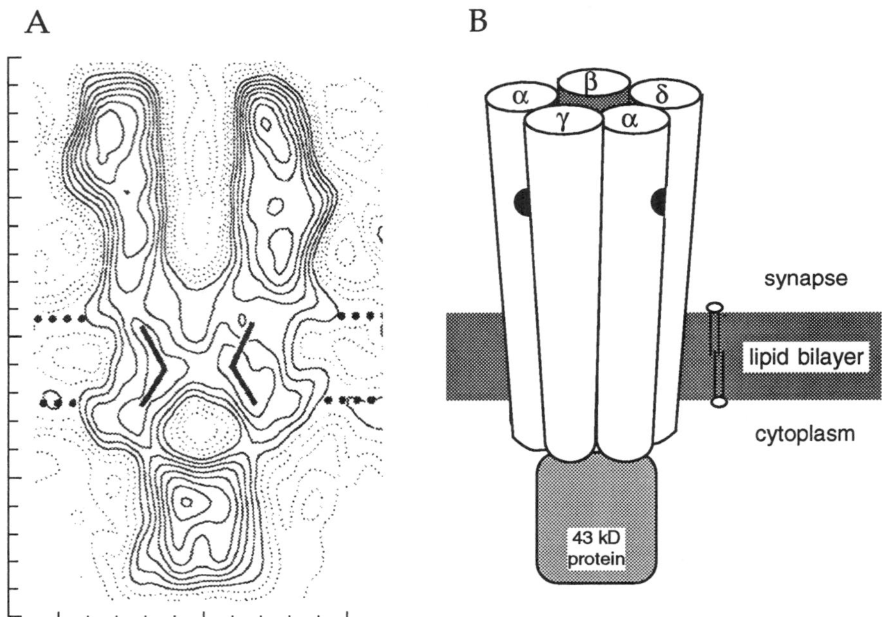

Figure 4. Cross-sectional side view of the AChR. **(A)** Electron-density map constructed from high-resolution electron microscopy of AChRs from the electric organ of *Torpedo*. The 43-kd protein on the cytoplasmic side is also visible. The grid markers are 10 Å apart. (From ref. 88, used with permission.) **(B)** Drawing of the topology of the AChR in the muscle membrane. The *black semicircles* represent the ACh-binding sites at the α-γ and α-δ- subunit interfaces.

organic cations as they approach the narrowest part of the pore. The narrowest part of the pore extends for about 3 to 6 Å along the axis of the pore (19).

The AChR undergoes several conformational changes after ACh binds. The results of these changes are (a) an increase in the binding affinity for ACh (ACh binds more tightly); (b) a change in the conformation of the pore from nonconducting (closed) to conducting (open); and (c) after a delay, a change in the conformation of the pore to one or more additional closed conformations known as desensitized states.

A likely site for the gate of the channel is a highly conserved leucine residue in the M2 region (*arrow* in Fig. 3, *bent lines* in Fig. 4A). There is a kink in α-helical structure of M2 at this point. The kink causes a bend in each M2 helix. It has been proposed (88) that when the channel is closed, the kink from each subunit is oriented toward the center of the pore, allowing the leucines to associate with each other and constricting the pore (Fig. 5). The channel opens when the M2 helices rotate so that the kinks are oriented tangentially around the ring of the pore. The leucines no longer associate with each other so that the constriction of the pore is released. The narrowest region of the open pore is 6 amino acids away from the leucines toward the cytoplasmic end of M2, the threonine ring mentioned above.

How does the binding of ACh induce the conformational change of channel gating? Comparison of the high-resolution structures of the closed and open conformations provide evidence for widespread changes in the protein. The following scenario is based on those changes and a bit of speculation (88). Binding of ACh causes distinct changes in the ligand-binding regions of the two α-subunits. These changes are coupled allosterically via the γ-subunit and induce small rotations of all of the subunits. Close to the surface of the membrane, the rotation of subunits is translated primarily to the M2 region. Rotation of M2 disrupts the association of the leucines at the kink and the obstruction is removed from the pore. The last step of this process, the click from closed to open, takes place in less than 10 μs (55). Modern high-resolution structural and functional techniques are providing us with a fascinating view of a complex piece of nature's machinery.

METABOLISM OF THE ACETYLCHOLINE RECEPTOR

The AChR subunits are synthesized separately from separate genes. They are assembled sequentially in the endoplasmic reticulum and undergo conformational changes during assembly (34,36). The α-subunit contains a sequence of 17 residues in the long cytoplasmic loop (Fig. 3) that are required for complete assembly (100). Phosphorylation of the γ-submit may regulate subunit assembly (35) but complete assembly can occur in the absence of γ-subunit phosphorylation (39).

The muscle-type AChR is phosphorylated both in vivo and in vitro. Phosphorylation is mediated by adenosine 3′,5′-cyclic

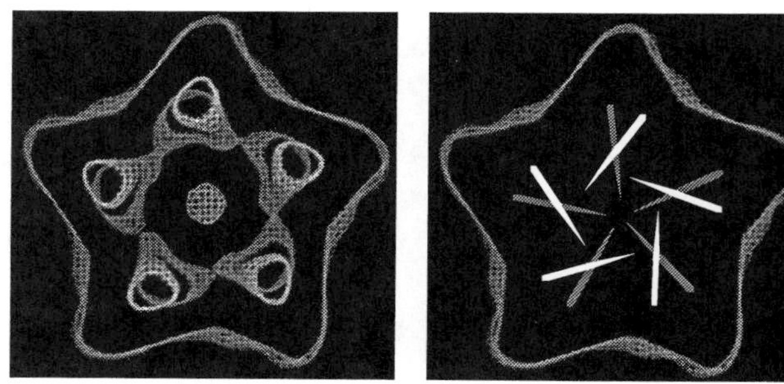

Figure 5. A comparison of the structure of the open and closed channel. **(A)** High-resolution view of the pore of the channel at the level of the kink in the M2 region (*arrow* in Fig. 3, *bent lines* in Fig. 4A). The *gray loops* are the five M2 subunits in their closed channel conformation. The *white loops* are the five M2 subunits in their open channel conformation. When the channel is open, the narrowest part of the pore is closer to the cytoplasmic end of the channel than the image shown here. The *light circle* in the center of the pore is not thought to be part of the channel structure, but rather, an image of ACh at its open channel blocking position. (From ref. 88, used with permission.) **(B)** A schematic drawing of part A using *gray tapered lines* to represent the orientation of the kink in the closed channel and *white tapered lines* to represent the orientation of the kink in the open channel.

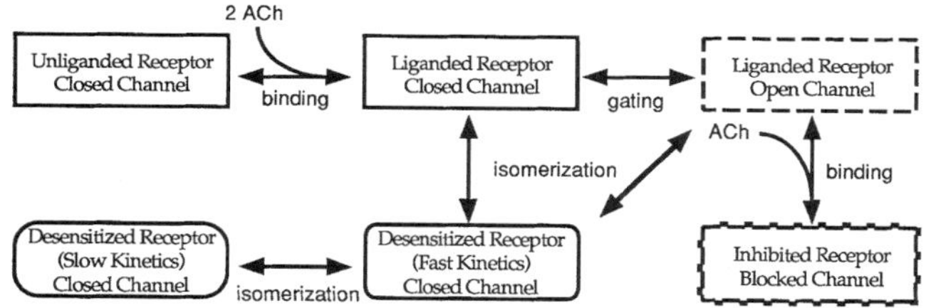

Figure 6. A block diagram of major conformational states of the muscle AChR. The processes of ligand binding, channel gating, channel block by agonist, and desensitization are shown. See text for details.

monophosphate (cAMP)-dependent protein kinase (PKA), protein kinase C (PKC), and protein tyrosine kinase. The PKA phosphorylation sites are serine residues found within the cytoplasmic loop between M3 and M4 on the γ- and δ-subunits (99). PKC phosphorylates the δ-subunit (59). The tyrosine kinase phosphorylation sites are on the β-, γ-, and δ-subunits (42).

After assembly, AChRs are transported to the muscle cell surface. As the muscle develops, the type, density, and turnover rate of AChRs changes (37). Initially, ααβγδ receptors are distributed uniformly at a moderate density throughout the muscle cell membrane. These receptors have a half-life of <1 day. When the muscle is innervated, ααβγδ receptors aggregate into clusters around the synapse. At about the same time, density of receptors away from the synapse decreases. Finally, the γ-subunit in the synaptic receptors is replaced by an ε-subunit. The receptors in this mature synapse have a longer metabolic half-life, about 8 days. The subunit composition and turnover time of the remaining receptors outside the synapse does not change. After a muscle is denervated or if there has been no synaptic activity for a few days, the clusters remain intact, but there is a reappearance of the γ-subunit. Physical or functional denervation also results in a 10- to 20-fold increase in the number of extrajunctional receptors that are diffusely distributed on the surface of the muscle. Reinnervation reverses the changes of denervation.

A number of proteins have been implicated in the formation and maintenance of clusters. Among these are the 43-kd protein, actin, spectrin, dystrophin-related protein, and agrin (27,73). The nerve clearly regulates receptor clustering (and, conversely, the muscle regulates the development of the nerve terminal) but the mechanisms are not fully understood.

ELECTROPHYSIOLOGY OF THE ACETYLCHOLINE RECEPTOR

Equilibrium

Figure 6 is a simplified state diagram of the AChR. It shows the six major conformations of the receptor: unliganded, closed liganded, open liganded, fast desensitized, slow desensitized, and a blocked conformation also known as the agonist self-inhibited state. Some transitions involve ligand (ACh) binding: unliganded to closed liganded (two separate ACh-binding steps), and agonist self-inhibition (the binding of a third ACh molecule to a completely different site). The other transitions involve a change in conformational state of the protein: channel gating between closed and open states, and desensitization isomerizations. A complete kinetic description of this ion channel protein must include (a) transitions between all pairs of conformations, (b) the binding of ACh to desensitized states, (c) the opening of unliganded and singly liganded closed channels, and (d) the voltage dependence of the transitions. The kinetic description for the muscle-type AChR is not complete (51), but it is quite detailed. This section focuses on this description. Presumably, similar models will be found to describe neuronal AChRs.

The probability of the channel being open, P_{open}, is a function of ligand concentration [ACh], time, and voltage. Figure 7 presents two [ACh]-P_{open} curves for the AChR at the resting potential of a muscle cell (–80 mV), one at times for which desensitization is not yet important (t = 1–5 ms after ACh is applied), and one at times for which fast desensitization dominates (t = 5 s after ACh is applied). Desensitization of the AChR is so profound that less than 1% of channels remain open after 5 s of continuous exposure to ACh. However, because ACh is removed from the synapse (by hydrolysis and diffusion) on the millisecond time scale, it is unlikely that either fast or slow desensitization plays any physiologic role in normal synaptic transmission. It is possible, however, that desensitization is important in the function of the muscle-type AChR in the presence of drugs or in pathologic states and in the function of the neuronal AChR.

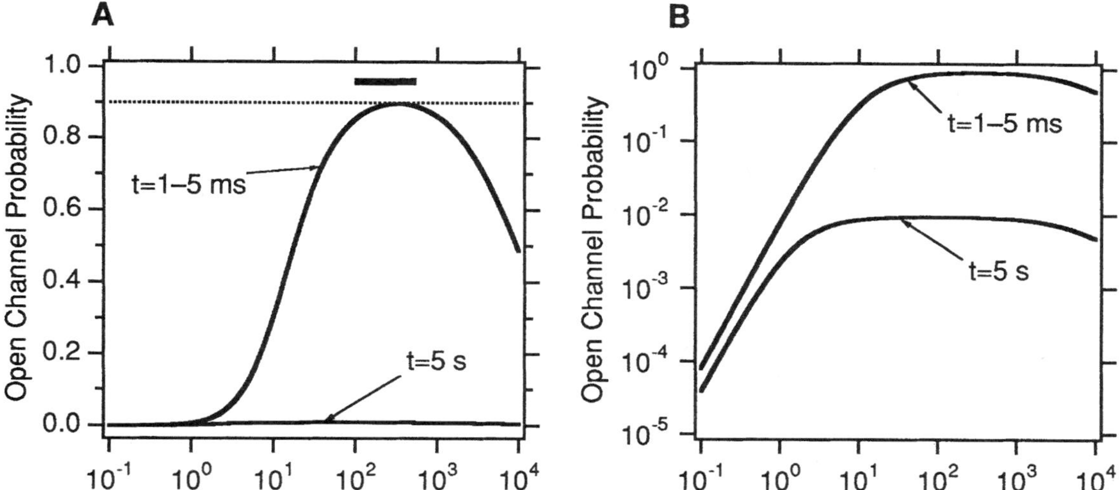

Figure 7. [ACh]-P_{open} (dose-response) curves for activation of the muscle AChR channel by ACh. **(A)** P_{open} vs log [ACh] at early (1–5 ms, before desensitization) and late (5 s, after fast desensitization) time periods. The *solid bar* indicates the range of ACh concentrations (100–500 μM) in the synaptic cleft during neuromuscular transmission. At these levels, activation of the channel is maximal. **(B)** The curves of A shown with a logarithmic P_{open} axis. This view presents a quantitative measure of the low levels of activation that occur after fast desensitization.

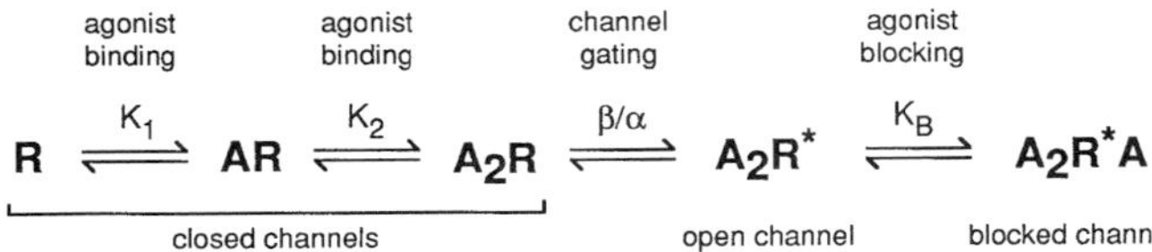

Figure 8. A five-state kinetic scheme often used to describe the equilibrium and kinetic behavior of the AChR channel before desensitization.

The nondesensitized [ACh]-P_{open} curve (Fig. 7) contains information about the number of states of the AChR and the equilibrium among them (technically, equilibrium is reached only after desensitization has completely developed; here, we are considering the quasi-equilibrium achieved after 1 to 5 ms). The minimal kinetic scheme required to describe the nondesensitized [ACh]-P_{open} curve is given in Fig. 8. The scheme has five states: unliganded receptor (R), singly liganded receptor (AR), doubly liganded receptor (A_2R), doubly liganded open state (A_2R^*), and blocked state (A_2R^*A). It is characterized by four equilibrium constants: two ACh agonist binding affinities (K_1, K_2), an isomerization (channel gating) constant (β/α, where β is the opening rate and α is the closing rate of the channel) and an ACh blocking affinity (K_B).

The [ACh]-P_{open} curve in Fig. 7 was constructed from the equilibrium constants $K_1 = 25$ μM, $K_2 = 100$ μM, $\beta/\alpha = 20$, $K_B =$ 10,000 μM. The receptor exhibits some negative cooperativity ($K_1<K_2$) in that the second agonist molecule is less tightly bound than the first. Negative cooperativity is advantageous for the AChR because it allows for a quick termination of the response after ACh is removed from the synapse (45). The large value of β/α means that the channel opening rate is 20 times greater than the closing rate and, when a channel is doubly liganded, it is 20 times more likely to be open than closed. This means that ACh is a very efficacious agonist. The binding of a third molecule of ACh to the channel blocking site is important only at concentrations higher than 1 mM ACh.

The physiologically important part of the [ACh]-P_{open} curve is the region of the nondesensitized curve between 100 and 500 μM ACh (Fig. 7, *solid bar*). In this region, the occupancy of the ligand-binding sites is high but channel blockade and desensitization are minimal. As a result, about 90% of the channels are opened when ACh is released from the nerve terminal.

Kinetics

The kinetics of the scheme of Fig. 8 are also important to the physiologic operation of the channel. The ligand-binding steps are probably diffusion limited. The channel opening rate is 20/ms and the closing rate is 1/ms. ACh dissociates from the closed, doubly liganded state, A_2R, at a rate of 20/ms. As a result, channels open with a time constant of 0.1 to 0.2 ms after 100 to 500 μM ACh is applied. Channels close with a time constant of 1 ms. The average channel opens 1.5 times before ACh dissociates from the ligand-binding site. P_{open} decreases with a time constant of about 1.5 ms after ACh is removed.

Although the AChR channel is gated by ligand-binding and not by voltage, the gate does have a small sensitivity to voltage. The channel closing rate, α, is about three times slower at −50 mV than at +50 mV (56) so that the channel stays open longer at −50 mV than at +50 mV. (This voltage sensitivity is considerably smaller than that of voltage-gated ion channels, which exhibit threefold changes in kinetics with a change in potential of a few mV). In contrast, the channel opening rate, β, does not vary significantly with voltage (54). As a result, the channel open probability, P_{open}, is greater −50 mV than at +50 mV. This effect is most pronounced at nonsaturating concentrations of ACh where the difference in P_{open} can be as large as threefold. However, in the physiologically important part of the [ACh]-P_{open} curve, the voltage-dependence of α decreases P_{open} from 0.9 to 0.83 with a 100 mV change in potential.

Neuronal AChR channels also exhibit a voltage-dependent channel closing rate such that channels close more quickly at positive potentials. The potential needed to change the closing rate by a factor of three varies among different types of neuronal receptor, ranging from 45 mV (98) to 140 mV (43).

Channel Block by ACh

The decrease in P_{open} at high concentrations of ACh is due to ACh binding to a site inside the pore of the channel and blocking the flow of ions through the channel. This process is voltage dependent: ACh binds more tightly to its blocking site at hyperpolarized potentials than at depolarized potentials (81). Channel block by ACh is an example of fast, open channel block (3). ACh can bind to the open channel only and ACh must dissociate from the blocking site before the channel can return to the closed state. (Note that this is in contrast to the action of ACh at the ligand-binding site. As indicated in Fig. 8, it is thought that the open channel must close before ACh dissociates from the ligand-binding site.) The average dwell time for ACh at the blocking site is <0.01 ms (66).

Desensitization

The desensitized states of the AChR have a higher binding affinity for ACh (77). The fast desensitized states bind ACh about 10 times more tightly than the undesensitized receptor; the slow desensitized states have an even higher affinity. Fast desensitization occurs on the 100 ms time scale and is not voltage dependent (23). This process appears to be regulated by the phosphorylation of serine residues on the γ- and δ-subunits (39). Mutant AChRs, in which these serines were replaced by alanines so that they could not be phosphorylated by PKA, desensitize more slowly than wild-type AChRs (39). Measurements of the kinetics of slow desensitization range from seconds to minutes, suggesting that there may be several different types of slow desensitization (65). It is not clear whether or not slow desensitization can also be regulated by phosphorylation (39,41,83).

Conductance

The pore of the muscle-type AChR channel is quite large and nonselective compared to the pores of voltage-gated K^+ and Na^+ channels. The AChR channel pore conducts Na^+ and K^+ with nearly equal permeability. The permeability sequence for monovalent metal cations is $Tl^+>Cs^+>Rb^+>K^+>Na^+>Li^+$ (1,16); this implies that monovalent cations move through the channel almost fully hydrated and have very little interaction with the walls of the channel. Divalent cations such as Ca^{2+} and Mg^{2+} also permeate the channel but do so less effectively (0.2 times the Na^+ permeability). This observation, along with the permeability sequence for divalent cations,indicates that these ions interact with charged groups as they move through the pore (1). In addition, the channel is permeable to many monovalent, organic cations (16,26). The permeability of the channel to glucosamine$^+$ (which requires a 7.4 Å-wide pathway) is about 0.03 times the Na^+ permeability (26). The permeability data suggest that the cross-sectional shape of the frog muscle pore can be approximated as a 6.5 × 6.5 Å square (1). Glucosamine$^+$ would pass through such a pore if it were aligned with its widest section along the diagonal of the square. A somewhat larger pore diameter, 8.4 Å, has been suggested for the mouse muscle AChR which is permeable to arginine (16). Even ACh^+ and other agonists can permeate the channel (81) but only under extremely nonphysiologic conditions of concentration (>1 mM ACh) and membrane potential (<−100 mV).

Under physiologic conditions, the current-voltage curve for single AChR channels is linear with a reversal potential near 0 mV (Fig. 9A, curve 1). At 0 mV, the inward flux of Na^+ is balanced by the outward flux of K^+ so there is no net flux. This is a consequence of the equal permeability for Na^+ and K^+ and the fact that the intracellular K^+ concentration is nearly the same as the extracellular Na^+ concentration. The slope of the single-channel current-voltage curve depends on the subunit composition of the muscle-type receptor (see below). The current-voltage curve produced by a large number of AChR channels activated by saturating concentrations of ACh has a small degree of outward rectification. That is, the slope of the current-voltage curve (conductance) is slightly less steep at positive potentials than at negative potentials (Fig. 9A, curve 2). This is due to the voltage dependence of channel gating (see Kinetics section, above). Although each channel produces a linear current-voltage curve, fewer channels are open at positive potentials than at negative potentials.

In contrast, neuronal AChRs have strongly inwardly rectifying single-channel current-voltage curves, but the reversal potential is still near 0 mV (Fig. 9B, curve 1). The reversal potential indicates the channel is nearly equally permeable to Na^+ and K^+, so rectification is not due to the inability of K^+ to flow through the channel. However, there is no rectification when Mg^{2+} is removed from the intracellular solution (Fig. 9B, curve 2). Thus, rectification is the result a voltage-dependent block of the channel by intracellular Mg^{2+} (43). At normal intracellular Mg^{2+} concentrations (1.3 mM, Fig. 9B curve 1), Mg^{2+} has a high affinity for binding within the pore and blocking the efflux of K^+. This decreases the slope of the current-voltage curve at potentials between 0 and +40 mV. At potentials more positive than +40 mV, there is enough energy for Mg^{2+} to go all the way through the pore and restore the pathway for K^+ efflux. The whole-cell current-voltage curve produced by a large number of neuronal AChR channels (43,98) has a greater degree of outward rectification than predicted from the single-channel current-voltage curve (Fig. 9B,curve 3). The additional rectification comes from the voltage-dependence of the channel closing rate as described in the section on kinetics.

Neuronal AChRs are considerably more permeable to divalent cations than are the muscle type AChRs. Estimates of the permeability of neuronal AChRs to Ca^{2+} range from 1.5 to 20 times the Na^+ permeability (68). This implies that a significant flux of Ca^{2+} enters the postsynaptic cholinergic neuron during synaptic transmission. The physiologic importance of this is not yet known. However, glutaminergic receptors that are also highly permeable to Ca^{2+} and blocked by Mg^{2+} are thought to be involved in long-term potentiation and memory (7).

End-Plate Currents and Potentials

At the neuromuscular junction, many channels are activated simultaneously upon release of ACh from the nerve terminal. The rise in ACh concentration is transient; it is rapidly hydrolyzed by AChE. If the muscle is voltage clamped, a current can be measured across the muscle cell membrane. During spontaneous release of ACh from a single synaptic vesicle in the nerve (one quantum), a miniature end-plate current (MEPC) is measured. An MEPC is the superposition of the currents of 1000 to 2000 single channels; it is several nanoamperes (nA) in amplitude. When the nerve is stimulated, hundreds of vesicles of ACh are released (the number of vesicles released is referred to as the quantal content). This results in an end-plate current (EPC) that may be hundreds of nA in amplitude.

Figure 10 shows the results of a simulation in which 100 single-channel current traces were generated. Ten of these individual current traces are shown in Fig. 10A along with the sum of the ten traces. Figure 10B shows the sum of all 100 traces—a simulated MEPC. As more traces are summed, the random openings and closings start to delineate the smooth onset and

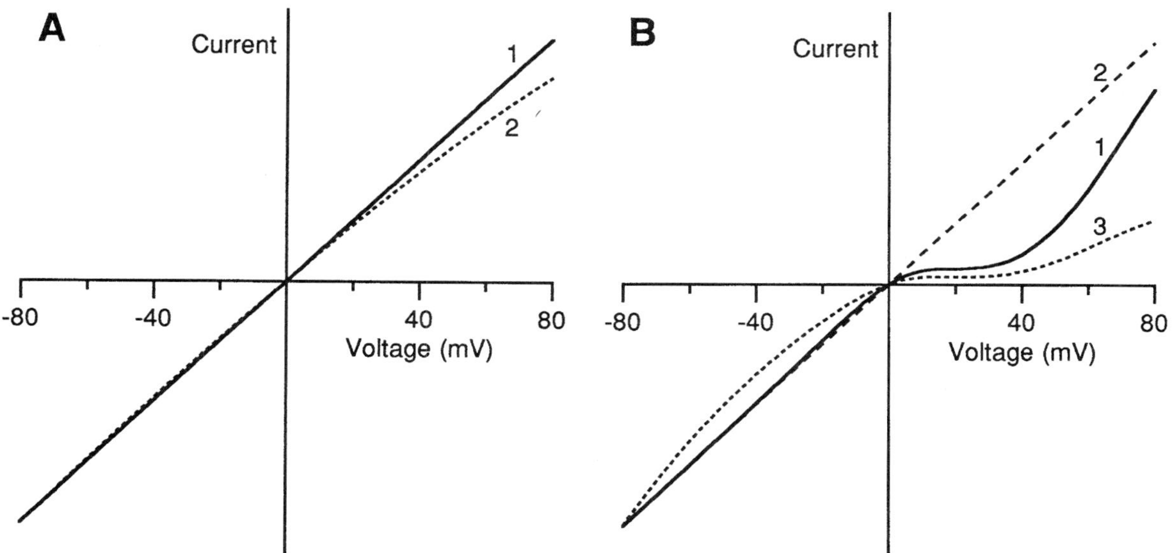

Figure 9. Current-voltage curves for AChR channels. The current scale is not shown because it is scaled by the number of active channels. The shape of the curves are discussed in the text. **(A)** Muscle AChR. Trace 1 is the single-channel current-voltage curve, trace 2 is the multichannel current-voltage curve. Calculation of the multichannel current-voltage curve was based on saturating concentrations of ACh (100 μM), current measurements made before desensitization, and a weakly voltage-dependent channel closing rate (threefold increase for 100 mV depolarization). Rectification of trace 2 is due to the voltage dependence of the closing rate. **(B)** Neuronal AChR. Trace 1 is the single-channel current-voltage curve obtained for an intracellular solution containing 1.8 mM Mg^{2+}. Trace 2 is the single-channel current-voltage curve obtained for an intracellular solution containing no Mg^{2+}. Trace 3 is the multichannel current-voltage curve. Calculation of the multichannel current-voltage curve was based on a low maximum open channel probability and a weakly voltage-dependent channel closing rate (threefold increase for 145 mV depolarization). Rectification of trace 1 is due to channel block by Mg^{2+}; rectification of trace 3 is due to channel block by Mg^{2+} and the voltage dependence of the closing rate.

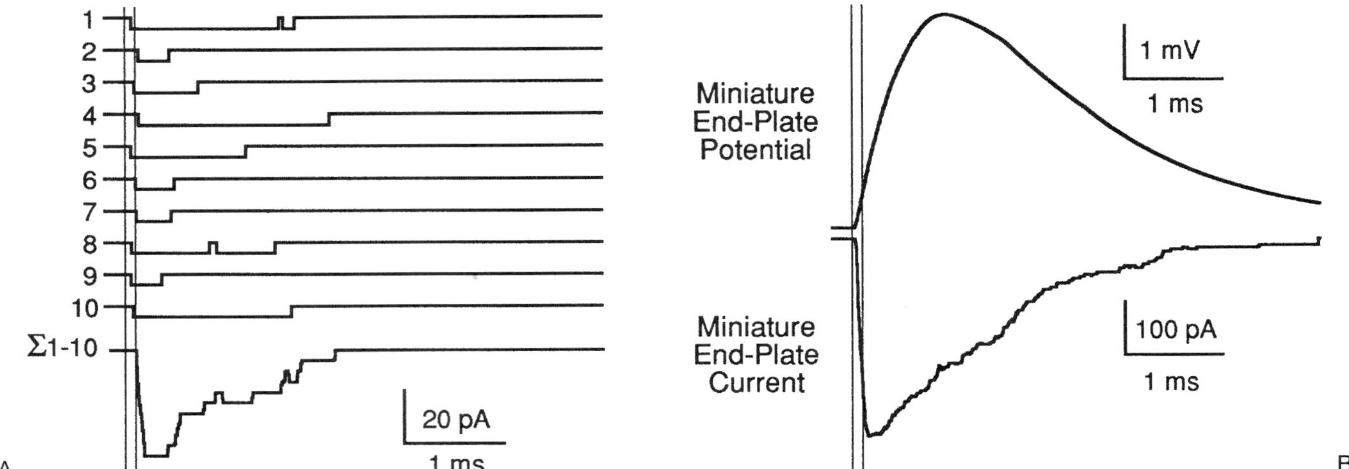

Figure 10. A simulation of the AChR channel activity occurring during spontaneous release of ACh from the nerve terminal. ACh is assumed to be present for the 0.1-ms time interval indicated by the *thin vertical lines.* **(A)** Ten simulated single-channel traces assuming a channel opening rate of 2 x 10^4/s, a closing rate of 10^3/s, and a 50% probability for the channel to reopen before ACh dissociates. The sum of these traces begins to take on the features of a miniature end-plate current (MEPC). **(B)** The lower curve is a simulated MEPC, the sum of 100 single-channel traces. The MEPC activates with a time constant of 0.1 ms and decays with a time constant of 1.6 ms. The upper curve is a simulated MEPP (miniature end-plate potential). It has a slower time course because of the capacitance charging time of the muscle cell membrane.

offset phases of the MEPC. The onset time constant (0.1 ms in this simulation) is a function of the rate at which the channels open after exposure to ACh. The offset time constant (1 ms) reflects the closing rate of the channels. More detailed modeling of neuromuscular transmission (49) indicates that three factors control the rise time of the MEPC (diffusion of ACh, hydrolysis of ACh, and channel gating time) and these three process occur at about the same rate (10/ms).

The membrane potential of a muscle cell in vivo is not clamped. The change in membrane permeability that results from opening AChR channels is converted into a change in membrane potential from its resting value of −80 mV. The inward flux of Na^+ through the channel produces a depolarizing end-plate potential (EPP). Release of a single quantum of ACh from the nerve produces a depolarization of about 1 mV (a miniature EPP). This is not nearly sufficient to reach the threshold for firing an action potential in the muscle cell (−55 mV). When the quantal content is high (when the nerve releases many vesicles upon stimulation), the depolarization exceeds the action potential threshold and may approach V = 0 as a limiting value (the reversal potential for the channel).

The time course of an EPP is somewhat slower than the corresponding EPC (Fig. 10B). This is because the membrane potential does not change instantaneously when Na^+ begins to enter the cell. The time course of the potential change is slower because of the time needed to charge and discharge the capacitance of the cell membrane. The EPP of Fig. 10B was calculated assuming a membrane charging time constant of 3 ms; the EPP onset is 0.3 ms and the EPP decay is 2 ms.

Junctional and Extrajunctional Muscle Receptors

The conductance and kinetics properties of extrajunctional/embryonic receptors (ααβγδ) differ from that of junctional/adult receptors (ααβεδ). The earliest observation (75) was that end-plate currents from extrajunctional receptors decay more slowly than those from junctional receptors (Fig. 11A). At the single-channel level, extrajunctional receptors have a smaller amplitude and a longer open duration. The extrajunctional receptor has a conductance of 40 pS, whereas the junctional receptor has a conductance of 60 pS (Fig. 11B). The mean open time of the extrajunctional receptor is about three times longer than that of the junctional receptor (Fig. 11C). The brief open time confers the fast end-plate current decay to the junctional receptor. If it were possible to compare end-plate currents recorded from equal numbers of junctional and extrajunctional receptors, the amplitude of the junctional receptor end-plate current would be larger than that of the extrajunctional current due to the larger conductance of the junctional receptor channel.

Normal Neuromuscular Transmission

The electrical and chemical events that occur during normal neuromuscular transmission are illustrated in Fig. 12. An action potential, propagated by voltage-gated Na^+ and K^+ channels in the presynaptic nerve axon, depolarizes the nerve terminal. This depolarization opens voltage-gated Ca^{2+} channels allowing the entry of Ca^{2+} into the terminal. Ca^{2+} entry promotes the fusion of synaptic vesicles with the presynaptic membrane and the release of ACh into the synapse. ACh diffuses across the synapse and binds to the ligand binding sites on the AChRs embedded in the muscle cell membrane. ACh binding opens the AChR channel and allows Na^+ to enter and depolarize the muscle cell (EPP). If the EPP reaches excitation threshold, an action potential is initiated in the muscle cell by voltage-gated Na^+ channels and is propagated by these and voltage-gated K^+ channels. When action potential reaches the transverse-tubule system of the muscle cell, it induces the release of Ca^{2+} from the sarcoplasmic reticulum. The muscle contracts when Ca^{2+} binds to troponin and causes the myofilaments to slide past each other. ACh dissociates from the AChR and is hydrolyzed by AChE into choline and acetate. Choline is transported into the nerve terminal, synthesized into ACh and packaged into synaptic vesicles.

Once released from the neuron, ACh molecules are subject to hydrolysis by AChE. AChE is a diffusion limited enzyme: it has a maximum rate of 10/ms and binds ACh with an affinity of 100 μM. About 80% of the of ACh molecules released manage to escape immediate hydrolysis and bind to an AChR. However, after they dissociate from the receptor, they will almost

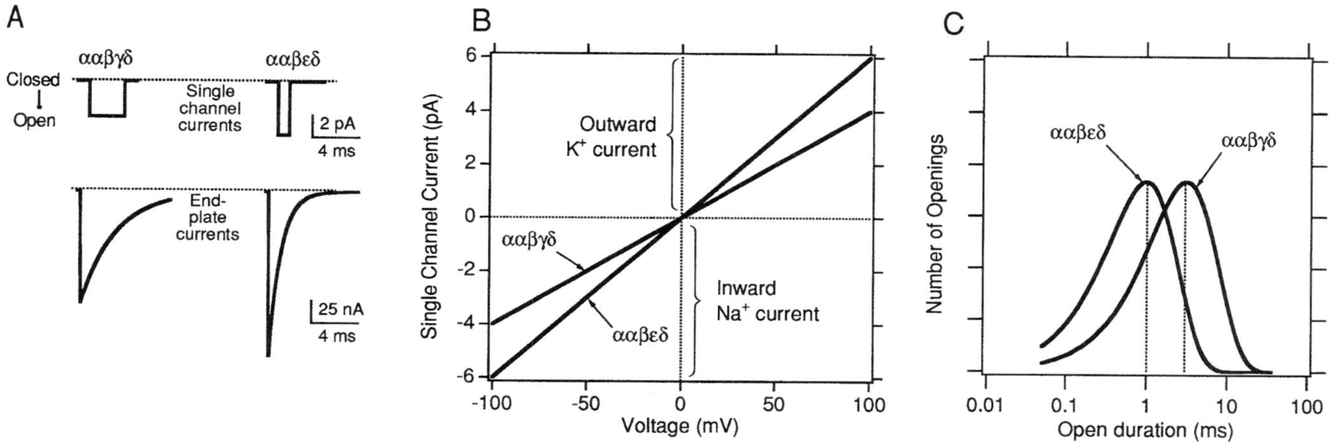

Figure 11. The gamma-epsilon subunit switch. Differences in the electrophysiology of extrajunctional (ααβγδ) and junctional (ααβεδ) isoforms of the muscle AChR. **(A)** Single channels from extrajunctional receptors are longer in duration, but smaller in amplitude than channels from junctional receptors. The same is true for end-plate currents. **(B)** Current voltage curves for the two isoforms of muscle AChRs. The extrajunctional receptors have the smaller conductance. **(C)** Open duration histograms (logarithmic time scale) for the two isoforms of muscle AChRs. The extrajunctional receptors have the longer open time.

certainly meet their hydrolytic fate. Only rarely will a molecule of ACh have the opportunity to bind to a receptor more than once (49).

The kinetic cycle of the voltage-gated Na^+ channels is highlighted in Fig. 12 because it is important in the discussion of depolarizing muscle relaxants in the next section. In normal neuromuscular transmission, the Na^+ channels undergo the activation transition (closed to open) when the muscle membrane is depolarized by an end-plate potential. At the peak of the muscle action potential, the Na^+ channels inactivate (open to inactivated). At the end of the action potential, the muscle membrane potential returns to its normal resting level allowing the Na^+ channels to recover from inactivation (inactivated to closed). The Na^+ channels are then primed to initiate another action potential when the end plate is depolarized again.

The initiation of an action potential is an all-or-none event. An EPP that reaches 0 mV fires the same action potential as an EPP that just barely depolarizes the membrane to the −55 mV threshold potential. The margin of safety of neuromuscular transmission is determined by the size of the EPP compared to the action potential threshold. Many muscles have a margin of safety as high as 80% (67). This means that neuromuscular transmission will function normally until 80% of the AChRs are inhibited or the amount of ACh released is reduced by 80%.

A high margin of safety ensures that synaptic transmission is protected against moderate changes in quantal content. A decrease in quantal content occurs when the nerve is stimulated at a high frequency (tetanus) because, for example, the number of vesicles near the active zone is decreased. An increase in quantal content may occur after a short delay following a tetanus (posttetanic potentiation) because the intracellular Ca^{2+} level is elevated and this appears to mobilize or increase the number of vesicles available for immediate release. One manifestation of the margin of safety is the constant train-of-four ratio seen in normal, unparalyzed muscle stimulated at 2 Hz. Although the four closely spaced (0.5 sec) nerve stimuli may cause some decrease in quantal content, this is not sufficient to cause synaptic transmission to fail. However, when many AChRs are blocked, the margin of safety is low and the decrease in quantal content during train-of-four stimulation may prevent the initiation of more than one muscle action potential.

During normal neuromuscular transmission, desensitization of the AChR does not occur. The desensitized receptor state is included in the diagram of Fig. 12 as a reminder that desensitization may be important in the presence of drugs and/or under pathologic conditions.

PHARMACOLOGY OF THE ACETYLCHOLINE RECEPTOR

The pharmacology of the AChR is complicated by the fact that there are at least five enzymes at the synapse (junctional AChR, extrajunctional AChR, AChE, Na^+-choline$^+$ cotrans-

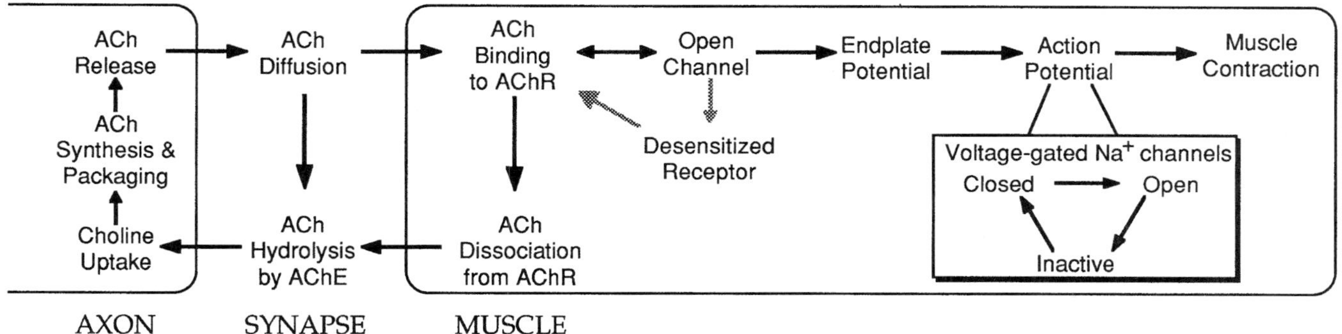

Figure 12. A diagram depicting the events during normal neuromuscular transmission. In this and the other diagrams, a *gray arrow* indicates transitions that do not occur in this particular situation.

porter, and presynaptic AChR) that recognize ACh or choline and drugs that work at the synapse. Many of these interactions are not highly specific. As a result, it is often hard to dissect the different actions that pharmacologic agents have at the NMJ. In addition, most our knowledge about AChR pharmacology is based on experiments with receptors from fish electric organ, amphibian muscle, and mouse embryonic muscle. Very few basic experimental studies have been done on the receptors that come from the most relevant tissues—human adult muscle and human neurons. It has been known since the 1950s that there are species differences in the interaction of muscle relaxants with adult mammalian muscle (101). The importance of differences in amino acid sequences and/or posttranslational modification among receptors from different animals has only begun to be determined.

Agonists

There are many derivatives of ACh that act as agonists on the AChR. Carbamycholine and suberyldicholine are commonly used in experimental studies because they are not hydrolyzed by AChE. The potency of an agonist is a function of two factors: binding affinity and efficacy (the ability of the agonist, once bound, to induce channel opening). At the muscle AChR, the rank order of agonist binding affinities is suberyldicholine >ACh>carbamylcholine , but all three agonists have a high efficacy (>90%).

Some compounds act as partial agonists on the AChR. A true partial agonist is one that has a low efficacy, that is, once it is bound to the receptor, its ability to open the channel is poor. In terms of the kinetic scheme (Fig. 8), a partial agonist is characterized by a channel opening rate that is smaller than the channel closing rate ($\beta<\alpha$). It is often hard to distinguish partial agonism from some other inhibitory action of the agonist on the channel (channel block, for example). Decamethonium has been shown to be a true partial agonist at the embryonic mouse muscle AChR (53).

Neuronal AChRs can be activated by the agonists ACh, nicotine, cytisine, and dimethylphenylpiperazinium. However, the relative potency of these agonists depends on the subunit composition of the neuronal receptor. Both the α- and β-subunits of the neuronal receptor help determine the sensitivity to different agonists (68). Because ACh is probably the only endogenous agonist for the receptor, differences in agonist potency must be a manifestation of some other property of the neuronal AChR.

Nondepolarizing Muscle Relaxants

A nondepolarizing muscle relaxant is a compound that is a competitive antagonist for the AChR. Curare (more precisely, d-tubocurarine, the active ingredient in curare) was the first nondepolarizing muscle relaxant (Fig. 13). Curare is a naturally occurring substance found in the South American vines of the species *Strychnos* and *Chondrodendron*. It is used as a dart poison in the Amazon. Metocurine is a synthetic derivative of curare containing three additional methyl groups. Some of the synthetic compounds commonly used nondepolarizing muscle relaxants are shown in Fig. 13. Pancuronium and its congeners, pipecuronium and vecuronium, are *bis*-quaternary ammonium steroids compounds that also bind to the α-subunit of the acetylcholine receptor. Atracurium is a member of the benzylisoquinolinium family of nondepolarizers that includes mivacurium and doxacurium. Gallamine, a representative of another series of synthetic substitutes for curare, has three quaternary ammonium groups.

Paralysis by nondepolarizing muscle relaxants is characterized by a slow onset (slower than for depolarizing muscle relaxants), decrement (fade) in the train-of-four ratio, and slow recovery. The mechanism of action of curare (as the representative nondepolarizer) is shown in Fig. 14. Curare competes with ACh for binding to the ligand-binding sites on the AChR, but once it is bound curare does not allow the channel to open. In other words, curare is a competitive antagonist at the AChR. As a result, there is no influx of Na^+, no EPP, no action potential, and no muscle contraction. The large, bulky, rigid structures nondepolarizing muscle relaxants suggest that when they are bound to the ligand-binding site on the α-subunit, they also attach to sites on neighboring subunits. This might stabilize the AChR in the closed state and make it difficult for the receptor to undergo the conformational change necessary for channel gating.

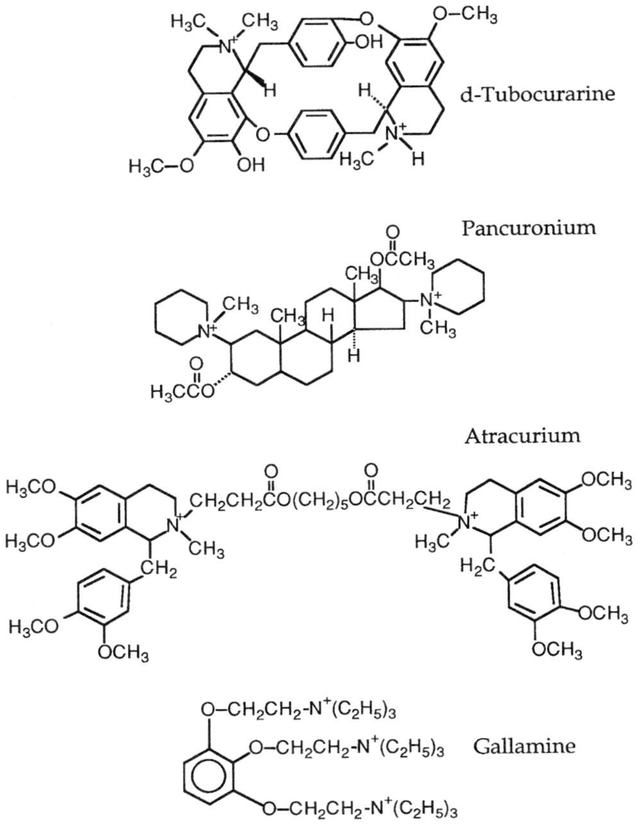

d-Tubocurarine

Pancuronium

Atracurium

Gallamine

Figure 13. The structure of some nondepolarizing muscle relaxants. The original nondepolarizing agent, curare, and representatives from three categories of synthetic agents are shown.

The force of contraction of a whole muscle is equal to the sum of the forces generated by each individual muscle fiber. When curare causes 50% paralysis (i.e., the amplitude of a single twitch is 50% of its normal value), half of the muscle fibers fail to fire an action potential and do not contract. The other half of the fibers do fire action potentials and contract normally. The fibers that do contract are operating with a very low margin of safety. Small changes in the amount of ACh released from the nerve will make a big difference in the probability that an action potential will fire.

Curare binds with higher affinity to the ligand-binding site at the α-γ-subunit interface than to the site at the α-δ-subunit interface (80). Most of the basic experimental studies were done with metocurine rather than curare. For mouse muscle receptors, the difference in affinity is nearly 100-fold, 0.3 and 28 μM (82). For human muscle receptors, the difference in affinity is only threefold, 0.2 and 0.6 μM (78). In both cases, the binding of curare to just one of the ligand-binding sites is sufficient to prevent channel opening by ACh (82).

When two nondepolarizing muscle relaxants are combined, the effect can usually be predicted by simple additivity of the

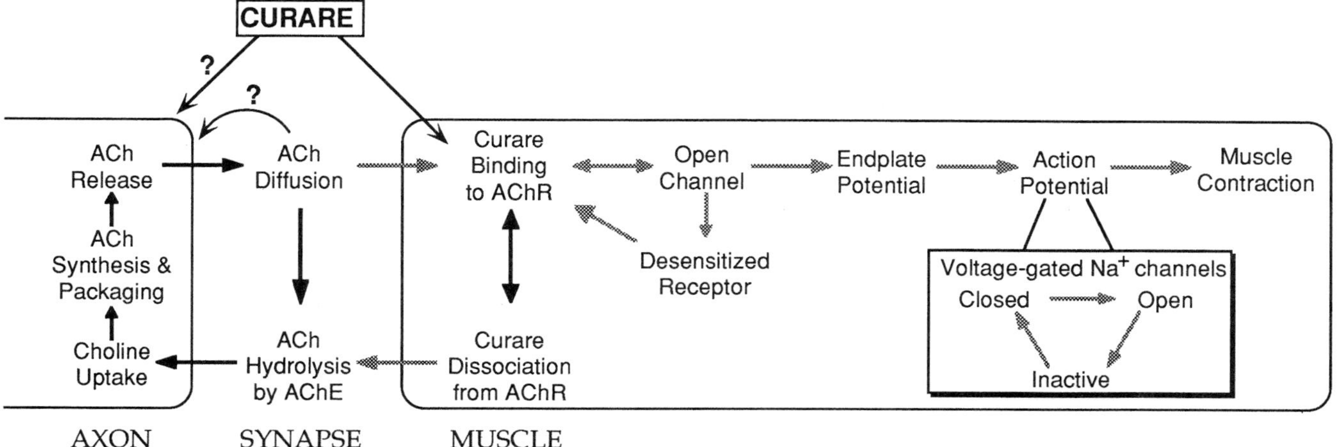

Figure 14. A diagram depicting the events during neuromuscular transmission in the presence of nondepolarizing muscle relaxants; curare is used as an example here. There is no consensus on the mechanism of train-of-four fade by curare; see text for details.

effects of the drugs individually. Some combinations of nondepolarizers administered to humans (e.g., metocurine plus pancuronium [50,94], and all combinations of atracurium, mivacurium, and vecuronium [46, 58]), however, show synergism and produce a larger than additive effect. Synergistic effects between two drugs usually indicate that there is more than one site of action for the drugs. One possibility is that one drug acts primarily at presynaptic AChRs, whereas the other acts primarily at postsynaptic AChRs. In one in vitro study, presynaptic effects were thought to be unimportant (94). One need look no further than the postsynaptic AChR itself to find two distinct binding sites for nondepolarizers. A mathematical analysis demonstrated that synergism could occur if the α-δ-subunit interface was the higher affinity site for one of the nondepolarizers and the α-ε-subunit interface (in the adult form of the receptor) was the higher affinity site for the other nondepolarizer (85,94). Thus far, this remains a plausible but untested explanation for synergism between nondepolarizers.

The mechanism by which curare reduces the amplitude of a single twitch is the least controversial issue in the pharmacology of muscle relaxants. The question of how curare produces decrement in the train-of-four ratio (or tetanic fade) is one of the most controversial issues. There are at least four viewpoints:

1. Tetanic fade is entirely due to actions of curare on the muscle AChR such as desensitization (12).
2. Tetanic fade is simply a manifestation of reduced quantal content (depletion of vesicles from the active zone) in the nerve due to frequent stimulation. It is seen because the muscle fibers are operating at a low margin of safety (18).
3. Tetanic fade is due to curare binding to AChRs in the presynaptic nerve. This interpretation presupposes that the function of presynaptic AChRs is to provide positive feedback to the nerve during high-frequency stimulation. When curare binds to these receptors, the feedback loop is broken. The nerve does not get the message that it should mobilize more vesicles and, as a result, there is a decrease in quantal content (9,86).
4. Tetanic fade is due to the action of adenosine (coming from hydrolysis of the ATP^{3-} that is released along with ACh^{+} from synaptic vesicles) on purine receptors in the nerve terminal membrane. This scheme postulates that the purine receptors provide a negative feedback control of quantal release (74). Curare unmasks this effect as in #2 above.

The currently best supported hypothesis is the third—tetanic fade arises from presynaptic actions of nondepolarizing drugs (9). The evidence favoring this hypothesis includes the observation that the decrement of the train-of-four ratio depends on the chemical structure of the nondepolarizer (reviewed in ref. 10). However, the issue is not likely to be completely resolved very quickly. In addition to the fact that not enough is known about the physiology of the various proteins that bind ACh and curare, there are other difficulties. There are inter- and intraspecies differences in AChRs and muscle fibers that may confound extrapolations from laboratory studies to the operating room. Moreover, neuromuscular transmission does not occur under equilibrium conditions of time or space (52,70), so we must turn to models and simulations to improve our conceptual understanding. Finally, there may be more than one mechanism for tetanic fade. One indication of this is that the decrement of the train-of-four ratio is much more pronounced during recovery from nondepolarizing muscle blockade than during the onset of block (69).

Nondepolarizing muscle relaxants differ in their speed of action. Moreover, the speed of action is correlated to the potency of the nondepolarizer: the higher the potency, the slower the onset of action (11). For example, at the ED_{95} of doxacurium (30 μg/kg), the time to maximum suppression is 10.2 minutes, whereas at the ED_{95} of pancuronium (100 μg/kg), the time to maximum suppression is 2.4 minutes (6). This phenomenon is probably not due to global pharmacokinetic factors because the inverse relationship between potency and onset time is also seen when the drugs are applied by iontophoresis to an in vitro muscle preparation (33). Two possibilities remain: onset is limited by binding kinetics at the AChR, or onset is limited by the time it takes for the drug to diffuse into the synapse. Diffusion into spaces as small as the synapse should take no more than a few milliseconds. However, when the drug reaches the edge of a synapse and encounters a high density of AChRs, its movement will be slowed because of the time it spends bound to these receptors. This process is known as buffered diffusion (2). In vitro onset times have a low sensitivity to temperature (33). Diffusional processes are characterized by a low-temperature sensitivity (less than a 40% change for a 10°C change in temperature). This supports the idea that the speed of action of nondepolarizing muscle relaxants is limited by diffusion of drug into the synapse.

Recovery from nondepolarizing muscle relaxation is a function of redistribution, metabolism and excretion. Curare, metocurine, gallamine and doxacurium are not appreciably metabolized so recovery is relatively slow and depends on redistribution and excretion. Recovery from pancuronium is also slow even though it is partially hydroxylated in the liver. Atracurium has an intermediate duration of action; it is hydrolyzed by plasma esterases into less-potent metabolites and undergoes spontaneous degradation by Hofmann elimination. Vecuronium undergoes substantial metabolism which results in a duration of action similar to that of atracurium. The short duration of action of mivacurium is partially due to its hydrolysis by plasma cholinesterase, but involves other metabolic mechanisms as well.

In addition to its competitive antagonist action, curare has several other actions on the AChR. In some muscle cells, curare is a weak partial agonist (84). The agonist efficacy of curare is so low that 1 μM curare opens no more than 0.05% of the AChR channels from BC3H-1 cells (*unpublished results* from the author's laboratory). It is unlikely that such a weak partial agonist action has any clinical significance. The degree of partial agonism has not yet been measured for other nondepolarizing muscle relaxants. Curare also acts as a high affinity open channel blocker of the AChR channel (17). Although the blocking affinity (0.12 μM) is within the range of clinical concentrations of curare, block by curare is not likely to be clinically important. The reason is that curare blocks only open channels and the antagonist action of curare prevents channels from reaching the open state. Channel block is also not a viable mechanism for tetanic fade because channel block is voltage-dependent (17) whereas fade is voltage-independent (9).

Depolarizing Muscle Relaxants

Depolarizing muscle relaxants are, by definition, compounds that are efficacious agonists for the muscle AChR. Succinylcholine (Sux, also known as suxamethonium) is the only depolarizing muscle relaxant currently in clinical use; decamethonium has been used in the past (Fig. 15). In contrast to the nondepolarizing muscle relaxants, the depolarizing muscle relaxants are slim and flexible. Sux is essentially two molecules of ACh joined at their acetyl ends, so it is not surprising that Sux binds to the ligand-binding site on the AChR and promotes channel opening. Sux differs from ACh in that it is not hydrolyzed by AChE. Thus, constant administration of Sux will result in a sustained level of the drug at the synapse.

There are two phases to the action of Sux as a muscle relaxant. Phase I is characterized by a fast onset time, muscle fasciculations, a constant train-of-four ratio and fast recovery. Figure 16 illustrates the action of Sux in phase I block. Sux competes with ACh for binding to the ligand-binding sites on the AChR and opens the ion channel. Although Sux has two quaternary ammonium groups, the 30 Å separation between the α-subunits (38) precludes one molecule of Sux from binding to both α-subunits simultaneously. Two molecules of Sux are required for

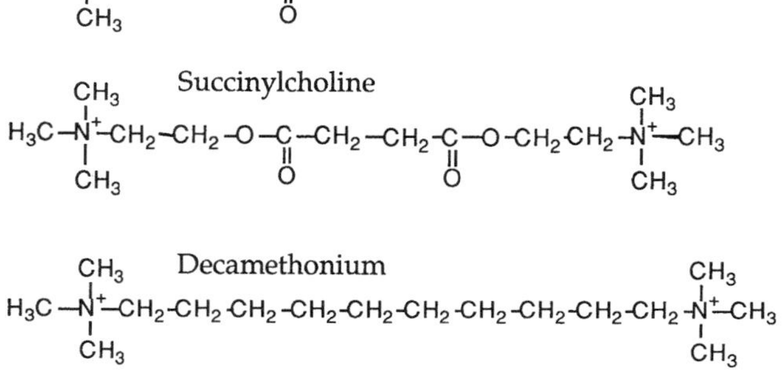

Acetylcholine

$H_3C{-}N^+(CH_3)_2{-}CH_2{-}CH_2{-}O{-}C({=}O){-}CH_3$

Succinylcholine

$H_3C{-}N^+(CH_3)_2{-}CH_2{-}CH_2{-}O{-}C({=}O){-}CH_2{-}CH_2{-}C({=}O){-}O{-}CH_2{-}CH_2{-}N^+(CH_3)_2{-}CH_3$

Decamethonium

$H_3C{-}N^+(CH_3)_2{-}CH_2{-}CH_2{-}CH_2{-}CH_2{-}CH_2{-}CH_2{-}CH_2{-}CH_2{-}CH_2{-}CH_2{-}N^+(CH_3)_2{-}CH_3$

Figure 15. The chemical structures of depolarizing compounds: acetylcholine, succinylcholine, and decamethonium.

channel opening (57). The influx of Na^+ through the channel into the muscle cell causes an EPP. An action potential will fire and the muscle will contract once or just a few times (the clinically observed fasciculation). Because it is not hydrolyzed, the level of Sux at the synapse remains high allowing Sux to equilibrate with the receptor-binding sites. Although this constant exposure to Sux induces AChR desensitization, enough channels remain open to produce a persistent depolarization of the muscle (18). Consider the consequence of a persistent depolarization of the muscle cell to the voltage-gated Na^+ channel. This will lock the Na^+ channel in its inactivated conformation. As a result, no more action potentials will fire and the muscle will not contract.

To summarize phase I block by Sux, the pharmacologic site of action of Sux is the AChR. However, the physiologically important event is inactivation of the Na^+ channel. The two are linked by the muscle cell membrane potential. Sux depolarizes the membrane, the depolarized membrane prevents the Na^+ channel from leaving the inactivated state.

Rapid reversal of phase I block occurs because of the hydrolysis of Sux by butyrylcholinesterase. Butyrylcholinesterase (also known as plasma cholinesterase and pseudo-cholinesterase) is a nonspecific cholinesterase found in the blood and liver. Butyrylcholinesterase hydrolyzes Sux into succinylmonocholine which has only a weak action at the AChR. When administration of Sux is stopped, the concentration of Sux in the blood decreases quickly. This produces a large concentration gradient of Sux between muscle and blood so there is a large flux of Sux away from the muscle.

The mechanism for the fast onset of action of Sux has not been studied in detail. There are several ways in which Sux differs from nondepolarizers that could contribute to its fast onset of action. Sux is less potent than all of the nondepolarizing muscle relaxants, so the buffered diffusion hypothesis would predict a fast onset of action for Sux (33). A second factor is that Sux has to bind to fewer receptors in order to induce paralysis. Thus, even if the diffusion of Sux through the synapse were slowed by binding to the AChR, it might be sufficient for Sux to bind to the receptors at the outer edge of the synapse. Third, Sux might induce muscle depolarization by binding to extrajunctional receptors on the surface of the muscle. Such binding would occur even before Sux diffused into the synapse.

There are several theories as to why Sux does not cause decrement of the train-of-four ratio. These parallel the hypotheses for tetanic fade by nondepolarizers. There is no need to present each one in detail because they are based on the agonist action of Sux in contrast to the antagonist action of curare. One theory does require some explanation, however. It notes that during phase I block by Sux, the margin of safety of the functioning muscle fibers is still quite high (the moderate amount of depolarization experienced by these fibers does not impair their ability to fire an action potential). Thus, the decrease in quantal content during high frequency stimulation has no effect (18).

Paralysis by Sux has several adverse effects: fasciculation, muscle pain, and increased intraocular and intragastric pressure. To minimize these effects while preserving the advantage of fast onset by Sux, anesthesiologists sometimes administer a small dose of a nondepolarizing muscle relaxant before giving Sux. For this precurization regimen to work, the dose of the nondepolarizer must be too small to produce paralysis (but may actually block 50% of the AChRs [95]) and the dose of Sux must be 1.5 to 2 times the standard dose (timing is important, too). If we assume that both drugs are competing for the same binding site (the postsynaptic AChR), it is difficult to understand how precurization could selectively blunt the adverse effects (e.g., fasciculation) and yet preserve the desired effect (paralysis). One problem is that the phenomenon occurs under nonequilibrium conditions of drug concentrations (95). In a qualitative, quasi-equilibrium analysis, Waud and Waud

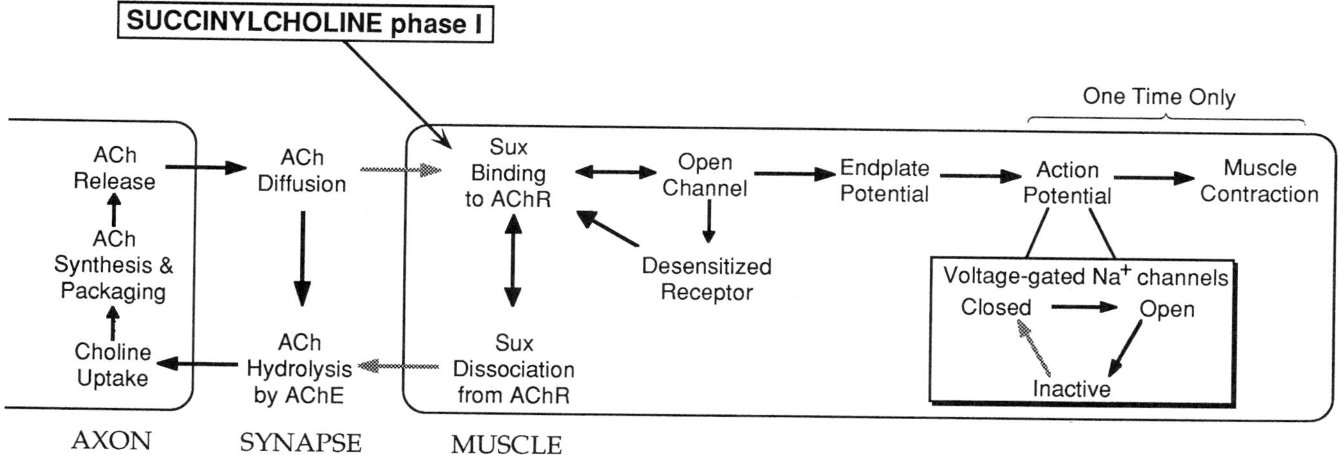

Figure 16. A diagram depicting the events during neuromuscular transmission in the presence of a depolarizing muscle relaxant, succinylcholine (Sux) during phase I.

(95) argued that the success of precurization is due to a diminution of all effects of Sux rather than a selective elimination of some effects.

The depolarization of a muscle by Sux opens voltage-gated K^+ channels in the muscle cell membrane. This leads to an efflux of K^+ from the muscle cell and a 0.5 mM increase in serum K^+ levels. Most patients will tolerate this increase. However, in patients whose serum K^+ levels are already elevated, the resulting hyperkalemia may lead to cardiac arrest. Depolarizing muscle relaxants are therefore contraindicated for patients with severe burns, muscle trauma, and diseases involving denervation.

Phase II block by Sux develops when Sux is used for periods greater than 30 min. It is characterized by a decrement in the train-of-four ratio and slow recovery. The mechanism for phase II block by Sux is another controversial question (Fig. 17). Phase II may be a result of some slowly developing change in the physiology of the NMJ brought about by the persistent depolarizing action of Sux. The change may be presynaptic, due to Sux binding to presynaptic AChRs, postsynaptic, or both. One idea is that persistent depolarization of either the nerve or muscle cell upsets the ionic balance of the cell (18,102). For example, as noted above the opening of voltage-gated K^+ channels will lead to an efflux of K^+ from the muscle cell. Another possibility is that depolarization causes changes in the concentrations of intracellular messengers or the phosphorylation state of an enzyme. When the anesthesiologist stops infusing Sux, Sux dissociates quickly from its binding sites on AChRs, diffuses away from the synapse, and is rapidly hydrolyzed by plasma cholinesterase. However, the nerve and/or muscle cell needs time to restore normal intracellular conditions. This becomes the rate-limiting step in recovery from phase II block.

Sux also has a voltage-dependent channel blocking effect on the AChR. The blocking affinity for Sux is 200 μM at −120 mV (57). Based on the voltage-sensitivity of block by ACh (81), we would expect that the blocking affinity would be 600 μM at −80 mV. The plasma concentration of Sux in paralyzed humans is about 20 μM (57). Thus, we would expect less than a 5% channel blocking effect by Sux during depolarizing muscle relaxation.

Anticholinesterases

Anticholinesterases are compounds that inhibit AChE, making it unavailable for hydrolysis of ACh. This increases the amount of time that the concentration of ACh remains high in the synapse. Some molecules of ACh will have the opportunity to bind repeatedly to the AChR before they diffuse out of the synapse; thus, the end-plate potential will be prolonged. If the

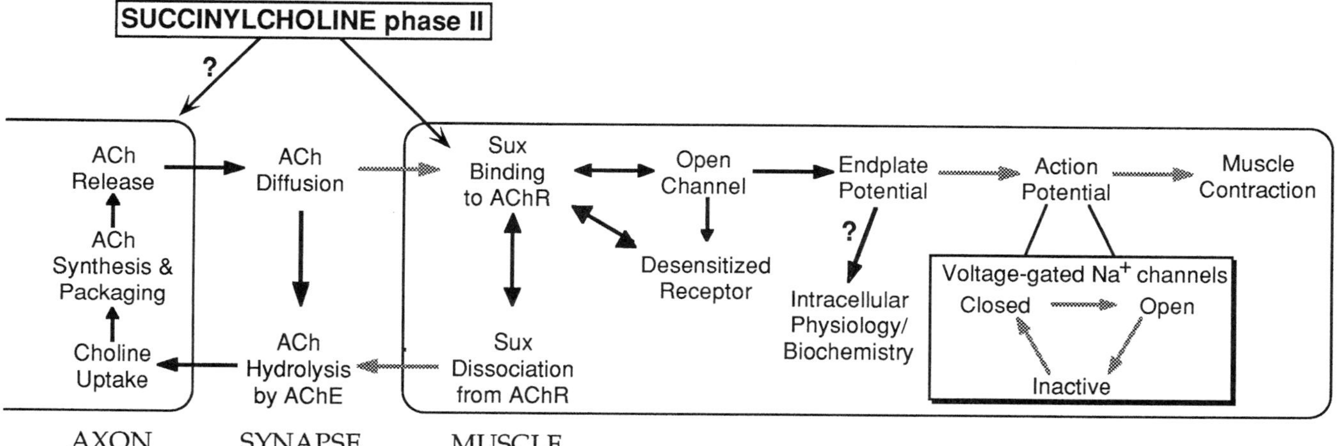

Figure 17. A diagram depicting some possible events during neuromuscular transmission in the presence of succinylcholine during phase II block. There is no consensus on the mechanism of phase II block, but it is likely to involve slowly developing changes in intracellular compartments in the muscle and/or nerve cell.

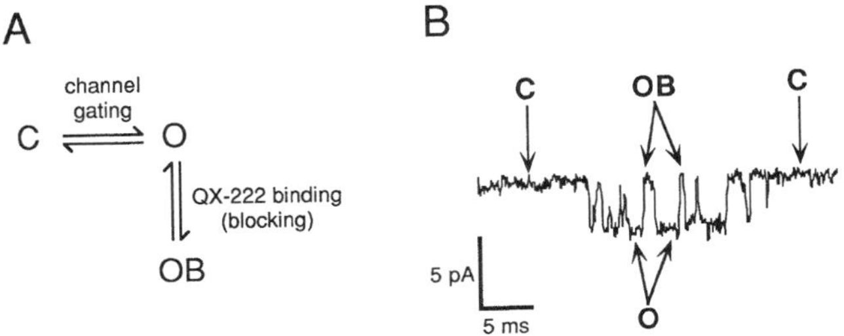

Figure 18. Open channel blockade of the AChR. **(A)** The open channel blocking model for interactions of local anesthetics and other noncompetitive inhibitors of the AChR. The three states are: C—a composite of the closed states (R, AR, A_2R), O—the open state (A_2R^*), OB—a nonconducting state in which the drug binds and blocks the open channel. **(B)** Flickering of a single AChR channel in the presence of 30 μM QX-222. The presumed state that is occupied at several times during this burst is indicated. (Unpublished data from the author's laboratory; 200 nM ACh, −100 mV.)

muscle is operating at a low margin of safety, such a prolongation keep the end-plate depolarized long enough to fire a muscle action potential.

Clinically useful anticholinesterases include physostigmine (eserine), neostigmine, and edrophonium. Edrophonium competes with ACh for the active site on AChE. Physostigmine and neostigmine, on the other hand, are hydrolyzed by AChE. After the hydrolysis reaction, AChE is carbamoylated and inactive. The carbamoylated AChE slowly reverts to active AChE by hydrolysis.

It is not surprising that compounds that recognize AChE also recognize the AChR. Physostigmine has both a channel blocking action (93) and an agonist action (71) on the AChR.

Local Anesthetics (Noncompetitive Inhibitors)

The anesthetic site of action of local anesthetics is the voltage-gated Na^+ channel in neurons. Local anesthetics also have actions on the AChR. These compounds are known as noncompetitive inhibitors of the AChR because they have an inhibitory action but do not compete with ACh at the ligand-binding site. The compounds include QX-222 (a permanently charged derivative of lidocaine), procaine, chlorpromazine, and phencyclidine. QX-222 is the best characterized of these compounds (14,62).

The action of QX-222 (at concentrations <40 μM) is well described by the open channel blocking model (3) illustrated in Fig. 18A. The three states are the closed (C), open (O), and blocked while open (OB). The activation of the AChR channel has been simplified to a single step (C→O) in this model. The blocker can bind only when the channel is open (O→OB) and must dissociate before the channel can close (OB→O→B). This model makes several predictions about the time course of end-plate currents and single-channel currents as a function of blocker concentration. At the single-channel level, a flickering channel behavior is observed as QX-222 molecules bind the pore of the channel and block the flow of current through the channel (Fig. 18B). A burst of channel activity consists of several O↔OB transitions before the gate of the channel closes (O→C). The brief closed times within the burst correspond to the dwell times of QX-222 at its blocking site. The evidence that the binding site of QX-222 is within the pore of the channel comes from site-directed mutagenesis studies. The duration of brief closures is affected by mutations within the M2 region of the AChR (14).

General Anesthetics

Before curare was used clinically, surgical muscle relaxation was achieved by using high doses of ether. This was the earliest evidence that general anesthetics have inhibitory actions on the AChR. These effects can be seen in the practice of anesthesiology today—the use of a volatile general anesthetic lowers a patient's requirement for muscle relaxants (30,60). Electrophysiologic and biochemical studies have shown that general anesthetics have several effects on the muscle AChR.

The most prominent effects of anesthetics on the AChR is an inhibitory effect that resembles the flickery channel block produced by QX-222. Single AChR channels exposed to various general anesthetics assume one of three patterns (Fig. 19). Channels exposed to ether have an amplitude that is noisy and smaller than normal. Channels exposed to isoflurane have a flickery appearance. Channels exposed to propofol have an open duration that is briefer than normal but do not exhibit either flickering or decreased amplitude. Similar effects are seen with intravenous anesthetics (91,92), alcohols (61), and barbiturates (8).

The kinetics of these effects are not completely consistent with the open channel blocking model used for QX-222. However, extension of the model to allow for blockade of both open and closed channels (Fig. 20) accounts for most of the observed data (21,22,24,61). This model has one additional state, CB, in which the anesthetic is bound while the gate of the channel is closed. Thus, anesthetic molecules can bind before the channel opens (C→CB) and the gate of the channel can close while the anesthetic is still bound (OB→CB).

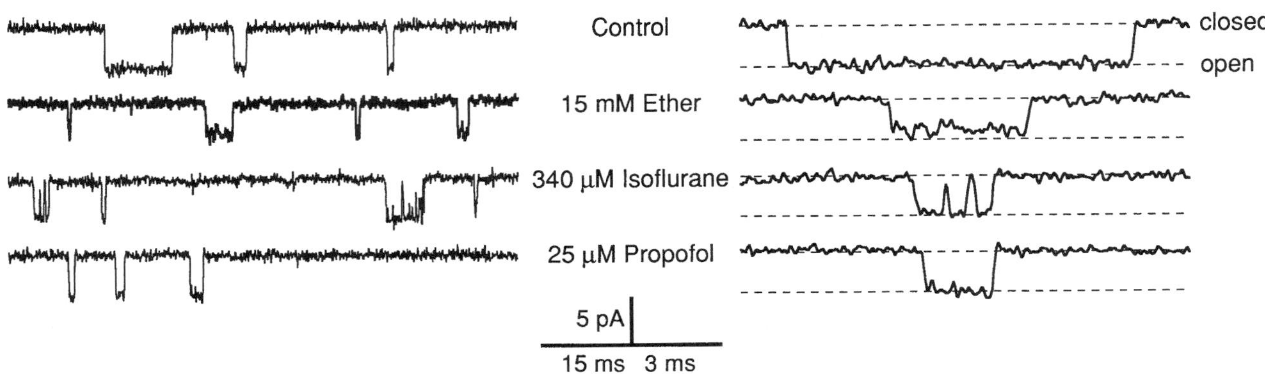

Figure 19. Inhibition of the AChR channel by general anesthetics. Single AChR channels in an excised patch were activated by 0.2 μM ACh and perfused with no drug (control) and the indicated concentration of anesthetic. Traces at the right show one burst for each condition on an expanded time scale. *Dashed lines* indicate the current amplitude in the control record. Patch potential was −100 mV. (From ref. 24, used with permission.)

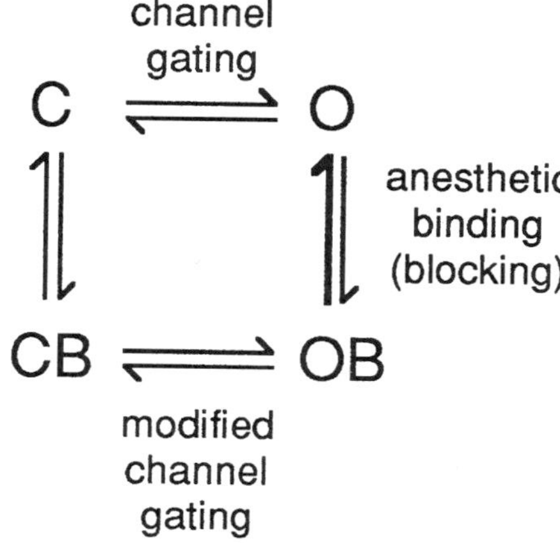

Figure 20. The open/closed channel blocking model that provides a good description of the effects of general anesthetics on the AChR channel. The states C, O, and OB are the three states found in the open channel blocking model (Fig. 18A). State CB is a nonconducting state in which the drug binds to the closed channel. General anesthetics differ in the rate at which anesthetics dissociate from the open/blocked state (OB→O, *bold arrow* in figure). For the anesthetics shown in Fig. 19, the rank order of dissociation rates is ether>isoflurane>propofol.

The three distinct patterns of activity can all arise from this model. It is assumed that there is a single general anesthetic binding (blocking) site on the AChR protein and that the three anesthetics have different rates for dissociation from this site. In this scenario, ether would have fast-binding kinetics—so fast that most of the individual binding events are too brief to be resolved. The kinetics of isoflurane would be slower so that most of the binding events are seen as brief gaps within a burst of channel activity. The kinetics of propofol would be slower still; most of the time, propofol would remain bound until after the gate of the channel has closed.

The most hydrophobic of the three anesthetics, propofol, has the highest affinity for the putative general anesthetic binding site. This suggests that the site has a hydrophobic or amphipathic chemical nature. It is clear that the channel, in particular the M2 region, contains hydrophobic residues and that hydrophobic molecules can bind to these residues (97). However, it remains to be determined whether general anesthetics block the AChR channel by binding within the pore or by binding to some allosteric site that induces a conformational change to a nonconducting state of the receptor (25).

REFERENCES

1. Adams DJ, Dwyer TM, Hille B. The permeability of endplate channels to monovalent and divalent metal cations. *J Gen Physiol* 1980; 75:493–510.
2. Adams PR. Drug interactions at the motor endplate. *Pflugers Arch* 1975;360:155–164.
3. Adams PR. Voltage jump analysis of procaine action at frog endplate. *J Physiol (Lond)* 1977;268:291–318.
4. Ballivet M, Patrick J, Lee J, Heinemann S. Molecular cloning of a cDNA coding for the γ subunit of *Torpedo* acetylcholine receptor in its membrane environment. *Proc Natl Acad Sci USA* 1982;79: 4466–4470.
5. Barchan D, Kachalsky S, Neumann D, Vogel Z, Ovadia M, Kochva E, Fuchs S. How the mongoose can fight the snake—the binding site of the mongoose acetylcholine receptor. *Proc Natl Acad Sci USA* 1992;89:7717–7721.
6. Basta SJ, Savarese JJ, Ali HH, Embree PB, Schwartz AF, Rudd GD, Wastila WB. Clinical pharmacology of doxacurium chloride. *Anesthesiology* 1988;69:478–486.
7. Bliss TVP, Collingridge GL. A synaptic model of memory: long-term potentiation in the hippocampus. *Nature* 1993;361:31–39.
8. Boguslavsky R, Dilger JP. Inhibition of ACh receptor channels by barbiturates. *Biophys J* 1995;68:A377.
9. Bowman WC, Marshall IG, Gibb AJ, Harborne AJ. Feedback control of transmitter release at the neuromuscular junction. *Trends Pharmacol Sci* 1988;9:16–20
10. Bowman WC. Prejunctional and postjunctional cholinoceptors at the neuromuscular junction. *Anesth Analg* 1980;59:935–943.
11. Bowman WC, Rodger IW, Houston J, Marshall RJ, McIndewar LI. Structure:action relationships among some desacetoxy analogues of pancuronium and vecuronium in the anesthetized cat. *Anesthesiology* 1988;69:57–62.
12. Bradley RJ, Sterz R, Peper K, Chau W-C, Zhang G. Evidence that postsynaptic effects of d-tubocurarine or α-toxin cause fade at the neuromuscular junction. *Ann NY Acad Sci* 1990;604:548–557.
13. Changeux J-P, Kasai M, Lee C-Y. Use of a snake venom toxin to characterize the cholinergic receptor protein. *Proc Natl Acad Sci USA* 1970;67:1241–1247.
14. Charnet P, Labarca C, Leonard RJ, Vogelaar NJ, Czyzyk L, Gouin A, Davidson N, Lester HA. An open-channel blocker interacts with adjacent turns of α-helices in the nicotinic acetylcholine receptor. *Neuron* 1990;2:87–95.
15. Chavez RA, Maloof J, Beeson D, Newsom-Davis J, Hall ZW. Subunit folding and αδ heterodimer formation in the assembly of the nicotinic acetylcholine receptor. Comparison of the mouse and human α subunits. *J Biol Chem* 1992;267:23028–23034.
16. Cohen BN, Labarca C, Davidson N, Lester HA. Mutations in M2 alter the selectivity of the mouse nicotinic acetylcholine receptor for organic and alkali metal cations. *J Gen Physiol* 1992;100:373–400.
17. Colquhoun D, Dreyer F, Sheridan RE. The actions of tubocurarine at the frog neuromuscular junction. *J Physiol* 1979;293:247–284.
18. Colquhoun D. On the principles of postsynaptic action of the neuromuscular blocking agents. In: Kharkevich DA, ed. *New neuromuscular blocking agents.* Berlin: Springer-Verlag, 1986;59–113.
19. Dani J. Open channel structure and ion binding sites of the nicotinic acetylcholine receptor channel. *J Neurosci* 1989;9:884–892.
20. Deneris ES, Connolly J, Rogers SW, Duvoisin R. Pharmacological and functional diversity of neuronal nicotinic acetylcholine receptors. *Trends Pharmacol Sci* 1991;12:34–40.
21. Dilger JP, Brett RS, Lesko LA. Effects of isoflurane on acetylcholine receptor channels. 1. Single channel currents. *Mol Pharmacol* 1992;41:127–133.
22. Dilger JP, Brett RS, Mody HI. Effects of isoflurane on acetylcholine receptor channels. 2. Currents elicited by rapid perfusion of acetylcholine. *Mol Pharmacol* 1993;44:1056–1063.
23. Dilger JP, Liu Y. Desensitization of acetylcholine receptors in BC3H-1 cells. *Pflugers Arch* 1992;420:479–485.
24. Dilger JP, Vidal AM, Mody HI, Liu Y. Evidence for direct actions of general anesthetics on an ion channel protein—a new look at a unified mechanism of action. *Anesthesiology* 1994;81:431–442.
25. Dilger JP, Vidal AM. Cooperative interactions between general anesthetics and QX-222 within the pore of the ACh receptor ion channel. *Mol Pharmacol* 1994;45:169–175.
26. Dwyer TM, Adams DJ, Hille B. The permeability of the endplate channel to organic cations in frog muscle. *J Gen Physiol* 1980;75: 469–492.
27. Ferns MJ, Hall ZW. How many agrins does it take to make a synapse? *Cell* 1992;70:1–3.
28. Ferrer-Montiel AV, Montal M. A negative charge in the M2 transmembrane segment of the neuronal-α-7 acetylcholine receptor increases permeability to divalent cations. *FEBS Lett* 1993;324: 185–190.
29. Fertuck HC, Salpeter MM. Quantitation of junctional and extrajunctional acetylcholine receptors by electron microscope autoradiography after ^{125}I-α-bungarotoxin binding at mouse neuromuscular junctions. *J Cell Biol* 1976;69:144–158.
30. Fogdall RP, Miller RD. Neuromuscular effects of enflurane, alone and combined with d-tubocurarine, pancuronium and succinylcholine, in man. *Anesthesiology* 1975;42:173–178.
31. Galzi JL, Devillers-Thiéry A, Hussy N, Bertrand S, Changeux J-P, Bertrand D. Mutations in the channel domain of a neuronal nicotinic receptor convert ion selectivity from cationic to anionic. *Nature* 1992,359:500–505.
32. Galzi JL, Revah F, Bessis A, Changeux J-P. Functional architecture of the nicotinic acetylcholine receptor—from electric organ to brain. *Annu Rev Pharmacol* 1991;31:37–72.
33. Glavinovic MI, Law Min JC, Kapural L, Donati F, Bevan DR. Speed of action of various muscle relaxants at the neuromuscular junc-

tion binding vs. buffering hypothesis. *J Pharmacol Exp Ther* 1993; 265:1181–1186.
34. Green WN, Claudio T. Acetylcholine receptor assembly: subunit folding and oligomerization occur sequentially. *Cell* 1993;74: 57–69.
35. Green WN, Ross AF, Claudio T. Acetylcholine receptor assembly is stimulated by phosphorylation of its γ subunit. *Neuron* 1991;7: 659–666.
36. Gu Y, Forsayeth JR, Verrall S, Yu XM, Hall ZW. Assembly of the mammalian muscle acetylcholine receptor in transfected COS cells. *J Cell Biol* 1991;114:799–807.
37. Hall ZW, Sanes JR. Synaptic structure and development—the neuromuscular junction. *Cell* 1993;72:99–121.
38. Herz JM, Johnson DA, Taylor P. Distance between the agonist and noncompetitive inhibitor sites on the nicotinic acetylcholine receptor. *J Biol Chem* 1989;264:12439–12448.
39. Hoffman PW, Ravindran A, Huganir RL. Role of phosphorylation in desensitization of acetylcholine receptors expressed in *Xenopus* oocytes. *J Neurosci* 1994;14:4185–4195.
40. Hucho F, Görne-Tschelnokow U, Strecker A. β-structure in the membrane-spanning part of the nicotinic acetylcholine receptor (or how helical are transmembrane helices?) *Trends Biochem Sci* 1994;19:383–387.
41. Huganir RL, Delcour AH, Greengard P, Hess GP. Phosphorylation of the nicotinic acetylcholine receptor regulates its rate of desensitization. *Nature* 1986;321:774–776.
42. Huganir RL, Greengard P. Regulation of receptor function by protein phosphorylation. *Trends Pharmacol Sci* 1987;8:472–477.
43. Ifune CK, Steinbach JH. Rectification of acetylcholine-elicited currents in PC12 pheochromocytoma cells. *Proc Natl Acad Sci USA* 1990;87:4794–4798.
44. Jackson MB, Imoto K, Mishina M, Konno T, Numa S, Sakmann B. Spontaneous and agonist-induced openings of an acetylcholine receptor channel composed of bovine muscle α-, β-, and δ-subunits. *Pflugers Arch* 1990;417:129–135.
45. Jackson MB. Perfection of a synaptic receptor: kinetics and energetics of the acetylcholine receptor. *Proc Natl Acad Sci USA* 1989;86: 2199–2203.
46. Jalkanen L, Meretoja OA, Taivainen T, Brandom BW, Dyanl B. Synergism between atracurium and mivacurium compared with that between vecuronium and mivacurium. *Anesth Analg* 1994;79: 998–1002.
47. Kehoe JS. Acetylcholine receptors in molluscan neurones. *Adv Pharmacol Ther* 1979;8:285–298.
48. Kullberg R, Owens JL, Camacho P, Mandel G, Brehm P. Multiple conductance classes of mouse nicotinic acetylcholine receptors expressed in *Xenopus* oocytes. *Proc Natl Acad Sci USA* 1990;87: 2067–2071.
49. Land BR, Salpeter EE, Salpeter MM. Kinetic parameters for acetylcholine interaction in intact neuromuscular junction. *Proc Natl Acad Sci USA* 1981;78:7200–7204.
50. Lebowitz PW, Ramsey FM, Savarese JJ, Ali HH. Potentiation of neuromuscular blockade in man produced by combinations of pancuronium and metocurine or pancuronium and d-tubocurarine. *Anesth Analg* 1980;59:604–609.
51. Lingle CJ, Maconochie D, Steinbach JH. Activation of skeletal muscle nicotinic acetylcholine receptors. *J Membr Biol* 1992;126: 195–217.
52. Lingle CJ, Steinbach JH. Neuromuscular blocking agents. In: Firestone LL, ed. *Molecular basis of drug action in anesthesia.* Boston: Little, Brown, 1988;288–301.
53. Liu Y, Dilger JP. Decamethonium is a partial agonist at the nicotinic acetylcholine receptor. *Synapse* 1993;13:57–62.
54. Liu Y, Dilger JP. Opening rate of acetylcholine receptor channels. *Biophys J* 1991;60:424–432.
55. Maconochie DJ, Fletcher GH, Steinbach JH. The conductance of the muscle nicotinic receptor channel changes rapidly upon gating. *Biophys J* 1995;68:483–490.
56. Magleby KL, Stevens CF. The effect of voltage on the time course of end-plate currents. *J Physiol* 1972;223:151–171.
57. Marshall CG, Ogden DC, Colquhoun D. The actions of suxamethonium (succinyldicholine) as an agonist and channel blocker at the nicotinic receptor of frog muscle. *J Physiol* 1990;428: 155–174.
58. Meretoja OA, Brandom BW, Taivainen T, Jalkanen L. Synergism between atracurium and vecuronium in children. *Br J Anaesth* 1993;71:440–442.
59. Miles K, Huganir RL. Protein phosphorylation of nicotinic acetylcholine receptors. *Mol Neurobiol* 1988;2:91–124.
60. Miller RD, Eger EI II, Way WL, Stevens WC, Dolan WM. Comparative neuromuscular effects of Forane and halothane alone and in combination with d-tubocurarine in man. *Anesthesiology* 1971;35: 38–42.
61. Murrell RD, Braun MS , Haydon DA. Actions of n-alcohols on nicotinic acetylcholine receptor channels in cultured rat myotubes. *J Physiol* 1991;437:431–448.
62. Neher E. The charge carried by single-channel currents of rat cultured muscle cells in the presence of local anaesthetics. *J Physiol* 1983;339:663–678.
63. Neubig RR, Cohen JB. Equilibrium binding of [^{3}H]tubocurarine and [^{3}H]acetylcholine by *Torpedo* postsynaptic membranes: stoichiometry and ligand interactions. *Biochemistry* 1979;18:5464–5475.
64. Noda M, Takahashi H, Tanabe T, Toyosato M, Kikyotani S, Furutani Y, Hirose T, Takashima H, Inayama S, Miyata T, Numa S. Structural homology of *Torpedo californica* acetylcholine receptor subunits. *Nature* 1983;302:528–532.
65. Ochoa ELM, Chattopadhyay A, McNamee MG. Desensitization of the nicotinic acetylcholine receptor: molecular mechanisms and effects of modulators. *Cell Mol Neurobiol* 1989;9:141–178.
66. Ogden DC, Colquhoun D. Ion channel block by acetylcholine, carbachol and suberyldicholine at the frog neuromuscular junction. *Proc R Soc Lond B* 1985;225:329–355.
67. Paton WDM, Waud DR. The margin of safety of neuromuscular transmission. *J Physiol (Lond)* 1967;l91:59–90.
68. Patrick J, Sequela P, Vernino S, Amador M, Luetje C, Dani JA. Functional diversity of neuronal nicotinic acetylcholine receptors. *Progr Brain Res* 1993;98:113–120.
69. Pearce AC, Casson WR, Jones RM. Factors affecting train of four fade. *Br J Anaesth* 1985;57:602–606.
70. Pennefather P, Quastel DMJ. Modification of dose-response curves by effector blockade and uncompetitive antagonism. *Mol Pharmacol* 1982;22:369–380.
71. Pereira EFR, Alkondon M, Tano T, Castro NG, Froesferrao MM, Rozental R, Aronstam RS, Schrattenholz A, Maelicke A, Albuquerque EX. A novel agonist binding site on nicotinic acetylcholine receptors. *J Recept Res* 1993;13:413–436.
72. Phillips WD, Kopta C, Blount P, Gardner PD, Steinbach JH, Merlie JP. ACh receptor-rich membrane domains organized in fibroblasts by recombinant 43-kilodalton protein. *Science* 1991;251:568–570.
73. Phillips WD, Merlie JP. Recombinant neuromuscular synapses. *Bioessays* 1992;14:671–679.
74. Redman RS, Silinsky EM. ATP released together with acetylcholine as the mediator of neuromuscular depression at frog motor nerve endings. *J Physiol (Lond)* 1994;477:117–127.
75. Sakmann B, Brenner HR. Change in synaptic channel gating during neuromuscular development. *Nature* 1978;276:401–402.
76. Sargent PB. The diversity of neuronal nicotinic acetylcholine receptors. *Annu Rev Neurosci* 1993;16:403–443.
77. Sine S, Taylor P. Functional consequences of agonist-mediated state transitions in the cholinergic receptor. Studies in cultured muscle cells. *J Biol Chem* 1979;254:3315–3325.
78. Sine S. Functional properties of human skeletal muscle acetylcholine receptors expressed by the TE671 cell line. *J Biol Chem* 1988;263:18052–18062.
79. Sine SM, Claudio T, Sigworth FJ. Activation of *Torpedo* acetylcholine receptors expressed in mouse fibroblasts. Single channel current kinetics reveal distinct agonist binding affinities. *J Gen Physiol* 1990;96:395–437.
80. Sine SM, Claudio T. γ-and δ-Subunits regulate the affinity and the cooperativity of ligand binding to the acetylcholine receptor. *J Biol Chem* 1991;266:19369–19377.
81. Sine SM, Steinbach JH. Agonists block currents through acetylcholine receptor channels. *Biophys J* 1984,46:277–284.
82. Sine SM, Taylor P. Relationship between reversible antagonist occupancy and the functional capacity of the acetylcholine receptor. *J Biol Chem* 1981;256:6692–6699.
83. Steinbach JH, Zempel J. What does phosphorylation do for the nicotinic acetylcholine receptor? *Trends Neurosci* 1987;10:61–64.
84. Takeda K, Trautmann A. A patch-clamp study of the partial agonist actions of tubocurarine on rat myotubes. *J Physiol* 1984;349: 353–374.
85. Taylor P. Are neuromuscular blocking agents more effective in pairs? *Anesthesiology* 1985;63:1–3.

86. Tian LJ, Prior C, Dempster J, Marshall IG. Nicotinic antagonist-produced frequency-dependent changes in acetylcholine release from rat motor nerve terminals. *J Physiol (Lond)* 1994;476:517–529.
87. Unwin N. Nicotinic acetylcholine receptor at 9 Å resolution. *J Mol Biol* 1993;229:1101–1124.
88. Unwin N. Acetylcholine receptor channel imaged in the open state. *Nature* 1995;373:37–43.
89. Valenzuela CF, Weign P, Yguerabide J, Johnson DA. Transverse distance between the membrane and the agonist binding sites on the *Torpedo* acetylcholine receptor—a fluorescence study. *Biophys J* 1994;66:674–682.
90. Villarroel A, Sakmann B. Threonine in the selectivity filter of the acetylcholine receptor channel. *Biophys J* 1992;62:196–208.
91. Wachtel RE, Wegrzynowicz ES. Kinetics of nicotinic acetylcholine ion channels in the presence of intravenous anaesthetics and induction agents. *Br J Pharmacol* 1992;106:623–627.
92. Wachtel RE. Ketamine decreases the open time of single-channel currents activated by acetylcholine. *Anesthesiology* 1988;68: 563–570.
93. Wachtel RE. Physostigmine block of ion channels activated by acetylcholine in BC3H1-cells. *Mol Pharmacol* 1993;44:1051–1055.
94. Waud BE, Waud DR. Interaction among agents that block end-plate depolarization competitively. *Anesthesiology* 1985;63:4–15.
95. Waud BE, Waud DR. Muscle relaxant interactions. In: Agoston S, Bowman WC, eds. *Muscle relaxants.* Amsterdam: Elsevier, 1990; 231–243.
96. Weill CL, McNamee MC, Karlin A. Affinity labeling of purified acetylcholine receptor from *Torpedo californica. Biochem Biophys Res Commun* 1974;61:997–1003.
97. White BH, Cohen JB. Agonist-induced changes in the structure of the acetylcholine receptor M2 regions revealed by photoincorporation of an uncharged nicotinic noncompetitive antagonist. *J Biol Chem* 1992;267:15770–15783.
98. Yawo H. Rectification of synaptic and acetylcholine currents in the mouse submandibular ganglion cells. *J Physiol* 1989;417:307–322.
99. Yee GH, Huganir RL. Determination of the sites of cAMP-dependent phosphorylation on the nicotinic acetylcholine receptor. *J Biol Chem* 1987;262:16748–16753.
100. Yu XM, Hall ZW. A sequence in the main cytoplasmic loop of the α subunit is required for assembly of mouse muscle nicotinic acetylcholine receptor. *Neuron* 1994;13:247–255.
101. Zaimis E. Motor end-plate differences as a determining factor in the mode of action of neuromuscular blocking substances. *J Physiol* 1953;122:238–251.
102. Zaimis E. The neuromuscular junction: areas of uncertainty. *Handbook Exp Pharmacol* 1976;42:1–21.

Anesthesia: Biologic Foundations, edited by
Tony L. Yaksh et al. Lippincott–Raven Publishers,
Philadelphia © 1997.

CHAPTER 15

ANESTHETIC ACTIONS ON EXCITATORY AMINO ACID RECEPTORS

ROBERT W. PEOPLES AND FORREST F. WEIGHT

Glutamate is now recognized as the neurotransmitter at the majority of excitatory synapses in the central nervous system. Glutamate mediates fast and slow neurotransmission via stimulation of three general classes of excitatory amino acid receptors: *N*-methyl-D-aspartate (NMDA) receptors, α–amino-3-hydroxy-5-methyl-4-isoxazolepropionic acid (AMPA)/kainate receptors, and metabotropic glutamate receptors. The importance of these receptors in subserving central nervous system excitatory neurotransmission makes these receptors likely target sites of sedative or anesthetic agents, as inhibiting the function of these receptors would be predicted to depress central nervous system excitability.

As a comprehensive review of the current state of knowledge of the seemingly exponentially expanding field of excitatory amino acid receptor structure and function is beyond the scope of this chapter, what follows is a brief summary of this field. For a more detailed treatment, several recent reviews are available (11,95,190,219,220,270,274).

NMDA RECEPTORS

Structure and Function

NMDA receptors are ligand-gated cation channels with several unusual features, which result in distinctive functional properties. NMDA receptor activity is strongly voltage dependent due to block by Mg^{2+} ions at negative membrane potentials (188,224), with the result that it contributes little to neuronal function except when the neuron is depolarized. The NMDA receptor is also highly permeable to Ca^{2+} ions (112,186), so that when it is stimulated under depolarizing conditions it allows the entry of Ca^{2+} into the cell. In addition, the NMDA receptor has complex ion channel gating kinetics, which produce synaptic currents that activate and deactivate relatively slowly (70,146,147). This permits temporal summation of synaptic inputs; that is, it allows for a longer interval in which two or more subthreshold synaptic impulses arriving at different times can together produce a threshold response. Finally, NMDA receptor activity is modulated by a large number of agents, including the coagonist glycine (118,130), Mg^{2+} (188,224), Zn^{2+} (237,317), Ca^{2+} (144,259,265,338), polyamines (198,251,289), oxidizing and reducing agents (2), protons (302,308), fatty acids (205,222,238,297), protein kinases (35,36,69,78,81,166,197,311), and phosphatases (149,310,311). These properties are believed to imbue the NMDA receptor with a number of unique information processing capabilities. In addition, functional studies have implicated NMDA receptors in a variety of neural phenomena such as certain types of learning and memory (22,50,213), motor coordination (33,66,323), and neurotoxicity and neurodegenerative isorders (64,143,152,330).

The NMDA receptor is thought to be a pentamer composed of at least two types of receptor subunits: NMDAR1 (212) (or ζ1 [333]) and NMDAR2 (110,209) (or ε [140,200]). NMDAR1 is widely distributed throughout the nervous system (212,219). NMDAR2 subunits are further subdivided into at least four subtypes, NMDAR2A to NMDAR2D (or ε1 to ε4), which differ in their distribution in the CNS (200,209), pattern of expression during development (312,313), and pharmacologic properties (140,200,209). In addition, at least nine variants of the NMDAR1 subunit and at least two variants of the NMDAR2 subunit may occur in vivo due to RNA splicing (57,58,93,110,217, 292); these splice variants differ in several functional properties, including sensitivity to agonists, antagonists, and modulators (57,93,217). Both types of subunits have a large extracellular domain, which, at least in the NMDAR1 subunit, is believed to contain the glutamate and glycine binding sites (212,333); whether the NMDAR2 subunit contributes to these sites is not known at present. By analogy to AMPA/kainate receptors (see below), each NMDA receptor subunit appears to have three membrane-spanning regions, TM1, TM3, and TM4 (Fig. 1), and a loop, TM2, that dips into the plane of the membrane from the cytoplasmic side but does not traverse the membrane (16,96,326). The *N*-terminal domain is located extracellularly, whereas the *C*-terminal domain is located in the cytoplasm (301). TM2 appears to line the ion channel pore; in addition, it contains an asparagine residue at the site analogous to the Q/R site of AMPA/kainate receptors (see below). In the NMDAR1 subunit, this site appears to control primarily Ca^{2+} permeability, whereas in the NMDAR2 subunit this site appears to affect primarily susceptibility to Mg^{2+} block (29,210,264).

Possible Role in Anesthesia

Noncompetitive NMDA receptor antagonists can induce an anesthetic state referred to as dissociative anesthesia (see below). Several investigators have also reported sedative and anesthetic effects of competitive NMDA receptor antagonists. France and colleagues (66) report that at high doses, the competitive NMDA receptor antagonist *cis*-4-phosphonomethyl-2-piperidine-carboxylic acid (CGS 19755) produced anesthesia as assessed by loss of righting reflex and loss of reactivity to painful stimulation in rhesus monkeys. Rabbani et al. (243) observed that the competitive NMDA antagonists CGP 37849 and CGP 39551 produced decreased motor activity and sedation in mice. Finally, Daniell (49) reported that NMDA antagonists administered intracerebroventricularly produce anesthesia. A caveat of these studies is that at the high doses of NMDA antagonists required to produce sedation and anesthesia, these agents could be less selective for NMDA receptors. Thus, it is unclear whether the large doses of NMDA antagonists were required to produce a certain percentage of inhibition of NMDA receptors, or to produce an action at another site.

AMPA AND KAINATE RECEPTORS

Structure and Function

Non-NMDA ionotropic glutamate receptors are a group of ligand-gated cation channels that are broadly classified as AMPA or kainate receptors based on their agonist sensitivity. Non-NMDA ionotropic glutamate receptors are distinguished from NMDA receptors by a number of characteristics. Unlike NMDA receptors, they have rapid channel gating kinetics,

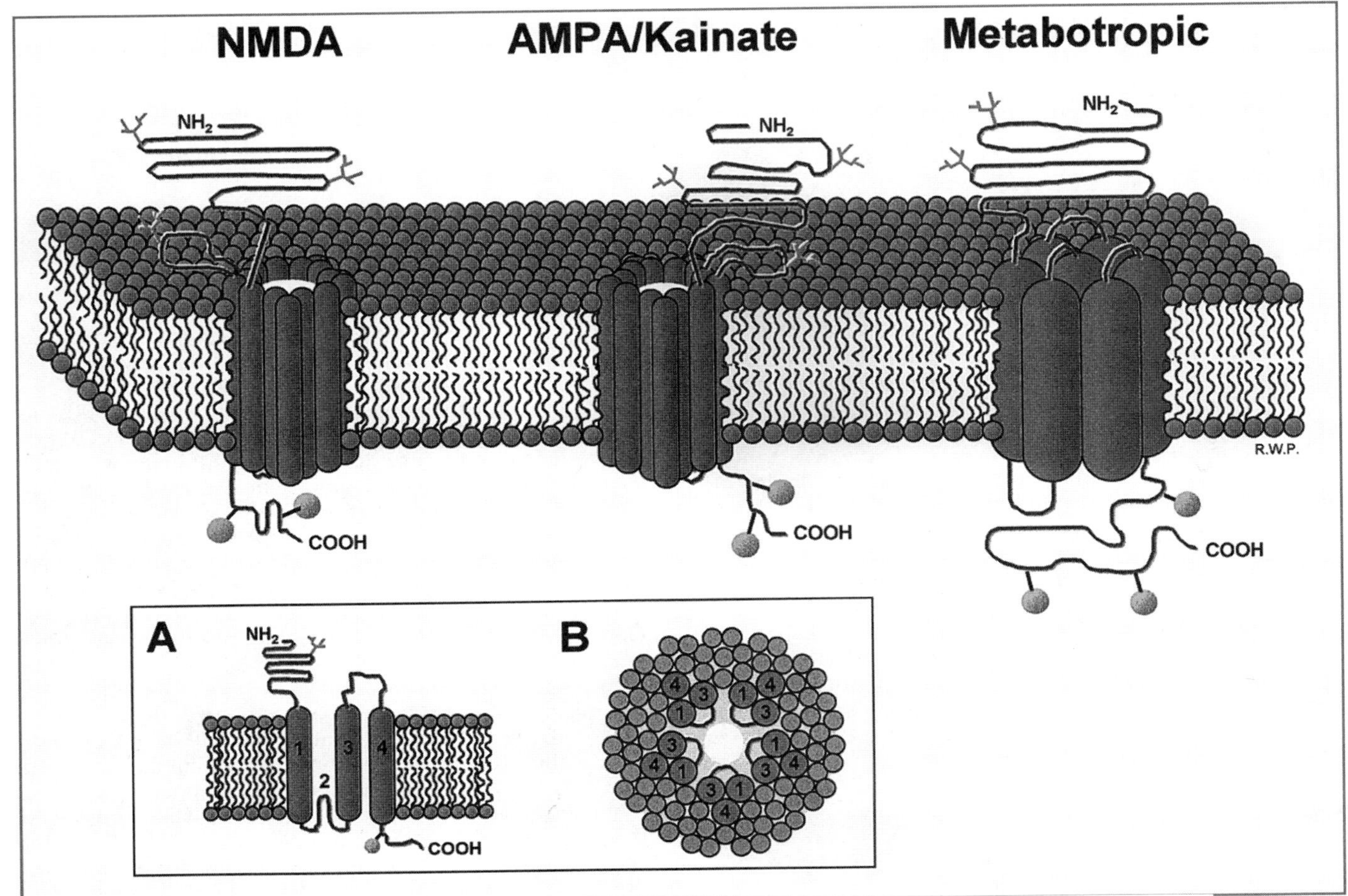

Figure 1. Proposed models of the subunit structure of the NMDA *(left)*, AMPA/kainate *(center)*, and metabotropic *(right)* glutamate receptors. Membrane-spanning domains are shown in *blue,* and other regions in *dark green.* Extracellular sites may be glycosylated, as indicated by the branched structures in *red,* and intracellular sites may be phosphorylated, as indicated by the *orange* spheres. In the models shown, NMDA and AMPA/kainate receptor subunits have three membrane-spanning domains (designated 1, 3, 4) and a loop (designated 2) that enters but does not traverse the plane of the membrane (**Inset,** A). NMDA and AMPA/kainate receptor-ion channels consist of groups of five subunits arranged around a central pore (shown in cross section in **Inset**, B). Metabotropic receptors are linked to intracellular second messenger systems and have seven membrane-spanning domains. Extracellular and intracellular domains of NMDA and AMPA/kainate receptors are shown on only one subunit for clarity. *(See color plate 1.)*

resulting in very fast synaptic currents (221,280,296,304), they have current-voltage relations that are linear or moderately outwardly rectifying (7,120,187) (apparently due to voltage dependence of desensitization [232]), they are (in general) impermeable to Ca^{2+} (106,120,186), and they are unaffected by most of the agents that modulate NMDA receptor function (e.g., they are insensitive to glycine, Mg^{2+}, oxidizing and reducing agents, and protons). Although these properties of AMPA/kainate receptors do not invest them with the integrative capabilities of NMDA receptors, they make them ideally suited for high-frequency impulse transmission.

Non-NMDA ionotropic glutamate receptors are also thought to be pentameric structures composed of one or more types of subunits. The subunit composition of the receptor determines its physiologic properties, such as agonist sensitivity and desensitization rate. At least nine subunits have been identified in mammalian brain, of which four, GluR1 to GluR4 (or GluRA to GluRD), are selective for AMPA, and five, GluR5 to GluR7 and KA-1 to KA-2, are selective for kainate (21,27,59,87,97,128,211, 218,262,263,288,316). Although kainate receptors are widely distributed in the brain, their role in CNS function remains to be determined (274). AMPA receptors, on the other hand, appear to mediate the majority of fast excitatory transmission in the CNS (274). AMPA/kainate receptor subunits appear to have a large extracellular *N*-terminal region containing the agonist binding site, three transmembrane domains, TM1, TM3, and TM4, a reentrant loop, TM2, that lines the ion channel pore, and an intracellular carboxy terminus (Fig. 1) (16,96,290,326). As mentioned above, the TM2 region of AMPA receptors contains the Q/R site, which dictates the Ca^{2+} permeability and voltage dependence of the ion channel. When this site contains a glutamine residue, as do the GluR1, GluR3, and GluR4 subunits, the resulting ion channels are highly permeable to Ca^{2+} and exhibit strong inward rectification, whereas when this site contains an arginine residue, as in the GluR2 subunit, the resulting ion channels resemble most of the native AMPA receptors, in that they are impermeable to Ca^{2+} and exhibit slight outward rectification (27,28,94,104, 306). Interestingly, the presence of Ca^{2+}-permeable AMPA receptors has been reported in hippocampal neurons and astrocytes (71,108). The Q/R site of kainate receptors appears to function in a similar, albeit more complex, manner (for discussion see ref. 274).

In the great majority of studies of anesthetic effects on non-NMDA glutamate receptors, the precise identity and subunit composition of the receptors was not determined. Thus, in the following discussion AMPA and kainate receptors will be considered together.

Possible Role in Anesthesia

As AMPA/kainate receptors are believed to mediate the majority of fast excitatory synaptic transmission in the brain, inhibition of these receptors would be predicted to have profound consequences for CNS excitability. These receptors would therefore be possible sites of action of anesthetics. Until relatively recently, however, investigation of the physiologic roles of non-NMDA glutamate receptors was hampered by the unavailability of highly selective and potent antagonists for these receptors. The synthesis by Honoré et al. (99) and Sheardown et al. (277) of the quinoxalinedione non-NMDA receptor antagonists was a significant breakthrough that has facilitated rapid progress in the field. One of the most selective of these agents for AMPA/kainate receptors is 2,3-dihydroxy-6-nitro-7-sulfamoyl-benzo(f)quinoxaline (NBQX) (277). Dall et al. (45) have communicated preliminary evidence that NBQX given intracerebroventricularly or intravenously at high doses induces anesthesia in rodents. In contrast, Juhász and colleagues (125) reported that 6-cyano-7-nitroquinoxaline-2,3-dione (CNQX) applied via microdialysis in the ventroposterolateral thalamic nuclei of cats reduced the number of episodes of wakefulness and enhanced the duration of episodes of slow-wave sleep, but did not produce evident behavioral effects. The failure of CNQX to produce anesthesia or sedation in this study may not necessarily negate a role of non-NMDA receptors in anesthesia, but may rather reflect the very limited region of the brain affected by CNQX applied in this manner. Support for this conclusion may be drawn from the observation that the NMDA antagonist 2-amino-5-phosphonovalerate (APV) failed to produce behavioral effects when administered by microdialysis to the same thalamic nuclei, although competitive NMDA antagonists administered by other methods in other studies have been shown to produce sedation and anesthesia (66,243). Further studies will thus be required to resolve this issue.

METABOTROPIC GLUTAMATE RECEPTORS

Structure and Function

Unlike the NMDA and AMPA/kainate receptors, the metabotropic glutamate receptors are not ion channels, but rather are coupled to various signal transduction systems via G proteins. These receptors mediate much slower responses than the ionotropic receptors, and consequently usually subserve neuromodulation rather than neurotransmission (220). Although the physiologic roles of metabotropic receptors remain largely uncharacterized, they appear to be involved in information processing in the visual (223) and olfactory (86) systems, and have been implicated in neurotoxicity (136,194, 195,261,271,279), and in forms of synaptic plasticity thought to underlie certain types of learning and memory (12,26, 256,257,337).

Eight metabotropic glutamate receptor subunits have so far been identified, which can be classified on the basis of their associated transduction systems and their agonist sensitivity. Two of the subunits, mGluR1 and mGluR5, stimulate the formation of inositol trisphosphate (1,5,101,185), while the remaining six subunits, mGluR2 to mGluR4 and mGluR6 to mGluR8, inhibit the synthesis of cyclic AMP (216,228,266,294, 295). Of the latter six subunits, mGluR2, mGluR3, and mGluR8 are most sensitive to *trans*-1-amino-cyclopentane-1,3-dicarboxylate (ACPD) (294,295), while mGluR4, mGluR6, and mGluR7 are most sensitive to L-2-amino-4-phosphonobutyrate (L-AP4) (216,228,266,295). Each of these subunits appears to have seven transmembrane domains, and a large extracellular *N*-terminal region thought to contain the ligand-binding site (225,293) (Fig. 1).

Possible Role in Anesthesia

Few studies have addressed the behavioral effects of metabotropic glutamate receptor agonists and antagonists, and of these, only a single study has addressed potential anesthetic effects of such agents. Miyamoto and colleagues (206) investigated the effects of intracerebroventricular injection of (2*S*,1'*R*,2'*R*,3'*R*)-2-(2,3-dicarboxycyclopropyl)glycine (DCG-IV), a selective agonist at mGluR2 and mGluR3 metabotropic glutamate receptors, in rats. These investigators reported that DCG-IV produced marked sedation, and increased the duration of halothane anesthesia (assessed by loss of righting reflex) by up to fivefold. The less selective metabotropic receptor antagonists (1*S*,3*R*)-ACPD and 2*S*,1'*S*,2'*S*)-2-(carboxycyclopropyl)glycine (L-CCG-I) also prolonged halothane anesthesia, but much less potently than DCG-IV. More detailed studies will be required to define the mechanism by which metabotropic receptor agonists prolong the action of anesthetics, and to determine whether metabotropic receptors have any role in producing the effects of anesthetics.

ACTIONS OF VARIOUS CLASSES OF ANESTHETICS ON EXCITATORY AMINO ACID RECEPTORS

Barbiturates

Barbiturates are among the most widely studied anesthetic agents, largely because they have a long history of extensive clinical use, and because their physical characteristics, particularly their relatively high aqueous solubility and their nonvolatility, are amenable to experimental investigation. Despite a large body of evidence for effects of anesthetics on excitatory amino acid receptors, the potential importance of excitatory amino acid receptors in contributing to or mediating the anesthetic state has been largely obscured by the more recent attention directed toward the γ-aminobutyric acid ($GABA_A$) receptor as a site of action of barbiturates. While barbiturate effects on the $GABA_A$ receptor are undoubtedly important, it is often overlooked that in many cases barbiturates affect $GABA_A$ receptors and excitatory amino acid receptors with equal potency.

NMDA Receptors

Behavioral Experiments Drug discrimination is an operant behavioral technique that allows the subjective effects of drugs to be compared in a quantitative manner (323). In drug discrimination procedures, an animal is trained to recognize whether it has been administered a particular drug (at a given dose) or vehicle, and to respond in a specified manner (e.g., pressing a lever) depending on which drug it has received. The extent to which the animal perceives a test drug to be like the drug it was trained to recognize (whether the test drug substitutes for the training drug) can then be estimated. In pigeons, the noncompetitive NMDA receptor antagonists ketamine and dextrorphan partially substituted for pentobarbital, suggesting that the subjective effects of these drugs are similar, but not identical to, those of barbiturates (88). Similarly, Willetts and colleagues (322, 324) reported that in rats, competitive (3-((±)-2-carboxypiperazin-4-yl) propyl-1-phosphonic acid [CPP] and 2-amino-4,5-(1,2-cyclohexyl)-7-phosphonoheptanoic acid [NPC 12626]) and noncompetitive (1-[1-phenylcyclohexyl]piperidine [phencyclidine] and [(+)-5-methyl-10,11-dihydro-5*H*-dibenzo[*a,d*]cyclohepten-5,10-imine maleate [MK-801]) NMDA receptor antagonists substituted for pentobarbital only partially. In mice, CPP substituted for pentobarbital, but at doses that reduced rates of responding, while MK-801 only partially substituted for pentobarbital (325). Koek and coworkers (133) observed that pentobarbital failed to substitute for phencyclidine, and failed to block the discriminative stimulus effects of NMDA in rats. The observation that pentobarbital appears to act as an NMDA receptor antagonist only partially at best in these studies may indicate either that barbiturates produce a complex discriminative stimulus through actions at several sites, including the NMDA receptor, or that CNS depressants acting at different sites may be perceived as being similar to some extent.

If NMDA receptors have a role in mediating the anesthetic effect of barbiturates, then antagonists of the NMDA receptor may be expected to increase, and NMDA agonists decrease, barbiturate anesthesia. Consistent with this hypothesis, the noncompetitive NMDA antagonists MK-801, phencyclidine, and ketamine, at subanesthetic doses, increased the duration of loss of righting reflex produced by pentobarbital in mice (46). Similarly, the competitive NMDA antagonist CGS 19755 increased the duration of pentobarbital-induced loss of righting reflex by up to twofold for pentobarbital (47). The polyamines spermine and spermidine, which at low concentrations enhance the activity of the NMDA receptor (198,258, 289), also increased the duration of loss of righting reflex produced by pentobarbital (48). As the interactions of polyamines with NMDA receptors are complex, however (18,198,258,289), and polyamines interact with multiple sites in vivo (272), this latter result does not necessarily implicate NMDA receptors as a site of action of barbiturates. Moreover, while the ability of NMDA antagonists to increase the duration of barbiturate anesthesia provides evidence for a role of the NMDA receptor in contributing to the anesthetic state, it does not by itself establish that the anesthetic effects of barbiturates are due to NMDA receptor inhibition. Other CNS depressants, such as clonidine, that do not interact with NMDA receptors can also increase the anesthetic potency of barbiturates (145).

The addictive liability of barbiturates is well known, and, in addition to their toxicity in high doses, is primarily responsible for their supersession in clinical use by the benzodiazepine sedative/hypnotics. The barbiturate withdrawal syndrome is characterized by generalized CNS excitation, which can result in life-threatening convulsions. In barbiturate-dependent rats, the NMDA receptor antagonists 2-amino-7-phosphonoheptanoic acid (AP7) or $MgSO_4$ reduced the incidence of barbiturate withdrawal-induced seizures when administered intracerebroventricularly (191,192). In addition, the selective competitive NMDA receptor antagonists CGP 39551 and CGP 37849, which cross the blood-brain barrier, reduced barbital withdrawal-induced seizures in mice (243). These results may indicate that barbiturate dependence produces an increase in NMDA receptor density or sensitivity in certain brain regions (see below), or may simply reflect the importance of the NMDA receptor in regulating CNS excitability. Whether the ability of NMDA antagonists to suppress the seizures elicited by withdrawal from barbiturates reflects a direct interaction of barbiturates with the NMDA receptor-ion channel cannot be determined from these studies.

Binding Experiments Martin and coworkers (184) reported that barbiturates inhibited the binding of the NMDA competitive antagonist [^{3}H]CGS 19755 and the NMDA noncompetitive antagonist [^{3}H]MK-801 in a rat brain membrane preparation. These investigators reported that pentobarbital and secobarbital inhibited [^{3}H]CGS 19755 binding with IC_{50} values of 6 and 3 mM, respectively, and [^{3}H]MK-801 binding with respective IC_{50} values of 2.5 and 1.5 mM. Martin et al. concluded that the mechanism of inhibition of [^{3}H]CGS 19755 binding was noncompetitive, as the barbiturates decreased the apparent density of binding sites but not the apparent affinity of binding, but that the mechanism of inhibition of [^{3}H]MK-801 binding was competitive, as barbiturates decreased the apparent affinity but not the apparent binding site density. These investigators further concluded that the differences in the IC_{50} values reflected dual, unrelated actions of the barbiturates. Honoré et al. (99) and Sheardown et al. (277) reported that the IC_{50} for pentobarbital inhibition of the binding of the competitive NMDA antagonist [^{3}H]CPP, if determinable, was above 1 mM. These investigators did not report, however, whether they observed any inhibition of [^{3}H]CPP binding by 1 mM pentobarbital. Similarly, Rabbani et al. (243) concluded that barbiturates do not interact with the dissociative anesthetic binding site on the NMDA receptor, because barbital did not displace [^{3}H]MK-801 binding in mouse cortical membranes or alter displacement of [^{3}H]MK-801 binding by the phencyclidine analogue thienylcyclohexylpiperidine (TCP). As barbital is nearly 25 times less hydrophobic than pentobarbital (137), and the potency of barbiturates is correlated with their hydrophobicity (30,80), the IC_{50} for barbital inhibition of [^{3}H]MK-801 binding would be predicted to be much higher than the pentobarbital IC_{50} of 2.5 mM (perhaps 50 mM or higher). Therefore, it is possible that Rabbani et al. may have failed to observe barbital displacement of [^{3}H]MK-801 binding because they tested the effect of barbital only at a concentration of 100 μM. Nevertheless, it should be noted that if, as reported by Martin et al., barbiturates do interact with the NMDA receptor, they may do so only at concentrations far in excess of those required to produce anesthesia (anesthetic concentrations of pentobarbital are considered to be 50 to 200 μM [255]).

Barbiturates administered repeatedly also appear to regulate the expression of NMDA receptors. Repeated administration of phenobarbital or barbital to mice resulted in an increase in the B_{max} (receptor density) of [^{3}H]MK-801 binding but no change in the K_d (affinity) in membranes from cerebral cortex, and no change in [^{3}H]MK-801 binding in hippocampus (243,278). While the upregulation of NMDA receptors in response to prolonged CNS depression by barbiturates is likely to represent an important compensatory mechanism, it is unclear whether it results from a direct effect of barbiturates on the NMDA receptor, or from an indirect effect (i.e., one mediated by a different receptor type), perhaps due to a decrease in glutamatergic neurotransmission.

Biochemical Experiments Teichberg and colleagues (299) reported that a series of barbiturates spanning a wide range of hydrophobicity and anesthetic potency (from barbital to secobarbital) did not inhibit efflux of $^{22}Na^+$ evoked by glutamate, aspartate, or NMDA in rat striatal slices. In contrast, subsequent studies have revealed effects of barbiturates on NMDA receptors. Martin et al. (184) reported that pentobarbital inhibited NMDA-stimulated $^{45}Ca^{2+}$ uptake into rat brain membrane vesicles with an IC_{50} of approximately 300 μM. Cai and McCaslin (31) found that thiamylal and secobarbital, but not pentobarbital or phenobarbital, blocked NMDA-induced elevations in intracellular Ca^{2+} in rat cerebellar granule cells in culture, and Daniell (49) recently reported that a series of barbiturates inhibited NMDA-evoked increases in Ca^{2+} in rat hippocampal membrane vesicles. The reasons for the discrepancy between the findings of these latter studies and those of Teichberg et al. are unclear. It is possible that Cai and McCaslin did not observe NMDA receptor inhibition by pentobarbital and phenobarbital because they tested each barbiturate at a concentration of 100 μM. However, this explanation cannot account for the results of Teichberg and colleagues, who tested each barbiturate at a concentration of 1 mM, at which concentration the more hydrophobic and potent barbiturates such as secobarbital and pentobarbital would be expected to produce an effect.

Interestingly, the upregulation of NMDA receptors by repeated administration of barbiturates has also been observed in vitro. In rat cerebellar granule neurons in culture, 4 days of exposure to thiamylal or phenobarbital followed by removal of barbiturates from the culture medium produced an enhanced intracellular Ca^{2+} response to NMDA (31). This result provides support for the view that barbiturates upregulate NMDA receptors by an action on the same neurons expressing NMDA receptors, rather than by acting on impinging neurons, but does not necessarily indicate a direct action of barbiturates on the NMDA receptors.

Electrophysiologic Experiments Some of the earliest electrophysiologic studies of anesthetic action addressed the effect of barbiturates on excitatory amino acid receptor-mediated synaptic events. This section, as well as the following sections discussing electrophysiologic experiments, will address anesthetic effects on responses to exogenous agonists. For a review of anesthetic effects on synaptic transmission, the reader is referred to Chapter 17.

Many of the early studies of barbiturate effects on responses mediated by excitatory amino acid receptors were performed prior to the discovery of the NMDA receptor and the elucidation of its physiology and pharmacology. These studies thus were not performed under conditions that would allow determination in retrospect of the relative contribution of NMDA receptors to the excitatory amino acid receptor-mediated events under investigation. For example, many of these studies used excitatory amino acid agonists, such as glutamate and D,L-homocysteic acid, which have little or no selectivity for NMDA vs. non-NMDA receptors, and most, if not all, of the early studies were performed using solutions containing Mg^{2+}, which blocks the NMDA receptor at negative membrane potentials (188,224). These studies will therefore be discussed in the section on AMPA/kainate receptors, and this convention will also be followed in subsequent sections.

A number of studies have addressed the effects of barbiturates on NMDA receptor-mediated responses in brain slice preparations. Pentobarbital at concentrations up to 300 μM failed to inhibit NMDA-evoked depolarization in rat cerebral cortical slices, despite significantly inhibiting responses to kainate and quisqualate (82). In contrast, in guinea pig hippocampal slices, pentobarbital blocked NMDA-evoked depolarization, although it blocked responses to glutamate, kainate, and quisqualate more potently (267). Collins and Anson (39) also observed inhibition of NMDA-induced depolarization in rat olfactory cortex slices by pentobarbital, phenobarbital, and thiopental, but found different patterns of sensitivity of the excitatory amino acid agonist responses to inhibition among the barbiturates tested. For example, while the apparent order of potency for pentobarbital was quisqualate ≥ kainate > NMDA, for thiopental the apparent order of potency was quisqualate > kainate = NMDA. Although Collins and Anson did not determine IC_{50} values for the barbiturates, the apparent NMDA receptor inhibitory potency of the barbiturates tested corresponded to their anesthetic potency. Other investigators have reported that both methohexital and thiopental inhibited NMDA- and AMPA-stimulated depolarization in mouse cortical slices to a similar extent (32,230).

Results of more recent experiments utilizing whole-cell patch-clamp recording in cultured neurons were not consistent with the majority of experiments performed in brain slices, in that they demonstrated little or no inhibition of NMDA receptors by barbiturates. In mouse hippocampal neurons in culture, the barbiturates pentobarbital and phenobarbital inhibited NMDA-activated current only at very high concentrations (e.g., the IC_{50} for pentobarbital inhibition of NMDA-activated current was ~ 1mM), despite potently inhibiting kainate- and quisqualate-activated current (314,315). Similarly, pentobarbital at a concentration of 100 μM significantly inhibited ion current activated by kainate and quisqualate, but not NMDA, in rat cortical neurons in culture (179).

Mechanism of Action Based upon results of ligand binding experiments, Martin et al. (184) concluded that barbiturates have dual actions on NMDA receptors: a direct interaction with the MK-801 binding site and another action resulting in a noncompetitive inhibition of binding to the NMDA/glutamate site. As other investigators did not report effects of barbiturates on ligand binding to the NMDA/glutamate (99,277) or MK-801 (243) sites, however, these conclusions have not been confirmed. Experimental techniques that yield the most information about mechanism of action of modulators of the NMDA receptor, such as whole-cell and single-channel patch-clamp recording, have not detected consistent effects of barbiturates at concentrations associated with anesthesia. Thus, the mechanism by which barbiturates inhibit the NMDA receptor-ion channel remains to be determined.

AMPA/Kainate Receptors

Behavioral Experiments As noted above, behavioral studies of the effects of non-NMDA excitatory amino acid antagonists and their interaction with various anesthetics have, until relatively recently, been hindered by the unavailability of potent and selective antagonists that gain access to the CNS. Dall and colleagues (45) have recently utilized the selective and centrally active non-NMDA receptor antagonist NBQX to provide evidence for an influence of AMPA/kainate receptor antagonism upon barbiturate anesthesia. NBQX administered by intravenous infusion increased, in a dose-dependent manner, the duration of the loss of righting reflex produced by hexobarbital in rats. The highest dose of NBQX that was tested (1.1 mg/kg/min) prolonged the duration of hexobarbital anesthesia by over fourfold. Dall et al. also reported that NBQX did not alter plasma concentrations of hexobarbital, and concluded that its effect on the duration of hexobarbital anesthesia is attributable to non-NMDA receptor inhibition rather than to an alteration in the pharmacokinetic disposition of hexobarbital. The enhancement of barbiturate anesthesia via inhibition of AMPA/kainate receptors observed in this study, along with evidence that barbiturates at anesthetic concentrations inhibit AMPA/kainate receptors in vitro, suggests that this mechanism also contributes to the CNS depression produced by barbiturates in vivo.

Binding Experiments Results from receptor binding studies indicate that pentobarbital does not alter the specific binding of [^{3}H]AMPA, [^{3}H]kainate, or the non-NMDA excitatory amino acid antagonist [^{3}H]CNQX (99,184,277). Thus, assuming first that the mechanism of action of pentobarbital does not differ qualitatively from that of other barbiturates, and second that each subtype of non-NMDA receptor was present and detectable in the receptor binding assays used in these studies, these results indicate that barbiturates do not interact with the ligand-binding site of AMPA/kainate receptors. If the above assumptions are valid, then effects of barbiturates on non-NMDA receptors would be expected to occur via a noncompetitive mechanism.

Biochemical Experiments Teichberg et al. (299) reported that a series of barbiturates (pentobarbital, phenobarbital, secobarbital, amobarbital, butabarbital, and barbital) blocked $^{22}Na^+$ efflux from rat striatal slices evoked by kainate or quisqualate. These investigators found that the potency of the various barbiturates for inhibition of responses to kainate or quisqualate was similar (~150 μM), but the efficacy of the various barbiturates differed significantly (from <10% for barbital to 70% to 80% for secobarbital), and generally corresponded to their anesthetic potency. Stated another way, these authors suggested that the higher the anesthetic potency (the dose or concentration necessary to produce anesthesia) of a given barbiturate, the greater the number of receptors inhibited at the maximal concentration (efficacy). It seems possible, however, that these investigators did not test full concentration ranges for each barbiturate, and consequently obtained low estimates for maximal inhibition.

Cai and McCaslin (31) observed inhibition by barbiturates of excitatory amino acid-stimulated increases in intracellular Ca^{2+}. In this study, the barbiturates pentobarbital, secobarbital, and thiamylal inhibited kainate- and quisqualate-evoked increases in intracellular Ca^{2+} in rat cerebellar granule neurons in primary culture. Although phenobarbital was reportedly without effect in this study, it was tested only at a concentration of 100 μM. As discussed above in relation to NMDA receptors, the lower anesthetic potency of phenobarbital relative to the other barbiturates requires the use of higher aqueous concentrations to produce a similar response.

Electrophysiologic Experiments Barbiturate inhibition of neuronal responses to nonselective excitatory amino acid agonists has been demonstrated in a number of studies. In an early study, Krnjevic and Phillis (138) reported that in cats anesthetized with DIAL (sodium diallylbarbiturate + urethane), the administration of pentobarbital and DIAL reduced the firing rate of cortical neurons activated by L-glutamate. Crawford and Curtis (44) and Crawford (43) obtained similar results using the excitatory amino acid agonist D,L-homocysteic acid. These investigators demonstrated that the barbiturates pentobarbital, phenobarbital, sodium diallylbarbiturate (in combination with urethane as DIAL), and sodium methylthioethyl-2-pentyl thiobarbiturate reduced D,L-homocysteic acid-stimulated action potential firing rates of cat cortical neurons. In decerebrate or nitrous oxide-anesthetized cats, intravenous thiopental (2.5 mg/kg) suppressed the increase in firing rate of cortical neurons produced by iontophoretically applied glutamate (117). Similar results were obtained by Richards and Smaje (254), who reported that pentobarbital at concentrations of 50 to 300 μM reduced the rate of action potential firing induced by glutamate in neurons of the guinea pig olfactory cortex. An exception to these studies is the study of Catchlove et al. (34), who found that L-glutamate-evoked firing in cortical neurons of cats anesthetized with nitrous oxide was increased, rather than decreased, by pentobarbital, methohexital, and DIAL. While the explanation for the effect of barbiturates in the experiments of Catchlove and colleagues is unclear, the inhibitory effects of barbiturates on excitatory amino acid receptors have been confirmed in a number of subsequent studies. In a series of investigations, Barker and colleagues demonstrated that barbiturates inhibited responses to glutamate in mouse embryonic spinal cord neurons grown in tissue culture (10,167,168,248, 249). Ransom and Barker (248,249) demonstrated that the depolarization evoked by iontophoretically applied glutamate was inhibited by pentobarbital applied either via iontophoresis or, at anesthetic concentrations (100 to 200 μM), via large-bore pipettes, and that this inhibition was concentration dependent and reversible. In a subsequent analysis, these authors showed that pentobarbital inhibited responses to glutamate in a noncompetitive manner, that pentobarbital did not alter the rate of decay of the glutamate response, and that pentobarbital affected responses to glutamate and GABA with equal potency (10). In addition, Macdonald and Barker (167,168) reported that iontophoretically applied phenobarbital inhibited responses to glutamate in a concentration-dependent and reversible manner, albeit with lower potency than pentobarbital, as would be predicted based on its anesthetic potency. Using intracellular recording from spinal cord motor neurons in decerebrate cats, Lambert and Flatman (142) observed that the depolarizations induced by iontophoretic application of homocysteate or glutamate were decreased by thiopental administered intravenously (5 to 10 mg/kg), or pentobarbital administered intravenously (4 to 15 mg/kg) or applied iontophoretically.

As mentioned previously, the agonists used in these studies, glutamate and D,L-homocysteic acid, appear to activate excitatory amino acid receptors nonselectively (231). L-Glutamate is less than ten times as potent an agonist at NMDA receptors as at non-NMDA receptors (231). In the case of D,L-homocysteic acid, although the L-isomer is over 35 times more potent an agonist at NMDA than non-NMDA receptors, it would selectively activate NMDA receptors only at low concentrations (231). In addition, the D-isomer of homocysteic acid appears to activate non-NMDA receptors more potently than NMDA receptors (89). Thus, the use of these agonists precludes precise determination of the relative contribution of NMDA receptors to the excitatory amino acidñevoked responses measured in these studies.

In more recent studies using agonists selective for excitatory amino acid receptor types, it has generally been found that barbiturates inhibit responses to kainate and quisqualate more potently than responses to NMDA, although this has depended somewhat on the experimental procedure employed. Investigators using the grease-gap technique, in which a slice of brain tissue is positioned to pass through the sealed boundary between two chambers, and the electrical potential resulting from the addition of drugs to one of the chambers is measured (described in Harrison and Simmonds [85]), have often failed to observe selectivity of barbiturates for non-NMDA receptors. An exception to this is an early study by Harrison (82), in which he reported that pentobarbital at a concentration of 100 μM inhibited the depolarizations evoked by kainate and quisqualate in rat cerebral cortical slices by 37% and 57%, respectively, but did not appreciably inhibit the depolarization produced by NMDA. Collins and Anson (39) also reported that pentobarbital inhibited responses to kainate and quisqualate more potently than those to NMDA, but found little or no selectivity of thiopental or phenobarbital for inhibition of non-NMDA receptor-mediated responses. In addition, thiopental inhibited depolarizations evoked by AMPA and NMDA in mouse cortical slices to a similar extent (32), and in rat cortical slices, methohexital inhibited the depolarizing response to kainate, but not AMPA, more potently than that to NMDA (230).

In contrast to the results obtained in experiments using grease-gap recording, selectivity of barbiturates for non-NMDA vs. NMDA receptors has been consistently observed in studies utilizing intracellular or patch-clamp recording from individual neurons in brain slices or in culture. Miljkovic and MacDonald (204) demonstrated that pentobarbital inhibited the ion current activated by kainate more potently than that activated by L-aspartate, an agonist for NMDA receptors (231), in mouse-cultured hippocampal neurons. In guinea pig hippocampal slices, pentobarbital applied by iontophoresis reduced the amplitude of depolarizations induced by glutamate, kainate, quisqualate, and, less potently, NMDA (267). Interestingly, pentobarbital was reportedly less potent in enhancing the activity of the $GABA_A$ receptor than in inhibiting non-NMDA glutamate receptors (267). In mouse cultured hippocampal neurons, pentobarbital, phenobarbital, secobarbital, and thiopental potently inhibited kainate- and quisqualate-activated current (314,315). In these experiments, pentobarbital inhibited kainate-activated current with an IC_{50} of 105 μM, but inhibited NMDA-activated current with an IC_{50} of 991 μM. Similarly, phenobarbital inhibited NMDA-activated current much less potently than quisqualate-activated current (IC_{50} values of 2050 and 553 μM, respectively). In rat cortical neurons in culture, pentobarbital inhibited kainate-activated current with an IC_{50} of 50 μM, but did not significantly inhibit NMDA-activated current at concentrations up to 100 μM (179).

The explanation for the discordant results obtained in studies using grease-gap recording and those using intracellular or patch-clamp recording is not immediately obvious, but several possible reasons may be suggested. First, the membrane potential across a brain slice is a global or averaged response that undoubtedly reflects the contribution of multiple types of receptors and transduction systems on many types of neurons (and perhaps other cell types, such as glia, as well), and the interactions of these cells, receptors, and transduction systems, whereas intracellular or patch-clamp recording measures the response of a single cell, the morphology and physiology of which can usually be determined. Thus, results obtained in grease-gap experiments may not represent effects of barbiturates on only the receptor of interest. Second, in grease-gap recording, agonists must be applied to brain slices via addition to the bathing solution, with the result that the time course of agonist-evoked responses is limited by diffusion through the bathing solution as well as through the slice itself. In contrast, the use of intracellular or patch-clamp recording permits any of several agonist application methods to be employed, including iontophoresis or multibarrel superfusion, which allow for much more rapid control of agonist delivery to the cell under investigation. Grease-gap experiments are therefore unable to detect effects on rapidly desensitizing receptors, or to distinguish between effects on peak and steady-state responses. Third, very few variables can be controlled or measured in grease-gap recording, while intracellular or patch-clamp recording allows for control or measurement of many variables, such as membrane potential and conductance, and concentrations of extracellular (in cultured cells) and intracellular constituents. Effects of barbiturates additional to those on the receptor of interest could thus produce misleading results in grease-gap experiments.

As non-NMDA glutamate receptors are a heterogeneous group of receptor subtypes composed of various combinations of subunits (68,95,219,274), these receptor subtypes might be predicted to differ in their sensitivity to barbiturates. This has recently been explored in part by Taverna and colleagues (298), who performed concentration-response analyses for pentobarbital inhibition of receptors composed of different combinations of the AMPA receptor subunits GluR1 to GluR4 expressed in *Xenopus* oocytes. These investigators reported that pentobarbital inhibited receptors containing the GluR2 subunit (GluR1/2 or GluR2/3) with IC_{50} values of ~180 to 200 μM, whereas pentobarbital inhibited receptors lacking the GluR2 subunit (GluR1, GluR1/3, GluR3) much less potently, with IC_{50} values of ~1.1 to 2 mM. Interestingly, the presence of the GluR2 subunit also decreased the slope factors of the concentration-response curves from values greater than 1 to values less than 1, but whether this represents the addition of a pentobarbital binding site (298), a decrease in the cooperativity of pentobarbital binding (40), greater ease of access of pentobarbital to its binding site (148), or some other effect, remains unclear.

Mechanism of Action The mechanism by which barbiturates inhibit non-NMDA receptor-mediated responses has not been conclusively established, but most probably involves physical occlusion of the ion channel (open-channel block). Concentration-response experiments revealed that barbiturates decrease the maximal response (efficacy) of non-NMDA agonists without altering their half-maximal inhibitory concentration (potency), which is consistent with a noncompetitive mechanism of inhibition (3,100). Miljkovic and MacDonald (204) reported that inhibition of excitatory amino acid-activated currents by pentobarbital is voltage dependent, which they interpreted as evidence that pentobarbital acts via an open-channel block mechanism. These investigators also concluded that, since pentobarbital is predominantly uncharged at physiologic pH, the voltage dependence must be due to an effect of the membrane electric field on the receptor-ion channel protein rather than on pentobarbital. In more recent experiments, we (233,314) and others (179) have not observed a voltage-dependent inhibition of kainate-activated current. However, these latter experiments provided strong evidence that barbiturates inhibit kainate-gated ion channels via an open-channel blocking mechanism. In these experiments, pentobarbital did not significantly inhibit kainate-gated ion channels unless agonist was present, and pentobarbital inhibition persisted in the absence of agonist (179,233,314). These observations have been interpreted as indicating that the barbiturate can inhibit the ion channel only in the open agonist-bound state. According to this model, the failure of pentobarbital to inhibit the ion channel in the absence of agonist is due to inaccessibility of its binding site within the channel in the absence of agonist, and the persistence of inhibition in the absence of agonist is due to closing of the ion channel following agonist dissociation, trapping the drug in the closed ion channel. Recovery from block occurs when agonist opens the channel, permitting the barbiturate to dissociate from its binding site. Consistent with this hypothesis, the rate constants for onset of and recovery from inhibition by pentobarbital increase with increasing agonist concentration (Peoples and Weight, *unpublished observations*). Preliminary results using the single-channel recording technique showed that pentobarbital decreased the frequency of opening; however, because of the small amplitude and short open time of these currents, the mechanism of this inhibition could not be determined (291).

Volatile Anesthetics

NMDA Receptors

Behavioral Experiments A number of studies have demonstrated modulation of volatile anesthetic potency by agents acting upon the NMDA receptor. Raja and coworkers (245) reported that the dissociative anesthetic phencyclidine, which is a noncompetitive NMDA antagonist, reduced the minimum alveolar concentration (MAC; concentration producing anesthesia in 50% of subjects) of cyclopropane by approximately 40% in rats. As phencyclidine affects multiple receptors and ion channels, however (154), this effect may not necessarily have resulted from NMDA receptor antagonism. Scheller and colleagues (268) found that the noncompetitive NMDA receptor antagonist MK-801 reduced the MAC of halothane required to produce anesthesia in rabbits in a dose-dependent manner. Daniell (46–48), in a series of studies, demonstrated that various competitive and noncompetitive antagonists of the NMDA receptor increased anesthetic potency in mice. In these studies, the MAC of halothane was substantially reduced by pretreatment with the noncompetitive NMDA receptor antagonists MK-801 and phencyclidine (46), by the competitive NMDA receptor antagonist CGS 19755 (47), and by spermine and spermidine, agonists at the polyamine modulatory site of the NMDA receptor (48). The enhancement of anesthetic potency by polyamines may seem paradoxical, since they enhance the activity of the NMDA receptor at low concentrations (198,258,289); however, at concentrations found in vivo (260,276), the predominant effect of polyamines on the NMDA receptor appears to be inhibitory (198,258,289). Interestingly, the anesthetic potency of diethyl ether was enhanced by MK-801 and phencyclidine, but not by CGS 19755 or polyamines (46–48). Kuroda and coworkers (139) observed that the anesthetic potency of isoflurane is also enhanced by NMDA receptor antagonists. A noncompetitive antagonist, MK-801, and two competitive antagonists, D-CPPene and CGS 19755, produced dose-dependent and substantial (up to approximately 60%) decreases in the MAC of isoflurane in rats. As discussed previously, these observations provide evidence that the NMDA receptor may contribute to the anesthetic state, but are not sufficient to establish that the NMDA receptor is the site of action of volatile anesthetics.

Binding Experiments The influence of volatile anesthetics on ligand binding to the NMDA receptor-ion channel complex has thus far not been thoroughly investigated. In a brief study, Martin and colleagues (183) reported that enflurane inhibited glutamate-stimulated [^{3}H]MK-801 binding to rat cortical membranes in a concentration-dependent manner. Enflurane, 1.1 mM, reduced the maximal response of the concentration-response curve for glutamate stimulation of [^{3}H]MK-801 binding, suggesting a noncompetitive mechanism of inhibition. Further evidence for a noncompetitive mechanism was provided by the observation that enflurane had no appreciable effect on specific binding of the competitive NMDA antagonist [^{3}H]CGS 19755. The authors suggested that enflurane may interact with the glycine modulatory site of the receptor, as increasing the glycine concentration reversed the effect of enflurane. However, glycine did not enhance control [^{3}H]MK-801 binding stimulated by 100 μM glutamate, suggesting that the concentration of background or contaminating glycine in the membrane suspension was quite high, which could produce effects additional to those on the NMDA receptor (see Peoples and Weight [234] and Woodward [331] for further discussion of this point in relation to alcohols). Further experiments will be required to resolve this issue.

Biochemical Experiments Puil and coworkers (241) have demonstrated that volatile anesthetics can depress excitatory amino acid-induced increases in intracellular Ca^{2+} in CNS neurons. In rat hippocampal neurons in primary culture, anesthetic concentrations of halothane and isoflurane reduced glutamate- and NMDA-evoked increases in intracellular Ca^{2+} as measured using the Ca^{2+}-sensitive dye fura-2. Under conditions selective for NMDA receptor activation, isoflurane inhibited the glutamate-evoked increase in intracellular Ca^{2+} with an IC_{50} of 1.2%. However, since the voltage-dependent Ca^{2+} channel antagonist verapamil also inhibited the glutamate-evoked increase in intracellular Ca^{2+} by up to 50%, a substantial part of the effect of glutamate appears to be mediated by voltage-gated Ca^{2+} channels. Thus, the reported IC_{50} value for isoflurane inhibition of the NMDA receptor may reflect a contribution of effects on voltage-gated ion channels.

Enflurane and halothane also inhibited glutamate- and NMDA-stimulated $^{45}Ca^{2+}$ uptake into a suspension of microvesicles (synaptoneurosomes and resealed membrane fragments resulting from brief homogenization) prepared from rat forebrain (6). In this study, enflurane and halothane reportedly inhibited $^{45}Ca^{2+}$ uptake evoked by 100 μM NMDA with IC_{50} values of 200 and 300 μM, respectively. The authors also reported that enflurane and halothane maximally inhibited the response to NMDA by 80% and 60%, respectively. However, replotting their concentration-response curves on a logarithmic scale (which greatly facilitates accurate measurement of concentration-response maxima), revealed that the true maxima approach or equal 100%. The reported IC_{50} values are thus probably slight underestimates; nevertheless, both anesthetics produced substantial inhibition of responses to NMDA at physiologic concentrations. The authors also reported that increasing the concentration of glycine reversed the effect of enflurane (but see the caveat discussed in the above section).

Electrophysiologic Experiments

Volatile anesthetics have also been observed to inhibit NMDA receptors in electrophysiologic experiments. In guinea pig cortical neurons, isoflurane (0.5 to 2.5 MAC) inhibited the depolarizations evoked by glutamate and NMDA in a concentration-dependent manner, with an IC_{50} for inhibition of responses to glutamate of 1.9 MAC (240). The IC_{50} for isoflurane inhibition of responses to NMDA was not reported, but was apparently 1.2 to 1.3 MAC, as concentrations in this range produced approximately 50% inhibition of NMDA-evoked depolarization. Halothane (2.5 MAC) also inhibited responses to glutamate, but its effect on NMDA-evoked depolarization was not tested. In acutely dissociated neurons from the rat nucleus tractus solitarius, enflurane and halothane (both at 2 mM) produced a small but significant inhibition of glutamate-activated current, and halothane (1 mM) inhibited NMDA-activated current by 10% to 20% (309). Because of the modest effects of the anesthetics on excitatory amino acid-activated currents observed in this study, the authors did not perform concentration-response experiments. In mouse hippocampal neurons in culture, concentration-response analysis revealed that volatile anesthetics inhibited NMDA receptors with low potency compared to their anesthetic potencies (235). Enflurane, halothane, and isoflurane inhibited NMDA-activated current with IC_{50} values of 5.9, 7.5, and 15.1 mM, respectively (compare these values with their respective MAC values of 0.46, 0.32, and 0.51 mM [121]). It should be noted that in some instances determination of these IC_{50} values involved slight extrapolation, since the highest concentrations of the anesthetics that could be tested produced less than 50% inhibition. Diethyl ether, in contrast, inhibited NMDA-activated current in mouse hippocampal neurons with an IC_{50} of 30 to 35 mM (158). More potent effects of anesthetics were observed in grease-gap recordings from mouse cortical slices (32). Although IC_{50} values were not determined in this study, halothane, 3 mM, isoflurane, 2 mM, and diethyl ether, 20 mM, produced 50% to 55% inhibition of the NMDA-evoked depolarization. Thus these concentrations may be taken as rough estimates of the IC_{50} values. Interestingly, chloroform, 5 mM, did not inhibit the response to NMDA, despite completely inhibiting the response to AMPA. Volatile anesthetics have also been demonstrated to inhibit neuronal NMDA receptors expressed in other cell types: enflurane, 1.8 mM, inhibited mouse brain NMDA receptors expressed in *Xenopus laevis* oocytes by 34% (151).

Mechanism of Action

Few studies have addressed the mechanism by which volatile anesthetics inhibit NMDA receptors. Lin and coworkers (151) reported that enflurane inhibition of mouse brain NMDA receptors expressed in *Xenopus* oocytes was independent of the concentrations of NMDA and glycine. Similar evidence was presented by Carlá and Moroni (32), who showed that isoflurane depressed the maximal response to NMDA without altering its potency, which is consistent with a noncompetitive mechanism of action. Thus, volatile anesthetics do not appear to interact with the NMDA or glycine binding sites of the NMDA receptor-ionophore. Single-channel analysis of NMDA-activated ion channels in rat hippocampal neurons in culture revealed complex effects of isoflurane (334). At physiologic concentrations (< 2 mM), isoflurane reduced the frequency of channel opening without producing the channel flickering (multiple, brief closings) characteristic of open-channel block, and without affecting the mean open time of the channel. At higher concentrations (2 to 8.5 mM), isoflurane produced channel flickering and markedly reduced the mean open time of the ion channel. These results may indicate that isoflurane inhibits the NMDA receptor-ion channel via multiple mechanisms, perhaps including channel block at high concentrations. Delineation of the precise mechanism of action of anesthetics on the NMDA receptor, particularly within the physiologic concentration range, will require further study.

AMPA/Kainate Receptors

Behavioral Experiments Despite the importance of non-NMDA excitatory amino acid receptors in mediating excitatory neurotransmission in the CNS, and their consequent potential as sites of action of anesthetics, to date only one behavioral study has addressed interactions between non-NMDA antagonists and volatile anesthetics. In this study, intravenous infusion of the non-NMDA antagonist NBQX reduced the anesthetic concentration (MAC) of halothane by up to nearly 60% in rats

(196). Moreover, there was a logarithmic relation between MAC for halothane and the plasma concentration of NBQX.

Biochemical Experiments In rat cultured hippocampal neurons, under conditions relatively selective for AMPA/kainate receptors (0.8 mM Mg^{2+} and no added glycine), glutamate induced an increase in intracellular Ca^{2+} that was depressed by halothane and isoflurane at physiologically relevant concentrations (241). Isoflurane inhibited the glutamate-evoked increase in intracellular Ca^{2+} with an IC_{50} of 1.7%, but this value may not represent an effect of isoflurane only on AMPA/kainate receptors. Because voltage-dependent Ca^{2+} channels were not blocked under these experimental conditions, these ion channels would be predicted to mediate all or part of the glutamate-stimulated increase in Ca^{2+}. An action of isoflurane on voltage-gated Ca^{2+} channels was in fact inferred in this study from the observation that isoflurane inhibited the K^+-evoked increase in intracellular Ca^{2+} by up to 60%. The potency of isoflurane in inhibiting the glutamate-stimulated increase in Ca^{2+} in this study therefore should not be taken as its potency for inhibiting AMPA/kainate receptors. Other experiments in which more of the variables were controlled should provide more accurate estimates of the potency of anesthetics for inhibition of non-NMDA receptors.

Electrophysiologic Experiments Initial studies of effects of volatile anesthetics on responses to excitatory amino acids yielded conflicting results. In an early study, Catchlove and colleagues (34) found that the volatile anesthetics cyclopropane, chloroform, ether, halothane, methoxyflurane, nitrous oxide, and trichloroethylene did not inhibit, and in some cases increased, L-glutamate induced action potential firing frequency in cortical neurons of nitrous oxide-anesthetized cats (34). Crawford and Curtis (44) and Crawford (43) reported that in decerebrate cats, anesthetic concentrations of halothane, but not trichloroethylene, methoxyflurane, or nitrous oxide, produced a slight reduction in the frequency of D,L-homocysteic acid-induced firing in cortical neurons. In contrast, Richards and Smaje (254) reported effects of anesthetics in slices of guinea pig olfactory cortex nearly opposite to those observed by Crawford and Curtis. In this study, ether, methoxyflurane, and trichloroethylene, at anesthetic concentrations, inhibited L-glutamate-evoked action potential firing, while halothane was effective only at high concentrations (>1%).

Although the explanation for the discordant results obtained in the previous studies is unclear, subsequent studies have generally found inhibitory effects of volatile anesthetics on non-NMDA excitatory amino acid receptors, although often only at relatively high concentrations. Enflurane at a concentration of 1.8 mM (3.9 MAC [121]) inhibited currents activated by AMPA and kainate by up to 33% and 27%, respectively, in *Xenopus* oocytes injected with mouse brain mRNA, and inhibited kainate-activated current in *Xenopus* oocytes injected with human brain mRNA by up to 29% (151). In mouse hippocampal neurons in primary culture, enflurane, halothane, and isoflurane inhibited kainate-activated ion current with IC_{50} values of 6.9, 3.4, and 10.9 mM, respectively (235). The percent inhibition of kainate-activated ion current at the MAC for each agent was enflurane 7%, halothane 16%, and isoflurane 9%. At 1.3 MAC (at which 99% of subjects are anesthetized [51]), the percent inhibition of kainate-activated ion current for each agent was enflurane 8%, halothane 19%, and isoflurane 11%; and at 2 MAC, the percent inhibition of kainate-activated ion current for each agent was enflurane 12%, halothane 23%, and isoflurane 15%. In neurons dissociated from the rat nucleus tractus solitarius, halothane appeared to inhibit kainate-activated current less potently than quisqualate-activated current (309). Although the investigators in this study did not determine IC_{50} values, 1 mM halothane inhibited currents activated by kainate and quisqualate by 8% and 40%, respectively. Carlá and Moroni (32) observed more potent effects of halothane and other anesthetics on AMPA-induced depolarization in mouse cortical slices. These investigators reported that responses to AMPA were inhibited by approximately 45% to 55% by 1 mM halothane, 1.5 mM isoflurane, 20 mM ether, and 3 mM chloroform. As the authors of this study employed grease-gap recording, however, the more potent effects of anesthetics they reported may result from actions of anesthetics upon multiple sites, as discussed previously.

Mechanism of Action The mechanism of action by which volatile anesthetics inhibit AMPA/kainate receptors has not been characterized. The only available evidence has been provided by Lin et al. (151) and by Carlá and Moroni (32). These investigators reported that volatile anesthetic inhibition of responses to AMPA and kainate was independent of agonist concentration, which supports a noncompetitive mechanism of inhibition. However, the precise mechanism and site of action of volatile anesthetics on non-NMDA receptor-ion channels remains to be determined.

Dissociative Anesthetics

Unquestionably the clearest evidence that an excitatory amino acid receptor is the site of action of an anesthetic is that regarding the actions of the dissociative anesthetics on the NMDA receptor. The dissociative anesthetics, phencyclidine, ketamine, MK-801 (dizocilpine), and related compounds, induce a state of atypical anesthesia characterized by a feeling of dissociation from the environment (42,178). Although whether MK-801 acts as a dissociative anesthetic in all species is open to question (129), because of its many similarities to the other agents in this class it will be considered as such for the purposes of this review. As dissociative anesthetics have been found not to affect the function of AMPA/kainate receptors, this area has been omitted from the present review.

NMDA Receptors

Behavioral Experiments In drug discrimination assays, ketamine, phencyclidine and its active analogues, and MK-801 have been shown to substitute for each other (8,13,17,67,111,133, 135,303,320). As might be expected of an NMDA antagonist, ketamine decreased the ability of rats to recognize the subjective effects of NMDA (15), and the NMDA competitive antagonists APV and AP7 substituted for phencyclidine in pigeons (134) and rats (303). In the majority of studies, however, dissociative anesthetics did not disrupt the NMDA discriminative stimulus (133,321), and NMDA competitive antagonists and dissociative anesthetics substituted for each other either only partially or not at all (23,38,61,67,72, 77,111,133,173,319,324).

The failure of dissociative anesthetics to behave like competitive NMDA antagonists has not generally been taken as an indication that the subjective effects of these agents are not due to NMDA receptor inhibition, but rather have been interpreted as indicating that dissociative anesthetics and competitive NMDA antagonists may produce different subjective effects (23,38,72, 111,133,173,319,322,324,325). This interpretation is consistent with observations that other classes of NMDA receptor antagonists, such as the atypical noncompetitive antagonists ifenprodil (111) and eliprodil (8), the glycine site antagonists HA-966 (281) and 5,7-dichlorokynurenic acid (41), and the ion channel blocker Mg^{2+} (124), did not produce subjective effects similar to those of dissociative anesthetics. In addition, other noncompetitive NMDA antagonists failed to block the discriminative stimulus effects of NMDA (133).

The conclusion that the NMDA receptor is the site through which dissociative anesthesia is produced is based on different lines of evidence, such as the potent effects of dissociative anesthetics on NMDA receptors in vitro (see below) and a strong correlation between anesthetic potency and NMDA receptor inhibitory potency for various dissociative anesthetics (135,201). Effects of NMDA agonists and competitive antagonists on dissociative anesthetic potency, however, have been examined in only a single study to date. In this study, Irifune and colleagues (109) demonstrated that NMDA, but not *N*-methyl-L-aspartate, its inactive isomer, or the non-NMDA agonists kainate and quisqualate, decreased the percentage of animals displaying loss of righting reflex and decreased the duration of loss of righting reflex in mice administered ketamine. In addition, the NMDA antagonists CPP and Mg^{2+} increased the duration of ketamine-induced loss of righting reflex and increased the percentage of animals displaying loss of righting reflex.

Binding Experiments Zukin and Zukin (339) and Vincent et al. (307) first demonstrated high affinity binding of radiolabeled phencyclidine in rat brain. Mendelsohn and colleagues (201) subsequently reported that the affinity of a series of drugs to displace specific binding of phencyclidine was highly correlated with their potency to produce catalepsy in pigeons, which was taken as an indication of the relevance of this site to dissociative anesthesia. Although the initial observations that dissociative anesthetics acted upon the NMDA receptor were made in electrophysiologic studies (see below), evidence obtained in binding studies confirmed that the dissociative anesthetic binding site was associated with the NMDA receptor-ion channel complex. Loo et al. (156) demonstrated that dissociative anesthetic binding in brain membranes was dependent on an endogenous excitatory amino acid, as it was reduced by extensive washing and restored by exogenous glutamate. Loo and colleagues also reported that the binding of dissociative anesthetics was increased by NMDA receptor agonists, as was also observed in other studies (60,65, 157,253). In addition, a number of investigators reported that dissociative anesthetic binding was decreased by the NMDA receptor antagonists APV, AP7, and CPP (65,114,116,157,253). Furthermore, agonists (25,119,252,253,285,300,328) and antagonists (282) at the glycine site of the NMDA receptor-ion channel complex also modulated binding of dissociative anesthetics. Results of subsequent studies, however, indicated that in these initial experiments the binding assays had not been performed at equilibrium (24,131,132), and thus the conclusions drawn from the initial studies that NMDA and glycine agonists and antagonists altered the affinity or density of the binding sites appeared questionable. Bonhaus, McNamara and colleagues (24,25), Kloog and colleagues (131), and Javitt and Zukin (115,116) delineated more fully the effects of NMDA agonists and antagonists and glycine agonists on the kinetics of dissociative anesthetic binding. These investigators showed that NMDA agonists (24,115,116,131) or glycine agonists (25, 115, 116,131) increase, and NMDA antagonists decrease (25,115, 116,131), the rates of association and dissociation of dissociative anesthetics without altering the binding site affinity or density (115,116,131). Kloog et al. additionally suggested that when the channel is closed, dissociative anesthetics might be able to gain access to their binding site in the channel with very slow kinetics, whereas Javitt and Zukin proposed a model in which this slow interaction would occur when the channel is singly liganded. Finally, several groups provided evidence that the dissociative anesthetic binding site was associated with the NMDA receptor-ion channel complex by demonstrating that the distribution in the CNS of binding sites for NMDA receptor ligands was similar to that of dissociative anesthetic binding sites (113,176,177,208).

Biochemical Experiments Dissociative anesthetics have been shown to inhibit the NMDA receptor-mediated release of neurotransmitters in a number of experiments. Lodge and Johnston (155) demonstrated that ketamine reduced the NMDA-stimulated efflux of [^{3}H]acetylcholine from rat cortical slices in an apparently noncompetitive manner. Similarly, Snell and Johnson (283,284) observed a similar inhibition of NMDA-evoked [^{3}H]acetylcholine and dopamine release from striatal slices by ketamine, phencyclidine, and related compounds. Additionally, these investigators reported a correlation between the potency of these compounds to inhibit acetylcholine release and their potency in a behavioral assay (283). Other investigators have demonstrated that dissociative anesthetics inhibit NMDA-stimulated release of GABA from cortical neurons (55), norepinephrine from hippocampus (122,141,269, 287) and cerebellum (335), dopamine from nucleus accumbens (123) and striatum (227), and acetylcholine from nucleus accumbens (123) and striatum (329). In a number of these studies, dissociative anesthetics were reported to inhibit the NMDA receptor in a stereoselective (141), noncompetitive or uncompetitive (122,141,227,329), and use-dependent manner (269).

Dissociative anesthetic inhibition of NMDA receptor-mediated effects on ionic fluxes and intracellular Ca^{2+} concentration has also been demonstrated. Pullan (242) reported that phencyclidine, ketamine, and MK-801 inhibited NMDA-stimulated efflux of $^{22}Na^+$ from rat hippocampal slices in a noncompetitive manner. Furthermore, the potency of drugs to inhibit NMDA-evoked $^{22}Na^+$ efflux was correlated with their affinity for the NMDA receptor determined in binding studies. Ransom and Stec (250) similarly observed that phencyclidine, phencyclidine analogues, and MK-801 inhibited NMDA-stimulated $^{22}Na^+$ efflux from rat hippocampal slices, and that the mechanism of inhibition was noncompetitive. O'Shaughnessy and Lodge (226) found that L-glutamate and NMDA stimulated the uptake of $^{45}Ca^{2+}$ into rat cortical slices and increased the Ca^{2+} concentration in rat cortical synaptosomes, and that these effects were blocked by ketamine and phencyclidine. Yuzaki and coworkers (336) observed a similar inhibition by MK-801 of the NMDA receptor-mediated increase in intracellular Ca^{2+} in mouse hippocampal neurons in culture. In this study, the recovery of the NMDA receptor from blockade by MK-801 exhibited pronounced use dependence.

Electrophysiologic Experiments The initial demonstration that dissociative anesthetics inhibit NMDA receptors was provided by Lodge and Anis (153). These investigators showed that phencyclidine, whether administered intravenously or iontophoretically, reduced the increase in firing rate evoked by *N*-methyl-DL-aspartate, but not kainate or quisqualate, in cat spinal cord neurons in vivo. In subsequent studies, Berry et al. (19,20) reported that the sigma opioid agonist *N*-allylnormetazocine (SKF 10,047) and two phencyclidine analogues exhibited stereoselective inhibition of responses to *N*-methyl-DL-aspartate, but not to kainate or quisqualate. Furthermore, the enantiomers that were more potent in displacing specific binding of phencyclidine and in eliciting phencyclidine-like behavioral effects were also more potent in inhibiting the NMDA receptor. These investigators also demonstrated that ketamine, as well as phencyclidine, blocked the response of cat or rat spinal neurons to *N*-methyl-DL-aspartate, glutamate, or aspartate, but had little or no effect on responses to quisqualate, kainate, or the inhibitory amino acids GABA or glycine (4). Effects of dissociative anesthetics on NMDA receptor-mediated responses in the brain were demonstrated by Harrison and Simmonds (85), who showed that ketamine inhibited NMDA-mediated depolarization in rat cortical slices, and by Duchen et al. (56), who reported that ketamine inhibited *N*-methyl-DL-aspartate-evoked depolarization and action potential firing in mouse hippocampal neurons. Harrison and Simmonds also found that ketamine increased the potency of the competitive NMDA antagonist APV, and concluded from this that ketamine inhibition is noncompetitive. Martin and Lodge (180) also provided evidence for a noncompetitive action of ketamine by demonstrating a similar interaction of ketamine and APV in frog spinal cord, and a Schild plot for ketamine of less than unity.

A number of studies have provided evidence that dissociative anesthetics inhibit NMDA receptors in a use-dependent manner, which is generally taken as an indication of an open-channel block mechanism of inhibition (see below). In an early study, Honey and coworkers (98) observed a progressive decrement in the amplitude of responses to L-aspartate in the presence of the dissociative anesthetics ketamine and phencyclidine, suggesting that the inhibition was agonist dependent. Wong et al. (327) reported that MK-801 produced a similar apparent use dependence of inhibition of NMDA-evoked depolarization in rat cortical slices. In addition, these investigators reported that the NMDA response did not recover completely upon removal of MK-801, even when the slices were washed in MK-801–free solution for 3 hours. Clear evidence of use-dependent inhibition of NMDA receptors by dissociative anesthetics was provided in several subsequent studies. Woodruff et al. (330) reported that prolonged exposure of rat cortical slices to MK-801 caused a decrement in responses to NMDA only when NMDA was repeatedly applied, and thus the inhibition was agonist dependent, rather than time dependent. MacDonald and colleagues (165) also observed that NMDA receptors did not recover from inhibition by ketamine unless agonist was present, and that the inhibition of NMDA receptors by ketamine increased as the magnitude of the NMDA-activated current increased. Similar observations of the agonist dependence of both the onset of, and recovery from, inhibition of NMDA receptors by dissociative anesthetics were reported by Huettner and Bean (103), Mayer et al. (189), Halliwell et al. (79), and MacDonald et al. (164).

Dissociative anesthetic inhibition of NMDA receptors is also regulated by membrane voltage. Ketamine and phencyclidine have been shown to markedly inhibit NMDA receptor-mediated current at negative, but not at positive, membrane holding potentials (79,98,103,164,165,189). In contrast, inhibition of NMDA receptors by MK-801 was reported in some cases to be independent of membrane potential (79,126). High concentrations of MK-801 were used in the latter studies, however, which would produce a substantial degree of block and thus could have obscured effects of membrane potential. At a lower concentration, MK-801 inhibition of NMDA receptors exhibited considerable voltage dependence (164). In addition, the equilibrium dissociation constant (K_d) for MK-801, estimated from the rate constants for onset and offset of inhibition, was shown to differ markedly at different membrane potentials (103).

Mechanism of Action Dissociative anesthetics have been demonstrated to inhibit NMDA receptors in a noncompetitive manner (85,155,180). In addition, dissociative anesthetic inhibition of NMDA receptor function exhibits use dependence, i.e., is dependent on the presence of agonist and persists in the absence of agonist (79,103,164,165,189,330). As described above for barbiturate inhibition of non-NMDA receptors, these observations have been interpreted as indicating that dissociative anesthetics can bind within the channel of the NMDA receptor only in the open agonist-bound state, and are trapped when the ion channel closes. This interpretation is also supported by results obtained in single-channel studies. Although preliminary, in these studies MK-801, phencyclidine, and two behaviorally active phencyclidine analogues, but not a behaviorally inactive analogue, decreased the frequency of opening and mean open time of the ion channel, which is consistent with an open-channel block mechanism (103,247). In addition, fluctuation analysis of NMDA-activated current revealed that ketamine markedly decreased the mean channel open time (189).

The voltage dependence of the dissociative anesthetic inhibition of NMDA-gated ion channels is also consistent with an open-channel blocking mechanism, although the basis for the voltage dependence appears unusual. Voltage-dependent inhibition of an ion channel is usually thought to arise from the effect of the membrane electrical field on the blocking agent, and perhaps occasionally on the ion channel itself (90). In the case of ketamine, and presumably the other dissociative anesthetics as well, it is the charged form of the dissociative anesthetic that is thought to inhibit NMDA receptor-ion channels (164). Despite this, membrane voltage does not appear to affect the onset rate of inhibition of NMDA-activated current, as would be predicted if the dissociative anesthetics were affected by the membrane potential (103,164, 189). Depolarization of the membrane, however, dramatically increases the rate of recovery from inhibition (103,164,189). As the accelerating effect of positive membrane potential on rate of recovery from block is not observed when impermeant ions are substituted on the intracellular side of the membrane, these observations have been interpreted as indicating that the increased efflux of permeant cations at positive membrane potentials increases the apparent dissociation rate of the blocking agent by enhancing its clearance from the ion channel lumen (164); this mechanism has been previously proposed for charybdotoxin block of voltage-dependent K^+ channels (169).

Recent studies have addressed the subunit and structural requirements for dissociative anesthetic inhibition of the NMDA receptor. Sakurada et al. (264) tested the effects of NMDA receptor antagonists on NMDA receptors composed of NMDAR1 subunits with single amino acid substitutions coexpressed with NMDAR2A subunits. These investigators reported that substitution of an asparagine residue in TM2 at the Q/R/N site, which determines Ca^{2+} permeability, with either glutamine or arginine decreased the sensitivity of the receptor to inhibition by Mg^{2+} and MK-801. Similarly, Kawajiri and Dingledine (127) demonstrated that replacing the asparagine at the Q/R/N site of the NMDAR1 subunit with serine reduced the potency of the phencyclidine analogue TCP to block the ion channel. Interestingly, Lynch and coworkers (162) found specific binding of MK-801 in cells coexpressing NMDAR1 and NMDAR2A subunits, but did not detect binding of MK-801 in cells expressing only NMDAR1 or NMDAR2A subunits, which may indicate that regions of both subunits constitute the dissociative anesthetic binding site.

Other Anesthetics

Anesthetic Steroids

Anesthetic steroids have, in some cases, been reported to inhibit excitatory amino acid receptor-mediated responses. Richards and Smaje (254) reported that the anesthetic steroid alphaxalone, at a concentration of 50 μM, decreased the rate of glutamate-stimulated action potential firing in guinea pig cortical neurons. Similar results were obtained by Puil and El-Beheiry (240), who observed that althesin (a mixture of alphaxalone and its inactive isomer alphadalone), at concentrations of 25 to 200 μM, had little effect on responses to GABA, but reduced the depolarizations induced by glutamate and NMDA in guinea pig cortical neurons. It should be noted, however, that the steroid concentrations used by these investigators were well above the anesthetic range (6 to 12 μM [273]). It has now been shown in several studies that at concentrations associated with anesthesia, alphaxalone, and other anesthetic steroids markedly potentiate $GABA_A$ receptor-mediated responses (9, 83,84,107,170,305). In addition, another anesthetic steroid, 5α-pregnane-3α,21-diol-20-one, also potentiates GABA-activated current (83,170) but does not inhibit currents activated by NMDA, kainate, or quisqualate even at concentrations above the anesthetic range (314).

Riluzole

Riluzole (2-amino-6-trifluoromethoxybenzothiazole) is an agent with anticonvulsant (207) and neuroprotective properties (171,172,239). Mantz and coworkers (174) have demonstrated that riluzole can also act as an anesthetic. At high doses (>15 mg/kg), riluzole induced loss of righting reflex in rats, while at a lower dose (5 mg/kg), riluzole prolonged the duration of ketamine- and thiopental-induced loss of righting reflex and decreased the anesthetic requirement for halothane. The neurochemical basis for the effects of riluzole remains unclear, but may result from inhibition of excitatory amino acid receptors, which has been demonstrated in several studies. Benavides et al. (14) reported that riluzole blocked *N*-methyl-DL-aspartate–stimulated release of acetylcholine in striatum and increases in cerebellar cyclic guanosine monophosphate (cGMP) induced by several excitatory amino acids, including *N*-methyl-DL-aspartate, kainate, and quisqualate. Debono and colleagues (52) found that in *Xenopus laevis* oocytes injected with rat brain mRNA, riluzole inhibited NMDA receptors more potently than AMPA/kainate receptors, and that this inhibition was not use dependent. In addition, these investigators reported that in radioligand binding assays, riluzole did not interact with the dissociative anesthetic or glycine sites of the NMDA receptor, or with the agonist binding site of AMPA/ kainate receptors. Hubert et al. (102) have also recently reported that riluzole inhibits NMDA-stimulated increases in intracellular Ca^{2+} concentration in cerebellar granule cells in culture. Riluzole has multiple actions, however, including inhibition of synaptic release of glutamate and aspartate (37,182) and inhibition of GABA uptake (175), any of which could mediate or contribute to its anesthetic effect. Further research will therefore be needed to determine the relative importance of each of these actions to the anesthetic effect of riluzole.

Alcohols

Although alcohols are not used clinically as anesthetics, they can produce an anesthetic state, and much research on anesthetic actions in the past century has been performed using alcohols (202,215,229,275). In addition, research into the effects of alcohols on excitatory amino acid receptors has yielded information of potential relevance to the mechanism of action of some anesthetics. In an early study, Teichberg and colleagues (299) reported that alcohols from methanol to 1-butanol inhibited excitatory amino acid-evoked $^{22}Na^{+}$ efflux in striatal slices, and that alcohols inhibited responses to kainate or quisqualate more potently than responses to NMDA. Lovinger et al. (159) demonstrated inhibition of NMDA-, kainate-, and quisqualate-activated ion current in mouse hippocampal neurons in culture by alcohols from methanol to isopentanol. In contrast to the findings of Teichberg et al., these investigators reported that alcohols inhibited current activated by NMDA more potently than that activated by kainate or quisqualate. These investigators also found that there was a significant linear relation between NMDA receptor inhibitory potency and intoxicating potency for the series of alcohols. Other investigators subsequently reported potent inhibition by alcohols of a number of NMDA receptor-mediated responses, including NMDA-gated single-channel currents (150,199), and NMDA-induced increases in neurotransmitter release (62,74–76,332), Ca^{2+} uptake and intracellular Ca^{2+} concentration (53,92), and cGMP levels (91,92). Other studies have confirmed that alcohols inhibit responses mediated by NMDA receptors more potently than responses mediated by AMPA/kainate receptors (63,161). Despite the large body of evidence for alcohol inhibition of NMDA receptors, studies designed to identify the molecular site of alcohol action on the NMDA receptor have been inconclusive to date. Although some studies have suggested that alcohols interact with the modulatory sites for glycine (54,92,244,286,332) or Mg^{2+} (181,203,214) on the NMDA receptor, in other studies interactions of alcohols with the glycine (160,234,318,331) or Mg^{2+} sites have not been observed (54,75,160). The reasons for the discrepant findings among these studies are not yet clear, but may be attributable to differences in experimental conditions and methods, or to differences in the subunit composition and/or biochemical state (e.g., phosphorylation) of

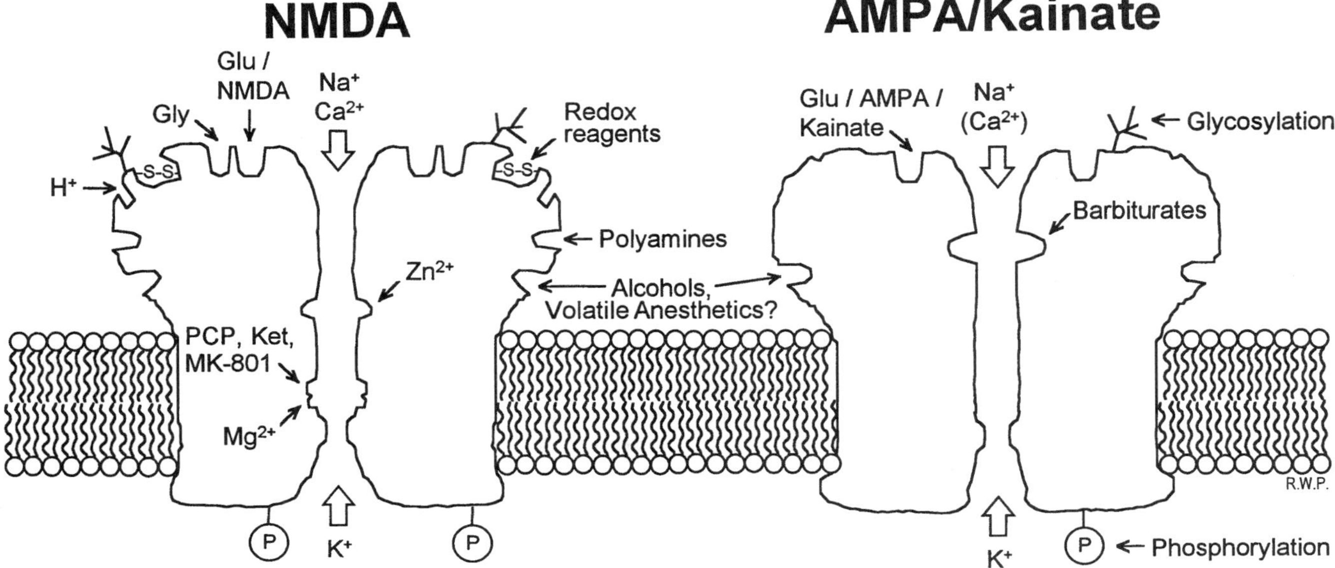

Figure 2. Diagram of the NMDA **(left)** and AMPA/kainate **(right)** glutamate receptors, showing proposed sites of action of agonists, modulatory agents, and anesthetics. Glu, glutamate; Gly, glycine; H+, proton; Ket, ketamine; PCP, phencyclidine.

the NMDA receptors among different preparations (203, 234,331).

Recent results from our laboratory have provided insight into the mechanism of action of alcohols on the NMDA receptor. For almost a century, it has been widely accepted that alcohols and anesthetics produce their CNS effects by acting on neuronal membrane lipids (73,105,163,193,202,215,229,246, 275). This lipid theory considers the effects of alcohols and anesthetics on membrane proteins, such as neurotransmitter receptors, to be secondary to their perturbation of membrane lipids. Our results, however, are difficult to reconcile with the most commonly proposed variant of such a mechanism, the hypothesis that alcohols act by disordering membrane lipids. This hypothesis predicts that the NMDA receptor inhibitory potency of various alcohols should closely follow their membrane disordering potency. We have found that this prediction holds true for aliphatic *n*-alcohols with fewer than six carbon atoms, but fails for *n*-alcohols with six or more carbon atoms (159,236). As the number of carbon atoms in an aliphatic *n*-alcohol is increased beyond six, NMDA receptor inhibitory potency reaches a maximum and then declines precipitously (236). This cutoff in potency is not explained by membrane disordering, because lipid solubility and membrane lipid disordering potency continue to increase in an exponential fashion as the number of carbon atoms in the alcohol is increased above six. In contrast, the cutoff for alcohol inhibition of NMDA receptors is consistent with an interaction of the alcohol with a hydrophobic pocket of fixed dimensions on the receptor protein. In addition, the potency of aliphatic *n*-alcohols for producing intoxication exhibited a cutoff that was similar to the cutoff for inhibition of NMDA receptors, suggesting that alcohol inhibition of NMDA receptors may contribute to alcohol intoxication.

SUMMARY AND CONCLUSIONS

Excitatory amino acids mediate the majority of excitatory neurotransmission in the CNS. Consequently, excitatory amino acid receptors would be predicted to be potential sites through which anesthetics could affect CNS excitability. This may be best illustrated by the observation that competitive and noncompetitive antagonists of NMDA and AMPA/kainate receptors have been reported to increase the duration of action or potency of various anesthetics, and to produce sedation and anesthesia. In regard to anesthetic action on excitatory amino acid receptors, there is compelling evidence that dissociative anesthetics act via NMDA receptor inhibition, and other anesthetics, such as barbiturates, inhibit AMPA/kainate receptors at concentrations associated with anesthesia. Thus, it is highly probable that inhibition of excitatory amino acid receptors mediates or contributes significantly to the CNS depressant effects of some anesthetic agents. On the other hand, the observation that some types of anesthetics, such as anesthetic steroids and many volatile anesthetics, produce little or no inhibition of excitatory amino acid receptors at concentrations associated with anesthesia argues against excitatory amino acid receptors as the sole site of action of all anesthetics. In addition, studies of the effects of various anesthetic agents on excitatory amino acid receptors indicate differences among types of anesthetics with respect to their specificity for excitatory amino acid receptor subtypes, site of action, and molecular mechanism of action (Fig. 2). Thus, although both dissociative anesthetics and barbiturates act via an open-channel block mechanism, dissociative anesthetics selectively inhibit NMDA receptors, while barbiturates selectively inhibit AMPA/kainate receptors. Volatile anesthetics, on the other hand, may inhibit excitatory amino acid receptor function by interacting with a hydrophobic pocket on the receptor protein that is similar, if not identical, to that associated with alcohol action on those receptors.

REFERENCES

1. Abe T, Sugihara H, Nawa H, Shigemoto R, Mizuno N, Nakanishi S. Molecular characterization of a novel metabotropic glutamate receptor mGluR5 coupled to inositol phosphate/Ca^{2+} signal transduction. *J Biol Chem* 1992;267:13361–13368.
2. Aizenman E, Lipton SA, Loring RH. Selective modulation of NMDA responses by reduction and oxidation. *Neuron* 1989; 2: 1257–1263.
3. Allott PR, Steward A, Flook V, Mapleson WW. Variation with temperature of the solubilities of inhaled anaesthetics in water, oil and biological media. *Br J Anaesth* 1973;45:294–301.
4. Anis NA, Berry SC, Burton NR, Lodge D. The dissociative anaesthetics, ketamine and phencyclidine, selectively reduce excitation of central mammalian neurones by N-methyl-aspartate. *Br J Pharmacol* 1983;79:565–575.
5. Aramori I, Nakanishi S. Signal transduction and pharmacological characteristics of a metabotropic glutamate receptor, mGluR1, in transfected CHO cells. *Neuron* 1992;8:757–765.
6. Aronstam RS, Martin DC, Dennison RL. Volatile anesthetics inhibit NMDA-stimulated ^{45}Ca uptake by rat brain microvesicles. *Neurochem Res* 1994;19:1515–1520.
7. Ascher P, Nowak L. Quisqualate- and kainate-activated channels in mouse central neurones in culture. *J Physiol (Lond)* 1988; 399: 227–245.
8. Balster RL, Nicholson KL, Sanger DJ. Evaluation of the reinforcing effects of eliprodil in rhesus monkeys and its discriminative stimulus effects in rats. *Drug Alcohol Depend* 1994;35:211–216.
9. Barker JL, Harrison NL, Lange GD, Owen DG. Potentiation of γ-aminobutyric-acid-activated chloride conductance by a steroid anaesthetic in cultured rat spinal neurones. *J Physiol (Lond)* 1987; 386:485–501.
10. Barker JL, Ransom BR. Pentobarbitone pharmacology of mammalian central neurones grown in tissue culture. *J Physiol (Lond)* 1978;280:355–372.
11. Barnes JM, Henley JM. Molecular characteristics of excitatory amino acid receptors. *Prog Neurobiol* 1992;39:113–133.
12. Bashir ZI, Bortolotto ZA, Davies CH, et al. Induction of LTP in the hippocampus needs synaptic activation of glutamate metabotropic receptors. *Nature* 1993;363:347–350.
13. Beardsley PM, Hayes BA, Balster RL. The self-administration of MK-801 can depend upon drug-reinforcement history, and its discriminative stimulus properties are phencyclidine-like in rhesus monkeys. *J Pharmacol Exp Ther* 1990;252:953–959.
14. Benavides J, Camelin JC, Mitrani N, et al. 2-Amino-6-trifluoromethoxy benzothiazole, a possible antagonist of excitatory amino acid neurotransmission-II. Biochemical properties. *Neuropharmacology* 1985;24:1085–1092.
15. Bennett DA, Bernard PS, Amrick CL. A comparison of PCP-like compounds for NMDA antagonism in two in vivo models. *Life Sci* 1988;42:447–454.
16. Bennett JA, Dingledine R. Topology profile for a glutamate receptor: three transmembrane domains and a channel-lining reentrant membrane loop. *Neuron* 1995;14:373–384.
17. Benvenga MJ, Wing AV, Del Vecchio RA. The discriminative stimulus effect of MK-801 in ketamine-trained rats. *Pharmacol Biochem Behav* 1991;38:211–213.
18. Benveniste M, Mayer ML. Multiple effects of spermine on *N*-methyl-D-aspartic acid receptor responses of rat cultured hippocampal neurones. *J Physiol (Lond)* 1993;464:131–163.
19. Berry SC, Burton NR, Anis NA, Lodge D. Stereoselective effects of two phencyclidine derivatives on N-methylaspartate excitation of spinal neurones in the cat and rat. *Eur J Pharmacol* 1983;96: 261–267.
20. Berry SC, Dawkins SL, Lodge D. Comparison of sigma- and kappa-opiate receptor ligands as excitatory amino acid antagonists. *Br J Pharmacol* 1984;83:179–185.
21. Bettler B, Boulter J, Hermans-Borgmeyer I, et al. Cloning of a novel glutamate receptor subunit, GluR5: expression in the nervous system during development. *Neuron* 1990;5:583–95.
22. Bliss TVP, Collingridge GL. A synaptic model of memory: long-term potentiation in the hippocampus. *Nature* 1993;361:31–39.
23. Bobelis DJ, Balster RL. Pharmacological specificity of the discriminative stimulus properties of 2-amino-4,5-(1,2-cyclohexyl)-7-phosphono-heptanoic acid (NPC 12626), a competitive *N*-methyl-D-aspartate receptor antagonist. *J Pharmacol Exp Ther* 1993;264: 845–853.
24. Bonhaus DW, McNamara JO. *N*-methyl-D-aspartate receptor regu-

lation of uncompetitive antagonist binding in rat brain membranes: kinetic analysis. *Mol Pharmacol* 1988;34:250–255.
25. Bonhaus DW, Yeh GC, Skaryak L, McNamara JO. Glycine regulation of the *N*-methyl-D-aspartate receptor-gated ion channel in hippocampal membranes. *Mol Pharmacol* 1989;36:273–279.
26. Bortolotto ZA, Collingridge GL. Activation of glutamate metabotropic receptors induces long-term potentiation. *Eur J Pharmacol* 1992;214:297–298.
27. Boulter J, Hollmann M, O'Shea-Greenfield A, et al. Molecular cloning and functional expression of glutamate receptor subunit genes. *Science* 1990;249:1033–1037.
28. Burnashev N, Monyer H, Seeburg PH, Sakmann B. Divalent ion permeability of AMPA receptor channels is dominated by the edited form of a single subunit. *Neuron* 1992;8:189–198.
29. Burnashev N, Schoepfer R, Monyer H, et al. Control by asparagine residues of calcium permeability and magnesium blockade in the NMDA receptor. *Science* 1992;257:1415–1419.
30. Butler TC. The delay in onset of action of intravenously injected anesthetics. *J Pharmacol* 1942;74:118–128.
31. Cai Z, McCaslin PP. Acute, chronic and differential effects of several anesthetic barbiturates on glutamate receptor activation in neuronal culture. *Brain Res* 1993;611:181–186.
32. Carlà V, Moroni F. General anaesthetics inhibit the responses induced by glutamate receptor agonists in the mouse cortex. *Neurosci Lett* 1992;146:21–24.
33. Carter AJ. Many agents that antagonize the NMDA receptor-channel complex in vivo also cause disturbances of motor coordination. *J Pharmacol Exp Ther* 1994;269:573–580.
34. Catchlove RFH, Krnjevic K, Maretic H. Similarity between effects of general anesthetics and dinitrophenol on cortical neurones. *Can J Physiol Pharmacol* 1972;50:1111–1114.
35. Cerne R, Jiang M, Randic M. Cyclic adenosine 3′5′-monophosphate potentiates excitatory amino acid and synaptic responses of rat spinal dorsal horn neurons. *Brain Res* 1992;596:111–123.
36. Chen L, Huang L-YM. Sustained potentiation of NMDA receptor-mediated glutamate responses through activation of protein kinase C by a mu opioid. *Neuron* 1991;7:319–326.
37. Chéramy A, Barbeito L, Godeheu G, Glowinski J. Riluzole inhibits the release of glutamate in the caudate nucleus of the cat in vivo. *Neurosci Lett* 1992;147:209–212.
38. Clissold DB, Pontecorvo MJ, Jones BE, et al. NPC 16377, a potent and selective sigma-ligand. II. Behavioral and neuroprotective profile. *J Pharmacol Exp Ther* 1993;265:876–886.
39. Collins GGS, Anson J. Effects of barbiturates on responses evoked by excitatory amino acids in slices of rat olfactory cortex. *Neuropharmacology* 1987;26:167–171.
40. Cooper JR, Bloom FE, Roth RH. *The biochemical basis of neuropharmacology*, 6th ed. New York: Oxford University Press, 1991.
41. Corbett R, Dunn RW. Effects of 5,7 dichlorokynurenic acid on conflict, social interaction and plus maze behaviors. *Neuropharmacology* 1993;32:461–466.
42. Corssen G, Domino EF. Dissociative anesthesia: further pharmacologic studies and first clinical experience with the phencyclidine derivative CI-581. *Anesth Analg* 1966;45:29–40.
43. Crawford JM. Anaesthetic agents and the chemical sensitivity of cortical neurones. *Neuropharmacology* 1970;9:31–46.
44. Crawford JM, Curtis DR. Pharmacological studies on feline Betz cells. *J Physiol (Lond)* 1966;186:121–138.
45. Dall V, Orntoft U, Schmidt A, Nordholm L. Interaction of the competitive AMPA receptor antagonist NBQX with hexobarbital. *Pharmacol Biochem Behav* 1993;46:73–76.
46. Daniell LC. The noncompetitive N-methyl-D-aspartate antagonists, MK-801, phencyclidine and ketamine, increase the potency of general anesthetics. *Pharmacol Biochem Behav* 1990;36:111–115.
47. Daniell LC. Effect of CGS 19755, a competitive *N*-methyl-D-aspartate antagonist, on general anesthetic potency. *Pharmacol Biochem Behav* 1991;40:767–769.
48. Daniell LC. Alteration of general anesthetic potency by agonists and antagonists of the polyamine binding site of the *N*-methyl-D-aspartate receptor. *J Pharmacol Exp Ther* 1992;261:304–310.
49. Daniell LC. Effect of anesthetic and convulsant barbiturates on *N*-methyl-D-aspartate receptor-mediated calcium flux in brain membrane vesicles. *Pharmacol* 1994;49:296–307.
50. Davis S, Butcher SP, Morris RGM. The NMDA receptor antagonist D-2-amino-5-phosphonopentanoate (D-AP5) impairs spatial learning and LTP in vivo at intracerebral concentrations comparable to those that block LTP in vitro. *J Neurosci* 1992;12:21–34.
51. de Jong RH, Eger EI. MAC expanded: AD_{50} and AD_{95} values of common inhalation anesthetics in man. *Anesthesiology* 1975;42: 384–389.
52. Debono M-W, Le Guern J, Canton T, Doble A, Pradier L. Inhibition by riluzole of electrophysiological responses mediated by rat kainate and NMDA receptors expressed in *Xenopus* oocytes. *Eur J Pharmacol* 1993;235:283–289.
53. Dildy JE, Leslie SW. Ethanol inhibits NMDA-induced increases in free intracellular Ca^{2+} in dissociated brain cells. *Brain Res* 1989;499: 383–387.
54. Dildy-Mayfield JE, Leslie SW. Mechanism of inhibition of *N*-methyl-D-aspartate-stimulated increases in free intracellular Ca^{2+} concentration by ethanol. *J Neurochem* 1991;56:1536–1543.
55. Drejer J, Honoré T. Phencyclidine analogues inhibit NMDA-stimulated [^{3}H]GABA release from cultured cortex neurons. *Eur J Pharmacol* 1987;143:287–290.
56. Duchen MR, Burton NR, Biscoe TJ. An intracellular study of the interactions of *N*-methyl-DL-aspartate with ketamine in the mouse hippocampal slice. *Brain Res* 1985;342:149–153.
57. Durand GM, Bennett MVL, Zukin RS. Splice variants of the *N*-methyl-D-aspartate receptor NR1 identify domains involved in regulation by polyamines and protein kinase C. *Proc Natl Acad Sci USA* 1993;90:6731–6735.
58. Durand GM, Gregor P, Zheng X, Bennett MV, Uhl GR, Zukin RS. Cloning of an apparent splice variant of the rat *N*-methyl-D-aspartate receptor NMDAR1 with altered sensitivity to polyamines and activators of protein kinase C. *Proc Natl Acad Sci USA* 1992;89: 9359–9363.
59. Egebjerg J, Bettler B, Hermans-Borgmeyer I, Heinemann S. Cloning of a cDNA for a glutamate receptor subunit activated by kainate but not AMPA. *Nature* 1991;351:745–748.
60. Fagg GE. Phencyclidine and related drugs bind to the activated *N*-methyl-D-aspartate receptor-channel complex in rat brain membranes. *Neurosci Lett* 1987;76:221–227.
61. Ferkany JW, Kyle DJ, Willetts J, et al. Pharmacological profile of NPC 12626, a novel, competitive *N*-methyl-D-aspartate receptor antagonist. *J Pharmacol Exp Ther* 1989;250:100–109.
62. Fink K, Göthert M. Inhibition of *N*-methyl-D-aspartate-induced noradrenaline release by alcohols is related to their hydrophobicity. *Eur J Pharmacol* 1990;191:225–229.
63. Fink K, Schultheiss R, Göthert M. Inhibition of *N*-methyl-D-aspartate- and kainate-evoked noradrenaline release in human cerebral cortex slices by ethanol. *Naunyn-Schmiedebergs Arch Pharmacol* 1992; 345:700–703.
64. Foster AC, Gill R, Kemp JA, Woodruff GN. Systemic administration of MK-801 prevents *N*-methyl-D-aspartate-induced neuronal degeneration in rat brain. *Neurosci Lett* 1987;76:307–311.
65. Foster AC, Wong EH. The novel anticonvulsant MK-801 binds to the activated state of the *N*-methyl-D-aspartate receptor in rat brain. *Br J Pharmacol* 1987;91:403–409.
66. France CP, Winger GD, Woods JH. Analgesic, anesthetic, and respiratory effects of the competitive *N*-methyl-D-aspartate (NMDA) antagonist CGS 19755 in rhesus monkeys. *Brain Res* 1990;526: 355–358.
67. France CP, Woods JH, Ornstein P. The competitive *N*-methyl-D-aspartate (NMDA) antagonist CGS 19755 attenuates the rate-decreasing effects of NMDA in rhesus monkeys without producing ketamine-like discriminative stimulus effects. *Eur J Pharmacol* 1989; 159:133–139.
68. Gasic GP, Hollmann M. Molecular neurobiology of glutamate receptors. *Annu Rev Physiol* 1992;54:507–536.
69. Gerber G, Kangrga I, Ryu PD, Larew JS, Randic M. Multiple effects of phorbol esters in the rat spinal dorsal horn. *J Neurosci* 1989;9: 3606–3617.
70. Gibb AJ, Colquhoun D. Glutamate activation of a single NMDA receptor-channel produces a cluster of channel openings. *Proc R Soc Lond [Biol]* 1991;243:39–45.
71. Glaum SR, Holzwarth JA, Miller RJ. Glutamate receptors activate Ca^{2+} mobilization and Ca^{2+} influx into astrocytes. *Proc Natl Acad Sci USA* 1990;87:3454–3458.
72. Gold LH, Balster RL. Effects of NMDA receptor antagonists in squirrel monkeys trained to discriminate the competitive NMDA receptor antagonist NPC 12626 from saline. *Eur J Pharmacol* 1993; 230:285–292.
73. Goldstein DB. The effects of drugs on membrane fluidity. *Annu Rev Pharmacol Toxicol* 1984;24:43–64.
74. Gonzales RA, Westbrook SL, Bridges LT. Alcohol-induced inhibi-

tion of N-methyl-D-aspartate-evoked release of [^{3}H]norepinephrine from brain is related to lipophilicity. *Neuropharmacology* 1991; 30:441–446.

75. Gonzales RA, Woodward JJ. Ethanol inhibits N-methyl-D-aspartate-stimulated [^{3}H]norepinephrine release from rat cortical slices. *J Pharmacol Exp Ther* 1990;253:1138–1144.
76. Göthert M, Fink K. Inhibition of N-methyl-D-aspartate (NMDA)- and L-glutamate-induced noradrenaline and acetylcholine release in the rat brain by ethanol. *Naunyn-Schmiedebergs Arch Pharmacol* 1989;340:516–521.
77. Grant KA, Colombo G. Discriminative stimulus effects of ethanol: effect of training dose on the substitution of N-methyl-D-aspartate antagonists. *J Pharmacol Exp Ther* 1993;264:1241–1247.
78. Greengard P, Jen J, Nairn AC, Stevens CF. Enhancement of the glutamate response by cAMP-dependent protein kinase in hippocampal neurons. *Science* 1991;253:1135–1138.
79. Halliwell RF, Peters JA, Lambert JJ. The mechanism of action and pharmacological specificity of the anticonvulsant NMDA antagonist MK-801: a voltage clamp study on neuronal cells in culture. *Br J Pharmacol* 1989;96:480–494.
80. Hansch C, Anderson SM. The structure-activity relationship in barbiturates and its similarity to that in other narcotics. *J Med Chem* 1967;10:745–753.
81. Harada K, Nagatsugu Y, Ito H, Shingai R. Intracellular cAMP regulates the response to NMDA in hippocampal neurons. *Neuroreport* 1991;2:673–676.
82. Harrison NL. Pentobarbitone as an excitatory amino acid antagonist in slices of rat cerebral cortex. *J Physiol (Lond)* 1985;360:38P.
83. Harrison NL, Majewska MD, Harrington JW, Barker JL. Structure-activity relationships for steroid interaction with the γ-aminobutyric acid$_A$ receptor complex. *J Pharmacol Exp Ther* 1987;241: 346–353.
84. Harrison NL, Simmonds MA. Modulation of the GABA receptor complex by a steroid anaesthetic. *Brain Res* 1984;323:287–292.
85. Harrison NL, Simmonds MA. Quantitative studies on some antagonists of N-methyl D-aspartate in slices of rat cerebral cortex. *Br J Pharmacol* 1985;84:381–391.
86. Hayashi Y, Momiyama A, Takahashi T, et al. Role of a metabotropic glutamate receptor in synaptic modulation in the accessory olfactory bulb. *Nature* 1993;366:687–690.
87. Herb A, Burnashev N, Werner P, Sakmann B, Wisden W, Seeburg PH. The KA-2 subunit of excitatory amino acid receptors shows widespread expression in brain and forms ion channels with distantly related subunits. *Neuron* 1992;8:775–785.
88. Herling S, Valentino RJ, Winger GD. Discriminative stimulus effects of pentobarbital in pigeons. *Psychopharmacology (Berl)* 1980; 71:21–28.
89. Herrling PL, Maeder J, Meier CL, Do KQ. Differential effects of (D)- and (L)-homocysteic acid on the membrane potential of cat caudate neurons in situ. *Neuroscience* 1989;31:213–217.
90. Hille B. *Ionic channels of excitable membranes,* 2nd ed. Sunderland, MA: Sinauer Associates, 1992.
91. Hoffman PL, Moses F, Tabakoff B. Selective inhibition by ethanol of glutamate-stimulated cyclic GMP production in primary cultures of cerebellar granule cells. *Neuropharmacology* 1989;28:1239–1243.
92. Hoffman PL, Rabe CS, Moses F, Tabakoff B. N-methyl-D-aspartate receptors and ethanol: inhibition of calcium flux and cyclic GMP production. *J Neurochem* 1989;52:1937–1940.
93. Hollmann M, Boulter J, Maron C, et al. Zinc potentiates agonist-induced currents at certain splice variants of the NMDA receptor. *Neuron* 1993;10:943–954.
94. Hollmann M, Hartley M, Heinemann S. Ca^{2+} permeability of KA-AMPA-gated glutamate receptor channels depends on subunit composition. *Science* 1991;252:851–853.
95. Hollmann M, Heinemann S. Cloned glutamate receptors. *Annu Rev Neurosci* 1994;17:31–108.
96. Hollmann M, Maron C, Heinemann S. N-Glycosylation site tagging suggests a three transmembrane domain topology for the glutamate receptor GluR1. *Neuron* 1994;13:1331–1343.
97. Hollmann M, O'Shea-Greenfield A, Rogers SW, Heinemann S. Cloning by functional expression of a member of the glutamate receptor family. *Nature* 1989;342:643–648.
98. Honey CR, Miljkovic Z, MacDonald JF. Ketamine and phencyclidine cause a voltage-dependent block of responses to L-aspartic acid. *Neurosci Lett* 1985;61:135–139.
99. Honoré T, Davies SN, Drejer J, et al. Quinoxalinediones: potent competitive non-NMDA glutamate receptor antagonists. *Science* 1988;241:701–703.
100. Horne AL, Simmonds MA. The pharmacology of quisqualate and AMPA in the cerebral cortex of the rat in vitro. *Neuropharmacology* 1989;28:1113–1118.
101. Houamed KM, Kuijper JL, Gilbert TL, et al. Cloning, expression, and gene structure of a G protein-coupled glutamate receptor from rat brain. *Science* 1991;252:1318–1321.
102. Hubert JP, Delumeau JC, Glowinski J, Prémont J, Doble A. Antagonism by riluzole of entry of calcium evoked by NMDA and veratridine in rat cultured granule cells: Evidence for a dual mechanism of action. *Br J Pharmacol* 1994;113:261–267.
103. Huettner JE, Bean BP. Block of N-methyl-D-aspartate-activated current by the anticonvulsant MK-801: selective binding to open channels. *Proc Natl Acad Sci USA* 1988;85:1307–1311.
104. Hume RI, Dingledine R, Heinemann SF. Identification of a site in glutamate receptor subunits that controls calcium permeability. *Science* 1991;253:1028–1031.
105. Hunt WA. Neuroscience research: How has it contributed to our understanding of alcohol abuse and alcoholism? A review. *Alcohol Clin Exp Res* 1993;17:1055–1065.
106. Iino M, Ozawa S, Tsuzuki K. Permeation of calcium through excitatory amino acid receptor channels in cultured rat hippocampal neurones. *J Physiol (Lond)* 1990;424:151–165.
107. Im WB, Blakeman DP, Davis JP, Ayer DE. Studies on the mechanism of interactions between anesthetic steroids and γ-aminobutyric acid$_A$ receptors. *Mol Pharmacol* 1990;37:429–434.
108. Ino M, Ozawa S, Tsuzuki K. Permeation of calcium through excitatory amino acid receptor channels in cultured rat hippocampal neurones. *J Physiol (Lond)* 1990;424:151–165.
109. Irifune M, Shimizu T, Nomoto M, Fukuda T. Ketamine-induced anesthesia involves the N-methyl-D-aspartate receptor-channel complex in mice. *Brain Res* 1992;596:1–9.
110. Ishii T, Moriyoshi K, Sugihara H, et al. Molecular characterization of the family of the N-methyl-D-aspartate receptor subunits. *J Biol Chem* 1993;268:2836–2843.
111. Jackson A, Sanger DJ. Is the discriminative stimulus produced by phencyclidine due to an interaction with N-methyl-D-aspartate receptors? *Psychopharmacology (Berl)* 1988;96:87–92.
112. Jahr CE, Stevens CF. Glutamate activates multiple single channel conductances in hippocampal neurons. *Nature* 1987;325:522–525.
113. Jarvis MF, Murphy DE, Williams M. Quantitative autoradiographic localization of NMDA receptors in rat brain using [^{3}H]CPP: comparison with [^{3}H]TCP binding sites. *Eur J Pharmacol* 1987;141: 149–152.
114. Javitt DC, Jotkowitz A, Sircar R, Zukin SR. Non-competitive regulation of phencyclidine/sigma-receptors by the N-methyl-D-aspartate receptor antagonist D-(-)-2-amino-5-phosphonovaleric acid. *Neurosci Lett* 1987;78:193–198.
115. Javitt DC, Zukin SR. Interaction of [^{3}H]MK-801 with multiple states of the N-methyl-D-aspartate receptor complex of rat brain. *Proc Natl Acad Sci USA* 1989;86:740–744.
116. Javitt DC, Zukin SR. Biexponential kinetics of [^{3}H]MK-801 binding: evidence for access to closed and open N-methyl-D-aspartate receptor channels. *Mol Pharmacol* 1989;35:387–393.
117. Johnson ES, Roberts MHT, Straughan DW. The responses of cortical neurones to monoamines under differing anaesthetic conditions. *J Physiol (Lond)* 1969;203:261–280.
118. Johnson JW, Ascher P. Glycine potentiates the NMDA response in cultured mouse brain neurons. *Nature* 1987;325:529–531.
119. Johnson KM, Sacaan AI, Snell LD. Equilibrium analysis of [^{3}H] TCP binding: effects of glycine, magnesium and N-methyl-D-aspartate agonists. *Eur J Pharmacol* 1988;152:141–146.
120. Jonas P, Sakmann B. Glutamate receptor channels in isolated patches from CA1 and CA3 pyramidal cells of rat hippocampal slices. *J Physiol (Lond)* 1992;455:143–171.
121. Jones MV, Brooks PA, Harrison NL. Enhancement of γ-aminobutyric acid-activated Cl^- currents in cultured rat hippocampal neurones by three volatile anaesthetics. *J Physiol (Lond)* 1992;449: 279–293.
122. Jones SM, Snell LD, Johnson KM. Phencyclidine selectively inhibits N-methyl-D-aspartate-induced hippocampal [^{3}H]norepinephrine release. *J Pharmacol Exp Ther* 1987;240:492–497.
123. Jones SM, Snell LD, Johnson KM. Inhibition by phencyclidine of excitatory amino acid-stimulated release of neurotransmitter in the nucleus accumbens. *Neuropharmacology* 1987;26:173–179.
124. Jortani SA, Willetts J, Balster RL. Systemic magnesium chloride administration fails to produce phencyclidine-like discriminative stimulus effects in rats. *Neurosci Lett* 1992;135:136–138.

125. Juhász G, Kékesi K, Emri Z, Soltesz I, Crunelli V. Sleep-promoting action of excitatory amino acid antagonists: a different role for thalamic NMDA and non-NMDA receptors. *Neurosci Lett* 1990; 114:333–338.
126. Karschin A, Aizenman E, Lipton SA. The interaction of agonists and noncompetitive antagonists at the excitatory amino acid receptors in rat retinal ganglion cells in vitro. *J Neurosci* 1988;8: 2895–2906.
127. Kawajiri S, Dingledine R. Multiple structural determinants of voltage-dependent magnesium block in recombinant NMDA receptors. *Neuropharmacology* 1993;32:1203–1211.
128. Keinänen K, Wisden W, Sommer B, et al. A family of AMPA-selective glutamate receptors. *Science* 1990;249:556–560.
129. Kelland MD, Soltis RP, Boldry RC, Walters JR. Behavioral and electrophysiological comparison of ketamine with dizocilpine in the rat. *Physiol Behav* 1993;54:547–554.
130. Kleckner NW, Dingledine R. Requirement for glycine in activation of NMDA-receptors expressed in Xenopus oocytes. *Science* 1988;241:835–837.
131. Kloog Y, Haring R, Sokolovsky M. Kinetic characterization of the phencyclidine-*N*-methyl-D-aspartate receptor interaction: evidence for a steric blockade of the channel. *Biochem* 1988;27: 843–848.
132. Kloog Y, Nadler V, Sokolovsky M. Mode of binding of [^{3}H]dibenzocycloalkenimine (MK-801) to the *N*-methyl-D-aspartate (NMDA) receptor and its therapeutic implication. *FEBS Lett* 1988; 230: 167–170.
133. Koek W, Woods JH, Colpaert FC. *N*-methyl-D-aspartate antagonism and phencyclidine-like activity: a drug discrimination analysis. *J Pharmacol Exp Ther* 1990;253:1017–1025.
134. Koek W, Woods JH, Jacobson AE, Rice KC. Phencyclidine (PCP)-like discriminative stimulus effects of metaphit and of 2-amino-5-phosphonovalerate in pigeons: generality across different training doses of PCP. *Psychopharmacology (Berl)* 1987;93:437–442.
135. Koek W, Woods JH, Winger GD. MK-801, a proposed noncompetitive antagonist of excitatory amino acid neurotransmission, produces phencyclidine-like behavioral effects in pigeons, rats and rhesus monkeys. *J Pharmacol Exp Ther* 1988;245:969–974.
136. Koh JY, Palmer E, Cotman CW. Activation of the metabotropic glutamate receptor attenuates *N*-methyl-D-aspartate neurotoxicity in cortical cultures. *Proc Natl Acad Sci USA* 1991;88:9431–9435.
137. Korten K, Miller KW. Erythrocyte ghost-buffer partition coefficients of phenobarbital, pentobarbital, and thiopental support the pH-partition hypothesis. *Can J Physiol Pharmacol* 1979;57: 325–328.
138. Krnjevic K, Phillis JW. Pharmacological properties of acetylcholine-sensitive cells in the cerebral cortex. *J Physiol (Lond)* 1963; 166:328–350.
139. Kuroda Y, Strebel S, Rafferty C, Bullock R. Neuroprotective doses of *N*-methyl-D-aspartate receptor antagonists profoundly reduce the minimum alveolar anesthetic concentration (MAC) for isoflurane in rats. *Anesth Analg* 1993;77:795–800.
140. Kutsuwada T, Kashiwabuchi N, Mori H, et al. Molecular diversity of the NMDA receptor channel. *Nature* 1992;358:36–41.
141. Lalies M, Middlemiss DN, Ransom R. Stereoselective antagonism of NMDA-stimulated noradrenaline release from rat hippocampal slices by MK-801. *Neurosci Lett* 1988;91:339–342.
142. Lambert JDC, Flatman JA. The interaction between barbiturate anaesthetics and excitatory amino acid responses on cat spinal neurones. *Neuropharmacology* 1981;20:227–240.
143. Leander JD, Lawson RR, Ornstein PL, Zimmerman DM. *N*-methyl-D-aspartic acid-induced lethality in mice: selective antagonism by phencyclidine-like drugs. *Brain Res* 1988;448:115–120.
144. Legendre P, Rosenmund C, Westbrook GL. Inactivation of NMDA channels in cultured hippocampal neurons by intracellular calcium. *J Neurosci* 1993;13:674–684.
145. Leslie K, Mooney PH, Silbert BS. Effect of intravenous clonidine on the dose of thiopental required to induce anesthesia. *Anesth Analg* 1992;75:530–535.
146. Lester RAJ, Clements JD, Westbrook GL, Jahr CE. Channel kinetics determine the time course of NMDA receptor-mediated synaptic currents. *Nature* 1990;346:565–567.
147. Lester RAJ, Jahr CE. NMDA channel behavior depends on agonist affinity. *J Neurosci* 1992;12:635–643.
148. Li H, Chen S, Zhao H. Fractal mechanisms for the allosteric effects of proteins and enzymes. *Biophys J* 1990;58:1313–1320.
149. Lieberman DN, Mody I. Regulation of NMDA channel function by endogenous Ca^{2+}-dependent phosphatase. *Nature* 1994;369: 235–239.
150. Lima-Landman MTR, Albuquerque EX. Ethanol potentiates and blocks NMDA-activated single-channel currents in rat hippocampal pyramidal cells. *FEBS Lett* 1989;247:61–67.
151. Lin L-H, Chen LL, Harris RA. Enflurane inhibits NMDA, AMPA, and kainate-induced currents in *Xenopus* oocytes expressing mouse and human brain mRNA. *FASEB J* 1993;7:479–485.
152. Lipton SA, Rosenberg PA. Mechanisms of disease: Excitatory amino acids as a final common pathway for neurologic disorders. *N Engl J Med* 1994;330:613–622.
153. Lodge D, Anis NA. Effects of phencyclidine on excitatory amino acid activation of spinal interneurones in the cat. *Eur J Pharmacol* 1982;77:203–204.
154. Lodge D, Johnson KM. Noncompetitive excitatory amino acid receptor antagonists. *Trends Pharmacol Sci* 1990;11:81–86.
155. Lodge D, Johnston GA. Effect of ketamine on amino acid-evoked release of acetylcholine from rat cerebral cortex in vitro. *Neurosci Lett* 1985;56:371–375.
156. Loo P, Braunwalder A, Lehmann J, Williams M. Radioligand binding to central phencyclidine recognition sites is dependent on excitatory amino acid receptor agonists. *Eur J Pharmacol* 1986;123: 467–468.
157. Loo PS, Braunwalder AF, Lehmann J, Williams M, Sills MA. Interaction of L-glutamate and magnesium with phencyclidine recognition sites in rat brain: evidence for multiple affinity states of the phencyclidine/*N*-methyl-D-aspartate receptor complex. *Mol Pharmacol* 1987;32:820–830.
158. Lovinger DM, Peoples RW. Actions of alcohols and other sedative/hypnotic compounds on cation channels associated with glutamate and 5-HT_3 receptors. In: Alling C, Diamond I, Leslie SW, Sun G, Wood WG, eds. *Alcohol, cell membranes, and signal transduction in brain.* New York: Plenum Press, 1993;157–167.
159. Lovinger DM, White G, Weight FF. Ethanol inhibits NMDA-activated ion current in hippocampal neurons. *Science* 1989;243: 1721–1724.
160. Lovinger DM, White G, Weight FF. Ethanol (EtOH) inhibition of NMDA-activated ion current is not voltage-dependent and EtOH does not interact with other binding sites on the NMDA receptor/ionophore complex. *FASEB J* 1990;4:A678.
161. Lovinger DM, White G, Weight FF. NMDA receptor-mediated synaptic excitation selectively inhibited by ethanol in hippocampal slice from adult rat. *J Neurosci* 1990;10:1372–1379.
162. Lynch DR, Anegawa NJ, Verdoorn T, Pritchett DB. *N*-methyl-D-aspartate receptors: different subunit requirements for binding of glutamate antagonists, glycine antagonists, and channel-blocking agents. *Mol Pharmacol* 1994;45:540–545.
163. Lyon RC, McComb JA, Schreurs J, Goldstein DB. A relationship between alcohol intoxication and the disordering of brain membranes by a series of short-chain alcohols. *J Pharmacol Exp Ther* 1981;218:669–675.
164. MacDonald JF, Bartlett MC, Mody I, et al. Actions of ketamine, phencyclidine and MK-801 on NMDA receptor currents in cultured mouse hippocampal neurones. *J Physiol (Lond)* 1991;432: 483–508.
165. MacDonald JF, Miljkovic Z, Pennefather P. Use-dependent block of excitatory amino acid currents in cultured neurons by ketamine. *J Neurophysiol* 1987;58:251–266.
166. MacDonald JF, Mody I, Salter MW. Regulation of *N*-methyl-D-aspartate receptors revealed by intracellular dialysis of murine neurones in culture. *J Physiol (Lond)* 1989;414:17–34.
167. Macdonald RL, Barker JL. Different actions of anticonvulsant and anesthetic barbiturates revealed by use of cultured mammalian neurons. *Science* 1978;200:775–777.
168. Macdonald RL, Barker JL. Enhancement of GABA-mediated postsynaptic inhibition in cultured mammalian spinal cord neurons: a common mode of anticonvulsant action. *Brain Res* 1979;167: 323–336.
169. MacKinnon R, Miller C. Mechanism of charybdotoxin block of the high-conductance, Ca^{2+}-activated K^+ channel. *J Gen Physiol* 1988;91:335–349.
170. Majewska MD, Harrison NL, Schwartz RD, Barker JL, Paul SM. Steroid hormone metabolites are barbiturate-like modulators of the GABA receptor. *Science* 1986;232:1004–1007.
171. Malgouris C, Bardot F, Daniel M, et al. Riluzole, a novel antiglutamate, prevents memory loss and hippocampal neuronal damage in ischemic gerbils. *J Neurosci* 1989;9:3720–3727.
172. Malgouris C, Daniel M, Doble A. Neuroprotective effects of riluzole on *N*-methyl-D-aspartate- or veratridine-induced neurotoxic-

ity in rat hippocampal slices. *Neurosci Lett* 1994;177:95–99.
173. Mansbach RS, Balster RL. Pharmacological specificity of the phencyclidine discriminative stimulus in rats. *Pharmacol Biochem Behav* 1991;39:971–975.
174. Mantz J, Chéramy A, Thierry A-M, Glowinski J, Desmonts J-M. Anesthetic properties of riluzole (54274 RP), a new inhibitor of glutamate neurotransmission. *Anesthesiol* 1992;76:844–848.
175. Mantz J, Laudenbach V, Lecharny JB, Henzel D, Desmonts JM. Riluzole, a novel antiglutamate, blocks GABA uptake by striatal synaptosomes. *Eur J Pharmacol* 1994;257:R7–8.
176. Maragos WF, Chu DC, Greenamyre JT, Penney JB, Young AB. High correlation between the localization of [^{3}H]TCP binding and NMDA receptors. *Eur J Pharmacol* 1986;123:173–174.
177. Maragos WF, Penney JB, Young AB. Anatomic correlation of NMDA and ^{3}H-TCP-labeled receptors in rat brain. *J Neurosci* 1988; 8:493–501.
178. Marshall BE, Longnecker DE. General anesthetics. In: Gilman AG, Rall TW, Nies AS, Taylor P, eds. *Goodman and Gilman's the pharmacological basis of therapeutics,* 8th ed. New York: Pergamon Press, 1990;285–310.
179. Marszalec W, Narahashi T. Use-dependent pentobarbital block of kainate and quisqualate currents. *Brain Res* 1993;608:7–15.
180. Martin D, Lodge D. Ketamine acts as a non-competitive *N*-methyl-D-aspartate antagonist on frog spinal cord in vitro. *Neuropharmacology* 1985;24:999–1003.
181. Martin D, Morrisett RA, Bian XP, Wilson WA, Swartzwelder HS. Ethanol inhibition of NMDA mediated depolarizations is increased in the presence of Mg^{2+}. *Brain Res* 1991;546:227–234.
182. Martin D, Thompson MA, Nadler JV. The neuroprotective agent riluzole inhibits release of glutamate and aspartate from slices of hippocampal area CA1. *Eur J Pharmacol* 1993;250:473–476.
183. Martin DC, Abraham JE, Plagenhoef M, Aronstam RS. Volatile anesthetics and NMDA receptors. Enflurane inhibition of glutamate-stimulated [^{3}H]MK-801 binding and reversal by glycine. *Neurosci Lett* 1991;132:73–76.
184. Martin DC, Dennison RL, Aronstam RS. Barbiturate interactions with *N*-methyl-d-aspartate (NMDA) receptors in rat brain. *Mol Neuropharmacol* 1992;2:255–259.
185. Masu M, Tanabe Y, Tsuchida K, Shigemoto R, Nakanishi S. Sequence and expression of a metabotropic glutamate receptor. *Nature* 1991;349:760–765.
186. Mayer ML, Westbrook GL. Permeation and block of *N*-methyl-D-aspartic acid receptor channels by divalent cations in mouse cultured central neurones. *J Physiol (Lond)* 1987;394:501–527.
187. Mayer ML, Westbrook GL. Mixed-agonist action of excitatory amino acids on mouse spinal cord neurones under voltage clamp. *J Physiol (Lond)* 1988;354:29–53.
188. Mayer ML, Westbrook GL, Guthrie PB. Voltage-dependent block by Mg^{2+} of NMDA responses in spinal cord neurones. *Nature* 1984;309:261–263.
189. Mayer ML, Westbrook GL, Vyklicky L. Sites of antagonist action on *N*-methyl-D-aspartic acid receptors studied using fluctuation analysis and a rapid perfusion technique. *J Neurophysiol* 1988; 60: 645–663.
190. McBain CJ, Mayer ML. *N*-methyl-D-aspartic acid receptor structure and function. *Physiol Rev* 1994;74:723.
191. McCaslin PP, Morgan WW. 2-Amino-7-phosphoheptanoic acid, a selective antagonist of *N*-methyl-D-aspartate, prevents barbital withdrawal-induced convulsions and the elevation of cerebellar cyclic GMP in dependent rats. *Neuropharmacology* 1987;26: 731–735.
192. McCaslin PP, Morgan WW. Anticonvulsive activity of several excitatory amino acid antagonists against barbital withdrawal-induced spontaneous convulsions. *Eur J Pharmacol* 1988;147:381–386.
193. McCreery MJ, Hunt WA. Physico-chemical correlates of alcohol intoxication. *Neuropharmacology* 1978;17:451–461.
194. McDonald JW, Fix AS, Tizzano JP, Schoepp DD. Seizures and brain injury in neonatal rats induced by 1*S*, 3*R*-ACPD, a metabotropic glutamate receptor agonist. *J Neurosci* 1993;13: 4445–4455.
195. McDonald JW, Schoepp DD. The metabotropic excitatory amino acid receptor agonist 1S,3R-ACPD selectively potentiates *N*-methyl-D-aspartate-induced brain injury. *Eur J Pharmacol* 1992; 215:353–354.
196. McFarlane C, Warner DS, Todd MM, Nordholm L. AMPA receptor competitive antagonism reduces halothane MAC in rats. *Anesthesiol* 1992;77:1165–1170.
197. McGlade-McCulloh E, Yamamoto H, Tan S-E, Brickey DA, Soderling TR. Phosphorylation and regulation of glutamate receptors by calcium/calmodulin-dependent protein kinase II. *Nature* 1993; 362:640–642.
198. McGurk JF, Bennett MVL, Zukin RS. Polyamines potentiate responses of *N*-methyl-D-aspartate receptors expressed in Xenopus oocytes. *Proc Natl Acad Sci USA* 1990;87:9971–9974.
199. McLarnon JG, Wong JHP, Sawyer D, Baimbridge K, G. The actions of intermediate and long-chain *n*-alkanols on unitary NMDA currents in hippocampal neurons. *Can J Physiol Pharmacol* 1991;69: 1422–1427.
200. Meguro H, Mori H, Araki K, et al. Functional characterization of a heteromeric NMDA receptor channel expressed from cloned cDNAs. *Nature* 1992;357:70–74.
201. Mendelsohn LG, Kerchner GA, Kalra V, Zimmerman DM, Leander JD. Phencyclidine receptors in rat brain cortex. *Biochem Pharmacol* 1984;33:3529–3535.
202. Meyer HH. Zur Theorie der Alkoholnarkose. I. Mitt. Welche Eigenschaft der Anästhetika bedingt ihre narkotische Wirkung? *Arch Exp Pathol Pharmakol* 1899;42:109–118.
203. Michaelis ML, Michaelis EK. Effects of ethanol on NMDA receptors in brain: Possibilities for Mg^{2+}-ethanol interactions. *Alcoholism (NY)* 1994;18:1069–1075.
204. Miljkovic Z, MacDonald JF. Voltage-dependent block of excitatory amino acid currents by pentobarbital. *Brain Res* 1986;376: 396–399.
205. Miller B, Sarantis M, Traynelis SF, Attwell D. Potentiation of NMDA receptor currents by arachidonic acid. *Nature* 1992;355: 722–725.
206. Miyamoto M, Ishida M, Kwak S, Shinozaki H. Agonists for metabotropic glutamate receptors in the rat delay recovery from halothane anesthesia. *Eur J Pharmacol* 1994;260:99–102.
207. Mizoule J, Meldrum B, Mazadier M, et al. 2-Amino-6-trifluoromethoxy benzothiazole, a possible antagonist of excitatory amino acid neurotransmissionól. Anticonvulsant properties. *Neuropharmacology* 1985;24:767–773.
208. Monaghan DT, Olverman HJ, Nguyen L, Watkins JC, Cotman CW. Two classes of *N*-methyl-D-aspartate recognition sites: differential distribution and differential regulation by glycine. *Proc Natl Acad Sci USA* 1988;85:9836–9840.
209. Monyer H, Sprengel R, Schoepfer R, et al. Heteromeric NMDA receptors: molecular and functional distinction of subtypes. *Science* 1992;256:1217–1221.
210. Mori H, Masaki H, Yamakura T, Mishina M. Identification by mutagenesis of a Mg^{2+}-block site of the NMDA receptor channel. *Nature* 1992;358:673–675.
211. Morita T, Sakimura K, Kushiya E, et al. Cloning and functional expression of a cDNA encoding the mouse β2 subunit of the kainate-selective glutamate receptor channel. *Mol Brain Res* 1992; 14:143–146.
212. Moriyoshi K, Masu M, Ishii T, Shigemoto R, Mizuno N, Nakanishi S. Molecular cloning and characterization of the rat NMDA receptor. *Nature* 1991;354:31–37.
213. Morris RGM, Anderson E, Lynch GS, Baudry M. Selective impairment of learning and blockade of long-term potentiation by an *N*-methyl-D-aspartate antagonist, AP5. *Nature* 1986;319:774–776.
214. Morrisett RA, Martin D, Oetting TA, Lewis DV, Wilson WA, Swartzwelder HS. Ethanol and magnesium ions inhibit *N*-methyl-D-aspartate-mediated synaptic potentials in an interactive manner. *Neuropharmacology* 1991;30:1173–1178.
215. Mullins LJ. Some physical mechanisms in narcosis. *Chem Rev* 1954; 54:289–323.
216. Nakajima Y, Iwakabe H, Akazawa C, et al. Molecular characterization of a novel retinal metabotropic glutamate receptor mGluR6 with a high agonist selectivity for L-2-amino-4-phosphonobutyrate. *J Biol Chem* 1993;268:11868–11873.
217. Nakanishi N, Axel R, Shneider NA. Alternative splicing generates functionally distinct *N*-methyl-D-aspartate receptors. *Proc Natl Acad Sci USA* 1992;89:8552–8556.
218. Nakanishi N, Shneider NA, Axel R. A family of glutamate receptor genes: evidence for the formation of heteromultimeric receptors with distinct channel properties. *Neuron* 1990;5:569–581.
219. Nakanishi S. Molecular diversity of glutamate receptors and implications for brain function. *Science* 1992;258:597–603.
220. Nakanishi S. Metabotropic glutamate receptors: synaptic transmission, modulation, and plasticity. *Neuron* 1994;13:1031–1037.
221. Nelson PG, Pun RY, Westbrook GL. Synaptic excitation in cultures

of mouse spinal cord neurones: receptor pharmacology and behaviour of synaptic currents. *J Physiol (Lond)* 1986;372:169–190.
222. Nishikawa M, Kimura S, Akaike N. Facilitatory effect of docosahexaenoic acid on *N*-methyl-D-aspartate response in pyramidal neurones of rat cerebral cortex. *J Physiol (Lond)* 1994;475:83–93.
223. Nomura A, Shigemoto R, Nakamura Y, Okamoto N, Mizuno N, Nakanishi S. Developmentally regulated postsynaptic localization of a metabotropic glutamate receptor in rat rod bipolar cells. *Cell* 1994;77:361–369.
224. Nowak L, Bregestovski P, Ascher P, Herbet A, Prochiantz A. Magnesium gates glutamate-activated channels in mouse central neurones. *Nature* 1984;307:462–465.
225. O'Hara PJ, Sheppard PO, Thøgersen H, et al. The ligand-binding domain in metabotropic glutamate receptors is related to bacterial periplasmic binding proteins. *Neuron* 1993;11:41–52.
226. O'Shaughnessy CT, Lodge D. *N*-methyl-D-aspartate receptor-mediated increase in intracellular calcium is reduced by ketamine and phencyclidine. *Eur J Pharmacol* 1988;153:201–209.
227. Ohmori T, Koyama T, Nakamura F, Wang P, Yamashita I. Effect of phencyclidine on spontaneous and *N*-methyl-D-aspartate (NMDA)-induced efflux of dopamine from superfused slices of rat striatum. *Neuropharmacology* 1992;31:461–467.
228. Okamoto N, Hori S, Akazawa C, et al. Molecular characterization of a new metabotropic glutamate receptor mGluR7 coupled to inhibitory cyclic AMP signal transduction. *J Biol Chem* 1994;269: 1231–1236.
229. Overton E. *Studien ¸ber die Narkose zugleich ein Beitrag zur allgemeinen Pharmakologie.* Jena: G. Fischer, 1901.
230. Palmer AJ, Zeman S, Lodge D. Methohexitone antagonises kainate and epileptiform activity in rat neocortical slices. *Eur J Pharmacol* 1992;221:205–209.
231. Patneau DK, Mayer ML. Structure-activity relationships for amino acid transmitter candidates acting at *N*-methyl-D-aspartate and quisqualate receptors. *J Neurosci* 1990;10:2385–2399.
232. Patneau DK, Vyklicky L Jr., Mayer ML. Hippocampal neurons exhibit cyclothiazide-sensitive rapidly desensitizing responses to kainate. *J Neurosci* 1993;13:3496–3509.
233. Peoples RW, Lovinger DM, Weight FF. Inhibition of excitatory amino acid currents by general anesthetic agents. *Soc Neurosci Abstr* 1990;16:1017.
234. Peoples RW, Weight FF. Ethanol inhibition of *N*-methyl-D-aspartate-activated ion current in rat hippocampal neurons is not competitive with glycine. *Brain Res* 1992;571:342–344.
235. Peoples RW, Weight FF. Inhibition of excitatory amino acid-activated ion currents by inhalational anesthetics. *Soc Neurosci Abstr* 1992;18:248.
236. Peoples RW, Weight FF. Cutoff in potency implicates alcohol inhibition of *N*-methyl-D-aspartate receptors in alcohol intoxication. *Proc Natl Acad Sci USA* 1995 (in press).
237. Peters S, Koh J, Choi DW. Zinc selectively blocks the action of *N*-methyl-D-aspartate on cortical neurons. *Science* 1987;236:589–593.
238. Petrou S, Ordway RW, Singer JJ, Walsh JV Jr. A putative fatty acid-binding domain of the NMDA receptor. *Trends Biochem Sci* 1993; 18:41–42.
239. Pratt J, Rataud J, Bardot F, et al. Neuroprotective actions of riluzole in rodent models of global and focal cerebral ischaemia. *Neurosci Lett* 1992;140:225–230.
240. Puil E, El-Beheiry H. Anaesthetic suppression of transmitter actions in neocortex. *Br J Pharmacol* 1990;101:323–326.
241. Puil E, El-Beheiry H, Baimbridge KG. Anesthetic effects on glutamate-stimulated increase in intraneuronal calcium. *J Pharmacol Exp Ther* 1990;255:955–961.
242. Pullan LM. Receptor specific inhibition of *N*-methyl-D-aspartate stimulated ^{22}Na flux from rat hippocampal slices by phencyclidine and other drugs. *Neuropharmacology* 1988;27:493–497.
243. Rabbani M, Wright J, Butterworth AR, Zhou Q, Little HJ. Possible involvement of NMDA receptor-mediated transmission in barbiturate physical dependence. *Br J Pharmacol* 1994;111:89–96.
244. Rabe CS, Tabakoff B. Glycine site-directed agonists reverse the actions of ethanol at the *N*-methyl-D-aspartate receptor. *Mol Pharmacol* 1990;38:753–757.
245. Raja SN, Moscicki JC, Woodside JR Jr., DiFazio CA. The effect of acute phencyclidine administration on cyclopropane requirement (MAC) in rats. *Anesthesiol* 1982;56:275–279.
246. Rall TW. Hypnotics and sedatives; ethanol. In: Gilman AG, Rall TW, Nies AS, Taylor P, eds. *The pharmacological basis of therapeutics,* 8th ed. Elmsford, New York: Pergamon Press, 1990;345–382.
247. Ramoa AS, Albuquerque EX. Phencyclidine and some of its analogues have distinct effects on NMDA receptors of rat hippocampal neurons. *FEBS Lett* 1988;235:156–162.
248. Ransom BR, Barker JL. Pentobarbital modulates transmitter effects on mouse spinal neurones grown in tissue culture. *Nature* 1975;254:703–705.
249. Ransom BR, Barker JL. Pentobarbital selectively enhances GABA-mediated post-synaptic inhibition in tissue cultured mouse spinal neurons. *Brain Res* 1976;114:530–535.
250. Ransom RW, Stec NL. Inhibition of *N*-methyl-D-aspartate evoked sodium flux by MK-801. *Brain Res* 1988;444:25–32.
251. Ransom RW, Stec NL. Cooperative modulation of [^{3}H]MK-801 binding to the *N*-methyl-D-aspartate receptor-ion channel complex by L-glutamate, glycine and polyamines. *J Neurochem* 1988;51: 830–836.
252. Reynolds IJ, Miller RJ. Multiple sites for the regulation of the *N*-methyl-D-aspartate receptor. *Mol Pharmacol* 1988;33:581–584.
253. Reynolds IJ, Murphy SN, Miller RJ. ^{3}H-labeled MK-801 binding to the excitatory amino acid receptor complex from rat brain is enhanced by glycine. *Proc Natl Acad Sci USA* 1987;84:7744–7748.
254. Richards CD, Smaje JC. Anaesthetics depress the sensitivity of cortical neurones to L-glutamate. *Br J Pharmacol* 1976;58:347–357.
255. Richter JA, Holtman JR Jr. Barbiturates: their in vivo effects and potential biochemical mechanisms. *Prog Neurobiol* 1982;18: 275–319.
256. Richter-Levin G, Errington ML, Maegawa H, Bliss TVP. Activation of metabotropic glutamate receptors is necessary for long-term potentiation in the dentate gyrus and for spatial learning. *Neuropharmacology* 1994;33:853–857.
257. Riedel G, Reymann K. An antagonist of the metabotropic glutamate receptor prevents LTP in the dentate gyrus of freely moving rats. *Neuropharmacology* 1993;32:929–931.
258. Rock DM, Macdonald RL. The polyamine spermine has multiple actions on *N*-methyl-D-aspartate receptor single-channel currents in cultured cortical neurons. *Mol Pharmacol* 1992;41:83–88.
259. Rosenmund C, Westbrook GL. Rundown of *N*-methyl-D-aspartate channels during whole-cell recording in rat hippocampal neurons: role of Ca^{2+} and ATP. *J Physiol (Lond)* 1993;470:705–729.
260. Sacaan AI, Johnson KM. Spermidine reverses arcaine's inhibition of *N*-methyl-D-aspartate-induced hippocampal [^{3}H]norepinephrine release. *J Pharmacol Exp Ther* 1990;255:1060–1063.
261. Sacaan AI, Schoepp DD. Activation of hippocampal metabotropic excitatory amino acid receptors leads to seizures and neuronal damage. *Neurosci Lett* 1992;139:77–82.
262. Sakimura K, Bujo H, Kushiya E, et al. Functional expression from cloned cDNAs of glutamate receptor species responsive to kainate and quisqualate. *FEBS Lett* 1990;272:73–80.
263. Sakimura K, Morita T, Kushiya E, Mishina M. Primary structure and expression of the γ2 subunit of the glutamate receptor channel selective for kainate. *Neuron* 1992;8:267–274.
264. Sakurada K, Masu M, Nakanishi S. Alteration of Ca^{2+} permeability and sensitivity to Mg^{2+} and channel blockers by a single amino acid substitution in the *N*-methyl-D-aspartate receptor. *J Biol Chem* 1993;268:410–415.
265. Sather W, Johnson JW, Henderson G, Ascher P. Glycine-insensitive desensitization of NMDA responses in cultured mouse embryonic neurons. *Neuron* 1990;4:725–731.
266. Saugstad JA, Kinzie JM, Mulvihill ER, Segerson TP, Westbrook GL. Cloning and expression of a new member of the L-2-amino-4-phosphonobutyric acid-sensitive class of metabotropic glutamate receptors. *Mol Pharmacol* 1994;45:367–372.
267. Sawada S, Yamamoto C. Blocking action of pentobarbital on receptors for excitatory amino acids in the guinea pig hippocampus. *Exp Brain Res* 1985;59:226–231.
268. Scheller MS, Zornow MH, Fleischer JE, Shearman GT, Greber TF. The noncompetitive N-methyl D-aspartate receptor antagonist MK-801 profoundly reduces volatile anesthetic requirements in rabbits. *Neuropharmacology* 1989;28:677–681.
269. Schmidt CJ, Taylor VL. Release of [^{3}H]norepinephrine from rat hippocampal slices by *N*-methyl-D-aspartate: comparison of the inhibitory effects of Mg^{2+} and MK-801. *Eur J Pharmacol* 1988;156: 111–120.
270. Schoepfer R, Monyer H, Sommer B, et al. Molecular biology of glutamate receptors. *Prog Neurobiol* 1994;42:353–357.
271. Schoepp DD, Sacaan AI. Metabotropic glutamate receptors and neuronal degenerative disorders. *Neurobiol Aging* 1994;15: 261–263.

272. Scott RH, Sutton KG, Dolphin AC. Interactions of polyamines with neuronal ion channels. *Trends Neurosci* 1993;16:153–160.
273. Sear JW, Prys-Roberts C. Plasma concentrations of alphaxalone during continuous infusion of Althesin. *Br J Anaesth* 1979;51: 861–865.
274. Seeburg PH. The TiPS/TINS lecture: the molecular biology of mammalian glutamate receptor channels. *Trends Pharmacol Sci* 1993;14:297–303.
275. Seeman P. The membrane actions of anesthetics and tranquilizers. *Pharmacol Rev* 1972;24:583–655.
276. Shaw GG, Pateman AJ. The regional distribution of the polyamines spermidine and spermine in brain. *J Neurochem* 1973; 20:1225–1230.
277. Sheardown MJ, Nielsen E , Hansen AJ, Jacobsen P, Honoré T. 2,3-Dihydroxy-6-nitro-7-sulfamoyl-benzo(F)quinoxaline: a neuroprotectant for cerebral ischemia. *Science* 1990;247:571–574.
278. Short KR, Tabakoff B. Chronic barbiturate treatment increases NMDA receptors but decreases kainate receptors in mouse cortex. *Eur J Pharmacol* 1993;230:111–114.
279. Siliprandi R, Lipartiti M, Fadda E, Sautter J, Manev H. Activation of the glutamate metabotropic receptor protects retina against N-methyl-D-aspartate toxicity. *Eur J Pharmacol* 1992;219:173–174.
280. Silver RA, Traynelis SF, Cull-Candy SG. Rapid-time-course miniature and evoked excitatory currents at cerebellar synapses in situ. *Nature* 1992;355:163–166.
281. Singh L, Menzies R, Tricklebank MD. The discriminative stimulus properties of (+)-HA-966, an antagonist at the glycine/N-methyl-D-aspartate receptor. *Eur J Pharmacol* 1990;186:129–132.
282. Sircar R, Frusciante MJ, Javitt DC, Zukin SR. Glycine reverses 7-chlorokynurenic acid-induced inhibition of [^{3}H]MK-801 binding. *Brain Res* 1989;504:325–327.
283. Snell LD, Johnson KM. Antagonism of N-methyl-D-aspartate-induced transmitter release in the rat striatum by phencyclidine-like drugs and its relationship to turning behavior. *J Pharmacol Exp Ther* 1985;235:50–57.
284. Snell LD, Johnson KM. Characterization of the inhibition of excitatory amino acid-induced neurotransmitter release in the rat striatum by phencyclidine-like drugs. *J Pharmacol Exp Ther* 1986; 238:938–946.
285. Snell LD, Morter RS, Johnson KM. Glycine potentiates N-methyl-D-aspartate-induced [^{3}H]TCP binding to rat cortical membranes. *Neurosci Lett* 1987;83:313–317.
286. Snell LD, Tabakoff B, Hoffman PL. Involvement of protein kinase C in ethanol-induced inhibition of NMDA receptor function in cerebellar granule cells. *Alcohol Clin Exp Res* 1994;18:81–85.
287. Snell LD, Yi SJ, Johnson KM. Comparison of the effects of MK-801 and phencyclidine on catecholamine uptake and NMDA-induced norepinephrine release. *Eur J Pharmacol* 1988;145: 223–226.
288. Sommer B, Burnashev N, Verdoorn TA, Keinänen K, Sakmann B, Seeburg PH. A glutamate receptor channel with high affinity for domoate and kainate. *EMBO J* 1992;11:1651–1656.
289. Sprosen TS, Woodruff GN. Polyamines potentiate NMDA induced whole-cell currents in cultured striatal neurons. *Eur J Pharmacol* 1990;179:447–478.
290. Stern-Bach Y, Bettler B, Hartley M, Sheppard PO, O'Hara PJ, Heinemann SF. Agonist selectivity of glutamate receptors is specified by two domains structurally related to bacterial amino acid-binding proteins. *Neuron* 1994;13:1345–1357.
291. Stockbridge LL. Pentobarbital interaction with single kainate channels in mouse cortical neurons. *Soc Neurosci Abstr* 1992;18: 653.
292. Sugihara H, Moriyoshi K, Ishii T, Masu M, Nakanishi S. Structures and properties of seven isoforms of the NMDA receptor generated by alternative splicing. *Biochem Biophys Res Comm* 1992;185: 826–832.
293. Takahashi K, Tsuchida K, Tanabe Y, Masu M, Nakanishi S. Role of the large extracellular domain of metabotropic glutamate receptors in agonist selectivity determination. *J Biol Chem* 1993;268: 19341–19345.
294. Tanabe Y, Masu M, Ishii T, Shigemoto R, Nakanishi S. A family of metabotropic glutamate receptors. *Neuron* 1992;8:169–179.
295. Tanabe Y, Nomura A, Masu M, Shigemoto R, Mizuno N, Nakanishi S. Signal transduction, pharmacological properties, and expression patterns of two rat metabotropic glutamate receptors, mGluR3 and mGluR4. *J Neurosci* 1993;13:1372–1378.
296. Tang C-M, Shi Q-Y, Katchman A, Lynch G. Modulation of the time course of fast EPSCs and glutamate channel kinetics by aniracetam. *Science* 1991;254:288–290.
297. Tang L-H, Aizenman E. Allosteric modulation of the NMDA receptor by dihydrolipoic and lipoic acid in rat cortical neurons in vitro. *Neuron* 1993;11:857–863.
298. Taverna FA, Cameron B-R, Hampson DL, Wang L-Y, MacDonald JF. Sensitivity of AMPA receptors to pentobarbital. *Eur J Pharmacol Mol Pharmacol* 1994;267:R3–R5.
299. Teichberg VI, Tal N, Goldberg O, Luini A. Barbiturates, alcohols and the CNS excitatory neurotransmission: specific effects on the kainate and quisqualate receptors. *Brain Res* 1984;291:285–292.
300. Thomas JW, Hood WF, Monahan JB, Contreras PC, O'Donohue TL. Glycine modulation of the phencyclidine binding site in mammalian brain. *Brain Res* 1988;442:396–398.
301. Tingley WG, Roche KW, Thompson AK, Huganir RL. Regulation of NMDA receptor phosphorylation by alternative splicing of the C-terminal domain. *Nature* 1993;364:70–73.
302. Traynelis SF, Cull-Candy SG. Proton inhibition of N-methyl-D-aspartate receptors in cerebellar neurons. *Nature* 1990;345: 347–350.
303. Tricklebank MD, Singh L, Oles RJ, Wong EH, Iversen SD. A role for receptors of N-methyl-D-aspartic acid in the discriminative stimulus properties of phencyclidine. *Eur J Pharmacol* 1987;141: 497–501.
304. Trussell LO, Zhang S, Raman IM. Desensitization of AMPA receptors upon multiquantal neurotransmitter release. *Neuron* 1993;10: 1185–1196.
305. Turner DM, Ransom RW, Yang JS-J, Olsen RW. Steroid anesthetics and naturally occurring analogs modulate the γ-aminobutyric acid receptor complex at a site distinct from barbiturates. *J Pharmacol Exp Ther* 1989;248:960–966.
306. Verdoorn TA, Burnashev N, Monyer H, Seeburg PH, Sakmann B. Structural determinants of ion flow through recombinant glutamate receptor channels. *Science* 1991;252:1715–1718.
307. Vincent JP, Kartalovski B, Geneste P, Kamenka JM, Lazdunski M. Interaction of phencyclidine ("angel dust") with a specific receptor in rat brain membranes. *Proc Natl Acad Sci USA* 1979;76: 4678–4682.
308. Vyklicky L Jr., Vlachov̂ V, Krusek J. The effect of external pH changes on responses to excitatory amino acids in mouse hippocampal neurones. *J Physiol (Lond)* 1990;430:497–517.
309. Wakamori M, Ikemoto Y, Akaike N. Effects of two volatile anesthetics and a volatile convulsant on the excitatory and inhibitory amino acid responses in dissociated CNS neurons of the rat. *J Neurophysiol* 1991;66:2014–2021.
310. Wang L-Y, Orser BA, Brautigan DL, MacDonald JF. Regulation of NMDA receptors in cultured hippocampal neurons by protein phosphatases 1 and 2A. *Nature* 1994;369:230–232.
311. Wang YT, Salter MW. Regulation of NMDA receptors by tyrosine kinases and phosphatases. *Nature* 1994;369:233–235.
312. Watanabe M, Inoue Y, Sakimura K, Mishina M. Distinct spatio-temporal distributions of the NMDA receptor channel subunit mRNAs in the brain. *Ann NY Acad Sci* 1993;707:463–466.
313. Watanabe M, Inoue Y, Sakimura K, Mishina M. Distinct distributions of five N-methyl-D-aspartate receptor channel subunit mRNAs in the forebrain. *J Comp Neurol* 1993;338:377–390.
314. Weight FF, Lovinger DM, White G, Peoples RW. Alcohol and anesthetic actions on excitatory amino acid-activated ion channels. *Ann NY Acad Sci* 1991;625:97–107.
315. Weight FF, Peoples RW. General anesthetic effects on excitatory amino acid activated ion channels in hippocampal neurons. *XXXII Congress IUPS Abstr* 1993;32:41.
316. Werner P, Voigt M, Keinänen K, Wisden W, Seeburg PH. Cloning of a putative high-affinity kainate receptor expressed predominantly in hippocampal CA3 cells. *Nature* 1991;351:742–744.
317. Westbrook GL, Mayer ML. Micromolar concentrations of Zn^{2+} antagonize NMDA and GABA responses of hippocampal neurons. *Nature* 1987;328:640–643.
318. White G, Lovinger DM, Peoples RW, et al. Analysis of ethanol (EtOH) interaction with glycine potentiation of NMDA-activated ion current. *Soc Neurosci Abstr* 1990;16:1041.
319. Willetts J, Balster RL. The discriminative stimulus effects of N-methyl-D-aspartate antagonists in phencyclidine-trained rats. *Neuropharmacology* 1988;27:1249–1256.
320. Willetts J, Balster RL. Phencyclidine-like discriminative stimulus properties of MK-801 in rats. *Eur J Pharmacol* 1988;146:167–169.
321. Willetts J, Balster RL. Effects of competitive and noncompetitive N-methyl-D-aspartate (NMDA) antagonists in rats trained to dis-

criminate NMDA from saline. *J Pharmacol Exp Ther* 1989;251: 627–633.
322. Willetts J, Balster RL. Pentobarbital-like discriminative stimulus effects of *N*-methyl-D-aspartate antagonists. *J Pharmacol Exp Ther* 1989;249:438–443.
323. Willetts J, Balster RL, Leander JD. The behavioral pharmacology of NMDA receptor antagonists. *Trends Pharmacol Sci* 1990;11: 423–428.
324. Willetts J, Bobelis DJ, Balster RL. Drug discrimination based on the competitive *N*-methyl-D-aspartate antagonist, NPC 12626. *Psychopharmacology (Berl)* 1989;99:458–462.
325. Willetts J, Tokarz ME, Balster RL. Pentobarbital-like effects of *N*-methyl-D-aspartate antagonists in mice. *Life Sci* 1991;48:1795–1798.
326. Wo ZG, Oswald RE. Transmembrane topology of two kainate receptor subunits revealed by N-glycosylation. *Proc Natl Acad Sci USA* 1994;91:7154–7158.
327. Wong EH, Kemp JA, Priestley T, Knight AR, Woodruff GN, Iversen LL. The anticonvulsant MK-801 is a potent *N*-methyl-D-aspartate antagonist. *Proc Natl Acad Sci USA* 1986;83:7104–7108.
328. Wong EH, Knight AR, Ransom R. Glycine modulates [^{3}H]MK-801 binding to the NMDA receptor in rat brain. *Eur J Pharmacol* 1987; 142:487–488.
329. Wood PL, Steel D, McPherson SE, Cheney DL, Lehmann J. Antagonism of *N*-methyl-D-aspartate (NMDA) evoked increases in cerebellar cGMP and striatal ACh release by phencyclidine (PCP) receptor agonists: evidence for possible allosteric coupling of NMDA and PCP receptors. *Can J Physiol Pharmacol* 1987;65: 1923–1927.
330. Woodruff GN, Foster AC, Gill R, Kemp JA, Wong EH, Iversen LL. The interaction between MK-801 and receptors for *N*-methyl-D-aspartate: functional consequences. *Neuropharmacology* 1987;26: 903–909.
331. Woodward JJ. A comparison of the effects of ethanol and the competitive glycine antagonist 7-chlorokynurenic acid on *N*-methyl-D-aspartic acid-induced neurotransmitter release from rat hippocampal slices. *J Neurochem* 1994;62:987–991.
332. Woodward JJ, Gonzales RA. Ethanol inhibition of *N*-methyl-D-aspartate-stimulated endogenous dopamine release from rat striatal slices: reversal by glycine. *J Neurochem* 1990;54:712–715.
333. Yamazaki M, Mori H, Araki K, Mori J, Mishina M. Cloning, expression and modulation of a mouse NMDA receptor subunit. *FEBS Lett* 1992;300:39–45.
334. Yang J, Zorumski CF. Effects of isoflurane on *N*-methyl-D-aspartate gated ion channels in cultured rat hippocampal neurons. *Ann NY Acad Sci* 1991;625:287–289.
335. Yi SJ, Snell LD, Johnson KM. Linkage between phencyclidine (PCP) and *N*-methyl-D-aspartate (NMDA) receptors in the cerebellum. *Brain Res* 1988;445:147–151.
336. Yuzaki M, Miyawaki A, Akita K, et al. Mode of blockade by MK-801 of *N*-methyl-D-aspartate-induced increase in intracellular Ca^{2+} in cultured mouse hippocampal neurons. *Brain Res* 1990;517:51–56.
337. Zheng F, Gallagher JP. Metabotropic glutamate receptors are required for the induction of long-term potentiation. *Neuron* 1992;9:163–172.
338. Zilberter Y, Uteshev V, Sokolova S, Khodorov B. Desensitization of *N*-methyl-D-aspartate receptors in neurons dissociated from adult rat hippocampus. *Mol Pharmacol* 1991;40:337–341.
339. Zukin SR, Zukin RS. Specific ^{3}H-phencyclidine binding in rat central nervous system. *Proc Natl Acad Sci USA* 1979;76:5372–5376.

Anesthesia: Biologic Foundations, edited by Tony L. Yaksh et al. Lippincott–Raven Publishers, Philadelphia © 1997.

CHAPTER 16

GABA$_A$ RECEPTORS AND ANESTHESIA

BERIT X. CARLSON, TIM G. HALES, AND RICHARD W. OLSEN

MECHANISM OF ANESTHETIC ACTION

Anesthetics play an integral role in the practice of modern medicine. Anesthetic agents are routinely and expertly administered daily. Despite the widespread use of sedatives and general anesthetics, the mechanisms by which these agents alter waking consciousness is not known. At the turn of the century, Meyer (111,112) and Overton (129) demonstrated that the solubility (measured as the partition coefficient) of an anesthetic in an olive oil/water mixture exhibited a linear correlation with the potency of general anesthetics. This finding led to the hypothesis that anesthetics exert their primary effects at a nonpolar site within neuronal membranes. Whether this nonpolar site is lipid or protein is still the subject of great debate. Hydrophobic sites on protein molecules are plausible candidates (48,113,183), and protein molecules, such as neuronal ion channels, have been shown to have their activity altered by general anesthetics (49,50). For further detail regarding the interaction of anesthetic agents with lipids, proteins, or other effector systems, please refer to preceding chapters in Section 1 of this text. The present chapter will present data supporting the hypothesis that sedation and anesthesia by certain general anesthetics are produced, at least in part, by enhancing neuronal inhibition at a ligand-gated ion channel, the γ-aminobutyric acid$_A$ (GABA$_A$) receptor.

GABA is the major inhibitory neurotransmitter in the mammalian CNS (147). GABAergic neurons are widely distributed throughout the brain (117), and most neurons receive inhibitory GABAergic input (44). GABA mediates neuronal inhibition by binding either to the GABA$_A$ or GABA$_B$ receptor. The latter receptor differs from the GABA$_A$ receptor primarily by its pharmacology and effector mechanisms (Table 1). Distinct ligands bind to these receptors. Muscimol is a specific GABA$_A$ agonist, and baclofen binds to GABA$_B$ receptors. The GABA$_B$ receptor also is insensitive to the GABA$_A$ antagonist bicuculline. The activation of GABA$_B$ receptors is thought to cause inhibition by enhancing potassium conductance or reducing calcium conductance via a G-protein-coupling system (15). Unlike GABA$_A$ receptors, general anesthetic agents have not been shown to interact with GABA$_B$ receptors (reviewed in ref. 16). This chapter focuses on the evidence supporting the GABA$_A$ receptor as a target for numerous depressant drugs, including general anesthetics (Fig. 1), and the implications that this evidence has for the role of GABA$_A$ receptors in mediating sedation and anesthesia. The next section of this chapter reviews the basic structure of GABA$_A$ receptors and the GABA$_A$-related actions of benzodiazepines, general anesthetics, and alcohols.

GABA$_A$ RECEPTOR: A PUTATIVE SITE OF ACTION FOR ANESTHETIC AGENTS

The GABA$_A$ receptor belongs to a superfamily of ligand-gated ion channels typified by the nicotinic acetylcholine receptor. In the case of the GABA$_A$ receptor, a chloride ion channel is formed from a heterooligomeric structure (Fig. 2), and the chloride channel is allosterically gated by GABA binding to its recognition site on the protein complex (reviewed in ref. 127). Thus, the binding of GABA to GABA$_A$ receptors induces an increase in chloride permeability, and this action in neurons is predominately inhibitory (149). The GABA$_A$ receptor also contains at least five putative binding sites that recognize drugs and endogenous ligands that act as positive and negative allosteric modulators (Fig. 2). The following section will present evidence in support of benzodiazepines and general anesthetics acting as positive allosteric modulators at GABA$_A$ receptors.

Table 1. GABA RECEPTORS

	GABA$_A$	GABA$_B$
Agonists	GABA Isoguvacine Muscimol THIP	GABA 1-Baclofen 3-Aminopropylphosphonic acid
Antagonists	Bicuculline Picrotoxin[a] TBPS	Saclofen Phaclofen 2-Hydroxysaclofen
Structure	Multisubunit chloride ion channel (ligand-gated ion channel)	7 transmembrane G-protein–linkedreceptor coupled to Ca^{2+} and/or K^+ channels
Effector pathways	Increase Cl^- current	Decrease Ca^{2+} or increase K^+ current via G proteins
Sensitivity to anesthetics	Yes	No

[a] Picrotoxin is a convulsant that is a plant toxin related to compounds used in insecticides and is a chloride ion channel blocker.

THIP, 4,5,6,7-tetrahydroisoxazolo[5,4-c]pyridin-3-ol; TBPS, t-butyl bicyclophosphorothionate (an analogue to picrotoxin).

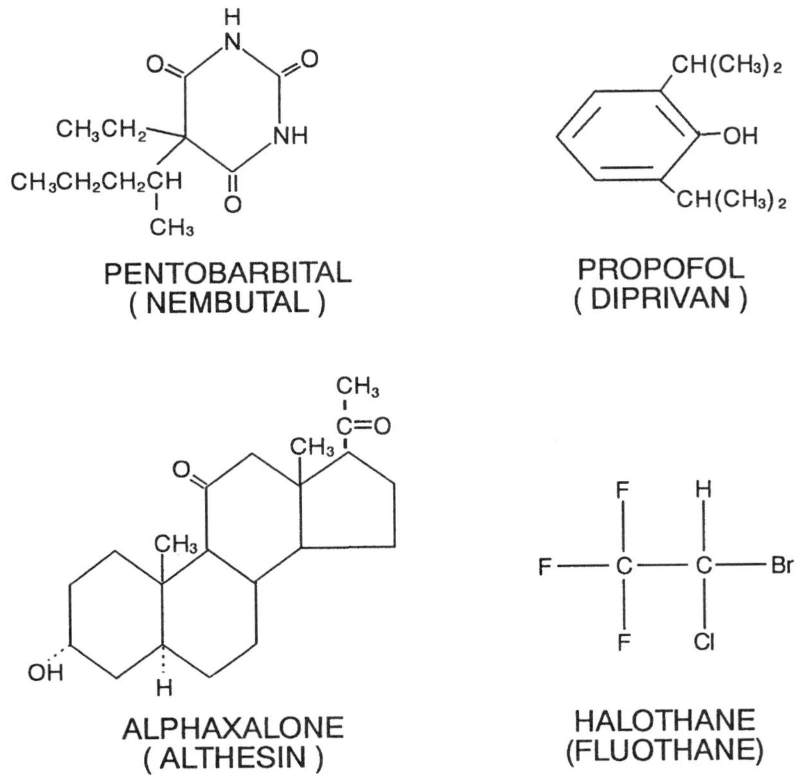

PENTOBARBITAL
(NEMBUTAL)

PROPOFOL
(DIPRIVAN)

ALPHAXALONE
(ALTHESIN)

HALOTHANE
(FLUOTHANE)

Figure 1. Structures of various anesthetic compounds. These general anesthetics have been used clinically and are known to modulate $GABA_A$ receptors.

$GABA_A$-Related Actions of Benzodiazepines and Anesthetic Agents

Benzodiazepines

Receptor Binding Benzodiazepines were first shown to have specific binding sites in the CNS using [^{3}H]diazepam (18,115). In 1978, Tallman et al. (173) demonstrated with cortical membrane homogenates that GABA modulates in vitro benzodiazepine binding by increasing the affinity of the benzodiazepine binding site. This modulation by GABA is reversed in the presence of the $GABA_A$ antagonist, bicuculline. Using [^{3}H]flunitrazepam, similar results also have been observed in intact primary cultured spinal neurons (108). Benzodiazepines also enhance GABA binding in a concentration-dependent manner, and this effect occurs by increasing the affinity of the

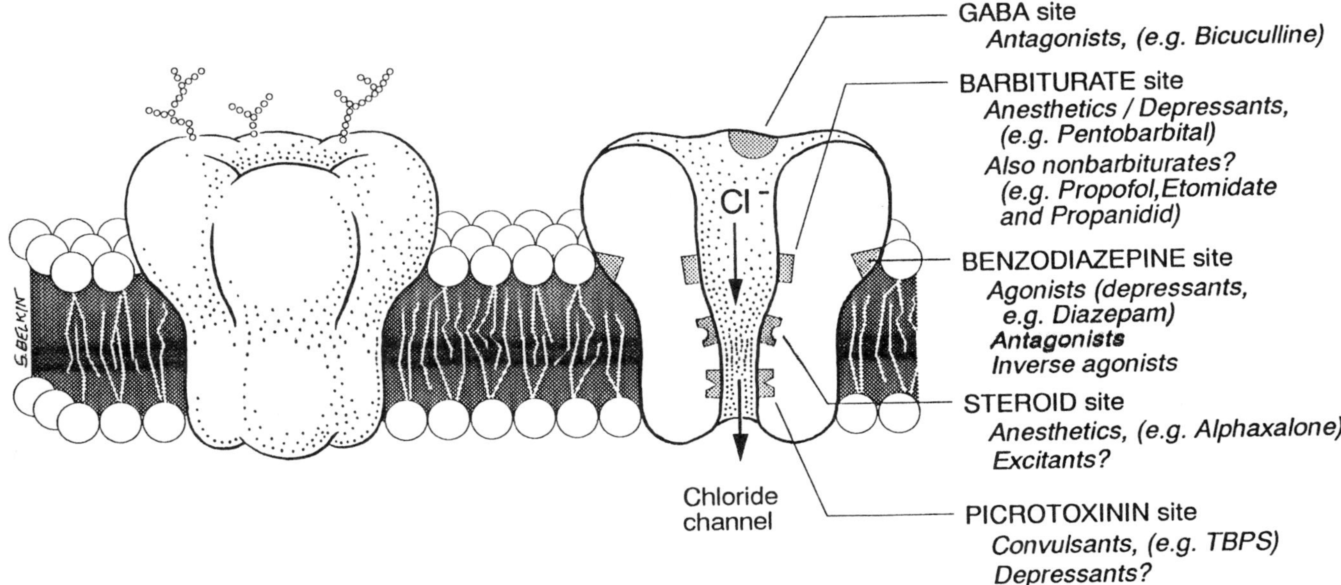

Figure 2. Schematic representation of $GABA_A$ receptor with modulatory sites. The hypothetical target sites of a number of agonists, antagonists, general anesthetics, and benzodiazepines are illustrated. This schematic is not intended to give an accurate representation of the location of these compounds within the receptor complex. (Reprinted, in adapted form, with permission from ref. 36.)

GABA binding site (166). The binding of the GABA$_A$ channel blocker t-butyl bicylcophosphorothionate (TBPS) is inhibited by benzodiazepines (29). These results all support the hypothesis that GABA$_A$ and benzodiazepine receptors are coupled. Thus, the sedative effects of benzodiazepines may be mediated, in part, by allosterically modulating binding at GABA$_A$ receptors, and the functional parameters of this modulation will be the focus of the next two sections in this chapter.

Electrophysiology In the mid-1970s, Dray and Straughan (40) were the first to report that benzodiazepines may act via a GABA receptor. They observed that chlordiazepoxide (Librium) decreased the firing rate of rat brain neurons, and this benzodiazepine-induced inhibition of neuronal activity was blocked by bicuculline and picrotoxin (40). Since then, electrophysiological studies have shown that benzodiazepines reversibly potentiate GABA-responses recorded from cultured neurons (28,98). This effect exhibits dose dependency (98) and is antagonized by a specific benzodiazepine receptor antagonist, flumazenil (77). In voltage-clamped mouse spinal neurons, fluctuation analysis suggested that benzodiazepines enhance chloride ion conductance by increasing the frequency of GABA-gated channel openings (169). Following the advent of the patch-clamp technique (62), this conclusion was confirmed by directly observing the effects of benzodiazepines on GABA-activated single channels in outside-out patches excised from mouse spinal cord neurons (105). Thus, at pharmacologically relevant concentrations, benzodiazepines positively modulate GABA$_A$ receptor function by increasing the frequency of GABA-evoked chloride channel openings.

Chloride Flux Radiolabeled chloride ($^{36}Cl^-$) flux studies performed in cortical synaptoneurosomes (neuronal membrane vesicles) and brain slices have demonstrated findings in support of single channel analyses. Benzodiazepines increase GABA or muscimol-stimulated $^{36}Cl^-$ flux in a concentration-dependent manner (124,196). This effect is blocked in the presence of flumazenil (124,196). These results indicate that benzodiazepine-enhanced GABA$_A$ chloride flux requires the binding of benzodiazepines to a specific site on neurons, shown by biochemical studies to be situated on GABA$_A$ receptors. Both electrophysiological and $^{36}Cl^-$ flux studies also have demonstrated that benzodiazepines alone, in the absence of GABA or muscimol, do not directly activate GABA$_A$ chloride channel gating (28,157,196). As will be noted in the sections about general anesthetics, direct activation of GABA-channel gating is a functional quality that separates sedatives from general anesthetic agents. The mechanism by which general anesthetics act may require direct receptor activation and will be discussed in further detail in the next two sections.

General Anesthetics: Intravenous Agents

Receptor Binding In vitro receptor binding studies have demonstrated that intravenous anesthetic agents have specific interactions with the GABA$_A$ receptor. In cortical homogenates, pentobarbital (Nembutal), etomidate (amidate), and alphaxalone (Althesin) enhance GABA or muscimol binding, apparently by increasing the number of binding sites, whereas propofol (Diprivan) presumably increases the affinity of the GABA binding site (67,130,176). Willow and Johnston (189), however, reported that pentobarbital increases the high-affinity component of the GABA binding site without any change with the low-affinity site. It seems that these drugs enhance the affinity of normally detectable as well as undetectable binding sites, the latter effect appearing to be an increase in the number of sites (126).

These intravenous anesthetic agents also modulate benzodiazepine binding. Potentiation of GABA or benzodiazepine binding by intravenous agents has been shown to be dose dependent, stereospecific, and antagonized by bicuculline or picrotoxin (66,89,167,176). Intravenous agents potentiate benzodiazepine binding by increasing the affinity of the benzodiazepine binding site (66,89,135,176). Barbiturates also allosterically inhibit the binding of benzodiazepine inverse agonists such as βCCM and of GABA antagonists such as bicuculline (193). This result suggests that the allosteric interactions in binding studies are probably related to the functional efficacy of the drugs. In addition, pentobarbital enhancement of GABA or benzodiazepine binding is dependent on the presence of chloride ions or other anions that penetrate GABA$_A$ chloride channels (7,89,126,188). It has been reported that the potentiation of benzodiazepine binding by different classes of barbiturates is directly related to their pharmacological potencies (87). It is interesting to note that in the presence of more than one anesthetic agent (e.g., pentobarbital and etomidate; or alphaxalone and pentobarbital) the enhancement in GABA and muscimol binding is additive (176,179). In addition, combinations of benzodiazepines and barbiturates produce a synergistic enhancement of muscimol binding (34). These results suggest that binding sites for different classes of intravenous anesthetic agents are distinct from each other as well as from benzodiazepine binding sites. Similarly to benzodiazepines, these intravenous agents also inhibit noncompetitively picrotoxin and TBPS binding (66,103,130,178,179). Even though some intravenous agents have been reported to modulate ligand binding on other ligand-gated ion channels, such as the nicotinic acetylcholine receptor (39), these data strongly support the conclusion that various types of intravenous agents at clinically relevant concentrations interact with the GABA$_A$ receptor.

Electrophysiology Electrophysiological studies have demonstrated that the receptor binding data, mentioned above, have functional significance. Extracellular recordings showed that inhibitory synaptic transmission in several areas of the CNS, now known to be mediated by GABA$_A$ receptors, is potentiated by barbiturates (119). Intracellular recordings from cultured mouse spinal neurons have shown that hypnotic barbiturates, such as pentobarbital, potentiate GABA responses (9,144). Also, it has been demonstrated that, under voltage-clamp conditions, GABA-evoked currents are potentiated by hypnotic barbiturates (148). Using fluctuation analysis, it appears that in contrast to benzodiazepines, which increase the frequency of GABA-activated channel openings, barbiturates augment GABA-mediated inhibition by increasing the duration of GABA-gated chloride channel open time (169). This effect has been confirmed in experiments using outside-out patches in which prolongation of channel open time by pentobarbital has been directly observed (99,181). The non-barbiturate anesthetics etomidate (140), propofol (56), propanidid (Epontol) (132), chlormethiazole (Heminevrin) (57), and the anesthetic steroids (8) also potentiate GABA-induced chloride currents. Like the barbiturates, propofol (Fig. 3), alphaxalone, and other neuroactive steroids have been shown to enhance GABA responses, primarily by increasing GABA-gated channel open time rather than increasing the frequency of openings (56,84,180).

Not all intravenous anesthetics enhance GABA-elicited chloride currents. For example, ketamine (Ketlar), the dissociative anesthetic, has been shown either to decrease GABA$_A$ activity or to potentiate GABA responses only at high concentrations, thus suggesting that this anesthetic mediates its actions at a different receptor, possibly the *N*-methyl D-aspartate-type excitatory amino acid receptor (52,91) (see Chapter 15). In contrast, potentiation of GABA responses by barbiturates, etomidate, and alphaxalone occurs at clinically relevant concentrations and demonstrates stereospecificity (8,9,42,46, 56,75). It should be noted that the foregoing intravenous agents do not have specific pharmacological antagonists, which makes difficult an emphatic demonstration of a protein site of action. However, intracellular application of intravenous agents at high concentrations does not affect GABA$_A$ receptor activity, suggesting that a simple lipid interaction is insufficient to describe the actions of intravenous agents at GABA$_A$ receptors (56,84). Together, these results provide

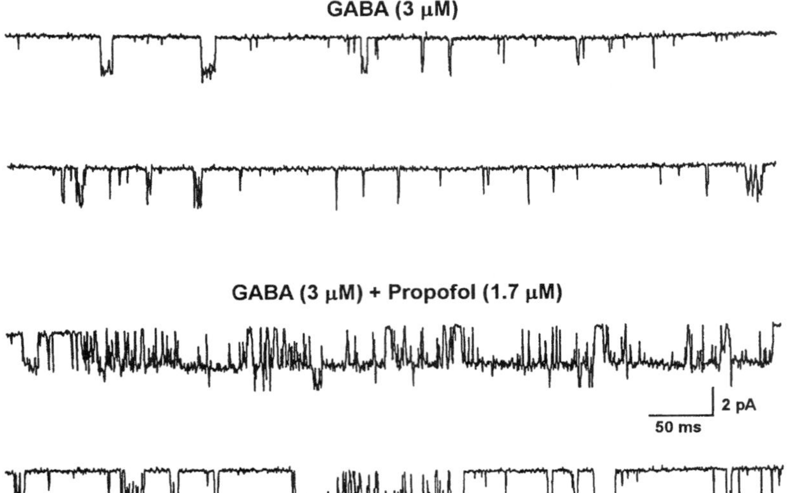

Figure 3. Modulation of GABA-activated single-channel activity by propofol. Top two traces illustrate channels opening (downward deflections) in the presence of GABA (3 μM). On addition of propofol (1.7 μM), GABA-activated channel openings appear to become markedly prolonged. This action of the general anesthetic propofol is similar to that of other intravenous general anesthetics such as pentobarbital, alphaxalone, and chlormethiazole. (Reprinted, in adapted form, with permission, from ref. 56.)

evidence for a specific interaction of general anesthetics with the $GABA_A$ receptor chloride ion channel complex.

Direct activation of chloride current in the absence of GABA has been observed with pentobarbital, etomidate, alphaxalone, chlormethiazole, and propofol at concentrations slightly higher than needed for potentiation of GABA-evoked currents (8,45,46,56,57,154). This direct action distinguishes these general anesthetics from the benzodiazepines, which are unable to activate $GABA_A$ receptors. It is interesting to note that the direct effects for some of these agents occur at clinically relevant concentrations, whereas the potentiating effects of $GABA_A$ receptor activity appear to be manifested at subanesthetic concentrations. It has been postulated that direct activation of $GABA_A$ receptors by intravenous anesthetics may be a mechanism by which anesthesia is produced. Potentiation of GABAergic synaptic transmission, on the other hand, may be responsible for the anxiolytic and anticonvulsant properties of these agents (154).

Chloride Flux In support of electrophysiological studies, intravenous anesthetics have also been shown to enhance $GABA_A$ receptor function using the $^{36}Cl^-$ flux assays. Barbiturates, alphaxalone, and propofol potentiate in a concentration-dependent manner GABA-stimulated (or muscimol-stimulated) $^{36}Cl^-$ flux in cortical synaptoneurosomes and brain slices, and bicuculline or picrotoxin antagonizes this enhancing effect (2,130,179,192). It also has been shown that the enhancing effect of barbiturates on $^{36}Cl^-$ flux is stereospecific (2,156,192). In agreement with electrophysiological studies demonstrating the direct activation of $GABA_A$ receptors by anesthetic barbiturates, these compounds activate $^{36}Cl^-$ flux in the absence of exogenously applied GABA or muscimol (155,192). A final piece of evidence for the pharmacological and clinical relevance of these $^{36}Cl^-$ flux assays is that the potencies of different anesthetic barbiturates in stimulating $^{36}Cl^-$ flux correlate linearly with their anesthetic potencies in vivo (76,155). This evidence provides strong support for the involvement of $GABA_A$ receptors in mediating anesthesia.

General Anesthetics: Volatile Agents

Receptor Binding Due to the lack of pharmacological antagonists and low-binding affinities, volatile anesthetics have not been demonstrated to have specific binding sites in the CNS. It has been reported, however, that volatile agents modulate ligand binding at various ligand-gated ion channels, including $GABA_A$ receptors. Volatile anesthetics have been shown to enhance GABA binding at clinically relevant concentrations (e.g., 1% halothane, Fluothane; 1.7% enflurane, Ethrane) (27). At concentrations that increase muscimol-stimulated chloride flux, $GABA_A$ receptor affinity for [^{3}H]muscimol is increased in a Ca^{2+}-independent manner by halothane (94). Likewise, halothane, enflurane, and isoflurane (Forane) potentiate benzodiazepine binding by increasing the affinity of the binding site for its ligand and augment benzodiazepine binding in the presence of GABA (65). Similarly to pentobarbital, etomidate, alphaxalone, and propofol, the volatile anesthetics, also inhibit TBPS binding (95,116). Thus, these data provide evidence in support of the hypothesis that volatile anesthetics interact with $GABA_A$ receptor ion channels.

Electrophysiology A functional interaction of volatile agents with $GABA_A$ receptors has been studied extensively using electrophysiological techniques. In rat embryonic cultured hippocampal neurons, halothane, isoflurane, and enflurane have been shown to enhance the amplitude and duration of GABA-induced chloride currents in a concentration-dependent and reversible manner (78). It should be noted that the anesthetic concentrations used in the Jones study (78) are equivalent to 1–1.5 MAC (minimum alveolar concentration), a clinically effective dose. Nakahiro et al. (118) demonstrated in voltage-clamped, rat dorsal root ganglion neurons that halothane, isoflurane, and enflurane at 2 MAC had a dual effect on GABA-mediated chloride currents. At low subsaturating GABA concentrations ($1–3 \times 10^{-6}$ M), the volatile agents significantly increased chloride current, and at high GABA concentrations ($10^{-5}–10^{-3}$ M), where desensitization is prevalent, the desensitized steady state current was suppressed by the inhalational anesthetics (118). From the same group, single-channel analysis has revealed that halothane prolonged GABA-gated channel open time, shortened the duration of interburst intervals (i.e., time between bursts), and lengthened the burst duration (197). As demonstrated by receptor binding studies, an increase in the affinity of the binding site for GABA appears to be a mechanism for the augmentation of GABA-evoked chloride currents by halothane and enflurane (185). Wakamori et al. (185) found that the dose-dependent potentiation of chloride currents has a Hill coefficient close to 2, suggesting that two molecules of either halothane or enflurane are needed to bind to $GABA_A$ receptors for enhancing chloride currents. Similarly to intravenous agents, halothane, isoflurane, and enflurane also appear to directly activate $GABA_A$ receptors (58,195). The volatile anesthetic-activated chloride current can be blocked by bicuculline and picrotoxin, indicating that the current is mediated by $GABA_A$ receptor activation (58,195). Taken together, these data have shown that a common action of three volatile agents is to enhance $GABA_A$ receptor responses. In addition, a mechanism by which volatile anesthetics may produce anesthesia is by directly opening GABA$_A$ receptor chloride ion channels, thus inducing neuronal inhibition.

Unlike the intravenous agents, it has been suggested that there is a role for intracellular Ca^{2+} in the potentiation of GABA$_A$ receptor activity by inhalation anesthetics. Patch-clamp recordings from hippocampal slices have shown that, in the presence of the intracellularly applied Ca^{2+} chelator BAPTA (1,2-bis [2-aminophenoxy] ethane-N,N,N'N''-tetraacetic acid) or the Ca^{2+} release inhibitor dantrolene, there was a significant partial reduction in halothane-enhanced GABA$_A$ spontaneous inhibitory postsynaptic currents (100,114). However, the presence of Ca^{2+} chelators in cultured hippocampal neurons did not appear to suppress potentiation of GABA-evoked currents in these neurons (78). In support of the latter study, Lin et al. (90) have demonstrated, using mouse cortical mRNA in the *Xenopus* oocyte expression system, that for some GABA$_A$ receptors their modulation by volatile anesthetics is not influenced by intracellular Ca^{2+}. The enhancing effects of halothane, isoflurane, and enflurane at clinically relevant concentrations were displayed in the absence and presence of the intracellularly injected Ca^{2+} chelator EGTA [ethylene glycol-bis (β-aminoethyl ether) N,N,N'N''-tetraacetic acid] (90). Thus, the role of intracellular Ca^{2+} in the modulatory effects of volatile agents at GABA$_A$ receptors is controversial.

Chloride Flux Chloride flux studies also have demonstrated that volatile anesthetics, such as halothane, enflurane, and methoxyflurane (Metofane), enhance muscimol-stimulated GABA$_A$ receptor function as well as directly activate GABA$_A$ channels in a concentration-dependent and picrotoxin-sensitive manner. In a cortical synaptoneurosome preparation, basal $^{36}Cl^-$ flux was enhanced, but muscimol-stimulated $^{36}Cl^-$ flux was not enhanced by enflurane (116). Longoni and Olsen (95), however, have demonstrated in rat cortical slices that halothane at clinically relevant concentrations potentiated muscimol-induced $^{36}Cl^-$ flux. The opposing results from the two studies may reflect the use of different techniques in measuring $^{36}Cl^-$ flux. In Longoni et al. (94), the Ca^{2+} dependency of the halothane effect on $^{36}Cl^-$ flux also was analyzed. Using either Ca^{2+}-free medium or blocking voltage-gated Ca^{2+} channels with cobalt reduced the direct $^{36}Cl^-$ flux enhancement by halothane seen in the absence of a GABA$_A$ agonist (94). Potentiation of muscimol-stimulated $^{36}Cl^-$ flux by volatile agents was found to be Ca^{2+}-independent (94). This result is consistent with the findings of Lin et al. (90) and Jones et al. (78), that volatile anesthetic enhancement of muscimol-induced chloride currents are not dependent on intracellular Ca^{2+}. The Longoni study (94) also suggests that the effects of inhalational anesthetics on GABA$_A$ receptors may involve both allosteric modulation of GABA$_A$ receptor activity and, in part, indirect effects mediated by other cellular systems.

Alcohols

Receptor Binding Ethanol exhibits some allosteric interactions that are similar to the intravenous anesthetics. Ethanol has been reported to potentiate in vitro benzodiazepine binding in whole rat brain membranes but only at high concentrations (100 mM) (177). On the contrary, TBPS binding in mouse whole brain microsacs is inhibited by in vitro ethanol, only at several times the lethal concentration, IC_{50} = 377 mM (76). A series of n-alcohols, methanol to decanol, also were shown to inhibit TBPS binding, and the potencies were directly related to chain length (i.e., the most potent was decanol) (76). In vivo administration of ethanol (0.5–4 g/kg p.o.) has been demonstrated to induce a dose-dependent inhibition of TBPS binding measured ex vivo in rat cerebral cortices, and this inhibition is blocked by the partial inverse agonist Ro15-4513 (29). The mechanism for ethanol-induced inhibition of TBPS binding was related to a decrease in the affinity of the binding site for TBPS. In the presence of in vivo diazepam (0.25 mg/kg), the effect of in vivo ethanol (0.5 g/kg) on ex vivo TBPS binding was enhanced (29). Unlike general anesthetics, ethanol has not been shown to enhance GABA or muscimol binding (177). The technique used by Concas et al. (29) demonstrates that under physiological conditions ethanol has significant effects on GABA$_A$ receptor channels, and these data are consistent with those observed in nonphysiological or in vitro conditions. Thus, the receptor binding data suggest that ethanol may modulate, possibly indirectly, GABA$_A$ receptor activity.

Electrophysiology Electrophysiological studies have provided functional evidence for the interaction of ethanol with GABA$_A$ receptors. In some, but not all, cultured mouse hippocampal and cortical neurons, ethanol at pharmacologically relevant concentrations potentiated GABA-activated chloride currents in a concentration-dependent, saturable, and reversible manner (1). Nishio and Narahashi (123) found in voltage-clamped, cultured dorsal root ganglion neurons that ethanol increased the amplitude of GABA-activated chloride currents in a concentration-dependent and reversible manner, whereas sustained currents induced by higher concentrations of GABA were not altered in the presence of ethanol. Ethanol was also reported to enhance GABA currents in cultured chick cortical neurons and certain cells in chick, rat, and mouse CNS (26,145). Numerous other workers have reported that ethanol does not affect GABA synapses or postsynaptic responses (128,165). Indeed, electrophysiological measurements show ethanol to enhance the actions of GABA in some areas, such as inferior colliculus and medial septum, but not in lateral septum (30). Proctor et al. (141) found ethanol to enhance some GABAergic synapses but not others. It appears that some GABA receptive cells are not sensitive to ethanol, while others are. In addition, the enhancement of GABA responses by ethanol may involve a modulation of desensitization rate and/or indirect effects on chloride channel activity. Nevertheless, electrophysiological evidence supports the view that ethanol may, in part, mediate sedation and loss of consciousness by enhancing GABA$_A$-activated neuronal inhibition, at least in some neurons. The heterogeneity of GABA$_A$ receptors may be responsible for the pharmacological heterogeneity.

Chloride Flux Using chloride flux assays, alcohols have been found by some laboratories to modulate GABA$_A$ receptors. Ethanol (10 mM) has been reported to potentiate muscimol and pentobarbital-induced $^{36}Cl^-$ ion flux in rat cerebral cortex synaptoneurosomes (3,171). At higher concentrations (20–50 mM), ethanol has demonstrated GABA-mimetic properties, and the enhancing effects of ethanol are antagonized by bicuculline and picrotoxin (171). Another study by Suzdak et al. (170) revealed that the potentiating effect of ethanol on GABA$_A$ receptor-mediated $^{36}Cl^-$ flux is blocked by the imidazodiazepine Ro15-4513, a benzodiazepine receptor ligand with partial inverse agonist activity. This effect may be a mechanism for the blockade of the anticonflict and intoxicating actions of ethanol by parenteral pretreatment with Ro15-4513 (3 mg/kg). The Ro15-4513 antagonism of ethanol's potentiating effects is reversed in the presence of the benzodiazepine antagonist flumazenil (170). These data indicate that the neurochemical and behavioral actions of ethanol may be associated with the benzodiazepine binding site on GABA$_A$ receptors.

Similar interactions of ethanol on the GABA$_A$ receptor-mediated $^{36}Cl^-$ flux have been observed in cultured mouse spinal cord neurons (109). In the Mehta and Ticku study (109), the enhancing and direct effects of ethanol on $^{36}Cl^-$ flux also were blocked by another partial inverse agonist, FG-7142. This antagonism by FG-7142, as with Ro15-4513, occurs at concentrations lower than those that demonstrate an inverse agonist effect on GABA-activated $^{36}Cl^-$ flux (109). Further evidence in support of the interaction of ethanol with GABA$_A$ receptors has been demonstrated using mice selectively bred for alcohol sensitivity (3). Allan and Harris(3) reported that muscimol-induced $^{36}Cl^-$ flux was greater in mice selected for ethanol sensitivity than in those not as sensitive to the hypnotic effects of ethanol. Thus, it appears that ethanol at pharmacologically relevant concentrations (20–50 mM) has positive modulatory actions on $GABA_A$ receptors.

Anatomical Correlates for $GABA_A$-Related Actions of Benzodiazepines and Anesthetic Agents

Receptor Binding

Benzodiazepines The benzodiazepine binding site on $GABA_A$ receptors has a complex pharmacology. Three different kinds of ligands can interact with the binding site: agonists, inverse agonists, and antagonists (Table 2). Briefly, agonists, such as benzodiazepines, and inverse agonists, like β-carbolines, have opposite effects on $GABA_A$ receptors. The former enhance the opening of the chloride channel, and the latter inactivate $GABA_A$ chloride channels. Antagonists, like flumazenil (Ro15-1788), block the actions of both agonists and inverse agonists. This unusual and extensive pharmacology led to the first documentation of $GABA_A$ receptor subtypes: types I and II (Table 3). By performing ligand binding analyses from different brain regions, Klepner et al. (81) first reported that type I (also termed BZ_1) benzodiazepine binding sites demonstrated high affinity for the benzodiazepine agonist CL218,872 (an anxiolytic triazolopyridazine), whereas type II (also termed BZ_2) binding sites displayed low affinity for CL218,872. A similar dichotomy in the pharmacology of the benzodiazepine binding site was also observed using the anxiogenic β-carbolines (17). Type I and II binding sites were distinguished by the high and low affinity, respectively, for these compounds. Although benzodiazepines such as diazepam (Valium) or flunitrazepam (Rohypnol) display equally high affinity for both subtypes (81,93,163), quazepam (Dormalin) displays a selectivity for the type I binding sites (162). In light of the extensive heterogeneity of $GABA_A$ receptors as revealed by molecular biology, it should be noted that this pharmacological dichotomy in $GABA_A$ receptors potentially represents various molecular subtypes.

Receptor autoradiography has been used to show that the pharmacological subtypes of the benzodiazepine binding site are distributed differentially across the CNS (92,120,125,198). The predominant pharmacological subtype, type I, revealed a high density of binding sites in the cortex (layer IV), cerebellar molecular layer, globus pallidus, and substantia nigra. Type II benzodiazepine receptors demonstrated a more limited distribution, with high densities located in the caudate-putamen, dentate gyrus, hippocampus (CA1), superior colliculus, and spinal cord. In vitro receptor binding using rat brain cerebral cortical and cerebellar homogenates has suggested that type I and not type II [^{3}H]flunitrazepam binding is preferentially stimulated by pentobarbital (121). A biochemical and an autoradiographic study have reported that barbiturate binding sites are effectively coupled to both type I and II benzodiazepine receptors, and that barbiturate-enhanced benzodiazepine binding is not strictly associated with the type I benzodiazepine binding site (24,88). In all, the differential distribution of type I and II benzodiazepine binding sites suggest that nonsedative triazolopyradizines and some benzodiazepine hypnotics target different regions of the brain, which may explain the therapeutic differences between the two drugs. Do the $GABA_A$-related actions of general anesthetics demonstrate a differential distribution across the brain? This topic will be discussed in the following section of this chapter.

Table 2. BENZODIAZEPINE BINDING SITE PHARMACOLOGY

	Ligands	Intrinsic activity
Agonists	Benzodiazepines, e.g., midazolam	+++
Partial agonists[a]	Clonazepam, alpidem, bretazenil, divaplon	+
Antagonists	Flumazenil (Ro15-1788)	None
Partial inverse agonists	Ro15-4513 (alcohol antagonist), FG-7142	-
Inverse agonists	DMCM	---

[a]Data from Haefely et al. (54).
DMCM, methyl 6,7-dimethoxy-β-carboline-3-carboxylate.

Table 3. PHARMACOLOGICAL SUBTYPES OF $GABA_A$ RECEPTORS

	Type I	Type II
High affinity for diazepam and flunitrazepam	Yes	Yes
High affinity for triazolopyridazine, CL218872	Yes	No
High affinity for zolpidem	Yes	Yes[a] or no
High affinity for β-carbolines	Yes	No

[a]Zolpidem has been considered as a type I specific ligand. Molecular biology has revealed that type II binding can be represented by three α subunit isoforms, two of which (α2 and α3) have a high affinity for zolpidem, whereas the third (α5) has low affinity for zolpidem (38).

General Anesthetics $GABA_A$ receptors from different brain regions demonstrate differential sensitivities to barbiturates and anesthetic steroids (21,23,24,88,126,150). This effect may be attributed to different subunit compositions of the $GABA_A$ receptor in distinct rat brain regions. Most of the receptor binding studies with anesthetic agents have been performed with brain homogenates, namely cerebral cortex. A recent study using semiquantitative receptor autoradiography has demonstrated that alphaxalone differentially enhances [^{3}H]muscimol binding throughout the rat brain (21). In the presence of alphaxalone, brain areas such as cerebral cortex, hippocampus, and the molecular layer of the cerebellum showed a greater enhancement of [^{3}H]muscimol binding than the thalamus, caudate-putamen, and granule layer of the cerebellum (21). The interaction of alphaxalone on [^{35}S]TBPS binding has also been studied using receptor autoradiography in the rat brain (150). In the presence of alphaxalone, the cerebellum demonstrated the greatest decrease in binding. Within the cerebral cortex, [^{35}S]TBPS binding was decreased in the superficial layers and increased within the deeper layers. In addition, alphaxalone (and GABA) increased [^{35}S]TBPS binding in the hindbrain reticular formation (150). These data suggest that $GABA_A$ chloride channel binding sites in the brainstem are allosterically connected to anesthetic binding sites in a different manner than in the cerebellum.

The modulation of [^{3}H]flunitrazepam binding by alphaxalone and pentobarbital also has been demonstrated using semiquantitative and quantitative receptor autoradiography (21,24). In a study by Bureau and Olsen (21), alphaxalone and pentobarbital augmented [^{3}H]flunitrazepam binding in most brain areas measured; however, a few brain areas (striatum, ventromedial hypothalamus, select thalamic nuclei, and the principal sensory trigeminal nucleus) displayed greater sensitivity (i.e., a greater enhancement of benzodiazepine binding) to alphaxalone than pentobarbital. These data suggest that $GABA_A$ receptors in the select nuclei mentioned above may be involved in the regulation of physiological functions that are depressed by steroid anesthetics but not by anesthetic barbiturates. In the study of Carlson et al. (24), pentobarbital-enhanced [^{3}H]flunitrazepam binding was measured in 133 discrete rat brain areas. The hypothesis that pentobarbital would enhance benzodiazepine binding in a site-specific manner across the rat brain was tested. The greatest percentage increases in [^{3}H]flunitrazepam binding occurred in medullary nuclei that control physiological functions, such as cardiopulmonary parameters, motor tone, and arousal, which are known to be depressed by systemically administered pentobarbital. In all, these autoradiographical findings reflect a heterogeneity of anesthetic binding sites on GABA$_A$ receptors. Would this heterogeneity also reflect a differential modulation of GABA$_A$ receptor function by anesthetic agents across brain regions?

Functional Studies

Only a few studies examining the interactions of benzodiazepines and anesthetic agents with GABA$_A$ receptor function have been performed using different brain regions. Chronic diazepam treatment in rats reduced the ability of GABA to stimulate $^{36}Cl^-$ flux in cortical slices, but no change occurred in the cerebellum (104). These data suggest that the behavioral effect of tolerance induced by chronic diazepam treatment appears to involve GABA$_A$ receptors in cortex more than in the cerebellum. Pentobarbital has been shown to differentially induce $^{36}Cl^-$ flux across different rat brain regions (155). In the presence of the barbiturate, GABA$_A$ receptors from the cerebellum, hippocampus, and cortex demonstrated a greater $^{36}Cl^-$ flux than in the striatum and hindbrain. These functional data are not consistent with the receptor binding data from Carlson et al. (24), which reported that the greatest effects of barbiturate-enhanced ligand binding occurred in the brainstem. It should be noted that the results from the study of Schwartz et al. (155) were highly correlated with the relative density of the distribution of TBPS binding sites, an indication of GABA-gated chloride channel density. This correlation would suggest that the effects of barbiturates are mediated by brain areas with a greater number of GABA$_A$ chloride channels. Ethanol enhancement of $^{36}Cl^-$ flux has been investigated across brain regions (64). No significant differences were apparent in the actions of ethanol between the mouse cerebral and cerebellar cortices (64). In mouse hippocampus, muscimol-stimulated $^{36}Cl^-$ flux, however, appeared to be insensitive to ethanol (3), suggesting that the behavioral and/or physiological effects of ethanol may not require the potentiation of GABA$_A$ receptor activity in the hippocampus. GABA$_A$ receptors in several other brain regions have been found to be relatively insensitive to ethanol (30,141,165). More studies will be needed in order to elucidate which brain areas, hence GABA$_A$ receptor subtypes, are important in mediating the actions of benzodiazepines and general anesthetics.

MOLECULAR BIOLOGY OF GABA$_A$ RECEPTORS AND ANESTHETIC ACTION

The previous section of this chapter reviewed the GABA$_A$-related actions of sedative and anesthetic agents and anatomical correlates for this interaction. This evidence supports the hypothesis that GABA$_A$ receptors are a putative site of action for sedative and general anesthetic agents. The GABA$_A$ receptor family is a potentially diverse group of ligand-gated ion channels comprised of various polypeptides. The following section will review (a) the molecular heterogeneity of GABA$_A$ receptors; (b) the interaction of anesthetic agents with specific GABA$_A$ subunits and subunit combinations; and (c) the differential localization of GABA$_A$ subunits in the brain.

Molecular Heterogeneity of GABA$_A$ Receptors

The original cloning of the GABA$_A$ receptor suggested that the oligomeric structure consists of two α and two β subunits (153). Each subunit contains four transmembrane polypeptide chains (M1–M4), an extracellular N-terminal end including consensus sites for glycosylation, an intracellular loop between M3 and M4, which for some subunits contain a consensus sequence for phosphorylation, and a short extracellular C-terminus (reviewed in ref. 182) (Fig. 4). Photoaffinity labeling has shown that the β subunit contained the high-affinity GABA binding site, and the α subunit contained the high-affinity benzodiazepine binding site (25,37,168). It has also been reported that β and α subunits may both contain binding sites for GABA and benzodiazepines, respectively (19). Radiation inactivation studies determined that binding sites for picrotoxin, barbiturates, and nonbarbiturate hypnotics were not resolved to a single subunit but rather located on an oligomeric structure, possibly within the channel lumen (102,122,158) (Fig. 2). Binding analyses revealed an analogous but distinct binding site for naturally occurring and synthetic anesthetic steroids (67,76,179).

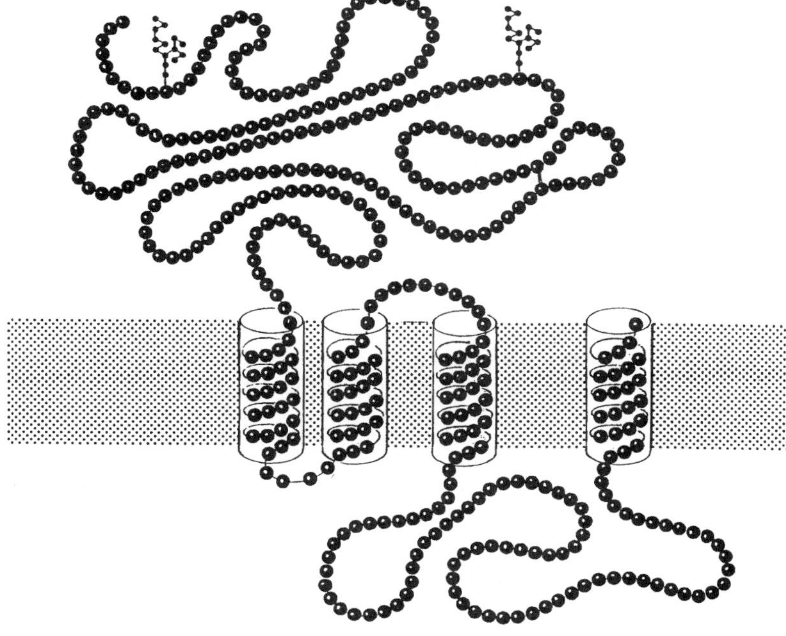

Figure 4. Generic topological structure of a GABA$_A$ receptor subunit. The N-terminal half of the polypeptide is suggested to be extracellular, with probable sites for glycosylation (polymeric, *black circles*) and a conserved cystine bridge between all members of the ligand-gated ion channel superfamily. Four putative membrane-spanning domains are shown as α-helixes within the cell membrane (*stippled*). Some subunits contain a C-terminal that is located at the extracellular end of the fourth membrane-spanning region. Potential phosphorylation sites in several subunit isoforms are present on the large putative intracellular loop between the third and fourth membrane-spanning regions. (Reprinted, in adapted form, with permission from ref. 127.)

More recent molecular cloning has identified three additional $GABA_A$ receptor subunits (γ, δ, ρ). The δ subunit contributes to high-affinity GABA binding, and the γ subunit is necessary for benzodiazepine binding and potentiation of chloride current (161). The ρ subunit is an integral part of $GABA_A$ receptors in the retina (32). To date, the stoichiometry and configuration of native $GABA_A$ receptors in the CNS is not known, but the $GABA_A$ receptor is believed to have a five-subunit configuration (reviewed in refs. 35 and 182) (Fig. 5), similar to the nicotinic acetylcholine receptor (184). Molecular cloning also has demonstrated polymorphism with four of the five subunits (α 1–6; β 1–4; γ 1–3; δ; ρ 1 and 2), and additional diversity can occur with alternative splicing (reviewed in refs. 22, 35, and 182). To date, RNA splice variants have been described for only the β2, β3, β4, and γ2 subunits (10,68,80,82,187). In all, a total of 16 distinct $GABA_A$ subunits have been isolated. This heterogeneity may be a factor that enables the interaction of structurally diverse sedative and anesthetic agents with the $GABA_A$ receptor family (reviewed in refs. 60 and 174). The sensitivity of specific $GABA_A$ subunit isoforms to sedative and general anesthetics will be reviewed in the following section of this chapter.

$GABA_A$ Receptor Subunit-Specificity for Anesthetic Action

Recent studies have concentrated on elucidating which subunits as well as which subunit compositions are essential for anesthetic sensitivity. Studies implementing the techniques of photoaffinity labeling and recombinant receptor pharmacology are reviewed here; these studies focus on the pharmacological and functional heterogeneity of $GABA_A$ receptors.

Protein Chemistry

Pharmacological heterogeneity of $GABA_A$ receptors has been shown at the polypeptide level using the technique of photoaffinity labeling. When allosteric modulators have been preincubated with specific radiolabeled ligands, prior to ultraviolet light exposure, specific polypeptides from purified $GABA_A$ receptors have revealed differential photoincorporation of the radiolabeled ligand (20,21). In the presence of pentobarbital, $[^3H]$muscimol binding was greater in the α1 and β2 polypeptide than the α2 and β3 subunits. Similarly, alphaxalone enhanced $[^3H]$flunitrazepam photolabeling to α1 and β2 subunits more than the α2 and β3 peptide bands (21). It should be noted that GABA enhancement of $[^3H]$flunitrazepam binding was more pronounced in the α2 than the α1 polypeptide (21). These data indicate that α1 and β2 subunits are more sensitive to anesthetic agents than α2 and β3 subunits. Thus, $GABA_A$ receptors containing α1 and β2 are potentially important components for anesthetic-sensitive $GABA_A$ receptors.

Recombinant Receptor Pharmacology

Recombinant $GABA_A$ receptors are expressed by (a) injecting cDNAs or mRNAs encoding specific subunits into *Xenopus* oocytes or (b) transfecting cDNAs for distinct $GABA_A$ polypeptides transiently or stably into cell lines. These expression systems contain the machinery for transcription and translation and for assembly of subunit-specific $GABA_A$ receptors. The ligand-sensitive ion channels can be characterized pharmacologically using electrophysiology or receptor binding. The expression of recombinant $GABA_A$ receptors has been useful in elucidating the subunit composition of functional $GABA_A$ receptors. The formation of functional GABA-gated chloride ion channels has been reported for certain homomeric receptors (14). The coexpression of α and β subunits comprise hetero-oligomer channels that display a more robust GABA response than homomeric receptors (139). Although the stoichiometry and subunit composition of native $GABA_A$ receptors is not known at this time, the heterooligomeric channels appear to demonstrate a closer likeness than homomeric channels to GABA-gated chloride channels found in situ. The interaction of benzodiazepines and anesthetic agents with recombinant receptors have provided important information regarding the subunit combinations exhibiting anesthetic sensitivity.

Benzodiazepines The α and γ subunits are essential for benzodiazepine pharmacology (138). High-affinity benzodiazepine binding appears to require α and γ subunits. Benzodiazepine potentiation of GABA-gated chloride currents only occurs in the presence of a γ subunit (59,134,138,161). The functional expression of recombinant $GABA_A$ receptors has shown that isoforms of the α subunit can be used to distinguish pharmacological subtypes of the $GABA_A$ receptor (i.e., type I and II) (136). Type I pharmacology was determined by the presence of an α1 subunit, and receptors containing α2, α3, and α5 polypeptides appeared to represent type II pharmacology. This study (136) as well as other investigations produced data demonstrating microheterogeneity of the recombinant receptors containing subunits in the type II class (53,106,137,143). For example, α5-containing recombinant receptors bound benzodiazepine-like ligands with a lower affinity than recombinant receptors containing α2 or α3 subunits (137). As a functional correlate to this binding data, diazepam potentiates GABA-elicited chloride currents with greater efficacy in $GABA_A$ receptors with α2 or α3 compared to those containing α5 subunits (143,164).

Using recombinant $GABA_A$ receptors, it has also been shown that the $GABA_A$ agonist muscimol binds with high affinity to the α4 and α6 subunits, and benzodiazepine agonists fail to bind to these two subunits (79,97,190). $GABA_A$ receptors containing α4 or α6 subunits have been characterized as benzodiazepine insensitive, and therefore, these $GABA_A$ receptors are most likely not essential for the sedative actions of benzodiazepines. It is interesting to note that a single amino acid substitution at position 100 in rat of the α6 subunit can alter the sensitivity to benzodiazepines (83). In this study, recombinant $GABA_A$ receptors with the point mutation on the α6 subunit produced GABA-activated chloride currents that were, unlike the wild-type α6, potentiated by diazepam (83). These functional studies using recombinant receptors have provided important evidence for elucidating the essential components of benzodiazepine binding sites on $GABA_A$ receptors.

Unlike the α subunit, the functional differences seen with the different β isoforms have not been correlated with pharmacologically defined subtypes of the $GABA_A$ receptor (e.g., type I and II). Benzodiazepine enhancement of GABA-induced chloride current was shown to be greater in recombinant $GABA_A$ receptors assembled with the β2 subunit than with the β1 isoform (164). This result suggests that $GABA_A$ receptors incorporating a β2 subunit provide a better allosteric modulatory site for benzodiazepines than β1 subunits. A recent study has analyzed the expression of α and γ cDNAs in the absence or presence of β2 cDNA, and this work has demonstrated that $GABA_A$ receptors with type I pharmacology can be constituted without a β subunit (194). It is not known whether this conclusion applies to native receptors.

Different γ subunits can differentially modulate responsiveness of α subunit-containing $GABA_A$ receptors to benzodiazepine agonists, inverse agonists, and antagonists (143,199). Recombinant receptors assembled with γ1 subunits are positively modulated by inverse agonists, as opposed to their normal negative modulation, but inhibited by benzodiazepine agonists, which typically potentiate GABA responses (143,199). Herb et al. (70) have demonstrated that the γ3 subunit lowers binding affinities for benzodiazepine agonists without altering the affinities for the antagonist and inverse agonists of the benzodiazepine binding site. These data indicate that the diverse pharmacology of benzodiazepines is dependent on the presence of specific γ isoforms as well as the α subunits.

Intravenous Anesthetics As discussed in the previous section, the γ2 subunit is an important component for the func-

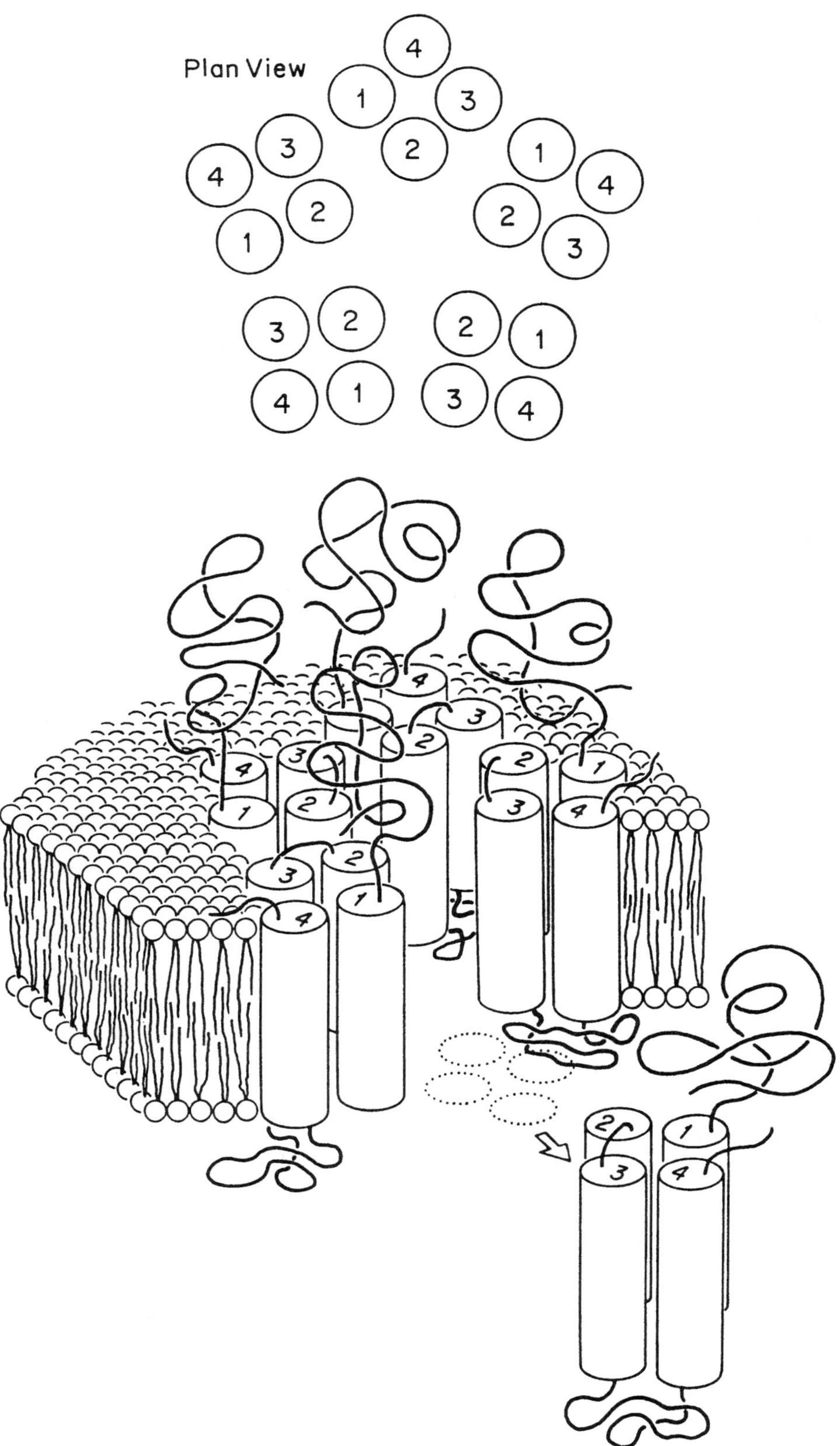

Figure 5. Model of the GABA$_A$ receptor/chloride ion channel protein complex. The ligand-gated ion channel is proposed to be a hetero-oligomer composed of five subunits of the type shown in Fig. 4. Each subunit has four membrane-spanning domains (cylinders 1–4), one or more of which contribute to the wall of the ion channel. The structure is patterned after the well-characterized nicotinic acetylcholine receptor. GABA$_A$ receptors are composed of various combinations of the α, β, γ, δ, and ρ polypeptides, but the exact subunit composition, stoichiometry, and number of subunits are not presently known. (Reprinted with permission from ref. 127.)

tional $GABA_A$-related properties mediated by benzodiazepines. It appears, however, that the actions of general anesthetics in enhancing $GABA_A$ receptors may not require a γ subunit. Electrophysiological recordings from the chinese hamster ovary (CHO) cell line, transfected with α1 and β1 $GABA_A$ receptor cDNAs, have shown that pentobarbital, an anesthetic steroid 5β-pregnan-3α-ol-20-one, etomidate, chlormethiazole, and propofol produce robust potentiations of GABA-evoked chloride currents (72). A similar effect has been observed in an immortalized hypothalamic neuronal line, GT1-7. GT1-7 cells express functional $GABA_A$ receptors that lack γ subunits (59). GABA-activated chloride currents recorded from voltage-clamped GT1-7 cells are augmented in a reversible manner by pentobarbital, the anesthetic steroid, 5α-pregnan-3α-ol-20-one, and propofol (55,59). The nonanesthetic stereoisomer, 5α-pregnan-3β-ol-20-one, however, did not alter the current elicited by GABA in these cells, indicating that $GABA_A$ receptors lacking γ subunits are sensitive to anesthetic steroids (59).

In mouse fibroblast cells transfected with α1, β1 or α1, β1, γ2L subunit combinations, Horne et al. (74) observed that pentobarbital and alphaxalone potentiated more effectively the maximal GABA responses without the γ2L subunit. These results indicate that the anesthetic agents modulated $GABA_A$ responses on receptors without γ subunits. Pentobarbital also potentiates GABA-evoked currents recorded from HEK-293 cells transfected with only α or β $GABA_A$ receptor cDNAs (139). In addition, $GABA_A$ receptors of HEK-293 cells transfected only with δ cDNA are sensitive to the barbiturate (161). These observations, however, must be treated with caution since HEK-293 cells contain β3 subunit mRNA (80). This endogenous subunit may combine with transfected subunits to produce functional, hetero-oligomeric $GABA_A$ channels in these cells.

Using *Xenopus* oocytes, ρ homomeric channels are gated by GABA and blocked by picrotoxin; however, these channels were insensitive to barbiturates as well as benzodiazepines and bicuculline (159). It has been suggested that GABA receptors comprised of the ρ subunit form a different subtype from bicuculline-sensitive receptors.

The electrophysiological studies reviewed so far suggest that most $GABA_A$ receptor combinations are modulated by intravenous anesthetics. There is however evidence that the potency of these compounds as $GABA_A$ receptor modulators may be influenced by subunit composition (61,74). This conclusion is supported by radioligand binding. For example, 5α-pregnan-3α-ol-20-one potentiation of [^{3}H]flunitrazepam binding was greater in the α3β1γ2 than the α1β1γ2 or α2β1γ2 combinations (85). A functional correlate to this finding was observed in *Xenopus* oocytes, and $GABA_A$ receptors containing α3 and α1 subunits demonstrated a greater enhancement of GABA-activated chloride currents by 5α-pregnan-3α-ol-20-one than $GABA_A$ receptors with α2 (160). It is interesting to note that steroid potency was increased with the addition of a γ2 subunit for $GABA_A$ recombinant receptors containing α1 and α2 subunits but not with the α3 subunit (160). In contrast, no subunit specificity was observed in HEK-293 cells for the actions of anesthetic steroids on GABA responses (142).

There is also evidence to support subunit selectivity for the direct activation of $GABA_A$ responses by intravenous anesthetics. For example, pentobarbital directly activates recombinant $GABA_A$ receptors in *Xenopus* oocytes injected with α1 or α5 subunits (plus a β and γ), and currents activated by the barbiturate were greater in oocytes expressing receptors containing α1 rather than α5 mRNA (164). Unlike native $GABA_A$ receptors of chromaffin cells (56) and hippocampal neurons (63), which are directly activated by propofol (<8 μM), receptors expressed by GT1-7 neurons are not activated even by high (100 μM) concentrations of the anesthetic (55). This observation suggests that GT1-7 cells lack one or more subunit(s) required for direct anesthetic activation of the $GABA_A$ receptor. Sensitivity of $GABA_A$ receptors to direct activation by anesthetics is apparently not conferred by the γ subunit, because α2β1 recombinant receptors in HEK-293 cells were activated by low concentrations of propofol (<2 μM). In fact, similar to the observation by Horne et al. (74), for pentobarbital, activation of $GABA_A$ receptors required higher concentrations of propofol in HEK-293 cells expressing α2β1γ2 receptors than in those expressing α2β1 receptors (61).

The majority of evidence suggests that there is subunit dependence to the actions of intravenous general anesthetics on the $GABA_A$ receptor. The nature of the subunit dependence of these agents is however complex and at present less well defined than that of the benzodiazepines.

Volatile Anesthetics Similar studies to those described above for the intravenous general anesthetics have been carried out to investigate the subunit specificity of $GABA_A$ receptor modulation by the volatile anesthetics. Using the oocyte expression system, recombinant $GABA_A$ receptors containing α1 and β1 subunits were more sensitive to the enhancing effects of enflurane than were recombinant receptors containing the α, β, and γ2S or γ2L subunits (91). In addition, Lin et al. (91) showed that the splice variants of the γ2 subunit did not differ in sensitivity to enflurane. GABA-gated chloride currents recorded from GT1-7 cells are also enhanced by the volatile agent isoflurane (58). It should be noted that direct activation of $GABA_A$ receptors with anesthetic concentrations of isoflurane is not observed in GT1-7 cells (58). This observation is similar to that reported for propofol (55) and suggests that the subunits required for direct activation by volatile anesthetics as well as intravenous anesthetics may be missing from GT1-7 cells.

Alcohols It has been proposed that a critical component for ethanol sensitivity is the γ2L subunit. The expression of α1, β1, and γ2S or γ2L mRNAs in *Xenopus* oocytes demonstrated that the alternatively spliced γ2L subunit was required for the potentiating actions of a low concentration of ethanol (186). The extra eight amino acids in the γ2L variant contain a protein kinase C phosphorylation site, suggesting that the actions of ethanol may involve phosphorylation. This evidence may help to explain the regional heterogeneity of the alcohol effects on the $GABA_A$ receptor reported by different laboratories. At present, more functional studies are needed to distinguish which subunits are essential for potent anesthetic and alcohol sensitivity.

Differential Brain Regional Localization of Subunit Isoforms

In combination with the data from recombinant receptor pharmacology, identification of brain areas containing $GABA_A$ receptor subtypes may help to localize discrete sites of anesthetic action in the brain and may provide insight into brain areas involved in regulating states of consciousness. The following sections will review present knowledge concerning localization of $GABA_A$ receptor subunits using the techniques of in situ hybridization and immunohistochemistry.

In Situ Hybridization

Molecular cloning of $GABA_A$ receptor subunits has shown that each subunit is represented by a family of genes. Each family of genes has considerable sequence homology, yet within families the genes encode subunits with distinct amino acid sequences. The native combinations of these gene products, which assemble into $GABA_A$ receptor subtypes in vivo, and the distribution of these subtypes in the brain are presently not known. In situ hybridization has been used to localize the mRNAs of specific subunits throughout the brain. Localizing the distribution of $GABA_A$ receptor subunit mRNAs has helped identify potential subunit combinations for $GABA_A$ receptor subtypes and possibly subtypes displaying anesthetic sensitivity.

Alpha Subunit mRNAs To date, six α subunits of the $GABA_A$ receptor have been isolated by molecular cloning. The genomic message of the α subunit isoforms has been mapped, demonstrating a differential distribution throughout the mammalian CNS and coexpression of several of the isoforms. For example, the α1 message has been shown to be ubiquitously distributed in the rat brain (86,101,131,191). The α2 and α3 mRNAs are expressed in high amounts in the spinal cord, nucleus accumbens, caudate-putamen, and parts of the amygdala, and the α2 message is especially enriched in olfactory bulb and hippocampus. The thalamic nuclei contain high amounts of α4 message and α1 message. The α5 mRNA is predominately expressed in the hippocampus, and the α6 message is confined to cerebellar granule cells. In the brainstem, α1 and α3 are the predominant mRNA transcripts, and α5 and α6 transcripts appear to be completely absent. The functional significance of these distributions is not presently understood.

The distribution of the α subunit mRNAs also has been compared to the localization of pharmacologically defined subtype receptor binding. Because the α1 subunit is a necessary component of the type I benzodiazepine receptor, and α2, α3, and α5 subunits exhibit type II benzodiazepine binding (reviewed in ref. 38), the mapping of specific α subunit genomic messages has shown that the α1 subunit and type I benzodiazepine binding display a comparable distribution in the mammalian CNS. The localization of α2 and α3 subunit genomic messages parallels the distribution of type II benzodiazepine ligand binding (86,120,131,133,191).

Beta Subunit mRNAs Three different encoding genes have been identified for the β subunit family in mammalian CNS (four in birds), and β subunit mRNAs demonstrate differential distributions (86,131,191,200). The β1 message is highly expressed in the hippocampal formation. The β2 transcript is the most widely distributed message and has been found in the olfactory bulb, neocortex, basal ganglia, thalamic nuclei, cerebellum, and brainstem/spinal cord. The expression of β3 transcripts has been localized to olfactory bulb, neocortex, hippocampus, hypothalamus, and cerebellum. The β1 and β3 transcripts are not as prevalent as the β2 transcript, but the β3 mRNA is more widespread than the β1 message. Unlike the α isoforms, the distribution of β subunit genomic messages does not strictly correlate with the localization of the pharmacologically defined subtypes and the GABA$_A$ agonist binding sites determined by receptor autoradiography.

Gamma Subunit mRNAs The γ subunit family contains three encoding genes. Similarly to the α and the β genomic messages, the distribution of γ subunit mRNA transcripts is heterogeneous throughout the rat brain (86,131,191). The γ1 encoding gene is prevalent in specific limbic areas such as the amygdala, hypothalamus, and septum (199). The γ2 transcript is the most common isoform in the mammalian CNS. The γ3 mRNA has a limited distribution in the mammalian CNS and is primarily localized in the cortex, claustrum, caudate-putamen, and medial geniculate of the thalamus (70).

Delta and Rho Subunit mRNAs To date, only one gene has been identified for the δ subunit class. The δ subunit transcript has a very limited distribution in the rat brain and is primarily localized in thalamic nuclei and cerebellar granule cells (86,131,161,191). In addition to containing δ subunit mRNA, thalamic nuclei and cerebellar granule cells have high-affinity [^{3}H]muscimol binding, low levels of benzodiazepine binding, and high amounts of α4 and α6 genomic messages, respectively. Taken together, these data suggest that δ subunits may associate with the α4 and/or α6 subunit(s) to form specific GABA$_A$ receptor subtypes that do not bind benzodiazepines.

Two cDNAs have been isolated for two subunits expressed in the retina, termed ρ1 and ρ2 (31,32). Both ρ mRNAs have been localized primarily in the mammalian retina. The transcripts are undetectable in bovine cerebral cortex; however, transcripts have been detected in the bovine cerebellum (32).

Immunohistochemistry

GABA$_A$ receptor subunit-specific antibodies have been used to localize the distribution of GABA$_A$ receptors throughout the mammalian CNS. Immunohistochemistry has provided an alternative approach to receptor autoradiography in the mapping of GABA$_A$ receptor proteins. The mapping of specific subunit isoforms with antibodies also is useful in verifying the expression of GABA$_A$ receptor gene products in brain areas, identified by in situ hybridization of mRNAs.

Mapping of the GABA$_A$ receptor using immunohistochemistry was first performed with monoclonal antibodies raised against the 55-kilodalton (kDa) β subunit, and the 50-kDa α subunit. The anti–55-kDa polypeptide recognized the β2 and β3 subunits, and the anti–50-kDa polypeptide was selective for the α1 subunit (47,146,152). Both α and β monoclonal antibodies produced a similar distribution of staining for GABA$_A$ receptor antigenic sites, which reconfirmed the presence of both α and β subunits in GABA$_A$ receptors. Another group produced a monoclonal antibody to β subunits and a polyclonal antibody to α subunits and observed similar results using immunohistochemistry (33). The immunohistochemical localization of these GABA$_A$ receptor antibodies was similar to the distribution to both [^{3}H]flunitrazepam and [^{3}H]muscimol binding sites (146,152). These results demonstrated that both the α and β subunits appeared to be components of the high-affinity benzodiazepine and GABA binding sites on the GABA$_A$ receptor. A limitation to this finding was the inability of these two monoclonal antibodies to distinguish between the high-affinity [^{3}H]flunitrazepam and the [^{3}H]muscimol binding sites, which are localized to distinct GABA$_A$ receptor populations as shown by receptor autoradiography (125).

Alpha and Beta Subunit Antibodies The development of antibodies directed against specific amino acid sequences of GABA$_A$ receptor subunit isoforms has been useful in mapping the regional distribution of GABA$_A$ receptor polypeptides. For example, antibodies directed against the α1, α2, and α3 subunits have demonstrated that the distribution of these proteins is similar to the heterogeneous distribution of the mRNAs (201). The mapping of immunoreactivity for α1 or α2 and α3 antipeptides also showed a similar localization with the type I and type II pharmacological subtypes, respectively (201). At present, the α4 subunit has not been resolved immunogenically.

Using α5 and α6 affinity-purified antibodies has revealed a pattern of distribution that parallels the anatomical localization of genomic transcripts (175). The α5 immunoreactivity was predominant in hippocampal CA3 region, and lower amounts of staining were predominant in cortical interneurons, anterior thalamic nucleus, and cerebellar Purkinje neurons. The α6 immunolabeling was strictly found in cerebellar granule cells. High-resolution microscopy has demonstrated that the subcellular distribution of α6 polypeptide is restricted to the postsynaptic plasma membrane of granule cell dendrites (11). Anti-α1 and β2/β3 polypeptide staining colocalize with α6 staining, suggesting that GABA$_A$ receptors containing α1 and α6 subunits are distributed at similar granule cell synaptic sites. It should be noted that the β2 and β3 subunits have not been resolved with distinct antibodies. Another immunohistochemical study that has identified five potential GABA$_A$ receptor subtypes by double and triple immunofluorescence staining demonstrated that not all GABA$_A$ receptor subtypes may contain β2/3 subunits (51). This result was specific to brainstem nuclei. Although it appears that most GABA$_A$ receptors likely contain a single α subunit isoform, immunohistochemical and immunoprecipitation studies have indicated that more than one α subunit isoform may be present in some GABA$_A$ heterooligomers (41,43,51,96,106,110).

Gamma and Delta Subunit Antibodies The localization of γ2 immunoreactivity in the brain corresponds to the distribution of γ2 mRNA (12). Double immunofluorescence labeling has

Table 4. POTENTIAL GABA$_A$ SUBUNITS MEDIATING ANESTHETIC ACTIONS IN DISTINCT BRAIN AREAS[a]

Brain area	Function	Sensitivity to anesthetics[b]	α2 (73,200,201)	α2 (191,201; Brecha and Sternini)
Lateral reticular nucleus	Cardiopulmonary	Receptor autoradiography (24)	-	-
Medullary reticular formation	Behavioral state	Receptor autoradiography (24)	(+) ++	-
Solitary nucleus	Cardiopulmonary	Receptor autoradiography (24)	+	-
Vestibular nuclei	Motor and balance	Receptor autoradiography (24)	±	-
Pontine reticular formation	Behavioral state	Receptor autoradiography (21,24)	+	-
Locus ceruleus	Behavioral state	Glucose metabolism (107,151)	-	±
Interpeduncular nucleus	Limbic	Glucose metabolism; acetylcholine release; receptor autoradiography (23,69,71,107,172)	-	ND
Medial habenula	Limbic	Glucose metabolism; receptor autoradiography (23,71,107)	(-) +	(+) ++
Lateral septal nucleus	Limbic	Receptor autoradiography (21,23)	(++) +	(++) +++

[a]These brain areas control physiological functions (e.g., cardiopulmonary, motor, behavioral state) that are depressed by general anesthetics. Anesthetic agents have been shown to have distinctive effects in each of the brain areas.

[b]Sensitivity to anesthetics is suggested by (a) receptor autoradiography, high increase in benzodiazepine binding; (b) glucose metabolism, spared or augmented regional glucose utilization; and/or (c) acetylcholine release, increased interstitial acetylcholine.

[c]Data are taken from studies using in situ hybridization (-, not detectable; ±, weakly positive; +, positive; ++, strongly positive; +++, intense staining; ND, no data) and immunohistochemistry (same code as in situ data but bracketed).

Brecha and Sternini, *unpublished results* of N. Brecha and C. Sternini, *personal communication*.

shown that γ2 antibodies colocalize, with most of the staining by α1 and α3 antibodies (51). This result is consistent with immunoprecipitation experiments demonstrating that the γ2 subunit is a frequent component of GABA$_A$ receptors that contain the α1 and β2 (or β3) subunits (12). In contrast to the γ subunit, δ subunit immunohistochemistry has been shown to be restricted to a few brain areas (13). The δ subunit identified using polyclonal antisera has been localized to brain areas that demonstrate high-affinity [^{3}H]muscimol binding, such as the cerebellar granule layer and certain thalamic nuclei (13). Antibodies for the δ subunit also immunoprecipitated some high-affinity benzodiazepine binding, which appears to be consistent with the immunoreactivity found in hippocampal dentate gyrus, a brain area with a high density of benzodiazepine binding sites (13). It also suggests that some receptors contain both γ and δ subunits (110).

Immunohistochemistry has demonstrated the regional localization and the neuronal localization (i.e., axodendritic, axosomatic, and pre- and postsynaptic anatomical sites) of various polypeptide GABA$_A$ subunit isoforms. It will be advantageous to develop subunit-specific antibodies against the remaining isoforms of each family of subunits in order to have a complete mapping of the proteins that comprise GABA$_A$ receptor subtypes. Immunohistochemistry and in situ hybridization have provided strategies for elucidating neuroanatomical sites of action between anesthetic agents and specific GABA$_A$ receptor subtypes.

CONCLUSION

This chapter has reviewed studies that provide evidence, at structural and functional levels, supporting the hypothesis that sedation and general anesthesia are produced, in part, by enhancing neuronal inhibition at GABA$_A$ receptors. The mechanism of anesthetic action has yet to be fully understood, yet a diverse group of anesthetic agents, such as hypnotic barbiturates, steroid anesthetics, and volatile anesthetics, have all been shown to enhance GABAergic transmission at clinically relevant concentrations. Thus, GABA$_A$ receptors are promising candidates for neuronal sites of anesthetic action. Knowledge of the subunit composition as well as the distribution of GABA$_A$ receptor subtypes in the brain may be important for targeting more efficacious anesthetics.

In Table 4, the distributions of GABA$_A$ receptor subunits are listed for specific brain areas known to control physiological functions depressed by anesthetic agents. Anesthetic agents have distinct effects in these brain areas (Table 4). Briefly, pentobarbital and alphaxalone have been shown to produce a greater enhancement of benzodiazepine binding in the brain areas listed in Table 4 as compared to more rostral brain regions (21,24). The measurement of glucose metabolism throughout the brain has demonstrated that general anesthetics depress glucose utilization in most brain areas except for select nuclei, such as the interpeduncular and medial habenular nuclei (69,71,107). In the presence of general anesthetics, these select nuclei were shown to have either spared or even augmented glucose metabolism. A functional correlate to these findings has been demonstrated by the measurement of increased interstitial acetylcholine in the interpeduncular nucleus in the presence of pentobarbital or halothane (172). Because there is evidence supporting the interaction of general anesthetic agents with GABA$_A$ receptors, one could postulate that a GABA$_A$ subtype may be involved in mediating these distinct effects of anesthetics in the brain areas listed in Table 4. For example, the α5, β3, and γ1 subunits, and possibly the α3, are present in the brain areas of interest. However, more research about the distribution of GABA$_A$ receptor polypeptides is needed in order to establish a receptor subtype involved in mediating the actions of anesthetic agents.

Presently, the exact subunit composition of native GABA$_A$ receptors is not known, however, recombinant receptors have been shown to share some of the native properties of neuronal GABA$_A$ receptors. Several investigators have proposed potential subunit combinations for GABA$_A$ receptor subtypes and the localization of these subtypes found in situ. Based on the patterns of mRNA expression and recombinant expression studies, Wisden et al. (191) have proposed that GABA$_A$ receptors comprised of the α1, β2, γ2 subunits most likely correspond to the type I pharmacological subtype of the GABA$_A$ receptor. The type II pharmacological subtype may coincide with three potential combinations of subunits: (a) α2, β3, γ2; (b) α3, βx (x = 1, 2, or 3), γ2; or (c) α5, β1, γ2. Several less abundant combinations of these subunits also occur. GABA$_A$ receptors express-

GABA$_A$ subunit isoforms[c]											
α3 (6,200,201)	**α4 (86,191)**	**α5 (6,175)**	**α6 (86,191)**	**β1 (200)**	**β2 (200)**	**β3 (51,200)**	**γ1 (4,51)**	**γ2 (5,51)**	**γ3 (191)**	**δ (13,86,191)**	**ρ (32)**
+	ND	(±) ++	-	±	±	++	-	++	ND	(-)	-
(+) +	ND	(±) ++	-	+	(+) ++	(+) ++	±	(+) +	ND	(-)	-
++	-	(±) ++	-	+	-	+	++	-	ND	(-)	-
++	-	(±) +	-	+	++	++	+	++	ND	(-)	-
+	-	(±) ++	-	+	+	+	±	±	ND	(-)	-
(+) ++	ND	+	-	+	-	+	++	(+) -	ND	(-)	-
++	ND	++	-	+	+	++	++	+	ND	(-)	-
(+) -	-	-	-	-	-	+	++	-	±	(-) -	-
(++) ++	+	(±) ++	-	+	+	++	++	+	±	(-) -	-

ing γ1 or γ3 subunits would represent additional GABA$_A$ receptor subtypes that have not been pharmacologically classified. Finally, the α4 and α6 subunit containing GABA$_A$ receptors would be constituents of GABA$_A$ receptors with no benzodiazepine binding site.

Fritschy et al. (51) have suggested from their work using immunohistochemistry five distinct patterns of subunit composition and localization. These patterns provide tentative suggestions of which subunits are frequently found together. The question whether any of these proposed GABA$_A$ receptor subtypes would mediate the actions of anesthetic agents is an important focus for future research. The answer may enable the development of subtype-specific anesthetic agents with higher therapeutic indices.

REFERENCES

1. Aguayo LG. Ethanol potentiates the GABA$_A$-activated Cl^- current in mouse hippocampal and cortical neurons. *Eur J Pharmacol* 1990;187:127–130.
2. Allan AM, Harris RA. Anesthetic and convulsant barbiturates alter γ-aminobutyric acid–stimulated chloride flux across brain membranes. *J Pharmacol Exp Ther* 1986;238:763–768.
3. Allan AM, Harris RA. γ-Aminobutyric acid and alcohol actions: Neurochemical studies of long sleep and short sleep mice. *Life Sci* 1986;39:2005–2015.
4. Araki T, Kiyama H, Tohyama M. The GABA$_A$ receptor γ1 subunit is expressed by distinct neuronal populations. *Mol Brain Res* 1992;15:121–132.
5. Araki T, Sato M, Kiyama H, Manabe Y, Tohyama M. Localization of GABA$_A$-receptor γ2-subunit mRNA-containing neurons in the rat central nervous system. *Neuroscience* 1992;47:45–61.
6. Araki T, Tohyama M. Region-specific expression of GABA$_A$ receptor α3 and α4 subunits mRNAs in the rat brain. *Mol Brain Res* 1992;12:293–314.
7. Asano T, Ogasawara N. Chloride-dependent stimulation of GABA and benzodiazepine receptor binding by pentobarbital. *Brain Res* 1981;225:212–216.
8. Barker JL, Harrison NL, Lange GD, Owen DG. Potentiation of γ-aminobutyric acid–activated chloride conductance by a steroid anaesthetic in cultured rat spinal neurones. *J Physiol* 1987;386:485–501.
9. Barker JL, Ransom BR. Pentobarbitone pharmacology of mammalian central neurones grown in tissue culture. *J Physiol* 1978;280:355–372.
10. Bateson AN, Lasham A, Darlison MG. γ-Aminobutyric acid$_A$ receptor heterogeneity is increased by alternative splicing of a novel β-subunit gene transcript. *J Neurochem* 1991;56:1437–1440.
11. Baude A, Sequier JM, McKernan RM, Olivier KR, Somogyi P. Differential subcellular distribution of the a6 subunit versus the α1 and β2/3 subunits of the GABA$_A$/benzodiazepine receptor complex in granule cells of the cerebellar cortex. *Neuroscience* 1992;51:739–748.
12. Benke D, Mertens S, Trzeciak A, Gillessen D, Möhler H. GABA$_A$ receptors display association of γ2-subunit with α1 and β2/3-subunits. *J Biol Chem* 1991;266:4478–4483.
13. Benke D, Mertens S, Trzeciak A, Gillessen D, Möhler H. Identification and immunohistochemical mapping of GABA$_A$ receptor subtypes containing the δ-subunit in rat brain. *FEBS Lett* 1991;283:145–149.
14. Blair LAC, Levitan ES, Marshall J, Dionne VE, Barnard EA. Single subunits of the GABA$_A$ receptor form ion channels with properties of the native receptor. *Science* 1988;242:577–579.
15. Bowery N. GABA$_B$ receptor pharmacology. *Annu Rev Pharmacol Toxicol* 1993;33:109–147.
16. Bowery NG, Price GW, Hudson AL, Hill DR, Wilkin GP, Turnbull MJ. GABA receptor multiplicity. *Neuropharmacology* 1984;23:219–231.
17. Braestrup C, Nielsen M. [^{3}H]Propyl β-carboline-3-carboxylate as a selective radioligand for the BZ$_1$ benzodiazepine receptor subclass. *J Neurochem* 1981;37:333–341.
18. Braestrup C, Squires RF. Specific benzodiazepine receptors in rat brain characterized by high-affinity [^{3}H]diazepam binding. *Proc Natl Acad Sci USA* 1977;74:3805–3809.
19. Bureau M, Olsen RW. γ-Aminobutyric/benzodiazepine receptor protein carries binding sites for both ligands on both two major peptide subunits. *Biochem Biophys Res Commun* 1988;153:1006–1011.
20. Bureau M, Olsen RW. Multiple distinct subunits of the γ-aminobutyric acid-A receptor protein show different ligand-binding affinities. *Mol Pharmacol* 1990;37:497–502.
21. Bureau MH, Olsen RW. GABA$_A$ receptor subtypes: ligand binding heterogeneity demonstrated by photoaffinity labeling and autoradiography. *J Neurochem* 1993;61:1479–1491.
22. Burt DR, Kamatchi GL. GABA$_A$ receptor subtypes: from pharmacology to molecular biology. *FASEB J* 1991;5:2916–2923.
23. Carlson BX, Baghdoyan HA. Pentobarbital differentially enhances the affinity of [^{3}H]flunitrazepam binding across brain regions *Pharmacology* 1994;49:1–10.
24. Carlson BX, Mans AM, Hawkins RA, Baghdoyan HA. Pentobarbital-enhanced [^{3}H]flunitrazepam binding throughout the rat brain: an autoradiographic study. *J Pharmacol Exp Ther* 1992;263:1401–1414.

25. Casalotti SO, Stephenson FA, Barnard EA. Separate subunits for agonist and benzodiazepine binding in the γ-aminobutyric $acid_A$ receptor oligomer. *J Biol Chem* 1986;261:15013–15016.
26. Celentano JJ, Gibbs TT, Farb DH. Ethanol potentiates GABA- and glycine-induced chloride currents in chick spinal cord neurons. *Brain Res* 1988;455:377–380.
27. Cheng SC, Brunner EA. Anesthetic effects on GABA binding. *Anesthesiology* 1984;61:A326.
28. Choi DW, Farb DH, Fischbach GD. Chlordiazepoxide selectively augments GABA action in spinal cord cell cultures. *Nature* 1977; 269:342–344.
29. Concas A, Sanna E, Serra M, Mascia MP, Santoro V, Biggio G. "Ex vivo" binding of ^{35}S-TBPS as a tool to study the pharmacology of $GABA_A$ receptors. In: Biggio G, Costa E, eds. *GABA and benzodiazepine receptor subtypes.* New York: Raven Press, 1990:89–108.
30. Criswell HE, Simson PE, Duncan GE, Morrow AL, Keir W, Breese GR. Ethanol enhancement of iontophoretically applied GABA: Association with type-1 benzodiazepine receptor binding. *Alcohol Clin Exp Res* 1992;16:376.
31. Cutting GR, Curristin S, Zoghbi H, O'Hara B, Seldin MF, Uhl GR. Identification of a putative γ-aminobutyric acid (GABA) receptor subunit ρ_2 cDNA and colocalization of the genes encoding ρ_2 (GABRR2) and ρ_1 (GABRR1) to human chromosome 6q14-q21 and mouse chromosome 4. *Genomics* 1992;12:801–806.
32. Cutting GR, Lu L, O'Hara BF, et al. Cloning of the γ-aminobutyric acid (GABA) ρ_1 cDNA: a GABA receptor subunit highly expressed in the retina. *Proc Natl Acad Sci USA* 1991;88:2673–2677.
33. De Blas AL, Vitorica J, Friedrich P. Localization of the $GABA_A$ receptor in the rat brain with a monoclonal antibody to the 57,000 M_r peptide of the $GABA_A$ receptor/benzodiazepine receptor/Cl^- channel complex. *J Neurosci* 1988;8:602–614.
34. DeLorey TM, Kissin I, Brown P, Brown GB. Barbiturate- benzodiazepine interactions at the $GABA_A$ receptor in rat cerebral cortical synaptoneurosomes. *Anesth Analg* 1993;77:598–605.
35. DeLorey TM, Olsen RW. γ-Aminobutyric $acid_A$ receptor structure and function. *J Biochem* 1992;267:16747–16750.
36. DeLorey TM, Olsen RW. GABA and glycine. In: Siegel GJ, et al., eds. *Basic neurochemstry: molecular, cellular, and medical aspects.* 5th ed. New York: Raven Press, 1994:389–399.
37. Deng L, Ransom RW, Olsen RW. [^{3}H]Muscimol photolabels the γ-aminobutyric acid receptor binding site on a peptide subunit distinct from that labeled with benzodiazepines. *Biochem Biophys Res Commun* 1986;138:1308–1314.
38. Doble A, Martin IL. Multiple benzodiazepine receptors: no reason for anxiety. *Trends Pharmacol Sci* 1992;13:76–81.
39. Dodson BA, Braswell LM, Miller KW. Barbiturates bind to an allosteric regulatory site on nicotinic acetylcholine receptor rich membranes. *Mol Pharmacol* 1987;32:119–126.
40. Dray A, Straughan DW. Benzodiazepines: GABA and glycine receptors on single neurons in the rat medulla. *J Pharm Pharmacol* 1976;28:314–315.
41. Duggan MJ, Pollard S, Stephenson FA. Immunoaffinity purification of $GABA_A$ receptor α-subunit iso-oligomers. *J Biol Chem* 1991; 266:24778–24784.
42. Dunwiddie TV, Worth TS, Olsen RW. Facilitation of recurrent inhibition in rat hippocampus by barbiturate and related nonbarbiturate depressant drugs. *J Pharmacol Exp Ther* 1986;238:564–575.
43. Endo S, Olsen RW. Antibodies specific for α-subunit subtypes of $GABA_A$ receptors reveal brain regional heterogeneity. *J Neurochem* 1993;60:1388–1398.
44. Enna SJ. GABA receptors. In: Enna SJ, ed. *The GABA receptors.* Clifton, NJ: Humana Press, 1993:1–23.
45. Evans RH, Hill RG. The GABA-mimetic action of etomidate. *Br J Pharmacol* 1977;61:484P.
46. Evans RH, Hill RG. GABA-mimetic action of etomidate. *Experientia* 1978;34:1325–1327.
47. Ewert M, Shivers BD, Lüddens H, Möhler H, Seeburg PH. Subunit selectivity and epitope characterization of mAbs directed against the $GABA_A$/benzodiazepine receptor. *J Cell Biol* 1990;110: 2043–2048.
48. Franks NP, Lieb WR. What is the molecular nature of general anaesthetic target sites? *Trends Pharmacol Sci* 1987;8:169–174.
49. Franks NP, Lieb WR. Volatile general anaesthetics activate a novel neuronal K^- current. *Nature* 1988;333:662–664.
50. Franks NP, Lieb WR. Stereospecific effects of inhalational general anesthetic optical isomers on nerve ion channels. *Science* 1991; 254:427–430.
51. Fritschy JM, Benke D, Mertens S, Oertel WH, Bach T, Möhler H. Five subtypes of type A γ-aminobutyric acid receptors identified in neurons by double and triple immunofluorescence staining with subunit-specific antibodies. *Proc Natl Acad Sci USA* 1992;89: 6726–6730.
52. Gage PW, Robertson BR. Prolongation of inhibitory postsynaptic currents by pentobarbitone, halothane, and ketamine in CA1 pyramidal cells in rat hippocampus. *Br J Pharmacol* 1985;85:675–681.
53. Hadingham KL, Wingrove P, Le Bourdelles B, Palmer KJ, Ragan CI, Whiting PJ. Cloning of cDNA sequences encoding human α2 and α3 γ-aminobutyric $acid_A$ receptor subunits and characterization of the benzodiazepine pharmacology of recombinant α1-, α2-, α3-, and α5-containing human γ-aminobutyric $acid_A$ receptors. *Mol Pharmacol* 1993;43:970–975.
54. Haefely W, Martin JR, Schoch P. Novel anxiolytics that act as partial agonists at benzodiazepine receptors. *Trends Pharmacol Sci* 1990;11:452–456.
55. Hales TG. Direct activation of $GABA_A$ receptors by propofol may be subunit dependent. *Anesthesiology* 1992;77:A695.
56. Hales TG, Lambert JJ. The actions of propofol on inhibitory amino acid receptors of bovine adrenomedullary chromaffin cells and rodent central neurones. *Br J Pharmacol* 1991;104:619–628.
57. Hales TG, Lambert JJ. Modulation of $GABA_A$ and glycine receptors by chlormethiazole. *Eur J Pharmacol* 1992;210:239–246.
58. Hales TG, Jones MV, Harrison NL. Evidence for subunit dependent direct activation of the $GABA_A$ receptor by isoflurane. *Anesthesiology* 1992;77:A697.
59. Hales TG, Kim H, Longoni B, Olsen RW, Tobin AJ. Immortalized hypothalamic GT1-7 neurons express functional γ-aminobutyric acid type A receptors. *Mol Pharmacol* 1992;42:197–202.
60. Hales TG, Olsen RW. Basic pharmacology of intravenous induction agents. In: Bowdle TA, Horita AH, Kharasch ED, eds. *The pharmacological basis of anesthesiology: basic science and clinical applications.* New York: Churchill Livingston, 1994:295–306.
61. Hales TG, Pritchett DB, Greenblatt EP, Harrison NL, Jones MV. The contribution of the γ2 subunit to modulation of the $GABA_A$ receptor by propofol. *Anesthesiology* 1993;79:A720.
62. Hamill OP, Marty A, Neher E, Sakmann B, Sigworth FG. Improved patch-clamp techniques for high-resolution current recording from cells and cell-free membrane patches. *Pflugers Arch* 1981;391:85–100.
63. Hara M, Ikemoto Y, Kai Y. Propofol activates the $GABA_A$ receptor-ionophore complex in dissociated hippocampal neurons of the rat. *Anesthesiology* 1992;77:A696.
64. Harris RA, Allan AM, Daniell LC, Nixon C. Antagonism of ethanol and pentobarbital actions by benzodiazepine inverse agonists: neurochemical studies. *J Pharmacol Exp Ther* 1988;247:1012–1017.
65. Harris B, Wong G, Skolnick P. Volatile anesthetics and barbiturates exhibit neurochemical similarities at $GABA_A$ receptors. *Anesthesiology* 1992;77:A697.
66. Harrison NL, Majewska MD, Harrington JW, Barker JL. Structure-activity relationships for steroid interaction with the γ-aminobutyric $acid_A$ receptor complex. *J Pharmacol Exp Ther* 1987;241: 346–353.
67. Harrison NL, Simmonds MA. Modulation of the GABA receptor complex by a steroid anaesthetic. *Brain Res* 1984;323:287–292.
68. Harvey RJ, Chinchetru MA, Darlison MG. Alternative splicing of a 51-nucleotide exon that encodes a putative protein kinase C phosphorylation site generates two forms of the chicken γ-aminobutyric $acid_A$ receptor β2 subunit. *J Neurochem* 1994;63:10–16.
69. Hawkins RA, Biebuyck JF. Regional brain function during graded halothane anesthesia. In: Fink BR, ed. *Molecular mechanisms of anesthesia.* New York: Raven Press, 1980:145–156.
70. Herb A, Wisden W, Lüddens H, Puia G, Vicini S, Seeburg PH. The third γ subunit of the γ-aminobutyric acid type A receptor family. *Proc Natl Acad Sci USA* 1992;89:1433–1437.
71. Herkenham M. Anesthetics and the habenulo-interpeduncular system: selective sparing of metabolic activity. *Brain Res* 1981;210: 461–466.
72. Hill-Venning C, Lambert JJ, Peters JA, Hales TG. The actions of neurosteroids in inhibitory amino acid receptors. In: Costa E, Paul SM, eds. *Neurosteroids and brain function.* New York: Fidia Research Foundation Symposium Series, 1991:77–87.
73. Hironaka T, Morita Y, Hagihira S, Tateno E, Kita H, Tohyama M. Localization of $GABA_A$-receptor α1 subunit mRNA-containing neurons in the lower brainstem of the rat. *Mol Brain Res* 1990;7: 335–345.

74. Horne AL, Harkness PC, Hadingham KL, Whiting P, Kemp JA. The influence of the γ2L subunit on the modulation of responses to GABA$_A$ receptor activation. *Br J Pharmacol* 1993;108:711–716.
75. Huang LYM, Barker JL. Pentobarbital: stereospecific actions of (+) and (−) isomers revealed on cultured mammalian neurons. *Science* 1980;207:195–197.
76. Huidobro-Toro JP, Bleck V, Allan AM, Harris RA. Neurochemical actions of anesthetic drugs on the γ-aminobutyric acid receptor-chloride channel complex. *J Pharmacol Exp Ther* 1987;242:963–969.
77. Hunkeler W, Möhler H, Pieri L, et al. Selective antagonists of benzodiazepines. *Nature* 1981;290:514–516.
78. Jones MV, Brooks PA, Harrison NL. Enhancement of γ-aminobutyric acid–activated Cl^- currents in cultured rat hippocampal neurones by three volatile anaesthetics. *J Physiol* 1992;449:279–293.
79. Kato K. Novel GABA$_A$ receptor α subunit is expressed only in cerebellar granule cells. *J Mol Biol* 1990;214:619–624.
80. Kirkness EF, Fraser CM. A strong promoter element is located between alternative exons of a gene encoding the human γ-aminobutyric acid-type A receptor β3 subunit (GABARB3). *J Biol Chem* 1993;268:4420–4428.
81. Klepner CA, Lippa AS, Benson DI, Sano MC, Beer B. Resolution of two biochemically and pharmacologically distinct benzodiazepine receptors. *Pharmacol Biochem Behav* 1979;11:457–462.
82. Kofuji P, Wang JB, Moss SJ, Huganir RL, Burt DR. Generation of two forms of the γ-aminobutyric acid$_A$ receptor γ2-subunit in mice by alternative splicing. *J Neurochem* 1991;56:713–715.
83. Korpi ER, Kleingoor C, Kettenmann H, Seeburg PH. Benzodiazepine-induced motor impairment linked to point mutation in cerebellar GABA$_A$ receptor. *Nature* 1993;361:356–359.
84. Lambert JJ, Peters JA, Sturgess NC, Hales TG. Steroid modulation of the GABA$_A$ receptor complex: electrophysiological studies. *Ciba Found Symp* 1990;153:56–71.
85. Lan NC, Gee KW, Bolger MB, Chen JS. Differential responses of expressed recombinant human γ-aminobutyric acid$_A$ receptors to neurosteroids. *J Neurochem* 1991;57:1818–1821.
86. Laurie DJ, Seeburg PH, Wisden W. The distribution of 13 GABA$_A$ receptor subunit mRNAs in the rat brain. II. Olfactory bulb and cerebellum. *J Neurosci* 1991;12:1063–1076.
87. Leeb-Lundberg F, Olsen RW. Interactions of barbiturates of various pharmacological categories with benzodiazepine receptors. *Mol Pharmacol* 1982;21:320–328.
88. Leeb-Lundberg F, Olsen RW. Heterogeneity of benzodiazepine receptor interactions with γ-aminobutyric acid and barbiturate receptor sites. *Mol Pharmacol* 1983;23:315–325.
89. Leeb-Lundberg F, Snowman A, Olsen RW. Barbiturate receptor sites are coupled to benzodiazepine receptors. *Proc Natl Acad Sci USA* 1980;77:7468–7472.
90. Lin LH, Chen LL, Zirrolli JA, Harris RA. General anesthetics potentiate γ-aminobutyric acid actions on γ-aminobutyric acid$_A$ receptors expressed by *Xenopus* oocytes: lack of involvement of intracellular calcium. *J Pharmacol Exp Ther* 1992;263:569–578.
91. Lin LH, Whiting P, Harris RA. Molecular determinants of general anesthetic action: role of GABA$_A$ receptor structure. *J Neurochem* 1993;60:1548–1553.
92. Lo MMS, Niehoff DL, Kuhar MJ, Snyder SH. Autoradiographic differentiation of multiple benzodiazepine receptors by detergent solubilization and pharmacologic specificity. *Neurosci Lett* 1983;39:37–44.
93. Lo MMS, Strittmatter SM, Snyder SH. Physical separation and characterization of two types of benzodiazepine receptors. *Proc Natl Acad Sci USA* 1982;79:680–684.
94. Longoni B, Demontis GC, Olsen RW. Enhancement of GABA$_A$ receptor function and binding by the volatile anesthetic halothane. *J Pharmacol Exp Ther* 1993;266:153–159.
95. Longoni B, Olsen RW. Studies on the mechanism of interaction of anesthetics with GABA$_A$ receptors. *Adv Biochem Psychopharmacol* 1992;47:365–378.
96. Lüddens H, Killisch I, Seeburg PH. More than one α variant may exist in a GABA$_A$/benzodiazepine receptor complex. *J Recept Res* 1991;11:535–551.
97. Lüddens H, Pritchett DB, Kohler M, et al. Cerebellar GABA$_A$ receptor selective for a behavioural alcohol antagonist. *Nature* 1990;346:648–651.
98. Macdonald R, Barker JL. Benzodiazepines specifically modulate GABA-mediated postsynaptic inhibition in cultured mammalian neurones. *Nature* 1978;271:563–564.
99. Macdonald RL, Twyman RE, Rogers CJ, Weddle MG. Pentobarbital regulation of the kinetic properties of GABA receptor chloride channels. *Adv Biochem Pyschopharmacol* 1988;45:61–71.
100. MacIver MB, Tanelian DL, Mody I. Two mechanisms for anesthetic-induced enhancement of GABA$_A$-mediated neuronal inhibition. *Ann N Y Acad Sci* 1991;625:91–96.
101. MacLennan AJ, Brecha N, Khrestchatisky M, et al. Independent cellular and ontogenetic expression of mRNAs encoding three α polypeptides of the rat GABA$_A$ receptor. *Neuroscience* 1991;43:369–380.
102. Maksay G, Nielsen M, Simonyi M. The enhancement of diazepam and muscimol binding by pentobarbital and (+)-etomidate: size of the molecular arrangement estimated by electron irradiation inactivation of rat cortex. *Neurosci Lett* 1986;70:116–120.
103. Maksay G, Ticku MK. Dissociation of [^{35}S]t- butylbicyclophosphorothionate binding differentiates convulsant and depressant drugs that modulate GABAergic transmission. *J Neurochem* 1985;44:480–486.
104. Marley RJ, Gallager DW. Chronic diazepam treatment produces regionally specific changes in GABA-stimulated chloride influx. *Eur J Pharmacol* 1989;159:217–223.
105. Mathers DA. The GABA$_A$ receptor: new insights from single-channel recording. *Synapse* 1987;1:96–101.
106. McKernan RM, Quirk K, Prince R, et al. GABA$_A$ receptor subtypes immunopurified from rat brain with α subunit-specific antibodies have unique pharmacological properties. *Neuron* 1991;7:667–676.
107. McQueen JK, Martin MJ, Hamar AJ. Local changes in cerebral 2-deoxyglucose uptake during alphaxalone anaesthesia with special reference to the habenulo-interpeduncular system. *Brain Res* 1984;300:19–26.
108. Mehta AK, Ticku MK. Characteristics of flunitrazepam binding to intact primary cultured spinal cord neruons and its modulation by GABAergic drugs. *J Neurochem* 1987;49:1491–1497.
109. Mehta AK, Ticku MK. Ethanol potentiation of GABAergic transmission in cultured spinal cord neurons involves γ-aminobutyric acid$_A$–gated chloride channels. *J Pharmacol Exp Ther* 1988;246:558–564.
110. Mertens S, Benke D, Möhler H. GABA$_A$ receptor populations with novel subunit combinations and drug binding profiles identified in brain by α5- and δ-subunit-specific immunopurification. *J Biol Chem* 1993;268:5965–5973.
111. Meyer H. Zur theorie der alkoholnarkose. I. Mitt. welche eigenschaft der anasthetika bedingt ihre narkotische wirkung? *Arch Exp Pathol Pharmakol* 1899;42:109.
112. Meyer H. The theory of narcosis. In: *The Harvey lectures.* Philadelphia: Lippincott, 1906:11–17.
113. Middleton AJ, Smith EB. General anaesthetics and bacterial luminescence: the effect of diethyl ether on the in vitro light emission of *Vibrio fischeri. Proc R Soc Lond B* 1976;193:173–190.
114. Mody I, Tanelian DL, MacIver MB. Halothane enhances tonic neuronal inhibition by elevating intracellular calcium. *Brain Res* 1991;538:319–323.
115. Möhler H, Okada T. Benzodiazepine receptor: demonstration in the central nervous system. *Science* 1977;198:849–851.
116. Moody EJ, Suzdak PD, Paul SM, Skolnick P. Modulation of the benzodiazepine/γ-aminobutyric acid receptor chloride channel complex by inhalational anesthetics. *J Neurochem* 1988;51:1386–1393.
117. Mugnaini E, Oertel WH. An atlas of the distribution of GABAergic neurons and terminals in the rat CNS as revealed by GAD immunohistochemistry. In: Bjorklund A, Hokfelt T, eds. *Handbook of chemical neuroanatomy, vol. 4: GABA and neuropeptides in the CNS, part 1.* New York: Elsevier, 1985:436–622.
118. Nakahiro M, Yeh JZ, Brunner E, Narahashi T. General anesthetics modulate GABA receptor channel complex in rat dorsal root ganglion neurons. *FASEB J* 1989;3:1850–1854.
119. Nicoll RA, Eccles JC, Oshima T, Rubia F. Prolongation of hippocampal inhibitory postsynaptic potentials by barbiturates. *Nature* 1975;258:625–627.
120. Niddam R, Dubois A, Scatton B, Arbilla S, Langer SZ. Autoradiographic localization of [^{3}H]zolpidem binding sites in the rat CNS: comparison with the distribution of[^{3}H]flunitrazepam binding sites. *J Neurochem* 1987;49:890–899.
121. Niehoff DL, Mashal RD, Kuhar MJ. Benzodiazepine receptors: preferential stimulation of type I receptors by pentobarbital. *Eur J Pharmacol* 1983;92:131–134.
122. Nielsen M, Honoré T, Braestrup C. Radiation inactivation of

brain [^{35}S]t-butylbicyclophosphorothionate binding sites reveals complicated molecular arrangements of the GABA/benzodiazepine receptor chloride channel complex. *Biochem Pharmacol* 1985;34:3633–3642.
123. Nishio M, Narahashi T. Ethanol enhancement of GABA- activated chloride current in rat dorsal root ganglion neurons. *Brain Res* 1990;518:283–286.
124. Obata T, Yamamura HI. The effect of benzodiazepines and β-carbolines on GABA-stimulated chloride influx by membrane vesicles from the rat cerebral cortex. *Biochem Biophys Res Commun* 1986;141:1–6.
125. Olsen RW, McCabe RT, Wamsley JK. $GABA_A$ receptor subtypes: autoradiographic comparison of GABA, benzodiazepine, and convulsant binding sites in the rat central nervous system. *J Chem Neuroanat* 1990;3:59–76.
126. Olsen RW, Snowman AM. Chloride-dependent enhancement by barbiturates of γ-aminobutyric acid receptor binding. *J Neurosci* 1982;2:1812–1823.
127. Olsen RW, Tobin AJ. Molecular biology of $GABA_A$ receptors. *FASEB J* 1990;4:1469–1480.
128. Osmanovic SS, Shefner SA. Enhancement of current induced by superfusion of GABA in locus coeruleus neurons by pentobarbital, but not ethanol. *Brain Res* 1990;517:324–329.
129. Overton E. *Studien uber die narkose.* Jena: Verlag von Gustav Fischer, 1901.
130. Peduto VA, Concas A, Santoro G, Biggio G, Gessa GL. Biochemical and electrophysiologic evidence that propofol enhances GABAergic transmission in the rat brain. *Anesthesiology* 1991;75:1000–1009.
131. Persohn E, Malherbe P, Richards JG. Comparative molecular neuroanatomy of cloned $GABA_A$ receptor subunits in the rat CNS. *J Comp Neurol* 1992;326:193–216.
132. Peters JA, Lambert JJ, Cottrell GA. An electrophysiological investigation of the characteristics and function of $GABA_A$ receptors on bovine adrenomedullary chromaffin cells. *Pflugers Arch* 1989;415:95–103.
133. Poulter MO, Barker JL, O'Carroll AM, Lolait SJ, Mahan LC. Differential and transient expression of $GABA_A$ receptor α-subunit mRNAs in the developing rat CNS. *J Neurosci* 1992;12:2888–2900.
134. Pregenzer JF, Im WB, Carter DB, Thomsen DR. Comparison of interactions of [^{3}H]muscimol, t-butyl bicyclophosphoro-[^{35}S] thionate, and [^{3}H]flunitrazepam with cloned γ-aminobutyric $acid_A$ receptors of the α1 β2 and α1 β2 γ2 subtypes. *Mol Pharmacol* 1993;43:801–806.
135. Prince RJ, Simmonds MA. Propofol potentiates the binding of [^{3}H]flunitrazepam to the $GABA_A$ receptor complex. *Brain Res* 1992;596:238–242.
136. Pritchett DB, Lüddens H, Seeburg PH. Type I and type II $GABA_A$-benzodiazepine receptors produced in transfected cells. *Science* 1989;245:1389–1392.
137. Pritchett DB, Seeburg PH. γ-Aminobutyric $acid_A$ receptor α5-subunit creates novel type II benzodiazepine receptor pharmacology. *J Neurochem* 1990;54:1802–1804.
138. Pritchett DB, Sontheimer H, Shivers BD, et al. Importance of a novel $GABA_A$ receptor subunit for benzodiazepine pharmacology. *Nature* 1989;338:582–585.
139. Pritchett DB, Sontheimer H, Gorman CM, Kettenmann H, Seeburg PH, Schofield PR. Transient expression shows ligand gating and allosteric potentiation of $GABA_A$ receptor subunits. *Science* 1988;242:1306–1308.
140. Proctor WR, Mynlieff M, Dunwiddie TV. Facilitatory action of etomidate and pentobarbital on recurrent inhibition in rat hippocampal pyramidal neurons. *J Neurosci* 1986;6:3161–3168.
141. Proctor WR, Soldo BL, Allan AM, Dunwiddie TV. Ethanol enhances synaptically evoked $GABA_A$ receptor-mediated responses in cerebral cortical neurons in rat brain slices. *Brain Res* 1992; 595:220–227.
142. Puia G, Santi M, Vicini S, et al. Neurosteroids act on recombinant human $GABA_A$ receptors. *Neuron* 1990;4:759–765.
143. Puia G, Vicini S, Seeburg PH, Costa E. Influence of recombinant γ-aminobutyric $acid_A$ receptor subunit composition on the action of allosteric modulators of γ-aminobutyric acid–gated Cl^- currents. *Mol Pharmacol* 1991;39:691–696.
144. Ransom BR, Barker JL. Pentobarbital modulates transmitter effects on mouse spinal neurones grown in tissue culture. *Nature* 1975;254:703–705.
145. Reynolds JN, Prasad A, MacDonald JF. Ethanol modulation of GABA receptor-activated Cl^- currents in neurons of the chick, rat and mouse central nervous system. *Eur J Pharmacol* 1992;224:173–181.
146. Richards JG, Schoch P, Haring P, Takacs B, Möhler H. Resolving $GABA_A$/benzodiazepine receptors: Cellular and subcellular localization in the CNS with monoclonal antibodies. *J Neurosci* 1987;7: 1866–1886.
147. Roberts E. GABA: The road to neurotransmitter status. In: Olsen RW, Venter JC, eds. *Benzodiazepine/GABA receptors and chloride channels: structural and functional properties.* New York: Alan R. Liss, 1986:1–39.
148. Robertson B. Actions of anesthetics and avermectin on $GABA_A$ chloride channels in mammalian dorsal root ganglion neurones. *Br J Pharmacol* 1989;98:167–176.
149. Sakmann B, Hamill OP, Bormann J. Patch-clamp measurements of elementary chloride currents activated by the putative inhibitory transmitters GABA and glycine in mammalian spinal neurons. *J Neural Transm Suppl* 1983;18:83–95.
150. Sapp DW, Witte U, Turner DM, Longoni B, Kokka N, Olsen RW. Regional variation in steroid anesthetic modulation of [^{35}S]TBPS binding to γ-aminobutyric $acid_A$ receptors in rat brain. *J Pharmacol Exp Ther* 1992;262:801–808.
151. Savaki HE, Desban M, Glowinski J, Besson MJ. Local cerebral glucose consumption in the rat. I. Effects of halothane anesthesia. *J Comp Neurol* 1983;213:36–45.
152. Schoch P, Richards JG, Haring P, et al. Co-localization of $GABA_A$ receptors and benzodiazepine receptors in the brain shown by monoclonal antibodies. *Nature* 1985;314:168–171.
153. Schofield PR, Darlison MG, Fujita N, et al. Sequence and functional expression of the $GABA_A$ receptor shows a ligand-gated receptor super-family. *Nature* 1987;328:221–227.
154. Schulz DW, Macdonald RL. Barbiturate enhancement of GABA-mediated inhibition and activation of chloride conductance: Correlation with anticonvulsant and anesthetic actions. *Brain Res* 1981;209:177–188.
155. Schwartz RD, Jackson JA, Weigert D, Skolnick P, Paul SM. Characterization of barbiturate-stimulated chloride efflux from rat brain synaptoneurosomes. *J Neurosci* 1985;5:2963–2970.
156. Schwartz RD, Skolnick P, Hollingsworth EB, Paul SM. Barbiturate and picrotoxin-sensitive chloride efflux in rat cerebral cortical synaptoneurosomes. *FEBS Lett* 1984;175:193–196.
157. Schwartz R, Skolnick P, Seale T, Paul S. Demonstration of GABA/barbiturate-receptor mediated chloride transport in rat brain synaptoneurosomes: a functional assay of GABA receptor-effector coupling. *Adv Biochem Psychopharmacol* 1986;41:33–49.
158. Schwartz RD, Thomas JW, Kempner ES, Skolnick P, Paul SM. Radiation inactivation studies of the benzodiazepine/γ-aminobutyric acid/chloride ionophore receptor complex. *J Neurochem* 1985;45: 108–115.
159. Shimada S, Cutting G, Uhl GR. γ-Aminobutyric acid A or C receptor? γ-Aminobutyric acid ρ1 receptor RNA induces bicuculline-, barbiturate-, and benzodiazepine-insensitive γ-aminobutyric acid responses in *Xenopus* oocytes. *Mol Pharmacol* 1992;41:683–687.
160. Shingai R, Sutherland ML, Barnard EA. Effects of subunit types of the cloned $GABA_A$ receptor on the response to a neurosteroid. *Eur J Pharmacol* 1991;206:77–80.
161. Shivers BD, Killisch I, Sprengel R, et al. Two novel $GABA_A$ receptor subunits exist in distinct neuronal subpopulations. *Neuron* 1989;3:327–337.
162. Sieghart W. Several new benzodiazepines selectively interact with a benzodiazepine receptor subtype. *Neurosci Lett* 1983;38:73–78.
163. Sieghart W, Schuster A. Affinity of various ligands for benzodiazepine receptors in rat cerebellum and hippocampus. *Biochem Pharmacol* 1984;33:4033–4038.
164. Sigel E, Baur R, Trube G, Möhler H, Malherbe P. The effect of subunit composition of rat brain $GABA_A$ receptors on channel function. *Neuron* 1990;5:703–711.
165. Siggins GR, Pittman QJ, French ED. Effects of ethanol on CA1 and CA3 pyramidal cells in the hippocampal slice preparations. *Brain Res* 1987;414:22–34.
166. Skerritt JH, Willow M, Johnston GAR. Diazepam enhancement of low affinity GABA binding to rat brain membranes. *Neurosci Lett* 1982;29:63–66.
167. Skolnick P, Rice KC, Barker JL, Paul SM. Interaction of barbiturates with benzodiazepine receptors in the central nervous system. *Brain Res* 1982;233:143–156.
168. Stephenson FA, Mamalaki C, Casalotti SO, Barnard EA. The $GABA_A$ receptor and its antibodies. *Biochem Soc Symp* 1986;52: 33–40.
169. Study RE, Barker JL. Diazepam and (−)-pentobarbital: fluctuation analysis reveals different mechanisms for potentiation of γ-amino-

butyric acid responses in cultured central neurons. *Proc Natl Acad Sci USA* 1981;78:7180–7184.
170. Suzdak PD, Glowa JR, Crawley JN, Schwartz RD, Skolnick P, Paul SM. A selective imidazobenzodiazepine antagonist of ethanol in the rat. *Science* 1986;234:1243–1247.
171. Suzdak PD, Schwartz RD, Skolnick P, Paul SM. Ethanol stimulates γ-aminobutyric acid receptor-mediated chloride transport in rat brain synaptoneurosomes. *Proc Natl Acad Sci USA* 1986;83:4071–4075.
172. Taguchi K, Andresen MJ, Hentall ID. Acetylcholine release from the midbrain interpeduncular nucleus during anesthesia. *Neuroreport* 1991;2:789–792.
173. Tallman JF, Thomas JW, Gallager DW. GABAergic modulation of benzodiazepine binding site sensitivity. *Nature* 1978;274:383–385.
174. Tanelian DL, Kosek P, Mody I, MacIver MB. The role of the GABA$_A$ receptor/chloride channel complex in anesthesia. *Anesthesiology* 1993;78:757–776.
175. Thompson CL, Bodewitz G, Stephenson FA, Turner JD. Mapping of GABA$_A$ receptor α5 and α6 subunit-like immunoreactivity in rat brain. *Neurosci Lett* 1992;144:53–56.
176. Thyagarajan R, Ramanjaneyulu R, Ticku MK. Enhancement of diazepam and γ-aminobutyric acid binding by (+)etomidate and pentobarbital. *J Neurochem* 1983;41:578-585.
177. Ticku MK, Davis WC. Evidence that ethanol and pentobarbital enhance [^{3}H]diazepam binding at the benzodiazepine-GABA receptor-ionophore complex indirectly. *Eur J Pharmacol* 1981;71: 521–522.
178. Ticku MK, Olsen RW. Interaction of barbiturates with dihydropicrotoxinin binding sites in mammalian brain. *Life Sci* 1978;22: 1643–1652.
179. Turner DM, Ransom RW, Yang JSJ, Olsen RW. Steroid anesthetics and naturally occurring analogs modulate the γ-aminobutyric acid receptor complex at a site distinct from barbiturates. *J Pharmacol Exp Ther* 1989;248:960–966.
180. Twyman RE, Macdonald RL. Neurosteroid regulation of GABA$_A$ receptor single-channel kinetic properties of mouse spinal cord neurons in culture. *J Physiol* 1992;456:215–245.
181. Twyman RE, Rogers CJ, Macdonald RL. Pentobarbital and picrotoxin have reciprocal actions on single GABA$_A$ receptor channels. *Neurosci Lett* 1989;96:89–95.
182. Tyndale RF, Olsen RW, Tobin AJ. GABA$_A$ receptors. In: North RA, ed. *CRC handbook of receptors and channels: ligand- and voltage-gated ion channels.* Boca Raton, FL: CRC Press, 1995:265–290.
183. Ueda I, Kamaya H. Kinetic and thermodynamic aspects of the mechanism of general anesthesia in a model system of firefly luminescence in vitro. *Anesthesiology* 1973;38:425–436.
184. Unwin N. The structure of ion channels in membranes in excitable cells. *Neuron* 1989;3:665–676.
185. Wakamori M, Ikemoto Y, Akaike N. Effects of two volatile anesthetics and a volatile convulsant on the excitatory and inhibitory amino acid responses in dissociated CNS neurons of the rat. *J Neurophysiol* 1991;66:2014–2021.
186. Wafford KA, Burnett DM, Leidenheimer NJ, et al. Ethanol sensitivity of the GABA$_A$ receptor expressed in *Xenopus* oocytes requires 8 amino acids contained in the γ2L subunit. *Neuron* 1991;7:27–33.
187. Whiting P, McKernan RM, Iversen LL. Another mechanism for creating diversity in γ-aminobutyrate type A receptors: RNA splicing expression of two forms of γ2 subunit, one of which contains a protein kinase C phosphorylation site. *Proc Natl Acad Sci USA* 1990;87:9966–9970.
188. Whittle SR, Turner AJ. Differential effects of sedative and anticonvulsant barbiturates on specific [^{3}H]GABA binding to membrane preparations from rat brain cortex. *Biochem Pharmacol* 1982; 31:2891–2895.
189. Willow M, Johnston GAR. Enhancement of GABA binding by pentobarbitone. *Neurosci Lett* 1980;18:323–327.
190. Wisden W, Herb A, Wieland H, Keinanen K, Lüddens H, Seeburg PH. Cloning, pharmacological characteristics and expression pattern of the rat GABA$_A$ receptor α4 subunit. *FEBS Lett* 1991;289: 227–230.
191. Wisden W, Laurie DJ, Monyer H, Seeburg PH. The distribution of 13 GABA$_A$ receptor subunit mRNAs in the rat brain. I. Telencephalon, diencephalon, mesencephalon. *J Neurosci* 1992;12: 1040–1062.
192. Wong EHF, Leeb-Lundberg LMF, Teichberg VI, Olsen RW. γ-Aminobutyric acid activation of $^{36}Cl^-$ flux in rat hippocampal slices and its potentiation by barbiturates. *Brain Res* 1984;303: 267–275.
193. Wong EHF, Snowman AM, Leeb-Lundberg LMF, Olsen RW. Barbiturates allosterically inhibit GABA antagonist and benzodiazepine inverse agonist binding. *Eur J Pharmacol* 1984;102:205–212.
194. Wong G, Sei Y, Skolnick P. Stable expression of type I γ-aminobutyric acid$_A$/benzodiazepine receptors in a transfected cell line. *Mol Pharmacol* 1992;42:996–1003.
195. Yang J, Isenberg KE, Zorumski CF. Volatile anesthetics gate a chloride current in postnatal rat hippocampal neurons. *FASEB J* 1992;6:914–918.
196. Yang JSJ, Olsen RW. γ-Aminobutyric acid receptor- regulated $^{36}Cl^-$ flux in mouse cortical slices. *J Pharmacol Exp Ther* 1987;241:677–685.
197. Yeh JZ, Quandt FN, Tanguy J, Nakahiro M, Narahashi T, Brunner EA. General anesthetic action on γ-aminobutyric acid–activated channels. *Ann NY Acad Sci* 1991;625:155–173.
198. Young WS, Niehoff D, Kuhar MJ, Beer B, Lippa AS. Multiple benzodiazepine receptor localization by light microscopic radiohistochemistry. *J Pharmacol Exp Ther* 1981;216:425–430.
199. Ymer S, Draguhn A, Wisden W, et al. Structural and functional characterization of the γ1 subunit of GABA$_A$/benzodiazepine receptors. *EMBO J* 1990;9:3261–3267.
200. Zhang J, Sato M, Tohyama M. Region-specific expression of the mRNAs encoding β subunits (β1, β2, β3) of GABA$_A$ receptor in the rat brain. *J Comp Neurol* 1991;303:637–657.
201. Zimprich F, Zezula J, Sieghart W, Lassmann H. Immunohistochemical localization of the α1, α2, and α3 subunit of the GABA$_A$ receptor in the rat brain. *Neurosci Lett* 1991;127:125–128.

Anesthesia: Biologic Foundations, edited by Tony L. Yaksh et al. Lippincott–Raven Publishers, Philadelphia © 1997.

CHAPTER 17

GENERAL ANESTHETIC ACTIONS ON TRANSMISSION AT GLUTAMATE AND GABA SYNAPSES

M. BRUCE MACIVER

Studies of general anesthetic effects at the cellular and synaptic levels have demonstrated a myriad of actions at several independent sites. Anesthetics can hyperpolarize neurons by increasing K^+ or Cl^- currents and by depressing Na^+ or Ca^{2+} currents (31,61,80). Many agents have been shown to enhance synaptic inhibition (33,113), depress excitatory transmission (84,91), or both. Anesthetic effects on synaptic transmission involve both pre- and postsynaptic actions (3,63,73,83,100). It is likely that most anesthetics depress the central nervous system (CNS) by a combination of actions at several synaptic and membrane sites (48,50,62,69). This chapter reviews studies of anesthetic effects on transmission at synapses mediated by glutamate and gamma aminobutyric acid (GABA).

The development of in vitro brain slice preparations facilitated detailed studies of synaptic transmission in the mammalian CNS. Transverse slices of hippocampal cortex have been the best characterized of these preparations, both physiologically and pharmacologically (81). The anatomy of this brain structure allows for the preservation of major synaptic pathways and local interneuron circuits in the transverse plane used for brain slices (Fig. 1A). The CA 1 region of the hippocampus has been useful for studies of synaptic responses because of the relatively simple arrangement of glutamate-mediated excitatory inputs and GABA inhibitory interneurons that form monosynaptic connections with pyramidal neurons (Fig. 1B). This arrangement of glutamate and GABA synapses, providing balanced excitation and inhibition, is repeated throughout higher brain structures and forms the vast majority (more than two thirds) of synaptic circuitry in the mammalian brain (103). Thus, anesthetic effects at glutamate or GABA synapses would have important and widespread consequences. Several investigators have used hippocampal brain slices to study anesthetic effects on the relatively simple and well-characterized CA 1 circuit (48). In Fig. 2A, a schematic diagram of the CA 1 circuitry is shown, illustrating how both excitatory and inhibitory synaptic inputs contribute to synaptically evoked discharge of CA 1 pyramidal neurons. The EC_{50} for anesthetic-induced depression of synaptically evoked CA 1 neuron discharge was shown to correlate closely ($r \geq 0.98$) with in vivo potencies for volatile anesthetics and barbiturates (66). The correlation was further improved ($r = 0.995$) (Fig. 2B) with the addition of data for methoxyflurane (69) and thiopental (57). Thus, block of CA 1 synaptic discharge occurs at clinically relevant anesthetic concentrations and could contribute to anesthesia, since the hippocampus is *required* for memory formation (2,12) and plays a role in ascending arousal systems and sensory-motor integration (9).

ANESTHETICS DEPRESS EXCITATORY SYNAPTIC TRANSMISSION

The first study to demonstrate synaptic depression produced by anesthetics was performed >40 years ago by Larrabee and Posternak (52). They showed that pentobarbital depressed synaptic transmission through sympathetic ganglia at concentrations two to five times lower than needed to block axonal conduction in transganglionic axons. Similar results were reported by Somjen and Gill (104) for thiopental and diethyl ether in the spinal cord. Numerous investigators have confirmed that excitatory synapses are an important target for anesthetics and have extended the findings to include depression of synaptic transmission in higher brain structures at clinically relevant concentrations (3,5,6,61,64,66,75,91,95, 122).

The mechanisms of action involved in anesthetic-induced depression of synaptic discharge are not known, and several possible actions could contribute (Fig. 3). These include (a) depression of action potential conduction in presynaptic fibers, (b) blockade at any of a number of sites involved in transmitter release, (c) reduced chemosensitivity of postsynaptic receptors, (d) uncoupling of receptors and ionic channels, and (e) depression of postsynaptic Na^+/Ca^{2+} currents or enhanced Cl^-/K^+ currents. Evidence exists for anesthetic effects on each of these processes. Evidence for multiple effects derives from studies utilizing a number of different preparations, and together with results from hippocampal slices this evidence provides strong support for concentration-dependent effects at several independent sites of action. Studies describing anesthetic effects at individual sites are reviewed below.

ANESTHETICS DEPRESS ACTION POTENTIAL DISCHARGE IN SMALL DIAMETER AXONS

General anesthetics have been shown to depress small diameter axons in the CNS, and this was one of the earliest mechanisms proposed (30) to account for a depression of excitatory synaptic transmission (102). Numerous studies have shown that the smallest diameter fibers and axon branch points are the most susceptible to anesthetic block (29,36,47, 78,89,105). Recent patch-clamp studies of single voltage-gated sodium channels isolated from human brain have also shown significant depressant effects produced by pentobarbital and propofol at clinical concentrations (117). This would provide a mechanism for the observed block of fiber conduction, because action potentials in CNS fibers require sodium channel activation. Midazolam and ketamine also blocked sodium channels in this same study, but only at concentrations higher than achieved during anesthesia. We have found that halothane and isoflurane produce marked alterations of Schaffer-collateral fiber conduction in hippocampal brain slices at clinically relevant concentrations (Fig. 4). In contrast, thiopental does not alter fiber conduction over its clinical concentration range. Thus, it is likely that depression of action potential conduction may play a role for some anesthetics, but not for all agents.

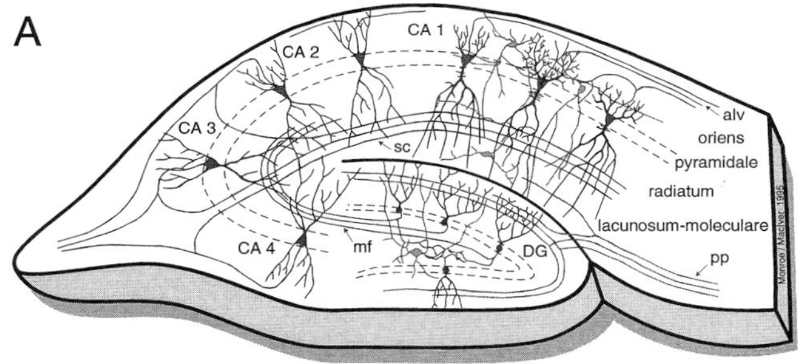

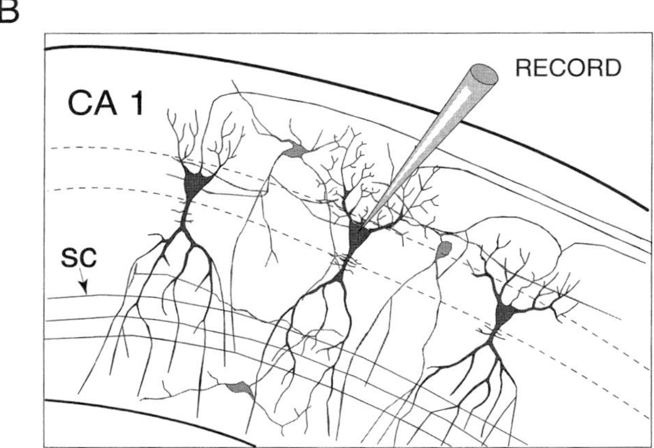

Figure 1. Transverse slices of hippocampal cortex preserve several synaptic pathways and interneuron circuits in 450-μM thick sections **(A)**. Perforant path (pp) fibers from entorhinal cortex form a major excitatory glutamate-mediated input to dentate granule (DG) neurons. Granule neurons project via the mossy fiber (mf) pathway to form glutamate-mediated synapses on CA 3 pyramidal neurons, which, in turn, provide glutamate-mediated excitation to the CA 1 area via Schaffer-collateral (sc) fibers. In all hippocampal areas, GABA inhibitory interneurons (*light gray*) modulate the excitatory inputs by providing feedforward and/or recurrent inhibition. CA 1 pyramidal neurons project to several cortical and lower brain regions via the alveus (alv) and form excitatory glutamate-mediated synapses on local GABA interneurons. Schaffer-collateral fibers also form excitatory glutamate-mediated synapses with some of these inhibitory interneurons **(B)**. By recording from CA 1 pyramidal neurons, it is possible to measure anesthetic effects on both glutamate and GABA-mediated synaptic inputs, as well as direct effects on pyramidal neuron excitability.

ANESTHETICS ENHANCE PRESYNAPTIC FIBER DISCHARGE

Anesthetic actions on fiber conduction may not only involve depression of action potentials, because anesthetic-induced excitation and mixed excitatory and depressant effects have also been reported. Volatile agents produce excitation of squid giant axon (28,41,42,117), crayfish giant axon (4), crayfish stretch receptor neurons (62,64), frog myelinated axons (11), and mammalian Aδ and C fiber nociceptor axons (67,114). In addition, halothane increased the discharge activity of nociceptors in monkeys (14) and increased conduction velocities in cat and human peripheral nerves (24,96). These excitatory effects occur at clinically relevant concentrations and could translate into increased depolarization of synaptic terminals, leading to greater release of neurotransmitter. Both ethanol and halothane produced burst discharge activity in GABA inhibitory fibers presynaptic to crayfish stretch receptor neurons (63), leading to a marked prolongation of synaptic inhibition. It is not known whether similar excitatory effects occur for axons in the mammalian CNS.

ANESTHETICS DEPRESS SCHAFFER-COLLATERAL PRESYNAPTIC FIBER DISCHARGE

Results from our laboratory indicate that halothane can depress presynaptic fiber volley amplitudes by as much as 20% at clinical concentrations (66). Richards et al. (90,93,95) have also observed a depression of fiber volley amplitudes produced by volatile and intravenous anesthetics in slices of olfactory and hippocampal cortex. These earlier studies are difficult to interpret because the fiber volley response was contaminated by the early part of synaptic potentials, which are also depressed by anesthetics. Recent studies eliminated this difficulty by examining anesthetic effects on isolated fiber volleys following block of synaptic potentials with specific antagonists of postsynaptic glutamate receptors (17,22,23). Under these conditions, halothane (1 MAC) was shown to depress fiber conduction by 18 ± 2.3%, whereas isoflurane (1 MAC) enhanced conduction by 12 ± 1.7%. These effects on Schaffer-collateral fiber conduction would contribute in opposite ways to the overall depression of CA 1 neuron synaptic discharge. Halothane-induced fiber volley depression would add to depression occurring at other sites, whereas the isoflurane excitatory effect partially reverses a cumulative depression at other sites in the circuit.

ANESTHETICS DEPRESS EXCITATORY SYNAPTIC TRANSMITTER RELEASE

Depression of excitatory synaptic transmission could result from a decrease in transmitter release. This has been postulated for a number of years based on results from electrophysiological studies (21,87). Weakly (118) was the first to demonstrate that anesthetics reduce the quantal content of motorneuron excitatory postsynaptic potentials (EPSP), but do not depress miniature EPSP amplitudes, indicating that a reduction in evoked transmitter output could occur. A number of CNS depressants have been shown to reduce acetylcholine release from preganglionic sympathetic nerve fibers (72), with the exception of isoflurane and desflurane (10). In the CNS, clinical concentrations of pentobarbital reduced the amount of L-glutamate and L-aspartate released from lateral olfactory tract fibers (18). Propofol also depressed glutamate release from rat synaptosomes (7); glutamate uptake and synaptosomal ATPase activity were also affected by low concentrations (2.5–35 μM) of propofol. Similar effects have been reported for several anesthetics on excitatory amino acid release from in vitro slices of thalamus (46,74,86). Thiopental, ketamine, and halothane have been shown to decrease glutamate levels in rat brain stem and cortex in vivo, but this could reflect an overall depression of neuronal activity associated with anesthesia (112). It should be noted that not all general anesthetics tested produced a depression of transmitter release (46), and it is not clear at present the extent to which this presynaptic action accounts for the overall depression of excitatory synapses produced by anesthetics (64,66,69,111). Although anesthetics are known to interfere with excitatory transmitter release, the mechanisms remain unknown, but direct actions on neurosecretory processes appear likely for some agents (34,84,85,91,108).

Presynaptic anesthetic actions at Schaffer-collateral fiber synapses on CA 1 pyramidal neurons were revealed using paired-pulse facilitation of EPSP responses as a measure. Paired-pulse facilitation is known to increase following manipulations that reduce calcium-mediated glutamate release from Schaffer-collateral fibers. For example, lowering the external calcium concentration produces a depression of CA 1 neuron EPSP amplitudes that results from a decrease in calcium influx through voltage-gated channels in presynaptic nerve terminals, secondary to a reduction in the driving force for calcium. This EPSP depression is inversely correlated with

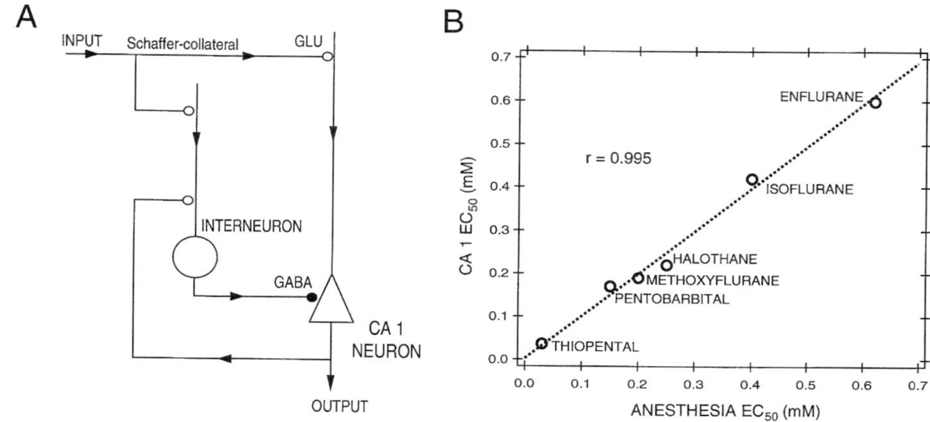

Figure 2. General anesthetics have been shown to depress synaptically evoked discharge in cortical circuits. A common synaptic circuit arrangement is evident in most cortical areas, where excitatory inputs are always balanced or modulated by inhibitory synapses. Cortical circuits use glutamate synapses for afferent excitation of pyramidal cells and interneurons. Feedforward and feedback inhibition is provided by GABA synapses. The major afferent input to CA 1 pyramidal neurons comes from CA 3 pyramidal neurons via the Schaffer-collateral fiber tract **(A)**. These afferents form glutamatergic (GLU) synapses on dendrites of CA 1 pyramidal neurons and local inhibitory interneurons. If afferent input is strong enough to cause CA 1 pyramidal neurons to discharge, then inhibitory interneurons are also excited by glutamatergic synapses from pyramidal axon collaterals. This excitation of interneurons provides feedback (recurrent) inhibition. The convergence of excitatory inputs to interneurons limits CA 1 neuron discharge by providing immediate GABA-mediated inhibition following synaptic activation. General anesthetics have been shown to depress synaptically evoked CA 1 neuron discharge at concentrations that correlate well with in vivo potencies **(B)**. Concentrations that produced half-maximal depression of population spike amplitudes (CA 1 EC_{50}) were plotted against half-maximal concentrations for producing anesthesia in rats (MAC for volatile agents and calculated free aqueous concentrations for barbiturates). Anesthesia was defined as a loss of tail clamp motor reflex. Note that the relationship yields a straight line close to unity (*dashed*), with a high correlation (0.995) when plotted on a linear-linear axis.

the degree of paired-pulse facilitation (53,73). Similarly, adenosine and NMDA are known to depress CA 1 neuron EPSP amplitudes by reducing a G-protein–linked calcium current in Schaffer-collateral nerve terminals, and this depression is also accompanied by an increase in paired-pulse facilitation (70). In contrast, manipulations that alter CA 1 neuron EPSPs via postsynaptic actions do not alter paired-pulse facilitation (70). Halothane and isoflurane also depress CA 1 neuron EPSPs (69), and this depression is accompanied by an increase in facilitation (Fig. 5), consistent with a presynaptic action to reduce glutamate release from Schaffer-collateral fiber terminals (83,100). Different effects on facilitation were evident comparing lowered extracellular calcium levels with effects produced by halothane and isoflurane. These differential actions on facilitation may indicate varying degrees of pre- and postsynaptic effects contributing to the synaptic depression produced by the two anesthetics. Recent studies showing anesthetic-induced depression of voltage activated calcium currents (particularly P- and N-type channels involved in transmitter release) provide one possible mechanism for anesthetic-induced depression of transmitter release (49,50,110).

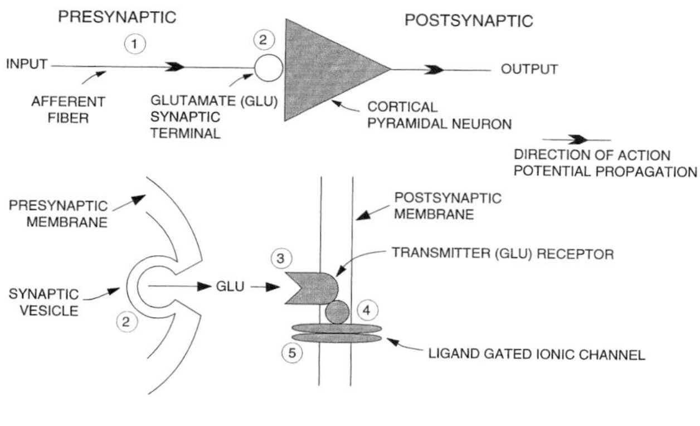

Figure 3. Possible sites of anesthetic action for depressing synaptic discharge of CA 1 pyramidal neurons. Anesthetics could depress (1) action potential conduction in afferent fibers, (2) glutamate release from nerve terminals, (3) glutamate receptor binding, (4) coupling between glutamate receptors and ionic channels, or (5) ionic channel conductance.

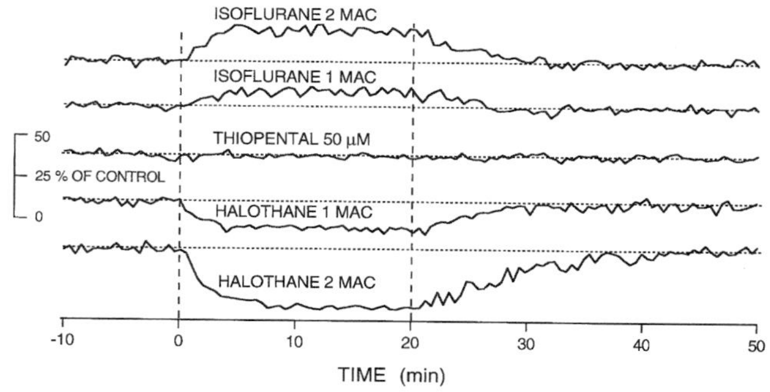

Figure 4. Anesthetics alter action potential conduction in presynaptic fibers. The five graphs show the concentration-dependent effects produced by three anesthetics on Schaffer-collateral fiber volley amplitudes, expressed as a percentage of control (preanesthetic; *dotted lines*) amplitudes. Each anesthetic was applied for 20 min (*dashed lines*) to achieve a steady state concentration-effect profile. Isoflurane increased fiber volley amplitudes, thiopental was without effect, and halothane depressed amplitudes (73).

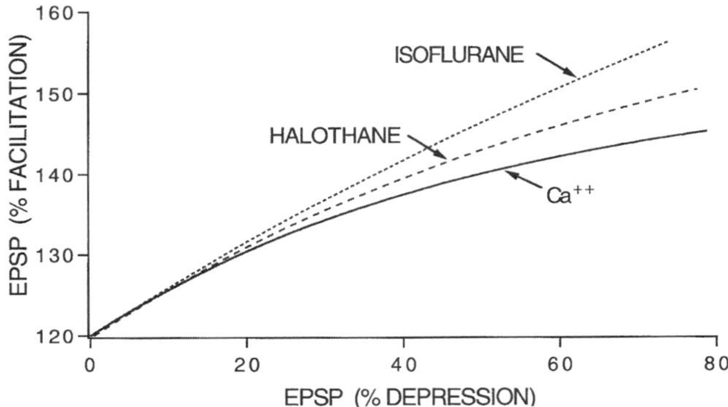

Figure 5. Anesthetics increase paired-pulse facilitation at glutamate-mediated synapses at concentrations that depress EPSP amplitudes. Facilitation was expressed as the percentage increase in amplitude of a test EPSP following a conditioning stimulus applied 120 ms before. In control (preanesthetic) conditions, there was no depression of EPSP amplitudes and a normal level of 120% facilitation was observed. In the presence of clinical concentrations of halothane and isoflurane (0.25–2 MAC), EPSP amplitude was progressively depressed to ~20% of control (80% depression). EPSP facilitation was increased to ~150% over this concentration range. A similar effect was produced by lowering the extracellular calcium concentration from 2.0 mM to 1.0 mM, showing the relationship between presynaptic calcium influx and synaptic responses (3).

ANESTHETICS DEPRESS POSTSYNAPTIC RESPONSES TO GLUTAMATE

Some anesthetics appear to depress glutamate-mediated synaptic responses by reducing chemosensitivity of the postsynaptic membrane (for futher details, see Chapter 15). Ether, methohexital, and pentobarbital depressed exogenous glutamate-evoked discharge at concentrations that depressed synaptic transmission (92,94). Pentobarbital also depressed glutamate-induced depolarization of cultured spinal neurons (88). Halothane, in contrast, did not affect responses to exogenous glutamate, even at concentrations higher than required to depress transmission (20,35,94). Postsynaptic glutamate receptor/ionophores exist as multiple subtypes, with two prominent classes being *N*-methyl-D-aspartate (NMDA) or α-amino-3-hydroxy-5-methyl-4-isoxazole priopionate (AMPA) selective. Glutamate receptors of the NMDA subtype may be particularly sensitive to some anesthetics (15,54), and depression of NMDA-mediated currents appears to play an important role for ketamine, ethanol, trichloroethanol, and some barbiturates (119). In mouse cortical neurons, halothane and chloroform preferentially depressed AMPA responses; thiopental, ether, and isoflurane antagonized both AMPA and NMDA responses, and ketamine selectively blocked NMDA responses (15). A similar profile of selective and differential effects on NMDA and AMPA receptors was also evident for a series of structurally related barbiturates (13). The effects produced by volatile anesthetics on postsynaptic sensitivity to glutamate and GABA at crab neuromuscular junctions also demonstrated that quite selective, nonsteric, effects occur that were related to solubility parameters for each anesthetic (51). As the solubility parameter for a series of volatile agents increased, effects on glutamate transmission increased, but actions on GABA receptors decreased (also see Fig. 9 below). This suggested that glutamate and GABA "gating molecules are housed in specific subregions of membrane" (51) with differing lipid solubilities or that anesthetics act directly on these proteins in a differential manner.

The volatile anesthetic enflurane also appears to act on glutamate synaptic transmission, but with effects opposite to those found with ketamine Enflurane has been shown to produce seizurelike discharges in the cortical EEG during anesthesia (8,109) and also promotes burst discharge activity of CA 1 neurons, similar to convulsants (65). The burst discharges do not come about via a depression of GABA inhibition, because enflurane increased inhibitory synaptic responses. They were not due to altered postsynaptic excitability (via K^+, Ca^{2+}, Na^+ or Cl^- channel alteration), since CA 1 neuron discharge in response to depolarizing current was also depressed by enflurane (61). Instead, enflurane increased CA 1 neuron excitability by enhancing glutamate transmission via NMDA receptors, similar to the convulsant effects of low Mg^{2+}, and enflurane-induced burst discharge was blocked by an NMDA receptor antagonist (61).

ANESTHETICS ENHANCE INHIBITORY SYNAPTIC TRANSMISSION

Nicoll et al. (79) were the first to demonstrate that general anesthetics enhance inhibition at gamma amino butyric acid (GABA) synapses. They found that pentobarbital prolonged the time course of inhibitory postsynaptic potentials (IPSPs) in hippocampal cortex, in vivo. This prolongation of IPSPs would result in enhanced inhibition and contribute to the barbiturate-induced CNS depression. Since that time, numerous studies have confirmed that barbiturates produce a profound increase in GABA-mediated inhibition (Fig. 6) and have extended earlier results by showing that enhanced inhibition is an action shared by most major chemical classes of anesthetics (5,37,82,113,121,123). In our laboratory, patch-clamp studies of anesthetic effects on GABA-mediated inhibitory postsynaptic currents (IPSCs) in hippocampal neurons have provided evidence for various mechanisms of action (Fig. 7) associated with volatile, barbiturate and alpha-adrenergic anesthetics (27,68, 76).

ANESTHETICS ENHANCE GABA INHIBITION VIA PRESYNAPTIC MECHANISMS

The alpha-adrenergic anesthetic, dexmedetomidine, has virtually no effect on hippocampal CA 1 neuron excitatory synaptic responses, resting membrane potential, or membrane conductance (26) (Fig. 8), yet dexmedetomidine can potentiate the depressant effects of isoflurane both in vivo and on hippocampal CA 1 neurons in the brain slice preparation (99). In addition, alpha-adrenergic agents including noradrenaline, do not increase postsynaptic responses at GABAergic synapses, like barbiturates and volatile agents do (25). Alpha-adrenergic agents, however, do produce a marked increase in the frequency of spontaneous IPSCs in hippocampal CA 1 neurons, but do not increase the frequency of action potential-independent miniature IPSCs (27). Thus, dexmedetomidine potentiation of isoflurane's actions appears to result from a presynaptic action (increased spike discharge activity in GABA interneurons) leading to increased GABA release. This presynaptic effect, together with the isoflurane-induced prolongation of GABA-mediated IPSCs (45), can account for the synergism observed for these two anesthetics (99).

Halothane, in contrast to alpha-adrenergic agents, produces an increase in the frequency of miniature IPSCs, indicating a direct effect on presynaptic GABA nerve terminals that is not dependent on action potential discharge activity in inhibitory interneurons, since the effect persists in the presence of tetrodotoxin (TTX) (I. Mody and M. B. MacIver, *unpublished observations,* 1993). Thus, halothane and alpha-adrenergic agents act at two independent presynaptic sites to increase the release of GABA. Halothane's presynaptic action, together with

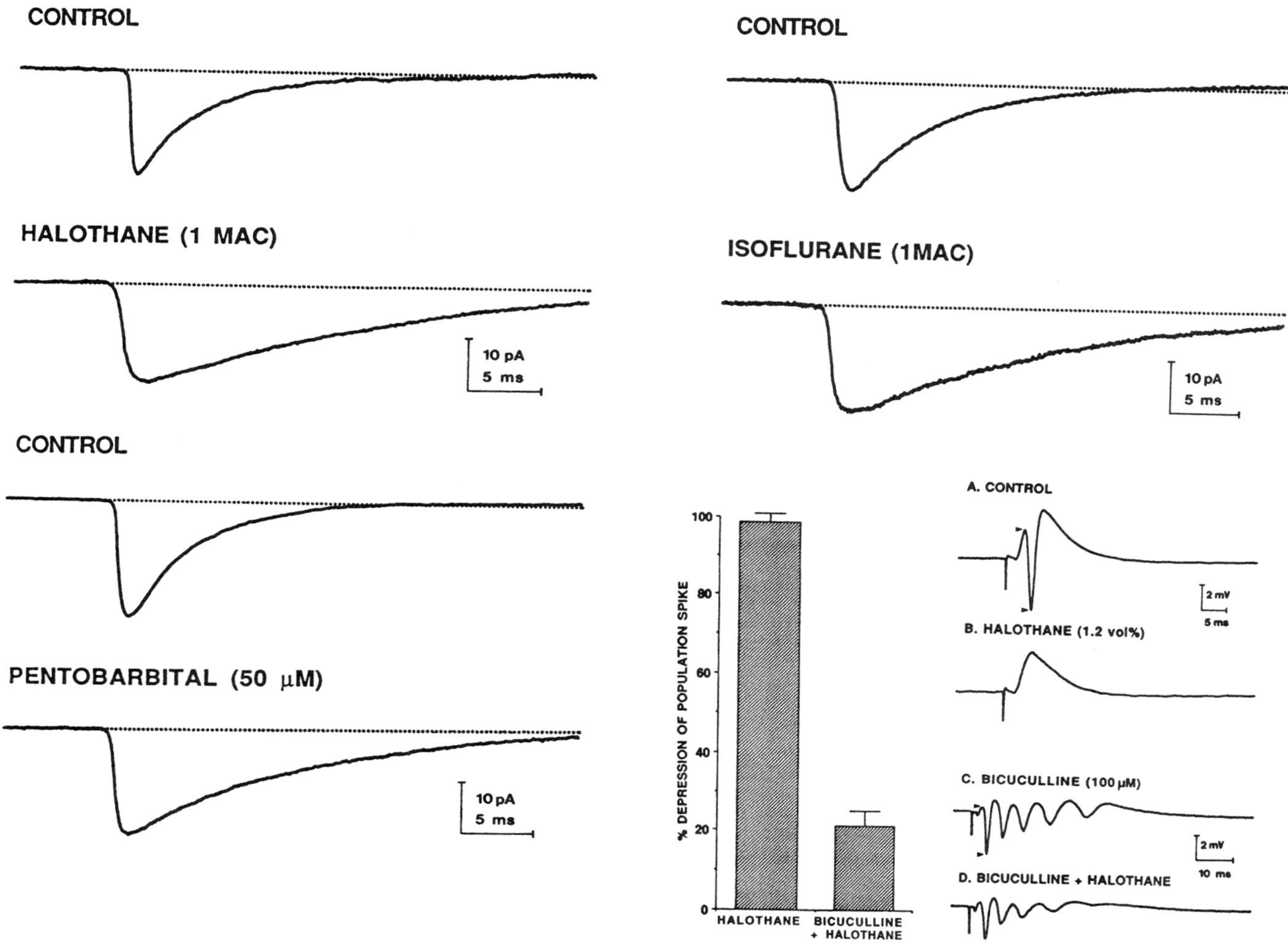

Figure 6. Anesthetics prolong GABA-mediated inhibitory postsynaptic currents (IPSCs) in hippocampal CA 1 neurons. Prolongation of miniature (TTX insensitive) IPSCs by clinically relevant concentrations of halothane, pentobarbital, and isoflurane are shown. The anesthetics produced a three- to fourfold increase in the decay times of these chloride currents. This would result in a dramatic increase in effective postsynaptic inhibition (>300%) even though IPSC amplitudes were unchanged, since inhibition is related to the integral (area) of the current trace. The extent to which this enhanced inhibition contributes to depression of synaptic discharge can be estimated by studying anesthetic-induced depression in the presence of a $GABA_A$ receptor antagonist (*lower right*). Halothane (1 MAC = 1.2 vol % in rats), like other anesthetics, produced ≈100% depression of evoked population spikes (control). The GABA antagonist, bicuculline, prevented most of the anesthetic-induced depression of CA 1 neuron synaptically evoked discharge (79 ± 4.7%; mean ± SD, n = 5), indicating that enhanced $GABA_A$ synaptic inhibition can contribute approximately three fourths of the overall depression of synaptic discharge (68,76).

the previously observed prolongation of IPSCs produced by halothane (45,68), can account for as much as 75% of the overall depression of CA 1 neuron responses produced by this anesthetic.

ANESTHETICS ENHANCE POSTSYNAPTIC RESPONSES TO GABA

The best-documented anesthetic effects on GABA-mediated inhibition involve postsynaptic actions on $GABA_A$-gated chloride channels. Different classes of anesthetics have been shown to bind at separate sites and to increase chloride channel flux via distinct mechanisms (for further details, see Chapter 16). Barbiturates and steroid anesthetics share the common actions of enhancing GABA binding, GABA-stimulated/channel opening frequency, and burst opening duration, but bind to separate sites on the receptor/channel complex (59,82,113). The barbiturates and steroids also directly activate chloride channels in the absence of GABA, whereas other classes of anesthetics require the presence of GABA to open chloride channels (1,60,71). Benzodiazepines, for example, enhance GABA binding and prolong chloride channel open times, but have no effect on conductance in the absence of GABA (58,101). The volatile anesthetics act via a mechanism that requires the presence of calcium (56), and the volatile anesthetic-induced prolongation of IPSCs can be blocked by intracellular administration of the calcium chelator BAPTA or calcium release inhibitor dantrolene (76). In contrast, the barbiturate-induced prolongation of IPSCs is not altered by these same manipulations of intracellular calcium (68). The calcium involvement for anesthetic-induced chloride current prolongation may be subunit and/or site specific, since BAPTA did not block halothane-induced prolongation in cultured hippocampal neurons (45). Similarly, halothane-induced chloride efflux in rat cortical slices was depressed by manipulations that blocked cal-

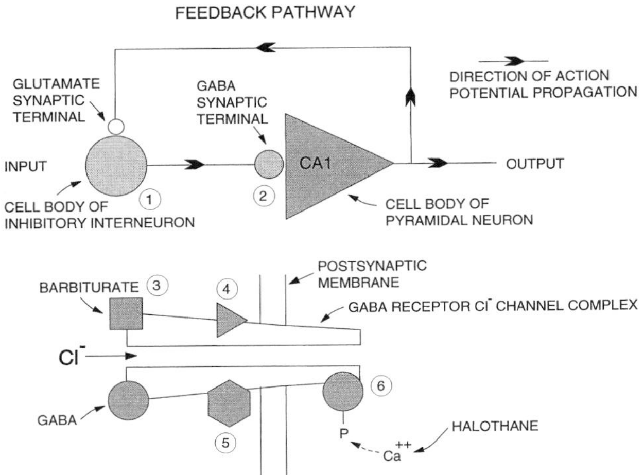

Figure 7. Possible anesthetic sites of action for increasing inhibitory GABA-mediated synaptic input to CA 1 pyramidal neurons. Anesthetics could increase (a) inhibitory neuron action potential discharge activity, (b) the release of GABA from nerve terminals, (c) GABA receptor binding, (d) chloride channel openings, (e) channel open time duration, and (f) intracellular regulatory activity (phosphorylation/dephosphorylation). The barbiturates, benzodiazepines, steroid anesthetics, and propofol have been shown to increase GABA binding to its receptor (3). Volatile anesthetics (e.g., halothane) can increase chloride channel activity in a calcium-dependent manner (6).

cium entry, but halothane-enhanced binding of the $GABA_A$ receptor agonist muscimol was calcium-independent (55).

ACTIONS AT THE $GABA_A$ COMPLEX PROVIDE EVIDENCE FOR ANESTHETIC-PROTEIN INTERACTIONS

Recent studies showing subunit specific and stereoselective anesthetic actions at the $GABA_A$ complex have provided some of the best evidence that anesthetics can interact directly with proteins, rather than through indirect actions secondary to alteration of membrane lipids. Anesthetics exhibit brain regional variations in binding to $GABA_A$ receptors (38,98), which can be accounted for by selective binding interactions with receptors composed of different heteromeric subunits (19,44). Similarly, potentiation of GABA inhibitory currents by anesthetics is also subunit specific, with $\alpha_1\beta_1\gamma_2$ being the most sensitive of the heteromeric $GABA_A$ complexes studied to date (40,54). Most homomeric and some heteromeric complexes are insensitive to anesthetics (16,40) (for more details, see Chapter 16). Such a high degree of anesthetic-selective effects on physicochemically similar proteins in common lipid/membrane environments implies direct, sterically constrained, protein/anesthetic interactions. The stereoselective actions of pentobarbital (43,64,97) and isoflurane (39,77) on the $GABA_A$ receptor/Cl^- channel complex provide further support for direct anesthetic/protein interactions. As pointed out by Franks and Lieb (33), stereoselective actions cannot be accounted for via actions on lipids, since stereoisomers are equipotent for depressing the phase transition temperature of phospholipid bilayers.

ACTIONS AT THE $GABA_A$ COMPLEX CONTRIBUTE TO ANESTHETIC-INDUCED CA 1 DEPRESSION

Clinically used concentrations of anesthetics have been shown to block CA 1 synaptic discharge, measured as a

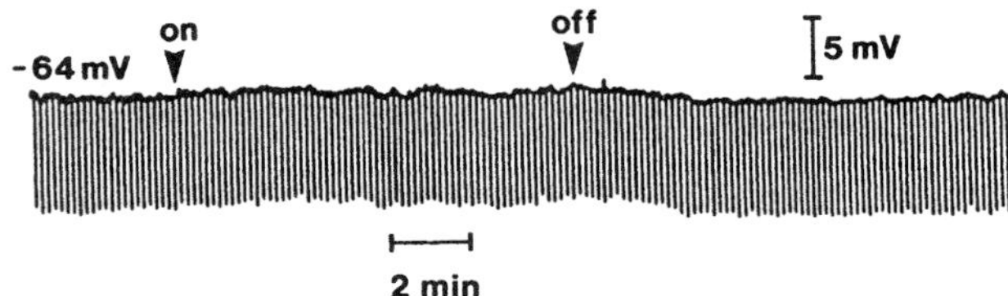

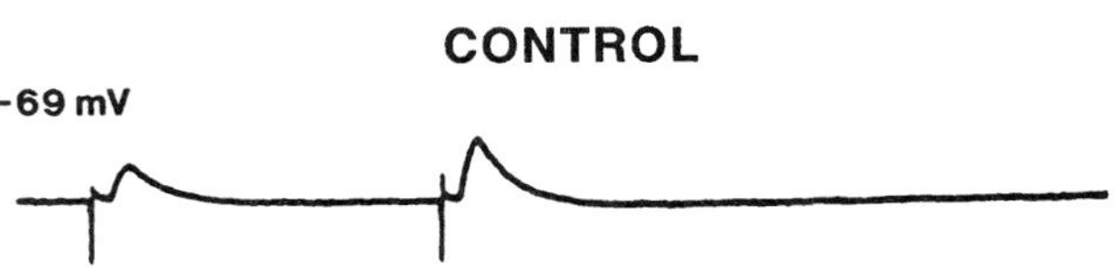

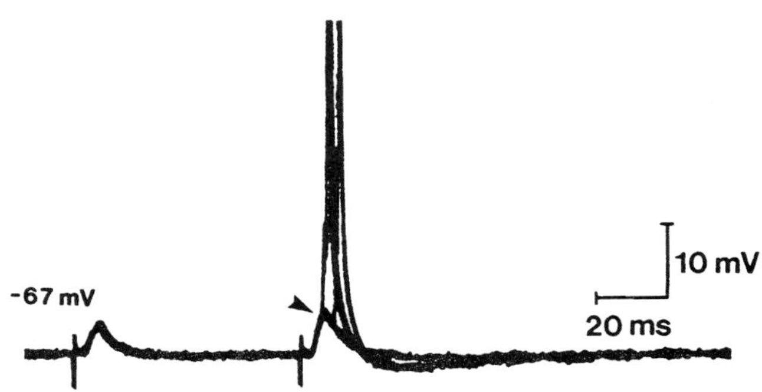

Figure 8. The alpha-adrenergic agonist dexmedetomidine does not depress synaptic discharge or alter postsynaptic membrane properties of CA 1 neurons. The recording on top shows the lack of effect of dexmedetomidine on the resting membrane potential and resistance of a CA 1 cell. Resistance was measured by applying brief hyperpolarizing current pulses through an intracellular microelectrode. A change in membrane resistance would have been evident as a change in amplitude of membrane voltage deflections resulting from the current pulses. Dexmedetomidine also did not depress glutamate-mediated synaptic excitation of CA 1 neurons and actually appeared to cause a slight increase in excitability, evident in the action potential discharges (*arrowheads*) seen in response to previously subthreshold stimulation. Thus, the synergistic interaction between dexmedetomidine and volatile anesthetics seen in vivo does not involve additive postsynaptic depression of neuronal excitability.

depression of population spike amplitude (Fig. 1). It was possible to determine the extent to which enhanced $GABA_A$-mediated inhibition contributed to the overall depression of CA 1 synaptic discharge by studying the ability of the $GABA_A$ receptor antagonist bicuculline to reverse anesthetic-induced population spike depression. Bicuculline reversed the thiopental-induced population spike depression almost completely (>90%) but was less effective against halothane-induced effects (Fig. 9). Enhanced $GABA_A$-mediated inhibition could account for most of the overall depression produced by barbiturate and halogenated alkane anesthetics. In contrast, the depression produced by isoflurane and enflurane was only modestly reversed by bicuculline, indicating that enhanced $GABA_A$-mediated inhibition contributes relatively little to the depressant effects of halogenated ethers. It

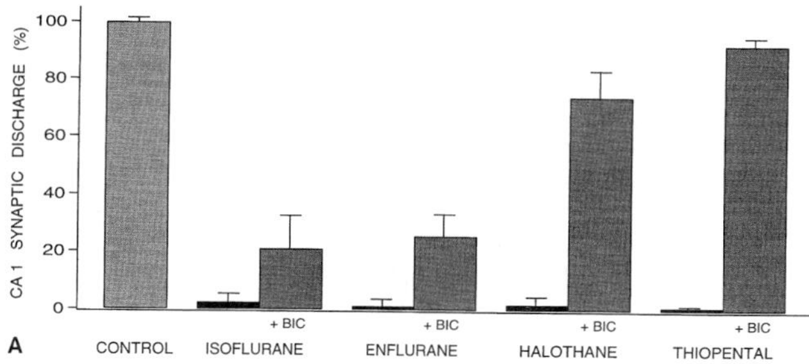

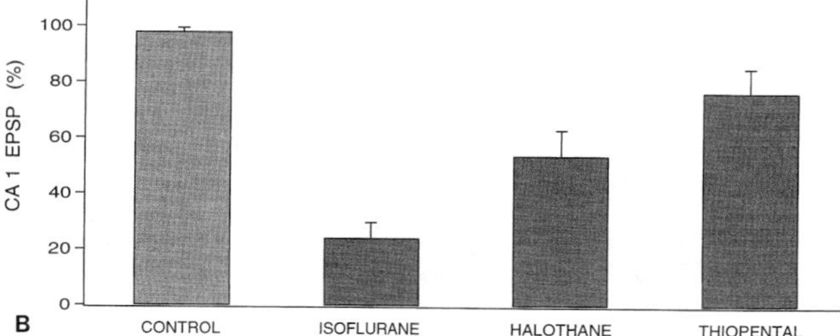

Figure 9. Effects on glutamate and GABA synapses can account for anesthetic-induced depression of CA 1 neurons. **(A)** The ability of bicuculline (BIC 10 μM) to reverse anesthetic-induced depression of synaptically evoked CA 1 population spike discharge is shown. Bicuculline was most effective at reversing thiopental-induced depression, followed by halothane > enflurane and isoflurane. Note that equieffective concentrations of each anesthetic were used, which also correspond to concentrations that produce surgical anesthesia in rats. In these experiments, anesthetic was applied first and bicuculline was then applied in the continued presence of anesthetic, to determine reversal. The bicuculline reversal of halothane-induced depression (74.2 ± 9.4%) agrees well with the value for the bicuculline prevention of halothane-induced depression (79 ± 4.7%) (Fig. 8). **(B)** Anesthetic-induced depression of field EPSP amplitudes. Clinical concentrations of isoflurane (1 MAC) were most effective at depressing EPSP amplitudes, followed by halothane (1 MAC) and thiopental (100 μM). Field EPSPs are known to be glutamate-mediated and are totally blocked in the presence of AMPA and NMDA receptor antagonists. Values presented are the mean ± SD for n ≥ 5 in both graphs, and were highly significant ($p < 0.005$, post-ANOVA Tukey test) for comparisons between control/anesthetic and anesthetic/bicuculline conditions. Data were compiled from Amagasu et al. (3) and Travis et al. (115).

is interesting that isoflurane was more effective at depressing glutamate-mediated synaptic excitation (EPSPs) (Fig. 9), and this effect could account for most of the overall depression of population spikes (see also refs. 51 and 69). Thiopental and halothane were less effective at depressing glutamate-mediated responses. Actions at both glutamate and GABA synapses were required to account for CA 1 population spike depression and the degree of effects at these sites was additive and anesthetic specific.

RELEVANCE TO CLINICAL ANESTHESIA AND THEORIES ON THE MECHANISM OF ANESTHETIC ACTION

It should be emphasized that anesthetic effects on glutamate and GABA synapses occur over clinically effective concentration ranges for barbiturate, benzodiazepine, steroid, and volatile agents. Several effects can occur simultaneously for an anesthetic acting at multiple pre- and postsynaptic sites. For some agents (e.g., halothane), presynaptic effects that enhance GABA release can add to postsynaptic actions (e.g., prolonged GABA-mediated IPSCs), resulting in potentiated synaptic inhibition, which, together with depressed glutamate synapses, contributes to the CNS depression associated with halothane anesthesia. For other anesthetics (e.g., dexmedetomidine and isoflurane), agent-specific actions at pre- and postsynaptic sites are required to account for synergistic interactions observed in vivo and in vitro. Such a complexity of anesthetic action is predicted by a Multisite Agent Specific (MAS) hypothesis (64,68), which states that anesthetics interact at many structurally selective sites in neuronal membranes and exhibit distinct patterns of activity at these sites. The MAS hypothesis is compatible with the Meyer-Overton rule of lipid solubility, since only hydrophobic sites in the membrane lipid/protein matrix may be involved (32,33,116), but recognizes that many distinct membrane proteins (ion channels, receptors, and enzymes) can provide distinct hydrophobic targets for anesthetics. The MAS hypothesis readily accounts for the agent specific clinical/behavioral/EEG profiles produced by different classes of anesthetics (106,107,120). Unitary and lipid theories are less convincing in this regard. Given the prevalence and importance of glutamate and GABA synapses in brain structures, together with the growing evidence of anesthetic actions on amino acid-mediated synaptic transmission, receptor-directed glutamate antagonists and GABA agonist/enhancers could become useful therapeutic agents for anesthesia.

Acknowledgment: I thank Frances Monroe for assistance preparing the manuscript and especially for help illustrating and designing the figures. Heath Lukatch, Shanti Amagasu, Anthony Mikulec, and Victoria Travis provided excellent technical assistance as well as helpful comments from critical reading of the manuscript. This work was supported by NIH GM49811.

REFERENCES

1. Allan AM, Harris RA. Anesthetic and convulsant barbiturates alter gamma-aminobutyric acid–stimulated chloride flux across brain membranes. *J Pharmacol Exp Ther* 1986;238:763–768.
2. Alvarez P, Squire LR. Memory consolidation and the medial temporal lobe: a simple network model. *Proc Natl Acad Sci USA* 1994; 91:7041–7045.
3. Amagasu SM, Mikulec AA, MacIver MB. Halothane-induced depression of axonal conduction in mammalian CNS fibers. *Anesthesiology* 1994;81:A1475.
4. Bean BP, Shrager P, Goldstein DA. Modification of sodium and potassium channel gating kinetics by ether and halothane. *J Gen Physiol* 1981;77:233–253.
5. Berg-Johnsen J, Langmoen IA. Changes in inhibitory synaptic transmission induced by isoflurane studied in rat hippocampal slices. *J Neurosurg Anesthesiol* 1993;5:36–40.
6. Berg-Johnson J, Langmoen IA. Mechanisms concerned in the direct effect of isoflurane on rat hippocampal and human neocortical neurons. *Brain Res* 1990;507:28–34.
7. Bianchi M, Battistin T, Galzigna L. 2,6-Diisopropylphenol, a general anesthetic, inhibits glutamate action on rat synaptosomes. *Neurochem Res* 1991;16:443–446.
8. Black GW. Enflurane. *Br J Anaesth* 1979;51:627–640.
9. Bland BH, Colom LV. Extrinsic and intrinsic properties underlying oscillation and synchrony in limbic cortex. *Prog Neurobiol* 1993; 41:157–208.
10. Boban N, McCallum JB, Schedewie HK, Boban M, Kampine JP, Bosnjak ZJ. Direct comparative effects of isoflurane and desflurane on sympathetic ganglionic transmission. *Anesth Analg* 1995; 80:127–134.
11. Butterworth JF, Raymond SA, Roscoe RF. Effects of halothane and enflurane on firing threshold of frog myelinated axons. *J Physiol* 1989;411:493–516.
12. Buzsaki G, Chen LS, Gage FH. Spatial organization of physiological activity in the hippocampal region: relevance to memory formation. *Prog Brain Res* 1990;83:257–268.
13. Cai Z, McCaslin PP. Acute, chronic and differential effects of sev-

eral anesthetic barbiturates on glutamate receptor activation in neuronal culture. *Brain Res* 1993;611:181–186.

14. Campbell JN, Raja SN, Meyer RA. Halothane sensitizes cutaneous nociceptors in monkeys. *J Neurophysiol* 1984;52:762–770.
15. Carla V, Moroni F. General anaesthetics inhibit the responses induced by glutamate receptor agonists in the mouse cortex. *Neurosci Lett* 1992;146:21–24.
16. Cestari IN, Li L, Uchida I, Yang J. Structural requirements of the $GABA_A$ β subunit for the agonist action of general anesthetics. *Anesthesiology* 1994;81:A796.
17. Collingridge GL, Herron CE, Lester RA. Synaptic activation of N-methyl-D-aspartate receptors in the Schaffer collateral-commissural pathway of rat hippocampus. *J Physiol* 1988;399:283–300.
18. Collins GGS. Release of endogenous amino acid neurotransmitter candidates from rat olfactory cortex: possible regulatory mechanisms and the effects of pentobarbitone. *Brain Res* 1980;190: 517–525.
19. Concas A, Santoro G, Mascia MP, Maciocco E, Dazzi L, Biggio G. Effects of propofol, pentobarbital and alphaxalone on t-[^{35}S]butylbicyclophosphorothionate binding in rat cerebral cortex. *Eur J Pharmacol* 1994;267:207–213.
20. Crawford JM. The sensitivity of cortical neurones to acidic amino acids and acetylcholine. *Brain Res* 1970;17:287–296.
21. Cutler RWP, Markowitz D, Dudzinski DS. The effect of barbiturates on (H^3)GABA transport in rat cerebral cortex slices. *Brain Res* 1974;81:189–197.
22. Davies CH, Davies SN, Collingridge GL. Paired-pulse depression of monosynaptic GABA-mediated inhibitory postsynaptic responses in rat hippocampus. *J Physiol* 1990;424:513–531.
23. Davies SN, Collingridge GL. Role of excitatory amino acid receptors in synaptic transmission in area CA 1 of rat hippocampus. *Proc R Soc (Lond)* 1989;236:373–384.
24. de Jong RH, Nace RA. Nerve impulse conduction and cutaneous receptor responses during general anesthesia. *Anesthesiology* 1967; 28:851–855.
25. Doze VA, Cohen GA, Madison DV. Synaptic localization of adrenergic disinhibition in the rat hippocampus. *Neuron* 1991;6: 889–990.
26. Doze VA, MacIver MB. Dexmedetomidine-induced excitation of rat hippocampal CA 1 neurons resembles the effects of opiate narcotics. *Anesthesiology* 1989;71:578.
27. Doze VA, Madison DV, MacIver MB. Hypnotic/anesthetic alpha-adrenergic agents enhance tonic $GABA_A$ synaptic inhibition of hippocampal CA 1 neurons. *IBRO Third World Congress Neurosci* 1991; 3:137.
28. Elliott AA, Elliott JR, Haydon DA. The effects of homologous series of anaesthetics on a resting potassium conductance of the squid giant axon. *Biochim Biophys Acta* 1989;978:337–340.
29. Fink BR, Cairnes AM. Differential slowing and block of conduction by lidocaine in individual afferent myelinated and unmyelinated axons. *Anesthesiology* 1984;60:111–120.
30. Frank GB, Sanders HD. A proposed common mechanism of action for general and local anaesthetics in the CNS. *Br J Pharmacol Chemother* 1965;21:1–9.
31. Franks NP, Lieb WR. Stereospecific effects of inhalational general anesthetic optical isomers on nerve ion channels. *Science* 1991;254: 427–430.
32. Franks NP, Lieb WR. Selective actions of volatile general anaesthetics at molecular and cellular levels. *Br J Anaesth* 1993;71:65–76.
33. Franks NP, Lieb WR. Molecular and cellular mechanisms of general anaesthesia. *Nature* 1994;367:607–614.
34. Fung S-C, Fillenz M. The actions of barbiturates on release of noradrenaline from rat hippocampal synaptosomes. *Neuropharmacology* 1984;23:1113–1116.
35. Galindo A. Effects of procaine, pentobarbital and halothane on synaptic transmission in the central nervous system. *J Pharmacol Exp Ther* 1969;169:185–195.
36. Gissen AJ, Covino BG, Gregus J. Differential sensitivities of mammalian nerve fibers to local anesthetic agents. *Anesthesiology* 1980; 53:467–474.
37. Hara M, Kai Y, Ikemoto Y. Enhancement by propofol of the gamma-aminobutyric acidA response in dissociated hippocampal pyramidal neurons of the rat. *Anesthesiology* 1994;81:988–994.
38. Harris B, Wong G, Skolnick P. Neurochemical actions of inhalational anesthetics at the $GABA_A$ receptor complex. *J Pharmacol Exp Ther* 1993;265:1392–1398.
39. Harris BD, Moody EJ, Basile AS, Skolnick P. Volatile anesthetics bidirectionally and stereospecifically modulate ligand binding to GABA receptors. *Eur J Pharmacol* 1994;267:269–274.
40. Harrison NL, Kugler JL, Jones MV, Greenblatt EP, Pritchett DB. Positive modulation of human gamma-aminobutyric acid type A and glycine receptors by the inhalation anesthetic isoflurane. *Mol Pharmacol* 1993;44:628–632.
41. Haydon DA, Simon AJ. Excitation of the squid giant axon by general anaesthetics. *J Physiol* 1988;402:375–389.
42. Haydon DA, Urban BW. The actions of some general anaesthetics on the potassium current of the squid giant axon. *J Physiol* 1986; 373:311–327.
43. Huang LY, Barker JL. Pentobarbital: stereospecific actions of (+) and (-) isomers revealed on cultured mammalian neurons. *Science* 1980;207:195–197.
44. Ito Y, Ho IK. Studies on picrotoxin binding sites of $GABA_A$ receptors in rat cortical synaptoneurosomes. *Brain Res Bull* 1994;33: 373–378.
45. Jones MV, Harrison NL. Effects of volatile anesthetics on the kinetics of inhibitory postsynaptic currents in cultured rat hippocampal neurons. *J Neurophysiol* 1993;70:1339–1349.
46. Kendall TJ, Minchin MC. The effects of anaesthetics on the uptake and release of amino acid neurotransmitters in thalamic slices. *Br J Pharmacol* 1982;75:219–227.
47. Kendig JJ, Grossman Y. Homogenous and branching axons: differing responses to anesthetics and pressure. In: Roth SH, Miller KW, eds. *Molecular and cellular mechanisms of anesthetics.* New York: Plenum Press, 1986:333–340.
48. Kendig JJ, MacIver MB, Roth SH. Anesthetic actions in the hippocampal formation. *Ann NY Acad Sci* 1991;625:37–53.
49. Kress HG, Muller J, Eisert A, Gilge U, Tas PW, Koschel K. Effects of volatile anesthetics on cytoplasmic Ca^{2+} signaling and transmitter release in a neural cell line. *Anesthesiology* 1991;74:309–319.
50. Krnjevic K. Cellular and synaptic actions of general anaesthetics. *Gen Pharmacol* 1992;23:965–975.
51. Landau EM, Richter J, Cohen S. Differential solubilities in subregions of the membrane: a nonsteric mechanism of drug specificity. *J Med Chem* 1979;22:325–327.
52. Larrabee MG, Posternak JM. Selective actions of anaesthetics on synapses and axons in mammalian sympathetic ganglia. *J Neurophysiol* 1952;15:91–114.
53. Leung LS, Fu XW. Factors affecting paired-pulse facilitation in hippocampal CA1 neurons in vitro. *Brain Res* 1994;650:75–84.
54. Lin LH, Whiting P, Harris RA. Molecular determinants of general anesthetic action: role of $GABA_A$ receptor structure. *J Neurochem* 1993;60:1548–1553.
55. Longoni B, Demontis GC, Olsen RW. Enhancement of gamma-aminobutyric acid A receptor function and binding by the volatile anesthetic halothane. *J Pharmacol Exp Ther* 1993;266:153–159.
56. Longoni B, Olsen RW. Studies on the mechanism of interaction of anesthetics with $GABA_A$ receptors. In: Biggio G, Concas A, Costa E, eds. *GABAergic neurotransmission.* New York: Raven Press, 1992: 365–378.
57. Lukatch HS, MacIver MB. Prolonged $GABA_A$ chloride currents underlie the thiopental induced slowing of EEG. *Anesthesiology* 1994;81:A798.
58. Macdonald R. Benzodiazepines specifically modulated GABA-mediated postsynaptic inhibition in cultured mammalian neurons. *Nature* 1978;271:564.
59. Macdonald RL, Olsen RW. GABAA receptor channels. *Annu Rev Neurosci* 1994;17:569–602.
60. Macdonald RL, Skerritt JH, Werz MA. Barbiturate and benzodiazepine actions on mouse neurons in cell culture. In: Roth SH, Miller KW, eds. *Molecular and cellular mechanisms of anesthetics.* Boston: Plenum Press, 1986:17–25.
61. MacIver MB, Kendig JJ. Anesthetic effects on resting membrane potential are voltage-dependent and agent-specific. *Anesthesiology* 1991;74:83–88.
62. MacIver MB, Roth SH. Anesthetics produce differential actions on the discharge activity of a single neuron. *Eur J Pharmacol* 1987;139: 43–52.
63. MacIver MB, Roth SH. Anesthetics produce differential actions on membrane responses of the crayfish stretch receptor neuron. *Eur J Pharmacol* 1987;141:67–77.
64. MacIver MB, Roth SH. Barbiturate effects on hippocampal excitatory synaptic responses are selective and pathway specific. *Can J Physiol Pharmacol* 1987;65:385–394.
65. MacIver MB, Roth SH. Enflurane-induced burst firing of hip-

pocampal CA 1 neurones. In vitro studies using a brain slice preparation. *Br J Anaesth* 1987;59:369–378.
66. MacIver MB, Roth SH. Inhalation anaesthetics exhibit pathway-specific and differential actions on hippocampal synaptic responses in vitro. *Br J Anaesth* 1988;60:680–691.
67. MacIver MB, Tanelian DL. Volatile anesthetics excite mammalian A-delta and C fiber nociceptor afferents recorded in vitro. *Anesthesiology* 1990;72:1022–1030.
68. MacIver MB, Tanelian DL, Mody I. Two mechanisms for anesthetic-induced enhancement of $GABA_A$-mediated neuronal inhibition. *Ann NY Acad Sci* 1991;625:91–96.
69. MacIver MB, Tauck DL, Kendig JJ. General anaesthetic modification of synaptic facilitation and long-term potentiation in hippocampus. *Br J Anaesth* 1989;62:301–310.
70. Manabe T, Nicoll RA. Long-term potentiation: evidence against an increase in transmitter release probability in the CA1 region of the hippocampus. *Science* 1994;265:1888–1892.
71. Mathers DA. The $GABA_A$ receptor: new insights from single-channel recording. *Synapse* 1987;1:96–101.
72. Matthews EK, Quilliam JP. Effects of central depressant drugs on acetylcholine release. *Br J Pharmacol Chemother* 1964;22:415–424.
73. Mikulec AA, Amagasu SM, Monroe FA, MacIver MB. Isoflurane and halothane produce opposite effects on facilitation of excitatory synaptic responses in CA 1 neurons. *Anesthesiology* 1994;81: A1476.
74. Minchin MCW. The effect of anaesthetics on the uptake and release of gamma-aminobutyrate and D-aspartate in rat brain slices. *Br J Pharmacol* 1981;73:681–693.
75. Miu P, Puil E. Isoflurane-induced impairment of synaptic transmission in hippocampal neurons. *Exp Brain Res* 1989;75:354–360.
76. Mody I, Tanelian DL, MacIver MB. Halothane enhances tonic neuronal inhibition by elevating intracellul calcium. *Brain Res* 1991; 538:319–323.
77. Moody EJ, Harris BD, Skolnick P. Stereospecific actions of the inhalation anesthetic isoflurane at the $GABA_A$ receptor complex. *Brain Res* 1993;615:101–106.
78. Nathon PW, Sears TA. Some factors concerned in differential nerve block by local anesthetics. *J Physiol* 1961;157:565–580.
79. Nicoll RA, Eccles JC, Oshima T, Rubia F. Prolongation of hippocampal inhibitory postsynaptic potentials by barbiturates. *Nature* 1975;258:625–626.
80. Nicoll RA, Madison DV. General anesthetics hyperpolarize neurons in the vertebrate central nervous system. *Science* 1982;217: 1055–1057.
81. Nicoll RA, Malenka RC, Kauer JA. Functional comparison of neurotransmitter receptor subtypes in mammalian central nervous system. *Physiol Rev* 1990;70:513–565.
82. Olsen RW, Sapp DM, Bureau MH, Turner DM, Kokka N. Allosteric actions of central nervous system depressants including anesthetics on subtypes of the inhibitory gamma-aminobutyric acid A receptor-chloride channel comples. *Ann NY Acad Sci* 1991;625: 145–154.
83. Perouansky M, Baranov D, Salman M, Yaari Y. Effects of halothane on glutamate receptor-mediated excitatory postsynaptic currents. *Anesthesiology* 1995;83:109–119.
84. Pocock G, Richards CD. Cellular mechanisms in general anaesthesia. *Br J Anaesth* 1991;66:116–128.
85. Pocock G, Richards CD. Anesthetic action on stimulus-secretion coupling. *Ann NY Acad Sci* 1991;625:71–81.
86. Potashner SJ, Lake N, Langlois EA, Ploffe L, Lecavalier D. Pentobarbital: differential effects on amino acid transmitter release. In: Fink BR, eds. *Molecular mechnanisms of anesthesia (progress in anesthesiology).* New York: Raven Press, 1980:469–482.
87. Quastel DMJ, Hackett JT, Okamoto K. Presynaptic action of central depressant drugs: inhibition of depolarization-secretion coupling. *Can J Physiol Pharmacol* 1972;50:279–287.
88. Ransom BR, Barker JL. Pentobarbital modulates transmitter effects on mouse spinal neurones grown in tissue culture. *Nature* 1975; 254:703–705.
89. Raymond SA, Shin HC, Steffensen SC. A role for changes in axonal excitability in general anesthesia. *Ann NY Acad Sci* 1991;625: 307–310.
90. Richards CD. On the mechanism of barbiturate anaesthesia. *J Physiol (Lond)* 1972;227:749–756.
91. Richards CD. Actions of general anaesthetics on synaptic transmission in the CNS. *Br J Anaesth* 1983;55:201–207.
92. Richards CD, Russell WJ, Smaje JC. The action of ether and methoxyflurane on synaptic transmission in isolated preparations of the mammalian cortex. *J Physiol* 1975;248:121–142.
93. Richards CD, Smaje JC. The actions of halothane and pentobarbitone on the sensitivity of neurones in the guinea-pig prepiriform cortex to iontophoretically applied L-glutamate. *J Physiol (Lond)* 1974;239:103–105.
94. Richards CD, Smaje JC. Anaesthetics depress the sensitivity of cortical neurones to L-glutamate. *Br J Pharmacol* 1976;58:347–357.
95. Richards CD, White AE. The actions of volatile anaesthetics on synaptic transmission in the dentate gyrus. *J Physiol* 1975;252: 241–257.
96. Rosner BS, Clark DL, Beck C. Inhalational anesthetics and conduction velocity of human peripheral nerve. *Electroencephalogr Clin Neurophysiol* 1971;31:109–114.
97. Roth SH, Tan KS, MacIver MB. Selective and differential effects of barbiturates on neuronal activity. In: Roth SH, Miller KW, eds. *Molecular and cellular mechanisms of anesthetics.* New York: Plenum Press, 1986:43–56.
98. Sapp DW, Witte U, Turner DM, Longoni B, Kokka N, Olsen RW. Regional variation in steroid anesthetic modulation of $[^{35}S]$TBPS binding to gamma-aminobutyric acid A receptors in rat brain. *J Pharmacol Exp Ther* 1992;262:801–808.
99. Savola MKT, MacIver MB, Doze VA, Kendig JJ, Maze MM. The alpha-2-adrenoceptor agonist dexmedetomidine increases the apparent potency of the volatile anesthetic isoflurane in rats *in vivo* and in hippocampal slice *in vitro. Brain Res* 1991;548:23–28.
100. Schlame M, Hemmings H. Inhibition by volatile anesthetics of endogenous glutamate release from synaptosomes by a presynaptic mechanism. *Anesthesiology* 1995;82:1406–1416.
101. Schwartz R, Skolnick P, Seale T, Paul S. Demonstration of GABA/ barbiturate-receptor mediated chloride transport in rat brain synaptoneurosomes: a functional assay of GABA receptor-effector coupling. *Adv Biochem Psychopharmacol* 1986;41:33–49.
102. Seeman P. The membrane actions of anesthetics and tranquilizers. *Pharmacol Rev* 1972;24:538–655.
103. Shepherd GM. *Neurobiolgoy.* New York: Oxford University Press, 1994.
104. Somjen GG, Gill M. The mechanism of the blockade of synaptic transmission in the mammalian spinal cord by diethyl ether and by thiopental. *J Pharmacol Exp Ther* 1963;140:19–30.
105. Staiman A, Seeman P. Conduction-blocking concentrations of anesthetics increase with nerve axon diameter: studies with alcohol, lidocaine and tetrodotoxin on single myelinated fibers. *J Pharmacol Exp Ther* 1977;201:340–349.
106. Stanski DR. Pharmacodynamic modeling of thiopental depth of anesthesia. In: D'Argenio, ed. *Advanced methods of pharmacokinetic and pharmacodynamic systems analysis.* New York: Plenum Press, 1991:79–85.
107. Stanski DR. Monitoring depth of anesthesia. In: Miller RD, ed. *Anesthesia.* New York: Churchill Livingstone, 1994:1127–1159.
108. Stern RC, Evers AS. The action of halothane on stimulus-secretion coupling in clonal (GH3) pituitary cells. *Ann NY Acad Sci* 1991;625:293–295.
109. Stevens JE, Fujinaga M, Oshima E, Mori K. The biphasic pattern of the convulsive property of enflurane in cats. *Br J Anaesth* 1984; 56:395–403.
110. Study RE. Isoflurane inhibits multiple voltage-gated calcium currents in hippocampal pyramidal neurons. *Anesthesiology* 1994;81: 104–116.
111. Sugiyama K, Muteki T, Shimoji K. Halothane-induced hyperpolarization and depression of postsynaptic potentials of guinea pig thalamic neurons *in vitro. Brain Res* 1992;576:97–103.
112. Suria A, Rasheed F. Evidence for involvement of amino acid neurotransmitters in anesthesia and naloxone induced reversal of respiratory paralysis. *Life Sci* 1994;54:2021–2033.
113. Tanelian DL, Kosek P, Mody I, MacIver MB. The role of the $GABA_A$ receptor/chloride channel complex in anesthesia. *Anesthesiology* 1993;78:757–776.
114. Tanelian DL, MacIver MB. Differential excitatory and depressant anesthetic effects on mammalia A-delta and C fiber sensory afferents. *Ann NY Acad Sci* 1991;625:273–275.
115. Travis VL, Lukatch HS, Monroe FA, MacIver MB. $GABA_A$ inhibition contributes more to the anesthetic actions of thiopental compared to halothane. *Anesthesiology* 1994;81:A801.
116. Trudell JR. A unitary theory of anesthesia based on lateral phase separations in nerve membranes. *Anesthesiology* 1977;46:5–10.
117. Urban BW, Frenkel C, Duch DS, Kauff AB. Molecular models of

anesthetic action on sodium channels, including those from human brain. *Ann NY Acad Sci* 1991;625:327–343.
118. Weakly JN. Effect of barbiturates on "quantal" synaptic transmission in spinal motoneurones. *J Physiol* 1969;204:63–77.
119. Weight FF, Aguayo LG, White G, Lovinger DM, Peoples RW. GABA- and glutamate-gated ion channels as molecular sites of alcohol and anesthetic action. *Adv Biochem Psychopharmacol* 1992; 47:335–347.
120. Winters WD. A review of the continuum of drug-induced states of excitation and depresssion. *Prog Drug Res* 1982;26:225–263.
121. Yeh JZ, Quandt FN, Tanguy J, Nakahiro M, Narahashi T, Brunner EA. General anesthetic action on gamma-aminobutyric acid-activated channels. *Ann NY Acad Sci* 1991;625:155–173.
122. Yoshimura M, Higashi H, Fujita S, Shimoji K. Selective depression of hippocampal inhibitory potentials and spontaneous firing by volatile anesthetics. *Brain Res* 1985;340:363–368.
123. Zimmerman SA, Jones MV, Harrison NL. Potentiation of gamma-aminobutyric acid A receptor Cl^- current correlates with *in vivo* anesthetic potency. *J Pharmacol Exp Ther* 1994;270: 987–991.

Anesthesia: Biologic Foundations, edited by
Tony L. Yaksh et al. Lippincott–Raven Publishers,
Philadelphia © 1997.

CHAPTER 18

PUMPS, EXCHANGERS, AND TRANSPORTERS

THOMAS J. J. BLANCK, HUGH C. HEMMINGS, JR.,
LEONARDO PAROLI, AND FANG XU

Communication and selective exchange between the extracellular and intracellular milieux are necessary for cell survival and organ function. Each organ is able to fulfill its evolved function because of its ability to respond to extracellular neuronal and hormonal signals and to selectively admit and exclude various molecular species to or from its intracellular environment. Within each cell making up an organ, the intracellular traffic of ions is also regulated to allow the appropriate cell response to occur at the appropriate time.

This chapter discusses examples of those molecules that are important in differentiating cellular and organ function. We discuss two important pumps: the Na^+K^+-ATPase (EC3.6.1.37) and the intracellular Ca^{2+}-ATPase (EC 3.6.1.38), the Na^+-Ca^{2+} exchanger, and neurotransmitter transporter family. Each of these are of physiologic significance. The Na^+,K^+-ATPase and Na^+-Ca^{2+} exchanger are found in the outer plasma membrane of most cells and perform universal functions of Na^+,Ca^{2+} homeostasis. The Ca^{2+}-ATPase, also called the calcium pump, is found inside the cell, imbedded in the sarcoplasmic reticulum or the endoplasmic reticulum. The neurotransmitter transporters are found at synaptic endings, integrated into the outer membrane of the synapse as well as in glia, where they are crucial for the reaccumulation of neurotransmitters.

NA^+,K^+-ATPASE

In 1941, Dean (29) described an unknown mechanism in the skeletal muscle membrane that could pump Na^+ out of or K^+ into the cell. In 1957, Skou (130) identified a membrane-bound enzyme that hydrolyzed ATP in the presence of Na^+, K^+ and Mg^{2+} that showed properties expected of the Na^+ pump described by Dean. This enzyme is now commonly called Na^+,K^+-ATPase (EC 3.6.1.37). Na^+,K^+-ATPase is an integral membrane protein found in the cells of all higher eukaryotes and is responsible for translocating Na^+ and K^+ ions across the cell membrane, utilizing ATP as the driving force. When it is working normally, the Na^+,K^+-ATPase pumps three Na^+ ions out of the cells and two K^+ ions into it for each molecule of ATP hydrolyzed. This transport produces both a chemical and an electrical gradient across the cell membrane, which allows the cell to perform a vast array of functions. The electrical gradient is essential for maintaining the resting potential of cells and for the excitable activity of nerve tissue and muscle. A number of transport processes, including the translocation of glucose, amino acids, and other nutrients into cells, are driven by the Na^+ gradient established by normal Na^+,K^+-ATPase activity. The physiological importance of the Na^+ pump is summarized in Table 1. It is estimated that ~23% of the ATP consumed in the human at rest is utilized by the Na^+ pump in maintaining the Na^+ gradient, the electrochemical energy of which supplies the wide array of cellular transport processes. The ATP consumed by the Na^+,K^+-ATPase reaches 40–50% of the total ATP used for maintaining the normal physiological activities of the brain (28). However, the high dependence on ATP availability also makes Na^+,K^+-ATPase vulnerable to traumatic events such as ischemia, hypoxia, and hypoglycemia, which result in impaired metabolism (77).

The Na^+,K^+-ATPase is a member of the so-called P-type ATPases, which include the sarcoplasmic reticulum and plasma membrane Ca^{2+}-ATPases (EC 3.6.1.38), the H^+,K^+-ATPase (EC 3.6.1.36) found in stomach and colon, and several prokaryotic transport enzymes (45,109). These enzymes share a similar catalytic cycle that involves a phosphorylated protein intermediate. However, Na^+,K^+-ATPase differs from the other members of this family in that it can be specifically inhibited by a class of drugs known as cardiac glycosides (e.g., ouabain, digoxin, digitoxin). These drugs bind to and inhibit the enzyme, resulting in an increase in intracellular Na^+ level, which is thought to decrease the outward transport of Ca^{2+} via an Na^+/Ca^{2+}-antiport protein. As a consequence, Ca^{2+} accumulates in the cell (15,16). The resulting increase in the intracellular concentration of Ca^{2+} is responsible for the positive inotropic action of these drugs on cardiac muscle. This is the basis for their extensive therapeutic use in the treatment of congestive heart failure (137).

Structure

Na^+,K^+-ATPase is composed of two subunits: an α- and β-subunit in a one-to-one stoichiometry (62). The α-subunit has a molecular mass of ~112 kDa and mediates the catalytic processes of the enzyme in that it contains binding site(s) for ATP, Na^+ and K^+ ions, and cardiac glycosides. The much smaller β-subunit is a glycosylated protein with the protein portion accounting for 35 kDa of the overall molecular mass of ~55 kDa after glycosylation in the Golgi apparatus (126). A clear understanding of the function of the β-subunit remains more elusive. However, evidence supports the hypothesis that the β-subunit facilitates the assembly and transport of the α-subunit into the

Table 1. CELL FUNCTIONS SUBSERVED DIRECTLY OR INDIRECTLY BY THE Na^+,K^+-ATPase[a]

Maintenance of transmembrane Na^+ and K^+ gradients
Regulation of cell volume
Transepithelial salt and water transport
Maintenance of resting potential
Maintenance of ion gradients required for electrical excitability
Electrogenic modulation of resting and action potentials
Protection against catastrophic firing
Regulation of intracellular $[Ca^{2+}]$ via Na^+-Ca^{2+} exchange
Regulation of intracellular pH via Na^+-H^+ or (Na^+, HCO_3^-)/(H^+, Cl^-) exchange
Coupled chloride movements via Na^+-K^+-$2Cl^-$ cotransport
Cotransport of sugars
Cotransport of amino acids and oligopeptides
Cotransport of vitamins (ascorbate, biotin, thiamine)
Recovery of neurotransmitters (e.g., GABA)
Renal (re)absorption of organic acids, including lactate and paraaminohippuric acid
Calorigenesis (?)
Vascular tone (?)

[a]Data from ref. 28.

plasma membrane (42,106). Recent evidence has also suggested the presence of a third 6.5-kDa γ-subunit associated with Na^+,K^+-ATPase, which has been cloned and sequenced (25,99).

Although it is still not completely certain whether the Na^+,K^+-ATPase exists in the membrane as a diprotomer, $(\alpha\beta)_2$ or in the form of a single αβ-unit, it is known that the single ab-unit is able to catalyze all the reactions and partial reactions that can be catalyzed by the intact Na^+ pump (44). In recent years, cDNA cloning techniques have revealed the entire primary sequences from a wide variety of organisms for many P-type ATPases, including the Na^+,K^+-ATPase (84,140).

Figure 1 is a cartoon of the topology of the Na^+ pump as well as the Ca^{2+} pump, the Na^+:Ca^{2+} exchanger, and a typical neurotransmitter transporter. The α-subunit of the Na^+,K^+-ATPase is composed of 10 transmembrane segments (H1–H10), and both N- and C- termini are located in the cytosol (36). Four strongly hydrophobic stretches of amino acids in the NH_2-terminal third of the Na^+,K^+-ATPase are conserved throughout the family of ion-transporting ATPases. These hydrophobic regions are predicted to cross the membrane as a-helices (H1–H4). The middle third of each ATPase, the part between H4 and H5 segments, has no hydrophobic stretches long enough to span the membrane and is assumed to be folded as a globular domain on the cytoplasmic surface of the membrane. Hydropathy-based predictions vary greatly with respect to the C-terminal third (H5–H10) of these ion pumps (82). The transmembrane segments form 40–50% of the total protein mass that is protected from intensive tryptic digestion by membrane lipids (63).

There is general agreement that the β-subunit (β1-isoform) spans the membrane a single time with 30–50 amino acids from its NH_2-terminus, which is located within the cytoplasm of the cell (96). The β-subunit also has three sites of *N*-glycosylation as well as three intrasubunit disulfide bridges in its ectodomain (72,100,135). The mature β-subunit is resistant to proteolysis in either the membrane-bound holoenzyme or as a detergent-purified polypeptide, suggesting that the polypeptide retains a compact tertiary structure even after denaturation. Those three disulfide bridges may be important in maintaining the stable tertiary structure of this polypeptide (96).

A complete ATPase pump cycle has four basic steps: (a) Binding of ATP and of three Na^+ ions to the cytoplasmic surface of the pump is followed by the transfer of a phosphoryl group from ATP to the pump and the trapping of the three Na^+ ions within the pump molecule. (b) These ions are released to the extracellular side; it is proposed that one of the Na^+ ions is released before the others and that this release is a electrogenic step. (c) The binding of two K^+ ions at the extracellular surface leads to transfer of the phosphor group from the pump to water (to form inorganic phosphate), and this is accompanied by the trapping of the two potassium ions. (d) A spontaneous step occurs at which the K^+ ions are released into the cytoplasm (Fig. 2). This cycle results in the transport of three Na^+ ions out of the cell and two K^+ ions into the cell for each ATP hydrolyzed. During part of this cycle, similar to the SERCA pumps, the cations are occluded and are inaccessible to either surface (44,82). Based on the observation that the occlusion of ions was not prevented either by the digestion of the β-subunit or by a prolonged treatment with trypsin that removed nearly all of the cytoplasmic segment, including the phosphorylation and ATP-binding site(s), and fragmented the remaining parts of the chain in the lipid, it is suggested that occlusion needs a relatively small fraction of the entire pump molecule (21,67,68).

A diagram by Glynn (1993) may give us a somewhat simpler and clearer picture about the ion occlusion and release during a Na^+,K^+-ATPase transport cycle (Fig. 3) (44). Glynne explained the diagram as follows: "There is a channel between some of the bunched transmembrane helices which, somewhere along its length, in the neighborhood of two carboxyl groups (from different helices), can occlude either two potassium ions or three sodium ions, which are, of course, smaller than potassium when unhydrated. Access from the occlusion sites to the inner and outer faces of the pump is controlled by two gates, and the opening and closing of these gates, as well as the relative affinities of the sites for sodium and potassium, are controlled by conformational changes that depend on events in the cytoplasmic loop, phosphorylation, dephosphorylation, and the binding of ATP."

The Na^+,K^+-ATPase is the receptor for cardiac glycosides that inhibit its activity. In recent years, a number of candidates for "endogenous ouabain" were identified in plasma, urine, and tissues, and were purified (140). Therefore, the different ouabain sensitivities found in different isoforms, different tissues, and different species may have functional significance. Cardiac glycosides inhibit the Na^+,K^+-ATPase by binding to the extracellular surface of the enzyme. The α-subunit has been identified as the primary site of binding (39). In site-directed mutagenesis experiments, construction of chimera between the C-terminal part of the ouabain-resistant rat α1 isoform and the N-terminal part of the ouabain-sensitive sheep or *Torpedo* α1 subunit demonstrated that the first half of the molecule, including the first transmembrane segments (H1–H4), contains the ouabain binding site (107,113).

A number of substitution experiments showed that amino acid residues that determine ouabain sensitivity are not restricted to the loop between the H1 and H2 transmembrane segments, but are also located in various regions of the α-subunit, such as Tyr-131, Ile-142, and Ser-147 (20,83). None of these substitutions could confer a complete ouabain resistance. This implies that the ouabain binding site is composed of multiple functional groups and that the loss of any one does not completely prevent binding. Nevertheless, the majority of the substitutions that affect ouabain binding are found in the first transmembrane and first extracellular regions (82).

Isoforms

Na^+,K^+-ATPase is now known to belong to a multigene family. Three distinct isoforms of the α-subunit (α1, α2, and α3) have been identified by using molecular genetic and immunologic techniques. The H^+,K^+-ATPase, which is 70% identical to the Na^+,K^+-ATPase and homologous along its entire length, can be considered to be a fourth isoform (132). Similarly, two isoforms for the β-subunit (β1 and β2) have been identified and, more recently, the existence of a third β-subunit isoform (β3) has been reported (59,84,139). The α and β isoform genes are expressed in a tissue- and cell-specific manner, and are subject to developmental and hormonal regulatory influences (43,84,132–134). The α1 isoform is found nearly everywhere, whereas the α2 isoform is predominant in skeletal muscle and is also detected in the brain (mostly in glia cells) and in the adult heart. The α3 isoform is limited essentially to neuronal cells and newborn cardiac tissue, but also found in ciliary epithelium, pineal, and in small amounts in kidney. Fambrough et al. (37) have recently reported that each of avian the isoforms has a direct homologue in mammals: the corresponding avian and mammalian β between different mammalian or the different avian a isoforms is only 82–83%. These results lead to the supposition that any unique functional roles they play arose early and were conserved through a substantial part of evolution.

A basic question arises: Why is there such a wide diversity of Na^+,K^+-ATPase subunits? One obvious advantage of the existence of different isoenzymes encoded by different genes is that their synthesis and degradation can be regulated independently. It also seems to be possible to target the different isoenzymes to different sites within a single cell. Another possible

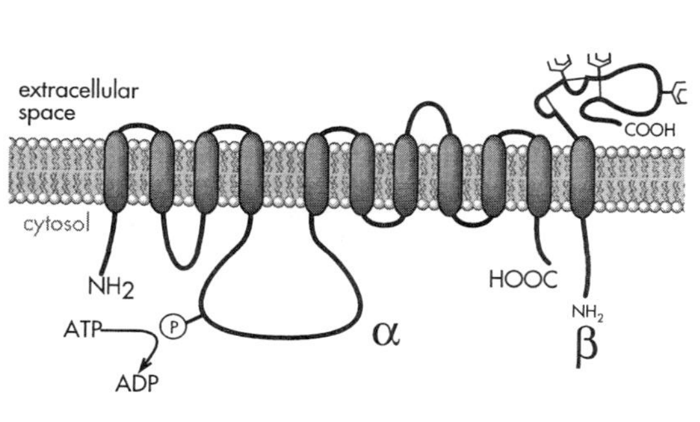

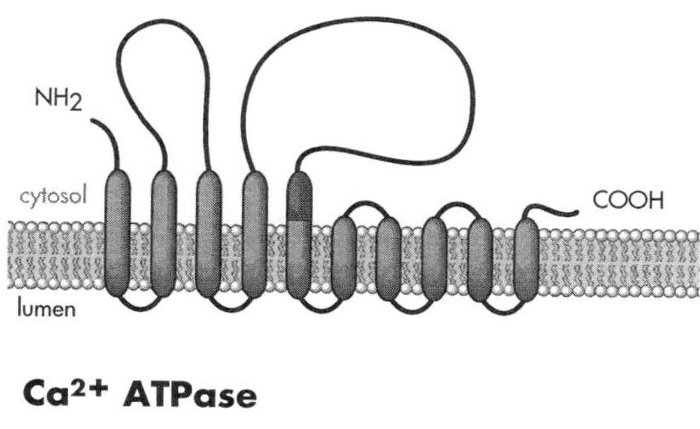

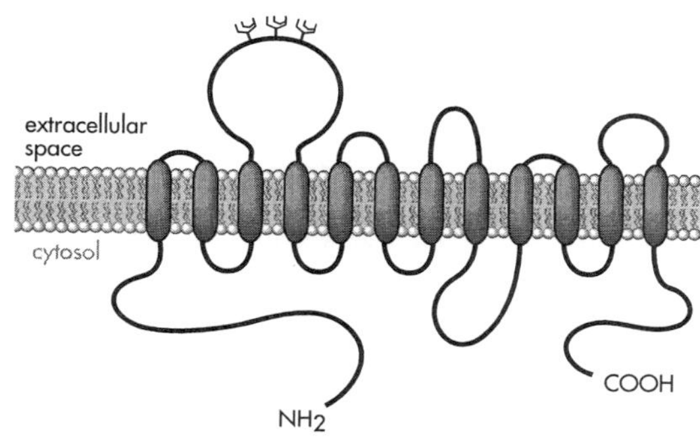

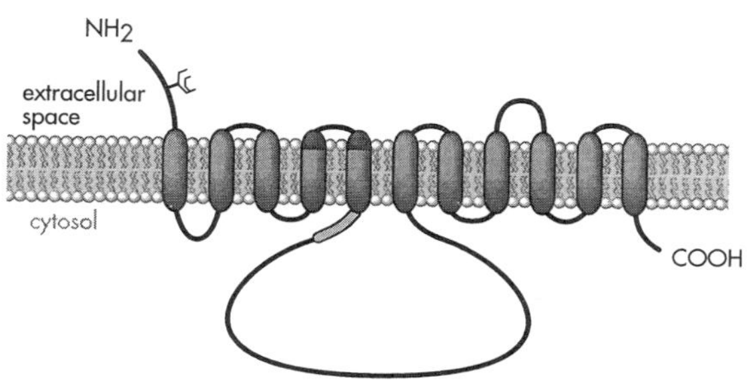

Figure 1. Schematic representation of the molecular structure of the following: (**A**) Na^+,K^+—ATPase. (Reprinted with permission from Fambrough DM, Lemas MV, Hamrick M, et al. Analysis of subunit assembly of the Na,K-ATPase. *Am J Physiol* 1994;266:C379–C589.) (**B**) Ca^{2+}-ATPase. (Reprinted with permission from MacLennan DH, et al. Nucleotide binding/hinge domain plays a crucial role in determining isoform-specific Ca^{2+} dependence of organellar Ca^{2+}-ATPase. *J Biol Chem* 1992;267:14492.) (**C**) Neurotransmitter transporter. (Reprinted with permission from Amara SG, Arriza JL. Neurotransmitter transporters: three distinct gene families. *Curr Opin Neurobiol* 1993;3:337–344.) (**D**) Na^+-Ca^{2+} exchanger. (Reprinted with permission from Philipson KD, Nicoll DA. Molecular and kinetic aspects of sodium-calcium exchange. *Int Rev Cytol* 1993;137C:199–227.)

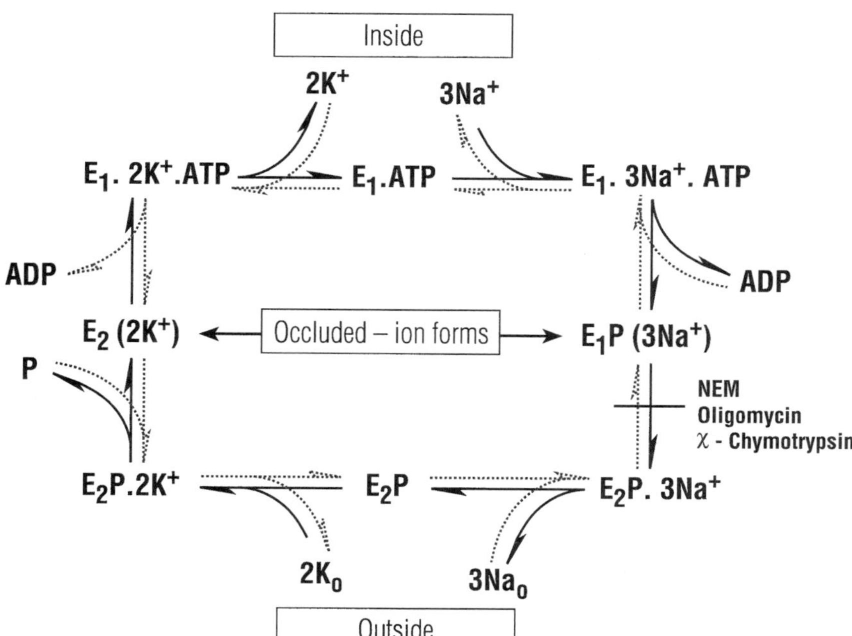

Figure 2. The normal pump cycle. The four basic steps of the pump cycle are depicted as follows: (a) the binding of ATP and 3 Na^+ ions on the cytoplasmic side followed by the transfer of the phosphoryl group to the enzyme and the occlusion of the Na^+ ions; (b) release of the Na^+ ions to the extracellular side; (c) the binding of 2 K^+ ions on the extracellular side and the transfer of the phosphoryl group to water; and (d) the release of K^+ ions into the cytoplasm. (Reprinted with permission from Glynn IM. Annual review prize lecture: all hands to the sodium pump. *J Physiol* 1993;462:1–30.)

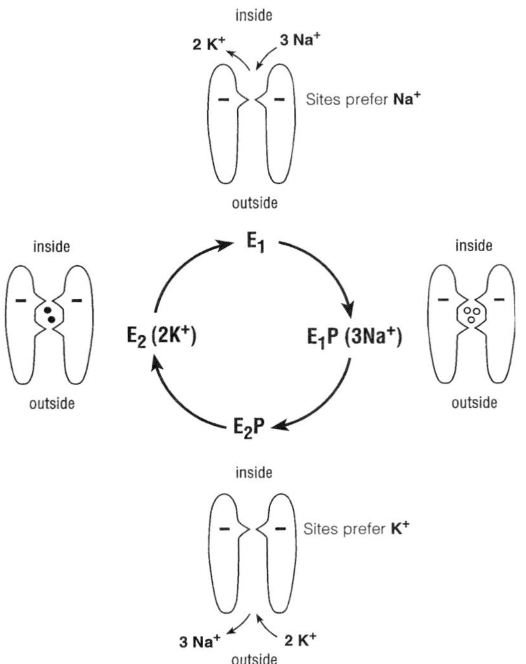

Figure 3. Diagram showing how the stages of the pump cycles can be related to different states of a doubly gated channel between the transmembrane helices. (Reprinted with permission from Glynn IM. Annual review prize lecture: all hands to the sodium pump. *J Physiol* 1993; 462:1–30.)

advantage is that their activities can be separately controlled. And the third possible advantage is that their properties might be tailored for different jobs (44).

It is well known that differences in cardiac glycoside sensitivity of the Na^+,K^+-ATPase isoforms exist not only between different species, but may also exist between the different isoforms from the same species. For example, the rat Na^+,K^+-ATPase is 1,000-fold more resistant to ouabain than Na^+,K^+-ATPase from other sources such as sheep and human. In the rat, α1 is of very low sensitivity, whereas α2 and α3 are of high sensitivity to ouabain. This is a species-specific phenomenon, because the α1-subunit of many species is very ouabain sensitive, despite 97–99% overall amino acid identity with rat α1 (134). Furthermore, the sensitivity to cardiac glycosides in different tissues obtained from the same animal was also shown to be different due to the tissue-specific distribution of a isoforms. In both rabbit and rat, the brain contains a Na^+,K^+-ATPase activity with higher ouabain sensitivity than that of kidney or heart (132).

Because of the identification of different endogenous ouabain-like factors, the differential sensitivities to cardiac glycosides are considered to play a significant role in regulatory mechanisms of Na^+,K^+-ATPase activity and cellular electrolyte homeostasis. In normal rats and in a range of cell types, chronic inhibition of Na^+,K^+-ATPase by ouabain induces an upregulation of both enzyme activity and its synthesis to restore the intracellular Na^+ level to preinsult condition (114, 115,142). In contrast, such homeostatic responses after chronic ouabain treatment could not be detected in cells of animals with a genetic defect in cellular homeostatic responses, such as in Dahl salt-sensitive rats or in cultured kidney cells cloned from these rats (B. M. Rayson and F. Xu, personal observation; and ref 114). This defect is considered as one of the possible causes for the volume contraction of hypertension. Because of the central role of Na^+,K^+-ATPase in Na^+ homeostasis and in providing the driving force for Na^+/Ca^{2+} exchange in muscle, alterations in enzyme activity or abundance could potentially alter vascular or cardiac contractility. A number of investigators have described a decrease in expression of the Na^+,K^+-ATPase α2 isoform, with or without a simultaneous increase of the α1 and isoforms, in cardiac tissue from rat models of hypertension (26,53).

Regulation of Activity

The activity of the Na^+,K^+-ATPase can be regulated through different mechanisms, including cations such as Na^+ and K^+, different hormones and neurotransmitters, and endogenous cardiac glycoside-like factors. The tissue-specific distribution of different subunit isoforms and their different affinities for ATP, Na^+, and cardiac glycosides can also contribute to the differential regulation of the enzyme activity (97,117). Regulation can be carried out directly and acutely without changing the biosynthesis rate of the enzyme (short-term regulation) or through the modulation caused by different hormones and neurotransmitters through either induction of Na^+,K^+-ATPase gene expression or posttranslational modification of preexisting enzymes (long-term regulation) (7,112,117).

Na^+,K^+-ATPase activity can be directly regulated by its substrates, Na^+, K^+, and ATP. Increased intracellular Na^+ elevates activity of existing pumps. Physiologically, this mechanism may be the most important controller of the rate at which the Na^+ pump functions. Extracellular K^+ is necessary for electrogenic pump function and can act as a noncompetitive antagonist of cardiac glycoside inhibition. ATP availability is likely to limit pump function only during anoxia and ischemia (31). Increased intracellular Na^+ is also able to stimulate transcription of pump subunit genes. However, the mechanism by which increased intracellular Na^+ leads to this change is still unknown (112).

Two of the catecholamines, dopamine and noradrenaline, appear to play a central role in the regulation of sodium homeostasis and blood pressure. Dopamine inhibits the Na^+,K^+-ATPase activity in kidney and decreases sodium retention, whereas noradrenaline stimulates the enzyme activity and decreases urinary sodium excretion, probably by regulating the state of phosphorylation of the catalytic α subunit (98). The inhibitory dopamine effect appears to require activation of both D1 and D2 receptor subtypes (8). Aldosterone, one of the mineralocorticoids, is another regulator of the Na^+,K^+-ATPase activity. A number of studies have shown that aldosterone can upregulate Na^+,K^+-ATPase activity by at least three routes: (a) a rapid Na^+-sensitive route, in which aldosterone increases the Na^+ permeability of the apical membrane in epithelial cells by activating the amiloride-sensitive Na^+ channels and so causes an increase of intracellular Na^+, which in turn stimulates the Na^+,K^+-ATPase activity; (b) a rapid direct induction of the subunits of the Na^+,K^+-ATPase by aldosterone at the genome level via a cytoplasmic receptor, with a delayed incorporation into the basolateral membrane; (c) in certain cells containing an aldosterone-sensitive Na^+/H^+ exchange mechanism, the resultant intracellular alkalosis could also enhance Na^+,K^+-ATPase subunit mRNA abundance and augment the pump activity over a longer time (56, 93). In different cell types, Na^+,K^+-ATPase expression has been found to be either increased or decreased by activation of cAMP-dependent protein kinase or protein kinase C, respectively.

Thyroid hormones and glucocorticoids are also important regulators of Na^+,K^+-ATPase, and both groups increase the enzyme activity. It is known that thyroid hormones bind to their specific nuclear receptor in target tissues with the possibility of modifying genetic expression, thereby inducing synthesis of specific mRNA leading to increased expression of the Na^+,K^+-ATPase (58,85).

The Na^+,K^+-ATPase is also activated by 5-hydroxytryptamine (5-HT, serotonin) in the CNS. In the raphe nuclei, brain areas where most serotonergic neuronal somas are contained, a very poor 5-HT activation of Na^+,K^+-ATPase was observed. In contrast, in target regions where 5-HT terminals are abundant, such as cerebral cortex, hippocampus, and striatum, 5-HT causes a significant dose-dependent activation of the Na^+ pump. Thus, 5-HT regulates brain Na^+,K^+-ATPase activity through the mediation of a specific receptor system (52,111).

Recently, Rodriquez de Lores Arnaiz (119) has characterized a soluble endogenous ouabain-like substance in the CNS, which is a Na^+,K^+-ATPase inhibitor. This substance can modify the regulatory function of insulin and certain neurotransmitters, including dopamine, noradrenaline, and 5-HT on synaptosomal membrane Na^+,K^+-ATPase. Noradrenaline was able to stimulate or inhibit the Na^+,K^+-ATPase activity, in rat cortex preparation, depending on the absence or presence of this soluble inhibitor. With the membrane alone, noradrenaline produced a significant decrease of Na^+,K^+-ATPase. In the presence of the soluble fraction, noradrenaline stimulated Na^+,K^+-ATPase. This stimulation, however, appears to be a direct effect on the enzyme and not mediated by cAMP or adrenergic receptors (118,121). A similar pattern of effects was also found for dopamine. In contrast, the stimulating effect of 5-HT on the Na^+,K^+-ATPase was independent of the presence of the soluble inhibitor of the Na^+ pump (3,120). Such ouabain-like endogenous Na^+,K^+-ATPase inhibitors have also been found in heart, skin, adrenal gland, and intestine (4,35,128, 136).

Anesthetic Effects

Despite the very active and extensive investigation of the Na^+,K^+-ATPase and the overall physiological importance of this enzyme, its role in anesthesia and the interaction between it and different anesthetics remain obscure. Although it is widely recognized that different membrane-bound proteins are involved in the anesthetic effects, there is very limited information about anesthetic effects on the Na^+,K^+-ATPase.

The general anesthetic thiopental strongly inhibits Na^+,K^+-ATPase purified from human placental tissue. However, this inhibitory effect on Na^+,K^+-ATPase activity was not observed in syncytiotrophoblast microvillus membrane from women anesthetized with thiopental or after in vitro addition of the anesthetic, probably due to a masking of a selective binding site of the anesthetic to Na^+,K^+-ATPase within the membrane (95). In crude rabbit heart membrane vesicle preparation, >50% of Na^+,K^+-ATPase activity was inhibited by volatile general anesthetics, including halothane, isoflurane, and enflurane (T. J. J. Blanck, 1986). Morphine strongly stimulates synaptosomal Na^+,K^+-ATPase activity and inhibits noradrenaline-release; stimulation of Na^+,K^+-ATPase by morphine can be antagonized by naloxone (104,105). It has been proposed that morphine may have some role in the suppression of membrane depolarization and/or the release of noradrenaline through its stimulatory action on the Na^+,K^+-ATPase activity.

Different general and local anesthetics can interact with cellular membranes and change the membrane fluidity (17,41,95,131,69), and the Na^+,K^+-ATPase activity is correlated with membrane fluidity (75). Therefore, it is possible that different anesthetics affect Na^+,K^+-ATPase activity indirectly through their influence on membrane fluidity.

CA^{2+} ATPASE

The Ca^{2+} pump was first described in skeletal muscle by Hasselbach and Makinose in 1961 (49); soon after, Ebashi and Lippman (32) also characterized a membrane fraction that had the ability to sequester Ca^{2+}. Ca^{2+} was recognized as the ion necessary for contraction in the heart and skeletal muscle. It was also recognized that the rapid regulation of Ca^{2+} ion concentration was necessary for the contraction-relaxation cycle to take place. This required a high-capacity, high-affinity system. The Ca^{2+} pump could fulfill these requirements, and was soon found to be ubiquitous in most cells with a well-developed sarcoplasmic reticulum (SR) or endoplasmic reticulum (ER). These proteins are encoded by at least three SERCA (sarcoplasmic, endoplasmic reticulum, calcium pumps) genes. Different isoforms are found in skeletal muscle, heart, brain, and other tissues. The function of the proteins encoded by the SERCA genes are essentially the same: to sequester Ca^{2+} and regulate Ca^{2+} concentration in the cytoplasm.

Structure

The generic Ca^{2+} pump protein is an integral membrane protein of 110 kDa with complex membrane and cytoplasmic domains (Fig. 1B). One model of the Ca^{2+} pump protein describes the molecule as having 10 transmembrane domains: four in the N-terminal end and six in the C-terminal (88,89). A cytoplasmic pear-shaped head attached to a stalk is constructed from extensions of the first five transmembrane domains. The ATP binding site and enzyme phosphorylation site are found in the extramembranous region of the Ca^{2+} pump protein, whereas the Ca^{2+} binding site appears localized to the transmembrane region. Mutation of six amino acid residues (Glu 309, Glu 771, Asp 800, Thr 799, Asn 796, Glu 908) in the transmembrane domain, in helices 4, 5, 6 and 8, interferes with activation of the enzyme by Ca^{2+} (57). These residues are found approximately halfway between the outer and inner membrane surfaces. The four helices mentioned have an amphiphilic character, with polar and charged residues facing one side of each helix and hydrophobic residues facing the surrounding membrane, forming a hydrophilic channel which can potentially bind and translocate Ca^{2+}. The ATP binding domain lies at least 6 nm from the membrane surface (47).

It was shown that 1 mol of Ca^{2+}-ATPase binds 2 mol of Ca^{2+} with high affinity in a sequential, cooperative manner (60). The bound Ca^{2+} is internalized, or occluded, upon addition of ATP and Ca^{2+}-ATPase phosphorylation. The Ca^{2+} remains occluded in the phosphoenzyme for a measurable period of time prior to translocation of Ca^{2+} into the lumen of the vesicle. A scheme for the catalytic translocation of Ca^{2+} and the hydrolysis of ATP is shown in Fig. 4. The movement, or active transport, of Ca^{2+} by and through the enzyme is by means of a very tight channel coupled to catalytic activity, which is substantially different from other ligand- and voltage-gated channels such as the voltage-dependent calcium channels. The voltage-dependent channels undergo a conformational change upon membrane depolarization, opening a channel which provides a free pathway for diffusion of a specific ion species. The active transport by the Ca^{2+}-ATPase provides a pathway for Ca^{2+} translocation, but the pathway always has part of its route obstructed throughout the catalytic cycle. The portion of the path for Ca^{2+} that is opened or closed depends upon the binding of the substrate, ATP, and its hydrolysis. Specifically, 2 mol of Ca^{2+} bind from the cytoplasmic side per 1 mol of enzyme. The 2 mol of Ca^{2+} are occluded, i.e., no longer exchangeable with the cytoplasm once ATP is bound and hydrolyzed to form a phosphoenzyme, but the Ca^{2+} then can dissociate into the lumen of the SR vesicle. The Ca^{2+} binding site of the phosphoenzyme has a dissociation constant in the millimolar range, much higher than the Ca^{2+} binding site of the nonphosphorylated enzyme, which has a dissociation constant in the micromolar range. This transformation of chemical catalysis into vectorial translocation is a general mechanism observed in all biological pump mechanisms.

Isoforms

Three separate genes encode the SERCA family of calcium pumps (88). They have a 75–85% sequence identity and similar hydropathy plots. The SERCA1, SERCA2, and SERCA3 genes expressed independently in COS-1 cells encoded and

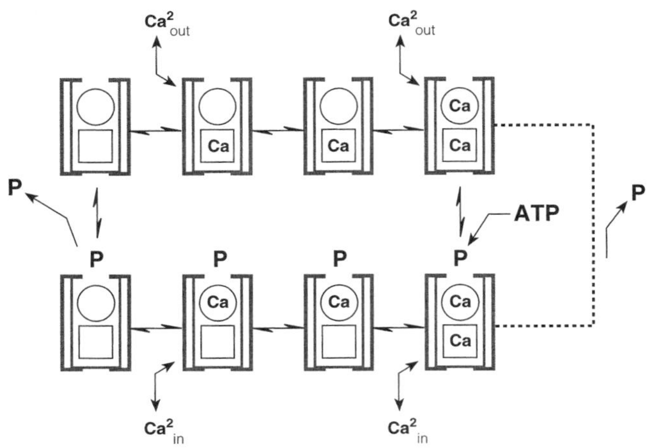

Figure 4. Diagram representing sequential steps for binding, occlusion, and translocations of Ca^{2+} by the Ca^{2+}-ATPase. Tight (*squares*) and very tight forms of binding (*circles*) are shown. The state immediately following phosphorylation represents the occluded state. (Reprinted with permission from Inesi G, Cantilina T, Yu X, Nikic D, Sagara Y, Kirtley ME. Long-range intramolecular linked functions in activation and inhibition of SERCA ATPases. *Ann NY Acad Sci* 1992;671:32–47.)

integrated intracellular Ca^{2+} pumps with similar transport capacities, similar ATP affinities, and similar Hill coefficients. The SERCA3 gene product, however, had a reduced affinity for Ca^{2+} and a different pH dependence than either SERCA1 or SERCA2. These results suggest different control levels of Ca^{2+} in cells expressing SERCA3. The tissue distribution of the SERCA3 gene and its protein product are at this time uncertain, but they appear to be found in nonmuscle cells (88). SERCA1 is exclusively expressed in fast-twitch skeletal muscle, while SERCA2 is expressed in slow-twitch skeletal, cardiac, and smooth muscle. The SERCA2 isoform of the Ca^{2+}-ATPase found in cardiac and slow-twitch muscle is often found in cells which coexpress phospholamban. Phospholamban, a homopentamer with subunits of 6000 d, imparts a reduced Ca^{2+} affinity to the Ca^{2+}-ATPase (138).

Two lines of investigation have recently led to new and exciting information regarding the role of phospholamban in the regulation of the Ca^{2+}-ATPase and contractility. Voss et al. (141) examined mouse atrial SR (MASR) from a tumor cell line that contains negligible amounts of phospholamban and compared it to mouse ventricular SR (MVSR) that contains phospholamban. They found, using time-resolved phosphorescence anisotropy, that the Ca^{2+}-ATPase in MASR was in a monomeric state allowing maximal mobility and catalytic activity, whereas MVSR, with unphosphorylated phospholamban, contained large aggregates of Ca^{2+}-ATPase in an unfavorable catalytic conformation. The phospholamban encouraged the formation of aggregates of the SR Ca^{2+}-ATPase, presumably resulting in a decreased mobility and decreased catalytic activity of the Ca^{2+}-ATPase and in its ability to sequester Ca^{2+}.

In a study of mice deficient in phospholamban achieved by targeted ablation of the phospholamban gene, Luo et al. (86) found that the Ca^{2+} uptake activity of heart homogenates had a greater sensitivity to Ca^{2+} than wild-type mice. They further showed that hearts of the phospholamban-deficient mice had greater contractile function than wild-type hearts under basal conditions and that the deficient mouse hearts did not respond to isoproterenol whereas wild type did. In the presence of maximal isoproterenol, the contractile function of the wild-type hearts could be raised to that of the phospholamban-deficient hearts. These studies suggest that phospholamban exerts a negative influence on the Ca^{2+} pump and contractile activity and that the major pathway by which isoproterenol stimulates contractility is through its phosphorylation of phospholamban.

The Ca^{2+} pump is a crucial part of the mechanism of relaxation in cardiac and skeletal muscle. Disease and extrinsic pathology of other systems (such as denervation of skeletal muscle, for example), exercise, and pressure overload of the myocardium can lead to alteration in both expression and function of the specific Ca^{2+} pump isoforms (65,124,125). The content of different isoforms of the Ca^{2+} pump appears to relate to three factors: (a) the efficiency of gene transcription and stability (fiber-type dependent), (b) the efficiency of translation and protein stability (muscle identity dependent), and (c) fiber composition (142). For example, denervated muscle demonstrates marked decreases in mRNA and protein expression of Ca^{2+} pump isoforms SERCA2a and SERCA1 (124). In Brody's disease, the Ca^{2+} pump function is markedly decreased, leading to problems of relaxation in humans (6). The expression of SERCA2 is decreased in the pressure overloaded heart, and relaxation is markedly impaired due to a lower density of Ca^{2+} pump proteins in the SR. In the stunned myocardium, where contractile dysfunction occurs, upregulation of the Ca^{2+}-ATPase leads to an increase in Ca^{2+} pumping.

The above results indicate that the synthesis and function of the Ca^{2+} pump protein in all cells is variable, depending on the particular function of the cell, the pump, and the physiologic or pathologic modulators of activity. Furthermore, direct and simple predictions appear unlikely in this complex regulatory system.

Anesthetic Effects

Examination of anesthetic effects on the SERCA Ca^{2+} pump have thus far been confined to those pumps extracted from either cardiac or skeletal muscle. Diamond and Berman (30) reported that halothane had no effect on skeletal SR Ca^{2+} transport at halothane concentrations of <5 mM. In 1981 and 1982, Blanck and Thompson (12,13), using isolated canine cardiac SR, demonstrated that halothane, enflurane, and isoflurane stimulated Ca^{2+} uptake into isolated SR vesicles. The data available suggest that the volatile anesthetics can stimulate Ca^{2+} pump activity at physiological pH and ATP concentration in cardiac SR, but that thiopental has no apparent effect on Ca^{2+} uptake activity (11). Changing assay conditions by varying the substrate concentration or altering the pH can result in a different response of the Ca^{2+} pump to anesthetics (12,23). At pH 7.2 and 5 mM ATP, the volatile anesthetics have little effect on Ca^{2+} uptake, suggesting that reports of decreased SR Ca^{2+} upon exposure to volatile anesthetics might result from an increased leak of Ca^{2+} out of the SR rather than from an inhibition of uptake (23,40). Similarly, several groups have reported stimulation by volatile anesthetics of Ca^{2+}-ATPase activity of the SERCA1 Ca^{2+} pump isolated from fast skeletal muscle SR, whereas others have reported inhibition but only at high anesthetic concentration (9,10,102). Karon and Thomas (69) have shown that halothane, at a high clinical concentration, activates the skeletal SR Ca^{2+}-ATPase. In temperature studies of Ca^{2+}-ATPase activity, halothane oligomerized the Ca^{2+}-ATPase at low temperature, but since at high temperature, the Ca^{2+}-

ATPase was already monomeric, activation by halothane was due to an increase in membrane fluidity (69). Little evidence exists indicating that these in vitro observations, which suggest acceleration of Ca^{2+}-ATPase and Ca^{2+} pump activity in vivo, actually change the physiologic function of either cardiac or skeletal muscle.

The important balance of Ca^{2+} uptake with Ca^{2+} leak and release by the SR results in greater or lesser availability of Ca^{2+} for contraction. If the Ca^{2+} pump is stimulated to take up more Ca^{2+}, yet the SR is also leakier, the total Ca^{2+} available for each beat is uncertain depending upon the relative magnitude of the two effects. Therefore, it is impossible to predict the overall effect of a drug on contractility based on in vitro measurements of isolated components unless all the organelles involved in Ca^{2+} homeostasis in the cell are taken into account in estimating the amount of Ca^{2+} available for contraction.

NA^{2+}-CA^{2+} EXCHANGER

Since the Na^+-Ca^{2+} exchanger was first described in guinea pig atria (116) almost 25 years ago, it has been recognized that the Na^+-Ca^{2+} exchanger plays a key role in maintaining intracellular Ca^{2+} levels in a wide variety of tissues. The Na^+-Ca^{2+} exchanger was thought to act primarily as a mechanism for extruding Ca^{2+} from cells. More recently, the Na^+-Ca^{2+} exchanger has been shown to regulate Ca^{2+} entry as well. Because of the importance of Ca^{2+} influx in controlling muscle contraction and in inducing release of neurotransmitters and hormones, interest in the exchanger has greatly intensified.

Anesthetics have been shown to affect fundamental mechanisms responsible for intracellular calcium homeostasis. Therefore, any effect of anesthetics on the Na^+-Ca^{2+} exchanger might augment the anesthetic-mediated perturbation of calcium homeostasis.

Structure

The cardiac exchanger is a 120-kDa protein consisting of two groups of transmembrane segments separated by a large intracellular loop. Figure 1C shows a tentative model of its arrangement in the sarcolemmal membrane (110). The model is based on the following evidence: (a) Hydropathy plots predict 11 transmembrane domains in the mature protein. (b) The asparagine at position 9 is glycosylated and assumed to be extracellular based on glycosylation sites in more fully described membrane proteins. (c) The region spanning membrane segments 4 and 5 has been modeled to be extracellular based on a 48% homology with an extracellular segment of the Na^+-K^+-ATPase. (d) A 520–amino acid hydrophilic segment occurs between membrane-spanning segments 5 and 6, and is the site at which the inhibitory peptide XIP acts.

XIP has been shown to act intracellularly; therefore, this hydrophilic region is modeled as an intracellular loop (110). This intracellular loop site is not essential for transport function but has attracted considerable interest because of its involvement in regulating intracellular Ca^{2+}. This regulatory site is a Ca^{2-}-binding domain (53,94) that resides near the center of the large intracellular hydrophilic loop of the exchanger comprising more than half of the exchanger protein. Deletion of a 124–amino acid segment from the loop completely abolishes secondary Ca^{2+} regulation (54). The intracellular high-affinity Ca^{2+} binding site is separate from the Ca transport site and selectively regulates Na^+-Ca^{2+} exchanger activity (94). The intracellular domain has been identified as the site of action of a newly designed peptide that is a selective inhibitor of the Na^+-Ca^{2+} exchanger (81).

The primary role of sarcolemmal Na^+-Ca^{2+} exchange is Ca^{2+} extrusion. Net efflux of Ca^{2-} is accomplished using the energy of the Na^+ gradient set up by the Na^+,K-ATPase. The stoichiometry for the exchange is 3 Na^+ to 1 Ca^{2+}. There is also a Na^+-Ca^{2+} exchanger on the mitochondrial membrane that was originally thought to involve a 2 Na^+ to 1 Ca^{2+} exchange carrier, though recently there is growing evidence that, similar to the sarcolemmal exchanger, it also operates with a 3 Na^+ to 1 Ca^{2+} ratio. The mitochondrial Na^+-Ca^{2+} exchanger has a low-affinity but a high-transport capacity for Ca^{2+}; therefore, it is active only after large increases in intracellular Ca^{2+} concentration.

The cardiac sarcolemmal Na^+-Ca^{2+} exchanger has a relatively high-affinity Ca^{2+} transport site at the intracellular membrane and a low-affinity Ca^{2+} transport site at the extracellular surface. The affinity for Na^+ (30 mM) and the current voltage relationship of the cardiac type and the brain type are similar (80).

Although the kinetic scheme of the cardiac type exchanger is not yet certain, evidence suggests a consecutive reaction mechanism. In this type of mechanism there is only one binding site that can bind either 1 Ca^{2+} or 3 Na^+ at one time and that is exposed only at one surface of the membrane. Na^+ or Ca^{2+} binds, moves across the membrane with the binding site, and is released. The exchanger binding site is then available to again bind Na^+ or Ca^{2+} to return across the membrane and complete the reaction cycle.

In addition to functioning as a transport site for Ca^{2+}, the cardiac Na^+-Ca^{2+} exchanger displays secondary regulation by Ca^{2+} and Na^+. Experimentally, secondary Ca^{2+} regulation has been observed as an activation of the exchange of extracellular Ca^{2+} for intracellular Na^+ [Na_i-Ca_o], the outward exchange current , secondary to a drop in internal Ca^{2+} or extracellular sodium. The significance of this autoregulatory mechanism is unclear. In the cardiac myocyte, Ca^{2+} entry through the voltage-dependent Ca^{2+} channel upon depolarization could increase Ca^{2+} binding to the exchanger regulatory site and activate Ca^{2+} influx through the exchanger during the early phase of the action potential. Alternatively, during diastole the Ca^{2+} regulatory site might act as a safety valve to prevent the exchanger from lowering cytoplasmic Ca^{2+} too far. Once $Ca^{2+}{}_i$ is reduced to <100 nM, the exchanger would inactivate to prevent further Ca^{2+} efflux. Both the cardiac and the brain type are secondarily regulated by intracellular Ca^{2+}, but the affinity of the brain type for regulatory Ca^{2+} (1.5 mM) upon initial application of Na^+, is lower than that of the cardiac type (0.3 mM) (54).

The Na^+-Ca^{2+} exchanger is also subject to Na^+-dependent inactivation (55). Experimentally this inactivation manifests as an exponential decay of the outward exchange current [$Na^+{}_i$-$Ca^{2+}{}_o$] in response to an increase in cytoplasmic Na^+. Both Ca^{2+} influx and efflux are affected by this process. The magnitude of decline is attenuated in rate and extent as the level of regulatory Ca^{2+} is increased (55). Thus, the activity of the exchanger appears to be regulated by an autoinhibitory domain.

Isoforms

The Na^+-Ca^{2+} exchanger has been found in a wide variety of tissues and in many species. Two different isoforms of Na^+-Ca^{2+} exchanger have been cloned: one in the heart (103), NCX1, and the other in the brain (80), NCX2. The canine cardiac Na^+-Ca^{2+} exchanger was cloned from canine myocytes (103) and expressed in *Xenopus* oocytes. Variants of the cardiac exchanger have been cloned from other tissues such as kidney, brain lung, smooth muscle and skeletal muscle. Alternatively spliced variants have also been described (73,77,127). In humans this gene is localized on chromosome 2p21-p23 (127). The second isoform, NCX2, present in rat brain cDNA library, is predicted to code for a protein of 921 amino acids and is the product of a different gene located on human chromosome 14.

The cardiac and the brain isoforms are 61% and 65% identical at the nucleotide and aminoacid level, respectively. In contrast to the cardiac Na^+-Ca^{2+} exchanger (NCX1), whose transcripts are distributed in various tissues, transcripts of the brain Na^+-Ca^{2+} exchanger are detected only in the brain and skeletal muscle. The NCX2 isoform is not present in cardiac muscle, which has the highest abundance of NCX1.

Physiology

Cardiac myocytes display an especially high Na^+-Ca^{2+} exchange activity and have been an ideal model for molecular studies. It has been demonstrated that the Na^+-Ca^{2+} exchanger is the dominant Ca^{2+} efflux mechanism in myocytes. This efflux is necessary in order for the muscle to relax; thus, the exchanger is essential for the diastolic phase of the cardiac cycle. The Na^+-Ca^{2+} exchanger directly affects intracellular Ca^{2+} homeostasis and is the main mechanism responsible for Ca^{2+} extrusion during Ca^{2+} overload (101). However, the exchanger itself may mediate Ca^{2+} overload as it has been shown during the period of posthypoxic reoxygenation (71).

Regulation of Ca^{2+} homeostasis implies Ca^{2+} efflux being equal to Ca^{2+} influx during each contraction cycle, and, since the Na^+-Ca^{2+} exchanger is involved in both the influx and efflux of Ca^{2+}, it can alter both the the systolic as well as the diastolic phase of the cardiac cycle.

The observation that dichlorobenzamil, an inhibitor of Na^+-Ca^{2+} exchange in sarcolemmal vesicles, causes a parallel reduction in contractile tension of guinea pig papillary muscles has prompted investigation into the mechanism by which Na^+-Ca^{2+} exchange may activate contraction (18,27,70,74,79,129). These data suggest that the Na^+-Ca^{2+} exchange activates contraction by contributing to the rise in $Ca^{2+}{}_i$ levels during depolarization. During depolarization, a transient rise in $(Na^+)_i$ would occur in the diffusion-restricted region near the intracellular opening of the Na^+ channel. This increase would cause reversal of the Na^+-Ca^{2+} exchanger and a consequent transient net influx of Ca^{2+} in the region of the sarcoplasmic feet. Contractile activation would follow as a result of Ca^{2+}-induced Ca^{2+} release. The intracellular Ca^{2+} pool from which release occurs has been identified as ionomycin sensitive (70). However, whole-cell voltage clamp experiments indicate that Ca^{2+}-induced Ca^{2+} release from the SR during depolarization results mainly from influx through L-type voltage-dependent Ca^{2+} channels rather than through a reverse of the Na^+-Ca^{2+} exchanger (79). In fact, treatment with the selective Na^+-Ca^{2+} exchanger inhibitor XIP or with the Na^+ channel blocker tetradotoxin (TTX) did not affect cardiac contraction.

The importance of Na^+-Ca^{2+} exchange as a regulator of the smooth muscle contractile state is highly controversial. The Na^+-Ca^{2+} exchanger has been identified in the arterial smooth muscle cell and less conclusively in arterial endothelial cell membranes (64). A hypothesis links the Na^+-Ca^{2+} exchanger of vascular smooth muscle to essential hypertension (14). This hypothesis has gained more attention since an endogenous Na^+ pump inhibitor has been isolated (48). This endogenous ouabain-like factor could cause a rise in the internal Na^+ concentration of vascular smooth muscle cells. The rise in Na^+ could increase internal Ca^{2+} via the Na^+-Ca^{2+} exchanger and lead to increased muscle tone.

The role of Ca^{2+} entry in the release of neurotransmitters and hormones is well known (123). The Na^+-Ca^{2+} exchange of neural tissue was initially described for the squid giant axon but has now been described in several preparations. The activity is moderately high compared with cardiac tissue and may account for the majority of Ca efflux from nerve terminals following excitation (122).

The exchanger has been localized to presynaptic nerve terminals ,concentrated mainly at the neuromuscular junction (87). The exchanger is also present in developing neurites and growth cones.

Anesthetic Effects

General anesthetics such as octanol and sodium pentobarbital inhibit Ca^{2+} uptake by the Na^+-Ca^{2+} exchanger (50). The concentrations of anesthetics found to be effective as inhibitors of Na^+-Ca^{2+} exchange are greater then those needed for anesthesia, but are comparable to those shown to have a negative inotropic effect on the heart. The 50% effective anesthetic doses of octanol and decanol are 60 and 13 mM. These are a factor of three to four less than the EC_{50} for inhibition of Na^+-Ca^{2+} exchange. The level of sodium pentobarbital reported to cause a 44% reduction in peak tension is comparable with the EC_{50} observed for inhibition of Na^+-Ca^{2+} exchange. This raises the possibility that the negative inotropic effect of general anesthetics may be related, in some way, to an inhibition of Na^+-Ca^{2+} exchange activity.

The effect of volatile anesthetics on Na^+-Ca^{2+} exchange activity are contradictory (5,51,108). Haworth and Goknur (51) have shown that the Na^+-Ca^{2+} exchanger is inhibited by volatile anesthetics in a dose-dependent fashion at clinically relevant concentrations. Their experiments were performed in Na^+-loaded myocytes using [$^{45}Ca^{2+}$] as a means of measuring Ca^{2+} uptake into isolated rat cardiac myocytes. Paroli and Blanck have employed the fura 2 fluorescence technique to measure the efflux of Ca^{2+} from single rat cardiac myocytes (108). They observed no effect of halothane on the Na^+-Ca^{2+} exchanger. Both sets of investigators measured the entry of Ca^{2+} into the cell secondary to a Na^+ gradient in which intracellular Na^+ exceeds extracellular Na^+, such that the Na^+-Ca^{2+} exchanger was examined in only one direction. However, Haworth et al. (50) showed that octanol was almost an order of magnitude more effective in inhibiting Na^+-Ca^{2+} exchange when extracellular Na^+ concentration was physiological. The experiments of Paroli and Blanck (108) were performed at $[Na^+]_o = 0$, a condition that might result in decreased sensitivity to anesthetics. Inhibition of the neonatal rabbit myocyte Na^+-Ca^{2+} exchanger by halothane has also been reported. Haworth and Goknur (51) suggest that, since the relative magnitude of the role of the exchanger on Ca^{2+} influx and efflux is uncertain, inhibition of the exchanger would lead to an uncertain inotropic effect. The implications of an inhibitory effect of halothane and isoflurane on the Na^+-Ca^{2+} exchanger on contractility will depend on a clear delineation of the overall contribution of the Na^+-Ca^{2+} exchanger to Ca^{2+} homeostasis during systole and diastole.

NEUROTRANSMITTER TRANSPORTERS

The distinct compositions of the intracellular and extracellular fluids are maintained by the selective diffusion and transport of various solutes across the cell membrane. A number of substances are taken up into or secreted from cells across the membrane against a large concentration gradient by the energy-dependent process of active transport. Active transport through the cell membrane is mediated by proteins known as pumps (e.g., Na^+,K^+-ATPase) or transporters (e.g., the glutamate transporter). These molecules play important roles in physiological regulation and are the targets of a number of drugs. This section will address the biochemical properties, physiological roles and pharmacology of transporter proteins and their relevance to anesthesiology. In contrast to pumps, which directly couple solute transport to ATP hydrolysis, most transporters concentrate substances by a cotransport (symport) or antiport process that couples transport to energy stored in transmembrane electrochemical gradients. For example, neurons and glia are able to take up neurotransmitters by Na^+-dependent cotransport that couples neurotransmitter uptake to the Na^+ gradient generated by the Na^+,K^+-ATPase. Although similar mechanisms are involved in the uptake and secretion of metabolites in most cells, the neurotransmitter transporters have come under intense scrutiny as a result of their important roles in neuropharmacology and cardiovascular pharmacology.

Recent studies have demonstrated the rich molecular diversity and pharmacologic importance of neurotransmitter uptake systems (2). The brain contains a number of uptake systems that are relatively specific for a specific neurotransmitter (Table 2). Pharmacological evidence indicates that transporters are an important mechanism for terminating synaptic transmission. For example, noradrenergic neurotransmission is potentiated by drugs that inhibit norepinephrine reuptake but not by inhibitors of norepinephrine metabolism, while norepinephrine overflow due to sympathetic stimulation can be detected in the presence, but not in the absence, of norepinephrine reuptake inhibitors. Similar experiments support the role of reuptake in terminating synaptic transmission mediated by most of the neurotransmitters listed in Table 1. An important exception from this list is acetylcholine, which is inactivated by cholinesterase-catalyzed hydrolysis. However, choline, the breakdown product as well as the precursor of acetylcholine, is taken up by a specific transporter.

Structure

A number of neurotransmitter transporters have been solubilized, purified, and reconstituted; the reconstituted transporters exhibit high-affinity binding and ion-dependent transport. Other transporters have been identified by expression cloning strategies that utilize *Xenopus* oocytes, a technique that has facilitated the identification and molecular characterization of low abundance transporters. The early molecular cloning of the mRNA encoding the GABA transporter and the norepinephrine transporter revealed a number of similar features that helped define the Na^+/Cl^--dependent plasma membrane neurotransmitter transporter gene family (1,2). These proteins have twelve transmembrane domains predicted by hydropathy analysis (Figs. 1D and 5). The highest degree of sequence identity exists among transmembrane domains 1, 2, and 4–8, which suggests that these domains may be of functional importance in transport activity. By taking advantage of the significant amino acid sequence similarities between the GABA and norepinephrine transporters, a number of members of this transporter family have been identified and characterized by molecular cloning techniques. These studies have revealed the existence of multiple transporter subtypes for a single neurotransporter, analogous to the multiple neurotransmitter receptor subtypes, which suggests a role for functional specialization.

The Na^+/K^+-dependent plasma membrane transporter family consists of three structurally related glutamate/aspartate transporters with distinct anatomical distributions. One member appears to encode a glial transporter, one an astrocytic transporter and one a peripheral epithelial and central neuronal transporter. The membrane topology of this family is controversial and has been proposed to consist of six to 10 transmembrane domains (Fig. 5).

The H^+-dependent vesicular transporter family consists of four distinct carriers that mediate neurotransmitter transport from the cytoplasm into the synaptic vesicle interior (33). These vesicular transporters function in series with the plasma membrane transporters to transport neurotransmitter from the cell exterior into the cell and then into vesicles. The energy for H^+-dependent transport is derived from the proton gradient generated by the vacuolar H^+-ATPase; the neurotransmitter is transported into the vesicle in exchange for one or more protons by an antiport mechanism. The membrane topology of these transporters is predicted to have twelve transmembrane domains.

Neurotransmitter transporter activity is subject to regulation by various signals acting through second messenger mediated protein phosphorylation pathways (2). Various first and second messengers have been shown to regulate the activities of a number of transporters, including the GABA, norepinephrine, dopamine, serotonin, and glutamate transporters. Furthermore, potential phosphorylation sites have been identified in the amino acid sequences of cytoplasmic domains of neurotransmitter transporters for which the sequence is known. Alterations in transmembrane electrochemical gradients due to ion channel or pump activation may indirectly regulate the activities of neurotransmitter transporters by affecting on the driving force for transport.

Physiology and Pharmacology

In addition to their distinct structural properties, the three neurotransmitter transporter families have distinct transport mechanisms (61). The Na^+/Cl^--dependent transporters are cotransporters (symporters) in which Na^+ and Cl^- are cotransported along with the neurotransmitter (Fig. 6). For the GABA transporter, whole cell voltage-clamp techniques have demonstrated the electrogenic nature of the transport process, which results in a net positive charge being transferred with each molecule of GABA. The transport of glutamate by its Na^+/K^+-dependent transporter requires extracellular Na^+ and intracellular K^+, and is also electrogenic. Recent studies suggest that the uptake of one glutamate molecule is coupled to the cotransport of two Na^+ and the countertransport of one K^+ and one OH^- (or HCO_3^-), which results in an inward current accompanied by intracellular acidification and extracellular alkalinization (19). The H^+-dependent vesicular transporters are antiporters in which neurotransmitter transport into the vesicle is coupled to the countertransport of one or more protons out of the vesicle.

A number of important drugs act on neurotransmitter transporters to produce their effects, including tricyclic antidepressants, amphetamines and other psychostimulants. Cocaine has been shown to block the reuptake of norepinephrine, serotonin and dopamine; these actions are in addition to its local anesthetic, antimuscarinic, and receptor effects (22). Blockade of dopamine reuptake by the dopamine transporter and potentiation of dopaminergic transmission is thought to underlie the euphorigenic and reinforcing properties of cocaine. Amphetamine also blocks the reuptake of norepinephrine, dopamine and serotonin, but additionally causes the release and ultimately the depletion of these biogenic amines from their presynaptic storage sites; amphetamines also inhibits monoamine oxidase. The mechanism of the neurotransmitter-releasing effects of amphetamine and its derivatives probably results from their ability to reverse neuronal plasma membrane and vesicular transport systems by plasma membrane transporter-mediated exchange and by dissipation of the vesicular transmembrane pH gradient (122). Reserpine also depletes vesicular monoamines, but does not affect the plasma membrane transporter. The high-affinity interaction of reserpine with

Table 2. NEUROTRANSMITTER TRANSPORTERS[a]

- Plasma membrane transporters
  - Na^+/Cl^--dependent
    - Dopamine
    - Norepinephrine/epinephrine
    - Serotonin
    - α-Aminobutyric acid (GABA)
    - Glycine
    - Choline
  - Na^+/K^+-dependent
    - Glutamate/aspartate
- Vesicular transporters
  - H^+-dependent
    - Monoamines
    - GABA/glycine
    - Glutamate
    - Acetylcholine

[a]Data from refs. 1 and 2.

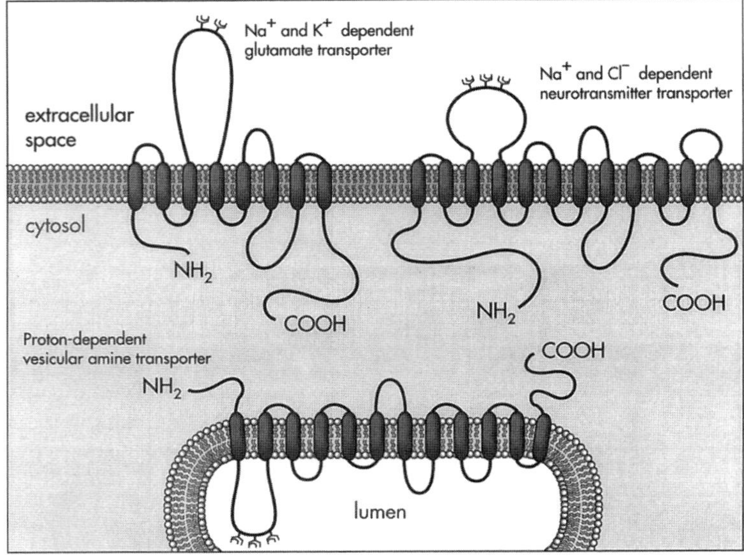

Figure 5. Schematic representations of the predicted transmembrane topologies for the three neurotransmitter transporter gene families. Potential N-linked glycosylation sites found in each protein family have been indicated. (Reprinted with permission from Amara SG, Arriza JL. Neurotransmitter transporters: three distinct gene families. *Curr Opin Neurobiol* 1993;3:337–344.)

synaptic vesicles leads to their destruction, which results in the inability of the nerve terminals to concentrate and store neurotransmitter.

Inhibition of Na^+/Cl^--dependent monoamine transport is the mechanism of action of the most widely used antidepressant drugs. The tricyclic antidepressants (which include imipramine, amitriptyline and their N-demethyl derivatives) block the neuronal uptake of norepinephrine, serotonin and, to a much lesser extent, dopamine by direct inhibition of their plasma membrane transporters. The potency and selectivity of the individual agents for specific transporters is variable. In general, the antidepressants are more effective in blocking norepinephrine and/or serotonin transport, while the stimulants (e.g., cocaine, amphetamine, methylphenidate) are more potent in blocking dopamine transport. The atypical antidepressants fluoxetine and trazodone are more specific inhibitors of the serotonin transporter. Many of these drugs have additional nontherapeutic effects as antagonists of various neurotransmitter receptors; these include muscarinic cholinergic, α adrenergic and H_1 and H_2 histaminergic receptors.

Anesthetic Effects

Several studies have examined the effects of general anesthetics on neurotransmitter transporters in vitro; however, a role for anesthetic action at this site in the clinical effects of general anesthetics has not been demonstrated. General anesthetics are known to affect synaptic transmission both presynaptically and postsynaptically, and anesthetic effects on transporters are a potential presynaptic site of action. Volatile anesthetics have been found to inhibit the transport of dopamine, serotonin and choline into presynaptic terminals, although the potency, efficacy, and kinetic mechanisms of the observed inhibition are variable. For example, halothane at clinical concentrations and to a lesser extent isoflurane, but not pentobarbital, inhibit dopamine uptake by a noncompetitive mechanism with full efficacy (34). Serotonin uptake is inhibited competitively by ketamine and halothane at clinical concentrations, and noncompetitively by isoflurane at higher concentrations (90–92). Halothane, enflurane, and isoflurane inhibit uptake of choline, the rate-limiting step in acetylcholine synthesis, by a noncompetitive mechanism with a maximal efficacy of 38% (46). In contrast, GABA uptake is not inhibited by halothane (24). The variability in potency and mechanism of the effects of anesthetics on neurotransmitter transport makes generalizations of anesthetic effects difficult even within transporter gene families. It is unlikely that inhibition of dopamine transport is an important component of general anesthetic action since other inhibitors have marked stimulatory, rather than depressant, effects on the central nervous system.

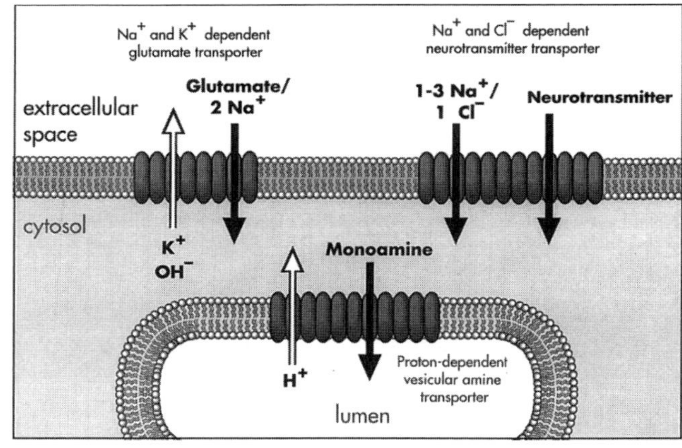

Figure 6. Neurotransmitter transport across cell membranes is coupled to the flow of ions down their concentration gradients. The distinct ionic requirements and the postulated stoichiometry of transport by each gene family have been illustrated schematically. The glutamate transporter gene family involves the cotransport of Na^+ and the countertransport of K^+ and a pH changing anion (OH^- or HCO_3^-) to drive glutamate movement across the plasma membrane. Cotransport of Na^+ and Cl^- are characteristic of the transporter gene family that mediates the transport of many neurotransmitters, including GABA, monoamines, glycine, and others. The transport of monoamines into synaptic vesicles is mediated by vesicular transporters that are coupled to proton antiport. (Reprinted with permission from Amara SG, Arriza JL. Neurotransmitter transporters: three distinct gene families. *Curr Opin Neurobiol* 1993;3:337–344.)

REFERENCES

1. Amara SG, Arriza JL. Neurotransmitter transporters: three distinct gene families. *Curr Opin Neurobiol* 1993;3:337–344.
2. Amara SG, Kuhar MJ. Neurotransmitter transporters: recent progress. *Annu Rev Neurosci* 1993;16:73–93.
3. Antonelli de Gomez de Lima M, Rodriguez de Lores Arnaiz G. Tissue-specificity of dopamine effects on brain ATPases. *Neurochem Res* 1981;6:969–977.
4. Araki K, Kuroki J, Ito O, Kuwada M, Tachibana S. Novel peptide inhibitor (SPAI) of Na^+,K^+-ATPase from porcine intestine. *Biochim Biophys Res Commun* 1989;164:496–502.
5. Baum VC, Wetzel GT. Sodium-calcium exchange in neonatal myocardium: reversible inhibition by halothane. *Anesth Analg* 1994; 78:1105–1109.
6. Benders AA, Veerkamp JH, Jongen PJ, et al. Ca^{2+} homeostasis in Brody's disease. A skeletal muscle and cultured muscle cells and the effects of dantrolene and verapamil. *J Clin Invest* 1994;94: 741–748.
7. Bertorello A, Aperia A. Short-term regulation of Na^+,K^+-ATPase activity by dopamine. *Am J Hypertens* 1990;3:51S–54S.
8. Bertorello AM, Katz AI. Short-term regulation of renal Na^+K-ATPase activity: physiological relevance and cellular mechanisms. *Am J Physiol* 1993;265:F743–F755.
9. Blanck TJ, Gruener R, Suffecool SL, Thompson M. Calcium uptake by isolated sarcoplasmic reticulum: examination of halothane inhibition, pH dependence, and Ca^{2+} dependence of normal and malignant hyperthermic human muscle. *Anesth Analg* 1981;60: 492–498.
10. Blanck TJJ, Peterson CV, Baroody B, Tegazzin V, Lou J. Halothane, enflurane, and isoflurane stimulate calcium leakage from rabbit sarcoplasmic reticulum. *Anesthesiology* 1991;76:813–821.
11. Blanck TJJ, Stevenson RL. Thiopental does not alter Ca^{2+} uptake by cardiac sarcoplasmic reticulum. *Anesth Analg* 1988;67:346–348.
12. Blanck TJJ, Thompson M. Calcium transport by cardiac sarcoplasmic reticulum: modulation of halothane action by substrate concentration and pH. *Anesth Analg* 1981;60:390–394.
13. Blanck TJJ, Thompson M. Enflurane and isoflurane stimulate calcium trnasport by cardiac sarcoplasmic reticulum. *Anesth Analg* 1982;61:142–145.
14. Blaustein MP, Ambesi A, Bloch RJ, et al. Regulation of vascular smooth muscle contractility: roles of the sarcoplasmic reticulum (SR) and the sodium/calcium exchanger. *Jpn J Pharmacol* 1992;S2: 107P–114P.
15. Blaustein MP. Sodium ions, calcium ions, blood pressure regulation, and hypertension: a reassessment and a hypothesis. *Am J Physiol* 1977;232:C167–C173.
16. Blaustein MP, Ashida T, Hamlyn JM. Sodium metabolism and hypertension: how are they linked? *Klin Wochenschr* 1987;65:21–32.
17. Boggs JM, Yoong T, Hsia JG. Site and mechanism of anesthetic action. *Mol Pharmacol* 1976;12:127–135.
18. Bouchard RA, Clark RB, Giles WR. Regulation of unloaded cell shortening by sarcolemmal sodium-calcium exchange in isolated rat ventricular myocytes. *J Physiol (Lond)* 1993;469:583–599.
19. Bouvier M, Szatkowski M, Amato A, Attwell D. The glial cell glutamate uptake carrier countertransports pH-changing anions. *Nature* 1992;360:471–474.
20. Cantley LG, Zhou XM, Cunha MJ, Epstein J, Cantley LC. Ouabain-resistant transfectants of the murine ouabain resistance gene contain mutations in the a-subunit of the Na,K-ATPase *J Biol Chem* 1992;267:17271–17278.
21. Capasso JM, Hoving S, Tal DM, Goldshleger R, Karlish SJD. Extensive digestion of Na^+,K^+-ATPase by specific and nonspecific proteases with preservation of cation occlusion sites. *J Biol Chem* 1992; 267:1150–1158.
22. Carroll FI, Lewin AH, Boja JW, Kuhar MJ. Cocaine receptor: biochemical characterization and structure-activity relationships of cocaine analogues at the dopamine transporter. *J Med Chem* 1992; 35:969–981.
23. Casella ES, Suite DA, Fisher YI, Blanck TJJ. The effect of volatile anesthetics on the pH dependence of calcium uptake by cardiac sarcoplasmic reticulum. *Anesthesiology* 1987;67:386–390.
24. Cheng S-C, Brunner EA. Inhibition of GABA metabolism in rat brain slices by halothane. *Anesthesiology* 1981;55:26–33.
25. Collins JH, Leszyck J. The "γ subunit" of Na^+,K^+-ATPase: a small amphiphilic protein with a unique amino acid sequence. *Biochemistry* 1987;26:8665–8668.
26. Crnkovic-Markovic R, Putnam DS, McDonough AA. Differential expression of Na,K-ATPase subunits in Sprague-Dawley rats with fructose induced hypertension and hyperinsulinemia. *Circulation* 1990;82:III-87.
27. Cyran SE, Phillips J, Ditty S, Baylen BG, Cheung J, La Noue K. Developmental differences in cardiac myocyte calcium homeostasis after steady-state potassium depolarization: mechanisms and implications for cardioplegia. *J Pediatr* 1993;122:S77–S83.
28. De Weer P. Cellular sodium-potassium transport. In: Seldin DW, Giebisch G, eds. *The kidney: physiology and pathophysiology* 2nd ed. New York: Raven Press, 1992:93–112.
29. Dean R. Theories of electrolyte equilibrium in muscle. *Biol Symp* 1941;3:331–348.
30. Diamond EM, Berman MC. The effect of halothane on the stability of Ca^{2+} transport activity of isolated fragmented sarcoplasmic reticulum. *Biochem Pharmacol* 1980;29:375–381.
31. Doris PA. Regulation of Na,K-ATPase by endogenous ouabain-like materials. *Proc Soc Exp Biol Med* 1994;205:202–212.
32. Ebashi S, Lippman F. Adenosine triphosphate-linked concentration of calcium ions in a particulate fraction of rabbit muscle. *J Cell Biol* 1962;14:389–400.
33. Edwards RH. The transport of neurotransmitters into synaptic vesicles. *Curr Opin Neurobiol* 1992;2:586–594.
34. El-Maghrabi EA, Eckenhoff RG. Inhibition of dopamine transport in rat brain synaptosomes by volatile anesthetics. *Anesthesiology* 1993;78:750–756.
35. Fagoo M, Godfraind T. Further characterization of cardiodigin, Na^+,K^+-ATPase inhibitor extracted from mammalian tissues. *FEBS Lett* 1985;184:150–154.
36. Fambrough DM, Lemas MV, Hamrick M, et al. Analysis of subunit assembly of the Na,K-ATPase. *Am J Physiol* 1994;266:C579–C589.
37. Fambrough DM, Wolitzky BA, Taormino JP, et al. A cell biologist's perspective on sites of Na,K-ATPase regulation. In: Kaplan JH, De Weer P, eds. *The sodium pump: structure, mechanism, and regulation.* New York: Rockefeller University Press, 1991:17–30.
38. Flier JS. Ouabain-like activity in total skin and its implications for endogenous regulation of ion transport. *Nature* 1978;274:285–286.
39. Forbush B III. Cardiotonic steroid binding to Na,K-ATPase. In: Hoffman JF, Forbush B III, eds. *Current topics in membranes and transport. Vol. 19.* New York: Academic Press, 1983:167–201.
40. Frazer MJ, Lynch C III. Halothane and enflurane effects on Ca^{2+} fluxes of isolated myocardial sarcoplasmic reticulum. *Anesthesiology* 1992;77:316–323.
41. Garcia-Martin E, Gutierrez-Merino C. Modulation of the Ca^{2+}, Mg^{2+}-ATPase activity of synaptosomal plasma membrane by the local anesthetics dibucaine and lidocaine. *J Neurochem* 1990;54: 1238–1246.
42. Geering K. Topical review: subunit assembly and functional maturation of Na^+,K^+-ATPase. *J Membr Biol* 1990;115:109–121.
43. Gick GG, Ismail-Beigi F, Edelman IS. Hormonal regulation of Na,K-ATPase. *Prog Clin Biol Res* 1988;268B:277–295.
44. Glynn IM. Annual review prize lecture: all hands to the sodium pump. *J Physiol* 1993;462:1–30.
45. Green NM. Evolutionary relationships within the family of P-type cation pumps. In: Scarpa A, Carafoli E, Papa S, eds. *Ion-motive ATPase: structure, function and regulation.* New York: New York Academy of Sciences, 1992:104–112.
46. Griffiths R, Greiff JMC, Boyle E, Rowbotham DJ, Norman RI. Volatile anesthetic agents inhibit choline uptake into rat synaptosomes. *Anesthesiology* 1994;81:953–958.
47. Gutierrez-Merino CFM, Mumkonge AM, Mata JM, et al. The position of the ATP binding site on the Ca^{2+}, Mg^{2+}-ATPase. *Biochim Biophys Acta* 1987;897:207–216.
48. Hamlyn JM, Blaustein MP, Bova S, et al. Identification and characterization of a ouabain-like compound from human plasma *Proc Natl Acad Sci USA* 1991;88:6259–6263.
49. Hasselbach W, Makinose M. Die Calciumpumpe der Erschlaffungs grana des Muskels and ihre Abh ngigkeit von der ATP-Spaltung. *Biochem Z* 1961;333:518–528.
50. Haworth RA, Goknur AB, Berkoff HA. Inhibition of Na-Ca exchange by general anesthetics. *Circ Res* 1989;65:1021–1028.
51. Haworth RA, Goknur AB. Inhibition of sodium/calcium exchange and calcium channels of heart cells. *Anesthesiology* 1995;82: 1255–1265.
52. Hernandez RJ. Na^+/K^+-ATPase regulation by neurotransmitters. *Neurochem Int* 1992;20:1–10.
53. Herrera V, Chobanian AV, Ruiz-Opazo N. Isoform-specific modula-

tion of Na,K-ATPase a subunit gene expression in hypertension. *Science* 1988;241:221–223.

54. Hilgemann DW, Collins A, Matsuoka S. Steady-state and dynamic properties of cardiac sodium-calcium exchange. Secondary modulation by cytoplasmic calcium and ATP. *J Gen Physiol* 1992;100: 933–961.
55. Hilgemann DW, Matsuoka S, Nagel GA, Collins A. Steady-state and dynamic properties of cardiac sodium-calcium exchange. Sodium-dependent inactivation. *J Gen Physiol* 1992;100:905–932.
56. Horisberger J-D, Rossier BC. Aldosterone regulation of gene transcription leading to control of ion transport. *Hypertension* 1992;19: 221–227.
57. Inesi G, Cantilina T, Yu X, Nikic D, Sagara Y, Kirtley ME. Long-range intramolecular linked functions in activation and inhibition of SERCA ATPases. *Ann NY Acad Sci* 1992;671:32–47.
58. Ismail-Beigi F. Regulation of Na^+,K^+-ATPase expression by thyroid hormone. *Semin Nephrol* 1992;12:44–48.
59. Jaunin P, Richter K, Corthesy I, Geering K. Posttranslational processing and basic properties of a putative β3-subunit of Na,K-ATPase. *J Gen Physiol* 1990;96:60A (abstr.).
60. Jencks WP. On the mechanism of ATP-driven Ca^{2+} transport by the calcium ATPase of sarcoplasmic reticulum. *Ann NY Acad Sci* 1992; 671:49–57.
61. Johnstone RM. Ion-coupled cotransport. *Curr Opin Cell Biol* 1990;2: 735–741.
62. Jorgensen PL. Mechanism of the Na,K-pump. *Biochim Biophys Acta* 1982;694:26–68.
63. Jorgensen PL. Functional domains of Na,K-ATPase; conformational transitions in the α-subunit and ion occlusion. *Acta Physiol Scand* 1992;146:89–95.
64. Juhaszova M, Ambesi A, Lindenmayer GE, Blocj RJ, Blaustein MP. Na^+-Ca^{2+} exchanger in arteries: identification by immunoblotting and immunofluorescence microscopy. *Am J Physiol* 1994;266: C234–C242.
65. Kandarian SC, Peters DG, Taylor JA, Williams JH. Skeletal muscle overload upregulates the sarcoplasmic reticulum slow calcium pump gene. *Am J Physiol* 1994;266:C1190–C1197.
66. Kanner BI, Schuldiner S. Mechanism of transport and storage of neurotransmitters. *CRC Crit Rev Biochem* 1987;22:1–38.
67. Karlish SJD, Goldshleger R, Tal DM, Stein WD. Structure of the cation binding sites of Na/K-ATPase. In: Kaplan JH, De Weer P, eds. *The sodium pump: structure, mechanism, and regulation.* New York: Rockefeller University Press, 1991:129–141.
68. Karlish SJD, Goldshleger R, Stein WD. A 19-kDa C-terminal tryptic fragment of the a chain of Na/K-ATPase is essential for occlusion and transport of cations. *Proc Natl Acad Sci USA* 1990;87:4566–4570.
69. Karon BS, Thomas DD. Molecular mechanism of Ca-ATPase activation by halothane in sarcoplasmic reticulum. *Biochemistry* 1993;32: 7503–7511.
70. Kiang JG, Smallridge RC. Sodium cyanide increases cytosolic free calcium: evidence for activation of the reversed mode Na^+/Ca^{2+} exchanger and Ca^{2+} mobilization from inositol triphosphate-insensitive pools. *Toxicol Appl Pharmacol* 1994;127:173–181.
71. Kihara Y, Sasayama S, Inoko M, Morgan JP. Sodium/calcium exchange modulates intracellular calcium overload during posthypoxic reoxygenation in mammalian working myocardium. Evidence from aequorin-loaded ferret ventricular muscles. *J Clin Invest* 1994;93:1275–1284.
72. Kirley TL. Determination of three disulfide bonds and one free sulfhydryl in the b-subunit of (Na,K)-ATPase. *J Biol Chem* 1989;264: 7185–7192.
73. Kofuji P, Hadley RW, Kieval RS, Lederer WJ, Schulze DH. Expression of the Na-Ca exchanger in diverse tissues: a study using the cloned human cardiac Na-Ca exchanger. *Am J Physiol* 1992;263: C1241–C1249.
74. Kohomoto O, Levi AJ, Bridge JH. Relation between reverse sodium-calcium exchange and sarcoplasmic reticulum calcium release in guinea pig ventricular cells. *Circ Res* 1994;74:550–554.
75. Le Grimellec C, Friedlander G, El Yandouzi EH, Zlatkine P, Giocondi M-C. Membrane fluidity and transport properties in epithelia. *Kidney Int* 1992;42:825–836.
76. LeBlanc N, Hume JR. Sodium current-induced release of calcium from cardiac sarcoplasmic reticulum. *Science* 1990;248:372–376.
77. Lee SL, Yu AS, Lytton J. Tissue-specific expression of Na^+-Ca^{2+} exchanger isoforms. *J Biol Chem* 1994;269:14849–14852.
78. Lees GJ. Inhibition of sodium-potassium-ATPase: a potentially ubiquitous mechanism contributing to central nervous system neuropathology. *Brain Res Rev* 1991;16:283–300.
79. Levi AJ, Spitzer KW, Kohmoto O, Bridge JH. Depolarization-induced Ca entry via Na-Ca exchange triggers SR release in guinea pig cardiac myocytes. *Am J Physiol* 1994;266:H1422–H1433.
80. Li Z, Matsuoka S, Hryshko LV, et al. Cloning of the NCX2 isoform of the plasma membrane Na^+-Ca^{2+} exchanger. *J Biol Chem* 1994;269: 17434–17439.
81. Li Z, Nicoll DA, Collins A, et al. Identification of a peptide inhibitor of the cardiac sarcolemmal Na^+-Ca^{2+} exhchanger. *J Biol Chem* 1991;266:1014–1020.
82. Lingrel JB, Kuntzweiler T. Na^+,K^+-ATPase. *J Biol Chem* 1994;269: 19659–19662.
83. Lingrel JB, Orlowski J, Price EM, Pathak BG. Regulation of the α-subunit genes of the Na,K-ATPase and determinants of cardiac glycoside sensitivity. In: Kaplan JH, De Weer P, eds. *The sodium pump: structure, mechanism, and regulation.* New York: Rockefeller University Press, 1991:1–16.
84. Lingrel JB, Orlowski J, Shull MM, Price EM. Molecular genetics of Na,K-ATPase. *Prog Nucleic Acid Res Mol Biol* 1990;38:37–89.
85. Lo CS, Klein LE. Thyroidal and steroidal regulation of Na^+,K^+-ATPase. *Semin Nephrol* 1992;12:62–66.
86. Luo W, Grupp IL, Harrer J, et al. Targeted ablation of the phospholamban gene is associated with markedly enhanced myocardial contractility and loss of β-agonist stimulation. *Circ Res* 1994;75: 401–409.
87. Luther PW, Yip RK, Bloch RJ, Ambesi A, Lindenmayer GE, Blaustein MP. Presynaptic localization of sodium/calcium exchangers in neuromuscular preparations. *J Neurosci* 1992;12:4898–4904.
88. Lytton J, Westlin M, Burk SE, Shull GE, MacLennan DH. Functional comparisons between isoforms of the sarcoplasmic reticulum or endoplasmic reticulum family of calcium pumps. *J Biol Chem* 1992;267:14483–14489.
89. MacLennan DH, Toyofuku T, Lytton J. Structure-function relationships in sarcoplasmic or endoplasmic reticulum type Ca^{2+} pumps. *Ann NY Acad Sci* 1992;671:1–10.
90. Martin DC, Adams RJ, Aronstam RS. The influence of isoflurane on the synaptic activity of 5-hydroxytryptamine. *Neurochem Res* 1990; 15:969–973.
91. Martin DC, Adams RJ, Introna RPS. Halothane inhibits 5-hydroxytryptamine uptake by synaptosomes from rat brain. *Neuropharmacology* 1990;29:9–16.
92. Martin DC, Introna RP, Aronstam RS. Inhibition of neuronal 5-HT uptake by ketamine, but not halothane, involves disruption of substrate recognition by the transporter. *Neurosci Lett* 1990;112:99–103.
93. Marver D. Regulation of Na^+,K^+-ATPase by aldosterone. *Semin Nephrol* 1992;12:56–61.
94. Matsuoka S, Nicoll DA, Reilly RF, Hilgeman DW, Philipson KD. Initial localization of regulatory regions of the cardiac sarcolemmal Na^+-Ca^{2+} exchanger. *Proc Natl Acad Sci USA* 1993;90:3870–3874.
95. Mazzanti L, Rabini RA, Staffolani R, Benedetti G, Cester N, Lenaz G. Modifications induced by general anesthetics on Na^+/K^+ ATPase obtained from human placenta. *Biochem Biophys Res Commun* 1990; 173:1248–1251.
96. McDonough AA, Geering K, Farley R. The sodium pump needs its subunit. *FASEB J* 1990;4:1598–1605.
97. McDonough AA, Hensley CB, Azuma KK. Differential regulation of sodium pump isoforms in heart. *Semin Nephrol* 1992;12:49–55.
98. Meister B, Aperia A. Molecular mechanisms involved in catecholamine regulation of sodium transport. *Semin Nephrol* 1993;13: 41–49.
99. Mercer RW, Biemesderfer D, Bliss DP Jr, Collins JH, Forbush B III. Molecular cloning and characterization of a γ subunit for the Na^+,K^+-ATPase. *J Physiol* 1990;96:4A–5A (abstr.).
100. Miller RP, Farley RA. All three potential *N*-glycosylation sites of the dog kidney (Na^+-K^+)-ATPase β-subunit contain oligosaccharide. *Biochim Biophys Acta* 1988;954:50–57.
101. Minezaki KK, Chapman RA. The role of the sodium pump and sodium-calcium exchange in recovery from calcium overload in guinea pig ventricular myocytes. *Exp Physiol* 1993;78:545–548.
102. Nelson TE, Sweo T. Ca^{2+} uptake and Ca^{2+} release by skeletal muscle sarcoplasmic reticulum: differing sensitivity to inhalational anesthetics. *Anesthesiology* 1988;69:571–577.
103. Nicoll DA, Longoni S, Philipson KD. Molecular cloning and functional expression of the cardiac sarcolemmal Na^+-Ca^{2+} exchanger. *Science* 1990;250:562–565.

104. Nishikawa T, Shimizu S-I. Inhibition of noradrenaline release from cerebrocortical synaptosomes and stimulation of synaptosomal Na^+,K^+-ATPase activity by morphine in rats. *J Pharm Pharmacol* 1990;42:68–71.
105. Nishikawa T, Teramoto T, Shimizu S-I. Effect of morphine on Na^+,K^+-ATPase from homogenate of synaptosomes and of synaptic mem brane of rat cerebral cortex. *Brain Res* 1990;510:92–96.
106. Noguchi SK, Higashi K, Kawamura M. A possible role of the β-subunit of Na,K-ATPase in facilitating correct assembly of the α-subunit into the membrane. *J Biol Chem* 1990;265:15991–15995.
107. Noguchi S, Ohta T, Takeda K, Ohtsubo M, Kawamura M. Ouabain sensitivity of a chimeric a subunit (*Torpedo*/Rat) of the (Na,K) ATPase expressed in *Xenopus* oocyte. *Biochem Biophys Res Commun* 1988;155:1237–1243.
108. Paroli L, Blanck TJJ. Effect of halothane on the Na^+-Ca^{2+}exchanger in isolated adult rat cardiac myocytes. *Anesth Analg* (in press).
109. Pedersen PL, Carafoli E. Ion motive ATPase. I. Uniquity, properties, and significance to cell function. *Trends Biochem Sci* 1987;12: 146–150.
110. Philipson KD, Nicoll DA. Molecular and kinetic aspects of sodium-calcium exchange. *Int Rev Cytol* 1993;137C:199–227.
111. Phillis JW. Na^+/K^+-ATPase as an effector of synaptic transmission. *Neurochem Int* 1992;20:19–22.
112. Pressley TA. Ionic regulation of Na^+,K^+-ATPase expression. *Semin Nephrol* 1992;12:67–71.
113. Price EM, Lingrel JB. Structure-function relationships in the Na,K-ATPase α subunit: site-directed mutagenesis of glutamine 111 to arginine and asparagine-122 to aspartic acid generates a ouabain-resistant enzyme. *Biochemistry* 1988;27:8400–8407.
114. Rayson BM. Rates of synthesis and degradation of Na^+-K^+-ATPase during chronic ouabain treatment. *Am J Physiol* 1989;256: C75–C80.
115. Rayson BM, Gupta RK. Steroids, intracellular sodium levels, and Na^+/K^+-ATPase regulation. *J Biol Chem* 1985;260:12740–12743.
116. Reuter H, Seitz N. The dependence of calcium efflux from cardiac muscle on temperature and external ion composition. *J Physiol (Lond)* 1968;195:451–470.
117. Rodrigo R, Novoa E. Is the renal (Na-K)-ATPase modulated by intracellular messengers? *Acta Physiol Pharmacol Ther Latinoam* 1992;42:87–104.
118. Rodriguez de Lores Arnaiz G. Neuronal Na^+,K^+-ATPase and its regulation by catecholamines. In: Caputto R, Ajmone Marsan C, eds. *Neural transmission, learning and memory.* New York: Raven Press, 1983:147–158.
119. Rodriguez de Lores Arnaiz G. In search of synaptosomal Na^+,K^+-ATPase regulators. *Mol Neurobiol* 1993;6:359–375.
120. Rodriguez de Lores Arnaiz G, Antonelli de Gomez de Lima M. The effect of several neurotransmitter substances on nerve ending membrane ATPase. *Acta Physiol Pharmacol Ther Latinoam* 1981; 31:39–44.
121. Rodriguez de Lores Arnaiz G, Mistrorigo de Pacheco M. Regulation of (Na^+,K^+) adenosine triphosphatase of nerve ending membranes: action of norepinephrine and a soluble factor. *Neurochem Res* 1978;3:733–744.
122. Rudnick G, Wall SC. The molecular mechanism of ecstasy [3,4-methylenedioxymethamphetamine (MDMA)]: serotonin transporters are targets for MDMA-induced serotonin release. *Proc Natl Acad Sci USA* 1992;89:1817–1821.
123. Sanchez-Armass S, Blaustein MP. Role of sodium-calcium exchange in regulation of intracellular calcium in nerve terminals. *Am J Physiol* 1987;252:C595–C603.
124. Schulte L, Peters D, Taylor J, Navarro J, Kandarian S. Sarcoplasmic reticulum Ca^{2+} pump expression in denervated skeletal muscle. *Am J Physiol* 1994;267:C617–C622.
125. Sharma HS, Verdouw PD, Lamers JM. Involvement of the sarcoplasmic reticulum calcium pump in myocardial contractile dysfunction: comparison between chronic pressure-overload and stunning. *Cardiovasc Drugs Ther* 1994;8:461–468.
126. Sherman J, Morimoto T, Sabatini DD. Biosynthesis of Na,K-ATPase in MDCK cells. *Curr Top Membr Transp* 1983;19:753–764.
127. Shieh BH, Xia Y, Sparkes RS, et al. Mapping of the gene for the cardiac sarcolemmal Na^+-Ca^{2+} exchanger to human chromosome 2p21-p23. *Genomics* 1992;12:616–617.
128. Shimoni Y, Gotsman M, Deutsch J, Kachalsky S, Lichtstein D. Endogenous ouabain-like compound increases heart muscle contractility. *Nature* 1984;307:369–371.
129. Siegl PK, Cragoe EJ Jr, Trumble MJ, Kaczorowski GJ. Inhibition of Na^+/Ca^{2+} exchange in membrane vesicle and papillary muscle preparations from guinea pig heart by analogs of amiloride. *Proc Natl Acad Sci USA* 1984;81:3238–3242.
130. Skou JC. The influence of some cations on an adenosine triphosphatase from peripheral nerves. *Biochim Biophys Acta* 1957;23: 394–401.
131. Staffolani R, Cester N, Magnanelli R, et al. Local anaesthetic effects on trophoblast membrane fluidity. *Biochem Mol Biol Int* 1993;29:527–530.
132. Sweadner KJ. Isozymes of the Na,K-ATPase. *Biochim Biophys Acta* 1989;988:185–220.
133. Sweadner KJ. Overview: subunit diversity in the Na,K-ATPase. In: Kaplan JH, De Weer P, eds. *The sodium pump: structure, mechanism, and regulation.* New York: Rockefeller University Press, 1991:63–76.
134. Sweadner KJ. Overlapping and diverse distribution of Na-K ATPase isozymes in neurons and glia. *Can J Physiol Pharmacol* 1991; 70:S255–S259.
135. Tamkun MM, Fambrough DM. The (Na^++K^+)-ATPase of chick sensory neurons: studies on biosynthesis and intracellular transport. *J Biol Chem* 1986;261:1009–1019.
136. Tamura M, Lam TT, Inagami T. Isolation and characterization of a specific endogenous Na^+,K^+-ATPase inhibitor from bovine adrenal. *Biochemistry* 1988;27:4244–4253.
137. Thomas R, Gray P, Andrews J. Digitalis: its mode of action, receptor, and structure-activity relationships. *Adv Drug Res* 1989;19: 311–561.
138. Toyofuku T, Kurzydloruski K, Tuda M, MacLennan DH. Identification of regions of the Ca^{2+}-ATPase of sarcoplasmic reticulum that affect functional association with phospholamban. *J Biol Chem* 1993;268:2809–2815.
139. Vasallo PM, Dackowski W, Emanuel JR, Levenson R. Identification of a putative isoform of the Na,K-ATPase beta subunit: primary structure and tissue specific expression. *J Biol Chem* 1989;264: 4613–4618.
140. Vasilets LA, Schwarz W. Structure-function relationships of cation binding in the Na^+/K^+-ATPase. *Biochim Biophys Acta* 1993;1154: 201–222.
141. Voss JC, Mahaney JE, Jones LR, Thomas DD. Molecular dynamics in mouse atrial tumor sarcoplasmic reticulum. *Biophys J* 1995;68: 1787–1795.
142. Wolitzky BA, Fambrough DM. Regulation of the $(Na^+$-$K^+)$-ATPase in cultured chick skeletal muscle. *J Biol Chem* 1986;261:9990–9999.
143. Wu KD, Lytton J. Molecular cloning and quantification of sarcoplasmic reticulum Ca^{2+}-ATPase isoforms in rat muscles. *Am J Physiol* 1993;264:C333–C341.

Anesthesia: Biologic Foundations, edited by Tony L. Yaksh et al. Lippincott–Raven Publishers, Philadelphia © 1997.

CHAPTER 19

MECHANISM OF SYNAPTIC TRANSMITTER RELEASE

CYNTHIA K. DAMER AND CARL E. CREUTZ

The transmission of the nerve impulse across chemical synapses is a physiologic function on which present and future anesthetics may act. To fully understand how anesthetic agents may influence neurotransmission in molecular terms it is essential to define the molecular basis of this process. This chapter summarizes recent advances in our understanding of exocytosis of neurotransmitter at the nerve terminal.

In the last several years a remarkable convergence of disparate research themes has occurred that sheds light on the protein molecules involved in exocytosis in neurons (for reviews see refs. 22,52,99,108,134,169). This convergence has involved research in four major areas that progressed independently during the past 15 years:

- Characterization of the protein components of synaptic vesicle membranes
- Biochemical analysis of the factors necessary for vesicular traffic in in vitro models of Golgi function
- Genetic analysis of the secretory pathway in yeast
- Functional analysis of the mechanism of action of clostridial neurotoxins

Proteins discovered in each of these areas of research have proven to be the same or homologous, thus providing powerful corroborating evidence for their involvement in the basic steps underlying neurotransmitter release. Although much remains to be learned about the molecular details of the interactions of these proteins, it seems clear that many of the essential players in neuroexocytosis have now been identified. This chapter reviews the discoveries made in these different research areas and indicates how they support the current, developing model for the mechanism of transmitter release.

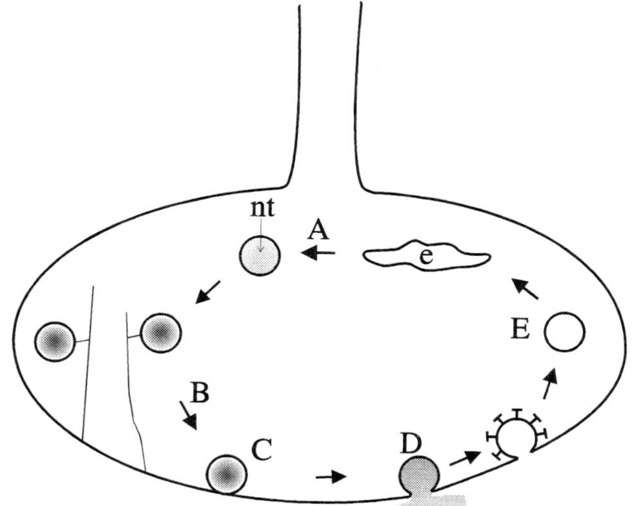

Figure 1. Life cycle of the synaptic vesicle. A: Vesicles bud off endosomal compartment (e) and are filled with neurotransmitter (nt). B: Vesicles are released from cytoskeleton and translocate to plasma membrane. C: Vesicles dock to plasma membrane. D: Vesicles fuse with plasma membrane discharging neurotransmitter into synaptic cleft. E: Vesicle membranes are endocytosed by clathrin-coated pits and recycled through the endosomal compartment. (Adapted from ref.52, with permission.)

OVERVIEW OF NEUROEXOCYTOSIS

Neurons exhibit one of the most complicated and intricately regulated secretory pathways (Fig. 1). Communication between neurons and their target cells takes place at synapses, where most synaptic transmission is mediated by an exocytotic release of neurotransmitter from the presynaptic cell. Neurotransmitters are stored in small electron-lucent synaptic vesicles in the presynaptic terminal. The current and longstanding model of synaptic vesicle exocytosis begins with the action potential reaching the nerve terminal, causing plasma membrane depolarization. Consequently, voltage-gated calcium channels open and produce a rise in intracellular calcium. The fusion of synaptic vesicles docked to the plasma membrane is triggered by the calcium influx and results in the release of transmitter into the synaptic cleft (106). Synaptic vesicle membranes are then recycled from the plasma membrane by endocytosis and ultimately refilled with neurotransmitter (107).

SYNAPTIC VESICLE PROTEINS

One of the key approaches to develop an understanding of the mechanism of neurotransmitter release has been to identify and characterize the proteins on the synaptic vesicles themselves. Many synaptic vesicle proteins have been identified. While some of these proteins have turned out to be transport proteins, such as channels and pumps necessary for uptake and storage of transmitter, several of those identified appear to function in the targeting, docking, and fusion of vesicles in synaptic vesicle exocytosis. These proteins are discussed in the sections below and illustrated schematically in Fig. 2.

Synapsin

Synapsins, a family of proteins first discovered as the major proteins phosphorylated in synaptic membrane fractions upon addition of adenosine 3',5'-cyclic monophosphate (cAMP) (101), are specific to synaptic vesicles in neurons (136) and bind to several proteins of the cytoskeleton (80). This has led to the proposed role of the synapsins in immobilizing synaptic vesicles in the cytoskeleton and regulating their availability for release. Synapsin I (a collective name for two nearly identical polypeptides, synapsin Ia and synapsin Ib) is composed of two major domains, a collagenase-resistant NH_2-terminal head domain rich in hydrophobic amino acids and a collagenase-sensitive COOH-terminal tail domain rich in proline and glycine (186). Molecular cloning of synapsins Ia and Ib led to the discovery of two more homologous proteins, synapsins IIa and IIb (186) (previously referred to as synaptic vesicle proteins IIIa and IIIb) (30). The messenger RNAs (mRNAs) of these four homologous proteins are generated by the differential splicing of two genes. Each synapsin has a common homologous amino-terminal domain and a distinct carboxyl-terminal domain (186).

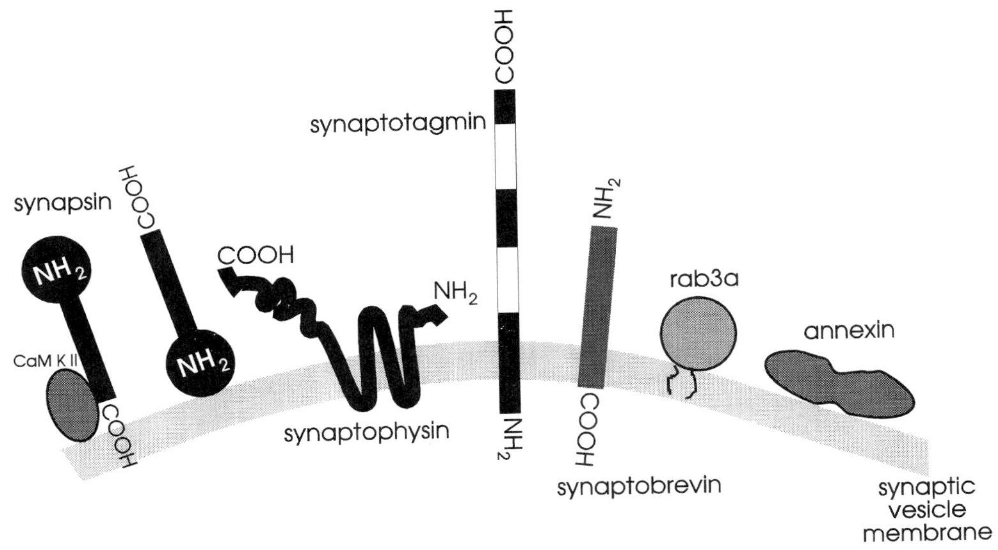

Figure 2. Synaptic vesicle membrane proteins. (Adapted from ref. 52, with permission.)

Synapsin I is found only in neurons (58), specifically associated with the cytoplasmic side of small synaptic vesicles (59,97), and absent from the large, dense-core vesicles (LDCVs) of neurons (136). Synapsins IIa and IIb are found in both neurons and the chromaffin cells of the adrenal medulla. Although subcellular fractionation studies localize synapsin II to the synaptic vesicle fraction in brain, further studies need to be done to determine its specific localization within the chromaffin cells (30). Immunostaining using monoclonal antibodies to the four synapsins produces a pattern that is similar for all of the synapsins; however, staining intensity of distinct nerve terminal populations in the brain are different for the four antisera (186).

All four synapsins have the same amino-terminal serine phosphorylation site for cAMP-dependent protein kinase and calcium/calmodulin protein kinase I (CaM kinase I) (51,186). Synapsins Ia/Ib have three additional phosphorylation sites in the carboxyl terminal domain: two different sites for the calcium/calmodulin protein kinase II (CaM kinase II) (96), and one site in the proline-rich tail for proline-directed protein kinase (84). All four synapsins are phosphorylated upon excitation of the nerve terminal (199), and synapsin II is phosphorylated in chromaffin cells upon stimulus-coupled catecholamine release (68).

Early studies report that synaptic vesicles contain a specific, saturable, and high-affinity site for synapsin I (174). This interaction was thought to be electrostatic in nature and to involve the tail region of synapsin I. Phosphorylation at the COOH-terminal sites resulted in a fivefold decrease in the binding affinity of synapsin I for synaptic vesicles (174). Consistent with these findings, quick-freeze deep-etch electron microscopy of the nerve terminal revealed short, fine strands linking synaptic vesicles to other synaptic vesicles, actin, and microtubules (89). In these micrographs, the synaptic vesicles appear to be linked, possibly by synapsin, to actin with the "head" on the actin and the "tail" on the synaptic vesicle.

In contrast, studies using synapsin I fragments obtained by cysteine-specific cleavage show that the head domain actively binds to acidic phospholipids and the tail domain does not significantly interact with phospholipids (15,16). Yet, the cysteine-specific cleavage tail fragment of synapsin I binds with relatively high affinity to synaptic vesicles (15). This binding is greatly decreased by phosphorylation in the tail region and abolished by high ionic strength. The data suggest the existence of two sites of interaction between synapsin I and small synaptic vesicles. The head domain interacts with vesicle phospholipids and the tail domain binds to a protein component on the vesicle membrane (15). Indeed, it has been reported that the binding of the tail domain of synapsin I to synaptic vesicles involves the regulatory domain of a synaptic-vesicle associated form of CaM kinase II (18). This suggests that a form of CaM kinase II not only functions to phosphorylate synapsin I, but also functions as a binding protein for synapsin I.

In vitro studies show synapsin I binds to several elements of the cytoskeleton, including spectrin, microtubules, and microfilaments (7,80). Synapsin I has actin bundling activity and phosphorylation appears to regulate the binding to actin filaments. The amount of synapsin I bound to filamentous actin (F-actin) as measured by co-sedimentation of actin and synapsin I is reduced with the phosphorylation of synapsin I by CaM kinase II at the COOH-terminal sites, while little effect is observed with the phosphorylation by cAMP-dependent protein kinase in the NH_2-terminal sites (6,158). Synapsin I has also been shown to cause a concentration-dependent increase in the formation of actin filaments in vitro (17). Synapsin I decreases the value of the critical concentration of actin in a dose-dependent fashion and has major effects on the kinetics of actin polymerization by suppressing the lag phase and increasing the initial rate of polymerization. This effect on actin polymerization is also present for the vesicle-bound form of synapsin I. Phosphorylation of synapsin I in the head region or the tail region abolishes its ability to increase the number of actin filaments. This is in contrast to the actin-bundling activity of synapsin I in which phosphorylation in the head region has no effect. Presumably synapsin I is able to bind actin filaments as characterized earlier (6,158), but, in addition, can bind actin monomers resulting in pseudonuclei that actively elongate (17). Considering function inside the cell, dephosphorylated synapsin I bound to synaptic vesicles may induce the growth of actin filaments from the vesicles, causing the vesicles to be embedded in an actin network, and therefore, not available for exocytosis (17).

The synapsins have been hypothesized to regulate the availability of synaptic vesicles for exocytosis in a phosphorylation-dependent manner. Phosphorylation of synapsins, by inhibiting new actin filament growth and decreasing the binding of synapsins to vesicles and actin filaments, would facilitate the release of vesicles from the cytoskeleton and make them available for exocytosis. Several microinjection studies provide evidence for this hypothesis. Presynaptic injection of dephosphorylated synapsin I inhibits neurotransmitter release in the squid giant synapse, while phosphorylation of the tail sites alone or head and tail sites prevents synapsin I from inhibiting release (120). CaM kinase II injected presynaptically facilitates transmitter release (120). Similarly, introduction of dephosphorylated synapsin I into rat brain synaptosomes decreases the K^+-induced release of glutamate, whereas introduction of synapsin I phosphorylated by CaM kinase II has no effect on glutamate release (139).

The goldfish Mauthner synapse has a large presynaptic axon that displays quantal synaptic transmission. Presynaptic injection of synapsin I into Mauthner axons results in a decrease in synaptic transmission and a significant decrease in the number of quantal units available for release, with no change in the probability of release or the amount of transmitter per quantum (83). Synapsin I could inhibit transmitter release by binding to synaptic vesicles and thereby removing them from the releasable pool.

In synaptosomes, the stoichiometry of phosphorylation of synapsin I is much higher in the soluble fraction than in the particulate fraction under resting conditions. Upon depolarization and the entry of calcium, there is a rapid translocation of synapsin I from the particulate to the cytosolic fraction and an accompanying twofold increase in the stoichiometry of phosphorylation of the soluble synapsin I (181). This is consistent with the hypothesis that upon depolarization synapsin I becomes phosphorylated and dissociates from the synaptic vesicles, leaving them free for fusion. In mouse retinal ganglion cells, synapsin I, moving along the axon with the slow component of axonal transport, is phosphorylated in vivo at both its head and tail regions (157). Once the synapsin I reaches the nerve endings, synapsin I exists predominantly in less phosphorylated forms. Phosphorylation could be functioning to prevent synapsin from binding to or forming actin filaments, which would restrict its movement. Once it arrives at the nerve terminal the phosphorylation of synapsin I may regulate the clustering of synaptic vesicles and their availability for exocytosis.

Although synapsin appears to have a role in neurotransmitter release, several facts argue against its role as an integral part of the machinery for rapid transmitter release. The onset of transmitter release in the squid giant synapse begins as soon as 180 μs following calcium entry and peaks at about 1 msec (121). However, the turnover rate for the phosphorylation of synapsin I by CaM kinase II is approximately 17 msec (119). This relatively slow phosphorylation reaction could not produce the time course associated with a postsynaptic potential. If synapsin is not directly involved in vesicular release, then why is calcium involved in its regulation? Llinás et al. (119) propose that calcium entry triggers two events. First, calcium could trigger fusion of vesicles already docked at the presynaptic membrane by binding to a protein. Second, a delayed effect independent of the release mechanism could occur after calcium had moved beyond the release site, by increasing the number of releasable vesicles following phosphorylation of synapsin I via activation of CaM kinase II. This delayed effect of calcium may be part of the phenomenon known as synaptic potentiation.

Synapsin has been implicated in a form of synaptic enhancement that resembles long-term potentiation (LTP) produced by norepinephrine (NE) (151). NE can produce an increase in transmitter release and enhance the phosphorylation of synapsin I and synapsin II in the dentate gyrus in hippocampal slices from young rats. Dentate slices from aged rats have shown a decreased sensitivity to NE and an impairment in their ability to exhibit LTP. NE does not stimulate synapsin phosphorylation in slices prepared from aged rats and the basal level of phosphorylation of synapsin is higher. This NE-stimulated phosphorylation of synapsin I and II in young rats may cause the increase in transmitter release produced by NE in the dentate, while the decrease in synapsin phosphorylation in aged rats may play some role in the deficits in plasticity seen in aged rats.

Mutant mice that do not express synapsin I have no apparent changes in overall nervous system structure and function (168). However, electrophysiologic studies on hippocampal slices from mutant mice reveal a significant enhancement of paired pulse facilitation, a decrease in paired pulse depression, and no changes in other synaptic parameters such as LTP. This suggests that synapsin I may function in short-term plasticity by limiting the increase in neurotransmitter caused by residual calcium after an initial stimulus (168).

Synaptophysin

Synaptophysin is a 38,000-dalton, glycosylated, integral membrane protein found on small synaptic vesicles (98,206). Synaptophysin has four membrane-spanning regions with both the amino and carboxyl termini cytoplasmic (103,111). Sequence comparisons among rat, bovine, and human synaptophysin reveal that only the intravesicular domains have a number of amino acid substitutions, while the transmembrane and the cytoplasmic sequences are highly conserved (103). The carboxyl terminus is a unique structure containing 9 or 10 copies of a tyrosine- and proline-rich tetrapeptide repeat (103,111). Originally, synaptophysin was reported to bind calcium on its cytoplasmic region (166); however, recently no calcium-binding ability has been detected (29).

Synaptophysin is expressed in neuronal and many endocrine cells. Although some controversy still remains, synaptophysin is thought to be absent from the large chromaffin granules and present on the small clear microvesicles (SLMVs) in chromaffin cells (72,122,137,145). Related proteins have been cloned, indicating the existence of a synaptophysin-like family of proteins. Synaptoporin, a 37-kd protein, displays 58% amino acid identity to synaptophysin, with highly conserved transmembrane regions and a divergent carboxyl terminal tail, although both proteins have tails with repeated amino acid sequences. This novel protein is also expressed in neurons and localized to synaptic vesicles (110), but has more of a restricted expression confined mainly to forebrain structures (125). A cDNA encoding a protein called HL-5 has been cloned from a human erythroleukemia cell cDNA library. The HL-5 clone has 54% sequence identity to synaptophysin, but lacks the C-terminal cytoplasmic tail (215). Monoclonal antibodies made to a transmembrane protein isolated from synaptic vesicles called p29 cross-react with synaptophysin, indicating that the two proteins have related epitopes (12). Like synaptophysin, p29 is tyrosine phosphorylated by an endogenous tyrosine kinase activity in intact vesicles and has similar tissue distribution. Two additional proteins have serologic cross-reactivity with synaptophysin; these have been named leukophysin and granulophysin and are expressed in leukocytes and dense granules of human platelets, respectively (3).

When isolated synaptic vesicles are allowed to undergo phosphorylation by endogenous kinases, tyrosines on synaptophysin are the major substrate phosphorylated (150). The tyrosine protein kinase $pp60^{c\text{-}src}$ is expressed in the central nervous system and is specifically associated with synaptic vesicles in neurons and synaptic-like vesicles in the endocrine PC12 cells (118). Recent evidence suggests synaptophysin is a physiologic substrate for $pp60^{c\text{-}src}$. The elimination of $pp60^{c\text{-}src}$ from vesicle extracts by immunoprecipitation abolishes tyrosine phosphorylation of synaptophysin and leaves phosphorylation of serine residues unchanged (10). CaM kinase II, which phosphorylates synapsin I, may be responsible for serine phosphorylation of synaptophysin (150,170). Depolarization of rat cerebrocortical slices and synaptosomes produces an rapid increase in serine phosphorylation of synaptophysin. The addition of calcium plus calmodulin to purified synaptic vesicles results in a fourfold increase in serine phosphorylation of synaptophysin. This phosphorylation can be inhibited by a peptide inhibitor of CaM kinase II. Purified rat brain CaM kinase II phosphorylates purified synaptophysin and vesicle-associated synaptophysin. The resulting chymotryptic phosphopeptide maps are similar to those maps obtained from synaptophysin phosphorylated in cerebrocortical slices, suggesting synaptophysin is a physiologic substrate for CaM kinase II (170).

A study of the interaction of synaptic vesicles with solubilized rat brain synaptosomes led to the identification of a 36-kd protein that binds to synaptic vesicles (189). This binding to synaptic vesicles can be inhibited competitively by synaptophysin, suggesting a specific interaction between the 36-kd protein and synaptophysin. Because of its affinity to synaptophysin, this newly identified protein was named physophilin. The interaction between vesicle-bound synaptophysin and solubilized physophilin is not affected by calcium ions, guanosine triphosphate (GTPγS), or adenosine triphosphate (ATP). Attempts to isolate physophilin by affinity chromatography using immobilized synaptophysin as a ligand have been unsuccessful. Indeed, physophilin may be part of a large complex of proteins and additional components may be needed for binding. Physophilin is present in the synaptic plasma membrane prepared from synaptosomes, but not in the synaptic vesicles themselves. After the identification of physophilin, syntaxins were discovered as proteins that bind to synaptotagmin (19). Syntaxins have a molecular weight of 35 kd and are also found in the plasma membrane. It is possible that physophilin and syntaxins are the same protein, which interacts with a complex containing synaptotagmin and synaptophysin.

Reconstitution of synaptophysin into planar lipid bilayers results in voltage-sensitive channel activity with an average conductance of 154 picosiemens (pS) (190). These studies, along with cross-linking studies, led to the proposal that synaptophysin is functionally similar to the gap junction protein, connexin. Connexin, like synaptophysin, spans the membrane four times with both its amino and carboxyl termini on the cytoplasmic surface and forms homo-oligomers; their similarities in topology led to the speculation that synaptophysin may form a transmembrane channel in the same way that connexin forms gap junctions. Cross-linking of synaptic vesicles produces a homodimer of synaptophysin, while cross-linking of purified synaptophysin results in homo-oligomeric structures containing three to six molecules (166,190). Thomas et al. (190) reported that cross-linking of synaptophysin resulted in a 220-kd adduct, formed by six synaptophysin molecules, similar to the hexameric configuration of gap junctions. Contrary to this, Johnston and Südhof (104) reported that purifying synaptophysin in the presence of detergents leads to intermolecular cross-linking through disulfide bonds not found in native synaptophysin. They argue that synaptophysin contains unstable intramolecular disulfide bonds that undergo disulfide exchange during solubilization, resulting in the covalent cross-linking of nearby synaptophysin molecules. They conclude that native synaptophysin does not form hexamers, as reported by Thomas et al., but that synaptophysin molecules isolated in nondenaturing conditions form tri- and tetrameric homopolymers linked by noncovalent forces. Südhof and Jahn (187) propose that synaptophysin does not function like a gap junction, but instead is involved in the formation of an unstable fusion pore like that described in mast cell exocytosis.

A novel technique has recently been utilized to study the function of synaptophysin inside the cell (4). *Xenopus* oocytes injected with total rat cerebellar mRNA are capable of secreting the excitatory neurotransmitter glutamate in a calcium-dependent manner. This may provide a convenient assay to study the molecular components necessary for neurotransmitter secretion. Synaptophysin was shown to be present in a punctate pattern in the oocyte cytoplasm by immunofluorescence and associated with small clear vesicles by immunoelectron microscopy. These vesicles were also present in control, uninjected oocytes; however, they were not labeled by synaptophysin antibodies. This is consistent with the findings that synaptophysin incorporates into preexisting vesicles in nonneuronal cells transfected with synaptophysin cDNA (38,102,112,117). When antisense oligonucleotides to synaptophysin message are co-injected with total mRNA, synaptophysin expression is blocked and calcium-dependent secretion is reduced to an average of 38% of that observed for oocytes injected with mRNA alone. Co-injection of synaptophysin antibody produces a reduction of secretion to 13% of control. This is the first experiment that provides evidence for a functional role for synaptophysin in transmitter secretion.

Synaptotagmin

Synaptotagmin is a 65-kd integral membrane protein, localized to secretory vesicles, that interacts with several proteins of the presynaptic membrane and binds phospholipids in a calcium-dependent manner. Several studies suggest that synaptotagmin is a key protein in the process of regulated exocytosis. Synaptotagmin has a small glycosylated amino-terminal intravesicular domain and a single transmembrane region. This is followed by a large cytoplasmic domain containing two copies of a sequence homologous to the C2-regulatory region of protein kinase C (PKC) and a small conserved carboxyl terminal domain. A small domain separating the transmembrane region from the two homologous repeats is predicted to form an amphipathic α-helix (153). The cytoplasmic region is conserved in evolution, most notably in the PKC-homologous repeats (153–155).

Synaptotagmin I appears to form multimers; Western blot analysis often results in the specific immunolabeling of a 130-kd protein, representing a synaptotagmin dimer partially resistant to SDS denaturation. On sucrose gradients, synaptotagmin I migrates in a nondenaturing detergent as a single peak with a high-molecular weight of approximately 220,000, suggesting synaptotagmin forms a complex of four subunits (153).

A single threonine located between the transmembrane region and the C2 domain repeats is phosphorylated by casein kinase II in vitro (56). Several lines of evidence suggest synaptotagmin is phosphorylated by casein kinase II in vivo. Casein kinase II can be immunoprecipitated with a synaptotagmin antibody from a synaptic vesicle-enriched fraction from rat brain. Affinity chromatography shows that casein kinase II interacts with synaptotagmin at the carboxyl terminal half of the cytoplasmic domain (21). Sequences around threonine-128 in rat synaptotagmin match the consensus sequence for casein kinase II (S/T-X-X-E/D). Casein kinase II activity can be inhibited by heparin and stimulated by polyamines. Yet, polylysine does not stimulate phosphorylation of synaptotagmin by casein kinase II. However, phosphorylation of a recombinant fragment not containing the polylysine region of synaptotagmin (11 lysines over 19 amino acids preceding the phosphorylation site) is stimulated by polylysine (56). This suggests that the polylysine region of synaptotagmin is a natural stimulatory site for casein kinase II. Casein kinase II is present in high concentrations in the hippocampus and has been shown to be rapidly activated during LTP (40). However, it has not yet been demonstrated that synaptotagmin is phosphorylated in vivo, nor whether the phosphorylation regulates synaptotagminís sensitivity to calcium, dimerization, or interactions with other proteins.

Several isoforms of synaptotagmin exist. Synaptotagmin I, II, and III are found in rat and have been cloned, and the two C2 domains are highly conserved among the isoforms (76,133,154). The three proteins have different distributions; synaptotagmin I is preferentially expressed in the cerebral cortex and hippocampus, synaptotagmin II is primarily expressed in phylogenetically old parts of the brain and absent from the adrenal medulla, and synaptotagmin III is expressed in both neuronal and endocrine cells (76,133). A fourth isoform has also been cloned from mouse brain (88), and the marine ray *Discopyge ommata* genome contains three synaptotagmin-related genes that are differentially expressed (202).

Immunocytochemical studies show that synaptotagmin I is widely distributed in nerve terminals of neuronal and neural secretory tissues and is probably present in every type of neuronal terminal. Synaptotagmin I is specifically localized to secretory vesicles including synaptic vesicles, large dense core vesicles in neurons, chromaffin granules, and small microvesicles in chromaffin cells (71,72,122,129).

Synaptotagmin interacts with several proteins localized to the presynaptic membrane suggesting that synaptotagmin, which is found on secretory vesicle membranes, is involved in docking the vesicle to the plasma membrane through protein-protein interactions. Synaptotagmin is reported to bind specifically to the plasma membrane receptor protein for α-latrotoxin (156). α-Latrotoxin is a vertebrate neurotoxin from black widow spider venom that binds to presynaptic nerve terminals and triggers massive neurotransmitter release. The binding of the α-latrotoxin receptor to synaptotagmin is calcium independent and of moderate affinity. Binding is mediated by a small 34-amino acid sequence at the highly conserved carboxyl terminus of synaptotagmin (152). Phosphorylation of synaptotagmin is potently inhibited by low concentrations of the α-latrotoxin receptor (156). The α-latrotoxin receptor is a member of a family of brain-specific cell surface proteins termed neurexins (195).

There are at least two different neurexin genes that produce multiple differentially spliced transcripts. Neurexins contain a single transmembrane region and an amino terminal extracellular domain that consists of repeats of sequences, each containing an epidermal growth factor (EGF) domain. These extracellular domains have homology with repeated sequences found in laminin A, slit, and agrin, which are extracellular matrix proteins implicated in axonal guidance and synaptogenesis (195). Given that neurexins have extracellular domains similar to extracellular matrix proteins, it is possible that neurexins align synaptic vesicles, through contacts with synaptotagmin, with structures in the extracellular matrix.

Two other proteins that interact with synaptotagmin have been identified by coimmunoprecipitation with a monoclonal antibody to synaptotagmin (19). These proteins, called syntaxins (also referred to as HPC-1) (212), are both 35 kd and are 85% identical to one another in sequence. The carboxyl terminal domain is very hydrophobic and serves as a transmembrane region, while the amino-terminus is cytoplasmic. Immunofluorescence microscopy of cultured hippocampal cells indicates syntaxins are localized to the synaptic plasma membrane concentrated at contacts between varicosities consistent with staining of active zones.

Since the initial identification of syntaxin A and B, several more isoforms have been cloned. A family of syntaxin-related proteins have been identified that shares 23% to 84% amino acid identity (20). These syntaxins display a broad tissue distribution and are targeted to distinct subcellular compartments. Syntaxin A and B [renamed syntaxin 1A and 1B(20)] are exclusively expressed in brain and syntaxins 2 and 5 are ubiquitously expressed. Syntaxin 3 is primarily expressed in heart, spleen, lung, and kidney, while syntaxin 4 is expressed in heart, skeletal muscle, and kidney. Four of the five syntaxins are localized to the plasma membrane, while syntaxin 5 appears to be targeted to cytoplasmic vesicles that are distinct from the endoplasmic reticulum (ER) and partially overlapping with the Golgi (20). Soluble fragments of syntaxin and syntaxin antibodies injected into PC12 cells significantly reduce granule exocytosis (20).

Synaptotagmin appears to also form a complex with calcium channels (114). Pathogenic antibodies in patients with Lambert-Eaton myasthenic syndrome (LEMS), an autoimmune disease of the neuromuscular junction, seem to down-regulate presynaptic calcium channels, causing reduced acetylcholine release and muscle weakness. Immunoglobulin G (IgG) fractions from LEMS patients immunoprecipitate a ω-conotoxin–labeled calcium channel complex solubilized from rat brain. The antigen in the complex was identified as synaptotagmin, indicating that synaptotagmin associates with ω-conotoxin-sensitive calcium channels to form a complex on the plasma membrane (114). However, a syntaxin antibody also immunoprecipitates ω-conotoxin–labeled N-type calcium channels from solubilized rat brain synaptosomes (19). Further investigation revealed that synaptotagmin is loosely bound to a more tightly interacting syntaxin-calcium channel complex (113).

Recently, it has been shown that synaptotagmin I is a high-affinity receptor for clathrin AP-2 in vitro (214). The fusion of synaptic vesicles during regulated exocytosis is followed by the rapid endocytosis of vesicle membranes mediated by clathrin coated pits. Coated pit assembly begins with the binding of the heterooligomeric protein complex, clathrin AP-2, to the inside surface of the plasma membrane. AP-2 binds with high affinity to a protein on the inside surface of fibroblasts. This binding site appears to recycle during receptor-mediated endocytosis. Investigators found that the AP-2 also binds with high affinity to synaptic vesicle membranes. This binding is mediated by synaptotagmin with the binding site in the second C2 domain. This study suggests that there may be other isoforms of synaptotagmin that are expressed outside the nervous system that function in coated pit assembly (214).

The large cytoplasmic domain of synaptotagmin is mostly composed of two repeats of sequences homologous to the C2 motif in protein kinase C (153). This C2 motif, found in several other proteins, including phospholipase A_2, *ras* guanosine triphosphatase (GTPase)-activating protein, phospholipase C, and rabphilin (209), has been proposed to be a calcium and phospholipid binding domain (42). Synaptotagmin does bind calcium and binds phospholipids in a calcium-dependent manner (29,154). Proteolytic fragments or recombinant fragments composed of only the cytoplasmic domain of synaptotagmin I bind to natural membranes and artificial liposomes containing negatively charged phospholipids (39,53,57). In addition, recombinant fragments composed of only the first C2 domain of synaptotagmin I can also bind to artificial liposomes made up of phosphatidylcholine with phosphatidylserine and phosphatidylinositol (39,53,57). Deletion of a highly conserved 9 amino acid sequence in the NH_2-terminal region of a fragment composed of only the first C2 domain abolishes calcium-dependent binding to phospholipid vesicles (39).

Several studies have been done to investigate synaptotagmin's proposed role in exocytosis in the cell (60,65,142,180). PC12 (pheochromocytoma) cell line variants that do not express synaptotagmin I or II are able to secrete catecholamines upon membrane depolarization with time courses and amounts similar to control cells. This led to the conclusion that synaptotagmin is not essential for exocytosis of the large dense core vesicles of PC12 cells (180). Yet, recently synaptotagmin III mRNA has been found in these PC12 clone variants, and this may explain why these cells can secrete (133). Antibodies to synaptotagmin and recombinant fragments composed of only the first C2 domain microinjected into PC12 cells decrease the K^+/Ca^{2+}-mediated secretion measured by dopamine hydroxylase surface staining, suggesting that synaptotagmin is important in PC12 secretion (65). Consistent with the idea that synaptotagmin is important in neurotransmitter release, peptides corresponding to conserved regions of the C2 domains of synaptotagmin injected into squid giant presynaptic terminals have been shown to produce a dramatic reduction in postsynaptic potential amplitude and rate of rise (26). Mutants in synaptotagmin have severely impaired synaptic transmission in *Drosophila* (60), *Caenorhabditis elegans* (142), and mice (78). It is clear from mutant studies that synaptotagmin has an important role in neurotransmitter release, but it is difficult to determine the specific role. The existence of other functioning isoforms further complicates the interpretation of these studies.

There are several hypotheses for the function of synaptotagmin in regulated exocytosis. First, synaptotagmin may regulate vesicle docking by keeping vesicles docked to the plasma membrane until fusion is triggered by the influx of calcium. This hypothesis is consistent with the *Drosophila* mutant studies, in which calcium-evoked junctional potentials are reduced, but the frequency of miniature potentials is increased. Second, synaptotagmin could function in the recycling of synaptic vesicles. This is consistent with the studies on the synaptotagmin mutant in *C. elegans,* where the number of synaptic vesicles in nerve terminals is vastly decreased. Alternatively, synaptotagmin may function as a low-affinity calcium receptor and promote calcium-triggered vesicle-plasma membrane fusion. This is consistent with results seen in the synaptotagmin I mutant mouse. In cultured hippocampal neurons from the mutant mice, the fast component of neurotransmitter release is decreased, with no effect on spontaneous miniature excitatory postsynaptic current frequency, and the number of synaptic vesicles in the terminals is not altered.

In summary, synaptotagmin may have multiple functions in the nerve terminal. Synaptotagmin interacts with several proteins localized to the presynaptic membrane (114,156,195), suggesting it may be involved in the regulation of vesicle docking. Yet, synaptotagmin binds phospholipids in a calcium-dependent manner, suggesting it may be involved in promoting membrane-membrane contact and fusion. Furthermore, clathrin AP-2 binds to synaptotagmin I, suggesting synaptotagmin is involved in vesicle membrane recycling.

Synaptobrevin

Synaptobrevin is an abundant synaptic vesicle integral membrane protein. Synaptobrevins were discovered independently in rat brain (11) and as a major component of cholinergic synaptic vesicles from marine rays where they are referred to as VAMPS (vesicle-associated membrane proteins) (192,193). This 18-kd protein can be divided into three domains: a cytoplasmic proline-rich amino terminus followed by a highly charged central region and a hydrophobic transmembrane carboxyl terminal region (185,192). Synaptobrevins in neurons and endocrine cells specifically associate with the secretory vesicles, including synaptic vesicles, SLMVs (11), and chromaffin granules (90). Originally, two isoforms of synaptobrevin were found to be expressed in the rat nervous system that differ slightly in their sequences in the amino and carboxyl termini (193). Later, a third isoform, named cellubrevin, was found to be ubiquitously expressed in all cell types (130). However, recently, synaptobrevin 1 and 2 have been reported to be not only expressed in neural tissues, but also found in nonneural cells including muscle, liver, and kidney, and as a component of the glucose transporter-containing vesicles in adipose tissue (36,165).

It has become clear from several different experimental fields that synaptobrevin and its isoforms are important not only in regulated exocytosis, but also in vesicle fusion events throughout the cell. Synaptobrevin is a part of the NSF/SNAP/SNARE fusion complex that is discussed below (183), is a substrate for several neurotoxins (172), and has homologues in yeast that are important for secretion all along the secretory pathway (22) (see below).

Rab3a

Several lines of evidence indicate that GTP hydrolysis is an essential step in cell secretion and that small GTP-binding proteins have a direct role in mediating transport of vesicles through the intracellular protein secretory pathway. These proteins, which have been described to function as molecular switches, exist either in a GTP- or guanosine diphosphate (GDP)-bound conformation, with each form being associated with a particular activity (27). The addition of a nonhydrolyzable analogue of GTP (GTPγS) to an in vitro intra-Golgi transport assay inhibits transport between the *cis* and medial Golgi compartments, causing a fivefold increase in the number of vesicles associated with the Golgi (131). In mammalian semi-intact cells, GTPγS inhibits transport between the ER and the *cis* Golgi compartment (13).

Several small GTP-binding proteins with homology to two yeast proteins necessary for protein secretion have been recently identified in mammals (213). These proteins make up the rab gene family that appears to be involved in intracellular vesicle transport. Sixteen rab family genes have now been cloned (64,127,191,213), and many of their gene products have been localized to exocytotic and endocytotic compartments (41). For example, rab2, is associated with a compartment between the ER and Golgi apparatus, rab5 is located on the cytoplasmic surface of the plasma membrane and early endosomes, and rab7 is found on late endosomes. There are four members of the rab3 subfamily (a,b,c, and d) (8,127), which are specifically expressed in cells that exhibit regulated exocytosis. Rab3a is expressed in neural, endocrine, and exocrine cells and localized to synaptic vesicles or synaptic-like vesicles and chromaffin granules (34,54,69,132). Rab3b, with 78% sequence identity to Rab3a, is the major form found in rat pituitary gland. Antisense nucleotides to rab3b introduced into pituitary cells inhibit calcium-dependent exocytosis (115). Rab3c is expressed in brain, adrenal medulla, testis, heart, and adipocytes (184), while Rab3d is mainly expressed in adipocytes and poorly expressed in brain (8).

Rab3a contains the four consensus domains involved in GTP/GDP binding and GTPase activity, but has an unique carboxyl terminus sequence, Cys-X-Cys, different from the rest of the members of the *ras* superfamily (213). Biochemical studies suggest this carboxyl terminal sequence is posttranslationally modified by two geranylgeranyl moieties and by carboxyl methylation (66). Rab3a exists in both soluble and membrane-bound forms (34), and the hydrophobic modification mediates the attachment of Rab3a to synaptic vesicles. Rab3a associates with synaptic vesicles in neurons and microvesicles in cultured chromaffin cells only after these organelles leave the Golgi complex, and it dissociates from vesicles before their return to the Golgi area (128).

In synaptosomes, rab3a dissociates from the synaptic vesicle membrane fraction during calcium-dependent exocytosis and can be partially restored to synaptic vesicles during recovery after stimulation (70). To investigate whether rab3a dissociates from synaptic vesicle membranes before or after their fusion with the plasma membrane, nerve terminals from the frog neuromuscular junction were treated with black widow spider venom to stimulate exocytosis. When this treatment is done in the absence of calcium to block subsequent endocytosis, it results in a massive exocytosis with depletion of synaptic vesicles and an increase in the plasma membrane area. After treatment, rab3a immunoreactivity was found to outline the profile of the nerve terminal that had increased in width, suggesting that rab3a remains associated with the synaptic vesicle membranes during fusion (128). Since rab3a becomes associated with synaptic vesicles only after vesicles have left the Golgi, translocates to the plasma membrane with exocytosis, and dissociates after fusion, rab3a is probably involved in steps after formation of vesicles and before endocytotic recycling of vesicles.

The conversion between the GDP- and GTP-bound states of rab3a is catalyzed by several different proteins. A novel regulatory protein for rab3a has been cloned and characterized (5,126). This protein, first named smgp25A GDP dissociation inhibitor (GDI) and later named rab GDI because of its ability to interact with all rabs (194), regulates the GDP/GTP exchange reaction by inhibiting the dissociation of GDP, thereby inhibiting binding of GTP. GDI forms a complex with the GDP-bound form of rab3A, but not with the GTP-bound form or the guanine nucleotide free form. Rab GDI inhibits the binding of the GDP-bound form of rab3a to membranes and induces the dissociation of the GDP-bound form from membranes. Two isoforms of rab GDI have been cloned: one is brain-specific, while the other is ubiquitously expressed (141). The discovery of this GDI protein suggests that the membrane removal of rab3a is triggered by GTP hydrolysis. A GTPase activating protein (GAP) has been detected in brain extracts (33). GTPase activating activity is present in particulate and cytosol fractions and is distinct from p21ras-specific GAP, which has no effect on rab3a GTPase activity. Another protein that has been detected biochemically is rab3a-GRF (guanine nucleotide releasing factor), a factor that stimulates the off-rate of GDP by tenfold (32). In addition, the mammalian protein, Mss4, the homologue of the yeast protein Dss4, acts as a suppressor to sec4 and has been shown to enhance GDP dissociation from several rab proteins, including rab3a (35).

A protein that interacts with rab3a has been detected by using a chemical cross-linker (179). When GTPγS-bound rab3a was incubated with a crude brain membrane fraction and the cross-linker, disuccinimidyl suberate, a complex of rab3a and another molecule of 86 kd was formed. A cDNA encoding this 86-kd protein has been isolated from a bovine brain library and sequenced. The sequence reveals the existence of two repeats homologous to the C2 domain of protein kinase C, similar to the repeats also seen in synaptotagmin. The 86-kd protein, called rabphilin-3a, does not appear to have any transmembrane regions, but is found in the membrane fraction and requires detergent for extraction. Rabphilin-3a complexes only with the GTP-bound form of rab3a and not the GDP-bound form (178). Rabphilin-3a has two functionally distinct domains: the C-terminal region, which contains the C2 domains and binds calcium and phospholipids, and the N-terminal region, which binds to rab3a (209). Rab3a (GTP bound form) binding to rabphilin-3a does not affect the phospholipid and calcium-binding properties of rabphilin-3a. Rabphilin-3a does strongly inhibit the rab3a GAP-stimulated GTPase activity of rab3a (109) and calcium/phospholipids show no effect on this activity. Rabphilin-3a may act as another rab3a regulatory protein that functions to keep rab3a in the GTP-bound active form.

One of the conserved domains among the rab proteins corresponds to the domain in *ras* proteins that is essential for the regulation of GTP hydrolysis and the interaction of p21*ras* with GAP (GTPase activating protein) (161). Synthetic peptides corresponding to part of this effector domain in rab3a inhibit ER to Golgi and intra-Golgi transport in vitro (161). Interestingly, these synthetic peptides stimulate exocytotic degranulation in mast cells (146) and stimulate exocytosis in permeabilized pancreatic acinar cells and chromaffin cells (149,177). In addition, these peptides injected into giant synapses formed between contacting somata of cultured neurons increase spontaneous frequency of miniature synaptic currents, but do not affect action potential–evoked neurotransmitter release. The proposed theory is that rab3a peptides may mimic the rab3a protein and activate the effector protein that is directly involved in exocytosis. However, these studies are called into question by a study showing that the rab3a peptides promote fusion between zymogen granules and plasma membranes in vitro, yet this fusion still persists even when the peptide sequence is scrambled (123). Also, rab3a antibodies that recognize a protein of the correct size on zymogen granules do not affect the fusion. The authors of this report suggest that the positive charges on the rab3a peptides enhance fusion, but not through any interaction with an effector protein.

Studies with mast cells have shown that intracellular perfusion with GTPγS can trigger complete exocytotic degranulation in the absence of known intracellular messengers (67), which is the opposite effect of GTPγS on intracellular vesicle transport (131). These studies in which GTPγS stimulates exocytosis suggest that GTP hydrolysis is not necessary for the actual fusion event, but for some other step in vesicle transport, and that GTPγS leads to the sustained action of rab3a, causing the subsequent activation of an effector protein. Yet, recent studies using the squid giant synapse show that GTPγS irreversibly inhibited neurotransmitter release and reduced the number of synaptic vesicles at the active zone, but did not affect the number of synaptic vesicles docked at the plasma membrane (87). Therefore, these results suggest that GTP hydrolysis follows docking and precedes neurotransmitter release. It is possible that in the mast cell studies, GTPγS was activating heterotrimeric G proteins that may also regulate exocytosis.

Two recent studies suggest that rab3a acts as a negative regulator of exocytosis. Overexpression of rab3a in cultured chromaffin cells inhibits regulated secretion (91). Moreover, overexpression of rab3a mutants that are defective in GTP hydrolysis inhibited exocytosis in PC12 cells, and injection of purified rab3a mutants in chromaffin cells also inhibited exocytosis. Chromaffin cells with injected antisense nucleotides to rab3a exhibited an increasing potential to respond to repetitive stimulation, while control cells exhibited desensitization (100). The authors of both of these studies concluded that rab3a is a regulatory factor that prevents exocytosis from occurring unless secretion is triggered.

Transgenic mice that do not express rab3a seem phenotypically normal at a gross level. However, electophysiologic recordings in hippocampal CA1 pyramidal cells of these mutants indicate that while most synaptic parameters are normal, synaptic depression after short trains of repetitive stimuli is significantly increased. Also in these mutant mice, levels of rabphilin-3a are decreased 70%, possibly due to the instability of the protein caused by the absence of rab3a (77).

Annexins

The annexins are a family of calcium-dependent membrane-binding proteins found in a variety of tissues. They have several proposed functions including phospholipase inhibition, blood anticoagulation, and membrane fusion (47). Although many functions have been attributed to different members of this family, several of their characteristics suggest their involvement in regulated exocytosis. Annexins are able to bind phospholipids in a calcium-dependent manner, to aggregate membrane vesicles and promote their fusion, and to form a channel or pore in a phospholipid bilayer.

The annexins have four homologous domains about 70 amino acids long with each domain containing a 17 amino acid conserved sequence. The N-termini are unique and in some cases contain phosphorylation sites. Annexins have no sequence similarities with any other proteins, in particular, with either the "EF-hand" family of calcium-binding proteins or the calcium and phospholipid binding proteins, PLA_2 and PKC.

The crystal structure of annexin V, an effective anticoagulant, has been determined (94). Because of the high degree of homology among the annexins, the annexin V structure may serve as a prototype for the other annexins. The four repeats are folded into compact domains consisting of five approximately parallel α-helices. The domains are arranged to form tight modules creating a twofold symmetry around a central hydrophilic pore or channel. The molecule is nearly planar with the calcium binding sites located on the side of the molecule suggested to be the membrane contact area. The N-terminal tail present on the opposite face of the molecule seems to hold the first domain to the fourth, maintaining the circular arrangement. Both lipocortin (annexin I) and calpactin (annexin II) have tyrosine and serine phosphorylation sites in their N-terminal tails and the phosphorylation of these proteins may be important in their regulation (105,200).

Subcellular localization studies demonstrate that specific annexins have unique subcellular distributions even within the same cell type (63). Calelectrin, isolated from the electric organ of *Torpedo marmorata,* is localized to the nerve ending and associates with cholinergic synaptic vesicles and presynaptic membrane fractions in a calcium-dependent manner in vitro (197). Immunofluorescence studies show that calpactin (annexin II) is localized to the inner face on the plasma membrane, closely associated with the cortical cytoskeleton in chromaffin cells (135). Immunoelectron microscopy on frozen ultrathin sections of stimulated chromaffin cells show that calpactin is closely associated with the inner face of the plasma membrane especially between the membrane and docked chromaffin granules (135). This localization suggests that calpactin may behave as a docking protein cross-linking granules to the plasma membrane after stimulation.

Synexin, the first annexin hypothesized to have a role in exocytosis, was isolated from the adrenal medulla as a protein that initiated in vitro chromaffin granule aggregation in the presence of calcium (48). Since then, most of the annexins have been shown to have similar activity (62). Synexin was found to bind to chromaffin granules at 5 to 10 μM calcium (50), but calcium concentrations on the order of 200 μM were required for half-maximal granule aggregation (48). Additional investigation demonstrated that synexin undergoes rapid self-association with the same calcium dependence as the granule aggregation reaction (49). This led to the hypothesis that synexin molecules on one membrane interact with synexin molecules on another membrane to bring the membranes into contact.

Distinct from other annexins, calpactin (annexin II) is able to aggregate chromaffin granules at low concentrations of calcium, about 0.1 μM (62). This may be due to the fact that calpactin is a tetramer made up of two annexin molecules, p36, which each bind to one subunit of a dimer of S-100 family molecules, called p10. This tetrameric molecule may be able to bind two membranes simultaneously. Phosphorylation of lipocortin and calpactin by protein kinase C does not significantly change their ability to bind membranes, but does strongly inhibit their membrane aggregating activity (105, 200).

In the presence of small amounts of unesterified, *cis*-unsaturated fatty acids, annexin-aggregated chromaffin granules will fuse. This suggests that the regions of contact between granules formed by annexins break, leading to fusion and the formation of larger vesicles (46,62). Arachidonic acid is the most effective at mediating fusion of annexin-aggregated granules and may be made available inside the cell during stimulation by the action of a phospholipase.

The hydrophilic central pore of annexin V evident in the crystal structure of this protein appears to possess properties like that of transmembrane ion channels. Indeed, annexin V and synexin have been shown to form voltage-dependent ion channels across synthetic phospholipid bilayers (31,167). The conductivity of these channels is on the order of 50 pS (162). This could indicate that annexins may not work alone and that other proteins are necessary to form a fusion pore during exocytosis and drive the fusion of two membranes. Because annexins are activated by calcium and can aggregate vesicles, they may be involved in bringing secretory vesicles in close contact with the plasma membrane during secretion. Alternatively, because of their wide distribution, they may be involved in more general membrane trafficking events within cells.

INSIGHTS FROM GOLGI FUSION PROCESSES: THE NSF/SNAP/SNARE COMPLEX

N-ethylmaleimide-sensitive fusion protein (NSF) is a soluble homotrimer (205) of 76-kd subunits that was purified on the basis of its ability to restore intercisternal Golgi transport in a cell-free assay (25). When NSF is withheld from incubations with Golgi stacks in the cell-free assay, uncoated vesicles accumulate and intra-Golgi transport does not occur (124). NSF has also been shown to be necessary for ER to Golgi transport in mammalian semi-intact cells (14) and endocytic vesicle fusion in a cell-free assay (61). NSF does not directly bind membranes, but requires additional factors to attach to Golgi membranes (201). Three soluble proteins, termed α-, β-, and γ-SNAPs (soluble NSF attachment proteins) have been purified from brain (44) and can promote vesicle transport between Golgi membranes (43). The β-SNAP is a brain-specific isoform that is almost identical to α-SNAP (204).

SNAPs bind to distinct sites on the Golgi membranes and NSF only interacts with SNAPs that are attached to membranes; NSF and SNAPs do not interact in solution (203). α-SNAP and β-SNAP compete for the same binding site on the NSF/membrane complex, while γ-SNAP binds to a noncompetitive site. NSF, SNAPs, and detergent extracts from Golgi membranes form a large multisubunit complex with a velocity coefficient of 20 S (207). Both α-SNAP and γ-SNAP are part of the same complex (203). The 20-S particle disassembles in the presence of Mg-ATP, but is stable in the presence of ATP and ethylenediaminetetraacetic acid (EDTA), and ATPγS, suggesting ATP hydrolysis is necessary for particle disassembly (207). NSF exhibits ATPase activity and has two ATP binding sites. Hydrolysis of ATP is required for membrane fusion catalyzed by NSF (205).

Initial cross-linking experiments suggested that a-SNAP interacts with a membrane protein of 30 to 40 kd (203). To further purify SNAP membrane receptors (SNAREs), the assembly and disassembly of the 20-S particle was used as the basis for an affinity purification technique (183). To isolate SNAP receptors (SNAREs), the 20-S particle was assembled using bovine brain extracts, recombinant NSF with an epitope tag, and recombinant SNAPs in the presence of ATPγS and EDTA. The complex was then attached to a solid matrix by means of an antibody to the epitope attached to the NSF. Because the 20-S particle dissociates in the presence of Mg-ATP, proteins specifically bound to the solid matrix were eluted with Mg-ATP (183).

Interestingly, the SNARE proteins isolated from brain were found to be proteins associated with the synapse, syntaxin 1A and 1B, synaptobrevin-2, and SNAP-25 (synapotosomal-associated protein of 25 kd). SNAP-25 is a brain-specific protein that is not an integral membrane protein, but is tightly associated with membrane components of the nervous system and localized to presynaptic terminals in specific neuronal cell types (148). There appear to be two isoforms of SNAP-25 that are generated by alternative splicing; these isoforms differ in only nine amino acids, which contain a fatty acid acylation site (9).

The fact that SNAP-25 and syntaxins are found in the plasma membrane and synaptobrevin-2 is found on the synaptic vesicles led to the hypothesis that these integral membrane proteins act as attachment sites for the NSF/SNAPS fusion complex (Fig. 3). The SNAREs also specifically associate with each other. For example, synaptobrevin 1 and 2 bind to syntaxins 1A and 4, but not 2 or 3, suggesting that synaptobrevin and syntaxin contribute to the specificity of vesicle targeting (37). Specific binding experiments show that synaptobrevin binding to syntaxin 1A is enhanced in the presence of SNAP-25. SNAP-25 binds preferentially to syntaxin 1A and 4.

A recent study reports that in the absence of NSF and SNAPS, SNAREs form a stable complex that can bind synaptotagmin (182). Synaptotagmin can be displaced from the com-

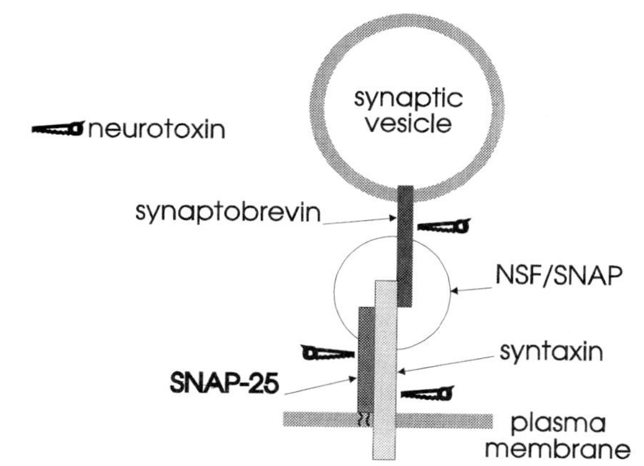

Figure 3. The 20-S docking and fusion particle. NSF and SNAP proteins bind to SNAREs (synaptobrevin in the synaptic vesicle and syntaxin and SNAP-25 in the plasma membrane). All three SNAREs are targets for neurotoxins.

plex by α-SNAP, suggesting that these two proteins share a common binding site. It has therefore been hypothesized that synaptotagmin acts as clamp to prevent fusion until the proper signal, then SNAP and NSF bind to promote fusion. Yet, calcium does not regulate any of these protein interactions. It may be that NSF and SNAPs are required for a prefusion step, which is reached upon ATP hydrolysis and dissociation of the NSF and SNAP; then synaptotagmin associates with the complex in a conformation that is regulated by calcium to trigger membrane fusion (144). Another study reports that SNAP-25, synaptobrevin-2, syntaxins 1A and 1B, and rab3a all form a complex in the absence of NSF and SNAPs (93).

Since the identification of SNAP receptors in brain tissue, studies looking at NSF tissue expression have shown that NSF is preferentially expressed in the nervous system, with low and uniform expression in all non-neural cells (92,164). In addition, NSF has been found to be associated with synaptic vesicles and is not released by Mg-ATP (92). This further suggests that some of the proteins involved in intracellular vesicle fusion events in all eukaryotic cells are the same as those necessary for synaptic vesicle exocytosis (183).

INSIGHTS FROM YEAST SECRETORY MUTANTS

The isolation of temperature-sensitive yeast secretion (*sec*) mutants has led to the discovery of many proteins important in protein secretion in yeast (Fig. 4). A number of these proteins have proven to be homologues of proteins present in the synapse, thus implicating the synaptic proteins in the process of exocytosis. At their restrictive temperature the *sec* mutants have blocked cell surface protein secretion, with an intracellular accumulation of secretory vesicles, or an exaggeration of one of the secretory organelles (143). Twenty-three temperature-sensitive secretory mutants were first characterized. These mutants have been classified into groups that exhibit defects in either ER to Golgi transport, budding from the Golgi complex, or those that accumulate secretory vesicles between the Golgi and the plasma membrane.

One of these *sec* mutants, *sec4,* inhibits protein secretion and causes cells to accumulate secretory vesicles between the Golgi apparatus and the plasma membrane. The *sec4* gene product was subsequently identified as a 23-kd, small, GTP-binding protein with homology to the *ras* proteins (171). The highest degree of sequence identity is in the regions of the *ras* protein implicated in GTP binding and GTPase activity. *sec4* protein binds GTP and exists in soluble and membrane-bound forms that rapidly associate with secretory vesicles and the plasma membrane in yeast (81). A mutation in the *sec4* gene that lowers the intrinsic GTP hydrolysis rate results in a slowing of secretion and an accumulation of secretory vesicles indicating that the ability of *sec4p* to cycle between its GTP- and GDP-bound forms is important for its function in vesicular transport (198). Another temperature-sensitive secretory mutant, *ypt1,* has transport blocked between the ER and Golgi apparatus, resulting in the buildup of ER membranes at restrictive temperatures. The *YPT1* gene product is also a 23-kd GTP-binding protein with 45% identity with the *sec4* protein (175). These studies suggest that small GTP-binding proteins are involved in regulating the transport of proteins through the different compartments of the constitutive secretory pathway in yeast. The mammalian homologues of these yeast proteins are the rab proteins. Rab3a has the highest sequence identity to *sec4p.*

SNC1, a gene isolated from the yeast *Saccharomyces cerevisiae,* encodes a homologue of vertebrate synaptobrevin (79). This gene was isolated by its ability to suppress the loss of *cap* (cyclase-associated protein) function in strains possessing an activated allele of *ras2.* The *ras* proteins in yeast, which are highly homologous to the *ras* mammalian oncogene products, are required to activate adenylyl cyclase. The *cap* protein copurifies with a *ras*-responsive adenylyl cyclase complex, and the C-terminal function of the *cap* protein is required for normal cellular morphology and responsiveness to nutrient extremes. *SNC1* was isolated as a gene that on multicopy plasmids is capable of suppressing the loss of the C-terminal function of *cap* in *cap* mutant cells. Expressing the rat synaptobrevin genes in yeast does not complement the defects in these *cap* mutant cells, and disruption of the *SNC1* locus does not cause a distinguishable phenotype. However, a second yeast gene that encodes another synaptobrevin homologue, *SNC2,* has been identified, and disruption of both genes results in defective secretion and the accumulation of post-Golgi vesicles (163). *SNC1p* was found to be localized to the post-Golgi vesicles. This suggests that *SNC1* and *SNC2* may function similarly to synaptobrevin in mammalian cells.

Isolation of genes that suppress or complement secretory mutants have identified several proteins necessary for secretion. For example, genetic studies have shown that multicopy expression plasmids carrying the genes that encode for SLY2 and SLY12 are able to suppress the loss of YPT1 function (147). The SLY2/BET1 and SLY12/SEC22 proteins have structural homology to synaptobrevin, and limited sequence homology. These proteins, similar to synaptobrevin, have hydrophobic carboxyl-terminal domains providing a membrane anchor, with the rest of the protein cytoplasmic (55,138). This suggests that rab and synaptobrevin families are involved in membrane trafficking at two stages of yeast transport and in the nerve terminal. This also indicates that rab proteins interacting with synaptobrevin-like proteins may be part of the conserved machinery for vesicular docking and/or fusion.

Several genes, including SED5, PEP12, SSO1, and SSO2, have been identified that encode proteins with a carboxyl-terminal membrane anchor and significant homology to syntaxins over a 70 amino acid region near the membrane anchor. SED5, a gene required for ER to Golgi transport, is a multicopy suppressor of the loss of ERD2 function (85). ERD2 is the ER retention receptor that functions in the retrieval of ER resident proteins from the Golgi (176). PEP12 is required for proper targeting of proteins to the yeast vacuole (22). SSO1 and SSO2 are multicopy suppressors of the *sec1* mutant and other late-acting *sec* genes, including *sec3, sec5, sec9,* and *sec15.* The SSO1 and SSO2 genes encode proteins that are 72% identical in sequence. Either gene can be disrupted without a detectable phenotype, but when both genes are disrupted the yeast is inviable. In yeast strains where SSO2 is disrupted and SSO1 is expressed from a galactose-induced GAL1 promoter, shifting the strain from galactose to glucose causes the yeast to

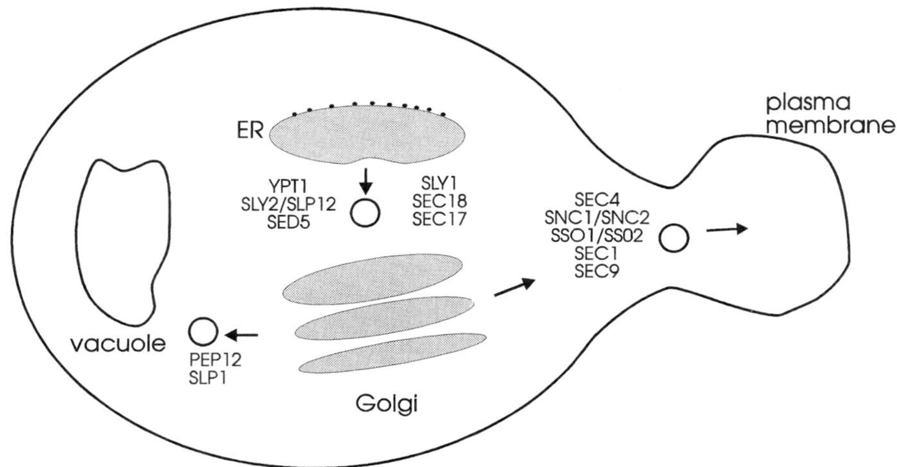

Figure 4. Genetic analysis of yeast secretion. Many genes that encode proteins homologous to synaptic proteins are necessary for different steps along the intracellular vesicular transport pathway in yeast.

cease to grow and results in the accumulation of large numbers of vesicles. SSO1/SSO2 are both localized to the yeast plasma membrane, like syntaxins in mammalian nerve terminals (28).

sec1 is required for vesicular transport from the Golgi to the plasma membrane. SLY1 (147) and SLP1 (196), two proteins with sequence similarity to *sec1* (2), are required for transport from the ER to the Golgi and from the Golgi to the vacuole, respectively. The yeast homologues of syntaxin, SSO1 and SSO2, are high copy suppressors of the mutation in the *sec1* gene (1). Recently, the mammalian homologue of *sec1*, munc-18/*n-sec1* has been identified by its ability to bind syntaxin (74,86,90,160). Munc-18/*n-sec1* is the mammalian homologue of the *Drosophila* protein, ROP, and the *C. elegans* protein, unc-18. Mutations in the unc-18 gene in *C. elegans* are characterized by a phenotype with defective neurotransmitter release (75). Munc-18 is a 67-kd protein found in rat brain that has no apparent transmembrane region (86). *msec1*, with almost identical sequence to Munc-18, was identified in bovine chromaffin cells by its association with syntaxin 1A. This 67-kd protein appears to be associated with chromaffin granules and can be removed by a high salt wash (90).

n-sec1 binds syntaxins 1,2, and 3, but not 5, and does not interact with either synaptobrevin or SNAP-25. *n-sec1* binding to syntaxin 1A inhibits the binding of synaptobrevin to syntaxin 1A, but *n-sec1* does not affect binding of synaptobrevin to syntaxin 4, which it does not bind. *n-sec1* also inhibits binding of SNAP-25 to syntaxin. These data suggest that *n-sec1* associates with syntaxin and regulates vesicle docking by preventing synaptobrevin and SNAP-25 from binding to syntaxin (159). In yeast, genetic experiments show the interaction of *sec1* and SSO, while in mammalian systems biochemical experiments show a direct interaction between syntaxin and munc-18/*n-sec1*.

The mammalian counterpart to *sec9* has turned out to be SNAP-25 (28). *sec9* is a potent high copy suppressor of a *sec4* effector domain mutant. The *sec9* gene product is required for exocytosis and is found in the yeast plasma membrane and not in the Golgi vesicles. In addition, *sec9p* appears to be physically associated with SNC and SSO (28). Overexpression of *SNCp* partially suppresses the temperature sensitivity of the *sec9* mutant and an *snc* null combined with *sec9* results in inviability (45). Again, genetic evidence in yeast, along with biochemical evidence in mammalian systems, indicates that SNAP-25, syntaxin, and synaptobrevin interact to form part of the fusion machinery.

The *sec18* yeast protein has 48% identity to NSF, and can replace NSF in the mammalian cell-free Golgi transport assay (208). *sec18* is required for vesicle transport from ER to Golgi, through Golgi compartments and from the Golgi to the cell surface (82). *SEC17* encodes a protein that is 34% and 33% identical to α-SNAP and β-SNAP, respectively (204). γ-SNAP can restore mammalian Golgi transport activity to cytosol prepared from *sec17* mutant yeast. *Sec17* mutants, like *sec18*, accumulate vesicles between the ER and Golgi and transport is blocked (43).

Recently, investigators have used *sec18* mutants to explore the protein complexes formed on the ER-derived transport vesicles. *Sec18* yeast mutants accumulate ER vesicles docked to Golgi cisternae. SED5p antibodies were used to immunoprecipitate proteins from *sec18* mutant whole-cell extracts prepared in nonionic detergents. Several previously identified proteins coimmunoprecipitated with SED5p, including SLP1p, *sec17*, BOS1p, SEC22p, and BET1p, along with three undescribed proteins of molecular masses of 28 kd, 26 kd, and 14 kd. This study provides evidence for the idea that different isoforms of SNAREs interact throughout the vesicle transport pathway to form a multisubunit complex involved in docking and fusion of vesicles. The inactivation of YPT1p, the rablike protein necessary for ER to Golgi transport, at the restrictive temperature prevented the accumulation of this SNARE-containing complex observed in the *sec18* mutants. This suggests that rab proteins are necessary for the assembly of the SNARE complex (188).

INSIGHTS FROM CLOSTRIDIAL NEUROTOXINS

The bacteria *Clostridium tetani* and *Clostridium botulinum* produce several structurally related neurotoxins that are potent inhibitors of neurotransmitter release. Recently, these toxins have been shown to be zinc peptidases that cleave specific proteins in the nerve terminal (Fig. 3). It turns out that these proteins are all part of the putative fusion machinery at the nerve terminal, as described in the sections above. Therefore, these toxins have become a powerful tool in identifying those proteins involved in neurotransmitter release and their particular functions. These neurotoxins are synthesized by bacteria as a single chain and are proteolytically cleaved to produce a heavy chain and a light chain attached by a disulfide bond. The heavy chain controls the targeting of toxins to the nerve cells and translocation of the light chain into the cytosol. The light chain becomes active once released from the heavy chain and acts as a zinc-dependent protease (172).

There are seven serotypes of the botulinum toxins that act on peripheral motoneurons and block neurotransmitter release. Tetanus toxin undergoes retrograde transport in the central nervous system and blocks release of inhibitory neurotransmitters. Each one of these toxins selectively proteolyzes proteins in the nerve terminal. Tetanus toxin (TeTx), botulinum neurotoxin A (BoNT/A), botulinum neurotoxin D (BoNT/D, and botulinum neurotoxin F (BoNT/F) cleave synaptobrevin-2 (172,210,211). Botulinum neurotoxins A and E selectively cleave SNAP-25 (23,173), while botulinum neurotoxin C1 cleaves syntaxin (24). It has also been reported that synaptotagmin is a receptor, not a target, for the heavy chain of botulinum neurotoxin B (140).

Neurotoxins have been used to determine the function of synaptobrevin and cellubrevin in different systems. Cellubrevin is specifically localized to microvesicles, including those that contain transferrin receptors, and is also cleaved by the light chain of tetanus toxin. One study looked at whether the cleavage of cellubrevin by tetanus toxin influenced the fusion of early endosomes in vitro. This fusion process that is ATP dependent and *N*-ethylmaleimide sensitive requires NSF, ATP, and other cytosolic factors, but is not affected by tetanus toxin, even though cellubrevin is proteolyzed (116). This suggests the cellubrevin is not necessary for endosome fusion but does not rule out the possibility of other isoforms of synaptobrevin functioning in this fusion process. Tetanus toxin treatment of CHO cells does result in the cleavage of cellubrevin and an inhibition of exocytosis of transferrin-receptor containing vesicles (73), sug-

Table 1. PROTEINS INVOLVED IN NEUROTRANSMITTER RELEASE

Protein names	Molecular weight	Tissue localization	Cellular localization	Phosphorylation	Characteristics	Proposed function
Synapsin Ia Synapsin IIb	86 80	Neural	Cytosolic, associated with SVs	Substrate for cAMP-dependent kinase, CaM kinase I, CaM kinase II, proline-directed kinase	Binds actin, spectrin, and microtubules	Regulates availability of SVs; synaptic potentiation
Synapsin IIa Synapsin IIb	74 55	Neural, adrenal medulla	Cytosolic, associated with SVs and SLMVs	Substrate for cAMP-dependent kinase CaM kinase I	—	—
Synaptotagmin I	65	Neural, endocrine	Integral, SVs, SLMVs, and secretory granule membranes	Substrate for casein kinase II	Binds calcium and phospholipids; interacts with neurexins and syntaxins	Docking, fusion, and recycling of secretory vesicles
Synaptophysin	38	Neural, endocrine	Integral, SVs and SLMVs membranes	Substrate for $pp60^{c\text{-}src}$ and CaM kinase II	Forms pore	—
Synaptobrevin	18	Neural, endocrine	Integral, SVs and secretory granule membranes	—	Interacts with NSF/SNAPs	Confers specificity of docking and fusion; recycling of vesicles
Rab3a	25	Neural, endocrine, and exocrine	Cytosolic, associated with SVs and secretory granules	—	Intrinsic GTPase activity	Targeting of secretory vesicles
Annexins	32.5–68	Wide tissue distribution	Cytosolic, associated with intracellular membranes	Substrate for $pp60^{c\text{-}src}$, EGF receptor kinase, and PKC (annexin I and II)	Forms channel, "bivalent" membrane interactions	Docking and fusion of secretory vesicles
NSF	76	Ubiquitous, neural	Soluble, associated with intracellular membranes	—	ATPase, forms complex with SNAPs/SNAREs	Membrane fusion
α–SNAP	35	Ubiquitous	Soluble, associated with intracellular membranes	—	Forms complex with NSF/SNAREs	Membrane fusion
γ–SNAP	39	Ubiquitous				
β–SNAP	36	Neural				
Syntaxin 1 A/B	35	Neural	Integral, plasma membrane	Substrate for casein kinase II	Forms complex with NSF/SNAPS, interacts with synaptotagmin and n-sec1	Confers specificity of docking and fusion of vesicles
SNAP-25	25	Neural	Attached to plasma membrane	—	Forms complex with NSF/SNAPs	Docking and fusion of secretory vesicles
Munc-18/n-sec1	67	Neural	Cytosolic, associated with chromaffin granule	—	Interacts with syntaxin	Regulates SNARE interactions

gesting that cellubrevin is involved in vesicle-plasma membrane exocytosis.

Another system that has been used to look at the function of synaptobrevin in nerve cells is the squid giant axon. The squid synaptobrevin is 65% to 68% identical to mammalian synaptobrevins and is also cleaved by tetanus and botulinum toxins. Injection of either toxin into the squid presynaptic terminal causes a slow and irreversible inhibition of neurotransmitter release, without affecting the calcium signal that triggers release (95). Electron microscopy of toxin-treated terminals shows that the number of both docked and undocked synaptic vesicles is increased. This suggests that synaptobrevin is not necessary for docking of vesicles to the plasma membrane, but is necessary for fusion.

CONCLUSIONS

The details of the ways in which the proteins described in this chapter (summarized in Table 1) work together to promote neurotransmitter release have yet to be defined. One limitation in this field of research is that a cell-free model for neuroexocytosis has not been developed that would permit further in vitro investigation of the protein-protein and protein-lipid interactions involved. Nonetheless, due to the convergence of the areas of research outlined above, there are now clear hypotheses for the roles of some of these essential proteins. The availability of the vesicles for release may be controlled by the synapsins. The complex formed by NSF, the SNAP proteins, and the SNARE proteins (e.g., syntaxin and synaptobrevin) may catalyze membrane fusion. In the nerve terminal the activity of this complex may be regulated by calcium through synaptotagmin, which may be a brake on the process, through rabphilin, which in concert with rab3a, might chaperone interactions between the proper membrane partners, and possibly through the annexins that would assist in bringing membranes into close apposition so that fusion can proceed. Additionally, the annexins and synaptophysin may participate in the formation of the initial fusion pore in the vesicle and plasma membranes. Although little is presently known about the influence of anesthetic agents on any of these proteins, they may be influenced directly by anesthetics or indirectly through alterations in their lipid environment due to anesthetics. In addition, these proteins appear to present attractive targets for the future development of novel anesthetic agents that would act by blocking neurotransmission.

ACKNOWLEDGMENT

Portions of this chapter were adapted from ref. 52, with permission from the publisher.

REFERENCES

1. Aalto MK, Ronne H, Keränen S. Yeast syntaxins Sso1p and Sso2p belong to a family of related membrane proteins that function in vesicular transport. *EMBO J* 1993;12:4095–4101.
2. Aalto MK, Ruohonen L, Hosono K, Keranen S. Cloning and sequencing of the yeast *Saccharomyces cerevisiae* SEC1 gene localized on chromosome IV. *Yeast* 1992;8:587–588.
3. Abdelhaleem MM, Hatskelzon L, Dalal BI, Gerrard JM, Greenberg AH. Leukophysin: A 28-kDa granule membrane protein of leukocytes. *J Immunol* 1991;147:3053–3059.
4. Alder J, Lu B, Valtorta F, Greengard P, Poo M. Calcium-dependent transmitter secretion reconstituted in *Xenopus* oocytes: requirement for synaptophysin. *Science* 1992;257:657–661.
5. Araki S, Kikuchi A, Hata Y, Isomura M, Takai Y. Regulation of reversible binding of smg p25A, a ras p21-like GTP-binding protein, to synaptic plasma membranes and vesicles by its specific regulatory protein, GDP dissociation inhibitor. *J Biol Chem* 1990;265: 13007–13015.
6. Bahler M, Greengard P. Synapsin I bundles f-actin in a phosphorylation-dependent manner. *Nature* 1987;326:704–707.
7. Baines AJ, Bennett V. Synapsin I is a spectrin-binding protein immunologically related to erythrocyte protein 4.1. *Nature* 1985; 315:410–413.
8. Baldini G, Hohl T, Lin HY, Lodish HF. Cloning of a rab3 isotype predominately expressed in adipocytes. *Proc Natl Acad Sci USA* 1992;89:5049–5052.
9. Bark IC, Wilson MC. Human cDNA clones encoding two different isoforms of nerve terminal protein SNAP-25. *Gene* 1994;139:291–292.
10. Barkenow A, Jahn R, Schartl M. Synaptophysin: a substrate for the protein tyrosine kinase pp60$^{c\text{-}src}$ in intact synaptic vesicles. *Oncogene* 1990;5:1019–1024.
11. Baumert M, Maycox PR, Navone F, De Camilli P, Jahn R. Synaptobrevin: an integral membrane protein of 18,000 daltons present in small synaptic vesicles of rat brain. *EMBO J* 1989;8:379–384.
12. Baumert M, Takei K, Hartinger J, et al. P29: a novel tyrosine-phosphorylated membrane protein present in small clear vesicles of neurons and endocrine cells. *J Cell Biol* 1990;110:1285–1294.
13. Beckers CJM, Balch WE. Calcium and GTP: essential components in vesicular trafficking between the endoplasmic reticulum and Golgi apparatus. *J Cell Biol* 1989;108:1245–1256.
14. Beckers CJM, Block MR, Glick BS, Rothman JE, Balch WE. Vesicular transport between the endoplasmic reticulum and the Golgi stack requires the NEM-sensitive fusion protein. *Nature* 1989;339: 397–398.
15. Benfenati F, Bahler M, Jahn R, Greengard P. Interactions of synapsin I with small synaptic vesicles: distinct sites in synapsin I bind to vesicle phospholipids and vesicle proteins. *J Cell Biol* 1989; 108:1863–1872.
16. Benfenati F, Greengard P, Brunner J, Bahler M. Electrostatic and hydrophobic interactions of synapsin I and synapsin fragments with phospholipid bilayers. *J Cell Biol* 1989;108:1851–1862.
17. Benfenati F, Valtorta F, Chieregatti E, Greengard P. Interaction of free and synaptic vesicle-bound synapsin I with F-actin. *Neuron* 1992;8:377–386.
18. Benfenati F, Valtorta F, Rubenstein JL, Gorelick FS, Greengard P, Czernik AJ. Synaptic vesicle-associated Ca^{2+}/calmodulin-dependent protein kinase II is a binding protein for synapsin I. *Nature* 1992;359:417–420.
19. Bennett MK, Calakos N, Scheller RH. Syntaxin: a synaptic protein implicated in docking of synaptic vesicles at presynaptic active zones. *Science* 1992;257:255–259.
20. Bennett MK, Garcia-Arrarás JE, Elferink LA, et al. The syntaxin family of vesicular transport receptors. *Cell* 1993;74:863–873.
21. Bennett MK, Miller KG, Scheller RH. Casein kinase II phosphorylates the synaptic vesicle protein p65. *J Neurosci* 1993;13:1701– 1707.
22. Bennett MK, Scheller RH. The molecular machinery for secretion in conserved from yeast to neurons. *Proc Natl Acad Sci USA* 1993; 90:2559–2563.
23. Binz T, Blasi J, Yamasaki S, et al. Proteolysis of SNAP-25 by types E and A botulinal neurotoxins. *J Biol Chem* 1994;269:1617–1620.
24. Blasi J, Chapman ER, Yamasaki S, Binz T, Niemann H, Jahn R. Botulinum neurotoxin C1 blocks neurotransmitter release by means of cleaving HPC-1/syntaxin. *EMBO J* 1993;12:4821–4828.
25. Block MR, Glick BS, Wilcox CA, Wieland FT, Rothman JE. Purification of an *N*-ethylmaleimide-sensitive protein catalyzing vesicular transport. *Proc Natl Acad Sci USA* 1988;85:7852–7856.
26. Bommert K, Charlton MP, DeBello WM, Chin GJ, Betz H, Augustine GJ. Inhibition of neurotransmitter release by C2-domain peptides implicates synaptotagmin in exocytosis. *Nature* 1993;363: 163–165.
27. Bourne HR. Do GTPases direct membrane traffic in secretion? *Cell* 1988;53:669–671.
28. Brennwald P, Kearns B, Champion K, Keränen S, Bankaitis Y, Novick P. Sec9 is a SNAP-25-like component of a yeast SNARE complex that may be the effector of Sec4 function in exocytosis. *Cell* 1994;79:245–258.
29. Brose N, Petrenko AG, Südhof TC, Jahn R. Synaptotagmin: a calcium sensor on the synaptic vesicle surface. *Science* 1992;256: 1021–1025.
30. Browning MD, Huang C-K, Greengard P. Similarities between protein IIIa and protein IIIb, two prominent synaptic vesicle-associated phosphoproteins. *J Neurosci* 1987;7:847–853.
31. Burns AL, Magendzo K, Shirvan A, et al. Calcium channel activity of purified human synexin and structure of the human synexin gene. *Proc Natl Acad Sci USA* 1989;86:3798–3802.

32. Burnstein ES, Macara IG. Characterization of a guanine nucleotide-releasing factor and a GTPase-activating protein that are specific for the ras-related protein $p25^{rab3A}$. *Proc Natl Acad Sci USA* 1992;89:1154–1158.
33. Burstein E, Linko-Stentz K, Lu Z, Macara IG. Regulation of the GTPase activity of the ras-like protein $p25^{rab3A}$. *J Biol Chem* 1991; 266:2689–2692.
34. Burstein E, Macara IG. The ras-like protein $p25^{rab3A}$ is partially cytosolic and is expressed only in neural tissue. *Mol Cell Biol* 1989; 9:4807–4811.
35. Burton J, Roberts D, Montaldi M, Novick P, De Camilli P. A mammalian guanine-nucleotide-releasing protein enhances function of yeast secretory protein Sec4. *Nature* 1993;361:464–467.
36. Cain CC, Trimble WS, Lienhard GE. Members of the VAMP family of synaptic vesicle proteins are components of glucose transporter-containing vesicles from rat adipocytes. *J Biol Chem* 1992; 267:116681–11684.
37. Calakos N, Bennett MK, Peterson KE, Scheller RH. Protein-protein interactions contributing to the specificity of intracellular vesicular trafficking. *Science* 1994;263:1146–1149.
38. Cameron PL, Südhof TC, Jahn R, De Camilli P. Colocalization of synaptophysin with transferrin receptors: implications for synaptic vesicle biogenesis. *J Cell Biol* 1991;115:151–164.
39. Chapman ER, Jahn R. Calcium-dependent interaction of the cytoplasmic region of synaptotagmin with membranes. *J Biol Chem* 1994;269:5735–5741.
40. Charriaut-Marlangue C, Otani S, Creuzet C, Ben-Ari Y, Loeb J. Rapid activation of hippocampal casein kinase II during long-term potentiation. *Proc Natl Acad Sci USA* 1991;88:10232–10236.
41. Chavier P, Parton RG, Hauri HP, Simons K, Zerial M. Localization of low molecular weight GTP binding proteins to exocytic and endocytic compartments. *Cell* 1990;62:317–329.
42. Clark JD, Lin L, Kriz RW, et al. A novel arachidonic acid-selective cytosolic PLA_2 contains a Ca^{2+}-dependent translocation domain with homology to PKC and GAP. *Cell* 1991;65:1043–1051.
43. Clary DO, Griff IC, Rothman JE. SNAPs, a family of NSF attachment proteins involved in intracellular membrane fusion in animals and yeast. *Cell* 1990;61:709–721.
44. Clary DO, Rothman JE. Purification of three related peripheral membrane proteins needed for vesicular transport. *J Biol Chem* 1990;265:10109–10117.
45. Couve A, Gerst JE. Yeast Snc proteins complex with sec9. *J Biol Chem* 1994;269:23391–23394.
46. Creutz CE. cis-Unsaturated fatty acids induce the fusion of chromaffin granules aggregated by synexin. *J Cell Biol* 1981;91:247–256.
47. Creutz CE. The annexins and exocytosis. *Science* 1992;258:924–931.
48. Creutz CE, Pazoles CJ, Pollard HB. Identification and purification of an adrenal medullary protein (synexin) that causes calcium-dependent aggregation of isolated chromaffin granules. *J Biol Chem* 1978;253:2858–2866.
49. Creutz CE, Pazoles CJ, Pollard HB. Self-association of synexin in the presence of calcium. *J Biol Chem* 1979;254:553–558.
50. Creutz CE, Sterner DC. Calcium dependence of the binding of synexin to isolated chromaffin granules. *Biochem Biophys Res Commun* 1983;114:355–364.
51. Czernik AJ, Pang DT, Greengard P. Amino acid sequences surrounding the cAMP-dependent and calcium/calmodulin-dependent phosphorylation sites in rat and bovine synapsin I. *Proc Natl Acad Sci USA* 1987;84:7518–7522.
52. Damer CK, Creutz CE. Secretory and synaptic vesicle membrane proteins and their possible roles in regulated exocytosis. *Prog Neurobiol* 1994;43:511–536.
53. Damer CK, Creutz CE. Synergistic membrane interactions of the two C2 domains of synaptotagmin. *J Biol Chem* 1994;269:31115–31123.
54. Darchen F, Zahraoui A, Hammel F, Monteils M-P, Tavitian A, Scherman D. Association of the GTP-binding protein Rab3A with bovine adrenal chromaffin granules. *Proc Natl Acad Sci USA* 1990; 87:5692–5696.
55. Dascher C, Ossig R, Gallwitz D, Schmitt HD. Identification and structure of four yeast genes (SLY) that are able to suppress the functional loss of YPT1, a member of the RAS superfamily. *Mol Cell Biol* 1991;11:872–885.
56. Davletov B, Sontag J-M, Hata Y, et al. Phosphorylation of synaptotagmin I by casein kinase II. *J Biol Chem* 1993;268:6816–6822.
57. Davletov BA, Südhof TC. A single C_2 domain from synaptotagmin I is sufficient for high affinity Ca^{2+}/phospholipid binding. *J Biol Chem* 1993;268:26386–26390.
58. De Camilli P, Cameron R, Greengard P. Synapsin I (protein I), a nerve terminal-specific phosphoprotein. I. Its general distribution in synapses of the central and peripheral nervous system demonstrated by immunofluorescence in frozen and plastic sections. *J Cell Biol* 1983;96:1337–1354.
59. De Camilli P, Harris SM, Huttner WB, Greengard P. Synapsin I (protein I), a nerve terminal-specific phosphoprotein. II. Its specific association with synaptic vesicles demonstrated by immunocytochemistry in agarose-embedded synaptosomes. *J Cell Biol* 1983; 96:1355–1373.
60. DiAntonio A, Parfitt KD, Schwarz TL. Synaptic Transmission persists in synaptotagmin mutants of *Drosophila*. *Cell* 1993;73: 1281–1290.
61. Diaz R, Mayorga LS, Weidman PJ, Rothman JE, Stahl P. Vesicle fusion following receptor-mediated endocytosis requires a protein active in Golgi transport. *Nature* 1989;339:398–400.
62. Drust DS, Creutz CE. Aggregation of chromaffin granules by calpactin at micromolar levels of calcium. *Nature* 1988;331:88–91.
63. Drust DS, Creutz CE. Differential subcellular distributions of p36 (the heavy chain of calpactin I) and other annexins in the adrenal medulla. *J Neurochem* 1991;56:469–478.
64. Elferink LA, Anzai K, Scheller RH. rab15, a novel low molecular weight GTP-binding protein specifically expressed in rat brain. *J Biol Chem* 1992;267:5768–5776.
65. Elferink LA, Peterson MR, Scheller RH. A role for synaptotagmin (p65) in regulated exocytosis. *Cell* 1993;72:153–159.
66. Farnsworth CC, Kawata M, Yoshida Y, Takai Y, Gelb MH, Glomset JA. C terminus of the small GTP-binding protein smg p25A contains two geranylgeranylated cysteine residues and a methyl ester. *Proc Natl Acad Sci USA* 1991;88:6196–6200.
67. Fernandez JM, Neher E, Gomperts BD. Capacitance measurements reveal stepwise fusion events in degranulating mast cells. *Nature* 1984;312:453–455.
68. Firestone JA, Browning MD. Synapsin II phosphorylation and catecholamine release in bovine adrenal chromaffin cells: additive effects of histamine and nicotine. *J Neurochem* 1992;58:441–447.
69. Fischer von Mollard G, Mignery GA, Baumert M, et al. Rab3 is a small GTP-binding protein exclusively localized to synaptic vesicles. *Proc Natl Acad Sci USA* 1990;87:1988–1992.
70. Fischer von Mollard G, Südhof TC, Jahn R. A small GTP-binding protein dissociates from synaptic vesicles during exocytosis. *Nature* 1991;349:79–81.
71. Floor E, Feist BE. Most synaptic vesicles isolated from rat brain carry three membrane proteins, SV2, synaptophysin, and p65. *J Neurochem* 1989;52:1433–1437.
72. Fournier S, Novas ML, Trifaro J-M. Subcellar distribution of 65,000 calmodulin-binding protein (p65) and synaptophysin (p38) in adrenal medulla. *J Neurochem* 1989;53:1043–1049.
73. Galli T, Chilcote T, Mundigl O, Binz T, Niemann H, De Camilli P. Tetanus toxin-mediated cleavage of cellubrevin impairs exocytosis of transferrin receptor-containing vesicles in CHO cells. *J Cell Biol* 1994;125:1015–1024.
74. Garcia EP, Gatti E, Butler M, Burton J, De Camilli P. A rat brain Sec1 homologue related to Rop and UNC18 interacts with syntaxin. *Proc Natl Acad Sci USA* 1994;91:2003–2007.
75. Gengyo-Ando K, Kamiya Y, Yamakawa A, et al. The *C. elegans unc-18* gene encodes a protein expressed in motor neurons. *Neuron* 1993;11:703–711.
76. Geppert M, Archer BT, III, Südhof TC. Synaptotagmin II. *J Biol Chem* 1991;266:13548–13552.
77. Geppert M, Bolshakov VY, Siegelbaum SA, et al. The role of rab3a in neurotransmitter release. *Nature* 1994;369:493–497.
78. Geppert M, Goda Y, Hammer RE, et al. Synaptotagmin I: a major Ca^{2+} sensor for transmitter release at a central synapse. *Cell* 1994; 79:717–727.
79. Gerst JE, Rodgers L, Riggs M, Wigler M. SNC1, a yeast homolog of the synaptic vesicle-associated membrane protein/synaptobrevin gene family: genetic interactions with the RAS and CAP genes. *Proc Natl Acad Sci USA* 1992;89:4338–4342.
80. Goldenring JR, Lasher RS, Vallano ML, et al. Association of synapsin with neuronal cytoskeleton. *J Biol Chem* 1986;261: 8495–8504.
81. Goud B, Salminen A, Walworth NC, Novick PJ. A GTP-binding protein required for secretion rapidly associates with secretory vesicles and the plasma membrane in yeast. *Cell* 1988;53: 753–768.
82. Graham TR, Emr SD. Compartmental organization of Golgi-specific protein modification and vacuolar protein sorting events

defined in a yeast *sec*18 (NSF) mutant. *J Cell Biol* 1991;114: 207–218.
83. Hackett JT, Cochran SL, Greenfield LJ Jr, Brosius DC, Ueda T. Synapsin I injected presynaptically into goldfish mauthner axons reduces quantal synaptic transmission. *J Neurophys* 1991;63: 701–706.
84. Hall FL, Mitchell JP, Vulliet PR. Phosphorylation of synapsin I at a novel site by proline-directed protein kinase. *J Biol Chem* 1990; 265:6944–6948.
85. Hardwick KG, Pelham HRB. *SED5* encodes a 39-kD integral membrane protein required for vesicular transport between the ER and the Golgi complex. *J Cell Biol* 1992;119:513–521.
86. Hata Y, Slaughter CA, Südhof TC. Synaptic vesicle fusion complex contains *unc-18* homologue bound to syntaxin. *Nature* 1993; 366:347–351.
87. Hess SD, Doroshenko PA, Augustine GJ. A functional role for GTP-binding proteins in synaptic vesicle cycling. *Science* 1993; 259:1169–1172.
88. Hilbush BS, Morgan JI. A third synaptotagmin gene, *syt3*, in the mouse. *Proc Natl Acad Sci USA* 1994;91:8195–8199.
89. Hirokawa N, Sobue K, Kanda K, Harada A, Yorifuji H. The cytoskeletal architecture of the presynaptic terminal and molecular structure of synapsin I. *J Cell Biol* 1989;108:111–126.
90. Hodel A, Schäfer T, Gerosa D, Burger MM. In chromaffin cells, the mammalian Sec1p homologue is a syntaxin 1A-binding protein associated with chromaffin granules. *J Biol Chem* 1994;269: 8623–8626.
91. Holz RW, Brondyk WH, Senter RA, Kuizon L, Macara IG. Evidence for the involvement of rab3a in Ca^{2+}-dependent exocytosis from adrenal chromaffin cells. *J Biol Chem* 1994;269:10229–10234.
92. Hong R-M, Mori H, Fukui T, et al. Association of *N*-ethylmaleimide-sensitive factor with synaptic vesicles. *FEBS Lett* 1994; 350:253–257.
93. Horikawa PM, Saisu H, Ishizuka T, et al. A complex of rab3a, SNAP-25, VAMP/synaptobrevin-2 and syntaxins in brain synaptic terminals. *FEBS Lett* 1993;330:236–240.
94. Huber R, Berendes R, Burger A, Schneider M, Karshikov A, Luecke H. Crystal and molecular structure of human annexin V after refinement. *J Mol Biol* 1992;223:683–704.
95. Hunt JM, Bommert K, Charlton MP, et al. A post-docking role for synaptobrevin in synaptic vesicle fusion. *Neuron* 1994;12:1269–1279.
96. Huttner WB, Degennaro LJ, Greengard P. Differential phosphorylation of multiple sites in purified protein I by cyclic AMP-dependent and calcium-dependent protein kinases. *J Biol Chem* 1981;265:1482–1488.
97. Huttner WB, Schiebler W, Greengard P, De Camilli P. Synapsin I (protein I), a nerve terminal-specific phosphoprotein. III. Its association with synaptic vesicles studied in a highly purified synaptic vesicle population. *J Cell Biol* 1983;96:1374–1388.
98. Jahn R, Schiebler W, Ouimet C, Greengard P. A 38,000-dalton membrane protein (p38) present in synaptic vesicles. *Proc Natl Acad Sci USA* 1985;82:4137–4141.
99. Jahn R. Südhof TC. Synaptic vesicles and exocytosis. *Annu Rev Neurosci* 1994;17:19–46.
100. Johannes L, Liedo P, Roa M, Vincent J, Henry J, Darchen F. The GTPase Rab3a negatively controls calcium-dependent exocytosis in neuroendocrine cells. *EMBO J* 1994;13:2029–2037.
101. Johnson EM, Ueda T, Maeno H, Greengard P. Adenosine 3′,5-monophosphate-dependent phosphorylation of a specific protein in synaptic membrane fractions from rat cerebrum. *J Biol Chem* 1972;247:5650–5652.
102. Johnston PA, Cameron PL, Stukenbrok H, Jahn R, De Camilli P, Südhof TC. Synaptophysin is targeted to similar microvesicles in CHO and PC12 cells. *EMBO J* 1989;8:2863–2872.
103. Johnston PA, Jahn R, Südhof TC. Transmembrane topography and evolutionary conservation of synaptophysin. *J Biol Chem* 1989; 264:1268–1273.
104. Johnston PA, Südhof TC. The multisubunit structure of synaptophysin. *J Biol Chem* 1990;265:8869–8873.
105. Johnstone SA, Hubaishy I, Waisman DM. Phosphorylation of annexin II tetramer by protein kinase C inhibits aggregation of lipid vesicles by the protein. *J Biol Chem* 1992;267:25976–25981.
106. Katz B. *Nerve, muscle, and synapse.* New York: McGraw-Hill, 1966.
107. Kelly RB. The cell biology of the nerve terminal. *Neuron* 1988;1: 431–438.
108. Kelly RB. Storage and release of neurotransmitters. *Cell* 1993;72 Suppl:43–53.
109. Kishida S, Shirataki H, Sasaki T, Kato M, Kaibuchi K, Takai Y. Rab3a GTPase-activating protein-inhibiting activity of rabphilin-3a, a putative rab3a target protein. *J Biol Chem* 1993;268: 22259–22261.
110. Knaus P, Marqueze-Pouey B, Scherer H, Betz H. Synaptoporin, a novel putative channel protein of synaptic vesicles. *Neuron* 1990;5: 453–462.
111. Leube RE, Kaiser P, Seiter A, et al. Synaptophysin: molecular organization and mRNA expression as determined from cloned cDNA. *EMBO J* 1987;6:3261–3268.
112. Leube RE, Wiedenmann B, Franke WW. Topogenesis and sorting of synaptophysin: synthesis of a synaptic vesicle protein from a gene transfected into neuroendocrine cells. *Cell* 1989;59:433–446.
113. Leveque C, El Far O, Martin-Moutot N, et al. Purification of the N-type calcium channel associated with syntaxin and synaptotagmin. *J Biol Chem* 1994;269:6306–6312.
114. Leveque C, Hoshino T, Pascale D, et al. The synaptic vesicle protein synaptotagmin associates with calcium channels and is a putative Lambert-Eaton myasthenic syndrome antigen. *Proc Natl Acad Sci USA* 1992;89:3625–3629.
115. Liedo P-M, Vernier P, Vincent J-D, Mason WT, Zorec R. Inhibition of rab3b expression attenuates Ca^{2+}-dependent exocytosis in rat anterior pituitary cells. *Nature* 1993;364:540–544.
116. Link E, McMahon H, Fischer von Mollard G, et al. Cleavage of cellubrevin by tetanus toxin does not affect fusion of early endosomes. *J Biol Chem* 1993;268:18423–18429.
117. Linstedt AD, Kelly RB. Synaptophysin is sorted from endocytotic markers in neuroendocrine PC12 cells but not transfected fibroblasts. *Neuron* 1991;7:309–317.
118. Linstedt AD, Vetter ML, Bishop JM, Kelly RB. Specific association of the proto-oncogene product $pp60^{c\text{-}src}$ with an intracellular organelle, the PC12 synaptic vesicle. *J Cell Biol* 1992;117:1077–1084.
119. Llinás R, Gruner JA, Sugimori M, Mcguiness TL, Greengard P. Regulation by synapsin I and Ca^{2+}-calmodulin-dependent protein kinase II of transmitter release in squid giant synapse. *J Physiol* 1991;436:257–282.
120. Llinás R, Mcguiness TL, Leonard CS, Sugimori M, Greengard P. Intraterminal injection of synapsin I or calcium/calmodulin-dependent protein kinase II alters neurotransmitter release at the squid giant synapse. *Proc Natl Acad Sci USA* 1985;82:3035–3039.
121. Llinás R, Steinberg IZ, Walton K. Relationship between presynaptic calcium current and postsynaptic potential in squid giant synapse. *Biophys J* 1981;33:323–352.
122. Lowe AW, Maddeddu L, Kelly RB. Endocrine secretory granules and neuronal synaptic vesicles have three integral membrane proteins in common. *J Cell Biol* 1988;106:51–59.
123. MacLean CM, Law GJ, Edwardson JM. Stimulation of exocytotic membrane fusion by modified peptides of the rab3 effector domain: re-evaluation of the role of rab3 in regulated exocytosis. *Biochem J* 1993;294:325–328.
124. Malhotra V, Orci L, Glick BS, Block MR, Rothman JE. Role of an N-ethylmaleimide-sensitive transport component in promoting fusion of transport vesicles with cisternae of the Golgi stack. *Cell* 1988;54:221–227.
125. Marqueze-Pouey B, Wisden W, Malosio ML, Betz H. Differential expression of synaptophysin and synaptoporin mRNAs in the postnatal rat central nervous system. *J Neurosci* 1991;11:3388–3397.
126. Matsui Y, Kikuchi A, Araki S, et al. Molecular cloning and characterization of a novel type of regulatory protein (GDI) for smg p25A, a ras p21-like GTP-binding protein. *Mol Cell Biol* 1990;10: 4116–4122.
127. Matsui Y, Kikuchi A, Kondo J, Hishid T, Teranishi Y, Takai Y. Nucleotide and deduced amino acid sequences of a GTP-binding protein family with molecular weights of 25,000 from bovine brain. *J Biol Chem* 1988;263:11071–11074.
128. Matteoli M, Takei K, Cameron R, et al. Association of Rab3A with synaptic vesicles at late stages of the secretory pathway. *J Cell Biol* 1991;115:625–633.
129. Matthew WD, Tsavaler L, Reichardt LF. Identification of a synaptic vesicle-specific membrane protein with a wide distribution in neuronal and neurosecretory tissue. *J Cell Biol* 1981;91:257–269.
130. McMahon HT, Ushkaryov YA, Edelmann L, et al. Cellubrevin is a ubiquitous tetanus-toxin substrate homologous to a putative synaptic vesicle fusion protein. *Nature* 1993;363:346–349.
131. Melancon P, Glick BS, Malhotra V, et al. Involvement of GTP-binding "G" proteins in transport through the Golgi stack. *Cell* 1987; 51:1053–1062.

132. Mizoguchi a, Kim S, Ueda T, et al. Localization and subcellular distribution of smg p25A, a ras p21-like GTP-binding protein, in rat brain. *J Biol Chem* 1990;265:11872–11879.
133. Mizuta M, Inagaki N, Nemoto Y, Matsukura S, Takahashi M, Seino S. Synaptotagmin III is a novel isoform of rat synaptotagmin expressed in endocrine and neuronal cells. *J Biol Chem* 1994;269:11675–11678.
134. Monck JR, Fernandez JM. The exocytotic fusion pore and neurotransmitter release. *Neuron* 1994;12:707–716.
135. Nakata T, Sobue K, Hirokawa N. Conformational change and localization of calpactin I complex involved in exocytosis as revealed by quick-freeze, deep-etch electron microscopy and immunocytochemistry. *J Cell Biol* 1990;110:13–25.
136. Navone F, Greengard P, De Camilli P. Synapsin I in nerve terminals: selective association with small synaptic vesicles. *Science* 1984;226:1209–1210.
137. Navone F, Jahn R, Di Gioia G, Stukenbrok H, Greengard P, De Camilli P. Protein p38: An integral membrane protein specific for small vesicles of neurons and neuroendocrine cells. *J Cell Biol* 1986;103:2511–2527.
138. Newman AP, Shim J, Ferro-Novick S. BET1, BOS1, and SEC22 are members of a group of interacting yeast genes required for transport from the endoplasmic reticulum to the Golgi complex. *Mol Cell Biol* 1990;10:3405–3414.
139. Nichols RA, Chilcote TJ, Czernik AJ, Greengard P. Synapsin I regulated glutamate release from rat brain synaptosomes. *J Neurochem* 1992;58:783–785.
140. Nishiki T, Kamata Y, Nemoto Y, et al. Identification of protein receptor for *Clostridium botulinum* type B neurotoxin in rat brain synaptosomes. *J Biol Chem* 1994;269:10498–10503.
141. Nishimura N, Nakamura H, Takai Y, Sano K. Molecular cloning and characterization of two rab GDI species from rat brain: brain-specific and ubiquitous types. *J Biol Chem* 1994;269:14191–14198.
142. Nonet ML, Grundahl K, Meyer BJ, Rand JB. Synaptic function is impaired but not eliminated in *C. elegans* mutants lacking synaptotagmin. *Cell* 1993;73:1291–1305.
143. Novick P, Field C, Schekman R. Identification of 23 complementation groups required for post-translational events in the yeast secretory pathway. *Cell* 1980;21:205–215.
144. O'Conner V, Augustine GJ, Betz H. Synaptic vesicle exocytosis: molecules and models. *Cell* 1994;76:785–787.
145. Obendorf D, Schwarzenbrunner U, Fischer-Colbrie R, Laslop A, Winkler H. In adrenal medulla synaptophysin (protein p38) is present in chromaffin granules and in a special vesicle population. *J Neurochem* 1988;51:1573–1580.
146. Oberhauser AF, Monck JR, Balch WE, Fernandez JM. Exocytotic fusion is activated by Rab3A peptides. *Nature* 1992;360:270–273.
147. Ossig R, Dascher C, Trepte H-H, Schmitt HD, Gallwitz D. The yeast SLY gene products, suppressors of defects in the essential GTP-binding ypt1 protein, may act in endoplasmic reticulum-to-Golgi transport. *Mol Cell Biol* 1991;11:2980–2993.
148. Oyler GA, Higgins GA, Hart RA, et al. The identification of a novel synaptosomal-associated protein, SNAP-25, differentially expressed by neuronal subpopulations. *J Cell Biol* 1989;109:3039–3052.
149. Padfield PJ, Balch WE, Jamieson JD. A synthetic peptide of the rab3a effector domain stimulates amylase release from permeabilized pancreatic acini. *Proc Natl Acad Sci USA* 1992;89:1656–1660.
150. Pang DT, Wang JKT, Valtorta F, Benfenati F, Greengard P. Protein tyrosine phosphorylation in synaptic vesicles. *Proc Natl Acad Sci USA* 1988;85:762–766.
151. Parfitt KD, Hoffer BJ, Browning MD. Norepinephrine and isoproterenol increase the phosphorylation of synapsin I and synapsin II in dentate slices of young but not aged Fisher 344 rats. *Proc Natl Acad Sci USA* 1991;88:2361–2365.
152. Perin MS. The COOH terminus of synaptotagmin mediates interaction with the neurexins. *J Biol Chem* 1994;269:8576–8581.
153. Perin MS, Brose N, Jahn R, Südhof TC. Domain structure of synaptotagmin (p65). *J Biol Chem* 1991;266:623–629.
154. Perin MS, Fried VA, Mignery GA, Jahn R, Südhof TC. Phospholipid binding by a synaptic vesicle protein homologous to the regulatory region of protein kinase C. *Nature* 1990;345:260–263.
155. Perin MS, Johnston PA, Ozcelik T, Jahn R, Francke U, Südhof TC. Structural and functional conservation of synaptotagmin (p65) in *Drosophila* and humans. *J Biol Chem* 1991;266:615–622.
156. Petrenko AG, Perin MS, Davletov BA, Ushkaryov YA, Geppert M, Südhof TC. Binding of synaptotagmin to the alpha-latrotoxin receptor implicates both in synaptic vesicle exocytosis. *Nature* 1991;353:65–68.
157. Petrucci TC, Macioce P, Paggi P. Axonal transport kinetics and posttranslational modification of synapsin I in mouse retinal ganglion cells. *J Neurosci* 1991;11:2938–2946.
158. Petrucci TC, Morrow JS. Synapsin I: an actin-bundling protein under phosphorylation control. *J Cell Biol* 1987;105:1355–1363.
159. Pevsner J, Hsu S, Braun JEA, et al. Specificity and regulation of a synaptic vesicle docking complex. *Neuron* 1994;13:353–361.
160. Pevsner J, Hsu SC, Scheller RH. n-Sec1: a neural-specific syntaxin-binding protein. *Proc Natl Acad Sci USA* 1994;91:1445–1449.
161. Plutner H, Schwaninger R, Pind S, Balch WE. Synthetic peptides of the Rab effector domain inhibit vesicular transport through the secretory pathway. *EMBO J* 1990;9:2375–2383.
162. Pollard HB, Guy HR, Arispe N, et al. Calcium channel and membrane fusion activity of synexin and other members of the annexin gene family. *Biophys J Biophys Soc* 1992;62:15–18.
163. Protopopov V, Govindan B, Novick P, Gerst JE. Homologs of the synaptobrevin/VAMP family of synaptic vesicle proteins function on the late secretory pathway in S. cerevisiae. *Cell* 1993;74:855–861.
164. Püschel AW, O'Connor V, Betz H. The N-ethylmaleimide-sensitive fusion protein (NSF) is preferentially expressed in the nervous system. *FEBS Lett* 1994;347:55–58.
165. Ralston E, Beushausen S, Ploug T. Expression of the synaptic vesicle proteins VAMPs/synaptobrevin 1 and 2 in non-neural tissues. *J Biol Chem* 1994;269:15403–15406.
166. Rehm H, Wiedenmann B, Betz H. Molecular characterization of synaptophysin, a major calcium-binding protein of the synaptic vesicle membrane. *EMBO J* 1986;5:535–541.
167. Rojas E, Pollard HB, Haigler HT, Parra C, Burns AL. Calcium-activated endonexin II forms calcium channels across acidic phospholipid bilayer membranes. *J Biol Chem* 1990;265:21207–21215.
168. Rosahl TW, Geppert M, Spillane D, et al. Short-term synaptic plasticity is altered in mice lacking synapsin I. *Cell* 1993;75:661–670.
169. Rothman JE. Mechanisms of intracellular protein transport. *Nature* 1994;372:55–63.
170. Rubenstein JL, Greengard P, Czernik AJ. Calcium-dependent serine phosphorylation of synaptophysin. *Synapse* 1993;13:161–172.
171. Salminen A, Novick PJ. A ras-like protein is required for a post-Golgi event in yeast secretion. *Cell* 1987;49:527–538.
172. Schiavo G, Benfenati F, Poulain B, et al. Tetanus and botulinum-B neurotoxins block neurotransmitter release by proteolytic cleavage of synaptobrevin. *Nature* 1992;359:832–835.
173. Schiavo G, Santucci A, DasGupta BR, et al. Botulinum neurotoxins serotypes A and E cleave SNAP-25 at distinct COOH-terminal peptide bonds. *FEBS Lett* 1993;335:99–103.
174. Schiebler W, Jahn R, Doucet J-P, Rothlein J, Greengard P. Characterization of synapsin I binding small synaptic vesicles. *J Biol Chem* 1986;261:8383–8390.
175. Segev N, Mullohand J, Botstein D. The yeast GTP-binding YPT1 protein and a mammalian counterpart are associated with the secretory machinery. *Cell* 1988;52:915–924.
176. Semenza JC, Hardwick KG, Dean N, Pelham HRB. *ERD2*, a yeast gene required for the receptor-mediated retrieval of luminal ER proteins from the secretory pathway. *Cell* 1990;61:1349–1357.
177. Senshyn J, Balch WE, Holz RW. Synthetic peptides of the effector-binding domain of rate enhance secretion from digitonin-permeabilized chromaffin cells. *FEBS Lett* 1992;309:41–46.
178. Shirataki H, Kaibuchi K, Sakoda T, et al. Rabphilin-3A, a putative target protein for smg p25A/rab3A p25 small GTP-binding protein related to synaptotagmin. *Mol Cell Biol* 1993;13:2061–2068.
179. Shirataki H, Kaibuchi K, Yamaguchi Y, Wada K, Horiuchi H, Takai Y. A possible target protein for smg-25A/rab3A small GTP-binding protein. *J Biol Chem* 1992;267:10946–10949.
180. Shoji-Kasai Y, Yoshida A, Sato K, et al. Neurotransmitter release from synaptotagmin-deficient clonal variants of PC12 cells. *Science* 1992;256:1820–1823.
181. Sihra TS, Wang JKT, Gorelick FS, Greengard P. Translocation of synapsin I in response to depolarization of isolated nerve terminals. *Proc Natl Acad Sci USA* 1989;86:8108–8112.
182. Söllner T, Bennett MK, Whiteheart SW, Scheller RH, Rothman JE. A protein assembly-disassembly pathway in vitro that may correspond to sequential steps of synaptic vesicle docking, activation, and fusion. *Cell* 1993;75:409–418.
183. Söllner T, Whiteheart SW, Brunner M, et al. SNAP receptors implicated in vesicle targeting and fusion. *Nature* 1993;362:318–324.
184. Su Y, Kao L, Chu Y, Liang Y, Tsai M, Chern Y. Distribution and reg-

ulation of rab3c, a small molecular weight GTP-binding protein. *Biochem Biophys Res Commun* 1994;200:1257–1263.
185. Südhof TC, Baumert M, Perin MS, Jahn R. A synaptic vesicle membrane protein is conserved from mammals to *Drosophila. Neuron* 1989;2:1475–1481.
186. Südhof TC, Czernik AJ, Kao H-T, et al. Synapsins: mosaics of shared and individual domains in a family of synaptic vesicle phosphoproteins. *Science* 1989;245:1474–1480.
187. Südhof TC, Jahn R. Proteins of synaptic vesicles involved in exocytosis and membrane recycling. *Neuron* 1991;6:665–677.
188. Spgaard M, Tani K, Ye RR, et al. A rab protein is required for the assembly of SNARE complexes in the docking of transport vesicles. *Cell* 1994;78:937–948.
189. Thomas L, Betz H. Synaptophysin binds to physophilin, a putative synaptic plasma membrane protein. *J Cell Biol* 1990;111:2041–2052.
190. Thomas L, Hartung K, Langosch D, et al. Identification of synaptophysin as a hexameric channel protein of the synaptic vesicle membrane. *Science* 1988;242:1050–1053.
191. Touchet N, Chardin P, Tavitian A. Four additional members of the ras gene superfamily isolated by an oligonucleotide strategy: molecular cloning of YPT-related cDNAs from a rat brain library. *Proc Natl Acad Sci USA* 1987;84:8210–8214.
192. Trimble WS, Cowan DM, Scheller RH. VAMP-1: a synaptic vesicle-associated integral membrane protein. *Proc Natl Acad Sci USA* 1988;85:4538–4542.
193. Trimble WS, Gray TS, Elferink LA, Wilson MC, Scheller RH. Distinct patterns of expression of two VAMP genes within the rat brain. *J Neurosci* 1990;10:1380–1387.
194. Ullrich O, Stenmark H, Alexandrov K, et al. Rab GDP dissociation inhibitor as a general regulator for the membrane association of rab proteins. *J Biol Chem* 1993;268:18143–18150.
195. Ushkaryov YA, Petrenko AG, Geppert M, Südhof TC. Neurexins: synaptic cell surface proteins related to the o-latrotoxin receptor and laminin. *Science* 1992;257:50–56.
196. Wada Y, Kitamoto K, Kanbe T, Tanaka K, Anraku Y. The *SLP1* gene of *Saccharomyces cerevisiae* is essential for vacuolar morphogenesis and function. *Mol Cell Biol* 1990;10:2214–2223.
197. Walker JH. Isolation from cholinergic synapses of a protein that binds to membranes in a calcium-dependent manner. *J Neurochem.* 1982;39:815–823.
198. Walworth NC, Brennwald P, Kabcenell AK, Garrett M, Novick P. Hydrolysis of GTP by Sec4 protein plays an important role in vesicular transport and is stimulated by a GTPase-activating protein in *Saccharomyces cerevisiae. Mol Cell Biol* 1992;12:2017–2028.
199. Wang JKT, Walaas SI, Greengard P. Protein phosphorylation in nerve terminals: comparison of calcium/calmodulin-dependent and calcium/diacylglycerol-dependent. *J Neurosci* 1988;8:281–288.
200. Wang W, Creutz CE. Regulation of the chromaffin granule aggregation activity of annexin I by phosphorylation. *Biochemistry* 1992; 31: 9934–9939.
201. Weidman PJ, Melançon P, Block MR, Rothman JE. Binding of an *N*-ethylmaleimide-sensitive fusion protein to Golgi membranes requires both a soluble protein(s) and an integral membrane receptor. *J Cell Biol* 1989;108:1589–1596.
202. Wendland B, Miller KG, Schilling J, Scheller RH. Differential expression of the p65 gene family. *Neuron* 1991;6:993–1007.
203. Whiteheart SW, Brunner M, Wilson DW, Wiedmann M, Rothman JE. Soluble *N*-ethylmaleimide-sensitive fusion attachment proteins (SNAPs) bind to a multi-SNAP receptor complex in Golgi membranes. *J Biol Chem* 1992;267:12239–12243.
204. Whiteheart SW, Griff IC, Brunner M, et al. SNAP family of NSF attachment proteins includes a brain-specific isoform. *Nature* 1993;362:353–355.
205. Whiteheart SW, Rossnagel K, Buhrow SA, Brunner M, Jaenicke R, Rothman JE. *N*-ethylmaleimide-sensitive fusion protein: a trimeric ATPase whose hydrolysis of ATP is required for membrane fusion. *J Cell Biol* 1994;126:945–954.
206. Wiedenmann B, Franke WW. Identification and localization of synaptophysin, an integral membrane glycoprotein of M_r 38,000 characteristic of presynaptic vesicles. *Cell* 1985;41:1071–1028.
207. Wilson DW, Whiteheart SW, Wiedmann M, Brunner M, Rothman JE. A multisubunit particle implicated in membrane fusion. *J Cell Biol* 1992;117:531–538.
208. Wilson DW, Wilcox CA, Flynn GC, et al. A fusion protein required for vesicle-mediated transport in both mammalian cells and yeast. *Nature* 1989;339:355–359.
209. Yamaguchi T, Shirataki H, Kishida S, et al. Two functionally different domains of rabphilin-3A, Rab3A/smgp25A-binding and phospholipid- and Ca^{2+}-binding domains. *J Biol Chem* 1993;268: 27164–27170.
210. Yamasaki S, Baumeister A, Binz T, et al. Cleavage of members of the synaptobrevin/VAMP family by types D and F botulinal neurotoxins and tetanus toxin. *J Biol Chem* 1994;269:12764–12772.
211. Yamasaki S, Hu Y, Binz T. et al. Synaptobrevin/vesicle-associated membrane protein (VAMP) of *Aplysia californica:* structure and proteolysis by tetanus toxin and botulinal neurotoxins type D and F. *Proc Natl Acad Sci USA* 1994;91:4688–4692.
212. Yoshida A, Oho C, Omori A, Kuwahara R, Ito T, Takahashi M. HPC-1 is associated with synaptotagmin and omega-conotoxin receptor. *J Biol Chem* 1992;267:24925–24928.
213. Zahraoui A, Touchet N, Chardin P, Tavitian A. The human Rab genes encode a family of GTP-binding proteins related to yeast YPT1 and SEC4 products involved in secretion. *J Biol Chem* 1989; 264:12394–12401.
214. Zhang JZ, Davletov BA, Sudhof TC, Anderson RGW. Synaptotagmin I is a high affinity binding receptor for clathrin AP-2: implications for membrane recycling. *Cell* 1994;78:751–760.
215. Zhong C, Hayzer DJ, Runge MS. Molecular cloning of a cDNA encoding a novel protein related to the neuronal vesicle protein synaptophysin. *Biochim Biophys Acta* 1992;1129:235–238.

Anesthesia: Biologic Foundations, edited by
Tony L. Yaksh et al. Lippincott–Raven Publishers,
Philadelphia © 1997.

CHAPTER 20

CYTOKINES AND GROWTH FACTORS

PAUL R. KNIGHT

The ancient Greek physicians believed that health and disease were determined by the harmony of the basic elements of air, fire, water, earth, and the four humors of blood, phlegm, yellow bile, and black bile (5). Through the work of Aristotle and Galen this paradigm dominated diagnostic and interventional thinking into the eighteenth century. For example, a disease that was cold and dry was believed to be associated with an imbalance in black bile and could be treated by therapies that were hot and wet such as blood letting. Thus, cupping, purging, cathartics, and many other therapeutic techniques of historical interest were justified on the basis of returning the humors to their proper balance. The recent discovery of the actions of cytokines in health and disease has led to an interesting parallel between these compounds and what the ancients would have recognized as "humoral." Imbalances in cytokines levels appear to be central in the pathogenesis of many different human illnesses. These peptides, secreted in the body in response to a number of stimuli, are responsible for normal cell-to-cell communication, cell differentiation, and proliferation, as well as being associated with the pathologic processes and generalized symptoms of many illnesses, e.g., fever, shaking chills, headache, and malaise. Fortunately, treatment strategies to counter the untoward consequences of a pathologic imbalance of these "humors" appear to be more promising than those historically used.

The first selective cytokine-mediated biologic response identified, other than the nonspecific symptomatology associated with infectious disease, was a result of increased tumor necrosis factor (TNF) activity (43). About a century ago it was noted that in some patients tumors regressed during bacterial infections. Clinical experimentation at this time, which tried to take advantage of this bedside observation, was performed by giving cancer patients a concoction prepared from filtrates of a streptococcus/serratia nutrient broth. Unfortunately, this treatment was not successful due to both the severe toxic systemic reactions associated with the filtered broth and a lack of susceptibility of most tumors to the therapy. In 1975 the factor responsible for producing tumor necrosis following endotoxin injection in mice primed with bacille Calmette-Guérin (BCG) vaccine was isolated. This factor was found to be identical to another agent responsible for weight loss and muscle wasting in cattle and rabbits with chronic parasitic infections termed cachectin (16,37). Interferon (IFN), however, was the first transferable agent capable of cell-to-cell communication to be demonstrated (92). This cytokine, which is produced by cells in response to a viral infection, prevents virus replication in other cells. The discovery of IFN followed the clinical demonstration of bacterial-induced tumor regression, but proceeded by 23 years the experimental identification of TNF as the cytokine responsible for cachexia and tumor necrosis.

Cytokines as a class represent a diverse group of proteins and peptides that are released by cells for the primary purpose of cellular communication. These agents control a wide range of functions including cellular activation, growth, and differentiation, and, in addition, regulate both physiologic and pathologic cellular interactions locally as well as systematically. For example, a cytokine may affect the cell from which it was released (autocrine), influence cells that are in close proximity (paracrine), or bring about changes at more distant sites (endocrine/hormonal) (148,162). Cytokines have multiple biologic responses, depending on which cell type is being stimulated (pleiotrophic), and two or more different cytokines may produce the same response in a given population of cells (176). Furthermore, a specific cytokine may affect a given cell type differently depending on what other cytokines have previously influenced the cell (148). Because of these interactions and overlaps in functions, the term *cytokine networks* has been coined to describe the cumulative effects of the multiple cytokines working in concert to produce a particular biologic function (e.g., wound healing, differentiation of cellular components of the blood). Unfortunately, the lack of a complete knowledge base of the interplay of the various cytokines that may form a network makes understanding the role of each cytokine in the biologic response difficult. For example, how a specific cytokine functions within a network in vivo does not necessarily coincide with any of its demonstrated action in vitro. Deciphering these in vivo interrelated functions of cytokine networks remains an important challenge for investigators in the future.

The cytokines of greatest interest to the anesthesiologist are probably those that play a major role in inflammation and the immune response. These cytokines are involved in the pathogenesis of many of the untoward complications that we, as physicians, would like to avoid but occasionally must deal with in the perioperative period (67). This pathologic role for cytokines during surgery include the development of (a) adult respiratory distress syndrome (ARDS) following aspiration of gastric contents, multiple transfusions (with and without hypotension secondary to hypovolemia), or fat embolization; (b) reperfusion injuries to various organs such as the central nervous system, kidneys, and myocardium; (c) postoperative infection (particularly pneumonia and sepsis), and (d) systemic inflammatory response syndrome (SIRS), which is associated with sepsis, trauma, burns, hemorrhagic shock, and/or pancreatitis. The role of cytokines in the pathogenesis of these severe problems as well as therapeutic strategies targeted at cytokine networks involved in their etiology are discussed in more detail in the following sections. Besides the major pathologic processes, inflammatory cytokines may also be involved in the catabolic state and general malaise that follow anesthesia and surgery (67). Attempts to decrease the production of cytokines and/or the negative biologic responses associated with these agents may represent new methods of decreasing hospitalization stay and the time required before returning to work following surgery. Evidence exists for this in recent outcome studies of postsurgical patients aggressively treated for pain (194). The use of specific anesthetic techniques to decrease the stress response of the patient, as determined by intraoperative and postoperative corticosteroid and catecholamine levels, is associated with decreased morbidity following surgery. Interestingly, elevated steroid levels are only one facet of the overall response to trauma and represent inhibitory homeostatic feedback control to injurious sequelae associated with the acute reaction following surgery, and caused in part by the release of proinflammatory cytokines (162).

This chapter explores the role of cytokine networks in both health and disease, particularly as it may pertain to the anesthesiologist. The complexity of the interaction of these agents can be confusing to the nonspecialist who would like to attain a working knowledge in the field. While it not possible to avoid technical jargon in describing this potent group of biologic regulators, our aim is to present the material in a way that we hope is easy to interpret. The chapter does not cover all the cytokines identified to date; it discusses cytokine groups and focuses on those individual agents that are believed to play major roles in health and disease.

OVERVIEW

The term *cytokine* describes a large group of protein mediators that function to facilitate cell-to-cell communication. To date numerous cytokines have been described, characterized, and produced in recombinant form. Cytokines usually range from 15 to 25 kd and may contain carbohydrate moieties (7). Originally these agents were called lymphokines or monokines to denote nonantibody mediators of inflammation and/or immunity produced by lymphocytes or macrophages respectively. However, with the demonstration that other cells, includ-

Table 1. CYTOKINES

Cytokine	Primary sources	Stimulation	Inhibition	Synergy	Targets and major effects
IL-1 α, β	Macrophages, APCs, endothelium, lymphocytes, many other cell types produce small amounts	Noxious physiologic stimuli (LPS), tissue injury products, C5a, TNF, CSF-1, TGF-β, IL-1 (autocrine)	IL-1ra, soluble receptors, IL-4 (induces IL-1ra), IL-6, IL-10, TGF-β, PGE_2, cortisol	TNF, IL-6, CSFs, cortisol (hepatic)	*Endothelium:* ↑ ICAM, ↑ PGE_2, ↑ procoagulant activity, ↑ IL-8; *Macrophages:* ↑ IL-1, IL-6, IL-8, TNF, ↑ PGE_2, ↑ cytotoxicity; *Bone marrow:* ↑ CSF activity, ↑ neutrophil activation and release; *Lymphocytes:* ↑ B-cell numbers and activity, ↑ T-cell activation; *CNS:* Fever, malaise, somnolence, anorexia, ↑ ACTH release; *Hepatic:* ↑ Acute phase proteins; *Bone:* ↑ Resorption; *Other:* changes in trace metal concentrations
IL-2	T-lymphocyte	APCs, T-cell receptor cross linkage, T-lymphocyte activators	TGF-β, IL-4	INF-γ, IL-1, IL-9, IL-12, IL-4	Activation and proliferation of T helper cells and effector cells of the immune system including B, NK, TIL, and LAK cells, CTLs, and macrophages; ↑ IL-1, IL-3, IL-4, IL-5, GM-CSF, TNF-α and β, INF-γ, and TGF-β production and IL-2R expression; bone resorption, ↑ ACTH, ↓ erythropoiesis
IL-4	T-lymphocyte and basophils	T-cell receptor cross-linkage and IgE binding to basophils	INF-γ, TGF-β	G-CSF, IL-6, EPO, IL-5, IL-9	↑ B cell development and enhances proliferation; ↑ Th2 cells and ↓ Th1 cells (favors humoral over cell-mediated response); IgG subgroups and IgE switching; inhibits most IL-2-mediated B- and T-cell actions; ↑ CTL differentiation; ↑ APC functions but ↓ macrophage oxidant, TNF, IL-1, IL-8, and PGE_2 production; enhances myeloid and erythroid development
IL-5	T-lymphocyte	T-cell receptor cross-linkage		IL-4	↑ Eosinophil and plasma cell differentiation; ↑ Ig production
IL-6	Macrophages, fibroblasts, T-lymphocyte, endothelial cells, bone marrow stromal cells	IL-1, TNF	IL-10, cortisol, estrogen	IL-1, TNF, IL-4, CSFs, EPO, cortisol (hepatic)	Comitogen for B and T cell, plasma cell maturation, ↑ Ig, ↑ NK cell and CTL cytotoxicity, ↑ IL-2R expression; ↑ monocytic and granulocytic proliferation and differentiation, ↑ megakaryocyte maturation; neutrophil priming; ↑ acute-phase proteins; fever, ↑ ACTH; antiviral activity; bone resorption; cachexia
IL-10	T-helper lymphocyte type 2 (Th2), other lymphocytes, macrophages, keratinocytes	APCs, T-cell receptor cross-linkage	INF-γ	IL-3, IL-4	Inhibit cytokine production by Th1 cells, some IL-2 actions on T-lymphocytes and macrophages, ↓ TNF, IL-1, IL-6, IL-8, GM-CSF, G-CSF, and NO production, ↑ IL-1ra; ↑ B-cell proliferation, differentiation, activation, and Ig production, ↑ thymocytes, IL-2– and IL-4–stimulated T cells, and CTL precursors proliferation
TNF-α, β	Macrophage, lymphocytes, many other cell types produce small amounts	Noxious physiologic stimuli (LPS), viruses, interferon-γ, GM-CSF, IL-1, CSF-1, TNF (autocrine)	Soluble receptors, IL-6, IL-10, PGE_2, cortisol	IL-1, IL-6, interferon-β, GM-CSF, CSF-1, cortisol (hepatic)	*Endothelium:* ↑ ICAM, PGE_2, IL-8, procoagulant activity; *Macrophages:* ↑ IL-1, IL-6, IL-8, TNF, and PGE_2, ↑ cytotoxicity; *Neutrophils:* ↑ bone marrow release, activation, attachment, and migration; *Lymphocytes:* ↑ TNF-β and interferon-γ release, ↑ IL-2R expression, B-cell proliferation and Ig production; *CNS:* fever, anorexia; malaise; *Hepatic:* ↑ acute phase proteins, ↑ lipogenesis, ↑ amino acid uptake; *Muscle:* ↑ protein catabolism, glucose uptake, and glycogen breakdown, ↑ ferritin; *Bone:* ↑ resorption; *Other:* shock (NO induction) ↑ cytotoxicity, ↑ vascular leak-edema, ↓ lipoprotein lipase, ↑ fibroblast proliferation, angiogenesis

(continued)

ing epithelial and endothelial cells, neutrophils, and fibroblasts, could also release these compounds, the name *cytokine* has gained more popularity.

Cytokines are divided into six major groups: interleukins, tumor necrosis factors, interferons, chemotactic factors (chemokines), colony stimulating factors, and growth factors (Table 1) (7,148,176). Interleukins, which represent the largest group, were named, at a meeting held at Interlaken, Switzerland, for a group of compounds that promote communication between leukocytes. While we now know these agents may have biologic effects not involving leukocytes, the name has persisted. Other groups of cytokines were also named for the biologic activity with which they were originally associated; however, as previously stated, these peptides are now known to be pleiotropic, many having overlapping biologic activities, and may be released by different cell types that are not derived from bone marrow.

Interleukins

Currently there are 15 members of this group that are designated interleukin-1 to -15 (IL-1 through IL-15). IL-8 also belongs to the chemokine group while IL-3 also belongs to the colony stimulating factors (CSF). In addition, IL-1 has three forms: (a) IL-1α; (b) IL-1β; (c) IL-1ra (ra, receptor antagonist), which binds to the receptor but does not activate signal transduction, thereby blocking IL-1α- or IL-1β-mediated cellular changes (70). This group of cytokines has been intimately associated with the cells responsible for nonadaptive defense responses and inflammation as well as the development and regulation of both cellular and humoral limbs of the immune response. While these cytokines were originally believed to be exclusively responsible for molecular communication between leukocytes (monocyte/macrophage, granulocytes, and lymphocytes), it is now known that the interleukins are also released by a variety of cell types including cells of the integument (keratinocytes), endothelial cells, astrocytes, and fibroblasts (155). In addition, several members of the group (e.g., IL-1, IL-6) may function in a hormonal manner producing biologic responses in a wide variety of cells, many of which are not leukocytes (e.g., hepatocytes) (162).

Tumor Necrosis Factors

Only two members make up this important group of cytokines; TNF-α and TNF-β (lymphotoxin) (177,187). Although these

Table 1. CYTOKINES *(continued)*

Cytokine	Primary sources	Stimulation	Inhibition	Synergy	Targets and major effects
INF-γ	T-lymphocyte and NK cells	T-lymphocyte antigen binding, IL-2, activates macrophages and NK cells	IL-10, IL-4	IL-2, TGF-β, GM-CSF	Antiviral; activates macrophages to produce oxidants, IL-1, IL-6, IL-8, TNF, NO, and ↑ APC functions; ↑ Th1 cells and ↓ Th2 cells (enhances cell-mediated immunity over humoral), ↑ complement binding IgG; ↑ CTL and NK cell cytotoxicity, ↓ myelopoiesis
IFN-α, β	INF-α: macrophages, lymphocytes; IFN-β: fibroblasts, and other cell types	Viruses, other microbes and microbial products, CSF-1, PDGF		Growth factors	*Lymphocytes:* antiproliferative, ↑ NK cell cytotoxicity; *Macrophages:* ↑ APC function, ↑ IL-1 and TNF production, antiviral, ↓ mitogenic activity of many growth factors
Chemokines, e.g., IL-8, RANTES, MIPs, and MCPs	Monocytes, neutrophils, fibroblasts, endothelial, lymphocytes, platelets, keratinocytes	IL-1, TNF, IFN-γ, IL-3, PDGF, viruses, particles, endotoxin, platelet activators	IL-8	IL-1, IL-6, TNF	Acute and chronic inflammatory facilitation by neutrophil, basophil, macrophage, or lymphocyte chemotaxis and activation; ↑ integrin expression; ↑ fibroblast and keratinocyte growth, granulocyte degranulation; some members of this group are also involved in modulation of myelopoiesis
TGF-β	Lymphocytes, platelets, several cell types of the thymus and bone marrow, placenta, macrophages	Glucocorticoids, IL-2, PDGF	IFN-γ	IL-1, IL-6, TNF	↑ Fibroblast proliferation and antiproliferative for other cells including bone marrow stem cells; ↑ collagen and collagenase synthesis, angiogenesis (scar formation and remodeling); suppresses antibody production, macrophage, NK, CTL, and LAK cell activation, and counteracts IL-1, IL-2, TNF, and induces IL-1ra (immune suppression); induces IL-1, IL-6, TNF, and PDGF, chemotactic for neutrophils, monocytes, T-lymphocytes, induces integrins (proinflammatory), ↑ IgA secretion; induces Th1 generation
CSFs, IL-3, and EPO	Stroma cells	Anemia and hypoxia, TNF, other CSFs, IL-1	TGF-β, INF-γ, TNF	IL-1, IL-2, IL-5, IL-6, IL-7, TNF, other CSFs	Myeloid, erythroid, lymphoid and megakaryocyte, proliferation, differentiation, and maturation, ↑ APC proliferation and activity
Growth factors: e.g., PDGF, EGF, FGF, NGF, and insulin-like growth factors	Platelets, endothelial cells, fibroblasts, macrophages, smooth muscle cells, and other cell types	Cytokines and other factors that activate cells (e.g, platelet adhesion)	TGF-β, INF-γ	TGF-β (fibroblast)	Very selective for mitogenic effect and activation, (e.g., fibroblasts, neuroblasts), some are proinflammatory: chemotactic, neutrophil activation, INF-γ production

cytokines share a common receptor and there is some homology in their amino acid sequences, these different forms of TNF are distinct. TNF-α is produced primarily by cells of the macrophage lineage in response to viruses, noxious stimuli, physiologic stress, and other cytokines. Other immune effector cells, for example mast cells and several lymphocyte subtypes as well as endothelial cells, can also release this cytokine, but only in limited amounts. TNF-β was originally believed to be involved exclusively with cytolytic T-lymphocyte (CTL) activity; however, we now know that this agent has other immune regulatory activity following T-cell activation. Furthermore, TNF-α can also function as a cytolytic agent. Indeed, since both forms of the cytokine work via the same receptor, it appears the major determining factor regarding the biologic role of these two forms of TNF is the stimuli that control their release and the microenvironment into which they are released. TNF-α is intricately involved with the inflammatory response, as described later. This cytokine is also important in thermoregulation and in the modulation of many immune/inflammatory functions (67). Due to its proinflammatory action, TNFα is also involved in the pathogenesis of many diseases.

Interferons

This group of cytokines is represented by three distinct classes. IFN-α and -β are acid-stable, while IFN-γ is acid labile (156). IFN-α is produced by a variety of cells including macrophages and B cells. There are at least 14 varieties of this cytokine. IFN-β is secreted primarily from fibroblasts and epithelial cells, while IFN-γ is produced primarily by pulmonary macrophages and T- and natural killer (NK) lymphocytes. All classes of IFN induce cellular resistance to viral infection and immune regulatory activity involving increasing NK lymphocyte cytotoxicity and/or controlling B-cell proliferation, maturation, and/or antibody secretion. IFN-γ is very important in intensifying the inflammatory response by promoting the transformation of monocytes into macrophages (131). Neutrophil activation is also enhanced by this cytokine (15). IFNs also have myelosuppressive and tumoricidal properties. These properties provide the rationale for clinical trials now being conducted to treat malignancy as well as multiple sclerosis.

Chemokines

This new group of low-molecular-weight (8 to 10 kd) compounds has been described just recently (143). The chemokines are predominantly chemotactic factors and can be further subdivided into the α and β subgroups. The α chemokines are primarily involved in neutrophil chemotaxis. Representatives of this group include IL-8, macrophage inflammatory proteins (MIP-1, -2), and neutrophil-activating proteins (NAP-1, -2). This subgroup is also chemotactic for lymphocytes. The β subgroup includes the monocyte chemotactic proteins (MCP-1, -2, -3) and RANTES, which is chemotactic for monocytes as well as lymphocytes. Chemokines do not as a rule induce expression of other cytokines and appear to be more specific and less pleiotrophic than other cytokines. Intensive studies are now being carried out to investigate the role of these agents in the inflammatory response and how to control this response via agonists and modulators of the chemokines. Control and modulation of chemokine biologic responses represent opportunities for therapeutic interventions involving inflammatory disease processes in the future.

Colony Stimulating Factors

CSFs are involved primarily in hematopoiesis, although several members of this group may play a role in the inflammatory response and wound healing (67,178). Major representatives of this group include GM-CSF, G-CSF, and M-CSF (G, granulocyte; M, macrophage) as well as IL-3 (multicolony-CSF), leukemia inhibitory factor (LIF), and erythropoietin. These cytokines are primarily responsible for differentiation and proliferation of pluripotential stem cells of the bone marrow into erythrocytes, granulocytes, monocytes, platelets, and lymphocytes. Other cytokines also play a role in the differentiation of these cellular blood elements and may act synergistically with one or more of the CSFs during hematopoiesis as well as outside the bone marrow in other biologic functions. The role of these cytokines produced outside the bone marrow probably reflects a feedback mechanism for signaling the body's need for more of a particular cell type.

Growth Factors

This final group includes the factors that promote the growth of a wide variety of cell types (36,100,109,151). These cytokines, which are usually targeted to a specific cell type, include epidermal growth factor (EGF), endothelial cell growth factor (ECGF), platelet-derived growth factor (PDGF), fibroblast growth factor (FGF), nerve growth factor (NGF), transforming growth factor (TGF), and insulin-like growth factor (IGF). The growth factors are a diverse group of proteins that are produced by a variety of cells that affect the replication and differentiation of cells by themselves or in concert with other cytokines. Some forms of cancer and atherosclerosis may reflect an abnormal response to these growth factors (7). Many of these cytokines are also involved in chemotaxis and cell migration as well as alterations in cellular metabolism. Furthermore, several of these cytokines, notably PDGF and TGF-β, are also involved in the inflammatory response and subsequent healing process that occurs afterward.

NATURAL CONTROL OF CYTOKINE ACTION

Cytokines are extremely potent and many have profound systemic as well as local toxic effects. Furthermore, as mentioned previously in the introduction, these compounds may be involved in the pathogenesis of many disease states. Therefore, cytokine production and activity must be tightly controlled by regulation of their biosynthesis and release as well as by mechanisms that limit their biologic responses. Femptomolar (10^{-15}M) concentrations are usually all that is required to elicit a physiologic response. Since most cytokines function in a paracrine rather than a systemic fashion, the low concentrations required for activity serve to limit the desired action locally. These small local concentrations can be rapidly terminally diluted as the cytokine molecules enter the vascular system, preventing any untoward systemic responses.

The biosynthesis and release of cytokines are also closely regulated by the levels of other cytokines and/or biologic mediators. The activity of these agents is finely controlled following discharge from the stimulated cells. Proteolysis of the cytokine, up- or downregulation of cellular receptors, modulation of the response by the action of other cytokines, and enhancement or inhibition of signal transduction by a variety of agents may all affect the duration and the nature of the biologic response to a given cytokine. Naturally occurring receptor antagonists and soluble receptors are also released by the same stimuli that stimulate the cytokines. Structurally similar receptor antagonists (e.g., IL-1ra) can competitively block cytokine bioactivity by binding to the specific receptors (70). These homologues, however, are unable to elicit a biologic response. Soluble receptors may act as a sink to bind cytokines and eliminate their bioactivity. Several authors have proposed that these mechanisms act as neutralizing buffers to limit systemic action but allow the cytokine to continue to work at the local level in a paracrine manner (70)

CYTOKINE RECEPTORS

Cytokine receptors are very selective and, as previously stated, usually have a high affinity for their ligand (126). Cellular distribution of cytokine receptors appears variable. For example, IL-1 and TNF are present on a wide variety of cells (6,52). Conversely receptors for IL-2 and IL-4 are present only on the surface of selective cell types (e.g., lymphocytes) (77,114). The differences in cell distribution relate to the functions of the different cytokines. In many cases the cell must be primed or activated, usually by other cytokines, before binding of the cytokine to receptors on the cell surface can elicit a response. Alternatively, the target cell of a specific cytokine may express very few or no receptors on the surface in the quiescent state. After stimulation or activation of these cells, receptor density is increased by an increase in the messenger RNA (mRNA) transcription, subsequent protein synthesis, and membrane incorporation, so that the cells become responsive to the binding of a specific cytokine. The IL-2 receptor on lymphocytes is a example of this type of control in the mediation of cytokine responses (77). Cytokine receptors have been divided into different categories based on structural characteristics (126).

The Hematopoietic Family

This group includes receptors for IL-2, IL-3, IL-4, IL-6, IL-7, erythropoietin, G-CSF, and GM-CSF as well as the receptors for prolactin and growth hormone (7,157). Although these receptors are structurally very different, this group is characterized by having a similar amino acid sequence at the amino terminal end and at the carboxyl terminus of the protein. In addition to their other actions, all members of this diverse group of receptors can stimulate cell division.

The Immunoglobulin Family

Many cells involved in the immune/inflammatory response express different classes of immmuoglobulin molecules on their cell surface. Receptors for M-CSF, PDGF, IL-6, IL-7, and the α and β receptors of IL-1 have a three-dimensional structure similar to immunoglobulins (7,126,157). Other noncytokine ligands also use receptors with this structure, making this group a large superfamily of receptors.

Other Distinguishable Cytokine Receptor Families

Other distinct groups of receptors include the NGF receptor group that also constitutes the TNFs, and the IFN receptor group (7,157). The IFN receptors are the only group that appear to be strictly species specific (7). Uniquely, the receptor for IL-8 belongs to the G-protein–linked receptor family that is characterized by seven-transmembrane α-helices (7). Interestingly, certain cytokine receptors show a great deal of sequence homology to oncogenes. For example, one amino acid substitution in the erythropoietin receptor can constitutively activate the receptor and lead to tumor development (195).

As stated previously, soluble receptors have been isolated for almost all cytokines (136). In most cases the soluble receptors probably originate from proteolysis of the extracellular domain of the cellular receptor protein. However, since distinct cDNAs have been identified for soluble receptors to IL-4 and IL-7, these may represent different gene products. The soluble forms of the cytokine receptors can inhibit the biologic response to a specific agent and probably act as "homeostatic sinks" to limit the biologic activity of the cytokines at the systemic level as well as in specific microenvironments.

The exact mechanisms of how signal transduction occurs following binding of a cytokine to a receptor is an area of intense study. Receptor occupancy by itself is usually not sufficient to induce cell activation (148). Phosphorylation of proteins following tyrosine kinase activation is involved in the mitogenic response following receptor binding of most growth factors such as PDGF and EGF (193). IL-2, IL-3, IL-4, IL-5, IL-6, IL-7, G-CSF, GM-CSF, and erythropoietin all increase tyrosine kinase activity (126). However, the exact method by which tyrosine kinase is activated has not been established. The receptors do not appear to have intrinsic tyrosine kinase activity themselves; therefore, a separate enzyme must associate with the receptors by some mechanism.

Phospholipase C, phosphatidyl-inositol 3-kinase, and guanosine triphosphatase (GTPase)-activating protein also appear to be involved in some of these signal transduction processes (126). Activation of G proteins, adenylate cyclase, and protein kinase C have also been demonstrated in several cases (148). Some cytokine receptors have secondary events that must occur in addition to ligand binding in order to activate the intracellular second message. For example, interaction of the receptor with a specific non-ligand-associated protein following binding, but prior to signal transduction, is required in a number of cases (7). Control of the expression of these proteins and subsequent membrane association with the appropriate receptor may reflect areas of regulation of the biologic response to cytokines.

Several cytokine receptors undergo endocytosis following ligand binding (157). Subsequently, the receptor is recycled to the cell surface minus the cytokine. Receptor-mediated endocytosis may serve several functions. Lysosomal degradation of the cytokine is a means of terminating ligand-receptor action and a way of recycling receptors. More interestingly, internalization of the ligand-receptor complex may be required to initiate the signal. Ligand internalization would be expected if there was a requirement for the ligand to be delivered to the nuclear compartment and become involved in transcription control at some level. EGF, NGF, IL-1, and IL-2 have all been detected in the nucleus following ligand internalization (157). Although no specific nuclear receptors have been demonstrated, it appears that IL-1 delivery to the nucleus is an important step in IL-1 signal transduction (157). Migration of TNF to the nucleus has not been studied. However, since NGF and TNF receptors belong to the same distinct family, direct involvement of TNF in transcription is a plausible hypothesis.

CYTOKINE NETWORKS

Key to comprehending how cytokines function is understanding the concept of the cytokine network. As previously stated, this can be extremely difficult since we do not currently know the complete picture in the more involved networks, even ones that have been extensively studied. A good model for illustrating the role of the cytokine network is the inflammatory reaction and subsequent healing that occurs following tissue injury, such as a skin wound. The steps or phases are similar to those involved with the genesis and resolution of an inflammatory lung injury that may be initiated by a number of stimuli (Fig. 1). The evolution of this process is usually well controlled and orchestrated by the timely release of different groups of cytokines at the appropriate phases of the injury and repair. Functionally, cytokines can be placed in the inflammatory network based on their role in (a) recognition of the injury and initiation of the cytokine cascade; (b) chemotaxis or recruitment of the appropriate effector cell types required to actually start the process; (c) upregulation and maintenance of effector cell activity in order to "clean up" or remove foreign substances, microorganisms, and tissue debris from the injured area; and (d) repair of the injured site by cell growth and deposition and remodeling of new matrix material.

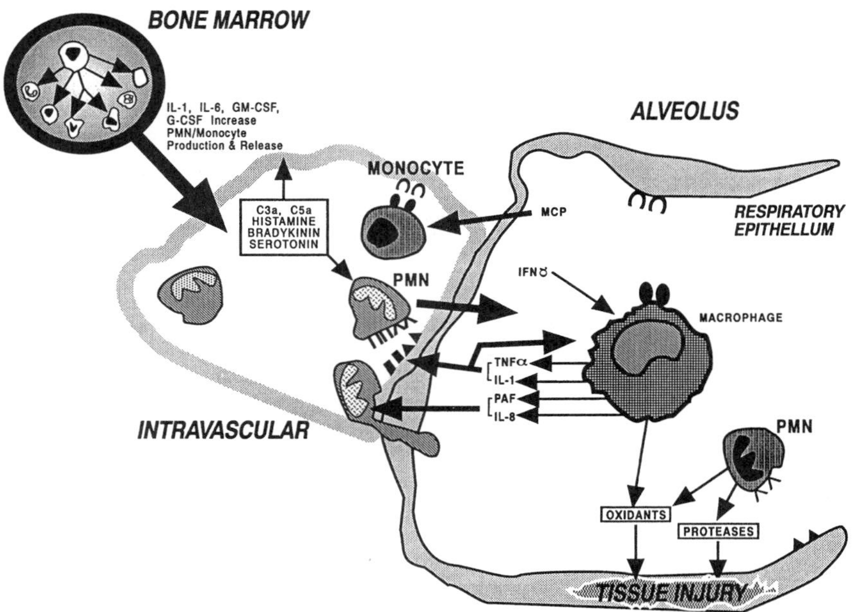

Figure 1. The putative role of several important proinflammatory cytokines in the recruitment and activation of effector cells associated with inflammatory lung injury.

IL-1 and TNF are the prototypical initiation cytokines involved in the early inflammatory response (23,54). While the production of most cytokines requires derepression of specific genes and subsequent transcription and translation, these cytokines are stored preformed in the membrane of tissue macrophages bound to precursor molecules and released in response to various stimuli such as PDGF discharged from platelets undergoing aggregation in response to tissue damage (148). The availability of IL-1 and TNF to be readily released from macrophages underscores their early recognition function (148). These early release cytokines interact with the neighboring cells in an autocrine or paracrine manner (187). In the lung these cells include macrophages, epithelial and endothelial cells, fibroblasts, and other resident immune cells that make up the alveolar wall. The subsequent cytokine cascade, stimulated by increased TNF and IL-1 levels, leads to the infiltration of inflammatory cells by the generation of chemotactic factors from contiguous resident cells. For example, neutrophils can be activated and recruited by the action of IL-8 while macrophages are attracted to the area of injury by cytokines such as the MCP (143). The recognition cytokines, IL-1 and TNF, also upregulate expression of cell adhesion molecules (e.g., ICAM-1, ELAM-1, and VCAM-1) on endothelial cells that serve as ligands for the integrins on inflammatory cells (e.g., neutrophils, macrophages, and lymphocytes), facilitating attachment of the effector cell prior to migration to the site having the higher chemotactic factor concentration (101,134,158,188).

Chemotactic agents are generated in response to exogenous irritants, TNF, and IL-1 as well as PDGF and IFN-γ (143). The ability of resident cells to produce chemotactic cytokines allows the inflammatory cells to migrate to the area where the inflammatory stimulus is localized. In addition to the chemokine subgroup of cytokines such as IL-8 and MCP-1, other noncytokine

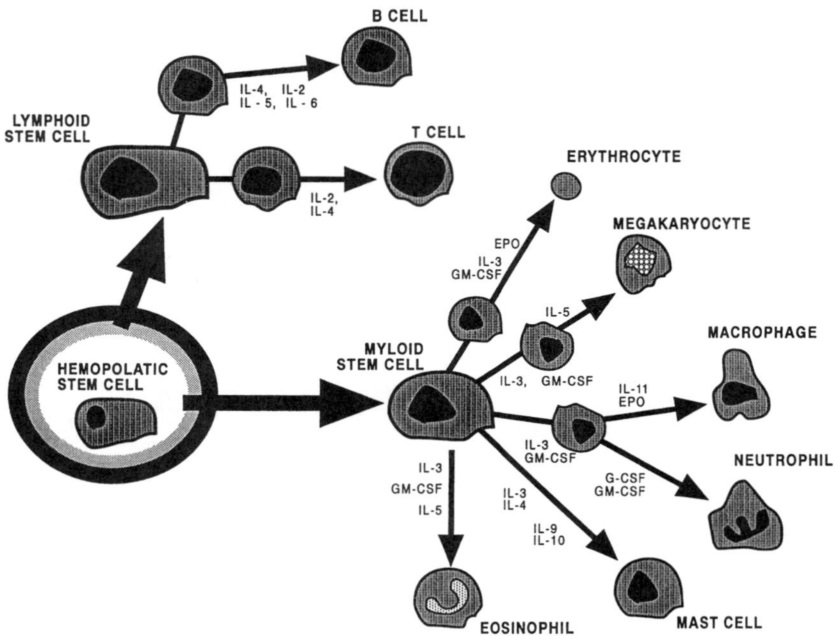

Figure 2. Schematic of the cytokine network involvement in hematopoiesis.

compounds may also be chemotactic for leukocytes. These substances are relatively nonspecific in their chemotactic role and include leukotriene B_4, platelet activating factor (PAF), components of the complement cascade (e.g., $C5_a$), and other substances released by cell injury such as polyamines and formyl peptides [e.g., f-Met-Leu-Phe (fMLP)] (35). However, only the chemokines possess a high degree of cellular specificity for recruitment of selective effector cells into the site of inflammation. As mentioned previously, the chemokines have recently become an area of intense study due to the potential for therapeutic control of the acute inflammatory pathologic process.

Following chemotaxis, other cytokines are secreted to fully activate the effector cells and maintain this increased level of activity. These cytokines continue to be released until the inciting stimulus (e.g., cellular debris) is removed. Of this group IFN-γ is central. This cytokine promotes the activation and differentiation of monocytes into macrophages, which increases the cells ability to phagocytize and digest the cellular debris and any other foreign material (e.g., bacteria or dirt particles), thereby increasing their removal so that repair can proceed (131). The oxidant activity is also increased in these cells as well as in neutrophils (15). Other cytokines including IFN-γ are also involved in the recruiting and activation of other effector cells such as lymphocytes to participate in this cleanup stage. These include the CSFs, IL-2, IL-4, IL-5, and IL-6. Changes in the microenvironment as well as the ability of the initial responses to be successful in cleaning up the injured site dictate which cytokines and effector cells are mobilized to participate in this process.

Cytokines involved in the reparative phase of the injury are responsible for normal healing after the initiating agent and/or damaged tissue is removed. These cytokines are important in the orchestration of cell growth and interstitial matrix deposition, neovascularization, fibrosis, and tissue remodeling following an injury (104). They are also important in inhibiting the inflammatory (and immune) responses that must precede this phase in order to prepare the microenvironment for subsequent reparative processes. PDGF, EGF, FGF, and TGF-β are all instrumental in directing the proliferation of resident cells to reestablish normal tissue architecture after injury. Cytokines secreted during the repair phase also stimulate neovascular development (angiogenesis) to reestablish blood flow to the injured area. IL-1, TNF, TGF-β, and FGF have all been demonstrated to have this property experimentally (7). Excessive scarring results from an exuberant or overly stimulated reparative process that can lead to keloid formation in the skin. When this occurs in the pulmonary system, it can result in fibrosis and restrictive lung disease.

Several models have been developed to illustrate the interaction of cytokine networks in acute inflammatory injury. The rodent model of antigen-antibody complex lung injury is one of the best-characterized examples of the role of these agents in experimental pulmonary disease (96). In this model immunoglobulin G (IgG) directed against bovine serum albumin is injected intratracheally and bovine serum is injected intravenously. The resultant injury is characterized histologically by neutrophilic infiltration, alveolar hemorrhage, and epithelial and endothelial cell damage. Leakage of protein into the alveoli can be used to quantify the severity of the resultant lung injury that directly correlates to the histologic picture morphometrically (97). Leakage of protein across the alveolar capillary border decreases following selective depletion of neutrophils or complement prior to injury (96). Therefore, the lung damage in this model requires the recruitment of neutrophils and activation of the complement cascade. Oxidants and proteases that are released from activated neutrophils and alveolar macrophages are the primary chemical mediators involved (97). In addition, endothelial cells are also active participants in the injury process, releasing PAF, cytokines, and oxidants, as well as upregulating the expression of adhesion molecules on their cells surface that serve as leukocyte attachment sites prior to migration into the alveoli (186). Most of these responses are cytokine mediated. A similar model of acute aspiration in rats has recently been developed, and although there are differences, many major parallels may be drawn between the inflammatory component of the acid-induced lung injury and the pathogenesis of the rodent antigen-antibody complex model (99,103).

Cytokines are intricately involved in the pathophysiology of this injury. As previous mentioned, alveolar macrophages are a reservoir of proinflammatory cytokines that may be released experimentally by many different types of stimuli. TNF activity increases manyfold during the development of the lung injury, and levels of this cytokine correlate with the severity of the capillary-alveolar protein leakage after 4 hours following instillation of the antigen. TNF induces the expression of endothelial adhesion molecules (e.g., ELAM-1), which plays a major role in neutrophil-endothelial interactions. PAF is also triggered by TNF. In addition, TNF causes the release of IL-8 and MCP-1 from endothelial as well as other cells. These cytokines are major selective chemotactic cytokines for neutrophils and macrophages, respectively. Antibodies directed against TNF can result in a marked reduction in alveolar permeability.

IL-1 plays a role similar to TNF in the pathogenesis of this lung injury model. This cytokine is also involved in neutrophil recruitment. IL-1, like TNF, induces ELAM-1 expression on endothelial cells and stimulates IL-8 and MCP-1 release (186). As previously mentioned, IL-1 and TNF represent the initial phase, recognition cytokines, and are responsible for the beginning of the cytokine cascade that leads to the recruitment and activation of the inflammatory effector cells and other cytokines involved in augmenting the acute inflammatory response, causing the development of the chronic inflammatory response (if the acute inflammatory reaction is unsuccessful in removing the stimulus), and the subsequent reparative processes.

CYTOKINES IN HEALTH

The Immune Response

The best-understood action of cytokines is their role in modulating the immune system. Most of the cytokines identified today are either directly or indirectly involved in the growth, differentiation, or activation of the different immune effector cells (9). Various cytokines can upregulate or downregulate the immune system depending on the cell type and its stage of differentiation. In addition, several cytokines (e.g., the INFs, TNFs, IL-1, and IL-6) also exhibit direct antiviral activity (7,13). Cell-mediated and humoral immunity are the primary mechanisms for attacking an infection (parasitic, bacterial, or viral), transplanted tissue, or tumor cells. Activation of this adaptive response requires a series of cellular activities, including cell-to-cell communication between lymphocytes and other monocytic cells via cytokines.

Mononuclear phagocytic cells, principally macrophages, are responsible for ingesting foreign antigens, as well as processing and presenting them in association with class I or class II major histocompatibility complexes (MHCs) to lymphocytes from both humoral and cell-mediated components of the immune response. In addition, these antigen-presenting cells (APCs) secrete IL-1, IL-6, and TNF, which activate and initiate the subsequent immunologic responses including proliferation of myeloid precursors in the bone marrow. These cytokines are also responsible for many of the systemic symptoms associated with infection. TNF activates macrophages in an autocrine fashion and increases TNF-β (lymphokine) production in lymphocytes (187). IL-1 is a potent cytokine in T-cell activation, TNF-β production, and macrophage activation (54). IL-6 enhances lymphocyte differentiation, B-lymphocyte proliferation and production of antibodies, and activation of T-lymphocytes (9). Phagocytosis, antigen presentation, expression of the MHC, and membrane-bound IL-1 activity are decreased by anesthesia and surgery in macrophages (45,58,141,165). Alterations in inhibitory and stimulatory cytokine secretion also occur in these cells following anesthesia and surgery (153).

Activation of effector cells (e.g., CTLs and antibody secreting plasma cells) specifically directed against an infectious organism or antigenically foreign cell requires presentation of specific antigens by APCs to T-helper cells (Th) as well as the potential effector cells. This activation also requires the synchronized release of cytokines from the APCs and Th cells (105). The cytokines released from macrophages have previously been described. Those released from Th cells include IL-2, IL-4, IL-10, and IFN-γ. IFN-γ increases the phagocytic properties and oxidant levels of macrophages and is key in the development of the delayed-type hypersensitivity (DTH) response (131). IL-2 specifically promotes the proliferation of clonally activated T-lymphocytes as well as enhancing lymphocyte-mediated cytotoxicity and TNF-β production (163). IL-2 is also involved in B-cell activation, specifically favoring the production of certain antibody subtypes. IL-4 in concert with IL-10 induces the secretion of antibody from B-lymphocytes and upregulates the expression of MHC class II antigens, enhancing the ability of B cells to interact with APCs (40,152). Other less clearly defined lymphocyte subsets modulate suppressor and augmentation activity, thereby controlling the intensity of the immune response to a specific stimulus. These immune modulating lymphocytes also function through the secretion of cytokines. For example, TGF-β and IL-10 may inhibit the production of other cytokines such as TNF and IL-1, which potentiate the inflammatory/immune response (134). TGF-β also has direct inhibitory effects on lymphocyte activity (7).

The interaction of IL-4 and IFN-γ is an excellent example of the role of cytokine networks in determining the response of the host to a foreign antigen. Experimentally, control of the immune response by restrictive production of cytokines results from stimulation of selective subsets of Th cells designated Th1 and Th2 (69). The interaction of these two different Th cell populations via the release of specific cytokines determines whether cell-mediated responses predominate and which pattern of humoral responses occur following exposure to a particular antigen. Th1 cells release IL-2 and IFN-γ, while Th2 cells appear to primarily release IL-4, IL-5, and IL-10. Th1-dominated immune responses to foreign antigens favor the cellular component, including DTH, but also increase B cell proliferation and production of selective subtypes of antibody. Th2-directed immune activities favor humoral responses and in particular IgE and other allergic reagents (127). IFN-γ profoundly inhibits IL-4 driven B-cell responses, while IL-4 and IL-10 inhibit IFN-γ-mediated lymphocyte responses. Interestingly, IL-10 is not depressed by cyclosporine or FK-506, two drugs used extensively in the maintenance phase of immune suppression for organ transplantation. Therefore, this cytokine may also be involved in the beneficial immune suppression in these patients.

Hematopoiesis

Hematopoiesis is a process in which a few self-renewing stem cells can differentiate and proliferate into all the cellular elements of the blood. The study of this important biologic function is very difficult since, as previously discussed, the direct or indirect (permissive, facilatory, additive, synergistic, antagonistic, etc.) effects in vivo cannot be differentiated simply by exogenous added cytokines. Furthermore, in vitro studies do not necessarily correlate with the in vivo findings. Selective use of monoclonal antibodies may help unravel some of these in vivo interactions in future experiments. Maturation of blood-forming cells must be tightly controlled. The intrinsic cytokines responsible for this control are termed hematopoietic growth factors. As would be expected, the development and release into the circulatory system of the cellular elements of blood and the immune response are closely integrated. Therefore, the cytokines involved in hematopoiesis include not only the three CSFs, IL-3, erythropoietin, and stem cell growth factor, but, not surprisingly, almost all of the ILs, TNFs, and IFNs (178). G-CSF is specific for stimulation of neutrophils, while M-CSF is involved with monocytes (178). Erythropoietin stimulates the proliferation and differentiation of red blood cells and the differentiation of megakaryocytes (29). In peripheral blood this is demonstrated by a reticulocytosis and thrombocytosis. GM-CSF and IL-3 enhance the proliferation of granulocytes, macrophages, and megakaryocytes, and are synergistic with erythropoietin in the production of RBCs (178). Furthermore, many of the cytokines whose primary role is hematopoiesis also play ancillary roles in inflammation and the immune response.

Other cytokines are also responsible of the growth, differentiation, maturation, and release of the blood-forming cellular elements in the bone marrow and other anatomic sites involved in hematopoiesis (e.g., lymph nodes, spleen, and other identifiable collections of reticuloendothelial cells, such as Peyer's patches). IL-1 produces lymphopenia, peripheral neutrophilia, and a mild myeloid hyperplasia after repeated doses (178). IL-2 produces lymphopenia followed by lymphocytosis (163). IL-5 causes eosinophil differentiation in vitro and is required for eosinophilia in response to experimental blood-borne parasite infection in mice (14). IL-6 enhances IL-3–dependent proliferation of granulocytes and macrophages (107). This cytokine also causes neutrophilia and lymphopenia and probably positively stimulates myeloid precursors. IL-6 also produces an indirect synergistic effect with erythropoietin, M-CSF, and G-CSF (107). IL-7 supports the growth of early B-cell precursors and T-lymphocytes (11). IL-8 results in an initial neutrophilia followed by neutropenia (178). The IFNs produce an antiproliferative action that suppresses the circulating numbers of neutrophils, monocytes, and lymphocytes (197). TNF may be either stimulatory or inhibitory to hematopoiesis depending on other cytokine levels and the cell being examined (149). The interactions of cytokines in the different stages of hematopoiesis are extremely complicated. Much more still needs to be learned before we can accurately define the important interactions between these physiologic modulators of the differentiation of the blood forming cells.

Other Properties

In addition to the biologic responses discussed above, cytokines are important in a number of other ways in maintaining health. Cytokines are critical determinants of local and systemic responses involving protection against injury and in stimulating the subsequent healing process. For example, recovery from small wounds, major trauma, hemorrhage, burns, poisoning, and cold exposure is all mediated by the action of cytokines. The local role of cytokines in the repair of a simple wound and lung injury has been described above. In addition, many of the systemic responses of cytokines are also directed toward protecting the injured patient. For example, TNF and IL-6 are responsible for many of the beneficial metabolic effects that are associated with injury (67). TNF promotes the mobilization of energy substrates and compounds required to synthesize protective proteins (e.g., lipids, amino acids) from the periphery to the liver. Following injury the liver is stimulated by TNF, IL-1, and IL-6 acting synergistically to produce acute-phase proteins that are acutely protective to the host during periods of intense stress (67). These include C-reactive protein, serum amyloid A, fibrinogen, α_1-antitrypsin, α_1-antichymotrypsin, and haptoglobulin. TNF and IL-1 also prepare the host to fight off an infection as previously described by increasing the proliferation, differentiation, and release of neutrophils and macrophages from the bone marrow, as well as activating these cells to be more cytocidal. Unfortunately, many of the beneficial roles of these proinflammatory cytokines may become detrimental when there is an exaggerated systemic release of these agents. Furthermore, the pathogenesis of many chronic diseases is associated with increased levels of these cytokines over extended periods of time.

A number of cytokines, particularly IL-1, IL-2, IL-6, and TNF, may be involved with normal hormonal homeostatic control mechanisms (162). Those hormonal properties most intensively studied include the neuroendocrine effects involving the release of adrenocorticotropic hormone (ACTH) as well as growth hormone, prolactin, LTH, β-endorphin, and corticotropic-releasing hormone. In addition, astrocytes in the brain may directly produce IL-1, IL-6, and TNF. As pyrogenic agents, IL-1, IL-6, and TNF are also involved in homeostatic control of temperature and circadian rhythms (102). In addition, many of the effects seen in the liver during periods of extreme stress may reflect the extreme response of otherwise normal control in nonstressful periods (162).

CYTOKINES IN DISEASE

Overview

Clinically, the role of cytokines in disease processes is best illustrated by their involvement in the pathogenesis of sepsis/SIRS. Sepsis continues to be a leading cause of death in the United States, with approximately 50% of the patients diagnosed as having septic shock progressing to a fatal outcome (38). The incidence of sepsis will increase as more patients are kept alive with severe debilitating illness or by treatment that results in significant clinical immune suppression. Surprisingly, in spite of more potent antibiotics, advanced monitoring, better mechanical ventilators, new inotropic agents, and improved nutritional support techniques, the mortality rate from sepsis and septic shock has not changed in 30 years (26,27,191). Death comes from the progression of a systemic response that is acutely characterized clinically by anorexia, fever, catabolism, and hemodynamic instability. Multisystem organ failure usually develops and heralds the patient's ultimate demise. A similar clinical picture is also seen in the absence of systemic infections, where severely injured or necrotic tissue replaces bacterial components as the initiating stimulus. The generalized inflammatory condition that develops from the intense systemic response to sepsis as well as other types of severe tissue injury, as previously mentioned, is known as SIRS (8). Other factors, besides infection, associated with the development of the clinical pictures of SIRS include massive trauma, extensive burns, prolonged and severe hemorrhagic shock, acute pancreatitis, and cardiopulmonary bypass. The final common pathway for these severe pathologic conditions appears to be widespread endothelial cell dysfunction leading to increased vascular permeability. Neutrophils and macrophages are activated and migrate into the surrounding tissues followed by the release of chemical mediators of inflammation (e.g., oxidants and proteases). These leukocyte-derived chemical effectors may produce massive tissue injury progressing to organ failure (28). This inflammatory response involves the interaction of a host of mediators whose roles are yet to be fully characterized. Although cytokines appear to play a central role in the pathogenesis of SIRS, other agents, including eicosanoids, complement factors, nitric oxide, and PAF, have all been implicated to some degree in the development of this unique injury pattern.

Proinflammatory cytokines, produced in response to infection or cell injury, that are involved as mediators in the pathogenesis of SIRS include TNF, IL-1, IL-6, IL-8, the CFSs, and IFN-γ. Many other cytokines have also been implicated in different aspects of the manifestation of this disease, but their exact roles are still undergoing investigation and are not completely defined. Intensive studies in many laboratories have now implicated these agents in the pathogenesis of the SIRS (21,22,39, 50,78,85,119,124,125,140).

The proinflammatory cytokines are produced both at the site of infection/injury as well as systemically. Furthermore, while the ability of the organism to respond to changes in the environment with small changes in TNF, IL-1, and IL-6 is important in homeostatic control and necessary in eliciting the immune response, the very high levels of these agents produced in response to pathologic stimuli can lead to the clinical picture of SIRS. Understanding the role of these proinflammatory cytokines in disease is important in developing new therapeutic strategies aimed at decreasing the morbidity and mortality of SIRS. These new therapies will be discussed later in the chapter; however, first it is important to understand the role of cytokines in the pathogenesis of SIRS as defined in both human and animal studies.

Cytokines and Infection

As previously stated, cytokines are important as mediators of the host immune defense against infection. However, the majority of the systemic damage resulting from sepsis is directly related to an exaggerated response leading to an increased release of endogenous proinflammatory cytokines. This is best demonstrated by the response of the organism to endotoxin, the lipopolysaccharide (LPS) component of the membrane wall of gram-negative bacteria. LPS is a potent stimulator of cytokine production in both animal and human models. Experimentally, plasma levels of TNF, IL-1, and IL-6 are increased following parental injection with either *Escherichia coli* or LPS (33,78,142). TNF plasma levels are also elevated in human volunteers given LPS and early in patients with known gram-negative and gram-positive bacteremia (46,71,124,183,185). Injection of LPS leads to a the development of SIRS, which appears to be mediated by sequential release of TNF, IL-1, and IL-6. Interestingly, parenterally administered TNF in man and experimental animals also produces the same pathophysiologic host responses as does LPS (64,132,172,174,180).

TNF levels also increase in response to many exogenous stimuli besides LPS. TNF levels are increased by malaria *(Plasmodium falciparum)* in human (170) and murine models (75). *Legionella pneumophila* (25) and influenza virus (19) also increase TNF induction. Human immunodeficiency virus increases TNF levels systemically (106) as well as following infection of isolated mononuclear cells (181) Influenza virus increases TNF-α and IL-1 levels locally as determined by bronchial alveolar washings in mice (168,179). TNF levels are elevated following myocardial infarction (121) and heart allograft rejection (41), and appear to be an important mediator associated with mortality and morbidity in graft versus host reaction (145).

Experimentally, most if not all of the characteristic physiologic sequelae of sepsis as well as end-organ injury can be attributed to TNF and its induction of the inflammatory cytokine cascade (21,175). Parenterally administered recombinant TNF produces the septic syndrome characterized by hypotension, acidosis, multisystem organ failure, and death in dogs (174) and rodent models (172). Histopathologic evidence of pulmonary congestion, adrenal necrosis, and bowel ischemia and necrosis are demonstrated in rodents following TNF administration (172). TNF induces a hemodynamic profile identical to the one associated with sepsis in canines (130) as well as depresses myocyte function in vitro (91). However, increased TNF levels alone are not responsible for the pathogenesis of septic shock (140). IL-1 has been implicated in the hemodynamic response associated with sepsis, and together with TNF, associated with the severity of end organ injury (140).

TNF also stimulates release of other cytokines, resulting in a cascade of mediators with complex and as yet not fully defined interactions. In this regard, TNF, as an early initiator of this cascade, has been extensively studied in experimental sepsis. Elevated levels of TNF are temporally associated with the release of other proinflammatory cytokines that in turn may potentiate or ameliorate the release and/or the biologic responses to TNF. TNF appears in the circulation within minutes after challenge with LPS, peaks within 2 hours, and returns to baseline by 4 hours (17,85). IL-1 peaks approximately 3 hours after LPS infusion and IL-6 levels continue to rise for up to 8 hours (66) (Fig. 3). TNF enhances both the release of IL-1 and IL-6 in this model of sepsis. Furthermore, these increases in IL-1 and IL-6 levels can be attenuated using TNF antibodies in an experimental model (66).

Specific examples of marked cytokine synergism and potentiation have been identified. For example, in rabbits, small amounts of TNF and IL-1 injected alone have no effect. However, when TNF and IL-1 are combined in the same dosages that had previously produced no symptoms, profound shock results, and there is histologic evidence of pulmonary edema, hemorrhage, and severe lung injury (140). IL-1 also potentiates the lethal affect of TNF-α in mice (184). Murine recombinant IFN-γ pretreatment of mice challenged with salmonella endotoxin increases TNF and IL-6 levels and mortality. Pretreatment with IFN-γ monoclonal antibody leads to increased survival in the same model (83).

In humans the interactions of the cytokine network during clinical sepsis are still being unraveled. Recently there has been an explosion of interest in the role of these cytokines in the pathogenesis of sepsis, since this represents an area of potential therapy for a disease of high morbidity and mortality. Not surprisingly, contradictory results have been reported. The reasons for these conflicting findings are readily apparent. Cytokines have short serum half-lives (182), resulting in sporadic detection in obviously septic patients, further causing difficulty in interpreting the data. Furthermore, temporal relationships of cytokine cascades that are very easy to control experimentally are very difficult to follow in patients in which the status of many of the confounding variables is not discernible. To confuse the issue even further, elevated levels of TNF-soluble receptors and the competitive IL-1 antagonist IL-1ra appear in the serum within minutes after a biologic stimulus to release the cytokine in an apparent attempt to attenuate the pathophysiologic responses of these agents (61). Moreover, downregulation of production of TNF, IL-1, IL-6, and IL-8 by IL-10 also occurs. Increases in the levels of IL-10 as well as several other cytokines (e.g., TGF-β) are associated with inhibition of the proinflammatory cytokines as well as the immune response in general. This inhibition may also account for some of the increased susceptibility to infectious complications that occur in these patients. The associated cytokine responses as well as the action of noncytokine mediators would obviously be important in the eventual outcome of the disease and may vary from patient to patient based on a number of factors such as age and physical status (2). Lastly, unknown species variation can make extrapolation of experimental findings difficult. Therefore, not surprisingly, TNF activity can be detected systemically in only a third of patients with septic shock (118).

Cytokines and Trauma/Hemorrhagic Shock

Increases in proinflammatory cytokines have been directly implicated as the mediators of the acute-phase response, leukocyte dysfunction, and immune/inflammatory changes that contribute to the potential development of ARDS and sepsis following hemorrhage and/or trauma (1). Thirty percent or more of severely traumatized patients develop ARDS, and many of these patients progress to SIRS with other organ dysfunction and death (59,68). The role cytokines play in SIRS following trauma and hemorrhagic shock differs from that of sepsis. Although TNF is strongly implicated in the pathophysiology of septic shock, its role in the initial acute inflammatory (146) or pathophysiologic response to trauma is not as readily apparent. Early TNF levels do not correlate with the injury severity score, Glasgow Coma Scale, presence of hemorrhagic shock, site of injury, or the need for emergent surgery. Likewise, TNF levels are not predictive of which patients go on to develop sepsis or multisystem organ failure (146). However, following traumatic injuries, patients do have elevated levels of TNF-soluble receptors when compared to nontraumatized patients (169). These intriguing results pose the question of whether traumatic injury causes just the elevation of TNF receptors or if an increase in TNF activity occurs acutely that is not detectable due to the increase in soluble receptors. Molecular techniques will help answer this question. However, in a murine hemorrhagic shock model, survival rates do not improve when TNF antibody is administered (49).

Other cytokines also appear to be involved in the systemic response to trauma, some very early, as evidenced by autopsy findings of ARDS-like changes present in as little as 24 hours following injury (137). Severe accidental trauma is associated with large systemic increases in IL-6 (56,90,167) and IL-8 shortly following injury (90). Both the magnitude and the duration of elevation of these two cytokines correlates directly with the severity of injury. In this same population IL-1 was not found in any patients and TNF levels were insignificant (90). Likewise, marked increases in IL-10 and smaller elevations of IL-4 are also seen following injury and hemorrhage. As previously mentioned, these cytokines have a major impact on downregulation of the cell-mediated immune response and, as a result of this, may be responsible for some of the immune

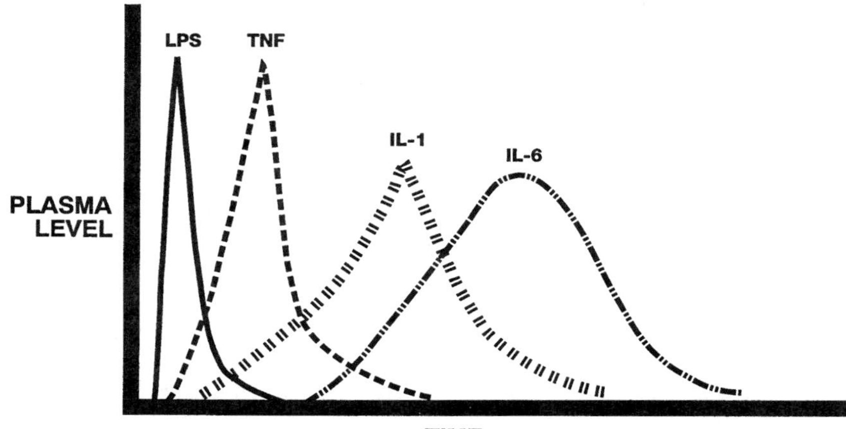

Figure 3. Sequential appearance of cytokines in plasma following endotoxin challenge.

suppression associated with trauma. Routine surgical operations also demonstrate increased systemic levels of these trauma-associated cytokines as well as immune suppression (44,135).

While TNF and IL-1 do not appear to have major roles in the pathophysiology following trauma and hemorrhage, depression of other cytokines following hemorrhage may alter the normal immune response and render the host susceptible to infection and sepsis. Hemorrhagic shock increases susceptibility to subsequent infection (1,12,112,117). Hemorrhagic shock results in decreased production of IL-1 (40), IL-2, IFN-γ (2,4), IL-3, and IL-5 (4). Similarly, in mice IL-2, IL-3, IFN-γ, and IL-6 are decreased following hemorrhage (122). IL-2 levels that are depressed following simple hemorrhage in an animal model remain depressed for 3 days despite adequate fluid resuscitation (164). IL-2 levels are also depressed for 48 hours in a murine hemorrhagic model, but increase twofold by 72 hours posthemorrhage (4). Patients with hemorrhage and trauma are also noted to have decreased IL-2 production by mononuclear cells, and this decrease correlates with the severity of injury and hemorrhage. Predictably, lymphocyte responses are also reduced, and correlate with the extent of injury (3). Interestingly, elevations in IL-10 levels that, as previously stated, are also associated with trauma may both inhibit the release and directly antagonize the actions of TNF, IL-1, IL-2, IL-6, and IFN-γ.

Cytokines and Cardiopulmonary Bypass

Multisystem organ failure following cardiopulmonary bypass may be similar to that seen following sepsis. The most common manifestation of SIRS after cardiopulmonary bypass is ARDS (123). This has caused attention to be focused on the role of proinflammatory cytokines as the mediators of organ dysfunction following cardiac surgery. TNF, IL-1, IL-6, and IL-8 have all been reported elevated after use of extracorporeal circulation.

Institution of cardiopulmonary bypass results in a transient increase in serum levels of endotoxin that are elevated a second time following unclamping of the aorta. This increase in serum endotoxin levels is associated with an elevation of serum TNF levels that peak approximately one hour post-bypass (95). In addition, TNF may be responsible for the endothelial dysfunction seen following myocardial ischemia and the reperfusion injury also associated with cardiac surgery (108). Furthermore, use of extracorporeal circulation is also associated with an increase in systemic IL-1 levels (47,79). IL-1 and IL-8 are also increased in circulating leukocytes. These cell-associated cytokine levels peak at 24 hours postbypass. Interestingly, IL-8 is not found free in the plasma (98). IL-6 levels are also reported elevated in the immediate post–cardiopulmonary bypass period (30). These findings suggest a presumptive cause for the ARDS-like picture that patients occasionally present following cardiac surgery.

Cytokines and Burns

Clinical data following major thermal injuries reveal that, unlike trauma, TNF may play a role in the pathogenesis of the systemic response. Systemic TNF levels are increased following severe thermal injury; however, they do not correlate with burn size or outcome (34,150). IL-1 levels are also elevated following thermal injury, peaking during the first week. However, unlike TNF, IL-1 levels do correlate with burn size (53,192). Conversely, IL-2 levels are suppressed following thermal injury, and the degree and duration of suppression correlates inversely with the size of the burn (192). Suppression of IL-2 production inhibits the cellular immune response to infection, which may be reversed by administering recombinant IL-2. Experimentally, IL-2, given to burned mice, offers increased protection against bacterial challenge (74).

Acute thermal injury also results in systemic elevation of IL-6 and IL-8 levels (53,150). However, increases in systemic levels of these cytokines as well as TNF do not correlate with mortality, organ failure, or the incidence of infection. Interestingly, IL-8 serum levels do correlate with the size and depth of the burn, suggesting that IL-8 may be used as a systemic marker for determining the extent of tissue damage associated with the thermal injury (150). In the same report, acute thermal injury resulted in an increase in the local production of IL-6 and IL-8, including lung as well as both burned and unburned skin. The pulmonary injury that appears following the burn does correlate with the generation of IL-8 in the resident cells of the lung (150). As previously stated, increased systemic levels of both IL-1 and TNF may be responsible for the local production of both IL-6 and IL-8. Since IL-8 appears to be the major cytokine generated by the lung following thermal skin injury, its role in ARDS in these patients needs further defining.

Other Diseases

Cytokine imbalances have also been indicated in the etiology of a number of acute and chronic diseases representing not only the lung but most other organ systems. While it is not within the purview of this chapter to expand upon these interesting areas, a brief mention illustrates the scope of the possible roles of cytokines in disease processes. Not unexpectedly, TNF, IL-1, IL-2, IL-3, IL-4, IL-5, IL-6, IL-8, IFN-γ, TGF-β, and GM-CSF have all been reported altered in rheumatic diseases (48). Imbalances in the local levels of TNF-α, IFN-γ, IL-1, IL-2, IL-4, IL-6, IL-8, and TGF-α have been suggested as the causes of many skin diseases, for example, contact dermatitis, atopic dermatitis, and psoriasis (133). The role of cytokines in the pathogenesis of glomerulonephritis has been extensively studied. Renal tubular interstitial disease has been less intensively examined. Alterations in TNF, IL-1, IL-2, IL-6, IL-8, and IFN-γ have been implicated in the pathogenesis of both forms of renal disease (55). Finally, cytokine interactions in patients with AIDS, cancer, inflammatory intestinal diseases, necrotizing enterocolitis, as well as many types of parasitic infections have become areas of focused study. Investigations of the involvement of these cytokine networks may help provide new therapeutic strategies to deal with many of these difficult diseases in the future.

Cytokines as Prognostic and Diagnostic Indicators

Elevated systemic cytokine levels have significant diagnostic and prognostic value. TNF levels correlate with fatal outcome in patients with meningococcal disease (71,183,185) and with the severity of the disease in children with malaria (76). In children with gram-negative meningococcemia and purpura fulminans, IL-1 and INF-γ levels are also significantly higher in nonsurvivors than in survivors (71). Conflicting results have been reported regarding the ability of TNF to predict outcome in septic patients. Several investigators have reported that TNF is predictive (31,185). However, in a prospective multicenter study, TNF levels have not been prognostic of outcome in septic patients (62). Interestingly, the inability to produce IL-1 has been related to poor prognosis in severely septic patients (116). Finally, IFN-γ levels are not associated with outcome in septic shock (31).

Increases in IL-6 levels appear to be the most reliable predictor of disease severity and outcome. Increased IL-6 levels and their temporal profile are prognostic of fatal outcomes as revealed in a human sepsis prospective multicenter study (62). For example, failure of IL-6 levels to drop over the first 24 hours following anti-TNF antibody treatment is predictive of a fatal outcome and is a more reliable predictor than the initial IL-6 titers (62,93). IL-6 levels are also greater in nonsurvivors of burn injury (53). Finally, IL-6 levels may be a diagnostic sign of nosocomial infections (60).

CYTOKINE-DIRECTED THERAPY

SIRS and Infectious Disease Therapy

The explosion of knowledge regarding the role of proinflammatory cytokines in pathogenesis of sepsis has resulted in exciting therapeutic possibilities in dealing with the organ damage associated with SIRS. Most current research has been directed toward two general strategic approaches: (a) reducing the generation of proinflammatory cytokines or enhancing the production of cytokines that antagonize or reverse the untoward effects of the inflammatory agents, and (b) decreasing the pathologic responses of these agents by employing specific soluble receptors and monoclonal antibodies directed against specific cytokines.

Strategies aimed at reducing or altering cytokine production include limiting cellular production, and attempting to restore the beneficial balance between different cytokines. Corticosteroids are the best-known inhibitors of expression of proinflammatory cytokines. Corticosteroids block the translation of TNF specific mRNA (20), thereby decreasing the generation of TNF by LPS. Corticosteroids protect animals in septic shock models (87,94), and low-dose dexamethasone lowers cerebral spinal fluid levels of TNF and IL-1 and improves neurologic outcome in pediatric patients with meningitis (129,138). The dose of steroid used appears to be critical. While the use of low-dose steroids appears to be beneficial (72), administration of high doses is without advantage (25,115,171) and may actually be harmful due to immune suppressive effects.

Other promising drugs include diltiazem and drugs that increase intracellular adenosine 3',5'-cyclic monophosphate (cAMP). Diltiazem reverses the inhibition of proimmune lymphocyte-mediated cytokine production that is depressed in a hemorrhagic murine model (122). Pentoxifylline increases intracellular cAMP, which results in increased TNF mRNA turnover (80,166), thereby reducing the generation of TNF in both animal models (154) and human volunteers (196). Pentoxifylline is beneficial in the resuscitation of experimental hemorrhagic shock (189) and prevents TNF-induced lung injury (110). Amrinone also inhibits TNF production via the cAMP mechanism (73). Dobutamine and other β-agonists may likewise decrease TNF production via cAMP (72). However, abrupt discontinuation of agents that increase cAMP have been shown to result in cellular hyperresponsiveness to LPS (73).

Nutritional factors may also affect cytokine production. Replacement of dietary N-6 fatty acids with N-3 fatty acids may depress TNF and IL-1 synthesis (24). Oral feedings also decrease TNF production as compared with intravenous feedings as a result of decreasing translocation of gut bacteria, thereby decreasing the amount of endotoxin reaching the systemic circulation (65).

The experimental evidence for the role of TNF in the pathogenesis of sepsis has led several investigators to examine the therapeutic effectiveness of anti-TNF monoclonal antibodies in the treatment of SIRS. Such therapy attempts to interrupt the initiation of the proinflammatory cytokine cascade. Unfortunately, the results to date on the efficacy of TNF monoclonal antibody therapy are inconsistent. TNF monoclonal antibody therapy decreases the mortality following (a) a lethal injection of LPS in rats (18) and nonhuman primates (88,173), (b) gram-negative sepsis in primates (125), (c) *Pseudomonas aeruginosa* infections in rats (142), and (d) *Staphylococcus aureus* infections in primates (89). However, TNF monoclonal antibodies do not protect against *Streptococcus pyogens*-induced sepsis in a murine model, in spite of the significant TNF elevations associated with the infection (190). In one large prospective multicenter study 80 patients with severe sepsis have received monoclonal TNF antibody without survival benefit (62). The results of this multicenter study indicate that the timing of anti-TNF therapy may be critical. Early intervention appears to be required, as once the septic state has developed TNF antibodies do not appear to be effective. This could be predicted based on overwhelming data supporting the paradigm that TNF is an initiating cytokine and promotes generation of other proinflammatory cytokines (e.g., IL-1, IL-6, IL-8, IFN-γ) that are required for inflammatory cell activation and recruitment as well as maintenance of the inflammatory response. Therefore, consistent with experimental results, TNF monoclonal antibody therapy has limitations (28). Supporting this hypothesis, TNF activity is found elevated in only one-third of septic shock patients (118), and studies have shown that TNF levels alone are not sufficient to produce shock (159). Furthermore, TNF monoclonal antibodies may not be effective in treating all causes of sepsis if different cytokine profiles are involved. For example, while anti-TNF therapy is efficacious in a murine model of *E. coli* infection, there is no protection against *Klebsiella pneumoniae* (160). Finally, blocking TNF activity with monoclonal antibodies may also inhibit the beneficial role of TNF in the immune response. For example, mice are more susceptible to the lethal effects of *Listeria* (82) and malarial parasites (75) following TNF antibody administration.

Although it may appear to be beneficial to block certain cytokines such as TNF, administration of other cytokines may be beneficial. IFN-γ administration improves outcome of bacterial infections in hemorrhagic and traumatized mice (57,84,112,117). This is most likely due to the ability of IFN-γ to promote the cell-mediated immune response, including increased macrophage effector function as well as neutrophil activity that have been depressed possibly as a result of increased inhibitory cytokine levels such as IL-10 or TGF-β secondary to the physiologic insult.

Use of exogenous-administered, naturally occurring, cytokine receptor antagonists also holds promise as a therapeutic modality (72). IL-1ra, previously described, competitively binds to the same receptor as IL-1, but does not transduce a cellular signal (81). In animal models IL-1ra improves survival in cases of endotoxemia (10,51,139). IL-1ra also reduces the lethality of an endotoxin-induced shock in rabbits, and the therapeutic value is also observed even when given after onset of septic shock (139). In humans, endogenous IL-1ra is currently undergoing trials in a large-scale multicenter study in septic patients. The initial data indicate a dose-dependent decrease in mortality (63).

Whereas receptor antagonists to IL-1 appear therapeutic in improving outcome in sepsis, there is a down side to this treatment. IL-1 is still an important cytokine in the immune response to sepsis. For example, in a murine model of combined thermal injury and sepsis, improved survival and fewer positive blood cultures have been reported in mice receiving exogenous IL-1 (161). Interestingly, IL-1 preconditioning of rats for 48 hours also reduces the tissue damage following myocardial ischemia-reperfusion injury (120). This example illustrates a problem previously eluded to that may be associated with anticytokine therapy. Most of these agents are important in the natural response of the patient to the physiologic insult. As a result, inhibiting the untoward effects of a cytokine may cause iatrogenic problems that are unforeseen. This is particularly of concern since admittedly our understanding of the role of cytokine networks in health and disease is still in its infancy.

Naturally occurring cytokine-soluble receptors to most cytokines can be demonstrated. As previously stated, these agents probably are responsible for homeostatic limiting of the biologic activity of the corresponding cytokine. A recombinant, soluble receptor for TNF has recently been developed (86), and a TNF-receptor–IgG protein inhibitor that has the same affinity of a natural receptor but a much longer half-life has been synthesized (144). Clinical trials utilizing these strategies are forthcoming.

The best therapeutic promise probably lies with a combination of therapies that interrupt the inflammatory cascade at multiple levels. For example, in a septic pig model TNF antibody when combined with ibuprofen attenuates the hemodynamic dysfunction and reduces the acute lung injury induced by sepsis to a greater degree than either agent used separately (128). Studies are currently under way that treat sepsis with combinations of TNF antibodies, IL-ra, and monoclonal antibodies to LPS. These multilevel therapeutic strategies hold great promise in reducing the significant morbidity and mortality currently associated with SIRS.

Control of the Immune Response to Transplantation

Cyclosporine and FK-506 are structurally different agents that work by similar mechanisms (111). The efficacy of both agents correlates with their ability to inhibit IL-2 production by lymphocytes in response to antigen presentation by APCs. Following antigen presentation, lymphocytes specific for that antigen express receptors to IL-2 (IL-2R). It is these lymphocytes that are sensitive to the mitogenic effects of IL-2. Therefore, inhibition of IL-2 production prevents activation and clonal expansion of these primed (IL-2R bearing) effector lymphocytes. Cyclosporine and FK-506 inhibit IL-2 synthesis by binding to intracellular proteins (immunophillins) that purportedly inhibit calcium-mediated cell signal transduction (113). This intracellular pathway is also responsible for the production of several other cytokines involved in immune regulation. These other cytokines, released from Th cells (e.g., IFN-γ, IL-4), may also be responsible for some of the immune suppressive actions of cyclosporine and FK-506. Interestingly, neither of these drugs inhibits IL-10, a cytokine also released from Th lymphocytes. Increased IL-10 levels are associated with inhibition of the cell-mediated immune responses, particularly the lymphocyte-directed, macrophage-mediated, delayed-type hypersensitivity response.

Understanding the cytokine cascade by which antigens become immunogenic suggests several possibilities currently under investigation that may protect the transplanted organ from allograft rejection (32). For example, IL-1 and TNF are both early-recognition cytokines released from macrophages in response to foreign antigen exposure as well as the ischemia/reperfusion injury that may occur following removal of the organ from the donor but prior to reanastomosis of blood vessels in the recipient. These cytokines are involved in the early immune responses involving antigen recognition and presentation of the antigen to the lymphocyte. Antigen and IL-1 appear to be required for the release of IL-2 and IFN-γ from Th cells. In addition, as previously stated, IL-1 and TNF are also both involved in initiating the cytokine cascade responsible for both acute and chronic inflammation. Experimental evidence exists for prolonging graft life by inhibiting the biologic responses associated with elevated levels of these cytokines. Steroids are directly antagonistic to IL-1 release and this effect may explain some of their efficacy in preventing organ rejection. More specifically, monoclonal antibodies directed against IL-1, TNF, or IL-1ra are possible strategies for treatment. Inhibition of specific cytokines at different sites in the immune activational network may help us tailor the immune suppression required to prevent allograft rejection, yet allow the host to maintain an otherwise normal defense against pathogenic organisms.

CONCLUSION

Cytokines are important regulators of biologic responses. Our ability to understand the importance of cytokine networks in health and disease is just beginning. Understanding and controlling the biologic responses of these potent agents responsible for cellular communication has great promise for treating patients with a myriad of diseases as well as allowing for the development of therapeutic interventions previously unimagined. We predict that, in the future, opportunities will develop, based on strategies designed to control the in vivo effects of cytokines, that will allow us to decrease many of the complications associated with anesthesia and surgery.

REFERENCES

1. Abraham E. Host defense abnormalities after hemorrhage, trauma, and burns. *Crit Care Med* 1989;17:934– 939.
2. Abraham E. T- and B-cell function and their roles in resistance to infection. *New Horizons* 1993;1:28–36.
3. Abraham E, Regan RF. The effects of hemorrhage and trauma on interleukin-2 production. *Arch Surg* 1985;120:1341–1344.
4. Abraham E, Freitas AA. Hemorrhage produces abnormalities in lymphocyte function and lymphokine generation. *J Immunol* 1989; 142:899–906.
5. Ackerknecht EH. Greek medicine: physicians, priests, philosophers. In: Ackerknecht EH, ed. *A short history of medicine.* Baltimore: Johns Hopkins University Press, 1982;47–54.
6. Aggarwal BB, Eessalu TE, Hass PE. Characterization of receptors for human tumoe necrosis factor and their regulation by gamma interferon. *Nature* 1985;318:665–667.
7. Aggarwal BB, Pocsik E. Cytokines: from clone to clinic. *Arch Biochem Biophys* 1992;292:335–359.
8. American College of Chest Physicians/Society of Critical Care Medicine Consensus Conference. Definitions for sepsis and organ failure and guidelines for the use of innovative therapies in sepsis. *Crit Care Med* 1992;20:864–874.
9. Arai K, Lee F, Miyajima A, et al. Cytokines: coordinators of immune and inflammatory responses. *Annu Rev Biochem* 1990;59: 783.
10. Arend WP. Interleukin-1 receptor antagonist. *J Clin Invest* 1991;88: 1445–1451.
11. Armitage RJ, Namen AE, Sassenfeld HM, et al. Regulation of human T-cell proliferation by IL-7. *J Immunol* 1990;144:938–941.
12. Ayala A, Perrin MM, Wagner MA, et al. Enhanced susceptibility to sepsis after simple hemorrhage. Depression of Fc and C3b receptor-mediated phagocytosis. *Arch Surg* 1990;125:70–75.
13. Balkwill FR. Interferons. *Lancet* 1989;1:1060–1063.
14. Basten A, Beeson PB. Mechanism of eosinophilia. II. Role of lymphocyte. *J Exp Med* 1970;131:1288.
15. Berton G, Zeni L, Cassatella MA, et al. Gamma interferon is able to enhance the oxidative metabolism of human neutrophils. *Biochem Biophys Res Commun* 1986;138:1276–1282.
16. Beutler B, Greenwald D, Hulmes JD, et al. Identity of tumor necrosis factor and macrophage-secreted factor cachectin. *Nature* 1985;316:552–554.
17. Beutler BA, Milshark IW, Cerami A. Cachectin/tumor necrosis factor: production, distribution and metabolic fate in vivo. *J Immunol* 1985;135:3972–3977.
18. Beutler B, Milshark IW, Cerami AC. Passive immunization against cachectin/tumor necrosis factor protects mice from lethal effect of endotoxin. *Science* 1985;229:869.
19. Beutler B, Krochin N, Milshark IW, et al. Induction of cachectin (tumor necrosis factor) synthesis by influenza virus: deficient production by endotoxin-resistant (C3H/HeJ) macrophages. *Clin Res* 1986;34:491A.
20. Beutler B, Krochin N, Milshark IW, et al. Control of cachectin (tumor necrosis factor) synthesis: mechanism of endotoxin resistance. *Science* 1986;232:977–980.
21. Beutler B, Cerami AC. Cachectin: more than a tumor necrosis factor. *N Engl J Med* 1987;316:379–385.
22. Beutler B, Cerami AC. The common mediator of shock, cachexia and tumor necrosis. *Adv Immunol* 1988;42:213–231.
23. Beutler B, Cerami A. The biology of cachectin/TNF-a primary mediator of the host response. *Annu Rev Immunol* 1989;7:625–655.
24. Billiar TR, Bankey PE, Svingen BA, et al. Fatty acid intake and kupffer cell function: fish oil alters eiconsanoid and monokine production to endotoxin stimulation. *Surgery* 1988;104:343–349.
25. Blanchard DK, Djeu JY, Klein TW, et al. The induction of tumor necrosis factor (TNF) in murine lung tissue during infection with *Legionella pneumophila:* a potential productive role of TNF. *Abstr Lymphokine Res* 1987;6:1421.
26. Bone RC, Fischer CJ, Clemmer TP, et al. Sepsis syndrome. A valid clinical entity. *Crit Care Med* 1989;17:389–393.

27. Bone RC. A critical evaluation of new agents for the treatment of sepsis. *JAMA* 1991;266:1686–1691.
28. Bone RC. The pathogenesis of sepsis. *Ann Intern Med* 1991;115: 457–469.
29. Burstein SA, Ishibashi T. Erythropoietin and megakaryocytopoiesis. *Blood Cells* 1989;15:202–204.
30. Butler J, Chong GL, Baigrie RJ, et al. Cytokine response to cardiopulmonary bypass with membrane and bubble oxygenation. *Ann Thorac Surg* 1992;53:833–838.
31. Calandra T, Baumgartner JD, Grau GE, et al. Prognostic value of tumor necrosis factor-cachectin, interleukin-1 interferon-alpha, and interferon-gamma in the serum of patients with septic shock. *J Infect Dis* 1990;161:982–987.
32. Campbell DA, McCurry K, Colletti L, et al. Cytokine biology and transplantation. In: Kunkel SL, Remick DG, eds. *Cytokines in health and disease.* New York: Marcel Dekker, 1992;353–370.
33. Cannon JG, Tompkins RG, Gelfand JA, et al. Circulating interleukin-1 and tumor necrosis factor in septic shock and experimental endotoxin fever. *J Infect Dis* 1990;161:79–84.
34. Cannon JG, Friedberg JS, Gelfand JA, et al. Circulating interleukin-1 beta and tumor necrosis factor- alpha concentration after burn injury in humans. *Crit Care Med* 1992;20:1414–1419.
35. Carp H. Mitochondrial N-formylmethionyl proteins as chemoattractants for neutrophils. *J Exp Med* 1982;155:264–275.
36. Carpenter G, Cohne S. Epidermal growth factor. *J Biol Chem* 1990; 265:7709–7712.
37. Carswell EA, Old LJ, Kassel RL, et al. An endotoxin induced serum factor that causes necrosis of tumors. *Proc Soc Natl Acad Sci* 1975;72:3666–70.
38. Centers for Disease Control. Increase in national hospital discharge survey rates for septicemia - United States.9–1987. *MMWR* 1987;39:31–34.
39. Cerami AC, Beutler B. Role of cachectin TNF in endotoxin shock cachexia. *Immunol Today* 1988;9:28–31.
40. Chaudry IH, Ayala A, Ertel W, et al. Hemorrhage and resuscitation: immunological aspects. *Am J Physiol* 1990;259:R663–R678.
41. Chollet-Martin S, Depoix JP, Hvass U, et al. Raised plasma levels of tumor necrosis factor in heart allograft rejection. *Transplant Proc* 1990;22:283–286.
42. Coffman RL, Ohara J, Bond MW, et al. B cell stimulatory factor 1 enhances the IgE response of lipopolysaccharide-activated B cells. *J Immunol* 1986;136:4538–4541.
43. Coley WB. The treatment of malignant tumors by repeated inoculations of erysipelas; with a report of ten original cases. *Am J Med Sci* 1883;105:487.
44. Cruickshank AM, Fraser WD, Burns HJ, et al. Response of serum interleukin-6 in patients undergoing elective surgery of varying severity. *Clin Sci* 1990;79:161–165.
45. Dagan O, Segal S, Tzehoval E. Effect of anesthesia on the immune system: suppression of the immunogenic capacity of macrophages and of lymphocyte transformation. *Immunol Invest* 1989;18: 975–985.
46. Damas P, Reuter A, Gysen P, et al. Tumor necrosis factor and interleukin-1 serum levels during severe sepsis in humans. *Crit Care Med* 1989;17:975–978.
47. Datta S, Engelman RM, Low H, et al. Interleukin-1 expression and it regulation of oxygen-free radical production in patients undergoing cardiopulmonary bypass. *Surg Forum* 1991;42:280–282.
48. DeMarco D, Zurier RB. Cytokines and rheumatic diseases. In: Kunkel SL, Remick DG, eds. *Cytokines in health and disease.* New York: Marcel Dekker, 1992;371–395.
49. De Maria EJ, Pellicane JV, Lee RB. Hemorrhagic shock in endotoxin-resistant mice: improved survival unrelated to deficient production of tumor necrosis factor. *J Trauma* 1993;35:720–724.
50. Dietch EA. Multiple organ failure: pathophysiology and potential future therapy. *Ann Surg* 1992;216:117– 134.
51. Dinarello CA, Thompson RC. Blocking IL-1: interleukin-1 receptor antagonist in vivo and in vitro. *Immunol Today* 1991;12: 404–409.
52. Dower SK, Sims JE, Cerretti DP, et al. The interleukin-1 system: receptors, ligands and signals. *Chem Immunol* 1992;51:33–64.
53. Drost AC, Burleson DG, Cioffi WG, et al. Plasma cytokines following thermal injury and their relationship with patient mortality, burn size, and time postburn. *J Trauma* 1993;35:335–339.
54. Durum SK, Schmidt JA, Oppenheim JJ. Interleukin-1: an immunological perspective. *Annu Rev Immunol* 1985;3:263–287.
55. Emancipator SN, Sedor JR. Cytokines and renal diseases. In: Kunkel SL, Remick DG, eds. *Cytokines in health and disease.* New York: Marcel Dekker, 1992;467–488.
56. Ertel W, Faist E, Nestle C, et al. Kinetics of interleukin-2 and interleukin-6 synthesis following major mechanical trauma. *J Surg Res* 1990;48:622–628.
57. Ertel W, Morrison MH, Ayala A, et al. Interferon attenuates hemorrhage-induced suppression of macrophage and splenocyte functions and decreases susceptibility to sepsis. *Surgery* 1992;111: 177–187.
58. Everson NW, Neoptolemos JP, Scott DJ, et al. The effect of surgical operation on monocytes. *Br J Surg* 1981;68:257–260.
59. Faist E, Baue AE, Dittmer H, et al. Multiple organ failure in polytrauma patients. *J Trauma* 1983;23:775– 787.
60. Fassbender K, Parggen H, Muller W, et al. Interleukin-6 and acutephase protein concentrations in surgical intensive care unit patients: diagnostic signs in nosocomial infection. *Crit Care Med* 1993;21:1175– 1180.
61. Fischer E, Van Zee KJ, Marano MA, et al. Interleukin-1 receptor antagonist circulates in experimental inflammation and in human disease. *Blood* 1992;79:2196–2200.
62. Fisher CJ, Opal SM, Dhainaut JF, et al. Influence of an anti-tumor necrosis factor monoclonal antibody on cytokine levels in patients with sepsis. *Crit Care Med* 1993;21:318–327.
63. Fisher CJ, Slotman GJ, Opal SM, et al. Initial evaluation of human recombinant interleukin-1 receptor antagonist in the treatment of sepsis syndrome: a randomized, open-label, placebo-controlled multi- center trail. *Crit Care Med* 1994;22:12–21.
64. Flores EA, Bistrain BR, Pomposelli JJ, et al. Infusion of tumor necrosis factor/cachectin promotes muscle catabolism in the rat. A synergistic effect with interleukin-1. *J Clin Invest* 1989;83: 1614–1622.
65. Fong YM, Marano MA, Barber A, et al. Total parenteral nutrition and bowel rest modify the metabolic response to endotoxin in humans. *Ann Surg* 1989;210:449–456.
66. Fong Y Tracey KJ, Moldawer LL, et al. Antibodies to cachectin/ tumor necrosis factor reduce interleukin-1 B and interleukin-6 appearance during lethal bacteremia. *J Exp Med* 1989;170: 1627–1633.
67. Fong Y, Lowry SF. Cytokines and the cellular response to injury and infection. *Sci Am* 1992;1–22.
68. Fowler AA, Hamman RF, Good JT, et al. Adult respiratory distress syndrome: risk with common redispositions. *Ann Intern Med* 1983; 98:593–597.
69. Gajewski TF, Schell SR, Nau G, et al. Regulation of T cell activation: differences among T cell subnets. *Immunol Rev* 1989;111: 79–110.
70. Gehr G, Braun T, Lesslauer W. Cytokines, receptors, and inhibitors. *Clin Invest* 1992;70:64–69.
71. Girardin E, Grau GE, Dayer JM, et al. Tumor necrosis factor and interleukin-1 in the serum of children with severe infectious purpura. *N Eng J Med* 1988;319:397–400.
72. Giroir BP. Mediators of septic shock: new approaches for interrupting the endogenous inflammatory cascade. *Crit Care Med* 1993;21:780–789.
73. Giroir BP, BeutlerB. Effect of amrinone on tumor necrosis factor production in endotoxin shock. *Circ Shock* 1992;36:200–207.
74. Gough DB, Moss NM, Jordon A, et al. Recombinant interleukin-2 improves immune response and host resistance to septic challenge in thermally injured mice. *Surgery* 1988;104:292–300.
75. Grau GE, Farjardo, LF, Piguet PF, et al. Tumor necrosis factor (cachectin) as an essential mediator in murine cerebral malaria. *Science* 1987;237:1210–1212.
76. Grau GE, Taylor TE, Molyneux ME, et al. Tumor necrosis factor and disease severity in children with falciparum malaria. *N Engl J Med* 1989;320:1586–1591.
77. Greene WC, Leonard WJ. The human interleukin-2 receptor. *Annu Rev Immunol* 1986;4:69–95.
78. Hack CE, DeGroot ER, Felt-Bersma RJF, et al. Increased plasma levels of interleukin-6 in sepsis. *Blood* 1989;74:1704–1710.
79. Haeffner-Cavaillon N, Roussellier N, Ponzio O, et al. Induction of interleukin-1 production in patients undergoing cardiopulmonary bypass. *J Thorac Cardiovasc Surg* 1989;98:1100–1106.
80. Han J, Thompson P, Beutler B. Dexamethasone and pentoxifylline inhibit endotoxin-induced cachectin/tumor necrosis factor synthesis at separate points in the signalling pathway. *J Exp Med* 1990;172:391–394.
81. Hannum CH, Wilcox CJ, Arend WP, et al. Interleukin-1 receptor

antagonist activity of a human interleukin-1 inhibitor. *Nature* 1990; 343:336–340.
82. Havell EA. Evidence that tumor necrosis factor has an important role in antibacterial resistance. *J Immunol* 1989;143:2894–2899.
83. Heinzel FP. The role of interferon- in the pathology of experimental endotoxemia. *J Immunol* 1990;145:2920–2924.
84. Hershman MJ, Polk HC, Pietsch JD, et al. Modulation of infection by gamma interferon treatment following trauma. *Infect Immun* 1988;56:2412–2416.
85. Hesse DG, Tracey KJ, Fong Y, et al. Cytokine appearance in human endotoxemia and primate bacteremia. *Surg Gynecol Obstet* 1988; 166:147–153.
86. Himmler A, Maurer-Fogy I, Kronke M, et al. Molecular cloning and expression of human and rat tumor necrosis factor receptor chain (p60) and its soluble derivative, tumor necrosis factor-binding protein. *DNA Cell Biol* 1990;9:705–715.
87. Hinshwa LB, Archer LT, Beller-Todd BK, et al. Survival of primates in LD100 septic shock following steroid antibiotic therapy. *J Surg Res* 1980;:151–170.
88. Hinshaw LB, Tekamp-Olson P, Chang ACK, et al. Survival of primates in LD 100 septic shock following therapy with antibody to tumor necrosis factor (TNF). *Circ Shock* 1990;9–292.
89. Hinshaw LB, Enerson TE, Taylor FB, et al. Lethal staphylococcus aureus shock in primates. prevention of death with anti-TNF antibody. *J Trauma* 1992;33:568–573.
90. Hoch RC, Rodriguez R, Manning T, et al. Effects of accidental trauma on cytokine and endotoxin production. *Crit Care Med* 1993;21:839–845.
91. Hollenberg SM, Cunnion RE, Lawrence M, et al. Tumor necrosis factor depresses myocardial cell function: results using an in vivo assay of myocyte performance. *Clin Res* 1989;37:528A.
92. Isaacs A, Lindenmann J. Virus interference. I the interferon. *Proc Natl Acad Sci USA* 1957;147:258.
93. J5 Study Group Treatment of severe infectious purpura in children with human plasma from donor immunized with the *Escherichia coli* J5: a prospective double blind study. *J Infect Dis* 1992;165:695–701.
94. Jansen NJG, Van Oeveren W, Hoiting BH, et al. Methylprednisolone prophylaxis protects against endotoxin induced death in rabbits. *Inflammation* 1991;15:91–101.
95. Jansen NJG, Van Oeveren W, Gu YJ, et al. Endotoxin release and tumor necrosis factor formation during cardio pulmonary bypass. *Ann Thorac Surg* 1992;54:744–747.
96. Johnson KJ, Ward PA. Acute immunologic pulmonary alveolitis. *J Clin Invest* 1974;54:49–57.
97. Johnson KJ, Ward PA. Role of oxygen metabolites in immune complex injury lung. *J Immunol* 1981;126:1365–1368.
98. Kaflin RE, Engelman RM, Low H, et al. Induction of interleukin-8 expression during cardiopulmonary bypass. *Circulation* 1993;88: 401–406.
99. Kennedy TP, Johnson KJ, Kunkel R, et al. Acute acid aspiration lung injury in the rat: biphasic pathogenesis. *Anesth Analg* 1989;69: 87–92.
100. Klagsburn M, Edelman ER. Biological and biochemical properties of fibroblast growth factors. *Atherosclerosis* 1989;9:269–278.
101. Klebanoff SJ, Vados MA, Harlan JM, et al. Stimulation of neutrophils by tumor necrosis factor. *J Immunol* 1986;136:4220–4225.
102. Kluger MJ. Fever: role off pyrogens and cryogens. *Physiol Rev* 1991; 71:93–127.
103. Knight PR, Druskovich G, Tait AR, et al. The role of neutrophils, oxidants and proteases in the pathogenesis of acid pulmonary injury. *Anesthesiology* 1992;77:772–778.
104. Kovacs EJ. Fibrogenic cytokines: the role of immune mediators in the development of scar tissue. *Immunol Today* 1991;12:17–23.
105. Kupfer A, Singer SJ. Cell biology of cytotoxic and helper T cell functions: immunofluorescence microscope studies of single cells and cell couples. *Annu Rev Immunol* 1989;7:309–337.
106. Lahdevirta J, Maury CP, Teppo AM, et al. Raised circulating cachectin/tumor necrosis factor in patients with the acquired immunodeficiency syndrome. *Am J Med* 1988;86:289–291.
107. Le J, Vilcek J. Interleukin-6: a multifunctional cytokine regulating immune reactions and the acute phase protein response. *Lab Invest* 1989;61:588–602.
108. Lefer AM, Xin-Liang MA. Cytokines and growth factor in endothelial dysfunction. *Crit Care Med* 1993;21:S9–S14.
109. Levi-Montalcini R, Angeletti PU. Nerve growth factor. *Physiol Rev* 1968;48:534–569.
110. Lilly CM, Sandhu JS, Ishizaka A, et al. Pentoxifylline prevents tumor necrosis factor-induced lung injury. *Am Rev Respir Dis* 1989; 139:1361–1368.
111. Liu J. FK506 and cyclosporin: molecular probes for studying intracellular signal transduction. *Trends Pharmacol Sci* 1993;14:182–188.
112. Livingston DH, Malangoni MA. Interferon restores immune competence after hemorrhagic shock. *J Surg Res* 1988;45:37–43.
113. Lorber MI, Paul K, Harding MW, et al. Cyclophilin binding: a receptor-mediated approach to monitoring CsA activity following organ transplantation. *Transplant Proc* 1990;22:1240–1244.
114. Lowenthal JW, Castle BE, Christiansen J, et al. Expression of high affinity receptors for murine interleukin-4 (BSF-1) on hemopoietic and nonhemopoietic cells. *J Immunol* 1988;140:456–464.
115. Luce JM, Montgomery AB, Marks JD, et al. Ineffectiveness of high-dose methylprednisolone in preventing parenchymal lung injury and improving mortality in patients with septic shock. *Am Rev Respir Dis* 1988;138:62–68.
116. Luger A, Graf H, Schwartz HP, et al. Decreased serum interleukin-1 activity and monocyte interleukin- 1 production in patients with fatel sepsis. *Crit Care Med* 1986;14:458–461.
117. Malangoni MA, Livingston DH, Sonnenfeld G, et al. Interferon gamma and tumor necrosis factor alpha. Use in gram-negative infection after shock. *Arch Surg* 1990;125:444–446.
118. Marks JD, Marks CB, Luce JM, et al. Plasma tumor necrosis factor in patients with septic shock. *Am Rev Respir Dis* 1990;141:94–97.
119. Mathison JC, Wolfson E, Ulevitch RJ. Participation of tumor necrosis factor in the mediation of gram-negative bacterial lipopolysaccharide-induced injury in rabbits. *J Clin Invest* 1988;81: 1925–1937.
120. Maulik N, Engelman RM, Wei Z, et al. Interleukin-1 preconditioning reduces myocardial ischemia reperfusion injury. *Circulation* 1993;88:387–394.
121. Maury CP, Teppo AM. Circulating tumor necrosis factor - alpha (cachectin) in myocardial infarction. *J Intern Med* 1989;225: 333–336.
122. Meldrum DR, Ayala A, Perrin MM, et al. Diltiazem restores IL-2, IL-3, IL-6 and IFN-synthesis and decreases host susceptibility to sepsis following hemorrhage. *J Surg Res* 1991;51:158–164.
123. Messent M, Sullivan K, Keogh, et al. Adult respiratory distress syndrome following cardiopulmonary bypass: incidence and prediction. *Anesthesia* 1992;47:267–268.
124. Michie HR, Manogue KR, Spriggs DR, et al. Detection of circulating tumor necrosis factor after endotoxin administration. *N Engl J Med* 1988;318:1481–1486.
125. Michie HR, Spriggs DR, Manogue KR, et al. Tumor necrosis factor and endotoxin induce similar metabolic response in human beings. *Surgery* 1988;104:280–286.
126. Miyajima A, Kitamura T, Harada N, et al. Cytokine receptors and signal transduction. *Annu Rev Immunol* 1992;10:295–331.
127. Mosmann TR, Coffman RL. Th1 and Th2 cells: different patterns of lymphokine secretion lead to different functional properties. *Annu Rev Immunol* 1989;7:145–173.
128. Mullen PG, Windsor ACJ, Walsh CJ, et al. Combined ibuprofen and monoclonal antibody to tumor necrosis factor- attenuate hemodynamic dysfunction and sepsis- induced acute lung injury. *J Trauma* 1993;34:612–620.
129. Mustafa MM, Ramilo O, Saez-Llorens X, et al. Cerebrospinal fluid prostaglandins, interleukin-1 and tumor necrosis factor in bacterial meningitis. Clinical laboratory correlations in placebo-treated and dexamethasone-treated patients. *Am J Dis Child* 1990;144:883.
130. Natanson C, Eichenholz PW, Danner RL, et al. Endotoxin and tumor necrosis factor challenges in dogs stimulate the cardiovascular profile of human septic shock. *J Exp Med* 1989;169:823–832.
131. Nathan C. Interferon and Inflammation. In: Gallin JI, Goldstein IM, Snyderman R, eds. *Inflammation: basic principles and clinical correlates,* 2nd ed. New York: Raven Press, 1992;265–290.
132. Nawabi MD, Block KP, Chakrabarti MC, et al. Administration of endotoxin, tumor necrosis factor, or interleukin-1 to rats activates skeletal muscle branched-chain alpha-keto acid dehydrogenase. *J Clin Invest* 1990;85:256–263.
133. Nickoloff BJ. Cytokine networks in skin disease. In: Kunkel SL, Remick DG, eds. *Cytokines in health and disease.* New York: Marcel Dekker, 1992;413–432.
134. Nicod LP. Cytokines. 1. Overview. *Thorax* 1993;48:660–667.
135. Nishimoto N, Yoshizaki K, Tagoh H, et al. Elevation of serum interleukin-6 prior to acute phase proteins on the inflammation by surgical operation. *Clin Immunol Immunopathol* 1989;50:399–401.

136. Novick D, Engelmann H, Wallach D, et al. Soluble cytokine receptors are present in the human urine. *J Exp Med* 1989;170: 1409–1414.
137. Nuytinck HKS, Xavier JM, Offerman W, et al. Whole body inflammation in trauma patients: an autopsy study. *Arch Surg* 1988;123: 1519–1524.
138. Odio CM, Farngezicht I, Paris M, et al. The beneficial effects of early dexamethasone administration in infants and children with bacterial meningitis. *N Engl J Med* 1991;324:1525–1531.
139. Ohlsson K, Bjork P, Bergenfeldt M, et al. Interleukin-1 receptor antagonist reduces mortality from endotoxin shock. *Nature* 1990; 348:550–552.
140. Okusawa S, Gelfand JA, Ikejima T, et al. Interleukin-1 induces a shock-like state in rabbits. Synergism with tumor necrosis factor and the effect of cyclooxygenase inhibition. *J Clin Invest* 1988;81: 1162–1172.
141. Oladimeji M, Grimshaw AD, Baum M, et al. Effect of surgery upon monocyte function. *Br J Surg* 1982;69:145–146.
142. Opal SM, Cross AS, Kelly NM, et al. Efficacy of a monoclonal antibody directed against tumor necrosis factor in protecting neutropenic rats from lethal infection with pseudomonas aeruginosa. *J Infect Dis* 1990;161:1148–1152.
143. Oppenheim JJ, Zachariae CO, Mukaida N, et al. Properties of the novel proinflammatory supergene "intercrine" cytokine family. *Annu Rev Immunol* 1991;9:617–648.
144. Peppel K, Crawford D, Beutler B. A tumor necrosis factor (TNF) receptor-IgG heavy chain chimeric protein as a bivalent antagonist of TNF activity. *J Exp Med* 1991;174:1483–1489.
145. Piguet PF, Grau G, Allet B, et al. Tumor necrosis factor (TNF) is an important mediator of the mortality and morbidity induced by the graft-versus-host reaction (GVHR). *Abstr Immunobiol* 1987;175:27.
146. Rabinovici R, John R, Esser KM, et al. Serum tumor necrosis factor-alpha profile in trauma patients. *J Trauma* 1993;35:698–702.
147. Rampart M, van Damme J, Zonnekeyn L, et al. Granulocyte chemotactic protein/IL-8 induces plasma leakage and neutrophil accumulation in rabbit skin. *Am J Pathol* 1989;135:21–25.
148. Rees RC. Cytokines as biological response modifiers. *J Clin Pathol* 1992;45:93–98.
149. Remick DG, Kunkel RG, Larrick JW, et al. Acute in vivo effects of recombinant TNF. *Lab Invest* 1987;56:583–590.
150. Rodriguez JL, Miller CG, Garner WL, et al. Correlation of the local and systemic cytokine response with clinical outcome following thermal injury. *J Trauma* 1993;34:684–694.
151. Ross R, Raines EW, Bowen-Pope DF. The biology of platelet-derived growth factor. *Cell* 1986;464:155–159.
152. Rousset F, Malefyt RW, Slierendregt B, et al. Regulation of Fc receptor for IgE (CD23) and class IIMHC antigen expression of Burkitt's lymphoma cell lines by human IL-4 and IFN-gamma. *J Immunol* 1988;140:2625–2632.
153. Salo M. Effects of anesthesia and surgery on the immune response. *Acta Anaesthesiol Scand* 1992;36:201– 220.
154. Scade UF. Pentoxifylline increases survival in murine endotoxin shock and decreases formation of tumor necrosis factor. *Circ Shock* 1990;31:171–181.
155. Scales WE. Structure and function of interleukin-1. In: Kunkel SL, Remick DG, eds. *Cytokines in health and disease.* New York: Marcel Dekker, 1992;15–26.
156. Sen GC, Lengyel P. The interferon system. A bird's eye view of its biochemistry. *J Biol Chem* 1992;267:5017–5020.
157. Shepard VL. Cytokine receptors. In: Kunkel SL, Remick DG, eds. *Cytokines in health and disease.* New York: Marcel Dekker, 1992; 509–536.
158. Sherry B, Cerami A. Cachectin/tumor necrosis factor exerts endocrine, paracrine, and autocrine control of inflammatory responses. *J Cell Biol* 1988;107:1269–1277.
159. Silva AT, Applemelk BJ, Buurman WA, et al. Monoclonal antibody to endotoxin core protects mice from *Escherichia coli* sepsis by a mechanism independent of tumor necrosis factor and interleukin-6. *J Infect Dis* 1990;162:454–459.
160. Silva AT, Bayston KF, Cohen J. Prophylactic and therapeutic effects of monoclonal antibody to tumor necrosis factor-alpha in experimental gram-negative shock. *J Infect Dis* 1990;162:421–427.
161. Silver GM, Gamelli RL, O'Reilly M, et al. The effect of interleukin-1 on survival in a murine model of burn wound sepsis. *Arch Surg* 1990;125:922–935.
162. Smith EM. Hormonal activities of cytokines. Edited by Blalock JE. *Chem Immunol* 1992;52:154–169.
163. Smith KA. Interleukin-2. *Sci Am* 1990;262:50–57.
164. Stephan RN, Conrad PJ, Janeway CA, et al. Decreased interleukin-2 production following simple hemorrhage. *Surg Forum* 1986;37: 73–75.
165. Stephan RN, Saizawa M, Conrad PJ, et al. Depressed antigen presentation function and membrane interleukin-1 activity of peritoneal macrophages after laparotomy. *Surgery* 1987;102:147–154.
166. Strieter RM, Remick DG, Ward PA, et al. Cellular and molecular regulation of tumor necrosis factor- production by pentoxifylline. *Biochem Biophys Res Commun* 1988;155:1230–1236.
167. Szabo G, Kodys K, Miller Graziano CL. Elevated monocyte interleukin-6 (IL-6) production in immunosuppressed trauma patients. II. Downregulation by IL-4. *J Clin Immunol* 1991;11: 336–344.
168. Tait AR, Davidson BA, Johnson KJ, et al. Halothane inhibits the intraalveolar recruitment of neutrophils, lymphocytes, and macrophages in response to influenza virus infection in mice. *Anesth Analg* 1993;76:1106–1113.
169. Tan LR, Waxman K, Scannell G, et al. Trauma causes early release of soluble receptors for tumor necrosis factor. *J Trauma* 1993;34: 634–638.
170. Taverne J, Bate CA, Sarkar DA, et al. Human and murine macrophages produce TNF in response to soluble antigens of plasmodium falciparum. *Parasite Immunol* 1990;12:33–43.
171. The Veterans Administration Systemic Sepsis Cooperative Study Group. Effect of high-dose glucocorticoid therapy on mortality in patients with clinical signs of systemic sepsis. *N Engl J Med* 1987; 317:659–665.
172. Tracey KJ, Beutler B, Lowry SF, et al. Shock and tissue injury induced by recombinant human cachectin. *Science* 1986;234: 470–474.
173. Tracey KJ, Fong Y, Hesse DG, et al. Anti-cachectin/tumor necrosis factor monoclonal antibodies prevent septic shock during lethal bacteremia. *Nature* 1987;330:662–666.
174. Tracey KJ, Lowry SF, Fahey TJ, et al. Cachectin/tumor necrosis factor induces lethal shock and stress hormone responses in the dog. *Surg Gynecol Obstet* 1987;164:415–422.
175. Tracey KJ, Cerami A. Tumor necrosis factor: an updated review of its biology. *Crit Care Med* 1993;21:S415–S422.
176. Trotta PP. Cytokines: an overview. *Am J Reprod Immunol* 1991;25: 137–141.
177. Tsuji Y, Torti FM. Tumor necrosis factor structure and function. In: Kunkel SL, Remick DG, eds. *Cytokines in health and disease.* New York: Marcel Dekker, 1992;131–150.
178. Ulich TR. Hematological effects of cytokines in vivo. In: Kunkel SL, Remick DG, eds. *Cytokines in health and disease.* New York: Marcel Dekker, 1992;235–256.
179. Vacheron F, Rudert A, Perin S, et al. Production of interleukin-1 and tumor necrosis factor activities in bronchoalveolar washing following infection of mice by influenza virus. *J Gen Virol* 1990;71: 477–479.
180. Van der Poll T, Buller HR, Ten Cote H, et al. Activation of coagulation after administration of tumor necrosis factor to normal subjects. *N Engl J Med* 1990;322:1622–1627.
181. Vyakarnam A, McKeating J, Meager A, et al. Tumor necrosis factors (alpha, beta) induced by HIV-1 in peripheral blood mononuclear cells potentiate virus replication. *AIDS* 1990;4:21–27.
182. Waage A. Production and clearance of tumor necrosis factor in rats exposed to endotoxin and dexamethasone. *Clin Immunol Immunopathol* 1987;45:348–355.
183. Waage A, Halstensen A, Spevik T. Association between tumor necrosis factor in serum and fatal outcome in patients with meningococcal disease. *Lancet* 1987;1:355–357.
184. Waage A, Espevik T. Interleukin-1 potentiates the lethal effect of tumor necrosis factor-/cachectin in mice. *J Exp Med* 1988;167: 1987–1992.
185. Waage A, Brandtzag P, Halstensen A, et al. The complex pattern of cytokines in serum from patients with meningococcal septic shock. Association between interleukin-6, interleukin-1, and fatal outcome. *J Exp Med* 1989;169:333–338.
186. Warren JS. The role of cytokines in experimental lung injury. In: Kunkel SL, Remick DG, eds. *Cytokines in health and disease.* New York: Marcel Dekker, 1992;257–269.
187. Warren JS, Ward PA, Johnson KJ. Tumor necrosis factor: a plurifunctional mediator of acute inflammation. *Modern Pathol* 1988;1: 242–247.
188. Warren JS, Barton PA, Mandel DM, et al. Intrapulmonary tumor

necrosis factor triggers local platelet- activating factor production in rat immune complex alveolitis. *Lab Invest* 1990;63:746–745.

189. Waxman K, Clark L, Soliman MH, et al. Pentoxifylline in resuscitation of experimental hemorrhagic shock. *Crit Care Med* 1991;19: 728–731.
190. Wayte J, Silva AT, Krausz T, et al. Observation on the role of tumor necrosis factor- in a murine model of shock due to streptococcus pyogens. *Crit Care Med* 1993;21:1207–1212.
191. Wenzel RP, Andriole VT, Bartlett JG, et al. Anti-endotoxin monoclonal antibodies for gram-negative sepsis: guidelines from the Infectious Diseases Society of America. *Clin Infect Dis* 1992;14:973–976.
192. Wood JJ, Rodrick ML, O'Mahony JB, et al. Inadequate interleukin-2 production. A fundamental immunological deficiency in patients with major burns. *Ann Surg* 1984;200:311–320.
193. Yarden Y, Ulrich A. Growth factor receptor tyrosine kinases. *Annu Rev Biochem* 1988;57:443–478.
194. Yeager MP, Glass CC, Neff RK, et al. Epidural anesthesia and analgesia in high risk surgical patients. *Anesthesiology* 1987;66: 729–736.
195. Yoshimura A, D'Andrea AD, Lodish HF. Friend spleen focus-forming virus glycoprotein gp55 interacts with the erythropoietin receptor in the endoplasmic reticulum and affects receptor metabolism. *Proc Natl Acad Sci USA* 1990;87:4139–4143.
196. Zabel P, Wolter DT, Schonharting MM, et al. Oxpentifylline in endotoxaemia. *Lancet* 1989;2:1474–1477.
197. Zoumbos NC, Gascon P, Djeu JY, et al. Interferon is a mediator of the hematopoietic suppression in aplastic anemia in vitro and possibly in vivo. *Proc Natl Acad Sci USA* 1985;82:188–192.

B

TECHNIQUES OF CELL BIOLOGIC STUDY

Anesthesia: Biologic Foundations, edited by Tony L. Yaksh et al. Lippincott–Raven Publishers, Philadelphia © 1997.

CHAPTER 21

TECHNIQUES OF CELLULAR ELECTROPHYSIOLOGIC INVESTIGATION

JOSEPH J. PANCRAZIO

Evidence now exists supporting roles for the anesthetic-induced alterations of both voltage- and ligand-gated channels to produce the anesthetic state. Consequently, modern research in anesthetic mechanisms requires the use of tools capable of probing the electrophysiological behavior of membrane ion channels. The intent of this chapter is to review methods used in the measurement of ion channels for scientists interested in these increasingly common techniques. The commercial availability of amplifiers and bundled software-hardware data acquisition systems has contributed to the dramatic increase in the number of laboratories with a major effort in electrophysiologic investigation. By necessity, this chapter not only describes modern electrophysiological methods, but also discusses practical aspects of analysis, particularly in the case of single ion channels. The overall aim of this chapter is to provide a sturdy foundation for new or future investigator in electrophysiology.

CONCEPTS IN BIOPHYSICS

The majority of our understanding of ion channel behavior has been made through electrical measurements based on the movement or flow of charged ions. Electric charge is measured in Coulombs, C, where a proton or a positive charge yields 1.6 × 10^{-19} C. If one considers 1 mole of K^+ ions, the quantity of charge would be:

$$\frac{1 \text{ mole K}^+}{1} \cdot \frac{6.023 \times 10^{23}\text{ K}^+}{1 \text{ mole K}^+} \cdot \frac{1\text{ (+charge)}}{1\text{ K}^+} \cdot \frac{1.6 \times 10^{-19}\text{ C}}{1\text{ (+charge)}}$$

$$= 96{,}368 \text{ C}$$

Current, I, is defined as the movement or change in charge, q, over time; therefore:

$$I = \frac{dq}{dt} \sim \frac{\Delta q}{\Delta t} \qquad [1]$$

where q is charge in coulombs, t is time in units of sec, and I is in units of amperes, A, such that 1 ampere = 1 C/sec (Example 1).

In order to move a charge through an electrical field, which exists due to the voltage difference across the cell membrane, energy is required. The energy is supplied in the form of electrical potential in units of volts where 1 volt = 1 joule/C. By a convention attributed to Benjamin Franklin, the movement of positive charge flows from high potential to low potential and the difference between the high-potential and low-potential points is called a potential difference or voltage drop as shown in Fig. 1. Although individual potentials (V_A and V_B) can be schematically and algebraically denoted, it is the voltage difference $V_{AB} = V_A - V_B$ that enables the flow of charge. Ohm's Law states that the current flowing from node A to node B is proportional to V_{AB} by a constant resistance, R:

$$V_{AB} = IR \qquad [2]$$

Alternatively, we can consider the conductance, G, from node A to node B where $R = 1/G$ yielding:

$$I = GV_{AB} \qquad [3]$$

Electrical equivalent models of the cellular membrane characterize ion channels as conductors; and current carried by channels therefore may be described by Ohm's Law. However, the electrical potential is a function not only of the electrical gradient across the cell membrane, but also the concentration gradient for the permeating ion. The equilibrium or Nernst potential is the transmembrane voltage which balances the fluxes due to both the electrical and concentration gradients. Consequently, the electrochemical driving force is simply the difference between the transmembrane voltage, V_m, and the equilibrium potential, E_{ion}, yielding:

$$I = G(V_m - E_{ion}) \qquad [4]$$

By setting the total flux from both gradients, which is quantitatively described by the Nernst-Planck electrodiffusion equation, equal to 0, E_{ion} is found to be a function of the extracellular and intracellular ion concentrations C_{out} and C_{in}, respectively:

$$E_{ion} = \frac{RT}{zF}\ln\left(\frac{C_{out}}{C_{in}}\right) \qquad [5]$$

where RT/F is ~26 mV at 25°C and 27 mV at 37°C. If the ion conductance could be represented by a simple linear conductor, then the current-voltage (I–V) curve predicted by eq. 3

> Example 1. How many ions actually move when a channel opens?
>
> When open, ion channels permit charged ions to flow at rates ranging from 0.1 to 20 picoamps (pA = 10^{-12} C/sec). If we consider a single Ca^{2+} channel in a membrane that opens to permit 0.2 pA of current to enter the cell for 2 msec, we can calculate the number of Ca^{2+} ions that actually enter the cell:
>
> $$\frac{0.002\text{ sec}}{1} \cdot \frac{0.2 \times 10^{-12}\text{C}}{\text{sec}} \cdot \frac{1\text{ (+charge)}}{1.6 \times 10^{-19}\text{ C}} \cdot \frac{1\text{ Ca}^{2+}\text{ ion}}{2\text{ (+charges)}}$$
>
> $$= 1250\text{ Ca}^{2+}\text{ ions}$$

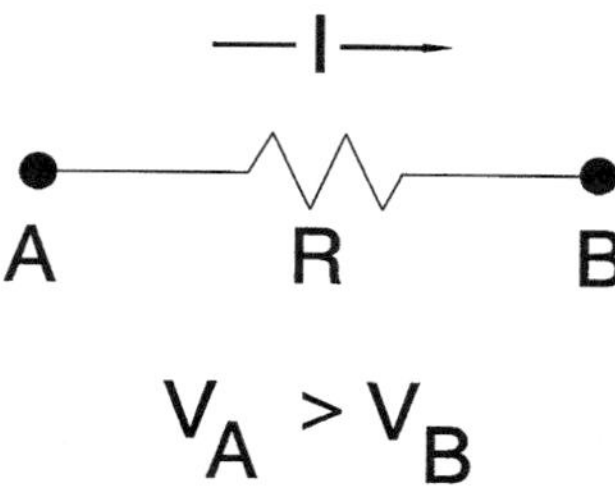

Figure 1. According to Ohm's law, the current, I, flowing through a resistance, R, from node A to node B, is proportional to the voltage difference across the resistor, $V_{AB} = V_A - V_B$.

would be linear with an x-intercept at E_{ion} and the slope to be constant, G. At a first approximation, single ion channels follow this ohmic behavior when open. Ionic current, which is the sum of the current through all of the randomly opening channels, is best described by a conductance term, G, which is a function of both time and voltage (Example 2).

Although we can model membrane channels as conductors, the lipid bilayer acts as an insulating layer to separate and store charge. This process of separating and storing charge results in the electrical equivalent of a parallel plate capacitor (Fig. 2). The capacitance, C_m, in units of Farads (C/V), is given by:

$$C_m = \frac{\varepsilon_r \varepsilon_o A}{d} \qquad [6]$$

where ε_o is the polarizability of free space equal to 8.85×10^{-12} CV^{-1} m^{-1} and ε_r is the dielectric constant of the material between the plates, A is the surface area (in m^2) of one of the identical plates, and d is the distance between the plates (in m). Although it is common to refer to the "membrane as a capacitor," this is not exactly true. Technically, it is the extracellular and intracellular electrolyte containing solutions which correspond to the parallel plates of the capacitor and the lipid bilayer serves as the dielectric of the capacitor. For biological membranes, the ε_r is ~3.2, and d, corresponding to the bilayer thickness, is ~30 nm yielding a capacitance/area of 1 μF/cm^2. As an example, consider mammalian neurons which have diameters of 10–20 μm. Assuming a spherical geometry, the membrane surface area provides capacitance levels of 3–12 pF. Due to membrane folding, cleft, or tubule networks, the actual capacitance may greatly exceed that approximated by the surface area.

The amount of charge, q, which the capacitor can store is proportional to the applied voltage difference:

$$q = C_m V \qquad [7]$$

Capacitive or displacement current, resulting from discharge of the capacitor is:

Example 2. A clear understanding of electrophysiology requires comprehension of Ohm's Law.

A mammalian neuron is voltage clamped at the resting potential of the cell, –83 mV, at 25°C. A voltage step to –30 mV evokes an outward K^+ current reaching a peak of 30 pA; a pulse to +50 mV triggers an outward current that reaches an amplitude of 1 nA. If the intracellular and extracellular K^+ concentrations are 150 mM and 5 mM, respectively, determine the maximum membrane K^+ conductance at each step potential.

$$E_K = 26 \ln\left(\frac{5}{150}\right) = -88 mV$$

Rearranging eq. 5:

$$G_K = \frac{I_K}{V - E_K}$$

For $V = -30$ mV and $I_K = 30$ pA:

$$G_K = \frac{30 \times 10^{-12} A}{(-30 - (-88)) \times 10^{-3} V} = 0.52\ nS$$

For $V = +50$ and $I_K = 1$ nA:

$$G_K = \frac{1 \times 10^{-9} A}{(+50 - (-88)) \times 10^{-3} V} = 7.25\ nS$$

Note that if the peak conductance was not a function of voltage such that G_K was equal to 0.52 nS regardless of the test potential, then the voltage step to +50 mV would evoke a maximum K^+ current of only 72 pA instead of 1 nA.

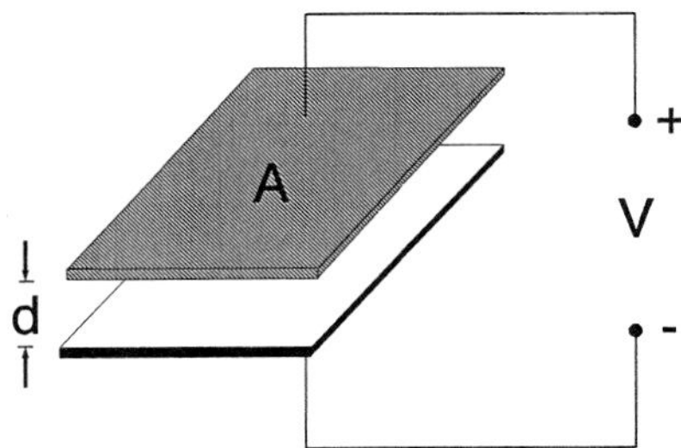

Figure 2. Cell membrane capacitance, C_m, due to the charge separation across the lipid bilayer, can be adequately modelled by a parallel plate capacitor where the amount of stored charge is proportional to C_m and the voltage difference, V. C_m is proportional to the surface area, A, of the plate and inversely proportional to the distance, d, between the plates.

$$I = \frac{dq}{dt} = C_m \frac{dV}{dt} \qquad [8]$$

Therefore, from a modelling point of view, the membrane consists of both a capacitor and one or more resistors connected in parallel (Fig. 3). In addition, a series resistance, R_s, must be incorporated to account for the electrical resistance of the means of access to the membrane interior. For example, in the case of injecting current into a cell via a standard glass microelectrode, R_s primarily represents the resistance of the glass microelectrode. The presence of a capacitor causes a voltage difference, $V_x(t)$, across the parallel resistor-capacitor (R-C) network to follow behind or lag while rapidly accumulating charge across the capacitor plates. This shunting effect across the capacitor diminishes exponentially with time so that the voltage drop across the R-C network will approach the steady-state condition as if the capacitor was absent. Under the experimental conditions most relevant to this chapter, we are concerned with the effect of a step voltage of magnitude V_o (Fig. 3, *upper right panel*) on the measured current. Initially, capacitive charging permits a current of magnitude V_o/R_s, which falls exponentially to a steady-state level equal to V_o/R (Fig. 3, *middle right panel*). As derived in the Appendix 1:

$$I(t) \approx \frac{V_o}{R} + \frac{V_o}{R_s} \exp(-t/\tau) \text{ and } \tau \approx R_s C \qquad [9]$$

Furthermore, the voltage across the R-C network, $V_x(t)$, will lag behind the command step potential (Fig. 3 *lower right panel*):

$$V_x(t) \approx V_o [1 - \exp(-t/\tau)] \qquad [10]$$

During the practical recording of membrane currents, the capacitive property of the membrane proves to be little more than an inconvenience necessitating the use of capacitive artifact subtraction to isolate ionic current entirely. Without artifact subtraction, the preferential use of step potentials to measure ionic current restricts the capacitive current to flow only during voltage transitions at the initiation and termination of the voltage step when $dV/dt \neq 0$. The spike artifact, given by the exponential decay component of eq. 10, becomes negligible for $t > 4\tau$. As we will see later in the chapter, with the use of whole-cell patch clamp methods, one can take advantage of the current contributed from the membrane capacitance to estimate changes in cell surface area as a measure of exocytotic secretion.

ELECTRICAL CIRCUIT MODEL OF A CELLULAR MEMBRANE

A complete circuit model depicted in Fig. 4 shows that the total membrane current, I_T, can be written using Kirchhoff's current law:

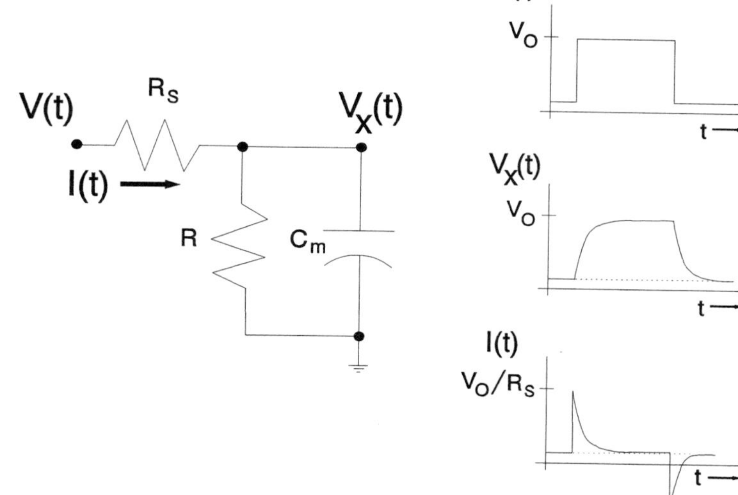

Figure 3. An equivalent circuit model relevant to voltage-clamp measurements. The parallel combination of a resistor, R, and a capacitor, C, models the membrane impedance, whereas an additional series resistance, R_s, models the electrical access to the membrane interior. Assuming that $R >> R_s$, a step depolarization of magnitude V_o applied at node $V(t)$ (*upper right panel*) results in a potential at $V_x(t)$ (*middle right panel*), which lags behind $V(t)$ with a time constant, $\tau = R_s C$ and a current $I(t)$ (*lower right panel*) with spikes of magnitude V_o/R_s at the beginning and termination of the voltage pulse.

$$I_T = C_m \frac{dV_m}{dt} + \sum_{i=1}^{n} G_i(V_m - E_i) \quad [11]$$

where there are n different types of selective ion channels with equilibrium potentials E_i (for $i = 1, \ldots, n$). With this equivalent circuit model, we can address how the individual conductances influence V_m. At rest, we expect $I_T = 0$ and V_m to be constant so $dV_m/dt = 0$, such that:

$$\sum_{i=1}^{n} G_i(V_m - E_i) = 0 \quad [12]$$

For a cell membrane which is permeable to only Na^+, K^+, and Cl^- under resting conditions:

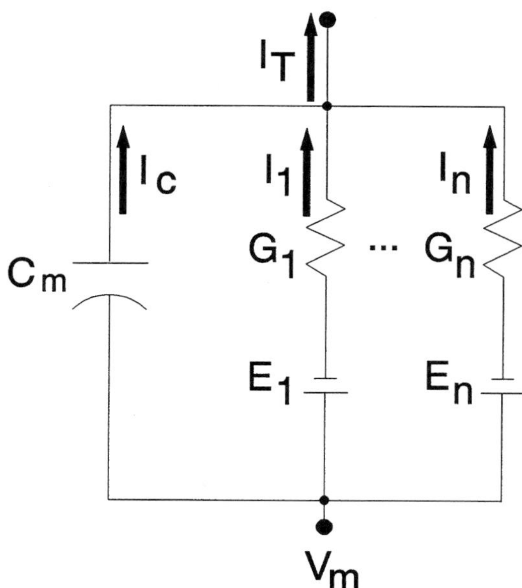

Figure 4. Complete membrane circuit model incorporating conductive and capacitive elements with n parallel conductances G_1 through G_n, associated equilibrium potentials, E_1 through E_n, and a capacitor, C. The interior of the modelled cell is at voltage, V_m, with respect to the extracellular media. The total current, I_T, is the sum of the currents through each parallel branch.

$$G_{Na}(V_m - E_{Na}) + G_K(V_m - E_K) + G_{Cl}(V_m - E_{Cl}) = 0 \quad [13]$$

Rearranging the terms to solve for V_m yields the Goldman equation:

$$V_m = \frac{G_{Na}E_{Na} + G_K E_K + G_{Cl}E_{Cl}}{G_{Na} + G_K + G_{Cl}} \quad [14]$$

The major interpretation of the Goldman equation is that V_m is primarily influenced by the equilibrium potential of the dominant conductance. When attempting to determine the influence of particular ion permeation pathways on the membrane potential, for example, increased G_{Cl}, it is tempting to consider the charge of the permeant ion and perform the mental exercise of following an imaginary ion into or out of a cell. The Goldman equation shows that we need only know the reversal potential, which carries information regarding the valence of the ion as z and its concentration difference, to predict the effect of changing G_{ion} on V_m. Furthermore, only the ratio of the ion conductances may be required to calculate V_m, if the ion equilibrium potentials are known (Example 3).

Example 3. The Goldman equation permits calculation of the steady-state transmembrane potential based on the conductances of permeant ions.

Assuming a cell with intracellular and extracellular ion concentrations in mM: $[K]_i = 150$, $[K]_o = 5$, $[Na]_i = 15$, $[Na]_o = 145$, $[Cl]_i = 20$, $[Cl]_o = 150$ at 37°C. Determine V_m if (a) the cell was exclusively selective for K^+; and (b) $G_{Na}/G_K = 0.04$ and $G_{Cl}/G_K = 0.25$.

(a)

$$V_m = E_K = 27 \ln \left(\frac{5}{150}\right) = -92 \text{ mV}$$

(b)

$$E_{Na} = 27 \ln \left(\frac{145}{15}\right) = +61 \text{ mV} \qquad E_{Cl} = -27 \ln \left(\frac{150}{20}\right) = -54 \text{ mV}$$

Using the Goldman equation, divide numerator and denominator by G_K to yield:

$$V_m = \frac{(0.04)(61) + (1)(-92) + (0.25)(-54)}{1 + 0.04 + 0.25} = -80 \text{ mV}$$

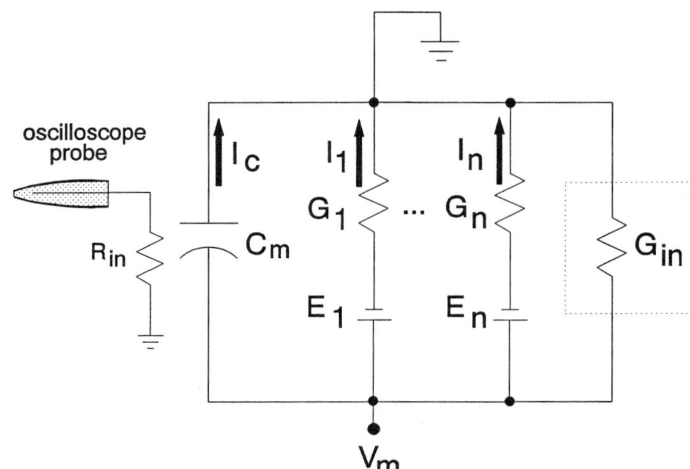

Figure 5. What if you could directly insert an oscilloscope probe into a cell? Addition of a low-resistance, R_{IN}, to ground representing an oscilloscope input, causes the membrane potential, V_m, predicted by eq. 15 to be dominated by $G_{IN} = 1/R_{IN}$ such that $V_m \sim 0$. By using a high-input impedance amplifier between the cell and the oscilloscope, G_{IN} becomes negligible, such that V_m is accurately assessed.

USE OF AMPLIFIERS IN THE MEASUREMENT OF BIOPOTENTIALS

Biopotentials in the mV range are of a voltage magnitude that can be easily monitored with a standard laboratory oscilloscope. Even if it was possible to plunge an oscilloscope probe into the interior of a cell, the measured potential would only be a fraction of the true cell membrane potential. Why? We can model the input of any device as an impedance, R_{in}, to ground, as illustrated in the left schematic of Fig. 5. The electrical equivalent of the insertion of the probe into the cell, depicted by the circuit model in Fig. 5, can be readily interpreted as the addition of another conductance pathway $G_{in} = 1/R_{in}$ to the membrane model with an equilibrium potential of 0 mV. Typically, R_{in} for oscilloscopes is 1 MΩ yielding G_{in} = 1 μS; an extremely large conductance which "shunts" the membrane potential toward 0 mV. This phenomenon is called *loading*.

Operational amplifiers (Op-amps), which are composed of transistors, resistors and capacitors, can be used as a high-input resistance buffer to measure biopotentials without loading. Utilizing a negative feedback configuration, op-amps can produce a virtually infinite input resistance such that practically no current can flow into the inputs. Another property of an op-amp circuit configured using negative feedback is that the voltages at both inputs are essentially equivalent.

VOLTAGE CLAMP METHODS

It was recognized >50 years ago that the bioelectrical phenomenon known as an action potential was associated with the time-dependent changes in the conductance of the membrane. The changes in potential across an excitable membrane, such as an action potential, are determined by the currents flowing across the membrane. The ionic currents, however, are determined by the membrane potential. This dynamic behavior can be attributed to the fact that some of the ion conductances of the membrane are both voltage and time dependent. A dynamic system like an excitable membrane can be analyzed only by fixing or clamping the transmembrane potential and measuring the ionic current which is proportional to the conductance. A required property of a voltage clamp is that there can be no substantial variations in the potential over the length of the membrane. Using a squid axon, Hodgkin and Huxley (24) achieved a spatially clamped implementation by use of the axial wire voltage clamp. As shown in Fig. 6, the membrane potential, V_m, is continuously monitored and compared to the command voltage, V_c. Current which is proportional to the voltage error, $V_c - V_m$, is then injected until the error is 0. This error correction is not instantaneous; instead, the clamp response time depends on the gain of the differential amplifier and the membrane capacitance.

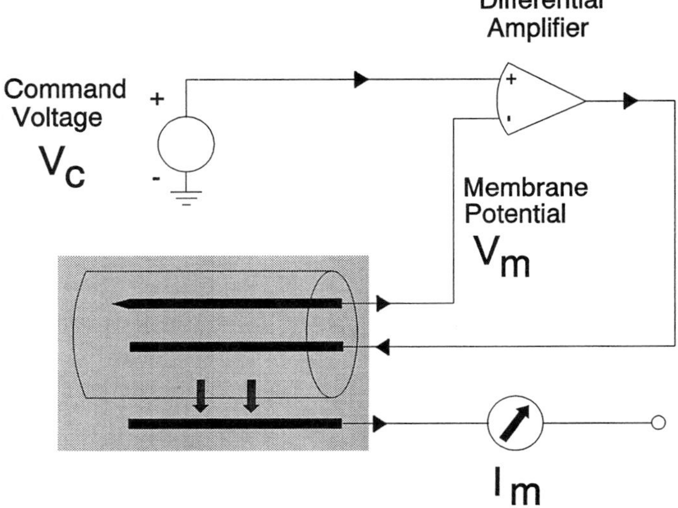

Figure 6. The axial wire voltage clamp, which is suitable for large-diameter cylindrical preparations like the squid giant axon, illustrates the major features of nearly all voltage-clamp implementations. Low-resistance wires running the length of the axon ensure spatial clamping of the entire membrane surface. A high-input impedance amplifier compares the membrane potential, V_m, with the command voltage, V_c, and injects a current proportional to the difference scaled by the differential amplifier gain, *A*. It is through the use of negative feedback that V_m closely follows V_c. The transmembrane current, I_m, is sensed with a third wire electrode in the bath.

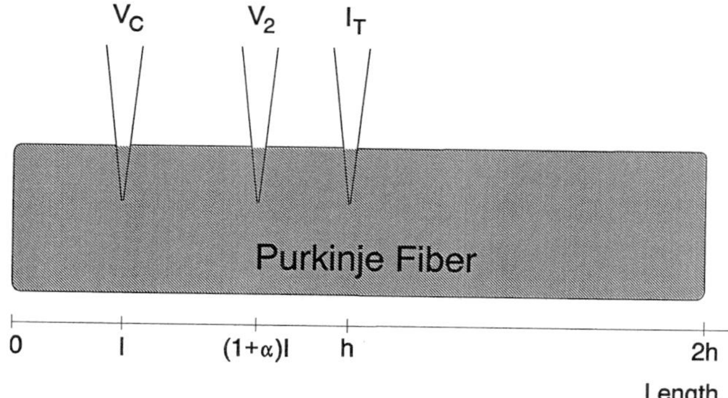

Figure 7. A cardiac Purkinje fiber is long and cylindrical; however, the diameter is far too narrow to permit insertion of axial wires for voltage clamping. Upon cutting a Purkinje fiber into short sections, the ends show an unusual and beneficial property of "healing over" such that each fiber segment behaves like a short cable terminated by a high resistance at each end. Adapting Adrian et al.'s (1) technique for three microelectrode clamping of skeletal muscle fibers, Kass et al. (30) determined optimal placement for electrodes V_c, V_2, and I_T. In contrast to the axial wire voltage clamp, the transmembrane voltage in this clamp arrangement does vary over the length of the fiber segment. The current injecting electrode, I_T, is located at a distance h from each sealed end. The positions of V_2 and V_c, separated by a distance αl, are adjusted to measure optimally inward or outward current. The voltage difference V_2 - V_c is proportional to the transmembrane current density at electrode V_c.

One key feature of nearly all voltage-clamp techniques is the ability to clamp an entire membrane surface area under investigation. A notable exception is the use of two and three microelectrodes to clamp long cylindrical cells which are far too slender (10–20 μm in diameter) for insertion of an axial wire. Adrian et al. (1) utilized three microelectrodes to voltage clamp a skeletal muscle fiber where the entire length of membrane under measurement is not at the same potential. Kass et al. (30) extended Adrian's work to cardiac Purkinje fibers (Fig. 7) and determined optimal placement for the two and three microelectrode arrangements. Under this recording condition, the command potential, V_c, is maintained at a set voltage with a current-injecting electrode, I_T, and the transmembrane current density, J_m, at electrode V_c is proportional to the voltage difference $V_2 - V_c$:

$$J_m = \frac{p(V_2 - V_c)}{\alpha(1 + \frac{\alpha}{2})l^2 r_i} \qquad [15]$$

where r_i is the cytoplasmic intracellular resistance and p is a correction factor which estimates the accuracy of the technique. The placement of the microelectrodes determines the value of p, which under ideal conditions is equal to 1. Analytical solutions for p, which are based on the application of the cable equation, depend on whether the membrane current of interest is inward or outward (29). For outward currents, p is a complicated function incorporating the hyperbolic cosine of $1/\lambda$; for inward currents, p includes the cosine of $1/\lambda$, where λ is the space constant.

Further discussion of specific voltage clamp methods will focus on the two modern techniques which are most used to characterize the properties of ion channels: the two-electrode voltage clamp and variations of the patch clamp technique. In the application of these techniques to the voltage clamp of isolated patches of membrane or spherical-like cells without processes, concerns about the spatial variations in V_m are negligible (4,16).

TWO-ELECTRODE VOLTAGE CLAMP

The two-electrode voltage clamp illustrated in Fig. 8 is well-suited for recording from extremely large cells such as *Xenopus* oocytes and tissues such as skeletal muscle. Oocytes, due to the low level of native ion channels and the abundance of protein synthesis machinery, have proved quite useful in the molecular characterization of channels. Injection of mRNA or cDNA encoding voltage-sensitive channel proteins results in high levels of channel expression. Oocytes, which are visible to the naked eye and are typically manipulated under a standard laboratory dissecting microscope, can exhibit a cell capacitance as high as 0.5 μF with current levels of some expressed channels exceeding 100 nA. Like the axial wire voltage clamp, one electrode, E_2, measures membrane potential, V_m, while a differential amplifier compares V_m with the command potential V_C, and outputs a voltage, V_o, proportional to the difference:

$$V_o = A(V_c - V_m) \qquad [16]$$

where A is the gain of the differential amplifier. By Ohm's law, the current, I_i, injected into the cell from the second electrode, E_1, is:

$$I_i = \frac{A(V_c - V_m)}{R_1} \qquad [17]$$

where R_1 is the resistance of electrode E_1. According to Kirchhoff's current law, the current flowing into the cell must be equal to the current flowing out, i.e., the transmembrane current, I_m, so:

$$I_m = \frac{A(V_c - V_m)}{R_1} = \frac{V_m}{Z} \qquad [18]$$

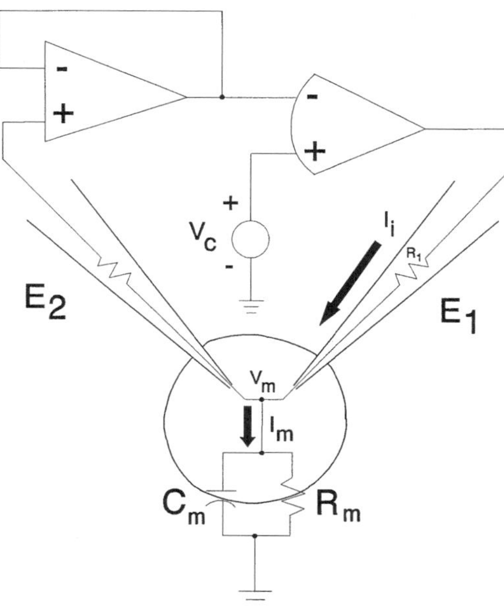

Figure 8. A two-electrode clamp that is conceptually similar to axial wire clamp permits voltage clamping of large spherical cells such as *Xenopus* oocytes. A microelectrode E_2 senses the membrane potential, V_m, which is first passed through a high-input impedance follower (triangle) with gain equal to 1. A differential amplifier compares the command voltage, V_C, with V_m and injects a current, I_i, which is proportional to the difference V_C - V_m through electrode E_1. Circuit analysis reveals that the time response of the voltage clamp circuit is related to the gain of the differential amplifier, the capacitance of the membrane, and the resistance of the microelectrode, R_1.

where Z is the impedance of the membrane, a function of the membrane resistance and capacitance, R_m and C_m, respectively. For a step voltage command input of magnitude V_o, assuming that $AR_m >> R_1$, it can be shown that:

$$V_m = V_c[1 - \exp(-t/\tau)] \quad [19]$$

where the time constant, τ:

$$\tau = \frac{R_1 C_m}{A} \quad [20]$$

Therefore, with a large differential amplifier gain, A, and a small resistance current-delivering electrode E_1, τ will be diminished resulting in a fast voltage-clamp response. Based on the circuit analyses above, electrodes of very low resistance would prove most ideal in terms of clamp speed. Unfortunately, lower-resistance electrodes tend to be more blunt, and thus, more damaging to the cell than higher-resistance electrodes.

PATCH CLAMP TECHNIQUE

Over the past 15 years, use of the patch clamp technique has generated the most insight into the function and pharmacology of ion channels. The patch clamp technique was introduced by Neher and Sakmann (43) with further enhancements reported by Hamill et al. (23). Although the initial intent of the patch clamp method was to isolate electrically a patch of membrane from the bathing solution to record unitary channel activity, a variation of the technique, the whole-cell recording mode, has permitted detailed analysis of membrane currents of smaller excitable cells typical of the mammalian nervous system.

A critical component to the success of the patch clamp method is the preparation of cells, usually requiring treatment with digestive enzymes to ensure a smooth membrane surface. In our experience with the isolation of mammalian cardiac ventricular myocytes, cell isolation as a science ranks somewhere between phrenology and alchemy. The results of cell isolation depend on a number of factors not least of which are enzyme lot and activity. With regard to central neurons, Edwards et al. (15) have described a technique where patch recordings can be accomplished from a thin brain slice, thus bypassing cell isolation procedures. Neurons, which can be visually identified in the slice, are locally cleaned with a closely positioned wide-tipped pipette containing physiological saline. The high flow rate through the wide-tipped pipette effectively blasts the cell surface clean to permit subsequent gigaohm seal formation with a second pipette.

PATCH ELECTRODE FABRICATION

Typically, patch electrodes are prepared with the use of a two-stage pipette puller. A glass capillary tube, which is threaded through the puller-heating filament, is held by each end under tension. During the first pull sequence, the maximum travel of the capillary tube is limited to 5–7 mm, resulting in the formation of a steep electrode taper to a diameter of 100–200 μm. After a brief cooling period, the filament is recentered to the middle of the electrode taper and the second pull is performed to separate the pair of electrodes with patch pipette tip of ~1 μm resulting in a resistance of between 1–10 MΩ when filled with saline solution. When recording at high gain for resolution of single-channel openings, a source of noise becomes apparent due to the separation of charge, ions in solution, across the glass wall of the pipette. Like the lipid bilayer, the pipette glass exhibits dielectric properties allowing electrolyte solutions of each side of the electrode wall to behave like a capacitor. By coating the exterior of the pipette, direct glass contact with the extracellular solution is diminished, and, consequently, the noise due to electrode capacitance is reduced. Sylgard 184, which is available from Dow Corning, forms an insulating layer of silicone rubber once it is cured, which has proven to be virtually ideal for patch clamp applications. To apply the sylgard to within 100 μm of the tip, a glass rod with a curved tip may be used. After coating the electrode, a hot-air jet is very useful for curing the sylgard layer. In general, the time-consuming process of coating electrodes is well worth the effort during single-channel recording; however, it is of less benefit during standard whole-cell recording.

To improve the likelihood of achieving a tight seal between the pipette tip and the cell membrane, electrode tips are often heat polished with the use of a microforge. A heating filament with a small glass bead mounted at the working distance of a microscope objective allows the annulus of the pipette to be smoothed while under constant microscopic evaluation. Heating the tip should be continued until there is a visible change in the tip diameter or color. For some types of glass, such as KIMAX-51, both a blackening and narrowing of the tip is readily observed upon fire polishing. Also, with certain types of glass, blunt and ragged tips can be carefully heated to produce a particular tip geometry (46).

GIGAOHM SEAL FORMATION: THE GLASS-CELL INTERFACE

Electrical isolation of the membrane patch is the key first step in the achievement of any of the patch clamp configurations. The degree of electrical isolation is reported as a seal resistance, R_{seal}, which is the resistance between the pipette electrode tip and the external bathing solution. Electrical isolation depends on the ability of the measurement system to reduce the inherent background current noise or "Johnson noise" which is related to the resistance by:

$$\sigma_i^2 = \frac{4kT\,BW}{R_{seal}} \quad [21]$$

where σ_i^2 is the current noise variance, BW is the recording frequency bandwidth, k is the Boltzmann constant, and T is the temperature. Clearly, as R_{seal} increases, σ_i^2 decreases to permit clearer observation of ionic currents.

As the fire-polished pipette tip makes contact with an enzymatically cleaned cell membrane surface, R_{seal} increases to the MΩ range. Fortunately, a small amount of vacuum applied at the other end of the pipette has been shown to increase dramatically R_{seal} to the gigaohm (GΩ, 10^9 ohms) level. The physical separation between the pipette tip annulus and the cell membrane is on the order of Å 10^{-10} m as would be expected for a chemical bond (13). Given that the extracellular matrix may rise hundreds of angstroms above the cell surface, it is surprising that the pipette tip can achieve such a close proximity to the cell membrane, especially in the case of gigaohm seal formation with cells not treated with enzymes. Milton and Caldwell (40) and Ruknudin et al. (48) have examined this issue in detail and have reported that, upon application of vacuum, lipid blebs form in the tip. They have proposed that it is these blebs, which consist of mobile lipids and channels, that allow gigaohm seal formation.

Regardless of the manner by which gigaohm seals are formed, the pipette glass is in extremely close contact with the cell membrane. Although a variety of glass will form gigaohm seals, differing electrical and thermal properties make some types of glass more or less appropriate for use (for review, see ref. 46). In addition, it has become apparent that some glass types may not be physiologically inert (12,14,21,47,51). Trace elements, including barium, lead, and aluminum, in some glass can be leached from the glass itself to alter channel activity. Consequently, it is advisable for each glass-channel system be examined for possible interfering effects.

PATCH CLAMP MODES OF RECORDING

Figure 9 illustrates the different recording configurations of the patch clamp technique. Once a GΩ seal has been achieved, unitary channel activity may be measured in the cell-attached mode. A major disadvantage of the cell-attached configuration is the lack of exact voltage control of the trans-patch potential which is the difference between V_m and the pipette potential, V_p, i.e., $V_m - V_p$. Under some recording conditions, the single-channel current under measurement can alter V_m, resulting in a distortion in the form of the single-channel currents (20). A major advantage, however, is that intracellular constituents which may be important for second messenger-mediated modulation of the ion channel are undisturbed. Withdrawal of the pipette from the cell often leaves the membrane patch intact so that the cytosolic side of the membrane patch faces the extracellular bathing solution (inside-out). The inside-out configuration is particularly useful in the study of channels which are affected by intracellular modulators such as ATP-dependent K^+ channels and Ca^{2+}-activated K^+ channels. Instead of withdrawing the pipette, a transient pulse of suction can be used to rupture the membrane patch to gain direct electrical access to the cell permitting the whole-cell recording configuration. Whole-cell recording, which is probably the most commonly employed variation of the patch clamp method, yields measurements of the sum of all of the functional ion channels in the entire cell. A particular advantage of the whole-cell recording technique is that upon rupture of the membrane patch, the solution contained within the patch pipette, which is a virtually infinite volume when compared to the intracellular volume, rapidly dialyses the interior of the cell. The time course of cell dialysis is depends on several factors, including the access resistance to the interior of the cell and molecular weight of the mobile molecule (44); ions the size of K^+ and Mg^{2+} achieve nearly complete dialysis in <30 sec. Cells can be dialyzed with solutions containing ions which do not permeate one or more types of channels, thus allowing a particular ionic current to be isolated for study. In addition, a fluorescent dye useful in the measurement of internal ion concentration may be included into the pipette solution, eliminating the need for membrane permeant forms of the dye (3,41). Unfortunately, dialysis may deplete intracellular components which are critical for maintained integrity of some classes of channels. This is particularly the case for Ca^{2+} channels, which are notorious for exhibiting "rundown" or "washout" (for example, see ref. 18).

From the whole-cell recording configuration, withdrawal of the pipette allows the membrane to reseal about the pipette tip such that the cytosolic side of the membrane faces the pipette solution and the extracellular side of the membrane faces the bathing solution (outside-out). The outside-out configuration is ideal for examining the activity of single ligand-gated channels, such as the $GABA_A$-linked Cl^- channel and the NMDA receptor. Note that after a pipette makes contact with the membrane of a cell, debris may adhere to the tip, making the use of this pipette with another cell less likely to achieve a gigaohm seal.

How does the patch clamp perform a voltage clamp of the membrane and measure ionic current with a single electrode? Consider the simple electrical model of the whole-cell recording mode shown in Fig. 10. Note that R_s is not equivalent to the pipette resistance; usually it is ~2–3 times as large (37), presumably due to partial clogging of the pipette tip during whole-cell recording. Assuming that the direction of the membrane current, I_m, is out the cell (carried by K^+ ions, for instance), by Kirchhoff's current law, the current flowing through the patch electrode across R_s is equal to I_m. This current is then split between the negative input of the op-amp and the feedback resistor, R_f. Recall that for op-amps, we expect the current flowing into the negative input to be 0, so that I_m is then equal to the I_f. The voltage difference across the feedback resistor, or equivalently, $V_o - V_c$, is proportional to I_m. To clamp the membrane voltage, recall another rule for negative feedback amplifiers: The voltages at the positive and negative inputs are equal. We can show using Ohm's law that:

$$V_m = V_c - I_m R_s \qquad [22]$$

Thus, if the voltage error which is the product of I_m and R_s is sufficiently small, i.e., <3 mV, then $V_m \approx V_C$. However, as R_s increases, the degree of voltage control is diminished resulting in a possible distortion of the ionic current. Figure 11 illustrates a simulated Na^+ current and associated membrane potential, V_m, evoked by a command voltage step from –80 to + 10 mV with $R_s = 1$ MΩ (*solid lines*) and $R_s = 30$ MΩ (*dashed lines*). Clearly, the lower value of R_s allows V_m to follow more closely V_C. The particular effect of increased R_s on V_m is dependent on the ionic current under measurement. One should not expect identical results if the ionic current was carried by delayed outward K^+ channels. In addition, we have demonstrated earlier with the two-electrode voltage clamp that for a command voltage step, V_m lagged behind with a time constant,

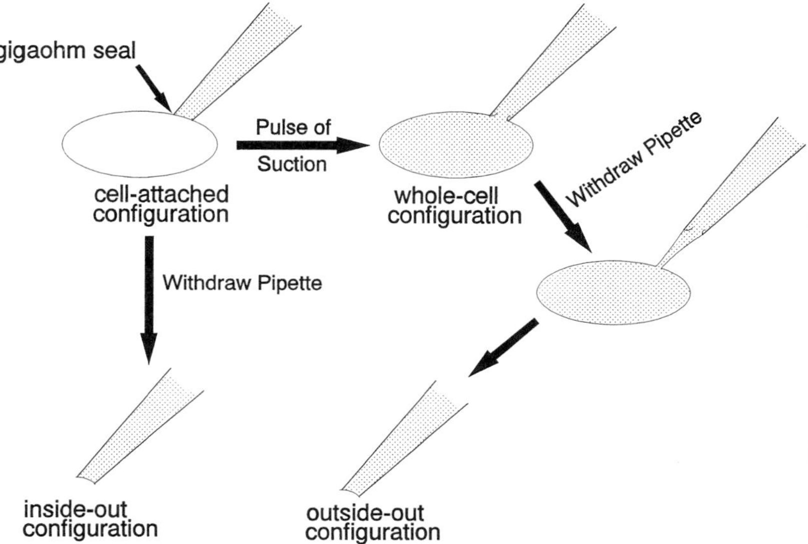

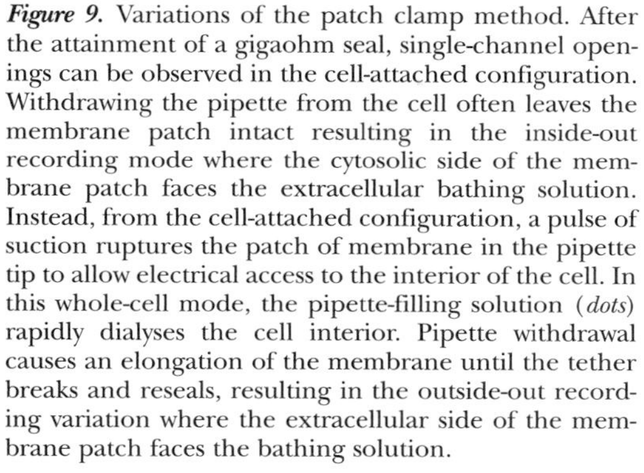
Figure 9. Variations of the patch clamp method. After the attainment of a gigaohm seal, single-channel openings can be observed in the cell-attached configuration. Withdrawing the pipette from the cell often leaves the membrane patch intact resulting in the inside-out recording mode where the cytosolic side of the membrane patch faces the extracellular bathing solution. Instead, from the cell-attached configuration, a pulse of suction ruptures the patch of membrane in the pipette tip to allow electrical access to the interior of the cell. In this whole-cell mode, the pipette-filling solution (*dots*) rapidly dialyses the cell interior. Pipette withdrawal causes an elongation of the membrane until the tether breaks and reseals, resulting in the outside-out recording variation where the extracellular side of the membrane patch faces the bathing solution.

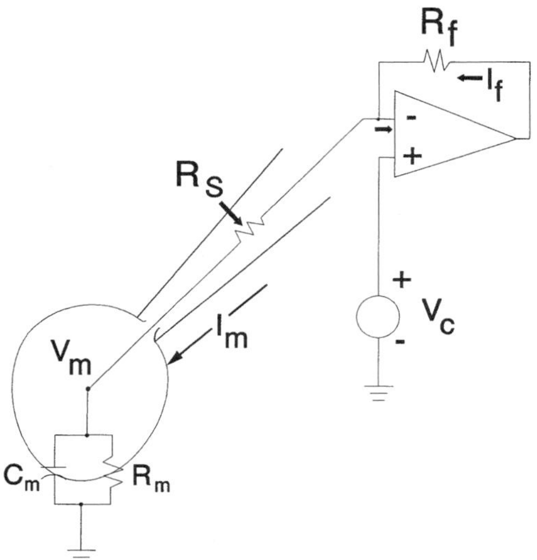

Figure 10. Whole-cell voltage-clamp and current measurement is accomplished with only one pipette electrode. Because the input impedance of the operational amplifier does not draw any current through the negative (or positive) input, by Kirchhoff's current law, we expect that the transmembrane current, I_m, will be equivalent to the current through the feedback resistor, R_f. Negative feedback sets the voltage at the positive and negative inputs equal so I_m is proportional to the voltage difference $V_o - V_c$. The error in the clamp voltage, $V_C - V_m$ is equal to the voltage drop across the series resistance, R_s. As shown in Fig. 4, V_m lags behind V_C with a time constant $\tau = R_sC_m$.

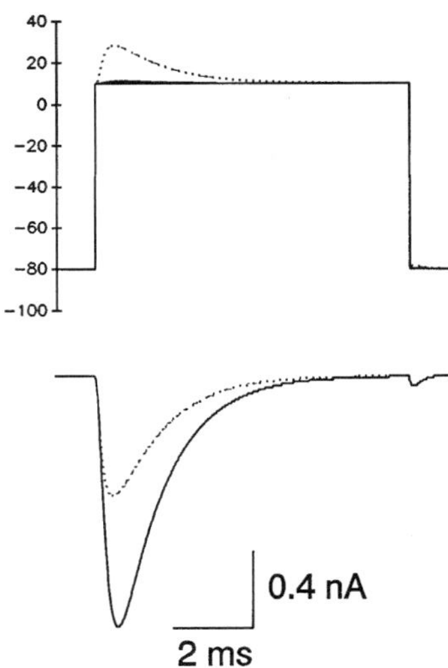

Figure 11. Under whole-cell voltage-clamp conditions, high series resistance, R_s, values distort the membrane voltage, V_m, and the form of the voltage-dependent current. While neglecting the effect of cell capacitance, the current shown was simulated digitally, based on a Hodgkin-Huxley representation of the rapid inward Na^+ current of mammalian thalamocortical relay neurons (38), assuming a maximum conductance of 100 nS. *Upper traces* show V_m, and the *lower traces* show the simulated current under conditions of $R_s = 1$ MΩ (*solid lines*) and $R_s = 30$ MΩ (*dashed lines*).

τ, proportional to membrane capacitance. For the whole-cell voltage clamp, the equivalent circuit is identical to that shown in Fig. 3. Consequently, when V_c is a step potential, eqs. 9 and 10 hold true (with $V_m = V_X$), indicating that actual membrane voltage, V_m, also lags behind the command voltage step with $\tau = R_sC_m$, and the whole-cell current, I_m, has capacitive spikes at the beginning and termination of the command step pulse.

MEASUREMENT OF CELL CAPACITANCE AS AN ASSAY FOR EXOCYTOSIS

During exocytosis in neurosecretory cells, intracellular vesicles containing neurotransmitter or hormone fuse with the cell membrane to release their intravesicular contents. Membrane fusion of a vesicle results in an increase in the effective surface area of the cell and, by eq. 6, a rise in cell capacitance, C_m. For adrenal chromaffin cells, the capacitance increase is very small, on the order of femtofarads (10^{-15} F). To detect such small changes, a sine wave rather than a voltage step was applied as the command input of a voltage-clamped cell. Linear systems analysis of the circuit shown in Fig. 3 reveals that the resulting current sinusoid, $I_m(t)$, will be of the same frequency as the command voltage reference signal. An elegant study by Neher and Marty (42) showed that by evaluating the magnitude of $I_m(t)$ at particular times or phase angles relative to the reference signal, the magnitudes of the circuit model elements can be estimated. To illustrate this concept, consider the simple case where the series resistance, R_s, is absent from the circuit model (Fig. 12A). In this instance, $I_m(t)$ will be equal to the sum of the currents through the parallel R-C network:

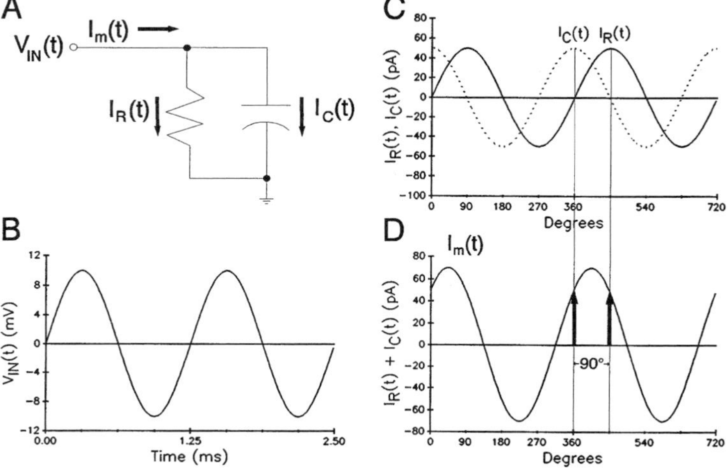

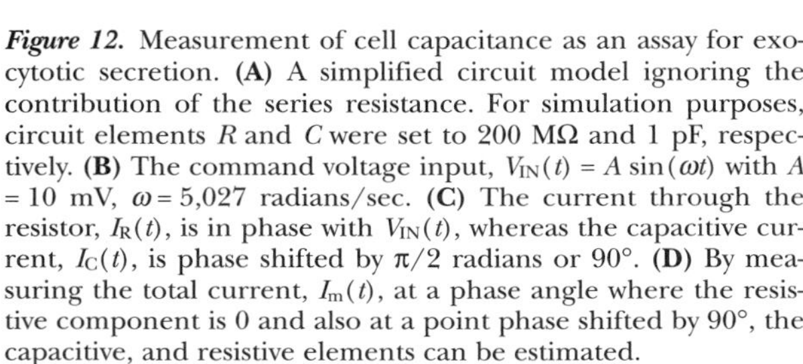

Figure 12. Measurement of cell capacitance as an assay for exocytotic secretion. **(A)** A simplified circuit model ignoring the contribution of the series resistance. For simulation purposes, circuit elements *R* and *C* were set to 200 MΩ and 1 pF, respectively. **(B)** The command voltage input, $V_{IN}(t) = A\sin(\omega t)$ with $A = 10$ mV, $\omega = 5{,}027$ radians/sec. **(C)** The current through the resistor, $I_R(t)$, is in phase with $V_{IN}(t)$, whereas the capacitive current, $I_C(t)$, is phase shifted by $\pi/2$ radians or 90°. **(D)** By measuring the total current, $I_m(t)$, at a phase angle where the resistive component is 0 and also at a point phase shifted by 90°, the capacitive, and resistive elements can be estimated.

$$I_m(t) = I_R(t) + I_c(t) \quad [23]$$

where $I_R(t)$ is the current through the resistance R and $I_C(t)$ is the capacitive current. For an input reference signal, $V_{IN}(t) = A \sin(\omega t)$ (Fig. 12B), we expect $I_R(t)$ (Fig. 12C, *solid line*) to be proportional and in phase or alignment with $V_{IN}(t)$. However, $I_C(t)$ (Fig. 12C, *dashed line*) will be $\pi/2$ radians (or 90°) out of phase with the reference signal since:

$$I_c(t) = C_m \frac{dV_{IN}(t)}{dt} = AC_m \omega \cos(\omega t) = AC_m \omega \sin\left(\omega t + \frac{\pi}{2}\right) \quad [24]$$

The sum of the two sine waves, $I_m(t)$ (Fig. 12D), yields a sine wave where the capacitive component is at a maximum at $t = 0$ when the resistive component is zero and visa-versa at $t = T/4$ or 90°, where T is the period of the sine wave. Therefore, by measuring $I_m(t)$ at $t = 0$ and $t = T/4$ (or at $t = T$ and $t = 5T/4$ as shown by the *arrows* in Fig. 12D, *lower right panel*), the magnitudes of C_m and R_m can be determined, respectively. In practice, a two-phase lock-in amplifier was originally used in combination with the patch clamp amplifier to generate output signals corresponding to R_m and C_m. Modern techniques utilize a computer to generate and acquire the sinusoidal waveforms (for example, see ref. 19).

The incorporation of R_s into the equivalent circuit introduces an additional phase shift which causes the exact time location, or phase angle, of capacitive and resistive maxima to become uncertain. Neher and Marty (42) searched for an appropriate phase angle by changing the effective capacitance of the circuit through compensation circuitry until no change in the signal corresponding to the resistance was observed. Such compensation circuitry is a standard feature among many of the commercially available patch clamp amplifiers. After determination of the appropriate phase angle and 90° later, R_m and C_m can be estimated, respectively. Large changes in R_m or C_m can alter the phase angle necessary for separation of the equivalent circuit elements (28), thus requiring a means of rapidly updating the phase angle. Fidler and Fernandez (19) modified the original phase angle detection technique by including a computer-controlled calibration resistance in series with the cell to automate the process.

WHOLE-CELL VOLTAGE CLAMP USING THE PERFORATED PATCH METHOD

As mentioned earlier, a major disadvantage of the whole-cell patch clamp technique is dialysis of intracellular constituents which may be critical to the maintenance of channel function or a modulatory pathway. By including the pore-forming antibiotic nystatin in the pipette solution, Horn and Marty (27) were able to gain electrical access to the cell interior within several minutes after establishing the cell-attached configuration. Nystatin-induced pores permit the diffusion of monovalent ions such as Cs^+ and Cl^-, but not divalent ions, Ca^{2+} and Mg^{2+}, or any larger molecules such as cAMP. Therefore, concern over the intracellular buffering of Ca^{2+} with either EGTA or BAPTA and the loss of intracellular constituents is alleviated. Although nystatin is capable of diffusing laterally in the membrane, it does not appear to able to cross outside of the glass-membrane seal (25). The perforated patch technique has proved particularly useful in the long duration study of Ca^{2+} currents, in particular the effect modulators (for review, see ref. 2). In addition, it has been applied to the measurement of cell capacitance as an estimate of exocytosis from adrenal chromaffin cells (22). When using the perforated patch method, it must be recognized that a Donnan equilibrium is established between the cell interior and the pipette solution (27). Consequently, the absence of negatively charged impermeant species in the pipette may lead to cell swelling (32). The major problem with the perforated patch recording is that the series resistance, R_s, achieved with nystatin pore is often greater (20–50 MΩ) than under standard whole-cell conditions (1–10 MΩ). As discussed earlier, a large R_s can manifest a substantial voltage error as well as affect the response time of the voltage clamp. Rae et al. (45) have reported that with refined electrode fabrication and the use of another antibiotic, amphotericin B, a much more suitable range of R_s can be attained (3–10 MΩ).

WHOLE-CELL CURRENT AND THE SINGLE-CHANNEL PROBABILITY OF OPENING, $P_O(t)$

As discussed earlier, the whole-cell current can be represented by Ohm's law with a conductance term, G, which is both voltage and time dependent. We can relate G to the number of ion channels, N, the single-channel conductance, γ, and $P_o(t)$:

$$G = N\gamma P_o(t) \quad [25]$$

Therefore, $I(t)$ can also be expressed as follows:

$$I(t) = NiP_o(t) \quad [26]$$

where i is the single-channel current. Note that the only time-dependent functions are $I(t)$ and $P_o(t)$ indicating that the whole-cell current reveals the form of $P_o(t)$ scaled by the constants N and i.

THEORETICAL ASPECTS OF ION CHANNEL GATING

The kinetic behavior of ion channel is usually considered to be a Markov process with two or more discrete states. For a Markov process, the transition rates leaving a state are independent of the time spent in that particular state. In a sense, ion channels are assumed to have no memory; i.e., the past and duration of the present occupation of a state has no bearing on the future state of the channel. Colquhoun, Hawkes, and Sigworth have made immense contributions to the theory and practical analysis of channel kinetics. To a large extent, the theory presented in the following sections can be considered a synthesis of their work.

The basic strategy of single-channel analysis is to construct a gating model consisting of as few states as possible. The notion among electrophysiologists that a membrane protein can be modelled by a few discrete states may be somewhat unreasonable given that some proteins exhibit thousands of energy minima (for example, see ref. 17), suggesting a continuum of conformational states rather than a discrete few. In recent years fractal models, which assume that transition rates are dependent on the time spent in a particular state, have been proposed as a more physiologically consistent interpretation of channel protein behavior (33–35). However, it is not known to what extent that protein conformational states correspond to conducting and nonconducting states of the channel. Consequently, both the usefulness and adequacy of fractal models have been questioned (31,39). Markov models do offer the advantage that pharmacological interactions may be readily modelled in a quantitative framework. Therefore, further discussions will assume that Markov processes underlie channel kinetics.

To relate $P_o(t)$ to channel gating, we assume that channels, like enzymes, are subject to the law of mass action which states that the rate of a chemical reaction is directly proportional to the product of the reactant concentrations at any given moment. Considering the simplest channel gating scheme where the channel protein can exist in only two measurable states closed, C, and open, O:

$$C \underset{\beta}{\overset{\alpha}{\rightleftarrows}} O$$

where α and β are rate constants. The probability of channel being open, $P_o(t)$, and closed, $P_c(t)$, at time t are related:

$$\frac{dP_o(t)}{dt} = -\beta P_o(t) + \alpha P_c(t) \qquad [27]$$

Clearly, if the channel is not open, it is closed, so:

$$P_o(t) + P_c(t) = 1 \qquad [28]$$

Therefore,

$$\frac{dP_o(t)}{dt} = -\beta P_o(t) + \alpha[1 - P_o(t)] = \alpha - (\alpha + \beta)P_o(t) \qquad [29]$$

We can solve this differential equation for a solution for $P_o(t)$:

$$P_o(t) = P_o(\infty) + [P_o(0) - P_o(\infty)]\exp(-\tfrac{t}{\tau}) \qquad [30]$$

where

$$P_o(\infty) = \frac{\alpha}{\alpha + \beta} \quad \text{and} \quad \tau = \frac{1}{\alpha + \beta} \qquad [31]$$

Mathematically, in order to convey voltage-dependence to $P_o(t)$, and subsequently to $I(t)$, we need only consider the rate constants to be functions of voltage. For most of the voltage-dependent channel gating models, the forward rate constants, e.g., α, increase with depolarization whereas the reverse reaction rates, e.g., β, decrease with depolarization. Figure 13 depicts $P_o(t)$ in response to a change in the voltage level with one set of rate constants ($\alpha = 10\ s^{-1}$; $\beta = 100\ s^{-1}$) to another voltage level with different rate constant levels ($\alpha = 100\ s^{-1}$; $\beta = 10\ s^{-1}$). Thus, for the simple two state gating scheme, fitting $I(t)$ to a single exponential and estimating $P_o(\infty)$ for a family of evoked currents would allow estimation of α and β from the whole-cell current records. However, for even slightly more complicated gating models, such as the presence of two closed states:

$$C_1 \underset{l}{\overset{k}{\rightleftarrows}} C_2 \underset{\beta}{\overset{\alpha}{\rightleftarrows}} O$$

curve fitting to estimate the rate constants is possible, however much more difficult (6).

In the case of most voltage-gated currents, curve fitting can be accomplished with the assumption of Hodgkin-Huxley (H-H) gating. This representation of ionic current, based on the classic work by Hodgkin and Huxley (24), is still used as a biophysical benchmark for comparison of channel types among various cell preparations. In the case of the delayed outward K^+ current of the squid axon, activation was quantitatively described by four independent gating particles where $n(t)$ is the probability that a gating particle is in the permissive state and $1\text{-}n(t)$ is the probability that the particle is in the nonpermissive state:

$$1 - n(t) \underset{\beta}{\overset{\alpha}{\rightleftarrows}} n(t)$$

where α is the forward reaction rate for the transition of the gating particle from nonpermissive to permissive and β for the reverse reaction. The expression for $n(t)$ is identical to that for $P_o(t)$ given in eqs. 32 and 33:

$$n(t) = n(\infty) + [n(0) - n(\infty)]\exp(-\tfrac{t}{\tau}) \qquad [32]$$

where

$$n(\infty) = \frac{\alpha}{\alpha + \beta} \quad \text{and} \quad \tau = \frac{1}{\alpha + \beta} \qquad [33]$$

Now, however, the probability that the K^+ channel opens is the product of each of the independent gating particles being in the permissive state, $n(t)^4$, thus:

$$I_K(t) = G_{K,max}(V - E_K)\,n(t)^4 \qquad [34]$$

where $G_{K,\,max}$ is the maximum delayed outward K^+ conductance. In a similar manner, Hodgkin and Huxley (24) developed an expression for the rapid inward Na^+ current, $I_{Na}(t)$:

$$I_{Na}(t) = G_{Na,max}(V - E_{Na})\,m(t)^3 h(t) \qquad [35]$$

where $m(t)$ and $h(t)$ describe activation and inactivation, respectively, and have the same solution as $n(t)$ as shown in eq. 36.

MEASUREMENT OF ACTIVATION AND INACTIVATION

By applying variable amplitude test potentials from a (usually very hyperpolarized) holding potential such that m_0 and n_0 are 0 and h_0 is 1, eqs. 38 and 39 can be simplified for estimation of τ for the H-H parameters using a curve-fitting program. Because activation and inactivation are considered the result of independent processes in the H-H model, each phase is often subjected to curve fitting separately. In the case of $I_K(t)$, n_∞ at each test potential can be assessed by:

$$n_\infty = \sqrt[4]{\frac{I_K(V)}{G_{K,max}(V - E_K)}} \qquad [36]$$

where $I_K(V)$ is the peak K^+ current at each test potential, V. To calculate h_∞, one must be concerned with the fact that inactivation cannot be observed without activation first; it is through activation that the current can be observed at all. With test potentials of sufficient amplitude to trigger a measurable I_{Na}, h_∞

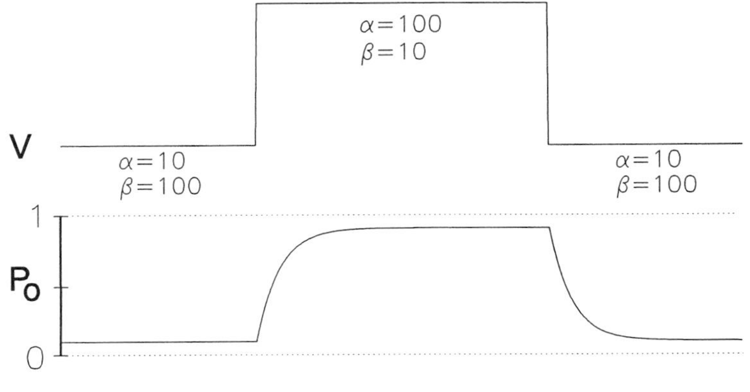

Figure 13. The probability of channel opening, $P_o(t)$, for a simple two-state model of channel gating with voltage-dependent rate constants α and β. With a voltage step, α transitions from 10 sec^{-1} to 100 sec^{-1}, whereas β decreases from 100 sec^{-1} to 10 sec^{-1}. Although the rate constants change immediately, $P_o(t)$ lags behind with a time constant $\tau = 1/(\alpha + \beta)$.

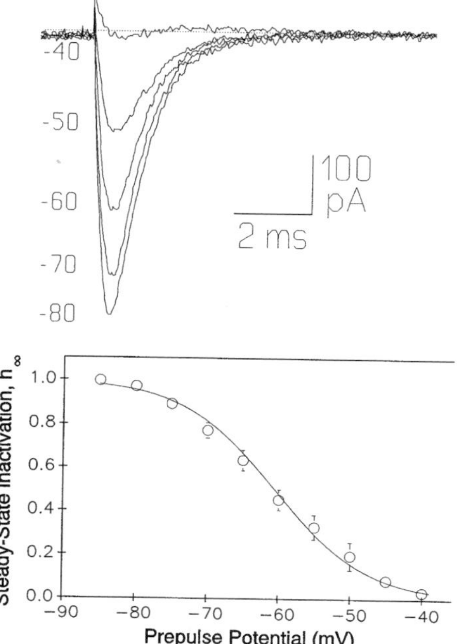

Figure 14. The voltage-dependence steady-state inactivation of I_{Na} recorded from a bovine adrenal chromaffin cell with the whole-cell patch clamp technique. The external solution contained (in mM): 140 NaCl, 5 KCl, 0.5 $CaCl_2$, 1 $CoCl_2$, 1 $MgCl_2$, 10 *N*-2-hydroxyethylpiperazine-*N'*-2-ethanesulfonic acid (HEPES), pH 7.4. The internal patch pipette solution contained (in mM): 120 CsCl, 30 CsOH, 10 HEPES, 10 ethylene glycol bis (β-aminoethyl ether)-*N,N,N',N'*-tetraacetic acid (EGTA), 5 Mg-ATP, pH 7.3. *Upper figure:* I_{Na} evoked by a test pulse to +10 mV from a 100-msec duration prepulse ranging from –80 mV to –40 mV. *Lower figure:* Steady-state inactivation, h_∞, calculated using eq. 41, was well-fitted by the Boltzmann function (see text) with $V_{½}$= 61 mV and κ' = –6.4 mV.

is quite close to 0, which is the reason why I_{Na} always appears as a transient current. To assess h_∞ over a wide range of potentials, a prepulse protocol is required where the magnitude of the prepulse voltage, but not the test potential, is varied. Since inactivation occurs more slowly than activation, one can simply measure peak I_{Na} as a function of the prepulse voltage, $I_{Na}(V_{pre})$ and calculate h_∞:

$$h_\infty = \frac{I_{Na}(V_{pre})}{I_{Na,max}(V_{pre})} \qquad [37]$$

where V_{pre} is the prepulse potential and $I_{Na,\,max}(V_{pre})$ is the maximum I_{Na} reached during the prepulse experiment. As shown with the data in Fig. 14, the voltage-dependence of h_∞ (as well as m_∞ and n_∞) can be well described by the Boltzmann function:

$$h_\infty = \frac{1}{1 + \exp(\frac{V_{½} - V'}{k'})} \qquad [38]$$

where V′ is the prepulse potential (or for m∞ and n∞, the test voltage), $V_{½}$ is the potential where $h_\infty = 0.5$, and k′ is the slope factor. The H-H representation is the simplest means by which to model voltage-clamp data; however, the requirement of independence of the activation and inactivation processes coupled with the inability to accommodate voltage-independent transitions can make the H-H model inappropriate for use in some instances. Throughout the electrophysiology literature, the Boltzmann function is commonly used to describe quantitatively activation and inactivation, even though an H-H model may not have been used to model the data. Detailed descriptions of channel gating with multiple closed and open states have been developed based on whole-cell records (for example, see ref. 8), although measurement and analysis of single-channel records is far more direct means of determining channel properties.

SINGLE-CHANNEL RECORDS (SUMMARY 1)

Single-channel data records exhibit a pattern quite unlike the whole-cell ionic current. The records contain small step-like current deflections of random time length, usually from fixed levels. The estimation of the amplitude of single ion channel openings is the least confusing aspect of single-channel analysis. When a channel is in the conducting state, the current, *i*, is related to the single-channel conductance, γ, by Ohm's law:

$$i = \gamma(V - E_{ion}) \qquad [39]$$

Unlike eq. 5 for the whole-cell current, γ is a constant that can be directly calculated from the slope of the *i*-*V* relation. In Fig. 15, the top three traces show inside-out patch clamp recordings from a membrane patch with two Ca^{2+}-dependent K^+ "BK" channels. The cytoplasmic side of the membrane was exposed to a solution containing ~150 mM K^+, with the level of free Ca^{2+} buffered to 500 nM, and the membrane patch was depolarized from a holding potential of –80 mV to +80 mV. The upward deflections represent channel openings and the downward deflections are channel closings. The ensemble average of the 64 sweeps, shown in the bottom trace of Fig. 15, is strongly representative of the contribution of these channels to the form of the whole-cell current. The analysis of single-channel open amplitude is relatively straightforward because channels open in an "all-or-none" manner. But the length of time that a

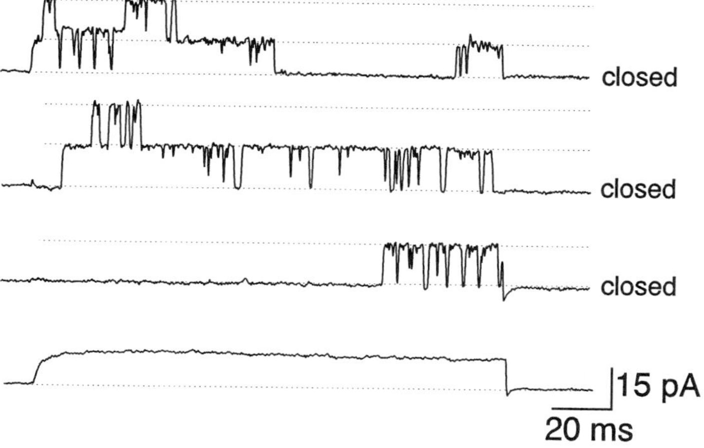

Figure 15. Excised patch inside-out recordings from the large conductance Ca^{2+}-dependent "BK" K^+ channels of bovine adrenal chromaffin cells. The bathing solution facing the cytosolic side of the membrane patch contained (in mM): 140 KCl, 2 $MgCl_2$, 5 HEPES, 0.08 EGTA, 0.067 $CaCl_2$, pH 7.3, yielding ~500 nM free Ca^{2+}. The pipette solution contained (in mM): 140 NaCl, 5 KCl, 2 $CaCl_2$, 1 $MgCl_2$, 10 HEPES, pH 7.4. Voltage steps to +80 mV from a holding potential of –80 mV were used to evoke BK channel openings (*upper three traces*). Multiple current levels, denoted by the *dashed lines*, indicate at least two BK channels are in the patch, and possibly, a subconductance level. *Bottom trace:* The ensemble average of 64 sweeps.

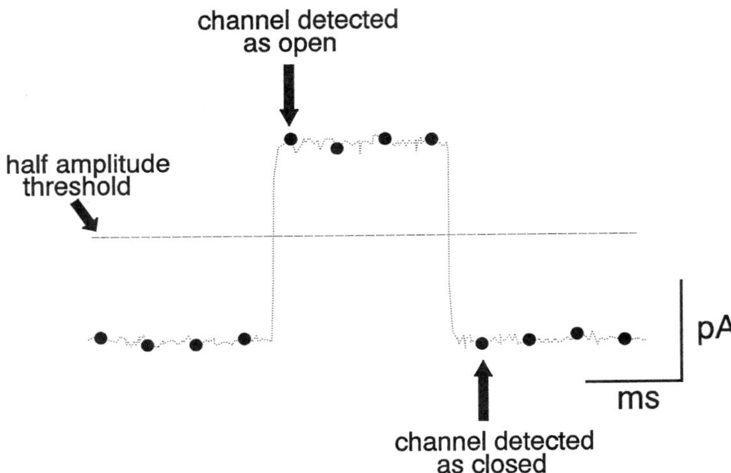

Figure 16. Half-amplitude threshold detection of channel openings. The *dotted line* represents the true single channel opening, whereas the *large dots* show the points digitized. The *dashed line* is the amplitude threshold, usually set by visual inspection of the data records. A channel is considered opened when the current signal exceeds the threshold for a user-specified number of points. Once the current signal falls below the threshold, the channel is considered closed.

channel spends in a given state, either closed or open, is probabilistic; i.e., its state is not absolutely known at any given moment. Since channel open and closed times are essentially random variables, some fundamental concepts in stochastic processes are reviewed in Appendix 2.

CHANNEL EVENT DETECTION

The technique most often used to distinguish channel openings is called half amplitude thresholding (49). Colquhoun and Sigworth (11) have examined the effects of filtering and noise on the threshold-driven event detection and concluded that 50% threshold crossing detection offers minimal errors in estimation of event duration. To illustrate this method, Fig. 16 shows a series of dots representing the digitized current trace. A channel opening is detected if the digitized current signal exceeds 50% of the expected amplitude of the channel opening. When the current signal falls below the half amplitude threshold, a channel closing occurs. Once an event has been identified, the open time is simply the duration of the event, and the amplitude is the peak or the average of the current during the open event. The current amplitude, open time, and previous closed time, can be added to an event list for further analysis.

Alternatively, an all-points histogram can be used to assess open channel amplitude. The advantage of this method is that is does not rely on a priori assumptions concerning the expected open channel amplitude. By sorting all of the digitized data points according to magnitude, both the baseline and open channel amplitudes will be apparent by the bell-shaped (gaussian) curves about the mean values. Another advantage of this technique is that the relative sizes of the bell-shaped curves can qualitatively convey the probability of the channel occupying the open state. Furthermore, the presence of multiple channel openings or rare subconductance states will be evident from the histogram. For example, the *upper trace* of Fig. 17 shows a current recording from 3 BK Ca^{2+}-dependent K^+ channels exposed to 1 μM free Ca^{2+} at the cytosolic side of the excised, inside-out, membrane patch. The all-points histogram (*lower panel* of Fig. 17) clearly shows a majority of data points centered about the zero baseline with peaks occurring every 8.2 pA, which is consistent with the simultaneous opening of up to 3 BK channels. In addition, a small subconductance state centered at 2.7 pA can be observed from the histogram.

ANALYSIS OF CHANNEL LIFETIMES

If we examine single-channel openings and closings in a patch, we can measure open and closed times to estimate channel transition rates. For the simple channel gating scheme with one closed and one open state:

$$\frac{dP_c(t)}{dt} = -\alpha P_c(t) = \beta P_o(t) \qquad [40]$$

For very small Δt such that the channel can make no more than one transition, the derivative can be approximated as:

$$\frac{P_c(t+\Delta t) - P_c(t)}{\Delta t} = -\alpha P_c(t) = \beta P_o(t) \qquad [41]$$

For open time analysis, we need only consider the transition of the channel from the open state at time t to the closed state at time $t + \Delta t$. Thus, we are interested in the conditional prob-

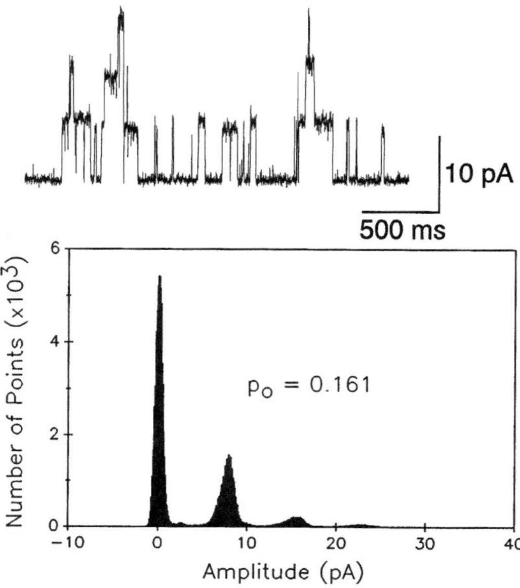

Figure 17. All-points histogram of a channel record does not rely on a priori assumptions concerning the expected open channel amplitude. *Upper trace:* Data recorded from an inside-out membrane patch containing three Ca^{2+}-dependent "BK" K^+ channels from an adrenal chromaffin cell held at +30 mV. The solution included in the patch pipette was identical to the bathing solution (in mM): 100 KCl, 42 KOH, 9.32 $CaCl_2$, 10 EGTA, 10 HEPES, pH 7.3, yielding ~1 μM free Ca^{2+}. Digitized data points are sorted according to amplitude and plotted in a histogram. The height of the peaks centered at current amplitudes qualitatively indicates the frequency of a particular event. For example, the histogram is dominated by 0 amplitude data points, suggesting that most often the channels were closed.

ability, $P_c^*(t+\Delta t)$, that the channel will be closed at time $t+\Delta t$ given that it was open at time t; therefore:

$$P_c^*(t+\Delta t) = \beta\Delta t \qquad [42]$$

At time $t+\Delta t$, the channel can either be open or closed, so the conditional probability, $P_o^*(t+\Delta t)$, that the channel will be open at time $t+\Delta t$ given that it was open at time t is:

$$P_o^*(t+\Delta t) = 1 - \beta\Delta t \qquad [43]$$

Up to this point, we can only make predictions of the channel state from one instant, Δt in duration, to the next. We define $\lambda(t)$ as the probability that the channel remains open for the entire duration from 0 to t. Then, $\lambda(t+\Delta t)$ is the probability $\lambda(t)$ combined with the conditional probability that the channel remains open at $t+\Delta t$ after having been open at t, i.e., $P_o^*(t+\Delta t)$. Because $\lambda(t)$ and $P_o^*(t+\Delta t)$ correspond to independent events, the probability of both events is simply the product:

$$\lambda(t+\Delta t) = \lambda(t)P_o^*(t+\Delta t) = \lambda(t)(1-\beta\Delta t) \qquad [44]$$

Rearranging the terms:

$$\frac{\lambda(t+\Delta t)-\lambda(t)}{\Delta t} = -\beta\lambda t \qquad [45]$$

Note that if one considers Δt approaching 0, then the left side of eq. 49 reduces to the derivative of $\lambda(t)$:

$$\frac{d\lambda(t)}{dt} = -\beta\lambda t \qquad [46]$$

The solution to this first order differential equation is:

$$\lambda(t) = \exp(-t\beta) \qquad [47]$$

Although experimental data can be reported in the form of $\lambda(t)$, data are most often given in the form of a frequency histogram, which is for all intents and purposes a list of possible open times on the x-axis with the number of corresponding observed channel openings plotted on the y-axis. How do we extend $\lambda(t)$ to open times? We must recognize that the event that a channel remains open from 0 to t is the same as the event in which the channel open time is greater than t. Hence, $\lambda(t) = P(\text{open time} > t)$, and more importantly:

$$P(\text{open time} \le t) = 1 - \lambda(t) \qquad [48]$$

By definition (see Appendix 2), $P(\text{open time} \le t)$ is the cumulative distribution function, and therefore, the probability density function (*pdf*) of the channel open time random variable is:

$$pdf = \frac{d}{dt}[1-\exp(-\beta t)] = \beta\exp(-\beta t) \qquad [49]$$

We can predict the size of each bin of the frequency histogram by calculating the product of the total number of events, N_T, and the probability of an open time ranging from t_1 to t_2:

$$N(t_1 \text{ to } t_2) = N_T\int_{t_1}^{t_2}\beta\exp(-\beta t)\,dt = N_T[\exp(-\beta t_1)-\exp(-\beta t_2)] \qquad [50]$$

Also, we can determine the mean open time, m_o, using the *pdf*:

$$m_o = \int_{-\infty}^{+\infty} t\,\beta\exp(-\beta t)\,dt = \frac{1}{\beta} \qquad [51]$$

Figure 18 illustrates the major steps in the identification of channel openings, sorting events, and analysis in the form of a histogram. Once single-channel openings have been identified in a digitized data set, lists of open and closed times can be prepared. For the open time list, bins spanning the range of the recorded open times are constructed and the data are sorted to construct a frequency histogram. Assignment of appropriate bin dimensions has been discussed in detail by Colquhoun and Sigworth (11). The midpoints of each bin, for example $(t_1 + t_2)/2$, and the corresponding number of events in each bin may then be fit to a single exponential decay function to estimate the rate constant leaving the open state, β, or in the case of multiple paths away from a single open state, the sum of the rate constants leaving the open state. Our discussion to this point has been limited to the simple situation where there is only one open state. If the data are better fit by the sum of two or more exponential functions, then one must consider the possibility of multiple open states. The relationship between the fitted time constants and the rate constants associated with the particular open states depends on the assumed gating model. General techniques for processing data of this nature have been examined by a number of investigators (5,7,9,26,36). The presence of multiple closed states is quite common and can sometimes be apparent from visual inspection of the data traces. Long quiescent periods may be punctuated by channel opening bursts, which are openings separated by brief closures, suggesting two or more closed states are necessary to characterize the results. Data from two

1. Acquire raw data.

2. Detect open events to form idealized records.

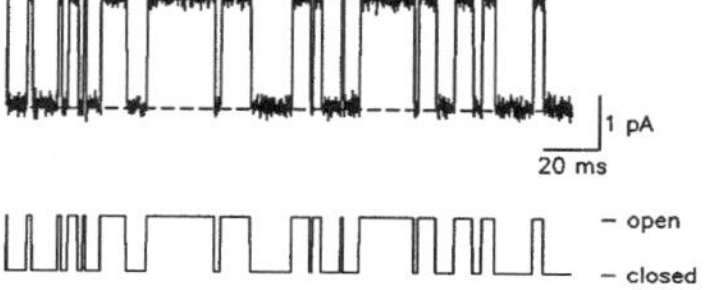

3. Sort openings by duration.

Open Time Range	Number of Events
0.0 - 0.4	475
0.4 - 0.8	432
0.8 - 1.2	402
1.2 - 1.6	324
1.6 - 2.0	312
. . .	. . .

4. Histogram and fit a curve to estimate rate constants.

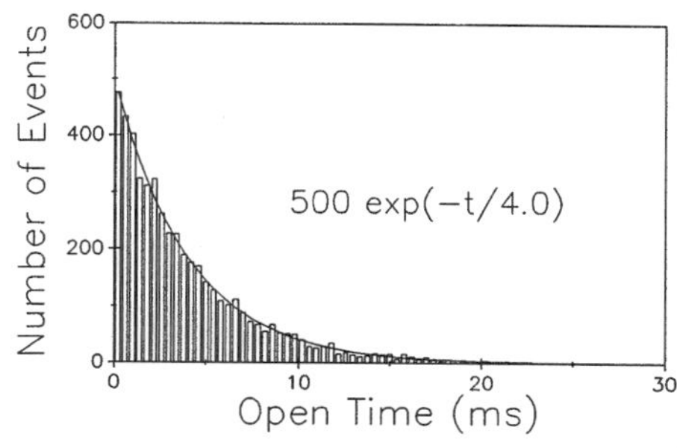

Figure 18. The basic steps involved in single channel kinetic analysis: (1) single channel data is digitized so that (2) open channel (and closed channel) events can be detected, usually by using a half-amplitude threshold scheme. From the list of open times, (3) the events are sorted into duration bins. (4) These results are plotted in a histogram and fitted to one or more exponential decay functions of the form: $A_i\exp(-t/\tau_i)$, where A_i is the amplitude and g_i is the time constant of ith component. In this example, $\tau = 4.0$ msec, which is equal to the inverse of the sum of the rate constants leaving this open state.

or more states which differ in average dwell time by several orders of magnitude pose a problem for the preparation of a histogram with a linear dwell time *x*-axis. Sine and Sigworth (50) have derived the form and necessary function for curve fitting for data histogrammed in terms of the square root of the number of events versus the log dwell time. Multiple states are readily distinguished by the presence of multiple humps in the transformed histogram.

A major assumption of channel kinetic analysis, which is often incorrectly ignored in the presentation of data, is that the analyzed records are due to a unitary ion channel. Under conditions where P_o is large, simultaneous openings become obvious to indicate more than one channel in the patch. In the case of multiple channels in a patch, the closed time histogram is greatly biased against long closures since we cannot determine which channel's closed time is terminated with an opening; only periods where both channels are closed can be considered. In contrast, as long as P_o is not too large, simultaneous openings may be discarded and the open time histogram can be constructed with only a slight bias against long duration openings, when the simultaneous openings are more likely to occur. For complete and accurate kinetic analysis, however, there should only be one channel in the patch during recording. Although simultaneous openings clearly indicate two or more channels, the lack of simultaneous openings must be regarded with caution, since when P_o is small, the likelihood of observing simultaneous openings over a brief observation time can be extremely low. For example, if the apparent P_o is 0.002 (perhaps two openings averaging 1 msec in duration occurring each second) and there are actually two homogenous, independent channels in the patch, then the true P_o is 0.001 and the probability of having both channels open simultaneously is $P_o^2 = 1 \times 10^{-6}$. Addressing this problem, Colquhoun and Hawkes (10) approximated the probability, P_1, that a data record from a patch with N channels will exhibit only single openings:

$$P_1 \approx \exp[-T(\frac{N-1}{N})\frac{m_o}{m_c^2}] \qquad [52]$$

where m_o is the mean open time, m_c is the mean closed time, and T is the observation time. For example, if only single openings averaging 1 msec in duration are observed at a rate of 1/sec for 10 min, can we then conclude that there is only one channel in the patch? Using eq. 52 to calculate the probability that there are still two or more channels in the patch yields 0.741, indicating that, based on the present data, there may well be more than one channel in the patch. In order to reduce P_1 to <0.05, an arbitrary level for statistical significance for rejecting the hypothesis of two or more channels, the observation time, T, for no double openings must be >100 min.

Modern methods in electrophysiology are capable of examining state transitions of the membrane proteins which form ion channels. Indeed, the tools available for investigating such bioelectrical processes are quite powerful, but not without limitations. Successful use of these techniques and the interpretation of electrophysiological data requires an understanding of these limitations.

> Summary: Major concepts in single-channel kinetics:
> - The probability that a channel remains in a state depends on the rate constants *leaving* that state.
> - For a single open state, the time constant, τ from fitting a single exponential decay is:
>
> $$\tau = \frac{1}{\sum \text{rate constants leaving that state}}$$
>
> The presence of other open states of the same conductance may be distinguished by the use of multiple exponential decay function to describe $\lambda(t)$.
> - The effects of pharmacologic agents on ion channels can be described quantitatively by (a) changes in single-channel conductance; (b) altered transition rates between states; or (c) the addition of one or more new states to the gating scheme.

APPENDIX 1

The Laplace transform method offers a means of solving differential equations typical in circuit analysis. Utilizing the Laplace domain, the total impedance, $Z(s)$, of the circuit can be written as:

$$Z(s) = R_s + \frac{R}{RCs+1} = \frac{R_sRCs + R_s + R}{RCs+1} \qquad [A1]$$

Since $I(s) = V(s)/Z(s)$ and $V(s) = V_o/s$, then:

$$I(s) = \frac{V_o}{s}\,\frac{RCs+1}{R_sRCs + R_s + R} = \frac{V_o(\frac{s}{R_s} + \frac{1}{R_sRC})}{s + \frac{R_s+R}{R_sRC}} \qquad [A2]$$

Using the partial fraction expansion method, $I(s)$ can be expressed as:

$$I(s) = \frac{A}{s} + \frac{B}{s + \frac{R_s+R}{R_sRC}} \qquad [A3]$$

Solving for A:

$$A = \frac{V_o(\frac{s}{R_s} + \frac{1}{R_sRC})}{s + \frac{R_s+R}{R_sRC}}\Big|_{s=0} = \frac{V_o}{R_s+R} \qquad [A4]$$

Solving for B:

$$B = \frac{V_o(\frac{s}{R_s} + \frac{1}{R_sRC})}{s}\Big|_{s=-\frac{R_s+R}{R_sRC}} = \frac{V_o}{R_s} - \frac{V_o}{R_s+R} \qquad [A5]$$

Applying the inverse Laplace transform:

$$I(t) = \frac{V_o}{R_s+R} + [\frac{V_o}{R_s} - \frac{V_o}{R_s+R}]\exp(-t/\tau) \quad \text{and} \quad \tau = \frac{R_s+R}{R_sRC} \qquad [A6]$$

The voltage drop across the R-C network, V_x:

$$V_x = V - IR_s \qquad [A7]$$

If V is a step potential of magnitude V_o, then:

$$V_x(t) = (V_o - \frac{V_oR_s}{R_s+R})[1 - \exp(-t/\tau)] \qquad [A8]$$

Under conditions where $R >> R_s$, eq. A6 reduces to:

$$I(t) \approx \frac{V_o}{R} + \frac{V_o}{R_s}\exp(-t/\tau) \quad \text{and} \quad \tau \approx R_sC \qquad [A9]$$

and eq. 64 becomes:

$$V_x(t) \approx V_o[1 - \exp(-t/\tau)] \qquad [A10]$$

APPENDIX 2

Probability Density Function (*pdf*)

The duration of a channel opening may be viewed as a continuous random variable. To illustrate the complexity of assigning probabilities to particular values of continuous random variables, consider a random number generator which outputs a real or noninteger number, x, between 0 and 1. Clearly, the probability that x will be equal to 0.5314592173 is, for all practical purposes, equal to 0. Instead, we have to consider the probability that x will be between a range of values. The probability density function (*pdf*) of x is a function such that when it is integrated over the entire range of possible values of x, it is equal to 1:

$$\int_{-\infty}^{+\infty} pdf(x)\ dx = 1 \qquad [A11]$$

Therefore, in order to determine the probability that x will fall within a specified interval bounded by x_1 and x_2:

$$P(x_1 < x \le x_2) = \int_{x_1}^{x_2} pdf(x)\ dx \qquad pdf(x) \ge 0 \text{ for all } x \qquad [A12]$$

Cumulative Distribution Function [$F(x)$]

For a random variable x, we can calculate the probability that x takes on the value x_1 or less, $P(x_1 \le x)$, which is defined as the cumulative distribution function:

$$F(x_1) = P(x_1 \le x) = \int_{-\infty}^{x_2} pdf(x)\ dx \qquad [A13]$$

There are two properties that are useful in the examination of channel kinetics. First, the derivative of the cumulative distribution function is equal to the *pdf*:

$$\frac{dF(x)}{dx} = pdf(x) \qquad [A14]$$

if the derivative exists. Second, mean of random variable x, μ_x, is related to the *pdf* of x:

$$\mu_x = \int_{-\infty}^{+\infty} x\ pdf(x)\ dx \qquad [A15]$$

REFERENCES

1. Adrian RH, Chandler WK, Hodgkin AL. Voltage clamp experiments in striated muscle fibres. *J Physiol (Lond)* 1970;208:607–644.
2. Akaike N, Harata N. Nystatin perforated patch recording and its application to analyses of intracellular mechanisms. *Jpn J Physiol* 1994;44:433–473.
3. Almers W, Neher E. The Ca signal from fura-2 loaded mast cells depends strongly on the method of dye-loading. *FEBS Lett* 1985; 192:13–18.
4. Armstrong CM, Gilly WF. Access resistance and space clamp problems associated with whole-cell patch clamping. In: Rudy B, Iverson LE, eds. *Methods in enzymology, volume 207. Ion channels.* San Diego: Academic Press, 1992:100–122.
5. Ball FG, Sansom MSP. Ion-channel gating mechanisms: model identification and parameter estimation from single channel recordings. *Proc R Soc Lond B* 1989;236:385–416.
6. Balser JR, Roden DM, Bennett PB. Global parameter optimization for cardiac potassium channel gating models. *Biophys J* 1990;57: 433–444.
7. Bauer RJ, Bowman BF, Kenyon, JL. Theory of the kinetic analysis of patch clamp data. *Biophys J* 1987;52:961–978.
8. Chen C, Hess P. Mechanism of gating of T-type calcium channels. *J Gen Physiol* 1990;96:603–630.
9. Colquhoun D, Hawkes AG. On the stochastic properties of single ion channels. *Proc R Soc Lond B* 1981;211:205–235.
10. Colquhoun D, Hawkes AG. The principles of the stochastic interpretation of ion channel mechanisms. In: Sakmann B, Neher E, eds. *Single channel recording.* New York: Plenum Press, 1983:135–175.
11. Colquhoun D, Sigworth FJ. Fitting and statistical analysis of single channel records. In: Sakmann B, Neher E, eds. *Single channel Recording* New York: Plenum Press, 1983:191–263
12. Copella J, Simon B, Segal Y, et al. Ba^{2+} release from soda glass modifies single maxi K^+ channel activity in patch clamp experiments. *Biophys J* 1991;60:931–941.
13. Corey DP, Stevens CF. Science and technology of patch-recording electrodes. In: Sakmann B, Neher E, eds. *Single channel recording.* New York: Plenum Press, 1983:53–68.
14. Cota G, Armstrong CM. Potassium channel "inactivation" induced by soft-glass patch pipettes. *Biophys J* 1988;53:107–109.
15. Edwards FA, Konnerth A, Sakmann B, Takahashi T. A thin slice preparation for patch clamp recordings from neurones of the mammalian central nervous system. *Pflugers Arch* 1989;414:600–612.
16. Eisenberg RS, Engel E. The spatial variation of membrane potential near a small source of current in a spherical cell. *J Gen Physiol* 1970;55:736–757.
17. Elber R, Karplus M. Multiple conformation states of proteins: a molecular dynamics analysis of myoglobin. *Science* 1987;235: 318–321.
18. Fenwick EM, Marty A, Neher E. Sodium and calcium channels in bovine chromaffin cells. *J Physiol (Lond)* 1982;331:599–635.
19. Fidler N, Fernandez JM. Phase-tracking: an improved phase detection technique for cell membrane capacitance measurements. *Biophys J* 1989;56:1153–1162.
20. Fischmeister R, Ayer RK, DeHaan RL. Some limitations of the cell-attached patch clamp technique: a two-electrode analysis. *Pflugers Arch* 1986;406:73–82.
21. Furman RE, Tanaka JC. Patch electrode glass composition affects ion channel currents. *Biophys J* 1988;53:287–292.
22. Gillis KD, Pun RYK, Misler S. Single cell assay of exocytosis from adrenal chromaffin cells using "perforated patch recording." *Pflugers Arch* 1991;418:611–613.
23. Hamill OP, Marty A, Neher E, Sakmann B, Sigworth FJ. Improved patch-clamp techniques for high resolution current recording from cells and cell-free membrane patches. *Pflugers Arch* 1981;391: 85–100.
24. Hodgkin AL, Huxley AF. A quantitative description of membrane current and its application to conduction and excitation in nerve. *J Physiol (Lond)* 1952;116:449–472.
25. Horn R. Diffusion of nystatin in plasma membrane is inhibited by a glass-membrane seal. *Biophys J* 1991;60:329–333.
26. Horn R, Lange K. Estimating kinetic constants from single channel data. *Biophys J* 1983;43:207–223.
27. Horn R, Marty A. Muscarinic activation of ionic currents measured by a new whole-cell recording method. *J Gen Physiol* 1988;92: 145–159.
28. Joshi C, Fernandez JM. Capacitance measurements: an analysis of the phase detector technique used to study exocytosis and endocytosis. *Biophys J* 1986;53:885–892.
29. Kass RS, Bennett PB. Microelectrode voltage clamp: the cardiac Purkinje fiber. In: Smith TG, Lecar H, Redman SJ, Gage PW, eds. *Voltage and patch clamping with microelectrodes* Baltimore: Williams & Wilkins, 1985:171–189.
30. Kass RS, Siegelbaum SA, Tsien RW. Three-microelectrode voltage-clamp experiments in calf cardiac Purkinje fibers: is slow inward current adequately measured? *J Physiol (Lond)* 1979;290:201–225.
31. Korn SJ, Horn R. Statistical discrimination of fractal and Markov models of single channel gating. *Biophys J* 1989;54:871–877.
32. Korn SJ, Marty A, Connor JA, Horn R. Perforated patch recording. In: Conn PM, ed. *Electrophysiology and microinjection.* San Diego: Academic Press, 1991:364–373.
33. Liebovitch LS, Fischbarg J, Koniarek JP. Ion channel kinetics: a model based on fractal scaling rather than Markov processes. *Math Biosci* 1987;84:37–68.
34. Liebovitch LS, Fischbarg J, Koniarek JP, Todorova I, Wang M. Fractal model of ion-channel kinetics. *Biochim Biophys Acta* 1987;896: 173–180.
35. Liebovitch LS, Sullivan JM. Fractal analysis of voltage-dependent potassium channel from cultured mouse hippocampal neurons. *Biophys J* 1987;52:979–988.

36. Magleby KL, Weiss DS. Identifying kinetic gating mechanisms for ion channels by using two-dimensional distributions of simulated dwell times. *Proc R Soc Lond B* 1990;241:220–228.
37. Marty A, Neher E. Tight-seal whole-cell recording. In: Sakmann B, Neher E, eds. *Single channel recording* New York: Plenum Press, 1983: 107–122.
38. McCormick DA, Huguenard JR. A model of the electrophysiological properties of thalamocortical relay neurons. *J Neurophysiol* 1992; 68:1384–1400.
39. McManus OB, Weiss DS, Spivak CE, Blatz AL, Magleby KL. Fractal models are inadequate for the kinetics of four different ion channels. *Biophys J* 1989;54:859–870.
40. Milton RL, Caldwell JH. How do patch clamp seals form? A lipid bleb model. *Pflugers Arch* 1990;416:758–765.
41. Neher E, Almers W. Patch pipettes used for loading small cells with fluorescent indicator dyes. *Adv Exp Med Biol* 1986;211:1–5.
42. Neher E, Marty A. Discrete changes of cell membrane capacitance observed under conditions of enhanced secretion in adrenal bovine adrenal chromaffin cells. *Proc Natl Acad Sci USA* 1982;79: 6712–6716.
43. Neher E, Sakmann B. Single channel currents recorded from membrane of denervated frog muscle fibres. *Nature* 1976;260: 799–802.
44. Pusch M, Neher E. Rates of diffusional exchange between small cells and a measuring patch pipette. *Pflugers Arch* 1988;411: 204–211.
45. Rae J, Cooper K, Gates P, Watsky M. Low access resistance perforated patch recordings using amphotericin B. *J Neurosci Methods* 1991;37:15–26.
46. Rae JL, Levis RA. Glass technology for patch clamp electrodes. In: Rudy B, Iverson LE, eds. *Methods in enzymology, volume 207. Ion channels.* San Diego: Academic Press, 1992:66–92.
47. Rojas L, Zuazaga C. Influence of the patch pipette glass on single acetylcholine channels recorded from *Xenopus* oocytes. *Neurosci Lett* 1988;88:39–44.
48. Ruknudin A, Song MJ, Sachs F. The ultrastructure of patch-clamped membranes: a study using high voltage electron microscopy. *J Cell Biol* 1991;112:125–134.
49. Sachs F, Neil J, Barkakati N. The automated analysis of data from single ionic channels. *Pflugers Arch* 1982;395:331–340.
50. Sine SM, Sigworth FJ. Data transformations for improved display and fitting of single-channel dwell time histograms. *Biophys J* 1987; 52:1047–1054.
51. Zuazaga C, Steinacker A. Patch-clamp recording of ion channels: interfering effects of patch pipette glass. *News Phys Sci* 1990;5: 155–158.

Anesthesia: Biologic Foundations, edited by Tony L. Yaksh et al. Lippincott–Raven Publishers, Philadelphia © 1997.

CHAPTER 22

MOLECULAR BIOLOGY TECHNIQUES

MARCEL E. DURIEUX

The techniques of molecular biology have produced a revolution in the biological sciences. Two decades have passed since the initial development of approaches to manipulate DNA (19). During this short time, we have seen not only an explosion of information about the structure and function of the genome and its products, but also a virtually unparalleled spread of the use of these techniques among the different branches of biological science. Far advanced beyond gene cloning, its initial core of methodology, molecular biology now provides a multitude of tools to the basic scientist as well as the clinician. These techniques have made it remarkably easier to obtain detailed views of the molecular structure of receptors, channels, enzymes, and other proteins. They have made possible the localization of these macromolecules within tissues and within cells, and they have allowed study of the effects of specifically induced alterations in their amino acid sequence. It is now simpler to deduce the amino acid sequence of a protein from the gene encoding it, rather than directly from the protein itself, and easier to synthesize a protein in vitro from cloned genetic material than to extract it from cells. The clinician has been helped in similar ways. An ever growing number of diseases (e.g., sickle cell anemia, cystic fibrosis, and to some degree malignant hyperthermia) can be diagnosed using molecular biology techniques; for others (e.g., the breast cancers caused by the breast cancer gene that recently received much media attention), the etiology has been elucidated using these tools. Recombinant DNA technology has made the production of insulin, growth hormone and other therapeutic proteins, as well as vaccines, more efficient and safer. Gene therapy for selected diseases, either by supplying a missing protein or blocking expression of a detrimental one, will soon be a reality.

Following this increase in applications has been a similarly remarkable simplification of the procedures. For many of the standard procedures in molecular biology, complete kits are commercially available, and rapid improvements in reagents and protocols have made a "cookbook" approach feasible for many routine applications. The introduction of nonradioactive labeling techniques has eliminated the hazards and regulatory burdens involved in the use of radioactive isotopes. Whereas gene cloning and similar complex procedures will probably remain the field of dedicated laboratories, procedures such as the polymerase chain reaction and mapping of mRNA distribution in tissues can be performed by almost any investigator. While this makes it possible for many researchers to apply this technology to their field of study with little formal training, a general understanding of the principles of molecular biology is still needed to evade the pitfalls present in these techniques.

This chapter provides an overview of the most common molecular biology procedures. A number of specific applications, with relevance to anesthesiology, are included in this chapter to demonstrate the use of these procedures in answering specific scientific questions.

Several excellent introductory texts are available for the interested reader. A well-written description of many techniques and practical applications has been provided by Watson et al. (17). Other publications provide more technical descriptions of procedures and protocols, and are invaluable in the laboratory setting (2,15).

TECHNIQUES

The essential invention of molecular biology is to use enzymes from living organisms to perform complex operations on DNA and RNA, rather than to manipulate these macromolecules in standard chemical ways. Progress in molecular biology has been commensurate with the number of enzymes that are known, and have been isolated and induced to perform their function in vitro. Molecular biology procedures, therefore, are largely imaginative applications of enzyme functions to new uses. The use of these biologic activities implies that most molecular biology reactions take place in aqueous solutions of close to neutral pH and proceed at temperatures rarely far removed from room temperature. This section provides an overview of these techniques, progressing from the basic building blocks to more complex procedures. The section on applications then demonstrates how these techniques are combined to answer specific research questions.

Analysis

Before addressing the issues relating to the preparation and modification or RNA and DNA, it is first necessary to describe how nucleic acids are physically identified and analyzed. This is not a trivial issue. Generally, only minute amounts of DNA and RNA (pg to μg) are obtained in experiments, and, in contrast to proteins, there is little or no difference in physicochemical characteristics between one gene and another. Therefore, sensitive methods, able to differentiate similar pieces of nucleic acid, needed to be developed. Over the past decades, a number of very elegant techniques have been designed that have solved these problems satisfactorily.

Restriction Enzymes

In the year 1953, the year that saw the development of the concept of the DNA double helix, the stage was also set for the analysis and manipulation of DNA. In that year, it was shown that some bacterial strains rapidly degrade foreign DNA introduced into these cells, whereas their own DNA is spared. It was shown that this DNA degradation results from the action of restriction nucleases: enzymes that cleave DNA at highly specific, palindromic sequences (a sequence and its inverted repeat linked together) (Fig. 1). The bacterial DNA is spared because nucleotides in restriction sequences are selectively methylated, making them immune to the nuclease. For the bacterium, restriction enzymes are a defense mechanism against invading bacteriophage DNA; for the molecular biologist, these enzymes provide, among many functions that will be discussed later, a way to tell apart pieces of DNA. If two DNA molecules, one of which contains a sequence sensitive to a restriction enzyme, are incubated with the enzyme, only one of the two will be cut. This principle can be considerably expanded on, as detailed in the section on restriction mapping, to allow sensitive and specific diagnosis of DNA.

The first restriction enzyme was isolated in 1970, and several hundred have been found since. Rather than extracting them laboriously from bacterial cultures, many are now prepared by the recombinant techniques they helped establish. Restriction enzymes are named in a standard way: an abbrevi-

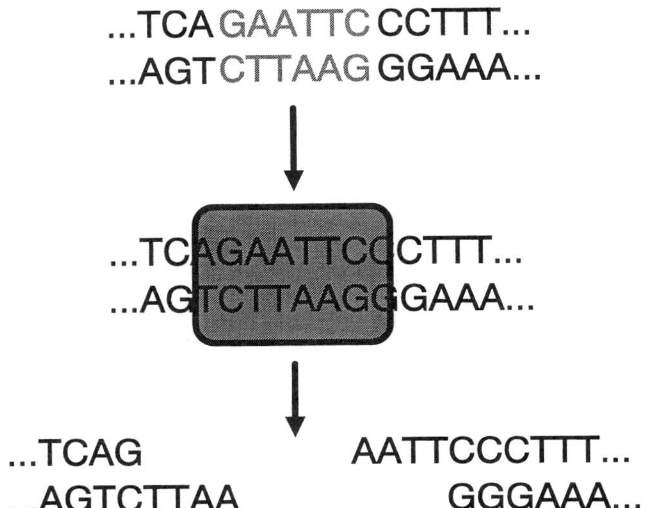

Figure 1. Restriction enzymes cleave DNA at specific, palindromic sequences. The highlighted area in the sequence indicates the restriction enzyme recognition site for the enzyme *Eco*RI. The enzyme recognizes this sequence and cuts it at positions indicated, leaving overhangs, or "sticky ends," on the DNA strands.

ation of the bacterial strain they were isolated from, followed by a sequential number in roman numerals. Thus, *Taq*I was the first restriction enzyme isolated from *Thermus aquaticus*, and *Eco*RV was the fifth one isolated from *Escherichia coli* strain R. Although all recognize palindromic sequences (a result of symmetry in the enzyme molecule), there are differences in not only the exact sequences recognized, but also in the length of the restriction recognition sequence and the necessity for an exact match. Table 1 shows restriction sequences for several common enzymes. Some recognize four bases, some six, and a few even eight. If bases were distributed randomly throughout DNA, which is an acceptable presumption for large pieces of DNA, a "4-cutter" will cleave every ~256 bases, a "6-cutter" every 4,096 bases, and an "8-cutter" will cleave only once every 65 kilobases (kb). *Not*I, an 8-cutter that in addition requires the infrequent CG sequence, fragments mammalian DNA in 1–1.5 million base pair pieces. As noted in Table 1, many restriction enzymes require an exact match, but some will accept any purine or any pyrimidine at one position, usually in the center of the sequence.

There are also differences among restriction enzymes in the type of DNA ends that are generated. Some enzymes create blunt ends; i.e., both strands of DNA are cut at the same position. Most enzymes, however, cut the two strands in different places, a few nucleotides apart. This results in so-called overhangs, or "sticky ends,"that can be either 3′ or 5′, depending on the enzyme. The generation of overhangs is almost as important to the molecular biologist as the specific cleavage site of the enzyme. If two fragments of DNA are cut with a restriction enzyme that creates overhangs, the resulting pieces will have complementary single-stranded ends (Fig. 2). Under the right conditions, these sticky ends can be made to base pair (anneal), allowing the investigator to link together previously separate DNA fragments. At this point, the two fragments are held together by hydrogen bonds between the bases only, but if after base pairing the reaction mixture is treated with DNA ligase, this enzyme will reconnect the sugar-phosphate backbone, creating a new covalently linked DNA molecule. Thus, restriction enzymes and ligases are powerful tools for removing, moving, and replacing fragments of DNA.

Table 1. RESTRICTION SEQUENCES OF SOME RESTRICTION ENZYMES

Enzyme	Sequence	Notes
*Taq*I	5′ . . . T↓CG A . . . 3′	4-bp recognition sequence
	3′ . . . A GC↑T . . . 5′	Creates 5′ overhang
*Dde*I	5′ . . . C↓TNA G . . . 3′	4-bp recognition sequence
	3′ . . . G ANT↑C . . . 5′	Allows any base in center
*Eco*RI	5′ . . . G↓AATT C . . . 3′	6-bp recognition sequence
	3′ . . . C TTAA↑G . . . 5′	Creates a 5′ overhang
*Pst*I	5′ . . . CT GCA↓G . . . 3′	6-bp recognition sequence
	3′ . . . GA↑CGT C . . . 5′	Creates a 3′ overhang
*Eco*RV	5′ . . . GAT↓ATC . . . 3′	6-bp recognition sequence
	3′ . . . CTA↑TAG . . . 5′	Creates blunt ends
*Not*I	5′ . . . GC↓GGC CGC . . . 3′	8-bp recognition sequence
	3′ . . . CG CCG↑CGC . . . 5′	Creates a 5′ overhang

Gel Electrophoresis

To analyze the fragments of DNA produced by the action of a restriction enzyme, a method had to be devised to separate DNA fragments by size. This was found in the method of gel electrophoresis. For many applications, horizontal agarose gels are used. When an electrical field is applied to the gel, DNA molecules introduced in the gel will move at a velocity inversely proportional to their size (Fig. 3). To obtain precise separation, DNA molecules must be linear, as supercoiling (i.e., twisting of the DNA double helix itself) of circular DNA will result in aberrant mobility in the gel. The concentration of agarose can be varied to allow separation of DNA fragments of quite different sizes, from several hundred base pairs to >10 kb. An adaptation of the technique, pulsed-field electrophoresis, can even separate fragments up to several thousand kb. DNA fragments of known length are used as size markers. After electrophoresis, the DNA fragments in the gel can be made visible by staining it with a dye such as ethidium bromide, which intercalates between the two strands of the DNA helix and fluoresces under

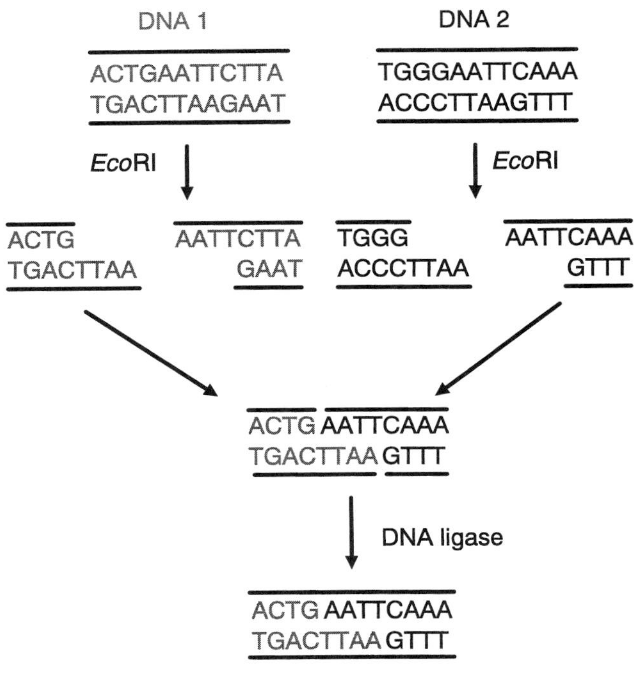

Figure 2. Two fragments of DNA are cut with the restriction enzyme *Eco*RI, resulting in short sticky ends on the cut fragments. When the fragments are mixed, the sticky ends will anneal. To reconstruct a covalently linked DNA molecule, the sugar-phosphate backbone must be reconnected, using the enzyme DNA ligase.

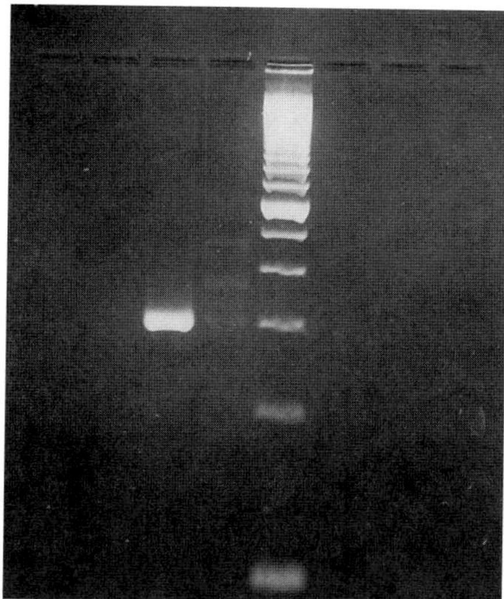

Figure 3. DNA fragments of different sizes can be separated by agarose gel electrophoresis. When a voltage potential is applied across the gel, the negatively charged DNA molecules will move toward the positive pole with a velocity proportional to their molecular weight, which, conveniently, is proportional to their length. DNA fragments thus separated can be visualized by staining with the intercalating agent ethidium bromide, which fluoresces under ultraviolet light.

ultraviolet light. Importantly, after size separation on an agarose gel the DNA can be eluted from the gel to be used in further experiments. This provides a very powerful system to fractionate nucleic acids.

RNA similarly can be analyzed by agarose gel electrophoresis, but because of its tendency to base pair within the molecule itself, it can exhibit a significant amount of secondary structure, rather than being linear as DNA is. Similar to the effects of supercoiled circular DNA, the secondary structure of RNA affects its behavior in a gel, and therefore separation is not as precise. The use of denaturing conditions (e.g., formaldehyde) can improve this, by limiting secondary structure formation. Also, the single strands of RNA do not allow intercalation of ethidium bromide, resulting in less optimal staining. Nonetheless, gel electrophoresis and size fractionation of RNA have their place in the molecular biology armamentarium.

For even more precise separation of small nucleic acid fragments (<1,000 bases) vertical acrylamide electrophoresis systems are employed. These allow separation of DNA fragments that differ in length by only a single base and are routinely employed for DNA sequencing.

Restriction Mapping

The ability of restriction enzymes to cut DNA in specific places and of agarose gel electrophoresis to separate DNA restriction fragments can be combined in the powerful method of DNA analysis termed restriction mapping (Fig. 4). Here, a fragment of DNA is cut with several restriction enzymes, and the reaction products are separated on an agarose gel. Each enzyme will cut the DNA to produce a specific series of fragments (bands), which, taken together, are diagnostic for the DNA fragment. Thus, the restriction map forms a signature of the DNA. Restriction mapping has found an important clinical application in the diagnostic technique of locating restriction fragment length polymorphisms.

Sequencing and Computer Sequence Analysis

For many purposes, diagnostic tests on DNA need to go beyond restriction maps. Complete sequencing of a DNA fragment is often necessary for the study of newly cloned genes or for the analysis of mutations. Several powerful DNA sequencing methods have been devised, of which the Sanger dideoxy method is most commonly used. Figure 5 describes the technique. Dideoxynucleotides are nucleotides in which the 3′ hydroxyl group has been removed. Although they can be incorporated normally into a growing DNA chain, it is not possible to link another nucleotide to a dideoxynucleotide, because the formation of a phosphodiester bond requires the presence of a 3′ hydroxyl group. Therefore, the dideoxynucleotides are chain elongation terminators. The AIDS drug azidothymidine (AZT), which consists of thymidine with the 3′ hydroxyl group replaced with an azido group, works in a similar way. In sequencing reactions, small amounts of a single type of dideoxynucleotide are added to a reaction mixture containing single-stranded DNA to be sequenced, DNA polymerase, a radioactively labeled primer (generally complementary to part of the vector in which the DNA has been incorporated, as discussed below), and normal nucleotides of all four kinds. The

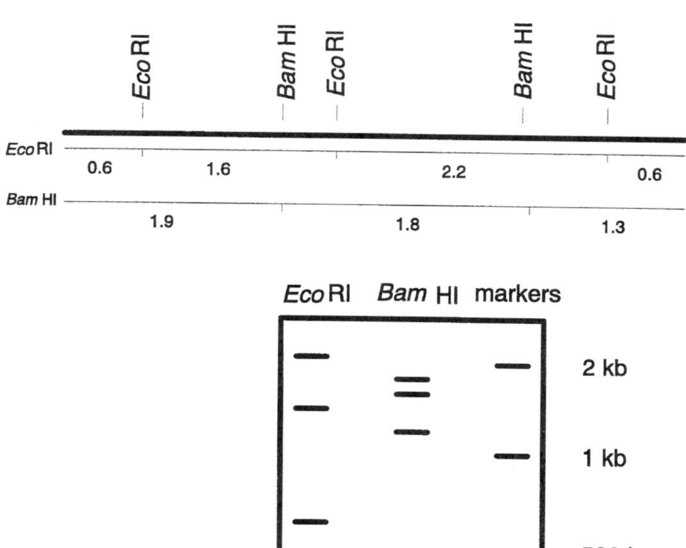

Figure 4. DNA fragments can be identified by their particular complement of restriction sites (*top*). The DNA is cut with several enzymes, and the products of the reactions are separated on agarose gel (*bottom*). The number and sizes of the resulting fragments form a signature of the particular piece of DNA.

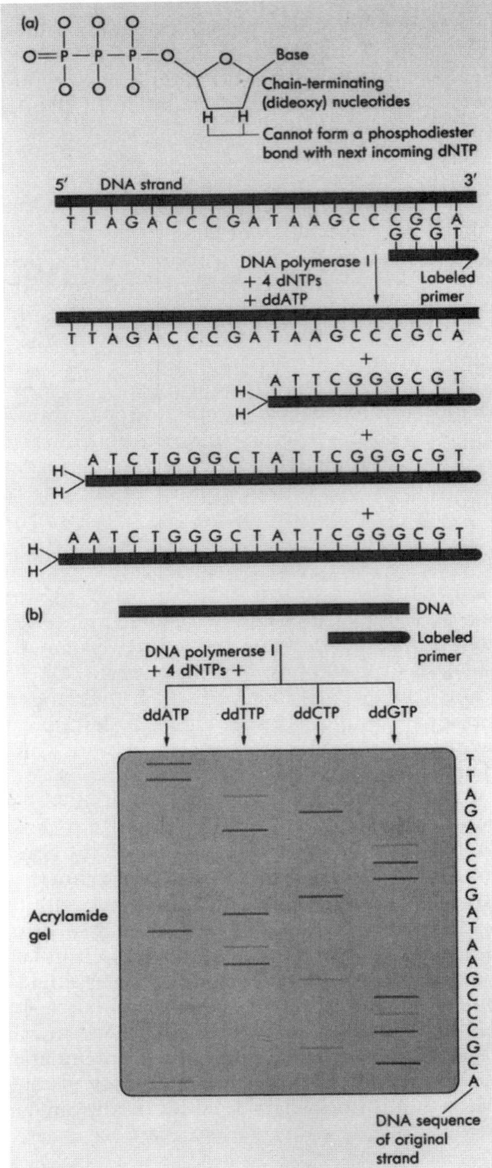

Figure 5. The Sanger dideoxy method provides a convenient way to sequence DNA. Dideoxynucleotides (*top*) are chain terminators: the absence of a 3′ hydroxy group makes it impossible to incorporate further bases after the dideoxynucleotide. When a DNA strand to be sequenced is incubated with a labeled primer, DNA polymerase, the four normal nucleotides (dNTPs), and a small amount of dideoxy-ATP (ddATP), the result will be a series of labeled DNA fragments that terminate at places where the dideoxynucleotide was incorporated (i.e., places corresponding to a T in the original strand). Similar reactions are run with the other three dideoxynucleotides, and the resulting fragments are separated on a denaturing acrylamide gel (*bottom*). The sequence of the original strand can be directly read from the autoradiogram of the gel. (Reprinted with permission from Watson JD, Gilman M, Witkowski J, Zoller M. *Recombinant DNA*. 2nd ed. New York: W. H. Freeman, 1992.)

polymerase synthesizes complementary strands on the DNA to be sequenced, starting with the double-stranded area where the primer has annealed. All products will therefore be radioactively labeled. Whenever a dideoxynucleotide rather than a normal nucleotide happens to be incorporated, DNA synthesis of that particular strand will stop. Assuming that dideoxyadenine was added, this sequencing reaction will result in a series of DNA chains of various length, each ending at a position where the original strand contained a thymine. These products are separated by acrylamide gel electrophoresis and visualized by autoradiography, next to the results of similar reactions using the three other dideoxynucleotides. The result is an autoradiogram from which the sequence of the original DNA strand can be read directly (for example, see Fig. 24).

DNA sequencing has become a routine technique. Automated systems are available that, rather than using four reactions in different lanes of a gel, run them all in a single lane and separate the products of the four reactions by using different fluorescent labels on each of the four primers. The results are analyzed automatically using photometric techniques and stored on computer. These systems are able to sequence large amounts of DNA very rapidly. Even if standard autoradiography is employed, several gel-reading systems allow rapid data entry into computer systems. Comprehensive software packages are available to analyze sequences (6). Translation into amino acid sequence, localization of restriction sites to predict restriction maps, and comparison with large databases such as Genbank using sophisticated search algorithms are just a few examples of the features of these systems.

Propagation of DNA

At times, individual fragments of DNA, such as those prepared by restriction digestion, are all that is needed for a specific experimental purpose. However, replication of DNA fragments, as well as a multitude of other cloning, selection, and expression procedures, which will be described later, are much easier to perform if the DNA is incorporated in a fragment of "utility DNA" called a vector.

Vectors

Many bacteria contain, apart from their main chromosomes, one to many small circular pieces of DNA named plasmids. Plasmids are autonomously replicating mini-chromosomes, a few thousand base pairs in size, that originally attracted interest because they carry bacterial antibiotic resistance genes. Plasmid DNA can be isolated easily from bacteria and is also introduced easily into plasmid-free bacteria, using any of a variety of methods. Some of the most common of these so-called transfection methods are calcium chloride treatment followed by heat shock and an electrical method called electroporation. It was realized that the autonomous nature of plasmids provides a convenient way to propagate foreign DNA through a process called cloning (Fig. 6). Plasmid DNA can be extracted, linearized with a restriction enzyme that has only one cleavage site in the circular plasmid DNA molecule, and mixed with DNA from a different source, cut with a restriction enzyme that creates the same overhangs. The overhangs of the cut plasmid and the cut DNA will anneal and can be linked with DNA ligase, resulting in plasmids containing fragments of foreign DNA. These plasmids can then be reintroduced into bacteria, where they can be indefinitely maintained and multiplied. Whereas the original experiments with this system used naturally occurring plasmids, significant improvements have been obtained by modifying the plasmids considerably. In fact, modern vectors, as these artificial constructs are called, show little resemblance to natural plasmids and are engineered from many pieces, each with a specific use for the investigator.

Figure 7A shows the structure of a generic cloning vector. Several features are noteworthy. An origin of replication is necessary to permit autonomous replication in bacteria. The presence of one or more drug resistance genes (as present on natural plasmids) allows easy selection of bacteria carrying the plasmid by growing them in a medium containing the selection antibiotic. The polylinker site consists of a series of restriction

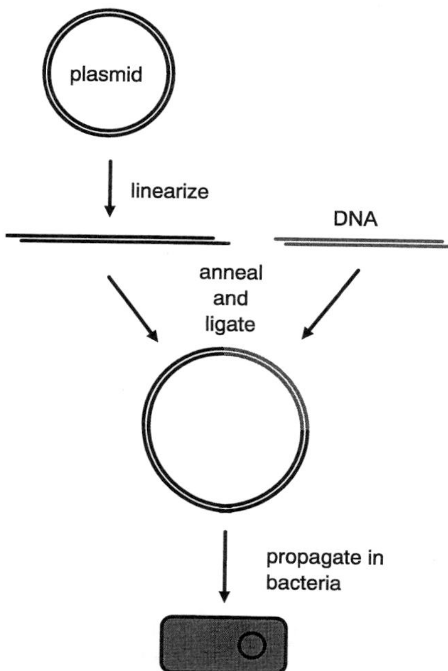

Figure 6. For ease of handling, DNA fragments are often inserted into fragments of "utility DNA," named vectors. This procedure is called cloning and is based on the method of linking DNA fragments discussed above. The plasmid as well as the DNA to be cloned are cut with a restriction enzyme leaving overhangs and then mixed together. The plasmid DNA and the DNA to be cloned will anneal and can be covalently linked using DNA ligase. The resulting vector and insert, as the cloned DNA is called, can then be easily propagated in bacteria.

sequences, a convenient one of which can be used to linearize the vector in order to introduce the foreign DNA. The polylinker is embedded within the *lacZ* gene, which encodes β-galactosidase. When the vector is propagated in bacteria, this enzyme is expressed and cleaves a colorless compound in the culture medium, X-gal, to a blue product. The presence of an uninterrupted *lacZ* gene in the plasmid, therefore, results in blue bacterial colonies on the culture plate. If, however, foreign DNA has been inserted into the polylinker site it will interrupt the *lacZ* gene and colonies will be white. This so-called blue-white selection system provides an easy selection marker for bacteria harboring vectors with foreign DNA. In vectors designed for expression, strong promoters for the bacteriophage RNA polymerases SP6 and T7 often flank the polylinker area, so that DNA introduced into the vector can be selectively transcribed from either direction.

A completely different type of vector is the phage vector, of which λt10 is an example (Fig. 7B). DNA introduced in phage vectors is not manipulated as easily as that in plasmid vectors, but library screening procedures are much simplified. The use of these vectors is based on the finding that much of the phage DNA sequence is not necessary for phage survival. Specifically, the central part can be removed, leaving only two phage arms. Foreign DNA can be introduced between these arms, using procedures similar to those described for cloning DNA into plasmid vectors. The phage are then packaged in a protein coat using lysates of infected bacteria, and the resulting phage particles can be used to infect new bacteria. On culture plates, phage are identified by the clear plaques on a lawn of bacteria, resulting from phage-induced bacterial lysis.

Bacteria

To propagate the cloned DNA, either in plasmid or in phage vectors, the vectors are introduced into bacteria, either by transfection or infection, and the bacteria are grown in standard culture. Universally, strains of the common bacterium *E. coli* are used for this purpose. For many years, this part of the cloning process has worried investigators and the lay public alike. The concern is that these bacteria would "escape" from the laboratory and infect humans. As *E. coli* is normally an innocuous bacterium, few immunological defense systems are present against it. However, the foreign DNA they harbor could conceivably turn these benign microbes into deadly organisms. Concern about this issue became particularly acute when attempts to clone genomic material from tumor viruses were considered.

Starting with the Asilomar conference of 1975 and continuing up to the present National Institutes of Health (NIH) guidelines for recombinant DNA research, this issue has been addressed thoroughly. Only strains of *E. coli* modified to such an extent that survival outside the laboratory environment is virtually impossible are now used for recombinant DNA research. For instance, the original cloning strain χ1776 (developed during the bicentennial of the American declaration of independence) is dependent for survival on the presence in the environment of diaminopimelic acid, a compound not present in the human intestinal tract. Similarly, it has a very fragile cell wall and is therefore intolerant of salt or even trace detergents. Strains similar to χ1776 are now used routinely for molecular biology studies.

Another issue of concern was the spread of antibiotic resistance through the use of antibiotics as selectable markers. This has been adequately addressed by using only very common antibiotics, such as ampicillin and tetracyclin, which are already spread widely through the environment, as markers in plasmids.

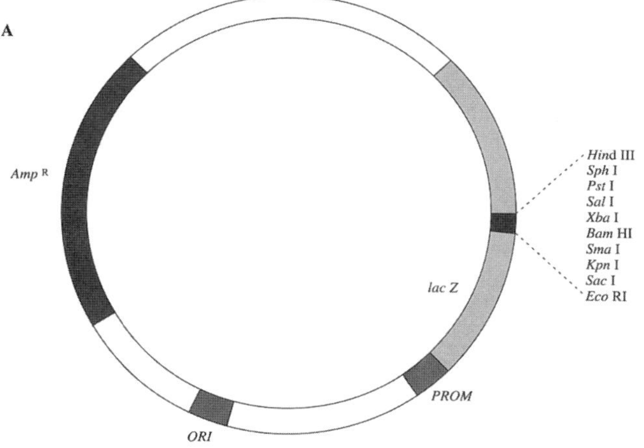

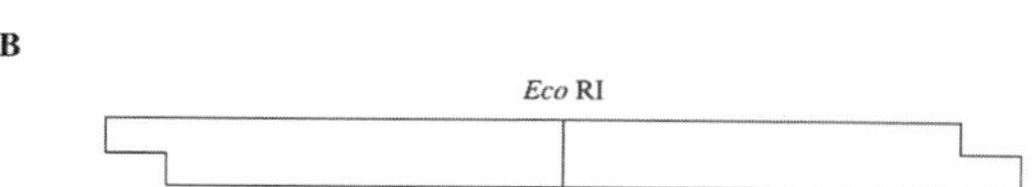

Figure 7. **(A)** pUC18, a typical plasmid-derived cloning vector. Note the presence of an origin of replication (ORI), allowing autonomous replication within bacteria; an ampicillin resistance gene (*Amp*[R]), allowing selection of bacteria harboring the vector; a polylinker consisting of a number of unique restriction sites, allowing convenient cloning of DNA into the vector; a *lacZ* gene and promoter (PROM), allowing easy color selection of bacteria harboring plasmids containing an insert. **(B)** λgt10, a typical phage vector. Note the two phage arms and a unique cloning site (*Eco*RI) in-between. The cohesive ends are necessary for phage replication in host bacteria.

It is of importance to note that current NIH guidelines require the establishment of a institutional biosafety committee, charged with overseeing recombinant techniques in the institution. Whereas routine molecular biology work generally does not require direct supervision of this committee, work with genes potentially dangerous to humans and particularly with vectors capable of infecting humans should not be initiated without prior review and approval of the committee.

Preparation of DNA and RNA

So far we have discussed methods for analyzing DNA and RNA, and procedures to propagate DNA in a form that is manipulated easily. However, we have not yet addressed the question where this DNA or RNA comes from. Originally, of course, it derives from living cells. In this section, we therefore discuss the methods in use for selectively extracting nucleic acids from tissues, followed by descriptions of common techniques used to prepare DNA and RNA in vitro.

DNA Extraction

Each cell in the body of a eukaryotic organism contains the full set of genomic material. Therefore, extracting DNA from tissue will in principle always generate the same set of genetic information, independent of the tissue used. For this reason, the choice of tissue for preparation of genomic DNA is determined primarily by ease of access and yield of DNA. Most often the liver is used. Whereas it might appear at first that selective isolation of nucleic acid from the myriad of cellular constituents would be a daunting task, the actual procedure is relatively straightforward. The tissue is homogenized to fracture the cells, and treated with proteinases and a detergent to allow access to the DNA in the nucleus. Separation from protein, the major cellular macromolecular constituent, is accomplished by extractions in phenol and chloroform. DNA will remain in the aqueous phase, whereas protein accumulates at the interface between water and the organic solvent. For further purification, the nucleic acid is selectively precipitated in ammonium acetate and ethanol, the precipitate is dried, and redissolved in water or a buffer. DNA is a very stable compound, as a carrier of genetic information should be, and can be stored indefinitely at −20°C. The amount of DNA prepared can be measured rapidly by spectroscopy at a wavelength of 260 nm. Whereas nucleic acids absorb primarily at this wavelength, proteins absorb at both 260 and 280 nm. Therefore, the amount of protein contamination in the sample can be determined by measuring absorption at both wavelengths and calculating a 260/280 ratio.

RNA Extraction

RNA extraction is performed for different reasons than DNA extraction. As stated above, the DNA of each cell holds a complete copy of the genome. mRNA, however, is only made when needed. Therefore, the mRNA present in a tissue will generally be a reflection of the proteins present in the cells, and, in fact, identification of the message for a particular protein is frequently the most straightforward way to determine the presence or absence of a protein in the tissue.

RNA is less stable chemically than DNA, which might have caused it to be selected against for long-term information storage. Also, because it is constantly produced and degraded, a number of ribonucleases (RNAses) are present in tissue. Because of these issues, RNA extraction is somewhat different from DNA extraction. The main goal of most procedures is the rapid inhibition of endogenous, and the avoidance of contamination with exogenous RNAses. For these reasons, all procedures are done in sterilized glass and plasticware, sterile solutions are used, and gloves are worn. Some investigators elect to treat their solutions with diethylpyrocarbonate (DEPC), a compound that avidly reacts with proteins and inactivates them, and subsequently decomposes spontaneously. Using these precautions, tissue is homogenized in the RNAse inhibitor guanidine thiocyanate as quickly as possible after removal from the body.

Further preparation involves the separation of the RNA from the large amount of DNA present in the cell. Several techniques are available to achieve this separation. A common approach is ultracentrifugation of the nucleic acid on a layer of cesium chloride solution. As the buoyant density of RNA in cesium chloride is much higher than that of other cell components, it will pass through the layer and form a pellet on the bottom of the centrifuge tube. A disadvantage of this method is the need for an ultracentrifuge. Another approach, circumventing this problem, makes use of the differential solubility of RNA and DNA in acid phenol. If the tissue homogenate is extracted with phenol equilibrated to a pH of 4, RNA will remain in the aqueous phase, but DNA will pass into the phenol phase, and the two can be separated easily. After separation from DNA, the RNA can be purified further by ethanol precipitation, and the amount obtained determined by spectroscopy.

The resulting RNA, however, is a mixture of mRNA, rRNA, tRNA, and small nuclear ribonucleotides. Further purification steps, such as poly-A selection and sucrose density centrifugation, can be employed to enrich for specific fractions of mRNA.

Poly-A Selection and Sucrose Density Centrifugation

mRNA forms only a small fraction of the total cellular RNA content: 1–5%, dependent on the cell type. As it is this fraction that is of primary interest to most investigators, a selection step for mRNA is very useful. This has been found in the method of poly-A selection. Eukaryotic mRNA receives a poly-A tail at the 3′ end. This feature can be used to enrich the mRNA fraction by affinity chromatography on a column containing short sequences of polydeoxythymidine attached to cellulose (oligo dT column) (Fig. 8). During passage over the column, poly-A tails will anneal with the oligo dT, whereas RNA not containing a poly-A tail will pass through. The enriched mRNA fraction can then be eluted from the column and is often recirculated for further selection. Generally, this protocol reduces the amount of RNA to 1–2% of the original amount, but this fraction is highly enriched in mRNA. Nonetheless, in expression

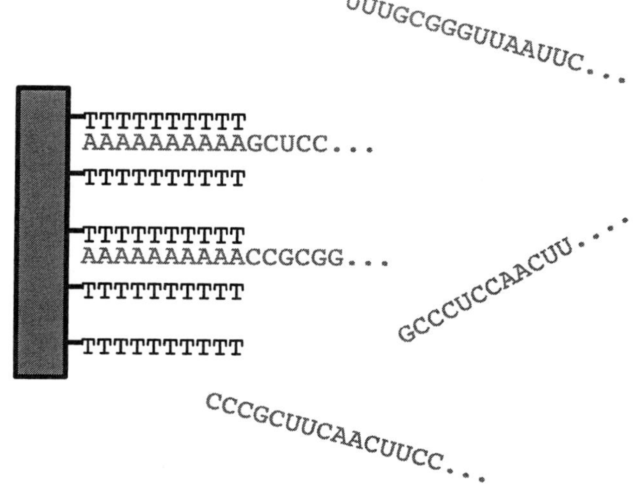

Figure 8. To separate the small fraction of mRNA from the remainder of cellular RNA, a procedure called poly-A selection is performed. Short poly-T sequences (oligo dT) are immobilized on cellulose in a column, and the total cellular RNA is passed through the column. Only mRNA with a poly-A tail will anneal to the oligo dT, whereas the remainder (tRNA and rRNA without a poly-A tail) will pass through. The mRNA can then be eluted separately.

experiments it has often been noted that the increase in activity when poly-A selected RNA is used is not commensurate with the amount of selection. In other words, a 100-fold reduction in RNA amount by poly-A selection might only result in a two- to ten-fold increase in activity per ng RNA.

Another way in which RNA can be fractionated further is by molecular weight. This is particularly useful if the size of the mRNA of interest is known, or can be estimated. When RNA is loaded onto a sucrose density gradient in a tube and centrifuged, it will separate by size. The different fractions can be isolated and studied individually. Although used less commonly, it is also possible to size-fractionate RNA by separating it using agarose gel electrophoresis, cutting out parts of the gel, and extracting the RNA.

The methods described so far in this section dealt with the extraction of nucleic acids from tissues. Often, however, these compounds are prepared in vitro, either completely synthetically or using natural nucleic acid as a template. These techniques will be discussed in the following sections.

Oligonucleotides

The automated preparation of short (10–100 nucleotides) synthetic DNA fragments (oligonucleotides) has made possible many new techniques in molecular biology. The use of these oligonucleotides in the polymerase chain reaction and as molecular probes will be detailed below. Oligonucleotides are generated completely synthetically. In fact, this is one of the very few procedures in molecular biology where manipulations on nucleic acids are performed by wholly chemical means. Although several techniques exist, all use the principle of attaching the first nucleotide to a solid support and, after protection of the appropriate groups, sequentially adding new nucleotide types to the reaction, which become attached to the growing chain. The support matrix is washed between each step. After the final nucleotide has been added the oligonucleotide is released from the support matrix and purified. Fully automated systems are now employed routinely, and have resulted in faster turnaround time and much less expense to the investigator.

An interesting variation in the production of synthetic oligonucleotides is the preparation of degenerate oligonucleotides. These are mixtures of oligonucleotides with different nucleotides at specified positions. Their use will be described below in the section on molecular cloning. Degenerate oligonucleotides can be prepared easily by adding a mixture of nucleotides, rather than a single type, at the specified point during the preparation. The growing chains will incorporate, at random, one of the nucleotides in the mixture, and the result will be a specifically defined mixture of oligonucleotides.

In Vitro Transcription

As DNA is much more stable than RNA and handled more easily through the incorporation in vectors, it is the preferred material for manipulation and cloning. However, for expression purposes, as described below, RNA is a necessary intermediate. This RNA must therefore be prepared in vitro from cloned DNA. As discussed above in the section on vectors, many vectors include promoters for bacteriophage RNA polymerase flanking the polylinker site where DNA is cloned. When such a vector is incubated in an appropriate buffer with the polymerase and the four ribonucleotides, the polymerase will transcribe RNA from the vector. Large amounts (up to 50 times the amount of template) can be produced in a few hours. Linearizing the vector by cutting it with a restriction enzyme downstream of the DNA to be transcribed enhances transcription, as the polymerase does not unnecessarily transcribe vector sequence beyond the DNA of interest. If desired, radioactively labeled nucleotide can be included in the mixture, resulting in radiolabeled RNA strands. If expression in a eukaryotic system is planned, a so-called capping analogue, consisting of two guanines, one methylated, linked by a triphosphate bond (^{7m}GpppG), can be used instead of regular G. Although with lesser efficiency, this G analogue is incorporated as a G by the polymerase, resulting in an artificial cap structure at the 5′ end, which enhances translation. Of course, unless the DNA template already contained a stretch of poly-T, the resulting RNA will not have a poly-A tail, but this does not affect translation.

Reverse Transcription

A process that is basically the reverse of in vitro transcription, and appropriately called "reverse transcription," is used to prepare DNA complementary to extracted RNA. Such DNA, termed cDNA, is very useful for many purposes in molecular biology. As mentioned, DNA is more stable than RNA and handled more easily, but in addition several important procedures require DNA as a substrate. Reverse transcription is accomplished using a retroviral enzyme, reverse transcriptase, that is able to synthesize double-stranded DNA on an RNA template. Synthesis takes place in two separate steps (Fig. 9). Reverse transcriptase needs a double-stranded region to start transcription. This region is conveniently created by mixing the mRNA with poly-T oligonucleotides. These will anneal to the poly-A tail and function as primers for transcription. The product is known as oligo-dT-primed cDNA. A single priming site may result in incomplete transcription of long mRNAs; therefore, an alternative technique employs short (six to 10 nucleotides in length) random nucleotide sequences that are mixed with the mRNA and will anneal at irregular intervals, initiating transcription at each site. The product of this procedure is known as random-primed cDNA. Either approach initially generates a DNA-RNA hybrid. For the second synthesis step, the RNA is removed enzymatically using RNAse H, an RNAse that digests the mRNA strand into a number of short fragments. Each fragment then becomes a primer to initiate DNA synthesis by DNA polymerase, which replaces the RNA fragments with DNA. The DNA fragments are then linked by DNA ligase, resulting in double-stranded cDNA. The fact that these two steps are separate makes it possible to prepare, depending on the application, either single- or double-stranded cDNA using this technique.

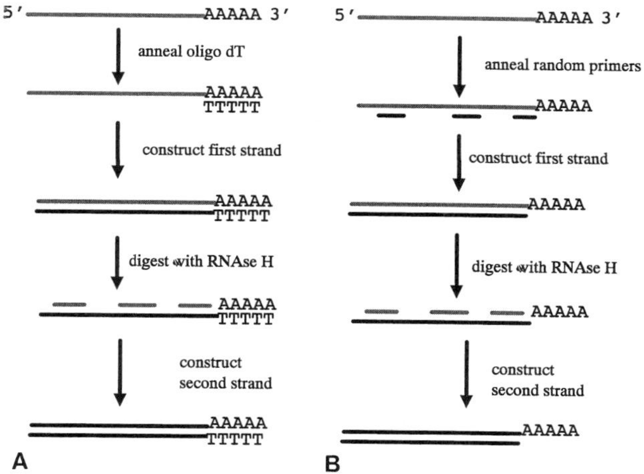

Figure 9. To create cDNA from extracted mRNA, the procedure of reverse transcription is employed. Two techniques exist, depending on the primer that is used for the polymerase. **(A)** To construct oligo-dT primer cDNA (*left*), the mRNA is mixed with short poly-T sequences. **(B)** To construct random-primed cDNA (*right*), short random sequences, which will anneal at random locations, are used as primers. After construction of the first strand the RNA template is digested away with RNAse H, which leaves short fragments of RNA that are used as primers for the construction of the second strand.

Libraries

For some purposes, the cDNA prepared can be studied directly, e.g., as a substrate for the polymerase chain reaction. However, if cloning and screening procedures are planned, this cDNA must first be incorporated into a vector. As the cDNA prepared as described above has blunt ends, it can not be inserted conveniently using the sticky end method. This problem is circumvented by the use of linkers, artificial restriction cleavage sites that are first ligated to the end of the cDNA and then cut with the appropriate enzyme. The vector is cut with the same enzyme, and the complementary sticky ends allow insertion of the cDNA into the vector. A novel modification of this cDNA preparation technique uses a vector that incorporates a tract of poly-T. This allows generation of the first cDNA strand directly on the vector, a procedure named vector-primed cDNA synthesis.

A collection of mRNA incorporated in vectors as cDNA is termed a cDNA library. Libraries generated from different organs or species will contain different complements of genetic material. In contrast, genomic libraries, created by incorporating extracted DNA directly into vectors, will contain the full genomic information of the species they are prepared from.

Once DNA or RNA has been prepared, it can be used for a variety of purposes. Often, one wants to determine the presence of a specific mRNA in a specific cell line, tissue or species, and to quantitate its presence. Frequently, such questions are answered most easily by annealing specific pieces of DNA to prepared nucleic acid in a process called hybridization.

Hybridization

The hybridization techniques described here are all based on a similar idea: a labeled nucleic acid fragment (probe) is allowed to anneal (hybridize) with a collection of RNA or DNA. Unbound probe is washed away, and techniques that visualize the bound, labeled probe (the hybrid) will then reveal the presence, amount, and, depending on the technique, size of the hybridizing species in the DNA or RNA. We will discuss the preparation of probes and the most commonly used hybridization techniques.

Probes and Hybridization

The standard approach for the preparation of labeled nucleic acid probes has been the incorporation of radioactive nucleotides (usually containing ^{32}P or ^{35}S) during preparation. The probe is prepared either synthetically or by using the procedures outlined for the generation of RNA or single-stranded DNA. However, over the past years, several new labeling systems have been developed that eliminate the need for radioactive materials. Several approaches exist, but all use modified nucleotides that can be visualized using a secondary molecule such as a fluorescent antibody. Although at present these techniques appear to be somewhat less sensitive than radiolabeled approaches, and possibly slightly less reliable, there seems to be little doubt that nonradioactive labeling procedures will soon be standard technology in molecular biology. For the remainder of this discussion, we presume the use of radioactive probes, as they are still used most commonly.

The avidity with which a probe anneals to DNA or RNA depends on several factors. Most important is the degree of match between the probe and the nucleic acid it anneals to. A perfect match will provide the best hybridization, and the more mismatched base pairs exist, the less avid the probe will anneal. The specific nucleotides involved in hybridization are important as well, as a GC base pair, due to its three hydrogen bonds, is more stable than an AT pair. A third factor, which can be manipulated by the investigator, is stringency. Basically, this is a measure of the degree to which the reaction conditions favor or disfavor hybridization. Although the chemical composition of the reaction mixture plays a role, temperature is most important in determining stringency: as the reaction temperature is increased, less of a mismatch between the probe and its target is tolerated before they will dissociate, and stringency is increased. Stringency is of great importance, as it determines to a large extent what targets will be found. If a probe that is known to be an exact match to its target is used to localize a specific nucleic acid fragment in a library, high-stringency conditions can be used to minimize hybridization to similar, but wrong, targets. Conversely, if a probe derived from a specific gene is used to search a cDNA library for subtypes of the gene, which will probably be similar but not identical, low-stringency hybridization is employed.

In the following sections, we discuss the use of labeled probes for the localization of nucleic acids in libraries (screening), in extracted RNA (Northern analysis) and DNA (Southern analysis), and directly in tissue (in situ hybridization).

Library Screening

The procedure of using a labeled probe to determine the presence of a complementary sequence in a cDNA or genomic library is called screening. It is a standard approach to cloning of novel genes. The sequence of the probe can either be derived from the amino acid sequence of the protein searched for, if sufficient protein has been purified to sequence a short amino acid segment, or derived from the DNA sequence of a related gene. Usually, phage libraries are used for screening. The first step in the screening technique is physically separating the clones in the library (Fig. 10). This is done by plating the phage on agar plates covered with host bacteria. Plaques develop, and these are replicated onto nitrocellulose or nylon paper. The phage DNA is bound to the paper and incubated under conditions of the desired stringency with the probe. If hybridization takes place, it will be revealed by autoradiography of the paper. The autoradiogram can then be lined up with the original plate to show which phage carry the sequence of interest, and these phage can be isolated and further amplified. Often, several rounds of plating and screening are necessary to obtain the desired sequence. This sequence is then isolated from the phage, transferred to a plasmid vector (a procedure called subcloning) and further analyzed by sequencing and expression.

Blotting

A common biological question is whether or not a specific protein is present in a tissue or cell type under certain conditions, and if so, how much. Purification of the protein is generally impractical. The technique named Northern analysis (in analogy to Southern analysis) bypasses protein purification by determining the amount of mRNA for the protein in the tissue. It is one of the most commonly used molecular biology techniques. Northern analysis is a combination of gel electrophoresis and hybridization (Fig. 11). RNA is extracted from the tissue of interest and separated by size on an denaturing agarose gel. The RNA in the gel is transferred to nitrocellulose or nylon paper placed on top of the gel (i.e., blotted), and bound tightly to the paper. The paper is than incubated with labeled probe at the desired stringency, washed to remove unhybridized probe, and afterwards exposed to x-ray film. If mRNA complementary to the probe is present in the RNA on the blot its presence and size will be revealed by a band on the film. The intensity of the band will be proportional to the amount of mRNA present in the tissue. In a procedure termed mapping, equal amounts of RNA from a variety of tissues are loaded in adjacent lanes on a gel and probed, providing a measure of the relative distribution of the RNA among various tissues.

A related technique named the nuclease protection assay or RNAse protection assay is more sensitive than regular Northern blotting because of reduced background signal. The technique employs hybridization in solution, rather than on a blot,

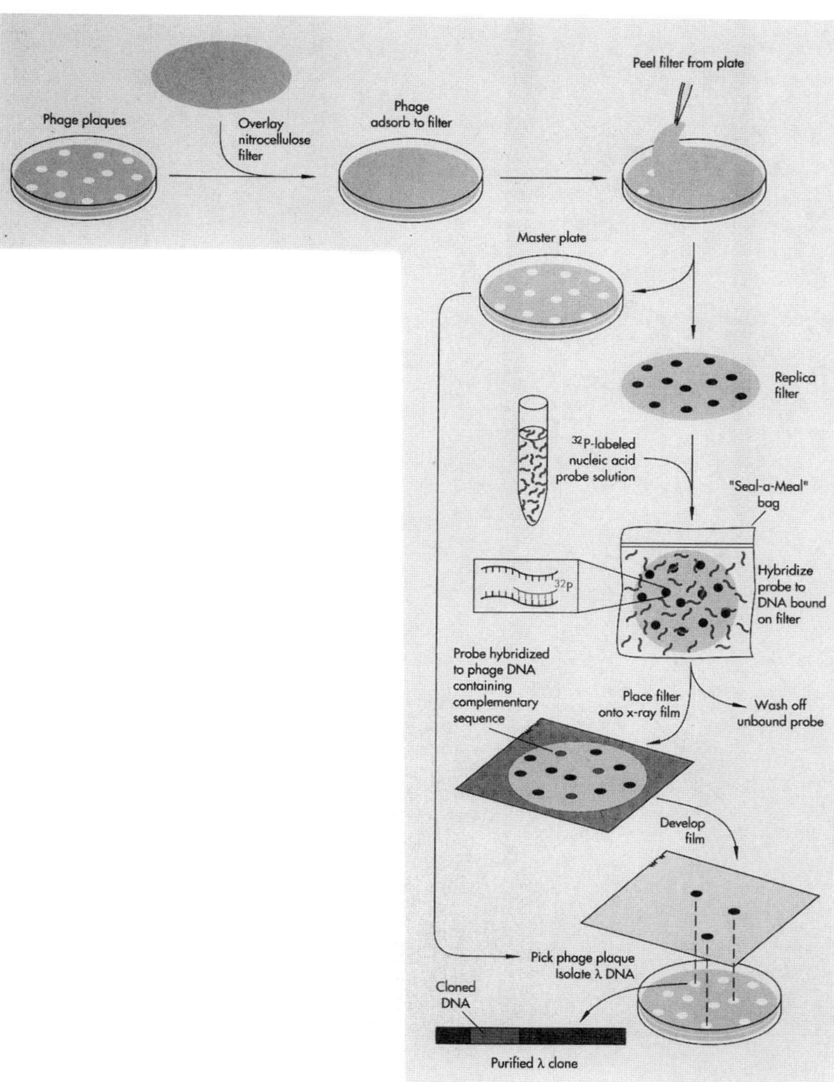

Figure 10. To isolate a DNA fragment from a library, a screening procedure with a labeled probe is used. The phage library is plated out on culture plates with confluent bacteria, and plaques develop due to lysis of the bacteria by infecting phage. Some of the phage DNA is transferred to a filter by simply overlaying the filter on the plate and removing it after absorption has taken place. This replica filter is then used for hybridization with a ^{32}P-labeled probe. After hybridization, excess probe is washed off and the filter is exposed to x-ray film. The probe will have hybridized to those places on the filter where complementary phage DNA was present, and these positions can be identified by autoradiography. The spots on the x-ray film are then lined up with the master culture plate to determine which plaques contained the correct DNA. (Reprinted with permission from Watson JD, Gilman M, Witkowski J, Zoller M. *Recombinant DNA.* 2nd ed. New York: W. H. Freeman, 1992.)

followed with digestion of the reaction with an RNAse that only cleaves single-stranded RNA. The remaining double-stranded hybrid, consisting of annealed probe and mRNA target, is then visualized by autoradiography after acrylamide gel electrophoresis.

The technique of blotting nucleic acids separated by gel electrophoresis was initially developed by E.M. Southern for DNA. Genomic DNA is fragmented by restriction enzyme digestion, separated by agarose gel electrophoresis, blotted and probed, a technique named Southern blotting after the inventor. Southern blotting is useful to determine the number of genes in the genome encoding a specific message, as well as for interspecies comparisons (using so-called zoo blots). Besides Northern and Southern blotting a Western blotting technique exists, where protein is separated on a gel and "probed" with a specific antibody, and even a Southwestern blot has been developed for the study of DNA-binding proteins.

In Situ Hybridization

Northern blotting techniques can provide useful information about the distribution of mRNA among organs or parts of organs, but the resolution is limited by the size of the organ part that can be dissected. Certainly it is not possible to localize mRNA to specific cells in an organ such as the brain. To accomplish this precise localization, a different technique exists, named in situ hybridization. Here tissue is removed from an animal and microscopic sections are prepared. These sections are then incubated with a labeled probe, which will hybridize with mRNA present in cells. The slides are coated with photographic emulsion and, after exposure, studied under the microscope. Silver grains will be visible over areas where the probe annealed, allowing highly detailed maps of mRNA distribution to be constructed.

The usefulness of many of these hybridization techniques is limited by the minimum amount of mRNA necessary to generate a visible signal. Particularly with low-abundance messages this can be a significant problem. When blotting techniques are used this can be partially compensated for by loading more nucleic aid on the gel; with in situ hybridization this is not an option. In situ reverse transcription has been used in an attempt to increase the amount of message present within the cell, but unfortunately the method has met with limited success.

The general problem of manipulating low-abundance messages has been solved to a large extent by a very successful methodology, the polymerase chain reaction.

Polymerase Chain Reaction

The development of the polymerase chain reaction (PCR) in the mid-1980s has revolutionized molecular biology. Many stud-

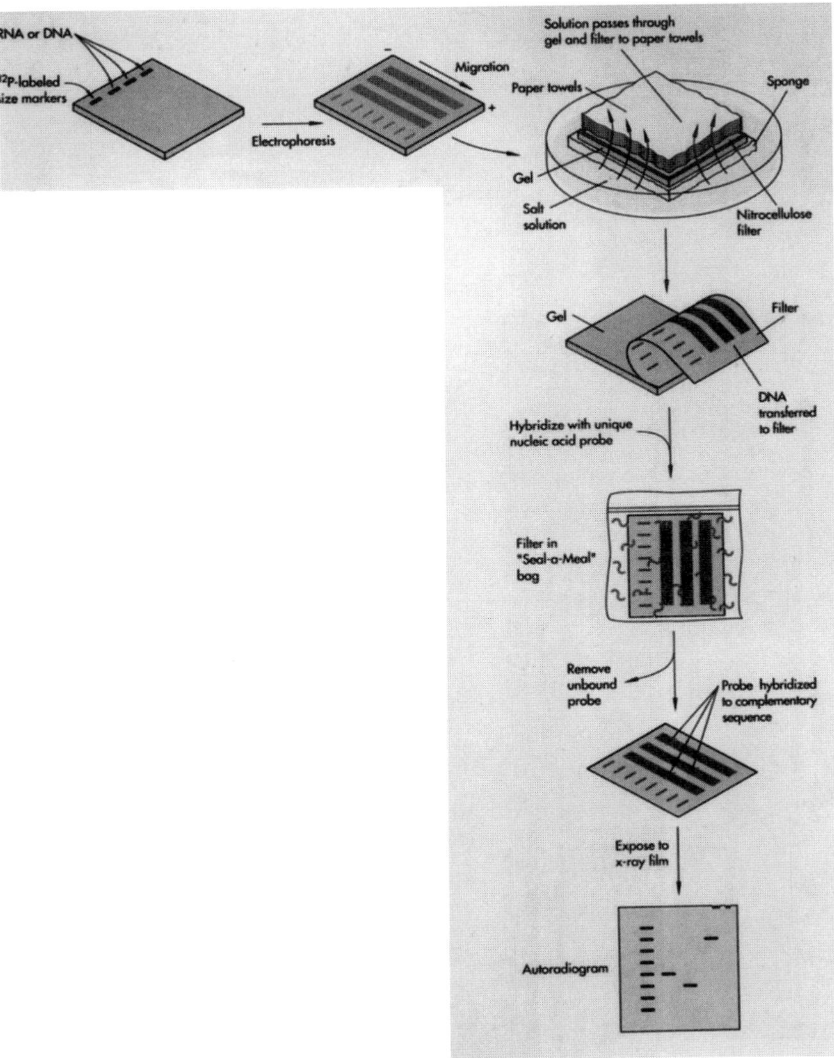

Figure 11. The presence of a particular DNA or RNA sequence in a sample can be ascertained through blotting procedures. Southern blotting is used to determine the presence of a sequence in genomic DNA, and Northern blotting is used to determine the presence of a sequence in mRNA. In both techniques, the nucleic acids are separated by gel electrophoresis and subsequently transferred to filter paper by capillary action, vacuum, or positive pressure. The filter is then hybridized with a labeled probe, which will hybridize to complementary sequence in the nucleic acid. The result can be visualized by autoradiography. (Reprinted with permission from Watson JD, Gilman M, Witkowski J, Zoller M. *Recombinant DNA*. 2nd ed. New York: W. H. Freeman, 1992.)

ies that were not even possible before its invention have become not only feasible, but even simple to perform. PCR technology has become immensely important because of two reasons: its ability to amplify selectively tiny amounts of DNA more than a million-fold and its ability to work from unprepared DNA, without the need for subcloning and vectors.

Basically, PCR is a clever modification of DNA replication allowing exponential multiplication of double-stranded DNA (Fig. 12). A PCR reaction consists of cycles of three steps: denaturing, annealing and extension. During the denaturing step the mixture is heated to 94°C, resulting in separation of the DNA strands. Two oligonucleotide primers, a few hundred base pairs apart, one complementary to each of the two strands, are present in the reaction. During the second step the temperature is decreased and these primers anneal to the now single-stranded DNA. The temperature used depends on the stringency desired, but is generally ~55°C. In the third step, the temperature is taken to 72°C, the optimum temperature for the DNA polymerase employed, which extends the primers, assembling a second strand on each single-stranded DNA molecule. Therefore, the total amount of DNA in the area flanked by the primers is now doubled. During the second cycle, this DNA will denature, anneal more primer, and again be doubled. The amount of DNA is therefore doubled per cycle, resulting in theoretical amplification after 22 cycles of more than a million-fold. Considering that each cycle only takes ~10 min, this is an almost unbelievable amount of amplification.

PCR became practical only after a DNA polymerase became available that could survive the denaturing step at 94°C. This was found in *Taq* polymerase, an enzyme from the microorganism *Thermus aquaticus* that lives in hot water vents at temperatures of ~75°C. Since then, several other heat-stable polymerases have been isolated, some with much lower error rates than the somewhat error-prone *Taq* polymerase. PCR has now been fully automated, with compact, programmable temperature cycling systems available at reasonable prices.

A major advantage of PCR is that the DNA used as a template does not need to be highly purified. Genomic DNA or cDNA can be used, but successful PCR is also possible using DNA released after simple boiling of cells and tissue. Because of the immense amplification power of PCR, only minute amounts are required. DNA from single hairs, from blood spots, and even from Egyptian mummies thousands of years old has been amplified by PCR. On the other hand, the extreme sensitivity of PCR makes it prone to artifacts. Even the smallest amount of contamination with foreign DNA may result in a band on a gel, a fact particularly important for forensic applications.

Applications of PCR will be described below.

Expression

So far we have discussed techniques focusing on the manipulation and analysis of nucleic acids. Often, however, investiga-

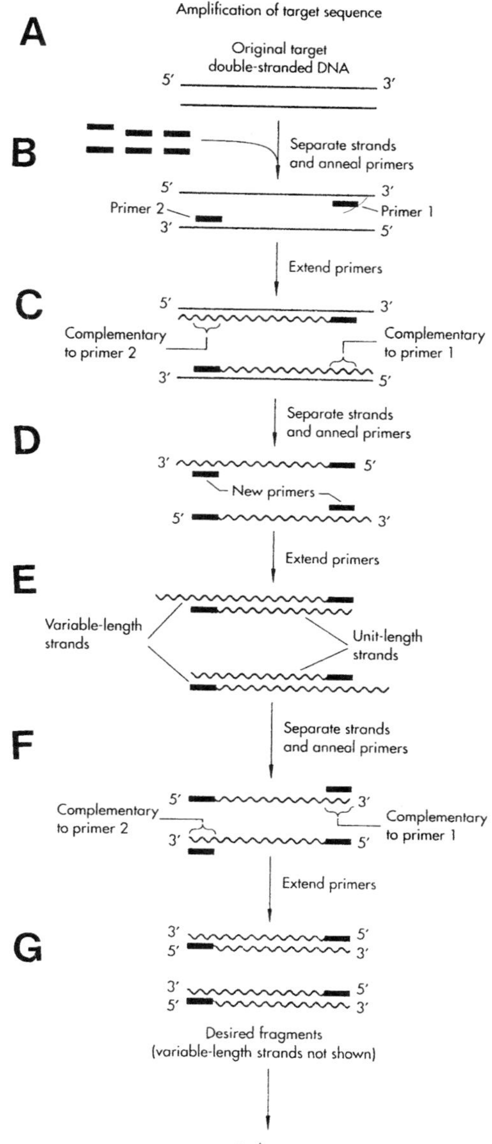

Figure 12. The polymerase chain reaction (PCR) allows amplification of DNA using two primers flanking the region to be amplified. The strands of target DNA are separated by heating **(A)**, and then the primers are annealed **(B)**. Note that the primers anneal to different strands. The primers are extended **(C)**, and a new strand of DNA is created that will contain the sequences complementary to the primers. These strands are then separated again **(D)**, and new primers will anneal to these newly created complementary sequences. These primers can be extended **(E)**. This time, however, unit-length strands will result, as template length is limited. This process of separation of the strands, annealing of primers **(F)** and extension **(G)**, can be continued for >30 cycles, resulting in over a million-fold amplification of the selected fragment. (Reprinted with permission from Watson JD, Gilman M, Witkowski J, Zoller M. *Recombinant DNA*. 2nd ed. New York: W. H. Freeman, 1992.)

tors are primarily interested in the proteins produced from these information-carrying molecules. Although procedures like Northern blotting can provide indirect information about the proteins encoded by the nucleic acids, often the direct study of receptors, channels and enzymes is more appropriate. Expression techniques allow the translation of mRNA in well-defined systems, so that the resulting proteins can be studied in isolation. In addition, these techniques can be used to prepare large amounts of recombinant protein to be used as immunogen for the preparation of polyclonal or monoclonal antibodies. We will review the most commonly used transient expression systems.

In Vitro Translation

As with most other procedures described in this chapter, the in vitro translation of mRNA into protein became possible by establishing the conditions under which natural enzymatic activity, in this instance of ribosomes, could be maintained outside the cell. Several standard systems are in use. Most commonly employed is the reticulocyte lysate system. The reticulocyte is a precursor of the red blood cell, primarily involved in the synthesis of hemoglobin. It has a highly active protein assembly system, which can be exploited for in vitro use. In vitro translation has limited application, as the amounts of protein synthesized are relatively small and not incorporated in a system where their function can be tested. Other expression systems are therefore more useful for the study of recombinantly expressed proteins.

Xenopus Oocytes

The oocytes of the African clawed toad *Xenopus laevis* have become of major importance in molecular biology, as they provide a powerful and easily assayed expression system, particularly for membrane proteins. These cells are extremely large, up to 1.5 mm in diameter, and can therefore be injected easily with foreign mRNA. As most of their size is due to accumulation of large amounts of yolk protein, they also have a highly active protein synthesizing system. In fact, in these oocytes part of the genome dealing with protein synthesis is selectively amplified to be able to provide the huge number of ribosomes needed for yolk synthesis. Injected mRNA, either extracted from tissues or synthesized and capped in vitro, is translated efficiently, the proteins are routed to their correct locations, and the appropriate post-translational modifications are made. Alternatively, cDNA in a vector containing an appropriate promotor can be injected directly into the germinal vesicle (the equivalent of the nucleus in the oocyte) and is transcribed into RNA and then translated into protein. An additional advantage is the relative lack of endogenous signaling systems that would interfere with expressed proteins. On the other hand, most of the intracellular pathways, such as G proteins, adenylate cyclase and the inositol system, are present. For all these reasons *Xenopus* oocytes have become a very common expression system. Their size makes electrophysiologic study very simple, and they have been used extensively for the study of ion channels. Ca^{2+}-mobilizing receptors can be studied electrophysiologically as well, as the oocyte membrane contains Ca^{2+}-activated Cl^- channels. Oocytes have also been used for cloning purposes and for the analysis of the effects of induced mutations.

COS Cells

Whereas *Xenopus* oocytes provide not only expression of the protein, but allow testing of its function, COS cells primarily generate massive amounts of protein. Their most useful role is for binding studies. COS cells are monkey kidney cells, carrying an integrated portion of the SV40 virus genome involved in viral replication. When vectors carrying the SV40 origin of replication are transfected into these cells, the plasmid is replicated to a very high copy number. This results in very high expression of DNA sequence carried on the vector, so high, in fact, that the cells can only sustain expression for a short period of time. The vast excess of protein often overwhelms intracellular signaling systems, so that functional studies are difficult, but membrane preparations from these cells are very useful for binding experiments. COS cells have played a major role in the cloning of many genes.

Yeast, Baculovirus, and Vaccinia Virus

Other systems have been developed for the expression of large amounts of recombinant proteins. Yeast is particularly useful because it performs many posttranslational modifications in ways very similar to mammalian cells and can be induced to secrete its products into the medium from where they can be isolated. Baculovirus is an insect virus that, during infection, produces extremely high levels of its coat protein. A system has been developed that allows substitution of the coat protein gene with recombinant DNA, resulting in very high expression levels after infection of insect cells in culture. The vaccinia expression system consists of a modified vaccinia virus that expresses a bacteriophage RNA polymerase. Cells infected with the vaccinia virus accumulate extremely high levels of this polymerase. Also, the virus shuts down host protein synthesis. As a result, introduction of a gene to be expressed on a vector carrying the promoter for the bacteriophage polymerase results in very high expression levels.

Cloning

Often, molecular biology is equated with gene cloning. Although originally a large part of the discipline was directed toward obtaining genetic material encoding proteins, much recent research has applied these techniques towards very different questions. In fact, it is unlikely that molecular cloning would be the primary application of molecular biology for investigators in anesthesiology. Nonetheless, a brief overview of the principal cloning techniques is included, not only because of their inherent interest, but also because cloning studies demonstrate how a number of different molecular biology techniques can be used together to solve a scientific problem. Most cloning strategies attempt to find a short fragment of the DNA of interest, which then can be used to obtain the full clone. Differences between the techniques are mainly in how this initial fragment is obtained. In contrast, expression cloning uses a completely different approach.

Cloning by Protein Sequencing

Although very laborious, often the only way a short fragment of DNA of the clone can be obtained is by purifying sufficient amounts of the protein encoded so that a short stretch of amino acids can be sequenced (Fig. 13). This amino acid sequence can then be back-translated to nucleotide sequence, using the genetic code. An oligonucleotide with this sequence is prepared and used as a probe to screen a library by hybridization. An example of such a cloning project will be described. Apart from the work involved, a major problem with this approach is the degeneracy of the genetic code. Almost always there are multiple codons for each amino acid, and although educated guesses can be made based on the distribution of codon usage in a species, there is no method to determine in advance which deduced nucleotide sequence will be the correct one. However, as the degeneracy of the genetic code is primarily in the third position of the codon degenerate oligonucleotides can be synthesized, together containing all possible codons for each amino acid. Alternatively, a unique "guessmer" can be synthesized, with a sequence based on the expected distribution of codon usage.

Cloning by Homology Screening

Many genes cluster in related groups, termed gene families, that appear to have developed evolutionary by gene duplication followed by divergence. Therefore, if one member of a gene family is known, it is often possible to clone other mem-

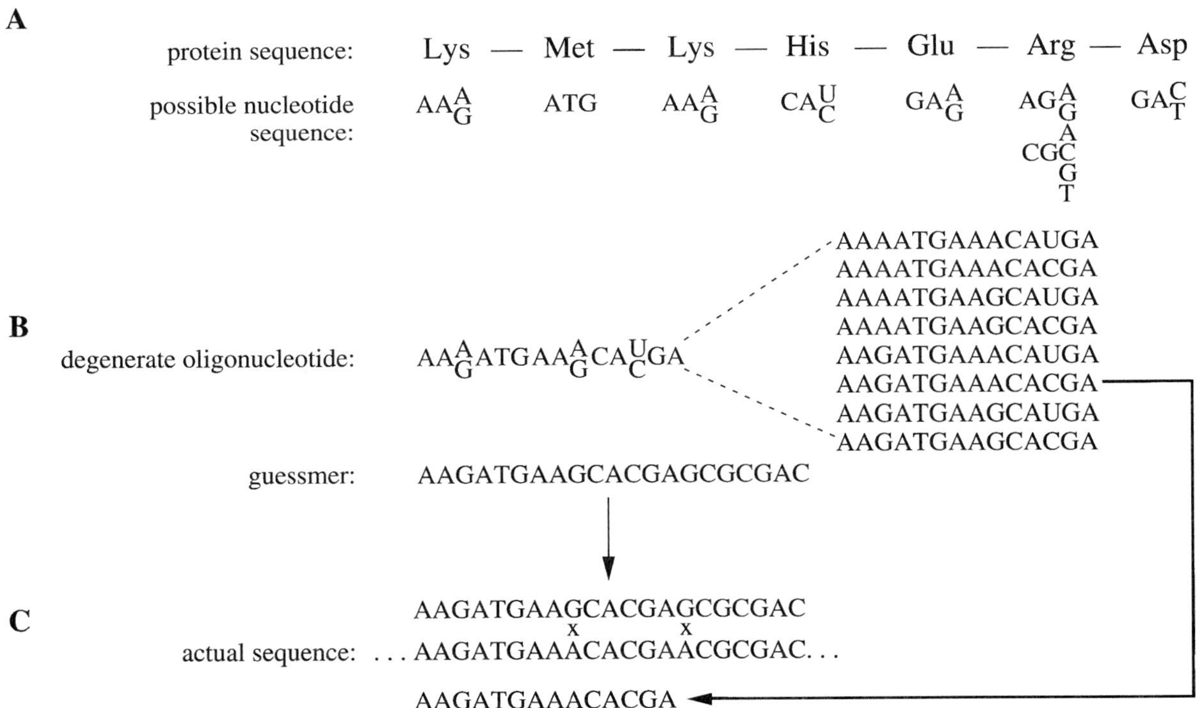

Figure 13. The protein of interest is purified in sufficient amounts to obtain fragments by proteolysis that can be partially sequenced. Using the obtained amino acid sequence, the underlying DNA sequence is deduced (**A**). As a result of the degeneracy of the genetic code, multiple DNA sequences can usually encode the same polypeptide. To create a DNA probe, either a degenerate probe is constructed, which is actually a mixture of sequences, or a unique guessmer is synthesized (**B**). The probe is then used to screen a library. Adjustment of the stringency allows occasional mismatches between the probe and the target sequence (**C**).

bers of the same family based on their homology, by screening a library at low stringency with a probe derived from the known member. This approach is decidedly easier than cloning by protein sequencing and has been very fruitful in finding subtypes of receptors and channels. An essential part of the approach is the demonstration that a cloned gene indeed encodes a functional member of the family. Many cDNAs have been cloned that, based on sequence similarity, are clear members of the family, but that are not expressed (pseudogenes), or to which no function has been assigned (orphans). As an example, in the large family of G-protein receptor genes so far ~50 cDNAs have been cloned for which no ligands are known.

Cloning by PCR

The advent of PCR has made homology cloning even easier. In PCR cloning, primers are designed based on a known subtype of a gene family, or on a consensus sequence determined from a computer alignment of multiple known sequences. These primers are then used in a PCR reaction at low stringency using as a substrate cDNA prepared from a tissue expected to express other subtypes of the gene. The resulting PCR product is subsequently used to screen a library to obtain the full-length clone. Even more than with homology screening, PCR cloning is prone to clone orphans or fragments of DNA without a function.

Expression Cloning

In contrast to the screening methods described above, expression cloning does not require a short DNA fragment of the clone (Fig. 14). mRNA is extracted from tissue, and a cDNA library is prepared. This cDNA is then expressed in an appropriate system, e.g., by expression in COS cells, or by in vitro transcription and injection of the RNA in *Xenopus* oocytes. The presence of a sign of expression of the clone of interest (binding, response to a ligand, or ion flux) is looked for. If a response is found, the clone is isolated from the cDNA library through a procedure called sib selection. The library is divided in a number of pools, which are tested individually for responses. The pool giving the largest response is presumed to hold the highest amount of message for the clone of interest. It is amplified by propagation in bacteria, again divided in pools, and these pools are tested individually. Presumably, the response will now have increased in some of the pools. Again, the pool with the best response is selected for further subdivision. This process is repeated until a single cDNA is obtained, which represents the clone. An example of expression cloning is provided below. Apart from being fairly labor intensive, a disadvantage of this system is that it is virtually impossible to clone multisubunit proteins, as their messages will usually be in separate pools.

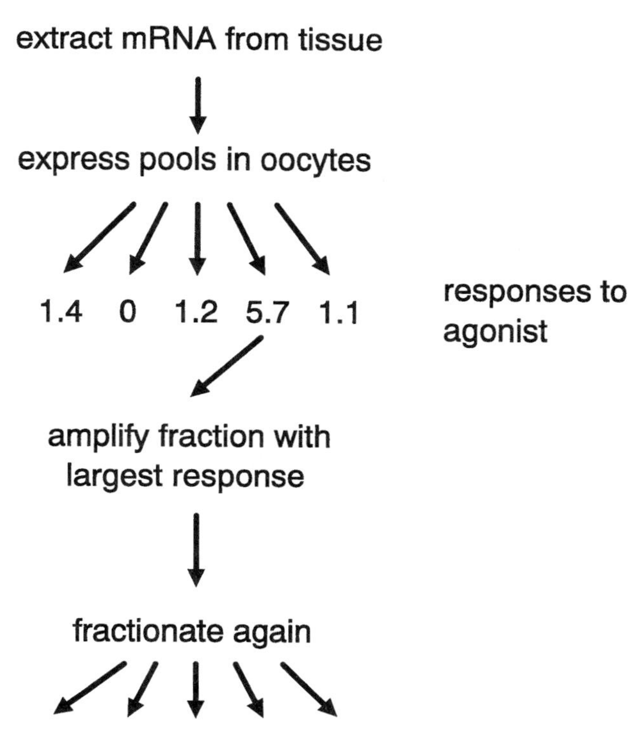

Figure 14. mRNA is extracted from tissue and divided into a number of pools. These pools are then individually tested for activity in a suitable assay system, such as the *Xenopus laevis* oocyte. The pool that yields the highest response is selected for further study. It is amplified, again divided into subpools and expressed again. This process is continued until the pure clone is obtained.

Mutagenesis

One of the most powerful techniques in molecular biology is mutagenesis, the ability to modify the amino acid sequence of proteins highly selectively and to study the effects of such induced changes. This type of functional study makes it possible to assign specific functions to parts of polypeptides and, in addition, provides, at least in theory, an approach to the repair of genetically determined diseases. We will discuss the most common forms of mutagenesis, as well as approaches to selectively direct expression of foreign genes in organisms.

Chimeras

Our knowledge of structure-function relationships of polypeptides is frequently limited, and therefore it can be difficult to decide where specific amino acid changes should be made. First, a protein's functional domains must be mapped. This is frequently done by the creation of chimeras, i.e., recombinant proteins consisting of fragments of different molecules connected together. This so-called domain swapping allows creation of molecules with properties of both parents, and the functions of these domains can be elucidated. For instance, chimeras of adrenergic receptors have been constructed that, when expressed in *Xenopus* oocytes, bound α_2-adrenergic agonists, but activated adenylate cyclase like β_2-adrenergic receptors (8). The most rapid technique for generating the fragments to construct chimeras is by PCR of selected areas of the parent cDNAs.

Random Mutagenesis

Another, less commonly used approach to determine the location of functional domains in a protein is the generation of random mutations in the cDNA. A number of methodologies exist, such as chemical modification of the cDNA in the vector, or the incorporation of wrong nucleotides during in vitro DNA synthesis by providing an excess of the incorrect nucleotide. The method has been largely supplanted by more selective approaches.

Site-Directed Mutagenesis

The improvements in synthetic oligonucleotide preparation have made site-directed mutagenesis, i.e., specific deletion, insertion, or modification of selected nucleotides in a sequence, a relatively simple procedure. This technique gives the experimenter full control over the resulting amino acid sequence of the protein under study.

Site-directed mutagenesis is based on the use of a mismatched primer for DNA synthesis (Fig. 15). An oligonucleotide is prepared that contains the desired mismatch flanked by 10–15 correctly matching nucleotides on both

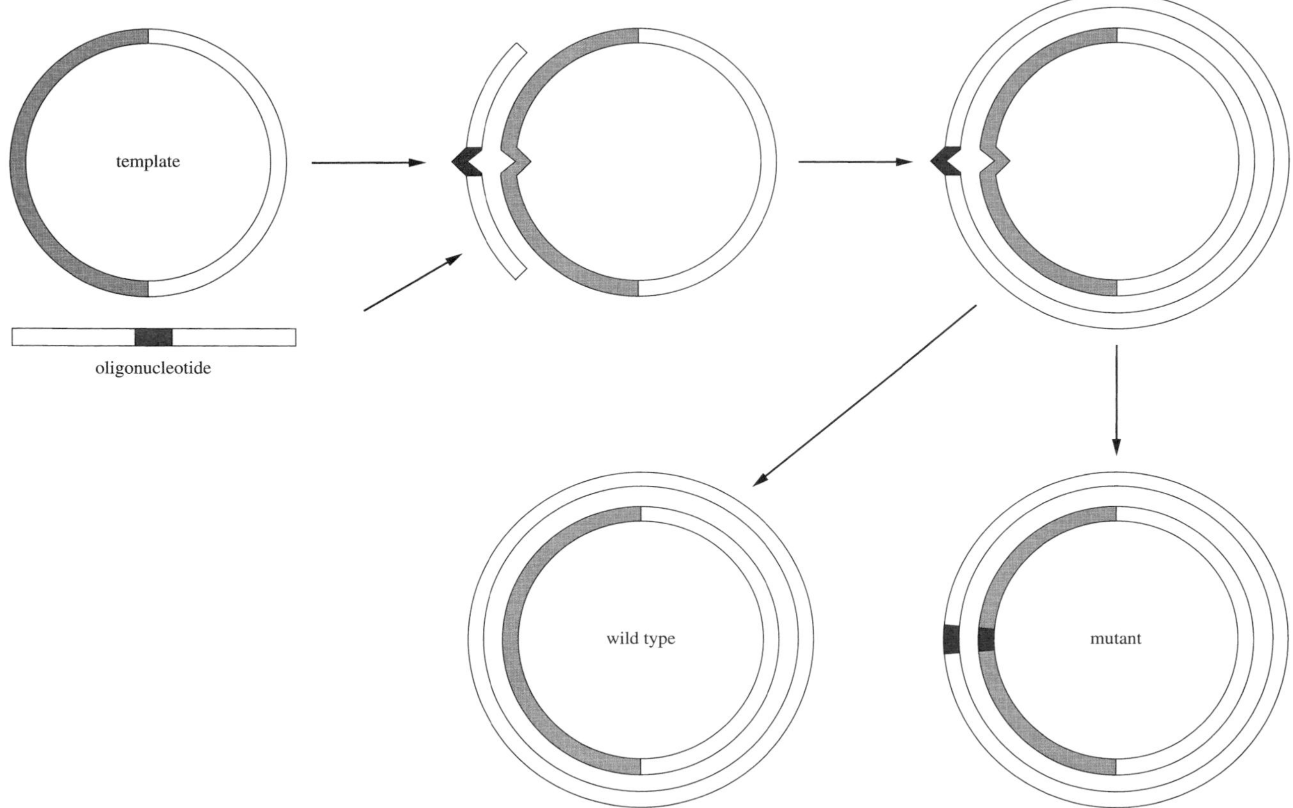

Figure 15. To induce selective mutations in a clone, a single-stranded DNA template is constructed. This DNA is annealed with an oligonucleotide carrying the mutation, flanked by 10–15 correctly matching nucleotides. This oligonucleotide is used as a primer for the synthesis of a second strand, which will contain the mutation. When completely synthesized, the ends of the new strand are ligated together, and the vectors are transfected into bacteria. DNA repair mechanisms will rapidly correct the mismatched base pair, so that either both strands are wild-type or both are mutated.

sides. This oligonucleotide is annealed under low-stringency conditions with a single-stranded vector containing the cDNA sequence of interest. Despite the mismatch, the oligonucleotide will anneal and is subsequently used as a primer for synthesis of a second DNA strand. Ligation will form a complete double-stranded vector, the cDNA insert of which contains the desired mutation in one strand.

Frequently, a whole series of mutations through a selected region is planned to study effects of small changes in protein structure. In such cases, it is useful to create so-called cassettes, oligonucleotides or mutated fragments of the cDNA that can replace a segment of the wild type using unique restriction sites (Fig. 16). If such restriction sites are not available naturally they can be created using site-directed mutagenesis. Computer programs can locate so-called silent restriction sites, i.e., places where sites can be created without changing the resulting amino acid sequence (a result of the degeneracy of the genetic code). After inserting the mutated cassette into the wild type, the cDNA can be expressed and tested for changes in function.

Transgenics

Site-directed mutagenesis has created enormous opportunities for the study of protein function. However, the techniques described so far limit study of the mutated protein to what have been called "in transfecto" assays, such as the *Xenopus* oocyte or COS cells. Ideally, one would like to express the mutated proteins in the appropriate location in animals and observe for effects in vivo. To a large extent, this has become feasible using transgenic techniques.

Mice are commonly used for the creation of transgenic animals (Fig. 17). Fertilized eggs are removed from females, and the cDNA of interest is injected into one of the two pronuclei. The eggs are then transferred to foster mothers. In a variable percentage of eggs, the DNA will become integrated into the genome and passed on during cell division: the cDNA has become a transgene. After birth offspring is checked for the presence of the transgene by PCR or Southern blotting, using as substrate a small amount of genomic DNA obtained from a tail biopsy. Transgenes can integrate in germ lines, so that stable lines expressing a particular transgene can be constructed.

A major disadvantage of this technique is the inability to control the location where the cDNA integrates. A different approach, using embryonic stem cells, circumvents this problem. Embryonic stem cells are cultured from mouse blastocysts, but retain their pluripotentiality. cDNA can be incorporated by various means, and its presence at the desired location in the genome can be confirmed before the cells are injected into blastocysts and develop into mice. This system even makes it possible to selectively replace a mutant gene with a corrected one using a process named homologous recombination. Here the flanking regions of a transgene exchange with identical flanking regions of the native gene, leading to exchange of the native gene for the transgene. Although the specifics of homologous recombination are not fully understood, the technique provides a powerful method for replacing genes in living systems.

Transgenes have been used for a variety of purposes. Specific organs can be targeted by linking the gene of interest to tissue-specific regulatory sequences, so that it will be expressed in the desired tissues only. When such tissue-specific sequences are

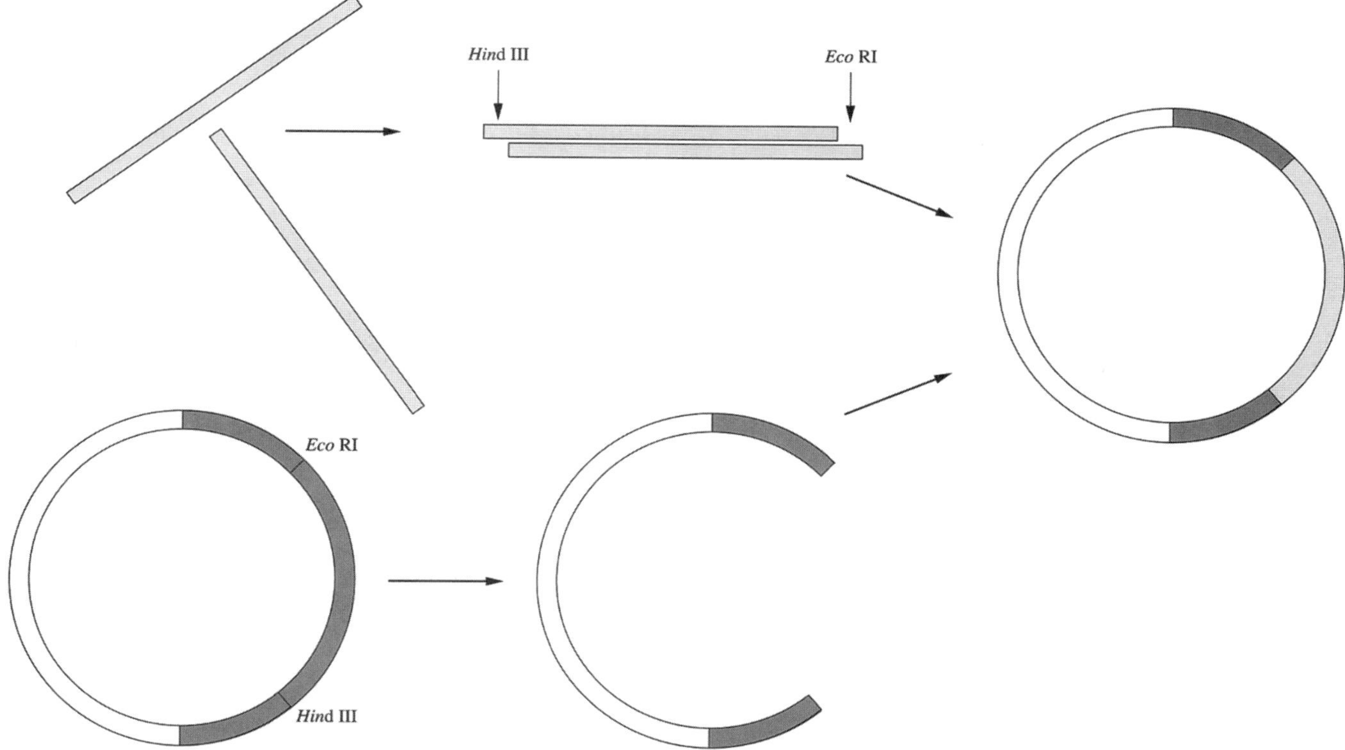

Figure 16. The replacement of a fragment of a cloned gene by a synthesized oligonucleotide containing a mutation is a useful method (known as cassette mutagenesis) if multiple mutations will need to be screened. The fragment is removed from the vector by digestion with restriction enzymes known to have only a single site (*bottom left*). Synthetic oligonucleotides are designed in a way that will yield overhangs when they are annealed (*top left*). This double-stranded oligonucleotide can then be ligated into the vector (*right*), which can subsequently be used to transform bacteria.

coupled to a gene encoding a toxin, specific cell lineages in the developing animal can be killed. A system that allows inducible killing of selected cells has been devised by coupling tissue-specific regulatory sequences to a gene that metabolizes a specific nucleotide into a toxic product. Injection of the nucleotide at a time determined by the investigator will result in death of the cells. Transgenic systems can also be used to destroy selectively the functioning of endogenous genes ("knock-out") and study the effects on development. This system is useful in ascertaining the necessity for, and role of, a gene product, although compensatory changes in expression by other genes can make interpretation of findings difficult. Finally, by inducing selective mutations, mouse models of human diseases have been created. New uses will no doubt arise as more experience is gained with the system.

APPLICATIONS OF MOLECULAR BIOLOGY

In contrast to some other scientific methodologies, it is rare that a single molecular biology technique will provide the answer to a scientific question. Most times a sequence of protocols has to be followed. As an example, mapping of mRNA in various organs will necessitate performing the following techniques in sequence: RNA extraction, poly-A selection, generation of a labeled probe, and finally Northern analysis. For this reason, a description of individual techniques, as provided above, is inadequate to convey a sense of the practice of molecular biology. This final section therefore illustrates the combined use of the techniques discussed so far by describing actual research applications in the area of molecular biology. Studies have been selected that yielded results of particular importance to the anesthesiologist. Several practical cloning examples will be discussed, followed by short descriptions of studies in the areas of diagnosis and treatment of diseases.

Cloning

Although the emphasis of this chapter is not on cloning, the combinations of techniques used in the cloning process illustrate well how a problem in molecular biology is solved by the sequential application of a series of procedures. We discuss three cloning studies exemplifying the three cloning approaches (protein sequencing, expression, and homology) discussed above. Although all studies were directed towards cloning members of the G-protein–coupled receptor family, it will be clear that a variety of approaches can be employed to attain this goal. The particular circumstances determine which technique is the most appropriate.

Cloning Using Protein Sequence: The β-Adrenergic Receptor

A thorough understanding of the adrenergic system is of enormous importance in the practice of anesthesiology. Pharmacologic studies have classified adrenergic receptors into several groups. First, the α and β receptors were shown to be pharmacologically distinct, and the development of new drugs led to the characterization of further subtypes within these classes. However, no data existed on the molecular structure of these receptors, or on the molecular basis for the difference in binding affinity between the subtypes. Such studies became feasible only with the cloning of the cDNA for these receptors.

In 1986, Dixon et al. reported molecular cloning of the β_2-adrenergic receptor from hamster lung (3). As this was the

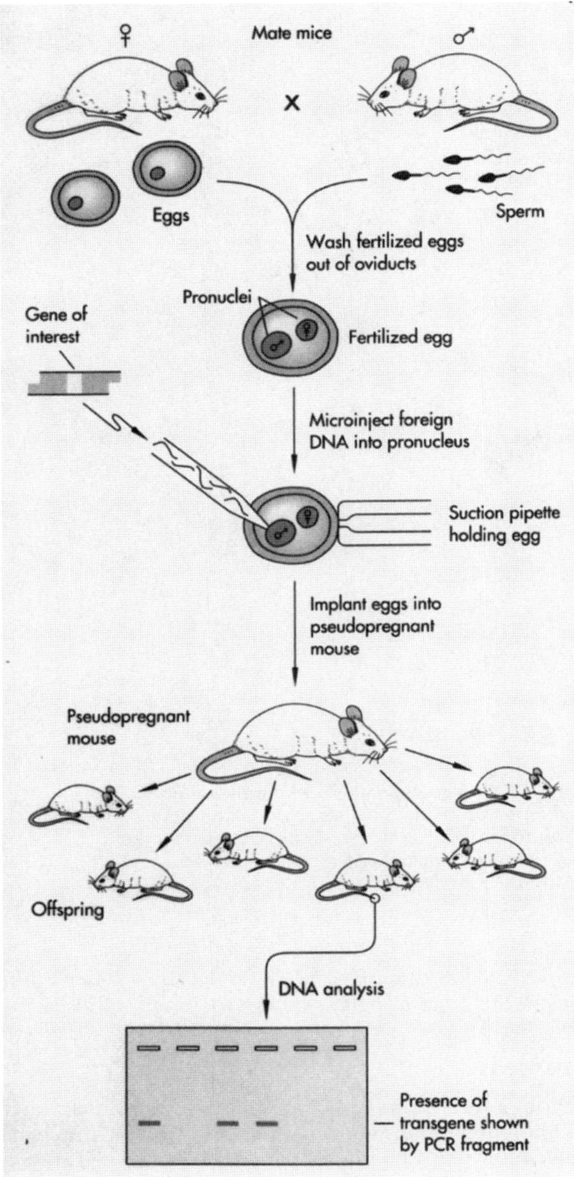

Figure 17. To create transgenic mice, fertilized eggs are washed out of the oviducts of mated, female mice. The gene of interest is injected into one of the pronuclei, and the eggs are implanted into pseudopregnant females (produced by mating females with vasectomized males). As indicated by Southern analysis of DNA obtained by tail biopsy, some of the offspring will carry the transgene. (Reprinted with permission from Watson JD, Gilman M, Witkowski J, Zoller M. *Recombinant DNA*. 2nd ed. New York: W. H. Freeman, 1992.)

first subtype of this class of receptors to be cloned, they employed partial protein sequencing as their technique (Fig. 18). The receptor was purified to homogeneity using affinity chromatography. The protein was then cleaved in a number of fragments, and the seven most prominent peptides were used to obtain partial amino acid sequences. One of these was used in the subsequent experiments. To verify that this peptide fragment was indeed part of the adrenergic receptor, antibodies were raised against it. This was done by synthesizing an oligonucleotide encoding the fragment and linking it to the sequence of a carrier protein, resulting in a so-called fusion protein sequence. The sequence was expressed in bacteria and the fusion protein injected into rabbits. The resultant antibodies were shown to bind to purified β-adrenergic receptor, indicating that the fragment was indeed part of the receptor.

Next, several oligonucleotides complementary to the deduced DNA sequence of this same peptide fragment were synthesized. These were first used on Southern blots with hamster genomic DNA and were shown to result in a single band on the blot, at a size of 5.2 kb. This indicated that a genomic sequence complementary to the oligonucleotide could be identified. This 5.2-kb fragment, however, must contain significantly more sequence than that encoding the receptor, as estimated from its molecular weight. A hamster genomic library was screened using the same oligonucleotide, and five clones were isolated. Restriction mapping of each of these clones showed that treatment with the restriction enzyme *Hin*dIII resulted in a fragment of 1.3 kb that still hybridized the oligonucleotide. This fragment, much closer to the predicted size of the receptor, was subcloned and sequenced, and was found to contain an area encoding a 435–amino acid protein. The sequences of all seven protein fragments mentioned above were contained within this sequence. The genomic clone had been isolated successfully.

However, the presence of a genomic sequence does not guarantee that the gene is actually expressed. Using the *Hin*dIII fragment as a probe, a hamster cDNA library was screened. Clones obtained from this library confirmed that the message encoded by the genomic clone was indeed expressed as mRNA and also demonstrated the absence of introns in the genomic sequence. Although this is unusual for mammalian genes in general, it has since been found that many G-protein–coupled receptor genes do not contain introns.

To analyze the sequence, a hydropathy plot was constructed (Fig. 19), which indicates areas of hydrophobicity within the protein and can localize putative membrane-spanning domains. The plot showed seven putative transmembrane areas, a configuration surprisingly similar to the rhodopsins, the light-transducing receptors in the eye. It is now known that the rhodopsins, the adrenergic receptors, the odorant receptors, and a multitude of other transducing systems coupled to G proteins all have this so-called heptahelical membrane configuration.

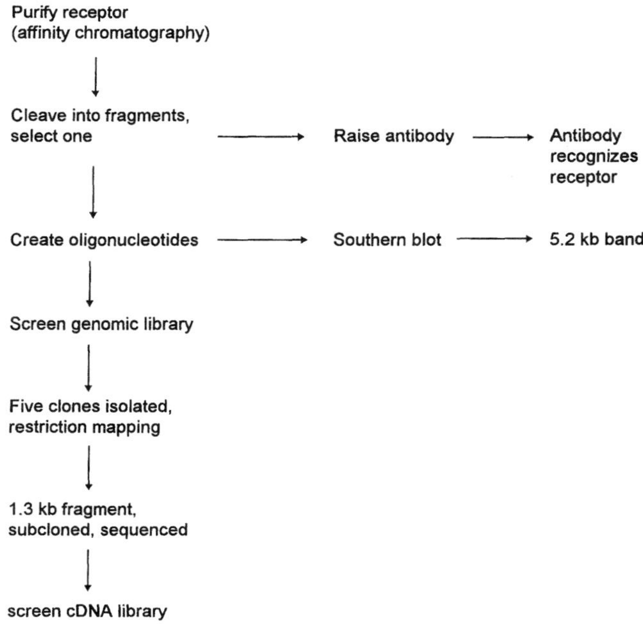

Figure 18. Cloning of the β-adrenergic receptor.

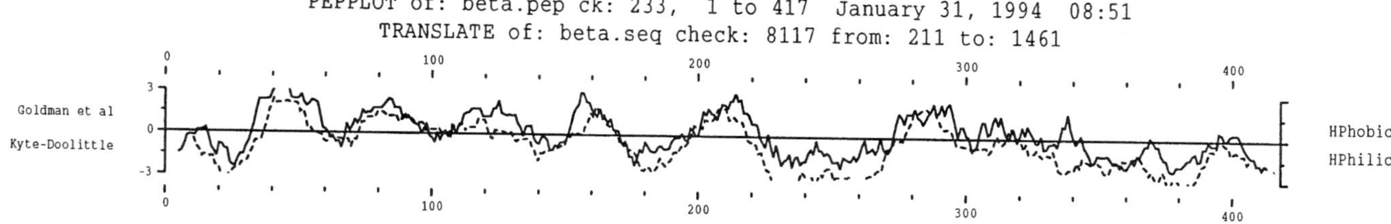

Figure 19. This hydropathy plot of the β-adrenergic receptor is based on the method of Kyte and Doolittle (10) and created with the Genetics Computer Group software package (6). It shows the amino acid number along the *x* axis and a measure of relative hydrophobicity or hydrophilicity on the *y* axis. To calculate each point the hydropathy measures of several amino acids (a window) are averaged and the result is plotted. The window then "slides" one amino acid and the process is repeated. The hydropathy plot of the β-adrenergic receptor shows seven hydrophobic areas (the seventh is less pronounced, a common feature in receptors of this family), presumed to indicate membrane-spanning regions.

Cloning Using Expression: The δ-Opioid Receptor

After the cloning of the first adrenergic receptor subtype, an explosion of homology screening and PCR cloning generated G-protein–coupled receptor cDNAs at high rate. In fact, several hundred different members of this superfamily are currently known. However, one receptor, of particular interest to anesthesiologists, defied cloning attempts: the opiate receptor. Clearly, it was not sufficiently closely related to other members to be cloned by homology, and expression cloning was hampered by the hydrophobicity of the available ligands (resulting in high nonspecific binding to membrane). It was not until the end of 1992 that successful cloning of an opioid receptor subtype was reported (7).

The δ-opioid receptor was cloned using an expression technique (Fig. 20). RNA was extracted from the neuronal cell line NG108-15, and, using random priming, a cDNA library was constructed in a vector suitable for expression. Fractions of cDNA were transfected into COS cells. After 72 h of culture, membranes were isolated, and a ^{3}H-labeled ligand was used to assay for specific binding to expressed receptor. Background binding was ~700 ± 250 dpm, and a single fraction was noted to give a signal consistently 10% above background (i.e., only one third of a SE different from background). This fraction was subdivided and again expressed, and one fraction now produced a signal 20% above background, that in addition disappeared in the presence of naloxone. Two more subdivisions led to a single clone.

As the ligand used was not selective for only a single subtype of opioid receptor, expressed receptor was bound with a number of ligands. The resulting rank order of potency showed that the clone encoded a δ-opioid receptor. A hydropathy plot revealed seven transmembrane areas, as expected.

An interesting problem in this project concerned the species of origin of this clone, as NG108-15 cells are hybrids of cell lines from two species: mouse N18TG neuroblastoma and rat C6Bu-1 glioma cells. To answer this question, oligonucleotide primers were prepared complementary to an area just outside the coding region, presumably less conserved among species. Therefore, the primers should only anneal to DNA of the species from which the clone was obtained. These primers were used in PCR reactions, with mouse and rat genomic DNA as templates. Only with mouse DNA was a single amplified product of the predicted size obtained, which was subcloned, sequenced, and shown to be an exact match to the corresponding area in the cDNA. Therefore, the receptor derived from mouse.

Since the δ-receptor cDNA was obtained, most other opioid receptor subtypes have been cloned by homology screening.

Cloning Using Homology: The Cannabinoid Receptor

Marijuana is a mixture of several neuroactive compounds, the cannabinoids, the most important of which is Δ^9-tetrahydrocannabinol (Δ^9-THC). Apart from its popularity as a recreational drug, Δ^9-THC has several properties that make it of interest to the anesthesiologist, including central nervous system depression as well as potent analgesic and antiemetic effects. It is a highly lipophilic drug and for long had been considered to exert its effect through a nonspecific interaction with cell membranes. Although the discovery of specific cannabinoid binding sites made this a less likely explanation of its mechanism of action, it was only with the cloning of a cannabinoid receptor of the G-protein–coupled receptor class that a specific action was fully accepted.

Matsuda et al. (13) reported the cannabinoid receptor cloning in 1990. This study was different from the two described above, as the cannabinoid receptor was not the specific goal of the project. Rather, it was a homology screening search for novel receptors. A cDNA library was prepared from rat cerebral cortex mRNA and was screened with an oligonucleotide based on a section of the G-protein–coupled receptor for substance K. A cDNA clone was found, encoding 473 amino acids, and with the hydropathy signature of a G-protein–coupled receptor. However, the clone was not sufficiently similar to any other member of the superfamily to assign it a ligand. In other words, it was an orphan. Therefore, a laborious search began, expressing the clone in *Xenopus* oocytes and mammalian cell lines, and testing for binding and changes in intracellular Ca^{2+} and cAMP after ligand application. A large number of potential ligands was screened, but without success. In

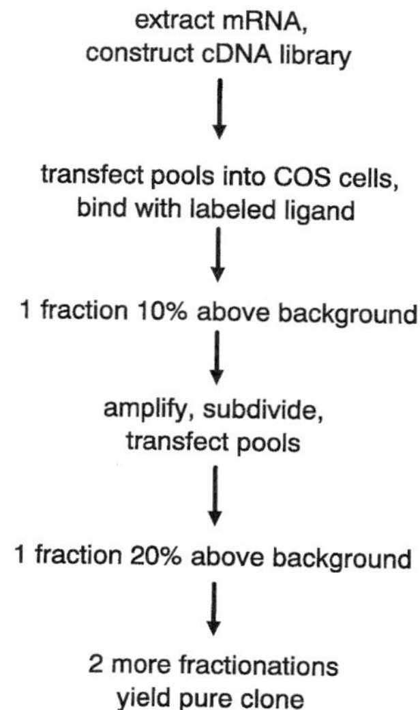

Figure 20. Cloning of the δ-opioid receptor.

addition, mRNA levels in different parts of the brain, as well as in several cell types, were mapped, in the hope that knowledge of the distribution of expression would give a hint about the ligand. In the end, it was the observation that mRNA of the clone colocalized with cannabinoid binding sites that spurred an attempt to test Δ^9-THC as a possible ligand. The clone had been integrated in the genome of a Chinese hamster ovary K1 cell line, and it was shown that in these cells expressing the clone addition of Δ^9-THC resulted in inhibition of forskolin-stimulated cAMP production. Experiments with related ligands confirmed that the clone encoded a cannabinoid receptor. Since then, the distribution of mRNA in the human brain has been mapped using in situ hybridization, and it has been shown to be primarily present in several layers of the cerebral cortex (as expected, because of the origin of the clone), the dentate gyrus and the hippocampus (12).

Diagnosis

A number of genetically determined disease states can now be diagnosed, often prenatally, using molecular biology techniques. For some of these, the defective gene has been cloned (hemophilia, cystic fibrosis and Duchenne muscular dystrophy are a few examples with relevance to the anesthesiologist), and the specific mutation is known. However, even if the gene has not yet been cloned, early diagnosis is often possible using a combination of molecular and genetic approaches. We will discuss three relevant examples of diseases diagnosed using molecular biology techniques: hemophilia, cystic fibrosis, and malignant hyperthermia. These diagnostic approaches have found application in a wide area, ranging from the genetic typing of tumors in order to determine therapy and prognosis, to genetic fingerprinting of individuals for forensic purposes.

Hemophilia

The application of PCR has made diagnosis of genetic diseases much easier. The small amounts of fetal DNA obtained from chorionic villus biopsy are more than sufficient for PCR, and extraction of the DNA is not even necessary. An example of this technique is the prenatal diagnosis of hemophilia A.

Hemophilia A is due to a defect in coagulation factor VIII, a complicated gene containing 26 exons. Kogan et al. (9) developed a rapid technique for prenatal screening for this disease. It uses PCR combined with a technique known as restriction fragment length polymorphism (RFLP) analysis (Fig. 21). RFLP analysis presupposes the existence of a marker sequence close to or in the gene of interest, so that the marker and gene will be co-inherited. The marker must contain a mutation that modifies a restriction site, so that either the presence or absence of the site is inherited with the mutation in the gene of interest. To test for the presence of the site, DNA is digested with the specific restriction enzyme, separated on a gel, and subsequently hybridized to a probe recognizing the marker sequence. This probing step is necessary to find the single copy of the marker in the background of DNA. The size of the resulting band on autoradiography (the restriction fragment length) will indicate whether or not the marker area was cut, and this will inform the investigator if the normal or diseased gene is present in the DNA. Alternatively, a selected area containing the RFLP can be amplified by PCR, digested with the enzyme, and analyzed by simple gel electrophoresis. The amplification step makes probing unnecessary. This was the approach used by Kogan et al.

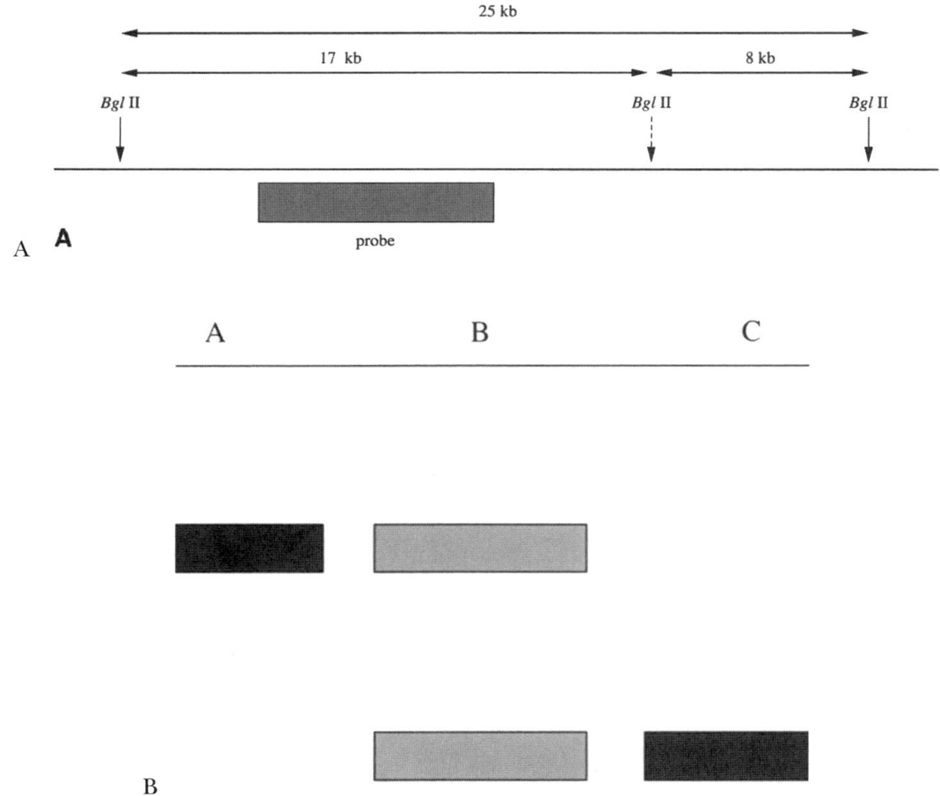

Figure 21. An RFLP of a hypothetical gene is shown. **(A)** The region can contain either two or three restriction sites for the enzyme *Bgl*II, so that digestion with *Blg*II followed by hybridization with the DNA probe will either result in a 17- or 25-kb labeled fragment. Absence of the polymorphic (*center*) restriction site is associated with an abnormality in the gene. **(B)** After digestion, hybridization and gel analysis, three configurations are possible, with the site present in neither (lane A), one (lane B), or both (lane C) chromosomes.

Several RFLPs are present within the factor VIII gene. Two of these RFLPs, for the restriction enzymes *BclI* and *XbaI*, were used as target sequences (Fig. 22). PCR primers were prepared flanking these regions, and DNA obtained from chorionic villi was used as substrate. The amplified fragment was digested with the enzyme and separated on gel, where, after staining with ethidium bromide, fragment sizes and thus carrier status could be determined directly.

Cystic Fibrosis

Cystic fibrosis is the most common severe autosomal recessive disorder affecting the white population (11). The gene involved has been cloned, and a deletion three nucleotides in length, removing a single phenylalanine residue, has been identified as being responsible for the disease in the majority of cases. Because of the poor prognosis of the disease, prenatal screening is of importance. Several methods, including amniotic fluid enzyme levels and RFLPs, are available. However, Lemna et al. (11) used oligonucleotides designed to anneal with either the normal or diseased allele to detect the mutation directly.

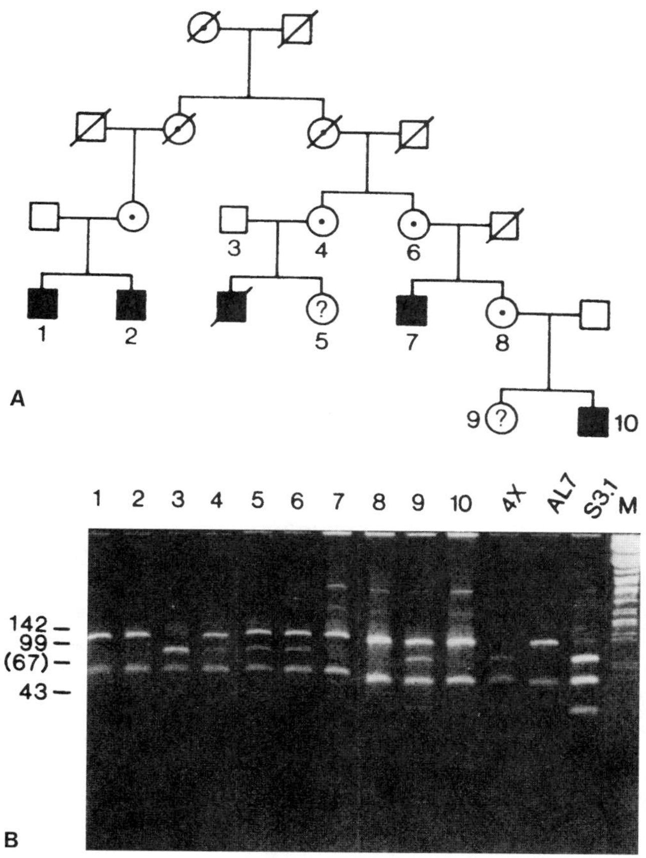

Figure 22. RFLP detection of hemophilia carriers is shown. **(A)** A pedigree analysis of a family carrying the hemophilia gene: males (*squares*), females (*circles*), subjects with hemophilia A (*filled symbols*), female carriers (*circles with dots*), and diseased family members (*diagonal lines*). **(B)** Gel electrophoresis of a PCR-amplified area carrying a polymorphic *BclI* site, after digestion with *BclI*. Absence of the site is linked to the hemophilia gene. Therefore, a 142-bp band indicates a chromosome carrying the disease, and a 99-bp plus a 43-bp band indicate a normal chromosome. Numbers indicate subjects in the family described in A. Not only homozygous patients, but also heterozygous carriers are easily detected. Note the verification of carrier status for subjects 5 and 9, and the homozygous state of subject 8. (Reprinted with permission from Kogan SC, Doherty M, Gitschier J. An improved method for prenatal diagnosis of genetic diseases by analysis of amplified DNA sequences; application to hemophilia A. *N Engl J Med* 1987;317: 985–990.)

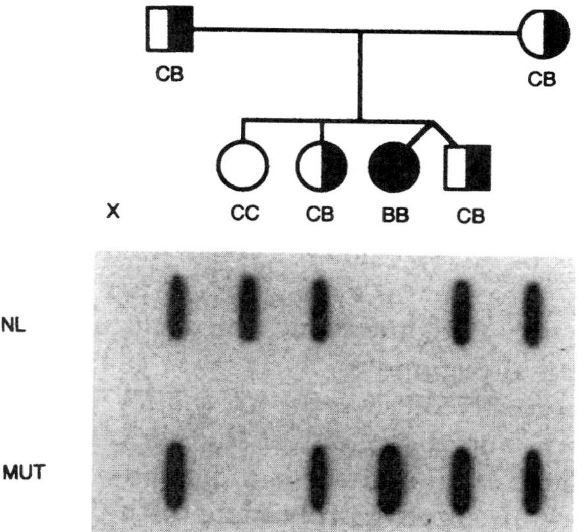

Figure 23. Detection of the cystic fibrosis gene with allele-specific probes. In the pedigree analysis, the following are shown: males (*squares*), females (*circles*), affected members (*solid symbols*), heterozygotes (*half-solid symbols*), and noncarriers (*open symbols*). DNA from these subjects was amplified by PCR and hybridized to allele-specific probes in a procedure named slot blotting. NL denotes the oligonucleotide complementary to the normal allele, MUT the mutant allele-specific nucleotide. A control where no DNA was added to the PCR reaction is indicated (*X*). The carrier status of all subjects is easily ascertained. (Reprinted with permission from Lemna WK, Feldman GL, Kerem B, et al. Mutation analysis for heterozygote detection and the prenatal diagnosis of cystic fibrosis. *N Engl J Med* 1990;322:291–296.)

PCR primers were constructed that flanked the area of the mutation, and these were used to amplify a fragment including the mutation site using DNA obtained from blood as substrate. This amplified DNA was then hybridized with the two allele-specific oligonucleotides. After autoradiography the carrier status of the individual could be read directly (Fig. 23). The use of PCR assures that only tiny amounts of DNA are needed, and the simplicity of the method allows its application in large-scale screening programs.

Localization of the mutation in the cystic fibrosis gene has led to attempts to correct this deletion. We will discuss one such study below.

Malignant Hyperthermia

Although the availability of dantrolene has significantly improved outcome of the malignant hyperthermia (MH) syndrome, an MH crisis remains one of the more dramatic, albeit uncommon, intraoperative events treated by the anesthesiologist. Research over the past years has attempted to locate the specific defect in this disease, and, although the general term MH might encompass several specific disease states, it appears that abnormalities in the skeletal muscle Ca^{2+} release channel (ryanodine receptor) play a major role. The gene for this channel has been cloned and localized to a specific section of human chromosome 19. In MH-susceptible pigs, a specific mutation (C at position 1843 to T, resulting in a change of one amino acid) appears responsible for halothane sensitivity (4), and a similar mutation has been observed in a single family of humans. The study by Gillard et al. (5) described here was performed to search for additional mutations linked to MH in humans.

mRNA was obtained from muscle biopsies of three individuals known to be susceptible to MH, and cDNA was prepared using random priming. The DNA was amplified using PCR,

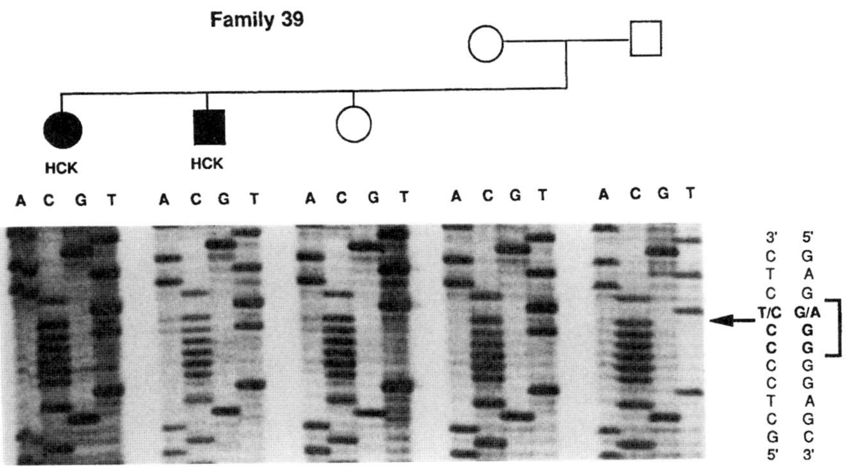

Figure 24. Mutations in a family with malignant hyperthermia. DNA from the RYR1 gene was amplified by PCR and sequenced in the region containing an Arg for Gly mutation. In the family tested, the mutation segregates with susceptibility to MH, as determined by halothane, caffeine, and halothane-caffeine tests (HCK). (Reprinted with permission from Gillard EF, Otsu K, Fujii J, et al. Polymorphisms and deduced amino acid substitutions in the coding sequence of the ryanodine receptor (RYR1) gene in individuals with malignant hyperthermia. *Genomics* 1992;13:1247–1254.)

sequenced, and the sequences obtained were tested for variants. Twenty-one changes from the normal gene sequence were noted in these three patients. Four of these nucleotide substitutions resulted in a change in amino acid sequence and could therefore play a causative role in the disease process. On the other hand, 13 of the changes resulted in the loss or gain of a restriction site and could therefore be used for RFLP analysis of MH. Both the amino acid substitutions and the RFLPs were studied separately.

Forty-five families with MH-susceptible members were studied to determine the presence or absence of the four amino acid substitutions and linkage of their presence to MH. As three of these substitutions also created an RFLP, their presence could easily be detected by PCR amplification of genomic DNA, followed by digestion with the appropriate restriction enzyme and gel electrophoresis. Presence or absence of the final substitution had to be determined by direct DNA sequencing. To this purpose, the sequence was amplified by PCR and the PCR product was sequenced. Only one of the mutations (Arg for Gly in position 248) segregated with MH-susceptibility in one of the 45 families (Fig. 24). Therefore, it could be a causative mutation in a selected group of patients. The other three mutations did not segregate with the disease in any family and must therefore be considered simple polymorphisms.

To study the 13 RFLPs, primers for use with PCR were synthesized flanking the region containing the variant. These were used to amplify these regions in members of MH-susceptible families, and the linkage between MH susceptibility and the RFLP was determined. Three of the RFLPs were found to be particularly useful for identifying MH-susceptible individuals and may be used for diagnostic purposes. This study therefore not only identified a potential causative mutation in a subgroup of MH patients, but also provided several new diagnostic tools.

Prevention and Treatment

Molecular biology not only plays a role in diagnosing diseases, but is becoming ever more prominent in treatment as well. Although attempts at gene therapy receive most news coverage, the role in the preparation of medications and vaccines is at the moment far more important. Gene therapy is still fraught with many problems. Although we have the capabilities to correct identified mutations in single cells, it is not clear at all how to target these corrected cells to the appropriate site in the body. In transgenic animals defective genes have been corrected successfully, but routine use in humans will need further study. Defects in the hematopoietic system are probably most easy to address, and, indeed, initial studies have corrected an immunodeficiency syndrome by removing lymphocytes from patients, infecting these cells with a modified virus carrying the corrected gene, and returning the cells to the patient. For other cell types, targeting therapy to the correct tissue will be much more difficult. We will discuss two examples of therapeutic uses of molecular biology: the preparation of hepatitis B vaccine and correction of the cystic fibrosis mutation in vitro.

Yeast Expression of Hepatitis B Vaccine

One of the concerns in vaccine preparation has always been the possibility of disease transmission through the vaccine. This problem can be solved by preparing so-called subunit vaccines, i.e. vaccines that consist only of the surface protein of the virus. When prepared recombinantly, such vaccines will carry no risk of infection.

Valenzuela et al. (16) reported synthesis of the surface antigen of the hepatitis B virus (HBsAg) in yeast cells (Fig. 25). The HBsAg sequence was isolated from the hepatitis B virus genome and subcloned into a yeast expression vector. The vector used was designed to be replicated to high copy number and contained a strong transcriptional promoter. Yeast cells were transfected and, after selection for uptake of the vector, grown to high density in fermentors. The yeast cells were isolated by centrifugation, and HBsAg particles could be isolated, which were shown to be antigenic. The yeast protein is now available as a commercial vaccine.

In Vitro Correction of Cystic Fibrosis

As mentioned above, the gene involved in cystic fibrosis has been cloned. Although its function is not completely clear at the moment, it appears to be involved in regulating Cl^- conductance across the cell membrane, and it is consequently termed the transmembrane conductance regulator. The result of a single amino acid deletion in this gene is disruption of Cl^- transport, leading to excessive viscosity of secretions. As the most disabling symptoms result from abnormal electrolyte transport in the airway epithelium, this has been an object of study for possible gene therapy. Although at present no effective therapy has been described, promising progress has been made. Several important problems, including the development of techniques to introduce genes stably into epithelial cells without causing alterations in gene expression, have been solved.

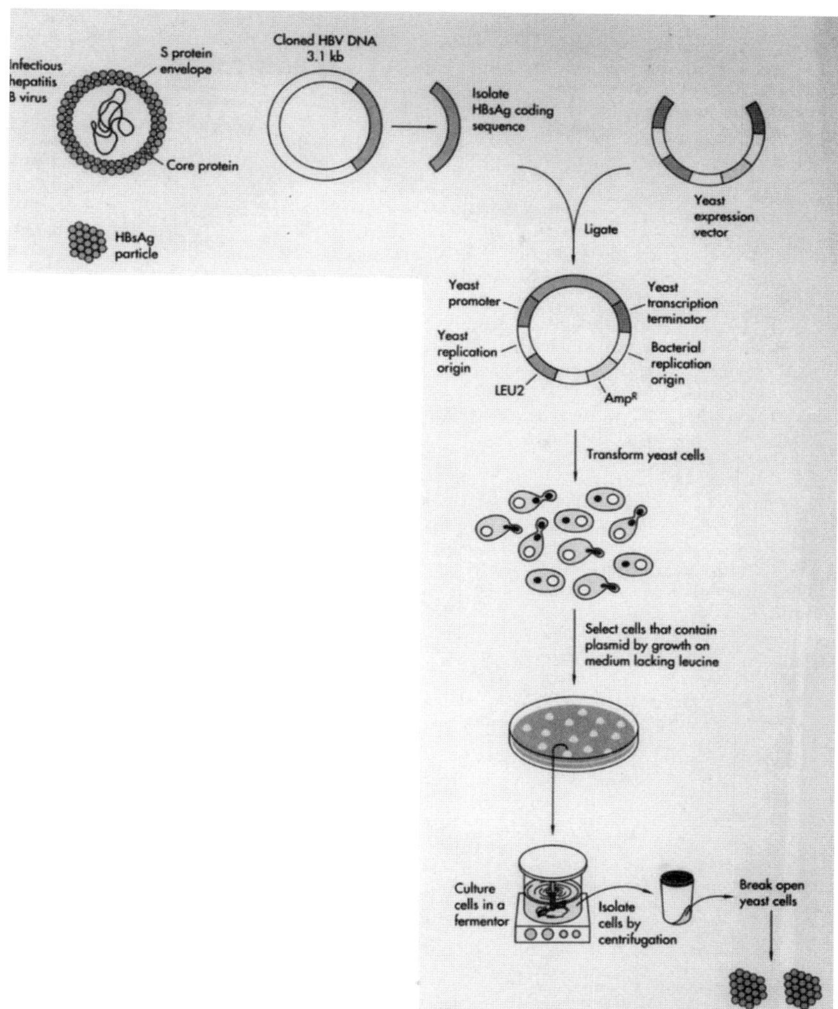

Figure 25. Recombinant preparation of a hepatitis B vaccine. The hepatitis B virus consists of a small genome encapsulated in core protein and an S protein envelope. The latter can form HBsAg particles in isolation. The HBsAg coding sequence was cloned into a yeast expression vector, between a strong promoter and a transcription terminator. Also present on the vector are both bacterial and yeast replication origins, to allow propagation in either host, and selection systems. The vector was used to transform yeast cells, isolated by its ability to grow in leucine-free media (induced by the LEU2 gene on the vector), and grown to high density in fermentors. The HBsAg particles could be extracted by centrifugation and were subsequently shown to be antigenic. (Reprinted with permission from Watson JD, Gilman M, Witkowski J, Zoller M. *Recombinant DNA.* 2nd ed. New York: W. H. Freeman, 1992.)

Rich et al. (14) described the correction of the cystic fibrosis (CF) defect in airway epithelial cells. A cDNA of the normal CF gene was constructed and introduced, using the vaccinia virus system, into a cell line carrying an abnormal CF gene. Cl^- conductance in response to adenylate cyclase activation was measured in these cells and was found to be comparable to that of normal human airway epithelial cells. Because the main pathologic findings in CF concern the airways, a straightforward method for targeting the gene to its site of action would be to deliver it by aerosol. CF patients could inhale aerosols carrying a functioning conductance regulator gene. This approach has been studied to a limited extent in transgenic animals and may one day be available to humans.

CONCLUSIONS

Molecular biology has affected many areas of biological research. Indeed, it is becoming increasingly difficult to follow the basic science literature without at least some understanding of molecular biology principles. The reason for the explosion of interest is clear: these techniques have not only allowed access to the genome, but have also made a large number of studies, particularly of proteins, much easier to perform. Molecular biology has several properties that set it apart from the remainder of science. It is a "modular" science. Experiments can take many weeks, with each step building on the results of the previous one. It is also a nonstatistical science, which can be unnerving to those of us used to seeing means and SEs. However, once the basics are understood, the easy availability of optimized protocols, the development of PCR, and the use of kits and nonradioactive labeling techniques should make these approaches accessible to almost all researchers.

REFERENCES

1. Alberts B, Bray D, Lewis J, Raff M, Roberts K, Watson JD. *Molecular biology of the cell.* 2nd ed. New York: Garland, 1989.
2. Ausubel FM, Brent R, Kungston RE, et al. *Current protocols in molecular biology.* Greene Publishing, 1989.
3. Dixon RAF, Kobilka BK, Strader DJ, et al. Cloning of the gene and cDNA for mammalian β-adrenergic receptor and homology with rhodopsin. *Nature* 1986;342:75–79.
4. Fujii J, Otsu K, Zorzato F, et al. Identification of a mutation in porcine ryanodine receptor associated with malignant hyperthermia. *Science* 1991;253:448–451.
5. Gillard EF, Otsu K, Fujii J, et al. Polymorphisms and deduced amino acid substitutions in the coding sequence of the ryanodine receptor (RYR1) gene in individuals with malignant hyperthermia. *Genomics* 1992;13:1247–1254.
6. Genetics Computer Group. *Program manual for the GCG package, version 7.* Madison, WI: Genetics Computer Group, 1991.
7. Kieffer NL, Befort K, Gaveriaux-Ruff C, Hirth CG. The δ-opioid receptor: isolation of a cDNA by expression cloning and pharmacological characterization. *Proc Natl Acad Sci USA* 1992;89: 12048–12052.

8. Kobilka BK, Kobilka TS, Daniel D, Regan JW, Caron MC, Lefkowitz RJ. 2-Adrenergic receptors: delineation of domains involved in effector coupling and ligand binding specificity. *Science* 1988;240: 1310–1316.
9. Kogan SC, Doherty M, Gitschier J. An improved method for prenatal diagnosis of genetic diseases by analysis of amplified DNA sequences; application to hemophilia A. *N Engl J Med* 1987;317: 985–990.
10. Kyte J, Doolittle RF. A simple method for displaying the hydropathic character of a protein. *J Mol Biol* 1982;157:105–132.
11. Lemna WK, Feldman GL, Kerem B, et al. Mutation analysis for heterozygote detection and the prenatal diagnosis of cystic fibrosis. *N Engl J Med* 1990;322:291–296.
12. Mailleux P, Parmentier M, Vanderhaeghen JJ. Distribution of cannabinoid receptor messenger RNA in the human brain: an in situ hybridization histochemistry with oligonucleotides. *Neurosci Lett* 1992;143:200–204.
13. Matsuda LA, Lolait SJ, Brownstein MJ, Young AC, Bonner TI. Structure of a cannabinoid receptor and functional expression of the cloned cDNA. *Nature* 1990;346:561–564.
14. Rich DP, Anderson MP, Gregory RJ, et al. Expression of cystic fibrosis transmembrane conductance regulator corrects defective chloride channel regulation in cystic fibrosis airway epithelial cells. *Nature* 1990;347:358–363.
15. Sambrook J, Fritsch EF, Maniatis T. *Molecular cloning, a laboratory manual.* 2nd ed. Cold Spring Harbor, NY: Cold Spring Harbor Laboratory Press, 1989.
16. Valenzuela P, Medina A, Rutter WJ, Ammerer G, Hall BD. Synthesis and assembly of hepatitis B virus surface antigen particles in yeast. *Nature* 1982;298:347–350.
17. Watson JD, Gilman M, Witkowski J, Zoller M. *Recombinant DNA.* 2nd ed. New York: W. H. Freeman, 1992.
18. Watson JD, Hopkins NH, Roberts JW, Steitz JA, Weiner AM. *Molecular biology of the gene.* 4th ed. Menlo Park, CA: Benjamin/Cummings, 1987.
19. Watson JD, Tooze J. *The DNA story: a documentary history of gene cloning.* New York: W. H. Freeman, 1981.

Anesthesia: Biologic Foundations, edited by
Tony L. Yaksh et al. Lippincott–Raven Publishers,
Philadelphia © 1997.

CHAPTER 23

USE OF NUCLEAR MAGNETIC RESONANCE AND ELECTRON PARAMAGNETIC RESONANCE IN ANESTHESIA RESEARCH

YAN XU AND LEONARD FIRESTONE

The invisible forces that cause certain objects to attract or repel each other have fascinated humanity since the dawn of civilization. In the ancient city of Magnesia (Manisa, Turkey), rocks were found that could orient themselves in a certain direction and regain that direction after being spun on their axes. This property was later termed magnetism after the name of the ancient city.

Magnetism exists also at the atomic level. The microscopic quantities related to the magnetic property of nuclei and electrons are, respectively, the nuclear and electron magnetic moments, often denoted by μ. In 1946, Bloch et al. (15) and Purcell et al. (184) discovered the phenomenon of magnetic resonance, in which magnetic moments were measured in an externally applied magnetic field, $\mathbf{B_0}$. When the nuclear magnetic moment is measured, the technique is called nuclear magnetic resonance (NMR). Similarly, when the electron magnetic moment is measured, the technique is electron magnetic resonance or, more commonly, electron paramagnetic resonance (EPR). The term paramagnetic emphasizes the fact that unpaired electrons are strongly attracted by the magnetic field.

Soon after their initial development in physics laboratories, NMR and EPR became widely used in other fields of science, particularly chemistry and material science. Unlike many other physical techniques, magnetic resonance, especially NMR, has a unique potential for the study of biologic samples, including humans. As early as the 1950s, not long after the discovery of NMR, Purcell and Hahn (99,146) tried the first biologic NMR experiments, and Singer (196) measured blood flow with NMR. Not until 1971, however, did NMR engage the medical community, when Damadian (34) found that healthy and diseased tissues differed in their NMR spectral characteristics. Two years later, Lauterbur (125) astonished the NMR community by using magnetic field gradients superimposed on $\mathbf{B_0}$ to image biologic samples. Since then, the field of magnetic resonance has rapidly expanded to include magnetic resonance imaging (MRI) for clinical diagnosis, and the technology of magnetic resonance has become an indispensable part of modern medicine. Research using new and improved NMR and EPR techniques has made it possible to answer an ever-increasing variety of clinical questions, including those in anesthesiology.

In this chapter, the basic principles common to NMR (including MRI) and EPR are discussed, followed by separate accounts of NMR and EPR techniques and their use in anesthesiology research. Because anesthesiology encompasses a broad area of drug action and physiology at molecular, cellular, tissue, and intact animal levels, the discussion is organized on the basis of the techniques used *and* on the complexity of the system studied.

BASIC PRINCIPLES OF MAGNETIC RESONANCE

Nuclear and Electron Spins

Directly related to the magnetic moment of nuclei and electrons is a basic physical quantity known as angular momentum. A classical example of angular momentum is a top spinning at an angle relative to the vertical line of gravity (Fig. 1A). Instead of tipping over, the spinning top precesses about the vertical line by virtue of interaction between the angular momentum, **P**, and the gravity, **G**. Although a full description of nuclear and electron angular momenta requires quantum mechanics, this classical analogy is so vivid that the intrinsic angular momentum of nuclei and electrons is referred to as nuclear spin (**I**) and electron spin (**S**), respectively (Fig. 1B).

Yet nuclear and electron spins differ from classical angular momentum in that they are quantized. This means that the spins, as vectors, can take only discrete numbers of directions relative to the external magnetic field $\mathbf{B_0}$. All electrons have a spin of 1/2 (i.e., $|\mathbf{S}| = 1/2$) and can take only two possible directions, denoted by +1/2 or −1/2, depending on the spin projection onto the direction of $\mathbf{B_0}$. For any given atom, a basic physical principle (the Pauli's exclusion principle) requires that no two electrons occupy exactly the same quantum state. Thus, the maximum number of electrons that can share the same orbital state is two, with the two spin projections being in the opposite directions. When this occurs, the two spins are paired and the resultant spin is zero. Only those molecular species with unpaired electrons are amenable to EPR. The observed total of electron spin depends on the number of unpaired electrons.

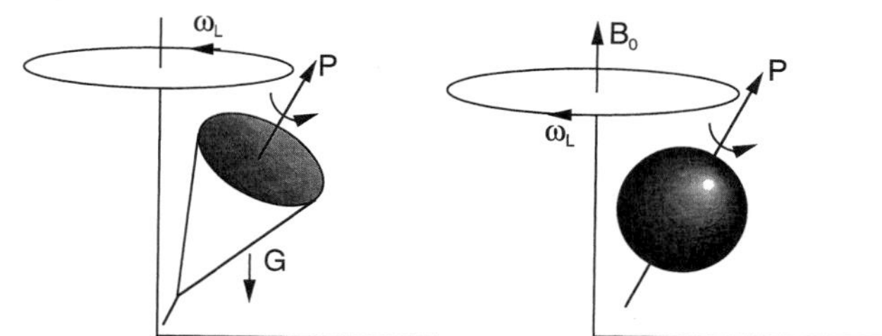

Figure 1. **A**: A spinning top does not tip over because of interaction between the spinning angular momentum, **P**, and gravity, **G**. This interaction exerts a torque perpendicular to both **P** and **G** to cause the top to precess about the vertical line at an angular speed, ω_L, called Larmor frequency. **B**: Analogous to the spinning top, nuclear or electron spins and the associated magnetic moments, μ, interact with the magnetic field, $\mathbf{B_0}$, to induce spin precession about $\mathbf{B_0}$. The precession frequencies for nuclei and electrons are $\omega_L = \gamma B_0$ and $\omega_L = g\mu_B B_0/\hbar$, respectively.

The situation is slightly more complicated with nuclei, which are composed of protons and neutrons. Each proton and neutron has a spin of 1/2. For nuclei of different elements or different isotopes of the same element, the observed total of nuclear spin depends on the internal construction of nuclei. General rules are as follows: (a) nuclei with an odd mass number have a half-integral spin (±1/2, ±3/2, . . .); (b) nuclei with an even mass number but an odd charge number have an integral spin (±1, ±2, . . .); and (c) nuclei with an even mass number and an even charge number have a zero spin. For example, ^{1}H, ^{13}C, ^{19}F, and ^{31}P have spin of 1/2; ^{23}Na, ^{35}Cl, and ^{39}K have spin of 3/2; ^{2}H and ^{14}N have spin of 1; and ^{12}C, ^{16}O, and ^{32}S have spin of 0. Only those nuclei with nonzero spins are amenable to NMR and MRI. Among nonzero spins, spin 1/2 and spin greater than 1/2 have different characteristics. The latter, called quadrupolar nuclei, have a nonspherical symmetry and can respond not only to a magnetic field, but also to electric field gradients to give rise to the so-called quadrupolar splitting and quadrupolar relaxation.

Origin of NMR and EPR Signals

A magnetic moment is generated when a charged particle, such as a nucleus or an electron, spins. This moment is given by $\mu = g\mu_B s$ for electrons and $\mu = g_N \mu_N I$ for nuclei. The quantities μ_B and μ_N, called the Bohr magneton and the nuclear magneton, are the unit measures for electron and nuclear magnetic moments, respectively ($\mu_B \approx 9.27 \times 10^{-24}$ JT^{-1} and $\mu_N \approx 5.05 \times 10^{-27}$ JT^{-1}, where J [joule] and T [tesla] are the SI units for energy and magnetic field induction, respectively). The proportional factors g and g_N are called the Landé slitting factor (or simply g-factor) and the nuclear g-factor, respectively. Because g_N is nucleus specific, it is customary in NMR to define another variable, the magnetogyric ratio γ, such that $\mu = \gamma\hbar$ **I** (or $\gamma = g_N\mu_N/\hbar$), where $\hbar$ is Planck constant ($\hbar \approx 1.05 \times 10^{-34}$ Js).

A magnetic moment μ in a magnetic field $\mathbf{B_0}$ has an energy E given by $E = -\mu \cdot \mathbf{B_0}$. Because the orientations of **I** and **S** are quantized, so is the energy calculated from this dot product (the projection). Figure 2 depicts a spin energy diagram for a single nucleus with I = 1/2 (such as ^{1}H) as a function of the magnetic field B_0. (For electrons or nuclei with negative γ, the energy diagram is similar except that the −1/2 projection has a lower energy.) Using the relationship between μ and **I** (or μ and **S**), it is easy to show that the energy difference between the two energy levels for nuclei and electrons are $\Delta E = g_N\mu_N B_0 = (\hbar\gamma B_0$ and $\Delta E = g\mu_B B_0$, respectively. For spins other than 1/2, the total number of energy levels is 2I + 1 (or 2S + 1). The energy difference between the adjacent levels is, again, given by these equations.

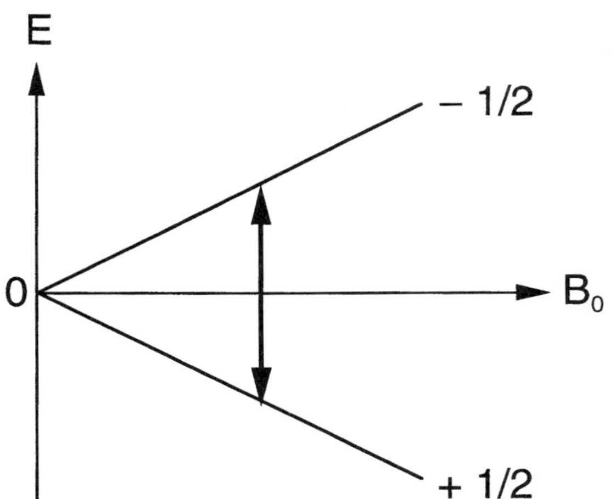

Figure 2. The nuclear spin energy for a single nucleus with I = 1/2 (such as ^{1}H) is plotted as a function of the magnetic field B_0. Transition between the two levels for a particular value of B_0 is indicated by the double-headed arrow. The length of the arrow represents the energy absorbed or emitted during the transition. NMR spectroscopy records such transitions.

In NMR or EPR experiments, energy in the form of electromagnetic radiation is applied perpendicular to $\mathbf{B_0}$. This energy is absorbed and emitted by nuclear or electron spins to induce transitions between the spin energy levels (i.e., flip-flop among the possible orientations). The condition that the absorbed energy matches the energy gap ΔE is called the resonance condition. Because radiation energy is given by $\hbar\omega$, where ω is 2π times the radiation frequency, u, the resonance condition for NMR and EPR are, respectively:

$$\omega = \gamma B_0 \quad [1]$$

and

$$\hbar\omega = h\upsilon = g\mu_B B_0 \quad [2]$$

where $h = 2\pi\hbar$. The w (or υ) values fulfilling these equations are called Larmor frequencies.

From equations [1] and [2] (also see Fig. 2), it is clear that the resonance condition is a function of B_0. For a typical clinical MRI scanner, B_0 is ~0.5–1.5 T; for a high-resolution NMR magnet, B_0 is ~2.3–17.4 T; and for a conventional X-band EPR, B_0 is ~0.3 T. Using the values of μ_N (or γ) and μ_B, it can be estimated that the energy under the resonance condition is on the order of magnitude of 10^{-25} J for NMR and MRI, and 10^{-23} J for EPR. The corresponding Larmor frequencies are in the radiofrequency range ($10–700 \times 10^6$ Hz) for NMR and MRI, and the microwave range ($1–4 \times 10^9$ Hz; wavelength of 3–0.8 cm) for EPR. (Note that μ_B is ~1.8×10^3 times larger than μ_N.)

These energies, however, are usually too weak to detect from individual spins. The signals measured in NMR and EPR result from the so-called resonance phenomenon, in which an ensemble of spins act coherently in response to the electromagnetic radiation. Because at thermal equilibrium, there are slightly more spins at the lower energy levels than at the higher energy levels (the Boltzmann distribution), the net excess in spin population of some orientations over others adds up to a macroscopic magnetic quantity called magnetization (denoted by **M**). The intensities of the coherence, and thus the NMR or EPR signal strengths, are determined by |**M**|.

NMR and EPR Spectrometers

Although technical implementation is different for NMR and EPR, the basic construction of NMR (including MRI) and EPR spectrometers is quite similar. A spectrometer typically has three main parts: a magnet; an operating console; and a transceiver, known as a probe for NMR and MRI or a cavity for EPR. Figure 3 shows a block diagram of an NMR or EPR spectrometer.

The need for a magnet is obvious. In modern NMR and MRI, superconducting magnets with a bore size ranging from a few cm up to 1 m in diameter are common. Most EPR spectrometers use either permanent or electric magnets, with associated power supplies and cooling systems.

A console usually consists of a pulse programmer (for NMR and MRI) or a microwave frequency generator (for EPR), one or more transmitters with power amplifiers, one or more receivers with analog-to-digital converters and digitizers, and a computer with associated human-machine interfaces and other input/output devices. A nuts-and-bolts discussion is beyond the scope of this chapter. Excellent texts on the topic are available (88,108).

A transceiver is a critical device that delivers the excitation energy to the sample and receives the resonance signal from the sample. In NMR and MRI, the probe may be of numerous designs. The most commonly used for in vivo studies are birdcage resonators and surface coil probes.

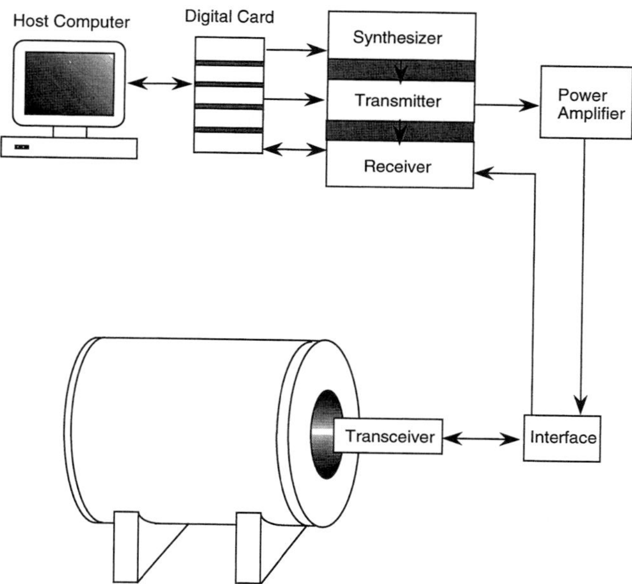

Figure 3. A block diagram of an NMR or EPR spectrometer.

NMR TECHNIQUES

Technical Overview

Free-Induction Decay and Fourier Transformation

It seems straightforward to match the resonance condition by sweeping the electromagnetic radiation frequency in the vicinity of the Larmor frequency ($\omega_L = \gamma B_0$) of a given nucleus. This frequency-domain method was used in the earlier years of NMR development, but proved inefficient because most time was spent sweeping the spectral baselines, which contain only noise. A truly revolutionary change for time-domain NMR acquisition was suggested in 1957 (140) and realized 9 years later (59). In the time domain, coherence occurs when an ensemble of spins respond to very strong RF pulses. Because a RF pulse with short time duration contains a wide band of frequencies (bandwidth ≈ 1/pulse-duration), it excites nuclei of different frequencies all at once. After excitation, spins are allowed to relax in the absence of pulses. This relaxation process, called free-induction decay (FID, meaning relaxation in the absence of pulses), emits nuclear spin energies that are recorded as a function of time by the NMR spectrometer. Figure 4A shows a representative FID of ^{19}F nuclei in isoflurane, a fluorinated volatile general anesthetic of clinical importance.

This time-domain FID contains rich frequency information. To reveal this information, a purely mathematical transformation, called Fourier transformation (FT), is carried out to convert time-domain decay into frequency-domain spectrum. For the FID seen in Fig. 4A, Fourier transformation yields the spectrum shown in Fig. 4B. The peaks in the spectrum can be assigned to different groups of ^{19}F nuclei in the isoflurane molecules (CF_3-CHCl-O-CHF_2).

Spectral Intensity

NMR peak intensities are measured by the areas under the peaks. These areas are proportional to the number of nuclei contributing to the peaks. For the spectrum seen in Fig. 4B, the ratio of the singlet to doublet is 3:2, indicating that the ^{19}F nuclei in the -CF_3 group are magnetically equivalent and combine to give rise to the singlet; whereas those in the -CHF_2 group give rise to the doublet. As will be discussed later, the proportional relationship between the NMR intensity and the number of nuclei contributing to the intensity is the basis for noninvasive NMR analysis of energy metabolism, anesthetic uptake and elimination, blood flow, and anesthetic distribution.

Chemical Shift and Relaxation Time

What makes NMR and MRI among the most powerful analytical and diagnostic tools is the high resolution achievable in probing the molecular environment of the observed nuclei. Resolution, referring to the ability to distinguish spectral differences, appears primarily as changes in resonance frequencies or in the lifetime of coherence.

The most commonly known frequency change in NMR spectroscopy is chemical shift, often measured in parts per million (ppm) relative to a standard sample or to the spectrometer frequency. Chemical shifts result from electron shielding of the external magnetic field. Movement of electrons about the nuclei generates a secondary field, which is superimposed on B_0. Because resonance frequency of a nucleus is proportional to the magnetic field actually sensed by the nucleus, the same kind of isotopes (e.g., ^{19}F of isoflurane in Fig. 4) in different chemical environments will experience slightly different electronic shielding, and thus resonate at different frequencies. For example, ^{19}F in the -CF_3 group in isoflurane experiences a different microenvironment from ^{19}F in the -CHF_2 group. This difference results in the chemical shifts for the singlet at -3.4 ppm (less electron shielding) and the doublet at -9.5 ppm (more electron shielding).

In addition to electron shielding, other interactions may also cause frequency changes. These include the so-called J-J coupling (coupling through chemical bonds), nuclear dipole-dipole interaction, nucleus-electron spin coupling, and interaction of quadrupolar nuclei with nonzero electric field gradient. For example, in Fig. 4B, the splitting of the doublet results from the J-J coupling between the two ^{19}F nuclei in the -CHF_2 group. Analysis of chemical shifts and spectral splitting allows for detailed characterization of the molecular environment, in which the nuclei under investigation reside.

The decaying profile of FID (Fig. 4A, *dashed lines*) is another spectral feature indicative of the nuclear microenvironment. The motion of an ensemble of spins, as quantified by the magnetization M, is characterized by two time constants: the longitudinal relaxation time, T_1, and transverse relaxation time, T_2. After M is driven to a nonequilibrium state, two processes can occur. In one, the spin energy is transferred into other forms of energy, which are collectively referred to as lattice energy. The T_1 time constant measures how fast this transfer proceeds. A period of T_1 is the time required for M to recover by 63% (i.e., $1 - e^{-1}$) from the nonequilibrium state. In the other process, the spin energy is exchanged and redistributed within the nuclear spin system. This process does not restore thermal equilibrium, but causes spins to lose their initial coherence. The T_2 time constant characterizes the rate of this process. A period of T_2 is the time after which 63% of the initial coherence is lost.

T_1 and T_2 reflect the motional characteristics of the molecules bearing the nuclei under investigation. In general, a long T_2 indicates a relatively free (or more mobile) microenvironment, whereas a short T_2 indicates a relatively bound (or less mobile) microenvironment.

In MRI, differences in T_1 or T_2 among various tissue types have been used to improve imaging contrast. For example, a region with longer T_1 requires a longer waiting time between consecutive pulses to avoid saturating the magnetization. If pulse repetition rate is manipulated such that tissues with long T_1 are not fully relaxed, these tissues will appear to have lower MRI intensity due to saturation. In contrast, regions with shorter T_1 will be hyperintensive. Numerous pulse schemes have been developed to take the advantage of the T_1 or T_2 distribution in living systems (207). Table 1 summarizes typical T_1 and T_2 values of water protons at 1 T in various tissues.

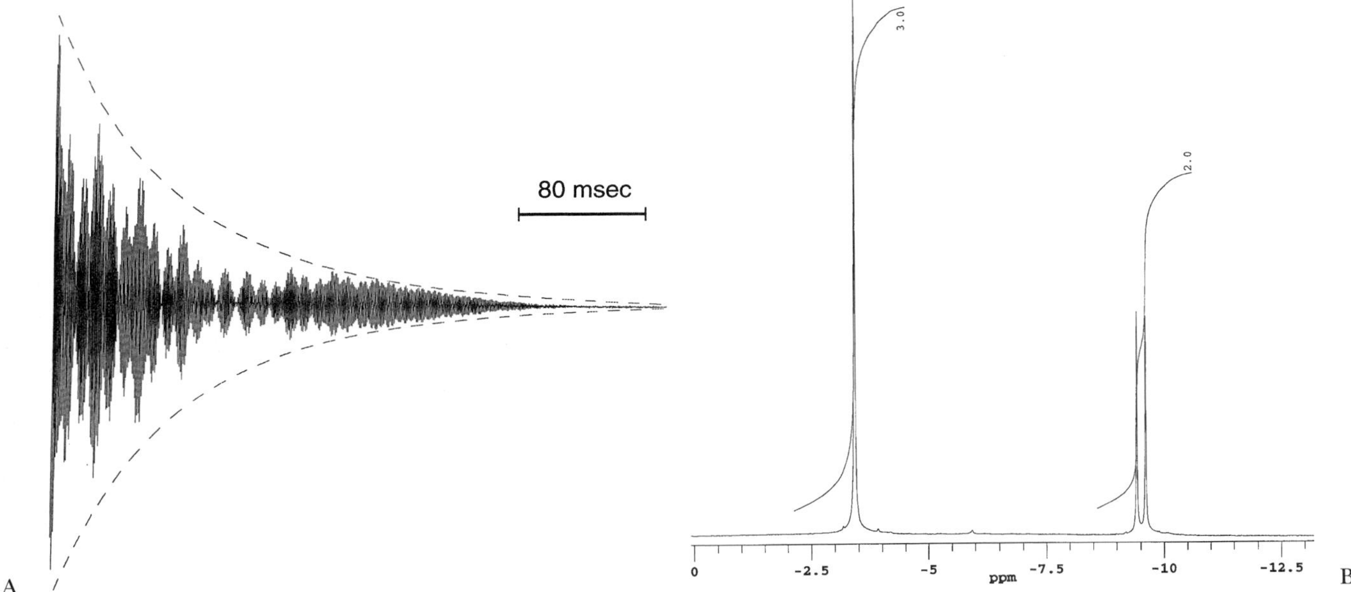

Figure 4. **A**: Representative ^{19}F free-induction decay (FID) of isoflurane dissolved in a Hepes buffer. The oscillation of the decay contains frequency information, whereas the profile (or envelope) of the decay is related to the lifetime (T_2) of the coherence. **B**: Resultant ^{19}F NMR spectrum of isoflurane after Fourier transformation of A.

Magnetic Gradient: A Bridge Between Frequency and Space

The concept of MRI stems from the most basic principle of NMR, that is, the proportional relationship between frequency and magnetic field strength. Imagine that an ensemble of nuclear spins, of exactly the same type, are distributed along a one-dimensional line. If these spins are in a homogeneous field B_0, they would all resonate at the same frequency. If, however, these spins are in a field whose strength increases linearly from one end of the line to the other, the spins at different segments on the line would experience different field strengths, and resonate at different frequencies. Thus, the location of the spins along the line is recorded as frequency changes in the form of a spectrum. In MRI terminology, this process is called frequency encoding. The magnetic field with its strength increasing linearly in space is called the magnetic field gradient. The encoding can be carried out in all three spatial dimensions, and an MRI scanner can decode and display the encoded information as images.

Table 1. APPROXIMATE T_1 AND T_2 VALUES FOR ^1H IN VARIOUS TISSUES AT 1 T[a]

Tissue type	T_1 (ms)	T_2 (ms)
Fat	180	90
Muscle	600	40
Liver	270	50
Spleen	480	80
White matter	390	90
Gray matter	520	100
Blood	800	180
Cerebrospinal fluid	2,000	300

[a]T_1 and T_2 of ^1H in pure water are ~2,500 ms.

NMR Studies of Mechanisms of General Anesthetic Action

Controversies

The century-long quest for the molecular and cellular mechanisms of general anesthesia continues to be one of the great scientific challenges. Two points of view prevail: according to one, anesthetic agents cause a generalized perturbation of neuronal membrane structure through a *nonspecific* interaction with membrane lipids (11,25,74,104,120,154); according to the other, anesthetics bind to sets of *specific* sites of appropriate molecular dimension on membrane proteins (64,65,79,82,84, 85,164,187). Some attempts have also been made to couple the colligative lipid effects to lipid-matrix-mediated modulations of membrane proteins without receptor binding (95,96). Although significant progress has been made along these lines, an unequivocal mechanism for general anesthesia has not yet been identified.

NMR is a unique and powerful technique to tackle some of the difficulties in resolving these controversies. The advantages of NMR methods come from the compatibility of the NMR time scale with that of anesthetic action. The effective concentrations (e.g., EC_{50}) of most general anesthetics are in the millimolar range, suggesting that anesthetics are in rapid exchange among different pools, including those considered as crucial sites of action. If the exchange is examined under the context of binding and dissociation, irrespective of lipid or protein action, the dissociation constants, K_D, must be in the range of 10^{-3} M or higher. A conventional biochemical determination of ligand binding relies on effective separation of bound from free ligand after an equilibrium is reached. Such a Scatchard type of analysis is accurate only when $K_D \leq 10^{-5}$ M. Pharmacologic competition of strong ligands with weak ones can potentially extend the range of measurable affinity to 10^{-4} M. The NMR approach, on the other hand, allows for analysis of low-affinity interactions ($K_D \geq 10^{-4}$ M) with great precision.

Anesthetic-Lipid Interaction

General anesthetics, which range from simple monatomic inert gases to complex steroids, share no structural commonality. It thus seems to be a natural conclusion, though more or less on a priori grounds, that general anesthetics exert their primary effects by dissolving in and perturbing the lipid bilayer of excitable membranes, rather than by fitting into a single cleft in proteins. The well-known Meyer-Overton rule provides evidence showing a strong correlation between the potency of an anesthetic agent and its ability to partition into a hydrophobic phase, such as olive oil. The molecular details of interaction between anesthetics and lipids thus became the focus of many early NMR investigations.

Trudell and Hubbell (211) carried out the pioneering work using ^{19}F-NMR to determine the location of the fluorinated anesthetic halothane in phospholipid membranes. Chemical shifts of ^{19}F nuclei in halothane molecules were measured separately in lipid, water, and hexane. Hexane was chosen to mimic the environment of the interior of a phospholipid bilayer. The authors' initial proposition was that if halothane molecules partitioned statically in the lipid and the surrounding aqueous environment, then they would resonate at two frequencies: one near the chemical shift due to hexane and the other at the chemical shift due to water. What they found, however, was a single chemical shift intermediate between the two expected frequencies, suggesting that the halothane molecules exchanged rapidly between the membrane interior and the aqueous environment. To further confirm this, they introduced stable free radicals at different locations in the membrane. These free radicals could broaden the resonance lines of halothane molecules located in the immediate proximity of the radicals. It was found again that rapid exchange caused equal broadening of spectral lines, irrespective of the location of the free radicals. The same conclusion was reached using paramagnetic ions, which would have been expected to broaden only peaks from halothane in the aqueous phase. It was concluded that molecular theories of anesthesia must include not only a fluid and rapidly exchanging membrane, but also anesthetic molecules in rapid exchange among different environments in the neuronal membranes.

Line broadening induced by free radicals or paramagnetic ions belongs to a more general effect, in which T_2 relaxation is enhanced. Compared with visual inspection of spectral linewidths, T_2 measurements can provide more accurate identification of linewidth components. Situations may exist in which different environments are indistinguishable in chemical shifts but appear as different components in the relaxation times. As will be shown later, this is often the case in vivo.

The existence of two or more T_2 components does not negate the conclusion of Trudell and Hubbell that anesthetics are in rapid exchange between different microenvironments. The rate of exchange is characterized by a statistically significant time, τ_{ex}, during which anesthetic can relocate from one environment to the other. A meaningful assessment of rapidity is to compare τ_{ex} with the characteristic time of the measurements. For chemical shift, the characteristic time can be estimated by $1/\Delta\upsilon$, where $\Delta\upsilon$ is the chemical shift difference between various microenvironments. Thus, if $\tau_{ex} << 1/\Delta\upsilon$, the exchange is considered rapid by the chemical shift standard. For example, for halothane in water and hexane, $\Delta\upsilon \approx 1.8$ ppm, corresponding to 170 Hz at 2.3 T. Therefore, τ_{ex} must be faster than 1 μs for the two resonance frequencies to coalesce into one. In contrast, a T_2 measurement has a time resolution on the order of 1~10 μs. If τ_{ex} is comparable to or slower than this, then different environments may appear as different components in T_2 relaxation.

Coalescence of chemical shifts due to rapid exchange has been used to study the subcellular distribution of general anesthetics. A two-site exchange between lipid and water is often assumed to simplify the theoretical consideration. The observed shifts are treated as weighted averages of two limiting shifts: that in the lipid and that in the water. If the lipid concentration is increased at a constant anesthetic concentration, then the resultant shift as a function of lipid concentration is indicative of anesthetic preference to different lipid environments. A knowledge of dynamic partitioning of anesthetic in lipid can thus be deduced (233). Conversely, if the anesthetic concentration is increased at a fixed lipid concentration, the effects of anesthetic molecules on membrane structure can be analyzed. Numerous studies have been carried out using these approaches (113,119,204,205,232,233). Of significance is the finding that the water/lipid partition coefficients differ for different moieties of the same anesthetic molecules (233), suggesting that interaction of general anesthetics with membrane is directed toward the lipid-water interface, with anesthetic molecules poised in specific orientations relative to the membrane surface.

Taking a different approach, Kelusky et al. (116,197–199) investigated anesthetic-lipid interaction using deuterium (^{2}H) NMR in a condensed (solid) phase of lipids. Deuterium (I = 1) is a quadrupolar nucleus, and hence subject to quadrupolar splitting and quadrupolar relaxation due to nonzero averaged electric field gradient in an ordered membrane. (Lipids have charge centers in the head group. In a solid state, which restricts motion, the electric fields generated by these charge centers do not average to zero; rather they combine to produce a steady-state electric field gradient inside and outside the membrane.) Without losing generality of the approach, Smith et al. (197) systematically studied the influence of a local anesthetic, tetracaine (TTC), on the order of lipids. Deuterium labels were separately introduced in the head and tail regions of phosphatidylcholine (PC) lipids, as well as at different positions in the TTC molecules. The quadrupolar splitting of the ^{2}H labels was used to calculate the so-called order parameter (195), which may have a value ranging from 0 (no order) to 1 (perfect order). It was found that TTC fluidized (i.e., disordered) the tail region of the lipid, and altered the orientation of the head group relative to the membrane surface. Moreover, when TTC was changed from a charged form (assumed at pH = 5.5) to a neutral form (assumed at pH = 9), its influence on the head and tail regions differed. It was concluded that in the neutral form, TTC was located deeper within the lipid bilayer, whereas in the charged form, it was located at the lipid-water interface.

Although chemical shifts and quadrupolar splitting are indicative of macroscopic perturbation by anesthetics to the bulk lipids, they offer only indirect information (e.g., through perturbation to selected labels) about the location of anesthetic molecules in the membrane. Attempts have been made to use the nuclear Overhauser effect (NOE) to determine site-specific interactions (231). Because of its dependence on nuclear dipole-dipole interaction, which is inversely proportional to the sixth power of the internuclear distance, NOE occurs only when the interacting nuclei are close to each other. When NOE is measured in a two-dimensional (2D) NOE spectroscopy (NOESY) experiment, nuclei are allowed to evolve in the absence of pulses in two distinct time periods. These two periods are separated by a third period called mixing time. If through NOE two nuclei interact during the mixing time, the resonance of one nucleus will modulate the other. This modulation will appear in the 2D NOESY spectrum as an off-diagonal peak (also called cross peak). In a ^{1}H-NOESY experiment (mixing time = 150 μs) using methoxyflurane in PC vesicles (231), a pair of weak cross peaks seemed to occur between the choline methyl protons of the PC and the hydrophobic methoxy protons of methoxyflurane. No other cross peaks were found. These results were claimed as a direct evidence showing that the probability of finding anesthetic molecules was highest at the interface.

NOESY data must be interpreted with caution, however. Unlike intramolecular NOE, intermolecular NOE, such as that between anesthetics and membrane, is difficult to detect. Rapid movement of anesthetic molecules relative to membrane reduces the efficiency of intermolecular NOE buildup; a long mixing time is thus required. This requirement, however, is opposed by the intrinsic T_1 relaxation and NOE between nuclei of the same species (142). Therefore, failure to detect cross peaks may result from insufficient detection sensitivity rather than absence of interaction.

In most NMR analyses of anesthetic-lipid interaction, extremely high anesthetic concentrations, often one to two orders of magnitude higher than the clinical concentration, must be used to detect any significant spectral changes (17,76,130,212). The question thus arises as to whether any of the detected changes are relevant to the action of general anesthetics. Indeed, many proposed perturbations and changes in bulk membrane by general anesthetics can be reproduced by increasing the membrane temperature by a few degrees. Moreover, a recent study in rats shows that changes in membrane physical properties persist after animals revive from anesthesia (193).

Thus, the investigative approach to the lipid theory of general anesthesia should consist of at least the following three steps: (a) identify the sites of interaction; (b) identify, among all sites of interaction, those sites where the interaction is consistent with the clinical response to general anesthetics (that is, identify the sites of action); and (c) determine how interaction at the sites of action can produce general anesthesia. Most NMR studies to date have been confined to the first step. More studies are needed to extend our knowledge beyond the current limitation.

Recently, a novel approach was taken by Tang and Xu (208,228), in which xenon, a noble gas having favorable general anesthetic properties (18,123,158), was used as a molecular probe to examine the site-specific interaction between anesthetics and phospholipid model membranes. Because of its chemical inertness and lack of structure, xenon offers a chemically unbiased assessment of the sites where strong anesthetic-membrane interactions are most likely to occur. Intermolecular, heteronuclear, truncated driven NOE, a method based not on coherent frequency change but on noncoherent NOE transfer, was used to determine the dipole-dipole interaction between xenon and selected protons in different membrane locations. At the clinical concentration of xenon, the most favorable location for xenon-membrane interaction was at the lipid head region. Involvement of interfacial water was also evident. Because xenon is extremely sensitive to its environment and at the same time is a weak anesthetic, coadministration of potent anesthetics at their clinical concentrations to compete for xenon binding sites can potentially alter the interaction pattern of xenon with the membrane. This competition method has the potential to be used as a pathfinder to accomplish the second step, described above.

Anesthetic-Protein Interaction

Protein theories of general anesthetic action are based on the key observation by Franks and Lieb (77) that the soluble (thus lipid-free) protein luciferase can be competitively inhibited by a diverse range of simple anesthetic agents at concentrations close to those causing general anesthesia. Subsequent studies also show that some important ligand-gated ion channels, e.g., nicotinic acetylcoline receptors (40,42,66,69) and $GABA_A$ receptors (110,131,133,168,216), are sensitive to volatile anesthetics at clinical concentrations. Because numerous examples exist wherein the activity of a protein is profoundly affected by a single small effector molecule, it is conceivable that the function of some crucial proteins in the central nervous system (CNS) can be altered by anesthetic binding (78,81,85). Although no protein in the CNS has yet been positively identified as the target site for general anesthesia, the concept of protein action has motivated extensive investigations to determine anesthetic-protein interactions (1,38,39,41–43,45,100,103,110,111,132,133,235), with a clear emphasis on the $GABA_A$ receptor, the primary inhibitory synaptic receptor in the CNS. Experimental tests of any protein theories, however, have proved difficult because any possible direct actions on proteins must be distinguished from indirect actions mediated by changes in the surrounding lipids (1,86).

Direct interaction between anesthetics and proteins can be analyzed using NMR relaxation measurements. As mentioned earlier, T_2 relaxation reflects the motional characteristics of the molecules bearing the nuclei under investigation. If anesthetic molecules become less mobile because of binding to proteins, the T_2 of the observable nuclei will become shorter. Shortening of T_2 (i.e., increase in T_2 relaxation) depends on equilibration of anesthetics in the free and bound states, and on how rapidly the binding and dissociation occur relative to how rapidly the T_2 is measured. Such dependence offers a means to link the T_2 measurements with determination of the apparent equilibrium binding constant, K_D, and the mean lifetime of the anesthetic in the bound state, τ_b.

An example of such an analysis is given by Dubois and Evers (45). Using ^{19}F-NMR, they studied the binding of isoflurane to bovine serum albumin (BSA), a soluble protein devoid of lipid. They showed that saturable and fatty acid replaceable binding sites for isoflurane did exist in BSA. The binding at these specific sites had a K_D of ~1 mM and a τ_b of ~250 μs. Other fluorinated anesthetics, such as halothane, sevoflurane, and methoxyflurane, can compete with isoflurane for the same specific binding sites (44). Although BSA plays no mechanistic role in general anesthesia, the demonstration that the K_D of anesthetic-protein binding is on the same order of magnitude as the clinical concentration of the anesthetic agents is striking. A τ_b of a few hundred microseconds, which suggests a fast dissociation rate, also has significant implications. If protein is indeed the primary target site for anesthetic action, and if such action is mimicked by the interaction in BSA, then a static view of an anesthetic molecule occupying certain clefts in a protein may be insufficient. The frequency at which anesthetic molecules bind to and dissociate from such clefts may be important as well (43).

An indirect test of protein theory is stereoselectivity associated with general anesthetics. Although chiral centers exist in pure and cholesterol-containing lipid bilayers, stereoselectivity is usually interpreted as *direct* and *specific* receptor-mediated action (53,83,85,100–102,141,162,163). When rats were anesthetized with optically pure isoflurane (141), the S(+) enantiomer appeared to be more potent than the R(–) enantiomer. Whether such stereoselectivity truly reflects action at the anesthetic target sites, or merely different physiologic responses to the enantiomers, warrants further investigation. To evaluate the intrinsic ability of anesthetic enantiomers to interact with pure proteins, Xu et al. (229) recently examined the binding of the two enantiomers of isoflurane to BSA, using the ^{19}F-NMR T_2 relaxation method and gas chromatography (GC). They found that the S(+) and R(–) isoflurane bound to the same specific (i.e., the fatty acid-replaceable) sites in the BSA, and that the K_D at these sites exhibited no stereoselectivity. Nonetheless, stereoselectivity was observed in dynamic binding parameters: the S(+) enantiomer bound with slower association and dissociation rates than the R(–). The differences in these rates, although small, may reemphasize the importance of the dynamic process in anesthetic-protein interaction. The dynamic association rate constant indicates the goodness of fit between an anesthetic and its protein target, whereas the dissociation rate constant reflects the strength of binding. Thus, although the effects of an anesthetic on a given protein depend on the equilibrium effective concentration (e.g., EC_{50}), the details of the anesthetic-protein interaction (contained in the

k_{on} and k_{off} individually) may be much more revealing. For example, the S(+) enantiomer could bind to a ligand-gated channel protein with longer duration (smaller k_{off}) to produce a stronger effect, even when the K_D appeared the same because of a slower association rate (smaller k_{on}). Differences in binding and dissociation rates have been suggested as the basis of a unitary mechanism of action of ether, isoflurane, and propofol on acetylcholine receptor channel conductance (43).

In Vivo ^{19}F-NMR of Anesthetic Uptake and Elimination

It was Wyrwicz et al. (224) who first demonstrated the use of ^{19}F-NMR in the study of uptake and elimination of fluorinated anesthetics in living animals. Fluorinated hydrocarbons represent a very important class of inhalational general anesthetics, including those in wide clinical use. ^{19}F-NMR has several advantages. First, the natural abundance (100%) of ^{19}F eliminates any need for isotopic enrichment or labeling. Second, ^{19}F exists only in trace (hence, nondetectable) amounts in living systems, so that exogenously administered fluorinated anesthetics can be observed and quantified without complication from unwanted background signals (unlike, say, ^{1}H-NMR, which yields a large signal from tissue water). Third, ^{19}F is one of the few nuclei with high NMR receptivity, having the third highest γ value of all nuclei. Recall that the nuclear spin energy gap is proportional to γ; the larger the γ, the stronger the NMR signal can be from the same amount of nuclei. Thus, if natural abundance is taken into account, ^{19}F is the second most sensitive nucleus for NMR.

The original study by Wyrwicz et al. (224) and many subsequent studies (22,134,139,159,221–223,227) are all based on one principle: that the NMR signal intensity is proportional to the number of nuclei contributing to the signal. In a silent background, the detected ^{19}F signal originates exclusively from the fluorinated anesthetics administered (and sometimes their breakdown products). Thus, the pharmacokinetics of anesthetic uptake and elimination can be measured continuously based on changes in NMR intensity as a function of uptake and elimination time. Moreover, if a volume of interest (e.g., brain) can be defined, as in the case of imaging, the signal intensity can be related to the anesthetic concentration in that volume.

In their initial study of rabbits anesthetized with 1% halothane, Wyrwicz et al. (224) found, in contrast to common belief, that a significant level of brain ^{19}F-NMR signal persisted for several days after a 30-min period of halothane anesthesia. This prolonged presence of the ^{19}F-NMR signal, originally assigned to halothane, was attributed to the presence of halothane metabolites. In a subsequent study (221), halothane was replaced with isoflurane, an anesthetic agent that undergoes negligible metabolism. A prolonged presence of ^{19}F-NMR signal in the head region was, again, detected after termination of a 90-min period of 1.5% isoflurane anesthesia. This slow elimination raised a serious concern as to whether patients after general anesthesia were being discharged too soon, as potentially dangerous amounts of anesthetic might persist in the brain.

More fundamentally, the slow elimination kinetics also challenges the view that anesthetic uptake and elimination in the brain are perfusion limited (57). Invasive but meticulous studies, including those using GC (206), radiochromatography, and autoradiography (28–30), all show that inhaled anesthetics are almost completely eliminated from the brain within a few hours after termination of general anesthesia.

This disagreement between invasive and noninvasive methods promoted several more refined in vivo NMR studies (134,139,159,222,227). These studies demonstrated that the anesthetic uptake and elimination kinetics measured with overall NMR signal intensities can vary depending on the technical implementation of the NMR method. When cerebral localization is achieved, by use of either spatially selective depth pulses (134) or smaller (diameter of <1 cm) surface coils placed directly above surgically exposed brain tissues, the rate of elimination from the brain approximates that measured by the invasive methods. For example, the half-time, $t_{1/2}$, for halothane elimination from rat brain is 34 ± 8 min (134), and that for isoflurane from rabbit brain is 36 ± 5 min (159). These values are similar to, although slightly longer than, the value estimated by the invasive method using GC ($t_{1/2}$ = 18 ± 5 min) (206). When larger NMR probes are used, elimination consists of two or more components with different elimination rates (159,222). The slower components can be attributed to NMR signals from extracranial tissues, primarily the vessel-poor (thus poorly perfused) adipose tissues. Careful examination of the results of several in vivo NMR studies reveals that the pharmacokinetics of anesthetic uptake and elimination in the brain are correctly defined by the invasive methods and can be correctly measured by in vivo NMR if precautions are taken to specify the volumes of detection.

The technical complexity and possible difficulties in interpreting pharmacokinetic data do not diminish the value of in vivo NMR spectroscopy. Many of its unique features are unparalleled by any of the invasive methods. Most important, it allows not only for assessment of anesthetic concentrations based on overall NMR intensity, but also for noninvasive analysis of the microenvironment of general anesthetics based on their T_2 values. In homogenized brain tissues of rats anesthetized with halothane, the ^{19}F-NMR signal exhibits at least two T_2 components: a fast component, T_{2fast}, of 3.6 ms, and a slow component, T_{2slow}, of 46 ms (64). Of great relevance to the mechanisms of general anesthetic action (80) is the finding that with increasing halothane concentration in spontaneously breathed gas, the T_{2fast} component of the NMR signal in brain homogenates appears to plateau, indicating some degree of saturation. If this were not physiologic in origin, it would suggest a specific action of anesthetic at a limited number of sites in the brain. The observation that only the T_{2fast} component is saturated further suggests a protein action, because T_{2fast} relaxation often reflects immobilization due to binding. Nevertheless, the initial enthusiasm over this correlation between saturation of the T_{2fast} component and anesthetic-protein interaction in brain tissue was tempered by subsequent studies (65,139,230), showing that such saturation was indeed physiologic in origin. The saturation was attributed to cardiac suppression by halothane in spontaneously breathing animals, and was not observed in animals anesthetized during mechanical ventilation (136,139).

As shown recently by Xu et al. (227), studies integrating the two types of experiments described above, namely, the pharmacokinetic studies of anesthetic uptake and elimination, and analyses of anesthetic microenvironments, can offer new insights into the action of general anesthetics in vivo. In mechanically ventilated rats anesthetized with 4% sevoflurane, the T_2 of ^{19}F in sevoflurane was measured continuously in consecutive time segments, 4.3 min each, during uptake and elimination. The overall ^{19}F-NMR intensity in each time segment was then decomposed based on the percentage of different T_2 compositions in that time segment. For comparison, two different NMR probes were used: a 2-cm diameter surface coil, which provided partial localization to the brain region, and a homogeneous head coil, which detected signals from the entire head. As the uptake time increased (up to 90 min), the ratio of the two T_2 components varied, with the percentage of the T_{2fast} component in the total intensity decreasing exponentially (although the absolute intensity increased without saturation). For example, the T_{2fast} component contributed initially to almost 60% of the total ^{19}F-NMR signal intensity in the head, as measured with the head coil (or 82%, as measured with the 2-cm surface coil). Ninety minutes later, this contribution decreased to <28% when measured with the head coil (or to ~55% with the surface coil). Such decrease was due not to absolute reduction in the T_{2fast} component, but to delayed increase in the T_{2slow} component. Moreover, in the same animals and at any given time during uptake and elimination, the signal measured with the surface coil contained more T_{2fast} component than that measured with the head coil, suggesting a different spatial distribution of the two T_2 components in the head. Apparently, the signal from vessel-rich brain tissue contributed mostly to the T_{2fast} component, whereas that from vessel-poor adipose tissue contributed mostly to the T_{2slow} component.

To illustrate the uniqueness of the integrated NMR method used by Xu et al. (227), Fig. 5 depicts representative washout kinetics of sevoflurane from the head region of rats after 67–89 min of 4% sevoflurane general anesthesia. The elimination of the overall intensity, characterized by two elimination rate constants, exemplifies what has been found in previous studies (134,139,159,221,222). Additional information on elimination from individual microenvironments is obtained by decomposing the overall intensity at each time point into T_{2fast} and T_{2slow} components. Clearly, sevoflurane molecules in the two microenvironments exhibit distinct elimination kinetics. From the molecular compartment where sevoflurane is relatively immobile, as characterized by T_{2fast}, the washout is a single exponential with a $t_{1/2}$ of 13 min. In contrast, from more mobile environments, as characterized by T_{2slow}, sevoflurane washout has two rates, with $t_{1/2}$ of 15 and 100 min, respectively. Thus, after 1 h of washout, sevoflurane is almost completely eliminated from the immobile environments; and after 2 h of washout, 99.8% of the total ^{19}F signal remaining in the rat head originates from the T_{2slow} component.

Taken together, these results suggest that three anesthetic environments are distinguishable by in vivo NMR spectroscopy. These environments are characterized phenomenologically by (a) $T_2 = T_{2fast} \approx 3\text{~}5$ ms and $t_{1/2} \approx 13$ min; (b) $T_2 = T_{2slow} \approx 105\text{~}130$ ms and $t_{1/2} \approx 15$ min; and (c) $T_2 = T_{2slow} \approx 105\text{~}130$ ms and $t_{1/2} = 100$ min, respectively. The rapid awakening observed after sevoflurane anesthesia would suggest that only sevoflurane molecules in the first and the second environments (i.e., with rapid elimination rates) are responsible for producing general anesthesia. However, the lack of a T_{2slow} component in brain tissue during the onset of anesthesia rules out the involvement of the second environment. Thus, it seems very likely that the relatively immobilized sevoflurane molecules are associated with anesthetic action. However, such immobilization may not be interpreted simply as protein binding. The molecular nature of immobilization in vivo has not been fully elucidated.

^{19}F-MRI of Anesthetic Distribution in the Brain

To date, no consensus has been reached on the macroscopic loci of general anesthetic action in the CNS. Whether the action involves occupation of certain sites in isolated region(s), or requires colligative activation of many regions, is yet to be determined. Although invasive measurements of general anesthetic distribution in the brain have been made (29), a meaningful correlation between functional activity of the brain and the regional anesthetic concentration requires noninvasive assessment in a timely fashion of the spatial distribution of general anesthetics. Naturally, ^{19}F-MRI of fluorinated general anesthetics has attracted much attention because of the successful use of ^{19}F-NMR spectroscopy in vivo.

Earlier attempts at imaging halothane distribution in animals (22,222,223) produced only silhouettes of the brain. The very short T_2 (~3–5 ms) of the ^{19}F signal in brain tissue is the cause of this failing. Conventional imaging techniques, widely used in clinical ^{1}H-MRI of tissue water, have proved inadequate for ^{19}F-MRI of general anesthetics, because the mandatory waiting time between the creation of coherence and the beginning of imaging acquisition is too long relative to the lifetime of the coherence (i.e., T_2) to yield sufficient signal for imaging. New and improved MRI pulsing techniques are needed to capture the rapidly decaying ^{19}F signal in the brain.

Using a three-dimensional and a specially designed 2D imaging technique, Xu et al. (227) recently obtained the first in vivo ^{19}F images of sevoflurane distribution in rat parenchyma. Figure 6A shows such an image, with an anatomic reference provided in Fig. 6B. These images represented a major advance toward mapping the anesthetic distribution in the CNS. A

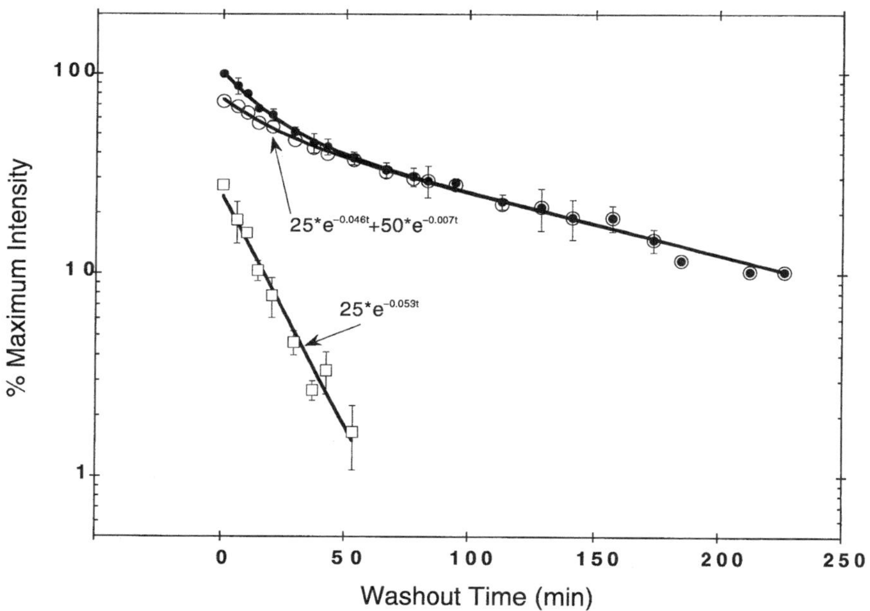

Figure 5. Elimination of sevoflurane from rat brain. The total wash-out intensity (*solid circle*) at each time point is weighted by the percentage of T_{2fast} and T_{2slow} components at that time point, resulting in separate elimination kinetics for the T_{2fast} (*open square*) and T_{2slow} (*open circle*) components. The *solid lines* are best fit to the data with single or double exponential functions, yielding elimination rate constants: $k_f = 0.053 \pm 0.004$ min^{-1}, $k_{s1} = 0.046 \pm 0.009$ min^{-1}, and $k_{s2} = 0.007 \pm 0.001$ min^{-1}. (Reprinted with permission from Xu Y, Tang P, Zhang W, Firestone L, Winter PM. ^{19}F-NMR imaging and spectroscopy of sevoflurane uptake, distribution and elimination in rat brain. *Anesthesiology* 1995;83:766–774.)

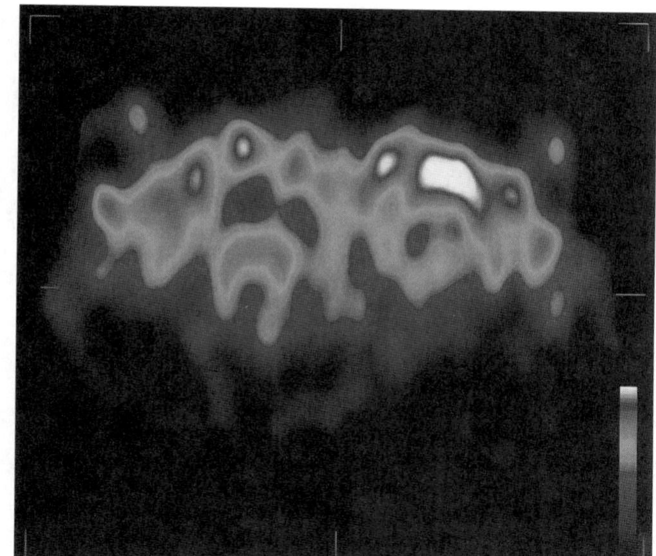

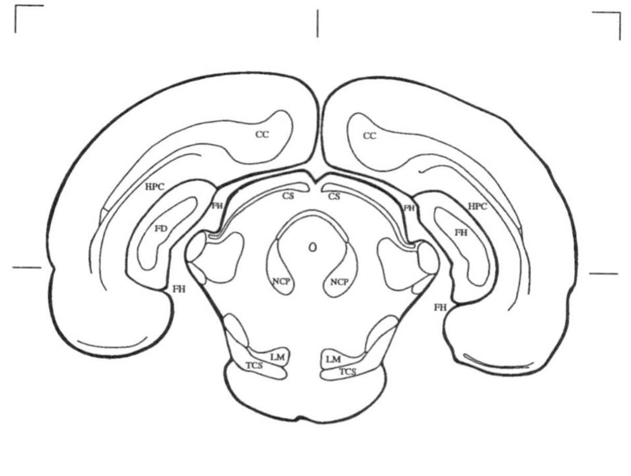

Figure 6. **(A)** A representative surface-coil ^{19}F image showing detailed distribution of sevoflurane in a rat brain. *(See color plate 2.)* **(B)** An anatomic schematic for A. The *frames* and *lines* are added as reference marks only and are not the margins of field-of-view. (Reprinted with permission from Xu Y, Tang P, Zhang W, Firestone L, Winter PM. ^{19}F-NMR imaging and spectroscopy of sevoflurane uptake, distribution and elimination in rat brain. *Anesthesiology* 1995;83:766–774.)

sequence of images acquired during sevoflurane uptake showed early abundance of the anesthetic in the vessel-rich brain tissue and delayed accumulation in the vessel-poor extracranial tissues. Moreover, as shown in Fig. 6A, anesthetic distribution in the brain is nonuniform. This may be attributed to either heterogeneous distribution, or difference in relaxation rates in various regions, or a combination of the two.

The ability to image anesthetics in the CNS has important implications (227). For example, if fluorinated anesthetics are administered by microdialysis and the affected regions visualized by ^{19}F-MRI with improved image quality, regional anesthetic concentrations can be correlated with neurophysiologic effects. A systematic investigation along these lines may shed new light on identifying the CNS sites of general anesthetic action. Another potential application of ^{19}F-MRI is to evaluate anesthetic distribution in the presence of abnormal cerebral blood flow (CBF), such as in head injury and stroke.

NMR Studies of Energy and Hydrocarbon Metabolism

With critical care medicine becoming an integral part of modern anesthesiology, it is worthwhile to mention two other important applications of in vivo NMR: noninvasive assessment of brain energy and hydrocarbon metabolism, and measurements of CBF. The past 15 years have produced numerous publications in these areas of research. Rather than attempt to review this literature, we will limit the discussion to fundamentals and a few examples. Several excellent reviews are available (19,127,169,181,183,213).

^{31}P-NMR Measurements of Bioenergetics and Intracellular pH

Among many naturally occurring and artificial metabolic probes, ^{31}P is one of the most commonly used nuclei for continuous and noninvasive observation of metabolic changes under various physiologic and pathophysiologic conditions. ^{31}P is 100% naturally abundant and has an NMR sensitivity approximately one-fifth that of ^{1}H. The ^{31}P chemical shift range of tissue metabolites is ~30 ppm, permitting spectral resolution of some very important intermediates of energy metabolism. Under normal experimental conditions, ^{31}P-NMR spectra of good signal-to-noise ratio can be obtained with a temporal resolution of a few minutes.

One of the most important uses of ^{31}P-NMR is to monitor the energy state of an organ or a tissue in vivo. Figure 7 depicts a typical ^{31}P-NMR spectrum of a rat brain, acquired noninvasively at 4.7 T. Several resonance peaks are discernible. A group of three peaks, labeled α, β, and γ, arise from nucleoside triphosphates, which are predominantly adenosine triphosphate (ATP) in the brain. Because the chemical environment of α- and γ-phosphates in ATP is very similar to that of α- and β-phosphates in adenosine diphosphate (ADP), respectively, the α and γ peaks also contain contributions from ADP and other nucleoside diphosphates. In addition, the α peak is overlapped by NAD/NADP signals. Only the β-phosphate resonance is free of contamination and is often used to quantify changes in ATP. The sharp resonance next to the γ-ATP peak arises from phosphocreatine (PCr). Other assignable peaks are inorganic phosphate (P_i), phosphomonoester (PME), and phosphodiester (PDE). Both PME and PDE peaks are poorly resolved. The former may contain contributions from denosine monophosphate (AMP), sugar phosphates (glucose-6-phosphate, fructose-6-phosphate), phosphocholine, and phosphoethanolamine, whereas the latter may be a combination of glycerophosphorylcholine and glycerophosphorylethanolamine. The large, broad component, which has been partially suppressed in this spec-

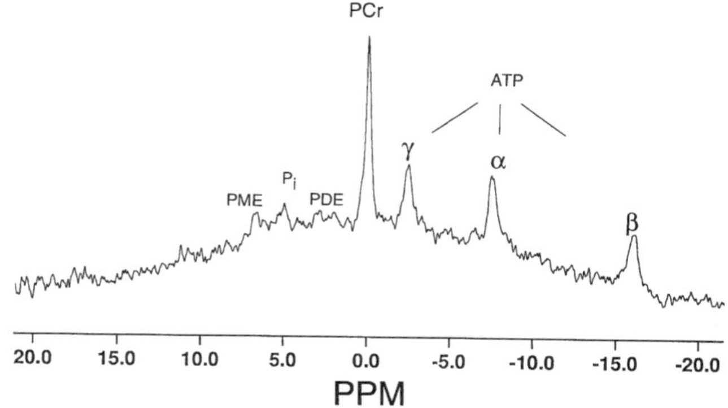

Figure 7. A representative in vivo ^{31}P-NMR spectrum of an adult rat brain. Peaks labeled are α-, β-, and γ-ATP, phosphocreatine (PCr), inorganic phosphate (P_i), phosphomonoester (PME), and phosphodiester (PDE).

trum by a presaturation pulse, is attributable to bone (3) and immobile membrane phospholipids (94).

Energy depletion and associated neuronal injury during and after cerebral ischemia have been the focus of many experimental stroke studies. Typically, the brain energy state is monitored continuously by measuring changes in PCr, ATP, and P_i levels as a function of time. It is often assumed that high PCr and ATP levels and low P_i level are indicative of the metabolic health and viability of the brain. Depletion of PCr and ATP and elevation of P_i are taken as signs of neuronal damage or death.

In addition to measuring changes in overall PCr, ATP, and P_i levels, in vivo ^{31}P-NMR has also been used to estimate the rate of energy metabolism by means of magnetization transfer (32,105,122). The magnetization transfer technique exploits a property of enzymatic reactions, $E + S \leftrightarrow ES \leftrightarrow EP \leftrightarrow E + P$, where S and P share the same magnetization-relaxation pool in the substrate-enzyme complexes (ES and EP). Thus, saturation of P magnetization will affect the relaxation rate of S, and vice versa. For the creatine-kinase (CK) catalyzed reaction (PCr + ADP + H $\leftrightarrow$ Cr + ATP), for example, it is assumed that the rate-determining step is the transfer of the phosphoryl group in the exchange PCr.(k_{for} and k_{rev}) [γ – P]ATP, where k_{for} and k_{rev} are the pseudo first-order forward and reverse rate constants. The change in PCr magnetization (and hence PCr intensity) depends not only on its own equilibrium magnetization level, M_0, but also on [γ-P]ATP magnetization. It can be shown that when [γ-P]ATP is saturated for a period t, the observed PCr intensity is a function of t, given by

$$M(PCr) = M_\infty + (M_0 - M_\infty)e^{-t/\tau} \qquad [3]$$

where $1/\tau = 1/T_1 + k_{for}$, and M_∞ is the limiting magnetization when $t >> \tau$. Thus, measurements of M(PCr) as a function of a series of saturation time t can be used to estimate k_{for}. A similar analysis for [γ-P]ATP magnetization, while PCr is saturated, can yield estimates for k_{rev}.

An added feature of ^{31}P-NMR spectroscopy is its utility for measuring intracellular pH (pH_i) and intracellular free magnesium (Mg_i^{2+}). The pH_i measurement is based on the chemical shift difference between P_i and PCr resonance. Whereas the chemical shift of PCr is relatively insensitive to physiologic pH, that of P_i is very sensitive, because the observed shift, δ_{obs}, is a weighted average of two shifts, δ_m and δ_d, corresponding respectively to monobasic ($H_2PO_4^-$) and dibasic (HPO_4^{2-}) phosphates. At a given pH, the equilibrium between mono- and dibasic phosphates obeys $pH = pK_a + \log[(\delta_{obs} - \delta_m)/(\delta_d - \delta_{obs})]$, where $pK_a = \log K_a$, and K_a is the proton dissociation constant for the monobasic phosphate. Values for pK_a, δ_m, and δ_d are 6.77, 3.29, and 5.68, respectively (180). Slightly different values have also been reported.

Hypoxia and ischemia are accompanied by intracellular acidosis, which has for some time been viewed as the cause of cellular injury. To evaluate the effects of low pH_i on neuronal injuries, a series of in vivo NMR investigations were carried out by Litt et al. (31,61,135,226). Hypercapnia of various degrees was used to lower the pH_i while maintaining adequate oxygenation. In an extreme case, an elaborate hyperbaric chamber was constructed (137,226) to permit elevation of P_aCO_2 to up to 760 mm Hg. Brain pH_i was monitored continuously with ^{31}P-NMR. It was found that intracellular acidosis, with pH_i values as low as 6.2 (a value commonly found during injurious stroke), was well tolerated by the rats, with no detectable neuronal injury. In short, these in vivo NMR studies showed unquivocally that low pH_i per se is not the cause of neuronal damage in hypoxia or ischemia. Other mechanisms, including excitotoxicity (26), have been the recent focus of in vivo and ex vivo NMR investigations (60,62,63).

The basis for determining Mg_i^{2+} from ^{31}P spectra is similar to pH_i determination (16,97), and it exploits the fact that biologically useful ATP occurs as Mg_i^{2+}-ATP. In ^{31}P NMR spectra, the presence of Mg_i^{2+} causes a pH-dependent modulation of the chemical shifts of the β- and γ-ATP resonance peaks. After first determining pH_i, it is possible to calculate the average free Mg_i^{2+} concentration based on in vitro calibration curves and the apparent dissociation constant of Mg_i^{2+}-ATP (166,219), given accurate determinations (±0.03 ppm) of the chemical shifts of the β- and γ-ATP peaks relative to the α-ATP peak. This method has been used, for example, to evaluate the effects of intracellular Mg_i^{2+} on brain protection in alcohol-induced hemorrhagic stroke (5) and on cardiac performance in perfused hearts (12).

^{1}H-NMR Spectroscopy In Vivo

^{1}H is the most sensitive naturally occurring NMR probe in biologic systems. The development of its use in vivo, however, has had a slow start. The difficulty of in vivo ^{1}H-NMR is twofold: (a) the presence of a very large number of proton-containing tissue metabolites, all of which resonate in a very small chemical shift range (≤15 ppm), leading to complicated spectra of widely overlapping broad peaks; and (b) the presence of an intense water proton signal (~80 M water proton concentration in most tissue), imposing technical limits (the so-called dynamic range problem) on detecting signals from millimolar concentrations of metabolites. To overcome these limitations, most in vivo ^{1}H-NMR experiments entail a water suppression technique combined with the spin-echo pulse sequence. Spectral editing by adjusting the spin-echo time can selectively enhance the detection of certain metabolites (19).

With the water signal suppressed, the readily detectable metabolites in vivo include inositols (Ins), choline (Cho), creatine and phosphocreatine (Cr/PCr), glutamate and glutamine (Glx), N-acetylaspartate (NAA), and lactate (Lac). A representative spectrum is shown in Fig. 8.

Lac is an important metabolic marker of hypoxic and ischemic neuronal injury. Improving its detection has been the focus of many in vivo studies. Spectral editing based on J-coupling between lactates β-CH_3 and α-CH is commonly used. Because the J-coupling constant is 7.0 Hz, a spin-echo delay of $1/2J \approx 71$ ms ensures maximum Lac detection. Under in vivo conditions, how-

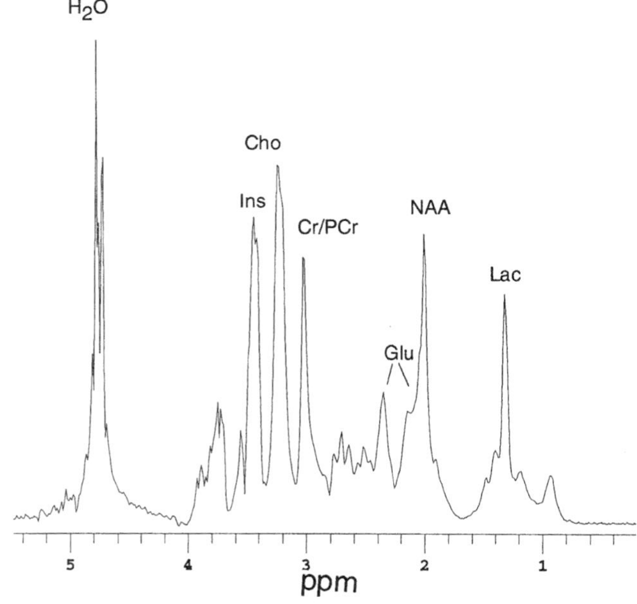

Figure 8. A representative water-suppressed ^{1}H-NMR spectrum of perfused (live) rat brain slices at 9.4T. Peaks assigned are inositols (Ins), choline (Cho), creatine and phosphocreatine (Cr/PCr), glutamate and glutamine (Glx), N-acetylaspartate (NAA), and lactate (Lac).

ever, the optimal delay is slightly less than 1/2J when the line width is large relative to the coupling constant. The most frequently used value is 68 ms or its multiples (31,106,190,220,226), although values as low as 60 ms have been reported (20).

NAA is one of the most abundant metabolites in adult brain. It is hypothesized to be a neuronal marker, and other neurobiologic roles have been speculated (14). Because the methyl resonance of the N-acetyl moiety of NAA is the most distinct peak in the ^{1}H-NMR spectra, it is conveniently used as an internal standard to observe changes in other metabolites, such as Lac (20,21). Recently, changes in NAA itself have been closely examined in kainate-induced status epilepticus in rats (52). Reliable and quantifiable spectroscopic changes, particularly the NAA/Cho and NAA/(Cho + Cr) ratios, are observed in epileptogenic regions.

Time-Shared Multinuclear NMR Spectroscopy

An important feature of in vivo NMR is the possibility of observing two or more nuclei almost simultaneously, permitting excellent time correlation of different physiologic processes characterized separately by different nuclei. Such interleaved NMR experiments exploit the property that the RF excitation and detection are nucleus specific, and can be applied to one element (e.g., ^{31}P) without perturbing other elements (e.g., ^{1}H, ^{19}F). The computer of the NMR spectrometer keeps track of which NMR acquisition belongs to which element, and at the end of each experiment, the NMR spectra are sorted and processed separately. Because data acquisition for each element takes place during the obligatory waiting period given for other elements to relax after their own excitations, the overall duration of a multinuclear NMR experiment, in which spectra are acquired for several nuclei, is not substantially longer than the time duration for acquiring spectra of only a single nucleus. ^{31}P/^{1}H interleaved NMR spectroscopy has been used to correlate Lac formation (from ^{1}H spectra) with energy depletion and intracellular acidosis (from ^{31}P spectra) (21,226). Recently, triple nuclear ^{1}H/^{19}F/^{31}P interleaved acquisition has been used (60) to study glutamate-induced neuronal toxicity in perfused rat cerebral cortical slices, which have been loaded with fluorinated calcium indicators for ^{19}F-NMR measurement of intracellular free calcium (8,10).

NMR Studies of CBF

CBF is of primary concern in critical care medicine. The metabolism, function, and viability of brain are exquisitely dependent on the minute-to-minute local blood supply (191). The ability to map noninvasively the perfusion in brain tissue not only can improve the accuracy of early diagnosis in such cases as stroke and head injury, but also can assist in the evaluation of treatment.

Although one of the earliest biologic applications of NMR was the measurement of blood flow velocity (196), mapping of CBF with MRI has a recent origin (213). The current emphasis in technical development is on either microcirculation (i.e., tissue perfusion), or NMR angiography, in which large vessels, often of several pixels in size, are mapped.

NMR Angiography

Methods for NMR angiography can be classified roughly into two broad categories: those based on time-of-flight phenomena and those based on gradient-modulated phase effects. In time-of-flight methods, flowing spins are tagged by RF excitation at one position, followed by later observation of this nonequilibrium magnetization at a different position. Different tagging methods have been proposed, including inversion of longitudinal magnetization (152), presaturation (73), and passive tag of in-flow of fully relaxed spins (6,150). Aside from tagging, the time-of-flight techniques are further classified according to the method of acquisition, including three-dimensional volumetric acquisition (33,147,149,150, 188,192), 2D sequential slice acquisition (56,75,115), traveling presaturation 2D acquisition (115), black-blood acquisition (54,55), and echo-planar imaging acquisition (70).

The phase methods are intellectually more challenging, and they offer better flow contrast (especially when flow is slow) and larger field of view than the time-of-flight methods. In simple terms, a phase refers to an angle spanned by precession in a given time period, and can be calculated by integrating the product of position and gradient over time:

$$\phi = \gamma \int_{D}^{t} x(t)G(t)dt \quad [4]$$

Because the position of a flowing spin depends on its initial position, x_0, velocity, v, acceleration, a, the derivative of acceleration (called jerk or pulsatility), j, and so on, a Taylor series: $x(t) = x_0 + vt + \frac{1}{2}at^2 + \frac{1}{6}jt^3 + \ldots$ is usually used to describe the time dependence of the position. The phase accumulated over time for a flowing spin can be made either dependent or independent of x_0, v, a, or j, depending on the integral of each term in the Taylor series and the arrangement of the gradients as a function of time.

The simplest gradient arrangement for flow encoding is a pair of gradients, identical in amplitude and duration but opposite in polarity. For stationary spins (the x_0 term in the series), the effects from the first half of the gradient pair are canceled by the second half, resulting in zero phase accumulation. Such cancellation, however, will not occur to the flowing spins, because in the second half, the flowing spins have already changed their position. A net phase, ϕ, is hence accumulated. If the same experiment is repeated with the polarity of the gradient pair reversed, the phase for the stationary spins will remain zero, but that for the flowing spins will become ϕ. Subtracting the results of the second experiment from that of the first, the stationary spins are canceled, and the flowing spins are left with a net advance in phase of 2ϕ. Maximum intensity for flowing spins is obtained when $\phi = \pi/2$ or $\phi = \pi$. Dumoulin et al. (46,47,49–51) were the first to combine this method with an otherwise conventional spin-warp gradient-echo imaging sequence for MR angiography. Many variations of this phase contrast method, including three-dimensional phase contrast (179,215) and velocity mapping (48,200), have now been used clinically.

Perfusion and Diffusion Measurements by NMR

The classical definition of perfusion, P, is a normalized volumetric flow rate of a freely diffusible tracer in an organ. Clinically, P is measured in units of ml/100 g/min. Numerous methods have been developed to measure P directly or indirectly in the brain. These methods can be categorized into three groups: (a) use of contrast agents, (b) use of traceable nuclei, and (c) manipulation of signal from water protons.

Contrast Agent Methods In dynamic perfusion studies using paramagnetic contrast agents, the agents are introduced into the bloodstream as a bolus. The flow of blood through the brain is measured by observing changes in image contrast as a function of time. Because most contrast agents are nondiffusible, strictly speaking, this method does not provide a precise measure of perfusion in the classical sense. However, since tissue water protons, which are used to form the images, diffuse rapidly through the inhomogeneous magnetic field gradients produced by the contrast agents (144), it is often assumed (71,93), especially when the intravascular concentration of the contrast agent is not too high, that the signal changes (i.e., the contrast) is proportional to the volume fraction of the capillaries, i.e., to the total blood volume, which in turn determines the brain tissue concentration of the agent. With this assumption, the perfusion be evaluated by

$$P = V/(MT) \quad [5]$$

where *V* is the total distribution volume of the contrast agent in the tissue (the total blood volume if the agent is nondiffusible), *M* is the total mass of brain tissue perfused, and *T* is the mean transit time of the bolus.

Commonly used paramagnetic contrast agents are chelated lanthanides, including Gd-DTPA and Dy-DTPA (DTPA is diethylene-triaminepentaacetic acid). Typical passage time of these agents through brain is in the range of 5–20 s. Clearly, fast imaging techniques are essential. FLASH (98) and echo-planar imaging (EPI) (145) are the two most frequently used ones.

Tracer Methods Tracers for CBF measurement may be of endogenous or exogeneous origin. Blood itself can be used as an endogenous contrast agent. This concept was first suggested independently by Xu et al. (225) and Ogawa et al. (173), and demonstrated by Ogawa et al. (170–173). The underlining mechanism of blood contrast is the bulk magnetic susceptibility effect (27,225). Because deoxyhemoglobin is paramagnetic, the magnetic susceptibility of the deoxygenated blood is different from that of the brain tissue and the fully oxygenated blood. Such susceptibility gradient across the vessel wall in the capillary bed generates a local magnetic field inhomogeneity, which in turn increases the T_2 relaxation of the water protons diffusing in the vicinity the these vessels.

The second endogenous tracer is blood water, which is freely diffusible in brain tissue. A method similar to that used in time-of-flight angiography has been proposed by Detre et al. (36,37,234) for perfusion mapping. Water protons in the blood are tagged by inversion or saturation pulses around the neck area. These tagged protons are imaged as they perfuse through the brain tissue. Perfusion images of very high quality have been obtained using this method. Most important, this method is completely noninvasive.

Foreign tracers are used mostly to measure global CBF based on tracer clearance, as in the anesthetic washout studies discussed earlier. The most thoroughly investigated tracers are ^{19}F and ^{2}H. Nontoxic, fluorinated refrigerants, such as FC 22 and FC 23, are commonly used (58) for ^{19}F measurement. Deuterated water, which is somewhat toxic, is used for ^{2}H measurements (2,118).

Manipulation of Water Signal for Perfusion and Diffusion Imaging In the capillary beds in the brain, especially in the gray matter, blood flow is slow, random, and isotropic, and can be viewed as a pseudodiffusive process (128). This intravoxel incoherent motion (IVIM) behaves very much like classical diffusion. As early as 1965, diffusion was the subject of NMR investigation (203). The standard procedure for diffusion measurements is to use a pair of gradients; the first gradient dephases the transverse magnetization, then the second one rephases it. For spins with incoherent movement, the initial phase will not be fully regained by the second gradient, resulting a signal loss in the images. The extent to which signal is lost depends on the strength of the gradient. When the signal loss is measured as a function of the gradient strength, a quantity called apparent diffusion constant (ADC) can be calculated.

A distinction has been made to separate the diffusion constant for pseudodiffusion in the capillary bed, D_p, from that for true diffusion in the tissue, D_s. Theory (127) has been developed to estimate perfusion, P, based on the knowledge of D_p, given that the mean blood traveling distance and the mean capillary length between arteriole and venule are known (177).

Probably the most exciting clinical application of diffusion measurements is the diffusion-weighted imaging (DWI) used for early detection of stroke and brain injury (89,121, 165,167,182). Among the physiologic signs, edema is one of the most sensitive indicators of ischemic insult. Cell edema results in intracellular accumulation of tissue water, which in turn restricts the movement of water molecules. When measured with DWI, this effect is evident as a marked reduction of ADC in the affected regions (194). Numerous experiments have been carried out using animals (9,35,91,92,143,178,186,214). The clinical use of this technique in humans has been evaluated (72) and implemented (23,129,217,218).

EPR TECHNIQUES

As described above, EPR spectroscopy is a method that detects unpaired electrons by their absorption of microwave energy (~10^{10} Hz) when in a strong magnetic field (~0.3 Tesla). Since the vast majority of biological molecules contain paired electrons, stable free radicals (so-called "spin labels") are introduced to act as probes in systems without intrinsic EPR signals. Transition metal ions such as Mn, Fe, Co, Cu, V, and Mo contain unpaired electrons, but the use of such intrinsic EPR signals has so far been minimal in anesthesia research. The origin of the EPR signal was discussed earlier.

Technical Overview

EPR Equipment

The EPR spectrometer (Fig. 9) consists of a hollow tube that conducts microwave radiation from a source ("klystron") to a sample cavity ("resonator") located between the pole caps of a water-cooled electromagnet. The dimensions of the conducting tube are determined by microwave wavelengths; the most commonly used system, called an X-band spectrometer, has a 3-cm width, corresponding to an operating frequency of 9,000 kHz (9 GHz). When a sample (containing spin label molecules) is placed in the cavity, the magnetic field strength is varied ("swept") through the resonance condition. The small absorption signal is then detected, amplified, and recorded. Detection is improved by having the cavity in one arm of a balanced network, and by modulating the magnetic field. Since the modulation is typically less than the linewidth of the absorption, and the detector is sensitive to phase, the signal (spectrum) appears as a derivative of the absorption line.

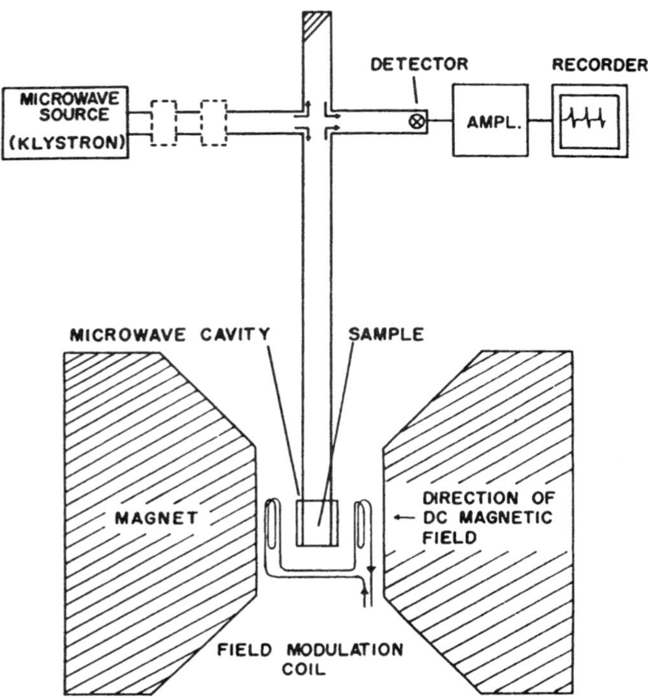

Figure 9. Schematic of EPR instrumentation. (Reprinted with permission from Jost P, Griffith OH. Instrumental aspects of spin labeling. In: Berliner LJ, ed. *Spin labeling theory and applications, vol. 2.* New York: Academic Press, 1979:251–272.)

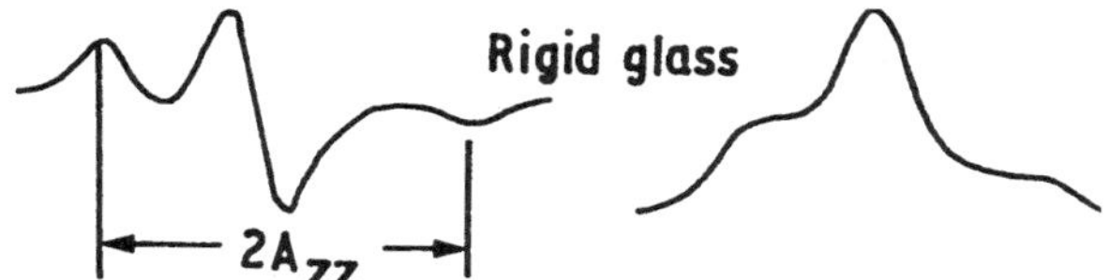

Figure 10. EPR spectrum. The 9.5-GHz first-derivative *(left)* and absorption spectrum *(right)* of a nitroxide spin label in a rigid matrix are depicted. This "rigid-glass," or powder spectrum, is obtained for any randomly oriented spin label, assuming absence of molecular motion. The characteristic three-line spectrum arises from interaction of the unpaired electron spin with the nuclear spin of nitrogen ($I = 1$). See text for definition of A_{zz}.

Unless unusual adjustments are made to the cavity, samples typically have volumes of 10–500 μL, and can be aqueous or solid. Flat quartz cells, or capillary tubes may be used to contain aqueous samples, provided they can be held rigidly in place in the cavity. A stream of anhydrous nitrogen flowing through the cavity is usually necessary to prevent sample heating by the microwave irradiation.

Spectral Parameters

The EPR signal (Fig. 10) is usually displayed as the first derivative of the absorption spectrum. The spectrum may be characterized by four main parameters: (a) intensity, (b) linewidth, (c) *g*-value, and (d) multiplet structure known as "splitting."

Intensity is defined as the integrated area under the energy absorption spectrum, and is usually proportional to the concentration of the unpaired spins that give rise to the spectrum. However, intensity may be inaccurate in the presence of quenching or saturation, limiting certain quantitative applications of EPR. Quenching occurs as a consequence of an excessively high concentration of paramagnetic species in solution. Saturation may be observed when energy is used in excess of that needed for the resonance condition.

The EPR linewidth is influenced by two main factors: the spin-lattice relaxation time (T_1) and broadening from field inhomogeneities. The spin-lattice relaxation time is a measure of the recovery rate of spin populations after experiencing fluctuating magnetic fields; shorter T_1s yield broader lines. Local magnetic fields are also slightly different at each molecule, leading to a spread in values for their resonance frequencies and inhomogeneous broadening. This is particularly relevant under conditions where molecules are either static, or tumbling unusually slowly (e.g., with spectroscopy at low temperature or in gel phases).

In EPR, the *g*-value reflects an electron's local magnetic field and thus will respond to different microenvironments (in NMR, the nuclear *g*-factor is constant for each given nucleus, and it is screening effects that alter the effective field at the nucleus). The *g*-value characterizes the position of a resonance, and is thus useful to identify an unknown signal. *g*-Values are anisotropic, that is, their value will vary according to the orientation of the molecule in the applied magnetic field. However, when motion is unrestricted, the local fields are continuously altering, and the measured *g*-value represents an average.

Analogous to NMR, multiplet structure occurs in EPR because resonances are split by "hyperfine" interactions between electron spins and nuclear spins. Specifically, nuclear spin I produces a local magnetic field at the electron. Since there are $(2I + 1)$ orientations of the nuclear spin, and the electron spin senses these different orientations, the EPR spectrum is split into $(2I + 1)$ lines of equal intensity. The magnitude of the splitting between the lines is called the hyperfine splitting constant, A. For the common nitroxide spin labels, the presence of nitrogen ($I = 1$) determines that the absorption signal will be split into three lines.

EPR Spectral Anisotropy: Effect of Orientation

A molecule's *g*-value (position) and *A*-value (hyperfine splitting) usually depend on the direction of the magnetic field relative to its axis and are thus "anisotropic." In principle, a fast rate of motion in all directions will average the anistropy, yielding "isotropic" *g*- and *A*-values. However, motional averaging is seldom ideal, thus spectra from biological samples are affected by such anisotropy.

The *g*-value anisotropy is characterized by three principal *g*-values, g_{xx}, g_{yy}, and g_{zz}, corresponding to the principal axes of the spin label moiety. In the case of axial symmetry, as is typical for spin labels, $g_{xx} = g_{yy}$. By convention, g_{zz} is defined as the *g*-value observed when the applied field is parallel to the symmetry axis, and it is designated $g_{\parallel}$. Thus g_{xx} and g_{yy} are designated $g_{\perp}$, which is the value when the applied field is perpendicular to the symmetry axis. In a crystal, the three principal *g*-values can be measured when the magnetic field is applied along the principal axes of the spin label molecule; thus, the angular variations of the *g*-values can give information on the orientation of the principal axes. In a liquid or frozen sample, the molecules will be randomly oriented, thus there will be a spread of *g*-values due to the individual absorptions of molecules. Characterization of anisotropy of the nuclear hyperfine interaction, A (sometimes known as T for tensor), is analogous to that for *g*-value anisotropy: there are three principal axes and with axial symmetry, $A_{\parallel} = A_{zz}$, while $A_{\perp} = A_{xx} = A_{yy}$. When nitroxide free radicals are used as spin labels, the unpaired electron is primarily localized to a 2*p*-electron orbital on the nitrogen. This orbital is anistropic, therefore the hyperfine interactions are also anisotropic. The nitroxide radical can be oriented in a rigid matrix; when the magnetic field is then applied along the principal axes of the nitroxide, the absorption spectrum and corresponding first-derivative interpeak distance ($2A_{zz}$) obtained are as shown in Fig. 10.

EPR Spectral Order Parameter: Quantifying Motion

The amplitude of spin label motion is determined by the restrictive characteristics of its microenvironment. The extent of fast-motional averaging of the anisotropy has been defined by an order parameter, S, which is the ratio of observed anisotropy to maximum anisotropy. The observed anisotropy is $A_{\parallel}\ A_{\perp}$, and the maximum anisotropy is $A_{zz} - 1/2(A_{xx} + A_{yy})$; these are the hyperfine splittings (interpeak distances) obtained when the label is rigidly oriented in a single crystal. Thus $S = 1$ for highly ordered systems, and $S = 0$ for totally isotropic motion.

Hyperfine interaction also depends on the unpaired electron density at the nitrogen atom. The polarity of the environment may influence this, by favoring certain electronic density forms of the spin label, thus changing A. The isotropic splitting constant, a_0, provides a relative index of polarity. In general, it is defined as:

$$a_0 = 1/3\ (A_{xx} + A_{yy} + A_{zz}) \qquad [6]$$

which is also the splitting measured for small molecules tumbling isotropically in solution. It is measured experimentally by comparing its value for a given label in different solvents. Since a_0 is independent of the amplitude of motion of the label, it can be used to probe the polarity profile of the microenvironment of interest. Further detailed discussion regarding appropriate interpretation of order parameters in spin labeled membranes and the effects of polarity can be found in Gaffney (90).

EPR Time Scale

If molecular motions are rapid enough, anisotropy is averaged. For example, in solution, the anisotropy of g is small, the tumbling rate is rapid (~10^{-10} s), and all that can be measured is an average *g*-value:

$$g_0 = 1/3\ (g_{xx} + g_{yy} + g_{zz}). \qquad [7]$$

In spin labeled biological systems, molecular motions occur somewhat more slowly (10^{-7} to 10^{-9} stime domain), broadening the major linewidths. EPR lines are also broadened by anisotropic hyperfine interactions (vide supra), and by exchange between two microenvironments (i.e., a spin-labeled ligand binding to a protein) where each is characterized by a different relaxation time.

Molecular motions that occur in the μsec time domain (e.g., rotations of motionally-restricted proteins in membranes), can be observed by the special technique known as saturation transfer EPR spectroscopy (for a review, see ref. 108).

EPR Studies of Anesthetic-Lipid Interactions

After Hubbell and McConnell (107) and Metcalfe et al. (153) reported that amphiphiles such as benzyl alcohol disordered the interior of lipid bilayers, Trudell et al. (210) demonstrated that the same was true for halothane and methoxyflurane (Fig. 11). Subsequently, gaseous (24), volatile (157), steroid (126), amine (157), and barbiturate (175) anesthetics were all shown to disorder spin-labeled lipid bilayers and biomembranes. Disordering effects of anesthetics are measurable by EPR spectroscopy at therapeutic concentrations (151), and when considered on a membrane concentration basis, a physicochemically diverse group of anesthetics can be shown to disorder membranes equipotently (176). Although the disordering effect is generally rather small (typically 0.5–1.5% decrease in lipid order parameter from control, depending on the position of the spin label) (Fig. 12), it is similar in magnitude to the volume change at anesthesia predicted by the critical volume hypothesis (for a discussion of this and other antecedents of the disordered lipid theory of anesthesia, see ref. 68).

For the most part, EPR has provided compelling support for the disordered lipid hypothesis, with demonstrations that (a) lipid disordering is reversed by pressure (as is anesthesia itself) (210); (b) the ability of the unbranched, primary alkanols to disorder lipid bilayers "cuts off" at tetradecanol (156) (Fig. 13) as does obtunding potency in tadpoles (4) (for an analogous study with the cycloalkanemethanols, see ref. 185); and (c) the intravenous anesthetic alphaxalone disorders lipid bilayers while its inactive isomer betaxolone does not disorder (126). However, not all evidence is consistent; although (+)-isoflurane is 50% more potent in rats than the (−) isomer when assayed by MAC (141), the optical isomers of the closely related halogenated anesthetic, halothane, do not differ in their ability to disorder lipid bilayers (117). Further analysis of EPR evidence pertaining to the disordered lipid hypothesis may be found in Janoff and Miller (109).

EPR of Anesthetic-Protein Interactions in Membranes

To investigate the relationship between anesthetic-induced lipid perturbations and functional effects on membrane proteins, Firestone et al. (66,69) studied acetylcholine receptor-rich membranes from *Torpedo* electroplax. Anesthetic concentrations required to desensitize receptors were compared to those that disordered bulk membrane lipid using 5-palmitate and 12-stearate spin labels (Fig. 14). It was found that anesthetic-induced bulk membrane disordering was strongly correlated with desensitization by the same agents (Fig. 15).

EPR has also been used to investigate anesthetic effects on the lipid domain immediately adjacent to, and in direct contact with integral membrane proteins, called the boundary lipid. The fraction of lipids in this microdomain, and their rotational dynamics, can be determined by spectral subtraction techniques (148). Specifically, a spectrum obtained from a protein-free, pure lipid system may be normalized, aligned and digitally subtracted from that obtained from a bilayer system containing the protein of interest. The difference spectrum then yields the component of the lipid immobilized by the presence of the protein, and double-integration can be used for quantitation. Alternatively, a lipid-alone spectrum may be incrementally added to the spectrum obtained from a purified, delipidated membrane protein,

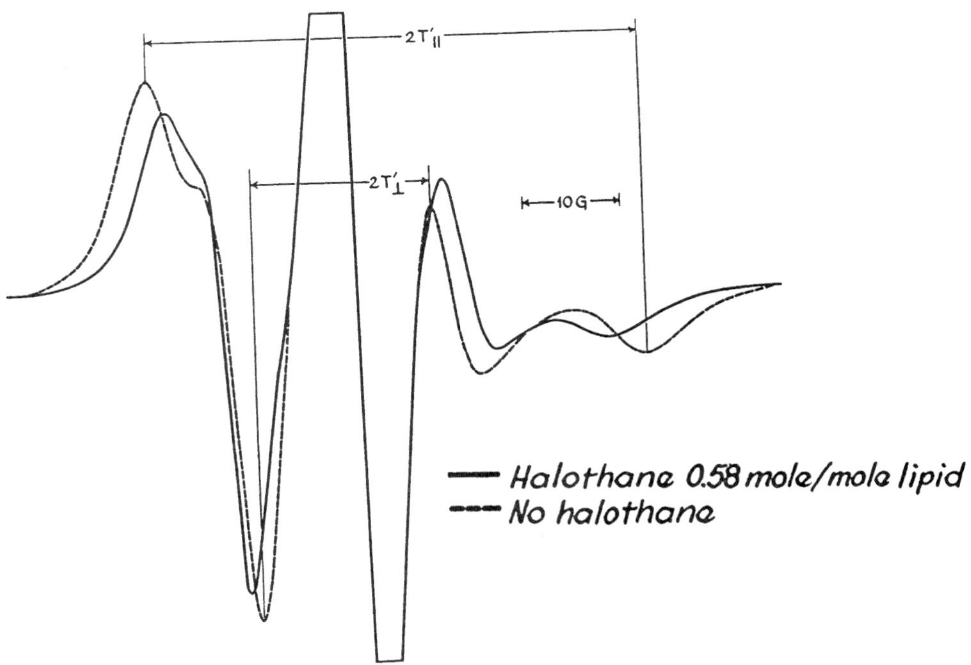

Figure 11. Effect of halothane on spin-labeled phosphtidylcholine-cholesterol vesicles. A phosphatidlycholine nitroxide spin probe (1% by weight) was used to label vesicles. Halothane reduces the hyperfine extremes, thus diminishes lipid order. The 58 mmoles of halothane per mole of lipid is close to the 30–60 mmoles/L predicted by the Meyer-Overton rule (174). (Reprinted with permission from Trudell JR, Hubbell WL, Cohen EN. Pressure reversal of inhalation anesthetic induced disorder in spin-labeled phospholipid vesicles. *Biochim Biophys Acta* 1973;291:335–340.)

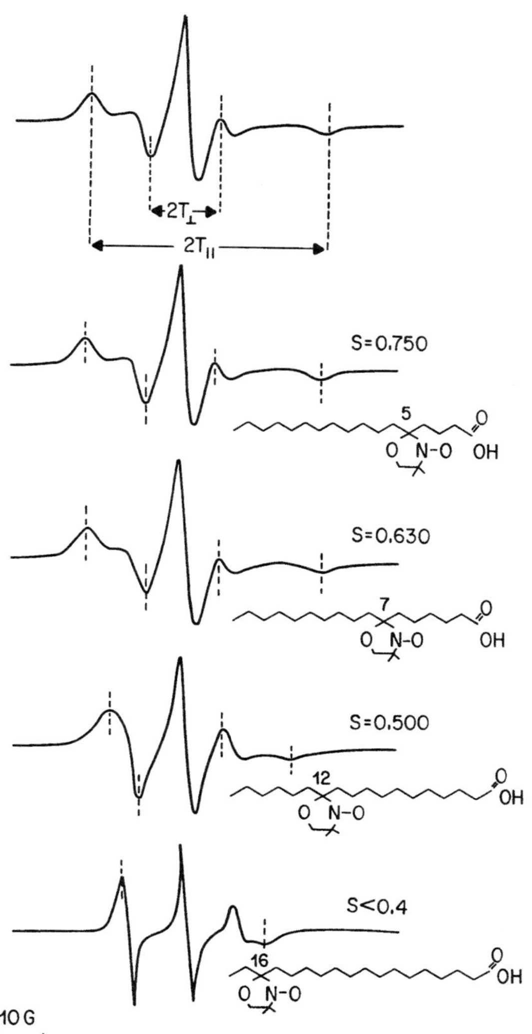

Figure 12. Order parameter (S)-dependence on position of the spin "reporter" on the spin probe molecule. EPR spectra, hyperfine splittings, and S are presented for 4 fatty acyl spin probes, whose spin reporters are positioned at varying distances from the carbonyl moiety (5, 7, 12, and 16 carbons, from top to bottom of figure). Because the carbonyl orients toward the aqueous interface, this series of spin reporters reflect the electronic environment at progressive depths in the membrane. S ranges from 0.750 (near the motionally restricted aqueous interface) to <0.4 (deep in the relatively less ordered hydrophobic membrane core), and consequently, anesthetic effects on S are depth-dependent (also see refs. 66 and 155). (Reprinted with permission from Firestone LL, Kitz RJ. Anesthetics and lipids: some molecular perspectives. *Semin Anesth* 1986;5:286–300.)

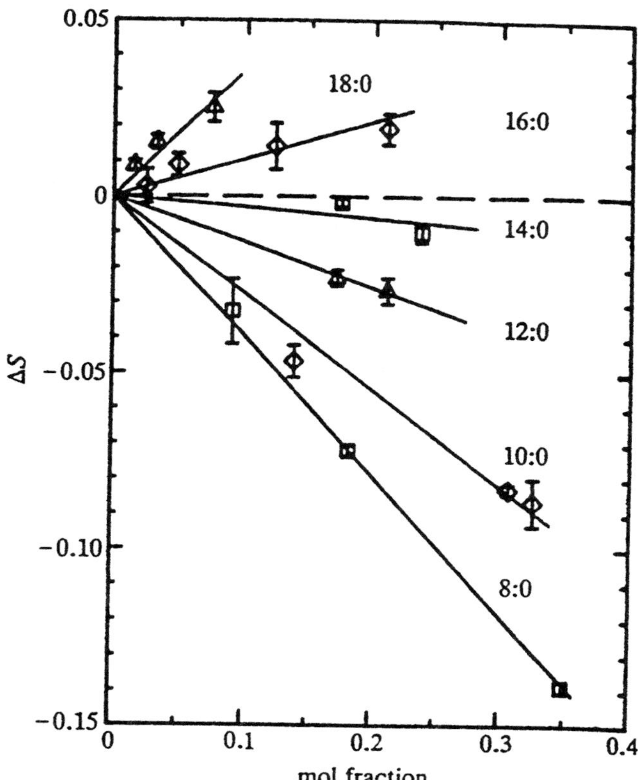

Figure 13. Cutoff in disordering potency among unbranched, primary alkanols. The change in lipid order parameter, S, is plotted as a function of mol fraction of alkanol in the membrane. S was measured from EPR spectra of a doxylstearic acid spin labeled on the 12th carbon. The membrane alcohol mol fraction [alkanol/(alkanol + lipid)] was established with ^{14}C-labeled alkanols, and the mol of lipid was taken as measured phospholipid plus 0.5 mol of cholesterol per phospholipid. *Lines* are least-squares fits; *points* are the mean of at least three samples in each of two experiments. Errors are SDs. Alkanol carbon chain lengths are listed to the right of each line (the absence of unsaturations is indicated by :0). In this alkanol series, disordering slopes gradually diminish with increasing alkanol molecular size; the slope for tetradecanol (14:0) is statistically the same as zero (i.e., the disordering effect "cuts off"). (Reprinted with permission from Miller KW, Firestone LL, Alifimoff JK, Streicher P. Nonanesthetic alcohols dissolve in synaptic membranes without perturbing their lipids. *Proc Natl Acad Sci USA* 1989;86:1084–1087.)

until the recombinant spectrum matches that of obtained from the native membrane. The boundary component then corresponds to [100% – (% lipid-alone)] (Fig. 16).

Applying such methodology to *Torpedo* electroplax membranes labeled with a C-14 spin-labeled phosphatidylcholine, Fraser et al. (86) reported that hexanol, urethane, diethyl ether, and ethanol decreased the percentage of motionally restricted lipid at the protein interface, in the case of hexanol from 33% to 20% at 7°C (Fig. 17), and prolonged the off-rates of exchange at the lipid-protein interface. However, such an effect required 16.7 mM hexanol, >20 times its obtunding potency, indicating the relative resistance of this lipid domain to anesthetics. Similar findings for ethanol, diethyl ether, halothane and octanol were reported by Firestone et al. (67) using both spectral subtraction, and the in-phase spectral saturation intensity method of Squier and Thomas (202), to distinguish the boundary component.

The Ca-ATPase from sarcoplamic reticulum (SR) has also been intensely studied as a model integral protein, and the effects on SR function of lipid disordering, protein rotational mobility, and protein aggregation state are well documented (201,209). For example, by spin labeling the Ca-ATPase protein, relations between its rotational dynamics (μs time domain) and boundary lipid mobility can be investigated by saturation transfer and conventional EPR, respectively (Fig. 18). Recently, Karon and Thomas (114) employed EPR to study the mechanism by which halothane activates the Ca-ATPase in SR from rabbit skeletal muscle. Using a stearic acid spin labeled at the C-5 position, halothane was shown to decrease lipid order in a manner analogous to heating, such that 311 mM (membrane) halothane reduced the order parameter to the same degree (19%) as an elevation of the temperature by 4°C. This amount disordering (or heating) was associated with a doubling of Ca-ATPase activity, probably on the basis of aggregation effects (Fig. 19). Qualitatively similar findings have been reported for the actions of diethyl ether on SR membranes (13).

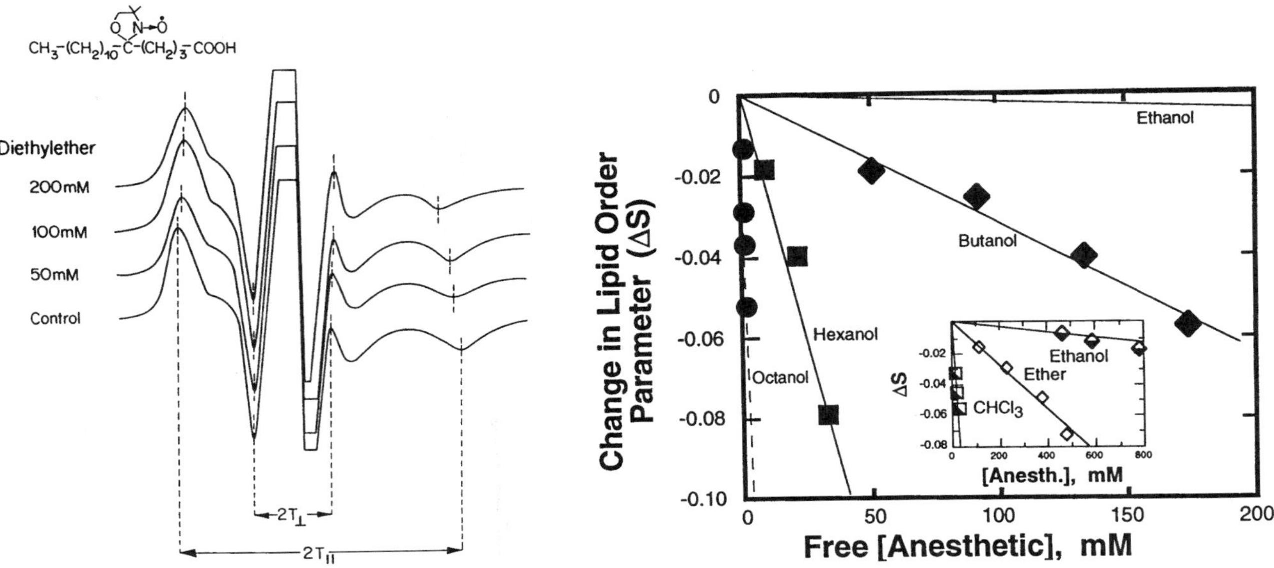

Figure 14. **(Left)** EPR spectra for *Torpedo* membranes labeled with a 5-palmitate spin label (*upper left*). Spectra obtained in the presence and absence of diethylether are vertically stacked; the hyperfine splittings are indicated by the *dashed lines.* The *x* axis is 100 Gauss; *y* axis is relative signal intensity. **(Right)** Anesthetic-induced change in lipid order parameter. Membranes were labeled as in the left panel; *lines* are least squares fit of data. **(Insert)** Data for an extended concentration range. (Reprinted with permission from Firestone LL, Alifimoff JK, Miller KW. Does general anesthetic-induced desensitization of the *Torpedo* acetycholine receptor correlate with lipid disordering? *Mol Pharmacol* 1994;46:508–515.)

EPR Studies of Other Relevant Physiologic Processes

Generation of free radicals, now known to play a pivotal role in microvascular control as well as the pathophysiology of ischemia and reperfusion injury, can be monitored by EPR. In the method known as spin trapping, a compound is used that can form a stable free radical after reacting covalently with an unstable free radical (Fig. 20), thus "trapping" it in a relatively long-lived form. Identification of a particular free radical depends on knowledge of the expected hyperfine splitting pattern ("fingerprint"), thus several different spin traps may be necessary for an unambiguous assignment. The effects of anesthetics, as well as numerous anesthesia-related physiologic perturbations, on free-radical generation during ischemia and reperfusion, is an area of active investigation by EPR.

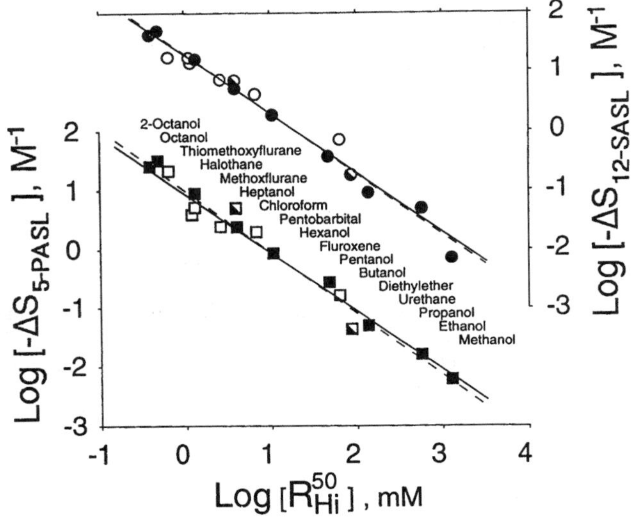

Figure 15. Correlation between anesthetic-induced receptor desensitization (*x* axis) and membrane disordering (both *y* axes). **(Upper plot)** Correlation using a spin label in the C-12 position (membrane interior). **(Lower plot)** C-5 spin label (near the aqueous interface). The *dashed lines* are free fits, whereas the *solid lines* are constrained to a slope of −1 (theoretical perfect correlation). The free fits do not differ from −1 ($p > 0.2$). (Reprinted with permission from Firestone LL, Alifimoff JK, Miller KW. Does general anesthetic-induced desensitization of the *Torpedo* acetycholine receptor correlate with lipid disordering? *Mol Pharmacol* 1994;46:508–515.)

Another example of EPR's utility when investigating the physiology of anesthesia involves the paramagnetic gas, nitric oxide. Nitric oxide has recently been shown to be a potent endogenous vasodilator, with modulatory effects on inflammation, thrombosis, immunity and neurotransmission (reviewed in refs. 160 and 161). Based on this, therapeutic trials are underway for both intravenous nitric oxide donors and nitric oxide synthase inhibitors (160), as well as for inhaled gaseous nitric oxide (87,189).

Under strict anaerobic conditions, nitric oxide binds reversibly to ferrous heme proteins to form nitrosyl hemes. Since nitrosylhemoglobins have EPR spectra that are easily observed at 77°K, with a characteristic hyperfine structure (Fig. 21) not seen when hemoglobin is exposed to other nitro compounds (e.g., NO_2^-, azide), hemoglobin can serve as a sensitive and specific spin trap. Thus the production of nitric oxide by many biologic systems was first observed by monitoring the appearance of the characteristic nitrosylhemoglobin hyperfine splittings at $g = \sim 2.00$ (reviewed in ref. 7).

Detection of nitrosylhemoglobin by EPR may also find use in the clinical realm. Based on the knowledge that iron-nitrosyl species appear during macrophage activation and sepsis, Lancaster et al. (124) investigated whether iron-nitrosyl EPR signals could be recognized in the blood of rats during rejection of

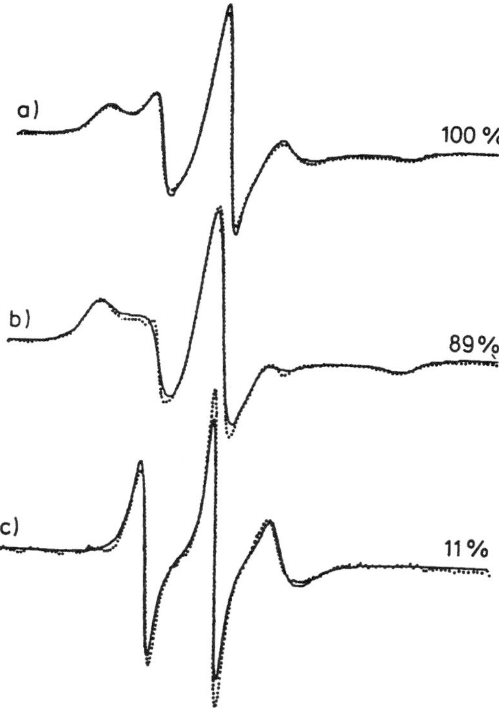

Figure 16. Identification of boundary lipid using spectral addition and subtraction. The *full lines* represent original EPR spectra: (a) integral membrane protein at a lipid/protein ratio of 12/1; (b) integral protein alone (note close correspondance of the outer hyperfine extrema with the spectrum in a; (c) lipid alone (note overall sharpened linewidths). The *dotted lines* represent summed or difference spectra: (a) 11% lipid-alone spectrum plus 89% protein-alone spectrum; (b) recombinant (*dotted*) spectrum "a" minus 11% lipid-alone spectrum (normalized); (c) recombinant (*dotted*) spectrum "a" minus 89% protein-alone spectrum. (Reprinted with permission from Marsh D. ESR spin label studies of lipid-protein interactions. In: Watts A, DePonts JM, eds. *Progress in protein-lipid interactions.* Amsterdam: Elsevier, 1985:143–172.)

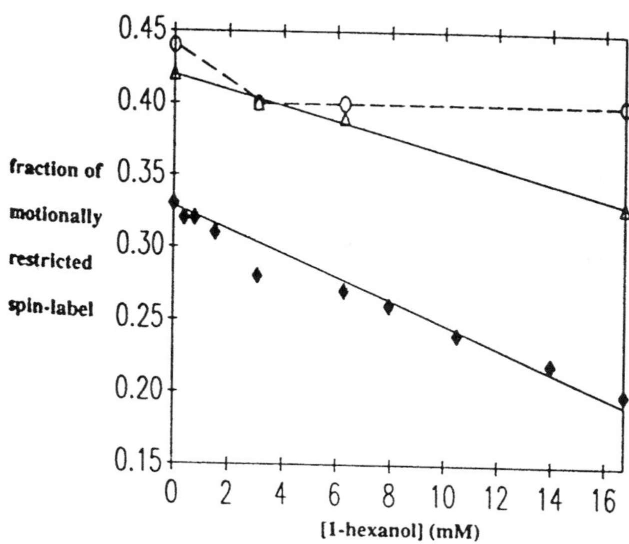

Figure 17. Effect of 1-hexanol on the fraction of motionally restricted spin label. Acetylcholine receptor rich membranes from *Torpedo* electroplax were spin labeled with a 14-stearic acid spin label (*circles*), a 14-phosphatidylcholine spin label (*diamonds*), or a 14-phosphatidylglycerol spin label (*triangles*). Spectral subtraction and simulation methods are described in detail elsewhere (86). (Reprinted with permission from Frasier DM, Louro SRW, Horvath LI, Miller KW, Watts A. A study of the effect of general anesthetics on lipid-protein interactions in acetylcholine receptor enriched membranes from *Torpedo nobiliana* using nitroxide spin labels. *Biochemistry* 1990;29: 2664–2669.)

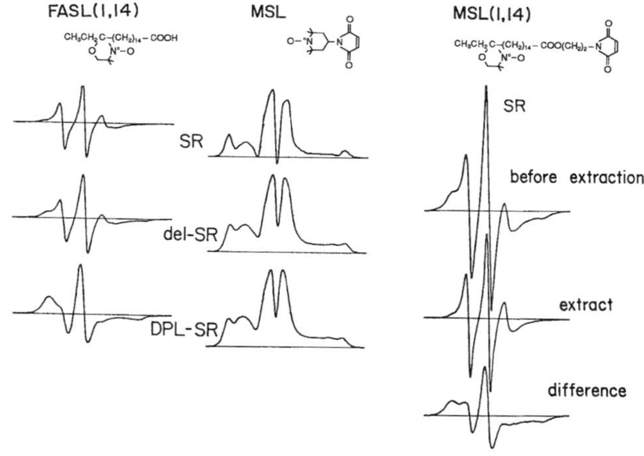

Figure 18. Effect of varying SR lipid content on lipid and Ca-ATPase dynamics. FASL(1,14): Conventional EPR spectra using fatty acid spin labeled at the C-14 position; note how the immobilized lipid component (outer hyperfine extrema) is enhanced in the partially delipidated SR (del-SR) and lipid-depleted SR (DPL-SR) compared to native membranes (SR). MSL: Saturation transfer EPR spectra using short chain maleimide spin label attached to the Ca-ATPase; note how progressive delipidation eliminates most of the μs mobility of the protein as reflected by the broadened linewidths and low field peak heights and ratio. MSL(1,14): Conventional EPR spectra using the long chain maleimide spin label attached to the Ca-ATPase, to probe the adjacent boundary lipid. The "extract" spectrum consists of lipid only, to correct for unreacted probe molecules in the SR lipid by subtraction from the native SR spectrum (before extraction). Thus, the difference spectrum represents the immobilized boundary component. (Reprinted with permission from Thomas DD, Bigelow DJ, Squier TC, Hidalgo C. Rotational dynamics of protein and boundary lipid in sarcoplasmic reticulum membrane. *Biophys J* 1982;37:217–225.)

allogeneic (but not syngeneic) heart grafts. They were able to directly demonstrate the formation of nitrosylhemoglobin during allograft rejection (Fig. 22), and its prevention by administration of the immunosuppressant, FK506. Early, noninvasive detection of human allograft rejection would clearly represent a significant therapeutic advance, and is one of many intriguing possibilities for future uses of EPR in anesthesia-related research.

Acknowledgment: This work was supported, in part, by grants from the National Institutes of Health (GM49202 to Y.X. for the NMR and MRI portion, and GM35900 to L.F. and GM15904 to the Harvard Anesthesia Center for the EPR portion), the Charles A. King Trust of Boston (to L.F.), and the Epilepsy Foundation of America (to Y.X.). Support from the Department of Anesthesia, Massachusetts General Hospital, the Department of Biological Chemistry and Molecular Pharmacology, Harvard Medical School, the Department of Anesthesiology and Critical Care Medicine, University of Pittsburgh, the Boston Biomedical Research Institute (for use of EPR equipment), and the University Anesthesiology and CCM Foundation of Pittsburgh is gratefully acknowledged. We also thank Richard J. Kitz, M.D., Jack Lancaster, Ph.D., Lawrence Litt, Ph.D., M.D., Keith W. Miller, D.Phil., Pei Tang, Ph.D., Peter M. Winter, M.D., Lisa Cohn, Maureen Di Battiste, and Melissa Sampson.

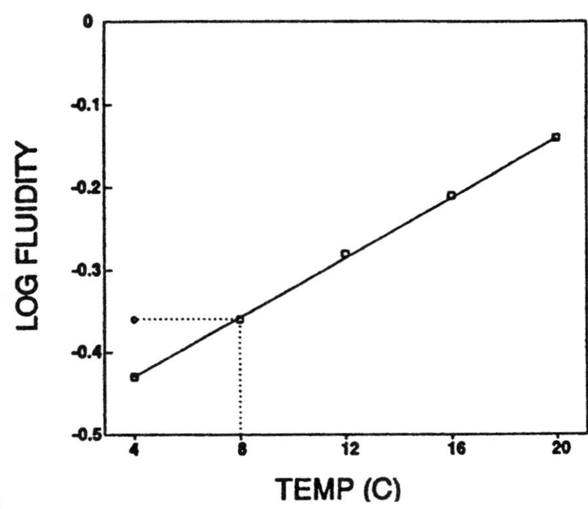

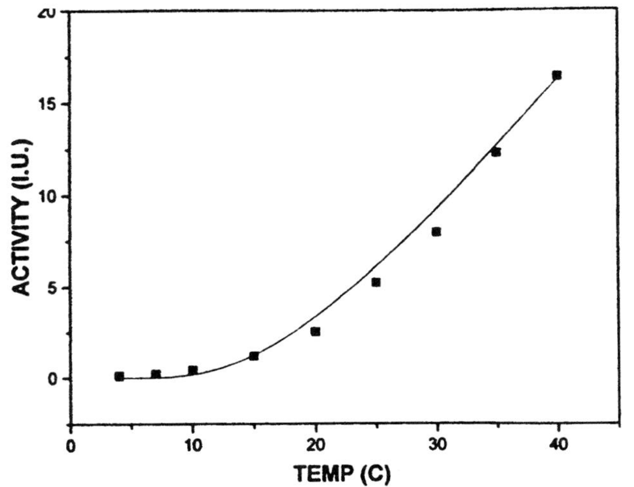

Figure 19. **A:** The effect of halothane and temperature on SR lipid disordering ("fluidity"). The fluidity of SR membrane with halothane 311 mM (membrane) is represented by the circle. The *dashed line* connecting it to the linear temperature relation illustrates that the increment in lipid fluidity produced by halothane is equivalent to that associated with a temperature elevation of 4°C. **B:** Experimental and simulated Ca-ATPase activity. Experimental data of Ca-ATPase activity at 4–40°C are represented by the *solid squares*; the *curve* is the activity predicted by lipid fluidity measurements in the same temperature range, using previous information relating SR lipid fluidity and Ca-ATPase aggregation state. The correspondence of fit supports a model where either temperature- or halothane-induced lipid disordering can shift the equilibrium of aggregates toward monomers and dimers, resulting in dramatic activation of the membrane-bound enzyme. (Reprinted with permission from Karon BS, Thomas DD. Molecular mechanism of Ca-ATPase activation by halothane in sarcoplasmic reticulum. *Biochemistry* 1993;32:7503–7511.)

CH_3 CH_3 $\overset{+}{N}$ O^- → CH_3 CH_3 $\overset{+}{N}$ O° H R

Figure 20. Spin trapping reaction. The nitrone compound 5,5-dimethylpyrroline-1-oxide (*left*), which is diamagnetic, may react in a free radical-generating reaction to form a paramagnetic adduct (*right*).

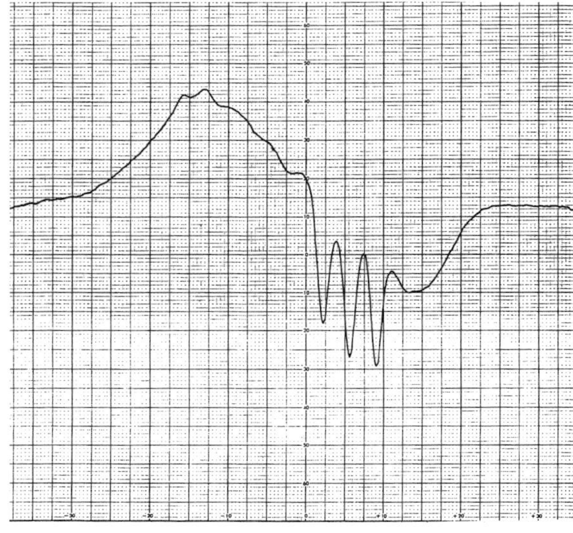

Figure 21. Characteristic spectrum of nitrosylhemoglobin at 77°K, derived from averaging 10 spectra. In this frozen state, a nine-line powder spectrum (a broad "triplet of triplets") results from the overlapping nitrogen contributions of the nitrosyl group and the proximal histidine. At physiologic pH, the low field peak is typically located at a *g* value of 2.04; the midfield triplet *g* is 2.00; and high field is 1.97. Spectrum was obtained on a Bruker ESP-300 spectrometer operating at 9.032 GHz, and digitized using the spectrometer's microcomputer running Bruker OS-9-compatible ESP 1600 spectral acquisition software. Instrumental parameters: 8 G modulation amplitude, 100 kHz modulation frequency, and 5 mW microwave power.

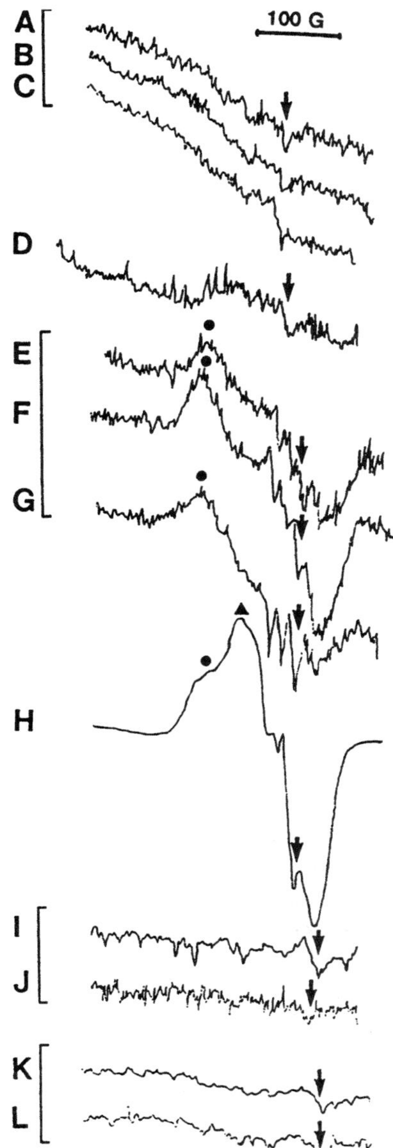

Figure 22. EPR spectra of packed rat erythrocytes under various conditions. Spectra A–C are from recipients of allogeneic hearts 3 days following the transplant operation; spectrum D is from untreated erythrocytes; spectra E–G are from recipients 5 days following heart transplantation; spectrum H is from erythrocytes treated with nitric oxide gas; spectra I and J are from recipients of syngeneic heart grafts 3 days following transplantation; spectra K and L are from recipients 5 days following transplantation. *Arrows* indicate $g = 2.00$; triangles indicate $g = 2.04$. (Reprinted with permission from Lancaster JR, Langrehr JM, Bergonia HA, Murase N, Simmons RL, Hoffman RA. EPR detection of heme and nonheme iron-containing protein nitrosylation by nitric oxide during rejection of rat heart allograft. *J Biol Chem* 1992;267: 10994–10998.)

REFERENCES

1. Abadji VC, Raines DE, Watts A, Miller KW. The effect of general anesthetics on the dynamics of phosphatidylcholine-acetylcholine receptor interactions in reconstituted vesicles. *Biochim Biophys Acta* 1993;1147:143–153.
2. Ackerman JJ, Ewy CS, Becker NN, Shalwitz RA. Deuterium nuclear magnetic resonance measurements of blood flow and tissue perfusion employing ^2H_2O as a freely diffusible tracer. *Proc Natl Acad Sci USA* 1987;84:4099–4102.
3. Ackerman JJ, Grove TH, Wong GG, Gadian DG, Radda GK. Mapping of metabolites in whole animals by ^{31}P NMR using surface coils. *Nature* 1980;283:167–170.
4. Alifimoff JK, Firestone LL, Miller KW. Anaesthetic potencies of primary alkanols: implications for the molecular dimensions of the anaesthetic site. *Br J Pharmacol* 1988;96:9–16.
5. Altura BM, Gebrewold A, Altura BT, Gupta RK. Role of brain $[Mg^{2+}]_i$ in alcohol-induced hemorrhagic stroke in a rat model: a ^{31}P-NMR *in vivo* study. *Alcohol* 1995;12:131–136.
6. Anderson CM, Saloner D, Tsuruda JS, Shapeero LG, Lee RE. Artifacts in maximum-intensity-projection display of MR angiograms. *AJR* 1990;154:623–629.
7. Archer S. Measurement of nitric oxide in biological models. *FASEB J* 1993;7:349–360.
8. Bachelard HS, Badar GR, Brooks KJ, Dolin SJ, Morris PG. Measurement of free intracellular calcium in the brain by ^{19}F-nuclear magnetic resonance spectroscopy. *J Neurochem* 1988;51: 1311–1313.
9. Back T, Hoehn BM, Kohno K, Hossmann KA. Diffusion nuclear magnetic resonance imaging in experimental stroke. Correlation with cerebral metabolites. *Stroke* 1994;25:494–500.
10. Badar GR, Ben YO, Dolin SJ, Morris PG, Smith GA, Bachelard HS. Use of 1,2-bis(2-amino-5-fluorophenoxy)ethane-N,N,N′,N′-tetraacetic acid (5FBAPTA) in the measurement of free intracellular calcium in the brain by ^{19}F-nuclear magnetic resonance spectroscopy. *J Neurochem* 1990;55:878–884.
11. Bangham AD, Hill W. The proton pump/leak mechanism of unconsciousness. *Chem Phys Lipids* 1986;40:189–205.
12. Barbour RL, Altura BM, Reiner SD, et al. Influence of Mg^{2+} on cardiac performance, intracellular free Mg^{2+} and pH in perfused hearts as assessed with ^{31}P nuclear magnetic resonance spectroscopy. *Magnes Trace Elem* 1991;10:99–116.
13. Bigelow DJ, Thomas DD. Rotational dynamics of lipid and the Ca-ATPase in sarcoplasmic reticulum. *J Biol Chem* 1987;262: 13449–13456.
14. Birken DL, Oldendorf WH. N-acetyl-L-aspartic acid: a literature review of a compound prominent in ^1H-NMR spectroscopic studies of brain. *Neurosci Biobehav Rev* 1989;13:23–31.
15. Bloch F, Hansen WW, Packard M. Nuclear induction. *Phys Rev* 1946;69:127.
16. Bock JL, Wenz B, Gupta RK. Changes in intracellular Mg adenosine riphosphate and ionized Mg^{2+} during blood storage—detection by ^{31}P nuclear magnetic resonance spectroscopy. *Blood* 1985;65: 1526–1530.
17. Boggs JM, Yoong T, Hsia JC. Site and mechanism of anesthetic action. I. Effect of anesthetics and pressure on fluidity of spin-labeled lipid vesicles. *Mol Pharmacol* 1976;12:127–135.
18. Boomsma F, Rupreht J, Man in 't Veld AJ, de Jong FH, Dzoljic M, Lachmann B. Haemodynamic and neurohumoral effects of xenon anaesthesia. *Anaesthesia* 1990;45:273–278.
19. Chang LH, James TL. NMR methods in studies of brain ischemia. *Biol Magn Reson* 1992;11:135–158.
20. Chang LH, Pereira BM, Weinstein PR, et al. Comparison of lactate concentration determinations in ischemic and hypoxic rat brains by *in vivo* and *in vitro* ^1H NMR spectroscopy. *Magn Reson Med* 1987; 4:575–581.
21. Chang LH, Shirane R, Weinstein PR, James TL. Cerebral metabolite dynamics during temporary complete ischemia in rats monitored by time-shared ^1H and ^{31}P NMR spectroscopy. *Magn Reson Med* 1990;13:6–13.
22. Chew W, Moseley ME, Mills PA, et al. Spin-echo fluorine magnetic resonance imaging at 2 T: *in vivo* spatial distribution of halothane in the rabbit head. *Magn Reson Imaging* 1987;5:51–56.
23. Chien D, Kwong KK, Gress DR, Buonanno FS, Buxton RB, Rosen BR. MR diffusion imaging of cerebral infarction in humans. *AJNR* 1992;13:1097–1102.
24. Chin JH, Trudell JR, Cohen EN. The compression-ordering and solubility-disordering effects of high pressure gases on phospholipid bilayers. *Life Sci* 1976;18:489–498.
25. Chiou JS, Ma SM, Kamaya H, Ueda I. Anesthesia cutoff phenomenon: interfacial hydrogen bonding. *Science* 1990;248:583–585.
26. Choi DW. Excitotoxic cell death. *J Neurobiology* 1992;23:1261–1276.
27. Chu SC, Xu Y, Balschi JA, Springer CJ. Bulk magnetic susceptibility shifts in NMR studies of compartmentalized samples: use of paramagnetic reagents. *Magn Reson Med* 1990;13:239–262.
28. Cohen EN. Metabolism of halothane-2 ^{14}C in the mouse. *Anesthesiology* 1969;31:560–565.

29. Cohen EN, Chow KL, Mathers L. Autoradiographic distribution of volatile anesthetics within the brain. *Anesthesiology* 1972;37:324–331.
30. Cohen EN, Hood N. Application of low-temperature autoradiography to studies of the uptake and metabolism of volatile anesthetics in the mouse. III. Halothane. *Anesthesiology* 1969;31:553–559.
31. Cohen Y, Chang LH, Litt L, et al. Stability of brain intracellular lactate and ^{31}P-metabolite levels at reduced intracellular pH during prolonged hypercapnia in rats. *J Cereb Blood Flow Metab* 1990; 10:277–284.
32. Corbett RJ, Laptook AR. Age-related changes in swine brain creatine kinase-catalyzed ^{31}P exchange measured *in vivo* using ^{31}P NMR magnetization transfer. *J Cereb Blood Flow Metab* 1994;14: 1070–1077.
33. Creasy JL, Price RR, Presbrey T, Goins D, Partain CL, Kessler RM. Gadolinium-enhanced MR angiography. *Radiology* 1990;175: 280–283.
34. Damadian R. Tumor detection by nuclear magnetic resonance. *Science* 1971;171:1151.
35. Dardzinski BJ, Sotak CH, Fisher M, Hasegawa Y, Li L, Minematsu K. Apparent diffusion coefficient mapping of experimental focal cerebral ischemia using diffusion-weighted echo-planar imaging. *Magn Reson Med* 1993;30:318–325.
36. Detre JA, Leigh JS, Williams DS, Koretsky AP. Perfusion imaging. *Magn Reson Med* 1992;23:37–45.
37. Detre JA, Zhang W, Roberts DA, et al. Tissue specific perfusion imaging using arterial spin labeling. *NMR Biomed* 1994;7:75–82.
38. Dickinson R, Franks NP, Lieb WR. Thermodynamics of anesthetic/protein interactions. Temperature studies on firefly luciferase. *Biophys J* 1993;64:1264–1271.
39. Dilger JP, Brett RS. Actions of volatile anesthetics and alcohols on cholinergic receptor channels. *Ann NY Acad Sci* 1991;625:616–627.
40. Dilger JP, Brett RS, Lesko LA. Effects of isoflurane on acetylcholine receptor channels. 1. Single-channel currents. *Mol Pharmacol* 1992;41:127–133.
41. Dilger JP, Brett RS, Mody HI. The effects of isoflurane on acetylcholine receptor channels: 2. Currents elicited by rapid perfusion of acetylcholine. *Mol Pharmacol* 1993;44:1056–1063.
42. Dilger JP, Liu Y. Desensitization of acetylcholine receptors in BC3H-1 cells. *Pflugers Arch* 1992;420:479–485.
43. Dilger JP, Vidal AM, Mody HI, Liu Y. Evidence for direct actions of general anesthetics on an ion channel protein. A new look at a unified mechanism of action. *Anesthesiology* 1994;81:431–442.
44. Dubois BW, Cherian SF, Evers AS. Volatile anesthetics compete for common binding sites on bovine serum albumin: a ^{19}F-NMR study. *Proc Natl Acad Sci USA* 1993;90:6478–6482.
45. Dubois BW, Evers AS. ^{19}F-NMR spin-spin relaxation (T_2) method for characterizing volatile anesthetic binding to proteins. Analysis of isoflurane binding to serum albumin. *Biochemistry* 1992;31: 7069–7076.
46. Dumoulin CL, Hart HJ. Magnetic resonance angiography. *Radiology* 1986;161:717–720.
47. Dumoulin CL, Souza SP, Feng H. Multiecho magnetic resonance angiography. *Magn Reson Med* 1987;5:47–57.
48. Dumoulin CL, Souza SP, Hardy CJ, Ash SA. Quantitative measurement of blood flow using cylindrically localized Fourier velocity encoding. *Magn Reson Med* 1991;21:242–250.
49. Dumoulin CL, Souza SP, Hart HR. Rapid scan magnetic resonance angiography. *Magn Reson Med* 1987;5:238–245.
50. Dumoulin CL, Souza SP, Walker MF, Wagle W. Three-dimensional phase contrast angiography. *Magn Reson Med* 1989;9:139–149.
51. Dumoulin CL, Souza SP, Walker MF, Yoshitome E. Time-resolved magnetic resonance angiography. *Magn Reson Med* 1988;6:275–286.
52. Ebisu T, Rooney WD, Graham SH, Weiner MW, Maudsley AA. N-acetylaspartate as an *in vivo* marker of neuronal viability in kainate-induced status epilepticus: ^{1}H magnetic resonance spectroscopic imaging. *J Cereb Blood Flow Metab* 1994;14:373–382.
53. Eckenhoff RG, Shuman H. Halothane binding to soluble proteins determined by photoaffinity labeling. *Anesthesiology* 1993;79:96–106.
54. Edelman RR, Mattle HP, Wallner B, et al. Extracranial carotid arteries: evaluation with "black blood" MR angiography. *Radiology* 1990;177:45–50.
55. Edelman RR, Wentz KU, Mattle H, et al. Projection arteriography and venography: initial clinical results with MR. *Radiology* 1989; 172:351–357.
56. Edelman RR, Wentz KU, Mattle HP, et al. Intracerebral arteriovenous malformations: evaluation with selective MR angiography and venography. *Radiology* 1989;173:831–837.
57. Eger EI II. *Anesthetic uptake and action.* Baltimore: Williams & Wilkins, 1974.
58. Eleff SM, Schnall MD, Ligetti L, et al. Concurrent measurements of cerebral blood flow, sodium, lactate, and high-energy phosphate metabolism using ^{19}F, ^{23}Na, ^{1}H, and ^{31}P nuclear magnetic resonance spectroscopy. *Magn Reson Med* 1988;7:412–424.
59. Ernst RR, Anderson WA. Application of fourier transform spectroscopy to magnetic resonance. *Rev Sci Instr* 1966;37:93.
60. Espanol MT, Litt L, Xu Y, et al. ^{19}F NMR calcium changes, edema and histology in neonatal rat brain slices during glutamate toxicity. *Brain Res* 1994;647:172–176.
61. Espanol MT, Litt L, Yang GY, et al. Tolerance of low intracellular pH during hypercapnia by rat cortical brain slices: a ^{31}P/^{1}H NMR study. *J Neurochem* 1992;59:1820–1828.
62. Espanol MT, Xu Y, Litt L, et al. Modulation of edema by dizocilpine, kynurenate, and NBQX in respiring brain slices after exposure to glutamate. *Acta Neurochir Suppl (Wien)* 1994;60:58–61.
63. Espanol MT, Xu Y, Litt L, et al. Modulation of glutamate-induced intracellular energy failure in neonatal cerebral cortical slices by kynurenic acid, dizocilpine, and NBQX. *J Cereb Blood Flow Metab* 1994;14:269–278.
64. Evers AS, Berkowitz BA, d'Avignon DA. Correlation between the anaesthetic effect of halothane and saturable binding in brain. *Nature* 1987;328:157–160.
65. Evers AS, Berkowitz BA, d'Avignon DA. Correlation between the anaesthetic effect of halothane and saturable binding in brain. *Nature* 1989;341:766.
66. Firestone LL, Alifimoff JK, Miller KW. Does general anesthetic-induced desensitization of the *Torpedo* acetylcholine receptor correlate with lipid disordering? *Mol Pharmacol* 1994;46:508–515.
67. Firestone LL, Ferguson C. Action of ethanol and volatile general anesthetics at boundary lipid. *Anesthesiology* 1990;72:A709.
68. Firestone LL, Kitz RJ. Anesthetics and lipids: some molecular perspectives. *Semin Anesth* 1986;5:286–300.
69. Firestone LL, Sauter J-F, Braswell LM, Miller KW. Actions of general anesthetics on acetylcholine receptor rich membranes from *Torpedo californica. Anesthesiology* 1986;64:694–702.
70. Firmin DN, Klipstein RH, Hounsfield GL, Paley MP, Longmore DB. Echo-planar high-resolution flow velocity mapping. *Magn Reson Med* 1989;12:316–327.
71. Fisel CR, Ackerman JL, Buxton RB, et al. MR contrast due to microscopically heterogeneous magnetic susceptibility: numerical simulations and applications to cerebral physiology. *Magn Reson Med* 1991;17:336–347.
72. Fisher M, Sotak CH, Minematsu K, Li L. New magnetic resonance techniques for evaluating cerebrovascular disease. *Ann Neurol* 1992; 32:115–122.
73. Foo TK, Perman WH, Poon CS, Cusma JT, Sandstrom JC. Projection flow imaging by bolus tracking using stimulated echoes. *Magn Reson Med* 1989;9:203–218.
74. Forman SA, Miller KW. Molecular sites of anesthetic action in postsynaptic nicotinic membranes. *Trends Pharmacol Sci* 1989;10: 447–452.
75. Frahm J, Merboldt KD, Hanicke W, Gyngell ML, Bruhn H. Rapid line scan NMR angiography. *Magn Reson Med* 1988;7:79–87.
76. Franks NP, Lieb WR. Where do general anaesthetics act? *Nature* 1977;274:339–342.
77. Franks NP, Lieb WR. Do general anaesthetics act by competitive binding to specific receptors? *Nature* 1984;310:599–601.
78. Franks NP, Lieb WR. Mapping of general anaesthetic target sites provides a molecular basis for cutoff effects. *Nature* 1985;316: 349–351.
79. Franks NP, Lieb WR. What is the molecular nature of general anaesthetic target sites? *Trends Pharmacol Sci* 1987;8:169–174.
80. Franks NP, Lieb WR. Anaesthetics on the mind. *Nature* 1987;328: 113–114.
81. Franks NP, Lieb WR. Volatile general anaesthetics activate a novel neuronal K^+ current. *Nature* 1988;333:662–664.
82. Franks NP, Lieb WR. Selective effects of general anesthetics on identified neurons. *Ann NY Acad Sci* 1991;625:54–70.
83. Franks NP, Lieb WR. Stereospecific effects of inhalational general anesthetic optical isomers on nerve ion channels. *Science* 1991; 254:427–430.
84. Franks NP, Lieb WR. Selective actions of volatile general anaesthetics at molecular and cellular levels. *Br J Anaesth* 1993;71:65–76.
85. Franks NP, Lieb WR. Molecular and cellular mechanisms of general anaesthesia. *Nature* 1994;367:607–614.

86. Frasier DM, Louro SRW, Horvath LI, Miller KW, Watts A. A study of the effect of general anesthetics on lipid-protein interactions in acetylcholine receptor enriched membranes from *Torpedo nobiliana* using nitroxide spin labels. *Biochemistry* 1990;29:2664–2669.
87. Frostell CG, Blomqvist H, Hedenstierna G, Lundberg J, Zapol WM. Inhaled nitric oxide selectively reverses human hypoxic pulmonary vasoconstriction without causing systemic vasodilation. *Anesthesiology* 1993;78:427–435.
88. Fukushima E, Roeder SBW. *Experimental pulse NMR: a nuts and bolts approach.* Addison-Wesley, Reading, MA, 1981.
89. Gadian DG, Allen K, van BN, Busza AL, King MD, Williams SR. Applications of NMR spectroscopy to the study of experimental stroke in vivo. *Stroke* 1993;24:157–159.
90. Gaffney BJ. Practical considerations for the calculation of order parameters for fatty acid or phospholipid spin labels in membranes. In: Berliner LJ, ed. *Spin labeling theory and applications, vol. 1.* New York: Academic Press, 1979:567–571.
91. Gill R, Sibson NR, Hatfield RH, et al. A comparison of the early development of ischaemic damage following permanent middle cerebral artery occlusion in rats as assessed using magnetic resonance imaging and histology. *J Cereb Blood Flow Metab* 1995;15: 1–11.
92. Gill SC, Perez TA, Xue M, Furlan AJ, Awad IA. Magnetic resonance diffusion-weighted imaging: sensitivity and apparent diffusion constant in stroke. *Acta Neurochir Suppl (Wien)* 1994;60:207–210.
93. Gillis P, Koenig SH. Transverse relaxation of solvent protons induced by magnetized spheres: application to ferritin, erythrocytes, and magnetite. *Magn Reson Med* 1987;5:323–345.
94. Gonzalez-Mendez R, Litt L, Koretsky AP, Von Colditz J, Weiner MW, James TL. Comparison of ^{31}P NMR Spectra of *in vivo* rat brain using convolution difference and saturation with a surface coil. Source of the broad component in the brain spectrum. *J Magn Reson* 1984;57:526–533.
95. Gruner SM. Stability of lyotropic phases with curved interfaces. *J Phys Chem* 1989;93:7562–7570.
96. Gruner SM, Shyamsunder E. Is the mechanism of general anesthesia related to lipid membrane spontaneous curvature? *Ann NY Acad Sci* 1991;625:685–697.
97. Gupta RK, Gupta P, Moore RD. NMR studies of intracellular metal ions in intact cells and tissues. *Annu Rev Biophys Bioeng* 1984;13: 221–246.
98. Haase A, Frahm AJ, Matthaei JD, Hnicke W, Merboltd KD. FLASH imaging. Rapid NMR imaging using low flip-angle pulses. *J Magn Reson* 1986;67:258–266.
99. Hahn EL. NMR and MRI in retrospect. *Philos Trans R Soc Lond A* 1990;333:403–411.
100. Hall AC, Lieb WR, Franks NP. Stereoselective and non-stereoselective actions of isoflurane on the GABAA receptor. *Br J Pharmacol* 1994;112:906–910.
101. Harris B, Moody E, Skolnick P. Isoflurane anesthesia is stereoselective. *Eur J Pharmacol* 1992;217:215–216.
102. Harris BD, Moody EJ, Basile AS, Skolnick P. Volatile anesthetics bidirectionally and stereospecifically modulate ligand binding to GABA receptors. *Eur J Pharmacol* 1994;267:269–274.
103. Harrison NL, Kugler JL, Jones MV, Greenblatt EP, Pritchett DB. Positive modulation of human gamma-aminobutyric acid type A and glycine receptors by the inhalation anesthetic isoflurane. *Mol Pharmacol* 1993;44:628–632.
104. Haydon DA, Elliott JR, Hendry BM. Effects of anesthetics on the squid giant axon, in Kleinzeller A, Baker PF (eds). *Curr Top Membr Transp* 1984;22:445–482, Academic Press, London.
105. Hemmer W, Wallimann T. Functional aspects of creatine kinase in brain. *Dev Neurosci* 1993;15:249–260.
106. Hetherington HP, Avison MJ, Shulman RG. ^{1}H homonuclear editing of rat brain using semiselective pulses. *Proc Natl Acad Sci USA* 1985;82:3115–3118.
107. Hubbell WL, McConnell HM. Spin label studies of the excitable membranes of nerve and muscle. *Proc Natl Acad Sci USA* 1968;61: 12–16.
108. Hyde JS, Dalton LR, Saturation transfer spectroscopy. In: Berliner LJ, ed. *Spin labeling theory and applications, Vol. 2.* New York: Academic Press, 1979:3–70.
109. Janoff A, Miller KW. A critical assessment of the lipid theories of general anaesthetic action. In: Chapman D, ed. *Biological membranes, vol. 4.* New York: Academic Press, 1982:417–476.
110. Jones MV, Brooks PA, Harrison NL. Enhancement of gamma-aminobutyric acid-activated Cl- currents in cultured rat hippocampal neurones by three volatile anaesthetics. *J Physiol (Lond)* 1992;449:279–293.
111. Jones MV, Harrison NL. Effects of volatile anesthetics on the kinetics of inhibitory postsynaptic currents in cultured rat hippocampal neurons. *J Neurophysiol* 1993;70:1339–1349.
112. Jost P, Griffith OH. Instrumental aspects of spin labeling. In: Berliner LJ, ed. *Spin labeling theory and applications, vol. 2.* New York: Academic Press, 1979:251–272.
113. Kaneshina S, Lin HC, Ueda I. Anisotropic solubilization of an inhalation anesthetic, methoxyflurane, into the interfacial region of cationic surfactant micelles. *Biochim Biophys Acta* 1981;647: 223–226.
114. Karon BS, Thomas DD. Molecular mechanism of Ca-ATPase activation by halothane in sarcoplasmic reticulum. *Biochemistry* 1993;32: 7503–7511.
115. Keller PJ, Drayer BP, Fram EK, Williams KD, Dumoulin CL, Souza SP. MR angiography with two-dimensional acquisition and three-dimensional display. Work in progress. *Radiology* 1989;173: 527–532.
116. Kelusky EC, Boulanger Y, Schreier S, Smith ICP. A ^{2}H-NMR study on the interactions of the local anesthetic tetracaine with membranes containing phosphatidylserine. *Biochim Biophys Acta* 1986; 856:85–90.
117. Kendig JJ, Trudell JR, Cohen EN. Halothane stereoisomers: lack of stereospecificity in two model systems. *Anesthesiology* 1973;39: 510–524.
118. Kim SG, Ackerman JJ. Multicompartment analysis of blood flow and tissue perfusion employing D_2O as a freely diffusible tracer: a novel deuterium NMR technique demonstrated via application with murine RIF-1 tumors. *Magn Reson Med* 1988;8:410–426.
119. Koehler L, Fossel ET, Koehler KA. Halothane fluorine-19 nuclear magnetic resonance in dipalmitoylphosphatidylcholine liposomes. *Biochemistry* 1977;16:3700–3707.
120. Krnjevic K. Cellular mechanisms of anesthesia. *Ann NY Acad Sci* 1991;625:1–16.
121. Kucharczyk J, Vexler ZS, Roberts TP, et al. Echo-planar perfusion-sensitive MR imaging of acute cerebral ischemia. *Radiology* 1993; 188:711–717.
122. Kupriyanov VV, Balaban RS, Lyulina NV, Steinschneider AYA, Saks VA. Combination of ^{31}P-NMR magnetization transfer and radioisotope exchange methods for assessment of an enzyme reaction mechanism: rate-determining steps of the creatine kinase reaction. *Biochim Biophys Acta* 1990;1020:290–304.
123. Lachmann B, Armbruster S, Schairer W, et al. Safety and efficacy of xenon in routine use as an inhalational anaesthetic. *Lancet* 1990; 335:1413–1415.
124. Lancaster JR, Langrehr JM, Bergonia HA, Murase N, Simmons RL, Hoffman RA. EPR detection of heme and nonheme iron-containing protein nitrosylation by nitric oxide during rejection of rat heart allograft. *J Biol Chem* 1992;267:10994–10998.
125. Lauterbur PC. Image formation by induced local interactions: examples employing nuclear magnetic resonance. *Nature* 1973; 242:190–191.
126. Lawrence DK, Gill EW. Structurally specific efects of some steroid anesthetics on spin labeled liposomes. *Mol Pharmacol* 1975;11: 280–286.
127. Le Bihan D. Molecular diffusion nuclear magnetic resonance imaging. *Magn Reson Q* 1991;7:1–30.
128. Le Bihan D, Breton E, Lallemand D, Grenier P, Cabanis E, Laval-Jeantet M. MR imaging of intravoxel incoherent motions: application to diffusion and perfusion in neurologic disorders. *Radiology* 1986;161:401–407.
129. Le Bihan D, Turner R, Douek P, Patronas N. Diffusion MR imaging: clinical applications. *AJR* 1992;159:591–599.
130. Lieb WR, Kovalycsik M, Mendelsohn R. Do clinical levels of general anaesthetics affect lipid bilayers? Evidence from Raman scattering. *Biochim Biophys Acta* 1982;688:388–398.
131. Lin LH, Chen LL, Zirrolli JA, Harris RA. General anesthetics potentiate gamma-aminobutyric acid actions on gamma-aminobutyric acidA receptors expressed by Xenopus oocytes: lack of involvement of intracellular calcium. *J Pharmacol Exp Ther* 1992;263:569–578.
132. Lin LH, Leonard S, Harris RA. Enflurane inhibits the function of mouse and human brain phosphatidylinositol-linked acetylcholine and serotonin receptors expressed in Xenopus oocytes. *Mol Pharmacol* 1993;43:941–948.
133. Lin LH, Whiting P, Harris RA. Molecular determinants of general anesthetic action: role of GABAA receptor structure. *J Neurochem* 1993;60:1548–1553.

134. Litt L, González-Méndez R, James TL, et al. An *in vivo* study of halothane uptake and elimination in the rat brain with fluorine nuclear magnetic resonance spectroscopy. *Anesthesiology* 1987;67:161–168.
135. Litt L, González-Méndez R, Severinghaus JW, et al. Cerebral intracellular changes during supercarbia: an *in vivo* ^{31}P nuclear magnetic resonance study in rats. *J Cereb Blood Flow Metab* 1985;5:537–544.
136. Litt L, Lockhart S, Cohen Y, et al. *In vivo* ^{19}F nuclear magnetic resonance brain studies of halothane, isoflurane, and desflurane. Rapid elimination and no abundant saturable binding. *Ann NY Acad Sci* 1991;625:707–724.
137. Litt L, Xu Y, Cohen Y, James TL. Nonmagnetic hyperbaric chamber for in vivo NMR spectroscopy studies of small animals. *Magn Reson Med* 1993;29:812–816.
138. Lockhart SH, Cohen Y, Yasuda N, et al. Cerebral uptake and elimination of desflurane, isoflurane, and halothane from rabbit brain: an *in vivo* NMR study. *Anesthesiology* 1991;74:575–580.
139. Lockhart SH, Cohen Y, Yasuda N, et al. Absence of abundant binding sites for anesthetics in rabbit brain: an in vivo NMR study. *Anesthesiology* 1990;73:455–460.
140. Lowe IJ, Norberg RE. Free induction decay in solids. *Phys Rev* 1957;107:46–61.
141. Lysko GS, Robinson JL, Casto R, Ferrone RA. The stereospecific effects of isoflurane *in vivo. Eur J Pharmacol* 1994;263:25–29.
142. Macura S, Ernst RR. Elucidation of cross-relaxation in liquids by two-dimensional nuclear magnetic resonance spectroscopy. *Mol Phys* 1980;41:95–117.
143. Maeda M, Itoh S, Ide H, et al. Acute stroke in cats: comparison of dynamic susceptibility-contrast MR imaging with T2- and diffusion-weighted MR imaging. *Radiology* 1993;189:227–232.
144. Majumdar S, Zoghbi SS, Gore JC. Regional differences in rat brain displayed by fast MRI with superparamagnetic contrast agents. *Magn Reson Imaging* 1988;6:611–615.
145. Mansfield P, Maudsley AA. Medical imaging by NMR. *Br J Radiol* 1977;50:188–194.
146. Mansfield P, Morris PG. NMR imaging in biomedicine. In: Waugh JS, ed. *Advances in magnetic resonance, supplement 2.* New York: Academic Press, 1982:2.
147. Marchal G, Bosmans H, Van FL, et al. Intracranial vascular lesions: optimization and clinical evaluation of three-dimensional time-of-flight MR angiography. *Radiology* 1990;175:443–448.
148. Marsh D. ESR spin label studies of lipid-protein interactions. In: Watts A, DePonts JM, eds. *Progress in protein-lipid interactions.* Amsterdam: Elsevier, 1985:143–172.
149. Masaryk TJ, Modic MT, Ross JS, et al. Intracranial circulation: preliminary clinical results with three-dimensional (volume) MR angiography. *Radiology* 1989;171:793–799.
150. Masaryk TJ, Modic MT, Ruggieri PM, et al. Three-dimensional (volume) gradient-echo imaging of the carotid bifurcation: preliminary clinical experience. *Radiology* 1989;171:801–806.
151. Mastrangelo CJ, Trudell JR, Edmunds HN, et al. Effects of clinical concentrations of halothane on phospholipid-cholesterol membrane fluidity. *Anesthesiology* 1973;39:518–524.
152. Matthaei D, Frahm J, Haase A, Merboldt KD, Hanicke W. Multipurpose NMR imaging using stimulated echoes. *Magn Reson Med* 1986;3:554–561.
153. Metcalfe JC, Seeman P, Burgen ASV. The proton relaxation of benzyl alcohol in erythrocyte membranes. *Mol Pharmacol* 1968;4: 87–95.
154. Miller KW. The nature of the sites of general anesthesia. *Int Rev Neurobiol* 1985;27:1–61.
155. Miller KW, Braswell LM, Firestone LL, et al. General anesthetics act both specifically and nonspecifically on acetylcholine receptors. In: Roth S, Miller KW, eds. *Molecular and cellular mechanisms of anesthetics.* New York: Plenum Press, 1986:125–138.
156. Miller KW, Firestone LL, Alifimoff JK, Streicher P. Nonanesthetic alcohols dissolve in synaptic membranes without perturbing their lipids. *Proc Natl Acad Sci USA* 1989;86:1084–1087.
157. Miller KW, Pang K-YY. General anesthetics can selectively perturb lipid bilayer membranes. *Nature* 1976;263:253–255.
158. Miller KW, Reo NV, Schoot Uiterkamp AJM, Stengle DP, Stengle TR, Williamson KL. Xenon NMR: chemical shifts of a general anesthetic in common solvents, protein, and membranes. *Proc Natl Acad Sci USA* 1981;78:4946–4949.
159. Mills PA, Sessler DI, Moseley M, et al. An *in vivo* ^{19}F nuclear magnetic resonance study of isoflurane elimination in the rabbit brain. *Anesthesiology* 1987;67:169–173.
160. Moncada S, Higgs EA. Molecular mechanisms and therapeutic strategies related to nitric oxide. *FASEB J* 1995;9:1319–1330.
161. Moncada S, Palmer RMJ, Higgs EA. Nitric oxide: physiology, pathophysiology and pharmacology. *Pharmacol Rev* 1991;43:109–141.
162. Moody EJ, Harris BD, Skolnick P. Stereospecific actions of the inhalation anesthetic isoflurane at the $GABA_A$ receptor complex. *Brain Res* 1993;615:101–106.
163. Moody EJ, Harris BD, Skolnick P. The potential for safer anaesthesia using stereoselective anaesthetics. *Trends Pharmacol Sci* 1994;15:387–391.
164. Morgan PG, Sedensky M, Mcneely PM. Multiple sites of action of volatile anesthetics in *Caenorhabditis elegans. Proc Natl Acad Sci USA* 1990;87:2965–2969.
165. Moseley ME, Wendland MF, Kucharczyk J. Magnetic resonance imaging of diffusion and perfusion. *Top Magn Reson Imaging* 1991;3:50–67.
166. Mosher TJ, Williams GD, Doumen C, LaNoue KF, Smith MB. Error in the calibration of the MgATP chemical shift limit: effects on the determination of free magnesium by ^{31}P NMR spectroscopy. *Magn Reson Med* 1992;24:163–169.
167. Muller TB, Haraldseth O, Jones RA, et al. Combined perfusion and diffusion-weighted magnetic resonance imaging in a rat model of reversible middle cerebral artery occlusion. *Stroke* 1995;26:451–458.
168. Nakahiro M, Yeh JZ, Brunner E, Narahashi T. General anesthetics modulate GABA receptor channel complex in rat dorsal root ganglion neurons. *FASEB J* 1989;3:1850–1854.
169. Neil JJ. The validation of freely diffusible tracer methods with NMR detection for measurement of blood flow. *Magn Reson Med* 1991;19:299–304.
170. Ogawa S, Lee TM. Magnetic resonance imaging of blood vessels at high fields: in vivo and in vitro measurements and image simulation. *Magn Reson Med* 1990;16:9–18.
171. Ogawa S, Lee TM, Barrere B. The sensitivity of magnetic resonance image signals of a rat brain to changes in the cerebral venous blood oxygenation. *Magn Reson Med* 1993;29:205–210.
172. Ogawa S, Lee TM, Kay AR, Tank DW. Brain magnetic resonance imaging with contrast dependent on blood oxygenation. *Proc Natl Acad Sci USA* 1990;87:9868–9872.
173. Ogawa S, Lee TM, Nayak AS, Glynn P. Oxygenation-sensitive contrast in magnetic resonance image of rodent brain at high magnetic fields. *Magn Reson Med* 1990;14:68–78.
174. Overton CE. *Studies of narcosis.* New York: Chapman and Hall, 1991.
175. Pang K-Y, Miller KW. Cholesterol modulates the effects of membrane perturbers in phospholipid vesicles and biomenbranes. *Biochim Biophys Acta* 1978;11:1–9.
176. Pang K-YY, Braswell LM, Chang L, et al. The perturbation of lipid bilayers by general anesthetics: a quantitative test of the disordered lipid hypothesis. *Mol Pharmacol* 1980;18:84–90.
177. Pawlik G, Rackl A, Bing RJ. Quantitative capillary topography and blood flow in the cerebral cortex of cats: an in vivo microscopic study. *Brain Res* 1981;208:35–58.
178. Perez TA, Xue M, Ng TC, et al. Sensitivity of magnetic resonance diffusion-weighted imaging and regional relationship between the apparent diffusion coefficient and cerebral blood flow in rat focal cerebral ischemia. *Stroke* 1995;26:667–674.
179. Pernicone JR, Siebert JE, Potchen EJ, Pera A, Dumoulin CL, Souza SP. Three-dimensional phase-contrast MR angiography in the head and neck: preliminary report. *AJR* 1990;155:167–176.
180. Petroff OA, Prichard JW, Behar KL, Alger JR, den Hollander JA, Shulman RG. Cerebral intracellular pH by ^{31}P nuclear magnetic resonance spectroscopy. *Neurology* 1985;35:781–788.
181. Pettegrew JW, ed. *NMR: principles and applications to biomedical research.* Berlin: Springer-Verlag, 1990.
182. Prichard JW. Nuclear magnetic resonance methods in stroke. *Stroke* 1993;24:170–171.
183. Prichard JW, Shulman RG. NMR spectroscopy of brain metabolism *in vivo. Annu Rev Neurosci* 1986;9:61–85.
184. Purcell EM, Torrey HC, Pound RV. Resonant absorption by nuclear magnetic moments in a solid. *Physiol Rev* 1946;69:37.
185. Raines DK, Korten SE, Hill AG, Miller KW. Anesthetic cutoff in cycloalkanemethanols. *Anesthesiology* 1993;78:918–927.
186. Reith W, Hasegawa Y, Latour LL, Dardzinski BJ, Sotak CH, Fisher M. Multislice diffusion mapping for 3-D evolution of cerebral ischemia in a rat stroke model. *Neurology* 1995;45:172–177.
187. Richards CD. The synaptic basis of general anaesthesia. *Eur J Anaesthesiol* 1995;12:5–19.

188. Ross JS, Masaryk TJ, Modic MT, Ruggieri PM, Haacke EM, Selman WR. Intracranial aneurysms: evaluation by MR angiography. *AJNR* 1990;11:449–455.
189. Rossaint R, Falke KJ, Lopez F, Slama K, Pison U, Zapol W. Inhaled nitric oxide for the adult respiratory distress syndrome. *N Engl J Med* 1993;328:399–405.
190. Rothman DL, Behar KL, Hetherington HP, Shulman RG. Homonuclear ^{1}H double-resonance difference spectroscopy of the rat brain in vivo. *Proc Natl Acad Sci USA* 1984;81:6330–6334.
191. Roy CS, Sherrington CS. On the regulation of the blood supply of the brain. *J Physiol* 1890;11:85–108.
192. Ruggieri PM, Laub GA, Masaryk TJ, Modic MT. Intracranial circulation: pulse-sequence considerations in three-dimensional (volume) MR angiography. *Radiology* 1989;171:785–791.
193. Sastry BVR, Franks JJ, Surber MJ. Halothane-induced alteration in the fluidity of rat brain synaptosomal membranes and its relationship to anesthesia. *Ann NY Acad Sci* 1991;625:433–437.
194. Seega J, Elger B. Diffusion- and T_2-weighted imaging: evaluation of oedema reduction in focal cerebral ischaemia by the calcium and serotonin antagonist levemopamil. *Magn Reson Imaging* 1993; 11:401–409.
195. Seelig J, Seelig A. Lipid conformation in model membranes and biological membranes. *Q Rev Biophys* 1980;13:19–61.
196. Singer JR. Blood flow rates by nuclear magnetic resonance measurements. *Science* 1959;130:1652–1653.
197. Smith ICP, Auger M, Jarrell HC. Molecular details of anesthetic-lipid interaction. *Ann NY Acad Sci* 1991;625:668–684.
198. Smith ICP, Butler KW. Location and dynamics of anesthetics in membranes: a magnetic resonance view. In: Covino BG, Fozzard HA, Rehder K, Strichartz G, eds. *Effects of anesthesia.* Baltimore: Waverly Press, 1985:1–11.
199. Smith ICP, Butler KW. Molecular details of anesthetic-lipid interaction as seen by nuclear magnetic resonance. In: Roth SH, Miller KW, eds. *Molecular and cellular mechanisms of anaesthetics.* New York: Plenum Press, 1986:309–318.
200. Spritzer CE, Pelc NJ, Lee JN, Evans AJ, Sostman HD, Riederer SJ. Rapid MR imaging of blood flow with a phase-sensitive, limited-flip-angle, gradient recalled pulse sequence: preliminary experience. *Radiology* 1990;176:255–262.
201. Squier TC, Bigelow DJ, Thomas DD. Lipid fluidity directly modulates the overall protein rotational mobility of the Ca-ATPase in sarcoplasmic reticulum. *J Biol Chem* 1988;263:9178–9186.
202. Squier TC, Thomas DD. Selective detection of the rotational dynamics of the protein-associated lipid hydrocarbon chains in sarcoplasmic reticulum membranes. *Biophys J* 1989;56:735–748.
203. Stejskal EO, Tanner JE. Spin diffusion measurements: spin echoes in the presence of a time dependent field gradient. *J Chem Phys* 1965;42:288–292.
204. Stengle TR, Hosseini SM, Basiri HG, Williamson KL. NMR chemical shifts of xenon in aqueous solutions of amphiphiles: a new probe of the hydrophobic environment. *J Solution Chem* 1984;13:779–787.
205. Stengle TR, Hosseini SM, Williamson KL. NMR chemical shifts of xenon in mixed aprotic solvents: a probe of liquid structure. *J Solution Chem* 1986;15:777–790.
206. Strum DP, Johnson BH, Eger EI II. Elimination of anesthetics from rabbit brain. *Science* 1986;234:1586–1587.
207. Sweitzer MC, Kramer DM. Standard MR pulse sequences: a closer look. In: Woodward P, Freimarck RD, eds. *MRI for technologists.* New York: McGraw-Hill, 1995:91–124.
208. Tang P, Xu Y. Probing sites of anesthetic interaction using xenon-129 NMR. *Anesthesiology* 1994;81:A413.
209. Thomas DD, Bigelow DJ, Squier TC, Hidalgo C. Rotational dynamics of protein and boundary lipid in sarcoplasmic reticulum membrane. *Biophys J* 1982;37:217–225.
210. Trudell JR, Hubbell WL, Cohen EN. Pressure reversal of inhalation anesthetic induced disorder in spin-labeled phospholipid vesicles. *Biochim Biophys Acta* 1973;291:335–340.
211. Trudell JR, Hubbell WL. Localization of molecular halothane in phospholipid bilayer model nerve membranes. *Anesthesiology* 1976; 44:202–205.
212. Turner GL, Oldfield E. Effect of a local anaesthetic on hydrocarbon chain order in membranes. *Nature* 1979;277:669–670.
213. Turner R, Keller P. Angiography and perfusion measurements by NMR. *Prog NMR Spectr* 1991;23:93–133.
214. van Gelderen P, de Vleeschouwer MHM, DesPres D, Pekar J, van Zijl PCM, Moonen CT. Water diffusion and acute stroke. *Magn Reson Med* 1994;31:154–163.
215. Wagle WA, Dumoulin CL, Souza SP, Cline HE. 3DFT MR angiography of carotid and basilar arteries. *AJNR* 1989;10:911–919.
216. Wakamori M, Ikemoto Y, Akaike N. Effects of two volatile anesthetics and a volatile convulsant on the excitatory and inhibitory amino acid responses in dissociated CNS neurons of the rat. *J Neurophysiol* 1991;66:2014–2021.
217. Warach S, Chien D, Li W, Ronthal M, Edelman RR. Fast magnetic resonance diffusion-weighted imaging of acute human stroke. *Neurology* 1992;42:1717–1723.
218. Warach S, Gaa J, Siewert B, Wielopolski P, Edelman RR. Acute human stroke studied by whole brain echo planar diffusion-weighted magnetic resonance imaging. *Ann Neurol* 1995;37: 231–241.
219. Williams GD, Mosher TJ, Smith MB. Simultaneous determination of intracellular magnesium and pH from the three ^{31}P NMR chemical shifts of ATP. *Anal Biochem* 1993;214:458–467.
220. Williams SR, Gadian DG. Tissue metabolism studied in vivo by nuclear magnetic resonance. *Q J Exp Physiol* 1986;71:335–360.
221. Wyrwicz AM, Conboy CB, Ryback KR, Nichols BG, Eisele P. *In vivo* ^{19}F-NMR study of isoflurane elimination from brain. *Biochim Biophys Acta* 1987;927:86–91.
222. Wyrwicz AM, Conboy CB, Nichols BG, Ryback KR, Eisele P. *In vivo* ^{19}F-NMR study of halothane distribution in brain. *Biochim Biophys Acta* 1987;929:271–277.
223. Wyrwicz AM, Conboy CB. Determination of halothane distribution in the rat head using ^{19}F NMR technique. *Magn Reson Med* 1989;9:219–228.
224. Wyrwicz AM, Pszenny MH, Schofield JC, Tillman PC, Gordon RE, Martin PA. Noninvasive observations of fluorinated anesthetics in rabbit brain by fluorine-19 nuclear magnetic resonance. *Science* 1983;222:428–430.
225. Xu Y, Balschi JA, Springer CJ. Magnetic susceptibility shift selected imaging: MESSI. *Magn Reson Med* 1990;16:80–90.
226. Xu Y, Cohen Y, Litt L, Chang LH, James TL. Tolerance of low cerebral intracellular pH in rats during hyperbaric hypercapnia. *Stroke* 1991;22:1303–1308.
227. Xu Y, Tang P, Zhang W, Firestone L, Winter PM. ^{19}F-NMR imaging and spectroscopy of sevoflurane uptake, distribution and elimination in rat brain. *Anesthesiology* 1995;83:766–774.
228. Xu Y, Tang P. Amphiphilic sites for anesthetic action? Evidence from ^{129}Xe-^{1}H intermolecular NOE. *Biochim Biophys Acta* 1997; 1323:154–162.
229. Xu Y, Tang P, Firestone L, Zhang TT. ^{19}F-NMR investigation of stereoselective binding of isoflurane to bovine serum albumin. *Biophysical J* 1996;70:532–538.
230. Yeh HJ, Moody EJ, Skolnick P. Halothane and anaesthesia. *Nature* 1990;346:227.
231. Yokono S, Ogli K, Miura S, Ueda I. 400 MHz two-dimensional nuclear Overhauser spectroscopy on anesthetic interaction with lipid bilayer. *Biochim Biophys Acta* 1989;982:300–302.
232. Yoshida T, Takahashi K, Kamaya H, Ueda I. ^{19}F-NMR study on micellar solubilization of a volatile anesthetic halothane: dose-related biphasic interaction. *J Colloid Interface Sci* 1988;124:177–185.
233. Yoshida T, Takahashi K, Ueda I. Molecular orientation of volatile anesthetics at the binding surface: ^{1}H- and ^{19}F-NMR studies of submolecular affinity. *Biochim Biophys Acta* 1989;985:331–333.
234. Zhang W, Williams DS, Detre JA, Koretsky AP. Measurement of brain perfusion by volume-localized NMR spectroscopy using inversion of arterial water spins: accounting for transit time and cross-relaxation. *Magn Reson Med* 1992;25:362–371.
235. Zimmerman SA, Jones MV, Harrison NL. Potentiation of gamma-aminobutyric acid$_A$ receptor Cl^- current correlates with *in vivo* anesthetic potency. *J Pharmacol Exp Ther* 1994;270:987–991.

Anesthesia: Biologic Foundations, edited by
Tony L. Yaksh et al. Lippincott–Raven Publishers,
Philadelphia © 1997.

CHAPTER 24

METHODS FOR MONITORING MODULATIONS IN INTRACELLULAR FREE CALCIUM CONCENTRATION

PAUL A. IAIZZO

MOBILIZATION OF Ca^{2+} FOR INTRACELLULAR SIGNALING

There is little need to expound on the important role that variation in intracellular free calcium concentration ($[Ca^{2+}]_i$) plays in the regulation of biochemical reactions essential not only for normal cell function, but also for the cell's response to external conditions or stimuli that may impose a stress (e.g., the presence of xenobiotics). Because the $[Ca^{2+}]_i$ is controlled by an elaborate system that is primarily membrane associated and because anesthetics can have profound membrane effects, there have been numerous investigations performed to examine closely the influence these agents have on regulation of $[Ca^{2+}]_i$. However, the intent of this chapter is not to critically evaluate the results of such investigations, but to provide an update on the methodologies commonly employed to monitor the activity of Ca^{2+} within a cell and to summarize a few of the potential complications that may arise when the effects of anesthetic agents on Ca^{2+} mobilization are studied.

Investigators interested in studying the modulation of $[Ca^{2+}]_i$ have numerous specific calcium indicators to choose from, and the list continues to expand. Likewise there are ever increasing novel methods described to: (a) introduce a specific indicator into the cell or a targeted subcellular compartment (including transinfecting a cell with an appropriate cDNA); (b) image the spatial modulations in $[Ca^{2+}]_i$ including those within specific organelles and with ever increasing temporal resolution (e.g., using confocal microscopy); and (c) gain new insights into the utility and limitations of each applied method.

Compartmentalization of Ca^{2+} in Various Cell Types

In general, eukaryotic cells contain ~10–20% of their total calcium content in the cytosol, but nearly all is bound to soluble binding proteins (e.g., calmodulin and parvalbumin) and membrane surfaces (102,119,129,162). Hence, the majority of a cell's Ca^{2+} pool is located within membrane-bound compartments, which include mitochondria, nuclei, endoplasmic reticulum, and perhaps the Golgi apparatus (for more details, see Chapter 9) (Fig. 1). In certain cell types, as the requirements of modulating Ca^{2+} become more specialized, both temporally and/or spatially, these basic cell structures can also become more extensive and/or complex (e.g., the incorporation of numerous regulatory systems). The complex architecture of many endomembrane systems can be determined solely by looking at the numerous types of Ca^{2+} channels incorporated within their membrane structures, each of which has unique kinetics that may also be modulated by membrane potential, receptors or second messengers (36,123). One well-known example of this great specialization is that of the sarcoplasmic reticulum in skeletal muscle. The membrane-bound storage sites may also contain specialized Ca^{2+} binding proteins (e.g., calsequestrins and calreticulins), which are important for maintaining Ca^{2+} levels exceeding those of the cytoplasm. Furthermore, for a given cell type, the dynamic release of Ca^{2+} can have very different modulatory functions, and the second messenger system in which Ca^{2+} is coupled is also predictably unique (for excellent reviews on this topic, see refs. 123,127). These differences are important to consider in the design and interpretation of experiments aimed at monitoring the regulation of $[Ca^{2+}]_i$.

Amplitudes and Durations of Transients

The mobilization of Ca^{2+} as a second messenger system normally involves a relatively brief rise in $[Ca^{2+}]_i$, on the order of milliseconds or seconds. Yet, it is known that many hormones, neurotransmitters, and growth factors can evoke oscillation in $[Ca^{2+}]_i$ in their target cells (10,127,156,158,163). However, it is also known that if an increase in $[Ca^{2+}]_i$ becomes sustained it activates in turn a cascade of potentially harmful events that may lead to irreversible damage: a 10-s duration of such a rise has been noted as being detrimental in certain cell types (30,62,65,86).

If the activity of intracellular Ca^{2+} is most commonly monitored by a molecule added to the internal environment, its presence will influence, to some extent, the concentration it is intended to indicate. For example, this has been a particular criticism in attempts to monitor resting $[Ca^{2+}]_i$ in normal and diseased skeletal muscle: if the concentration of the incorporated indicator becomes too great, it will mask any potential differences. On the other hand, any attempt to isolate an abnormal or diseased cell for $[Ca^{2+}]_i$ measurements can in itself induce artificial increases in resting levels or elicited responses

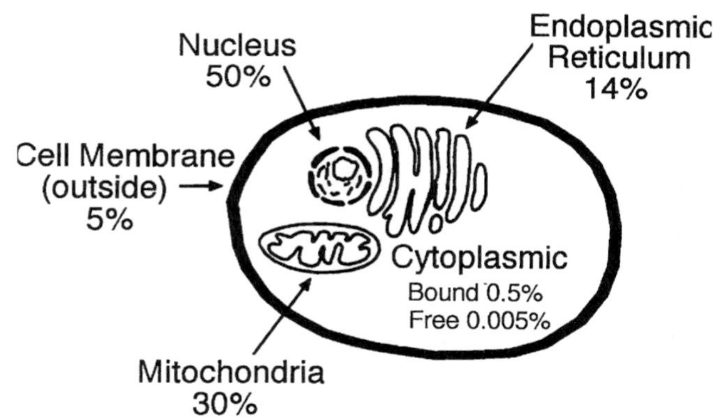

Figure 1. The relative Ca^{2+} distributions in a typical eukaryotic cell. The total cell Ca^{2+} content is ~2 mM with an average extracellular $[Ca^{2+}]$ of 2×10^{-3} M and an intracellular $[Ca^{2+}]$ of 1×10^{-7} M.

to administered agents. Such results are considered in part due to inherent increased sensitivities to injury which are exacerbated by experimental preparation methods (62,63,66).

TECHNIQUES USED TO STUDY THE MODULATION OF INTRACELLULAR [Ca^{2+}]

Radioisotopic Methods

No technique used for the study of Ca^{2+} homeostasis in intact living tissues is without experimental limitations. One of the more simplified approaches to study Ca^{2+} mobilization that is focused on the release of Ca^{2+} from endoplasmic reticulum is to determine the uptake and release of its gamma radiation-emitting isotope $^{45}Ca^{2+}$. In principle, a population of isolated cells, usually several million, are incubated in an uptake media containing $^{45}Ca^{2+}$, and then the relative uptake of radiolabled Ca^{2+} and subsequent release is monitored. Hence, the relative effects of various drugs (e.g., volatile anesthetics) on either uptake or release can be determined. In most studies, the isolated cells are also permeabilized and uptake by specific intracellular organelles is potentially blocked (e.g., mitochondria) in order to better study the dynamics of the flux of Ca^{2+} in and out of the endoplasmic reticulum (i.e., sarcoplasmic in muscle). The most commonly employed permeabilization procedure is to treat the cells with saponin, which is thought to selectively permeabilize only the surface plasma membrane. However, without the employment of such procedures one cannot be totally certain if the mobilization of Ca^{2+} originated from any number of potential storage organelles or via uncoupling from the cytoplasmic surfaces of each potential membrane system (Fig. 2). It should be mentioned that for skeletal muscle, the ability to mechanically remove (skin off) the surface membrane while preserving the cell's ability to release and store Ca^{2+} as well as to produce force, allows for a unique system to investigate $^{45}Ca^{2+}$ movement (e.g., see ref. 40).

The specifics of permeable cell preparation include incubation of isolated cells with an uptake medium containing ~100 nM free-$^{45}Ca^{2+}$ at either physiological (37°C) or room temperatures. Such media normally contain 5% polyethylene glycol, 0.5 mM 2,4-dinitrophenol, 16 M antimycin A, 2 g/ml oligomycin, 0.375 mM EGTA, 1.5 mM ATP, 3 mM creatine phosphate, 30 g/ml creatine phosphokinase, and 50 M $CaCl_2$. The antimycin and oligomycin are added to block mobilization of Ca^{2+} by mitochondria, whereas the high-energy phosphates are provided to maintain the function of active Ca^{2+} transport systems (24,64,115,116,122,135). Uptake curves for the various cell types under investigation are then normally determined by removing small aliquots of loaded cells at various predetermined time points (e.g., once a minute for 30 min). The removed cells are collected on a vacuum filter system using a glass filter and immediately washed numerous times with uptake buffer containing 1 mM $LaCl_3$. Subsequently, the individual filters are removed and placed in scintillation vials to which a tissue solubilizer (e.g., 0.5 M quaternary ammonium hydroxide in toluene) is added. Then the vials are dried, a liquid scintillation cocktail is added to each, and resultant radioactivity levels are determined. The effects of an anesthetic or any other agent of interest on $^{45}Ca^{2+}$ uptake are easily investigated by adding such an agent to the uptake buffer (64,66,67,116,122,134,135). However, there are known pitfalls with these methods that one must consider in interpreting $^{45}Ca^{2+}$ uptake and release data (18).

To optimally determine the effects of various agents on release of $^{45}Ca^{2+}$, one should derive from an uptake curve a relative time period during which $^{45}Ca^{2+}$ uptake is considered maximal. This value will vary from cell type to cell type and among different species. For example, the maximal uptake time for saponin-treated rat hepatocytes at 35°C was 13–16 min following incubation, whereas for treated hepatocyte isolated from swine at the same temperature it was between 8 and 9 min (64,66). It should be noted that the period of maximal uptake of $^{45}Ca^{2+}$ will also depend on whether or not cells have been exposed to a saponin pretreatment: i.e., the maximal uptake time in untreated rat hepatocytes was 9–13 min (64). Once a maximal uptake time period is chosen for a given experimental protocol, the effects of a putative releasing agent can be determined by preincubating a portion of the loaded cell population with the agent for a fixed period of time and subsequently isolating the treated and control cells for radioactivity determinations as mentioned above. An incubation period should be chosen that by itself causes minimal release and/or additional uptake of untreated cells. For example, in previous studies investigating the potential releasing effects of volatile anesthetics, an initial cell sample was removed from the incubation tube and filtered; 15 s later the various releasing agents were added, and exactly 2 min after the initial sample was filtered a second aliquot was processed. Two similar samples were

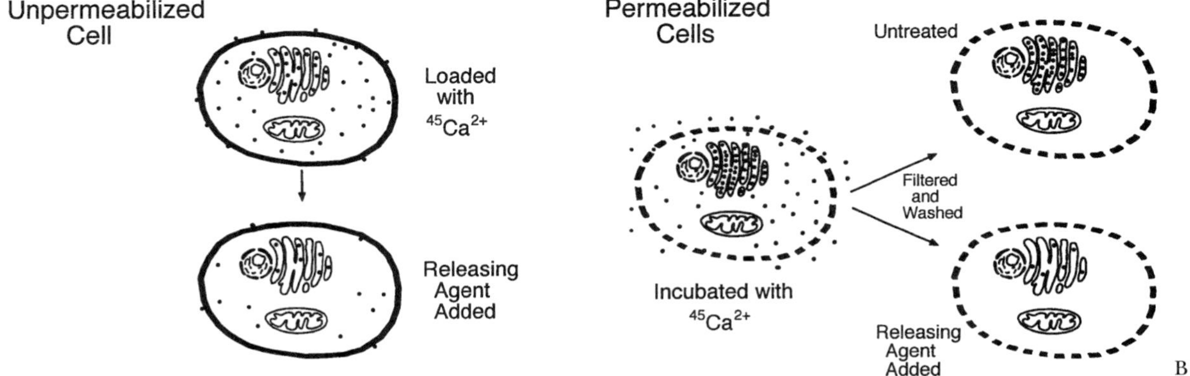

Figure 2. The diagrammatic representation of the effects of the administration of putative Ca^{2+} releasing agent on the flux of $^{45}Ca^{2+}$ out of intact cells or ones that have been permeabilized. The *dots* represent $^{45}Ca^{2+}$ molecules. Following the administration of a releasing agent in the unpermeabilized cells **(A)**, the subsequent cellular content of $^{45}Ca^{2+}$ decreases, which includes a decrease in the membrane-bound component as well as a release from storage sites. When cells are pretreated with a permeabilizing method, it is considered that the subsequent decrease in the detection of $^{45}Ca^{2+}$ is primarily due to release from the endoplasmic reticulum **(B)**. In most experimental protocols the relative effects of several releasing agents are determined by comparing the remaining radiation levels to matched controls (i.e., prepared in an identical fashion and of equal aliquots or cell numbers of the same preparation) without such agents added.

removed at the same time points, but without adding a putative releasing agent (i.e., to determine a control response) (64,66,67). To determine the absolute amount of $^{45}Ca^{2+}$ uptake by a given cell type, one can follow the calculation described by Gill and Chuen (46).

The exact mechanism of action of saponin on various cell types is uncertain, but it is thought that in most, the plasma membrane is made permeable by the removal of membrane-bound cholesterol (108). Membrane systems such as those of the endoplasmic reticulum or mitochondria have little or no cholesterol and, therefore, are considered to be unaffected by the saponin treatment. To support this notion, there is ample evidence that the Ca^{2+} uptake by sarcoplasmic reticulum in muscle is unaffected by saponin treatment, as is the Ca^{2+} uptake or release by microsomes or mitochondria from rat hepatocytes (8,24,98). Hence, saponin treatment is considered to yield model cell systems in which the internal function of the cell is intact while the cytosolic content can be readily controlled by the composition of the medium.

$^{45}Ca^{2+}$ continues to be utilized to investigate the mobilization of $[Ca^{2+}]_i$ by specific anesthetic agents in various cell types. The data presented in several reports have clearly indicated that at anesthetic concentrations, halothane, enflurane, sevoflurane and isoflurane caused the release of Ca^{2+} from internal storage sites (61,64,66,116). Presumably, the major storage site was the endoplasmic reticulum and not mitochondria because these measurements were made in the presence of mitochondrial inhibitors (24).

Although this review's focus is on Ca^{2+} mobilization in intact cells, mention is warranted concerning studies that have used radiolabled ryanodine to investigate potential defects of the so-called "ryanodine receptor," which is a calcium release channel within the sarcoplasmic reticulum. Much knowledge has been gained concerning normal and abnormal regulation of $[Ca^{2+}]_i$ by these channels, identified by means of investigations of the relative binding of [^{3}H]ryanodine (e.g., see refs. 51,103,104, 152). Ryanodine is a neutral plant alkaloid whose most striking effects are to cause irreversible contracture in skeletal muscle without depolarization and to have a negative inotropic effect on cardiac muscle (70). Ryanodine binds to its receptor when the calcium channel is open (101). The use of [^{3}H]ryanodine has not only been essential for the biochemical isolation of the calcium release channel, but it has also been used to identify the roles of putative activators or inhibitors of channels function in both normal and diseased muscle. In general, physiological investigations have determined how ryanodine binding, within the subfraction of heavy sarcoplasmic reticulum, is modulated by the composition of the ion solution or in the presence of potential channel modulators (e.g., halothane or caffeine) (95,103,104).

Ca^{2+}-Selective Microelectrodes

When two aqueous solutions of different ionic constituents are separated by a membrane exclusively permeable to one ion, an electrical potential will be established that reflects the concentration difference of the permeable ion. In Ca^{2+}-selective electrodes, a reagent or ligand that binds Ca^{2+} with high selectivity is incorporated into a water insoluble membrane. For cellular measurements, a short column of a water-immiscible organic solvent containing a Ca^{2+}-selective ligand or ionophor is placed in the tip of a glass micropipette and the rest of the pipette is filled with a solution of fixed, but not necessarily known, $[Ca^{2+}]$. Ca^{2+} diffuses down its concentration gradient until a potential difference between the inside and outside of the pipette is achieved that is defined by the Nerst equation (at 37°C): $V_{elec} = 31\ mV \cdot \log([Ca^{2+}]_x/[Ca^{2+}]_{elec})$, where x is the region where Ca^{2+} is measured. Such pipettes can be used to monitor changes in either extracellular or intracellular $[Ca^{2+}]$, depending on tip location: i.e., for intracellular monitoring the cell must be impaled by the electrode tip (for more details of fabrication and use of these electrodes, see refs. 2,14,83,89,93). Obviously, ligands that show little interference by other commonly occuring biologic cations must be used. When a Ca^{2+}-selective electrode is used in vitro, the potential difference detected across the ligand membrane is recorded through nonpolarizable junctions which make contact with the solutions inside and outside the electrode. When the tip of such an electrode is located within a living cell, the electrode measures the cell membrane potential as well as the potential established by the Ca^{2+} gradient. Consequently, the required reference potential takes the form of a conventional (voltage) microelectrode which is normally filled with 3 M KCl so that the intracellular Ca^{2+} signal is determined as the difference between the potentials recorded by the two different electrodes. Both electrodes need to be intracellular or the transmembrane potential of the cell will be added to the recorded Ca^{2+} potential (14). Furthermore, it is optimal if the placement of the tips of the two electrodes be in the same region of the same cell. If this is not the case, the measured difference between the potentials will become variable and bias the Ca^{2+} potential. In fact, by placing the two electrodes in two different cells with different resting membrane potentials, one could encounter either abnormally low or high resting $[Ca^{2+}]_i$. Double-barreled electrodes have been fabricated in which one barrel is filled with KCl and the other prepared as a Ca^{2+}-selective electrode; however, their use also has inherent problems: e.g., the larger tips may cause an increased leakage of Ca^{2+} through the impalement site (89). Typically, careful calibration in solutions of known $[Ca^{2+}]$ is employed prior to cell impalement.

Ca^{2+}-selective microelectrodes respond to the $[Ca^{2+}]$ in the immediate environment of their tips. This concentration is likely to be influenced by Ca^{2+} leakage at the site of impalement (14). Results with Ca^{2+}-selective microelectrodes must thus be interpreted with the suspicion that they may be biased in the direction of elevated $[Ca^{2+}]_i$. This may be further exacerbated when one uses this method to investigate $[Ca^{2+}]_i$ in cells known to have inherent increased sensitivities to injury stemming from either unknown causes or due to an identified altered surface membrane structural matrix (e.g., Duchenne muscular dystrophy or myotonic dystrophy) (44,62,63,86). Furthermore, constructed microelectrodes that subsequently provide uniform calibration curves tend to have large tip diameters, whereas those best suited for cell impalement (~0.5 μm or less) do not (14). Such electrodes have relatively high resistances (>100 MΩ) compared to standard KCl-filled microelectrodes (<15 MΩ), which means that the time constants of their responses to abrupt changes in $[Ca^{2+}]$ are predictably slow; this is regarded as one of their principal disadvantages over other methods (14). Although in the past the temporal resolution of Ca^{2+} electrodes was considered inadequate to track rapid changes in $[Ca^{2+}]_i$ in an appropriate physiological range of concentrations (e.g., in cardiac and skeletal muscle), new synthetic ligands continue to elicit improved detection limits (2,83).

Optical Methods

The techniques for monitoring modulation in $[Ca^{2+}]_i$ that allow for the most detailed examination of subcellular fluxes employ optical methods. This type of approach requires the introduction into the cell of a marker molecule that binds Ca^{2+}, which results in a change in a monitored optical signal. The Ca^{2+}-dependent optical signal depends upon the type of intracellular indicator molecule that binds Ca^{2+}: (a) photoproteins emit light; (b) fluorophores shift their fluorescent behavior; and (c) metallochromic dyes demonstrate an alteration of absorbence characteristics (color). The advantages and disadvantages of each approach or technique depend largely upon the binding affinity for Ca^{2+} of the chosen indicator molecule and the potential for interference by other optical signals in the biological tissue itself (e.g., autofluorescence). Each of the three major optical methods (i.e., photoproteins, absorbance dyes, and fluorescence dyes) may show particular advantages in certain tissues and/or types of studies.

The fluorescence and absorbance techniques rely on the fact that the concentration of Ca^{2+}-bound reporter molecule (C_b) will be proportional to the $[Ca^{2+}]_i$ by the following formula:

$$C_b = C_f \cdot [Ca^{2+}]/K_d$$

where C_f is the concentration of the unbound reporter molecule and K_d is the binding constant (148). If the K_d is much greater or much less than the $[Ca^{2+}]$ to be determined, the change in C_b versus C_f may not be detectible. Consequently, to accurately monitor mobilization $[Ca^{2+}]_i$, the K_d must be appropriate for the expected $[Ca^{2+}]$. For metallochromic dyes, due to the nonlinearity of the absorbance change, the $[Ca^{2+}]$ range of interest should be less than the K_d (131). For the fluorescent indicators, the effective range over which the $[Ca^{2+}]$ can be determined is 0.05–0.1, up to 10–20 times the K_d. The values for the commonly employed Ca^{2+} indicators are listed in Table 1.

Another consideration when utilizing any of these optical methods is that the binding of Ca^{2+} itself by these marker molecules may significantly buffer the $[Ca^{2+}]_i$, either prior to or during an active release, so that the physiological response under investigation will be abnormally attenuated. In addition, the binding of Ca^{2+} to certain indicator molecules may be inherently slow (e.g., 2–5 ms for arsenazo III) compared to the biologic process under study, and may prove unsuitable on that basis.

Table 1. CHARACTERISTICS OF INDICATORS COMMONLY USED FOR OPTICAL DETERMINATION OF $[Ca^{2+}]$[a]

Compound	K_d Ca^{2+}[b]	Effective range of $[Ca^{2+}]$ study	Wavelength of intensity measurement (nm)
Photoprotein aequorin	10 μM	0.01–1,000 μM	460
Metallochromic (absorbance) dyes			
Murexide	1–3 mM	5–500 μM	540–570
Arsenazo III	15–60 μM	<1–10 μM	675–685, 650–685[c]
Antipyrylazo III	95–380 μM	1–100 μM	670–690, 720–790[c]
Fluorescent indicators			
Fura-2	224 nM	0.01–4 μM	505 (excitation: 340 free), 380 (Ca^{2+} bound[d])
Fluo-3	316 nM	0.02–6 μM	525 (excitation: 488[d])
Quin-2	126 nM	0.005–2 μM	492 (excitation: 339[d])
Indo-1	250 nM	0.01–4 μM	483 (free), 400 (Ca^{2+} bound) (excitation 355[d])

[a]Data tabulated from refs. 52 and 132.
[b]K_d for Ca^{2+} for the various compounds may be influenced by ionic strength and pH.
[c]Wavelength pairs employed to reduce interference by other species.
[d]Excitation wavelength(s) required to produce the emitted (measured) wavelength are indicated parenthetically.

At present, fluorescence techniques are considered superior, because a lower concentration of probe molecules need to be internalized for detection purposes and because small changes in relative light intensities (i.e., emission levels in response to a given wavelength of excitation) are more easily detected against a dark background (48). In contrast, a small change in $[Ca^{2+}]_i$ may not be detected using an absorbance technique where the changes in intensity of a beam of light need to be measured and a higher concentration of dye molecules are required. However, the performance of a given fluorescence technique may also be compromised if there is a relatively intense constant background of fluorescence in the desired detection range (autofluorescence), which in turn markedly increases the signal-to-noise ratio. Absorbance techniques are far less susceptible to signal degradation of this type. It needs to be noted that the perhaps the major advantages of employing photoproteins for optical investigations are that they are typically active over a far wider $[Ca^{2+}]$ range and the nonlinearity of their luminescence can make signal detection less complicated.

Photoproteins

Photoproteins can be considered as conveniently packaged Ca^{2+} indicator systems containing all the ingredients required for the bioluminescent reaction, which gives them great biologic utility (13–15,17,124). Although there are several naturally occurring photoproteins, only two have been used widely as intracellular Ca^{2+} indicators: aequorin, isolated from jellyfish of the genus *Aequorea*, and obelin, from hydroids of the genus *Obelia*. All the components required for luminescence (the apoprotein, a low-molecular-weight chromophore, and oxygen) are bound together and they behave as single macromolecules. Aequorin is the more popular photoprotein, of which 15 kinds of recombinant semisynthetic and recombinant fluorescein-conjugated forms have been described (136). In addition, these photoproteins have now been expressed in mammalian cell lines within various organelles using molecular biologic techniques (23,25,28,124,126).

Photoproteins are consumed in the luminescent reaction; i.e., the chromophore is degraded and is not replenished. This behavior implies certain constraints on the manner in which these Ca^{2+} indicators are employed (15). Yet, in most cells, the rate of photoprotein consumption at rest is so low that it does not lead to rapid depletion. For example, activated Ca^{2+} transients (electrical stimulation) of several days' duration have been recorded in single frog skeletal muscle fibers following just one injection session. There was no significant change in activated luminescence intensity during the experimental period. It is common to activate such muscle cells numerous times with minimal change in intensity: ≤50 twitch and tetanic stimulations (e.g., at 100 Hz for 200 ms) (16,58–60,105). However, the rate of consumption in cardiac muscle is believed to be somewhat higher than in most other cell types; thus, the rate of consumption can become a limitation if the amount of photoprotein injected is low. No matter how much of a photoprotein is present within a cell, the changes in luminescence are best detected using a photomultiplier or a high gain image intensifier, with care taken to maximize optical efficiency. For example, light guides (e.g., fiberoptics) or reflective mirror systems are commonly employed to maximize the light emission into a photomultiplier (13–15,58). Nevertheless, signal averaging is often appropriate when the relative change in $[Ca^{2+}]_i$ is low and recorded from a single or relatively small population of cells.

The employment of photoproteins is extremely useful for the study of rapid Ca^{2+} transients, and they are much less prone than any other type of Ca^{2+} indicator to movement artifacts. These properties make them especially well suited to study the activity of Ca^{2+} within muscle cell in both skeletal and cardiac muscle (14). In many studies in which photoproteins have been used to monitor the effects of anesthetics on Ca^{2+} transients within a muscle cell, the photoprotein was microinjected either into a single cell or into a large number of superficial cells within an isolated biopsy (e.g., see refs. 20,21,56,84,139, 144). The intensity of luminescence of the photoprotein aequorin is a nonlinear function of $[Ca^{2+}]$ (13–15,124,165). Thus, as a minimal precaution when photoproteins are injected into a fairly large cell in which their diffusion may be limited, it is best to perform multiple injections (Fig. 3). If inhomogeneities in aequorin distribution exist or fluctuations of calcium concentration are regionalized, then errors in estimating mean $[Ca^{2+}]$ will occur (14,142,165). Yet, the advantage of such an approach is that contractile force and luminescence can be recorded simultaneously with few complications. It should be noted that injection of a photoprotein is not limited to those cells (e.g., muscle) with fairly large diameters. For example, Oakes et al. (113) have successfully microinjected cells with diameters as small as 10 μm and then used the same pipette as an electrode to record changes in membrane potential during the pharmacological activation of Ca^{2+} transients. In cells with small volumes, one should consider injecting a concentrated solution of photoprotein: this approach can greatly enhance the subsequent amount of luminescence recorded (31,32). Nevertheless, the degree of the difficulty related to the injection of a photoprotein should not be understated.

Fortunately, other approaches have been identified for the successful incorporation of photoproteins into living cells that are much easier to employ. These methods depend on altering the transport of substance through the surface membrane in a reversible fashion. They include (a) an EGTA-loading technique (107,145); (b) permeabilizing cells by brief exposures to a hypotonic solution (19,27,138); (c) a cultured cell detachment procedure (100); and (d) a centrifugation loading technique. It is this latter technique that is considered the easiest to use and has been utilized by this, and other authors, in numerous reports on the effects of anesthetics on Ca^{2+} mobilization in a variety of cell types (61,65–67,116). However, caution needs to be taken when using this approach for any molecule (even those up to 100 kD) that may be present in an incubation solution may potentially become internalized: i.e., one needs to consider this possibility in all centrifugation procedures that employ living cells (for more details, see below, where this approach will be described for the incorporation of fluorophores into cells).

The interaction of Ca^{2+} with a photoprotein is inhibited competitively by Mg^{2+}, which implies it is necessary to know the $[Mg^{2+}]$ in the immediate location of the indicator in order to accurately interpret the kinetics of the Ca^{2+} mobilization. It has been reported that if, for example, aequorin is preequilibrated with mM concentrations of Mg^{2+}, the response of this indicator to a step change in $[Ca^{2+}]$ is significantly slowed (14,105). To convert luminescence measurements recorded from living cells into an estimate of $[Ca^{2+}]$, it is necessary to refer to a Ca^{2+} concentration-effect curve that has been determined in vitro which mimics the same experimental conditions of temperature, ionic strength, and $[Mg^{2+}]_i$ (14). To determine the absolute Ca^{2+} concentration, the light intensity recorded from the cells has to be converted to the fractional luminescence in order to use a derived calibration curve. To determine the fractional luminescence, the light intensity (L) from an elicited response is divided by the maximal luminescence (L_{max}) that could be recorded from the given cell preparation under investigation. An estimate of L_{max} can be obtained if all the photoprotein in that preparation can be discharged fairly rapidly (within minutes) without changing the optical conditions used to obtain the physiological responses (14). The method most commonly used to accomplish this is lysis of the cell membranes with Triton X100 detergent (1–5%). This method is not only fairly simple, but is considered reliable because this detergent does not alter the quantum yield of the aequorin reaction in vitro (14,15).

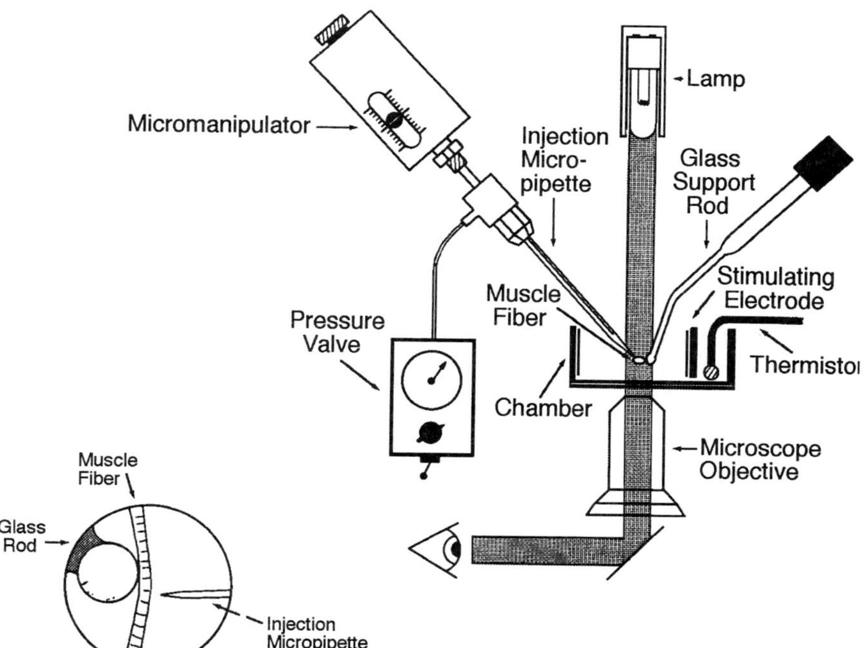

Figure 3. A typical setup for the injection of a photoprotein into an isolated muscle fiber. During the injection, the fiber is viewed using an inverted microscope. The fiber is stretched until it is somewhat taut (e.g., a sarcomere spacing of ≤2.4 μm) and stabilized against a small fire-polished support rod. A micromanipulator is used to position the injection micropipette; once the cell is impaled, pressure is gradually applied to the pipette until membrane swelling is observed. Care is taken not to overinject, because this will cause irreversible damage. The fiber is injected at several sites along its length. The *inset* at the *lower left* depicts the investigator's view. (Reprinted with permission from Iaizzo PA. Aequorin luminescence from stimulated skeletal muscle cells: relation between changes in intracellular calcium and contractile force [Dissertation]. Minneapolis: University of Minnesota, 1986.)

Both aequorin and obelin have been expressed in mammalian cell lines within various organelles using molecular biologic techniques (23,25,28,124,126). The apoprotein of obelin has been incorporated into the cytoplasm of living cells using a immunoliposome technique, after which the Ca^{2+}-activatible photoprotein has been reformed within the cell by the addition of synthetic coelenterazine (29). Several other reports have described the expression of the apoprotein of aequorin into various locations of a cell using recombinant DNA methods (23,25,124,126). The expressed apoprotein also needs to be reconstituted in the intact cells by incubation with purified coelenterazine. Both methods for apoprotein creation have been used successfully to produce an abundance of luminescent protein that has retained its Ca^{2+}-dependent properties. Thus, the advantages of molecular techniques over microinjection or permeabilization methods to incorporate appropriate concentrations of these photoproteins into cells will only increase their subsequent application. For more detail concerning the properties and use of these photoproteins, the reader is referred to the excellent publications available (e.g., 13–15,17,33,59, 105,124).

Metallochromic Dyes

Metallochromic dyes change color upon the binding of Ca^{2+}, and this property has made them useful for monitoring changes in $[Ca^{2+}]_i$ by monitoring changes in light absorbance. There are numerous metallochromic dyes that have been employed as Ca^{2+} indicators. They include antipyrlazo III, arsenaso III, Azo-l, dichlorophosphonazo III, 1,1′-dimethylpurpurate 3-3′ diacetic acid (DMPDAA), murexide, purpurate-3,3′ diacetic acid (PDAA), and tetramethylmurexide (5,6,13,14). Several studies have employed these dyes in various ways to study the effects of anesthetic agents on Ca^{2+} mobilization (e.g., see ref. 42).

The absorbance of a cellular preparation that includes a metallochromic dye is normally measured at two or more wavelengths: one at which Ca^{2+} binding has a major influence and one at which it does not. If the latter wavelength is one where the absorbance of the dye is appreciable, potential changes in these measurements (e.g., due to dye loss) can be used to estimate the concentration of the indicator within the cellular preparation and/or nonspecific changes in absorbance due to movement (14). The problem of motion artifacts is probably the most serious complication in using metallochromic dyes in any muscle or other cell that may alter its shape in response to the mobilization of Ca^{2+}. In skeletal muscle, this problem is partially overcome by stretching it beyond myofilament overlap (actin and myosin), thereby excluding the possibility of associating the changes in $[Ca^{2+}]_i$ with contractile events (75). In addition to these limitations, many of the metallochromic dyes have biophysical properties than may be of further detriment in certain applications. For example, arsenazo II, antipyrlazo III, and murexide have been reported to be reduced by rat liver microsomes to an azo anion radical, from which reoxidized byproducts are formed that are toxic active oxygen radicals (37).

Fluorescent Ca^{2+} Indicators

Changes in the fluorescent properties of Ca^{2+} binding reporter molecules such as chlortetracycline or calcein have been employed for a number of years as a means to assess changes in the concentration of this ion (17). More recently, largely through the developmental work of Tsien (148), a variety of fluorescent molecules have been synthesized which have been subsequently used to examine fluxes of a number of ionic constituents. These molecules elicit altered fluorescent optical characteristics upon binding of an ion with a selected high specificity (148).

In the early 1980s, the Ca^{2+} fluorophore Quin-2 was widely used as means to monitor changes in $[Ca^{2+}]_i$; in 1985, a new generation of fluorescent Ca^{2+} indicators was described, which included the commonly used Fura-2 and Indo-1 (48,149). These three indicators continue to have widespread use, and new methodologies to apply them continue to be reported. More recently, additional fluorescent Ca^{2+} indicators have been developed, Fluo-3 and Rhod-2, which can be excited by visible radiation (e.g., from lasers). This makes them well suited for study with confocal microscopes (111). Further modifications and suggested improvements of these and other probes will continue to increase the list of available indicators, e.g., Fura-Red, C18-Fura-2, and Calcium-Green (38,52). Thus, anyone interested in studying the mobilization of Ca^{2+} in a particular cell type needs to be aware of the advantages and disadvantages of each indicator prior to selection.

The commonly used fluorescent indicators are derivatives of the Ca^{2+} chelator EGTA and as such are highly charged (Fig. 4). Like this chelator, they have much higher affinities for Ca^{2+} than for Mg^{2+}. However, each indicator differs significantly in the nature of its excitation and emission spectra and in the way in which those spectra are altered upon its binding of Ca^{2+} or other ions. Yet each fluorophore emits visible light. Quin-2, Fura-2, and Indo-1 are best excited by ultraviolet (uV) light, which requires special optics (e.g., quartz lenses which transmit uV wavelengths accurately) (33). In contrast, other indicators, such as Fluo-3 and Rhod-2, have both their excitation and emission spectra within that of visible light. Upon binding Ca^{2+}, these fluorescent indicators either alter their intensity of fluorescence (e.g., Quin-2, Fluo-3, Rhod-2, Fura-Red) or undergo shifts in either the excitation or emission spectrum (e.g., Fura-2, Indo-1, furapta, C18-Fura-2). This property of the latter type permits the dyes to be used in a ratio mode; i.e., the concentration of dye and the thickness of the specimen are automatically corrected for. This is a major advantage in that the cell or cellular preparation does not have to be destroyed or its function interfered with to obtain an appropriate calibration curve (14,22,48,80,94,160)

Specifically, while Fura-2 emits the same wavelength of blue-green light (510 nm) after binding Ca^{2+}, the efficiency is greater when the exciting wavelength is shorter (its excitation spectrum changes upon the binding of Ca^{2+}, but its emission spectrum is unchanged). As with increasing $[Ca^{2+}]$, as a greater fraction of Fura-2 binds Ca^{2+}, its excitation spectrum shifts (Fig. 5A). It is common to measure the fluorescence intensity at the peak of the emission spectrum (~510 nm) while switching back and forth between two excitation wavelengths. One of these wavelengths is chosen such that when Ca^{2+} binds to Fura-2 the recorded fluorescence intensity rises (e.g., 340 nm), whereas for the other wavelength (e.g., 380 nm) the intensity falls (e.g., see refs. 62,63,146). From the ratio between the emission signals recorded following excitation at the two wavelengths, one can estimate the $[Ca^{2+}]$ from a derived calibration curve (14,33,48,62,69,121,138,140,149). The equation used for this purpose is commonly that described by Grynkiewicz et al. (48):

$$[Ca^{2+}] = K_d\ (R - R_{min}/R_{max} - R)\ (S_{f2}/S_{b2})$$

where K_d is the effective dissociation constant, R is the ratio of the total fluorescence intensities at the two excitation wavelengths, R_{min} is the limiting value that R can have at a zero $[Ca^{2+}]$, R_{max} is the ratio at a saturating $[Ca^{2+}]$, S_{f2} is the free dye proportionality coefficient for at least one of the excitation wavelengths, and S_{b2} is the proportionality coefficient of the dye bound to Ca^{2+} at that same wavelength (for more details, see ref. 48). It should be noted that many commercially available automated fluorescence detection systems, designed for use with Fura-2, have incorporated these equations into the sampling programs, thus representing obtained measurements in terms of $[Ca^{2+}]_i$.

A ratio approach has also been to utilize the fluorescent properties of Indo-1. In contrast to Fura-2, Indo-1 does not change its peak excitation wavelength on binding Ca^{2+}, but

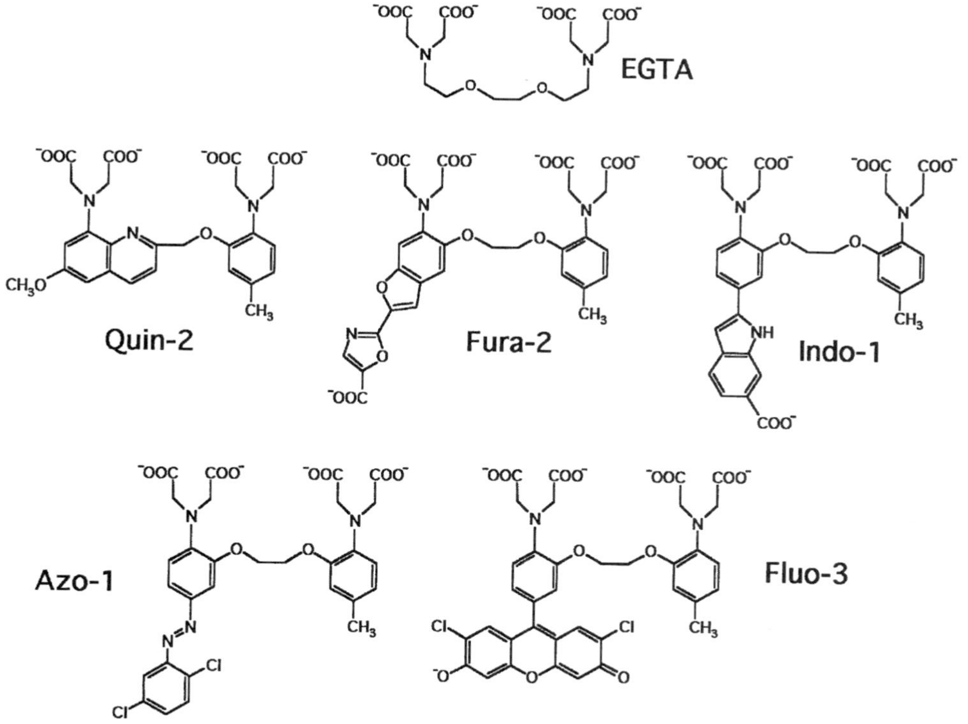

Figure 4. The structural formulas for EGTA and several derivatives which are popular Ca^{2+} indicators. Quin-2, Fura-2, Indo-1, and Fluo-3 are fluorescent dyes, whereas Azo-1 is a metallochromic indicator. (Reprinted, in adapted form, from Blinks JR. Intracellular [Ca^{2+}] measurements. In: Fozzard HA, Haber E, Jennings RB, Katz AM, Morgan HE, eds. *The heart and cardiovascular system.* New York: Raven Press, 1992:1171–1201.)

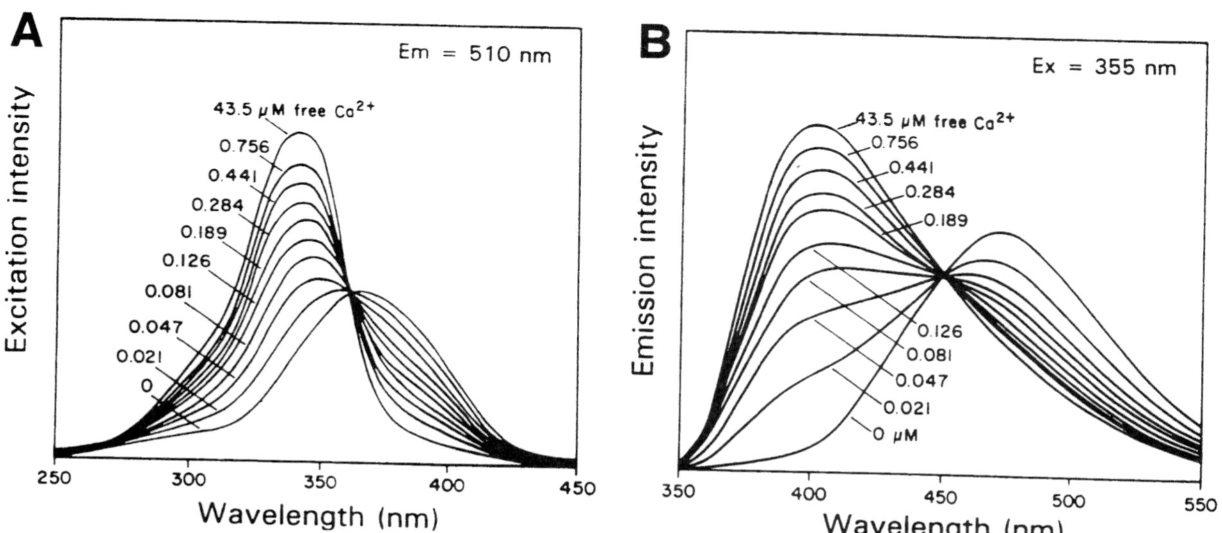

Figure 5. Fluorescence spectra of the Ca^{2+} indicator dyes with different Ca^{2+} concentrations. **A:** The fluorescence intensity of 1 μM Fura-2 measured at 510 nm, when the excitation wavelength is varied between 300 and 400 nm. At higher Ca^{2+} concentrations, which result in a greater fraction of Fura having bound Ca^{2+}, the light emission measured at 510 nm is enhanced when the exciting frequency shifts from 380 to 340 nm. The isosbestic excitation frequency is 365 nm, i.e., the wavelength at which Fura-2 and Fura-2 Ca^{2+} show equivalent emission intensity. **B:** The intensity of the emitted light at various wavelengths from 1 mM Indo 1 as the [Ca^{2+}] is altered. The excitation wavelength in this case is maintained at 460 nm. In contrast to Fura-2, the wavelength of emitted light varies upon binding of $Ca^{2+}$when the exciting wavelength is maintained constant. (Reprinted with permission from Haugland RP. *Handbook of fluorescent probes and research chemicals.* Eugene, OR: Molecular Probes, 1992.)

rather emits light with a lower peak wavelength (404 instead of 485 nm). Consequently, a single excitation wavelength is used and the emitted fluorescence is recorded at two wavelengths (33,48,121,149). Accurate ratiometric detection for Indo-1 requires emission at two different wavelengths, making this indicator more difficult to use for image analysis (14). On the other hand, this property is advantageous for monitoring changes in Ca^{2+} while employing flow cytometry (33,118,137).

Like photoproteins, fluorophores can be incorporated into cells via microinjection techniques or via methods which depend on altering the transport of substances through the surface membrane in a reversible fashion. In addition, most of these dyes can and have been made lipid-soluble by fabricating them into neutral esters. For example, in Fura-2-AM the five carboxyl groups are reacted to form acetoxymethyl esters. In such a neutral ester form, these dyes easily penetrate the surface membrane. Once inside the cell, these esters are hydrolyzed by cytoplasmic esterases, and the resultant negatively charged molecules become trapped within the cytoplasm. It should be noted that the mode by which a given dye is incorporated into the cytoplasm can greatly influence the fluorescence signals that are subsequently recorded (1,3,14,34,99, 114). The ester forms of the fluorescent dyes are cleaved by cytoplasmic esterases to yield the Ca^{2+}-sensitive forms of the dye, although in some cases several intermediates may also persist. Upon excitation at various wavelengths these partially hydrolyzed forms of the dye, having distinct fluorescence spectra, may fluoresce with differing intensities. Thus, successful application of the ratio method to estimate $[Ca^{2+}]_i$ may not be possible, for this requires that Fura-2 is the predominant fluorescent species present (33,48,114,130). The presence of various Fura-2-AM metabolites can be determined using HPLC as previously described (63,114). It was previously reported that the relative amount of fluorescent metabolites of Fura-2 AM and the half-time loss of Fura-2 were unique for three cell types investigated: in N1E-115 neuroblastoma cells, small amounts of at least four non-Fura-2 metabolites were present along with large amounts of unhydrolyzed Fura-2 AM, and the half-time loss of Fura-2 was estimated at 34 min; in human pulmonary artery endothelial cells, Fura-2 was not the predominant form of the dye after 60 min of incubation, and the half-time loss was estimated to be 74 min; and in rat hepatocytes, the Fura-2 concentration was maximal at 15 min and it was the predominant form in the cell, but was rapidly extruded from these cells (114). In contrast, for both swine or human skeletal muscle, the predominant hydrolyzed product is Fura-2, which remains within the cell for hours, and nonuniformity due to intermediates can be neglected (62,63,86,87) (Fig. 6). An additional disadvantage of fluorescent indicators is that they may be prone to problems due to movement artifacts (13,14).

Fura-2 and, potentially, the other Ca^{2+}-sensitive fluorophores may also be loaded into various cells using the aforementioned techniques to incorporate photoproteins into harvested cells. For example, it has been observed that Fura-2 could be loaded using a centrifugation technique into a suspension of fresh hepatocytes (P. A. Iaizzo, *unpublished data,* 1989). To do so, ~5 × 10^6 cells/ml were washed either two or three times by centrifuging at 1,500 RPM for 30 s in a buffer containing 135 mM NaCl, 4 mM KCl, 11 mM glucose, and 0.5 mM potassium phosphate at 4°C (pH 7.4). The buffer for the third wash also contained 1 mM EGTA. The washed cells were suspended in 0.5 ml of solution containing 200–500 mM Fura-2, 0.15 M KCl, and 50 mM HEPES, pH 7.4, and incubated with gentle shaking for 10 min at 4°C before being centrifuged at 1,500 RPM for 30 s. The Fura-2 solution can be reused for loading additional preparations of cells. The cells were then suspended in Krebs solution and either plated at 2 × 10^6 cells per coverslip within the culture dishes (used 1–3 h later) or placed directly on coverslips mounted on the microscope stage (i.e., as a multi-layer cell preparation). It has been observed that hepatocytes loaded

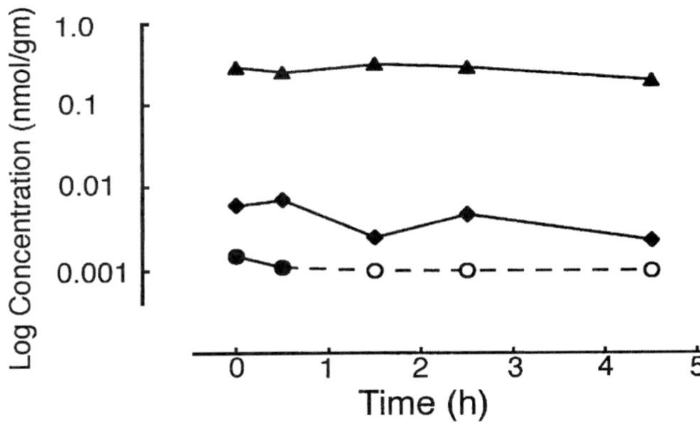

Figure 6. The time course of Fura-2 AM hydrolysis by human skeletal muscle into its metabolites. Time zero indicates the end of a 30-min loading period at 35°C. The relative concentrations of the remaining Fura-2 AM (◆), the formed Fura-2 (▲), and other metabolites (●) were estimated from 14 carefully dissected bundles of intact intercostal fibers which were obtained from the same biopsy. The *open circles* indicate nonquantifiable amounts of metabolites. Note the relative amounts of Fura-2 remain 50 times greater than all other forms combined. (Reprinted with permission from Iaizzo PA, Seewald M, Oakes SG, Lehmann-Horn F. The use of Fura-2 to estimate myoplasmic $[Ca^{2+}]$ in human skeletal muscle. *Cell Calcium* 1989;10:151–158.)

using Fura-2 AM resulted in "hot spots" of intensified fluorescence (observed using a video imaging system) (65). The contribution of fluorescence from such sites is also a potential problem when one tries to determine absolute $[Ca^{2+}]_i$ (65,141). Furthermore, the presence or absence of growth factors (i.e., serum versus serum-free medias) in the incubation and/or bathing solutions also modified the responsiveness of hepatocytes to either take up the dye, hydrolyze the ester form, or respond with changes in $[Ca^{2+}]_i$ to various drug exposure. In contrast, the fluorescence emitted from the cells that were loaded by centrifugation with Fura-2 appeared more uniform: "hot spots" were not obvious, and this mode of dye loading provided levels of fluorescence that were comparable to the Fura-2 AM incubations (two to three times that of the cell autofluorescence). However, rapid loss of dye from rat hepatocytes was noted with either loading technique.

Complications due to subsequent dye loss, a relative high intracellular Ca^{2+} buffering capacity by a fluorophore, or a significant heterogeneity in the responses of an investigated population of cells will abnormally bias the quantitation of actual $[Ca^{2+}]_i$ (12,26,65,74). It has been shown in several studies that a large fraction of a fluorophore may be bound to constituents of the cytoplasm and undergoes significant changes in its chemical and optical properties as a result (11,79). This limitation is not so restrictive as to preclude their use; however, the potential for error introduced by these alterations must be recognized. Numerous experiments have been performed to determine the relative changes in fluorescence in response to the administration of anesthetics, thereby providing important insights as to the effects of these substances on Ca^{2+} mobilization in a variety of cell types (e.g., see refs. 43,55,57,62,63,65, 68,71,76–78,81,92,158,164). In addition, several reports have investigated the correlation between relative changes in fluorescence with simultaneous changes in some other biophysical process. The relative changes in fluorescence and associated changes in contractile force following the application of anesthetic agents have been determined for cardiac, smooth and skeletal muscle (e.g., see refs. 39,56,62,63,71,72,150,151,164). In any such experiment, the interpretation of the data is made easier if one can show the reversibility of an anesthetic response (Fig. 7). However, the advantages of simultaneously recording associated biophysical processes and modulations in

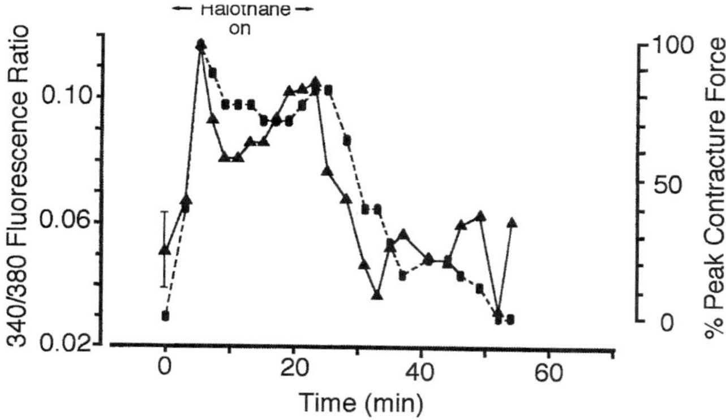

Figure 7. The reversible effects of halothane on ratioed Fura-2 fluorescence (▲, 340/380 nm) and force (●, %) elicited from intact intercostal fiber from a swine susceptible to malignant hyperthermia.

fluorescence can limit the system employed by which the measurements are obtained, i.e., using a microscope equipped for measuring nonimaged epifluorenscence (Fig. 8), versus a confocal microscope. It should be noted that studies have also been performed with fluorophores to investigate the modulation of [Ca^{2+}] within a specific cellular organelle (e.g., 35,47, 49,54,90). In a recent article, a droplet technique was described which allows one to investigate Ca^{2+} extrusion from a cell; in these experiments, Fura-2 was used as an intracellular indicator and Fluo-3 as the extracellular indicator in the solution droplet (146).

Measurements of [Ca^{2+}]$_i$ may strongly be affected by the relative pH within the cellular compartment which contains the optical probe; it has been reported that fluorescent Ca^{2+} indicators are sensitive to pH (97). It has been shown using the simultaneous measurement of intracellular pH and Ca^{2+}, using fluorophores SNARF-1 and Fura-2 respectively, that alterations in cellular pH have an apparent effect on the K_d of Fura-2 (97). Despite this observation, this phenomenon is frequently overlooked in the reports of studies purporting to determine the "absolute" [Ca^{2+}]$_i$; i.e., assurance of unchanging intracellular pH during a set of measurements is a prerequisite for accurately determining [Ca^{2+}]$_i$. When possible, knowledge of the relative intracellular pH will also provide important information as to the relative physiological responsiveness of a given cell type, for many Ca^{2+} regulatory processes, especially ATPase activities, are also pH sensitive. For additional details, the reader is referred to several excellent publications which discuss the limitations of utilizing these fluorophores (1,3,7,9,14, 33,41,53,65,91,106,120,125,128,157,161).

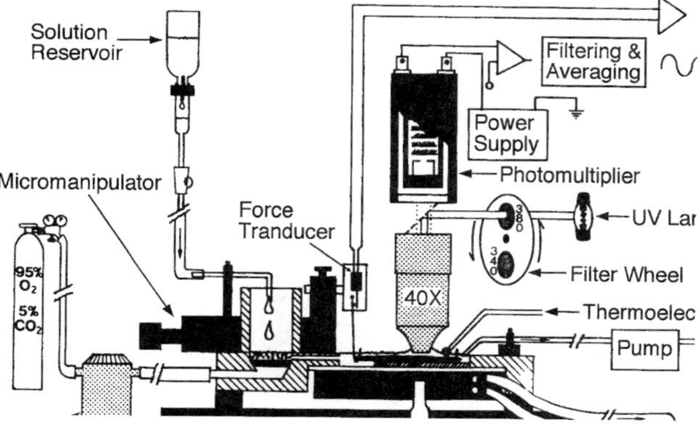

Figure 8. Schematic diagram of an experimental setup used to record Fura-2 fluorescence following excitation at either 340 or 380 nm and contractile force simultaneously. This system included a means to deliver a volatile anesthetic at various concentrations using continuous perfusion. Fluorescence emitted from the fibers passed through an interference filter (500 nm) and was from a circular area with a diameter of 40 μm (via the use of a pinhole filter). (Reprinted with permission from Iaizzo PA, Seewald M, Oakes SG, Lehmann-Horn F. The use of Fura-2 to estimate myoplasmic [Ca^{2+}] in human skeletal muscle. *Cell Calcium* 1989;10:151–158.)

Combination with Patch-Clamp Techniques One approach to incorporate Fura-2 into cells has been to combine its use with the whole cell patch-clamp technique: i.e., Fura-2 is incorporated into the internal solution of the patch electrode and diffuses into the cell (112). The time course of dye diffusion into the cell can be monitored by detecting fluorescence at 358 nm, a wavelength independent of [Ca^{2+}]$_i$, and thus changes in fluorescence are simply proportional to the amount of dye inside the cell. On the other hand, Fura-2 has been used to determine the relative contents of bleb preparations used for single channel recordings (88).

Confocal Microscopy and Fluorescent Ca^{2+} Indicators In conventional microscopy, while light from the plane of focus is accurately seen in the image, light from outside the plane of focus will not be accurately represented on the planar image field. When examining fluorescent sources, those images not in the plane of focus and not in vertical register with objects in the plane of focus, may contribute fluorescence and provide an inaccurate image of the distribution. In confocal microscopy, a smaller beam of light or a laser beam is employed to eliminate the object of interest. By employing a pinhole image window, fluorescent sources out of the vertical register of the plane of focus will not reach the light-sensitive image plane (Fig. 9). By this means, high spatial resolution within a focal plane can be achieved and the fluorescent behavior of indicators in microscopic subcellular compartments can be more clearly delineated.

A new method was recently described for ratiometric Ca^{2+} measurements using Fluo-3 and Fura-Red, which have excitation spectra in the visible wavelength range (91). A laser-scanning confocal microscopy was utilized to monitor changes in [Ca^{2+}]$_i$, which allowed for a high degree of temporal and spatial resolution. The fluorescent Ca^{2+} indicators were loaded into the cells utilizing the whole-cell patch-clamp technique which also allowed the investigators to follow membrane currents simultaneously. It was reported that the Fluo-3 showed an increase in fluorescence upon a rise in [Ca^{2+}]$_i$, whereas the Fura-Red fluorescence decreased. Because the fluorescence of Fluo-3 is about two times brighter than that of Fura-Red, the cells were loaded with a 1:2 mixture of these indicators, respectively. In a subsequent study, AM forms of these two dyes were used for cell loading and monitored by confocal microscopy with reported equal success (132). In a recent report, a novel UV laser-scanning confocal microscope for the measurement of [Ca^{2+}]$_i$ was described (82). Modification to the optics of a conventional confocal laser-scanning microscope were made which allowed imaging of intracellular Ca^{2+}-dependent fluorescence with a UV laser (excitation wavelengths of 351 or 364 nm) (82). The potential limitation to the use of confocal microscopy employing fluorophores have been recently reviewed (159).

Other Techniques

Other methodologies exist that are useful in determining the effect of anesthetic agents on the mobilization of intracellular Ca^{2+} but which do not employ Ca^{2+} indicators. These methods include nuclear magnetic resonance (for details on this, see Chapter 23), photolabile Ca^{2+} chelators, and electron probe x-ray microanalysis.

Photolable calcium chelators have been used to study intracellular Ca^{2+}-dependent processes (50,96). These "caged" Ca^{2+} compounds have been used to bypass rate limiting steps in excitation-contraction coupling in muscle (73,85,109,154,155).

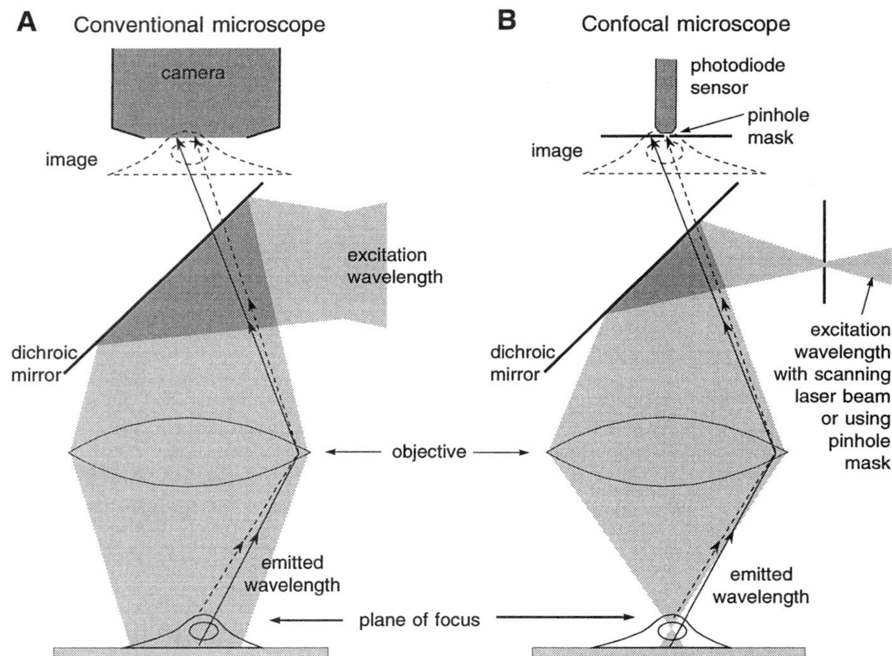

Figure 9. Comparison of the conventional **(A)** and confocal **(B)** epifluorescence microscopy, showing how confocal imaging discriminates against blurring from out-of-focus parts of the specimen. Excitation light, shown as *stippling*, enters from the right, reflects off the dichroic mirror, and passes downward through the schematized objective and specimen. In this example, the plane of focus is imagined to be the top of the cell. In conventional microscopy (A) the wide-open field stop allows fairly uniform illumination of the specimen; fluorescence emission from the desired plane (*solid lines*) focuses on the camera film or face plate, but emission from out-of-focus portions (*dashed lines*) also reaches the camera, causing an obscuring haze. In confocal microscopy (B), an intense illuminating beam is tightly focused at one point of the specimen. Other parts recieve much less intense excitation or none at all. Emission from the desired zone efficiently passes through another pinhole in front of the photodetector, whereas emission from out-of-focus planes is largely blocked. A complete *x,y* image is built up by scanning the two pinholes in synchrony or by moving the specimen.

Cells must be exposed to high-intensity ultraviolet light to release the Ca^{2+}. The minimum energy density required for photolysis in the past has required excitation by either a doubled ruby laser (with flash durations of 25 ns) or a xenon flash system (using longer flash durations; i.e., 4 ms), both of which are expensive to purchase (154). The photolysis of caged Ca^{2+} utilizing a low-cost flash unit with a 4-ms flash duration has been recently described, in which one flash on 1.00 nM Nitr5 (a commercially produced photolabile calcium chelator, Calbiochem) increased the free $[Ca^{2+}]$ in a cuvette from 10^{-7} to 1.1×10^{-5} M (154). The availability of such a system will likely increase the novel employment of this approach; however, one still has to consider the potential complications of exposing a given cellular preparation to high intensity UV radiation.

The location of Ca^{2+} in a cell during a given process can also be analyzed at fixed moments by rapid (<5 ms) freezing of tissue. Electron probe microanalysis can then be used to measure the content and distribution of elements in cells with a resolution of 0.2 μm (166). For example, a recent report described the use of electron probe x-ray microanalysis technique to monitor the movement of mass dense granules that contained high amount of Ca^{2+} in various developmental stages of an amoebae aggregate (133). Although the spatial and temporal resolution of such methods continues to improve, they still require the analysis of freeze-dried cryosections of rapid-frozen preparations (166). Nevertheless, they do offer an additional and unique approach, with increasingly high resolution, to monitor the mobilization of Ca^{2+} in certain situations.

Comparisons Among Methods

Numerous studies have been performed in which more than one method have been used to monitor the mobilization of $[Ca^{2+}]_i$ in a given cell type. Such investigations have involved one of three approaches designed to (a) substantiate a cellular response or pathomechanism; (b) determine how a specific cellular compartment or component modulates Ca^{2+} mobilization; or (c) specifically compare the relative dynamic responses, sensitivity limits or potential complications attributed to each indicator in that particular cell type.

One example of this latter study is that of Ozake and Kume (117), who found that in human neutrophils loaded with either Fura-2 or aequorin, ionomycin exposure caused a sharp rise in each indicator response. However, the decay of the Ca^{2+} signal in the Fura-2–loaded cells was extremely slow compared to the signal of the photoproteins (117). These findings suggested that extracellular Ca^{2+} influx is important in the ionomycin-induced $[Ca^{2+}]_i$ and that the more slowly decaying response observed for Fura-2 can be attributed in part to a relative buffering property. In similar experiments, the decay of Quin-2 fluorescence was noted to outlast that of Fura-2, probably due to its even stronger intracellular buffering of Ca^{2+}. The relative intracellular properties of Fura-2 and Indo-2 have been contrasted in several experiments. For example, both acetoxymethyl forms of these indicators were shown to be converted into their Ca^{2+}-dependent forms by mitochondria with rat hepatocytes (49); in another study, reduced PO_2 in bovine pulmonary artery endothelial cells caused a significant upward shift of in vivo calibration curves for both fluorophores (143).

A number of studies have compared the subsequent mobilization of loaded $^{45}Ca^{2+}$ to transients pharmacologically initiated in cells loaded with either a photoprotein or fluorophore (29,110,115,134). Several such studies performed by myself and my colleagues have involved similar protocols to gain insights as to the differential effects of volatile anesthetic agents on Ca^{2+} mobilization (65–67). In these studies, volatile anesthetics induced transient increases of $[Ca^{2+}]_i$ in a variety of cell types (cultured vascular smooth muscle, rat and swine hepatocytes, and Swiss 3T3 fibroblasts) in a dose-dependent manner, but with varying degrees of potency. Although the exact mechanisms of action were not identified, they appeared to be different for each of the agents: e.g., the amplitude of transients elicited in aequorin-loaded cells that were induced by isoflurane were more dependent on the presence of extracellular Ca^{2+} than those induced by halothane (61). Consistent with this difference, the release of $^{45}Ca^{2+}$ from optimally loaded, saponin-treated cells by halothane or enflurane was significantly greater than that by isoflurane, even at equivalent 1 MAC concentrations, thereby confirming that isoflurane has a lesser effect on releasing Ca^{2+} from intracellular storage sites (Fig. 10). In response to the administration of an anesthetic, the duration of the increases in $[Ca^{2+}]_i$ estimated for the Fura-2–loaded cells was somewhat longer than the durations of increased luminescence recorded from aequorin-loaded cells. This difference may be related to the previously discussed distinctions in the Ca^{2+} buffering characteristics of these methods (14,75,117).

POTENTIAL COMPLICATIONS IN MONITORING CA2+ MOBILIZATION ATTRIBUTED TO ANESTHETICS

To date, there is little or no information concerning the potential complications that anesthetic agents may induce on the measurement of the mobilization of $[Ca^{2+}]_i$ by radioisotopes, metallochromic dyes, or Ca^{2+}-selective microelectrodes. Intuitively, potential limitations come to mind only in relation to this latter method, for if a given anesthetic agent fluidizes a membrane, the potential for leakage around these electrodes increases as does the possibility for recording an exaggerated increase in $[Ca^{2+}]_i$. Nevertheless, limitations have also been reported for the use of both photoproteins and fluorophores in studies involving the administration of anesthetic agents (4,14,61–63,65).

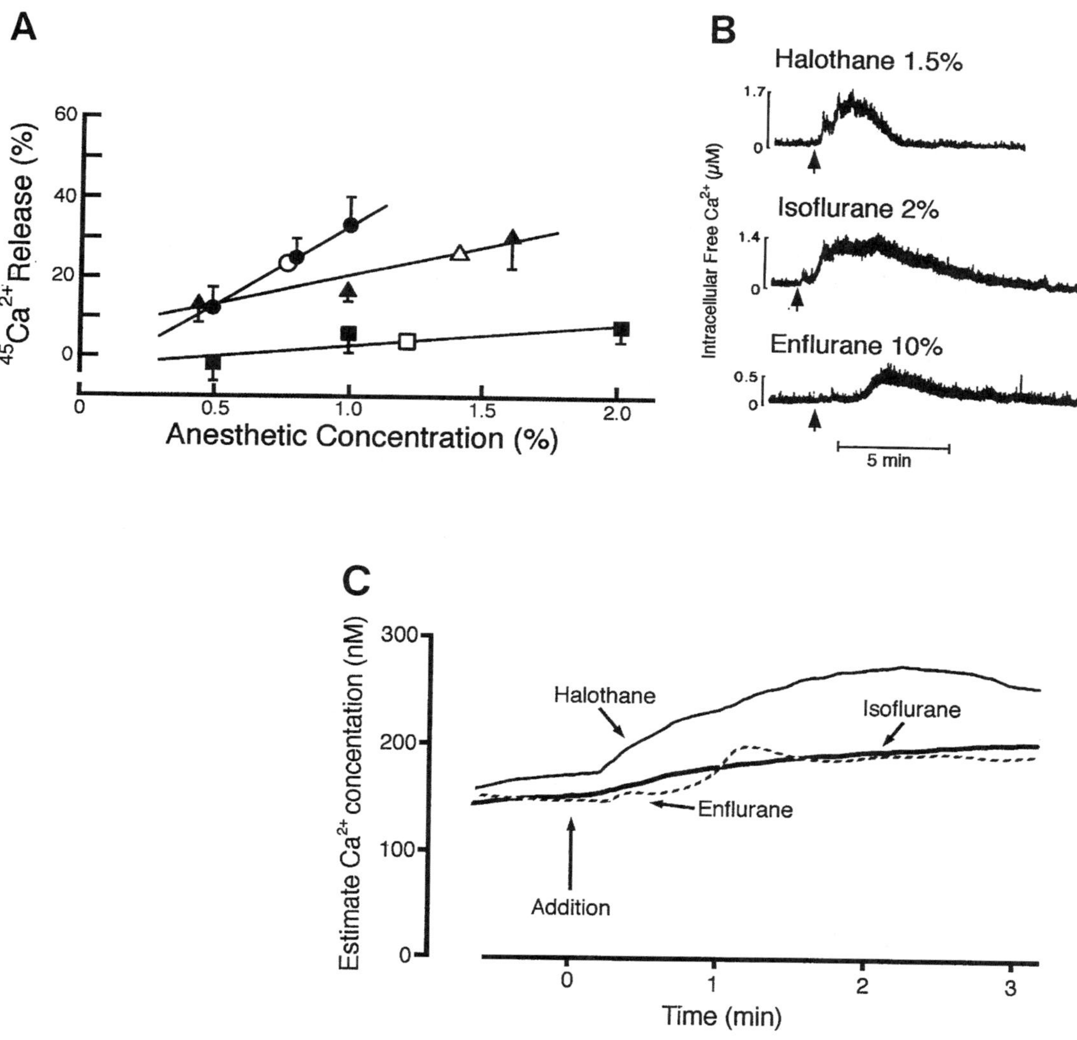

Figure 10. The relative effects of halothane, isoflurane and enflurane on Ca^{2+} mobilization in rat hepatocytes evaluated using three different methodologies. Shown in **(A)** is the dose-dependent release of $^{45}Ca^{2+}$ in saponin treated cells following the administration of halothane (●), enflurane (▲) and isoflurane(■) (*open symbols* indicate 1 MAC equivalents); **(B)** luminescence increases in cells loaded with aequorin; and **(C)** estimated changes in $[Ca^{2+}]_i$ using a Fura-2 ratiometric method following the administration of 1% concentrations of each agent at time 0 min.

A decrease in fluorescence from a cell preparation loaded with a fluorophore may result from (a) photobleaching, (b) quenching of fluorescence, and/or (c) an enhanced loss of dye by cell membrane leakage (1,33,65,106,114). Each of these processes may be accentuated by the application of a drug such as an anesthetic. Therefore, in any experiment in which the mobilization of $[Ca^{2+}]_i$ is monitored in conjunction with the application of an anesthetic agent, appropriate control experiments need to be performed. In certain cases, the effects of the anesthetic agent on either the cell to be investigated or on the probe used to monitor Ca^{2+} mobilization may be so dramatic that such experiments are rendered uninterpretable. On the other hand, the relative conditions of cell population or tissues under investigation may in turn influence the relative effect of an anesthetic one wishes to study. For example, the presence or absence of various growth factors in a cell culture media will modify the mobilization of $[Ca^{2+}]_i$ following the administration of anesthetic agents (61,65,122) (Fig. 11).

Enhanced Leakage of Membranes

The use of Fura-2 to study changes of $[Ca^{2+}]_i$ within cell suspensions of rat hepatocytes may be impractical due to the rapid extrusion of dye by these cells (65,114) (Fig. 12). The fluorescence contribution of the extracellular Fura-2 may eventually reach the levels emitted from the cells themselves (P. A. Iaizzo, *unpublished data,* 1989), and when the extracellular dye concentration becomes this large, one cannot distinguish between intracellular or extracellular changes in $[Ca^{2+}]_i$. In such a case, an investigator might misinterpret induced cell rupture as an induced increase in $[Ca^{2+}]_i$.

In a previous study, it was observed that this rapid movement of dye out of the hepatocytes was most probable in experiments dealing with cell suspensions (P. A. Iaizzo, *unpublished data,* 1989). The amount of dye located in the extracellular media became a major source of fluorescence; in some cases, this fluorescence was as high (same order of magnitude) as that originating from within the cells. In one set of experiments, loaded (and washed) cell suspensions remained within the observation cuvette (with continuous mixing in the absence of light) for 1 h. The hepatocytes in the suspension were then removed from the Krebs bathing media by centrifugation. The extracted media had an emitted fluorescence following excitation at 340 and 380 nm that was one half the intensity recorded when the cells were present. The addition of saturating Ca^{2+} and subsequently 1 mM EGTA to this cell-free media induced changes in fluorescence intensities that were as great as those induced by 10 µM ionomycin in cuvettes with cells present.

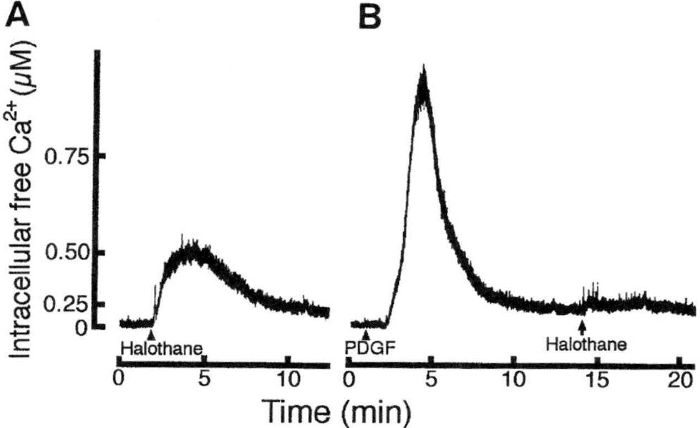

Figure 11. Inhibition by platelet-derived growth factor (PDGF) of the increase in $[Ca^{2+}]_i$ produced by halothane. Swiss 3T3 fibroblasts were loaded with aequorin 18 h prior to study and then serum deprived for 3 h. Halothane (1%) induced a transient increase in $[Ca^{2+}]_i$ **(A)**, but this response was not observed following the addition of 3.3×10^{-9} M PDGF **(B)**. Additions were made at the *arrows.* The external media contained 1.8 mM Ca^{2+}. (Reprinted, in adapted form, with permission from Olsen RA, Seewald MJ, Melder DC, Berggren M, Iaizzo PA, Powis G. Platelet-derived growth factor blocks the increase in intracellular free Ca^{2+} caused by calcium ionophores and a volatile anesthetic agent in Swiss 3T3 fibroblasts without altering toxicity. *Toxicol Lett* 1991;55:117–125.)

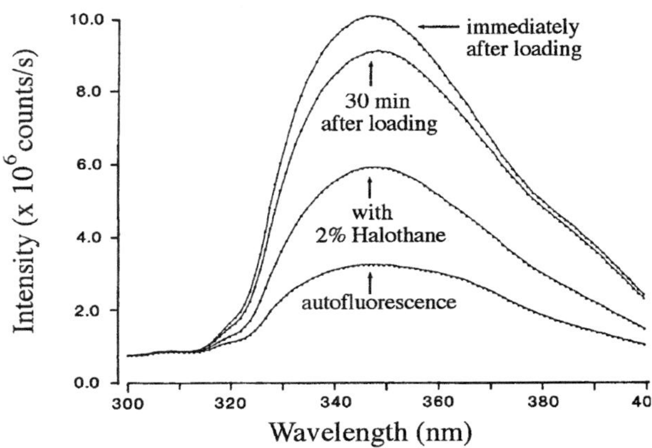

Figure 12. The effects of time and halothane on the fluorescence excitation spectrum of rat hepatocytes loaded with Fura-2. The field of cells from which all spectra was recorded was the same. The initial autofluorescence was recorded, and then the cells were incubated in 5×10^{-7} M Fura-2 AM for 1 h at 37°C. Subsequently, the extracellular dye was removed and an excitation spectrum immediately recorded. At 0.5 h later a third excitation spectrum was obtained and a decrease of fluorescence noted, which was due to a loss of cytoplasmic dye or a change in the fluorescent properties of the dye. Finally, the cells were exposed to halothane (2%) for 5 min, and a fourth spectrum was recorded. (Reprinted, in adapted form, with permission from Iazzo PA, Olsen RA, Seewald MJ, Powis G, Stier A, Van Dyke R. Transient increases of intracelleular Ca^{2+} induced by volatile anesthetics in rat hepatocytes. *Cell Calcium* 1990;11:515–524.)

Interactions Between the Indicator and the Anesthetic Administered

It has been suggested that halothane may enhance the photobleaching of Fura-2 in skeletal muscle fibers (62). In rat hepatocytes, a dramatic decrease of Fura-2 fluorescence occurred immediately following the administration of halothane and which was noted to require excitation of the preparation by light (65) (Fig. 13). An additional report has indicated that Fura-2 photobleaching was not equivalent to simply decreasing the intracellular concentration of the dye. If this were the case, then the effect could be corrected to some degree by the ratio method of analysis. The problem may be related to the production of a photobleaching decay product(s) that has different fluorescent characteristics and/or Ca^{2+} affinity than the parent compound (Fura-2). There is good reason to suspect that the multiple Fura-2 metabolites reported by Oakes et al. (114) may be in part the result of photobleaching and not entirely related to metabolism.

Halothane is an extremely electrophilic compound that has been shown to undergo reductive as well as oxidative metabolism (45,153). The first step of either metabolic pathway is the release of bromide from the halothane molecule, a consequence of the addition of an electron. This results in the formation of an intermediate radical which is quickly oxidized in the presence of oxygen, but under hypoxic conditions the radical will bind to adjacent molecules, e.g., unsaturated fatty acids (45,153). Although no direct evidence has been obtained that supports this type of reaction, it may be conjectured that free radical products contribute to Fura-2 breakdown. In support of this mechanism, perhaps, is the fact that neither isoflurane nor enflurane enhance photobleaching; these two agents produce

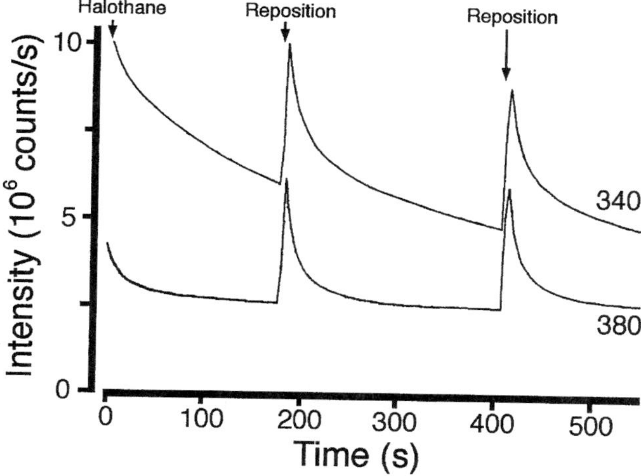

Figure 13. Enhanced photobleaching following exposure to halothane. A monolayer of rat hepatocytes was exposed to ~2% halothane at time zero. The cells exposed to alternating 340- and 380-nm light rapidly lost their ability to fluoresce. When the field of cells was changed to cells previously not subjected to light, the initial level of detected florescence was high, but photobleaching rapidly followed. Note that the rate of decreased fluorescence in the latter two fields was similar following excitation at either wavelength. Hence, it appears that both the Ca^{2+} bound and unbound forms of the dye are equally sensitive to the enhanced photobleaching which was detected following the administration of halothane. (Reprinted, in adapted form, with permission from Iaizzo PA, Olsen RA, Seewald MJ, Powis G, Stier A, Van Dyke R. Transient increases of intracellular Ca^{2+} induced by volatile anesthetics in rat hepatocytes. *Cell Calcium* 1990;11:515–524.)

the same effect on membrane stability as halothane, but do not form radical intermediates. It is possible that a number of other drugs or chemicals will contribute to photobleaching (as does halothane), but only if they are strong electrophiles which are associated with free radical formation.

It has been reported that the Ca^{2+} detection properties of the photoprotein aequorin may be altered by a variety of local anesthetics and urethane (4). Although another study has confirmed the effects of urethane on the Ca^{2+} sensitivity of aequorin, it was not able to identify any effect of local anesthetics on aequorin's detection properties (14). Housmans et al. (56) have determined that halothane, enflurane, and isoflurane have no effect on the Ca^{2+} concentration-effect curve for aequorin (also see P. Housmans, L. Wanek, and E. Carton, *personal communication,* 1990).

Contamination or Autofluorescent Properties

As with any pharmacological experiment, complications due to the addition of contaminated substance are a concern when one investigates changes in $[Ca^{2+}]_i$. Various tissue components themselves can have autofluorescent properties which will compromise the use of a given fluorophore for the estimation of $[Ca^{2+}]_i$. Thus, either the preparation needs to be modified to remove or minimize this factor, or the internalized, functional dye concentration needs to be increased until the autofluorescence is negligible in the final experimental estimation of $[Ca^{2+}]_i$. However, adding enough dye to overcome autofluorescent properties of the cellular preparation to be investigated may in turn lead to excessive buffering of $[Ca^{2+}]_i$, and thus alter the cellular response to give an unphysiological situation. One preparation in which autofluorescence, in the operational spectral range of Fura-2, can be of high enough magnitude to minimize the utility of this fluorophore, is mammalian skeletal muscle. Any appreciable amount of intermuscular adipose tissue and/or connective tissue has been considered to contribute to such a situation.

The cytoplasmic composition of cells can vary considerably. For example, skeletal muscle isolated from certain vertebrates (e.g., frogs) have extremely high concentration of the soluble Ca^{2+} binding protein parvalbumin (58,59). It would be of interest to determine if such unusually large amounts of such a constituent will interact with any molecular probe that might be internalized (Fig. 14). The in vitro presence of parvalbumin does not alter the properties of either aequorin or Fura-2 (58; and P. A. Iaizzo, *unpublished data,* 1986). If were to have an effect on a given probe, then the reaction kinetics for that molecule should be either corrected for appropriately or determined using an in vivo calibration technique.

There are several pharmacological agents other than anesthetics which have been shown to modulate the mobilization of Ca^{2+} and which have been intensely studied by anesthesia research laboratories. One such agent is dantrolene, a well-known treatment for the abnormal regulation of Ca^{2+} that can be induced by administration of volatile anesthetic agents in humans or swine susceptible to malignant hyperthermia (62–64,66,76–78,86,103,104,152). This substance has been reported to fluoresce in the same spectral region used to detect differences in the Ca^{2+}-bound and unbound states of Fura-2. Thus, other methodologies should be chosen to best determine the mode of action, such as $^{45}Ca^{2+}$ release, $[^3H]$ ryanodine binding, photoprotein luminescence, or Ca^{2+}-selective microelectrodes (64,93,103,104,152). This limitation is noted here in order to alert potential investigators in this field of the need to determine potential interactions or complications not only of the anesthetic agents they may administer to a given cellular preparation, but also those of any other modulator substance to be studied.

CONCLUSION

The number of investigative tools for studying the effects of anesthetics on the mobilization of intercellular Ca^{2+} and the identified methodologies to apply them have increased at a rapid pace. As would be the case for studying the pharmacological effects of a given substance on a particular cellular function, it is appropriate to seek confirmation of critical results by more than one method. With increased commercial interest in producing Ca^{2+} indicators and with the increased availability of affordable optical equipment to perform such studies, this goal is becoming a reality. Nevertheless, each new indicator or system design will have limitations as well as advantages that inves-

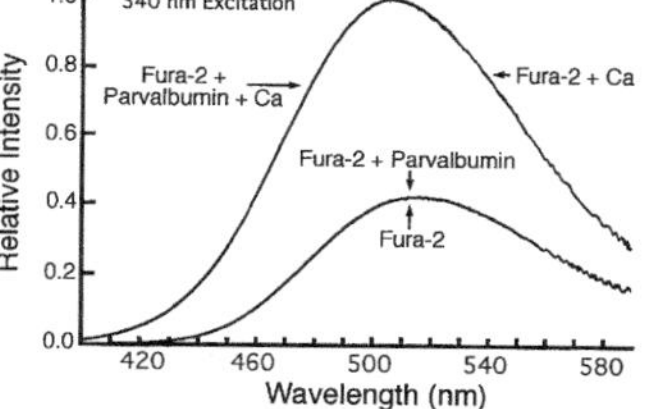

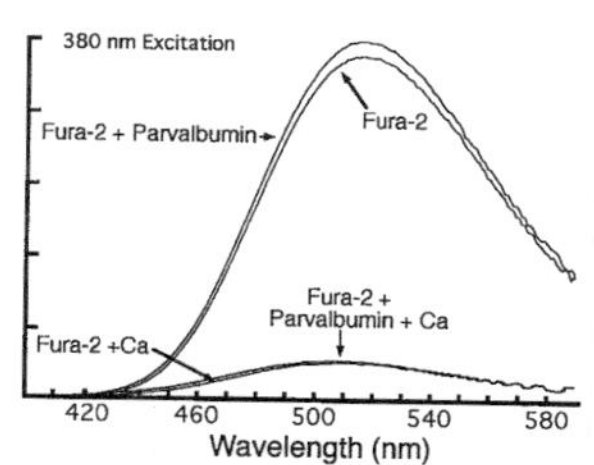

Figure 14. Emission spectra of steady-state fluorescence intensity of Fura-2 (10^{-5} M) preequillibrated with parvalbumin and/or Ca^{2+}. Spectra were recorded following excitation at either 340 or 380 nm. Each curve represents a single scan in which the monochromator was incremented in 1-nm steps with an acquisition rate of 1 Hz. The excitation and emission bandpass filters were 2 and 8 nm, respectively. The parvalbumins were from frog skeletal muscle (*Rana temporaria*), and the amount added was 0.3 mM, the approximate myoplasmic concentration in such muscle. The buffer solution contained 150 mM KCl, 5 mM PIPES (pH = 7.0) and is some cases a $[Ca^{2+}]$ of ~2 mM. The preequilibration of Fura-2 with parvalbumins has little or no effect on the fluorescent characteristics of this dye.

tigators need to recognize. For example, certain florophores in specific cell types have perhaps a more limited use than other indicator types when one is investigating the effects of volatile anesthetics on Ca^{2+} mobilization. The interpretation of data collected in any investigation monitoring modulations in $[Ca^{2+}]_i$ is made easier if (a) careful and thorough control experiments define all complicating factors; (b) a potential effect can be shown to have a dose dependency; (c) attempts are made to show that a recorded effect is reversible; and/or (d) associated changes in appropriately chosen biophysical phenomena are simultaneously monitored and recorded for a given cell type (e.g., membrane potential, pH changes, contractile force or secretion).

Acknowledgment: I would like to acknowledge the following colleagues and mentors who taught me a great deal about the mobilization of $[Ca^{2+}]_i$: J. R. Blinks, F. Lehmann-Horn, E. D. W. Moore, S. G. Oakes, R. A. Olsen, G. Powis, M. J. Seewald, S. R. Taylor, and R. A. Van Dyke.

REFERENCES

1. Almers W, Neher E. The Ca signal from fura-2–loaded mast cells depends strongly on the method of dye-loading. *FEBS Lett* 1985; 192:13–18.
2. Ammann D, Buhrer T, Schefer U, Muller M, Simon W. Intracellular neutral carrier-based Ca^{2+} microelectrode with subnanomolar detection limit. *Pflugers Arch* 1987;409:223–228.
3. Backx PH, ter Keurs HED. Fluorescent properties of rat cardiac trabeculae microinjected with fura-2 salt. *Am J Physiol* 1993;264: H1098–H1110.
4. Baker PF, Schapira AH. Anaesthetics increase light emission from aequorin at constant ionised calcium. *Nature* 1980;284: 168–169.
5. Baylor SM, Quinta FM, Hui CS. Comparison of isotropic calcium signals from intact frog muscle fibers injected with Arsenazo III or Antipyrylazo III. *Biophys J* 1983;44:107–112.
6. Baylor SM, Hollingworth S, Hui CS, Quinta FM. Properties of the metallochromic dyes Arsenazo III, Antipyrylazo III and Azol in frog skeletal muscle fibres at rest. *J Physiol* 1986;377:89–141.
7. Baylor SM, Hollingworth S. Fura-2 calcium transients in frog skeletal muscle fibres. *J Physiol* 1988;403:151–192.
8. Becker GL, Fiskum G, Lehninger AL. Regulation of free Ca^{2+} by liver mitochondria and endoplasmic reticulum. *J Biol Chem* 1980; 255:9009–9012.
9. Becker PL, Fay FS. Photobleaching of fura-2 and its effect on determination of calcium concentrations. *Am J Physiol* 1987;253: C613–C618.
10. Berridge MJ. Inositol trisphosphate and diacylglycerol: two interacting second messengers. *Annu Rev Biochem* 1987;56:159–193.
11. Blatter LA, Wier WG. Intracellular diffusion, binding, and compartmentalization of the fluorescent calcium indicators indo-1 and fura-2. *Biophys J* 1990;58:1491–1499.
12. Blatter LA, Blinks JR. Simultaneous measurement of Ca^{2+} in muscle with Ca electrodes and aequorin. Diffusible cytoplasmic constituent reduces Ca^{2+}-independent luminescence of aequorin. *J Gen Physiol* 1991;98:1141–1160.
13. Blinks JR. The use of photoproteins as calcium indicators in cellular physiology. *Techniq Cell Physiol* 1982;126:1–38.
14. Blinks JR. Intracellular $[Ca^{2+}]$ measurements. In: Fozzard HA, Haber E, Jennings RB, Katz AM, Morgan HE, eds. *The heart and cardiovascular system.* New York: Raven Press, 1992:1171–1201.
15. Blinks JR, Prendergast FG, Allen DG. Photoproteins as biological calcium indicators. *Pharmacol Rev* 1976;28:1–93.
16. Blinks JR, Rüdel R, Taylor SR. Calcium transients in isolated amphibian skeletal muscle fibres: detection with aequorin. *J Physiol* 1978;277:291–323.
17. Blinks JR, Wier WG, Hess P, Prendergast FG. Measurement of Ca^{2+} concentrations in living cells. *Prog Biophys Mol Biol* 1982;40:1–114.
18. Borle AB. Pitfalls of the ^{45}Ca uptake method. *Cell Calcium* 1981;2: 187–196.
19. Borle AB, Freudenrich CC, Snowdowne KW, A simple method for incorporating aequorin into mammalian cells. *Am J Physiol* 1986; 251:C323–C326.
20. Bosnjak ZJ, Supan FD, Rusch NJ. The effects of halothane, enflurane, and isoflurane on calcium current in isolated canine ventricular cells. *Anesthesiology* 1991;74:340–345.
21. Bosnjak ZJ, Aggarwal A, Turner LA, Kampine JM, Kampine JP. Differential effects of halothane, enflurane, and isoflurane on Ca^{2+} transients and papillary muscle tension in guinea pigs. *Anesthesiology* 1992;76:123–131.
22. Bright GR, Rogowska J, Fisher G, Taylor D. Fluorescence ratio imaging microscopy: temporal and spatial measurements in single living cells. *Bio Techniq* 1987;5:556–562.
23. Brini M, Murgia M, Pasti L, Picard D, Pozzan T, Rizzuto R. Nuclear Ca^{2+} concentration measured with specifically targeted recombinant aequorin. *EMBO J* 1993;12:4813–4819.
24. Burgress GM, McKinney JS, Fabiato A, Leslie BA, Putney JW Jr,. Calcium fluxes in saponin-permeabilized guinea pig hepatocytes. *J Biol* 1983;258:15336–15345.
25. Button D, Brownstein M. Aequorin-expressing mammalian cell lines used to report Ca^{2+} mobilization. *Cell Calcium* 1993;14: 663–671.
26. Byron KL, Villereal ML. Mitogen-induced $[Ca^{2+}]_i$ changes in individual human fibroblasts. Image analysis reveals asynchronous responses which are characteristic for different mitogens. *J Biol Chem* 1989;264:18234–18239.
27. Campbell AK, Dormer RL. The permeability to calcium of pigeon erythrocytes "ghosts" studied by using the calcium-activated luminescent protein, obelin. *Biochem J* 1975;152:255–265.
28. Campbell AK, Patel AK, Razavi ZS, McCapra F. Formation of the Ca^{2+}-activated photoprotein obelin from apo-obelin and mRNA inside human neutrophils. *Biochem J* 1988;252:143–149.
29. Chen WS, Lazar CS, Lund KA, et al. Functional independence of the epidermal growth factor receptor from a domain required for ligand-induced internalization and calcium regulation. *Cell* 1989; 59:33–43.
30. Choi DW. Glutamate neurotoxicity and diseases of the nervous system. *Neuron* 1989;1:623–634.
31. Cobbold PH, Cuthbertson KS, Goyns MH, Rice V. Aequorin measurements of free calcium in single mammalian cells. *J Cell Sci* 1983; 61:123–136.
32. Cobbold PH, Bourne PK. Aequorin measurements of free calcium in single heart cells. *Nature* 1984;312:444–446.
33. Cobbold PH, Rink TJ. Fluorescence and bioluminescence measurement of cytoplasmic free calcium. *Biochem J* 1987;248:313–328.
34. Connor JA. Intracellular calcium mobilization by inositol 1,4,5-trisphosphate: intracellular movements and compartmentalization. *Cell Calcium* 1993;14:185–200.
35. Davis MH, Altschuld RA, Jung DW, Brierley GP. Estimation of intramitochondrial pCa and pH by fura-2 and 2,7 biscarboxyethyl-5(6)-carboxyfluorescein (BCECF) fluorescence. *Biochem Biophys Res Commun* 1987;149:40–45.
36. Dawson AP, Comerford JG. Effects of GTP on Ca^{2+} movements across endoplasmic reticulum membranes. *Cell Calcium* 1989;10: 343–350.
37. Docampo R, Moreno SNJ, Mason RP. Generation of free radical metabolites and superoxide anion by the calcium indicators arsenaso III, antipyrlazo III, and murexide in rat liver microsomes. *J Biol Chem* 1983;258:14920–14925.
38. Etter EF, Kuhn MA, Fay FS. Detection of changes in near-membrane Ca^{2+} concentration using a novel membrane-associated Ca^{2+} indicator. *J Biol Chem* 1994;269:10141–10149.
39. Field M, Azzawi A, Styles P, Henderson C, Seymor A, Radda G. Intracellular Ca^{2+} transients in isolated perfused rat heart: measurement using the fluorescent indicator Fura-2/AM. *Cell Calcium* 1994;16:87–100.
40. Ford LE, Podolsky RJ. Intracellular calcium movements in skinned muscle fibers. *J Physiol* 1972;223:21–33.
41. Fralix TA, Heineman FW, Balaban RS. Effects of tissue absorbance on NAD(P)H and Indo-1 fluorescence from perfused rabbit hearts. *FEBS Lett* 1990;262:287–292.
42. Frazer MJ, Lynch C. Halothane and isoflurane effects on Ca^{2+} fluxes of isolated myocardial sarcoplasmic reticulum. *Anesthesiology* 1992;77:316–323.
43. Freeman LC, Li Q. Effects of halothane on delayed afterdepolarization and calcium transients in dog ventricular myocytes exposed to isoproterenol. *Anesthesiology* 1991;74:146–154.
44. Gailly P, Boland B, Himpens B. Critical evaluation of cytosolic calcium determination in resting muscle fibres from normal and dystrophic (mdx) mice. *Cell Calcium* 1993;14:473–483.
45. Gelman S, Van Dyke RA. Mechanism of halothane-induced hepa-

totoxicity: another step on a long path. *Anesthesiology* 1988;68: 3479–3482.
46. Gill DL, Chuen SH. An intracellular (ATP + Mg^{2+})-dependent calcium pump within the N1E-115 neuronal cell line. *J Biol Chem* 1985; 260:9289–9297.
47. Giovannardi S, Cesare P, Peres A. Rapid synchrony of nuclear and cytosolic Ca^{2+} signals activated by muscarinic stimulation in the human tumor line TE671/RD. *Cell Calcium* 1994;16:491–499.
48. Grynkiewicz G, Poenie M, Tsien RY. A new generation of Ca^{2+} indicators with greatly improved fluorescence properties. *J Biol Chem* 1985;260:3440–3450.
49. Gunter TE, Restrepo D, Gunter KK. Conversion of esterified fura-2 and indo-1 to Ca^{2+}-sensitive forms by mitochondria. *Am J Physiol* 1988;255:C304–C310.
50. Gurney AM, Tsien RY, Lester HA. Activation of a potassium current by rapid photochemically generated step increases of intracellular calcium in rat sympathetic neurons. *Proc Natl Acad Sci USA* 1987;84: 3496–3500.
51. Hamilton SL, Mejia Alvarev R, Fill M. [^{3}H]PN200-110 and [^{3}H]ryanodine binding and reconstitution of ion channel activity with skeletal muscle membrane. *Anal Biochem* 1989;183:31–41.
52. Haugland RP. *Handbook of fluorescent probes and research chemicals.* Eugene, OR: Molecular Probes, 1992.
53. Highsmith S, Bloebaum P, Snowdowne KW. Sarcoplasmic reticulum interacts with the Ca^{2+} indicator precursor fura-2-am. *Biochem Biophys Res Commun* 1986;138:1153–1162.
54. Himpens B, De Smedt H, Casteels R. Relationship between [Ca^{2+}] changes in nucleus and cytosol. *Cell Calcium* 1994;16:239–246.
55. Hoffmann P, Heinroth K, Richards D, Plews P, Toraason M. Depression of calcium dynamics in cardiac myocytes—a common mechanism of halogenated hydrocabon anesthetics and solvents. *J Mol Cell Cardiol* 1994;26:579–589.
56. Housmans P, Wanek L, Carton E. Halothane, Enflurane and Isoflurane decrease myofibrillar Ca^{2+} responsiveness in intact mammalian ventricular muscle. *Biophys J* 1990;57:554a.
57. Hossain MD, Evers AS. Volatile anesthetic-induced efflux of calcium from IP_3-gated stores in clonal (GH3) pituitary cells. *Anesthesiology* 1994;80:1379–1389.
58. Iaizzo PA. Aequorin luminescence from stimulated skeletal muscle cells: relation between changes in intracellular calcium and contractile force [Dissertation]. Minneapolis: University of Minnesota, 1985.
59. Iaizzo PA. The effects of temperature on relaxation in frog skeletal muscle: the role of parvalbumin. *Pflugers Arch* 1988;412:195–202.
60. Iaizzo PA. Histochemical and physiological properties of Rana temporaria tibialis anterior and lumbricalis IV muscle fibres. *J Muscle Res Cell Motil* 1990;11:281–292.
61. Iaizzo PA. The effects of halothane and isoflurane on intracellular Ca^{2+} regulation in cultured cells with characteristics of vascular smooth muscle. *Cell Calcium* 1992;13:513–520.
62. Iaizzo PA, Klein W, Lehmann-Horn F. Fura-2 detected myoplasmic calcium and its correlation with contracture force in skeletal muscle from normal and malignant hyperthermia susceptible pigs. *Pflugers Arch* 1988;411:648–653.
63. Iaizzo PA, Seewald M, Oakes SG, Lehmann-Horn F. The use of Fura-2 to estimate myoplasmic [Ca^{2+}] in human skeletal muscle. *Cell Calcium* 1989;10:151–158.
64. Iaizzo PA, Seewald MJ, Powis G, Van Dyke R. The effects of volatile anesthetics on Ca^{++} mobilization in rat hepatocytes. *Anesthesiology* 1990;72:504–509.
65. Iaizzo PA, Olsen RA, Seewald MJ, Powis G, Stier A, Van Dyke R. Transient increases of intracellular Ca^{2+} induced by volatile anesthetics in rat hepatocytes. *Cell Calcium* 1990;11:515–524.
66. Iaizzo PA, Seewald MJ, Olsen R, et al. Enhanced mobilization of intracellular Ca^{2+} induced by halothane in hepatocytes isolated from swine susceptible to malignant hyperthermia. *Anesthesiology* 1991;74:531–538.
67. Iaizzo PA, Seewald MJ, Powis G, Van Dyke R. The effects of sevoflurane on intracellular Ca^{2+} regulation in rat hepatocytes. *Toxicol Lett* 1993;66:81–88.
68. Iino M. Calcium-induced calcium release mechanism in guinea pig taenia caeci. *J Gen Physiol* 1989;94:363–383.
69. Jackson AP, Timmerman MP, Bagshaw CR, Ashley CC. The kinetics of calcium binding to fura-2 and indo-1. *FEBS Lett* 1987;216:35–39.
70. Jenden DJ, Fairhurst AS. The pharmacology of ryanodine. *Physiol Rev* 1969;21:1–25.
71. Jones KA, Wong GY, Lorenz RR, Warner DO, Seick GC. Effects of halothane on the relationship between cytosolic calcium and force in airway smooth muscle. *Am J Physiol* 1994;266:L199–L204.
72. Kakuyama M, Hatano Y, Nakamura K, et al. Halothane and enflurane constrict canine mesenteric arteries by releasing Ca^{2+} from intracellular Ca^{2+} stores. *Anesthesiology* 1994;80:1120–1127.
73. Kao JP, Harootunian AT, Tsien RY. Photochemically generated cytosolic calcium pulses and their detection by fluo-3. *J Biol Chem* 1989;264:8179–8184.
74. Kawanishi T, Blank LM, Harootunian AT, Smith MT, Tsien RY. Ca^{2+} oscillations induced by hormonal stimulation of individual fura-2–loaded hepatocytes. *J Biol Chem* 1989;264:12859–12866.
75. Klein MG, Simon BJ, Szucs G, Schneider MF. Simultaneous recording of calcium transients in skeletal muscle using high- and low-affinity calcium indicators. *Biophys J* 1988;53:971–988.
76. Klip A, Britt BA, Elliott ME, Walker D, Ramlal T, Pegg W. Changes in cytoplasmic free calcium caused by halothane. Role of the plasma membrane and intracellular Ca^{2+} stores. *Biochem Cell Biol* 1986;64:1181–1189.
77. Klip A, Britt BA, Elliott ME, Pegg W, Frodis W, Scott E. Anaesthetic-induced increase in ionised calcium in blood mononuclear cells from malignant hyperthermia patients. *Lancet* 1987;1: 463–466.
78. Klip A, Ramlal T, Walker D, Britt BA, Elliott ME. Selective increase in cytoplasmic calcium by anesthetic in lymphocytes from malignant hyperthermia-susceptible pigs. *Anesth Analg* 1987;66:381–385.
79. Konishi M, Olson A, Hollingworth S, Baylor SM. Myoplasmic binding of fura-2 investigated by steady-state fluorescence and absorbance measurements. *Biophys J* 1988;54:1089–1104.
80. Konishi M, Hollingworth S, Harkins AB, Baylor SM. Myoplasmic calcium transients in intact frog skeletal muscle fibers monitored with the fluorescent indicator furaptra. *J Gen Physiol* 1991;97: 271–301.
81. Kress HG, Muller J, Eisert A, Gilge U, Tas PW, Koschel K. Effects of volatile anesthetics on cytoplasmic Ca^{2+} signaling and transmitter release in a neural cell line. *Anesthesiology* 1991;74:309–319.
82. Kuba K, Hua S, Hayashi T. A UV laser-scanning confocal microscope for the measurement of intracellular Ca^{2+}. *Cell Calcium* 1994; 16:205–218.
83. Kubota T, Hagiwara N, Fujimoto M. Intracellular calcium measurements with PVC-resin Ca-selective microelectrodes in frog proximal tubules and sartorius muscle fibers. *Jpn J Physiol* 1990;40: 79–95.
84. Kurihara S, Konishi M, Miyagishima T, Sakai T. Effects of enflurane on excitation-contraction coupling in frog skeletal muscle fibers. *Pflugers Arch* 1984;402:345–352.
85. Lea TJ, Ashley CC. Ca^{2+} release from the sarcoplasmic reticulum of barnacle myofibrillar bundles initiated by photolysis of caged Ca^{2+}. *J Physiol* 1990;427:435–453.
86. Lehmann-Horn F, Iaizzo PA. Are myotonias and periodic paralyses associated with susceptibility to malignant hyperthermia? *Br J Anaesth* 1990;65:692–697.
87. Lehmann-Horn F, Iaizzo PA, Franke C. Hatt H, Spaans F. Schwartz-Jampel syndrome: II. Na^+ channel defect causes myotonia. *Muscle Nerve* 1990;13:528–535.
88. Lerche H, Fahlke Ch, Iaizzo PA, Lehmann-Horn F. Characterization of the high-conductance Ca^{2+}-activated K^+ channel in adult human skeletal muscle. *Pflugers Arch* 1995;429:738–747.
89. Levy S. Effect of intracellular injection of inositol trisphosphate on cytosolic calcium and membrane currents in Aphysia neurons. *J Neurosci* 1992;12:2120–2129.
90. Lin C, Hajnoczky G, Thomas A. Propagation of cytosolic calcium waves into the nuclei of hepatocytes. *Cell Calcium* 1994;16:247–258.
91. Lipp P, Niggli E. Ratiometric confocal Ca^{2+}-measurements with visible wavelength indicators in isolated cardiac myocytes. *Cell Calcium* 1993;14:359–372.
92. Loeb AL, Longnecker DE, Williamson JR. Alteration of calcium mobilization in endothelial cells by volatile anesthetics. *Biochem Pharmacol* 1993;45:1137–1142.
93. Lopez JR, Allen P, Alamo L, Ryan JF, Jones DE, Sreter F. Dantrolene prevents the malignant hyperthermic syndrome by reducing free intracellular calcium concentration in skeletal muscle in susceptible swine. *Cell Calcium* 1987;8:385–396.
94. Lückhoff A. Measuring cytosolic free calcium concentration in endothelial cells with indo-1: the pitfall of using the ratio of two fluorescence intensities recorded at different wavelengths. *Cell Calcium* 1986;7:233–248.
95. Lynch C III, Frazer MJ. Anesthetic alteration of ryanodine binding

by cardiac calcium release channels. *Biochim Biophys Acta* 1994; 1194:109–117.
96. Malenka RC, Kauer JA, Zucker RS, Nicoll RA. Postsynaptic calcium is sufficient for potentiation of hippocampal synaptic transmission. *Science* 1988;242:81–84.
97. Martínez-Zaguilán R, Martínez GM, Lattanzio F, Gillies RJ. Simultaneous measurement of intracellular pH and Ca^{2+} using fluorescence of SNARF-1 and fura-2. *Am J Physiol* 1991;429:C297–C307.
98. Martinosi A. Sarcoplasmic reticulum. V. The structure of sarcoplasmic reticulum membranes. *Biochim Biophys Acta* 1968;150:694–704.
99. McDonough PM, Button DC. Measurement of cytoplasmic calcium concentration in cell suspensions: correction for extracellular Fura-2 through use of Mn^{2+} and probenecid. *Cell Calcium* 1989;10: 171–180.
100. McNeil PL, Murphy RF, Lanni F, Taylor DL. A method for incorporating macromolecules into adherent cells. *J Cell Biol* 1984;98: 1556–1564.
101. Meissner G. Ryanodine activation and inhibition of the Ca^{2+} release channel of sarcoplasmic reticulum. *J Biol Chem* 1986;261: 6300–6306.
102. Meldolesi J, Madeddu L, Pozzan T. Intracellular Ca^{2+} storage organelles in non-muscle cells: heterogeneity and functional assignment. *Biochim Biophys Acta* 1990;1055:130–140.
103. Mickelson JR, Gallant EM, Litterer LA, Johnson KM, Rempel WE, Louis CF. Abnormal sarcoplasmic reticulum ryanodine receptor in malignant hyperthermia. *J Biol Chem* 1988;263: 9310–9315.
104. Mickelson JR, Letterer LA, Jacobson BA, Louis CF. Stimulation and inhibition of [^{3}H]ryanodine binding to sarcoplasmic reticulum from malignant hyperthermia susceptible pigs. *Arch Biochem Biophys* 1990;278:251–257.
105. Moore EDW. Properties of aequorin relavant to its use in the measurement of intracellular [Ca^{2+}] in skeletal muscle fibers [Dissertation]. Rochester: Mayo Clinic, 1986.
106. Moore EDW, Becker PL, Fogarty KE, Williams DA, Fay FS. Ca^{2+} imaging in single living cells: theoretical and practical issues. *Cell Calcium* 1990;11:157–179.
107. Morgan JP. Abnormal intracellular modulation of calcium as a major cause of cardiac contractile dysfunction. *N Engl J Med* 1991; 325:625–632.
108. Murphy E, Coll K, Rich TL, Williamson JR. Hormonal effects on calcium homeostasis in isolated hepatocytes. *J Biol Chem* 1980;255: 6600–6608.
109. Näbauer M, Morad M. Ca^{2+} induced Ca^{2+} release as examined by photolysis of caged Ca^{2+} in single ventricular myocytes. *Am J Physiol* 1990;258:C189–C193.
110. Nicotera P, McConkey DJ, Jones DP, Orrenius S. ATP stimulates Ca^{2+} uptake and increases the free Ca^{2+} concentration in isolated rat liver nuclei. *Proc Natl Acad Sci USA* 1989;86:453–457.
111. Niggli E, Lederer WJ. Real-time confocal microscopy development of a fluorescence microscope with high temporal and spatial resolution. *Cell Calcium* 1990;11:121–130.
112. Nüsse O, Lindau M. The calcium signal in human neutrophils and its relation to exocytosis investigated by patch-clamp capacitance and Fura-2 measurements. *Cell Calcium* 1993;14:255–269.
113. Oakes SG, Iaizzo PA, Richelson E, Powis G. Histamine-induced intracellular free Ca^{++}, inositol phosphates and electrical changes in murine N1E-115 neuroblastoma cells. *J Pharmacol Exp Ther* 1988;247:114–121.
114. Oakes SG, Martin WJ II, Lisek CA, Powis G. Incomplete hydrolysis of the calcium indicator precursor fura-2 pentaacetoxymethyl ester (fura-2 AM) by cells. *Anal Biochem* 1988;169:159–166.
115. Olsen R, Seewald M, Powis G. Contribution of external and internal Ca^{2+} to changes in intracellular free Ca^{2+} produced by mitogens in Swiss 3T3 fibroblasts: the role of dihydropyridine sensitive Ca^{2+} channels. *Biochem Biophys Res Commun* 1989;162:448–455.
116. Olsen RA, Seewald MJ, Melder DC, Berggren M, Iaizzo PA, Powis G. Platelet-derived growth factor blocks the increase in intracellular free Ca^{2+} caused by calcium ionophores and a volatile anesthetic agent in Swiss 3T3 fibroblasts without altering toxicity. *Toxicol Lett* 1991;55:117–125.
117. Ozaki Y, Kume S. Functional responses of aequorin-loaded human neutrophils. Comparison with fura-2-loaded cells. *Biochim Biophys Acta* 1988;972:113–119.
118. Ozhan M, Sill JC, Atagunduz P, Martin R, Katusic ZS. Volatile anesthetics and agonist-induced contractions in porcine coronary artery smooth muscle and Ca^{2+} mobilization in cultured immortalized vascular smooth muscle cells. *Anesthesiology* 1994;80: 1102–1113.
119. Pietrobon D, Di VF, Pozzan T. Structural and functional aspects of calcium homeostasis in eukaryotic cells. *Eur J Biochem* 1990;193: 599–622.
120. Poenie M. Alteration of intracellular Fura-2 fluorescence by viscosity: a simple correction. *Cell Calcium* 1990;11:85–91.
121. Poenie M, Tsien R. Fura-2: a powerful new tool for measuring and imaging [Ca^{2+}]$_i$ in single cells. *Prog Clin Biol Res* 1986;210:53–56.
122. Powis G, Seewald MJ, Sehgal I, Iaizzo PA, Olsen RA. Platelet-derived growth factor stimulates non-mitochondrial Ca^{2+} uptake and inhibits mitogen-induced Ca^{2+} signaling in Swiss 3T3 fibroblasts. *J Biol Chem* 1990;265:10266–10273.
123. Pozzan T, Rizzuto R, Volpe P, Meldolesi J. Molecular and cellular physiology of intracellular calcium stores. *Physiol Rev* 1994;74: 595–636.
124. Prendergast FG, Allen DG, Blinks JR. Properties of the calcium-sensitive bioluminescent protein aequorin. In: Wasserman RH, Corradino RA, Carafoli E, Kretsinger RH, MacLennan DH, Siegal FL, eds. *Calcium binding proteins and calcium function.* Amsterdam: Elsevier North-Holland, 1977:469–479.
125. Rink TJ, Pozzan T. Using quin-2 in cell suspensions. *Cell Calcium* 1985;6:133–144.
126. Rizzuto R, Simpson AW, Brini M, Pozzan T. Rapid changes of mitochondrial Ca^{2+} revealed by specifically targeted recombinant aequorin. *Nature* 1992;358:325–327.
127. Roche E, Prentki M. Calcium regulation of immediate-early response genes. *Cell Calcium* 1994;16:331–338.
128. Roe MW, Lemasters JJ, Herman B. Assessment of Fura-2 for measurements of cytosolic free calcium. *Cell Calcium* 1990;11:63–73.
129. Sachs G, Muallem S. Sites and mechanisms of Ca^{2+} movement in non-excitable cells. *Cell Calcium* 1989;10:265–273.
130. Scanlon M, Williams DA, Fay FS. A Ca^{2+}-insensitive form of fura-2 associated with polymorphonuclear leukocytes. Assessment and accurate Ca^{2+} measurement. *J Biol Chem* 1987;262:6308–6312.
131. Scarpa A. Measurements of cation transport with metallochromic indicators. In: Fleischer S, Iverson LE, eds. *Measurements of cation transport. Methods in enzymology LVI.* San Diego: Academic Press, 1979:301–339.
132. Schild D, Jung A, Schultens HA. Localization of calcium entry through calcium channels in olfactory receptor neurons using a laser scanning microscope and the calcium indicator dyes Fluo-3 and Fura-Red. *Cell Calcium* 1994;15:341–348.
133. Schlatterer C, Buravkov S, Zierold K, Knoll G. Calcium-sequestering organelles of *Dictyostelium discoideum*: changes in element content during early development as measured by electron probe x-ray analysis. *Cell Calcium* 1994;16:101–111.
134. Seewald MJ, Schlager JJ, Olsen RA, Melder DC, Powis G. High molecular weight dextran sulfate inhibits intracellular Ca^{2+} release and decreases growth factor-induced increases in intracellular free Ca^{2+} in Swiss 3T3 fibroblasts. *Cancer Comm* 1989;1: 151–156.
135. Seewald MJ, Olsen RA, Sehgal I, Melder DC, Modest EJ, Powis G. Inhibition of growth factor-dependent inositol phosphate Ca^{2+} signaling by antitumor ether lipid analogues. *Cancer Res* 1990;50: 4458–4463.
136. Shimomura O, Musicki B, Kishi Y, Inouye S. Light-emitting properties of recombinant semi-synthetic aequorins and recombinant fluorescein-conjugated aequorin for measuring cellular calcium. *Cell Calcium* 1993;14:373–378.
137. Sill JC, Uhl C, Eskuri S, Van Dyke R, Tarara J. Halothane inhibits agonist-induced inositol phosphate and Ca^{2+} signaling in A7r5 cultured vascular smooth muscle cells. *Mol Pharmacol* 1991;40: 1006–1013.
138. Snowdowne KW, Borle AB. Measurement of cytosolic free calcium in mammalian cells with aequorin. *Am J Physiol* 1984;247: C396–C408.
139. Sprung J, Stowe DF, Kampine JP, Bosnjak ZJ. Hypothermia modifies anesthetic effect on contractile force and Ca^{2+} transients in cardiac Purkinje fibers. *Am J Physiol* 1994;267:H725–H733.
140. Spurgeon HA, Stern MD, Baartz G, et al. Simultaneous measurement of Ca^{2+}, contraction, and potential in cardiac myocytes. *Am J Physiol* 1990;258:H574–H586.
141. Steinberg TH, Newman AS, Swanson JA, Silverstein SC. Macrophages possess probenecid-inhibitable organic anion transporters that remove fluorescent dyes from the cytoplasmic matrix. *J Cell Biol* 1987;105:2695–2702.

142. Stern MD. Bounds on the estimation of calcium by aequorin luminescence in the presence of inhomogeneity. *Biophys J* 1985;48: 853–857.
143. Stevens T, Fouty B, Cornfield D, Rodman DM. Reduced PO2 alters the behavior of Fura-2 and Indo-1 in bovine pulmonary artery endothelial cells. *Cell Calcium* 1994;16:404–412.
144. Stowe DF, Sprung J, Turner LA, Kampine JP, Bosnjak ZJ. Differential effects of halothane and isoflurane on contractile force and calcium transients in cardiac Purkinje fibers. *Anesthesiology* 1994; 80:1360–1368.
145. Sutherland PJ, Stephenson DG, Wendt IR. A novel method for introducing Ca^{++} -sensitive photoproteins into cardiac cells. *Proc Aust Physiol Pharmacol Soc* 11:160P.
146. Tepikin AV, Llopis J, Snitsarev VA, Gallacher DV, Peterson OH. The droplet technique: measurement of calcium extrusion from single isolated mammalian cells. *Pflugers Arch* 1994;428:664–670.
147. Timmerman MP, Ashley CC. Fura-2 diffusion and its use as an indicator of transient free calcium changes in single striated muscle cells. *FEBS Lett* 1986;209:1–8.
148. Tsien RY. Fluorescent probes of cell signaling. *Annu Rev Neurosci* 1989;12:227–253.
149. Tsien RY, Rink TJ, Poenie M. Measurement of cytosolic free Ca^{2+} in individual small cells using fluorescence microscopy with dual excitation wavelengths. *Cell Calcium* 1985;6:145–157.
150. Tsuchida H, Namba H, Yamakage M, Fujita S, Notsuki E, Namiki A. Effects of halothane and isoflurane on cytosolic calcium ion concentrations and contraction in the vascular smooth muscle of the rat aorta. *Anesthesiology* 1993;78:531–540.
151. Tsuchida H, Namba H, Seki S, Fujita S, Tanaka S, Namiki A. Role of intracellular Ca^{2+} pools in the effects of halothane and isoflurane on vascular smooth muscle contraction. *Anesth Analg* 1994; 78:1067–1076.
152. Valdvia HH, Hogan K, Coronado R. Altered binding site for Ca^{2+} in the ryanodine receptor of human malignant hyperthermia. *Am J Physiol* 1991;261:C237–C245.
153. Van Dyke RA, Wood CL. Binding of radioactivity from C-labeled halothane in isolated perfused rat livers. *Anesthesiology* 1973;38: 328–332.
154. Van Koeveringe KG, van Mastrigt MR. Excitatory pathways in smooth muscle investigated by phase-plot analysis of isometric force development. *Am J Physiol* 1991;261:R138–R144.
155. Van Koeveringe KG, van Mastrigt MR. Photolysis of caged calcium using a low-cost flash unit: efficacy analysis with a calcium selective electrode. *Cell Calcium* 1994;15:423–430.
156. Wakui M, Potter BV, Petersen OH. Pulsatile intracellular calcium release does not depend on fluctuations in inositol trisphosphate concentration. *Nature* 1989;339:317–320.
157. Wier WG, Cannell MB, Berlin JR, Marban E, Lederer WJ. Cellular and subcellular heterogeneity of $[Ca^{2+}]_i$ in single heart cells revealed by fura-2. *Science* 1987;235:325–328.
158. Wilde DW, Knight PR, Sheth N, Williams BA. Halothane alters control of intracellular Ca^{2+} mobilization in single rat ventricular myocytes. *Anesthesiology* 1991;75:1075–1086.
159. Williams DA. Mechanisms of calcium release and propagation in cardiac cells. Do studies with confocal microscopy add to our understanding? *Cell Calcium* 1993;14:724–735.
160. Williams DA, Fogarty KE, Tsien RY, Fay FS. Calcium gradients in single smooth muscle cells revealed by the digital imaging microscope using Fura-2. *Nature* 1985;318:558–561.
161. Williams DA, Fay FS. Intracellular calibration of the fluorescent calcium indicator Fura-2. *Cell Calcium* 1990;11:75–83.
162. Williams RJP. Calcium-binding proteins in normal and transformed cells. *Cell Calcium* 1994;16:339–346.
163. Woods NM, Cuthbertson KS, Cobbold PH. Repetitive transient rises in cytoplasmic free calcium in hormone-stimulated hepatocytes. *Nature* 1986;319:600–602.
164. Yamakage M, Kawamata T, Kohro S, Namiki A. Inhibitory effects of Halothane on high K^+-induced canine tracheal smooth muscle contraction and intracellular Ca^{2+} increment. *Acta Anaesthesiol* 1994;38:816–819.
165. Yue DT, Wier WG. Estimation of intracellular $[Ca^{2+}]$ by nonlinear indicators. A quantitative analysis. *Biophys J* 1985;48: 533–537.
166. Zierold K. Cryofixation methods for ion localization in cells by electron probe microanalysis: a review. *J Microsc* 1991;161: 357–366.

II

INTEGRATED SYSTEMS

A

BEHAVIORAL STATES

Anesthesia: Biologic Foundations, edited by Tony L. Yaksh et al. Lippincott–Raven Publishers, Philadelphia © 1997.

CHAPTER 25

INTEGRATED SYSTEMS

GARY R. STRICHARTZ AND JULIEN F. BIEBUYCK

Our knowledge of mechanisms of anesthetic action at the level of the central nervous system (CNS) depends on and thereby parallels the stages of development of the modern concepts of neurobiology. One of the major challenges of modern neuroscience is to relate behavior to cellular and molecular processes. Anesthesia is, by definition, a behavioral phenomenon. Various behavioral functions, many directly attributable to the normal activity of the CNS, are differentially altered by different anesthetic agents (13). Our ignorance of anesthetic mechanisms illustrates an epistemological gap; with varying potency and selectivity, different drugs produce analgesia, unconsciousness, and amnesia (emphatically, the second condition does not guarantee the third) (9). These same drugs are known to modify many of the growing number of newly identified molecular targets, including ion channels directly gated by gamma amino butyric acid (the inhibitory $GABA_A$ receptor) (11,21), by glutamate (excitatory NMDA- and non-NMDA-sensitive channels) (10,14,22,23), by acetylcholine (neuronal nicotinic acetylcholine receptors, or nAChR) (2,7), and by separate classes of transmitter activated G-protein-coupled receptors (6), as well as several types of voltage-gated calcium channels that are key players in neurosecretion (12,20). The challenge in understanding anesthetic mechanisms is to discover which of these molecular targets participate in a particular behavior, where in the nervous system this occurs, and the degree to which alteration of the target affects that behavior (8).

While we can formulate the epistemological question clearly, we are less perspicacious about the experimental approach. First, the primary properties of molecular targets themselves differ among different loci in the CNS. For example, the subunit composition of $GABA_A$ (16) and of nACh receptors (5) differs in anatomically distinct parts of the brain. Such structural differences effect different physiological and pharmacological properties. Interactions with cytoplasmic proteins that, for example, control receptor desensitization, may also vary among cells and the metabolic state of the cell is known to modulate receptor availability through redox-sensitive receptors (1,17).

Second, at microanatomic resolution, the distribution of receptors and channels on the cell surface is a major determinant of the influence of those elements on cellular excitability. In motoneurons, for example, excitatory synapses near the axon's initial segment provide a more effective current than those located on distal dendrites (19). One can imagine that the same degree of binding of anesthetic to receptor, producing the same degree of inhibition at receptor molecules, will have vastly different consequences for cellular activity due to different spatial distributions of the receptors.

A third complication is imposed by the complex connectivity of the CNS. Many neural centers in the brain and spinal cord are constantly under the influence of activity that is generated elsewhere. Often there is a reciprocal relationship between separate loci, which results in a balanced action and reaction. Within these constructs, an anesthetic agent may act directly at one locus, but its major, ramifying effects on behavior will occur through the projections into other neural centers.

For all three of the above reasons, the properties of the brain that control states of consciousness and behavior cannot be solely studied at the molecular or cellular level in any one isolated area of the brain. It has been elegantly pointed out (3) that the various research techniques currently available in neurobiology elicit new knowledge either by their temporal relationship to a neurological event, and/or by their reflection of molecular or behavioral functions (Fig. 1). Somewhat surprisingly, the electroencephalogram remains the most immediate source of information of cellular events during anesthesia (4), while PET scanning and functional MRI most accurately localize brain sites of behavioral control in the functioning human brain (18). This latter information has enabled researchers to focus on specific anatomical areas of the brain for the study of isolated molecular targets.

For almost a century, the quest for anesthetic mechanisms has encountered a series of unifying hypotheses. These have ranged from physicochemical theories of membrane perturbation and clathrate structures of membrane-adjacent water to the promotion of one type of specific receptor as the exclusive anesthetic target. At the present time, however, the existence of a unitary mechanism for general anesthesia seems unlikely (15). Because there are neither single classes of receptors for consciousness, memory, and pain, nor a single transmitter that subserves all three functions, the likelihood of one mechanism, shared by all effective clinical anesthetics, seems remote (13). However, the plurality of receptors, transmitters, and modes of

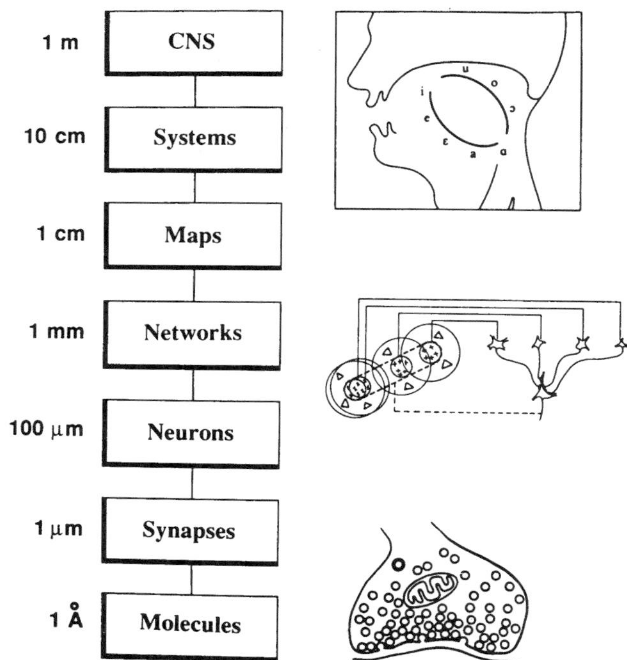

Figure 1. Structural levels of organization in the nervous system. The spatial scale at which anatomical organization can be identified varies over many orders of magnitude, from molecular dimensions to that of the entire CNS. The schematic diagrams on the right illustrate a typical chemical synapse (*bottom*), a proposed circuit for generating oriented receptive fields in visual cortex (*middle*), and part of the motor system that controls the production of speech sounds (*top*). (Reprinted with permission from Churchland PS, Koch C, Sejnowski TJ. What is computational neuroscience? In: Schwartz EL, ed. *Computational neuroscience.* Cambridge: MIT Press, 1990:46–55.)

coupling to ion channels admits the possibility of designing anesthetic drugs with selective actions as sedatives, amnesics, and analgesics. This potential promises to inform the gaps between molecular actions and behavioral consequences and to build bridges to advance knowledge of the brain and refine further the practice of anesthesia. The design of anesthetic drugs based on new scientific understanding of molecular events must also take into account our equivalent new knowledge of states of arousal, sleep, and neural control of respiration, cardiovascular functions, and thermal regulation. It is the object of this section to coordinate the new molecular and cellular knowledge outlined in the first volume and apply it to an understanding of the function of the whole brain and its control of states of consciousness and vital functions.

REFERENCES

1. Aizenman E, Lipton SA, Loring RH. Selective modulation of NMDA responses by reduction and oxidation. *Neuron* 1989;2: 1257–1263.
2. Brett RS, Dilger JP, Yland KF. Isoflurane causes flickering of the acetylcholine receptor channel. *Anesthesiology* 1988;69:161–170.
3. Churchland PS, Koch C, Sejnowski TJ. What is computational neuroscience? In: Schwartz EL, ed. *Computational neuroscience.* Cambridge: MIT Press, 1990:46–55.
4. Clark DK, Rosner BS. Neurophysiologic effects of general anesthetics. I. The electroencephalogram and sensory evoked response in man. *Anesthesiology* 1973;38:564–582.
5. Corriveau RA, Berg DK. Coexpression of multiple acetylcholine receptor genes in neurons: quantification of transcripts during development. *J Neurosci* 1993;13:2662–2671.
6. Dan'ura T, Kurokawa T, Yamashita A, Higashi K, Ishibashi S. Inhibition of brain adenylate cyclase by barbiturates through the effect on the interaction between guanine nucleotide-binding stimulatory regulatory protein and catalytic unit. *J Pharmacobiodyn* 1987; 10:98–103.
7. Dodson BA, Braswell LM, Miller KW. Barbiturates bind to an allosteric regulatory site on nicotinic acetylcholine receptor-rich membranes. *Mol Pharmacol* 1988;32:119–126.
8. Franks NP, Lieb WR. Molecular and cellular mechanisms of general anaesthesia. *Nature* 1994;367:607–614.
9. Ghoneim MM, Block RI. Learning and consciousness during general anesthesia. *Anesthesiology* 1992;76:279–305.
10. Gonzales JM, Loeb AL, Reichard PS, Irvine S. Ketamine inhibits glutamate-, *N* methyl-D-aspartate, and quisqualate-stimulated cGMP production in cultured cerebral neurons. *Anesthesiology* 1995;82: 205–213.
11. Jones MV, Brooks PA, Hrrison NL. Enhancement of γ-aminobutyric acid–activated Cl^- currents in cultured rat hippocampal neurones by three volatile anaesthetics. *J Physiol (Lond)* 1992;449:279–293.
12. Heyer EJ, MacDonald RL. Barbiturate reduction of calcium-dependent action potentials: correlation with anesthetic action. *Brain Res* 1982;236:157–171.
13. Kissin I. General anesthetic action: an obsolete notion? [Editorial]. *Anesth Analg* 1993;76:215–218.
14. Kullmann DM, Martin RL, Redman SJ. Reduction by general anaesthetics of group Ia excitatory postsynaptic potentials and currents in the cat spinal cord. *J Physiol* 1989;412:277–296.
15. MacIver MB, Roth SH. Inhalation anaesthetics exhibit pathway-specific and differential actions on hippocampal synaptic responses in vitro. *Br J Anaesth* 1988;60:680–691.
16. Olsen RW, Tobin AJ. Molecular biology of $GABA_A$ receptors. *FASEB J* 1990;4:1469–1480.
17. Pan Z-H, Bahring R, Grantyn R, Lipton SA. Differential modulation by sulfhydryl redox agents and glutathione of GABA- and Glycine-evoked currents in rat retinal ganglion cells. *J Neurosci* 1995;15:1384–1391.
18. Petersen SE, Fox PT, Snyder AZ, Raichle ME. Activation of extrastriate and frontal corticol areas by visual words and word-like stimuli. *Science* 1990;249:1041–1044.
19. Rall W. Distinguishing theoretical synaptic potentials computed for different soma-dendritic distributions of synaptic input. *J Neurophysiol* 1967;30:1138–1168.
20. Study RE. Isoflurane inhibits multiple voltage-gated calcium currents in hippocampal pyramidal neurons. *Anesthesiology* 1994;81: 104–116.
21. Tanelian DL, Kosek P, Mody I, MacIver MB. The role of the $GABA_A$ receptor/chloride channel complex in anesthesia. *Anesthesiology* 1993;78:757–776.
22. Teichberg VI, Tal N, Goldberg O, Luini A. Barbiturates, alcohols and the CNS excitatory neurotransmission: specific effects on the kainate and quisqualate receptors. *Brain Res* 1984;291:285–292.
23. Weight FF, Lovinger DM, White G, Peoples RW. Alcohol and anesthetic actions on excitatory amino acid-activated ion channels. *Ann NY Acad Sci* 1991;625:97–107.

Anesthesia: Biologic Foundations, edited by Tony L. Yaksh et al. Lippincott–Raven Publishers, Philadelphia © 1997.

CHAPTER 26

CONSCIOUSNESS: LESSONS FOR ANESTHESIA FROM SLEEP RESEARCH

J. ALLAN HOBSON

Such changes in conscious state as occur in anesthesia and sleep may be most effectively understood by exploring their underlying mechanisms at the level of the brain. Many of the details describing the state-dependent alterations in the activity of neuronal populations in individual brain cells and even, in particular, ion channels, constitute the main content of this book.

Before digging into this vast welter of microscopic facts, it may first be helpful to orient ourselves by defining conscious states and by analyzing the components of consciousness that change in both sleep and anesthesia. The specific strategy of this chapter is to focus upon the shared features of the natural state of sleep and the induced state of anesthesia. The fact that in sleep impressive reductions in pain can occur without the use of drugs is highly informative and suggests that naturalistic approaches to pain control could be sought in parallel with our biochemical investigations of anesthetic drug effects. In its most highly developed human form, waking consciousness comprises (a) the ability to create an accurate internal representation of the external world and (b) the ability to reflect upon that representation.

We assume that many animals other than humans make accurate representations of the world but that only humans possess the ability to reflect upon that representation (Fig. 1). We further suppose that the second, higher level of consciousness depends upon the human's unique capacity for linguistic and numerical abstraction. Thus, while many animals may indeed be perceptually and emotionally conscious, only we humans are conceptually conscious.

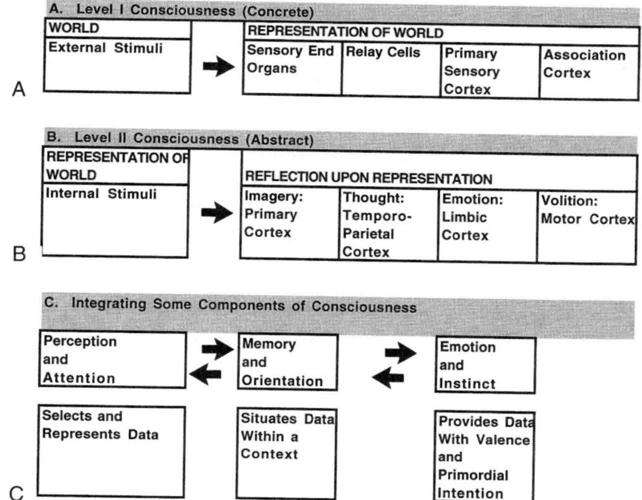

Figure 1. **(A, B)** The concrete and abstract levels of consciousness are depicted in parallel as the processing of external and internal information. Level I is the kind of consciousness experience we share with lower animals, whereas level II is the exclusive domain of humans. **(C)** Some of the components of consciousness listed in Table 1 are paried with respect to their functions in processing external and internal informants.

COMPONENTS OF CONSCIOUSNESS

The creation of an accurate representation of the world requires that sensory channels be open and that the signals that represent the physical world be conveyed from sensory endings to the central brain (Fig. 1A). Achieving this task requires that a certain level of activation be achieved within the brain and that competitive signaling arising from within the brain itself be restrained. Were it not for powerful internal restraint, our waking conscious experience would be as chaotic as it sometimes becomes in our dreams.

At the cognitive level, the two processes that are involved in high-fidelity representation of the world are perception and attention (Fig. 1C). If either fails, all other aspects of consciousness will be impaired. We assume that many animals share the primary perceptual and attentional groundwork of consciousness. This assumption is of more than academic interest because the use of animal models to investigate perception and attention is only valid only if this assumption holds. Perception and attention are essential foundations upon which all other aspects of consciousness depend.

For the content of perceived, attended information to be salient, the conscious subject must be able to relate its ongoing data processing to its current context and to its short- and long-range goals (Fig. 1B,C). Context is given by the representation of the three dimensions of orientation: time, place, and person. Fully conscious human subjects have a representation of themselves that is both richer and more abstract than that which we can now confidently attribute to any other species of animal. The oriented self depends upon an accurate memory of recent events (which a dog might show) and an internal narrative account of personal history (which we humans possess but are inclined to doubt in dogs or cats).

Orientation and memory are thus twin functions in the same sense as perception and attention (Fig. 1C). But whereas perception and attention are essential to the recognition and reception of sensory data, orientation and memory constitute the reference frame upon which the figuration of all input is traced (Fig. 1C).

Memory permits our conscious experience to assume both the immediate and remote meanings that inform our goals or intentions. The oriented conscious self knows who he or she is; knows who else is present; knows what time it is; and knows the place of the self and its action (Table 1). The orientational aspect of consciousness thus gives our action direction in terms of long- and short-term plans. If we lose either memory or orientation, our behavior is seriously disrupted.

Conscious experience not only integrates the data representing the continuously shifting present with the remembered representations of the past, but it adds to this unity both the value tinge of emotion and the impulse vector of instinctual drive (Fig. 1C). Emotional data thus confer a valence to the contents of consciousness. Our personal and situational context is felt to be safe or dangerous according to the net strength of such emotions as fear and affection. By means of fixed instinctual programs, these conscious signals also prepare us for action, to flee or to approach (in the case of fear and affec-

Table 1. DEFINITION OF COMPONENTS OF CONSCIOUSNESS

Component	Definition
Perception	Representation of the external world
Attention	Selection of data
Memory	Internal storage of representations
Orientation	Representation of times, places, and persons
Emotion	Feelings about situations
Instinct	Fixed action patterns
Thought	Representation of plans and goals
Volition	Decision to act
Consciousness	All of the above, working in concert

tion) or to emit threat displays or perform aggressive actions (in the case of anger). We feel quite confident that other animals share our conscious experience of emotion and of instinctual response.

THOUGHT AND ACTION

Among all species, only we humans have the unique capabilities of language and enumeration. Only we make the secondary abstract or symbolic representations of the perceptual, mnemonic, and instinctual representations of the primary level of consciousness (Fig. 1A,B). Put another way, we humans can think; we can form ideas (and even theories), and we can represent them to ourselves (via cognition) and to each other (via spoken or graphic written communication).

Utilizing our thoughts and ideas, we can consciously influence our actions; we can make decisions (including moral ones), and we are operationally possessed of free will. Although philosophers may endlessly debate the issue of free will and physiologists may persistently fail to see intention in an oscilloscope trace, no conscious human can deny his or her sense of voluntary control over thought and action. And no society can survive without instantiating this assumption in its laws. However constrained such volitional freedom may be by our particular historical experiences and by current social contexts, we are at every waking instant significantly capable of thoughtful, guided, and discriminative action.

CONSCIOUSNESS AND ANESTHESIA

When it comes to surgical intervention, many patients—and most doctors—would be happiest if nothing were felt (anesthesia) and nothing were remembered (amnesia). Complete unconsciousness is the goal of anesthesia, and for many patients and doctors complete unresponsiveness (atonia) is also desirable. But a few patients, some doctors, and many theorists would be satisfied if pain could be selectively eliminated (analgesia) without loss of consciousness. It would likewise be interesting if the pain experienced by some conscious patients could be unremembered (amnesia).

Notice that all of the clinical examples just mentioned evince dissociation of one component of consciousness from others: in conscious analgesia, the sensation or the perception of pain is dissociated from other components of consciousness; in amnesic pain, it is memory that is dissociated. Our subsequent examination of natural states of consciousness will be particularly sensitive to the natural dissociations of sensation, perception, and memory that occur in sleep. And we will be particularly keen to develop a description of the mechanisms that underlie such dissociations. A better understanding of how such selective alterations of consciousness are physiologically mediated could help us to evolve more effective behavioral and pharmacological strategies for manipulating and managing the pain of our patients.

The anesthetist's metaphor of "putting the patient to sleep" can be shown to be misleading in more ways than the irreversibility of the unconsciousness that is guaranteed by drug action. In fact, anesthesia is all too little like sleep. Yet as we will see, naturally sleeping subjects normally experience, especially in the rapid eye movement (REM) phase, all three desiderata of anesthesiology: analgesia, amnesia, and atonia. Meanwhile, in the delirium of our dreams, many other sensations and perceptions may actually be enhanced.

The analgesia of sleep is accompanied by a loss of attention. And attention is the component of consciousness most relevant to the pain control achieved in conscious analgesia. Indeed, hypnotic analgesia is achieved by the purposeful redirection of attention. This is a clear example of one dissociation of conscious state elements that is already appreciated by at least some anesthesiologists: those involved in dentistry and childbirth.

While there may be cardiorespiratory and other autonomically mediated instabilities in REM sleep, there is no hangover and no urinary retention when the natural state of sleep ends. The fact that REM sleep can now be experimentally induced by administering analogs of the natural neurotransmitter acetylcholine suggests that entirely new approaches to anesthesia should at least be considered.

STATES OF CONSCIOUSNESS

Consciousness undergoes a natural but dramatic succession of changes in state over the course of a normal day. Using the state of waking consciousness as a reference point, we can track these changes best by defining two other major states that occur in sleep (Fig. 1 and Table 2).

All living creatures alternate rest and activity each day under the direction of biological clocks. These clocks generate the circadian rhythm of ~24-h period length. In mammals, including humans, this circadian rest-activity cycle is directed by the suprachiasmatic nucleus (SCN) in the hypothalamus. The output of the SCN is linked to a sleep cycle clock in the pontine tegmentum whose periodic alternation of REM and non-REM (NREM) sleep varies in duration according to the size of the animal's brain. While the fixed rhythm of the hypothalamic circadian clock is not suppressed by anesthetic agents, the variable rhythm of the pontine NREM-REM clock is highly sensitive to such suppression.

In sighted animals, including humans, the tight link between the circadian rest-activity and sleep-wake cycles determines the marked diurnal fluctuations in our conscious state. Susceptibility to anesthesia is one of many functions that vary in a circadian fashion. Thus, it is probably true that the early morning, while optimal for anesthesiologists and surgeons, is the worst

Table 2. CHANCES IN CONSCIOUSNESS DURING SLEEP

Function	Wake	NREM	REM
Input		Low	Blocked
Attention		Poor	Poor
Perception		Weak	Strong (internal)
Memory		Poor	Poor
Orientation		Poor	Unstable
Thought		Perservative	Illogical
Insight		Poor	Delusional
Narrative		Poor	Confabulatory
Emotion		Episodically strong	Strong
Instinct		Episodically strong	Strong
Intentions		Weak	Confused
Volition		Poor	Episodically strong
Output		Low	Blocked

time for the patient. This is because brain activation levels are peaking at dawn and remain high throughout the morning when most surgery is being done. While it is all well and good that the surgeon is highly alert at this time of day, it might be better if the patient was at the low point of his or her circadian cycle. Perhaps patients should be rhythm shifted as well as—or instead of—premedicated.

But if anesthetic agents enhanced REM sleep mechanisms instead of suppressing them, the morning might be made optimal for patients undergoing surgery. This is because the probability that sleep will be REM actually peaks in the late morning (along with brain activation level). Compared to waking, REM sleep possesses three features of particular interest to anesthesiology: (a) active suppression of sensory input, (b) active blockade of motor output, and (c) intrinsic analgesia. All three functions are also present in NREM sleep (Fig. 2 and Table 2).

While the mechanisms of sensory input and motor output blockade in sleep are well understood (Fig. 3), the mechanism of the intrinsic analgesia is obscure. By intrinsic analgesia, I mean the marked and dramatic absence of reported pain in accounts of dreaming. In our dreams, we have sharp, though entirely fictive, sensations in most other modalities. So why not pain? And why not taste and smell? A definitive answer to these questions could be extremely enlightening.

Could the analgesia of REM sleep be due to the aminergic demodulation of the brain caused by the arrest of firing of the serotonergic raphe neurones known to be involved in pain control? And could this analgesia be enhanced or complimented by the arrest of firing of noradrenergic locus coeruleus neurones (known to be involved in attention, learning, and memory)? If this were so, we could link two desirable features of anesthesia, analgesia and amnesia, to a single cause, aminergic demodulation. This theory is attractive because much preanesthetic pain medication is directly targeted at these brain stem neuromodulatory systems.

And what about the REM sleep potentiation of the cholinergic system? Cholinergic brain processes are known to mediate conservative functions generally, and they too play a role in memory formation (Table 3). In this sense, those anesthetic premedications with anticholinergic properties could be doing double duty: inhibiting secretions (via their peripheral action) and mediating analgesia and amnesia (via their central effects). It must be considered significant that the microinjection of cholinergic agonists can induce either immediate and short-lived REM enhancement (when the paramedian pons is the target) or delayed and long-lasting REM enhancement (when the far lateral peribrachial area is the target). We will describe these dramatic drug effects in a subsequent section.

Recent studies suggest that gabaergic processes may mediate the aminergic demodulation (perhaps causing analgesia and amnesia), whereas glycinergic mechanisms may mediate the atonia. Because all of these mechanisms can be set in motion by cholinergic agonists, it is the more the pity that so many anesthetics actually shut off the central cholinergic system. In doing so, they weaken or eliminate desirable central cholinergic effects.

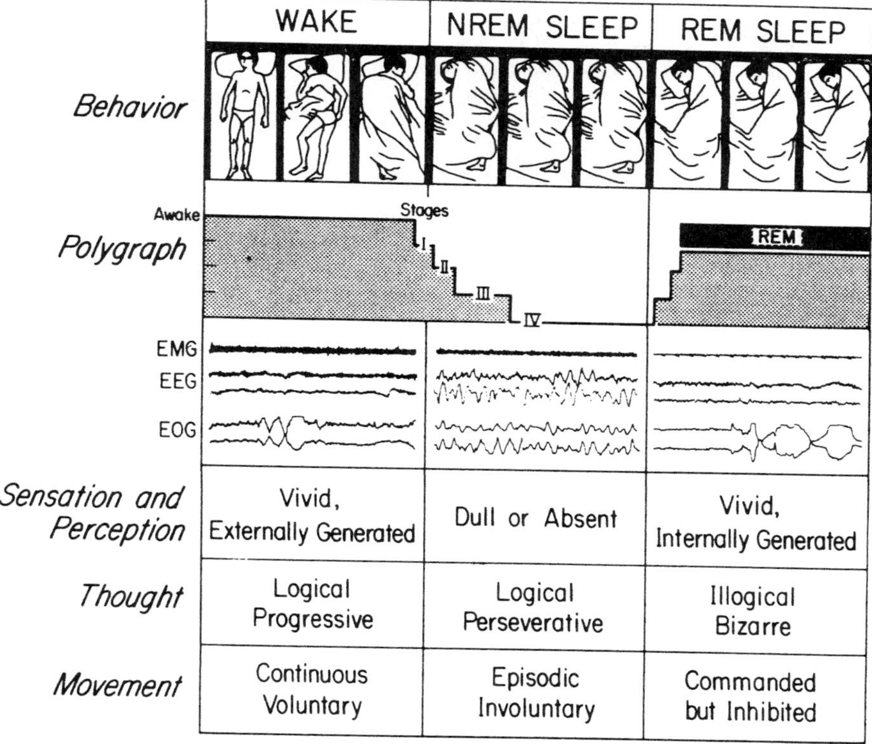

Figure 2. Behavioral states in humans. States of waking, NREM sleep, and REM sleep have behavioral, polygraphic, and psychological manifestations. In behavior channel, posture shifts (detectable by time-lapse photography or video) can occur during waking and in concert with phase changes of sleep cycle. Two different mechanisms account for sleep immobility: disfacilitation (during stages I—IV of NREM sleep) and inhibition (during REM sleep). In dreams, we imagine that we move but we do not. Sequence of these stages represented in polygraph channel. Sample tracings of three variables used to distinguish state are also shown: electromyogram (EMG), which is highest in waking, intermediate in NREM sleep, and lowest in REM sleep; and electroencephalogram (EEG) and electrooculogram (EOG), which are both activated in waking and REM sleep and inactivated in NREM sleep. Each sample record is 20 s. Three lower channels describe other subjective and objective state variables. (Reprinted with permission from Hobson JA, McCarley RW. The brain as a dream state generator: an activation-synthesis hypothesis of the dream process. *Am J Psychiatry* 1977;134:1335–1348.)

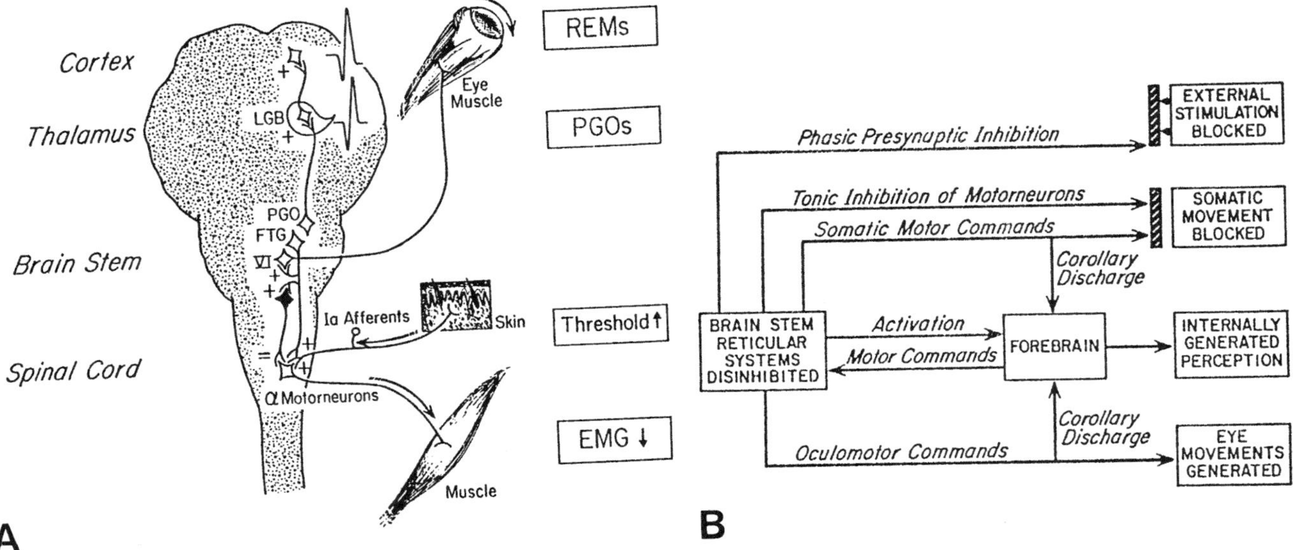

Figure 3. **(A)** Three mechanisms underlying state-dependent changes in sensorimotor gating are shown. (a) Efferent copy: During REM sleep, neurons of the pontine reticular formation (FTG) are activated. When they fire in bursts, ipsiversive REMs are generated, and ipsilateral PGO waves are triggered in the LGB and posterolateral cortex. (b) Presynaptic inhibition: Via axons descending from the FTG, the primary afferent terminals of the group 1a cutaneous afferents are depolarized, making them less responsive to incoming volleys from the skin. In this way, sensory thresholds are raised. (c) Postsynaptic inhibition: Cells of the medullary reticular formation are also excited by volleys from the pons, but they convey inhibitory signals to the anterior horn motoneurons and muscle tone is suppressed (EMG). In this way, the threshold to motor activation is raised. **(B)** Systems model. As a result of disinhibition caused by cessation of aminergic neuronal firing, brain stem reticular systems autoactivate. Their outputs have effects including depolarization of afferent terminals causing phasic presynaptic inhibition and blockade of external stimuli, especially during the bursts of REM; postsynaptic hyperpolarization causes tonic inhibition of motoneurons, which effectively counteract concomitant motor commands so that somantic movement is blocked. Only the oculomotor commands are read out as eye movements because the motoneurons are not inhibited. The forebrain, activated by the reticular formation and also aminergically disinhibited, receives efferent copy or corollary discharge information about somatic motor and oculomotor commands from which it may synthesize such internally generated perceptions as visual imagery and the sensation of movement, both of which typify dream mentation. The forebrain may, in turn, generate its own motor commands that help to perpetuate the process via positive feedback to the reticular formation.

Table 3. PHYSIOLOGICAL BASIS OF DIFFERENCES BETWEEN WAKING AND DREAMING

Function	Nature of difference	Casual hypothesis
Sensory input	Blocked	Presynaptic inhibition
Perception	Enhanced (internal)	Cholinergic activation
Attention	Diminished	Aminergic demodulation
Memory	Remote increased	Cholinergic activation
	Recent diminished	Aminergic demodulation
Orientation	Unstable	Aminergic demodulation/ cholinergic activation
Thought	Ad hoc/nonsequential	Aminergic demodulation/ cholinergic activation
Insight	Poor	Aminergic demodulation/ cholinergic activation
Narrative	Confabulatory	Aminergic demodulation/ cholinergic activation
Emotion	Episodically strong	Aminergic demodulation/ cholinergic activation
Instinct	Episodically strong	Aminergic demodulation/ cholinergic activation
Intention	Weak	Aminergic demodulation/ cholinergic activation
Output	Blocked	Aminergic demodulation/ cholinergic activation

SLEEP AS NATURAL ANESTHESIA

In the balance of this book, the reader may be guided by the three criteria for anesthesia that derive from the neurophysiology of conscious state control: analgesia, amnesia, and atonia. We now consider, in more detail, how analgesia, amnesia, and atonia are physiologically mediated during the states of sleep (Table 4).

Table 4. ASPECTS OF ANESTHESIA SIMULATED BY REM SLEEP

Phenomenon simulated	Possible mechanisms
Amnesia	Despite abundance of activation plasticity cannot occur without NE and 5HT
Atonia	Motorneurones subjected to: glycinergic hyperpolarization (10 MV), serotonergic disfacilitation, noradrenergic disfacilitation
Analgesia	Aminergic demodulation, cholinergic hypermodulation, hyperpolarization of 2° relay cells, presynaptic inhibition of 1° afferent cells

NREM SLEEP

Sleep onset is associated with what we might call a functional decortication. As the reciprocal thalamocortical neuronal systems change from the wake to the NREM sleep mode, they become incapable of conveying information from incoming sensory channels to the cortex. This functional blockade (which is well simulated by barbiturate anesthesia) appears to involve the following: (a) diminished firing of brain stem aminergic and cholinergic neurones, which leads to (b) disfacilitation of the gabaergic neurones of the reticularis nucleus, which causes (c) hyperpolarization of thalamic relay cells and a change in their firing mode from (d) the tonic pattern of waking to the burst-silence mode of sleep, and this, in turn, results in (e) the cortical EEG spindles and slow waves that are stigmatic of NREM sleep and most other deeply unresponsive brain states.

It is no wonder that sleep is so often sought as a natural anodyne for the relief of pain. But unfortunately sleep is not equal to the task. As patients with fibromyalgia will attest, sleep analgesia may not be adequate to quell musculoskeletal pain. The stigmatic alpha-delta EEG pattern that is recorded in their sleep indicates that the thalamocortical system is dissociated. As a result, the brain is of two minds: one awake (alpha, in response to pain stimuli) and the other asleep (delta, in response to a sleep signal from the hypothalamus). If a drug could induce a strong, but reversible NREM sleep state, could such noxious stimuli be totally blocked? And might operative surgery then be possible? It is at least a theoretically realistic suggestion.

The practically total amnesia for our conscious experience in NREM sleep is not surprising under the circumstances. As with anesthesia, there is, however, some evidence that high-level processing (and even learning) can go on. When subjects are experimentally aroused from NREM sleep, they usually give very brief and garbled reports of antecedent mental activity. Because sleep persists in subsequent waking epochs, they perform badly on tests of cognition. If they have previously been sleep deprived, graduate students in mathematics cannot perform several one-digit subtractions because of this sleep inertia. All of these amnesic phenomena could be a consequence of the prolonged decrease in aminergic and cholinergic modulation. An ideal anesthesia agent might thus block *both* aminergic and cholinergic neurotransmission.

As for the atonia, the muscle relaxant effect of NREM sleep appears to be due mainly to a disfacilitatory mechanism. There is a decrease in input from both primary afferent and secondary relay cells, which mirrors the diminution of cholinergic and aminergic output that deafferents the thalamus. At the same time, the alpha and gamma motorneurones show parallel decreases in excitability. Muscle tone declines, often to zero. This disfacilitation raises problems for airway patency as the sleep apnea syndrome so clearly demonstrates.

REM SLEEP

The fact that analgesia, amnesia, and atonia are all maintained (or are even intensified) in the face of the dramatic brain activation of REM sleep is clear proof that we do not need to knock people out to achieve significant reductions in pain sensation, memory, and muscle tone. In REM sleep, the brain accomplishes all three of the major goals of anesthesia on its own simply by further changing the aminergic-cholinergic balance away from the wake state mode.

By completely shutting down the noradrenergic locus coeruleus and the serotonergic raphe and by simultaneously increasing the output of the LDT/PPT cholinergic system, the brain has been chemically transformed so that (a) remote and recent memories are activated and experienced, but the experience is not itself memorized; (b) visual, auditory, somesthetic, motor, and postural sensations are simulated, but pain is not; and (c) none of the imagined motor acts of our dreams occur because the commands of upper brain motor centers are blocked at the level of the final common path motoneurones.

The cellular and molecular neurobiology of REM sleep has been successfully studied in part because of this set of built-in anesthesia-like mechanisms (Fig. 4).

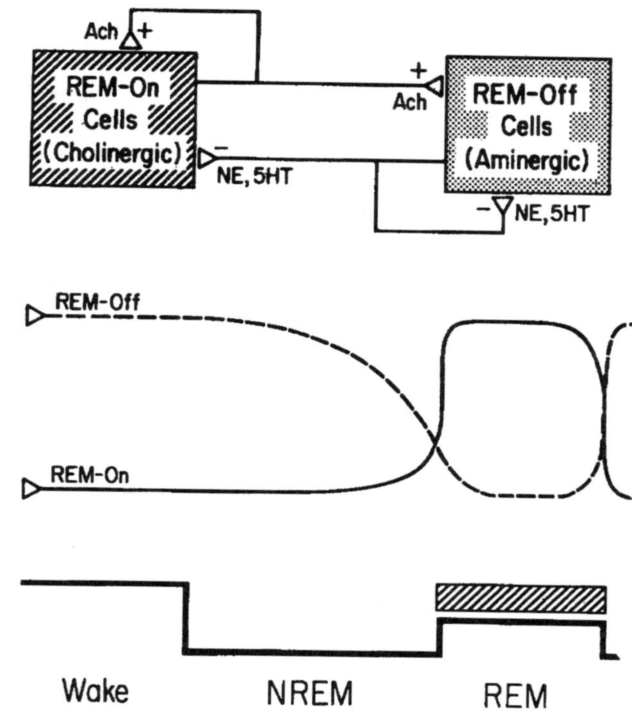

Figure 4. Physiological mechanisms determining alterations in activation level A. **(A)** Structural model of reciprocal interaction. REM-on cells of the pontine reticular formation are cholinoceptively excited and/or cholinergically excitatory (ACH+) at their synaptic endings (*open boxes*). Pontine REM-off cells are noradrenergically (NE) or serotonergically (5HT) inhibitory (-) at their synapses (*filled boxes*). **(B)** Dynamic model. During waking, the pontine aminergic (*filled box*) system is tonically activated and inhibits the pontine cholinergic (*open box*) system. During NREM sleep, aminergic inhibition gradually wanes and cholinergic excitation reciprocally waxes. At REM sleep onset, aminergic inhibition is shut off and cholinergic excitation reaches its high point. **(C)** Activation level A. As a consequences of the interplay of the neuronal systems shown in A and B, the net activation level of the brain (A) is at equally high levels in waking and REM sleep, and at about half this peak level in NREM sleep. (Reprinted with permission from Hobson JA. A new model of brain state: activation level, input source and mode of processing (AIM). In: Antrobus J, Bertini M, eds. *The neuropsychology of dreaming sleep.* 1992:227–245.)

CHOLINERGIC REM SLEEP INDUCTION AS A MODEL OF ANESTHESIA

Because an experimental model now compliments the natural state of REM sleep, anesthesia research can be approached more physiologically now than previously. The ability to induce REM sleep at will provides a controllable and natural substrate for the investigation of analgesia, amnesia, and atonia. To date, only a few neurophysiologists have appreciated this model, and none has been directly engaged in anesthesia research. That this situation may be changing is suggested by recent increases in communication between sleep and anesthesia research, including Chapter 27 in this volume.

Table 5. CHEMICAL INDUCTION OF REM SLEEP

	Natural REM	Artificial REM short term	Artificial REM long term
Molecular species	Acetylcholine	Carbachol Neostigmine (Ach) Bethanechol Pilocarpine	Carbachol Neostigmine (Ach)
Anatomical locus	Distributed network PRF (on) LC, DRN (off) LDT, PPR (on)	Paramedian Anterodorsal pons (near but not in LC, DR, LDT)	Lateral mid pons (near but not in PPT, VN)
Conscious state alterations	Dreaming Amnesia Analgesia Atonia	Dreaming Amnesia Analgesia Atonia	Not done in humans Not done in humans Not done in humans Atonia

Of course, neither the short- nor the long-term enhancement of REM sleep by cholinergic agonists is truly physiological because a drug is used to get each phenomenon going (Table 5). But the most effective drug, carbachol, is an analog of naturally occurring neurotransmitters acetylcholine, and other effective drugs, like neostigmine, increase the efficacy of endogenous acetylcholine. While the drug acts on a highly localized and discrete endogenous brain system, the global effects, including those causing the analgesia, amnesia, and atonia, occur at a distance and are, without doubt, mediated in a physiological manner.

CHOLINERGIC HYPOTHESIS OF REM SLEEP GENERATION

The cholinergic hypothesis of REM sleep generation was articulated by Hernandez-Peon et al. (10) and Jouvet (18) on the basis of lesion and pharmacology studies. These pioneers postulated a pontine brain stem locus of control and a widely distributed neuronal effector population. Extensive confirmation of these findings (9) and further specification of the concept of state control by reciprocal neuromodulatory influences of cholinergic and aminergic pontine brain stem neurons (15,16 22) have sparked the development of more precise chemical microstimulation experiments. This approach has been used to selectively activate (or inactivate) chemically specific brain stem neuronal populations and thereby to change the balance between the aminergic and cholinergic systems in the brain.

This strategy has recently culminated in the short latency induction of REM sleep by microinjecting a variety of cholinergic drugs into a restricted paramedian zone of the anterodorsal pontine tegmentum (2,3,16,32,36). At this sensitive site, a very high proportion of neurons is strongly activated by carbachol (37). The cholinergic drugs that are effective in acutely enhancing REM sleep signs share muscarinic acetylcholine receptor agonist properties (33), and all are blocked, in a dose-dependent manner, by muscarinic receptor blockers (3,34).

Opposing this cholinoceptive REM sleep induction system and responsible for activating the forebrain in waking are the neuronal populations of the locus coeruleus and raphe nuclei, which use the modulatory biogenic amines norepinephrine and serotonin to inhibit the cholinergic and cholinoceptive REM sleep generator network (1,6,17,23).

The fact that the enhancement of REM sleep signs obtained with neostigmine (2,4,5) is as potent as that seen with carbachol indicates that enhanced endogenous acetylcholine release is probably a key step in physiological REM sleep induction, a supposition that has recently been supported by the direct measurement of increased acetylcholine release in the pontine tegmentum during naturally occurring REM sleep (19) and during cholinergically induced REM (20).

Because the paramedian reticular site for the short-latency cholinergic microstimulation of REM sleep has been found to be devoid of cholinergic neurons (29), it has been postulated that the source of cholinergic input to the paramedian trigger zone is either the dorsolateral tegmentum (Ch6) and/or the pedunculopontine tegmentum (Ch5) cholinergic cell groups, both of which show dramatic state-specific increases in firing during REM sleep (7,25,28,30,31) and both of which project axons into the paramedian brain stem (24,26).

The pedunculopontine cholinergic neurons that are located in the peribrachial region are of particular interest because they have been identified as part of a local network of neuronal origin and as transferring elements of phasic activations of the lateral geniculate body (LGB) and occipital cortex, recorded in REM sleep as pontogeniculooccipital (PGO) waves (25,27,28, 31). Thus, the pedunculopontine cholinergic cell group is a candidate structure for both the direct mediation of distinctive REM sleep signs (the PGO waves), and for releasing acetylcholine at brain stem and thalamic target sites so as to shift the neuromodulatory balance in those structures in the cholinergic direction.

From previous pilot studies (35), we had good reason to suppose that the cholinergic PGO burst cells and PGO waves could be activated by the peribrachial microinjection of carbachol without any immediate effect upon REM sleep. But we first needed to replicate these findings. In addition to confirming the immediate triggering of PGO activity first observed by Vivaldi et al. (35), we were surprised also to notice a delayed but massive and prolonged increase in REM sleep. This delayed but massive REM sleep increase reached its peak of 3–400% 24–48 h following carbachol microinjection and thereafter declined to baseline level only gradually over the subsequent ten days. The long-term REM sleep enhancement suggested that carbachol activation of the cholinergic population in this pontine site might produce a sustained and widespread increase in the efficacy of cholinergic neurotransmission, both in the brain stem and in the thalamic postsynaptic domain of the cholinergic neurons.

CHOLINERGIC REM SLEEP INDUCTION: THE LONG-TERM ENHANCEMENT SITE

Within a few minutes after carbachol is microinjected into the peribrachial region of the pontine brain stem (Pb), state-independent PGO waves are observed in the ipsilateral LGB (Fig. 5). Consonant with demonstrated projections from the peribrachial area to the paramedian reticular formation (26), these ipsilateral PGO waves are associated with small ipsiversive

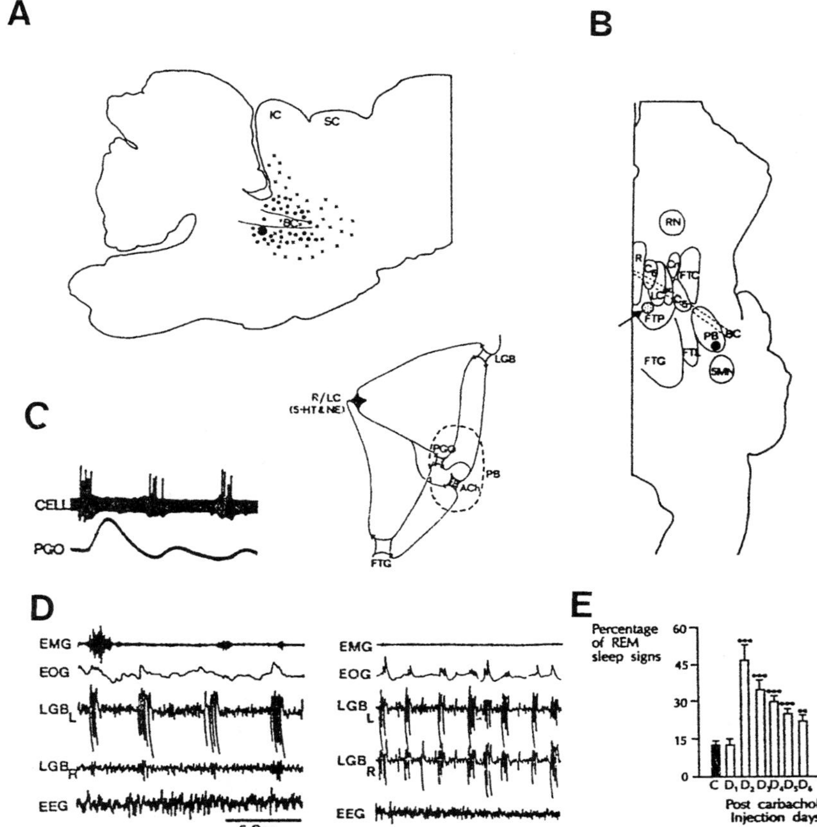

Figure 5. Relationship of PGO burst cells to cholinergic REM induction sites. **(A)** *Filled circle* indicates site of injection of carbachol into peribrachial pons. *Small dots* indicate location of cholinergic cells and crosses location of PGO burst cells. **(B)** Location of peribrachial long-term (**filled circle**) and paramedian short-term (**open circle with dots**) REM induction sites. **(C)** On the left is an extracellular unit recording of a PGO burst cell and PGO waves in the ipsilateral LGB. On the right is a hypothetical wiring diagram of the PGO trigger zone (PB) elements (PGO and ACh) with modulatory aminergic raphe (R) and locus coeruleus (LC), thalamic (LGB), and paramedian pontine reticular cells (FTG). **(D)** Injections of carbachol at the PB site shown in A and B produce immediate PGO waves in the ipsilateral LGB. **(E)** After 24 h, REM triples and remains elevated for 6 days; this is the long-term REM effect. Reticular tegmental nuclei (FTG, FTP, FTL, FTC), aminergic nuclei (R, LC), and cholinergic nuclei (C5, C6) are shown. Reference structures shown are red nucleus (RN), trigeminal motor nucleus (MN), and brachium conjuctivum (BC). (Reprinted with permission from Hobson JA. Sleep and dreaming: induction and mediation of REM sleep by cholinergic mechanisms. *Curr Opin Neurobiol* 1992;2:759–763.)

eye movements (as if the oculomotor systems were being driven by the PGO-related neuronal discharge instead of the reverse, which we imagine to be the case under physiological conditions). But this direct input is apparently neither sufficiently strong nor properly targeted to trigger the REM sleep network, as occurs readily when the carbachol is placed in the paramedian reticular formation. At these paramedian short-term enhancement sites, the PGO waves are always recruited only secondarily (as part of the whole REM sleep syndrome) and bilaterally (5,32,36).

The ipsilateral PGO wave enhancement that follows Pb injection continues for 24 h, much longer than the expected duration of carbachol action, which, in the paramedian reticular formation is only 4–6 h (5,32,36). Thus, we must consider either that carbachol binding is much stronger to the receptors of the Pb (which seems unlikely) or that some sort of self-perpetuating cascade mechanism has already been established in the peribrachial network by the end of day 1. This "cascade" hypothesis is attractive to us because on day 2 the normal amount of REM sleep increases three- to fourfold and is still active on days 3–10, when REM sleep levels remain significantly elevated.

To flesh out the cascade idea, our working hypothesis is that the membrane activation of a relatively discrete network (the PGO burst-cholinergic neuron ensemble) somehow primes the more widely distributed REM sleep generator network. We speculate that this priming process is mediated intracellularly, perhaps via a chain reaction that connects cyclic GMP to G protein leading ultimately to the synthesis of choline acetyltransferase. A chain reaction of this kind could play a further role in altering the cell's short-term behavior (through enzymatic events) and long-term behavior (through genetic events) and thus control how the cell propagates neural signals to remote target areas. A nonexclusive alternative is that the excitability of local Pb circuits is enhanced and increases the excitatory drive upon remote REM generator neurons.

As with our earlier work on the paramedian short-latency REM induction site, it is now essential to demonstrate that these carbachol effects are physiologically meaningful and biochemically specific. Encouraging preliminary evidence comes from the replication of the two-phase response to carbachol by neostigmine (indicating that the response can be triggered by preventing the breakdown of endogenous acetylcholine) and from our ability to completely block the two-phase response to carbachol by pretreatment of a documented PbN "hot site" with methoctramine indicating that activation of M2 receptors mediates the effect (8).

IMPLICATIONS OF THE DIFFERENCES BETWEEN SHORT- AND LONG-TERM REM SLEEP ENHANCEMENT

There is a striking and informative contrast between the effects of cholinergic chemical microstimulation of the paramedian reticular formation (where the REM enhancement is sudden but short-lived) and the peribrachial complex (where the REM enhancement is delayed but persistent). Two implications of this contrast are as follows:

1. While the paramedian reticular network can directly mediate all REM phenomena, including PGO waves, the peribrachial complex directly mediates only the PGO waves. This suggests that the paramedian site is at the center of a triggering or execute neuronal network for REM.

2. While the peribrachial PGO generator has delayed and prolonged priming effect upon the paramedian reticular system, no such long-term consequences are seen following activation of the paramedian executive network. This suggests that the Pb has a regulatory or level-setting function for the executive network.

From this it follows that projections from the paramedian reticular system to the peribrachial PGO complex are functionally strong and obligatory (relatively "hard-wired"), whereas the peribrachial to reticular projections are weak and facultative (relatively "loosely-coupled") such that their influence is cumulative, and delayed. Why should evolution have formed this apparent division of neuronal labor? Our intuitive answer is that it assures two important desiderata for REM sleep: (a) reliability of immediate triggering (once certain local network conditions are met) and (b) reliability of long-term regulation (via remote and diffuse neurochemical processes that affect the metabolism of the brain at large).

CONCLUSION

While currently available anesthetic alterations of consciousness are adequate, they are not ideal and they sometimes run counter to the brain's own anesthetic propensities. In the hope of stimulating scientifically inclined anesthesiologists to consider more physiological approaches, I have advanced the heuristic argument that the ways in which the brain produces the analgesia, atonia, and amnesia during natural REM sleep may provide guidelines for innovative thinking and new research in anesthesia.

Following a definition and discussion of the components of consciousness, I show how pain perception, memory, and motor output models of waking consciousness are dramatically altered during REM sleep. Since a diminution in these three consciousness modules is the goal of anesthesia, it follows that their artificial chemical induction by anesthetic agents might do well to mimic this natural neurophysiology. The most basic underlying neurobiological change mediating these natural events appears to be a shift in balance between the aminergic and cholinergic neuronal populations that constitute the pontine brain stem oscillator for the sleep-wake cycle. When the aminergic population is dominant, we are awake: we feel pain, we remember it, and we move to avoid it. When the cholinergic population is dominant, we dream: we feel no pain (even when injured), we forget most of our distress, and we cannot move a muscle to avoid it.

Pointing the way to a practical program, I review the experimental means by which REM sleep can be enhanced in cats. Microinjection of cholinergic agonists produces either short-term (6 h) or longer-term (12 days) REM sleep augmentation according to the brain stem target site. It is an unproven assumption that these experimental interventions could alter consciousness in humans, but anesthetic preanesthetic agents that are cholinergic and/or antiaminergic should be particularly attractive to the scientific anesthesiologist.

Acknowledgment: This work was supported by NIH Grants MH 13,923 and MH 48,832 and the Mind-Body Network of the MacArthur Foundation.

REFERENCES

1. Aston-Jones G, Bloom FE. Activity of norepinephrine-containing locus coeruleus neurons in behaving rats anticipates fluctuations in the sleep-waking cycle. *J Neurosci* 1981;1:876–886.
2. Baghdoyan HA, Lydic R, Callaway CW, Hobson JA. Increased ponto-geniculo-occipital (PGO) wave frequency following central administration of neostigmine. *Neurosci Lett* 1987;82:287–294.
3. Baghdoyan HA, Lydic R, Callaway, Hobson JA. The carbachol-induced enhancement of desynchronized sleep signs is dose dependent and antogonized by centrally administered atropine. *Neuropsychopharmacology* 1989;2:67–79.
4. Baghdoyan HA, Monaco AP, Rodrigo-Angulo ML, Assens F, McCarley RW, Hobson JA. Microinjection of neostigmine into the pontine reticular formation of cats enhances desynchronized sleep signs. *J Pharmacol Exp Ther* 1984;231:173–180.
5. Baghdoyan HA, Rodrigo-Angulo ML, McCarley RW, Hobson JA. Site-specific enhancement and suppression of desynchronized sleep signs following cholinergic stimulation of three brainstem regions. *Brain Res* 1984;306:39–52.
6. Chu N, Bloom FE. Norepinephrine-containing neurons: changes in spontaneous discharge patterns during sleeping and waking. *Science* 1973;179:908–910.
7. Datta S, Kumar VM, Singh B. The role of reticular activating system in altering medial preoptic neuronal activity in anesthetized rats. *Brain Res* 1989;22:1031–1037.
8. Datta S, Quattrochi JJ, Hobson JA. Effect of specific muscarinic M2 receptor antagonist on carbachol-induced long-term REM sleep. *Sleep* 1993;16:8–14.
9. George R, Haslett WL, Jenden DJ. A cholinergic mechanism in the brainstem reticular formation: induction of paradoxical sleep. *Int J Neuropharmacol* 1964;3:541–552.
10. Hernandez-Peon R, Chavez-Ibarra G, Morgane PJ, Timo-Iaria C. Cholinergic pathways for sleep, alertness and rage in the limbic midbrain circuit. *Acta Neurol Latinoamerica* 1962;8:93–96.
11. Hobson JA. Sleep and dreaming: induction and mediation of REM sleep by cholinergic mechanisms. *Curr Opin Neurobiol* 1992;2:759–763.
12. Hobson JA. A new model of brain-mind state: activation level, input source and mode of processing (AIM). In: Antrobus J, Bertini M, eds. *The neuropsychology of sleep and dreaming.* Hillsdale, New Jersey: Lawrence Erlbaum Associates, Publishers, 1992:227–245
13. Hobson JA, McCarley RW. The brain as a dream state generator: an activation-synthesis hypothesis of the dream process. *Am J Psychiatry* 1977;134:1335–1348.
14. Hobson JA, McCarley RW, Freedman, Pivik. Time course of discharge rate changes by cat pontine brain stem neurons during sleep cycle. *J Neurophysiol* 1974;37:1297–1309.
15. Hobson JA, McCarley RW, Wyzinki PW. Sleep cycle oscillation: reciprocal discharge by two brainstem neuronal groups. *Science* 1975;189:55–58.
16. Hobson JA, Steriade M. The neuronal basis of behavioral state control: internal regulatory systems of the brain. In: Bloom FE, ed. *Handbook of physiology—the nervous system, vol. IV.* Bethesda: American Physiological Society, 1986:701–823.
17. Jacobs BL, Asher R, Henricksen SJ, Dement WC. Electroencephalographic and behavioral effects of stimulation of the raphe nuclei in cats. *Sleep Res* 1972;1:23.
18. Jouvet M. Recherche sur les structures nerveuses et les mechanismes responsables des differentes phases du sommeil physiologiaue. *Arch Ital Biol* 1962;100:125—206.
19. Kodama T, Takahashi Y, Honda Y. Enhancement of acetylcholine release during paradoxical sleep in the dorsal tegmental field of the cat brain. *Neurosci Lett* 1990;114:277–282.
20. Lydic R, Baghdoyan HA. Cholinergic pontine mechanisms causing state-dependent respiratory depression. American Physiological Society.
21. McCarley RW, Hobson JA. The neurobiological origins of psychoanalytic theory. *Am J Psychiatry* 1977;134:1211–1221.
22. McCarley RW, Hobson JA. Neuronal excitability modulation over the sleep cycle: a structural and mathematical model. *Science* 1975;189:58–60.
23. McGinty RW, Harper RM. Dorsal raphe neurons: depression of firing during sleep in cats. *Brain Res* 1976;101:569–575.
24. Mitani A, Ito K, Mitani Y, et al. The laterodorsal and pedunculopontine tegmental nuclei are sources of cholinergic projections to the pontine gigantocellular tegmental field in the cat. *Sleep Res* 1988;16:10.
25. Nelson JP, McCarley RW, Hobson JA. REM sleep burst neurons, PGO waves, and eye movement information. *J Neurophysiol* 1983;50:784–797.
26. Quattrochi JJ, Mamelak A, Madison R, Macklis J, Hobson JA. Mapping neuronal inputs to REM sleep induction sites with carbachol-fluorescent microspheres. *Science* 1989;245:984–986.
27. Sakai K, Jouvet M. Bainstem PGO-on cells projecting directly to the cat dorsal lateral geniculate nucleus. *Brain Res* 1980;194:500–505.
28. Sakai K, Yoshimoto Y, Luppi PH, et al. Lower brainstem afferents to the cat posterior hypothalamus: a double-labeling study. *Brain Res* 1990;24:437–455.
29. Shiromani PJ, Armstrong DM, Berkowitz A, Jeste DV, Gillin JC. Distribution of choline acetyltransferase immunoreactive somata in the feline brainstem: implications for REM sleep generation. *Sleep* 1988;11:1–16.
30. Steriade M, Datta S, Pare D, Oakson G, Curro Dossi R. Neuronal activities in brain-stem cholinergic nuclei related to tonic activation processes in thalamocortical systems. *J Neurosci* 1990;10:2541–1559.
31. Steriade M, Pare D, Datta S, Oakson G, Curro Dossi R. Different cellular types in mesopontine cholinergic nuclei related to ponto-geniculo-occipital waves. *J Neurosci* 1990;10:2560–2579.

32. Vanni-Mercier G, Sakai K, Lin JS, Jouvet M. Mapping of cholinoceptive brainstem structures responsible for the generation of paradoxical sleep in the cat. *Arch Ital Biol* 1989;127:133–164.
33. Velazquez-Moctezuma J, Gillin JC, Shiromani PJ. Effect of specific M1, M2 muscarinic receptor agonists on REM sleep generation. *Brain Res* 1989;503:128–131.
34. Velazquez-Moctezuma J, Shalauta M, Gillin JC, Shiromani PJ. Cholinergic antagonists and REM sleep generation. *Brain Res* 1991; 543:175–179.
35. Vivaldi, McCarley RW, Hobson JA. Evocation of desynchronized sleep signs by chemical microstimulation of the pontine brain stem: reticular formation revisited. 1980;513–529.
36. Yamamoto K, Mamelak AN, Quattrochi JJ, Hobson JA. A cholinoceptive desynchronized sleep induction zone in the anterodorsal pontine tegmentum: locus of the sensitive region. *Neuroscience* 1990;39: 279–293.
37. Yamamoto K, Mamelak AN, Quattrochi JJ, Hobson JA. A cholinoceptive desynchronized sleep induction zone in the anterodorsal pontine tegmentum: spontaneous and drug-induced neuronal activity. *Neuroscience* 1990;39:295–304.

Anesthesia: Biologic Foundations, edited by Tony L. Yaksh et al. Lippincott–Raven Publishers, Philadelphia © 1997.

CHAPTER 27

CHOLINERGIC CONTRIBUTIONS TO THE CONTROL OF CONSCIOUSNESS

R. LYDIC AND HELEN A. BAGHDOYAN

Anesthesia and sleep are distinctly different states of consciousness. These states, however, exhibit many similar physiological and behavioral traits. Motor atonia, cardiopulmonary dysregulation, stereotypic eye movements, diminished responsiveness to the environment, hallucinoid mentation, changes in the electroencephalogram (EEG), and altered neuronal excitability are some of the characteristics common to sleep and anesthesia. The thesis of this chapter is that the neuronal networks which have evolved to regulate sleep are preferentially involved in generating at least some traits comprising at least some anesthetically induced states. A logical corollary of this working hypothesis is that the discipline of sleep neurobiology has the potential to help elucidate the mechanisms by which some anesthetic molecules eliminate wakefulness. Likewise, data concerning the mechanisms by which anesthesia causes the loss of waking consciousness are uniquely poised to advance sleep neurobiology.

To date, the exchange between neuroscientists interested in sleep and investigators interested in anesthesia has focused largely on the control of breathing (57,82,167). Respiratory control continues to provide a fruitful interface for the dialogue between sleep and anesthesia. Recent investigations have shown that cholinergic and cholinoceptive neurons known to be involved in rapid eye movement (REM) sleep generation (12) also contribute to state-dependent respiratory depression (for reviews, see refs. 113,115). Cholinergic neurotransmission in the pontine reticular formation appears particularly relevant for efforts to understand some of the cellular and molecular mechanisms generating sleep and anesthesia. For example, acetylcholine (ACh) release in the medial pontine reticular formation increases during REM sleep (15,108), and ACh release in the pons recently has been shown to be inhibited by morphine (122), halothane (86), and ketamine (116).

This chapter aims to achieve two goals. The first is to provide a brief overview of the recency with which sleep and anesthesia have been studied from a neuroscience perspective. The conceptual importance of differentiating sites versus mechanisms of anesthetic action and of seeking a systematic nosology of anesthetically induced states is emphasized. The second goal is to selectively review evidence that cholinergic and cholinoceptive mechanisms in the brain stem reticular formation play a major role in regulating behavioral states, breathing, and motor tone, and in modulating pain sensation.

ANESTHESIA AND SLEEP: HISTORICAL AND CONCEPTUAL PERSPECTIVES

The discoveries of REM sleep and anesthesia are recent additions to the cartography of human behavioral states. It is curious that the study of behavioral states developed so recently and with such apparent torpor. The time-span from Morton's (189) 1846 demonstration of successful anesthesia to Aserensky and Kleitman's (4) discovery of REM sleep was 107 years. For comparative purposes, only 66 years separated the first flight by the Wright brothers in 1903 and the first humans landing on the moon. Most of us will never experience microgravity, but all humans have direct knowledge of pain and different states of consciousness.

Brains and Membranes

There is presently a better understanding of how anesthetic molecules affect cells than how anesthetics cause the loss of waking consciousness. The focus on cellular effects of anesthetics was stimulated by Meyer and Overton's (134) important discoveries in the early 1900s, showing the positive correlation between solubility of an anesthetic in olive oil and potency for causing unconsciousness. The critical influence of lipid solubility on anesthetic potency now is appreciated to reflect the fact that anesthetics alter neuronal membranes which are comprised of lipid bilayers containing a large variety of imbedded proteins (171,172). In addition to the difficulty of linking studies of consciousness to studies of lipid bilayers, four other factors make it difficult to understand how anesthetics eliminate wakefulness (5). First, anesthetic agents have widely varying chemical structures, so it is difficult to elucidate structure-activity relationships. Second, there are no specific antagonists of general anesthetics, which suggests that anesthetic molecules do not act on a single class of cellular receptor. Third, the molecular sites at which anesthetics act remain incompletely understood. Fourth, the brain mechanisms that generate natural states of consciousness also are incompletely understood.

Why has an understanding of the neural mechanisms generating states of sleep and anesthesia been so long delayed? Conceptual and practical impediments continue to challenge the application of reductionistic techniques to the study of behavioral states. Conceptually, there is a long-standing, pejorative view leading some investigators to eschew any study of behavior. Natural sleep can be viewed as a behavior, and minimum alveolar anesthetic concentration (MAC) is, in fact, a behavioral measure of anesthetic potency (47,161,176). Although general anesthetics and opioids disrupt sleep (93,94,106), the relationship between anesthesia, sleep, awareness, and other states of consciousness has not been extensively studied. With few exceptions (70), contemporary textbooks of anesthesia contain no discussion of sleep stages and their underlying neuronal substrates (13,24,90,134,147,170). Neither "sleep" or "wakefulness" are found in the index to volumes on the molecular and cellular mechanisms of anesthetics (171,172). Such omissions are not unique to anesthesia, and textbooks on sleep (98,130,178,187) do not consider mechanisms by which anesthetics produce altered states of consciousness, except rarely (22). Nevertheless, we concur with Papper (151) that "the study of consciousness and awareness could be one of the most fruitful and ambitious areas of research in anaesthesia for the near and long-term future."

Much of the research on anesthetics can be grouped under two different research paradigms. Miller (133) has elegantly described one paradigm: "Ignorance of the physiology of consciousness forces these seekers of the molecular mechanisms of general anaesthesia to study simple but arbitrarily chosen model systems, such as lipid bilayers or pure proteins, in the hope that eventually the behavior of the whole may be reconstructed by the sum of its parts." A second paradigm incorporates the view that the science of behavior is part of biology (184) and that states of consciousness, and their physiological traits, are generated as emergent processes (32) by anatomically distributed neuronal networks (72,121,187). Thus, factors causing a physiological trait such as state-dependent motor atonia are not reducible solely to hyperpolarization of an individual spinal alpha motoneuron. Instead, state-dependent loss of muscle tone emerges, in part, as a synaptic consequence of complex ponto-medullo-spinal networks. Consistent with this latter view, it has been postulated that "each anaesthetic agent has a unique action, the end result of which is to produce a state of anaesthesia" (2).

Study of the cellular action of anesthetics has a long and distinguished history. Although Morton's demonstration of anesthesia and the discovery of REM sleep are products of the New World, these discoveries soon attracted the attention of leading European laboratories. Of particular relevance are the mid-19th century experiments of Claude Bernard who systematically studied the effects of anesthetic molecules on a large variety of plants and animals. Interestingly, ongoing controversies about sites versus mechanisms of anesthetic action recapitulate concepts which Bernard sought to clarify. Fink's (16) recent translation of Bernard's work from the late 1870s shows the current relevance of Bernard's concepts. Bernard concluded that "The irritability of the protoplasm of brain cells is impaired by ether and henceforth conscious sensation is abolished. Similarly, when the protoplasm of the spinal cord and ganglion cells becomes impaired, unconscious sensitivity will be abolished in the corresponding nervous mechanisms. In sum, sensitivity is a function, irritability is a property." Bernard's notion about cell "irritability" clearly corresponds to modern work on sites of anesthetic action (i.e., membrane lipids and proteins). "Sensitivity" to Bernard was "only a higher degree of a simpler property existing everywhere." Bernard's concept of sensitivity as a function, therefore, corresponds to the contemporary idea of emergent processes generating complex behavioral states.

Existing Evidence Fails to Support the Unitary Hypothesis of Anesthetic Action

States of consciousness are operationally defined by their particular constellation of physiological and behavioral traits. Mechanistic studies of sleep and anesthesia are united by the need to understand the brain mechanisms through which a diverse collection of autonomic and behavioral traits are organized into a behavioral state (121). As we have noted elsewhere (115), no single neurotransmitter, population of neurons, or brain region causes the constellation of physiological and behavioral traits that comprise naturally occurring states such as REM sleep. To the best of our knowledge, this same caveat also applies to anesthesia, because no single, unitary action of an anesthetic molecule can cause the complex constellation of physiological and behavioral traits comprising any anesthetically induced state (44,164).

A scholarly review of the multiplicity of effects on neurons exerted by anesthetic molecules is available elsewhere (95). Selected examples, however, easily illustrate the diverse actions of anesthetics. For >20 years, biochemical data have shown that anesthetic agents increase brain cyclic 3′-5′ adenosine monophosphate (cAMP) (41). More recently, halothane has been shown to significantly alter protein phosphorylation in the growth cone tips of developing neurites (177). For some neurons, hyperpolarization has been shown to be a common effect caused by a variety of anesthetic molecules that increase potassium conductance (146). Nonsynaptically mediated membrane hyperpolarization, however, has not been demonstrated—as required to satisfy the unitary hypothesis of anesthetic action—to generate all of the physiological and behavioral traits comprising an anesthetic state. Volatile anesthetics also have been shown to hyperpolarize vertebrate neurons by mechanisms other than potassium conductance. Examples include the ability of anesthetics to cause increased chloride ion conductance and by the ability of anesthetics to accentuate the activity of transmission at γ-aminobutyric $acid_a$ ($GABA_a$) synapses (203).

Neurobiological studies that include objective measures of behavioral states emphasize the heterogeneity of neuronal activity associated with different arousal states. For example, cell glucose metabolism during REM sleep has been shown to significantly decrease or not change in some brain nuclei, and to significantly increase in brain stem regions known to be involved in REM sleep generation (117). A large body of data collected since the late 1960s has identified REM sleep-specific changes in neuronal excitability throughout the brain and spinal cord (187). Additional lines of evidence also argue against a unitary site or mechanism by which anesthetic molecules alter consciousness. Regional differences in brain energy metabolism have been shown to result from a diverse assortment of compounds, including the steroid anesthetic althesin (38), etomidate (39), one MAC concentrations of halothane and isoflurane (96), and ketamine (40). Different, rather than unitary, mechanisms of anesthetic action also are suggested by many studies demonstrating species-specific and interstrain differences in anesthetic susceptibility (reviewed in 174). Taken together, these data are consistent with the view that "there is no single mechanism by which all anaesthetics produce their effects" (164).

The present inability to confirm that a single cellular mechanism causes all states of anesthesia is not a failure, but a scientific advancement with important clinical implications. Anesthesia is difficult to define but includes lack of patient movement in response to surgical incision, blunting of hemodynamic and endocrine responses, and a lack of awareness and memory (175). In addition to anesthetics having nonuniform effects on cells, recent data demonstrate differential anesthetic effects on the brain and spinal cord (3,89,162). Emphasis on brain stem mediation of anesthetic states (162) is consistent with our working hypothesis that brain stem regions involved in regulating sleep are preferentially involved in mediating some anesthetic states. The clinical relevance of data showing nonuniform anesthetic effects arising from different brain regions, derives from the potential for regional anesthetic intervention. For cases during which patient movement is spinal in origin and elicited by painful surgical stimulation, such movements may be amenable to elimination with spinal administration of anticholinergics (175). Subsequent sections describe cholinoceptive mechanisms in the medial pontine reticular formation that modulate motor tone by altering spinal α-motoneuron excitability.

States Are Operationally Defined by a Constellation of Traits

The introduction to this chapter noted that although sleep and anesthesia share a number of common physiological and behavioral traits, they are distinctly different states. In the mid-1940s, preclinical studies used the trait of motor control (loss of righting reflex) to provide an operational definition for potency of a volatile anesthetic (166). Loss of righting reflex has been referred to as "sleep time" in some anesthesia studies to indicate the amount of time required for induction of an anesthetic state. It is imprecise and inaccurate to equate loss of motor tone with an altered state of consciousness. For example, although the state of REM sleep is characterized by the trait of motor atonia, it is possible to pharmacologically dissociate the motor atonia from the loss of wakefulness and to produce a state of waking with atonia (137,192). Thus, loss of righting reflex cannot be equated with sleep or with anesthesia. Controlled sedation also has been described as "light sleep" (163). The need for reemphasizing that sedation and anesthesia are not equivalent to sleep is illustrated by the following quote from a recent chapter on nonopioid intravenous anesthetics: "The terms sleep, hypnosis, and unconsciousness are used interchangeably in anesthesia literature to refer to the state of artificially induced (i.e., drug-induced) sleep" (58). Given these terminological inaccuracies, it is perhaps not surprising that there are controversies over the existence of anesthetic states (76,91,160), and whether anesthesia causes loss of consciousness (102).

Behavioral arousal and cortical EEG arousal also can be pharmacologically dissociated (97). A classic example from the sleep literature is the effect of systemically administered atropine, which produces a state of wakefulness characterized by a synchronized, non-REM (NREM) sleep-like EEG (80). Dissociated states of consciousness represent an important clinical concern for sleep disorders medicine (126) and for anesthesia. Numerous dissociated states have been documented during which a patient appears to be anesthetized and surgery proceeds on a paralyzed but otherwise conscious patient (63,78,102,109,138). Systematic classification schemes developed for the diagnosis of disorders of sleep and arousal emphasize the multiplicity of naturally occurring states of consciousness (169,191). Efforts to develop systematic, operational definitions of complex anesthetic states demonstrate the importance of such an undertaking (194). The reductionistic elegance of membrane biophysics and the resolving power of molecular biological techniques will be grossly mismatched to the study of anesthesia in the absence of systematically developed classifications of states of consciousness caused by anesthetic agents.

RELEVANCE OF THE RETICULAR FORMATION FOR SLEEP AND ANESTHESIA

Contemporary textbooks of neuroscience (81) make clear that the brain stem reticular formation mediates four major functions relevant for generating sleep and anesthetically induced states. These four functions include: (a) generating behavioral states, (b) cardiopulmonary control, (c) control of somatic motor tone, and (d) modulation of pain sensation. These reticular functions originate from distinct but interacting groups of brain stem neurons that extend from the midbrain to the caudal medulla. A large part of the art and science of clinical anesthesia is devoted to abolishing behavioral arousal and pain sensation without causing excessive cardiopulmonary depression. The complexity of this clinical task is due, in part, to the extensive structural overlap and functional interaction among brain stem reticular neurons. The four sections below describe recent progress in specifying the role of cholinergic and cholinoceptive reticular neurons in relation to regulation of behavioral states, breathing, motor tone, and pain sensation.

Cholinergic Modulation of Behavioral States

The human sleep cycle is comprised of two major phases: REM sleep and NREM sleep. During the REM phase of sleep, the brain is metabolically (117) and electrically active, the EEG is desynchronized (as it is during wakefulness), muscles become atonic, there is cardiopulmonary dysregulation, the subjective experience is of dreaming, and there are numerous endocrine changes (98,115). Natural sleep is actively generated by the brain and not simply the loss of wakefulness due to sensory deafferentation. As we have noted previously (72), the presence of a waking-like EEG pattern during REM sleep originally led Jouvet to name this state "paradoxical sleep," to accentuate the paradox of behavioral sleep accompanied by an activated EEG.

REM sleep comprises ~20% of total sleep time for humans ranging in age from the second through sixth decade. During a typical night of human sleep, REM sleep alternates with NREM sleep, occurring about every 90 min. The length of this REM and NREM cycle exhibits species-specific rhythmicity. The rhythmic nature of REM sleep is observed in all terrestrial, placental mammals (28). In addition to showing a high degree of temporal organization, REM sleep is homeostatically regulated. REM sleep deprivation provides an example of this homeostatic control. Analogous to the tachypnea that follows breath holding, REM sleep inhibition always is followed by a rebound increase in the percentage of total sleep time spent in the REM phase (42). The ultradian (<<24 h) rhythm of NREM/REM cycles and the homeostatic properties of REM sleep have long suggested that brain stem central pattern generating neurons regulate REM sleep (111). Circadian (≈24 h) rhythms are generated by the hypothalamic suprachiasmatic nuclei (for a review, see ref. 1), and circadian control systems can influence the timing of wakefulness and the ultradian NREM/REM cycle (46). But what brain regions, cells, membrane properties, receptors, neurotransmitters, and signal transduction systems generate REM sleep?

Attention was directed towards the pons as a brain region involved in controlling behavioral states by Moruzzi and Magoun's (144) discovery that electrical stimulation of the brain stem reticular formation could alter more rostral thalamocortical circuits generating the EEG. Reticular stimulation caused the high-voltage, low-frequency (i.e., synchronized) EEG, typical of sleep and some anesthetic states, to be converted to the low-voltage, high-frequency (desynchronized) EEG characteristic of both wakefulness and REM sleep. Focus on the reticular formation was further refined by Jouvet's discovery that the pontine reticular formation played a key role in REM sleep generation (79). As recently reviewed (115), there are presently at least nine lines of converging evidence showing that cholinergic and cholinoceptive pontine reticular neurons play a key role in REM sleep generation. The discussion of ACh in the present chapter is limited to recent data concerning the role of cholinergic neurotransmission within the medial pontine reticular formation in the generation of sleep and anesthesia.

Through the work of Yaksh et al. (197,200), the power of intracranial drug administration for elucidating the sites and mechanisms of opioid analgesia has long been appreciated. Studies involving intracranial drug delivery also have made a major contribution to sleep neurobiology. In the 1960s, it was shown that microinjecting microgram quantities of cholinergic agonists into the pontine reticular formation of intact, unanesthetized cat caused these animals to enter a REM sleep-like state (14,34,62). Animals receiving these pontine microinjections appeared to be asleep and they exhibited all of the polygraphic features of REM sleep: motor atonia, EEG desynchrony, and rapid eye movements. Detailed behavioral studies (11), neuroanatomical mapping (10,11,193), dose-response studies (7), and evocation of the REM sleep-like state by the acetylcholinesterase inhibitor neostigmine (9) have now convincingly demonstrated this state to provide a valid and reliable model of REM sleep. The conclusion that the cholinergically induced REM sleep-like state offers an important tool for understanding brain stem control of states of consciousness is supported by data from many laboratories (for example, see ref. 66 and Table 4 of ref. 12). Today, we know that the cholinergically induced REM sleep-like state is site-dependent within the pons, dose-dependent, and blocked by atropine (12). These studies have led to the conclusion that the cholinergically induced REM sleep-like state provides a phenomenologically adequate model of naturally occurring REM sleep (67).

As an experimental tool, the success of the cholinergic model of REM sleep is difficult to overemphasize. The cholinergic model has advanced our understanding of state-dependent changes in spinal motoneuron excitability (142), and has characterized cholinergic contributions to sleep-dependent respiratory depression (113). The model also has made it possible to map changes in proto-oncogene expression in cholinergic (181) and cholinoceptive (201) reticular formation regions compared to *c-fos* expressed during natural REM sleep (132). Recently, this cholinergic model has made it possible to reveal that the REM sleep-like state and respiratory depression evoked from the pons are mediated by pertussis toxin-sensitive G proteins (182).

All of the work noted above was derived from cat, and for many years successful evocation of the REM sleep-like state in rat has been more difficult to obtain. The dose and injection site parameters for reliable evocation of a REM sleep-like state in rat only recently have been derived (25). This important discovery will make the cholinergic model of REM sleep even more accessible as a tool for elucidating the cholinergic control of sleep and anesthesia. Recent data have identified new compounds that can promote sleep, and it will be important to explore their contributions to states of anesthesia. For example, brain lipids comprising a group of fatty acid primary amides recently have been shown to be sleep-inducing (35), but their interaction with cholinergic neurotransmission and their response to anesthetic molecules has not yet been reported. In many areas of brain the neurotrophin nerve growth factor (NGF) co-localizes in cholinergic cell bodies or terminals, and preliminary data have shown that NGF microinjected into the pontine reticular formation can cause a REM sleep-like state (202). The effect of volatile anesthetics on NGF levels in the pontine brain stem remains to be investigated.

Acetylcholine and States of Consciousness

What data suggest that ACh is causally related to the generation of sleep and anesthesia? As early as 1949, ACh content of whole brain was shown to vary as a function of arousal state (165). Cortical ACh release was noted to decrease with increasing depth of anesthesia (136), and ACh was the first cortical neurotransmitter for which levels of release were shown to significantly change across the sleep/wake cycle (29). These pioneering studies were consistent with the view advanced in the late 1960s that diminished arousal induced by some anesthetic molecules may result, in part, from alterations in ACh release (97).

The continued development of microdialysis and high pressure liquid chromatography (HPLC) has revolutionized neurochemistry (168), making it possible to measure ACh release from localized brain regions during states of wakefulness, sleep, and anesthesia. The following data review recent work using microdialysis and HPLC to test the hypothesis that cholinergic neurotransmission in the pons varies during REM sleep and during anesthesia. This discussion will focus on two pontine regions. One is the medial pontine reticular formation, the cholinoceptive area from which the REM sleep-like state is produced by microinjecting cholinomimetics. The second pontine region includes the laterodorsal and pedunculopontine tegmental (LDT/PPT) nuclei. The LDT/PPT nuclei contain the cholinergic neurons that send projections (135,180) and release ACh (114) in the medial pontine reticular formation. Microdialysis data reviewed below show that ACh release in the medial pontine reticular formation is increased over waking levels during REM sleep and decreased below waking levels during anesthetic states induced by morphine, halothane, and ketamine.

We first performed microdialysis studies in the LDT/PPT terminal field of the medial pontine reticular formation in order to measure ACh release during states of quiet wakefulness, NREM sleep, and the REM sleep-like state caused by injecting the contralateral pons with the cholinergic agonist carbachol (118,122). The results (Fig. 1) showed that the cholinergically induced REM sleep-like state was always accompanied by a statistically significant increase in ACh release.

When carbachol was injected into the pons, but outside the medial pontine reticular formation region known to cause the REM sleep-like state, there was no increase in ACh release and no signs of the REM sleep-like state. The ability of unilateral pontine carbachol administration to significantly increase ACh release in the contralateral medial pontine reticular formation also varied as a function of the carbachol dose.

Because the brain itself contains no pain receptors, it is possible to perform these dialysis experiments using unanesthetized animals that spontaneously sleep and wake. Figure 2 illustrates ACh release during 200 min of simultaneous measurement of breathing and multiple polygraphic variables used for objectively scoring states of sleep and wakefulness. Note, in Fig. 2, the pattern of EEG desynchrony (low voltage, high frequency) typical of wakefulness. During REM sleep, the EEG also is desynchronized, and for this reason the right hand portion of Fig. 2 refers to the carbachol-induced REM sleep-like state as DCarb. The black histograms at the bottom of Fig. 2 illustrate ACh release in one side of the medial pontine reticular formation following a microinjection of 4.0 μg carbachol into the contralateral medial pontine reticular formation.

Both the microinjection data (for a review, see ref. 12) and direct measures using in vitro biochemical (6) and autoradiographic techniques (8) demonstrate that the feline pontine reticular formation contains muscarinic cholinergic receptors. It is reemphasized, however, that the medial pontine reticular formation neurons do not produce ACh. This raised the still unanswered question: By what mechanism does administration of carbachol on one side of the medial pontine reticular formation cause increased ACh release in the contralateral reticular formation during the REM sleep-like state?

We were stimulated by the anatomical data showing that cholinergic neurons in the LDT/PPT project to the medial pontine reticular formation (135,180) to test the hypothesis that ACh release in the medial pontine reticular formation is regulated by LDT/PPT neurons. Therefore, we electrically stimulated the LDT/PPT nuclei while dialyzing the terminal projection field in the medial pontine reticular formation (Fig. 3). The results showed that electrical stimulation of the LDT/PPT caused a monotonic increase in ACh release within the medial pontine reticular formation (Fig. 4).

These results were an important contribution to our understanding of cholinergic mechanisms regulating the control of consciousness. These data showed for the first time that ACh release in the medial pontine reticular formation was regulated by cholinergic LDT/PPT neurons.

These ACh release data directly support the hypothesis that pontine cholinergic neurotransmission is critically important for regulating REM sleep and, as we have now demonstrated and describe below, states of consciousness caused by anesthetic molecules. The ACh release data illustrated by Fig. 4 also are consistent with previous data showing that REM sleep is associated with increased energy metabolism in LDT/PPT and medial pontine reticular formation neurons (117). Furthermore, increased ACh release evoked by LDT/PPT stimulation extends the important finding that LDT/PPT neurons exhibit increased discharge rates that phase-lead the onset of REM sleep (48,49).

Morphine, Halothane, and Ketamine Eliminate REM Sleep and Decrease Pontine ACh Release

When we observed the results summarized by Fig. 4, we immediately recognized that the ability to study ACh release evoked by LDT/PPT stimulation provided us with an important

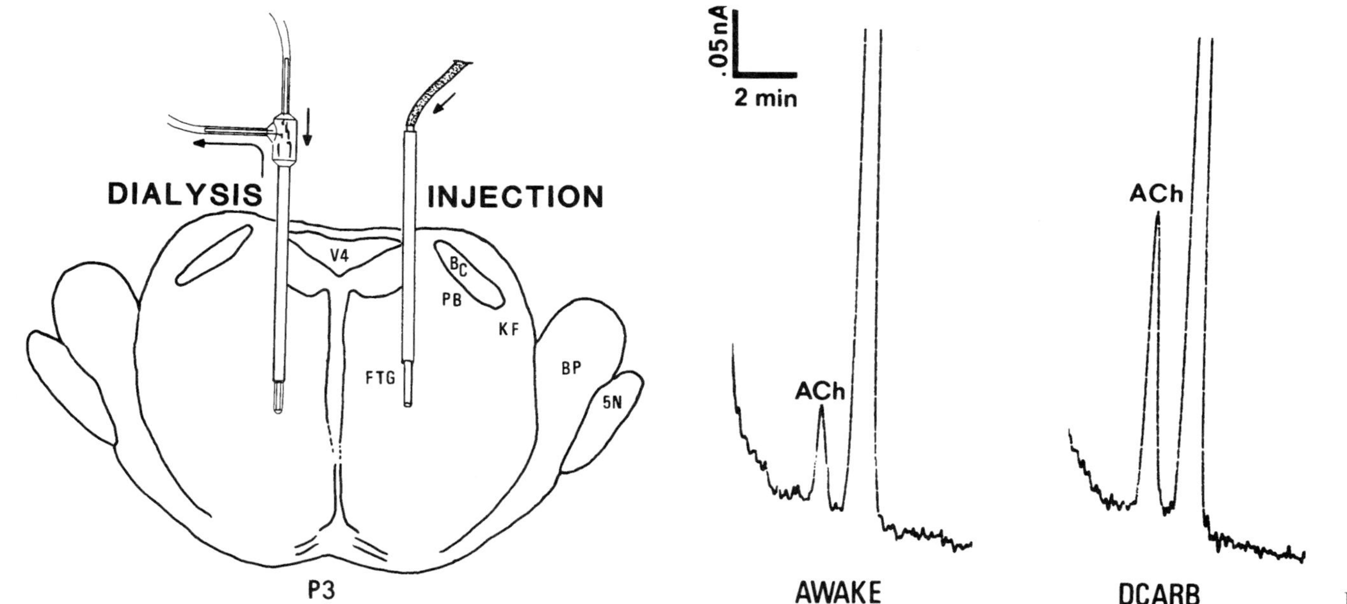

Figure 1. Schematic drawing of a coronal section through cat pons showing a microinjection cannula (INJECTION) and a microdialysis probe (DIALYSIS) placed in the medial pontine reticular formation **(A)** Chromatograms obtained by HPLC analysis of microdialysis samples collected from the medial pontine reticular formation **(B)** The peaks labeled ACh indicate the amount of acetylcholine measured during wakefulness (AWAKE) and show the increase during the REM sleep-like state produced by microinjecting carbachol into the medial pontine reticular formation (DCARB). (Reprinted with permission from Lydic R, Baghdoyan HA, Lorinc Z. Microdialysis of cat pons reveals enhanced acetylcholine release during state-dependent respiratory depression. *Am J Physiol* 1991;261:R766–R770.)

tool for our continuing efforts to understand opioid effects on states of consciousness. We hypothesized that systemically administered morphine sulfate (MSO_4) would cause decreased ACh release in the medial pontine reticular formation (122). This prediction was based on two lines of evidence. First, clinical observations have made it clear that patients receiving morphine do not have normal REM sleep (85) and exhibit rebound increases in REM sleep when opioid therapy is withdrawn (93). Second, our animal studies showed that microinjecting morphine sulfate into the medial pontine reticular formation causes REM sleep inhibition (87). The advantage of being able to study evoked ACh release is illustrated by the Fig. 2 histograms. That figure makes clear that basal levels of ACh release in the medial pontine reticular formation typically average 0.3–0.4 pmol/10 min dialysis. These ACh release levels are near the lower end of detectability. Since the existing data led us to hypothesize that morphine sulfate would decrease ACh release, we anticipated that systemic morphine might make ACh detection impossible. This limitation was circumvented by studying the effect of systemically administered morphine on ACh release in the pontine reticular formation evoked by electrical stimulation of the LDT/PPT (122). Figure 5 illustrates the large increase in ACh release caused by LDT/PPT stimulation and the significant decrease in this evoked ACh release caused by systemically administered morphine.

The finding that microinjection of morphine sulfate into specific pontine sites blocked REM sleep (87), combined with results of Fig. 5, identified for the first time a brain region (the medial pontine reticular formation) and one possible mechanism (decreased ACh release) by which systemically administered opioids inhibit REM sleep. Since opioid-induced REM sleep inhibition is recognized as an undesirable opioid side effect with potential life-threatening complication (for a review, see ref. 36) these basic studies have potential clinical significance for the development of effective countermeasures. The fact that opioid-induced REM sleep inhibition was site-dependent within the medial pontine reticular formation, dose-dependent, and blocked by naloxone (87) was consistent with the possibility that opioid receptors in the medial pontine reticular formation mediate REM sleep inhibition. These results raised the question: Which opioid receptor subtype in the medial pontine reticular formation mediates REM sleep inhibition? The pontine distribution of μ, δ, and κ opioid receptors in cat is less well understood than in rodent (128). Microinjection of subtype selective opioid agonists into the medial pontine reticular formation was, therefore, used to test the hypothesis that a particular opioid receptor caused REM sleep inhibition. The results (Fig. 6) showed that REM sleep inhibition was attributable to opioid receptors of the μ subtype (36).

One important question for the future will be to characterize the differential effects of subtype selective opioid agonists on ACh release within the medial pontine reticular formation. It will also be important to quantify the extent to which morphine decreases pontine ACh release by acting on cholinergic cell bodies in the LDT/PPT versus actions exerted on LDT/PPT cholinergic terminals within the medial pontine reticular formation. Considered together, the three lines of evidence reviewed above (36,87,122) are consistent with our hypothesis that pontine cholinergic mechanisms regulating naturally occurring states of consciousness may contribute to generating some anesthetic-induced states.

Perhaps decreased ACh release in the medial pontine reticular formation could be caused only by opioid compounds. Alternatively, if our working hypothesis is generalizable, one would predict similar effects on cholinergic neurotransmission and REM sleep caused by a very different class of anesthetic agents. Therefore, as a continuing test of these concepts, we next investigated the effects on ACh release in the medial pontine reticular formation of the halogenated alkane halothane.

Recent reviews concerning the effect of anesthetics on transmitter uptake, synthesis, and release note that ACh plays a key role in regulating states of consciousness but that few studies

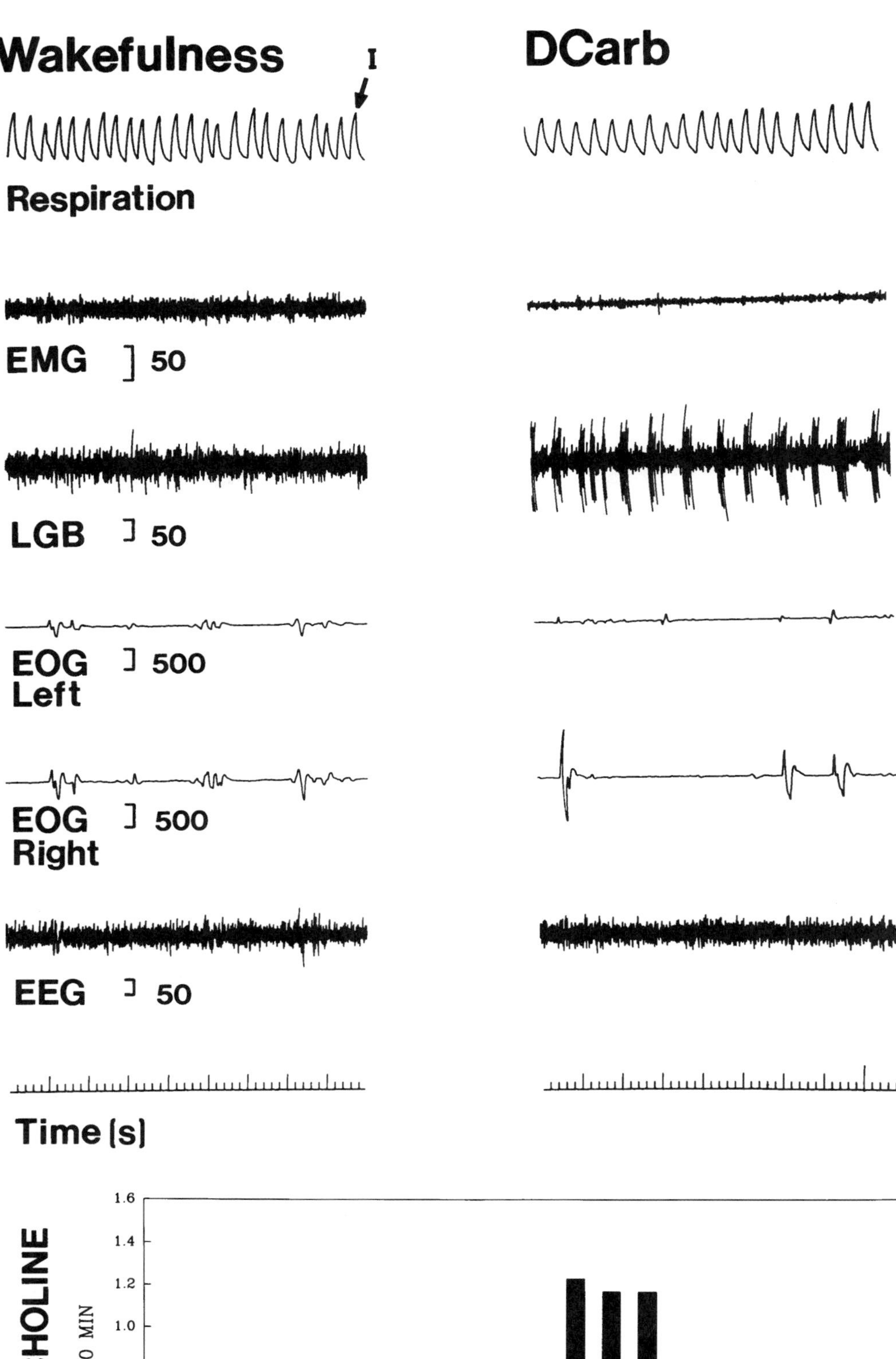

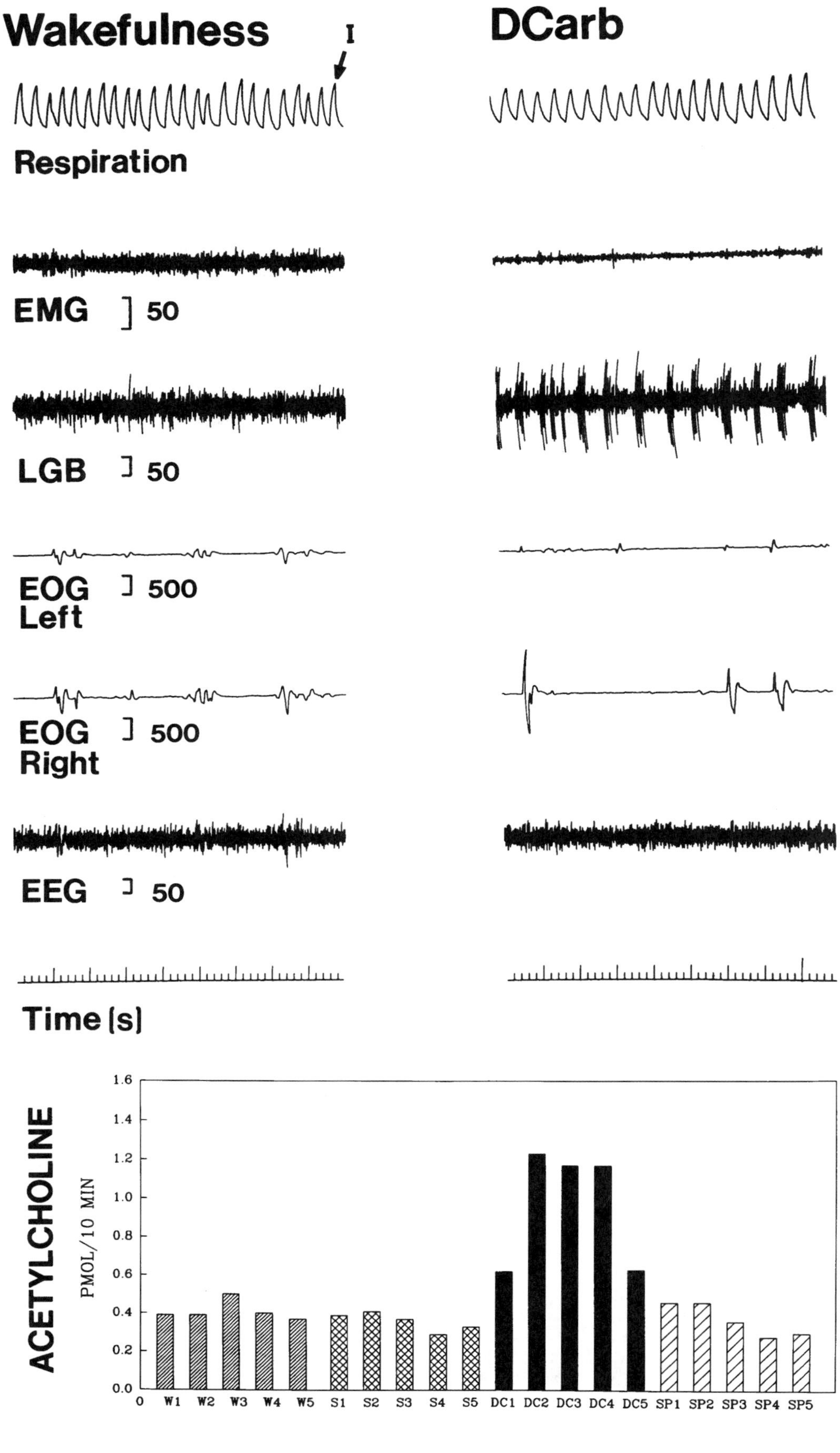

Figure 2. Simultaneous measurement of breathing, states of consciousness, and acetylcholine release. **Left column:** Polygraphic recordings during wakefulness. **Right column:** Polygraphic recordings during the carbachol-induced REM sleep-like state (DCarb). Bar graph shows acetylcholine release from the medial pontine reticular formation. Each histogram represents a 10-min dialysis sample taken during wakefulness (W), synchronized or non-REM sleep (S), the cholinergically induced REM sleep-like state (DC), and during a dissociated state characterized by the presence of EEG spindles (S) and PGO waves (P) recorded from the lateral geniculate body of the thalamus. Note that ACh release was increased only during the REM sleep-like state (DC). EMG, neck electromyogram; LGB, lateral geniculate body recording; EOG, eye movement potentials; EEG, electroencephalogram. (Reprinted with permission from Lydic R, Baghdoyan HA. Pedunculopontine stimulation alters respiration and increases ACh release in the pontine reticular formation. *Am J Physiol* 1993;264:R544–R554.)

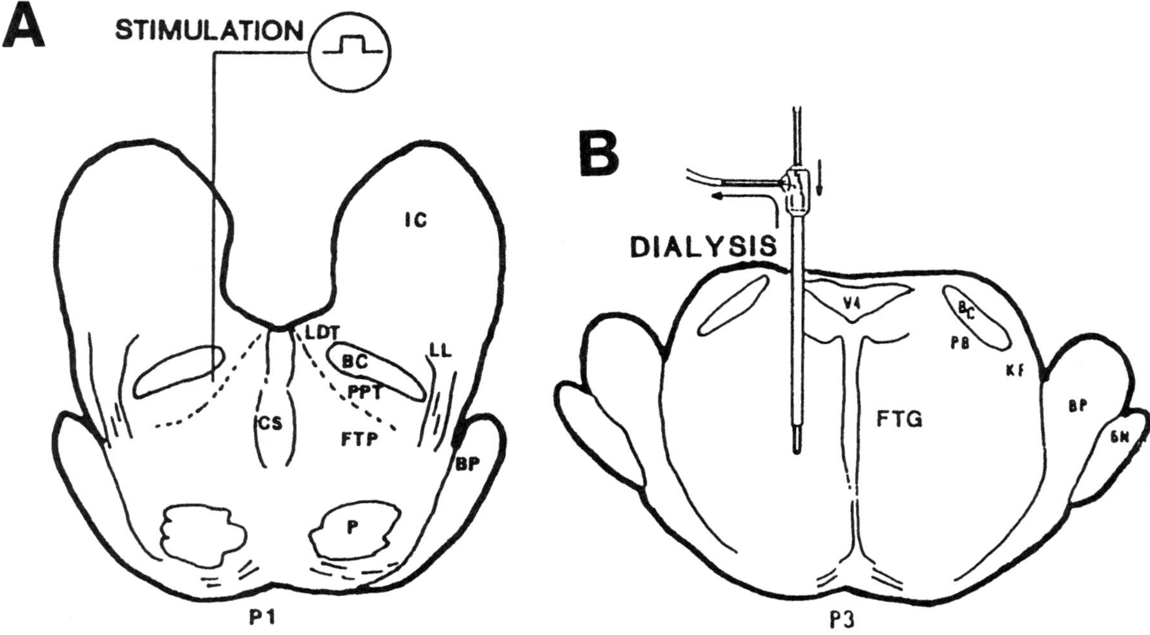

Figure 3. Schematic drawings of coronal sections through cat pons showing the technique for placement of a stimulating electrode in the cholinergic laterodorsal tegmental and pedunculopontine tegmental (LDT/PPT) nuclei **(A)** Simultaneous placement of a microdialysis probe in the medial pontine reticular formation, also referred to as gigantocellular tegmental field (FTG), is illustrated **(B)** With this procedure it was possible to electrically stimulate the cholinergic LDT/PPT neurons which have axons projecting to the FTG region of the medial pontine reticular formation and, therefore, study evoked ACh release. (Reprinted with permission from Lydic R, Baghdoyan HA. Pedunculopontine stimulation alters respiration and increases ACh release in the pontine reticular formation. *Am J Physiol* 1993;264:R544–R554.)

have been performed examining the effects of anesthetics on ACh release (68). We hypothesized that halothane would depress ACh release in the medial pontine reticular formation (86). In order to test this hypothesis, cats were anesthetized with halothane and the medial pontine reticular formation was dialyzed (Fig. 3B) for measuring ACh release. The end-tidal halothane concentration was 1.2%, previously shown to correspond to the 1 MAC value for cats. After acquiring multiple dialysis samples, administration of halothane was discontinued while continuing to measure ACh release during emergence and during wakefulness. The results showed that 1 MAC halothane significantly decreased ACh release in the medial pontine reticular formation (Fig. 7) and abolished all polygraphic signs of REM sleep (86).

Subsequent studies have shown that the volatile anesthetics isoflurane and enflurane also significantly decreased ACh release in the medial pontine reticular formation (88). Regional brain differences in ACh release in response to halothane have been reported in recent microdialysis studies. In the interpeduncular nucleus, ACh release increased in response to 3% halothane (190), but in the striatum halothane decreased ACh release (37). The cellular and molecular mechanisms through which these volatile anesthetics decreased pontine ACh release are not presently known. These varied effects of halothane on ACh release negate the possibility that halothane uniformly alters ACh release throughout the brain (for a review, see ref. 95).

Halothane anesthesia is known to cause spindle activity in the human EEG (204) and 1 MAC halothane in cat caused EEG spindles (Fig. 8) that were not significantly different in waveform, amplitude, or number from the EEG spindles of NREM sleep (88).

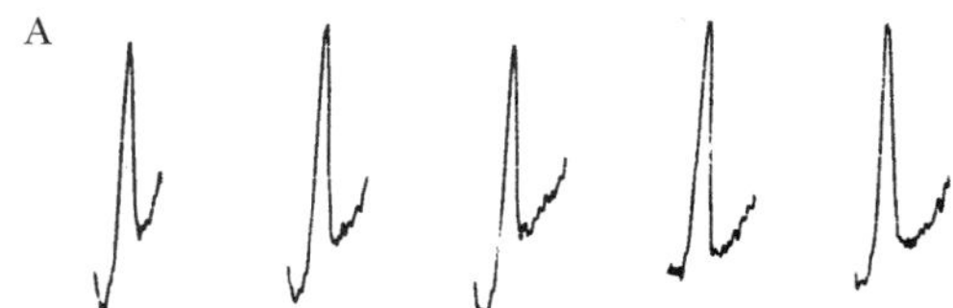

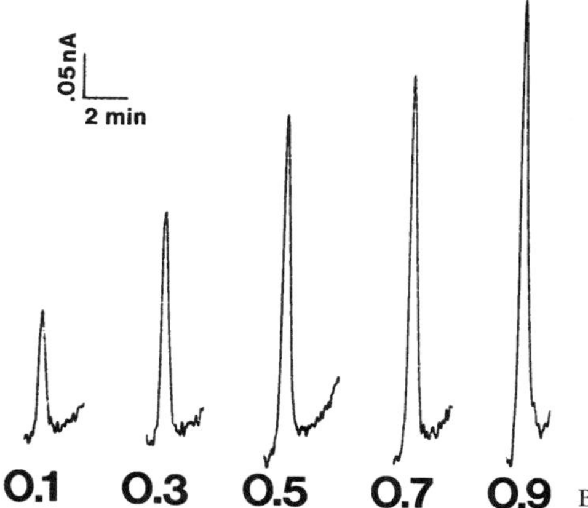

Figure 4. Chromatograms representing ACh measurement in the medial pontine reticular formation. **(A)** Five consecutive, 10-min microdialysis samples of ACh under control conditions, before electrical stimulation of LDT/PPT. **(B)** Monotonic increase in ACh release produced by increasing current amplitude (mA) stimulating LDT/PPT. The results shown in B provided the first functional evidence that ACh release in the medial pontine reticular formation is regulated by LDT/PPT neurons. (Reprinted with permission from Lydic R, Baghdoyan HA. Pedunculopontine stimulation alters respiration and increases ACh release in the pontine reticular formation. *Am J Physiol* 1993;264:R544–R554.)

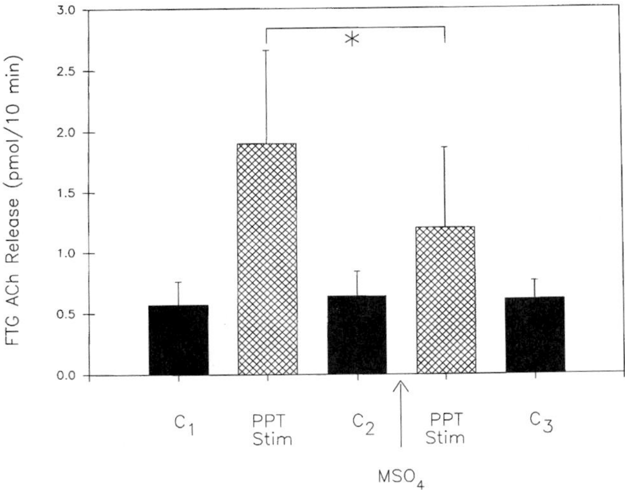

Figure 5. Histograms showing average ACh release in medial pontine reticular formation (FTG) before and after systemic administration of morphine sulfate. Mean and standard deviation ACh release are plotted on the ordinate and experimental conditions are shown on the abscissa. The histograms labeled C_1, C_2, and C_3 indicate control ACh release, without electrical stimulation of LDT/PPT. The histograms labeled "PPT Stim" indicate significant increases in ACh release evoked by electrical stimulation of LDT/PPT. To the right of the C_2 histogram, the arrow indicates systemic administration of morphine sulfate (MSO_4) (500 μg/kg^{-1}). Note that MSO_4 significantly decreased ACh release evoked from the LDT/PPT. (Reprinted with permission from Lydic R, Keifer JC, Baghdoyan HA, Becker L. Microdialysis of the pontine reticular formation reveals inhibition of acetylcholine release by morphine. *Anesthesiology* 1993;79:1003–1012.)

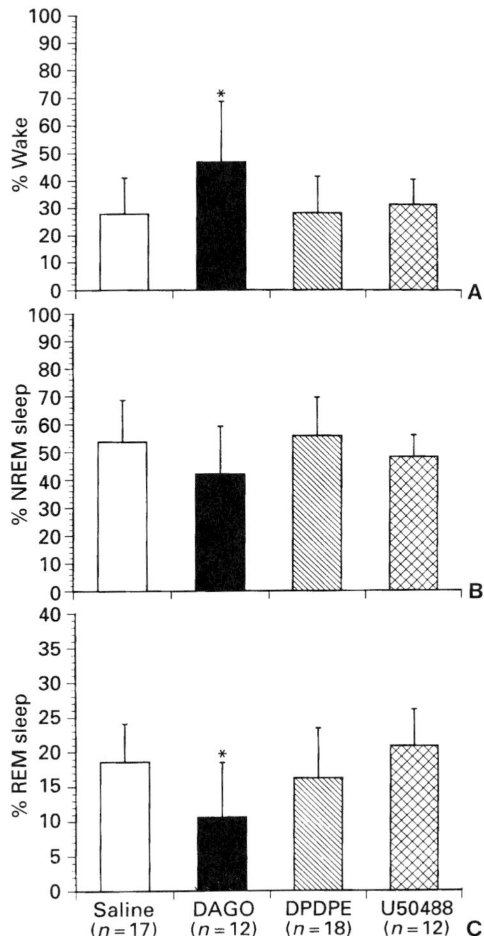

Figure 6. Effect of opioid microinjection into the medial pontine reticular formation on the amount of time spent in wakefulness **(A)**, NREM sleep **(B)**, and REM sleep **(C)**. All drugs were microinjected into the medial pontine reticular formation of intact, unanesthetized cat, and only the μ-specific agonist DAGO (D-Ala[2], N-Me-Phe[4], Gly-ol[5]-enkephalin) significantly inhibited REM sleep. These results suggest that opioid-induced REM sleep inhibition is mediated by μ receptors within the medial pontine reticular formation. (Reprinted with permission from Cronin A, Keifer JC, Baghdoyan HA, Lydic R. Narcotic inhibition of rapid eye movement sleep induced by a specific mu receptor agonist. *Br J Anaesth* 1995;74:188–192.)

Similar to the ACh release data of Fig. 7, these EEG spindle data are consistent with our hypothesis that cholinergic brain stem mechanisms regulating naturally occurring states generate physiological traits comprising some anesthetic states. In addition to providing cholinergic input to the medial pontine reticular formation (114), the cholinergic peribrachial neurons of LDT/PPT (Fig. 3) also provide cholinergic input to the thalamus. Recent data have shown that decreased discharge of LDT/PPT cholinergic neurons projecting to the thalamus is involved in EEG spindle generation (188). Microdialysis of the medial thalamus in rat has revealed that ACh release originating from LDT/PPT neurons is essentially the same during the EEG activation characteristic of waking and REM sleep and significantly reduced with the onset of NREM sleep spindles (196). Along with these previous data (188), the results summarized by Figs. 7 and 8 suggest that halothane anesthesia causes decreased LDT/PPT cholinergic input to the thalamus resulting in generation of EEG spindles (86,88).

Ketamine is a phencyclidine that produces a dissociative anesthetic state and also inhibits REM sleep. Therefore, ketamine offers yet another class of anesthetic agent with which to test the hypothesis that ACh release in the medial pontine reticular formation varies with ketamine-induced changes in state of consciousness. A preliminary report (116) showed that following 15.0 mg/kg ketamine, pontine ACh release was significantly less than ACh release during REM sleep. At higher doses of ketamine (33.3 mg/kg), ACh release was not significantly different from ACh release during REM sleep. These data show for the first time that ACh release in the pontine reticular formation is altered in a dose-dependent manner during ketamine anesthesia. Since ketamine is known to block *N*-methyl-D-aspartate (NMDA) channels, these data suggest a role for pontine reticular NMDA receptors in the regulation of consciousness. Furthermore, these data comprise another line of evidence suggesting that cholinergic mechanisms in the medial pontine reticular formation play a key role in mediating the loss of wakefulness caused by a third type of anesthetic agent.

State-Dependent Respiratory Depression Can Be Evoked from the Cholinoceptive Pontine Reticular Formation

State-dependent respiratory depression is a key concern for anesthesiology and pulmonary medicine. Sleep apnea is a poorly understood disorder characterized by periodic cessation of breathing (apnea) and a failure to ventilate normally while asleep (131,157). Sleep apnea presently has no fixed definition; but, if one uses ≥5 apneas/h and daytime hypersomnolence as diagnostic criteria, then the disease has been estimated in the United States to affect 4% of adult males and 2% of adult females (205). In 1990 alone, the estimated economic cost of sleep apnea in the United States was $275 million (43). Sleep apnea has four major pathophysiological sequelae, including (a) systemic and pulmonary hypertension, (b) cardiac arrhythmia, (c) behavioral morbidity such as sleepiness leading to

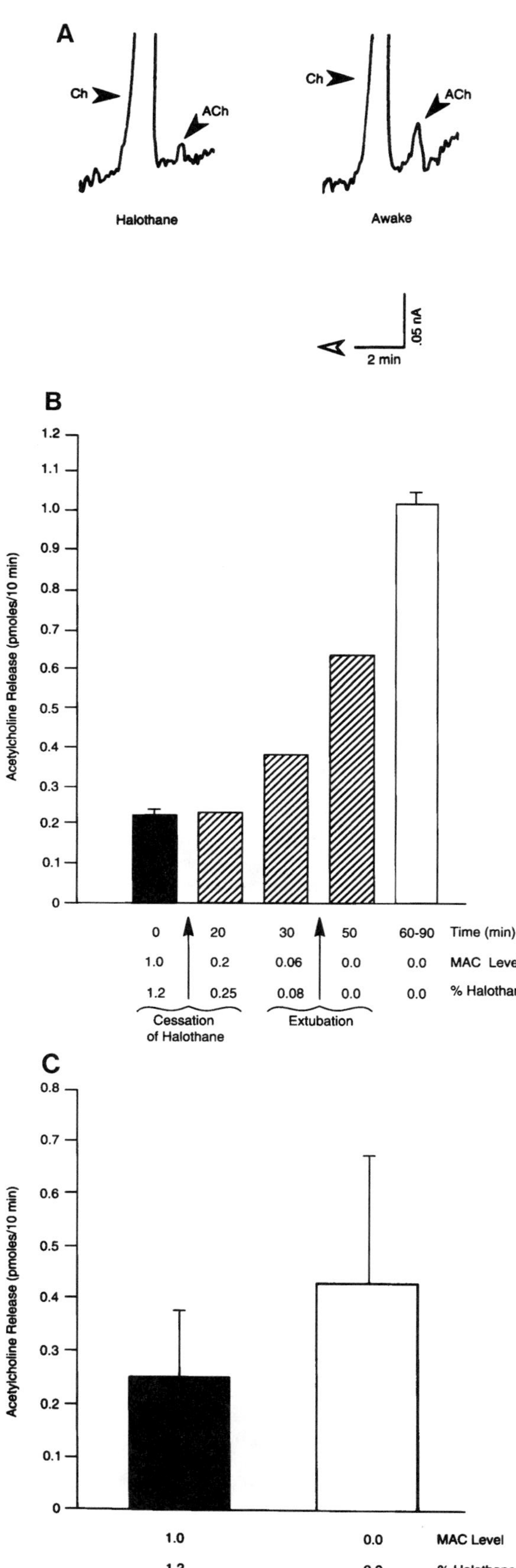

Figure 7. ACh release in the medial pontine reticular formation during halothane anesthesia and during wakefulness. **(A)** Individual chromatograms for ACh and choline (Ch). **(B)** ACh release plotted for one experiment. Note that with decreasing concentrations of halothane, there was a progressive increase in the amount of ACh. **(C)** Group data summarizing multiple measurements of ACh release in the medial pontine reticular formation during halothane anesthesia (*solid histogram*) and during wakefulness (*open histogram*). Administration of 1.2% halothane significantly decreased ACh release in the medial pontine reticular formation. (Reprinted with permission from Keifer JC, Baghdoyan HA, Becker L, Lydic R. Halothane decreases pontine acetylcholine release and increases EEG spindles. *NeuroReport* 1994;5:577–580.)

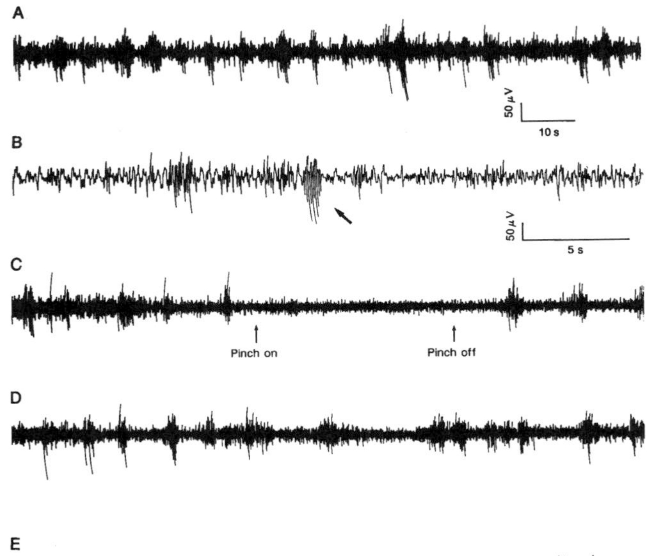

Figure 8. Polygraphic recordings of the EEG illustrating the ability of halothane to evoke EEG spindles identical to the EEG spindles of non-REM sleep. **(A)** EEG spindles induced by 1.2% halothane. **(B)** EEG recording at a faster chart speed in order to visualize the 10-Hz spindle waveform. **(C)** During 1.2% halothane administration, painful stimuli caused a loss of EEG spindles and behavioral arousal. **(D)** When painful stimulation was discontinued, EEG spindles returned. **(E)** Desynchronized EEG characteristic of wakefulness. (Reprinted with permission from Keifer JC, Baghdoyan HA, Becker L, Lydic R. Halothane decreases pontine acetylcholine release and increases EEG spindles. *NeuroReport* 1994;5:577–580.)

increased frequency of accidents, and (d) neuropsychological deficits such as altered affect and diminished problem-solving ability (for reviews, see refs. 98,131). Anesthesia causes respiratory depression, and, in the United States alone, ~19 million patients are anesthetized each year (113). Patients with sleep apnea require special anesthetic management (33), but maintaining upper airway patency and adequate ventilation is a key concern for every anesthetic induction and extubation.

Anesthesiologists have long been aware that the loss of waking consciousness is accompanied by respiratory depression. Fink et al. (54–56) described the respiratory-facilitator effect of behavioral arousal as a "wakefulness stimulus for breathing." In the late 1970s, pulmonary biologists (148) and pulmonologists (155,156) recognized that Fink's concepts had explanatory value for efforts to understand neuronal mechanisms contributing to sleep-disordered breathing. Stimulation provided by these concepts and recognition of the need for quantitative and mechanistic analyses (75) have led to considerable progress in characterizing the cellular and molecular mechanisms that contribute to state-dependent respiratory depression. This section is limited to a brief overview of data relating cholinergic control of behavioral states to the control of breathing. Detailed reviews are available elsewhere (113,115,150).

As recently as the late 1980s, the first studies appeared showing that respiratory depression could be evoked from cholinoceptive regions in the medial pontine reticular formation known to be involved in REM sleep generation (112,120). Since these pontine reticular regions contain no major clusters of premotor or upper motor respiratory neurons, this discovery was unique in demonstrating respiratory depression from a nonrespiratory region of the brain. Without an understanding of the mechanisms generating states of consciousness, studies of state-dependent respiratory depression will remain incomplete. Therefore, application of the cholinergic model of REM sleep to the study of state-dependent respiratory depression offers three key advantages. First, the cholinergic model has made it possible to specify a brain region (the medial pontine reticular formation) and a receptor system (muscarinic cholinergic) causing state-dependent respiratory depression. Second, since pontine microinjection of cholinomimetics causes a REM sleep-like state and causes respiratory depression, the cholinergic model of REM sleep is ideal for testing causal, rather than merely correlational, hypotheses. Advances in neuroscience now make it possible to acquire cellular and intracellular data from intact, unanesthetized animals during naturally occurring states of sleep and wakefulness (for reviews, see refs. 149,187). Therefore, a third advantage is that sleep and respiratory studies can be conducted in the same animal during both natural REM sleep and during the REM sleep-like state caused by pontine administration of cholinomimetics. Such combined studies permit direct observation of the cellular mechanisms causing state-dependent respiratory depression.

Microinjecting cholinomimetics directly into the pontine reticular formation of intact, conscious cat causes a state that resembles naturally occurring REM sleep (for a review, see ref. 12). Similar to REM sleep, the cholinergically induced REM sleep-like state is accompanied by upper airway muscle hypotonia (120) and diminished minute ventilation (112). During the cholinergically evoked REM sleep-like state, as in natural REM sleep, cats also revealed a diminished ventilatory response to hyperoxic hypercapnia (119). Following administration of the cholinergic agonist, these respiratory effects occurred with a short latency suggesting synaptic mediation.

Neuroanatomical studies made it possible to test the hypothesis that the medial pontine reticular formation has synaptic connections to brain stem respiratory nuclei. Pseudorabies virus was used as a transsynaptic marker to examine connections between the medial pontine reticular formation and the laryngeal abductor muscles. Injection of pseudorabies virus into the posterior cricoarytenoid muscle of the larynx produced labeled cells, as expected in the nucleus ambiguus, and in the pontine reticular formation (50). Such transsynaptic labeling demonstrates polysynaptic pathways connecting the pons and the posterior cricoarytenoid muscles. Additional neuroanatomical studies (105) used retrograde fluorescent tracers to examine the connections between the medial pontine reticular formation and cells within the pontine, ventral, and dorsal respiratory nuclei (51). The results showed that cholinoceptive regions of the medial pontine reticular formation involved in REM sleep generation have reciprocal monosynaptic connections with the pontine respiratory nuclei and receive monosynaptic projections from both the dorsal and ventral respiratory nuclei (105).

Electrophysiological experiments also were performed to test the hypothesis that cholinergic pontine reticular mechanisms could alter the activity of neurons that discharge in-phase with breathing. Such cells are referred to as respiratory neurons, and the aim was to record breathing and the discharge of these respiratory neurons during REM sleep and during the REM sleep-like state caused by pontine microinjections of cholinergic agonists. The results (Fig. 9) showed that, as in REM sleep, the discharge of pontine respiratory neurons was significantly decreased during the cholinergically evoked REM sleep-like state (64).

The decreased discharge of parabrachial neurons was observed during the cholinergically induced REM sleep-like state caused by pontine administration of carbachol or evoked by microinjecting the pons with neostigmine (64). These results, combined with the neuroanatomical tracing studies (50,105), convincingly demonstrate synaptically mediated modulation of premotor respiratory neurons evoked from cholinoceptive pontine regions known to play a role in REM sleep generation.

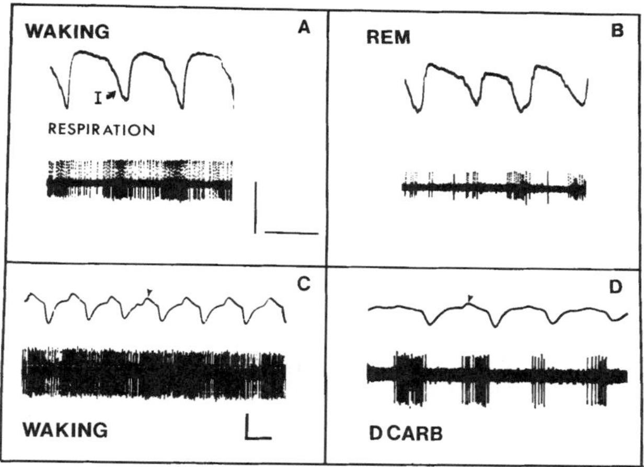

Figure 9. Parabrachial respiratory neuron discharge recorded from cat during wakefulness **(A)** natural REM sleep **(B)** wakefulness **(C)** and the carbachol-induced REM sleep-like state **(D).** In each frame the upper waveform indicates respiration with an *arrow* marking the inspiratory (I) portion of the respiratory cycle. The extracellular discharge of a single respiratory neuron is shown below the airflow trace. Note that with the transition from wakefulness to REM sleep (A versus B), there was a decrease in parabrachial respiratory neuron discharge. C and D show that with the transition from wakefulness to the carbachol-induced REM sleep-like state, respiratory neuron discharge also diminished. These results indicate that for some respiratory neurons, cell excitability during the cholinergically induced REM sleep-like state parallels cell excitability changes that occur during natural REM sleep. (Reprinted with permission from Gilbert KA, Lydic R. Pontine cholinergic reticular mechanisms cause state-dependent changes in the discharge of parabrachial neurons. *Am J Physiol* 1994;266:R136–R150.)

During our microdialysis studies of the relationship between pontine ACh release and states of consciousness, we also quantified the relationship between ACh release and rate of breathing. The results revealed that during the cholinergically induced REM sleep-like state, ACh release in the medial pontine reticular formation accounted for 86% of the variance in respiratory frequency (118). These findings encouraged us to examine the respiratory effect of electrically stimulating cholinergic cells in the LDT/PPT that are known to provide ACh to the medial pontine reticular formation. Consistent with the earlier finding of a significant correlation between respiratory rate depression and ACh release (118), increasing levels of LDT/PPT stimulation caused increasing depression of rate of breathing while increasing the release of ACh in the medial pontine reticular formation (114).

These microdialysis and breathing studies suggest that it would be worthwhile to obtain a better understanding of the transmembrane signal transduction processes regulating ACh release in the pons. Our understanding of respiratory depression during sleep and anesthesia would be advanced if we knew more about the cellular mechanisms that cause LDT/PPT neurons to increase their discharge frequency and thereby increase pontine ACh release during REM sleep. It is known that the cholinergic neurons in the LDT/PPT stain positively for the enzyme NADPH-diaphorase. It is also known that in many brain regions neuronal NADPH-diaphorase is a reliable marker for nitric oxide synthase (NOS). Nitric oxide is a diffusible cellular messenger produced when NOS converts L-arginine to L-citrulline. These facts (for citations, see ref. 108) encouraged us to test the hypothesis that NOS participates in regulating ACh release within the medial pontine reticular formation.

Our initial test of this hypothesis used microdialysis to deliver the NOS inhibitor N^G-nitro-L-arginine (NLA) to the pontine reticular formation and to simultaneously measure ACh release. The results (Fig. 10) show that the NOS inhibitor NLA

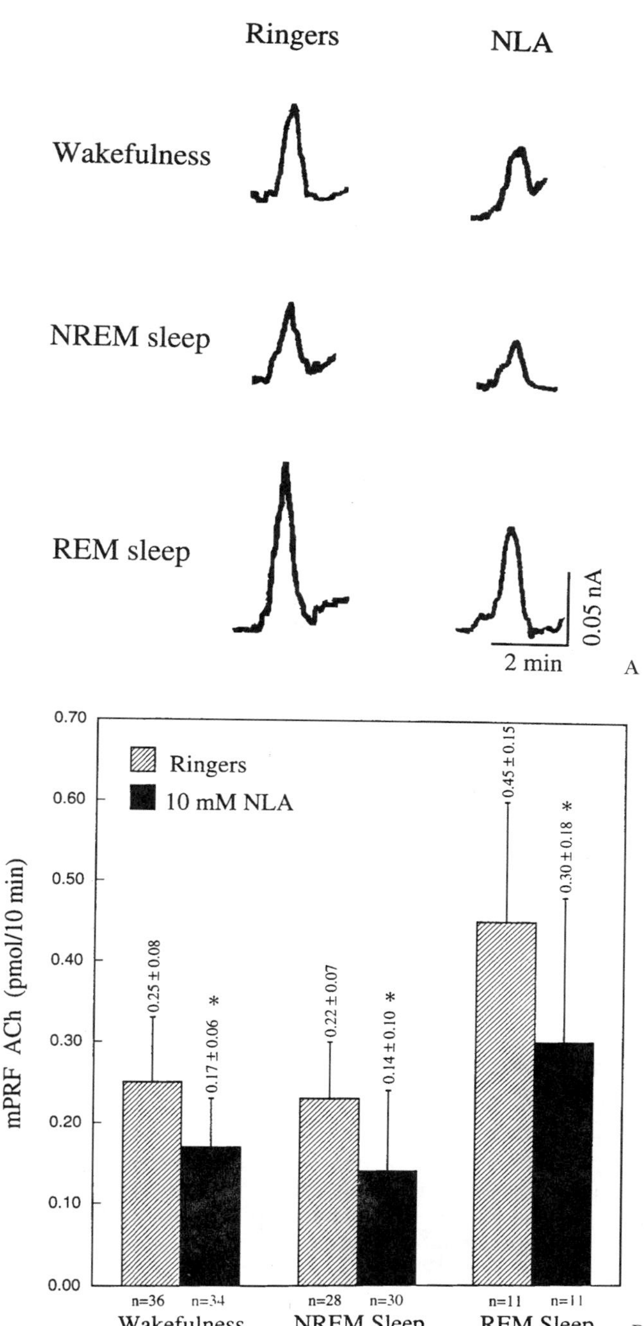

Figure 10. **(A)** Chromatograms represent ACh release in the medial pontine reticular formation during wakefulness, non-REM (NREM) sleep, and REM sleep during dialysis with Ringers alone (control) and with Ringers containing 10 mM N^G-nitro-L-arginine (NLA), a known nitric oxide synthase (NOS) inhibitor. **(B)** Bar graph shows mean and standard deviation acetylcholine release in the medial pontine reticular formation (mPRF) during sleep and wakefulness without (Ringers) and with (NLA) inhibition of nitric oxide synthase. These data indicate that nitric oxide is involved in regulating acetylcholine release in the medial pontine reticular formation. (Reprinted with permission from Leonard TO, Lydic R. Nitric oxide synthase inhibition decreases pontine acetylcholine release. *NeuroReport* 1995;6:1525–1529.)

significantly decreased ACh release in the medial pontine reticular formation (108).

Because pontine ACh is known to be involved in REM sleep generation, the results in Fig. 10 identify for the first time a brain region (the medial pontine reticular formation) and components of a transmembrane signal transduction pathway (NOS-nitric oxide-ACh) through which nitric oxide might contribute to the control of sleep and wakefulness. These results also encourage future studies designed to determine if nitric oxide plays a role in modulating state-dependent respiratory depression caused by pontine cholinergic mechanisms.

Cholinergic Initiation of Motor Atonia

REM sleep is characterized by pronounced motor atonia. The atonia of REM sleep is present in all somatic muscles except for extraocular and some respiratory muscles. During the motor atonia of REM sleep, intracellular recordings from spinal α-motoneurons have revealed bombardment by inhibitory postsynaptic potentials (IPSPs) (140). Microinjection of cholinergic agonists into the medial pontine reticular formation has long been known to cause atonia, and electrically stimulating the pontine reticular formation during REM sleep hyperpolarizes lumbar motoneurons (61). Neurons in the medial pontine reticular formation activate medullary inhibitory neurons in nucleus gigantocellularis which, in turn, provide an inhibitory input to spinal α-motoneurons (30, 103). Microinjection of carbachol into the medial pontine reticular formation also has been shown to cause IPSPs that are indistinguishable from the IPSPs recorded from α-motoneurons during natural REM sleep (142).

Many anesthetic agents decrease muscle tone, and a better understanding of the mechanisms causing state-dependent inhibition of motor tone also has potential clinical relevance for sleep apnea and narcolepsy. These clinical implications have stimulated considerable research aiming to specify the neurons and neurotransmitter systems causing state-dependent atonia. This research aims to determine whether atonia results from active postsynaptic inhibition versus the removal of excitatory input, a process referred to as disfacilitation. Active inhibition is thought to be the mechanism by which spinal motoneurons are inactivated during REM sleep. Spinal α-motoneurons are known to receive inhibitory input from a group of spinal interneurons called Renshaw cells. Since Renshaw cells also are inhibited during the cholinergically induced REM sleep-like state, Renshaw cells are unlikely to contribute to state-dependent hyperpolarization of α-motoneurons (141). The inhibitory amino acid glycine has been shown to mediate the lumbar spinal IPSPs of REM sleep (31, 186). In contrast, data have been presented indicating that postsynaptic inhibition during cholinergically induced atonia is not observed for hypoglossal motoneurons (99). State-dependent decreases in hypoglossal neuron excitability were suggested to result from removal of serotonergic excitatory drive, or disfacilitation (101).

Two important findings have come from efforts to understand cholinergically induced postsynaptic hyperpolarization of motoneurons. First, is the finding that active inhibition also is observed in digastric jaw-opener motoneurons which, like hypoglossal motoneurons, provide nonantigravity functions distinctly different from lumbar motoneurons (153). These and additional data suggest that pontine cholinoceptive reticular neurons activate parvocellular, medullary reticular formation neurons which provide glycinergic inhibition of brain stem and spinal motoneurons. Furthermore, state-dependent motoneuron hyperpolarization is likely to result from two processes: postsynaptic inhibition as well as disfacilitation (for a review, see ref. 153).

A second important finding concerns advances in understanding the role of serotonin (5-HT) as a modulator of both arousal state and motoneuron excitability. Serotonergic raphe neurons in the brain stem have excitatory effects on spinal motoneurons (60). Serotonin enhances motoneurons innervating the upper airway (for a review, see ref. 150), and these 5-HT effects are likely to be relevant for efforts to understand mechanisms regulating airway patency during anesthesia. Multiple lines of evidence suggest that one such mechanism facilitating respiratory motoneurons is serotonergic neurotransmission. Serotonin containing neurons in the pontine and medullary raphe nuclei exhibit firing rates that are positively correlated with arousal, and serotonergic neurons in the dorsal raphe nucleus cease discharging during REM sleep (187). This fact led to the suggestion some years ago that loss of aminergic drive during REM sleep could contribute to sleep apnea syndrome (see Table 4 of ref. 72). Of direct relevance to the concept of a wakefulness stimulus for breathing, was the prediction that "a leading candidate for neurons that mediate the stimulating effect of wakefulness on respiration includes serotonin-containing cells in the brain stem raphe nuclei" (110). As reviewed in detail elsewhere (150), electrophysiological recordings (99,101) and direct neurochemical measurements (100) now have demonstrated facilitatory effects of serotonin on upper airway motoneurons. Figure 11 illustrates the ability of microinjecting cholinergic agonists into the medial pontine reticular formation to cause decreased hypoglossal 5-HT release and decreased motor tone.

The likelihood that state-dependent hyperpolarization of motoneurons is the result of both active inhibition (glycinergic IPSPs) and disfacilitation (decreased 5-HT) also is consistent with the finding that motoneuron hyperpolarization occurred in temporal association with ponto-geniculo-occipital (PGO) waves (153). PGO waves are high-amplitude (300 μV, 100 ms) field potentials recorded from the thalamus. PGO waves appear as single spikes during NREM sleep just before REM sleep onset, and bursts of PGO waves (8/s) are one of the hallmark electrographic signs of REM sleep (27). Studies quantifying the firing rate of neurons in the serotonergic dorsal raphe nucleus have shown the time-course of raphe discharge to be inversely correlated with the onset of PGO waves (124,125). Thus, the association in time between motoneuron hyperpolarization and the occurrence of PGO waves (153) is consistent with evidence suggesting that motoneuron disfacilitation during REM sleep is due to reductions in serotonergic drive. It will be important for future studies to determine how the foregoing data concerning mechanisms of REM sleep atonia are similar to, and different from, anesthetically induced mechanisms causing motor atonia.

Cholinergic Modulation of Pain

Reticular formation regulation of pain sensation is humbling in its complexity, beyond the scope of this chapter, and addressed elsewhere (20,52,53,69,159). Within the spinal cord, >50 neurotransmitters and peptides have been localized and ACh is present in primary afferent fibers, intrinsic spinal neurons, and in descending fibers of supraspinal origin (19). The purpose of this section is to highlight evidence demonstrating the functional interaction between cholinergic modulation of nociception and cholinergic regulation of behavioral states.

Cholinergic brain mechanisms have long been known to modulate pain perception and to interact with opioids (154,183). Electrophysiological data demonstrate that opioids inhibit the excitability of peribrachial cholinergic neurons in the pedunculopontine tegmental nuclei (179). These are the same cells described above (see LDT/PPT) for their role in regulating ACh release, sleep, and state-dependent respiratory depression (114). Additional reviews note that it has been >50 years since the first demonstration that administering the acetylcholinesterase inhibitor physostigmine increases pain threshold in humans (71). Intrathecal administration of the cholinergic

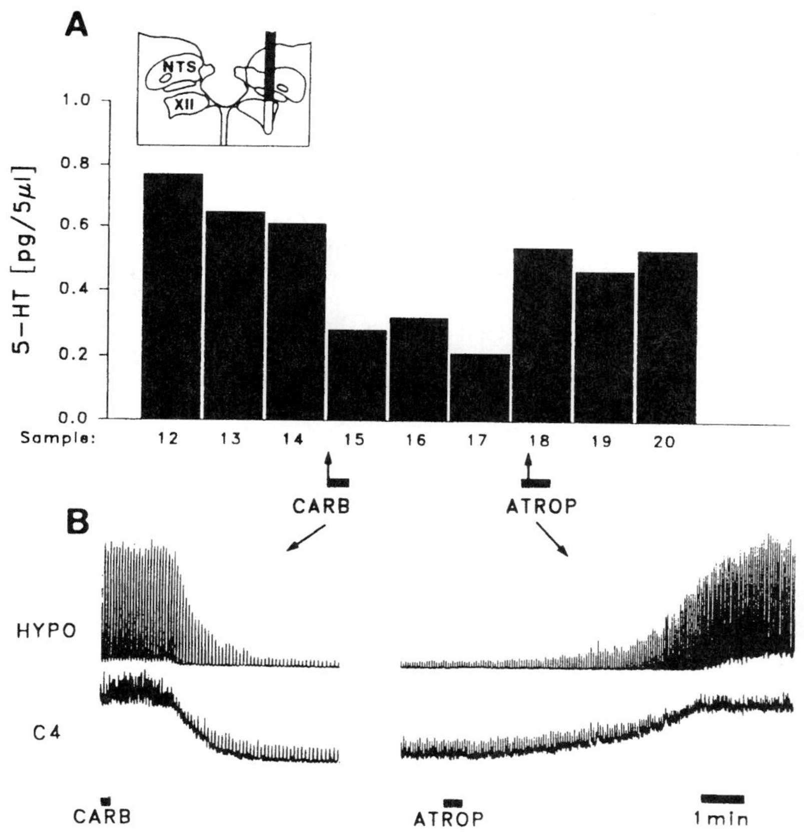

Figure 11. Serotonin (5-HT) levels in the hypoglossal XII nucleus **(A)** and electrical activity from hypoglossal (HYPO) and postural C4 nerve **(B).** Note that pontine microinjection of carbachol (CARB) decreased 5-HT release in XII nucleus and nerve traffic in XII nerve and nerve (C4) to postural muscles. The muscarinic cholinergic antagonist atropine (ATROP) when injected in pons restored XII nerve activity. These data emphasize the importance of 5-HT as a contributor to state-dependent depression of upper airway muscle activity. [Reprinted, in adapted form, with permission from (100)].

agonist carbachol (65,198), and spinal delivery of the acetylcholinesterase inhibitor neostigmine have been shown to produce analgesia and sedation (74,199). The ability of cholinergic agents to modulate nociception offers the potential clinical benefit of improved analgesia, while minimizing undesirable side effects such as opioid-induced respiratory depression (185,195). Clearly the effect of acetylcholinesterase inhibitors depends on the site of administration since studies noted above have shown that microinjecting neostigmine into the medial pontine reticular formation causes a REM sleep-like state (9).

Textbooks on pain management acknowledge the clinically important interaction between pain and sleep disruption. In discussing the physiological and behavioral effects of chronic pain, Bonica notes that "sleep disturbances are the most common complaint among patients with continuous chronic pain" (23). This follows from a fact understood by anyone who has experienced unrelenting discomfort: pain creates a unique behavioral state known to significantly disrupt normal states of consciousness (143,159).

A particularly exciting area for future research concerns efforts to better understand the interaction between cholinergic modulation of nociception, affective states, and sleep. We have previously reviewed evidence showing that some forms of depression appear to result from increased cholinergic and/or decreased aminergic activity (72). Depressed affect is a well-known problem associated with chronic pain and the severity of pain has been shown to predict future depression (173). Furthermore, the causal relationship between behavioral state control and nociception is reciprocal since depression and negative emotional states also have been shown to exacerbate the perception of pain (107).

One of the best examples of efforts to understand the interaction between pain and natural sleep comes from studies of fibromyalgia. The syndrome of fibromyalgia is characterized by musculoskeletal pain with local tenderness elicited at sensitive points of palpation. Fibromyalgia patients exhibit a nonrestorative sleep pattern characterized by feeling unrefreshed and fatigued following a night of sleep. Moldofsky et al. (139) have shown the EEG of fibromyalgia patients to be characterized by intrusion of fast frequency EEG into the slow frequency EEG of normal NREM sleep. Nonrestorative sleep syndrome can be triggered or exacerbated by interference with the immune system, acute febrile illness, and stress (139), all common in the perioperative setting. Interestingly, some fibromyalgia patients have been reported to have altered serotonin metabolism, although the central nervous system contributions to this syndrome remain poorly understood (for a review, see ref. 129).

The suggested relevance of serotonin in fibromyalgia also is of interest because of long-standing hypotheses that the ratio of aminergic-to-cholinergic neurotransmission contributes to NREM/REM sleep cycle generation (for reviews, see refs. 72,187). Stimulation of 5-HT–containing neurons causes EEG and behavioral arousal, and electrophysiological studies of the dorsal raphe have shown that the loss of waking consciousness parallels the cessation of raphe neuron discharge (123–125). Measurement of 5-HT in dorsal raphe recently has shown that the DRN discharge profiles are directly paralleled by extracellular 5-HT concentration (158). Thus, in contrast to acetylcholine levels, which are higher during waking and during REM sleep, 5-HT levels are elevated only during waking and reach their lowest values during REM sleep. In addition to data showing a clear relationship between 5-HT and state of consciousness, microinjection of the cholinergic agonist carbachol into the serotonergic raphe produces antinociception from pontine raphe dorsalis (92) and hypoalgesia via spinally projecting neurons in medullary raphe magnus (26). These findings are illustrative of many studies showing that bulbospinal serotonergic (18) and noradrenergic (21) systems play a major role in analgesia. Thus, efforts to systematically characterize the cholinergic reticular modulation of pain and behavioral states must also consider the role of monoamines.

Parabrachial regions of the pontine brain stem contain catecholaminergic and cholinergic neurons known to modulate sleep and breathing (64). Parabrachial neurons are adjacent to and intermingled with peribrachial cholinergic neurons modulating the generation of EEG sleep spindles (188). As noted elsewhere (127), converging lines of evidence suggest that cholinergic mechanisms in the parabrachial pons also mediate the interaction between respiration and pain. Increased rate of breathing is a common response to painful stimuli (45) and pain-induced changes in respiratory rate are likely to be influenced by the parabrachial nuclei (17). Clinical evidence has shown that electrical stimulation of the parabrachial region in humans produces relief from morphine-resistant pain (83) and parabrachial administration of cholinergic agonists elicits analgesia in cat (84).

Considered together, these data emphasize the importance of future studies designed to specify the role of muscarinic cholinergic receptor subtypes in the reticular formation contributing to the regulation of pain perception. The finding that muscarinic receptors mediate the analgesia resulting from spinal cholinesterase administration (145), provides a rather clear answer to questions of whether muscarinic receptor subtypes have a place in clinical anesthesia (104). Efforts to localize muscarinic cholinergic receptor subtypes in brain stem regions regulating states of consciousness (8) and breathing (127) have been successful. Most recently, receptor binding studies are showing the presence of M2, M3, and M4, but not M1, muscarinic receptor subtypes in the dorsal horn of rat thoracic spinal cord (73). Muscarinic receptor subtype localization also encourages ongoing and future efforts to elucidate the mechanism of transmembrane cell signaling that contribute to the cholinergic control of consciousness (108,182) and sensation of pain (77).

CONCLUSION

The information conveyed in this chapter has sought to deemphasize the artificial choice between reductionistic (restricting the study of consciousness to the level of cell membranes) and integrative (seeking to understand the assortment of neuronal mechanisms generating complex behavioral states) neuroscience. A pluralistic incorporation of both reductionistic and integrative research paradigms appears most productive for elucidating the brain mechanisms regulating sleep and anesthesia. Such an approach is incorporative rather than exclusionary and conceptually liberalizing rather than restrictive. The appropriateness of a pluralistic approach also is supported by the literature showing that studies of the mechanisms of anesthetic action (2) are neither synonymous or at odds with studies of the sites of anesthetic action (59). All experimental models have a limited domain of validity. Appreciating the distinction between sites and mechanisms of behavioral state control offers the potential for unifying reductionistic and integrative experimental models. Such a unification, through a mechanistic deconstruction of states into their component traits, has two key advantages. First, it acknowledges the humbling complexity of behavioral states. Second, applying the armamentaria of neuroscience to the study of physiological and behavioral traits offers a viable alternative to monoideational, and we believe naive, attempts to discover a single mechanism regulating consciousness.

Parallels and distinctions are both appropriate when considering sleep and anesthesia. We hypothesize that brain mechanisms which have evolved to regulate naturally occurring loss of wakefulness are preferentially involved in generating some of the physiological and behavioral traits comprising anesthetically induced loss of waking consciousness. This chapter has summarized some of the data in support of this hypothesis. Furthermore, this chapter has asserted that the foregoing hypothesis is compatible with the fact that sleep and anesthesia are distinctly different states. Equating sleep and anesthesia belies the complexity of behavioral state control, as is easily illustrated. Subtle trait differences can produce drastically different states (78,126), yet two very different states of consciousness can have similar physiological traits. The EEG of wakefulness, for example, is indistinguishable from the EEG of REM sleep (72,187). Equating sleep and anesthesia also denigrates the complex clinical skills required for the practice of anesthesia. Patients are commonly misinformed that "anesthesia will put them to sleep," while in veterinary medicine "having one's pet put to sleep" is euthanasia. Patients, other health professionals, and anesthesia as a discipline, are not well served by euphemisms. Modern anesthesia includes the obliteration of consciousness but, more impressively, maintenance of all life support systems followed by restoration of normal, waking consciousness. This indemnification against pain and suffering, followed by revitalization, is more accurately conveyed by the French description of *anesthésie et réanimation* and by Italian departments with names like *Instituto di Anesthesiologia e Rianimazione.*

This chapter has focused on the regulation of behavioral states by cholinergic neurotransmission within the pontine reticular formation. All evidence to date suggests that no state of consciousness is generated by any single brain region or neurotransmitter. There is widespread agreement, however, that pontine cholinergic neurotransmission plays a major role in regulating states of consciousness. Understanding how ACh interacts with other transmitters to generate physiological traits offers an exciting opportunity for future studies aiming to elucidate the control of behavioral states. And it could be, as Paton suggested (152), "that the analysis of the action of that group of drugs that selectively suspends consciousness may turn out to be the path to understanding the neurological substrate of consciousness itself."

Acknowledgment: We gratefully acknowledge the support of J. F. Biebuyck and the Department of Anesthesia. For expert secretarial assistance, we thank P. Myers. Original work described in this chapter was made possible by grant support from the National Institutes of Health MH-45361 (HAB) and HL-40881 (RL).

REFERENCES

1. Albers EA, Liou SY, Stopa EG, Zoeller RT. Neurotransmitter colocalization and circadian rhythms. *Prog Brain Res* 1992;92:289–307.
2. Angel A. Central neuronal pathways and the process of anaesthesia. *Br J Anaesth* 1993;71:148–163.
3. Antognini JF, Schwartz K. Exaggerated anesthetic requirements in the preferentially anesthetized brain. *Anesthesiology* 1993;79:1244–1249.
4. Aserinsky E, Kleitman N. Regularly occurring periods of eye motility, and concomitant phenomena, during sleep. *Science* 1953;118:273–274.
5. Baghdoyan HA. Anesthesia. In: Carskadon MA, eds. *Encyclopedia of sleep and dreaming.* New York: Macmillan, 1993:35–37.
6. Baghdoyan HA, Carlson BX, Roth MT. Pharmacological characterization of muscarinic receptors in cat pons and cortex. *Pharmacology* 1994;48:77–85.
7. Baghdoyan HA, Lydic R, Callaway CW, Hobson JA. The carbachol-induced enhancement of desynchronized sleep signs is dose-dependent and antagonized by centrally administered atropine. *Neuropsychopharmacology* 1989;2:67–79.
8. Baghdoyan HA, Mallios VJ, Duckrow RB, Mash DC. Localization of muscarinic receptor subtypes in brain stem areas regulating sleep. *NeuroReport* 1994;5:1631–1634.
9. Baghdoyan HA, Monaco AP, Rodrigo-Angulo ML, Assens ML, McCarley RW, Hobson JA. Microinjection of neostigmine into the pontine reticular formation of cats enhances desynchronized sleep signs. *J Pharmacol Exp Ther* 1984;231:173–180.
10. Baghdoyan HA, Rodrigo-Angulo ML, McCarley RW, Hobson JA. Site-specific enhancement and suppression of desynchronized sleep signs following cholinergic stimulation of three brain stem regions. *Brain Res* 1984;396:39–52.

11. Baghdoyan HA, Rodrigo-Angulo ML, McCarley RW, Hobson JA. A neuroanatomical gradient in the pontine tegmentum for the cholinoceptive induction of desynchronized sleep signs. *Brain Res* 1987;414:245–261.
12. Baghdoyan HA, Spotts JL, Snyder SG. Sleep cycle alterations following simultaneous pontine and forebrain injections of carbachol. *J Neurosci* 1993;13:227–240.
13. Barash PG, Cullen BF, Stoelting RK, eds. *Clinical anesthesia.* 2nd ed. Philadelphia: Lippincott, 1992.
14. Baxter BL. Induction of both emotional behavior and a novel form of REM sleep by chemical stimulation applied to cat mesencephalon. *Exp Neurol* 1969;23:220–229.
15. Becker L, Baghdoyan HA, Lydic R. Acetylcholine release in the medial pontine reticular formation (mPRF) increases during natural rapid eye movement (REM) sleep. *Soc Neurosci Abstracts* 1994; 20:82.
16. Bernard C. *Lectures on anesthetics and on asphyxia.* Park Ridge, IL: Wood Library-Museum/Paris: Bailliere, 1989.
17. Bernard JF, Besson J-M. The spino(trigemino)pontoamygdaloid pathway: electrophysiological evidence for an involvement in pain processes. *J Neurophysiol* 1990;63:473–490.
18. Besson J-M, ed. *Serotonin and Pain.* Elsevier: Excerpta Medica, 1990.
19. Besson J-M. The pharmacology of pain: twenty-five years of hope, despair, and hope. In: Gebhart GF, Hammond DL, Jensen TS, eds. *Proceedings of the 7th World Congress on Pain.* Seattle: IASP Press, 1994: 23–39.
20. Besson J-M, Chaouch A. Peripheral and spinal mechanisms of nociception. *Physiol Rev* 1987;67:67–186.
21. Besson J-M, Guilbaud G, eds. *Towards the use of noradrenergic agonists for the treatment of pain.* Elsevier: Excerpta Medica, 1992.
22. Biebuyck JF. Anesthesia and sleep: a search for mechanisms and research approaches. In: Lydic R, Biebuyck JF, eds. *Clinical physiology of sleep.* Bethesda: American Physiological Society, 1988: 221–228.
23. Bonica JJ. General considerations of chronic pain. In: Bonica JJ, ed. *The management of pain.* 2nd ed. Philadelphia: Lea & Febiger, 1990: 180–196.
24. Bonica JJ, McDonald JS, eds. *Principles and practice of obstetric analgesia and anesthesia.* Baltimore: Williams & Wilkins, 1995.
25. Bourgin P, Escourrou P, Gaultier C, Adrien J. Induction of rapid eye movement sleep by carbachol infusion into the pontine reticular formation in the rat. *NeuroReport* 1995;6:532–536.
26. Brodie MS, Proudfit HK. Hypoalgesia induced by the local injection of carbachol into the nucleus raphe magnus. *Brain Res* 1984; 291:337–342.
27. Callaway CW, Lydic R, Baghdoyan HA, Hobson JA. Pontogeniculooccipital waves: spontaneous visual system activity during rapid eye movement sleep. *Cell Mol Neurobiol* 1987;7:105–149.
28. Campbell SS, Tobler I. Animal sleep: a review of sleep duration across phylogeny. *Neurosci Biobehav Rev* 1984;8:269–300.
29. Celesia GG, Jasper HH. Acetylcholine released from cerebral cortex in relation to state of activation. *Neurology* 1966;16:1053–1064.
30. Chase MH. Synaptic mechanisms and circuitry involved in motoneuron control during sleep. *Int Rev Neurobiol* 1983;24: 213–258.
31. Chase MH, Soja PJ, Morales FR. Evidence that glycine mediates the postsynaptic potentials that inhibit lumbar motoneurons during the atonia of active sleep. *J Neurosci* 1989;9:743–751.
32. Churchland PS. *Neurophilosophy: toward a unified science of the mind-brain.* Cambridge: MIT Press, 1986.
33. Connolly LA. Anesthetic management of obstructive sleep apnea patients. *J Clin Anesth* 1991;3:461–469.
34. Cordeau J, Moreau A, Beaulnes A, Laurin C. EEG and behavioral changes following microinjections of acetylcholine and adrenaline in the brain stem of cats. *Arch Ital Biol* 1963;101:30–47.
35. Cravatt BF, Prospero-Garcia O, Siuzdak G, Gilala NB, Henriksen SJ, Boger DL, Lerner RA. Chemical characterization of a family of brain lipids that induce sleep. *Science* 1995; 268:1506–1509.
36. Cronin A, Keifer JC, Baghdoyan HA, Lydic R. Narcotic inhibition of rapid eye movement sleep induced by a specific mu receptor agonist. *Br J Anaesth* 1995;74:188–192.
37. Damsma G, Fibiger HC. The effects of anaesthesia and hypothermia on interstitial concentrations of acetylcholine and choline in rat striatum. *Life Sci* 1991;48:2469–2474.
38. Davies DW, Hawkins RA, Mans AM, Hibbard LS, Biebuyck JF. Regional cerebral glucose utilization during althesin anesthesia. *Anesthesiology* 1984;61:362–368.
39. Davies DW, Mans AM, Biebuyck JF, Hawkins RA. Regional brain glucose utilization in rats during etomidate anesthesia. *Anesthesiology* 1986;64:751–757.
40. Davies DW, Mans AM, Biebuyck JF, Hawkins RA. The influence of ketamine on regional brain glucose use. *Anesthesiology* 1988;69: 199–205.
41. Dedrick DF, Scherer YD, Biebuyck JF. Use of a rapid brain-sampling technique in a physiologic preparation: effects of morphine, ketamine, and halothane on tissue energy intermediates. *Anesthesiology* 1975;42:651–657.
42. Dement W, Henry P, Cohen H, Ferguson J. Studies on the effect of REM deprivation in humans and animals. *Res Publications ARNMD* 1965;45:456–468.
43. Dement WC, Mitler M. It's time to wake up to the importance of sleep disorders. *JAMA* 1993;269:1548–1550.
44. Dilger JP, Firestone LL. More models described for molecular "target" of anesthetics and alcohols. *Trends Pharmacol* 1990;11: 431–432.
45. Duranti R, Pantaleo T, Belinni F, Bongianni F, Scano G. Respiratory responses induced by the activation of somatic nociceptive afferents in humans. *J Appl Physiol* 1991;71:2440–2448.
46. Edgar DM, Dement WC, Fuller CA. Effect of SCN lesions on sleep in squirrel monkeys: evidence for opponent process in sleep-wake regulation. *J Neurosci* 1993;13:1065–1079.
47. Eger EI, Saidman LJ, Brandstater B. Minimum alveolar anesthetic concentration: a standard of anesthetic potency. *Anesthesiology* 1965;26:756–763.
48. El Mansari M, Sakai K, Jouvet M. Unitary characteristics of presumptive cholinergic tegmental neurons during the sleep-waking cycle in freely moving cats. *Exp Brain Res* 1989;76:519–529.
49. El Mansari M, Sakai K, Jouvet M. Responses of presumed cholinergic mesopontine tegmental neurons to carbachol microinjections in freely moving cats. *Exp Brain Res* 1990;83:115–123.
50. Fay R, Gilbert KA, Lydic R. Pontomedullary neurons transsynaptically labeled by laryngeal pseudorabies virus. *NeuroReport* 1993;5: 141–144.
51. Feldman JL. Neurophysiology of breathing in mammals. In: *Handbook of physiology. The nervous system. Intrinsic regulatory systems of the brain. Sect. 1, vol. IV.* Bethesda, MD: American Physiological Society, 1986:463–524.
52. Fields HL, Besson J-M, eds. *Pain modulation.* Amsterdam: Elsevier, 1988.
53. Fields HL, Liebeskind JC, eds. *Pharmacological approaches to the treatment of chronic pain: new concepts and critical issues.* Seattle: International Association for the Study of Pain, 1994.
54. Fink BR. Influence of cerebral activity in wakefulness on regulation of breathing. *J Appl Physiol* 1961;16:15–20.
55. Fink BR, Hanks EC, Ngai SH, Papper EM. Central regulation of respiration during anesthesia and wakefulness. *Ann NY Acad Sci* 1963;109:892–900.
56. Fink BR, Katz R, Reinhold H, Schoolman A. Suprapontine mechanisms in regulation of respiration. *Am J Physiol* 1962;202:217–220.
57. Fitzgerald RS, Gautier H, Lahiri S, eds. *The regulation of respiration during sleep and anesthesia.* New York: Plenum Press, 1978.
58. Fragen RJ, Avram MJ. Nonopioid intravenous anesthetics. In: Barash PG, Cullen BF, Stoelting RK, eds. *Clinical anesthesia.* 2nd ed. Philadelphia: Lippincott, 1992:385–412.
59. Franks NP, Lieb WR. Molecular and cellular mechanisms of general anaesthesia. *Nature* 1994;367:607–614.
60. Fung SJ, Barnes CD. Raphe-produced excitation of spinal cord motoneurons in the cat. *Neurosci Lett* 1989;103:185–190.
61. Fung SJ, Boxer P, Morales FR, Chase M. Hyperpolarizing membrane responses induced in lumbar motoneurons by stimulation of the nucleus reticularis pontis oralis during active sleep. *Brain Res* 1982;248:267–273.
62. George R, Haslett WL, Jenden DL. A cholinergic mechanism in the brain stem reticular formation: induction of paradoxical sleep. *Int J Neuropharmacol* 1964;3:541–552.
63. Ghoneim MM, Block RI. Learning and consciousness during general anesthesia. *Anesthesiology* 1992;76:279–305.
64. Gilbert KA, Lydic R. Pontine cholinergic reticular mechanisms cause state-dependent changes in the discharge of parabrachial neurons. *Am J Physiol* 1994;266:R136–R150.
65. Gillberg PG, Gordh T, Hartvig P, Jansson I, Pettersson J. Characterization of the antinociception induced by intrathecally administered carbachol. *Pharmacol Toxicol* 1989;64:340–343.
66. Gillin JC, Salin-Pascual R, Velazquez-Moctezuma J, Shiromani P,

Zoltoski R. Cholinergic receptor subtypes and REM sleep in animals and normal controls. *Prog Brain Res* 1993;98:379–387.
67. Greene RW, Hass HL, Gerber U, McCarley RW. Cholinergic activation of medial pontine reticular formation neurons in vitro. In: Frotscher M, Misgeld U, eds. *Central cholinergic synaptic transmission.* Boston: Birkhauser, 1989:123–137.
68. Griffiths R, Norman RI. Effects of anaesthetics on uptake, synthesis, and release of transmitters. *Br J Anaesth* 1993;71:96–107.
69. Guilbaud G, Bernard JF, Besson J-M. Brain areas involved in nociception and pain. In: Wall PD, Melzack R, eds. *Textbook of pain.* 3rd ed. Edinburgh: Churchill Livingstone, 1994:113–128.
70. Hanning CD, Aitkenhead AR. Sleep, depth of anaesthesia and awareness. In: Nimmo WS, Rowbotham DJ, Smith G, eds. *Anaesthesia.* Oxford: Blackwell Scientific, 1994:3–20.
71. Harvig P, Gillberg PG, Gordh T, Post C. Cholinergic mechanisms in pain and analgesia. *Trends Pharmacol Sci* 1989;10:75–79.
72. Hobson JA, Lydic R, Baghdoyan HA. Evolving concepts of sleep cycle generation: from brain centers to neuronal populations. *Behav Brain Res* 1986;9:371–448.
73. Hoglund AU, Baghdoyan HA. M2, M3 and M4 but not M1 muscarinic receptor are in rat thoracic spinal cord *J Pharmacol Exp Ther* 1997;281:470–477.
74. Hood DD, Eisenach JC, Tuttle R. Phase I safety assessment of intrathecal neostigmine methylsulfate in humans. *Anesthesiology* 1995;82:331–343.
75. Hornbein T. Anesthetics and ventilatory control. In: Covino BG, Fozzard HA, Rehder K, Strichartz G, eds. *Effects of anesthetics.* Bethesda: American Physiological Society, 1985:75–80.
76. Hug CG. Does opioid "anesthesia" exist? *Anesthesiology* 1990;73: 1–4.
77. Iwamoto ET, Marion L. Pharmacologic evidence that spinal muscarinic analgesia is mediated by an L-argine/nitric oxide/cyclic GMP cascade in rats. *J Pharmacol Exp Ther* 1994;271:601–608.
78. Jones JG. Memory of intraoperative events. *Br Med J* 1994;15: 967–968.
79. Jouvet M. Recherches sur les structures nerveuses et les mechanismes responsables des differentes phases du sommeil physiologique. *Arch Ital Biol* 1962;100:125–206.
80. Jouvet M. The role of monoamines and acetylcholine containing neurons in the regulation of the sleep waking cycle. *Rev Physiol* 1972;64:225.
81. Kandel ER, Schwartz JH, Jessell TM. *Principles of neural science.* 3rd ed. New York: Elsevier, 1991.
82. Karczewski WA, Grieb P, Kulesza J. *Control of breathing during sleep and anesthesia.* New York: Plenum Press, 1988.
83. Katayama Y, Tsubokawa T, Hirayama T, Yamamoto T. Pain relief following stimulation of the pontomesencephalic parabrachial region in humans: brain sites for nonopiate-mediated pain control. *Appl Neurophysiol* 1985;48:195–200.
84. Katayama Y, Watkins LR, Becker DP, Hayes RL. Non-opiate analgesia induced by carbachol microinjection into the pontine parabrachial region of the cat. *Brain Res* 1984;269:263–283.
85. Kay DC, Eisenstein RB, Jasinski DR. Morphine effects on human REM state, waking state, and NREM sleep. *Psychopharmacologia* 1969;14:404–416.
86. Keifer JC, Baghdoyan HA, Becker L, Lydic R. Halothane decreases pontine acetylcholine release and increases EEG spindles. *NeuroReport* 1994;5:577–580.
87. Keifer JC, Baghdoyan HA, Lydic R. Sleep disruption and increased apneas after pontine microinjection of morphine. *Anesthesiology* 1992;77:973–982.
88. Keifer JC, Baghdoyan HA, Lydic R. Pontine cholinergic mechanisms modulate the cortical EEG spindles of halothane anesthesia. *Anesthesiology* 1996;84:945–954.
89. Kendig JJ. Spinal cord as a site of anesthetic action. *Anesthesiology* 1993;79:1161–1162.
90. Kirby RP, Gravenstein N, eds. *Clinical anesthesia practice.* Philadelphia: Saunders, 1994.
91. Kissin I. General anesthetic action: an obsolete notion? *Anesth Analg* 1993;76:215–218.
92. Klamt JG, Prado WA. Antinociception and behavioral changes induced by carbachol microinjected into identified sites of the rat brain. *Brain Res* 1991;549:9–18.
93. Knill RL, Moote CA, Skinner MI, Rose EA. Anesthesia with abdominal surgery leads to intense REM sleep during the first postoperative week. *Anesthesiology* 1990;73:52–61.
94. Knill RL, Novick T, Vandervoort MK. Postoperative nightmares relate to perioperative opioid therapy. *Can J Anaesth* 1994;41:A24.
95. Koblin D. Mechanisms of action. In: Miller RD, ed. *Anesthesia.* New York: Churchill Livingstone, 1994:67–99.
96. Kofke WA, Hawkins RA, Davies DW, Biebuyck JF. Comparison of the effects of volatile anesthetics on brain glucose metabolism in rats. *Anesthesiology* 1987;66:810–813.
97. Krnjevic K. Chemical transmission and cortical arousal. *Anesthesiology* 1967;28:100–105.
98. Kryger MH, Roth T, Dement WC. *Principles and practice of sleep medicine.* 2nd ed. Philadelphia: WB Saunders, 1994.
99. Kubin L, Kimura H, Tojima H, Davies RO, Pack AI. Suppression of hypoglossal motoneurons during the carbachol-induced atonia of REM sleep is not caused by fast synaptic inhibition. *Brain Res* 1993; 611:300–312.
100. Kubin L, Reignier C, Tojima H, Taguchi O, Pack AI, Davies RO. Changes in serotonin level in the hypoglossal nucleus region during carbachol-induced atonia. *Brain Res* 1994;645:291–302.
101. Kubin L, Tojima H, Davies RO, Pack AI. Serotoninergic excitatory drive to hypoglossal motoneurons in the decerebrate cat. *Neurosci Lett* 1992;139:243–248.
102. Kulli J, Koch C. Does anaesthesia cause loss of consciousness? *Trends Neurosci* 1991;14:6–10.
103. Lai YY, Siegel JM. Medullary regions mediating atonia. *J Neurosci* 1988;8:4790–4796.
104. Lambert DG, Appadu BL. Muscarinic receptor subtypes: do they have a place in clinical anaesthesia? *Br J Anaesth* 1995;74:497–499.
105. Lee LH, Friedman DB, Lydic R. Respiratory nuclei share synaptic connectivity with pontine reticular regions regulating REM sleep. *Am J Physiol* 1995;268:L251–L262.
106. Lehmkuhl P, Prass D, Pichlmayr I. General anesthesia and postnarcotic sleep disorders. *Neuropsychobiology* 1987;18:37–42.
107. Leino P, Magni G. Depressive and distress symptoms as predictors of low back pain, neck-shoulder pain and other musculoskeletal morbidity: a 10-year follow-up of mental industry employees. *Pain* 1993;53:163–169.
108. Leonard TO, Lydic R. Nitric oxide synthase inhibition decreases pontine acetylcholine release. *NeuroReport* 1995;6:1525–1529.
109. Liu D, Thorp S, Aitkenhead AR. Incidence of awareness with recall during general anaesthesia. *Anaesthesia* 1991;46:435–437.
110. Lydic R. State-dependent aspects of regulatory physiology. *FASEB J* 1987;1:6–15.
111. Lydic R. Central pattern-generating neurons and the search for general principles. *FASEB J* 1989;3:2457–2478.
112. Lydic R, Baghdoyan HA. Cholinoceptive pontine reticular mechanisms cause state-dependent changes in respiration. *Neurosci Lett* 1989;102:211–216.
113. Lydic R, Baghdoyan HA. Cholinergic pontine mechanisms causing state-dependent respiratory depression. *News Physiol Sci* 1992; 7:220–224.
114. Lydic R, Baghdoyan HA. Pedunculopontine stimulation alters respiration and increases ACh release in the pontine reticular formation. *Am J Physiol* 1993;264:R544–R554.
115. Lydic R, Baghdoyan HA. The neurobiology of rapid-eye-movement sleep. In: Saunders NA, Sullivan CE, eds. *Sleep and breathing.* 2nd ed. New York: Marcel Dekker, 1994:47–78.
116. Lydic R, Baghdoyan HA, Becker L, Biebuyck JF. Systemic ketamine causes dose-dependent alterations in acetylcholine (ACh) release within the medial pontine reticular formation (mPRF). *Soc Neurosci Abstracts* 1994;20:82.
117. Lydic R, Baghdoyan HA, Hibbard L, Bonyak EV, DeJoseph MR, Hawkins RA. Regional brain glucose metabolism is altered during rapid eye movement sleep in the cat. *J Comp Neurol* 1991;304: 517–529.
118. Lydic R, Baghdoyan HA, Lorinc Z. Microdialysis of cat pons reveals enhanced acetylcholine release during state-dependent respiratory depression. *Am J Physiol* 1991;261:R766–R770.
119. Lydic R, Baghdoyan HA, Wertz R, White DP. Cholinergic reticular mechanisms influence state-dependent ventilatory response to hypercapnia. *Am J Physiol* 1991;261:R738–R746.
120. Lydic R, Baghdoyan HA, Zwillich CW. State-dependent hypotonia in posterior cricoarytenoid muscles of the larynx caused by cholinergic reticular mechanisms. *FASEB J* 1989;3:1625–1631.
121. Lydic R, Biebuyck JF. Sleep neurobiology: relevance for mechanistic studies of anaesthesia. *Br J Anaesth* 1994;72:506–508.
122. Lydic R, Keifer JC, Baghdoyan HA, Becker L. Microdialysis of the pontine reticular formation reveals inhibition of acetylcholine release by morphine. *Anesthesiology* 1993;79:1003–1012.
123. Lydic R, McCarley RW, Hobson JA. Forced activity alters sleep cycle

periodicity and dorsal raphe discharge rhythm. *Am J Physiol* 1984;247:R135–R145.

124. Lydic R, McCarley RW, Hobson JA. Serotonin neurons and sleep. I. Long term recordings of dorsal raphe discharge frequency and PGO waves. *Arch Ital Biol* 1987;125:317–343.
125. Lydic R, McCarley RW, Hobson JA. Serotonin neurons and sleep. II. Time course of dorsal raphe discharge, PGO waves, and behavioral states. *Arch Ital Biol* 1987;126:1–28.
126. Mahowald MW, Schenck CH. Dissociated states of wakefulness and sleep. *Neurology* 1992;42:44–52.
127. Mallios VJ, Lydic R, Baghdoyan HA. Muscarinic receptor subtypes are differentially distributed across brain stem respiratory nuclei. *Am J Physiol* 1995;268:L941–L949.
128. Mansour A, Watson SJ. Anatomical distribution of opioid receptors in mammalians: an overview. In: Herz A, Akil H, Simon EJ, eds. *Handbook of experimental pharmacology. Vol. 104/I. Opioids I.* Berlin: Springer-Verlag, 1993:79–106.
129. McCain GA. Fibromyalgia and myofacial pain. In: Wall PD, Melzack R, eds. *Textbook of pain.* 3rd ed. Edinburgh: Churchill Livingstone, 1994:475–493.
130. McGinty DJ, Drucker-Colin R, Morrison A, Parmeggiani PL, eds. *Brain mechanisms of sleep.* New York: Raven Press, 1985.
131. McNamara SG, Cistulli PA, Sullivan CE, Strohl KP. Clinical aspects of sleep apnea. In: Saunders NA, Sullivan C, eds. *Sleep and breathing.* 2nd ed. New York: Marcel Dekker, 1994:493–528.
132. Merchant-Nancy H, Vazquez J, Aguilar-Roblero R, Drucker-Colin R. c-fos proto-oncogene changes in relation to REM sleep duration. *Brain Res* 1992;579:342–346.
133. Miller KW. Models of consciousness. *Nature* 1986;323:584.
134. Miller RD, ed. *Anesthesia.* 4th ed. New York: Churchill Livingstone, 1994.
135. Mitani A, Ito K, Hallanger AH, Wainer BH, Kataoka K, McCarley RW. Cholinergic projections from the laterodorsal and pedunculopontine tegmental nuclei to the pontine gigantocellular tegmental field in the cat. *Brain Res* 1988;451:397–402.
136. Mitchell JF. The spontaneous and evoked release of acetylcholine from the cerebral cortex. *J Physiol (Lond)* 1963;163:98–116.
137. Mitler MM, Dement WC. Cataplectic-like behavior in cats after microinjections of carbachol in pontine reticular formation. *Brain Res* 1974;68:335–343.
138. Moerman M, Bonke B, Oosting J. Awareness and recall during general anesthesia. *Anesthesiology* 1993;79:454–464.
139. Moldofsky H. Sleep, neuroimmune and neuroendocrine functions in fibromyalgia and chronic fatigue syndrome. *Adv Neuroimmunol* 1995;5:39–76.
140. Morales FR, Boxer P, Chase MH. Behavioral state-specific inhibitory postsynaptic potentials impinge on cat lumbar motoneurons during active sleep. *Exp Neurol* 1987;98:418–435.
141. Morales FR, Engelhardt JK, Pereda AE, Yamuy J, Chase MH. Renshaw cells are inactive during motor inhibition elicited by the pontine microinjection of carbachol. *Neurosci Lett* 1988;86: 289–295.
142. Morales FR, Englehardt JK, Soja PA, Pereda AE. Motoneurons properties during motor inhibition produced by microinjection of carbachol into the pontine reticular formation of the decerebrate cat. *J Neurophysiol* 1987;57:1118–1129.
143. Morris DB. *The culture of pain.* Berkeley: University of California, 1991.
144. Moruzzi G, Magoun HW. Brain stem reticular formation and activation of the EEG. *Electroencephalogr Clin Neurophysiol* 1949;1: 455–473.
145. Naguib M, Yaksh TL. Antinociceptive effects of spinal cholinesterase inhibition and isobolographic analysis of the interaction with μ and α2 receptor systems. *Anesthesiology* 1994;80: 1338–1348.
146. Nicoll RA, Madison DV. General anesthetics hyperpolarize neurons in the vertebrate central nervous system. *Science* 1982;217: 1055–1057.
147. Nunn JF, Utting JE, Brown BR, eds. *General anaesthesia.* London: Buttersworth, 1989.
148. Orem J. Breathing during sleep. In: Davies DG, Barnes CD, eds. *Regulation of ventilation and gas exchange.* New York: Academic Press, 1978:131–166.
149. Orem J. Respiratory neurons and sleep. In: Kryger MH, Roth T, Dement WC, eds. *Principles and practice of sleep medicine.* 2nd ed. Philadelphia: WB Saunders, 1994:177–193.
150. Pack AI. Changes in respiratory motor activity during rapid eye movement sleep. In: Dempsey JA, Pack AI, eds. *Regulation of breathing.* 2nd ed. New York: Marcel Dekker, 1995:983–1010.
151. Papper EM. The state of consciousness: some humanistic considerations. In: Rosen M, Lunn JN, eds. *Consciousness, awareness and pain in general anaesthesia.* London: Butterworth, 1987:10–11.
152. Paton WDM. How far do we understand the mechanism of anaesthesia? *Eur J Anaesthesiol* 1984;1:93–103.
153. Pedroarena C, Castillo P, Chase MH, Morales FR. The control of jaw-opener motoneurons during active sleep. *Brain Res* 1994;653: 31–38.
154. Pert A. Cholinergic and catecholaminergic modulation of nociceptive reactions: interactions with opiates. *Pain Headache* 1987;9: 1–63.
155. Phillipson EA. Regulation of breathing during sleep. *Am Rev Respir Dis* 1977;115:217–224.
156. Phillipson EA. Arousal: the forgotten response to respiratory stimuli. *Am Rev Respir Dis* 1978;118:807–809.
157. Phillipson EA. Sleep apnea a major public health problem. *N Engl J Med* 1993;328:1271–1273.
158. Portas CM, McCarley RW. Behavioral state-related changes of extracellular serotonin concentration in the dorsal raphe nucleus: a microdialysis study in the freely moving cat. *Brain Res* 1994;648: 306–312.
159. Price DD. *Psychological and neural mechanism of pain.* New York: Raven Press, 1988.
160. Prys-Roberts C. Anaesthesia: a practical or impractical construct? *Br J Anaesth* 1987;59:1341–1345.
161. Quasha AL, Eger EI, Tinker JH. Determination and application of MAC. *Anesthesiology* 1980;53:315–334.
162. Rampil IJ, Mason P, Singh H. Anesthetic potency (MAC) is independent of forebrain structures in the rat. *Anesthesiology* 1993;78: 707–712.
163. Ramsay MAE, Savege TM, Simpson BRJ, Goodwin R. Controlled sedation with alphaxalone-alphadolone. *Br Med J* 1974;2:656–659.
164. Richards CD. In search of the mechanisms of anaesthesia. *Trends Neurosci* 1980;3:9–13.
165. Richter D, Crossland J. Variation in acetylcholine content of the brain with physiological state. *Am J Physiol* 1949;159:247–255.
166. Robbins BH. Preliminary studies of the anesthetic activity of fluorinated hydrocarbons. *J Pharmacol Exp Ther* 1946;86:197–204.
167. Robinson RW, Zwillich CW. Sleep breathing disorders. In: Kryger MH, Roth T, Dement WC, eds. *Principles and practice of sleep medicine.* Philadelphia: WB Saunders, 1994:603–620.
168. Robinson TE, Justice JB, eds. *Microdialysis in the neurosciences.* New York: Elsevier, 1991.
169. Roffwarg HP. Diagnostic classification of sleep disorders. *Sleep* 1979;2:5–137.
170. Rogers MC, Tinker JH, Covino BG, Longnecker DE, eds. *Principles and practice of anesthesiology.* St. Louis: CV Mosby, 1993.
171. Roth SH, Miller KW, eds. *Molecular and cellular mechanisms of anesthetics.* New York: Plenum Press, 1986.
172. Rubin E, Miller KW, Roth SH, eds. *Molecular and cellular mechanisms of alcohol and anesthetics.* New York: New York Academy of Sciences, 1991.
173. Rudy TE, Kerns RD, Turk DC. Chronic pain and depression: Towards a cognitive-behavioral mediation model. *Pain* 1988;35: 129–140.
174. Russell GB, Graybeal JM. Differences in anesthetic potency between Sprague-Dawley and Long-Evans rats for isoflurane but not nitrous oxide. *Pharmacology* 1995;50:162–167.
175. Saidman LJ. Anesthesiology. *JAMA* 1995;273:1661–1662.
176. Saidman LJ, Eger EI, Munson ES, Babad AA, Muallem M. Minimum alveolar concentrations of methoxyflurane, halothane, ether and cyclopropane in man: correlation with theories of anesthesia. *Anesthesiology* 1967;28:994–1002.
177. Saito S, Fujita T, Igarashi M. Effects of inhalational anesthetics on biochemical events in growing neuronal tips. *Anesthesiology* 1993; 79:1338–1347.
178. Saunders NA, Sullivan CE, eds. *Sleep and breathing.* 2nd ed. New York: Marcel Dekker, 1994.
179. Serafin M, Khateb A, Muhlenthaler M. Opiates inhibit pedunculopontine neurones in guinea pig brainstem slices. *Neurosci Lett* 1990;119:125–128.
180. Shiromani PJ, Armstrong DM, Gillin JC. Cholinergic neurons from the dorsolateral pons project to the medial pons: a WGA-HRP and choline acetyltransferase immunohistochemical study. *Neurosci Lett* 1988;95:19–23.

181. Shiromani PJ, Kilduff TS, Bloom FE, McCarley RW. Cholinergically induced REM sleep triggers fos-like immunoreactivity in dorsolateral pontine regions associated with REM sleep. *Brain Res* 1992;580:351–357.
182. Shuman SL, Capece ML, Baghdoyan HA, Lydic R. Pertussis toxin-sensitive G proteins mediate carbachol-induced REM sleep and respiratory depression. *Am J Physiol* 1995;269:R308–R317.
183. Sitaram N, Gillin JC. Acetylcholine: possible involvement in sleep and analgesia. In: Davis KL, Berger PA, eds. *Brain acetylcholine and neuropsychiatric disease.* New York: Plenum Press, 1979:311–343.
184. Skinner BF. The steep and thorny way to a science of behavior. *Am Psychol* 1975;30:42–49.
185. Snir-Mor I, Weinstock M, Davidson JT, Bahar M. Physostigmine antagonizes morphine-induced respiratory depression in human subjects. *Anesthesiology* 1983;59:6–9.
186. Soja PJ, Lopez-Rodriguez F, Morales FR, Chase MH. The postsynaptic inhibitory control of lumbar motoneurons during the atonia of active sleep: effect of strychnine on motoneuron properties. *J Neurosci* 1991;11:2804–2811.
187. Steriade M, McCarley RW. *Brainstem control of wakefulness and sleep.* New York: Plenum Press, 1990.
188. Steriade M, McCormick DA, Sejnowski TJ. Thalamocortical oscillations in the sleeping and aroused brain. *Science* 1993;262: 679–785.
189. Sykes WS. *Essays on the first hundred years of anaesthesia. Vol. 1.* Huntington, NY: Krieger, 1972.
190. Taguchi K, Andersen MJ, Hentall ID. Acetylcholine release from the midbrain interpeduncular nucleus during anesthesia. *NeuroReport* 1991;2:789–792.
191. Thorpy MJ, ed. *International Classification of Sleep Disorders: diagnostic and coding manual.* Rochester, MN: American Sleep Disorders Association, 1990.
192. Van Dongen PAM. Locus coeruleus region: effects on behavior of cholinergic, noradrenergic and opiate drugs injected intracerebrally into freely moving cats. *Exp Neurol* 1980;67:52–78.
193. Vanni-Mercier G, Sakai K, Lin JS, Jouvet M. Mapping of cholinoceptive brainstem structures responsible for the generation of paradoxical sleep in the cat. *Arch Ital Biol* 1989;127: 133–164.
194. White DC. Anaesthesia: a privation of the senses. An historical introduction and some definitions. In: Rosen M, Lunn JN, eds. *Consciousness, awareness and pain in general anaesthesia.* London: Butterworth, 1987:1–9.
195. Willette RN, Boorley BM, Sapru HN. Activation of cholinergic mechanisms in the medulla oblongata reverse intravenous opioid-induced respiratory depression. *J Pharmacol Exp Ther* 1987;240: 352–358.
196. Williams JA, Comisarow J, Day J, Fibiger HC, Reiner PB. State-dependent release of acetylcholine in rat thalamus measured by in vivo microdialysis. *J Neurosci* 1994;14:5236–5242.
197. Yaksh TL. Sites of action of opiates in production of analgesia. *Prog Brain Res* 1988;77:371–394.
198. Yaksh TL, Dirksen R, Harty GJ. Antinociceptive effects of intrathecal cholinomimetic drugs in the rat and cat. *Eur J Pharmacol* 1985; 117:81–88.
199. Yaksh TL, Grafe MR, Malkmus S, Rathbun ML, Eisenach JC. Studies on the safety of chronically administered intrathecal neostigmine methylsulfate in rats and dogs. *Anesthesiology* 1995;82: 412–427.
200. Yaksh TL, Rudy TA. Narcotic analgesics: CNS cites and mechanisms of action as revealed by intracerebral injection techniques. *Pain* 1978;4:299–359.
201. Yamuy J, Mancillas JR, Morales FR, Chase MH. C-fos expression in the pons and medulla of the cat during carbachol-induced active sleep. *J Neurosci* 1993;13:2703–2718.
202. Yamuy J, Morales FR, Chase MH. Induction of rapid eye movement sleep by microinjection of nerve growth factor into the pontine reticular formation of the cat. *Neuroscience* 1995;66:9–13.
203. Yang J, Isenberg KE, Zorumski CF. Volatile anesthetics gate a chloride current in postnatal rat hippocampal neurons. *FASEB J* 1992; 6:914–918.
204. Yli-Hankala A, Eskola H, Kaukinen S. EEG spectral power during halothane anaesthesia: a comparison of spectral bands in the monitoring of anaesthesia level. *Acta Anaesthesiol Scand* 1989;33: 304–308.
205. Young T, Palta M, Dempsy J, Skatrud J, Weber S, Badr S. The occurrence of sleep-disordered breathing among middle-aged adults. *New Engl J Med* 1993;328:1230–1235.

Anesthesia: Biologic Foundations, edited by
Tony L. Yaksh et al. Lippincott–Raven Publishers,
Philadelphia © 1997.

CHAPTER 28

MEMORY AND RECALL

RANDALL C. CORK, LAWRENCE J. COUTURE,
AND JOHN F. KIHLSTROM

Among the most important clinical indices of general anesthesia is the patient's inability to remember, postoperatively, the events that transpired during his or her surgery. Patients who cannot remember such events, including sensations of pain and other experiences of distress, are held to have been adequately anesthetized. The central role played by memory in assessments of the adequacy of anesthesia lends great importance to understanding the nature of this mental faculty. This is especially the case, in view of emerging evidence that conscious recollection is not all there is to memory. The possibility that surgical events may be encoded in memory and expressed in postsurgical experience, thought and action, albeit outside of phenomenal awareness, poses both a special challenge and a special opportunity for anesthesiology. (For additional coverage of the literature on anesthesia and memory, see refs. 3,8,9,44,88,89,91,120,125,126,143,160. A great deal of related literature on awareness and depth of anesthesia is collected in refs. 101,116,169. Of special interest are the proceedings of the first and second international symposia on Memory and Awareness in Anesthesia, refs. 31,181. The third such symposium was held in Amsterdam in 1995.)

PSYCHOLOGY OF MEMORY

Memory refers to a mental faculty by which organisms form, retain, and use mental representations of the past. (For thorough treatments of the psychology of memory, see refs. 11,64,76,96,180,188; also see the periodic reviews appearing in the *Annual Review of Psychology*. For comprehensive treatments of cognitive psychology, see refs. 6,13,141. For a discussion of memory in a neuroscientific context, see refs. 87,175.) Put another way, memory refers to the means by which organisms encode, store, and retrieve knowledge acquired through experience. There is an intimate relationship between memory, perception, learning, and thought. Perception forms mental representations of current events; memory stores knowledge gleaned from the present for use in the future, when stored knowledge is retrieved and mental representations of past events are reconstructed. It is by means of learning that organisms acquire new knowledge and store it in memory. In the course of thinking, organisms use stored knowledge, retrieved from memory, in the service of judgment, reasoning, inference, and problem-solving.

Classification of the Contents of Memory

Not all stored knowledge is of the same type. Intuitively, there are qualitative differences among one's knowledge of English grammar or of the way to tie a Windsor knot, the meaning of words like hegemony or leitmotif, that Columbus landed in America in 1492 and that ether was introduced by Morton in 1846, one's first kiss and what one ate for dinner last Tuesday. In accordance with these intuitions, as well as a great deal of experimental evidence, psychologists often classify the knowledge stored in memory in terms of the hierarchy displayed in Fig. 1.

At the highest level of the hierarchy is the distinction between procedural and declarative knowledge (5,218). Declarative knowledge consists of facts or beliefs about the nature of the world: it can be represented in propositions, sentence-like statements consisting of two nouns (or noun phrases) and a verb (or verb phrase) expressing some relation between the noun phrases—for example, "The surgeon grasped the scalpel." Procedural knowledge, by contrast, consists of the skills, rules, and strategies by which we manipulate and transform declarative knowledge: it can be represented in productions, "if-then" statements consisting of a goal, a condition, and an action by which that goal can be achieved under that condition—for example, "If you want to tie a Windsor knot, then begin by bringing the long end of the tie in front of the short end; then bring the long end up through the loop."

The difference between declarative and procedural knowledge is the difference between knowing that and knowing how (170). Procedural knowledge can be further classified into cognitive skills (such as performing long division or taking square roots) and motor skills (such as playing piano or tennis). Some procedural knowledge is innate, but much of it is acquired through repeated practice. Once acquired, however, productions are executed automatically when their constituent goals and conditions are instantiated, without any conscious intent on the part of the person, and without consuming any attentional capacity. Once engaged, productions cannot be controlled until they have been discharged, and further, the person may be entirely unaware of their execution.

Declarative knowledge can be further classified into episodic and semantic forms (203). Episodic memory consists of autobiographical information: the individual's knowledge of specific events that have transpired in his or her lifetime. Semantic knowledge is the individual's mental dictionary (and encyclopedia) of abstract and categorical information about the world. Both episodic and semantic knowledge can be represented in propositions. But in the case of episodic knowledge, the proposition contains more or less concrete reference to the specific time and place at which an event occurred, as well as reference to the rememberer as the agent or experiencer of that event. Thus, our knowledge that Columbus landed in America in 1492 is a fragment of semantic memory; by contrast, our knowledge of the circumstances under which we acquired that bit of knowledge is a piece of episodic memory. Most, if not all, of our declarative knowledge is acquired through experience; but as the circumstances under which that knowledge is acquired

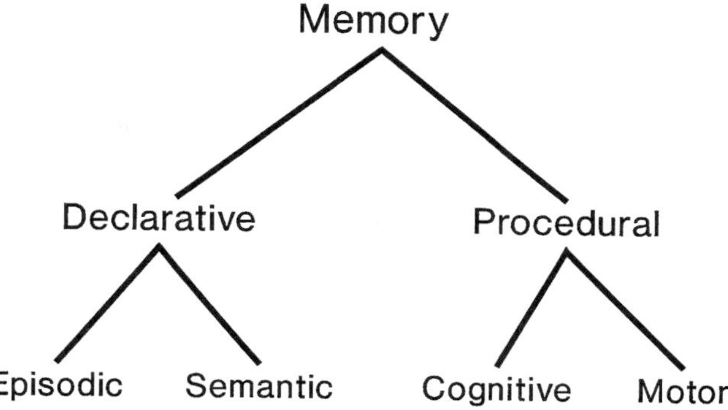

Figure 1. Hierarchical classification of knowledge stored in memory.

begin to blur and fade, episodic memories are transformed into semantic ones.

Consider the following report from the annals of neurology. While greeting a patient suffering amnesia from alcoholic Korsakoff's syndrome, Claparede (53; and for a discussion, see ref. 122) pricked her palm with a pin hidden in his hand. Claparede left the ward while the patient was placated, after which he returned and greeted her again. The patient had no memory for having met Claparede before, but declined to shake his proffered hand. When asked to justify her refusal, she replied only that people sometimes hide pins in their hands. Knowledge that people sometimes hide pins in their hands is a piece of semantic information, presumably acquired through direct or vicarious experience; knowledge of the occasion on which the patient was herself pricked is a piece of episodic information, representing the experience itself.

Processing of Memory

The distinctions between declarative and procedural knowledge, and between episodic and semantic knowledge, are highly relevant to the question of postoperative memory. When we ask whether a patient was adequately anesthetized, we ask whether he or she has any recollection of events (e.g., conversations among members of the surgical team) and experiences (e.g., feelings of pain) that transpired while he or she was in surgery. That is to say, we ask questions about the person's episodic memory. Understanding why certain events are remembered, and why others have been forgotten, has been a central task of cognitive psychology since the scientific psychology of memory began with the work of Ebbinghaus (70). This literature can be summarized as a series of nine principles governing remembering and forgetting (for more extended treatment of these principles, see ref. 123).

The analysis of memory is governed by an overarching framework known as the stage principle (64).

1. The stage principle. Any instance of forgetting can be attributed to a failure of encoding, storage, or retrieval, either alone or in combination.

Encoding is the process by which a trace of current experience is laid down in memory; storage, that by which an encoded memory trace remains available over time; and retrieval, the process of recovering information from storage for use in ongoing cognitive activity. In strictly logical terms, a memory cannot be retrieved from storage unless it was encoded in the first place, or if it was lost from storage after being encoded.

The encoding process itself is governed by two principles, elaboration (7,60,61) and organization (36,138).

2. The elaboration principle. The memorability of an event increases when that event is related to preexisting knowledge available at the time of encoding.

3. The organization principle. The memorability of an event increases when that event is related to other events occurring at the time of encoding.

Events are remembered to the extent that they were encoded at the time they occurred. Proper encoding does not occur automatically, but rather requires active, cognitive effort. This effort takes two forms (103): relating individual items to the base of preexisting knowledge already stored in memory (elaboration, or item-specific processing), and relating individual items to each other (organization, or relational processing).

Once a memory has been encoded, it is, at least in principle, available for subsequent retrieval and use. However, in practice memories seem to fade over time, an observation that has been enshrined in another principle (70):

4. The time-dependency principle. The memorability of an event declines as the length of the storage interval (i.e., the time between encoding and retrieval) increases.

Of course, there are instances in which knowledge appears to be preserved in rich detail over long periods of time, as in so-called "flashbulb" memories for emotionally arousing events (216), and the "permastore" of factual knowledge (12). But these are the exceptions that test the rule, and in any event careful studies have shown that many flashbulb memories are highly inaccurate, and the notion of a permastore generally refers to semantic rather than episodic memory.

The experimental literature does contain a number of studies of so-called hypermnesia, in which memory appears to grow rather than fade with time (77,123,156). This phenomenon appears to contradict the time-dependency principle, but in fact it is consistent with the elaboration, organization, and time-dependency principles. Hypermnesia occurs when items were subject to elaborative and organizational activity at the time of encoding, and most hypermnesia is accomplished on the first few attempts at retrieval, relatively soon after encoding has taken place.

The retrieval process itself is governed by a large set of principles, all of which follow from the general distinction between the availability and accessibility of items in memory storage (204):

5. The accessibility principle. An item that is available in memory storage is not necessarily accessible on every retrieval attempt.

For example, accessibility varies with the means by which retrieval is attempted. By and large, recognition tests produce more memory than recall tests, and cued recall produces more memory than free recall. This leads to another principle, directly governing the accessibility of items available in memory storage (202):

6. The cue-dependency principle. The memorability of an event increases with the amount of information supplied by the retrieval cue.

Remembering usually begins with some kind of cue that provides some information about the event which is to be remembered. Cues that are highly informative are more likely to contact available memory traces than those that are not. In some respects, encoding and retrieval are in a complementary relationship: access to well-encoded memories generally requires fewer retrieval cues, and a rich retrieval environment can promote access even to very poorly encoded memories.

Cues are important, but they must also supply the right kind of information, not just the right amount (206):

7. The encoding specificity principle. The memorability of an event increases when the information processed at the time of retrieval was also processed at the time of encoding.

The manner in which an event is encoded—the meaning of the event, how it is perceived, interpreted, and categorized—determines which retrieval cues will be successful in gaining access to that event. Encoding specificity appears to underlie the phenomenon of state-dependent memory—whether "state" is defined in physiological, emotional, or environmental terms.

Memory is also determined by the degree to which an event conforms to our expectations and beliefs (100):

8. The schematic processing principle. The memorability of an event increases when that event is relevant to expectations and beliefs about that event.

The general principle is straightforward enough, but the details may be a little surprising. If memory is plotted as a function of the degree to which the target events can be predicted on the basis of preexisting knowledge (represented in the form of organized knowledge structures known as schemata), it turns out that events that are highly congruent with expectations are also highly memorable; but events that are highly incongruent with active schemata are even more memorable. Events which are irrelevant to our expectations are generally unmemorable. The U-shaped function apparently reflects the operation of two different principles: events that are inconsistent with preexisting schemata are surprising and draw more attention, and thus receive more elaborative and organizational activity at the time of encoding; and at the time of retrieval, the relevant schema provides additional cue information that can facilitate access to relevant memories. Events that are irrelevant to the schema get neither advantage, and so are poorly remembered.

The role of cognitive schemata is also underscored by another principle (14):

9. The reconstruction principle. The memory of an event reflects a blend of information retrieved from specific traces encoded at the time of that event, with knowledge, expectations, and beliefs derived from other sources.

In describing how memory works, we often resort to the metaphor of a library: memory traces are books that must be purchased and catalogued; the prospective user must look up the book in the catalog in order to know where to find it; and in order for the search to succeed, the book must not have been eaten by worms, or displaced by a careless user. The library metaphor will take us a long way, but the notion of memory retrieval obscures the fact that memories can be distorted, biased, and otherwise altered by changes in perspective and other events that occur after the time of encoding. In the final analysis, memory is not so much like reading a book as it is like writing one from fragmentary notes. The reconstruction principle is of utmost importance in the present context, because it means that any particular memory is only partly derived from trace information encoded at the time of the event: in the process of remembering, trace information combines with knowledge, beliefs, and inferences derived from other sources.

Several of these principles of remembering and forgetting are directly relevant to the question of postanesthetic memory. For example, the accessibility and cue-dependency principles lead us to worry about the degree to which the usual tests of memory employed by anesthesiologists adequately assess any information patients have acquired during their surgical experience. To what extent is patients' performance on memory tests administered immediately after surgery affected by their incomplete recovery from general anesthesia, or the clouding of consciousness produced by postsurgical administration of analgesics such as morphine? Would the same test, administered after a delay, produce different results? In adequately anesthetized patients, tests of free recall generally yield nothing; but what might be revealed by other tests, such as cued recall and recognition? But if patients seem to remember more under conditions of cued recall and recognition than free recall, we have to worry about the reconstruction principle: to what extent do the patients' reports reflect the actual retrieval of memories, compared to plausible reconstructions based on information supplied in the investigator's queries?

The encoding specificity principle, which states that encoding conditions constrain the effectiveness of retrieval cues, has a number of implications for postsurgical memory. Consider first the principles governing memory encoding. The formation of a well-encoded (and thus long-lasting and easily retrievable) memory trace depends on elaboration and organization. These processes require the active deployment of attention—a degree of cognitive activity that is likely to be precluded by adequate general anesthesia. At the same time, however, the schematic processing principle holds that encoding is likely to be enhanced for events that are unexpected, personally relevant, and highly salient—which, in the surgical context, would seem most likely to include mishaps, accidents, and remarks about the patient. Accordingly, any memories retained from surgery are probably more likely to be negative (and litigable) than positive in character.

The encoding specificity principle raises the further, and somewhat disconcerting, question of whether memory for intraoperative events might not be state-dependent—that is, whether memories encoded during general anesthesia might be inaccessible in the normal waking state, but fully accessible if the patient is subsequently anesthetized. Beginning with the classic studies of Overton (154), a large empirical literature has documented state-dependent learning and memory (SDM) effects associated with a wide variety of psychoactive drugs including alcohol, barbiturates, caffeine, and marijuana (for reviews, see refs. 72,75,211). That is, if encoding takes place under the influence of a particular pharmacological substance, retrieval is more effective when the subject is under the influence of that same drug (or one with highly similar pharmacological properties). Could such a thing happen under anesthesia as well? This theoretical possibility would seem impossible to test, given the inability of adequately anesthetized patients to communicate with others (and thus complete memory tests) during surgery. Moreover, it should be remembered that most drugs which produce SDM also impair encoding and retrieval processes. Thus, even when both encoding and retrieval occur in the drugged state, memory is not as good as it would be in the absence of drugs. Thus, the practical consequences of state-dependent memory in general anesthesia would seem to be minimal. However, the possibility of state-dependency should not be discounted in cases where patients undergo surgery under lighter planes of anesthesia.

Explicit and Implicit Expressions of Episodic Memory

When we ask questions about postoperative memory, we usually ask about the patient's conscious ability to recollect intraoperative events. However, as Claparede's (53) case of Korsakoff's syndrome shows, it is possible for information relating to an episode to be retained in memory, and influence subsequent behavior, even though the episode itself is not remembered.

The influence of past experience on present behavior, in the absence of conscious recollection of that experience, is manifested on more formal tests performed on amnesic patients. For example, the patient H.M., who underwent surgical excision of the medial portion of his temporal lobes as a desperate treatment for intractable epilepsy, remembers nothing that has occurred since the date of his operation (57,146,179). Yet, he retains a number of perceptual-motor skills, including mirror drawing and pursuit-rotor learning, which were taught to him after his operation. Studies of other amnesic patients show similar selective effects on memory: in each case, procedural knowledge is acquired and retained, although declarative-episodic memory for the learning experience is lost. However, the fact that the skill has been retained means that some trace of the learning episode has been preserved as well.

The selective effects of amnesia can be demonstrated within the declarative domain itself. In a typical experiment, amnesic patients are asked to study a list of familiar words, such as motel or assassin. After a short period of distraction, they are unable to remember any of the words that appeared on the list. At this point, they are presented with stems (e.g., mot—) or fragments (e.g., a—a—in) and asked to complete them with the first word that comes to mind. In the case of word stems, which have many possible completions, amnesic patients are more likely to fill in the blanks with study items than are control subjects, who never encountered the list; in the case of word fragments, which have only a single possible solution, amnesic subjects are more likely to produce the target than controls. These outcomes (for example, see refs. 95,210) are generically known as priming effects. In fact, amnesics generally show the same degree of priming as normal subjects who remember the study list perfectly well.

Priming is most frequently observed on semantic memory tasks: subjects are asked to retrieve items from their mental lexicons rather to remember items that they have studied. However, not all priming is mediated by semantic knowledge. In repetition priming, presentation of an item at study facilitates the processing of that same item at test; in semantic priming, presentation of an item at study facilitates the processing of a semantically related item at test (there are also other forms of priming). Regardless of the nature of the priming, however, the effect is clearly attributable to the prior presentation of list items: thus, when priming occurs, it is because something of the episode has been preserved in memory.

The ability of amnesic patients to capitalize on prior episodes of study or learning, in the absence of any recollection of the episodes themselves, motivates a distinction between two expressions of memory: explicit and implicit (171–173). Explicit memory refers to conscious recollection, as indicated by the ability to recall or recognize an event from the past; in fact, explicit memory tasks require just such conscious recollection. Implicit memory, on the other hand, refers to any change in experience, thought, or action, such as priming effects, that is attributable to past events; in formal terms, implicit memory tasks do not require conscious recollection of the past. In fact, a large amount of evidence has accumulated that explicit and implicit memory can be dissociated in both amnesic patients and normals. That is, implicit memory can be spared even though explicit memory is grossly impaired.

Current theoretical accounts of implicit memory come in three basic forms, each with a number of variants (for fuller discussion, see refs. 94,114,134,164–167,171–173). According to the activation view, perceptual processing of an event activates preexisting internal representations of knowledge corresponding to the features of that event. This activation persists for some time after the event has passed, forming the basis for priming effects. According to the multiple systems view, explicit and implicit expressions of memory are supported by different physical systems in the brain. For example, explicit but not implicit memory may require involvement of the hippocampus. According to the processing view, explicit and implicit memory result from different kinds of operations performed on perceptual inputs. For example, explicit memory may require that the meaning of an event be processed, while implicit memory may require analysis only in terms of its physical properties.

Each of these views makes its own particular assumptions about how memory is structured. For example, the activation and processing views tend to assume that memory is a unitary storehouse of knowledge, whereas the multiple systems view assumes that there are many different kinds of memory. In addition, the activation view assumes that new events are encoded by recombining preexisting knowledge, while the multiple systems and processing views allow for the encoding of entirely new representations in memory. In principle, these sorts of differences create the possibility that experimental tests could indicate which view is correct, but in practice this sort of evidence has been difficult to produce. Moreover, some versions of each view include elements of one or more other views, making decisive tests difficult to conduct. For present purposes, it is the explicit-implicit distinction itself that is more important, because it raises the possibility that memories of surgical events may be encoded, retained, and expressed outside of awareness. The specific characteristics of implicit memory are important in interpreting the literature on implicit memory in surgical anesthesia, however, so we will return to this issue at the end of the chapter.

From Implicit Memory to Implicit Perception

In the usual case, implicit memory occurs for events that were consciously perceived at the time they originally occurred. Amnesic patients, for example, are aware of the target items at the time they study them, even if they forget them quite quickly thereafter. However, it is also possible to observe priming effects when the events were never perceived in the first place. In such cases, implicit memory provides evidence for implicit perception: a change in experience, thought, or action that is attributable to an event in the current environment, independent of conscious perception of that event (124). A great deal of evidence, involving both brain-damaged patients and intact subjects, shows that explicit and implicit perception can be dissociated in much the same way as explicit and implicit memory.

For example, patients suffering damage to the striate cortex report an inability to see objects presented in their scotoma; yet, in at least some cases, they are able to make "guesses" about the visual properties of stimuli that are more accurate than would be expected by chance—a phenomenon dubbed "blindsight" (212). Similarly, patients with lesions in the temporoparietal region of the right hemisphere fail to attend to objects in their left visual field; yet, again at least in some cases, their choice behavior is guided by information available in the neglected area. Among intact subjects, interest in so-called subliminal perception has been revived by compelling demonstrations of priming effects attributable to stimuli that are presented at intensities that are too low, or durations too short, to be consciously perceived (35,49,97,142,152).

One piece of evidence supporting the concept of implicit perception is a form of the mere exposure effect (222). In the typical mere exposure experiment, subjects receive repeated presentations of a list of unfamiliar items (e.g., pseudowords, nonsense drawings, or foreign words). They are then presented with list items, paired with previously unpresented control items, and asked to indicate which they prefer. On average, subjects prefer those items to which they had been previously exposed. The mere exposure effect is an expression of implicit memory, because the previous exposures have changed the person's response to the list items. Interestingly, the mere exposure effect occurs even if the initial presentation of the items was subliminal (129; for a review, see ref. 34). Because memory for an event requires that the event be perceived in the first place, in this case implicit memory simultaneously provides evidence for implicit perception: the subject's experience, thought, and action is influenced by visual events in the absence of conscious perception of those events.

The implication of the literature on implicit memory is that assessments of memory should go beyond what the person can consciously recall or recognize, to examine the possibility of remembering without awareness (71,107). In the same manner, the implication of the literature on implicit perception is that unperceived events can also leave traces in memory that affect subsequent behavior. Therefore, the possibility remains that, even though adequately anesthetized patients do not explicitly perceive surgical events (at least by the most generally accepted accounts of anesthesia) and, in any event, lack explicit memory for such events, careful testing might show that implicit memories of surgical events have been preserved.

This possibility is strengthened by the fact that at least some forms of implicit memory are not affected by the same sorts of factors (e.g., elaboration and organization) that govern the encoding of consciously accessible memories (171–173,205). Thus, implicit memory may occur even when a patient is unable to perform the kinds of cognitive operations usually considered necessary for the formation of an explicit memory. In the remainder of this chapter, we survey a rapidly developing literature which assumes that explicit memory is impaired by adequate anesthesia (as indeed it must be, by definition), and proceeds to inquire into the fate of implicit memory.

Notes on the Neuroscience of Memory

From a psychological point of view, an episodic memory may be described as a bundle of features, or a set of propositions, that describe some event or experience. A basic question for neuroscience concerns how such knowledge is encoded in the nervous system (for comprehensive reviews, see refs. 186,187,189). This question has been approached at a number of different levels. For example, studies of conditioning and learning in the marine mollusk aplysia have shed a great deal of light on the molecular basis of memory (117). Despite their very simple nervous systems, aplysia are capable of both nonassociative (habituation, sensitization) and associative (classical conditioning, and instrumental conditioning) forms of learning (for example, see ref. 43). The fact that aplysia neurons are both relatively few in number and relatively large in size permits detailed analysis of synaptic changes (known as short-term and long-term potentiation) occurring as a result of learning. Similar analyses have been carried out in a wide variety of species, suggesting that some physiological mechanisms of learning and memory are common to vertebrates and invertebrates.

Of course, studies of nonhuman animals cannot inform us of the biological substrates of conscious recollection, because we have no way of knowing whether, or to what degree, such animals are aware of what they have learned. However, such evidence is now available from two sources: neuropsychological studies of brain-damaged patients who display a dense anterograde amnesia known as the amnesic syndrome (182); and behavioral studies of monkeys and other primates in whom experimentally induced lesions seem to produce deficits in learning and memory analogous to those observed in the amnesic syndrome (147). The organic amnesic syndrome comes in two general forms: patients displaying Korsakoff's syndrome, such as the woman described by Claparede (53), have suffered damage to the midline portion of the diencephalon, including the dorsomedial thalamic nuclei and the mammillary bodies; in other cases, such as the patient H.M. (57,146,179), the damage is to the medial area of the temporal lobe, including the hippocampus, amygdala, and other adjacent areas. Diencephalic patients usually show damage to the frontal lobes and diffuse cortical atrophy as well, giving their amnesia special properties, such as anosognosia, confabulation, and metamemory deficits (149,183).

Once the memory deficit in question has been thoroughly described, anatomical and brain-imaging studies can be performed to determine which brain areas are involved. Recently, for example, Squire and Zola-Morgan (191; see also ref. 189) have offered evidence for a memory system located in the medial portions of the temporal lobe, which is important for the encoding and storage of declarative knowledge, both semantic and episodic. The system consists of the hippocampus, entorhinal cortex, perirhinal cortex, and the parahippocampal cortex. When these structures are damaged, perception and short-term memory are unaffected, but long-term memory is grossly impaired. Moreover, the long-term impairment affects explicit memory, but not implicit memory. The medial-temporal lobe system is not where memories are permanently stored: this purpose is served by the cortex. Squire and Zola-Morgan (191) propose that memory for an event is distributed across a number of different cortical sites, each representing a different aspect of the event, and that the medial-temporal lobe memory system serves to bind these different sites together, forming a unified representation. The characteristic failure of explicit memory in amnesic patients presumably reflects the lack of this binding function: given a retrieval cue, patients cannot use links (that would have been established by an intact hippocampus) to retrieve associated memories. However, event-related information supported by the several cortical sites is sufficient to support performance on tests of implicit memory.

AWARENESS, MEMORY, AND SURGICAL ANESTHESIA

Prior to the introduction of surgical anesthesia in the 19th century, pain and explicit memory of it were considered a normal part of the surgical procedure (158). Although extensive efforts were made to alleviate pain with hypnosis, ingestion of alcohol, herbs, botanical extracts, and the local application of pressure or ice on nerves, surgery was generally a painful and memorable experience. It is interesting that in South America the Incan priests were quite successful at pain relief for trephination simply by allowing cocaine-saturated saliva to drip into the wound. Still, one might expect that those who underwent this procedure were aware of it at the time and remembered it later.

The distinction between awareness and memory was made very early in the history of the practice of surgical anesthesia. In January 1845, Horace Wells attempted the first public demonstration of nitrous oxide as a general anesthetic. The patient, undergoing removal of an impacted tooth, screamed and struggled throughout the procedure, and Wells was jeered by the audience. Despite this apparent failure of anesthesia, the patient later claimed to have no memory for the procedure. Thus, the patient was aware of the procedure, and in obvious pain during it, but remembered nothing of it later. This is in contrast to the first public demonstration of ether by William Morton in 1846. Morton anesthetized Edward Gilbert Abbott, a young printer, for the surgical repair of a congenital venous malformation in his left cervical triangle. The demonstration was a success: the patient showed no obvious evidence of awareness or pain during the procedure, and no memory of pain afterwards.

The subsequent development of the clinical practice of anesthesia was haunted by the risk of inadequate depth, resulting in awareness and/or recall (for a review of the assessment of anesthetic depth, see ref. 199). Moreover, this risk underwent an abrupt increase when neuromuscular blocking agents were introduced into the practice of anesthesia in the 1940s (98). These drugs made lighter planes of anesthesia possible, thus decreasing the risk of morbidity. However, as Cherkin and Harroun (50,99) and Crile (63) warned, they effectively prevented inadequately anesthetized patients from communicating their awareness to the anesthesiologist, and obtaining relief. Thus, the muscle relaxants effectively increased the risk of surgical awareness.

Incidence of Surgical Awareness

The incidence of surgical awareness is thankfully low: the highest incidence reported is 2–4% and this under very light planes of anesthesia (4,40,41,62,178,208). Hutchinson (104) reported only 1.2% incidence of any sort of recall; Faithfull (83) recorded only five instances of postoperative recall in a series of 1,328 surgical patients; Wilson et al. (215) estimated an incidence of 1%; Moerman and Porcelijn (148) reported only two such incidents among 557 patients who had undergone a total of 1,000 surgical procedures, and Liu et al. (136) gave an estimate of 0.2%. However, Winterbottom's (219) classic case does have its contemporary counterparts: Tracy (200) has provided an especially vivid example from her own experience as a patient. Of course, not all cases of awareness and memory can be attributed to improperly administered anesthetic. Awareness is especially common in situations where relatively light planes of anesthesia are the standard of care: caesarian sections, trauma surgery, and cardiopulmonary bypass surgery. Even the possibility of intraoperative awareness and postoperative memory can cause preoperative anxiety. Cases where awareness and memory occur unexpectedly can result in posttraumatic stress disorder for the patient, and a lawsuit for the practitioner.

During postoperative interviews, patients are frequently surprised to learn that during their stay in the postanesthesia care unit, immediately after surgery, they were alert and talkative, sometimes carrying on long conversations with the staff. They were certainly aware of themselves and their surroundings at the time, but they no longer remember this episode in their lives.

Anesthesiologists have often wondered if their patients were in fact aware during surgery, even though they do not remember their awareness later (a question somewhat analogous to whether a tree falling in a forest makes a sound if no one hears it). One way of approaching this question is through the isolated forearm technique, in which an arm tourniquet is applied prior to administration of neuromuscular blockers. With a prearranged hand-signal, the patient is able to communicate if he or she is aware. This technique was introduced by Tunstall (207) as an aid to assessing anesthetic depth during caesarian sections (see also ref. 39). A recent study of this procedure, involving 30 patients (128), yielded some disturbing findings: at the time of skin incision, 97% of patients signaled awareness and pain; this figure dropped to 77% for awareness and 63% for pain 1 min later, and 20% for awareness and 7% for pain 2 min later; one patient remained aware at 3 min. During postoperative interviews, none of the patients remembered experiencing any pain, or making any signals. Apparently, the tree falling does, indeed, make a sound.

IMPLICIT MEMORY AFTER GENERAL ANESTHESIA

For the first 100 years of general anesthesia, physicians and patients were primarily concerned with whether the technique worked as advertised to prevent concurrent and retrospective awareness of surgical events. The idea that memory for intraoperative events might be preserved outside awareness came only later. Apparently Cheek (46–48) was the first to seriously raise this possibility. Cheek studied a group of patients with poor postsurgical outcome. None of the patients had any explicit memory of surgical events. But when hypnotized, many of them were able to remember negative statements that had been made about them, during surgery, by members of the surgical team. Cheek suggested that these memories unconsciously influenced the patients' postoperative course.

Other clinicians have made similar observations (for example, see refs. 81,82), although the patients' reported memories are not always easy to verify. Goldmann et al. (93) elicited memories of intraoperative events from seven of 33 patients, sometimes with the aid of hypnosis, but only three of these memories were corroborated by the operating room records.

At about the same time, Levinson (130) reported a case of a woman who suffered from a severe depression after plastic surgery on her face. When interviewed under hypnosis, she repeated the words of her surgeon, describing what he thought was a malignant tumor inside her mouth. Because the mass proved benign, the episode was never mentioned to the patient postoperatively. Nevertheless, Levinson (130) concluded that the patient had learned of the possibility of cancer during her surgery, and that this knowledge had unconsciously affected her postoperative mood. This case directly motivated one of most notorious studies in the history of medicine (131). (For other accounts of this study and its context, see refs. 132,133.) By prior arrangement with the surgeon, Levinson (130) staged a mock surgical crisis for each of 10 patients. The patients were anesthetized with a combination of nitrous oxide, oxygen, and ether (there was no muscle relaxant). At a particular point, the anesthesiologist stopped the operation, and announced that the patient had turned blue and might die; shortly thereafter, the anesthesiologist declared that the patient was out of danger and permitted the surgery to proceed. None of the patients had any conscious recollection of this episode. One month later, however, when hypnotized and age-regressed to the time of the surgery, four patients repeated the words of the anesthesiologist verbatim, while four more reported that something bad had happened but they did not know what it was. The remaining two patients recalled nothing at all. Although there is no evidence that the patients' postoperative course was influenced by the mock crisis, the results of the hypnotic interviews indicated to Levinson (130) that the event had been processed and maintained in memory, albeit outside of awareness.

Cheek's and Levinson's reports languished in the literature for two decades. In a review of anesthetic awareness and memory, Trustman et al. (201) concluded that anesthetized patients processed surgical events to the extent that they were awake—an echo of the famous conclusion of Simon and Emmons (185) about the possibility of sleep learning (for updates, see refs. 1,73). There the matter probably would have rested, had it not been for two factors: the conviction of some physicians and psychologists that some degree of information-processing, if not frank awareness, continued during anesthesia; and mounting evidence of spared implicit memory in brain-damaged patients and others who were densely amnesic on tests of explicit memory. The current revival of interest in awareness and memory in anesthesia may be traced to this fortuitous combination of clinical concern and experimental results.

Intraoperative Instructions for Postsurgical Behavior

Credit for rekindling the question of surgical awareness and postsurgical memory goes to Bennett (21; also see refs. 15–18,20). Bennett (21) instructed anesthetized patients that, when interviewed postsurgically, they should pull on their ears to indicate that they had heard his message during surgery. Compared to control patients who heard only operating room conversation through their earphones, a significant number of patients in the experimental group displayed the instructed behavior, even though none of them had any conscious recollection of the contents of the tape (thus, they did not appreciate the significance of their behavior, or experience it as an intentional act). Moreover, patients in the experimental group spent more time touching their ears than those in the control group. These findings were substantially replicated in a subsequent study, which compared four different motor behaviors, only one of which had been targeted by the instructions (22; see also ref. 18). Similar results were obtained by Goldmann et al. (93). These investigators were unsuccessful in inducing patients to pull on their ears, although they were successful when patients were instructed to touch their chins! Although Merikle and Rondi (143) have raised questions about the statistical analysis of this study, Block et al. (26) also obtained an instructed motor effect. Their study compared two behaviors: one targeted by the intraoperative instruction and the other never mentioned intraoperatively.

However, not all attempts to replicate Bennett's findings have been successful. Jansen et al. (109) failed to find any difference in instructed ear touching between experimental and control groups in a study which followed a standard anesthetic protocol involving enflurane, and included pre- and postoperative testing of the target behavior. Three other studies also found no evidence of the behavior suggested during surgery (23,24,140). Finally, two studies in which Bennett himself was a co-investigator found no difference between experimental and control conditions (51,69); a third study found the effect under nitrous oxide but not under isoflurane (68).

In principle, positive response to intraoperative instructions fits the formal definition of implicit memory: a change in experience, thought, or action (e.g., ear-touching behavior) that is attributable to a past event (delivery of the instruction) in the absence of conscious recollection of that event. Bennett's initial study (21) helped set the stage for subsequent work on implicit memory, but it has also been criticized on methodological grounds (144,214; for a reply, see ref. 17). For example, the statistical significance of the instruction effect may have been carried by two patients who showed extraordinarily high levels of ear touching; when these two subjects are eliminated, there is no difference between the experimental and control subjects. This problem confronts the study of Block et al. (26) as well as Ghoneim and Block (88), although, apparently, the overall effect was not entirely carried by a few outliers. In addition, Merikle and Rondi (143) have raised questions about Goldmann et al.'s (93) statistical analysis. At present, then, the suggestion that patients can respond postoperatively to intraoperative instruction for motor behavior remains a tantalizing possibility, but one which has not received adequate experimental support to date.

FORMAL STUDIES OF IMPLICIT MEMORY FOLLOWING GENERAL ANESTHESIA

Recent years have seen an explosion of studies employing more conventional implicit-memory paradigms of a sort familiar in cognitive psychology. In these experiments, adequately anesthetized patients are presented with auditory stimulus material, and then complete postoperative tests of explicit and implicit memory. The goal of these studies has been to search for functional dissociations between explicit and implicit memory analogous to those observed in cases of amnesia. The general hypothesis of this research is that while explicit memory for intraoperative events (recall and recognition) is grossly impaired (as indeed it should be) under at least some conditions of adequate anesthesia implicit memory (such as priming) will be spared.

Priming Effects

By far, the greatest portion of the literature on implicit memory following anesthesia involves priming effects of one sort or another. That is, the investigators seek evidence of improved performance on some perceptual-cognitive task that is attributable to the patient's surgical experience, in the absence of conscious recollection of that experience. In most of these experiments, performance on some priming test of implicit memory is compared with a free recall or recognition test of explicit memory.

The first experiment of this type yielded negative results. Eich et al. (74) presented anesthetized patients with a tape recorded list of items consisting of a homophone (e.g., ATE or EIGHT, PIECE or PEACE) and a disambiguating context (e.g., Dinner at EIGHT; War and PEACE). Ordinarily, such an experience will bias the subject's spelling of these words on a later test, regardless of whether the list items themselves are remembered—clear evidence of priming, and thus of implicit memory. Among patients who heard the tape preoperatively, Eich et al. (74) obtained the expected priming effect on spelling performance. When the tape was presented intraoperatively, however, they found no evidence of either explicit or implicit memory.

In contrast, the next study yielded positive results. Kihlstrom et al. (127) prepared two lists of paired-associates of the form OCEAN-WATER; one of these was presented to patients anesthetized with isoflurane, and the second list, carefully matched to the first in terms of normative cue-target probability, served as a control. Anesthesia was induced by thiopental and maintained with isoflurane, and the critical tape was played from the first incision to the last stitch. On an initial interview in the recovery room, the patients remembered nothing of the list. The left-hand panel of Fig. 2 shows the results of explicit and implicit memory testing. For the explicit memory test, the patients were presented with the cue terms from both lists of paired-associates and asked to recall the response term with which each cue had been paired. Obviously, this is possible only for the list actually presented for study. Nevertheless, there was no difference in the proportion of targets recalled from the critical and neutral list. For the implicit memory test, the subjects were presented with the cues and asked simply to respond with the first word that came to mind. Here, the patients showed a significant priming effect: they were more likely to produce targets as free associates to critical than neutral cues. Taken together, these results indicate that while the patients had no explicit memory for items presented during surgery, implicit memory for these items was preserved to some degree. (The order of explicit and implicit tests was counterbalanced across subjects, and there was greater priming observed when free association preceded cued recall.)

In a subsequent experiment, Cork et al. (55) repeated this procedure with patients whose anesthesia was maintained by sufentanil and nitrous oxide in oxygen (for a direct comparison of the two experiments, see ref. 56). In order to examine implicit memory in the absence of explicit memory, a few patients who showed some recall of intraoperative events on an initial interview were excluded from further consideration. The right-hand panel of Fig. 2 shows the results of cued recall and free association memory testing in the remaining patients. In

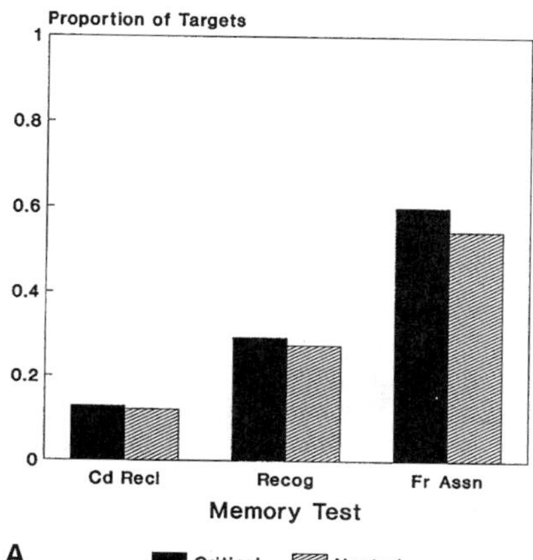

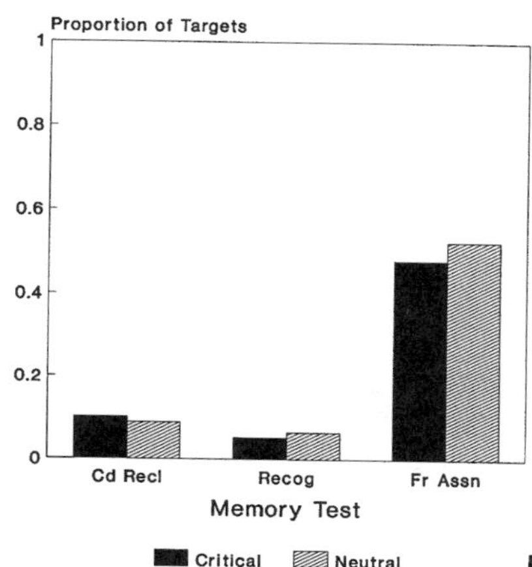

Figure 2. Performance on explicit and implicit memory tests following general anesthesia with isoflurane (127) (**A**) and sufentanil/nitrous oxide (55) (**B**). Cd Recl, cued recall; Recog, recognition; Fr Assn, free association.

this experiment, there was evidence of neither explicit nor implicit memory, regardless of the order of testing. Thus, explicit and implicit memory were dissociated with isoflurane anesthesia, but not with sufentanil/nitrous oxide.

A similar pattern of results had been obtained earlier in a pair of studies reported by Couture et al. (59; see also refs. 196,197). In the first study (196), surgical patients were randomized to one of two groups. Anesthesia was induced with thiopental and maintained with isoflurane. During surgery, patients in the experimental group heard a list of six low-frequency words (e.g., CORUSCATE, TERGIVERSATION) repeated a total of 19 times; controls heard a list of six pseudowords. Within 48 h of their operation, the patients were asked to listen to a tape recording of 36 words, including the six words presented to the experimental group, and to circle on a list any words which seemed familiar. Figure 3 shows the results. The patients in the experimental group were much more likely than their counterparts in the control group to identify the six target words as familiar, even though they had no memory that any of the words had been presented during surgery. The effect of exposure on familiarity judgments is a priming effect indicative of implicit memory. Still, a subsequent experiment (197), in which anesthesia was induced by thiopental but maintained with fentanyl and nitrous oxide in oxygen, showed no difference between experimental and control groups. The results are also presented in Fig. 3. Thus, as in the studies by Cork et al. (54–56), explicit and implicit memory were dissociated with an inhalant anesthetic but not with an opioid derivative.

Following on these studies, a large number of investigations have compared postsurgical explicit and implicit memory in patients receiving general anesthesia. These experiments have employed a wide variety of paradigms, and they have produced a mix of positive and negative results (see also refs. 8,9,19,52,88,89,121,143).

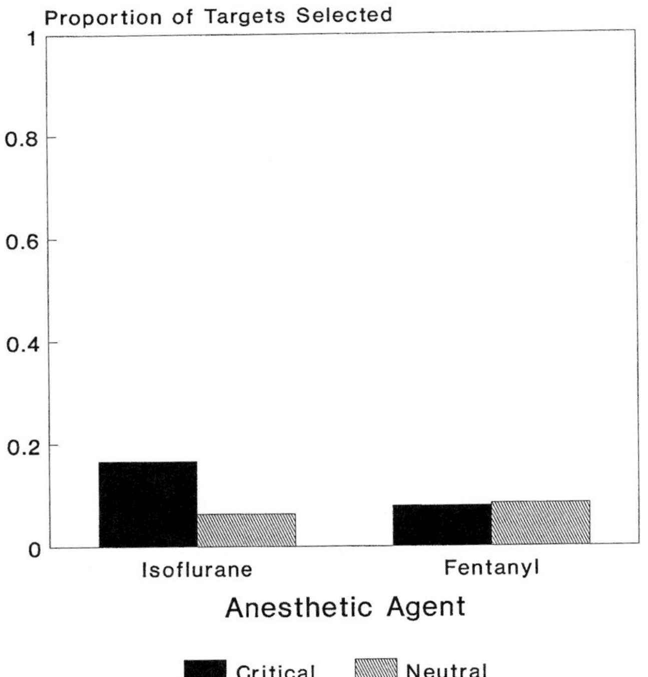

Figure 3. Performance on familiarity judgments following general anesthesia with isoflurane and sufentanil/nitrous oxide. (Reprinted, in adapted form, with permission from Couture LJ, Stolzy, SL, Edmonds HL. Postoperative evidence of intraoperative implicit perception of words: a comparison of two anesthetic techniques (submitted)

Homophone Spelling

Using the homophone-spelling paradigm employed by Eich et al. (74), Westmoreland et al. (213) also failed to obtain evidence of implicit memory.

Free Association

Humphreys et al. (102) combined the free-association and homophone-spelling paradigms. They presented homophones in a disambiguating context, as Eich et al. (74) had done. Instead of asking subjects to spell the homophones, however, they collected free associations to the ambiguous words. Scoring of these associations indicated that they were influenced by the context in which the cues had been presented during surgery. This effect held only for items presented at a very light plane of anesthesia (<1.2% end-tidal concentrations of isoflurane); although it should be understood that the patients were adequately anesthetized throughout the procedure.

Employing a more conventional free-association procedure, Bethune et al. (23) presented their patients with target words and sentences of the form, “Tar makes a mark,” at the rate of 20 times/h during surgery. Later, subjects were presented with the sentences frames, and asked to report the first word which came to mind. Subjects whose anesthesia was induced with fentanyl and maintained with propofol produced more list items than those who received fentanyl followed by methohexitone.

Schwender et al. (177) employed fentanyl in combination with benzodiazepine, isoflurane, or propofol, in three separate groups of ten patients. During surgery, the patients were read the Robinson Crusoe story; 3–5 days later, they were asked to free-associate to the word “Friday.” Half the patients in the benzodiazepine group responded with “Robinson Crusoe,” whereas only one in each of the other groups did so (in a control group which did not hear the tape, none responded with “Robinson Crusoe9). Interestingly, these investigators also monitored the mid-latency auditory event-related potential (MLAERP), an EEG component that occurs 20–100 ms after auditory stimulation. The MLAERP was preserved in the benzodiazepine group, but suppressed in the isoflurane and propofol groups. (In the studies reviewed in this chapter, spared implicit memory provides indirect evidence of cognitive processing during anesthesia. The ERP, whether elicited by auditory or tactile stimulation, provides such evidence directly; see refs. 120,126. For example, evidence that the middle or, especially, late components of the ERP are preserved would indicate that anesthetized patients are performing rather complex cognitive operations on environmental stimuli, regardless of whether these events are subsequently remembered; for reviews of this research, see refs. 159,176,194,198,199.)

Category Generation

A variant on free association is category generation, in which subjects are asked to give instances of taxonomic categories such as ARTICLE OF CLOTHING or FOUR-FOOTED ANIMAL. In the first study of this type, Roorda-Hrdlickova et al. (168) presented the words YELLOW BANANA, GREEN PEAR during surgery under nitrous oxide and isoflurane; later, the patients were asked to generate instances of the categories VEGETABLES, FRUIT, AND COLORS. In this study, patients who heard the list during surgery were more likely to produce target items than were those who heard a tape of neutral sounds. These findings were replicated by Jelicic et al. (112), employing nitrous oxide and fentanyl or sufentanil as the anesthetic agent. Evidence of priming was also obtained by Brown et al. (42). In this case, however, the evidence was of negative priming: target items were significantly less likely than neutral items to be produced as category instances.

Despite these positive results, other investigations have failed to obtain evidence of priming on category-generation tasks (10,26,29,45,52,192,209,213).

Perceptual Identification

A common finding in the priming literature is that previously presented words are more readily identified under conditions of degraded input, such as brief visual presentation, or following a printed word with a pattern mask (for example, see ref. 105). Charlton et al. (45) employed such a task, in which critical and neutral items were presented auditorily against a background of white noise. The patients were more likely to identify critical than neutral items. However, when these words were presented clearly to subjects for an explicit recognition task, subjects were unable to distinguish critical from neutral items. Thus, implicit memory as represented by the lexical identification task was dissociated from explicit memory as represented by the recognition task.

Stem Completion

Another popular task in the implicit-memory literature is word-stem completion. Block et al. (26) found a small effect evidence of priming on this task, but the anesthetized patients' initial exposure to the words was necessarily auditory, while the test was presented visually. This is a problem because implicit memory is often modality specific—i.e., that implicit memory is preserved only when the modality of test matches the modality of study (for example, see ref. 105). Therefore, a shift in modality between presentation and test might have depressed any effect. Recently, Bonebakker et al. (30) carried out a similar study with an auditory stem-completion test, and obtained a significant priming effect. This kind of study requires pronounceable word stems; for this reason, a study of word-fragment completion following auditory presentation of whole words is probably impossible.

Affective Judgments

A few researchers have sought evidence of postoperative implicit memory in the mere exposure effect, by which exposure to an item increases a subject's preference for that item (222). As noted earlier, the mere exposure effect occurs with subliminal as well as supraliminal stimulus presentation (34), raising the possibility that it might occur for stimuli processed during anesthesia as well. So far, four studies have been performed, yielding conflicting results. (Insofar as the affective judgments are mediated by exposure, the familiarity-rating task employed by Couture et al. may be another instance of this genre; for this work, see ref. 59.) Block et al. (26) did find a marginal increase in preferences for pseudowords presented during anesthesia. Items which had been presented 16 times were preferred over those which had been played 0–8 times. On the other hand, Winograd et al. (217) played a tape recording of unfamiliar melodies (actually, non-Western folk music) three times to patients anesthetized with a combination of nitrous oxide and oxygen, isoflurane, and sufentanil. On postoperative testing, there was no evidence of a mere exposure effect; by contrast, melodies which had been played three or 12 times to a control group were preferred over those which had not been played previously. Caseley-Rondi et al. (44), in a study involving preference for Japanese melodies played eight times, also failed to find an exposure effect. In a study of children, Bonke et al. (33) played a tape consisting of 20 repetitions of the sentence THE CHILD IS PLAYING WITH THE __ BALL, with the blank filled in with the color orange or green. Later, when the children were given an opportunity to color a picture of a ball, their color selections were unrelated to the tape which had been played.

A variant on the mere exposure paradigm is the "false fame effect" discovered by Jacoby et al. (106,108). These investigators found that presentation of an unfamiliar name increases the likelihood that this name will be judged famous on a subsequent test; apparently, the misattribution of fame is mediated by priming effects, and a feeling of familiarity, similar to those observed in the mere exposure paradigm. Interestingly, the false fame effect is independent of subjects' ability to remember the names which they had studied; and amnesic patients show the effect even though they cannot remember the study trial (190). Thus, misattributions of fame constitute evidence of implicit memory. Jelicic et al. (113) obtained a false fame effect for names presented to anesthetized patients, but they failed to replicate themselves in a subsequent experiment (110).

Fact Learning

Another line of research bearing on the question of preserved implicit memory comes from experiments in which patients are presented with obscure "trivia" information during surgery. Of course, adequately anesthetized patients will have no memory for the learning experience itself. However, studies of other forms of amnesia have indicated that patients and subjects can acquire new semantic knowledge, even if they do not remember the episode in which that knowledge is acquired—a phenomenon termed source amnesia (80,174,184). Source amnesia reflects implicit memory because it is a change in behavior—the ability to answer certain factual questions—attributable to a past experience (e.g., hearing the answers to these questions over an audiotape) in the absence of conscious recollection of the learning experience.

A study informally reported by Goldmann (92) was the first to demonstrate source amnesia following adequate anesthesia. During surgery, the patients were played a tape containing a number of trivia questions and their answers (e.g., "What is the blood pressure of an octopus?). The patients' knowledge of these answers (tested by recognition) improved from pretest to posttest, although few if any of the patients had awareness that they had been taught the answers during surgery. More recent attempts to replicate this finding have yielded mixed results (68,69,110,113).

Conditioning

In classical (or Pavlovian) conditioning, the repeated pairing of a stimulus (the unconditioned stimulus, US) which routinely elicits a reflexive response (the unconditioned response, UR) with a neutral stimulus (the conditioned stimulus) leads to the appearance of a new response (the conditioned response, CR) to the CS which resembles the UR. Classical conditioning is ubiquitous, in that it can be observed in some form in almost every species with a nervous system (163). Of course, experiments on nonhuman animals clearly show that CRs can be acquired during anesthesia, and preserved after recovery, so long as the URs can be elicited by the USs. Because, in strictly logical terms, an organism need not consciously recollect the acquisition trials in order to give CRs to CSs, conditioning counts as an expression of implicit memory. Ghoneim et al. (90) failed to obtain evidence of classical conditioning in patients anesthetized with isoflurane and nitrous oxide, but this may have occurred because the anesthetic agents prevented the US from eliciting the UR in the first place.

Recognition Memory Redux

By definition, adequate general anesthesia renders a patient unable to consciously remember surgery. This assumption is confirmed by a number of experimental studies which fail to find evidence of either recall or recognition of intraoperative events (for example, see refs. 55,74,127,137,155,209). This is so even when recollection is attempted while the patient is hypnotized (18,21,93). The recognition results are especially reassuring, because recognition is generally considered to be a very sensitive test of explicit memory.

It is important to note, however, that most studies of recognition after anesthesia have used a yes/no procedure, in which subjects were asked to examine test items, including both targets and lures, and to indicate whether each had been presented previously. In another type of recognition test, known as forced-choice, subjects are presented with pairs (or larger sets) of items, one critical and one or more neutral, and required to select the one which had been previously presented—guessing if necessary. Employing such a test, Dubovsky and Trustman (67) found no evidence of recognition; Block et al. (26) obtained evidence of recognition for nonsense syllables, but not words, presented during surgery. Actually, however, there are reasons to think that forced-choice recognition might be spared, to at least some degree, if implicit memory is also spared. Mandler (139) has argued that recognition is a judgment of prior occurrence which can be made on the basis of two sorts of information: (a) a feeling of familiarity, such as occurs when a name or face "rings a bell," or (b) retrieval of the circumstances under which we previously encountered the object or person. From Mandler's (139) point of view, the "bell-ringing" recognition by familiarity is mediated by the same activation of prior knowledge which (according to his view) mediates priming. Forced to choose, subjects strategically rely on perceptual salience, or other phenomenal qualities which accompany priming effects, to construct inferences, or make informed guesses, about study items which are right more often then they are wrong. It should be understood, however, that priming-based recognition by familiarity does not compromise the postoperative amnesia which is part and parcel of the definition of adequate anesthesia. This is because the recognition is largely inferential; unless they are forced to choose or encouraged to guess, adequately anesthetized patients will rarely if ever recognize intraoperative events as such.

In fact, Bonebakker et al. (30) have obtained evidence of forced-choice recognition (explicit memory) as well as priming in word-stem completion (implicit memory). In accounting for this result, it is important to note that the procedure employed by these investigators differed from its predecessors in important respects. They presented the patients with two lists of words, one preoperatively and one intraoperatively; after surgery, the patients were tested on both lists. Recognition for a list of words presented intraoperatively was grossly impaired compared to recognition of a list presented preoperatively, but for the intraoperative list there were significantly more hits than false alarms. Anesthesia has no retrograde effect on memory, so it is not surprising that the patients were able to recognize some items from the preoperative list; this, in turn, may have created a mental set in which they were able to make better-than-chance recognition judgments about items from the intraoperative list. Similarly, in studies discussed below, Evans and Richardson (78) and Casely-Rondi et al. (44) found that, forced to choose, patients could guess with above-chance accuracy which of two tapes had been played to them during surgery; however, Bethune et al. (24) did not get this effect. Earlier, Millar and Watkinson (145), employing a signal-detection procedure in which patients were encouraged to guess, found significant yes/no recognition of words presented during surgery. (For a discussion of this experiment and its implications for implicit memory, see ref. 126.)

It would be interesting to know whether the patients could distinguish between the two sets of items; perhaps they incorrectly attributed items from the intraoperative list to the preoperative list. In any event, the above-chance levels of forced-choice recognition does not imply that the patients were inadequately anesthetized; rather, it suggests that the preserved implicit memory indicated by the stem-completion test served as the basis for "informed guessing"—the recognition-by-familiarity of Mandler (139)—on the recognition test.

EFFECTS OF INTRAOPERATIVE THERAPEUTIC SUGGESTIONS

Some practitioners, apparently inspired by the positive evidence of intraoperative information processing, or at least convinced of its possibility, have suggested that therapeutic suggestions, analogous to those administered in hypnosis, might be effective in relieving postsurgical pain and improving postoperative recovery. Following some uncontrolled clinical observations of therapeutic suggestion, Pearson (157) was the first to attempt a controlled, double-blind study. He found that patients who received therapeutic suggestions during surgery were discharged sooner than those who were played only music or a blank tape. However, the two groups did not differ in terms of their need for postoperative narcotic analgesia or rated course of recovery. Although no memory tests of any kind were administered in Pearson's study, the effects on postoperative release fit the formal definition of implicit memory: a change in experience, thought, or action that is attributable to some past event, independent of conscious recollection of that event.

The findings of Pearson's (157) pioneering study have been supported in some, but not all, subsequent investigations (for example, see refs. 2,24,25,28,32,44,58,78,79,85,86,111,135, 140, 151,195,220,221). Evaluation of this body of literature is made difficult by the wide variety of surgical procedures, anesthetic agents, and outcome measures employed (8,44,143). Moreover, many studies employ multiple measures of outcome, not all of which yield the same results; because multiple measures can capitalize on chance, interpretation of these studies is ambiguous.

Still, some of the findings in this literature are extremely provocative. For example, in a double-blind study of patients receiving total abdominal hysterectomy, Evans and Richardson (78) found that patients who heard a tape containing suggestions for postoperative comfort, lack of pain and nausea, etc., were discharged from the hospital an average of 1 day earlier than those who heard a blank control tape. They also showed less pyrexia and less difficulty with their bowels. Bethune et al. (24), studying angina patients receiving elective coronary artery bypass surgery, found a difference of 2 days in duration of hospital stay. McClintock et al. (140) placed a group of hysterectomy patients on patient-controlled analgesia (PCA); those who were played a tape of therapeutic suggestions during their surgery showed a 23% reduction in morphine consumption over the next 24 h. Steinberg et al. (195) obtained similar results in a study of patients undergoing hysterectomy or breast reconstruction. Caseley-Rondi et al. (44) also obtained a significant effect on PCA, in a study of patients receiving hysterectomy or oophorectomy. This study is especially significant for its introduction of a novel control group: some patients heard suggestions, while others heard soothing melodies; others heard both, while the rest heard neither. The discharge and PCA effects are particularly interesting, because they are behavioral in nature, and thus not vulnerable to the criticisms often directed at self-reports.

With respect to memory and recall, the positive effects of intraoperative therapeutic suggestion are of interest because they fit the formal definition of implicit memory: an effect of a past event on subsequent experience, thought, and action, independent of conscious awareness of that event. Positive results clearly indicate that information from the tape was encoded and stored in memory. It should be understood, however, that negative results are equivocal with respect to implicit memory. This is because positive response requires that the suggestion be both processed and executed. Consider an analogy to hypnosis: positive response to hypnotic suggestions obviously indicates that the subject has heard them; but negative response may be due merely to the fact that the subject lacks the degree of hypnotizability needed to respond positively. Similarly, intraoperative therapeutic suggestions may be encoded in memory, but remain unexpressed because the patient lacks the capacity to execute them. Intraoperative therapeutic suggestions are modeled on hypnotic suggestions, and it has sometimes been suggested that hypnotizability might mediate their outcomes. Although hypnotizability does seem to mediate the somatic outcomes of hypnotic suggestion (37,38), Casely-Rondi et al. (44) found no such effect for intraoperative suggestion. Studies of therapeutic suggestions which yield null results should not count as evidence against implicit memory following general anesthesia.

CONSCIOUS SEDATION

In cases where awareness is possible or cannot be prevented, as in trauma surgery or the modern practice of conscious sedation, administration of benzodiazepines can result in an anterograde amnesia for surgical events (91,153,160). However, it should be understood that the anterograde amnesia covers only explicit expressions of memory. Implicit memory is relatively spared by benzodiazepines (this is also the case for nitrous oxide) (27). In a study by Fang et al. (84), volunteer subjects (not surgical patients) who had heard a list of words while sedated with diazepam performed more poorly on a test of free recall (explicit memory) than control subjects who were not drugged. On a second test, the subjects were presented with three-letter stems that could be completed by list items. Subjects in the two groups were equally likely to produce list items on this test of implicit memory. Similar findings were obtained by Danion et al. (66), although exactly the reverse—explicit memory spared, implicit memory impaired—were obtained in a study reported by Danion et al. (65). A series of studies by Polster et al. (161,162) also documented dissociations between explicit and implicit memory produced by midazolam and propofol.

The sparing of implicit memory under propofol was recently confirmed by Cork et al. (54) in the first study of memory following conscious sedation to involve actual patients rather than volunteer subjects. Patients scheduled for ambulatory surgery received an intravenous bolus of propofol and fentanyl prior to surgery; during the operation, propofol was constantly infused, with supplemental boluses under the control of either the anesthesiologist or the patients themselves. At the last skin stitch, an audiotape presented a list of 15 paired associates of the sort employed by Kihlstrom et al. (127) and Cork et al. (55). After 1 h in the recovery area, the patients completed a series of free recall, free association, cued recall, and recognition tests for the critical and neutral lists (those patients showing any free recall were removed from subsequent analyses). Figure 4 shows that on tests of cued recall and recognition there was no advantage for the critical over the neutral list; that is, the patients had essentially no explicit memory for the items which they had studied during surgery. In the free association test, however, they were much more likely to give the targeted response to cues from the critical list than to cues from the control list; in other words, the patients showed significant priming on this test, indicating that implicit memory had been preserved to some degree.

In general anesthesia, adequately anesthetized patients lack both concurrent and retrospective awareness of surgery: they are not cognizant of these events as they occur, and they have no memory of them afterward. Conscious sedation separates these two functions: the patient is aware of what is happening, but has no memory afterwards. Apparently, sedative drugs prevent adequate encoding of surgical experiences, leading to a failure of explicit memory. However, implicit memory is largely independent of elaborative and organizational activity at the time of

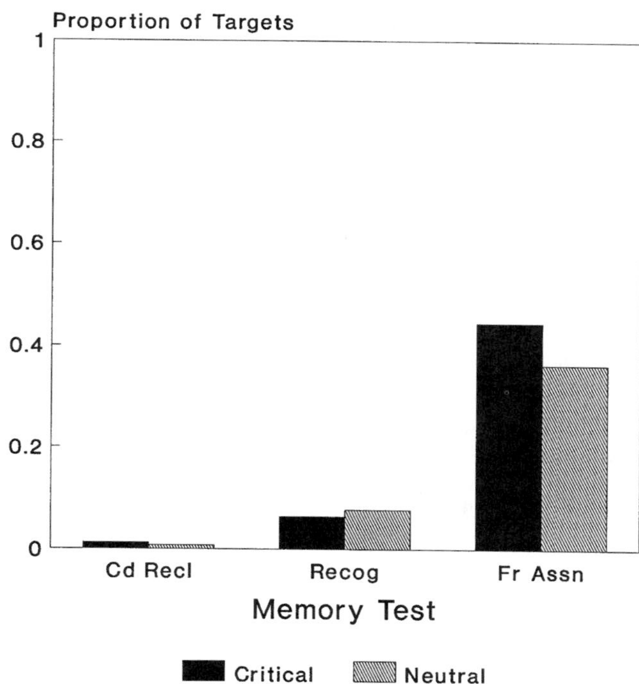

Figure 4. Performance on explicit and implicit memory tests following conscious sedation with propofol (54). Cd Recl, cued recall; Recog, recognition; Fr Assn, free association. (Reprinted, in adapted form, with permission from Cork RC, Friley KA, Heaton JF, Campbell CE, Kihlstrom JF. Effect of sedation with propofol on implicit memory (submitted).

encoding. The sparing of implicit memory has obvious implications for the use of benzodiazepines and other agents to control memory in both conscious sedation and general anesthesia. Although administration of sedatives may produce a dense amnesia in terms of conscious recollection, surgical events may nonetheless influence the patient's postsurgical experience, thought, and action outside of phenomenal awareness.

There have been no studies of the effect of therapeutic suggestions administered during conscious sedation. In view of mounting evidence that preoperative psychosocial interventions can facilitate recovery from surgery (for example, see ref. 150), experiments with therapeutic suggestions administered during conscious sedation would seem to be in order.

FACTORS AFFECTING IMPLICIT MEMORY AFTER GENERAL ANESTHESIA

Table 1 summarizes the results of those formal studies of implicit memory, published through the end of 1994, which have employed standard laboratory tasks. The studies of therapeutic suggestion have been excluded, because (for reasons noted above) negative results are ambiguous with respect to the question of implicit memory. Scientific understanding is advanced by producing an effect reliably; it can also be advanced by making it go away reliably. Thus, the mix of positive and negative results reviewed displayed in this table is not disconcerting, provided that some pattern is discernable. Unfortunately, no such pattern is discernable yet, perhaps because this line of research is in its infancy. For this reason, too, we have not performed a metanalysis of the available literature. Still, some comments may help direct future studies in this area to the point where systematic metaanalyses might be very fruitful.

For example, it is clear that progress in this area can only be made when the patients enrolled in these experiments receive standardized anesthetic regimes. Unless this occurs, positive

Table 1. FORMAL STUDIES OF IMPLICIT MEMORY FOLLOWING GENERAL ANESTHESIA: SUMMARY BY PARADIGM SINCE 1985

Positive results	Negative results
Behavioral response	
Bennett and Boyle, 1986 (20)	McClintock et al., 1990 (140)
Goldmann et al., 1987(93)	Jansen et al., 1991 (109)
Bennett et al., 1988 (22)	Bethune et al., 1992 (23)
Block et al., 1991 (25)	Dwyer et al., 1992 (68)
Dwyer et al., 1992 (68)	Dwyer et al., 1992 (69)
	Bethune et al., 1993 (24)
	Chortkoff et al., 1993 (51)
Homophone spelling	
	Eich et al., 1985 (74)
	Westmoreland et al., 1993 (213)
Free association	
Kihlstrom et al., 1990 (127)	Cork et al., 1992 (55)
Bethune et al., 1992 (23)	
Humphreys et al., 1993 (102)	
Schwender et al., 1994 (177)	
Category generation	
Roorda-Hrdlickova et al., 1990 (168)	Standen et al., 1987 (192)
	Block et al., 1991 (25)
Jelicic et al., 1992 (112)	Bonebakker et al., 1993 (29)
Brown et al., 1992 (42)	Charlton et al., 1993 (45)
	Chortkoff et al., 1993 (51)
	Villemure et al., 1993 (209)
	Westmoreland et al., 1993 (213)
	Andrade et al., 1994 (10)
Perceptual identification	
Charlton et al., 1993 (45)	
Stem completion	
Block et al., 1991 (25)	
Bonebakker et al., 1994 (30)	
Familiarity/fame judgments	
Stolzy et al., 1986 (196)	Stolzy et al., 1987 (197)
Jelicic et al., 1992 (113)	Jelicic et al., 1993 (110)
Affective judgments	
Block et al., 1991 (25)	Winograd et al., 1991 (217)
	Bonke et al., 1993 (33)
	Caseley-Rondi et al., 1994 (44)
Fact learning	
Goldmann, 1987 (92)	Dwyer et al., 1992 (68)
Jelicic et al., 1992 (113)	Dwyer et al., 1992 (69)
	Jelicic et al., 1993 (110)
Conditioning	
	Ghoneim et al., 1992 (90)

effects obtained with one agent (or class of agents) may be obscured by the negative effects of others. Careful control also needs to be exercised over preoperative and postoperative medication. Furthermore, investigators should repeat their experiments across a wide range of anesthetic agents, in order to determine the generalizability of positive (and, for that matter, negative) results. Of course, comparison is made difficult by the task of insuring that patients given different agents are all anesthetized to the same depth; for this reason, further research is also needed to develop techniques for monitoring the depth of anesthesia (116,193). Studies of both patients and volunteers clearly indicate that the effects on memory vary as a function of anesthetic depth (for example, see refs. 10,51,68). However, it should be understood that, in the experiments summarized here, all patients were adequately anesthetized according to standard clinical criteria.

Such comparisons are theoretically important because the amnestic properties of various agents may be related to their biochemical mechanisms of action. The inhalants are nonspecific anesthetics, which apparently act on the neuronal membrane to block the sodium channel; by inhibiting depolarization, they prevent synaptic transmission. By contrast, the opioids, benzodiazepines, and ketamine exert selective blocking effects on the receptors of particular neurotransmitters. In this light, it is interesting that both Couture et al. (59) and Cork et al. (55) found that implicit memory is spared when subjects receive inhalant anesthesia (isoflurane), but not when they receive a nitrous-narcotic preparation (fentanyl or sufentanil). On the other hand, Block et al. (26) obtained evidence of spared implicit memory on one test (stem-completion) under both sorts of conditions, while Schwender et al. (177) found the reverse. Obviously, further research is needed on this topic.

Similarly, careful attention also must be given to the means by which implicit memory is tested. It is easy, and fun, to invent implicit memory tasks. But if research in this area is to progress, it is important to use tasks which have been extensively studied under standard laboratory conditions. Otherwise the investigator risks studying one unknown with another. Unfortunately, many of the best-studied implicit memory tasks (e.g., word-stem- and word-fragment-completion) generally require visual presentation and testing. However, others (e.g., free-association, category generation, homophone-spelling, preference judgments) do not, and some tasks (e.g., perceptual identification and lexical decision) exist in both visual and auditory forms.

Even among these tasks, however, certain characteristics may be critical to the success or failure of the research. For example, the homophone-spelling task requires the subjects to process the meaning of the stimulus word (as implied by its sentence context), and it may well be that such complex cognitive processes are beyond the powers of the anesthetized patient (97,118–121). If patients cannot analyze the meaning of a word at the time of initial presentation, they cannot use semantic information to bias spelling performance at the time of test. There are good reasons for thinking that implicit memory in anesthetized patients, to the extent that it exists at all, is mediated by a perceptual representation system which analyzes the form and structure, but not the meaning, of objects and events (172,175,205).

Accordingly, tests which require subjects to process the semantic properties of stimuli may fail to reveal implicit memory which would be uncovered by tests which require them only to process perceptual properties. In this respect, the successful studies of Kihlstrom et al. (127) and Bethune et al. (23) may seem anomalous, because the priming of free associations would ordinarily seem to require processing of semantic links. However, this is not the case in these studies. In the former study, the whole paired associate, including cue and target, was presented during surgery, as were the targets and their sentence frames in the latter. This is a situation very close to repetition, rather than semantic, priming. Under these circumstances, priming could have been mediated by perceptual rather than semantic representations of the stimuli in question. Other variants on the free-association task, in which the cue and the target were not presented together during surgery, probably would have yielded negative results.

This consideration of the cognitive requirements of different implicit memory tasks is important. Individuals who are unconscious are not able to deploy attention, and engage in complex cognitive activities, such as elaboration and organization, in the way that their conscious counterparts are. Semantic analysis, or at least the elaborative and organizational processing described earlier, appears to be necessary for explicit memory; and the fact that explicit memory is abolished in anesthesia supports the idea that these processes are unavailable to adequately anesthetized patients. However, elaboration, organization, and semantic analysis are not necessary for implicit memory—at least for those forms of implicit memory which are mediated by a perceptual representation system. Thus, implicit memory may well be spared, provided that it is based on a presemantic perceptual representation system. (It should be noted that the involvement of perceptual representations in postoperative implicit memory places limits on the effectiveness of intraoperative therapeutic suggestions, insofar as understanding such suggestions requires semantic processing.) Nevertheless, the sparing of implicit memory, to the extent that it occurs at all, does not mean that the patient was conscious during surgery or was in any sense inadequately anesthetized. Implicit memory in general anesthesia is theoretically interesting precisely because it tests the limits of information-processing outside of conscious awareness and control.

RECOMMENDATIONS FOR CLINICAL PRACTICE

Despite our currently limited knowledge about perioperative awareness and postsurgical implicit memory, there are certain basic, common-sense precautions which clinicians can take to protect patients against explicit memory—and, if intraoperative suggestion actually works, to exploit implicit memory to the patient's advantage.

It has been well documented that preoperative explanation of anesthesia and surgery can take the place of a significant amount of medication in allaying patient fear and anxiety. The anesthesiologist should talk to the patient about the potential for explicit and implicit memory following anesthesia, and offer the patient the opportunity to have something placed over his or her ears during surgery. Alternatives include simple earplugs, designed to take away loud or distracting operating room noises, audiocassette earphones for music that the patient likes, or even positive suggestions recorded by the patient, the anesthesiologist, the surgeon, or anyone else the patient wants. We may not know whether the patient is hearing or will remember anything, but the precautions are so simple and the repercussions for failing to take them so unsavory that it would make sense to provide something for the patient's ears.

In the holding area and prior to the induction of anesthesia, the patient may be in a very terrified state, and the sound environment is important to proper management. Instruments crashing, radios playing, and surgeons conducting detailed conversations about the patient's pathology should be stopped. Again, earphones with taped music or suggestions should be an option.

During anesthesia, derogatory remarks about the patient, as well as negative comments about pathology, should be forbidden. Of course, we do not know that music or taped suggestions improve outcome, but they may keep patients from hearing partial or inadvertent comments. If you do not provide the patient with cassette players and earphones, at least provide earplugs.

The same rules apply to emergence and recovery. Environmental noise and conversation should be controlled. Be prepared to repeat, the next day, postoperative conversations held immediately after the surgery: the patient is likely not to remember them. If the patient is an outpatient, make sure that any explanations or instructions are carefully given to whomever is responsible for taking the patient home.

Admittedly, these are aggressive measures to take to prevent a problem that may never occur. We recommend them, however, because they are easy to accomplish and help protect both the patient and the physician from an unhappy experience. They do no harm, and they may well do some good.

Acknowledgment: Preparation of this paper was supported in part by a grant from the McDonnell-Pew Cognitive Neuroscience Program to the University of Arizona, and by Grant MH-35856 from the National Institute of Mental Health to John F. Kihlstrom. We thank Melissa Birren, Michael Cyphers, Jennifer Dorfman, Elizabeth Glisky, Martha Glisky, Heather Law, Victor Shames, Michael Valdisseri, Susan Valdisseri, and Michele Wright for their comments.

REFERENCES

1. Aarons L. Sleep-assisted instruction. *Psychol Bull* 1976;83:1–40.
2. Abramson M, Greenfield I, Heron W. Response to or perception of auditory stimuli under deep surgical anesthesia. *Am J Obstet Gynecol* 1966;96:584–585.
3. Adam N. Disruption of memory functions associated with general anesthetics. In: Kihlstrom JF, Evans FJ, eds. *Functional disorders of memory.* Hillsdale, NJ: Erlbaum, 1979:219–238.
4. Agarwal G, Sikh SS. Awareness during anaesthesia: a prospective study. *Br J Anaesth* 1977;49:835–838.
5. Anderson JR. *Language, memory, and thought.* Hillsdale, NJ: Erlbaum, 1976.
6. Anderson JR. *Cognitive psychology and its implications.* 3rd ed. San Francisco: Freeman, 1990.
7. Anderson JR, Reder LM. An elaborative processing explanation of depth of processing. In: Cermak LS, Craik FIM, eds. *Levels of processing in human memory.* Hillsdale, NJ: Erlbaum, 1979:385–403.
8. Andrade J. Learning during anaesthesia: a review. *Br J Psychol* (in press).
9. Andrade J, Baddeley AD. Human memory and anesthesia. *Int Anesthesiol Clin* 1993;31:39–51.
10. Andrade J, Munglani R, Jones JG, Baddeley AD. Cognitive performance during anesthesia. *Conscious Cogn* 1994;3:148–165.
11. Baddeley AD. *Human memory: theory and practice.* Boston: Allyn and Bacon, 1990.
12. Bahrick HP. Semantic memory content in permastore: 50 years of memory for Spanish learned in school. *J Exp Psychol Gen* 1984;113:1–29.
13. Barsalou LW. *Cognitive psychology: an overview for cognitive scientists.* Hillsdale, NJ: Erlbaum, 1992.
14. Bartlett FC. *Remembering: a study in experimental and social psychology.* Cambridge: Cambridge University Press, 1932.
15. Bennett H. Response to intraoperative conversation. *Br J Anaesth* 1986;58:134–135.
16. Bennett HL. Learning and memory in anaesthesia. In: Rosen M, Lunn JN, eds. *Consciousness, awareness and pain in general anaesthesia.* London: Butterworth, 1987:132–149.
17. Bennett HL. Unconscious perception during general anaesthesia. *Br J Anaesth* 1987;59:1335–1337.
18. Bennett HL. Perception and memory for events during adequate general anesthesia for surgical operations. In: Pettinati HM, ed. *Hypnosis and memory.* New York: Guilford, 1988:193–231.
19. Bennett HL. Memory for events during anesthesia does occur: a psychologist's viewpoint. In: Sebel PS, Bonke B, Winograd E, eds. *Memory and awareness in anesthesia.* Englewood Cliffs, NJ: PTR Prentice Hall, 1993:459–466.
20. Bennett HL, Boyle WA. Selective remembering: anaesthesia and memory. *Anesth Analg* 1986;65:988–989.
21. Bennett HL, Davis HS, Giannini JA. Non-verbal response to intraoperative conversation. *Br J Anaesth* 1985;57:174–179.
22. Bennett HL, DeMorris RN, Willits NH. Acquisition of auditory information during different periods of anesthesia. *Anesth Analg* 1988;67: S12.
23. Bethune DW, Ghosh S, Bray B, et al. Learning during general anaesthesia: implicit recall after methohexitone or propofol infusion. *Br J Anaesth* 1992;69:197–199.
24. Bethune DW, Ghosh S, Walker IA, Carter A, Kerr L, Sharples LD. Intraoperative positive therapeutic suggestions improve immediate postoperative recovery following cardiac surgery. In: Sebel PS, Bonke B, Winograd E, eds. *Memory and awareness in anesthesia.* Englewood Cliffs, NJ: PTR Prentice Hall, 1993:154–161.
25. Block RI, Ghoneim MM, Sum Ping ST, Ali MA. Efficacy of therapeutic suggestions for improved postoperative recovery presented during general anesthesia. *Anesthesiology* 1991;75:746–55.
26. Block RI, Ghoneim MM, Sum Ping ST, Ali MA. Human learning during general anaesthesia and surgery. *Br J Anaesth* 1991;66:170–178.
27. Block RE, Ghoneim MM, Pathak D, Kumar V, Hinrichs JV. Effects of a subanesthetic concentration of nitrous oxide on overt and covert assessments of memory and associative processes. *Psychopharmacology* 1988;96:324–331.
28. Boeke S, Bonke B, Bouwhuis-Hoogerwerf ML, Bovill JG, Zwaveling A. Effects of sounds presented during general anaesthesia on postoperative course. *Br J Anaesth* 1988;60:697–702.
29. Bonebakker AE, Bonke B, Klein J, Wolters G, Hop WCJ. Implicit memory during balanced anaesthesia. *Anaesthesia* 1993;48:657–660.
30. Bonebakker AE, Bonke B, Klein J, et al. Information-processing in

balanced anesthesia: evidence for unconscious memory (submitted).
31. Bonke B, Bovill JG, Moerman N, eds. *Memory and awareness in anaesthesia III.* Assen, The Netherlands: Van Gorcum, 1996.
32. Bonke B, Schmitz PIM, Verhage F, Zwaveling, A. Unconscious perception during general anaesthesia. *Br J Anaesth* 1987;59: 1335–1336.
33. Bonke B, VanDam ME, VanKleef F, Slijper FME. Implicit memory tested in children with inhalational anaesthesia. In: Sebel PS, Bonke B, Winograd E, ed. *Memory and awareness in anesthesia.* Englewood Cliffs, NJ: PTR Prentice Hall, 1993:48–56.
34. Bornstein RB. Exposure and affect: overview and meta-analysis of research. *Psychol Bull* 1989;106:265–289.
35. Bornstein RB, Pittman TS, eds. *Perception without awareness: Cognitive, clinical, and social perspectives.* New York: Guilford, 1992.
36. Bower GH. Organizational factors in memory. *Cogn Psychol* 1970;1: 18–46.
37. Bowers KS. Hypnosis: an informational approach. *Ann NY Acad Sci* 1977;296:222–237.
38. Bowers KS, Kelly P. Stress, disease, psychotherapy, and hypnosis. *J Abnorm Psychol* 1979;88:490–505.
39. Breckenridge JL, Aitkenhead AR. Isolated forearm technique for detection of wakefulness during general anaesthesia. *Br J Anaesth* 1981;53:665–666.
40. Breckenridge JL, Aitkenhead AR. Awareness during anesthesia: a review. *Ann R Coll Surg* 1983;65:93–96.
41. Brice DD, Hetherington RR, Uting JE. A simple study of awareness during anaesthesia. *Br J Anaesth* 1970;42:535–542.
42. Brown AS, Best MR, Mitchell DB, Hagggard LC. Memory under anesthesia: evidence for response suppression. *Bull Psychon Soc* 1992;30:244–246.
43. Carew TJ, Sahley CL. Invertebrate learning and memory: from behavior to molecules. *Annu Rev Neurosci* 1986;9:435–487.
44. Caseley-Rondi, G Merikle PM, Bowers KS. Unconscious cognition in the context of general anesthesia. *Conscious Cogn* 1994;3: 166–195.
45. Charlton PFC, Wang M, Russell IF. Implicit and explicit memory for word stimuli presented during general anesthesia without neuromuscular blockade. In: Sebel PS, Bonke B, Winograd E, eds. *Memory and awareness in anesthesia.* Englewood Cliffs, NJ: PTR Prentice Hall, 1993:64–73.
46. Cheek DB. Unconscious perception of meaningful sounds during surgical anesthesia as revealed under hypnosis. *Am J Clin Hypn* 1959;1:101–113.
47. Cheek DB. Surgical memory and reaction to careless conversation. *Am J Clin Hypn* 1964;6:237.
48. Cheek DB, LeCron LM. *Clinical hypnotherapy.* New York: Grune & Stratton, 1968.
49. Cheesman J, Merikle PM. Distinguishing conscious from unconscious perceptual processes. *Can J Psychol* 1986;40:343–367.
50. Cherkin A, Harroun P. Anesthesia and memory processes. *Anesthesiology* 1971;34:469–474.
51. Chortkoff BS, Bennett HL, Eger EI. Subanesthetic concentrations of isoflurane suppress learning as defined by the category-example task. *Anesthesiology* 1993;79:16–22.
52. Chortkoff BS, Eger EI. Memory for events during anesthesia has not been demonstrated: an anesthesiologist's viewpoint. In: Sebel PS, Bonke B, Winograd E, eds. *Memory and awareness in anesthesia.* Englewood Cliffs, NJ: PTR Prentice Hall, 1993:467–475.
53. Claparede E. Recognition and me-ness. In Rapaport D, ed. *Organization and pathology of thought: selected sources.* New York: Columbia University Press, 1950:58–75.
54. Cork RC, Friley KA, Heaton JF, Campbell CE, Kihlstrom JF. Is there implicity memory after propofol sedation? *Br J Anaesth* 1996; 76:492–498.
55. Cork RC, Kihlstrom JF, Schacter DL. Absence of explicit or implicit memory in patients anesthetized with sufentanil/nitrous oxide. *Anesthesiology* 1992;76:892–898.
56. Cork RC, Kihlstrom JF, Schacter DL. Implicit and explicit memory with isoflurane compared to sufentanil/nitrous oxide. In: Sebel PS, Bonke B, Winograd E, eds. *Memory and awareness in anesthesia.* Englewood Cliffs, NJ: PTR Prentice Hall, 1993:74–80.
57. Corkin S. Lasting consequences of bilateral medial temporal lobectomy: clinical course and experimental findings in H.M. *Semin Neurol* 1984;4:249–259.
58. Couture LJ, Kihlstrom JF, Cork RC, Behr SE, Hughes S. Therapeutic suggestions presented during isoflurane anesthesia: preliminary report. In: Sebel PS, Bonke B, Winograd E, eds. *Memory and awareness in anesthesia.* Englewood Cliffs, NJ: PTR Prentice Hall, 1993: 182–186.
59. Couture LJ, Stolzy SL, Edmonds HL. Postoperative evidence of intraoperative implicit perception of words: a comparison of two anesthetic techniques (submitted).
60. Craik FIM, Lockhart RS. Levels of processing: a framework for memory research. *J Verb Learn Verb Behav* 1972;11:671–684.
61. Craik FIM, Tulving E. Depth of processing and the retention of words in episodic memory. *J Exp Psychol Gen* 1975;11:268–294.
62. Crawford JS. Awareness during operative obstetrics under general anaesthesia. *Br J Anaesth* 1971;43:179–182.
63. Crile G. *An autobiography.* Philadelphia: Lippincott, 1947.
64. Crowder RG. *Principles of learning and memory.* Hillsdale, NJ: Erlbaum, 1976.
65. Danion J-M, Peretti S, Grange D. Effects of chlorpromazine and lorazepam on explicit memory, repetition priming, and cognitive skill learning in healthy volunteers. *Psychopharmacology* 1992;108: 345–351.
66. Danion J-M, Zimmerman M-A, Willard-Schroeder D, Grange D, Singer L. Diazepam produces a dissociation between explicit and implicit memory. *Psychopharmacology* 1989;99:238–243.
67. Dubovsky SL, Trustman R. Absence of recall after general anesthesia: implications for theory and practice. *Anesth Analg* 1976;55: 696–701.
68. Dwyer R, Bennett HL, Eger EI, Heilbron D. Effects of isoflurane and nitrous oxide in subanesthetic concentrations on memory and responsiveness in volunteers. *Anesthesiology* 1992;77:888–898.
69. Dwyer R, Bennett HL, Eger EI, Peterson N. Isoflurane anesthesia prevents unconscious learning. *Anesth Analg* 1992;75:107–112.
70. Ebbinghaus H. *Memory: a contribution to experimental psychology [1885].* New York: Teachers College, Columbia University, 1913.
71. Eich E. Memory for unattended events: remembering with and without awareness. *Mem Cogn* 1984;12:105–111.
72. Eich E. Theoretical issues in state dependent memory. In: Roediger HL, Craik FIM, eds. *Varieties of memory and consciousness: essays in honour of Endel Tulving.* Hillsdale, NJ: Erlbaum, 1989:331–354.
73. Eich E. Learning during sleep. In: Bootzin R, Kihlstrom JF, Schacter DL, eds. *Cognition and sleep.* Washington, DC: American Psychological Association, 1990:88–108.
74. Eich E, Reeves JL, Katz RL. Anesthesia, amnesia, and the memory/awareness distinction. *Anesth Analg* 1985;64:1143–1148.
75. Eich JE. The cue-dependent nature of state-dependent retrieval. *Mem Cogn* 1980;8:157–173.
76. Ellis HC, Hunt RR. Fundamentals of human memory and cognition. Dubuque, IA: Brown, 1989.
77. Erdelyi MH. The recovery of unconscious (inaccessible) memories: laboratory studies of hypermnesia. In: Bower GH, ed. *The psychology of learning and motivation, vol. 18.* New York: Academic Press, 1984: 95–127.
78. Evans C, Richardson PH. Improved recovery and reduced postoperative stay after therapeutic suggestions during general anaesthesia. *Lancet* 1988;8609:491–493.
79. Evans C, Richardson PH. Reply to D. S. Mackie. *Lancet* 1988;8617: 955–956.
80. Evans FJ. Contextual forgetting: posthypnotic source amnesia. *J Abnorm Psychol* 1979;88:556–563.
81. Ewen DM. Hypnosis in surgery and anesthesia. In: Wester WC, Smith AH, eds. *Clinical hypnosis: a multidisciplinary approach.* Philadelphia: Lippincott, 1984:210–235.
82. Ewen DM. Hypnotic technique for recall of sounds heard under general anaesthesia. In: Bonke B, Fitch W, Millar K, eds. *Memory and awareness in anaesthesia.* Amsterdam: Swets and Zeitlinger, 1990: 226–232.
83. Faithfull NS. Awareness during anaesthesia. *Br Med J* 1969;2:117.
84. Fang JC, Hinrichs JV, Ghoneim MM. Diazepam and memory: evidence for spared memory function. *Pharmacol Biochem Behav* 1987; 28:347–352.
85. Furlong M. A randomized double blind study of positive suggestions presented during anaesthesia. In: Bonke B, Fitch W, Millar K, eds. *Memory and awareness in anaesthesia.* Amsterdam: Swets and Zeitlinger, 1990:170–175.
86. Furlong M, Read C. Therapeutic suggestions during general anesthesia. In: Sebel PS, Bonke B, Winograd E, eds. *Memory and awareness in anesthesia.* Englewood Cliffs, NJ: PTR Prentice Hall, 1993: 166–175.
87. Gazzaniga MS, ed. *The cognitive neurosciences.* Cambridge: MIT Press, 1995.

88. Ghoneim MM, Block RI Learning and consciousness during general anesthesia. *Anesthesiology* 1992;76:279–305.
89. Ghoneim MM, Block RI. Memory for events during anesthesia does occur: an anesthesiologist's viewpoint. In: Sebel PS, Bonke B, Winograd E, eds. *Memory and awareness in anesthesia*. Englewood Cliffs, NJ: PTR Prentice Hall, 1993:452–458.
90. Ghoneim MM, Block RI, Fowles DC. No evidence of classical conditioning of electrodermal responses during anesthesia. *Anesthesiology* 1992;76:682–688.
91. Ghoneim MM, Mewaldt SP. Benzodiazepines and human memory: a review. *Anesthesiology* 1990;2:926–938.
92. Goldmann L. Further evidence for cognitive processing under general anaesthesia. In: Rosen M, Lunn JN, eds. *Consciousness, awareness and pain in general anaesthesia*. London: Butterworth, 1987: 132–149.
93. Goldmann L, Shah M, Hebden M. Memory of cardiac anaesthesia: psychological sequelae of cardiac patients to intraoperative suggestions and operating theatre conversation. *Anaesthesiology* 1987;42: 596–603.
94. Graf P, Masson MEJ, eds. *Implicit memory: new directions in cognition, development, and neuropsychology*. Hillsdale, NJ: Erlbaum, 1993.
95. Graf P, Squire LR, Mandler G. The information that amnesic patients do not forget. *J Exp Psychol Learn Mem Cogn* 1984;10:164–178.
96. Greene RL. *Human memory: paradigms and paradoxes*. Hillsdale, NJ: Erlbaum, 1992.
97. Greenwald AG. New look 3: unconscious cognition reclaimed. *Am Psychol* 1992;47:766–790.
98. Griffith HR, Johnson GE. Use of curare in general anesthesia. *Anesthesiology* 1942;3:418–420.
99. Harroun P, Beckert FE, Fisher CW. The physiologic effects of curare and its use as an adjunct to anesthesia. *Surg Gynecol Obstet* 1947;84:491–498.
100. Hastie R. Schematic principles in human memory. In: Higgins ET, Herman CP, Zanna MP, eds. *Social cognition: The Ontario Symposium. Vol. 1*. Hillsdale, NJ: Erlbaum, 1981:39–88.
101. Hindmarch I, Jones JG, Moss E. *Aspects of recovery from anaesthesia*. Chichester, UK: John Wiley, 1987.
102. Humphreys KJ, Asbury AJ, Millar K. Investigation of awareness by homophone priming during computer-controlled anaesthesia. In: Bonke B, Fitch W, Millar K, eds. *Memory and awareness in anaesthesia*. Amsterdam: Swets and Zeitlinger, 1990:101–109.
103. Hunt RR, Einstein GO. Relational and item-specific information in memory. *J Verb Learn Verb Behav* 1981;20:497–514.
104. Hutchinson R. Awareness during surgery: a study of its incidence. *Br J Anaesth* 1960;33:463–469.
105. Jacoby LL, Dallas M. On the relationship between autobiographical memory and perceptual learning. *J Exp Psychol Gen* 1981;110: 306–340.
106. Jacoby LL, Kelley CM, Brown J, Jasechko J. Becoming famous overnight: limits on the ability to avoid unconscious influences of the past. *J Pers Soc Psychol* 1989;56:326–338.
107. Jacoby LL, Witherspoon D. Remembering without awareness. *Can J Psychol* 1982;36:300–324.
108. Jacoby LL, Woloshyn V, Kelley CM. Becoming famous without being recognized: unconscious influences of memory produced by dividing attention. *J Exp Psychol Gen* 1989;118:115–125.
109. Jansen CK, Bonke B, Klein J, van Desselaar N, Hop WCJ. Failure to demonstrate unconscious perception during balanced anesthesia by postoperative motor response. *Acta Anaesth Scand* 1991; 35:407–410.
110. Jelicic M, Asbury AJ, Millar K, Bonke B. Implicit learning during enflurane anesthesia in spontaneously breathing patients? *Anaesthesia* 1993;48:766–768.
111. Jelicic M, Bonke B, Millar K. Different intra-anesthetic suggestions and their effect on postoperative course. In: Sebel PS, Bonke B, Winograd E, eds. *Memory and awareness in anesthesia*. Englewood Cliffs, NJ: PTR Prentice Hall, 1993:176–181.
112. Jelicic M, Bonke B, Wolters G, Phaf RH. Implicit memory for words presented during anaesthesia. *Eur J Cogn Psychol* 1992;4: 71–80.
113. Jelicic M, de Roode A, Bovill JG, Bonke B. Unconscious learning during anaesthesia. *Anaesthesia* 1992;47:835–837.
114. Johnson MK, Hasher L. Human learning and memory. *Annu Rev Psychol* 1987;38:631–668.
115. Jones, J.G. Use of evoked responses in EEG to measure depth of anaesthesia. In: Rosen M, Lunn JN, eds. *Consciousness, awareness and pain in general anaesthesia*. London: Butterworth, 1987: 132–149.
116. Jones JG, ed. Depth of anaesthesia. *Baillieres Clin Anaesthesiol* 1989;3.
117. Kandel ER. *Cellular basis of behavior*. San Francisco: Freeman, 1976.
118. Kihlstrom JF. The cognitive unconscious. *Science* 1987;237: 1445–1452.
119. Kihlstrom JF. The psychological unconscious. In: Pervin L, ed. *Handbook of personality: theory and research*. New York: Guilford, 1990: 445–464.
120. Kihlstrom JF. The continuum of consciousness. *Conscious Cogn* 1993;2:334–354.
121. Kihlstrom JF. Implicit memory function during anesthesia. In: Sebel PS, Bonke B, Winograd E, eds. *Memory and awareness in anesthesia*. New York: Prentice Hall, 1993:10–30.
122. Kihlstrom JF. Memory and consciousness: an appreciation of Claparède and his "Recognition et Moiïte." *Conscious Cogn* (in press).
123. Kihlstrom JF, Barnhardt TM. The self-regulation of memory: for better and for worse, with and without hypnosis. In: Wegner DM, Pennebaker JW, eds. *Handbook of mental control*. Englewood Cliffs, NJ: Prentice Hall, 1993:88–125.
124. Kihlstrom JF, Barnhardt TM, Tataryn DJ. Implicit perception. In: Bornstein RF Pittman TS, eds. *Perception without awareness*. New York: Guilford, 1992:17–54.
125. Kihlstrom JF, Couture LJ. Awareness and information processing in general anesthesia. *Br J Psychopharmacol* 1992;6:410–417.
126. Kihlstrom JF, Schacter DL. Anaesthesia, amnesia, and the cognitive unconscious. In: Bonke B, Fitch W, Millar K. *Memory and awareness in anaesthesia*. Amsterdam: Swets and Zeitlinger, 1990: 21–44.
127. Kihlstrom JF, Schacter DL, Cork RC, Hurt CA, Behr SE. Implicit and explicit memory following surgical anesthesia. *Psychol Sci* 1990; 1:303–306.
128. King H, Ashley S, Braithwaite D, Decayette J, Wooten DJ. Adequacy of general anesthesia for cesarean section. *Anesth Analg* 1993;77: 84–88.
129. Kunst-Wilson WR, Zajonc RB. Affective discrimination of stimuli that cannot be recognized. *Science* 1980;207:557–558.
130. Levinson BW. States of awareness under general anaesthesia. A case history. *Med Proc S Afr* 1965:243–5.
131. Levinson BW. States of awareness during general anaesthesia. *Br J Anaesth* 1965;67:544–566.
132. Levinson BW. The states of awareness in anaesthesia in 1965. In: Bonke B, Fitch W, Millar K, eds. *Memory and awareness in anaesthesia*. Amsterdam: Swets and Zeitlinger, 1990:11–18.
133. Levinson BW. Quo vadis. In: Sebel PS, Bonke B, Winograd E, eds. *Memory and awareness in anesthesia*. Englewood Cliffs, NJ: PTR Prentice Hall, 1993:498–500.
134. Lewandowsky S, Dunn JC, Kirsner K, eds. *Implicit memory: theoretical issues*. Hillsdale, NJ: Erlbaum, 1989.
135. Liu WHD, Standen PJ, Aitkenhead AR. Liu WHD, Standen P, Aitkenhead AR. Therapeutic suggestions during general anaesthesia in patients undergoing hysterectomy. *Br J Anaesth* 1992;68: 277–81.
136. Liu WHD, Thorp TAS, Graham SG, Aitkenhead AR. Incidence of awareness with recall during general anesthesia. *Anesthesiology* 1991;46:435–437.
137. Loftus E, Schooler J, Loftus G, Glauber D. Memory for events occurring under anesthesia. *Acta Psychol* 1985;59:123–128.
138. Mandler G. Organization and memory. In: Spence KW, Spence JT, eds. *The psychology of learning and motivation, vol. 1*. New York: Academic Press, 1967:327–372.
139. Mandler G. Recognizing: the judgment of prior occurrence. *Psychol Rev* 1980;87:252–271.
140. McClintock TTC, Aitken H, Downie CFA, Kenny GNC. Post-operative analgesic requirements in patients exposed to positive intra-operative suggestions. *Br Med J* 1990;301;788–790.
141. Medin DL, Ross BH. *Cognitive psychology*. Fort Worth, TX: Harcourt Brace Jovanovich, 1992.
142. Merikle PM, Reingold EM. Measuring unconscious processes. In: Bornstein RF, Pittman TS, eds. *Perception without awareness: cognitive, clinical, and social perspectives*. New York: Guilford, 1992:55–80.
143. Merikle PM, Rondi G. Memory for events during anesthesia has not been demonstrated: a psychologist's viewpoint. In: Sebel PS, Bonke B, Winograd E, eds. *Memory and awareness in anesthesia*. Englewood Cliffs, NJ: PTR Prentice Hall, 1993:476–497.
144. Millar K. Unconscious perception during general anaesthesia. *Br J Anaesth* 1987;59:1334–1335.
145. Millar K, Watkinson N. Recognition of words presented during general anaesthesia. *Ergonomics* 1983;26:585–594.

146. Milner B, Corkin S, Teuber H-L. Further analysis of the hippocampal amnestic syndrome: 14-year follow-up of H.M. *Neuropsychology* 1968;6:215–234.
147. Mishkin M. A memory system in the monkey. *Philos Trans R Soc Lond* 1982;298:85–92.
148. Moerman N, Porcelijn T. The patient's view of anaesthesia: a report of 1000 anaesthetics noted by the anaesthetist. In: Bonke B, Fitch W, Millar K, eds. *Memory and awareness in anaesthesia.* Amsterdam: Swets and Zeitlinger, 1990:233–235.
149. Moscovitch, M. Confabulation and the frontal systems: strategic versus associative retrieval in neuropsychological theories of memory. In: Roediger HL, Craik FIM, eds. *Varieties of memory and consciousness: essays in honour of Endel Tulving.* Hillsdale, NJ: Erlbaum, 1989:133–160.
150. Mumford E, Schlesinger HJ, Glass G. The effect of psychological intervention on recovery from surgery and heart attacks: an analysis of the literature. *Am J Public Health* 1982;72:141–151.
151. Münch F, Zug HD. Do intraoperative suggestions prevent nausea and vomiting in thyroidectomy patients? An experimental study. In: Bonke B, Fitch W, Millar K, eds. *Memory and awareness in anaesthesia.* Amsterdam: Swets and Zeitlinger, 1990:185–188.
152. Niedenthal PM. Affect and social perception: on the psychological validity of rose-colored glasses. In: Bornstein RF, Pittman TS, ed. *Perception without awareness: cognitive, clinical, and social perspectives.* New York: Guilford, 1992:211–235.
153. O'Boyle C. Benzodiazepine-induced amnesia and anaesthetic practice: a review. In: Hindmarch I, Ott H, eds. *Benzodiazepine receptor ligands, memory, and information processing.* Berlin: Springer-Verlag, 1988:146–165.
154. Overton DA. Dissociated learning in drug states (state-dependent learning). In: Efron DH, Cole JO, Levine J, Wittenborn R, eds. *Psychopharmacology: a review of progress, 1957–1967.* Washington, DC: U.S. Government Printing Service, 1968:918–930.
155. Parker CJR, Oates JDL, Boyd AH, Thomas SD. Memory for auditory material presented during anaesthesia. *Br J Anaesth* 1994;72: 181–184.
156. Payne DG. Hypermnesia and reminiscence in recall: a historical and empirical review. *Psychol Bull* 1987;101:5–27.
157. Pearson RE. Response to suggestions given under general anesthesia. *Am J Clin Hypn* 1961;4:106–114.
158. Pernick MS. *A calculus of suffering: pain, professionalism, and anesthesia in nineteenth-century America.* New York: Columbia University Press, 1985.
159. Plourde G, Picton TW. Long-latency auditory evoked potentials during general anesthesia: N1 and P3. *Anesth Analg* 1991;72: 342–350.
160. Polster MR. Drug-induced amnesia: implications for cognitive neuropsychological investigations of memory. *Psychol Bull* 1993; 114:477–493.
161. Polster MR, Gray PA, O'Sullivan G, McCarthy RA, Park GR. A comparison of the sedative and amnesic effects of midazolam and propofol. *Br J Anesth* 1993;70:612–616.
162. Polster MR, McCarthy RA, O'Sullivan G, Gray P, Park G. Midazolam-induced amnesia: implications for the implicit/explicit memory distinction. *Brain Cogn* 1993;22:244–265.
163. Razran G. Recent Soviet phyletic comparisons of classical and of operant conditioning: experimental designs. *J Comp Physiol Psychol* 1961;54:357–367.
164. Richardson-Klavehn A, Bjork RA. Measures of memory. *Annu Rev Psychol* 1988;39:475–543.
165. Roediger HL. Implicit memory: a commentary. *Bull Psychonom Soc* 1990;28:373–380.
166. Roediger HL. Implicit memory: retention without remembering. *Am Psychol* 1990;45:1043–1056.
167. Roediger HL, McDermott KB. Implicit memory in normal human subjects. In: Boller F, Graffman J, eds. *Handbook of neuropsychology, vol. 8.* Amsterdam: Elsevier, 1993:63–131.
168. Roorda-Hrdlickova V, Wolters G, Bonke B, Phaf RH. Unconscious perception during general anaesthesia, demonstrated by an implicit memory task. In: Bonke B, Fitch W, Millar K, eds. *Memory and awareness in anaesthesia.* Amsterdam: Swets and Zeitlinger, 1990:150–155.
169. Rosen M, Lunn JN, eds. *Consciousness, awareness, and pain in general anaesthesia.* London: Butterworths, 1987.
170. Ryle G. *The concept of mind.* London: Hutchinson, 1949.
171. Schacter DL. Implicit memory: history and current status. *J Exp Psychol Learn Mem Cogn* 1987;13:501–518.
172. Schacter DL. Implicit memory: a new frontier for cognitive neuroscience. In: Gazzaniga MA, ed. *The cognitive neurosciences.* Cambridge, MA: MIT Press, 1995:815–824.
173. Schacter DL, Chiu C-YP, Ochser, KN. Implicit memory: a selective review. *Annu Rev Neurosci* 1993;16:159–182.
174. Schacter DL, Harbluk JL, McLachlan DR. Retrieval without recollection: an experimental analysis of source amnesia. *J Verb Learn Verb Behav* 1984;23:593–611.
175. Schacter DL, Tulving E, eds. *Memory systems 1994.* Cambridge, MA: MIT Press, 1994.
176. Schwender D, Klasing S, Madler C, Pöppel E, Peter K. Midlatency auditory evoked potentials and cognitive function during general anesthesia. *Int Anesthesiol Clin* 1993;31:89–106.
177. Schwender D, Madler C, Klasing S, Peter K, Pöppel E. Anesthetic control of 40-hz brain activity and implicit memory. *Conscious Cogn* 1994;3:129–147.
178. Scott SM. Awareness during general anaesthesia. *Can Anaesth Soc J* 1972;19:173–183.
179. Scoville WB, Milner B. Loss of recent memory after bilateral hippocampal lesions. *J Neurol Neurosurg Psychiatr* 1957;20:11–21.
180. Searleman A, Herrmann D. *Memory from a broader perspective.* New York: McGraw-Hill, 1994.
181. Sebel PS, Bonke B, Winograd E, eds. *Memory and awareness in anesthesia.* Englewood Cliffs, NJ: PTR Prentice Hall, 1993.
182. Shimamura AP. Disorders of memory: the cognitive science perspective. In: Boller F, Grafman J, eds. *Handbook of neuropsychology, vol. 3.* Amsterdam: Elsevier, 1989:35–73.
183. Shimamura AP. Memory and frontal lobe function. In: Gazzaniga MS, ed. *The cognitive neurosciences.* Cambridge, MA: MIT Press, 1995:803–813.
184. Shimamura AP, Squire LR. A neuropsychological study of fact learning and source amnesia. *J Exp Psychol Learn Mem Cogn* 1987; 13:464–474.
185. Simon CW, Emmons WH. Learning during sleep? *Psychol Bull* 1955;52:328–342.
186. Squire LR. Mechanisms of memory. *Science* 1986;232:1612–1619.
187. Squire LR. *Memory and brain.* New York: Oxford University Press, 1987.
188. Squire LR, ed. *Encyclopedia of learning and memory.* New York: Macmillan, 1992.
189. Squire LR, Knowlton B, Musen G. The structure and organization of memory. *Annu Rev Psychol* 1993;44:453–495.
190. Squire LR, McKee R. Influence of prior events on cognitive judgments in amnesia. *J Exp Psychol Learn Mem Cogn* 1992;18:106–115.
191. Squire LR, Zola-Morgan S. The medial temporal lobe memory system. *Science* 1991;253:1380–1386.
192. Standen PJ, Hain WR, Hosker KJ. Retention of auditory information presented during anaesthesia: a study of children who received light general anaesthesia. *Anaesthesia* 1987;42:604–608.
193. Stanski DR. Monitoring depth of anesthesia. In: Miller RD, ed. *Anesthesia.* 3rd ed. New York: Churchill Livingstone, 1990: 1001–1029.
194. Stark JA, Fitzgerald WJ, Rayner PJW. Electroencephalogram and evoked potentials analysis: a model-based approach. *Int Anesthesiol Clin* 1993;31:121–141.
195. Steinberg ME, Hord AH, Reed B, Sebel PS. Study of the effect of intraoperative suggestions on postoperative analgesia and well-being. In: Sebel PS, Bonke B, Winograd E, eds. *Memory and awareness in anesthesia.* Englewood Cliffs, NJ: PTR Prentice Hall, 1993: 205–208.
196. Stolzy S, Couture, LJ, Edmonds HL. Evidence of partial recall during general anesthesia. *Anesth Analg* 1986;65:S154.
197. Stolzy S, Couture LJ, Edmonds HL. A postoperative recognition test after balanced anesthesia. *Anesth Analg* 1987;67:A377.
198. Thornton C. Evoked potentials in anaesthesia. *Eur J Anesthesiol* 1991;8:89–107.
199. Thornton C, Jones JG. Evaluating depth of anesthesia: review of methods. *Int Anesthesiol Clin* 1993;39:67–88.
200. Tracy J. Awareness in the operating room: a patient's view. In: Sebel PS, Bonke B, Winograd E, eds. *Memory and awareness in anesthesia.* Englewood Cliffs, NJ: PTR Prentice Hall, 1993:349–353.
201. Trustman R, Dubovsky S, Titley R. Auditory perception during general anesthesia: myth or fact? *Int J Clin Exp Hypn* 1977;25: 88–105.
202. Tulving E. Cue-dependent forgetting. *Am Sci* 1974;62:74–82.
203. Tulving E. *Elements of episodic memory.* Oxford: Oxford University Press, 1983.

204. Tulving E, Pearlstone Z. Availability versus accessibility of information in memory for words. *J Verb Learn Verb Behav* 1966;5:381–391.
205. Tulving E, Schacter DL. Priming and human memory systems. *Science* 1990;247:301–306.
206. Tulving E, Thomson DM. Encoding specificity and retrieval processes in episodic memory. *Psychol Rev* 1973;80:352–373.
207. Tunstall ME. Detecting wakefulness during general anaesthesia for caesarean section. *Br Med J* 1977;1:1321.
208. Utting JE. Awareness: clinical aspects. In: Rosen M, Lunn JN, eds. *Consciousness, awareness, and pain in general anaesthesia.* London: Butterworths, 1987:171–183.
209. Villemure C, Plourde G, Lussier I, Normandin N. Auditory processing during isoflurane anesthesia: a study with an implicit memory task and auditory evoked potentials. In: Sebel PS, Bonke B, Winograd E, eds. *Memory and awareness in anesthesia.* Englewood Cliffs, NJ: PTR Prentice Hall, 1993:99–106.
210. Warrington EK, Weiskrantz L. New method of testing long-term retention with special reference to amnesic patients. *Nature* 1968; 217:972–974.
211. Weingartner H. Human state dependent learning. In: Ho BT, Richards DW, Chute DL, eds. *Drug discrimination and state dependent learning.* New York: Academic Press, 1978:361–382.
212. Weiskrantz L. *Blindsight: a case study and implications.* Oxford: Oxford University Press, 1986.
213. Westmoreland C, Sebel MB, Winograd E, Goldman WP. Indirect memory during anesthesia: effect of midazolam. *Anesthesiology* 1991;75:A192.
214. Wilson ME, Spiegelhalter D. Unconscious perception during general anaesthesia. *Br J Anaesth* 1987;59:1333.
215. Wilson SL, Vaughn RW, Stephen CR. Awareness, dreams and hallucinations associated with general anaesthesia. *Anesth Analg* 1975; 54:609–617.
216. Winograd E, Neisser U, eds. *Flashbulb memories. Emory Symposia in cognition, vol. 4.* Cambridge: Cambridge University Press, 1992.
217. Winograd E, Sebel PS, Goldman WP, Clifton CL. Indirect assessment of memory for music during anesthesia. *J Clin Anesth* 1991; 3:276–279.
218. Winograd T. Frame representations and the procedural-declarative controversy. In: Bobrow D, Collins A, eds. *Representation and understanding: studies in cognitive science.* New York: Academic Press, 1975:185–210.
219. Winterbottom EH. Insufficient anaesthesia. *Br Med J* 1950;1: 247–248.
220. Woo R, Seltzer JL, Marr A. The lack of response to suggestion under controlled surgical anesthesia. *Acta Anaesthesiol Scand* 1987; 31:567–571.
221. Wood WE, Gibson W, Longo D. Moderation of morbidity following tonsillectomy and adenoidectomy: a study of awareness under anesthesia. *Int J Pediatr Otorhinolaryngol* 1990;20:93–105.
222. Zajonc RB. Attitudinal effects of mere exposure. *J Pers Soc Psychol Mon* 1968;9:1–28.

B

PAIN

Anesthesia: Biologic Foundations, edited by Tony L. Yaksh et al. Lippincott–Raven Publishers, Philadelphia © 1997.

CHAPTER 29

AN INTRODUCTORY PERSPECTIVE ON THE STUDY OF NOCICEPTION AND ITS MODULATION

TONY L. YAKSH

The pervasive impact of pain and its consequences upon the human endeavor is mirrored in every page of human history. Much as the basic needs of hunger and sleep drive our daily existence, escape from the pain state provides one referent for the interactions that define the framework for our experience. The importance of this imperative has made it a focus for the philosophers and serves to effectively highlight the relationship that exists between the mental experience made possible by the neural substrate and the physical environment.

PAIN AS A CONCEPT USEFUL FOR RESEARCH

Because pain is a descriptor of a conscious experience to which the outside observer is not privy, and because this emotional state can be induced by a wide variety of events to which the human is exposed, it has been necessary to provide some operational definition for the event we wish to consider. Thus, the death of a close friend or failure in a lifelong endeavor may cause us "pain," or having a rib removed (the first recorded surgical procedure, which was performed upon Adam by God) may cause us to have pain. It is the context of the third condition, tissue injury, that serves as the focus of our interest. It is possible at this instant to verify that the "pain state" has at least two principal components: (a) the stimulus with its immediate consequences on system function, and (b) the higher order processing that is the mind or state of mental activity that we define as consciousness. In the case of Adam, God, the first surgeon, saw fit to place Adam in a deep sleep, presumably to spare Adam the consequences of this traumatic intervention. (This, not incidentally, made God the first anesthesiologist.) Accordingly, Adam had no conscious experience of the tissue intervention and did not experience a pain state. As will be considered in later chapters, it is possible to alter the immediate consequences of the tissue-injuring stimulus from consciousness (as in the case of spinal anesthesia or opiates) and conversely to prevent the perceptual corollaries of tissue injury without altering the immediate consequences (as with volatile anesthetics).

The systematic investigation of the substrate that mediates the consequences of a tissue injury (or a stimulus that activates components of the pathway activated by tissue injury) has served as an important organizing focus of investigation. This emphasis on the stimulus and its immediate consequences is formally recognized by the use of the word "nociception" coined by Sherrington (68) (ca. 1906). At its simplest level of organization, "nociception" may be considered as the activity in the sensory afferent. At higher levels it may be the reflex evoked by that stimulus (as systematically studied by Sherrington). At yet higher levels, it may be the response evoked by such stimuli that are organized at the brainstem level (such as cardiovascular or hormonal responses). As Sherrington (68) noted, "Pain is a nociceptive reflex with a psychical component."

The nexus of the second part of the postinjury pain state (where or what is the "psychical component of the nociceptive reflex") continues to elude us. It can be seen, however, that as we engage in investigations related to the higher levels of behavioral organization of responses evoked by tissue-injuring stimuli, we move progressively closer to levels of organization that likely define components of a conscious state (see below). I suspect that a review of this field within the next 10 years will in fact provide a union of substrates that influence pain behavior, because of the role played by those structures in the emotive and perceptual components of sensory processing.

TOOLS THAT HAVE PERMITTED ADVANCES IN PAIN RESEARCH

It may be opined that advances in the neurobiology of nociception, reflected by the followint chapters in this volume, have occurred because of fundamental insights into the structure, function and biochemistry of related systems.

The formal definition of structure is characterized by the development of detailed anatomic observations of dissected materials, as typified by the organized compendia of Galen (ca. 200 A.D.), the evolution of the microscope, and subsequently the appearance of specialized fixation and staining techniques. This permitted the definition of cell bodies and axons, which, coupled with the prescient observations of Waller (8), allowed the tracing of tracts by axonal degeneration. The evolution of functional insights arose from (a) precise anatomic-functional correlates provided by experiments of nature, and (b) the correlation between systematic interventions such as stimulation and lesions, and function in animal models. Also, there has been an evolving biochemistry of neural function, with the evolution of our understanding of the actions of agents that selectively block pain and the definition of the pharmacology of synaptic transmission. Through these systematic approaches and the experimental method, major streams of investigation have coalesced to provide the basis for the insights on which our current understanding of the pain state is based. Finally, perhaps the most important tool for advances in pain research has been the evolution of the theoretical perspective, outlined in the preceding section, that permits one to address the issue of "nociception" without having to advance in a single step to the highest order of complexity, e.g., the state of consciousness.

AN OVERVIEW OF ORGANIZING PRINCIPLES IN PAIN RESEARCH

For organizational purposes, I believe it is possible to consider that the current thinking about pain is broadly based on five classes of insights. In the following sections, I discuss these areas and provide a brief historical perspective of each. This approach is not intended as a detailed history, but rather an attempt to provide the reader with a heuristic outline that defines the thinking that has led to the underlying organization of the present volume.

Two Components of Tissue Injury

The pain state generated by a tissue injury is considered in terms of two components: a specific intensity-related component that maps the pain report in terms of the intensity and location of an effective stimulus (sensory-discriminative), and a component of perceptual processing defining environmental context and complex behavioral attributes such as emotion and anxiety (affective-motivational).

From a practical perspective, it is common experience that a state we define as painful can be evoked by physical injury. The report of a sentient observer exposed to such a stimulus reflects on the time course (when it starts and when it stops), the location of the injury, and the intensity of the stimulus event. Humans and animals, in the face of such stimuli, have been shown to be capable of defining differences in stimulus intensities and in the case of verbal organisms, assigning specific descriptors to those events. In this regard, the tissue damage inducing a pain event possesses characteristics of other physical interventions that generate a "sensation."

Philosophically, the constructs that embody the usage of the word *pain,* however, also reflect on the undesirable nature of the pain state and the ability of that state to induce suffering or a negative emotional state. Suffering is a perspective that is mediated by the context in which the sentient organism views the stimulus. As such, suffering, a negative emotional state, is believed to require life experience and the neurologic substrate that permits the ability to establish remembered relationships and consequences. While any stimulus may be used to condition a learned association that leads to suffering, a persistent activation of the substrate that is otherwise activated by a tissue-injuring stimulus can lead to a state of suffering without such conditioning. Thus, classical conditioning of a light with an intense shock can lead to a state in which simple presentation of the light will lead to behavior in animals suggesting a tissue-damaging (e.g., elevated blood pressure, increased gastric acid secretion) stimulus. In contrast, simple, uncued exposure of the animal to shock will lead to that state without additional learning. Accordingly, suffering (the negative emotional state) induced by a tissue-injuring stimulus can have the ability to exaggerate the manifestations of the response to a given stimulus. Conversely, the obverse is also true. If learning and experience cues a positive emotional state,[1] the nature of the response manifested to the injurious stimulus will be accordingly lessened. In this light, it can be appreciated that the magnitude of the observed response, e.g., the index of processes unknowable by the external observer, will be dependent on these internal states.

The above separation of components into the initiating stimulus and into the higher organization that impacts on its ability to generate behavior (including an emotive verbalization) has been a component of the thinking of behaviorists. In this century, the formal expression of this concept was made manifest by a large number of observers, such as Livingston (48) in 1943 and Beecher (6) in 1959. The best expression of the components has been provided in terms of the dimensions of sensory-discriminative and affective-motivational (56).

The utility of this separation is supported not only by the experiential issues outlined above, but also by the investigations into the underlying mechanisms. Thus, as will be reviewed below, during the last 100 years or so the greatest success has been with an evolving appreciation of the substrates through which the afferent activity generated by tissue-injuring stimuli passes. The insights into reflex, so clearly outlined by Sherrington (68) in 1906, has served to provide insights that parallel the organized behaviors evoked by tissue-injuring stimuli in the intact organism. This provides substantial support for the sensory discriminative function. There has been less insight into the underlying substrate that regulates the affective-motivational component of the state generated by tissue injury. Nevertheless, there is the continued appreciation of the differences between pain and suffering, where the observed behavioral state is clearly defined by elements of the sensory message and the emotional component.

In the current approaches to pain management, the impact of both components on the pain state are clear. The blockade of the afferent message, as with local anesthetics and various drugs, is a primary goal in pain management. Nevertheless, it is clear that the emotional component contributes pervasively to the behavioral impact of the afferent message. Substantive confirmation of the duality of the structural components associated with pain in humans is supported by the observation that lesions of the forebrain or their connections with the thalamus lead to states in which the affective component associated with pain appeared to be lost and prefrontal lobotomies were implemented on occasion for this purpose. In such instances, the patients indicated that they felt the pain, but with a typical lack of affect, reported that it did not bother them (82). The effects of such lesions, the potent role played by the positive psychological state induced by various pharmaceutical agents (such as systemic opiates), and the insights into the role played by forebrain/limbic structures in emotionality suggest that this area can be considered discretely in addition to those systems that process the afferent message.

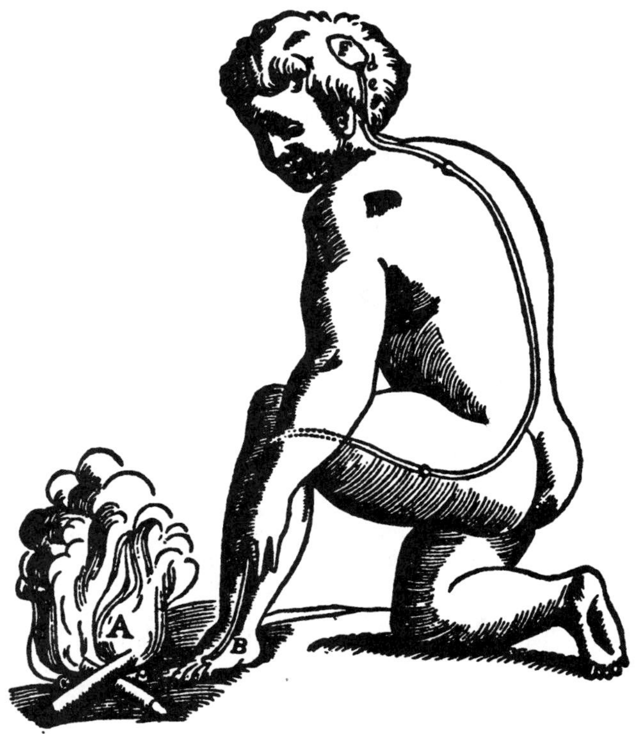

Figure 1. Cartoon of boy with toe in fire. The stimulus activates humors that travel up the nerve in the thigh to the spinal cord and thence to the brain where it terminated in the pineal gland. (Presented by Descartes in 1644, *L'Homme.*)

[1]"Negative" and "positive" are not employed to imply good or bad, but simply emotional states of contrasting impact.

Sensations Leading to a Pain State Are Transmitted by Anatomically Defined Pathways

The notion of pain being a specific sensation that could be ascribed to some role played by parts specific to the sensorium is clearly manifested in the cartoon by Descartes of the boy with his toe in the fire. Here an effective stimulus makes its way to the brain by the movement of neural humors (Fig. 1). This specificity of the sensation was a logical consequence of the thinking by Johannes Mueller in 1842 in his proposition of specific nerve energies. That is to say, it was recognized that injury provided a sensation interpreted as painful *because* it activated a specific pathway. The evolving appreciation of the role of the dorsal roots in the transmission of sensory information (Charles Bell and Francois Magendie, ca. 1800; Fig. 2), and the observation of the sensory loss after cord hemisections (Charles-Edouard Brown-Sequard, ca. 1850) (7) reinforced the concept of afferent systems that were responsible for the movement of information from the periphery to sites within the central nervous system. The concept of specific tracts for information leading to a pain state is embedded in the studies of physiology in the late 19th century. For example, William Gower (26) reported that a ventrolateral quadrant lesion in a man (caused by a misdirected gunshot wound) resulted in a contralateral pain deficit (emphasizing the importance of a crossed pathway), without a change in tactile sensitivity. In contrast, it was appreciated that the syndrome of locomotor ataxia associated with late-stage syphilis was characterized by massive degeneration in the dorsal spinal cord (the dorsal columns) and this state was associated with an ipsilateral loss of proprioception and touch, but not pain. Those observations and their implications were confirmed by Spiller who diagnosed prospectively a spinal lesion from observing sensory deficits, by Martin, who performed the first cordotomy for pain, and Beer, in 1912, for the pain of a sacral metastasis (76).

Spinal Organization

At the spinal level, the observations by Kuru (41) in 1949 showed the contralateral degeneration in dorsal horn neurons in the gelatinosa and in the marginal layer after ventrolateral lesions and he correlated this with the analgesia produced by such lesions. The systematic studies by Rexed (65) in 1952 provided an appreciation for the laminar organization that has dominated our thinking regarding spinal anatomy and physiology.

The anatomic organization of the afferent system provided a substrate, but demonstration of the role of that substrate by defining its physiologic properties provided the experimental basis for defining the properties of its function. Sherrington (68), at the turn of the century in his Silliman lectures, provided a mechanistic basis for the physiologic structuring of pain processing in his work on the integrative function of the nervous system and in his coining of the concept and jargon of the "nociceptive" reflex. Subsequently, the early recording by Adrian (1) in 1928 and later by Zotterman (100) in 1939 from peripheral nerves provided the recognition that small, slowly conducting axons were activated by a high-intensity, potentially tissue damaging stimulus, and the nerves and the role of such small afferents in these nociceptive reflexes provided the physiologic basis for functionally defining the properties of a nociceptive pathway.

Electrophysiologic studies have provided prominent insights into the characteristics of the ascending links and the nature of

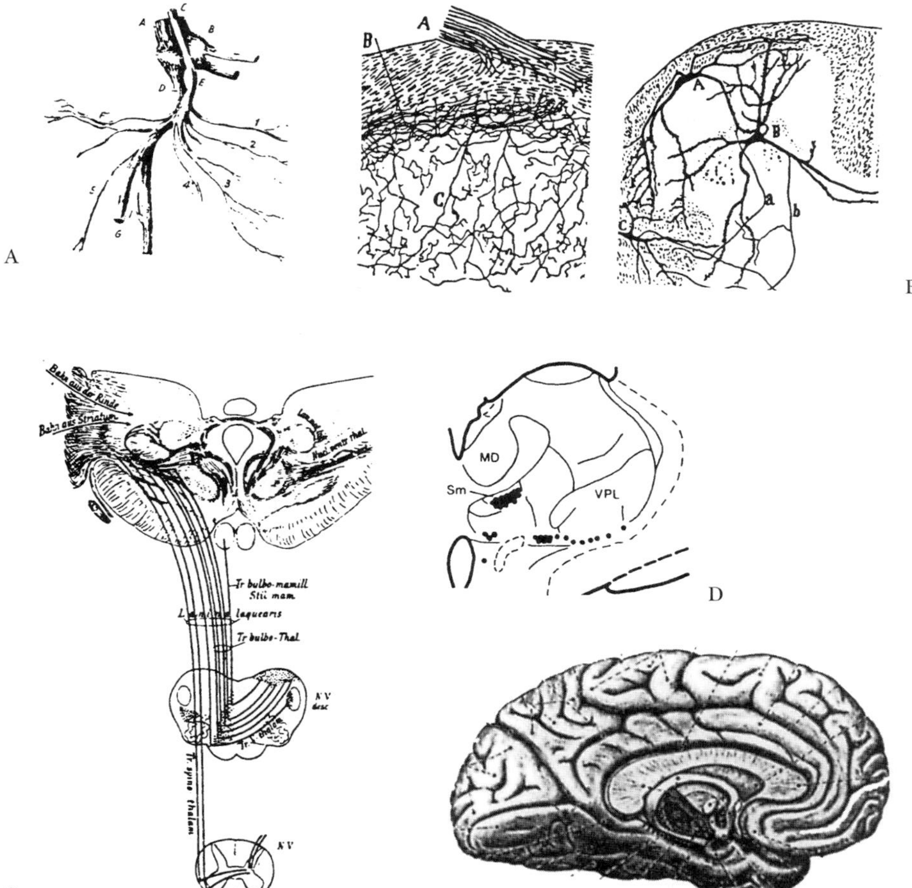

Figure 2. **(A)** Bell's (1811) representation of the Gasserian ganglion (B) with the posterior dorsal root (A) and anterior dorsal root (C) clearly shown (from ref. 39). **(B)** Ramón y Cajal's 1909 presentation of spinal dorsal horn, showing the penetration of afferent fibers into the substantia gelatinosa (from ref. 8). **(C)** Edinger's 1904 drawing of the, crossed spinothalamic tract in 1904 (from ref. 39). **(D)** Craig's 1987 presentation of the location of the n. submedius that receives marginal cell input (14). **(E)** Anterior cingulate. Representation of the location of changes in blood flow, defined by PET scan, that is activated by noxious thermal stimuli applied to the contralateral arm. See text for discussion (71).

the encoding processes involved. The early single unit recording from the spinal cord (40,78) provided the basis for the identification of the process by which afferent input was encoded into a spinofugal message. It now seems certain that at the least, there are cell systems that are largely selective for high intensity input (e.g., nociceptive specific) (11) and that correspond to the large marginal cells identified by Kuru. On the other hand, there are yet larger populations of neurons, as described electrophysiologically, that receive convergent input and appear to respond with increasing frequency as the intensity of the stimulus rises, recruiting first low-threshold and then high-threshold afferents (83). In this manner, it appeared increasingly plausible that spinofugal traffic generated by small afferent input could be defined as (a) that which encodes intensity and location with a great deal of precision, and (b) that which provides an all-or-nothing response, with the effective stimulus being noxious in character.

Supraspinal Organization

Anatomic and electrophysiologic studies consistent with the early dissections of the anatomists have revealed that many of these spinal neurons displayed complex projections to brainstem and diencephalic sites. Several points began to evolve during the late 19th and early 20th centuries. First, a large body of work began to describe the tract by which spinal systems might gain access to higher centers. Thus, tracing by dissection and degeneration led to the appreciation of the projections by Ludwig Edinger (1855–1918) (23) of the crossed fibers into the thalamic nuclei of the diencephalon. Second, aside from the long projections that made their way directly to the thalamus, it was appreciated that the spinal projections could arrive direct at higher centers by multiple links (e.g., the spinothalamic) as well as indirectly, perhaps via the "nuclei of the formation reticularis." Anatomic-behavioral correlates established by Dejerine and Roussy (18) in 1906 with vascular infarcts emphasized that the thalamus, being the site of termination of the secondary sensory pathways and the source of projection to the cortex, played an important relay role. Anatomists such as Ramón y Cajal (8) had indeed provided strong evidence for significant cortical complexity and localization work by experimentalists and clinicians such as David Ferrier and Hughling Jackson (99) suggested the existence of sensory and motor centers being organized at this level. Such connectivity and functional corollaries provided substantial evidence for a Cartesian model of afferent processing with increasing complexity of organization as one ascended in the neuraxis. This concept of increasing functional complexity at rostral centers was rationally compatible with a variety of observations, including the systematic transections of the neuraxis by C. Legallois (1770–1814) and by the systematic ablation studies of Pierre Flourens (1794–1867). By such ablations, Flourens demonstrated that the cerebrum was the organ necessary for volition and coordination. Importantly, while these studies provide strong support for the role of cortical interactions, the ability of Frederic Goltz in 1874 (25), for example, to evoke aggressive behavior by strong pinches in the decorticated animal emphasized that the ability to manifest components of a pain behavior could be organized at the subcortical level.

An important intellectual concept formulated in the early 20th century was the formal introduction of the organizational complexity at the higher centers. It had been emphasized by the work of von Monakow (1853–1930) that the cortex received thalamic projections and it reciprocally projected back to the thalamus (39, p. 127). Henry Head (1861–1940) (31), on the basis of the work by Roussy with the thalamic syndrome, considered that the thalamus was not only a relay station for information flow to the cortex, but that it served to move information to other areas within the thalamus proper and itself was the recipient of feedback from cortical centers. He and his colleagues proposed that the thalamus thus served to establish the pleasantness or unpleasantness of the sensation and it did so by its interactions with input from the cortex. While other examples may be cited, this thinking provides the backdrop for later concepts that relate to the endowment by the neural systems of a higher order overlay on the emotional significance of stimuli interpreted as painful. Thus, for example, William Penfield (63) in 1952 suggested that afferent input was conveyed by classical sensory projections to the cortex where it was then reprojected to other higher order centers such as the temporal cortex for comparison with past experiences, and to the precentral gyrus where voluntary actions are initiated.

Search for the "Specific" Pathway

The issues outlined above regarding the elucidation of the ascending pathways, as most popularly demonstrated by the cartoon presented by Descartes, has been the search for two defining characteristics: functional specificity and site of "perception." In terms of specificity, the anatomic and functional physiology have provided some suggestion that at the spinal level the degree of specificity declines as one ascends in the neuraxis. At higher levels, there is a specific component of the afferent traffic evoked by tissue-damaging stimuli that maps the identity of the stimulus onto specific thalamic (e.g., ventrobasal complex) and cortical (somatosensory cortex) sites, providing a basis for the ability to define the precise mapping of a stimulus event and its intensity (a corollary perhaps with an "epicritic" characteristic as defined by Head [31]). In this regard, one might argue that the sensation of "pain" is essentially a continuum with other thermal or mechanical sensations. The possibility that there are "specific" sites at higher levels of neural organization that respond only to high intensity or potentially tissue damaging stimuli has proven elusive. Some evidence has begun to evolve that raises the possibility of such loci even at higher centers. For example in cats, such a current site is reported to be the nucleus submedius (15). Such a site might serve to map less specifically the discriminative components of the message (e.g., it tends to receive nociceptive-specific input from nociceptive-specific spinal neurons), but links the ascending systems into components of the limbic forebrain that are functionally defined for their apparent association with emotive components of behavior.

Recent studies using positron emission tomography (PET) scanning revealed that nonnoxious stimuli would increase cerebral blood flow in regions of the specific somatosensory system. Increasing the stimulus intensity to an intensity reported as painful by the observer revealed an unexpected activity in the anterior cingulate gyrus, a region known to receive input from the N. submedius of the thalamus (10,71). Limbic forebrain structures are widely believed to provide the substrate for the emotional context of an afferent stimulus. Description of at least a simple linkage between a designated diencephalic projection site for high-threshold afferent input and such limbic forebrain structures provides an important rationale for defining a substrate mediating a component of the affective-motivational component of the response to a noxious stimulus.

With regard to the locus of pain perception, again, the cartoon of Descartes serves to illuminate the nature of the grail, a site at which the impact of a tissue-damaging stimulus comes to have conscious significance. In the drawing of the Cartesian machine, the twitches of the midline pineal gland served to define the ultimate site of decoding of the message. To the extent that we perceive consciousness as having a locus, then ideally such a site would have access to the highest level of organization. On the other hand, to the extent that we perceive consciousness to be the result of the activity in a distributed state, e.g., being defined by the common activity present in a network of supratentorial nuclear groups, then the issue of such a "pain center" involved in the consciousness related to "pain" is irrelevant.

The Processing or Encoding of Afferent Input is Subject to Dynamic Influences that Alter the Input-Output Relationship

Importantly, popular thinking regarding the organization of systems excited by noxious input implicitly assumed an immutable relationship between input and output. This is implicitly portrayed in the Descartes cartoon of the boy with his toe in the fire. This effective pain stimulus gives rise to the movement of vital humors from the spinal cord to the pineal gland and thence to the manifestation of the facial signs reflective of the pain state. Nevertheless, after the turn of the century, numerous instances emphasized that the relationship between stimulus and response at both the neural and behavioral levels was subject to significant alteration. Brown-Sequard, in his spinal hemisection studies, noted that after such lesions, "the sensibility seems to be much increased in the posterior limb on the side of the section, while it seems to be lost...on the opposite side." Thus, early studies on dorsal lateral spinal lesions resulted in a hyperpathia and a role for descending suppression of afferent traffic was recognized as early as the 1930s by the German neurosurgeon Forester.

The accumulating knowledge suggesting an underlying plasticity was formalized by Melzack and Wall (58) in 1965 in the gate control theory. This synthesis, based on an extensive line of thinking that could be dated to the mid-1800s, was both insightful and timely. Importantly, this plasticity is manifested in virtually all physiologic indices of spinal function.[2]

Downregulation of Small Afferent Evoked Activity

Stimulation of descending spinal pathways suppressed spinal afferent processing (9,28) and produced analgesia (67). The block of descending input conversely displayed an increase in the response properties of dorsal horn neurons (77). Stimulation of large afferent collaterals in the dorsal column would suppress nociceptive input and yield a behaviorally defined analgesia (80).

Upregulation of Small Afferent Evoked Activity

Early work by Thomas Lewis (1881–1945) demonstrated that repetitive stimulation of the sensory nerves would lead to a local hyperalgesic state, as defined by human sensory thresholds (46). These observations likely reflect both a peripheral effect releasing active factors from sensory (5) terminals to induce a local sensitization of nerve terminals (5) as well as a central sensitization due to repetitive activation of dorsal horn neurons (59). The development of animal models has led to the appreciation of the importance of this facilitated component as a common element in the postinjury pain state (Fig. 3).

Alterations in Larger Afferent Evoked Activity

The development of the concept of specific pain systems was based on the premise that potentially tissue damaging stimuli were nociceptive and that these systems acted through small afferents. Clinical observations, however, dating back to the first systematic report by Weir-Mitchell and colleagues (81) in 1864 emphasized that after nerve injury a pain state could be evoked by a low-threshold mechanical stimuli. Current evidence now suggests that the allodynic state may reflect a sprouting of large afferents into spinal regions that originally had received input from small afferents (e.g., the substantial gelatinosa) (85), and an acute loss of a tonic inhibition because of a loss of small interneurons in the dorsal horn (69). Trigeminal neuralgia associated with a paroxysmal pain state evoked by tactile stimulation of a trigger point was described clearly by Chaucier (ca. 1810) (66). Animal models in which such states can be systematically demonstrated are a recent achievement and have served to demonstrate the contribution of different mechanisms to the persistent changes associated with nerve injury.

In each of the above cases, the relationship between the input and output functions could be shown to be altered under a variety of physiologic conditions. In this manner, the definition of an effective stimulus, e.g., one that is defined as noxious, could be altered. In one case, the intensity required to produce escape was elevated (e.g., a hypoalgesia), in another it was lowered (e.g., a hyperalgesia), and in a third, innocuous stimuli were observed to result in a pain state (e.g., allodynia).

Injury to the Nervous System can Induce Long-Term Changes in Connectivity and Organization

The clearly defined organization of the nervous system and the perceived importance of connectivity argues that meaningful encoding requires immutable connectivity. Lesions to linkages of the systems lead to a loss of input. This consideration was consistent with the observed effects of nerve section and spinal injury. An important insight that has arisen over the last 50 years has been that considerable plasticity in the organization of the central nervous system can be demonstrated after injury. In the late 1800s, an insistent controversy related to the question of whether the nervous system was a continuous syncytium, as espoused by Camillo Golgi in the 1870s, or composed of discrete units (neurons), as argued by Wilhelm Waldeyer. An important determinant in favor of the discrete elements was the observation that injury to one element led to a limited loss, e.g., the entire system did not disappear. Thus, it followed that a peripheral nerve injury would effect the organization at the peripheral site. Nevertheless, it has been long appreciated that cut axons could display significant arborization (8). Early studies by Liu and Chambers (47) suggested that long track sprouting could occur within the spinal cord. It is now apparent that injury to one link leads to progressive changes at elements central to the injury. In the spinal cord, peripheral injuries can lead to prominent changes in the apparent functionality of dorsal horn neurons. Whether these changes reflect a loss of local trophic factors is not known. The loss, however, is believed to reflect a change in the processing of afferent input. In addition to the change in postsynaptic morphology, injury to the peripheral nervous system can lead to a reorganization of central terminals of the injured axon (arborization) (8). Thus, it is now appreciated that large afferents may sprout into laminae I and II, sites originally innervated by small, high-threshold afferents (85). Similarly, such peripheral lesions are now known to induce sympathetic

[2]An important footnote to the investigation of the relationship between a stimulus and higher levels of organization is the oft-cited variability in the response generated by a tissue-injuring stimulus. This variation is often cited as an indication that the system is for practical purposes unknowable. Nevertheless, this conundrum appears to arise only if we fail to recognize that the neural system at every level has the ability to regulate its processing and that the output function of any component is always state dependent. This state dependency is thus part of the set of experimental variables that may be an implicit, and thus unrecognized, part of the experimental model. Thus, the evoked firing of a cell in the spinal cord of an anesthetized animal does not reflect the simple firing of that cell induced by a stimulus applied to the sciatic nerve, but the composite of the anesthetic state, the ongoing barrage of afferent input from the incision and laminectomy, the input from the vagal afferents activated by the volume depletion of the animals, etc. In intact behaving systems, yet higher order processes may alter our organized response to a tissue injuring stimulus. Commonly cited instances where the stimulus and organized response are dissociated are conditions of overwhelming joy, religious ecstasy, and the stress of battle or competition (55,57). These again represent knowable variables, if we are so inclined to consider their influence. The complexity of the systems may be daunting. Yet, the advances to be noted below have reflected the parallels in the advance in experimental technology and an increased ability to control a plethora of variables.

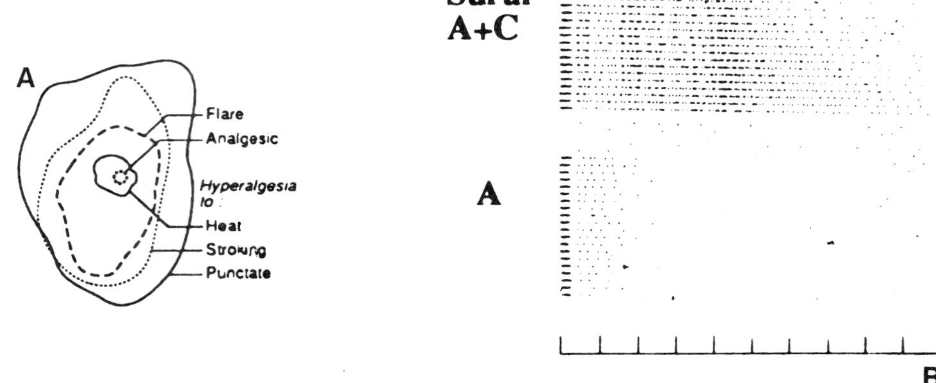

Figure 3. Plasticity: alterations in input–output function. **(A)** Peripheral injury induced by a mild burn or the local injection of capsaicin leads to a regional change in sensory threshold indicating a hyperalgesia or nocifensor tenderness. **(B)** Repetitive activation of A- and C-fiber afferents leads to a protracted facilitation of the discharge of the dorsal horn wide dynamic range neuron (59). Figure is a "dot-raster" in which each point indicates a single discharge of the cell. The sensory beware is a stimulated approximately 1/sec. The response of the cell to each stimulus is indicated by the line of dots extending from the left axis.

sprouting into the ganglion cell of the injured axon (53). Finally, the injury may induce the insertion of channels and receptors into the membrane of the injured axon (19). The net effect of such alterations is to induce (a) increased spontaneous activity in the injured axons, (b) coupling of sympathetic activity to activity in the injured afferent, and (c) and the ability of low-threshold afferent input to drive pain behavior.

The Transmitter and Receptor Pharmacology of Anatomically and Functionally Defined Systems Relevant to Nociceptive Processing is Sufficiently Unique as to Allow Specific Modification of the Transmission and Encoding Process

The development of insights into the anatomic pathways for nociception continued for literally hundreds of years prior to the appreciation that the mechanism of transmission was the action potential and then, with the evolution of the neuronal doctrine by Waldeyer and Ramon y Cajal in the late 19th century, that a method of communication could arise that involved the release of an active factor that acted upon a recognition site, e.g., a receptor (54). Several representative lines of research leading to the current areas will be considered.

Afferent Neurotransmitters

Because of its accessibility, perhaps the first component of the system for which neurotransmission could be defined was the primary afferent. Early work by Bayliss (4) described the observation that antidromic stimulation of the sensory nerve would cause reddening of the skin, indicative of vasodilatation. This phenomenon was defined as neurogenic antidromic vasodilatation. This was addressed again by Lewis (46), who described the hyperalgesia associated with such stimulation, and both authors in effect attributed the activity to the release from the stimulated axons. It was not until 1950 that Lembeck (44) suggested that the active substance resembled that bioassayable material that had originally been isolated by von Euler and Gaddum (74) and designated as substance P. The presence of substance P was then identified by laborious extraction and identified in the spinal cord. Lembeck (44) accordingly suggested that this polypeptide was an afferent transmitter. The isolation of and preparation of an antibody for the peptide sP by Leeman et al. (43) then permitted the localization of this immunoreactivity in the substantia gelatinosa and in small dorsal root ganglion cells, both signs indicating unmyelinated afferents (43,61). Subsequent work demonstrated that this material could be released from the spinal cord (62) by C fiber stimulation (92) (Fig. 4). It is now appreciated that small afferents may release sP peripherally (accounting for the neurogenic antidromic effects observed by Bayliss) and centrally, where it serves to encode in part the orthodromic evoked excitation of dorsal horn neurons produced by high-threshold stimuli (see Chap. 33). Since those studies, the number of peptide transmitters so identified has risen greatly (see Chap. 34). Of additional importance, it was early appreciated that at the electron microscopic level, dendrites displayed synaptic vesicles that differed in their morphology and staining characteristics (60). This led to the appreciation that multiple transmitters may in fact be released from the same terminal. Current work has in fact emphasized such co-containment as a common feature of synaptic transmission (see Chap. 34) (a fact earlier suggested by Dale [17] in 1935).

Modulatory Neurochemical Systems

Bulbospinal Pathways The observations noted above in the early 1950s led to the appreciation that descending pathways could regulate spinal function. Studies in spinally transected animals led to the appreciation that increasing catecholaminergic terminal activity could inhibit flexor reflex afferent activity (2). Subsequent demonstration that these effects could be blocked by serotonergic and noradrenergic systems coincided with the demonstration that cell systems in the brainstem gave rise to bulbospinal projections of 5HT (caudal raphe) and noradrenaline (locus coeruleus) (16). These studies thus provided an important model for targeting the mechanisms whereby spinal processing of nociceptive information could be altered by supraspinal systems (see Chap. 38).

Opiates The alcoholic extract of the poppy (laudanum) was widely used in the 17th and 18th centuries. Morphine was extracted and its structure characterized as early as 1806 by Serturner, and synthetic chemistry was working with the basic ring structure to form novel molecules as early as the turn of the century. Molecular analogues of the basic structure (N-allylnorcodeine) that had no effect on behavior or physiology but that could prevent and reverse the effects of morphine, e.g., antagonists were reported as early as 1914 by Pohl. Early efforts were clearly directed at preventing some of the important recognized side effects of this class of agents, notably the craving that developed with the use of the agent. During the 1930s, a large series of molecules (meperidine and methadone) was developed as opiate substitutes. In the early 1960s, synthetic chemistry at Janssen Pharmaceutica led to the development of extraordinarily potent and clinically useful molecules—the anilinopiperidines. The potency and specificity of these agents on nociception and the reliable structure activity relationship led inexorably to the conclusion that opiates were acting at specific sites within the brain. Importantly, the early appreciation that opiates induced a change in affect led to the conclusion that they were acting on "higher" centers. Yet, early studies in spinally transected animals revealed that the Sherringtonian nociceptive reflex could be blocked by opiates. This model in the transected dog later formed the basis for the pivotal studies by Martin et al. (52) in which they defined the mu and kappa opioid subtypes. Binding subsequently confirmed the existence of a high-affinity site (64) that had been routinely suggested by the more precise pharmacologic studies with a variety of bioassays (27). It was to this list of receptors that the delta receptor was added by Kosterlitz's group (49) after the isolation and characterization of the endogenous opioids. Work in the 1970s led to the targeting of specific brainstem and spinal sites and to the location of brainstem and spinal receptors that were relevant to the analgesic actions of the opiates (94). The elucidation of the actions of opiates led to the appreciation of the modulatory circuits that regulated afferent processing. Thus, based on its action in the brain, it seemed certain that these receptor interactions led to the activation of bulbospinal pathways that could regulate sensory evoked activation (86). The nature of the relevant transmitters emphasized the probable role of aminergic systems in this action. In the spinal cord, the observation of a specific effect on afferent processing led to the appreciation that the selective effect on nociceptive input related to the association of opiate receptors with the small afferent terminals, preventing the release of sP (92). Similarly, it was appreciated that opiates were coupled by cyclic guanosine monophosphate (cGMP) to the K channels, and this led to a hyperpolarization that depressed the excitability of the cell. These joint effects in the spinal cord appeared to account for the potent antinociceptive action that could be demonstrated in animal and human pain states (88).

Salicylates The extract of the willow bark was found to contain an active product, salicylic acid. The acetylated version of this product was created by Charles Gerhard in 1852 and antipyrine was created in 1883 (66). Mechanistically, these agents were noted to have a powerful effect, reducing the magnitude of the inflammation and fever. Accordingly, they were referred to as antipyretic analgesics. It was discovered in the early 1950s and in the 1960s that inflammatory exudate contained algogenic substances that were lipidic acids, synthesized by a cyclooxygenase enzyme. The discovery that these agents served to block that enzyme accounted for their ability to alter certain types of postinjury pain, but not acute pain states (24,73). It was not until the mid-1980s that it was appreciated that these agents could exert a spinal action (87), because of the role played by central prostanoids as hormones released by protracted afferent stimulation that led to a facilitated release of other neurohormones (50).

EVOLVING AREAS OF PAIN RESEARCH

In the above discussion I have given a brief overview of what I believe are the major trends that have led us to the current state of application of the physiology and pharmacology of nociception. The rapid pace at which this work evolves mirrors the major advances that are occurring in neuroscience as a whole. At a minimum, several points reflect some of the directions that this frenzied advance may take.

Definition of the Encoding Process

Even though considerable insights have been garnered into the anatomy and function organization of the ascending systems, there is little information available as to the paradigm

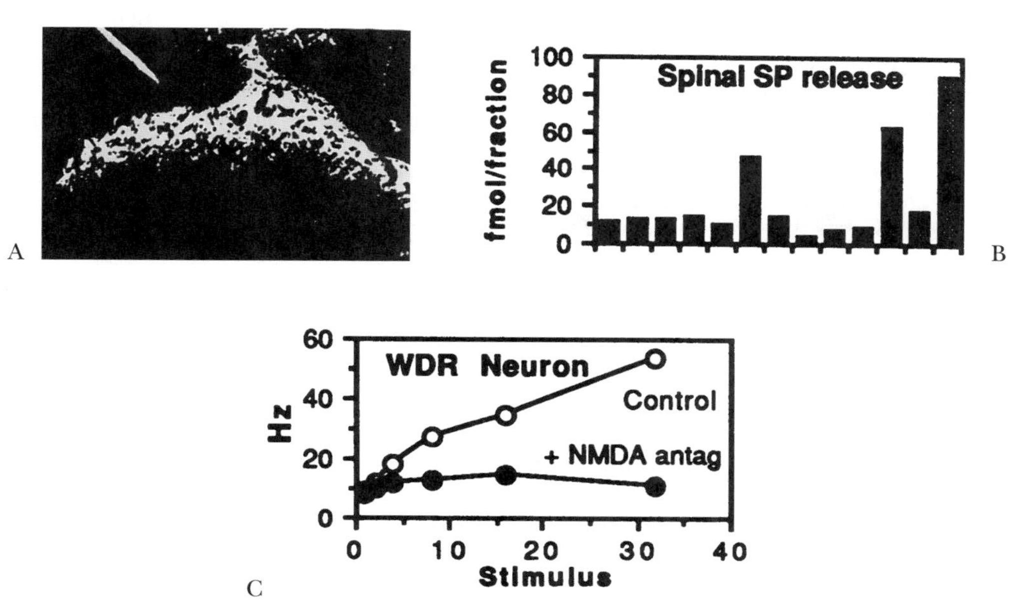

Figure 4. Transmitters and receptors: afferent excitation. **(A)** The distribution of substance P immunoreactivity in the dorsal horn of the rat. The light portion outlines the substantia gelatinosa. **(B)** The release of substance P from the spinal cord of the cat by C-, but not A-afferent stimulation of the sciatic nerve and capsaicin. The release evoked by C-fiber stimulation was blocked by the addition of morphine to the infusion fluid. **(C)** Schematic showing that sequential small afferent stimulation in the halothane anesthetized rat will produce an increase in activity that increases with each subsequent stimulus. The addition of an NMDA receptor antagonist presents the wind up, but does not block the initial discharge (see text for details).

that is employed by the nervous system that permits the encoding of the afferent message. Thus, while it is clear that the intensity of the afferent message out of the spinal cord is related to its stimulus intensity, it is not clear what is the role of the total pattern of the output. Thus, after a single stimulus, it is possible to recognize that if information is concurrently traveling in a time-locked fashion via both ipsilateral and contralateral pathways, and that even the high-threshold input generates activity in the lemniscal systems. It seems probable that the nature of the message decoded at supraspinal sites is a complex function of that pattern of input received at the mesencephalic and diencephalic levels.

Pharmacology of the Peripheral Terminal and the Transduction Process

Injury leads to traffic in small afferents. The translation of the physical state to the action potential may involve direct mechanical stimulation, but more often it is mediated by hormonal intermediary released by the injury or by the inflammatory process generated by the injury. The current efforts focused on the transduction process will likely provide important ways to prevent that transduction. This may occur as we define the nature of the active intermediaries, such as interleukins, kinins, and prostanoids. There is an appreciation that in nerve injury there is development of spontaneous activity, likely related to the time insertion of sodium channels in the regenerating membrane (19,20). The growing appreciation of multiple sodium channel subtypes and the potential development of agents with high affinity for those sites may lead to appropriate local anesthetics that target depolarizing terminals with the appropriate sodium channel type, e.g., fiber-specific local anesthetics (72).

Work in the early 1950s emphasized that products released by injuries could induce activity in small afferents and evoke a pain state. The developing chemistry of the peripheral site revealed the importance of local pH, a variety of peptides, such as bradykinin (BK) and the lipidic acids (e.g., the prostanoids), and, more recently, a plethora of cytokines such as interleukins (29,45). These products can induce activity in the normally quiescent afferents and facilitate their discharge in response to lower intensity stimuli. The development of specific receptor antagonists for the sites has provided an important link in preventing the initiation of the afferent activity that signals a state of tissue injury.

Importantly, aside from the simple definition of the afferent transmitter systems, it is becoming increasingly clear that these terminals also display a common property of neurotransmission system, e.g., activity-dependent changes in linkages. Thus, after peripheral injury, kinins are believed to play a role in activating the peripheral terminal. Under resting conditions, BK may interact with one of two sites (BK2). However, after inflammation, there may be an upregulation of the BK1 site and it may serve as the primary transducer (77). In the spinal cord, repetitive afferent input or peripheral nerve injury may serve to upregulate the levels of immediate early genes and lead to the expression of additional transmitters and receptors (32,33,36). Such findings may lead to practical insights relevant to the control of the transduction process.

Elucidation of Higher Order Function in Pain Processing

While tissue injury may lead to a characteristically encoded afferent traffic, there is little doubt that attributes of consciousness contribute ultimately to the expression of the pain state. Depression, anxiety, euphoria, expectation, and other components of consciousness are known to influence the manner in which we respond to a stimulus. Agents that alter these attributes have an important role in pain management. Yet, our utilization of these agents reflects the manner in which narcotics were used prior to the 1950s and 1960s. At present, while preclinical scientists can discuss in great detail the pathways and influences regulating afferent traffic, we are clearly less able to define the experimental variables influencing the impact of higher function on that processing. While a widescale attack on the mechanisms of consciousness may be a daunting task, there are elements that suggest potential directions of advance. Thus, as reviewed above, there are now anatomic and functionally defined linkages that may relate components of the somatosensory systems with forebrain systems that are classically associated with emotionality (for example: marginal cell → n. submedius → anterior cingulate) (15), vegetative function (spinal cord → hypothalamus) (12) and fear (spinal cord → mesencephalic periaqueductal gray (PAG) and reticular formation) (3). Many of these forebrain sites are considered essential for linkages into substrates that support emotive behaviors in animals and humans. The complexity of these systems is clear and the relevance of these circuits will in fact depend largely on the development of appropriate preclinical models that can define as functional variables constructs such as anxiety or depression (learned helplessness). The actions of opiates have often in the past served to elucidate underlying pathways. They may continue to do so here. Thus, as noted above, opiates have long been held to change the affective component of nociception. In the mesencephalon they are known to activate bulbospinal monoaminergic projections. Importantly, ascending aminergic projections to limbic forebrain arise from anatomically contiguous sites and it seems likely that PAG morphine could readily serve to influence forebrain function via such rostral projections. Thus, aside from whatever is the direct action of morphine at forebrain sites, such ascending aminergic projections activated by a focal brain stem action of morphine could exert powerful effects on emotional tone.

In this regard, while considerable data exist as to the identity of the transmitters in the unmyelinated primary afferent, little is known regarding the transmitter in the larger afferents and virtually nothing about the pharmacology of the ascending systems. The nature of the transmitters and receptors that constitute the spinofugal pathways has not been widely investigated, with few exceptions. It will be of primary importance to define these systems. The ability to target the excitation produced by these ascending systems will be of particular importance in the evolution of future therapy.

Alteration in the Central Systems After Peripheral Nerve Injury and Persistent Afferent Input

As reviewed above, there is little doubt that prominent changes in organization may occur with peripheral nerve injury. The mechanisms whereby those changes are evoked are unclear, but are of undoubted importance and demand characterization. The triggering mechanisms for such changes as sprouting and postterminal degeneration may arise from factors that are transported by the injured axons (98). Those factors may lead to the sympathetic sprouting that occurs after nerve injury. Identification of those factors and the blockade of their transport or the use of growth factor antagonists and/or treatments to prevent the expression of these systems might serve to minimize the appearance of sympathetically dependent states.

The current state of knowledge in pain research has benefited from the ability to alter the postterminal effects of various transmitters. The continuing development of the nature of such coupled receptors and how these receptors function will remain an integral component of research and therapy.

Facilitatory Pharmacology

Since the time that the role played by substance P was defined, there has been a significant increase in the number of probable transmitters for unmyelinated afferents, including additional peptides and excitatory amino acids, many co-contained and released from the same terminal (93). The recognition of tachykinins such as sP or calcitonin gene-related peptides such as C-fiber transmitters and the development of antagonists selective for the several receptors raise the possibility that they may serve to selectively block spinal excitation evoked by such afferent traffic. Excitatory amino acids are found in the primary afferent and are believed to mediate a direct postsynaptic effect through a non–*N*-methyl-D-aspartate (NMDA) receptor. The spinal delivery of these agents has been shown to have a modest effect on acute pain states, but can serve to prevent the development of a facilitated state (13,22,97). With the excitatory amino acids, development of specific antagonists for these sites revealed that the facilitated state induced by repetitive small afferent input was in part mediated by activation of the NMDA receptor. Thus, the spinal facilitation that was observed after protracted small afferent input was not due to a simple change resulting from the repetitive firing of the cell (e.g., as an elevated extracellular K), but that it had a specific pharmacology. This observation led to the appreciation that at the least, the postinjury events that evoked a pain state could be separated into acute and chronic components. Thus, brief activation of specific systems by small afferents led to an evoked pain state that is proportional to the stimulus intensity and time linked to stimulus duration. On the other hand, brief extensions of this stimulus exposure led to a facilitated state (21,88,89). The systematic elucidation of the events associated with the facilitated state has now revealed that the protracted stimulus triggers the initiation of a cascade of events that involves the release of messengers, such as prostanoids, nitric oxide, and free radicals, which could exert longer term influences upon the excitability of the neuron (93). Accordingly, a blockade of the formation of these products is now believed to prevent the evolution of the facilitated state of processing and by that degree diminishes the postinjury pain state.

It is now clear that the pharmacology of the systems that process information generated by nociception may display changes in the face of continued afferent input. Aside from the acute alterations induced by transmitter release (leading, for example, to a transient facilitated state), the nature of the receptor systems that might modulate function may also change over time. An example of this is the observation that repetitive afferent barrage may yield a time-dependent upregulation of several enzymes such as phospholipase and cyclooxygenase. Such induction may occur in the periphery and in the brain. Importantly, the pharmacology of these induced enzymes may vary substantially from the enzyme of the constitutive form (70,95) (see Chap. 34) .

Modulatory Systems

As noted above, there is evidence that the traffic through the spinal cord may be subject to regulation by a variety of systems. Elucidation of the pharmacology of these modulatory systems has led to the appreciation of the ability of specific receptors to regulate nociceptive processing, the best known being the receptor systems acted on by the opioids. However, as noted, some of the action of systemic opioids may be mediated by the activation of bulbospinal pathways that contain and release amines such as noradrenaline or peptides such as neuropeptide Y (NPY). Accordingly, spinal injections of α_2-adrenoceptor agonists can alter nociceptive transmission by local interaction at dorsal horn α_2-receptor sites (91). Our current appreciation of receptor systems that regulate afferent traffic has expanded prominently. Thus, muscarinic, adenosine, γ-aminobutyric acid (GABA), and somatostatin receptors have been shown to influence nociceptive processing as measured electrophysiologically or behaviorally (93).

Delivery Systems

A technical issue is to get the drug to the site of action with minimal intervention and in a way that minimizes side effects. For centrally acting agents that are targeted at a mechanism (receptor, channel, or enzyme) that is mechanistically associated only with transmission and that freely passes the blood-brain barrier, topical or oral delivery is ideal. While such delivery is clearly preferable, other approaches with minimal impact include sublingual and transcutaneous approaches. The utilization of the charge of the molecule to delivery agents transdermally may be useful in developing a rapid plasma level with little hysteresis. Delivery by the airway can take advantage of the high blood flow and large surface area of the airway and the nasal mucosa. While these approaches do not represent particularly novel approaches, the efficient utilization of an existent technology can literally revolutionize a therapy. The development of oral morphine is one such example. Failure of penetration or unacceptable systemic side effects leads to the need for more targeted technologies. The spinal cord will likely continue to be an important target of drug delivery because of the important role it plays in sensory encoding (or miscoding) and the ease with which it can be addressed. The use of spinal delivery systems has, however, shown surprisingly little useful advances. There is little systematic work targeted on the actual delivery systems themselves. The nature of the biomechanical interface that leads to local reactions is not understood. The lack of a foolproof externalization system that does not require repeated percutaneous penetration and is not subject to local inflammation or reaction is not available, and the problems reflect the complexities of the biologic-material interface. Such developments could render the spinal targeting of drugs as routine as a transdermal patch.

Molecular Approaches

There is little doubt that the developments in pharmacology will lead to clearer insights into the pharmacology of these relevant receptors, ion channels, and transmitters. Such knowledge coupled with targeted drug synthesis directed by active site analysis and combinatorial techniques make it probable that increasingly selective agents will be obtained. In addition, molecular approaches to cell function will likely become of equal or greater value in changing cell function for extended periods. One such technique is the use of antisense for mRNA (75). To the degree that the physiologist and pharmacologist can identify certain transmitters (substance P), receptors (NK/NMDA), and channels (sodium channels in the injured afferent axon) as linkages in the postinjury pain state, or even the growth factors responsible for large afferent sprouting, a partial reduction in their expression could serve to minimize their impact on subsequent function. The use of antisense for mRNA prevents the expression of the respective protein sequence. Receptors, channels, and transmitter prohormones are known to undergo turnover. The blockade of the ability of the mRNA to express that protein means a temporary downregulation of that receptor or channel (see Chap. 34). While current antisense approaches suffer from lack of efficiency, the development of transfection systems that employ, for example, nonreplicating adenoviruses (38) may improve the transfer of products that could alter the expression for a brief interval of days to weeks of the complement of receptors that a cell might express.

CONCLUSION

This short overview represents an effort to provide a perspective for research leading to advances in our understanding of nociceptive processing.

Our understanding of pain as a physiologic process has been integrally tied to the evolving developments in neurobiology. Such cross-fertilization is not uncommon. Consider that in the 1980s many researchers interested in membrane processes associated with neurotransmission focused on the hippocampus, learning, and memory (a presumptive function of that structure). Important insights, including the concept of long-term potentiation (LTP), glutamate receptor function, the role of nitric oxide, and so on, arose in part from those lines of investigation. I would argue that many who studied learning and memory in the context of LTP, nitric oxide (NO), or glutamate were not particularly interested in learning and memory per se, but found the hippocampus to be a structure with a function of sufficient complexity and definition that it served their scientific purpose to focus in that area. It would seem now that nociception and its various components have reached such a state of rich complexity to warrant the attention of many neurobiologists with diverse interests. Accordingly, our concepts of facilitated processing, receptor down-regulation, the role of lipidic acids, nitric oxide, and excitatory amino acids (see Chaps. 34 and 36) arose in part because of the mechanistic parallels revealed in the hippocampal work with LTP. Peptides such as substance P and vasoactive intestinal polypeptide were first studied in the gut and smooth muscle. The work on such systems paved the way for the insights relating these systems to transmission in the primary afferent and the presynaptic regulation of such excitability (see Chap. 34). The impact of the diverse lines of research in physiology, pharmacology, and molecular biology on our appreciation of nociceptive processing will doubtless have explosive consequences of great benefit and show us things of which today we can only dream.

REFERENCES

1. Adrian ED. *The basis of sensation.* London:Christophers, 1928.
2. Anden N-E, Jukes MGM, Lundberg A. The effect of DOPA on the spinal cord. 2. A pharmacological analysis. *Acta Physiol Scand* 1966; 67:387–397.
3. Bandler R, Carrive P, Zhang SP. Integration of somatic and autonomic reactions within the midbrain periaqueductal grey, viscerotopic, somatotopic and functional organization. *Progr Brain Res* 1991;87:269–305.
4. Bayliss WM. On the origin from the spinal cord of the vasodilator fibres of the hindlimb and on the nature of these fibers. *J Physiol* 1901;26:173–209.
5. Bayliss WM. *The vasomotor system.* London: 1923.
6. Beecher HK. *Measurement of subjective response.* New York:Oxford University Press, 1959.
7. Brown-Sequard CE. Course of lectures on the physiology and pathology of the central nervous system, Philadelphia:Collins, 1860. In: Keele KD, ed. *Anatomies of pain.* Springfield, IL: Charles C. Thomas, 1957;112.
8. Cajal, Ramon y S. *Degeneration and regeneration in the central nervous system.* Oxford University Press, 1928.
9. Carpenter D, Engberg I, Lundberg. Differential subspinal control of inhibitory and excitatory actions from the FRA to ascending spinal pathways. *Acta Physiol Scand* 1965;63:103–110.
10. Casey KL, Minoshima S, Berger KL, Koeppe RA, Morrow TJ, Frey KA. Positron emission tomographic analysis of cerebral structures activated specifically by repetitive noxious heat stimuli. *J Neurophysiol* 1994;71(2):802–807.
11. Christensen BN, Perl ER. Spinal neurons specifically excited by noxious or thermal stimuli: marginal zones of the dorsal horn. *J Neurophysiol* 1970;33:293–307.
12. Cliffer KD, Burstein R, Giesler GJ Jr. Distributions of spinothalamic, spinohypothalamic, and spinotelencephalic fibers revealed by anterograde transport of PHA-L in rats. *J Neurosci* 1991;11(3): 852–868.
13. Coderre TJ, Melzack R. The contribution of excitatory amino acids to central sensitization and persistent nociception after formalin-induced tissue injury. *J Neurosci* 1992;12:3665–3670.
14. Craig AD, Burton H. Spinal and medullary lamina I projection to nucleus submedius in medial thalamus: a possible pain center. *J Neurophysiol* 1981;45:443–466.
15. Craig AD, Bushnell MC, Zhang ET, Blomqvist A. A thalamic nucleus specific for pain and temperature sensation. *Nature* 1994; 372(6508):770–773.
16. Dahlstrom A, Fuxe K. Evidence for the existence of monamine neurons in the central nervous system. II. Experimentally induced changes in the intraneuronal amine levels of the bulbospinal neuron system. *Acta Physiol Scand Suppl* 1965;247:1–36.
17. Dale HH. Pharmacology of nerve endings. *Proc R Soc Med* 1935;28: 319–332.
18. Dejerine J, Roussy G. Le syndrome thalamicque. *Rev Neurol* 1906; 531–532.
19. Devor M, Govrin-Lippmann R, Angelides K. Na+ channel immunolocalization in peripheral mammalian axons and changes following nerve injury and neuroma formation. *J Neurosci* 1993; 13(5):1976–1992.
20. Devor M, Wall PD, Catalan N. Systemic lidocaine silences ectopic neuroma and DRG discharge without blocking nerve conduction. *Pain* 1992;48:261–268.
21. Dickenson AH. A cure for wind up: NMDA receptor antagonists as potential analgesics. *Trends Pharmacol Sci* 1990;11(8):307–309.
22. Dickenson AH, Sullivan AF. Evidence for a role of the NMDA receptor in the frequency dependent potentiation of deep rat dorsal horn nociceptive neurones following C fibre stimulation. *Neuropharmacology* 1987;26(8):1235–1238.
23. Edinger L. Vorlesungen uber den Bau der Nervosen Zentralorgane, Leipzig, 1904. In: Keele KD, ed. *Anatomies of pain.* Springfield, IL: Charles C. Thomas, 1957;118.
24. Ferreira SH, Moncada S, Vane JR. Prostaglandins and the mechanism of analgesia produced by aspirin-like drugs. *Br J Pharmacol* 1973;49(1):86–97.
25. Goltz FL. *Pflugers Arch Ges Physiol* 1874;8:460. In: Keele KD, ed. *Anatomies of pain.* Springfield, IL: Charles C. Thomas, 1957;171.
26. Gower WR. *Manual of diseases of the nervous system.* Philadelphia: 1888.
27. Gyand EA, Kosterlitz HW. Agonist and antagonist actions of morphine-like drugs on the guinea-pig isolated ileum. *Br J Pharmacol* 1966;27(3):514–527.
28. Hagbarth KE, Kerr DIB. Central influences on spinal afferent conduction. *J Neurophysiol* 1954;17:295–307.
29. Handwerker HO, Reeh PW. Pain and inflammation. *Pain Res Clin Manage* 1991;4:59–70.
30. Head H. Sensory disturbances from cerebral lesions. *Brain* 1911; 34:102–254.
31. Head H. *Studies in neurology.* London:Hodder and Stoughton, 1920.
32. Herdegen T, Fiallos-Estrada C, Schmid W, Bravo R, Zimmermann M. The transcription factor CREB, but not immediate-early gene encoded proteins, is expressed in activated microglia of lumbar spinal cord following sciatic nerve transection in the rat. *Neurosci Lett* 1992;142:57–61.
33. Herdegen T, Fiallos-Estrada CE, Schmid W, Bravo R, Zimmermann M. The transcription factors c-JUN, JUN D and CREB, but not FOS and KROX-24, are differentially regulated in axotomized neurons following transection of rat sciatic nerve. *Mol Brain Res* 1992;14:155–165.
34. Hingtgen CM, Vasko MR. Prostacyclin enhances the evoked-release of substance P and calcitonin gene-related peptide from rat sensory neurons. *Brain Res* 1994;655:51–60.
35. Hokfelt T, Kellerth JO, Nilsson G, Pernow B. Substance P: localization in the central nervous system and in some primary sensory neurons. *Science* 1975;190(4217):889–890.
36. Jenkins R, McMahon SB, Bond AB, Hunt SP. Expression of c-Jun as a response to dorsal root and peripheral nerve section in damaged and adjacent intact primary sensory neurons in the rat. *Eur J Neurosci* 1993;5(6):751–759.
37. Jessell TM, Iversen LL. Opiate analgesics inhibit substance P release from rat trigeminal nucleus. *Nature* 1977;268(5620): 549–551.
38. Kass-Eisler A, Falck-Pedersen E, Alvira M, Riviera J, Buttrick PM, Wittenberg BA, Cipriana L, Leinwand LA. Quantitative determination of adenovirus-mediated gene delivery to cardiac myocytes in vitro and in vivo. *Proc Natl Acad Sci USA* 1993;90:11498–1150.

39. Keele KD. *Anatomies of pain.* Springfield, IL: Charles C. Thomas, 1957.
40. Kolmodin G, Skogland CR. Analysis of spinal interneurons activated by tactile and nociceptive stimulation. *Acta Physiol Scand* 1960;50:337–355.
41. Kuru M. Sensory paths in the spinal cord and brainstem of Man. Tokyo and Osaka (Sogensya): 1949 (*personal communication* F.W.L. Kerr).
42. LaMotte RH, Lundberg LE, Torebjork HE. Pain, hyperalgesia and activity innociceptive C units in humans after intradermal injection of capsaicin. *J Physiol* 1992;448:749–764.
43. Leeman SE, Mroz EA. Substance P. *Life Sci* 1974;15(12): 2033–2044.
44. Lembeck F. Zur Frage der zentralen Ubertragung afferenter Impulse. III Mitteilung. Das Vollkommenund die Bedeutung der Substanz P in den dorsalen Wurzeln des Ruckenmarks. *Nauyn Schmiedebergs Arch Pharmacol* 1953;219:197–213.
45. Levine JD, Fields HL, Basbaum AI. Peptides and the primary afferent nociceptor. *J Neurosci* 1993;13:2273–2286.
46. Lewis T. *Pain.* New York:Macmillan, 1942.
47. Liu CN, Chambers WW. Intraspinal sprouting of dorsal root axons. *Arch Neurol Psychiat* 1958;79:46–61.
48. Livingston WK. *Pain mechanisms.* New York:Macmillan, 1943.
49. Lord JA, Waterfield AA, Hughes J, Kosterlitz HW. Endogenous opioid peptides: multiple agonists and receptors. *Nature* 1977; 267(5611):495–499.
50. Malmberg AB, Yaksh TL. Cyclooxygenase inhibition and the spinal release of prostaglandin E2 and amino acids evoked by paw formalin injection: a microdialysis study in anesthetized rats. *J Neurosci* 1995;15:2768–2776.
51. Mantyh PW, DeMaster E, Malhotra A, Ghilardi JR, Rogers SD, Mantyh CR, Liu H, Basbaum AI, Vigna SR, Maggio JE, et al. Receptor endocytosis and dendrite reshaping in spinal neurons after somatosensory stimulation. *Science* 1995;268(5217): 1629–1632.
52. Martin WR, Eades CG, Thompson WO, Thompson JA, Flanary HG. Morphine physical dependence in the dog. *J Pharmacol Exp Ther* 1974;189(3):759–771.
53. McLachlan EM, Janig W, Devor M, Michaelis M. Peripheral nerve injury triggers noradrenergic sprouting within the dorsal root ganglia. *Nature* 1993;363:543–546.
54. McLennon H. *Synaptic transmission.* Philadelphia: WB Saunders, 1970.
55. Melzack R. Pain perception. *Assoc Res Nerv Ment Dis* 1970;48: 272–285.
56. Melzack R, Caesy K. Sensory, motivational and central control determinants of pain: a new conceptual model. In: Kenshalo D, ed. *The skin senses.* Springfield, IL: Charles C. Thomas, 1968; 423–443.
57. Melzack R, Chapman CR. Psychologic aspects of pain. *Postgrad Med* 1973;53:69–75.
58. Melzack R, Wall PD. Pain mechanisms: a new theory. *Science* 1965; 150(699):971–979.
59. Mendell LM, Wall PD. Responses of single dorsal cord cells to peripheral cutaneous unmyelinated fibers. *Nature* 1965;206: 97–99.
60. Narotzky RA, Kerr FWL. Marginal neurons of the spinal cord: types, afferent synaptology and functional considerations. *Brain Res* 1978;139:1–20.
61. Nilsson G, Hokfelt T, Pernow B. Distribution of substance P-like immuno-reactivity in the rat central nervous system as revealed by immunohistochemistry. *Med Biol* 1974;52(6):424.
62. Otsuka K, Konishi S. Substance P, an excitatory transmitter of primary sensory neurons. *Cold Spring Harbor Symp Quant Biol* 1976;40: 135–143.
63. Penfield W. *Res Publ Assoc Nerv Ment Dis* 1952;30:513.
64. Pert CB, Snyder SH. Opiate receptor: demonstration in nervous tissue. *Science* 1973;179(77):1011–1014.
65. Rexed B. The cytoarchitectonic organization of the spinal cord in the cat. *J Comp Neurol* 1952;96:415–495.
66. Rey R. *History of pain.* Paris: Editions La Decouverte, 1993.
67. Reynolds DV. Surgery in the rat during electrical analgesia induced by focal brain stimulation. *Science* 1969;164(878): 444–445.
68. Sherrington CS. *The integrative action of the nervous system.* New Haven, CT: Yale University Press, 1906.
69. Sugimoto T, Bennett GJ, Kajander KC. Transsynaptic degeneration in the superficial dorsal horn after sciatic nerve injury: effects of a chronic constriction injury, transection, and strychnine. *Pain* 1990;42:205–213.
70. Swierkosz TA, Mitchell JA, Warner TD, Botting RM, Vane JR. Co-induction of nitric oxide synthase and cyclo-oxygenase: interactions between nitric oxide and prostanoids. *Br J Pharmacol* 1995; 114:1335–1342.
71. Talbot JD, Marrett S, Evans AC, Meyer E, Bushnell MC, Duncan GH. Multiple representations of pain in human cerebral cortex. *Science* 1991;251:1355–1358.
72. Thalhammer JG, Raymond SA, Popitz-Bergez FA, Strichartz GR. Modality-dependent modulation of conduction by impulse activity in functionally characterized single cutaneous afferents in the rat. Somatosens Mot Res 1994;11(3):243–257.
73. Vane JR. Inhibition of prostaglandin synthesis as a mechanism of action for aspirin-like drugs. *Nature New Biol* 1971;231(25): 232–235.
74. Von Euler US, Gaddum JH. An unidentified depressor substance in certain tissue extracts. *J Physiol Lond* 1931;72:74–87.
75. Wagner RW. The state of the art in antisense research. *Nature Med* 1995;1:1116–1118.
76. Walker AE. *A history of neurological surgery.* London: 1951
77. Walker K, Perkins M, Dray A. Kinins and kinin receptors in the nervous system. *Neurochem Int* 1995;26(1):1–16.
78. Wall PD. Cord cells responding to touch, damage and temperature of skin. *J Neurophysiol* 1960;23:197–210.
79. Wall PD. The laminar organization of dorsal horn and effects of descending impulses. *J Physiol (Lond)* 1967;188:403–423.
80. Wall PD, Sweet WH. Temporary abolition of pain in man. *Science* 1967;155(758):108–109.
81. Weir-Mitchell S, Morehouse GR, Keen WW. *Gunshot wounds and other injuries of nerves.* Philadelphia: Lippincott, 1864.
82. White JC, Sweet WH. *Pain and the neurosurgeon.* Baltimore: University Park Press, 1969.
83. Willis WD, Coggeshall RE. *Sensory mechanisms of the spinal cord.* New York: Plenum Press, 1978.
84. Willis WD Jr. Dorsal horn neurophysiology of pain. *Ann NY Acad Sci* 1988;531:76–89.
85. Woolf CJ, Shortland P, Coggeshall RE. Peripheral nerve injury triggers central sprouting of myelinated afferents. *Nature* 1992; 355:75–78.
86. Yaksh TL. Direct evidence that spinal serotonin and noradrenaline terminals mediate the spinal antinociceptive effects of morphine in the periaqueductal gray. *Brain Res* 1979;160:180–185.
87. Yaksh TL. Central and peripheral mechanisms for the antialgesic action of acetylsalicylic acid. In: Barnet JM, Hirsh J, Mustard JF, eds. *Acetylsalicylic acid:* new uses for an old drug. New York: Raven Press, 1982;137–152.
88. Yaksh TL. The spinal actions of opioids. In: Herz A, ed. *Handbook of experimental pharmacology,* vol 104/II. Berlin Heidelberg: Springer-Verlag, 1993;53–90.
89. Yaksh TL. The spinal pharmacology of facilitation of afferent processing evoked by high-threshold afferent input of the postinjury pain state. *Curr Sci* 1993;6:250–256.
90. Yaksh TL. Preclinical models for analgesic drug study. In: Goldberg AM, Zutphen LFM, eds. *Alternative methods in toxicology and the life sciences, II: The World Congress on Alternatives and Animal Use in the Life Sciences: education, research, testing.* New York: Mary Ann Liebert, 1995.
91. Yaksh TL, Jage J, and Takano Y. Pharmacokinetics and pharmacodynamics of medullar agents. The spinal actions of α_2-adrenergic agonists as analgesics. In: Aitkenhead AR, Benad G, Brown BR, Cousins MJ, Jones JG, Strunin L, Thomson D, Van Aken H, eds. *Baillière's clinical anaesthesiology,* vol 7, no. 3. London: Baillière Tindall, 1993;597–614.
92. Yaksh TL, Jessell TM, Gamse R, Mudge AW, Leeman SE. Intrathecal morphine inhibits substance P release from mammalian spinal cord *in vivo. Nature* 1980;286:155–156.
93. Yaksh TL, Malmberg AB. Central pharmacology of nociceptive transmission. In: Melzack R, Wall P, eds. *Textbook of pain,* 3rd ed. Edinburgh, UK: Churchill Livingstone, 1993;165–200.
94. Yaksh TL, Rudy TA. Narcotic analgesics: CNS sites and mechanisms of action as revealed by intracerebral injection techniques. *Pain* 1978;4:299–359.
95. Yamagata K, Andreasson KI, Kaufmann WE, Barnes CA, Worley PF. Expression of a mitogen-inducible cyclooxygenase in brain neurons: regulation by synaptic activity and glucocorticoids. *Neuron* 1993;11:371–386.
96. Yamamoto T, Yaksh TL. Stereospecific effects of a nonpeptidic

NK1 selective antagonist, CP-96,345: antinociception in the absence of motor dysfunction. *Life Sci* 1991;49:1955–1963.

97. Yamamoto T, Yaksh TL. Comparison of the antinociceptive effects of pre and post treatment with intrathecal morphine and MK801, an NMDA antagonist on the formalin test in the rat. *Anesthesiology* 1992;77:757–763.
98. Yamamoto T, Yaksh TL. Effects of colchicine applied to the peripheral nerve on the thermal hyperalgesia evoked with chronic nerve constriction. *Pain* 1993,55:227–233.
99. Young RM. The functions of the brain: Gall to Ferrier (1808–1886). *Isis* 1968;59:251–268.
100. Zotterman Y. Touch, pain, and tickling: an electrophysiological investigation on cutaneous sensory nerves. *J Physiol (Lond)* 1939; 95:1–28.

Anesthesia: Biologic Foundations, edited by Tony L. Yaksh et al. Lippincott–Raven Publishers, Philadelphia © 1997.

CHAPTER 30

MORPHOLOGY OF THE PERIPHERAL NERVOUS SYSTEM AND ITS RELATIONSHIP TO NEUROPATHIC PAIN

ROBERT R. MYERS

This chapter describes and illustrates the morphology of the distal aspects of the sensory nervous system. In addition to providing a structural context for many of the physiologic discussions in the book, this chapter presents a perspective on the relationship between abnormal nerve structure and function, highlighting some structural aspects of the peripheral nervous system that are believed to be related to the pathogenesis of chronic pain states caused by nerve injury. The discipline of pathology is concerned with the relationship between cellular structure and function, especially the changes caused by disease. Experimental neuropathologic investigations that correlate behavioral function with basic pathologic mechanisms such as nerve ischemia, altered axoplasmic transport, or wallerian degeneration of injured nerve fibers should provide insights into disease mechanisms causing neuropathic pain and, from that, the design of effective therapy.

Before discussing these relationships, however, the development of the primary afferent system and the structural hallmarks of first-order sensory neurons should be considered. This background in the development and organization of the peripheral nervous system is useful in establishing the importance of chemotactic factors in guiding nerve terminals to their end-organs and in evaluating the changes in neuronal function associated with axonal sensing of the local chemical environment. The morphology of the axon is described next at the resolution of both the light and electron microscopes. In this section, the nature of axonal transport is stressed because of its relevance to the maintenance of the normal axon and to axonal regeneration following nerve injury. We now believe that retrograde axonal transport of substances from sites of peripheral nerve injury play an important role in the pathogenesis of neuropathic pain. This concept permeates the discussion of glial cells and other cells that support axonal functions and the homeostasis of nerve bundles. These cells are presented in relationship to their immunopathologic function, highlighting changes in the expression of cytokines and trophic factors that may contribute to the pathogenesis of pain. In contrast to the extensive literature on axons and Schwann cells, there is relatively little known about the morphology of peripheral sensory receptors. However, new techniques in anatomy and neuropathology are being used to study free nerve endings and this information is presented with electron micrographs of specialized nerve terminals in skin. Details of the ultrastructure of the peripheral afferent system are available in up-to-date reference volumes (60,275) and are reviewed here to the extent that their pathologic variations are thought to relate to anesthesia or painful syndromes.

Whenever possible, the micrographs are from human tissue. Several illustrations from experimental procedures in rodents are also included because of superior fixation and focused neuropathologic changes that could not be illustrated clearly in human biopsy or autopsy material.

DEVELOPMENT OF THE PRIMARY AFFERENT SYSTEM

The nervous system of vertebrates derives from the ectoderm, the outer embryonic layer of cells that eventually gives rise to skin structures, the nervous system, sensory organs, the pineal gland, and part of the pituitary and suprarenal glands. The neural plate forms in the midregion of the ectoderm and subsequently becomes the neural groove and then the neural tube as its lateral ridges close. The neural tube develops into the brain and spinal cord. The peripheral nervous system develops entirely from cells of the neural crest, located at the top of the neural tube. The neural crest was originally referred to as the ganglion crest by German authors who noted that it was the origin of spinal and dorsal root ganglia. It is now known that in addition to generating sensory, sympathetic, parasympathetic, and enteric neurons, the neural crest gives rise to Schwann cells, satellite cells, and nonneural structures such as melanocytes of the skin, connective tissues, and skeletal and endocrine cells. The adrenal medulla is also derived from the neural crest. These insights have come from detailed studies using amphibians and embryotic quail chicks in which neural crest cells were labeled or transplanted before following them to their final locations and identifying their terminal differential state (322).

Several congenital disorders with clinically diverse findings and symptoms affecting different organs and tissues can be related to abnormalities in embryonic development of the neural crest (322). These so-called neurocristopathies (26) can affect diffuse cell lines that would seem to be unrelated apart from their similar embryonic origin. von Recklinghausen neurofibromatosis and other syndromes caused by pathologic abnormalities of neural crest derivatives have been identified and several experimental models have been developed to explore these problems in more detail (118,182,291). It is thought that the susceptibility of neural crest cells to dysplasia may be related to their extreme plasticity and migratory capacity (322). The migratory capacity of cells derived from the neural crest is one of the most remarkable features of these cells. Precursors of Schwann cells lining peripheral nerves and enteric ganglion and glial cells travel the greatest distances, migrating first longitudinally along the neural crest and then laterally and dorsoventrally (272). Developing limb buds attract both sensory and motor axons to form a nerve plexus. Neurites from motor neurons grow before processes of sensory neurons and these "pioneer" neurites provide guidance for later emerging neurites from sensory neurons, but the existence of this interaction is not a requirement for the development of a normal pattern of innervation (53). Cutaneous sensory nerves, in particular, do not require motor axons for guidance since normal innervation occurs in limbs deprived of motor axons (253). The capability of cutaneous sensory axons to reach their precise target fields seems to be programmed from the outset

(252) but then lost after maturation. Although the direction of axonal outgrowth and its patterns of dendritic branching seem to be genetically determined, there are important guiding mechanisms that help control the final destination of growth cones. While these mechanisms are not entirely clear, it is thought that various adhesive molecules and growth factors (see below) assist in the process of neurite guidance.

There is great variability in axonal length from neuron to target. However, at least in cranial sensory ganglia, there is a direct intrinsic relationship between growth rate and target distance, i.e., axons grow at a faster rate to distal targets (54). At the terminal end of elongating neurites is the growth cone that has a high concentration of growth-associated protein 43 (GAP-43) in its membrane. GAP-43 may interact with cytoskeletal proteins and modulate intracellular signaling by calcium (257). Calcium ion concentration regulates growth cone motility and neurite outgrowth and therefore may have a role in determining the transition from neurite growth to functional activity of the terminal. The growth cone is characterized morphologically by conical swelling with a thickened cytoplasmic core and thin, irregular filopodia containing a fine filamentous matrix. The growth cone also contains numerous endoplasmic reticulum, vesicles, mitochondria, and collections of fine filaments (Fig. 1). Tissue culture studies have shown that actin-containing microfilaments are responsible for growth cone movements and that neurite elongation is dependent on microtubules

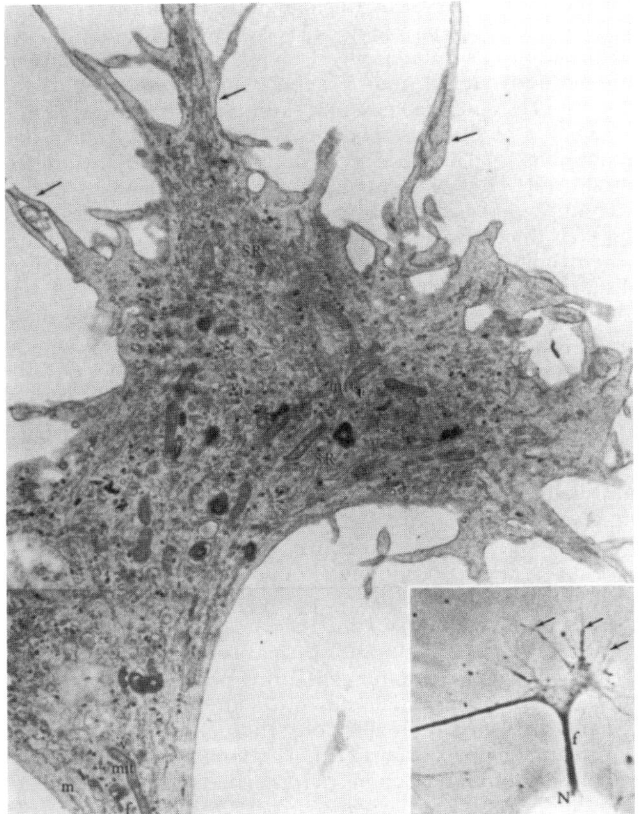

Figure 1. Growth cone from sympathetic neuron in tissue culture. *Insert* is phase contrast micrograph showing fibers (f) extending from perikaryon (N) of a neuron. Filopodia *(arrows)* extend from growth cone. The electron micrograph from the same growth cone shows filopodia and numerous cytoplasmic particles, including elongated mitochondria (mit), smooth endoplasmic reticulum (SR), vesicles (v), vesicles with dense contents (v1), and microtubules (m). Original magnification × 1400 for EM, × 1350 for phase contrast micrograph. (From ref. 213a, with permission.)

(299). The continuous production of new membrane structures and the development of the infrastructure for anterograde and retrograde transport of axoplasmic constituents require substantial substrate and metabolic energy for their functional organization.

There are physicochemical mechanisms through which the growth cone senses its environment. This has been demonstrated with tracer techniques in which vesicles located at the leading edge of growth cones were shown to be involved in endocytosis of proteins and tracers from the environment before being transported proximally (33). These guidance signals are also of great interest in the adult because of their relevance to neural regeneration. As early as 1934, Hamburger (98) demonstrated that extirpation of a limb bud decreased the number and size of neurons innervating that target. Others showed that the addition of extra target tissue during embryonic development increased innervation. This research led to the discovery of nerve growth factor (NGF) that is now studied intensively in tissue culture preparations (145). It has been known since 1975 that retrograde transport of NGF from the distal terminal to the cell body is important in the development of adrenergic neurons (209) and more recently that changes in NGF and NGF receptor transport following nerve injury are important signals to the cell body that modulate its function (104,119). NGF is the best-understood polypeptide growth factor among an increasing number of polypeptides that promote growth. Polypeptides with some sequence homology to NGF include brain-derived neuronotrophic factor (BNDF) (15,112), which plays a role in the earliest stages of sensory neuron development (315) but is primarily a factor supporting motor neuron development, and neurotropin-3 (NT-3) (156) and NT-4 (116), which have important effects on the differentiation and maintenance of cultured hippocampal neurons. Additional factors will undoubtedly be identified. A variety of soluble extracts from peripheral nerve have also been demonstrated to have neural growth-promoting activities. Ciliary neuronotrophic factor (CNTF) is one such factor that promotes parasympathetic neuronal growth (4). It is important to note that the physiologic roles and anatomic location of these compounds are not necessarily related to their names. Their growth-promoting effects cross several cell types, and their expression and function can be different during periods of development, maturation, disease, and neural regeneration (40,165,258).

Much of the present understanding of the physiologic role of nerve growth factor comes from tissue culture studies, yet the mechanisms by which NGF induces growth in neurons is almost completely unknown. NGF treatment alters cell adhesional molecules, which are known to be important in nervous system development (236) but little is known about the mechanisms of this process (168). Cultured anterior horn cells and parasympathetic ganglion cells do not require or respond to NGF, although anterior horn cells are able to bind, internalize, and retrogradely transport NGF (318). Sympathetic and dorsal root ganglion (DRG) cells require NGF for survival in culture if the progenitor cells are removed from the embryo. After maturation, these cells are less dependent on NGF. Small- and medium-sized DRG neurons have a higher density of NGF receptor on their surfaces than the large DRG neurons. These small neurons give rise to the smaller sensory nerve fibers that express substance P (SP) and calcitonin gene-related peptide (CGRP). Retrograde transport of CNTF also occurs (50). However, in transvector experiments that eliminated the CNTF gene, anterior horn neurons developed normally but then degenerated at a postnatal age of about 28 weeks, presumably due to lack of trophic support from Schwann cells that normally contain a high concentration of CNTF (159).

Nerve growth factor receptor (NGFR) is a membrane receptor with both high- and low-affinity forms (270) that is thought to specifically bind NGF. When occupied, the NGFR-NGF complex is internalized within the axon in a membrane-bound vesicle that is retrogradely transported to the cell body where it presumably promotes cell survival and modulates the process of growth (119). NGFR expression on sympathetic and sensory ganglia is generally high during development and growth but is downregulated when contact is made with the target. However, after transection of an adult axon, there is a significant increase in NGFR expression on the Schwann cells of injured nerve. Interestingly, Schwann cells increase production of NGFR when they have lost contact with the axons, and this may be an important mechanism promoting and guiding axonal regeneration (312). The presence of NGFR in normal sensory corpuscles of human digital skin has recently been investigated using monoclonal antibodies to human NGFR (290). NGFR immunoreactivity (NGFR-IR) was noted primarily in Meissner and pacinian corpuscles. In Meissner's corpuscles NGFR-IR was found in the lamellar cells, whereas in the pacinian corpuscles NGFR-IR was seen in the inner core, outer core, and capsule.

NEURONS OF THE PERIPHERAL NERVOUS SYSTEM

Sympathetic Chain and Enteric Ganglia

Neurons in the peripheral nervous system support sympathetic, parasympathetic, enteric, and sensory function and are organized in numerous ganglia along the vertebral column and in the vicinity of major visceral organs. The sympathetic trunk is a collection of ganglia extending from the base of the cranium to the coccyx located adjacent to, but outside the spinal column. In the cervical region, the trunk lies ventral to the transverse processes of the vertebrae and dorsal to the carotid arteries, whereas in the thorax the trunk lies ventral to the neck of the ribs. From the lumbar segment to the sacral prominence, it follows the medial border of the psoas muscle and then the ventral surface of the sacrum in the pelvis. Major ganglia outside this chain include the ciliary, sphenopalatine, otic, and submandibular ganglia in the cervical region and the celiac, and superior and inferior mesenteric ganglia in the body core. Other autonomic ganglia are located in the walls of visceral organs and in nerve plexuses closely associated with the visceral organs they innervate. The enteric nervous system is a unique division of the autonomic nervous system responsible for gastrointestinal function whose ganglionated plexuses are embedded throughout the length of the gut wall.

Several structural features characterize these ganglia and their neurons that distinguish them from sensory neurons in the DRGs. For instance, the sympathetic and parasympathetic ganglion cells are multipolar, whereas DRG cells are pseudounipolar with a single axon leaving the cell body and no true dendrites (296). This axon extends for a variable distance from the cell body and then bifurcates into a central and peripheral process. In myelinated fibers, this occurs at a node of Ranvier. Cell bodies of the autonomic ganglion tend to be smaller than DRG cell bodies and range between 20 and 60 μm. Although enteric neurons are organized in ganglia, they are not encapsulated but lie in the connective tissue framework between muscle layers or in the submucosa. The enteric nervous system is a rich source of cytochemical factors with neurotransmitter features and has been a useful source for collecting and purifying putative neurotransmitters (275a). A complete description of the anatomy, pharmacology, and function of these ganglia is beyond the scope of this chapter but is available elsewhere (39,62,105,183,275).

Dorsal Root Ganglia

The perikarya of dorsal root ganglion cells range in diameter from 20 to 100 μm and their axons may be more than 1 m in length. There is general acceptance that DRG neurons can be divided into two groups based on size (57,245), although some investigators describe intermediate-sized cells (136,284) and early histograms of human DRG diameters were said to have three peaks (125). Based on cytologic correlations, however, the convention of two major cell populations has prevailed (309). Using basic stains, DRG cells appear either light (clear) or dark (Fig. 2). Lightly staining cells tend to be large (A cells) but can be of any size while darkly staining cells are always small (B cells) (149). The selective immunostaining of large, clear cells with the RT97 antibody that recognizes neurofilaments also supports this major division (141). Several authors have attempted to refine this classification using other cytologic markers or electrophysiologic criteria (57,117,224,262), but there has not been general acceptance of these schemes.

Continued attempts at correlating structure and function have shifted to using morphologic markers to identify subpopulations of DRG cells. Willis and Coggeshall (309) summarize the extensive literature on the localization of immunocytochemical peptides in DRG cells; this is also covered in detail elsewhere in this book. Thirteen individual peptides ranging alphabetically from α-neo-endorphin to vasopressin differentially label between 2% and 63% of DRG cells. Calcitonin gene-related peptide, vasopressin, and oxytocin each label more than 30% of the total DRG population, while substance P labels between 10% and 30% of DRG neurons. The other peptides label less than 10% of the cells. Most of these labeled cells are from the small-diameter DRG cell population giving rise to unmyelinated fibers. Colocalizations of peptides are extensive but difficult to rationalize from a functional neurotransmitter

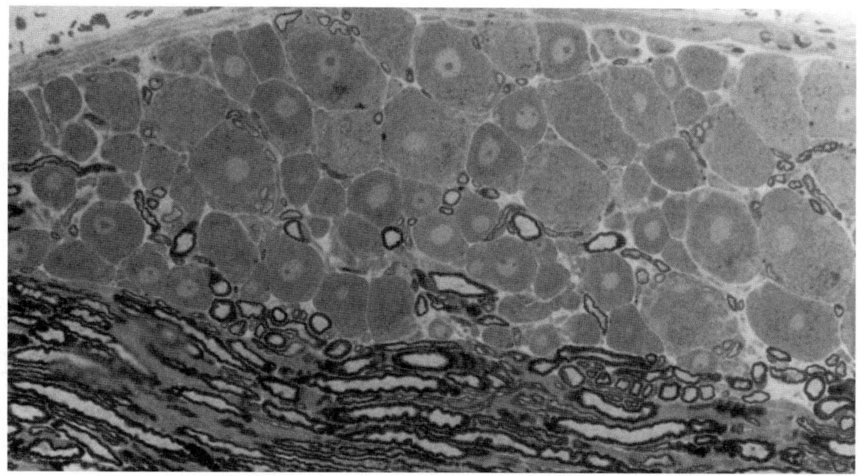

Figure 2. Photomicrograph of section of L5 dorsal root ganglia from control rat. Note differential staining of A and B DRG cells. Lightly staining cells tend to be large while darkly staining cells are always small B cells. Normal cells have centrally located nuclei with prominent nucleoli. Myelinated fiber profiles are seen primarily in longitudinal sections at bottom of micrograph and in transverse sections intermingled with DRG cells.

point of view (309). The most prevalent colocalization is sP and CGRP. Almost all SP cells contain CGRP, but many CGRP neurons do not contain SP.

A second biochemical scheme for classification of DRG cells is based on their enzyme content (127). The hydrolase, fluoride-resistant acid phosphatase (FRAP), in particular, seems to be a useful marker of small DRG neurons. FRAP labeling is also found in the dorsal horn of the spinal cord and in sensory but not motor axons (162) at the periphery. It is generally accepted that FRAP is made in the cell body and transported both proximally and distally (128), although its function is not clear. FRAP reaction product is lost following axotomy but subsequently returns (55).

The ultrastructure of dorsal root and autonomic neurons is similar (273). The small and large neurons of the DRG contain the same types of cytoplasmic organelle, but the numbers and distribution differ. This probably accounts for their differences in staining. Thus, the density of Nissl granules, the Golgi network, mitochondria, neurofibrillae, and pigment granules differ between neurons as does the pattern and intensity of the basophilic Nissl staining. The small, dark neurons have very fine Nissl particles densely distributed throughout their cytoplasm. Larger cells have clumps of Nissl substance separated by pale areas of cytoplasm. It is well known that the Nissl substance stained with cresyl violet corresponds to granular endoplasmic reticulum and that ribosomes, or clusters of ribosomes called polyribosomes, are responsible for basophilic staining (208, 273).

The Golgi complex is usually a conspicuous organelle. It consists of closely packed saccules and vesicles that may be curved into a C-shape configuration (273). Coated vesicles having a spiked outer surface are found in the Golgi region where they may sometimes coalesce with saccules.

Single membrane-bound dense bodies, multivesicular bodies, multilaminar bodies, and lipofuscin granules can be found throughout the cell. Many of these organelles may be involved with intracellular degradation since they exhibit acid phosphatase activity (113). Dense-core granules associated with the Golgi apparatus can also be found in the processes of DRG and sympathetic neurons, suggesting that they are transported to these distal regions.

Neurofilaments and microtubules located in the perikaryon and cell processes may be the structural substrate for the two-way axonal transport of substances between cell body and distal terminal. Neurofilaments appear in high concentration in the axon hillock and initial segment of the axon. They are about 10 nm in diameter with a hollow core and spine-like projections from their surfaces. Microtubules are scattered among the neurofilaments in the perikarya of DRG cells and are more abundant in sympathetic neurons. Microtubules are about 20 nm in diameter and circular in cross section with a core of low density, although they sometimes contain a central dot (273). Additional ultrastructural detail and electron micrographs of various ganglia are available elsewhere (35,75,161,273).

Chromatolysis

Chromatolysis is the term given by Marinesco (157) to Nissl's description of the morphologic changes in nerve cells following axotomy (184) (Fig. 3). The process has also been referred to as primary irritation (185) and the axonal reaction (164). Chromatolysis is the dissolution of the neuronal chromophil substance (Nissl bodies) and is an important early pathologic finding in perikarya. That the perikarya should reflect injuries to its processes is not surprising, given that there is continuity of cytoplasm between the cell body and axon and active biochemical communication between the distal terminal and the protein synthesizing machinery in the DRG. Brattgård and coworkers (28) demonstrated that the process of chromatolysis is not merely degenerative, but primarily anabolic, in that active metabolic processes are involved in reorganization of the organelle, presumably in preparation for regeneration. After axotomy there is an increase in ornithine decarboxylase activity (274) that is considered to be involved in the regulation of DNA and RNA synthesis leading to elevated levels of nucleic acids and proteins in chromatolytic cell bodies (167,294,295). Within 24 hours after axotomy, there is also an increase in the uptake of 2-deoxyglucose by the cell bodies (132). Following the initial period of degeneration-like changes in cell structure, there is an increase in the amount of smooth endoplasmic reticulum and neurofilaments in the cell body as well as a substantial increase in the number, size, and internal complexity of

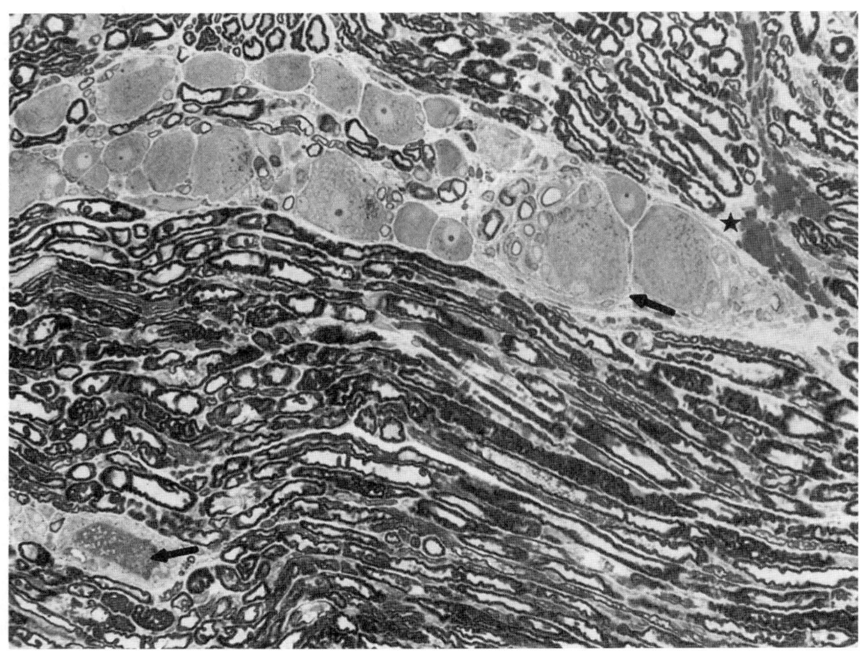

Figure 3. Photomicrograph of section of rat L5 DRG that had been compressed with microforceps. Note hemorrhage (*) in the interstitial space among the nerve cell bodies. Chromatolysis has occurred in several of the cell bodies *(arrows)* in response to the traumatic injury and is indicated by margination of the nucleus and dispersion of Nissl material. Note injury to myelinated fibers seen in longitudinal section within the ganglion. Early disruption and clumping of myelin is seen here within 2 hours of crush injury, which increased endoneurial fluid pressure 2.5-fold in this compartmentalized tissue.

lysosome-like dense bodies (160). This shift in synthetic activity in chromatolytic cells is necessary to supply the regenerating fiber with structural substrate. Correspondingly, there is a reduction in compounds such as acetylcholinesterase (AChE) that participate in synaptic processes, since this function is diminished in regenerating fibers (120).

The most striking feature of chromatolysis is the disappearance of Nissl bodies, which are initially replaced by a finely granular material (275a). This change starts near the axon hillock at the center of the cell 2 to 3 days after axotomy. Small cells in sensory ganglia are the first to respond and may display more intense changes than large neurons (148). A maximum intensity is reached in 1 to 3 weeks after the lesion, after which the Nissl substance begins to be reconstituted. Nissl body recovery occurs during the period of regeneration but it is not necessary for the axon to make appropriate functional connections with an end organ since similar signs of recovery are seen in cells whose axons terminate in a neuroma. Another characteristic feature of chromatolytic cells is that their nuclei become eccentric (281) and, in motor neurons, migrate to the pole opposite the hillock (41). Both the nucleus and nucleolus increase in volume.

Several factors can influence the process of chromatolysis. Axonal injury in immature animals results in cell death (137), while in old animals there is a relative delay in restoration of function (269) compared to younger animals. An important factor in the rapidity of the response, in the intensity of the reaction, and in the extent of cell degeneration is the proximity of the lesion to the cell body (275a). In sensory neurons of the DRG, whose unipolar axon bifurcates into a central and peripheral projection, there is no chromatolysis following transection of the central branch (47,148). Sheen and Chung (255) note that signs of neuropathic pain appear only when injury occurs at a part of the peripheral nerve distal to the dorsal root ganglion. While the pathogenic mechanisms of neuropathic pain are not clear (see below), the magnitude and duration of chromatolysis following axonal injury may influence the development of hyperalgesia.

Not all sensory cells survive injury to their axons. Cell death occurs when there is extreme chromatolysis with nuclear disintegration and extrusion (148). Sensory ganglion cells that disappear are replaced by knots of satellite cells that have proliferated in response to the neuronal failure (12). These have a characteristic appearance and are called nodules of Nageotte.

THE AXON

Morphology

Axons are extensions of the cell body and contain a continuous channel of neuronal cytoplasm. Axons provide communication with the periphery by both electrical and chemical means. Electrical impulses travel at a rate of approximately 1 m/sec in mammalian unmyelinated axons and considerably faster in myelinated fibers. Bidirectional chemical communication occurs via an internal axonal transport system in which substances and organelles are translocated at rates varying from 1 mm/day to over 400 mm/day. In addition to supporting the metabolic maintenance and growth of these very long cellular processes, orthograde axonal transport delivers neurotransmitters to distal terminals. Retrograde axonal transport provides biochemical signals from the periphery that modulate the function of the primary afferent neuron. Details of axonal transport are presented later in the text. Details of electrophysiologic function in axons are provided elsewhere in this book.

This section presents the morphologic characteristics of axons, considering first the unmyelinated axons and then the myelinated axons. Schwann cells invest every peripheral axon but myelinate only some (Fig. 4). This complex cell is considered separately because of its importance to conduction in myelinated fibers, its susceptibility to ischemic injury, its role in producing neurotrophic factors, and its purported osmoregulatory functions. The morphology and function of other cells in the endoneurial space of nerve fibers will also be discussed since they assist in regulating the specialized environment of nerve fibers. By common usage, the term *nerve fiber* has come to mean the combination of the axon and Schwann cell as a functional unit and this convention will be employed here. There are several excellent reviews of the microscopic anatomy of nerve fibers (275), particularly myelinated fibers and their complex relationship to the axon (82,84,138).

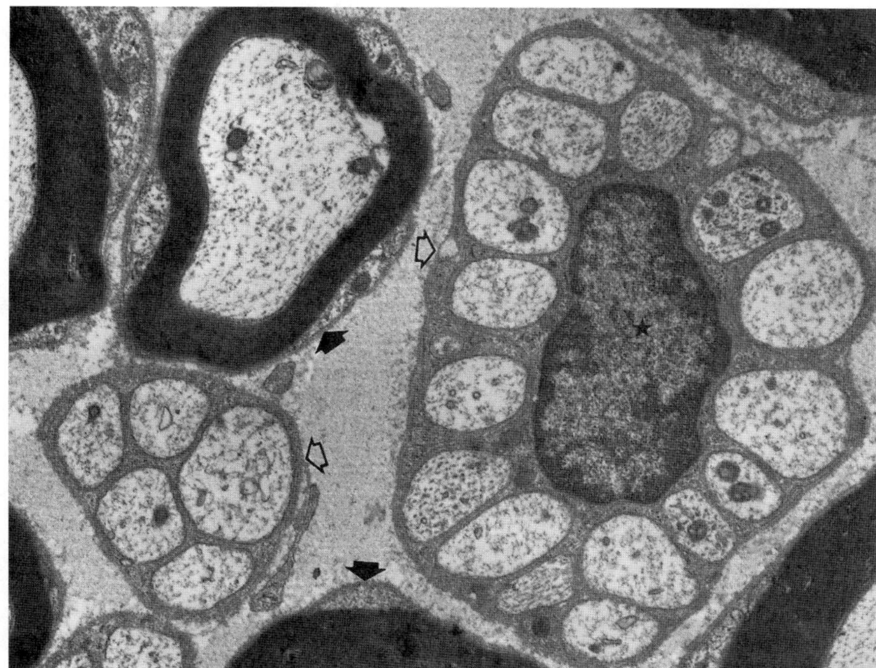

Figure 4. Myelinated and unmyelinated fibers are seen in transverse section surrounded by Schwann cell cytoplasm. Several unmyelinated fibers are contained within the basal lamina of single Schwann cells *(open arrowheads),* while larger, myelinated fibers are individually invested by separate Schwann cells *(closed arrowheads).* Note Schwann cell nucleus in unmyelinated nerve bundle (*).

Unmyelinated Axons

The axoplasm has a viscosity about five times that of water (94) and is surrounded by the axolemma that is separated from the adaxonal membrane of the Schwann cell by an extracellular gap of approximately 10 nm (Fig. 5). This gap is known as the periaxonal space. Tracer studies visualized with electron microscopy suggest tight junctions between these two membranes, but freeze-fracture studies have been unable to confirm this impression (275). At high magnification the axolemma appears as a three-layered membrane about 8 nm thick, and by freeze-fracture is seen to be invested with intramembranous particles, some of which may represent voltage-gated Na^+ channels (265).

As a fluid compartment, the axoplasm contains suspended formed elements. These elements include mitochondria, endoplasmic reticulum, dense lamellar bodies, multivascicular bodies, membranous tubes and vesicles, and the cytoskeleton but not ribosomes or the Golgi apparatus seen in the cytoplasm of the cell body (Fig. 5).

Mitochondria

Mitochondria are 0.1 to 0.2 μm in diameter, 0.5 to 0.8 μm in length, and are divided into outer and inner compartments. The outer compartment contains monoamine oxidase, which is responsible for degradation of catecholamines, and binding sites for interacting with the kinesthetic machinery of axonal transport (158). The inner compartment, bounded by highly infolded membranes called cristae, contains the respiratory electron transport and energy transport enzymes and coenzymes involved in the Krebs cycle. The nucleotides adenosine triphosphate (ATP) and adenosine diphosphate (ADP) are also contained in the intracellular compartment. The concentration of mitochondria is greater in smaller axons. They are probably formed in the cell body, although the association of their outer membranes with agranular reticulum suggests that they may be generated within the axon (263). Mitochondria are usually randomly located throughout the axon; some are stationary but there is also bidirectional transport at the rate of other organelle (69). By intravital microscopy in large axons, mitochondria can be seen to rapidly move along the axon in spurts of different temporal duration interrupted by periods of quiescence (46,69). It is hypothesized that mitochondria use the same mechanisms of transport as smaller organelle but that occasionally they "drop off" the transport carrier for reasons that are not understood (197). This unitary hypothesis of axonal transport is discussed below.

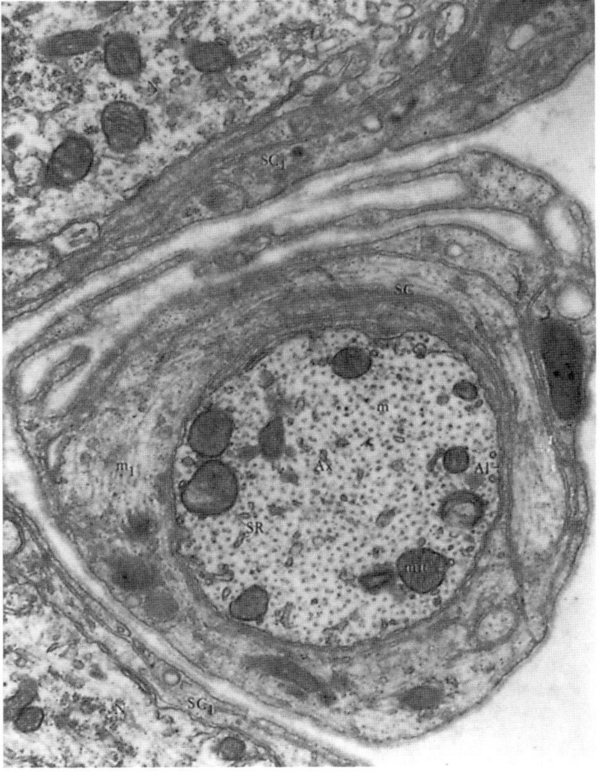

Figure 5. Electron micrograph of transverse section from mouse ganglion cell axon. The axolemma (Al) is the boundary of the axoplasm and is surrounded by Schwann cell processes (SC) containing microtubules (m1). Within the axoplasm, microtubules (m) are homogeneously dispersed. Mitochondria (mit) and tubular profiles of smooth endoplasmic reticulum (SR) are also seen in this section. Original magnification × 26,000. (From ref. 213a, with permission.)

Axoplasmic Reticulum

As a specialization of endoplasmic reticulum, the axoplasmic reticulum is a system of membranous tubules that extend lengthwise throughout the axon (275). It connects to the rough endoplasmic reticulum of the soma at the axon hillock via transitional endoplasmic reticulum (150). Two subdivisions exist: a major inner central component with links to a singular layer of membranous sacs and tubes in the subaxolemma space. While the function of the axoplasmic reticulum is not entirely understood, it is thought to be a vector in slow anterograde transport (150) and as a reservoir for Ca^+ ions (58).

While it is generally believed that the proteins of the nerve endings are synthesized on the endoplasmic reticulum and polyribosomes in the perikarya and eventually delivered to distal presynaptic terminals by axonal flow (Graftstein), a recent report suggests that in the squid neurofilament proteins are synthesized in nerve endings (48). Using Western blot analysis and immunoabsorption methods, Crispino et al. (49) reported that translation products of the squid synaptosomal fraction included neurofilament proteins that were different from perikarya-generated proteins. Their experiments excluded the possibility that these distal neurofilament proteins were assembled fractions of proteins synthesized in the cell body and strengthened the hypothesis that the axon contains a local system for protein synthesis (86,130).

Dense Lamellar and Multivesicular Bodies

These have a variety of shapes up to 0.5 μm in diameter and are found predominantly in the vicinity of the node of Ranvier (80). Their location and acid hydrolase content suggest a lysosomal function.

Microtubules

Microtubules and neurofilaments form the major cytoskeletal elements of the axon and are the major physical conduits for bidirectional axonal transport (102). The microtubules are between 100 and 800 μm in length, 25 nm thick, and extend longitudinally in the axon as individual elements or in small bundles. Their numbers vary inversely with axonal diameter, ranging from $40/\mu m^2$ for small axons to approximately $10/\mu m^2$ for large axons (275).

Neurofilaments

Neurofilaments also run longitudinally in the axon, but often in a spiral course. Their length is uncertain and their diameter is less than one-half that of microtubules, but their density is far greater than microtubules, averaging between 150 to $200/\mu m^2$. The fact that their density does not vary with axonal size has suggested that neurofilaments are the major determinant of axon size (109,283). In the pathologic condition known as giant axonal neuropathy (20), large accumulations of neurofilaments focally distend axons to diameters of 50

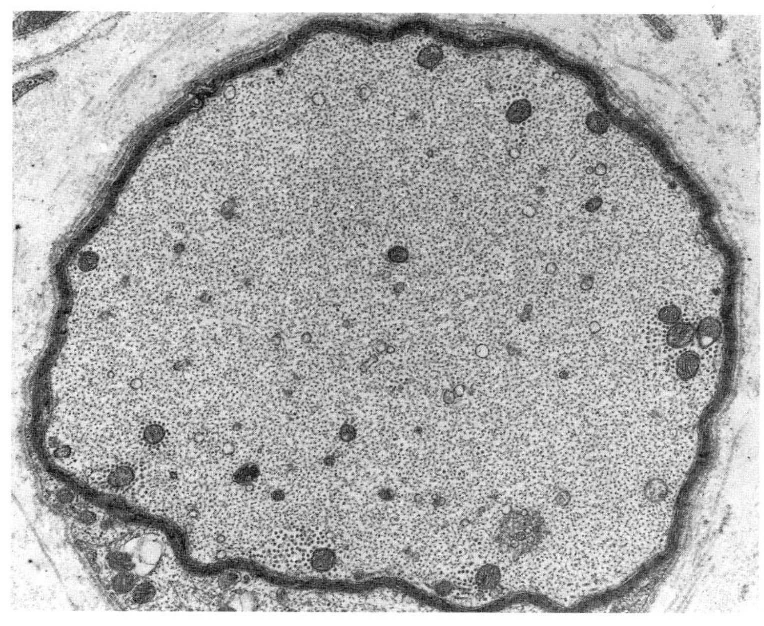

Figure 6. Giant axonal neuropathy in mouse sciatic nerve following experimental intoxication with 2,5–hexanedione. Note segregation of mitochondria and microtubules at periphery of axoplasm. The remainder of the axon is filled with neurofilaments. Original magnification × 10,000. (From ref. 220, with permission.)

μm or more (Fig. 6). This is a rare finding in humans, presenting as an idiopathic childhood disorder (129), presumably via autosomal recessive inheritance, although it has also been described in a case of vitamin B_{12} deficiency (248) and in experimental intoxication of laboratory animals with 2,5-hexanedione (220). It is a generalized disorder of cytoplasmic intermediate filaments for which no treatment is effective (206).

While there is debate about the stability of performed cross-links between the shafts of neurofilaments and microtubules (the microtrabecular lattice) within the axoplasm (63,107, 232), recent biochemical studies have shown that microtubule-associated proteins have only weak interactions with neurofilaments, membranous organelles, and microtubules (287). A popular view is that the structure of the axoplasm appears to consist of proteins in solution interspersed between the cytoskeletal organelles, that is, two different domains rather than a cross-linked matrix (30). The former view that the cytoskeleton is a unitary structure that slowly moves down the axon has been challenged by the idea that it is essentially a stationary structure with its components locally assembled following transportation of precursor proteins from the cell body (194).

Myelinated Axons

Myelin provides insulation for the rapid electrical propagation of action potentials, changing the propagation mechanics from passive, continuous conduction, to saltatory conduction between gaps in the myelin (27,76). The simple functional concept that the only difference between unmyelinated and myelinated axons is the presence of myelin does not hold with respect to the ultrastructural organization of these axons. The presence of myelin affects the physical shape of the axon, the distribution of axoplasmic organelle and neurofilaments, and the local density of ion channels in the axon. These changes further support the enhanced electrophysiologic function of myelinated axons.

Schwann cells periodically invest axons and, unlike oligodendrocytes of the central nervous system, myelinate a portion of only a single axon. The Schwann cell forms myelin as a spiral process in proportion to the axonal diameter (18) (Fig. 7). That is, the thicker the axon, the thicker its myelin sheath. This is, of course, a generalization since the ratio of axonal diameter to nerve fiber diameter (g-ratio) changes during development (249) and varies between species (275). Nevertheless, the g-ratio is a useful morphologic feature in identifying remyelinating nerves since these nerves have inappropriately thin myelin sheaths that gradually thicken during the process of remyelination. In myelinated nerves, myelin is formed individually from adjacent Schwann cells, leaving short unmyelinated segments (the nodes of Ranvier) between myelinated segments of axons. The internodal length of myelinated segments varies from 0.2 to 1.8 mm in adult human nerves and is directly related to the diameter of the axon (292), although internodal length may be considerably shorter in branched skin plexuses of certain species (305).

The paranodal region is approximately 100 μm long and in transverse section can be recognized by its irregular myelin sheath contour and large area of Schwann cell cytoplasm. In many mammalian species the paranodal myelin sheath appears crenated around a correspondingly fluted axon (308). It is within this region that the myelin sheath terminates. Terminating myelin lamella split into leaflets containing Schwann cell cytoplasm, forming a so-called terminal cytoplasmic pocket (275). This axon–Schwann cell network may help regulate the local axonal environment. The paranodal region of the axon is exceptionally rich in mitochondria and lysosomal bodies (80) and the corresponding Schwann cell compartment contains membranous debris and residual bodies. Thus, the axon–Schwann cell network may have the ability to disintegrate axonal constituents as a means of regulating the nodal environment. Because of the relatively high metabolic requirements of the node-paranode, this region is susceptible to pathologic change. Schwann cells are particularly sensitive to ischemic injury and ischemic demyelination may occur without injury to the axon (172,188,221). Early structural changes in myelin often appear in the paranodal region exposing K^+ channels that otherwise would not be in direct contact with the interstitium. Paranodal demyelination increases the capacitance and reduces the radial resistance of the axon (76). In terms of signal transmission, these effects are complementary in slowing and reducing the propagated signal. The adjacent node will be charged more slowly and to a lesser level than normal and may not reach threshold. Complete demyelination of three adjacent internodes blocks conduction.

The node of Ranvier is approximately 0.3 μm long and is the most highly specialized segment of myelinated axons (Fig. 8). The axon is severely constricted at the node or Ranvier with

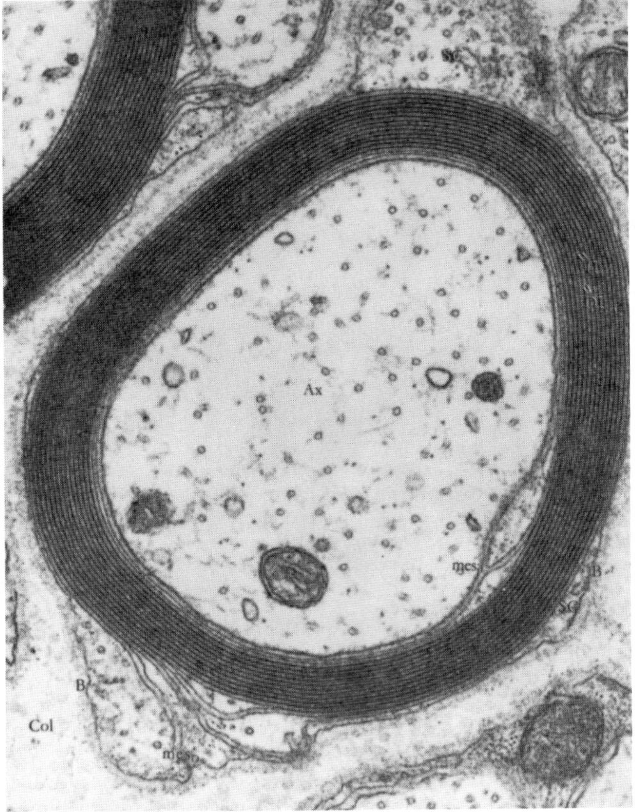

Figure 7. The transversely sectioned axon (Ax) from an adult rat is surrounded by a myelin sheath composed of lamellae formed from the spiraled plasma membrane of a Schwann cell. In the myelin sheath, the alternating major dense lines (DL) and intraperiod lines (IL) are visible. The spiral of the lamellae starts on the inside of the sheath at the internal mesaxon (mes\d\s-2i\s0\u) where the outer faces of the plasma membrane of the Schwann cell come together to form an intraperiod line, and ends on the outside of the sheath at the outer mesaxon (mes\d\s-2o\s0\u). The major dense line is formed by apposition of the cytoplasmic faces of this membrane. Surrounding the myelin is a thin rim of Schwann cell cytoplasm (SC). Outside the Schwann cell is a basal lamina (B) and beyond this the collagen fibers (Col) of the endoneurium. Original magnification × 100,000. (From ref. 213a, with permission.)

more than 50% of neurofilaments interrupted in the paranodal-nodal region (275). The node contains high concentrations of cell adhesional molecules of both the neuron-glial and neuronal types and of the extracellular matrix protein cytotactin in the nodal axoplasm and axolemma (231). Unmyelinated axons lack cytotactin and have a uniform distribution of cell adhesional molecules. The abnormal presentation of adhesional molecules in mouse mutants with defects in cell interactions affecting myelination suggest that surface modulation of cell adhesional molecules may be important in establishing and maintaining nodes of Ranvier (231). The node is rich in Na^+ channels, slow (TEA-blocked) K^+ channels and Na K^+–adenosine triphosphatase (ATPase) (10) but relatively devoid of fast (4-AP–blocked) K^+ channels that appear in higher concentration in the paranodal region (25). This high concentration of functional substrate makes the node particularly sensitive to artifacts in fixation including distortion of the nodal gaps by dehydration.

Following injury to myelinated fibers, regenerating sprouts form at the nodes of Ranvier. The process begins within 3 hours after crush injury, and after 12 hours sprouts can be seen at nodes 1 to 1.5 mm proximal to the lesion (278). These sprouts contain clear vesicles about 50 nm in diameter, multivesicular bodies, and vacuoles measuring 100 to 200 nm in diameter (Fig. 9).

Important communications between the axon and Schwann cell occur by transmural passage across the axolemma to regulate Schwann cell proliferation and myelin production (29,37,93,143). If lipid precursors such as $[^3H]$-glycerol are injected into the dorsal root ganglia, they can be found in Schmidt-Lanterman incisures and inner myelin lamellae following axonal transport from the DRG (56). Conversely, myelin components can be carried by retrograde axonal transport to cell bodies for utilization of their molecular components (199). In nerve injuries in which there is damage to the axon, an unknown axonal signal initiates the immunologic cascade leading to wallerian degeneration. The absence of this signal in the OLA mouse mutant (154) delays the onset of wallerian degeneration and the magnitude of the resultant hyperalgesia (180). Also, it has been shown that blocking retrograde axonal transport with topical application of colchicine to the nerve between the nerve lesion and cell body eliminates the development of hyperalgesia (317). This occurs presumably through the ability of colchicine to dissemble microtubules in dividing cells (131) and block axonal transport of factor(s) generated at the lesion site, which influences the function of central neurons.

Nerve Fiber Morphometry

Quantitative morphology, or morphometry, of nerve biopsies can be a useful aid in the diagnosis of peripheral neuropathies that assists the pathologist in interpreting histologic sections of nerve by supplementing qualitative analysis and providing numerical evaluations of microscopic images. It is especially useful in determining the severity of a neuropathy and the rate of nerve fiber recovery (60). Modern techniques are computer-based and use video microscopy and image processing to measure several pathologic variables. An excellent general-purpose image analysis program for Macintosh computers is in the public domain (226).

Determination of the distribution of nerve fiber sizes is a useful first step in quantitative analysis. This can be done for the fiber as a whole and for the axon separately if the g-ratio is of interest. Figure 10 shows the distributions of fiber diameters, myelin area, and axon area for a normal sciatic nerve and a nerve that had been axotomized 24 months earlier, and demonstrates the changes in the distribution of these variables during the process of nerve regeneration. Note that the distribution of myelinated fiber diameters in normal nerve is bimodal, but that regenerating nerve is characterized by an increase in the number of small fibers and a corresponding reduction in large diameter fibers. This change is also reflected in the distribution of axon and myelin areas as a shift to the left in the peak histogram values. These are the classical morphometric changes associated with nerve fiber regeneration. The absolute numerical values for any particular nerve, however, may differ from this human example, depending on factors such as the nerve being analyzed, age, species, and technique of tissue preparation. It is important to note that although nerve fiber diameters and conduction velocity change after injury, the function of the neuronal unit does not change, although its sensitivity to stimuli may be altered. What once were classified as A-β fibers may now appear as C or A-δ fibers if sorted by morphologic or electrophysiologic criteria. Thus, strict classification of fibers by these criteria may not correlate with neuronal function until the regeneration process is complete, and even then there will be subtle differences in morphometry including a shift to smaller diameter fibers and shorter internodal lengths in myelinated fibers. This latter change correlates directly with myelin thickness, which is also reduced in regenerated nerve fibers (259).

The density of cellular elements within the endoneurial space, the ratio of normal to abnormal fibers, and the volume

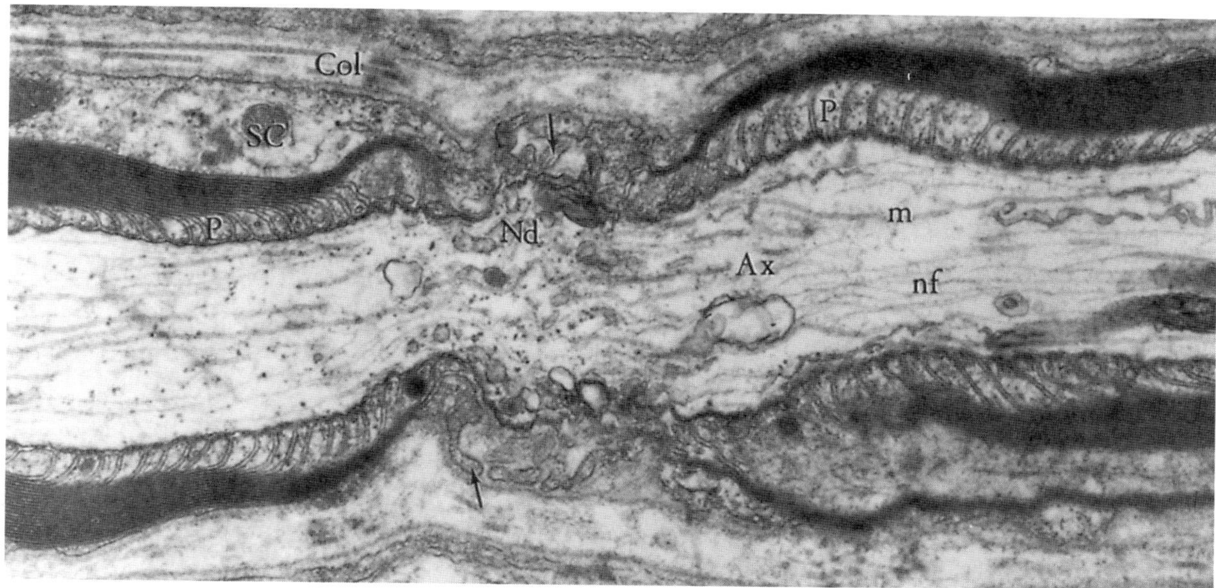

Figure 8. Longitudinal section of the nodal region of a myelinated axon (Ax). As the adjacent lengths of myelin approach the nodal region (Nd), the successive lamellae terminate to enclose pockets of paranodal cytoplasm (P). Processes *(arrows)* from the Schwann cells (SC) cover the nodal region of the axon. In addition to the longitudinally oriented microtubules (m) and neurofilaments (nf) in the axon, note arrangement of the collagen fibers (Col) in the endoneurium. Original magnification × 36,000. (From ref. 213a, with permission.)

of extracellular space can be determined statistically by superimposing a grid over the microscope image and identifying structures beneath grid intersections (122). Human sural nerves contain as many as 65,000 fibers/μm^2, and this sampling technique eliminates the need to characterize each fiber.

Axonal Transport

Throughout the preceding discussion, there has been reference to the role of axonal transport in maintaining the structural integrity of the axon, in providing neurotransmitters to the synaptic terminal, and in regulating neuronal function by the retrograde transport of substances from the periphery to the cell body. We now consider in more detail the hypothesized mechanisms for the bidirectional transport of materials and substances within the axoplasm and the role of axonal transport in nerve disease. Several detailed reviews of these subjects are available (88,194,195,301).

The process of axonal transport is operative in all viable axons, both myelinated and unmyelinated (191,198). The transport rate is sensitive to temperature and slows progressively as temperature declines until it is blocked at a critical temperature near 11°C (200). Fast axonal transport is absolutely dependent on ATP energy stores (192,196,239) and can be readily interrupted by anoxia (196). When ATP is depleted, particle movement stops (3). In a nitrogen environment, both transport and action potentials are blocked within 10 to 30 minutes, although these changes are reversible if the anoxic/ischemic duration is less than 5 to 7 hours and sufficient time is allowed for recovery (144).

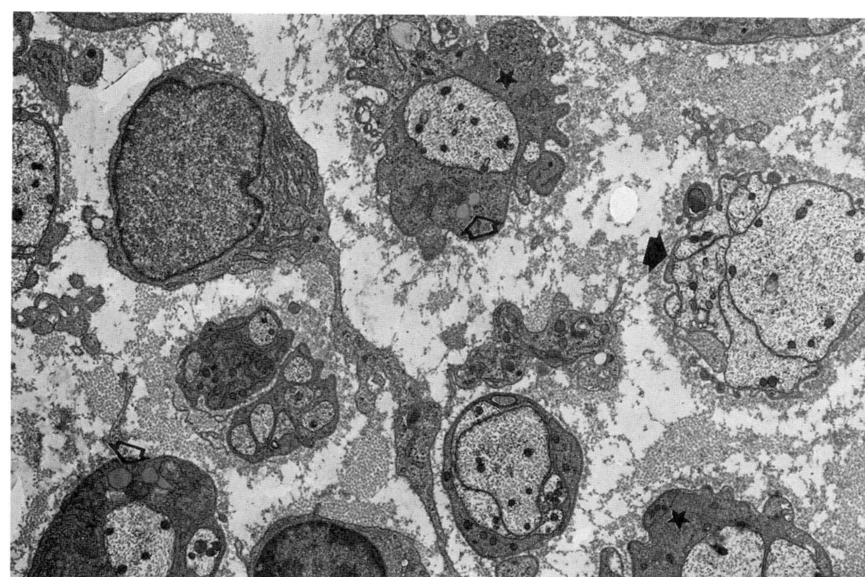

Figure 9. Unmyelinated nerve sprouts *(closed arrowhead)* are seen in this electron micrograph of rat sciatic nerve 14 days after placement of several loose ligatures proximally to produce the chronic constriction injury model of neuropathic pain. Demyelinated axons are also seen surrounded by hydropic Schwann cells (*) with lightly staining lipid inclusions *(open arrowheads).*

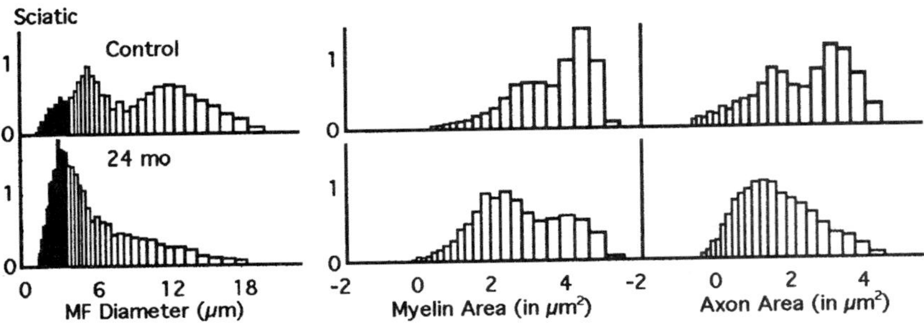

Figure 10. Composite histograms of myelinated fiber diameters *(left)*, myelin areas *(middle)*, and axon areas *(right)* of control *(top)* and transected cat sciatic nerve *(bottom)* demonstrating altered size distribution 24 months after axotomy. (From ref. 60, with permission.)

Using radiolabeled precursors injected into the vicinity of cell bodies and two-dimensional sodium dodecyl sulfate–polyacrylamide gel electrophoresis (SDS-PAGE) to separate proteins by their different isoelectric points and molecular weight, more than 1000 differently labeled proteins can be resolved (310). These can be separated into five different groups based on transport rate (Table 1) (306,307).

Fast anterograde transport of neurotransmitters such as norepinephrine, dopamine, serotonin, and substance P, and neurotransmitter-related compounds such as AChE occur at a rate between 400 and 430 mm/day (31,51,193,251). These compounds resupply vesicles in the nerve terminal (101). Several such cycles of transmitter release and resupply occur before empty vesicles are transported back to the cell body. Some unused proteins are also turned around at the terminal and carried back toward the cell body by retrograde transport at rates approaching that for anterograde transport. Additionally, exogenous substances in the terminal environment are delivered to the cell body by retrograde transport (133). In fact, retrograde axonal transport is an extremely important mechanism for communication between the periphery and cell body, although it is also a vector for some viral and toxic diseases of the neuron. For example, tetanus toxin, and herpes simplex and polio viruses are taken up at the peripheral terminal and transported retrogradely to the cell body (134,223). This mechanism of peripheral uptake and retrograde transport can be exploited experimentally to trace axonal pathways and identify the corresponding cell bodies. Horseradish peroxidase (HRP) is widely used for this purpose since its small molecular size (40 kd) and the electron density of its enzyme reaction product make it an ideal tracer. Retrograde transport is dependent on adequate supplies of ATP, but, unlike anterograde transport, can be inhibited with erythro-9 [3-2(hydroxy-3-nonyl)] adenine (68).

A separate mechanism for slow anterograde axonal transport of proteins was inferred from observations of what appeared to be bulk flow of neurofilament proteins and tubulins of 57 and 53 kd at 1.0 mm/day (110). The mechanism postulated that proteins were assembled into a fixed structural matrix within the cell body and that this continuing process pushed the matrix down the axon at a rate known as slow component "a." Calcium-activated proteases solubilized the matrix at the terminal end (140). As mentioned earlier, however, there is now considerable evidence that the matrix is not fixed and that structural proteins are assembled at the terminal site after being transported in soluble form from the cell body. Tubulin in particular can be seen by intravital microscopy being assembled into microtubules in growth cones of axons (241). Other experiments in which localized application of microtubule blocking agents were used in culture also supports this view (14).

What, then, controls the variable rate of protein transport? Ochs (190) proposed a unitary hypothesis based on a single transport system in which some proteins made in the cell body are delivered uninterrupted at the fast transport rate to the distal terminal, while other proteins and organelles use similar carriers but drop off occasionally and thus appear to be moving more slowly when measured by accumulation methods over a long period of time.

Since the development of this hypothesis there has been direct evidence for organelle movement along the microtubules (3,70) and the discovery that kinesin was necessary to support anterograde transport (229,286). Kinesin is composed of two heavy chains of 124 kd and two light chains of 64 kd (106). There is effectively a hinge in the heavy chain that permits translocation of the terminal light chains, attached to the organelle, from the globular head of the heavy chains attached to the microtubules. There is a cyclic binding and unbending of kinesin from microtubules that is dependent on the presence of ATP (285) and that may be the molecular motor for axonal transport (8). These observations are consistent with the transport filament hypothesis since transport carriers could also be moved by this molecular motor, at least in the anterograde direction. Retrograde axonal transport requires a separate motor and it is postulated that a dynein protein serves this purpose (288). While the precise mechanisms of axonal transport are speculative and the control of precursor uptake, drop-off, and routing (5) of specific proteins to terminal locations is even less well understood, the unitary hypothesis provides a foundation for understanding pathologic changes in transport function producing neuropathy.

Figure 11 illustrates the numerous sites at which axonal transport can be adversely affected. Obviously, interference

Table 1. CLASSIFICATION OF AXOPLASMIC PROTEINS BY TRANSPORT RATE

Group	Velocity	Substances
I	>240 mm/day	membrane constituents and transmitter vesicles: glycoproteins glycolipids lipids cholesterol acetylcholine norepinephrine serotonin substance P other putative transmitters associated enzymes
II	40 mm/day	mitochondrial components fodrin
III-IV	2-8 mm/day	actin myosin-like proteins glycolytic enzymes calmodulin clathrin some additional fodrin
V	1mm/day	cystoskeleton proteins neurofilament proteins

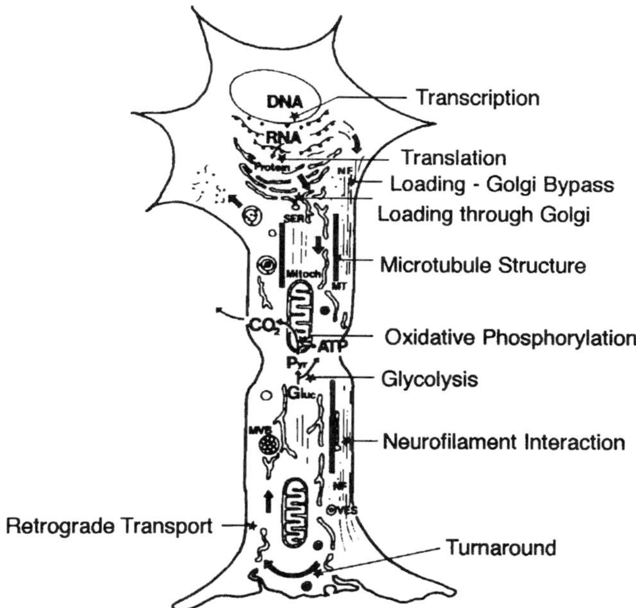

Figure 11. Diagram of the stages in rapid axonal transport and sites at which interruption of transport can take place. The stages include transcription, translation, and loading of transported proteins in the cell body and then their energy-dependent movement along the axon. Turnaround of proteins and retrograde transport of proteins and other substances at the axon terminal play important roles in regulating neuronal protein production. (Modified from ref. 195, with permission.)

with loading of proteins onto transport carriers will affect the quantity transported to the periphery, but other factors including protein transcription rates, microtubule dissociation, and efficiency of turnaround will also affect cellular functions. Much of the knowledge about the mechanisms of axonal transport has come from studies of neurotoxicity (163) in which numerous agents have been shown to have a selective toxic affect on a particular aspect of axonal transport. These insights have been helpful in understanding disease mechanisms (195).

It is interesting to speculate on the role of axonal transport in sensory function and pain. Little is known of a direct relationship except that colchicine topically applied to a peripheral nerve between a focal lesion site and corresponding DRG prevented the expected development of thermal hyperalgesia in the cutaneous distribution of the nerve (317). Colchicine applied to normal nerves in the same dose did not affect the latency to withdrawal from a noxious thermal source or motor function, so it is unlikely that normal sensory function was affected directly by colchicine during the 7-day period of observation. Rather, we have hypothesized that colchicine-induced disruption of retrograde axonal transport prevented some factor liberated at the lesion site from gaining access to the afferent neuron and signaling pain (180a,316). As discussed below, there is evidence to suggest that a cytokine, or a substance generated secondary to an effect of a cytokine, could be responsible for this signaling (180).

SUPPORT CELLS

Schwann Cells

The cell of Schwann (250) is ubiquitous in the peripheral nervous system; approximately 90% of all endoneurial cells are Schwann cells (12). Every peripheral nerve axon is ensheathed from the root zone to the distal axonal termination by a continuous basal lamina from sequentially placed Schwann cells. Schwann cells isolated in culture do not form basal lamina, although in the presence of nerve cells basal lamina will be generated (45). Additionally, the presence of fibroblasts are required for Schwann cell basal lamina deposition and ensheathment of unmyelinated sympathetic neurites in culture (189). The presence of ascorbic acid is required for expression of Schwann cell basal lamina, and basal lamina is required for myelination (61) along with the adhesional molecule L1. Antibody inhibition of L1 does not block basal lamina formation but strongly blocks myelin formation (314). The basal lamina is composed primarily of type IV collagen with lesser amounts of laminen and fibronectin that is present particularly at nodes of Ranvier (207,244).

The presence of basal lamina distinguishes Schwann cells from fibroblasts, macrophages, and mast cells. Basal lamina is preserved when Schwann cells degenerate, and with repeated Schwann cell injuries duplicate basal lamina are formed by new Schwann cells, presenting an onion bulb appearance when viewed ultrastructurally (Fig. 12). The basal lamina is thus an important diagnostic feature, both in identifying endoneurial cells and in establishing the pathogenesis of the nerve injury. Additionally, because the basal lamina degenerates very slowly after Schwann cell death (234), the basal lamina has a critical function in axonal regeneration where it serves as a conduit for nerve fiber regrowth in those lesions in which the nerve has not been transected. This provides for appropriate connection between axons and their original target organs, whereas in transected nerves axons are guided only by neurotrophic factors in the general direction of end organs, although this may occur through remnant basal lamina tubes used previously by another axon. Schwann cells not in contact with axons express nerve growth factor and NGF receptor on their surfaces, and this may also assist in guiding axons down remnant basal lamina tubes in which mitotic activity produces new Schwann cells. For this reason, we prefer to freeze nerves rather than to transect them for neurolytic management of pain following thoracotomy because this produces the desired functional deficit while assuring successful regeneration (175). Freeze-treated allogeneic nerve grafts are used experimentally to bridge the gap between transected ends of nerve since this procedure eliminates host cellular elements but preserves Schwann cell basal lamina and is more effective in promoting axons to bridge the gap than are other allogeneic grafts (205).

The Schwann cell itself is thought of as a flat, trapezoidal-shaped cell that is spirally wrapped around the axon. At the center of one end is the nucleus that contains clumped peripheral chromatin and is elongated in the length of the axon. Adjacent cytoplasmic organelles include rough endoplasmic reticulum, Golgi membranes, centroids, lipid vacuoles, mitochondria, and Reich granules. The protogon (pi) granules of Reich are approximately 1 μm long, membrane-bound, lamellated bodies that stain metachromatically (186,276). The role of Reich granules may be lysosomal since they are associated with acid phosphatase activity (303). Their numbers increase with age.

The Schwann cell plasmalemma is a three-layered membrane like the axolemma but it is symmetric with uniform thickness of its leaflets. The inner mesaxon is the surface membrane of the Schwann cell where it forms the first spiral loop around the axon (79,214). A small amount of adaxonal Schwann cell cytoplasm lies adjacent to the inner mesaxon. The growth rate of Schwann cells increases exponentially during development and the formation of the first four to six spiral layers of myelin and then remains relatively constant as the spiral sheet enlarges and becomes more compact (298). While the detailed relationships between membrane growth and spiral wrapping are poorly understood, it has been suggested that as the number of spiral turns increases, the external mesaxon and nucleus move around the axon; rotation of the sheath and internal mesaxon may occur in the opposite direction (299).

The myelin sheath appears as compact spiral lamellae that are alternately light and dark when viewed in osmicated, trans-

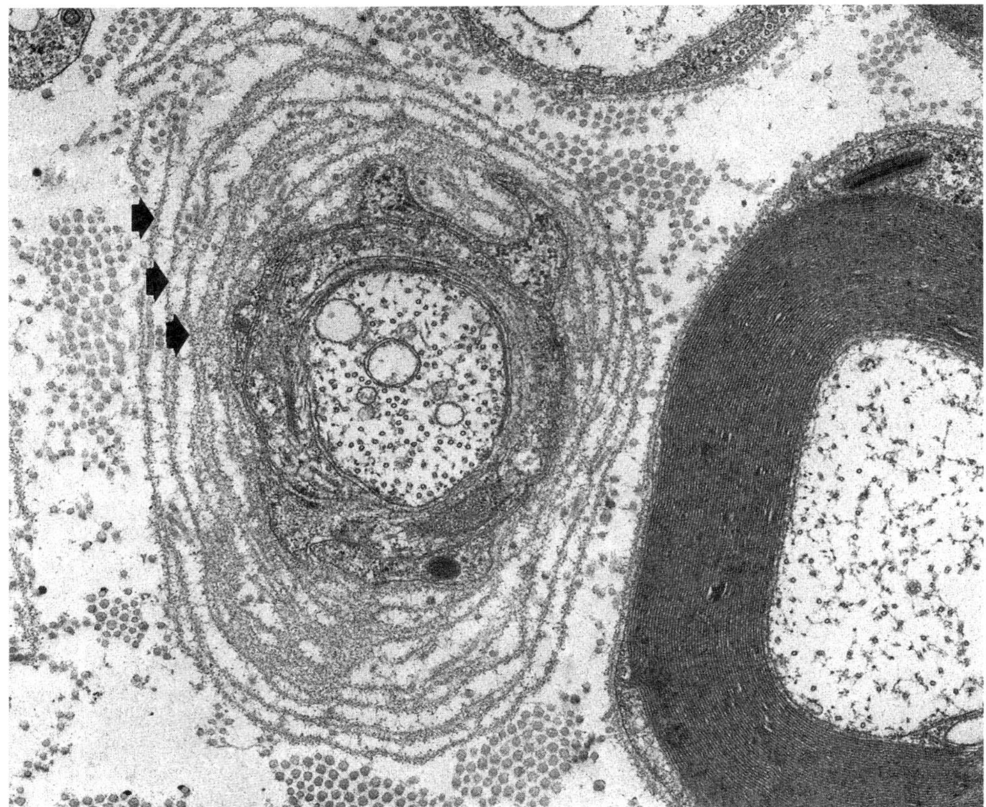

Figure 12. Duplicated Schwann cell basal lamina *(arrowheads)* surrounding an otherwise normal-appearing axon. Repeated ischemic injury to the Schwann cell or schwannopathy from other causes produces these loosely concentric layers of basal lamina that develop when new Schwann cells associate with the axon. The basal lamina appear as an onion bulb would in cross section and are often referred to by that descriptive name. Note normal myelinated axon adjacent. (From ref. 220, with permission.)

verse section by electron microscopy (Fig. 7). The light lines, or intraperiod lines, are formed by the approximation of the external membrane surfaces of the Schwann cell. At high power, both membranes can be seen with an extracellular water space of 5 nm between them (275). The dark, or major dense lines, are formed by the approximation of the inner cytoplasmic surfaces of Schwann cell surface membranes. X-ray diffraction studies show the dense line as two distinct membranes separated by 4 nm, but after fixation and osmication they appear as a single major dense line in electron micrographs. Freeze-fracture studies have provided additional information on the intramembranous particulate organization of myelin lamellae (275). The linear periodicity of these lines in compact myelin is about 15 nm in aldehyde-fixed specimens. This morphology is easily disrupted by incomplete fixation, producing artifacts that appear as focal bubbles in otherwise compact segments of myelin. These are not to be confused with pathologic alterations in structure caused primarily by neurotoxic agents that selectively split myelin lamellae (Fig. 13).

Schmidt-Lanterman incisures (73,139,274) in the myelin sheath are clefts in which the major dense lines open to enclose granular cytoplasm of the Schwann cell (96). They occur predominantly in the internodal region (297) and may extend through the whole myelin sheath or only a few lamellae in either dimension of the Schwann cell. As many as 25 incisures are present per internode in large fibers of the rat sciatic nerve (108) with fewer numbers in thinner myelin sheaths (74). Their role is unknown. During wallerian degeneration most myelinated fibers show segmentation at incisures to form myelin ovoids (83,85). There is not an increase in the number of incisures as some reports have suggested, but rather an increase in their dilation during wallerian degeneration (83). There are conflicting reports on the metabolic activity of incisures and their role in passage of tracers from axon to Schwann cell, even though incisures have been shown to have acid phosphatase activity (71), to take up certain tracers (256), and to be associated with coated smooth-wall vesicles in the Schwann cell cytoplasm (96). Their increased number in developing, regenerating, and remyelinating nerves and their failure to elongate in remyelinated adult nerves (83,108) suggest that they may have a role in the longitudinal growth of developing nerves (43).

Apart from its role in myelination, the Schwann cell may help control the hydration of nerve fibers by regulating the osmotic environment of the endoneurial space. The Schwann cell has a high concentration of aldose reductase (AR), the first enzyme in the polyol pathway that converts hexose sugars to polyhydric alcohols. AR is expressed in differentiated or mature Schwann cells (313) and has been implicated in the pathogenesis of neuropathy in metabolic disorders such as diabetes (279). Aldose reductase inhibitors are a promising experimental therapy for the early complications of diabetes relating to exaggerated flux through the polyol pathway (280) and the associated increase in osmolytes that leads to endoneurial edema (169,170). Recent studies in renal cell cultures (13,16,38) and other tissues (111,124) have shown that induction of AR messenger RNA (mRNA), enzyme activity, and production of polyol serve to maintain cellular volume in response to changing extracellular tonicity. The specific localization of aldose reductase to paranodal cytoplasm, Schmidt-

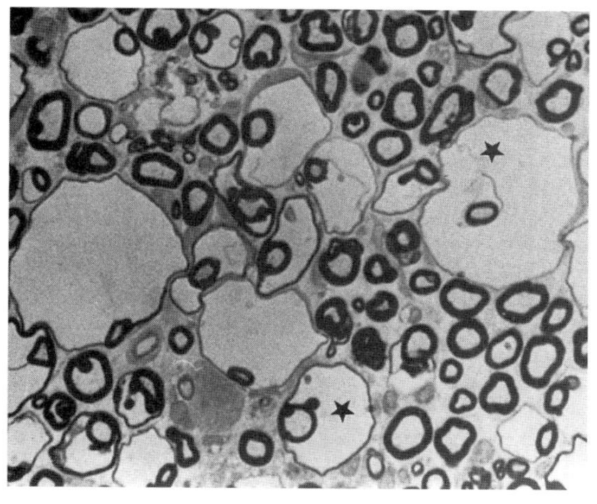

Figure 13. Ingestion of hexachlorophene produces a neuropathy characterized by splitting of the myelin sheath at the intraperiod line, giving rise to wide separation of myelin lamellae. Hexachlorophene interferes with enzymes that regulate cation exchange and causes a permeability disorder in myelin such that the myelin swellings are fluid filled. This, in turn, causes an increase in endoneurial fluid pressure. Large intramyelinic vacuoles (*) are seen in this example from a rat sciatic nerve 14 days after starting a diet containing 1000 parts per million of hexachlorophene.

Lanterman incisures, and the outer and inner glial loops of myelinated Schwann cells (218) may also reflect a volume regulatory role in a cell with a complex and compacted cytoarchitecture that requires the maintenance of cytoplasmic channels (169).

In experimental studies of nerve blood flow in which an ischemic insult can be varied and quantified, several investigators have been impressed with the vulnerability of the Schwann cell to ischemic injury (172,187,188,221). Using several different techniques for measuring local nerve blood flow, we have concluded that moderate levels of nerve ischemia cause Schwann cell injury and demyelination, while severe ischemia causes axonal injury, wallerian degeneration, and neuropathic pain (180a,188,221). Local anesthetics can also reduce nerve blood flow, especially when epinephrine is used as an adjuvant (173), and it may be through this mechanism that nerve injury occasionally occurs during procedures requiring local anesthesia (174). In related studies with local anesthetics, it has been shown that the Schwann cells of unmyelinated fibers are selectively vulnerable to the neurotoxic effects of high concentrations of local anesthetics (219) and that pathologic changes in Schwann cells occur early in the course of ischemic nerve injuries (123).

Finally, Schwann cells have been shown to have a phagocytic role in neuropathy (23,178,217,264,266) (Fig. 14) and to express low levels of major histocompatibility complex (MHC) class I molecules that are markedly increased following exposure to interferon-γ (243,282). Whether Schwann cells can act as antigen-presenting cells in vivo is unclear (89,246), although they play an important role in immune reactions in the peripheral nervous system (100). In tissue culture studies with interferon-γ Schwann cells will express MHC class II antigens and present antigen to T cells (242,302), although in experimental autoimmune neuritis, the primary class II–positive cells are macrophages (246,320). The release of interleukin-1 (IL-1) from activated macrophages in the endoneurial space stimulates the synthesis of nerve growth factor by Schwann cells, as we have already seen, and peripheral nerve regeneration is impeded in the presence of an IL-1 receptor antagonist (32,92). The importance of understanding the complex relationships among macrophages, Schwann cells, and mast cells that function normally

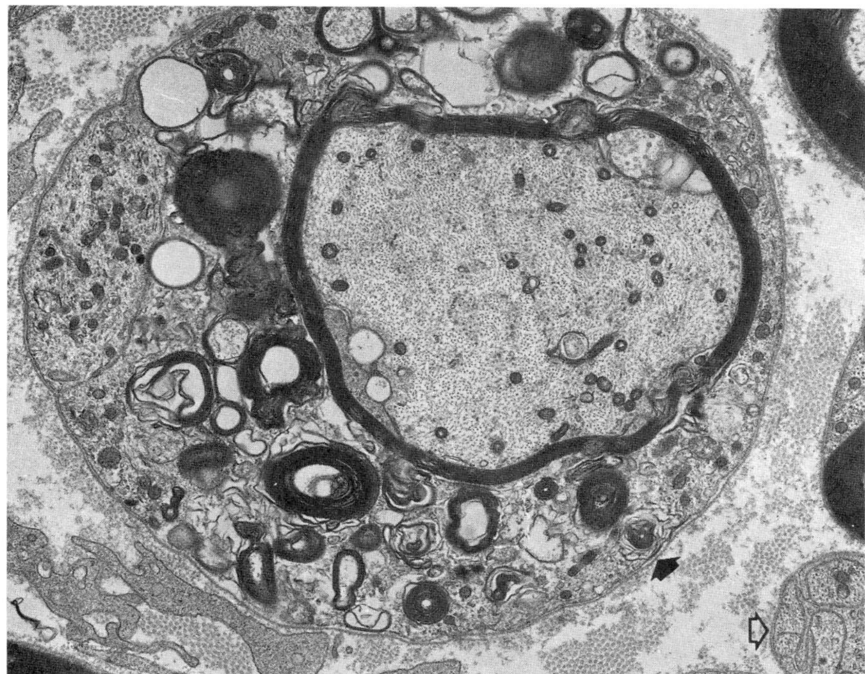

Figure 14. Schwann cell phagocytosis observed 7 days after ischemic injury to rat peripheral nerve. Note cytoplasmic inclusion of myelin and other lipid debris contained within the basal lamina *(solid arrowhead)* boundary of the Schwann cell. Splitting and disruption of remaining myelin is also evident around axon that is displaying dystrophic changes. Note intact unmyelinated nerve fiber bundle in lower right *(open arrowhead).*

to regulate the immune reactions of nerve fibers to foreign antibodies is heightened by the several clinical diseases like Guillain-Barré syndrome in which it is thought that autoimmune processes cause macrophages to attack normal myelin (Fig. 15). Demyelination can be either primary or secondary and an extrinsic or intrinsic event affecting Schwann cells or myelin. Apart from autoimmune-induced demyelination, numerous toxins can disrupt the integrity of established myelin sheaths or the metabolic machinery of Schwann cells such that the insulating function of myelin is lost. If this is limited to single Schwann cells or randomly affects isolated segments of the nerve fiber, then segmental demyelination is said to have occurred. Although the axon may remain intact, and remyelination may begin concurrently, demyelination significantly affects nerve function by altering impulse propagation through the demyelinated segment (27). Segmental demyelination of three consecutive nodes produces conduction block (67).

Mast Cells

Mast cells are normal constituents of the peripheral nervous system but are seen more frequently in the endoneurial interstitium of cat, mouse, and rat than in man (12,78,203). Mast cells appear rounded or elliptical and have numerous filopodia but no basal lamina (Fig. 16). They are filled with membrane-bound, intracytoplasmic granules that are osmophilic and stain metachromatically. The fact that the granules contain various biogenic amines and heparin suggests that they play a role in nerve hydration (227). Several studies have shown that mast cell numbers increase after nerve trauma and during wallerian degeneration (64,202). During injury, the granules are released by exocytosis and degranulate to liberate heparin, histamine, and serotonin (Fig. 16). The classical experimental agent used to liberate mast cell granules is Compound 48/80 (204). Injection of Compound 48/80 or histamine, but not serotonin or heparin, into rat peripheral nerves is associated with increases in endoneurial edema and endoneurial fluid pressure (222).

Activation of mast cells may be an important initial factor in immune responses and macrophage recruitment to peripheral nerve by altering the permeability of the blood-nerve barrier to permit extravasation of T-lymphocytes and macrophages into the endoneurial space (100). Recent reports indicate that mast cells produce cytokines including tumor necrosis factor-α (TNF-α), IL-1, IL-3, IL-4, IL-6, and granulocyte-macrophage colony stimulating factor (GM-CSF) (9,87), suggesting a "mast cell-leukocyte cytokine cascade" (77) that modulates the biologic process of inflammation. IgE-dependent mast cell activation results in the rapid release of preformed stores of TNF-α followed by the synthesis and sustained release of large quantities of newly formed TNF-α (87). In an important observation that may have special relevance to the pathogenesis of neuropathic pain, it has recently been shown that substance P selectively activates TNF-α gene expression in murine mast cells (9) and triggers release of histamine, but not IL-1, -3, -4, -6, or GM-CSF. It does this in a dose-dependent manner. This neuropeptide-induced mast cell cytokine release may be the initial factor in the inflammatory cascade associated with focal injuries to peripheral nerve causing hyperalgesia. The sequence of events may include:

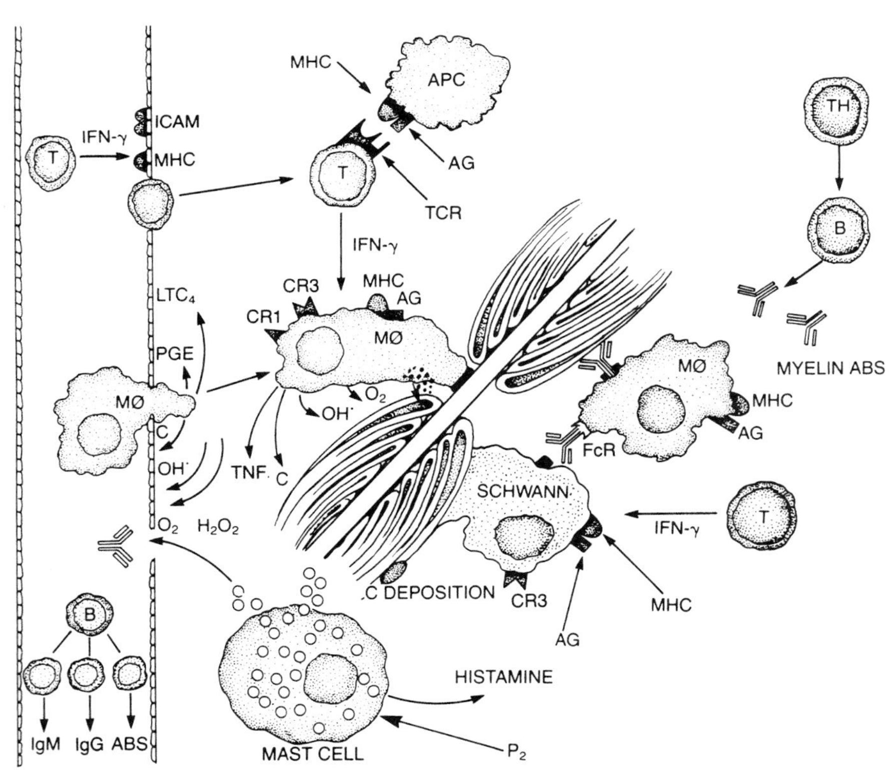

Figure 15. Synoptic view of cellular and humoral immunity in experimental autoimmune neuritis (EAN) and Guillain-Barré syndrome (GBS), acute neuropathies in which the myelin sheath is attacked by macrophages. Local immune circuitry in the nerve is composed of macrophages, antigen-presenting cells (APC, macrophages and/or Schwann cells), Schwann cells, T-lymphocytes (T, TH), B-lymphocytes/plasma cells (B), and mast cells. The initial event leading to autoimmunization currently remains elusive. Circulating activated T cells cross the blood-nerve barrier, possibly facilitated by interferon-γ (IFN-γ), and interact via their T-cell receptor (TCR) with antigen-presenting cells that display on their surface the putative autoantigen(s) (AG) in association with major histocompatibility complex (MHC) class II gene products. Activated T cells, via the release of interferon-γ, recruit macrophages that either directly attack the myelin sheath through phagocytosis or release injurious effector molecules, e.g., oxygen free radicals: superoxide anion, hydroxyl radical, arachidonic acid metabolites such as prostaglandin E (PGE); hydrolytic enzymes; or complement components (C). Exactly how macrophages are attracted to nerve and gain target specificity is unclear. A cooperative action with antimyelin antibodies (ABS) via the Fc receptor may guide them to the myelin sheath. An interaction of the macrophage complement type 3 (CR3) with opsonized myelin could likewise be involved. Finally, mast cells may also contribute to the amplification/effector phase by synthesizing chemoattractants and vasoactive amines that enhance permeation of inflammatory cells through the blood-nerve barrier. (From ref. 100, with permission.)

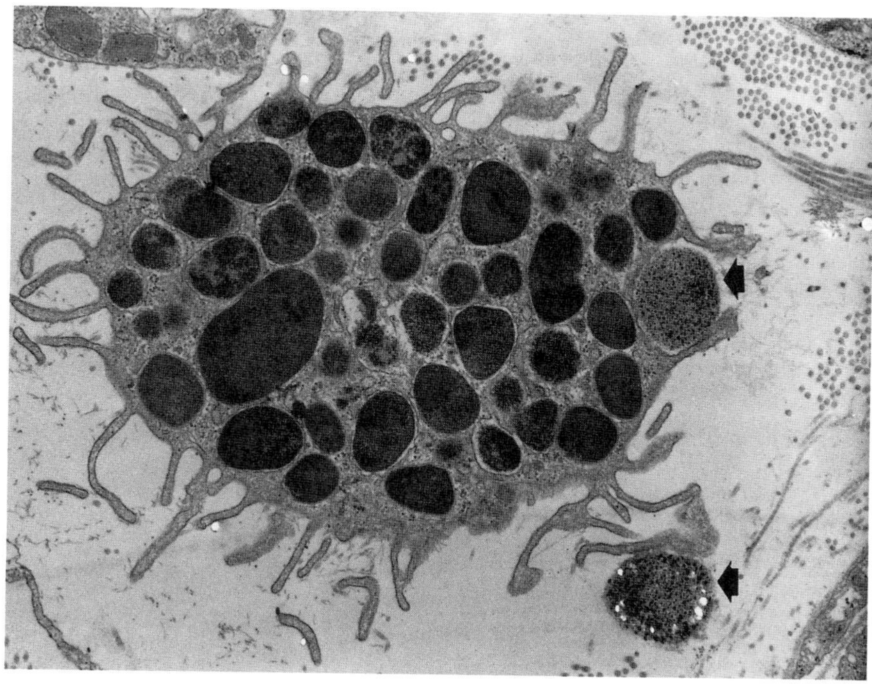

Figure 16. Endoneurial macrophage showing characteristic filopodia and lack of basal lamina. Intact, membrane-bound, intracytoplasmic granules contain biogenic amines and stain darkly. This activated mast cell is in the process of releasing granules by exocytosis. Activated, degranulated mast cells reveal a reticular pattern with fine punctate densities *(arrowheads).*

1. substance P release from injured sensory nerves,
2. activation of mast cells,
3. mast cell release of TNF-α and biogenic amines that assist in the recruitment of macrophages by altering the permeability of the blood-nerve barrier to permit extravasation of immune cells recruited to the injury site,
4. activation of hematogenous macrophages by complement opsonization of myelin fragments,
5. macrophage release of IL-1 and other cytokines that influence Schwann cells to alter production of NGF, and
6. retrograde axonal transport of NGF, cytokines, or other products released or generated locally at the injury site that alter the function of afferent neurons leading to hyperalgesia in the presence of ectopic electrophysiologic activity.

Thus, in combination with resident macrophages (see below), mast cells aid in policing the endoneurial environment of nerve fibers, responding rapidly to elevated concentrations of sensory neuropeptides and trafficking of specialized immune cells to nerve injury sites.

Macrophages

Macrophages are found as resident cells in the endoneurial space of peripheral nerves, accounting for 2% to 4% of the intrafascicular nuclei (11,201). In normal nerves they are located predominantly in the perivascular space surrounding endoneurial venules and are actively renewed from circulating cells (289). They are found in higher concentration in sensory and sympathetic ganglia (66) where there is a less substantial blood-nerve barrier. Resident macrophages are elongated cells that are frequently ramified and oriented in the longitudinal axis of the nerve (89,171). Phenotypic macrophage markers are diagnostic in neuropathology (114). Macrophages express complement receptor 3, low levels of CD4, and the Fc receptor, and are faintly positive for MHC class II antigens (66,90,171). Rat macrophages stain positively with the ED2 monoclonal antibody.

The role of macrophages in regulating the immunologically privileged space of the peripheral nervous system via presentation of antigens to other cells in the immune system and their phagocytic role following nerve injury has only recently been recognized (91,212). While macrophages are the dominant Schwann cell phagocytes in demyelinating and autoimmune neuritis, macrophages play an essential role in the pathology of nerve injuries involving the integrity of the axon (Fig. 17). The pathology of these injuries, frequently caused by nerve transection, crush, or severe ischemia, was originally described by Augustus Waller in 1850 (293) and includes an initial reaction at the site of injury and then degeneration and phagocytosis of myelin and axons distal to the injury. Following nerve injury, nonresident, hematogenous macrophages invade the injury site, their numbers peaking during the intense period of phagocytic activity associated with wallerian degeneration (213,266,267). In 1984 Beuche and Friede (21) demonstrated that nonresident macrophages are the primary effector cell in wallerian degeneration by showing that severed nerves did not degenerate when they were isolated in a millipore chamber that excluded the entry of macrophages. Additional insights into the relationship between nerve degeneration and macrophage activity have been significantly advanced by the chance discovery of a mouse mutant (C57BL/OLA) in which there is delayed recruitment of hematogenous macrophages to the site of nerve injury (154). This is associated with delayed wallerian degeneration (154) and reduced neuropathic pain (180). Although it has been shown that wallerian degeneration can be inhibited by preventing the recruitment of macrophages with a monoclonal antibody against their complement type 3 receptor (240), this is apparently not the reason for delayed recruitment of macrophages to injured nerve in OLA animals. Rather, there appears to be an absence in the required chemotactic signal from injured axons or Schwann cells (211). Macrophage function per se is normal in OLA animals since macrophages respond appropriately to injuries outside the nervous system.

The mechanisms by which macrophages potentiate wallerian degeneration are not known, although it is thought that cytokine signaling and secretion of proteases play a central role. A key element in the mechanism is macrophage activation (2). Activated macrophages show profound differences in membrane proteins and cytoskeletal protein regulation and transcription that alter the synthesis, expression, and location of cell-bound and secre-

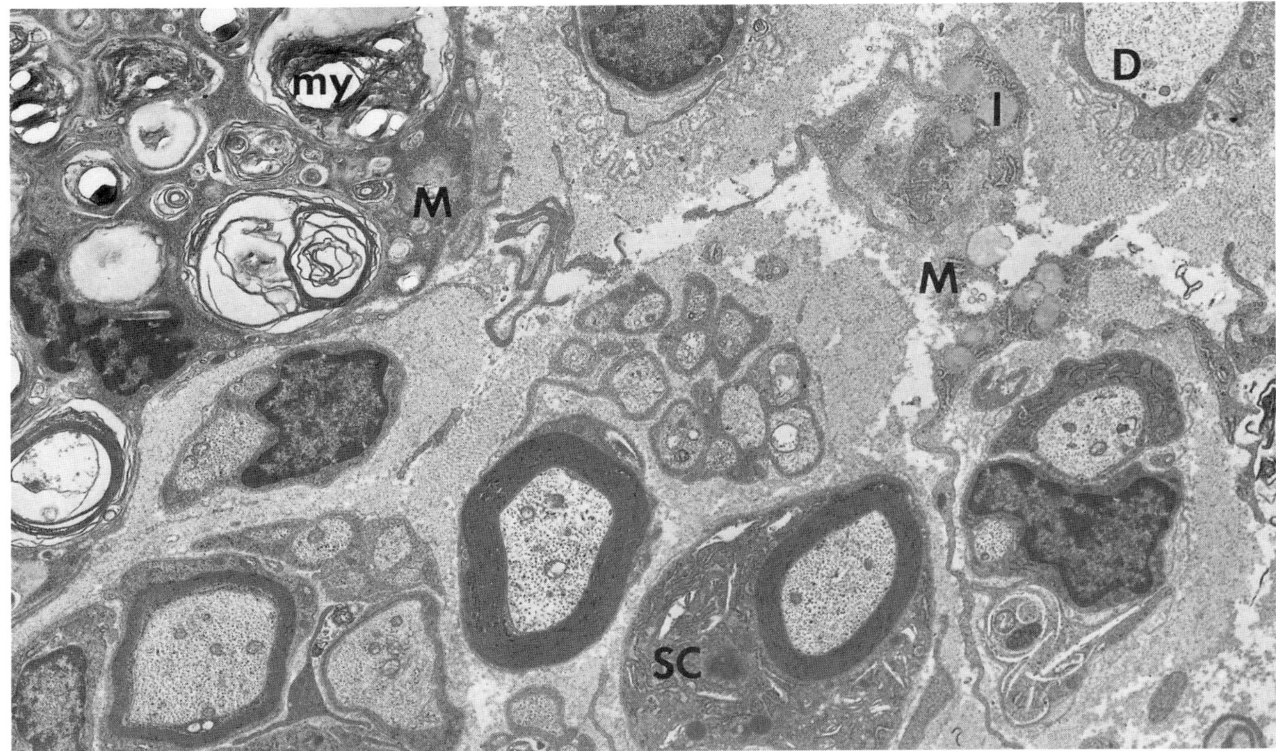

Figure 17. Macrophage invasion of endoneurium 7 days after peripheral nerve injury. Macrophages (M) are identifiable as phagocytic cells lacking a basal lamina and can be seen here with ingested lipid (l) and myelin (my) debris. Note filopodia probing the periphery of degenerating nerve fiber on the right edge of the electron micrograph and demyelinated axon (D) with ruffled basal lamina of associated Schwann cell. Dystrophic Schwann cell (SC) with intact myelinated axon may eventually undergo wallerian degeneration with macrophage phagocytosis.

tory proteins (1). Activated macrophages secrete components of the complement cascade, coagulation factors, proteases, hydrolases, inteferons, tumor necrosis factor, and other cytokines (1). The cascade of events is complex and may be dependent initially on other cells in the endoneurium including mast cells and Schwann cells that are driven by interferon-γ to express class II antigens. Recent reports suggest that resident macrophages may start the cascade by recognizing the release of sensory neuropeptides in the setting of axonal injury (22). This may be associated with a similar or complementary effect in mast cells (see above). IL-1 or other cytokines secreted from activated macrophages after nerve injury may have a key role in altering central neuronal function leading to chronic neuropathic pain. It has been shown that there are changes in plasma cytokines associated with peripheral nerve injury (304) and these circulating factors may directly influence neuronal function. More likely, however, would be an effect mediated by retrograde axonal transport of higher concentrations of cytokines from the nerve injury site, or by retrograde transport of other factors stimulated by local cytokine release. In this regard, we have already seen that IL-1 stimulates Schwann cells to express nerve growth factor on their surfaces, and that retrograde transport of NGF from the injury site is an important signal affecting the function of dorsal root ganglia neurons. Recently some authors have suggested that NGF or an octapeptide of NGF is painful when injected peripherally, but it is not clear by what mechanism this may be mediated (147,271). Tumor necrosis factor liberated from activated macrophages may also have a role in the pathogenesis of neuropathic pain since TNF-α has been shown to induce axonal degeneration when injected into rat nerves (240). TNF-α is a mediator of leukocyte recruitment (6), and we believe that it is associated with the pathologic alterations in the endoneurial

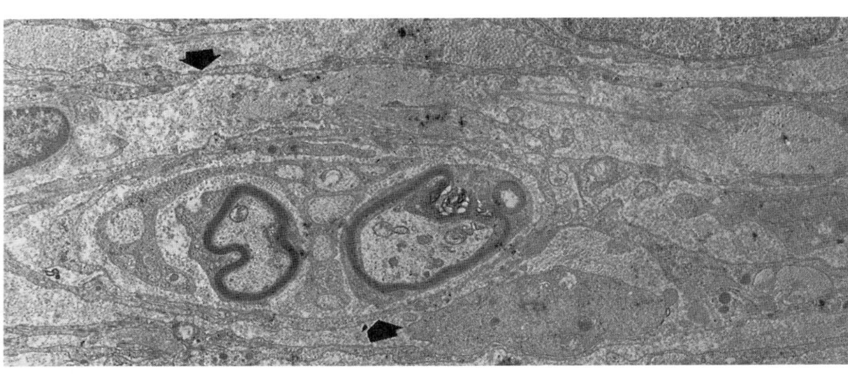

Figure 18. Remyelinated axons following peripheral injury. Fibroblasts are numerous and their processes *(arrowheads)* have begun to encase these two axons in what may become a minifascicle in which differentiated fibroblasts form a perineurium-like barrier either within the endoneurium or outside the original perineurium if it has been injured.

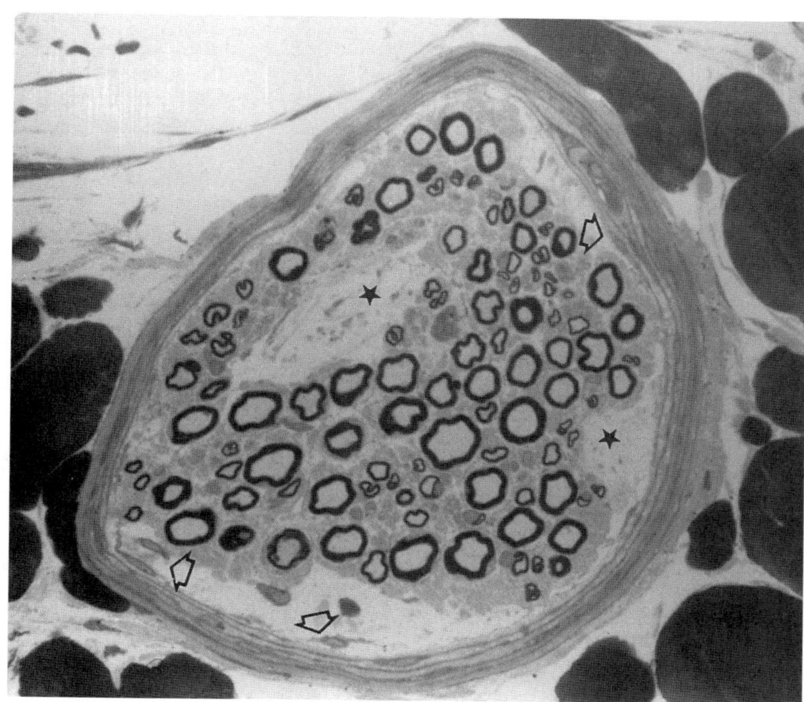

Figure 19. Reanut bodies (*) in pig spinal nerve roots. These space-occupying lesions can appear in some species normally but may be more prevalent in nerves that have been chronically compressed. They are composed of loosely organized fibroblasts. Fat cells surround the thickened perineurium. Note numerous fibroblasts in subperineurial space *(arrowheads).*

endothelial cells in the Bennett and Xie (19) rat model of neuropathic pain (180a,260). It has recently been demonstrated that inhibition of TNF-α by thalidomide reduces the hyperalgesia associated with this model (261).

Fibroblasts

Fibroblasts are normal constituents of the endoneurium, appearing predominantly in the subperineurial region and in endoneurial septa as long tenuous processes without basal lamina. The cytoplasm is rich in rough endoplasmic reticulum and ribosomes. As mentioned previously, fibroblasts are required for production of basal lamina by Schwann cells. In cultures consisting of only Schwann cells and fibroblasts, Schwann cells become enclosed in a basal lamina-like structure (36). Fibroblasts provide lamina, type IV collagen, and heparan sulfate proteoglycan for the production of Schwann cell basal lamina and other unknown factors necessary for the deposition of Schwann cell basal lamina (36,126). Thus, fibroblasts appear to be able to substitute for neurons in promoting basal lamina deposition on the surface of Schwann cells (34).

Fibroblasts proliferate following nerve injury and are an early finding in the subperineurial space associated with endoneurial edema. Reactive changes in this environment may lead to epineurial fibrosis that can affect the long-term recovery of nerves. In experimental compression injuries of peripheral nerve producing wallerian degeneration and injury to the perineurium, and in other traumatic nerve injuries, nerve fibers may venture into new tissue areas and become surrounded by consecutive layers of elongated fibroblasts or perineurial cells thought to be differentiated fibroblasts (Fig. 18). These minifascicles are a distinctive feature of aberrant regeneration (142,260).

In chronic nerve entrapment, large accumulations of fibroblasts are seen in whorled bundles with randomly oriented collagen and fine fibrillary material (Fig. 19). In a recent study, Weis et al. (300) used immunohistochemical methods to identify the oxytalan component of elastic fibers in Renaut's bodies (230) in addition to type IV collagen, laminin, and s-laminin. These authors concluded that Renaut's bodies are composed of fibroblasts that show perineurial differentiation. Renaut's bodies also occur occasionally in normal human nerves where their pathologic significance is unknown. They are more prominent in horses and donkeys, and we have noted a high incidence in mini-pig spinal nerves.

PERIPHERAL SENSORY RECEPTORS

Peripheral sensory receptors are terminal specializations of afferent axons that are normally classified in terms of their physiologic functions (Fig. 20) (Table 2) (149a). Details of the correlation between sensory stimuli and the electrophysiologic activity of single nerve fibers are given elsewhere in the text and are summarized in other recent reviews (149a,321). We will consider the morphologic aspects of sensory receptors, although there is less than a complete understanding of the relationship between sensory function and terminal receptor morphology. In some cases, sensory functions have not been correlated with morphologic specializations (Table 2), although there have been early and persistent attempts to correlate function with fiber specialization, beginning with the work of von Frey (71,72), who compared the density of specialized cutaneous nerve terminals with detailed observations on the nature of discrete skin locations for sensing pressure, cold, warmth, and pain. von Frey's work led to the teaching that Meissner corpuscles and Merkel cells transduced touch, Ruffini endings transduced warmth, Krause end-bulbs transduced cold, and "free" nerve endings transduced pain. Although it is now recognized that the same receptor may be used for different functions, the general concept of specificity of afferent fibers (155) is still the approach that guides modern research.

The following morphologic criteria, proposed by Andres and Düring (7), have been used to identify terminal receptors:

1. Afferent input to DRG or cranial nerve ganglia is present.
2. Receptor terminal exhibits clear and dense core vesicles and a fine filamentous ground substance (the receptor matrix) beneath the axonal membrane, in addition to the axoplasmic organelle described earlier for all axons.
3. Receptor terminal is devoid of a myelin sheath.

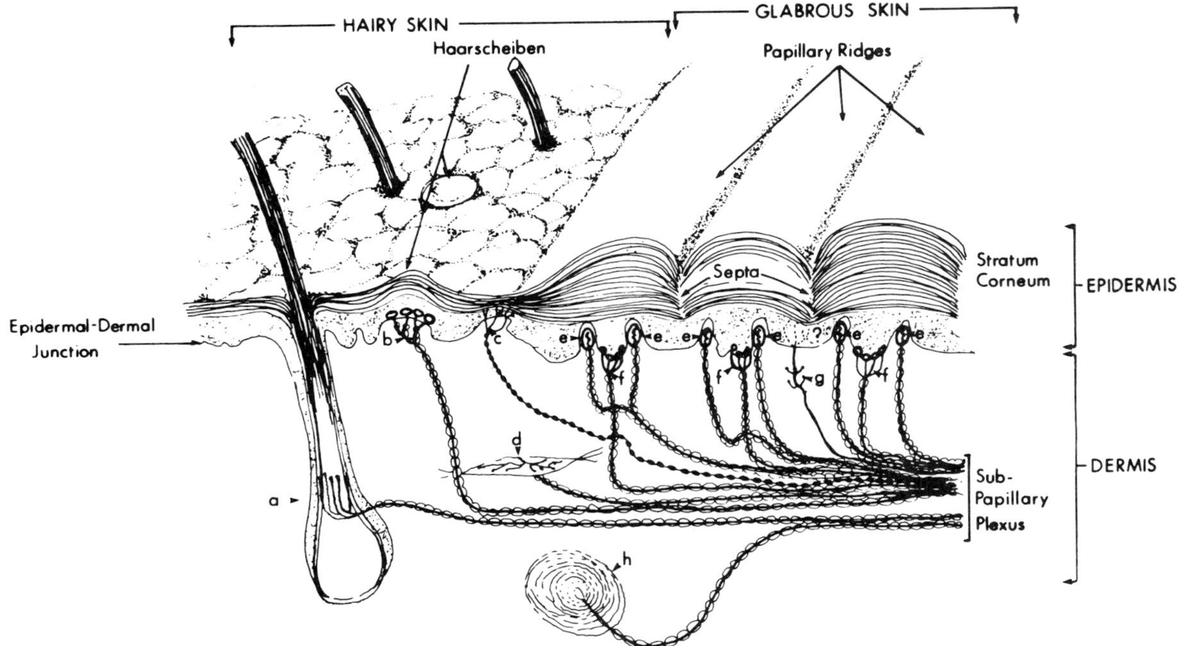

Figure 20. Schematic drawing showing the location of various receptors in hairy and glabrous skin of primate. **a:** Hair follicle with "palisade" endings (G1, G2 hair). **b:** Haarscheibe ("touch dome") neurite complex terminating on Merkel cells (type I). **c:** "Free" nerve ending (actually coated by Schwann cell) penetrating basal lamina and terminating among keratinocytes (myelinated nociceptor; cooling receptor?). **d:** Ruffini ending (type II; SA II). **e:** Meissner corpuscle found in dermal papillae (RA glabrous skin receptor; field receptor). **f:** Merkel cell-neurite complex found on intermediate ridge of dermal papillae (SA I). **g:** "Free nerve ending stemming from unmyelinated axon (C polymodal?; cooling?; warming?). **h:** Pacinian corpuscle (pacinian corpuscle receptor). (From ref. 149a, with permission.)

4. Specializations of the Schwann cell covering are present.
5. Topography and location of the receptor terminal are ubiquitous, restricted, or associated with hairs or glands.
6. Differentiation of associated perineurial and endoneurial sheaths is present.

With these criteria and limitations in mind, the terminal morphologic basis for each major category of sensory function, namely, low-threshold mechanoreception, thermoreception, and nociception, is summarized below.

Low-Threshold Mechanoreceptors

Several specialized terminal receptors have been associated with transduction of mechanical stimuli and these have been further subdivided into receptors signaling (a) tissue displacement, (b) velocity of displacement, and (c) vibration (Table 2). These receptors have in common an intimate contact with tissue-supporting structures such as epidermal cells or connective tissue compartments, fingerlike protrusions of the axon into surrounding tissues, and the lack of an intimate Schwann cell covering so that the axonal membrane interacts

Table 2. CHARACTERISTICS OF CUTANEOUS SENSORY UNITS

Category	Subcategory	Physiologic Name	Morphologic Receptor
Low-threshold mechanoreceptors	Signaling displacement	Type I	Haarscheibe "touch spot"
		SA I	Merkel cell neurite complex
		Type II and SA II	Ruffini ending
	Velocity of displacement	G_2 hair	Hair follicle "palisade ending"
		RA (Rapidly Adapting)	Meissner corpuscle
		Field receptor	?
		D hair	?
		C low-threshold mechanoreceptor	?
	Vibration	Pacinian corpuscle	Pacinian corpuscle
		G_1 hair	Hair follicle
Thermoreceptors	Cooling	Cold receptor	Unmyelinated neurite complex
	Warming	Warm receptor	?
Nociceptors	Myelinated	Myelinated nociceptor	Unmyelinated neurite-Schwann cell complex
	Unmyelinated	C-polymodal nociceptor	?

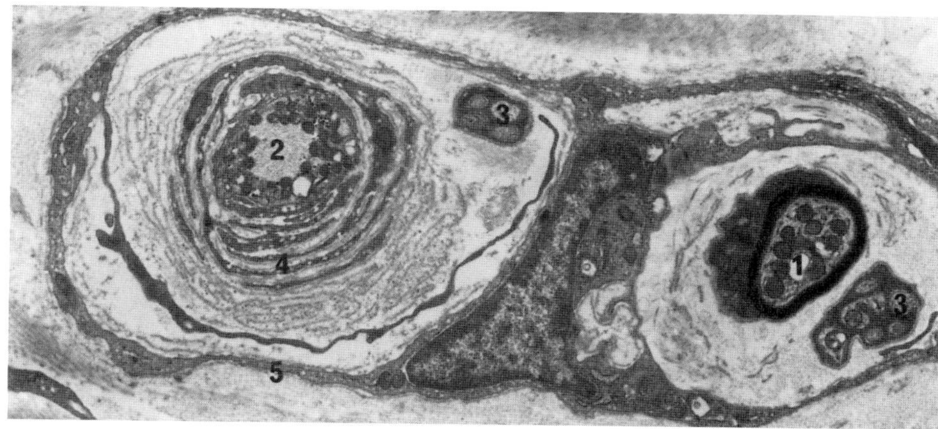

Figure 21. Small lamellated corpuscle in a nerve fascicle from the cone skin of the nose of the kowari in section perpendicular to the skin surface. 1, myelinated afferent axon; 2, nerve terminal of the lamellated corpuscle; 3, nonmyelinated axons in a nerve fascicle; 4, cytoplasmic lamellae of the terminal Schwann cell; 5, perineural capsule cells. Original magnification × 4000. (From ref. 95a, with permission.)

directly with the tissue in which it is embedded (Figs. 21 and 22). It is hypothesized that these characteristics permit mechanical stimuli to act directly on protein receptors in the axonal membrane, reversibly altering their configuration and transforming the mechanical stimulus into electrical depolarization (7).

The simplest mechanoreceptor for sensing displacement is the free stretch receptor. It is an unmyelinated terminal of a myelinated fiber in which the nodal segment can measure up to 50 μm in length. The length of the total receptor may extend to 300 μm and have several arborizations. These free nerve endings are found in the connective tissue of the papillary layer of the dermis and basal parts of the granular and adhesive ridges (42).

The Haarscheibe touch spot (215) is an epidermal dome 80 to 100 μm high and 100 to 300 μm in diameter at the base of which is a concentration of up to 50 Merkel cells. The Merkel cell receptor (115) is differentiated from stratified squamous epithelial cells (65) and is characterized by finger-like cell processes invading local epithelial cells. Dense core vesicles and afferent nerve terminals from large myelinated fibers form a disk below the cell. While the biologic function of the Merkel

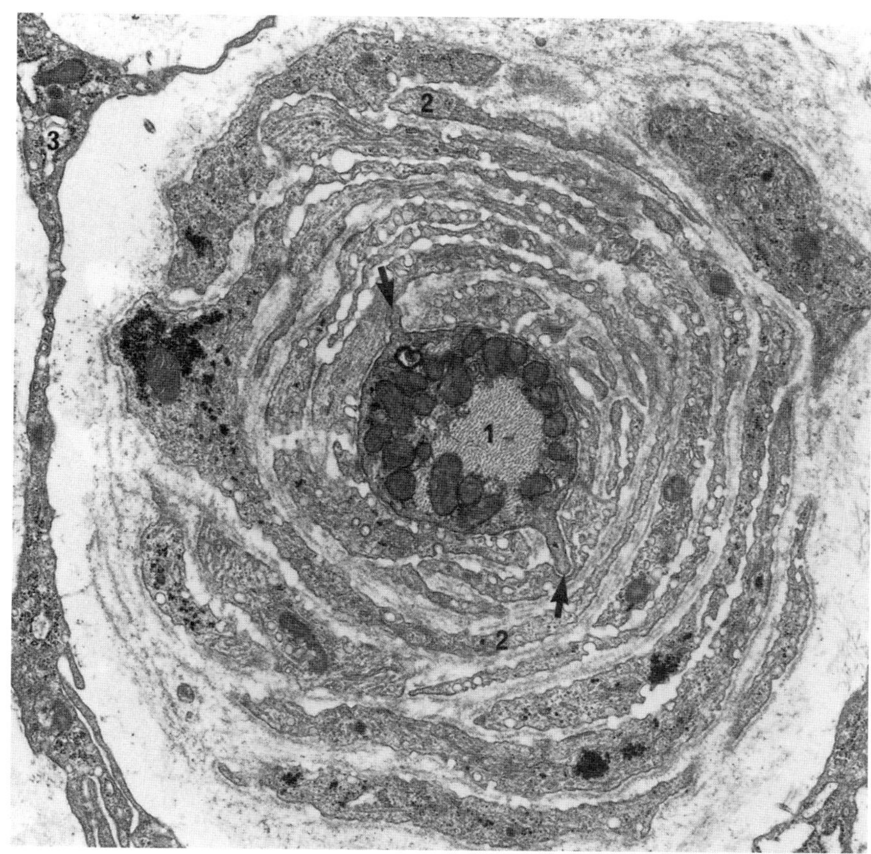

Figure 22. Small lamellated corpuscle from the cone skin of the nose of the kowair in section perpendicular to the skin surface. 1, nerve terminal with accumulations of mitochondria *(arrows)*, fingerlike protrusions of the nerve terminal (spikes); 2, cytoplasmic lamellae of the terminal Schwann cell; 3, fibroblast from the subcapsular space. Original magnification × 20,000. (From ref. 95a, with permission.)

cell remains obscure, the presence of synaptic contacts with afferent nerve terminals and multiple messenger candidates have led some investigators to conclude that these cells modulate or mediate local free stretch receptors (7,99).

The Ruffini ending is an encapsulated structure in the dermis having the same axonal structural organization as free stretch receptors (44,235). The receptor complex is in a fluid-filled space approximately 0.5 to 2 mm by 40 to 150 μm in size that is encapsulated by three to five perineurial cell layers except at the pole where collagen bundles enter the spindle. The unbundled collagen fibers anchor nerve terminals within the capsule, consistent with the view that the Ruffini ending is a stretch receptor.

The Meissner and the Krause corpuscles represent another class of mechanoreceptors in that they are integrated with differentiated Schwann cells (Figs. 23 and 24). These corpuscles consist of one to five unmyelinated receptor axons (from myelinated fibers) that are coiled in combination with loose cytoplasmic lamellae of Schwann cells. Collagen fibrils run in the fissures of Schwann cell lamellae. The axons assume the shape of oval disks and lie parallel to the surface of the epidermis. A perineurial capsule sometimes envelopes the corpuscle.

Pacinian corpuscles are located deep in the dermis and consist of a myelinated afferent axon, an inner core and a perineurial capsule (210). The terminal axon is unmyelinated and slightly thickened. The inner cone consists of 20 to 60 cytoplasmic lamellae of Schwann cells. Pacinian corpuscles can occasionally be found in the perineurial sheath (Fig. 25).

The Tastscheibe of the hairy skin, also known as the Pinkus corpuscle (215), is composed of an epithelial rise near groups of hair follicles in which there are Merkel cells and terminal axonal thickenings (268). These hairs are often longer and thicker than normal and may transmit mechanical stimuli to the Tastscheibe.

Thermoreceptors

While there is some uncertainty in the morphologic identification of thermal receptors, the following criteria are useful in distinguishing temperature receptors from mechanoreceptors:

1. The exposed nerve terminals are close to the skin surface.
2. There is an absence of mechanical structures linking the axon to the tissue matrix.

It is thought that warm receptors in mammals are unmyelinated C fibers terminating in the subcutaneous layer (321). Infrared receptors in snakes are better characterized and give rise to myelinated axons from the scales or groves in the head (59). The cold receptor is a group of several free nerve terminals in the basal layer of the epidermis supplied by a myelinated nerve fiber (103). The receptors lack desmosomes and are not attached to epidermal membranes.

Nociceptors

By definition, nociceptors are sensory endings that respond to tissue-damaging stimuli. They include several morphologic types including mechanical receptors with A-δ electrophysiologic characteristics and C-polymodal receptors responding, as the name implies, to several categories of stimuli including mechanical, thermal, and chemical. The morphology of A-δ mechanical nociceptors includes Schwann cell-ensheathed terminals invading the epidermis (135). The unmyelinated extensions of myelinated axons in the papillary layer are accompanied by thin Schwann cell processes to the epidermal basal lamina. At the site of epidermal penetration, the axons contain both clear and large, dense-core vesicles. Kruger et al. (135) suggest that these complexes are the sense organs initiating prickling pain.

C-polymodal nociceptors are more difficult to identify morphologically, since it is almost impossible to distinguish efferent from afferent unmyelinated fibers on structural criteria. As in most studies of peripheral sensory receptor morphology, it is necessary to use special electrophysiologic techniques to help locate and identify these receptors (166). With selected tissue sampling of receptive sites, the afferent C fibers have been described as fibers that exhibit a filamentous receptor matrix and one or two mitochondria per cross section and, at selected sites, an axonal membrane that lacks a Schwann cell covering and, occasionally, a basal lamina. These fibers are distributed in the epidermis and in the connective tissue of the papillary and reticular layer of the dermis.

Visualization of unmyelinated nerve fibers is done best with electron microscopy techniques, but these techniques require specialized tissue processing and are necessarily limited to small tissue samples, which makes surveys of cutaneous fiber density difficult to perform. A detailed immunohistologic study of sensory and autonomic innervation (24) using antisera against neurofilaments, neuron-specific enolase, myelin basic protein, protein S-100, substance P, neurokinin A, neuropeptide Y, tyrosine hydroxylase, and vasoactive intestinal peptide, when analyzed in total, has helped classify receptors and their afferent fibers, but has also demonstrated that no known single marker can uniquely identify the sensory unit. A new technique

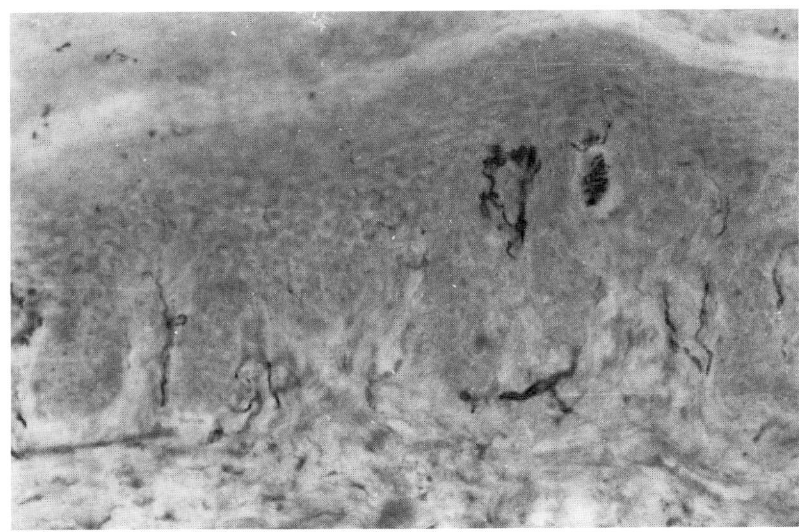

Figure 23. Numerous immunoreactive structures are present in the epidermis and dermis using the anti–protein gene product (PGP) 9.5 method of staining. In particular, three corpuscles are clearly evident in the dermal papillae. Original magnification ×300. (From ref. 225, with permission.)

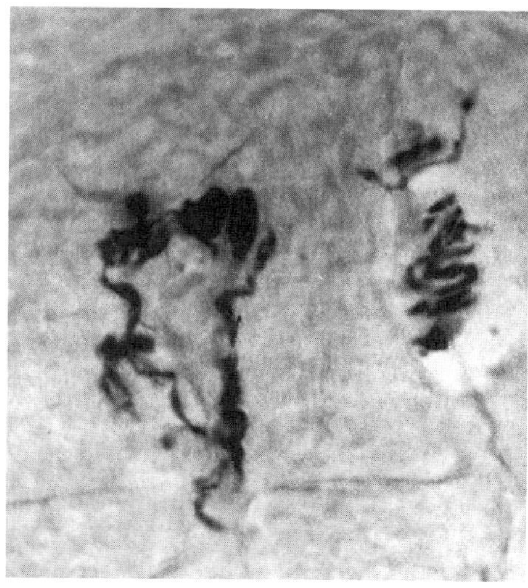

Figure 24. A higher magnification of Fig. 23 shows the details of a Meissner's corpuscle and of two couples simple coiled corpuscles. Anti-PGP. Original magnification × 1000. (From ref. 225, with permission.)

using polyclonal immunocytochemistry of protein gene product 9.5 (PGP 9.5) on tissue embedded in paraffin extends this survey and is a promising technique for assessing unmyelinated fiber density (225,311). PGP 9.5 stains neurons and nerve fibers at all levels of the central and peripheral nervous system. In properly prepared tissue, the reaction product extends beyond the axoplasm and it is this feature that makes unmyelinated fibers visible at the level of the light microscope. Myelinated fibers can be easily distinguished from unmyelinated fibers. In the cutaneous nerves of laboratory animals and human diabetics, the technique has been useful in correlating innervation density with neuropeptide activity (52,146).

What role might cutaneous sensory receptors have in nerve injuries producing neuropathic pain with hyperalgesia and mechanical allodynia? While there are no morphologic data suggesting altered structure of the receptor as a cause of hypersensitivity to sensory stimuli, Na et al. (181) hypothesize that sympathetically driven dysfunction of cutaneous mechanoreceptors is responsible for signaling mechanical allodynia. They report an abnormality in rapidly adapting mechanoreceptors producing low and irregular static discharges during a maintained mechanical stimulus. While these receptors may have modified functional sensitivity, it is possible that they may be newly formed mechanoreceptors resulting from collateral sprouting of intact afferent nerve fibers into skin territories denervated by the previous nerve injury. Continued studies with morphologic end points will be useful in exploring this possibility further and in supplementing our knowledge of the relationship between sensory terminal structure and function.

THE PRIVILEGED ENVIRONMENT OF NERVE FIBERS

The peripheral nervous system functions in a protected environment maintained by specialized endothelial and perineurial cells that limit the permeability of macromolecules from vascular and systemic interstitial spaces. Since the endoneurial environment of the peripheral nervous system lacks lymphatic channels, the free macromolecule concentration in nerve directly influences tissue hydration, which, in turn, is reflected in the magnitude of the tissue fluid pressure in nerve fascicles. This endoneurial fluid pressure (EFP) is normally slightly positive but can increase during nerve injuries and disease to levels that compromise tissue blood flow (176,177). The clinical importance of increased EFP is analogous to the compartment syndromes recognized in other tissues. While it has been well known from clinical experience that transient ischemia of nerves can cause analgesia and then pain on reperfusion, the mechanisms of these relationships have not been understood completely. Advances in the methods used in experimental neuropathology have led to new insights into the role of endoneurial fluid pressure and ischemia in the pathogenesis of nerve injury and neuropathic pain. In the following sections we consider the importance of connective tissues, especially the perineurium, in creating a privileged endoneurial environment for normal functioning of nerve fibers and the structural and physiologic characteristics of the nerve circulation that regulate nerve hydration and the chemistry of the nerve fiber environment.

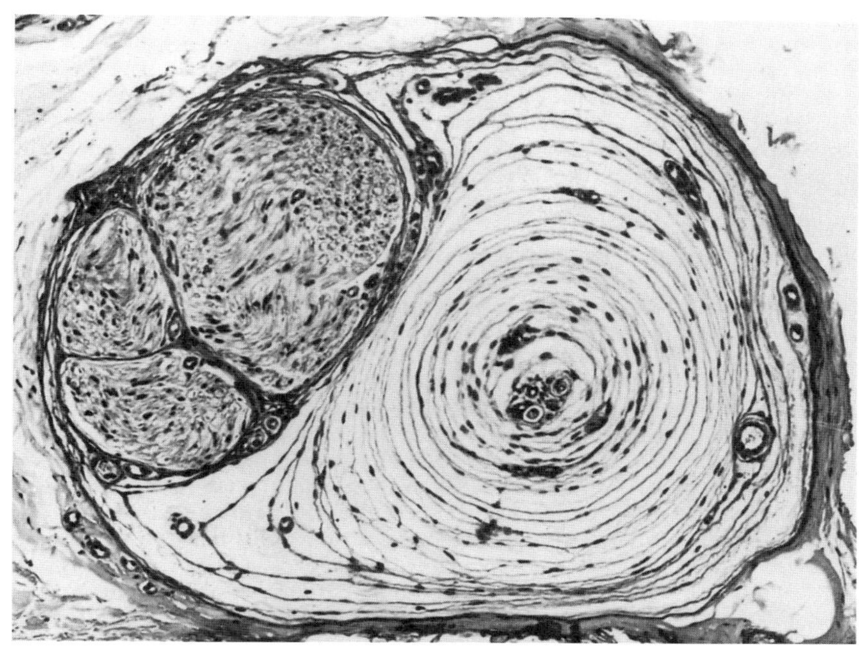

Figure 25. Transverse section through pacinian corpuscle within the perineurium of a fascicle in human sural nerve. Periodic acid-Schiff stain. Original magnification × 140. (From ref. 275, with permission.)

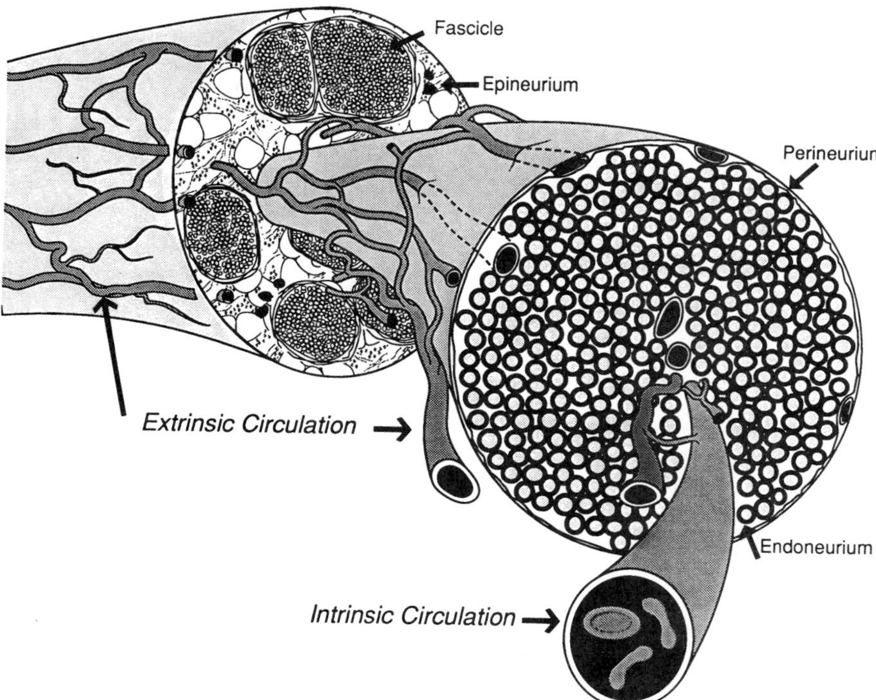

Figure 26. Schematic illustration of the circulation in peripheral nerve and the connective tissue sheaths that contribute to regulation of the specialized environment of nerve fibers. The relationship between the extrinsic epineurial vessels and the intrinsic endoneurial vessels is emphasized. Numerous branching vessels form a rich anastomotic network on the surface of the fascicles. These vessels are connected to the intrinsic vasculature by transperineurial vessels that are vulnerable to compressive forces acting from within or on the external surface of the nerve sheath.

Connective Tissue

The three connective tissues in peripheral nerve—the epineurium, perineurium, and endoneurium—are anatomically separate and contribute differently to the function and biomechanics of the nerve (Fig. 26). The connective tissues of the nerve have an important mechanical function in providing tensile strength to the nerve bundle. Nerves can be stretched approximately 10% before structural injury, but ultimately stretching is inhibited by collagen, which contributes significantly to the tensile strength of the nerve along its longitudinal axis. Histologic and biomechanical studies show that the major tensile strength of whole nerve resides in the perineurium, which ruptures catastrophically when loading forces are steadily increased (95,238,319). Each connective tissue is described separately in the following text.

The epineurium is a loose collection of areolar connective tissue with longitudinally oriented collagen fibrils approximately 80 nm in diameter that surrounds single fascicles and multifascicular nerve bundles. Collagen is relatively sparse, and there is a great amount of potential space for movement and stretching of the nerve. Elastic fibers are seen in the epineurium adjacent to the perineurium (277). At the proximal end of peripheral nerves, the epineurium is in continuity with the dura mater and is separated from the perineurium at the subarachnoid angle (97), which represents an anatomic barrier through which molecules in CSF space may pass (237).

The epineurium contains important cellular, vascular, and lymphatic components that affect the response to injury. Epineurial fat cells help cushion the nerve from compression injury, and their reduced numbers in diabetics may be a reason for an increased incidence of compression injuries in these individuals. Fibroblasts are present in the epineurium and proliferate following injury, with resulting fibrosis limiting mobility of the nerve and predisposing it to stretch and compression injuries.

The perineurium is the connective tissue sheath that defines a fascicle by surrounding groups of nerve fibers and consists of a laminated arrangement of flattened polygonal cells as many as 15 layers thick bounded by a basal lamina that is thickened in diabetes and aging (121) (Fig. 27). Perineurial cells are thought to be specialized fibroblasts, as suggested by the proliferation of fibroblasts adjacent to injured perineurium and by morphologic analysis of regenerating nerves in which fibroblasts initially encircle groups of sprouting nerves to form what is known as minifascicles (Fig. 18). Four weeks after loose ligature compression injury to peripheral nerve in which the perineurium and nerve fibers have been damaged, axonal sprouts can be seen growing outside the perineurium, even across the ligatures, and organizing in minifascicles. These are well developed in the segments of tissue under the ligatures and have reached the distal segments by 6 to 12 weeks. These minifascicles lack a conduit for reconnection to the original target tissue and may eventually form neuromas (260).

As in the epineurium, collagen is oriented longitudinally in the perineurium and is seen in bundles between the layers of perineurial cells. Collagen fibril diameter is less than in the epineurium, averaging approximately 65 nm. Because of closely aggregated filaments similar in appearance to the myofilaments of smooth muscle, it has been suggested that the perineurium has contractile elements (233), although this has not yet been substantiated with rigorous biomechanical tests. The perineurium is under tension longitudinally, as demonstrated by the shortening of nerve segments following transection.

There are some differences in the structure of the perineurial layers. The outer lamellae have a high density of endocytotic vesicles that diminishes toward the inner lamellae. Glucose transporters have been reported to exist within the perineurium (81); previously they were thought to occur only in the endothelial cells of endoneurial microvessels. The inner few lamellae have tight junctions between contiguous cells in which the extracellular space is obliterated. This normally blocks the intercellular transport of macromolecules, but an increase in intercellular perineurial permeability occurs following topical application of local anesthetics (174).

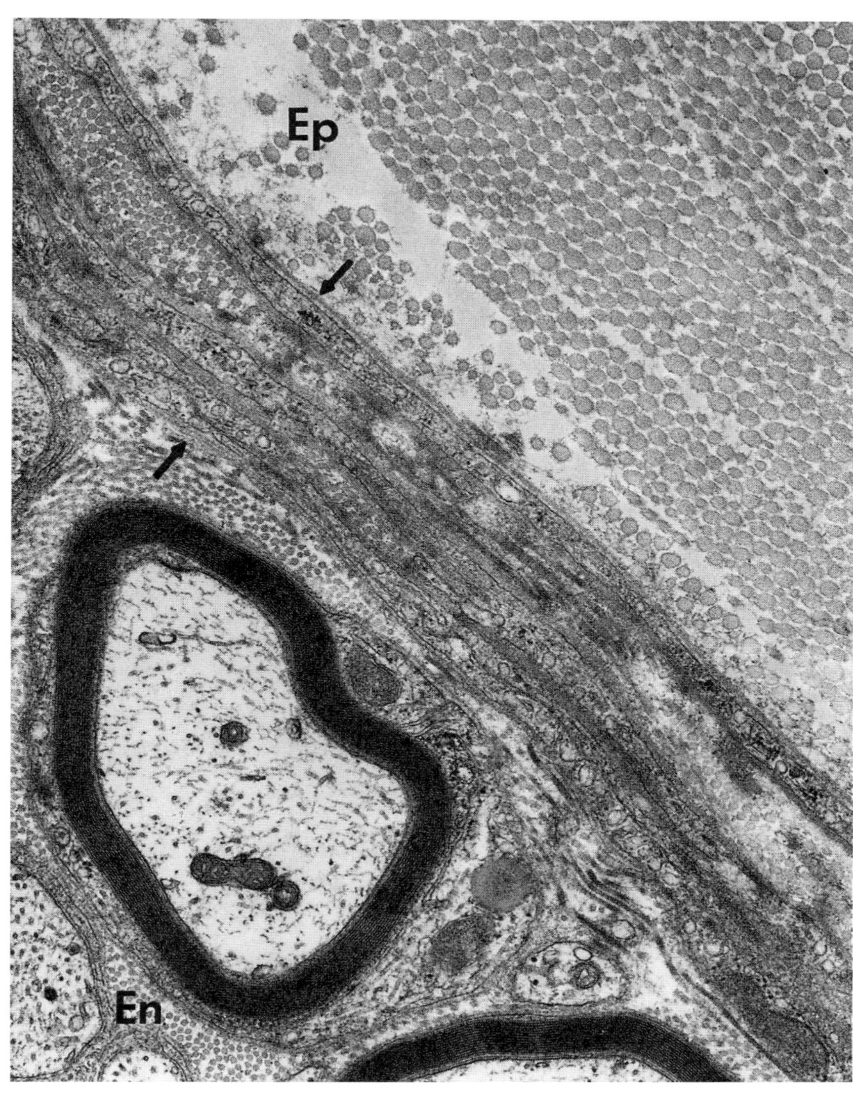

Figure 27. Electron micrograph of the perineurium (between *arrows*) also showing the epineurial (Ep) and endoneurial (En) connective tissues of peripheral nerve. Note the basal lamina immediately beneath the arrows on the inner and outer boundaries of the perineurium and the difference in diameter of collagen fibers in these three connective tissues. Normal myelinated and unmyelinated fibers are also visible in this transverse section from normal rat sciatic nerve.

This component of the blood-nerve barrier can also be opened with osmotic manipulation of the local fluid environments, which can shrink the volume of perineurial cells and break their tight junctions.

These morphologic features suggest that the perineurium is functionally a semielastic and semipermeable membrane that has a major role in regulating the endoneurial environment. The perineurium is a compliant membrane that stretches circumferentially in response to endoneurial edema or other mass-occupying lesions contained by it (151,178). The perineurium is normally under tension circumferentially because it contains an interstitial environment with a slightly positive fluid pressure, unlike most tissue fluid spaces that have a zero or slightly negative interstitial fluid pressure. When the integrity of the perineurium is breached, nerve fibers herniate through the defect as a consequence of the positive endoneurial fluid pressure, causing demyelination secondary to local nerve fiber ischemia (187).

Lastly, the endoneurium consists of intrafascicular connective tissue appearing as a matrix of collagen fibrils throughout the interstitial spaces as well as partitions of dense connective tissue that develop between diverging fascicles that eventually become perineurium when the fascicles separate. The collagen fibrils are smaller in diameter than in the other nerve connective tissues, longitudinally oriented, and grouped around nerve fibers and capillaries. The interstitial matrix is deficient in the immediate subperineurial space, which explains why edema accumulates preferentially in this region. As has been implied in the preceding text, the terms *endoneurium* and *endoneurial* are taken also to mean the fascicular contents bounded by the perineurium. Thus, endoneurial fluid pressure is the same as interstitial fluid pressure within the fascicle. Since the endoneurium lacks lymphatic channels, the presence of endoneurial osmolytes, including albumin and other proteins leaked from vessels in the dorsal root ganglia (216) and transported distally by convection, controls tissue hydration and endoneurial fluid pressure. There is a proximodistal gradient in endoneurial fluid pressure from the dorsal root ganglia to the distal terminations of the perineurium at the neuromuscular junctions where the perineurium is loosely attached (179). This provides the driving force for the turnover of endoneurial fluid that is transported along the pressure gradient.

Nerve Vasculature and Blood Flow

There are several components to the vasculature of peripheral nerve that differ in structure and physiologic function. The extrinsic circulation within the epineurium consists of a longitudinal plexus of arterioles and venules supplied by regional arteries from the systemic circulation (Fig. 26). Blood flow in these microvessels is affected by adrenergic

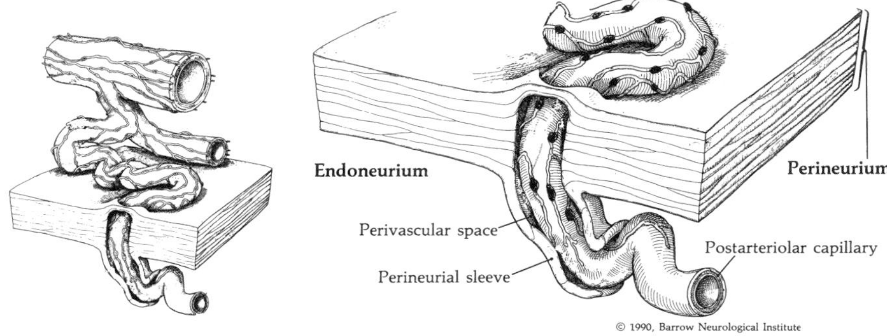

Figure 28. Some transperineurial arterioles pass directly through the perineurium; others take a tangential route. Vessels entering the endoneurium retain a perineurial sleeve for variable distances. The innervating unmyelinated nerve fibers usually diminish in density as the arteriole gains access to the perineurium. Darkened areas represent axonal varicosities. (From ref. 17, with permission.)

stimulation (153), topical application of epinephrine and local anesthetics (173,254), and, to a minor degree, by arterial CO_2 tension (228). These vessels anastomose with the endoneurial capillary circulation by traversing the perineurium (17) where they are susceptible to focal compression in edematous neuropathies with increased endoneurial fluid pressure (176) (Fig. 28). Both the transperineurial and epineurial vessels are innervated by plexuses of unmyelinated axons, but this autonomic innervation is lost as the transperineurial vessels anastomose with the intrinsic circulation of the endoneurium. Beggs et al. (17) have shown abnormal innervation of the vasa nervorum in human diabetics and suggest that the loss of arteriolar control may lead to or aggravate endoneurial ischemia or hypoxia in diabetic patients with neuropathy.

The intrinsic circulation within the endoneurium is formed mainly by large capillaries with tight endothelial junctions. This represents the second structural component of the blood-nerve barrier. There are also larger vessels within the endoneurium, especially in the central core of fascicles, and these also have tight endothelial junctions (Figs. 29 and 30). Blood flow in the intrinsic circulation is not autoregulated and responds passively to changes in systemic pressure (152).

As suggested previously, several lines of experiments using pharmacologic, mechanical, or surgical manipulations to selectively interfere with specific components of the vasculature indicate that a functional epineurial circulation is necessary for the survival of endoneurial nerve fibers in the subperineurial space. Devascularization of the epineurium over a 2-cm length in the rat sciatic-tibial nerve produces edema, subperineurial demyelination, and to a lesser extent, axonal degeneration. This procedure is associated with a 58% reduction in local nerve-blood flow and a corresponding 38% reduction in subperineurial oxygen tension, indicating that ischemia is the pathogenic mechanism of demyelination. A consensus of findings in these studies support the concept that mild levels of ischemia cause endoneurial edema, while moderate levels of ischemia produce demyelination and severe ischemia produces wallerian degeneration, initiating the cascade of immunologic events that contributes to the pathogenesis of neuropathic pain.

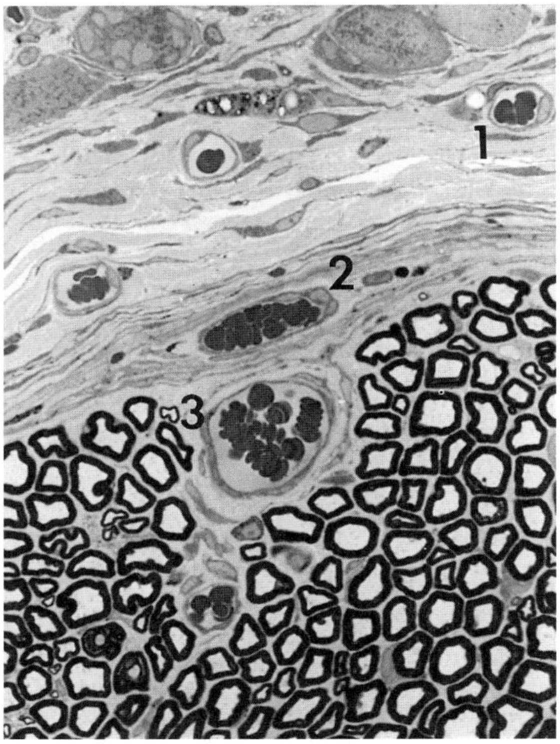

Figure 29. Transverse section of rat sciatic nerve showing epineurial (1), perineurial (2), and endoneurial vessels (3).

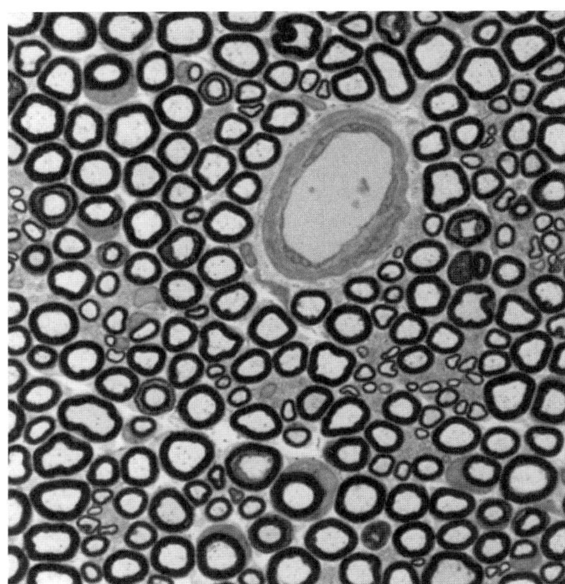

Figure 30. Transverse section of rat sciatic nerve showing normal central arteriole.

ACKNOWLEDGMENT

Henry Powell, M.D., Chief of Anatomic and Neuropathology at University of California–San Diego, and Claudia Sommer, M.D., neurologist at the Neurologische Klinik, Aachen, Germany, collaborated in the experimental studies and kindly contributed electron micrographs.

REFERENCES

1. Adams DO, Hamilton TA. Phagocytic cells: cytotoxic activities of macrophages. In: Gallin JI, Goldstein M, Snyderman R, eds. *Inflammation: basic principles and clinical correlates.* New York: Raven Press, 1988;471–492.
2. Adams DO, Hamilton TA. The cell biology of macrophage activation. *Annu Rev Immunol* 1984;2:283–311.
3. Adams RJ. Organelle movement in axons depends on ATP. *Nature* 1982;297:327–329.
4. Adler R, Landa K, Manthorpe M, Varon S. Cholinergic neuronotropic factors—intraocular distribution of trophic activity for ciliary neurons. *Science* 1979; 204:1434–1436.
5. Aletta JM, Goldberg J. Routing of transmitter and other changes in fast axonal transport after transection of one branch of the bifurcate axon on an identified neuron. *J Neurosci* 1984;4:1800–1808.
6. Andersson PB, Perry VH, Gordon S. Intracerebral injection of proinflammatory cytokines or leukocyte chemotaxins induces minimal myelomonocytic cell recruitment to the parenchmya of the central nervous system. *J Exp Med* 1992;176:255–259.
7. Andres KH, Düring MV. Comparative and functional aspects of the histological organization of cutaneous receptors in vertebrates. In: Zenker W, Neuhuber WL, eds. *The primary afferent neuron.* New York: Plenum Press, 1990.
8. Andrews SB, Gallant PE, Leapman RD, Schnapp BJ, Reese TS. Single kinesin molecules crossbridge microtubules in vitro. *Proc Natl Acad Sci USA* 1993;90:6503–6507.
9. Ansel JC, Brown JR, Payan DG, Brown MA. Substance P selectively activates TNF-α gene expression in murine mast cells. *J Immunol* 1993;150:4478–4485.
10. Ariyasu RG, Nichol JA, Ellisman MH. Localization of sodium/potassium adenosine triphosphatase in multiple cell types of the murine nervous system with antibodies raised against the enzyme from kidney. *J Neurosci* 1985;5:2581–2596.
11. Arvidson B. Cellular uptake of exogenous horseradish peroxidase in mouse peripheral nerve. *Acta Neuropathol* 1977;37:35–41.
12. Asbury AK, Johnson PC. *Pathology of peripheral nerve.* Philadelphia: WB Saunders, 1978;246–249.
13. Bagnasco SM, Murphy HR, Bedford JJ, Burg MB. Osmoregulation by slow changes in aldose reductase and rapid changes in sorbitor flux. *Am J Physiol* 1988;254:C788–792.
14. Bamburg JR, Bray D, Chapman K. Assembly of microtubules at the tip of growing axons. *Nature* 1986;321:788–790.
15. Barde Y-A, Edgar D, Thoenen H. Purification of a new neurotrophic factor from mammalian brain. *EMBO J* 1982;1: 549–553.
16. Bedford JJ, Bagnasco SM, Kador PF, Harris HW, Burg MB. Characterization and purification of a mammalian osmoregulatory protein, aldose reductase, induced in renal medullary cells by high extracellular NaCl. *J Biol Chem* 1987;262:14255–14259.
17. Beggs J, Johnson PC, Olafsen A, Watkins CJ. Innervation of the vasa nervorum: changes in human diabetics. *J Neuropathol Exp Neurol* 1992;51:612–629.
18. Behse F. Morphometric studies on the human sural nerve. *Acta Neurol Scand (Suppl)* 1990;132:1–38.
19. Bennett GJ, Xie YK. A peripheral mononeuropathy in the rat that produces disorders of pain sensation like those seen in man. *Pain* 1988;33:87–107.
20. Berg BO, Rosenberg S, Asbury AK. Giant axonal neuropathy. *Pediatrics* 1972;49:894–899.
21. Beuche W, Friede RL. The role of non-resident cells in wallerian degeneration. *J Neurocytol* 1984;13:767–796.
22. Bienenstock J, Blennerhassett M, Tomioka M, Marshall J, Perdue MH, Stead RH. Evidence of mast cell-nerve interactions. In: Goetzl EJ, Spector NH, eds. *Neuroimmune networks:* physiology and diseases. New York: Alan R. Liss, 1989;149.
23. Bigbee JW, Yoshino JE, DeVries GH. Morphological and proliferative responses of cultured Schwann cells following rapid phagocytosis of a myelin-enriched fraction. *J Neurocytol* 1987;16: 487–496.
24. Björklund H, Dalsgaard C-J, Jonsson C-E, Hermansson A. Sensory and autonomic innervation of non-hairy and hairy human skin. An immunohistochemical study. *Cell Tissue Res* 1986;243:51–57.
25. Black JA, Kocsis JD, Waxman SG. Ion channel organization of the myelinated fiber. *Trends Neurosci* 1990;13:48–54.
26. Bolande RP. The neurocristopathies. A unifying concept of disease arising in neural crest maldevelopment. *Hum Pathol* 1974;5: 409–429.
27. Bostock H. Impulse propagation in experimental neuropathy. In: Dyck PJ, Thomas PK, Griffin JW, Low PA, Poduslo JF, eds. *Peripheral neuropathy.* Philadelphia: WB Saunders, 1993;109–120.
28. Brattgård S-O, Edström J-E, Hydn H. The chemical changes in regenerating neurons. *J Neurochem* 1957;1:316–325.
29. Bray GM, Rasminsky M, Aguayo AJ. Interactions between axons and their sheath cells. *Annu Rev Neurosci* 1981;4:127–162.
30. Bridgman P. Structure of cytoplasm as revealed by modern electron microscopy techniques. *Trends Neurosci* 1987;10:321–329.
31. Brimijoin S, Dyck PJ. Axonal transport of dopamine-β-hydroxylase and acetylcholinesterase in normal and abnormal human sural nerves. *Exp Neurol* 1979;66:467–478.
32. Brown MC, Perry VH, Lunn ER, Gordon S, Heumann R. Macrophage dependence of peripheral sensory nerve regeneration: possible involvement of nerve growth factor. *Neuron* 1991;6: 359–370.
33. Bunge MB. Initial endocytosis of peroxidase or ferritin by growth cones of cultured nerve cells. *J Neurocytol* 1977;6:407–439.
34. Bunge MB. Schwann cell regulation of extracellular matrix biosynthesis and assembly. In: Dyck PJ, Thomas PK, Griffin JW, Low PA, Poduslo JF, eds. *Peripheral neuropathy.* Philadelphia: WB Saunders, 1993;299–316.
35. Bunge MB, Bunge RP, Peterson ER, Murray MR. A light and electron microscope study of long-term organized cultures of rat dorsal root ganglia. *J Cell Biol* 1967;32:439–466.
36. Bunge MB, Wood PM. Basal lamina deposition on Schwann cells cultured with fibroblasts in the absence of neurons. *Soc Neurosci Abstr* 1989;15:689.
37. Bunge R, Moya F, Bunge M. Observations on the role of Schwann cell secretion in Schwann cell-axon interactions. In: Martin JB, Reichlin S, Bick KL, eds. *Neurosecretion and brain peptides.* New York: Raven Press, 1981;229–242.
38. Burg MB. Role of aldose reductase and sorbitol in maintaining the medullary intracellular milieu. *Kidney Int* 1988;33:635–641.
39. Burnstock G, Hoyle CHV. *Autonomic neuroeffector mechanisms.* Philadelphia: Harwood Academic, 1992.
40. Calcutt NA, Muir D, Powell HC, Mizisin AP. Reduced ciliary neuronotrophic factor-like activity in nerves from diabetic or galactose-fed rats. *Brain Res* 1992;575:320–324.
41. Cammermeyer J. Peripheral chromatolysis after transection of mouse facial nerve. *Acta Neuropathol (Berl)* 1963;2:213–230.
42. Cauna N. Fine morphological characteristics and microtopography of the free nerve endings of the human digital skin. *Anat Rec* 1980;198:643–656.
43. Celio MR. The Schmidt-Lantermann incisures of the myelin sheath of Mauthner axons: places of longitudinal growth of myelin? *Brain Res* 1976;108:221–235.
44. Chambers MR, Andres KH, Von Duering M, Iggo A. The structure and function of the slowly adapting type II mechanoreceptor in hairy skin. *Q J Exp Physiol* 1972;57:417–445.
45. Clark MB, Bunge MB. Cultured Schwann cells assemble normal-appearing basal lamina only when they ensheath axons. *Dev Biol* 1989;133:393–404.
46. Cooper PD, Smith RS. The movement of optically detectable organelles in myelinated axons of *Xenopus laevis. J Physiol (Lond)* 1974;242:77–97.
47. Cragg BG. What is the signal for chromatolysis? *Brain Res* 1970; 23:1–21.
48. Crispino M, Capano CP, Kaplan BB, Giuditta A. Neurofilament proteins are synthesized in nerve endings from squid brain. *J Neurochem* 1993;61:1144–1146.
49. Benech J, Crispino M, Chan JT, Kaplan BB, Giuditta A. Protein synthesis in nerve endings from squid brain: modulation by calcium ions. *Biol Bull* 1994;187:269.
50. Curtis R, Adryan KM, Zhu Y, Harkness PJ, Lindsay RM, Distefano PS. Retrograde axonal transport of ciliary neurotrophic factor is increased by peripheral nerve injury. *Nature* 1993;365:253–255.

51. Dahlström A. Axoplasmic transport (with particular respect to adrenergic neurons). *Philos Trans R Soc Lond (Biol)* 1971;261: 325–358.
52. Daranth SS, Springall DR, Kuhn DM, Levene MM, Polar JM. An immunocytochemical study of cutaneous innervation and the distribution of neuropeptides and protein gene product 9.5 in man and commonly employed laboratory animals. *Am J Anat* 1991;19: 369–383.
53. Davies AM. The development of primary sensory neurons. In: Zenker W, Neuhuber WL, eds. *The primary afferent neuron.* New York: Plenum Press, 1990;109–117.
54. Davies AM, Lumsden A. Ontogeny of the somatosensory system: origins and early development of primary sensory neurons. *Annu Rev Neurosci* 1990;13:61–73.
55. Devor M, Claman D. Mapping and plasticity of acid phosphatase afferents in the rat dorsal horn. *Brain Res* 1980;190:17–28.
56. Droz B, Giamberardino L, Koenig HL. Contribution of axonal transport to the renewal of myelin phospholipids in peripheral nerves. I. Quantitative radioautographic study. *Brain Res* 1981; 219:57–71.
57. Duce IR, Keen P. An ultrastructural classification of the neuronal cell bodies of rat dorsal root ganglion using zinc iodine-osmium impregnation. *Cell Tissue Res* 1977;185:263–277.
58. Duce IR, Keen P. Can neuronal smooth endoplasmic reticulum function as a calcium reservoir? *Neuroscience* 1978;3:837–848.
59. Düring VM, Miller MR. Sensory nerve endings of the skin and deeper structures. In: Gans C, ed. *Biology of the reptilia,* vol 9, Neurology A. New York: Academic Press, 1978.
60. Dyck PJ, Giannini C, Lais A. Pathologic alterations of nerves. In: Dyck PJ, Thomas PK, Griffin JW, Low PA, Poduslo JF, eds. *Peripheral neuropathy.* Philadelphia: WB Saunders, 1993;514–595.
61. Eldridge CF, Bunge MB, Bunge RP. Differentiation of axon-related Schwann cells in vitro: II. Control of myelin formation by basal lamina. *J Neurosci* 1989;9:625–638.
62. Elfvin L-G. *Autonomic ganglia.* New York: John Wiley, 1983.
63. Ellisman MH, Porter KR. Microtrabecular structure of the axoplasmic matrix: visualization of cross-linked structures and their distribution. *J Cell Biol* 1980;87:464– 479.
64. Enerback L, Olsson Y, Sourander P. Mast cells in normal and sectioned peripheral nerve. *Z Zellerforsch Mikrosk Anat* 1965;66: 596–608.
65. English KB, Burgess PR, Norman DK. Development of rat Merkel cells. *J Comp Neurol* 1980;194:475–496.
66. Esiri MM, Reading MC. Macrophages, lymphocytes and major histocompatibility complex (HLA) class II antigens in adult human sensory and sympathetic ganglia. *J Neuroimmunol* 1989;23: 187–193.
67. Fink BR. Mechanism of differential epidural block. *Anesth Analg* 1986;65:325–329.
68. Forman DS, Brown KJ, Promersberger ME. Selective inhibition of retrograde axonal transport by erythro-9 [3–(2–hydroxy-nonyl)] adenine. *Brain Res* 1983;272:194–197.
69. Forman DS, Lunch KJ, Smith RS. Organelle dynamics in lobster axons: anterograde, retrograde and stationary mitochondria. *Brain Res* 1987;412:96–106.
70. Forman DS, Padjen AL, Siggins GR. Axonal transport of organelles visualized by light microscopy: cinemicrographic and computer analysis. *Brain Res* 1977;136:197–213.
71. von Frey M. Beiträge zur Physiologie des Schmerzsinns. *Konigl Sachs Ges Wiss Math-Phys Kl* 1894;46:185–196.
72. von Frey M. Untersuchungen über die Sinnesfunctionen der Menschlichen Haut. I. Druckempfindung und Schmerz. *Konigl Sachs Ges Wiss Math-Phys Kl* 1896;23:175– 264.
73. Friede RL, Samorajski T. The clefts of Schmidt-Lantermann: a quantitative electron microscopic study of their structure in developing and adult sciatic nerves of the rat. *Anat Rec* 1969;165: 89–101.
74. Friede RL, Samorajski T. Myelin formation in sciatic nerve of the rat. A quantitative electron microscopic, histochemical and radioautographic study. *J Neuropathol Exp Neurol* 1968;27:546–570.
75. Gabella G. Ganglia of the autonomic nervous system. In: Landon DN, ed. *The peripheral nerve.* New York: John Wiley, 1976;355–395.
76. Galbraith JA, Myers RR. Impulse conduction. In: Gelberman RH, ed. *Operative nerve repair and reconstruction.* New York: JB Lippincott, 1991;19–45.
77. Galli SJ, Gordon JR, Wershil BK. Mast cell cytokines in allergy and inflammation. *Agents Actions Suppl* 1993;43:209–220.
78. Gamble HJ, Goldby S. Mast cells in peripheral nerve trunks. *Nature* 1961;189:766–767.
79. Gasser HS. Properties of dorsal root unmedullated fibers on the two sides of the ganglion. *J Gen Physiol* 1955;38:709–728.
80. Gatzinsky KP, Berthold C-H, Rydmark M. Acid phosphatase activity at nodes of Ranvier in alpha-motor and dorsal root ganglion neurons of the cat. *J Neurocytol* 1988;17:531–544.
81. Gerhart DZ, Drewes LR. Glucose transporters at the blood-nerve barrier are associated with perineurial cells and endoneurial microvessels. *Brain Res* 1990;508:46–50.
82. Ghabriel MN, Allt G. Incisures of Schmidt-Lanterman. *Prog Neurobiol* 1981;17:25–58.
83. Ghabriel MN, Allt G. Schmidt-Lanterman incisures. I. A quantitative teased fibre study of remyelinating peripheral nerve fibers. *Acta Neuropathol (Berl)* 1980;52:85–95.
84. Ghabriel MN, Allt G. The node of Ranvier. *Prog Anat* 1982;2: 137–160.
85. Ghabriel MN, Allt G. The role of Schmidt-Lanterman incisures in wallerian degeneration. II. An electron microscopic study. *Acta Neuropathol* 1979;48:95–103.
86. Giuditta A, Menichini E, Castigli E, Perrone CC. Protein synthesis in the axonal territory. In: Giuffrida SAM, de Vellis J, Perez PR, eds. *Regulation of gene expression in the nervous system.* New York: Alan R. Liss, 1990;205–218.
87. Gordon JR, Galli SJ. Mast cells as a source of both preformed and immunologically inducible TNF-α/cachectin. *Nature* 1990; 346:274–276.
88. Grafstein B, Forman DS. Intracellular transport in neurons. *Physiol Rev* 1980;60:1167–1283.
89. Griffin JW, George R, Ho T. Macrophage systems in peripheral nerves. A review. *J Neuropathol Exp Neurol* 1993;52:553–560.
90. Griffin JW, George R, Lobato C, Tyor WR, Li CY, Glass JD. Macrophage responses and myelin clearance during wallerian degeneration: relevance to immune-mediated demyelination. *J Neuroimmunol* 1992;40:153–166.
91. Griffin JW, Stoll G, Li CY, Tyor W, Cornblath DR. Macrophage responses in inflammatory demyelinating neuropathies. *Ann Neurol* 1990;27(suppl):S64.
92. Guenard V, Dinarello CA, Weston PJ, Aebischer P. Peripheral nerve regeneration is impeded by interleukin-1 receptor antagonist released from a polymeric guidance channel. *J Neurosci Res* 1991;29:396–400.
93. Gupta SK, Poduslo JF, Dunn R, Roder J, Mezei C. Myelin-associated glycoprotein C gene expression in the presence and absence of Schwann cell-axonal contact. *Dev Neurosci* 1990;12: 22–33.
94. Haak RA, Kleinhauys FW, Ochs S. The viscosity of mammalian nerve axoplasm measured by electron spin resonance. *J Physiol (Lond)* 1976;263:115–137.
95. Haftek J. Stretch injury of peripheral nerve. Acute effects of stretching on rabbit peripheral nerve. *J Bone Joint Surg* 1970;52: 354–365.
95a. Halata Z. Sensory innervation of the hairless and hairy skin in mammals including humans. *J Invest Derm* 1993;101:755–815.
96. Hall SM, Williams PL. Studies on the "incisures" of Schmidt and Lanterman. *J Cell Sci* 1970;6:767–791.
97. Haller FR, Low FN. The fine structure of the peripheral nerve root sheath in the subarachnoid space in the rat and other laboratory animals. *Am J Anat* 1970;131:1–20.
98. Hamburger V. The effects of wind bud extirpation on the development of the central nervous system in chick embryos. *J Exp Zool* 1934;68:449–494.
99. Hartschuh W, Weihe E. Multiple messenger candidates and marker substances in the mammalian Merkel cell-axon complex: a light and electron microscopic immunohistochemical study. In: Hamann W, Iggo A, eds. *Progress in brain research. Transduction and cellular mechanisms in sensory receptors,* vol 74. Amsterdam: Elsevier Science, 1988.
100. Hartung H-P, Stoll G, Toyka KV. Immune reactions in the peripheral nervous system. In: Dyck PJ, Thomas PK, Griffin JW, Low PA, Poduslo JF, eds. *Peripheral neuropathy.* Philadelphia: WB Saunders, 1993;418–444.
101. Helland L. Rapid retrograde transport of dopamine-β-hydroxylase as examined by the stop-flow technique. *Brain Res* 1976;102: 217–228.
102. Hellenbeck PJ. The transport and assembly of the axonal cytoskeleton. *J Cell Biol* 1989;108:223–227.

103. Hensel H, Andres KH, Düring VM. Structure and function of cold receptors. *Pflugers Arch* 1974;352:1–10.
104. Heumann R, Lindholm D, Bandtlow C. Differential regulation of mRNA encoding nerve growth factor and its receptors in rat sciatic nerve during development, degeneration, and regeneration: role of macrophages. *Proc Natl Acad Sci USA* 1987;84:8735–8739.
105. Heym C. *Histochemistry and cell biology of autonomic neurons and paraganglia*. Berlin: Springer-Verlag, 1987.
106. Hirokawa N. Cross-linker system between neurofilaments, microtubules, and membranous organelles in frog axons revealed by the quick-freeze, deep-etching method. *J Cell Biol* 1982;94:129–142.
107. Hirokawa N, Pfister KK, Yorifuji H, Wagner MC, Brady ST, Bloor GS. Submolecular domains of bovine brain kinesin identified by electron microscopy and monoclonal antibody decoration. *Cell* 1989;56:867–878.
108. Hiscoe HB. Distribution of nodes and incisures in normal and regenerated nerve fibers. *Anat Rec* 1947;99:447–475.
109. Hoffman PN, Cleveland DW, Griffin JW, Landes PW, Cowan NJ, Price DL. Neurofilament gene expression: a major determinant of axonal caliber. *Proc Natl Acad Sci USA* 1987;84:3472–3476.
110. Hoffman PN, Lasek RJ. The slow component of axonal transport. Identification of major structural polypeptides of the axon and their generality among mammalian neurons. *J Cell Biol* 1975;66:351–366.
111. Hohman TC, Carper D, Dasgupta S, Kaneko M. Osmotic stress induces aldose reductase in glomerular endothelial cells. *Adv Exp Med Biol* 1991;284:139–152.
112. Hohn A, Leibrock J, Bailey K, Barde Y-A. Identification and characterization of a novel member of the nerve growth factor/ brain-derived neurotrophic factor family. *Nature* 1990;344:339–341.
113. Holtzman E, Novikoff AB, Villaverde H. Lysomes and GERL in normal and chromatolytic neurons of the rat ganglion nodosum. *J Cell Biol* 1967;33:419–435.
114. Hulette CM, Downey BT, Burger PC. Macrophage markers in diagnostic neuropathology. *Am J Surg Pathol* 1992;16:493–499.
115. Iggo A, Muir AR. The structure and function of a slowly adapting touch corpuscle in hairy skin. *J Physiol (Lond)* 1969;200:763–796.
116. Ip NY, Li Y, Yancopoulos GD, Lindsay RM. Cultured hippocampal neurons show responses to BDNG, NT-3, and NT-4, but not NGF. *J Neurosci* 1993;13:3394–3405.
117. Jacobs J, Carmichael N, Cavanagh JB. Ultrastructural changes in the dorsal root and trigeminal ganglia of rats poisoned with methyl mercury. *Neuropathol Appl Neurobiol* 1975;1:1–19.
118. Jensen NA, Rodriguez ML, Garvey JS, Miller CA, Hood L. Transgenic mouse model for neurocristopathy: schwannomas and facial bone tumors. *Proc Natl Acad Sci USA* 1993;90:3192–3196.
119. Johnson EM, Taniuchi M, Clark HB. Demonstration of the retrograde transport of nerve growth factor receptor in the peripheral and central nervous system. *J Neurosci* 1974;7:923–929.
120. Johnson JL. Changes in acetylcholinesterase, acid phosphatase, and beta glucuronidase proximal to a nerve crush. *Brain Res* 1970;18:427–440.
121. Johnson PC, Brendel K, Meezan E. Human diabetic perineurial cell basement membrane thickening. *Lab Invest* 1981;44:265–270.
122. Kalichman MW, Myers RR, Heckman HM, Powell HC. Quantitative histologic analysis of local anesthetic-induced injury to rat sciatic nerve. *J Pharmacol Exp Ther* 1989;250:406–413.
123. Kalichman MW, Myers RR, Powell HC. Pathology of local anesthetic-induced nerve injury. *Acta Neuropathol* 1988;75:583–589.
124. Kaneko M, Carper D, Nishimura C, Millen J, Bock M, Hohman TC. Induction of aldose reductase expression in rat kidney mesangial cells and Chinese hamster ovary cells under hypertonic conditions. *Exp Cell Res* 1990;188:135–140.
125. Kawamura J, Dyck PJ. Evidence for 3 populations by size in L5 spinal ganglion in man. *J Neuropathol Exp Neurol* 1978;37:269–272.
126. Kleinman HC, McGarvey ML, Hassell JR, Star VL, Cannon FB, Laurie GW, Martin GR. Basement membrane complexes with biological activity. *Biochemistry* 1986;25:312–318.
127. Knyihár E. Fluoride resistant acid phosphatase system of nociceptive dorsal root afferents. *Exp Brain Res* 1971;26:73–87.
128. Knyihár-Csillik E, Csillik B. FRAP: histochemistry of the primary sensory nociceptive neuron. *Prog Histochem Cytochem* 1981;14:1–137.
129. Koch T, Schultz P, Williams R, Lampert PW. Giant axonal neuropathy: a childhood disorder of neurofilaments. *Ann Neurol* 1977;1:438–451.
130. Koenig E. Local synthesis of axonal proteins. In: Lajtha A, ed. *Handbook of neurochemistry*. New York: Plenum Press, 1984;315–340.
131. Kreutzberg GW. Neuronal dynamics and axonal flow IV. Blockage of intra-axonal enzyme transport by colchicine. *Proc Natl Acad Sci USA* 1969;62:722–728.
132. Kreutzberg GW, Emmert H. Glucose utilization of motor nuclei during regeneration: a [14C] 2-deoxyglucose study. *Exp Neurol* 1980;70:712–716.
133. Kristensson K. Retrograde transport of macromolecules in axons. *Annu Rev Pharmacol Toxicol* 1978;18:97–110.
134. Kristensson K, Lycke E, Sjöstrand J. Spread of herpes simplex virus in peripheral nerves. *Acta Neuropathol (Berl)* 1971;19:44–53.
135. Kruger L, Perl ER, Sedivec MJ. Fine structure of myelinated mechanical nociceptor endings in cat hairy skin. *J Comp Neurol* 1981;198:137–154.
136. Kuwayama Y, Terenghi G, Polak JM, Trojanowski JQ, Stone RA. A quantitative correlation of substance P-, calcitonin gene-related peptide- and cholecystokinin-like immunoreactivity with retrogradely labeled trigeminal ganglion cells innervating the eye. *Brain Res* 1987;405:220–226.
137. La Velle A, Sechrist JW. Immature and mature reaction patterns in neurons after axon section. *Anat Rec* 1970;166:335.
138. Landon DN. Structure of normal peripheral myelinated nerve fibers. In: Waxman SG, Ritchie JM, eds. *Demyelinating disease: basic and clinical electrophysiology*. New York: Raven Press, 1981.
139. Lanterman AJ. Über den feineren Bau der markhaltigen Nervenfasern. *Arch Mikrosk Anat Entwicklungsmech* 1877;13:1–8.
140. Lasek RJ, Katz MJ. Mechanisms at the axon tip regulate metabolic processes critical to axonal elongation. *Prog Brain Res* 1987;71:49–60.
141. Lawson SN, Harper AA, Harper EI, Garson JA, Anderton BH. A monoclonal antibody against neurofilament protein specifically labels a subpopulation of rat sensory neurons. *J Comp Neurol* 1984;228:263–272.
142. LeBeau JM, Ellisman M, Powell HC. Ultrastructural and morphometric analysis of long term peripheral nerve regeneration in silicone tubes. *J Neurocytol* 1988;17:161–172.
143. Lemke G, Chao M. Axons regulate Schwann cell expression of the major myelin and NGF receptor genes. *Development* 1988;102:499–504.
144. Leone J, Ochs S. Anoxic block and recovery of axoplasmic transport and electrical excitability of nerve. *J Neurobiol* 1978;9:229–245.
145. Levi-Montalcini R, Angeletti PU. The nerve growth factor. *Physiol Rev* 1968;48:534–569.
146. Levy DM, Karanth SS, Springall DR, Polak JM. Depletion of cutaneous nerves and neuropeptides in diabetes mellitus: an immunocytochemical study. *Diabetologia* 1989;32:427–433.
147. Lewin GR, Ritter AM, Mendell LM. Nerve growth factor-induced hyperalgesia in the neonatal and adult rat. *J Neurosci* 1993;2136–2148.
148. Lieberman AR. The axon reaction. A review of the principal features of perikaryal responses to axon injury. *Int Rev Neurobiol* 1971;14:49–124.
149. Lieberman AR. Sensory ganglia. In: Landon DN, ed. *The peripheral nerve*. London: Chapman and Hall, 1976;188–278.
149a. Light AR, Perl ER. Peripheral sensory systems. In: Dyck PJ, Thomas PK, Griffin JW, Low PA, Poduslo JF, eds. *Peripheral neuropathy*. Philadelphia: WB Saunders, 1993;149–165.
150. Lindsey JD, Ellisman MH. The neuronal endomembrane system. III. The origins of their axoplasmic reticulum and discrete axonal cisternae at the axon hillock. *J Neurosci* 1985;5:3135–3144.
151. Low PA, Dyck PJ, Schmelzer JD. Mammalian peripheral nerve sheath has unique responses to chronic elevations of endoneurial fluid pressure. *Exp Neurol* 1980;70:300–306.
152. Low PA, Tuck RR. Effect of changes in blood pressure, respiratory acidosis and hypoxia on blood flow in rat sciatic nerve. *J Physiol* 1984;347:513–524.
153. Lundborg G. Ischemic nerve injury. *Scand J Plast Reconstr Surg* 1970;6(suppl):11.
154. Lunn ER, Perry VH, Brown MC, Rosen H, Gordon S. Absence of wallerian degeneration does not hinder regeneration in peripheral nerve. *Eur J Neurosci* 1989;1:27–33.
155. Müller J. *Handbuch der Physiologie des Menschen,* vol 2. Coblenz: J Hölscher, 1841;249–503.
156. Maisonpierre PC, Belluscio L, Squinto S, Ip NY, Furth ME, Lind-

say RM, Yancopoulos GD. Neurotrophin-3: a neurotrophic factor related to NGF and BNDF. *Science* 1990;247:1446–1451.

157. Marinesco G. Des lésions primitives et les lésions secondaire de la cellule nerveuse. *CR Soc Biol* 1896;3:106.
158. Martz D, Lasek RJ, Brady ST, Allen RD. Mitochondrial motility in axons: membranous organelles may interact with the force generating system through multiple surface binding sites. *Cell Motil* 1984;4:89–101.
159. Masu Y, Wolf E, Holtmann B, Sendtner M, Brem G, Thoenen H. Disruption of the CNTF gene results in motor neuron degeneration. *Nature* 1993;365:27–32.
160. Matthews MR, Raisman G. A light and electron microscopic study of the cellular response to axonal injury in the superior cervical ganglion of the rat. *Proc R Soc Lond (Biol)* 1972;181:43–79.
161. Matthews MR, Raisman G. The ultrastructure and somatic efferent synapses of small granule-containing cells in the superior cervical ganglion. *J Anat* 1969;105:255–282.
162. McMahon SB. The localization of fluoride-resistant acid phosphatase (FRAP) in the pelvic nerves and sacral spinal cord of rats. *Neurosci Lett* 1986;64:305–310.
163. Mendell JR, Sahenk Z. Interference of neuronal processing and axoplasmic transport by toxic chemicals. In: Spencer PS, Schaumburg HH, eds. *Experimental and clinical neurotoxicology.* Baltimore: Williams & Wilkins, 1980;139–160.
164. Meyer A. On parenchymatous systemic degenerations mainly in the central nervous system. *Brain* 1901;24:47–115.
165. Meyer M, Matsuoka I, Wetmore C, Olson L, Thoenen H. Enhanced synthesis of brain- derived neurotrophic factor in the lesioned peripheral nerve: different mechanisms are responsible for the regulation of BDNF and NGF mRNA. *J Cell Biol* 1992;119: 45–54.
166. Meyer RA, Campbell JA. A novel electrophysiological technique for locating cutaneous nociceptive and chemospecific receptors. *Brain Res* 1988;441:81–86.
167. Miani N, Rizzoli A, Bucciante G. Metabolic and chemical changes in regenerating neurons. I. In vitro rate and incorporation of amino acids into proteins of the nerve cell perikaryon of the C8 spinal ganglion of rabbit. *J Neurochem* 1961;7:161–173.
168. Mitchison T, Kirschner M. Cytoskeletal dynamics and nerve growth. *Neuron* 1988;1:761–772.
169. Mizisin AP, Kalichman MW, Calcutt NA, Myers RR, Powell HC. Decreased endoneurial fluid electrolytes in normal rat sciatic nerve after aldose reductase inhibition. *J Neurol Sci* 1993;116: 67–72.
170. Mizisin AP, Powell HC, Myers RR. Edema and increased endoneurial sodium in galactose neuropathy: reversal with an aldose reductase inhibitor. *J Neurol Sci* 1986;74:35–43.
171. Monaco S, Gehrmann J, Raivich G, Kreutzberg GW. MHC-positive, ramified macrophages in the normal and injured rat peripheral nervous system. *J Neurocytol* 1992;21:623–634.
172. Myers RR, Heckman HM, Galbraith JA, Powell HC. Subperineurial demyelination associated with reduced nerve blood flow and oxygen tension after epineurial vascular stripping. *Lab Invest* 1991; 64:41–50.
173. Myers RR, Heckman HM. Effects of local anesthetics on nerve blood flow: studies using lidocaine with and without epinephrine. *Anesthesiology* 1989;71:757–762.
174. Myers RR, Kalichman MW, Reisner LS, Powell HC. Neurotoxicity of local anesthetics: altered perineurial permeability, edema and nerve fiber injury. *Anesthesiology* 1986;64:29–35.
175. Myers RR, Katz J. Neuropathology of neurolytic and semidestructive agents. In: Cousins MJ, Bridenbaugh PO, eds. *Neural blockade in clinical anesthesia and management of pain.* Philadelphia: JB Lippincott, 1987;1031–1051.
176. Myers RR, Murakami H, Powell HC. Reduced nerve blood flow in edematous neuropathies—a biomechanical mechanism. *Microvasc Res* 1986;32:145–151.
177. Myers RR, Powell HC. Endoneurial fluid pressure in peripheral neuropathies. In: Hargens AR, ed. *Tissue fluid pressure and composition.* Baltimore: Williams & Wilkins, 1981;193–208.
178. Myers RR, Powell HC, Shapiro HM, Costello ML, Lampert PW. Changes in endoneurial fluid pressure, permeability, and peripheral nerve ultrastructure in experimental lead neuropathy. *Ann Neurol* 1980;8:392–401.
179. Myers RR, Rydevik BL, Heckman HM, Powell HC. Proximodistal gradient in endoneurial fluid pressure. *Exp Neurol* 1988;102: 368–370.
180. Myers RR, Sommer C, Powell HC. The role of wallerian degeneration in the pathogenesis of neuropathic pain: studies with OLA mice. *J Neuropathol Exp Neurol* 1993;52:310.

180a. Myers RR, Yamamoto T, Yaksh TL, Powell HC. The role of focal nerve ischemia and wallerian degeneration in peripheral nerve injury producing hyperesthesia. *Anesthesiology* 1993;78:308–316.

181. Na HS, Leem JW, Chung JM. Abnormalities of mechanoreceptors in a rat model of neuropathic pain: possible involvement in mediating mechanical allodynia. *J Neurophysiol* 1993;70:522–528.
182. Nakamura T, Hara M, Kasuga T. Transplacental induction of peripheral nervous tumor in the Syrian golden hamster by N-nitroso-N-ethylurea. A new animal model for von Recklinghausen's neurofibromatosis. *Am J Pathol* 1989;135:251–259.
183. Netter FH. *Nervous system. The Ciba collection of medical illustrations.* New York: Ciba Pharmaceutical, 1962;80–99.
184. Nissl F. Über die Veränderungen der Ganglienzellen am Facialiskern des Kaninchens nach Auszeissung der Nerven. *Allg Z Psychiat* 1892;48:197.
185. Nissl F. Mittheilungen zur Anatomie der Nervenzelle. *Allg Z Psychiat* 1894;50:370.
186. Noback CR. The protagon (p) granules of Reich. *J Comp Neurol* 1953;99:91–101.
187. Nukada H, Powell HC, Myers RR. Perineurial window: demyelination in nonherniated endoneurium with reduced nerve blood flow. *J Neuropathol Exp Neurol* 1992;51:523–530.
188. Nukada H, Powell HC, Myers RR. Spatial distribution of nerve injury after occlusion of individual major vessels in rat sciatic nerves. *J Neuropathol Exp Neurol* 1993;52:452–459.
189. Obremski VJ, Johnson MI, Bunge MB. Fibroblasts are required for Schwann cell basal lamina deposition and ensheathment of unmyelinated sympathetic neurites in culture. *J Neurocytol* 1993;22: 102–117.
190. Ochs S. Calcium requirement for axoplasmic transport and the role of the perineurial sheath. In: Jewett DL, McCarroll HR Jr, eds. *Nerve repair and regeneration.* St Louis: CV Mosby, 1980;77–89.
191. Ochs S. Effect of maturation on aging on the rate of fast axoplasmic transport in mammalian nerve. *Prog Brain Res* 1973;40: 349–362.
192. Ochs S. Local supply of energy to the fast axoplasmic transport mechanism. *Proc Natl Acad Sci USA* 1971;68:1279–1282.
193. Ochs S. Rate of fast axoplasmic transport in mammalian nerve fibers. *J Physiol (Lond)* 1972;227:627–645.
194. Ochs S. *Axoplasmic transport and its relation to other nerve functions.* New York: Wiley-Interscience, 1982.
195. Ochs S, Brimijoin WS. Axonal transport. In: Dyck PJ, Thomas PK, Griffin JW, Low PA, Poduslo JF, eds. *Peripheral neuropathy.* Philadelphia: WB Saunders, 1993;331–360.
196. Ochs S, Hollingsworth D. Dependence of fast axoplasmic transport in nerve on oxidative metabolism. *J Neurochem* 1971;18: 107–114.
197. Ochs S, Jersild RA Jr, Li J-M. Slow transport of freely movable cytoskeletal components shown by beading partition of nerve fibers in the cat. *Neuroscience* 1989;33:421–430.
198. Ochs S, Jersild RA Jr. Fast axoplasmic transport in nonmyelinated mammalian nerve fibers shown by electron microscopic radioautography. *J Neurobiol* 1974;5:373–377.
199. Ochs S, Jersild RA Jr. Myelin intrusions in beaded nerve fibers. *Neuroscience* 1990;36:553–567.
200. Ochs S, Smith CB. Low temperature slowing and cold-block of fast axoplasmic transport in mammalian nerves in vitro. *J Neurobiol* 1975;6:85–102.
201. Oldfors A. Macrophages in peripheral nerves. An ultrastructural and histochemical study on rats. *Acta Neuropathol (Berl)* 1980:49: 43–49.
202. Olsson Y. Degranulation of mast cells in peripheral nerve injuries. *Acta Neurol Scand* 1967;43:365–374.
203. Olsson Y. Mast cells in the nervous system. *Int Rev Cytol* 1968;24: 27–70.
204. Olsson Y. The effect of the histamine liberator, Compound 48/80 on mast cells in sectioned peripheral nerves. *Acta Pathol Microbiol Scand* 1966;68:575–584.
205. Osawa T, Tohyama K, Ide C. Allogeneic nerve grafts in the rat, with special reference to the role of Schwann cell basal laminae in nerve regeneration. *J Neurocytol* 1990;19:833–849.
206. Ouvrier RA. Giant axonal neuropathy. A review. *Brain Dev* 1989; 11:207- 214.
207. Paetau M, Mellström K, Vaheri A, Haltia M. Distribution of a

major connective tissue protein, fibronectin, in normal and neoplastic human nerve tissue. *Acta Neuropathol (Berl)* 1980;51:47–51.

208. Palay SL, Palade GE. The fine structure of neurons. *J Biophys Biochem Cytol* 1955;1:69–92.
209. Paravicini U, Stoeckel K, Thoenen H. Biological importance of retrograde axonal transport of nerve growth factors in adrenergic neurons. *Brain Res* 1975;84:279–291.
210. Pease DC, Quilliam TA. Electron microscopy of the pacinian corpuscle. *J Biophys Biochem Cytol* 1956;3:331–342.
211. Perry VH, Brown MC, Lunn ER, Gordon S. Evidence that very slow wallerian degeneration is C57BL/OLA mice is an intrinsic property of the peripheral nerve. *Eur J Neurosci* 1990;2:802–812.
212. Perry VH, Gordon S. Macrophages and the nervous system. *Int Rev Cytol* 1991;125:203–244.
213. Perry VH, Gordon S. Modulation of CD4 antigen on macrophages and microglia in rat brain. *J Exp Med* 1987;166:1138–1143.

213a. Peters A, Parlay SL, Webster H de F. *The fine structure of the nervous system.* Philadelphia: WB Saunders, 1976.

214. Peters A, Vaughn JE. Morphology and development of the myelin sheath. In: Davison AN, Peters A, eds. *Myelination.* Springfield, IL: Charles C Thomas, 1970.
215. Pinkus F. Über Hautsinnesorgane neben den menschlichen Haar (Haarscheiben) und ihre vergleischend anatomische Bedeutung. *Arch Mikrosk Anat Entwmech* 1904;65:121–179.
216. Poduslo JF. Albumin and the blood-nerve barrier. In: Dyck PJ, Thomas PK, Griffin JW, Low PA, Poduslo JF, eds. *Peripheral neuropathy.* Philadelphia: WB Saunders, 1993;446–452.
217. Powell HC, Braheny SL, Myers RR, Rodriguez M, Lampert PW. Early changes in experimental allergic neuritis. *Lab Invest* 1983; 48:332–338.
218. Powell HC, Garrett RS, Kador PF, Mizisin AP. Fine-structural localization of aldose reductase and ouabain-sensitive, K^+-dependent *p*-nitrophenylphosphatase in rat peripheral nerve. *Acta Neuropathol* 1991;81:529–539.
219. Powell HC, Kalichman MW, Garrett RS, Myers RR. Selective vulnerability of unmyelinated fiber Schwann cells in nerves exposed to local anesthetics. *Lab Invest* 1988;59:271–280.
220. Powell HC, Koch T, Garrett R, Lampert PW. Schwann cell abnormalities in 2,5-hexanedione neuropathy. *J Neurocytol* 1978;7: 517–528.
221. Powell HC, Myers RR. Pathology of experimental nerve compression. *Lab Invest* 1986;55:91–100.
222. Powell HC, Myers RR, Costello ML. Increased endoneurial fluid pressure following injection of histamine and Compound 48/80 into rat peripheral nerves. *Lab Invest* 1980;43:564–572.
223. Price DL, Griffin J, Young A, Peck K, Stocks A. Tetanus toxin: direct evidence for retrograde intraaxonal transport. *Science* 1975;88:945–947.
224. Rambourg A, Clermont Y, Beaudet A. Ultrastructural features of six types of neurons in rat dorsal root ganglia. *J Neurocytol* 1983; 12:47–66.
225. Ramieri G, Stella M, Calcagni M, Teich-Alasia S, Cellino G, Panzica GC. Morphology of corpuscular receptors in hairy and nonhairy human skin as visualized by an antiserum to protein gene produce 9.5 compared to anti-neuron-specific enolase and anti-S-100 protein. *Acta Anat* 1992;144:343–347.
226. Rasband W. Personal Communication. Computer Morphometry. The NIH Image morphometry program is in the public domain, and is available electronically, including documentation and source code, by anonymous FTP from zippy.nimh.nih.gov.
227. Read GW, Kiefer EF. Benzyalkonium chloride: selective inhibitor of histamine release induced by Compound 48/80 and other polyamines. *J Pharmacol Exp Ther* 1979;211:711–715.
228. Rechthand E, Sato S, Oberg PA, Rapoport SI. Sciatic nerve blood flow response to carbon dioxide. *Brain Res* 1988;446:61–66.
229. Reese TS. The molecular basis of axonal transport in the squid giant axon. In: Kandel ER, ed. *Molecular neurobiology in neurology and psychiatry.* New York: Raven Press, 1987;65:89–102.
230. Renaut J. Recherche sur quelques points particuliers d'histologie des nerfs. *Arch Physiol (Paris)* 1881;8:180–190.
231. Rieger F, Daniloff JK, Pincon-Raymond M, Crossin KL, Grumet M, Edelman CM. Neuronal cell adhesion molecules and cytotactin are colocalized at the node of Ranvier. *J Cell Biol* 1986;103: 379–391.
232. Ris H. The cytoplasmic filament system in critical point-dried whole mounts and plastic-embedded sections. *J Cell Biol* 1985; 100:1474–1487.
233. Ross MH, Reith EJ. Perineurium: evidence for contractile elements. *Science* 1969; 165:604–606.
234. Roytta M, Salonen V. Long-term endoneurial changes after nerve transection. *Acta Neuropathol* 1988;76:35–45.
235. Ruffini A. Di un nuovo organo nervoso terminale e sulla presenza dei corpuscoli di Golgi-Mazzoni nel connettive sottocutaneo dei polpastrelli della dita del' uomo. *Atti Acad Naz Lincei Mem* 1891;7:398–410.
236. Rutishauser U, Jessell TM. Cell adhesion molecules in vertebrate neural development. *Physiol Rev* 1988;68:819–857.
237. Rydevik B, Holm S, Brown MD, Lundborg G. Diffusion from the cerebrospinal fluid as a nutritional pathway for spinal nerve roots. *Acta Physiol Scand* 1990;138:247– 248.
238. Rydevik BL, Kwan MK, Myers RR, Brown RA, Triggs KJ, Woo SL-Y, Garfin SR. Effects of acute stretching on rabbit tibial nerve: an in vitro mechanical and histological study. *J Orthop Res* 1990;8: 694–701.
239. Sabri MI, Ochs S. Relation of ATP and creatine phosphate to fast axoplasmic transport in mammalian nerve. *J Neurochem* 1972;9: 2821–2828.
240. Said G, Hontebeyrie-Joskowicz M. Nerve lesions induced by macrophage activation. *Res Immunol* 1992;143:589–599.
241. Sammak PJ, Borisy GG. Direct observation of microtubule dynamics in living cells. *Nature* 1988;332:724–726.
242. Samuel NM, Jessen KR, Grange JM, Mirsky R. Gamma interferon, but not Mycobacterium leprae, induces major histocompatibility class II antigens on cultured rat Schwann cells. *J Neurocytol* 1987;16:281–287.
243. Samuel NM, Mirsky R, Grance JM, Jessen KR. Expression of major histocompatibility complex class I and class II antigens in human Schwann cell cultures and effects of infection with *Mycobacterium leprae. Clin Exp Immunol* 1987;68:500–509.
244. Schiff R, Rosenbluth J. Ultrastructural localization of laminin in rat sensory ganglia. *J Histochem Cytochem* 1986;34:1691–1699.
245. Schmalbruch H. The number of neurons in dorsal root ganglia L4-L6 of the rat. *Anat Rec* 1987;219:315–322.
246. Schmidt B, Stoll G, Hartung HP, Heininger K, Schafer B, Toyka KV. Macrophages but not Schwann cells express Ia antigen in experimental autoimmune neuritis. *Ann Neurol* 1990;28:70–77.
247. Schmidt HC. On the construction of the dark or double-bordered nerve fibre. *Mon Microsc J (Lond)* 1874;11:200–221.
248. Schochet SS, Chesson AL. Giant axonal neuropathy. Possibly secondary to vitamin B_{12} malabsorption. *Acta Neuropathol (Berl)* 1977;40:79–83..
249. Schröder JM, Bohl J, Brodda K. Changes in the ratio between myelin thickness and axon diameter in the human developing sural nerve. *Acta Neuropathol (Berl)* 1978;43:169–178.
250. Schwann T. *Microscopical researches into the accordance in the structure and growth of animals and plants.* Translated by Henry Smith. London: Sydenham Society, 1847.
251. Schwartz JH, Goldman JE, Ambron RT, Goldberg DJ. Axonal transport of vesicles carrying [3H]-serotonin in the metacerebral neuron of Aplysia californica. *Cold Spring Harbor Symp Quant Biol* 1975;40:83–92.
252. Scott SA. Skin sensory innervation patterns in embryonic chick hind limbs deprived of motoneurons. *Dev Biol* 1988;126:362–374.
253. Scott SA. The development of the segmental pattern of skin sensory innervation in embryonic chick hind limb. *J Physiol (Lond)* 1982;330:203–230.
254. Selander D, Mansson LG, Karlsson L, Svanvik J. Adrenergic vasoconstriction in peripheral nerves of the rabbit. *Anesthesiology* 1985;62:6–10.
255. Sheen K, Chung JM. Signs of neuropathic pain depend on signals from injured nerve fibers in a rat model. *Brain Res* 1993;610: 62–68.
256. Singer M, Drishnan N, Fyfe DA. Penetration of ruthenium red into peripheral nerve fibers. *Anat Rec* 1972;173:375–389.
257. Skene JHP, Jacobson RD, Snipes GJ, et al. A protein induced during growth (GAP-43) is a major component of growth-cone membranes. *Science* 1986;233:783.
258. Smith GM, Rabinovsky ED, McManaman JL, Shine HD. Temporal and spatial expression of ciliary neurotrophic factor after peripheral nerve injury. *Exp Neurol* 1993;121:239–247.
259. Smith KJ, Blakemore WF, Murray JA, Patterson RC. Internodal myelin volume and axon surface area: a relationship determining myelin thickness? *J Neurol Sci* 1982;55:231–246.
260. Sommer C, Galbraith JA, Heckman HM, Myers RR. Pathology of

experimental compression neuropathy producing hyperesthesia. *J Neuropathol Exp Neurol* 1993;52:223– 233.

261. Sommer C, Myers RR. Thalidomide inhibition of TNF reduces hyperalgesia in neuropathic rats. *Reg Anaesth* 1994;19:1.
262. Sommer EW, Kazimierczak J, Droz B. Neuronal subpopulations in the dorsal root ganglion of the mouse as characterized by combination of ultrastructural and cytochemical features. *Brain Res* 1985; 346:310–326.
263. Spacek J, Lieberman AR. Relationships between mitochondrial outer membranes and agranular reticulum in nervous tissue: ultrastructural observations and a new interpretation. *J Cell Sci* 1980;46: 129–147.
264. Steinhoff U, Golecki JR, Kazda J, Kaufmann SHE. Evidence for phagosome lysome fusion in *Mycobacterium leprae* infected murine Schwann cells. *Infect Immunol* 1989;57:1008–1010.
265. Stolinski C, Breathnach AS. Freeze-fracture replication of mammalian peripheral nerve—a review. *J Neurol Sci* 1982;57:1–28.
266. Stoll G, Griffin JW, Li CY, Trapp BD. Wallerian degeneration in the peripheral nervous system: participation of both Schwann cells and macrophages in myelin degradation. *J Neurocytol* 1989;18:671–683.
267. Stoll G, Muller HW. Macrophages in the peripheral nervous system and astroglia in the central nervous system of rat commonly express apolipoprotein E during development but differ in their response to injury. *Neurosci Lett* 1986;72:233–238.
268. Straile WE. Sensory hair follicles in mammalian skin: the tylotrich follicle. *Am J Anat* 1960;106:133–148.
269. Sunderland S. *Nerve and nerve injuries.* Edinburgh: Churchill Livingstone, 1968.
270. Sutter A, Riopelle RJ, Harris-Warrick RW, Shooter EM. Nerve growth factor receptors. Characterization of two distinct classes of binding sites on chick embryo sensory ganglia cells. *J Biol Chem* 1979;254:5972–5982.
271. Taiwo YO, Levine JD, Burch RM, Woo JE, Mobley WC. Hyperalgesia induced in the rat by the amino-terminal octapeptide of nerve growth factor. *Proc Natl Acad Sci USA* 1991;88:5144–5148.
272. Teillet MA, Kalcheim C, Le Douarin NM. Formation of the dorsal root ganglia in the avian embryo: segmental origin and migratory behavior of neural crest progenitor cells. *Dev Biol* 1987;120: 329–347.
273. Tennyson VM, Gershon MD. Light and electron microscopy of dorsal root, sympathetic, and enteric ganglia. In: Dyck PJ, Thomas PK, Lambert EH, Bunge R, eds. *Peripheral neuropathy.* Philadelphia: WB Saunders, 1984;121–155.
274. Tetzlaff W, Kreutzberg GW. Ornithine decarboxylation in motoneurons during regeneration. *Exp Neurol* 1985;89:679–688.
275. Thomas PK, Berthold C-H, Ochoa J. Microscopic anatomy of the peripheral nervous system. In: Dyck PJ, Thomas PK, Griffin JW, Low PA, Poduslo JF, eds. *Peripheral neuropathy.* Philadelphia: WB Saunders, 1993;28–91.

275a. Thomas PK, Scaravilli F, Belai A. Pathologic alterations in cell bodies of peripheral neurons in neuropathy. In: Dyck PJ, Thomas PK, Griffin JW, Low PA, Poduslo JF, eds. *Peripheral neuropathy.* Philadelphia: WB Saunders, 1993;476–513.

276. Thomas PK, Slatford J. Lamellar bodies in the cytoplasm of Schwann cells. *J Anat* 1964;98:691.
277. Thomas PK. The connective tissue of peripheral nerve: an electron microscope study. *J Anat* 1963;97:35–44.
278. Tomatsuri M, Okajima S, Ide C. Sprout formation at nodes of Ranvier of crush-injured peripheral nerves. *Restorative Neurol Neurosci* 1993;5:275–282.
279. Tomlinson DR. Aldose reductase inhibitors and the complications of diabetes mellitus. *Diabetic Med* 1993;10:214–230.
280. Tomlinson DR. The pharmacology of diabetic neuropathy. *Diabetes Metab Rev* 1992;8:67–84.
281. Torvik A, Heding A. Histological studies on the effect of actinomycin D on retrograde cell reaction in the facial nucleus of mice. *Acta Neuropathol (Berl)* 1967;9:146–157.
282. Tsai CP, Pollard JD, Armati PJ. Interferon-γ inhibition suppresses experimental allergic neuritis: modulation of major histocompatibility complex expression on Schwann cells in vitro. *J Neuroimmunol* 1991;31:133–145.
283. Tsukita S, Usukura J, Tsukita S, Ishikawa H. The cytoskeleton in myelinated axons: a freeze-etch replica study. *Neuroscience* 1982;7: 2135–2147.
284. Tuchscherer MM, Seybold VS. Immunohistochemical studies of substance P, cholecystokinin-octapeptide and somatostatin in dorsal root ganglia of the rat. *Neuroscience* 1985;14:593–605.
285. Vale RD. Intracellular transport using microtubule-based motors. *Annu Rev Biol* 1987;3:347–378.
286. Vale RD, Schnapp BJ, Mitchison T, Steuer E, Reese TS, Sheetz MP. Different axoplasmic proteins generate movement in opposite directions along microtubules in vitro. *Cell* 1985;43:623–632.
287. Vallee RB. Molecular characterization of high molecular weight microtubule-associated proteins: some answers, many questions. *Cell Motil Cytoskeleton* 1990;15:204–209.
288. Vallee RB, Shpetner HS, Paschal BM. The role of dynein in retrograde axonal transport. *Trends Neurosci* 1989;12:66–70.
289. Vass K, Hickey WF, Schmidt RE, Lassmann H. Bone marrow-derived elements in the peripheral nervous system: an immunohistochemical and ultrastructural investigation in chimeric rats. *Lab Invest* 1993;69:275–282.
290. Vega JA, Del Valle ME, Calzada HB, Suarez-Garnacho S, Malinovsky L. Nerve growth factor receptor immunoreactivity in Meissner and Pacinian corpuscles of the human digital skin. *Anat Rec* 1993;236:730–736.
291. Verloes A, Elmer C, Lacombe D, et al. Ondine-Hirschsprung syndrome (Haddad syndrome). Further delineation in two cases and review of the literature. *Eur J Pediatr* 1993;152:75–77.
292. Vizoso AD. The relationship between internodal length and growth in human nerves. *J Anat* 1950;84:342–353.
293. Waller A. Experiments on the section of the glossopharyngeal and hypoglossal nerves of the frog and observations of the alterations produced thereby in the structure of their primitive fibers. Philos *Trans R Soc Lond (Biol)* 1850;140:423–438.
294. Watson WE. An autoradiographic study of the incorporation of nucleic-acid precursors by neurons and glia during nerve regeneration. *J Physiol (Lond)* 1965;180:741–753.
295. Watson WE. Observations on the nucleolar and total cell body nucleic acid of injured nerve cells. *J Physiol (Lond)* 1968;196: 655–676.
296. Waxman SG. Regional differentiation of the axon: a review with special reference to the concept of the multiplex neuron. *Brain Res* 1972;47:269–288.
297. Webster H de F. Relationship between Schmidt-Lantermann incisures and myelin segmentation during wallerian degeneration. *Ann NY Acad Sci* 1965;122:29–38.
298. Webster H de F. The geometry of peripheral myelin sheaths during their formation and growth in rat sciatic nerves. *J Cell Biol* 1971;48:348–367.
299. Webster H de F. Development of peripheral nerve fibers. In: Dyck PJ, Thomas PK, Griffin JW, Low PA, Poduslo JF, eds. *Peripheral neuropathy.* Philadelphia: WB Saunders, 1993;243–266.
300. Weis J, Alexianu ME, Heide G, Schröder JM. Renaut bodies contain elastic fiber components. *J Neuropathol Exp Neurol* 1993;52: 444–451.
301. Weiss DG, Seitz-Tutter D, Langford GM, Allen RD. The native microtubule as the engine for bidirectional organelle movements. In: Smith RS, Bisby MA, eds. *Axonal transport.* New York: Alan R. Liss, 1987.
302. Wekerle H, Schwab M, Linington C, Meyermann R. Antigen presentation in the peripheral nervous system. Schwann cells present endogenous myelin autoantigens to lymphocytes. *Eur J Immunol* 1986;16:1551–1557.
303. Weller RO, Herzog I. Schwann cell lysosomes in hypertrophic neuropathy and in normal human nerves. *Brain* 1970;93:347–356.
304. Wells MR, Racis SP Jr, Vaidya U. Changes in plasma cytokines associated with peripheral nerve injury. *J Neuroimmunol* 1992;39: 261–268.
305. Whitear M. Internode length in the skin plexuses of fish and the frog. *Q J Miscrosc Sci* 1952;93:307–313.
306. Willard M, Cowan WM, Vagelos PR. The polypeptide composition of intra-axonally transported proteins: evidence for four transport velocities. *Proc Natl Acad Sci USA* 1974:71:2183–2187.
307. Willard MB, Hulebak KL. The intra-axonal transport of polypeptide H: evidence for a fifth (very slow) group of transported proteins in the retinal ganglion cells of the rabbit. *Brain Res* 1977;36:289–306.
308. Williams PL, Landon DN. Paranodal apparatus of peripheral nerve fibres of mammals. *Nature (Lond)* 1963;198:670–673.
309. Willis WD, Coggeshall RE. *Sensory mechanisms of the spinal cord.* New York: Plenum Press, 1991.
310. Wilson DR. Two-dimensional polyacrylamide gel electrophoresis of proteins. In: Lajtha A, ed. *Handbook of neurochemistry,* vol 2. New York: Plenum Press, 1982;146.
311. Wilson PO, Barber PC, Hamid QA, Power BF, Dhillon AP, Rode

J, Day IN, Thompson RJ, Polak JM. The immunolocalization of protein gene product 9.5 using rabbit polyclonal and mouse monoclonal antibodies. *Br J Exp Pathol* 1988;69:91–104.

312. Windeband AJ. Neuronal growth factors in the peripheral nervous system. In: Dyck PJ, Thomas PK, Griffin JW, Low PA, Poduslo JF, eds. *Peripheral neuropathy.* Philadelphia: WB Saunders, 1993;377–388.
313. Wong E, Mizisin AP, Garrett RS, Miller AL, Powell HC. Changes in aldose reductase after crush injury of normal rat sciatic nerve. *J Neurochem* 1992;58:2212–2220.
314. Wood PM, Schachner M, Bunge RP. Inhibition of Schwann cell myelination in vitro by antibody to the L1 adhesion molecule. *J Neurosci* 1990;10:3635–3645.
315. Wright EM, Vogel KS, Davies AM. Neurotrophic factors promote the maturation of developing sensory neurons before they become dependent on these factors for survival. *Neuron* 1992;9:139–150.
316. Yaksh TL, Yamamoto T, Myers RR. Pharmacology of nerve compression-evoked hyperesthesia. In: Willis W, ed. *Hyperalgesia and allodynia.* New York: Raven Press, 1991;245–258.
317. Yamamoto T, Yaksh TL. Effects of colchicine applied to the peripheral nerve on the thermal hyperalgesia evoked with chronic nerve constriction. *Pain* 1993;55:227–233.
318. Yan W, Snider WD, Pinzone JJ, Johnson EM. Retrograde transport of nerve growth factor (NGF) in motoneurons of developing rats: assessment of potential neurotrophic effects. *Neuron* 1988;1:335–343.
319. Yoshimura M, Amaya S, Tyujo M, Nomura S. Experimental studies on the traction injury of peripheral nerves. *Neuro Orthop* 1989;7:1–7.
320. Yu LT, Rostami A, Silvers WK, Larossa D, Hickey WF. Expression of major histocompatibility complex antigens on inflammatory peripheral nerve lesions. *J Neuroimmunol* 1990;30:145.
321. Zenker W, Neuhuber WL. *The primary afferent neuron. A survey of recent morpho-functional aspects.* New York: Plenum Press, 1990.
322. Ziller C, Le Douarin NM. The neural crest in nerve development. In: Dyck PJ, Thomas PK, Griffin JW, Low PA, Poduslo JF, eds. *Peripheral neuropathy.* Philadelphia: WB Saunders, 1993; 230–242.

Anesthesia: Biologic Foundations, edited by
Tony L. Yaksh et al. Lippincott–Raven Publishers,
Philadelphia © 1997.

CHAPTER 31

TRANSDUCTION PROPERTIES OF THE SENSORY AFFERENT FIBERS

SRINIVASA N. RAJA, RICHARD A. MEYER,
AND JAMES N. CAMPBELL

A vital protective function of the nervous system is to provide information about the occurrence or threat of injury. Injury to tissues can be induced by trauma, either accidentally or through surgical intervention, or it can result from inflammation following a variety of disease states. By its inherent aversive nature, the sensation of pain serves as a warning of tissue injury. This chapter discusses the properties of a subset of sensory afferent fibers that responds to noxious (injurious or potentially injurious) stimuli, thus providing a signal to alert the organism of potential injury.

Recent studies on the origin and modulation of pain from somatic tissues have led to the hypothesis that pain is signaled by a specialized apparatus of sensors and conduction pathways and processed at multiple specific sites in the central nervous system. This neural apparatus must be capable of responding to the multiple energy forms that result in tissue injury (e.g., heat, mechanical, and chemical stimuli). In addition, this subgroup of primary afferent fibers must provide information to the central nervous system regarding the location and intensity of noxious stimuli.

This chapter focuses on peripheral nociceptive processing in somatic tissues and discusses in detail the nociceptive apparatus associated with skin and joints because these have been the most extensively studied tissues. (Properties of visceral afferent fibers are discussed in Chap. 39.) Cutaneous sensibility has been studied by single nerve fiber recordings in a number of species, including humans. This is done by first identifying the receptive field (i.e., the area of tissue responsive to the applied stimulus) of single fibers. A variety of stimuli are then applied to the receptive field and the characteristics of the neural response are noted. This analysis is particularly powerful in understanding the physiology of pain when combined with correlative psychophysical studies, in which the magnitude of pain induced by identical stimuli is rated by human subjects.

SPECIFICITY OF SENSORY AFFERENT FIBER FUNCTION IN NORMAL SKIN

Peripheral nerves are composed of varying combinations of sensory, motor, and autonomic fibers. The sensory nerve fibers are the axons of the primary afferent neurons that are located in the dorsal root ganglion. The primary afferent fibers are either myelinated or unmyelinated and have a wide range of diameters and conduction velocities. These specialized sensory fibers, alone or in concert with other specialized fibers, provide information to the central nervous system about the environment as well as about the state of the organism itself. For example, the skin has the capacity to detect a wide variety of cutaneous stimuli that may evoke the sensations of cooling, warmth, or touch. Sensory fibers that are selectively sensitive to these stimuli have been identified. Warm fibers, which are predominantly unmyelinated fibers, are exquisitely sensitive to gentle warming of their punctate receptive fields (Fig. 1). These fibers have the ability to signal exclusively the quality and intensity of warmth sensation (30,31,64,72). Similarly, the sense of cooling is encoded by a subpopulation of the thinly myelinated, Aδ-fibers that respond selectively to gentle cooling stimuli (29). Different classes of mechanoreceptive afferent fibers that are exquisitely sensitive to deformations of the skin encode the sense of touch. These low-threshold mechanoreceptors convey information that relates to the detection of texture and shape.

A class of cutaneous receptors is distinguished by their relatively high threshold for activation by heat, mechanical, or cooling stimuli. Because these receptors respond preferentially and in a graded fashion to noxious stimuli, they are termed nociceptors (139). Nociceptors are subclassified based on (a) presence or absence of myelination, i.e., unmyelinated (C-fiber) versus myelinated (A-fiber) parent nerve fiber; (b) the types of stimuli that evoke a response; and (c) the characteristics of the response (see 125 and 162 for reviews).

Once tissue is damaged, a cascade of events results in enhanced pain to natural stimuli, termed hyperalgesia. A corresponding increase in the responsiveness of nociceptors, called sensitization, occurs. The characteristics of hyperalgesia and its neurophysiologic counterpart, sensitization, are discussed at the end of this chapter.

RESPONSE PROPERTIES OF NOCICEPTORS IN NORMAL SKIN

A primary function of nociceptors is to transduce external stimuli. Transduction is the transfer of one form of energy (e.g., mechanical, thermal) to electrical impulses (action potentials). Many nociceptors respond to multiple stimulus modalities, including mechanical, heat, cold, and chemical stimuli (5,11,147,164). Hence, these receptors are labeled as polymodal nociceptors. However, in most systematic neurophysiologic studies of nociceptors, only heat and mechanical stimuli have been used. Therefore, the nomenclature of CMH and AMH has been adopted to refer to C-fiber mechano-heat–sensitive nociceptors and A-fiber mechano-heat–sensitive nociceptors, respectively.

Nociceptive afferent fibers do not generate spontaneous action potentials under ambient conditions. Thresholds for activation of nociceptors by heat and mechanical stimuli are considerably higher than those of thermoreceptors (warm and cold fibers) and low-threshold mechanoreceptors.

Nociceptor Responses to Heat Stimuli

C-Fiber Mechano-Heat Nociceptors (CMHs)

The heat threshold of CMHs in a number of species, including primates, is typically greater than 38°C, but less than 50°C. The response of CMHs in primates increases monotonically with stimulus intensity over the 41 to 49°C temperature range that encompasses the pain threshold in humans (Fig. 1). In contrast, a second class of primary afferents called "warm fibers" responds to gentle warming but exhibits a nonmonotonic response to temperature near pain threshold (Fig. 1B).

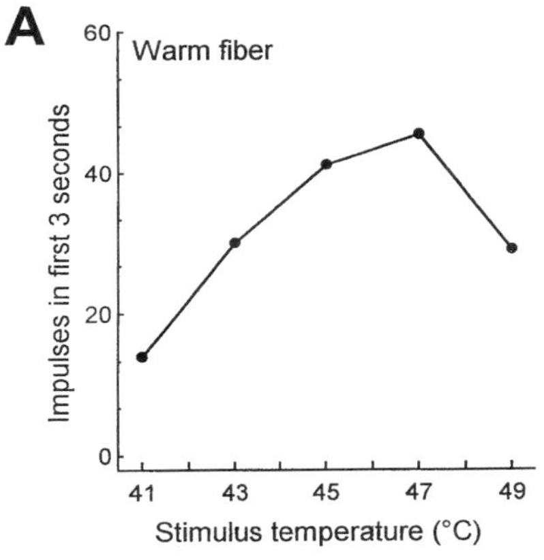

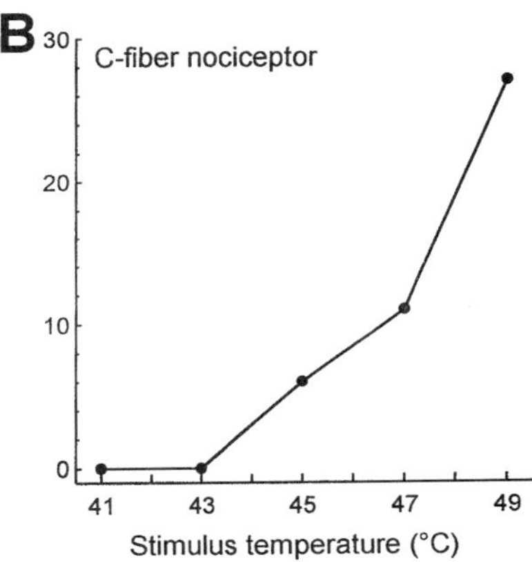

Figure 1. Heat response properties of two different types of C-fiber afferents that innervate glabrous skin. *Left panel* shows a typical warm fiber and the *right panel* a C-fiber nociceptor. Three second duration heat stimuli, ranging from 41-49°C, were presented in random order to the glabrous skin of the monkey hand. Base temperature was 38° C. **A.** Nonmonotonic response of a warm fiber to heat stimuli in the noxious range (45-49°C). Warm fibers are, therefore, unlikely to code for pain to heat stimuli. **B.** Monotonic stimulus-response function of C-fiber nociceptor to heat stimuli in the noxious range. C-fiber nociceptors are likely candidates that code for the intensity of pain induced by noxious heat stimuli. (Adapted with permission from ref. 80).

The response of CMHs is strongly influenced by the stimulus history. As in other sensory systems, the repeated presentation of a suprathreshold stimulus or the exposure to a stimulus of long duration often leads to a reduction in the response of the nociceptor. This phenomenon is termed "fatigue" or "habituation." Another unique property of nociceptors is that under certain circumstances the prior presentation of noxious stimuli may enhance the response to subsequent stimuli, a phenomenon termed "sensitization." Both fatigue and sensitization are observed in CMHs. Fatigue is dependent on the time between stimuli, with full recovery taking more than 10 minutes (154). A similar reduction in the pain intensity of repeated heat stimuli is observed in human subjects (80). The enhanced response, or sensitization, that may occur in CMHs after tissue injury is described below (see Primary and Secondary Hyperalgesia).

A-Fiber Mechano-Heat Nociceptors (AMHs)

Two types of AMHs have been identified (23,35). Type I AMHs have very high heat thresholds under normal circumstances, and, because of this, have been labeled as high-threshold mechanoreceptors (HTMs) by some investigators (16,17,121). The majority have thresholds of 53°C or greater, although some may respond to temperatures below 50°C. However, when a heat stimulus of sufficient intensity and duration is delivered, most HTMs respond to heat (Fig. 2). Type I AMHs are particularly prevalent on the glabrous skin of the hand in monkeys (19) and have also been described in other species (39,129). Type I AMHs in monkeys have a mean conduction velocity of 30 m/sec but some fibers may conduct at velocities as high as 55 m/sec. Thus, by the Erlanger/Glasser classification of fibers based on conduction velocity, type I AMHs fall into both the Aδ and Aβ fiber categories.

The second type of AMHs, type II AMHs, was first characterized on the monkey face (35), but has since been observed in other hairy skin areas of monkeys and human (1,160). Type II AMHs, however, have not been found on the glabrous skin of the hand. Type II AMHs are distinguished by a substantially lower threshold for activation by heat and a lower mean conduction velocity, (15 m/sec) than that of type I AMHs. As will be discussed later, type II AMHs are considered to signal first pain sensation.

The typical responses of the two types of AMHs to a heat stimulus is shown in Fig. 2. Type II AMHs have a much shorter receptor utilization time (time between stimulus onset and activation of the receptor) than the type I AMHs. In addition, type II AMHs exhibit a burst of activity at the onset of a step heat stimulus. In contrast, the response of type I AMHs does not adapt quickly (160).

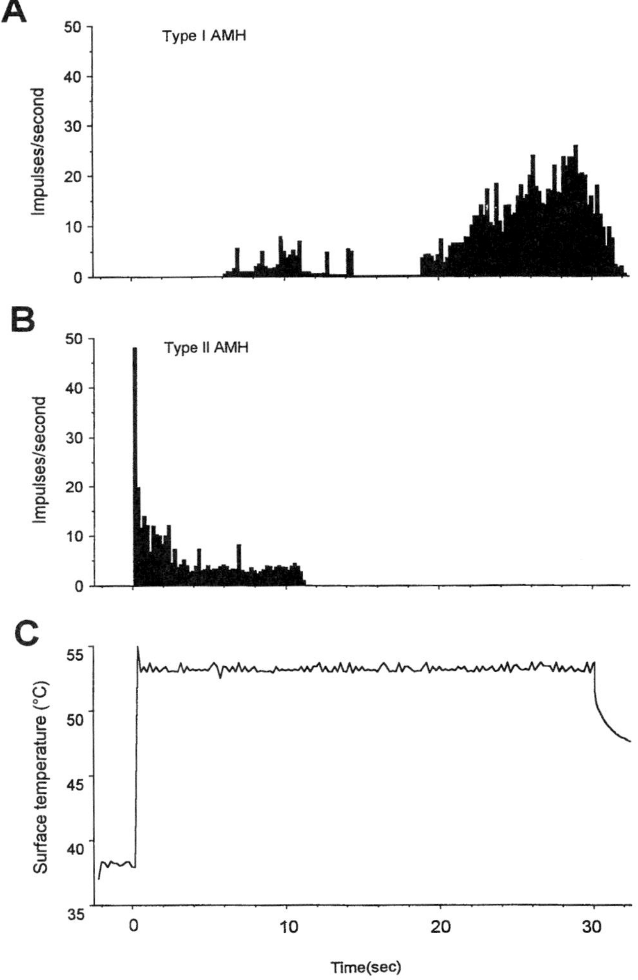

Figure 2. Typical responses of a type I and a type II AMH to a stepped heat stimulus (53°C, 30 sec). **A:** The type I AMHs have a longer receptor utilization time (time from onset of stimulus to first action potential) with a peak discharge frequency near the end of the stimulus. **B:** The type II AMHs have a short receptor utilization time and adapt quickly to stepped heat stimuli. **C:** Stimulus waveform—the type I AMHs play an important role in hyperalgesia to heat, while the type II AMHs are likely candidates for signaling first pain sensation (Adapted from ref. 160, with permission.)

Nociceptor Response to Mechanical Stimuli

In comparison to the detailed studies of the response properties of nociceptors to heat stimuli, studies on the response of nociceptors to mechanical stimuli are fewer and less well controlled. The main limiting factor is the lack of well-controlled mechanical stimulators that are capable of providing adequate stimuli that can excite nociceptors.

CMHs and AMHs

The commonly studied nociceptors (CMHs and AMHs, described above) respond to both heat and mechanical stimuli (Figs. 2-3). The area of the receptive field that responds to mechanical stimuli is similar to the site that responds to heat stimuli (161). However, it appears that the transducer elements that account for mechanosensitivity are likely different from those responsible for heat. Following the application of capsaicin, the active ingredient of hot chili pepper, to the skin of humans, analgesia to heat but not mechanical stimuli was observed (32,142). Similarly, when capsaicin was administered to C-fiber polymodal nociceptors in the cornea, their response to heat and chemical stimuli was eliminated, but they still responded to mechanical stimuli (9). Thus, probably the mechanical and heat transducer mechanisms are different.

Mechanically Insensitive Afferents

A class of cutaneous nociceptors has been recently reported that is relatively unresponsive to mechanical stimuli. Neurophysiologic studies suggest that about 50% of the cutaneous Aδ fiber nociceptors and 30% of the cutaneous C-fiber nociceptors either have very high mechanical thresholds (>6 bar=600 KPa=60 g/mm^2) or are unresponsive to mechanical stimuli (Fig. 4) (51,73,109). These nociceptors are referred to as mechanically insensitive afferents (MIAs), and as "silent" or "sleeping" nociceptors. These afferent fibers have also been found in knee joint (137), viscera (54), and cornea (150).

The physiologic role of the MIAs is still uncertain. Some cutaneous MIAs may be chemospecific receptors (33,73,81,108, 109) (Fig. 5). Others respond to intense cold or heat stimuli (73,82,109). In the knee joint, MIAs become responsive to mechanical stimuli following inflammation (44). Similar sensitization to mechanical stimuli has been observed in cutaneous MIAs after administration of inflammatory agents, or after cutaneous injury (33,51,109).

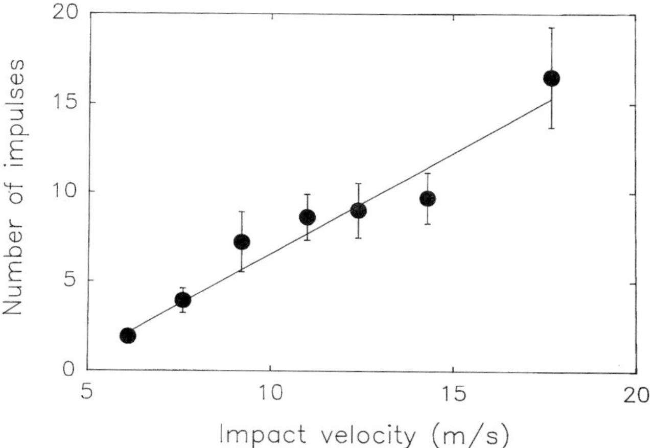

Figure 3. Response of C-fiber nociceptors in humans to noxious mechanical stimuli. A metal cylinder (0.3 g) was shot perpendicular to the skin at different velocities. Note that the response of the fibers increases monotonically with increasing stimulus intensity. The mean pain threshold during parallel psychophysical studies in awake humans was 11 m/sec (Adapted from ref. 70, with permission.)

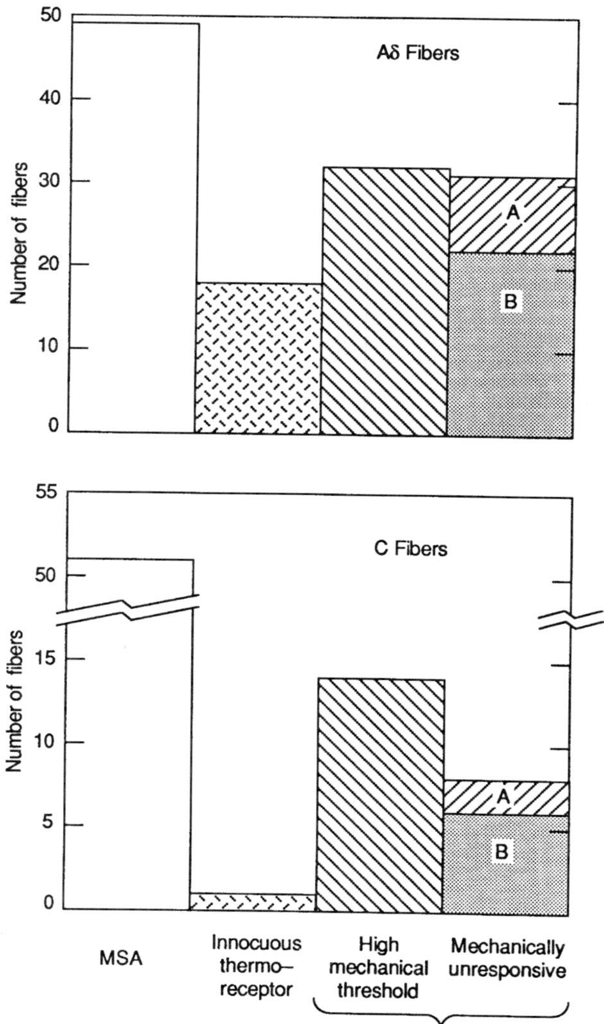

Figure 4. Histogram showing relative proportion of mechanically sensitive and mechanically insensitive afferent fibers in cutaneous nerves that innervate hairy skin in monkey. Mechanically sensitive afferents (MSAs) had thresholds to mechanical stimulation with von Frey hairs of less than 6 bars (=600 kPA=60 g/mm^2). Mechanically insensitive afferents (MIAs) had mechanical thresholds greater than 6 bars or were unresponsive to mechanical stimuli. MIAs can be further subdivided into receptors sensitive to chemical or intense thermal stimuli **(A)** or fibers for which no response to natural stimuli could be elicited **(B)**. (From ref. 109, with permission.)

Chemosensitivity of Nociceptors

The neural mechanisms of pain to noxious chemical stimuli is not well understood. For example, the response of nociceptors to chemical irritants such as capsaicin is low in comparison to the pronounced magnitude of pain induced by the agent (78). This discrepancy has prompted the suggestion that other receptor types may exist in the skin that are yet to be characterized. Potential candidate chemonociceptors may

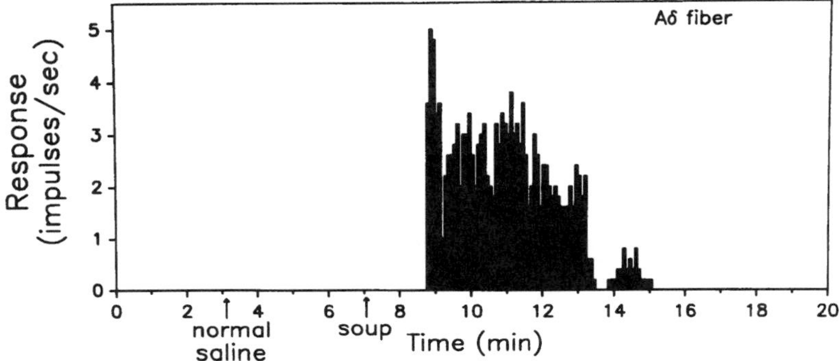

Figure 5. An example of a chemosensitive nociceptor. This Aδ fiber nociceptor was a mechanically insensitive afferent (MIA) that did not respond to heat or mechanical stimuli or to injections of saline. This MIA responded vigorously to the intradermal injection of a soup of inflammatory mediators containing bradykinin, prostaglandin E1, serotonin, and histamine. (From ref. 109, with permission.)

include a subset of the mechanically insensitive afferents described above (Fig. 5).

The response of CMHs and AMHs to a number of chemicals, released locally following injury, that may mediate or facilitate the inflammatory process has been studied. These inflammatory mediators include bradykinin, prostaglandins, leukotrienes, serotonin, histamine, substance P, thromboxanes, platelet-activating factor, protons, and free radicals. Some of these chemicals activate nociceptors and therefore are directly involved in producing pain, while others lead to a sensitization of the nociceptor response to natural stimuli and therefore play a role in primary hyperalgesia. A brief description of agents capable of activating nociceptors is given in this section. (See Chap. 33 for further discussion.)

Bradykinin

Bradykinin is released upon tissue injury and is present in inflammatory exudates (34,100,130). Bradykinin induces pain

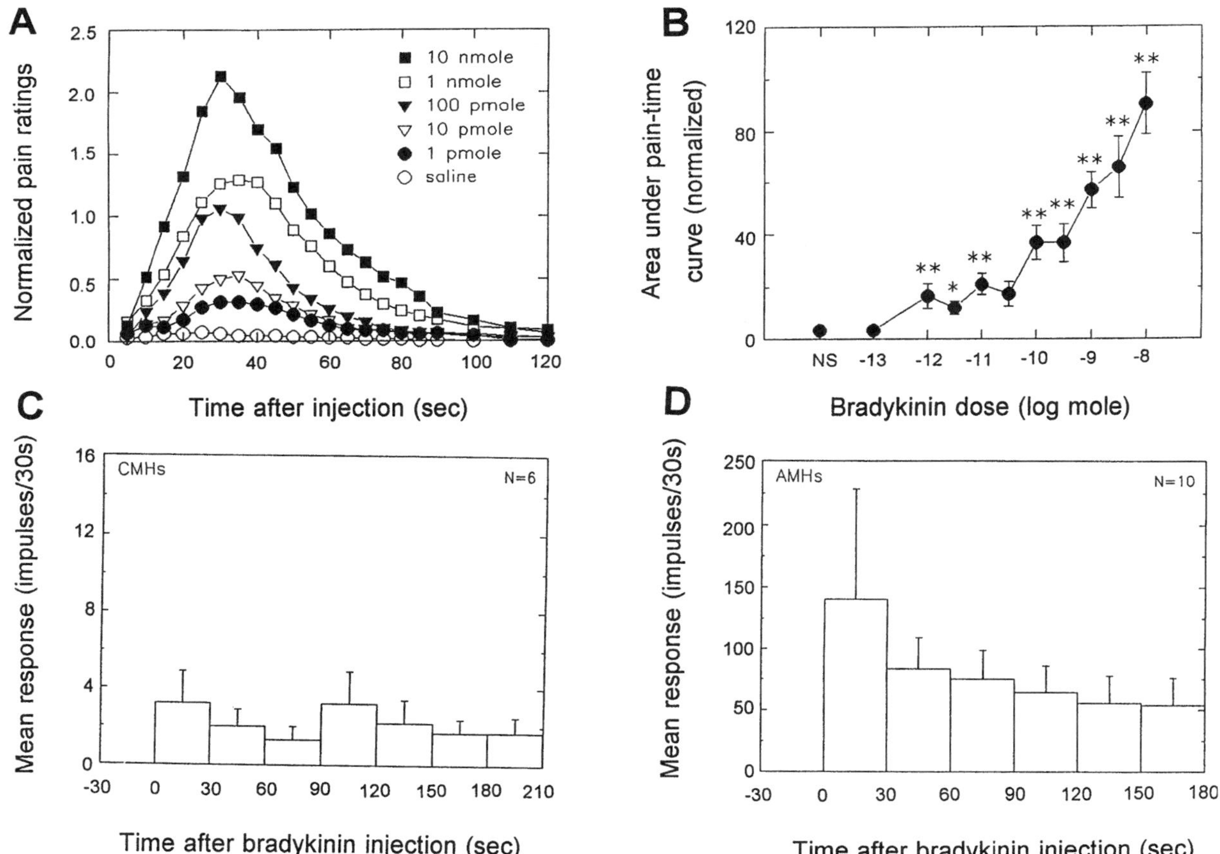

Figure 6. Bradykinin-induced pain in humans and evoked response in cutaneous nociceptors. **A:** Time course of bradykinin-evoked pain. Varying doses of bradykinin were injected in a 10-μl volume intradermally in volunteers. Ratings of pain intensity were obtained every 5 sec after injection. Pain ratings were normalized by dividing that subject's rating to a 45°C, 1 sec stimulus delivered at the beginning of the session. **B:** Bradykinin-evoked pain is dose related. Mean values for the integrated area under the curves in A is plotted against the dose of bradykinin injected. **C and D:** Bradykinin-evoked activity in C-fiber and A-fiber nociceptors (CMHs and AMHs) following the intradermal injection of 10 nmol bradykinin to their receptive fields. In C, the mean response of CMHs (6 of 10) that responded to the injection is plotted; in D, the mean evoked response in AMHs (10 of 17). These nociceptors are normally quiescent and are activated only by external stimuli. (Adapted from refs. 66 and 96, with permission.)

in man when given intradermally (Fig. 6A,B),intraarterially, or intraperitoneally (26,28,37,38,45,93,96). In addition to evoking pain, intradermal injection of bradykinin produces hyperalgesia to heat stimuli as well (96).

Bradykinin administered in the region of the receptive field of CMHs and AMHs results in an evoked response in the fibers (Fig. 6C,D) (6,49,50,66,83,112). However, a pronounced tachyphylaxis of the evoked response is observed following repeated administrations of bradykinin. The bradykinin-induced transient sensitization of the response of nociceptors to heat stimuli (66,71,75) correlates with the transient hyperalgesia to heat observed in humans.

Protons

The tissue pH at sites of inflammation is acidotic. This has led to the hypothesis that low pH levels may contribute to the pain and hyperalgesia associated with inflammation. Continuous administration of low pH solutions in humans causes pain and hyperalgesia to mechanical stimuli (146). This correlates with the recent observation that protons selectively activate nociceptors and produce a sensitization of nociceptors to mechanical stimuli (145).

Serotonin

Mast cells, upon degranulation, release platelet-activating factor. The latter, in turn, leads to serotonin release from platelets. Serotonin evokes pain when applied topically to a human blister base (128) and can activate nociceptors (41,83). Serotonin can also potentiate the pain induced by bradykinin (41,128,140) and enhance the response of nociceptors to bradykinin (40,60,83,102,113).

Nociceptors and Cold Pain Sensation

The commonly studied CMHs and AMHs in general respond meagerly to cooling stimuli. Thus, these nociceptors are less likely to be responsible for cold induced pain. Klement and Arndt (69) demonstrated that cold pain could be evoked by cold stimuli applied in the lumen of veins of human subjects. A local anesthetic applied within the vein, but not in the overlying skin, abolished the cold pain sensibility. Cold pain may, therefore, be signaled by vascular or perivascular afferents.

CORRELATION OF NOCICEPTOR ACTIVITY WITH PAIN SENSATIONS

Glabrous Skin

C-Fiber Mechano-Heat Nociceptor (CMHs)

In normal glabrous skin of the hand, heat stimuli at temperatures near the pain threshold in humans (i.e., around 45°C) activate two types of fibers, the CMH nociceptors (not AMHs) and the warm fibers. Hence, the warm fibers and CMHs are potential candidates for encoding information about noxious heat stimuli. Warm fibers respond vigorously to gentle warming of the skin (31,72). The response of warm fibers to stimuli in the noxious heat range, however is not monotonic over this temperature range (Fig. 1). In the example shown in Fig. 1, the total evoked response at 49°C was less than that at 45°C. Psychophysical studies done in man demonstrate that pain increases monotonically with stimulus intensities between 40 and 50°C (80). The warm fibers do not encode for stimulus intensity across this range of noxious stimuli. In contrast, the responses of CMHs increase monotonically over this temperature range (Fig. 1). CMHs are therefore the most likely candidates to signal the sensation of heat pain from the glabrous skin of the hand (80).

Other lines of evidence further support a role of CMHs in pain sensation. Human judgments of intensity of pain to stimuli over the range of 41° to 49°C correlate well with the activity of CMH nociceptors over this range (Fig. 7)(111). The latency to pain sensation (i.e., time from onset of stimulus to detection of pain) on glabrous skin following a step increase in temperature change is long and consistent with input from the slowly conducting CMHs (21). Selective ischemic or local anesthetic blocks of peripheral nerves indicate that C-fiber function is essential for thermal pain perception near the pain threshold (143,158). Stimulus interaction effects observed in psychophysical studies (80) are also observed in recordings from CMHs. Finally, in patients with congenital insensitivity to pain, examination of the peripheral nerves indicates an absence of C fibers (13).

Microneurographic Recordings in Human

Microneurography involves percutaneous insertion of a microelectrode into fascicles of nerves such as the superficial radial or median nerves at the wrist. This technique has been used to record from nociceptive afferents in awake humans. These studies have confirmed that the properties of nociceptors in man and monkey are similar (48,118). A distinct advantage of the microneurographic studies is that it allows direct correlations between the discharges of nociceptors and the reported sensations of the awake subject. In some experiments, the microelectrode has also been used to stimulate the identified, single nerve fiber evoking specific sensations.

Multiple lines of evidence from microneurographic studies in humans demonstrates the capacity of activity in CMHs to signal pain (Fig. 8A).Intraneural electrical stimulation of presumed single identified CMHs in humans elicits pain (155). In awake humans, the threshold for activation of CMHs by heat stimuli is just below the pain threshold (46,164). In addition, a

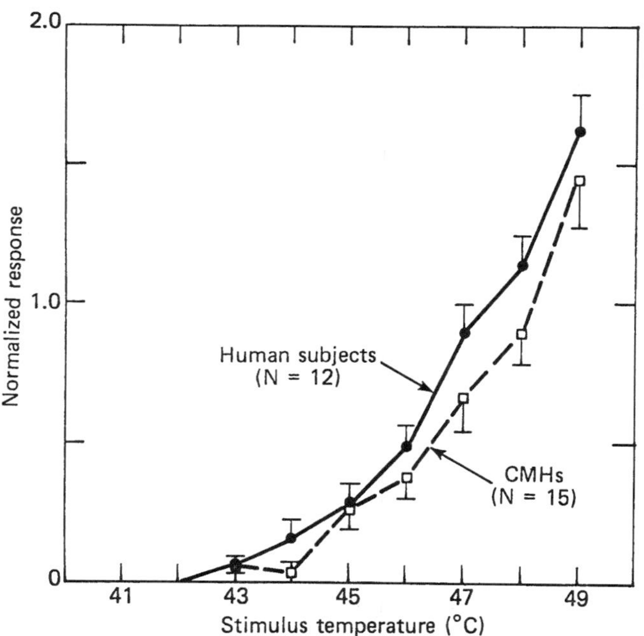

Figure 7. Correlation of C-fiber nociceptor response in monkey with pain ratings of human subjects. The close match between the curves supports a role of C-fiber nociceptors in heat pain sensation from the glabrous skin. The heat sequence consisted of an initial 45°C stimulus followed by a random sequence of nine stimuli that ranged from 41°C to 49°C in 1°C increments. Human judgments of pain were measured with a magnitude-estimation technique: Subjects assigned an arbitrary number (the modulus) to the magnitude of pain evoked by the first 45°C stimulus and judged the painfulness of all subsequent stimuli as a ratio of this modulus. The response to a given stimulus was normalized by dividing by the modulus for each human subject or by the average response to the first 45°C stimulus for the CMHs. (From ref. 111, with permission.)

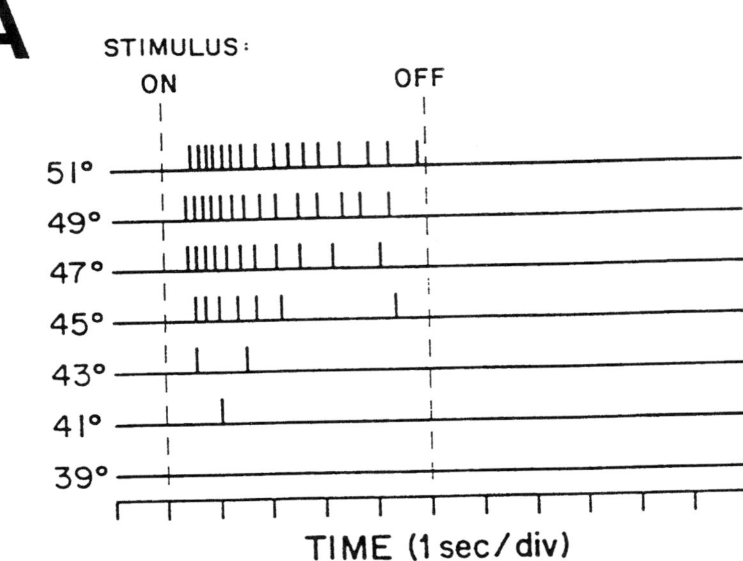

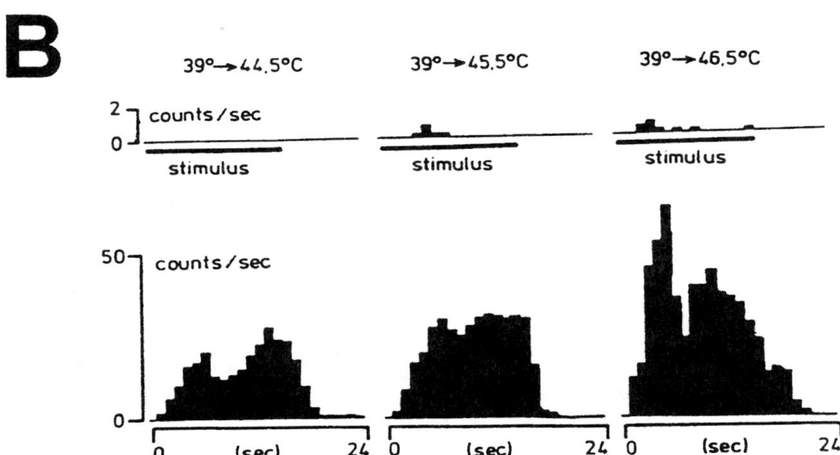

Figure 8. Microneurographic recordings of C-fiber and A-fiber nociceptors (CMH and AMH) in humans. **A:** Responses of CMH to graded heat stimuli. The receptive field of this unit was located on the dorsum of the foot. Each vertical line represents an action potential. Stimuli were delivered in ascending order at 30-sec intervals. The left and right *dashed lines* represent the onset and the offset of the heat stimuli (Reproduced with permission from ref. 156). **B:** Response of two AMHs to radiant heat stimuli. Note the relatively low discharge and prolonged latency to activation of the fiber in the *top panel* and the high discharge frequency and relatively short latency to activation after the onset of the heat stimulus in the fiber in the *bottom panel.* The *top panel* may represent a type I AMH, while the *bottom panel* may be a type II AMH. (Adapted from ref. 1, with permission.)

linear relationship exists between responses of CMHs and ratings of pain over the temperature range of 39° to 51°C (156).

AMHs and Pain

A prolonged heat stimulus to the glabrous skin of the hand in human subjects evokes substantial pain for the duration of the stimulus. While CMHs have a prominent discharge during the early phase of the stimulus, this response adapts within seconds to a low frequency of firing. In contrast, type I AMHs are initially unresponsive, but then discharge vigorously. Therefore, type I AMHs likely contribute to the pain during a sustained high-intensity heat stimulus (110).

Hairy Skin

Unlike glabrous skin, when the hairy skin in human is briefly touched with a hot object or when the skin temperature is rapidly increased (e.g., with a laser stimulator) a double pain sensation is evoked. An initial perception of a sharp pricking sensation is followed by a burning feeling that occurs after a brief delay during which no sensation is perceived (38a) (Fig. 9). The initial sensation, termed "first pain," is elicited with a short latency of approximately 400 msec (15,21,90). The delayed sensation is called "second pain." Myelinated afferent fibers must signal the first pain, since the conduction velocities of CMHs are too slow to account for latency of response to first pain (21). The receptor activation latency (time between stimulus onset and receptor activation) to heat stimuli of type I AMHs is too long to account for the short latency of the "first pain" sensation (Fig. 8B). The type II AMHs described earlier are ideally suited to signal the first pain sensation (Figs. 2 and 8B). Type II AMHs have thermal thresholds near the threshold temperature for eliciting first pain (35). Also, the receptor activation of these AMHs is short (160). Finally, type II AMHs often exhibit a burst of activity at the onset of the heat stimulus that is consistent with the perception of a momentary pricking sensation. The failure to find type II AMHs on the glabrous skin of the hand in monkey correlates with the absence of a first pain sensation to heat stimuli applied to the glabrous skin of the human hand (21).

Discrepancies Between Nociceptor Responses and Sensations of Pain

There are certain discrepancies between the response properties of nociceptors and the subjective sensations of pain. The nociceptor thresholds are, in general, lower than psychophysical pain thresholds (2,7,14,161,162,164). Thus, low levels of activity in nociceptors may not always lead to the sensation of pain. It is likely that a summation of nociceptor

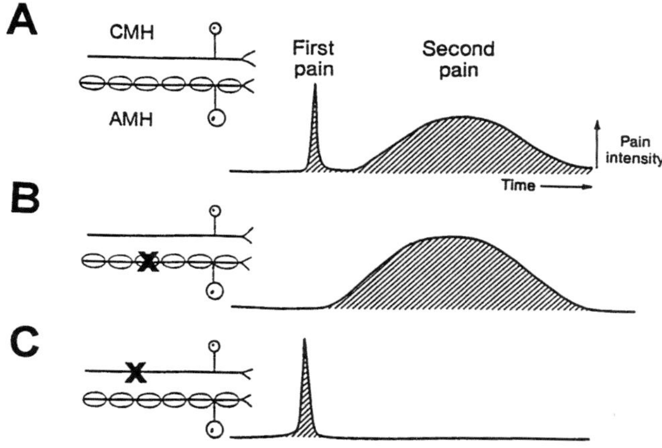

Figure 9. Schematic representation of first pain and second pain sensations following a noxious stimulus to the hairy skin (**A**). The first pain sensation is abolished when the A fibers are blocked (**B**), while the second pain sensation is abolished when the C fibers are blocked (**C**). (From ref. 38a, with permission.)

input is necessary for sensory detection (122). Both spatial and temporal summation of nociceptor input at central levels may contribute to the overall sensation of pain under most circumstances. Central mechanisms for attention quite obviously play a crucial role in whether and how much nociceptor activity leads to the perception of pain. It is also probable that receptors other than nociceptor signal pain in certain circumstances. For example, the pain to light touch that occurs after certain nerve injuries or with tissue injury appears to be signaled by activity in low-threshold mechanoreceptors (20, 123).

Another paradox with regard to mechanically induced pain is that a mechanical stimulus that evokes the same level of activity in a C-fiber nociceptor as a heat stimulus evokes less pain than the heat stimulus (164). In addition, the mechanical threshold for activating nociceptors is well below the pain threshold. This apparent discrepancy could be due to the spatial summation (i.e., recruitment of more nociceptors) associated with the larger area of heat stimuli compared to the commonly used mechanical stimuli. Alternatively, the coactivation of low-threshold mechanoreceptors with the mechanical, but not the heat, stimulus could result in suppression of pain via a "gate-control" mechanism (101).

Nociceptive afferents are often vigorously activated by mechanical stimuli that are reported to be nonpainful (46,164). As shown in Fig. 3, C-fiber nociceptors in humans display a monotonically increasing response for short-duration mechanical stimuli ranging from the innocuous into the noxious range. In this study, the mechanical stimulus was a light metal cylinder (0.3 g) that was shot at the skin at different velocities. All of the C fibers studied responded to stimuli that were not rated as painful by human subjects. At the mean pain threshold (11 m/sec), the mean evoked response was nine action potentials (70).

For long-duration mechanical stimuli, the response of nociceptors to suprathreshold stimuli adapt with time. However, when similar long-duration mechanical stimuli are applied to human subjects, pain increases throughout the stimulus (3). A hypothesis postulated for this apparent discrepancy is that recruitment of activity in nociceptors that innervate nearby skin might contribute to the increased pain with time (127). This hypothesis is based on the observation that when a stimulus was applied outside the receptive field of A-fiber nociceptors, the evoked response began several seconds after the stimulus onset and did not adapt.

RESPONSE PROPERTIES OF NOCICEPTORS IN INJURED SKIN

An unique characteristic of the nociceptor system is the enhanced sensitivity to pain following tissue injury. This phenomenon of hyperalgesia is characterized by a leftward shift of the stimulus-response function that relates magnitude of pain to stimulus intensity. The psychophysical observations are a lowered threshold for pain and an enhanced pain to suprathreshold stimuli (see Chap. 41). Hyperalgesia may also be associated with ongoing or spontaneous pain, i.e., pain in the absence of an external stimulus. Hyperalgesia is a common clinical feature in neuropathic conditions such as postherpetic neuralgia, diabetic neuropathy, and certain cases of traumatic nerve injury.

Primary and Secondary Hyperalgesia

Classic studies on the sensory consequences of cutaneous injury led to the description of two types of hyperalgesia based on the location relative to the injury site (52,91). Hyperalgesia at the site of injury is termed primary hyperalgesia. The hyperalgesia that occurs in the undamaged skin that surrounds the injury site is termed secondary hyperalgesia (89,91). Primary and secondary hyperalgesia differ both in their sensory characteristics and their underlying neural mechanisms.

Nociceptor Sensitization: Role in Primary Hyperalgesia

When the glabrous skin of the hand is burned, marked hyperalgesia to heat develops at the site of cutaneous injury (110). The hyperalgesia is manifest as a leftward shift of the stimulus-response function that relates magnitude of pain to stimulus intensity (Fig. 10). For example, a low heat stimulus (41°C) after injury was as painful as a high stimulus (49°C) prior to injury.

There is considerable evidence to support the concept that the primary hyperalgesia to heat stimuli that develops at the site of a burn injury is mediated by sensitization of nociceptors (77,110). Sensitization is a neurophysiologic phenomenon that corresponds to the psychophysical phenomenon of hyperalgesia. Sensitization is characterized by a lowering in threshold, an increased response to suprathreshold stimuli, and ongoing spontaneous activity (5,8,11).

Sensitization of nociceptors to heat stimuli has been extensively studied and is thought to be the peripheral neural mechanism of primary hyperalgesia to heat. Several different injury stimuli, e.g., heat, mechanical, inflammation and exogenous chemicals such as mustard oil, have been used to invoke sensitization of AMHs and CMHs. The stimulus response functions of AMH and CMH nociceptors that innervated glabrous skin obtained before and after a cutaneous burn injury to their receptive fields are shown in Fig. 10.

The relative roles of AMHs and CMHs in primary heat hyperalgesia varies with the skin type. In hairy skin, both AMHs and CMHs are sensitized to heat stimuli following an injury. Psychophysical studies indicate that in hairy skin CMHs may play a dominant role in the heat hyperalgesia (77) (Fig. 11). In the glabrous skin, AMHs (most of which are not initially responsive to mild noxious heat stimuli), develop pronounced heat sensitivity following injury (19,110). In contrast to the hairy skin, the CMHs in glabrous skin show an increased threshold and a decreased response to suprathreshold stimuli after injury (Fig. 10). These observations suggest that AMHs, not CMHs, code for the thermal hyperalgesia in the primary zone that results from thermal injuries to the glabrous skin.

It was initially assumed that sensitization of nociceptors to mechanical stimuli might parallel the sensitization to heat stimuli and account for the mechanical hyperalgesia in the zone of primary hyperalgesia. However, sensitization to mechanical stimuli was not observed in either CMHs or AMHs following heat or mechanical injury (19,20,152).

The development of mechanical sensitivity in a subgroup of afferents that are initially insensitive to mechanical stimuli may contribute to hyperalgesia to mechanical stimuli (33). Such a mechanism would be similar to the mechanism of heat hyperalgesia in glabrous skin, where AMHs that are initially unresponsive to heat stimuli become sensitized. An alternate peripheral mechanism that may account for primary hyperalgesia to mechanical stimuli may be expansion of the receptive field of a nociceptor into an adjacent area of injury. The receptive fields of AMH fibers as well as some CMH fibers expand into the area of an adjacent heat (152) or mechanical (127) injury. As a consequence of this expansion, heat or mechanical stimuli delivered after the injury will activate a greater number of fibers. This spatial summation provides a mechanism for primary hyperalgesia. The mechanical thresholds within the expansion areas, however, are similar to those in the original receptive fields (152). Hence, this form of sensitization may not account for the marked decrease in threshold observed psychophysically.

Another possible mechanism of mechanical hyperalgesia in the primary zone is the loss of central inhibition. Under usual circumstances, the production of pain from activation of nociceptors with mechanical stimuli is inhibited in the central nervous system by the concurrent activation of low-threshold mechanoreceptors (164). There is evidence that a cutaneous injury results in a decreased responsiveness of low-threshold mechanoreceptors (5). Hyperalgesia to mechanical stimuli in the primary zone could therefore be due to suppression of input from low-threshold mechanoreceptors, which would lead to a central disinhibition of nociceptor input and result in enhanced pain (viz., hyperalgesia).

Although a burn injury does not lead to a reduction in mechanical threshold for nociceptors, exposure of nociceptors to certain mediators of inflammatory pain nevertheless may cause nociceptors to become sensitized to mechanical as well as heat stimuli (33,97). Aδ fiber nociceptors can be sensitized to mechanical stimuli after exposure to a mixture of algesic inflammatory mediators (bradykinin, histamine, serotonin, and prostaglandin E_1) (33).

Secondary Hyperalgesia

The increased painfulness of stimuli applied to the uninjured region outside an area of injury is termed secondary hyperalgesia. In contrast to primary hyperalgesia, secondary hyperalgesia is characterized by enhanced pain to only mechanical stimuli and not to heat stimuli. There also is no hyperalgesia to cooling stimuli. The distinction between primary and secondary hyperalgesia to mechanical stimuli is to some extent artificial. Mechanisms that account for hyperalgesia to mechanical stimuli in the secondary zone may also account for mechanical hyperalgesia in the primary zone.

The Peripheral vs. Central Controversy

The question of how hyperalgesia spreads from the site of injury to surrounding undamaged tissue is of considerable

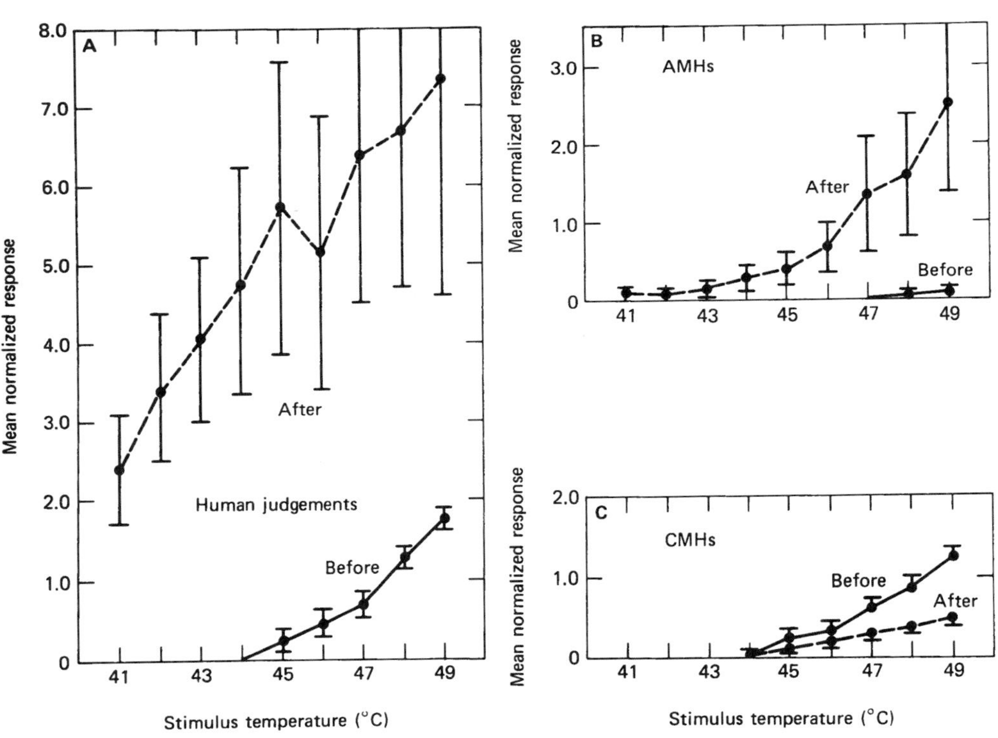

Figure 10. Primary hyperalgesia and sensitization of A-fiber nociceptors after a cutaneous injury to the glabrous skin. Responses to heat stimuli were obtained 5 min before and 10 min after a 53°C, 30-sec burn to the glabrous skin of the hand. The burn resulted in increases in the magnitude of pain (hyperalgesia) in human subjects that were matched by enhanced responses (sensitization) in type I AMHs in monkey. In contrast, CMHs exhibited decreased sensitivity after the burn. **A:** Human judgments of pain (n=8). **B:** Responses of A-fiber nociceptive afferents (type I AMHs) in monkeys (n=14). **C:** Responses of C-fiber nociceptive afferents (CMHs) in monkeys (n=15). The heat sequence and normalization is similar to that described in Fig. 7. Because the AMHs did not respond to the 45°C stimulus before the burn, the AMH data were normalized by dividing by the response to the first 45°C after the burn. (From ref. 110, with permission.)

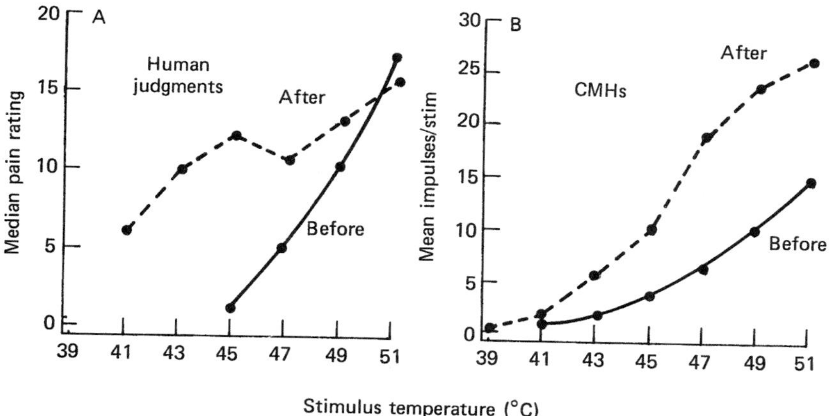

Figure 11. Hyperalgesia and sensitization of C-fiber nociceptors after a burn to the hairy skin. Responses to heat stimuli were obtained immediately before and 10 min after a 50°C, 100-sec burn to the forearm of human volunteers and anesthetized monkey. The burn resulted in a decrease in the pain threshold and an increase in the painfulness to mild heat stimuli (e.g., 41–45°C), but not to intense heat stimuli. In contrast, the burn resulted in an enhanced response of the C-fiber nociceptor to all temperatures. **A:** Median maximum pain ratings in human subjects (*n*=13). **B:** Mean total number of impulses per stimulus in C-fiber nociceptors (*n*=12). (Adapted from ref. 77a, with permission.)

importance in the neurobiology of pain. Earlier hypotheses based on the monumental works of Lewis (91) and Hardy et al. (52) were conflicting. Both investigators proposed that sensitization is initiated by the generation of action potentials in nociceptive afferents. The proposed mechanisms, however, differed in their emphasis on the relative importance of the peripheral and central nervous systems. While Lewis proposed that the local, antidromic spread of action potentials from the peripheral terminals of one nociceptor to another was instrumental in the spread of hyperalgesia, Hardy et al. postulated that secondary hyperalgesia was due to the orthodromic conduction of impulses resulting in a spreading sensitization in the spinal cord.

Peripheral Mechanisms

The evidence for a peripheral mechanism for secondary hyperalgesia, possibly via the local release of neuropeptides, is not convincing. For example, heat injury to one half of the receptive field of nociceptors does not alter sensitivity of the other half to heat stimuli (153). In addition, an injury adjacent to the receptive field of nociceptors fails to alter the responses of CMHs in monkey (20) and rat (126).

Although most injuries (e.g., cuts, burns, and certain chemical injuries) applied adjacent to receptive fields do not sensitize nociceptors, one type of injury does appear to lead to spreading sensitization. Reeh et al. (127) reported that a prolonged, intense, pressure stimulus applied immediately adjacent to mechanically sensitive A-fiber, but not C-fiber nociceptors leads to a lowered mechanical threshold within the receptive field.

Central Mechanisms

If peripheral mechanisms do not provide a satisfactory explanation for secondary hyperalgesia, central mechanisms need to be examined. Indeed, enhanced responsiveness of spinal dorsal horn neurons to mechanical stimuli have been demonstrated after cutaneous injury (141). Substantial evidence clearly indicates that the peripheral signal for pain does not reside exclusively with nociceptors. Under pathologic circumstances, other receptor types, such as low-threshold

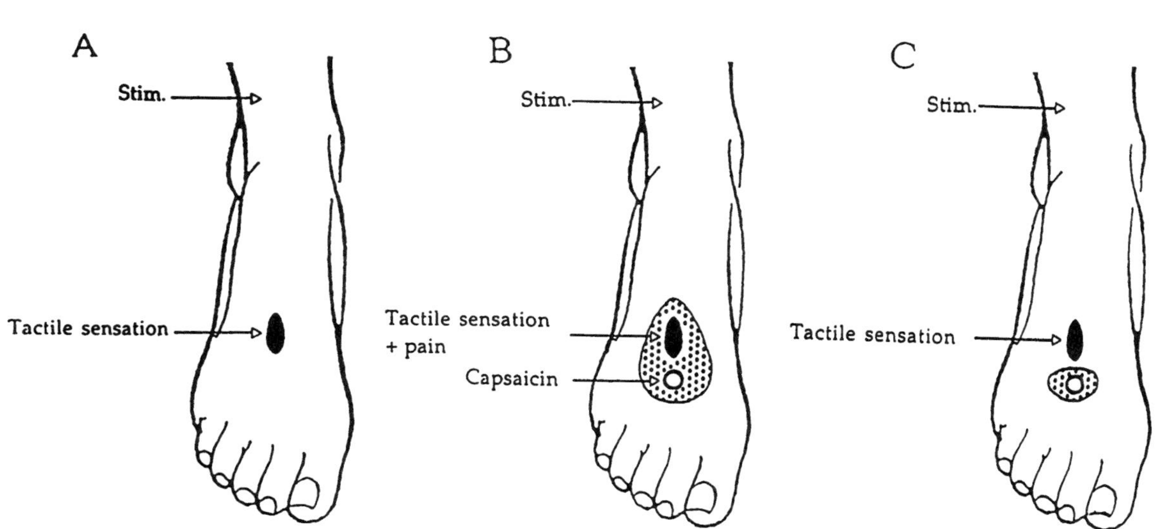

Figure 12. Microneurographic evidence that large-diameter myelinated fibers signal the pain to light touch in the zone of secondary hyperalgesia. **A:** Intraneural electrical stimulation of the superficial peroneal nerve at a low intensity evoked a purely tactile (nonpainful) sensation projected to a small skin area on the dorsum of the foot *(black area).* **B:** Following intradermal injection of capsaicin (100 μg in 10 μl) adjacent to the projected zone (at the site indicated by the *open circle),* a zone of secondary hyperalgesia developed that overlapped the sensory projection field *(stipled area).* Now, intraneural stimulation at the same intensity and frequency as in A was perceived as a tactile sensation accompanied by pain. **C:** During recovery, when the zone of secondary hyperalgesia no longer overlapped the sensory projection field, the intraneural stimulation was now perceived as purely tactile, without any pain component. (From ref. 157, with permission.)

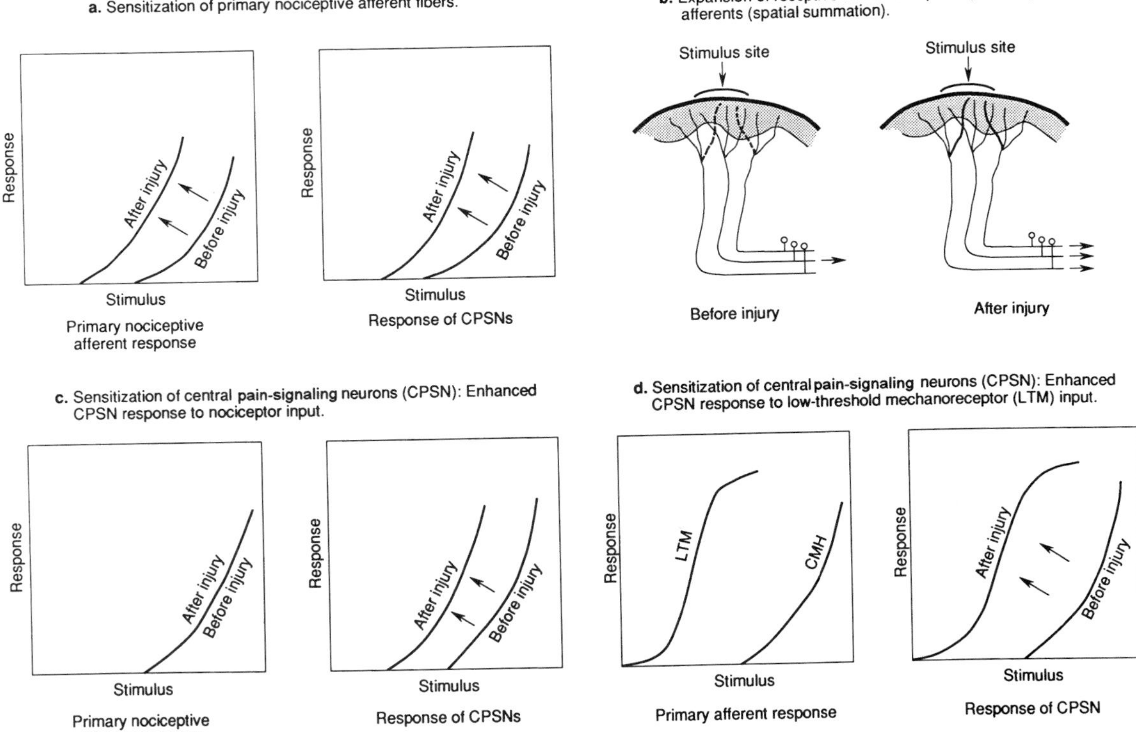

Figure 13. Schematic models for possible neural mechanisms of primary and secondary hyperalgesia. **a:** Sensitization of primary nociceptive afferents probably resulting from the injury-induced release of several chemical mediators. Primary afferent sensitization is characterized by a leftward shift in the stimulus-response function that relates neural discharge to stimulus intensity. This peripheral change will also result in a similar shift in the stimulus-response function of the central neurons. **b:** Expansion of the receptive field area of primary afferent nociceptors toward the region of an adjacent cutaneous injury. Now stimulation of the injury site leads to activation of branches of afferents that were nonresponsive before the injury *(dashed lines)*. This activation of a greater number of afferents can lead to an increased sensory response (i.e., spatial summation) from the injured peripheral site. Such a mechanism may play a role in primary hyperalgesia to heat and mechanical stimuli. **c:** Central neurons concerned with pain sensation (CPSNs) become sensitized to nociceptor input. With this mechanism there is no requirement for primary afferent sensitization. This mechanism may explain the hyperalgesia to mechanical stimuli at the primary and secondary hyperalgesia zones. **d:** CPSNs may develop an enhanced response to afferents other than nociceptors (e.g., low-threshold mechanoreceptors). This mechanism does not require peripheral sensitization. A leftward shift of the stimulus response function of CPSNs occurs. Such a mechanism may play a role in secondary hyperalgesia and in neuropathic pain. (From ref. 162, with permission.)

mechanoreceptors that are normally associated with the sensation of touch, acquire the capacity to evoke pain. This phenomenon is termed central sensitization. This principle applies not only to secondary hyperalgesia, but also to neuropathic pain states in general.

Central sensitization may result from several possible mechanisms. One possibility is that input from nociceptors may be facilitated. Alternately, central pain signaling neurons develop enhanced synaptic efficacy such that input from the normally ineffective low-threshold mechanoreceptors is now capable of activating the central neurons. Both direct recordings and indirect methods of studying the response properties of spinal neurons have supported a central mechanism for secondary hyperalgesia (27,141,167). Chapter 9 provides further details on plasticity of the central neurons that signal pain.

To determine the relative importance of peripheral and central sensitization in secondary hyperalgesia, LaMotte and colleagues (79) performed a number of experiments with intradermal capsaicin injections in volunteers. Capsaicin produces a pronounced zone of secondary hyperalgesia. A proximal nerve block prior to the intradermal injection of capsaicin prevented the development of secondary hyperalgesia in the period after recovery from the local anesthetic, 1 to 3 hours later. In contrast, in control experiments secondary hyperalgesia lasted for more than 3 hours after the capsaicin injection. Thus, when the CNS is spared the input of nociceptors at the time of the acute insult, the hyperalgesia is sharply curtailed. Central sensitization, therefore, plays a major role in secondary hyperalgesia. These studies also provide an experimental basis for the concept of preemptive analgesia in clinical practice.

The peripheral nervous system, however, plays a critical role in the maintenance of the central sensitization. When the capsaicin injection site is cooled or anesthetized after the injection, signs of secondary hyperalgesia are either eliminated or substantially reduced (79). Thus, to maintain the secondary hyperalgesia, input from the sensitized nociceptive neurons in the zone of primary hyperalgesia is essential.

Another line of evidence for central mechanisms in secondary hyperalgesia was reported by Torebjörk and colleagues (157). They performed intraneural microstimulation in awake human subjects. A microelectrode was placed within the nerve, and the electrical stimulus adjusted to evoke tactile paresthesias referable to a particular cutaneous area. Capsaicin was then injected adjacent to this area such that secondary hyperalgesia was created in the area of referred paresthesias. When the same electrical stimulus was repeated, it now evoked pain (Fig. 12). Thus, stimulation of primary afferent fibers normally concerned with tactile sensibility evoked pain when (but not before) secondary hyperalgesia was produced.

Possible neural mechanisms for primary and secondary hyperalgesia are summarized in a schematic form in Fig. 13.

NOCICEPTORS IN OTHER SOMATIC TISSUES

A principal reason for the major advances in our understanding of nociception in the skin is the relative ease with which parallel psychophysical studies in humans and neurophysiologic studies in animals can be conducted. Such correlative studies of nociceptor function in organs other than the skin, however, have proved to be difficult.

For many tissues (i.e., tooth pulp and cornea), pain is the only sensation that can be evoked. Thus, the afferent fibers that innervate these structures can be considered as nociceptors that signal pain. In the case of other deep tissues, such as muscle, fascia, joints, and bone, diverse perceptual possibilities complicate analysis. While some of the afferents from deep tissues may be involved in pain, other fibers may play a role in normal organ function or may be involved in sensations other than pain.

Behavioral and clinical studies indicate that there are important differences between cutaneous and deep pain. For example, unlike cutaneous pain, deep pain is diffuse and poorly localized. Deep pain may be associated with strong autonomic responses such as sweating, changes in heart rate, blood pressure, and respiration.

Joint

Much of what is known about joint afferent fibers is based on studies in cat by Schmidt and coworkers (for reviews see 55,134,138). The knee joint of the cat is primarily innervated by two nerves, the medial and the posterior articular nerves (MAN and PAN) (Table 1). Each nerve contains approximately 650 afferent fibers, the majority of which belong to group III (thinly myelinated) and group IV (unmyelinated) fibers (42,84,144). Nociceptors in the joint are located in the joint capsule and ligaments, bone, periosteum, articular fat pads, and perivascular sites, but probably not in the joint cartilage. The sensory endings of the group III and IV nerve fibers are unmyelinated and are not surrounded by perineurium. The branched, terminal tree of these fibers have a string-of-beads appearance that may represent multiple receptive sites in the nerve endings (55,58).

Afferent fibers that innervate the knee joint have been classified into five categories based on their sensitivities to pressure and joint movements. Classes 1 and 2 are low-threshold units that are excited strongly or weakly, respectively, by innocuous pressure and movements of the knee joint. Class 3 is high-threshold units that are activated only by noxious pressure or movements exceeding the working range of the joint. Class 4 units respond to strong pressure to the knee, but not to movement. Class 5 consists of units that do not react to any mechanical stimulus to the normal joint. These afferents are referred to as "silent nociceptors" (132). In the normal joint, the high-threshold units are thought to signal pain evoked by extreme joint movement (44,135,136).

Experimentally induced arthritis results in dramatic changes in the response properties of joint afferents (56,57, 137). Sensitization is observed in all types of afferent fibers. The increased responsiveness may be present as afferent activation of high-threshold units by movements in the working range, activation by pressure, or an induction or increase in resting discharges. The composition of the articular nerves in cat has been analyzed histologically and the discharge properties of individual fine afferents characterized. These studies have enabled investigators to estimate the number of impulses reaching the spinal cord in response to simple movements of the knee joint under both normal and inflamed conditions (55). These estimates indicate that following inflammation there is more than a sixfold increase in impulses that enter the spinal cord (Table 2). This increase in afferent signals is the result of both an increase in the percentage of fibers having resting activity and an increase in their mean discharge frequency. Chemical mediators of inflammation, such as bradykinin, prostaglandins, leukotrienes, potassium ions, serotonin, and possibly interleukins, are considered to play an important role in the sensitization of joint afferent fibers (Fig. 14) (56,59,133). Thus, the enhanced pain that accompanies arthritis is likely the results of inflammation-induced sensitization of articular afferents. Studies by Levine and coworkers (87,88) have suggested that peptides such as substance P released from the peripheral terminals of small diameter afferent fibers may contribute to the severity of joint injury. In addition, articular tissues are innervated by sympathetic efferents. A modulatory role for the sympathetic fibers via a prostaglandin-mediated mechanism has been suggested in arthritis (4).

Cornea

The primary afferent fibers that innervate the cornea have an activation threshold that is comparable to that of low-threshold mechanoreceptors in skin (10,151). This is reasonable since what would be considered mild mechanical stimuli elsewhere may induce injury when applied to the cornea. Low-intensity stimuli to the cornea can certainly induce pain.

Although pain is generally considered to be the only sensation that can be elicited from stimulation of the cornea, studies indicate that thermal and mechanical stimuli can be differentiated (12,65,85). There are, however, no obvious specialized sense organs in the cornea. Sensory terminals end in the intraepithelial tissue as unmyelinated fibers with an innervation density that is 300 to 600 times greater than in skin (131). The mechanical receptive fields of the nociceptors are uniformly sensitive and broad, covering as much as 20% of the corneal surface.

Tooth Pulp

Pain is the predominant sensation evoked by stimulation of the tooth pulp. The tooth pulp and dentin are innervated by Aδ and C fibers (18,53) that terminate as free nerve endings.

Table 1. COMPOSITION OF THE CAT'S ARTICULAR NERVES

Fibers (group)	Medial articular nerve (MAN)	Posterior articular nerve (PAN)
I	–	27 (4%)
II	59 (9%)	149 (22%)
III	131 (21%)	94 (14%)
IV	440 (70%)	410 (60%)
Afferents	630 (100%)	680 (100%)
Sympathetic	500	515

Table 2. INFLUENCE OF AN ACUTE INFLAMMATION ON AFFERENT IMPULSES REACHING THE SPINAL CORD

	Joint		
Medial articular nerve	Normal	Inflamed	Change
Resting activity (impulses/30 sec)	1,800	11,100	× 6.2
Low-threshold units	240 fibers	550 fibers	× 2.3
Movement (impulses/30 sec)	4,400	30,900	× 7.0

The receptors are polymodal, i.e., they respond to chemical, thermal, and mechanical stimuli (36,43,47,98). Single fiber recordings suggest that Aδ fibers are responsible for dentinal pain, whereas C fibers may be responsible for pain originating from the pulp (114,115,163).

Muscle

Muscle pain often results from strenuous exercise, direct trauma, inflammation, and during sustained muscle spasms (for reviews, see 103 and 104). Electrical stimulation of nerve fascicles in awake humans demonstrates that deep muscle pain is dependent on activation of small-diameter afferent fibers (156). Receptors for the muscle's nociceptive afferents are free nerve endings found in the connective tissue of the muscle, between muscle fibers, in blood vessel walls, and in tendons.

Two groups of fibers, groups III and IV, are thought to be responsible for signaling nociception in muscles. The small myelinated group III fibers have conduction velocities from 2.5 to 20 m/sec (119). The unmyelinated group IV fibers have conduction velocities less than 2.5 m/sec (41,60,105). Of all of the group III and IV fibers, 40% are thought to be nociceptors.

Groups III and IV muscle afferent fibers have been characterized by their vigorous response to endogenous chemicals such as bradykinin, serotonin, histamine, and potassium. Bradykinin-responsive fibers are selectively sensitive to high-intensity mechanical stimuli (120). Muscle nociceptors may also be sensitized by catecholamines (67) and by changes in the biochemical environment resulting from hypoxia and impaired metabolism. The local tenderness often associated with muscle trauma or unaccustomed exercise may result from sensitization of muscle nociceptors by endogenously released chemicals.

OTHER FUNCTIONS OF NOCICEPTORS

A large proportion of peripheral nerve fibers are unmyelinated. Cutaneous nerves have more than a fourfold higher number of small diameter Aδ and C fibers than the larger, myelinated Aβ fibers (25,117). In addition, only about 20% of the C fibers in cutaneous nerves are sympathetic efferents. The

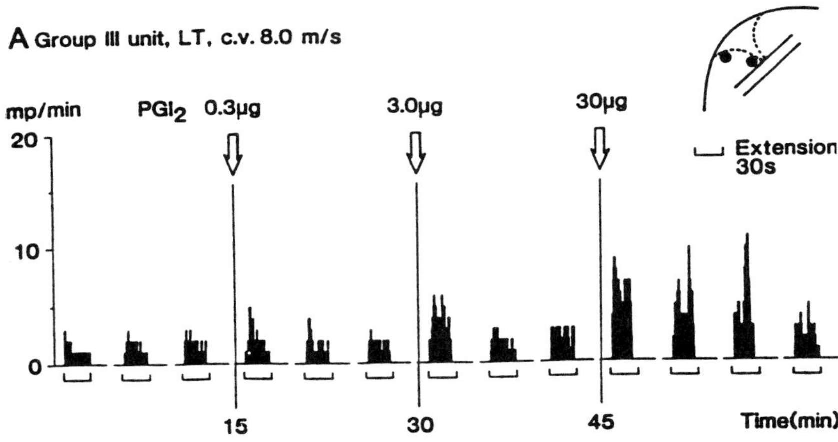

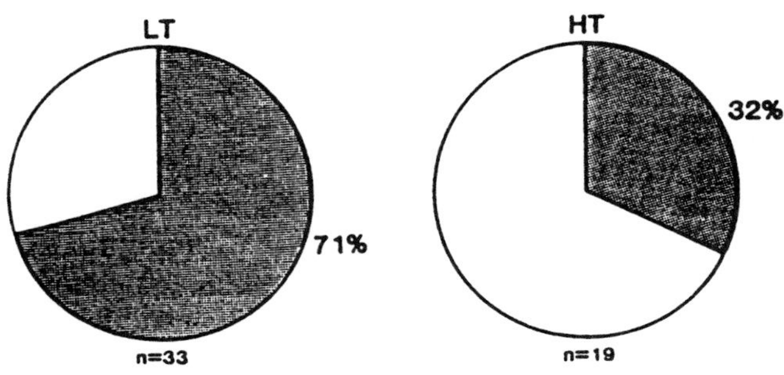

Figure 14. Prostaglandin I_2 (PGI_2)-induced sensitization of afferents from the knee joint to passive movements of the knee. **A:** Responses to movements in a low-threshold group III unit with two receptive fields in the knee joint (displayed as impulses per second) showing increasing response following injection of three different doses of PGI_2 **B:** Proportions of low-threshold (LT) and high-threshold (HT) group III and group IV units sensitized (*shaded area*) to movement by PGI_2. (Adapted from ref. 137a, with permission.)

majority of small fibers in peripheral nerves are hence afferents. One needs to explain why the rarely activated nociceptive system requires such a high number of signal lines in comparison to the mechanoreceptor system that provides information for the more commonly utilized and complex tactile detection system. A possible explanation is that nociceptors, apart from signaling pain, serve other regulatory and trophic functions (74,99).

Lewis (90) demonstrated that nociceptors likely account for the flare that surrounds an acute injury. C fibers may serve several other effector functions, such as regulation of blood flow and vascular permeability; trophic functions, such as maintenance and repair of skin integrity; and immunologic processes, such as emigration of leukocytes at sites of tissue injury (68,116). Small afferent fibers are also considered to play a role in the regulation of activity of autonomic ganglia and visceral smooth muscles (for reviews see 61,95,148).

Several lines of evidence indicate that capsaicin-sensitive C-fiber afferents are involved in antidromic vasodilatation, neurogenic inflammation, and axon reflex flare (24,62,63,149). The mechanism for flare is different from the mechanisms for pain. First, the size of the flare does not correlate with the intensity of pain induced by the stimulus. In humans, observations that low-firing frequencies of nociceptors may not be associated with any pain (46) may offer an explanation for flare not always being associated with pain. Second, strong mechanical stimulation adequate to excite most polymodal C fibers does not cause neurogenic vasodilation (94). Thus, flare and pain may represent two independent aspects of cutaneous small fiber function.

Flare is due to some form of a peripheral axon reflex. A noxious stimulus that activates one branch of a nociceptor results in the antidromic invasion of action potentials into adjacent branches of the receptor. This antidromic invasion, in turn, causes the release of vasoactive substances from the terminals of the nociceptor. However, the extent of the flare far exceeds the receptive field size of conventional nociceptors (7,8,22,76,124). Possible explanations for this incongruity might include the following: (a) Flare is mediated by a subpopulation of chemosensitive nociceptive fibers with large receptive fields (90). While C fibers with large, complex receptive fields have been observed (109), the time course of spread of flare from the stimulus site is too slow to be accounted for by conduction within terminal arborizations of single afferent neurons (94). (b) Axoaxonal ephaptic coupling between small fibers may be responsible for the spread of the flare reaction (98,107). (c) Flare may result from spreading depolarization along adjacent nociceptive terminals via a daisy-chain cascade mechanism (86).

ACKNOWLEDGMENTS

We appreciate the editorial assistance of J. L. Turnquist and T. V. Hartke. This research was supported by NIH grants NS-14447 and NS-26363. R. A. Meyer was supported, in part, by the U.S.Navy (N00039-92-C-0001).

REFERENCES

1. Adriaensen H, Gybels J, Handwerker HO, Van Hees J. Response properties of thinly myelinated (A-delta) fibers in human skin nerves. *J Neurophysiol* 1983;49:111–122.
2. Adriaensen H, Gybels J, Handwerker HO, Van Hees J. Suppression of C-fiber discharges upon repeated heat stimulation may explain characteristics of concomitant pain sensations. *Brain Res* 1984;302:203–211.
3. Adriaensen H, Gybels J, Handwerker HO, Van Hees J. Nociceptor discharges and sensations due to prolonged noxious mechanical stimulation—a paradox. *Hum Neurobiol* 1984;3:53–58.
4. Basbaum AI, Levine JD. The contribution of the nervous system to inflammation and inflammatory disease. *Can J Physiol Pharmacol* 1991;69:647–651.
5. Beck PW, Handwerker HO, Zimmermann M. Nervous outflow from the cat's foot during noxious radiant heat stimulation. *Brain Res* 1974;67:373–386.
6. Beck PW, Handwerker HO. Bradykinin and serotonin effects on various types of cutaneous nerve fibers. *Pflugers Arch* 1974;347:209–222.
7. Beitel RE, Dubner R. Fatigue and adaptation in unmyelinated (C) polymodal nociceptors to mechanical and thermal stimuli applied to the monkey's face. *Brain Res* 1976;112:402–406.
8. Beitel RE, Dubner R. Response of unmyelinated (C) polymodal nociceptors to thermal stimuli applied to monkey's face. *J Neurophysiol* 1976;39:1160–1175.
9. Belmonte C, Gallar J, Pozo MA, Rebollo I. Excitation by irritant chemical substances of sensory afferent units in the cat's cornea. *J Physiol (Lond)* 1991;437:709–725.
10. Belmonte C, Giraldez F. Responses of cat corneal sensory receptors to mechanical and thermal stimulation. *J Physiol (Lond)* 1981;321:355–368.
11. Bessou P, Perl ER. Response of cutaneous sensory units with unmyelinated fibers to noxious stimuli. *J Neurophysiol* 1969;32:1025–1043.
12. Beuerman RW, Tanelian DL. Corneal pain evoked by thermal stimulation. *Pain* 1979;7:1–14.
13. Biseoff A. Congenital insensitivity to pain with anhidrosis. A morphometric study of sural nerval and cutaneous receptors in the human prepuce. In: *Advances in pain research and therapy*. New York: Raven Press, 1979;3:53–65.
14. Bromm B, Jahnke MT, Treede RD. Response of human cutaneous afferents to CO2 laser stimuli causing pain. *Exp Brain Res* 1984;55:158–186.
15. Bromm B, Treede RD. Human cerebral potentials evoked by CO2 laser stimuli causing pain. *Exp Brain Res* 1987;67:153–162.
16. Burgess PR, Petit D, Warren RM. Receptor types in cat hairy skin supplied by myelinated fibers. *J Neurophysiol* 1968;31:833–848.
17. Burgess PR, Perl ER. Myelinated afferent fibres responding specifically to noxious stimulation of the skin. *J Physiol (Lond)* 1967;190:541–562.
18. Byers MR. Dental sensory receptors. *Int Rev Neurobiol* 1984;25:39–94.
19. Campbell JN, Meyer RA, LaMotte RH. Sensitization of myelinated nociceptive afferents that innervate monkey hand. *J Neurophysiol* 1979;42:1669–1679.
20. Campbell JN, Khan AA, Meyer RA, Raja SN. Responses to heat of C-fiber nociceptors in monkey are altered by injury in the receptive field but not by adjacent injury. *Pain* 1988;32:327–332.
21. Campbell JN, LaMotte RH. Latency to detection of first pain. *Brain Res* 1983;266:203–208.
22. Campbell JN, Meyer RA. Sensitization of unmyelinated nociceptive afferents in the monkey varies with skin type. *J Neurophysiol* 1983;49:98–110.
23. Campbell JN, Meyer RA. Primary Afferents and Hyperalgesia. In: Yaksh TL, ed. *Spinal afferent processing*. New York: Plenum Press, 1986;59–81.
24. Carpenter SE, Lynn B. Vascular and sensory responses of human skin to mild injury after topical treatment with capsaicin. *Br J Pharmacol* 1981;73:755–758.
25. Carter DA, Lisney SJW. The number of unmyelinated and myelinated axons in normal and regenerated rate saphenous nerve. *J Neurol Sci* 1987;80:163–171.
26. Coffman JD. The effect of aspirin on pain and hand flow responses to intra-arterial injection of bradykinin in man. *Clin Pharmacol Ther* 1966;7:26–37.
27. Cook AJ, Woolf CJ, Wall PD, McMahon SB. Dynamic receptive field plasticity in rat spinal cord dorsal horn following C-primary afferent input. *Nature* 1987;325:151–153.
28. Cormia FE, Dougherty JW. Proteolytic activity in development of pain and itching: Cutaneous reactions to bradykinin and kallikrein. *J Invest Dermatol* 1960;35:21–26.
29. Darian-Smith I, Johnson KO, Dykes R. "Cold" fiber population innervating palmar and digital skin of the monkey: Responses to cooling pulses. *J Neurophysiol* 1973;36:325–346.
30. Darian-Smith I, Johnson KO, LaMotte C, Kenins P, Shigenaga P, Ming VC. Coding of incremental changes in skin temperature by single warm fibers in the monkey. *J Neurophysiol* 1979;5:1316–1331.
31. Darian-Smith I, Johnson KO, LaMotte C, Shigenaga Y, Kenins P, Champness P. Warm fibers innervating palmar and digital skin of

the monkey: Responses to thermal stimuli. *J Neurophysiol* 1979;42: 1297–1315.
32. Davis KD, Meyer RA, Turnquist JL, Pappagallo M, Filloon TG, Campbell JN. Cutaneous injection of the capsaicin analog, NE-21610, produces analgesia to heat but not to mechanical stimuli. *Pain* 1995;62:373–378.
33. Davis KD, Meyer RA, Campbell JN. Chemosensitivity and sensitization of nociceptive afferents that innervate the hairy skin of monkey. *J Neurophysiol* 1993;69:1071–1081.
34. DiRosa M, Giroud JP, Willoughby DA. Studies of the mediators of the acute inflammatory response induced in rats in different sites by carrageenan and turpentine. *J Pathol* 1971;104:15–29.
35. Dubner R, Price DD, Beitel RE, Hu JW. Peripheral neural correlates of behavior in monkey and human related to sensory-discriminative aspects of pain. In: Anderson DJ, Mathews B, eds. *Pain in the trigeminal region.* Amsterdam: Elsevier Science, 1977; 57–66.
36. Dubner R. Neurophysiology of pain. *Dental Clin North Am* 1978; 22:11–30.
37. Ferreira SH, Moncada S, Vane JR. Indomethacin and aspirin abolish prostaglandin release from the spleen. *Nature* 1971;231: 237–239.
38. Ferreira SH. Peripheral and central analgesia. In: Bonica JJ, Lindblom U, Iggo A, eds. *Advances in pain research and therapy.* New York: Raven Press, 1983;5:627–634.
38a. Fields HL. The peripheral pain sensory system. In: *Pain.* New York: McGraw-Hill, 1987;13–40.
39. Fitzgerald M, Lynn B. The sensitization of high threshold mechanoreceptors with myelinated axons by repeated heating. *J Physiol* 1977;265:549–563.
40. Fjallbrant N, Iggo A. The effect of histamine, 5-hydroxytryptamine and acetylcholine on cutaneous afferent fibres. *J Physiol* 1961;156:578–590.
41. Fock S, Mense S. Excitatory effects of 5-hydroxytryptamine, histamine and potassium ions on muscular group IV afferent units: A comparison with bradykinin. *Brain Res* 1976;105:459–469.
42. Freeman MAR, Wyke B. The innervation of the knee joint. An anatomical and histological study in the cat. *J Anat* 1967;101: 505–532.
43. Funakoshi M, Zotterman Y. A study in the excitation of dental nerve fibers. In: Anderson DJ, ed. *Sensory mechanism in dentine.* Oxford: Pergamon Press, 1963.
44. Grigg P, Schaible HG, Schmidt RI. Mechanical sensitivity of group III and IV afferents from posterior articular nerve in normal and inflamed cat knee. *J Neurophysiol* 1986;55:635–643.
45. Guzman F, Braun C, Lim RKS. Visceral pain and the pseudoaffective response to intra-arterial injection of bradykinin and other algesic agents. *Arch Int Pharmacodynam* 1962;136:353–384.
46. Gybels J, Handwerker HO, Van Hees J. A comparison between the discharges of human nociceptive nerve fibers and the subjects ratings of his sensations. *J Physiol (Lond)* 1979;292:193–206.
47. Haegerstam G, Olgart L, Edwall L. The excitatory action of acetylcholine on intradental sensory units. *Acta Physiol Scand* 1975;93:113–18.
48. Hagbarth KE, Vallbo AB. Mechanoreceptor activity recorded percutaneously with semimicroelectrodes in human peripheral nerves. *Acta Physiol Scand* 1967;69:121–122.
49. Handwerker HO. Pharmacological modulation of the discharge of nociceptive C fibers. In: Zotterman Y, ed. *Sensory functions of the skin in primates.* Oxford: Pergamon Press, 1976;427–439.
50. Handwerker HO. Influences of algogenic substances and prostaglandins on the discharges of unmyelinated cutaneous nerve fibers identified as nociceptors. In: Bonica JJ, Albe-Fessard D, eds. *Advances in pain research and therapy.* New York: Raven Press, 1976;1:41–45.
51. Handwerker HO, Kilo S, Reeh PW. Unresponsive afferent nerve fibres in the sural nerve of the rat. *J Physiol* 1991;435:229–242.
52. Hardy JG, Wolff HG, Goodell H. Experimental evidence on the nature of cutaneous hyperalgesia. *J Clin Invest* 1950;29:115–140.
53. Harris R, Griffin CJ. Fine structure of nerve endings in the human dental pulp. *Arch Oral Biol* 1968;13:773–778.
54. Häbler H-J, Jänig W, Koltzenburg M. A novel type of unmyelinated chemosensitive nociceptor in the acutely inflamed urinary bladder. *Agents Actions* 1988;25:219–221.
55. Hanesh U, Heppelman B, Messlinger K, Schmidt RF. Nociception in normal and arthritic joints, structural and functional aspects. In: Willis WD Jr, ed. *Hyperalgesia and allodynia.* New York: Raven, 1992;81–106.
56. Heppelman B, Schaible HG, Schmidt RF. Effects of prostaglandins E1 and E2 on the mechanosensitivity of group III afferents from normal and inflamed cat knee joints. In: Fields HL, Dubner R, Cervero F, eds. *Advances in pain research and therapy.* New York: Raven Press, 1985;9:91–102.
57. Heppelman B, Hebert MK, Schaible HG, Schmidt RF. Morphological and physiological characteristics of the innervation of cats normal and arthritic knee joint. In: Pubols LS, Sessle BJ, Liss AR, eds. *Effects of injury in trigeminal and spinal somatosensory system.* New York: Alan R. Liss, 1987;19–27.
58. Heppelman B, Messlinger K, Neiss WF, Schmidt RF. Ultrastructural three-dimensional reconstruction of group III and group IV sensory nerve endings ("free nerve endings") in the knee joint capsule of the cat: evidence for multiple receptive sites. *J Comp Neurol* 1990;292:103–166.
59. Herbert MD, Schmidt RF. Activation of normal and inflamed fine articular afferent units by serotonin. *Pain* 1992;50:79–80.
60. Hiss E, Mense S. Evidence for the existence of different receptor sites for algesic agents at the endings of muscular group IV afferent units. *Pflugers Arch* 1976;362:141–146.
61. Holzer P. Local effector functions of capsaicin-sensitive sensory nerve endings: Involvement of tachykinins, calcitonin gene-related peptide and other neuropeptides. *Neuroscience* 1988;24: 739–768.
62. Jancso N, Jansco-Gabor A, Szolcsányi J. The role of sensory nerve endings in neurogenic inflammation induced in human skin and in the eye and paw of the rat. *J Pharmacol Chemother* 1968;32:32–41.
63. Jansco N, Jansco-Gabor A, Szolcsányi J. Direct evidence for neurogenic inflammation and its prevention by denervation and by pretreatment with capsaicin. *Br J Pharmacol Chemother* 1967;31: 138–151.
64. Johnson KO, Darian-Smith I, LaMotte C, Johnson B, Oldfield S. Coding of incremental changes in skin temperature by a monkey: correlation with intensity discrimination in man. *J Neurophysiol* 1979;42(5):1332–1353.
65. Kenshalo DR. Comparison of thermal sensitivity of the forehead, lip, conjunctiva, and cornea. *J Appl Physiol* 1960;15:987–991.
66. Khan AA, Raja SN, Manning DC, Campbell JN, Meyer RA. The effects of bradykinin and sequence-related analogs on the response properties of cutaneous nociceptors in monkeys. *Somatosens Motor Res* 1992;9:97–106.
67. Kieschke J, Mense S, Prabhakar NR. Influence of adrenaline and hypoxia on rat muscle receptors in vitro. In: Hamann W, Iggo A, eds. *Progress in brain research.* Amsterdam: Elsevier Science, 1988; 91–97.
68. Kjartansson J, Dalsgaard CJ, Jonsson CE. Decreased survival of experimental critical flaps in rats after sensory denervation with capsaicin. *Plast Reconstruct Surg* 1987;79:218–221.
69. Klement W, Arndt JO. The role of nociceptors of cutaneous veins in the mediation of cold pain in man. *J Physiol (Lond)* 1992;449: 73–83.
70. Koltzenburg M, Handwerker, HO. Differential ability of human cutaneous nociceptors to signal mechanical pain and to produce vasodilation. *J Neurosci* 1994;14:1756–1765.
71. Koltzenburg M, Kress M, Reeh PW. The nociceptor sensitization by bradykinin does not depend on sympathetic neurons. *Neuroscience* 1992;46:465–473.
72. Konietzny F, Hensel H. Warm fiber activity in human skin nerves. *Eur J Physiol* 1975;359:265–267.
73. Kress M, Koltzenburg M, Reeh PW, Handwerker HO. Responsiveness and functional attributes of electrically localized terminals of cutaneous C-fibers in vivo and in vitro. *J Neurophysiol* 1992;68: 581–595.
74. Kruger L. Morphological features of thin sensory afferent fibers: A new interpretation of `nociceptor' function. In: Hamann W, Iggo A, eds. *Progress in brain research.* Amsterdam: Elsevier, 1988; 253–257.
75. Kumazawa T, Mizumura K, Minagawa M, Tsujii Y. Sensitizing effects of bradykinin on the heat responses of the visceral nociceptor. *J Neurophysiol* 1991;66:1819–1824.
76. Kumazawa T, Perl ER. Primate cutaneous sensory units with unmyelinated (C) afferent fibers. *J Neurophysiol* 1977;40: 1325–1338.
77. LaMotte RH, Thalhammer JG, Torebjörk HE, Robinson CJ. Peripheral neural mechanisms of cutaneous hyperalgesia following mild injury by heat. *J Neurosci* 1982;2:765–781.
77a. LaMotte RH, Thalhammer JG, Robinson CJ. Peripheral neural correlates of magnitude of cutaneous pain and hyperalgesia: a

comparison of neural events in monkey with sensory judgements in human. *J Neurophysiol* 1983;50:1–26.
78. LaMotte RH, Simone DA, Baumann TK, Shain CN, Alreja M. Hypothesis for novel classes of chemoreceptors mediating chemogenic pain and itch. Pain. In: Dubner R, Gebhart GF, Bond MR, eds. *Proceedings of the Vth World Congress on Pain.* Amsterdam: Elsevier Science, 1988;529–535.
79. LaMotte RH, Shain CN, Simone DA, Tsai E-FP. Neurogenic hyperalgesia: psychophysical studies of underlying mechanisms. *J Neurophysiol* 1991;66:190–211.
80. LaMotte RH. Campbell JN. Comparison of responses of warm and nociceptive C-fiber afferents in monkey with human judgements of thermal pain. *J Neurophysiol* 1978;41:509–528.
81. LaMotte RH, Simone DA, Ngeow JYF, Whitehouse J, Becerra-Cabal L, Putterman AJ. The magnitude and duration of itch produced by intracutaneous injections of histamine. *Somatosens Res* 1987;5:81–92.
82. LaMotte RH, Thalhammer JG. Response properties of high-threshold cutaneous cold receptors in the primate. *Brain Res* 1982; 244:279–287.
83. Lang E, Novak A, Reeh PW, Handwerker HO. Chemosensitivity of fine afferents from rat skin in vitro. *J Neurophysiol* 1990;63: 887–901.
84. Langford LA, Schmidt RF. Afferent and efferent axons in the medial and posterior articular nerves of the cat. *Anat Rec* 1983; 206:71–78.
85. Lele PP, Weddell G. Sensory nerves of the cornea and cutaneous sensibility. *Exp Neurol* 1959;1:334–359.
86. Lembeck F, Gamse R. Substance P in peripheral sensory processes. *Ciba Found Symp* 1982;91:35–54.
87. Levine JD, Clark R, Devor M, Helms C, Moskowitz MA, Basbaum AI. Intraneuronal substance P contributes to the severity of experimental arthritis. *Science* 1984;226:547–549.
88. Levine JD, Dardick SJ, Basbaum AI, Scipio E. Reflex neurogenic inflammation. I. Contribution of the peripheral nervous system to spatially remote inflammatory responses that follow injury. *J Neurosci* 1985;5:1380–1386.
89. Lewis T. Experiments relating to cutaneous hyperalgesia and its spread through somatic fibres. *Clin Sci* 1935;2:373–423.
90. Lewis T. The nocifensor system of nerves and its reactions. *Br Med J* 1937;431–435.
91. Lewis T. *Pain.* New York: Macmillan, 1942.
92. Lewis T, Pochin EE. The double pain response of the human skin to a single stimulus. *Clin Sci* 1937;3:67–76.
93. Lim RKS, Miller DG, Guzman F, Rodgers DW, Wang RW, Chao SK, Shih TY. Pain and analgesia evaluated by intraperitoneal bradykinin-evoked pain method in man. *Clin Pharmacol Ther* 1967; 8:521–542.
94. Lynn B, Cotsell B. Blood flow increases in the skin of the anaesthetized rat that follow antidromic sensory nerve stimulation and strong mechanical stimulation. *Neurosci Lett* 1992;137:249–252.
95. Maggi CA, Meli A. The sensory-efferent function of capsaicin-sensitive sensory neurons. *Gen Pharmacol* 1988;19:1–43.
96. Manning DC, Raja SN, Meyer RA, Campbell JN. Pain and hyperalgesia after intradermal injection of bradykinin in humans. *Clin Pharmacol Ther* 1991;50:721–729.
97. Martin HA, Basbaum AI, Kwiat GC, Goetzl EJ, Levine JD. Leukotriene and prostaglandin sensitization of cutaneous high-threshold C- and A-delta mechanonociceptors in the hairy skin of rat hindlimbs. *Neuroscience* 1987;22:651–659.
98. Mathews B. Responses of intradental nerves to electrical and thermal stimulation of teeth in dogs. *J Physiol (Lond)* 1977;264: 641–664.
99. McMahon SB, Koltzenburg M. Novel classes of nociceptors: beyond Sherrington. *Trends Neurosci* 1990;13:199–201.
100. Melmon KL, Webster ME, Goldfinger SE, Seegmiller JE. The presence of a kinin in inflammatory synovial effusion from arthritides of varying etiologies. *Arthritis Rheum* 1967;10:13–20.
101. Melzack R, Wall PD. Pain mechanism: a new theory. *Science* 1965; 150:971–979.
102. Mense S. Sensitization of group IV muscle receptors to bradykinin by 5-hydroxytryptamine and prostaglandin E2. *Brain Res* 1981;225: 95–105.
103. Mense S. Physiology of nociception in muscles. In: Fricton JR, Awad EA, eds. *Advances in pain research and therapy.* New York: Raven Press, 1990;17:67–85.
104. Mense S. Considerations concerning the neurobiological basis of muscle pain. *Can J Physiol Pharmacol* 1991;69:610–616.
105. Mense S, Schmidt RF. Activation of group IV afferent units from muscle by algesic agents. *Brain Res* 1974;72:305–310.
106. Meyer RA, Campbell JN, Raja SN. Peripheral neural mechanisms of cutaneous hyperalgesia. In: Fields HL, Dubner R, Cervero F, eds. *Advances in pain research and therapy.* New York: Raven Press, 1985;9:53–71.
107. Meyer RA, Raja SN, Campbell JN. Coupling of action potential activity between unmyelinated fibers in the peripheral nerve of monkey. *Science* 1985;227:184–187.
108. Meyer RA, Campbell JN, Raja SN. Antidromic nerve stimulation in monkey does not sensitize unmyelinated nociceptors to heat. *Brain Res* 1988;441:168–172.
109. Meyer RA, Davis KD, Cohen RH, Treede R-D, Campbell JN. Mechanically insensitive afferents (MIAs) in cutaneous nerves of monkey. *Brain Res* 1991;561:252–261.
110. Meyer RA, Campbell JN. Myelinated nociceptive afferents account for the hyperalgesia that follows a burn to the hand. *Science* 1981; 213:1527–1529.
111. Meyer RA, Campbell JN. Peripheral neural coding of pain sensation. *Johns Hopkins Appl Phys Lab Tech Dig* 1981;2:164–171.
112. Mizumura K, Minagawa M, Tsujii Y, Kumazawa T. The effects of bradykinin agonists and antagonists on visceral polymodal receptor activities. *Pain* 1990;40:221–227.
113. Nakano T, Taira N. 5-Hydroxytryptamine as a sensitizer of somatic nociceptors for pain-producing substances. *Eur J Pharmacol* 1976; 38:23–29.
114. Narhi MVO. Dentin sensitivity: a review. *J Biol Buccale* 1985;13: 75–96.
115. Narhi MVO. The characteristics of intradental sensory units and their responses to stimulation. *J Dental Res* 1985;64:564–571.
116. Nilsson J, von Euler AM, Dalsgaard C-J. Stimulation of connective tissue cell growth by substance P and substance K. *Nature* 1985; 315:61–63.
117. Ochoa J, Mair WGP. The normal sural nerve in man. I. Ultrastructure and numbers of fibres and cells. *Acta Neuropathol (Berl)* 1969;13:197–216.
118. Ochoa JL, Torebjörk HE. Sensations evoked by intraneural microstimulation of single mechanoreceptor units innervating the human hand. *J Physiol (Lond)* 1983;342:633–654.
119. Paintal AS. Functional analysis of group III afferent fibers of mammalian muscle. *J Physiol (Lond)* 1960;152:250–270.
120. Paintal AS. Participation by pressure-pain receptors of mammalian muscles in the flexion reflex. *J Physiol (Lond)* 1961;156:498–514.
121. Perl ER. Myelinated afferent fibres innervating the primate skin and their response to noxious stimuli. *J Physiol (Lond)* 1968;197: 593–615.
122. Price DD, McHaffie JG, Larson MA. Spatial summation of heat-induced pain: Influence of stimulus area and spatial separation on perceived pain sensation intensity and unpleasantness. *J Neurophysiol* 1989;62:1270–1279.
123. Price DD, Bennett GJ, Rafii A. Psychophysical observations on painful peripheral neuropathies that are relieved by a sympathetic block. *Pain* 1989;36:273–288.
124. Raja SN, Campbell JN, Meyer RA. Evidence for different mechanisms of primary and secondary hyperalgesia following heat injury to the glabrous skin. *Brain* 1984;107:1179–1188.
125. Raja SN, Meyer RA, Campbell JN. Peripheral mechanisms of somatic pain. *Anesthesiology* 1988;68:571–590.
126. Reeh PW, Kocher L, Jung S. Does neurogenic inflammation alter the sensitivity of unmyelinated nociceptors in the rat? *Brain Res* 1986;384:42–50.
127. Reeh PW, Bayer J, Kocher L, Handwerker HO. Sensitization of nociceptive cutaneous nerve fibers from the rat tail by noxious mechanical stimulation. *Exp Brain Res* 1987;65:505–512.
128. Richardson BP, Engel G. The pharmacology and function of 5-HT3 receptors. *Trends Neurosci* 1986;9:424–427.
129. Roberts WJ, Elardo SM. Sympathetic activation of A-delta nociceptors. *Somatosens Res* 1985;3:33–44.
130. Rocha e Silva M, Rosenthal SR. Release of pharmacologically active substances from the rat skin in vivo following thermal injury. *J Pharmacol Exp Ther* 1961;132:110–116.
131. Rozsa AJ, Beuerman RW. Density and organization of free nerve endings in the corneal epithelium of the rabbit. *Pain* 1982;14: 105–120.
132. Schaible H-G, Schmidt RF. Time course of mechanosensitivity changes in articular afferents during a developing experimental arthritis. *J Neurophysiol* 1988;60:2180–2195.
133. Schaible H-G, Schmidt RF. Excitation and sensitization of fine

articular afferents from cat's knee joint by prostaglandin E2. *J Physiol (Lond)* 1988;403:91–104.
134. Schaible HG, Neugebauer V, Schmidt RF. Osteoarthritis and pain. *Semin Arthritis Rheum* 1989;18:30–34.
135. Schaible HG, Schmidt RF. Activation of groups III and IV sensory units in medial articular nerve by local mechanical stimulation of knee joint. *J Neurophysiol* 1983;49:35–44.
136. Schaible HG, Schmidt RF. Responses of fine medial articular nerve afferents to passive movements of knee joint. *J Neurophysiol* 1983;49:1118–1126.
137. Schaible HG, Schmidt RF. Effects of an experimental arthritis on the sensory properties of fine articular afferent units. *J Neurophysiol* 1985;54:1109–1122.
137a. Schepelmann K, MeBlinger K, Schaible H-G, Schmidt RF. Inflammatory mediators and nociception in the joint excitation and sensitization of slowly conducting afferent fibers of cat's knee by prostaglandin I_2. *Neuroscience* 1992;50:237–247.
138. Sessle BJ, Hu JW. Mechanisms of pain arising from articular tissues. *Can J Physiol Pharmacol* 1991;69:617–626.
139. Sherrington CS. *The integrative action of the nervous system.* New York: Scribner, 1906.
140. Sicuteri F, Fanciullacci M, Franchi G, Del Bianco PL. Serotonin-bradykinin potentiation on the pain receptors in man. *Life Sci* 1965;4:309–316.
141. Simone DA, Sorkin LS, Oh U, Chung JM, Owens C, LaMotte RH, Willis WD. Neurogenic hyperalgesia: Central neural correlates in responses of spinothalamic tract neurons. *J Neurophysiol* 1991;66: 228–246.
142. Simone DA, Ochoa J. Early and late effects of prolonged topical capsaicin on cutaneous sensibility and neurogenic vasodilatation in humans. *Pain* 1991;47:285–294.
143. Sinclair DC, Hinshaw JR. A comparison of the sensory dissociation produced by procaine and by limb compression. *Brain* 1950;73: 480–498.
144. Skoglund S. Anatomical and physiological studies of knee joint innervation in the cat. *Acta Physiol Scand* 1956;36(suppl 124):1–101.
145. Steen KH, Reeh PW, Anton F, Handwerker HO. Protons selectively induce long lasting excitation and sensitization to mechanical stimulation of nociceptors in rat skin, in vitro. *J Neurosci* 1992;1:86–95.
146. Steen KH, Reeh PW. Sustained graded pain and hyperalgesia from harmless experimental tissue acidosis in human skin. *Neurosci Lett* 1993;154:113–116.
147. Szolcsányi J. Effect of pain-producing chemical agents on the activity of slowly conducting afferent fibres. *Acta Physiol Acad Sci Hung* 1980;56:86.
148. Szolcsányi J. Capsaicin and neurogenic inflammation: History and early findings. In: Chahl LA, Szolcsányi J, Lembeck F, eds. *Antidromic vasodilatation and neurogenic inflammation.* Budapest: Akademiai Kiado, 1984;7–25.
149. Szolcsányi J. Antidromic vasodilation and neurogenic inflammation. *Agents Actions* 1988;23:4–11.
150. Tanelian DL. Cholinergic activation of a population of corneal afferent nerves. *Exp Brain Res* 1991;86:414–420.
151. Tanelian DL, Beuerman RW. Responses of rabbit corneal nociceptors to mechanical and thermal stimulation. *Exp Neurol* 1984; 84:165–178.
152. Thalhammer JG, LaMotte RH. Spatial properties of nociceptor sensitization following heat injury of the skin. *Brain Res* 1982;231: 257–265.
153. Thalhammer JG, LaMotte RH. Heat sensitization of one-half of a cutaneous nociceptor's receptive field does not alter the sensitivity of the other half. In: Bonica JJ, Lindblom U, Iggo A, eds. *Advances in pain research and therapy.* New York: Raven Press, 1983; 5:71–75.
154. Tillman DB. Heat response properties of unmyelinated nociceptors. [Doctoral dissertation]. Johns Hopkins University, Baltimore, MD, 1992.
155. Torebjörk E, Ochoa J. Specific sensations evoked by activity in single identified sensory units in man. *Acta Physiol Scand* 1980;110: 445–447.
156. Torebjörk HE, LaMotte RH, Robinson CJ. Peripheral neural correlates of magnitude of cutaneous pain and hyperalgesia: simultaneous recordings in humans of sensory judgments of pain and evoked responses in nociceptors with C-fibers. *J Neurophysiol* 1984; 51:325–339.
157. Torebjörk HE, Lundberg LER, LaMotte RH. Central changes in processing of mechanoreceptive input in capsaicin-induced secondary hyperalgesia in humans. *J Physiol (Lond)* 1992;448:765–780.
158. Torebjörk HE, Hallin RG. Perceptual changes accompanying controlled preferential blocking of A and C fibre responses in intact human skin nerves. *Exp Brain Res* 1973;16:321–332.
159. Treede R -D, Meyer RA, Campbell JN. Classification of primate A-fiber nociceptors according to their heat response properties. *Pflugers Arch* 1991;418(suppl 1):R42.
160. Treede R-D, Meyer RA, Raja SN, Campbell JN. Evidence for two different heat transduction mechanisms in nociceptive primary afferents innervating monkey skin. *J Physiol* 1995;483:747–758.
161. Treede RD, Meyer RA, Campbell JN. Comparison of heat and mechanical receptive fields of cutaneous C-fiber nociceptors in monkey. *J Neurophysiol* 1990;64:1502–1513.
162. Treede RD, Meyer RA, Raja SN, Campbell JN. Peripheral and central mechanisms of cutaneous hyperalgesia. *Prog Neurobiol* 1992;38: 397–421.
163. Trowbridge HO. Intradental sensory units: Physiological and clinical considerations. *J Endodontics* 1985;11:489–498.
164. Van Hees J, Gybels JC. Nociceptor activity in human nerve during painful and nonpainful skin stimulation. *J Neurol Neurosurg Psychiatry* 1981;44:600–607.
165. Wall PD, McMahon SB. Microneurography and its relation to perceived sensation. A critical review. *Pain* 1985;21:209–229.
166. White DM, Taiwo YO, Coderre TJ, Levine JD. Delayed activation of nociceptors: Correlation with delayed pain sensations induced by sustained stimuli. *J Neurophysiol* 1991;66:729–734.
167. Woolf CJ, King AE. Dynamic alteration in the cutaneous mechanoreceptor fields of dorsal horn neurons in the rat spinal cord. *J Neurosci* 1990;10:2717–2726.

Anesthesia: Biologic Foundations, edited by Tony L. Yaksh et al. Lippincott–Raven Publishers, Philadelphia © 1997.

CHAPTER 32

AFFERENT ACTIVITY IN INJURED AFFERENT NERVES

MARY G. GARRY AND DARRELL L. TANELIAN

Under normal conditions, the afferent axon is notably silent, e.g., it manifests little spontaneous activity. Application of an adequate physical or chemical stimulus to the distal terminal will lead to a generator potential and the production of a local action potential. Typically such application of this stimulus at sites mid-axon fails to evoke such a regenerative potential, short of inducing an acute deformation or injury to the axon. At such times, the axon may yield several discharges and then lapses into silence. It is now widely appreciated that over the ensuing period of time, there are prominent morphologic and biochemical changes that appear at the site of axon injury as well as in the dorsal root ganglion and the dorsal horn. Some of these local changes have been reviewed elsewhere (see Chap. 3). These changes may lead to the appearance of an anomalous spontaneous activity and the evolution of the ability of the axon to transduce chemical and physical stimuli at the site of injury.

Such anomalous afferent activity can result from numerous types of injury or disease and can cause or contribute to neuropathic pain syndromes. For example, abnormalities in sensory neurons are believed to be involved in pain syndromes that occur in association with neural trauma, diabetes (17,90), herpes zoster (137), limb amputation (37), tooth extraction (100,161), burn injuries (100), and, more recently, HIV infection (99,104,171). The prevalence of afferent abnormalities in so many neuropathic pain syndromes makes understanding the functional consequences of this aberrant activity, as well as the underlying mechanisms, essential in order to effectively treat such debilitating pain.

This chapter reviews anomalous afferent activity that occurs during neuropathic pain and discusses (1) anatomical, (2) electrophysiologic, and (3) neurochemical characteristics of peripheral neuronal injury. It should be noted that while changes in the central nervous system (CNS) have been clearly demonstrated to contribute to many pain states, consideration of these factors is not within the scope of this chapter (see Chaps. 40 and 56).

CONSEQUENCE OF NERVE INJURY

The clinical presentation of neuropathic pain varies considerably, yet has some landmark characteristics such as hyperalgesia and allodynia (6,60,127,132; see Chap. 28). Hyperalgesia, characterized by a decreased threshold and an enhanced response to a noxious stimuli, is frequently observed. Allodynia, the perception of pain following normally innocuous stimulation, is commonly reported by patients who are diagnosed with neuropathic pain. Many patients report that "guarding" is one method of pain reduction. Commonly, patients will wrap and protect the affected site from external stimuli (even gentle breezes are reported as painful in some cases). Nail grooming is often avoided.

Several animal models are available that mimic these human behaviors during neuropathic pain. Such similarities between human reports of pain and animal models of pain are derived by measuring behavioral responses to various stimuli (noxious or innocuous). In animals, both hyperalgesia and allodynia can be measured quantitatively. Guarding behaviors are often observed in animal models and, while this behavior is difficult to measure in a quantitative fashion, it may be indicative of spontaneous pain. Vocalization may also be correlated with spontaneous pain. Finally, though it is a controversial issue, autotomy (self-mutilation) is often considered a nociceptive behavior and a measure of pain.

Early animal studies have emphasized that crush or severance of the nerve will induce changes in behavior that suggest parallels with the postnerve injury pain state in humans. Guarding of the injured limb or autotomy is believed to be driven by an anomalous discharge from the injured nerve. Many of the animal models that are used for the study of abnormal activity have employed nerve severance or crush since selective and controlled lesions ensue following this type of injury.

In the last several years, however, a number of specific nerve injury models have been developed and characterized. Three models that have been widely examined are indicated in Fig. 1. In all of these models, these interventions have been shown to have specific behavioral consequences including varying degrees of hot and cold hyperalgesia and tactile allodynia. In addition, the spinal nerve model is characterized by having a tactile allodynia that is reversed by sympathectomy. The pain states induced in these different models each have a distinct pharmacology. These pharmacologic properties are reviewed in Chap. 40.

The behavioral consequences of these nerve injuries emphasize that these animal models yield predictable changes in behavior that are in close parallel with the effects of injuries in humans. Accordingly, such investigations into the altered function of the peripheral nerve after local injury are believed to provide mechanistic insights into the corresponding pain states in humans.

ANATOMICAL CHARACTERISTICS OF AXONAL INJURY

Normal Anatomy

The primary afferent neuron is a pseudounipolar neuron with a stem process that bifurcates into a central process that enters the dorsal horn of the spinal cord, and a peripheral process that travels to a target tissue via a peripheral nerve. These neuronal processes can be myelinated or unmyelinated and correspond to the alpha and beta or C-fiber classes of sensory fibers, respectively. In myelinated fibers, myelin is interrupted along the axon, forming the nodes of Ranvier that facilitate the propagation of electrical signals along the axon. Supporting Schwann cells are located in a paranodal position. Disruption of axonal myelination can lead to aberrant conduction or excitability along the axon. The axonal cytoplasm is composed of a cytoskeletal matrix that maintains the axonal shape and facilitates the transport of cellular products to, and away from, the cell body. Axonal transport is important for the maintenance and repair of axonal processes. Likewise, disruption of these transport processes can result in alteration of both the axon and change the expression of neuronal peptides following nerve injury (see Chap. 30 for a detailed discussion of axon morphology).

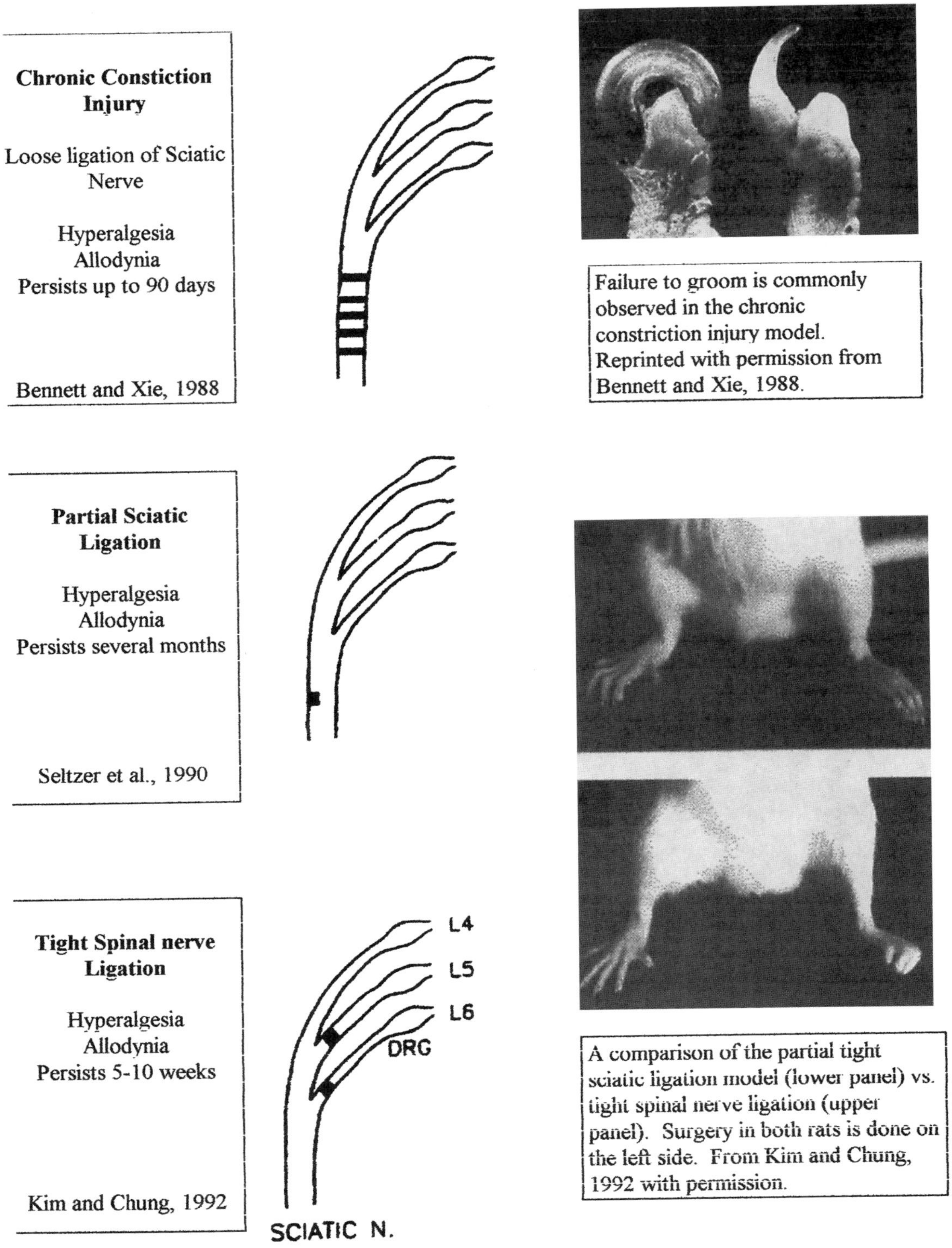

Chronic Constiction Injury

Loose ligation of Sciatic Nerve

Hyperalgesia
Allodynia
Persists up to 90 days

Bennett and Xie, 1988

Failure to groom is commonly observed in the chronic constriction injury model. Reprinted with permission from Bennett and Xie, 1988.

Partial Sciatic Ligation

Hyperalgesia
Allodynia
Persists several months

Seltzer et al., 1990

Tight Spinal nerve Ligation

Hyperalgesia
Allodynia
Persists 5-10 weeks

Kim and Chung, 1992

L4
L5
L6
DRG
SCIATIC N.

A comparison of the partial tight sciatic ligation model (lower panel) vs. tight spinal nerve ligation (upper panel). Surgery in both rats is done on the left side. From Kim and Chung, 1992 with permission.

Figure 1. The three principal nerve injuries that are commonly employed to induce nerve injury. First is the chronic constriction injury model. This involves placement of loose, chromic gut ligatures around the sciatic nerve at the level of the popliteal fossa (Bennett and Xie, 10). A similar model was developed by Maves et al. (102), who apposed chromic gut to the sciatic nerve. Second is the partial sciatic ligation model. In this model, a tight ligature is placed around half of the sciatic nerve proximal to the ischeal notch (Seltzer et al., 143). Third, Kim and Chung (85) introduced the tight ligation of the spinal nerve model. In this model, the L5/L6 nerves just distal to the vertebral body are tightly ligated.

Alterations in Nerve Anatomy Following Nerve Injury

Following injury to a peripheral nerve, the proximal and distal segments of the axon rapidly lose axoplasm but are capable of "sealing off" the injured site by fusion of the axonal membrane. Frequently, the distal portion of the remaining intact axon will swell and result in the formation of a neuroma (end bulb swelling). This swelling is believed to result from ongoing axonal transport that carries membrane-bound organelles such as mitochondria, lysosomes, and electron-dense vesicles to the neuronal terminals in the periphery (55). Large intramembranous particles have also been observed in this segment following injury when compared to intact axons (55).

In the rat sciatic nerve, a consistent finding is that in the afferent neuroma, the endings are free of compact myelin (55). These demyelinated regions have been observed to be enveloped with one or more thin sheetlike wrappings of Schwann cell cytoplasm following nerve section or chronic constriction injury (CCI) (26,55). The mechanism of this demyelination is not clear, although several theories exist. Early studies suggested that decreased blood flow or direct mechanical injury may enhance the breakdown of myelin following nerve ligation (51). More recently, it has been suggested that macrophages, which invade the site of nerve injury, may contribute to the demyelination of the axon following injury. It has been proposed that macrophages phagocytose myelin debris from degenerating axons and that such scavenging of myelin impairs the ability of the axon to regenerate since it has been shown that axonal membrane regeneration is largely dependent on recycled, as opposed to newly synthesized, myelin (56,57). Additional support for the macrophage's role in demyelination comes from studies demonstrating demyelination following peripheral axotomy can be blocked by the inhibition of tumor necrosis factor, which is produced by macrophages (148). These studies suggest that demyelination may occur in response to several events, independent or coupled, that ensue following injury. The contribution of demyelination to neuropathic pain remains the subject of current research, since demyelination that occurs in the absence of axoplasmic swelling, Schwann cell proliferation, and mast cell invasion does not produce a significant hyperalgesic state (115; see Chap. 30).

Axonal Number Following Injury

Following nerve injury, the number of sensory axons decreases distal to the lesion (8,26,125,141). This decrease is due, primarily, to a massive loss of large myelinated fibers (26,31,80,125). These anatomical data are supported by electrophysiologic data from animals with CCI which indicate that 85% to 89% and 55% to 65% of the Aβ and A-δ fibers are lost, respectively. In contrast, C fibers often appear to be spared. For example, it has been estimated that 30% to 92% of the C fibers remain following CCI (8,26,80). What remains unclear is whether a change in the myelinated fiber composition is required for the initiation and/or maintenance of hyperalgesia. In the CCI model, the onset of abnormal afferent activity coincides with the onset of nociceptive behavior. For example, following CCI, Aβ and Aδ fibers display increased spontaneous activity which occurs in approximately the same time frame as the appearance of hyperalgesia, allodynia, and possibly spontaneous pain (80,81).

Several studies have been directed at determining if certain types of postnerve injury nociceptive phenomena are associated with specific afferent fiber populations. It has been observed that neonatal capsaicin treatment, prior to tight or loose ligation of the sciatic nerve, prevents the development of the thermal hyperalgesia that typically occurs in this injury model (110,145), suggesting that capsaicin-sensitive fibers may mediate thermal hyperalgesia. Moreover, it was demonstrated that neonatal capsaicin has no effect on either mechanical allodynia or mechanical hyperalgesia (145), suggesting that different neuronal populations mediate these sensory alterations. In contrast, intrathecal capsaicin in adult rats does not block the exaggerated sensitivity in the lesioned paw, but results in a thermal hypoalgesia in the normal paw (173), suggesting that small capsaicin-sensitive afferents may not be responsible for the thermal hyperalgesia..

Death of sensory neurons in the dorsal root ganglion (DRG) has been reported following nerve lesioning. The extent of neuronal cell death in the DRG may be dependent on the age of the animal. For example, Schmalbruch (141) demonstrated a 50% to 90% perikaryal deficit in the L4-L6 DRG following lesion of the sciatic nerve in neonatal rats. In contrast, only a 30% loss of L4-L6 DRG neurons was observed following sciatic nerve lesion in the adult rat (174). These results are consistent with the observation that cell death in the DRG is considerably greater following sciatic nerve lesion in the kitten when compared to adult cats (3). However, it has been demonstrated that while more sensory neurons initially degenerate in neonatal mammals, neuronal regeneration is better in these animals when compared to regeneration in the adult mammal (66a). This enhanced recovery in neonatal animals is believed to be the result of growth factors that are present in the neonatal period. In addition to age dependence, cell death may be species dependent. This hypothesis is supported by data that indicate that there is a greater loss of cells in the DRG of rats when compared to the DRG of cats (40,154,174).

When injury occurs to a peripheral nerve, greater cell loss appears when the lesion is distal to the DRG compared with injury to the dorsal roots (70,116,121). Consistent with these findings is the observation that mortality of sensory neurons following a peripheral injury may be due to deprivation of target-derived trophic factors, such as apolipoprotein E, epidermal growth factor, and nerve growth factor (32,76,134,155, 156). The effects of deprivation of target-derived trophic factors is discussed in greater detail later in this chapter.

Neuronal Size in Dorsal Root Ganglia

Several studies have evaluated the effect of nerve injury on cell size within the DRG. Following crush of the sciatic nerve in rat, it has been demonstrated that initially there is a decrease in the size of the DRG cell bodies followed by a subsequent increase in their size (166). In contrast, several studies report that there is no change in the size of perikaryal within the DRG following injury (43,68,70,120). The discrepancy between these studies may depend on species, the severity of the injury, or the time of sacrifice following injury. Additional changes are observed as well, such as prolonged eccentricity of the nucleus (166). The functional significance of these alterations in cell size or morphology are unclear. Nonetheless, it has been demonstrated that morphologic changes are temporally correlated with metabolic changes in the DRG (166).

Axonal Sprouting

Following injury, sensory axons are capable of regeneration. It is believed that the success or failure of the regeneration process may dictate whether normal sensory recovery or neuropathic pain occurs following injury or during disease. The process of regeneration involves debris removal from the site of injury, the formation of axonal growth cones, the elongation of axons through the injured area, and reinnervation of the peripheral target tissue. Regeneration can be altered by physical or chemical factors in the surrounding tissue. Successful regeneration of injured peripheral nerves appears to be dependent on the presence of regeneration-promoting substances in the outgrowth region. Soluble factors having such properties include nerve growth factor (NGF) and apolipoprotein E. The former is known to promote the survival of some nerve cells (155), whereas the latter has been ascribed a role in the myelinization of newly grown axons (74). These substances are believed to be produced and secreted from Schwann cells in the outgrowth region. In addition, recent radiolabeling studies have demonstrated that axons are also capable of releasing various proteins (134) and that nontoxic inhibition of their release stunted axonal outgrowth. Together, these studies suggest that both the intrinsic and extrinsic neural environment supply substances that stimulate regeneration following injury.

Not only do injured axons undergo regeneration, but sensory fibers from neighboring intact nerves expand into the area previously innervated by the lesioned nerve (16,44,48,94,131). This phenomenon is termed collateral sprouting. A schematic illustrating the phenomenon of collateral sprouting is presented in Fig. 2. Such sprouting is reported to contribute to the early return of sensation in the rat foot following sciatic nerve severance (44). Moreover, the local application of capsaicin to the injured nerve trunk can prevent this collateral sprouting from adjacent noninjured neurons. Since capsaicin affects primarily nonmyelinated fibers, it has been suggested that healthy myelinated fibers remaining in the injured nerve are capable of preventing sprouting from the neighboring intact neurons (131). In addition, following CCI, where myelinated fibers in the sciatic nerve are primarily damaged, it has been demonstrated that severance of the saphenous nerve (within a week of sciatic nerve ligation) abolishes pain behaviors. It may be that the early hyperalgesia that develops in this model is due to collateral sprouting of the saphenous nerve (135).

An important consideration is that regenerating fibers can on occasion form connections with inappropriate target tissues. For example, it has been shown that muscle receptors can be reinnervated by cutaneous afferents, and the reverse is also true (87). Additionally, low-threshold cutaneous receptors can be reinnervated by nociceptive afferent neurons (87). Aside from this atypical peripheral reinnervation, central alterations in mechanoreceptor input to certain areas of the brain following injury and regeneration can also occur (129). It has been hypothesized that these aberrant central connections could also contribute to the development of pain following nerve injury.

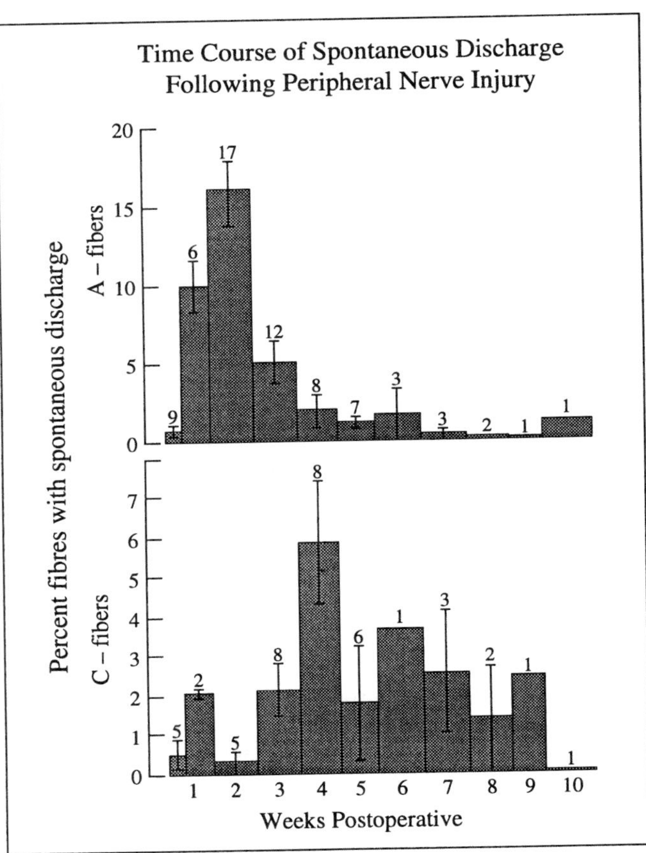

Figure 2. The appearance of spontaneous activity after the focal injury of the sciatic nerve. The incidence of spontaneously active myelinated (A) and unmyelinated (C) fibers in experimental neuromas in the sciatic nerve during the first 10 weeks after nerve section. The number of experiments performed at each time interval is indicated over the *bars.* (From ref. 38, with permission.)

ELECTROPHYSIOLOGIC CHARACTERISTICS OF POSTNERVE INJURY ACTIVITY

Normal Electrophysiology

Thermal and mechanical energy can impinge on the peripheral terminal of the primary afferent neuron. This energy is transduced into a generator potential that is then converted into an action potential and then propagated centrally along the axon to the spinal cord. Normally, most nociceptors are not tonically active, but respond only following stimulation or injury (53,130; see Chap. 31). In response to noxious stimulation, a nociceptive afferent typically responds by firing an action potential that is in phase with the stimulus, and the frequency of which is proportional to stimulus intensity (for review, see ref. 50). These impulses are then conducted anterogradely through the dorsal roots and into the dorsal horn.

Postnerve Injury Potentials

Alterations in Conduction Velocity

Following mid-axon injury, a decrease in the conduction velocity of both A and C fibers has been reported (38,147). This reflects changes in Schwann cell density and distribution and the state of remyelination as well as axon diameter. A positive correlation has been demonstrated between decreasing conduction velocity in C fibers and increasing age of the neuroma (165). Since regenerating fibers (as opposed to surviving fibers) often have slower conduction velocities than do normal fibers, the electrophysiologic classification of fiber types following nerve injury can be complicated and sometimes inaccurate.

Ephaptic Transmission

Normal intact nerves transmit impulses through well-insulated channels. Following nerve injury, this insulation can be disrupted, and the impulses carried in one nerve fiber may be transmitted to a neighboring fiber. Ephaptic communication or "cross-talk" has been demonstrated following stimulation of adjacent afferent fibers in the same nerve trunk (12). Ephaptic communication between fibers typically occurs immediately following nerve injury and then dissipates (37). It has been demonstrated that a second phase of ephaptic transmission emerges several weeks following injury (142). As a result of this cross-talk, the CNS is no longer able to receive accurate coding of the intensity of a given stimulus. Since the same peripheral stimulus can now result in the activation or recruitment of additional nerves following injury, a previously mild and perhaps innocuous stimulation could result in a larger than normal afferent barrage that the CNS interprets as being due to higher-intensity stimulation.

Ectopic Discharge at the DRG

A small percentage of normal DRGs exhibit spontaneous activity (41). This discharge is increased substantially following chronic nerve injury (41). Most injured afferents fire rhythmically and at high frequency. However, ectopic discharges that

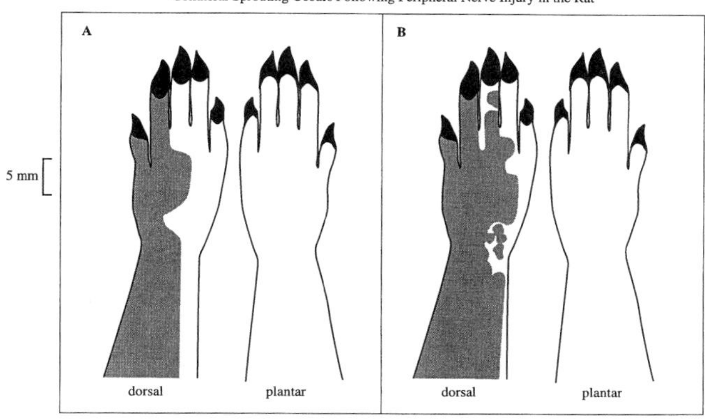

Figure 3. Schematic showing the appearance of collateral sprouting following sciatic nerve section. Diagrams of the dorsal and plantar surfaces of the feet in the right hindlimbs of a control animal **(A)**, and an animal in which the right sciatic nerve had been sectioned and capped 2 months previously **(B)**. The area delineated by plasma extravasation following saphenous nerve stimulation is shaded. These data suggest that the innervation of the saphenous nerve has increased following sciatic nerve section. (From ref. 16, with permission.)

occur at the DRG are slow and irregular (20,81). Nerve transection is reported to evoke spontaneous discharges from the cell bodies of myelinated fibers at the level of the dorsal root ganglia, but not from the cell bodies of unmyelinated axons (162). Moreover, the extent to which spontaneous discharge originates from the DRG seems to vary with the type of injury. For example, following nerve lesion and neuroma formation, only 6% of the injury-induced spontaneous activity appeared to be generated at the DRG (20,162). In contrast, Kajander et al. (81) demonstrated that nearly all of the spontaneous afferent activity observed following CCI was generated at the DRG. In addition to spontaneous activity, it has been demonstrated that chronic injury of the sural nerve produces a marked increase in mechanical sensitivity of the DRG in rabbits (73). Such sensitivity has been postulated to contribute significantly to the radicular pain that follows disk herniation.

Aberrant Spontaneous Activity

In contrast to normal sensory axons, as shown in Fig. 3, after injury, primary afferent axons develop ongoing or spontaneous activity (20,21,36,37,80). Most tonic activity occurs at a low-discharge rate, but some fibers have been observed to develop high-firing rates (80). Importantly, not all afferents develop spontaneous activity with an equal likelihood after injury. There is considerable variability in the occurrence of ongoing activity in A and C fibers.

Several factors appear to influence the appearance of afferent activity: (a) fiber type, (b) species, (c) time, and (d) specific nerve injured. Thus, following neuroma formation, up to 30% of the myelinated fibers and very few unmyelinated fibers develop spontaneous activity in the rat (165). Likewise, following CCI in rat, only 3% of C fibers developed spontaneous activity, whereas 35% and 15% of the A-beta and A-delta fibers displayed ongoing activity, respectively (80). In contrast, 4% to 13% of all afferent fibers evaluated developed spontaneous activity in the cat following neuroma formation. The majority of these active fibers were unmyelinated (13). With regard to time, it has been observed that myelinated fibers are among the earliest of the afferent population that display spontaneous activity after injury, whereas the C-fiber response is observed after some delay (13,37,80,165). A summary of the onset of spontaneous activity in certain fiber types is illustrated in Fig. 3.

With regard to the nerve injured, the occurrence of spontaneous discharge is dependent on the specific nerve. For example, a severed sciatic nerve has significantly more fibers (both A- and C-fiber types) that develop spontaneous firing when compared to a severed infraorbital nerve (151). It is interesting to consider the factors that may "protect" certain fibers from developing such firing patterns. It has been suggested that the differences between the trigeminal nerves and the somatic nerves involve the local milieu in which the axon is cut or possibly the density of sympathetic fibers (see below) surrounding a given nerve type (151).

Aberrant-Evoked Activity

Altered responsiveness to mechanical, chemical, and thermal stimulation can occur in the injured or regenerating nerve.

Mechanical Stimulation

It is well established that in or around the site of injury, damaged axons become sensitive to mechanical stimulation following neuroma formation. In cats with a neuroma of the peroneal nerve, 19% to 33% of fibers in the neuroma are responsive to probing with blunt glass rods (13). In rats with a saphenous nerve neuroma, 13% of C fibers and 25% of A-delta fibers are mechanically sensitive to von Frey hairs or blunt glass probes (165). Similar responses have been recorded in baboon (113) and mice (140), although the percentages of mechanically responsive fibers and the type of fiber involved varied with species.

Thermal Stimulation

Afferent nociceptors that respond to noxious heat have been well defined (for review, see ref. 170). Upon injury, their threshold for thermal activation is lower when compared to control animals (47). Ligation of the sciatic nerve yields a pronounced thermal hyperalgesia (9,10,150), which is believed to contribute to painful neuropathies in humans since human psychophysical studies of thermal hyperalgesia in patients with reinnervated skin correlate with the physiologic studies obtained in animals (126).

Chemical Stimulation

Prostanoids and Kinins A variety of substances are released into the tissue after local tissue injury (see Chap. 61). Certain algesic compounds are potent activators and sensitizing agents when present at the terminal of the normal, uninjured primary afferent. Typically, compounds such as bradykinin, histamine, prostaglandins (PGs), and leukotrienes (LTs) are only active at the terminals (and not the axons) of intact afferent neurons (165). Importantly, under normal conditions, such agents applied mid-axon are without significant effect. However, following injury, axons develop responsiveness to the application of these algesic compounds. For example, PGI_2 and 8,15-HETE evoke an increase in the discharge of C fibers in a mid-axonal region proximal to a mature neuroma (46). In a rat neuroma, 22% of spontaneously active fibers are responsive to local application of bradykinin while relatively insensitive to histamine (165). Consistent with these data is the observation that algesic compounds such as bradykinin, PGE_2, and histamine enhance the release of neuroactive peptides from capsaicin-sensitive afferent fibers in an in vitro dental pulp preparation (65a). One study, however, has documented that neuromas appear to be insensitive to the NK-1 and NK-3 tachykinin receptor agonists (46). The failure of these agonists to stimulate ectopic neuronal activity in neuromas suggests that these peptides may be inactive in the periphery following nerve injury. In general, these results support the concept that injured afferent neurons develop the ability to respond to algesic compounds. This response to algesic compounds may play a role in the development or maintenance of hyperalgesia following injury (see Chap. 33).

Parallel lines of evidence indicate that algesic compounds are produced and released locally following nerve injury. Blockade of the synthesis of, or the receptors for, these algesic compounds has been shown to reduce aberrant afferent firing and induce analgesia (34,66,112). Recently, through the use of microdialysis, the local release of bradykinin, PGE_2, and LTB_4 from tooth sockets following third molar extraction in humans (a "nerve injury" that is also capable of neuroma formation) has been demonstrated (136,149). These results indicate that the release of these algesic compounds occurs at the site of injury. Moreover, the rise in the concentration of these algesic compounds has been shown to correlate with patients reports of pain (149). These studies suggest that the local release of chemical mediators may contribute to the ectopic neuronal hyperexcitability that occurs at the site of nerve injury.

Adrenergic Sensitivity Discharge of afferent fibers has been observed following stimulation of sympathetic nerve fibers in the same nerve trunk (39). Electrophysiologic studies demonstrate that epinephrine and norepinephrine can stimulate afferent fibers that end in a neuroma (139,163). Moreover, adrenergic antagonists can block sensory discharge following sympathetic stimulation (39,139). Sympathetic communication with afferent neurons is hypothesized to be the result of an increase in α_2-adrenergic receptors on damaged primary afferent axons (88,139). The development of adrenergic chemosensitivity is variable. In rats with mature neuromas (>8.5 months), afferent fibers are activated by low-frequency stimulation of the sympathetic supply, but this response is not duplicated by administration of i.v. adrenaline (75). In contrast, fibers in cat neuromas respond weakly to i.v. adrenaline and noradrenaline (13). This variability in the response of afferent fibers to sympathetic agents may provide the basis for the clinical observation that there are sympathetically maintained and sympathetically independent pain syndromes (33,60,160). In addition to alterations in adrenergic receptor expression, a recent study indicates that axotomy causes a sprouting of sympathetic fibers that invade the DRG to form functional synapses (106). These sprouting fibers contain catecholamines, and it has been demonstrated that ectopic discharges may originate at the DRG by direct innervation from these sympathetic fibers that form basket-like structures around large diameter cell bodies in the DRG. Therefore, these studies indicate that sympathetic nerve fibers can invade the DRG following injury and may contribute to pain.

Sympathectomy can alleviate some chronic pain behaviors that occur following nerve injury. Attal et al. (5) has shown that sympathectomy prior to or immediately after nerve injury alleviates nociceptive behavioral syndromes in rats. It has also been demonstrated that surgical sympathectomy produces a lasting abolition of mechanical allodynia (pain evoked by innocuous mechanical stimulation) following nerve ligation (84). Guanethidine treatment (which depletes sympathetic neurotransmitters) reduces heat and cold allodynia following peripheral neuropathy in rats, but has little effect on mechanical allodynia (117).

INJURY-INDUCED ALTERATIONS IN ION CHANNELS

It is proposed that the excitability of afferent axonal membranes is altered following injury, resulting in a hyperexcitable membrane. This condition is believed to be the result of changes in ion channel proteins and their distribution. Several points have been marshaled in support of this theory. First, an increase in the occurrence of large intramembranous particles was observed in axons with neuromas when compared to intact axons (55). It is hypothesized that these particles are surface proteins such as receptors or channel proteins. Second, it has been demonstrated that membrane properties at the regenerating tip of an axon differ from those of the normal membrane (107). Thus, there is a disappearance of the Na^+-dependent action potential, and an increase in the resting membrane conductance to K^+, Na^+, and Ca^{2+} (107). In addition, the emergence of a calcium-dependent action potential was observed (62,107,172). The predominant membrane conductance of Ca^{2+} is believed to play a role in axonal growth and elongation since this type of conductance is also prominent during embryonic development (95,146). These studies clearly demonstrate that ionic conductances are altered in the regenerating axon. The changes in specific ion channels are considered below.

Sodium Channels

It has recently been demonstrated that injury causes a local increase in the concentration of Na^+ channels in rat axons. Specifically, sciatic nerve section evoked an increase in the concentration of Na^+ channels at the site of neuroma formation (42) (see Fig. 4). This increase in the concentration of Na^+ channels in the axon correlates with the occurrence of peak ectopic discharge following neuroma formation. It has been proposed that the absence of myelination near the neuroma permits the invasion of sodium channels that are transported along the axon. This theory is supported by previous studies that demonstrate that sites of demyelination have been observed to be sites of spontaneous discharge (19,25). Therefore, it is believed that the formation of Na^+ channel-rich

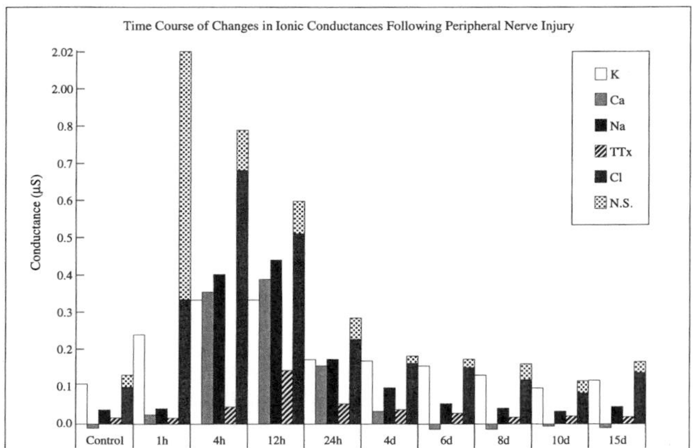

Figure 4. Time-dependent changes in resting membrane conductance after nerve injury. Resting ionic conductances measured at the tip of a giant axon from the nerve cord of the cockroach *Periplaneta americana*. The *bars* indicate the change (decrease) in membrane conductance after sequential removal of specific ionic conductances as indicated [potassium (K), calcium (Ca), sodium (Na), tetrodotoxin (TTX), chloride (Cl), and nonspecific (N.S). One hour to 4 days after sectioning, conductance was decreased after the removal of Ca, indicating an increasing fraction of Ca conductance from the total membrane conductance. After 6 days, the removal of calcium produced the same effect as in the controls. (From ref. 107, with permission.)

regions contribute to ectopic activity at the site of the neuroma. Collectively, these data suggest that alterations in the conductance of sodium through the axoplasmic membrane contribute to the anomalous activity that is observed in the afferent axon following injury.

Ectopic neuronal discharge is reduced by sodium channel blockers applied directly to the nerve or administered systemically (28,30,45,152). These drugs include local anesthetics, anticonvulsants, and antiarrhythmics that inhibit the opening of Na^+ channels in a use-dependent fashion (27,69). It has been demonstrated that local anesthetics, such as lidocaine, act by reducing ongoing ectopic discharge in peripheral nerves and in the dorsal root ganglion (1,30,45,46,152). Clinically there are numerous reports of these drugs reducing neuropathic pain (29,61,82,137).

Intrasynovial corticosteroids are widely used clinically in the treatment of certain types of inflammatory and neuropathic pains. Direct axonal application of corticosteroids has been observed to reduce the percent of fibers that display spontaneous discharge following injury (43). It has been suggested that direct nerve application of corticosteroids acts to stabilize axonal membranes by hyperpolarization of the nerve secondary to activation of an electrogenic sodium pump (43,65).

Potassium Channels

Potassium conductance is also important in the electrophysiology of injured nerve fibers (22,107). It has been demonstrated that agents that block potassium conductance and increase the concentration of intracellular potassium increase the firing rate of sensory neurons following injury (22,35,80). Following CCI, K^+ channel blockers are observed to induce activity in previously silent fibers or increase the rate of spontaneous firing of 50% of the A and 19% of the A-delta fibers. This effect appears to be limited to myelinated fibers, since there is no effect of K^+ channel blockers on C-fiber activity (80). It has also been demonstrated that regenerating, and not degenerating, nerve fibers are observed to have increased concentrations of endoneurial potassium (96). Such increases in extracellular K^+ may serve to increase spontaneous activity.

INJURY-INDUCED CHANGES IN NEUROACTIVE AGENTS

It is believed that sensory neurons in the DRG respond to injury by altering the proteins that they synthesize in an attempt to support and regenerate the injured neurons. The discussion of neuroactive substances following injury focuses on the neurochemical alterations that occur in the cell bodies of these afferent neurons in the DRG and trigeminal ganglion, since the identification of afferent fibers in the peripheral nerve is not always possible.

As reviewed elsewhere (see Chaps. 34 and 35), a variety of agents, notably peptides, have been found in the central and peripheral terminals of primary afferents, and these peptides are synthesized in the cell body and transported to the terminals (see Chap. 3). Current data indicate that injury to the peripheral afferent will lead to changes in the synthesis and transport of these peptides.

Substance P

It has been observed that there is a decrease in the number of cell bodies that are immunoreactive for SP in the DRG following major peripheral nerve injury (11,49,77,124,159,175). Likewise, the levels of SP immunoreactivity in peripheral sensory axons decrease following injury (63). This decrease in SP immunoreactivity correlates with decreases in preprotachykinin mRNA in the DRG (52,67,118,119,122,159,175). In contrast, noninjurious noxious stimulation of the rat hindpaw evokes an increase in the synthesis of tachykinins in the DRG (120).

Calcitonin Gene-Related Peptide (CGRP)

Like SP, CGRP is generally reported to decrease in the DRG following major nerve injury (49,123,175). In tooth pulp, CGRP-like immunoreactivity increases in sensory axons following mild injury (86,153), but is reduced or abolished following more severe injury (23,63,83). Decreases in the levels of CGRP mRNA and immunoreactivity are reported to occur in all sizes of cells in the DRG following severe injury such as peripheral axotomy (49,123,175). These alterations in the levels of CGRP mRNA in the DRG reflect decreases in both alpha- and beta-CGRP (123).

Vasoactive Intestinal Peptide (VIP)

In contrast to the general decreases in CGRP and SP, VIP immunoreactivity is increased in both the DRG and the trigeminal ganglion following lesion of the sciatic or mandibular nerves, respectively (4,144). Likewise, there is a reciprocal increase in the levels of VIP mRNA in the DRG following nerve resection (118,119,122). This is particularly remarkable since VIP is normally not expressed in these neurons in the uninjured animal. The increase in VIP immunoreactivity and mRNA may be species dependent, since there was no induction of VIP immunoreactivity or VIP mRNA in the DRG of monkey following sciatic nerve lesion (175).

Galanin

Like VIP, galanin immunoreactivity, synthesis, and galanin mRNA increase in the DRG following injury or disease (68,71,159,175). These alterations in the levels of galanin mRNA and immunoreactivity are primarily confined to small cells within the DRG (71,159,175).

Nitric Oxide

It has recently been demonstrated that the novel neuronal messenger nitric oxide may be involved in the primary afferent response to injury. In previous studies, it was observed that very few cells in the lumbar DRG are positive for a marker of the nitric oxide synthesizing [NOS] enzyme (2). Following transection of the sciatic nerve in rats, however, there is a marked increase in the number of NOS mRNA-positive cells in the L4-L6 DRG (158). The mechanisms that drive this increase are unclear; however, many of the cells that were positive for NOS mRNA were also immunoreactive for galanin and VIP. The results of these studies suggest that certain populations of cells alter their expression of nitric oxide in response to injury. The functional significance of these findings has not yet been elucidated.

FUNCTIONAL SIGNIFICANCE OF CHANGES IN THE AFFERENT TRANSMITTER

In the periphery, both SP and CGRP are excitatory peptides that play a critical role in the phenomenon known as neurogenic inflammation, which is characterized by enhanced blood flow and leakage of plasma constituents into the extracellular space. CGRP is known to be a potent endogenous agent that mediates vasodilation (15). Substance P has been demonstrated to evoke capillary leakage and the resulting plasma extravasation (91; for review see ref. 54). When both peptides are applied together, CGRP facilitates SP-induced plasma extravasation (14,57). Such facilitation is also observed in the central nervous system, since CGRP enhances SP-evoked hyperalgesia at the level of the spinal cord (128). There may also be an additional trophic role for SP and CGRP in peripheral target tissues (64,78,133,144).

In contrast to these excitatory peptides, galanin is generally an inhibitory peptide. In the spinal cord of normal rats, galanin has a biphasic effect on the flexor reflex (hyperalgesia at low doses, analgesia at high doses) (169). In axotomized rats, however, the analgesic effect of galanin occurs at much lower doses. Moreover, galanin inhibits the excitatory effects of SP and CGRP both in the CNS and PNS (168).

Vasoactive intestinal peptide is believed to facilitate neuronal regeneration by altering neuronal metabolism. For example, VIP has been demonstrated to stimulate glycogenolysis, increase glucose utilization, and increase blood flow (97,98, 105,138). Normally, VIP is not expressed in the DRG of primary afferent neurons and the expression of this peptide is induced following injury (118,119,122), further supporting the role of this peptide as a neurotrophic factor.

It is generally believed that alteration in the regulation of peptide synthesis that occurs following injury is an attempt to promote regeneration of injured afferent axons and to invoke endogenous analgesic systems (7,72,89,92). However, it has recently been determined that the upregulated VIP, present only after injury, assumes a "transmitter-like" role similar to SP. However, it has been postulated that the concurrent upregulation of galanin may counteract the excitatory actions of VIP, allowing the peptide to function primarily as a trophic factor. The precise roles that these neuropeptides play in the postinjury state remain to be elucidated.

Mechanism of Altered Neuropeptide Content Following Injury

The mechanisms that dictate the alterations in peptide synthesis and expression following injury are not completely known. However, it has been determined that the synthesis of SP and CGRP in primary afferent neurons is dependent on the target-derived trophic factor, nerve growth factor (NGF) (93,103). NGF is taken up by sensory terminals in peripheral tissues and transported to the DRG (18) where it binds to high- and low-affinity binding sites for NGF within the DRG neurons (157,167). Therefore, when nerves are injured to the point of impairing retrograde transport of NGF, there is a generalized decrease in the immunoreactivity and synthesis of CGRP and SP in the DRG neurons (24,93). Conversely, following mild injury, with no axonal disruption, it has been speculated that the sprouting of CGRP and SP containing axons may be the result of enhanced levels and transport of NGF following injury (24). Collectively, these studies suggest that the increases or decreases in CGRP and SP immunoreactivity that occur following injury are dictated by the availability of NGF to the DRG.

The factors that determine increases in VIP and galanin in primary afferent neurons following injury are also not clear. Little or no immunoreactivity or mRNA for either of these peptides is observed in the lumbar DRG of normal animals (4,58,118,119,122,144). Therefore, it is believed that an induction mechanism is activated following injury as opposed to an increase in the ongoing synthesis of these peptides. Interestingly, it has been observed that some of the VIP immunoreactive cells (up to 50%) are also immunoreactive for CGRP (49,79). These studies suggest that peptide containing cells within the DRG alter their genetic expression in an attempt to respond to the stresses on the cell.

CONCLUSION

Anomalous afferent activity may be generated in a number of ways: demyelination, alteration in ion channels and/or their conductances, alterations in the production of neuropeptides and neurotransmitters, and ectopic regeneration and connectivity of sensory and sympathetic fibers. Injury to the axon may lead to time-dependent changes in the afferent phenotype and in the expression of several neurotransmitters. The appearance of spontaneous activity in the otherwise quiescent axon clearly has a prominent role in altering the postnerve injury response characteristics of the afferent processing systems. The growing appreciation of the factors that lead to this activity including the appearance of increased channel density and coupled receptors at the injury site may offer targets for rational intervention. The role of this afferent activity and the role played by transported trophic factors in altering the central connectivity and excitatory efficacy of these afferent systems will likely provide considerable insight into the anomalous pain states that are frequently generated by such discrete nerve injuries.

REFERENCES

1. Abram SE, Yaksh TL. Systemic lidocaine blocks nerve injury-induced hyperalgesia and nociceptor-driven spinal sensitization in the rat. *Anesthesiology* 1994;80:383–391.
2. Aimi Y, Fujimura M, Vincent SR, Kimura H. *J Comp Neurol* 1991; 306: 382–392.
3. Aldskogius H, Risling M. Effect of sciatic neurectomy on neuronal number and size distribution in the L7 ganglion of kittens. *Exp Neurol* 1981;74: 597–604.
4. Atkinson ME, Shehab SAS. Peripheral axotomy of the rat mandibular trigeminal nerve leads to an increase in VIP and decrease of other primary afferent neuropeptides in the spinal trigeminal nucleus. *Regul Pept* 1986;16:69–82.
5. Attal N, Kayser V, Jazat F, Guilbaud G. Behavioural evidence for a bidirectional effect of systemic naloxone in a model of experimental neuropathy in the rat. *Brain Res* 1989;494:276–284.
6. Backonja M, Arndt G, Gombar KA, Check B, Zimmermann M. Response of chronic neuropathic pain syndromes to ketamine: a preliminary study. *Pain* 1994;56:51–57.
7. Barron KD. In: Kao CC, Bunge RP, Reier PJ, eds. Spinal cord reconstruction. New York: Raven Press, 1983;7–40.
8. Basbaum AI, Gautron M, Jazat F, Mayes M, Guilbaud G. The spectrum of fiber loss in a model of neuropathic pain in the rat: an electron microscopic study. *Pain* 1991;47:359–367.
9. Bennett GJ. An animal model of neuropathic pain: a review. *Muscle Nerve* 1993;16:1040–1048.
10. Bennett GJ, Xie Y-K. A peripheral mononeuropathy in rat that produces disorders of pain sensation like those seen in man. *Pain* 1988;33:87–107.
11. Bisby MA, Keen P. Regeneration of primary afferent neurons containing substance P-like immunoreactivity. *Brain Res* 1986;365: 85–95.
12. Blumberg H, Janig W. Activation of fibers via experimentally produced stump neuromas of skin nerves: ephaptic transmission or retrograde sprouting? *Exp Neurol* 1982;76(3):468–482.
13. Blumberg H, Janig W. Discharge pattern of afferent fibers from a neuroma. *Pain* 1984;20(4):335–353.
14. Brain SD, Williams TJ. Inflammatory oedema induced by synergism between calcitonin gene-related peptide (CGRP) and mediators of increased vascular permeability. *Br J Pharmacol* 1985;86:855–860.
15. Brain SD, Williams TJ, Tippins JR, Morris HR, MacIntyre I. Calcitonin gene-related peptide is a potent vasodilator. *Nature* 1985; 313:54–56.
16. Brenan A. Collateral reinnervation of skin by C-fibers following nerve injury in the rat. *Brain Res* 1986;385:152–155.
17. Britland ST, Young RJ, Sharma AK, Clarke BF. Acute and remitting painful diabetic polyneuropathy: a comparison of peripheral nerve fiber pathology. *Pain* 1992;48:361–370.
18. Brunso-Bechtold JK, Hamburger V. Retrograde transport of nerve growth factor in chicken embryo. *PNAS* 1979;76:1494–1496.
19. Burchiel KJ. Ectopic impulse generation in focally demyelinated trigeminal nerve. *Exp Neurol* 1980;69:423–429.
20. Burchiel KJ. Effects of electrical and mechanical stimulation on two foci of spontaneous activity which develop in primary afferent neurons after peripheral axotomy. *Pain* 1984;18:249–265.
21. Burchiel KJ. Carbamazepine inhibits spontaneous activity in experimental neuromas. *Exp Neurol* 1988;102:249–253.
22. Burchiel KJ, Russell LC. Effects of potassium channel-blocking

agents on spontaneous discharges from neuromas in rats. *J Neurosurg* 1985;63(2):246–249.
23. Byers M, Taylor P, Khayat B, Kimberly C. Effects of injury and inflammation on pulpal and periapical nerves. *J Endodontics* 1990; 16:78–84.
24. Byers MR, Wheeler EF, Bothwell M. Altered expression of NGF and P75 NGF-receptor by fibroblasts of injured teeth precedes sensory nerve sprouting. *Growth Factors* 1992;6:41–52.
25. Calvin WH, Devor M, Howe JF. Can neuralgias arise from minor demyelination? Spontaneous firing, mechanosensitivity, and afterdischarge from conducting axons. *Exp Neurol* 1982;75:755–763.
26. Carlton SM, Dougherty PM, Power CM, Coggeshall RE. Neuroma formation and numbers of axons in a rat model of experimental peripheral neuropathy. 1991;131:88–92.
27. Catteral WA. Common modes of drug action on Na+ channels: local anesthestics, antiarrhythmics and anticonvulsants. *TIPS* 1987;8:57–65.
28. Chabal C, Jacobson L, Burchiel KJ. Pain responses to perineuromal injection of normal saline, gallamine, and lidocaine in humans. *Pain* 1989;36:321–325.
29. Chabal C, Jacobson L, Mariano A, Chaney E, Britell CW. The use of oral mexiletine for the treatment of pain after peripheral nerve injury. *Anesthesiology* 1992;76:513–517.
30. Chabal C, Russell LC, Burchiel KJ. The effect of intravenous lidocaine, tocaninide, and mexiletine on spontaneously active fibers originating in rat sciatic neuromas. *Pain* 1989;38:333–338.
31. Coggeshall RE, Dougherty PM, Pover CM, Carlton SM. Is large myelinated fiber loss associated with hyperalgesia in a model of experimental peripheral neuropathy in the rat? *Pain* 1993;52: 233–242.
32. Curtis R, Averill S, Priestley JV, Wilkin GP. The distribution of GAP-43 in normal rat spinal cord. *J Neurocytol* 1993;22(1):39–50.
33. Davis KD, Treede RD, Raja SN, Meyer RA Campbell JN. Topical application of clonidine relieves hyperalgesia in patients with sympathetically maintained pain. *Pain* 1991;47:309–317.
34. Dawson W, Willoughby D. Inflammation—mechanisms and mediators. In: Lombardino J, ed. *Nonsteroidal antiinflammatory drugs.* New York: John Wiley, 1985.
35. Devor M. Potassium channels moderate ectopic excitability of nerve-end neuromas in rats. *Neurosci Lett* 1984;40:181–186.
36. Devor M. The pathophysiology of damaged peripheral nerves. In: Wall PD, Melzack R, eds. *Textbook of pain,* 2nd ed. Edinburgh: Churchill Livingstone, 1989.
37. Devor M. Neuropathic pain and injured nerve: peripheral mechanisms. *Br Med Bull* 1991;47:619–630.
38. Devor M, Govrin-Lippmann R. Spontaneous neural discharge in neuroma C-fibers in rat sciatic nerve. *Neurosci Lett Suppl* 1995;22: 532.
39. Devor M, Janig W. Activation of myelinated afferents ending in a neuroma by stimulation of the sympathetic supply in the rat. *Neurosci Lett* 1981;24:43–47.
40. Devor M, Wall PD. Effect of peripheral nerve injury on receptive fields of cells in the cat spinal cord. *J Comp Neurol* 1981;199: 277–291.
41. Devor M, Wall PD. Cross-excitation in dorsal root ganglia of nerve-injured and intact rats. *J Neurophysiol* 1990;64:1733–1746.
42. Devor M, Gorvin-Lippmann R, Angelides K. Na+ channel immunolocalization in peripheral mammalian axons and changes following nerve injury and neuroma formation. *J Neurosci* 1993;13: 1976–1992.
43. Devor M, Govrin-Lippmann R, Raber P. Corticosteroids suppress ectopic neural discharge originating in experimental neuromas. *Pain* 1985;22:127–137.
44. Devor M, Schonfield D, Seltzer Z, Wall PD. Two modes of cutaneous reinnervation following peripheral nerve injury. *J Comp Neurol* 1979;185:211–220.
45. Devor M, Wall PD, Catalan N. Systemic lidocaine silences ectopic neuroma and DRG discharge without blocking nerve conduction. *Pain* 1992;48:261–268.
46. Devor M, White DM, Goetzl EJ, Levine JD. Eicosanoids, but not tachykinins, excite C-fiber endings in rat sciatic nerve-end neuromas. *NeuroReport* 1992;3:21–24.
47. Dickhaus H, Zimmermann M, Zottermann Y. The development in regenerating cutaneous nerves of C-fiber receptors Responding to noxious heating of the skin. In: Zottermann Y, ed. *Sensory function of the skin in primates.* New York: Pergamon Press, 1976.
48. Doucette R, Diamond J. Normal and precocious sprouting of heat nociceptors in the skin of adult rats. *J Comp Neurol* 1987;261: 592–603.
49. Doughty SE, Atkinson ME, Shehab SAS. A quantitative study of neuropeptide immunoreactive cell bodies of primary afferent sensory neurons following rat sciatic nerve peripheral axotomy. *Regul Pept* 1991;35:59–72.
50. Dubner R, Bennett GJ. Spinal and trigeminal mechanisms of nociception. *Annu Rev Neurosci* 1983;6:381–418.
51. Dyck PJ, Lais AC, Giannini C, Engelstad JK. Structural alterations of nerve during cuff compression. *Proc Natl Acad Sci USA* 1990; 87(24):9828–9832.
52. Ernfors P, Rosario CM, Merlio J-P, Grant G, Aldskogius H, Persson H. Expression of mRNAs for neurotrophin receptors in the dorsal root ganglion and spinal cord during development and following peripheral or central axotomy. *Mol Brain Res* 1993;17:217–226.
53. Fitzgerald M, Lynn B. The sensitization of high threshold mechanoreceptors with myelinated axons by repeated heating. *J Physiol* 1977;265(2):549–563.
54. Foreman JC, Jordan CC. Neurogenic inflammation. *TIPS* 1984; 5:116–119.
55. Fried K, Govrin-Lippmann R, Rosenthal F, Ellisman MH, Devor M. Ultrastructure of afferent axon endings in a nEuroma. *J Neurocytol* 1991;20:682–701.
56. Frisen J, Risling M, Fried K. Distribution and axonal relations of macrophages in a neuroma. *Neuroscience* 1993;55:1003–1013.
57. Gamse R, Saria A. Potentiation of tachykinin-induced plasma protein extravasation by calcitonin gene-related peptide. *Eur J Pharmacol* 1985;114:61–66.
58. Garry MG, Miller KE, Seybold VS. Lumbar dorsal root ganglia of the cat: a quantitative study of peptide immunoreactvity and cell size. *J Comp Neurol* 1989;284:36–47.
59. Goodrum JF, Earnhardt T, Goines N, Bouldin TW. Fate of myelin lipids during degeneration and regeneration of peripheral nerve: an autoradiographic study. *J Neurosci* 1994;14(1):357–367.
60. Gracely RH, Lynch SA, Bennett GJ. Painful neuropathy: altered central processing maintained dynamically by peripheral input. *Pain* 1992;51:175–194.
61. Graubard DJ, Peterson MC. Therapeutic uses of intravenous procaine. *Anesthesiology* 1949;7:175–187.
62. Grinvald A, Farber IC. Optical recording of calcium potentials from growth cones of cultured neurons with a laser microbeam. *Science* 1981;212(4499):1165–1167.
63. Grutzner EH, Garry MG, Hargreaves KM. Effect of injury on pulpal levels of immunoreactive substance P and immunoreactive calcitonin gene-related peptide. *J Endodontics* 1992;18:553–557.
64. Haegerstrand A, Dalsgaard CJ, Jonzon B, Larsson O, Nilsson J. Calcitonin gene-related peptide stimulates proliferation of human endothelial cells. *Proc Natl Acad Sci USA* 1990;87(9): 3299–3303.
65. Hall ED. Glucocorticoid effects on central nervous excitability and synaptic transmission. *Int Rev Neurobiol* 1982;23:165–195.
65a. Hargreaves KM, Swift JQ, Roszkowski MT, Bowles W, Garry MG, Jackson DL. Pharmacology of peripheral neuropeptide and inflammatory mediator release. *Oral Surg Oral Med Oral Pathol* 1994;78:503–510.
66. Hargreaves KM, Troullos E, Dionne R, et al. Bradykinin is increased during acute and chronic inflammation: therapeutic implications. *Clin Pharmacol Ther* 1988;44:613–619.
66a. Heath DD, Coggeshall RE, Hulsebosch CE. Axon and neuron numbers after forelimb amputation in neonatal rats. *Exp Neurol* 1986;92:220–233.
67. Henken DB, Martin JR. Herpes simplex virus induces a selective increase in the proportion of galanin positive neurons in mouse sensory ganglia. *Exp Neurol* 1992;118:195–205.
68. Henken DB, Battisti WP, Chesselet MF, Murray M, Tessler A. Expression of B-preprotachykinin mRNA and tachykinins in rat dorsal root ganglion cells following peripheral or central axotomy. *Neuroscience* 1990;39:733–742.
69. Hille B. Local anesthetics: hydrophilic and hydrophobic pathways for the drug-receptor reaction. *J Gen Physiol* 1977;69:497–515.
70. Himes BT, Tessler A. Death of some dorsal root ganglion nEurons and plasticity of others following sciatic nerve section in adult and neonatal rats. *J Comp Neurol* 1989;284(2):215–230.
71. Hokfelt T, Wiesenfeld-Hallin Z, Villar M, Melander T. Increase of galanin-like immunoreactivity in rat dorsal root ganglion cells after peripheral axotomy. *Neurosci Lett* 1987;83:217–220.
72. Hokfelt T, Zhang X, Wiesenfeld-Hallin Z. Messenger plasticity in

primary sensory neurons following axotomy and its functional implications. *TINS* 1994;17:22–30.
73. Howe JF, Loeser JD, Calvin WH. Mechanosensitivity of dorsal root ganglia and chronically injured axons: a physiological basis for the radicular pain of nerve root compression. *Pain* 1977;3:25–41.
74. Ignatius MJ, Gebicke-Harter PJ, Skene JH, Schilling JW, Weisgraber KH, Mahley RW, Shooter EM. Expression of apolipoprotein E during nerve degeneration and regeneration. *Proc Natl Acad Sci USA* 1986;83(4):1125–1129.
75. Janig W. Activation of afferent fibers ending in an old neuroma by sympathetic stimulation in the rat. *Neurosci Lett* 1990;111(3): 309–314.
76. Johnson EM, Yip HK. Central nervous system and peripheral nerve growth factor provide trophic support critical to mature sensory nEuronal survival. *Nature* 1985;314:751–752.
77. Jones K, LaVelle A. Differential effects of axotomy on immature and mature hamster facial neurons: a time course study of initial nucleolar and nuclear changes. *J Neurocytol* 1986;15:197–206.
78. Jones MA, Marfurt CF. Calcitonin gene-related peptide and corneal innervation: a developmental study in the rat. *J Comp Neurol* 1991;313(1):132–50.
79. Ju G, Hokfelt T, Brodin E, Fahrenkrug J, Fischer JA, Frey P, Elde RP, Brown JC. Primary sensory neurons of the rat showing calcitonin gene-related peptide immunoreactivity and their relation to substance P-, somatostatin-, galanin-, vasoactive intestinal polypeptide- and cholecystokinin-immunoreactive ganglion cells. *Cell Tissue Res* 1987;247:417–431.
80. Kajander KC, Bennett GJ. Onset of a painful peripheral nEuropathy in rat: a partial and differential deafferentation and spontaneous discharge in AB and AD primary afferent neurons. *J Neurophysiol* 1992;68:734–744.
81. Kajander KC, Wakisaka S, Bennett GJ. Spontaneous discharge originates in the dorsal root ganglion at the onset of a painful peripheral neuropathy in rat. *Neurosci Lett* 1992;138:225–228.
82. Kastrup J, Petersen P, Dejgard A, Angelo HR, Hilsted J. Intravenous lidocaine infusion—a new treatment of chronic painful diabetic neuropathy? *Pain* 1987;28:69–75.
83. Khayat B, Byers M. Responses of nerve fibers to pulpal inflammation and periapical lesion in rat molars demonstrated by calcitonin gene-related peptide immunocytochemistry. *J Endodontics* 1988;14:577–87.
84. Kim SH, Chung JM. Sympathectomy alleviates mechanical allodynia in an experimental animal model for neuropathy in the rat. *Neurosci Lett* 1991;134:131–134.
85. Kim SH, Chung JM. An experimental model for peripheral nEuropathy produced by segmental spinal nerve ligation in the rat. *Pain* 1992;50:355–360.
86. Kimberly C, Byers M. Inflammation of rat molar pulp and periodontum causes increased calcitonin gene related peptide and azonal sprouting. *Anat Rec* 1988;222:289–300.
87. Koerber HR, Seymour AW, Mendell LM. Mismatches between peripheral receptor type and central projections after peripheral nerve regeneration. *Neurosci Lett* 1989;99:67–72.
88. Korenman EMD, Devor M. Ectopic adrenergic sensitivity in damaged peripheral nerve axons in the rat. *Exp Neurol* 1981;72:63–81.
89. Kreutzberg GW. In: Nicholls JG, ed. *Repair and regeneration of the nervous system.* New York: Springer-Verlag, 1982;57–69.
90. Lanting P, Faes TJC, Ijff GA, Betelsmann FW, Heimans JJ, van der Veen EA. Autonomic and somatic peripheral nerve function and the correlation with neuropathic pain in diabetic patients. *J Neurol Sci* 1989;94:307–317.
91. Lembeck F, Holzer P. Substance P as neurogenic mediator of antidromic vasodilation and neurogenic plasma extravasation. *Naunyn Schmiedebergs Arch Pharmacol* 1979;310(2):175–183.
92. Lieberman AR. The avon reaction: a review of the principal features of perikayal responses to axon injury. *Int Rev Neurobiol* 1971; 14:49–124.
93. Lindsay RM, Lockett C, Sternberg J, Winter J. Neuropeptide expression in cultures of adult sensory neurons: modulation of substance P and calcitonin gene-related peptide levels by nerve growth factor. *Neuroscience* 1989;33(1):53–65.
94. Livingston WK. Evidence of active invasion of denervated areas by sensory fibers from neighbouring nerves in man. *J Neurosurg* 1947;4:140–145.
95. Llinas R, Sugimori M. Calcium conductances in Purkinje cell dendrites: their role in development and integration. *Prog Brain Res* 1979;51:323–334.
96. Low P. Endoneurial potassium is increased and enhances spontaneous activity in regenerating mammalian nerve fibers—implication for neuropathic positive symptoms. *Muscle Nerve* 1985;8: 27–33.
97. Magistretti PJ, Schroder M. VIP and noradrenaline act synergistically to increase cyclic AMP in cerebral cortex. *Nature* 1984;308: 280–282.
98. Magistretti PJ, Morrison JH, Shoemaker WJ, Sapin V, Bloom FE. Vasoactive intestinal polypeptide induces glycogenesis in mouse cortical slices: a possible regulatory mechanism for the local control of energy metabolism. *Proc Natl Acad Sci USA* 1981;78:6535–6539.
99. Mah V, Vartavarian LM, Akers MA, Vinters HV. Abnormalities of peripheral nerve in patients with human immunodeficiency virus infection. *Ann Neurol* 1988;24(6):713–717.
100. Marbach JJ. Is phantom tooth pain a deafferentation (neuropathic) syndrome? *Oral Surg Oral Med Oral Pathol* 1993;75:95–105.
101. Marquez S, Turley JJE, Peters WJ. Neuropathy in burn patients. *Brain* 1993;116:471–483.
102. Maves TJ, Pechman PS, Gebhart GF, Meller ST. Possible chemical contribution from chromic gut sutures produces disorders of pain sensation like those seen in man. *Pain* 1993;54:57–69.
103. Mayer N, Lembeck F, Goedert M, Otten U. Effects of antibodies against nerve growth factor on the postnatal development of substance P-containing sensory neurons. *Neurosci Lett* 1982;29 (1): 47–52.
104. McArthur JC. Neurologic manifestations of AIDS. *Medicine* 1987; 66:407–37.
105. McCullock J, Kelly PAJ. A functional role for vasoactive intestinal polypeptide in anterior cingulate gyrus. *Nature* 1983;304:438–440.
106. McLachlan EM, Jnig W, Devor M, Michaelis M. Peripheral nerve injury triggers noradrenergic sprouting within dorsal root ganglia. *Nature* 1993;363:543–546.
107. Meiri J, Spira ME, Parnas I. Membrane conductance and axon potential of a regenerating axonal tip. *Science* 1981;211:709–711.
108. Meller ST, Gebhart GP. Nitric oxide (NO) and nociceptive processing in the spinal cord. *Pain* 1993;52:127–136.
109. Meller ST, Dykstra C, Gebhart CF. Production of endogenous nitric oxide and activation of soluble guanylate cyclase are required for *N*-methyl-D-asparate-produced facilitation of the nociceptive tailnick reflex. *Eur J Pharmacol* 1992;214:93–96.
110. Meller ST, Gebhart GF, Maves TJ. Neonatal capsaicin treatment prevents the development of the thermal hyperalgesia produced in a model of neuropathic pain in the rat. *Pain* 1992;51:317–321.
111. Meller ST, Pechman PS, Gebhart GF Maves TJ. Nitric oxide mediates the hermal hyperalgesia produced in a model of neuropathic pain in the rat. *Neuroscience* 1992;50:7–10.
112. Mense S. Sensitization of group IV muscle receptors to bradykinin by 5-hydroxytryptamine and prostaglandin E2. *Brain Res* 1981;225: 95–104.
113. Meyer RA, Srinivasa NR, Cambell JN, MacKinnon S, Dellon AL. Neural activity originating from a neuroma in baboon. *Brain Res* 1985;325:255–260.
114. Mikulec AA, Monroe FA, MacIver MB, Tanelian DL. EGF and CGRP increase in vitro corneal epithelial wound healing. *Invest Ophthalmol Vis Sci* 1993;34:1376(3323).
115. Myers RR, Yamamoto T, Yaksh TL, Powell HC. The role of focal nerve ischemia and Wallerian degeneration in peripheral nerve injury producing hyperesthesia. *Anesthesiology* 1993;78:308–316.
116. Nam SC, Kim KJ, Leem JW, Chung KS, Chung JM. Fiber counts at multiple sites along the rat ventral root after neonatal peripheral neurectomy or dorsal rhizotomy. *J Comp Neurol* 1989;290(3): 336–342.
117. Neil A, Attal N, Guilbaud G. Effects of guanethidine on sensitization to natural stimuli and self-mutilating behaviour in rats with a peripheral neuropathy. *Brain Res* 1991;565:237–246.
118. Nielsch U, Keen P. Reciprocal regulation of tachykinin- and vasoactive intestinal peptide-gene expression in rat sensory neurones following cut and crush injury. *Brain Res* 1989;481:25–30.
119. Nielsch U, Bisby MA, Keen P. Effect of cutting or crushing the rat sciatic nerve on synthesis of substance P by isolated L5 dorsal root ganglia. *Neuropeptides* 1987;10:137–145.
120. Noguchi K, DeLeon M, Nahin RL, Senba E, Ruda MA. Quantification of axotomy-induced alteration of neuropeptide mRNAs in dorsal root ganglion neurons with special reference to neuropeptide Y mRNA and the effects of neonatal capsaicin treatment. *J Neurosci Res* 1993;35(1):54–66.
121. Noguchi K, Dubner R, De Leon M, Senba E, Ruda MA. Axotomy

induces preprotachykinin gene expression in a subpopulation of dorsal root ganglion neurons. *J Neurosci Res* 1994;37:596–603.

122. Noguchi K, Senba E, Morita Y, Sato M, Tohyama M. Prepro-VIP and preprotachykinin mRNAs in the rat dorsal root ganglion cells following peripheral axotomy. *Mol Brain Res* 1989;6:327–330.
123. Noguchi K, Senba E, Morita Y, Sato M, Tohyama M. Alpha-CGRP and beta-CGRP mRNAs are differentially regulated in the rat spinal cord and dorsal root ganglion. *Brain Res* 1990;7(4):299–304.
124. Nothias F, Tessler A, Murray M. Restoration of Substance P and calcitonin gene related peptide in dorsal root ganglia and dorsal horn after neonatal sciatic nerve lesion. *J Comp Neurol* 1993;334: 370–384.
125. Nuytten D, Kupers R, Lammens M, Dom R, Van Hees J, Gybels J. Further evidence for myelinated as well as unmyelinated fiber damage in a rat model of neuropathic pain. *Exp Brain Res* 1992; 91:73–78.
126. Ochoa JL. The newly recognized painful ABC syndrome: thermographic aspects. *Thermology* 1986;2:65–107.
127. Ochoa JL, Yarnitsky D. Mechanical hyperalgesias in neuropathic pain patients: dynamic and static subtypes. *Ann Neurol* 1993;33: 465–472.
128. Oku R, Satoh M, Fujii N, Otaka A, Yajima H, Takagi H. Calcitonin gene-related peptide promotes mechanical nociception by potentiating release of substance P from the spinal dorsal horn in rats. *Brain Res* 1987;403:350–354.
129. Paul RL, Goodman H, Merzenich M. Alterations in mechanoreceptor input to Brodman's areas 1 and 3 of the postcentral hand area of Macaca mulatta after nerve section and regeneration. *Brain Res* 1972;39:1.
130. Perl ER. Myelinated afferent fibers innervating the primate skin and their response to noxious stimuli. *J Physiol* 1968;197(3): 593–615.
131. Pertovarra A. Collateral sprouting of nociceptive C-fibers after cut or capsaicin treatment of the sciatic nerve in adult rats. *Neurosci Lett* 1988;90:248–253.
132. Price DD, Bennett GJ, Rafii A. Psychophysical observations on patients with neuropathic pain relieved by a sympathetic block. *Pain* 1989;36:273–288.
133. Reid TW, Murphy CJ, Iwashashi CK, Foster BA, Mannis MJ. Stimulation of epithelial cell growth by the neuropeptide substance P. *J Cell Biochem* 1993;52(4):476–485.
134. Remgard P, Edbladh M, Ekstrom PAR, Edstrom A. Growth cones of regenerating adult sciatic sensory axons release axonally transported proteins. *Brain Res* 1992;572:139–145.
135. Ro LS, Jacobs JM. The role of the saphenous nerve in experimental sciatic nerve mononeuropathy produced by loose ligatures: a behavioral study. *Pain* 1993;52(3):359–369.
136. Roszkowski MT, Swift JQ, Hargreaves KM. Local tissue release of immunoreactive substance P, bradykinin, PGE2, and LTB4 in a model of surgically induced inflammation. *Soc Neurosci Abst* 1993; 19:521.
137. Rowbotham MC, Reisner-Keller LA, Fields HL. Both intravenous lidocaine and morphine reduce the pain of postherpetic neuralgia. *Neurology* 1991;41:1024–1028.
138. Said SI, Mutt V. Polypeptide with broad biological activity: isolation from small intestine. *Science* 1970;169:1217–1218.
139. Sato J, Perl ER. Adrenergic excitation of cutaneous pain receptors induced by peripheral nerve injury. *Science* 1991;251(5001): 1608–1610.
140. Scadding JW. Development of ongoing activity, mechanosensitivity, and adrenaline sensitivity in severed peripheral nerve axons. *Exp Neurol* 1981;73:345–364.
141. Schmalbruch H. Loss of sensory neurons after sciatic nerve section in the rat. *Anat Rec* 1987;219:323–329.
142. Seltzer Z, Devor M. Ephatic transmission in chronically damaged peripheral nerves. *Neurology* 1979;29:1061–1064.
143. Seltzer Z, Dubner R, Shir Y. A novel behavioral model of neuropathic pain disorders produced in rats by partial sciatic nerve injury. *Pain* 1992;43:205–218.
144. Shehab SAS, Atkinson ME. Vasoactive intestinal polypeptide increases in areas of the dorsal horn of the spinal cord from which other neuropeptides are depleted following peripheral axotomy. *Exp Brain Res* 1986;62:422–430.
145. Shir Y, Seltzer Z. A-fibers mediate mechanical hyperesthesia and allodynia and C-fibers mediate thermal hyperalgesia in a new model of causalgiaform pain disorders in rats. *Neurosci Lett* 1990;115:62–67.
146. Spitzer NC. Ion channels in development. *Annu Rev Neurosci* 1979; 2:363–397.
147. Stohr M, Schumm F, Reill P. Retrograde changes in motor and sensory conduction velocity after nerve injury. *J Neurosci* 1977; 214(4)281–287.
148. Stoll G, Jung S, Jander S, van der Meide P, Hartung HP. Tumor necrosis factor-alpha in immune-mediated demyelination and Wallerian degeneration of the rat peripheral nervous system. *J Neuroimmunol* 1993;45:175–82.
149. Swift JQ, Garry MG, Roszkowski MT, Hargreaves KM. Effect of flurbiprofen on tissue levels of immunoreactive bradykinin and acute postoperative pain. *J Oral Maxillofac Surg* 1993;51(2):112–116.
150. Tal M, Bennett GJ. Dextrorphan relieves neuropathic heat-evoked hyperalgesia in the rat. *Neurosci Lett* 1993;151:107–110.
151. Tal M, Devor M. Ectopic discharge in injured nerves: comparison of trigeminal and somatic afferents. *Brain Res* 1992;579(1):148–151.
152. Tanelian DL, MacIver MB. Analgesic concentrations of lidocaine suppress tonic A-delta and C fiber discharges produced by acute injury. *Anesthesiology* 1991;74:934–936.
153. Taylor P, Byers M, Redd P. Sprouting of CGRP nerve fibers in response to dentin injury in rat molars. *Brain Res* 1988;461: 371–376.
154. Tessler A, Himes BT, Krieger NR, Murray M, Goldberger ME. Sciatic nerve transection produces death of dorsal root ganglion cells and reversible loss of substance P in spinal cord. *Brain Res* 1985;332:209–218.
155. Thornena H, Barde Y-A. Physiology of nerve growth factor. *Physiol Rev* 1980;60:1284–1335.
156. Toma JG, Pareek S, Barker P, Mathew TC, Murphy RA, Acheson A, Miller FD. Spatiotemporal increases in epidermal growth factor receptors following peripheral nerve injury. *J Neurosci* 1992;12(7): 2504–2515.
157. Verge VMK, Riopelle RJ, Richardson PM. Nerve growth factor receptors on normal and injured sensory neurons. *J Neurosci* 1989;9:914–922.
158. Verge VM, Xu Z, Xu XJ, Wiesenfeld-Hallin Z, Hokfelt T. Marked increase in nitric oxide synthase mRNA in rat dorsal root ganglia after peripheral axotomy: in situ hybridization and functional studies. *Proc Natl Acad Sci USA* 1992;89(23):11617–11621.
159. Villar MJ, Cortes R, Theordorsson E, Wiesenfeld-Hallin Z, Schalling M, Fahrenkrug J, Emson PC, Hokfelt T. Neuropeptide expRession in rat dorsal root ganglion cells and spinal cord after peripheral nerve injury with special reference to galanin. *Neuroscience* 1989;33:587–604.
160. Wahren LK, Torebjork E. Quantitative sensory tests in patients with neuralgia 11 to 25 years after injury. *Pain* 1992;48(2):237–244.
161. Wall PD. The biological function and dysfunction of different pain mechanisms. In: Sicuteri F, Terenius L, Vecchiet L, eds. *Advances in pain therapy*. New York: Raven Press, 1992;19–28.
162. Wall PD, Devor M. Sensory afferent impulses originate from dorsal root ganglia as well as from the periphery in normal and nerve injured rats. *Pain* 1983;17:321–339.
163. Wall PD, Gutnick M. Properties of afferent nerve impulses originating from a neuroma. *Nature (Lond)* 1974;248:740–743.
164. Wall PD, Gutnick M. Ongoing activity in peripheral nerves: the physiology and pharmacology of impulses originating from a neuroma. *Exp Neurol* 1974;43:580–593.
165. Welk E, Leah JD, Zimmermann M. Characteristics of A- and C-fibers ending in a sensory nerve neuroma in the rat. *J Neurophysiol* 1990;11:759–766.
166. Wells MR, Vaidya U. Morphological alterations in dorsal root ganglion neurons after peripheral axon injury: association with changes in metabolism. *Exp Neurol* 1989;104:32–38.
167. Wetmore C, Bygdeman M, Olson L. High and low affinity NGF receptor mRNAs in human foetal spinal cord and ganglia. *Neuroreport* 1992;3:689–692.
168. Wiesenfeld-Hallin Z, Bartfai T, Hokfelt T. Galanin in sensory neurons in the spinal cord. *Front Neuroendocrinol* 1992;13:319–343.
169. Wiesenfeld-Hallin Z, Xu XJ, Villar MJ, Hokfelt T. The effect of intrathecal galanin on the flexor reflex in rat: increased depression after sciatic nerve section. *Neurosci Lett* 1989;105:149–154.
170. Willis WD. The Pain System. The neural basis of noniceptive transmission in the mammalian nervous system. *Pain and Headache* 1985;8:1–346.
171. Winer JB, Bang JRB, Clarke JR, Knox K, Cook TJ, et al. A study of neuropathy in HIV infection. *Q J Med* 1992;83:473–488.
172. Xie YK, Xiao WH, Li HQ. Relationship between new ion channels

and ectopic discharges from a region of nerve injury. *Sci China* 1993;36:68–74.

173. Yamamoto T, Yaksh TL. Effects of intrathecal capsaicin and an NK-1 antagonist, CP,96-345, on the thermal hyperalgesia observed following unilateral constriction of the sciatic nerve in the rat. *Pain* 1992;51:329–334.

174. Ygge J. Neuronal loss in lumbar dorsal root ganglia after proximal compared to distal sciatic nerve resection: a quantitative study in rat. *Brain Res* 1989;478:193–195.

175. Zhang X, Ju G, Elde R, Hokfelt T. Effect of peripheral nerve cut on neuropeptides in dorsal root ganglia and the spinal cord of monkey with special reference to galanin. *J Neurocytol* 1993;22:342–381.

Anesthesia: Biologic Foundations, edited by
Tony L. Yaksh et al. Lippincott–Raven Publishers,
Philadelphia © 1997.

CHAPTER 33

PHARMACOLOGY OF PERIPHERAL AFFERENT TERMINALS

ANDY DRAY

All tissues are innervated by afferent fibers, but the properties of these fibers differ markedly depending on whether they are somatic afferents (innervating skin, joints, muscles) or visceral afferents (innervating cardiovascular or respiratory tissues, the gastrointestinal tract, or renal and reproductive systems). Certain intense, unconditioned physical or chemical stimuli applied to somatic or visceral receptive fields will evoke an organized escape response and verbalization or vocalization consistent with discomfort, e.g., nociception. Two organizing principles should be considered. First, in the context of afferent populations mediating the response to these nociceptive stimuli, electrophysiologic studies have emphasized the role of fine, slowly conducting afferent fibers (C and A-δ fibers), rather than the rapidly conducting afferents for which low-threshold proprioceptive or mechanoreceptive stimuli serve as adequate stimuli (190,206) (see Chap. 31). Current work has emphasized that the family of fine fibers referred to as C-polymodal nociceptors is believed to constitute the principal class of afferent nociceptors. These afferents respond to increasing stimulus intensities with an increasing discharge frequency (see Chap. 4). Second, there is increasing evidence that tissue damage and inflammation result in local release of a wide variety of active factors, such as ions, amines, cytokines peptides, and enzymes, and will provoke several important events summarized in Fig. 1. These include changes in local blood flow and vascular permeability, and in activation and migration of immune cells. Furthermore, as will be reviewed below, local application of a variety of these products to the skin, vasculature, or viscera will yield pain behavior in humans and animal models. These agents applied to the distal terminal of the sensory afferent can have a series of profound actions including induction of activity in the quiescent C polymodal afferent, enhancement of the responsiveness of the afferent to otherwise ineffective stimuli, and altering the phenotype of the dorsal root ganglion cell. The importance of this humoral action is evidenced by the observation that a number of C-fiber terminals appear to be uniquely chemosensitive (72). Normally fibers or a terminal branch of the afferent axon appears unresponsive, even to intense physiologic stimuli. When influenced by inflammatory mediators, or following the administration of irritants, they may exhibit spontaneous activity or become sensitized and responsive to mechanical stimulation (68,72,169,173). These properties emphasize the probable pathophysiologic significance to afferent function played by humoral factors released during tissue damage and inflammation. This chapter discusses these factors and the current thinking on the pharmacology of the peripheral terminal.

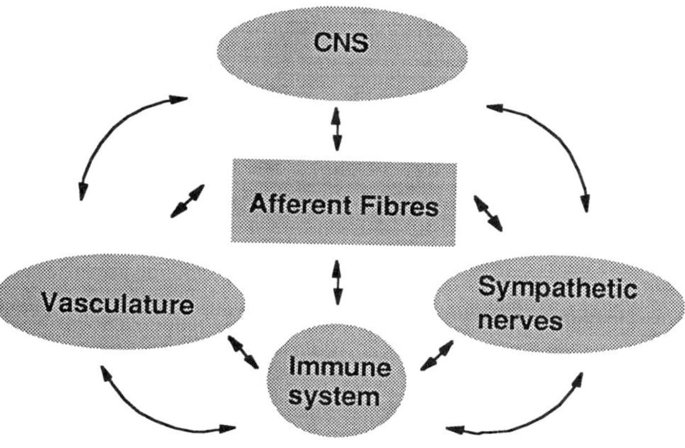

Figure 1. Tissue injury and inflammation trigger a cascade of interactions in which several systems—vascular, immune cells, sympathetic nerves and the CNS—interact. A variety of chemical mediators affects the activity of afferent fibers via interactions with pharmacologically defined receptors. Afferent fibers also exert reflex neurogenic influences on these systems.

COMPONENTS OF CHEMICAL TRANSDUCTION IN THE AFFERENT TERMINAL

Because of the technical difficulties of recording activity from fine afferent fibers, much of our understanding of the molecular signaling events in afferents has been obtained from studies of their cell bodies in sensory ganglia. Chemical mediators usually act via membrane receptors, which can be characterized using pharmacologically selective agents and by molecular biologic methods.

Many of the families of agents to be discussed below serve to interact with the excitability of the afferent terminal by interacting with a specific receptor complex that alters membrane ion permeability (e.g., the receptor is an ionophore, such as the nicotinic receptor or the receptor may be coupled to intracellular elements such as G proteins or other second messengers). This repertoire of cellular regulatory intermediates (G proteins, second messengers) may additionally be coupled to a number of ion channels that regulate membrane ion permeability (Fig. 2). Diverse signals produced by different chemicals can be amplified or attenuated by adjustments of common biochemical pathways or by stimulating the production of other mediators. For example, receptor coupled activation or inhibition of adenosine 3′,5′-cyclic monophosphate (cAMP) is a common mechanism by which membrane excitability is regulated through altered potassium conductance. Increased membrane K^+ conductance evoked by activation of a G_i protein results in a hyperpolarization of the membrane and depressed membrane excitability. Conversely, decreased K^+ permeability evoked by coupling to a G_s protein leads to an increased excitability of the membrane.

As in other excitable cells sensory neurons and their terminals express a diversity of ion channels (144). Several representative examples are cited in the following subsections.

Sodium Channels

Nerve fibers possess voltage-gated Na^+ channels that are important for nerve conduction and that can be blocked with the puffer-fish toxin tetrodotoxin. A large number of fine

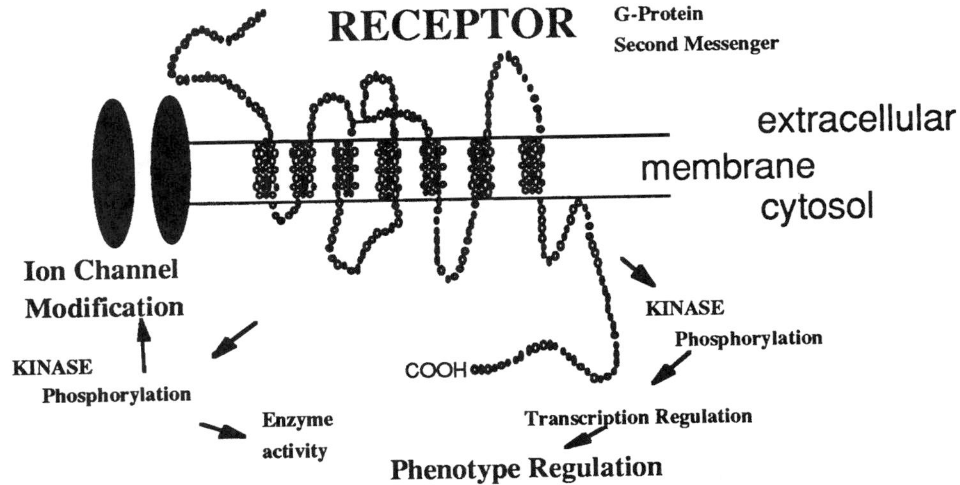

Figure 2. Chemical signal transduction by afferent fibers. Receptors are either coupled directly with ion channels or more commonly they are coupled via G proteins. Receptor activation induces changes in ionic conductance and thereby nerve excitability via phosphorylation of membrane ion channel proteins. Phosphorylation also alters the activity of enzymes or regulators of gene transcription to alter cell phenotype and thereby the synthesis of receptors and enzymes.

afferents fibers can be distinguished by having tetrodotoxin-resistant Na^+ channels that may be differentially regulated by inflammatory mediators (1). Most recently nerve growth factor (NGF) has been shown to promote the expression of a gene for the PN1 type of Na^+ channel, which is found only in peripheral afferent nerves and sympathetic fibers (138). The significance of this is not yet understood, although it may be related to increased afferent excitability and hyperalgesia caused by NGF (99).

Potassium Channels

Sensory neurons also possess calcium-activated potassium channels through which several proinflammatory mediators affect excitability and may thereby induce hyperalgesia (198).

Calcium Channels

As in other neurons, voltage-dependent T-, N-, and L-calcium channels contribute to the excitability of sensory neurons, but N-channels are particularly important as they control the release of neurochemicals from peripheral and central terminals of sensory neurons. N- and L-channels can be blocked by a number of drugs (dihydropyridines), or their opening prevented by several chemical transmitters (opioids, γ-aminobutyric acid [GABA], neuropeptide Y [NPY]) to prevent nociceptive signaling (47a,98). Abnormal calcium channel activity has been implicated in the ectopic discharges of sensory ganglion cells after peripheral nerve transection. Thus spontaneous discharges could be blocked by verapamil and a number of N-channel, ω–conotoxin derivatives (207,211).

NONNEURONAL FACTORS RELEASED SECONDARY TO TISSUE DAMAGE

A variety of substances are released upon damage to cells while others are synthesized during the events that follow tissue injury. These families of products have a profound impact on the production of inflammation and on afferent fiber activity.

Reactive Oxygen Species

Reactive oxygen species (ROS) include, H_2O_2, superoxide ($-O_2^{\cdot}$), and hydroxyl ($-OH^{\cdot}$), which are normal products of cellular electron transfer reactions, often involving xanthine oxidase activity. The production of ROS is finely controlled since cellular oxygenation is very important for the regulation of enzyme activity. Thus, ROSs are effectively neutralized by the antioxidative activity of superoxide desmutase and catalase. During ischemia, which follows the immediate vasoconstriction response upon tissue injury, there is a lack of oxygen, resulting in hypoxia or anoxia, and a fall in intracellular levels of ROS to unphysiologically low levels. This switches off antioxidant activity. Following this, reperfusion of injury creates a cellular oxidative stress in which oxygen and nitrogen species are produced in abundance. The above-normal levels of ROS produce a number of effects. There is a counteractive ROS-mediated induction of cellular transcription factors such as NF-kB and the *fos/jun* dimer, AP-1 (128). These activate the production of a second wave of gene products encoding enzymes with radical scavenging (catalase) and tissue repair activity (collagenase, stromelysin) as well as genes encoding cytokines, cell surface receptors, cell adhesion molecules, and hemopoietic growth factors. High levels of ROS, sufficient to be cytotoxic, result from a combination of events including ROS production by stimulated leukocytes, particularly neutrophils, and by oxidative stress induced by cytokine stimulation. Interestingly, aspirin has been shown to inhibit NF-kB production (92a), which may be relevant to its antiinflammatory activity.

Clearly, ROSs can make an important contribution to inflammation, but their effects on sensory neurons and the induction of hyperalgesia are largely unknown as few studies have been done. However, in vitro exposure of nociceptors to high concentrations of H_2O_2 did not evoke marked activation, although the effects of a number of inflammatory mediators (bradykinin, PGE_2) were significantly enhanced (93). However, it is well known that accidental application of H_2O_2, the contact lens sterilizing solution, to the corneal surface produces remarkable pain (Dray, *unpublished data*).

Protons

Proton activation of unmyelinated afferent fibers is likely to contribute to the sensation of aching and discomfort following tissue acidosis after muscle exercise. Indeed, direct activation of nociceptors accounts for the sharp stinging pain produced by local injections of acidic solutions. Such observations suggest that protons may have a pathophysiologic role in hypoxia/anoxia as well as in inflammation (36,121) in which the pH of the extracellular environment is known to fall. In addition, pain would result from direct nociceptor activation and from enhancing the effects of other inflammatory mediators (91).

Two types of proton-induced depolarization have been seen in sensory neurons. One type is associated with a rapid increase in membrane cation permeability evoked by pH changes in the normal physiologic range. The second type, associated with a more prolonged increase in membrane permeability, is evoked by lower extracellular pH, similar to that which gives rise to sustained nerve activation (14) and is responsible for enhanced afferent mechanosensitivity (177). It is likely that protons activate and depolarize nociceptors by acting on the external surface of the nerve membrane. However, CO_2-induced activation of nociceptors can be abolished by carbonic anhydrase inhibition, suggesting that activation could also occur following the intracellular generation of protons (177).

It is significant that protons and the agent capsaicin produce a similar activation of afferent nerves that may involve identical mechanisms (12,14). Capsaicin is an important pungent principally obtained from *Capsicum* peppers, with highly specific actions on polymodal nociceptors (13,49). Capsaicin activates nociceptors via a specific membrane receptor that can be distinguished by the competitive antagonist, capsazepine (15,47). Interestingly, following nociceptor activation, the increased membrane permeability to cations, particularly calcium ions, leads to membrane inexcitability. The consequences of this are that noxious stimuli are no longer effective in producing membrane desensitization; indeed, the release of sensory neuropeptides from the terminals is also prevented. Capsaicin can thus produce a selective analgesia and prevent neurogenic inflammation resulting form the local release of neuropeptides from the peripheral C-fiber terminal. The occurrence of a capsaicin receptor has also suggested that there may be an endogenous ligand for this site (Fig. 3). However, it is unclear whether protons are the most likely endogenous candidate, as capsazepine has no effect on proton-induced activation of sensory neurons (16,49). Other studies, however, show that proton-induced membrane changes in trigeminal neurons (101) and proton-induced neuropeptide release from visceral sensory neurons (heart, trachea) were inhibited by capsazepine (103,165). One explanation for this discrepancy is that protons induce the release of a capsaicin-like molecule or that visceral and somatic fibers differ in their mechanism of activation by protons. Recent studies favor the hypothesis that protons directly activate visceral afferents and that this is antagonized by capsazepine (59), suggesting heterogeneous mechanism for proton induced activation of afferent fibers. Finally, however, capsaicin and proton sensitivity is regulated in a similar manner since responsiveness is controlled by the presence of NGF (16a,201a) .

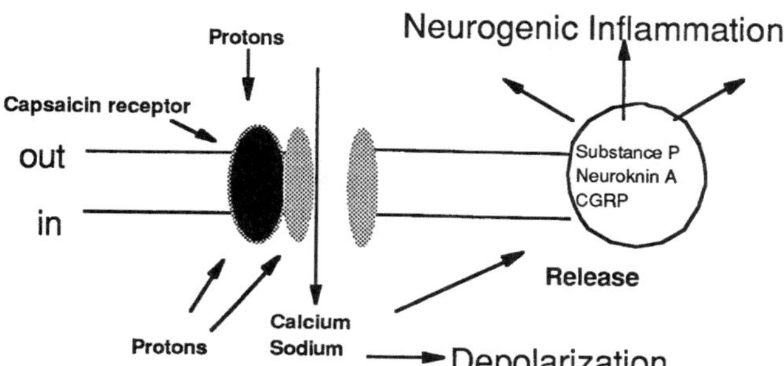

Figure 3. The membrane of an afferent terminal showing the capsaicin receptor. This receptor is coupled with an ion channel that allows entry of cations and induces depolarization. Calcium entry via this channel as well as calcium entry through voltage activated channels triggers peptide release and the activation of a number of calcium dependent enzymes. Proton-induced depolarization occurs via the capsaicin receptor or another proton sensitive site. The effect of capsaicin and protons (in some afferents) can be antagonized by capsazepine.

Nitric Oxide (NO)

NO Synthesis and Localization

NO is a readily diffusible and reactive molecule that is important in intercellular communication between many types of tissues, including cells of peripheral and central nociceptive pathways. NO is formed from L-arginine following the activation of the constitutive enzyme, nitric oxide synthase (cNOS), by calcium and other cofactors. NO then alters cellular processes mainly via the activation of guanylate cyclase and the production of cyclic guanosine monophosphate (GMP) (133) (See Chap. 10). cNOS is thought to be highly regulated through phosphorylation by a number of kinases (32). Small and medium-sized sensory neurons are able to make NO (2,193) and it is possible that they release NO, since an increase in cyclic GMP occurs in satellite cells in the DRG upon administration of NO donors (135).

During inflammation, a calcium-independent form of NOS (i-NOS) can be induced in a number of immune cell types including macrophages (133) and in microglia cells in the CNS. In addition, following peripheral nerve injury, NOS is also induced in many small sensory neurons that are likely to be involved in nociception (193). The i-NOS in immune cells can produce high concentrations of NO, sufficient to induce a number of systemic pathologic effects (e.g., hypotension, vascular leakage) including cytotoxicity, especially when combined with other ROS to form peroxynitrite.

Membrane Action of NO

Under normal physiologic conditions, there is little evidence for direct activation of sensory neuron by NO (120), although intradermal injection of NO dissolved in phosphate buffer induced a delayed burning pain in man (78), and NO donors have been postulated to activate cerebral sensory fibers directly, causing release of the vasodilator CGRP (197). Indeed, NO has been suggested to contribute to migraine and other types of head pain (146). However, NO can also alter the excitability of sensory neurons indirectly by changing their responsiveness to inflammatory chemicals such as bradykinin (24,120,160). The details of this interaction are not known but may be produced through a cyclic GMP–dependent regulation of bradykinin receptor-effector coupling mechanism.

Inducible NOS also has an important role in the regulation of an inducible form of cyclooxygenase COX-2 activity (162) and hence the production of proinflammatory prostanoids. It is also possible that NO formation contributes to the ectopic discharges induced by peripheral nerve lesions as the increased sensory neuronal excitability is reduced by NOS inhibitors (193). Indeed, NOS inhibitors have been shown to produce antinociception in neuropathic (126,193) and chemically induced pain (134). It was concluded that the effects were mostly centrally mediated by the inhibition of NO-induced activation of glutamate release and thence *N*-methyl-D-aspartate (NMDA) receptors or by counteracting the effects of NO released from spinal cells (109,110,126). Since few inhibitors are selective for the specific form of NOS that occurs in neurons (7-nitroindazole), it is conceivable that vasoconstriction may have been a contributing factor to the effects of many nonspecific NOS inhibitors.

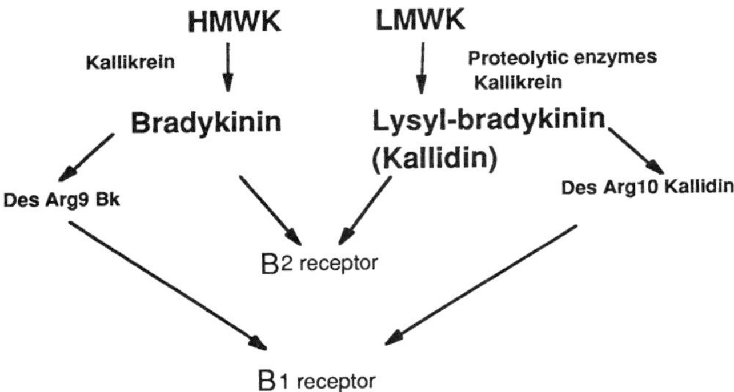

Figure 4. Kinin synthesis is stimulated during blood clotting and following tissue damage. The actions of kallikrein and other proteolytic enzymes form bradykinin and kallidin from high-molecular-weight kininogen (HMWK) and low-molecular-weight kininogen (LMWK) precursors, respectively. Both bradykinin and kallidin act predominantly on B2 receptors. Metabolism of these kinins by the enzyme kininase I forms des Arg^{9}Bk and des Arg^{10}kallidin, respectively. These metabolites act on B1 receptors. Enzyme activity at other cleavage sites produces inactive metabolites.

Kinins

Kinin Synthesis

There are two major biochemical cascades that produce kinins, one that occurs within the blood and a second in other tissues. In the plasma, bradykinin is formed as part of the blood-clotting cascade from high–molecular-weight kininogen precursor, by the enzymatic action of kallikrein or other proteolytic enzymes. In other tissues, the precursor for kinin production is a low-molecular-weight kininogen. This is degraded by tissue kallikrein and by proteolytic enzymes liberated during tissue damage to form kallidin (Lysyl-bradykinin) (8,17). Kinin production may also occur without kallikrein activity since kinins can be formed by immune cells (mast cells, basophils) associated with acute inflammatory reactions following the release of cellular proteases. Both bradykinin and kallidin are rapidly degraded by kininases to generate the active metabolites desArg^{9}bradykinin or desArg^{10}kallidin, respectively (Fig. 4).

Kinin Receptors

The effects of kinins are mediated via two main receptors, B1 and B2, although B3 receptors have been hypothesized to exist in the airways (69). The B1 (127) and B2 receptor (119) belong to the super family of G-protein–coupled receptors with seven transmembrane spanning domains, but there appears to be little sequence homology between these kinin receptors. The preferred agonist for the B2 receptor is bradykinin, but kallidin also acts here. A number of selective antagonists with high affinity for the B2 receptor are available including the peptide analogues NPC567, NPC16731 (Hoe 140; 69,77), dimeric peptides such as CP-0127 (31), and the nonpeptide antagonist WIN 64338 (163) (Fig. 5). The pharmacology of the B1 receptor has not been as extensively characterized, but this receptor is preferentially activated by the kinin metabolites des-Arg^{9}-bradykinin or desArg^{10}kallidin whereas des-Arg^{9}-Leu^{8}-bradykinin has been used as the prototypic antagonist at this site (Fig. 5).

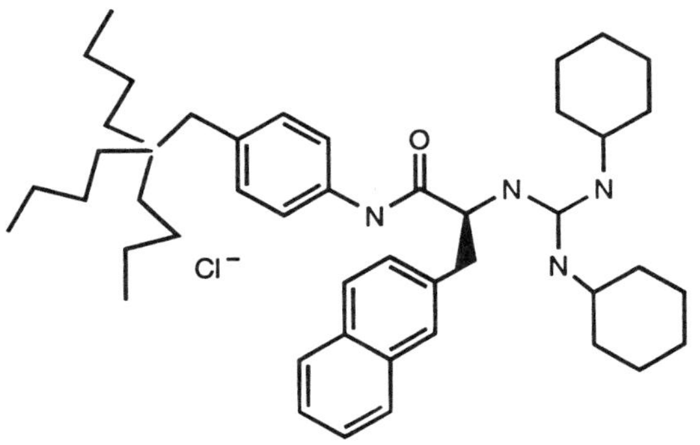

B1 receptors are constitutively expressed in certain tissues such as arterial smooth muscle. In general, they are encountered infrequently under normal conditions. However, B1 receptor expression is increased rapidly during inflammation or infection. This is due to the influence of immune cell products such as certain cytokines, interleukin (IL)-1β in particular (60). Although this may involve the synthesis of new receptor, it is also highly likely that unmasking of existing receptors or the facilitation of receptor-effector coupling can also occur.

Figure 5. Structures of peptidergic B2 receptor antagonists ranging from the earlier D-Phe7 substituted analogues to more recent analogues like Icatibant and Bradycor. WIN 64338 is the only nonpeptidergic antagonist to be described.

Kinin Membrane Effects

Of the kinins, bradykinin has received closest attention and exerts a number of proinflammatory effects: plasma extravasation; the release of prostaglandins, cytokines, and free radicals from a variety of cells; stimulation of postganglionic sympathetic neurons to affect blood vessel caliber and to release prostanoids; and the degranulate of mast cells to release histamine and other inflammatory mediators. Bradykinin, however, is a potent algogenic substance and induces pain by directly stimulating B2 receptors in skin, joint, and muscle afferents, as well as by sensitizing them to other stimuli including heat and mechanical stimulation (152a). Indeed, there is a strong synergism between the actions of bradykinin and other algogenic substances, e.g., prostaglandins and 5-hydroxytryptamine. Sympathetic neurons, which are activated by B2 kinin receptors, may also be involved in bradykinin-mediated mechanical hyperalgesia (183), although in the skin the mechanism for this is unclear as sympathectomy did not alter heat hyperalgesia induced by bradykinin (92,129).

Other studies support bradykinin as an important mediator of pain, since selective antagonists, especially Hoe 140, show that blockade of B2 receptors significantly attenuates pain and hyperalgesia in a number of conditions (74,149). These data indicate that B2 antagonists are likely to be useful analgesics in the future.

The mechanism of B2-receptor–induced activation of sensory neurons requires the activation of phospholipase C. This generates two intracellular second messengers, 1,4,5-inositoltrisphosphate (IP_3) and diacylglycerol (DAG) following cleavage of membrane phospholipids. IP_3 stimulates the release of calcium from intracellular stores, producing a rise in free calcium concentration within the cell. The effect of DAG is to activate protein kinase C (PKC) and to phosphorylate cellular proteins including membrane receptors and ion channels. PKC plays a key role in the excitation of afferent fibers by bradykinin (52) and this is associated with an inward ionic current in sensory neurons and an increase in membrane conductance, mainly to sodium ions (27,120,122) (Fig. 6). Bradykinin can also induce calcium influx (140,187) into sensory neurons. This is responsible for the secondary release of neuropeptides such as substance P and for stimulating arachidonic acid production via the activation of phospholipase C or alternatively by metabolism of DAG (153). However, in visceral sensory neurons (nodose ganglion cells), increased excitability is often associated with the inhibition of a long-lasting spike afterhyperpolarization (slow-AHP) that is regulated by a cAMP-dependent, calcium-activated potassium conductance mechanism. The slow-AHP, following a single action potential, produces a state of inexcitability that limits the number of action potentials that can be evoked upon stimulation (198). Prostaglandins and bradykinin (through prostanoid formation) inhibit the slow-AHP by stimulating cAMP formation, thus allowing the cell to fire repetitively following depolarization (Fig. 6). This mechanism may be common to a number of hyperalgesic substances and can account for sensitization of sensory neurons. Cyclic GMP also regulates B2 receptors on sensory neurons. Thus, bradykinin-induced IP_3 production and activation of sensory neurons is reduced in the presence of cGMP, possibly via desensitization of the B2 receptor (24,120,160). An important mechanism of desensitization is initiated via NO production, since inhibitors of NOS activity attenuated bradykinin-induced desensitization in sensory neurons and peripheral nociceptors (120,160).

As noted above, during inflammation there is an increase in the expression of B1 receptors. The practical significance of this effect is not entirely clear, but during inflammation or IL-1 administration, B1 receptors make an important contribution to hyperalgesia, as B1 receptor antagonists produce analgesia (40,43,50). Since there is little evidence for a direct activation of sensory neurons by B1 receptors, it is likely that B1-receptor–mediated hyperalgesia is mediated indirectly via release of other mediators (e.g., prostaglandins) from macrophages and leukocytes (43).

Arachidonic Acid Metabolites: Prostanoids

Prostanoid Synthesis

Prostanoids are synthesized upon the release of cell-membrane–derived arachidonic acid by the activation of phospholipase A. (164) (See Chap. 8). Membrane-bound enzymes lipoxygenase (145), or cyclooxygenase (164), act on these substrates to synthesize the leukotrienes and the prostanoids from arachidonic acid in the course of inflammatory diseases such as rheumatoid arthritis or after experimental inflammation. Thus, measurement of the extravascular, extracellular fluid, e.g., as in blister fluid, burn exudate, or knee joint fluid, reveals significant levels of a number of these lipidic acids including PGE_2, TXA_2, PGI_2 (65,71,201,202). Various agents, including norepinephrine and dopamine, stimulate synthesis of cellular phospholipids by releasing nonesterified free fatty acid precursors (58). Local intraarterial bradykinin will enhance the formation and release of prostaglandins (89,121).

Membrane Effects

COX products, notably TXA_2, PGI_2, PGD_2, $PGF_{2\alpha}$, and PGE interact with their own respective receptors, and PGE is believed to have at least three subtypes (64,70,154). Thus, prostaglandin PGD_2 interacts with the DP sites, PGE_2 with the EP sites, the FP receptor with the PGF_{2a} site, the IP receptor with the PGI_2 sites, and the TP sites with the TXA_2. Extensive

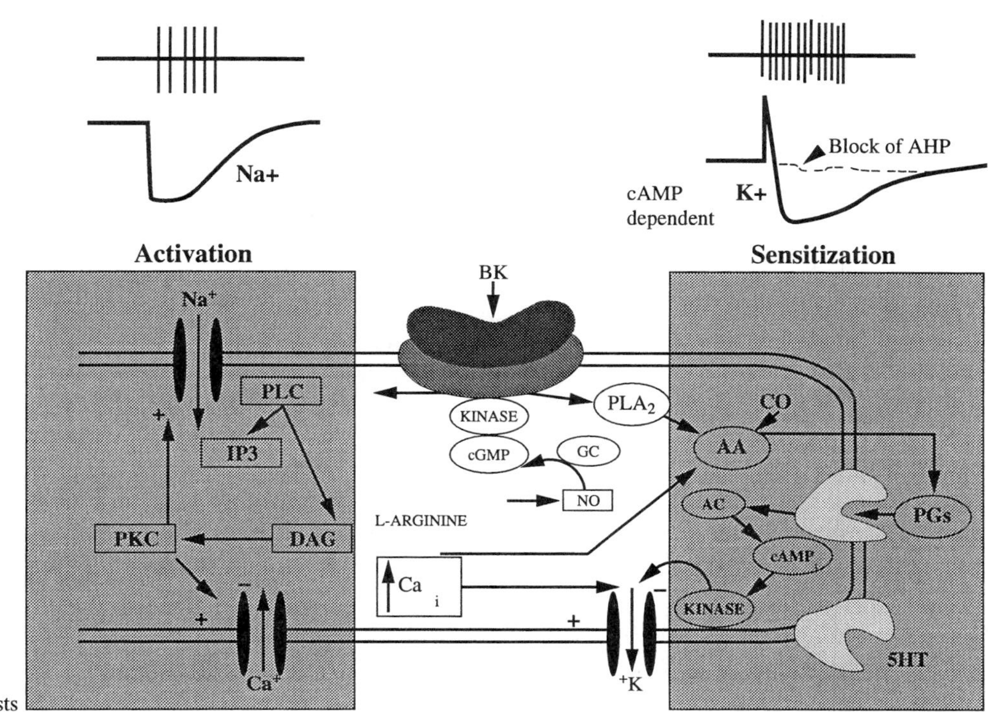

Figure 6. The afferent nerve terminal showing that B2 receptor activation generates PKC activity and increases Na^+ conductance that produces action potentials *(above)*. B2 receptor activation also generates arachidonic acid (AA) and prostanoids from phospholipase A_2 (PLA_2) activity. Bradykinin and prostanoids block cAMP-dependent potassium conductance to inhibit a long-lasting postspike afterhyperpolarization (AHP) and to facilitate cell firing *(shown above)*. This may be a mechanism for peripheral nociceptor sensitization during inflammatory hyperalgesia and may be shared by several mediators including 5-HT and prostanoids. Calcium-induced activation of NOS produces NO and the formation of cGMP via guanylate cyclase (GC). This may desensitize the bradykinin receptor.

literature has evolved reflecting upon the prostaglandins receptor effects; these actions include stimulation of inositol triphosphate (210), activation of PLC (20), stimulation of adenylate cyclase (164), and increases in [Ca] (204). Conversely, inhibitory effects by several prostanoids on cAMP production have been reported and are inhibited by a pertussis toxin-sensitive mechanism (125,141). The EP_3 receptor subtype, a G-protein–coupled receptor linked with adenylate cyclase, has been identified in the majority of sensory neurons, and is particularly linked with small diameter cells (181a).

Prostaglandins have been thought not to activate sensory neurons directly since they do not evoke pain when injected intradermally into human skin (39). In some circumstances, however, prostaglandins appear to produce a direct activation of sensory neurons since PGE_1 and prostacyclin (PGI_2) increased the activity of nociceptors in rat articular nerves (21,169), and PGE_2 stimulated the release of substance P from sensory neurons in culture (143). These direct excitatory effects may be due to an increased membrane Na^+ conductance (151). Some, but not all, families of prostaglandins serve to sensitize sensory neurons to other stimuli, thus contributing to mechanisms of peripheral hyperalgesia (21,132 170,172). PGE_2 and PGI_2 commonly induce sensitization, but PGD_2 does not (159). Sensitization by prostaglandins involves cAMP production (56), and agents that elevate cAMP may also induce hyperalgesia (182). The mechanisms of sensitization have not yet been fully elucidated but may involve a lowering of the threshold for the firing of action potentials in sensory neurons (142). In visceral afferent neurons, prostaglandins increase excitability via cAMP-mediated inhibition of the slow spike-AHP as described earlier with bradykinin.

Enzyme Inhibitors

Prevention of prostaglandin generation by inhibition of cyclooxygenase (COX) is believed to be one of the principal mechanisms for the antihyperalgesic and antiinflammatory actions of nonsteroidal anti-inflammatory drugs (NSAIDs) (see Chap. 34). Both the constitutive form of COX (COX-1) and a form induced during inflammation COX-2 (15) are susceptible to NSAIDs. Some NSAIDs (aspirin, indomethacin), however, act more potently against COX-1 than COX-2. Such findings have suggested that the therapeutic antiinflammatory and analgesic benefits of NSAIDs are derived from inhibition of COX-2, and the side effects attributed to inhibition of the constitutive enzyme COX-1 that normally synthesizes a number of prostanoids having an essential tissues protective function (23,131,174). However, there are other mechanisms by which NSAIDs produce their effects involving direct inhibition of afferent fiber excitability (178) or by inhibiting the formation of NFkB, an important activator of gene transcription, which is involved in the induction of immune-cell products and COX-2 (92a).

Other products of the arachidonic acid cascade, including leukotriene B_4 (a product of the 5-lipoxygenase pathway) or 8R,15S-di-hydroxyeicosatetraenoic acid (HETE) (a product of the 15-lipoxygenase pathway) decrease the mechanical and thermal thresholds for nociception after intradermal injection (97,106,115,152). The action of LTB_4 is unaffected by block of cyclooxygenase activity and appears to be mediated indirect via the release of 8R,15S-diHETE from polymorphonuclear leukocytes (97). 8R,15S-diHETE, however, appears to produce hyperalgesia directly, by decreasing the mechanical and thermal thresholds of C fibers (114). The hyperalgesic effect of 8R,15S-diHETE and LTB_4 can be inhibited by the isomer 8S,15S-diHETE (97), indicating that there may be complex inhibitory as well as facilitory interactions of prostanoids and nociceptor sensitivity.

Adenosine Triphosphate and Adenosine

Adenosine triphosphate (ATP) is released by tissue damage (153) where it can act on the local terminals of C fibers to produces a sharp, transient pain. Sensory neuron activation by ATP is due to an increase in Na^+ and Ca^{2+} ion permeability and can be blocked by purinergic P_2 receptor antagonists, such as suramin (10a,93a).

Adenosine, formed by the breakdown of ATP, also provokes pain when administered intradermally, intravenously, or onto a blister base (22,181b,186). The effects of adenosine are complex. The activation of A_2 receptors on sensory neurons induces hyperalgesia most probably via the activation of adenylate cyclase and production of AMP (186). As indicated earlier cAMP-induced changes in ion channel permeability account for the afferent hyperexcitability. On the other hand A_1 receptors are negatively coupled to cAMP activation, which reduces afferent excitability by blocking Ca^{2+} conductance or increasing K^+ permeability (104). Adenosine-mediated analgesia can occur both centrally or peripherally as agonists are efficacious when administered at either location (90,186). However, others have failed to show that A_1 or A_2 receptor ligands influence the activation of mechanoreceptive afferent fibers in normal or arthritic ankle joints in the rat (6), suggesting further direct studies are necessary.

Serotonin (5-HT)

Localization

In the circulation, serotonin is found in high concentrations in mast cells and platelets and these stores are released by degranulation and clotting (54). Platelets do not synthesize this amine, but possess the active uptake systems that allow them to avidly accumulate the molecule from the plasma and tissue.

Membrane Actions

Serotonin (5-HT) interacts with a diverse family of membrane receptors, many of which have been identified and cloned. Thus, at present 14 separate 5-HT receptors have evolved, which can be divided into seven main families (113,150,157).

Electrophysiologic studies have shown that 5-HT can excite dorsal root ganglion cells by several mechanisms, interacting with $5\text{-}HT_2$ and $5\text{-}HT_3$ sites. The activation of sensory neurons via $5\text{-}HT_2$ receptors is mediated by G proteins to close potassium channels, leading to membrane depolarization and neuronal firing (189). The $5\text{-}HT_3$ receptor binding site is part of a cation (Na^+) selective ion channel (112), and agonist occupancy of this site leads to depolarization and activation of sensory neurons. Finally, 5-HT may sensitize nociceptors and lower their threshold to heat and pressure stimuli (11). This action is mediated by activation of a cAMP-dependent kinase system. Thus, 5-HT–induced sensitization of nociceptors was blocked by Rp-cAMPS (an inhibitor of cAMP), and augmented by phosphodiesterase inhibition (185). Indeed, it has been proposed that 5-HT increases sensory neural excitability by a cAMP-mediated reduction of K^+ permeability. This mechanism attenuates the slow-AHP that follows the action potential and provokes repetitive firing (33).

Applications of serotonin to a blister base evokes mild and transient pain (155), and a similar direct excitation of sensory neurons is believed to occur when serotonin is released from platelets and mast cells during injury or inflammation. The algogenic effect of serotonin is believed to be due to an excitatory action at the $5\text{-}HT_3$ receptor activation, e.g., it is antagonized by $5HT_3$ receptor blockers (155,156).

Clearly, the molecular actions of 5-HT, to produce pain and hyperalgesia, are complex and involve a number of receptor subtypes. Sensitization and hyperalgesia appear to involve both 5-HT_1 and 5-HT_2 receptors (158,185), while the 5-HT–induced activation and the enhancement of bradykinin-evoked pain in the human blister base was blocked by ICS 205.930 (155), which appears to be 5-HT_3 receptor-mediated. Although ICS 205.930 may also act to block a 5-HT_4 receptor, so far this receptor has not been independently implicated in the effects of 5-HT on afferent nerves.

It is important to note that 5-HT_{1D}-like receptors, which are located on fine afferent fibers innervating the dura mater of the brain, have also been proposed to *reduce* afferent excitability, thereby reducing pain as well as the plasma extravasation and vasodilatation brought about by local sensory neuropeptide release. Such receptors may be important in ameliorating migraine headache, as a number of antimigraine agents including sumatriptan can prevent migraine by interacting as an agonist at these sites (28,29,84) (see Chap. 50).

Cytokines

Several cytokines are released by phagocytotic and antigen presenting cells of the immune system (See Chap. 20). These peptides are important cell regulators that stimulate the synthesis and release of a variety of agents (NO, PGs, SP) that trigger inflammation and thereby influence sensory neuron excitability.

Injection of IL-1β and IL-6 will induce a thermal and mechanical hyperalgesia. This effect may not be direct on the afferent as it is blocked by indomethacin and may be due in part to the release of prostaglandins from monocytes and fibroblasts (41–43,57,59a). In contrast, the hyperalgesia produced by IL-8 is blocked by β-adrenoceptor and dopamine (D_1) antagonists, and by the sympathetic neuron blocking drug, guanethidine, suggesting that the effects of IL-8 involve sympathetic nerves (41). On the other hand IL-1β has also been reported to activate and sensitize afferent fiber directly (59a).

Tumor necrosis factor (TNF-α) also induces mechanical hyperalgesia that can be attenuated, but not abolished, by antisera to IL-1, IL-6, and IL-8 (42). The effects of TNF-α are also attenuated by Lys-D-Pro-Thr, indomethacin, and a β-adrenergic receptor antagonist, indicating similarities between its actions and those of other cytokines against which these agents are effective. Other studies however give little support for the efficacy of TNF-α in producing hyperalgesia (43). It is not known whether TNF-α has direct actions on afferents since its hyperalgesic effects appear to be mediated in large part via the release of other cytokines.

The effects of some cytokines may be selective since hyperalgesia can be attenuated by specific antibodies, and in the case of IL-1, by the endogenous receptor antagonists of IL-1. In addition a-melanocyte-stimulating hormone and tripeptides related to Lys-D-Pro-Thr attenuate IL-1β- and IL-6- but not IL-8-induced hyperalgesia (41,57). It is also significant that the hyperalgesia induced by carrageenan, LPS, and UV irradiation of the skin was attenuated by Hoe 140 and by des Arg^8Leu^8 Bk indicating that kinin B2 and B1 receptors, respectively, were important for inducing hyperalgesia and may have been a primary stimulus for cytokine production(42,43,147: 148).

Neurotrophic Factors (Neurotrophins)

Origin

Nerve growth factor (NGF) is produced by peripheral target tissues for afferent fibers and by supporting cells including fibroblasts, Schwann cells, and keratinocytes (see Chap. 2).

Membrane Action

Dimeric NGF acta preferentially on one specific tyrosine kinase receptor, trkA, on sensory neurons. Following receptor activation, the NGF is transported to the cell body coupled with a low-affinity receptor complex, p75. Here it facilitates phosphorylation of special transcription factors such as Oct-2 (203) to interact with gene promoter regions and enhance gene transcription.

Under normal circumstances, NGF is essential for the survival and development of sensory neurons and for maintaining their phenotype (99,100). During inflammation increased amounts of NGF have been measured, in pleurisy, in the synovial fluid from patients with rheumatoid arthritis (3), in blister fluid, and in skin injured with UV irradiation. NGF has a number of functions, including to stimulate growth and differentiation of peripheral fibers as well as to release a number of mediators including histamine and LTC_4 from mast cells and leukocytes. On the other hand the synthesis of NGF is stimulated by cytokines such as IL-1β and TNF-α.

In sensory neurons, NGF induces mRNA for the neuropeptide precursors of tachykinins and CGRP. In addition the axoplasmic transport and release of sensory neuropeptides substance P and CGRP are enhanced (48). NGF also selectively regulates a number of other important proteins in afferent neurons such as the capsaicin receptor (201a), proton-activated ion channels (12), and the tetrodotoxin (TTX)-resistant Na^+ channel (1). Since NGF also promotes axonal sprouting at the periphery it can increase the receptive field of sensory fibers (46). As a result of these effects NGF induces prolonged increases in chemosensitivity and synaptic efficacy seen during inflammatory hyperalgesia. Consistent with this are studies showing that inflammatory mediators, or the injection of NGF, increases sensitivity to noxious stimuli. On the other hand anti-NGF antibodies reduce the hyperalgesia produced by NGF as well as that following inflammation (99,206). Anti-NGF antibodies also prevent the increase in mRNA for sensory neuropeptides seen after NGF treatment or inflammation (206). Interestingly, peripheral axotomy, which removes the target tissue source of NGF, induces a reduction of neurokinin and CGRP synthesis, whereas dorsal rhizotomy increases synthesis, indicating that the neurochemistry of sensory neurons is also regulated by other centrally derived neurotrophins whose identity is not known (85,194).

NGF is also an important trophic regulator for sympathetic neurons. Overexpression of NGF induces proliferation of sympathetic fibers to increase the innervation of perivascular areas and to innervation DRG neurons, which do not normally receive a sympathetic fiber input (44). The consequences of these effects are presently unclear but may be important in the production of hyperalgesia and causalgia in inflammatory and neuropathic pain conditions. Clearly, further studies of adrenergic receptors on afferent fibers are important in order to determine whether these are also changed by trophic factors or by pathophysiologic conditions.

NEURONAL FACTORS RELEASED SECONDARY TO TISSUE DAMAGE

In the preceding section, the appearance of several active factors secondary to local tissue injury was reviewed. Now we consider the role played by several specific neuronal elements that release products secondary to local tissue insult: the primary afferent terminal and the sympathetic nerve terminal.

Afferent Neuropeptides

It has long been appreciated that antidromic activation can induce peripheral changes suggestive of an efferent function

(9,10). Accordingly , it has been shown that the peripheral terminal of small, capsaicin-sensitive sensory afferents contains vesicularly stored pools of transmitters, such as substance P and CGRP (67) and that these transmitters may be locally released from the peripheral terminal secondary to local depolarization in a variety of tissues, including the eye (18), skin (130,199), knee joint (208), pia (137), and a variety of smooth muscle sites (83). This depolarization-evoked release can be induced by antidromic invasion of the terminal or by a local action of an agent on specific terminal receptor (such as bradykinin, or nicotine) or by the opening of a family of channels (such as for calcium or for protons) (80–82). This release is typically calcium dependent and displays all of the properties of excitatory-secretion coupling expected with neurotransmission (98).

Effects of Neurokinin Release

There is little evidence that the neurokinins directly affect afferent fibers excitability. However, direct depolarization of DRG neurons by substance P has been described (52a), and NK1 receptors on primary afferents have been postulated (108). Thus, it remains an intriguing possibility that presynaptic actions of NKs may be important for regulating spinal excitability. On the other hand, postsynaptic receptors for neurokinins have been more extensively characterized in the spinal cord where neurokinins play an essential role with glutamate to enhance the excitability of dorsal horn neurons following repetitive stimulation of peripheral nociceptive C fibers (191).

While the afferent peptides may not have a potent direct effect on afferent terminal activation, there is ample evidence to indicate that the peripheral release of neuropeptides (neurokinins, CGRP) from the peripheral endings of sensory nerves is believed to have an important function related to efferent and trophic activities as well as to the regulation of the immune system (reviewed in refs. 79,106a,197). They contribute to neurogenic inflammation and hyperalgesia in the periphery, while their release from central terminals in the spinal cord is involved in the transmission of pain signals and changes in excitability in the dorsal horn.

Substance P, NKA, and CGRP contribute to inflammation and hyperalgesia in a number of ways and in a number of systems (Fig. 7). As noted above, substance P and CGRP release from peripheral terminals has been demonstrated in a number of tissues. This local release can exert a number of trophic influences. Several examples may be cited: (a) Substance P can stimulate (via NK1 receptors) calcium-dependent NO synthesis from vascular endothelium, thereby causing vasodilation. In addition, substance P–induced contraction of endothelial cells causes plasma extravasation, via a specific NK1 receptor action (107). Stimulation of cytokine production from monocytes (102) leads to the activation of adhesion molecules necessary for the interaction of leukocytes with the vascular endothelium. Substance P may degranulate mast cells, allowing the release of inflammatory mediators, but this interaction does not involve an NK-receptor activation. CGRP does not produce plasma extravasation but is a powerful arteriolar vasodilator and by increasing blood flow into venules acts synergistically with substance P to enhance plasma extravasation (25,61). (b) Peripheral sensory terminals, and particularly those involved in substance P release, play a critical role in joint inflammation and in the etiology of rheumatoid arthritis. Thus, depletion of substance P by capsaicin can attenuate the development of animal models of inflammatory arthritis (94,96). (c) NK1 receptor–induced plasma extravasation may have special significance in cerebral inflammation and in the etiology of migraine and vascular headache. Thus, NK1 receptor antagonists, like other antimigraine drugs, potently attenuate the plasma extravasation induced by sensory nerve stimulation (139,176). It will be important to discover whether NK1 receptor antagonists have clinical antimigraine activity.

Tachykinin Receptors

The effects of neurokinins are mediated through the activation of one of several neurokinin receptors—NK1, NK2, or NK3, at which SP, NKA, and NKB, respectively, are the preferred naturally occurring ligands (107). From studies to date, tachykinin actions via NK1 and NK2 receptors have been considered to be responsible for the proinflammatory and

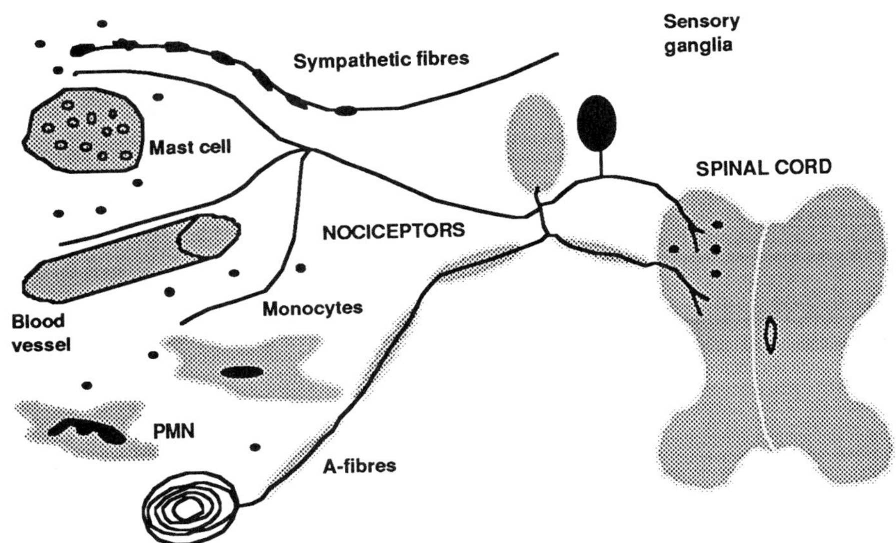

Figure 7. Neurogenic effects of afferent fibers are produced by the release of a number of peptides including neurokinins (substance P and neurokinin A) and CGRP. In the periphery, the neurokinins activate sympathetic fibers, and induce vasodilatation and plasma extravasation. They also stimulate immune cells and degranulating mast cells. These peptides are also released in the spinal dorsal horn to transmit nociceptive information and induce long-lasting changes in spinal excitability. Release of CGRP acts as a powerful arteriolar vasodilator.

hyperalgesic effects of neurokinins (98). Little work has been done related to NK3 receptors, and their involvement in afferent fiber activity or pain mechanisms is unclear. However, NK3 receptors are upregulated in the spinal cord following peripheral inflammation (118).

Neurokinin receptors belong to the family of G-protein–coupled receptors with a seven transmembrane spanning domain (140). The NK1 and NK2 receptors have been the most extensively characterized due to the development of a number of nonpeptide NK1 antagonists (CP99994, RP67580, SR140333), but a number of peptide and nonpeptide antagonists are also available for the NK2 receptor (e.g., MEN10,376, FK888, SR48,968) (196). Molecular studies using constructs of chimeric NK1 receptors have given some remarkable insights into the way in which ligands and receptors interact. Thus, important species differences have been identified in the binding epitopes for NK1 antagonists while point mutations of single amino acids in the NK1 receptor indicate that there are a few binding domains contained in TM5 and TM6 that are critical for nonpeptide antagonist binding (63). Such studies indicate that receptor-ligand modeling will facilitate the rational design of highly specific ligands for these binding epitopes.

Regulation of Afferent Neurokinin Activity and Effects

Given the importance of the peripherally released neuropeptides, it is important to note that their presence and postterminal actions are regulated by a variety of influences at the cellular and functional levels. As an example for general consideration, the economy of substance P will be presented.

At the cellular level, during inflammation neuropeptide content of sensory nerves is initially reduced, due to neural activation and increased release (63a). Following this, however, a number of changes occur. These include an increase in mRNA for neurokinin precursors, pre-proneurokinins, and, in the content of SP, NKA and a genomically unrelated peptide, CGRP (63a). Sprouting of sensory fibers may also occur, and NGF is an important intermediary for these effects. Normally, NGF is released from target tissues, e.g., fibroblasts, and provides an important trophic stimulus for maintaining the expression of some sensory neuropeptides. However, during inflammation greater amounts of NGF are secreted from a variety of cell types under the influence of cytokines (48). NGF then acts to increase mRNA for precursor peptides via the activation of specific transcription activators, e.g., Oct-2. Sympathetic neurons may also express substance P under the influence of cytokines, particularly leukemia inhibitory factor (LIF), which is generated during inflammation (87). These actions have indirect consequences for hyperalgesia since a number of cytokines have been implicated in the production of inflammatory hyperalgesia (43,50).

At the functional level, other sensory peptides such as galanin and somatostatin may reduce neurogenic inflammation since they decrease afferent excitability and thereby reduce substance P release from sensory fibers (62). In arthritis, pain relief has been obtained by injections of somatostatin, also contained in primary afferents, into the joint (117). These effects may be physiologically important for locally regulating neurogenic inflammation, although these interactions have not been studied in detail.

Sympathetic Neurons

A number of inflammatory mediators including bradykinin (7), serotonin, as well as neurokinins released from activated sensory neurons stimulate postganglionic sympathetic fibers to alter vascular caliber, induce changes in local blood flow, and indirectly affect plasma extravasation. In keeping with this, sympathectomy reduces the plasma extravasation induced by noxious stimulation (34) or that produced by the administration of inflammatory mediators. In the knee joint, however, the sympathetic transmitters noradrenaline and neuropeptide Y reduced plasma extravasation (66), probably due to an inhibition of calcium permeability necessary for neuropeptide release (55). Direct interactions of sympathetic nerves or sympathetic transmitters with afferent fibers have not been easy to demonstrate (95,124,190) except after peripheral nerve damage or inflammation. In support of this, afferent fibers can be sensitized during inflammation to induce hyperalgesia, by the release of prostanoids from sympathetic fibers (183). In addition, sympathetic nerve stimulation, or the direct administration of noradrenaline, excited some C-fiber afferents after a partial injury to a sensory nerve trunk (166) or after sciatic nerve transection (45). These effects could be attenuated by phentolamine block of α-adrenergic receptors that are presumed to be expressed on C fibers (166) as well as on large A fiber afferents (45). However, further characterization of the specific a receptor(s) expressed on C fibers is necessary.

There may be a specific role for NPY receptors on sensory neurons and afferent fibers in the pain response following nerve injury. Thus, Y1 and Y2 receptors have been located in small DRG neurons, but are unaffected by nerve injury (111,212). Interestingly, these receptor subtypes may have different functions, as Y1 receptors are limited to the cell body and are not transported, whereas Y2 receptors are transported to the afferent terminals (212). Since large-diameter DRG neurons express NPY and are likely to release it after injury (86,195), NPY receptors may be activated via large afferents or via NPY release from sympathetic fibers that sprout around sensory neurons following injury (123). This would be predicted to increase DRG excitability, as Y1 receptors activate calcium conductance, but Y2 receptor activation on sensory neuron or afferent terminals may inhibit calcium conductance and transmitter release (35).

PERIPHERAL ANTI-INFLAMMATORY AND ANALGESIC FACTORS

In the above sections, emphasis has been placed on the release of local factors that serve to stimulate or facilitate the excitation of the peripheral afferent. Yet, it is clear that there are peripheral factors that may serve to downregulate the powerful forces that enhance the peripheral excitability of the afferent system.

Classically, it is known that adrenocorticotrophin serves in an anti-inflammatory capacity and is released from the adrenal cortex as a function of stress to serve to suppress proinflammatory influences. Thus, inducible forms of NOS and COX activity are enhanced by inflammation over a 24-hour period (192). These changes are under regulatory control by glucocorticoids. Thus, upregulation of COX2 and NOS is suppressed by glucocorticoids (116,209).

Inflammation induces an increase in opioid peptides synthesis by immune cells and increases the expression of opioid receptors (μ, δ, κ) in peripheral cutaneous nerve fibers (73, 180). These receptors may be important for changing the excitability of afferents after the exogenous administration of opioids and for regulating afferent function by endogenously released opioids, as was recently shown with IL-1 or corticotrophin releasing factor (CRF) (168). In keeping with this, opioids produce analgesia and suppress neurogenic inflammation (88,161), in part by directly depressing activity in peripheral afferent fibers (4) (see Chap. 58). Clearly, this represents an important mechanism for producing selective peripheral analgesia and avoiding the central complications of systemic opioid therapy. In addition, opioids decrease sympathetic fiber activity (184), thereby reducing the release of several neurogenic factors described earlier that contribute to hyperalgesia and plasma extravasation. Depression of neural excitability is mediated by μ, δ, and κ receptors via receptor-coupled activation of a G protein and inhibition of adenylate cyclase. This reduces membrane excitability by reducing calcium permeability and/or by increasing potassium ion conductance (38,175).

SUMMARY

Fine peripheral afferent fibers detect and respond to a range of physical and chemical stimuli. In particular, their activity and metabolism is altered by chemical mediators generated by tissue injury and inflammation. Increasingly fine afferents are recognized as crucial elements necessary for the integration of the variety of inflammatory signals and to orchestrate the interactions of damaged tissue, the vascular system, the sympathetic nervous systems, and immune tissues that are important for tissue repair and restoration of normal functions after injury. Symptomatic of these interactions is the production of pain and hyperalgesia, which has been viewed as the more obvious role of afferent fibers following injury. This has been highlighted by the need and development of more efficacious and safer analgesics and anti-inflammatory agents. Ongoing pharmacologic and molecular studied aided by the introduction of novel antagonists for a variety of receptors (bradykinin, neurokinins) have helped to characterize the role of chemical mediators in the regulation of afferent fiber function and have added support for the importance of various mediators in inflammatory hyperalgesia. Studies of pathophysiologic sequelae of nerve injury and chronic inflammation have also highlighted dynamic aspects of these processes in which the neurochemistry, pharmacology, and morphology of afferent fibers and their signaling capabilities can alter. Emerging from these findings is the concept that the expression of new receptors (B1, NK1), enzymes (COX-2, i-NOS), and ion channels (Na^+) can be selectively targeted for treatment of pain and inflammation. This will be aided by further information about the pharmacology of afferents under physiologic and pathologic conditions.

REFERENCES

1. Aguayo LG, White G. Effects of nerve growth factor on TTX- and capsaicin-sensitivity in adult rat sensory neurones. *Brain Res* 1992;570:61–67.
2. Aimi Y, Fujimura M, Vincent SR, Kimura H. Localization of NADPH-diaphorase-containing neurons in sensory ganglia of the rat. *J Comp Neurol* 1991;306:382–392.
3. Aloe L, Tuveri MA, Carcassi U, Levi-Montalcini R. Nerve growth factor in the synovial fluid of patients with chronic arthritis. *Arthritis Rheum* 1992;35:351–355.
4. Andreev N, Dray A. Opioids suppress activity of polymodal nociceptors in rat paw skin induced by ultraviolet radiation. *Neuroscience* 1994;58:793–798.
5. Andrews PV, Helm RD, Thomas KL. NK1 receptor mediation of neurogenic plasma extravasation in the rat skin. *Br J Pharmacol* 1989;97:1232–1238.
6. Asghar AUR, McQueen DS, Macdonald AE. Absence of effect of adenosine on the discharge of articular mechanoreceptors in normal and arthritic rats. *Br J Pharmacol* 1992;105:309P.
7. Babbedge R, Dray A, Urban L. Bradykinin depolarises the isolated superior cervical ganglion via B2 receptor activation. *Br J Pharmacol* 1995;193:161–164.
8. Bathon JM, Proud D. Bradykinin antagonists. *Annu Rev Pharmacol Toxicol* 1991;31:129–162.
9. Bayliss WM. Further researches on the antidromic nerve impulse. *J Physiol* 1902;28:276–299.
10. Bayliss WM. On the origen from the spinal cord of the vasodilator fibers of the hindlimb and on the nature of these fibers. *J Physiol* 1901;26:173–209.
10a. Bean B, Williams CA, Ceelen PW. ATP-activated channels in rat and bullfrog sensory neurons: current-voltage relation and single-channel behavior. *J Neurosci* 1990;10: 11–19.
11. Beck PW, Handwerker HO. Bradykinin and serotonin effects on various types of cutaneous nerve fibers. *Pflugers Arch* 1974;347: 209–222.
12. Bevan SJ, Geppetti P. Protons: small stimulants of capsaicin-sensitive sensory nerves. *TINS* 1994;17:509–512.
13. Bevan S, Szolcsanyi J. Sensory neuron-specific actions of capsaicin: mechanisms and applications. *Trends Pharmacol Sci* 1990; 11:330–333.
14. Bevan S, Yeats J. Protons activate a cation conductance in a subpopulation of rat dorsal root ganglion neurons. *J Physiol* 1991;433:145–161.
15. Bevan S, Hothi S, Hughes G, James IF, Rang HP, Shah K, Walpole CSJ, Yeats JC. Capsazepine: a competitive antagonist of the sensory neurone excitant capsaicin. *Br J Pharmacol* 1992;197:44–552.
16. Bevan S, Rang HP, Shah K. Capsazepine does not block the proton induced activation of rat sensory neurons. *Br J Pharmacol* 1992;107:235P.
16a. Bevan S, Winter J. Nerve growth factor (NGF) differentially regulates the chemosensitivity of adult rat cultured sensory neurons. *J Neurosci* 1995;15:4918–4926.
17. Bhoola KD, Figueroa CD, Worthy K. Bioregulation of kinins: kallikreins, kininogens, and kininases. *Pharmacol Rev* 1992;44: 1–80.
18. Bill A, Stjernschantz J, Mandahl A, Brodin E, Nilsson G. Substance P: release on trigeminal nerve stimulation, effects in the eye. *Acta Physiol Scand* 1979:106:371–373.
19. Birch PJ, Harrison SM, Hayes AG, Rogers H, Tyers MB. The non-peptide NK1 receptor antagonist, (±) - CP -96,345, produces antinociception and anti-oedema effects in the rat. *Br J Pharmacol* 1992;105:508–510.
20. Birnbaumer L, Abramowitz J, Brown AM. Receptor-effector coupling by G proteins. *Biochim Biophys Acta* 1990;1031:163–224.
21. Birrell GJ, McQueen DS, Iggo A, Coleman RA, Grubb BD. PGI_2-induced activation and sensitization of articular mechanoceptors. *Neurosci Lett* 1991;124:5–8.
22. Bleehan T, Keele GA. Observations on the algogenic actions of adenosine compounds on the human blister base preparation. *Pain* 1977;3:367–377.
23. Boyce S, Chan C-C, Gordon R, Li C-S, Rodgers IW, Webb JK, Rupniak NMJ, Hill RG. L-745,337: a selective inhibitor of cyclooxygenase-2 elicits antinociceptive but not gastric ulceration in rats. *Neuropharmacology* 1994;33:1609–1611.
24. Bradley C, Burgess G. A nitric oxide synthase inhibitor reduces desensitisation of bradykinin-induced activation of phospholipase C in sensory neurones. *Trans Biochem Soc* 1993;21:4353.
25. Brain SD, Williams TJ. Inflammatory oedema induced by synergism between calcitonin gene related peptide and mediators of increased vascular permeability. *Br J Pharmacol* 1985;86:855–860.
26. Burgess GM, Mullaney I, McNeill M, Coote PR, Minhas A, Wood JN. Activation of guanylate cyclase by bradykinin in rat sensory neurones is mediated by calcium influx: possible role of the increase in cyclic GMP. *J Neurochem* 1989;53:1212–1218.
27. Burgess GM, Mullaney J, McNeil M, Dunn P, Rang HP. Second messengers involved in the action of bradykinin on cultured sensory neurons. *J Neurosci* 1989;9:3314–3325.
28. Buzzi MG, Moskowitz MA. The antimigraine drug sumatriptan (GR43175), selectively blocks neurogenic plasma extravasation from blood vessels in dura mater. *Br J Pharmacol* 1990;99:202–206.
29. Buzzi MG, Moskowitz MA, Peroutka SJ, Byun B. Further characterization of the putative 5HT receptor which mediates blockade of neurogenic plasma extravasation in rat dura mater. *Br J Pharmacol* 1991;103, 1421–1428.
30. Cervero F. Sensory innervation of the viscera: peripheral basis of visceral pain. *Physiol Rev* 1994;74:95.
31. Cheronis JC, Whalley ET, Nguyen KT, et al. A new class of bradykinin antagonists: synthesis and in vitro activity of bissuccinimidoalkane peptide dimers. *J Med Chem* 1992;35:1563–1572.
32. Choi D. Nitric oxide: foe or friend to the injured brain? *Proc Natl Acad Sci USA* 1993;90:9741–9743.
33. Christian EP, Taylor GE, Weinreich D. Serotonin increases excitability of rabbit C-fiber neurons by two distinct mechanisms. *J Appl Physiol* 1989;67:584–591.
34. Coderre TJ, Basbaum AI, Levine JD. Neural control of vascular permeability; interaction between primary afferents, mast cells, and sympathetic efferents. *J Neurophysiol* 1989;62:48–58.

35. Colmers WF, Bleakman D. Effects of neuropeptide Y on the electrical properties of neurons. *Trends Neurosci* 1994;17:373–379.
36. Corbe SM, Poole-Wilson PA. The time of onset and severity of acidosis in myocardial ischaemia. *J Mol Cell Cardiol* 1980;12: 745–760.
37. Courteix C, Lavarenne J, Eschalier A. RP-67580, a specific tachykinin NK1 receptor antagonist, relieves chronic hyperalgesia in diabetic rats. *Eur J Pharmacol* 1993;241:267–270.
38. Crain SM, Shen K-F, Opioids can evoke direct receptor-mediated excitatory effects on sensory neurons. *Trends Pharmacol Sci* 1990; 11:77–81.
39. Crunkhorn P, Willis AL. Cutaneous reaction to intradermal prostaglandins. *Br J Pharmacol* 1971;41:49–56.
40. Cruwys SC, Garrett NE, Perkins MN, Blake DR, Kidd BL. The role of bradykinin B1 receptors in the maintenance of intra-articular plasma extravasation in chronic antigen-induced arthritis. *Br J Pharmacol* 1994;113:940–944.
41. Cunha FQ, Lorenzetti BB, Poole S, Ferreira SH. Interleukin-8 as a mediator of sympathetic pain. *Br J Pharmacol* 1991;104: 765–767.
42. Cunha FQ, Poole S, Lorenzetti BB, Ferreira SH. The pivotal role of tumor necrosis factor α in the development of inflammatory hyperalgesia. *Br J Pharmacol* 1992;107:660–664.
43. Davis AJ, Perkins MN. The involvement of bradykinin B_1 and B_2 receptor mechanisms in cytokine-induced mechanical hyperalgesia in the rat. *Br J Pharmacol* 1994;113:63–68.
44. Davis BM, Katz DM, Seroogy KB, Albers KM. Overexpression of NGF in transgenic mice induces novel sympathetic projections to primary sensory neurons. *Soc Neurosci* 1994;20:1090.
45. Devor M, Janig W, Michaelis M. Modulation of activity in dorsal root ganglion neurons by sympathetic activation in nerve-injured rats. *J Neurophysiol* 1994;71:38–47.
46. Diamond J, Holmes M, Coughlin M. Endogenous NGF and nerve impulses regulate the collateral sprouting of sensory axons in the skin of the adult rat. *J Neurosci* 1992;12:1454–1466.
47. Dickenson AH, Dray A. Selective antagonism of capsaicin by capsazepine: evidence for a spinal receptor site in capsaicin-induced antinociception. *Br J Pharmacol* 1991;104:1045–1049.
47a. Dolphin AC. G protein modulation of calcium currents in neurons. *Annu Rev Physiol* 1990;52:243–255.
48. Donnerer J, Schuligoi R, Stein C. Increased content and transport of substance P and calcitonin gene-related peptide in sensory nerves innervating inflamed tissue: evidence for a regulatory function of nerve growth factor *in vivo*. *Neuroscience* 1992;49:693–698.
49. Dray A. Neuropharmacological mechanisms of capsaicin and related substances. *Biochem Pharmacol* 1992;44:611–615.
49a. Dray A. Inflammatory mediators of pain. *Br J Anaesth* 1995;75(2): 125–131.
50. Dray A, Perkins M. Bradykinin and inflammatory pain. *Trends Neurosci* 1993;16:99–104.
51. Dray A, Patel I, Naeem S, Rueff A, Urban L. Studies with capsazepine on peripheral nociceptor activation by capsaicin and low pH: evidence for a dual effect of capsaicin. *Br J Pharmacol* 1992;107:236P.
52. Dray A, Patel IA, Perkins MN, Rueff A. Bradykinin-induced activation of nociceptors: receptor and mechanistic studies on the neonatal rat spinal cord-tail preparation in vitro. *Br J Pharmacol* 1992:107:1129–1134.
52a. Dray A, Pinnock RD. Effects of substance P on adult rat sensory ganglion neurones in vitro. *Neurosci Lett* 1982;33(1):61–66.
53. Dray A, Urban L, Dickenson A. Pharmacology of chronic pain. *Trends Pharmacol Sci* 1994;15:190–197.
54. Essman WB. Serotonin distribution in tissues and fluids. In: Essman WB, ed. *Availability, localization and disposition,* vol 1. Serotonin in health and disease. New York: Spectrum, 1968;15–178.
55. Ewald DA, Matthies JG, Perney TM, Walker MW, Miller RJ. The effect of down regulation of protein kinase C on the inhibition of dorsal root ganglion neuron Ca^{2+} currents by neuropeptide Y. *J Neurosci* 1988;8:2447–2451.
56. Ferreira SH, Nakamura M. Prostaglandin hyperalgesia: the peripheral analgesic activity of morphine, enkephalin and opioid-antagonists. *Prostaglandins* 1979;18:191–200.
57. Ferreira SH, Lorenzetti BB, Bristow AF, Poole S. Interleukin 1b as a potent hyperalgesic agent antagonized by a tripeptide analogue. *Nature* 1988;334:698–700.
58. Flower RJ. Steroidal anti-inflammatory drugs as inhibitors of phospholipase A2. In: Galli C, Galli G, Porcellati G, eds. *Advances in prostaglandin thromboxane research,* vol 3. New York: Raven Press, 1978;105–112.
59. Fox AJ, Urban L, Barnes PJ, Dray A. Effects of capsazepine against capsaicin- and proton-evoked excitation of single airway C-fibers and vagus nerve from the guinea-pig. *Neuroscience* 1995;67(3):741–752.
59a. Fukuoka H, Kawatani M, Hisamitsu T, Takeshige C. Cutaneous hyperalgesia induced by peripheral injection of interleukin-1 beta in the rat. *Brain Res* 1994;657(1-2):133–140.
60. Galizzi JP, Bodinier MC, Chapelain B, Ly SM, Coussy L, Giraoud S, Neliat G, Jean T. Up-regulation of [^{3}H]des-Arg^{10}-kallidin binding to the bradykinin B1 receptor by interleukin-1β in isolated smooth muscle cells: correlation with B1 agonist induced PGI_2 production. *Br J Pharmacol* 1994;113:389–394.
61. Gamse R, Saria A.Potentiation of tachykinin-induced plasma protein extravasation by calcitonin gene-related peptide. *Eur J Pharmacol* 1985;114:61–66.
62. Gazelius B, Brodin E, Olgart L, Panopoulos P. Evidence that substance P is a mediator of antidromic vasodilatation using somatostatin as a release inhibitor. *Acta Physiol Scand* 1981;113:155–159.
63. Gether U, Johansen TE, Snider RM, Lowe III JA, Nakanishi S, Schwartz TW. Different binding epitopes on the NK1 receptor for substance P and non-peptide antagonist. *Nature* 1993;362: 345–348.
63a. Gillardon F, Morano I, Zimmermann M. Ultraviolet irradiation of the skin attenuates calcitonin gene-related peptide mRNA expression in rat dorsal root ganglion cells. *Neurosci Lett* 1991; 124:144–147.
64. Goureau O, Tanfin Z, Marc S, Harbon S. Diverse prostaglandin receptors activate distinct signal transduction pathways in rat myometrium. *Am J Physiol* 1992;263:C257–265.
65. Greaves MW, Sodergaard J, McDonald-Gibson W. Recovery of prostaglandins in human cutaneous inflammation. *Br Med J* 1971;2:258–260.
66. Green PG, Luo J, Heller P, Levine JD. Modulation of bradykinin-induced plasma extravasation in the rat knee joint by sympathetic co-transmitters. *Neuroscience* 1993;52:451–458.
67. Gulbenkian S, Merighi A, Wharton J, Varndell IM, Polak JM. Ultrastructural evidence for the coexistence of calcitonin gene-related peptide and substance P in secretory vesicles of peripheral nerves in the guinea pig. *J Neurocytol* 1986;15:535–542.
68. Habler HJ, Janig W, Kolzenburg M. Activation of unmyelinated afferent fibers by mechanical stimuli and inflammation of the urinary bladder in the cat. *J Physiol* 1990;425:545–562.
69. Hall JM. Bradykinin receptors: pharmacological properties and biological roles. *Pharmacol Ther* 1992;56:131–190.
70. Halushka PV, Mais DE, Mayeux PR, Morinelli TA. Thromboxane, prostaglandin and leukotriene receptors. *Annu Rev Pharmacol Toxicol* 1989;29:213–239.
71. Hamberg M, Jonsson CE. Increased synthesis of prostaglandins in the guinea pig following scalding injury. *Acta Physiol Scand* 1973;87:240–245.
72. Handwerker HO, Kilo S, Reeh PW. Unresponsive afferent nerve fibers in the sural nerve of the rat. *J Physiol* 1991;435:229–242.
73. Hassan AHS, Ableiter A, Stein C, Herz A. Inflammation of the rat paw enhances axonal transport of opioid receptors in the sciatic nerve and increases their density in the inflamed tissue. *Neuroscience* 1993;55:185–195.
74. Heapy CG, Shaw JS, Farmer SC. Differential sensitivity of antinociceptive assays to rge bradykinin antagonist Hoe 140. *Br J Pharmacol* 1993;108:209–213.
75. Hepplemann B, Messlinger K, Neiss WF, Schmidt RF. Ultrastructural three-dimensional reconstruction of Group III and Group IV sensory nerve endings ("free nerve endings") in the knee joint capsaule of the cat: evidence for multiple receptive sites. *J Comp Neurol* 1990;292:103–116.
76. Hla T, Nielson K. Human cyclooxygenase-2 cDNA. *Proc Natl Acad Sci USA* 1992;89:7389–7388.
77. Hock FJ, Wirth K, Albus U, et al. Hoe140 a new potent long acting bradykinin antagonist: in vitro studies. *Br J Pharmacol* 1991; 102:769–774.
78. Holthusen H, Arndt JO. Nitric oxide evokes pain in humans on intracutaneous injection. *Neurosci Lett* 1994;165:71–74.
79. Holzer P. Local effector functions of capsaicin-sensitive sensory nerve endings: involvement of tachykinins, calcitonin gene-related peptide, and other neuropeptides. *Neuroscience* 1988;24: 739–768.
80. Hua X-Y, Yaksh TL. Pharmacology of the effects of bradykinin,

serotonin, and histamine on the release of calcitonin gene-related peptide from C-fiber terminals in the rat trachea. *J Neurosci* 1993;13:1947–1953.
81. Hua X-Y, Yaksh TL. Release of calcitonin gene-related peptide and tachykinins from the rat trachea. *Peptides* 1992;13:113–120.
82. Hua X-Y, Jinno S, Back SM, Tam EK, Yaksh TL. Multiple mechanisms for the effects of capsaicin, bradykinin and nicotine on CGRP release from tracheal afferent nerves: Role of prostaglandins, sympathetic nerves and mast cells. *Neuropharmacology* 1994;33:1147–1154.
83. Hua XY. Tachykinins and calcitonin gene-related peptide in relation to peripheral functions of capsaicin-sensitive sensory neurons. *Acta Physiol Scand Suppl* 1986;551:1–45.
84. Humphrey PPA, Feniuk W. Mode of action of the anti-migraine drug sumatriptan. *TIPS* 1991;12:444–446.
85. Inaishi Y, Kashihara Y, Sakaguchi M, Nawa H, Kuno M. Cooperative regulation of calcitonin gene-related peptide levels in rat sensory neurons via their central and peripheral processes. *J Neurosci* 1992;12:518–524.
86. Itotagawa T, Yamanaka H, Wakisaka S, et al. Appearance of neuropeptide-Y like immunoreactivity in the rat trigeminal ganglion following dental injuries. *Arch Oral Biol* 1993;38:725–728.
87. Jonakait GM. Neural-immune interactions in sympathetic ganglia. *Trends Neurosci* 1993;10:419–423.
88. Joris J, Costello A, Dubner R, Hargreaves KM. Opiates suppress carrageenan-induced edema and hyperthermia at doses that inhibit hyperalgesia. *Pain* 1990;43:95–103.
89. Juan H. Mechanism of action of bradykinin-induced release of prostaglandin E. *Naunyn Schmiedebergs Arch Pharmacol* 1977;300: 77–85.
90. Karlsten R, Gordh T, Hartvig P, Post C. Effects of intrathecal injection of the adenosine receptor agonist R-phenylisopropyl-adenosine and N-ethylcarboxamide-adensosine on nociception and motor function in the rat. *Anesth Analg* 1990;71:60–64.
91. Kessler W, Kirchoff Ch, Reeh PW, Handwerker HO. Excitation of cutaneous afferent nerve endings in vitro by a combination of inflammatory mediators and conditioning effect of substance P. *Exp Brain Res* 1992;91:467–476.
92. Kolzenburg M, Kress M, Reeh PW. The nociceptor sensitization by bradykinin does not depend on sympathetic neurons. *Neuroscience* 1992;46:465–473.
92a. Kopp E, Ghosh S. Inhibition of NF-kB by sodium salicilate and aspirin. *Science* 1994;265:956–959.
93. Kress M, Riedl B, Reeh PW. Reactive oxygen species do not play a major role in acute hyperalgesia. *Soc Neurosci* 1992;18:134.
93a. Krishtal OA, Marchenko SM, Obukhov AG. Cationic channels activated by extracellular ATP in rat sensory neurons. *Neuroscience* 1988;27:995–1000.
94. Lam FY, Ferrell WR. Neurogenic component of different models of acute inflammation in the rat knee joint. *Ann Rheum Dis* 1991; 50:747–751.
95. Lang E, Nowak A, Reeh P, Handwerker HO. Chemosensitivity of fine afferents from rat skin in vitro. *J Neurophysiol* 1990;63: 887–901.
96. Levine JD, Clark R, Devor M, Helms C, Moskowitz MA, Basbaum AI. Intraneuronal substance P contributes to the severity of experimental arthritis. *Science* 1984;226:547–549.
97. Levine JD, Lam D, Taiwo YO, Donatoni P, Goetzl EJ. Hyperalgesic properties of 15-lipoxygenase products of arachidonic acid. *Proc Natl Acad Sci USA* 1986;83:5331–5334.
98. Levine JD, Fields HL, Basbaum AI. Peptides and the primary afferent nociceptor. *J Neuroscience* 1993;13:2273–2286.
99. Lewin GR, Mendell LM. Nerve growth factor and nociception. *TINS* 1993;16:353–358.
100. Lewin GR, Mendell LM. Regulation of cutaneous C-fiber heat nociceptors by nerve growth factor in the developing rat. *J Neurophysiol* 1993;71:941–949.
101. Liu L, Simon SA. A rapid capsaicin-activated current in rat trigeminal ganglion neurons. *Proc Natl Acad Sci USA* 1994; 91:738–741.
102. Lotz M, Vaughan JH, Carson DA. Effects of neuropeptides on production of inflammatory cytokines by human monocytes. *Science* 1988;241:1218–1221.
103. Lou Y-P, Lundberg JM. Inhibition of low pH evoked activation of airway sensory nerves by capsazepine, a novel capsaicin-receptor antagonist. *Biochem Biophys Res Commun* 1992;189:537–544.
104. MacDonald RL, Skerritt JH, Werz MA. Adenosine agonists reduce voltage dependent calcium conductance of mouse sensory neurones in cell culture. *J Physiol* 1986;370:75–90.
105. MacIver MB, Tanelian DL. Structural and functional specialization of Aδ and C fiber free nerve endings innervating rabbit corneal epithelium. *J Neurosci* 1993;13:4511–4524.
106. Madison S, Whitsel EA, Siarez-Roca H, Maixner W. Sensitizing effects of leukotriene B4 on intradental primary afferents. *Pain* 1992;49:99–104.
106a. Maggi CA, Meli A. The sensory-efferent function of capsaicin-sensitive sensory neurons. *Gen Pharmacol* 1988;19(1):1–43.
107. Maggi CA, Patacchini R, Rovero P, Giachetti A. Tachykinin receptors and tachykinin receptor antagonists. *J Auton Pharmacol* 1992;13:23–93.
108. Malcangio M, Bowery NG. Effect of tachykinin NK1 receptor antagonist, RP 67580 and SR 140333, on electrically evoked substance P release from rat spinal cord. *Br J Pharmacol* 1994;113: 635–641.
109. Malmberg AB, Yaksh TL. Spinal nitric oxide synthesis inhibition blocks NMDA-induced thermal hyperalgesia and produces antinociception in the formalin test in rats. *Pain* 1993;54:291–300.
110. Malmberg AB, Yaksh TL. Cyclooxygenase inhibition and the spinal release of prostaglandin E_2 and amino acids evoked by paw formalin injection: a microdialysis study in anesthetized rats. *J Neurosci* 1995;15:2768–2776.
111. Mantyh PW, Allen CJ, Rogers S, et al. Some sensory neurones express neuropeptide Y receptors: potential paracrine inhibition of primary afferent nociceptors following peripoharal nerve injury. *J Neurosci* 1994;14:3958–3968.
112. Maricq AV, Peterson AS, Brake AJ, Meyers RM, Julius D. Primary structure and functional expression of the 5HT3 receptor, a serotonin-gated ion channel. *Science* 1991;254:432–437.
113. Martin GR, Humphrey PP. Receptors for 5-hydroxytryptamine: current perspectives on classification and nomenclature. *Neuropharmacology* 1994;33(3-4):261–273.
114. Martin HA. Leukotriene B_4 induced decrease in mechanical and thermal thresholds of C-fiber mechanociceptors in rat hairy skin. *Brain Res* 1990;509:273–279.
115. Martin HA, Basbaum AI, Kwiat GC, Goetzl EJ, Levine JD. Leukotriene and prostaglandin sensitization of cutaneous high threshold C- and A-delta mechanoreceptors in the hairy skin of rat hindlimbs. *Neuroscience* 1987;22:651–659.
116. Masferrer JL, Seibert K, Zweifel B, Needleman P. Endogenous glucocorticoids regulate an inducible cyclooxygenase enzyme. *Proc Natl Acad Sci USA* 1992;89:3917–3921.
117. Matucci C, Marabini S. Somatostatin treatment for pain in rheumatoid arthritis: a double blind versus placebo study in knee involvement. *Med Sci Res* 1988;16:223–234.
118. McCarson KE, Krause JE. NK-1 and NK-3 type tachykinin receptor mRNA expression in the rat spinal cord dorsal horn is increased during adjuvant or formalin induced nociception. *J Neurosci* 1994;14:712–720.
119. McEaschern AE, Shelton ER, Bhakta S, et al. Expression cloning of a rat B2 bradykinin receptor. *Proc Natl Acad Sci USA* 1991;88: 7724–7728.
120. McGehee DS, Goy MF, Oxford GS. Involvement of the nitric oxide-cyclic GMP pathway in the desensitization of bradykinin responses of cultured rat sensory neurons. *Neuron* 1992;9: 315–324.
121. McGiff JC, Terragno NA, Malik KU, Lonigro AJ. Release of a prostaglandins E–like substance from canine kidney by bradykinin. *Circ Res* 1972;31:36–43.
122. McGuirk SM, Dolphin AC. G-protein mediation in nociceptive signal transduction: an investigation into excitatory action of bradykinin in a subpopulation of cultured sensory neurons. *Neuroscience* 1992;49:117–128.
123. McLachlan EM, Janig W, Devor M, Michaelis M. Peripheral nerve injuries triggers noradrenergic sprouting within dorsal root ganglia. *Nature* 1993;363:543–546.
124. McMahon SB. Mechanisms of sympathetic pain. *Br Med Bull* 1991;47:584–600.
125. Melien O, Winsnes R, Refsnes M, Gladhaug IP, Christoffersen T. Pertussis toxin abolishes the inhibitory effects of prostaglandins E1, E2, I2 and F2 alpha on hormone-induced cAMP accumulation in cultured hepatocytes. *Eur J Biochem* 1988;172:293–297.
126. Meller ST, Gebhart GF. Nitric oxide (NO) and nociceptive processing in the spinal cord. *Pain* 1993;52:127–136.

127. Menke JG, Borkowski JA, Bierilo K, et al. Expression cloning of a human B1 bradykinin receptor. *J Biol Chem* 1994;269: 21583–21586.
128. Meyer M, Schreck R, Baeuerle PA. H_2O_2 and antioxidants have opposite effects on activation of NF-kB and AP-1 in intact cells: AP-1 as secondary antioxidant-responsive factor. *EMBO J* 1993; 12:2005–2015.
129. Meyer RA, Davis KD, Raja SN, Campbell JN. Sympathectomy does not abolish bradykinin induced cutaneous hyperalgesia in man. *Pain* 1992;51:323–327.
130. Mirzai THM, Yaksh TL. Studies on the release of CGRP into the skin blister base. In: Besson JM, Guilbaud G, Ollat H, eds. *Peripheral neurons in nociception: physio-pharmacological aspects.* Paris: John Libbey Eurotext, 1994;125–136.
131. Mitchell JA, Akarasereenont P, Thiemermann C, Flower RJ, Vane JR. Selectivity of nonsteroidal antiinflammatory drugs as inhibitors of constitutive and inducible cyclooxygenase. *Proc Natl Acad Sci USA* 1993;90:11693–11697.
132. Mizumura K, Sato J, Kumazawa T. Effects of prostaglandins and other putative chemical intermediaries on the activity of canine testicular polymodal receptors studied in vitro. *Pflugers Arch* 1987;408:565–572.
133. Moncada S, Palmer RM, Higgs EA. Nitric oxide: physiology, pathophysiology, and pharmacology. *Pharmacol Rev* 1991; 43:109–142.
134. Moore PK, Oluyomi AO, Babbedge P, Wallace P, Hart SL. L-N^G-nitro arginine methyl ester exhibits antinociceptive activity in the mouse. *Br J Pharmacol* 1991;102:198–202.
135. Morris R, Southam E, Braid DJ, Garthwaite J. Nitric oxide may act as a messenger between dorsal root ganglion neurones and their satellite cells. *Neurosci Lett* 1992;137;29–32.
136. Moskowitz MA, Brody M, Liu-Chen LY. In vitro release of immunoreactive substance P from putative afferent nerve endings in bovine pia arachnoid. *Neuroscience* 1983;9:809–814.
137. Moskowitz MA, Brody M, Liu-Chen LY. In vitro release of immunoreactive substance P from putative afferent nerve endings in bovine pia arachnoid. *Neuroscience* 1983;9:809–814.
138. Moss BL, Rueff A, Tonra JR, Medell LM, Mendel G. NGF induces expression of a peripheral nerve sodium channel gene in vivo *Soc Neurosci* 1994;20:671.
139. Moussaoui SM, Phillipe L, Le Prado N, Garret C. Inhibition of neurogenic inflammation in the meninges by a non-peptide NK-1 receptor antagonists RP 67580. *Eur J Pharmacol* 1993; 238:421–424.
140. Nagy I, Pabla R, Matesz C, Dray A, Woolf CJ, Urban L. Cobalt uptake enables identification of capsaicin-and bradykinin-sensitive subpopulation of rat dorsal root ganglion cells in vitro. *Neuroscience* 1993;56:241–246.
140a. Nakanishi S. Mammalian tachykinin receptors. *Annu Rev Neurosci* 1991;14:123–136.
141. Negishi M, Ito S, Hayaishi O. Prostaglandin E receptors in bovine adrenal medulla are coupled to adenylate cyclase via Gi and to phosphoinositide metabolism in a pertussis toxin-insensitive manner. *J Biol Chem* 1989;264:3916–3923.
142. Nicol GD, Cui M. Enhancement by prostaglandin E_2 of bradykinin activation of embryonic rat sensory neurones. *J Physiol* 1994;480:485–492.
143. Nicol GD, Klingberg DK, Vasko MR. Prostaglandin E_2 increases calcium conductance and stimulates release of substance P in avian sensory neurons. *J Neurosci* 1992;12:1917–1927.
144. Nowycky M. Voltage gated ion channels in dorsal root ganglion neurons. In: Scott SA, ed. *Sensory neurons: diversity, development and plasticity.* New York: Oxford University Press, 1992.
145. Nugteren DH. Arachidonate lipoxygenase. In: Silver M, Smith, BJ, Kocsis, eds. *Prostaglandins in hematology.* New York: Spectrum, 1977;11–25.
146. Olesen J, Thomsen LL, Iversen H. Nitric oxide is a key molecule in migraine and other vascular headaches. *Trends Pharmacol Sci* 1994;15:149–153.
147. Perkins MN, Kelly D. Induction of bradykinin B1 receptors in vivo in a model of ultra-violet irradiation-induced thermal hyperalgesia in the rat. *Br J Pharmacol* 1994;110:1441–1444.
148. Perkins MN, Kelly D. Interleukin-1β induced-des Arg^9 bradykinin-mediated thermal hyperalgesia in the rat. *Neuropharmacology* 1994;33:657–660.
149. Perkins MN, Campbell E, Dray A. Anti-nociceptive activity of the B_1 and B_2 receptor antagonists $desArg^9Leu^8Bk$ and HOE 140, in two models of persistent hyperalgesia in the rat. *Pain* 1993;53: 191–197.
150. Peroutka SJ. Molecular biology of serotonin (5-HT) receptors. *Synapse* 1994;18(3):241–260.
151. Puttick RM. Excitatory action of prostaglandin E_2 on rat neonatal cultured dorsal root ganglion cells. *Br J Pharmacol* 1992;105:133P.
152. Rackham A, Ford-Hutchinson AW. Inflammation and pain sensitivity: effects of leukotrienes D_4, B_4 and prostaglandin E_1 in the rat paw. *Prostaglandins* 1983;25:193–203.
152a. Rang HP, Bevan S, Dray A. Chemical activation of nociceptive peripheral neurones. *Br Med Bull* 1991;47(3):534–548.
153. Rang HP, Bevan SJ, Dray A. Nociceptive peripheral neurones: cellular properties. In: Wall PD, Melzack R, ed. *Textbook of pain.* Edinburgh: Churchill Livingstone, 1994;57–78.
154. Reilly M, Fitzgerald GA. Cellular activation by thromboxane A2 and other eicosanoids. *Eur Heart J* 1993;suppl K:88–93.
155. Richardson BP, Engel G, Donatsch P, Stadler PA. Identification of serotonin M-receptor subtypes and their specific blockade by a new class of drugs. *Nature* 1985;316:126–131.
156. Robertson B, Bevan S. Properties of 5-hydroxytryptamine$_3$ receptor-gated currents in adult dorsal root ganglion neurones. *Br J Pharmacol* 1991;102:272–276.
157. Roth BL. Multiple serotonin receptors: clinical and experimental aspects. *Ann Clin Psychiatry* 1994;6(2):67–78.
158. Rueff A, Dray A. 5-Hydroxytryptamine-induced sensitization and activation of peripheral fibers in the neonatal rat are mediated via different 5-hydroxytryptamine-receptors. *Neuroscience* 1992; 50:899–905.
159. Rueff A, Dray A. Sensitization of peripheral afferent fibers in the in vitro neonatal rat spinal cord-tail by bradykinin and prostaglandins. *Neuroscience* 1993;54:527–535.
160. Rueff A, Patel IA, Urban L, Dray A. Regulation of bradykinin sensitivity in peripheral sensory fibers of the neonatal rat by nitric oxide and cyclic GMP. *Neuropharmacology* 1994;33: 1139–1145.
161. Russell N, Jamieson A, Callen T, Rance M. Peripheral opioid effects upon neurogenic plasma extravasation and inflammation. *Br J Pharmacol* 1985;86:788P.
162. Salvemini D, Misko TP, Masferrer JL, Seibert K, Cuiire MG, Needleman P. Nitric oxide activates cyclooxygenase enzymes. *Proc Natl Acad Sci USA* 1993;90:7240–7244.
163. Salvino JM, Seoane PR, Douty BD, et al. *J Med Chem* 1993;36: 2583–2584.
164. Samuelsson B, Goldyne M, Granstrom E, Hamberg M, et al. Prostaglandins and thromboxanes. *Annu Rev Biochem* 1978;47: 997–1029.
165. Santicioli P, Del Bianco E, Giachetti AM, Maggi CA. Capsazepine inhibits low pH-and capsaicin-induced release of calcitonin gene-related peptide (CGRP) from rat soleus muscle. *Br J Pharmacol* 1992;107:464P
166. Sato J, Perl ER. Adrenergic excitation of cutaneous pain receptors induced by peripheral nerve injury. *Science* 1991; 251:1608–1610.
167. Sawynok J, Sweeney MI. The role of purines in nociception. *Neuroscience* 1989;32:557–569.
168. Schafer M, Carter L, Stein C. Interleukin-1β and corticotrophin releasing factor inhibit pain by releasing opioids from immune cells in inflamed tissue. *Proc Natl Acad Sci USA* 1994;.
169. Schaible H-G, Schmidt RF. Excitation and sensitization of fine articular afferents from cat's knee joint by prostaglandin E_2. *J Physiol* 1988;403:91–104.
170. Schaible H-G, Schmidt RF. Time course of mechanosensitivity changes in articular afferents during a developing experimental arthritis. *J Neurophysiol* 1988;60:2180–2195.
171. Schaible H-G, Jarrott B, Hope PJ, Duggan AW. Release of immunoreactive substance P in the spinal cord during development of acute arthritis in the knee joint of the cat: a study with antibody microprobes. *Brain Res* 1990;529:214–223.
172. Schepelmann K, Messlinger K, Schaible H-G, Schmidt RF. Inflammatory mediators and nociception in the joint: excitation and sensitization of slowly conducting afferent fibers of cat's knee by prostaglandin I2. *Neuroscience* 1992;50(1):237–247.
173. Schmelz M, Schmidt R, Ringkamp M, Handwerker HO, Torebjork HE. Sensitization of insensitive branches of C nociceptors in human skin. *J Physiol* 1994;480:389–394.
174. Seibert K, Zhang Y, Leahy K, et al. Pharmacological and biochem-

ical demonstration of the role of cyclooxygenase 2 in inflammation and pain. *Proc Natl Acad Sci USA* 1994;91:12013–12017.
175. Shen K-F, Crain SM. Dynorphin prolongs the action potential of mouse sensory ganglion neurons by decreasing a potassium conductance whereas another specific kappa opioid does so by increasing a calcium conductance. *Neuropharmacology* 1990;29:343–349.
176. Shepheard SL, Williamson DJ, Hill RG, Hargreaves RJ. The non-peptide neurokinin-1 antagonist RP67580 blocks neurogenic plasma extravasation in the dura mater of rats. *Br J Pharmacol* 1993; 108:11–12.
177. Steen KH, Reeh PW, Anton F, Handwerker HO. Protons selectively induce lasting excitation and sensitization to mechanical stimuli of nociceptors in rat skin, in vivo. *J Neurosci* 1992;12:86–95.
178. Stefanidis D, Reeh PW, Kreysel HW, Steen KH. Acetylsalicilic and salicilic acid suppress pH induced excitation of rat nociceptors in vitro. *Soc Neurosci* 1994;20:15.
179. Stein C. Peripheral analgesic actions of opioids. *Pain Sympt Manage* 1991;6:119–124.
180. Stein C, Hassan AHS, Przewlocki R, Gramsch C, Peter K, Herz A. Opioids from immunocytes react with receptors on sensory nerves to inhibit nociception in inflammation. *Proc Natl Acad Sci USA* 1990;87:5935–5939.
181. Steranka RR, Manning D, DeHass CJ, et al. Bradykinin as a pain mediator: receptors are localized to sensory neurons, and antagonists have analgesic actions. *Proc Natl Acad Sci USA* 1988;85: 3245–3249.
181a.Sugimoto Y, Shigemoto R, Namba T, Negishi M, Mizuno N, Narumiya S, Ichikawa A. Distribution of the messenger RNA for the prostaglandin E receptor subtype EP3 in the mouse nervous system. *Neuroscience* 1994; 62(3):919–928.
181b.Sylven C, Jonzon B, Fredholm BB, Kaijser L. Adenosine injection into the brachial artery produces ischaemia like pain or discomfort in the forearm. *Cardiovasc Res* 1988;22(9):674–678.
182. Taiwo YO, Levine JD. Further confirmation of the role of adenyl cyclase and of cAMP-dependent protein kinase in primary afferent hyperalgesia. *Neuroscience* 1991;44:131–135.
183. Taiwo YO, Levine JD. Characterization of the arachidonic acid metabolite mediating bradykinin and norepinephrine hyperalgesia. *Brain Res* 1988;492:397–399.
184. Taiwo YO, Levine JD. κ- and δ-Opioids block sympathetically dependent hyperalgesia. *J Neurosci* 1991;11: 928–932.
185. Taiwo YO, Heller PH, Levine JD. Mediation of serotonin hyperalgesia by the cAMP second messenger system. *Neuroscience* 1992; 48:479–483.
186. Taiwo YO, Levine JD. Direct cutaneous hyperalgesia induced by adenosine. *Neuroscience* 1990;38:757–762.
187. Thayer ST, Ewald DA, Perney TM, Miller RJ. Regulation of calcium homeostasis is sensory neurons by bradykinin. *J Neurosci* 1988;8:4089–4097.
188. Thompson SWN, Dray A, Urban L. Injury-induced plasticity of spinal reflex activity: NK1 neurokinin receptor activation and enhanced A- and C-fiber mediated responses in the rat spinal cord in vitro. *J Neurosci* 1994;14:3672–3687.
189. Todorovic S, Anderson EG. 5-HT2 and 5-HT3 receptors mediate two distinct depolarizing responses in rat dorsal root ganglion neurons. *Brain Res* 511, 71–79.
190. Treede R-D, Meyer RA, Raja SN, Campbell JN. Peripheral and central mechanisms of cutaneous hyperalgesia. *Progr Neurobiol* 1990;38:397–421.
191. Urban L, Thompson SWN, Dray A. Modulation of spinal excitability: cooperation between neurokinin and excitatory amino acid transmission. *Trends Neurosci* 1994;17:432–438.
192. Vane JR, Mitchell JA, Appleton I, Tomlinson A, Bishop-Bailey D, Croxtall J, Willoughby DA. Inducible isoforms of cyclooxygenase and nitric-oxide synthase in inflammation. *Proc Natl Acad Sci USA* 1994;91:2046–2050.
193. Verge VMK, Xu Z, Xu X-J, Wiesenfelt-Hallin Z, Hokfelt T. Marked increase in nitric oxide synthase mRNA in rat dorsal root ganglia after peripheral axotomy: in situ hybridization and functional studies. *Proc Natl Acad Sci USA* 1992;89:11617–11621.
194. Villar MJ, Wiesenfelt-Hallin Z, Xu X-J, Theodorsson E, Emson PC, Hokfelt T. Further studies on galanin-, substance P-, and CGRP-like immunoreactivities in primary sensory neurons and spinal cord: effects of dorsal rhizotomies and sciatic nerve lesions. *Exp Neurol* 1991;112:29–39.
195. Wakisaka S, Kajander KC, Bennett GJ. Effects of peripheral nerve injuries and tissue inflammation on the levels of neuropeptide Y-like immunoreactivity in rat primary afferent neurons. *Brain Res* 1992;598:349–352.
196. Watling KJ. Neuropeptide antagonists herald new era in tachykinin research. *Trends Pharmacol Sci* 1992;13:266–269.
197. Wei P, Moskowitz MA, Boccalini P, Kontos HA. Calcitonin gene-related peptide mediates nitroglycerin and sodium nitroprusside-induced vasodilatation in feline cerebral arterioles. *Circ Res* 1992;70:1313–1319.
198. Weinreich D, Wonderlin WF. Inhibition of calcium-dependent spike after-hyperpolarization increases excitability of rabbit visceral sensory neurons. *J Physiol* 1987;394:415–427.
199. White DM, Helme RD. Release of substance P from peripheral nerve terminals following electrical stimulation of the sciatic nerve. *Brain Res* 1985;336:27–31.
200. White DM, Helme RD. Release of substance P from peripheral nerve terminals following electrical stimulation of the sciatic nerve. *Brain Res* 1985;336:27–31.
201. Willis AL. Release of histamine, kinin and prostaglandin during carragheenin-induced inflammation in the rat. In: Montegazza P, Horton EW, eds. *Prostaglandins, peptides and amines.* London: Academic Press, 1969:31–38.
201a.Winter J, Forbes CA, Sterberg J, Lindsay JM. Nerve growth factor (NGF) regulates adult rat cultured dorsal root ganglion neuron responses to capsaicin. *Neuron* 1988;1:973–981.
202. Wittenberg RH, Willburger RE, Kleemeyer KS, Schleberger R. Prostaglandin and leukotriene release of synovial tissue in various joint diseases. *Z Orthop Ihre Grenzgeb* 1991;129(6):531–536.
203. Wood JN, Lillycrop KA, Dent KL, et al. Regulation of expression of the neuronal POU protein Oct-2 by nerve growth factor. *J Biol Chem* 1992;267:17787–17791.
204. Woodward DF, Fairbairn CE, Goodrum DD, Krauss AH, Ralston TL, Williams LS. Ca^{2+} transients evoked by prostanoids in Swiss 3T3 cells suggest an FP-receptor mediated response. *Adv Prostaglandin Thromboxane Leukotriene Res* 1991;21A:367–370.
205. Woolf CJ, Doubell TP. The pathophysiology of chronic pain—increased sensitivity to low threshold Aβ-fiber inputs. *Curr Biol* 1994;4:525–534.
206. Woolf CJ, Safieh-Garabedian B, Ma Q-P, Crilly P, Winter J. Nerve Growth factor contributes to the generation of inflammatory sensory hypersensitivity. *Neuroscience* 1994;62:327–331.
207. Xiao W-H, Bennett GJ. Inhibition of neuropathic pain by N-type calcium channel blockade with omega-conopeptides applied to the site of nerve injury. *Soc Neurosci* 1994;20:559.
208. Yaksh TL. Substance P release from knee joint afferent terminals: modulation by opioids. *Brain Res* 1988;458:319–324.
209. Yamagata K, Andreasson KI, Kaufmann WE, Barnes CA, Worley PF. Expression of a mitogen-inducible cyclooxygenase in brain neurons: regulation by synaptic activity and glucocorticoids. *Neuron* 1993;11:371–386.
210. Yousufzai SY, Chen AL, Abdel-Latif AA. Species differences in the effects of prostaglandins on inositol trisphosphate accumulation, phosphatidic acid formation, myosin light chain phosphorylation and contraction in iris sphincter of the mammalian eye: interaction with the cyclic AMP system. *J Pharmacol Exp Ther* 1988;247:1064–1072.
211. Zhang JM, Kitabata LM, LaMotte RH. Verapamil inhibits the spontaneous activities originating in dorsal root ganglion cells after chronic nerve constriction in rats. *Soc Neurosci* 1994;20:760.
212. Zhang X, Bao L, Xu Z-Q, Kopp J, Arvidsson U, Elde R, Hokfelt T. Localization of neuropeptide Y Y1 receptors in the rat nervous system with special reference to somatic receptors on small dorsal root ganglion neurons. *Proc Natl Acad Sci USA* 1994;91: 11738–11742.

Anesthesia: Biologic Foundations, edited by Tony L. Yaksh et al. Lippincott–Raven Publishers, Philadelphia © 1997.

CHAPTER 34

PHARMACOLOGY OF SPINAL AFFERENT PROCESSING

GEORGE L. WILCOX AND VIRGINIA SEYBOLD

The neurotransmission of pain in the dorsal horn of the spinal cord relies on many of the same transmitters and receptors subserving neurotransmission in other areas of the central and peripheral nervous systems. On the surface, this commonality might indicate that dorsal horn pharmacology would be much the same as pharmacology at other CNS cites. However, the unique combination of neurotransmitters involved and the modes of interactions among them make the dorsal horn of the spinal cord an attractive opportunity for selective blockade of excitatory transmission or enhancement of inhibitory transmission to produce analgesia.

This chapter presents an exploration of current research concerning the neurotransmission between nociceptive primary afferent neurons and secondary neurons in the dorsal horn of the spinal cord. This chapter addresses the transmitters released from primary afferent sensory neurons, the modes of modulation of this release, and the consequences of transmitter interaction with particular receptors. The transmitters, numbering about ten, include simple molecules such as glutamate, with actions largely confined to the millisecond time frame, as well as complex molecules such as peptides, which produce actions lasting seconds to minutes. The receptors for these transmitters, numbering more than 30, mediate a wide variety of cellular actions. These cellular actions in turn determine the neural response to the synaptic input. Anesthetics and analgesics share sites of action at the axonal conduction, synaptic transmission, and cellular signaling phases of this neurotransmission. This chapter describes the action of these therapeutic agents within the context of the cellular processes involved in neurotransmission.

TRANSMITTERS RELEASED FROM PRIMARY AFFERENT NOCICEPTORS

As reviewed, high intensity thermal and mechanical or certain chemical stimuli (high [H^+], bradykinin, prostaglandins) induce escape behavior and a "pain" state (see Chaps. 4 and 6). These stimuli activate in a selective fashion populations of small lightly myelinated or unmyelinated primary afferents (see Chap. 3). Accordingly, attention has been paid to the transmitters that are released at the spinal synapses of these afferent fibers.

Little is known concerning the neurotransmitters involved in nociception in humans. It is generally assumed that data from primates approximate the biology of humans. Correlates between physiologic data for nociception in monkeys and psychophysical studies of pain in humans provide some validation of this assumption (see Chap. 31). In addition, the rat is frequently used to study nociception and mechanisms of analgesia (and a high level of predictability has been noted) (Chaps. 13 and 30). Therefore, this section summarizes data obtained from primates and rodents in order to provide a context for understanding the actions of anesthetics and analgesics used to treat pain in humans.

To facilitate the appreciation of the complex substrate represented by the spinal afferent-dorsal horn systems, several organizing points need to be noted. First, electrophysiologic studies have largely emphasized the fact that the interaction between the first-order (primary afferent) and second-order neuron is excitatory. There is typically no suggestion that there is a "monosynaptic" inhibition.

Second, current work has supported the concept that the afferent axon may release several transmitters. Such speculation is supported by two classes of observations: (a) At the electron microscopic level, a terminal can display multiple, morphologically distinct populations of synaptic vesicles (e.g., large, dense core, and small, clear core). This difference suggests multiple transmitters (106). (b) In in-vitro preparations, synaptically evoked potentials may show an early short-lasting excitatory postsynaptic potential (EPSP) and a delayed long-lasting one, the result of two different neurotransmitters being released from a single afferent axon (80,275). These observations jointly support the notion that afferent evoked synaptic activity reflects release from the same terminal. In the following section, several of the major classes of putative transmitters are reviewed.

Excitatory Amino Acids (EAA)

Glutamate is the neurotransmitter most consistently associated with the fast excitatory neurotransmission between nociceptors and spinal neurons (see ref. 290 for review). About one half of the neurons in dorsal root ganglia in monkeys, and a somewhat larger proportion in rats, exhibit glutamate-like immunoreactivity (19). Aspartate immunoreactivity is colocalized with glutamate immunoreactivity in many dorsal root ganglion neurons (271). Most sensory neurons exhibiting glutamate immunoreactivity have small perikarya. Because small neurons typically give rise to small diameter fibers (Aδ and C-fibers) (154), and 70% to 80% of C-fibers are nociceptive (155,165), it is likely that some glutamate-immunoreactive neurons are nociceptive.

Physiologic and pharmacologic data also link glutamate with nociceptive transmission in the spinal cord. Capsaicin, the chemical in hot chile peppers that evokes pain, selectively activates C-polymodal nociceptors. Capsaicin has been used experimentally to induce pain and clinically to inhibit pain (see below). Capsaicin stimulates the release of glutamate from primary afferent neurons in culture, and this suggests that glutamate is released from C-polymodal nociceptors in vivo (125). Recovery of glutamate and aspartate in microdialysates of the dorsal spinal cord in vivo is increased severalfold after injection of noxious chemicals in the periphery (171,178,250,254), providing additional support for the hypothesis that glutamate and aspartate are released from nociceptors, although other cellular sources of excitatory amino acids cannot be excluded in these studies. The data that are most convincing in establishing a role of excitatory amino acids in nociception are observations that selective antagonists of excitatory amino acid receptors block responses of dorsal horn neurons to noxious thermal, mechanical, and chemical stimuli applied to the skin (56,94). Importantly, antagonists of non–*N*-methyl-D-aspartate (NMDA) receptors (especially antagonists of AMPA-type receptors) are effective in blocking responses of dorsal horn neurons to acute noxious mechanical and thermal stimuli in normal animals (56,141), whereas antagonists of NMDA receptors are effective in attenuating the increased excitability of dorsal horn neurons that accompanies hyperalgesia (186,227) (see Chap. 36). Together, these observations support the hypothesis that glutamate is the fast-acting neurotransmitter released from nociceptors at the termination of their central processes in the spinal cord.

Peptides

Although substance P was hypothesized to be "the pain transmitter" more than 20 years ago because of its occurrence in capsaicin-sensitive, small-diameter, primary afferent neurons, it is now clear that a variety of other peptides also meet these criteria. The list of peptides includes substance P (SP), calcitonin gene-related peptide (CGRP), somatostatin (SOM), vasoactive intestinal polypeptide (VIP), galanin, neuropeptide Y (NPY), gastrin releasing peptide, dynorphin, and enkephalin (see ref. 152 for review).

These peptides are most likely co-contained with glutamate in terminals of primary afferent neurons (44) as well as with each other (272). Although the coexistence of peptides with small molecule neurotransmitters is a common phenomenon in the mammalian nervous system, the two classes of transmitters appear to be distributed among different compartments in the same axon terminal. Peptides are stored in large, dense core vesicles and not in the small, clear vesicles that are associated with fast synaptic transmission. One of the functional consequences of the different storage pools is that peptides and small molecule neurotransmitters are preferentially released in response to different firing patterns of the axon. Whereas small molecule neurotransmitters, such as glutamate, are released in response to a brief stimulus that results in a few action potentials, release of peptides from primary afferent neurons generally requires a prolonged train of action potentials, such as that which results from a persistent stimulus of high intensity. Thus, the quality of the chemical transmission varies depending on the pattern of firing of the sensory neuron in response to the stimulus. It is also noteworthy that neurosecretory pools of peptides and probably excitatory amino acids occur in peripheral as well as central terminals of primary afferent neurons. Release of peptides from peripheral terminals of primary afferent neurons contributes to neurogenic inflammation (109). As will be considered below, peptides released from the central terminals may contribute to the changes in spinal cord excitability that occur in states of persistent pain. Therefore, it is important to consider not only what peptides are present in primary afferent neurons of normal animals, but whether there is any relation of a particular peptide to a sensory modality or target tissue, and whether expression of a peptide changes during a pathologic condition. A discussion of these functional issues follows a short description of the peptides that occur most frequently in mammalian primary afferent neurons.

Calcitonin Gene-Related Peptide (CGRP)

This peptide was one of the first products of the technology of molecular biology. Two forms of CGRP, which differ in one to three amino acids depending on the species, are encoded in two variants of messenger RNA (mRNA) (α and β) that are spliced from the same gene that encodes calcitonin (10). The two mRNAs are expressed differentially among populations of primary afferent neurons (204). However, the peptides that arise from the different mRNAs are generally not differentially detected by receptors for CGRP or by antisera directed against CGRP. CGRP occurs in the highest frequency in dorsal root ganglion cells among the species studied. Approximately 45% of all neurons in rat lumbar DRG exhibit CGRP-like immunoreactivity (181), and 70% to 80% of dorsal root ganglion cells in monkey synthesize the peptide (281,314). Dorsal root ganglion neurons of all sizes express the peptide, but small cells are most intensely labeled by immunohistochemistry or in situ hybridization, suggesting they synthesize the highest levels of CGRP. Primary afferent neurons appear to be the sole source of CGRP in the dorsal horn of the spinal cord (272).

Although experimentally difficult, it is important to relate peptides to functional classes of primary afferent neurons, because purely anatomical associations may have little bearing on the functional role of peptide-containing fibers vis-à-vis nociception. Correlation of peptide immunoreactivity with the axonal conduction velocity of individual neurons in rat lumbar dorsal root ganglia partially satisfies this need. In rats, 46% of primary afferent neurons with C fibers contain CGRP, 33% with Aδ fibers, and 17% with Aβ fibers (181). Thus, the majority of CGRP-containing neurons could be classified as nociceptive on the basis of conduction velocity since approximately 70% to 80% of C fibers in rat peripheral nerves are C-polymodal nociceptors (155,165). In addition, however, it is important to characterize fibers with respect to their coding of natural noxious stimuli. CGRP-like immunoreactivity has been visualized in individual perikarya that were characterized by electrophysiologic recording to have A-fibers and to respond to intense mechanical stimuli (105). The relationship of CGRP with nociceptors is further established by data that immunoreactive CGRP is released from the central processes of primary afferent neurons following peripheral application of noxious thermal, mechanical, and chemical stimuli (76,193). Therefore, it is highly likely that CGRP is contained in and released from some primary afferent nociceptors in both rodents and primates. Although CGRP may be an exclusive label of primary afferent neurons in the dorsal horn of the spinal cord, it should not be assumed that CGRP has an exclusive relationship with nociceptors.

Substance P (SP) and Neurokinin A (NKA)

After CGRP, SP is the most widely distributed peptide among dorsal root ganglion neurons: 40% of cells in monkey lumbar DRG synthesize mRNA for SP (314). The gene that encodes SP (preprotachykinin A) gives rise to three different mRNAs (α, β, γ). All three mRNAs encode SP, but only two encode neurokinin A (β, γ) (100). The mRNA for the preprotachykinin A gene occurs in small- and medium-sized cells of rats (21), and a similar pattern occurs in monkeys (314), but the extent to which neurokinin A is colocalized with SP is not known. Since the β and γ forms of preprotachykinin A mRNA predominate in most tissues (29), it is likely that coexistence of the two tachykinins in primary afferent neurons would be extensive.

On the basis of measures of conduction velocity, about 50% of C fibers and 20% of Aδ fibers contain SP (180); thus, it is likely that some nociceptors contain SP and release the peptide upon activation. In fact, several different experimental approaches have demonstrated that extracellular levels of SP in the spinal cord rise in response to noxious peripheral stimuli. Perfusion methods have been used to show that SP is released from the spinal cord by C-fiber activation (86,300), by direct stimulation of central C fiber terminals by the local delivery of capsaicinoid agents (128), and during acute, noxious mechanical (147,209) and cold stimuli (269). Using a clever adaptation of the principles of a radioimmunoassay, Duggan's group (62) has shown that SP is released within the superficial laminae of the cat dorsal horn in response to noxious thermal, mechanical, and chemical stimuli. It is noteworthy that SP release is not consistently associated with a particular noxious stimulus; compare data of Kuraishi et al. (147) and Ohkubo et al. (208). SP release centrally may be more closely correlated with peripheral stimuli that cause tissue damage and inflammation. Although only 70% of SP-immunoreactive varicosities in the superficial laminae of the dorsal horn of the rat are estimated to arise from primary afferent neurons (272), the release of the peptide from nociceptors is further supported by data that bradykinin evokes the release of SP from primary cultures of rat dorsal root ganglia (279).

Since NKA is synthesized from some of the same precursor proteins that give rise to SP, it is not surprising that NKA is released in response to the same mechanical, thermal, and chemical stimuli that release SP (53,63). However, the degradation of NKA in the extracellular fluid appears to be considerably slower than that of SP, which suggests that NKA may have effects on neurotransmission that persist for much longer than those of SP.

Somatostatin (SOM)

Whereas SP and CGRP are believed to be released from some primary afferent neurons with A-fibers, SOM is most likely expressed only in dorsal root ganglion cells with C-fibers (152). SOM-immunoreactivity is restricted to only the population of small cells in rats (206) and monkeys (314). In monkey dorsal root ganglia, mRNA for SOM is distributed in about 10% of the neurons. Differential release of SOM in the spinal cord in response to noxious thermal but not noxious mechanical stimuli (148,149,194,269) suggests that SOM may be preferentially involved in thermal nociception. However, SOM is unique among the primary afferent peptide transmitter candidates in that its known receptors couple to inhibitory cellular signaling systems. The significance of this atypical coupling is not known at this time, but one would expect that secondary spinal cord neurons would be inhibited after activation of primary afferent sensory fibers containing SOM.

Vasoactive Intestinal Polypeptide (VIP)

Although VIP-immunoreactive neurons are scarce in lumbar ganglia, they are numerous in primary afferent neurons of thoracic and particularly sacral spinal nerves as well as in cranial nerves that innervate viscera in a variety of species (100,110, 134,146,301). Afferent stimulation, but not spinal capsaicin, has been shown to release VIP from spinal cord (264,298). Although physiologic effects of VIP on spinal neurons have received little attention, the peptide is believed to play an important role in the regulation of immune function.

Galanin (GAL)

Galanin immunoreactivity is present in spinal cord (188) in approximately 15% of dorsal root ganglion neurons from rats (152), and a comparable percentage of cells from monkey lumbar dorsal root ganglia express mRNA for GAL (314). Expression of the peptide occurs primarily in small cells, but neither the caliber of the fibers associated with GAL-containing neurons nor the stimuli to which they respond have been characterized as nociceptive or nonnociceptive. The physiologic stimuli that evoke the release of galanin in the spinal cord of normal animals also remain to be identified. GAL does not appear to be released in normal feline spinal cord in response to noxious, peripheral thermal or mechanical stimuli (193).

Within the spinal cord, the density of GAL-immunoreactive varicosities in the superficial laminae of the dorsal horn is about one-third that of CGRP-immunoreactive varicosities and one-half that of SP (272). About 40% of the GAL-immunoreactive varicosities in the superficial dorsal horn of normal animals are derived from primary afferent neurons (272). In normal animals, a low dose of GAL facilitates the flexor reflex in response to a noxious peripheral stimulus (289), but at higher doses, GAL causes depression of the reflex (289). Thus, at low levels of release, GAL may facilitate nociceptive neurotransmission, but the peptide may inhibit pain under conditions in which synthesis and release of the peptide is increased (see section on plasticity, below).

Modality and Target Tissue Specificity

Although some relationship of CGRP (105), SP, and somatostatin (153) with nociceptors has been described, it is not likely that neuroactive peptides are limited to primary afferent neurons with nociceptive properties.

CGRP has been localized to primary afferent neurons with Aβ fibers, and SP and SOM have also been identified in perikarya of primary afferent neurons that respond to innocuous thermal and mechanical stimuli (153). There may be a greater relationship between peptide immunoreactivity and the target tissue innervated by the primary afferent neuron.

As noted above, VIP may be preferentially distributed among visceral afferents. Similarly, CGRP and SP are expressed in a high proportion of spinal afferents that project to abdominal viscera (88) and in trigeminal neurons that project to visceral targets (104).

CGRP and SP are expressed in lower percentages of fibers that innervate the skin (approximately 50% and 20%, respectively) (152,206). In contrast, in rats many SOM-immunoreactive primary afferent neurons appear to project to skin, few to muscle, and none to viscera (206). Experimental evidence suggests that the target tissue affects the peptide expressed by the primary afferent neuron (184).

Plasticity in Expression of Peptides

Spinal Peptide Levels

The above description of the occurrence of peptides in primary afferent neurons has been based primarily on observations in normal animals. It is now clear that time dependent changes in the expression of peptides by sensory neurons occurs in animal models of persistent pain. The expression of SP and CGRP increases in primary afferent neurons during peripheral inflammation (55), and these changes are associated with an increase in mRNA encoding each of these peptides (54,75). Importantly, the expression of CGRP, for example, apparently is not induced in a novel population of neurons but is upregulated in neurons that synthesize the peptide under normal conditions. Conversely, the expression of SP and CGRP in primary afferent neurons decreases following axotomy (127,204), but the expression of other peptides is increased.

The synthesis of GAL is upregulated following axotomy in both rats (283) and monkeys (314). In this case, the expression of the peptide is induced in medium-sized and large neurons as well as upregulated in small neurons (203), such that almost 80% of neurons in monkey DRG synthesize mRNA for GAL after peripheral nerve axotomy (314).

It is noteworthy that the expression of peptides not normally present in sensory neurons of monkeys and rats, such as cholecystokinin-8 (CCK-8) and neuropeptide Y (NPY), occurs following nerve injury (281,284). Changes in the expression of these peptides after nerve injury vary, however, among species. The mRNA for CCK (281) is induced in rat DRG following nerve injury but not in monkey (314). Similarly, expression of VIP is increased in response to nerve injury in rats (182,245), but not in monkeys (315). Furthermore, the changes in peptide expression are specific to certain cell populations. Increased synthesis of mRNA for VIP occurs in small cells in rat dorsal root ganglia, whereas the increased synthesis of mRNA for NPY occurs in medium-sized to large neurons.

Whether the changes in peptide expression occur in neurons responding to a specific sensory modality remains to be determined. Nonetheless, the inhibitory activity of NPY and GAL on neurotransmission of primary afferent neurons and the increased expression of these peptides after nerve injury suggests the need for a closer examination of the roles of these peptides in nociception and neuropathic pain.

Role of Growth Factors

The changes in the expression of peptides by primary afferent neurons, either in response to inflammation or peripheral nerve injury reflect, in part, the availability of growth factors. Cells of the immune system as well as Schwann cells provide peripheral sources of nerve growth factor (NGF) and other growth factors as well (see Chap. 2).

High-affinity receptors for NGF have been localized to primary afferent neurons that also express CGRP and SP (280), and the expression of CGRP and SP in adult neurons is regulated by NGF (158). Increased synthesis of mRNA for SP and CGRP during peripheral inflammation is correlated with increased levels of NGF in synovial fluid of patients with rheumatoid arthritis (8) and increased content of NGF in the sciatic nerve of rats ipsilateral to an inflamed hind limb (55). Conversely, decreased transport of NGF after axotomy or peripheral nerve injury is most likely responsible for decreased expression of CGRP and SP in primary afferent neurons in these conditions.

Overall, the levels of peptide expressed in sensory neurons most likely reflect a balance between growth factors that have positive and negative regulatory effects. Two cytokine-related proteins, ciliary neurotrophic factor (CNTF) and leukemia inhibitory factor (LIF), partially antagonize the effects of NGF on levels of SP and CGRP in cultures of adult dorsal root ganglion neurons (196). In the case of VIP, NGF may inhibit the expression of VIP (196), which would be consistent with the increase in levels of VIP in sensory neurons following peripheral nerve lesion.

The relationship of specific receptors for growth factors to targets of sensory neurons is beginning to be elucidated (183). The TrkA receptor, which has selective affinity for NGF, is expressed by a high proportion of visceral afferents; this is consistent with the high proportion of visceral afferents that express SP and CGRP. In contrast, the TrkC receptor, which exhibits high affinity for the growth factor neurotrophin 3 (NT-3), is expressed most frequently among muscle afferents. Among cutaneous afferents, TrkA and TrkC receptors are expressed by different populations of neurons. Any relationship of neurotrophic receptors with sensory neurons of a specific modality remains to be resolved, but growth factors and their receptors may prove to be of profound importance in the development of neuropathic pain. In addition, modulation of the expression of neuropeptides by growth factors may influence the degree to which neurogenic inflammation participates in nonpathologic pain states as well.

EFFECTORS MEDIATING PAIN TRANSMISSION

Pain transmission can be modulated or inhibited primarily at two sites: a drug or neurotransmitter can bind to receptors located on nociceptive primary afferent fibers or terminals, altering the release of the excitatory transmitter released by those afferent fibers; and a drug or signaling agent can bind to a receptor located on secondary neurons in spinal cord dorsal horn and interfere with the excitatory effect of the transmitter released from the primary afferent terminal. Often, a given type of modulatory receptor is located both pre- and postsynaptically. The following sections describe the common intracellular coupling mechanisms shared by most of these intercellular signaling systems.

Cellular Effector Systems in Postsynaptic Neurons in Dorsal Horn

The release of multiple nociceptive neurotransmitters, some co-contained in and co-released by the same terminals, spawn multiple excitatory events that begin simultaneously. In the following discussion, the effects of EAA and neurokinins are employed as an example of the complex effects observed in the dorsal horn. EAA and neurokinin agonists are co-released from primary afferent neurons upon noxious stimulation and initiate several signaling processes with widely different time courses (290). The cell surface receptors activated by these neurotransmitters fall into two major classes: ionotropic receptors, which contain an ion channel that opens upon ligand binding; and G protein–coupled receptors (GPCR or metabotropic), which couple to other channel or enzyme molecules via G proteins.

At least three transmitter-receptor components, AMPA and NMDA which are activated by EAA and NK, receptors which are activated by SP are thought to interact in the production of neuronal excitation leading to the transmission of pain information from the nociceptive primary afferent fibers into the dorsal horn and then rostrally to the brain. Ionotropic EAA-mediated excitation AMPA receptors followed by NMDA initiates the temporal cascade of excitation depolarization between 1 and 100 ms after transmitter release. This is followed by slower depolarization mediated by NK_1 and metabotropic glutamate (mGluR) receptor activation (Fig. 1). Other primary afferent transmitters interact with other excitatory GPCR to modulate responses on these longer time scales. In addition, most of the analgesic neurotransmitter systems act through inhibitory GPCR to reduce transmission through the dorsal horn.

Ionotropic Effector Systems

The ligand-gated ion channels activated by EAA agonists are all thought to be cation channels: most AMPA- and kainate-operated channels admit monovalent cations (Na^+ and K^+), whereas NMDA-operated channels admit divalent cations as well (167); some variant AMPA and kainate receptors also admit Ca^{2+} ions. The effect of activation of these nonselective cation channels is to depolarize neural processes possessing them; synaptically released glutamate causes an excitatory postsynaptic potential ranging from 5 to 50 ms in duration. In addition, the admission of Ca^{2+} through these channels can initiate several intracellular events by increasing intracellular concentrations of Ca^{2+} and activating such signaling systems as calcium-calmodulin kinase (CaM-Kinase II). The admission of Mg^{2+} gives the NMDA receptor channel a contingency termed voltage-dependent block. This block can be overcome by prior depolarization with another excitatory agent, such as AMPA or SP. Thus, NMDA-receptor activation is contingent upon a prior depolarizing event (Fig. 2). Such contingent activation may be important in the "wind-up" observed after repeated C-fiber strength stimulation (52,163,187,267) and to the occurrence of long-term potentiation of synaptic efficacy in dorsal horn (161).

G Protein Coupling

G proteins are thought to transduce ligand-receptor binding to various effects on cell function by liberating an activated subunit of G_α (82); in addition, the $\beta\gamma$ subunits released upon activation are also thought to mediate some of the effects of G proteins. The activated α subunits and/or the $\beta\gamma$ subunits are thought to interact with enzymes or ion channels in neurons to alter their response to other inputs. Different subtypes of G proteins associate with and mediate the effects of different G protein–coupled (GPC) neurotransmitter receptors, creating a rich array of possible effects that are detailed below (see Chap. 5).

Neurokinin (NK_1 and NK_2) and metabotropic glutamate receptors (mGluRs) couple ligand binding through G proteins to a diverse array of intracellular signaling systems. Most GPCR-mediated excitatory effects of neurokinin and EAA agonists involve activation of phospholipase C (PLC) via a G protein subtype called G_q. G_q, like all G proteins, is composed of three subunits called α, β, and γ. Upon ligand-receptor binding, the α subunit takes on a molecule of GTP, dissociates from the $\beta\gamma$ subunit, and serves as an activated, locally effective, intracellular messenger. Activation of G_q causes production of inositol triphosphate (IP_3) and diacyl glycerol (DAG) (20). IP_3 opens Ca^{2+} channels in endoplasmic reticulum, releasing intracellular stores of Ca^{2+} into the cytosol, where it could activate CaM kinase II and/or pro-

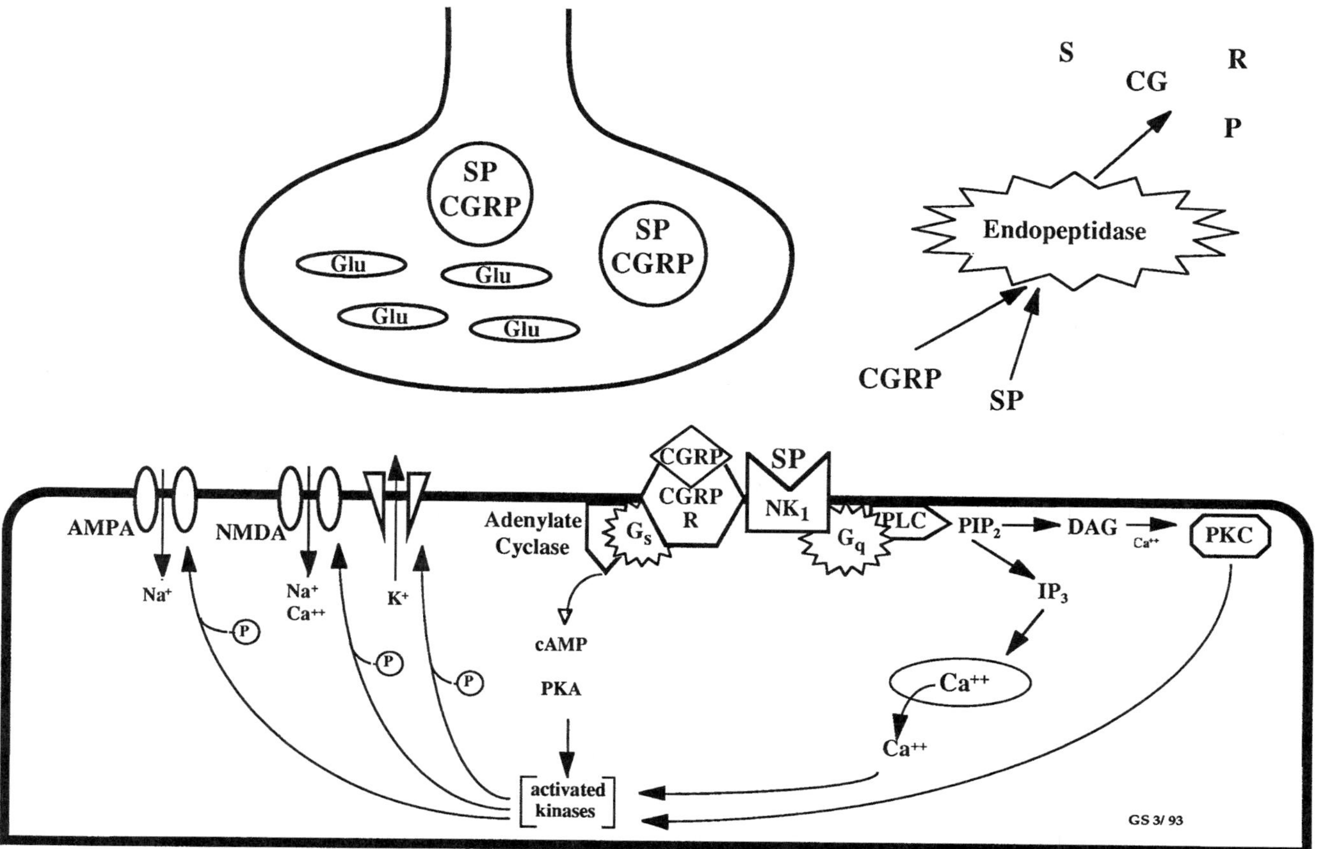

Figure 1. An examination of the intracellular signaling systems invoked by excitatory neurotransmitters involved in nociceptive neurotransmission in the dorsal horn of the spinal cord. The terminal at the top represents a presynaptic, primary afferent nociceptive terminal. The *rectangular shape* at the bottom represents a postsynaptic neuron in the dorsal horn. The diagram shows the inositol phosphate and adenylyl cyclase pathways activating kinases, which may alter the function of ligand-gated and voltage-gated channels.

mote neurotransmitter release. DAG may diffuse less in the cell, but its action may persist for several minutes or longer. DAG is thought to activate protein kinase C (PKC), which can affect several other signaling systems, including enhancing NMDA-receptor channel conductance (140). Conceivably, an appropriate combination of several afferent excitatory messages with an appropriate temporal distribution leading to ongoing changes in spinal synaptic activity (through changes in release, receptor number, and coupling) could explain progressive development of abnormalities in certain pain states, including acute postsurgical pain, joint pain, cutaneous hyperalgesia, and causalgiaform allodynia (see Chaps. 36 and 40).

G_i proteins are thought to transduce ligand-receptor binding to mostly inhibitory effects by liberating an activated subunit of G_i, α_i (73,82); in addition, the $\beta\gamma$ subunits released upon activation are also thought to mediate some of the effects of G_i. The activated α_i subunit inhibits the enzyme adenylyl cyclase, responsible for the synthesis of the diffusible second messenger molecule, cyclic adenosine monophosphate (cAMP); this action decreases the levels of cAMP inside cells, including, presumably, nerve terminals (89). Elevated levels of cAMP are commonly thought to activate protein kinase A (PKA), an enzyme that phosphorylates other cellular proteins including ion channels and enzymes (31,32). Subsequent effects in the cascade are less well understood, but phosphorylation of K^+ channels is thought to decrease their conductance or open time (11) while phosphorylation of Ca^{2+} channels increases their conductance or open time (31). Therefore, cAMP is generally thought to be an excitatory intracellular messenger facilitating transmitter release, and there are numerous examples of cAMP-induced increases in transmitter release or neuronal excitability (17,89,226).

An equally important mode of G protein–coupled modulation of neuronal excitability is via either G_i or G_o proteins, collectively labeled $G_{i/o}$. $G_{i/o}$ proteins mediate many of the direct (i.e., not involving a diffusible second messenger like cAMP) inhibitory actions of opioids and other analgesics on neuronal excitability (102,144,205,246,259). As in the case of G_i, this coupling transduces ligand-receptor binding to the liberation of an activated subunit of $G_{i/o}$, $\alpha_{i/o}$ (73,102,242). This activated subunit can encourage opening of a nearby K^+ channel (either voltage-gated K^+ channels (162) or G protein–coupled inwardly rectifying (GIRK) channels (145,205,246) or decrease the opening of voltage-gated Ca^{2+} channels (probably of the N type) (144,259,287,288). Similar to the cAMP-mediated actions discussed above, these more direct actions would decrease release of SP or glutamate from nociceptive terminals (205), inhibiting nociceptive transmission presynaptically.

SPINAL RECEPTORS MEDIATING PAIN TRANSMISSION

AMPA and Kainate Receptors—Rapid, Noncontingent Activation

The AMPA/kainate family of glutamate receptors is involved in nociceptive neurotransmission, particularly in neuropathic pain states. However, their involvement in synaptic transmis-

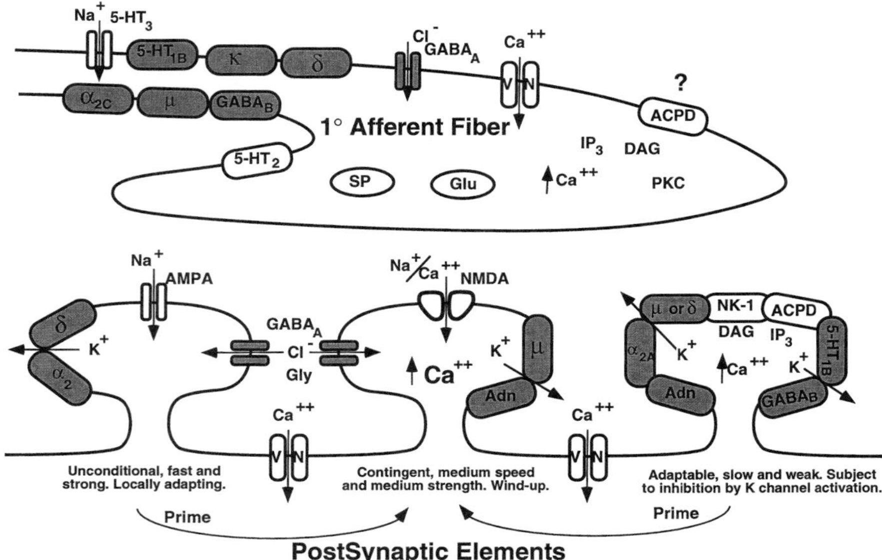

Figure 2. A hypothetical spatial arrangement of various excitatory *(clear)* and inhibitory *(shaded)* receptors, channels, and transmitters in and on pre- and postsynaptic structures in the dorsal horn of the spinal cord. Receptors grouped on a substructure have been observed to interact with one another in behavioral and/or electrophysiologic experiments.

sion from nonnociceptive afferent fibers is thought to be more important in nonpathologic states. AMPA receptors are localized in the most superficial band of the dorsal horn (laminae I–II), and the general view is that they are located on postsynaptic neurons in the dorsal horn. Exogenously applied agonists at AMPA receptors can mimic noxious stimulation (2,3,47,223) and decrease the threshold for activation of nociceptive neurons; such decreased thresholds would be expected to accompany an allodynic state. Electrophysiologically, these receptors when occupied by an agonist will yield a strong depolarization. In this sense, their activation is not dependent upon concurrent activity. Accordingly, this process is said to be "noncontingent." This is in contrast to "contingent" systems that are reviewed below.

A multiplicity of receptor subunits for AMPA and kainate have been cloned (107), and many of these have been localized by in situ hybridization in dorsal horn (207,270). Two nomenclatures are used for these receptors by different groups: GluR-1-4 correspond to GluR-A-D, and GluR 5–7 are used by both groups. Messenger RNAs for GluR-A and -B are preferentially located in superficial dorsal horn, whereas GluR-C and -D subunits are localized more in ventral horn. By contrast, mRNAs coding for kainate receptors were not apparent in these studies. Immunocytochemical localization of GluR subunits is limited by antibodies selective for GluR-1, GluR-2/3, and GluR-4 (74). The functional consequences of the presence of these receptors on dorsal horn neurons have been studied in both behavioral and electrophysiologic studies, the latter conducted both in vivo and in vitro. Common observations across most of these studies are that (a) application of the agonist AMPA decreases the threshold for activation of nociceptive neurons (290), and (b) blockade of AMPA receptors with nonselective (γ-D-glutamylglycine or kynurenate) or selective (CNQX) antagonists reduces synaptic activation of dorsal horn neurons by all afferent fibers and most peripheral stimuli (56).

Blockade of AMPA receptors attenuates responses of dorsal horn neurons to all kinds of stimuli (nonnoxious and noxious, including thermal, mechanical, and chemical) over both acute and chronic time scales. This lack of selectivity extends beyond the dorsal horn and multiple sensory modalities to encompass motor systems as well. Thus, spinal administration of AMPA antagonists produces paralysis at doses at or near those doses with antinociceptive effects (see Chap. 40).

NMDA Receptors—Slower Activation, Contingent on Prior Depolarization

NMDA receptors are more directly involved in responses of dorsal horn neurons to intense noxious stimuli. NMDA receptors are localized in superficial dorsal horn, but their distribution beyond substantia gelatinosa is more extensive than that of AMPA receptors. Conventional thought also places a majority of NMDA receptors postsynaptically, but recent evidence places receptors on presynaptic, primary afferent profiles in dorsal horn (160). The former location would account for afferent fiber- or NMDA-induced activation of dorsal horn neurons, whereas the presynaptic receptors would likely mediate release of transmitter from primary afferent fibers. The latter role suggests the existence of a positive feedback circuit mediated by glutamate released from primary afferent fibers acting upon those same fibers to release more transmitter.

A multiplicity of NMDA receptor subtypes has also been cloned and sequenced (107). NR1 subunits are thought to combine with NR2A, NR2B, NR2C, or NR2D, each of which confers different temporal characteristics of desensitization and different susceptibility to modulation by kinases. In situ hybridization shows intense labeling for NR1 subunits throughout the dorsal and ventral gray matter, accompanied by light staining in superficial layers by NR2B and NR2D subunits (270). It is unclear at this time if homomeric NR1 expression has higher incidence in dorsal horn neurons than heteromeric expression of NR1 and NR2 subunits. Results from dissociated dorsal horn neurons, however, indicate that responses to NMDA application are subject to positive modulation by PKC, suggesting that subunits with PKC phosphorylation sites are common (251).

The NMDA-operated channel can also be blocked by dissociative anesthetics, including phencyclidine (PCP), ketamine, MK-801, and related compounds (12). On the other hand, glycine at concentrations in the nanomolar range profoundly potentiates NMDA responses (151) in spinal cord. Finally, competitive antagonists selective for both the AMPA and NMDA receptors have been developed; CNQX and NBQX (111,244) selectively block AMPA receptors, and D-2-amino-phosphonovaleric acid (D-APV or AP5) selectively blocks NMDA receptors. Application of either APV or CNQX decreases nociceptive responses, suggesting that both EAA components must be intact for complete transmission. Whereas AMPA seems to decrease the threshold for activation of nociceptive neurons, NMDA enhances responses to intense stimuli without altering threshold (1). Interestingly, μ-opioid agonists block the effect of NMDA but not that of AMPA (290), reinforcing the idea that opioids act selectively on hyperalgesia and that hyperalgesia is a predominantly NMDA-mediated action.

Exogenously applied NMDA mimics noxious stimulation and, unlike AMPA agonists, induces a state of hyperalgesia (3). Single neuron recordings show that NMDA selectively excites nociceptive neurons (1,57,58) and NMDA antagonists can block behavioral and neuronal responses to intense nociceptive stimulation (56). This action is most evident in situations where afferent nociceptors are tonically activated by chemical stimuli and least evident in rapid reflexive tests such as the tail flick test (36,37,39,59,228) (see Chap. 40). These characteristics are consistent with the biophysical character of the NMDA receptor cation channel: blockade of the channel by Mg^{2+} at resting potential prevents ligand gating of channel conductance; depolarization of the plasma membrane removes this Mg^{2+} block, allowing subsequent ligand-gated conductances. Removal of this Mg^{2+} block may underlie the participation of this receptor in the "wind-up" phenomenon recruited by greater than 0.3 Hz activation of C-fibers (51,52).

Intense activation of primary afferent nociceptors is thought to release sufficient glutamate to depolarize postsynaptic neurons via postsynaptic AMPA receptors, enabling subsequent enhanced responses mediated by NMDA receptors (179).

Finally, NMDA receptors are critical participants in the induction of acute (formalin) and chronic (chronic constriction injury, CCI) hyperalgesia (38,299,304) (see Chaps. 32 and 40). Interestingly, the expression of this hyperalgesia is mediated partly by AMPA receptors. This characteristic is similar to that seen in hippocampal long-term potentiation. The net result of ionotropic EAA receptors on nociception is that both NMDA and AMPA receptors are important for dorsal horn neuronal responses to noxious stimuli and that antagonism of either receptor can have profound effects on nociceptive responses. Because the activity induced by occupancy of these receptors is dependent on temporarily contiguous membrane activity, their activation is said to be "contingent."

Neurokinin Receptors

Neurokinin receptors NK_1, NK_2, and NK_3 have the highest affinity for SP, neurokinin A (NKA), and neurokinin B (NKB), respectively. NK_1 receptors are densely distributed on the somata and dendrites of many superficial dorsal neurons as well as on some neurons in the deeper dorsal horn (159,257). SP evokes prolonged EPSPs after a long latency in spinal neurons and only excites nociceptive neurons (235). Furthermore, SP-responsive neurons are apposed by nerve terminals that contain SP (45) and NK_1 receptor immunoreactivity is internalized following peripheral injection of a noxious chemical stimulus (177). Application of exogenous SP produces behaviors suggestive of nociception (118,243) and causes hyperalgesia (171,212,309). The availability of nonpeptide antagonists for NK_1 receptors that also cross the blood-brain barrier has facilitated studies of the role of NK_1 receptors in nociception. Whereas the current perception is that NK_1 receptors are not involved in nociception, activation of NK_1 receptors may contribute to hyperalgesia. Antagonists of the NK_1 receptor decrease the afterdischarge that occurs in nociceptive neurons in response to an intense noxious stimulus (221) and attenuate the hyperalgesia that occurs in response to persistent noxious heat and administration of a noxious chemical (306,308). However, NK_1 receptors may not contribute to thermal hyperalgesia in neuropathic pain (307).

The role of NK_1 receptors in hyperalgesia may be mediated by modulation of the excitability of NMDA receptors in that SP potentiates neuronal responses to NMDA (57,58,224). The mechanism of action most likely involves coupling of NK_1 receptors to phospholipase C (213) and an intracellular pathway involving activation of protein kinase C (33,232). Figure 3 presents the activation of PKC by metabotropic and NK receptors leading to phosphorylation of NMDA receptors. NK_2 receptors also contribute to long latency responses following activation of C fibers (268) as well as to increased excitability of the spinal cord (266) by a pathway involving protein kinase C (276).

Metabotropic EAA Receptors

Metabotropic receptors for glutamate (mGluR), which couple to intracellular signaling systems similar to those activated by NK_1 receptors (258), have recently been implicated in nociceptive transmission (123,199,210). Intrathecal administration of an agonist at mGluRs, ACPD, elicits behaviors similar to those elicited by SP, and these behaviors show similar susceptibility to intrathecally administered analgesic agents. However, the effects of mGluR agonists on traditional nociceptive tests have not been studied extensively. Metabotropic receptors have been shown to participate in the hyperexcitable state following inflammation of the knee joint, suggesting that they are involved in more tonic forms of nociception (199,313).

It is important to recognize the heterogeneity of mGluRs and of their coupling to intracellular signaling systems. Five subtypes have been cloned (mGluR1–5), and early mapping stud-

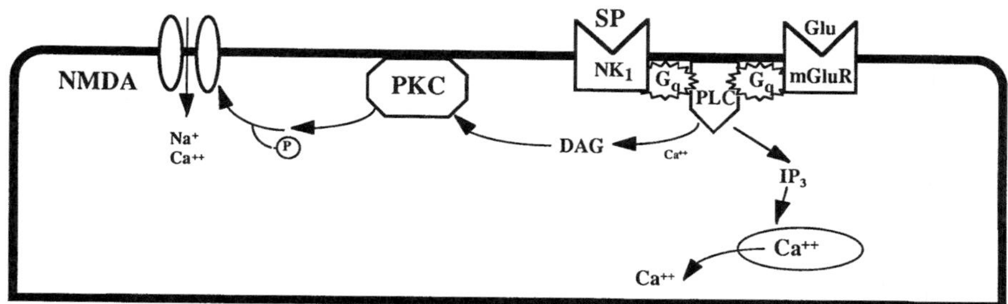

Figure 3. Either metabotropic glutamate receptors, mGluR, or neurokinin receptors, NK_1, can activate phospholipase C (PLC) via the G protein, G_q. Activated PLC enables release of Ca^{2+} from intracellular stores via production of IP_3. In the presence of Ca^{2+}, PLC produces diacyl glycerol, DAG, which can activate protein kinase C (PKC). PKC is thought to phosphorylate NMDA receptors, increasing their activity and conductance. EAAs and substance P release in spinal cord can therefore enhance subsequent responses mediated by NMDA receptors.

ies indicate that at least one subtype (mGluR 5) is localized on soma and dendrites in the dorsal horn (207,282). In addition to coupling through G_q (activating phospholipase C, as do neurokinin receptors), several subtypes of mGluRs can couple via G_i to inhibit adenylyl cyclase or open K^+ channels as do analgesic receptors such as opioid receptors. Therefore, the actions of glutamate or other nonselective agonists like ACPD at mGluRs is expected to be complex, having both excitatory and inhibitory components (123).

Nitric Oxide (NO)

The enzyme that synthesizes NO from arginine, nitric oxide synthase (NOS), is localized in some neurons in the dorsal horn and is activated by Ca^{2+} via calcium-calmodulin and CaM kinase II (CaMK-II). NO has characteristics unique among neuronal signaling molecules. It is a free radical that is freely permeable to aqueous and lipid barriers. Therefore, a neuronal point source of NO will have effects on other neurons and blood vessels within a sphere whose radius is determined by the diffusion coefficient of NO and by its half-life. Modeling suggests that the range expected is on the order of 200 μm, and this has been supported by experimental work in hippocampus. Inhibition of NOS by such drugs as L-N^G-nitro arginine methyl ester (L-NAME) block behavioral and electrophysiologic responses to noxious stimuli (intraplantar injections of formalin or carrageenan) and exogenous NMDA. The extracellular diffusion as a mode of NO access to relevant structures is supported by the efficacy of hemoglobin, which is thought to remain outside cells, in inhibiting putative NO-mediated effects.

Nitric oxide synthase (NOS), the enzyme responsible for synthesis of NO in neurons, has recently been localized in a subpopulation of small, presumably γ-aminobutyric acid (GABA)-ergic interneurons in the dorsal horn (277,278). Two studies showed that inhibition of NOS reduced responses to intradermal injections of formalin (93,95,191), and two studies showed that hyperalgesia induced by NMDA could be blocked by interrupting NO synthesis or removing it from the extracellular space (142,172,173,185). The action of NO produced by neurons in hippocampus (22,93,95,172,173) and spinal cord (142,185) resulting in, activation of postsynaptic NMDA receptors in influx of Ca^{2+} and activation of NOS leads to production of NO, which may feed back to the presynaptic neuron and enhance synaptic efficacy. This development of enhanced synaptic efficacy has been linked with the activation of guanylate cyclase by NO (66,67). Consistent with this hypothesis, spinal injection of NMDA or the injection of formalin into the paw is associated with an increase in the spinal release of citrulline, a stoiciometrically created by-product of NO synthesis (172,252).

Given the similar dependence of hippocampal LTP (40), NOS activation, and enhanced spinal nociceptive responses (43, 52,94,294) on NMDA receptor activation, the observation of NMDA-induced NO-mediated reinforcement of nociceptive transmission was not, in retrospect, surprising (93,95,173,185, 191). These studies together show consistently that inhibition of NOS with inhibitors or removal of extracellular NO with hemoglobin reduces or blocks stimulation-induced plasticity. In addition, elevation of NO with exogenous NO generators produce long-lasting hyperalgesia indicative of enhanced synaptic efficacy in the spinal cord (142). Whereas these studies consistently found little or no attenuation of "normal" transmission (i.e., not strong or tetanizing), recent report indicate that the NOS inhibitor L-NAME blocks responses to noxious thermal stimuli and to iontophoretically applied NMDA and SP (25,222) (see Chap.40.)

A number of caveats must be added to the retrograde hypothesis of NO action in spinal cord:

1. There is no evidence that projection neurons are the predominant producers of NO in dorsal horn. Rather, inhibitory interneurons appear to contain NOS (277,278). Thus, neuronal NO may be produced mostly by inhibitory interneurons in superficial dorsal horn that monitor and control firing of the projection neurons activated by the noxious stimulation. NO from interneurons would then influence afferent fiber transmitter release or projection neuron responsivity by a parallel rather than by a retrograde route.
2. NOS is in dorsal root ganglion neurons. NO produced in these cells presumably signals satellite cells, but the significance of this signaling is unclear at present (192). The ultimate target of NO from this source, however, may include the dorsal horn terminals of these neurons. If NO production is enhanced in these terminals, then this NO could affect transmission in the dorsal horn in an orthograde fashion.
3. The action of NO is not solely facilitative: NO-induced oxidation of sulfhydryls on the extracellular surface of NMDA receptors downregulates them (156). Thus, regardless of the source of NO, its effects may include enhancement of synaptic efficacy in association with a compensatory decrease in subsequent NMDA receptor activation.
4. Any of these neuronal sources of NO could affect the spinal cord vasculature in preparations where the tissue is maintained by vascular perfusion, and this vascular effect could have impact on spinal neuronal function in unknown ways. This is particularly true of nonspecific NOS inhibitors that might alter the spinal vascular bed. Deleterious effects have in fact been reported (310).

"Novel" Spinal Receptor Systems

The rapid developments in neurobiology almost daily provide insights into new or novel components of the pharmacology of dorsal horn transmission. It is difficult to classify some of these receptor systems in the categories above.

Electrophysiologic evidence indicates that adenosine triphosphate (ATP), perhaps acting at P_2 purinergic receptors, depolarizes dorsal horn neurons (121,236), suggesting a postsynaptic location. P_{2X} receptor subtypes have recently been cloned from dorsal root ganglia and characterized as ligand-gated cation channels (30,157), suggesting a presynaptic location.

A nonneurokinin receptor class seems to mediate responses to the N-terminal seven amino acid degradation product of substance P, SP(1–7). Activation of this receptor by exogenously applied SP(1–7) inhibits nociceptive responses by an as yet undetermined mechanism (112).

Prostaglandin synthesis is invoked by strong synaptic activation of spinal cord dorsal horn; subsequently, prostaglandin receptors located either presynaptically or postsynaptically probably enhance spinal nociceptive transmission (175). Spinal EP antagonists can diminish the response evoked by the injection of formalin into the paw (170). Conversely, activation of EP_2 receptors by PGE_2 promotes nociceptive neurotransmitter release from primary afferent fibers via G_s-mediated activation of adenylyl cyclase, elevation of cAMP and activation of PKA, whereas activation of EP_3 receptors by $PGF_{2\alpha}$ increases postsynaptic responsiveness via G_q-mediated activation of PLC, production of DAG, and activation of PKC (189). (See Chap. 61 for additional discussion of the role of cyclooxygenase products.)

Antialgesic Action of Capsaicin

Capsaicin excites a selective population of C fibers in adult animals. Whereas capsaicin excites C-polymodal nociceptors, it does not excite mechanoreceptors or cold receptors, and A-fibers are generally not responsive to capsaicin (with the possible exception of Aδ mechano-heat nociceptors (263); (see ref. 164 and Chap. 33 for review). Based on an emerging pharmacology, capsaicin appears to bind to a specific binding site that opens a nonselective cation channel that is voltage-independent (see ref. 169 and Chap. 33 for review) and induces an increase in intracellular calcium and other cations. The increase in intracellular calcium results in the release of peptides from the peripheral terminals of primary afferent neurons, and the increase in intracellular cations results in the depolarization of the nerve terminal. The depolarization of the nerve terminal results in the generation of action potentials and initiation of nociception as well as the release of peptides from other peripheral processes of the fiber by axon reflexes. Treatment of adult neurons with capsaicin results in desensitization of nerve fibers to subsequent applications of the substance, and the magnitude and duration of the effect is dose related (164). At low doses, there is selective desensitization of capsaicin receptors (also termed vanilloid receptors) (261), but at high doses, activation of the C-fiber by other stimuli is also impaired (60). The nonselective desensitization is believed to be related to the neurotoxicity that results from high concentrations of intracellular calcium (122).

Whereas systemic treatment with capsaicin is undesirable because of its widespread activation of C-polymodal nociceptors, there may be therapeutic value in desensitization of nociceptors following local application of capsaicin-related compounds. Such compounds could be analgesic as well as antiinflammatory under conditions of neurogenic inflammation. In addition to blocking excitation of the terminal, the compounds may decrease the synthesis of peptides by the primary afferent neurons (166) as a secondary effect. Thus, a secondary effect of capsaicin may be to deplete the central release of peptides that may contribute to central mechanisms of neuronal excitability that accompany persistent pain. There is interest in the development of vanilloids (capsaicin-like compounds), such as resiniferatoxin, which are more potent than capsaicin in causing desensitization of C-fibers but less excitatory (262). There has been some success with this approach, although the data are biased by the lack of true double-blind studies unless the algogenic effects of the drug are blocked. Neuropeptides may also contribute to tissue repair (143); therefore, treatment with capsaicin may *decrease* wound healing.

INHIBITORY RECEPTOR SYSTEMS REGULATING DORSAL HORN PROCESSING

Afferent processing through the spinal cord has been typically shown to be subject to a powerful regulation by a wide variety of spinal receptor systems. In this section, the location and coupling of a variety these receptor systems to membrane function are considered. Importantly, such modulation of nociceptive afferent processing would be hypothesized to alter the organized response of the animal and lead to an attenuation of pain behavior, e.g., analgesia. In this regard the effects of manipulating these systems in the unanesthetized animal by spinal drug delivery provides measures of the relevance of these several receptors systems to nociception. Further discussion of drug action and animal models is provided in Chap. 40.

Opioid Receptors

Opioid receptors have been shown to exert a powerful regulation of the processing of afferent-evoked activity at the spinal level in animal and human (see Chap. 58). The organization of these receptors will be briefly reviewed.

Early binding studies emphasized that opioid binding sites could be identified on primary afferent terminals and on membranes that were not primary afferent (see below). The two sites and their underlying mechanisms are often generically termed "presynaptic" and "postsynaptic," respectively.

Opioid Receptors on Primary Afferents: Central Terminals

The occurrence of opioid receptors on primary afferent neurons has been confirmed by morphologic studies and electrophysiologic studies in vitro. Using receptor autoradiography, μ–opioid binding sites have been localized to approximately 8% of the neurons in monkey dorsal root ganglia. The binding of the radio labeled opioid ligand is limited to the small cells within the population of dorsal root ganglion cells (202), and the location of opioid receptors on capsaicin-sensitive primary afferent neurons suggests their occurrence on C-polymodal nociceptors (150). With the cloning of opioid receptors and the deduction of the primary sequence of the subtypes of opioid receptor proteins, antisera generated against peptide fragments of the receptor are providing increased resolution of the distribution of opioid receptor subtypes among populations of dorsal root ganglion neurons.

Initial studies have localized μ- and δ-opioid receptors to small-diameter primary afferent neurons (13–15). The subtype of δ receptor that has been cloned and against which the antisera have been produced appears to be one that is only expressed presynaptically (41). The generation of antibodies to specific subtypes of opioid receptors makes it possible to correlate the occurrence of opioid receptors with other neurochemical characteristics or primary afferent neurons, such as peptide content or response characteristics. Initial evidence based on receptor autoradiography suggests that 20% of neurons in monkey dorsal root ganglia that express SP also express opioid receptors (201). This association appears even more striking in immunocytochemical studies showing near-complete colocalization of δ-opioid receptors with SP in terminals in the dorsal horn of the rat (230).

Physiologic Effects on Spinal Afferent Terminals

Current work has indicated that the effects of opiates on central afferent terminals may be characterized by both inhibitory and excitatory effects.

Inhibitory Effects Opioid receptors on terminals of primary afferent neurons inhibit the release of transmitter (86,168,195, 300) as well as transduction of the noxious stimulus in sensory neurons that innervate inflamed tissue (234,255).

Although there appears to be agreement that opioids do not modulate resting ion conductances in primary afferent neurons and that multiple opioid receptor subtypes occur on individual primary afferent neurons, the mechanisms underlying the inhibitory action of opioid receptors are not fully understood. The effects of opioids on ion conductances in primary afferent neurons have been studied on cell bodies of mouse and rat dorsal root ganglion neurons. In primary cultures of mouse fetal dorsal root ganglion neurons (287,288), μ– and δ-opioid receptors decrease somatic calcium-dependent action potentials by increasing potassium conductance, which results in a shortening of the duration of the action potential and an increase in the afterhyperpolarization. Activation of κ receptors, however, results in a direct suppression of calcium currents. In contrast, the effect of opioid agonists on cell bodies of acutely dissociated, adult rat dorsal root ganglion neurons suggests that opioids primarily modulate calcium conductances (4), most likely by inhibiting a common pool of N- and P-type calcium channels (190).

In spinal cord slices from young animals, opioid agonists usually reduce the size of excitatory postsynaptic potentials or currents without direct effects on the postsynaptic cell, suggesting a primarily presynaptic site of action (84,92). The differences in the actions of opioids in these models most likely reflect differences in membrane components (ion channels as well a G proteins) in immature and adult neurons. Although differences in membrane components may also occur between the cell body and the nerve terminal, it seems likely that opioids inhibit transmitter release by similar modulation of ion channels in the nerve terminal since N- and P-type channels have been implicated in the release of excitatory amino acids and peptides from primary afferent neurons.

Excitatory Effects Excitatory effects of low concentrations of opioids have also been described under special circumstances. Nanamolar concentrations of selective μ–, δ–, and κ–opioid agonists are reported to increase membrane excitability in explants of fetal mouse dorsal root ganglion neurons when certain populations of potassium channels are blocked (247). This effect, however, is not observed at low concentrations of opiates on cell bodies of adult rat dorsal root ganglion cells (190), raising the possibility that the excitatory effect is specific to particular experimental conditions. Since hyperalgesia in response to low doses of morphine has been observed in arthritic rats (135), the possibility that excitatory effects of opioids may occur in conjunction with pathologic states must be considered.

G Protein Coupling The G proteins and second messenger systems involved in mediating the action of opioid receptors in primary afferent neurons also remain to be resolved. Generally, the inhibitory actions of opioids on primary afferent neurons have been shown to be mediated by a pertussis-toxin–sensitive G protein, suggesting the involvement of either G_i or G_o. Inhibition of calcium channels may be a function of G_o since the α–subunit of G_o is more potent than G_i in restoring δ-opioid receptor–mediated inhibition of calcium conductance in a neuroblastoma cell line (102). It is also likely that opioid receptors on primary afferent neurons are negatively coupled to an adenylyl cyclase/cAMP pathway as has been demonstrated for postsynaptic receptors on central neurons (11).

In dorsal root ganglion neurons, an increase in cAMP results in increased excitability (89) and increased release of transmitter. Opioid receptors may counteract these effects via G_i-mediated inhibition of adenylyl cyclase. Thus, this pathway may only emerge in conjunction with sensitization of primary afferent neurons. Another mode of G protein coupling, activation of PKC presumably by G_q and DAG, has been implicated in the inhibition of calcium channels by opioids in dorsal root ganglion neurons (16,225). However, downregulation of PKC after phorbol ester treatment also blocks the inhibition of Ca^{2+} currents by κ opioids and α_2-adrenergic agonists, complicating the interpretation of these phenomena (16).

The fact that δ receptors have been shown to increase intracellular calcium in neuroblastoma cells by release of calcium from intracellular stores suggests that δ opioid receptors may be linked (possibly via G_q) to generation of inositol phosphates in primary afferent neurons under certain conditions (129). The relationship between these different modes of coupling is complex and remains to be elucidated.

Opioid Receptors on Peripheral Afferent Terminals

Opioid inhibition of sensory transduction in nociceptors (at the peripheral terminal) appears to occur only when nociceptors are sensitized, as in peripheral tissue injury. There is electrophysiologic evidence that local injection of opiates decreases the spontaneous firing of small-diameter primary afferent neurons that innervate an inflamed joint in cats (234) and prevents the antidromic release of SP into the knee joint (296). There are also behavioral studies that demonstrate analgesic effects of opioids injected directly into inflamed tissue. Injection of opiates into the plantar surface of inflamed hind paws in rats decreases, in a dose-dependent manner, the hyperalgesia exhibited in response to thermal (130) and mechanical stimuli (256) in the pain and compression of the inflamed knee joint (197).

The hyperalgesia can be reversed by agonists that are selective for μ–, κ–, and perhaps δ–opioid receptors, consistent with the occurrence of multiple opioid receptors on individual sensory neurons (255). That the effects are due to a local action of the opiate is supported by evidence that no changes in nociceptive threshold occur in the contralateral, normal paw, and no effect is observed after systemic injection of the same dose of opiate. Interestingly, profound analgesia occurs in animals that exhibit a persistent inflammation, e.g., 4 days after injection of complete Freund's adjuvant into the hindpaw (256), compared to attenuation of hyperalgesia during acute inflammation, e.g., 4 hours after injection of carrageenan into the hindpaw (130).

The effect of opiates on the hyperalgesia accompanying inflammation could be due to physiologic antagonism of the increased generation of cAMP by prostaglandins generated in the inflammatory response (see Chap. 33) or to increased peripheral transport of opiate receptors by sensory neurons during peripheral inflammation. The development of an analgesic response to the local injection of opiates over the course of inflammation (256) suggests that a direct inhibitory mechanism may emerge. The inhibition may be mediated by increased expression of opioid receptors on sensory neurons that innervate the inflamed tissue (98). However, it is also possible that changes in the milieu of the sensory terminal as a result of the inflammatory response (e.g., pH) may contribute to the unmasking of functional opioid receptors.

Postsynaptic Opioid Receptors

Opioid receptors also participate in neurotransmission in spinal dorsal horn, and μ and κ receptors have postsynaptic localizations on dorsal horn neurons, both somata and dendrites (13–15). Many studies document the participation of μ receptors in postsynaptic inhibition of neurons activated by primary afferent fiber stimulation. However, few studies clearly show that κ receptors have similar effects. In fact, a large fraction of studies using κ agonists report pronociceptive effects (61,117). A majority of studies further shows that postsynaptic effects are rarely seen for δ opioid agonists (84).

All three opioid receptor subtypes couple preferentially through G_i or G_o proteins to inhibitory effectors that cause inhibition of adenylyl cyclase or Ca^{2+} influx, or to G proteins that directly activate K^+ efflux. Postsynaptically, these actions tend to hyperpolarize neurons, impairing depolarization and rostrad propagation of nociceptor-driven action potentials (92). However, some evidence points to excitatory coupling of some opioid receptor subtypes. Postsynaptically, μ-opioid agonists enhanced NMDA-induced currents in dissociated dorsal horn neurons via activation of protein kinase C (PKC) through the phospholipase C–diacyl glycerol (PLC-DAG) pathway (32,115). This action would directly increase nociceptor-driven excitation incident on dorsal horn neurons. In addition, throughout the neuraxis μ receptors are often found on GABAergic interneurons. An inhibitory effect of μ-opioid receptor activation on these neurons could indirectly activate dorsal horn neurons through disinhibition. Either mechanism could account for observations of excitatory effects of opioid agonists in vivo (290).

A large number of studies have investigated the action of opioid agonists on nociceptive neurotransmission in vivo. Behavioral and clinical studies have identified antinociceptive and analgesic effects of intrathecally applied opioid agonists directed at all three receptor subtypes; however, pronociceptive effects have also been reported for κ agonists, notably in rats (117). In vivo electrophysiologic studies have extended these observations to the single cell level, and for the most part inhibitory effects of opioid agonists are highly correlated with behaviorally defined analgesia (120), with the exception that κ agonists produce pronociceptive effects in some neurons and laboratories (117). In spinal cord slices from young animals, opioid agonists are sometimes observed to directly hyperpolarize postsynaptic dorsal horn neurons (92,124), supporting the postsynaptic localization of opioid receptors. In dissociated spinal cord neurons, μ-opioid agonists hyperpolarize about half the cells, an action consistent with both physiologic and anatomic observations of postsynaptic μ-opioid receptors (13–15). In addition, however, μ-opioid agonists enhance NMDA-induced responses in most cells; this action is apparently mediated by atypical coupling of μ-opioid receptors to PKC (32,233). Nonetheless, the predominant postsynaptic effect of μ-opioid agonists is to inhibit postsynaptic neurons in slices and in vivo, decreasing responses to excitatory inputs as well.

α_2-Adrenergic Receptors

Early work on bulbospinal pathways revealed that large populations of these projections contained and released noradrenaline, and, by an action upon spinal α_2-adrenergic receptor subtypes, the receptors could regulate nociceptive processing (see Chaps. 58 and 59). Subsequent work revealed that these spinal receptors could produce a powerful analgesia in humans and animal models (see Chaps. 40 and 59). The locations and coupling of these spinal α_2 sites are considered below.

Presynaptic α_2-Adrenergic Receptors

α_2-Adrenergic receptors have been linked to primary afferent neurons and inhibition of sensory neurotransmission. A decrease in binding of α_2-adrenergic agonists in the spinal cord after dorsal rhizotomy (113) provided early morphologic evidence that α_2-adrenergic receptors occur on primary afferent neurons. Subsequent studies of the distribution of mRNAs for subtypes of α_2-adrenergic receptors in rats revealed a sparse distribution of neuronal cell bodies labeled with a probe for the α_{2A} receptor by in situ hybridization and considerably more cells labeled with a probe for the α_{2C} receptor. No cells were labeled with a probe for the α_{2B} receptor (200). α_2-Adrenergic receptors have been implicated in inhibition of transmitter release from primary afferent neurons (86,148,149,211), and inhibition of secretion appears to be mediated by a pertussis toxin–sensitive G protein [G_i or G_o; (108)]. It is most likely that the effect is mediated by G_o, as with opioid receptors, since α_{2C} receptors have been shown to couple with G_i to inhibit stimulated adenylate cyclase only at high receptor densities (64).

Paradoxically, peripheral α_2-adrenergic receptors have been linked to the hyperalgesia that accompanies peripheral nerve injury. Under normal conditions, norepinephrine and sympathetic nerve stimulation do not excite sensory neurons directly. In fact, sympathetic nerve stimulation blocks sensitization of C-polymodal nociceptors to heat. However, after peripheral nerve injury, norepinephrine excites a subpopulation of C-polymodal nociceptors via an α_2 receptor (238). The change in response to norepinephrine may be mediated by induction of a different α_2 receptor subtype, increased expression of the same receptor subtype, or a change in the population of G proteins. In a cell line transfected with the α_{2C}-adrenergic receptor, the α_2 agonist-mediated inhibition of adenylyl cyclase activity at low concentrations of agonist, but stimulation of the enzyme occurred at higher concentrations. The inhibitory activity was mediated by a pertussis toxin–sensitive G protein, whereas the excitatory activity was mediated by a cholera toxin–sensitive G protein (G_s) (65).

Postsynaptic α_2-Adrenergic Receptors

Recent studies have begun to identify the location of several $G_{i/o}$-coupled receptors in the spinal dorsal horn. Functional studies have shown that α_2 agonists inhibit dorsal horn neuronal responses to noxious stimulation apparently via a $G_{i/o}$ protein–mediated pathway (71,103). In situ hybridization shows α_{2A}-receptor mRNA in secondary neurons in dorsal horn, whereas α_{2C}-receptor mRNA is in primary afferent neurons (200). The therapeutic significance of this apparent separation is unclear because agents selective for one or the other receptor are not available. However, the functional significance of this differential localization may reside in the coupling of these α_{2A} receptors to inwardly rectifying potassium channels (GIRK), the opening of which may mediate a large part of the antinociceptive effect of α_2 agonists. In vitro electrophysiology has shown that, like μ-opioid–mediated postsynaptic inhibition, α_2-adrenergic agonists inhibit dorsal horn neurons by hyperpolarization, probably mediated by K^+ channels (126). The coupling of α_{2A} receptors to either ion channels or adenylyl cyclase (274) may contribute to the analgesic effects of α_2-receptor agonists. It is unclear which mode of coupling contributes to the synergistic interaction observed between opioid and adrenergic agonists (see below).

GABA Receptors

Presynaptic GABA Receptors

Synapses of GABAergic terminals onto functionally identified nociceptors have been resolved in monkey and cat spinal cord (9). These receptors may mediate inhibition of transmitter release by mechanisms similar to α_2 and opioid receptors since the effect of GABA is mediated by a pertussis toxin–sensitive G protein (108). It is not clear at this time whether $GABA_A$ (23,211) and/or $GABA_B$ receptors (108,220) mediate the effect, although the pertussis toxin sensitivity strongly supports the involvement of $GABA_B$ receptors. Little direct evidence can place either of the two receptor types on pre- vs. postsynaptic terminals in dorsal horn, but the analgesic efficacy of $GABA_B$ agonists together with the observed presynaptic actions of $GABA_B$ agonists lead most investigators to assert that $GABA_B$ receptors inhibit release of transmitter from primary sensory afferent fibers (101). The coupling of $GABA_B$ receptors to Ca^{2+} channels appears to be mediated by G_o proteins (28). It is noteworthy that GABA receptors may be differentially distributed across populations of peptide-containing primary afferent neurons since GABA inhibits the release of CGRP but not SP from spinal cord in rat (23,211). The $GABA_B$ agonist baclofen is reported to be more efficacious against chronic neuropathic pain (97,295) than the $GABA_A$ agonist muscimol (see Chaps. 40 and 62).

Postsynaptic GABA Receptors

Postsynaptic $GABA_A$ sites, which are ligand-gated anion channels selective for Cl^-, likely mediate attenuation of dorsal horn neuronal responses to peripheral activation (6). Therefore, their activation would be expected to hyperpolarize dorsal horn neurons or hold them near resting potential by a shunting action. Serotonin released from axons that descend from the brainstem may stimulate release of GABA from interneurons, which in turn inhibits other neurons. $GABA_A$ antagonists elevate responses to EAA agonists and block the inhibition produced by 5-HT_3 agonists. It is notable, however, that anesthetics and antianxiety agents like barbiturates and benzodiazepines, which act as potentiators of GABA at these receptors, fail to produce analgesia. It is conceivable that the temporal characteristics of $GABA_A$ receptors (i.e., inhibitory potential durations of several milliseconds) reduce the analgesic efficacy of these agents.

Glycine Receptors

Glycine receptors, like $GABA_A$ receptors, are ligand-gated anion channels selective for Cl^-; therefore, their activation would be expected to hyperpolarize dorsal horn neurons or hold them near resting potential by a shunting action. However, their temporal characteristics may also interfere with the production of analgesic effects.

While GABA agonists (see above) and glycine do not appear to exert a marked effect upon nociceptive processing, they represent a family of receptors that clearly plays a major role in regulating the ongoing encoding of afferent stimuli. This role is revealed by the effects on behavior of spinally delivered antagonists to $GABA_A$ (not $GABA_B$) and glycine (strychnine) receptors. Such injections lead to a powerful increase in the ability of low-threshold mechanical stimuli (touch) to evoke increases in pain behavior (248,249,297). These observations suggest that these inhibitory receptors control the encoding of low-threshold mechanoreceptive input. In the absence of that modulation, the otherwise innocuous input is perceived as highly aversive. Further consideration of the relevance of this to nociceptive processing is provided elsewhere (see Chaps. 9 and 28).

The observation that intrathecally applied strychnine invokes allodynia and pain-reactive behavior in rodents suggests the involvement of glycine receptors in dorsal horn nociceptive processing. Intrathecal application of strychnine in awake rats produces a behavioral syndrome suggesting allodynia: rats respond to normally innocuous stimuli like air puff and light stroking with vocalizations and aggressive protection (248). In anesthetized rats treated with strychnine, similar stimuli evoke increases in blood pressure suggestive of nociception and sympathetic activation.

Serotonin Receptors

The contribution of serotonin to descending inhibition of spinal pain transmission has received much attention (18). Blockade of reuptake of serotonin may account for some of the analgesic activity of such tricyclic antidepressants as amytriptylline and fluoxetine (116,136). Intrathecally administered serotonin can either inhibit (42,119,241,286,302) or stimulate (35,119) nociceptive reflexes depending on the dose and species tested. In addition, stimulation of nucleus raphe magnus (NRM), which is thought to release serotonin in the spinal cord, elicits both excitation (35,311) and inhibition (81). Three distinct serotonin receptor subtypes probably account for this multiplicity of effects: 5-HT_1, 5-HT_2, and 5-HT_3 receptors, with 5-HT_1 receptors further differentiated into A, B, C, and D subtypes (214,217). Most researchers concur that the 5-HT_{1B} (rat) and $5HT_{1D}$ (human) receptor subtypes mediate selective inhibition of nociceptive neurons (7,68), whereas 5-HT_{1A} agonists facilitate nociceptive responses (7).

The 5-HT_2 receptor subclass (which now includes what used to be known as the 5-HT_{1C} receptor renamed as 5-HT_{2C} (131,132), mediates neuronal excitation by a mechanism similar to SP and may be important in migraine headaches (72). Spinal 5-HT_2 receptors are also involved in the serotonergic modulation of nociception, and both pro- (119,291) and antinociceptive (5,303) actions have been observed. $5HT_2$ receptors may mediate primary pronociceptive serotonergic effects that are followed by secondary antinociceptive effects. Serotonin and SP share behavioral effects after spinal administration (70,119) and receptor coupling mechanisms (IP_3-Ca^{2+}-DAG intracellular messenger coupling) (293).

The role of 5-HT_3 receptors in the antinociceptive effects of serotonin has not been investigated as thoroughly as that of 5-HT_1 and 5-HT_2 receptors. This is largely because 5-HT_3 receptors were originally identified in the periphery, because 5-HT_3 receptors contribute to excitation of primary afferent sensory fibers, and because 5-HT_3 antagonists reduce pain in persons suffering from migraine headaches (229). The peripheral excitatory function of 5-HT_3 receptors involves the ligand-gated cation channel nature of these receptors (49). 5-HT_3 receptors are also present in the central nervous system, including spinal cord (83,85,96). Spinal 5-HT_3-mediated analgesia involves both $GABA_B$ and $GABA_A$ receptors, probably through excitation of GABAergic interneurons (6).

P_1 Adenosine Receptors

Behavioral studies have supported both A1 and A2 adenosine receptor involvement in spinally mediated antinociception (239), but the current work supports A1 adenosine receptors as the primary receptor-mediating adenosine analogue induced antinociception (133) (see Chap. 13). Investigations using radioligand binding and receptor autoradiography have also localized adenosine receptors in the region of the substantia gelatinosa (34,77,87). Pharmacologic and surgical manipulations appear to confirm that most adenosine receptors at spinal sites are localized on intrinsic neurons (34,77). Localization of adenosine receptors postsynaptic to primary afferent fibers is further supported by behavioral studies in which intrathecally administered adenosine analogues inhibit behaviors induced by coadministration of putative excitatory nociceptive neurotransmitters (47,48) and is highly effective in models of neuropathic pain where glutamate is believed to play a mediating role (154,305,306).

Activation of intrinsic adenosine receptors appears to mimic the actions of an endogenous purinergic system that may tonically modulate nociceptive input. In addition to adenosine receptors, adenosine deaminase (79), nucleoside transporters (78), and adenosine-like immunoreactivity (24) have been localized at spinal sites. Opioid-stimulated release of adenosine at spinal sites has also been shown (260), as well as adenosine interactions with opioid and nonopioid systems modulating nociceptive input (46,239). Pharmacologic inhibition of mechanisms responsible for clearance of endogenous adenosine induces antinociception (137,139), while intrathecally administered adenosine antagonists with methylxanthines increases behavioral responsiveness to noxious stimuli (240) and induces biting and scratching behavior similar to that observed following administration of putative pain neurotransmitters (138). Investigations to date suggest that adenosine is most effective as an inhibitor of spinal neuronal activation mediated through non-NMDA or substance P receptors (138).

Peptide Receptors

Receptors for neuropeptide Y (NPY) are found on DRG neurons of many species, including monkeys (176). In normal rats, receptors for NPY occur primarily on small cells (176,314), but the distribution shifts to include larger cells after peripheral nerve axotomy (314). It is noteworthy that although NPY in the spinal cord of normal animals is contained largely in axons of neurons that descend from the brainstem, the expression of NPY in sensory neurons is also induced by peripheral nerve injury (see section Plasticity in Expression of Peptides, above). NPY receptors are of interest in analgesic mechanisms because NPY has been shown to block the release of SP from cultured neurons by inhibiting calcium currents (285). NPY inhibition of calcium currents in DRG cells may be mediated more by the α subunit of G_o than by the α subunit of G_i (69). Spinal delivery of NPY has been shown to be a potent analgesic (114).

Presynaptic Regulation by Blockade of Voltage-Gated Ion Channels

Sodium Channels

It is commonly appreciated that the blockade of a sufficient fraction of sodium channels in an afferent axon broadens the action potential and reduces its ability to follow a given frequency and then ultimately leads to conduction failure (26). There is now growing appreciation that the biophysics of the membrane are such that alterations in transduction and conduction at the terminals may be particularly sensitive and reduce the ability of the afferent fiber to release transmitter. Thus, as the local or plasma concentration of the channel blocker is increased, disruption of function progresses as follows: (a) blockade of spontaneous firing in the ganglion cell of an injured axon (most sensitive) (50); (b) blockade of spontaneous firing of neuroma (50); (c) blockade of spontaneous firing of axon innervating an injured region of tissue (265); (d) blockade of conduction in injured axon (least sensitive) (see Chap. 32).

Other factors that may define the ability of sodium channel blockade to alter pain processing is the likelihood that the safety factor is not the same along the normal axon. Thus, conduction safety factor is reduced with branching (90,91). In the dorsal root entry zone, the afferent axon undergoes considerable branching, and it is possible that concentrations of anesthetics leading to a given level of sodium channel blockade may in fact selectively prevent the invasion of the action potential into the distal dendrite, from which the transmitter is released. Such an occurrence would explain the results in which behaviorally ineffective intrathecal doses of lidocaine would synergize with the analgesic actions of spinal morphine (215). Further considerations of sodium channel blockade are presented elsewhere (see Chap. 63).

Inhibition of the repetitive firing of C fibers that occurs during tissue injury may have important consequences in blocking the increased excitability of spinal neurons that accompanies this repetitive firing (see Chap. 36). Repetitive firing increases the percentage of voltage-gated Na^+ channels in the persistently open state; this state is susceptible to block by several anticonvulsant agents such as the anticonvulsant lamotrigine, which are relatively poor fast blockers of these channels, decreasing local anesthetic side effects (198). Blockade of action potentials at the site of tissue injury or along nerve trunks may also block axon reflexes and the peripheral release of peptides from primary afferent neurons. Inhibition of transmitter release from peripheral processes of primary afferent neurons may have an important role in decreasing neurogenic inflammation (see above).

Calcium Channels

Another target for voltage-gated channel blockade is Ca^{2+} channels in terminals of primary afferent fibers. Synaptic neurotransmission from primary afferent neurons is thought to require the arrival of action potentials at nerve terminals, which triggers the opening of voltage-gated calcium channels, increases cytoplasmic calcium, and initiates exocytotic release of transmitter. N-type calcium channels have been implicated in the release of peptides from primary afferent neurons (216,237) and P- and Q-type channels are involved in the release of glutamate from central neurons (218,219,273). Attenuation of nociceptive reflexes has been observed following intrathecal administration of N- and P-type calcium channel blockers (174), supporting the role of these Ca^{2+} channels in nociceptive neurotransmission.

ORGANIZING SUMMARY

Afferent Linkage

We have discussed aspects of the transmitters that are released from primary afferent fibers. Importantly, these transmitters are released from both the central and peripheral terminals to exert actions both in close proximity to the synaptic cleft and at receptor sites potentially distant from the point of release. Release of transmitter from a nerve terminal results in volumetric diffusion of transmitter, a spatial decrease in extracellular concentration (inversely proportional to the cube of the diffusion radius), and the ability to influence distal membranes. The central release is most evidently associated with the generation of the excitatory message, which is the first link between the environment and the spinal projection neurons. The peripheral release can exert powerful local effects on the vasculature and on local inflammatory cells that themselves possess receptors for the transmitters and can secrete active products (see Chaps. 30 and 33).

The ability of the afferent fiber to release multiple agents (e.g., an excitatory amino acid and a peptide or peptides) suggests that this is an important part of the encoding process, although its significance is at present poorly understood.

A number of receptor systems are thought to be localized primarily on postsynaptic neurons in dorsal horn and, therefore, to exert their excitatory or inhibitory effects postsynaptically. Because few of these receptor systems act exclusively postsynaptically, this separation must be viewed as somewhat artificial. These postsynaptic receptor systems are thought to fall into two major classes: ionotropic receptor systems with fast but short-lived action, and metabotropic receptor systems with slow onset and long duration of action.

Modulation of Afferent Traffic

Importantly, the release of transmitter from the central and peripheral terminals of these primary afferent fibers is subject to both acute and persistent regulatory influences.

Acutely, both the central and peripheral terminals of these primary afferent fibers express receptors that are so coupled as to permit the regulation of the excitability of that terminal, serving to increase or decrease the resting or evoked release of its contents. In Chap. 36, it was emphasized that a variety of agents could exert a powerful stimulatory effect through specific afferent receptors. It is possible that such facilitatory influences may enhance central release, e.g., the presynaptic NMDA receptor. Aside from the acute excitation, these terminals similarly possess receptors that reduce terminal excitability. The most clearly defined example is the opiates, which, by their coupling to G proteins, are able to prevent the release of transmitters otherwise evoked by the opening of voltage-sensitive calcium channels. Other such regulators include agonists for α_2-adrenoceptors and the neuropeptide Y receptor. Importantly, agents that appear to regulate the preterminal excitability of small afferent fibers tend to have a significant therapeutic ratio. Thus, while there are μ and α_2 receptors in the ventral horn on motor neurons, the spinal delivery of these agents has little effect on motor function at doses that alter the pain behavior. This observation likely reflects the importance of the presynaptic effect on the afferent fiber to reduce the excitatory drive and the postsynaptic action that hyperpolarizes projection neurons. Agents such as adenosine A1 or $GABA_B$ agonists, which do not influence small afferent fiber release as strongly as do opioid or α_2 agonists, show a greater likelihood of producing motor dysfunction at doses required to produce analgesia (see Chap. 40).

Chronically, the primary afferent terminal is subject to powerful influences that clearly serve to regulate the transmission of the sensory message. Thus, protracted afferent activity can result in changes in the expression of messenger RNA that defines the availability of the levels of releasable transmitter. Such activity-dependent adjustment in transmitter systems is widely found in the brain and periphery. In addition, injury to the axon will also lead to differential alterations in the expression of message and translation of that message into channel and receptor protein and into elements for transmitter synthesis. Again, although poorly understood, it is clear that these manipulations do not uniformly affect all transmitter systems. As noted, injury may lead to a reduction in substance P and an increase in galanin levels. These changes are symptomatic of the dynamic relationship that exists between the system and its local environment.

Interactions Among Postsynaptic Receptors

Excitatory

Multiple neurotransmitters are released from primary afferent fibers upon activation by peripheral noxious stimulation. The actions of these transmitters are not singular events because the transmitters interact with multiple receptors, and the receptor systems activated interact to alter the activity of spinal cord neurons. Interactions between excitatory transmitter-receptor systems, for example, NK_1 and NMDA receptors, appear to be importantly involved in the responses of dorsal horn neurons to noxious stimuli, and some synergy may exist between the two receptor systems. In view of the high probability that glutamate and SP are co-released from primary afferent terminals upon activation by nociceptive stimuli, this positive and excitatory interaction figures prominently in the overall responses of neurons to pain-driven input to the dorsal horn. One might predict that parallel transmission systems would render analgesic interruption of one of them ineffective. However, the aforementioned positive cooperativity at the receptor level may provide a mechanism explaining why some analgesic manipulations with selectivity for one or the other receptor system produce analgesia at all.

Inhibitory

Endogenous analgesic systems are similarly coactivated upon activation of nociceptive pathways or in situations of stress. As with the excitatory transmitters above, the inhibitory transmitters also activate multiple receptors, and the effects of receptor coactivation underlie the observed analgesic effects. Interactions between inhibitory transmitter-receptor systems are also prominent in spinal nociceptive processing. Both clinical and mechanistic studies have documented the synergistic interaction between opioid and α_2-adrenergic agonists; the presence of low levels of one agonist class can reduce the amount of the other agonist required for full analgesic effect by tenfold or more (231,292). Mechanistic studies indicate that adenosine and opioid agonists interact similarly (46). However, it is unclear at this time whether two postsynaptically acting analgesic agonists can interact synergistically or whether access to both pre- and postsynaptic locations is required. Exploiting such synergistic pairs of spinally active analgesic agents may yield therapeutic regimens in the future with markedly reduced side-effect profiles.

REFERENCES

1. Aanonsen LM, Lei S, Wilcox GL. Excitatory amino acid receptors and nociceptive neurotransmission in rat spinal cord. *Pain* 1990; 41:309–321.
2. Aanonsen LM, Wilcox GL. Phencyclidine selectively blocks a spinal action of N-methyl-D-aspartate in mice. *Neurosci Lett* 1986; 67:191–197.
3. Aanonsen LM, Wilcox GL. Nociceptive action of excitatory amino acids in the mouse: effects of spinally administered opioids, phencyclidine and σ agonists. *J Pharmacol Exp Ther* 1987;243:9–19.
4. Akins PT, McCleskey EW. Characterization of potassium currents in adult rat sensory neurons and modulation by opioids and cyclic AMP. *Neuroscience* 1993;56:759–769.
5. Alhaider AA, Kitto KF, Wilcox GL. Nociceptive modulation by intrathecally administered 5-HT_{1A} and 5-HT_{1B} agonists in mice. *FASEB J* 1990;4:A988.
6. Alhaider AA, Lei S, Wilcox GL. Spinal 5-HT_3 receptor-mediated antinociception: possible release of GABA. *J Neurosci* 1991;11: 1881–1888.
7. Alhaider AA, Wilcox GL. Differential roles of 5-HT_{1A} and 5-HT_{1B} receptor subtypes in modulating spinal nociceptive transmission in mice. *J Pharmacol Exp Ther* 1993;265(1):378–385.
8. Aloe L, Tuveri MA, Carcassi U, Levi-Montalcini R. Nerve growth factor in the synovial fluid of patients with chronic arthritis. *Arthritis Rheum* 1992;35:351–355.
9. Alvarez FJ, Kavookjian AM, Light AR. Synaptic interactions between GABA-immunoreactive profiles and the terminals of functionally defined myelinated nociceptors in the monkey and cat spinal cord. *J Neurosci* 1992;12:2901–2917.
10. Amara SG, Jonas V, Rosenfeld MG, Ong ES, Evans RM. Alternative RNA processing in calcitonin gene expression generates mRNAs encoding different polypeptide products. *Nature* 1982;298:240–244.
11. Andrade R, Aghajanian GK. Opiate- and alpha 2-adrenoceptor-induced hyperpolarizations of locus ceruleus neurons in brain slices: reversal by cyclic adenosine 3′:5′-monophosphate analogues. *J Neurosci* 1985;5:2359–2364.
12. Anis NA, Berry SC, Burton NR, Lodge D. The dissociative anesthetics, ketamine and phencyclidine, selectively reduce excitation of central neurons by N-methyl-aspartate. *Br J Pharmacol* 1983;79: 565–575.
13. Arvidsson U, Dado RJ, Riedl M, Lee JH, Law PY, Loh HH, Elde R, Wessendorf MW. Delta-opioid receptor immunoreactivity: distribution in brain stem and spinal cord and relationship to biogenic amines and enkephalin. *J Neurosci* 1995;15:1215–1235.
14. Arvidsson U, Riedl M, Chakrabarti S, Lee J-H, Nakano A, Dado RJ, Loh HH, Law PY, Wessendorf MW, Elde R. Distribution and targeting of a μ-opioid receptor (MORI) in brain and spinal cord. *J Neurosci* 1995;15(5):3328–3341.
15. Arvidsson U, Riedl M, Chakrabarti S, Vulchanova L, Lee J-H, Nakano AH, Lin X, Loh HH, Law P-Y, Wessendorf MW, Elde R. The kappa-opioid receptor is primarily postsynaptic: combined immunohistochemical localization of the receptor and endogenous opioids. *Proc Natl Acad Sci USA* 1995;92:5062–5066.
16. Attali B, Nah S-Y, Vogel Z. Phorbol ester pretreatment desensitizes the inhibition of Ca^{2+} channels induced by κ-opiate, α_2-adrenergic, and muscarinic receptor agonists. *J Neurochem* 1991;57: 1803–1806.
17. Axelrod J, Reisine TD. Stress hormones: their interaction and regulation. *Science* 1984;224:452–459.
18. Basbaum AI, Fields HL. Endogenous pain control mechanisms: review and hypothesis. *Ann Neurol* 1978;4:451–462.
19. Battaglia G, Rustioni A. Coexistence of glutamate and substance P in dorsal root ganglion neurons of the rat and monkey. *J Comp Neurol* 1988;277:302–312.
20. Berridge MJ. Inositol trisphosphate and diacylglycerol: two interacting second messengers. *Annu Rev Biochem* 1987;56:159–193.
21. Boehmer CG, Norman J, Catton M, Fine LG, Mantyh PW. High levels of mRNA coding for substance P, somatostatin and a-tubulin are expressed by rat and rabbit dorsal root ganglia neurons. *Peptides* 1989;10:1179–1194.
22. Böhme GA, Bon C, Stutzmann J-M, Doble A, Blanchard J-C. Possible involvement of nitric oxide in long-term potentiation. *Eur J Pharmacol* 1991;199:379–381.
23. Bourgoin S, Pohl M, Benoliel JJ, Mauborgne A, Collin E, Hamon M, Cesselin F. γ-Aminobutyric acid, through $GABA_A$ receptors, inhibits the potassium-stimulated release of calcitonin gene-related peptide but not that of substance P-like material from rat spinal cord slices. *Brain Res* 1992;583:344–348.
24. Braas KM, Newby AC, Wilson VS, Snyder SH. Adenosine-containing neurons in the brain localized by immunocytochemistry. *J Neurosci* 1986;6:1952–1961.
25. Budai D, Wilcox GL, Larson AA. Effects of nitric oxide availability on responses of spinal wide dynamic range neurons to excitatory amino acids. *Eur J Pharmacol* 1995;278:39–47.
26. Butterworth J4, Strichartz GR. Molecular mechanisms of local anesthesia: a review. [Review]. *Anesthesiology* 1990;72(4):711–734.
27. Cacciuttolo G, Bosler O, Nieoullon A. GABA neurons in the cat red nucleus: a biochemical and immunohistochemical demonstration. *Neurosci Lett* 1984;52:129–134.
28. Campbell V, Berrow N, Dolphin AC. GABAB receptor modulation of Ca2+ currents in rat sensory neurones by the G protein G(0): antisense oligonucleotide studies. *J Physiol* 1993;470:1–11.
29. Carter MS, Krause JE. Structure, expression, and some regulatory mechanisms of the rat preprotachykinin gene encoding substance P, neurokinin A, neuropeptide K, and neuropeptide γ. *J Neurosci* 1990;10:2203–2214.
30. Chen CC, Akopian AN, Sivilotti L, Colquhoun D, Burnstock G, Wood JN. A P_{2X} purinoceptor expressed by a subset of sensory neurons. *Nature* 1995;377:428–431.
31. Chen GG, Chalazonitis A, Shen KF, Crain SM. Inhibitor of cyclic AMP-dependent protein kinase blocks opioid-induced prolongation of the action potential of mouse sensory ganglion neurons in dissociated cell cultures. *Brain Res* 1988;462(2):372–377.
32. Chen L, Huang LY. Sustained potentiation of NMDA receptor-mediated glutamate responses through activation of protein kinase C by a mu opioid. *Neuron* 1991;7:319–326.
33. Chen L, Huang LY. Protein kinase C reduces Mg^{2+} block of NMDA-receptor channels as a mechanism of modulation. *Nature* 1992;356(6369):521–523.
34. Choca JI, Green RD, Proudfit HK. Adenosine A_1 and A_2 receptors of the substantia gelatinosa are located predominantly on intrin-

sic neurons: an autoradiographic study. *J Pharmacol Exp Ther* 1988; 247:757–764.
35. Clatworthy A, Williams JH, Barasi S. Intrathecal 5-HT and electrical stimulation of the nucleus raphe magnus in rats both reduce the antinociceptive potency of intrathecally administered noradrenaline. *Brain Res* 1988;455:300–306.
36. Coderre TJ. The role of excitatory amino acid receptors and intracellular messengers in persistent nociception after tissue injury in rats. [Review]. *Mol Neurobiol* 1993;7(3–4):229–246.
37. Coderre TJ, Empel IV. The utility of excitatory amino acid (EAA) antagonists as analgesic agents. 2. Assessment of the antinociceptive activity of combinations of competitive and non-competitive NMDA antagonists with agents acting at allosteric-glycine and polyamine receptor sites. *Pain* 1994;59:353–359.
38. Coderre TJ, Katz J, Vaccarino AL, Melzack Contribution of central neuroplasticity to pathological pain—review of clinical and experimental evidence. *Pain* 1993;52:259–285.
39. Coderre TJ, Melzack R. The contribution of excitatory amino acids to central sensitization and persistent nociception after formalin-induced tissue injury. *J Neurosci* 1992;12:3665–3670.
40. Collingridge GL, Singer W. Excitatory amino acid receptors and synaptic plasticity. *Trends Pharmacol Sci* 1990;11:290–296.
41. Dado RJ, Law PY, Loh HH, Elde R. Immunofluorescent identification of a delta-opioid receptor on primary afferent nerve terminals. *NeuroReport* 1993;5:341–344.
42. Davies JE, Roberts MHT. 5-Hydroxytryptamine reduces substance P responses on dorsal horn interneurones: a possible interaction of neurotransmitters. *Brain Res* 1981;217:399–404.
43. Davies SN, Lodge D. Evidence for involvement of N-methylaspartate receptors in `wind-up' of class 2 neurons in the dorsal horn of the rat. *Brain Res* 1987;424:402–406.
44. De Biasi S, Rustioni A. Glutamate and substance P coexist in primary afferent terminals in the superficial laminae of spinal cord. *Proc Natl Acad Sci USA* 1988;85:7820–7824.
45. DeKoninck Y, Riberio-da-Silva A, Henry JL, Cuello AC. Spinal neurons exhibiting a specific nociceptive response receive abundant substance P-containing synaptic contacts. *Proc Natl Acad Sci USA* 1992;89:5073–5077.
46. DeLander GE, Keil GJ. Antinociception induced by intrathecal coadministration of selective adenosine receptor and selective opioid receptor agonists in mice. *J Pharmacol Exp Ther* 1994;268: 943–951.
47. Delander GE, Wahl JJ. Behavior induced by putative nociceptive neurotransmitters is inhibited by adenosine or adenosine analogs coadministered intrathecally. *J Pharmacol Exp Ther* 1988; 246(2):565–570.
48. DeLander GE, Wahl JJ. Descending systems activated by morphine (ICV) inhibit kainic acid (IT)- induced behavior. *Pharmacol Biochem Behav* 1991;39(1):155–159.
49. Derkach V, Surprenant A, North RA. 5-HT3 receptors are membrane ion channels. *Nature* 1989;339(6227):706–709.
50. Devor M, Wall PD, Catalan N. Systemic lidocaine silences ectopic neuroma and DRG discharge without blocking nerve conduction. *Pain* 1992;48(2):261–268.
51. Dickenson AH. A cure for wind-up: NMDA receptor agonists as potential analgesics. *Trends Pharmacol Sci* 1990;11:307–309.
52. Dickenson AH, Sullivan AF. Evidence for a role of the NMDA receptor in the frequency dependent potentiation of deep rat dorsal horn nociceptive neurons following C fiber stimulation. *Neuropharmacology* 1987;26:1235–1238.
53. Diez Guerra FJ, Zaidi M, Bevis P, MacIntyre I, Emson PC. Evidence for release of calcitonin gene-related peptide and neurokinin A from sensory nerve endings in vivo. *Neuroscience* 1988; 25:839–846.
54. Donaldson LF, Harmar AJ, McQueen DS, Seckl, JR. Increased expression of preprotachykinin, calcitonin gene-related peptide, but not vasoactive intestinal peptide messenger RNA in dorsal root ganglia during the development of adjuvant monoarthritis in the rat. *Mol Brain Res* 1992;16:143–149.
55. Donnerer J, Schuligoi R, Stein C. Increased content and transport of substance P and calcitonin gene-related peptide in sensory nerves innervating inflamed tissue: evidence for a regulatory function of nerve growth factor in vivo. *Neuroscience* 1992;49: 693–398.
56. Dougherty PM, Palecek J, Paleckova V, Sorkin LS, Willis WD. The role of NMDA and non-NMDA excitatory amino acid receptors in the excitation of primate spinothalamic tract neurons by mechanical, chemical, thermal, and electrical stimuli. *J Neurosci* 1992; 12(8):3025–3041.
57. Dougherty PM, Willis WD. Enhancement of spinothalamic neuron responses to chemical and mechanical stimuli following combined micro-iontophoretic application of N-methyl-D-aspartic acid and substance P. *Pain* 1991;47:85–93.
58. Dougherty PM, Willis WD. Modification of the responses of primate spinothalamic neurons to mechanical stimulation by excitatory amino acids and an N-methyl-D-aspartate antagonist. *Brain Res* 1991;542:15–22.
59. Dougherty PM, Willis WD. Enhanced responses of spinothalamic tract neurons to excitatory amino acids accompany capsaicin-induced sensitization in the monkey. *J Neurosci* 1992;12(3): 883–894.
60. Dray A, Bettaney J, Forster P. Capsaicin desensitization of peripheral nociceptive fibres does not impair sensitivity to other noxious stimuli. *Neurosci Lett* 1989;99(50–54):
61. Dubner R, Ruda MA. Activity-dependent neuronal plasticity following tissue injury and inflammation. [Review]. *Trends Neurosci* 1992;15(3):96–103.
62. Duggan AW, Hendry IA, Morton CR, Hutchison WD, Zhao ZQ. Cutaneous stimuli releasing immunoreactive substance P in the dorsal horn of the cat. *Brain Res* 1988;451:261–273.
63. Duggan AW, Hope PJ, Jarrott B, Schaible, H-G, Fleetwood-Walker SM. Release, spread and persistence of immunoreactive neurokinin A in the dorsal horn of the cat following noxious cutaneous stimulation. Studies with antibody microprobes. *Neuroscience* 1990;35:195–202.
64. Duzic E, Coupry I, Downing S, Lanier SM. Factors determining the specificity of signal transduction by guanine nucleotide-binding protein-coupled receptors. I. Coupling of alpha 2-adrenergic receptor subtypes to distinct G-proteins. *J Biol Chem* 1992;267(14): 9844–9851.
65. Eason MG, Kurose H, Holt BD, Raymond JR, Liggett SB. Simultaneous coupling of a2-adrenergic receptors to two G-proteins with opposing effects. *J Biol Chem* 1992;267:15795–15801.
66. East SJ, Garthwaite J. Nanomolar N^G-nitroarginine inhibits NMDA-induced cyclic GMP formation in rat cerebellum. *Eur J Pharmacol* 1990;184:311–313.
67. East SJ, Garthwaite J. NMDA receptor activation in rat hippocampus induces cyclic GMP formation through the L-arginine-nitric oxide pathway. *Neurosci Lett* 1991;123:17–19.
68. El-Yassir N, Fleetwood-Walker SM, Mitchell R. Heterogeneous effects of serotonin in the dorsal horn of rat: the involvement of $5\text{-}HT_1$ receptor subtypes. *Brain Res* 1988;456:147–158.
69. Ewald DA, Pang I-H, Sternweis PC, Miller RJ. Differential G protein-mediated coupling of neurotransmitter receptors to Ca^{2+} channels in rat dorsal root ganglion cells in vitro. *Neuron* 1989;2: 1185–1193.
70. Fasmer OB, Berge O-G, Hole K. Similar behavioral effects of 5-hydroxytryptamine and substance P injected intrathecally in mice. *Neuropharmacology* 1983;22:485–487.
71. Fleetwood-Walker SM, Mitchell R, Hope PJ, Molony V, Iggo A. An $\alpha_2$receptor mediates the selective inhibition by noradrenaline of nociceptive responses of identified dorsal horn neurons. *Brain Res* 1985;334:243–254.
72. Fozard, JR. 5-Hydroxytryptamine in the pathophysiology of migraine. In: Beven JA, Godfraind T, Maxwell RA, Stoclet JC, Worcel M, eds. *Vascular neuroeffector mechanisms.* Amsterdam: Elsevier Science, 1985;321–328.
73. Freissmuth M, Casey PJ, Gilman AG. G proteins control diverse pathways in transmembrane signalling. *FASEB J* 1989;3:2125–2131.
74. Furuyama T, Kiyama H, Sato K, Park HT, Maeno H, Takagi H, Tohyama M. Region-specific expression of subunits of ionotropic glutamate receptors (AMPA-type, KA-type, and NMDA receptors) in the rat spinal cord with special reference to nociception. *Mol Brain Res* 1993;18:141–151.
75. Galeazza MT, Garry MG, Yost HJ, Strait KA, Hargreaves KM, Seybold VS. Plasticity in the synthesis and storage of substance P and calcitonin gene-related peptide in primary afferent neurons during peripheral inflammation. *Neuroscience* 1995;66:443–458.
76. Garry MG, Hargreaves KM. Enhanced release of immunoreactive CGRP and substance P from spinal dorsal horn slices occurs during carrageenan inflammation. *Brain Res* 1992;582:139–142.
77. Geiger JD, LaBella FS, Nagy JI. Characterization and localization of adenosine receptors in rat spinal cord. *J Neurosci* 1984;4: 2303–2310.

78. Geiger JD, Nagy JI. Localization of [^{3}H]nitrobenzylthioinosine binding sites in rat spinal cord and primary afferent neurons. *Brain Res* 1985;347:321–327.
79. Geiger JD, Nagy JI. Distribution of adenosine deaminase activity in rat brain and spinal cord. *J Neurosci* 1986;6:2707–2714.
80. Gerber G, Randic M. Excitatory amino acid-mediated components of synaptically evoked input from dorsal roots to deep dorsal horn neurons in the rat spinal cord slice. *Neurosci Lett* 1989; 106:211–9.
81. Giesler GJ, Menetrey D, Basbaum AI. Differential origins of spinothalamic tract projections to medial and lateral thalamus in the rat. *J Comp Neurol* 1979;184:107–126.
82. Gilman AG. Regulation of adenylyl cyclase by G proteins. *Adv Second Messenger Phosphoprotein Res* 1990;24:51–57.
83. Glaum SR, Anderson EG. Identification of 5-HT3 binding sites in rat spinal cord synaptosomal membranes. *Eur J Pharmacol* 1988; 156(2):287–90.
84. Glaum SR, Miller RJ, Hammond DL. Inhibitory actions of delta 1-, delta 2-, and mu-opioid receptor agonists on excitatory transmission in lamina II neurons of adult rat spinal cord. *J Neurosci* 1994; 14(8):4965–71.
85. Glaum SR, Proudfit HK, Anderson EG. 5-HT3 receptors modulate spinal nociceptive reflexes. *Brain Res* 1990;510:12–16.
86. Go VLW, Yaksh TL. Release of substance P from the cat spinal cord. *J Physiol* 1987;391:141–167.
87. Goodman RR, Snyder SH. Autoradiographic localization of adenosine receptors in the rat brain using [3H]cyclohexyladenosine. *J Neurosci* 1982;2:1230–1241.
88. Green T, Dockray GJ. Characterization of the peptidergic afferent innervation of the stomach in the rat, mouse and guinea-pig. *Neuroscience* 1988;25:181–193.
89. Grega DS, Macdonald RL. Activators of adenylate cyclase and cyclic AMP prolong calcium-dependent action potentials of mouse sensory neurons in culture by reducing a voltage-dependent potassium conductance. *J Neurosci* 1987;7(3):700–707.
90. Grossman Y, Parnas I, Spira ME. Differential conduction block in branches of a bifurcating axon. *J Physiol* 1979;295:283–305.
91. Grossman Y, Parnas I, Spira ME. Mechanisms involved in differential conduction of potentials at high frequency in a branching axon. *J Physiol* 1979;295:307–22.
92. Grundt TJ, Williams JT. μ-Opioid agonists inhibit spinal trigeminal substantia gelatinosa neurons in guinea pig and rat. *J Neurosci* 1994;14(3 Pt 2):1646–1654.
93. Haley JE, Dickenson AH, Schachter M. Electrophysiological evidence for a role of nitric oxide in prolonged chemical nociception in the rat. *Neuropharmacology* 1992;31:251–258.
94. Haley JE, Sullivan AF, Dickenson AH. Evidence for spinal N-methyl-D-aspartate receptor involvement in prolonged chemical nociception in the rat. *Brain Res* 1990;518:218–226.
95. Haley JE, Wilcox GL, Chapman PF. The role of nitric oxide in hippocampal long-term potentiation. *Neuron* 1992;8:211–216.
96. Hamon M, Collin E, Chantrel D, Daval G, Verge D, Bourgoin S, Cesselin F. Serotonin receptors and the modulation of pain. In: Hamon M, ed. *Serotonin and pain.* Amsterdam: Excerpta Medica, 1990;53–72.
97. Hao JX, Xu XJ, Yu YX, Seiger A, Wiesenfeld HZ. Baclofen reverses the hypersensitivity of dorsal horn wide dynamic range neurons to mechanical stimulation after transient spinal cord ischemia; implications for a tonic GABAergic-inhibitory control of myelinated fiber input. *J Neurophysiol* 1992;68:392–396.
98. Hassan AHS, Ableitner A, Stein C, Herz A. Inflammation of the rat paw enhances axonal transport of opioid receptors in the sciatic nerve and increases their density in the inflamed tissue. *Neuroscience* 1993;55:185–195.
99. Helke CJ, Hill KM. Immunohistochemical study of neuropeptides in vagal and glossopharyngeal afferent neurons in the rat. *Neuroscience* 1988;26:539–551.
100. Helke CJ, Krause JE, Mantyh PW, Couture R, Bannon MJ. Diversity in mammalian tachykinin peptidergic neurons: multiple peptides, receptors, and regulatory mechanisms. *FASEB J* 1990;4: 1606–1615.
101. Henry JL. Effects of intravenously administered enantiomers of baclofen on functionally identified units in lumbar dorsal horn of the spinal cat. *Neuropharmacology* 1982;21:1073–1083.
102. Hescheler J, Rosenthal W, Trautwein W, Schultz G. The GTP-binding protein, G_o, regulates neuronal calcium channels. *Nature* 1987;325:445–447.
103. Hoehn K, Reid A, Sawynok J. Pertussis toxin inhibits antinociception produced by intrathecal injection of morphine, noradrenaline and baclofen. *Eur J Pharmacol* 1988;146(1):65–72.
104. Hogan K, Kooy vd. Visceral target specific calcitonin gene-related peptide and substance P enrichment in trigeminal afferent projections. *J Neurosci* 1992;12:1135–1143.
105. Hoheisel U, Mense S, Scherotzke R. Calcitonin gene-related peptide-immunoreactivity in functionally identified primary afferent neurones in the rat. *Anat Embryol* 1994;189:41–49.
106. Hökfelt T. Neuropeptides in perspective. *Neuron* 1991;7:867–879.
107. Hollman M, Heinemann S. Cloned glutamate receptors. *Annu Rev Neurosci* 1994;17:31–108.
108. Holz GG4, Kream RM, Spiegel A, Dunlap K. G proteins couple alpha-adrenergic and GABA-B receptors to inhibition of peptide secretion from peripheral sensory neurons. *J Neurosci* 1989;9: 657–666.
109. Holzer P. Local effector functions of capsaicin-sensitive sensory nerve endings: involvement of tachykinins, calcitonin gene-related peptide and other neuropeptides. *Neuroscience* 1988;24: 739–768.
110. Honda CN, Rethelyi M, Petrusz P. Preferential immunohistochemical localization of vasoactive intestinal polypeptide (VIP) in the sacral spinal cord of the cat: light and electron microscopic observations. *J Neurosci* 1983;3:2183–2196.
111. Honoré T, Davies SN, Drejer J, Fletcher EJ, Jacobsen P, Lodge D, Neilsen FE. Quinoxalinediones: potent competitive non-NMDA glutamate receptor antagonists. *Science* 1988;241:701–703.
112. Hornfeldt CS, Sun X, Larson AA. The NH_2-terminus of substance P modulates NMDA-induced activity in the mouse spinal cord. *J Neurosci* 1994;14:3364–3369.
113. Howe JR, Yaksh TL, Go VLW. The effect of unilateral dorsal root ganglionectomies or ventral rhizotomies on α2-adrenoceptor binding to, and the substance P, enkephalin, and neurotensin content of, the cat lumbar spinal cord. *Neuroscience* 1987;21: 385–394.
114. Hua XY, Boublik JH, Spicer MA, Rivier JE, Brown MR, Yaksh TL. The antinociceptive effects of spinally administered neuropeptide Y in the rat: systematic studies on structure-activity relationship. *J Pharmacol Exp Ther* 1991;258:243–248.
115. Huang LM. The excitatory effects of opioids. *Neurochem Int* 1992; 20(4):463–468.
116. Hwang AS, Wilcox GL. Analgesic properties of intrathecally administered heterocyclic antidepressants. *Pain* 1987;28:343–355.
117. Hylden JL, Nahin RL, Traub RJ, Dubner R. Effects of spinal kappa-opioid receptor agonists on the responsiveness of nociceptive superficial dorsal horn neurons. *Pain* 1991;44:187–193.
118. Hylden JLK, Wilcox GL. Intrathecal substance P elicits a caudally-directed biting and scratching behavior in mice. *Brain Res* 1981; 217:212–215.
119. Hylden JLK, Wilcox GL. Intrathecal serotonin in mice: analgesia and inhibition of a spinal action of a spinal action of substance. *Life Sci* 1983;33:789–795.
120. Hylden JLK, Wilcox GL. Antinociceptive effect of morphine on rat spinothalamic tract and other dorsal horn neurons. *Neuroscience* 1986;19:393–402.
121. Jahr CE, Jessell TM. ATP excites a subpopulation of rat dorsal horn neurones. *Nature* 1983;304:730–733.
122. Jancso G, Karcsu S, Kiraly E, Szebeni A, Toth L, Bacsy E, Joo F, Parducz A. Neurotoxin-induced nerve cell degeneration: possible involvement of calcium. *Brain Res* 1984;295:211–216.
123. Jane DE, Jones PL, Pook PC, Tse HW, Watkins JC. Actions of two new antagonists showing selectivity for different sub-types of metabotropic glutamate receptor in the neonatal rat spinal cord. *Br J Pharmacol* 1994;112(3):809–816.
124. Jeftinija S. Enkephalins modulate excitatory synaptic transmission in the superficial dorsal horn by acting at mu-opioid receptor sites. *Brain Res* 1988;460:260–268.
125. Jeftinija S, Jeftinija K, Liu F, Skilling SR, Smullin DH, Larson AA. Excitatory amino acids are released from rat primary afferent neurons in vitro. *Neurosci Lett* 1991;125:191–194.
126. Jeftinija S, Korade Z. Mechanism of inhibitory action of enkephalins, norepinephrine, (-)-baclofen and somatostatin in the spinal dorsal horn: an in vitro study. In: Bond MR, Charlton JE, Woolf CJ, eds. *Proceedings of the VIth World Congress on Pain.* Amsterdam: Elsevier Science, 1991;151–158.
127. Jessell T, Tsunoo A, Kanazawa I, Otsuka M. Substance P: depletion in the dorsal horn of rat spinal cord after section of the peripheral

processes of primary sensory neurons. *Brain Res* 1979;168:247–259.

128. Jhamandas K, Yaksh TL, Harty G, Szolcsanyi J, Go VLW. Action of intrathecal capsaicin and its structural analogues on the content and release of spinal substance P: selectivity of action and relationship to analgesia. *Brain Res* 1984;306:215–225.
129. Jin W, Lee NM, Lob HH, Thayer SA. Opioids mobilize calcium from inositol 1,4,5-trisphosphate-sensitive stores in NG108-15 cells. *J Neurosci* 1994;14:1920–1929.
130. Joris JL, Dubner R, Hargreaves KM. Opioid analgesia at peripheral sites: A target for opioids released during stress and inflammation. *Anesth Analg* 1987;66:1277–1281.
131. Julius D, Huang KN, Livelli TJ, Axel R, Jessell TM. The $5HT_2$ receptor defines a family of structurally distinct but functionally conserved serotonin receptors. *Proc Natl Acad Sci USA* 1990;87: 928–932.
132. Julius D, MacDermott AB, Axel R, Jessell TM. Molecular characterization of a functional cDNA encoding the serotonin 1c receptor. *Science* 1988;241:558–564.
133. Karlsten R, Post C, Hide I, Daly JW. The antinociceptive effect of intrathecally administered adenosine analogs in mice correlates with the affinity for the A_1-adenosine receptor. *Neurosci Lett* 1991; 121:267–270.
134. Kawatani M, Nagel J, DeGroat WC. Identification of neuropeptides in pelvic viscera and pudendal nerve afferent pathways to the sacral spinal cord of the cat. *J Comp Neurol* 1986;249:117–132.
135. Kayser V, Besson JM, Guilbaud G. Paradoxical hyperalgesic effect of exceedingly low doses of systemic morphine in an animal model of persistent pain (Freund's adjuvant-induced arthritic rats). *Brain Res* 1987;414:155–157.
136. Kehl LJ, Wilcox GL. Antinociceptive effect of tricyclic antidepressants following intrathecal administration. *Anesth Prog* 1984;31: 82–84.
137. Keil GJ II, DeLander GE. Adenosine kinase and adenosine deaminase inhibition modulate spinal adenosine- and opioid agonist-induced antinociception in mice. *Eur J Pharmacol* 1994a;271: 37–46.
138. Keil GJ II, DeLander GE. Nociceptive and antinociceptive behaviors in mice following manipulation of spinal endogenous adenosine levels. *Am Pain Soc* 1994;(abstr).
139. Keil GJ II, DeLander GE. Time dependent antinociceptive interactions between opioids and nucleoside transport inhibitors. *J Pharmacol Exp Ther* 1995;274:1387–1392.
140. Kelso SR, Nelson TE, Leonard JP. Protein kinase C-mediated enhancement of NMDA currents by metabotropic glutamate receptors in *Xenopus* oocytes. *J Physiol (Lond)* 1992;449:705–718.
141. King AE, Lopez-Garcia JA. Excitatory amino acid receptor-mediated neurotransmission from cutaneous afferents in rat dorsal horn in vitro. *J Physiol* 1993;472:443–57.
142. Kitto KF, Haley JE, Wilcox GL. Involvement of nitric oxide in spinally mediated hyperalgesia in the mouse. *Neurosci Lett* 1992; 148:1–5.
143. Kjartansson J, Dalsgaard C-J, Jonsson C-E. Decreased survival of experimental critical flaps in rats after sensory denervation with capsaicin. *Plast Reconstruct Surg* 1987;79:218–221.
144. Kleuss C, Hescheler J, Ewel C, Rosenthal W, Schultz G, Wittig B. Assignment of G-protein subtypes to specific receptors inducing inhibition of calcium currents. *Nature* 1991;353(6339):43–48.
145. Kubo Y, Reuveny E, Slesinger PA, Jan YN, Jan LY. Primary structure and functional expression of a rat G-protein-coupled muscarinic potassium channel [see comments]. *Nature* 1993;364: 802–806.
146. Kuo DC, Kawatani M, De Groat WC. Vasoactive intestinal polypeptide identified in the thoracic dorsal root ganglia of the cat. *Brain Res* 1985;330:178–182.
147. Kuraishi Y, Hirota N, Sato Y, Hanashima N, Takagi H, Satoh M. Stimulus specificity of peripherally evoked substance P release from the rabbit dorsal horn in situ. *Neuroscience* 1989;30:241–250.
148. Kuraishi Y, Hirota N, Sato Y, Hino Y, Satoh M, Takagi H. Evidence that substance P and somatostatin transmit separate information related to pain in the spinal dorsal horn. *Brain Res* 1985;325: 294–298.
149. Kuraishi Y, Hirota N, Sato Y, Kaneko S, Satoh M, Takagi H. Noradrenergic inhibition of the release of substance P from the primary afferents in the rabbit spinal dorsal horn. *Brain Res* 1985;359: 177–182.
150. Laduron PM. Axonal transport of opiate receptors in capsaicin-sensitive neurones. *Brain Res* 1984;294:157–160.
151. Larson AA, Beitz AJ. Glycine potentiates strychnine-induced convulsions: role of NMDA receptors. *J Neurosci* 1988;8:3822–3826.
152. Lawson SN, Perry MJ, Prabhakar E, McCarthy PW. Primary sensory neurones: neurofilament, neuropeptides, and conduction velocity. *Brain Res Bull* 1993;30:239–243.
153. Leah JD, Cameron AA, Snow PJ. Neuropeptides in physiologically identified mammalian sensory neurons. *Neurosci Lett* 1985;56: 257–263.
154. Lee YW, Yaksh TL. Pharmacology of the spinal adenosine receptor which mediated the antiallodynic action of intrathecal adenosine agonists. *J Pharmacol Exp Ther* 1996;277:1642–1648.
155. Leem JW, Willis WD, Chung JM. Cutaneous sensory receptors in the rat foot. *J Neurophysiol* 1993;69:1684–1699.
156. Lei SZ, Pan Z-H, Aggarwal SK, Chen, H-SV, Hartman J, Sucher NJ, Lipton SA. Effect of nitric oxide production on the redox modulatory site of the NMDA receptor-channel complex. *Neuron* 1992; 8:1087–1099.
157. Lewis C, Neidhart S, Holy C, North RA, Buell G, Surprenant A. Co-expression of $P_{2\times2}$ and $P_{2\times3}$ receptor subunits can account for ATP-gated currents in sensory neurons. *Nature* 1995;377:432–435.
158. Lindsay RM, Lockett C, Sternberg J, Winter J. Neuropeptide expression in cultures of adult sensory neurons: modulation of substance P and calcitonin gene-related peptide levels by nerve growth factor. *Neuroscience* 1989;33:53–65.
159. Liu H, Brown JL, Jasmin L, Maggio JE, Vigna SR, Mantyh PW, Basbaum AI. Synaptic relationship between substance P and the substance P receptor: light and electron microscopic characterization of the mismatch between neuropeptides and their receptors. *Proc Nat Acad Sci USA* 1994;91:1009–1013.
160. Liu H, Wang H, Sheng M, Jan LY, Jan YN, Basbaum AI. Evidence for presynaptic N-methyl-D-aspartate autoreceptors in the spinal cord dorsal horn. *Proc Natl Acad Sci USA* 1994;91(18):8383–8387.
161. Liu XG, Sandkuhler J. Long-term potentiation of C-fiber-evoked potentials in the rat spinal dorsal horn is prevented by spinal N-methyl-D-aspartic acid receptor blockage. *Neurosci Lett* 1995;191: 43–46.
162. Lledo PM, Homburger V, Bockaert J, Vincent JD. Differential G Protein-mediated coupling of D2 Dopamine receptors to K^+ and Ca^{2+} currents in rat anterior pituitary cells. *Neuron* 1992;8:455–463.
163. Lodge D, Davies S. Evidence for involvement of N-methylaspartate receptors in 'wind-up' of class 2 neurons in the dorsal horn of the rat. *Brain Res* 1987;424:402–406.
164. Lynn B. Capsaicin: actions on nociceptive C-fibres and therapeutic potential. *Pain* 1990;41:61–69.
165. Lynn B, Carpenter SE. Primary afferent units from the hairy skin of the rat hind limb. *Brain Res* 1982;238:29–43.
166. Lynn B, Shakhanbeh J. Substance P content of the skin, neurogenic inflammation and numbers of C-fibres following capsaicin application to a cutaneous nerve in the rabbit. *Neuroscience* 1988; 24:769–775.
167. MacDermott AB, Mayer ML, Westbrook GL, Smith SJ, Barker JL. NMDA-receptor activation increases cytoplasmic calcium concentration in cultured spinal cord neurones. *Nature* 1986;321:519–522.
168. Macdonald RL, Nelson PG. Specific opiate-induced depression of transmitter release from dorsal root ganglia cells in culture. *Science* 1978;199:1449–1451.
169. Maggi CA. Capsaicin and primary afferent neurons: from basic science to human therapy? J *Auton Nerv Sys* 1991;33:1–14.
170. Malmberg AB, Rafferty MF, Yaksh TL. Antinociceptive effect of spinally delivered prostaglandin E receptor antagonists in the formalin test on the rat. *Neurosci Lett* 1994;173:193–6.
171. Malmberg AB and Yaksh TL. Hyperalgesia mediated by spinal glutamate or substance P receptor blocked by spinal cyclooxygenase inhibition. *Science* 257:1276–1279, 1992.
172. Malmberg AB, Yaksh TL. Spinal nitric oxide synthesis inhibition blocks NMDA-induced thermal hyperalgesia and produces antinociception in the formalin test in rats. *Pain* 1993;54(3): 291–300.
173. Malmberg AB and Yaksh TL. Spinal nitric oxide synthesis inhibition blocks NMDA-induced thermal hyperalgesia and produces antinociception in the formalin test in rats. *Pain* 1993;54(3): 291–300.
174. Malmberg AB, Yaksh TL. Voltage-sensitive calcium channels in spinal nociceptive processing: blockade of N- and P-type channels inhibits formalin-induced nociception. *J Neurosci* 1994;14: 4882–4890.
175. Malmberg AB, Yaksh TL. Cyclooxygenase inhibition and the spinal

release of prostaglandin E_2 and amino acids evoked by paw formalin injection: a microdialysis study in anesthetized rats. *J Neurosci* 1995;15:2768–776.

176. Mantyh PW, Allen CJ, Rogers S, Demaster E, Ghilardi JR, Mosconi T, Kruger L, Mannon PJ, Taylor IL, Vigna SR. Some sensory neurons express neuropeptide Y receptors: potential paracrine inhibition of primary afferent nociceptors following peripheral nerve injury. *J Neurosci* 1994;14:3958–3968.
177. Mantyh PW, DeMaster E, Malhotra A, Ghilardi JR, Rogers SD, Mantyh CR, Liu H, Basbaum AI, Vigna SR, Maggio JE, et al. Receptor endocytosis and dendrite reshaping in spinal neurons after somatosensory stimulation. *Science* 1995;268:1629–1632.
178. Marsala M, Malmberg AB, Yaksh TL. The spinal loop dialysis catheter: characterization of use in the unanesthetized rat. *J Neurosci Meth* 1995;62:43–53.
179. Mayer ML, Westbrook GL. The physiology of excitatory amino acids in the vertebrate central nervous system. *Prog Neurobiol* 1987; 28:197–276.
180. McCarthy PW, Lawson SN. Cell type and conduction velocity of rat primary sensory neurons with substance P-like immunoreactivity. *Neuroscience* 1989;28:745–753.
181. McCarthy PW, Lawson SN. Cell type and conduction velocity of rat primary sensory neurons with calcitonin gene-related peptide-like immunoreactivity. *Neuroscience* 1990;34:623–632.
182. McGregor GP, Gibson SJ, Sabate IM, Blaske MA, Christofides ND, Wall PD, Polak JM, Bloom SR. Effect of peripheral nerve section and nerve crush on spinal cord neuropeptides in the rat: increased VIP and PHI in the dorsal horn. *Neuroscience* 1984;13:207–226.
183. McMahon SB, Armanini MP, Ling LH, Phillips HS. Expression and coexpression of Trk receptors in subpopulations of adult primary sensory neurons projecting to identified peripheral targets. *Neuron* 1994;12:1161–1171.
184. McMahon SB, Gibson S. Peptide expression is altered when afferent nerves reinnervate inappropriate tissue. *Neurosci Lett* 1987;73: 9–15.
185. Meller SJ, Dykstra C, Gebhart GF. Production of endogenous nitric oxide and activation of soluble guanylate cyclase are required for N-methyl-D-aspartate-produced facilitation of the nociceptive tail flick reflex. *Eur J Pharmacol* 1992;214:93–96.
186. Meller ST, Dykstra CL, Gebhart GF. Acute mechanical hyperalgesia is produced by coactivation of AMPA and metabotropic glutamate receptors. *Neuroreport* 1993;4:879–82.
187. Mendell LM. Physiological properties of unmyelinated fiber projection to the spinal cord. *Exp Neurol* 1966;16:316–332.
188. Michener SR, Aimone LD, Yaksh TL and Go VLW. Distribution of galanin-like immunoreactivity in the pig, rat and human central nervous system. *Peptides* 1990;11:1217–1233.
189. Minami T, Uda R, Horiguchi S, Ito S, Hyodo M, Hayaishi O. Allodynia evoked by intrathecal administration of prostaglandin E2 to conscious mice. *Pain* 1994;57:217–223.
190. Moises HC, Rusin KI, Macdonald RL. μ- and κ-Opioid receptors selectively reduce the same transient components of high-threshold calcium current in rat dorsal root ganglion sensory neurons. *J Neurosci* 1994;14:5903–5916.
191. Moore PK, Oluyomi AO, Babbedge RC, Wallace P, Hart SL. L-N^G-nitro arginine methyl ester exhibits antinociceptive activity in the mouse. *Br J Pharmacol* 1991;102:198–202.
192. Morris R, Southam E, Braid DJ, Garthwaite J. Nitric oxide may act as a messenger between dorsal root ganglion neurons and their satellite cells. *Neurosci Lett* 1992;137:29–32.
193. Morton CR, Hutchison WD. Release of sensory neuropeptides in the spinal cord: studies with calcitonin gene-related peptide and galanin. *Neuroscience* 1989;31:807–815.
194. Morton CR, Hutchison WD, Hendry IA, Duggan AW. Somatostatin: evidence for a role in thermal nociception. *Brain Res* 1989; 488:89–96.
195. Mudge AW, Leeman SE, Fischbach GD. Enkephalin inhibits release of substance P from sensory neurons in culture and decreases action potential duration. *Proc Natl Acad Sci USA* 1979;76: 526–530.
196. Mulderry PK. Neuropeptide expression by newborn and adult rat sensory neurons in culture—effects of nerve growth factor and other neurotrophic Factors. *Neuroscience* 1994;59:673–688.
197. Nagasaka H, Awad H, Yaksh TL. Peripheral and spinal actions of opioids in the blockade of the autonomic response evoked by compression of the inflamed knee joint. *Anesthesiology* 1996;85:808–816.
198. Nakamura-Craig M, Follenfant RL. Effect of lamotrigine in the acute and chronic hyperalgesia induced by PGE2 and in the chronic hyperalgesia in rats with streptozotocin-induced diabetes. *Pain* 1995;63:33–37.
199. Neugebauer V, Lucke T, Schaible HG. Requirement of metabotropic glutamate receptors for the generation of inflammation-evoked hyperexcitability in rat spinal cord neurons. *Eur J Neurosci* 1994;6(7):1179–86.
200. Nicholas AP, Pieribone V, Hokfelt T. Distributions of mRNAs for alpha-2 adrenergic receptor subtypes in rat brain: an in situ hybridization study. *J Comp Neurol* 1993;328:575–594.
201. Ninkovic M, Hunt SP. Opiate and histamine H1 receptors are present on some substance P-containing dorsal root ganglion cells. *Neurosci Lett* 1985;53:133–137.
202. Ninkovic M, Hunt SP, Gleave JRW. Localization of opiate and histamine H1-receptors in the primary sensory ganglia and spinal cord. *Brain Res* 1982;241:197–206.
203. Noguchi K, De León M, Nahin RL, Senba E, Ruda MA. Quantification of axotomy-induced alteration of neuropeptide mRNAs in dorsal root ganglion neurons with special reference to neuropeptide Y mRNA and the effects of neonatal capsaicin treatment. *J Neurosci Res* 1993;35:54–66.
204. Noguchi K, Senba E, Morita Y, Sato M, Tohyama M. α-CGRP and β-CGRP mRNAs are differently regulated in the rat spinal cord and dorsal root ganglion. *Mol Brain Res* 1990;7:299–304.
205. North RA. Opioid receptor types and membrane ion channels. *Trends Neurosci* 1986;9:114–117.
206. O'Brien C, Woolf CJ, Fitzgerald M, Lindsay RM, Molander C. Differences in the chemical expression of rat primary afferent neurons which innervate skin, muscle or joint. *Neuroscience* 1989;32: 493–502.
207. Ohishi H, Shigemoto R, Nakanishi S, Mizuno N. Distribution of the mRNA for a metabotropic glutamate receptor (mGluR3) in the rat brain: an in situ hybridization study. *J Comp Neurol* 1993; 335:252–66.
208. Ohkubo T, Shibata M, Takahashi H, Inoki R. Roles of substance P and somatostatin on transmission of nociceptive information induced by formalin in spinal cord. *J Pharmacol Exp Ther* 1990;252: 1261–1268.
209. Oku R, Satih M, Takagi H. Release of substance P from the spinal dorsal horn is enhanced in polyarthritic rats. *Neurosci Lett* 1987;74: 315–319.
210. Palecek J, Paleckova V, Dougherty PM, Willis WD. The effect of trans-ACPD, a metabotropic excitatory amino acid receptor agonist, on the responses of primate spinothalamc tract neurons. *Pain* 1994;56:261–269.
211. Pang IH, Vasko MR. Morphine and norepinephrine but not 5-hydroxytryptamine and gamma-aminobutyric acid inhibit the potassium-stimulated release of substance P from rat spinal cord slices. *Brain Res* 1986;376:268–279.
212. Papir-Kricheli D, Frey J, Laufer R, Gilon C, Chorev M, Selinger Z, Devor M. Behavioral effects of receptor-specific substance P agonists. *Pain* 1987;31:263–276.
213. Parsons AM, EE El-Fakahany, VS Seybold. Tachykinins alter inositol phosphate formation, but no cAMP levels, in neonatal rat spinal neurons through activation of neurokinin receptors. *Neuroscience* 1995;68:855–865.
214. Pedigo NW, Yamamura HI, Nelson DL. Discrimination of multiple [^{3}H]5-hydroxytryptamine binding sites by the neuroleptic spiperone in rat brain. *J Neurochem* 1981;36:220–226.
215. Penning JP, Yaksh TL. Interaction of intrathecal morphine with bupivacaine and lidocaine in the rat. *Anesthesiology* 1992;77: 1186–2000.
216. Perney TM, Hirning LD, Leeman SE, Miller RJ. Multiple calcium channels mediate neurotransmitter release from peripheral neurons. *Proc Natl Acad Sci USA* 1986;83:6656–6659.
217. Peroutka SJ. Pharmacological differentiation and characterization of 5-HT1A, 5-HT1B, and 5-HT1C binding sites in rat frontal cortex. *J Neurochem* 1986;47:529–540.
218. Piser TM, Lampe RA, Keith RA, Thayer SA. Omega-Grammotoxin blocks action potential-induced Ca2+ influx and whole-cell Ca^{2+} current in rat dorsal root ganglion neurons. *Pflugers Arch Eur J Physiol* 1994;426:214–220.
219. Pocock JM, Nicholls DG. A toxin (Aga-GI) from the venom of the spider *Agelenopsis aperta* inhibits the mammalian presynaptic Ca^{2+} channel coupled to glutamate exocytosis. *Eur J Pharmacol* 1992;226: 343–350.
220. Price GW, Wilkin GP, Turnbull MJ, Bowery NG. Are baclofen-sensi-

tive $GABA_B$ receptors on primary afferent terminals of the spinal cord? *Nature* 1984;307:71–74.
221. Radhakrishnan V, Henry JL. Novel Substance-P antagonist, CP-96,345, blocks responses of cat spinal dorsal horn neurons to noxious cutaneous stimuli and to substance P. *Neurosci Lett* 1991;132:39–43.
222. Radhakrishnan V, Henry JL. L-NAME blocks responses to NMDA, Substance-P and noxious cutaneous stimuli in cat dorsal horn. *Neuroreport* 1993;4:323–326.
223. Raigorodsky G, Urca G. Intrathecal N-methyl-D-aspartate (NMDA) activates both nociceptive and antinociceptive systems. *Brain Res* 1987;422:158–162.
224. Randic M, Hecimovic H, Ryu PD. Substance P modulates glutamate-induced currents in acutely isolated rat spinal dorsal horn neurones. *Neurosci Lett* 1990;117:74–80.
225. Rane SG, Dunlap K. Kinase C activator 1,2-oleoylacetylglycerol attenuates voltage-dependent calcium current in sensory neurons. *Proc Natl Acad Sci USA* 1986;83:184–188.
226. Reisine TD, Heisler S, Hook VY, Axelrod J. Activation of beta 2-adrenergic receptors on mouse anterior pituitary tumor cells increases cyclic adenosine 3′:5′-monophosphate synthesis and adrenocorticotropin release. *J Neurosci* 1983;3:725–32.
227. Ren K, Dubner R. NMDA receptor antagonists attenuate mechanical hyperalgesia in rats with unilateral inflammation of the hindpaw. *Neurosci Lett* 1993;163:22–26.
228. Ren K, Williams GM, Hylden JL, Ruda MA, Dubner R. The intrathecal administration of excitatory amino acid receptor antagonists selectively attenuated carrageenan-induced behavioral hyperalgesia in rats. *Eur J Pharmacol* 1992;219:235–43.
229. Richardson BP, Engel G. The pharmacology and function of $5\text{-}HT_3$ receptors. *Trends Pharmacol Sci* 1986;7:424–428.
230. Riedl M, Arvidsson U, Dado RJ, Lee J-H, Wessendorf MW, Loh HH, Law P-Y, Elde R. Colocalization of substance P and A delta opioid receptor in the rat central nervous system. *Soc Neurosci Abst* 1994;20:1729.
231. Roerig S, Lei S, Kitto K, Hylden JLK, Wilcox GL. Spinal interactions between opioid and noradrenergic agonists in mice: multiplicitivity involves δ and α_2 receptors. *J Pharmacol Exp Ther* 1992;262:365–374.
232. Rusin KI, Jiang MC, Cerne R, Randic M. Interactions between excitatory amino acids and tachykinins in the rat spinal dorsal horn. *Res Bull* 1993;30:329–338.
233. Rusin KI, Randic M. Modulation of NMDA induced currents by μ opioid receptor agonist DAMGO in acutely isolated rat spinal dorsal horn neurons. *Neurosci Lett* 1991;124:208–212.
234. Russell NJW, Schaible H-G, Schmidt RF. Opiates inhibit the discharges of fine afferent units from inflamed knee joint of the cat. *Neurosci Lett* 1987;76:107–111.
235. Salter MW, Henry JL. Responses of functionally identified neurones in the dorsal horn of the cat spinal cord to substance P, neurokinin A and physalaemin. *Neuroscience* 1991;4:601–610.
236. Salter MW, Hicks JL. ATP-evoked increases in intracellular calcium in neurons and glia from the dorsal spinal cord. *J Neurosci* 1994;14:1563–1575.
237. Santicioli P, Del Bianco E, Tramontana M, Geppetti P, Maggi CA. Release of calcitonin gene-related peptide like-immunoreactivity induced by electrical field stimulation from rat spinal afferents is mediated by conotoxin-sensitive calcium channels. *Neurosci Lett* 1992;136:161–164.
238. Sato J, Perl ER. Adrenergic excitation of cutaneous pain receptors induced by peripheral nerve injury. *Science* 1991;251:1608–1610.
239. Sawynok J, Sweeney MI. The role of purines in nociception. *Neuroscience* 1989;32:557–569.
240. Sawynok J, Sweeney MI, White TD. Classification of adenosine receptors mediating antinociception in the rat spinal cord. *Br J Pharmacol* 1986;88:923–930.
241. Schmauss C, Hammond DL, Ochi JW, Yaksh TL. Pharmacological antagonism of the antinociceptive effects of serotonin in the rat spinal cord. *Eur J Pharmacol* 1983;90:349–357.
242. Schultz G, Rosenthal W, Hescheler J, Trautwein W. Role of G proteins in calcium channel modulation. *Annu Rev Physiol* 1990;52:275–292.
243. Seybold VS, Hylden JLK, Wilcox GL. Intrathecal substance P and somatostatin in rats: behaviors indicative of sensation. *Peptides* 1982;3:49–54.
244. Sheardown MJ, Nielsen EO, Hansen AJ, Jacobsen P, Honore T. 2,3-Dihydroxy-6-nitro-7-sulfamoyl-benzo(F)quinoxaline: a neuroprotectant for cerebral ischemia. *Science* 1990;247:571–574.
245. Shehab SAS, Atkinson ME, Payne JN. The origins of the sciatic nerve and changes in neuropeptides after axotomy: a double labelling study using retrograde transport of true blue and vasoactive intestinal polypeptide immunohistochemistry. *Brain Res* 1986;376:180–185.
246. Shen K-Z, North RA, Surprenant A. Potassium channels opened by noradrenaline and other transmitters in excised membrane patches of guinea-pig submucosal neurones. *J Physiol* 1992;445:581–599.
247. Shen KF, Crain SM. Dual opioid modulation of the action potential duration of mouse dorsal root ganglion neurons in culture. *Brain Res* 1989;491:227–242.
248. Sherman SE, Loomis CW. Morphine insensitive allodynia is produced by intrathecal strychnine in the lightly anesthetized rat. *Pain* 1994;56:17–29.
249. Sivilotti L, Woolf CJ. The contribution of $GABA_A$ and glycine receptors to central sensitization: disinhibition and touch-evoked allodynia in the spinal cord. *J Neurophysiol* 1994;72(1):169–179.
250. Skilling SR, Smullin DH, Beitz AJ, Larson AA. Extracellular amino acid concentration in dorsal spinal cord of freely moving rats following veratridine and nociceptive stimulation. *J Neurochem* 1988;51:127–132.
251. Song YM, Huang LY. Protein kinase C reduces Mg2+ block of NMDA-receptor channels as a mechanism of modulation. *Nature* 1990;348:242–245.
252. Sorkin LS. NMDA evokes an L-NAME sensitive spinal release of glutamate and citrulline. *Neuroreport* 1993;4(5):479–82.
253. Sorkin LS, McAdoo DJ. Amino acids and serotonin are released into the lumbar spinal cord of the anesthetized cat following intradermal capsaicin injections. *Brain Res* 1993;607:89–98.
254. Sorkin LS, Westlund KN, Sluka KA, Dougherty PM, Willis WD. Neural changes in acute arthritis in monkeys. IV. Time-course of amino acid release into the lumbar dorsal horn. *Brain Res* 1992;17:39–50.
255. Stein C. Peripheral mechanisms of opioid analgesia. *Anesth Analg* 1993;76:182–191.
256. Stein C, Millan MJ, Shippenberg TS, Peter K, Herz A. Peripheral opioid receptors mediating antinociception in inflammation. Evidence for involvement of mu, delta and kappa receptors. *J Pharmacol Exp Ther* 1989;248:1269–1275.
257. Stucky CL, Galeazza MT, Seybold VS. Time-dependent changes in Bolton-Hunter-labeled ^{125}I-substance P binding in rat spinal cord following unilateral adjuvant-induced peripheral inflammation. *Neuroscience* 1993;57:397–409.
258. Sugiyama H, Ito I, Hirono C. A new type of glutamate receptor linked to inositol phospholipid metabolism. *Nature* 1987;325:531–533.
259. Surprenant A, Shen KZ, North RA, Tatsumi H. Inhibition of calcium currents by noradrenaline, somatostatin and opioids in guinea-pig submucosal neurones. *J Physiol (Lond)* 1990;431:585–608.
260. Sweeney MI, White TD, Jhamanday KH, Sawynok J. Morphine releases endogenous adenosine from the spinal cord in vivo. *Eur J Pharmacol* 1987;141:169–170.
261. Szallasi A. The vanilloid (capsaicin) receptor: receptor types and species differences. *Gen Pharmacol* 1994;25:223–243.
262. Szallasi A, Blumberg PM. Mechanisms and therapeutic potential of vanilloids (capsaicin-like molecules). *Adv Pharmacol* 1993;24:123–155.
263. Szolcsanyi J, Anton F, Reeh PW, Handwerker HO. Selective excitation by capsaicin of mechano-heat sensitive nociceptors in rat skin. *Brain Res* 1988;446:262–268.
264. Takano M, Takano Y, and Yaksh TL. Release of calcitonin gene-related peptide (CGRP), substance P (SP), and vasoactive intestinal polypeptide (VIP) from rat spinal cord: modulation by α_2 agonists. *Peptides* 1993;14:371–378.
265. Tanelian DL, MacIver MB. Analgesic concentrations of lidocaine suppress tonic A-delta and C fiber discharges produced by acute injury. *Anesthesiology* 1991;74(5):934–936.
266. Thompson SW, Dray A, Urban L. Injury-induced plasticity of spinal reflex activity: NK1 neurokinin receptor activation and enhanced A- and C-fiber mediated responses in the rat spinal cord in vitro. *J Neurosci* 1994;14:3672–3687.
267. Thompson SWN, King AE, Woolf CJ. Activity dependent changes in rat ventral horn neurons in vitro: summation of prolonged afferent evoked postsynaptic depolarizations produce a D-APV sensitive windup. *Eur J Neurosci* 1990;2:638–649.

268. Thompson SW, Woolf CJ, Sivilotti LG. Small-caliber afferent inputs produce a heterosynaptic facilitation of the synaptic responses evoked by primary afferent A-fibers in the neonatal rat spinal cord in vitro. *J Neurophysiol* 1993;69:2116–2128.
269. Tiseo PJ, Adler MW, Liu-Chen L-Y. Differential release of substance P and somatostatin in the rat spinal cord in response to noxious cold and heat; effect of dynorphin A(1–17). *J Pharmacol Exp Ther* 1990;252:539–545.
270. Tolle TR, Berthele A, Zieglgansberger W, Seeburg PH, Wisden. The differential expression of 16 NMDA and non-NMDA receptor subunits in the rat spinal cord and in periaqueductal gray. *J Neurosci* 1993;13:5009–5028.
271. Tracey DJ, De Biasi S, Phend K, Rustioni A. Aspartate-like immunoreactivity in primary afferent neurons. *Neuroscience* 1991;40:673–686.
272. Tuchscherer MM, Seybold VS. A quantitative study of the coexistence of peptides in varicosities within the superficial laminae of the dorsal horn of the rat spinal cord. *J Neurosci* 1989;9:195–205.
273. Turner TJ, Adams ME, Dunlap K. Calcium channels coupled to glutamate release identified by w-Aga-IVA. *Science* 1992;258:310–313.
274. Uhlen S, Wikberg JES. α_2-Adrenoceptors mediate inhibition of cyclic AMP production in the spinal cord after stimulation of cyclic AMP with forskolin but not after stimulation with capsaicin or vasoactive intestinal peptide. *J Neurochem* 1989;52:761–767.
275. Urban L, Randic M. Slow excitatory transmission in rat dorsal horn: possible mediation by peptides. *Brain Res* 1984;290:336–41.
276. Urban L, Thompson S, Dray A. Modulation of spinal excitability: co-operation between neurokinin and excitatory amino acid neurotransmitters. *TINS* 1994;17:432–438.
277. Valtschanoff JG, Weinberg RJ, Rustioni A. NADPH diaphorase in the spinal cord of rats. *J Comp Neurol* 1992;321:209–222.
278. Valtschanoff JG, Weinberg RL, Rustioni A, Schmidt HHHW. Nitric-oxide synthase and GABA colocalize in lamina-II of rat spinal-cord. *Neurosci Lett* 1992;148:6–10.
279. Vasko MR, Campbell WB, Waite KJ. Prostaglandin E2 enhances bradykinin-stimulated release of neuropeptides from rat sensory neurons in culture. *J Neurosci* 1994;14:4987–4997.
280. Verge VMK, Richardson PM, Benoit R, Riopelle RJ. Histochemical characterization of sensory neurons with high-affinity receptors for nerve growth factor. *J Neurocytol* 1989;18:583–591.
281. Verge VMK, Wiesenfeld-Hallin Z, Hökfelt T. Cholecystokinin in mammalian primary sensory neurons and spinal cord: In situ hybridization studies in rat and monkey. *Eur J Neurosci* 1993;5: 240–250.
282. Vidnyanszky Z, Hamori J, Negyessy L, Ruegg D, Knopfel T, Kuhn R, Gorcs TJ. Cellular and subcellular localization of the mGluR5A metabotropic glutamate receptor in rat spinal cord. *Neuroreport* 1994;6:209–13.
283. Villar MJ, Cortes R, Theodorsson E, Wiesenfeld-Hallin Z, Schalling M, Fahrenkrug J, Emson PC, Hokfelt T. Neuropeptide expression in rat dorsal root ganglion cells and spinal cord after peripheral nerve injury with special reference to galanin. *Neuroscience* 1989;33: 587–604.
284. Wakisaka S, Kajander KC, Bennett GJ. Effects of peripheral nerve injuries and tissue inflammation on the levels of neuropeptide Y-like immunoreactivity in rat primary afferent neurons. *Brain Res* 1992;598:349–352.
285. Walker MW, Ewald DA, Perney TM, Miller RJ. Neuropeptide Y modulates neurotransmitter release and Ca^{2+} currents in rat sensory neurons. *J Neurosci* 1988;8:2438–2446.
286. Wang JK. Antinociceptive effect of intrathecally administered serotonin. *Anesthesiology* 1977;47:269–271.
287. Werz MA, Grega DS, MacDonald RL. Actions of mu, delta and kappa opioid agonists and antagonists on mouse primary afferent neurons in culture. *J Pharmacol Exp Ther* 1987;243:258–63.
288. Werz MA, Macdonald RL. Dynorphin and neoendorphin peptides decrease dorsal root ganglion neuron calcium-dependent action potential duration. *J Pharmacol Exp Ther* 1985;234:49–56.
289. Wiesenfeld-Hallin Z, Villar MJ, Hökfelt T. Intrathecal galanin at low doses increases spinal reflex excitability in rats more to thermal than mechanical stimuli. *Exp Brain Res* 1988;71:663–666.
290. Wilcox GL. Excitatory neurotransmitters and pain. In: Bond M, Woolf CJ, Charlton JE, eds. *Pain research and clinical management: Proceedings of the Sixth World Congress on Pain.* Amsterdam: Elsevier Science (Biomedical Division), 1991;97–117.
291. Wilcox GL, Alhaider AA. Nociceptive and antinociceptive action of serotonin agonists administered intrathecally. In: Besson J-M, ed. *Serotonin and pain.* Amsterdam: Elsevier Science, 1990; 205–219.
292. Wilcox GL, Carlsson K.-H, Jochim A, Jurna I. Mutual potentiation of antinociceptive effects of morphine and clonidine in rat spinal cord. *Brain Res* 1987;405:84–93.
293. Womack MD, Macdermott AB, Jessell TM. Sensory transmitters regulate intracellular calcium in dorsal horn neurons. *Nature* 1988;334:351–353.
294. Woolf CJ, Thompson SWN. The induction and maintenance of central sensitization is dependent on N-methyl-D-aspartic acid receptor activation; implications for the treatment of post-injury pain hypersensitivity states. *Pain* 1991;44:293–299.
295. Xu XJ, Hao JX, Aldskogius H, Seiger A, Wiesenfeld HZ. Chronic pain-related syndrome in rats after ischemic spinal cord lesion: a possible animal model for pain in patients with spinal cord injury. *Pain* 1992;48:279–290.
296. Yaksh TL. Substance P release from knee joint afferent terminals: modulation by opioids. *Brain Res* 1988;458:319–324.
297. Yaksh TL. Behavioral and autonomic correlates of the tactile evoked allodynia produced by spinal glycine inhibition: effects of modulatory receptor systems and excitatory amino acid antagonist. *Pain* 1989;37:111–123.
298. Yaksh TL, Abay E II, Go VL. Studies on the location and release of cholecystokinin and vasoactive intestinal peptide in rat and cat spinal cord. *Brain Res* 1982;242:279–290.
299. Yaksh TL, Chaplan SR, Malmberg AB. Future directions in the pharmacological management of hyperalgesic and allodynic pain states: the NMDA receptor. In: Chiang CN, Finnegan LP, eds. *Medications development for the treatment of pregnant addicts and their infants.* NIDA Research Monograph Series #149. Rockville, MD: US Dept. of Health and Human Services, 1995.
300. Yaksh TL, Jessell TM, Gamse R, Mudge AW, Leeman SE. Intrathecal morphine inhibits substance P release from mammalian spinal cord in vivo. *Nature* 1980;286:155–157.
301. Yaksh TL, Michener SR, Bailey JE, Harty GJ, Lucas DL, Nelson DK, Roddy DR, Go VL. Survey of distribution of substance P, vasoactive intestinal polypeptide, cholecystokinin, neurotensin, Met-enkephalin, bombesin and PHI in the spinal cord of cat, dog, sloth and monkey. *Peptides* 1988;9:357–372.
302. Yaksh TL, Rudy TA. Chronic catheterization of the spinal subarachnoid space. *Physiol Behav* 1976;17:1031–1036.
303. Yaksh TL, Wilson PR. Spinal serotonin terminal system mediates antinociception. *J Pharmacol Exp Ther* 1979;208:446–453.
304. Yaksh TL, Yamamoto T, and Myers RR. Pharmacology of nerve compression-evoked hyperesthesia. In: Willis WD Jr, ed. *Hyperalgesia and allodynia.* New York: Raven Press, 1992;245–258.
305. Yamamoto T, and Yaksh TL. Stereospecific effects of a nonpeptidic NK1 selective antagonist, CP-96,345: antinociception in the absence of motor dysfunction. *Life Sci* 1991;49:1955–1963.
306. Yamamoto T, Yaksh TL. Spinal pharmacology of thermal hyperesthesia induced by incomplete ligation of sciatic nerve. I. Opioid and nonopioid receptors. *Anesthesiology* 1991;75:817–826.
307. Yamamoto T, Yaksh TL. Effects of intrathecal capsaicin and an NK-1 antagonist, CP,96–345, on the thermal hyperalgesia observed following unilateral constriction of the sciatic-nerve in the rat. *Pain* 1992;51:329–334.
308. Yashpal K, Radhakrishnan V, Coderre TJ, Henry JL. CP-96,345, but not its stereoisomer, CP-96,344, blocks the nociceptive responses to intrathecally administered substance-P and to noxious thermal and chemical stimuli in the rat. *Neuroscience* 1993;52: 1039–1047.
309. Yashpal K, Wright DM, Henry JL. Substance P reduces tail flick latency: implication for chronic pain syndromes. *Pain* 1982;15: 155–167.
310. Yezierski RP, Liu S, Ruenes GL, Busto R, Dietrich D. Neuronal damage following the intraspinal injection of a nitric oxide synthase inhibitor in the rat. *J Cereb Blood Flow Metab* 1996;16: 996–1004.
311. Yezierski RP, Wilcox TK, Willis WD. The effects of serotonin antagonists on the inhibition of primate spinothalamic tract cells produced by stimulation in nucleus raphe magnus or periaqueductal gray. *J Pharmacol Exp Ther* 1982;220:266–277.

Anesthesia: Biologic Foundations, edited by
Tony L. Yaksh et al. Lippincott–Raven Publishers,
Philadelphia © 1997.

CHAPTER 35

SPINAL ANATOMY AND PHARMACOLOGY OF AFFERENT PROCESSING

LINDA S. SORKIN AND SUSAN M. CARLTON

The first-order link of the pathway through which information generated by a physical stimulus is projected to higher centers occurs at the spinal cord level. From the earliest days of Ramón y Cajal, large volumes of work have focused on the anatomical complexity of this linkage. By the turn of the century, anatomical diagrams were available that clearly displayed the connectivity of the afferent in the ipsilateral dorsal horn and the subsequent crossed projection to the brainstem and thalamus (e.g., 164). This consideration of the spinal cord resembles remarkably those diagrams published in medical school texts today, over 90 years later. The primary organizational principles of spinal function were thus defined in terms of the segmental somatotypy (based on the anatomical distribution of the sensory roots), the distribution of low-threshold input into the dorsal columns, and the crossed pathways for pain and temperature that traveled in the ventrolateral quadrant and the long tracts to the brainstem. Implicit in this organization was the stereotyped processing of the input. The Sherringtonian reflex with its invariant linkages was clearly a model for such an organization (479). In the past 20 years, there has been an evolving appreciation that the linkages can display a surprising level of modifiability in the input-output relationship and that these changes in the input-output function have predictable effects on pain behavior.

GENERAL ORGANIZING PRINCIPLES OF SPINAL AFFERENT PROCESSING[1]

As reviewed in Chap. 41, it is readily appreciated that the stimulus environment gives rise to a pattern of afferent traffic in afferent axons characterized by specific transduction characteristics. The primary function of the spinal cord is thus to encode the spatial and temporal characteristics of the excitation evoked in the dendritic fields of these labeled lines. The basis of this encoding reflects multiple organizing characteristics associated with the respective systems. The following discussion reflects a general overview of several properties that characterize the encoding process.

Spontaneous Versus Evoked Activity

Recording from the peripheral sensory axon reveals that large populations of axons have little or no spontaneous activity under normal conditions. In contrast, application of an "adequate" stimulus will lead to a significant increase in axonal discharge, with the frequency of discharge or bursts. Thus, afferent input has a high signal-to-noise ratio under normal circumstances. In addition, as reviewed previously (Chap. 31), the discharge frequency of many afferents are monotonically related to stimulus intensity over some range of intensities.

Modality Specificity of Afferent Input

The appreciation that different stimuli might be passed through specific pathways was hypothesized in the formalization of the concept of "specific nerve energies" by Mueller in 1842 (278a). This concept is an important component of the thinking regarding the manner in which the sensory environment can be encoded into the binomial information flow entering the dorsal horn. The subsequent appreciation that small afferents were responsible for the sensory experience of nociception became widely accepted in the early part of the 20th century. Single-unit recording revealed an explosion of functionally defined categories, e.g., temperature sensitive, high-threshold thermal, mechanosensitive, polymodal, and so on (see Chap. 4). The important concept is that an afferent axon possesses certain properties of transduction, and the context of that message possesses significance for the encoding process. It is now clear that the transduction properties can be altered transiently and permanently. Transient changes in the chemical milieu can alter transduction properties. Thus, certain afferents exist that are activated if at all only by exceedingly high-threshold input, but become spontaneously active and show an evoked activity profile associated with moderate intensity stimuli following injury (215). Permanent changes occur when alterations are made in the peripheral terminal environment (e.g., suturing a nerve to a novel target) (317) or following the delivery of growth factors (439).

Anatomical Connectivity

The fixed connectivity of the system is manifested in several properties. First, there is a prominent segmental organization, e.g., sensory afferents arising from the lateral aspect of the foot projects to the medial portion of the dorsal horn of the L5/6 spinal segment of the rat, which provides a local sign as to the somatotopic origin of the input. As reviewed in Chap. 37, the nervous system retains a significant, but not absolute, adherence to somatotopic organization along the projection axis. Second, as will be reviewed below, within any given level of segmental organization, there is a prominent segregation of small unmyelinated afferents and large myelinated afferents termination. Thus, the small afferents terminate in the dorsal most region of the dorsal horn (laminae I and II), while the large afferents terminate more deeply in the nucleus proprius (see below). Third, there is a tendency for some separation by somatomotor versus visceromotor afferents.

It will be stressed that the nature of the connectivity can be altered by physical injury and perhaps neural activity. Thus, peripheral nerve injury may lead to a loss of dorsal horn neurons (274) and to extensive sprouting of the primary afferent (578). Because the nervous system evidently depends on the anatomical sign, such sprouting and cell loss must influence the nature of the encoding process. With regard to neural activity, it has been shown that afferent inputs leading to the release of substance P (SP) will cause a change in dendritic morphology (340). Such alterations may be transient, but reflect upon changes that could be more enduring.

Second-Order Excitation

Electrophysiology has emphasized that the principal effect at the primary afferent synapse is excitation. There has been no

[1]This section was contributed by Tony L. Yaksh, Ph.D.

report of a monosynaptic inhibition from the primary afferent (240); see also reviews of dorsal horn function (318). Inhibition in the dorsal horn is driven by primary afferents, but at the minimum is believed to be disynaptic in nature.

Multiple Transmitters in a Terminal

Dorsal horn primary afferents (and other terminal systems in the dorsal horn) may contain and release multiple transmitters (see below; also see Chap. 34). A commonly cited example is the co-release of an excitatory amino acid (such as glutamate) and a peptide (such as substance P) (132,228). The characteristics of their postsynaptic action is to evoke a rapid short-lasting depolarization and a delayed, long-lasting depolariztion, respectively (186,287,529,592). As the release of the two products may be subject to the frequency of terminal depolarization or to the polarization state of the terminal (as influenced by axoaxonic synapses) the nature of the postsynaptic excitation induced by a given afferent input can be substantially altered and this release may be differentially regulated by the frequency of the terminal depolarization .

Point Versus Field Effects of a Released Transmitter

The classic vision of a transmitter within the CNS is its affiliation with a local action within the synapse from which it is released. It has been appreciated by those who collect spinal superfusates that substantial quantities of material may appear at some distance in the extravascular-extracellular space from which it is released (200). Using antibody-coated microelectrode probes, it has been shown that peptides may diffuse a considerable distance from the presumed point of afferent termination (153). Using the downregulation of the receptor as a method of determining the presence of a transmitter, SP has been shown to diffuse from a point of release in the substantial gelatinosa (where C fibers terminate) to a considerable distance within the dorsal horn (340). This emphasizes that transmitter changes in excitability can be induced by a local release. It would be presumed that as the kinetics of such diffusion must be at least first order, the longer or more intense the stimulus, the further the released material will influence distant receptor sites. Conditioning stimuli can thus influence the excitability of relatively large volumes of spinal cord.

Complex System Interactions

An important component of the entire encoding process is the presence of well-defined connectivity and transmitter interactions that can serve to predictably alter the excitability of the afferent processing system. Intrinsic and bulbospinal connections can have several functional aspects: (a) depress C-fiber input, (b) enhance C-fiber–evoked output, (c) depress A-fiber-evoked output, and (d) increase or decrease the size of the receptive field for a given dorsal horn neuron. This "plasticity" will be considered further below, and will be discussed in greater detail in Chap. 9. The high level of spinospinal and bulbospinal connectivity and transmitter multiplicity provides the substrates by which the encoding process may be dynamically modified to alter the input-output relationships of the spinal projection systems that feed into the supraspinal systems. The complexity of these local spinal systems mirrors the high level of organization required to produce the encoding of the barrage of input generated by the peripheral milieu. Such organization thus provides the systems whereby complex psychophysical responses are mediated.

In the following sections, the anatomical organization of dorsal horn systems and components of their ascending projections are considered. The organization follows anatomically the linkages that are initially defined by the primary afferent input. As will be seen, the anatomical distribution of these pathways and their projections provides a useful framework on which the complexity of spinal sensory organization can be hung. The net result of the spinal encoding of afferent input is communicated by the several long spinofugal tracts. The supraspinal linkages of these ascending pathways are considered in Chap. 37. For additional details on the pharmacology of sensory afferents, see Chaps. 33 and 34, and on the organization of bulbospinal pathways, see Chap. 38. For additional comments on the organization of visceral input, see Chap. 37.

DORSAL ROOT ENTRY ZONE

Organization of the Peripheral Root

The collective central processes of dorsal root ganglion cells, the dorsal roots, approach the spinal cord and divide into a series of rootlets. There are considerably more axons in each dorsal root than there are dorsal root ganglia cells (106,313); this supports the contention that a significant percentage of the primary afferents branch proximal to the ganglia. In the peripheral portion of the rootlets and up to within a few millimeters from their entry into the spinal cord, the distribution of the unmyelinated and myelinated fibers appears to be totally random (280,491) (Fig. 1). Closer to the entry zone, small-caliber myelinated and unmyelinated fibers bunch at the periphery of the rootlet and actually outline the individual fascicles. In the primate, but not the cat, both the small myelinated and unmyelinated axons then shift to the ventrolateral and ventral

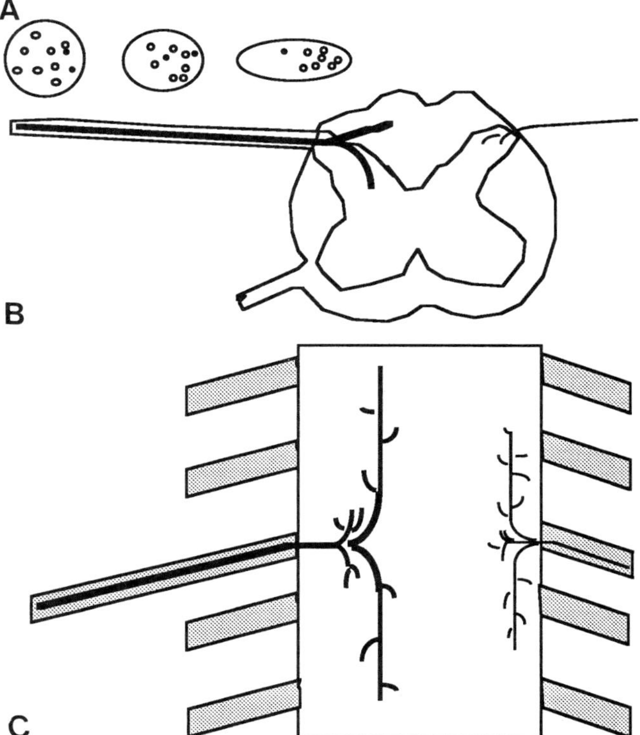

Figure 1. ***A:*** Schematic displaying the cross section of the distribution of the myelinated fibers (*open circles*) and unmyelinated profiles (*small dark circles*) as the root approaches the dorsal root entry zone. ***B:*** Schematic displaying the ramification of C fibers (*right*) into the coronal plane of the dorsal horn and collateralization into the tract of Lissauer and of Aβ fibers (*left*) into the dorsal columns and into the dorsal horn. ***C:*** Schematic showing the rostrocaudal distribution of the large (*left*) and small (*right*) fibers in the dorsal columns and the tract of Lissauer, respectively.

borders of the rootlet; the large myelinated fibers are excluded from these zones.

Distribution of Fibers by Size in the Dorsal Horn

There are several general organizing principles that describe the termination of the primary afferents after they penetrate the spinal cord:

1. Upon entry into the spinal cord, primary afferents may (a) send a primary projection into the dorsal horn of the segment of entry, and (b) form collaterals that project out of the segment rostrally and/or caudally for distances as short as one to three segments or as far in some cases as the dorsal column nuclei. In each case, these several collaterals may themselves send projections that terminate in specific laminae of the underlying gray matter.
2. The tracts followed by these afferent collaterals will typically be in the dorsal columns (large myelinated afferents) running medially, or in the Lissauer tract (small myelinated or unmyelinated afferents) that travels laterally to the dorsal columns
3. The distribution of the afferent terminals in the underlying spinal parenchyma dorsal horn may be defined in terms of the size of afferent (e.g., myelinated versus unmyelinated) and in terms of the type of afferent (e.g., visceral versus somatic). These points are schematically summarized in Fig. 1. Details reflecting these several general principles are discussed below.

Rostrocaudal Distribution of Afferent and Afferent Collaterals

Small unmyelinated afferents distribute laterally in the entry zone. The axons in this ventrolateral division merge with and become indistinguishable from Lissauer's tract, a white matter wedge located at the dorsolateral border of the spinal gray matter. In the primate, about 80% of the axons in Lissauer's tract are primary afferent fibers; the remainder are part of a propriospinal system originating from the substantia gelatinosa. In contrast to the popular notion that the dorsal columns is composed principally of large myelinated collaterals, C-primary afferent fibers (or their collaterals) can also ascend long distances through the dorsal columns (413,518,519), from the lumbar enlargement to the upper cervical spinal cord and/or the dorsal column nuclei. Unmyelinated axons (C fibers) have been estimated to compose about 20% of the total fiber population in the fasciculus gracilis in the subhuman primate (183), and calcitonin gene-related peptide immunoreactivity, considered a marker for small-diameter primary afferent fibers, has been demonstrated in the dorsal column nuclei (110). A second population of small myelinated fibers, presumably Aδ, also travels in Lissauer's tract and terminates in the dorsal horn (91,305). Degeneration and orthograde transport studies following highly selective lesions of Lissauer's tract or the medial or lateral divisions of the dorsal rootlets confirm the segregation of the dorsal rootlets according to fiber diameter (305,321). Segregation of the small fibers associated with signaling pain and temperature within the dorsal root is of more than anatomical interest; it has been the basis for performing selective dorsal rhizotomies and Lissauer's tractotomies to treat intractable pain (388,483). These surgeries are reported to be successful for some types of pain, in particular, pain arising from brachial plexus avulsions.

Large myelinated fibers predominate medially in the fascicles in the entry zone and directly approach the dorsal columns. At their entry point, they bifurcate into ascending and descending branches and send off collaterals to terminate in the underlying nucleus proprius and ventral horn.

Local Somatotopic Mapping of Afferent Input onto the Dorsal Horn

Different subclasses of primary afferents have anatomically distinct terminations within the spinal cord. In general, the afferent projection from specific regions of the body surface will display specific somatotopic affiliations organized rostrocaudally by segments. These have been most readily defined by defining the location of the input that excited specific spinal segments after the adjacent three or four roots have been sectioned (e.g., the spared root model). Within any given segment, well-defined laterality (ipsilateral vs. contralateral) and three-dimensional organization (rostrocaudal, mediolateral, dorsoventral) of the afferent terminations are frequently noted. The precise organization of these terminations is determined by two factors: (a) receptive field location of the primary afferent fiber, and (b) by the modality of the peripheral receptor. Since function is determined not only by the characteristics of the receptor but also by the central connections made by the neuron, both of these patterns influence central processing of afferent input.

With regard to laterality, somatic afferents essentially have an exclusively ipsilateral projection. Visceral, but not somatic, afferent terminations frequently extend to the contralateral deep dorsal horn and the area around the central canal (499,500).

The rostrocaudal and mediolateral organization of the dorsal horn in the lumbar and cervical enlargements can be interpreted in terms of the embryologic development of the limb (73). As the limb bud elongates and rotates medially, the simple dermatomal pattern is altered. Primary afferent projections and cells in the medial dorsal horn have receptive fields located on the anterior surface of the limbs; those located in the lateral dorsal horn have receptive fields located on the posterior surface (67,68,292,492). This pattern has also been demonstrated for afferent projections within the thoracic spinal cord (208). However, while cells recorded from the lateral dorsal horn of the thoracic spinal cord in the cat have receptive fields on the dorsal body surface, cells with fields on the anterior body surface do not appear to be differentially distributed (95). Within a given vertical column through the dorsal horn, receptive field locations are similar. Before specifically describing the terminal distribution of each modality, the laminar organization of the spinal cord will be reviewed.

LAMINAR ORGANIZATION OF THE SPINAL CORD

The spinal cord was classically divided in the coronal plane into the white and gray matter. The dorsal gray matter was organized according to its general anatomical appearance into a marginal layer (the outer layer of the dorsal horn); the substantia gelatinosa (the clear fragment that lies just ventral to the marginal layer); the nucleus proprius (the gray matter that lies under the substantia gelatinosa and constitutes the remainder of the dorsal horn); the region around the central canal; and the ventral horn.

Rexed (433,434) in the early 1950s recognized that in the coronal plane the spinal cord could be organized at each level into a series of layers that were essentially homologous from the sacral to the cervical cord. Of fundamental importance was the organizing principle that the spinal gray matter was best described, not as a series of discrete nuclei, but as specific laminae that were essentially continuous. Accordingly, based on the local cytoarchitecture (cell types, density, and myelination), he divided the gray matter of the spinal cord into 10 largely horizontal laminae (433,434). Most of these laminae are present along the entire length of the spinal cord, although minor variations exist (Fig. 2). The anatomical correlates of these laminae

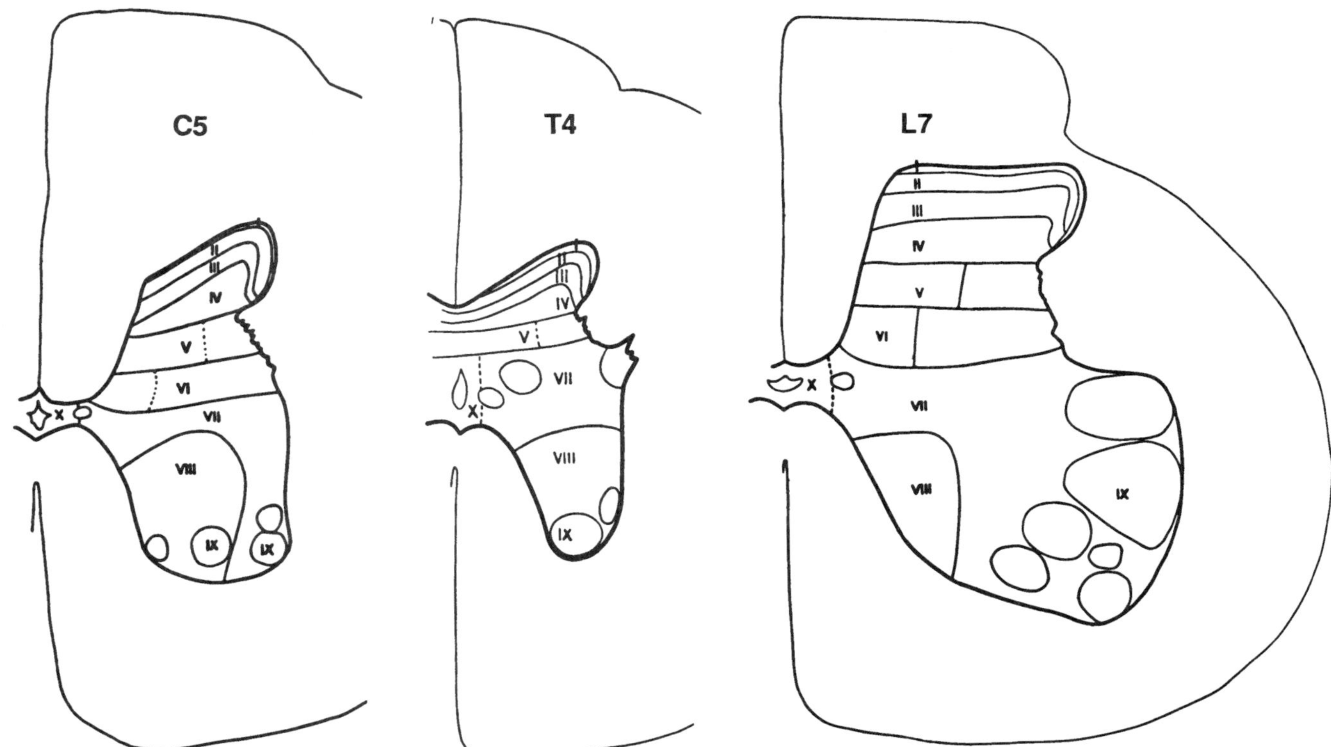

Figure 2. Diagrammatic representation of the 10 laminae of Rexed illustrated at three levels of the spinal cord within the lumbar (L7) and cervical (C5) enlargements and in the midthoracic cord (T4). Note the absence of lamina VI and the addition of the intermediate horn in the thoracic spinal cord. (From ref. 434.)

are summarized in Fig. 3. Laminae I to VI compose the dorsal horn, laminae VII to IX the ventral horn, and lamina X is the substantia grisea centralis or gray matter surrounding the central canal. Details of spinal organization by lamina are presented below.

Lamina I: Marginal Zone

The marginal layer is a thin band capping the gray matter. Laterally, it bends to form one border of the superficial dorsal horn (laminae I–III). It contains the large marginal cells of Waldeyer (108,427,544) in addition to several subdivisions of smaller neurons (38). The dendrites of the Waldeyer cells lie in the horizontal plane, are markedly elongated in the rostrocaudal direction, and thus resemble flattened oval disks (323,325,326,576). Since the original descriptions of these large cells, many classification systems have been devised for them, depending on axonal destination (387), the presence or absence of dendritic spines (202), organization of dendritic arborization (35,36,325,328), and cell soma shape and orientation (326,501). Although the majority of dendrites of marginal as well as other lamina I cells arborize in lamina I, some do reach down into deeper laminae (249,323,325,576). In humans, the dendrites of a population of lamina I cells extend ventrally into lamina II (465). Although several attempts have been made, convincing evidence of a correlation between dendritic morphology and cell function or response properties for lamina I cells has not been found (250, 323,429,496,576). However, new studies examining neurons within lamina I have concluded that there is a correlation between physiologic function and specific neuronal and dendritic morphology (213). A recent immunohistochemical study suggests that morphologic classification of lamina I cells may also indicate neurochemical content (324).

Retrograde axonal transport studies demonstrate that many marginal cells are projection neurons, contributing to the lateral spinocervical (57,121,376,522,571), spinoreticular (326, 327,361,501,587,590) and spinothalamic tracts (218,329,520, 595). Additionally, there are projections to the periaqueductal gray (218,326,330,339,563), the parabrachial nucleus (326, 412), and the nucleus submedius (116). In a study by Bennett

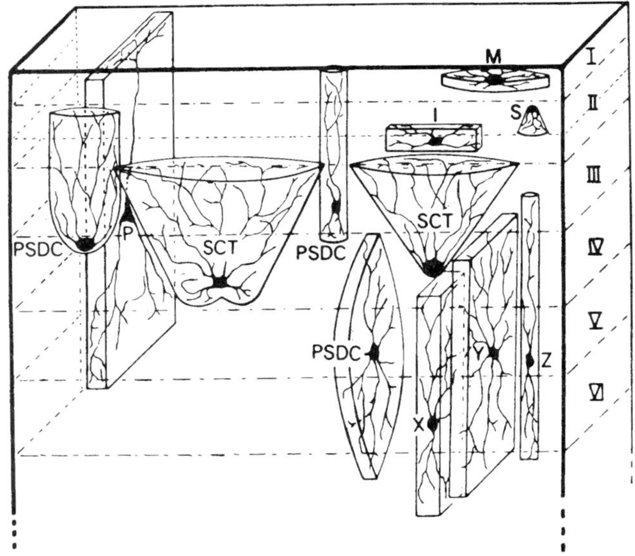

Figure 3. Diagrammatic representation of the cell body locations and dendritic tree organizations in the dorsal horn, as viewed in a parasagittal block of tissue. I, islet cell; M, marginal cell; P, pyramidal cell; PSDC, the three main types of neurons sending axons through the dorsal columns; S, stalked cell; SCT, spinocervical tract cell; X, Y, and Z, interneurons of laminae V and VI. (From ref. 65.)

et al. (38), some intracellularly injected lamina I neurons had axons with dense collaterals confined to lamina I.

Lamina II: Substantia Gelatinosa

Lamina II is deep to lamina I and medial to its lateral border. Frequently, it has been divided into two parts: II outer (IIo) and II inner (IIi). Collectively this region is called the substantia gelatinosa (SG), a term coined by Rolando to describe the clear gelatinous appearance resulting from the composition of the neuropil (97). This region contains a densely packed concentration of small neurons and has an absence of myelinated axons. The classical descriptions of cell types in the SG refer to limiting (limitrophe) cells and central cells (427). Following Gobel's (203,204) descriptive analysis of lamina II, stalked cells became the modern equivalent of limiting cells, and the appellation *islet cells* replaced the term *central cells*. Although the laminar boundaries and terminology used by Gobel have led to some confusion, the neurocircuitry revealed in his studies constitute a very important contribution to the field.

Stalk cells have short, stalklike spines and are located in IIo, particularly at the I–IIo border. Golgi studies indicate that the dendrites of these cells extend ventrally through laminae II to IV, forming a cone shape (Fig. 1) (65,203). However, following intracellular injection of stalk cells, Bennett et al. (38) described these cells as having a fanlike shape. The axons of stalk cells have their major ramification in lamina I (35,204), although projections into deeper laminae have also been observed (320,465). Islet cells are found mainly in IIi and their dendritic trees are oriented in the longitudinal direction within lamina II and flattened in the mediolateral plane (203,465). The axons of islet cells arborize mainly in lamina II (Fig. 1) (65,203). The suggestion has been made that islet cells are inhibitory cells (203) and indeed it has been demonstrated that cells with similar morphology contain the inhibitory neurotransmitter γ-aminobutyric acid (GABA) (512). One important characteristic of these cells is that their dendrites contain vesicles and form both dendroaxonic and dendrodendritic synapses (203). At this time, the neurocircuitry appears to be unique to this cell type in the dorsal horn since no other cell type, including stalk cells, has been identified as having vesicle containing dendrites as a major characteristic. Other cell types in lamina II that have not been as widely studied include arboreal cells, II–III border cells, and spiny cells (203,205). These cell types differ from islet cells in that axons arising from these cell populations distribute not only to lamina II, but also to laminae I and III (205). As an historical aside, it was once thought that the SG was a closed system. This concept was generated by Szentagothai (502), who suggested that the axons arising from SG neurons terminated exclusively within lamina II. Hence, information relayed by these neurons was thought to be not directly transmitted outside of the SG by axons, but exclusively by synaptic transmission onto dendrites that invaded this lamina. This theory is no longer tenable since intracellular injections of lamina II neurons demonstrated axonal arborizations in laminae IV to VI, with branches extending into both the ipsilateral dorsolateral funiculus and contralateral ventral funiculus (320). Furthermore, Willis et al. (572) demonstrated that some lamina II cells projected to the contralateral thalamus, although physiologically these might be considered displaced lamina I cells (89).

Lamina III

Lamina III forms a broad band across the dorsal horn and also has a ventrally pointed lateral border; the cell bodies are on average larger and less densely packed than in the substantia gelatinosa (433,434). At one time, lamina III was considered to be part of the substantia gelatinosa due to the fact that neurons in this lamina were similar to those in lamina II with respect to dendritic patterns, axonal projections (502), and physiologic characteristics (546). Although these facts remain true, in addition to the presence of myelinated axons in lamina III (426), it is now clear from histo- and cytochemical stains that major differences exist in the neurochemical content of these laminae. Now, lamina III, as well as laminae IV and V, is considered to be part of the nucleus proprius.

Cells in lamina III have been described as spindle shaped with relatively little cytoplasm (427,434). The dendritic patterns of lamina III cells are similar to those in lamina II, with a slightly greater extension (414,427,461,502). Upon reconstruction of Golgi-labeled neurons in lamina III, it was determined that the main orientation of the dendritic arbor was in the rostrocaudal plane, with a slightly flattened arbor in the mediolateral direction (35,337). Cells at the origin of two major ascending tracts involved in transmission of nociceptive information, the spinocervical tract (SCT) and the postsynaptic dorsal column (PSDC) pathway, have been localized to lamina III (39,65). Brown (65) documents that each cell type has a characteristic morphology; however, Bennett et al. (39) report that the dendritic patterns of both cell types are similar. The former study states that the dendritic arbors of SCT cells are oriented mainly in the longitudinal plane, and the dendrites do not reach up into lamina IIo and I (Fig. 1) (65). Dendrites of PSDC cells, on the other hand, are not flattened in the mediolateral direction and have some dendrites that travel into lamina I and II, and thus, unlike SCT cells, could receive monosynaptic input from fine-caliber primary afferent fibers (60,65). Other lamina III cells, which are neither SCT nor PSDC, have dendrites that extend dorsally into laminae I and II and ventrally into laminae IV and V (65). With such extensive dendritic arborizations, these lamina III cells could receive input from all types of primary afferent fibers. Most anatomical studies of lamina III consistently report two different cell types based on patterns of dendritic arborization (37,48,347,465).

Golgi studies indicate that some lamina III neurons have axons that collateralize locally in lamina III (37,48,342,347, 465). However, in addition to containing cell bodies of origin of PSDC and SCT projection pathways (39,58,62,65), lamina III also contains some cells that project into laminae IV, V, and VI (342). Other branches of lamina III axons terminate in laminae I and IV (337).

Laminae IV to VI

Laminae IV to VI make up the remainder of the dorsal horn. Lamina IV is a thick layer extending across the dorsal horn; the cells are heterogeneous with respect to size and less densely packed than those in lamina III due to increased numbers of nerve fibers passing through this space (434). Although they make up a small proportion of the total cell population in laminae IV and V, large cells with long spiny dendrites oriented in the dorsal, medial, lateral, and ventral planes have received particular attention (427,461,502). Due to the extensive dendritic arborizations in several planes, these cells are undoubtedly involved in the integration of a variety of synaptic inputs. Rethelyi and Szentagothai (430) and Proshansky and Egger (422) have distinguished at least three classes of neurons in lamina IV based on dendritic projection patterns (Fig. 1). Identified projection cells in lamina IV include SCT and PSDC cells (39,65). Another cell type described by Brown (65) has dendritic fields similar to SCT and PSDC cells, but its axons terminate locally rather than project out of the spinal cord. A fourth cell type has large dorsally directed dendrites with cranially directed axons. The axonal termination is unknown. Somas of spinothalamic tract (STT) cells are also found in lamina IV (2,17,18,85,119,196,571).

Lamina V traverses the narrowest part or neck of the dorsal horn. The cells are even more diverse than those in lamina IV; the general orientation of their dendrites is vertical, toward the more superficial laminae. In the lateral part, there is a preponderance of longitudinally oriented myelinated axons, giving this area a distinctive reticulated appearance, and the cells tend to be larger than in the medial zone. Scheibel and Scheibel (461), in discussing laminae V through IV, emphasize that there is a shift in the orientation of axons and dendrites in the lamina V neuropil. These investigators report that the dendrites of lamina V cells have little or no extension in the longitudinal plane of the cord, but instead radiate out in the dorsoventral and mediolateral planes. Proshansky and Egger (422) also note the radial arrangement of lamina V cells dendritic fields. Following serial reconstruction of several lamina V cells, Mannen (336) reported that the dendritic trees of these cells are not necessarily restricted, but spread out in all directions. Intracellular injection into lamina V neurons demonstrates that the dendritic trees are restricted in the longitudinal plane as originally reported by the Scheibels (65). That the dendritic fields increase in size from lamina IV to lamina V is agreed upon by most investigators (422). In an attempt to relate cell structure with function, Ritz and Greenspan (440) demonstrate a positive correlation between mediolateral dendritic spread and the responsivity of the cell to innocuous stimuli. As was true for lamina IV, cell bodies in lamina V contribute to three projection pathways—the SCT (Fig. 1) (39,65), PSDC, and STT pathways—with STT cells being the most plentiful (2,17,18,76,85,119,196,218,571). Matsushita (343) describes local axon collaterals emerging from some lamina V neurons and ramifying in laminae III, IV, and V.

Lamina VI makes up the base of the dorsal horn and is present only within the cervical and lumbar enlargements. Data relating specifically to lamina VI cells and their morphology are rare. For the most part, cells in this lamina are very similar to those in lamina V, having dendrites that extend in the dorsoventral and mediolateral planes with limited extension in the longitudinal plane (461). These cells are smaller and more regular in their appearance than those in lamina V. Brown (65) states that dendrites of lamina VI never reach into laminae I and II and thus would not sample primary afferent input to these regions (Fig. 3). Labeling experiments indicate that the axons of a few lamina VI cells contribute to the STT and SCT pathways; however, it is believed that the majority of cells in this lamina are propriospinal. Golgi studies indicate that cells in this lamina have not only recurrent axon collaterals that terminate in the vicinity of the parent cell body, but additional collaterals that project into laminae IV, V, and VII (342).

Laminae VII and VIII are not part of the dorsal horn, but they do contain cells that contribute to several of the fiber tracts thought to be involved in pain transmission, particularly the medial projection systems: medial STT, spinomesencephalic, and spinoreticular tracts. Lamina VII occupies an irregular space in the central portion of the spinal gray matter. In the lumbar and cervical enlargements, lamina VIII encompasses the medial half of the ventral horn with the exception of large islands of motor cells; throughout the remainder of the spinal cord it appears as a band across the middle of the ventral horn. Rexed (434) defines the lateral boundaries of lamina X as being indistinct, but placed somewhere in the region where the central gray matter begins to widen. Most of the cells are small; the majority are fusiform, pyramidal, or stellate shaped (384). Many possess a large number of short axon collaterals with a dense pattern of ramifications, often extending bilaterally (239). Cells with small to medium-sized soma and dendritic arbors that are restricted to the gray matter surrounding the central canal tend to have small receptive fields. Cells with larger perikarya and more wide-ranging dendritic spread are more likely to have large often discontinuous receptive fields (238). For the most part, cells in lamina X participate in propriospinal systems (376). A small number of projection cells in this region terminate in both the paramedian medullary and pontine reticular formations (339,384). There is also a projection to periaqueductal gray (384) and thalamus (33,571).

Primary Afferent Fibers: Organization and Terminal Distribution

Primary afferent fiber projections entering the dorsal horn are derived from receptors in the skin, subcutaneous tissues, muscle, joint capsules, and viscera. Numerous methods have been used to study the termination pattern of afferent fibers, and these are reviewed by Fitzgerald (174). The majority of the techniques used allow one to visualize groups or populations of primary afferent fibers. The finer details of individual afferent fiber patterns are revealed by studies using the Golgi technique (431) and more recently by studies employing intraaxonal injection of tracers such as horseradish peroxidase (HRP). The latter technique provides not only a detailed look at the intricacies of afferent distribution in the spinal cord, but also insight into the fiber type (group I, II, Aβ, Aδ, or C) and the adequate stimulus for its associated receptor.

The general termination pattern of large- and small-diameter fibers is revealed by the use of HRP conjugated to choleragenoid (the binding subunit of cholera toxin, CT-HRP) and wheat germ agglutinin (WGA-HRP), respectively (312,441). Each substance is preferentially transported by a particular fiber type and the result is the striking map shown in Fig. 4 in which CT-HRP was injected into the left sciatic nerve and WGA-HRP was injected into the right. The findings from these HRP studies leave little doubt that there is a high degree of segregation between large and small fibers in the dorsal horn. A more refined look at the distribution of particular classes of myelinated fibers is gained from intraaxonal injection into individual fibers. Reviews of this literature can be found in Brown (65,66), Fyffe (182), Rethelyi (432), and Fitzgerald (174).

Aβ Fiber Terminations

The classic literature describes large-diameter primary afferent fibers as entering the dorsal spinal cord through the medial division of the dorsal root and either descending through the medial part of lamina I or II, or curving around the medial edge of the dorsal horn to enter the horn ventrally (427). In either case, upon reaching the deeper laminae (laminae IV and V) these fibers turn and ascend into laminae III and IV, where they undergo repeated subdivisions and terminate in a characteristic "flame-shaped arbor" (461). There is significant overlap between arborizations of adjacent collaterals within the sagittal plane. These arbors, observed end on in a transverse section, actually

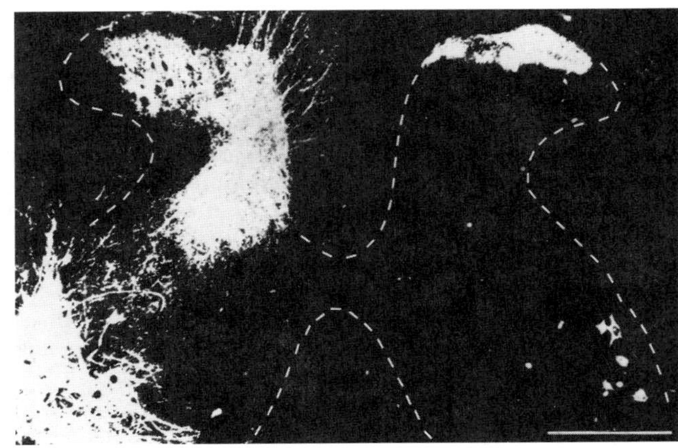

Figure 4. Polarized darkfield micrograph of the L5 spinal cord segment from a rat demonstrating the difference in fiber labeling following choleragenoid-HRP (CT-HRP) injection into the left sciatic nerve and WGA-HRP in the right sciatic nerve. CT-HRP–labeled axons and terminals are observed in laminae I, III–V, the intermediate gray, and in motoneurons in the ventral horn. In contrast, WGA-HRP–labeled axons and terminals are observed only in laminae I and II and in some motoneurons. *Bar* = 0.25mm. (From ref. 312.)

form longitudinally oriented sheets or columns of terminal fields in the dorsal horn (Fig. 3) (461), and this has been confirmed in HRP labeling studies of single afferent fibers (65,66). It is now known that this pattern of termination is characteristic of axons arising from hair follicle receptors (61,322,480,580). Axons from type I slowly adapting mechanoreceptors (Merkel disks) also enter the gray matter at the dorsal border of the dorsal horn and descend without branching to lamina IV or V; collaterals then turn and ascend in a C-shaped arc (as seen in the mediolateral plane) before turning once more and arborizing within the space circumscribed by the parent axon in laminae III to V. In contrast, axons from type II slowly adapting mechanoreceptors (field receptors) descend through the superficial dorsal horn and then form dense, transversely oriented plates of arborizations extending from lamina III through the dorsal portion of lamina VI. The plates are limited to 100 to 300 μm in the rostrocaudal plane. Several generalities concerning primary afferent fiber organization have been derived from studying single-afferent fibers. These include the fact that the pattern of termination for each type of cutaneous or muscle afferent is specific and unique (Fig. 5) (66); the distribution of the terminal arbor in the dorsal horn is somatotopically organized and related to the peripheral receptive field of the afferent unit (69,480); the more distal the receptive field, the smaller it is (67,526), and the terminal fields of the large-diameter afferents are restricted to the deeper laminae, with little or no incursion into laminae I and II (65,66,481,580). Recent data demonstrate, however, that following peripheral nerve transection, large myelinated axons sprout to terminate within the superficial laminae (578).

Aδ Fiber Terminations

Results of orthograde HRP transport studies and Golgi staining in the cat indicate that fine, myelinated axons are distributed to lamina I (201). However, a detailed analysis of the organization of terminal fields arising from small myelinated fibers was made possible by studies of Light and Perl (322); they injected HRP intraaxonally into functionally identified afferents innervating D-hair receptors or high-threshold mechanoreceptors in the cat. Not unexpectedly, each finely myelinated fiber type has a distinct and characteristic pattern of termination. Boutons arising from the D-hair afferents distribute mainly to lamina III, with a small contribution to the most ventral part of lamina II (IIi). The projection is exclusively ipsilateral. The high-threshold mechanoreceptors distribute to laminae I, IIo, and V. Branches are also seen crossing the midline, distributing to the contralateral lamina V, to the reticulated portion in particular. Nociceptive fibers from deep tissues (muscle and joint) with conduction velocities in the Aδ range have at least two patterns of termination: terminals distribute either exclusively to lamina I, or mainly to laminae IV and V, with a minor projection to lamina I (362). These patterns are similar to those previously described in investigations of fine fiber distribution using the Golgi technique (34,212).

C-Fiber Terminations

Studies using Golgi stains (201,431), degeneration techniques (205,305,425), and HRP transport (201) indicate that unmyelinated primary afferent fibers terminate in the superficial dorsal horn (reviewed in refs. 174 and 574). They have been described as forming a longitudinally oriented plexus over the marginal zone (280,502) or forming bushy arbors within the substantia gelatinosa (431). What is not agreed upon is whether the terminal arborizations of C fibers are relegated exclusively to lamina II, or whether they include both laminae I and II. Once again, intraaxonal injections of physiologically identified C fibers have been instrumental in elucidating dorsal horn anatomy. Analysis of the terminal patterns of C fibers identified as being connected to cold nociceptors, polymodal nociceptors, high-threshold mechanoreceptors, or low-threshold mechanoreceptors reveals that in a fashion similar to large myelinated fibers, the termination patterns are distinctive for each type of functionally defined C fiber. Lamina II appears to be the main termination zone for unmyelinated fibers from the skin, with some extensions into lamina I (499,500). Alvarez et al. (6) confirm these findings in the primate, demonstrating that the terminal arborizations of two intraaxonally injected C fibers are located in both laminae I and IIi. The only C-fiber unit with terminal arborizations deep to lamina II (i.e., in laminae III and IV) was a polymodal nociceptor described in the guinea pig (499). At this time it is safe to conclude that the *main* area of termination for cutaneous C fibers is lamina II, while that for Aδ fibers is lamina I.

Visceral Afferent Terminations

Transganglionic transport of HRP demonstrates that afferents arising from receptors in viscera distribute to laminae I, II, V to VII, and X of the sacral spinal cord (137,277,378,380,381). Visceral afferents entering the thoracic cord from the splanchnic nerve distribute mainly to laminae I and V with some terminals entering into lamina IIo (87,88,396). Following intracellular injection of *Phaseolus vulgaris* into guinea pig dorsal root ganglion cells, Sugiura et al. (500) observed terminations from individual C fibers in laminae I, II, IV, and X on the ipsilateral side and laminae V and X on the contralateral side (Fig. 6). In this study, it is noted that visceral C fibers never form the dense nests of concentrated terminations that have previously been noted for somatic C fibers. Furthermore, in contrast to somatic C fibers, which have a rostrocaudal extension of approximately 400 μm, visceral C fibers can extend rostocaudally up to five spinal segments (500). This latter finding certainly is contributory to the poor localization of visceral pain and its frequent referral to other body regions.

Muscle Afferent Terminations

Input from muscle is relayed from stretch receptors by group Ia, Ib, and II fibers, and from pressure-pain endings with either small myelinated (group III) or unmyelinated (group IV) afferent fibers (29). The group Ia afferents bifurcate upon entering the cord. Emerging collaterals descend vertically through the dorsal horn to lamina V or VI before subdividing. Upon ramification, terminal branches are observed in laminae VI, VII, and IX. Group Ib afferents follow a course similar to that described above; however, these fibers terminate mainly in medial lamina VI, with occasional branches in laminae V and VII. Hongo et al. (241) also demonstrated Ib fibers with terminations in lamina IX. Group II afferents arborize in laminae III and IV as well as in the lateral portion of laminae V to VII, and in lamina IX. A study that compares the central terminations of a pure muscle nerve (sternomastoid nerve) with a pure cutaneous nerve (cutaneous R. dorsalis) demonstrates that the former distributes mainly to laminae I and III with lesser terminations in IV and V (594).

Ventral Root Afferent Terminations

Anatomical (111,113,114,548) and electrophysiologic (114, 144,275,453) techniques confirm the existence of myelinated and unmyelinated sensory afferents in ventral roots. The available data suggest that the majority of these sensory afferents end blindly, never reaching the ventral horn (211,574). However, stimulation of ventral roots produces pain (180) and an increase in blood pressure (331), suggesting that these fibers may play some role in relaying noxious information.

HISTOCHEMISTRY OF DORSAL HORN NEURONAL SYSTEMS

With the advent of immunohistochemical techniques, there is virtually no limit to the number of substances that can be visualized in nervous tissue. The ever-changing field is in constant need of being updated. The following discussion on dorsal horn neurochemistry focuses on those substances that are

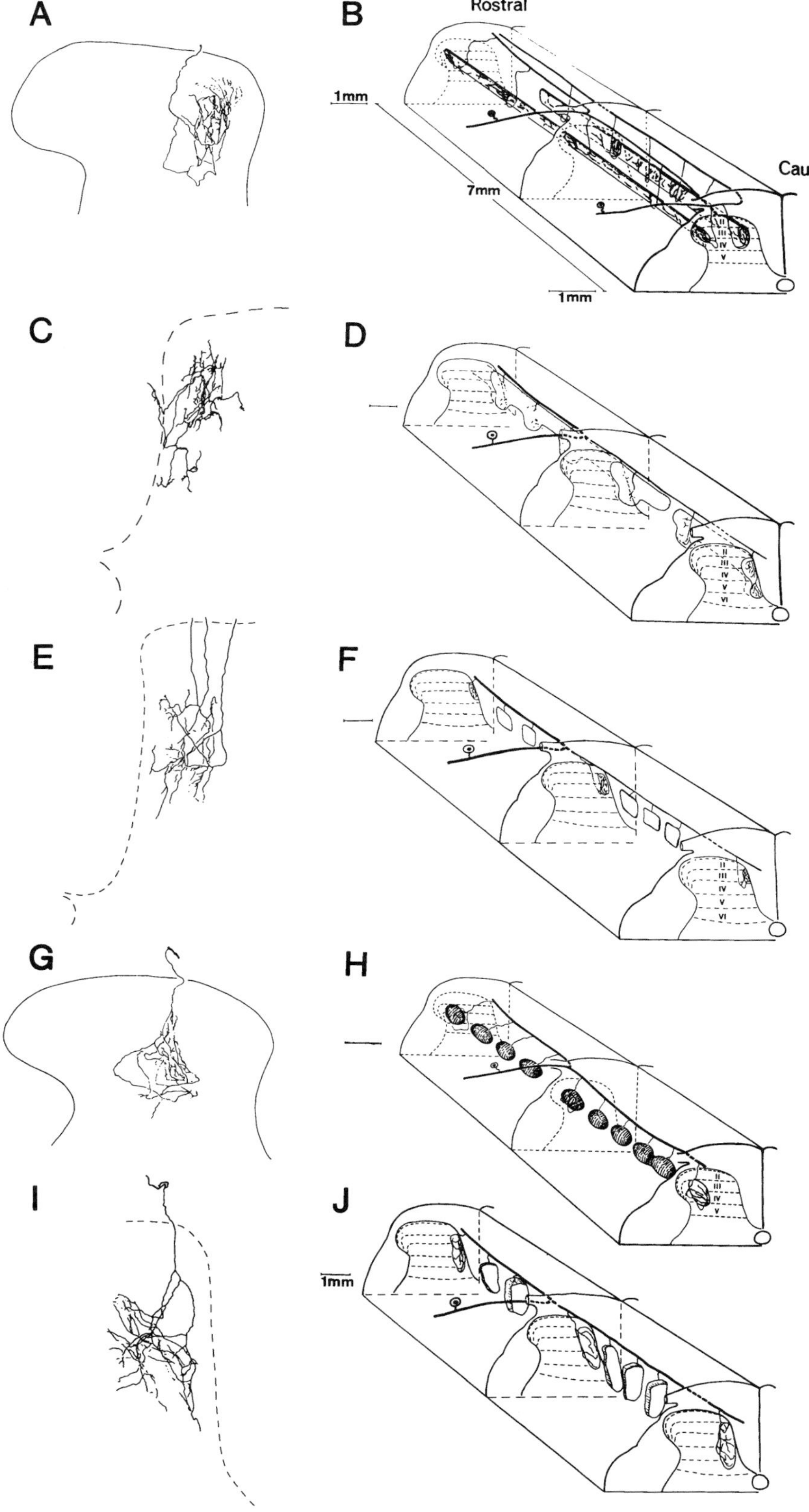

Figure 5. Demonstration of the pattern and extent of distribution of intraaxonal injected fibers in the cat dorsal horn: hair follicle afferent. (From ref. 65.) A, B: C, D: Pacinian corpuscle; E, F: Rapidly adapting mechanoreceptor; G, H: Type I mechanoreceptor; I, J: Type II mechanoreceptor.

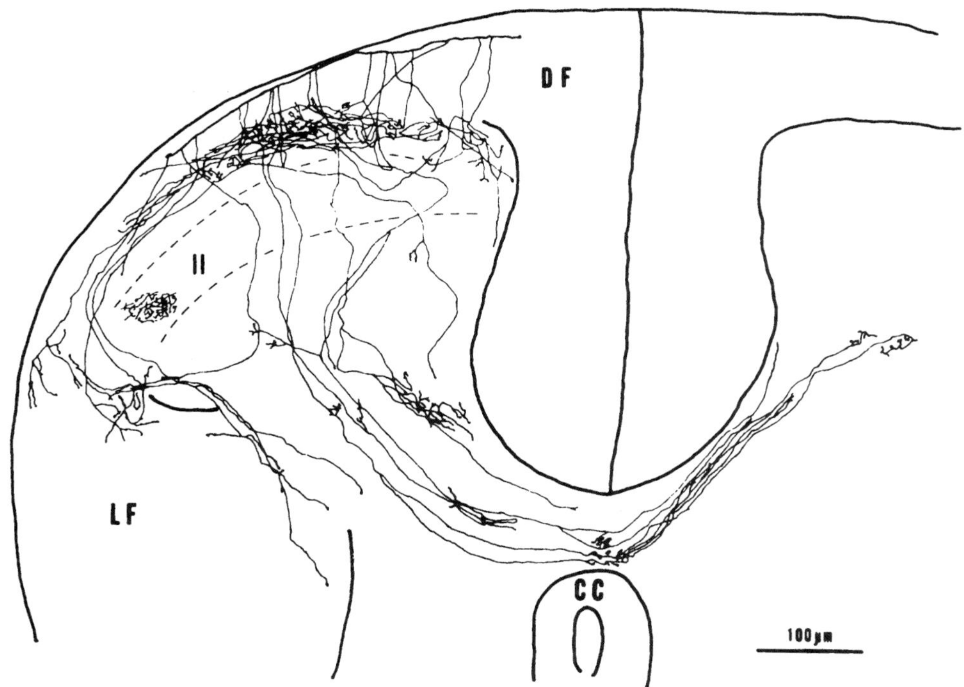

Figure 6. Transverse reconstruction of the central projection of a visceral C-afferent fiber from a guinea pig, labeled with *Phaseolus vulgaris* leucoagglutinin (PHA-L) following intracellular injection into a DRG cell. (From ref. 500.)

proven to be important in the functioning of the dorsal horn and the processing of sensory input.

Amino Acids

Glutamate (GLU)

This amino acid is localized in dorsal root ganglion (DRG) cells (151,271,517), dorsal roots (559), and in cell bodies and terminals in the superficial dorsal horn (271,366,370,551). Some GLU cells are involved in spinal cord local neurocircuitry, projecting three to five segments in the rostrocaudal direction (451); others are projection neurons, sending their axons to the thalamus (333). GLU-containing fibers and terminals are present in laminae I to IV and in the ventral horn (366). The majority of these terminals arise from primary afferent neurons (53,530); however, supraspinal sources have also been described (197,341,398,532). Double- and triple-labeling studies indicate that GLU is colocalized with SP and/or CGRP (32,133,366) and neurotensin (513). Double labeling in the DRG indicates that GLU is colocalized with some aspartate-containing cells, suggesting that some primary afferent terminals also contain both amino acids (517; however, see 366). Westlund et al. (558) have demonstrated that 50% of the terminals on spinothalamic tract (STT) cells contain GLU.

Aspartate (ASP)

This amino acid has been localized in DRG cells (271,517), dorsal root axons (560), and in cell bodies, axons, and terminals in laminae I to III (366,451,530). Analysis of the coexistence of ASP and GLU in terminals indicates that these amino acids are present in separate populations (366). These data are in contrast to the colocalization of ASP and GLU reported in the DRG cells (517). ASP is colocalized with synaptophysin (366). In addition to arising from primary afferent fibers, corticospinal fibers may also contribute ASP-labeled terminals to the cord (197). GLU and ASP are both considered to be fast neurotransmitters and their concentration in the superficial dorsal horn suggests that they are important in nociceptive transmission. A population of GLU insensitive cells in superficial dorsal horn are depolarized by *N*-methyl-D-aspartate (NMDA) (389); although ASP was not tested, it is the most likely endogenous neurotransmitter.

γ-Aminobutyric Acid (GABA)

The majority of the GABA terminals observed in the spinal cord arise from interneurons, with a small contribution from descending tracts (373). GABA terminals are concentrated in the superficial dorsal horn (28,79,246,351). GABAergic interneurons are present in all laminae except lamina IX (Fig. 7) (27,79) and are particularly concentrated in laminae I to III (181,246,334,512). Several other substances may coexist in GABAergic neurons including glycine (515), somatostatin and neurotensin (423), met-ENK (514), parvalbumin (15,303), nitric oxide synthase (303, 531), neuropeptide Y and acetylcholine (303), and thyrotropin-releasing hormone (175). Iontophoretic application of GABA results in inhibition of dorsal horn neurons (129,600), including STT cells (568). Confirming the latter findings, Carlton et al. (84) demonstrate GABAergic contacts on primate STT cells. GABA is involved in primary afferent depolarization (156,158–162; see reviews in 316,399, 463), a phenomenon that is believed to have axoaxonic synapses as its morphologic basis. Several examples of GABAergic terminals presynaptic to primary afferent terminals have been documented (6,28,30,79,344,346,511). However, the most prevalent arrangement appears to be GABAergic dendrites postsynaptic to primary afferent terminals (79,220). This anatomic arrangement indicates that primary afferents are in the position to act as a driving force for a GABAergic system (86). This inhibitory system could modify sensory input at the spinal cord level, before it is transmitted to higher cognitive centers. This afferent-mediated inhibition could be disrupted following peripheral nerve injury, dorsal rhizotomy, evulsions, etc., and could result in sensory abnormalities.

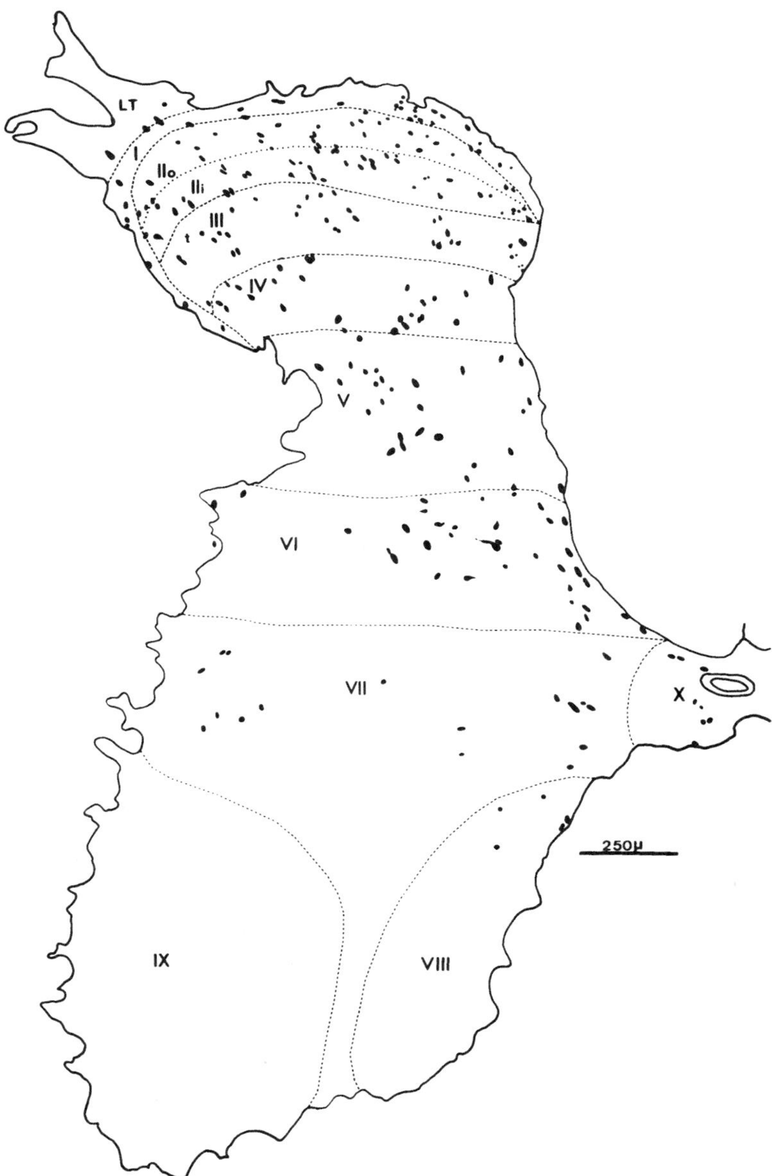

Figure 7. A section through the lumbar enlargement of the monkey spinal cord, showing the distribution of GABA-immunolabeled cell bodies. (From ref. 79.)

Glycine (GLY)

GLY-immunoreactivity has been localized in laminae I to III, VI, and VII (78,232,436,516,534). Todd and Sullivan (515) demonstrated that nearly all GLY-labeled cells in laminae I to III also contain GABA. Furthermore, GLY-labeled cells may also contain somatostatin (423). Iontophoretic application of this amino acid results in inhibition of dorsal horn neurons (70,126–128, 552,553,601), including identified STT cells (568). However, GLY acting at non–strychnine-sensitive receptors potentiates excitatory NMDA amino acid receptor response (265).

Taurine (TAU)

TAU is present in cell bodies in the superficial dorsal horn and is an inhibitory neurotransmitter/neuromodulator candidate (349,406, 472). TAU is believed to play a role in antinociception in the spinal cord (42,300,488,489).

Peptides

Substance P (SP)

There are numerous reports of SP-containing neurons in the superficial dorsal horn, with an emphasis on their concentration in lamina II (138,192,225,231,246,276,382,470,473,508). Messenger RNA encoding for this peptide is also found in the same region (547). Based on findings from rhizotomy (244, 338,507) and spinal transection studies (367), it is believed that approximately one half of the SP terminal population in the dorsal horn arises from intrinsic neurons, and the other half arises from primary afferent fibers. A subpopulation of STT neurons located in both laminae I and V, with a lesser number in the more ventral laminae, are SP positive (33), suggesting that SP-containing neurons are involved in the rostral transmission of nociceptive information. Almost all SP-containing neurons also contain enkephalin (ENK) (276,471).

Cholecystokinin (CCK)

In addition to being present in primary afferent neurons, CCK is also located in dorsal horn neurons in laminae II, IV, and V (181,467), some of which project to the thalamus (270). In normal primates, the majority of the receptors in spinal cord are of the CCK-A subtype, while in rats and rabbits CCK-B is the predominant receptor subtype (188,222). In the rat, neonatal capsaicin causes a substantial decrease in CCK binding sites in the superficial dorsal horn, indicating that the majority of binding sites are on primary afferent fibers (188). There is a specific upregulation of both mRNA for CCK-B receptors and CCK in rat DRG cells after peripheral axotomy (596). CCK may antagonize opiate analgesia (188), and morphine increases CCK release from spinal cord (599). Iontophoresis of CCK results in excitation of many of the neurons tested in laminae I to VII (260).

Thyrotropin-Releasing Hormone (TRH)

TRH immunoreactive fibers and terminals are located in laminae II and III, the intermediolateral cell column, around the central canal, and in ventral horn motor nuclei. TRH cell bodies are observed in II through IV (24,112,217,528). Iontophoretic application of TRH facilitates the responses of wide dynamic range and high-threshold neurons in laminae II to V to glutamate (256).

Corticotropin-Releasing Factor (CRF)

A limited population of CRF-containing cells have been described in the superficial dorsal horn (365). The CRF-labeled fibers and terminals in laminae I, II, and V may arise from these intrinsic neurons or from DRG cells (177,363,365, 408,462,485,487).

Galanin (GAL)

Sources of GAL to the dorsal horn include primary afferent fibers (23,98,269,486,524,537), spinal cord neurons including interneurons (98,269,354,442), and projection neurons (270, 354), and fibers arising from supraspinal sites (23). In the spinal cord, GAL-labeled cells are observed in laminae II, III, and X (23), with a dense axonal plexus in laminae I and II (23,296,524,537,538). Galanin-labeled terminals in laminae I and II may also contain SP, calcitonin gene-related peptide and CCK (597), and nitric oxide synthase (598). Galanin appears to have analgesic properties based on the observations that intrathecal GAL not only potentiates the effects of morphine (566), but also produces a dose-dependent increase in reaction time in the tail flick test (123). GAL immunoreactivity in the dorsal horn decreases following dorsal rhizotomy (224,538) and following sciatic nerve stimulation (289); however, it increases in the DRG and dorsal horn following sciatic nerve transection (235,537,538). The precise functional role of GAL following nerve injury is unknown; however, it has been hypothesized that GAL serves as an inhibitory factor in axotomized neurons, preventing the release of the principal transmitter(s), thus blocking the flow of abnormal and/or noxious sensory input (537).

Neurotensin (NT)

NT-containing cells are located primarily in lamina II, with smaller populations in laminae I, III, and V (Fig. 8) (142,143, 192,262,474,475,527,584). Fibers and terminals are concentrated in laminae I to III (142,192,262,335,473,584) and may colocalize with glutamate (513). The source of these fibers and terminals is most likely not primary afferent neurons, since rhizotomy and neonatal treatment with capsaicin do not affect NT content in the dorsal horn (257,400). Although not present in DRG cells, NT is released following stimulation of the sciatic nerve (584). Iontophoretic application of NT excites both nociceptive and nonnociceptive neurons in laminae I to III, but has little effect on neurons in deeper laminae (369,495).

Calcitonin Gene-Related Peptide (CGRP)

A dense plexus of CGRP-containing fibers and terminals is present in laminae I, II, V, and X (82,83,191,219,353). This peptide has been localized in unmyelinated (6) and small-diameter myelinated fibers (353). Most agree that CGRP-labeled terminals are of primary afferent origin, since extensive rhizotomies (107,191,518,519) result in an almost complete loss of CGRP staining in the dorsal horn. There is evidence of colocalization of CGRP and serotonin in terminals in the ventral horn; it is believed that these fibers arise from medullary sources (22). CGRP is colocalized with numerous other peptides in the DRG (269) and is considered to be a neuromodulator involved in the processing of noxious input. Nociceptive spinal reflexes (123,487,579) and the scratching/biting behavior produced by intrathecal SP and SOM (565,567) are potentiated by intrathecal application of CGRP.

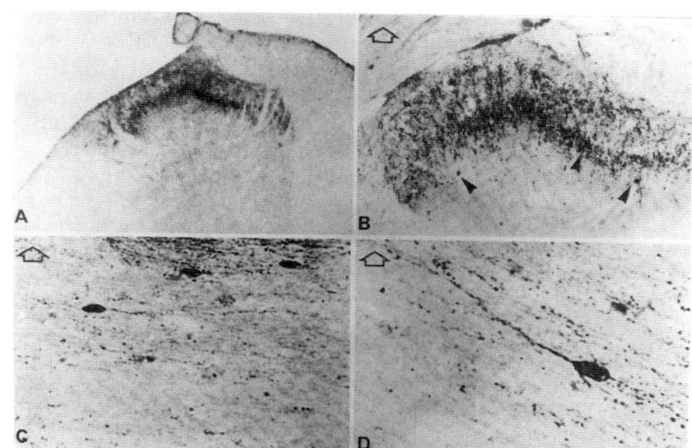

Figure 8. **A:** NT-immunoreactivity observed in the L4 dorsal horn of the rat. **B:** Higher magnification shows a dense band of immunostaining in lamina II and NT-immunoreactive cell bodies in lamina IIo and III *(arrows)*. **C,D:** Parasagittal section demonstrating NT-labeled cell bodies and their processes in laminae IIo and III. (From ref. 192.)

Opiate Peptides

Enkephalin (ENK) ENK-containing neurons are distributed throughout laminae I to V, with a concentration in laminae I and II (Fig. 9) (21,125,167,171,192,198,199,229,231,247,308, 364,372,457,471,482,494). The ENK-labeled terminals in the same region are believed to arise mainly from these dorsal horn neurons, with a small contribution coming from medullary cells (234). ENK has been localized in neurons projecting to the thalamus (385) and the parabrachial region (494). Iontophoretic studies show that ENK or its analogue met-enkephalinamide produces a selective inhibition of nociceptive dorsal horn neurons (148–150,152,428,459,602), including identified spinothalamic tract cells (569,570), which can be blocked by naloxone. Consistent with this finding, ENK-containing terminals have been demonstrated on STT cells (447,450). The enkephalinergic inhibitory actions are mediated by δ and μ receptors

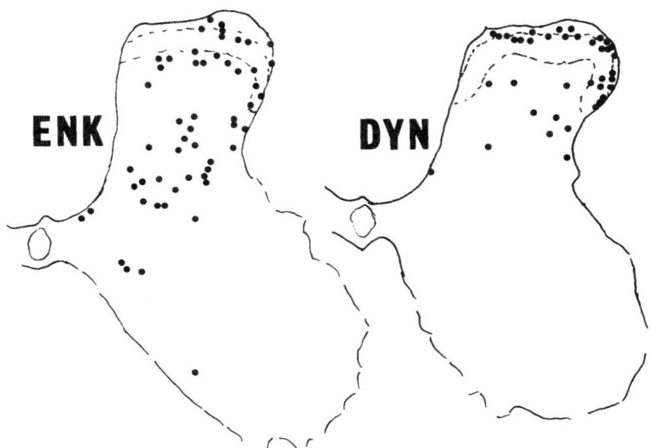

Figure 9. Schematic representation of the distribution of ENK- and DYN-labeled neurons in the cat spinal cord. Compared to DYN, ENK-labeled neurons are more widely distributed. (From ref. 125.)

(140,261). A greater concentration of ENK-containing cells is located in those segments receiving visceral as well as somatic afferents, suggesting that opiates also play an important role in the modulation of visceral input (371). Several studies indicate that ENK is colocalized with SP (276,438,471) or GABA (303) in dorsal horn neurons.

Dynorphin (DYN) Cells that contain another opiate peptide, DYN, are located mainly in laminae I, IIo, and V (Fig. 9) (100, 101,283,449,539,549). Some DYN cells in lamina I project to the parabrachial nucleus (494), while DYN cells located in deeper laminae project to the thalamus (386). Similar to ENK, a higher concentration of DYN cells are located in segments receiving visceral input (371). Mixed results are obtained when DYN is iontophoresed onto dorsal horn cells, producing either excitation or inhibition (290,570). The number of DYN-containing cells has been shown to increase in the dorsal horn following peripheral nerve and/or dorsal root transection (100,101), peripheral inflammation (253,403,549), and peripheral neuropathy (272,543). Interestingly, this increase is usually bilateral. Double-labeling studies indicate that the increase occurs in both interneurons and projection neurons (383). These documented changes in DYN are intriguing; however, to date it is unclear how these anatomical changes relate to the sensory abnormalities observed in inflammation and neuropathy models (147). Regardless, these observations serve to reinforce the opinion that DYN is intimately involved in primary afferent processing.

Somatostatin (SOM)

SOM-labeled neurons are observed in laminae I and II (131,172,225,246,264,374,443,464,468,473,540). In lamina II, synaptic contact has been demonstrated between SOM-containing fibers and cells (216). Laminae I and II also contain SOM terminals arising from primary afferent fibers (230,437) and intrinsic neurons. The proportion arising from each source is unknown. Terminals containing somatostatin immunoreactivity are also found in lamina X (306). Iontophoresis of SOM onto nociceptive neurons causes inhibition (428). SOM administered intrathecally or as a superfusion has no effect on A- (456) or C-fiber–evoked neuronal responses or wind up in the dorsal horn (99). However, responses to noxious thermal stimuli (456) as well as both the first and second phase of the neuronal response to intraplantar formalin (99) are suppressed by SOM.

Neuropeptide Y (NPY)

NPY-containing cells, fibers, and terminals are located in laminae I to III, V, and VI (5,104,139,189,233,245,297,458, 478). This peptide colocalizes with ENK and catecholamines (245) and with GABA (444). There are few investigations elucidating the functional role(s) of NPY; however, it is believed to play a role in the processing of sensory input (146), including nociception (263).

Vasoactive Intestinal Peptide (VIP)

The majority of the VIP fiber and terminal labeling is found in Lissauer's tract, laminae I, V, X, and the lateral collateral pathway in the sacral cord; other spinal cord levels have considerably less VIP label (12,31,135,192,237,277,310). There is some disagreement concerning whether VIP fibers extend into lamina II. VIP terminals arise mainly from primary afferent fibers (269,537), although a small population of VIP-containing neurons have been observed in the dorsal horn (190,310). VIP has been localized in a small population of STT cells (386). In a manner similar to GAL, VIP immunostaining increases in DRG cells and in the dorsal horn following peripheral nerve injury (25,124,350,476,477,537). C-fiber stimulation of the sciatic nerve also increases VIP immunostaining; however, it is limited to areas outside of the direct sciatic nerve terminations (289). Although the functional significance of these increases is unknown, intrathecal administration of VIP results in a dose-dependent decrease in tail flick reaction time to noxious radiant heat, suggesting that VIP may act as an excitatory agent in the processing of nociceptive input (123).

Monoamines

Dopamine (DOPA)

To date, a small population of DOPA-containing cells (visualized with an antibody to tyrosine hydroxylase) has been demonstrated in lamina I of the sacral spinal cord (379). The function of these cells is unknown; however, their location suggests they play a role in processing nociceptive information.

Noradrenaline (NE)

The enzyme used to localize NE is dopamine-β-hydroxylase (DβH). To date, no DβH-positive cells have been localized in the spinal cord. The DβH-labeled terminals in laminae I, II, and V arise from supraspinal sites (466,484,555,556). Approximately 5.6% of the terminal population on STT cell bodies are DβH-containing terminals (557). This population is most likely the basis for the NE-induced inhibition of STT cells to noxious input and to iontophoresed glutamate (568).

Epinephrine (EPI)

Antibodies raised against the enzyme phenylethanolamine-N-methyltransferase (PMNT) have been used to identify EPI-containing profiles. Although no PNMT-containing cell bodies are observed in the spinal cord, labeled fibers and terminals, arising from brainstem cells, are present at all spinal levels and are concentrated in the superficial dorsal horn, the intermediolateral cell column, and lamina X (80,81). Inhibition of glutamate-induced firing results from iontophoretic application of EPI onto STT cells (81).

Serotonin (5-HT)

The majority of 5-HT in the spinal cord arises from supraspinal sources (446); however, a small population of 5-HT-containing neurons has been described in the superficial dorsal horn and in lamina X (47,311,397). 5-HT has not been localized in DRG cells. Dense terminal labeling is present in laminae I and II (130,293,294,309,319,345,448,497). 5-HT colocalizes with SP (503,554) and ENK (504). 5-HT-labeled terminals have been observed synapsing on dorsal horn neurons including STT cells (227,250,307,368,401). There are multiple 5-HT receptor subtypes in the spinal cord, and understanding their respective actions has become a quagmire of conflicting findings. Iontophoretic administration of 5-HT is generally agreed to depress neuronal responses, including those of spinothalamic tract cells, to noxious stimulation (268). However, 5-HT1a agonists applied iontophoretically increase responsiveness of dorsal horn cells to noxious stimulation (4). In contrast, their antagonists block the antinociceptive actions produced by raphe stimulation (166). 5-HT3 agonists given spinally decrease responsiveness to noxious stimuli, but may do so by causing GABA release (3). 5-HT inhibits spinal release of presumptive primary afferent SOM (299).

Purines

Adenosine

Adenosine-containing neurons (51) and adenosine receptors (102,185,207,586) have been identified in lamina II. Consequently, this purine has been implicated as a potential neuromodulator in the processing of noxious input.

Others

Acetylcholine

The use of antibodies that recognize choline acetyltransferase (ChAT), demonstrate cholinergic cells bodies in laminae II to IV (243,286,415,416). It is believed that these interneurons give rise to the cholinergic system in the dorsal horn since ChAT has not been localized in DRG cells (26,46) nor does spinal cord transection affect the levels of ChAT staining in the cord (236). Ultrastructural studies demonstrate that ChAT-labeled terminals are both pre- and postsynaptic to central terminals in glomerular complexes, indicating that cholinergic mechanisms are intimately involved in sensory processing (435).

Calbindin and Parvalbumin

These are two calcium-binding proteins that have been localized in laminae I to III, although the two populations do not seem to overlap (585,591). Parvalbumin does not colocalize with peptides, but has been colocalized with GABA and GLY (303); calbindin coexists with NT and SP (591). The concentration of these proteins in the superficial dorsal horn indicates that they may be important in processing noxious input.

Nitric Oxide (NO)

Originally localized in endothelial tissue, where it has potent vasodilator effects (411), NO has recently been localized in neural tissue, where it acts as an intracellular messenger and/or neuromodulator (184,490). Visualization of NO is done indirectly by demonstrating the presence of nitric oxide synthase (NOS), the enzyme that generates NO from L-arginine (377). NOS can be localized with an antigen-antibody reaction or it can be demonstrated through histochemical methods for reduced nicotinamide adenine dinucleotide phosphate (NADPH) diaphorase (242). Using these two methods, NOS-labeled neurons have been localized in the DRG (1,542), and diffusely scattered throughout the dorsal gray matter of the spinal cord with a concentration at the laminae II–III border, in lamina X, and in the preganglionic sympathetic and parasympathetic nuclei (Fig. 10) (13,71,154,506,533). A dense plexus of stained fibers is present in laminae I and II and in the intermediolateral cell column (533). Following injury to the central nervous system (581,582), dorsal rhizotomy (541), or peripheral nerve injury (1,169,535,598), NADPH diaphorase staining and/or NOS immunoreactivity in the DRG and spinal cord increases. It is hypothesized that NO has a role in the processing of nociceptive input in the spinal cord and may contribute to the induction of hyperalgesia (288,355,356). This theory is supported by the fact that 10% of the STT cells in the region of the central canal are positive for NOS and approximately 40% of superficial dorsal horn cells that express Fos in response to noxious stimulation are in apposition to or in close proximity to NOS-labeled neuronal processes (315). NOS has been colocalized with GABA, GLY, and acetylcholine in the dorsal horn (493,531) and with CGRP, SP, and GAL in the DRG (598).

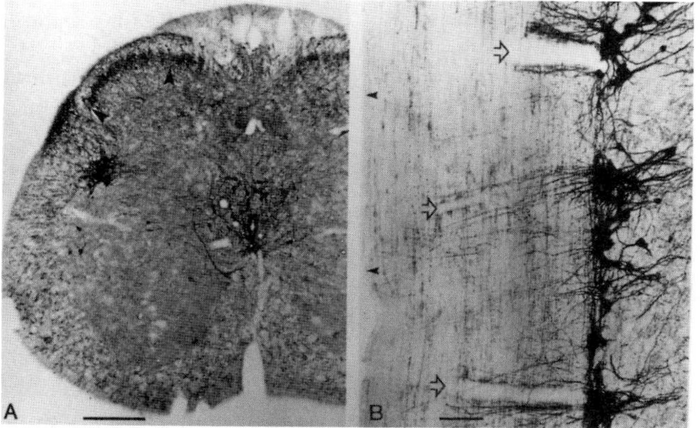

Figure 10. **A:** NADPHd-positive neurons and fibers in rat sacral cord. A dense plexus of fibers is present in lamina II (*arrows*). The main groups of stained cells are located at the laminae II–III border, in lamina X, and in the intermediolateral cell column (IMLCC). *Bar* = 250 μm. **B:** A horizontal section through the thoracic cord, demonstrating NADPHd-positive neurons in the IMLCC (*arrowheads* indicate lateral pial surface, *open arrows* indicate blood vessels). *Bar* = 100μm. (From ref. 533.)

DORSAL HORN SENSORY NEURONS

Primary afferent fibers discussed in previous sections relay sensory information to different populations of neurons upon entering the spinal cord. In the simplest formulation, one can consider that there are three categories of dorsal horn neurons:

1. Interneurons are typically small-diameter cells with axons terminating in the vicinity of the parent cell body. They serve as relays and participate in local processing and integration of information and are frequently subdivided into excitatory and inhibitory types.
2. Propriospinal neurons have longer axons that can extend over several spinal segments. They participate in heterosegmental reflexes and interactions among stimuli administered to separate loci.
3. Projection neurons send axons out of the spinal cord to terminate in supraspinal centers. Thus, they participate in the rostral transmission of sensory information.

All three components are essential for processing of sensory input, allowing the organism to make organized and appropriate responses. Some neurons, via axon collaterals, may serve in more than one capacity. Beyond this, neurons are further grouped based on their responses to natural peripheral stimuli, their projection site, laminar location of the cell body, or neurochemical content (155; see ref. 574 for review). Complete classification systems have proved to be cumbersome and are not commonly used for naming purposes. Common nomenclature is based on the characteristics of the stimuli that will evoke activity in the cell. In many cases, the response of the cell can be envisioned to be a function of the nature of the afferent input (e.g., low-threshold vs. high-threshold afferents). In other situations, the net response of the cell appears to reflect the complex excitatory/inhibitory milieu in which the cell is situated in the dorsal horn. These cells may thus show complex activity patterns (e.g., complex receptive field neurons and substantia gelatinosa neurons). These several categories are discussed below.

Intensity-Dependent Categorization

Class 1: Low-Threshold (LT) Cells

Low-threshold cells, also called class 1 cells, respond maximally to light touch, pressure, hair movement, and/or vibratory stimuli. Stimulation of their receptive fields within the noxious range produces no increase in firing frequency (Fig. 11). The majority of their input is mediated by large myelinated Aβ fibers, with the remainder composed of other mechanosensitive afferents (92,214,255). Receptive fields for these as well as most dorsal horn cells are larger than those of the primary afferent fibers due to convergence. This class has frequently been subdivided into touch (including hair movement) or class 1A neurons and touch-pressure class 1B neurons (358,360,418, 421). Low-threshold mechanoreceptive cells are thought by most laboratories not to respond to noxious heat or chemical stimuli; however, spinocervical tract cells with no high-threshold mechanical input do appear to respond selectively to noxious levels of thermal stimulation (55,56). This phenomenon has been characterized in the primate. Willis's group (145)

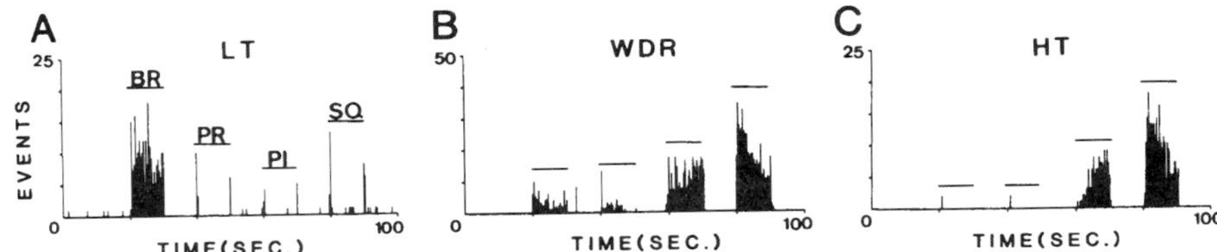

Figure 11. The panels display the number of action potentials emitted by three cells of different response categories to a series of mechanical stimuli applied to the most sensitive portion of their receptive fields. **A:** LT cells respond maximally to innocuous brushing (BR). This stimulus activates all hair follicles as well as many other low-threshold mechanoreceptors. **B:** WDR cells respond modestly to BR and to firm pressure (PR) and respond more vigorously to a maintained noxious pinch (PI) and a more intense squeeze (SQ). **C:** HT cells respond selectively to the two stimuli within the noxious range. (From ref. 492.)

found that low-threshold mechanoreceptive SCT cells respond to noxious heat, but their evoked responses to heating are lower than cells that also receive nociceptive mechanical input (145). LT cells are concentrated in laminae III and especially IV of the dorsal horn throughout the length of the spinal cord. For this reason, LTs have been referred to as "lamina IV-type cells"; however, this nomenclature is no longer used. Projection cells of this type are common in the SCT (56,64) and PSDC pathways (14,193) and are present, but less common, in the STT (410,573).

Class 2: Multireceptive Cell

In class 2, wide dynamic range (WDR) and multireceptive cells are common names for cells that receive both low- and high-threshold input via the convergence of afferent input from both large-diameter myelinated (Aβ) and small-diameter lightly myelinated and unmyelinated (Aδ and C) fibers (214,358,360). Implicit in the name and definition of wide dynamic range, but not multireceptive cells, is the fact that their output differentially codes for the intensity of the stimulus (358). WDR cells fire at a higher frequency as afferent stimulus intensity increases over a range comprising innocuous and noxious levels. Although multireceptive (WDR) cells are usually classified based on their response to mechanical stimuli, frequently they exhibit parallel differential responsiveness to innocuous warming and noxious heat. In addition, WDR cells often respond to noxious cold and receive convergent high-threshold input from muscle and viscera (178,179,417). The highest concentrations of WDR cells are centered around lamina V, with other smaller populations found in laminae I and X; they are located with lesser frequency in the remainder of the dorsal horn. This is not surprising, taking into account the distribution of primary afferent fiber types. Receptive fields of WDR cells tend to be larger than those of narrow dynamic range cells (223,546), although classically they are restricted to one limb or body part. In many cases receptive fields appear to be mixed, with a central or distal portion that responds to a range of inputs, from gentle touch to pinch, and a less sensitive surround that is activated only by high-intensity input (223) (Fig. 12). Projection cells of this type are common in the STT (410,573), spinomesencephalic (SMT) (587–589), spinoreticular (SRT), SCT (56,59,63), and spinohypothalamic (SHT) (75) tracts. At least within the lamina I STT cell population, axon diameter (conduction velocity) and probably cell size is larger for WDR cells than for high-threshold cells (168).

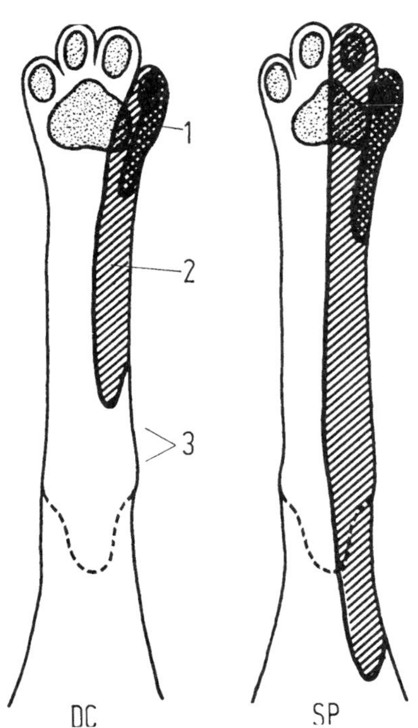

Figure 12. These panels illustrate the receptive-field organization of a lamina V cell. In the decerebrate animal (DC, *left*), as in the intact anesthetized one, there are three zones of differential responsiveness. Distally in zone 1 the cell responds to both innocuous and noxious cutaneous stimulation. In zone 2, only noxious stimulation was sufficient to activate the cell. Surrounding the excitatory field in zone 3, mechanical stimulation inhibited neuronal firing. The same cell in the spinalized state (SP, *right*) showed enlarged excitatory receptive fields and the inhibitory field disappeared, indicating brainstem involvement in tonic inhibition. (From ref. 223.)

Class 3: Nociceptive-Specific Cell

Class 3, high threshold (HT) and nociceptive specific, refers to a second class of narrow dynamic range cells that respond exclusively to mechanical stimuli within the noxious range (92,255,360). Iggo (255) stipulates that the effective stimulus "is not less than the threshold of pain in man." These have been divided by Cervero et al. (92) into class 3A, cells that are excited principally by Aδ nociceptors and respond almost exclusively to noxious mechanical stimulation, and class 3B, cells that receive input from both Aδ and C fibers. The majority of cells within this category are nocithermoreceptive as well as mechanosensitive and respond to noxious intensities of heat, but not to innocuous warming. Frequently, cells in this class respond to cold. Many have convergent input from muscle (group III and IV afferent fibers) as well as from skin (92). The highest concentration of high-threshold cells is in lamina I (103,118), with lower numbers found in laminae V (573) and X (239,384). Receptive fields are relatively small, but still larger than those of primary afferent fibers. Evoked activity in high-threshold cells is graded in proportion to stimulus intensity and is an indication that nociceptors have been stimulated. Thus, these cells code for both stimulus location and magnitude. These cells are common in the spinothalamic (168,410), spinomesencephalic (251), and spinohypothalamic (75) tracts.

Class 4: Deep Cells

Class 4 is composed of deep cells that respond maximally to stimulation or manipulation of subcutaneous structures such as muscles or joints (360,573). Often these cells also have convergent cutaneous and/or visceral input. Recent efforts have been made to classify cells in a more objective manner using a multivariate statistical analysis of the responses to several mechanical stimuli (105). This system has not achieved common use. However, the approach has led to the realization that dorsal horn cells divide into groupings based not only on adequate stimulus, but also according to the absolute quantity (maximum firing capacity) of their poststimulus discharge (410). This factor undoubtedly contributes to subsequent processing and final perception.

Complex Response Cells

Complex Receptive Field Cells

Complex WDR and HT cells have been described in the spinoreticular (454) and spinomesencephalic (589,588) tracts with large, frequently discontinuous, excitatory receptive fields; often their input is bilateral. In some cases these cells also have extensive inhibitory receptive fields (454,588,589); frequently, the inhibitory fields are distant and noncontiguous with the excitatory fields. Within each projection pathway, cells with complex receptive fields are most often found in the deeper laminae. In one study, almost all (94%) STT cells in the lumbosacral enlargement had this kind of inhibitory field (187). Common elements for inhibition among the different complex cell types are lack of continuity with the excitatory field, and inhibition arising only from noxious intensities of stimulation to either muscle or skin and not from activation of large myelinated fibers.

There is a long and ongoing debate about the function of multireceptive neurons that signal both light touch and potential tissue damage. How can activation of neurons that provide dual messages signal pain? It is probable that singly WDR neurons cannot make this distinction, but interpretation of the population response can result in the perception of pain. The frequency of action potentials evoked in individual neurons, in combination with the total number and pattern of dorsal horn cells activated, probably contributes to the perceived intensity and quality of somatic sensations and participates in the discrimination between noxious and innocuous stimuli. Significantly, there is evidence that selective activation of WDR neurons is sufficient to produce a sensation of pain in humans (348,421).

Substantia Gelatinosa

The vast majority of cells in substantia gelatinosa have response profiles that do not match any of those described (89–91). In the acutely prepared, anesthetized animal these cells maintain a high degree of background activity in the absence of stimulation to their receptive field. The three most prevalent classes of SG cells, inverse classes 1 to 3, are inhibited by input that excites the more "typical" dorsal horn cells. Inverse class 1 cells are inhibited by low-threshold stimulation of their receptive fields. Conversely, nociceptive stimulation of any kind applied to the same area of skin increases the firing of these cells (Fig. 13A). Inverse class 2 cells, the most common type, are inhibited by innocuous and noxious intensity mechanical stimulation of their receptive fields. While some cells of this type are excited by noxious thermal stimulation, the majority are inhibited. Inverse class 3 cells separate into two groups of about equal frequency: inverse 3A cells are inhibited by noxious mechanical (Fig. 13B), and inverse 3B cells are inhibited by both noxious mechanical and thermal activation of their receptive fields. Both types are excited by low-threshold stimulation. These inverse cell types are not commonly found in the surrounding laminae. Electrophysiologic studies indicate that these cells receive monosynaptic excitatory input from Aδ and C fibers (91,593). These cells do not appear to be subject to tonic descending modulation (94), but have been implicated in tonic inhibition of neurons in other spinal laminae (89). This function is consistent with the conceptual ideas, but not the anatomical detail of gate control (357).

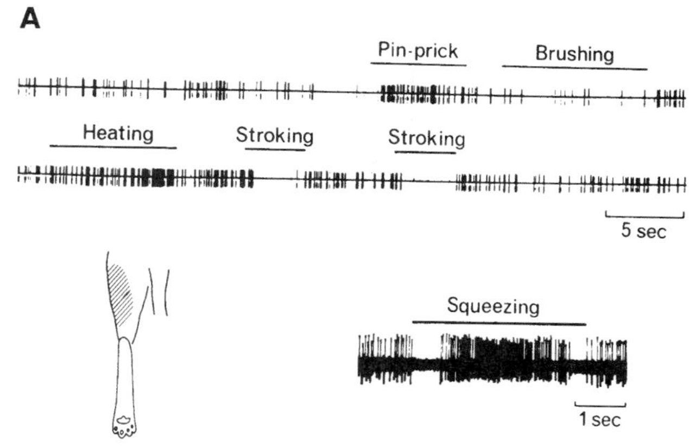

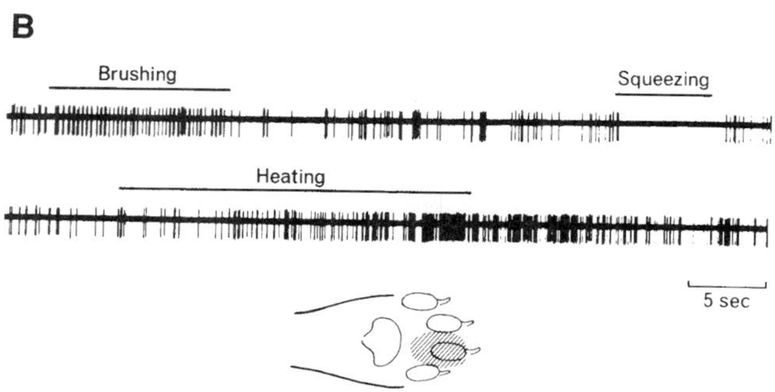

Figure 13. Receptive field organization of two substantia gelatinosa cells. **A:** Inverse class 1 cells are inhibited by low-threshold mechanical input and excited by noxious stimulation. Squeezing the receptive field with forceps results in excitation during the noxious phase and inhibition when the forceps are applied and removed from the skin. **B:** Inverse class 3 cells are inhibited by noxious mechanical stimuli, but excited by low-threshold mechanical and thermal stimulation of their receptive fields. (From ref. 91.)

Modality-Related Cells

In the preceding section, the principal organizing consideration has been the somatic input generated by mechanical stimuli. Input may be further encoded in dorsal horn neurons according to the modality of the connecting afferent.

Viscera

Viscerosomatic neurons have excitatory input from visceral afferent fibers in addition to the usual somatic input. They are found most commonly in the thoracic, lumbar, and sacral portions of the spinal cord, throughout laminae I and IV through VII, as well as in lamina X (10,239,352,384,392,417,469). In most cases, especially in cells recorded in the middle and lateral dorsal horn, cells that respond to visceral stimulation also have cutaneous receptive fields (43,44,96,417). Thus, visceral sensation is frequently mediated via convergent somatosensory pathways. Convergence of visceral and sensory input onto the same neuron within the sensory transmission system provides a solid basis for the convergence-projection theory of referred pain first proposed by Ruch (445). A small minority of cells (206,238,291) respond selectively to visceral stimulation. With infrequent exceptions, most neurons with visceral input exhibit convergence from multiple nerves and/or viscera (395). In almost all cases, visceral inputs appear to be exclusively nociceptive (mediated via Aδ and/or C fibers). Classification according to the convergent somatic input can be as LT, HT, and WDR. However, there is a very small percentage of LT cells and the HT/WDR ratio is much higher than for cells with exclusive somatic input (7,43,44). Low-threshold viscerosomatic cells appear to not receive Aβ input, as tested electrophysiologically (7). Comparable to the inverse cells found in SG, subtypes of viscerosomatic cells can have either superimposed inhibitory and excitatory receptive fields to different stimuli (44) or differing responses to somatic and visceral stimulation (43,44,239,393,394). Foreman's group first described HTi cells with excitatory responses resulting from visceral and nociceptive cutaneous input and inhibition during light brushing of the same cutaneous field (Fig. 14). It has been proposed that as the distance between a spinal viscerosomatic neuron and the level of afferent input increases, the greater the probability that the input will result in neuronal inhibition. This appears to be true for both somatic and visceral input (226, 393). Many cells with visceral input project to supraspinal levels and contribute to the spinothalamic (7,43,44) and spinoreticular (7,43,226) pathways. Further discussion on the organization of visceral input can be found in Chap. 39.

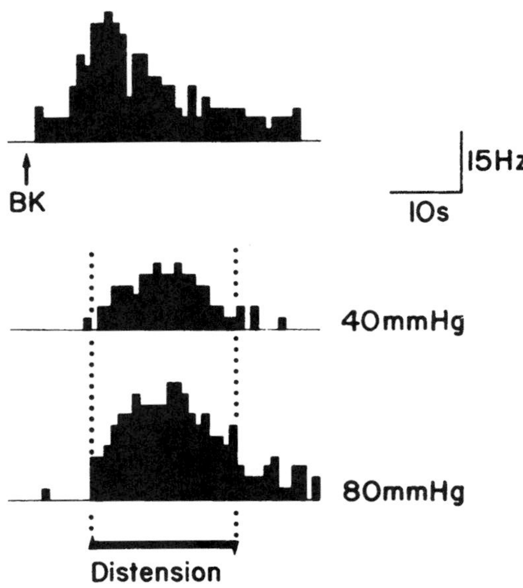

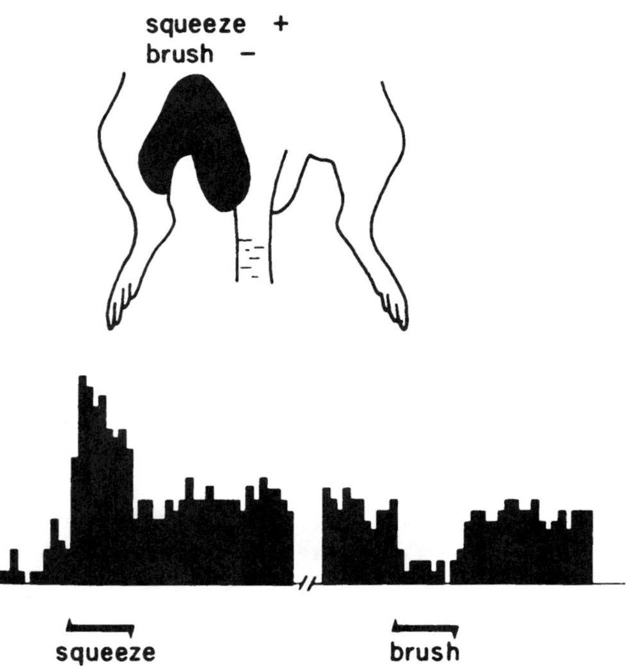

Figure 14. Responses of a viscerosomotic cell in the lumbosacral spinal cord of a rat. The cell fired in response to intraarterial bradykinin (BK) and in a dose-related manner to colorectal distention. Noxious stimulation of its cutaneous receptive field (*center*) also caused the cell to fire. However, low-threshold stimulation of the same cutaneous field initiated inhibition of ongoing activity. (From ref. 392.)

Temperature

Other response categories have been defined based on thermal stimuli. Neurons responding exclusively to either innocuous warming or cooling are found in lamina I and to a lesser extent in laminae III to V (221,298); others, in particular a subclass of lamina I spinothalamic and spinomesencephalic tract cells, respond exclusively to noxious heat and cold (103,118, 254,419). Evoked activity in the majority of cold-specific lamina I STT cells has recently been shown to be enhanced rather than depressed by systemic morphine (117).

ASCENDING PROJECTION SYSTEMS

After processing in the dorsal horn, sensory messages are relayed to supraspinal sites. Postmortem examination of lesions indicates that in humans, rostral transmission of nociceptive events leading to pain transmission is correlated with integrity of the contralateral anterolateral quadrant of the spinal cord (404). In animal studies, major percentages of cells projecting through several neuronal tracts, located in both the ventral and dorsal funiculi, respond exclusively or differentially to noxious stimulation. One explanation for the return of pain following cordotomy is that alternate pathways "learn" to take over the functions of the lesioned tracts. This section discusses some of the key properties of the several spinofugal systems. Figure 15 presents a schematic summary of these several systems.

Spinothalamic Tract

The spinothalamic tract is almost synonymous with the pain pathway in much of the literature. Based on the results of spinal cord lesions, it has been concluded that the STT in primates, including humans, is essential for transmission of information relating to nociceptive and thermal activation of receptive fields (176,404,536). In humans, pain transmission is most strongly correlated with integrity of the contralateral anterolateral quadrant (404); anterolateral cordotomy produces at least short-term relief of noncentral pain in 70% to 80% of patients (390,561). The STT also mediates some tactile sensation. In primates, thalamic targets for dorsal horn cells include the ventral posterior lateral (VPL) nucleus, the medial part of the posterior complex, and portions of the intralaminar complex (especially the central lateral nucleus) and the nucleus submedius (41,45,50). Prototypical response properties of cells that project to different thalamic nuclei are distinct. However, as in most dorsal horn physiology, there is overlap between properties of the parallel systems. Some of the duplication of function may be due to collateral projections participating in multiple pathways. In the rat, nearly 20% and 15% of cells projecting to nuclei in the medial and lateral thalamus, respectively, project to both (282). These numbers are probably slightly lower in the cat (498) and primate (119). Collectively, spinothalamic tract cells are located throughout the gray

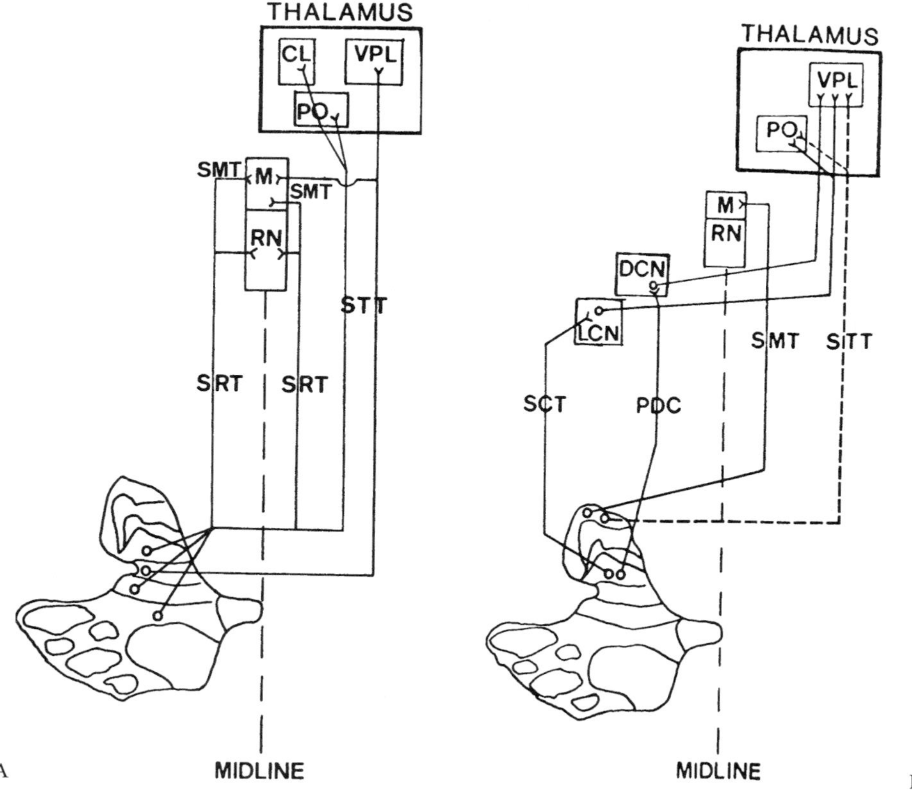

Figure 15. Illustrations of the major ventral **(A)** and dorsal **(B)** pathways taken by nociceptive information. (See text for abbreviations and descriptions.)

matter of the spinal cord, primarily laminae I and V through VII (17,18,76,85,119,571). The proportion of lamina I STT cells increases at more rostral segmental levels; in the cervical enlargement more than half of all STT cells are in lamina I (85,119,266). Twice as many lamina I cells project to both the medial and lateral nuclei as from any other lamina (119). In the rat, more than 80% of lamina I STT cells projecting through the DLF have collaterals contributing to the spinoreticular (parabrachial) tract (248). STT cells projecting to different nuclei are physiologically a heterogeneous mixture, usually resembling other cells in their lamina more than each other (196). Below the upper cervical cord, axons from approximately 90% of STT cells decussate in the anterior commissure and do so within one segment of the cell body, leaving a small ipsilateral projection. Cells in C_{1-2} have a much stronger ipsilateral projection than cells located throughout the remainder of the spinal cord (85,119). Axons within the ascending tract in the ventrolateral quadrant are arranged somatotopically (20).

Kuru (301), examining the results of retrograde chromatolysis in fixed human spinal cord, distinguishes separate anteromedial and dorsolateral spinothalamic tracts. This has been confirmed experimentally in the last few years. The dorsal lateral portion of the STT in the cat has been localized to the dorsolateral funiculus (266,267) and in the middle of the lateral funiculus at the level of the central canal (122). Studies in the primate have placed it in the dorsal lateral funiculus (16,18,19) and at the level of the denticulate ligament (424). There is general agreement that axons from cells in the superficial dorsal horn (primarily lamina I) project mainly through the dorsolateral division, dorsal to and separate from axons from cells found in the deeper laminae, which project exclusively through the anteromedial spinothalamic tract in the ventral quadrant (18,122,424). The functional relevance of the dorsolateral pathway is highlighted by Moffie (375), who presented case reports in which lesions restricted to the posterolateral funiculus result in complete analgesia and thermanesthesia; however, see Nathan (391).

Many lamina I STT cells are HT class 3 cells. A significant percentage are class 2 or WDR cells; virtually none are low threshold. In addition to responding differentially to noxious mechanical stimuli, lamina 1 STT cells can code for graded noxious heat stimuli (103,118,168,279). Receptive fields of lamina I cells tend to be smaller than those for lamina V STT cells (575) and they are somatotopically organized (573). Most electrophysiology studies in the primate have identified STT cells by stimulation in ventral posterior lateral thalamus; however, recent work indicates that a more prominent thalamic termination site for lamina I is in the medial part of the posterior complex (120,424), although Apkarian and Hodge (19) see only small differences between STT termination sites originating from different laminae. Thus, it is likely that representative samples of lamina I cells in primate have not been sampled.

It has been proposed that the lamina I projection to the suprageniculate-limitans/posterior complex consists of primarily HT cells (120,424); this is supported by extrapolations from cat data (118). In the primate, cells that project laterally to the ventral posterior lateral (VPL) nucleus of the thalamus, the major sensory relay nucleus of the thalamus, are concentrated in lamina V, but are scattered throughout the other laminae, including a significant population in lamina I (18,168,571). Cells projecting to both the VPL and the intralaminar complex are located laterally in lamina V and medially in laminae VI and VII. Cells terminating in the VPL are responsive to noxious stimulation of their receptive fields; the majority in the lumbar enlargement are WDRs (55%), a significant fraction are classified as high threshold (32%), and the remainder are either deep (11%) or low threshold (2%). Receptive fields are ipsilateral, are usually excitatory, and range from encompassing a single digit to most of a limb (20,168,575). Most lamina V STT cells are located laterally, in the reticulated region, and somatotopic organization is lost (575). Throughout the length of the spinal cord, STT cells are found with convergent input from muscle and other deep structures (7,178,395). Frequently, the cutaneous receptive field overlies the deep field. Viscerosomatic STT cells in the thoracic and sacral cord correspond to the distribution of autonomic afferents. Accordingly, responsiveness to cardiopulmonary stimulation, including intracardiac bradykinin and occlusion of a coronary artery, are characteristic of STT cells in the upper thoracic cord (43,44). Interestingly, responses to occlusion are frequently delayed, indicating that the effective stimulus is the development of cardiac ischemia (43). Laterally projecting STT cells with a given visceral input have cutaneous receptive fields within a restricted distribution (7,43). The locations of the cutaneous fields correspond to the distribution of referred pain for that particular organ system. Approximately 10% of the STT neurons in lamina X contain nitric oxide synthase, thus implicating NO in rostral transmission via the spinothalamic tract (315). The VPL projects to sensory cortex; thus, cells with localized receptive fields with responses that code for stimulus intensity are thought to be part of the classic sensory-discriminative pain system.

Cells that project to the medial nuclei, including the medial dorsal, central lateral, and posterior complex are concentrated in the deeper laminae (VII and VIII), but their lamina I component is equal to those projecting to VPL thalamus (2,194,571). The majority are high threshold, with large multilimb or whole-body receptive fields (8,196). After section of the cervical spinal cord of all but the contralateral ventral funiculus, the receptive field shrinks and includes only excitatory input from an ipsilateral segmental distribution. This implicates supraspinal structures in the control of their receptive field characteristics. Many exhibit a prominent afterdischarge for several seconds or more after the cessation of the stimulus (196). Cells that project to both lateral and medial thalamus most resemble the laterally projecting cells. Output of the medial system is to limbic areas, as well as frontal and parietal cortex. Thus, cells whose activation presumably leads to arousal have little spatial and temporal specificity, but instead signal the presence or absence of real or impending tissue damage.

Spinoreticular Tract

The spinoreticular tract refers collectively to spinal neurons that project to any of several reticular nuclei, including the lateral reticular nucleus, nucleus reticularis gigantocellularis, nucleus reticularus pontis caudalis and oralis, nucleus paragigantocellularis dorsalis, and lateralis and nucleus subcoeruleus (49,52,409). In the primate, spinoreticular tract (SRT) cells from the lumbar enlargement mainly project to the contralateral brainstem with a minor ipsilateral projection. In the cervical enlargement, however, the projection is strongly bilateral (281). In some cases neurons may have dual projections to the reticular formation and thalamus (282). The cells of origin are found primarily in the deep dorsal horn, although there are minor projections from laminae I and X, and in this way the cells resemble medially projecting STT cells. Receptive fields are large, frequently bilateral, and have complex excitatory and inhibitory components with cutaneous, deep, and/or visceral inputs (509,510). Cells respond to graded nociceptive visceral input in a dose-related manner (11). Although Thies and Foreman (509) reported that half of their sample of SRT cells had background firing rates of 1 Hz or less, many have high-background firing rates but no demonstrable excitatory input from the periphery, and are inhibited by low-threshold stimulation (210,454) (Fig. 16). Other SRT neurons have response properties and receptive field characteristics that resemble either medially or laterally projecting STT cells. The spinoreticular tract has recently been proposed as the ascending limb of the diffuse noxious inhibitory control or counterirritation system in man (134).

Spinomesencephalic Tract

The spinomesencephalic tract (SMT) is a collection of several discrete pathways projecting from the spinal cord to the midbrain. The projection extends from the superior colliculus to the rostral periaqueductal gray. The strongest projection is from lamina I with additional input from laminae IV through VIII and X (339,361,522,564). The lamina I component of the SMT appears to be larger than that of the STT (248). As was found for the STT, cells from the lumbar enlargement have a predominantly contralateral projection, while those from the upper cervical spinal cord project bilaterally. In the primate, approximately 15% of the cells projecting to the midbrain send a collateral to the lateral thalamus (595). Cells from lamina I selectively project to the lateral periaqueductal gray; in contrast, cells from the deeper laminae terminate in both the

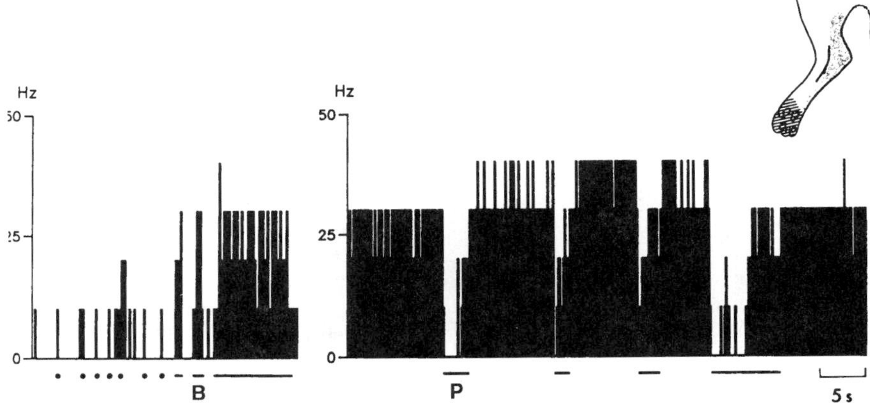

Figure 16. Peristimulus histograms illustrating the excitatory and inhibitory components of a deep-complex receptive field of a SRT neuron. Brushing the proximal foot and ankle (*stippled area, B*) excited the cell, while pinch applied to the distal paw (*hatched area P*) inhibited the discharge evoked by intracellular depolarizing current injection. (From ref. 454.)

lateral and medial portions (339). The lamina I SMT projection travels in the dorsolateral funiculus with the STT from the superficial dorsal horn.

Lamina I SMT cells are primarily nociceptive specific; only a few are of wide dynamic range and their receptive fields tend to be small (252,587,589). Those from the deeper laminae are more often WDRs; none are low threshold. The WDR cells generally have convergent input from subcutaneous tissues and fall into two categories. Some, including most of the cells that send collaterals to the lateral thalamus, have restricted excitatory receptive fields with prominent inhibitory input (588,589). Others, similar to the SRT cells, have complex, often discontinuous, excitatory and inhibitory fields encompassing most of the body. Many of these complex cells exhibit a prolonged afterdischarge following nociceptive stimulation. Some SMT cells, particularly those from lamina X, have a descending spinal projection as well as an ascending one to the midbrain (590). This implies a strong proprioceptive involvement.

Spinohypothalamic Tract

The spinohypothalamic tract (SHT) is a recently discovered direct projection transmitting primarily nociceptive information (48% WDR, 39% HT) from the spinal cord dorsal horn to the hypothalamus (74,75). As such it provides another route of activating the motivational-affect component of pain and initiating autonomic and neuroendocrine responses. Cells of origin are located throughout the dorsal horn with a significant fraction (37%) found in the superficial laminae. Receptive fields are generally small. Axons ascend in the contralateral dorsal or ventral lateral funiculi; the majority of SHT axons cross back to the side ipsilateral to their cell bodies within the supraoptic decussation of the hypothalamus before terminating (74,109), but there is a component that remains contralateral. This results in a bilateral projection.

Spinocervical Tract

Spinocervical tract cells, located in laminae I, III, and IV, project via the ipsilateral dorsal lateral funiculus to the lateral cervical nucleus (LCN), a nuclear group located ventrolateral to the dorsal horn within the C_1 to C_3 segments (57,115,121). The lamina I component terminates exclusively in the medial LCN, and the deeper cell bodies project to the lateral portions (115). The axons of most LCN cells decussate and continue to the lateral and posterior thalamus as well as to the midbrain. In humans, the existence of the LCN is controversial; its development varies among individuals (523). An alternate theory is that the LCN is present in humans it is just indistinct from the dorsal horn in many. There is spatial overlap in the thalamus among the terminations of the spinocervicothalamic tract, the STT, and axons from the dorsal column nuclei (41). Additionally, collaterals from cervicothalamic tract axons are thought to terminate in the mesencephalon in the monkey. Spinocervical tract cells have small cutaneous excitatory receptive fields; the major input comes from hair follicles. Many respond to nociceptive intensities of thermal stimulation (55,56,64,145), although this input can be excitatory or inhibitory (90). Small inhibitory fields responding to innocuous stimuli are eccentric to the excitatory field, while noxious stimulation in limbs distant to the excitatory field is also inhibitory. There is no evidence of visceral input. While many of the cells in both cat and monkey respond to nociceptive input, they rarely are excited exclusively by it (72,90). In the LCN, receptive fields are larger, and interestingly a greater percentage (7.5%) appear to be nociceptive specific. In the nonhuman primate, slightly more than half of the LCN cells respond differentially or exclusively to nociceptive stimuli (145). The spinocervicothalamic tract appears not to be of major significance as a sensory pathway in humans (574).

Postsynaptic Dorsal Column Pathway

In the monkey, cells of origin of the PSDC pathway are concentrated in laminae IV to VI (40,452); in the cervical enlargement these cells cluster in the medial dorsal horn, but in the lumbar enlargement they are found in the lateral dorsal horn. The axons ascend primarily through the dorsal columns to the ipsilateral dorsal column nuclei (DCN); axons originating from cervical levels give rise to a minor projection through the dorsal lateral funiculus also projecting to the DCN (195). Conduction velocity studies indicate that all axons are myelinated (14,58,526). The termination pattern of the PSDC axons within the DCN is separate and distinct from that of the primary afferent fibers (302). In the cat, the majority of the cells are multireceptive; they possess small inhibitory receptive fields usually proximal to the excitatory field (54,58). Inhibitory postsynaptic potentials are exclusively mediated by activation of low-threshold cutaneous afferents (259). Cells in the cat, but not the rat, code for nociceptive thermal input; however, it appears to be mediated by Aδ- and not C-polymodal nociceptors (193,273). Although these cells have not been studied electrophysiologically in the monkey, Vierck and Luck (536), using behavioral measures in the primate, have shown that section of the dorsal columns reduces responsiveness to strong nociceptive stimuli without changing responses to near threshold stimuli (536). This indicates a functional role for the PSDC pathway in the organized response to pain.

SEGMENTAL CONTROLS

In the preceding section, there is a clear organization that relates afferent input to the spinofugal outflow. This organization, however, leads to a perception that there is an unalterable relationship between stimulus intensity and the outflow of the system. In fact, the psychophysical data in humans (see Chap. 41) and animals (see Chap. 40) emphasize that the encoding process is extraordinarily plastic. The modifiability of the processing systems by bulbospinal (see Chap. 38) and by a variety of intrinsic (see Chaps. 34 and 36) systems is reviewed in detail elsewhere. However, a number of points should be noted at this point as regards the general organization of the modulatory influences that govern local traffic through the dorsal horn.

1. It is clear that modulation may be constituted by either an inhibition or suppression of the evoked or spontaneous activity of a cell, or it could reflect upon a facilitation of the response by that cell to excitatory input.
2. Modulation may influence afferent traffic by a number of neuronal mechanisms that involve interactions pre- and postsynaptic to the sensory afferent.
3. While a large historical literature has made modulation synonymous with an endogenous analgesic system, the function of these systems is not necessarily to render the animals nonresponsive to high-threshold stimuli, but to participate in the sensory encoding process.

Several examples are noted in the following subsections that reflect the above organizing comments.

Low-Threshold Afferent-Evoked Inhibition

An inhibition of spinal neurons can be initiated by the activation of large-diameter primary afferent fibers or their collaterals through the posterior columns. This includes a circuit initiated by activity in low-threshold afferents, resulting in primary afferent depolarization (157,295,545) and presynaptic inhibition of other primary afferents (258), including C fibers (77,173; for review see ref. 463). Primary afferent depolarization is thought to reduce the amount of neurotransmitter released by primary afferent fibers in response to a given afferent stimulus (163,463). In psychophysical experiments, natural activation of large myelinated fibers by application of vibratory stimuli produces a reduction of chronic pain (332) as well as an increase in pain thresholds in normal volunteers (165).

High-Threshold Afferent-Evoked Inhibition

Nociceptive stimulation, i.e., activation of fine primary afferent fibers, can activate inhibitory influence on dorsal horn neurons. Gerhardt et al. (187) demonstrated inhibition of evoked activity in WDR spinothalamic tract cells by high-intensity, but not low-intensity, stimulation of much of the body surface remote from the excitatory receptive field of spinal dorsal horn neurons. Spinal transection in the upper cervical spinal cord had only minimal effects, and a strong inhibition of the excitatory field remained. This finding indicates the presence of effective propriospinal inhibitory pathways. Similar spinal mechanisms are responsible for distant inhibitory receptive fields seen for viscerosomatic neurons. Distant noxious cutaneous stimulation inhibits visceral evoked nociceptive neurons (394), and conversely visceral stimulation distant from an excitatory cutaneous receptive field is also inhibitory (393). The strength of the inhibition is directly related to the intensity of the inhibitory stimulus. Both types of inhibition are present in spinal preparations, but spinalization has been shown to reduce the effect. Wide dynamic range neurons are more susceptible to heterosegmental inhibition than are nociceptive specific neurons; in one study 92% of WDR vs. 10% of HT cells were inhibited by distant nociceptive conditioning stimuli (394). Bulbospinal systems that release spinal monoamines (noradrenaline/serotonin) by a spino-bulbospinal loop have been shown to be activated by C-fiber stimulation (525). Spinal monoaminergic tone has been shown to exert a powerful inhibitory effect over small afferent-evoked activity (see Chaps. 36 and 38).

Bulbospinal-Mediated Inhibition

Tonic inhibition from the brainstem can shift cells from one cell response type to another (546), decrease receptive field size (223,402), and mask C-fiber input (214,304). Some of these tonic effects are mediated by 5-HT, as methysergide, a 5-HT antagonist administered to awake cats, increases receptive field size and sensitivity to noxious stimuli as well as converts some LT cells to WDRs (455). Thermal sensitivity in dorsal horn neurons is also decreased by tonic descending modulatory effects (141). Laird and Cervero (304) have estimated that over half of the WDR neurons and all of the high-threshold neurons are subject to tonic descending inhibition. Chronic pain states, such as arthritis, increase the ongoing level of descending inhibition (460), reaching dorsal horn projection cells, and increase the monoamine content of the spinal cord (550). A lower proportion of cells is influenced by a tonic supraspinal excitation (141,304). Low-threshold cells are the least influenced by tonic supraspinal modulation, either inhibitory or excitatory. Viscerosomatic cells are subject to both tonic inhibition and excitation, but the visceral component appears to be the focus of greater modulation (505). The majority of viscerosomatic cells in lamina V are tonically inhibited; however, overall a significantly larger percent of viscerosomatic cells than somatic cells is subject to descending excitation. Further discussion of the effects of and role played by the bulbospinal systems can be found in Chap. 38.

Small Afferent-Evoked Facilitation

As noted above, populations of cells refereed to as wide dynamic range neurons receive convergent input from large (A) and small (C) afferents. Early work by Mendell (358) describing these convergent neurons also noted that repetitive small afferent input would yield a facilitated discharge that was described as "wind up." This facilitated state is characterized by an enhanced response to a moderately intense stimulus and increases the receptive field size of the neuron (577). This phenomenon has been shown to have behavioral prominence as a likely mechanism underlying the state of hyperalgesia in humans (see Chap. 41) and animals (see Chap. 40). The pharmacology of this state suggests an important role for a number of spinal neurohumoral-receptor systems, including those for glutamate (see Chap. 60), cyclooxygenase products (see Chap. 61), and nitric oxide (see Chap. 36).

Interneurons and Large Afferent Input

An important component in the encoding process is the frequent assumption that information generated by high-threshold afferents can evoke a pain response, while input from a low-threshold mechanoreceptive afferent does not. This suggests an intrinsic aspect of the organization of the spinal afferent processing. It is clear, however, that the "nonnoxious" character of the encoding process is not a simple function of the connectivity. It has been shown that the spinal delivery of a $GABA_A$ or a glycine receptor antagonist can induce an exaggerated response to low-threshold mechanical stimuli (284,583; Puig and Sorkin, *unpublished observation*). Loss of glycinergic binding in certain mutant animal models gives a similar behavioral correlate (209,562). These observations suggest that the spinal GABAergic and glycinergic interneurons in the dorsal horn (see references provided above) systems have a high level of tonic or evoked activity. Accordingly, transient blockade of their function yields a spinal processing system in which low-threshold afferent input is responded to as if noxious. This mechanisms may play an important role in certain postnerve injury pain states in which central changes may occur leading to the clinical syndrome of causalgia (see Chaps. 36 and 56).

REFERENCES

1. Aimi Y, Fujimura M, Vincent SR, Kimura H. Localization of NADPH-diaphorase-containing neurons in sensory ganglia of the rat. *J Comp Neurol* 1991;306:382–392.
2. Albe-Fessard D, Boivie J, Grant G, Levante A. Labelling of cells in the medulla oblongata and the spinal cord of the monkey after injections of horseradish peroxidase in the thalamus. *Neurosci Lett* 1975;1:75–80.
3. Alhaider AA, Lei SZ, Wilcox GL. Spinal 5-HT3 receptor-mediated antinociception: possible release of GABA. *J Neurosci* 1991;11: 1881–1888.
4. Ali Z, Wu G, Kozlov A, Barasi S. The actions of 5HT1 agonists and antagonists on nociceptive processing in the rat spinal cord: results from behavioural and electrophysiological studies. *Brain Res* 1994; 661:83–90.
5. Allen JM, Gibson SJ, Adrian TE, Polak JM, Bloom SR. Neuropeptide Y in human spinal cord. *Brain Res* 1984;308:145–148.
6. Alvarez FJ, Kavookjian AM, Light AR. Ultrastructural morphology, synaptic relationships, and CGRP immunoreactivity of physiologically identified C-fiber terminals in the monkey spinal cord. *J Comp Neurol* 1993;329:472–490.
7. Ammons WS. Electrophysiological characteristics of primate spinothalamic tract cells with renal and somatic inputs. *J Neurophysiol* 1989;61:1121–1130.
8. Ammons WS, Girirdot M-N, Foreman RD. T_2-T_5 spinothalamic neurons projecting to medial thalamus with viscerosomatic input. *J Neurophysiol* 1985;54:73–89.
9. Ammons WS. Characteristics of spinoreticuler and spinothalamic neurons with renal input. *J Neurophysiol* 1987;50:480–495.
10. Ammons WS. Renal afferent input to thoracolumbar spinal neurons of the cat. *Am J Physiol* 1986;250:R435–R443.
11. Ammons WS. Responses of spinoreticular cells to graded increases in renal venous pressure. *Am J Physiol* 1991;260:R27–31.
12. Anand P, Gibson SJ, McGregor GP, Blank MA, Ghatei MA, Bacarese-Hamilton AJ, Polak JM, Bloom SR. A VIP-containing system concentrated in the lumbosacral region of human spinal cord. *Nature* 1983;305:143–145.

13. Anderson CR. NADPH diaphorase-positive neurons in the rat spinal cord include a subpopulation of autonomic preganglionic neurons. *Neurosci Lett* 1992;139:280–284.
14. Angaut-Petit D. The dorsal column system II. Functional properties and bulbar relay of the postsynaptic fibres of the cat's fasciculus gracilis. *Exp Brain Res* 1975;22:471–493.
15. Antal M, Polgar E, Chalmers J, Minson JB, Llewellyn-Smith I, Heizmann CW, Somogyi P. Different populations of parvalbumin- and calbindin-D28k-immunoreactive neurons contain GABA and accumulate ^{3}H-D-aspartate in the dorsal horn of the rat spinal cord. *J Comp Neurol* 1991;314:114–124.
16. Apkarian AV, Hodge CJ. A dorsolateral spinothalamic tract in macaque monkey. *Pain*;1989:37:323–333.
17. Apkarian AV, Hodge CJ. Primate spinothalamic pathways: I. A quantitative study of the cells of origin of the spinothalamic pathway. *J Comp Neurol* 1989;288:447–473.
18. Apkarian AV, Hodge CJ. Primate spinothalamic pathways: II. The cells of origin of the dorsolateral and ventrolateral pathways. *J Comp Neurol* 1989;288:474–492.
19. Apkarian AV, Hodge CJ. Primate spinothalamic pathways: III. Thalamic terminations of the dorsolateral and ventral spinothalamic pathways. *J Comp Neurol* 1989;288:493–511.
20. Applebaum EA, Beall JE, Foreman RD, Willis WD. Organization and receptive fields of primate spinothalamic tract neurons. *J Neurophysiol* 1975;38:572–586.
21. Aronin N, Difiglia M, Liotta A, Martin J. Ultrastructural localization and biochemical features of immunoreactive leu-enkephalin in monkey dorsal horn. *J Neurosci* 1981;1:561–577.
22. Arvidsson U, Schalling M, Cullheim S, Ulfhake B, Terenius L, Verhofstad A, Hökfelt T. Evidence for coexistence between calcitonin gene-related peptide and serotonin in the bulbospinal pathway in the monkey. *Brain Res* 1990;532:47–57.
23. Arvidsson U, Ulfhake B, Cullheim S, Bergstrand A, Theodorsson E, Hökfelt T. Distribution of ^{125}I-galanin binding sites, immunoreactive galanin, and its coexistence with 5-hydroxytryptamine in the cat spinal cord: biochemical, histochemical, and experimental studies at the light and electron microscopic level. *J Comp Neurol* 1991;308:115–138.
24. Arvidsson U, Ulfhake B, Cullheim S, Shupliakov O, Brodin E, Franck J, Bennett GW, Fone KC, Visser TJ, Hökfelt T. Thyrotropin-releasing hormone (TRH)-like immunoreactivity in the grey monkey (Macaca fascicularis) spinal cord and medulla oblongata with special emphasis on the bulbospinal tract. *J Comp Neurol* 1992;322:293–310.
25. Atkinson ME, Shehab SAS. Peripheral axotomy of the rat mandibular trigeminal nerve leads to an increase in VIP and decrease of other primary afferent neuropeptides in the spinal trigeminal nucleus. *Reg Peptides* 1986;16:69–82.
26. Barber RP, Phelps PE, Houser CR, Crawford GD, Salvaterra PM, Vaughn JE. The morphology and distribution of neurons containing choline acetyltransferase in the adult rat spinal cord: an immunocytochemical study. *J Comp Neurol* 1984;229:329–346.
27. Barber RP, Vaughn JE, Roberts E. The cytoarchitecture of gabaergic neurons in rat spinal cord. *Brain Res* 1982;238:305–328.
28. Barber RP, Vaughn JE, Saito K, McLaughlin BJ, Roberts E. GABAergic terminals are presynaptic to primary afferent terminals in the substantia gelatinosa of the rat spinal cord. *Brain Res* 1978;141: 35–55.
29. Barker D. The structure and distribution of muscle receptors. In: Barker D, ed. *Symposium on muscle receptors.* Hong Kong: Hong Kong University Press, 1962;227–240.
30. Basbaum AI, Glazer EJ, Oertel W. Immunoreactive glutamic acid decarboxylase in the trigeminal nucleus caudalis of the cat: A light- and electron-microscopic analysis. *Somatosensory Res* 1986; 4:77–94.
31. Basbaum AI, Glazer EJ. Immunoreactive vasoactive intestinal polypeptide is concentrated in the sacral spinal cord: A possible marker for pelvic visceral afferent fibers. *Somatosensory Res* 1983;1: 69–82.
32. Battaglia G, Rustioni A. Coexistence of glutamate and substance P in dorsal root ganglion neurons of the rat and monkey. *J Comp Neurol* 1988;277:302–312.
33. Battaglia G, Rustioni A. Substance P innervation of the rat and cat thalamus II. Cells of origin in the spinal cord. *J Comp Neurol* 1992; 315:473–486.
34. Beal JA, Bicknell HR. Primary afferent distribution pattern in the marginal zone (lamina I) of adult monkey and cat lumbosacral spinal cord. *J Comp Neurol* 1981;202:255–263.
35. Beal JA, Cooper MH. The neurons in the gelatinosal complex (laminae II and III) of the monkey (Macaca mulatta): a Golgi study. *J Comp Neurol* 1978;179:89–122.
36. Beal JA, Penny JE, Bicknell HR. Structural diversity of marginal (lamina I) neurons in the adult monkey (Macaca mulatta) lumbosacral spinal cord: a Golgi study. *J Comp Neurol* 1981; 202:237–254.
37. Beal JA, Russell CT, Knight DS. Morphological and development characterization of local circuit neurons in lamina III of rat spinal cord. *Neurosci Lett* 1988;86:1–5.
38. Bennett GJ, Abdelmoumene M, Hayashi H, Hoffert MJ, Dubner R. Spinal cord layer I neurons with axon collaterals that generate local arbors. *Brain Res* 1981;209:421–426.
39. Bennett GJ, Nishikawa N, Lu GW, Hoffert MJ, Dubner R. The morphology of dorsal column postsynaptic (DCPS) spinomedullary neurons in the cat. *J Comp Neurol* 1984;224:568–578.
40. Bennett GJ, Seltzer Z, Lu GW, Nishikawa N, Dubner R. The cells of origin of the dorsal column postsynaptic projection in the lumbosacral enlargements of cats and monkeys. *Somatosens Res* 1983;1: 131–149.
41. Berkley KJ. Special relationships between the terminations of somatic sensory and motor pathways in the rostral brainstem of cats and monkeys. 1. Ascending somatic sensory inputs to lateral diencephalon. *J Comp Neurol* 1980;186:283–317.
42. Beyer C, Banas C, Gomora P, Komisaruk BR. Prevention of the convulsant and hyperalgesic action of strychnine by intrathecal glycine and related amino acids. *Pharmacol Biochem Behav* 1988;29:73–78.
43. Blair RW, Ammons WS, Foreman RD. Responses of thoracic spinothalamic and spinoreticular cells to coronary artery occlusion. *J Neurophysiol* 1984;51:636–648.
44. Blair RW, Weber RN, Foreman RD. Characteristics of primate spinothalamic tract neurons receiving viscerosomatic convergent inputs in the T_3-T_5 segments. *J Neurophysiol* 1981;46:797–811.
45. Boive J. An anatomical reinvestigation of the termination of the spinothalamic tract in monkey. *J Comp Neurol* 1979;186:343–370.
46. Borges LF, Iversen SD. Topography of choline acetyltransferase immunoreactive neurons and fibers in the rat spinal cord. *Brain Res* 1986;362:140–148.
47. Bowker RM. Instrinsic 5HT-immunoreactive neurons in the spinal cord of the fetal non-human primate. *Dev Brain Res* 1986;28: 137–143.
48. Bowsher D, Abdel-Maguid TE. Superficial dorsal horn of the adult human spinal cord. *Neurosurgery* 1984;15:893–899.
49. Bowsher D, Westman J. The gigantocellular reticular region and its spinal afferents: a light and electron microscopic studying the cat. *J Anat* 1970;106:23–36.
50. Bowsher D. The termination of secondary somatosensory neurons within the thalamus of *Macaca mulatta*: an experimental degeneration study. *J Comp Neurol* 1961;117:213–227.
51. Braas KM, Newby AC, Wilson VS, Snyder SH. Adenosine-containing neurons in the brain localized by immunocytochemistry. *J Neurosci* 1986;6:1952–1961.
52. Brodal A. *The reticular formation of the brain stem. Anatomical aspects and functional correlations.* Edinburgh: Oliver and Boyd, 1957.
53. Broman J, Anderson S, Ottersen OP. Enrichment of glutamate-like immunoreactivity in primary afferent terminals throughout the spinal cord dorsal horn. *Eur J Neurosci* 1993;5:1050–1061.
54. Brown AG, Brown PB, Fyffe REW, Pubols LM. Receptive field organization and response properties of spinal neurones with axons ascending the dorsal columns in the cat. *J Physiol* 1983;337: 575–588.
55. Brown AG, Franz DN. Patterns of response in spinocervical tract neurones to different stimuli of long duration. *Brain Res* 1970;17: 156–160.
56. Brown AG, Franz DN. Responses of spinocervical tract neurones to natural stimulation of identified cutaneous receptors. *Exp Brain Res* 1969;7:231–249.
57. Brown AG, Fyffe REW, Noble R, Rose PK, Snow PJ. The density, distribution and topographical organization of spinocervical tract neurones in the cat. *J Physiol* 1980;300:409–428.
58. Brown AG, Fyffe REW. Form and function of dorsal horn neurones with axons ascending the dorsal columns in cat. *J Physiol* 1981;321: 31–47.
59. Brown AG, Hamann WC, Martin HF. Effects of activity in non-myelinated afferent fibres on the spinocervical tract. *Brain Res* 1975;98:719–738.
60. Brown AG, Noble R, Riddell JS. Relations between spinocervical

and postsynaptic dorsal column neurones in the cat. *J Physiol* 1986; 381:333–349.

61. Brown AG, Rose PK, Snow PJ. Morphology of hair follicle afferent fibre collaterals in the cat spinal cord. *J Physiol (Lond)* 1977;272: 770–797.
62. Brown AG, Rose PK, Snow PJ. The morphology of spinocervical tract neurones revealed by intracellular injection of horseradish peroxidase. *J Physiol* 1977b;270:747–764.
63. Brown AG. Ascending and long spinal pathways: dorsal columns spinocervical tract and spinothalamic tract. In: Iggo A, ed. *Somatosensory system*, vol 2. Berlin, Heidelberg, New York: Springer-Verlag, 1973;315–338.
64. Brown AG. Effects of descending impulses on transmission through the spinocervical tract. *J Physiol* 1971;219:103–125.
65. Brown AG. *Organization in the spinal cord: The anatomy and physiology of identified neurones.* New York: Springer-Verlag, 1981.
66. Brown AG. The terminations of cutaneous nerve fibres in the spinal cord. *Trends Neurosci* 1981;4:64–67.
67. Brown PB, and Koerber HR. Cat hindlimb tactile dermatomes determined with single unit recordings. *J Neurophysiol* 1978;41: 260–267.
68. Brown PB, Fuchs JL. Somatotopic representation of hindlimb skin in cat dorsal horn. *J Neurophysiol* 1975;38:1–9.
69. Brown PB, Gladfelter WE, Culberson JL, Covalt-Dunning D, Sonty RV, Pubols LM, Millecchia RJ. Somatotopic organization of single primary afferent axon projections to cat spinal dorsal horn. *J Neurosci* 1991;11:289–309.
70. Bruggencate GT, Engberg I. Analysis of glycine actions on spinal interneurons by intracellular recording. *Brain Res* 1968; 11:446–450.
71. Bruning G. Localization of NADPH diaphorase, a histochemical marker for nitric oxide synthase, in the mouse spinal cord. *Acta Histochem* 1992;93:397–401.
72. Bryan RN, Coulter JD, Willis WD. Cells of origin of the spinocervical tract in the monkey. *Exp Neurol* 1974;42:574–586.
73. Bryan RN, Trevino DL, Coulter JD, Willis WD. Location and somatotopic organization of the cells of origin of the spino-cervical tract. *Exp Brain Res* 1973;17:177–189.
74. Burstein R, Cliffer KD, Giesler GJ Jr. Direct somatosensory projections from the spinal cord to the hypothalamus and telencephalon. *J Neurosci* 1987;7:4159–4164.
75. Burstein R, Dado RJ, Cliffer KD, Giesler GJ Jr. Physiological characterization of spinohypothalamic tract neurons in the lumbar enlargement of rats. *J Neurophysiol* 1991;66:261–284.
76. Burstein R, Dado RJ, Giesler GJ. The cells of origin of the spinothalamic tract of the rat: a quantitative reexamination. *Brain Res* 1990;511:329–337.
77. Calvillo O, Madrid J, Rudomin P. Presynaptic depolarization of unmyelinated primary afferent fibers in the spinal cord of the cat. *Neurosci* 1982;7:1389–1400.
78. Campistron G, Buijs RM, Geffard M. Glycine neurons in the brain and spinal cord. Antibody production and immunocytochemical localization. *Brain Res* 1986;376:400–405.
79. Carlton SM, Hayes ES. Light microscopic and ultrastructural analysis of GABA-immunoreactive profiles in the monkey spinal cord. *J Comp Neurol* 1990;300:162–182.
80. Carlton SM, Honda CN, Denoroy L, Willis WD. Descending pheylethanolamine-N-methyltransferase projections to the monkey spinal cord: an immunohistochemical double labeling study. *Neurosci Lett* 1987;76:133–139.
81. Carlton SM, Honda CN, Willcockson WS, Lacrampe M, Zhang D, Denoroy L, Chung JM, Willis WD. Descending adrenergic input to the primate spinal cord and its possible role in modulation of spinothalamic cells. *Brain Res* 1991;543:77–90.
82. Carlton SM, McNeill DL, Chung K, Coggeshall RE. A light and electron microscopic level analysis of calcitonin gene-related peptide (CGRP) in the spinal cord of the primate: an immunohistochemical study. *Neurosci Lett* 1987;82:145–150.
83. Carlton SM, McNeill DL, Chung K, Coggeshall RE. Organization of calcitonin gene-related peptide-immunoreactive terminals in the primate dorsal horn. *J Comp Neurol* 1988;276:527–536.
84. Carlton SM, Westlund KN, Zhang D, Willis WD. GABA-immunoreactive terminals synapse on primate spinothalamic tract cells. *J Comp Neurol* 1992;322:528–537.
85. Carstens E, Trevino DL. Laminar origins of spinothalamic projections in the cat as determined by the retrograde transport of horseradish peroxidase. *J Comp Neurol* 1978;182:151–166.
86. Castro-Lopes LM, Tavares I, Coimbra A. GABA decreases in the spinal cord dorsal horn after peripheral neurectomy. *Brain Res* 1993;620:287–291.
87. Cervero F, Connell LA. Distribution of somatic and visceral primary afferent fibres within the thoracic spinal cord of the cat. *J Comp Neurol* 1984;230:88–98.
88. Cervero F, Connell LA. Fine afferent fibers from viscera do not terminate in the substantia gelatinosa of the thoracic spinal cord. *Brain Res* 1984;294:370–374.
89. Cervero F, Iggo A, Molony V. An electrophysiological study of the neurones in the substantia gelatinosa Rolandi of the cat's spinal cord. *Q J Exp Physiol* 1979;64:297–314.
90. Cervero F, Iggo A, Molony V. Responses of spinocervical tract neurones to noxious stimulation of the skin. *J Physiol* 1977;267: 537–558.
91. Cervero F, Iggo A, Molony V. Segmental and intersegmental organization of neurones in the substantia gelatinosa Rolandi of the cat's spinal cord. *Q J Exp Physiol* 1979;64:315–326.
92. Cervero F, Iggo A, Ogawa H. Nociceptor driven dorsal horn neurones in the lumbar spinal cord of the cat. *Pain* 1976;2:5–24.
93. Cervero F, Molony V, Iggo A. Extracellular and intracellular recordings from neurons in the substantia gelatinosa Rolandi. *Brain Res* 1977;136:565–569.
94. Cervero F, Molony V, Iggo A. Supraspinal linkage of substantia gelatinosa neurones: effects of descending impulses. *Brain Res* 1979;175:351–355.
95. Cervero F, Tattersall JEM. Cutaneous receptive fields of somatic and viscerosomatic neurones in the thoracic spinal cord of the cat. *J Comp Neurol* 1985;237:325–332.
96. Cervero F. Somatic and visceral inputs to the thoracic spinal cord of the cat: effects of noxious stimulation of the biliary system. *J Physiol* 1983;337:51–67.
97. Cervero, F., Iggo, A. The substantia gelatinosa of the spinal cord. A critical review. *Brain* 1980.
98. Ch'ng JLC, Christofides ND, Anand P, Gibson SJ, Allen YS, Su HC, Tatemoto K, Morrison JFB, Polak JM, Bloom SR. Distribution of galanin immunoreactivity in the central nervous system and the responses of galanin-containing neuronal pathways to injury. *Neuroscience* 1985;16:343–354.
99. Chapman V, Dickenson AH. The effects of sandostatin and somatostatin on nociceptive transmission in the dorsal horn of the rat spinal cord. *Neuropeptides* 1992;23:147–152.
100. Cho HJ, Basbaum AI. Increased staining of immunoreactive dynorphin cell bodies in the deafferented spinal cord of the rat. *Neurosci Lett* 1988;84:125–130.
101. Cho HJ, Basbaum AI. Ultrastructural analysis of dynorphin B-immunoreactive cells and terminals in the superficial dorsal horn of the deafferented spinal cord of the rat. *J Comp Neurol* 1989;281: 193–205.
102. Choca JI, Green RD, Proudfit HK. Adenosine A1 and A2 receptors of the substantia gelatinosa and located predominantly on intrinsic neurons: an autoradiograph study. *J Pharmacol Exp Ther* 1988; 247:757–764.
103. Christensen BN, Perl ER. Spinal neurons specifically excited by noxious or thermal stimuli: marginal zone of the dorsal horn. *J Neurophysiol* 1970;33:293–307.
104. Chronwall BM, DiMaggio DA, Massari VJ, Pickel VM, Ruggiero DA, O'Donohue TL. The anatomy of neuropeptide-Y-containing neurons in rat brain. *Neuroscience* 1985;15:1159–1181.
105. Chung JM, Surmeier DJ, Lee KH, Soirkin LS, Honda CN, Tsong Y, Willis WD. Classification of primate spinothalamic and somatosensory thalamic neurons based on cluster analysis. *J Neurophysiol* 1986;56:308–327.
106. Chung K, Coggeshall RE. The ratio of dorsal root ganglion cells to dorsal root axons in sacral segments of the cat. *J Comp Neurol* 1984;225: 24–30.
107. Chung K, Lee WT, Carlton SM. The effects of dorsal rhizotomy and spinal cord isolation on calcitonin gene-related peptide-labeled terminals in the rat lumbar dorsal horn. *Neurosci Lett* 1988; 90:27–32.
108. Clarke JL. Further researches on the grey substance of the spinal cord. *Philos Trans R Soc Lond* 1959;149:437–467.
109. Cliffer KD, Burstein R, Giesler GJ Jr. Distribution of spinothalamic, spinohypothalamic and spinotelencephalic fibers revealed by anterograde transport of PHA-L in rats. *J Neurosci* 1991;11: 852–868.
110. Cliffer KD, Cameron AA, Dougherty PM, Willis WD, Carlton SM. Histochemical changes in gracile nucleus following experimental peripheral neuropathy in the sciatic nerve of rats. *Neurosci Abs* 1991b;17:436.

111. Clifton GL, Coggeshall RE, Vance WH, Willis WD. Receptive fields of unmyelinated ventral root afferent fibres in the cat. *J Physiol* 1976;256:573–600.
112. Coffield JA, Miletic V, Zimmermann E, Hoffert MJ, Brooks BR. Demonstration of thyrotropin-releasing hormone immunoreactivity in neurons of the mouse spinal dorsal horn. *J Neurosci* 1986;6:1194–1197.
113. Coggeshall RE, Coulter JD, Willis WD. Unmyelinated axons in the ventral roots of the cat lumbosacral enlargement. *J Comp Neurol* 1974;153:39–58.
114. Coggeshall RE, Ito H. Sensory fibres in ventral roots L7 and S1 in the cat. *J Physiol* 1977;267:215–235.
115. Craig AD, Broman J, Blomqvist A. Lamina I spinocervical terminations in the medial part of the lateral cervical nucleus in the cat. *J Comp Neurol* 1992;322:99–110.
116. Craig AD, Burton H. Spinal and medullary lamina I projection to nucleus submedius in medial thalamus: a possible pain center. *J Neurophysiol* 1981;45:443–466.
117. Craig AD, Hunsley SJ. Morphine enhances the thermoreceptive cold-specific Lamina I spinothalamic neurons in the cat. *Brain Res* 1991;558:93–97.
118. Craig AD, Kniffki KD. Spinothalamic lumbosacral lamina I cells responsive to skin and muscle stimulation in the cat. *J Physiol* 1985;365:197–221.
119. Craig AD, Linington AJ, Kniffki KD. Cells of origin of spinothalamic projections to medial and/or lateral thalamus in the cat. *J Comp Neurol* 1989;289:568–585.
120. Craig AD. Organization of lamina I terminations in the posterior thalamus of the cynomolgus monkey. *Neurosci Abs* 1992;18:385.
121. Craig AD. Spinal and medullary input to the lateral cervical nucleus. *J Comp Neurol* 1978;181:729–744.
122. Craig AD. Spinal distribution of ascending lamina I axons anterogradely labeled with Phaseolus vulgaris leucoagglutinin (PHA-L) in the cat. *J Comp Neurol* 1991;131:377–393.
123. Cridland RA, Henry JL. Effects of intrathecal administration of neuropeptides on a spinal nociceptive reflex in the rat: VIP, galanin, CGRP, TRH, somatostatin, and angiotensin II. *Neuropeptides* 1988;11:23–32.
124. Crowe R, Burnstock G. An increase of vasoactive intestinal polypeptide-, but not neuropeptide Y-, substance P- and catecholamine-containing nerves in the iris of the streptozotocin-induced diabetic rat. *Exp Eye Res* 1988;263:539–562.
125. Cruz L, Basbaum AI. Multiple opioid peptides and the modulation of pain: immunohistochemical analysis of dynorphin and enkephalin in the trigeminal nucleus caudalis and spinal cord of the cat. *J Comp Neurol* 1985;240:331–348.
126. Curtis DR, Hösli L, Johnston GAR, Johnston IH. Glycine and spinal inhibition. *Brain Res* 1967;5:112–114.
127. Curtis DR, Hösli L, Johnston GAR. A pharmacological study of the depression of spinal neurones by glycine and related amino acids. *Exp Brain Res* 1968;6:1–18.
128. Curtis DR, Hösli L, Johnston GAR. Inhibition of spinal neurones by glycine. *Nature* 1967;215:1502–1503.
129. Curtis DR, Phillis JW, Watkins JC. The depression of spinal neurones by gamma-aminobutyric acid and β-alanine. *J Physiol* 1959;146:185–203.
130. Dahlstrom A, Fuxe K. Evidence for the existence of monoamine neurons in the central nervous system. II. Experimentally induced changes in the intraneuronal amine levels of bulbospinal neuron systems. *Acta Physiol Scand* 1965;64:1–36.
131. Dalsgaard CJ, Hökfelt T, Johansson O, Elde R. Somatostatin immunoreactive cell bodies in the dorsal horn and the parasympathetic intermediolateral nucleus of the rat spinal cord. *Neurosci Lett* 1981;27:335–339.
132. De Biasi S, Rustioni A. Glutamate and substance P coexist in primary afferent terminals in the superficial laminae of spinal cord. *Proc Natl Acad Sci USA* 1988;85:7820–7824.
134. De Broucker T, Cesaro P, Willer JC, Le Bars D. Diffuse noxious inhibitory controls in man. Involvement of the spinoreticular tract. *Brain* 1990;113:1223–1234.
135. DeGroat WC, Kawatani M, Hisamitsu T, Lowe I, Morgan C, Roppolo J, Booth AM, Nadelhaft I. The role of neuropeptides in the sacral autonomic reflex of the cat. *J Auton Nerv Syst* 1983;7:339–350.
136. DeGroat WC, Nadelhaft I, Milne RJ, Booth AM, Morgan C, Thor K. Organization of the sacral parasympathetic reflex pathways to the urinary bladder and large intestine. *J Auton Nerv Syst* 1981;3:135–160.
137. DeGroat WC, Nadelhaft I, Morgan C, Schauble T. Horseradish peroxidase tracing of visceral efferent and primary afferent pathways in the sacral spinal cord of the cat using benzidine processing. *Neurosci Lett* 1978;10:103–108.
138. Del Fiacco M, Cuello AC. Substance P- and enkephalin-containing neurons in the rat trigeminal system. *Neuroscience* 1980;5:803–815.
139. DeQuidt ME, Emson PC. Distribution of neuropeptide Y-like immunoreactivity in the rat central nervous system. II. Immunohistochemical analysis. *Neuroscience* 1986;18:545–618.
140. Dickenson AH, Sullivan A, Feeney C, Fournie-Zaluski MC, Roques BP. Evidence that endogenous enkephalins produce delta-opiate receptor mediated neuronal inhibitions in rat dorsal horn. *Neurosci Lett* 1986;72:179–182.
141. Dickhaus H, Pauser G, Zimmermann M. Tonic descending inhibition affects the intensity coding on nociceptive responses in spinal dorsal horn neurones in the cat. *Pain* 1985;23:145–158.
142. Difiglia M, Aronin N, Leeman SE. Immunocytochemical study of neurotensin localization in the monkey spinal cord. *Ann N Y Acad Sci* 1982;400:405–408.
143. Difiglia M, Aronin N, Leeman SE. Ultrastructural localization of immunoreactive neurotensin in the monkey superficial dorsal horn. *J Comp Neurol* 1984;225:1–12.
144. Dimsdale JA, Kemp JM. Afferent fibres in ventral nerve roots in the rat. *J Physiol (Lond)* 1966;187:25–26.
145. Downie JW, Ferrington DG, Sorkin LS, Willis WD. The primate spinocervicothalamic pathway: responses of cells in the lateral cervical nucleus and spinocervical tract to innocuous and noxious stimuli. *J Neurophysiol* 1988;59:861–885.
146. Doyle CA, Maxwell DJ. Light- and electron-microscopic analysis of neuropeptide Y-immunoreactive profiles in the cat spinal dorsal horn. *Neuroscience* 1994;61:107–121.
147. Dubner R, Ruda MA. Activity-dependent neuronal plasticity following tissue injury and inflammation. *TINS* 1992;15:96–102.
148. Duggan AW, Hall JG, Headley PM. Enkephalins and dorsal horn neurones of the cat: effects on responses to noxious and innocuous skin stimuli. *Br J Pharmacol* 1977;61:399–408.
149. Duggan AW, Hall JG, Headley PM. Morphine, enkephalin and the substantia gelatinosa. *Nature* 1976;264:456–458.
150. Duggan AW, Johnson SM, Morton CR. Differing distributions of receptors for morphine and met5-enkephalinamide in the dorsal horn of the cat. *Brain Res* 1981;229:379–387.
151. Duggan AW, Johnston GAR. Glutamate and related amino acids in cat spinal roots, dorsal root ganglia and peripheral nerves. *J Neurochem* 1970;17:1205–1208.
152. Duggan AW, North RA. Electrophysiology of opioids. *Pharmacol Rev* 1984;35:219–281.
153. Duggan AW;Schaible HG; Hope PJ; Lang CW. Effect of peptidase inhibition on the pattern of intraspinally released immunoreactive substance P detected with antibody microprobes. *Brain Res* 1992;579:261–269.
154. Dun NJ, Dun SL, Forstermann U, Tseng LF. Nitric oxide synthase immunoreactivity in rat spinal cord. *Neurosci Lett* 1992;147:217–220.
155. Eccles JC, Eccles RM, Lundberg A. Types of neurons in and around the intermediate nucleus of the lumbosacral cord. *J Physiol* 1960;154:89–114.
156. Eccles JC, Kostyuk PG, Schmidt RF. Central pathways responsible for depolarization of primary afferent fibres. *J Physiol* 1962;161:237–257.
157. Eccles JC, Krnjevic K. Potential changes recorded inside primary afferent fibres within the spinal cord. *J Physiol* 1959;149:250–273.
158. Eccles JC, Magni F, Willis WD. Depolarization of central terminals of group I afferent fibres from muscle. *J Physiol* 1962;160:62–93.
159. Eccles JC, Schmidt R, Willis WD. Pharmacological studies on presynaptic inhibition. *J Physiol* 1963;168:500–530.
160. Eccles JC, Schmidt RF, Willis WD. Depolarization of central terminals of group Ib afferent fibers of muscle. *J Neurophysiol* 1963;26:1–27.
161. Eccles JC, Schmidt RF, Willis WD. Depolarization of the central terminals of cutaneous afferent fibers. *J Neurophysiol* 1963;26:646–661.
162. Eccles JC, Schmidt RF, Willis WD. The location and the mode of action of the presynaptic inhibitory pathways on to group I afferent fibers from muscle. *J Neurophysiol* 1963;26:506–522.
163. Eccles JC. *The physiology of synapses.* New York: Springer, 1964.
164. Edinger, L. Vorlesungen uber der Bau der nervosen Zentralorgane, Leipzig, vol 1. 1904. In: Keele, KD, ed. *Anatomies of pain.* Charles Thomas, Springfield, IL. 1957;119.

165. Ekblom A, Hansson P. Effects of conditioning vibratory stimulation on pain threshold of the human tooth. *Acta Physiol Scand* 1982;114:601–604.
166. El-Yassar N, Fleetwood-Walker SM, A 5HT-1 receptor mediates the antinociceptive effect of nucleus raphe magnus stimulation in the rat. *Brain Res* 1990;523:92–99.
167. Elde R, Hökfelt T, Johansson O, Terenius L. Immunohistochemical studies using antibodies to leucine-enkephalin: Initial observations on the nervous system of the rat. *Neurosci* 1976;1: 349–350.
168. Ferrington DG, Sorkin LS, Willis. Responses of spinothalamic tract cells in the superficial dorsal horn of the primate lumbar spinal cord. *J Physiol* 1987;388:681–703.
169. Fiallos-Estrada CE, Kummer W, Mayer B, Bravo R, Zimmermann M, Herdegen T. Long-lasting increase of nitric oxide synthase immunoreactivity, NADPH-diaphorase reaction and c-JUN co-expression in rat dorsal root ganglion neurons following sciatic nerve transection. *Neurosci Lett* 1993;150:169–173.
170. Fields HL, Clanton CH, Anderson SD. Somatosensory properties of spinoreticular neurons in the cat. *Brain Res* 1977;120:49–66.
171. Finley JCW, Maderdrut JL, Petrusz P. The immunocytochemical localization of enkephalin in the central nervous system of the rat. *J Comp Neurol* 1981;198:541–565.
172. Finley JCW, Maderdrut JL, Roger LJ, Petrusz P. The immunocytochemical localization of somatostatin-containing neurons in the rat central nervous system. *Neurosci* 1981;6:2173–2192.
173. Fitzgerald M, Woolf CJ. Effects of cutaneous and intraspinal conditioning on C-fibre afferent terminal excitability in decerebrate spinal rats. *J Physiol* 1981;318:25–39.
174. Fitzgerald M. The course and termination of primary afferent fibers. In: Wall PD, Melzack R, eds. *Textbook of pain.* New York: Churchill Livingstone, 1989;46–62.
175. Flemming AA, Todd AJ. Thyrotropin-releasing hormone- and GABA-like immunoreactivity coexist in neurons in the dorsal horn of the rat spinal cord. *Brain Res* 1994;638:347–351.
176. Foerster O, Gagal O. Die Vorderseitenstrangdurchschneidung beim Menschen. Eine klinisch-patho-physiologisch-anatomische Studie. *Z Gasamte Neurol Psychiatr* 1932;138:1–92.
177. Foote SL, Cha CI. Distribution of corticotropin-releasing factor-lime immunoreactivity in brainstem of two monkey species (Saimiri sciureus and Macaca fascicularis): an immunocytochemical analysis. *J Comp Neurol* 1988;276:239–264.
178. Foreman RD, Hancock MB, Willis WD. Responses of spinothalamic tract cells in the thoracic spinal cord of the monkey to cutaneous and visceral inputs. *Pain* 1981;11:149–162.
179. Foreman RD, Schmidt RF, Willis WD. Convergence of muscle and cutaneous input onto primate spinothalamic tract neurons *Brain Res* 1977;124:555-560.
180. Frykholm R, Hyde J, Norlen G, Skoglund CR. On pain sensations produced by stimulation of ventral roots in man. *Acta Physiol Scand* 1953;29:455–469.
181. Fuji K, Senba E, Fujii S, Nomura I, Wu J-Y, Ueda Y, Tohyama M. Distribution, ontogeny and projections of cholecystokinin-8, vasoactive intestinal polypeptide and gamma-aminobutyrate-containing neuron systems in the rat spinal cord: an immunohistochemical analysis. *Neurosci* 1985;14:881–894.
182. Fyffe REW. Afferent fibers. In: Davidoff RA, ed. *Handbook of the spinal cord.* New York: Dekker, 1984;79–136.
183. Garrett L, Coggeshall RE, Patterson JT, Chung K Numbers and proportions of unmyelinated axons at cervical levels in the fasciculus gracilis of monkey and cat. *Anat Rec* 1992;232:301–304.
184. Garthwaite J, Charles SL, Chess-Williams R. Endothelium-derived relaxing factor release on activation of NMDA receptors suggests a role for an intercellular messenger in the brain. *Nature* 1988; 336:385–388.
185. Geiger JD, Nagy JI. Localization of [^{3}H] nitrobenzylthionosine binding sites in rat spinal cord and primary afferent neurons. *Brain Res* 1985;347:321–327.
186. Gerber G, Randic M 1989 Excitatory amino acid-mediated components of synaptically evoked input from dorsal roots to deep dorsal horn neurons in the rat spinal cord slice. *Neurosci Lett* 106: 211–219
187. Gerhardt KD, Yezierski RP, Giesler GJ Jr, Willis WD. Inhibitory receptive fields of primate spinothalamic tract cells. *J Neurophys* 1981;46:1309–1325.
188. Ghilardi JR, Allen CJ, Vigna SR, McVey DC, and Mantyh PW. Trigeminal and dorsal root ganglion neurons express CCK receptor binding sites in the rat, rabbit and monkey: possible site of opiate-CCK analgesic interactions. *J Neuroscience* 1992;12: 4854–4866.
189. Gibson SJ, Polak JM, Allen JM, Adrian TE, Kelly JS, Bloom SR. The distribution and origin of a novel brain peptide, neuropeptide Y, in the spinal cord of several mammals. *J Comp* Neurol 1984;227: 78–91.
190. Gibson SJ, Polak JM, Anand P, Blank MA, Morrison JFB, Kelly JS, Bloom SR. The distribution and origin of VIP in the spinal cord of six mammalian species. *Peptides* 1984;5:201–207.
191. Gibson SJ, Polak JM, Bloom SR, Sabate IM, Mulderry PM, Ghatei MA, McGreagor GP,, Morrison JF, Kelly JS, Evans RM, Rosenfeld MG. Calcitonin gene-related peptide immunoreactivity in the spinal cord of man and eight other species. *J Neurosci* 1984;4: 3101–3111.
192. Gibson SJ, Polak JM, Bloom SR, Wall PD. The distribution of nine peptides in rat spinal cord with special emphasis on the substantia gelatinosa and on the area around the central canal (lamina X). *J Comp Neurol* 1981;201:65–79.
193. Giesler GJ, Cliffer KD. Postsynaptic dorsal column pathway in the rat. II. Evidence against an important role in nociception. *Brain Res* 1985;326:347–356.
194. Giesler GJ, Menétrey D, Basbaum AI. Differential origins of spinothalamic tract projections to medial and lateral thalamus in the rat. *J Comp Neurol* 1979;184:107–126.
195. Giesler GJ, Nahin RL, Madsen AM. Postsynaptic dorsal column pathway of the rat. I. Anatomical studies. *J Neurophysiol* 1984;51: 260–275.
196. Giesler GJ, Yezierski RP, Gerhart KD, Willis WD. Spinothalamic tract neurons that project to medial and/or lateral thalamic nuclei: evidence for a physiologically novel population of spinal cord neurons. *J Neurophysiol* 1981;46:1285–1308.
197. Giuffrida R, Rustioni A. Glutamate and aspartate immunoreactivity in corticospinal neurons of rats. *J Comp Neurol* 1989;288: 154–164.
198. Glazer EJ, Basbaum AI. Immunohistochemical localization of leucine-enkephalin in the spinal cord of the cat: enkephalin-containing marginal neurons and pain modulation. *J Comp Neurol* 1981;196:377–389.
199. Glazer EJ, Basbaum AI. Opioid neurons and pain modulation: an ultrastructural analysis of enkephalin in cat superficial dorsal horn. *Neuroscience* 1983;10:357–376.
200. Go, V.L.W. and Yaksh, T.L.: Release of substance P from the cat spinal cord. J. Physiol. 391:141–167, 1987.
201. Gobel S, Falls WM, Humphrey E. Morphology and synaptic connections of ultrafine primary axons in lamina I of the spinal dorsal horn: candidates for the terminal axonal arbors of primary neurons with unmyelinated (C) axons. *J Neurosci* 1981;1: 1163–1179.
202. Gobel S. Golgi studies of the neurons in layer I of the dorsal horn of the medulla (trigeminal nucleus caudalis). *J Comp Neurol* 1978; 180:375–394.
203. Gobel S. Golgi studies of the neurons in layer II of the dorsal horn of the medulla (trigeminal nucleus caudalis). *J Comp Neurol* 1978; 180:395–414.
204. Gobel S. Golgi studies of the substantia gelatinosa neurons in the spinal trigeminal nucleus of the adult cat. *Brain Res* 1975;83: 333–338.
205. Gobel S. Neural circuitry in the substantia gelatinosa of Rolando: anatomical insights. *Adv Pain Res Ther* 1979;3:175–195.
206. Gokin AP, Kostyuk PG, Preobrazhensky NN. Neuronal mechanisms of interactions of high-threshold visceral and somatic afferent influences in spinal cord and medulla. *J Physiol (Paris)* 1977; 73:319–33.
207. Goodman RR, Snyder SH. Autoradiographic localization of adenosine receptors in rat brain using [^{3}H]cyclohexyladenosine. *J Neurosci* 1982;2:1230–1241.
208. Grant G, Ygge J. Somatotopic organization of the thoracic spinal nerve in the dorsal horn demonstrated with transganglionic degeneration. *J Comp Neurol* 1981;202:357–364.
209. Gundlach A L, Dodd P R, Grabara Watson WEJ, Johnston GAR, Harper PAW, Dennis JA, Healy PJ Deficits of spinal cord glycine / strychnine receptors in inherited myoclonius of poll Hereford calves. *Science* 1988;241:1807–1810.
210. Haber LH, Moore BD, Willis WD. Electrophysiological response properties of spinoreticular neurons in the monkey. *J Comp Neurol* 1982;207:75–84.
211. Habler HJ, Janig W, Koltzenburg M, McMahon SB. A quantitative

study of the central projection patterns of unmyelinated ventral root afferents in the cat. *J Physiol* 1990;422:265–287.

212. Hamano K, Mannen H, Ishizuka N. Reconstruction of trajectory of primary afferent collaterals in the dorsal horn of the cat spinal cord, using Golgi-stained serial sections. *J Comp Neurol* 1978;181: 1–16.
213. Han Z-S, Craig AD. Morphological characteristics of physiologically identified lamina I cells in cats. *Neuroscience Abs* 1994;20:547.
214. Handwerker HO, Iggo A, Zimmermann M. Segmental and supraspinal actions on dorsal horn neurones responding to noxious and non-noxious stimuli. *Pain* 1975;1:147–165.
215. Handwerker HO, Reeh PW. Pain and inflammation. *Pain Res Clin Manage* 1991;4:59–70.
216. Hannan LJ and Ho RH. Anatomical evidence for interactions between somatostatin neurites in lamina II of the rat spinal cord. *Peptides* 1992;13:329–337.
217. Harkness DH, Brownfield MS. A thyrotropin-releasing hormone-containing system in the rat dorsal horn separate from serotonin. *Brain Res* 1986;384:323–333.
218. Harmann PA, Carlton SM, Willis WD. Collaterals of spinothalamic tract cells to the periaqueductal gray: a fluorescent double-labeling study in the rat. *Brain Res* 1988;441:87–97.
219. Harmann PA, Chung K, Briner RP, Westlund KN, Carlton SM. Calcitonin gene-related peptide (CGRP) in the human spinal cord: a light and electron microscopic analysis. *J Comp Neurol* 1988;269: 371–380.
220. Hayes ES, Carlton SM. Primary afferent interactions: analysis of calcitonin gene-related peptide-immunoreactive terminals in contact with unlabeled and GABA-immunoreactive profiles in the monkey dorsal horn. *Neurosci* 1992;47:873–896.
221. Hellon RF, Misra NK. Neurones in the dorsal horn responding to scrotal skin temperature changes . *J Physiol* 1973;232:375–388.
222. Hill DR, Woodruff GN. Differentiation of central cholecystokinin receptor binding sites using the non-peptide antagonists MK-329 and L-365,260. *Brain Res* 1990;526:276–283.
223. Hillman P, Wall PD. Inhibitory and excitatory factors influencing the receptive fields of lamina 5 spinal cord cells. *Exp Brain Res* 1969;9:284–306.
224. Hirakawa M, Kawata M. Changes of chemoarchitectural organization of the rat spinal cord following ventral and dorsal root transection. *J Comp Neurol* 1992;320:339–352.
225. Ho RH. Widespread distribution of substance P-and somatostatin-immunoreactive elements in the spinal cord of the neonatal rat. *Cell Tissue Res* 1983;232:471–486.
226. Hobs SF, Oh UT, Brennan TJ, Chandler MJ, Kim KS, Foreman RD. Urinary bladder and hindlimb stimuli inhibit T1-T6 spinal and spinoreticular tract cells. *Am J Physiol* 1990;258:R10–20.
227. Hoffert MJ, Miletic V, Ruda MA, Dubner R. Immunocytochemical identification of serotonin axonal contacts on characterized neurons in laminae I and II of the cat dorsal horn. *Brain Res* 1983; 267:361–364.
228. Hökfelt T. Neuropeptides in perspective. *Neuron* 1991;7: 867–879.
229. Hökfelt T, Elde K, Johansson O, Terenius L, Stein L. The distribution of enkephalin immunoreactive cell bodies in the rat central nervous system. *Neurosci Lett* 1977;5:25–31.
230. Hökfelt T, Elde R, Johansson O, Luft R, Arimura A. Immunohistochemical evidence for the presence of somatostatin, a powerful inhibitory peptide, in some primary sensory neurons. *Neurosci Lett* 1975;1:231–235.
231. Hökfelt T, Ljungdahl Å, Terenius L, Elde R, Nilsson G. Immunohistochemical analysis of peptide pathways possibly related to pain and analgesia: enkephalin and substance P. *Proc Natl Acad Sci USA* 1977;74:3081–3085.
232. Hökfelt T, Ljungdahl A. Light and electron microscopic autoradiography on spinal cord slices after incubation with labeled glycine. *Brain Res* 1971;32:189–194.
233. Hökfelt T, Lundberg JM, Terenius L, Jancso G, Kimmel J. Avian pancreatic polypeptide (APP) immunoreactive neurons in the spinal cord and spinal trigeminal nucleus. *Peptides* 1981;2:81–87.
234. Hökfelt T, Terenius L, Kuypers HGJM, Dann O. Evidence for enkephalin immunoreactive neurons in the medulla oblongata projecting to the spinal cord. *Neurosci Lett* 1979;14:55–60.
235. Hökfelt T, Wiesenfeld-Hallin Z, Villar MJ, Melander T. Increase of galanin-like immunoreactivity in rat dorsal root ganglion cells after peripheral axotomy. *Neurosci Lett* 1987;83:217–220.
236. Holzer-Petsche U, Rinner I, Lembeck F. Distribution of choline acetyltransferase activity in rat spinal cord-influence of primary afferents? *J Neural Trans* 1986;66:85–92.
237. Honda CN, Rethelyi M, Petrusz P. Preferential immunohistochemical localization of vasoactive intestinal polypeptide (VIP) in the sacral spinal cord of the cat: Light and electron microscopic observations. *J Neurosci* 1983;3:2183–2196.
238. Honda CN. Visceral and somatic afferent convergence onto neurons near the central canal in the sacral spinal cord of the cat *J Neurophysiol* 1985;53:1059–1078.
239. Honda CN, Perl ER. Functional and morphological features of neurons in the midline region of the caudal spinal cord of the cat. *Brain Res* 1985;340:285–295.
240. Hongo T, Jankowska E, Lundberg A. Postsynaptic excitation and inhibition from primary afferents in neurones of the spinocervical tract. *J Physiol (Lond)* 1968;199:569–592.
241. Hongo T, Kudo N, Sasaki S, Yamashita M, Yoshida K, Ishizuka N, Mannen H. Trajectory of group Ia and Ib fibers from the hindlimb muscles at the L3 and L4 segments of the spinal cord of the cat. *J Comp Neurol* 1987;262:159–194.
242. Hope BT, Michael GL, Knigge KM, Vincent SR. Neuronal NADPH-diaphorase is a nitric oxide synthase. *Proc Natl Acad Sci USA* 1991;88:2811–2814.
243. Houser CR, Crawford GD, Barber RP, Salvaterra PM, Vaughn JE. Organization and morphological characteristics of cholinergic neurons: an immunocytochemical study with s monoclonal antibody to choline acetyltransferase. *Brain Res* 1983;266:97–119.
244. Howe JR, Zieglgansberger W. Responses of rat dorsal horn neurons to natural stimulation and to iontophoretically applied norepinephrine. *J Comp Neurol* 1987;225:1–17.
245. Hunt SP, Emson PC, Gilbert R, Goldstein M, Kimmell JR. Presence of avian pancreatic polypeptide-like immunoreactivity in catecholamine and methionine-enkephalin-containing neurones within the central nervous system. *Neurosci Lett* 1981;21: 125–130.
246. Hunt SP, Kelly JS, Emson PC, Kimmel JR, Miller RJ, Wu JY. An immunohistochemical study of neuronal populations containing neuropeptides or gamma-aminobutyrate within the superficial layers of the rat dorsal horn. *Neurosci* 1981;6:1883–1898.
247. Hunt SP, Kelly JS, Emson PC. The electron microscopic localization of methionine-enkephalin within the superficial layers (I and II) of the spinal cord. *Neuroscience* 1980;5:1871–1890.
248. Hylden JL, Anton F, Nahin RL. Spinal lamina I projection neurons in the rat: collateral innervation of parabrachial area and thalamus. *Neuroscience* 1989:28:27–37.
249. Hylden JLK, Hayashi H, Bennett GJ, Dubner R. Spinal lamina I neurons projecting to the parabrachial area of the cat midbrain. *Brain Res* 1985;336:195–198.
250. Hylden JLK, Hayashi H, Bennett GJ. Lamina I spinomesencephalic neurons in the cat ascend via the dorsolateral funiculi. *Somatosens Res* 1986;4:31–41.
251. Hylden JLK, Hayashi H, Dubner R, Bennett GJ. Physiology and morphology of the lamina I spinomesencephalic projection. *J Comp Neurol* 1986;247:505–515.
252. Hylden JLK, Hayashi H, Ruda MA, Dubner R. Serotonin innervation of physiologically identified lamina I projection neurons. *Brain Res* 1986;370:401–404.
253. Iadarola MJ, Douglass J, Civelli O, Naranjo JR. Differential activation of spinal cord dynorphin and enkephalin neurons during hyperalgesia: evidence using cDNA hybridization. *Brain Res* 1988; 455:205–212.
254. Iggo A, Ramsey RL. Thermosensory mechanisms in the spinal cord of monkeys. In: Zotterman Y, eds. *Sensory functions of the skin in primates with special reference to man.* Oxford: Pergamon, 1976; 285–304.
255. Iggo A. Activation of cutaneous nociceptors and their actions on dorsal horn neurones. *Adv Neurol* 1974;4:1–9.
256. Jackson DA, White SR. Thyrotropin releasing hormone (TRH) modifies excitability of spinal cord dorsal horn cells. *Neurosci Lett* 1988;92:171–176.
257. Jancso G, Hökfelt T, Lundberg JM, Kiraly E, Halasz N, Nilsson G, Terenius L, Rehfeld J, Steinbusch H, Verhofstad A, elder R, Said S, Brown M. Immunohistochemical studies on the effect of capsaicin on spinal and medullary peptide and monoamine neurons using antisera to substance P, gastrin/CCK, somatostatin, VIP enkephalin, neurotensin and 5 hydroxytryptamine. *J Neurocytol* 1981;10:963–980.
258. Jänig W, Schmidt RF, Zimmermann M. Two specific feedback pathways to the central afferent terminals of phasic and tonic mechanoreceptors. *Exp Brain Res* 1968;6;116–129.
259. Jankowska E, Rastad J Zarzecki P. Segmental and supraspinal

input to cells of origin of nonprimary fibres in the feline dorsal columns. *J Physiol* 1979;290:185–200.
260. Jeftinija S, Miletic V, Randic M. Cholecystokinin octapeptide excites dorsal horn neurons both in vivo and in vitro. *Brain Res* 1981;213:231–236.
261. Jeftinija S. Enkephalins modulate excitatory synaptic transmission in the superficial dorsal horn by acting at μ-opioid receptor sites. *Brain Res* 1988;460:260–268.
262. Jennes L, Stumpf WE, Kalivas PW. Neurotensin: topographical distribution in rat brain by immunohistochemistry. *J Comp Neurol* 1982;210:211–224.
263. Ji RR, Zhang X, Wiesenfeld-Hallin Z, Hökfelt T. Expression of neuropeptide Y and neuropeptide Y (Y1) receptor mRNA in rat spinal cord and dorsal root ganglia following peripheral tissue inflammation. *J Neurosci* 1994;14:6423–6434.
264. Johansson O, Hökfelt T, Elde R. Immunohistochemical distribution of somatostatin-like immunoreactivity in the central nervous system of the adult rat. *Neurosci* 1984;13:265–339.
265. Johnson JW, Ascher P. Glycine potentiates the NMDA response in cultured mouse brain neurons. *Nature* 1987;325:529–531.
266. Jones MW, Apkarian AV, Stevens RT, Hodge CJ. The spinothalamic tract: an examination of the cells of origin of the dorsolateral and ventral spinothalamic pathways in cats. *J Comp Neurol* 1987;260:349–361.
267. Jones MW, Hodge CJ, Apkarian AV, Stevens RT. A dorsolateral spinothamic pathway in cat. *Brain Res* 1985;335:188–193.
268. Jordan LM, Kenshalo Jr DR, Martin RF, Haber LH, Willis WD. Depression of spinothalamic tract neurons by iontophoretic application of 5-hydroxytryptamine. *Pain* 1978;5:135–142.
269. Ju G, Hökfelt T, Brodin E, Fahrenkrug J, Fischer JA, Frey P, Elde RP, Brown JC. Primary sensory neurons of the rat showing calcitonin gene-related peptide immunoreactivity and their relation to substance P-, somatostatin-, galanin-, vasoactive intestinal polypeptided- and cholecystokinin- immunoreactive ganglion cells. *Cell Tissue Res* 1987;247:417–431.
270. Ju G, Melander T, Ceccatelli S, Hökfelt T, Frey P. Immunohistochemical evidence for a spinothalamic pathway co-containing cholecystokinin- and galanin-like immunoreactivity in the rat. *Neuroscience* 1987;20:439–456.
271. Kai-Kai MA, Howe R. Glutamate-immunoreactivity in the trigeminal and dorsal root ganglia, and intraspinal neurons and fibres in the dorsal horn of the rat. *Histochem J* 1991;23:171–179.
272. Kajander KC, Sahara Y, Iadarloa MJ, Bennett GJ. Dynorphin increases in the dorsal spinal cord in rats with a painful peripheral neuropathy. *Peptides* 1990;11:719–728.
273. Kamogawa H, Bennett GJ. Dorsal column postsynaptic neurons in the cat are excited by myelinated nociceptors. *Brain Res* 1986;364: 386–390.
274. Kapadia SE, LaMotte CC. Deafferentation-induced alterations in rat dorsal horn: I Comparison of peripheral nerve injury vs. rhizotomy effects on presynaptic, post-synaptic and glial processes. *J Comp Neurol* 1987;266:183–197.
275. Kato M, Hirata Y. Sensory neurons in the spinal ventral roots of the cat. *Brain Res* 1968;7:479–482.
276. Katoh S, Hisano S, Kawano H, Kagotani Y, Daikoku S. Light- and electron-microscopic evidence of costoring of immunoreactive enkephalins and substance P in dorsal horn neurons of rat. *Cell Tissue Res* 1988;253:297–303.
277. Kawatani M, Lowe IP, Nadelhaft I, Morgan C, DeGroat WC. Vasoactive intestinal polypeptide in visceral afferent pathways to the sacral spinal cord of the cat. *Neurosci Lett* 1983;42:311–316.
278. Kawatani M, Takeshige C, DeGroat WD. Central distribution of afferent pathways from the uterus of the cat. *J Comp Neurol* 1990; 302:294–304.
278a. Keele KD. *Anatomies of pain.* Springfield, IL: Charles C. Thomas Press, 1957.
279. Kenshalo DR Jr, Leonard RB, Chung JM, Willis WD. Responses of primate spinithalamic neurons to graded and to repeated noxious heat stimuli. *J Neurophysiol* 1979;42:1370–1389.
280. Kerr FWL. Neuroanatomical substrates of nociception in the spinal cord. *Pain* 1975;1:325–356.
281. Kevetter GA, Haber LH, Yezierski RP, Martin RF, Willis WD. Cells of origin of the spinoreticular tract in the monkey. *J Comp Neurol* 1982;207:61–74.
282. Kevetter GA, Willis WD. Spinothalamic cells in the rat lumbar cord with collaterals to the medullary reticular formation. *Brain Res* 1982;22:181–185.
283. Khachaturian H, Watson SJ, Lewis ME, Coy D, Goldstein A, Akil H. Dynorphin immunocytochemistry in the rat central nervous system. *Peptides* 1982;3:941–954.
284. Khayyat GF, Yu YJ, King RB. Response patterns to noxious and non-noxious stimuli in rostral trigeminal relay nuclei. *Brain Res* 1975;97:47–60.
285. Khayyat GF, Yu YJ, King RB. Response patterns to noxious and non-noxious stimuli in rostral trigeminal relay nuclei. *Brain Res* 1975;97:47–60.
286. Kimura H, McGeer PL, Peng JH, McGeer EG. The central cholinergic system studied by choline acetyltransferase immunohistochemistry in the cat. *J Comp Neurol* 1981;200:151–201.
287. King AE, Thompson SW, Urban L, Woolf CJ. An intracellular analysis of amino acid induced excitations of deep dorsal horn neurones in the rat spinal cord slice. *Neurosci Lett* 1988;89: 286–292.
288. Kitto KF, Haley JE, Wilcox GL. Involvement of nitric oxide in spinally mediated hyperalgesia in the mouse. *Neurosci Lett* 1992; 148:1–5.
289. Klein CM, Coggeshall RE, Carlton SM, Sorkin LS. The effects of A- and C-fiber stimulation on patterns of neuropeptide immunostaining in the rat superficial dorsal horn. *Brain Res* 1992;580: 121–128.
290. Knox RJ, Dickenson AH. Effects of selective and non-selective kappa-opioid receptor agonists on cutaneous C-fibre-evoked responses of rat dorsal horn neurones. *Brain Res* 1987;415:21–29.
291. Knuepfer MM, Akeyson EW, Schramm LP. Spinal projections of renal afferent nerves in the rat. *Brain Res* 1988;446:17–25.
292. Koerber, HR. Somatotopic organization of cat brachial spinal cord. *Exp Neurol* 1980;481–492.
293. Kojima M, Takeuchi Y, Goto M, Sato Y. Immunohistochemical study of the distribution of serotonin fibers on the spinal cord of the dog. *Cell Tissue Res* 1982;226:477–491.
294. Kojima M, Takeuchi Y, Goto M, Sato Y. Immunohistochemical study on the localization of serotonin in fibers and terminals in the spinal cord of the monkey. *Cell Tissue Res* 1983;229:23–36.
295. Kopketsu K. Intracellular potential changes of primary afferent nerve fibers in spinal cords of cats. *J Neurophysiol* 1956;19:375–392.
296. Kordower JH, Le HK, Mufson EJ. Galanin immunoreactivity in the primate central nervous system. *J Comp Neurol* 1992;319: 479–500.
297. Krukoff TL. Neuropeptide Y-like immunoreactivity in cat spinal cord with special reference to autonomic areas. *Brain Res* 1987; 415:300–308.
298. Kumazawa T, Perl ER, Burgess PR, Whitehorn D. Ascending projections from marginal zone (lamina I) neurons of the spinal cord *J Comp Neurol* 1975;162:1–12.
299. Kuraishi Y, Minami M, Satoh M. Serotonin, but neither noradrenaline nor GABA, inhibits capsaicin-evoked release of immunoreactive somatostatin from slices of rat spinal cord. *Neuroscience Res* 1991;9:238–245.
300. Kuriyama K, Yoneda Y. Morphine induced alterations of gamma amino butyric acid and taurine contents and L-glutamate decarboxylase activity in rat spinal cord and thalamus: Possible correlations with analgesic actions of morphine. *Brain Res* 1978;148: 163–179.
301. Kuru M. *Sensory paths in the spinal cord and brain stem of man.* Tokyo: Sogensya, 1949.
302. Kuypers HGJM, Tuerck JD. The distribution of the cortical fibers within the nuclei cuneatus and gracilis in the cat. *J Anat* 1964;98: 143–162
303. Laing I, Todd AJ, Heizmann CW, Schmidt HH. Subpopulations of GABAergic neurons in laminae I-III of rat spinal dorsal horn defined by coexistence with classical transmitters, peptides, nitric oxide synthase or parvalbumin. *Neuroscience* 1994;61:123–132.
304. Laird JMA, Cervero F. Tonic descending influences on receptive field properties of nociceptive dorsal horn neurons in sacral spinal cord of rat. *J Neurophysiol* 1990;63:1022–1032.
305. LaMotte C. Distribution of the tract of Lissauer and the dorsal root fibers in the primate spinal cord. *J Comp Neurol* 1977;172: 529–562.
306. LaMotte CC and Shapiro CM. Ultrastructural localization of substance P, met-enkephalin, and somatostatin immunoreactivity in lamina X of the primate spinal cord. *J Comp Neurol* 1991;306: 290–306.
307. LaMotte CC, Carlton SM, Honda CN, Surmeier DJ, Willis WD. Innervation of identified primate spinothalamic tract neurons:

ultrastructure of serotonergic and other synaptic profiles. *Neurosci Abstr* 1988;14:852. (Abstract)
308. LaMotte CC, deLanerolle NC. Ultrastructure of chemically defined neuron systems in the dorsal horn of the monkey. II. Methionine-enkephalin immunoreactivity. *Brain Res* 1983;274: 51–63.
309. LaMotte CC, deLanerolle NC. Ultrastructure of chemically defined neuron systems in the dorsal horn of the monkey. III. Serotonin immunoreactivity. *Brain Res* 1983;274:65–77.
310. LaMotte CC, deLanerolle NC. VIP terminals, axons, and neurons: distribution throughout the length of monkey and cat spinal cord. *J Comp Neurol* 1986;249:133–145.
311. LaMotte CC, Johns DR, deLanerolle NC. Immunohistochemical evidence of indolamine neurons in monkey spinal cord. *J Comp Neurol* 1982;206:359–370.
312. LaMotte CC, Kapadia SE, Shapiro CM. Central projections of the sciatic, saphenous, median, and ulnar nerves of the rat demonstrated by transganglionic transport of choleragenoid-HRP (B-HRP) and wheat germ agglutinin-HRP (WGA-HRP). *J Comp Neurol* 1991;311:546–562.
313. Langford LA, Coggeshall RE. Branching of sensory axons in the dorsal root and evidence for the absence of dorsal efferent fibers. *J Comp Neurol* 1979;184:193–204.
314. LeBars D, Dickenson AH, Besson JM. Diffuse noxious inhibitory controls' (DNIC). I. Effects on dorsal horn convergent neurones in the rat. *Pain* 1979;6:283–304.
315. Lee J-H, Price RH, Williams FG, Mayer B, Beitz AJ. Nitric oxide synthase is found in some spinothalamic neurons and in neuronal processes that appose spinal neurons that express Fos induced by noxious stimulation. *Brain Res* 1993;608:324–333.
316. Levy RA. The role of GABA in primary afferent depolarization. *Prog Neurobiol* 1977;9:211–267.
317. Lewin GR, McMahon SB. Physiological properties of primary sensory neurons appropriately and inappropriately innervating skin in the adult rat. *J Neurophysiol* 1991;66:1205–1231.
318. Light AR. The organization of nociceptive neurons in the spinal grey matter. In: Light AL, ed. *The initial processing of pain and its descending control:* spinal and trigeminal system. Basel: Karger, 1992;109–168.
319. Light AR, Kavookjian AM, Petrusz P. The ultrastructure and synaptic connections of serotonin-immunoreactive terminals in spinal laminae I and II. *Somatosensory Res* 1983;1:33–50.
320. Light AR, Kavookjian AM. Morphology and ultrastructure of physiologically identified substantia gelatinosa (lamina II) neurons with axons that terminate in deeper dorsal horn laminae (III-V). *J Comp Neurol* 1988;267:172–189.
321. Light AR, Perl ER. Differential termination of large-diameter and small-diameter primary afferent fibers in the spinal dorsal gray matter as indicated by labeling with horseradish peroxidase. *Neurosci Lett* 1977;6:59–63.
322. Light AR, Perl ER. Spinal termination of functionally identified primary afferent neurons with slowly conducting myelinated fibres. *J Comp Neurol* 1979;186:133–150.
323. Light AR, Trevino DL, Perl ER. Morphological features of functionally defined neurons in the marginal zone and substantia gelatinosa of the spinal dorsal horn. *J Comp Neurol* 1979;186: 151–172.
324. Lima D, Avelino A, Coimbra A. Morphological characterization of marginal (lamina I) neurons immunoreactive for substance P, enkephalin, dynorphin and gamma-aminobutyric acid in the rat spinal cord *J Chem Neuroanat* 1993;6:43–52.
325. Lima D, Coimbra A. A Golgi study of the neuronal population of the marginal zone (lamina I) of the rat spinal cord. *J Comp Neurol* 1986;244:53–71.
326. Lima D, Coimbra A. Morphological types of spinomesencephalic neurons in the marginal zone (lamina I) of the rat spinal cord, as shown after retrograde labeling with cholera toxin subunit B. *J Comp Neurol* 1989;279:327–339.
327. Lima D, Coimbra A. Structural types of marginal (Lamina I) neurons projecting to the dorsal reticular nucleus of the medulla oblongata. *Neurosci* 1990;34:591–606.
328. Lima D, Coimbra A. The neuronal population of the marginal zone (lamina I) of the rat spinal cord. A study based on reconstructions of serially sectioned cells. *Anat Embryol* 1983;167: 273–288.
329. Lima D, Coimbra A. The spinothalamic system of the rat: structural types of retrogradely labeled neurons in the marginal zone (lamina I). *Neurosci* 1988;27:215–230.
330. Liu RP. Laminar origins of spinal projections to the periaqueductal gray of the rat. *Brain Res* 1983;264:118–122.
331. Longhurst JC, Mitchell JH, Moore MB. The spinal cord ventral root: an afferent pathway of the hind-limb pressor reflex in cats. *J Physiol* 1980;301:467–476.
332. Lundeberg T, Nordemar R, Ottoson D. Pain alleviation by vibratory stimulation. *Pain* 1984;20:25–44.
333. Magnusson KR, Clements JR, Larson AA, Madl JE, Beitz AJ. Localization of glutamate in trigeminothalamic projection neurons: A combined retrograde transportimmunohistochemical study. *Somatosensory Res* 1987;4:177–190.
334. Magoul R, Onteniente B, Geffard M, Calas A. Anatomical distribution and ultrastructural organization of the GABAergic system in the rat spinal cord. An immunocytochemical study using anti-GABA antibodies. *Neurosci* 1987;3:1001–1009.
335. Mai JK, Triepel J, Metz J. Neurotensin in the human brain. *Neurosci* 1987;22:499–524.
336. Mannen H. Reconstruction of axonal trajectory of individual neurons in the spinal cord using Golgi-stained serial sections. *J Comp Neurol* 1975;159:357–374.
337. Mannen N, Sugiura Y. Construction of neurons of dorsal horn proper using Golgi-stained serial sections. *J Comp Neurol* 1976;168: 303–312.
338. Mantyh PW, Hunt SP. The autoradiographic localization of substance P receptors in the rat and bovine spinal cord and the cat spinal trigeminal nucleus pars caudalis and the effects of neonatal capsaicin. *Brain Res* 1985;332:315–324.
339. Mantyh PW. The ascending input to the midbrain periaqueductal gray of the primate. *J Comp Neurol* 1982;211:50–64.
340. Mantyh PW, DeMaster E, Malhotra A, Ghilardi JR, Rogers SD, Mantyh CR, Liu H, Basbaum AI, Vigna SR, Maggio JE, et al. Receptor endocytosis and dendrite reshaping in spinal neurons after somatosensory stimulation. *Science* 1995;268:1629–1632.
341. Matsumoto M, Takayama K, Miura M. Distribution of glutamate- and GABA-immunoreactive neurons projecting to the vasomotor center of the interomediolateral nucleus of the lower thoracic cord of Wistar rats: a double-labeling study. *Neurosci Lett* 1994;174: 165–168.
342. Matsushita M. Some aspects of the interneuronal connections in cat's spinal grey matter. *J Comp Neurol* 1969;136:57–80.
343. Matsushita M. The axonal pathways of spinal neurons in the cat. *J Comp Neurol* 1970;138:391–418.
344. Maxwell DJ, Christie WM, Short AD, Brown AG. Direct observations of synapses between GABA-immunoreactive boutons and muscle afferent terminals in lamina VI of the cat's spinal cord. *Brain Res* 1990;530:215–222.
345. Maxwell DJ, Leranth C, Vertrofstad AA. Fine structure of serotonin containing axons in the marginal zone of the rat spinal cord. *Brain Res* 1983;266:253–259.
346. Maxwell DJ, Noble R. Relationships between hair-follicle afferent terminations and glutamic acid decarboxylase-containing boutons in the cat's spinal cord. *Brain Res* 1987;408:308–312.
347. Maxwell DJ. Combined light and electron microscopy of Golgi-labelled neurons in lamina III of feline spinal cord. *J Anat* 1985; 141:155–169.
348. Mayer DJ, Price DD, Becker DP. Neurophysiological characterization of the anterolateral spinal cord neurons contributing to pain perception in man. *Pain* 1975;1:51–58.
349. McBride WJ, Frederickson CA. Taurine as a possible inhibitory transmitter in the cerebellum. *Fed Proc* 1980;39:2701–2705.
350. McGregor GP, Gibson SJ, Sabate IM, Blank MA, Christofides ND, Wall PD, Polak JM, Bloom SR. Effect of peripheral nerve section and nerve crush on spinal cord neuropeptides in the rat: increased VIP and PHI in the dorsal horn. *Neurosci* 1984;13: 207–216.
351. McLaughlin BJ, Barber R, Saito K, Roberts E, Wu JY. Immunocytochemical localization of glutamate decarboxylase in rat spinal cord. *J Comp Neurol* 1975;164:305–322.
352. McMahon SB, Morrison JFB. Two groups of spinal interneurons that respond to stimulation of the abdominal viscera of the cat. *J Physiol* 1982;322:21–34.
353. McNeill DL, Coggeshall RE, Carlton SM. A light and electron microscopic study of calcitonin gene-related peptide in the spinal cord of the rat. *Exp Neurol* 1988;99:699–708.
354. Melander T, Hökfelt T, Rokaeus A. Distribution of galaninlike immunoreactivity in the rat central nervous system. *J Comp Neurol* 1986;248:475–517.

355. Meller ST, Gebhart GF. Nitric oxide (NO) and nociceptive processing in the spinal cord. *Pain* 1993;52:127–136.
356. Meller ST, Pechman PS, Gebhart GF, Maves TJ. Nitric oxide mediates the thermal hyperalgesia produced in a model of neuropathic pain in the rat. *Neurosci* 1992;50:7–10.
357. Melzack R, Wall PD. Pain mechanisms: a new theory. *Science* 1965; 150:971–979.
358. Mendell L. Physiological properties of unmyelinated fiber projections to the spinal cord. *Exp Neurol* 1966;16:316–322.
359. Menétrey D, Chaouch A, Besson JM. Location and response properties of dorsal horn neurons at origin of spinoreticular tract in lumbar enlargement of the rat. *J Neurophysiol* 1980;44:862–877.
360. Menétrey D, Giesler GJ, Besson JM. Analysis of response profiles of spinal cord dorsal horn neurones to nonnoxious and noxious stimuli in the spinal rat. *Exp Brain Res* 1977;27:15–33.
361. Menétrey, D, Chaouch A, Binder D, Besson JM. The origin of the spinomesencephalic tract in the rat: an anatomical study using the retrograde transport of horseradish peroxidase. *J Comp Neurol* 1982;206:193–207.
362. Mense S, Prabhakar NR. Spinal termination of nociceptive afferent fibres from deep tissues in the cat. *Neurosci Lett* 1986;66: 169–174.
363. Merchenthaler I, Hynes MA, Vigh S, Shally AV, Petrusz P. Immunocytochemical localization of corticotropin releasing factor (CRF) in the rat spinal cord. *Brain Res* 1983;275:373–377.
364. Merchenthaler I, Maderdrut JL, Altschuler RA, Petrusz P. Immunocytochemical localization of proenkephalin-derived peptides in the central nervous system of the rat. *Neurosci* 1986;17: 325–348.
365. Merchenthaler I. Corticotrophin releasing factor (CRF)-like immunoreactivity in the rat central nervous system. Extrahypothalamic distribution. *Peptides* 1984;5:53–69.
366. Merighi A, Polak JM, Theodosis DT. Ultrastructural visualization of glutamate and aspartate immunoreactivities in the rat dorsal horn, with special reference to the co-localization of glutamate, substance P and calcitonin-gene related peptide. *Neurosci* 1991; 40:67–80.
367. Micevych PE, Stoink A, Yaksh T, Go VLW. Immunochemical studies of substance P and cholecystokinin octapeptide recovery in dorsal horn following unilateral lumbosacral ganglionectomy. *Somatosensory Res* 1986;33:239–260.
368. Miletic V, Hoffert MJ, Ruda MA, Dubner R, Shigenaga Y. Serotoninergic axonal contacts on identified cat spinal dorsal horn neurons and their correlation with nucleus raphe magnus stimulation. *J Comp Neurol* 1984;228:129–141.
369. Miletic V, Randic M. Neurotensin excites cat spinal neurones located in laminae I-III. *Brain Res* 1979;169:600–604.
370. Miller KE, Clements JR, Larson AA, Beitz AJ. Organization of glutamate-like immunoreactivity in the rat superficial dorsal horn: light and electron microscopic observations. *Synapse* 1988;2: 28–36.
371. Miller KE, Seybold VS. Comparison of met-enkephalin, dynorphin A, and neurotensin immunoreactive neurons in the cat and rat spinal cords: II. Segmental differences in the marginal zone. *J Comp Neurol* 1989;279:619–628.
372. Miller KE, Seybold VS. Comparison of met-enkephalin-, dynorphin A-, and neurotensin-immunoreactive neurons in the cat and rat spinal cords: I. Lumbar cord. *J Comp Neurol* 1987;255:293–304.
373. Millhorn DE, Hökfelt T, Seroogy K, Oertel W, Verhofstad AAJ, Wu JY. Immunohistochemical evidence for colocalization of gamma-aminobutyric acid and serotonin in neurons of the ventral medulla oblongata projecting to the spinal cord. *Brain Res* 1987;410:179–185.
374. Mizukawa K, Otsuka N, McGeer PL, Vincent SR, McGeer EG. The ultrastructure of somatostatin-immunoreactive cell bodies, nerve fibers and terminals in the dorsal horn of rat spinal cord. *Arch Histol Cytol* 1988;51:443–452.
375. Moffie D. Spinothamic fibers, pain conduction and cordotomy. *Clin Neurol Neurosurg* 1975;78:261–268.
376. Molenaar I, Kuypers HGJM. Cells of origin of propriospinal fibers and of fibers ascending to supraspinal levels. A HRP study in cat and rhesus monkey. *Brain Res* 1978;152:429–450.
377. Moncada S, Palmer RMJ, Higgs EA. Nitric oxide: physiology, pathophysiology and pharmacology. *Pharmacol Rev* 1991;43: 109–142.
378. Morgan C, Nadelhaft I, DeGroat WC. The distribution of visceral primary afferents from the pelvic nerve to Lissauer's tract and the spinal gray matter and its relationship to the sacral parasympathetic nucleus. *J Comp Neurol* 1981;201:415–440.
379. Mouchet P, Manier M, Dietl M, Feuerstein C, Berod A, Arluison M, Denoroy L, Thibault J. Immunohistochemical study of catecholaminergic cell bodies in the rat spinal cord. *Brain Res Bull* 1986;16:341–353.
380. Nadelhaft I, Booth AM. The location and morphology of the preganglionic neurons and the distribution of visceral afferents from the rat pelvic nerve: a horseradish peroxidase study. *J Comp Neurol* 1984;226:238–245.
381. Nadelhaft I, Roppolo J, Morgan C, DeGroat WC. Parasympathetic preganglionic neurons and visceral primary afferents in monkey sacral spinal cord revealed following application of horseradish peroxidase to pelvic nerve. *J Comp Neurol* 1983;216:36–52.
382. Nagy JI, Hunt SP. Biochemical and anatomical observations on the degeneration of peptide containing primary afferent neurons after neonatal capsaicin. *Neurosci* 1981;6:1923–1934.
383. Nahin RL, Hylden JLK, Iadarola MJ, Dubner R. Peripheral inflammation is associated with increased dynorphin immunoreactivity in both projection and local circuit neurons in the superficial dorsal horn of the rat lumbar spinal cord. *Neurosci Lett* 1989;96: 247–252.
384. Nahin RL, Madsen AM, Giesler GJ. Anatomical and physiological studies of the gray matter surrounding the spinal cord central canal. *J Comp Neurol* 1983;220:321–335.
385. Nahin RL, Micevych PE. A long ascending pathway of enkephalin-like immunoreactive spinoreticular neurons in the rat. *Neurosci Lett* 1986;65:271–276.
386. Nahin RL. Immunocytochemical identification of long ascending, peptidergic lumbar spinal neurons terminating in either the medial or lateral thalamus in the rat. *Brain Res* 1988;443:345–349.
387. Narotzky RA, Kerr FW. Marginal neurons of the spinal cord: types, afferent synaptology and functional considerations. *Brain Res* 1978;139:1–20.
388. Nashold BS, Urban B, Zorub DS. Phantom relief by focal destruction of substantia gelatinosa of Rolando. In: Bonica JJ, Albe-Fessard D, eds. *Advances in pain research and therapy*, vol 1. New York: Raven Press, 1976;959–963.
389. Näsström JB, Schneider SP, Perl ER. *N*-methyl-D-aspartate (NMDA) depolarizes glutamate-insensitive neurones in the superficial dorsal horn. *Acta Physiol Scand* 1992;144:483–484.
390. Nathan PW. Results of antero-lateral cordotomy for pain in cancer. *J Neurol Neurosurg Psychiatry* 1963;26:353–362.
391. Nathan PW. Comments on "A dorsolateral spinothalamic tract in macaque monkey" by Apkarian and Hodge. *Pain* 1990;40: 239–240.
392. Ness TJ, Gebhart GF. Characterization of neuronal responses to noxious visceral and somatic stimuli in the medial lumbosacral spinal cord of the rat. *J Neurophysiol* 1987;57:1867–1892.
393. Ness TJ, Gebhart GF. Interactions between visceral and cutaneous nociception in the rat. I. Noxious cutaneous stimuli inhibit nociceptive neurons and reflexes. *J Neurophysiol* 1991;66:20–28.
394. Ness TJ, Gebhart GF. Interactions between visceral and cutaneous nociception in the rat. II. Noxious visceral stimuli inhibit cutaneous nociceptive neurons and reflexes. *J Neurophysiol* 1991;66: 29–39.
395. Ness TJ, Gebhart GF. Visceral pain: a review of experimental studies. Pain 1990;41:167–234.
396. Neuhuber WL, Sandoz PA, Fryscak T. The central projections of primary afferent neurons of greater splanchnic and intercostal nerves in the rat: a horseradish peroxidase study. *Anat Embryol (Berl)* 1986;174:123–144.
397. Newton BW, Hamill RW. The morphology and distribution of rat serotoninergic intraspinal neurons: an immunohistochemical study. *Brain Res Bull* 1988;20:349–360.
398. Nicholas AP, Pieribone VA, Avridsson U, Hökfelt T. Serotonin-, substance P- and glutamate/aspartate-like immunoreactivities in medullo-spinal pathways of rat and primate. *Neurosci* 1992;48: 545–559.
399. Nicoll RA, Alger BE. Presynaptic inhibition: transmitter and ionic mechanisms. *Int Rev Neurobiol* 1979;21:217–258.
400. Ninkovic M, Hunt SP, Kelly JS. Effect of dorsal rhizotomy on the autoradiographic distribution of opiate and neurotensin receptors and neurotensin-like immunoreactivity within the rat spinal cord. *Brain Res* 1981;230:111–119.
401. Nishikawa N, Bennett GJ, Ruda MA, Lu GW, Dubner R. Immunocytochemical evidence for a serotoninergic innervation of dorsal column postsynaptic neurons in cat and monkey: light- and electron-microscopic observations. *Neurosci* 1983;10:1333–1340.

402. Noble R, Riddell JS. Descending influences on the cutaneous receptive fields of postsynaptic dorsal column neurones in the cat. *J Physiol* 1989;408:167–183.
403. Noguchi K, Kowalski K, Traub R, Solodkin A, Iadarola MJ, Ruda MA. Dynorphin expression and Fos-like immunoreactivity following inflammation induced hyperalgesia are colocalized in spinal cord neurons. *Mol Brain Res* 1991;10:227–233.
404. Noordenbos W, Wall PD. Diverse sensory functions with an almost totally divided spinal cord. A case of spinal cord transection with preservation of part of one anterolateral quadrant. *Pain* 1976;2: 185–195.
405. Nyberg G, Blomqvist A. The somatotopic organization of forelimb cutaneous nerves in the brachial dorsal horn. An anatomical study in the cat. *J Comp Neurol* 1985;242:28–39.
406. Oja SS, Lahdesmaki . Is taurine an inhibitory neurotransmitter? *Med Biol* 1974;52:138–143.
407. Oku R, Satoh M, Fuji N, Otaka A, Uajima H, Takagi H. Calcitonin gene-related peptide promotes mechanical nociception by potentiating release of substance P from the spinal dorsal horn in rats. *Brain Res* 1987;403:350–354.
408. Olschowka JA, O'Donohue TL, Mueller GP, Jacobowitz DM. The distribution of corticotrophin releasing factor-like immunoreactive neurons in rat brain. *Peptides* 1982;3:995–1015.
409. Olszewski J. The cytoarchitecture of the human reticular formation. In: Adrian ED, Bremer F, Jasper HH, eds. *Brain mechanisms and consciousness.* Oxford: Blackwell, 1954;54–76.
410. Owens CM, Zhang D, Willis WD. Changes in the response states of primate spinothalamic tract cells caused by mechanical damage of the skin or activation of descending controls. *J Neurophysiol* 1992; 67:1509–1527.
411. Palmer RMJ, Ferrige AG, Moncada S. Nitric oxide release accounts for the biological activity of endothelium-derived relaxing factor. *Nature* 1987;327:324–326.
412. Panneton WM, Burton H. Projections from the paratrigeminal nucleus and the medullary and spinal dorsal horns to the peribrachial area in the cat. *Neurosci* 1985;15:779–797.
413. Patterson JT, Head PA, McNeil DL, Chung K Coggeshall RE. Ascending unmyelinated primary afferent fibers in the dorsal funiculus. *J Comp Neurol* 1989;290:384–390.
414. Pearson AA. Role of gelatinous substance of spinal cord in conduction of pain. *Arch Neurol Psychiat* 1952;68:515–529.
415. Phelps PE, Barber RP, Houser CR, Crawford GD, Salvaterra PM, Vaughn JE. Postnatal development of neurons containing choline acetyltransferase in rat spinal cord: an immunocytochemical study. *J Comp Neurol* 1984;229:347–361.
416. Phelps PE, Barber RP, Vaughn JE. Generation patterns of four groups of cholinergic neurons in rat cervical spinal cord: a combined tritiated thymidine autoradiographic and choline actyltransferase immunocytochemical study. *J Comp Neurol* 1988;273: 459–472.
417. Pomeranz B, Wall PD, Weber WV. Cord cells responding to fine myelinated afferents from viscera, muscle and skin. *J Physiol* 1968; 199:511–532.
418. Price DD, Browe AC. Responses of spinal cord neurons to graded noxious and non-noxious stimuli. *Brain Res* 1973;64:425–429.
419. Price DD, Dubner R. Neurons that subserve the sensory-discriminative aspect of pain. *Pain* 1977;3:307–338.
420. Price DD, Hayes RL, Ruda MA, Dubner R. Spatial and temporal transformations of input to spinothalamic tract neurons and their relation to somatic sensation. *J Neurophysiol* 1978;41:933–947.
421. Price DD, Mayer DJ. Neurophysiological characterization of the anterolateral quadrant neurons subserving pain in *M. Mulatta.* Pain 1975;1:59–72.
422. Proshansky E, Egger MD. Dendritic spread of dorsal horn neurons in cat. *Exp Brain Res* 1977;28:153–166.
423. Proudlock F, Spike RC, Todd AJ. Immunocytochemical study of somatostatin, neurotensin, GABA and glycine in rat spinal dorsal horn. *J Comp Neurol* 1993;327:289–297.
424. Ralston HJ III, Ralston DD. The primate dorsal spinothalamic tract: evidence for a specific termination in the posterior nuclei (Po/SG) of the thalamus. *Pain* 1992;48:107–118.
425. Ralston HJ, Ralston DD. The distribution of dorsal root axons in laminae I, II and III of the macaque spinal cord: a quantitative electron microscope study. *J Comp Neurol* 1979;184:643–684.
426. Ralston HJ. The fine structure of laminae I, II and III of the macaque spinal cord. *J Comp Neurol* 1979;184:619–642.
427. Cajal Ramon y S. *Histologie du systeme nerveux de l'homme et des vertebres.* Madrid: Institute Cajal, 1909;1:908–911.
428. Randic M, Miletic V. Depressant actions of methionine-enkephalin and somatostatin in cat dorsal horn neurones activated by noxious stimuli. *Brain Res* 1978;152:196–202.
429. Rethelyi M, Light AR, Perl ER. Synaptic ultrastructure of functionally and morphologically characterized neurons of the superficial spinal dorsal horn of cat. *J Neurosci* 1989;9(6):1846–1863.
430. Rethelyi M, Szentagothai J. Distribution and connections of afferent fibres in the spinal cord. In: Iggo A, ed. *Handbook of sensory physiology.* New York: Springer-Verlag, 1973;207–252.
431. Rethelyi M. Preterminal and terminal axon arborizations in the substantia gelatinosa of cat's spinal cord. *J Comp Neurol* 1977;172: 511–528.
432. Rethelyi M. Synaptic connectivity in the spinal dorsal horn. In: Davidoff A, ed. *Handbook of the spinal cord.* New York: Dekker, 1984; 137–175.
433. Rexed B. A cytoarchitectonic atlas of the spinal cord of the cat. *J Comp Neurol* 1954;100:297–351.
434. Rexed B. The cytoarchitectonic organization of the spinal cord in the rat. *J Comp Neurol* 1952;96:415–466.
435. Ribeiro-Da-Silva A, Claudio Cuello A. Choline acetyltransferase-immunoreactive profiles are presynaptic to primary sensory fibers in the rat superficial dorsal horn. *J Comp Neurol* 1990;295:370–384.
436. Ribeiro-Da-Silva A, Coimbra A. Neuronal uptake of [^{3}H]GABA and [^{3}H]glycine in laminae I-III (substantia gelatinosa Rolandi) of the rat spinal cord. An autoradiographic study. *Brain Res* 1980; 188:449–464.
437. Ribeiro-Da-Silva A, Cuello AC. Ultrastructural evidence for the occurrence of two distinct somatostatin-containing systems in the substantia gelatinosa of rat spinal cord. *J Chem Neuroanat* 1990;3: 141–153.
438. Ribeiro-Da-Silva A, Pioro EP, Cuello AC. Substance P- and enkephalin-like immunoreactivities are colocalized in certain neurons of the substantia gelatinosa of the rat spinal cord: An ultrastructural double-labeling study. *J Neurosci* 1991;11:1068–1080.
439. Ritter AM, Lewin GR, Mendell LM. Regulation of myelinated nociceptor function by nerve growth factor in neonatal and adult rats. *Brain Res Bull* 1993;30:245–249.
440. Ritz LA, Greenspan JD. Morphological features of lamina V neurons receiving nociceptive input in cat sacrocaudal spinal cord. J Comp Neurol 1985;238:440–452.
441. Robertson B, Grant G. A comparison between wheat germ agglutinin-and choleragenoid-horseradish peroxidase as anterogradely transported markers in central branches of primary sensory neurones in the rat with some observations in the cat. *Neuroscience* 1985;14:895–905.
442. Rökaeus A, Melander T, Hökfelt T, Lundberg JM, Tatemoto K, Carlquist M, Mutt V. A galanin-like peptide in the central nervous system and intestine of the rat. *Neurosci Lett* 1984;47:161–166.
443. Rosenthal BM, Ho RH. An electron microscopic study of somatostatin immunoreactive structures in lamina II of the rat spinal cord. *Brain Res Bull* 1989;22:439–451.
444. Rowan S, Todd AJ, Spike RC Evidence that neuropeptide Y is present in GABAergic neurons in the superficial dorsal horn of the rat spinal cord. *Neuroscience* 1993;53:537–545.
445. Ruch TC. Pathophysiology of pain. In: Ruch TC, Patton HD, Woodbury JW, Towe AL, eds. *Neurophysiology.* Philadelphia: WB Saunders, 1961;350–368.
446. Ruda MA, Bennett GJ, Dubner R. Neurochemistry and neural circuitry in the dorsal horn. In: Emson PC, Rossor MN, Tonyama M, eds. *Progress in brain research.* Amsterdam: Elsevier, 1986;219–268.
447. Ruda MA, Coffield J, Dubner R. Demonstration of postsynaptic opioid modulation of thalamic projection neurons by the combined techniques of retrograde horseradish peroxidase and enkephalin immunocytochemistry. *J Neurosci* 1984;4:2117–2132.
448. Ruda MA, Coffield J, Steinbusch HWM. Immunohistochemical analysis of serotonergic axons in lamina I and II of the lumbar spinal cord of the cat. *J Neurosci* 1982;2:1660–1671.
449. Ruda MA, Iadarola MJ, Cohen LV, Young WS. In situ hybridization histochemistry and immunocytochemistry reveal an increase in spinal dynorphin biosynthesis in a rat model of peripheral inflammation and hyperalgesia. *Proc Natl Acad Sci USA* 1988;85:622–626.
450. Ruda MA. Opiates and pain pathways: Demonstration of enkephalin synapses on dorsal horn projection neurons. *Science* 1982;215:1523–1525.
451. Rustioni A, Cuenod M. Selective retrograde transport of d-aspartate in spinal interneurons and cortical neurons of rats. *Brain Res* 1982;236:143–155.

452. Rustioni A, Hayes NL, O'Neill S. Dorsal column nuclei and ascending spinal afferents in macaques. *Brain* 1979;102:95–125.
453. Ryall RW, Piercey MF. Visceral afferent and efferent fibers in sacral ventral roots in cats. *Brain Res* 1970;97:57–65.
454. Sahara Y, Xie Y-K, Bennett GJ. Intracellular records of the effects of primary afferent input in lumbar spinoreticular tract neurons in the cat. *J Neurophys* 1990;64:1791–1800.
455. Saito Y, Collins JG, Iwasaki H. Tonic 5-HT modulation of spinal dorsal horn neuron activity evoked by both noxious and non-noxious stimuli: a source of neuronal plasticity. *Pain* 1990;40:205–219.
456. Sandkuhler J, Fu QG, Helmchen C. Spinal somatostatin superfusion in vivo affects activity of cat nociceptive dorsal horn neurons: comparison with spinal morphine. *Neuroscience* 1990;34:565–576.
457. Sar M, Stumpf WE, Miller RJ, Chang KJ, Cuatrecasas P. Immunohistochemical localization of enkephalin in rat brain and spinal cord. *J Comp Neurol* 1978;96:415–495.
458. Sasek CA, Elde RP. Distribution of neuropeptide Y-like immunoreactivity and its relationship to FMRF-amide-like immunoreactivity in the sixth lumbar and first sacral spinal cord segments of the rat. *J Neurosci* 1985;7:1729–1739.
459. Sastry BR, Goh JW. Actions of morphine and met-enkephalineamide on nociceptor driven neurones in substantia gelatinosa and deeper dorsal horn. *Neuropharmacology* 1983;22:119–122.
460. Schaible H-G, Neugebauer V, Cervero F, Schmidt RF. Changes in tonic descending inhibition of spinal neurons with articular input during the development of acute arthritis in the cat. *J Neurophys* 1991;66:1021–1032.
461. Scheibel ME, Scheibel AB. Terminal axon patterns in cat spinal cord. II: The dorsal horn. *Brain Res* 1968;9:32–58.
462. Schipper J, Steinbuch WM, Vermes I, Tildes FJH. Mapping of CRF-immunoreactive nerve fibers in the medulla oblongata and spinal cord of the rat. *Brain Res* 1983;267:145–150.
463. Schmidt RF. Presynaptic inhibition in the vertebrate central nervous system. *Ergeb Physiol* 1971;63:20–101.
464. Schoenen J, Lotstra F, Vierendeels G, Reznik M, Vanderhaeghen JJ. Substance P, enkephalins, somatostatin, cholecystokinin, oxytocin, and vasopressin in human spinal cord. *Neurology* 1985;35: 881–890.
465. Schoenen J. The dendritic organization of the human spinal cord: the dorsal horn. *Neuroscience* 1982;7:2057–2087.
466. Schroder HD, Skagerberg G. Catecholamine innervation of the caudal spinal cord in the rat. *J Comp Neurol* 1985;242:358–368.
467. Schroder HD. Localization of cholecystokinin-like immunoreactivity in the rat spinal cord, with particular reference to the autonomic innervation of the pelvic organs. *J Comp Neurol* 1983;217: 176–186.
468. Schroder HD. Somatostatin in the caudal spinal cord: an immunohistochemical study of the spinal centers involved in the innervation of pelvic organs. *J Comp Neurol* 1984;223:400–414.
469. Selzer M, Spencer WA. Convergence of visceral and cutaneous afferent pathways in the lumbar spinal cord. *Brain Res* 1968;14: 331–348.
470. Senba E, Shiosaka S, Hara Y, Inagaki S, Sakanaka M, Takatsuki K, Kawai Y, Tohyama M. Ontogeny of the peptidergic system in the rat spinal cord: immunohistochemical analysis. *J Comp Neurol* 1982;208:54–66.
471. Senba E, Yanaihara C, Yanaihara N, Tohyama M. Co-localization of substance P and Met-enkephalin-Arg^6-Gly^7-Leu^8 in the intraspinal neurons of the rat, with special reference to the neurons in the substantia gelatinosa. *Brain Res* 1988;453:110–116.
472. Serrano JS, Serrano MI, Guerrero MR, Ruiz MR, Polo J. Antinociceptive effect of taurine and its inhibition by naloxone. *Pharmacologist* 1990;21:333–336.
473. Seybold VS, Elde RP. Immunohistochemical studies of peptidergic neurons in the dorsal horn of the spinal cord. *J Histochem Cytochem* 1980;28:367–370.
474. Seybold VS, Elde RP. Neurotensin immunoreactivity in the superficial laminae of the dorsal horn of the rat. I. Light microscope studies of cell bodies and proximal dendrites. *J Comp Neurol* 1982; 205:89–100.
475. Seybold VS, Maley B. Ultrastructural study of neurotensin immunoreactivity in the superficial laminae of the dorsal horn of the rat. *Peptides* 1984;5:1179–1189.
476. Shehab SAS, Atkinson ME. Vasoactive intestinal polypeptide (VIP) increases in the spinal cord after peripheral axotomy of the sciatic nerve originate from primary afferent neurons. *Brain Res* 1986;372:37–44.
477. Shehab SAS, Atkinson ME. Vasoactive intestinal polypeptide increases in areas of the dorsal horn of the spinal cord from which other neuropeptides are depleted following peripheral axotomy. *Exp Brain Res* 1986;62:422–430.
478. Shen WZ, Luo CB, Dong L, Chan WY, Yew DT. Distribution of neuropeptide Y in the developing human spinal cord. *Neuroscience* 1994;62:251–256.
479. Sherrington C. *The integrative action of the nervous system.* Yale University Press, New Haven, CT:1906.
480. Shortland P, Woolf CJ, Fitzgerald M. Morphology and somatotopic organization of the central terminals of hindlimb hair follicle afferents in the rat lumbar spinal cord. *J Comp Neurol* 1989;289: 416–433.
481. Shortland P, Woolf CJ. Morphology and somatotopy of the central arborizations of rapidly adapting glabrous skin afferents in the rat lumbar spinal cord. *J Comp Neurol* 1993;329:491–511.
482. Simantov R, Kuhar MJ, Uhl GF, Snyder SH. Opioid peptide enkephalin: Immunohistochemical mapping in rat central nervous system. *Proc Natl Acad Sci USA* 1977;74:2167–2171.
483. Sindou M, Fischer G, Mansuy L. Posterior spinal rhizotomy and selective posterior rhizidiotomy. *Prog Neurol Surg* 1976;7:210–250.
484. Skagerberg G, Björklund A, Lindvall O, Schmidt RH. Origin and termination of the diencephalo-spinal dopamine system in the rat. *Brain Res Bull* 1982;9:237–244.
485. Skofitsch G, Insel TR, Jacobowitz DM. Binding sites for corticotropin releasing factor in sensory areas of the rat hindbrain and spinal cord. *Brain Res Bull* 1985;15:519–522.
486. Skofitsch G, Jacobowitz DM. Galanin-like immunoreactivity in capsaicin sensitive sensory neurons and ganglia. *Brain Res Bull* 1985;15:1–195.
487. Skofitsch G, Zamir N, Helke C, Savitt J, Jacobowitz D. Corticotropin releasing factor-like immunoreactivity in sensory ganglia and capsaicin sensitive neurons of the rat central nervous system: colocalization with other neuropeptides. *Peptides* 1985;6:307–318.
488. Smullin DH, Schamber CD, Skilling SR, Larson AA. A possible role for taurine in analgesia. In: Pasantes-Morales H, del Rio M, Shane W, eds. *Functional neurochemistry of taurine.* New York: Wiley-Liss, 1990;129–132.
489. Smullin DH, Skilling SR, Larson AA. Interactions between substance P, calcitonin gene-related peptide, taurine and excitatory amino acids in the spinal cord. *Pain* 1990;42:93–101.
490. Snyder SH. Nitric oxide: first in a new class or neurotransmitters? *Science* 1992;257:494–496.
491. Snyder, R. The organization of the dorsal root entry zone in cats and monkeys. *J Comp Neurol* 1977;174:47–70.
492. Sorkin, LS, Ferrington, DG, Willis, WD. Somatotopic organization and response characteristics of dorsal horn neurons in the cervical spinal cord of the cat *Somatosens Res* 1986;3:323–338.
493. Spike RC, Todd AJ, Johnston HM. Coexistence of NADPH diaphorase with GABA, glycine, and acetylcholine in rat spinal cord. *J Comp Neurol* 1993;335:320–333.
494. Standaert DG, Watson SJ, Houghten RA, Saper CB. Opioid peptide immunoreactivity in spinal and trigeminal dorsal horn neurons projecting to the parabrachial nucleus in the rat. *J Neurosci* 1986;6:1220–1226.
495. Stanzione P, Zieglgänsberger W. Action of neurotensin on spinal cord neurons in the rat. *Brain Res* 1983;268:111–118.
496. Steedman WM, Molony V, Iggo A. Nociceptive neurons in the superficial dorsal horn of cat lumbar spinal cord and their primary afferent input. *Exp Brain Res* 1985;58:171–182.
497. Steinbusch HWM. Distribution of serotonin-immunoreactivity in the central nervous system of the rat cell bodies and terminals. *Neurosci* 1981;6:557–618.
498. Stevens RT, Hodge CJ, Apkarian AV. Medial, intralaminar, and lateral terminations of lumbar spinothalamic tract neurons: a fluorescent double-label study. *Somatosens Motor Res* 1989;6: 285–308.
499. Sugiura Y, Lee CL, Perl ER. Central projections of identified, unmyelinated (C) afferent fibers innervating mammalian skin. *Science* 1986;234:358–361.
500. Sugiura Y, Terui N, Hosoya Y. Difference in distribution of central terminals between visceral and somatic unmyelinated (C) primary afferent fibers. *J Neurophysiol* 1989;62:834–840.
501. Swett JE, McMahon SB, Wall PD. Lond ascending projections to the midbrain from cells of lamina I and nucleus of the dorsolateral funiculus of the rat spinal cord. *J Comp Neurol* 1985;238: 401–416.

502. Szentagothai J. Neuronal and synaptic arrangement in the substantia gelatinosa Rolandi. *J Comp Neurol* 1964;122:219–239.
503. Tashiro T, Ruda MA. Immunocytochemical identification of axons containing coexistent serotonin and substance P in the cat lumbar spinal cord. *Peptides* 1988;9:383–391.
504. Tashiro T, Satoda T, Takahashi O, Matsushima R, Mizuno N. Distribution of axons exhibiting both enkephalin- and serotonin-like immunoreactivities in the lumbar cord segments: and immunohistochemical study in the cat. *Brain Res* 1988;440:357–362.
505. Tattersall JEH, Cervero F, Lumb BM. Effects of reversible spinalization on the visceral input to viscerosomatic neurons in the lower thoracic spinal cord of the cat. *J Neurophysiol* 1986;56: 785–796.
506. Terenghi G, Riveros-Moreno V, Hudson LD, Ibrahim NBN, Polak JM. Immunohistochemistry of nitric oxide synthase demonstrates immunoreactive neurons in spinal cord and dorsal root ganglia of man and rat. *J Neurol Sci* 1993;
507. Tessler A, Gazer E, Artymyshyn R, Murray M, Goldberger ME. Recovery of substance P in the cat spinal cord after unilateral lumbosacral deafferentation. *Brain Res* 1980;191:459–470.
508. Tessler A, Himes BT, Artymyshyn R, Murray M, Goldberger ME. Spinal neurons mediate return of substance P following deafferentation of cat spinal cord. *Brain Res* 1981;230:263–281.
509. Thies R, Foreman RD. Inhibition and excitation of thoracic spinoreticular neurons by electrical stimulation of vagal afferent nerves. *Exp Neurol* 1983;82:1–16.
510. Thies R. Activation of lumbar spinoreticular neurons by stimulation of muscle, cutaneous and sympathetic afferents. *Brain Res* 1985;333:151–155.
511. Todd AJ, Lochhead V. GABA-like immunoreactivity in type I glomeruli of rat substantia gelatinosa. *Brain Res* 1990;514:171–174.
512. Todd AJ, McKenzie J. GABA-immunoreactive neurons in the dorsal horn of the rat spinal cord. *Neuroscience* 1989;31:799–806.
513. Todd AJ, Spike RC, Price RF, Neilson M. Immunocytochemical evidence that neurotensin is present in glutamatergic neurons in the superficial dorsal horn of the rat. *J Neurosci* 1994;14:774–784.
514. Todd AJ, Spike RC, Russell G, Johnston HM. Immunohistochemical evidence that Met-enkephalin and GABA coexist in some neurones in rat dorsal horn. *Brain Res* 1992;584:149–156.
515. Todd AJ, Sullivan AC. Light microscope study of the coexistence of GABA-like and glycine-like immunoreactivities in the spinal cord of the rat. *J Comp Neurol* 1990;296:496–505.
516. Todd AJ. An electron microscope study of glycine-like immunoreactivity in laminae I-III of the spinal dorsal horn of the rat. *Neuroscience* 1990;39(2):387–394.
517. Tracey DJ, De Biasi S, Phend K, Rustioni A. Aspartate-like immunoreactivity in primary afferent neurons. *Neuroscience* 1991; 40: 673–686.
518. Traub RJ, Iadarola MJ, Ruda MA. Effect of multiple dorsal rhizotomies on calcitonin gene-related peptide-like immunoreactivity in the lumbosacral dorsal spinal cord of the cat: a radioimmunoassay analysis. *Peptides* 1989;10:979–983.
519. Traub RJ, Solodkin A, Ruda MA. Calcitonin gene-related peptide immunoreactivity in the cat lumbosacral spinal cord and the effects of multiple rhizotomies. *J Comp Neurol* 1989;287:225–237.
520. Trevino DL, Carstens E. Confirmation of the location of spinothalamic neurons in the cat and monkey by the retrograde transport of horseradish peroxidase. *Brain Res* 1975;98:177–182.
521. Trevino DL, Coulter, JD, Willis WD. Location of cells of origin of spinothalamic tract in lumbar enlargement in the monkey. *J Neurophysiol* 1973;36:750–761.
522. Trevino DL. The origin and projections of a spinal nociceptive and thermoregulative pathway. In: Zotterman Y, ed. *Sensory functions of the skin in primates, with special reference to man,* vol 27. New York: Pergamon Press, 1976;367–376.
523. Truex RC, Taylor MJ, Smythe MQ, Gildenberg PL. The lateral cervical nucleus of cat, dog and man. *J Comp Neurol* 1970;139:93–104.
524. Tuchscherer MM, Seybold VS. A quantitative study of the coexistence of peptides in varicosities within the superficial laminae of the dorsal horn of the rat spinal cord. *J Neurosci* 1989;9:195–205.
525. Tyce GM, Yaksh TL. Monoamine release from cat spinal cord by somatic stimuli: an intrinsic modulatory system. *J Physiol (Lond)* 1981;314:513–529.
526. Uddenberg N. Functional organization of long, second-order afferents in the dorsal funiculus. *Exp Brain Res* 1968;4:377–382.
527. Uhl GR, Goodman RR, Snyder SH. Neurotensin-containing cell bodies, fibers and nerve terminals in the brain stem of the rat: immunohistochemical mapping. *Brain Res* 1979;167:77–91.
528. Ulfhake B, Arvidsson U, Cullheim S, Hökfelt T, Visser TJ. Thyrotropin-releasing hormone (TRH)-immunoreactive boutons and nerve cell bodies in the dorsal horn of the cat L7 spinal cord. *Neurosci Lett* 1987;73:3–8.
529. Urban L, Randic M. Slow excitatory transmission in rat dorsal horn: possible mediation by peptides. *Brain Res* 1984;290: 336–341.
530. Valtschanoff JG, Phend KD, Bernardi PS, Weinberg RJ, Rustioni A. Amino acid immunocytochemistry of primary afferent terminals in rat dorsal horn. *J Comp Neurol* 1994;346:237–252.
531. Valtschanoff JG, Weinberg RJ, Rustioni A, Schmidt HHHW. Nitric oxide synthase and GABA colocalize in lamina II of rat spinal cord. *Neurosci Lett* 1992;148:6–10.
532. Valtschanoff JG, Weinberg RJ, Rustioni A. Amino acid immunoreactivity in corticospinal terminals. *Exp Brain Res* 1993;93:95–103.
533. Valtschanoff JG, Weinberg RJ, Rustioni A. NADPH diaphorase in the spinal cord of rats. *J Comp Neurol* 1992;321:209–222.
534. van den Pol AN, Gorcs T. Glycine and glycine receptor immunoreactivity in brain and spinal cord. *J Neurosci* 1988;8(2):472–492.
535. Verge VMK, Xu Z, Xu X-J, Wiesenfeld-Hallin Z, Hökfelt T. Marked increase in nitric oxide synthase MRNA in rat dorsal root ganglia after peripheral axotomy: *in situ* hybridisation and functional studies. *Proc Natl Acad Sci USA* 1992;89:11617–11621.
536. Vierck CJ Jr, Luck MM. Loss and recovery of reactivity to noxious stimuli in monkeys with primary spinothalamic cordotomies, followed by secondary and tertiary lesions of other cord sectors. *Brain* 1979;102:233–248.
537. Villar MJ, Cortes R, Theodorsson E, Wiesenfeld-Hallin Z, Schalling M, Fahrenkrug J, Emson PC, Hökfelt T. Neuropeptide expression in rat dorsal root ganglion cells and spinal cord after peripheral nerve injury with special reference to galanin. *Neuroscience* 1989;33:587–604.
538. Villar MJ, Wiesenfeld-Hallin Z, Xu X-J, Theodorsson E, Emson PC, Hökfelt T. Further studies on galanin-, substance P-, and CGRP-like immunoreactivities in primary sensory neurons and spinal cord: effects of dorsal rhizotomies and sciatic nerve lesions. *Exp Neurol* 1991;112:29–39.
539. Vincent SR, Hökfelt T, Christensson I, Terenius L. Dynorphin-immunoreactive neurons in the central nervous system of the rat. *Neurosci Lett* 1982;33:185–190.
540. Vincent SR, McIntosh CHS, Bueham AMJ, Brown JC. Central somatostatin systems revealed with monoclonal antibodies. *J Comp Neurol* 1985;238:169–186.
541. Vizzard MA, Erdman SL, de Groat WC. The effect of rhizotomy on NADPH diaphorase staining in the lumbar spinal cord of the rat. *Brain Res* 1993;607:349–353.
542. Vizzard MA, Erdman SL, Erickson VL, Stewart RJ, Roppolo JR, De Groat WC. Localization of NADPH diaphorase in the lumbosacral spinal cord and dorsal root ganglia of the cat. *J Comp Neurol* 1994; 339:62–75.
543. Wagner R, DeLeo JA, Coombs DW, Willenbring S, Fromm C. Spinal dynorphin immunoreactivity increases bilaterally in a neuropathic pain model. *Brain Res* 1993;339:62–75.
544. Waldeyer H. Das Gorilla-Rueckenmark. *Akad Wissensch* 1888; 147(abstr).
545. Wall PD. Excitability changes in afferent fibre terminations and their relation to slow potentials. *J Physiol* 1958;142:1–21.
546. Wall PD. The laminar organization of dorsal horn and effects of descending impulses. *J Physiol* 1967;188:403–423.
547. Warden MK, Young WS. Distribution of cells containing mRNAs encoding substance P and neurokinin B in the rat central nervous system. *J Comp Neurol* 1988;272:90–113.
548. Wee BEF, Emery DG, Blanchard JL. Unmyelinated fibers in the cervical and lumbar ventral roots of the cat. *Am J Anat* 1985;172: 307–316.
549. Weihe E, Hohr D, Millan MJ, Stein C, Muller S, Gramsch C, Herz A. Peptide neuroanatomy of adjuvant-induced arthritic inflammation in rat. *Agents Actions* 1988;25:255–259.
550. Weil-Fugazza J, Godefroy F, Manceau V, Besson JM. Increased norepinephrine and uric acid levels in the spinal cord of arthritic rats. *Brain Res* 1986;374:190–194.
551. Weinberg RJ, Conti F, Van Eyck SL, Petrusz P, Rustioni A. Glutamate immunoreactivity in the superficial laminae of rat dorsal horn and spinal trigeminal nucleus. In: Hicks TP, Lodge D, McLennan H, eds. *Excitatory amino acid transmission, neurology and neurobiology.* New York: Liss, 1987;126–133.
552. Werman R, Aprison MH. Glycine: the search for a spinal cord

inhibitory transmitter. In: von Euler C, Skoglund S, Soderberg U, eds. *Structure and function of inhibitory neural mechanisms.* Oxford: Pergamon, 1968;473–486.

553. Werman R, Davidoff RA, Aprison MH. Inhibitory action of glycine of spinal neurons in the cat. *J Neurophysiol* 1968;31:81–95.
554. Wessendorf MW, Elde R. The coexistence of serotonin- and substance P-like immunoreactivity in the spinal cord of the rat as shown by immunofluorescent double labeling. *J Neurosci* 1987;7: 2352–2363.
555. Westlund KN, Bowker RM, Ziegler MG, Coulter JD. Noradrenergic projections to the spinal cord of the rat. *Brain Res* 1983;263: 15–31.
556. Westlund KN, Bowker RM, Ziegler MG, Coulter JD. Origins of spinal noradrenergic pathways demonstrated by retrograde transport of antibody to dopamine-β-hydroxylase. *Neurosci Lett* 1981; 25:243–249.
557. Westlund KN, Carlton SM, Zhang D, Willis WD. Direct catecholaminergic innervation of primate spinothalamic tract neurons. *J Comp Neurol* 1990;299:178–186.
558. Westlund KN, Carlton SM, Zhang D, Willis WD. Glutamate-immunoreactive terminals synapse on primate spinothalamic tract cells. *J Comp Neurol* 1992;322:519–527.
559. Westlund KN, McNeill DL, Coggeshall RE. Glutamate immunoreactivity in rat dorsal roots. *Neurosci Lett* 1989;96:13–17.
560. Westlund KN, McNeill DL, Patterson JT, Coggeshall RE. Aspartate immunoreactive axons in normal rat L4 dorsal roots. *Brain Res* 1989;489:347–351.
561. White JC, Sweet WH, Hawkins R, Nilges RG. Anterolateral cordotomy: results, complications and causes of failure. *Brain* 1950;73: 346–367.
562. White WF, Heller AH. Glycine receptor alteration in the mutant mouse spastic. *Nature* 1982;298:655–657.
563. Wiberg M, Blomqvist A. The spinomesencephalic tract in the cat: its cells of origin and termination pattern as demonstrated by the intraaxonal transport method. *Brain Res* 1984;291:1–18.
564. Wiberg M, Westman J, Blomqvist A. Somatosensory projection to the mesencephalon: An anatomical study in the monkey. *J Comp Neurol* 1987;264:92–117.
565. Wiesenfeld-Hallin Z, Hökfelt T, Lundberg JM, Forssmann WG, Reinecke M, Tschopp FA, Fischer JA. Immunoreactive calcitonin gene-related peptide and substance P coexist in sensory neurons to the spinal cord and interact in spinal behavioral responses of the rat. *Neurosci Lett* 1984;52:199–204.
566. Wiesenfeld-Hallin Z, Xu X-J, Villar MJ, Hökfelt T. Intrathecal galanin potentiates the spinal analgesic effect of morphine: electrophysiological and behavioural studies. *Neurosci Lett* 1990;109: 217–221.
567. Wiesenfeld-Hallin Z. Somatostatin and calcitonin gene-related peptide synergistically modulate spinal sensory and reflex mechanisms in the rat: behavioral and, electrophysiological studies. *Neurosci Lett* 1986;67:319–323.
568. Willcockson JM, Chung JM, Hori Y, Lee KH, Willis WD. Effects of iontophoretically released amino acids and amines on primate spinothalamic tract cells. *J Neurosci* 1984;4(3):732–740.
569. Willcockson WS, Chung JM, Hori Y, Lee KH, Willis WD. Effects of iontophoretically released peptides on primate spinothalamic tract cells. *J Neurosci* 1984;4:741–750.
570. Willcockson WS, Kim J, Shin HK, Chung JM, Willis WD. Actions of opioids on primate spinothalamic tract neurons. *J Neurosci* 1986; 6(9):2509–2520.
571. Willis WD, Kenshalo DR Jr, Leonard RB. The cells of origin of the primate spinothalamic tract. *J Comp Neurol* 1979;188:543–574.
572. Willis WD, Leonard RB, Kenshalo DR Jr, Spinothalamic tract neurons in the substantia gelatinosa *Science* 1978;202:986–988.
573. Willis WD, Trevino DL, Coulter JD, Mauntz RD. Responses of primate spinothalamic tract neurons to natural stimulation of the hindlimb. *J Neurophysiol* 1974;40:968–981.
574. Willis WD Jr, Coggeshall RE. *Sensory mechanisms of the spinal cord.* New York: Plenum Press, 1991.
575. Willis WD. Neural mechanisms of pain discrimination. In: Lund JS, ed. *Sensory processing in the mammalian brain.* New York: Oxford University Press, 1989;130–143.
576. Woolf CJ, Fitzgerald M. The properties of neurones recorded in the superficial dorsal horn of the rat spinal cord. *J Comp Neurol* 1983;221:313–328.
577. Woolf CJ, King AE. Dynamic alterations in the cutaneous mechanoreceptive fields of dorsal horn neurons in the rat spinal cord. *J Neurosci* 1990;10:2717–2726.
578. Woolf CJ, Shortland P, Coggeshall RE. Peripheral nerve injury triggers central sprouting of myelinated afferents. *Nature* 1992; 355:75–81.
579. Woolf CJ, Wiesenfeld-Hallin Z. Substance P and calcitonin gene-related peptide synergistically modulate the gain of the nociceptive flexor withdrawal reflex in the rat. *Neurosci Lett* 1986;66: 319–323.
580. Woolf CJ. Central terminations of cutaneous mechanoreceptive afferents in the rat lumbar spinal cord. *J Comp Neurol* 1987;261: 105–119.
581. Wu W, Liuzzi FJ, Schinco FP, Depto AS, Li Y, Mong JA, Dawson TM, Snyder SH. Neuronal nitric oxide synthase is induced in spinal neurons by traumatic injury. *Neuroscience* 1994;61: 719–726.
582. Wu W. Expression of nitric-oxide synthase (NOS) in injured CNS neurons as shown by NADPH diaphorase histochemistry. *Exp Neurol* 1993;120:153–159.
583. Yaksh TL. Behavioral and autonomic correlates of the tactile evoked allodynia produced by spinal glycine inhibition: effects of modulatory receptor systems and excitatory amino acid antagonists. *Pain* 1989;37:111–122.
584. Yaksh TL, Schmauss C, Micevych PE, Abay EO, Go VLW. Pharmacological studies on the application, disposition, and release of neurotensin in the spinal cord. *Ann NY Acad Sci* 1982;400: 228–243.
585. Yamamoto T, Carr PA, Baimbridge KG, Nagy JI. Parvalbumin- and calbindin D28K-immunoreactive neurons in the superficial layers of the spinal cord dorsal horn of rat. *Brain Res Bull* 1989;23: 493–508.
586. Yamamoto T, Geiger JD, DaDonna PE, Nagy JI. Subcellular, regional and immunohistochemical localization of adenosine deaminase in various species. *Brain Res Bull* 1987;19:473–484.
587. Yezierski RP, Broton JG. Functional properties of spinomesencephalic tract (SMT) cells in the upper cervical spinal cord of the cat. *Pain* 1991;45:187–196.
588. Yezierski RP, Schwartz RH. Response and receptive-field properties of spinomesencephalic tract cells in the cat. *J Neurophysiol* 1986;55:76–96.
589. Yezierski RP, Sorkin LS, Willis WD. Response properties of spinal neurons projecting to midbrain or midbrain-thalamus in the monkey. *Brain Res* 1987;437:165–170.
590. Yezierski RP. Spinomesencephalic tract: projections from the lumbosacral spinal cord of the rat, cat, and monkey. *J Comp Neurol* 1988;267:131–146.
591. Yoshida S, Senba E, Kubota Y, Hagihira S, Yoshiya I, Emson PC, Tohyama M. Calcium-binding proteins calbindin and parvalbumin in the superficial dorsal horn of the rat spinal cord. *Neuroscience* 1990;37:839–848.
592. Yoshimura M, Jessell TM. Primary afferent evoked synaptic response and slow potential generation in rat substantia gelatinosa neurons in vitro. *J Neurophysiol* 1989;622:96–108.
593. Yoshimura M, Jessell T. Amino acid-mediated EPSPs at primary afferent synapses with substantia gelatinosa neurones in the rat spinal cord. *J Physiol* 1990;430:315–335.
594. Zenker W, Groh V, Mysicka A. Mapping of muscle and skin primary afferents central projections from the rats neck region. An HRP study. *Neurosci Lett (Suppl)* 1980;5:S486.
595. Zhang D, Carlton SM, Sorkin LS, Willis WD. Collaterals of primate spinothalamic tract neurons to the periaqueductal gray. *J Comp Neurol* 1990;296:277–290.
596. Zhang X, Dagerlind A, Elde RP, Castel MN, Broberger C, Wiesenfeld-Hallin Z, Hökfelt T. Marked increases in cholecystokinin B receptor messenger RNA levels in rat dorsal root ganglia after peripheral axotomy. *Neuroscience* 1994;57:227–233.
597. Zhang X, Nicholas AP, Hökfelt T. Ultrastructural studies on peptides in the dorsal horn of the spinal cord I. Co-existence of galanin with other peptides in primary afferents in normal rats. *Neuroscience* 1993;57:365–384.
598. Zhang X, Verge V, Wiesenfeld-Hallin Z, Ju G, Bredt D, Snyder SH, Hökfelt. Nitric oxide synthase-like immunoreactivity in lumbar dorsal root ganglia and spinal cord of rat and monkey and effect of peripheral axotomy. *J Comp Neurol* 1993;335:563–575.
599. Zhou Y, Sun, YH Zhang ZH and Han JS. Increased release of

immunoreactive cholecystokinin octapeptide by morphine and potentiation of mu-opioid analgesia by CCKB receptor antagonist L-365-260 in rat spinal cord. *Eur J Pharmacol* 1993;234: 147–154.
600. Zieglgänsberger W, Puil EA. Actions of glutamic acid on spinal neurones. *Exp Brain Res* 1973;17:35–49.
601. Zieglgänsberger W, Sutor B. Responses of substantia gelatinosa neurons to putative neurotransmitters in an in vitro preparation of the adult rat spinal cord. *Brain Res* 1983;279:316–320.
602. Zieglgänsberger W, Tulloch IF. The effects of methionine- and leucine-enkephalin on spinal neurones of the cat. *Brain Res* 1979; 167:53–64.

Anesthesia: Biologic Foundations, edited by
Tony L. Yaksh et al. Lippincott–Raven Publishers,
Philadelphia © 1997.

CHAPTER 36

RESPONSE PROPERTIES OF DORSAL HORN NEURONS: PHARMACOLOGY OF THE DORSAL HORN

ANTHONY H. DICKENSON, LOUISE C. STANFA,
VICTORIA CHAPMAN, AND TONY L. YAKSH.

High-intensity stimulation yields activity in specific subclasses of primary afferents. The magnitude of the activity is typically proportional to the intensity of the stimulus impressed upon the afferent terminal. It is clear however that the encoding schema underlying the processing of such input is extraordinarily nonlinear. As reviewed in Chap. 1, it has been appreciated since the turn of the century that the mapping of the response to the stimulus is subject to modification. The appreciation of this organization was described in the exposition by Melzack and Wall (117) that led to the formalization referred to as the gate theory of pain. The proposed schema recognized the fact that the output of dorsal horn wide dynamic range (WDR) neurons (see Chap. 35) was under an ongoing regulation by local segmental circuits and by activity in extraspinal projections. Consequently, activity in spinal motoneurons (as in nociceptive reflexes) is not likely to reflect a simple function of primary afferent activity. Moreover, given that the nature (frequency and patterning) of the spinopetal traffic defines in part the psychophysical characteristics of the organized behavior (see Chaps. 31 and 41), the modifiability of the input-output function of these spinal projection neurons emphasizes that the psychophysics of the pain state evoked by a given stimulus may be significantly and predictably altered. Of particular significance has been the evolving appreciation that these specific systems possess a definable pharmacology. This chapter focuses on the dynamic properties of several of these spinal systems.

DORSAL HORN ORGANIZATION

As reviewed in detail in Chaps. 35 and 37, retrograde labeling and antidromic stimulation have amply illustrated that the dorsal horn contains two major classes of neurons contributing to the ascending tracts. Broadly speaking, these neurons are concentrated in two areas of the dorsal horn, in the superficial laminae I and II and deep in the neck of the dorsal horn, approximately in and around lamina V and the central canal (lamina X). Although anatomical techniques cannot resolve the functional responses of the neurons, it is clear from electrophysiologic recording from these areas that a large proportion of neurons in these zones respond to high-intensity peripheral stimuli and receive inputs from C fibers (see Chap. 35).

The superficial nociceptive neurons often correspond to the elongated Waldeyer cells, whereas the deeper lamina nociceptive neurons have a more disparate morphology. Staining of the deep cells in the lamina V zone shows that these cells have variable dendritic trees, some of which extend dorsally to penetrate the superficial laminae (149). As will be noted, electrophysiologic evidence has emphasized that both shallow and deep neurons receive excitatory C-fiber input (191). The superficial nociceptive neurons are probably directly contacted by C-fiber terminals. These deep neurons receive excitatory C-fiber input (see Chap. 35). However, as the bulk of the C-fiber input terminates in the outer layers of the superficial dorsal horn (see Chaps. 34 and 35), the linkage of afferent neurons with C-fiber–evoked excitation likely reflects upon the contact of C fibers with this dorsal spreading dendritic tree and by polysynaptic (indirect) input (e.g., all deep cells do not show such a dendritic tree). Conversely, as the majority of nociceptive neurons in the dorsal horn also receive inputs from low-threshold A fibers, it is thought that deep cells are located in a position to receive large A-fiber afferent inputs close to their somata, whereas superficial cells will be indirectly excited by interneuronal pools.

Although some cells within the substantia gelatinosa do project supraspinally, neurons within this region typically appear to form a closed system that projects within the segment and to neighboring segments (56,101). It should be noted that the neurons in the substantia gelatinosa have a density that equals the most densely packed areas seen elsewhere in the central nervous system. Although the original electrophysiologic recordings from neurons in this area were confusing due to different anesthetic protocols altering neuronal responses, it is now generally accepted that the bulk of the neurons in this zone receive convergent afferent inputs from both large and small afferent fibers. However, it is also clear that the cells in this area have a tendency to respond in a more prolonged fashion than the output cells in the adjoining laminae. In addition there are at least two morphologically distinct types of neurons in this area and evidence suggests that this may reflect their function. Thus, the islet cells that send axons ventrally to the lamina V area are thought to be inhibitory interneurons, whereas the stalked cells with a more restricted projection zone are probably excitatory (56).

Many populations of spinal dorsal horn neurons, which are immediately postsynaptic to the primary afferent, will display positive covariance between increasing stimulus intensity and output (see Chap. 35). This relationship reflects upon an increased terminal depolarization and an increased release of afferent transmitter. Factors attenuating that input-output function would change the magnitude of the pain behavior evoked by a given stimulus. Several mechanisms have been shown to alter the relationship of the stimulus-response relationship at the spinal level.

FACTORS INFLUENCING AFFERENT-EVOKED EXCITATION OF A LOCAL NEURON

As reviewed in Chap. 35, discrete classes of dorsal horn neurons can be functionally characterized in terms of (a) the effective stimulus that evokes their activity and (b) the characteristics (size and composition) of the receptive field within which a stimulus may be applied to evoke activity in a given neuron. The intrinsic organization of the dorsal horn system emphasizes that these characteristics will be subject to considerable flexibility. Several factors influence the relationship between the stimulus and the response: (a) anatomical connectivity, e.g., the hardwiring; and (b) factors that influence the excitability of the afferent linkages and cellular excitability.

Connectivity

After entering the spinal cord at the dorsal root entry zone, afferents collateralize, and the principal branch enters the spinal gray to terminate dorsally (small afferents) or more deeply, below lamina II (large myelinated afferents). In addition, the collaterals may enter the dorsal columns (large afferents) or the lateral Lissauer tract (small afferents). These collaterals may then reenter the dorsal horn at distal segments to make contact with neurons that lie outside the segment of entry (Fig. 1). Thus, electrophysiologically, neurons that may lie as many as several segments distally from the stimulated root may display excitatory postsynaptic potentials (EPSPs). These neurons display increasingly more modest excitatory responses as the distances from the segment of entry increases (Fig. 1 and Chap. 35). These extrasegmental excitatory inputs into a single neuron are consistent with the fact that the size of the receptive field of a spinal neuron may be larger than the peripheral distribution of the respective root.

Efficiency of Synaptic Connections and Cell Excitability

The efficacy of the synaptic connection can be altered by a number of mechanisms that can be considered in terms of being either pre- or postterminal. Preterminally, changes in the postsynaptic action could occur as a result of reduced release of primary afferent transmitter. This may occur by (a) changes in the releasable pool of transmitter, (b) altered ability of a invading action potential to depolarize the terminal, and/or (c) open voltage-sensitive Ca channels to mobilize transmitter release. Postsynaptically, increasing K or Cl conductance may

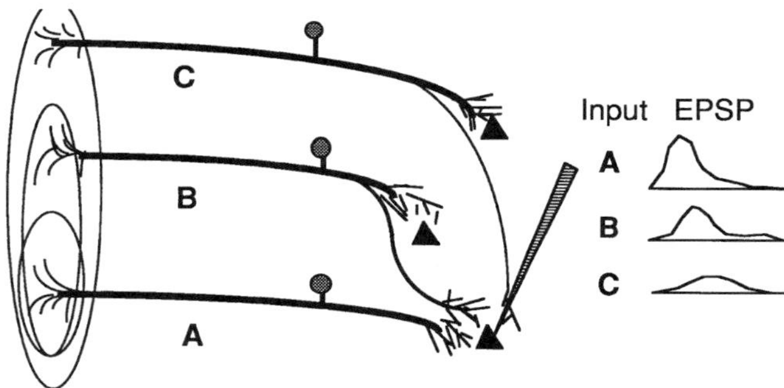

Figure 1. Schematic displaying receptive field (RF) of three afferent axons projecting principally to three neurons with branching collaterals. As indicated, the segmental input yields the strongest excitatory postsynaptic potentials (EPSPs) with the shortest latency as measured by an intracellular electrode, with the EPSP from axon C in the distal segment having only modest and delayed excitatory input. If the input from axons A and B, but not C, are sufficient to depolarize the neuron, then that neuron would have a receptive field as indicated by RF 1 and 2. If the excitability of the synaptic connections are decreased, as by a hyperpolarization of the recorded cell (as by an increase in K^+ or Cl^- conductance) or by a presynaptic effect that reduces transmitter release (as with a reduction in terminal depolarization and/or a decrease in the opening of voltage-sensitive Ca channels), then the receptive field of the cell will be limited to RF 1 or none. Conversely, if the excitability of the cell is enhanced by a partial depolarization of the cell, as with a decrease in K^+ or Cl^- conductance, then the modest input from axon C might yield a depolarization adequate to discharge the neuron. In this case, the receptive field of the recorded neurons will be as large as 3. Alterations in the ongoing excitatory or inhibitory input into the respective segments would accordingly lead to predictable changes in the receptive fields of a neuron.

serve to hyperpolarize or shunt the membrane, resulting in hyperpolarization of the cell, making it refractory to depolarization. Conversely, decreasing K conductance or increasing Na conductance will serve to enhance the excitability of the cell and increase the likelihood that a subliminal input might evoke a depolarization.

It can be appreciated that factors altering the efficacy of synaptic connections into the dorsal horn can have profound effects on afferent processing. Those inputs arriving from distal segments to evoke a modest depolarization of the cell may become effective if the excitability of the cell is altered. This would be reflected in an increase in the size of the receptive field of the cell. Conversely, decreasing the excitability of the cell or reducing afferent terminal excitability would serve to depress the input from afferents that contribute to the margins of the receptive field of the cell and the size of the receptive field would correspondingly decrease.

As noted, in the above section, and in Chap. 34, classes of neurons in the dorsal horn show an excitation evoked by large (low-threshold) and small (high-threshold) primary afferents. Each cell displays a principal excitatory drive from a relatively limited dermatome. However, as noted, afferents display significant extrasegmental projections that exert a progressively smaller postsynaptic effect at the more distal segments. This organization, though simplified, suggests how prominent changes in responsiveness can be induced by a variety of influences at the brainstem and spinal level that either depress or facilitate the postsynaptic responsiveness of local circuits. It is the flow of excitation and inhibition that provides the dynamic quality of the system. In the following section, the transmitter pharmacology of local substrates that decrease (inhibit) or increase (facilitate) the excitability of this system are considered.

INHIBITORY SYSTEMS

Stimulation of several physiologically defined elements will depress spinal circuit excitability.

1. Dorsal column stimulation antidromically activates the collaterals of large primary afferents and reduces the activity in dorsal horn nociceptors (72). These results led to the clinical use of dorsal column stimulation for the relief of pain (129,186). The neuronal pathways that mediate the mechanisms of inhibition of the cord are not well understood.
2. Stimulation of the lateral Lissauer tract (a presumed outflow of gelatinosa neurons) results in the development of segmental dorsal root potentials (187) and a concurrent inhibition of the polysynaptic ventral root reflex, as well as the discharge of dorsal horn neurons evoked by noxious stimulation (185). In contrast, a lesion of the Lissauer tract results in an increased receptive field size (31).
3. Bulbospinal projections diminish the slope of the response (frequency of discharge) versus stimulus intensity curve of dorsal horn neurons, as well as shift the stimulus intensity intercept of the stimulus-response curve to the right, indicating an increase in the threshold stimulus intensity necessary to evoke activity in the cell (53,54).

PHYSIOLOGIC MODULATION OF DORSAL HORN RESPONSIVENESS

Virtually every pathway carrying nociceptive information, including the spinoreticular (73) and spinothalamic (189), are under modulatory control of bulbospinal projections. These pathways originate in a variety of brainstem nuclei including the midline raphe, the lateral tegmentum, and the locus coeruleus complex. These pathways descend in the dorsolateral funiculus to terminate within the spinal parenchyma (6,27; see Chap. 38).

Electrical stimulation or microinjections of excitatory amino acids in mesencephalon and medulla inhibit the discharge of spinal neurons (16,53,54) and inhibit nociceptive reflex function (18,80,82). Such observations emphasize the role of spinopetal systems in controlling spinal nociceptive processing. Brainstem stimulation has been observed to have a potent and relatively selective effect upon the discharge of dorsal horn neurons evoked by high-threshold, but not low-threshold input. Systematic studies have shown that bulbospinal input results in a right shift of the stimulus response curve of dorsal horn neurons and a reduction in the slope of that curve (53,54). Extensive discussion of the organization of this bulbospinal system and the linkages of brainstem systems that regulate the activity in the bulbospinal loop is provided in Chap. 38.

The mechanisms underlying this descending inhibition have been a subject of considerable investigation. It is apparent that much of this bulbospinal modulation may be mediated by monoaminergic transmission. Evidence for this may be briefly summarized:

1. Bulbospinal projections originating in the midline raphe contain serotonin, while locus coeruleus and lateral tegmentum cells systems contain noradrenaline (6,27).
2. Electrical stimulation or microinjections of opiates at brainstem sites such as the periaqueductal gray or the nucleus gigantocellularis inhibit nociceptive reflexes, and this effect is antagonized by the intrathecal administration of serotonergic or noradrenergic antagonists, or both (13,61,81).
3. Focal stimulation in the medulla or periaqueductal gray that alters nociceptive thresholds are associated with an increased release of serotonin or norepinephrine in the spinal cord (60,140).
4. Spinal application of adrenergic or serotonergic agonists by iontophoresis or by intrathecal administration will antagonize Aδ–/C-fiber–evoked activity in dorsal horn neurons (see Table 1 in Chap. 40).
5. Serotonin and norepinephrine are released in spinal cord by high- but not low-intensity stimulation of afferent input (178), an effect mediated by a spinobulbospinal loop.
6. Although the principal interest is focused on spinopetal aminergic pathways, other neurotransmitter systems have been shown to project to the spinal cord and become released by bulbospinal activation (20), including dopamine (105), substance P (120,172), thyrotropin-releasing hormone, (5) and neuropeptide Y (126,177). The complexity of this system is emphasized further by the fact that a number of these agents may be co-contained, such as substance P and serotonin (135) and enkephalin and serotonin (146; see Chaps. 34 and 35). The role of these several systems has yet to be ascertained, but they provide additional substrates whereby brainstem systems may interact with spinal cord sensorimotor processing.

PHARMACOLOGY OF SPINAL INHIBITORY RECEPTORS

Pharmacologic investigations have revealed that the activation of a variety of spinal receptor systems will depress the discharge of dorsal horn neurons that is evoked by small high-intensity/small afferent-mediated input. As reviewed in Chap. 34 and in Table 3 in Chap. 40, certain receptor classes, including those for the μ, δ opioid and α_2-adrenergic, produce a powerful suppression of the excitation of the activation of dorsal horn neurons produced by the activation of populations of small afferents and yield a selective inhibition of the animals response to a strong threshold after spinal delivery (see Chap. 40). The mechanisms by which these several modulatory receptor systems exert their surprisingly selective effect on afferent-evoked excitation and pain behavior are several:

1. Presynaptic actions. As indicated in Chap. 40, Table 3, several of the receptor systems display binding that is presynaptic on primary afferents, as defined by binding in gelatinosa or on dorsal root ganglion cells, and, given the selective effects of capsaicin as a C-fiber neurotoxin (44), some of these binding sites appear to be largely on small fibers (see Chap. 6). Consistent with the presynaptic locus of binding, agonist occupancy of these receptors has been shown to diminish the depolarization-evoked release of spinal excitatory amino acids (glutamate) and peptide (substance P and calcitonin gene-related peptide [CGRP]) (110,111,171,180,183).
2. Postsynaptic actions. While rhizotomy may diminish significantly the binding for a number of the receptor systems, none shows a reduction of greater than 50%. This suggests that there is additional binding that is not on the primary afferent. A variety of studies have shown that many of these receptors exert their effect by increasing K^+ conduction through a $G_{i/o}$-coupled protein. This results in a hyperpolarization that serves to depress excitability of the respective postafferent neuron (137).

It is thus considered that agents that possess a joint pre- and postsynaptic action may exert their powerful modulatory influence by a selective effect on small input and a coincidental postsynaptic action (198; see Chap. 58).

The behavioral relevance of these inhibitory receptor systems for pain is emphasized by the observation that the spinal delivery of the appropriate agonists serves to powerfully regulate the animals response to mechanical, thermal, and chemical stimuli that would otherwise evoke indices of pain behavior in animals (e.g., escape, vocalization) and humans. Thus, as summarized in Table 4 in Chap. 40, the spinal delivery of μ, δ opioid and α_2-adrenoceptor agonist, neuropeptide Y, and agonists for several 5-HT receptors are able to produce a powerful antinociceptive effect. Where examined, these actions have been substantiated in humans as with the spinal actions of μ, δ, and α_2-adrenoceptor agonists (198,200). Such behavioral observations substantiate the powerful role played by these receptor systems in the regulation of afferent traffic evoked by a high-intensity stimulus.

ENDOGENOUS INHIBITORY SYSTEMS

The presence of these receptors and the powerful effects of exogenously administered adrenoceptor and opiate agonists on spinal nociceptive functioning lead to the question of what are the *endogenous* systems that normally act on these receptors and what normally activates those systems. As summarized in Table 3 in Chap. 40, the several transmitters with which these several receptors are associated are found in descending (bulbospinal pathways), such as those for the amines (noradrenaline, dopamine, and serotonin) and intrinsic interneurons, such as the enkephalins.

Several populations of endorphins have been identified (41), including those deriving from the pre/prohormones of proopiomelanocortin (21,69,90), pre/proenkephalin (10,76, 150), and pre/prodynorphin (79). Products of the latter two populations such as met- and leu-enkephalin, and various extended peptides such as $Phe^7Arg^6Met^5$-enkephalin and extended chains of leu-enkephalin (yielding dynorphins) have been identified in dorsal horn neurons. Importantly, these several classes of opioids have been shown to possess a differential receptor preference (196). These intrinsic systems have been shown to be activated by a variety of conditions. Thus, both the bulbospinal pathways (amines) (178) and the intrinsic spinal neurons (endorphins and enkephalins) are released from spinal cord in animal models by high-intensity but not low-intensity stimulation and irritant stimuli (19,102,166,199,203). It should be stressed that while these systems clearly have the potential of regulating the afferent traffic as indicated by the powerful effects of the exogenously delivered receptor agonists, there is surprisingly little support for the thesis that these systems play a significant ongoing role in the regulation of C-fiber–evoked activity. Thus, with few exceptions, antagonists for these several systems such as naloxone (all opiate receptors) or phentolamine (α–adrenoceptor antagonist) fail to produce evident hyperalgesia (197).

FACILITATORY SYSTEMS

Dynamic Properties of the Response of Dorsal Horn Neurons to Afferent Input

Focal stimuli applied to the exteroceptors excite specific populations of primary afferents, and these afferents retain a significant degree of precision with respect to the region of the body surface from which the excitation may be elicited and the magnitude (e.g., frequency) of the response evoked by a given physical stimulus. However, it is clear from the foregoing commentary, that the relationship between the stimulus and the response may be significantly altered. This alteration may be dependent on (a) characteristics of the afferent input and (b) activity in dorsal horn systems that regulate the excitability of the synaptic activity of the dorsal horn neurons.

Response Properties as a Function of the Afferent Message

As reviewed in Chap. 34, populations of dorsal horn neurons may be excited in a modality-specific fashion, as by low-threshold Aβ mechanoreceptors or by high-threshold Aδ afferents. Other populations of afferents may receive convergent input from large low-threshold as well as fine high-threshold afferents. Early studies by Mendell and Wall (119) revealed such convergent excitatory input. Low-frequency electrical stimulation activating large and small afferents would lead to a reliable neuronal response showing the excitation evoked by the early-arriving fast-conducting afferent and the subsequent delayed discharge associated with the more slowly conducing Aδ and C afferents. Such a typical response is presented in Fig. 2.

As noted in Fig. 2 these cells have complex receptive fields the were composed in overlapping regions in which light touch, pressure, and pinch would evoke increasingly robust responses. Of import is the observation that the repetition of a constant intensity C-fiber stimulus would evoke a progressive enhancement of the cells response to a subsequent stimulus. This progressive response augmentation, shown in Fig. 3, was named "wind-up" (118).

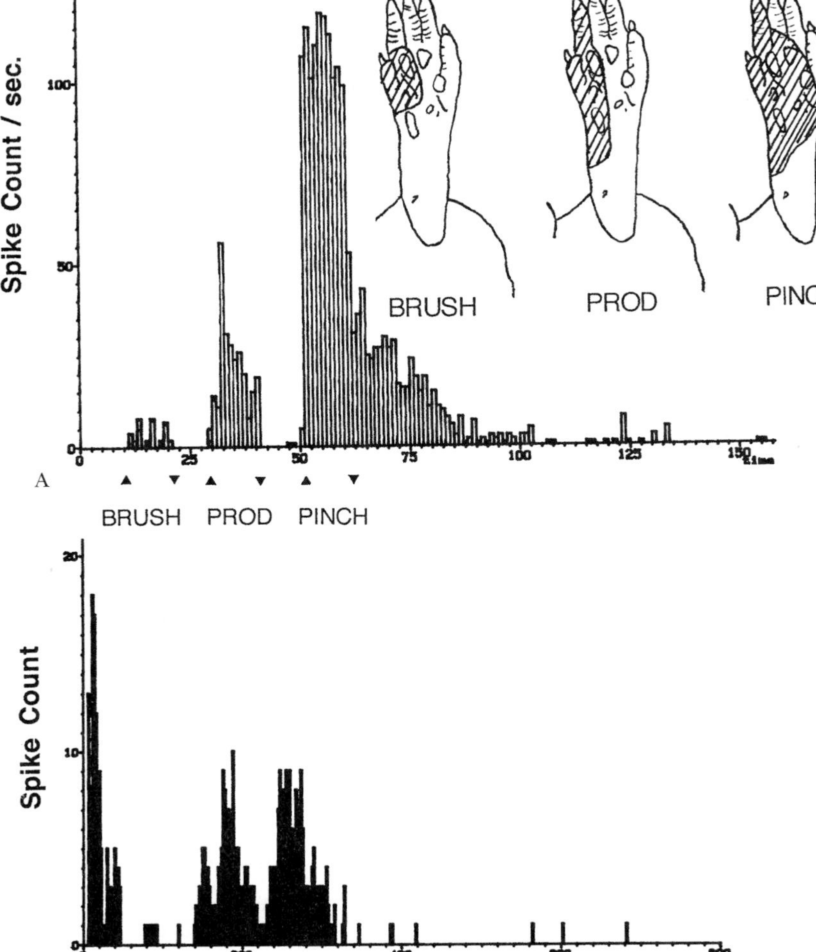

Figure 2. Electrophysiologic recording of the spontaneous activity in a single identified dorsal horn neuron and the response of that neuron to light touch, brush, and pinch applied to a cutaneous receptive field. As indicated, there are overlapping areas in which touch, brush, and pinch a may evoke a progressively increasing response frequency of neurons located in the ipsilateral dorsal horn decerebrate spinal unanesthetized rat. In the bottom portion, the poststimulus time histogram presents the response of the cell to electrical stimuli applied to the sural nerve at electrical intensities that induce activity in large and small afferents. This leads to a multiphasic appearance of activity in the recorded cell. The initial discharge represents the early activity generated by rapidly conducting A fibers, while the later discharge reflects the activity evoked by more slowly conducting Aδ and C fibers as well as some of the natural repetitive activity of the cell.

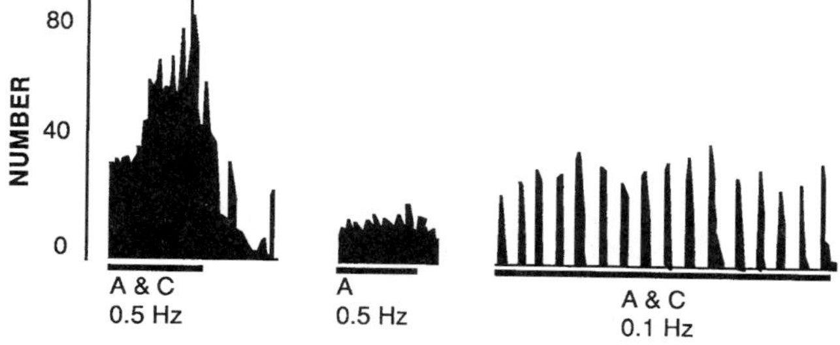

Figure 3. Response of a dorsal horn neuron being activated by an electrical stimulus applied to the sural nerve at an intensity that activates A and C fibers. *Right,* the stimulus is presented at a rate of 0.1 Hz. Each stimulus results in a subsequent barrage of activity in that cell. *Left,* the stimulus is presented at a rate of 0.5 Hz. At this higher frequency, it can be seen that the cell displays a progressive augmentation in its discharge pattern in response to each stimulus. This augmented response to each stimulus is referred as "wind-up." The receptive field of this cell will be markedly increased by this repetitive conditioning barrage. Stimulating a high frequency at an intensity that activated only large myelinated afferents is ineffective *(middle trace).* (Adapted from ref. 38.)

This phenomenon has been widely studied and is known to possess several specific properties:

1. Small (C-fiber), but not large (A-fiber) afferent input induce the enhanced response (38). Increases in the magnitude of the cell responses are produced to a marked degree so that tenfold increases in activity are common.
2. This augmentation in responding is typically induced by input from somatic and muscle afferents.
3. The response augmentation is dependent on afferent barrages that are delivered with frequencies in excess of 0.5 Hz.
4. WDR (wide dynamic range) neurons showing wind-up will continue to respond for minutes after the cessation of the peripheral input (38,39,118).
5. Measurement of the somatic receptive field reveals a pronounced increase in the size of the skin surface from which cellular activity can be evoked in facilitated cells (72,191).
6. This property of an afferent-evoked wind-up is largely limited to cells that display convergent input and that lie within deeper laminae. Superficial cells, such as those in lamina I, do not show wind-up (38).
7. Convergent neurons in the facilitated state induced by repetitive C-fiber input similarly display an augmented response to low-threshold primary afferents (42,43).

Facilitation Produced by Natural Stimuli

Augmentation of spinal neuronal responses has indeed been demonstrated in a number of animal models after the induction of an injury state, such as after knee joint inflammation (155,156) or the injection of irritant into the skin (38,43). These models are typically characterized by unexpectedly high levels of spinal neuronal activity in the face of relatively modest ongoing activity in the respective afferents (Fig. 4). In the case of the formalin model and of the knee joint, after the initial state of activation, blockade of afferent input by the use of a local nerve block typically results in a reduction in the measured neuronal activity (23,37). This observation emphasizes that the ongoing neuronal activity is dependent in large part on the afferent drive associated with the postinjury state and on a component of central facilitation that serves to enhance the response of the neuron to the otherwise nominal input. An important consideration is that some component of the stimulus serves to condition the spinal cord to produce an exaggerated response to subsequent input. In the case of the formalin injection, the initial intense barrage is believed to provide that stimulus. Thus, in that model, block of the afferent input by a local anesthetic during phase 1 attenuates the subsequent response observed during phase 2. These studies suggest the primary drive for the spinal cord neurons during the second phase of the formalin response is the peripheral input and that this impinges on central neurons that are sensitized by the conditioning barrage. The studies do not support the idea of a central state operating independently of afferent drive.

The electrophysiologic data outlined above are mirrored by the behavioral syndromes evoked in the animal. Thus, in the case of the injection of an irritant, such as formalin, the phenomenon observed in the second phase appears to reflect an exaggerated response to the otherwise modest afferent barrage (Fig. 4). Other examples, such as the hyperalgesic component observed after the creation of an inflamed knee joint (127,153; see Chap. 40) in animals or the injection of capsaicin in the skin of a human observer (97) or after an experimental burn (124), emphasize that this phenomenon has clear relevance to the behavior of the intact animal and human observed after an acute or protracted small afferent barrage. Importantly, in the behavioral models, the transient blockade of the afferent input during the first phase, as with local anesthetics or with intrathecal opiates (which serve to block small afferent input), diminishes the magnitude of the subsequent facilitated component (1,2,23). As will be discussed below, this facilitated response is characterized by a unique transmitter/receptor pharmacology.

This property of repetitive afferent input yielding a facilitated state of processing has great functional significance. As

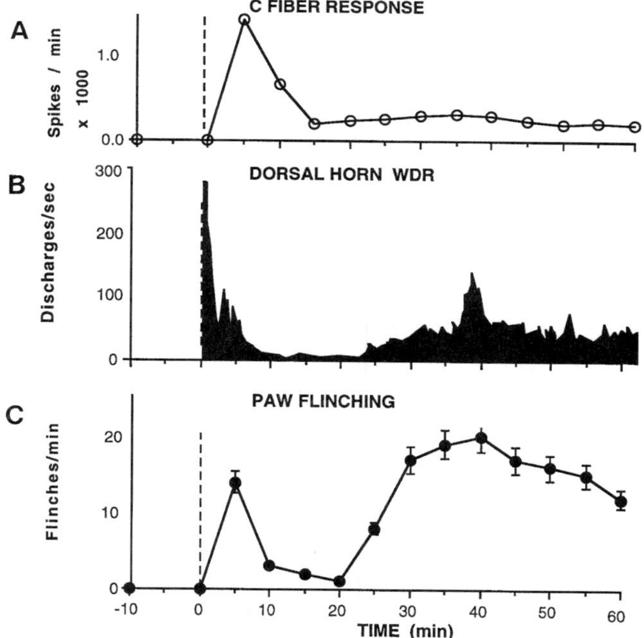

Figure 4. **A:** Discharge rate of multiple axons recorded in the saphenous nerve of the rat after the injection of formalin in the paw. (Adapted from ref. 67.) **B:** Firing frequency histogram of dorsal horn wide dynamic range neuron after the injection of formalin into the paw of the halothane-anesthetized rat. (Adapted from ref. 38.) **C:** Incidence of licking and flinching of the injected paw in the unanesthetized rat. (Adapted from ref. 109.) Note the input generated by the formalin injection with an initial peak declining to low, but nonzero, levels. In contrast, both the firing of the dorsal horn neuron and the coincident behavior in the unanesthetized rat shows an initial response (phase 1) consistent with the input and after some delay a second phase of discharge activity and behavior (phase 2).

reviewed in Chap. 32, after injury, the typical patterning of the afferent input is one of a relatively high level of tonic discharge (in contrast to the comparative silence of the uninjured state) interspersed with intervals of high-frequency discharges. Such high-frequency activity suggests that the standard condition of postinjury spinal processing involves this facilitated component.

PHARMACOLOGY OF SPINAL NEURONAL FACILITATION

Studies on the pharmacology of the spinal system that alter the facilitated state have employed electrophysiologic and behavioral indices where the agents are delivery topically to the spinal cord during the investigation. Using models involving protracted afferent input of small afferents, it has been possible to begin to separate the configuration of the transmitter/receptor systems that regulate the excitability of the dorsal horn evoked by small afferent input. The pharmacology of the afferent terminals and some of their postsynaptic consequences have been reviewed in Chaps. 34 and 35. It is clear that these terminals can release a variety of products including peptides such as substance P (SP), and amino acids such as glutamate. Several specific spinal systems will be discussed in the context of these facilitated states.

Substance P (SP)

SP and other tachykinins (known as neurokinin A and B) are contained in small dorsal root ganglion cells and contained in spinal terminals present in the substantia gelatinosa (46). These peptides are released by high-intensity but not low-intensity stimulation (47,55,96,201). Postsynaptically, SP may act on one of several tachykinin receptors: neurokinin-1, -2, and -3 receptors. SP has been shown to be the preferred tachykinin at the neurokinin-1 (NK1) receptor (68), whereas neurokinin A and B act on the NK2 and NK3 receptors. These receptors are located postsynaptically to the afferent fiber terminals, in laminae I, II, and X of the dorsal horn of the spinal cord (86).

NK1 antagonists have been shown to block slow excitatory postsynaptic potentials induced by noxious cutaneous stimulation and repetitive C-fiber stimulation, and to reduce noxious heat neuronal responses without affecting innocuous inputs (143,173,175). In addition, intrathecal NK1 antagonists have been shown to inhibit SP and C-fiber–induced reflex facilitation but not the unconditioned flexor reflex (22,75,208). Intrathecal NK1 antagonists produce a marked inhibition of the facilitated state observed after the knee joint (134). Importantly, these agents have little effect on the baseline escape latencies of animals that are not hyperalgesic (144,207). This is consistent with the observation that these agents do not block the acute response of the second-order neuron to the primary afferent stimulus.

Excitatory Amino Acids

Glutamate and aspartate are frequently used by spinal neurons as excitatory. Anatomical studies indicate a large proportion of peripheral sensory fibers including both small and large fibers contain glutamate and aspartate (9,114). This, together with the observations that up to 90% of substance P containing C fibers also contain glutamate (9,121), makes the point that there is significant cotransmission in C fibers, making it likely that a noxious stimulus releases both peptides and excitatory amino acids from the afferent nociceptive fibers. As the excitatory amino acids and peptides are found in different vesicles in the terminals (121), a differential release may occur under certain circumstances. During activation of the large-diameter innocuous fibers, which do not contain peptides, a release of glutamate has been demonstrated (85). With a noxious stimulus, amino acids are released after both acute (85,162) and prolonged (110,111) stimulation. In the case of the peptides as discussed earlier, SP may only be released when the stimulus is sufficiently long (142). Early electrophysiologic studies on dorsal horn neurons showed that nonselective antagonism of glutamate, in contrast to the antagonism of the peptides, blocked both the C- and large A-fiber–evoked activity of nociceptive neurons. The point was thus made that in the absence of transmission by excitatory amino acids, the actions of the peptides on the dorsal horn neurons are insufficient to cause excitation. Consequently, the long slow depolarizations produced by SP and other peptides provide excitation that acts cooperatively with that caused by amino acids.

As reviewed in Chap. 34, there are two major subtypes of glutamate receptors: ionotrophic and metabotrophic. The ionotrophic classes are reflected by the two principal classes, known as the AMPAl and (NMDA) *N*-methyl-D-aspartate sites [(RS)-α-amino-3-hydroxy-5-methyl-4-isoxazole proprionic acid]. AMPA receptor antagonism can block miniature end-plate potentials in superficial dorsal horn neurons (74) and attenuate C-fiber–evoked excitation of dorsal horn neurons (174). Pre- and postspinal administration of non-NMDA antagonists inhibits the formalin-evoked dorsal horn neuronal responses and behavioral measures (130).

The NMDA receptor, serving as a calcium ionophore (see Chap. 60), has been shown to be critical for several facilitatory processes in the CNS, including induction of long-term potentiation (LTP) in the hippocampus, and in rhythmic motor function at spinal levels are also well established (66).

There is now good evidence that the membrane effect mediated by the NMDA receptor plays a key role in mediating components of spinal excitability. At doses that do not block the initial discharge of the cell, agents that prevent the agonist evoked increase in the NMDA channel opening also prevent the evolution of the enhanced excitability otherwise produced by the repetitive small afferent stimulus. Thus, wind-up has been shown to be sensitive to spinally delivered NMDA receptor antagonists (2-amino-5-phosphono-valeric acid (AP5)), to drugs that act as channel blockers (MK-801 and ketamine) and to antagonists at the glycine site (29,36,38,40). The enhanced flexion reflex has also been shown to be sensitive to MK-801 (193). Similar results have been demonstrated for spinal neuronal activity evoked by peripheral injury and inflammation. Thus, as noted, the injection of formalin into the paw of the rat (36,59) or the generation of an inflamed knee joint (154) induces an ongoing afferent barrage and a state of persistent activity in dorsal horn neurons. The systemic or spinal delivery of NMDA receptor antagonists significantly reduces the persistent activity otherwise observed during the second phase of the formalin test (38) and after knee joint inflammation (132,133).

With regard to the behavioral state, intrathecally injected NMDA antagonists have little effect on acute nociceptive thresholds (such as the hot plate), but diminish the hyperalgesic components produced by protracted nociceptive afferent stimulation. Thus, the behavioral hyperalgesia as assessed in the formalin flinching model (205), the thermal hyperalgesia induced by carrageenan inflammation of the paw (148), ischemia of the hind limb (158), and the hyperalgesia induced by knee joint inflammation (127) are reduced toward baseline thresholds by the intrathecal delivery of these agents.

It should be emphasized that the role of the NMDA receptor in inflammation is not restricted to hyperalgesia. Detailed studies of the changes in neuronal activity induced by carrageenan inflammation reveal both increased and decreased responses in a large neuronal population (167). The direction of the changes in both the C- and Aβ-fiber responses of the neurons were dependent on the initial degree of wind-up in the cell (see Fig. 1). Since the NMDA receptor is excitatory, at first sight it would seem paradoxical that postcarrageenan responses in some cells were reduced and furthermore these were the cells that exhibited the most wind-up prior to carrageenan. However, NMDA receptor activation could also influence inhibitory interneurons in the spinal cord. There is some evidence for this proposition since it has been demonstrated that intrathecal NMDA activates both nociceptive and antinociceptive systems (123,145), and there is indirect evidence from studies in the hippocampus (15,45). An increase in glutamic acid decarboxylase in the rat dorsal horn after inflammation has been demonstrated (128) and this increase in γ-aminobutyric acid (GABA) may be responsible for some of the inhibition of the C-fiber–evoked responses seen following the carrageenan injection.

Physiology of Spinal SP and Glutamate Terminals

The above observations suggest that the activation of spinal afferents leads to the release of SP and glutamate, and that the subsequent activation of an SP or glutamate receptor leads to a hyperalgesic state. Iontophoretic delivery of SP, NMDA, and AMPA evokes background firing and increases the response of spinal dorsal horn neurons to thermal and mechanical stimuli (42). Similarly, intrathecal (it)-SP, AMPA, and NMDA evoke thermal and mechanical hyperalgesia lasting about 15 to 30 min (24,107) as well as an exaggerated response to light touch (allodynia) (Chaplan and Bach, *unpublished data* 1996). In these studies, it-delivery of the respective antagonists *before* it-injection of these agonists prevents thermal hyperalgesia or tactile allodynia, while delivery 5 min *after* the agonist has no effect on the hyperalgesic state (107; Chaplan and Bach, *unpublished data*). Thus, a relatively brief spinal NK1/excitatory amino acid agonist receptor occupancy can initiate a clear and transient facilitation of afferent processing.

MECHANISMS OF DORSAL HORN FACILITATION

Several intervening mechanisms that may account for these sustained states of facilitation have been identified. Depolarization of neurons or the activation of the NMDA receptor leads to an increase in intracellular Ca^{2+} (190), which evokes a cascade of biochemical events. The contributions of two elements of this cascade, prostaglandins and nitric oxide, are considered below.

Prostaglandins

Increased intracellular Ca^{2+} activates phospholipase A_2, leading to the appearance of cytosolic arachidonic acid and formation of cyclooxygenase (COX) and lipoxygenase products (100). COX immunoreactivity is distributed in brain and spinal neurons and to a lesser degree in glia or microvessels (11,204). In vivo, it-, K^+, -CAP (capsaicin), and -NMDA increase prostaglandin E_2 (PGE_2) levels in spinal perfusates or dialysates (162,195). Strong thermal stimulation (23) and subcutaneous (SC) formalin (111) evoke an acute and modestly sustained increase in spinal PGE_2 release. In contrast, knee joint arthritis evokes a progressive and sustained (>24 hour) increase in spinal PGE_2 release (207). Importantly, the PGE_2 release evoked by SC formalin or knee joint arthritis is reduced by morphine and spinal NMDA antagonism (111). These extracellular lipidic acids can (a) facilitate the depolarization evoked increases in Ca^{2+} conductance in dorsal root ganglion cells, and increase secretion of primary afferent peptides (136); and (b) evoke a thermal hyperalgesia after spinal delivery (179). Also, spinal cyclooxygenase inhibitors suppress the thermal hyperalgesia induced by spinally injected SP or NMDA (107) and the behavioral hyperalgesia resulting from peripheral tissue injury (108). Thermal hyperalgesia induced by it-SP, AMPA, and NMDA is reduced by it-nonsteroidal anti-inflammatory drugs (NSAIDs) (107). These effects of it-NSAIDs are stereospecific and display a structure activity relationship parallel to that for COX inhibition. Consistent with a role for spinal COX products, it-PGE antagonists diminish formalin Ph2 (106), while it-prostaglandins (PGs), including PGE_2, $PGF_{2\alpha}$, thromboxane A_2 (TXA_2), and PGI_2, produce a thermal and mechanical hyperalgesia (122,179). These results suggest that (a) spinal action of these prostanoids through one or more of the PG-receptors (r) sustain a hyperalgesic state, (b) activation of spinal NK/NMDA/AMPA receptors evokes the release of COX products, and protracted afferent input must evoke a sustained release of spinal PGs. For additional discussion on the role of central prostanoids in hyperalgesia, see Chap. 61.

Nitric Oxide

Nitric oxide (NO) formation is induced by NMDA receptor-mediated increases in Ca^{2+} (52). Nitric oxide synthase (NOS) is a cytosolic enzyme that catalyzes formation of NO through an interaction with the terminal guanidine nitrogen of L-arginine. This reaction leads to a stoichiometric formation of citrulline (CIT) (125). NOS (or reduced nicotinamide adenosine dinucleotide phosphate [NADPH]-diaphorase activity) is located in (a) DRG cells (182,211), (b) spinothalamic neurons, and (c) neurons containing GABA/glycine (98,181); it-NMDA, -CAP, and the injection of SC formalin have been shown to increase spinal CIT release. This release is reduced by NOS inhibitors and increased by L-Arg, emphasizing its covariance with NO synthesis (163). As defined in the hippocampus, NO diffuses from the site of formation to adjacent cells to increase intracellular cyclic guanosine monophosphate (cGMP) (164) and GLU release (138). In the spinal cord, NOS inhibition decreases GLU and PGE_2 release (162,163). This effect is in accord with reports that COX activity may be mediated by NOS activation (152). The hyperalgesia induced by spinal NMDA (107,116) or the second phase of the formalin test can be blocked by spinal injection of a inhibitor of NO synthesis (109). While these studies reflect the probable role of glutamate and substance P, the large number of afferent transmitters strongly suggests that a variety of these candidate transmitters may subserve roles similar to those defined above for excitatory amino acids and SP.

DYNAMIC INFLUENCES ON THE ENCODING OF LOW-INTENSITY INPUT

Definition of components of systems that mediate a "pain state" has typically evolved from the association of activity evoked by small-afferent input (Aδ/C) and the failure to evoke such states with large afferent (A) input (see Chap. 14). An extensive literature exists in which low-threshold, otherwise nonaversive, stimulation evokes a clearly defined pain state. Two conditions appear commonly associated with this change in the encoding process: (a) As reviewed in Chap. 18, after the protracted afferent activation of C fibers, as in the injection of intradermal capsaicin in humans, a pain state may be evoked by low-threshold mechanoreceptive stimuli applied to an extended area around the injection site. This allodynia may be prevented by the prior blockade of the afferents from the injection site. This argues that processes generated by the repetitive small-afferent barrage will alter dorsal horn processing. (b) After peripheral nerve injury, animals and humans may develop a condition in which a low-threshold mechanical stimulus evokes a pain state. The psychophysics of this state clearly emphasize that the state is mediated by the activation of low-threshold Aβ mechanoreceptors. In the following sections, several components of this dynamic reorganization are considered.

GABA/Glycine Systems and Aloydynia

Low-threshold afferents terminate ventral to the substantia gelatinosa and converge on lamina V wide-dynamic-range neurons. As noted in the preceding sections, these cells are also activated by small afferents and are believed to play a role in the encoding of the pain message. Early studies revealed that the local inhibition of GABA and glycine receptors systems in the vicinity of the primary afferent terminals (using bicuculline or strychnine, respectively) would (a) significantly enhance the discharge evoked by Aβ afferents, but only modestly the input generated by high-threshold afferents (91,209); and (b) permit light tactile stroking of the skin to evoke a well-defined pain state as defined by autonomic and behavioral criteria (159, 197). These simple observations suggest that the encoding of low-intensity mechanical stimuli as innocuous depends on the ongoing presence of tonically active intrinsic glycine and or GABAergic neurons. Such neurons are found within the dorsal horn (17,176), and glycine (8,210) and GABA (160) binding in the dorsal horn has been demonstrated. These GABA-containing terminals are frequently presynaptic to the large central afferent terminal complexes and may form reciprocal synapses (7). GABAergic axosomatic connections on spinothalamic cells have also been identified (17).

The relevance of these inhibitory amino acid systems in regulating behavior generated by low-threshold afferent transmission is suggested by (a) mouse (188) and bovine (58) results showing a prominent somatic sensitivity display up to a tenfold decrease in glycine binding; (b) strychnine intoxication in man, which is characterized by a hypersensitivity to light touch (3); and (c) spinal cord ischemia, which is known to destroy amino acid containing interneurons, yields a tactile allodynia (62–64,112).

Post–Nerve Injury and Allodynia

In the human state, allodynic conditions are frequently observed after peripheral nerve compression or injury (139,141; see Chap. 56). Animal studies have evolved several models in which peripheral nerve compression will lead to a state of hyperalgesia or tactile allodynia (92,197; see Chap. 40). Pursuit of the changes that are induced by such nerve injury has provided some insights into the systems that may be involved in the evolution of the post–nerve injury allodynia. Following peripheral nerve ligation or section, several events occur, signaling long-term changes in peripheral and central processing:

1. Peripheral changes in terminal sensitivity are noted. The sprouted terminals display a characteristic growth cone that possesses transduction properties that were not possessed by the original axon. These include significant mechanical and chemical sensitivity. Thus, these sprouted endings may have sensitivity to a number of humoral factors, such as PGs, catecholamines, and cytokines (35). In addition, it is known that these regenerating terminals have significant densities of various ion channels, notably those for sodium (32). Increased ionic conductance may result in the increase in spontaneous activity that develops in a sprouting axon (32,113).
2. Persistent small afferent fiber activity originates after an interval of days to weeks from the lesioned site (neuroma) and from the dorsal root ganglion (DRG) of the injured nerve (12, 34).
3. Prominent changes in the morphology of the DRG cells is observed. Recent data for example has indicated that following peripheral lesion, there is a hyper-innervation of the type A ganglion cells by sympathetic terminals (115) and cross talk between A and C fibers develops in the ganglion (33).
4. Morphologic changes are seen in the ipsilateral spinal dorsal horn. While the mechanism of these changes is not clear, it is likely that enduring changes result secondary to the chronic afferent barrage or to a change in factors transported from the lesioned site. Transsynaptic changes include the appearance of immediate early gene products, such as *C-fos*; an increase in message for specific neurotransmitter, such as substance P; and "dark staining" neurons in the spinal dorsal horns (14,50,51, 70,71,169). These alterations clearly signal changes in dorsal horn function.
5. After peripheral nerve lesions, large primary afferent (Aβ) axons have been shown to sprout and to send terminals dorsally into the overlying substantia gelatinosa (192). As previously discussed, small afferents typically project only into the substantia gelatinosa, and there appears to be a fine demarcation into the projection fields of the several fiber classes. This sprouting thus places the large afferents into close proximity with systems that were originally only impacted by small afferents. While the precise significance of this is not known, it appears reasonable that such anomalous projections may underlie some of the connectivity required to explain the phenomenon of low-threshold afferents driving a pain state.

PHARMACOLOGY OF THE ALLODYNIC STATE

The evolution of the several preclinical models in which allodynia plays an important role in the behavioral syndrome leads naturally to the question of what regulates this behavior. Table 4 in Chap. 40 summarizes some of the pharmacology that appears to regulate the animal's allodynic response.

A common factor that has permeated the preclinical allodynia studies has been the probable importance of the release of glutamate. Thus, spinal NMDA antagonists appear to be particularly potent in reversing the allodynia observed in a number of nerve injury–allodynia animal models (see Table 4 in Chap. 40). Direct measurement of the release of glutamate from the spinal cord has indicated the appearance of an ongoing elevation in glutamate levels after peripheral tissue injury (110,209). As noted previously, direct activation of the glutamate receptor by spinal drug delivery evokes a hyperalgesic/allodynic state. It thus seems probable that at least a component of the allodynia following nerve injury may be the consequence of an increased spontaneous release of glutamate. Importantly, agents thought to regulate glutamate release such as the adenosine A_1 receptor (28,49) also display a potent antiallodynic effect in animals (99), reduce the facilitated discharge of dorsal horn neurons (147), and reduce allodynia in humans (87). This role of enhanced glutamatergic activity may reflect a change in the postsynaptic coupling (e.g., more receptors) or an enhanced release, perhaps occurring secondary to the spontaneous activity originating from the neuroma or the dorsal root ganglion cell. In this regard, case reports in human patients suffering from significant allodynia secondary to a presumed nerve injury can be blocked by local anesthetic injections into the injured region (57). This argues that whatever changes may have occurred within the neuraxis, the appearance of the pain state requires the ongoing input from the periphery. Furthermore, it is interesting to note that some allodynic states may be driven. Thus, brushing an area of dysesthesia (e.g., driving large afferent input) may evoke a widespread area of tactile allodynia (95). The diminished effect of spinal opiates on neuropathic pain in man (4) and in the animal models (see above) is consistent with electrophysiologic observations that spontaneous activity in dorsal horn neurons that is generated following brachial plexus lesion is poorly sensitive to opiates, and with the clinical reports suggesting mixed effects of opiates on neuropathic pain states. Alternately, the marginal effect of opiates in the neuropathic pain models as compared to the acute thermal response model (hot plate) is consistent with the probable role of C fibers in the acute pain models and A fibers in the neuropathic models. In recent work, it was shown that spinal α_2-agonists have a potent antiallodynic effect in post–nerve injury models (202). This effect was believed to be mediated in part by the sympatholytic effects of spinal α_2-agonists.

It appears likely that the allodynic state that follows nerve injury may have several mechanisms: (a) changes in spinal cord connectivity after nerve injury (e.g., sprouting of large afferents; sprouting of the sympathetic efferent into the neuroma and dorsal root ganglia); (b) the loss of intrinsic modulatory systems that alter the subsequent encoding of afferent evoked excitation (e.g., dark-staining neurons); (c) an upregulation of excitatory processes (e.g., dorsal horn NK receptors among others); and (d) dynamic processes that are reflected by tonic afferent input generated by the appearance of spontaneous activity arising from the neuroma and the dorsal root ganglion cell. It is important to appreciate that as acute pain states have many components, it is similarly true that all neuropathic pain is not the same and will likely display distinct mechanisms. This can be intuited from the simple case reports noted above. In a patient suffering from a spontaneous dysesthesia, brushing the dysesthetic region evoked a large area of tactile allodynia. Both reflected components of a neuropathic pain state. However, intrathecal NMDA receptor antagonism attenuated only the evoked tactile allodynia; the area of spontaneous dysesthesia was not attenuated. Further discussion on the mechanisms of the post–nerve injury pain state may be found in Chap. 56.

DYNAMIC EFFECTS OF AFFERENT TRAFFIC ON RECEPTOR FUNCTION

Thus far, this chapter has provided a framework on which excitatory events, mediated by excitatory amino acids and peptides, can interact to produce pain events that will vary depending on the particular systems that are active at that time. We can start to see how pain states may possess a distinct pharmacology depending on different relative roles of these excitatory systems. Consider the following example. Behavioral studies have shown that after an injection of a proinflammatory agent such as carrageenan, edema rapidly develops, followed by a period of hyperalgesia that peaks at 3 to 4 hours following inoculation, and is largely resolved 24 to 72 hours later (65,89). An increased antinociceptive effect of systemically administered opiate agonists has been reported in animals following the induction of peripheral inflammation (83,88,131). This had previously been attributed to additional actions of these drugs at opiate receptors in the periphery, which become functional within the inflamed tissue (84,168). However in a behavioral study, Hylden et al. (77) have demonstrated an increase in the antinociceptive effect of opioids following intrathecal administration, suggesting that central changes also play a role. Similarly, in carrageenan inflamed rats, μ, δ, and κ opioids applied onto the spinal cord exhibit an increased antinociceptive potency (167). The enhancement of opioid actions at the spinal level, seen in both the behavioral study of Hylden et al. (77) and in electrophysiologic studies (167), has been shown to occur within 2 hours of the onset of the inflammation.

This enhanced activity may result from several mechanisms: (a) There could be an enhanced opioid binding, but no such changes have been observed (30,78). (b) A variety of inflammatory states are associated with elevated levels of opioid gene transcripts, and peptides in the spinal cord, particularly dynorphin, have been found (78,151). (c) Dynorphin and other synthetic κ ligands such as U-50,488H and U69593 have been shown to produce both inhibitions and excitations of dorsal horn nociceptive neurons when administered intrathecally (77,94,170). There was a close correlation between the magnitude of change in the neuronal responses after inflammation and the effects of norbinaltophimine (nBNI). Those cells with the greatest changes in their activity after inflammation were the most sensitive to nBNI. Since the magnitude of changes in the neuronal responses correlates with the wind-up of the cells, this provides evidence for a chain of events in the spinal cord following peripheral inflammation. The developing inflammation activates peripheral afferents that in turn activate spinal NMDA receptors. Cells with relatively low-NMDA participation in their responses exhibit increased responses, whereas those with high-NMDA drive are inhibited. In addition to driving the neuronal changes, the NMDA activation enhances κ opioid function in the cord, but the relevance of this to transmission and modulation remains unknown (166).

Potential Mechanisms for Alterations in Receptor Sensitivity

Cholecystokinin (CCK) and FLFQPQRF amide, found within intrinsic spinal cord neurons with an additional descending contribution, reduce μ but not δ opioid actions in chronic inflammatory models (104) and in behavioral tests (48). An increase in μ opioid efficacy could then be predicted if there was a depletion or a reduced release of these nonopioid peptides. Klein et al. (93) have demonstrated alterations in the levels of spinal peptides, including CCK, following peripheral nerve damage, and so it is conceivable that the peripheral inflammatory state could also induce modifications in these spinal peptides. Since the two peptides have the ability to reduce morphine analgesia in normal animals, it can be predicted that a reduction in their actions either due to reduced release or receptor changes would lead to an increase in the efficacy of morphine. The former seems to be the situation in inflammation, since based on the use of agonists and antagonists there are no CCK-B receptor changes in the spinal cord, but there is evidence for a reduced release of the peptide, which in turn removes the limitation on the effects of morphine, which results in the enhanced effects of the opioid.

It has been suggested that the greater enhancement in the potency of μ opiates compared to that seen with selective δ and κ agonists following carrageenan inflammation may be explained by increased activity of the noradrenergic descending controls possibly producing altered α_2-adrenoceptor number or function. Many studies have reported that synergism occurs between the spinal antinociceptive actions of morphine and those of selective α_2-agonists such as clonidine and dexmedetomidine (165). The selective and potent α_2-agonist dexmedetomidine is able to specifically potentiate the antinociceptive actions of morphine but not those of δ agonists when given by the intrathecal route. This, together with the finding that the turnover of noradrenaline in the spinal cord is increased following inflammation forms a basis for the theory that noradrenaline is involved in the enhanced actions of morphine following carrageenan-induced inflammation.

RELEVANCE OF SPINAL FACILITATORY STATES

Perhaps no issue has served to alter our thinking about the organization of afferent processing so significantly in the past 15 years as the growing appreciation that the afferent input generated is subject to a prominent modulation, although in the 1970s to 1980s the emphasis was on a downregulation of afferent processing (e.g., the endogenous modulatory systems). The current perspective reflects more on the fact that the systems are subject to a pronounced upregulation in the face of the injury response of the peripheral afferent. The important issue here is that low-threshold Aβ afferents can initiate a pain state. Specific studies in this area reviewed above and in other chapters in this volume have revealed that the electrophysiology and biochemistry of these changes in processing have a complex pharmacology. The preclinical studies reviewed elsewhere (see Chap. 40) have begun to provide important insights into the behavioral relevance of that upregulation and the respective pharmacology. Importantly, where thus far examined, the preclinical insights appear to have close parallels to those changes that occur in human nociceptive processing during the postinjury pain state (see Chap. 41). This reregulation results in an enhanced signal that appears to require greater inhibitory input (e.g., opiates to regulate that processing) (194), and the enhancement may occur even under conditions of surgical planes of anesthesia (1). Thus, as reviewed elsewhere (see Chap. 43), there is controversy as to whether anesthetic concentrations of volatile anesthetics alone may not block the initiation of a facilitated state. Accordingly, an effective management of a postinjury pain state may require greater emphasis on methods that frankly block afferent input, diminish C-fiber drive, or prevent the evolution of the facilitated state.

REFERENCES

1. Abram SE, Yaksh TL. Morphine, but not inhalation anesthesia, blocks post-injury facilitation. The role of preemptive suppression of afferent transmission. *Anesthesiology* 1993;78:713–721.
2. Abram SE, Yaksh TL. Systemic lidocaine blocks nerve injury-induced hyperalgesia and nociceptor-driven spinal sensitization in the rat. *Anesthesiology* 1994;80:383–891.
3. Arena JM. *Poisoning toxicology, symptoms, treatments,* 4th ed. Springfield, IL: Charles C. Thomas, 1970.
4. Arner S, Meyerson BA. Lack of analgesic effect of opioids on neuropathic and idiopathic forms of pain. *Pain* 1988;33:11–23.
5. Arvidsson U, Ulfhake B, Cullheim S, Shupliakov O, Brodin E, Franck J, Bennett GW, Fone KC, Visser TJ, Hokfelt T. Thyrotropin-releasing hormone (TRH)-like immunoreactivity in the grey monkey (Macaca fascicularis) spinal cord and medulla oblongata with special emphasis on the bulbospinal tract. *J Comp Neurol* 1992;322:293–310.
6. Azmitia EC, Gannon PJ. The primate serotonergic system: a review of human and animal studies and a report on Macaca fascicularis. *Adv Neurol* 1986;43:407–468.
7. Barber RP, Vaughn JE, Saito K, McLaughlin BJ, Roberts E. Gabaergic terminals are presynaptic to primary afferent terminals in the substantia gelatinosa of the rat spinal cord. *Brain Res* 1978;141:35–55.
8. Basbaum AI. Distribution of glycine receptor immunoreactivity in the spinal cord of the rat: cytochemical evidence for a differential glycinergic control of lamina I and V nociceptive neurons. *J Comp Neurol* 1988;278:330–336.
9. Battaglia G, Rustioni A. Coexistence of glutamate and substance P in dorsal root ganglion neurons of the rat and monkey. *J Comp Neurol* 1988;277:302–312.
10. Borsook D, Hyman SE. Proenkephalin gene regulation in the neuroendocrine hypothalamus: a model of gene regulation in the CNS. *Am J Physiol* 1995;269:E393–408.
11. Breder CD, Smith WL, Raz A, Masferrer J, Seibert K, Needleman P, Saper CB. Distribution and characterization of cyclooxygenase Immunoreactivity in the ovine brain. *J Comp Neurol* 1992;322:409–438.
12. Burchiel KJ. Spontaneous impulse generation in normal and denervated dorsal root ganglia: sensitivity to alpha adrenergic stimulation and hypoxia. *Exp Neurol* 1984;85:257–272.
13. Camarata PJ, Yaksh TL. Characterization of the spinal adrenergic receptors mediating the spinal effects produced by the microinjection of morphine into the periaqueductal gray. *Brain Res* 1985;336: 133–142.
14. Cameron AA, Cliffer KD, Dougherty PM, Willis WD, Carlton SM. Changes in lectin, GAP-43 and neuropeptide staining in the rat superficial dorsal horn following experimental peripheral neuropathy. *Neurosci Lett* 1991;131:249–252.
15. Capek R, Esplin B. Attenuation of hippocampal inhibition by a NMDA (N-methyl-D-aspartate) receptor antagonist. *Neurosci Lett* 1991;129:145–148.
16. Carlton SM, Honda CN, Willcockson WS, Lacrampe M, Zhang D, Denoroy L, Chun JM, Willis WD. Descending adrenergic input to the primate spinal cord and its possible role in modulation of spinothalamic cells. *Brain Res,* 1991;543:77–90.
17. Carlton SM, Westlund KN, Zhang D, Willis WD. GABA-immunoreactive terminals synapse on primate spinothalamic tract cells. *J Comp Neurol* 1992;322:528–537.
18. Carstens E, Hartung M, Stelzer B, Zimmermann M. Suppression of a hind limb flexion withdrawal reflex by microinjection of glutamate or morphine into the periaqueductal gray in the rat. *Pain* 1990;43:105–112.
19. Cesselin F, Bourgoin S, Artaud F, Hamon M. Basic and regulatory mechanisms of in vitro release of Met-enkephalin from the dorsal zone of the rat spinal cord. *J Neurochem* 1984;43:763–774.
20. Chalmers J, Kapoor V, Mills E, Minson J, Morris M, Pilowsky P, West M. Do pressor neurons in the ventrolateral medulla release amines and neuropeptides? *Can J Physiol Pharmacol* 1987;65:1598–1604.
21. Chang AC, Cochet M, Cohen SN. Structural organization of human genomic DNA encoding the pro-opiomelanocortin peptide. *Proc Natl Acad Sci USA* 1980;77:4890–4894.
22. Chapman V, Dickenson AH. The effect of intrathecal administration of RP67580, a potent neurokinin 1 antagonist on nociceptive transmission in the rat spinal cord. *Neurosci Lett* 1993;157:149–152.
23. Coderre TJ, Gonzales R, Goldyne ME, West J, Levine JD. Noxious stimulus-induced increase in spinal prostaglandin E2 is noradrenergic terminal-dependent. *Neurosci Lett* 1990;115:253–258.
24. Coderre TJ, Melzack R. The contribution of excitatory amino acids to central sensitization and persistent nociception after formalin-induced tissue injury. *J Neurosci* 1992;12:3665–3670.
25. Coderre TJ, Vaccarino AL, Melzack R. Central nervous system plasticity in the tonic pain response to subcutaneous formalin injection. *Brain Res* 1990 535:155–158.
26. Coderre TJ, Yashpal K. Intracellular messengers contributing to persistent nociception and hyperalgesia induced by L-glutamate and substance P in the rat formalin pain model. *Eur J Neurosci* 1994; 6:1328–1334.
27. Coote JH, Lewis DI. Bulbospinal catecholamine neurones and sympathetic pattern generation. *J Physiol Pharmacol* 1995;46:259–271.
28. Corradetti R, Lo Conte G, Moroni F, Passani MB, Pepeu G. Adenosine decreases aspartate and glutamate release from rat hippocampal slices. *Eur J Pharmacol* 1984;104:19–26.
29. Davies SN, Lodge D. Evidence for involvement of N-methylaspartate receptors in 'wind-up' of class 2 neurones in the dorsal horn of the rat. *Brain Res* 1987;424:402–406.
30. Delay-Goyet P, Kayser V, Zajac JM, Guilbaud G, Besson JM, Roques BP. Lack of significant changes in mu, delta opioid binding sites and neutral endopeptidase EC 3.4.24.11 in the brain and spinal cord of arthritic rats. *Neuropharmacology* 1989;28:1341–1348.
31. Denny-Brown D, Kirk EJ, Yanagisawa N. The tract of Lissauer in relation to sensory transmission in the dorsal horn of spinal cord in the macaque monkey. *J Comp Neurol* 1973;151:175–200.
32. Devor M, Govrin-Lippmann R, Angelides K. Na+ channel immunolocalization in peripheral mammalian axons and changes following nerve injury and neuroma formation. *J Neurosci* 1993;13:1976–1992.
33. Devor M, Wall PD. Cross-excitation in dorsal root ganglia of nerve-injured and intact rats. *J Neurophysiol* 1990;64:1733–1746.
34. Devor M, Wall PD, Catalann N. Systemic lidocaine silences ectopic neuroma and DRG discharge without blocking nerve conduction. *Pain* 1992;48:261–268.
35. Devor M, White DM, Goetzl EJ, Levine JD. Eicosanoids, but not tachykinins, excite C-fiber endings in rat sciatic nerve-end neuromas. *Neuroreport* 1992;3:21–24.
36. Dickenson AH, Aydar E. Antagonism at the glycine site on the NMDA receptor reduces spinal nociception in the rat. *Neurosci Lett* 1991;121:263–266.
37. Dickenson AH, Sullivan AF. Peripheral origins and central modulation of subcutaneous formalin-induced activity of rat dorsal horn neurones. *Neurosci Lett* 1987;83:207–211.
38. Dickenson AH, Sullivan AF. Evidence for a role of the NMDA receptor in the frequency dependent potentiation of deep rat dorsal horn nociceptive neurones following C fibre stimulation. *Neuropharmacology* 1987;26:1235–1238.
39. Dickenson AH, Sullivan AF. Differential effects of excitatory

amino acid antagonists on dorsal horn nociceptive neurones in the rat. *Brain Res* 1990;506 31–39.
40. Dickenson AH, Sullivan AF, Stanfa LC, McQuay HJ. Dextromethorphan and levorphanol on dorsal horn nociceptive neurones in the rat. *Neuropharmacology* 1991 30:1303–1308.
41. Dores RM, Akil H, Watson SJ. Strategies for studying opioid peptide regulation at the gene, message and protein levels. *Peptides* 1984;5(suppl 1):9–17.
42. Dougherty PM, Palecek J, Zorn S, Willis WD. Combined application of excitatory amino acids and substance P produces long-lasting changes in responses of primate spinothalamic tract neurons. Brain Res. *Brain Res Rev* 1993;18:227–246.
43. Dougherty PM, Willis WD. Enhanced responses of spinothalamic tract neurons to excitatory amino acids accompany capsaicin-induced sensitization in the monkey. *J Neurosci* 1992;12:883–894.
44. Dray A. Mechanism of action of capsaicin-like molecules on sensory neurons. *Life Sci* 1992;51:1759–1765.
45. Dudek SM, Bear MF. Homosynaptic long-term depression in area CA1 of hippocampus and effects of N-methyl-D-aspartate receptor blockade. Proc Natl Acad Sci USA 1992;89:4363–4367.
46. Duggan AW, Hendry LA. Laminar localization of the sites of release of immunoreactive substance P in the dorsal horn with antibody-coated microelectrode. *Neurosci Lett* 1986;68:134–140.
47. Duggan AW, Hendry LA, Morton CR, Hutchison WD, Zhao ZO. Cutaneous stimuli releasing immunoreactive substance P in the dorsal horn of the cat. *Brain Res* 1988;451:261–273.
48. Faris PL, Komisaruk BR, Watkins LR, Mayer DJ. Evidence for the neuropeptide cholecystokinin as an antagonist of opiate analgesia. *Science* 1983;219:310–312.
49. Fredholm BB, Fastbom J, Lindgren E. Effects of N-ethylmaleimide and forskolin on glutamate release from rat hippocampal slices. Evidence that prejunctional adenosine receptors are linked to N-proteins, but not to adenylate cyclase. *Acta Physiol Scand* 1986;127: 381–386.
50. Garrison CJ, Dougherty PM, Kajander KC, Carlton SM. Staining of glial fibrillary acidic protein (GFAP) in lumbar spinal cord increases following a sciatic nerve constriction injury. *Brain Res* 1991;565:1–7.
51. Garry MG, Kajander KC, Bennett GJ. Seybold VS. Quantitative autoradiographic analysis of [^{125}I]-human CGRP binding sites in the dorsal horn of rat following chronic constriction injury or dorsal rhizotomy. *Peptides* 1991;12:1365–1373.
52. Garthwaite J, Garthwaite G, Palmer RM, Moncada S. NMDA receptor activation induces nitric oxide synthesis from arginine in rat brain slices. *Eur J Pharmacol* 1989;172:413–416.
53. Gebhart GF, Sandkuhler J, Thalhammer JG, Zimmermann M. Quantitative comparison of inhibition in spinal cord of nociceptive information by stimulation in periaqueductal gray or nucleus raphe magnus of the cat. *J Neurophysiol* 1983;50:1433–1445.
54. Gebhart GF, Sandkuhler J, Thalhammer JG, Zimmermann M. Inhibition in spinal cord of nociceptive information by electrical stimulation and morphine microinjection at identical sites in midbrain of the cat. *J Neurophysiol* 1984;51:75–89.
55. Go VL, Yaksh TL. Release of substance P from the cat spinal cord. *J Physiol* 1987;391:141–167.
56. Gobel S, Falls WM, Bennett GJ, Abdelmoumene M, Hayashi H, Humphrey E. An EM analysis of the synaptic connections of horseradish peroxidase-filled stalked cells and islet cells in the substantia gelatinosa of adult cat spinal cord. *J Comp Neurol,* 1980; 194:781–807.
57. Gracely RH, Lynch SA, Bennett GJ. Painful neuropathy: altered central processing maintained dynamically by peripheral input. *Pain* 1992;51:175–194.
58. Grundlach AL, Dodd PR, Grabara-Watson WEJ, et al. Deficits of spinal cord glycine / strychnine receptors in inherited myoclonius of poll Hereford calves. *Science* 1988;241:1807–1810.
59. Haley JE, Sullivan AF, Dickenson AH. Evidence for spinal N-methyl-D-aspartate receptor involvement in prolonged chemical nociception in the rat. *Brain Res* 1990;518:218–226.
60. Hammond DL, Tyce GM, Yaksh TL. Efflux of 5-hydroxytryptamine and noradrenaline into spinal cord superfusates during stimulation of the rat medulla. *J Physiol* 1985;359:151–162.
61. Hammond DL, Yaksh TL. Antagonism of stimulation-produced antinociception by intrathecal administration of methysergide or phentolamine. *Brain Res* 1984;298:329–337.
62. Hao JX, Xu XJ, Aldskogius H, Seiger A, Wiesenfeld-Hallin Z. Allodynia-like effects in rat after ischaemic spinal cord injury photochemically induced by laser irradiation. *Pain* 1991;45:175–185.
63. Hao JX, Xu XJ, Yu YX, Seiger A, Wiesenfeld-Hallin Z. Transient spinal cord ischemia induces temporary hypersensitivity of dorsal horn wide dynamic range neurons to myelinated, but not unmyelinated, fiber input. *J Neurophysiol* 1992;68:384–383.
64. Hao JX, Xu XJ, Yu YX, Seiger A, Wiesenfeld-Hallin Z. Baclofen reverses the hypersensitivity of dorsal horn wide dynamic range neurons to mechanical stimulation after transient spinal cord ischemia, implications for a tonic GABAergic inhibitory control of myelinated fiber input. *J Neurophysiol* 1992;68:392–396.
65. Hargreaves K, Dubner R, Brown F, Flores C, Joris J. A new and sensitive method for measuring thermal nociception in cutaneous hyperalgesia. *Pain* 1988;32:77–88.
66. Headley PM, Grillner S. Excitatory amino acids and synaptic transmission: the evidence for a physiological function. *Trends Pharmacol Sci* 1990;11:205–211.
67. Heapy CG, Jamieson A, Russell NJW. Afferent C-fiber and A-delta activity in models of inflammation. *Br J Pharmacol* 1987;90:164P.
68. Henry JL. Participation of substance P in spinal physiological responses to peripheral aversive stimulation. *Regul Pept* 1993;46: 138–143.
69. Herbert E, Birnberg N, Civelli O, Lissitzky JC, Uhler M, Durrin L. Regulation of genetic expression of pro-opiomelanocortin in pituitary and extrapituitary tissues of mouse and rat. *Adv Biochem Psychopharmacol* 1982;33:9–18.
70. Herdegen T, Fiallos-Estrada C, Schmid W, Bravo R, Zimmermann M. The transcription factor CREB, but not immediate-early gene encoded proteins, is expressed in activated microglia of lumbar spinal cord following sciatic nerve transection in the rat. *Neurosci Lett* 1992;142:57–61.
71. Herdegen T, Fiallos-Estrada CE, Schmid W, Bravo R, Zimmermann M. The transcription factors c-JUN, JUN D and CREB, but not FOS and KROX-24, are differentially regulated in axotomized neurons following transection of rat sciatic nerve. *Mol Brain Res* 1992;14: 155–165.
72. Hillman P, Wall PD. Inhibitory and excitatory factors influencing the receptive fields of lamina 5 spinal cord cells. *Exp Brain Res* 1969;9:284–306.
73. Holmqvist B, Lundberg A, Oscarsson O. Supraspinal inhibitory control of transmission to three ascending spinal pathways influenced by the flexion reflex afferents. *Arch Ital Biol* 1960;98:60–80.
74. Hori Y, Endo K. Miniature postsynaptic currents recorded from identified rat spinal dorsal horn projection neurons in thin-slice preparations. *Neurosci Lett* 1992;142:191–195.
75. Hosoki R, Yanagisawa M, Guo JZ, Yoshioka K, Maehara T, Otsuka M. Effects of RP 67580, a tachykinin NK1 receptor antagonist, on a primary afferent-evoked response of ventral roots in the neonatal rat spinal cord. *Br J Pharmacol* 1994;113:1141–1146.
76. Howells RD, Kilpatrick DL, Bhatt R, Monahan JJ, Poonian M, Udenfriend S. Molecular cloning and sequence determination of rat preproenkephalin cDNA: sensitive probe for studying transcriptional changes in rat tissues. *Proc Natl Acad Sci USA* 1984;81: 7651–7655.
77. Hylden JL, Thomas DA, Iadarola MJ, Nahin RL, Dubner R. Spinal opioid analgesic effects are enhanced in a model of unilateral inflammation/hyperalgesia: possible involvement of noradrenergic mechanisms. *Eur J Pharmacol* 1991;194:135–143.
78. Iadarola MJ, Brady LS, Draisci G, Dubner R. Enhancement of dynorphin gene expression in spinal cord following experimental inflammation: stimulus specificity, behavioral parameters and opioid receptor binding. *Pain* 1988;35:313–326.
79. James IF, Fischli W, Goldstein A. Opioid receptor selectivity of dynorphin gene products. *J Pharmacol Exp Ther* 1984;228:88–93.
80. Janss AJ, Gebhart GF. Brainstem and spinal pathways mediating descending inhibition from the medullary lateral reticular nucleus in the rat. *Brain Res* 1988;440:109–122.
81. Jensen TS, Yaksh TL. Examination of spinal monoamine receptors through which brainstem opiate-sensitive systems act in the rat. *Brain Res* 1986;363:114–127.
82. Jones SL, Gebhart GF. Inhibition of spinal nociceptive transmission from the midbrain, pons and medulla in the rat: activation of descending inhibition by morphine, glutamate and electrical stimulation. *Brain Res* 1988;460:281–296.
83. Joris J, Costello A, Dubner R, Hargreaves KM. Opiates suppress carrageenan-induced edema and hyperthermia at doses that inhibit hyperalgesia. *Pain* 1990;43:95–103.
84. Joris JL, Dubner R, Hargreaves KM. Opioid analgesia at peripheral sites: a target for opioids released during stress and inflammation? *Anesth Analg* 1987;66:1277–1281.

85. Kangrga I, Randic M. Outflow of endogenous aspartate and glutamate from the rat spinal dorsal horn in vitro by activation of low- and high-threshold primary afferent fibers. Modulation by mu-opioids. *Brain Res* 1991;553:347–352.
86. Kar S, Quirion R. Neuropeptide receptors in developing and adult rat spinal cord: an in vitro quantitative autoradiography study of calcitonin gene-related peptide, neurokinins, mu-opioid, galanin, somatostatin, neurotensin and vasoactive intestinal polypeptide receptors. *J Comp Neurol* 1995;354:253–281.
87. Karlsten R, Gordh T Jr. An A1-selective adenosine agonist abolishes allodynia elicited by vibration and touch after intrathecal injection. *Anesth Analg* 1995;80:844–847.
88. Kayser V, Guilbaud G. The analgesic effects of morphine, but not those of the enkephalinase inhibitor thiorphan, are enhanced in arthritic rats. *Brain Res* 1983;267:131–138.
89. Kayser V, Guilbaud G. Local and remote modifications of nociceptive sensitivity during carrageenin-induced inflammation in the rat. *Pain* 1987;28:99–107.
90. Keightley MC, Funder JW, Fuller PJ. Molecular cloning and sequencing of a guinea-pig pro-opiomelanocortin cDNA. *Mol Cell Endocrinol* 1991;82:89–98.
91. Khayyat GF, Yu YJ, King RB. Response patterns to noxious and non-noxious stimuli in rostral trigeminal relay nuclei. *Brain Res* 1975; 97:47–60.
92. Kim SH, Chung JM. An experimental model for peripheral neuropathy produced by segmental spinal nerve ligation in the rat. *Pain* 1992;50:355–363.
93. Klein CM, Guillamondegui O, Krenek CD, La Forte RA, Coggeshall RE. Do neuropeptides in the dorsal horn change if the dorsal root ganglion cell death that normally accompanies peripheral nerve transection is prevented? *Brain Res* 1991;552:273–282.
94. Knox RJ, Dickenson AH. Effects of selective and non-selective kappa-opioid receptor agonists on cutaneous C-fibre-evoked responses of rat dorsal horn neurones. *Brain Res* 1987;415:21–29.
95. Kristensen JD, Svensson B, Gordh T Jr. The NMDA-receptor antagonist CPP abolishes neurogenic 'wind-up pain' after intrathecal administration in humans. *Pain* 1992;51(2):249–253.
96. Kuraishi Y, Hirota N, Sato Y, Hanashima N, Takagi H, Satoh M. Stimulus specificity of peripherally evoked substance P release from the rabbit dorsal horn in situ. *Neuroscience* 1989;30: 241–250.
97. LaMotte RH, Lundberg LE, Torebjörk HE. Pain, hyperalgesia and activity in nociceptive C units in humans after intradermal injection of capsaicin. *J Physiol* 1992;448:749–764.
98. Lee JH, Price RH, Williams FG, Mayer B, Beitz AJ. Nitric oxide synthase is found in some spinothalamic neurons and in neuronal processes that appose spinal neurons that express Fos induced by noxious stimulation. *Brain Res* 1993;608:324–333.
99. Lee Y-W, Yaksh TL. Pharmacology of the spinal adenosine receptor which mediates the antallodynic action of intrathecal adenosine agonists. *J Pharmacol Exp Ther* 1996;277:1642–1648.
100. Leslie JB, Watkins WD. Eicosanoids in the central nervous system. *J Neurosurg* 1985;63:659–668.
101. Light AR, Kavookjian AM. Morphology and ultrastructure of physiologically identified substantia gelatinosa (lamina II) neurons with axons that terminate in deeper dorsal horn laminae (III–V). *J Comp Neurol* 1988;267:172–189.
102. Lucas D, Yaksh TL. Release in vivo of Met-enkephalin and encrypted forms of Met-enkephalin from brain and spinal cord of the anesthetized cat. *Peptides* 1990;11:1119–1125.
103. Ma QP, Woolf CJ. Involvement of neurokinin receptors in the induction but not the maintenance of mechanical allodynia in rat flexor motoneurones. *J Physiol* 1995;486(pt 3):769–777.
104. Magnuson DS, Sullivan AF, Simonnet G, Roques BP, Dickenson AH. Differential interactions of cholecystokinin and FLFQPQRF-NH2 with mu and delta opioid antinociception in the rat spinal cord. *Neuropeptides* 1990;16:213–218.
105. Maisky VA, Doroshenko NZ. Catecholamine projections to the spinal cord in the rat and their relationship to central cardiovascular neurons. *J Auton Nerv Sys* 1991;34:119–128.
106. Malmberg AB, Rafferty MF, Yaksh TL. Antinociceptive effect of spinally delivered prostaglandin E receptor antagonists in the formalin on the rat. *Neurosci Lett* 1994;173:193–196.
107. Malmberg AB, Yaksh TL. Hyperalgesia mediated by spinal glutamate or substance P receptor blocked by spinal cyclooxygenase inhibition. *Science* 1992;257:1276–1279.
108. Malmberg AB, Yaksh TL. Antinociceptive actions of spinal non-steroidal anti-inflammatory agents on the formalin test in the rat. *J Pharmacol Exp Ther* 1992;263:136–146.
109. Malmberg AB, Yaksh TL. Spinal nitric oxide synthesis inhibition blocks NMDA-induced thermal hyperalgesia and produces antinociception in the formalin test in rats. *Pain* 1993;54:291–300.
110. Malmberg AB, Yaksh TL. Cyclooxygenase inhibition and the spinal release of prostaglandin E2 and amino acids evoked by paw formalin injection: a microdialysis study in unanesthetized rats. *J Neurosci* 1995;15:2768–2776.
111. Malmberg AB, Yaksh TL. The effect of morphine on formalin-evoked behavior and spinal release of excitatory amino acids and prostaglandin E_2 using microdialysis in conscious rats. *Br J Pharmacol* 1995;114:1069–1075.
112. Marsala M, Yaksh TL. Transient spinal ischemia in the rat: characterization of behavioral and histopathological consequences as a function of the duration of aortic occlusion. *J Cereb Blood Flow Metab* 1994;14:526–535.
113. Matzner O, Devor M. Na+ conductance and the threshold for repetitive neuronal firing. *Brain Res* 1992;597:92–98.
114. Maxwell DJ, Christie WM, Ottersen OP, Storm-Mathisen J. Terminals of group Ia primary afferent fibres in Clarke's column are enriched with L-glutamate-like immunoreactivity. *Brain Res* 1990; 510:346–350.
115. McLachlan EM, Jang W, Devor M, Michaelis M. Peripheral nerve injury triggers noradrenergic sprouting within dorsal root ganglia. *Nature* 1993;363:543–546.
116. Meller ST, Dykstra C, Gebhart GF. Production of endogenous nitric oxide and activation of soluble guanylate cyclase are required for N-methyl-D-aspartate-produced facilitation of the nociceptive tail-flick reflex. *Eur J Pharmacol* 1992;214:93–96.
117. Melzack R, Wall PD. Pain mechanisms: a new theory. *Science* 1965; 150:971–979.
118. Mendell LM. Physiological properties of unmyelinated fiber projections to the spinal cord. *Exp Neurol* 1966;16:316–332.
119. Mendell LM, Wall PD. Responses of single dorsal cord cells to peripheral cutaneous unmyelinated fibers. *Nature* 1965;206: 97–99.
120. Menetrey D, Basbaum AI. The distribution of substance P-, enkephalin- and dynorphin-immunoreactive neurons in the medulla of the rat and their contribution to bulbospinal pathways. *Neuroscience* 1987;23:173–187.
121. Merighi A, Polak JM, Theodosis DT. Ultrastructural visualization of glutamate and aspartate immunoreactivities in the rat dorsal horn, with special reference to the co-localization of glutamate, substance P and calcitonin-gene related peptide. *Neuroscience* 1991;40:67–80.
122. Minami T, Uda R, Horiguchi S, Ito S, Hyodo M, Hayaishi O. Allodynia evoked by intrathecal administration of prostaglandin F2 alpha to conscious mice. *Pain* 1992;50:223–229.
123. Mjellem-Joly N, Lund A, Berge OG, Hole K. Intrathecal co-administration of substance P and NMDA augments nociceptive responses in the formalin test. *Pain* 1992;51:195–198.
124. Moiniche S, Dahl JB, Kehlet H. Time course of primary and secondary hyperalgesia after heat injury to the skin. *Br J Anaesth* 1993; 71:201–205.
125. Moncada S, Palmer RM, Higgs EA. Nitric oxide: physiology, pathophysiology, and pharmacology. *Pharmacol Rev* 1991;43:109–142.
126. Morris MJ, Pilowsky PM, Minson JB, West MJ, Chalmers JP. Microinjection of kainic acid into the rostral ventrolateral medulla causes hypertension and release of neuropeptide Y-like immunoreactivity from rabbit spinal cord. *Clin Exp Pharmacol Physiol* 1987;14:127–132.
127. Nagasaka H, Awad H, Yaksh TL. Peripheral and spinal actions of opioids in the blockade of the autonomic response evoked by compression of the inflamed knee joint. *Anesthesiology* 1996; 85:808–816.
128. Nahin RL, Hylden JL. Peripheral inflammation is associated with increased glutamic acid decarboxylase immunoreactivity in the rat spinal cord. *Neurosci Lett* 1991;128:226–230.
129. Nashold BS Jr, Friedman N. Dorsal column stimulation for control of pain. Preliminary report on 30 patients. *J Neurosurg* 1972;36: 590–597.
130. Nasstrom J, Karlsson U, Post C. Antinociceptive actions of different classes of excitatory amino acid receptor antagonists in mice. *Eur J Pharmacol* 1992;212:21–29.
131. Neil A, Kayser V, Gacel G, Besson JM, Guilbaud G. Opioid receptor types and antinociceptive activity in chronic inflammation:

both kappa- and mu-opiate agonistic effects are enhanced in arthritic rats. *Eur J Pharmacol* 1986;30:203–208.
132. Neugebauer V, Lucke T, Schaible HG. N-methyl-D-aspartate (NMDA) and non-NMDA receptor antagonists block the hyperexcitability of dorsal horn neurons during development of acute arthritis in rat's knee joint. *J Neurophysiol* 1993;70:1365–1377.
133. Neugebauer V, Lucke T, Schaible HG. Differential effects of N-methyl-D-aspartate (NMDA) and non-NMDA receptor antagonists on the responses of rat spinal neurons with joint input. *Neurosci Lett* 1993;155:29–32.
134. Neugebauer V, Weiretter F, Schaible HG. Involvement of substance P and neurokinin-1 receptors in the hyperexcitability of dorsal horn neurons during development of acute arthritis in rat's knee joint. *J Neurophysiol* 1995;73:1574–1583.
135. Nevin K, Zhuo H, Helke CJ. Neurokinin A coexists with substance P and serotonin in ventral medullary spinally projecting neurons of the rat. *Peptides* 1994;15:1003–1011.
136. Nicol GD, Klingberg DK, Vasko MR. Prostaglandin E2 increases calcium conductance and stimulates release of substance P in avian sensory neurons. *J Neurosci* 1992;12:1917–1927.
137. North RA, Williams JT, Suprenant A, Christie MJ. μ and δ Receptors belong to a family of receptors that are coupled to potassium channels. *Proc Natl Acad Sci USA* 1987;84:5487–5491.
138. O'Dell TJ, Hawkins RD, Kandel ER, Arancio O. Tests of the roles of two diffusable substances in long-term potentiation: Evidence for nitric oxide as a possible early retrograde messenger. *Proc Natl Acad Sci USA* 1991;88:11285–11289.
139. Payne R. Neuropathic pain syndromes, with special reference to causalgia and reflex sympathetic dystrophy. *Clin J Pain* 1986;2: 59–73.
140. Pilowsky PM, Kapoor V, Minson JB, West MJ, Chalmers JP. Spinal cord serotonin release and raised blood pressure after brainstem kainic acid injection. *Brain Res* 1986;366:354–357.
141. Portenoy RK. Management of Neuropathic pain. In: Chapman CR, Foley KM, eds. *Current and emerging issues in cancer pain.* New York: Raven Press, 1993;351–369.
142. Radhakrishnan V, Henry JL. Novel substance P antagonist, CP-96,345, blocks responses of cat spinal dorsal horn neurons to noxious cutaneous stimulation and to substance P. *Neurosci Lett* 1991;132:39–43.
143. Radhakrishnan V, Henry JL. Antagonism of nociceptive responses of cat spinal dorsal horn neurons in vivo by the NK-1 receptor antagonists CP-96,345 and CP-99,994, but not by CP-96,344. *Neuroscience* 1995;64:943–958.
144. Radhakrishnan V, Yashpal K, Hui-Chan CW, Henry JL. Implication of a nitric oxide synthase mechanism in the action of substance P: L-NAME blocks thermal hyperalgesia induced by endogenous and exogenous substance P in the rat. *Eur J Neurosci* 1995;7:1920–1925.
145. Raigorodsky G, Urca G. Intrathecal N-methyl-D-aspartate (NMDA) activates both nociceptive and antinociceptive systems. *Brain Res* 1987;422:158–162.
146. Reddy VK, Cassini P, Ho RH, Martin GF. Origins and terminations of bulbospinal axons that contain serotonin and either enkephalin or substance-P in the North American opossum. *J Comp Neurol* 1990;294:96–108.
147. Reeve AJ, Dickenson AH. The roles of spinal adenosine receptors in the control of acute and more persistent nociceptive responses of dorsal horn neurons in the anaesthetized rat. *Br J Pharmacol* 1995;116:2221–2228.
148. Ren K, Hylden JL, Williams GM, Ruda MA, Dubner R. The effects of a non-competitive NMDA receptor antagonist, MK-801, on behavioral hyperalgesia and dorsal horn neuronal activity in rats with unilateral inflammation. *Pain* 1992;50:331–344.
149. Ritz LA, Greenspan JD. Morphological features of lamina V neurons receiving nociceptive input in cat sacrocaudal spinal cord. *J Comp Neurol* 1985;238:440–452.
150. Rosen H, Douglass J, Herbert E. Isolation and characterization of the rat proenkephalin gene. *J Biol Chem* 1984;259: 14309–14313.
151. Ruda MA, Iadarola MJ, Cohen LV, Young WS III. In situ hybridization histochemistry and immunocytochemistry reveal an increase in spinal dynorphin biosynthesis in a rat model of peripheral inflammation and hyperalgesia. *Proc Natl Acad Sci USA* 1988;85: 622–626.
152. Salvemini D, Misko TP, Masferrer JL, Seibert K, Currie MG, Needleman P. Nitric oxide activates cyclooxygenase enzymes. *Proc Natl Acad Sci USA* 1993;90:7240–7244.
153. Sato A, Sato Y, Schmidt RF. Changes in blood pressure and heart rate induced by movements of normal and inflamed knee joints. *Neurosci Lett* 1984;52:55–60.
154. Schaible HG, Neugebauer V, Cervero F, Schmidt RF. Changes in tonic descending inhibition of spinal neurons with articular input during the development of acute arthritis in the cat. *J Neurophysiol* 1991;66:1021–1032.
155. Schaible HG, Schmidt RF, Willis WD. Responses of spinal cord neurones to stimulation of articular afferent fibres in the cat. *J Physiol* 1986;372:575–593.
156. Schaible HG, Schmidt RF, Willis WD. Convergent inputs from articular, cutaneous and muscle receptors onto ascending tract cells in the cat spinal cord. *Exp Brain Res* 1987;66:479–488.
157. Sher GD, Mitchell D. Intrathecal N-methyl-D-aspartate induces hyperexcitability in rat dorsal horn convergent neurones. *Neurosci Lett* 1990;119:199–202.
158. Sher G, Mitchell D. N-methyl-D-aspartate mediates responses of rat dorsal horn neurons to hind limb ischemia. *Brain Res* 1990; 522:55–62.
159. Sherman SE, Loomis CW. Morphine insensitive allodynia is produced by intrathecal strychnine in the lightly anesthetized rat. *Pain* 1994;56:17–29.
160. Singer E, Placheta P. Reduction of ^{3}H-muscimol binding sites in rat dorsal spinal cord after neonatal capsaicin treatment. *Brain Res* 1980;202:484–487.
161. Sorkin LS, McAdoo DJ. Amino acids and serotonin are released into the lumbar spinal cord of the anesthetized cat following intradermal capsaicin injections. *Brain Research* 1993;607:89–98.
162. Sorkin LS. Intrathecal ketorolac blocks NMDA-evoked spinal release of prostaglandin E_2 and thromboxane B_2. *Anesthesiology* 1993;79:A909.
163. Sorkin LS. NMDA evokes an L-NAME sensitive spinal release of glutamate and citrulline. *Neuroreport* 1993;4:479–482.
164. Southam E, Garthwaite J. Comparative effects of some nitric oxide donors on cyclic GMP levels in rat cerebellar slices. *Neurosci Lett* 1991;130:107–111.
165. Stanfa LC, Dickenson AH. Enhanced alpha-2 adrenergic controls and spinal morphine potency in inflammation. *Neuroreport* 1994; 5:469–472.
166. Stanfa LC, Dickenson AH. Electrophysiological studies on the spinal roles of endogenous opioids in carrageenan inflammation. *Pain* 1994;56:185–191.
167. Stanfa LC, Sullivan AF, Dickenson AH. Alterations in neuronal excitability and the potency of spinal mu, delta and kappa opioids after carrageenan induced inflammation. *Pain* 1992;50:345–354.
168. Stein C, Millan MJ, Shippenberg TS, Peter K, Herz A. Peripheral opioid receptors mediating antinociception in inflammation. Evidence for involvement of mu, delta and kappa receptors. *J Pharmacol Exp Ther* 1989;248:1269–1275.
169. Sugimoto T, Bennett GJ, Kajander KC. Transsynaptic degeneration in the superficial dorsal horn after sciatic nerve injury: effects of a chronic constriction injury, transection, and strychnine. *Pain* 1990;42:205–213.
170. Sullivan AF, Dickenson AH. Electrophysiologic studies on the spinal antinociceptive action of kappa opioid agonists in the adult and 21-day-old rat. *J Pharmacol Exp Ther* 1991;256:1119–1125.
171. Takano M, Takano Y, Yaksh TL. Release of calcitonin gene-related peptide (CGRP), substance P (SP), and vasoactive intestinal polypeptide (VIP) from rat spinal cord: modulation by alpha 2 agonists. *Peptides* 1993;14:371–378.
172. Takano Y, Martin JE, Leeman SE, Loewy AD. Substance P immunoreactivity released from rat spinal cord after kainic acid excitation of the ventral medulla oblongata: a correlation with increases in blood pressure. *Brain Res* 1984;291:168–172.
173. Thompson SW, Dray A, Urban L. Injury-induced plasticity of spinal reflex activity: NK1 neurokinin receptor activation and enhanced A- and C-fiber mediated responses in the rat spinal cord in vitro. *J Neurosci* 1994;14:3672–3687.
174. Thompson SW, Gerber G, Sivilotti LG, Woolf CJ. Long duration ventral root potentials in the neonatal rat spinal cord in vitro;the effects of ionotropic and metabotropic excitatory amino acid receptor antagonists. *Brain Res* 1992;595:87–97.
175. Thompson SW, Urban L, Dray A. Contribution of NK1 and NK2 receptor activation to high threshold afferent fibre evoked ventral root responses in the rat spinal cord in vitro. *Brain Res* 1993;625: 100–108.
176. Todd AJ, Sullivan AC. Light microscopic study of the coexistence

of GABA-like and glycine-like immunoreactivities in the spinal cord of the rat. *J Comp Neurol* 1990;296:496–505.
177. Tseng CJ, Lin HC, Wang SD, Tung CS. Immunohistochemical study of catecholamine enzymes and neuropeptide Y (NPY) in the rostral ventrolateral medulla and bulbospinal projection. *J Comp Neurol* 1993;334:294–303.
178. Tyce GM, Yaksh TL. Monoamine release from cat spinal cord by somatic stimuli: an intrinsic modulatory system. *J Physiol (Lond)* 1981;314:513–529.
179. Uda R, Horiguchi S, Ito SM, Hayaishi O. Nociceptive effects by intrathecal administration of prostaglandin D2, E2 or F2a to conscious mice. *Brain Res* 1990;510:26–32.
180. Ueda M, Oyama T, Kuraishi Y, Akaike A, Satoh M. Alpha 2-adrenoceptor-mediated inhibition of capsaicin-evoked release of glutamate from rat spinal dorsal horn slices. *Neurosci Lett* 1995;188: 137–139.
181. Valtschanoff JG, Weinberg RJ, Rustioni A, Schmidt HH. Nitric oxide synthase and GABA colocalize in lamina II of rat spinal cord. *Neurosci Lett* 1992;148:6–10.
182. Vizzard MA, Erdman SL, Erickson VL, Stewart RJ, Roppolo JR, De Groat WC. Localization of NADPH diaphorase in the lumbosacral spinal cord and dorsal root ganglia of the cat. *J Comp Neurol* 1994; 339:62–75.
183. Walker MW, Ewald DA, Perney TM, Miller RJ. Neuropeptide Y modulates neurotransmitter release and Ca2+ currents in rat sensory neurons. *J Neurosci* 1988;8:2438–2446.
184. Wall PD. The laminar organization of dorsal horn and effects of descending impulses. *J Physiol* 1967;188:403–423.
185. Wall PD, Merrill EG, Yaksh TL. Responses of single units in laminae 2 and 3 of cat spinal cord. *Brain Res* 1979;160:245–260.
186. Wall PD, Sweet WH. Temporary abolition of pain in man. *Science* 1967;155:108–109.
187. Wall PD, Yaksh TL. The effect of Lissauer tract stimulation on activity in dorsal and ventral roots. *Exp Neurol* 1978;60:570–583.
188. White WF, Heller AH. Glycine receptor alteration in the mutant mouse spastic. *Nature* 1982;298:655–657.
189. Willis WD, Haber LH, Martin RF. Inhibition of spinothalamic tract cells and interneurons by brainstem stimulation in the monkey. *J Neurophysiol* 1977;40:968–998.
190. Womack MD, MacDermott AB, Jessell TM. Sensory transmitters regulate intracellular calcium in dorsal horn neurons. *Nature* 1988;334:351–353.
191. Woolf CJ, King AE. Physiology and morphology of multireceptive neurones with C-afferent fibre inputs in the deep dorsal horn of the rat lumbarspinal cord. *J Neurophysiol* 1987;58:460–479.
192. Woolf CJ, Shortland P, Coggeshall RE. Peripheral nerve injury triggers central sprouting of myelinated afferents. *Nature* 1992; 355:75–78.
193. Woolf CJ, Thompson SW. The induction and maintenance of central sensitization is dependent on N-methyl-D-aspartic acid receptor activation;implications for the treatment of post-injury pain hypersensitivity states. *Pain* 1991;44:293–299.
194. Woolf CJ, Wall PD. Morphine-sensitive and morphine-insensitive actions of C-fibre input on the rat spinal cord. *Neurosci Lett* 1986; 64:221–225.
195. Yaksh TL. Central and peripheral mechanisms for the antialgesic action of acetylsalicylic acid. In: Barnet JM, Hirsh J, Mustard JF, eds. *Acetylsalicylic acid: new uses for an old drug*. New York: Raven Press, 1982;137–152.
196. Yaksh TL. Multiple opioid receptor systems in brain and spinal cord. Part 2. *Eur J Anaesthesiol* 1984;1:171–243.
197. Yaksh TL. Behavioral and autonomic correlates of the tactile evoked allodynia produced by spinal glycine inhibition: effects of modulatory receptor systems and excitatory amino acid antagonists. *Pain* 1989;37:111–123.
198. Yaksh TL. The spinal actions of opioids. In: Herz A, ed. *Handbook of experimental pharmacology*, vol 104/II. Berlin, Heidelberg: Springer-Verlag, 1993;53–90.
199. Yaksh TL, Elde RP. Factors governing release of methionine enkephalin-like immunoreactivity from mesencephalon and spinal cord of the cat in vivo. *J Neurophysiol* 1981;46:1056–1075.
200. Yaksh TL, Jage J, Takano Y. Pharmacokinetics and pharmacodynamics of medullar agents. c. The spinal actions of α_2-adrenergic agonists as analgesics. In: Aitkenhead AR, Benad G, Brown BR, et al. eds. *Baillière's clinical anaesthesiology*, vol 7, no. 3. London: Baillière Tindall, 1993;597–614.
201. Yaksh TL, Jessell TM, Gamse R, Mudge AW, et al. Intrathecal morphine inhibits substance P release from mammalian spinal cord in vivo. *Nature* 1980;286:155–156.
202. Yaksh TL, Pogrel JW, Lee YW, Chaplan SR. Reversal of nerve ligation-induced allodynia by spinal alpha-2 adrenoceptor agonists. *J Pharmacol Expr Ther* 1995;272:207–214.
203. Yaksh TL, Terenius L, Nyberg F, Jhamandas K, Wang JY. Studies on the release by somatic stimulation from rat and cat spinal cord of active materials which displace dihydromorphine in an opiate-binding assay. *Brain Res* 1983;268:119–128.
204. Yamagata K, Andreasson KI, Kaufmann WE, Barnes CA, Worley PF. Expression of a mitogen-inducible cyclooxygenase in brain neurons: regulation by synaptic activity and glucocorticoids. *Neuron* 1993;11:371–386.
205. Yamamoto T, Yaksh TL. Studies on the spinal interaction of morphine and the NMDA antagonist MK-801 on the hyperesthesia observed in a rat model of sciatic mononeuropathy. *Neurosci Lett* 1992;135:67–70.
206. Yamamoto T, Yaksh TL. Effects of intrathecal capsaicin and an NK-1 antagonist, CP,96-345, on the thermal hyperalgesia observed following unilateral constriction of the sciatic nerve in the rat. *Pain* 1992;51:329–334.
207. Yang, Ln Ch, Marsala, M, Yaksh, TL. Characterization of the time course of spinal amino acids citrulline and PGE2 release after carrageenan/kaolin induced knee joint inflammation: a chronic microdialysis study. *Pain* 1996;67:345–354.
208. Yashpal K, Radhakrishnan V, Coderre TJ, Henry JL. CP-96,345, but not its stereoisomer, CP-96,344, blocks the nociceptive responses to intrathecally administered substance P and to noxious thermal and chemical stimuli in the rat. *Neuroscience* 1993;52:1039–1047.
209. Yokota T, Nishikawa N, Nishikawa Y. Effects of strychnine upon different classes of trigeminal subnucleus caudalis neurons. *Brain Res* 1979;168:430–434.
210. Zarbin MA, Wamsley JK, Kuhar MJ. Glycine receptor: light microscopic autoradiographic localization with [^{3}H]strychnine. *J Neurosci* 1981;1:532–547.
211. Zhang X, Verge V, Wiesenfeld-Hallin Z, Ju G, Bredt D, Synder SH, Hokfelt T. Nitric oxide synthase-like immunoreactivity in lumbar dorsal root ganglia and spinal cord of rat and monkey and effect of peripheral axotomy. *J Comp Neurol* 1993;335:563–575.

Anesthesia: Biologic Foundations, edited by Tony L. Yaksh et al. Lippincott–Raven Publishers, Philadelphia © 1997.

CHAPTER 37

PROCESSING OF NOCICEPTIVE INFORMATION AT SUPRASPINAL LEVELS

A. D. CRAIG AND J. O. DOSTROVSKY

This chapter summarizes basic knowledge regarding supraspinal projections and substrates that are associated with the processing of information leading to the expression of the pain state. Our knowledge of the functional anatomy of central pain pathways has increased substantially in recent years. The origins, terminations, and physiologic characteristics of ascending pathways that carry nociceptive activity have been studied anatomically and electrophysiologically in primates, cats, and rats. Evidence in the human has been obtained with modern imaging techniques that enlarge greatly upon the experimental work. These recent insights build upon long-standing inferences based on clinical findings.

HISTORICAL CONTEXT

The concept that ascending pathways activated by noxious peripheral stimuli reach higher centers and that information carried by these pathways comes into consciousness has long been appreciated as a philosophical construct. The conceptualization that spinofugal projections carried relevant information to higher centers where the appreciation of the aversive quality of a potentially injurious stimulus comes into consciousness was emphasized in the cartoon of Descartes (see Chap. 1). The concept of a specific spinofugal pathway through which pain-evoked information would ascend originated with the prescient animal studies of Brown-Sequard (43b), who demonstrated the crossed nature of nociceptive transmission observation. Early observations by Gowers (126a) of a patient in whom an attempted suicide caused a unilateral ventral quadrant lesion of the spinal cord resulted in the patient displaying a contralateral analgesia with light touch being preserved at levels below the spinal injury.

The basis of the current rational appreciation of the role of higher centers in pain processing derives in part from the original observations of the French neurologist Dejerine who with Roussy in 1906 first described the sensory deficits and chronic dysesthetic pain that can occur following thrombosis of the thalamogeniculate artery, that results in destruction of the posterolateral thalamus and/or its projections to cortex (96). These observations coincided with the recognition that the most rostral distribution of spinofugal projections is the thalamus and led to the concept of the thalamus as a sensory center in the late 19th century. In the early 20th century the work of the Queen's Square neurologists Head and Holmes (137) provided the outline of our current thinking regarding the specific involvement of the thalamus in pain and pain disorders. Based on clinical observations, they inferred that the sensory aspects of pain are mediated by a specific substrate in the lateral thalamus and that the affective (emotional) aspects of pain are mediated by the medial ("essential") thalamus. This concept was developed phylogenetically by investigators such as Bishop (33), and it was formalized and popularized in more recent times by Melzack and Casey (203). Although this concept may be an oversimplification, it is now widely accepted by researchers in the field (1,117,226,278). Recent advances have begun to demonstrate the thalamocortical substrates predicted by these workers.

SUPRASPINAL PROJECTIONS OF NOCICEPTIVE PATHWAYS

As reviewed in Chap. 35, noxious stimuli activate specific populations of spinal neurons that project via ascending spinofugal pathways to supraspinal sites. The pathways by which these neurons reach higher centers may be considered in terms of their general localization in the spinal white matter or by the target to which they project. The association of these pathways with nociceptive processing may be made on the basis of the response properties of identified projecting cells or by the effects observed when these pathways or terminal regions are lesioned.

Several afferent pathways from the spinal cord to the brain may be considered with respect to the central processing of nociceptive information: (a) direct projections to the brainstem, e.g., spinobulbar (spinoreticular [SRT] and spinomesencephalic [SMT] tracts); (b) direct projections to the thalamus (the spinothalamic tract [STT]); (c) direct projections to the hypothalamus/ventral forebrain (spinohypothalamic tract [SHT]); and (d) indirect ascending pathways that are integrated and relayed by intervening stations, viz., the postsynaptic dorsal column (PSDC) system, the spinocervicothalamic (SCT) pathway, and the spinoparabrachial pathways.

While the names of these pathways specifically denote spinofugal connections, homologues of these pathways are also present that originate from the trigeminal sensory nuclei in the medulla (see Chap. 53), and these are included with the descriptions of the spinal projections. The characteristics of the cells of origin, the locations of the ascending axons, and the distribution of terminations are described in this section for each of these pathways. Comprehensive reviews of these substrates have been provided by several authors (43,117,278,279). See Chap. 35 of this volume for discussions of other particular issues relevant to the physiology and pharmacology of the spinal cells of origin of these pathways.

Spinothalamic Projections

The direct spinothalamic (and trigeminothalamic) projection is most closely associated with pain and temperature sensation; lesions at various levels of this pathway clinically result in analgesia or hyperalgesia that is almost always accompanied by thermanesthesia (78,220,275,278). Accordingly, considerable efforts have been made to uncover the functional anatomy of this pathway.

Cells of Origin

Spinothalamic tract (STT) cells have been identified with retrograde anatomical tracers, such as horseradish peroxidase (HRP), wheat germ agglutinin (WGA)-HRP, and fast blue, which label the neuronal cell bodies from their axonal termination sites in the thalamus. The STT cells are primarily located in three regions of the spinal gray matter (Fig. 1) in the monkey, cat, and rat (5,46,56,87,280):

1. the marginal zone, or lamina I, at the most superficial aspect of the dorsal horn (or equivalently, of the trigeminal nucleus caudalis);

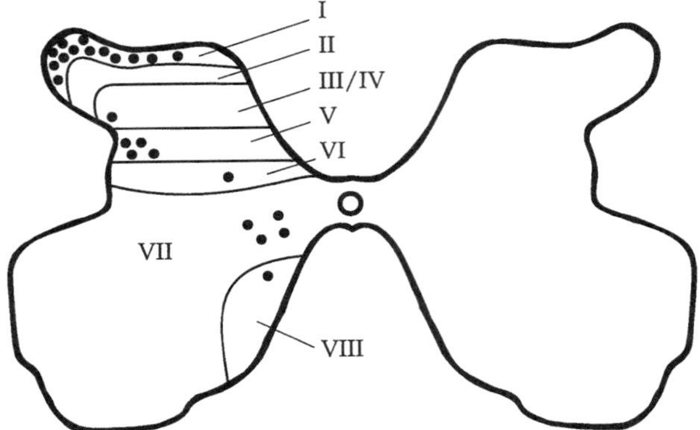

Figure 1. Location of spinofugal neurons. Spinal neurons with long ascending axons that project to the brainstem and the thalmus are concentrated in laminae I and V of the dorsal horn and in lamina VII in the intermediate zone, as shown in this schematic of a transverse section of the spinal gray matter.

2. the lateral neck of the dorsal horn, or laminae IV to V (or equivalently, the base of the trigeminal n. caudalis);
3. the intermediate zone, or lamina VII, between the dorsal and ventral horns (the trigeminal equivalent may be part of the lateral medullary reticular formation or the n. interpolaris).

About one half of STT cells are located in lamina I, about one-quarter are found in lamina V, and another quarter in lamina VII. In addition, a large population of STT cells is located bilaterally throughout the C1-2 spinal gray matter.

As discussed in Chap. 35, each of these three populations of spinal cord neurons is characterized by a different set of primary afferent fibers, and thus each displays a different general pattern of physiologic activity (183,278,279). Briefly, lamina I neurons receive small-diameter (Aδ and C) primary afferent fiber input. Lamina V neurons receive direct input from large-diameter fibers and polysynaptic input from small-diameter fibers. Lamina VII cells generally receive convergent input from large-diameter deep (muscle, joint) inputs and other (polysynaptic) cutaneous, deep, and visceral inputs.

Physiologic experiments have accordingly revealed that there are several basic types of STT cells. In such experiments, individual STT cells are identified by antidromic activation from their termination sites in the thalamus and then they are characterized with natural stimuli. These types of STT cells are each more or less localized to one of the three spinal regions that contain STT cells (117,226,278,281). These may be summarized as follows:

1. Nociceptive-specific (NS) cells respond within a small receptive field to noxious mechanical or noxious thermal stimuli or both, but not to innocuous stimulation. These cells are concentrated in lamina I. Two additional types of STT cell are found exclusively in lamina I, viz., thermoreceptive-specific ("cold") cells that are excited by innocuous cooling and inhibited by warming of the skin, and HPC (heat, pinch, and cold) cells that respond in a polymodal fashion to noxious cold and also to noxious heat and pinch (64,83,86). Thus, activity in lamina I STT cells is specifically related to both pain and temperature stimulation. The fundamental role of lamina I may be to distribute modality selective afferent input related to the physiologic status of the tissues of the body.
2. Wide dynamic range (WDR) cells respond to both innocuous and noxious stimuli over a larger receptive field in a graded manner. They often receive convergent deep and visceral input. The magnitude of the response is typically monotonically correlated with stimulus intensity and thus, although these cells are modality-ambiguous, they show their strongest response to noxious stimulation. These cells predominate in lamina V, and they may serve as cumulative integrators of the entire spectrum of somatic afferent inflow.
3. Complex cells respond to innocuous or noxious stimulation within large, bilateral, or widely separated somatic regions. They can have large inhibitory fields and can respond differently to different modes of stimulation, often including proprioceptive inputs. These cells, which are usually located in lamina VII, may serve to integrate somatic and visceral afferent and motoric interneuronal activity.

The correspondence between cell type and laminar location is not exclusive, for example, WDR cells can be located in lamina I and NS cells can be found in lamina V. Noxious stimulation of deep (muscle, joint) tissues or visceral tissues can activate cells in any of these locations. Nociceptive cells that receive visceral or deep activation usually, but not always (86,212), receive cutaneous input as well.

Anatomical Organization of Ascending STT Axons

Ascending axons of STT cells generally cross in the ventral commissure to the contralateral side within one to two segments of the cell of origin. While crossed STT fibers predominate, 10% to 15% of STT cells project ipsilaterally to the thalamus (5,77,87,200,280).

Within the ventrolateral quadrant, ascending STT axons are concentrated in two locations: the middle of the lateral funiculus (the classical "lateral" spinothalamic tract), and the middle of the anterior (ventral) funiculus (the classical "anterior" spinothalamic tract). The STT axons in the lateral funiculus originate predominantly from lamina I cells, whereas the ascending STT axons in the anterior funiculus originate from laminae V and VII cells (6,77). There is, nonetheless, considerable dispersion and individual variability within this pattern.

Consideration of the trajectory of the STT reveals that there is a crude somatotopy. At the spinal level, the crossing fibers displace ascending axons laterally, resulting in a tendency for axons from the caudal body regions to be located most laterally and superficially in the white matter and those from the rostral segments more medially (proximal to midline). At the spinomedullary junction the ascending STT fibers are located in the ventrolateral aspect of the medulla, where they course through the catecholamine cell groups in the ventrolateral medulla (201,273). Trigeminal axons (the medullary homologue of the SST) join the medial aspect of the STT at this level. At the caudal end of the pons the STT shifts dorsally to pass the parabrachial region and occupy a position ventrolateral to the inferior colliculus. It ascends in this region through the midbrain to the diencephalon.

STT Projection Sites

The STT terminates in six major regions of the primate (and presumably human) thalamus (1,7,23,40,47,76,200): (a) the ventral posterior nuclei (VPL, VPM, and VPI); (b) the posterior portion of the ventral medial n. (VMpo); (c) the ventral lateral n. (VL); (d) the central lateral n. (CL); (e) the parafascicular n. (Pf); and (f) the ventral caudal portion of the medial dorsal n. (MDvc). The overall disposition of these regions is presented in Fig. 2.

These regions defined in the primate are generally named similarly in the human, but atlases may vary significantly (135,140,155,200). The posterior inferior region called VMpo in the monkey, for example, is anatomically part of the suprageniculate or posterior complex in earlier work (79,227), and it may be functionally equivalent to the V.c.pc. (parvicellular

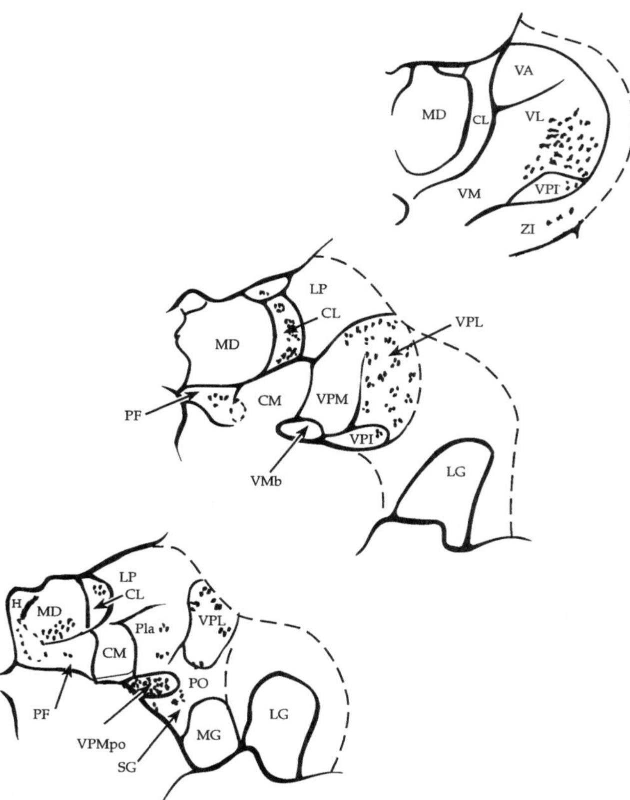

Figure 2. Organization of thalamic projection of spinal neurons. Spinothalamic terminations in the primate are located in both lateral and medial thalamus in particular sites, as shown in these three representative frontal levels (*lower left,* most posterior; *upper right,* most anterior). Abbreviations for nuclei: CL, central lateral; CM, center median; H, habenula; LG, lateral geniculate; LP, lateral posterior; MD, medial dorsal; MG, medial geniculate; PF, parafascicular; Pla, anterior pulvinar; PO, posterior; VA, ventral anterior; VL, ventral lateral; VM, ventral medial; VMb, basal part of VM; VMpo, posterior part of VM; VPI, ventral posterior inferior; VPL, ventral posterior lateral; VPM, ventral posterior medial; ZI, zona inserta.

part of the ventral caudal nucleus) of Hassler (135).The characteristics of these anatomical linkages are considered in the following subsections.

Ventral Posterior Nuclei The pronounced clusters of STT terminations (classically termed "archipelago") that appear scattered throughout VP (i.e., VPM and VPL) are historically the first STT termination observed (1,38,40,47,68,195,200,265, 271). These clusters are particularly dense in the dorsal portion of VP and near the fiber laminae that subdivide VP. They are topographically organized in the mediolateral direction in parallel with the precise somatopy of VP, that is, trigeminothalamic cells project to VPM, cervical STT cells project to medial VPL, and lumbar STT cells project to lateral VPL. The STT terminations in VP originate primarily from cells in laminae IV to V (1,7,38,227). These terminations are associated with VP cells immunopositive for calbindin, whereas VP cells that receive lemniscal inputs (from the dorsal column nuclei and the principal trigeminal nucleus) are instead immunoreactive for parvalbumin (229). While the significance of this distinction is not appreciated, such differences emphasize the likelihood that these tracts are associated with neuronal systems with a distinguishable pharmacology and biochemistry. STT-recipient VP cells project to the primary somatosensory cortex (SI), possibly to its superficial layers only (126,229). Lamina I and probably laminae IV to V STT terminations also occur in VPI, which projects to the second somatosensory cortex (79,118). STT input to VP probably subserves aspects of discriminative pain, as the physiology described below indicates. STT input to VL, rostral to VP, which overlaps with projections from the deep cerebellar nuclei (1,11,23), probably originates from lamina V and particularly lamina VII cells and is likely associated with somatomotor integration.

Ventral Medial Nucleus (VMpo) The primary projection target of lamina I STT cells in the primate is VMpo, where a dense termination field is present (76,79,227) (Fig. 3). This projection is organized topographically in the anteroposterior direction, with input from lumbar dermatomes found most posteriorly and cervical, and trigeminal input found successively more anteriorly.

The lamina I termination site in VMpo is characterized by a dense field of fibers immunopositive for calbindin (79), reflecting the strong calbindin immunoreactivity of lamina I cells (10). Ultrastructural findings indicate that the lamina I STT terminations in VMpo are glutamatergic (115).

The VMpo probably serves as a specific thalamocortical relay nucleus for lamina I STT cells, and thus, for specific pain and temperature sensibility. VMpo projects to the dorsal part of the anterior insular cortex buried in the lateral sulcus (49,89a,118) (Fig. 3). The insula is associated in general with visceral sensory activity and with the integration of somatosensory and limbic activity (4,119,282). The cortical projection of VMpo to the insula may reflect the relationship of pain and temperature sensibility to the physiologic processes necessary for the maintenance of the tissues of the body (81). Together with the adjacent insular projection of visceral afferents related to vagal and gustatory (parasympathetic) input, this cortical area forms the basis for a sense of the condition of the body. Infarcts in this region that produced hypalgesia and thermanesthesia have been reported (see below). The buried location of the insular cortex means that superficial cortical lesions (i.e., from physical wounds) would rarely affect it, which perhaps explains why the role of the cortex in pain was not appreciated by early neurologists.

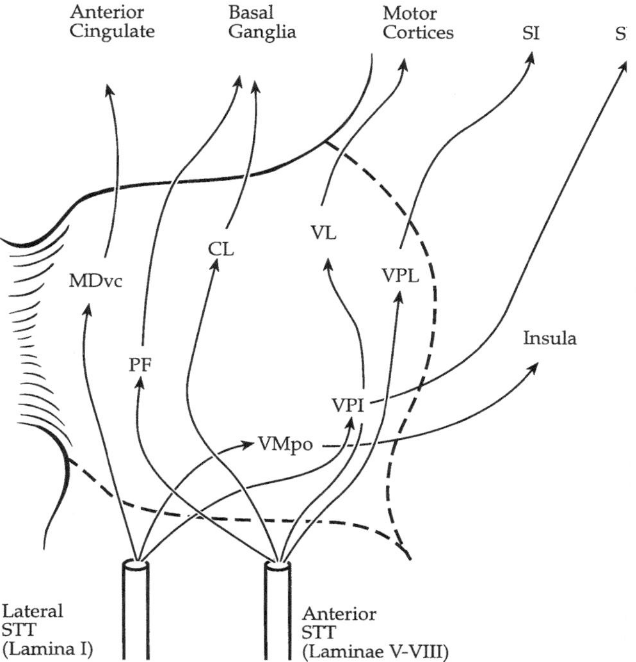

Figure 3. Organization of cortical projections of spinothalamic targets. The main spinothalamic termination sites, identified in Fig. 2, project to the cortical targets indicated. Abbreviations as for Fig. 2.

Central Lateral Nuclei (CL) The dense STT input to the caudal portion of CL arises primarily from lamina VII STT cells (7, 9,87,123,124). This projection does not appear to have a simple topography; rather, several individual clusters of CL cells may receive STT input from different portions of the spinal cord (85). Some cells in this portion of the intralaminar thalamus project to the basal ganglia and others project to the superficial and deep layers of motor and posterior parietal cortices (155).

Parafascicular Nucleus (Pf) There is a weak projection from lamina I and lamina V STT cells to Pf. Cells in Pf project to the basal ganglia or to the motor cortex (155,240,242).

Medial Dorsal Nucleus (MD) STT neurons project to the ventral caudal part of MD with an anteroposterior topography, the trigeminal input being located most posteriorly (76). This STT projection originates from lamina I cells (2,76); it is only of moderate density in comparison with the strong lamina I STT projection to VMpo. Cells in MDvc appear to project to the anterior cingulate cortex rather than to the prefrontal cortex (229a; A. D. Craig, *unpublished data*).

Species Considerations It is important to remember that anatomic studies are carried out in a variety of species, and systematic observations have shown distinguishable differences. In most cases, the relevance of these differences is not presently known, but as more sophisticated insights into behavior and physiology are acquired, such comparative anatomical differences may provide important clues to the association of different projections with different functions.

In the cat, STT projections differ from those in the monkey (1,23,84,85)—the major termination sites are caudal PO, the ventral aspect of VP (including VPI), and the ventral aspect of the basal part of the ventral medial n. (VMb), Pf, CL, VL, and n. submedius (Sm) in the medial thalamus. In stark contrast to the monkey, there are few STT terminations within VP in the cat. Dense, topographic terminations in Sm originate from lamina I STT cells; this region may be similar to the lamina I projection to MDvc in the primate, since Sm is a developmental offshoot of the pronucleus of MD. However, Sm in the cat (and the rat) projects to ventrolateral orbitofrontal cortex (VLO) (71,89,292), and STT input to the anterior cingulate in the cat passes instead through the ventral aspect of VP (209,283). Moderately dense and weakly topographic lamina I STT terminations occur in ventral VP and ventral VMb (78); it is not yet clear whether these may form a primordial homologue of the lamina I STT projection to VMpo in the primate. As in the monkey, the STT projections to VL and CL originate from laminae V and VII cells, and the projection to Pf is sparse.

In the rat, STT terminations differ from both monkey and cat (70,199,221); the major targets are VP, ventral VMb (called VPMpc and VPLpc in this species), CL, Sm, and Pf. The major difference is that STT terminations occur throughout VP. The sources of STT input to Sm differ from the cat; trigeminal cells are found in the most rostral part of n. caudalis, as well as in lamina I, and in interpolaris, and lumbar STT cells that project to Sm are located predominantly in lamina VI (92,293). All types of STT cells (i.e., in laminae I, V, and VII) project to VP in the rat, which may reflect the broad overlap of the somatosensory and motor cortices in this species.

Spinobulbar Projections

Spinobulbar projections are important not only for the integration of nociceptive activity with the processes of homeostasis that are subserved in the brain stem (see Chap. 38), but also because indirect projections of nociceptive activity to the forebrain via the brain stem may be important for the conscious experience of pain. Identification of the cells of origin of spinal projections to the brain stem is still incomplete due to the technical difficulty imposed by the ascending STT fibers of passage.

The presently available information indicates that the overall distribution of spinoreticular (SRT) and spinomesencephalic (SMT) cells is quite similar to the distribution of STT cells. That is, they are also found in laminae I, V, and VII in monkey, cat, and rat (219,276,277,285,286). In addition, the same physiologic response categories as STT cells have been described (151,184,287,288), with the exception that few thermoreceptive SRT or SMT cells have yet been identified (184). These similarities suggest that STT and spinobulbar projections may originate from the same populations of cells; however, few STT cells have been shown by means of retrograde double-labeling or antidromic activation to have collateral projections to regions in the brain stem (149,151,184,219,286,295). These pathways probably originate largely (80% to 90%) from different spinal neurons. This provides the opportunity for differential descending control of spinofugal input to different rostral targets. The location of the spinal axons that ascend and terminate in the brain stem overlaps with the course of STT axons, albeit spinal input to the brain stem is bilateral rather than strictly contralateral (Fig. 4). Further details on the physiology and pharmacology of SRT and SMT cells can be found in Chap. 9 of this volume.

Anatomical evidence indicates that spinofugal terminations in the brain stem are concentrated in four major areas (81a,199,201,273,276,277): (a) the regions containing the catecholamine cell groups in the ventrolateral medulla (A1, C1, A5), the nucleus of the solitary tract (A2), the locus coeruleus (A6), and the subcoerulear and Kölliker-Füse regions in the dorsolateral pons (A7); (b) the parabrachial n. (PB); (c) the periaqueductal gray (PAG); and (d) the brain stem reticular formation.

Retrograde and anterograde tracer studies indicate that lamina I cell terminations occur in the first three sites, but not in the reticular formation (35,48,81a,273). Retrograde tracer studies have shown that the terminations of spinal laminae V and VII cells probably occur in the PAG, the solitary n., and the reticular formation, but are weak in PB (35,62,150,165,166, 204,285).

Catecholamine Cell Groups

The brain stem catecholamine cell groups (see Chap. 38) that receive spinal input are well-known integration sites for cardiorespiratory and autonomic function. Cells in these regions give rise to descending spinopetal projections that terminate throughout the spinal gray, including particularly the thoracolumbar sympathetic intermediolateral cell column. Cells in these catecholamine groups also project rostrally to the hypothalamus or locally to autonomic integration sites in the brain stem (186; see Chap. 38). Thus, spinal input to these catecholamine cell groups presumably engages integrative cardiorespiratory and other autonomic functions, including spino-bulbospinal sympathetic reflex arcs and spino-bulbohypothalamic endocrine mechanisms (250).

Lamina I input to cells in the dorsolateral pons is of particular interest, because the catecholamine A7 cells appear to provide the major source of descending noradrenergic modulation of nociceptive dorsal horn activity (67,272,273,294). Other descending spinopetal cells in this region that are enkephalinergic may also receive spinofugal input (36a). Projections from the locus coeruleus (A6) include the entire neuraxis; its overall role is thought to be in vigilance and attention. Thus, lamina I input to this nucleus may be integrated in such processes (80).

Periaqueductal Gray

The PAG is a major integration site for homeostatic control and limbic motor output and has both ascending and descending projections. The SMT input to the PAG is concentrated in its lateral and ventrolateral portions and it is topographically organized rostrocaudally in a trigeminal, cervical, lumbar progression (35,81a). Stimulation of these portions of the PAG can simultaneously elicit aversive behaviors, cardiovascular changes,

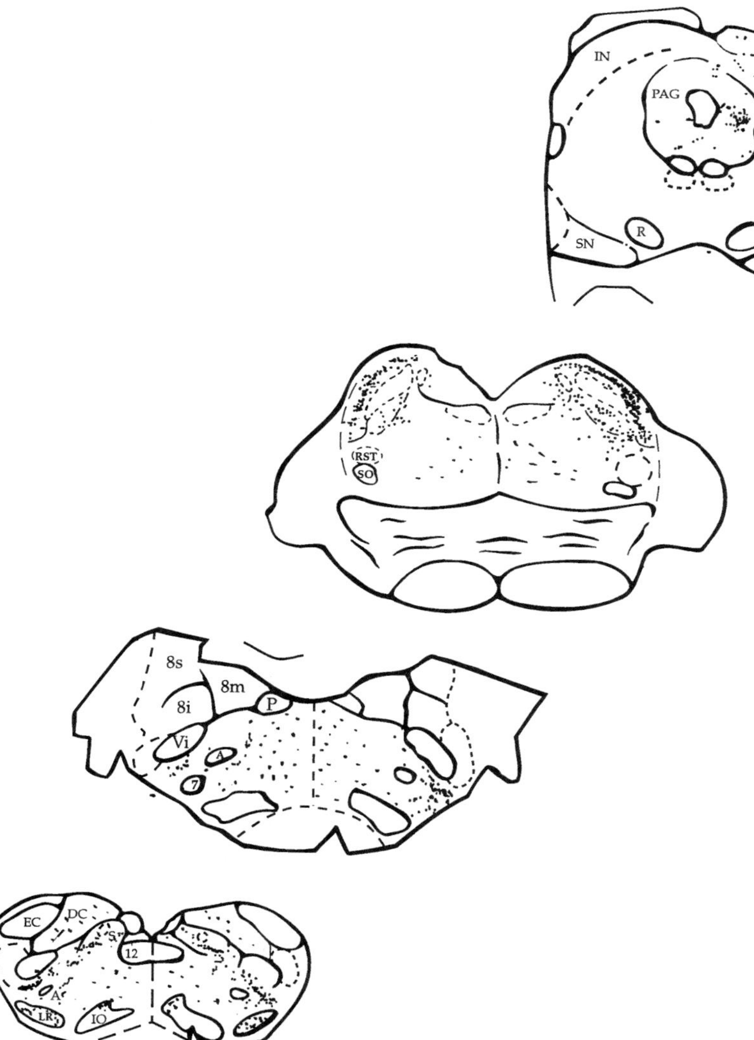

Figure 4. Organization of brainstem projections of spinal neurons. Spinobulbar terminations in the primate are concentrated in the ventrolateral medulla, the dorsolateral pons, and the midbrain periaqueductal gray, with scattered terminations through the brain stem reticular formation, as shown in these four representative transverse levels from posterior *(left)* to anterior *(right).* Abbreviations for nuclei: A, ambiguous; DC, dorsal column nuclei; EC, external cuneate; IN, intercollicular; IO, inferior olive; LR, lateral reticular; P, preapositus hypoglossi; PAG, periaqueductal gray; R, red nucleus; RST, rubrospinal tract; S, solitary; SO, superior olive; Vi, interpolar trigeminal; 7, motor nucleus of the seventh nerve (facial); 8i, 8m, 8s, inferior, medial, and superior vestibular nuclei; 12, hypoglassal motor.

and antinociceptive modulation (14; see Chap. 11). These efferent actions appear to be topographically integrated in an appropriate manner for different behavioral states (14,97). Thus, SMT input to the PAG could be integrated with descending modulatory feedback to the spinal cord, via the raphe and the ventromedial reticular formation (16,117). Notably, these same portions of the PAG also have ascending projections to the hypothalamus and to the thalamus (191,202,230,236), specifically to the reticular n., Pf, and the center median (CM). Thus, SMT input to the PAG may simultaneously affect brain stem modulation of diencephalic processes. The SMT-PAG-thalamic pathway could also provide an indirect alternative pathway for nociceptive sensory activity to reach the thalamus. In this regard, it is important to note that lesions studies have suggested that opioid binding may be presynaptic on the spinofugal projections in the PAG and medullary core (227a), and opiates in this region may be involved in regulating either directly (blocking excitatory input into the midbrain) or indirectly the activation of efferent modulatory circuits (see Chap. 58).

Parabrachial Nuclei (PB)

The PB receives a dense input from lamina I that is concentrated in the lateral part but that overlaps partially in the medial and ventrolateral parts with general visceral afferent input from the solitary n. (26,36,48,62,81a,121,201,219). There is one report of topography (115a). The PB has numerous interconnections with cell groups in the pontine and medullary reticular formation (including the catecholamine cell groups), appropriate for its role in homeostasis and cardiovascular integration (63,122,138,141). It also projects to the hypothalamus, to the amygdala, to Sm (in rats), and to a portion of the ventrobasal thalamus (the basal portion of VM) that likely serves as a relay for general and special visceral sensory activity to the insular cortex (27,29,61,133,171,249,292). This pathway is strongly associated with several peptides, most notably calcitonin gene-related peptide (CGRP) (192,284). Nociceptive neurons recorded in PB have been antidromically activated from the amygdala and the hypothalamus (28). The lamina I input to PB thus serves as an indirect pathway for nociceptive activity to reach the forebrain (28,187), as well as a pathway for general integration of tissue status with homeostatic mechanisms.

Reticular Formation

The reticular formation receives scattered spinal terminations that have only been observed with silver techniques (199,201,265); these have not been well studied with modern methods. Nociceptive neurons have been recorded in the reticular formation, some of which apparently project back to the spinal cord (see section V.a) and could modulate sensory or motor activity. Because many neurons in the brain stem project to the thalamus, the possibility that some of these relay nociceptive activity to the thalamus must also be considered. Such a so-called spinoreticulothalamic pathway has long been hypothesized and purported to serve the motivational aspect of pain (33,41,203). Unfortunately, the distribution of brain stem neurons that project to the thalamus shows little overlap with the distribution of spinal input to the brain stem (34,55,199), suggesting that SMT inputs to the PAG and to PB may be the only routes for indirect spinal access to the thalamus via the brain stem. Nonetheless, recent studies have revealed that neurons in the dorsomedial medullary reticular formation (the subnucleus reticularis dorsalis [SRD]) probably receive direct input from laminae I and V cells, display nociceptive-specific response characteristics, and may project to the thalamus as well as back to the spinal cord (31,239,270,273). The role of such cells in pain has not been determined.

Spinohypothalamic Pathway

Recent evidence indicates a massive spinal projection to the lateral hypothalamus in the rat that originates from cells in laminae I, V, and X over the entire length of the cord (46,70). These cells include nociceptive neurons. Nonetheless, in the cat a much weaker projection has been reported that originates nearly entirely from the sacral spinal segments (160), and there is little evidence of a direct spinal input to the hypothalamus in the primate. The role played by these specific projections is unclear. Nevertheless, such systems provide direct access by nociceptive input to vegetative centers related to regulation of the hypothalamopituitary axis (see Chap. 42).

Other Indirect Pathways

In addition to the indirect spinofugal pathways to the forebrain that can relay in the brain stem, there are two other indirect pathways that relay in the spinal cord itself. These are the postsynaptic dorsal column (PSDC) system and the spinocervicothalamic pathway (SCTP). The PSDC originates from second-order cells in the spinal dorsal horn, primarily in laminae IV to V, that project via the dorsal columns and the dorsolateral funiculus to the dorsal column nuclei. These axons terminate within the ventral and rostral portions of the dorsal column nuclei, which project to motor-related portions of the brain stem and the thalamus (24). The SCTP originates from a similar, overlapping population of second-order cells in laminae IV to V of the spinal dorsal horn that project via the dorsolateral funiculus to the lateral cervical nucleus in the C1-2 spinal segments (39). Lateral cervical neurons project to VP in the thalamus. Nociceptive neurons have been recorded in both the PSDC and SCTP pathways (88,107,116,159). Nonetheless, activity in both of these pathways is overwhelmingly dominated by low-threshold mechanoreceptor stimulation, and their functional contributions to pain sensation are unknown.

Functional Role of Anterolateral Tract Axons

The physiologic characteristics of anatomically defined spinofugal projections described in the above sections make it clear that several defined pathways exist through which afferent information relevant to nociceptive processing and pain sensation may travel. The precise relevance of these several individual pathways remains obscure. However, the importance of the ascending activity in the anterolateral quadrant is emphasized by (a) consideration of the parallels between activity in the systems and pain behavior, (b) effects of lesions, and (c) effects of direct stimulation on pain behavior.

Correlated Activity in Anterolateral Tract Axons and Pain Behavior Insofar as acute heat and mechanical nociception are concerned, increases in stimulus intensity are associated with monotonic increases in the discharge of many spinofugal neurons and in the magnitude of the reported pain state (see Chap. 41). Multiunit records obtained from axons in the ventrolateral quadrant prior to cordotomy in humans have shown close parallels between the frequency of neuronal activity, the pain report, and the noxious stimulus applied to the appropriate dermatome (196). Close correlations have been reported between the discharge activity of projection neurons in the medullary dorsal horn and the discriminative responses of awake, behaviorally trained monkeys to noxious heat stimuli applied to the face (52,108). In cases of hyperalgesia, as after burn or repetitive C-fiber stimulation, an augmented pain report is observed in humans (see Chap. 41) and animals (see Chap. 40), and WDR neurons (see Chap. 36) that project out of the spinal cord show a corollary increase in discharge rate (174,218,255).

Anterolateral Tract Stimulation Stimulation of the anterolateral quadrant in pain patients during a percutaneous cordotomy procedure results in reports of thermal (warm, less often cool) and sometimes painful sensations referred to contralateral dermatomes at levels below the segments of stimulation (125,263,275). Stimulation parameters (intensity and frequency) that induce reports of referred pain in cordotomy patients (who are under local anesthesia but have ongoing pain) can be correlated in part with the physiologic characteristics of ascending STT fibers in the monkey (196).

Anterolateral Tract Lesions Lesions in the middle of the lateral funiculus have been most closely associated with the production of analgesia and thermanesthesia (173,211,214,275). As noted, classical observations indicated that these lesions resulted in a contralateral deficit in dermatomes that were one to two segments below the level of the lesion. Further support for the role of crossed projection systems is provided by the observation that midline section along the longitudinal axis of the spinal cord can produce a bilateral analgesia in pain patients. Psychophysical studies carried out in primates with a variety of spinal lesions have revealed findings similar to those observed in humans (269a). Thus, the distribution of the referred pain induced by focal ventrolateral quadrant stimulation and the organization of analgesia produced by lesions of the anterolateral quadrant support the historical concept that ascending pain-related activity is a "crossed" pathway.

It is clear that the anterolateral quadrant contains projection systems that are integral to the perception of pain evoked by a strong stimulus in the contralateral body, but it must be stressed that this biologic system is redundant, plastic, and not a singular, hard-wired substrate. Thus, Noordenbos and Wall (1976) observed that severance of all but a fragment of the anterolateral quadrant left a patient with an intact sense of pain, but surprisingly there was bilateral sensitivity. Furthermore, lesions that produce analgesia in humans and primates will result, over intervals of 6 to 12 months, in the emergence of a central, dysesthetic pain condition in about half the cases (196,269). These observations emphasize the complexity of the spinal-supraspinal linkages involved in pain perception.

FUNCTIONAL CHARACTERISTICS OF SUPRASPINAL NOCICEPTIVE NEURONS

The supraspinal structures that receive ascending nociceptive spinofugal projections are presumed to be relevant to afferent nociceptive processing. These projection targets will now be considered.

Thalamus

Nociceptive neurons have been identified physiologically in several nuclei in both the medial and the lateral thalamus. In the following discussion, particular emphasis is placed on the regions that receive direct STT input, not all of which have been well characterized. Detailed anatomical descriptions of the several nuclei are available elsewhere (155).

Ventral Posterior Nuclei

Functional Correlates These somatosensory nuclei contain the major somatotopic representation of the body, by virtue of their lemniscal input from the dorsal column nuclei and the principal trigeminal nucleus. The face is represented medially in VPM and the forelimb and hindlimb are represented successively more laterally in the medial and lateral parts of VPL (155).

Stimulation within VP in humans generally evokes a report of topographically localized paresthesia and rarely a report of a painful sensation (155,180,263). Reports of pain are somewhat more common with VP stimulation in central pain patients (95, 103,177). However, chronic electrical stimulation of VP is commonly used to alleviate certain pain conditions (131,172,253). Some neurons in regions of VP that have been deafferented in humans display bursting discharges that may or may not be related to deafferentation pain (178). Lidocaine injections into VPM can impair behavioral discrimination of noxious heat and innocuous cool in the awake monkey if a sufficiently large region is injected, probably including the region posterior and inferior to VP (see below) (110).

Neuronal Activity Nociceptive neurons can be found among the many low-threshold neurons in the VP nuclei in the monkey, generally in register with the topography of VP (60,66, 163). These neurons presumably receive direct STT input (66, 163). The responses of these cells are graded with mechanical and heat stimuli and they discharge to low-threshold and, more vigorously, to noxious stimuli, i.e., they are wide dynamic range (WDR) neurons. Their responses can be affected by the state of arousal (208). Some of these WDR cells respond phasically to cooling (53). These cells tend to have receptive fields of moderate size; that is, they may respond to stimuli over a third of the face or over the entire hand or arm. The stimulus-response functions of these cells are consistent with the discriminative ability of behaviorally trained monkeys (53). Some WDR cells in VP have been antidromically activated from primary somatosensory cortex (163). WDR cells have also been recorded in VPI, the portion of ventrobasal thalamus that projects to the second somatosensory cortex (8).

In the cat, the organization of nociceptive neurons differs markedly. In contrast to the primate, there are few, if any, nociceptive cells within VP in the cat. Nociceptive neurons have been identified in the dorsal and ventral aspects of VP, including VPI (142,168,289,290). These are NS and WDR cells that can encode stimulus intensity in the noxious range. They are crudely topographically organized, with trigeminal cells located medially, and cervical and lumbar cells located successively more laterally. They can be activated by stimulation of skin, muscle, tooth pulp, viscera, or cranial vasculature (12,44, 94,144,168,291). Some of these cells project to somatosensory cortex or the anterior cingulate cortex (167,283). Lesions of the VPM that also encompass Sm (see below) in the cat can produce hypalgesia to tooth pulp stimulation (158). In the rat, nociceptive cells are found throughout VP intermixed (in topographic register) with low-threshold neurons (130,223). Both NS and WDR cells have been reported that encode stimulus intensity and that generally have large, often bilateral, receptive fields. In rats with experimentally induced arthritis or neuropathies, many more WDR cells are reported in VP that project to the somatosensory cortex (128,129). Modulation by stimulation of the PAG or the raphe in the brain stem has been observed (143,170).

Posterior Region

Functional Correlates The presence of nociceptive neurons posterior to VP has been the subject of much debate in nonprimate studies (cited below). The earliest study in the human thalamus by Hassler (135) indicated that reports of painful sensations can be elicited by electrical stimulation of the region posterior and inferior to VP, which he called V.c.pc. Recent studies have confirmed this observation (106,132,180) and support the original Head and Holmes (137) hypothesis that a specific pain nucleus may be located in the posterolateral thalamus. Such stimulation is complicated by the presence of ascending STT fibers in this region (40,263); nonetheless, recent physiologic data in the primate and the human (described below) and the anatomical demonstration of the lamina I spinothalamocortical pathway through VMpo (summarized above) provide strong corroboration for this hypothesis. Hassler's report of a mediolateral topography for pain referral from this region, however, has not been confirmed.

Infarcts or thromboses in this general region of the human thalamus can result in hypalgesia and thermanesthesia. In some individuals the paradoxical thalamic pain syndrome develops, in which burning, dysesthetic pain occurs within the zone of thermanesthesia and hypalgesia (137,176,216). These findings are all consistent with the presence of a specific nociceptive sensory relay nucleus.

Neuronal Activity In the cynomolgus monkey, nociceptive and thermoreceptive neurons have been physiologically identified in VMpo, the region in which dense lamina I STT terminations occur (50,89b). Almost all of these cells are modality-specific. Their stimulus-response functions show graded response magnitudes to noxious or thermal stimuli. Receptive fields for the majority of VMpo neurons are small (3 cm^2 or less) and they are topographically distributed rostrocaudally, corresponding with the anatomical findings in the monkey. Nociceptive-specific neurons have been reported posterior to VP in the squirrel monkey as well (8). In the human, recordings have recently been reported from nociceptive neurons in the region posterior and inferior to the main somatosensory representation, i.e., in the region of VMpo. Both WDR and NS neurons were recorded. Stimulation in this region produces pain or cold sensations (179).

In the cat, an early study indicated that more than half of PO units were nociceptive, but this could not be confirmed in later work (91,225). Nonetheless, some recent studies have reported nociceptive cutaneous and visceral responses in the region of PO (42,57). The portion of PO found dorsal to VP differs from the portion found caudal to VP, since it projects to area 5a (262), but it also seems to contain nociceptive cells (44,148, 213). In the rat, PO receives convergent descending input from VP via the somatosensory cortex (99), thus it similarly contains neurons responsive to noxious stimulation. A recent study in the rat indicates that nociceptive cells with visceral input are located not only within VP but also on its borders (25).

Intralaminar Nuclei

Functional Correlates The CM-Pf complex is a large, clearly visible region in the human thalamus that for several years was thought to receive STT input and was therefore associated with pain in the literature and in textbooks. However, modern tracing studies show that there are essentially no STT terminations in CM and only weak input to Pf. The dominant inputs to this region originate from the cerebellum, pallidum, tectum, and brain stem, and the major efferent projections from CM and Pf are to the basal ganglia. Lesions were made in this region in many neurosurgical studies in the 1950s to alleviate chronic pain, with mixed success (259); large lesions may have involved VMpo and MDvc. Lesions in the region of CL in the human reportedly do not cause analgesia or thalamic pain syndrome (37).

Neuronal Activity Neurons responsive to noxious stimuli have been recorded in most areas of the medial thalamus in the primate, but because CL and Pf receive STT input, these intralaminar nuclei are of particular interest with respect to pain. Nociceptive intralaminar neurons have been identified in awake monkeys (51,58). Most had large receptive fields. Stimulus coding properties of these neurons have not been well studied, but some show clearly graded responses to noxious heat

(51). Many CL neurons discharge with eye movements (251), consistent with the dominant ascending inputs to CL from the cerebellum and the superior colliculus.

In the cat and the rat, a large number of studies have reported nociceptive neurons in the intralaminar nuclei (3,20, 101,215,222,232,257,296). Most of these investigations relied on responses to strong electrical stimuli, but some responses to natural noxious stimulation have been reported (105,222). The data indicate that such neurons are widely scattered throughout the medial thalamus, with no apparent localization. Some neurons with graded responses have been observed, and modulation by stimulation of various brain regions, primarily motor related, has been reported (182).

Medial Dorsal Nucleus

Functional Correlates The presence of lamina I STT input to the ventral caudal part of MD indicates that nociceptive neurons may be found there. It is noteworthy that many of the neurosurgical lesions made in the CM-Pf region or in posterior CL for the purpose of alleviating chronic pain probably involved the ventral caudal part of MD (78,153,233,235).

Neuronal Activity There is little physiologic evidence to date regarding the nociceptive responsiveness of MDvc cells in the primate. The medial thalamic nucleus submedius (Sm) in the cat and the rat receives lamina I input, just as MDvc does, and may be functionally similar. Nociceptive-specific neurons have been recorded in Sm in the cat (75,84), and primarily nociceptive and a few low-threshold cells have been found there in the rat (104,161,207). In the rat, inputs from cutaneous and deep tissues have also been recorded. In the cat, both nociceptive and thermoreceptive lamina I STT cells project to Sm (82), but no cells excited by cold have been observed in Sm, raising the possibility that cold-induced inhibition of nociceptive processing could occur there (78). In the arthritic rat, many Sm cells are responsive to innocuous joint movements (104). Noxious stimulation can produce increased gene transduction (c-Fos activity) in Sm and in several midline nuclei not related to STT terminations in the rat (45). It should also be noted that several studies have focused on the possibility that the habenula (adjacent to MD) may be involved in pain modulation (21, 74,100,189,264), but the significance of this is unclear.

Cortex

A variety of cortical lesions have been attempted to alleviate pain. Prefrontal lobectomies, amydalectomies, capsulotomies, and cingulotomies have been reported to alter the human or animal response to strong stimuli, but these effects may have been due to global alterations in the response to the environment and were not selective for pain. Lesions of the primary sensory cortex have been shown to produce an anesthetic action, but generally do not produce selective effects upon nociceptive responding (220). Lesions of the parieto-insular cortex or the underlying internal capsule have been associated with hypalgesia, thermanesthesia, central pain syndrome, and pain asymbolia (32,127,176). Given the intimate, organized, and reciprocal interconnections that exist between thalamus, cortex, and these various areas, mixed evidence for both localization and general interactions should be expected.

Imaging (positron emission tomography [PET]) studies in humans indicate several discrete regions of cortex that are activated by noxious stimulation (see Chap. 23). These include the first and second somatosensory cortices (SI and SII), the anterior insula, and the anterior cingulate cortex (59,154,260). It appears likely that the regions activated in the PET studies receive their nociceptive thalamic inputs from the STT termination sites described above: SI from VP; SII from VPI; insula from VMpo; and anterior cingulate from MDvc. Physiologic EEG recordings of laser-induced pain indicate activation of SI, a midline (vertex) region, and a region in the area of the lateral sulcus (43a). These functional studies provide strong evidence that regions of the cortex may be the target of information generated by noxious input.

Somatosensory Cortex (SI/SII)

Functional Correlates Available clinical evidence suggests that lesions of SI cortex have minimal effects on pain sensation, and that stimulation of the postcentral gyrus does not cause pain in humans (220).

Neuronal Activity There is physiologic evidence in the monkey indicating the presence of nociceptive neurons in SI and in the region of SII (102,164). Such nociceptive cortical neurons include both NS and WDR cells in several cortical layers of areas 3b and 1 of SI. In addition, nociceptive neurons have been recorded in area 7 of the lateral parietal cortex (102).

In the cat, recordings of nociceptive cortical neurons have been obtained from cells responsive to tooth pulp stimulation in the coronal gyrus or SI (152,194,238). In the rat, nociceptive cells have been recorded in all layers of SI cortex (120).

Insula

Functional Correlates The insula is thought to provide the substrate for generation of an image of the body that underlies the basic emotional states associated with maintenance of the integrity of the body (93a). Lesions of the anterior insula have been reported to produce analgesia and thermanesthesia, whereas lesions of the posterior insula (and the overlying parietal cortex) may produce pain asymbolia (31a).

Neuronal Activity Nociceptive neurons have not yet been physiologically identified in the insula.

Anterior Cingulate

Functional Correlates In PET imaging studies, the anterior cingulate cortex is activated by painful but not innocuous stimuli (59,154,260); however, it can be activated by attention-related somatosensory tasks (49a). Lesions of the anterior cingulate can have significant but variable effects on pain (259).

Neuronal Activity Nociceptive neurons have been recorded in the anterior cingulate in the human (147) and in the rabbit (254). These were mostly NS neurons with large receptive fields. Analogous recordings have been obtained in the ventrolateral orbital (VLO) cortex, which receives input from Sm (see above) in the cat and the rat (13,256). The VLO neurons were excited or inhibited by noxious cutaneous stimulation; some showed persistent aftereffects from single stimuli, and acute pain increased glucose utilization in VLO cortex in the cat (267).

Other Telencephalic Structures

Amygdala

Functional Correlates Lesions of the amygdala in primates can cause memory deficits, but effects on pain sensibility apparently have not been observed. Increased glucose metabolism in the amygdala has been observed in a neuropathic pain model in the rat (193). The amygdala may be significant for the analgesic effects of systemic morphine (137a).

Neuronal Activity Nociceptive neurons have been identified in the central nucleus of the amygdala only in the rat; these studies confirm the efficacy of the nociceptive PB neurons that project there (30,146).

Basal Ganglia

Functional Correlates Clinical lesions of the basal ganglia and diseases that affect these structures (e.g., Parkinson's or Huntington's) may have some effect on pain perception (reviewed in ref. 65).

Neuronal Activity Nociceptive neurons have been recorded in these presumably motor-related structures in the rat (30,65), but not in the cat or the primate. Nociceptive responses have also been obtained in the substantia nigra that are sensitive to systemic morphine (15,19).

Hypothalamus

Functional Correlates In humans, lesions of the periventricular gray, involving the posterior hypothalamus, have been used to alleviate pain (259).

Neuronal activity Nociceptive neurons have not been well studied in the hypothalamus, but cells that respond to visceral or tooth pulp stimulation have been recorded in the rat (134).

PHARMACOLOGIC CHARACTERISTICS OF SUPRASPINAL NOCICEPTIVE NEURONS

In comparison with primary afferents and spinal cord terminal systems, relatively little is known concerning the neurotransmitters and receptors utilized by nociceptive neurons or by the modulatory inputs to these neurons at the thalamic and cortical levels. Even our knowledge of the pharmacology of nonnociceptive transmission at these levels is rudimentary (156,256a). Most of the work that is available has been performed in the rat. In view of the paucity of information, this review also summarizes information relating to nonnociceptive transmission, as it is quite likely that both systems utilize similar pharmacologic mechanisms. It is also useful to review data obtained from the better-studied visual system (see review by McCormick [197]).

General consideration of the nature of the transmitters that mediate the effects of the primary spinofugal input suggests that the identity of the relevant agents would be supported by (a) presence in the cell bodies of projecting neurons, (b) presence in the terminal fields of the projecting neurons, (c) mimicry of the effects of physiologic stimulation when the exogenous receptor agonist is applied in the terminal region, and (d) a comparable antagonist pharmacology for blocking the effects of the physiologic stimulus and the exogenously administered agonist.

As reviewed above, the primary postsynaptic effect of ascending afferent traffic is a powerful excitation. However, as in all neural circuits, there is a considerable amount of sculpting of the neuronal output by local feedback circuits. As will be considered below, it is generally assumed at this time that the excitatory amino acids, i.e., glutamate and aspartate, constitute the principal excitatory mediators involved in signal transmission and processing at the thalamic and cortical levels, whereas the inhibitory amino acids γ-aminobutyric acid (GABA) and glycine, the monoamines (norepinephrine [NE], serotonin [5-HT], and dopamine [DA]), acetylcholine (ACh), and histamine are utilized by modulatory systems that control the overall excitability of the thalamocortical systems in a state-dependent manner (197,256a).

An important point in the interpretation of work defining these central systems is the need to limit drug action to the region of interest. The systemic delivery of agents in complex models involving supraspinal processing systems and the potential multiple sites of drug action severely limit the ability to interpret mechanisms with respect to the effects of systemically delivered drug on single-unit activity or behavior (22,54).

Excitatory Amino Acids

Spinofugal neurons have been identified as containing glutamate or glutamate synthesizing enzymes (114b,188). It is thus likely that these projection neurons release these excitatory amino acids at their terminals in brain stem and thalamus. This has been demonstrated for spinothalamic lamina I terminals in the monkey (36b). The pioneering studies of Curtis and Johnston (91a) first demonstrated that thalamic neurons were excited by iontophoretically applied excitatory amino acids.

Local iontophoretic delivery into the terminal regions of the spinofugal projections have shown that both *N*-methyl-D-aspartate (NMDA) and non-NMDA glutamate receptors are involved in mediating innocuous somatosensory inputs (112–114,243, 244,246–248). Short duration stimuli appear to activate primarily non-NMDA receptors (251a,247), whereas prolonged stimuli lead to activation of NMDA receptors. Of particular interest are the findings of recent studies that suggest that the synaptic response to noxious stimulation is mediated by group I metabotropic glutamate receptors and NMDA receptors. This combination of receptors is different from that involved in mediating the excitatory inputs from nonnoxious inputs but similar to those involved in mediating corticothalamic excitation (114a,248a). Responses of VB nociceptive neurons are blocked by NMDA but not non-NMDA receptor antagonists (113; however, see 268).

Thalamic projection neurons probably also release glutamate from their terminals in cortex. There is anatomical evidence that thalamocortical neurons contain glutamate within their cortical terminals (165a,224a), and that they excite cortical neurons through AMPA receptors (224a). Corticothalamic neurons also utilize glutamate and aspartate (156,241) and the excitation evoked by activity in that system is mediated by both NMDA and non-NMDA receptors (98).

The intracerebral microinjection of glutamate into the medial mesencephalon (periaqueductal gray), but not in the regions throughout the thalamus was shown to produce "pain behavior" in the unanesthetized rat. This effects was mediated by an NMDA, but not a kainate-sensitive receptor (153a). Pain behavior was not evoked by glutamate agonists microinjected throughout the thalamus in the rat.

Since NMDA receptors may be important in inducing long-term changes in synaptic efficacy, it has been proposed that they may be important in mediating changes occurring in chronic pain states. Dissociative anesthetics, such as ketamine, are NMDA receptor antagonists. Accordingly, it is possible that the antihyperalgesic analgesic properties of these agents may be due in part to an action at these receptors at the thalamic level (243). However, NMDA receptors are likely involved in many circuits and are not selective for nociceptive transmission.

Inhibitory Amino Acids–GABA

It is well established that GABA plays a major role as an inhibitory neurotransmitter in thalamus. All major anesthetic agents appear to act in part though an effect mediated by the $GABA_A$ ionophore (261). The intrinsic interneurons of the thalamus as well as the neurons of the thalamic reticular nucleus (TRN) that innervate the thalamus are GABAergic (145,155,241). Iontophoretically applied bicuculline, a GABA antagonist, has been shown to reduce the inhibition of nonnociceptive neurons in rat and cat VB (245) and increase the duration of stimulus-induced thalamic responses (139). There is evidence that at least in the anesthetized state, nonnociceptive neurons are under tonic GABAergic inhibition (268). More recent studies have implicated the $GABA_A$ receptor in mediating afferent-induced inhibitory effects (237). In addition, the short latency IPSP elicited in thalamic relay neurons by stimulation of the TRN is mediated primarily by $GABA_A$ receptors (175a,266), whereas longer latency inhibition is mediated by $GABA_B$ receptors (175a). Release of GABA from these terminals can be reduced by activation of presynaptic glutamate metabotropic receptors (248b).

Although all these findings pertain to nonnociceptive neurons, it is likely that GABAergic neurons also project onto thalamic nociceptive neurons. As an example, nucleus submedius (Sm) in the rat receives a dense projection from the TRN (292). Since TRN neurons are reported to be entirely GABAergic (145) and Sm contains many nociceptive neurons (104, 161), this suggests a GABAergic control of nociceptive activity. Similar connections of TRN with VP also exist and thus it is likely that nociceptive neurons in VP also receive GABAergic inputs. Not surprisingly, iontophoretic application of GABA and the GABA agonist tetrahydroisoxazolopyridinol (THIP) inhibited the spontaneous activity and responses of nociceptive neurons in rat Pf (231). Of considerable interest, injections of these drugs into Pf increased withdrawal latency as ascertained by the tail-immersion assay. It has also been shown that picrotoxin, a $GABA_A$ antagonist, partially reverses dorsal column stimulation-induced inhibition of nociceptive responses of nociceptive neurons in cat thalamus (215a).

It has been suggested that thalamic GABA receptors may be involved in mediating plasticity and deafferentation pain at the VP level (237). Following chronic deafferentation (C2–C4 rhizotomies) in primates, a downregulation of $GABA_A$ receptors has been shown (228). This suggests that release from inhibition may contribute to the marked changes in the thalamic somatotopic representation observed in these animals and may also be responsible for the development of chronic deafferentation pain syndromes.

Monoamines

The thalamus, like most other brain regions, receives projections from serotoninergic and noradrenergic neurons in the brain stem (90,205,224,258). Although limited, there are some indications, as described below, suggesting their involvement in nociceptive processing at the thalamic level. Furthermore, there is evidence from animal studies that monoamines can modulate bursting activity in thalamic neurons that is associated with calcium spikes (224). There is some data suggesting that calcium spike associated activity is increased in chronic pain (153,178,266a). Tricyclic antidepressants that are effective in the treatment of chronic pain (e.g., amitriptyline) enhance monoamine terminal activity by blocking reuptake (234). It has thus been suggested that they may act in part at the thalamic level to reduce central deafferentation pain (178).

Noradrenaline

Both axonal terminals and receptors for noradrenaline have been demonstrated in VP and in medial thalamic regions associated with pain processing (157,217,224,258,274). Most of the projections arise from the locus coeruleus (LC) (274). The projection is particularly dense in the lateral thalamus including VP, Sm, and CM-Pf (224). The thalamus contains a high density of α_1-adrenoreceptors (157). The TRN is densely innervated by noradrenergic axons. Both electrical stimulation of the LC and direct application of NE onto TRN cells cause excitation via α_1-receptors (162). The effects of manipulating the noradrenergic system and in particular of lesions or stimulation of the LC have been shown to have mixed effects on pain perception. Given the rostral and caudal projection of these axons, however, it is not possible to appreciate whether these effects reflect an effect on forebrain and/or spinal cord processing.

Serotonin

The main source of serotoninergic innervation of the thalamus is from the dorsal raphe nucleus and both VP and medial thalamic regions implicated in pain receive inputs. The highest levels of 5-HT1 and 5-HT2 receptors were reported to be in the medial thalamus, in particular in dorsal Sm, CM-Pf (224) in rat, and in VPL in monkey (274). In the rat, the dorsal Sm in which ascending STT terminations are concentrated receives a denser serotonin innervation than the ventral region. Whether this serotoninergic input is inhibitory or excitatory (depending on the local class of serotoninergic receptor: 5-HT1 is inhibitory, and 5-HT2 is excitatory) is not known, but reflects the likelihood of a modulatory effect on the afferent input to that thalamic nucleus. The TRN receives a moderate to dense serotoninergic innervation (90). In contrast to its action on thalamic relay neurons, iontophoretic application of 5-HT onto TRN neurons results in strong excitation, probably by activation of 5-HT2 receptors (198). Because of the probable release of GABA by this system (see above), the ultimate effect on relay of sensory transmission would still be inhibitory.

Stimulation of the dorsal raphe region has long been known to produce analgesia. Although most work has focused on descending pain inhibitory mechanisms, some recent work has suggested that ascending pathways may also be involved in analgesia. Stimulation of the dorsal raphe in the cat has been shown to inhibit the responses of nociceptive neurons in the periphery of VPL (143). The effect could also be observed on responses elicited by stimulation of the ventrolateral funiculus, suggesting an action at the thalamic level. However, whether the inhibition was due to 5-HT release was not tested. Dorsal raphe stimulation has also been shown to inhibit the nociceptive responses of neurons in the rat intralaminar nuclei, an effect blocked by 5-HT depletion (93). Iontophoretic application of serotonin inhibits about 50% of medial thalamic neurons responding to nociceptive stimulation (112).

Dopamine

There have been very few studies concerning the role of dopamine in thalamus. However, dopamine receptors have been observed in the thalamus and dopamine metabolites measured (224). The source of this innervation has not been established. Recent data suggest that cocaine-induced analgesia is mediated by a supraspinal action at dopamine D1 or D2 receptors, although the sites remain unclear (185). It has also been shown that systemically administered cocaine inhibits medial thalamic nociceptive neurons, an effect blocked by a D2 receptor antagonist (252), and that lesions of Pf attenuate the analgesic effects of cocaine in the formalin test. These findings suggest a role for dopamine in thalamic mechanisms of nociception.

Acetylcholine

The thalamus receives cholinergic input from the nucleus basalis and the pontomesencephalic reticular formation, the former supplying primarily the TRN. Cholinergic innervation of VP is light, but medial thalamic structures implicated in nociception, including the dorsal Sm, are well innervated (181). Although there have been reports of analgesia following intraventricular injections of cholinergic agonists, the involvement of thalamus in these effects has not been examined. Direct application of ACh to thalamic neurons produces predominantly excitatory responses in relay neurons and inhibition of TRN neurons (197; but see 193a), but there has been no direct data on thalamic nociceptive neurons and the pharmacology of this effect has not been well defined. Of interest, however, is the dense innervation of the TRN and the fact that iontophoretically applied ACh inhibits TRN neurons. This latter effect is to disinhibit the GABAergic inhibition of sensory transmission and may be related to arousal and attention.

Opioids

Although the concentration of opiate peptides is generally quite low in the thalamus, and major opioid projections have not been described, it is possible that opiate peptides have a depressant action on thalamic nociceptive neurons. Autoradiographic binding studies indicate dense concentrations of μ, δ, and κ receptors, particularly in the medial thalamus and in Sm (190). In general, morphine inhibits the activity of medial thalamic neurons (93,109,252). Coffield and Miletic (72,206) reported that some enkephalin-containing spinal and trigeminal projection neurons terminate in Sm and that micropressure injections of enkephalin inhibit the majority of the nociceptive neurons in rat Sm (73). He et al. (136) iontophoretically applied etorphine and naloxone on rabbit thalamic neurons. They demonstrated that etorphine blocked some excitatory responses of nociceptive neurons and that the effects were antagonized by naloxone. Naloxone alone potentiated the responses of some nociceptive neurons, suggesting the existence of tonic opioidergic modulation of thalamic neurons. Naloxone was also shown to antagonize the acupuncture-induced depression of nociceptive neurons. Microinjection studies in this region have been surprisingly negative with μ, δ, and κ agonists having little effect on acute electrical or thermal escape latencies. It is possible, however, that such models may not reveal subtle effects on nociceptive processing that are associated with protracted afferent stimuli (such as in models of inflammation or nerve injury). A recent study has revealed the presence of prepro-enkephalin messenger RNA (mRNA) expressing neurons in rat thalamus, including some in regions of medial thalamus that are known to contain nociceptive neurons and are believed to be involved in nociception (138a).

Adenosine and Histamine

The thalamus contains high levels of adenosine receptors (175). Iontophoresis of adenosine on thalamic neurons produces inhibition (169). The inhibition of lateral geniculate neurons (LGNs) is mediated by A1 receptors (197).

The thalamus is innervated by histaminergic fibers, apparently arising from the tuberomamillary nucleus of the hypothalamus, and contains H1 and H2 receptors. Histamine produces a slow depolarization of LGNs (197). There is no information on the role of these substances in thalamic mechanisms of pain.

Thyrotropin-Releasing Hormone (TRH)

Clarke and Djourhi (69) showed that a TRH analogue reverses the depressant effects of anesthetics on the responses of neurons in the rat VPL. They proposed that anesthesia depresses the transmission of sensory information through thalamus primarily by an action on TRN neurons.

Peptides

There have also been many immunohistochemical studies revealing the locations of various peptides in thalamus (e.g., CCK, dynorphin, enkephalin, NPY, SP, somatostatin, neurotensin, somatotropin-release inhibiting factor [SRIF]). In general, these have not been related to afferent fiber systems. Substance P labeling has been associated with STT projections in the cat and the rat (18,114b); they have similar distributions, and the SP labeling can be greatly diminished by cordotomy. Similarly, CGRP has been associated with the parabrachial terminations in VMb (192) and lamina I STT terminations in VMpo. STT neurons have also been shown to include cells that contain enkephalin, dynorphin, and vasoactive intestinal polypeptide (17,72,192,210). There has also been a study demonstrating the existence of many different peptides (e.g., SP, NPY, CGRP, galanin, CCK) in brain stem neurons projecting to medial and lateral thalamus, including thalamic sites likely to be involved in nociception (174a). CCK has recently been demonstrated to exist in about 80% of corticothalamic neurons projecting to the rat ventrolateral nucleus (251b). The function of the peptides in thalamic terminations is unknown (156).

Nitric Oxide

Not much is known yet about the role of NO in thalamic function. However, the thalamus is known to show NADPH-diaphorase activity (215b,269b), which is thought to be a marker for the enzyme NO synthase. It has also been shown that arginine, the NO precursor, is released in rat VP by vibrissal stimulation and that its iontophoretic release facilitates sensory synaptic transmission, possibly by promoting synthesis of NO (99a).

CONCLUSIONS

A complex organization occurs with neural traffic, suggesting the complexity of the organization that is anticipated in the processing mechanisms that may be brought into play in decoding the information generated by high-intensity somatic stimuli that activate small-diameter nociceptive sensory afferents. It is important to realize that the outlining of anatomical connectivity may not emphasize the fact that a high-intensity peripheral stimulus will concurrently activate Aβ, Aδ, and C afferents that in turn generate a complex pattern of neural traffic that ascends by several well-defined and discretely organized pathways that project to a number of supraspinal sites that are themselves joined by internuclear linkages. Thus, organizationally, we can see that the "encoding" of an afferent message arising from a given dermatome involves:

1. Frequency profile of the afferent traffic in the ascending system (increasing stimulus intensity will be encoded as an increased frequency of discharge in ascending sensory pathways).
2. The specific anatomical projections of adjacent spinofugal pathways originating from the same spinal level (e.g., input from spinothalamic projections to the medial vs ventrobasal thalamus vs the submedius).
3. The supraspinal convergence between the several spinofugal tracts (e.g., ventrobasal excitation evoked by large afferents through the dorsal column and thence via the lemniscal connections and by spinothalamic input from the same spinal level);
4. The temporal ordering of the arrival of the afferent traffic (e.g., input through paucisynaptic systems such as the spinothalamic will arrive at the ventrobasal complex prior to the input from the spinomesencephalic-thalamic linkages).

The role of this encoding process is to provide an algorithm whereby the sensory environment can be mapped onto neural networks. It seems likely that these systems by their organizational complexity provide the framework for interactions with processes that coincide with higher order systems that relate that environment to patterns providing linkages to emotion and memory. Such processes are considered to be mediated by limbic and cortical systems. The exciting lines of investigation that open to us now are the understanding of the connectivity and the nature of the functional interactions that lead to the "perception of the pain state."

REFERENCES

1. Albe-Fessard D, Berkley KJ, Kruger L, Ralston HJ III, Willis WD Jr. Diencephalic mechanisms of pain sensation. *Brain Res Rev* 1985;9: 217–296.
2. Albe-Fessard D, Boivie J, Grant G, Levante A. Labelling of cells in the medulla oblongata of the monkey after injections of horseradish peroxidase in the thalamus. *Neurosci Lett* 1975;1:75–80.
3. Albe-Fessard D, Kruger L. Duality of unit discharges from cat centrum medianum in response to natural and electrical stimulation. *J Neurophysiol* 1962;25:3–20.
4. Allen GV, Saper CB, Hurley KM, Cechetto DF. Organization of vis-

ceral and limbic connections in the insular cortex of the rat. *J Comp Neurol* 1991;311:1–16.

5. Apkarian AV, Hodge CJ. Primate spinothalamic pathways: I. A quantitative study of the cells of origin of the spinothalamic pathway. *J Comp Neurol* 1989;288:447–473.
6. Apkarian AV, Hodge CJ. Primate spinothalamic pathways: II. The cells of origin of the dorsolateral and ventral spinothalamic pathways. *J Comp Neurol* 1989;288:474–492.
7. Apkarian AV, Hodge CJ. Primate spinothalamic pathways: III. Thalamic terminations of the dorsolateral and ventral spinothalamic pathways. *J Comp Neurol* 1989;288:493–511.
8. Apkarian AV, Shi T, Stevens RT, Kniffki K-D, Hodge CJ. Properties of nociceptive neurons in the lateral thalamus of the squirrel monkey. *Soc Neurosci Abstr* 1991;17:838.
9. Applebaum AE, Leonard RB, Kenshalo DR Jr, Martin RF, Willis WD. Nuclei in which 1979;188:575–586.
10. Aronin N, Chase K, Folsom R, Christakos S, DiFiglia M. Immunoreactive calcium-binding protein (calbindin-D28k) in interneurons and trigeminothalamic neurons of the rat nucleus caudalis localized with peroxidase and immunogold methods. *Synapse* 1991;7: 106–113.
11. Asanuma C, Thach WT, Jones EG. Distribution of cerebellar terminations and their relation to other afferent terminations in the ventral lateral thalamic region of the monkey. *Brain Res Rev* 1983;5: 237–265.
12. Asato F, Yokota T. Responses of neurons in nucleus ventralis posterolateralis of the cat thalamus to hypogastric inputs. *Brain Res* 1989;488:135–142.
13. Backonja M, Miletic V. Responses of neurons in the rat ventrolateral orbital cortex to phasic and tonic nociceptive stimulation. *Brain Res* 1991;557:353–355.
14. Bandler R, Carrive P, Zhang SP. Integration of somatic and autonomic reactions within the midbrain periaqueductal grey: viscerotopic, somatotopic and functional organization. In: Holstege G, ed. *Progress in brain research,* vol 87. New York: Elsevier, 1991; 269–305.
15. Barasi S. Responses of substantia nigra neurones to noxious stimulation. *Brain Res* 1979;171:121–130.
16. Basbaum AI, Fields HL. Endogenous pain control mechanisms: review and hypothesis. *Ann Neurol* 1978;4:451–462.
17. Battaglia G, Spreafico R, Rustioni A. Substance P–immunoreactive fibers in the thalamus from ascending somatosensory pathways. In: Bentivoglio M, Spreafico R, eds. *Cellular thalamic mechanisms.* Elsevier Science, 1988;365–374.
18. Battaglia G, Spreafico R, Rustioni A. Substance P innervation of the rat and cat thalamus. I. Distribution and relation to ascending spinal pathways. *J Comp Neurol* 1992;315:457–472.
19. Baumeister AA, Nagy M, Hebert G, Hawkins MF, Vaughn A, Chatellier MO. Further studies of the effects of intranigral morphine on behavioral responses to noxious stimuli. *Brain Res* 1990;525: 115–125.
20. Belczynski CR Jr, Pertovaara A, Morrow TJ, Casey KL. The effect of systemic cocaine on spontaneous and nociceptively evoked activity of neurons in the medial and lateral thalamus. *Brain Res* 1990;517: 344–346.
21. Benabid AL, Jeaugey L. Cells of the rat lateral habenula respond to high threshold somatosensory inputs. *Neurosci Lett* 1989;96: 289–294.
22. Benoist JM, Kayser V, Gautron M, Guilbaud G. Low dose of morphine strongly depresses responses of specific nociceptive neurones in the ventrobasal complex of the rat. *Pain* 1983; 15:333–344.
23. Berkley KJ. Spatial relationships between the terminations of somatic sensory and motor pathways in the rostral brain stem of cats and monkeys. I. Ascending somatic sensory inputs to lateral diencephalon. *J Comp Neurol* 1980;193:283–317.
24. Berkley KJ, Budell RJ, Blomqvist A, Bull M. Output systems of the dorsal column nuclei in the cat. *Brain Res Bull* 1986;11:199–225.
25. Berkley KJ, Guilbaud G, Benoist JM, Gautron M. Responses of neurons in and near the thalamic ventrobasal complex of the rat to stimulation of uterus, cervix, vagina, colon, and skin. *J Neurophysiol* 1993;69:557–568.
26. Berkley KJ, Scofield SL. Relays from the spinal cord and solitary nucleus through the parabrachial nucleus to the forebrain in the cat. *Brain Res* 1990;529:333–338.
27. Bernard JF, Alden M, Besson JM. The organization of the efferent projections from the pontine parabrachial area to the amygdaloid complex: a *Phaseolus vulgaris* leucoagglutinin (PHA-L) study in the rat. *J Comp Neurol* 1993;329:201–229.
28. Bernard JF, Besson JM. The spino(trigemino)pontoamygdaloid pathway: electrophysiological evidence for an involvement in pain processes. *J Neurophysiol* 1990;63:473–490.
29. Bernard JF, Carroué J, Besson JM. Efferent projections from the external parabrachial area to the forebrain: a *Phaseolus vulgaris* leucoagglutinin study in the rat. *Neurosci Lett* 1991;122:257–260.
30. Bernard JF, Huang GF, Besson JM. Nucleus centralis of the amygdala and the globus pallidus ventralis: electrophysiological evidence for an involvement in pain processes. *J Neurophysiol* 1992;68: 551–569.
31. Bernard JF, Villanueva L, Carroué J, Le Bars D. Efferent projections from the subnucleus reticularis dorsalis (SRD): a *Phaseolus vulgaris* leucoagglutinin study in the rat. *Neurosci Lett* 1990;116: 257–262.
31a. Berthier ML, Starkstein SE, Leiguarda RC. Asymbolia for pain:a sensory-limbic disconnection syndrome. *Ann Neurol* 1988;24:41–49.
32. Biemond A. The conduction of pain above the level of the thalamus opticus. *Arch Neurol Psychiatr* 1956;75:231–244.
33. Bishop GH. The relation between nerve fiber size and sensory modality: phylogenetic implications of the afferent innervation of cortex. *J Nerv Ment Dis* 1959;128:89–114.
34. Blomqvist A, Berkley KJ. A reexamination of the spino-reticulo-diencephalic pathway in the cat. *Brain Res* 1992;579:17–31.
35. Blomqvist A, Craig AD. Organization of spinal and trigeminal input to the PAG. In: Depaulis A, Bandler R, eds. *The midbrain periaqueductal gray matter.* New York: Plenum Press, 1991;345–363.
36. Blomqvist A, Ma W, Berkley KJ. Spinal input to the parabrachial nucleus in the cat. *Brain Res* 1989;480:29–36.
36a. Blomqvist A, Hermanson O, Ericson H, Larhammar D. Activation of a bulbospinal opioidergic projection by pain stimuli in the awake rat. *NeuroReport* 1994;5:461–464.
36b. Blomqvist A, Ericson AC, Craig AD, Broman J. Evidence for glutamate as a neurotransmitter in spinothalamic tract terminals in the posterior region of owl monkeys. *Exp Brain Res* 1996;in press.
37. Bogousslavsky J, Regli F, Uske A. Thalamic infarcts: clinical syndromes, etiology, and prognosis. *Neurology* 1988;38:837–848.
38. Boivie J. An anatomical reinvestigation of the termination of the spinothalamic tract in the monkey. *J Comp Neurol* 1979;186: 343–370.
39. Boivie J. Anatomic and physiologic features of the spino-cervico-thalamic pathway. In: Macchi G, Rustioni A, Spreafico R, eds. *Somatosensory integration in the thalamus.* Amsterdam: Elsevier, 1983; 63–106.
40. Bowsher D. The termination of secondary somatosensory neurons within the thalamus of *Macaca mulatta: an experimental degeneration study.* J Comp Neurol 1961;117:213–227.
41. Bowsher D. Diencephalic projections from the midbrain reticular formation. *Brain Res* 1975;95:211–220.
42. Brinkhus HB, Carstens E, Zimmerman M. Encoding of graded noxious skin heating by neurons in posterior thalamus and adjacent areas in the cat. *Neurosci Lett* 1979;15:37–42.
43. Brodal A. *Neurological anatomy.* New York: Oxford, 1982.
43a. Bromm B, Treede RD. Human cerebral potentials evoked by CO2 laser stimuli causing pain. *Exp Brain Res* 1987;67:153–162.
43b. Brown-Sequard CE. Course of lectures on the physiology and pathology of the nervous system, Philadelphia, 1860.
44. Brüggemann J, Vahle-Hinz C, Kniffki K-D. Representation of the urinary bladder in the lateral thalamus of the cat. *J Neurophysiol* 1993;70:482–491.
45. Bullitt E. Expression of C-fos-like protein as a marker for neuronal activity following noxious stimulation in the rat. *J Comp Neurol* 1990; 296:517–530.
46. Burstein R, Dado RJ, Giesler GJ Jr. The cells of origin of the spinothalamic tract of the rat: a quantitative reexamination. *Brain Res* 1990;511:329–337.
47. Burton H, Craig AD Jr. Spinothalamic projections in cat, raccoon and monkey: a study based on anterograde transport of horseradish peroxidase. In: Macchi G, Rustioni A, Spreafico R, eds. *Somatosensory integration in the thalamus.* New York: Elsevier, 1983; 17–41.
48. Burton H, Craig AD Jr, Poulos DA, Molt J. Efferent projections from temperature sensitive recording loci within the marginal zone of the nucleus caudalis of the spinal trigeminal complex in the cat. *J Comp Neurol* 1979;183:753–788.
49. Burton H, Jones EG. The posterior thalamic region and its corti-

cal projection in new world and old world monkeys. *J Comp Neurol* 1976;168:249–302.

49a. Burton H, Videen TO, Raichle ME. Tactile-vibration-activated foci in insular and parietal-opercular cortex studied with positron emission tomography: mapping the second somatosensory area in humans. *Somatosens Mot Res* 1993;10:297–308.

50. Bushnell MC, Craig AD. Nociceptive—and thermoreceptive—specific neurons in a discrete region of the monkey lateral thalamus. *Soc Neurosci Abstr* 1993;19:1073.

51. Bushnell MC, Duncan GH. Sensory and affective aspects of pain perception: is medial thalamus restricted to emotional issues. *Exp Brain Res* 1989;78:415–418.

52. Bushnell MC, Duncan GH, Dubner R, He LF. Activity of trigeminothalamic neurons in medullary dorsal horn of awake monkeys trained in a thermal discrimination task. *J Neurophysiol* 1984;52:170–187.

53. Bushnell MC, Duncan GH, Tremblay N. Thalamic VPM nucleus in the behaving monkey. I. Multimodal and discriminative properties of thermosensitive neurons. *J Neurophysiol* 1993;69:739–752.

54. Carlsson KH, Monzel W, Jurna I. Depression by morphine and the non opioid analgesicetamizol (dipyrone), lysine acetylsalicylate, and paracetamol, of activity agents, min rat thalamus neurones evoked by electrical stimulation of nociceptive afferents. *Pain* 1988;32:313–326.

55. Carstens E, Leah J, Lechner J, Zimmermann M. Demonstration of extensive brain stem projections to medial and lateral thalamus and hypothalamus in the rat. *Neuroscience* 1990;35:609–626.

56. Carstens E, Trevino DL. Laminar origins of spinothalamic projections in the cat as determined by the retrograde transport of horseradish peroxidase. *J Comp Neurol* 1978;182:151–166.

57. Carstens E, Yokota T. Viscerosomatic convergence and responses to intestinal distension of neurons at the junction of midbrain and posterior thalamus in the cat. *Exp Neurol* 1980;70:392–402.

58. Casey KL. Unit analysis of nociceptive mechanisms in the thalamus of the awake squirrel monkey. *J Neurophysiol* 1966;29:727–750.

59. Casey KL, Minoshima S, Berger KL, Koeppe RA, Morrow TJ, Frey KA. PET analysis of brain structures differentially activated by noxious thermal stimuli. *Soc Neurosci Abstr* 1992;18:833.

60. Casey KL, Morrow TJ. Ventral posterior thalamic neurons differentially responsive to noxious stimulation of the awake monkey. *Science* 1983;221:675–677.

61. Cechetto DF, Saper CB. Evidence for a viscerotopic sensory representation in the cortex and thalamus in the rat. *J Comp Neurol* 1987;262:27–45.

62. Cechetto DF, Standaert DG, Saper CB. Spinal and trigeminal dorsal horn projections to the parabrachial nucleus in the rat. *J Comp Neurol* 1985;240:153–160.

63. Chamberlin NL, Saper CB. Topographic organization of cardiovascular responses to *J Comp Neurol* 1992;326:245–262.

64. Christensen BN, Perl ER. Spinal neurons specifically excited by noxious or thermal stimuli: marginal zone of the dorsal horn. *J Neurophysiol* 1970;33:293–307.

65. Chudler EH, Sugiyama K, Dong WK. Nociceptive responses in the neostriatum and globus pallidus of the anesthetized rat. *J Neurophysiol* 1993;69:1890–1903.

66. Chung JM, Lee KH, Surmeier DJ, Sorkin LS, Kim J, Willis WD. Response characteristics of neurons in the ventral posterior lateral nucleus of the monkey thalamus. *J Neurophysiol* 1986;56: 370–390.

67. Clark FM, Proudfit HK. The projection of noradrenergic neurons in the A7 catecholamine cell group to the spinal cord in the rat demonstrated by anterograde tracing combined with immunocytochemistry. *Brain Res* 1991;547:279–288.

68. Clark WE, Gros LE. The termination of ascending tracts in the thalamus of the macaque monkey. *J Anat* 1936;71:7–40.

69. Clarke KA, Djourhi L. TRH analogue antagonizes anaesthetic induced depression of information transfer through the ventrobasal thalamus of the rat. *Neuropeptides* 1991;18:193–200.

70. Cliffer KD, Burstein R, Giesler GJ Jr. Distributions of spinothalamic, spinohypothalamic, and spinotelencephalic fibers revealed by anterograde transport of PHA L in rats. *J Neurosci* 1991;11: 852–868.

71. Coffield JA, Bowen KK, Miletic V. Retrograde tracing of projections between the nucleus submedius, the ventrolateral orbital cortex, and the midbrain in the rat. *J Comp Neurol* 1992;321: 488–499.

72. Coffield JA, Miletic V. Immunoreactive enkephalin is contained within some trigeminal and spinal neurons projecting to the rat medial thalamus. *Brain Res* 1987;425:380–383.

73. Coffield JA, Miletic V. Responses of rat nucleus submedius neurons to enkephalins applied with micropressure. *Brain Res* 1993; 630:252–261.

74. Cohen SR, Melzack R. The habenula and pain: Repeated electrical stimulation produces prolonged analgesia but lesions have no effect on formalin pain or morphine analgesia. *Behav Brain Res* 1993;54:171–178.

75. Craig AD. Lamina I trigeminothalamic projections in the monkey. *Soc Neurosci Abstr* 1990;16:1144.

76. Craig AD. Nociceptive neurons in the nucleus submedius (Sm) in the medial thalamus of the cat. *Pain* 1990;suppl 5:S492.

77. Craig AD. Supraspinal pathways and mechanisms relevant to central pain. In: Casey KL, ed. *Pain and central nervous system disease:* the central pain syndromes. New York: Raven Press, 1991; 157–170.

78. Craig AD. Spinal distribution of ascending lamina I axons anterogradely labeled with Phaseolus vulgaris leucoagglutinin (PHA-L) in the cat. *J Comp Neurol* 1991;313:377–393.

79. Craig AD. Organization of lamina I terminations in the posterior thalamus of the cynomolgus monkey. *Soc Neurosci Abstr* 1992;18: 385.

80. Craig AD. Spinal and trigeminal lamina I input to the locus coeruleus anterogradely labeled with Phaseolus vulgaris leucoagglutinin (PHA-L) in the cat and the monkey. *Brain Res* 1992;584: 325–328.

81. Craig AD. Propriospinal input to thoracolumbar sympathetic nuclei from cervical and lumbar lamina I neurons in the cat and the monkey. *J Comp Neurol* 1993;331:517–530.

81a. Craig AD. Distribution of brain stem projections from spinal lamina I neurons in the cat and the monkey. *J Comp Neurol* 1995;361: 225–248.

82. Craig AD, Dostrovsky JO. Thermoreceptive lamina I trigeminothalamic neurons project to the nucleus submedius in the cat. *Exp Brain Res* 1991;85:470–474.

83. Craig AD, Hunsley SJ. Morphine enhances the activity of thermoreceptive cold-specific lamina I spinothalamic neurons in the cat. *Brain Res* 1991;558:93–97.

84. Craig AD Jr, Burton H. Spinal and medullary lamina I projection to nucleus submedius in medial thalamus: a possible pain center. *J Neurophysiol* 1981;45:443–466.

85. Craig AD Jr, Burton H. The distribution and topographical organization in the thalamus of anterogradely transported horseradish peroxidase after spinal injections in cat and raccoon. *Exp Brain Res* 1985;58:227–254.

86. Craig AD Jr, Kniffki K-D. Spinothalamic lumbosacral lamina I cells responsive to skin and muscle stimulation in the cat. *J Physiol (Lond)* 1985;365:197–221.

87. Craig AD Jr, Linington AJ, Kniffki K-D. Cells of origin of spinothalamic tract projections to the medial and lateral thalamus in the cat. *J Comp Neurol* 1989;289:568–585.

88. Craig AD Jr, Tapper DN. Lateral cervical nucleus in the cat: functional organization and characteristics. *J Neurophysiol* 1978;41: 1511–1534.

89. Craig AD Jr, Wiegand SJ, Price JL. The thalamocortical projection of nucleus submedius in the cat. *J Comp Neurol* 1982;206:28–48.

89a. Craig AD, Krout K, Zhang ET. Cortical projections of VMpo, a specific pain and temperature relay in primate thalamus. *Soc Neurosci Abstr* 1995;21:1165.

89b. Craig AD, Bushnell MC, Zhang ET, Blomqvist A. A thalamic nucleus specific for pain and temperature sensation. *Nature* 1994; 372:770–773.

90. Cropper EC, Eisenman JS, Azmitia EC. An immunocytochemical study of the serotonergic innervation of the thalamus of the rat. *J Comp Neurol* 1984;224:38–50.

91. Curry MJ. The exteroceptive properties of neurones in the somatic part of the posterior group (PO). *Brain Res* 1972;44: 439–462.

91a. Curtis DR, Johnston GAR. Amino acid transmitters in the mammalian central nervous system. *Ergeb Physiol* 1974;69:97–188.

92. Dado RJ, Giesler GJ Jr. Afferent input to nucleus submedius in rats: retrograde labeling of neurons in the spinal cord and caudal medulla. *J Neurosci* 1990;10:2672–2686.

93. Dafny N, Reyes-Vazquez C, Qiao JT. Modification of nociceptively identified neurons in thalamic parafascicularis by chemical stimulation of dorsal raphe with glutamate, morphine, serotonin and

focal dorsal raphe electrical stimulation. *Brain Res Bull* 1990;24: 717–723.

93a. Damasio AR. *Descartes' error:* emotion, *reason, and the human brain.* New York: Putnam, 1993.

94. Davis KD, Dostrovsky JO. Properties of feline thalamic neurons activated by stimulation of the middle meningeal artery and sagittal sinus. *Brain Res* 1988;454:89–100.

95. Davis KD, Dostrovsky JO, Tasker RR, Kiss ZK, Hutchison WD. Increased incidence of pain evoked by thalamic stimulation in post-stroke patients. *Soc Neurosci Abstr* 1993;19:1572.

96. Dejerine J, Roussy G. La syndrome thalamique. *Rev Neurol* 1906; 14:521–532.

97. Depaulis A, Keay KA, Bandler R. Longitudinal neuronal organization of defensive reactions in the midbrain periaqueductal gray region of the rat. *Exp Brain Res* 1992;90:307–318.

98. Deschênes M, Hu B. Electrophysiology and pharmacology of the corticothalamic input to lateral thalamic nuclei: an intracellular study in the cat. *Eur J Neurosci* 1990;2:140–152.

99. Diamond ME, Armstrong-James M, Budway MJ, Ebner FF. Somatic sensory responses in the rostral sector of the posterior group (POm) and in the ventral posterior medial nucleus (VPM) of the rat thalamus: Dependence on the barrel field cortex. *J Comp Neurol* 1992;319:66–84.

99a. Do K-Q, Binns KE, Salt TE. Release of the nitric oxide precursor, arginine, from the thalamus upon sensory afferent stimulation, and its effect on thalamic neurons in vivo. *Neuroscience* 1994;60: 581–586.

100. Dong WQ, Wilson OB, Skolnick MH, Dafny N. Hypothalamic, dorsal raphe and external electrical stimulation modulate noxious evoked responses of habenula neurons. *Neuroscience* 1992;48: 933–940.

101. Dong WK, Ryu H, Wagman IH. Nociceptive responses of neurons in medial thalamus and their relationship to spinothalamic pathways. *J Neurophysiol* 1978;41:1592–1613.

102. Dong WK, Salonen LD, Kawakami Y, Shiwaku T, Kaukoranta EM, Martin RF. Nociceptive responses of trigeminal neurons in SII-7b cortex of awake monkeys. *Brain Res* 1989;484:314–324.

103. Dostrovsky JO, Davis KD, Wells FEB, Tasker RR. Pain evoked by microstimulation in the thalamus of chronic pain patients. *Soc Neurosci Abstr* 1992;18:832.

104. Dostrovsky JO, Guilbaud G. Noxious stimuli excite neurons in nucleus submedius of the normal and arthritic rat. *Brain Res* 1988; 460:269–280.

105. Dostrovsky JO, Guilbaud G. Nociceptive responses in medial thalamus of the normal and arthritic rat. *Pain* 1990;40:93–104.

106. Dostrovsky JO, Wells FEB, Tasker RR. Pain evoked by stimulation in human thalamus. In: Inoka R, Shigenaga Y, Tohyama M, eds. *Processing and inhibition of nociceptive information.* International Congress Series 989. Amsterdam: Excerpta Medica, 1992;115–120.

107. Downie JW, Ferrington DG, Sorkin LS, Willis WD Jr. The primate spinocervicothalamic pathway: responses of cells of the lateral cervical nucleus and spinocervical tract to innocuous and noxious stimuli. *J Neurophysiol* 1988;59:861–885.

108. Dubner R, Kenshalo DR Jr, Maixner W, Bushnell MC, Oliveras J-L. The correlation of monkey medullary dorsal horn neuronal activity and the perceived intensity of noxious heat stimuli. *J Neurophysiol* 1989;62:450–457.

109. Duggan AW, Hall JG. Morphine, naloxone and the responses of medial thalamic neurones of the cat. *Brain Res* 1977;122:49–57.

110. Duncan GH, Bushnell MC, Oliveras J-L, Bastrash N, Tremblay N. Thalamic VPM nucleus in the behaving monkey. III. Effects of reversible inactivation by lidocaine on thermal and mechanical discrimination. *J Neurophysiol* 1993;70:2086–2096.

112. Eaton SA, Salt TE. Modulatory effects of serotonin on excitatory amino acid responses and sensory synaptic transmission in the ventrobasal thalamus. *Neuroscience* 1989;33:285–292.

113. Eaton SA, Salt TE. Thalamic NMDA receptors and nociceptive sensory synaptic transmission. *Neurosci Lett* 1990;110:297–302.

114. Eaton SA, Salt TE. Membrane and action potential responses evoked by excitatory amino acids acting at N-methyl-D-aspartate receptors and non-N-methyl-D-aspartate receptors in the rat thalamus in vivo. *Neuroscience* 1991;44:277–286.

114a. Eaton SA, Salt TE. The role of excitatory amino acid receptors in thalamic nociception. In: Besson J-M, ed. *Pain in forebrain areas.* Paris: John Libbey Eurotext, 1996.

114b. Ericson A-C, Blomqvist A, Craig AD, Ottersen OP, Broman J. Evidence for glutamate as neurotransmitter in trigemino- and spinothalamic tract terminals in the nucleus submedius of cats. *Eur J Neurosci* 1995;7:305–317.

115a. Feil K, Herbert H. Topographic organization of spinal and trigeminal somatosensory pathways to the rat parabrachial and Kölliker-Fuse nuclei. *J Comp Neurol* 1995;353:506–528.

116. Ferrington DG, Downie JW, Willis WD Jr. Primate nucleus gracilis neurons: responses to innocuous and noxious stimuli. *J Neurophysiol* 1988;59:886–907.

117. Fields HL. *Pain.* New York: McGraw Hill, 1987.

118. Friedman DP, Murray EA. Thalamic connectivity of the second somatosensory area and neighboring somatosensory fields of the lateral sulcus of the macaque. *J Comp Neurol* 1986;252: 348–373.

119. Friedman DP, Murray EA, O'Neill JB, Mishkin M. Cortical connections of the somatosensory fields of the lateral sulcus of macaques: evidence for a corticolimbic pathway for touch. *J Comp Neurol* 1986;252:323–347.

120. Fu Q-G, Chandler MJ, McNeill DL, Foreman RD. Vagal afferent fibers excite upper cervical neurons and inhibit activity of lumbar spinal cord neurons in the rat. *Pain* 1992;51:91–100.

121. Fulwiler CE, Saper CB. Subnuclear organization of the efferent connections of the parabrachial nucleus in the rat. *Brain Res Rev* 1984;7:229–259.

122. Gang S, Mizuguchi A, Kobayashi N, Aoki M. Descending axonal projections from the medial parabrachial and Kölliker-Fuse nuclear complex to the nucleus raphe magnus in cats. *Neurosci Lett* 1990;118:273–275.

123. Giesler GJ Jr, Menetrey D, Basbaum AI. Differential origins of spinothalamic tract projections to medial and lateral thalamus in the rat. *J Comp Neurol* 1979;184:107–126.

124. Giesler GJ Jr, Yezierski RP, Gerhart KD, Willis WD. Spinothalamic tract neurons that project to medial and/or lateral thalamic nuclei: evidence for a physiologically novel population of spinal cord neurons. *J Neurophysiol* 1981;46:1285–1308.

125. Gildenberg PL. Physiologic observations concerned with percutaneous cordotomy. In: Somjen G, ed. *Neurophysiology studied in man.* Amsterdam: Elsevier, 1972;231–236.

126. Gingold SI, Greenspan JD, Apkarian AV. Anatomic evidence of nociceptive inputs to primary somatosensory cortex: relationship between spinothalamic terminals and thalamocortical cells in squirrel monkeys. *J Comp Neurol* 1991;308:467–490.

126a. Gowers WR. *Manual of diseases of the nervous system.* London: 1886.

127. Greenspan JD, Winfield JA. Reversible pain and tactile deficits associated with a cerebral tumor compressing the posterior insula and parietal operculum. *Pain* 1992;50:29–39.

128. Guilbaud G, Benoist JM, Jazat F, Gautron M. Neuronal responsiveness in the ventrobasal thalamic complex of rats with an experimental peripheral mononeuropathy. *J Neurophysiol* 1990;64: 1537–1554.

129. Guilbaud G, Neil A, Benoist JM, Kayser V, Gautron M. Thresholds and encoding of neuronal responses to mechanical stimuli in the ventro basal thalamus during carrageenin induced hyperalgesic inflammation in the rat. *Exp Brain Res* 1987;68:311–318.

130. Guilbaud G, Peschanski M, Gautron M, Binder D. Neurones responding to noxious stimulation in VB complex and caudal adjacent regions in the thalamus of the rat. *Pain* 1980;8:303–318.

131. Gybels JM, Sweet WH. *Neurosurgical treatment of persistent pain. Physiological and pathological mechanisms of human pain. Pain and headache,* vol 11. Basel: Karger, 1989.

132. Halliday AM, Logue V. Painful sensations evoked by electrical stimulation in the thalamus. In: Somjen GG, ed. *Neurophysiology studied in man.* Amsterdam: Excerpts Medica, 1972;221–230.

133. Halsell CB. Organization of parabrachial nucleus efferents to the thalamus and amygdala in the golden hamster. *J Comp Neurol* 1992; 317:57–78.

134. Hamba M, Hisamitsu H, Muro M. Nociceptive projection from tooth pulp to the lateral hypothalamus in rats. *Brain Res Bull* 1990; 25:355–364.

135. Hassler R. Dichotomy of facial pain conduction in the diencephalon. In: Hassler R, Walker AE, eds. *Trigeminal neuralgia.* Philadelphia: Saunders, 1970;123–138.

136. He L, Dong W, Wang M. Effects of iontophoretic etorphine and naloxone, and electroacupuncture on nociceptive responses from thalamic neurones in rabbits. *Pain* 1991;44:89–95.

137. Head H, Holmes G. Sensory disturbances from cerebral lesions. Brain 1911;34:102–254.

137a. Helmstetter FJ, Bellgowan PS, Tershner SA. Inhibition of the tail

flick reflex following microinjection of morphine into the amygdala. *NeuroReport* 1993;4:471–474.
138. Herbert H, Moga MM, Saper CB. Connections of the parabrachial nucleus with the nucleusof the solitary tract and the medullary reticular formation in the rat. *J Comp Neurol* 1990;293:540–580.
138a. Hermanson O, Hallbeck M, Blomqvist A. Preproenkephalin mRNA-expressing neurones in the rat thalamus. *Neuroreport* 1995; 6:833–836.
139. Hicks TP, Metherate R, Landry P, Dykes RW. Bicuculline induced alterations of response properties in functionally identified ventroposterior thalamic neurones. *Exp Brain Res* 1986;63:248–264.
140. Hirai T, Jones EG. A new parcellation of the human thalamus on the basis of histochemical staining. *Brain Res Rev* 1989;14:1–34.
141. Holstege G. Anatomical evidence for a strong ventral parabrachial projection to nucleus raphe magnus and adjacent tegmental field. *Brain Res* 1988;447:154–158.
142. Honda CN, Mense S, Perl ER. Neurons in ventrobasal region of cat thalamus selectively responsive to noxious mechanical stimulation. *J Neurophysiol* 1983;49:662–673.
143. Horie H, Pamplin PJ, Yokota T. Inhibition of nociceptive neurons in the shell region of nucleus ventralis posterolateralis following conditioning stimulation of the periaqueductal grey of the cat. Evidence for an ascending inhibitory pathway. *Brain Res* 1991;561: 35–42.
144. Horie H, Yokota T. Responses of nociceptive VPL neurons to intracardiac injection of bradykinin in the cat. *Brain Res* 1990;516: 161–164.
145. Houser CR, Vaughn JE, Barber RP, Roberts E. GABA neurons are the major cell type of the nucleus reticularis thalami. *Brain Res* 1980;200:341–354.
146. Huang G-F, Besson J-M, Bernard J-F. Intravenous morphine depresses the transmission of noxious messages to the nucleus centralis of the amygdala. *Eur J Pharmacol* 1993;236:449–456.
147. Hutchison WD, Dostrovsky JO, Davis KD, Lozano AM. Single unit responses and microstimulation effects in cingulate cortex of an awake patient. *Abstracts of the 7th World Congress on Pain* 1993;461.
148. Hutchison WD, Lühn MAB, Schmidt RF. Knee joint input into the peripheral region of the ventral posterior lateral nucleus of cat thalamus. *J Neurophysiol* 1992;67:1092–1104.
149. Hylden JLK, Anton F, Nahin RL. Spinal lamina I projection neurons in the rat: collateral innervation of parabrachial area and thalamus. *Neuroscience* 1989;28:27–37.
150. Hylden JLK, Hayashi H, Bennett GJ, Dubner R. Spinal lamina I neurons projecting to the parabrachial area of the cat midbrain. *Brain Res* 1985;336:195–198.
151. Hylden JLK, Hayashi H, Dubner R, Bennett GJ. Physiology and morphology of the lamina I spinomesencephalic projection. *J Comp Neurol* 1986;247:505–515.
152. Iwata K, Tsuboi Y, Muramatsu H, Sumino R. Distribution and response properties of cat SI neurons responsive to changes in tooth temperature. *J Neurophysiol* 1990;64:822–834.
153. Jeanmonod D, Magnin M, Morel A. Thalamus and neurogenic pain: physiological, anatomical and clinical data. *Neuroreport* 1993; 4:475–478.
153a. Jensen TS, Yaksh TL. Brain stem excitatory amino acid receptors in nociception: Microinjection mapping and pharmacological characterization of glutamate-sensitive sites in the brain stem associated with algogenic behavior. *Neuroscience* 1992;46:535–547.
154. Jones AKP, Brown WD, Friston KJ, Qi LY, Frackowiak RSJ. Cortical and subcortical localization of response to pain in man using positron emission tomography. *Proc R Soc Lond [Biol]* 1991;244: 39–44.
155. Jones EG. *The thalamus.* New York: Plenum Press, 1985.
156. Jones EG. Immunocytochemical studies on thalamic afferent transmitters. In: Besson J-M, Guilbaud G, Peschanski M, eds. *Thalamus and pain.* Amsterdam: Excerpta Medica, 1987;83–109.
157. Jones LS, Gauger LL, Davis JN. Anatomy of brain alpha 1-adrenergic receptors: in vitro autoradiography with [125I]-HEAT. *J Comp Neurol* 1985;231:190–208.
158. Kaelber WW, Mitchell CL, Yarmat AJ, Afifi AK, Lorens SA. Centrum medianum-parafascicularis lesions and reactivity to noxious and non-noxious stimuli. *Exp Neurol* 1975;46:282–290.
159. Kajander KC, Giesler GJ Jr. Responses of neurons in the lateral cervical nucleus of the cat to noxious cutaneous stimulation. *J Neurophysiol* 1987;57:1686–1704.
160. Katter JT, Burstein R, Giesler GJ Jr.. The cells of origin of the spinohypothalamic tract in cats. *J Comp Neurol* 1991;303:101–112.
161. Kawakita K, Dostrovsky JO, Tang JS, Chiang CY. Responses of neurons in the rat thalamic nucleus submedius to cutaneous, muscle and visceral nociceptive stimuli. *Pain* 1993;55:327–338.
162. Kayama Y, Negi T, Sugitani M, Iwama K. Effects of locus coeruleus stimulation on neuronal activities of dorsal lateral geniculate nucleus and perigeniculate reticular nucleus of the rat. *Neuroscience* 1982;7:655–666.
163. Kenshalo DR Jr, Giesler GJ Jr, Leonard RB, Willis WD. Responses of neurons in primate ventral posterior lateral nucleus to noxious stimuli. *J Neurophysiol* 1980;43:1594–1614.
164. Kenshalo DR Jr, Isensee O. Responses of primate SI cortical neurons to noxious stimuli. *J Neurophysiol* 1983;50:1479–1496.
165. Kevetter GA, Haber LH, Yezierski RP, Chung JM, Martin RF, Willis WD. Cells of origin of the spinoreticular tract in the monkey. *J Comp Neurol* 1982;207:61–74.
165a. Kharazia VN, Weinberg RJ. Glutamate in thalamic fibers terminating in layer IV of primary sensory cortex. *J Neurosci* 1994;14: 6021–6032.
166. Kitamura T, Yamada J, Sato H, Yamashita K. Cells of origin of the spinoparabrachial fibers in the rat: a study with fast blue and WGA HRP. *J Comp Neurol* 1993;328:449–461.
167. Kniffki K-D, Craig AD Jr. The distribution of nociceptive neurons in the cat's lateral thalamus: the dorsal and ventral periphery of VPL. In: Rowe M, Willis WD, eds. *Development, organization and processing in somatosensory pathways.* New York: Alan Liss, 1985; 375–382.
168. Kniffki K-D, Mizumura K. Responses of neurons in VPL and VPL-VL regions of the cat to algesic stimulation of muscle and tendon. *J Neurophysiol* 1983;49:649–661.
169. Kostopoulos GK, Phillis JW. Purinergic depression of neurons in different areas of the rat brain. *Exp Neurol* 1977;55:719–724.
170. Koyama N, Yokota T. Ascending inhibition of nociceptive neurons in the nucleus ventralis posterolateralis following conditioning stimulation of the nucleus raphe magnus. *Brain Res* 1993;609: 298–306.
171. Krukoff TL, Harris KH, Jhamandas JH. Efferent projections from the parabrachial nucleus demonstrated with the anterograde tracer *Phaseolus vulgaris* leucoagglutinin. *Brain Res Bull* 1993;30: 163–172.
172. Kupers RC, Gybels JM. Electrical stimulation of the ventroposterolateral thalamic nucleus (VPL) reduces mechanical allodynia in a rat model of neuropathic pain. *Neurosci Lett* 1993;150:95–98.
173. Kuru M. *The sensory paths in the spinal cord and brain stem of man.* Tokyo: Sogensya, 1949.
174. LaMotte RH, Lundberg LER, Torebjörk HE. Pain, hyperalgesia and activity in nociceptive C units in humans after intradermal injection of capsaicin. *J Physiol (Lond)* 1992;448:749–764.
174a. Lechner J, Leah JD, Zimmermann M. Brain stem peptidergic neurons projecting to the medial and lateral thalamus and zona incerta in the rat. *Brain Res* 1993;603:47–56.
175. Lee KS, Reddington M. Autoradiographic evidence for multiple CNS binding sites for adenosine derivatives. *Neuroscience* 1986;19: 535–549.
175a. Lee SM, Friedberg MH, Ebner FF. The role of GABA-mediated inhibition in the rat ventral posterior medial thalamus. II. Differential effects of GABAA and GABAB receptor antagonists on responses of VPM neurons. *J Neurophysiol* 1994;71:1716–1726.
176. Leijon G, Boivie J, Johansson I. Central post stroke pain Neurological symptoms and pain characteristics. Pain 1989;36:13–25.
177. Lenz FA. Ascending modulation of thalamic function and pain. In: Sicuteri F, ed. *Advances in pain research and therapy,* vol 20. New York: Raven Press, 1992;177–196.
178. Lenz FA, Kwan HC, Dostrovsky JO, Tasker RR. Characteristics of the bursting pattern of action potentials that occurs in the thalamus of patients with central pain. *Brain Res* 1989;496:357–360.
179. Lenz FA, Seike M, Lin YC, Baker FH, Rowland LH, Gracely RH, Richardson RT. Neurons in the area of human thalamic nucleus ventralis caudalis respond to painful heat stimuli. *Brain Res* 1993; 623:235–240.
180. Lenz FA, Seike M, Richardson RT, Lin YC, Baker FH, Khoja I, Jaeger CJ, Gracely RH. Thermal and pain sensations evoked by microstimulation in the area of human ventrocaudal nucleus. *J Neurophysiol* 1993;70:200–212.
181. Levey AI, Hallanger AE, Wainer BH. Choline acetyltransferase immunoreactivity in the rat thalamus. *J Comp Neurol* 1987;257: 317–332.
182. Li J, Ji Y-P, Qiao J-T, Dafny N. Suppression of nociceptive responses

in parafascicular neurons by stimulation of substantia nigra: an analysis of related inhibitory pathways. *Brain Res* 1992;591: 109–115.
183. Light AR. *The initial processing of pain and its descending control: spinal and trigeminal systems.* Basel: Karger, 1992.
184. Light AR, Sedivec MJ, Casale EJ, Jones SL. Physiological and morphological characteristics of spinal neurons projecting to the parabrachial region of the cat. *Somatosens Mot Res* 1993;10: 309–326.
185. Lin Y, Morrow TJ, Kiritsy-Roy JA, Terry LC, Casey KL. Cocaine: evidence for supraspinal, dopamine-mediated, non-opiate analgesia. *Brain Res* 1989;479:306–312.
186. Loewy AD, Spyer KM. *Central regulation of autonomic functions.* New York: Oxford, 1990.
187. Ma W, Blomqvist A, Berkley KJ. Spino diencephalic relays through the parabrachial nucleus in the cat. *Brain Res* 1989;480:37–50.
188. Magnusson KR, Clements JR, Larson AA, Madl JE, Beitz AJ. Localization of glutamate in trigeminothalamic projection neurons: a combination retrograde transport immunohistochemical study. *Somatosens Res* 1987;4:177–190.
189. Mahieux G, Benabid AL. Naloxone reversible analgesia induced by electrical stimulation of the habenula in the rat. *Brain Res* 1987; 406:118–129.
190. Mansour A, Khachaturian H, Lewis ME, Akil H, Watson SJ. Autoradiographic differentiation of mu, delta, and kappa opioid receptors in the rat forebrain and midbrain. *J Neurosurg* 1987;7(8): 2445–2464.
191. Mantyh PW. Connections of midbrain periaqueductal gray in the monkey. I ascending efferent projections. *J Neurophysiol* 1983;49: 567–581.
192. Mantyh PW, Hunt SP. Neuropeptides are present in projection neurones at all levels in visceral and taste pathways: from periphery to sensory cortex. *Brain Res* 1984;299:297–311.
193. Mao J, Mayer DJ, Price DD. Patterns of increased brain activity indicative of pain in a rat model of peripheral mononeuropathy. *J Neurosci* 1993;13:2689–2702.
193a. Marks GA, offwarg HP. Cholinergic responsiveness of neurons in the ventroposterior thalamus of the anesthetized rat. *Neuroscience* 1993;54:391–400.
194. Matsumoto N, Sato T, Suzuki TA. Characteristics of the tooth pulp-driven neurons in a functional column of the cat's somatosensory cortex (SI). *Exp Brain Res* 1989;74:263–271.
195. May WP. The afferent path. *Brain* 1906;29:742–803.
196. Mayer DJ, Price DD, Becker DP. Neurophysiological characterization of the anterolateral spinal cord neurons contributing to pain perception in man. *Pain* 1975;1:51–58.
197. McCormick DA. Neurotransmitter actions in the thalamus and cerebral cortex and their role in neuromodulation of thalamocortical activity. *Prog Neurobiol* 1992;39:337–388.
198. McCormick DA, Wang Z. Serotonin and noradrenaline excite GABAergic neurones of the guinea pig and cat nucleus reticularis thalami. *J Physiol (Lond)* 1991;442:235–255.
199. Mehler WR. Some neurological species differences—a posteriori. *Ann NY Acad Sci* 1969;167:424–468.
200. Mehler WR. Central pain and the spinothalamic tract. In: Bonica JJ, ed. *Advances in neurology—International Symposium on Pain.* New York: Raven Press, 1974.
201. Mehler WR, Feferman ME, Nauta WJH. Ascending axon degeneration following anterolateral cordotomy. An experimental study in the monkey. *Brain* 1960;83:718–750.
202. Meller ST, Dennis BJ. Efferent projections of the periaqueductal gray in the rabbit. *Neuroscience* 1991;40:191–216.
203. Melzack R, Casey KL. Sensory, motivational, and central control determinants of pain. In: Kenshalo DR, ed. *The skin senses.* Springfield, IL: Charles C. Thomas, 1968;423–443.
204. Menetrey D, Basbaum AI. Spinal and trigeminal projections to the nucleus of the solitary tract: a possible substrate for somatovisceral and viscerovisceral reflex activation. *J Comp Neurol* 1987;255: 439–450.
205. Mesulam M-M, Mufson EJ, Wainer BH, Levey AI. Central cholinergic pathways in the rat: an overview based on an alternative nomenclature (Ch1-Ch6). *Neuroscience* 1983;4:1185–1201.
206. Miletic V, Coffield JA. Enkephalin-like immunoreactivity in the nucleus submedius of the cat and rat thalamus. *Somatosens Res* 1988;5:325–334.
207. Miletic V, Coffield JA. Responses of neurons in the rat nucleus submedius to noxious and innocuous mechanical cutaneous stimulation. *Somatosens Mot Res* 1989;6:567–588.
208. Morrow TJ, Casey KL. State-related modulation of thalamic somatosensory responses in the awake monkey. *J Neurophysiol* 1992;67:305–317.
209. Musil SY, Olson CR. Organization of cortical and subcortical projections to anterior cingulate cortex in the cat. *J Comp Neurol* 1988; 272:203–218.
210. Nahin RL. Immunocytochemical identification of long ascending, peptidergic lumbar spinal neurons terminating in either the medial or lateral thalamus in the rat. *Brain Res* 1988;443:345–349.
211. Nathan PW, Smith MC. Clinico-anatomical correlation in anterolateral cordotomy. In: Bonica JJ, ed. *Advances in pain research and therapy*, vol 3. New York: Raven Press, 1979;921–926.
212. Ness TJ, Gebhart GF. Visceral pain: a review of experimental studies. *Pain* 1990;41:167–234.
213. Nomura T, Nishikawa N, Yokota T. Intracellular HRP study of nociceptive neurons within the ventrobasal complex of the cat thalamus. *Brain Res* 1992;570:323–332.
214. Norrsell U. Behavioural thermosensitivity after unilateral, partial lesions of the lateral funiculus in the cervical spinal cord of the cat. *Exp Brain Res* 1989;78:369–373.
215. Olausson B, Shyu B-C, Rydenhag B, Andersson S. Thalamic nociceptive mechanisms in cats, influenced by central conditioning stimuli. *Acta Physiol Scand* 1992;146:49–59.
215a. Olausson B, Xu Z-Q, Shyu B-C. Dorsal column inhibition of nociceptive thalamic cells mediated by gamma-aminobutyric acid mechanisms in the cat. *Acta Physiol Scand* 1994;152:239–247.
215b. Otake K, Ruggiero DA. Monoamines and nitric oxide are employed by afferents engaged in midline thalamic regulation. *J Neurosci* 1995;15:1891–1911.
216. Pagni CA. Central pain due to spinal cord and brain stem damage. In: Wall PD, Melzack R, eds. *Textbook of pain.* New York: Churchill Livingstone, 1984;481–491.
217. Palacios JM, Wamsley JK. Catecholamine receptors. In: Bjorklund A, Hokfelt T, Kuhar MJ, eds. *Handbook of chemical neuroanatomy, vol 3: Classical transmitters and transmitter receptors in the CNS, Part II.* New York: Elsevier Science, 1984;325–351.
218. Palecek J, Dougherty PM, Kim SH, Palecková V, Lekan H, Chung JM, Carlton SM, Willis WD. Responses of spinothalamic tract neurons to mechanical and thermal stimuli in an experimental model of peripheral neuropathy in primates. *J Neurophysiol* 1992;68: 1951–1966.
219. Panneton WM, Burton H. Projections from the paratrigeminal nucleus and the medullary and spinal dorsal horns to the peribrachial area in the cat. *Neuroscience* 1985;15:779–797.
220. Perl ER. Pain and nociception. In: Darian-Smith I, ed. *Handbook of physiology, section 1, The nervous system, vol 3, Sensory processes.* Bethesda: American Physiological Society, 1984;915–975.
221. Peschanski M. Trigeminal afferents to the diencephalon in the rat. *Neuroscience* 1984;12:465–487.
222. Peschanski M, Guilbaud G, Gautron M. Posterior intralaminar region in rat: neuronal responses to noxious and non-noxious cutaneous stimuli. *Exp Neurol* 1981;72:226–238.
223. Peschanski M, Guilbaud G, Gautron M, Besson J-M. Encoding of noxious heat messages in neurons of the ventrobasal thalamic complex of the rat. *Brain Res* 1980;197:401–413.
224. Peschanski M, Weil-Fugazza J. Aminergic and cholinergic afferents to the thalamus: experimental data with reference to pain pathways. In: Besson J-M, Guilbaud G, Peschanski M, eds. *Thalamus and pain.* Amsterdam: Excerpta Medica, 1987;127–154.
224a. Pirot S, Jay TM, Glowinski J, Thierry A-M. Anatomical and electrophysiological evidence for an excitatory amino acid pathway from the thalamic mediodorsal nucleus to the prefrontal cortex in the rat. *Eur J Neurosci* 1994;6:1225–1234.
225. Poggio GF, Mountcastle VB. A study of the functional contributions of the lemniscal and spinothalamic systems to somatic sensibility. *Bull Johns Hopkins Hosp* 1960;106:266–316.
226. Price DD. *Psychological and neural mechanisms of pain.* New York: Raven Press, 1988.
227. Ralston HJ III, Ralston DD. The primate dorsal spinothalamic tract: Evidence for a specific termination in the posterior nuclei (Po/SG) of the thalamus. *Pain* 1992;48:107–118.
227a. Ramberg DA, Yaksh TL. Effects of cervical spinal hemisection of dihydromorphine binding in brain stem and spinal cord in cat. *Brain Res* 1989;483:61–67.

228. Rausell E, Cusick CG, Taub E, Jones EG. Chronic deafferentation in monkeys differentially affects nociceptive and nonnociceptive pathways distinguished by specific calcium-binding proteins and down-regulates gamma aminobutyric acid type A receptors at thalamic levels. *Proc Natl Acad Sci USA* 1992;89:2571–2575.
229. Rausell E, Jones EG. Chemically distinct compartments of the thalamic VPM nucleus in monkeys relay principal and spinal trigeminal pathways to different layers of the somatosensory cortex. *J Neurosci* 1991;11:226–237.
229a. Ray JP, Price JL. The organization of projections from the mediodorsal nucleus of the thalamus to orbital and medial prefrontal cortex in macaque monkeys. *J Comp Neurol* 1993;337:1–31.
230. Reichling DB, Basbaum AI. Collateralization of periaqueductal gray neurons to forebrain or diencephalon and to the medullary nucleus raphe magnus in the rat. *Neuroscience* 1991;42:183–200.
231. Reyes-Vazquez C, Dafny N. Microiontophoretically applied THIP effects upon nociceptive responses of neurons in medial thalamus. *Appl Neurophysiol* 1983;46:254–260.
232. Reyes-Vazquez C, Qiao J-T, Dafny N. Nociceptive responses in nucleus parafascicularis thalami are modulated by dorsal raphe stimulation and microiontophoretic application of morphine and serotonin. *Brain Res Bull* 1989;23:405–411.
233. Richardson DE. Thalamotomy for intractable pain. *Confinia Neurol* 1967;29:139–145.
234. Richelson E. The newer antidepressants: structures, pharmacokinetics, pharmacodynamics, and proposed mechanisms of action. *Psychopharmacol Bull* 1984;20:213–223.
235. Rinaldi PC, Young RF, Albe-Fessard D, Chodakiewitz J. Spontaneous neuronal hyperactivity in the medial and intralaminar thalamic nuclei of patients with deafferentation pain. *J Neurosurg* 1991;74:415–421.
236. Rinvik E, Wiberg M. Demonstration of a reciprocal connection between the periaqueductal gray matter and the reticular nucleus of the thalamus. *Anat Embryol* 1990;181:577–584.
237. Roberts WA, Eaton SA, Salt TE. Widely distributed GABA-mediated afferent inhibition processes within the ventrobasal thalamus of rat and their possible relevance to pathological pain states and somatotopic plasticity. *Exp Brain Res* 1992;89:363–372.
238. Roos A, Rydenhag B, Andersson S. Activity in cortical cells after stimulation of tooth pulp afferents in the cat. Extracellular analysis. *Pain* 1983;16:61–72.
239. Roy J-C, Bing Z, Villanueva L, Le Bars D. Convergence of visceral and somatic inputs onto subnucleus reticularis dorsalis neurones in the rat medulla. *J Physiol (Lond)* 1992;458:235–246.
240. Royce GJ, Bromley S, Gracco C, Beckstead RM. Thalamocortical connections of the rostral intralaminar nuclei: An autoradiographic analysis in the cat. *J Comp Neurol* 1989;288:555–582.
241. Rustioni A, Schmechel DE, Spreafico R, Cheema S, Cuenod M. Excitatory and inhibitory amino acid putative neurotransmitters in the ventralis posterior complex: an autoradiographic and immunocytochemical study in rats and cats. In: Machhi G, Rustioni A, Spreafico R, eds. *Somatosensory integration in the thalamus.* Amsterdam: Elsevier, 1983;365–383.
242. Sadikot AF, Parent A, Smith Y, Bolam JP. Efferent connections of the centromedian and parafascicular thalamic nuclei in the squirrel monkey: A light and electron microscopic study of the thalamostriatal projection in relation to striatal heterogeneity. *J Comp Neurol* 1992;320:228–242.
243. Salt TE. Mediation of thalamic sensory input by both NMDA receptors and non NMDA receptors. *Nature* 1986;322:263–265.
244. Salt TE. Excitatory amino acid receptors and synaptic transmission in the rat ventrobasal thalamus. *J Physiol (Lond)* 1987;391: 499–510.
245. Salt TE. Gamma-aminobutyric acid and afferent inhibition in the cat and rat ventrobasal thalamus. *Neuroscience* 1989;28:17–26.
246. Salt TE. Modulation of NMDA receptor-mediated responses by glycine and D serine in the rat thalamus in vivo. *Brain Res* 1989; 481:403–406.
247. Salt TE, Eaton SA. Function of non NMDA receptors and NMDA receptors in synaptic responses to natural somatosensory stimulation in the ventrobasal thalamus. *Exp Brain Res* 1989;77:646–652.
248. Salt TE, Eaton SA. Sensory excitatory postsynaptic potentials mediated by NMDA and non NMDA receptors in the thalamus in vivo. *Eur J Neurosci* 1991;3:296–300.
248a. Salt TE, Eaton SA. The function of metabotropic excitatory amino acid receptors in synaptic transmission in the thalamus: Studies with novel phenylglycine antagonists. *Neurochem Int* 1994;24: 451–458.
248b. Salt TE, Eaton SA. Distinct presynaptic metabotropic receptors for L-AP4 and CCG1 on GABAergic terminals: pharmacological evidence using novel -methyl derivative mGluR antagonists, MAP4 and MCCG, in the rat thalamus in vivo. *Neuroscience* 1995;65:5–13.
249. Saper CB, Loewy AD. Efferent connections of the parabrachial nucleus in the rat. *Brain Res* 1980;197:291–317.
250. Sato A, Schmidt RF. Somatosympathetic reflexes: Afferent fibers, central pathways, discharge characteristics. *Physiol Rev* 1973;53: 916–947.
251. Schlag J, Schlag-Rey M. Role of the central thalamus in gaze control. *Prog Brain Res* 1986;64:191–201.
251a. Schwarz M, Block F. Visual and somatosensory evoked potentials are mediated by excitatory amino acid receptors in the thalamus. *Electroencephalogr Clin Neurophysiol* 1994;91:392–398.
251b. Senatorov VV, Trudeau VL, Hu B. Expression of cholecystokinin mRNA in corticothalamic projecting neurons: a combined fluorescence in situ hybridization and retrograde tracing study in the ventrolateral thalamus of the rat. *Mol Brain Res* 1995;30: 87–96.
252. Shyu BC, Kiritsy-Roy JA, Morrow TJ, Casey KL. Neurophysiological, pharmacological and behavioral evidence for medial thalamic mediation of cocaine-induced dopaminergic analgesia. *Brain Res* 1992;572:216–223.
253. Siegfried J. Stimulation of thalamic nuclei in human: sensory and therapeutical aspects. In: Besson J-M, Guilbaud G, Peschanski M, eds. *Thalamus and pain.* Amsterdam: Excerpta Medica, 1987; 271–278.
254. Sikes RW, Vogt BA. Nociceptive neurons in area 24 of rabbit cingulate cortex. *J Neurophysiol* 1992;68:1720–1732.
255. Simone DA, Sorkin LS, Oh U, Chung JM, Owens C, LaMotte RH, Willis WD. Neurogenic hyperalgesia: Central neural correlates in responses of spinothalamic tract neurons. *J Neurophysiol* 1991;66: 228–246.
256. Snow PJ, Lumb BM, Cervero F. The representation of prolonged and intense, noxious somatic and visceral stimuli in the ventrolateral orbital cortex of the cat. *Pain* 1992;48:89–99.
256a. Steriade M, Jones EG, Llinas RR. Thalamic oscillations and signalling. New York: John Wiley, 1990.
257. Sugiyama K, Ryu H, Uemura K. Identification of nociceptive neurons in the medial thalamus: Morphological studies of nociceptive neurons with intracellular injection of horseradish peroxidase. *Brain Res* 1992;586:36–43.
258. Swanson LW, Hartman BK. The central adrenergic system. An immunofluorescence study of the location of cell bodies and their efferent connections in the rat utilizing dopamine-beta-hydroxylase as a marker. *J Comp Neurol* 1975;163:467–506.
259. Sweet WH. Cerebral localization of pain. In: Thompson RA, Green JR, eds. *New perspectives in cerebral localization.* New York: Raven Press, 1982;205–242.
260. Talbot JD, Marrett S, Evans AC, Meyer E, Bushnell MC, Duncan GH. Multiple representations of pain in human cerebral cortex. *Science* 1991;251:1355–1358.
261. Tanelian DL, Kosek P, Mody I, MacIver MB. The role of the GABAA receptor / chloride channel complex in anesthesia. *Anesthesiology* 1993;78:757–776.
262. Tanji DG, Wise SP, Dykes RW, Jones EG. Cytoarchitecture and thalamic connectivity of third somatosensory area of cat cerebral cortex. *J Neurophysiol* 1978;41:268–284.
263. Tasker RR. Stereotaxic surgery. In: Wall PD, Melzack R, eds. *Textbook of pain.* Edinburgh: Churchill Livingstone, 1984;639–655.
264. Terenzi MG, Prado WA. Antinociception elicited by electrical or chemical stimulation of the rat habenular complex and its sensitivity to systemic antagonists. *Brain Res* 1990;535:18–24.
265. Thiele FH, Horsley V. A study of the degenerations observed in the central nervous system in a case of fracture dislocation of the spine. *Brain* 1901;24:519–531.
266. Thomson AM. Inhibitory postsynaptic potentials evoked in thalamic neurons by stimulation of the reticularis nucleus evoke slow spikes in isolated rat brain slices I. *Neuroscience* 1988;25:491–502.
266a. Tsoukatos J, Kiss ZHT, Tasker RR, Lozano AM, Davis KD, Dostrovsky JO. Distinct patterns of bursting activity in the human medial and lateral thalamus. *Soc Neurosci Abstr* 1995;21:109.
267. Tsubokawa T, Katayama Y, Ueno Y, Moriyasu N. Evidence for the involvement of frontal cortex in pain related cerebral events in

cats: increase in local cerebral blood flow by noxious stimuli. *Brain Res* 1981;217:179–185.
268. Vahle-Hinz C, Hicks TP, Gottschaldt K-M. Amino acids modify thalamo cortical response transformation expressed by neurons of the ventrobasal complex. *Brain Res* 1993;
269. Vierck CJ Jr, Greenspan JD, Ritz LA, Yeomans DC. The spinal pathways contributing to the ascending conduction and the descending modulation of pain sensations and reactions. In: Yaksh TL, ed. *Spinal afferent processing.* New York: Plenum Press, 1986;275–329.
269a.Vierck CJ Jr, Greenspan JD, Ritz LA. Long-term changes in purposive and reflexive responses to nociceptive stimulation following anterolateral chordotomy. *J Neurosci* 1990;10:2077–2095.
269b.Vincent SR. Nitric oxide: a radical neurotransmitter in the central nervous system. *Prog Neurobiol* 1994;42:129–160.
270. Villanueva L, de Pommery J, Menetrey D, Le Bars D. Spinal afferent projections to subnucleus reticularis dorsalis in the rat. *Neurosci Lett* 1991;134:98–102.
271. Walker AE. The spinothalamic tract in man. *Arch Neurol Psychiatr* 1940;43:284–298.
272. Westlund KN, Bowker RM, Ziegler MG, Coulter JD. Origins and terminations of descending noradrenergic projections to the spinal cord of monkey. *Brain Res* 1984;292:1–16.
273. Westlund KN, Craig AD. Spinal cord lamina I terminations in brain stem catecholamine cell groups. *Soc Neurosci Abstr* 1993;19:517.
274. Westlund KN, Sorkin LS, Ferrington DG, Carlton SM, Willcockson HH, Willis WD. Serotoninergic and noradrenergic projections to the ventral posterolateral nucleus of the monkey thalamus. *J Comp Neurol* 1990;295:197–207.
275. White JC, Sweet WH. *Pain and the neurosurgeon: a forty year experience.* Springfield, IL: Charles C. Thomas, 1969.
276. Wiberg M, Blomqvist A. The spinomesencephalic tract in the cat: its cells of origin and termination pattern as demonstrated by the intraaxonal transport method. *Brain Res* 1984;291:1–18.
277. Wiberg M, Westman J, Blomqvist A. Somatosensory projection to the mesencephalon: an anatomical study in the monkey. *J Comp Neurol* 1987;264:92–117.
278. Willis WD. *The pain system.* Basel: Karger, 1985.
279. Willis WD, Coggeshall RE. *Sensory mechanisms of the spinal cord.* New York: Plenum, 1978.
280. Willis WD, Kenshalo DR Jr, Leonard RB. The cells of origin of the primate spinothalamic tract. *J Comp Neurol* 1979;188:543–574.
281. Willis WD, Trevino DL, Coulter JD, Maunz RA. Responses of primate spinothalamic tract neurons to natural stimulation of hindlimb. *J Neurophysiol* 1974;37:358–372.
282. Yasui Y, Breder CD, Saper CB, Cechetto DF. Autonomic responses and efferent pathways from the insular cortex in the rat. *J Comp Neurol* 1991;303:355–374.
283. Yasui Y, Itoh K, Kamiya H, Ino T, Mizuno N. Cingulate gyrus of the cat receives projection fibers from the thalamic region ventral to the ventral border of the ventrobasal complex. *J Comp Neurol* 1988; 274:91–100.
284. Yasui Y, Saper CB, Cechetto DF. Calcitonin gene-related peptide immunoreactivity in the visceral sensory cortex, thalamus, and related pathways in the rat. *J Comp Neurol* 1989;290:487–501.
285. Yezierski RP. Spinomesencephalic tract: projections from the lumbosacral spinal cord of the rat, cat, and monkey. *J Comp Neurol* 1988;267:131–146.
286. Yezierski RP, Mendez CM. Spinal distribution and collateral projections of rat spinomesencephalic tract cells. *Neuroscience* 1991;44: 113–130.
287. Yezierski RP, Schwartz RH. Response and receptive-field properties of spinomesencephalic tract cells in the cat. *J Neurophysiol* 1986;55:76–96.
288. Yezierski RP, Sorkin LS, Willis WD. Response properties of spinal neurons projecting to midbrain or midbrain-thalamus in the monkey. *Brain Res* 1987;437:165–170.
289. Yokota T, Asato F, Koyama N, Masuda T, Taguchi H. Nociceptive body representation in nucleus ventralis posterolateralis of cat thalamus. *J Neurophysiol* 1988;60:1714–1727.
290. Yokota T, Koyama N, Matsumoto N. Somatotopic distribution of trigeminal nociceptive neurons in ventrobasal complex of cat thalamus. *J Neurophysiol* 1985;53:1387–1400.
291. Yokota T, Koyama N, Nishikawa Y, Hasegawa A. Dual somatosensory representation of the periodontium in nucleus ventralis posteromedialis of the cat thalamus. *Brain Res* 1988;475:187–191.
292. Yoshida A, Dostrovsky JO, Chiang CY. The afferent and efferent connections of the nucleus submedius in the rat. *J Comp Neurol* 1992;324:115–133.
293. Yoshida A, Dostrovsky JO, Sessle BJ, Chiang CY. Trigeminal projections to the nucleus submedius of the thalamus in the rat. *J Comp Neurol* 1991;307:609–625.
294. Young RF, Tronnier V, Rinaldi PC. Chronic stimulation of the Kölliker Fuse nucleus region for relief of intractable pain in humans. *J Neurosurg* 1992;76:979–985.
295. Zhang D, Carlton SM, Sorkin LS, Willis WD. Collaterals of primate spinothalamic tract neurons to the periaqueductal gray. *J Comp Neurol* 1990;296:277–290.
296. Zhi-Hua Z, Yi-Fang X, Jian-Tian Q. Effects of stimulation of superior colliculus on nociceptive unit discharges in parafascicular neurons and nocifensive reflex of hind limb in rat. *Brain Res* 1991;542:248–253.

Anesthesia: Biologic Foundations, edited by Tony L. Yaksh et al. Lippincott–Raven Publishers, Philadelphia © 1997.

CHAPTER 38

ORGANIZATIONAL CHARACTERISTICS OF SUPRASPINALLY MEDIATED RESPONSES TO NOCICEPTIVE INPUT

MARY M. HEINRICHER

In considering the organization of the sensory pathways, it has been emphasized that afferent traffic is encoded at the level of the dorsal horn and gains access to supraspinal systems via long ascending tracts. These ascending projections provide input to several brainstem regions, and to structures as far rostral as the thalamus and hypothalamus (see Chaps. 35 and 37). Two points may be made. First, it should be appreciated that the rostral levels of the neuraxis provide the integrative and organizational capacity to mediate increasingly complex behavioral patterns. Input from spinal and various supraspinal systems may thus converge at more than one level to generate behavioral patterns conditioned by the stimulus environment. Second, it is clear that the encoding of afferent traffic is shaped dynamically by modulatory systems that alter the input-output function at each level, and that are themselves regulated by ascending afferent input. It should be evident that such regulation becomes yet more complex when sensory processing is considered in the context of higher centers.

As reviewed in Chap. 36, such regulation occurs first at the level of the dorsal horn. Early studies by Hagbarth and Kerr (97a) and later studies by Anden and colleagues (6a) demonstrated that descending pathways, some of which were likely catecholaminergic, could regulate spinal traffic. In a complementary approach, Wall (255a) showed that activity of dorsal horn neurons was much increased by high spinal section, thus demonstrating a potent descending inhibition acting upon these neurons. In a pivotal observation, Reynolds (218) demonstrated that electrical stimulation of the periaqueductal gray matter (PAG) surrounding the cerebral aqueduct in the midbrain inhibited behavioral responses to noxious stimulation in awake rats, thus confirming the behavioral relevance of modulatory systems. Inasmuch as PAG stimulation was subsequently shown to be capable of blocking spinal nociceptive reflexes, and also to produce inhibition of dorsal horn neurons, it seemed likely that the behavioral effects might involve descending projections from brainstem to the spinal cord dorsal horn (see below). Although a number of sites have now been implicated in descending modulation (33,92), the best characterized is a system with links in the rostral ventromedial medulla (RVM) as well as the PAG.

In this section we consider some aspects of the organization of systems in the medial core of the brainstem, with a particular focus on this PAG-RVM system (Fig. 1). The PAG-RVM system receives inputs from ascending spinal afferent systems (including spinoreticular and spinomesencephalic tracts, as well as collaterals from spinothalamic tract axons) that converge with inputs from a wide range of supraspinal sites. In terms of outflow, the RVM is the source of an extensive bulbospinal projection, and the PAG in particular has substantial, although functionally less well characterized, rostral projections to diencephalic and limbic sites. This connectivity will be considered further below, but it should be evident that this system is ideally situated to mediate a complex integration of sensory traffic with higher order, particularly limbic, influences.

The primary focus of the present chapter is on:

1. the organization of modulatory circuitry within the brainstem, with the emphasis being on the properties of the PAG-RVM–spinal cord network;
2. how this intrinsic circuitry is activated, both pharmacologically (for example, by opioid analgesics) and by environmental stimuli (most notably under conditions of environmental threat); and
3. the role played by these midbrain systems in integrating complex behavioral responses to noxious stimuli.

PERIAQUEDUCTAL GRAY

Local Organization and Connections of the PAG

The PAG is a cell-rich region surrounding the cerebral aqueduct, extending from the caudal aspect of the third ventricle to the opening of the aqueduct into the fourth ventricle. This region is sometimes considered to be a caudal extension of the limbic system into the midbrain (124). A number of neurotransmitters and neuropeptides, including γ-aminobutyric acid (GABA), serotonin, neurotensin, enkephalins, substance P, vasoactive intestinal peptide, and cholecystokinin are concentrated in this region (27,29,53,192,193,214,215,238,268). Although both the intrinsic and extrinsic connectivity of the PAG is unquestionably very complex, this structure can be organized into dorsomedial, dorsolateral, and lateral columns that are aligned along its rostrocaudal axis.

Afferents to the PAG originate from widespread areas of the neuraxis. Rostrally, forebrain (prefrontal and insular cortex, central nucleus of the amygdala, and bed nucleus of the stria terminalis) and hypothalamus send projections into the PAG. More caudally, deep layers of the superior colliculus, the nucleus cuneiformis and parabrachial area, and pontomedullary reticular formation including locus coeruleus, send projections into the PAG. Direct spinomesencephalic inputs to the PAG derive primarily from lamina I and from laminae IV and V contralaterally (see Chaps. 35 and 37) (26,37, 219,220,236). Importantly, the spinomesencephalic projection has an additional, somatotopic organization, with fibers originating at cervical levels projecting to the rostral aspect, and those originating at lumbar levels terminating more caudally in the lateral columns.

The terminal fields of many of these inputs are known to be highly organized, respecting the rostrocaudal columnar organization already mentioned (Fig. 2). For example, the projections from prefrontal and cingulate cortex project to the dorsolateral column, while those from the amygdala and hypothalamus tend to project to the dorsomedial column (see ref. 11 for a complete review of connections of the PAG).

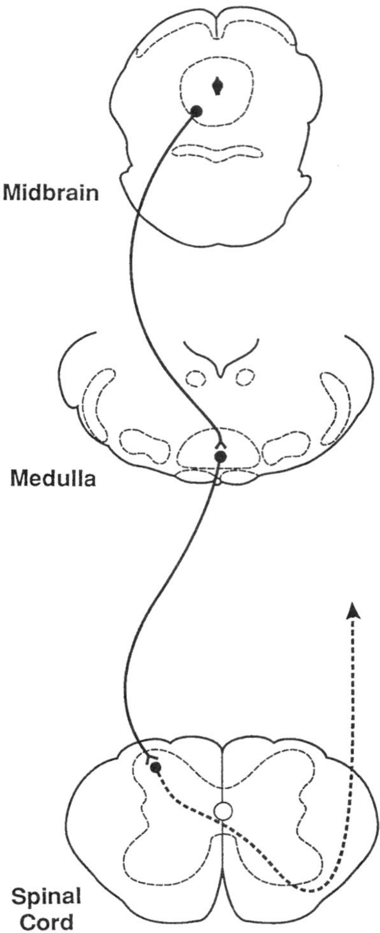

Figure 1. Schematic diagram of descending modulatory circuit involving midbrain periaqueductal gray and rostral ventromedial medulla (RVM). Activation of neurons in either site produces inhibition of dorsal horn and behavioral responses to noxious stimuli. This is in large part through a descending inhibitory action exerted at the level of the spinal cord. The anatomical substrate for this is a large projection to the dorsal horn from the RVM. It travels through the dorsolateral funiculus, and terminates in dorsal horn laminae involved in nociception. The PAG itself has only a sparse projection to the spinal cord, and its influence on the cord is indirect, through its connection with the RVM.

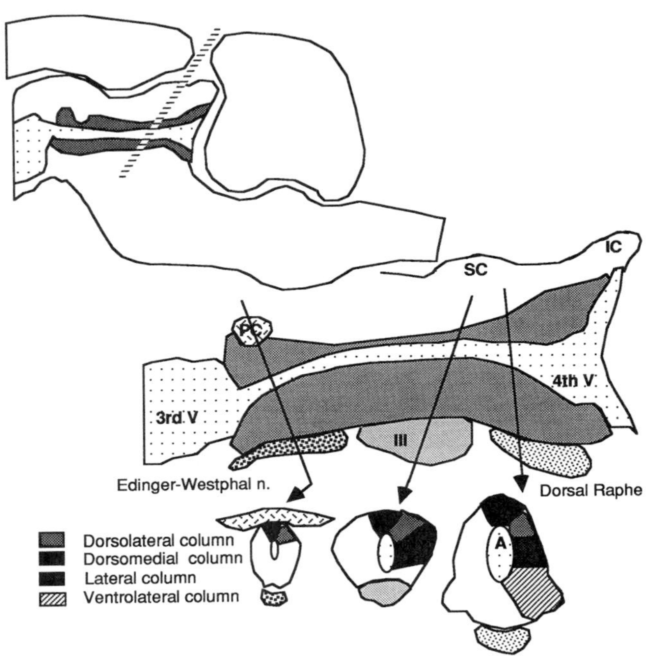

Figure 2. General schematic summary of organization of the periaqueductal gray along its rostrocaudal axis.

Cells within the PAG project caudally into the rostral ventromedial medulla (see below) and rostrally into the diencephalon, hypothalamus, and limbic forebrain. As with the afferent input, there is a tendency for these projections to show a rostrocaudally oriented columnar organization. Thus, for example, the strong projections into the rostroventral medulla tend to arise from the ventrolateral aspects of the PAG. Perhaps the most important consideration with regard to the efferent connections of the PAG is that this region does not project to the spinal cord in any substantial way (124). Thus, the modulation of spinal function resulting from manipulations of PAG neurons appears to be largely mediated via relays in the rostral ventromedial medulla (Fig. 1) (84).

Function of PAG in Modulating Nociception

The PAG is known to be involved in a variety of functions, including reproductive behaviors, vocalization, and defense responses (59), and with the demonstration that electrical stimulation in this area produced a potent antinociception, the PAG was the first brain region to be implicated in supraspinal modulation of nociception (218). This finding was subsequently confirmed and extended to other species, with inhibition of spinal nociceptive reflexes and of supraspinally mediated responses elicited by noxious stimuli (178,270). PAG stimulation was also shown to produce analgesia in humans (12). Antinociception is obtained with stimulation throughout the PAG, but the lowest threshold is found ventrolaterally (152). The fact that microinjection of the neuroexcitant glutamate is similarly antinociceptive indicates that electrical stimulation-produced antinociception in the PAG is due to local excitation of neuronal cell bodies or dendrites, and not only of fibers of passage (19,132).

Opioid Activation of PAG Outflow

The PAG is also an important substrate for opioid analgesia, with a dense concentration of opioid peptides and receptors (58,86,174,193). Microinjection of morphine or opioid peptides into the PAG produces a dose-dependent, naloxone-reversible antinociception (129,152,274,276). The caudal ventrolateral aspect of the PAG is reported to be the most sensitive to the effects of local opioid application (277), and there is evidence that this antinociception is mediated by an action at the μ-opioid receptor (130,240). Localization of opiate action and the pharmacology of these effects have been reviewed in additional detail in Chap. 58.

In view of the fact that direct activation of PAG neurons using electrical stimulation or microinjection of neuroexcitant agents such as glutamate produces antinociception, whereas lesions of the PAG do not (68,270,275), it can be inferred that opioid administration within the PAG must, in some manner, activate an antinociceptive output from the region (277). The considerable overlap in the distributions of sites at which morphine and glutamate microinjections produce antinociception adds further weight to this inference (132,152), as does the observation that multiunit activity recorded in the PAG in

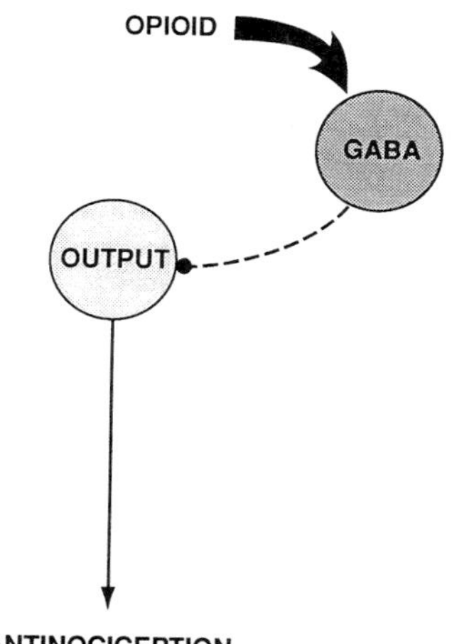

Figure 3. Opioid disinhibition of output neuron that exerts a net antinociceptive effect. Direct effects of opioids within the central nervous system are generally inhibitory, suggesting that the activation of PAG neurons by opioids must be via disinhibition, likely through inhibiting the activity of a GABAergic inhibitory interneuron.

awake rats is increased following systemic administration of morphine (249). However, the *direct* cellular effects of opioids in the central nervous system are generally inhibitory (196,197), and the majority of neurons recorded in the PAG slice exhibit a naloxone-reversible hyperpolarization and decrease in firing following bath application of met-enkephalin. A subset of neurons do, however, show an excitation (20), and this excitation is blocked by addition of a high concentration of magnesium to the bathing medium to interfere with synaptic transmission. Considered collectively, these data indicate that opioids activate a significant number of PAG neurons, but through an indirect mechanism, by directly inhibiting the firing of an inhibitory, most likely GABA-containing, interneuron (Fig. 3).

The evidence that the opioid-sensitive interneuron within this PAG opioid-sensitive circuit is GABAergic is as follows. GABA is abundant in the PAG, with the densest concentrations of terminals around the aqueduct and in the ventrolateral region (214; see above). Synaptic contacts from GABA-containing terminals onto PAG neurons projecting to the medulla have been demonstrated, providing direct anatomical evidence for GABA-mediated control over the efferent projection from this region (215,269). Several lines of evidence suggest that opiate actions within the PAG may be mediated by an action on GABA-containing elements. First, GABA release within the PAG is decreased following systemic administration of morphine (217). Second, GABA agonists applied within the PAG attenuate, whereas $GABA_A$ receptor antagonists enhance, the antinociception resulting from microinjection of morphine at the same site (63,182) (see Chap. 62). Third, blocking GABA transmission in the PAG using $GABA_A$ receptor antagonists leads to increased activity in many PAG neurons recorded in vitro (21). Fourth, microinjection of GABA antagonists in the PAG mimics the behavioral effects of opioid application in producing an antinociception (182,233,234).

The above observations would be most parsimoniously explained if the interneurons inhibited by opioids were to contain GABA. Inhibition of this interneuron would in turn disinhibit a PAG output neuron. Activation of the output neuron would ultimately give rise to an inhibitory effect upon spinal nociceptive transmission (by means of a relay in the rostral ventromedial medulla, see below).

ROSTRAL VENTROMEDIAL MEDULLA

Relay of Descending Actions of PAG within Rostral Ventromedial Medulla

The effectiveness of electrical stimulation in the midbrain PAG in suppressing both spinally and supraspinally organized responses to noxious stimuli is thought to result in large part from the inhibition of nociceptive transmission at the level of the spinal cord dorsal horn. Thus, electrical stimulation of the PAG profoundly inhibits both noxious-evoked activity of dorsal horn neurons and spinally mediated nocifensor reflexes (178,270). However, insofar as the PAG itself has only sparse direct projections to the spinal cord (124), these effects require an intervening link. Indeed, the descending inhibition resulting from activation of PAG neurons is largely mediated through a relay in the RVM (Fig. 4), a region including the nucleus raphe magnus, the laterally adjacent nucleus reticularis gigantocellularis *pars alpha,* and the juxtafacial portion of the nucleus reticularis paragigantocellularis lateralis (Pgi) (84). The RVM receives a large projection from the PAG (1,25,27,47,89,250), which arises from the dorsal, as well as lateral and ventrolateral, aspects (1,250). Distinct but intermingled subsets of neurons within each PAG region send axons to each of the individual cytoarchitecturally defined nuclei within the RVM (28). Electrical stimulation in the PAG excites the great majority of RVM neurons, including identified medullospinal neurons (165,177,205,252,272). Indeed, the threshold current for activation of RVM neurons using PAG stimulation is indistinguishable from that required to produce a behaviorally measurable antinociception (252). The RVM in turn projects via the dorsolateral funiculus to the spinal cord where its targets include (but are not restricted to) dorsal horn laminae implicated in nociception (16, 125,241).

An important role for the RVM in mediating antinociception from the PAG is further supported by lesion studies. Inactivation of the RVM, using electrolytic lesions or a local anesthetic, attenuates descending inhibition from the PAG (3,19, 93,162,191,209,231,283). The entire RVM, including nucleus raphe magnus and the adjacent reticular formation, must

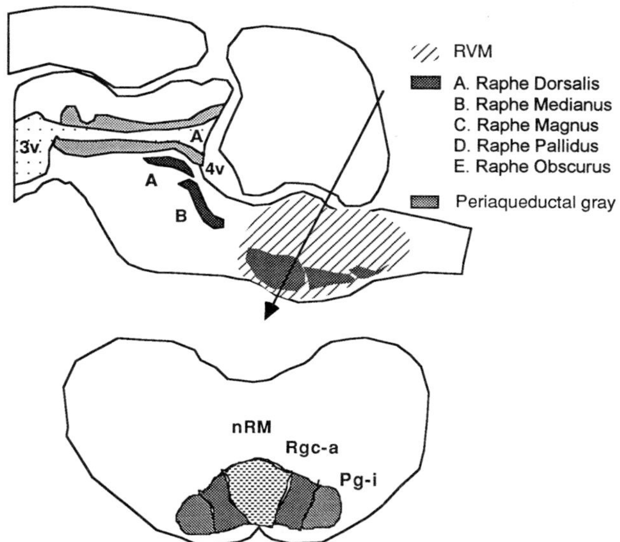

Figure 4. General schematic organization of the brain stem axis. The RVM and its relation to cytoarchitectonically defined nuclei of the ventral medulla are depicted.

apparently be inactivated in order to completely block the antinociceptive action of PAG stimulation (3,93,231; although see 162). This finding is consistent with anatomical studies demonstrating an overlapping projection from both dorsal and lateral/ventrolateral PAG across the entire mediolateral extent of the RVM (250). These observations, in conjunction with the connections of the RVM reviewed above, suggest that the RVM could provide an important functional link for descending brainstem modulation of spinal afferent processing.

Functional Role of RVM in Nociceptive Modulation

RVM involvement in nociceptive modulation is confirmed by the fact that nonselective activation of neurons in this region using electrical stimulation or glutamate microinjection depresses activity of nociceptive neurons in the dorsal horn, inhibits spinal nocifensive reflexes, and reduces supraspinally organized responses to noxious stimulation (3,132,163,178, 230,235,270,288). The convergent effects of electrical stimulation and neuroexcitant injection emphasize that the effects of electrical stimulation are not merely due to activation of a distant region by activating local fibers of passage. Microinjection of morphine or opioid peptides in the RVM is also antinociceptive (5,8,64,72,129,151,274). Thus, like the PAG, the RVM is a sufficient substrate for opioid antinociception, and it is likely to contribute to the antinociceptive action of systemically administered opioids.

Physiologic Analysis of RVM Circuitry

The functional observations outlined above pointed to a significant role for the RVM in nociceptive modulation, but early analyses of the circuitry within this region were complicated by the diversity of its constituent neurons in terms of physiology, pharmacology, morphology, and neurochemistry (83,84). Inhibitory as well as excitatory responses to noxious somatic or visceral stimulation can be obtained in RVM, and many neurons exhibit multisensory convergence when examined in awake animals (83,199,200). Pharmacologic response properties are similarly heterogeneous. Most significantly, RVM neurons show both excitatory and inhibitory responses to systemically administered opioids (90).

Thus, to identify neuronal mechanisms through which RVM regulates spinal nociceptive processes, studies have been carried out examining the activity of single RVM neurons in lightly anesthetized rats. These experiments reveal two classes of RVM neurons that display abrupt changes in activity beginning just *prior* to execution of the tail flick (Fig. 5) (82). These cell classes, termed *off-cells* and *on-cells,* possess distinct pharmacologies (14,51,106,107,109), and are likely to have opposing roles in nociceptive modulation (83).

Off-Cells

These cells are characterized by an abrupt pause in firing that begins just prior to a nociceptive response elicited by application of a noxious stimulus (e.g., a tail flick reflex evoked by application of a heat stimulus to the tail). This inhibition of activity is not considered a "sensory" response coding intensity of the noxious stimulus, because the onset of the pause is much more closely correlated with reflex occurrence than with tail temperature. Since nonselective excitation of RVM neurons is known to inhibit the tail flick (see above), the very fact that off-cells pause at the time of the reflex means that these neurons are likely to inhibit nociception under normal conditions. That is, the pause in firing permits the nociceptive reflex to occur.

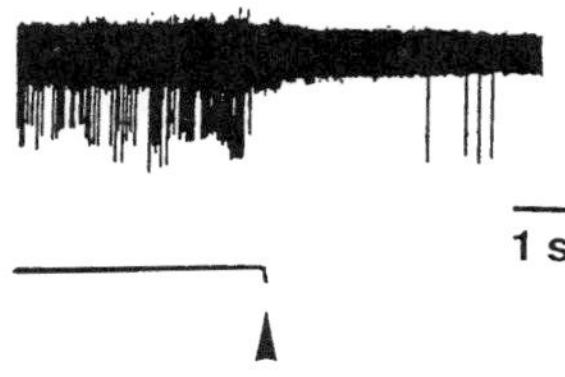

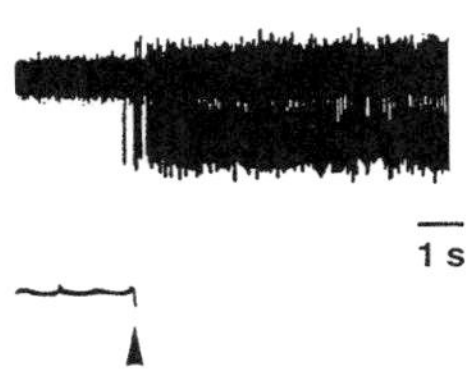

Figure 5. Changes in activity that are temporally linked with the occurrence of nocifensor reflexes such as the tail flick can be used to characterize RVM neurons physiologically. *Upper traces* of two single 10-s oscilloscope sweeps show sudden cessation in firing (off-cell) and burst of firing (on-cell) beginning just before the occurrence of the tail flick, which is indicated by deflection in tail position monitor output (*triangle* on *lower trace* of each sweep).

Indeed, if off-cells are induced to cease firing by delivery of a noxious stimulus to a body region remote from the tail, the withdrawal reflex elicited by application of noxious heat to the tail can subsequently be elicited at a lower stimulus temperature (213).

On-Cells

Other RVM neurons are called "on-cells" because they show a sudden burst of activity beginning just before the execution of the tail flick (and other nociceptive reflexes). Again, changes in cell activity are correlated with reflex execution, rather than with stimulus intensity (e.g., skin temperature). Moreover, the fact that the tail flick occurs during a burst of on-cell firing indicates that these neurons cannot have a potent inhibitory influence on nociception. Rather, the reflex-related burst of activity suggests a pronociceptive role, i.e., on-cells are likely to permit or even facilitate nociceptive transmission.

Neutral Cells

Finally, a third class of neurons identified in the RVM has been termed "neutral cells" because these neurons show no change in activity associated with the execution of nocifensive reflexes (82). Their role, if any, in nociceptive modulation, is not immediately obvious. For example, neutral cells are unaffected by morphine given systemically, microinjected into the PAG, or applied by iontophoresis (14,51,109). Nevertheless, there is anatomical evidence that some subset of neutral cells contains serotonin (206). In view of the evidence implicating medullospinal serotonergic projections in descending inhibition of nociception (17,32), it seems that further examination of this cell class is in order.

Role of On- and Off-Cell Classes in Nociceptive Modulation

Additional evidence that both on- and off-cells play a role in nociceptive modulation derives from a number of complementary experimental approaches. As would be expected from the circuit diagram in Fig. 1, both on- and off-cells are excited by electrical stimulation of the PAG, and at least some cells of each class can be shown using antidromic activation methods to project to the spinal cord (252,253). Moreover, under almost all conditions examined, elimination of the reflex-related off-cell pause is associated with inhibition of nociceptive responses. This is most clearly seen in investigations of the role of these two cell classes in opioid analgesia. On- and off-cells show predictable and differential responses when opioid administration (whether systemic, intrathecal, or microinjected into the PAG) produces an antinociception (as measured by inhibition of reflex responses to noxious stimulation). Off-cells invariably become continuously active, with no cessation of activity during noxious stimulation under these conditions. In contrast, on-cells uniformly become silent (51,85,105,187,224).

In general, elimination of the off-cell pause is associated with an inhibition of nocifensor reflexes, whereas activation of on-cells is associated with normal or increased nociceptive responsiveness (18,104,121,185,186,213,245). (However, see Thurston and Randich [244] for one instance in which an inverse correlation was obtained, and Heinricher and Tortorici [112] for a more complete discussion of this issue.)

Off-Cells: Disinhibition of Spinopetal Inhibition

Significantly, the same changes in on- and off-cell activity produced by systemic morphine administration are also seen when an opioid is microinjected directly into the RVM itself to produce antinociception (110) (Fig. 6). The suppression of on-cell firing is likely a direct effect, since on-cells are also inhibited when morphine is applied directly using iontophoresis. On the other hand, the activation of off-cells by opioids must be indirect, since these neurons are not responsive when opioids are applied directly (109).

A simple circuit that can account for the activation of off-cells by opioids is shown in Fig. 7. There are a number of observations that support this model. First, the existence of an opioid-sensitive GABAergic inhibitory mechanism within the RVM has been demonstrated in the RVM slice preparation, where local electrical stimulation elicits GABA-mediated synaptic potentials in a subset of neurons. These locally evoked synaptic potentials are blocked by addition of an opioid to the bath (203). Second, there is strong evidence that the off-cell pause is mediated by GABA (107). Third, interfering with GABAergic transmission within the RVM by local application of $GABA_A$ receptor antagonists produces an antinociceptive effect (69,108), and this behavioral antinociception can be attributed to a disinhibition of off-cells (112).

In addition, it can reasonably be inferred that at least some on-cells function as inhibitory interneurons within the RVM. If inhibitory neurons responsible for the off-cell pause are located within the RVM, they would, by definition, be on-cells in that they would show a burst of activity during the off-cell pause, that is, at the time of the tail flick. Moreover, on-cells are the only RVM neurons known to be directly sensitive to opioids. Consequently, the opioid inhibition of on-cells would release off-cells from inhibitory control, and this would have a net antinociceptive effect. Thus, as was the case in the PAG, disinhibition appears to be a central mechanism in nociceptive modulation within the RVM.

It should also be noted that a substantial number of on-cells project to the spinal cord. Assuming that the net effect of on-cell firing at spinal levels is to facilitate nociception, and to the extent that on-cells are active at any given moment, opioid inhibition of medullospinal on-cells would reinforce the antinociceptive effect of activating off-cells. However, this second aspect of opioid action on on-cells would not by itself be sufficient to produce complete suppression of nociceptive responses, since lesions of the RVM do not produce analgesia (162,210,211,231,283).

On-Cells: Spinopetal Facilitation

Evidence for a descending facilitatory influence of on-cells has been provided by Fields and coworkers (81), who found that a period of lowered nociceptive threshold that occurs during acute naloxone-induced reversal of morphine analgesia is associated with an increase in firing of on-cells, and a concurrent decrease in the firing of off-cells (18). They further demonstrated that this hyperalgesia is attenuated by local inactivation of RVM using lidocaine microinjection. This finding indicates that the hyperalgesia does not represent a pas-

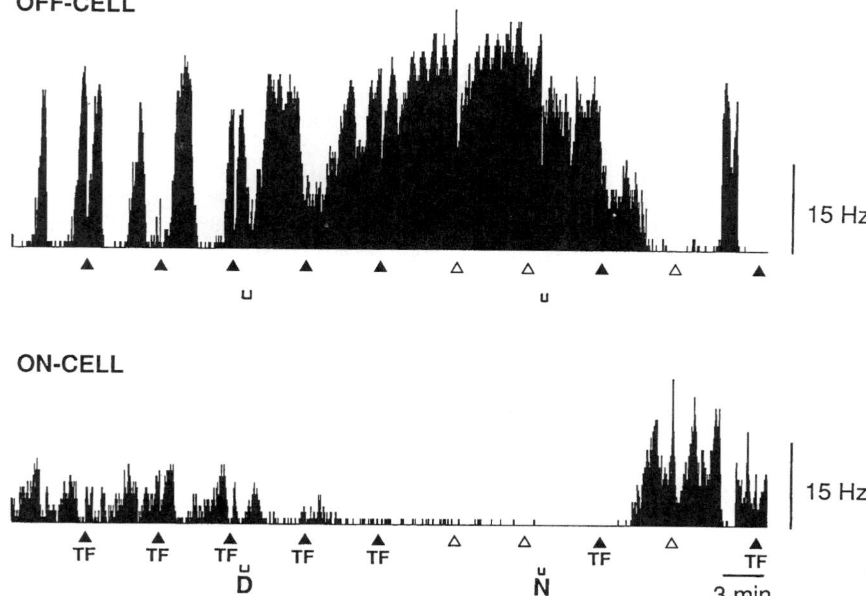

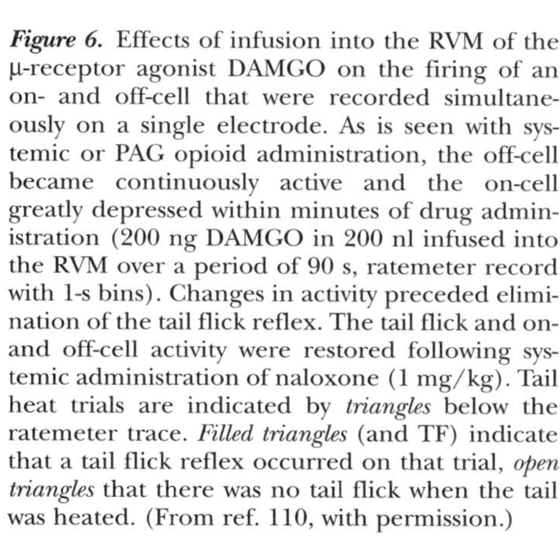

Figure 6. Effects of infusion into the RVM of the µ-receptor agonist DAMGO on the firing of an on- and off-cell that were recorded simultaneously on a single electrode. As is seen with systemic or PAG opioid administration, the off-cell became continuously active and the on-cell greatly depressed within minutes of drug administration (200 ng DAMGO in 200 nl infused into the RVM over a period of 90 s, ratemeter record with 1-s bins). Changes in activity preceded elimination of the tail flick reflex. The tail flick and on- and off-cell activity were restored following systemic administration of naloxone (1 mg/kg). Tail heat trials are indicated by *triangles* below the ratemeter trace. *Filled triangles* (and TF) indicate that a tail flick reflex occurred on that trial, *open triangles* that there was no tail flick when the tail was heated. (From ref. 110, with permission.)

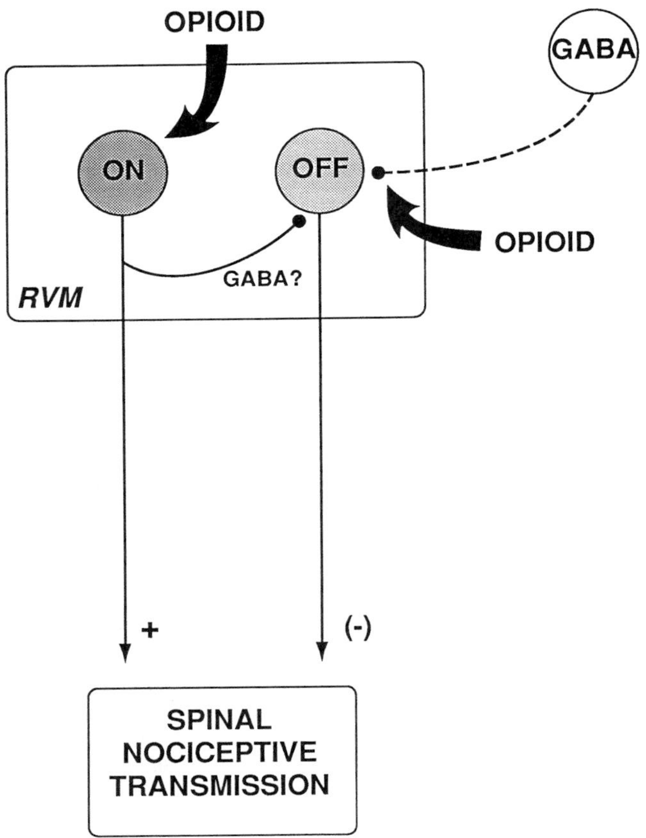

Figure 7. Indirect opioid activation of off-cells via inhibition of a GABAergic inhibitory interneuron. On-cells are the only RVM neurons known to respond to opioids directly. Some on-cells may contain GABA and function as inhibitory interneurons within the RVM. Thus, antinociception results when these neurons are inhibited with an opioid, or if their inhibitory effect on the off-cell is blocked by local application of a $GABA_A$ receptor antagonist. An additional possibility, that opioids act presynaptically to inhibit GABA release from terminals entering the RVM from some other site, is also shown.

sive response resulting from a withdrawal of descending inhibition (i.e., the decrease in off-cell firing), but rather is an active facilitatory process that is mediated by recruitment of some descending projection originating in or passing through the RVM (135). Activation of on-cells is also likely to be involved in the facilitation of some nocifensive reflexes that can result from prolonged noxious stimulation applied to a second body region (186,188).

Thus, the weight of evidence is that the opposing firing patterns exhibited by on- and off-cell populations are, at least under some conditions, responsible for substantial alterations in nociceptive responsiveness. The existence of two classes of modulatory neurons with complementary properties is particularly significant, as it provides a potential basis for bidirectional modulation of nociception from the RVM (70,81,91, 259). The fact that electrical stimulation in RVM typically produces an antinociception does not argue against a dual outflow from this region, because electrical stimulation would activate both facilitatory and inhibitory efferent streams, and because the relative effectiveness of inhibiting and facilitating influences on dorsal horn processing could be very different. We have recently shown that disinhibition of off-cells is sufficient to inhibit the tail flick reflex irrespective of whether activity of on-cells is increased or decreased (112). Moreover, electrical or chemical stimulation in the RVM has been reported to produce a facilitation of nociceptive reflexes and an increase in the activity of dorsal horn neurons under some conditions (91,142,160,243). Indeed, Zhuo and Gebhart (285–287) have demonstrated, in a series of careful studies, that many stimulation sites in RVM support an intensity-dependent biphasic effect, with facilitation followed by inhibition as current intensity is increased.

It should be recognized that controls mediated by the RVM are not called into play only at the extremes of nociceptive hypo- and hyperresponsiveness (as exemplified by the effects of exogenous morphine administration or naloxone-precipitated withdrawal). It has in fact been shown that RVM outflow exerts a tonic control over nociceptive responses (69,108). Furthermore, there is evidence that moment-to-moment variations in nociceptive threshold are related to shifts in the balance of ongoing discharges between on- and off-cell populations (104). To add to the complexity of the situation, the balance of ongoing discharges between on- and off-cell populations is itself under the influence of afferent input (105,186,188, 213). Thus, brainstem modulation of nociceptive processing is not an extraordinary control superimposed upon normal neuronal afferent traffic. Rather, it should be considered a continuing and integral aspect of afferent processing of nociceptive information under physiologic conditions.

PAG AND RVM LINKAGES: NEUROTRANSMITTERS AND PHARMACOLOGY

The functional significance of the connection between the PAG and RVM is firmly grounded in data obtained using nonselective lesion and electrical stimulation approaches. Nonetheless, a full elucidation of the circuitry linking these two regions has not been straightforward. This is in large part because the various physiologically and neurochemically distinct cell populations are intermingled within each region in a way that precludes a full analysis using these nonselective methods. This consideration has prompted a more selective approach, in which pharmacologic tools, such as microinjection of selective agonists and antagonists or microiontophoresis, are used to activate or interfere with the function of a pharmacologically distinct subset of neurons within each region. Among the neurotransmitters that have been identified in PAG-RVM projection neurons are excitatory amino acids, neurotensin, serotonin, and somatostatin (27,29,53, 265).

Excitatory Amino Acid Neurotransmitters

Several avenues of investigation have suggested an important role for excitatory amino acid transmission in the PAG projection to the RVM. Neurons immunoreactive for glutamate and aspartate are found throughout the PAG, with the most concentrated distribution in the dorsal and lateral subdivisions (53). Many of these neurons are undoubtedly involved in local connections within the PAG, but a substantial number likely project to the RVM, as indicated by retrograde transport of D-[^{3}H]aspartate (265). Beitz and Williams (30) have shown that chemical stimulation of PAG neurons using focal application of D, L-homocysteic acid leads to an increase in release of aspartate and glutamate in RVM, and the functional significance of this release has been confirmed in behavioral experiments. Thus, microinjection of nonselective excitatory amino acid antagonists into the RVM significantly increases the current required to inhibit the tail flick using PAG stimulation, and attenuates the increase in tail flick latency produced by PAG morphine microinjection (3,251). Moreover, iontophoretic application of nonselective excitatory amino acid antagonists (γ-D-glutamylglycine and kynurenate) attenuates the short-latency excitation of RVM neurons evoked by PAG stimulation

(265). Viewed collectively, these observations favor the idea that excitatory amino acid–containing neurons are important in the connection between the PAG and RVM.

Neurotensin

The role of neurotensin in the relation between PAG and RVM is of particular interest. This thirteen amino acid peptide is widely distributed throughout the PAG, with a high concentration in the ventrolateral subdivision (238). Neurotensin excites PAG neurons, both in vivo and in vitro (22,24), and microinjection of neurotensin within the PAG produces an antinociception that is mediated through the RVM (6,22).

Within the RVM, the effects of neurotensin are apparently more complex than in the PAG. Microinjection of neurotensin within the RVM has a dose-related biphasic effect, with lower doses facilitating responses on several tests of nociception (247), and higher doses producing a dose-related antinociception (73,247). The physiologic mechanisms that would account for such a dose-response relation for exogenous neurotensin are not clear. Microinjection of a neurotensin antagonist or neurotensin antibody has no effect on baseline tail flick latencies, and thus rules out a hypoalgesic effect of ongoing neurotensin release within the RVM. However, interference with neurotensin transmission within the RVM does enhance the antinociceptive efficacy of morphine microinjected into the PAG. This facilitation is specific for the PAG outflow activated by morphine, since a similar facilitation of the antinociceptive actions of β-endorphin does not occur (247,248). Thus, morphine acting within the PAG produces a dual effect within the RVM, with both analgesic and antianalgesic influences, the latter mediated by release of neurotensin. This finding therefore extends to the PAG-RVM axis the idea of "antianalgesia peptides," the spinal release of which has been proposed to be coordinated with, and in functional opposition to, that of analgesia-promoting substances (66,173).

Sources of neurotensin afferents to the RVM include the nucleus reticularis paragigantocellularis (Pgi) caudal to the facial nucleus, and cells in the A1 and A5 regions, as well as the PAG itself (27). Thus, one possibility is that morphine acting within the PAG disinhibits PAG-RVM projection neurons, some of which contain neurotensin. Activation of this subset of the PAG output would partially counteract the effects of the antinociceptive PAG outflow to the RVM. Indirect connections (via Pgi or the A5 region for example) are another possibility (250).

Serotonin

The role of serotonin (5-HT) in the connection between the PAG and RVM is clearly important, yet poorly understood. It has been demonstrated that interfering with serotonin transmission within the RVM greatly attenuates the antinociceptive effect of PAG morphine microinjections (138). 5-HT_{1C} and/or 5-HT_2 as well as 5-HT_3 receptors seem to be involved in this effect (139). Moreover, microinjection of serotonin itself within the RVM has been reported to produce an antinociception (127,161; but see 3). However, the origin of the relevant serotonergic inputs and the serotonin pharmacology of different RVM cell populations have not been determined.

The dorsal raphe and PAG are a significant source of serotonergic inputs to the RVM (27), but it is not known whether these neurons are activated by morphine microinjected into the PAG, or whether PAG morphine leads to activation of serotonergic neurons within the RVM itself. A substantial number of RVM neurons contain serotonin. Although many serotonergic neurons in RVM project to the spinal cord, some may have local collaterals within the RVM, and other serotonergic neurons may serve as local interneurons (43,239).

Electrophysiologic studies in which iontophoretic techniques were utilized have demonstrated that many RVM neurons respond to serotonin. Unfortunately, a consistent picture has not emerged, with a predominant excitation (161), inhibition (202,266), or opposing effects on different neurons (120,262) reported in different studies. It has been proposed that excitatory effects of serotonin in this region are mediated by an action at a 5-HT_2 receptor, whereas inhibitory effects are due to an action at a 5-HT_1-like receptor (55,56) (see Bobker and Williams [38] for review of ionic mechanisms associated with activation of different receptor subtypes in vertebrate CNS). Interestingly, investigations of the extent to which the physiologically characterized cell classes in RVM show distinct responses to serotonin indicate that individual neurons of on-, off-, and neutral cell classes can be both excited and inhibited by serotonin agonists acting at different serotonin receptor subtypes (111). In view of the behavioral evidence demonstrating an important role for serotonin within the RVM, these electrophysiologic results suggest that serotonin has a rather broad neuromodulatory role in controlling RVM circuitry.

Opioids

The antinociception resulting from PAG morphine microinjection is attenuated by microinjection of a μ– or δ-opioid antagonist within the RVM (140). Because there is evidently no physiologically relevant tonic opioidergic control over RVM circuitry (3,140), this observation implies that administration of an exogenous opioid within the PAG provokes release of an endogenous opioid within the RVM. Consistent with this inference is the fact that on-cells, which are the only RVM neurons known to be directly sensitive to opioids, are inhibited when morphine is microinjected into the PAG (51,187). Indeed, the suppression of on-cell firing following PAG morphine microinjection is indistinguishable from that seen following local application of an opioid agonist within the RVM itself (110).

Few enkephalin-immunoreactive neurons in the PAG project directly to the RVM (25,268), and the direct projection from the PAG to both on- and off-cells in RVM is predominantly excitatory (146,170,252). Thus, the inhibition of RVM on-cells by PAG morphine is most likely accomplished through activation of opioidergic neurons that project to the RVM from some other site. Enkephalin-containing neurons that project to the medial aspect of the RVM have been identified in nucleus cuneiformis and the dorsal parabrachial region, as well as within the RVM itself (25). The latter projection is potentially quite interesting as it may involve off-cells. Off-cells are excited by electrical stimulation of the PAG (252), activated following PAG morphine microinjection (51), and have been shown to have axon collaterals within the RVM (176). Thus, it is an intriguing possibility that a subset of off-cells are themselves opioidergic, and that activation of these off-cells contributes to the inhibition of on-cells following PAG morphine microinjection.

This analysis of the circuitry linking the PAG with the RVM fits well with the observations of Rossi et al. (226), who reported that concurrent administration of morphine in the PAG and RVM produced an antinociception that was greater than the sum of effects obtained from each site individually. Moreover, inactivation of the PAG (using local application of a local anesthetic agent) abolishes the antinociceptive effect of opioid application in the lateral RVM (225). Thus, the well-established idea of a synergistic relationship between spinal and supraspinal opioid analgesia substrates (181,223,282) can be extended to include interactions within the brain itself. Indeed, the PAG-RVM axis appears to be linked with opioid-sensitive sites in forebrain, among them nucleus accumbens and the amygdala, which have direct as well as indirect (e.g., via the habenula) reciprocal connections with the PAG and with each other (26,96,97,145,154–156,194,201, 219,237). Significantly, some PAG neurons projecting to nucleus

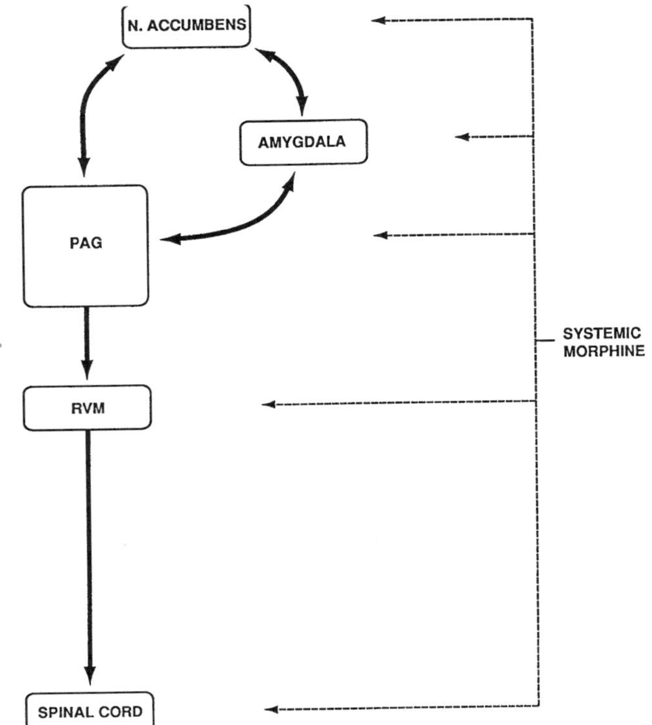

Figure 8. Schematic diagram of connections among opioid-sensitive sites at multiple levels of the neuraxis that are likely to contribute to the antinociceptive potency of opioids given systemically. The synergy between spinal and supraspinal opioid-sensitive sites is well established. Recent evidence now suggests a synergistic opioidergic relationship between the PAG and RVM, and connections linking PAG, amygdala, and nucleus accumbens have been proposed to form an opioid-dependent "mesolimbic loop."

accumbens and amygdala are enkephalin-immunoreactive (153,155). Both nucleus accumbens and amygdala show substantial levels of opioid peptides and receptors (58,95,174), and local microinjection of opioids at either site produces an antinociception (67,102,116,246). (However, the antinociceptive effects of morphine microinjected into the nucleus accumbens should be interpreted with caution, as these microinjections also elicit significant catalepsy [67].) Moreover, Ma and Han's team (167–169) has provided evidence for an opioid-dependent "mesolimbic loop" connecting the PAG with nucleus accumbens and amygdala. Thus, the antinociceptive potency of morphine administered systemically most likely reflects its ability to simultaneously activate elements of an interconnected opioidergic network whose elements span the neuraxis, from forebrain to spinal cord (Fig. 8).

Relation of Pontine Noradrenergic Cell Groups to the PAG-RVM Axis

There is substantial evidence that the release of noradrenaline at spinal levels contributes to the antinociception induced by stimulating neurons within the RVM. RVM stimulation–produced antinociception is diminished by intrathecal application of (α-adrenergic antagonists (4,13,101,128,131,227,273), and stimulation in the RVM releases noradrenaline (NA) into superfusates collected from the spinal cord (100). Since noradrenaline-containing cell bodies are not found within the RVM (150), the antinociception elicited from midline structures must, in part, be mediated by activation of pontospinal noradrenergic neurons.

One mechanism that has been proposed to underlie a recruitment of noradrenergic systems by RVM stimulation is antidromic activation of brainstem collaterals of spinally projecting catecholamine-containing neurons. Spinally projecting neurons of the A5 cell group are reported to send axon collaterals into the RVM (15). Thus, electrical stimulation in either one of these regions could activate A5 neurons antidromically. However, this cannot be a complete explanation for how norepinephrine comes to contribute to the antinociception elicited from the RVM, since norepinephrine is also implicated in the antinociception resulting from microinjection of glutamate or morphine (128,131). An alternative explanation would be that neurons in the RVM project to and activate pontine cells that contain noradrenaline. Both A7 and A5 regions receive a substantial projection from the RVM, with that to the A7 area being the more dense (52). The projection from the RVM to A7 has been shown to include substance P (280), but not serotonin (52). Microinjection of substance P into the A7 region produces a bilateral antinociception that is attenuated by intrathecal application of (ga>$_2$-adrenergic antagonists (281). Although not conclusive, these data suggest that activation of substance P–containing neurons in RVM could excite A7 noradrenergic neurons that project to the dorsal horn and exert an antinociceptive effect (279,280).

In addition to mediating some of the spinal effects resulting from activation of RVM, norepinephrine also modulates the activity of RVM neurons. The RVM receives a noradrenergic input (99), although the source of this input is not entirely clear (15,45). Local microinjection of the nonselective α-adrenergic antagonist phentolamine into the RVM produces an increase in nociceptive threshold as measured using the tail flick and hot plate tests (98,99). An analysis of the receptor subtypes involved in this effect revealed opposing roles for norepinephrine acting at α_1- and α_2-adrenergic receptors in RVM, with the α_1-receptor facilitating, and the α_2-receptor inhibiting, nociception. Thus, in awake rats, microinjection of the selective α_1-antagonist prazosin produced antinociception, whereas the α_2-selective antagonist yohimbine enhanced nociceptive responsiveness. The opposing behavioral consequences of α_1- and α_2-receptor activation within RVM were confirmed using microinjection of selective agonists: microinjection of the α_2-selective agonist clonidine yielded antinociception, and the α_1-selective compound phenylephrine yielded hyperalgesia (103,228).

Although iontophoretic application of norepinephrine itself has been reported to exert both excitatory and inhibitory effects on RVM neurons (23,262,266), the opposing behavioral effects can be most easily explained by opposing effects of α_1- and α_2-receptor activation on one class of RVM neuron, the on-cells. On-cells, but not off-cells or neutral cells, respond to iontophoretic application of norepinephrine and selective receptor agonists. The response to norepinephrine applied by iontophoresis is a slow, long-lasting facilitation that is blocked by the α_1-receptor antagonist prazosin, but not the α_2-receptor antagonists yohimbine or idazoxan, indicating an α_1-mediated excitation of this cell class. The α_2-receptor agonist clonidine produced an α_2-mediated inhibitory action in these same neurons (106).

Thus, like opioids, α_2-adrenergic agonists exert a selective suppressive effect on the firing of on-cells when applied using iontophoresis, and a behaviorally measurable antinociception when microinjected into the RVM (103,109,110,228). This antinociception is mediated in part by release of norepinephrine at spinal levels (99,227,229), indicating that suppression of on-cell firing in some way permits increased activity of pontospinal noradrenergic neurons. One possibility is that suppression of on-cell firing disinhibits substance P–containing neurons projecting from the RVM to the A7 cell group (279, 280).

ASCENDING MODULATION INVOLVING THE PAG-RVM AXIS

Role in Noxious-Evoked Behaviors

The preceding discussion has emphasized that modulation of nociception operates at very early stages in central transmission, with an impact on first-order neurons or even primary afferent terminals in the dorsal horn (17,33). Clearly, it would be of considerable value to regulate the earliest steps in processing, so as to preempt spinally organized reflexes that could interfere with higher priority defensive behaviors. However, responses to noxious stimulation are not limited to reflexive withdrawal from the source of painful input. Individuals are capable of discriminating the location, intensity, and duration of noxious stimuli, and of making judgments about their affective qualities (180), processes that require that supraspinal centers be engaged. There is evidence that these later stages of nociceptive processing are themselves subject to modulation. The effects of PAG or RVM activation on supraspinally organized responses have been characterized in a number of behavioral studies. In these experiments, the effectiveness of PAG or RVM activation in inhibiting supraspinally organized nociceptive responses was sometimes spared under conditions in which descending inhibition was removed. For example, intrathecal administration of amine antagonists eliminated the ability of intracerebral morphine or stimulation in the PAG or RVM to inhibit spinal withdrawal reflexes, but did not block inhibition of supraspinally organized responses (128,273). Further evidence in support of an ascending influence from PAG was provided by Morgan et al. (189), who demonstrated that a lesion that transected the caudally directed outflow from the PAG, thus abolishing the antinociceptive effects of PAG stimulation on the spinally mediated tail flick reflex, did not disrupt stimulation-produced inhibition of the supraspinally organized response on the hot plate test.

Ascending Circuitry

The circuitry involved in the ascending control mechanisms inferred from these behavioral studies has received relatively little attention, in part because the potential targets for ascending modulation are so numerous, but also because our understanding of the supraspinal mechanisms of nociceptive processing is still very incomplete. The PAG is known to have extensive rostral projections, with targets in both diencephalic and telencephalic regions implicated in nociception (50,54,71,175,219). Projections to medial thalamus are particularly dense, and may be important in modulating affective aspects of pain sensation (44). One particularly intriguing observation is that some PAG neurons have axon collaterals directed both caudally, to the RVM, and rostrally, to the medial thalamus or hypothalamus. Activation of neurons making such bifurcating ascending and descending connections would potentially be able to influence both thalamic and spinal nociceptive processing simultaneously (216). The RVM itself also has ascending projections, including targets in medial thalamus (50,204).

Electrophysiologic approaches to this problem are complicated by the fact that any change in central processing may be secondary to descending modulation of ascending spinal input. This is a particular weakness in many electrophysiologic studies in which electrical or chemical stimulation of PAG or RVM was shown to alter noxious-evoked activity at supraspinal sites. For instance, in both rat and cat, stimulation in the PAG has been shown to block noxious-evoked activity of neurons in medial thalamus (7,212). Unfortunately, there were no controls that would have ensured that the observed central changes were not simply a reflection of changes at the spinal level, so these results must be interpreted with caution. However, other experiments provide more convincing evidence in favor of an ascending influence. In one experiment in cat, nociceptive neurons in the shell region of nucleus ventralis posterolateralis (VPL) were shown to be inhibited by PAG stimulation (126). This depression of VPL activity was not eliminated by lesions of the descending outflow from the RVM in the spinal dorsolateral funiculus, thus implicating an ascending pathway. Electrical stimulation in the RVM was also shown to inhibit nociceptive neurons in VPL, but the interpretation of this result is complicated by the fact that glutamate microinjection at the same site was ineffective (143). This raises the question as to whether the effect of electrical stimulation in RVM may have been mediated by an antidromic activation of PAG-RVM projection neurons that have collateral projections to the diencephalon (216). Electrical stimulation in the RVM was also demonstrated to attenuate cortical potentials evoked by foot shock or stimulation in VPL, but to have no effect on visual-evoked potentials (87). These effects were not blocked by lesions of the spinal cord dorsolateral funiculus, again implicating an ascending pathway that would influence thalamic or thalamocortical processing. Thus, much work clearly remains to be done, yet the convergence of behavioral, anatomical, and physiologic evidence suggests an important role for ascending modulatory systems.

FUNCTIONAL SIGNIFICANCE OF NOCICEPTIVE MODULATION FROM PAG AND RVM

Antinociception as a Component of Defensive Responses

It is well documented that the analgesia resulting from stimulation in the PAG can be associated with overt behavioral reactions. These can include flight, jumping, freezing, gnawing, or vocalization, depending on the region stimulated (80, 134,179,183,207,278). Various interpretations of these behaviors have been advanced:

1. Response to an aversive state generated by the stimulus. Fardin et al. (80) have suggested that the motor responses are indications of an aversive state produced by the stimulation. This was presumed to provoke a "stress-induced analgesia" through some unspecified mechanism. However, others have shown that stress-induced analgesia cannot account for the observed antinociception, since the motor and antinociceptive effects of PAG stimulation can be dissociated pharmacologically (184).
2. Behavior generated by activating PAG neurons receiving input from ascending nociceptive pathways. Jensen and Yaksh (133,134) suggest that the coordinated behaviors evoked by PAG stimulation represent a pain-like state resulting from activation of PAG neurons that receive nociceptive spinomesencephalic inputs. However, these authors acknowledge that stimulation in other sites that receive nociceptive input does not produce similar behaviors, suggesting that this also cannot be a sufficient explanation.
3. Component of a defense response. Behaviors evoked by PAG stimulation closely resemble behavioral components of the defensive responses that are normally elicited by threatening or fear-inducing stimuli in the environment (75,183). Many of the behaviors produced by PAG stimulation are also seen in rats confronted with a potential predator. The specific response provoked in a given situation shows an orderly relationship with the immediacy of the threat

and possibilities for escape. For example, when a rat encounters a potential predator at a distance of several meters or more, the most likely response is flight. If an escape route is not available, the animal is likely to "freeze," entering a state of alert immobility. Freezing presumably helps the animal escape the attention of the predator. However, if the predator does approach more closely, "defensive threat," in which the rat faces its attacker and vocalizes, is followed by "defensive attack," which includes jumping and biting (35,36). Thus, the flight, freezing, vocalization, and jump-attack elicited by stimulation in discrete areas of the PAG very likely represent behavioral components of specific defense responses.

Role of PAG-RVM Axis in Defense Responses

This conclusion that PAG stimulation evokes components of defense reactions is further strengthened by the observation that various autonomic changes considered to be important elements of defensive responding are also produced by PAG stimulation (11,166,198,278). In general, activation of neurons in the region lateral to the cerebral aqueduct provokes a sympathoexcitation, with an increase in blood pressure, inhibition of arterial baroreflexes, and a redirection of the cardiac output from the viscera to skeletal muscle. Interestingly, the pressor response evoked by activation of neurons in the caudal third of the PAG is associated with an increase in blood flow to skeletal muscle of the hindlimb. In contrast, activation of more rostral sites within this lateral column leads to an increase in flow to the face and head (48) (Fig. 9). These two distinct patterns of altered blood flow parallel specific defensive behaviors obtained with stimulation at equivalent sites in awake animals. In the cat, stimulation at caudal sites elicits running and attempts to escape, whereas more rostral placements elicit a forward-oriented, but stationary, threat display, with hissing and howling (9,284). Thus, as shown schematically in Fig. 9, the differential patterns of altered blood flow resulting from stimulation at caudal and intermediate levels of the lateral PAG are organized to support the somatomotor components of defense that are elicited from those sites.

A similar rostrocaudal organization of defensive responses within the lateral PAG has been also been demonstrated in the rat (60,61). Microinjections of small volumes of kainic acid generally elicit an immobility or freezing response in which the animal remains motionless if undisturbed. However, introduction of another rat evokes distinct patterns of defensive behaviors in the PAG-stimulated animals, which vary depending on the rostrocaudal location of the microinjection. In the intermediate lateral PAG, kainic acid microinjection leads to a "backing defense," in which the stimulated animal faces toward the intruder. With more caudal placements, introduction of a partner causes a "forward defense," in which the stimulated animal shows bursts of forward movement. Kainic acid stimulation at these more caudal sites is also associated with ultrasonic vocalizations and enhanced responses to innocuous tactile stimulation of the contralateral body. Although patterns of altered blood flow have not been examined in this paradigm, microinjections at equivalent sites in the lateral PAG of decerebrated rats evoke increases in blood pressure and heart rate (61). Thus, within the lateral PAG of both cats and rats, stimulation at different rostrocaudal levels evokes distinct defensive responses, and there is a close coordination of the behavioral and vasomotor components of the response evoked from each site.

More ventrally, in the ventrolateral aspect of the caudal PAG, stimulation produces a suppression of movement in both cats and rats (10,75,183,284), and has a depressor effect (49,164). The implication of this phenomenon for defensive responding has been a matter of debate, with two very different functions

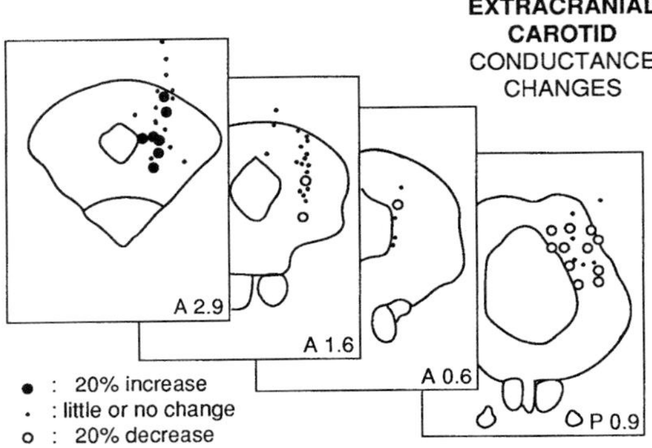

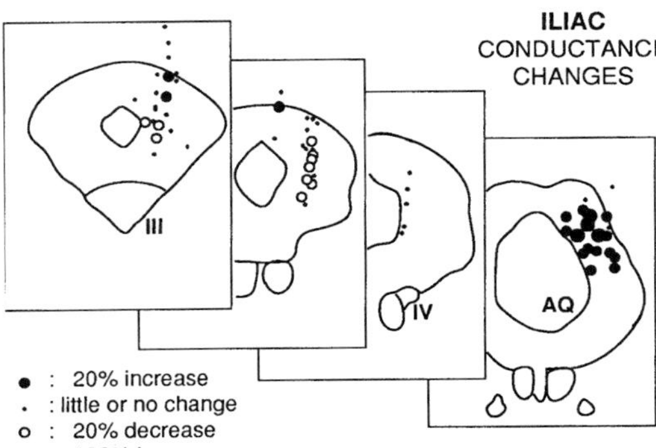

Figure 9. Sites in the lateral PAG at which microinjection of the neuroexcitant D,L-homocysteic acid resulted in changes in extracranial carotid and iliac blood flow. Vasodilator and vasoconstrictor sites, characterized by a greater than 20% change in conductance, are indicated by *filled* and *open circles,* respectively. Increased flow to the hindlimb, resulting from an increase in iliac conductance, was obtained from sites in the caudal third of the lateral PAG. Increased flow to the face and head was obtained from more rostral sites. AQ, cerebral aqueduct; III, oculomotor nucleus; IV, trochlear nucleus. (From ref.48, with permission.)

proposed. On the one hand, the antinociception, immobility, and sympathoinhibition have been argued to represent a state of behavioral inhibition and recuperation, or even relaxation, that follows an injury or episode of intense exertion (11,49,62, 137,166). On the other hand, several lines of evidence suggest a second interpretation. First, recovery following an injury or illness is commonly thought to be associated not with analgesia, but with an enhanced nociceptive responsiveness (39,263,264, 271). Moreover, freezing (i.e., immobility) is a well-characterized antipredator defensive behavior, at least in rodents. It is in fact the dominant response in situations in which the threat is relatively distant but there is no opportunity to escape (35,36). In addition, fear-associated freezing is blocked by lesions of the caudal ventrolateral PAG (149,159). Finally, in various species of wild rodents, freezing elicited in response to a visual threat is accompanied by a fall in blood pressure (123). These considerations suggest that, like the behaviors and sympathoexcitation elicited from the lateral PAG, the immobility and sympathoinhibition produced by stimulation in the ventrolateral PAG also represent elements of a specific, active defense reaction. Further work will clearly be needed to resolve this issue.

In any case, it should be clear that activation of neurons in different regions of the PAG yields characteristic patterns of behavioral and physiologic effects that mimic the specific defensive reactions elicited by different environmental threats (Fig. 10). This realization leads to the current view of PAG function in nociceptive modulation, which is that this region is

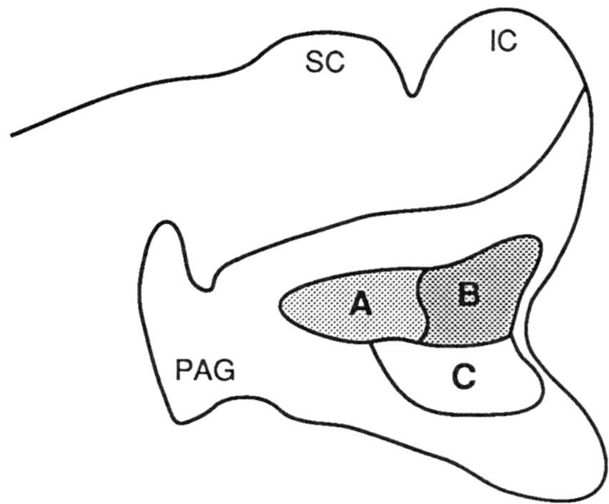

Figure 10. Schematic representation of a sagittal section of the PAG summarizing the coordination of behavioral and vasomotor aspects of defensive responding with the antinociception obtained from different regions of the lateral and ventrolateral PAG. PAG, periaqueductal gray; SC, superior colliculus; IC, inferior colliculus. (From ref. 10, with permission.

important in integrating and coordinating responses needed for survival in a range of stressful and threatening situations. From this perspective, nociceptive modulation can be considered an important element in various forms of defensive responding that are integrated within the PAG.

ACTIVATION OF PAG-RVM SYSTEMS IN BEHAVING ANIMALS

The discussion up to now has focused on experimental manipulations of brainstem nociceptive modulatory circuitry using electrical or chemical stimulation, including opiates. This work has been quite fruitful in delineating connections between the PAG and RVM, and the role of descending projections from the RVM in modulating nociceptive transmission at the level of the spinal cord. However, our understanding of how these systems come to be activated in behaving animals is still fragmentary.

Activation by Noxious Inputs: A Negative-Feedback Loop

Much early work in this area was based on the idea of a negative-feedback loop in which descending inhibition was invoked directly by nociceptive information conveyed to the PAG and/or RVM over spinoreticular and spinomesencephalic systems, and via collaterals of axons continuing to more rostral sites (17). This view that "pain inhibits pain" was grounded in the well-documented ability of one noxious stimulus to alter responses to a second noxious stimulus applied to a distant region of the body. Numerous illustrations of this potent heterosegmental inhibition have been provided, with noxious-evoked activity in the dorsal horn and nocifensive reflexes usually depressed by a remote noxious stimulus. Pain experienced by human subjects is also susceptible to this form of inhibition (144,147,190,242,258,267).

However, although the ability of one noxious stimulus to alter responses to another noxious stimulus is well supported, it has become increasingly apparent that activation of the PAG-RVM axis does not have a unique or primary role in this form of nociceptive regulation. Thus, using a lesion approach, Watkins and colleagues (257,261) demonstrated that the PAG is not required for the unconditioned analgesia that occurs for a short period (2 to 4 min) immediately following an episode of intense forepaw shock, although this analgesia is blocked by lesions of the RVM. In addition, the antinociceptive effect of hindpaw shock on the tail flick reflex does not involve brainstem circuits, since this form of antinociception is not abolished following transection of the thoracic spinal cord (258).

Similarly, the PAG-RVM system does not appear to have a critical role in the heterosegmental inhibition of nociceptive neurons in the dorsal horn elicited by application of a noxious stimulus applied to a second, distant, region of the body (147,188,195). This is a well-characterized effect that has been termed diffuse noxious inhibitory control (DNIC) (147), and has been advanced as a neurophysiologic model for counterirritation phenomena. Although early studies indicated that DNIC was blocked by lesions of the RVM (65), more recent work demonstrates that this is not the case (40,41,188). It is now thought that DNIC is mediated in large part by neurons in the subnucleus reticularis dorsalis (SRD) in the caudal medulla (42). Neurons in the SRD have properties that would be consistent with a role in DNIC. They are excited by noxious thermal, mechanical, and visceral stimulation applied to large areas of the body (254,255), and have descending projections to the spinal cord via the dorsolateral funiculus, with terminations in laminae V, VI, VII, and X (31). In addition, the possibility that propriospinal connections with neurons at the C1-C2 level play an important role in heterosegmental inhibition is also receiving increasing attention (46,94,122,232).

There is thus an important involvement of connections through the caudal medulla and within the spinal cord, but not the PAG and RVM, in the heterosegmental inhibition of nociception produced by application of a different noxious stimulus. Although heterosegmental inhibition may form the basis for various counterirritation therapies that have been part of pain treatment for centuries, a physiologic role of such inhibitory interactions is still undetermined. Indeed, heterosegmental facilitation of nociception is obtained in some paradigms (188,213,263). One recent proposal is that heterosegmental inhibition is important in coordinating protective reflexes and organizing motor responses in situations where noxious inputs are impinging on multiple regions of the body (208). There is, however, no direct evidence that this is the case.

Role of Fear in Activation of the PAG-RVM System

A very different approach to the physiologic function of the PAG-RVM system is to consider nociceptive modulation within the larger context of integrating and organizing defensive responses to noxious or threatening aspects of the environment (10,75,166). Presumably the value of suppressing nociception in potentially dangerous circumstances is that it lessens the likelihood that the distress or overt behaviors that would otherwise be evoked by a painful stimulus might diminish the likelihood of an effective response (see Bolles and Fanselow [39] for discussion).

Investigators taking this approach have shown that antinociception can be produced by biologically relevant threat stimuli, such as an attacking conspecific or potential predator (75,79, 136,157,222). Antinociception is also elicited as a conditioned response to previously neutral cues that have been paired in a classical conditioning paradigm with noxious or aversive events (74). This latter phenomenon, termed conditional hypoalgesia, has been of particular interest, in part because the eliciting stimuli are not themselves intrinsically noxious. Conditional hypoalgesia is blocked by lesions of the PAG or the RVM (119, 141,257). An involvement of endogenous opioids in conditional hypoalgesia is shown by the finding that it can be blocked by opiate receptor antagonists (76,158,256). Moreover, opioid transmission within the PAG is specifically implicated, since microinjection of naltrexone into the ventrolateral PAG also attenuates conditional hypoalgesia (118). It should, however, be noted that the effectiveness of opioid antagonists in preventing conditioned hypoalgesia can be overcome by increasing the severity of the conditioning procedures (158).

Stimuli that elicit conditional hypoalgesia apparently gain access to modulatory circuitry of the PAG and RVM at least in part by means of fear-related processes organized in the amygdala (113–115,260). The amygdala, a structure with a well-documented role in fear (2,57), has dense reciprocal connections with the PAG. These connections are organized in a rostrocaudally oriented columns that overlap the regions in which PAG neurons projecting to the RVM are also found (219). Direct experimental manipulations of the amygdala lead to parallel alterations in measures of fear and conditional hypoalgesia. Thus, lesions of the amygdala, or microinjection of a benzodiazepine anxiolytic agent prevent both fear (as measured by freezing) and, in parallel, the hypoalgesia conditioned to stimuli paired with shock (113,115,148,172,260). Amygdala lesions also attenuate freezing and analgesia in rats exposed to a cat (34,88). It has been demonstrated that pharmacologic manipulations that would be expected to modify fear also alter at least some forms of conditional analgesia. For instance, systemic administration of anxiolytic agents such as diazepam or midazolam attenuates both freezing and conditioned hypoalgesia elicited by shock-associated cues (77,171), as does direct local application of diazepam in the amygdala (114). Conversely, inverse agonists at the benzodiazepine receptor, which would be expected to have an anxiogenic or fear-promoting effect, yield a hypoalgesia after either intracerebral or systemic administration (78,117,221). Furthermore, lesions of the ventral PAG can block expression of conditional fear as well as hypoalgesia (75,119,141,149). Taken together, the above findings suggest that one way in which the modulatory circuitry of the PAG and RVM could be activated physiologically in behaving animals is through fear elicited by signals for danger, whether learned or innate.

Hyperalgesia Associated with Illness

Although the primary focus of investigators interested in pain modulation has been on mechanisms of pain inhibition, it has become clear that endogenous mechanisms of pain facilitation also exist in the central nervous system. It has been proposed that a mechanism by which sensitivity to pain could be enhanced would be useful under conditions of injury or illness. Such a mechanism would facilitate recuperation by promoting quiescence and protection of injured parts (39). Indeed, administration of substances that provoke nonspecific symptoms of illness in rats leads to a long-lasting, centrally mediated hyperalgesia, with decreases in tail flick latencies and enhanced responding on the formalin test. Responses to innocuous pressure are not increased under these conditions. In addition, just as decreased nociceptive responsiveness can be conditioned to neutral stimuli associated with aversive events, augmented sensitivity can be conditioned to tastes that have been paired with illness-inducing agents (264).

Explorations of the neural mechanisms underlying this form of hyperalgesia have only recently begun, but there is some anatomical overlap with PAG-RVM systems already implicated in inhibition of nociception (259). Thus, illness-induced hyperalgesia is blocked by lesions of the medial portion of the RVM and by bilateral transections of the dorsolateral funiculi, which suggests that some medullospinal neurons within the RVM can act to facilitate nociception under these conditions. A role for the RVM is further supported by the observation that this form of hyperalgesia is associated with an increase in the medial RVM of Fos-like immunoreactivity, generally considered a marker for neuronal activation. This proposal is consistent with other evidence indicating that the RVM exerts pronociceptive as well as antinociceptive effects (81).

Additional experiments demonstrate that illness-induced hyperalgesia is abolished by cutting the hepatic branch of the vagus, and by decerebration (259). Thus, the afferent branch of this circuit involves fibers traveling to the nucleus tractus solitarius (NTS) via the vagus. Although pathways subsequent to the NTS are as yet unclear, the RVM is evidently activated via a multisynaptic circuit that includes sites rostral to the middle mesencephalon. Activation of RVM neurons (possibly on-cells, which have been implicated in descending facilitation on other grounds) then leads to enhanced nociceptive responsiveness by means of a descending influence on spinal nociceptive circuitry (173,259).

CONCLUSION

An underlying theme of this chapter has been that modulation is an integral part of the processing of nociceptive information under physiologic conditions. A number of brain sites have been implicated in nociceptive modulation using stimulation, microinjection, and lesion techniques, but the most extensively studied to date has been an opioid-sensitive system with important elements in the PAG and RVM. This system is now known to augment, as well as diminish, nociceptive processing and to influence nociceptive responses organized at both spinal and supraspinal levels. Recent studies of the circuitry of the PAG and RVM reveal that GABA-mediated inhibition has a pivotal role in the pain-modulating function of each region, and that activation of these systems by exogenous opioids involves a disinhibition. Links between the PAG and RVM and other opioid-sensitive sites in brain and spinal cord likely contribute to the potent analgesic action of systemically administered opioids.

Activation of the PAG-RVM system under physiologic conditions in behaving animals remains an area of intense investigation. The PAG, in particular, is now thought to play an important role in integrating and coordinating behavioral and autonomic aspects of defensive responses to noxious or otherwise threatening aspects of the environment. From this vantage point, antinociception, mediated in large part by neurons in RVM, can be viewed as an important element in various forms of defensive responding.

ACKNOWLEDGMENTS

I wish to thank Michael M. Morgan for helpful criticism of this manuscript. This work is supported by grants from NIDA (DA05608) and from the National Headache Foundation.

REFERENCES

1. Abols IA, Basbaum AI. Afferent connections of the rostral medulla of the cat: a neural substrate for midbrain-medullary interactions in the modulation of pain. *J Comp Neurol* 1981;201:285–297.
2. Aggleton JP. *The amygdala. Neurobiological aspects of emotion, memory and mental dysfunction.* New York: Wiley-Liss, 1992.
3. Aimone LD, Gebhart GF. Stimulation-produced spinal inhibition from the midbrain in the rat is mediated by an excitatory amino acid neurotransmitter in the medial medulla. *J Neurosci* 1986;6: 1803–1813.
4. Aimone LD, Jones SL, Gebhart GF. Stimulation-produced descending inhibition from the periaqueductal gray and nucleus raphe magnus in the rat: mediation by spinal monoamines but not opioids. *Pain* 1987;31:123–136.
5. Akaike A, Shibata T, Satoh M, Takagi H. Analgesia induced by microinjection of morphine into, and electrical stimulation of, the nucleus reticularis paragigantocellularis of rat medulla oblongata. *Neuropharmacology* 1978;17:775–778.
6. al-Rodhan NR, Richelson E, Gilbert JA, McCormick DJ, Kanba KS, Pfenning MA, Nelson A, et al. Structure-antinociceptive activity of

neurotensin and some novel analogues in the periaqueductal gray region of the brainstem. *Brain Res* 1991;557:227–235.

6a. Anden NE, Jukes GM, Lundberg A, Vyklicky L. the effects of L-DOPA on the spinal cord. *Acta Physiol Scand* 1966;67:373–386.

7. Andersen E. Periaqueductal gray and cerebral cortex modulate responses of medial thalamic neurons to noxious stimulation. *Brain Res* 1986;375:30–36.
8. Azami J, Llewelyn MB, Roberts MH. The contribution of nucleus reticularis paragigantocellularis and nucleus raphe magnus to the analgesia produced by systemically administered morphine, investigated with the microinjection technique. *Pain* 1982;12:229–246.
9. Bandler R, Carrive P. Integrated defence reaction elicited by excitatory amino acid microinjection in the midbrain periaqueductal grey region of the unrestrained cat. *Brain Res* 1988;439:95–106.
10. Bandler R, DePaulis A. Midbrain periaqueductal gray control of defensive behavior in cat and rat. In: DePaulis A, Bandler R, eds. *Midbrain periaqueductal gray matter.* New York: Plenum Press, 1991; 175–198.
11. Bandler R, Shipley MT. Columnar organization in the midbrain periaqueductal gray: modules for emotional expression? *Trends Neurosci* 1994;17:379–389.
12. Barbaro NM. Studies of PAG/PVG stimulation for pain relief in humans. *Prog Brain Res* 1988;77:165–173.
13. Barbaro NM, Hammond DL, Fields HL. Effects of intrathecally administered methysergide and yohimbine on microstimulation-produced antinociception in the rat. *Brain Res* 1985;343:223–229.
14. Barbaro NM, Heinricher MM, Fields HL. Putative pain modulating neurons in the rostral ventral medulla: reflex-related activity predicts effects of morphine. *Brain Res* 1986;366:203–210.
15. Basbaum AI. Anatomical studies of the noradrenergic projection to the spinal cord dorsal horn. In: Besson JM, Guilbaud G, eds. *Towards the use of noradrenergic agonists for the treatment of pain.* Amsterdam: Elsevier, 1992;77–89.
16. Basbaum AI, Clanton CH, Fields HL. Three bulbospinal pathways from the rostral medulla of the cat: an autoradiographic study of pain modulating systems. *J Comp Neurol* 1978;178:209–224.
17. Basbaum AI, Fields HL. Endogenous pain control systems: brainstem spinal pathways and endorphin circuitry. *Annu Rev Neurosci* 1984;7:309–338.
18. Bederson JB, Fields HL, Barbaro NM. Hyperalgesia during naloxone-precipitated withdrawal from morphine is associated with increased on-cell activity in the rostral ventromedial medulla. *Somatosens Mot Res* 1990;7:185–203.
19. Behbehani MM, Fields HL. Evidence that an excitatory connection between the periaqueductal gray and nucleus raphe magnus mediates stimulation produced analgesia. *Brain Res* 1979;170: 85–93.
20. Behbehani MM, Jiang M, Chandler SD. The effect of [Met]enkephalin on the periaqueductal gray neurons of the rat: an in vitro study. *Neuroscience* 1990;38:373–380.
21. Behbehani MM, Jiang MR, Chandler SD, Ennis M. The effect of GABA and its antagonists on midbrain periaqueductal gray neurons in the rat. *Pain* 1990;40:195–204.
22. Behbehani MM, Pert A. A mechanism for the analgesic effect of neurotensin as revealed by behavioral and electrophysiological techniques. *Brain Res* 1984;324:35–42.
23. Behbehani MM, Pomeroy SL, Mack CE. Interaction between central gray and nucleus raphe magnus: role of norepinephrine. *Brain Res Bull* 1981;6:361–364.
24. Behbehani MM, Shipley MT, McLean JH. Effect of neurotensin on neurons in the periaqueductal gray: an in vitro study. *J Neurosci* 1987;7:2035–2040.
25. Beitz AJ. The nuclei of origin of brain stem enkephalin and substance P projections to the rodent nucleus raphe magnus. *Neuroscience* 1982;7:2753–2768.
26. Beitz AJ. The organization of afferent projections to the midbrain periaqueductal gray of the rat. *Neuroscience* 1982;7:133–159.
27. Beitz AJ. The sites of origin brain stem neurotensin and serotonin projections to the rodent nucleus raphe magnus. *J Neurosci* 1982; 2:829–842.
28. Beitz AJ, Mullett MA, Weiner LL. The periaqueductal gray projections to the rat spinal trigeminal, raphe magnus, gigantocellular pars alpha and paragigantocellular nuclei arise from separate neurons. *Brain Res* 1983;288:307–314.
29. Beitz AJ, Shepard RD, Wells WE. The periaqueductal gray-raphe magnus projection contains somatostatin, neurotensin and serotonin but not cholecystokinin. *Brain Res* 1983;261:132–137.
30. Beitz AJ, Williams FG. Localization of putative amino acid transmitters in the PAG and their relationship to the PAG-raphe magnus pathway. In: DePaulis A, Bandler R, eds. *Midbrain periaqueductal gray matter.* New York: Plenum Press, 1991;305–327.
31. Bernard JF, Villanueva L, Carroue J, Le Bars D. Efferent projections from the subnucleus reticularis dorsalis (SRD): a *Phaseolus vulgaris* leucoagglutinin study in the rat. *Neurosci Lett* 1990;116: 257–262.
32. Besson JM. *Serotonin and pain.* Amsterdam: Excerpta Medica, 1990.
33. Besson JM, Chaouch A. Peripheral and spinal mechanisms of nociception. *Physiol Rev* 1987;67:67–186.
34. Blanchard DC, Blanchard RJ. Innate and conditioned reactions to threat in rats with amygdaloid lesions. *J Comp Physiol Psychol* 1972; 81:281–290.
35. Blanchard RJ, Blanchard DC, Rodgers J, Weiss SM. The characterization and modelling of antipredator defensive behavior. *Neurosci Biobehav Rev* 1990;14:463–472.
36. Blanchard RJ, Flannelly KJ, Blanchard DC. Defensive behavior of laboratory and wild Rattus norvegicus. *J Comp Psychol* 1986;100: 101–107.
37. Blomqvist A, Craig AD. Organization of spinal and trigeminal input to the PAG. In: DePaulis A, Bandler R, eds. *Midbrain periaqueductal gray.* New York: Plenum Press, 1991;345–363.
38. Bobker DH, Williams JT. Ion conductances affected by 5-HT receptor subtypes in mammalian neurons. *Trends Neurosci* 1990;13: 169–173.
39. Bolles RC, Fanselow MS. A perceptual-defensive-recuperative model of fear and pain. *Behav Brain Sci* 1980;3:291–301.
40. Bouhassira D, Bing Z, Le Bars D. Studies of the brain structures involved in diffuse noxious inhibitory controls: the mesencephalon. *J Neurophysiol* 1990;64:1712–1723.
41. Bouhassira D, Bing Z, Le Bars D. Studies of brain structures involved in diffuse noxious inhibitory controls in the rat: the rostral ventromedial medulla. *J Physiol* 1993;463:667–687.
42. Bouhassira D, Villanueva L, Le Bars D. Effects of systemic morphine on diffuse noxious inhibitory controls: role of the periaqueductal grey. *Eur J Pharmacol* 1992;216:149–156.
43. Bowker RM, Westlund KN, Coulter JD. Origins of serotonergic projections to the spinal cord in rat: an immunocytochemical-retrograde transport study. *Brain Res* 1981;226:187–199.
44. Bushnell MC, Duncan GH. Neurophysiological correlates of the affective-motivational dimension of pain. *APS Journal* 1992;1: 240–242.
45. Byrum CE, Guyenet PG. Afferent and efferent connections of the A5 noradrenergic cell group in the rat. *J Comp Neurol* 1987;261: 529–542.
46. Cadden SW, Villanueva L, Chitour D, Le Bars D. Depression of activities of dorsal horn convergent neurones by propriospinal mechanisms triggered by noxious inputs; comparison with diffuse noxious inhibitory controls (DNIC). *Brain Res* 1983;275:1–11.
47. Carlton SM, Leichnetz GR, Young EG, Mayer DJ. Supramedullary afferents of the nucleus raphe magnus in the rat: a study using the transcannula HRP gel and autoradiographic techniques. *J Comp Neurol* 1983;214:43–58.
48. Carrive P, Bandler R. Control of extracranial and hindlimb blood flow by the midbrain periaqueductal grey of the cat. *Exp Brain Res* 1991;84:599–606.
49. Carrive P, Bandler R. Viscerotopic organization of neurons subserving hypotensive reactions within the midbrain periaqueductal grey: a correlative functional and anatomical study. *Brain Res* 1991; 541:206–215.
50. Carstens E, Leah J, Lechner J, Zimmermann M. Demonstration of extensive brainstem projections to medial and lateral thalamus and hypothalamus in the rat. *Neuroscience* 1990;35:609–626.
51. Cheng ZF, Fields HL, Heinricher MM. Morphine microinjected into the periaqueductal gray has differential effects on 3 classes of medullary neurons. *Brain Res* 1986;375:57–65.
52. Clark FM, Proudfit HK. Projections of neurons in the ventromedial medulla to pontine catecholamine cell groups involved in the modulation of nociception. *Brain Res* 1991;540:105–115.
53. Clements JR, Madl JE, Johnson RL, Larson AA, Beitz AJ. Localization of glutamate, glutaminase, aspartate and aspartate aminotransferase in the rat midbrain periaqueductal gray. *Exp Brain Res* 1987;67:594–602.
54. Coffield JA, Bowen KK, Miletic V. Retrograde tracing of projections between the nucleus submedius, the ventrolateral orbital cortex, and the midbrain in the rat. *J Comp Neurol* 1992;321: 488–499.

55. Davies M, Wilkinson LS, Roberts MH. Evidence for depressant 5-HT_1-like receptors on rat brainstem neurones. *Br J Pharmacol* 1988;94:492–499.
56. Davies M, Wilkinson LS, Roberts MHT. Evidence for excitatory 5-HT_2-receptors on rat brainstem neurones. *Br J Pharmacol* 1988;94: 483–491.
57. Davis M. The role of the amygdala in fear and anxiety. *Annu Rev Neurosci* 1992;15:353–375.
58. Delfs JM, Yu L, Ellison GD, Reisine T, Chesselet MF. Regulation of mu-opioid receptor mRNA in rat globus pallidus: effects of enkephalin increases induced by short- and long-term haloperidol administration. *J Neurochem* 1994;63:777–780.
59. Depaulis A, Bandler R. *Midbrain periaqueductal gray matter.* New York: Plenum Press, 1991.
60. Depaulis A, Bandler R, Vergnes M. Characterization of pretentorial periaqueductal gray matter neurons mediating intraspecific defensive behaviors in the rat by microinjections of kainic acid. *Brain Res* 1989;486:121–132.
61. Depaulis A, Keay KA, Bandler R. Longitudinal neuronal organization of defensive reactions in the midbrain periaqueductal gray region of the rat. *Exp Brain Res* 1992;90:307–318.
62. Depaulis A, Keay KA, Bandler R. Quiescence and hyporeactivity evoked by activation of cell bodies in the ventrolateral midbrain periaqueductal gray of the rat. *Exp Brain Res* 1994;99:75–83.
63. Depaulis A, Morgan MM, Liebeskind JC. GABAergic modulation of the analgesic effects of morphine microinjected in the ventral periaqueductal gray matter of the rat. *Brain Res* 1987;436:223–228.
64. Dickenson AH, Le Bars D, Besson JM. An involvement of nucleus raphe magnus in diffuse noxious inhibitory controls (DNIC) in the rat. *Neurosci Lett* 1979;suppl. 5:S375.
65. Dickenson AH, Le Bars D, Besson JM. Diffuse noxious inhibitory controls (DNIC). Effects on trigeminal nucleus caudalis neurones in the rat. *Brain Res* 1980;200:293–305.
66. Dickenson AH, Stanfa LC. The segmental control of pain. In: Besson JM, Guilbaud G, eds. *Towards the use of noradrenergic agonists for the treatment of pain.* Amsterdam: Elsevier, 1992;27–46.
67. Dill RE, Costa E. Behavioral dissociation of the enkephalinergic systems of nucleus accumbens and nucleus caudatus. *Neuropharmacology* 1977;16:323–326.
68. Dostrovsky JO, Deakin JFW. Periaqueductal gray lesions reduce morphine analgesia in the rat. *Neurosci Lett* 1977;4:99–103.
69. Drower EJ, Hammond DL. GABAergic modulation of nociceptive threshold: effects of THIP and bicuculline microinjected in the ventral medulla of the rat. *Brain Res* 1988;450:316–324.
70. Dubner R. Central nervous system facilitation and increased pain. *APS Journal* 1992;1:82–84.
71. Eberhart JA, Morrell JI, Krieger MS, Pfaff DW. An autoradiographic study of projections ascending from the midbrain central gray, and from the region lateral to it, in the rat. *J Comp Neurol* 1985;241:285–310.
72. Fang FG, Haws CM, Drasner K, Williamson A, Fields HL. Opioid peptides (DAGO-enkephalin, dynorphin A(1-13), BAM 22P) microinjected into the rat brainstem: comparison of their antinociceptive effect and their effect on neuronal firing in the rostral ventromedial medulla. *Brain Res* 1989;501:116–128.
73. Fang FG, Moreau JL, Fields HL. Dose-dependent antinociceptive action of neurotensin microinjected into the rostroventromedial medulla of the rat. *Brain Res* 1987;420:171–174.
74. Fanselow MS. Conditioned fear-induced opiate analgesia: a competing motivational state theory of stress analgesia. *Ann N Y Acad Sci* 1986;467:40–54.
75. Fanselow MS. The midbrain periaqueductal gray as a coordinator of action in response to fear and anxiety. In: DePaulis A, Bandler R, eds. *The midbrain periaqueductal gray matter.* New York: Plenum Press, 1991;151–173.
76. Fanselow MS, Calcagnetti DJ, Helmstetter FJ. Role of mu and kappa opioid receptors in conditional fear-induced analgesia: the antagonistic actions of nor-binaltorphimine and the cyclic somatostatin octapeptide, $Cys^2Tyr^3Orn^5Pen^7$-amide. *J Pharmacol Exp Ther* 1989;250:825–830.
77. Fanselow MS, Helmstetter FJ. Conditional analgesia, defensive freezing, and benzodiazepines. *Behav Neurosci* 1988;102:233–243.
78. Fanselow MS, Kim JJ. The benzodiazepine inverse agonist DMCM as an unconditional stimulus for fear-induced analgesia: implications for the role of $GABA_A$ receptors in fear-related behavior. *Behav Neurosci* 1992;106:336–344.
79. Fanselow MS, Sigmundi RA. Species-specific danger signals, endogenous opioid analgesia, and defensive behavior. *J Exp Psychol [Anim Behav]* 1986;12:301–309.
80. Fardin V, Oliveras JL, Besson JM. A reinvestigation of the analgesic effects induced by stimulation of the periaqueductal gray matter in the rat. I. The production of behavioral side effects together with analgesia. *Brain Res* 1984;306:105–123.
81. Fields HL. Is there a facilitating component to central pain modulation. *APS Journal* 1992;1:71–78.
82. Fields HL, Bry J, Hentall I, Zorman G. The activity of neurons in the rostral medulla of the rat during withdrawal from noxious heat. *J Neurosci* 1983;3:2545–2552.
83. Fields HL, Heinricher MM. Anatomy and physiology of a nociceptive modulatory system. *Philos Trans R Soc Lond [Biol]* 1985;308: 361–374.
84. Fields HL, Heinricher MM, Mason P. Neurotransmitters in nociceptive modulatory circuits. *Annu Rev Neurosci* 1991;14:219–245.
85. Fields HL, Vanegas H, Hentall ID, Zorman G. Evidence that disinhibition of brain stem neurones contributes to morphine analgesia. *Nature* 1983;306:684–686.
86. Finley JC, Maderdrut JL, Petrusz P. The immunocytochemical localization of enkephalin in the central nervous system of the rat. *J Comp Neurol* 1981;198:541–565.
87. Follett KA, Gebhart GF. Modulation of cortical evoked potentials by stimulation of nucleus raphe magnus in rats. *J Neurophysiol* 1992;67:820–828.
88. Fox RJ, Sorenson CA. Bilateral lesions of the amygdala attenuate analgesia induced by diverse environmental challenges. *Brain Res* 1994;648:215–221.
89. Gallagher DW, Pert A. Afferents to brain stem nuclei (brain stem raphe, nucleus reticularis pontis caudalis and nucleus gigantocellularis) in the rat as demonstrated by microiontophoretically applied horseradish peroxidase. *Brain Res* 1978;144:257–275.
90. Gebhart GF. Opiate and opioid peptide effects on brain stem neurons: relevance to nociception and antinociceptive mechanisms. *Pain* 1982;12:93–140.
91. Gebhart GF. Can endogenous systems produce pain? *APS Journal* 1992;1:79–81.
92. Gebhart GF, Randich A. Brainstem modulation of nociception. In: Klemm WR, Vertes RP, eds. *Brainstem mechanisms of behavior.* New York: John Wiley, 1990;315–352.
93. Gebhart GF, Sandkuhler J, Thalhammer JG, Zimmermann M. Inhibition of spinal nociceptive information by stimulation in midbrain of the cat is blocked by lidocaine microinjected in nucleus raphe magnus and medullary reticular formation. *J Neurophysiol* 1983;50:1446–1459.
94. Gerhart KD, Yezierski RP, Giesler G Jr., Willis WD. Inhibitory receptive fields of primate spinothalamic tract cells. *J Neurophysiol* 1981;46:1309–1325.
95. Gray TS, Cassell MD, Kiss JZ. Distribution of pro-opiomelanocortin-derived peptides and enkephalins in the rat central nucleus of the amygdala. *Brain Res* 1984;306:354–358.
96. Gray TS, Magnuson DJ. Peptide immunoreactive neurons in the amygdala and the bed nucleus of the stria terminalis project to the midbrain central gray in the rat. *Peptides* 1992;13:451–460.
97. Groenewegen HJ, Russchen FT. Organization of the efferent projections of the nucleus accumbens to pallidal, hypothalamic, and mesencephalic structures: a tracing and immunohistochemical study in the cat. *J Comp Neurol* 1984;223:347–367.
97a. Hagbarth & Kerr, 1954.
98. Hammond DL, Levy RA, Proudfit HK. Hypoalgesia following microinjection of noradrenergic antagonists in the nucleus raphe magnus. *Pain* 1980;9:85–101.
99. Hammond DL, Levy RA, Proudfit HK. Hypoalgesia induced by microinjection of a norepinephrine antagonist in the raphe magnus: reversal by intrathecal administration of a serotonin antagonist. *Brain Res* 1980;201:475–479.
100. Hammond DL, Tyce GM, Yaksh TL. Efflux of 5-hydroxytryptamine and noradrenaline into spinal cord superfusates during stimulation of the rat medulla. *J Physiol* 1985;359:151–162.
101. Hammond DL, Yaksh TL. Antagonism of stimulation-produced antinociception by intrathecal administration of methysergide or phentolamine. *Brain Res* 1984;298:329–337.
102. Han JS, Xuan YT. A mesolimbic neuronal loop of analgesia: I. Activation by morphine of a serotonergic pathway from periaqueductal gray to nucleus accumbens. *Int J Neurosci* 1986;29:109–117.
103. Haws CM, Heinricher MM, Fields HL. α–Adrenergic receptor agonists, but not antagonists, alter the tail-flick latency when

microinjected into the rostral ventromedial medulla of the lightly anesthetized rat. *Brain Res* 1990;533:192–195.
104. Heinricher MM, Barbaro NM, Fields HL. Putative nociceptive modulating neurons in the rostral ventromedial medulla of the rat: firing of on- and off-cells is related to nociceptive responsiveness. *Somatosens Mot Res* 1989;6:427–439.
105. Heinricher MM, Drasner K. Lumbar intrathecal morphine alters activity of putative nociceptive modulatory neurons in rostral ventromedial medulla. *Brain Res* 1991;549:338–341.
106. Heinricher MM, Haws CM, Fields HL. Opposing actions of norepinephrine and clonidine on single pain-modulating neurons in rostral ventromedial medulla. In: Dubner R, Gebhart GF, Bond MR, eds. *Pain research and clinical management.* Amsterdam: Elsevier, 1988;590–594.
107. Heinricher MM, Haws CM, Fields HL. Evidence for GABA-mediated control of putative nociceptive modulating neurons in the rostral ventromedial medulla: iontophoresis of bicuculline eliminates the off-cell pause. *Somatosens Mot Res* 1991;8:215–225.
108. Heinricher MM, Kaplan HJ. GABA-mediated inhibition in rostral ventromedial medulla: role in nociceptive modulation in the lightly anesthetized rat. *Pain* 1991;47:105–113.
109. Heinricher MM, Morgan MM, Fields HL. Direct and indirect actions of morphine on medullary neurons that modulate nociception. *Neuroscience* 1992;48:533–543.
110. Heinricher MM, Morgan MM, Tortorici V, Fields HL. Disinhibition of off-cells and antinociception produced by an opioid action within the rostral ventromedial medulla. *Neuroscience* 1994;63: 279–288.
111. Heinricher MM, Roychowdhury SM. Iontophoretic application of serotonergic agonists produces both excitation and inhibition of physiologically characterized putative pain modulating neurons in the rostral ventromedial medulla of lightly anesthetized rats. *Soc Neurosci Abstr* 1994;20:962.
112. Heinricher MM, Tortorici V. Interference with GABA transmission in the rostral ventromedial medulla: disinhibition of off-cells as a central mechanism of nociceptive modulation. *Neuroscience* 1994;63:533–546.
113. Helmstetter FJ. The amygdala is essential for the expression of conditional hypoalgesia. *Behav Neurosci* 1992;106:518–528.
114. Helmstetter FJ. Stress-induced hypoalgesia and defensive freezing are attenuated by application of diazepam to the amygdala. *Pharmacol Biochem Behav* 1993;44:433–438.
115. Helmstetter FJ, Bellgowan PS. Lesions of the amygdala block conditional hypoalgesia on the tail flick test. *Brain Res* 1993;612: 253–257.
116. Helmstetter FJ, Bellgowan PS, Tershner SA. Inhibition of the tail flick reflex following microinjection of morphine into the amygdala. *Neuroreport* 1993;4:471–474.
117. Helmstetter FJ, Calcagnetti DJ, Fanselow MS. The beta-carboline DMCM produces hypoalgesia after central administration. *Psychobiology* 1990;18:293–297.
118. Helmstetter FJ, Landeira-Fernandez J. Conditional hypoalgesia is attenuated by naltrexone applied to the periaqueductal gray. *Brain Res* 1990;537:88–92.
119. Helmstetter FJ, Tershner SA. Lesions of the periaqueductal gray and rostral ventromedial medulla disrupt antinociceptive but not cardiovascular aversive conditional responses. *J Neurosci* 1994;14: 7099–7108.
120. Hentall ID, Andresen MJ, Taguchi K. Serotonergic, cholinergic and nociceptive inhibition or excitation of raphe magnus neurons in barbiturate-anesthetized rats. *Neuroscience* 1993;52: 303–310.
121. Hernandez N, Lopez Y, Vanegas H. Medullary on- and off-cell responses precede both segmental and thalamic responses to tail heating. Pain 1989;39:221–230.
122. Hobbs SF, Oh UT, Chandler MJ, Fu QG, Bolser DC, Foreman RD. Evidence that C1 and C2 propriospinal neurons mediate the inhibitory effects of viscerosomatic spinal afferent input on primate spinothalamic tract neurons. *J Neurophysiol* 1992;67: 852–860.
123. Hofer MA. Cardiac and respiratory function during sudden prolonged immobility in wild rodents. *Psychosom Med* 1970;32: 633–647.
124. Holstege G. Descending pathways from the periaqueductal gray and adjacent areas. In: DePaulis A, Bandler R, eds. *The midbrain periaqueductal gray matter.* New York: Plenum Press, 1991;239–265.
125. Holstege G, Kuypers HG. The anatomy of brain stem pathways to the spinal cord in cat. A labeled amino acid tracing study. *Prog Brain Res* 1982;57:145–175.
126. Horie H, Pamplin PJ, Yokota T. Inhibition of nociceptive neurons in the shell region of nucleus ventralis posterolateralis following conditioning stimulation of the periaqueductal grey of the cat. Evidence for an ascending inhibitory pathway. *Brain Res* 1991; 561:34–42.
127. Inase M, Nakahama H, Otsuki T, Fang JZ. Analgesic effects of serotonin microinjection into nucleus raphe magnus and nucleus raphe dorsalis evaluated by the monosodium urate (MSU) tonic pain model in the rat. *Brain Res* 1987;426:205–211.
128. Jensen TS, Yaksh TL. Spinal monoamine and opiate systems partly mediate the antinociceptive effects produced by glutamate at brainstem sites. *Brain Res* 1984;321:287–297.
129. Jensen TS, Yaksh TL. Comparison of antinociceptive action of morphine in the periaqueductal gray, medial and paramedial medulla in rat. *Brain Res* 1986;363:99–113.
130. Jensen TS, Yaksh TL. Comparison of the antinociceptive action of mu and delta opioid receptor ligands in the periaqueductal gray matter, medial and paramedial ventral medulla in the rat as studied by the microinjection technique. *Brain Res* 1986;372: 301–312.
131. Jensen TS, Yaksh TL. Examination of spinal monoamine receptors through which brainstem opiate-sensitive systems act in the rat. *Brain Res* 1986;363:114–127.
132. Jensen TS, Yaksh TL. Comparison of the antinociceptive effect of morphine and glutamate at coincidental sites in the periaqueductal gray and medial medulla in rats. *Brain Res* 1989;476: 1–9.
133. Jensen TS, Yaksh TL. The antinociceptive activity of excitatory amino acids in the rat brainstem: an anatomical and pharmacological analysis. *Brain Res* 1992;569:255–267.
134. Jensen TS, Yaksh TL. Brainstem excitatory amino acid receptors in nociception: microinjection mapping and pharmacological characterization of glutamate-sensitive sites in the brainstem associated with algogenic behavior. *Neuroscience* 1992;46:535–547.
135. Kaplan H, Fields HL. Hyperalgesia during acute opioid abstinence: evidence for a nociceptive facilitating function of the rostral ventromedial medulla. *J Neurosci* 1991;11:1433–1439.
136. Kavaliers M. Brief exposure to a natural predator, the short-tailed weasel, induces benzodiazepine-sensitive analgesia in white-footed mice. *Physiol Behav* 1988;43:187–193.
137. Keay KA, Clement CI, Owler B, Depaulis A, Bandler R. Convergence of deep somatic and visceral nociceptive information onto a discrete ventrolateral midbrain periaqueductal gray region. *Neuroscience* 1994;61:727–732.
138. Kiefel JM, Cooper ML, Bodnar RJ. Inhibition of mesencephalic morphine analgesia by methysergide in the medial ventral medulla of rats. *Physiol Behav* 1992;51:201–205.
139. Kiefel JM, Cooper ML, Bodnar RJ. Serotonin receptor subtype antagonists in the medial ventral medulla inhibit mesencephalic opiate analgesia. *Brain Res* 1992;597:331–338.
140. Kiefel JM, Rossi GC, Bodnar RJ. Medullary mu and delta opioid receptors modulate mesencephalic morphine analgesia in rats. *Brain Res* 1993;624:151–161.
141. Kinscheck IB, Watkins LR, Mayer DJ. Fear is not critical to classically conditioned analgesia: the effects of periaqueductal gray lesions and administration of chlordiazepoxide. *Brain Res* 1984; 298:33–44.
142. Knuepfer MM, Holt IL. Effects of electrical and chemical stimulation of nucleus raphe magnus on responses to renal nerve stimulation. *Brain Res* 1991;543:327–334.
143. Koyama N, Yokota T. Ascending inhibition of nociceptive neurons in the nucleus ventralis posterolateralis following conditioning stimulation of the nucleus raphe magnus. *Brain Res* 1993;609: 298–306.
144. Kraus E, Le Bars D, Besson JM. Behavioral confirmation of "diffuse noxious inhibitory controls" (DNIC) and evidence for a role of endogenous opiates. *Brain Res* 1981;206:495–499.
145. Krettek JE, Price JL. Amygdaloid projections to subcortical structures within the basal forebrain and brainstem in the rat and cat. *J Comp Neurol* 1978;178:225–254.
146. Lakos S, Basbaum AI. An ultrastructural study of the projections from the midbrain periaqueductal gray to spinally projecting, serotonin-immunoreactive neurons of the medullary nucleus raphe magnus in the rat. *Brain Res* 1988;443:383–388.
147. Le Bars D, Villanueva L. Electrophysiological evidence for the

activation of descending inhibitory controls by nociceptive afferent pathways. *Prog Brain Res* 1988;77:275–299.
148. LeDoux JE, Cicchetti P, Xagoraris A, Romanski LM. The lateral amygdaloid nucleus: sensory interface of the amygdala in fear conditioning. *J Neurosci* 1990;10:1062–1069.
149. LeDoux JE, Iwata J, Cicchetti P, Reis DJ. Different projections of the central amygdaloid nucleus mediate autonomic and behavioral correlates of conditioned fear. *J Neurosci* 1988;8:2517–2529.
150. Levitt P, Moore RJ. Origin and organization of brainstem catecholamine innervation in the rat. *J Comp Neurol* 1979;186: 505–528.
151. Levy RA, Proudfit HK. Analgesia produced by microinjection of baclofen and morphine at brain stem sites. *Eur J Pharmacol* 1979; 57:43–55.
152. Lewis VA, Gebhart GF. Evaluation of the periaqueductal gray (PAG) as a morphine-specific locus of action and examination of morphine-induced and stimulation-produced analgesia at coincident PAG loci. *Brain Res* 1977;124:283–303.
153. Li YQ, Jia HG, Rao ZR, Shi JW. Serotonin-, substance P- or leucine-enkephalin-containing neurons in the midbrain periaqueductal gray and nucleus raphe dorsalis send projection fibers to the central amygdaloid nucleus in the rat. *Neurosci Lett* 1990;120:124–127.
154. Li YQ, Rao ZR, Shi JW. Collateral projections from the midbrain periaqueductal gray to the nucleus raphe magnus and nucleus accumbens in the rat. A fluorescent retrograde double-labelling study. *Neurosci Lett* 1990;117:285–288.
155. Li YQ, Rao ZR, Shi JW. Midbrain periaqueductal gray neurons with substance P- or enkephalin-like immunoreactivity send projection fibers to the nucleus accumbens in the rat. *Neurosci Lett* 1990;119:269–271.
156. Li YQ, Takada M, Mizuno N. Demonstration of habenular neurons which receive afferent fibers from the nucleus accumbens and send their axons to the midbrain periaqueductal gray. *Neurosci Lett* 1993;158:55–58.
157. Lichtman AH, Fanselow MS. Cats produce analgesia in rats on the tail-flick test: naltrexone sensitivity is determined by the nociceptive test stimulus. *Brain Res* 1990;533:91–94.
158. Lichtman AH, Fanselow MS. Opioid and nonopioid conditional analgesia: the role of spinal opioid, noradrenergic, and serotonergic systems. *Behav Neurosci* 1991;105:687–698.
159. Liebman JM, Mayer DJ, Liebeskind JC. Mesencephalic central gray lesions and fear-motivated behavior in rats. *Brain Res* 1970;23: 353–370.
160. Light AR, Casale EJ, Menetrey DM. The effects of focal stimulation in nucleus raphe magnus and periaqueductal gray on intracellularly recorded neurons in spinal laminae I and II. *J Neurophysiol* 1986;56:555–571.
161. Llewelyn MB, Azami J, Roberts MHT. Effects of 5-hydroxytryptamine applied into nucleus raphe magnus on nociceptive thresholds and neuronal firing rate. *Brain Res* 1983;258:59–68.
162. Lovick TA. Ventrolateral medullary lesions block the antinociceptive and cardiovascular responses elicited by stimulating the dorsal periaqueductal grey matter in rats. *Pain* 1985;21: 241–252.
163. Lovick TA. Analgesia and the cardiovascular changes evoked by stimulating neurones in the ventrolateral medulla in rats. *Pain* 1986;25:259–268.
164. Lovick TA. Inhibitory modulation of the cardiovascular defence response by the ventrolateral periaqueductal grey matter in rats. *Exp Brain Res* 1992;89:133–139.
165. Lovick TA. Midbrain influences on ventrolateral medullo-spinal neurones in the rat. *Exp Brain Res* 1992;90:147–152.
166. Lovick TA. Integrated activity of cardiovascular and pain regulatory systems: role in adaptive behavioural responses. *Prog Neurobiol* 1993;40:631–644.
167. Ma QP, Han JS. Neurochemical studies on the mesolimbic circuitry of antinociception. *Brain Res* 1991;566:95–102.
168. Ma QP, Han JS. Naloxone blocks opioid peptide release in periaqueductal gray and amygdala elicited by morphine injected into N. accumbens. *Peptides* 1992;13:261–265.
169. Ma QP, Shi YS, Han JS. Naloxone blocks opioid peptide release in N. accumbens and amygdala elicited by morphine injected into periaqueductal gray. *Brain Res Bull* 1992;28:351–354.
170. Maciewicz R, Sandrew BB, Phipps BS, Poletti CE, Foote WE. Pontomedullary raphe neurons: intracellular responses to central and peripheral electrical stimulation. *Brain Res* 1984;293:17–33.
171. Maier SF. Diazepam modulation of stress-induced analgesia depends on the type of analgesia. *Behav Neurosci* 1990;104: 339–347.
172. Maier SF, Grahn RE, Kalman BA, Sutton LC, Wiertelak EP, Watkins LR. The role of the amygdala and dorsal raphe nucleus in mediating the behavioral consequences of inescapable shock. *Behav Neurosci* 1993;107:377–388.
173. Maier SF, Wiertelak EP, Watkins LR. Endogenous pain facilitatory systems. Antianalgesia and hyperalgesia. *APS Journal* 1992;1: 191–198.
174. Mansour A, Khachaturian H, Lewis ME, Akil H, Watson SJ. Anatomy of CNS opioid receptors. *Trends Neurosci* 1988;11:308–314.
175. Mantyh PW. Connections of midbrain periaqueductal gray in the monkey. I. Ascending efferent projections. *J Neurophysiol* 1983;49: 567–581.
176. Mason P, Fields HL. Axonal trajectories and terminations of on- and off-cells in the cat lower brainstem. *J Comp Neurol* 1989;288: 185–207.
177. Mason P, Strassman A, Maciewicz R. Pontomedullary raphe neurons: monosynaptic excitation from midbrain sites that suppress the jaw opening reflex. *Brain Res* 1985;329:384–389.
178. Mayer DJ, Price DD. Central nervous system mechanisms of analgesia. *Pain* 1976;2:379–404.
179. Mayer DJ, Wolfe TL, Akil H, Carder B, Liebeskind JC. Analgesia from electrical stimulation in the brainstem of the rat. *Science* 1971;174:1351–1354.
180. Melzack R, Casey KL. Sensory, motivational and central control of determinants of pain. In: Kenshalo D, ed. *The skin senses.* Springfield, IL: Charles C. Thomas, 1968;423–439.
181. Miyamoto Y, Morita N, Kitabata Y, Yamanishi T, Kishioka S, Ozaki M, Yamamoto H. Antinociceptive synergism between supraspinal and spinal sites after subcutaneous morphine evidenced by CNS morphine content. *Brain Res* 1991;552:136–140.
182. Moreau JL, Fields HL. Evidence for GABA involvement in midbrain control of medullary neurons that modulate nociceptive transmission. *Brain Res* 1986;397:37–46.
183. Morgan MM. Differences in antinociception evoked from dorsal and ventral regions of the caudal periaqueductal gray matter. In: DePaulis A, Bandler R, eds. *The midbrain periaqueductal gray matter.* New York: Plenum Press, 1991;139–150.
184. Morgan MM, Depaulis A, Liebeskind JC. Diazepam dissociates the analgesic and aversive effects of periaqueductal gray stimulation in the rat. *Brain Res* 1987;423:395–398.
185. Morgan MM, Fields HL. Activity of nociceptive modulatory neurons in the rostral ventromedial medulla associated with volume expansion-induced antinociception. *Pain* 1993;52:1–9.
186. Morgan MM, Fields HL. Pronounced changes in the activity of nociceptive modulatory neurons in the rostral ventromedial medulla in response to prolonged thermal noxious stimuli. *J Neurophysiol* 1994;72:1161–1170.
187. Morgan MM, Heinricher MM, Fields HL. Circuitry linking opioid-sensitive nociceptive modulatory systems in periaqueductal gray and spinal cord with rostral ventromedial medulla. *Neuroscience* 1992;47:863–871.
188. Morgan MM, Heinricher MM, Fields HL. Inhibition and facilitation of different nocifensor reflexes by spatially remote noxious stimuli. *J Neurophysiol* 1994;72:1152–1160.
189. Morgan MM, Sohn JH, Liebeskind JC. Stimulation of the periaqueductal gray matter inhibits nociception at the supraspinal as well as spinal level. *Brain Res* 1989;502:61–66.
190. Morton CR, Du HJ, Xiao HM, Maisch B, Zimmermann M. Inhibition of nociceptive responses of lumbar dorsal horn neurones by remote noxious afferent stimulation in the cat. *Pain* 1988;34: 75–83.
191. Morton CR, Duggan AW, Zhao ZQ. The effects of lesions of medullary midline and lateral reticular areas on inhibition in the dorsal horn produced by periaqueductal grey stimulation in the cat. *Brain Res* 1984;301:121–130.
192. Moss MS, Basbaum AI. The peptidergic organization of the cat periaqueductal gray. II. The distribution of immunoreactive substance P and vasoactive intestinal polypeptide. *J Neurosci* 1983;3: 1437–1449.
193. Moss MS, Glazer EJ, Basbaum AI. The peptidergic organization of the cat periaqueductal gray. I. The distribution of immunoreactive enkephalin-containing neurons and terminals. *J Neurosci* 1983; 3:603–616.
194. Nauta WJH, Smith GP, Faull RLM, Domesick VB. Efferent con-

nections and nigra afferents of the nucleus accumbens septi in the rat. *Neuroscience* 1978;3:385–401.

195. Ness TJ, Gebhart GF. Interactions between visceral and cutaneous nociception in the rat. I. Noxious cutaneous stimuli inhibit visceral nociceptive neurons and reflexes. *J Neurophysiol* 1991;66: 20–28.
196. Nicoll RA, Malenka RC, Kauer JA. Functional comparison of neurotransmitter receptor subtypes in mammalian central nervous system. *Physiol Rev* 1990;70:513–565.
197. North RA. Opioid actions on membrane ion channels. In: Herz A, ed. *Opioids*. I. Berlin: Springer-Verlag, 1992;773–797.
198. Nosaka S, Murata K, Inui K, Murase S. Arterial baroreflex inhibition by midbrain periaqueductal grey in anaesthetized rats. *Pflugers Arch* 1993;424:266–275.
199. Oliveras JL, Martin G, Montagne J, Vos B. Single unit activity at ventromedial medulla level in the awake, freely moving rat: effects of noxious heat and light tactile stimuli onto convergent neurons. *Brain Res* 1990;506:19–30.
200. Oliveras JL, Vos B, Martin G, Montagne J. Electrophysiological properties of ventromedial medulla neurons in response to noxious and non-noxious stimuli in the awake, freely moving rat: a single-unit study. *Brain Res* 1989;486:1–14.
201. Ottersen OP. Afferent connections to the amygdaloid complex of the rat with some observations in the cat. III. Afferents from the lower brain stem. *J Comp Neurol* 1981;202:335–356.
202. Pan ZZ, Wessendorf MW, Williams JT. Modulation by serotonin of the neurons in rat nucleus raphe magnus in vitro. *Neuroscience* 1993;54:421–429.
203. Pan ZZ, Williams JT, Osborne PB. Opioid actions on single nucleus raphe magnus neurons from rat and guinea-pig in vitro. *J Physiol* 1990;427:519–532.
204. Peschanski M, Besson JM. Diencephalic connections of the raphe nuclei of the rat brainstem: an anatomical study with reference to the somatosensory system. *J Comp Neurol* 1984;224:509–534.
205. Pomeroy SL, Behbehani MM. Physiologic evidence for a projection from periaqueductal gray to nucleus raphe magnus in the rat. *Brain Res* 1979;176:143–147.
206. Potrebic SB, Fields HL, Mason P. Serotonin immunoreactivity is contained in one physiological cell class in the rat rostral ventromedial medulla. *J Neurosci* 1994;14:1655–1665.
207. Prado WA, Roberts MH. An assessment of the antinociceptive and aversive effects of stimulating identified sites in the rat brain. *Brain Res* 1985;340:219–228.
208. Price DD, McHaffie JG. Effects of heterotopic conditioning stimuli on first and second pain: a psychophysical evaluation in humans. *Pain* 1988;34:245–252.
209. Prieto GJ, Cannon JT, Liebeskind JC. N. raphe magnus lesions disrupt stimulation-produced analgesia from ventral but not dorsal midbrain areas in the rat. *Brain Res* 1983;261:53–57.
210. Proudfit HK. Reversible inactivation of raphe magnus neurons: effects on nociceptive threshold and morphine-induced analgesia. *Brain Res* 1980;201:459–464.
211. Proudfit HK. Time-course of alterations in morphine-induced analgesia and nociceptive threshold following medullary raphe lesions. *Neuroscience* 1981;6:945–951.
212. Qiao JT, Dafny N. Dorsal raphe stimulation modulates nociceptive responses in thalamic parafascicular neurons via an ascending pathway: further studies on ascending pain modulation pathways. *Pain* 1988;34:65–74.
213. Ramirez F, Vanegas H. Tooth pulp stimulation advances both medullary off-cell pause and tail flick. *Neurosci Lett* 1989;100: 153–156.
214. Reichling DB, Basbaum AI. Contribution of brainstem GABAergic circuitry to descending antinociceptive controls: I. GABA-immunoreactive projection neurons in the periaqueductal gray and nucleus raphe magnus. *J Comp Neurol* 1990;302:370–377.
215. Reichling DB, Basbaum AI. Contribution of brainstem GABAergic circuitry to descending antinociceptive controls: II. Electron microscopic immunocytochemical evidence of GABAergic control over the projection from the periaqueductal gray to the nucleus raphe magnus in the rat. *J Comp Neurol* 1990;302:378–393.
216. Reichling DB, Basbaum AI. Collateralization of periaqueductal gray neurons to forebrain or diencephalon and to the medullary nucleus raphe magnus in the rat. *Neuroscience* 1991;42:183–200.
217. Renno WM, Mullett MA, Beitz AJ. Systemic morphine reduces GABA release in the lateral but not the medial portion of the midbrain periaqueductal gray of the rat. *Brain Res* 1992;594:221–232.
218. Reynolds DV. Surgery in the rat during electrical analgesia induced by focal brain stimulation. *Science* 1969;154:444–445.
219. Rizvi TA, Ennis M, Behbehani MM, Shipley MT. Connections between the central nucleus of the amygdala and the midbrain periaqueductal gray: topography and reciprocity. *J Comp Neurol* 1991;303:121–131.
220. Rizvi TA, Ennis M, Shipley MT. Reciprocal connections between the medial preoptic area and the midbrain periaqueductal gray in rat: a WGA-HRP and PHA-L study. *J Comp Neurol* 1992;315:1–15.
221. Rodgers RJ, Randall JI. Benzodiazepine ligands, nociception and "defeat" analgesia in male mice. *Psychopharmacology* 1987;91: 305–315.
222. Rodgers RJ, Randall JI. Environmentally induced analgesia: situational factors, mechanisms and significance. In: Rodgers RJ, Cooper SJ, eds. *Endorphins, opiates and behavioral processes*. New York: John Wiley, 1988;107–144.
223. Roerig SC, Fujimoto JM. Multiplicative interaction between intrathecally and intracerebroventricularly administered mu opioid agonists but limited interactions between delta and kappa agonists for antinociception in mice. *J Pharmacol Exp Ther* 1989;249: 762–768.
224. Rosenfeld JP, Huang KH, Xia LY. Effects of single and simultaneous combined nanoinjections of Met-enkephalin into rat midbrain and medulla on activity of differentially nociresponsive ventral medullary neurons. *Brain Res* 1990;508:199–209.
225. Rosenfeld JP, Xia LY. Reversible tetracaine block of rat periaqueductal gray (PAG) decreases baseline tail-flick latency and prevents analgesic effects of met-enkephalin injections in nucleus paragigantocellularis (PGC). *Brain Res* 1993;605:57–66.
226. Rossi GC, Pasternak GW, Bodnar RJ. Synergistic brainstem interactions for morphine analgesia. *Brain Res* 1993;624:171–180.
227. Sagen J, Proudfit HK. Hypoalgesia induced by blockade of noradrenergic projections to the raphe magnus: reversal by blockade of noradrenergic projections to the spinal cord. *Brain Res* 1981; 223:391–396.
228. Sagen J, Proudfit HK. Evidence for pain modulation by pre- and postsynaptic noradrenergic receptors in the medulla oblongata. *Brain Res* 1985;331:285–293.
229. Sagen J, Winker MA, Proudfit HK. Hypoalgesia induced by the local injection of phentolamine in the nucleus raphe magnus: blockade by depletion of spinal cord monoamines. *Pain* 1983;16: 253–263.
230. Sandkühler J, Gebhart GF. Characterization of inhibition of a spinal nociceptive reflex by stimulation medially and laterally in the midbrain and medulla in the pentobarbital-anesthetized rat. *Brain Res* 1984;305:67–76.
231. Sandkühler J, Gebhart GF. Relative contributions of the nucleus raphe magnus and adjacent medullary reticular formation to the inhibition by stimulation in the periaqueductal gray of a spinal nociceptive reflex in the pentobarbital-anesthetized rat. *Brain Res* 1984;305:77–87.
232. Sandkühler J, Stelzer B, Fu QG. Characteristics of propriospinal modulation of nociceptive lumbar spinal dorsal horn neurons in the cat. *Neuroscience* 1993;54:957–967.
233. Sandkühler J, Willmann E, Fu QG. Blockade of $GABA_A$ receptors in the midbrain periaqueductal gray abolishes nociceptive spinal dorsal horn neuronal activity. *Eur J Pharmacol* 1989;160:163–166.
234. Sandkühler J, Willmann E, Fu QG. Characteristics of midbrain control of spinal nociceptive neurons and nonsomatosensory parameters in the pentobarbital-anesthetized rat. *J Neurophysiol* 1991;65:33–48.
235. Satoh M, Oku R, Akaike A. Analgesia produced by microinjection of L-glutamate into the rostral ventromedial bulbar nuclei of the rat and its inhibition by intrathecal alpha-adrenergic blocking agents. *Brain Res* 1983;261:361–364.
236. Semenenko FM, Lumb BM. Projections of anterior hypothalamic neurones to the dorsal and ventral periaqueductal grey in the rat. *Brain Res* 1992;582:237–245.
237. Shinonaga Y, Takada M, Mizuno N. Topographic organization of collateral projections from the basolateral amygdaloid nucleus to both the prefrontal cortex and nucleus accumbens in the rat. *Neuroscience* 1994;58:389–397.
238. Shipley MT, McLean JH, Behbehani MM. Heterogeneous distribution of neurotensin-like immunoreactive neurons and fibers in the midbrain periaqueductal gray of the rat. *J Neurosci* 1987;7: 2025–2034.
239. Skagerberg G, Bjorklund A. Topographic principles in the spinal

projections of serotonergic and non-serotonergic brainstem neurons in the rat. *Neuroscience* 1985;15:445–480.
240. Smith DJ, Perrotti JM, Crisp T, Cabral ME, Long JT, Scalzitti JM. The mu opiate receptor is responsible for descending pain inhibition originating in the periaqueductal gray region of the rat brain. *Eur J Pharmacol* 1988;156:47–54.
241. Strack AM, Sawyer WB, Platt KB, Loewy AD. CNS cell groups regulating the sympathetic outflow to adrenal gland as revealed by transneuronal cell body labeling with pseudorabies virus. *Brain Res* 1989;491:274–296.
242. Talbot JD, Duncan GH, Bushnell MC, Boyer M. Diffuse noxious inhibitory controls (DNICs): psychophysical evidence in man for intersegmental suppression of noxious heat perception by cold pressor pain. *Pain* 1987;30:221–232.
243. Tattersall JE, Cervero F, Lumb BM. Viscerosomatic neurons in the lower thoracic spinal cord of the cat: excitations and inhibitions evoked by splanchnic and somatic nerve volleys and by stimulation of brain stem nuclei. *J Neurophysiol* 1986;56:1411–1423.
244. Thurston CL, Randich A. Effects of vagal afferent stimulation on ON and OFF cells in the rostroventral medulla: relationships to nociception and arterial blood pressure. *J Neurophysiol* 1992;67: 180–196.
245. Tortorici V, Vanegas H. "Off" and "on" cells of the medulla oblongata as possible mediators of analgesia produced by mesencephalic and diencephalic stimulation in rats. *Acta Cient Venez* 1990;41:317–326.
246. Tseng LF, Wang Q. Forebrain sites differentially sensitive to beta-endorphin and morphine for analgesia and release of Met-enkephalin in the pentobarbital-anesthesized rat. *J Pharmacol Exp Ther* 1992;261:1028–1036.
247. Urban MO, Smith DJ. Role of neurotensin in the nucleus raphe magnus in opioid-induced antinociception from the periaqueductal gray. *J Pharmacol Exp Ther* 1993;265:580–586.
248. Urban MO, Smith DJ. The non-peptide neurotensin antagonist, SR4869, reveals the antianalgesic action of neurotensin neuronal projections from the PAG to the RMg. *Can J Physiol Pharmacol* 1994 (in press).
249. Urca G, Liebeskind JC. Electrophysiological indices of opiate action in awake and anesthetized rats. *Brain Res* 1979;161: 162–166.
250. Van Bockstaele EJ, Aston-Jones G, Pieribone VA, Ennis M, Shipley MT. Subregions of the periaqueductal gray topographically innervate the rostral ventral medulla in the rat. *J Comp Neurol* 1991;309: 305–327.
251. van Praag H, Frenk H. The role of glutamate in opiate descending inhibition of nociceptive spinal reflexes. *Brain Res* 1990;524: 101–105.
252. Vanegas H, Barbaro NM, Fields HL. Midbrain stimulation inhibits tail-flick only at currents sufficient to excite rostral medullary neurons. *Brain Res* 1984;321:127–133.
253. Vanegas H, Barbaro NM, Fields HL. Tailflick-related activity in medullospinal neurons. *Brain Res* 1984;321:135–141.
254. Villanueva L, Bing Z, Bouhassira D, Le Bars D. Encoding of electrical, thermal, and mechanical noxious stimuli by subnucleus reticularis dorsalis neurons in the rat medulla. *J Neurophysiol* 1989; 61:391–402.
255. Villanueva L, Bouhassira D, Bing Z, Le Bars D. Convergence of heterotopic nociceptive information onto subnucleus reticularis dorsalis neurons in the rat medulla. *J Neurophysiol* 1988;60: 980–1009.
255a. Wall PD. The laminar organization of dorsal horn and effects of descending impulses. *J Physiol* 1967;188:403–423.
256. Watkins LR, Cobelli DA, Mayer DJ. Classical conditioning of front paw and hind paw footshock induced analgesia (FSIA): naloxone reversibility and descending pathways. *Brain Res* 1982;243: 119–132.
257. Watkins LR, Kinscheck IB, Mayer DJ. The neural basis of footshock analgesia: the effect of periaqueductal gray lesions and decerebration. *Brain Res* 1983;276:317–324.
258. Watkins LR, Mayer DJ. Organization of endogenous opiate and nonopiate pain control systems. *Science* 1982;216:1185–1192.
259. Watkins LR, Wiertelak EP, Goehler LE, Mooney-Heiberger K, Martinez J, Furness L, Smith KP, et al. Neurocircuitry of illness-induced hyperalgesia. *Brain Res* 1994;639:283–299.
260. Watkins LR, Wiertelak EP, Maier SF. The amygdala is necessary for the expression of conditioned but not unconditioned analgesia. *Behav Neurosci* 1993;107:402–405.
261. Watkins LR, Young EG, Kinscheck IB, Mayer DJ. The neural basis of footshock analgesia: the role of specific ventral medullary nuclei. *Brain Res* 1983;276:305–315.
262. Wessendorf MW, Anderson EG. Single unit studies of identified bulbospinal serotonergic units. *Brain Res* 1983;279:93–103.
263. Wiertelak EP, Furness LE, Horan R, Martinez J, Maier SF, Watkins LR. Subcutaneous formalin produces centrifugal hyperalgesia at a non-injected site via the NMDA-nitric oxide cascade. *Brain Res* 1994;649:19–26.
264. Wiertelak EP, Smith KP, Furness L, Mooney-Heiberger K, Mayr T, Maier SF, Watkins LR. Acute and conditioned hyperalgesic responses to illness. *Pain* 1994;56:227–234.
265. Wiklund L, Behzadi G, Kalen P, Headley PM, Nicolopoulos LS, Parsons CG, West DC. Autoradiographic and electrophysiological evidence for excitatory amino acid transmission in the periaqueductal gray projection to nucleus raphe magnus in the rat. *Neurosci Lett* 1988;93:158–163.
266. Willcockson WS, Gerhart KD, Cargill CL, Willis WD. Effects of biogenic amines on raphe-spinal tract cells. *J Pharmacol Exp Ther* 1983;225:637–645.
267. Willer JC, De Broucker T, Le Bars D. Encoding of nociceptive thermal stimuli by diffuse noxious inhibitory controls in humans. *J Neurophysiol* 1989;62:1028–1038.
268. Williams FG, Beitz AJ. Ultrastructural morometric analysis of enkephalin-immunoreactive terminals in the ventrocaudal periaqueductal gray: analysis of their relationship to periaqueductal gray-raphe magnus projection neurons. *Neuroscience* 1990;38: 381–394.
269. Williams FG, Beitz AJ. Ultrastructural morphometric analysis of GABA-immunoreactive terminals in the ventrocaudal periaqueductal grey: analysis of the relationship of GABA terminals and the $GABA_A$ receptor to periaqueductal grey-raphe magnus projection neurons. *J Neurocytol* 1990;19:686–696.
270. Willis W Jr. Anatomy and physiology of descending control of nociceptive responses of dorsal horn neurons: comprehensive review. *Prog Brain Res* 1988;77:1–29.
271. Willis WD. *Hyperalgesia and allodynia.* New York: Raven Press, 1992.
272. Willis WD, Gerhart KD, Willcockson WS, Yezierski RP, Wilcox TK, Cargill CL. Primate raphe- and reticulospinal neurons: effects of stimulation in periaqueductal gray or VPLc thalamic nucleus. *J Neurophysiol* 1984;51:467–480.
273. Yaksh TL. Direct evidence that spinal serotonin and noradrenaline terminals mediate the spinal antinociceptive effects of morphine in the periaqueductal gray. *Brain Res* 1979;160:180–185.
274. Yaksh TL, Al-Rodhan NR, Jensen TS. Sites of action of opiates in production of analgesia. *Prog Brain Res* 1988;77:371–394.
275. Yaksh TL, Plant RL, Rudy TA. Studies on the antagonism by raphe lesions of the antinociceptive action of systemic morphine. *Eur J Pharmacol* 1977;41:399–408.
276. Yaksh TL, Rudy TA. Narcotic analgetics: CNS sites and mechanisms of action as revealed by intracerebral injection techniques. *Pain* 1978;4:299–359.
277. Yaksh TL, Yeung JC, Rudy TA. Systematic examination in the rat of brain sites sensitive to the direct application of morphine: observation of differential effects within the periaqueductal gray. *Brain Res* 1976;114:83–103.
278. Yardley CP, Hilton SM. The hypothalamic and brainstem areas from which the cardiovascular and behavioural components of the defence reaction are elicited in the rat. *J Auton Nerv Syst* 1986;15: 227–244.
279. Yeomans DC, Clark FM, Paice JA, Proudfit HK. Antinociception induced by electrical stimulation of spinally projecting noradrenergic neurons in the A7 catecholamine cell group of the rat. *Pain* 1992;48:449–461.
280. Yeomans DC, Proudfit HK. Projections of substance P-immunoreactive neurons located in the ventromedial medulla to the A7 noradrenergic nucleus of the rat demonstrated using retrograde tracing combined with immunocytochemistry. *Brain Res* 1990;532: 329–332.
281. Yeomans DC, Proudfit HK. Antinociception induced by microinjection of substance P into the A7 catecholamine cell group in the rat. *Neuroscience* 1992;49:681–691.
282. Yeung JC, Rudy TA. Multiplicative interaction between narcotic agonisms as revealed by concurrent intrathecal and intracerebroventricular injections of morphine. *J Pharmacol Exp Ther* 1980; 215:633–642.
283. Young EG, Watkins LR, Mayer DJ. Comparison of the effects of ventral medullary lesions on systemic and microinjection morphine analgesia. *Brain Res* 1984;290:119–129.

284. Zhang SP, Bandler R, Carrive P. Flight and immobility evoked by excitatory amino acid microinjection within distinct parts of the subtentorial midbrain periaqueductal gray of the cat. *Brain Res* 1990;520:73–82.
285. Zhuo M, Gebhart GF. Characterization of descending inhibition and facilitation from the nuclei reticularis gigantocellularis and gigantocellularis pars alpha in the rat. *Pain* 1990;42:337–350.
286. Zhuo M, Gebhart GF. Spinal cholinergic and monoaminergic receptors mediate descending inhibition from the nuclei reticularis gigantocellularis and gigantocellularis pars alpha in the rat. *Brain Res* 1990;535:67–78.
287. Zhuo M, Gebhart GF. Characterization of descending facilitation and inhibition of spinal nociceptive transmission from the nuclei reticularis gigantocellularis and gigantocellularis pars alpha in the rat. *J Neurophysiol* 1992;67:1599–1614.
288. Zorman G, Hentall ID, Adams JE, Fields HL. Naloxone-reversible analgesia produced by microstimulation in the rat medulla. *Brain Res* 1981;219:137–148.

Anesthesia: Biologic Foundations, edited by Tony L. Yaksh et al. Lippincott–Raven Publishers, Philadelphia © 1997.

CHAPTER 39

ORGANIZATION OF VISCERAL INPUT

ROBERT D. FOREMAN

Information concerning the status of visceral organs in thoracic and abdominal cavities as well as vasculature is transmitted to the central nervous system by afferent fibers. These fibers may travel with sympathetic nerves, have their cell bodies in the dorsal root ganglia, and project to specific spinal cord segments (e.g., sympathetic afferents), or travel with the vagus nerve and have their cell bodies in the nodose ganglia, and terminate in the brainstem (e.g., vagal afferents). Common experience tells us that intense pain states may be evoked as a result of certain injuries, inflammatory events, or distention of the viscera.

Even though diseases of the viscera cause numerous types of acute and chronic pain, the central and peripheral functional organization of visceral afferent fibers and their inputs is understood much less than that which arises from cutaneous inputs. Several reasons can account for this disparity. The most logical explanation is that cutaneous receptors are much more accessible and produce more predictable stimulus responses and psychophysical properties. In fact, early in the 20th century there was a belief that viscera do not contain afferent fibers that elicit pain. Several investigators elicited no responses in conscious patients under local anesthesia when structures in the heart, abdomen, and pelvic region were pinched, cut, stretched, and manipulated (see Lewis [146] for references and details). These observations led MacKenzie (152) to argue that all visceral pain occurs because impulses relaying innocuous information ascended from visceral organs to the spinal cord. These afferent impulses spread to sensory tracts, generated an "irritable focus" in the spinal cord, and then created pain that was referred to the peripheral distribution of the somatic nerve from the overlying skin and caused muscular spasm. This hypothesis never received full acceptance because several scientists were convinced that pain may arise directly from the viscera (146). While numerous studies exist to demonstrate that pain can be generated from visceral structures, only two examples from work of White (264) will be used to illustrate this point. Stimulation of the central end of cut splanchnic nerves in patients elicits a deep, diffuse, poorly localized painful sensation that is referred primarily to the abdomen. Electrical stimulation of the upper thoracic ganglia evokes pain in the precordium, deep in the chest and back, and extends down the arm for variable distances. This pain mimics angina pectoris and aneurysm of the aorta arch.

This chapter discusses receptor properties, arrangement and distribution of afferent input, and central organization and processing of visceral information, especially noxious information. The major focus of the chapter is on spinal cord organization and processing and to a lesser extent on the supraspinal pathways. The discussion is divided into the organization of input traveling with the sympathetic afferents and that traveling with the vagus. Organization of visceral input centers on the cardiopulmonary system, as this area has been studied in detail and provides an organizing focus for the input originating from other visceral structures.

ENCODING OF SENSORY RECEPTORS

Certain characteristics of visceral sensation set it apart from cutaneous sensation. Cutaneous sensation results from the existence of three separate categories of peripheral receptors that respond specifically to different stimulus modalities. The three modalities are (1) mechanoreceptors that transmit information about tactile stimulation, (2) nociceptors designed to signal noxious or potentially noxious events that result in the perception of cutaneous pain, and (3) thermoreceptors transmitting information about cold and warm temperatures. These stimuli applied to discrete regions of the body evoke "pain sensations," with the magnitude of the reported sensation proportional to stimulus intensity. These localized sensations are referenced to the site of stimulus exposure of reflexes with a local sign (e.g., nociceptor reflexes).

Visceral sensation has several characteristics that make it more complicated than cutaneous sensation (60): (1) Internal organs are innervated with many receptors whose activation does not appear to evoke a conscious experience, but produces reflexes. The nature of adequate stimuli is difficult to determine for these receptors. (2) Activation of receptors located in internal organs produces a limited range of sensation that often results in discomfort and pain. (3) Some visceral organs generate visceral sensation (e.g., bladder fullness or gastric distention) that is sensed initially as nonpainful, but if the stimulus persists, sensation can become progressively unpleasant and painful without changing the quality of the stimulus. (4) Sensation of visceral pain in some cases can start as a unique and extremely painful sensory experience, and is the only sensation elicited from certain organs such as the heart and gallbladder. (5) Visceral sensation in most forms is poorly localized or is referred to somatic structures most commonly in the physical proximity to the threatened visceral organ. (6) Approximately 16,000 primary visceral neurons conduct information from visceral organs to the spinal cord. Of the total population of spinal visceral neurons, only 20% of these axons transmit afferent information. In the dorsal root these afferent fibers comprise only 2% of the total number of somatic and visceral afferent fibers. A more detailed account of spinal innervation of the viscera can be found in Cervero (58), Jänig and Morrison (127), and Ness and Gebhart (190). One can conclude, therefore, that innervation density of fibers from the viscera is much less than the somatic population.

Intensity Versus Specificity in Stimulus Transduction

In recent years, major advances have been made to understand encoding of the visceral receptors. For many years one group of scientists has proposed the specificity theory and another group has proposed the pattern or intensity theory to explain encoding noxious events, e.g., these stimuli producing escape behavior on pain reports by visceral afferent fibers (Fig. 1). Specificity theory is used to describe receptor encoding systems that respond only to specific stimulus intensities. In this theory one population of receptors responds to low-intensity innocuous stimuli and another population is excited only by high-intensity noxious stimuli often with the frequency of the output function being proportional to stimulus intensity (see Chapter 9). One group of laboratories that studied the heart, biliary system, ureter, uterus, and testes argues that the visceral

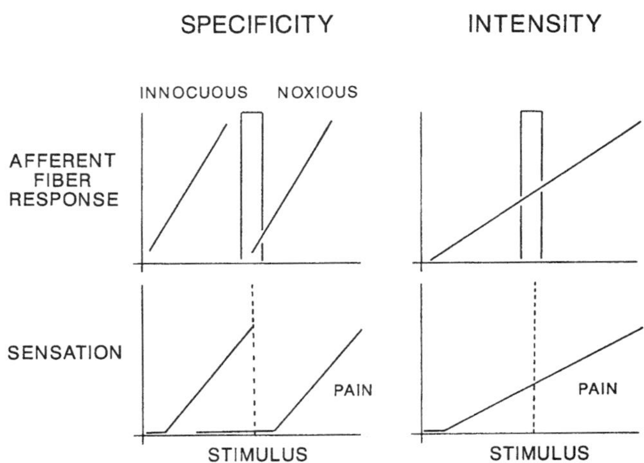

Figure 1. Schematic diagram illustrating classic specificity and intensity theories to describe response characteristics visceral afferent receptors. Diagrams are based on encoding of action potentials transmitted in visceral afferent fibers during innocuous and noxious stimulation. (Modified from ref. 60.)

receptors fit the specificity definition of visceral nociceptors (22,33,55,63,137). The researchers classified them in this manner because a group of receptors responded only to noxious intensities of visceral stimulation.

Other groups of investigators have provided evidence to support the intensity theory. The intensity theory states that receptors respond to a wide range of stimulus intensities. Receptors in organs such as the heart, colon, and urinary bladder encode for intensity of the visceral stimulus (19,43,126,159). Threshold for activation of those receptors occurs in the innocuous range, but provides pain sensation at higher intensities.

Investigators supporting these two different theories argue for their respective perspectives based on their interpretations of the data (61). Recent findings, however, provide evidence to argue that both mechanisms may be operating in visceral organ systems. Studies on afferent innervation of the esophagus show that both specific nociceptors and intensity encoding receptors exist together and their afferent fibers are found to travel in sympathetic and vagal afferent nerves (230,231). Threshold, encoding ability, and pathways used for projecting information to the brainstem or spinal cord can be used to differentiate these receptors into categories. One group of sympathetic afferent fibers (e.g., axons, the cell bodies of which are in the dorsal root ganglia and which travel with the sympathetic efferent fibers) can be classified as intensity coding because these receptors become active in the physiological range and then intensify their discharge pattern throughout the distention range (Fig. 2). In the esophagus balloon, distention beyond 60 mm Hg generally creates discomfort and pain in animal and human subjects (151). In contrast, another group of sympathetic afferents has receptors with thresholds around 40 mm Hg distention pressure and the frequency of the action potentials in their axons continue to increase as the stimulus is intensified. Thus, both specific and intensity encoding receptors are operating in the same organ and within the same afferent pathway. Further support for nociceptive specific afferents comes from studies showing that a small number of unmyelinated afferents responds only to noxious stimuli (63,109). These afferent fibers exist in a population of fibers that also demonstrates intensity encoding activity.

In addition to receptors found in the sympathetic afferent system, a group of afferent fibers is found in the vagus that respond only to distention pressure in the physiologic range (230). These receptors have a very low threshold and operate at much higher frequencies throughout the range of graded stimuli.

Some concerns need to be raised regarding the functional classification of visceral receptors. While separation of the sympathetic afferents into exclusive intensity and specificity categories is appealing, curves of individual receptors typically show a continuum of responses when each stimulus response curve was plotted on a graph (230,231). An examination of the individual curves leads to the conclusion that intensity coding could explain the information. It should be pointed out, however, that the pressure required to activate part of the population was substantially higher than the pressures needed for the other group. A second concern is that the number of nociceptive-specific fibers appears to be far less than the number of receptors that are part of the intensity coding.

Silent Nociceptors

An important subcategory of receptors that may contribute to pain sensation are those referred to as "silent" nociceptors. Oftentimes distention of a visceral organ does not produce any sensation until the disease process causes inflammation of the organ. The presence of "silent" nociceptors may be the key for producing pain sensation in this situation. The concept of silent nociceptors originates from work in the joint, in which certain populations of nociceptors are not activated until joints become inflamed (73,226,227). Receptors with these properties have also been found in the urinary bladder (109,110). Unmyelinated and small myelinated bladder afferent fibers responded very weakly, if at all, to intense bladder distention, but the discharge frequency increased greatly after the urinary bladder was rendered acutely inflamed (109,110,165). These observations provide evidence that different classes of nociceptors can signal the state of the visceral organ in the presence of acute and noxious stimuli, and that the encoding of the stimu-

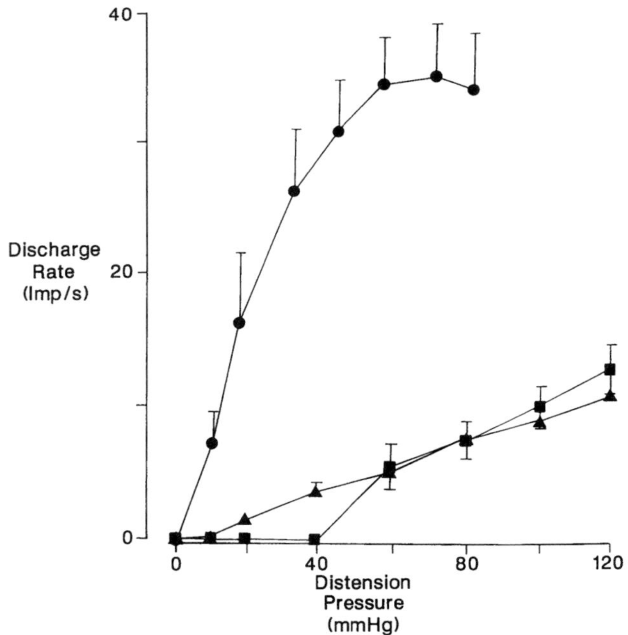

Figure 2. Stimulus-response characteristics of three classes of afferent fibers arising from the opossum esophagus. Specificity encoding can describe the stimulus response characteristics of the low-threshold vagal afferent fibers (LT, *circles;* $n = 41$) that discharged primarily in the physiologic range and the high-threshold spinal visceral afferents fibers (HT, *squares;* $n = 35$) encode only in the noxious range. Intensity encoding described a group of fibers (LTi, *triangles;* $n = 21$) that responded to both low-intensity and high-intensity stimuli. Responses are given as means ±1 SEM. (Modified from ref. 231.)

lus is accomplished from the outset by the population of fibers activated and by the rate they discharge.

These explanations cannot stand alone without incorporating characteristics of the central processing of nociceptive information. This information will be provided following a discussion about the functional and anatomical organization of central processing of visceral information.

SYMPATHETIC AFFERENT ORGANIZATION

Information from heart or other visceral organs is carried to cell bodies located in dorsal root ganglia of spinal segments. Cell bodies of visceral afferent axons tend to be smaller than the overall cell population in the dorsal root ganglia (253). This agrees with the observation that most spinal visceral afferent fibers are unmyelinated C-fiber axons, with a few being small myelinated A-δ axons (127,142).

Segmental Distribution

Visceral organs from thoracic, abdominal, and pelvic structures (Fig. 3) have afferent fibers entering different segments of the spinal cord. Afferent fibers arising from each organ enter primarily at one or two adjacent segments of the spinal cord, but ramify rosterally and caudally to cause overlap among populations of afferent fibers having different peripheral distribution. Cardiopulmonary nerves have their maximum innervation in the T2 and T3 segments (123,141,195,253). Renal, lumbar colonic, and hypogastric afferent fibers are found primarily in the second, third, and fourth lumbar dorsal root ganglia, respectively (23–25,140,181). The pelvic nerve contains visceral afferent fibers that enter the second sacral segment (182).

Spinal segments receiving information from the heart are distinct from those of the gallbladder, kidney, and urinary bladder (16,71,123,125), but considerable overlap exists when visceral organs are found in the same region of the body. For example, spinal projections of afferent input from the esophagus (72,77,136) overlaps not only with input from cardiac afferents but also with gallbladder input. This overlap of afferent input contributes to the confusion that results from efforts to explain various forms of chest pain; however, it may not be the only explanation.

Spinal visceral afferent inputs can extend for several segments in the rostrocaudal direction. This observation was made by injecting a neuroanatomical tracer into single visceral afferent C fibers and showing that these afferent axons can ascend and descend for several segments before they terminate in the gray matter (236). As a visceral afferent axon traverses several segments, collaterals periodically leave the parent branch to terminate in laminae I, II, V, and X. In addition, some fibers project contralaterally to laminae V and VII. In contrast, rostrocaudal distributions of somatic afferent fibers are much more limited and focused.

Spinal Cord Organization

Axons from neurons in dorsal root ganglia cells of the upper thoracic segments penetrate the spinal cord and convey afferent information to cells located in the gray matter of the spinal cord (141). These afferent axons enter the tract of Lissauer and terminate in the same segment where they enter the spinal cord or they ascend and descend a few segments. In general, visceral afferent axons take two different routes to enter the gray matter (59) (Fig. 4). Some afferent axons course over the dorsal surface of the gray matter and terminate primarily in lamina I, whereas others slip along the lateral edge of the gray matter and then terminate primarily in laminae V, VII, and X. In addition, termination sites are located in or near the cells in the intermediolat-

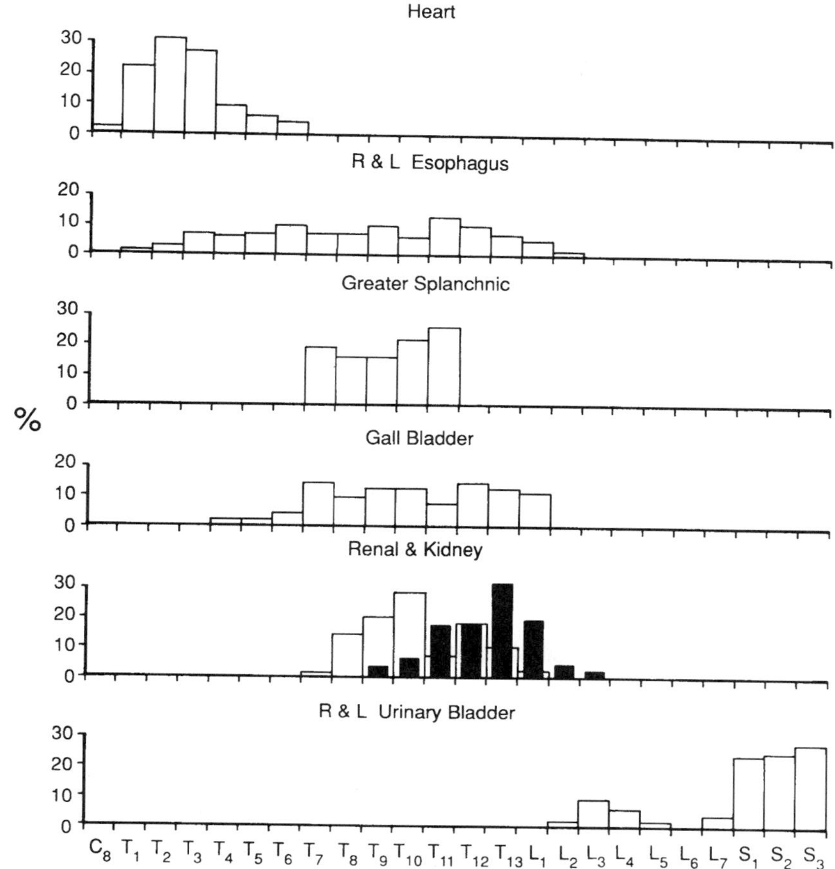

Figure 3. Histogram showing segmental distribution of dorsal root ganglia of sympathetic afferent fibers originating from different visceral organs or visceral nerves. Ganglia were retrogradely labeled with horseradish peroxidase after injections were made into visceral organs or nerves. Abscissa indicates the spinal segment and the ordinate shows percentage of the total number of labeled cells for each segment. *Open bars* in the renal and kidney histogram represent injections made on the left side; *solid bars* are from the right side (97).

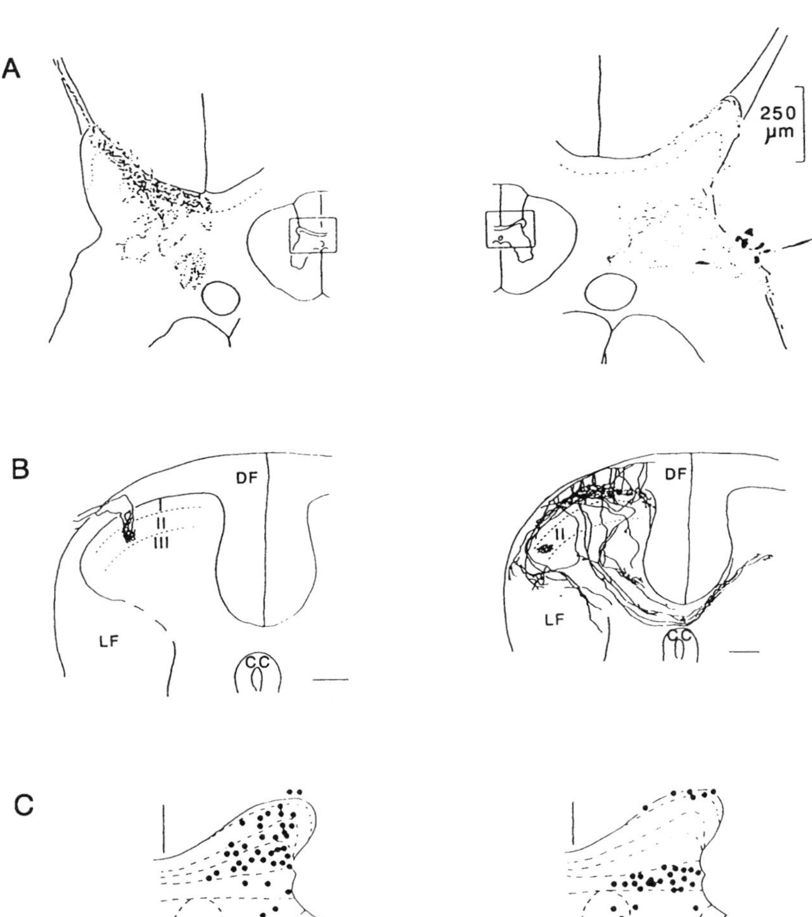

Figure 4. Spinal organization of primary afferent fibers and location of spinal neurons receiving afferent input. The panels on the *left* represent somatic afferent input and those on the *right* represent spinal visceral afferent input. **A:** Reconstructions from serial sections of projections of somatic (*left*) and visceral (*right*) afferent fibers to the T9 segment in cat. Horseradish peroxidase was applied to the intercostal nerve (*left*) of the T9 spinal nerve and to the splanchnic nerve (*right*). (From ref. 59, with permission.) **B:** Transverse reconstructions of central projections of a single somatic C fiber (*left*) and a single visceral afferent C fiber (*right*). (From ref. 236, with permission.) **C:** Locations of recording sites of somatic (*left*) and viscerosomatic (*right*) spinal neurons. Responses of spinal neurons were determined by manipulation of the somatic receptive field (*left*) and electrical stimulation of splanchnic nerve (*right*). (From ref. 57, with permission.)

eral cell column. This pattern of afferent distribution is observed for visceral afferents in the lower thoracic (59,139), lumbar (181,192), and sacral (185) segments of the spinal cord.

A few spinal visceral afferent axons appear to terminate directly in the substantia gelatinosa (lamina II) (236). In contrast to visceral distribution patterns, somatic afferent axons terminate primarily in the substantia gelatinosa (lamina II) and, to a much less extent, in other laminae of the gray matter (59,236). The density of visceral termination sites is much less than those of somatic afferent fibers.

The diffuse and poorly localized nature of visceral sensations may depend on two characteristics of the visceral spinal system. First, of the total number of afferent fibers transmitting various information, spinal visceral afferent axons make up only a small percentage that mediate visceral pain and arise from most of the thoracic and upper abdominal viscera, including the heart and gastrointestinal tract. Second, the wide rostrocaudal distribution of the visceral afferent fibers innervates second-order neurons in several segments, thus causing the diffuse and poorly localized nature of the visceral pain. In general, somatic afferent axons terminate in very localized regions of the gray matter of the spinal cord. Thus, it is not surprising that visceral sensations are diffuse and more difficult to localize precisely than cutaneous sensations.

Visceral afferent fibers terminate either directly or indirectly on cells located primarily in the dorsal horn of the gray matter. These cells, in general, are located in the marginal zone of the dorsal horn (lamina I and the outer part of laminae II, V, and VI, and to a much less extent lamina IV), and deeper in primarily the medial zone (including the base of the dorsal horn, the intermediate zone or lamina VII, and lamina VIII in the ventral horn) (64) (Fig. 4). A common feature of these neurons is that they most commonly receive both visceral and somatic afferent inputs. The majority of neurons that respond only to somatic afferent input are found in laminae II, III, IV, and V of the dorsal horn. However, the spinothalamic tract (STT) cells in the C7 and C8 segments of the cervical cord (118) and the L5 and L6 segments of the lumbar cord (120) receive primarily somatic input from distal somatic structures.

Part of the total population of cells in the gray matter is the origin of ascending pathways that transmit visceral information to areas of the brain to process sensory information (Fig. 5). Axons of cells of origin generally cross over to the contralateral side within one or two segments and then travel in the anterolateral quadrant. Recent observations also have shown that some of the axons remain on the ipsilateral side and some are carried in the dorsolateral quadrant (15). It should be pointed out that to date no ascending pathways convey only visceral afferent information; they usually carry viscerosomatic convergent information.

The spinothalamic tract (STT) is the most studied system for transmitting visceral afferent information to the brain (Fig. 5). Visceral afferent information ascends in pathways to both the lateral and medial thalamus (11,12,40,41,100,176). The lateral thalamus receiving visceral information is composed of the ventral posterior lateral and ventral posterior medial nucleus (31,50,67). Cells of the lateral thalamus then projects to the primary (SI) somatosensory cortex and possibly the secondary (SII) somatosensory cortex. Scanty and preliminary data exist about the processing of visceral information in the somatosensory cortex. A few cells in the somatosensory cortex have been shown to receive visceral input (14,95), and thalamic cells with visceral as well as somatic input have been activated antidromically from the SI cortex (67). Based on this information coupled with findings that noxious somatic input excites SI cells, one can assume that visceral input reaches at least the SI area (70,107,133,134,143–145,254). Information processed in these regions appears to be important for the sensory-discriminative nature of pain that refers to the capacity to analyze location, intensity, and duration of the nociceptive stimulus (170,207). Ascending axons with visceral and somatic input also project to the medial thalamus, which is composed primarily of the centralis lateralis and centrum medianum-parafascicularis nuclei (45,168). Axons from these nuclei project to the association cortex, which includes primarily the insular cortex, amygdala, and cingulate gyrus (29,30,116,224), but no direct functional evidence about the transmission of visceral information from the medial thalamus to the association cortex exists. Based on behavioral responses, one can assume that visceral information reaches these areas of the cortex. The association cortex appears to be primarily responsible for motivational-affective components of pain, including autonomic adjustments (3,53,169,170; however, see 52).

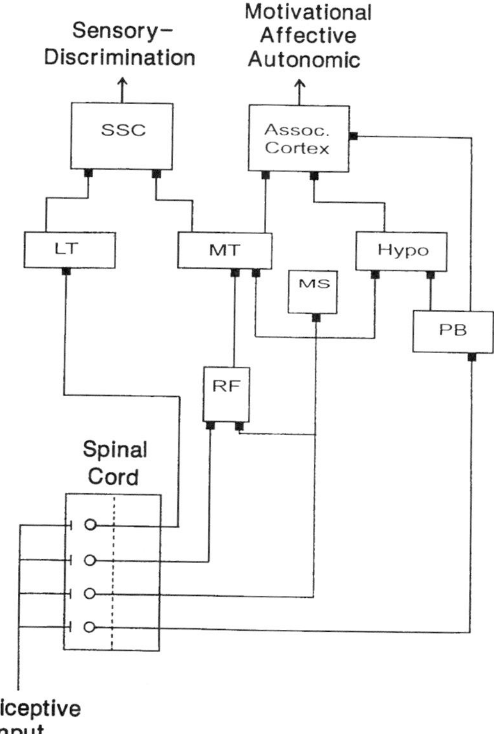

Figure 5. Schematic diagram showing general organization of ascending pathways and their sites of termination that participate in processing nociceptive information from spinal visceral afferent inputs. Assoc. Cortex, association cortex; Hypo, hypothalamus; LT, lateral thalamus; MS, mesencephalon; MT, medial thalamus; PB, parabrachial-nucleus; RF, reticular formation; SSC, somatosensory cortex.

In addition to the spinothalamic pathway system, the spinoreticular pathway has also been shown to receive visceral input, but usually in conjunction with somatic input (98) (Fig. 5). The reticular formation may mediate motor responses to visceral pain as well as motor responses associated with escape and alerting behavior; in addition, sympathetic function may be modulated by collaterals that descend to the intermediolateral cell column or to interneurons (36–39). Other pathways such as the spinomesencephalic (269,270), spinosolitary (171), and spinohypothalamic (51,129) also may convey visceral information, but much less information is known about the visceral responsiveness of these pathways.

Recently it has been shown that the parabrachial region of the pons may serve as an important relay for processing viscerosomatic nociceptive information (Fig. 5). The parabrachial area is composed of a group of cells that surrounds the brachium conjunctivum in the dorsolateral pons and extends to the mesencephalic tegmentum (102). The lateral parabrachial area receives a major projection of axons originating from lamina I (42,54,166,203) and to a lesser extent from laminae V and X of the spinal cord (172). Nociceptive spinovisceral as well as somatic information projects from the parabrachial area to the amygdala (34) and the ventromedial nucleus and the retrochiasmatic area of the hypothalamus (35). It is speculated that this system might be involved with emotional-affective, behavioral, and autonomic reactions to noxious events. To date, this pathway has been described for the rat but has not been studied in any detail in other species. Future studies need to address similarities and differences of the information that is transmitted via the parabrachial relay versus the medial thalamic relay nuclei.

Functional Organization of Visceral-Evoked Afferent Processing

In the preceding sections, the anatomical distribution of segmental afferent input was described. While clear, such connectivity does not reveal the organizational complexity that is involved in the encoding of input which derives from visceral afferents. Three principles should be considered to form the thesis for the following discussion:

1. Spatial organization of projections is part of the encoding processing that provides organizational "meaning" to the output function of a neuron (e.g., the input comes from site X). To the extent that the input from an organ projects uniquely to specific population of cells within a segment and to the extent that these cells project supraspinally to alter organized behavioral components or to motor neuron pools to evoke a reflex, the input can be said to have a local sign. However, it is clear from the preceding sections that visceral afferents (as do somatic afferents) may enter one segment to make synaptic contact and to send collaterals extrasegmentally, and correspondingly activate neurons that are themselves believed to receive primary input from afferents of other segments. Moreover, local axons can potentially project intraspinally to other segments to excite projection neurons. To the extent that this divergence of input occurs, the processing loses its "local sign" and the spatial linkage is less determinable between input and output.
2. Cells may receive convergence from several classes of afferents. To the extent that these several afferents have the same postsynaptic effect (e.g., excitation), then the cell is less able to discriminate between the modalities transduced by each afferent fiber. Such convergence leads to the inability to readily discriminate and creates confusion as to the origin anticipated.
3. As is appreciated from somatic input, the first-order synapse for the primary afferent is uniformly believed to

be excitatory in nature. However, an important principle of neural organization is the existence of inhibitory systems that serve to depress the excitability of the cells. Thus, an afferent excitation may induce a second-order inhibition, either by directly accessing inhibitory interneurons (e.g., a spinospinal inhibition) or it may access long loop systems that serve to produce a local effect through the activation of spinobulbospinal reflex arcs. Such linkages serve to sculpt response properties of the output neuron, leading to a limiting of input properties to which the cell will respond or to regulate frequency response characteristics of the output neuron.

These several modulatory processes are thus essential in considering the nature of the process by which afferent input in general and visceral afferent input in particular is encoded, and governs the response evoked by these systems. Such information provides a neural basis for explaining and defining the organization of visceral sensation and for defining mechanisms of referred pain. One primary example where significant information has been garnered in visceral processing is with respect to the spinal systems activated by cardiopulmonary afferent fiber (for review see ref. 96). Such systems are believed to provide the basis for a number extremely important sympathetic reflex functions (see Chapter 42). This system also provides a model to explain referred pain associated with angina pectoris specifically and serves as a model for referred pain states in general.

Anatomical evidence shows that cardiopulmonary afferent fibers enter the spinal cord primarily in segments T1 to T4 (253), although retrograde HRP transport after cardiopulmonary nerve injections has shown a few dorsal root ganglion cells of C6 and C7 segments to also be filled (123).

Electrophysiologic studies have shown that electrical stimulation of cardiopulmonary afferent axons evokes a strong and widespread excitation of identified STT cells in the T1 and T2 segments (Fig. 6C), with 80% of the population of cells recorded in these spinal segments being activated. Excited cells typically increase their activity on average 72% above control (118).

Cardiopulmonary afferent stimulation has little, if any, effect on the activity of the cells in the C7 and C8 segments that innervate the distal forelimb and hand. This lack of responsiveness of C7–C8 neurons (Fig. 6B) to visceral input is consistent with the anatomical data and agrees with clinical observations showing that anginal pain and other thoracic visceral pain generally are not referred to the hand and the distal forelimb (115,208, 225). A study of C3–C6 STT cells reveals that approximately 60% of these cells are excited following cardiopulmonary afferent stimulation (118) (Fig. 6A).

Electrophysiologic studies and to a lesser extent anatomical studies thus support cardiopulmonary excitation of cells in cervical cord segments. These findings raise the issue about how information from cardiopulmonary afferent fibers of the upper thoracic segments project to the STT cells of these "distal" segments. Electrical stimulation of the inferior cardiac nerve that originates from the heart produces neuronal potentials that are recorded on the dorsal surface of C6 and C8 segments (193). Transection of the T2 and T3 dorsal roots abolishes these potentials, but they remain unchanged after cutting the C8 and T1 dorsal roots. Thus, cardiopulmonary afferent fibers activate a propriospinal pathway that directly or indirectly contacts STT cells in the cervical cord. Alternatively, it is also possible that branches of sympathetic afferent fibers in the T2 to T3 segments travel in or near the zone of Lissauer for several segments (236). If these long projecting fibers produce these effects, then it is unclear why they do not make many contacts with STT cells of the C7 and C8 segments.

Characteristics of Referred Pain

Visceral afferent activity arising from abdominal visceral organs and input from overlying somatic structures converge onto neurons in the lower thoracic (1,56,57,100,113), thoracolumbar (4), or lumbosacral (32,176,187–189) segments (for review, see 190). Until recently a common assumption was that visceral input primarily excited neurons limited to the spinal

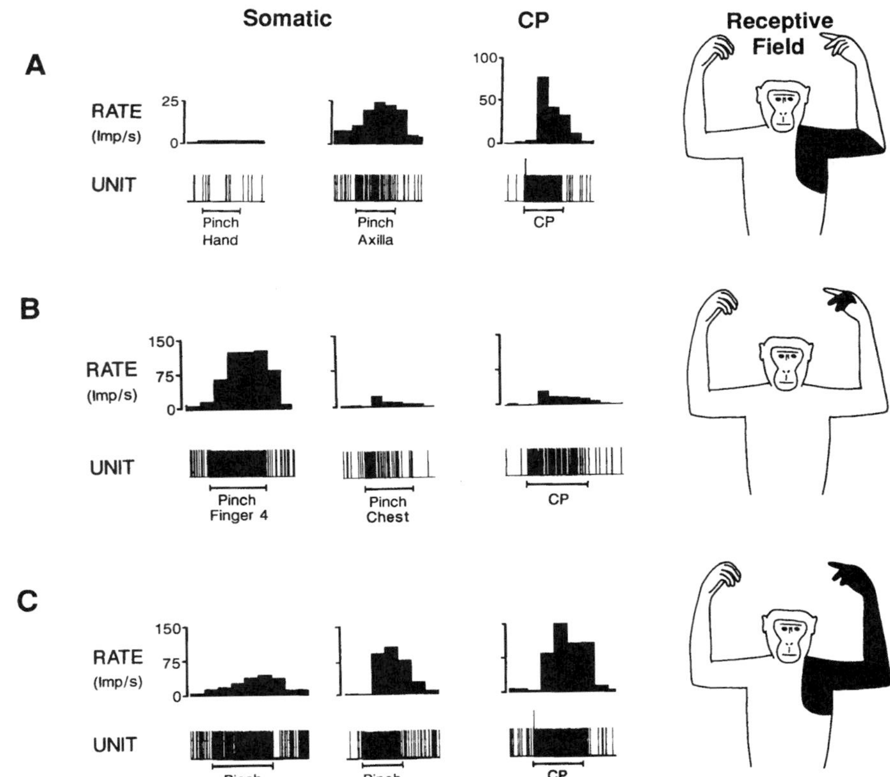

Figure 6. Cervical and thoracic segmental organization of spinothalamic tract (STT) cells in the C5 **(A)**, C8 **(B)**, and T1 **(C)** segments. Responses are to somatic and cardiopulmonary (CP) afferent fiber stimulation and to location of somatic receptive fields. Upper tracings in each panel show discharge rate of cells in impulses per second (Imp/s). Action potentials were collected in one-second bins; thus, a one-second delay occurred between rate and unit activity. *Vertical lines* on lower tracings represent extracellular action potentials after being fed through a window discriminator. The stimulus is represented as a *horizontal bar* under each panel. Illustrations of monkeys with blackened areas show locations of somatic receptive fields. (Modified from ref. 118, with permission.)

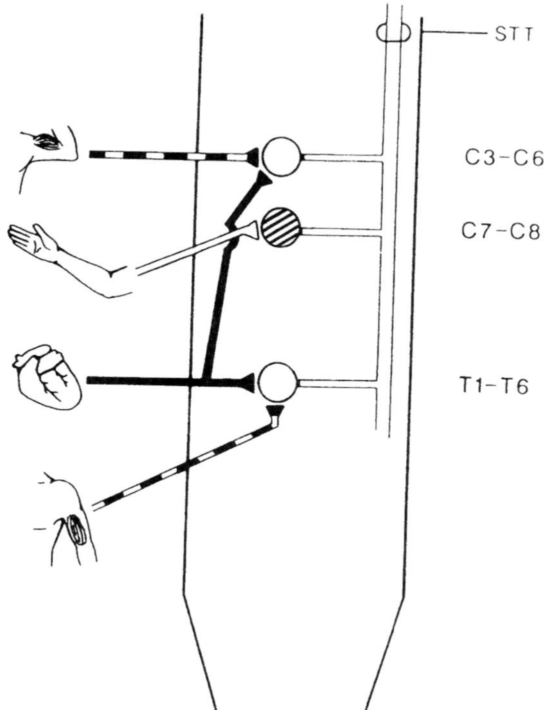

Figure 7. Diagrammatic representation of neural mechanisms to explain characteristics of referred pain associated with angina pectoris. Spinothalamic tract is represented as *circles* with *horizontal lines* extending to the right and the *large vertical bar* represents different segments of the spinal cord. *Open circles* are STT cells with somatic and visceral input. *Slashed circle* represents STT cells with primarily somatic input. Muscle drawn in the upper arm indicates that muscle afferent fibers provide the largest somatic input. *Hashed lines* extending from the upper chest and proximal and distal arm and the heart represent somatic afferent fibers and the *filled lines* represent the sympathetic afferent fibers.

segments innervating tissue overlying the organs and had little if any excitatory effect on the activity of neurons located in distant spinal segments. This convergence of somatic and visceral input onto discrete populations of dorsal horn projection neurons provides an important concept in the phenomenon of referred pain. It is widely appreciated that activation of visceral afferents from a specific organ can yield a system that is "referred" to specific regions on the body surface. Three evident characteristics of referred pain are exemplified by angina pectoris, and the clinical characteristics can be explained using the response properties of the STT cells (Fig. 7): (1) In general, pain originating from the heart and other visceral organs is referred primarily to overlying or adjacent somatic areas (223). The neural basis for this characteristic can be supported by the evidence that STT cells receive convergent input from both the heart and overlying somatic structures (11,12,40,41,118). (2) Anginal pain is referred most commonly to the proximal and axial body, but generally does not involve the extremities (46). It was found that STT cells with proximal receptive fields and not distal fields were strongly activated by cardiopulmonary afferent stimulation (118). (3) Angina pain and visceral pain in general are described as deep, suffering-like pain, not superficial or cutaneous pain (146). The STT cells responses supported this observation because neurons with predominantly cutaneous input exhibited little response to cardiopulmonary stimulation, but cells with predominantly muscle input were strongly excited by cardiopulmonary stimulation (118). The preference for convergence of visceral input to STT cells with muscle input could provide a reason for the fact that visceral sensation is similar to muscle pain (131,132).

Central Sensitization of Visceral Afferent Fibers

Central mechanisms, in addition to peripheral mechanisms, that may provide the functional substrate for hyperalgesic states resulting from injury to the skin, somatic tissues, and visceral organs is currently of considerable interest. A recent review has been written to address the somatic components and central sensitization (267), but very little information is available for visceral effects. It should be pointed out, however, that central sensitization may occur after strong visceral stimulation. Repeated painful distentions with a balloon in the colorectal region in conscious humans elicited increased pain sensitivity and enlarged the area of pain referral to the overlying superficial somatic areas of the body (191). Experimental studies in the animal model support the findings observed in humans. Responses of neurons in the gray matter of the spinal cord that might be involved with processing this information about sensitization in the central nervous system were studied by examining the effects of gallbladder distention (62). Noxious stimulation of the gallbladder enlarges the size of the somatic receptive fields only of spinal neurons that receive this visceral input. Thus, the conditioning visceral stimulus is selective because only those cells responding to the stimulated visceral afferent fibers change their sensitization to the somatic input. Another interesting feature of these responsive cells is that the changes in the somatic referral of visceral pain tended to outlast the duration of the noxious visceral stimulus. This observation correlates well with the clinical experience. These observations may help to explain the anomalous pains states that often are associated with acute and chronic visceral diseases.

Cardiovascular Reflexes

Electrical and natural stimulation of cardiac receptors and their afferent fibers activate a variety of cardiocardiac reflexes. Electrical stimulation of afferent cardiac sympathetic nerves increases arterial pressure (205), myocardial contractility (163), and heart rate (162) primarily through spinal reflexes. Chemosensitive receptors are implicated as epicardial administration of bradykinin activates cardiac sympathetic afferent fibers in anesthetized animals and this input evokes cardiovascular reflexes (92,148,149,186,234,235). In conscious animals, chemical injections of bradykinin into the coronary circulation (200) or the pericardium (88) produce increases in arterial blood pressure, left ventricular pressure, dp/dt, and heart rate. Cardiovascular reflex responses also occur when receptors in the heart are activated with natural stimuli. For example, occlusion of the left coronary artery produces myocardial ischemia that increases activity in preganglionic and postganglionic sympathetic efferent axons coursing to the heart (49,90,91,158,163,164). These reflexes are enhanced if the spinal cord is transected in the cervical region or if sinoaortic denervation and/or vagotomy are done in these animals. While the vagotomy and sinoaortic denervation reveal removal of end-organ regulatory influences, the transection reveals the probable role of modulatory bulbospinal projections activated by ascending input (see Chapter 38) and elicits significant increases in left ventricular pressure, LV dp/dt, and mean arterial pressure (147).

The output generated by cardiac afferent input evokes postganglionic excitation that reflects activation of both local loop and spinobulbospinal reflex arcs. Thus, cardiac sympathetic afferent nerve stimulation after vagotomy and/or sinoaortic denervation most commonly excites adrenal, gastrohepatic, hindlimb muscle, renal, and splenic vasoconstrictor nerves (178, 209,217,257–260). Bulbospinal projections to preganglionic neurons are discussed elsewhere (Chapter 38). Coronary arterial occlusion also increases renal nerve activity (257), which most likely results from activation of receptors located on the superficial epicardial layers of the left ventricle (177).

Corresponding to the influence of afferent input from the heart on other systems, these systems can also alter cardiac performance. Thus, the heart responds to changes that occur in abdominal and pelvic organs (150). Thus, stimulation of mechanical and chemical receptors located in different visceral organs produces cardiorespiratory reflex responses and activates cardiopulmonary preganglionic neurons (69,93,108,197, 198,201). Organizationally, this will be reviewed in greater detail in the next section.

Blood Vessel Innervation and Reflexes

Afferent innervation and sensation, including pain, originating from blood vessels of the extremities have not been addressed either scientifically or clinically to any great extent in recent literature. This sensory innervation of blood vessels in diseased limbs is not taken into consideration as contributing to the disease process and pain sensation. Yet the potential for involving peripheral vasculature and the nervous system in disease processes should be reevaluated. For example, the sensation of dull and aching pain elicited during arterial punctures in patients is particularly unpleasant (26,179). Pseudoaffective reactions attributed to the presence of pain occurs when irritants are injected into the arteries of lightly anesthetized animals (179). All arteries can evoke these reactions, but it is argued that arteries located in the extremities have receptors that are more sensitive to noxious stimuli than those found in the viscera (180).

Sensory nerves and their endings are located with the perivascular plexuses that run in the adventitia of distal blood vessels (117,174,251,266). Nociceptive signals are most likely transmitted in the unmyelinated nerve endings that are found in the adventitia. Afferent information originating from the arteries of the hind limb in animals and the legs in humans enters the spinal cord above the level of entrance of the segmental spinal nerves supplying this region (124,138,206,232). In fact, lumbar sympathectomy eliminated sensations, which led to the conclusion that afferent fibers in the sympathetic trunk mediated this information (87,138,249,255,265).

Sensory afferent fibers from the blood vessels not only may have a role in sensation but also may be important for producing reflex responses that change the diameter of the blood vessels and modulate blood flow (161). This suggestion is based on studies that examined the effects of distending the descending aorta (157). Mechanical and chemical stimulation of the aorta increases the discharge rate of action potentials carried in the sympathetic afferent fibers of the second to the sixth thoracic sympathetic rami communicantes (160,252). This activity produced in these afferent fibers may be important for producing cardiovascular reflex responses to aortic distention in conscious dogs (199). Each animal was instrumented with a stainless steel tube surrounded by an inflatable rubber cylinder that was inserted into the aorta between the T7 and T10 segments. This cannula was designed so that the walls of the thoracic aorta could be stretched without impeding aortic blood flow. Distention of the aorta in this manner produced significant increases in mean aortic pressure and heart rate. Thus, a positive feedback sequence is set in motion because aortic distention produces a potent pressor sympathetic reflex. If these types of reflexes can occur in the aorta, then one can speculate that this type of positive feedback might also occur in the peripheral blood vessels. Such a mechanism could contribute to, or even initiate, events associated with peripheral vascular diseases of the extremities. This type of mechanism is not taken into account to any great extent in the clinical literature (44,46,173). Research in this area might produce important results that would contribute to our understanding about the underlying mechanisms associated with the complex etiologies of these diseases.

SPINAL INTERACTIONS FROM DIVERSE VISCERAL ORGAN SYSTEMS

In the following sections, characteristics of multiorgan interaction will be considered in terms of convergence between somatic (skin/muscle) and visceral, and between cardiac and several representative noncardiac visceral afferent systems. The significance of such organ system interactions may be considered in terms of the effects on sensory perception (e.g., referred pain states) and in terms of evoked (reflex) autonomic outflow.

As summarized in Fig. 3, afferent innervation of different visceral organ systems are mapped onto the spinal cord at discrete spinal levels. As inputs arriving through different segments may demonstrate a functional interaction with populations of cells in adjacent systems, it can be appreciated that this spatial relationship may reflect upon the characteristics of the interaction that exists when afferent input arrives at the spinal level from different visceral organ systems.

Visceral Organ System Interactions

In this section afferent inputs from the gallbladder and urinary bladder are described to illustrate how sensory input from the heart can be modulated by input generated in other distant visceral organs. These organs are chosen for discussion because most of the research done in this area has focused on interactions between these organs and the heart. Furthermore, affer-

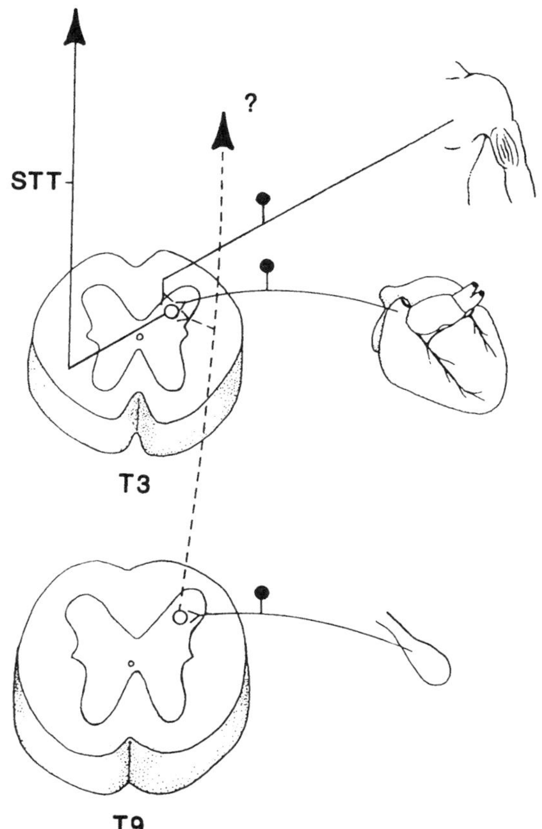

Figure 8. Schematic diagram showing viscero-visceral interactions between the gallbladder and the heart. Spinothalamic tract cell in T3 spinal segment receives somatic and cardiac input and also received excitatory input originating from afferent fibers of the gallbladder projecting to the T9 spinal segment. A propriospinal pathway represented by the *broken line* transmits information to the upper thoracic segments and either terminates there or gives off collaterals as it ascends to supraspinal regions.

ent input from the gallbladder and the urinary bladder affect afferent and efferent pathways of the heart in different ways.

Gallbladder

Gallbladder disease can cause referred pain that mimics angina pectoris (112,175,215,216). In addition, mechanical and/or chemical stimuli applied to the gallbladder can affect the electrical activity and contractile properties of the heart (197) as well as blood pressure (10). Anginal-like pain resulting from gallbladder disease may depend, at least in part, on activation of STT cells in the T1 to T5 segments. Electrical stimulation of the splanchnic nerve excites approximately 75% of the T1 to T5 STT cells and, in addition, these same cells receive excitatory inputs from cardiopulmonary afferent axons as well as somatic afferent information from the upper forearm and chest (8) (Fig. 8). Propriospinal pathways and, to a much lesser extent, the sympathetic chain are most likely responsible for transmitting splanchnic information to upper thoracic segments (20,81,82). Approximately 20% of the T1 to T4 STT cell activity resulting from splanchnic stimulation is removed after the sympathetic chain is cut between segments T5 and T6. The remainder of the activity is abolished when lateral and ventrolateral funiculi are disrupted at the T5 segment (8). Thus, lower and upper thoracic segments are connected with a propriospinal pathway directly or through a pathway that may project to the upper cervical and/or supraspinal levels.

Gallbladder distention has proved to be an effective tool to demonstrate that natural stimuli also activate upper thoracic STT cells and lower thoracic spinal neurons (7,8,10,57). Pressures ranging between 10 and 100 mm Hg are used to distend the gallbladder. The average threshold pressure needed to activate STT cells is 50 mm Hg, a pressure that coincides with gallbladder pressures that occur in acute cholecystitis (79). High-pressure requirements support the argument that these inputs are noxious.

Distention of the gallbladder and electrical stimulation of the cardiopulmonary afferent axons converge with excitatory input on approximately one third of the STT cells in the upper thoracic segments. An interesting finding is that of these responsive cells, 90% respond to intracardiac injections of bradykinin, whereas 55% of cells that do not receive inputs from the gallbladder respond to these chemical injections (7). In addition, bradykinin injections cause greater responses in the gallbladder-responsive neurons than in the cells that do not receive gallbladder input. Thus, in the clinical setting, referred pain of gallbladder origin, which is similar to the pain resulting from myocardial ischemia, may depend on this subpopulation of upper thoracic STT cells. This information, however, does not explain why the gallbladder pain is referred to the abdomen in some patients and to the chest and arm in other patients.

Gallbladder stimulation using mechanical and chemical interventions also can produce cardiovascular changes. Blood pressure increases in a sigmoid fashion when the gallbladder is mechanically distended between 20 and 100 mm Hg in the cat (10). Average distention threshold for initiating a change in arterial pressure is 27 mm Hg. Chemical stimulation of the gallbladder by placing bradykinin on its surface increases heart rate, left ventricular end-diastolic pressure, and left ventricular dp/dt in the cat (196). Bilateral input from splanchnic nerves, but not from the vagus nerves, is necessary to produce these reflexes.

Urinary Bladder

The urinary bladder also can induce interactions between a distant organ and the heart. In contrast to the increased heart rate and cardiac contractility elicited by gallbladder stimulation, the most common responses of the heart to urinary bladder distention are *decreased* rate and cardiac output (18). Decreased heart rate may result from a general decrease in thoracic sympathetic preganglionic efferent neuronal activity (228). Thus, both urinary bladder distention and spontaneous contractions reduce activity in cervical sympathetic preganglionic neurons.

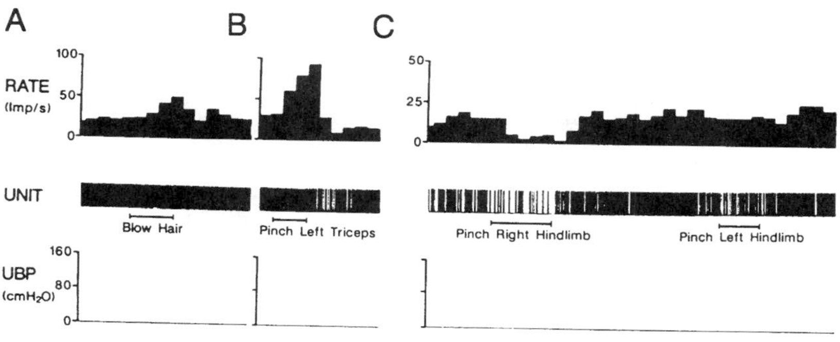

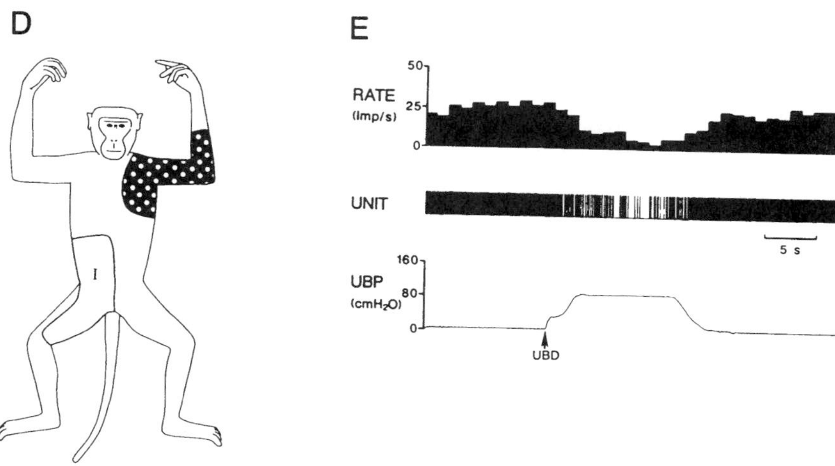

Figure 9. Experimental observations showing inhibitory effects of urinary bladder distention on activity of thoracic STT cells that receive cardiopulmonary afferent input. **A:** Blowing hair of upper arm increased cell activity. *Upper tracing* in each of the panels is the output of rate meter in impulses per second (Imp/s). *Middle tracing* is unit activity of extracellular action potentials after being fed through a window discriminator. Rate meter delays unit activity by one second. UBP = urinary bladder pressure (cm H_2O). **B:** Cell response during pinch of the skin and muscle of the left triceps region. **C:** Cell response during pinch of the hamstring region of the right and left hindlimb. **D:** Somatic receptive field represented as the black background with white dots are excited during noxious pinch of the skin and muscle and during hair movement. I = somatic field where pinching inhibited cell activity. This cell also responded to stimulation of the cardiopulmonary afferent fibers. (Modified from ref. 48, with permission.)

Urinary bladder distention can also modulate afferent evoked excitation of neurons in the upper thoracic segments. Spontaneous and evoked activity of STT cells, spinoreticular tract cells, and spinal neurons of the T1 to T5 segments are inhibited during urinary bladder distention (Fig. 9) (48,119). These bladder-responsive cells are often also excited by afferent input from the heart (119). This suppression occurring as a result of bladder distention may be important for coding intensity and location of noxious visceral and somatic stimuli, as well as for organizing the appropriate sequence of motor responses when multiple noxious stimuli are present.

Decreases in cardiovascular function, efferent sympathetic activity, and suppression of STT cell activity during urinary bladder distention may require the involvement of supraspinal and possibly upper cervical neurons. Supraspinal mechanisms are implicated because blood pressure increases markedly during urinary bladder distention (184) after acute spinal transection at the C8 to T1 segments. It also appears that heart rate either remains unchanged or increased when the urinary bladder has distended. This finding contrasts with the decreased responses observed in the intact animal (18). Furthermore, urinary bladder distention increases blood pressure and elicits inotropic responses in patients who are spinalized above the T1 segment (268), but has little effect on the cardiovascular system in normal individuals (240). Absence of inhibitory responses after spinal transection supports the idea that supraspinal pathways might be required to suppress activity in intact animals and humans. Effects of urinary bladder distention on the cardiovascular reflexes have focused on supraspinal pathways, but recent studies also suggest that propriospinal pathways also may participate in these reflexes.

Intraspinal Inhibitory Neural Mechanisms

Supraspinal nuclei are known to inhibit the activity of STT cells in the spinal cord that receive visceral input (9,13,47), but much less is understood about intraspinal inhibition. Noxious stimulation of the forelimb can inhibit neuronal activity of most lumbosacral STT cells (103), but those inhibitory responses are sometimes present even after spinal cords are transected between the C2 and C4 segments. Evidence that local inhibitions evoked by altered input may persist in spinalized preparations suggests there are local inhibitory interactions. Intraspinal inhibitory mechanisms can thus operate through propriospinal pathways that descend directly and/or indirectly to lumbar and sacral segments. Hobbs et al. (122) demonstrated that stimulation of cardiopulmonary nerves or manipulation of forelimb somatic structures effectively suppresses STT cell activity both before and after transection of the spinal cord at the C1 segment (Fig. 10). In marked contrast, however, inhibitory effects of the same visceral and somatic stimuli before transection are abolished after spinal cord transections are made at or below the C3 segment (Fig. 10). These observations indicate that neuronal mechanisms located in the C1 and C2 segments of the spinal cord participate in intraspinal inhibitory effects. In this scenario propriospinal neurons in the C1 and C2 segments could process and integrate afferent information and then transmit the resultant information to cells in the lumbosacral spinal cord.

Anatomically, it has been shown that cells located in the medial part of the lateral cervical nucleus in these upper cervical segments have axons that project to distant segments of the spinal cord (94,237). Noxious somatic and visceral stimuli acti-

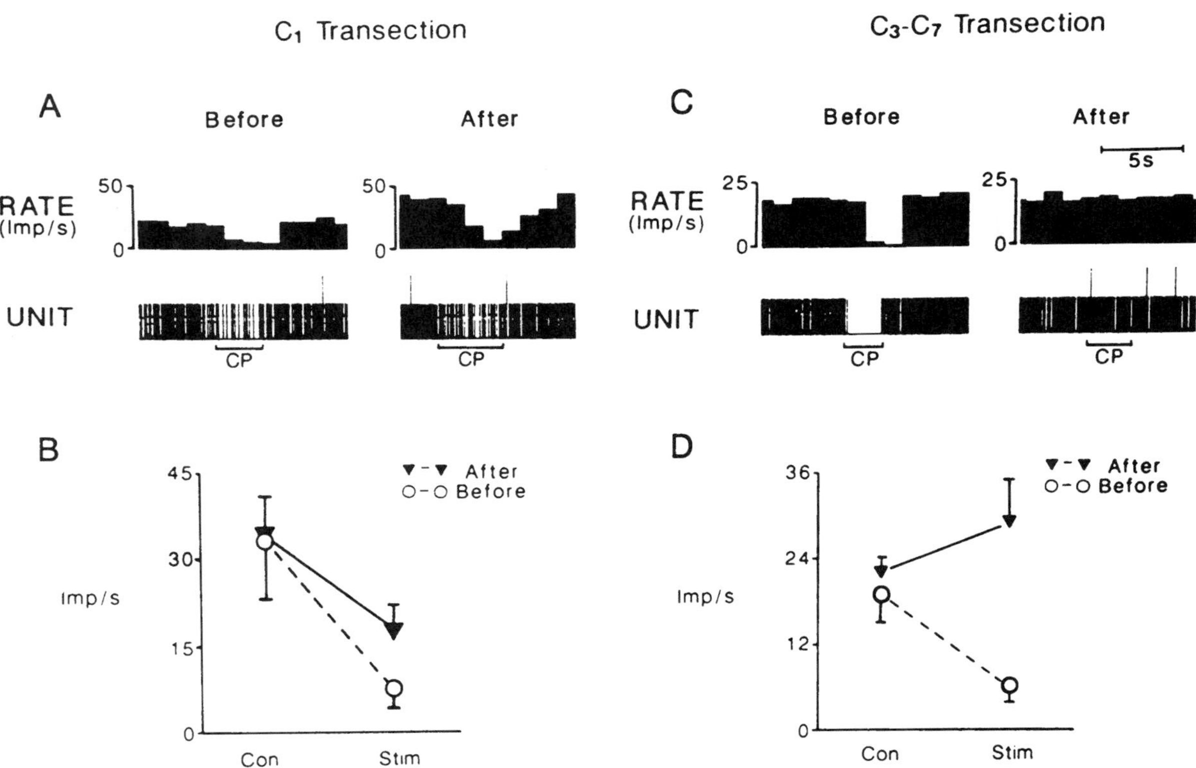

Figure 10. Experimental evidence showing effects of inhibitory responses on lumbosacral STT cells during electrical stimulation of cardiopulmonary afferent fibers. Cardiopulmonary inputs were tested before and after spinal transections at C1 **(A)** and between C3 and C7 segments **(C)**. Tracings are the same as those described in Fig. 9. Inhibitory responses before and after C1 transection in A were similar. However, the inhibitory response before transection was abolished after a transection was made below the C2 segment in a different animal (C). **(B** *and* **D)** Average control (Con) activity and activity during electrical stimulation (Stim) of cardiopulmonary afferent fibers before and after spinal transection. Activity (Imp/s) was reduced significantly before and after C1 transections in five of five animals. Inhibition was abolished after transections between the C3–C7 segments were made in seven of seven animals in another set of experiments. (Modified from ref. 122, with permission.)

vate neurons of this nucleus (78). Studies are now required to identify and characterize response characteristics of the propriospinal cells that may be involved with the intraspinal inhibitory reflex discussed above. A preliminary report has shown that cells with axons projecting to the thoracic and lumbosacral segments are excited by stimulation of cardiopulmonary afferents (68).

At least two mechanisms can be diagrammed to explain how C1–C2 propriospinal neurons might participate in the inhibition of STT neurons (122): (1) Afferent information coming from the cardiopulmonary region or related somatic structures might ascend to the C1–C2 segments (Fig. 11A). This afferent information directly or indirectly activates cells having axons that descend down the spinal cord and suppress activity of STT cells directly or indirectly via inhibitory interneurons. (2) C1–C2 propriospinal neurons could tonically excite inhibitory circuits to provide a constant brake on the activity of lumbosacral STT cells (Fig. 11B). To explain this inhibition, cardiopulmonary afferent input might activate propriospinal neurons located in the upper thoracic spinal gray matter that project down the cord to further excite the same lumbar spinal inhibitory interneurons that also are excited by tonically active propriospinal neurons from the C1–C2 segments. In this scheme, spinal sections below the C2 segment most likely would abolish the tonic excitatory input impinging on the propriospinal inhibitory interneuron circuit. Reduced excitatory input would reduce or abolish the ability of cardiopulmonary activation but by itself would not be sufficient to activate the spinal inhibitory circuit and therefore would not inhibit STT cells. These two schemes might not be mutually exclusive, but

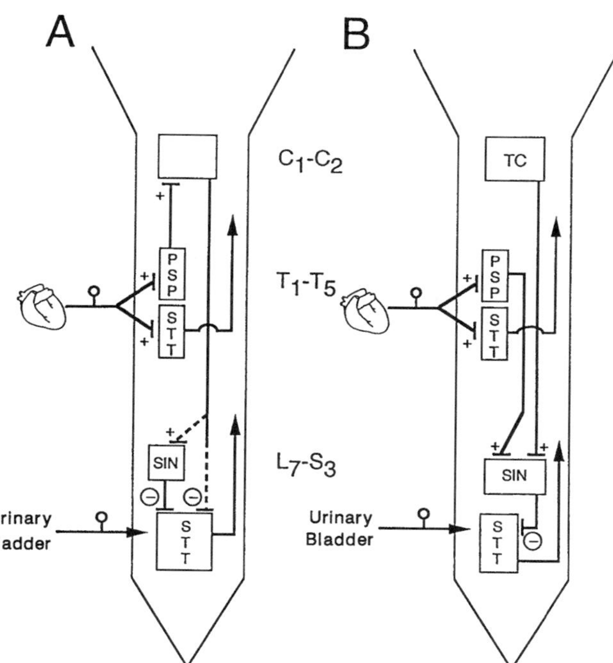

Figure 11. Schematic diagrams are illustrated to explain intraspinal inhibitory neural mechanisms. **A:** Cardiopulmonary afferent information may ascend from thoracic segments to the C1–C2 segments, activate propriospinal neurons that descend down the spinal cord and inhibit STT activity directly or indirectly through spinal inhibitory neurons. **B:** The C1–C2 propriospinal neurons may tonically excite spinal inhibitory neurons. These neurons sustain a constant level of STT cell inhibition. In this paradigm, cardiopulmonary afferent fibers excite propriospinal neurons in thoracic segments that project down to the spinal inhibitory neurons and further suppress STT cell activity. (From ref. 97, with permission.) PSP, propriospinal pathway; SIN, spinal inhibitory neurons; STT, spinothalamic tract; TC, tonic center.

at this time insufficient information exists to describe the functional organization of the C1–C2 propriospinal neurons that inhibit STT neuronal activity.

Intrasegmental inhibition may function to enhance the signal-to-noise ratio of sensory information that is generated by noxious stimuli. A diseased organ increases activity of STT cells in overlying segments. This information is carried to cells located in the ventral posterior lateral thalamus that are somatotopically related to ascending input. In contrast, this increased afferent information from the diseased organ suppresses activity of STT cells located in distant segments. In turn, a sharply reduced amount of information is transmitted to the regions of the ventral posterior lateral thalamus that surround the group of excited thalamic cells. The ability of a person to precisely locate the sensory stimulus may depend on a comparison of activities of thalamic cells excited by a stimulus with the activity of surrounding cells located in the same nucleus that decrease their activities (86). This comparison could increase the signal-to-noise ratio in the thalamus. Increased signal-to-noise ratio could then result in greater ability to differentiate location and intensity of the stimulus.

VAGAL AFFERENT ORGANIZATION

Afferent fibers contained in vagus nerves also participate in regulation of several visceral organs, but this discussion focuses primarily on the cardiovascular system. Vagal afferent activation decreases sympathetic efferent activity and hemodynamic responses (135,229,241,246,248). This section reviews the role of the vagal afferent fibers in modulating sensory information, more specifically noxious information. In addition to reflex effects, activation of vagal afferent fibers may also modulate pain sensitivity (5,6,99,153,155,212). Vagal afferent pathways appear to be involved in decreasing pain sensitivity in conscious animals (214). Hypertensive rats exhibit a lower pain sensitivity that increases after vagotomy (271). Right cervical vagotomy in spontaneously hypertensive rats reverses opioid-mediated analgesia using hot plate assays of pain sensitivity. Right cervical vagotomy also reduces stress-induced analgesia resulting from intermittently shocking the foot of rat (155,156). It is important to note that humans who have borderline or essential hypertension experience increased sensory and pain thresholds to tooth pulp stimulation (104,222,272).

Decreased pain sensitivity most likely results from suppression of noxious information in pain pathways during vagal afferent stimulation. Studies performed in rats, cats, and monkeys show that vagal stimulation reduces the number of action potentials to noxious stimuli in spinothalamic tract and spinoreticular tract neurons (5,66,121,221,244) and in dorsal horn neurons (218,243).

Vagal suppression of pain sensitivity has gained interest in light of reports about silent ischemia. Although several mechanisms have been proposed (17), the ability of increased vagal activity to decrease pain sensitivity, increase pain thresholds, and suppress spinothalamic tract cell activity has led to the suggestion that the vagus may play a role in asymptomatic myocardial ischemia and possibly in unrecognized myocardial infarction (5,83,99). In the following sections details about the vagus and its effects are described. Then a more detailed discussion about silent ischemia and the role of the vagus nerve is presented.

Vagal Afferent Fibers and Terminals

Small myelinated and unmyelinated vagal afferent fibers transmit action potentials from the heart to the brainstem. Receptors with myelinated fibers originate primarily from the atria and venoatrial junction (76,202,248). Fewer myelinated fibers originate from receptors located in the ventricle and coronary arteries (75,80). In contrast, unmyelinated fibers have sensory endings distributed to all regions of the heart (21,75,

183,233,247,248). Although studies of this type yield information regarding distribution of afferent fibers, they do not provide an accurate picture about the density of afferents originating from receptors in different regions of the heart.

Receptor endings associated with unmyelinated fibers are separated primarily into chemosensitive or mechanosensitive responders. Chemosensitive endings do not appear to discharge with a cardiac rhythm (130) and are unresponsive to all but extreme vascular distentions. Afferent traffic in these endings increases when the endogenous, potentially algesic chemical bradykinin is injected into the left atrium or is applied to the surface of the heart (130). Prostaglandin E_2 markedly increases activity of vagal afferents that fire irregularly and are relatively insensitive to increased ventricular pressure. Exogenous chemicals, such as capsaicin, phenylbiguanide, nicotine, and veratrum alkaloid, also excite these afferents (21). Afferent impulses in fibers with mechanosensitive endings in control conditions commonly display a more regular discharge pattern; usually one or two impulses occur with each cardiac cycle (21,247). Increased activity with a rhythmic discharge pattern in these endings occurs when the ventricular volume is increased during venous infusion or aortic occlusion endings (247). In addition nicotine and veratrum alkaloids activate many of these afferents (194,233). However, in contrast to chemosensitive endings, capsaicin, phenylbiguanide, bradykinin, and prostaglandins do not appear to stimulate mechanosensitive endings (21,130).

Myocardial ischemia generated during coronary artery occlusion increases activity of unmyelinated vagal afferent fibers (245,246). In general, myocardial bulging and changes in the S-T segment of the ECG occur before afferent activity of vagal fibers increases. Initially increased activity usually displays cardiac rhythm, but the discharge pattern becomes continuous as the occlusion is maintained. These afferents appear to have mechanosensitivity, but responses of afferents with chemosensitive endings have not been studied systematically during myocardial ischemia. It is likely that chemosensitive and mechanosensitive afferents increase their discharge rate during coronary artery occlusion. The assumption, however, that chemosensitive afferents are excited is based on the observation that chemicals released during ischemia excite them; actual experiments to demonstrate this have not been done.

Vagal Afferents and Their Effects on Central Sensory Processing

Since vagal stimulation inhibits activity of neurons that affect cardiovascular and other responses, it is possible that vagal stimulation also suppresses sensory processing by inhibiting the activity of neurons involved with integrating of nociceptive information, i.e., STT cells. Stimulation of the left thoracic vagus markedly inhibits the increased STT cell activity that follows bradykinin injections (Fig. 12A). These effects are eliminated after transection of the cervical vagi (Fig. 12B) (6). Vagal stimulation also markedly reduces evoked activity of STT cells that results from applying a noxious pinch to somatic receptor fields located on the left shoulder, chest, and left arm. These results support the possibility that activation of vagal afferent fibers can suppress potentially noxious sympathetic cardiac afferent input that activates STT cells in upper thoracic segments.

Vagal afferents originating in the cardiopulmonary region are primarily responsible for suppressing primate STT cell activity. This finding is based on evidence that electrical stimulation of the thoracic vagus above the heart or cervical vagus suppresses activity of primate STT cells; but no significant inhi-

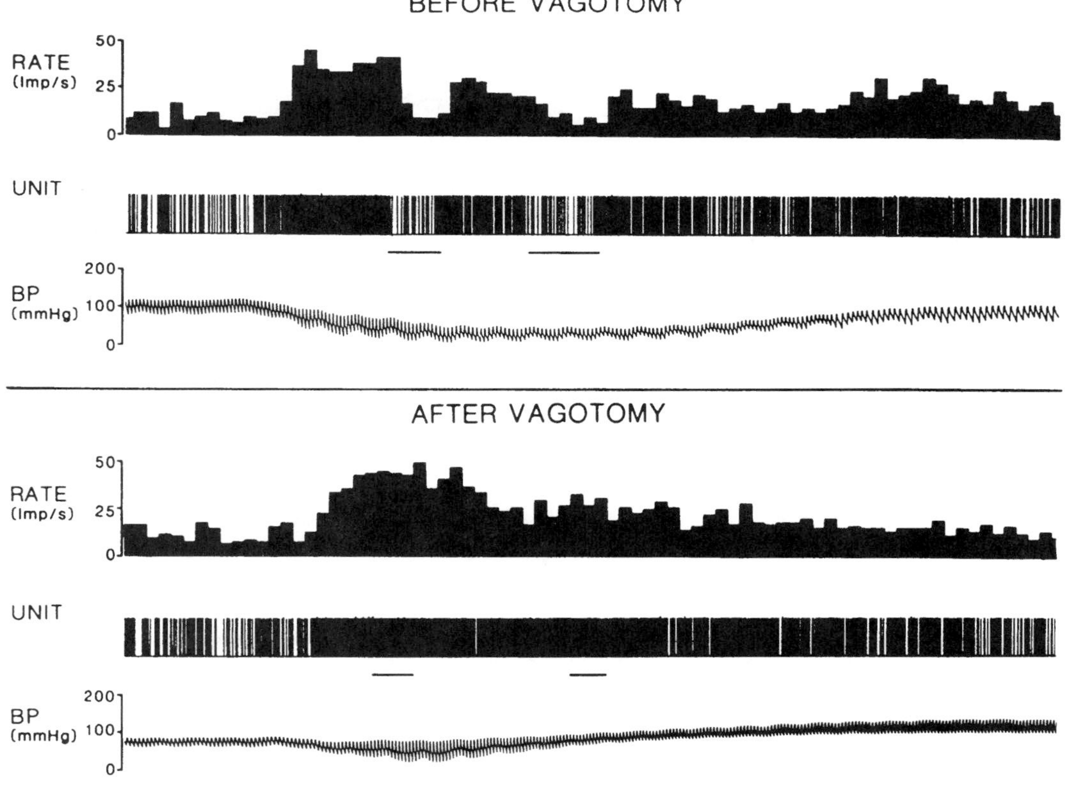

Figure 12. Vagal inhibition of STT cell activity. Vagal stimulation inhibited activity of an STT cell to an intracardiac injection of bradykinin before, but not after, bilateral cervical vagotomy. Period of left thoracic vagal stimulation (6.9 V, 2 ms, 20 Hz) is marked by *bars* below second trace in each panel. Tracings from top to bottom are rate of cell discharge (rate), output of the window discriminator (unit; each deflection represents one cell spike), and blood pressure (BP). (Modified from ref. 6, with permission.)

bition is produced when the vagus is stimulated between the heart and diaphragm (5,121). In addition, stimulation of the cardiac branch of the vagus reduces the discharge rate of STT cells in a manner similar to the inhibition observed for thoracic vagal stimulation, demonstrating that afferents in the cardiac branch make the major contribution for the inhibitory responses of the thoracic vagus (5). Thus, these results provide support that vagal afferent fibers from the cardiopulmonary region and more specifically the heart are critical for inhibiting STT cell activity.

Although studies on the primate STT cells show that stimulation of the abdominal vagus does not affect spontaneous or evoked activity of STT cells, these results are not in full agreement with vagal stimulation studies reported in the rat (250). In rats, the tail flick reflex and dorsal horn cells in lumbar spinal cord are inhibited during electrical stimulation of abdominal vagal afferent fibers. Differences might exist because different species were studied, different anesthetic was used, or different pathways were involved.

Inhibition of STT cell activity is the predominant effect resulting from electrical stimulation of thoracic vagal afferent fibers. Left thoracic vagal stimulation suppresses approximately 60% of STT cells (5); however, about 10% are excited or are excited and then inhibited. The remainder of the cells are unresponsive to vagal stimulation. Overall cell activity decreased significantly when the responses of all cells tested for vagal stimulation are compared to control spontaneous activity. Again, observations made in rats (218,221) differ somewhat from the primate studies in that a larger percentage of rat STT cells and spinal neurons are facilitated during cervical vagal stimulation. It should be pointed out that vagal stimulation facilitated the evoked noxious response of the cells, but the stimulus did not directly produce excitation of the cell without the noxious input. Low-intensity stimulation applied during a noxious stimulation facilitates activity of approximately 25% of the cells, and higher intensities inhibit noxious responses in rats. In the primate STT studies lower stimulus intensities were not examined routinely; therefore, this facilitatory response might have been missed. Another complicating factor is that stimulation of the cervical vagus may activate nonvagal fibers that produce facilitation (155), whereas thoracic vagal stimulation may produce less facilitation of cells. In summary, the predominant effect of vagal stimulation is suppression of somatic and cardiac input to STT cells, which provides a mechanism for increasing pain threshold and decreasing pain sensitivity.

Vagal afferent stimulation causes a general inhibitory effect on STT neurons at most levels of the spinal cord. Spontaneous and evoked activities of STT cells at the lower cervical, thoracic, and lumbosacral segments of the spinal cord are suppressed during vagal stimulation (5,66,121). Similar findings also are observed in lumbosacral spinal neurons and STT cells of the rat (218,221).

Central Integration

Supraspinal pathways and nuclei that might be involved in the suppression of sensory processing of STT cells by vagal stimulation are discussed in this section. Although a number of candidate regions of the brainstem have been implicated, anatomical, behavioral, and physiologic evidence suggests that the subcoeruleus parabrachial (SC-PB)/locus coeruleus region of the pons may be one of the important relays for producing vagal suppression of STT cells.

Vagal afferent fibers terminate primarily in the caudal medulla of the brainstem (28). The contralateral nucleus tractus solitarius (NTS) also receives afferent fibers that cross the midline. Physiologic evidence in the rat shows that vagal suppression of spinal neuronal activity is dependent on the NTS (219).

The caudal part of the NTS is important in primates because neurons from this region send a large number of their axons to the medial and lateral parabrachial nuclei (27). Since the vagus terminates primarily in the caudal NTS, one could argue that vagal information is carried in this pathway to the SC-PB region. In the SC-PB region a population of cells sends axons to the spinal cord (114,239,262,263). To continue the argument, information originating from the vagus most likely is processed in this population of cells and then sends a volley of activity down these axons and either directly or indirectly suppresses STT cell activity.

To demonstrate that neurons of the SC-PB region can suppress sensory processing, electrical stimulation of ipsilateral and contralateral sites in the SC-PB region strongly inhibits increased STT cell activity after bradykinin is injected into the

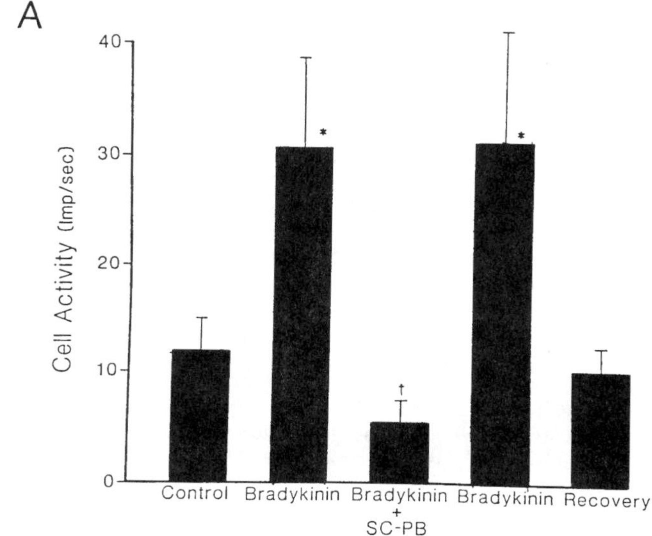

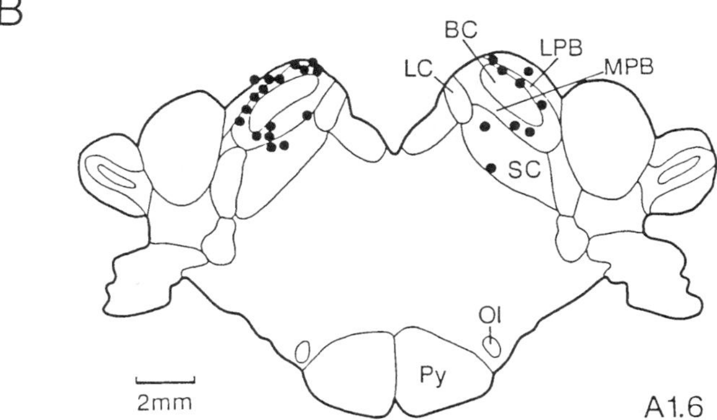

Figure 13. Electrical stimulation of subcoeruleus parabrachialis (SC-PB) suppresses increased STT cell activity in response to noxious visceral stimuli. **A:** Increase in cell activity following intracardiac bradykinin injections (4 μg/kg) was significantly greater than control (p<.05). SC-PB stimulation decreased cell activity below the bradykinin values (p<.05). Three bradykinin bars were obtained by measuring STT cell activity at three different times during the response to a single injection of bradykinin. First bradykinin bar was measured just before and the second one was measured just after the SC-PB stimulation. **B:** SC-PB stimulation sites producing suppression of STT cell activity are marked by *black dots* on one brainstem section of the monkey drawn from the atlas of Szabo and Cowan (238) and modified according to Westlund et al. (262). The left side is ipsilateral to the spinothalamic tract cell. BC, brachium conjunctivium; LPB, lateral parabrachial nucleus; MPB, medial parabrachial nucleus; SC, nucleus subcoeruleus; LC, nucleus locus coeruleus; Py, pyramid; OI, inferior olivary nucleus. (From ref. 47, with permission.)

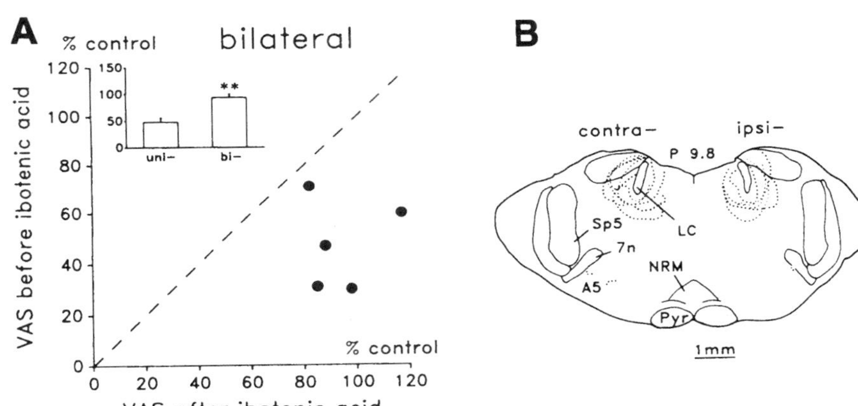

Figure 14. Experimental observations showing that the dorsolateral pons modulates spinal nociceptive transmission resulting from vagal stimulation. **A:** Effects of vagal stimulation (VAS) at the same intensity on spinal neurons that responded to heating of skin before and after ibotenic acid is microinjected bilaterally into the dorsolateral pons. Values in the abscissa and ordinate are expressed as a percentage of control response to heating. Each *dot* represents total number of impulses in 22 s. *Inset* illustrates mean data after unilateral and bilateral microinjections of ibotenic acid. **B:** *Dotted lines* outline the extent ibotenic acid produced lesions. A5, cell group; contra-, contralateral to spinal recording site; P9.8, brain stem section 9.8 mm posterior to the bregma in the rat; LC, locus coeruleus; ipsi-, ipsilateral to spinal recording site; NRM, nucleus raphe magnus; Pyr, pyramidal tract; 7n, facial nerve; Sp5, spinal trigeminal nucleus. (From ref. 220, with permission.)

heart (Fig. 13) (47) and during noxious stimulation of the somatic receptive fields (105). This showed the efficacy of inhibition from the region, but did not directly show if the vagus could activate these neurons and then produce the inhibition. A study in the rat more directly linked the vagus, the SC-PB region, and the neurons of the spinal cord (220). Bilateral injection of ibotenic acid, a selective neurotoxin for cell bodies, into the locus coeruleus/subcoeruleus region significantly attenuates suppression of nociceptive spinal activity when the vagus is stimulated (Fig. 14). These studies taken together suggest excitation of the vagal afferents activates neurons in the subcoeruleus and parabrachial region, and possibly the locus coeruleus, to produce modulation of pain.

Behavioral and pharmacologic studies also support the argument that the SC-PB is important for modulation of spinal nociceptive transmission. Basal nociceptor thresholds of the tail-flick or hot-plate test are not altered after lesions are made in the medial parabrachial nucleus, but the lesions do attenuate morphine analgesia (111). Nociceptive responses also are markedly suppressed when the muscarinic antagonist carbachol is injected in the vicinity of the SC-PB (128). Additional supraspinal nuclei such as the nucleus raphe magnus and rostral ventrolateral medulla may suppress neuronal activity during vagal stimulation (10,211,213,219,220). These studies have not been emphasized because their anatomical connections with the vagus nerve and NTS have not been described to any great extent.

While the emphasis for vagal inhibition has focused on supraspinal mechanisms, propriospinal neuronal mechanisms in the upper cervical segments of the spinal cord may also process information that might produce inhibition. Recent experimental evidence provides support for this suggestion. At least a small number of vagal afferent fibers enter the brainstem and descend to these cervical segments without synapsing first in the NTS of the medulla (167). In general, vagal afferent stimulation suppresses cardiocardiac and cardiosympathetic reflexes, the activity of STT cells below the C2 segment of the spinal cord (5,6,66,121), and cells in the trigeminal nucleus of the medulla (154). In marked contrast, however, vagal stimulation strongly excites spinal neurons (101) and STT cells (65) of the C1–C2 spinal segments (Fig. 15).

In addition, vagal afferent stimulation excites cells in the C1 to C3 segments that have axons projecting to the thoracic and lumbar segments (68). These propriospinal neurons may be the ones participating in the inhibition of STT cells in the distant segments of the spinal cord (122). Since vagal afferent input suppresses spinal visceral reflexes, one could argue that this inhibition is, in part, dependent on inhibitory mechanisms that involve the cervical spinal cord. Vagal input could directly or indirectly excite cells in the upper cervical segments and then send information down the spinal cord to suppress activity of autonomic neurons and sensory neurons directly and/or through spinal inhibitory mechanisms. The proposal for a cervical inhibitory pathway does not exclude involvement of a supraspinal mechanism. It is even possible that supraspinal mechanisms could set the bias to maintain the balance between excitatory and inhibitory inputs. An important goal is to explain how the central nervous system maintains the balance between inhibitory and excitatory processing in normal physiologic situations and how it alters this balance in pathologic conditions.

Vagal Afferents and Silent Ischemia

Clinical Description

Silent myocardial ischemia is the term used to describe a situation where the diagnostic information about the status of the heart predicts that angina pectoris should be felt in the patient, and yet none of the anginal symptoms is present. The symptoms of silent myocardial ischemia result from a transient imbalance between myocardial oxygen supply and demand. This imbalance mobilizes a series of metabolic, mechanical, hemodynamic, and electrocardiographic events that can be documented objectively (17) and is usually associated with angina pectoris. Yet in silent myocardial ischemia these events occur in the absence of chest pain or the usual angina equivalents such as arm or jaw pain and numbness. Patients are classified into two categories based on the presence or absence of angina pectoris in the face of myocardial ischemia (74). They are categorized as symptomatic if angina pectoris is experienced during myocardial ischemia and asymptomatic if episodes of ischemia occur without the associated pain. Silent myocardial ischemia can be separated into three types: type I patients are asymptomatic and have no history of myocardial infarction or angina pectoris, type II patients are asymptomatic but have had a myocardial infarction, and type III patients experience angina pectoris but also experience episodes of silent myocardial ischemia (74). Asymptomatic ischemic events occur approximately 60% to 80% of the time (17).

Clinical Correlations of Vagal Afferents and Silent Ischemia

Three theories have been outlined to explain the lack of anginal symptoms during episodes of significant myocardial ischemia (17): (1) global deficiency in pain perception, (2) anatomic changes in pain receptors and nerves, and (3) quantitative theory of silent myocardial ischemia. This last theory is based on the suggestion that myocardial ischemia is quantita-

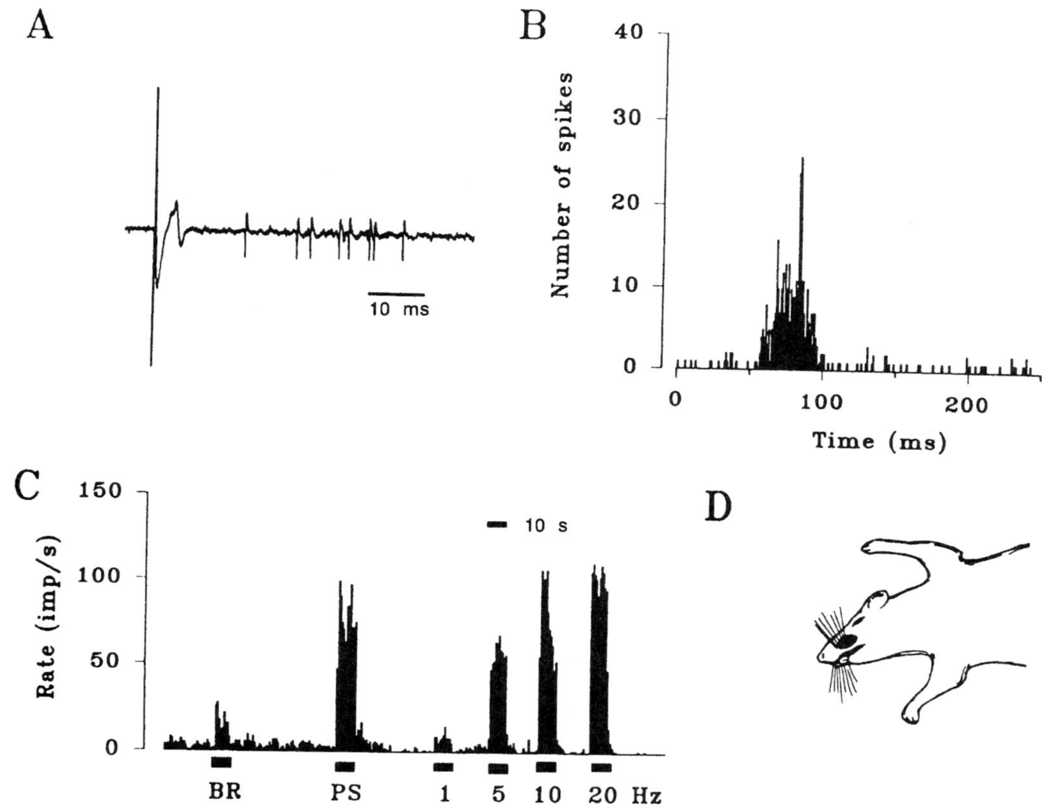

Figure 15. Excitatory effects of ipsilateral cervical vagal stimulation (ICVS) on the activity of a wide dynamic range cell in the C1 segment. **A:** A single oscilloscopic tracing showing the response to electrical stimulation of vagus nerve (33 V, 0.1 ms). Extracellular action potentials of cell occur approximately 12 ms after stimulus artifact (first large deflection). **B:** Peristimulus histogram (50 stimulus repetitions) of the cell response to ICVS. Stimulus delay was 50 ms and bin width was 1 ms. **C:** Tracing is output from a rate meter rate (imp/s) showing the response to somatic stimuli (BR, brushing hair; PS, pinching skin) and to ICVS at four frequencies (1–20 Hz). *Solid horizontal bars* mark the period of stimulus. **D:** *Blackened area* on the snout illustrates the excitatory somatic receptive field for this cell. (From ref. 101, with permission.)

tively less when it is associated with silent ischemia than with angina pectoris. Each of these or all three together may be needed to explain all aspects of silent myocardial ischemia, but the discussion in this section addresses the mechanisms related to global deficiency in pain perception. This theory is highlighted because vagal modulation of sensory processing can be hypothesized as one of the mechanisms that can lead to silent ischemia and produce pain deficiency.

Uneven distribution of vagal afferent fiber endings on the heart may contribute to silent ischemic episodes. Myocardial ischemia activates both sympathetic and vagal afferent fibers. An imbalance in the activity of these afferent fibers may lead to angina pectoris or silent ischemia depending on which population of afferent fibers are stimulated more intensely. This imbalance may occur because vagal afferent fibers have varying densities of receptors in different regions of the heart; vagal afferents are more concentrated in the inferior-posterior wall of the left ventricle (90,256), whereas sympathetic afferents appear to have a more general distribution in the heart (178). Hemodynamic studies show that myocardial infarction of the inferior wall of the ventricle often results in bradycardia and hypotension, responses that usually are associated with activation of vagal reflexes (210,261). In contrast, anterior myocardial infarction results more often in tachycardia and hypertension, responses that often are associated with activation of sympathetic reflexes (210,261). Vagal reflexes are evoked more effectively during experimental occlusion of the left circumflex artery than during occlusion of the left anterior descending artery (242). It is known that excitation of sympathetic afferent fibers by electrical stimulation and coronary artery occlusion significantly increases activity of the STT cells, whereas activation of vagal afferents in general can suppress STT activity. Since vagal and sympathetic afferent fibers to the heart are distributed unequally, a strong vagal input may suppress STT cell activities and thereby prevent information from reaching areas of the brain regions involved with pain perception. In contrast, strong excitation of sympathetic afferent fibers would increase STT cell activity, resulting in the symptoms of angina pectoris.

Silent myocardial ischemia more likely occurs in patients who experience ischemia in the inferior-posterior regions of the left ventricle. Preferential distribution of vagal afferent fibers and vagal reflexes to the inferior-posterior regions of the left ventricle may contribute to asymptomatic nature of these ischemic episodes. Further evidence is provided from a study showing that abnormalities in left ventricular wall movement localized to the inferior-posterior regions are related more significantly to asymptomatic patients (84). Thus, differential effects of sympathetic and vagal afferent input to STT cells may provide a possible neural basis for episodes of angina pectoris or silent myocardial ischemia. Right coronary artery stenosis or left circumflex stenosis is more frequently found in asymptomatic patients, but stenosis of the left anterior descending artery is more often observed in symptomatic patients. These findings, combined with the vagal distribution, leads to the proposal that myocardial ischemia localized in the inferior-posterior region of the heart tends to be asymptomatic because vagal afferent fibers are activated preferentially (84). Strong activation of the vagal afferents could activate the pathways that suppress activity of the STT cells. Their decreased discharge rate would not activate pain perception areas of the brainstem and the cortex. As a result, patients could experience ischemia episodes without angina symptoms.

Asymptomatic patients also are more likely to exhibit a higher threshold for perceiving somatic pain even though the significant ST-segment depression observed during exercise stress testing is similar to that in patients who experience symptoms (83,85,89,106,204). Altered pain perception appears not to result from destruction of specific myocardial nociceptive pathways because frequency of prior infarction, extent of multivessel coronary disease, and diseases such as diabetes and alcoholism that alter nociceptive capabilities are similar for both groups of patients. Different types of nociceptive modalities including electric shock, cold pressor stimulation, and tourniquet-induced forearm ischemia reveal that patients with silent myocardial ischemia experience a higher pain threshold and greater tolerance for these types of somatic pain than those with angina pectoris. Our finding that the vagus also suppresses activity arising from somatic structures supports the possibility that increased vagal activity may lead to higher pain thresholds and greater pain tolerance. Since asymptomatic patients can demonstrate decreased pain sensitivity even when there is no myocardial ischemic episode, tonic vagal activity may generally suppress STT cell activity. This aspect of the puzzle has not been clarified experimentally.

Conceptual Description of Physiologic and Clinical Mechanisms

A conceptual model based on physiologic and clinical studies is provided to describe how vagal afferents may play a role in asymptomatic patients. The information described in the previous sections is summarized in Fig. 16. Mechanosensitive and chemosensitive receptors of vagal afferents are preferentially excited during ischemic episodes in the inferior-posterior wall of the left ventricle. Sympathetic afferent fibers may be activated from this region at the same time, but the vagal afferent input predominates. Increased vagal afferent activity transmitted through the nodose ganglion makes excitatory synaptic connections on cells in the caudal nucleus tractus solitarius and/or projects directly to the upper cervical spinal cord. The NTS has fibers that project to the SC-PB/locus coeruleus region, and excite cells that send their axons down the spinal cord. The information is transmitted in this descending pathway and the potential pathway if the upper cervical spinal cord either directly or indirectly suppresses the activity of STT cells. Thus, the reduced activity of STT cells might result in silent ischemia.

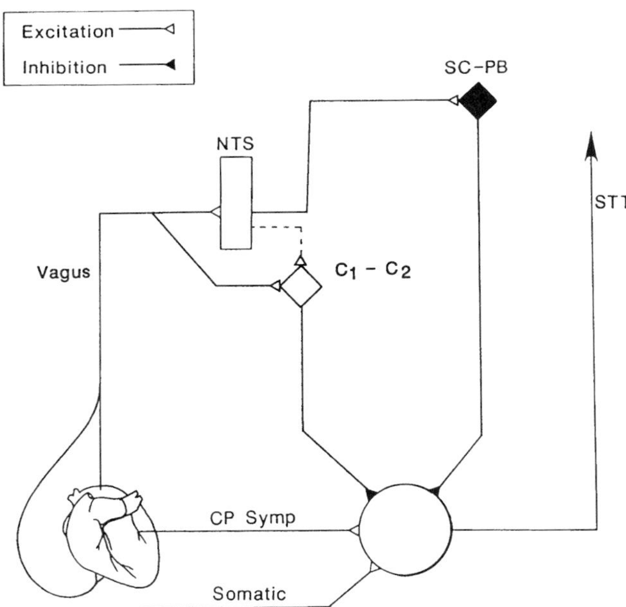

Figure 16. Schematic diagram illustrating the neural pathway that may modulate STT activity by vagal stimulation. *Filled diamond* highlights the possible supraspinal region for integration of vagal inhibition. *Open diamond* represents a possible spinal mechanism that may participate in vagal inhibition of STT cells. *Continuous lines* represent known pathways and *interrupted lines* represent indirect pathways. Connections between input and representative cell nucleus or region may be monosynaptic or polysynaptic. Inhibition from descending pathways may be presynaptic or postsynaptic. CP Symp, cardiopulmonary sympathetic afferent fibers; NTS, nucleus tractus solitarius; NRM, nucleus raphe magnus; Somatic, somatic afferent fibers; STT, spinothalamic tract system; SC-PB, subcoeruleus-parabrachial region.

ACKNOWLEDGMENTS

The author's studies were supported by Public Health Service Grant HL22732, and grants from the Presbyterian Health Foundation, Oklahoma Center for Advancement of Science and Technology, and the American Heart Association, Oklahoma Affiliate. The author is grateful for the important scientific contributions of W. S. Ammons, R. W. Blair, D. C. Bolser, T. J. Brennan, M. J. Chandler, Q.-G. Fu, M.-N. Girardot, S. F. Hobbs, R. N. Weber, U. T. Oh, and Jianhua Zhang, who were postdoctoral fellows or graduate students in his laboratory. These studies were accomplished because of their hard work, commitment, creativity, and devotion. A special word of appreciation to D. Holston for providing technical assistance, making the illustrations, and taking the photographs, and to C. Hulka for typing the manuscript.

REFERENCES

1. Akeyson EW, Knuepfer MM, Schramm LP. Splanchnic input to thoracic spinal neurons and its supraspinal modulation in the rat. *Brain Res* 1990;536:30–40.
2. Albe-Fessard D, Berkley KJ, Kruger L, Ralston HJ III, Willis WD Jr. Diencephalic mechanisms of pain sensation. *Brain Res Rev* 1985;9: 217–296.
3. Albe-Fessard D, Besson JM. Convergent thalamic and cortical projections. The non-specific system. In: Iggo A, ed. *Handbook of sensory physiology*. Berlin: Springer-Verlag, 1973;489–560.
4. Ammons W S. Responses of primate spinothalamic tract neurons to renal pelvic distention. *J Neurophysiol* 1989;62:778–788.
5. Ammons WS, Blair RW, Foreman RD. Vagal afferent inhibition of primate thoracic spinothalamic neurons. *J Neurophysiol* 1983;50: 926–940.
6. Ammons WS, Blair RW, Foreman RD. Vagal afferent inhibition of spinothalamic cell responses to sympathetic afferents and bradykinin in the monkey. *Circ Res* 1983;53:603–12.
7. Ammons WS, Blair RW, Foreman RD. Responses of primate T_1–T_5 spinothalamic neurons to gallbladder distention. *Am J Physiol* 1984;247:R995–R1002.
8. Ammons WS, Blair RW, Foreman RD. Greater splanchnic excitation of primate T1–T5 spinothalamic neurons. *J Neurophysiol* 1984; 51:592–603.
9. Ammons WS, Blair RW, Foreman RD. Raphe magnus inhibition of primate T_1–T_4 spinothalamic cells with cardiopulmonary visceral input. *Pain* 1984;20:247–260.
10. Ammons WS, Foreman RD. Cardiovascular and T_2–T_4 dorsal horn cells responses to gallbladder distention in the cat. *Brain Res* 1984; 321:267–277.
11. Ammons WS, Girardot M-N, Foreman RD. T_2–T_5 spinothalamic neurons projecting to medial thalamus with viscerosomatic input. *J Neurophysiol* 1985;54:73–89.
12. Ammons, WS, Girardot M-N, Foreman RD. Effects of intracardiac bradykinin on T_2–T_5 medial spinothalamic cells. *Am J Physiol* 1985; 249:R147–R152.
13. Ammons WS, Girardot M-N, Foreman RD. Periventricular gray

inhibition of thoracic spinothalamic cells projecting to medial and lateral thalamus. *J Neurophysiol* 1986;55:1091–1103.

14. Apkarian AV, Brüggemann JST, Airapetian LR. A thalamic model for true and referred visceral pain. In: Gebhart GF, ed. *Visceral pain, progress in pain research and management,* vol 5. Seattle: IASP Press, 1995;217–259.
15. Apkarian AV, Hodge CJ Jr. Primate spinothalamic pathways II. The cells of origin of the dorsolateral and ventral spinothalamic pathways. *J Comp Neurol* 1989;288:474–492.
16. Applebaum AE, Vance WH, Coggeshall RE. Segmental localization of sensory cells that innervate the bladder. *J Comp Neurol* 1980;192:203–209.
17. Assey ME. The recognition and treatment of silent myocardial ischemia. In: Hurst JW, ed. *The heart, arteries and veins.* New York: McGraw-Hill Information Services, 1990;1079–1086.
18. Baccelli G, Giuseppe M, Alberto DB, Albertini R, Zanchetti A. Cardiovascular changes during spontaneous micturition in conscious cats. *Am J Physiol* 1979;237:H213–H217.
19. Bahns E, Ernsherger U, Jänig W, Nelke A. Functional characteristics of lumbar visceral afferent fibres from the urinary bladder and the urethra in the cat. *Pflugers Arch* 1986;407:510–518.
20. Bain WA, Irving JT, McSwiney BA. The afferent fibres from the abdomen in the splanchnic nerves. *J Physiol (Lond)* 1935;84: 323–333.
21. Baker DG, Coleridge HM, Coleridge JCG. Vagal afferent C fibres from the ventricle. In: Hainsworth R, Kidd C, Linden RJ, eds. *Cardiac receptors.* Cambridge: Cambridge University Press, 1979; 117–137.
22. Baker DG, Coleridge HM, Coleridge JCG, Nerdrum T. Search for a cardiac nociceptor: stimulation by bradykinin of sympathetic afferent nerve endings in the heart of cat. *J Physiol (Lond)* 1980; 306:519–536.
23. Baron R, Jänig W, McLachlan EM. The afferent and sympathetic components of the lumbar spinal outflow to the colon and pelvic organs in the cat I: I. The hypogastric nerve. *J Comp Neurol* 1985;238:135–146.
24. Baron R, Jänig W, McLachlan EM. The afferent and sympathetic components of the lumbar spinal outflow to the colon and pelvic organs in the cat: II. The lumbar splanchnic nerves. *J Comp Neurol* 1985;238:147–157.
25. Baron R, Jänig W, McLachlan EM. The afferent and sympathetic components of the lumbar spinal outflow to the colon and pelvic organs in the cat: III. The colonic nerves, incorporating an analysis of all components of the lumbar prevertebral outflow. *J Comp Neurol* 1985;238:158–168.
26. Bazett HC, McGlone B. Note on pain sensations which accompany deep puncture. *Brain* 1928;51:18–23.
27. Beckstead RM, Morse JR, Norgren R. The nucleus of the solitary tract in the monkey: projections to the thalamus and brainstem nuclei. *J Comp Neurol* 1980;190:259–282.
28. Beckstead RM, Norgren R. An autoradiographic examination of the central distribution of the trigeminal, facial, glossopharyngeal, and vagal nerves in the monkey. *J Comp Neurol* 1979; 184:455–472.
29. Bentivoglio M, Macchi C, Albanese A. The cortical projections of the thalamic intralaminar nuclei as studies in cat and rat with the multiple-fluorescence retrograde tracing technique. *Neurosci Lett* 1981;26:5–10.
30. Berendse HW, Groenewengen VH. Restricted cortical termination fields of the midline and intralaminar thalamic nuclei in the rat. *Neuroscience* 1991;42:73–102.
31. Berkley KJ, Guilbaud G, Benoist J-M, Gautron M. Responses of neurons in and near the thalamic ventrobasal complex of the rat to stimulation of uterus, cervix, vagina, colon, and skin. *J Neurophysiol* 1993;69:557–568.
32. Berkley KJ, Hubscher CH, Wall PD. Neuronal responses to stimulation of the cervix, uterus, colon, and skin in the rat spinal cord. *J Neurophysiol* 1993;69:545–556.
33. Berkley KJ, Robbins A, Sato Y. Afferent fibers supplying the uterus in the rat. *J Neurophysiol* 1988;59:142–163.
34. Bernard JF, Huang GF, Besson JM. The parabrachial area: electrophysiological evidence for an involvement in visceral nociceptive processes. *J Neurophysiol* 1994;71:1646–1660.
35. Bester H, Menendez L, Besson JM, Bernard JF. Spino (trigemino) parabrachiohypothalamic pathway: electrophysiological evidence for an involvement in pain processes. *J Neurophysiol* 1995;73:568–585.
36. Blair RW. Noxious cardiac input onto neurons in medullary reticular formation. *Brain Res* 1985;326:335–346.
37. Blair RW. Cardiac input to medullary reticular formation: neuronal responses to CAO. *Am J Physiol* 1986;251:R670–R679.
38. Blair RW. Cardiac input to medullary reticular formation: neuronal responses to mechanical stimuli. *Am J Physiol* 1986;251: R680–R689.
39. Blair RW. Responses of feline medial medullary reticulospinal neurons to cardiac input. *J Neurophysiol* 1987;58:1149–1167.
40. Blair RW, Weber RN, Foreman RD. Characteristics of primate spinothalamic tract neurons receiving viscerosomatic convergent inputs in T_3–T_5 segments. *J Neurophysiol* 1981;46:797–811.
41. Blair RW, Weber RN, Foreman RD. Responses of thoracic spinothalamic neurons to intracardiac injection of bradykinin in the monkey. *Circ Res* 1982;51:83–94.
42. Blomqvist A, Ma W, Berkley KJ. Spinal input to the parabrachial nucleus in the cat. *Brain Res* 1989;480:29–36.
43. Blumberg H, Haupt P, Jänig W, Kohler W. Encoding of visceral noxious stimuli in discharge patterns of visceral afferent fibres of the colon. *Pflugers Arch* 1983;398:33–40.
44. Blumberg H, Jänig W. Clinical manifestations of reflex sympathetic dystrophy and sympathetically maintained pain. In: Wall PD, Melzack R, eds. *Textbook of pain.* Edinburgh: Churchill Livingstone, 1994;685–698.
45. Boivie J. An anatomical reinvestigation of the termination of the spinothalamic tract in the monkey. *J Comp Neurol* 1979;186:343–370.
46. Bonica JJ. *Management of pain.* London: Lea & Febiger, 1990; 133–179,211–244.
47. Brennan TJ, Oh U-T, Girardot M-N, Ammons WS, Foreman RD. Inhibition of cardiopulmonary input to thoracic spinothalamic tract cells by stimulation of the subcoeruleus-parabrachial region in the primate. *J Auton Nerv Sys* 1987;18:61–72.
48. Brennan TJ, Oh UT, Hobbs SF, Garrison DW, Foreman RD. Urinary bladder and hindlimb afferent input inhibits activity of primate T_2–T_5 spinothalamic tract neurons. *J Neurophysiol* 1989;61:573–588.
49. Brown AM, Malliani A. Spinal sympathetic reflexes initiated by coronary receptors. *J Physiol (Lond)* 1971;212:685–705.
50. Brüggemann J, Shi T, Apkarian AV. Squirrel monkey lateral thalamus. II. Viscerosomatic convergent representation of urinary bladder, colon, and esophagus. *J Neurosci* 1994;14:6796–6814.
51. Burstein R, Dado RJ, Cliffer KD, Giesler GJ Jr. Physiological characteristics of spinohypothalamic tract neurons in the lumbar enlargement of rats. *J Neurophys* 1991;66:261–284.
52. Buschnell MC, Duncan GH. Sensory and affective aspects of pain perception: is medial thalamus restricted to emotional issues? *Exp Brain Res* 1989;78:415–418.
53. Casey KL, Jones EG. Supraspinal mechanisms: an overview of ascending pathways: brainstem and thalamus. *Neurosci Res Prog Bull* 1978;16:103–118.
54. Cechetto, DF, Standaert, DG, Saper, CB. Spinal and trigeminal dorsal horn projections to the parabrachial nucleus in the rat. *J Comp Neurol* 1985;240:153–160.
55. Cervero F. Afferent activity evoked by natural stimulation of the biliary system in the ferret. *Pain* 1982;13:137–151.
56. Cervero F. Supraspinal connections of neurones in the thoracic spinal cord of the cat: ascending projections and effects of descending impulses. *Brain Res* 1983;275:251–261.
57. Cervero F. Somatic and visceral inputs to the thoracic spinal cord of the cat: effects of noxious stimulation of the biliary system. *J Physiol* (Lond) 1983;337:51–67.
58. Cervero, F. Sensory innervation of the viscera: Peripheral basis of visceral pain. *Physiol Rev* 1994;74:95–138.
59. Cervero F, Connell LA. Distribution of somatic and visceral primary afferent fibres within the thoracic spinal cord of the cat. *J Comp Neurol* 1984;230:88–98.
60. Cervero F, Foreman RD. Sensory innervation of the viscera. In: *Central regulation of autonomic functions.* In: Loewy AD, Spyer KM, eds. New York: Oxford University Press, 1990;104–125.
61. Cervero F, Jänig W. Visceral nociceptors: a new world order. *Trends Neurosci* 1992;15:374–378.
62. Cervero F, Laird JMA, Pozo MA. Selective changes of receptive field properties of spinal nociceptive neurones induced by visceral noxious stimulation in the cat. *Pain* 1992;51:335–342.
63. Cervero F, Sann H. Mechanically evoked responses of afferent fibres innervating the guinea-pig's ureter: an in vitro study. *J Physiol (Lond)* 1989:412:245–266.
64. Cervero F, Tattersall JEH. Somatic and visceral sensory integration in the thoracic spinal cord. In: Cervero F, Morrison JFB, eds. *Progress in Brain Research.* Amsterdam: Elsevier, 1986;67:189–205.
65. Chandler MJ, Zhang J, Foreman RD. Vagal, sympathetic and

somatic sensory inputs to upper cervical (C1–C3) spinothalamic tract neurons in monkeys. *J Neurophys* 1996;76:2555–2567.
66. Chandler MJ, Hobbs ST, Bolser DC, Foreman RD. Effects of vagal afferent stimulation on cervical spinothalamic tract neurons in monkeys. *Pain* 1991;44:81–87.
67. Chandler MJ, Hobbs SF, Fu Q-G, Kenshalo DR, Blair RW, Foreman DR. Responses of neurons in ventroposterolateral nucleus of primate thalamus to urinary bladder distention. *Brain Res* 1992;571:26–34.
68. Chandler MJ, Zhang J, Foreman RD. Vagal and sympathetic afferent inputs excite upper cervical (C_1–C_3) descending propriospinal neurons in monkeys. *Soc Neurosci* 1994;20(233.4).
69. Chernicovskiy VN. *Interoceptors* (Lindsley DB, ed. of English translation). Washington, DC: American Psychological Association, 1967.
70. Chudler EH, Anton F, Dubner R, Kenshalo DR Jr. Responses of nociceptive SI neurons in monkeys and pain sensation in humans elicited by noxious thermal stimulation: effect of interstimulus interval. *J Neurophys* 1990;63:559–569.
71. Cirello J, Calaresu FR. Central projections of afferent renal fibers in the rat: an anterograde transport study of horseradish peroxidase. *J Auton Nerv Syst* 1983;8:273–286.
72. Clerc N. Afferent innervation of the lower esophageal sphincter of the cat: an HRP study. *J Auton Nerv Syst* 1983;9:623–636.
73. Coggeshall RE, Hong KA, Langford LA, Schaible, HG, Schmidt RF. Discharge characteristics of fine medial articular afferents at rest and during passive movements of inflamed knee joints. *Brain Res* 1983;272:185–188.
74. Cohn PF. *Silent myocardial ischemia and infarction.* New York: Marcel-Dekker, 1989; 1–4.
75. Coleridge HM, Coleridge JCG, Kidd C. Cardiac receptors in the dog with particular reference to two types of endings in the ventricular wall. *J Physiol (Lond)* 1964;174:323–339.
76. Coleridge JCG, Hemingway A, Holmes RL, Linden RJ. The location of atrial receptors in the dog: a physiological and histological study. *J Physiol (Lond)* 1957;136:174–197.
77. Collman PI, Tremblay L, Diamant NE. The distribution of spinal and vagal sensory neurons that innervate the esophagus of the cat. *Gastroenterology* 1992;103:817–822.
78. Craig AD Jr, Tapper DN. Lateral cervical nucleus in the cat functional organization and characteristics. *J Neurophysiol* 1978;41: 1511–1534.
79. Csendes A, Sepulveda A. Intraluminal gallbladder pressure measurements in patients with chronic or acute cholecystites. *Am J Surg* 1980;13:383–385.
80. Donald DE, Shepherd JT. Reflexes from the heart and lungs; physiological curiosities or important regulatory mechanisms. *Cardiovasc Res* 1978;12:449–469.
81. Downman CBB. Skeletal muscle reflexes of splanchnic and intercostal nerve origin in acute spinal and decerebrate cats. *J Neurophysiol* 1955;18:217–235.
82. Downman CBB, Evans MH. The distribution of splanchnic afferents in the spinal cord of the cat. *J Physiol (Lond)* 1957;137:66–79.
83. Droste C, Greenlee MW, Roskamm H. A defective angina pectoris pain warning system: experimental findings of ischemic and electrical pain test. *Pain* 1986;26:199–209.
84. Droste C, Greenlee MW, Ruf G, Roskamm H. Localization of a coronary stenosis, left ventricular function, and pain perception during myocardial ischemia in patients with one-vessel disease. *J Cardiovasc Electrophysiol* 1991;2:S68–S75.
85. Droste C, Roskamm H. Experimental pain measurement in patients with asymptomatic myocardial ischemia. *J Am Coll Cardiol* 1983;1:940–945.
86. Eccles JC. *The inhibitory pathways of the central nervous system.* Springfield, IL: Charles C.Thomas, 1969;46–52.
87. Echlin F. Pain responses on stimulation of the lumbar sympathetic trunk under local anesthesia. *J Neurosurg* 1949;6:530–533.
88. Euchner-Wamser I, Meller ST, Gebhart GF. A model of cardiac nociception in chronically instrumented rats: behavioral and electrophysiological effects of pericardial administration of algogenic substances. *Pain* 1994;58:117–128.
89. Falcone C, Sconocchia R, Guasti L, Codega S, Monetmartini C, Specchia G. Dental pain threshold and angina pectoris in patients with coronary artery disease. *J Am Coll Cardiol* 1988;12:348–352.
90. Felder RB, Thames MD. Interaction between cardiac receptors and sinoaortic baroreceptors in the control of efferent cardiac sympathetic nerve activity during myocardial ischemia in dogs. *Circ Res* 1979;45:728–736.
91. Felder RB, Thames MD. The cardiocardiac sympathetic reflex during coronary occlusion in anesthetized dogs. *Circ Res* 1981;48:685–692.
92. Felder RB, Thames MD. Responses to activation of cardiac sympathetic afferents with epicardial bradykinin. *Am J Physiol* 1982; 242 (Heart Circ. Physiol 11):H148–H153.
93. Ferreira SH, Moncada S, Vane JR. Prostaglandins and the mechanism of analgesia produced by aspirin like drugs. *Br J Pharmacol* 1973;49:86–97.
94. Flink R, Svensson BA. Fluorescent double-labelling study of ascending and descending neurones in the feline lateral cervical nucleus. *Exp Brain Res* 1986;62:479–485.
95. Follett KA, Hadley R, Gebhart GF. Cerebral cortical neurons response to noxious visceral stimulation. *Soc Neurosci* 1991:292.
96. Foreman RD. Organization of the spinothalamic tract as a relay for cardiopulmonary sympathetic afferent fiber activity. In: Ottoson, D, ed. *Progress in sensory physiology.* Heidelberg: Springer-Verlag, 1989;1–51.
97. Foreman RD. Spinal cord neuronal regulation of the cardiovascular system. In: Armour JA, Ardell JL, eds. *Neurocardiology.* New York: Oxford University Press, 1994;245–276.
98. Foreman RD, Blair RW, Weber RN. Viscerosomatic convergence onto T2–T4 spinoreticular, spinoreticular-spinothalamic, and spinothalamic tract neurons in the cat. *Exp Neurol* 1984;85: 597–619.
99. Foreman RD, Chandler MJ. Vagal afferent modulation of cardiac pain. In: Levy MN, Schwartz PJ, eds. *Vagal control of the heart: experimental basis and clinical implications.* New York: Futura, 1994; 345–368.
100. Foreman RD, Hancock MB, Willis WD. Responses of spinothalamic tract cells in the thoracic spinal cord of the monkey to cutaneous and visceral inputs. *Pain* 1981;11:149–162.
101. Fu Q-G, Chandler MJ, McNeill DL, Foreman RD. Vagal afferent fibers excite upper cervical neurons and inhibit activity of lumbar spinal cord neurons in the rat. *Pain* 1992;51:91–100.
102. Fulwiler CE, Saper CB. Subnuclear organization of the efferent connections of the parabrachial nucleus in the rat. *Brain Res Rev* 1984;7:229–259.
103. Gerhart KD, Yezierski RP, Giesler GJ Jr, Willis WD. Inhibitory receptive fields of primate spinothalamic tract cells. *J Neurophysiol* 1981;46:1309–1325.
104. Ghione S, Rosa C, Mezzasalma L, Panattoni E. Arterial hypertension is associated with hypalgesia in humans. *Hypertension* 1988; 12:491–497.
105. Girardot M-N, Brennan TJ, Ammons WS, Foreman RD. Effects of stimulating the subcoeruleus-parabrachial region on the non-noxious and noxious responses of T_2–T_4 spinothalamic tract neurons in the primate. *Brain Res* 1987;409:19–30.
106. Glazier JJ, Chierchia S, Brown MJ, Maseri A. Importance of generalized defective perception of painful stimuli as a cause of silent myocardial ischemia in chronic stable angina pectoris. *Am J Cardiol* 1986;58:667–672.
107. Guilbaud G, Benoist JM, Levante A, Gautron M, Willcer JC. Primary somatosensory cortex in rats with pain-related behaviors due to a peripheral mononeuropathy after moderate ligation of one sciatic nerve: neuronal responsivity to somatic stimulation. *Exp Brain Res* 1992;92:227–245.
108. Guzman F, Braun C, Lim RKS. Visceral pain and the pseudoaffective response to intra-arterial injection of bradykinin and other algesic agents. *Arch Int Pharmacodyn Ther* 1962;136:353–383.
109. Häbler H-J, Jäng W, Koltzenburg M. Activation of unmyelinated afferent fibres by mechanical stimuli and inflammation of the urinary bladder in the cat. *J Physiol* 1990;425:545–562.
110. Häbler H-J, Jänig W, Koltzenburg M. Receptive properties of myelinated primary afferents innervating the inflamed urinary bladder of the cat. *J Neurophysiol* 1993;69:395–405.
111. Hammond DL, Proudfit HK. Effects of locus coeruleus lesions on morphine-induced antinociception. *Brain Res* 1980;188:79–91.
112. Hampton AG, Beckwith JR, Wood JE Jr. The relationship between heart disease and gallbladder disease. *Ann Intern Med* 1959; 50:1135–1148.
113. Hancock MB, Foreman RD, Willis WD. Convergence of visceral and cutaneous input onto spinothalamic tract cells in the thoracic spinal cord of the cat. *Exp Neurol* 1975;47:240–248.
114. Hancock MB, Fougerousse CL. Spinal projections from the nucleus locus coeruleus and nucleus subcoeruleus in the cat and monkey as demonstrated by the retrograde transport of horseradish peroxidase. *Brain Res Bull* 1976;1:229–234.
115. Harrison TR, Reeves TJ. Patterns and causes of chest pain. In:

Principles and problems of ischemic heart disease. Chicago: Year Book Medical, 1968;197–204.
116. Herkenham M. Laminar organization of thalamic projections to the rat neocortex. *Science* 1980;207:532–535.
117. Hinsey JC. Observations on the innervation of blood vessels in skeletal muscle. *J Comp Neur* 1928–29;47:23–60.
118. Hobbs SF, Chandler MJ, Bolser DC, Foreman RD. Segmental organization of visceral and somatic input onto C_3–T_6 spinothalamic tract cells of the monkey. *J Neurophysiol* 1992;68:1575–1588.
119. Hobbs SF, Oh UT, Brennan TJ, Chandler MJ, Kim KS, Foreman RD. Urinary bladder and hindlimb stimuli inhibit T_1–T_6 spinal and spinoreticular cells. *Am J Physiol* 1990;258:R10–R20.
120. Hobbs SF, Oh UT, Chandler MJ, Foreman RD. Differential effects of visceral spinal afferent input on lumbosacral spinothalamic tract (STT) cells in the monkey. *Soc Neurosci* 1987;13(pt 1)582(164.11).
121. Hobbs SF, Oh UT, Chandler MJ, Foreman RD. Cardiac and abdominal vagal afferent inhibition of primate T_9–S_1 spinothalamic cells. *Am J Physiol* 1989;257:R889–R895.
122. Hobbs SF, Oh UT, Chandler MJ, Fu QG, Bolser DC, Foreman RD. Evidence that C_1 and C_2 propriospinal neurons mediate the inhibitory effects of viscerosomatic spinal afferent input on primate spinothalamic tract neurons. *J Neurophysiol* 1992;67:852–860.
123. Hopkins DA, Armour JA. Ganglionic distribution of afferent neurons innervating the canine heart and cardiopulmonary nerves. *J Auto Nerv Sys* 1989;26:213–222.
124. Hyndman OR, Wolkin S. The sympathetic nervous system: Influence on sensibility to heat and cold and certain types of pain. *Arch Neurol Psychiatr* 1941;46:1006–1016.
125. Iwamoto GA, Waldrop TG, Longhurst JC, Ordway GA. Localization of the cells of origin for primary afferent fibers supplying the gallbladder of the cat. *Exp Neurol* 1984;84:709–714.
126. Jänig W, Koltzenburg M. Receptive properties of sacral primary afferent neurons supplying the colon. *J Neurophysiol* 1991;65: 1067–1077.
127. Jänig W, Morrison JFB. Functional properties of spinal visceral afferents supplying abdominal and pelvic organs, with special emphasis on visceral nociception. In: Cervero F, Morrison JFB, eds. *Visceral sensation. Progress in brain research,* vol 67. Amsterdam: Elsevier, 1986;87–113.
128. Katayama Y, Watkins LR, Becker DP, Hayes, RL. Non-opiate analgesia induced by carbacol microinjection into the pontine parabrachial region of the cat. *Brain Res* 1984;296:262–283.
129. Katter JT, Burstein R, Giesler J Jr. The cells of origin of the spinohypothalamic tract in cats. *J Comp Neurol* 1991;303:101–112.
130. Kaufman MP, Baker DG, Coleridge HM, Coleridge JC. Stimulation by bradykinin of afferent vagal C-fibers with chemosensitive endings in the heart and aorta of the dog. *Circ Res* 1980;46:476–484.
131. Kellgren JH. Observations on referred pain arising from muscle. *Clin Sci* 1937–1938;3:175–190.
132. Kellgren JH. Somatic simulating visceral pain. *Clinical Science* 1940;4:303–309.
133. Kenshalo DR, Isensee O. Responses of primate SI cortical neurons to noxious stimuli. *J Neurophysiol* 1983;50:1479–1496.
134. Kenshalo DR Jr, Chudler EH, Anton F, Dubner R. SI nociceptive neurons participate in the encoding process by which monkeys perceive the intensity of noxious thermal stimulation. *Brain Res* 1988;454:378–382.
135. Kezdi P, Kordenat RK, Misra SN. Reflex inhibitory effects of vagal afferents in experimental myocardial infarction. *Am J Cardiol* 1974;33:853–860.
136. Khurana PK and Petras JM. Sensory innervation of the canine esophagus, stomach, and duodenum. *Am J Anat* 1991;192:293–306.
137. Kumazawa T. Sensory innervation of reproductive organs. In: Cervero F, Morrison JFB, eds. *Visceral sensation. Progress in brain research,* vol 67. Amsterdam: Elsevier, 1986;115–131.
138. Kuntz A. Afferent innervation of peripheral blood vessels through sympathetic trunks—its clinical implications. *South Med J* 1951; 44:673–678.
139. Kuo DC, de Groat WC. Primary afferent projections of the major splanchnic nerve to the spinal cord and gracile nucleus of the cat-an anatomical study using transganglionic transport of horseradish peroxidase. *J Comp Neurol* 1985;231:421–434.
140. Kuo DC, Nadelhaft I, Hisamitsu T, de Groat WC. Segmental distribution and central projections of renal afferent fibers in the cat studied by transganglionic transport of horseradish peroxidase. *J Comp Neurol* 1983;216:162–174.
141. Kuo DC, Oravitz JJ, de Groat WC. Tracing of afferent and efferent pathways in the left inferior cardiac nerve in the cat using retrograde and transport of horseradish peroxidase. *Brain Res* 1984; 321:111–118.
142. Kuo DC, Yang GCH, Yamasaki DS, Krauthamer GM. A wide field electron microscopic analysis of the fiber constituents of the major splanchnic nerve in cat. *J Comp Neurol* 1982;210:49–58.
143. Lamour Y, Guilbaud G, Willer JC. Altered properties and laminar distribution of neuronal responses to peripheral stimulation in the SmI cortex of the arthritic rat. *Brain Res* 1983;273:183–187.
144. Lamour Y, Guilbaud G, Willer JC. Rat somatosensory (SmI)-cortex: II. Laminar and columnar organization of noxious and non-noxious inputs. *Exp Brain Res* 1983;49:46–54.
145. Lamour Y, Willer JC, Guilbaud G. Rat somatosensory (SmI) cortex: I. Characteristics of neuronal responses to noxious stimulation and comparison with responses to non-noxious stimulation. *Exp Brain Res* 1983;49:35–45.
146. Lewis T. *Pain.* New York: Macmillan, 1942.
147. Lombardi F, Della Bella P, Casalone C, Malfatto G, Malliani A. A sympathetic pressor reflex elicited by coronary occlusion in cats. In: *8th Cong Int Soc Hypertension, 31st May–3rd June, 1981. Ricerca Scientifica, suppl 19,* Milan, 1981.
148. Lombardi F, Della Bella P, Casati R, Malliani A. Effects of intracoronary administration of bradykinin on the impulse activity of afferent sympathetic unmyelinated fibers with left ventricular endings in cats. *Circ Res* 1981;48:69–75.
149. Lombardi F, Patton CP, Della Bella P, Pagani M, Malliani A. Cardiovascular and sympathetic responses reflexly elicited through the excitation with bradykinin of sympathetic and vagal cardiac sensory endings in the cat. *Cardiovasc Res* 1982;16:57–65.
150. Longhurst JC. Reflex effects from abdominal visceral afferents. In: Zucker IH, Gilmore JP, eds. *Reflex control of circulation.* Boston: CRC Press, 1991; 551–577.
151. Lynn RB. Mechanisms of esophageal pain. *Am J Med* 1992;92(5A): 11S–19S.
152. MacKenzie J. *Symptoms and their interpretation.* London: Shaw, 1909.
153. Maixner W. Interactions between cardiovascular and pain modulatory systems: Physiological and pathophysiological implications. *J Cardiovasc Electrophysiol* 1991;2:S3–S12.
154. Maixner W, Bossut DF, Whitsel EA. Evaluation of vagal afferent modulation of the digastric reflex in cats. *Brain Res* 1991;560: 55–62.
155. Maixner W, Randich A. Role of the right vagal nerve trunk in antinociception. *Brain Res* 1984;298:374–377.
156. Maixner W, Touw KB, Brody MJ, Gebhart GF, Long JP. Factors regulating the altered pain perception in the spontaneously hypertensive rat. *Brain Res* 1982;237:137–145.
157. Malliani A. Cardiovascular and sympathetic afferent fibers. *Rev Physiol Biochem Pharmacol* 1982;94:11–74.
158. Malliani A, Brown AM: Reflexes arising from coronary receptors. *Brain Res* 1970; 24:352–355.
159. Malliani A, Lombardi F. Consideration of the fundamental mechanisms eliciting cardiac pain. *Am Heart J* 1982;103:575–578.
160. Malliani A, Pagani M. Afferent sympathetic nerve fibres with aortic endings. *J Physiol* 1976;263:157–169.
161. Malliani A, Pagani M, Recordati G, Schwartz PJ. Spinal sympathetic reflexes elicited by increases in arterial blood pressure. *Am J Physiol* 1971;220:128–134.
162. Malliani A, Parks M, Tuckett RP, Brown AM. Reflex increases in heart rate elicited by stimulation of afferent cardiac sympathetic nerve fibers in the cat. *Circ Res* 1973;32:9–14.
163. Malliani A, Peterson DF, Bishop VS, Brown AM. Spinal sympathetic cardio-cardiac reflexes. *Circ Res* 1972;30:158–166.
164. Malliani A, Schwartz PJ, Zanchetti A. A sympathetic reflex elicited by experimental coronary occlusion. *Am J Physiol* 1969;217:703–709.
165. McMahon SB, Abel C. A model for the study of visceral pain states: chronic inflammation of the chronic decerebrate rat urinary bladder by irritant chemicals. *Pain* 1987;28:109–127.
166. McMahon SB, Wall PD. Electrophysiological mapping of brainstem projections of spinal cord lamina I cells in the rat. *Brain Res* 1985;333:19–26.
167. McNeill DL, Chandler MJ, Fu Q-G, Foreman RD. Projection of nodose ganglion cells to the upper cervical spinal cord in the rat. *Brain Res Bull* 1991;27:151–155.
168. Mehler WR, Feferman ME, Nauta WJH. Ascending axon degeneration following anterolateral cordotomy. An experimental study in the monkey. *Brain* 1960;83:718–751.
169. Melzack R, Casey KL. Sensory, motivational and central control determinants of pain. In: Kenshalo DR, ed. *The skin senses.* Springfield, IL: Charles C. Thomas, 1968;423–443.

170. Melzack R, Wall PD. *The challenge of pain*. New York: Basic Books, 1982.
171. Menétrey D, Basbaum AI. Spinal and trigeminal projections to the nucleus of the solitary tract: A possible substrate for somatovisceral and viscerovisceral reflex activation. *J Comp Neurol* 1987;255:439–450.
172. Menétrey D, DePommery J. Origins of spinal ascending pathways that reach central areas involved in visceroception and visceronociception in the rat. *Eur J Neurosci* 1991;3:249–259.
173. Meyer RA, Campbell JN, Raja SR. Peripheral neural mechanisms of nociception. In: Wall PD, Melzack R, eds. *Textbook of pain*. Edinburgh: Churchill Livingstone, 1994;13–44.
174. Millen JW. Observations on the innervation of blood vessels. *J Anat* 1948;82:68–80.
175. Miller HR. The interrelationship of disease of coronary arteries and gallbladder. *Am Heart J* 1942;24:579–587.
176. Milne RJ, Foreman RD, Giesler GJ, Willis WD. Convergence of cutaneous and pelvic visceral nociceptive inputs onto primate spinothalamic neurons. *Pain* 1981;11:163–183.
177. Minisi AJ, Thames MD. Activation of cardiac sympathetic afferents during coronary occlusion. *Circulation* 1991;84:357–367.
178. Minisi AJ, Thames MD. Distribution of left ventricular sympathetic afferents demonstrated by reflex responses to transmural myocardial ischemia and to intracoronary and epicardial bradykinin. *Circulation* 1993;87:240–246.
179. Moore RM, Moore RE. Studies on the pain-sensibility of arteries. I. Some observations on the pain sensibilities of arteries. *Am J Physiol* 1933;104:259–265.
180. Moore RM, Singleton AO. Studies on the pain sensibility of arteries. II. Peripheral paths of afferent neurons from the arteries of the extremities and of the abdominal viscera. *Am J Physiol* 1933;104:267–275.
181. Morgan C, de Groat WC, Nadelhaft I. The spinal distribution of sympathetic preganglionic and visceral primary afferent neurons that send axons into the hypogastric nerves of the cat. *J Comp Neurol* 1986;243:23–40.
182. Morgan C, Nadelhaft I, de Groat WC. The distribution of visceral primary afferents from the pelvic nerve to Lissauer's tract and the spinal gray matter and its relationship to the sacral parasympathetic nucleus. *J Comp Neurol* 1981;201:415–440.
183. Muers MF, Sleight P. Action potentials from ventricular mechanoreceptors stimulated by occlusion of the coronary sinus in the dog. *J Physiol (Lond)* 1972;221:283–309.
184. Mukherjee SR. Effect of bladder distention on arterial blood pressure and renal circulation in acute spinal cats. *J Physiol* 1957;138:300–306.
185. Nadelhaft I, Roppolo J, Morgan C, de Groat WC. Parasympathetic preganglionic neurones and visceral primary afferent in monkey sacral spinal cord revealed following application of horseradish peroxidase to pelvic nerve. *J Comp Neurol* 1983;216:36–52.
186. Nerdrum T, Baker DG, Coleridge HM, Coleridge JCG. Interaction of bradykinin and prostaglandin E_1 on cardiac pressor reflex and sympathetic afferents. *Am J Physiol* 1986;250:R815–R822.
187. Ness TJ, Gebhart GF. Characterization of neuronal responses to noxious visceral and somatic stimuli in the medial lumbosacral spinal cord of the rat. *J Neurophysiol* 1987:57:1867–1892.
188. Ness TJ, Gebhart GF. Characterization of neurons responsive to noxious colorectal distention in the T13–L2 spinal cord of the rat. *J Neurophysiol* 1988;60:1419–1438.
189. Ness TJ, Gebhart GF. Differential effects of morphine and clonidine upon visceral and cutaneous nociceptive transmission in the rat. *J Neurophysiol* 1989;62:220–230.
190. Ness TJ, Gebhart GF. Visceral pain: a review of experimental studies. *Pain* 1990;41:167–234.
191. Ness TJ, Metcalf AM, Gebhart GF. A psychophysiological study in humans using phasic colonic distention as a noxious visceral stimulus. *Pain* 1990;43:377–386.
192. Neuhuber W. The central projections of visceral primary afferent neurones of the inferior mesenteric plexus and hypogastric nerve and the location of the related sensory and preganglionic sympathetic cell bodies in the rat. *Anat Embryol (Berl)* 1982;164:413–425.
193. Nowicki D, Szulczyk P. Longitudinal distribution of negative cord dorsum potentials following stimulation of afferent fibres in the left inferior cardiac nerve. *J Auton Nerv Syst* 1986;17:185–197.
194. Oberg B, Thóren P. Circulatory responses to stimulation of medullated and non-medullated afferents in the cardiac nerve of the cat. *Acta Physiol Scand* 1972;87:121–132.
195. Oldfield BJ, McLachlan EM. Localization of sensory neurons traversing the stellate ganglion of the cat. *J Comp Neurol* 1978;182:915–922.
196. Ordway GA, Boheler KR, Longhurst JC. Stimulating intestinal afferents reflexly activates the cardiovascular system in cats. *Am J Physiol* 1988;23:H354–H360.
197. Ordway GA, Longhurst JC. Cardiovascular reflexes arising from the gallbladder of the cat. *Circ Res* 1983;52:26–35.
198. Ordway GA, Longhurst JC, Mitchell JH. Stimulation of pancreatic afferents reflexly activates the cardiovascular system in cats. *Am J Physiol* 1984;245:R820–R826.
199. Pagani M, Pizzinelli P, Bergamaschi M, and Malliani A. A positive feedback sympathetic pressor reflex during stretch of the thoracic aorta in conscious dogs. *Circ Res* 1982;50:125–132.
200. Pagani M, Pizzinelli P, Furlan R, Guzzetti S, Rimoldi O, Sandrone G, Malliani A. Analysis of the pressor sympathetic reflex produced by intracoronary injections of bradykinin in conscious dogs. *Circ Res* 1985;56:175–183.
201. Pagani M, Schwartz PJ, Banks R, Lombardi F, Malliani A. Reflex responses of sympathetic preganglionic neurones initiated by different cardiovascular receptors in spinal animals. *Brain Res* 1974;68:215–225.
202. Paintal AS. Vagal sensory receptors and their reflex effects. *Physiol Rev* 1973;53:159–227.
203. Panneton WM, Burton H. Projections from the paratrigeminal nucleus and the medullary and spinal dorsal horn to the peribrachial area in the cat. *Neuroscience* 1985;15:779–798.
204. Pedersen F, Pieterson A, Madsen JK, Ballegaard S, et al. Elevated pain threshold in patients with effort-induced angina pectoris and asymptomatic myocardial ischemia during exercise test. *Clin Cardiol* 1989;12:639–642.
205. Peterson DF, Brown AM. Pressor reflexes produced by stimulation of afferent cardiac nerve fibres in the cardiac sympathetic nerves of the cat. *Circ Res* 1971;28: 605–610.
206. Polley EH. The innervation of blood vessels in striated muscle and skin. *J Comp Neurol* 1955;103:253–267.
207. Price DD, Dubner R. Neurons that subserve the sensory-discriminative aspects of pain. *Pain* 1977;3:307–338.
208. Procacci P, Zoppi M. Heart Pain In: *Textbook of pain*. Edinburgh: Churchill Livingstone, 1989; 410–419.
209. Purtock R V, von Colditz JH, Seagard JL, Igler FO, Zuperku EJ, Kampine JP. Reflex effects of thoracic sympathetic afferent nerve stimulation on the kidney. *Am J Physiol* 1977;233:H580–H586.
210. Randall WC, Hasson DM, Brady JV. Acute cardiovascular consequences of anterior descending coronary artery occlusion in unanesthetized monkey. *Proc Soc Exp Biol Med* 1978;58:135–140.
211. Randich A, Aicher SA. Medullary substrates mediating antinociception produced by electrical stimulation of the vagus *Brain Res* 1988;445:68–76.
212. Randich A, Maixner W. Interactions between cardiovascular and pain regulatory systems. *Neurosci Biobehav Rev* 1984;8:343–367.
213. Randich A, Ren K, Gebhart GF. Electrical stimulation of cervical vagal afferents. II. Central relays for behavioral antinociception and arterial blood pressure decreases. *J Neurophysiol* 1990;64:1115–1124.
214. Randich A, Thurston CL. Antinociceptive states and hypertension *J Cardiovasc Electrophysiol* 1991;Vol 2 (Suppl):S54–S58.
215. Ravdin IS, Fitz-Hugh T Jr, Wolferth CC, Barbieri EA, Ravdin RG. Relation of gallstone disease to angina pectoris. *Arch Surg* 1955; 70:333–342.
216. Ravdin IS, Royster HP, Sanders GB. Reflexes originating the common duct giving rise to pain simulating angina pectoris. *Ann Surg* 1942;115:1055–1062.
217. Reimann KA, Weaver LC. Contrasting reflexes evoked by chemical activation of cardiac afferent nerves. *Am J Physiol* 1980;239: H316–H325.
218. Ren K, Randich A, Gebhart GF. Vagal afferent modulation of spinal nociceptive transmission in the rat. *J Neurophysiol* 1989;62: 401–415.
219. Ren K, Randich A, Gebhart GF. Modulation of spinal nociceptive transmission from nuclei tractus solitary: a relay for effects of vagal afferent stimulation *J Neurophysiol* 1990;63:971–986.
220. Ren K, Randich A, Gebhart GF. Electrical stimulation of cervical vagal afferents. I. Central relays for modulation of spinal nociceptive transmission. *J Neurophysiol* 1990;64:1098–1114.
221. Ren K, Randich A, Gebhart GF. Effects of electrical stimulation of vagal afferents on spinothalamic tract cells in the rat. *Pain* 1991; 44:311.

222. Rosa C, Chione S, Panattoni E, Mezzasalma L, et al. Comparison of pain perception in normotensives and borderline hypertensives by means of a tooth pulp-stimulation test. *J Cardiovasc Pharmacol* 1986;8(suppl 5):S125–S127.
223. Ruch TC. Pathophysiology of pain. In: Ruch TC, Patton HD, Woodbury JW, Towe AL, eds. *Neurophysiology*. Philadelphia: WB Saunders, 1961;350–368.
224. Sadikot AF, Parent A, Francois C. The center median and parafascicular thalamic nuclei project respectively to the sensorimotor and associate limbic striatal territories in the squirrel monkey. *Brain Res* 1990;510:161–165.
225. Sampson JJ, Cheitlin MD. Pathophysiology and differential diagnosis of cardiac pain. *Prog Cardiovasc Dis* 1971;23:507–531.
226. Schaible H-G, Schmidt RF. Effects of an experimental arthritis on the sensory properties of fine articular afferent units. *J Neurophysiol* 1985;54:1109–1122.
227. Schaible H-G, Schmidt RF. Time course of mechanosensitivity changes in articular afferents during a developing experimental arthritis. *J Neurophysiol* 1988;60:2180–2195.
228. Schondorf R, Laskey W, Polosa C. Upper thoracic sympathetic neuron responses to input from urinary bladder afferents. *Am J Physiol* 1983;245:R311–R320.
229. Schwartz PJ, Pagani M, Lombardi F, Malliani A, Brown AM. A cardiocardiac sympathovagal reflex in the cat. *Circ Res* 1973;32: 215–220.
230. Sengupta JN, Kauvar D, Goyal RK. Characteristics of vagal esophageal tension-sensitive afferent fibers in the opossum. *J Neurophys* 1989;61:1001–1010.
231. Sengupta JN, Saha JK, Goyal RK. Stimulus-response function studies of esophageal mechanosensitive nociceptors in sympathetic afferents of opossum. *J Neurophysiol* 1990;64:796–812.
232. Slaughter RF. Relief of causalgia-like pain in isolated extremity by sympathectomy; case report. *J Med Assoc Ga* 1938;27:253–256.
233. Sleight P, Widdicombe JG. Action potentials in fibres from receptors in the epicardium and myocardium of the dog's left ventricle *J Physiol* (Lond) 1965;181:235–258.
234. Staszewska-Barczak J, Dusting GJ. Sympathetic cardiovascular reflex initiated by bradykinin-induced stimulation of cardiac pain receptors in the dog. *Clin Exp Pharmacol Physiol* 1977;4: 443–452.
235. Staszewska-Barczak J, Ferreira SH, Vane JR. An excitatory nociceptive cardiac reflex elicited by bradykinin and potentiated by prostaglandins and myocardial ischemia. *Cardiovasc Res* 1976;10: 314–327.
236. Sugiura Y, Terul N, Hosoya Y. Difference in distribution of central terminals between visceral and somatic unmyelinated (C) primary afferent fibers. *J Neurophysiol* 1989;62:834–840.
237. Svensson BA, Westman J, Rostad J. Light and electron microscopic study of neurones in the feline lateral cervical nucleus with a descending projection. *Brain Res* 1985;361:114–124.
238. Szabo J, Cowan WMA. A stereotaxic atlas of the brain of the cynomolgus monkey *(Macaca fascicularis)*. *J Comp Neurol* 1984;222:2 65–300.
239. Takeuchi Y, Uemura M, Matsuda K, Matsushima R, Mizuno N. Parabrachial nucleus neurons projecting to the lower brainstem and the spinal cord. A study in the cat by the Fink-Heimer and the horseradish peroxidase methods. *Exp Neurol* 1980;70:403–413.
240. Taylor DEM. Cardiovascular disturbances in acute retention of urine. *Lancet* 1963;2:1033–1035.
241. Thames MD, Abboud FM. Inhibition of renal sympathetic nerve activity during myocardial ischemia mediated by left ventricular receptors with vagal afferents in dogs. *J Clin Invest* 1979;63: 395–402.
242. Thames MD, Klopfenstein HS, Abboud FM, Mark AL, Walker JL. Preferential distribution of inhibitory cardiac receptors with vagal afferents to the inferoposterior wall of the left ventricle activated during coronary occlusion in the dog. *Circ Res* 1978;43: 512–519.
243. Thies R, Foreman RD. Descending inhibition of spinal neurons in the cardiopulmonary region by electrical stimulation of vagal afferent nerves. *Brain Res* 1981;207:178–183.
244. Thies R, Foreman RD. Inhibition and excitation of thoracic spinoreticular neurons by electrical stimulation of vagal afferent nerves. *Exp Neurol* 1983;82:1–16.
245. Thóren PN. Left ventricular receptors activated by severe asphyxia and by coronary artery occlusion. *Acta Physiol Scand* 1972;85: 455–463.
246. Thóren PN. Activation of left ventricular receptors with nonmedullated vagal afferent fibers during occlusion of a coronary artery in the cat. *Am J Cardiol* 1976;37:1046–1051.
247. Thóren PN. Characteristics of left ventricular receptors with nonmedullated vagal afferents in cats. *Circ Res* 1977;40:415–421.
248. Thóren PN. Role of cardiac vagal C-fibers in cardiovascular control. *Rev Physiol Biochem Pharmacol* 1979;86:1–94.
249. Threadgill FD, Solnitzky C. Anatomical studies of afferency within the lumbosacral sympathetic ganglia. *Anat Rec Suppl* 1949;103:96.
250. Thurston L, Randich A. Acute increases in arterial blood pressure produced by occlusion of the abdominal aorta induces antinociception: Peripheral and central substrates. *Brain Res* 1990;519:12–22.
251. Truex RC. Sensory nerve terminations associated with peripheral blood vessels. *Proc Soc Exp Biol* 1936;34:699.
252. Uchida Y. Afferent aortic nerve fibers with their pathways in cardiac sympathetic nerves. *Am J Physiol* 1975;228(4):990–995.
253. Vance WH, Bowker RC. Spinal origins of cardiac afferents from the region of the left anterior descending artery. *Brain Res.* 1983; 258:96–100.
254. Vin-Christian K, Benoist JM, Gautron M, Levante A, Guilbaud G. Further evidence for the involvement of SmI cortical neurons in nociception: Modifications of their responsiveness over the early stage of a carrageenan-induced inflammation in the rat. *Somatosens Mot Res* 1992;9:245–261.
255. Walker AE, Nulsen F. Electrical stimulation of the upper thoracic portion of the sympathetic chain in man. *Arch Neurol Psychiatr 1948;*59:559–560.
256. Walker JL, Thames MD, Abboud FM, Mark AL, Klopfenstein HS. Preferential distribution of inhibitory cardiac receptors in left ventricle of the dog. *Am J Physiol* 1978;235:H188–H192.
257. Weaver LC, Danos LM, Oehl RS, Meckler RL. Contrasting reflex influences of cardiac afferent nerves during coronary occlusion. *Am J Physiol* 1981;240:H620–H629.
258. Weaver LC, Fry HK, Meckler RL, Oehl RS. Multisegmental spinal sympathetic reflexes originating from the heart. *Am J Physiol* 1983;245:R345–R352.
259. Weaver LC, Macklem LJ, Reimann KA, Meckler RL, Oehl RS. Organization of thoracic sympathetic afferent influences on renal nerve activity. *Am J Physiol* 1979;237:H44–H50.
260. Weaver LC, Meckler RL, Frey HK, Donoghue S.. Widespread neural excitation initiated from cardiac spinal afferent nerves. *Am J Physiol* 1983;245:R241–R250.
261. Webb SW, Adgey AA, Pantridge JF. Autonomic disturbances at onset of acute myocardial infarction. *Br Med J Clin Res* 1972; 3:89–92.
262. Westlund KN, Bowker RM, Ziegler MG, Coulter JD. Origins and terminations of descending noradrenergic projections to the spinal cord of the monkey. *Brain Res* 1984;292:1–16.
263. Westlund KN, Coulter JD. Descending projections of the locus coeruleus and subcoeruleus/medial parabrachial nuclei in the monkey: axonal transport studies and dopamine hydroxylase neurocytochemistry. *Brain Res Rev* 1980;2:235–264.
264. White JC. Conduction of pain in man: observations on its afferent pathways within the spinal cord and visceral nerves. In: *AMA archives of neurology and psychiatry*, vol 71. Boston: American Medical Association, 1954;1–23.
265. White JD, Smithwick HH. *The autonomic nervous system.* New York: Macmillan, 1941;37:131–147.
266. Woollard HH. The innervation of blood vessels. *Heart* 1926;13: 319–336.
267. Woolf CF. The dorsal horn: state-dependent sensory processing and the generation of pain. In: Wall PD, Melzack R, eds. *Textbook of pain.* Edinburgh: Churchill Livingstone, 1994:101–112
268. Wurster RD, Randall WC. Cardiovascular responses to bladder distention in patients with spinal transection. *Am J Physiol* 1975; 228:1288–1292.
269. Yezierski RP, Broton JG. Functional properties of spinomesencephalic tract (SMT) cells in the upper cervical spinal cord of the cat. *Pain* 1991;45:187–196.
270. Yezierski RP, Schwartz RH. Response and receptive-field properties of spinomesencephalic tract cells in the cat. *J Neurophysiol* 1986;55:76–96.
271. Zamir N, Segal M. Hypertension-induced analgesia: changes in pain sensitivity in experimental hypertensive rats. *Brain Res* 1979;160:170–173.
272. Zamir N, Shuber E. Altered pain perception in hypertensive humans. *Brain Res* 1980;201:471–474.

Anesthesia: Biologic Foundations, edited by Tony L. Yaksh et al. Lippincott–Raven Publishers, Philadelphia © 1997.

CHAPTER 40

PRECLINICAL MODELS OF NOCICEPTION

TONY L. YAKSH

As reviewed in Chapter 1 of this volume, the Sherringtonian definition of certain classes of stimuli as being nociceptive reflect their ability to generate certain constellations of behavioral (escape, vocalization) and physiological responses (blood pressure heart rate, hormone secretion). These constellations of behavior observed in nonverbal animals are hypothesized to mirror the human state referred to as "pain." In previous chapters, emphasis has been on the pathways and systems through which activity generated by such stimuli reach higher centers in the neuraxis. In this chapter, the behavioral consequences of these stimuli and the pharmacology of the systems regulating these effects in the intact and unanesthetized animal will be considered.

There are three reasons why such studies in intact animal models are required to advance our understanding of pain.

1. Research into the connectivity of systems, as in single unit activity or anatomical tract tracing studies, can define linkages, but the behavioral relevance of these linkages to pain or nociception can only be assessed in the context of the intact and unanesthetized organism. In the present example, the role played by a particular linkage in the pain state can be assessed only in the presence of the other elements of that system. For example, the relevance to pain of an afferent input that evokes a spinal reflex, depends upon whether that input also activates a supraspinal projection.
2. A systematic study of behavior in well-defined paradigms can provide insights that are not obvious in the complexity of human behavior. Such mechanistic dissection in animal models can reveal elements that are important components to the overall pain behavior (e.g., the presence of distinct systems for acute and facilitated components of nociceptive processing). In effect, the use of agents to systematically alter nociceptive behavior is a method to examine the pharmacology of systems that regulate the processing of afferent information, which, because it is being considered in the intact organism, is a measure of the relevance of that pharmacological system on the processing of nociceptive information.
3. To the extent that the animal models provide insight into mechanisms, they also provide a tool for defining the pharmacology of the systems, and they serve as a means for predicting the analgesic actions of drugs. In this sense, the animal models serve as a bioassay for antinociception.

PRECLINICAL MODELS OF NOCICEPTION

In a general sense, models of nociception can be grouped according to several defining characteristics.

Stimulus

The stimulus may be operationally defined in terms of the modality, intensity, and duration. Transient thermal (>42°C) stimuli, mechanical distortion, or changes in the local chemical milieu (e.g., pH of <5.0; K^+; capsaicin, irritants such as formalin) at the peripheral sensory terminal will (a) evoke the verbal report of pain in humans and efforts to escape in animals and (b) increase activity in the sympathetic pituitary axis (151,316) (see Chapters 14,41,72). The intensity of the stimulus is defined in terms of temperature, pressure or concentration, for thermal, mechanical and chemical stimuli, respectively. The question of intensity is often confounded with the time of onset of the stimulus. Thus, with a temperature probe applied to the skin, the stepwise increase in probe temperature from normal (~28°C) to –60°C versus 50°C, will not only result in a higher subcutaneous temperature at equilibrium, but also a more rapid increase in temperature from baseline to 50°C, than a stimulus temperature of 50°C. As noted in Chapter 14, rapidly rising stimulus intensities will be perceived as being more intense than the same change occurring over an extended interval. Mechanistically, this could reflect (a) the role of adaptation that may be mediated at the terminal or by a central mechanism, and (b) the concurrency with which activity is induced in a population of afferents and, accordingly, the uniformity with which the afferent barrage reaches the membrane of the second order neuron in the spinal cord. (Concurrently arriving input would generate a greater net EPSP and a stronger stimulus for depolarization; see ref. 468.)

It should be emphasized that the designation of a stimulus as noxious is dependent upon the demonstration that the stimulus is in fact able to evoke the expected behavior. If that behavior evoked by a given stimulus occurs at a lower intensity or at a shorter latency, or displays a greater magnitude (response strength) than would be predicted based on that stimulus intensity, the system is said to be hyperalgesic.

Response

The morphology of the response may be considered in terms of the behavior observed, e.g., escape (such as withdrawal of the paw or tail, a jerk of the jaw, a twitch of the skin), a characteristic autonomic response (such as a change in blood pressure or heart rate) (342), or a vocalization (70,214). Licking of the paw is typically considered to reflect a form of escape in that it provides a counter stimulus, although this has not been systematically studied.

The interpretation of the response as an index of a "pain" state is considered to be validated by several characteristics: (a) the response has a somatotopic sign, e.g., the response is directed towards the anatomic origin of the stimulus; (b) the response is contiguous with the onset of the stimulus, e.g., it occurs after the physical stimulus has been applied; and (c) the magnitude of the measured response parameter covaries monotonically over a range of stimulus intensities. For example, in the hot plate test, the hindpaws of the animal are in contact with the thermal surface and the response to such a stimulus is licking of the hind paw (e.g., it is somatotopically directed). Such licking is rarely, if ever, observed in the absence of an intense thermal stimulus and typically occurs after the stimulus has been presented. Finally, the latency to respond varies inversely with the intensity of the stimulus. Thus, increasing stimulus intensities will decrease the latency. In contrast to the hind paw licking response, in a stressful situation, the rodents will groom by licking their forepaws, independent of the thermal stimulus and, thus, direct their response towards a tissue site not receiving the primary stimulus. In other models, the response index may be assessed as an increase in the magnitude or strength of the response (e.g., an increase in motor horn outflow) or in vocalization intensity (214,276,400,403). In the case of a repetitive response, such as the licking of a paw after the injection of an irritant, the frequency or time of licking is proportional to concentration (411).

Level of Neural Organization Underlying Stimulus-Response Relationship

The classic separation of mechanisms related to physiological and behavioral consequences of strong stimuli relates to the question of spinal versus supraspinal levels of organization (Fig. 1). The Sherringtonian Reflex, a simple withdrawal response, evoked by a thermal stimulus or a forcible pinch reflects a segmental neuronal arc. This response is typically somatotopically organized and has a local sign (e.g., the pinched paw displays the withdrawal). More complex behaviors, such as the licking of the hind paw, vocalization and signs of coordinated agitation, as observed when the animal is on a hot surface, require an intact spinal pathway and a supraspinal level of organization. Lesion studies have shown that decerebrated animals will display prominent sham rage and well-defined nocifensive reactions in the face of a strong mechanical or thermal stimulus (319,417,465). In this sense, a sufficient component of the coordinated response involves a suprasegmental projection to the brainstem. However, coordinated motor responses and the precision of motor control normally anticipated require the engagement of the entire neuraxis. From an experimental perspective, the observation of a coordinated, unconditioned behavioral response to a strong stimulus is evidence that the afferent input has engaged behaviors which require the contribution and organizational role of higher centers. Conversely, the absence of that response is taken as an indication that transmission has been changed or that the relationship between the stimulus and the organized escape response has been altered. As the human response to a strong stimulus is mediated by the perceptions generated in part by the ascending message, this ability in the animal model to confirm that certain manipulations have abolished the stimulus-evoked supraspinal response without altering the general motor function of the animal is strong evidence that the manipulation has impacted on the processing of the stimulus message. In contrast, with spinal reflexes it is more difficult to exclude the possibility that the intervention has not altered the ability to express the motor response, therefore yielding an increased latency or a decreased response strength. For example, hyperpolarization of the motor horn cell or a loss of inhibition between the extensor and flexor pools of motor horn cells could block a reflex, suggesting changes in nociception in the absence of a real change in afferent processing.

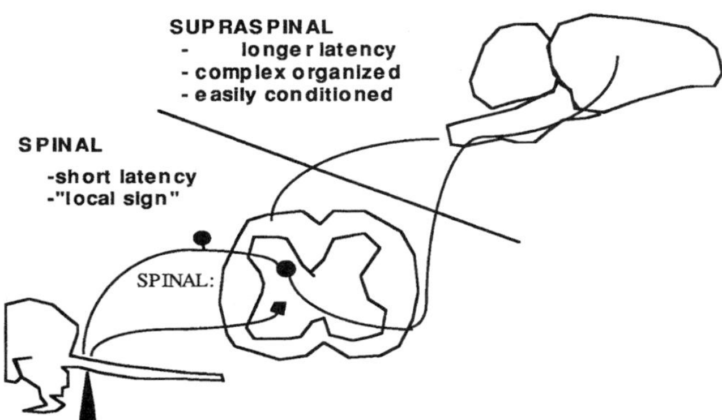

Figure 1. Levels of organization of the response evoked by a locally applied high-intensity thermal stimulus. In certain effector systems, a polysynaptic reflex that is segmentally organized will mediate observed response of the effector systems (In this case the tail). The same effector systems may similarly be activated secondary to the activation of an ascending system that through corticospinal projections then produces a stimulus-evoked movement of the tail. This would be referred to as a supraspinally organized response.

Hypothesized Organization of Processing Substrate

In the preceding section, it was emphasized that the organization of the response to a strong, nociceptive stimulus could be considered in terms of a spinal or supraspinal organization. At a more complicated level, our growing appreciation of the mechanisms whereby afferent information is processed has led to the ability to consider nociceptive modeling in terms of more precise mechanistic substrates. Thus, as reviewed in detail below, it is possible to consider nociceptive states in terms of several principal subdivisions according to the mechanisms which are believed to mediate the behavioral or physiological responses.

1. Responses generated by the acute delivery of transient high-intensity stimuli. This involves responses which are dependent upon the transient activation of pathways which are normally activated by the peripheral stimuli applied to the terminal (e.g., thermal or mechanical, or by a local chemical stimulus) or along their axis of conduction (e.g., electrical stimulation of the sensory axon).
2. Responses generated by stimuli subsequent to persistent small afferent input. As will be indicated, this condition may occur in the face of continued stimulus exposure or by the terminal application of a chemical stimulus to which the afferent terminal is sensitive, or by tissue injury. Such persistent input serves to condition the system, leading to an activity-dependent alteration in the processing of subsequent stimuli. These models typically reflect the initiation of a facilitated state in which allodynia and hyperalgesia are observed.
3. "Spontaneous behaviors" or evoked responses generated by stimuli in animals with a defined afferent nerve injury.

MECHANISTIC DIVISIONS OF PRECLINICAL MODELS OF NOCICEPTION

The following sections are organized in terms of the three principal sections outlined above. As reviewed below, these three functional divisions reflect a rational separation of models based on our current understanding of mechanisms and pharmacology. Importantly, the ability to assign mechanism allows the formulation of predictive hypotheses as to the physiology and pharmacology of the linkages mediating the behavioral profile. These systems are summarized in Table 1. It is stressed that although these divisions are based on the reasoning outlined elsewhere in this volume and have validity based on convergent lines of investigation, such separations are employed here primarily for their heuristic value, to assist in the organization of a large body of observations. Additional subdivisions and realignments, particularly in the categories of post nerve injury pain, will occur as further insights into their organization are obtained.

Acute High-Intensity Stimuli

Somatic and autonomic reflexes and organized escape behavior can be evoked by the acute and transient excitation of small Aδ/C primary afferent fibers (126,178,342,389) (see Chapter 35).

Mechanisms

In general, the organization of the systems which mediates the response evoked by the acute exposure of the organism to

Table 1. HYPOTHESIZED COMPONENTS OF PRECLINICAL PAIN MODELS

Pain state models	Stimulus	Time course	Afferent	Spinal system
Acute				
Hot plate Tail flick Paw pressure	High-intensity thermal/mech Chemical	Acute (s)	Aδ/C	Dorsal horn nociceptive specific/wide dynamic range/response proportional to frequency and fiber class of afferent message
Persistent/posttissue injury	Low-intensity thermal/mech	Ongoing afferent input (min, h)	Aβ /Aδ/C	Acute dorsal horn nociceptive specific/wide dynamic range/response to afferent input enhanced by conditioning stimuli
Formalin (Ph 2) Inflamed KJ/paw burn		Ongoing afferent input (min, h, days)		Induction of reorganization of biochemistry of dorsal horn receptors, channels transmitters/enzymes
Post-nerve injury	Low-intensity thermal/mech	Ongoing afferent input (h to days)	Aβ/Aδ/C	Changes in central transport of trophic factor Central sprouting of large afferents into lamina II
Sciatic, loose lig Sciatic, partial lig Sciatic, freeze L5/L6 nerve lig Diabetic rat IT strychnine		(days to weeks)		Peripheral terminal sprout and DRG changes lead to persistent spon activity Transynaptic degeneration Changes in terminal transmitter/receptor synthesis Sympathetic sprouting into neuroma/DRG

h, hours; KJ, knee joint; lig, ligation; mech, mechanical; min, minutes; s, seconds; spon, spontaneous

a high-intensity stimulus may be considered in terms of the afferent limb and the central organization.

Afferent Limb Acute stimulation of Aδ and C fibers by heat, cold or mechanical stimuli will evoke afferent activity which is proportional to the intensity of the stimulus (see Chapter 3). Because of the practical inability to distinguish between the response properties of high-threshold Aδ and C fibers, the precise role played by each is difficult to assess. However, several pharmacological manipulations have provided some insights. First, intrathecal or systemic capsaicin is believed to selectively inactivate C fibers. Accordingly, the ability of intrathecal or systemic capsaicin to significantly elevate thermal escape latencies (as in the hot plate and tail flick tests) or diminish the organized response induced by the injection of local irritants (435,172a) suggests that at least a component of these responses may be secondary to activity in C fibers. Second, it is believed that spinally delivered μ agonists exert a significant component of their effect upon spinal C-fiber terminals and will selectively diminish C-fiber-evoked dorsal horn wide dynamic range discharges (182,207) (see Chapters 34 and 58). Inflammation is believed to increase the sensitivity of C fibers to mechanical and thermal stimuli (see Chapter 33). Under such conditions, the doses of opiates required to significantly increase the response threshold are decreased (147).

Central Organization High-intensity stimuli activating small sensory afferents will lead to an augmented release of dorsal horn peptides and amino acid transmitters (134,202,241,372) (see Chapter 34), and postsynaptic activation of dorsal horn neurons which project segmentally and supraspinally (see Chapter 35). This output is correlated with the appearance of transient somatic and autonomic reflexes and organized escape behavior. For a given modality, increasing stimulus intensity yields (a) a greater frequency of discharge in dorsal horn wide dynamic range neurons and nociceptive-specific neurons (such as the marginal cell and wide dynamic range neurons) (see Chapter 35), and (b) a decreased behavioral response latency (94,102,105) (see Chapter 41) and an increased strength of the behavioral response (403). Systematic in vivo studies in unanesthetized chronically instrumented animals has in fact demonstrated a close covariance of dorsal horn neuronal response and behavioral escape characteristics in the same animal (102,230,291) (see Chapters 31 and 41). Conversely, treatments such as spinal μ agonists, which have been shown to produce a dose-dependent reduction in the discharge of dorsal horn wide dynamic range neurons, will produce a similar dose-dependent reduction in the magnitude of the escape measure or increase in response latency (see below).

Properties of Evoked Response Measures

These acute models of nociception have a number of common characteristics: (a) The stimulus is assumed to be unconditioned. Thus, efforts are made to avoid developing a classical conditioned response in which the test environment will evoke (or cue) the behavior independent of the strength of the stimulus. (b) All models have a practical "cutoff" parameter that serves to prevent the production of tissue injury. To the extent that the stimulus produces an injury state, the injury will likely lead to subsequent changes in threshold (i.e., see section below on protracted afferent input). This cutoff parameter may be the maximum time of stimulus exposure or the maximum amount of pressure. This results in a truncation of the response score. (c) Baseline response latencies are believed to reflect the intensity of the stimulus. Typically, the more intense the stimulus, the smaller the interanimal variation, but the less sensitive the test is to a drug treatment (see below).

Animal Models

Several models of acute high-intensity stimulus delivery that are commonly employed are considered below.

Tail Flick The tail of the rat or mouse is placed over an aperture through which a high-intensity bulb is shown. Initiation of the stimuli results in rapid removal of the tail by the animal (75). The latency covaries with stimulus intensity (276). Several variables can influence the nature of the response, including placement on the tail (282) and initial skin temperature (25,216). In the absence of a response, the tail is removed at some interval that precludes injury to the tail. An important component of the tail flick is that it may be mediated by spinal as well as supraspinal mechanisms, e.g., the response persists in the spinally transected animal (see above).

Tail Dip The immersion of the tail into water at varying temperatures, from warm to hot (44–60°C) (179,226) and cool to cold (4–10°C) (5,395) results in a brisk reflex jerk or flick of the tail in rodents and in primates (105). In a variant of that model, carotid artery blood pressure is measured in halothane-anesthetized rats. The tail is immersed 4 cm into a small container of water regulated at a temperature of 52–60°C for 15 s. The tail reflex latency and the blood pressure response are noted. The stimulus results in a short latency somatomotor reflex and a progressive elevation in blood pressure (autonomic), the magnitude at which responses correlate with water temperature (333).

Hot Plate The animal is placed on a metal surface (surrounded by a clear barrier). The temperature of the surface is regulated at some specific level typically at 48–60°C. Within several seconds, depending upon the surface temperature, the animal will display a species-specific response evoked by a thermal surface: licking of one of the hindpaws (419). If no response occurs within a certain time period, usually 20–60 s, the animal is removed and that cutoff time is assigned as the response latency. As intensity rises, response latency is typically reduced (see below).

A variant on the hot plate (HP) test described above was first described by Hargreaves and colleagues in 1988 (157). In this model, the rodent was placed upon a glass surface and a focused projection bulb was maneuvered under one of the hindpaws. The latency to withdrawal after initiation of the stimulus is the measure.

Skin Twitch The application of a small probe, maintained at 50-65°C, to the skin of the lower back will evoke an acute contraction of the local cutaneous musculature in the cat (433), dog (330,413) and guinea pig (L. Crone and T. L. Yaksh, unpublished observations, 1991). Systematic study of this response in the rat has indicated that it is mediated by capsaicin-sensitive C-polymodal nociceptors and represents a polysynaptic spinally mediated nociceptive reflex (96).

Paw Pressure The animal is lightly restrained and the paw placed between a surface and a device which produces a progressive increase in pressure (PP). The pressure is increased automatically at a fixed rate until the animal withdraws or a maximum pressure (cutoff) is reached. Alternatively, the animal is exposed to a fixed pressure and the latency to withdrawal is noted (56,317,390). Thresholds may vary considerably between laboratories, but they are typically in excess of 70-200 grams of weight exerted on the paw through a small probe tip. The stimulus is likely stimulating deep muscle or joint nerve endings.

Cold Plate The animal is placed on a cold surface and the time it takes to lift one of the hindpaws is recorded (208,304).

Foot Shock Threshold Brief shock applied to the grind upon which a rat is standing will evoke a flinch and then at a slightly higher intensity the animal will jump (114). In complex behavioral paradigms such as the shock titration, brief shocks have been used to assess thresholds. In these models, it has been shown that the animal (rats and primates) will press a manipulandum or display a response in response to the shock, such as jumping from one side of the operant chamber to the other to escape the shock stimulus. The programming is arranged such that a response causes the stimulus to be lowered by a fixed increment, while the absence of a response serves to increment the stimulus by one step. This permits control by the organism over the intensity of the stimulus. In this manner, the threshold and the effects of drug manipulations can be established. Different paradigms have involved the selection of continuous versus discrete shock titration and alter the relationship between the number of responses required to regulate the shock level (104,306,408,425).

Visceral Distention The distention of the colon will lead to an increase in abdominal tone and a rise in blood pressure (280). The mechanism of this is related to the activation of high-threshold mechanoreceptors in the hollow viscera, which leads to the acute activation of thoracolumbar neurons in the dorsal horn (274).

Tooth Pulp Stimulation Electrodes are embedded through the tooth enamel. The current is elevated until one of several end points are observed, including licking, chewing or a jaw-opening reflex (JOR), in several species including the cat, dog or primate (308,366). Tooth pulp is innervated largely by small myelinated and unmyelinated fibers (see Chapter 47). The JOR is believed to be a segmentally organized response (225, 355). Technically, it is believed that the threshold sensations of tooth pulp stimulation are noxious in character (see Chapter 47). On the other hand, the JOR is not capsaicin-sensitive, emphasizing that components of the response are not likely mediated by C fibers (394).

Pharmacology of Acute Pain States

The ability to alter the processing of acutely evoked activity in small primary afferents has been widely examined. The common paradigms such as the hot plate and tail flick tests reflect some of the earliest nociceptive bioassays. A summary of the effects of selective classes of agents delivered either systemically or into the intrathecal space is presented in Table 2.

The mechanisms associated with the actions of several of these classes of agents are discussed in subsequent chapters. In brief, however, several synthesizing issues can be presented based on the profile of activity outlined in Table 1 and summarized in Fig. 2.

Table 2. EFFECTS OF RECEPTOR CLASSES ON ACUTE NOCICEPTIVE END POINTS

	Acute nociception		
Drug class	IP/IV/SC	IT	References
Agonists			
Opioid			
μ	++	++	267,446
δ	(/)	++	237
κ	+	+	212,349
Adrenergic (α_2)	++	++	365,392
Serotonin	(/)	+M	449
Adenosine (A1)	0M	±M	166,373
GABA			
A	0M	0M	95,343
B	+M	+M	343,416
Cholinergic			
Muscarinic	+M	++	19,433
Nicotinic	+(M)	+(M)	335
Neuropeptide Y	(/)	++	172
Neurotensin	(/)	+	448
Antagonists			
Glutamate NMDA	0M	0M	63,150
Tachykinin NK-1	0	0/+M	452
Enzyme inhibitors			
Cholinesterase (muscarinic)	+	++	74,272
Cyclooxygenase	0	0	233,234
Nitric oxide synthase	±	0	238,264
Enkephalinase	+	+	219,295
Local anesthetic	0M	0/M	3,303
Capsaicin	+	+	273,435

Data reflect effects upon hot plate and tail flick, and phase 1 of formalin test.

(/), not tested, peptide; 0, no discernible antinociception; +, mild antinociception; ++, maximum antinociception; M, behavioral dysfunction impeding measurement of nociception.

Spinal receptors:	μ/∂/ α2 NPY/Mus	GABA A/B Aden A1
Binding: Subs Gelat	++	+
N proprius	+	+
Presynaptic		
C fiber binding	+	+/-
↓sP/CGRP release	+	-
Post synaptic		
↑pK -> ↓hyperpol	+	+
WDR neurons		
Therapeutic Ratio	++	+/-

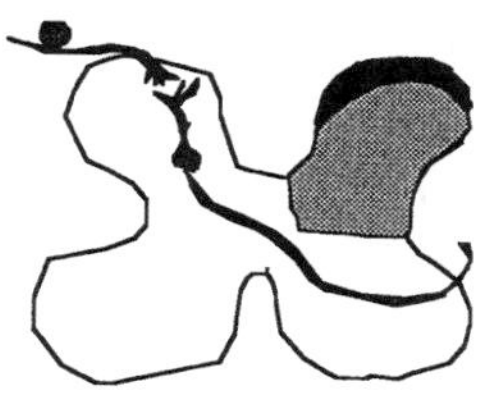

Figure 2. Modulation of acute afferent processing. Summarization of the properties (location of binding) and physiology (effect of C-fiber transmitter release and ability to hyperpolarize dorsal horn neurons) of several classes of spinal receptors that have been shown to regulate the response to acute nociceptive stimuli. The therapeutic ratio reflects the ability of the agent to block a thermal nociceptive end point without altering motor function. Large therapeutic ratios indicate a greater sensory versus motor selectivity.

Alteration in C-Fiber Terminal Excitability Based on the premises outlined above, models in which afferent processing is mediated by the activation of populations of lightly myelinated or unmyelinated primary afferents should be particularly sensitive to systems which regulate the central excitability of those terminals. Families of receptors which have been shown to have a potent presynaptic inhibitory effect on central C-fiber terminals, as defined (a) by the presence of receptor binding on the terminals of C fibers, and/or (b) by their ability to inhibit the release of C-fiber transmitters such as substance P(SP) or calcitonin gene-related peptide (CGRP) (Table 3), have been shown to alter the animal's response to an acute, high-intensity stimulus at doses which do not impact greatly on motor function. Such families of agents include μ and δ opioids (see Chapter 58), α_2 agonists (see Chapter 59); and neuropeptide Y (172). In the case of these agents, they also have been shown to be coupled to G protein and to serve to increase potassium conductance. This joint effect, serving to reduce the excitatory input and concurrently diminishing the postsynaptic excitability, would appear to maximize the likelihood of a selective effect upon acute nociceptive processing (Fig. 1). Agents such as adenosine A1 agonists have been shown to reduce C-fiber transmitter release, but to date their effects have been obscured by significant motor dysfunction (82,345,373). This, however, may reflect concurrent effects on other receptors (such as adenosine A2), which may be responsible for the motor activity (211).

Motor Effects Receptors that bind in the dorsal horn, and which increase K conductance leading to a hyperpolarization of the dorsal horn cell, but do not reliably modulate the dorsal horn release of SP or CGRP (439), tend to have a potent effect upon spinal nociceptive processing evoked by an acute high-intensity stimulus, however, their actions tend to occur at doses that may induce motor dysfunction. This class of agonists includes the GABA-A and GABA-B agonists (see Chapter 62), benzodiazepines (354,459). Alterations in motor function do not exclude the likelihood that a given agent may alter sensory transmission. Nevertheless, in the presence of motor dysfunction, such behavioral indices become questionable.

Postsynaptic Antagonism of Afferent Transmitters Importantly, agents which block the postsynaptic sites of glutamate and substance P tend to have a poor therapeutic ratio in terms of acute nociceptive measures. Thus, AMPA and Neurokinin 1 (NK1) receptors are believed to mediate at least some components of the postsynaptic effects of C fibers (see Chapters 34 and 35), yet the systemic or spinal delivery of NK antagonists (352,452) or glutamate antagonists (7,63,455–457) will often lead to significant motor weakness at doses which block the acute pain. As noted previously, failure to see a behaviorally defined analgesia does not necessarily exclude the agents from interacting with the components of nociceptive processing, but indicates that such effects if present occur at doses that are limited by motor dysfunction.

Inhibition of Metabolism of Endogenous Principals There are a number of endogenous systems known to alter spinal transmission. In a number of cases, the activity of these systems can be

Table 3. SUMMARY OF NONAFFERENT SPINAL RECEPTOR SYSTEMS WHICH MODULATE NOCICEPTIVE PROCESSING

Receptor		Location of spinal binding		Spinal effects	
				SP release[a]	WDR[b]
	δ	Pre/post (124,204)	D > V (265)	Dep (134)	Dep (117,179)
	κ	Pre/post (124,204)	D > V (65)	NE (134)	Dep (117,179)
Adrenergic	α_2	Pre/post (171)	D > V (298)	Dep (134,292)	Dep (118)
Serotonin	5-HT			NE (134)	Dep (113)
	5-HT_{1A}	Pre/post (78)	D > V (78,300a)	?	Dep (113)
	5-HT_{1B}	?	D > V (300a)	?	Dep (113)
	5-HT_2	?	D > V (300)	?	NC (113)
	5-HT_3	Pre/post (149)	D > V (149)	↑(341)	Dep (11)
Adenosine	(AI)	Post (127)	D > V (29)	Dep (336)	Dep (336)
GABA	A	Pre/post	D > V (396)	Dep (134)	Dep (11)
	B	Pre/post	D > V (314)	NE (134)	Dep (90)
Cholinergic	MI	Pre/post (133)	D ≈ V (132)	?	Dep (268)
	Nicotinic	?	D ≈ V (132)		
Neuropeptide Y	(?)	Pre/post (185)	D > V (185)	Dep (103)	?
Neurotensin	(?)	D > V (116)	?	?	Fac (259)
Glutamate	(NMDA)	Pre/post (79,218)	D > V (123)	↑[c]	Fac (351)

[a]Effect by agonist on the release of substance P from the spinal cord.
[b]Effect by full agonist on the discharge of wide dynamic range neuron in spinal dorsal horn.
[c]X.-Y. Hua and T. L. Yaksh, unpublished data.
References for data are in parentheses. SP, substance P; WDR, wide dynamic range; D, dorsal; V, ventral; pre, binding presynaptic (on primary afferent); post, binding postsynaptic (not on primary afferent); dep, depression; ↑, increase; NE, no effect; fac, facilitation; NC, no change.

substantially influenced by the use of inhibitors of either synthesis or degradation.

The potent effect of spinal cholinesterase (2,272) and enkephalinase (10,295) inhibition likely reflects upon the fact that afferent traffic evoked by acute high-intensity stimuli leads to the release of spinal acetylcholine (I. Khan, P. Taylor, and T. L. Yaksh, unpublished observations, 1996) and enkephalinoid products (434) which, acting though muscarinic (272) and μ/δ opioid receptors (92), respectively, serve to regulate spinal afferent processing. These products are metabolically labile and the blockade of their enzymatic processing will yield elevated levels of extracellular acetylcholine (I. Khan, unpublished observations, 1996) and a number of enkephalin products (28,219,432,447).

Agents which serve as inhibitors of cyclooxygenase and nitric oxide typically only modestly effect the animalís response to acute nociceptive stimuli. This modest action suggests that neither prostanoids nor nitric oxide play a detectable role in the processing generated by an acute nociceptive stimulus (see below).

C-Fiber Neurotoxins Agents such as capsaicin have been shown to produce a long-lasting (e.g., after systemic-neonatal treatment) and acute (as after acute systemic or intrathecal) thermal hypoalgesia. The mechanisms of this are believed to reflect a desensitization or a frank neurotoxic action upon spinal terminals of small afferents (35). Current evidence indicates that the site of capsaicin action is a specific recognition site on the C-fiber terminal (see Chapter 33). Recent work with the nicotinic receptor suggests that under certain conditions it may also exert a local desensitizing effect on some spinal link in nociceptive processing (190). Importantly, nicotine can directly stimulate C-fiber terminals and leads to their acute inactivation (181). Whether this action accounts for the central effects remains to be seen.

Facilitated Processing: Hyperalgesia

The psychophysics of the acute pain state generated by a transient stimulus have indicated that there is a close relationship between the reported intensity of the stimulus, the discharge evoked in the peripheral afferent and the magnitude of the reported pain. It is, however, appreciated that there are situations in which the magnitude of the afferent traffic and the pain response may be dissociated from the magnitude of the physical stimulus. Such conditions may be loosely referred to as reflecting a state of hyperalgesia. Such a state of hyperalgesia may be present in the tissue surrounding a local injury. Thus, in the area of a mild burn, there is a decreased nociceptive threshold to heat (a thermal hyperalgesia), an increased response to pinch or pin prick (mechanical hyperalgesia), and an exaggerated pain response generated by light touch (tactile allodynia), both inside and outside of the area of burn (76,215,261) (see Chapter 41). Importantly, at least one component of this hyperalgesia reflects upon activity in small afferents. The intradermal injection of small amounts of capsaicin, an agent known to selectively activate C fibers, can induce a secondary hyperalgesia/allodynia, and flare (due to antidromic activation of local C-fiber collaterals) (204,399) (see Chapter 33). This altered sensory condition persists after the termination of the pain produced by the capsaicin injection and extends anatomically beyond the local site in which the capsaicin was shown to exert an effect.

Mechanisms

Peripheral Mechanisms Classically, the interpretation of these psychophysics of the pain states observed after injury has focused on the peripheral injury and inflammation. The early appreciation that the products released by injury, such as bradykinin and prostanoids, could cause pain (e.g., activate small fibers) led models of inflammation to be interpreted primarily in terms of persistence of the peripheral afferent transduction characteristics (217). The correlation between such afferent sensitization and changes in the escape latency is typified in Fig. 3.

Central Mechanisms While focal injury can induce sensitization of the peripheral terminal such that low-intensity stimuli can activate an enhanced discharge and yield a behaviorally defined "hyperalgesia," several lines of evidence indicate that the peripheral sensitization alone is not adequate to explain the characteristics of such sensitization: (a) Components of the sensitization extend beyond the area of injury and erethema and appear to involve terminals not directly influenced by the injury. (b) Allodynia is believed to arise from low-threshold mechanoreceptor afferents and allodynia would not likely arise from an additional local sensitization. (c) The hyperalgesia can be induced by repetitive local electrical stimulation and this occurs in a manner not likely mediated by local inflammation (71,313). (d) The subsequent hyperalgesia/allodynia induced by intradermal capsaicin can be prevented by transient local blockade of the site of injection with local anesthetic (399). These observations strongly support the contention that an important component of the pain state generated by a persistent postinjury discharge, presumably in small afferents, may involve the activation of a central substrate which leads to an alteration in the processing of afferent input from adjacent dermatomes.

Electrophysiological studies have emphasized that the periodic (e.g., 0.1 Hz) electrical stimulation of sensory nerves will evoke a stable and repeatable response in dorsal horn wide dynamic range neurons. However, repetitive electrical stimulation at slightly higher frequencies (e.g., 0.5–1 Hz) will induce a

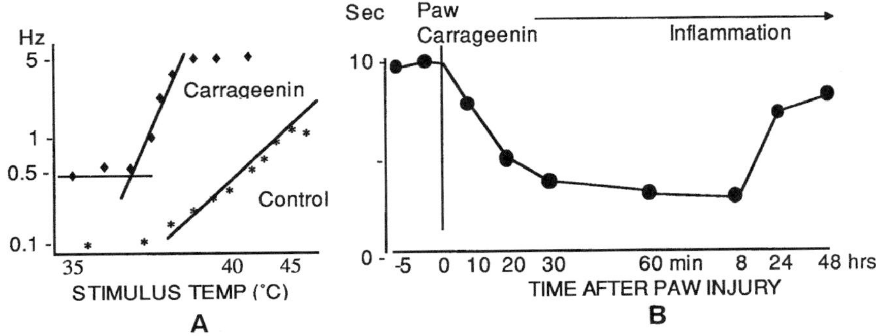

Figure 3. **A:** Typical stimulus C-fiber response relationship for a small slowly conducting primary afferent (for example, see refs. 150,151,206). The figure emphasizes several points: (a) minimal resting activity in a C-fiber innervating uninjured skin of the foot, (b) increasing skin temperatures above 45°C results in a monotonic increase in discharge activity, and (c) in the face of a local inflammation, the C fiber displays an ongoing discharge, an increase in discharge rat at a lower temperature (40°C) and a somewhat steeper slope. **B:** Response latency of the rat in response to a thermal stimulus applied to a paw which had been subjected to the injection of the proinflammatory agent carrageenin into the paw at time zero. This reduced latency reflects a thermal hyperalgesia and is in part the presumed consequence of the sensitized C fiber (M. Marsala and T. L. Yaksh, unpublished observation, 1996.)

profound facilitation of the response of the dorsal horn. In this phenomena, defined as "wind-up" (257), repetitive small (C fiber), but not large (A fiber), input evokes (a) a progressive facilitation in the spinal neuron's response to large and small afferent input and (b) an increase in the peripheral receptive field of the cell (297,397) (see Chapter 36). The importance of this observation of afferent-evoked facilitation is emphasized by the fact that in the postinjury state, the discharge properties of the peripheral afferent are characterized by a rapid and ongoing bursting discharge in classes of small afferents innervating the injury field (see Chapters 31 and 32). Such persistent activation would thus be considered to be physiologically adequate to induce a marked state of facilitated processing. This facilitated component could provide the substrate for mediating the exaggerated activity that underlies the behaviorally defined hyperalgesic state.

The mechanisms underlying the central facilitation have been discussed elsewhere in this volume (see Chapters 35 and 36). In brief, however, it should be emphasized that at the spinal level, both anatomical connectivity and dynamic elements are clearly involved. Thus, anatomically small afferents collateralize in the lateral Lissauer tract and may make excitatory connections as far as several segments rostrally and caudally. Under normal circumstances, these distant projections have only a modest effect. However, it is believed that after conditioning stimuli these connections may become more effective and account in part for the increasing size of the receptive field observed after tissue injury. In terms of the dynamic components, repetitive stimulation (through tachykinin and glutamatergic receptors) brings into play a number of pharmacological mechanisms which can induce and sustain a facilitated state. These issues will be considered again below in the discussion of the pharmacology of several aspects of facilitated pain models. A schematic representation of the spinal components of the organization leading to a facilitated state is presented in Fig. 4.

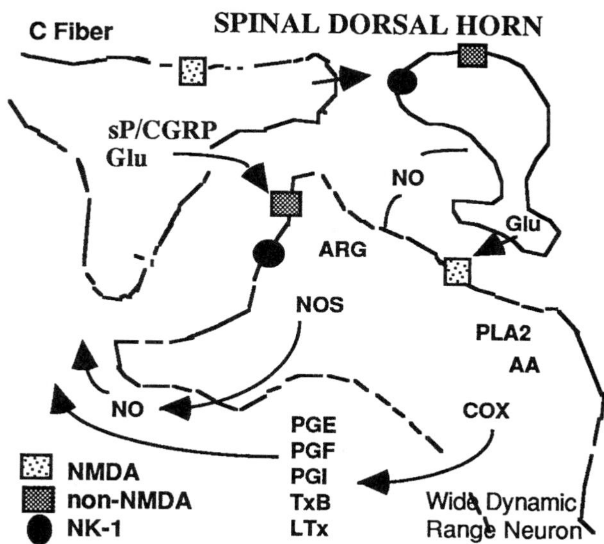

Figure 4. Summary of organization of dorsal horn systems leading to facilitated processing in the face of protracted afferent input. *(1)* Afferent initiation of facilitated states by release of SP and excitatory amino acids (Glutamate: GLU). *(2)* Excitatory amino acids (EAA) and SP interact with AMPA and NK1 sites postsynaptic to the primary afferent. *(3)* NK1, non-NMDA, and NMDA receptor occupancy lead to the release of a family of prostanoids (PG) and nitric oxide (NO). *(4)* Extracellular prostanoids interact with PG receptors to increase depolarization-evoked Ca flux and enhance transmitter release. *(5)* Increased NO facilitates GLU release. *(6)* Extracellular levels of GLU act presynaptically on NMDA receptors on afferent terminal to enhance release. *(7)* Presynaptic actions of $\mu/\alpha 2$ receptors depress release of SP/glutamate. *(8)* Repetitive activation of EAA /NK-1 receptor evokes induction of spinal NOS and COX isozymes. (9) Spontaneous release of pituitary ACTH is enhanced by spinofugal projections to increase release of corticosterone from adrenal cortex which tonically suppresses NOS/COX induction. +, excitation.

Properties of Models

The above discussions are jointly in accord with the proposition that a conditioning barrage or a protracted ongoing input such as that which occurs in the postinjury state will produce a marked facilitation. This facilitation causes the spinal response and the corresponding behavior to be greater than would be anticipated, or the same magnitude of escape behavior can be evoked by a much smaller stimulus. This property is referred to as hyperalgesia.

A variety of models have been developed that are believed to engage this mechanism of central facilitation. The common characteristics of these models are the initiation of an injury (as with a burn or an incision) or an inflammatory state (as with the local injection of carrageenin or Freunds adjuvant), or the injection of an agent that produces a persistent discharge of the sensory axon (such as capsaicin or formalin). It should be stressed that the presumptive mechanisms for such a hyperalgesia could be due to either a sensitization of the peripheral terminal and/or facilitation within the neuraxis. In the former case, it would seem that the central pharmacology of the postinjury pain state and that associated with the acute afferent barrage should be identical. In many instances, this is not the case (reviewed later), indicating that at least several postinjury hyperalgesic states are not due simply to a peripheral sensitization, but involve central changes.

Facilitated Models

Formalin Test Using mice, rats or guinea pigs, a small volume of irritant is injected into one of the hind paws. Upon recovery, the animal will favor the injected paw and display periodic flinches in the injected limb. Several measures have been employed: flinches are periodically counted; at the time the paw is licked, the paw is held elevated; or a number of "pain behaviors" are assessed in epochs for typically up to an hour, with the response during the first phase being distinguished from those in the second phase (62,233,410). At this time, the animal is sacrificed. While a variety of materials have been considered (411), formalin has been widely employed and characterized. Typically, each animal will display a two-phase response, the first (phase 1) lasting ~5–10 min, at which time the animal becomes quiescent. After ~10 min, the animal will begin to show flinching responses again and this second phase (phase 2) lasts ~40–50 min (411). Lower concentrations of formalin appear to represent a less imperative stimulus, leading to more modest flinching during both phases (12; also A. B. Malmberg and N. A. Calcutt, unpublished observations, 1996).

Treatment with the C-fiber neurotoxin capsaicin will reduce significantly the response to the irritant injected into the paw (435) and the second phase of the formalin test (98), suggesting a role for small afferents.

There is considerable evidence to support the proposition that phase 2 of the formalin test is related to a facilitated state. This presumption depends on the observation that the injection of an irritant such as formalin into the paw will evoke an initial burst of activity in saphenous afferents, followed by a prolonged, low-level of small afferent activity (160). Examination of single unit activity in dorsal horn projection neurons has revealed, in contrast to the afferent input but in accord with the observed flinching behavior, that there is a significant level of activity and behavior (flinching of the injected paw) during phases 1 and 2. It is believed that the first phase corresponds to the initial afferent burst of activity, but the second phase appears exaggerated in view of the low level of afferent drive. This has suggested that the second phase reflects an augmented response. It is important to note that the second phase is dependent upon the sustained (but low level) afferent input during Phase 2. Thus, local anesthetic blockade during the second phase will reduce dorsal horn neuron activity (91) and the display of flinching behavior to zero (77,165).

The pharmacology of the formalin test has been a subject of considerable investigation. Agents may be functionally considered in two classes, those that will completely reduce phase 2 (the facilitated component) and those that appear to exert a significant effect but one which is plateau limited. To date, all agents which are effective upon acute pain processing fall into the first category. These include opiate and α_2 agents (237) (see below). Agents which fall in the second class include NMDA (455) and NK1 receptor antagonists (289, 454), adenosine A1 agonists (187), GABA-A/B agonists (95, 288), cyclooxygenase inhibitors (237), and enkephalinase inhibitors (385).

Persistent Inflammation and Paw Mechanical/Thermal Threshold The injection of agents such as Freunds adjuvant (37) or carrageenan (157,379) will result in a local inflammation that evolves over an interval of several hours to days. Measurement of afferent activity in small afferents reveals that the ongoing discharge evolves over a corresponding interval and displays an increasing stimulus-response relationship (24,195). This treatment yields a significant reduction in the thermal escape latency and the strength of the mechanical stimulus required to evoke withdrawal (157). Single unit recording in rats prepared with Freunds adjuvant revealed a significant increase in spontaneous activity and evidence for an increased receptive field size and enhanced response properties (321).

The thermal hyperalgesia has been shown to be sensitive to systemic and intrathecally delivered opioid agonists (157): α_2 agonists (176), NMDA antagonists (112,320,321); cyclooxygenase inhibitors (296) and nitric oxide synthase inhibitors (254).

Joint Inflammation Injection of an inflammatory agent, such as urate crystals (64,290) or kaolin and carrageenan (348,367) into the knee or ankle joints, will induce a swelling of the joint, the appearance of inflammatory cells, and the elaboration of a variety of inflammatory products (346). This results in a reduction in weight-bearing of the injected limb and increases the pain behavior produced by compression of the injected joint (271). The knee joint inflammation is innervated by afferents in the articular nerve. Under normal circumstances, these afferents have no spontaneous activity and display an exceedingly high threshold, being activated only by severe distention of the joint (346). After generation of an inflammatory response with the injection of carrageenin, the articular afferent displays significant spontaneous activity and an exaggerated response to modest distention of the knee (348). This activity is accompanied by an increased release of peptides (170,347), excitatory amino acids and prostaglandins (462) from the spinal cord.

The physiological signs of hyperalgesia (spinal single unit activity or autonomic responses) have been shown to be diminished by systemic and spinally delivered opioids (271), cyclooxygenase inhibitors (283), Neurokinin (NK)–1 antagonists (285), and NMDA antagonists (284; H. Awad and T. L. Yaksh, unpublished observations, 1996).

Abdominal Irritants The intraperitoneal injections of a number of irritants, such as phenylbenzoquinone, acetylcholine, or acetic acid in the rodent will induce a characteristic response which involves a dorsoflexion of the back , extension of the hindlimbs and a strong contraction of the abdominal musculature (162,224,281,349). The syndrome typically displays an immediate onset and persists for intervals in excess of 1 h. The neural substrate involved in this syndrome is not well characterized. However, it is likely that these irritants may excite afferents terminating in the viscera well as in the wall of the peritoneal cavity.

The abdominal writhing test has been widely studied for its sensitivity to a variety of systemic and intrathecally delivered agents including opioid agonists (349,401) α_2-receptor agonists (227), cholinesterase inhibitors (74), enkephalinase inhibitors (55), and cyclooxygenase inhibitors (356) (for review, see ref. 281).

Bladder Irritation Mild distention of the bladder typically has little effect on the behavior of the rat. However, the induction of an inflammatory state by the injection of an irritant into the bladder such as turpentine will result in a condition where a mild bladder distention will lead to a prominent guarding response and hypersensitivity to noxious stimuli applied to the tail or caudal abdomen (252). The origin of this pain state is believed to be the bladder afferents that travel with the pelvic plexus in the hypogastric nerve that display enhanced spontaneous activity and increased sensitivity to distention following induction of inflammation, such as that which occurs after the intravesical application of agents such as turpentine (146). This model may serve as a model for the syndrome of interstitial cystitis (251).

The pain behavior/hyperreflexia is significantly reduced by the spinal delivery of NMDA antagonists (323) and nitric oxide synthase inhibitors (322).

Ureteric Calculosis A small volume of liquid dental acrylic is injected into the ureter. Behavioral analysis reveals that shortly after surgery, the animals begin to display incidences of stereotypic behavior that includes contraction of the left abdominal musculature, stretching, and elements resembling the "writhing" response induced by abdominal irritants (see above) (131). The incidence was highest during the first 3-4 days and declined over the ensuing 10 days, by which time the calculus is typically passed. In addition, electrical stimulation of the obliqus externus musculature induces spontaneous vocalization. This threshold is significantly lower in rats with the ureteral calculus. This resembles the phenomena of nocifensor tenderness in which percussion of the abdominal musculature in humans with a local visceral inflammation (as in acute pancreatitis, kidney infection, or appendicitis) will be reported to be painful by the patient (see Chapter 39). The behavioral and physiological effects of ureteral distention appear paralleled by autonomic responses (increased blood pressure) and increasing activity in the convergent dorsal horn neurons (203,328). The pain behaviors associated with ureteral distention are significantly diminished by antispasmolytics, nonsteroidal antiinflammatory agents (130) and opiates (328).

Pharmacology of Post-tissue Injury/Inflammation-Induced Pain Models

In Table 4, the effects of systemic and intrathecal agents on several models believed to reflect facilitated processing are indicated. Inspection of the effects of a variety of agents on postinjury-induced behaviors and hyperalgesia merit several general comments.

Components of Postinjury Pain State As reviewed above, the mechanisms of the postinjury pain state represent at least two essential components: a persistent afferent barrage generated by the peripheral milieu at the injury site and by changes in the central processing induced by the persistent barrage. The observation that spinally delivered drugs can "normalize" the nociceptive threshold at doses that are considerably less than those necessary for a systemic effect emphasizes a likely central effect. This is particularly noteworthy for agents such as the cyclooxygenase inhibitors, where the peripheral role of prostanoids in nociceptor sensitization is well-defined (see Chapters 33 and 61). The converse is not true, e.g., that a spinal effect of the drug precludes a peripheral action of the agent .

Multiple Sites of Drug Action Given potential peripheral and central multiple sites of action, it can be appreciated that systemically delivered agents may interact at one or both sites. In considering the effects of opiates and cyclooxygenase

Table 4. SUMMARY OF DRUG EFFECTS AS A FUNCTION OF PRECLINICAL PAIN MODELS

		Facilitated		Neuropathic				
Drug	Acute HP/TF	Formalin (flinching—phase 2)	Inflamed paw or knee (thermal injury/pressure)	Bennett (thermal hyperalgesia)	Chung (tactile allodynia)	Intrathecal strychnine (tactile allodynia)	Streptozocin diabetes (tactile allodynia)	Spinal ischemia (tactile allodynia)
Agonist								
Opioid								
μ	+ (430)	+ (237)	+ (157,378,450)	+ (213, 453)	0 (209,443)	0 (358,428)	+ (48,73)	0 (421)
δ	+ (430)	+[a]	+ (157,378,450)	+ (213,453)		0 (358,428)		
κ	+ (430)	+ (237,301)	+ (157,378,450)	+ (213,453)		0 (358,428)		
ACH								
Muscarinic	+ (177,433)	+[b]						
Nicotinic	+ (461)							
Adrenergic-α_2	+ (437)	+ (240)	+ (176,377)	+ (213,453)	+ (433)	0 (358,428)	+ (48,73)	0 (421)
GABA								
A	+[c]	+ (95)	+[d]	+ (368,453)			0 (155)	
B	+ (148,416)	+ (95)	+[d]	+ (368,453)		(358,428)		+ (155)
5-HT	+ (449)		+[d]					
Adenosine								
A1	+ (344,373)	+ (240)		+ (453)	+ (211)	+ (374)		
Neuropeptide								
Y	+ (172)							
Antagonist								
NMDA	0 (63)	+ (61,198,457)	+ (112,320,321)	+ (243,244,456)	+ (50)	+ 358	+ (48,73)	0 (422)
AMPA	0 (63)	+ (63,274)	+ (112,320,321)	+ (243)	+ (50)			+ (422)
NK1	0 (307)	+ (452)	+ (450,451)	0 (456)			+ (48,73)	
Inhibitor								
COX	0 (240)	+ (233)	+ (296)				+ (48,73)	
NOS	0 (197)	+ (238)	+ (254)	+ (255)				+ (153)
ACHase	+ (272)	+[e]						
Enk-ase	+ (295)	+ (93)	+ (378)					
Channels								
Intravenous								
sodium	0 (3)	+ (3)		+ (3)	+[e]		+ (48,73)	+ (156,421)
Calcium								
L	0 (145,240)	+ (145,240)			0 (49)			
N	0 (145,240)	0+ (145,240)			+ (49)			
P	0 (145,240)	+ (145,240)			0 (49)			

[a]H. Umeno and T. L. Yaksh, unpublished data
[b]M. Naguib and T. L. Yaksh, unpublished data.
[c]T. L. Yaksh, unpublished data.
[d]Awad and T. L. Yaksh, unpublished data.
[e]Spath and T. L. Yaksh, unpublished data.
References for data are in parentheses. HP, hot plate; TF, tail flick.

inhibitors there are two well-defined examples of the potential role played by both the central and peripheral sites. Thus, it has been shown that after local inflammation, as in the skin or knee joint, μ and κ agonists given spinally can diminish the observed hyperalgesia. In addition, these agonists given at the site of inflammation can similarly reduce the hyperalgesic components (271,379). The central effects are believed to be due to the alteration in central release, while the peripheral action is believed to attenuate the enhanced transduction properties and spontaneous activity of the terminal in the inflammatory milieu produced by the adjuvant or carrageenin (see Chapter 30). These observations are consistent with early literature which indicated that opioids which crossed the blood-brain barrier poorly could diminish the writhing response (369,370). With NSAIDS, it has been shown that both the systemic and intrathecal actions can alter the hyperalgesic state associated with the formalin test and with the thermal hyperalgesia as induced by carrageenin (see Chapter 61). The peripheral action is indicative of the role played by prostaglandins at the site of injury leading to sensitized nerve terminals, while the central effects represent the activation of prostaglandin releasing systems in the face of persistent small afferent input (as generated by the peripheral injury or inflammation). Given that the classes of agents (opiates and NSAIDs) which are as mechanistically well defined can possess both peripheral and central sites of action in postinjury hyperalgesia, one must retain considerable reservation in assessing the site of other less defined classes of agents. Importantly, in the early literature the activity of diverse classes of agents in the writhing test (as compared to the hot plate) was taken as a sign of nonspecificity of the test. It is now clear that this diversity probably represents the complexity of the system.

Effects of Agents Which Reduce Afferent Terminal Excitability Agents that are known to block transmitter release from C fibers are able to abolish pain behavior in the postinjury/inflammation state (Table 2). Thus, μ, δ, and α_2 agonists are potent inhibitors of the second phase of the formalin model and reduce the hyperalgesic response induced by inflammation of the knee or skin. The hyperalgesic state may represent an augmentation of the small primary afferent traffic evoked by a given stimulus and/or reflects an enhanced spinal response to a given degree of small primary afferent traffic. In either

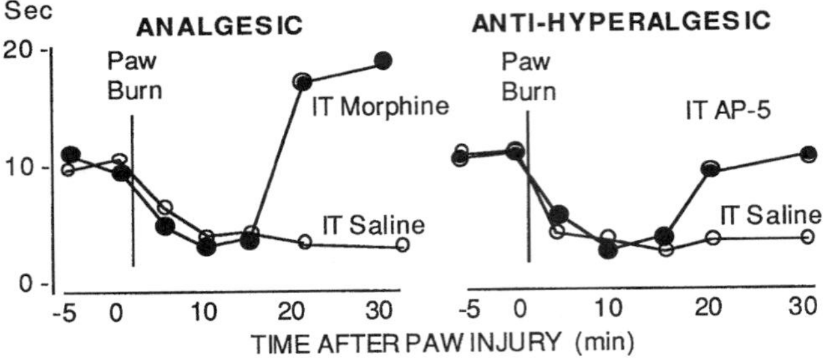

Figure 5. Paw with withdrawal latency in seconds plotted versus time after a thermal stimulus (52°C, 45 s) evoking an erythema was applied at T = 1 min in rats prepared with chronic intrathecal (IT) catheters. At the time indicated, one group of animals received intrathecal saline, IT morphine (10 μg, a μ opioid agonist) or IT AP-5 (3 μg, an NMDA receptor antagonist). As indicated, the injury resulted in a persistent thermal hyperalgesia as indicated by the decreased response latency. There was no change in the latency of the contralateral paw (data not shown). The injection of morphine resulted in a near complete block of the thermal escape response (e.g., maximum response latency = 20 s). The animal receiving AP-5 at a maximum usable dose resulted in a response latency not different from the preinjury baseline. (J. Jun and T. L. Yaksh, unpublished observations, 1997.)

case, it is presumed that an agent that blocks small afferent input will be similarly able to block the excitatory input generated by such stimulation. Such agents retain the ability to produce a maximum blockade of the stimulus-evoked pain behavior.

Antihyperalgesic Versus Analgesic Agents Consideration of the action of agents such as the NMDA receptor antagonists or cyclooxygenase inhibitors reveals that agents such as these appear to normalize the hyperalgesic component of the behavior to a level that corresponds to the preinjury/preinflammation response characteristics. Accordingly, these centrally acting agents are not precisely analgesics, but are in fact antihyperalgesics. This distinction is presented in Fig. 5 for morphine and the NMDA antagonist, MK801. As suggested in Table 3, agents such as GABA-A and -B agonists, adenosine A1 agonists, cyclooxygenase and nitric oxide synthase inhibitors appear to fall more clearly in the category of antihyperalgesics as defined by these models.

Triggering Effects of Phase 1 Inspection of the formalin test reveals that the two distinct phases (phases 1 and 2) are sequentially linked. Pretreatment during the phase 1 response will prevent the evolution of the phase 2 response, whereas treatment between phases 1 and 2 may fail to reduce the phase 2 response. An important example of this response pattern is seen with NMDA and NK-1 antagonists (454,457). This observation suggests that events mediated by NMDA and NK-1 receptor activation are initiated in phase 1 and that these events are required for the evolution of the phase 2 facilitated state (see Chapter 36).

Post Nerve Injury Models of Pain Behavior

Following peripheral nerve injury, anomalous pain syndromes have been reported in humans. These include a combination of the following elements: (a) spontaneous pain states referred to the distribution of the nerve injury, also called causalgia (from *causis*, burning/*algia*,pain); (b) pain reports evoked by low-intensity mechanical stimuli mediated by the activation of myelinated, low-threshold mechanoreceptors (41); (c) thermal hyperalgesia in which a moderate warm or cool stimulus may be reported as noxious; and (d) a coupling of activity in the sympathetic nervous systems with a sensory pain state (referred to as a complex regional pain syndrome type 2, or reflex sympathetic dystrophy). This sensory component has been widely documented to be an important component of the pain syndromes broadly classified as complex regional pain syndromes (36,309) (see Chapter 28). Of particular importance, the composite pain states reflected by these post nerve injury conditions are often said to display components for which typical analgesic regimens, notably using opiates, frequently display less efficacy (337) (see Chapter 56).

Mechanisms

We are not certain of all the mechanisms underlying these pain states which are observed after nerve injury. However, in brief, several points appear to contribute.

Spontaneous Afferent Traffic An injured peripheral nerve results in the development of spontaneous activity in both the injured portion of the nerve (the neuroma) and in the dorsal root ganglion cells (87). The spontaneous activity may be due to altered ion channel distribution in the neuroma (86,87) or the appearance of coupled receptors (see below).

Chemosensitivity of Neuroma Neuromas develop sensitivity to a variety of pharmacological stimuli, including epinephrine, prostaglandins, hydrogen ions and potassium (87) (see Chapters 32 and 33).

Inflammatory Cells Local products of injury may derive from the injury site or local cells such as macrophages drawn to the site as a result of the injury (122) (see Chapter 20).

Sympathetic Sprouting Increased sympathetic innervation is observed in the neuroma and the dorsal root ganglion cell of the injured axon. (249). Sympathetic stimulation leads to activity which originates in the neuroma and the dorsal root ganglion cell.

Central Afferent Sprouting Myelinated afferents which originally innervated deeper spinal lamina (III/IV) sprout to regions previously innervated primarily by small, high-threshold afferents (418).

Central Reorganization Following peripheral nerve lesions there is a major reorganization of spinal connectivity and function, including appearance of several immediate early genes (53,54,163,164), alterations in cellular markers (42), and the appearance of dark staining neurons (384). (For further discussion on these processes, see Chapters 30, 32, and 56.)

Factors Initiating Reorganization The initiation of the cascade outlined above appears to be dependent on several components, including (a) the initial burst of activity from the injury; (b) the ongoing spontaneous activity in the nerve injury site and DRG (53,54); and (c) the impact of growth factors that may be transported centrally from the site of nerve injury (458) arising from the inflammatory cells and Schwann cells that are proliferating as a function of the injury (253) (see Chapter 30).

Post-Nerve Injury Pain Models

Several models of nerve injury-induced hyperalgesia and allodynia have been reported. These will be reviewed below. (For additional discussion of these nerve injury models, see Chapter 32.)

Neurectomy-Autotomy Model Section of the sciatic nerve at the level of the popliteal fossa has been shown to result in an increased incidence of autotomy of the digits and paw of the lesioned limb. This develops over time (days to weeks) and may be mild to severe (requiring sacrifice) (407). The origin of this spontaneous behavior is believed to be due in part to the spontaneous activity which originates from the injured nerve or its dorsal root ganglion during the post nerve injury period (see Chapter 30).

Chronic Sciatic Nerve Constriction (Bennett Model) In this model, the sciatic nerve is loosely ligated unilaterally at the level of the popliteal fossa with 4 loose ligatures (Fig. 2). Rats so prepared will display (a) an exaggerated response to mechanical pinch; (b) a vocalization to light; (c) a vigorous escape response to temperatures as low as 46°C and as high as 10°C (hot and cold allodynia, respectively) and a faster response of the ligated paw to cutaneous thermal stimuli latency (16,23). In addition, the animals tend to display a characteristic positioning of the ligated paw, periodically elevating it above the surface. The hyperalgesia may appear ~4–6 days after placement of the ligatures and can persist for ~20 days.

Specific measurements of skin temperature reveal that in comparison with the nonligated paw, the ligated paw of the group displays a clear evolution over the course of 30 days after injury, transitioning from being abnormally warm to abnormally cold (406). Surgical (84) and chemical (guanethidine) sympathectomy. Treatment with guanethidine diminishes heat and cold sensitization, but has only a modest effect on mechanical sensitization (275,304). Studies focused on the pharmacology of this pain state is presented in Table 3.

Freeze Model The sciatic nerve is exposed at the level of the popliteal fossa. A low-temperature freeze probe is placed in apposition to the exposed nerve and the nerve is briefly subjected to a freeze-thaw cycle. This treatment initially yields a hypoesthesia that recovers over an interval of several weeks. Shortly after lesion, autotomy of the injured paw is noted to peak at 14 days. The onset of autotomy appears to occur when the limb is regaining sensitivity (83,404,405). Thus, within 14–21 days, the limb displays significant bilateral touch-evoked allodynia, but not thermal hyperalgesia (415). Measurement of axon profiles reveals an initial loss followed by regrowth over the ensuing 28-day interval. Unlike ligature models, the freezing model serves to disrupt the axon, but generally preserves the perineural sheath. Because of this preservation, there is an increased efficiency of the sprouting mechanisms. Sympathectomy does not alter the tactile allodynia observed following lesion (414).

Partial Ligation (Shir and Seltzer Model) A ligature is passed through half of one sciatic nerve, proximal to the ischeal notch, and ligated. Rats reliably developed a tactile allodynia and thermal hyperalgesia (359). Chemical sympathectomy has been shown to reverse the hyperpathia (359).

L5/L6 Nerve Ligation (Chung Model) The L5 and L6 nerves are unilaterally ligated just proximal to the vertebral bodies. This results in a highly reliable thermal hyperalgesia, cold allodynia and a tactile allodynia (57,192) (Fig. 6), with the effect being more robust when performed in young animals (59). Systematic studies have indicated that a stable allodynia is observed beginning approximately the second day after nerve ligation and lasting ~50 days (49). A variety of surgical interventions have emphasized that the behaviors are reversed by sympathectomy (57,193) and that the behavioral state is dependent upon signals entering the spinal cord from the injured fibers or the dorsal root ganglion (357). Studies on the nature of the afferent transduction properties have suggested that after ligation, a novel mechanoreceptor was observed over time in the injured paw. The response characteristics were normalized after systemic α-adrenergic receptor blockade (269). Studies focusing on the pharmacology of this pain state are presented in Table 3.

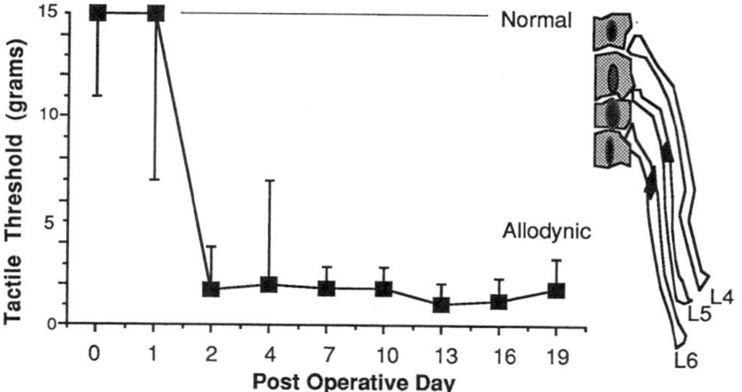

Figure 6. Graph presents the tactile threshold as assessed over days with von Frey hairs in a group of rats prepared with unilateral L5/L6 nerve ligations on day 0 and tested periodically. (Reprinted, in adapted form, with permission from Chaplan SR, Pogrel JW, Yaksh TL. Role of voltage-dependent calcium channel subtypes in experimental tactile allodynia. *J Pharmacol Exp Ther* 1994;269:1117–1123.)

Spinal Ischemia Focal spinal ischemia was induced by focal irradiation of the cord through a laminectomy after the intravenous delivery of a photosensitive dye (152) or by the transient ischemia of the spinal cord induced by reversible occlusion of the descending aorta (246). In these models, tactile stroking in the dermatones corresponding to the ischemic spinal segments will evoke vocalization and evidence of significant agitation. In the focal ischemia models, animals exhibit allodynia and aversive responses to mechanical and cold stimulation of the caudal body (areas innervated by the ischemic segments) (152,154,420). Single unit recording has shown that the focal ischemia results in an exaggerated response by wide dynamic range neurons to large, but not small, afferent input (155). The mechanisms of this allodynia are not clear, however, incomplete or reversible ischemia has been shown to have a prominent effect upon populations of small neurons in the dorsal and ventral spinal cords. Such interneurons are believed to contain GABA and/or glycine (328) and to serve a modulatory role on the activity evoked by low-threshold afferent input (428). Focal spinal ischemia has been shown to reduce GABA-positive cells in laminae I–III within days (167). With aortic occlusion, not only the spinal cord becomes ischemic, but the lower body as well. It has been shown that such ischemia of the tail can lead to spontaneous afferent activity, an enhanced discharge and "modality-specific hypersensitivity" of dorsal horn neurons and nociception (128,129).

Diabetic Neuropathy Subcutaneous injection of streptozotocin in rats induces hyperglycemia and glucosuria which are detectable within 24 h of injection. Examination of the morphology of the nerve reveals significant morphological changes which may be due in part to increases in endoneural pressure and reduced nerve perfusion (see Chapters 30 and 54). These physiological changes are accompanied by (a) a decrease in mechanical nociceptive threshold as defined by paw pressure (8,73); (b) an increased allodynia (low intensity tactile stimulation) (39,242) of the hindpaw; and (c) an increase in activity during the phase 1/phase 2 interphase of the formalin test (40) was detected, typically within 1 week. When examined, many of these changes were prevented by the concurrent delivery of therapeutic doses of insulin and aldose reductase inhibitors (39,40), but not by sympathectomy (8). The mechanisms underlying the observed dysfunction are not known. Recording for peripheral afferents has revealed that in streptozotocin rats, mechanical thresholds for C fibers are unaltered, but there was a significant afterdischarge (9). Studies focused on the pharmacology of this pain state are presented in Table 3.

Intrathecal Strychnine/Bicuculline The spinal inhibition of glycine or GABA-A receptor sites with strychnine or bicuculline/picrotoxin, respectively, will yield a state in which the application of a light tactile stimulus will evoke prominent organized pain behavior and a stimulus-dependent hypertension (358,428), as shown in Fig. 7. The effective stimulus site is limited to the spinal dermatomes upon which the intrathecal agent is acting (e.g., lower back and hind limbs). The sensory anomaly appears limited to a tactile stimulus, as thermal escape latencies are otherwise unaltered (428; T. L. Yaksh, unpublished observations, 1997). These behavioral and autonomic results are coincident with the electrophysiological observation that application of strychnine to the dorsal medullary will lead to augmentation of the low, but not high, threshold afferent-evoked component of trigeminal (191,463), and spinal (363) wide dynamic range neurons. Results of studies which focused on the pharmacology of this pain state are presented in Table 3.

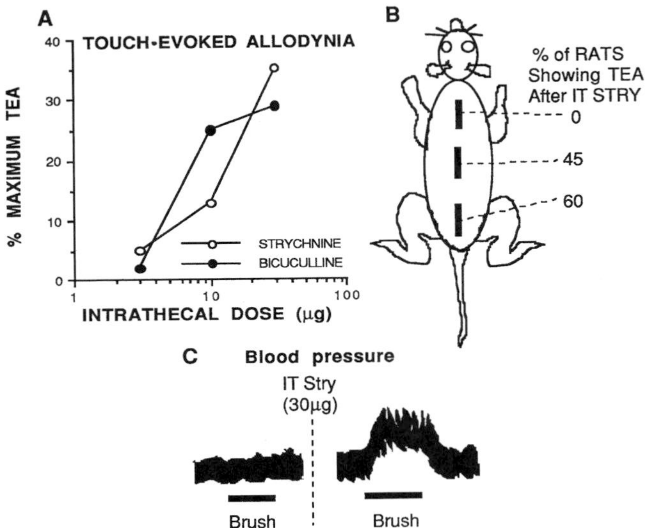

Figure 7. Intrathecal delivery of bicuculline and strychnine will produce a touch-evoked allodynia. **A:** Magnitude of the touch-evoked agitation response (TEA) evoked in the unanesthesized rat by tactile brushing of the flank in the presence of increasing doses of strychnine or bicuculline is dose dependent. **B:** The TEA is evoked by tactile brushing at or near the dermatomes associated with the spinal segments acted upon by the spinal strychnine. **C:** In anesthetized rats, after intrathecal strychnine, light brushing has no effect upon blood pressure in the normal rats, but will evoke a stimulation-dependent hypertension after intrathecal strychnine. (Reprinted, in adapted form, with permission from Yaksh TL. Behavioral and autonomic correlates of the tactile evoked allodynia produced by spinal glycine inhibition: effects of modulatory receptor systems and excitatory amino acid antagonists. *Pain* 1989;37:111–123.)

Pharmacology of the Post Nerve Injury Pain Models

The field related to the neuropathic models is clearly evolving. It is increasingly certain that alterations that occur after nerve injury will evoke significant changes in the manner in which afferent information is encoded at the spinal and higher levels. The most notable of these changes are (a) the development of a spontaneous dysesthesia, (b) the appearance of states in which pain is evoked by low-intensity tactile stimuli (e.g., allodynia), and (c) the appearance of heat, cold, and mechanical hyperalgesia. The pharmacology of these systems has just begun to be defined. Some of the related literature is summarized in Table 3.

As further insights into the organization of these systems evolve, it is probable that mechanistic differences, for example, between heat hyperalgesia and cold allodynia, or mechanical hyperalgesia and tactile allodynia, will become more evident. Accordingly, while there is insufficient evidence to make such a distinction at present, it is not trivial to consider, for example, the importance of data derived from the paw pressure test (reflecting mechanical hyperalgesia) and the threshold defined by using von Frey hairs (and reflecting tactile allodynia) as being potentially distinctive in terms of their pharmacology.

A number of comments may be drawn from several aspects of the current literature concerning the pharmacology of the post nerve injury pain state.

Glutamatergic Systems A compelling observation in the present series of studies is the prominence of the role played by spinal glutamatergic receptors. Several points should be noted:

1. All components of the allodynic and hyperalgesic states that are produced by a wide range of lesions ranging from frank nerve injury (Bennett and Chung nerve lesion models) to metabolic changes and ischemia are reversed by the systemic or spinal delivery of a variety of agents which block the NMDA receptor ionophore, including competitive (2-amino 5-phosphonovalorate) and noncompetitive (MK801) antagonists and glycine site antagonists (7-chlorokynurenate (431).

2. The behavioral results of the antagonists are consistent with the observation that intrathecal NMDA can induce a prominent tactile allodynia and thermal hyperalgesia (234).

3. The results of the antagonist studies suggest that in these nerve injury states, there may be an increase in the release of spinal glutamate or aspartate. In microdialysis studies of the spinal cord, using the Bennett model, there are marked and maintained increases in the extracellular levels of spinal glutamate and aspartate (247) and in diabetic rats (A. B. Malmberg and N. A. Calcutt, unpublished observations, 1996).

These results point to a surprisingly homogenous role for glutamatergic terminals in the spinal dorsal horn being in a state of exaggerated release. At present there are at least three mechanisms that may be relevant: (a) Repetitive small afferent input can induce the glutamate release from the rat spinal cord and induce the facilitated state that is believed to support the postinjury induced hyperalgesia, which has been discussed above. (b) There may be loss of regulation of extracellular levels of glutamate that occurs secondary to transynaptic changes associated with peripheral nerve injury, e.g., enhanced synthesis or reduced clearance. (c) Glutamate releasing terminals may be normal, but there may be a loss of extrinsic regulation in the dorsal horn. The observation that acute spinal GABA and glycine receptor antagonism can induce a prominent state of tactile allodynia (but not thermal hyperalgesia) and that this effect is reversed by the spinal delivery of NMDA antagonism and not by opiates or α_2 agonists (428) argues that changes in such intrinsic regulation secondary to nerve injury may be in part accountable.

The primacy of the glutamatergic system may serve to provide some degree of explanation as to the antiallodynic actions of a variety of agents shown to be effective in the preclinical models. Thus, agents thought to regulate glutamate release, such as the adenosine A 1 receptor (72,121), also display a potent antiallodynic effect (211,374).

GABA/Glycine Systems Transient blockade of GABA-A and glycinergic receptors yields a prominent allodynia and enhances low- but not high-threshold afferent-evoked discharge (see above for references). These observations suggest that the encoding of low-intensity mechanical stimuli as innocuous, depends upon the presence of a tonic activation of intrinsic glycine and/or GABAergic neurons. Such neurons and the respective binding are found within the dorsal horn (43,397), glycine (20,466), and GABA (361). GABA-containing terminals are frequently presynaptic to the large central afferent terminal complexes and may form reciprocal synapses (18). GABAergic axosomatic connections on spinothalamic cells have also been identified (43). The relevance of these inhibitory amino acid systems in regulating behavior generated by low-threshold afferent transmission is suggested by mouse (412) and bovine (143) models show a prominent somatic sensitivity, having a ten-fold decrease in spinal glycine binding; strychnine intoxication in humans is characterized by a hypersensitivity to light touch (13), and spinal cord ischemia known to destroy amino acids containing interneurons will yield a tactile allodynia (152,155,246). These observations thus provide the potential for an important clue to the component of the system reorganization that may lead to the altered encoding in which a low-intensity mechanical stimulus may lead to an allodynic state. It is interesting to note that while spinal GABA agonists have a positive effect, their action typically occurs at concentrations in which some degree of motor side effects are noted (see references in Table 3). Recent work has shown the antiallodynic efficacy of gabapentin (174), which, though its structure, suggests a GABA-like action, does not bind at common sites with which GABA may interact (386). The drug has been shown, however, to augment GABA current (196,386). This may occur through an increase in GABA release (140). Importantly, current data suggests a marked dissociation between the time of peak effect and the earlier peak in the extracellular drug concentrations. Accordingly, the likelihood of some intracellular action on GABA mobilization has been postulated (409).

Opiate Agonists The action of opiates in postnerve injury pain states in models of allodynia are variable. As noted in Table 3, for example, the hyperpathia in the Bennett model and the Streptozocin model is attenuated by opiates. In contrast, the tactile allodynia in the Chung model is relatively refractory to spinal morphine. This likely reflects the differences in the respective organization of the two models. Though unclear at present, the marginal effect of spinal opiates in the tactile allodynia neuropathic pain model as compared to the acute thermal response models (such as the hot plate or tail flick models) is consistent with the probable role of C fibers in the acute pain models and A fibers in the neuropathic models (Fig. 6). Current thinking emphasizes the probable presynaptic action of opiates in such somatic pain processing (430). Importantly, different anatomical systems may have distinguishable actions. Thus, while opiates given spinally do not influence the Chung model, supraspinal injection or systemic delivery can in fact attenuate the allodynia (209).

α_2 Agonists α_2 Agonists (such as clonidine) have been reported to be effective after spinal delivery in animals and humans. Thus, α_2 receptors may act presynaptically to reduce sympathetic terminal release. Spinally, α_2 agonists are known to depress preganglionic sympathetic outflow. In either case, to the degree that pain states were driven by sympathetic input, these states would be diminished accordingly. Interestingly, this consideration provides some explanation as to why opiates do not exert a potent effect upon the allodynia observed after nerve injury. As summarized above and in Fig. 8, neither μ nor α_2 agonists alter large afferent input. Yet, α_2 agonists may reduce allodynia. This differential action may result from the fact that opiates, unlike the α_2 agents, do not alter sympathetic outflow (as indicated by the lack of effect of spinal opiates on resting blood pressure). As noted, the Chung model possesses a significant sympathetic dependency (see above).

Blockers of Voltage-Sensitive Ion Channels At present, systematic studies have indicated that a variety of agents known to exert a blockade of several voltage-sensitive ion channels, notably those for sodium and several for calcium, can prevent the hyperpathy that occurs secondary to nerve injury. Important considerations relate to the question of whether the effects are mediated by a central or a peripheral site. Moreover, because many of these channels must be considered to be ubiquitous, the issue of selectivity is paramount.

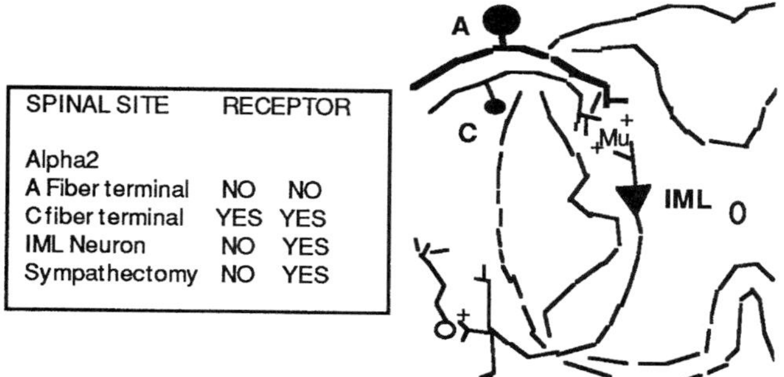

Figure 8. Spinal μ and α-2 receptors: somatic versus preganglionic sympathetic effects. Both opiates and α_2 agonists can reduce C-fiber evoked excitation, but neither block A-fiber excitation. The antiallodynic action of spinal α_2 agonists thus appears to depend upon the fact that spinal a_2 but not opiates inhibit preganglionic sympathetic outflow (443).

Sodium Channel The behavioral data have emphasized that intravenous lidocaine at steady state plasma concentrations that that do not yield motor dysfunction can reverse the allodynia and hyperpathia otherwise observed in several models of allodynia and hyperalgesia (Table 3). Although a number of "use-dependent" local anesthetics been employed, including mexilethine and tocainamide, in different preclinical models with comparable results (46), there is at present an inadequate structure activity relationship to precisely define the nature of the channel that is being influenced. Reports of antiallodynic effects that appear to result form the actions of peripheral lidocaine metabolites have been reported and the mechanisms of such effects are not clear. It is widely appreciated that many of the agents classified as sodium channel blockers can have a variety of potent effects, including blocking actions upon other channels (21,30). An important question is at which sites do these agents exert their antiallodynic actions? As reviewed in Chapter 36, there are considerable data to indicate that systemic lidocaine can reduce spontaneous activity at several links in the afferent system. Thus, after nerve injury in the rat, the ordering of sensitivity to blockade of afferent activity by iv lidocaine is: DRG (1–3 μg/ml) > central glutamate-evoked activity estimated to be (1–3 μg/ml) > neuroma (3–5 μg/ml) > injured terminal (5–10 μg/ml) >>> axon conduction. At concentrations of 1–2 μg/ml in the rat, the allodynia in the Chung Model is completely blocked (47). Importantly, this effect occurs at concentrations which do not affect general sensory or motor functions.

Calcium Channels Current work has shown that the spinal delivery of N channel blockers, to a lesser degree P channel blockers, and least of all L channel blockers are able to reverse the hyperpathic state observed after nerve injury (Table 4). Systemic delivery of these agents to the lesions site is typically without effect (49). The mechanisms of such a spinal action remain undefined, but the potential role of N-type calcium channels in the release of afferent transmitters, notably glutamate, is a tenable hypothesis (144). N-channel sites are found on dorsal root ganglion cells and are elevated in the spinal dorsal horn (135).

PRECLINICAL MODELS AS PREDICTORS OF THE HUMAN PAIN RESPONSE

There are two issues that will be considered in this section: (a) What can be said about the information provided by the preclinical models that are in general use? (b) What is the relationship between those preclinical models and the human pain state? Both questions relate to the issue of validation. As old models are being interpreted in terms of new insights into mechanisms, or when new preclinical models are defined, the characterization of the model in terms of the effects of various drugs or manipulations constitutes efforts to validate the predictive ability of the models for other preclinical pain models and for clinical pain states.

Mechanistic Validation of Preclinical Models

Preclinical models are used to define the activity (efficacy) of an agent prior to initiating trial studies in humans. The use of a nonhuman model to define the potential activity of an agent in humans implicitly assumes some relationship between the effect of the drug in the test model and its action in the target (human) model. This relationship requires "validation" of the model. Validation of drug action in the test model with respect to human analgesia may be based on three approaches.

Empirical Correlation

Empirical correlation is the demonstration of a statistical covariance between the model and the predicted outcome. The model requires no underlying assumptions but requires significant experimental data to permit definition of the degree of predicative ability. Moreover, the model cannot be safely used to predict elements that have not been studied. For example, it is known that after injury, the animal may display an immobility in an "open field" situation (119). The mechanism of this suppression is not known. It may be speculated, however, that a drug treatment that increases spontaneous behavior after injury might thus reflect a reduced pain state and an analgesic action of the drug. However, it is intuitively clear that various manipulations may increase spontaneous behavior without altering the pain state.

Face Validity

Face validity is a preclinical model that involves some sort of tissue injury (e.g., local formalin) or a local joint inflammation and a measure that involves "favoring" the injured part might be considered to provide a "pain state" that is equivalent to that observed in humans after surgery or in arthritis, respectively. In either case, there is an injury and an appropriate behavioral response. These apparent similarities suggest face validity. On the other hand, the identity of the afferent classes underlying the behavior generated by the experimental stimuli are not known and may differ in composition from those generated in the post-surgical state. Alternatively, the formalin test reflects a system that is activated for up to an hour, whereas the human postoperative state reflects events that may evolve over hours or days.

Rational Validity

With respect to rational validity, if mechanisms underlying a stimulus-response relationship are known, then models employing the same mechanism might provide information on the pharmacology and drug action relevant to pain transmission. Two examples will be noted. First, hippocampal long-term potentiation is mediated by NMDA receptor activation (81); spinal wind-up is mediated by an NMDA receptor (91). Thus, the two models may reflect common underlying mechanisms and what works in one will work in the other. Second, it is known that the contractions of the guinea pig ileum are blocked by an opiate receptor of the μ class. The potency of a variety of μ opiates corresponds closely with the clinical potency of μ opiates as analgesics (430) (see Chapter 58). Thus, the guinea pig ileum and several other smooth muscle models are good predictors of mu opiate efficacy. Those models do not, however, predict the side effect profile that might be defined in the in vivo model (e.g., pruritis, respiratory depression, urinary retention).

Convergent Validity

With respect to convergent validity, from a practical standpoint, as the effects of different manipulations are examined in several models, it is anticipated that the results will reveal parallels in drug activity in the independent models and that these results will covary with the effects of the drugs in the target system (the human pain state), e.g., convergent validation.

Parallels Between Mechanistic Substrates of Preclinical Models and Clinical States

The mechanisms of human clinical pain have not been comparably defined as in the preclinical pain states. Accordingly, mechanistic parallels have been largely limited to face validity. Such validations will thus be subject to discrepancies that cannot be assessed until studies permitting convergent validation are accomplished (see below). However, Table 5 outlines components of several human pain states based on the presumed substrates that are believed to underlie the respective syndrome. It is clear that most clinical pain states are not unidimensional. Thus, postoperative pain clearly has an acute component that reflects the acute activation of small afferents due to movement and the local activation release of agents that can stimulate C fibers. In addition, there is the component that reflects upon the augmented processing that results from the persistent afferent barrage. Syndromes such as cancer present yet additional dimensions that include not only the acute input generated by tumor bulk and the facilitation resulting from the persistent input, but the likelihood of a developing postinjury pain state. Other syndromes, such as those associated with burn, may have a neuropathic component that develops after

Table 5. HYPOTHESIZED COMPONENTS OF HUMAN PAIN STATES

Pain state	Acute	Persistent (posttissue injury)	Neuropathic (postnerve injury)		See for references and discussion
			Dysesthesia	Hyperpathia	
Experimental					Chapter 41
	Thermal threshold		X		
	Intradermal Capsaicin	X	X		
	Repetitive electrical stimulation of digit		X	X	
Postoperative	X	X			Chapter 43
Burn	X	X	?	?	Chapter 44
Arthritis	X	X			Chapter 49
Postherpetic neuralgia	X	X	X	X	Chapter 55
Fibromyalgia	X?	X?			Chapter 57
Cancer					Chapter 48
	Early stage	X	X		
	Late stage	X	X		
	Surgical debulking				Chapter 52
Radiation/chemotherapy					
Nerve section			X	X	Chapters 41, 51, and 56
Causalgia/RSD			X	X	Chapters 41, 51, and 56

the burn state has progressed. Syndromes such as fibromyalgia remain to be defined in terms of their afferent pathways or the physiology and pharmacology of their initiating stimulus.

Assessment of the Activity of Drug Classes in Human Pain States

The preceding sections have emphasized the relationship between the mechanism believed to underlie the behavioral substrate for the preclinical models and the effects of pharmacological interventions targeted at the linkages which are believed to account for the stimulus-response relationships defined by the respective pain models. To further define the underlying relationship to the human pain models, we could presume that some evidence of covariance of drug efficacy in various clinical pain states should correspondingly assist in determining the role played by one or more of the mechanisms believed on the basis of the preclinical studies to be sensitive to the respective drug action. An overview of the effects of the major drug classes that have been examined in a number of humans pain states is presented in Table 6. Additional agents are considered below.

Several specific comments may be considered regarding the association of preclinical drug efficacy with the several clinical state. For further discussion, see the several chapters on specific pain states.

Experimental Pain With respect to experimental pain, the psychophysics of the acute nociceptive thresholds are closely paralleled with the electrophysiologically defined response of small (Aδ/C) sensory axons (see Chapters 31 and 41). The enlarged and persistent receptive fields of tactile allodynia observed after capsaicin is parallel to the animal studies emphasizing the role of repetitive afferent input in evoking conditioning of the spinal cord, leading to enhanced excitability of neurons receiving otherwise marginally effective input from adjacent spinal dermatomes. The ability of repetitive electrical stimulation of C fibers to induce more pain that is progressively augmented is considered as an additional example of a developing centrally mediated facilitated state. As reviewed above, such well-defined sensory phenomena in humans emphasize that in the face of such repetitive small afferent input, humans will indeed display the anomalous, nonlinear encoding of the afferent message as predicted by the preclinical models (see above).

The pharmacology of the acute experimental sensory components have shown that the acute pain threshold in an experimental pain model which has been induced by heat, mechanical and electrical stimuli are increased by epidural opiates (morphine, alfentanil, sufentanil) in a naloxone-reversible fashion (31,60) (see Chapter 2).

The likelihood that the mechanisms underlying elements of the experimental human pain models possess facilitated components similar to those characterized in the preclinical models is supported by parallels in their pharmacology. Thus, in the human studies, systemic dextromethorphan, an NMDA antagonist, is able to selectively attenuate the facilitated component of the electrical stimulation model (312) (see Chapter 2). Similarly, intravenous lidocaine has shown that capsaicin-evoked hyperalgesia is significantly reduced in the human at plasma concentrations that do not block sensory transmission (M. Wallace, personal communication, 1996). These results are in accord with the pharmacology described for the preclinical models such as in the formalin test (Table 4). After experimental burn, the decrease in heat pain detection and tolerance thresholds within the area of injury (area of primary hyperalgesia), as well as the allodynia for brush and pinprick surrounding the injury (area of secondary hyperalgesia), was reversed by epidural morphine in a naloxone reversible fashion (32).

Postoperative/Injury Pain State The postoperative pain state is clearly dependent upon the mechanical injury to tissues associated with the surgical intervention. It is believed that postoperative pain which persists for intervals up to several days (see Chapter 15) implies the presence of, first, an ongoing afferent drive and, secondly, a state of central facilitation.

The role of acute nociceptive drive in the human postinjury pain state is emphasized by the fact that (a) local anesthetic blockade after surgery will completely obviate the postinjury pain state, and (b) the human postinjury pain state has been demonstrated to be sensitive to spinal opiates and α_2 agonists. These families of agents have been shown preclinically to attenuate acute small afferent evoked transmitter release, spinal dorsal horn excitation, and to block preclinical models of acute nociceptive processing (see Chapters 58 and 59).

The role of facilitated processing in the human postinjury pain state is based on (a) postinjection hyperalgesia and the expanded receptive field associated with intradermal capsaicin; (b) the ability to block the enhanced pain state with afferent blockade; and (c) the clinical reports indicating that regional blockade with local anesthetics may reduce the postsurgical opiate requirement, e.g., preemptive analgesia (see Chapter 15). Pharmacologically, the human postinjury pain state has

Table 6. SUMMARY OF RESPONSE OF HUMAN PAIN STATES TO DRUG THERAPY

Pain state	Opiate agonist	α_2 agonist	COX-I inhibition	NMDA-antagonism	IV-local anesthesia	TCA
Experimental						
Thermal threshold	Y (S)				N (S)	
Intradermal capsaicin					Y (S)	
Repetitive electrical stimulation of digit	Y (S)			Y (S)	Y (S)	
Postoperative	Y (I,E,S)	Y (E)	Y (S)	Y (E, S)	Y (S)	Y (S)
Burn	Y (E,S)		Y (S)			
Arthritis	Y (S)		Y (S)			
Postherpetic neuralgia	N (S)		N (S)		Y (S)	Y (S)
Fibromyalgia	Y (S)					
Cancer						
Early stage	Y (S)	Y (E)	Y (S)			Y (S)
Late stage	Y (I,E,S)	Y (E)	Y (S)		Y (S)	Y (S)
Surgical debulking	Y					
Radiation/chemotherapy	Y-N (S)					
Nerve section	N (S)					
Causalgia/RSD	Y-N (E,S)	Y (E)	N (S)	Y (E)	Y (S)	Y (S)
See the following Chapters	41,48,56,58	56,59	44,48,49,61	41,56,60	41,43,51,52,55,63	55,56,64

been shown to be markedly attenuated by the use of systemic cyclooxygenase inhibitors such as ketorolac or acetaminophen, which have only modest antiinflammatory effects, suggesting a probable central action (see Chapter 61), and by the use of epidural ketamine, an agent with putative NMDA antagonists properties (see Chapter 60). Preclinical studies have shown that spinal NMDA receptor occupancy may lead to a state of facilitated processing mediated in part by the spinal release of cyclooxygenase products (see Chapter 36). The above considerations thus render it likely that the postinjury pain state in humans possesses a facilitated component that resembles that observed in the postinjury preclinical models.

Cancer As reviewed in Chapter 48, the pain state that is present secondary to cancer is a complex syndrome. It clearly depends on the nature of the cancer (e.g., local bulk, versus highly invasive), its intrinsic biology (e.g., secretory) and its target organs. Nevertheless, in a generic fashion it is possible to consider the multiple elements that comprise the components that yield a cancer-affiliated pain state.

Acute pain components may arise from the tumor bulk leading to distention of soft tissue or inexpansible substrates, such as fascia or bone. The decalcification of the bone by invasive tumors is exceedingly painful. The lytic processes that are associated with such invasiveness may lead to the formation of active products. Thus, aside from mechanical stimuli, the cancer itself or though its interaction with host tissue may result in the release of active factors (such as cytokines) that can acutely stimulate and sensitize small afferents. These factors likely lead to acute pain components. The role of the ongoing stimulus presented by the cancer often can be deduced by the almost immediate loss of pain that accrues secondary to ameliorative therapies that reduce tumor mass. Thus, following treatments which shrinks the tumor (surgical debulking, steroids, hormones, or radiation), analgesic requirement may be reduced (see Chapter 48). The efficacy of spinal μ (115,310) and δ (266,293) opiates as well as α_2 (108) agonists in the cancer pain state provides support for the role played by the acute activation of small afferents.

In addition to the acute activation of small afferents, the cancer pain state is almost certainly associated with a persistent afferent traffic that can result in a state of facilitated processing, as in the postinjury pain state outlined in the preceding section. The efficacy of cyclooxygenase inhibitors in these states (as promulgated in the World Health Organization guidelines) provides additional support for the contributions of a facilitated pain states. Though a component of this action may be mediated by the peripheral antiinflammatory actions of agents such as aspirin and ibuprofen, limited observations by Devoghel (85) demonstrated a spinal action of lysine acetylsalicylate, which suggests that in the cancer pain patient as in the preclinical model, persistent afferent input may lead to a facilitated state of central.

The complexity of the cancer pain state and the multiple components will be present. As reviewed previously, different mechanisms will display differential sensitivity to different drug approaches. Thus, in cancer patients with spinal metastases and direct invasion of the sacral plexus, spinal bone pain was controlled adequately with morphine, whereas the sciatica requires larger dosages and the pain may be difficult to control (464). Similarly, in the pain states defined as "nociceptive" versus "neuropathic," relief achieved with fixed doses of morphine or heroin is greatest in the groups with "nociceptive" pain and least for those with "neuropathic" components (52). Similar results are obtained with spinally administered morphine (338). It is intriguing to speculate that in progressive syndromes such as cancer, as the pain component associated with an Aβ-evoked element increases, the reported pain syndrome will show an increasing refractoriness to opiate actions.

The continuous presence of an overlying tumor may lead to chronic nerve compression. The invasion by the tumor of nerves may yield changes in nerve function, while radiation, chemotherapy and nerve section in the course of surgical debulking may yield direct effects upon nerve integrity and function. Growing evidence suggests that postmastectomy pain syndrome may result from a section of branches of the intercostal nerves, the extensive radiation of the brachial plexus, and chemotherapy (see Chapter 20).

Pharmacologically, the likelihood that a post nerve injury component is relevant is suggested by the observation that components of cancer pain may be diminished by systemic NMDA receptor antagonism (258). Other agents shown to be effective in animal models of neuropathic and persistent pain states are intrathecal N-type calcium channels (Table 4) and somatostatin (51,58; but also see ref. 125). Limited trials thus far have shown efficacy for both SNX-111 (33) and somatostatin (263,302) after spinal delivery in humans.

As indicated in Tables 4 and 5, intravenous local anesthetics have been shown to be effective in neuropathic states in humans and animal models. Components of cancer pain have been shown to be in part relieved by the use of intravenous agents believed to interfere with sodium channel function (34,270).

Neuropathic Pain The current data regarding the pharmacology of human neuropathic pain is limited for several reasons. First, in most cases, the clinical syndrome of the presenting patient is often poorly defined and, second, it appears certain that as our understanding of the pharmacology of the human post nerve injury pain syndrome improves, we will be more aware of the multiple states which constitute the neuropathic pain syndromes. Because there is frequently a lack of distinction in many neuropathic cases, one is often forced to rely on a global indicator (i.e., "more or less pain") and not whether one or more components of the pain state are differentially altered by the particular treatment. Nevertheless, there are a number of examples which may be considered.

An important element of the neuropathic state is the allodynia which may be observed in such patients. Animal studies have emphasized that tactile allodynia is resistant to spinal opiates. This distinction is also believed to be the case in humans (14). It should be stressed that while opiates may not uniformly affect all aspects of a neuropathic pain syndrome, the complexity of such syndromes precludes a systematic statement as to their practical utility in any given patient. As emphasized in those patient suffering from cancer, components of their pain state may be readily managed by opiates, while other components may be more resistant. With appropriate systematic testing, it will probably develop that such is the case for different neuropathic pain syndromes. The issue of what fraction of patients display such components and to what extent do they contribute to the overall pain rating remains to be systematically defined. Thus, some syndromes such as postheretic neuralgia are indeed sensitive to opiate action (106,327), and there have been case studies in which spinal morphine was reported to be effective (175).

The preclinical models have emphasized the importance of several systems in altering in a relatively selective fashion the facilitated components of processing generated by persistent afferent input as well as the processing observed after nerve injury. In three such families of agents, effects which have been observed in humans are briefly considered.

1. *NMDA Antagonist:* The common role played by the NMDA receptor antagonism in preclinical models is consistent with the observation that systemic ketamine reduces the allodynia, hyperalgesia and after-sensation present in patients with peripheral nerve injury, and the magnitude of the relief is, in general, proportional to dose (17,194,248,305). Systemic ketamine has been effective in treating postherpetic neuralgia (206). The NMDA antagonist CPP was observed to significantly reduce the dynamic component of a post nerve injury pain state after spinal delivery (200).

2. *Adenosine Agonists:* In neuropathic pain models, these have been shown to be effective (Table 4). Systemic delivery of adenosine has been shown to reduce spontaneous pain and increase touch-evoked pain (22). Intrathecal delivery of a selective Adenosine A1 agonist was shown to abolish the allodynia otherwise observed in a neuropathic patient (186).

3. *Systemic Local Anesthetic:* The preclinical studies have shown that intravenous lidocaine at doses that do not block conduction will in fact alter the allodynic and hyperalgesic components. Intravenous lidocaine in humans has been shown to reduce spontaneous pain and mechanical hyperalgesia in nerve injury pain patients (245,270) and in patients with postherpetic neuralgia (270,327).

Human and Animal Correlations of "Analgesic" Drug Action

As indicated in this chapter in the sections on human clinical pain, it is certain that multiple mechanisms may be relevant. Accordingly, it is not adequate to ask whether an agent is an "analgesic" in the absence of qualifying statements about the pain states under investigation.

Inspection of Tables 4 and 6 and the comments outlined in the preceding section emphasizes that activity in the rat on acute nociceptive end points (such as the hot plate and tail flick) will predict the ability of classes of agents to display efficacy in a variety of postinjury pain states whether given by systemic or spinal delivery. Table 7 reflects a selected extraction of several principal classes of agents which have shown efficacy following systemic or spinal delivery in several human pain states and this is linked to the types of animal models in which the respective agent was observed to be active. Two important issues should be noted. First, agents which were classically active in the acute pain models (e.g., hot plate and tail flick) uniformly can have an impact on the human states that appear to have an injury component (e.g., postoperative pain, cancer). In contrast, activity in those models was not a reliable predictor of the efficacy of the agents in the neuropathic states. This appears best exemplified by the contrast between opiates and α_2 agonists. Secondly, agents that were active in either the postinjury pain models (e.g., formalin) or the neuropathic pain models (Bennett or Chung) were frequently noted to be effective in the postoperative state and in other tissue injury states. This incidence of activity is a likely indicator of the role routinely played by facilitated processing after injury. While there are relatively few examples, the incidence of positive effects from agents which might otherwise be unanticipated to be effective (based on their results in acute pain model) is notable. Importantly, one of the close alliances that has thus far arisen has been the parallel between the spinal action of agents in animal models and that observed in clinical pain states. Previous reviews have emphasized the correlation between potency in rodent and primate models and activity observed in humans (see Chapter 58). In addition, as indicated in Table 7, the current screening technologies have elucidated the activity of agents which were developed on the basis of preclinical investigations. This advance has occurred in part because of the development of robust methods of defining spinal drug safety. The importance of such intermediary investigations in the human implementation of novel drug classes should not be under estimated.

This predictive ability noted in the preceding paragraph leaves us with two insights. First, the parallels provide an important validation of the animal models that have been proposed to reflect the role played by certain spinal and peripheral transmitter/receptors systems. Second, the results reviewed in this chapter provide some sense of the maturity of the insights that have been garnered regarding the substrates that encode the nociceptive message. It is clear that there is much to learn, but the demonstration of the relevance of these pharmacological systems in both humans and animals suggests that the animal models, at least at the current level of analysis, provide useful information that can be employed to predict human drug activity. The evolving insights into the mechanisms of pain processing can be expected to yield even greater rewards.

BRIEF CONSIDERATIONS OF SEVERAL FACTORS RELEVANT TO THE PRECLINICAL ASSESSMENT OF CLINICALLY IMPORTANT ANALGESIA

Importance of In Vivo Models

Current understanding has permitted us to define the nature of neuronal systems that are activated by high-threshold stimuli which can evoke escape behavior in animals and verbal

Table 7. CORRELATION BETWEEN DRUG EFFICACY IN ANIMAL MODELS AND HUMAN STATES

Drug classes	Animal models[a]	Human pain states	Human drugs	References (see text and the following chapters)
μ opiates-spinal	A/P	Postop, cancer	β-endorphin, morphine, fentanyl, etc.	Chapter 58
δ opiates-spinal		Cancer	DADL	Chapter 58
α_2-spinal	A/P/N	Postop, cancer, neuropathic	Clonidine	Chapter 59
ACHase inhibit-spinal	A/P	Postop, cancer	Neostigmine	(168)
COX inhibition	P	Postop, cancer	Ketorolac, ibuprofen, etc.	Chapter 61
Adenosine agonist-spinal	P/N	Neuropathic	R-PIA	(186)
GABA (unknown)	P/N	Neuropathic	GABApentin	(256)
IV local anesthetic	P/N	Cancer, neuropathic	Lidocaine	Chapter 63
Spinal N-type channel blocker-spinal	P/N	Cancer	SNX-111	
NMDA antagonist-spinal	P/N	Postop, neuropathic	Ketamine, CPP	Chapter 60
Tricyclic antidepressants	P/N	Neuropathic	Amitryptiline	Chapter 64

[a]A, acute pain models (hot plate/tail flick); P, persistent pain states (formalin, inflamed knee joint /paw); N, neurpathic pain models (Bennett/Chung models). See text for further details regarding drug action and references.

responses of discomfort in humans. Such knowledge can be used to assess the effects of drugs on that neuronal activity. Similarly, binding studies can define the nature of the membrane interaction of the agent with the receptor site. However, none of these electrophysiological or biochemical technologies can permit one to assess whether the effects of a drug are relevant to pain processing. Such interpretation presumes that we know the functional significance of the activity evoked in that cell by noxious stimulation. To define the role of a given receptor in modulating the "pain state," we must ultimately assess the role of manipulation of the respective systems in the bioassay which defines a pain state, i.e., the behavior of the unanesthetized and intact animal. Thus, combining the various pain states induced by specific and well-defined stimuli, with efforts to assess the pharmacology of the receptors that exist in the terminal regions of the links in the tracts through which information generated by such a high-intensity stimuli project, the behavioral relevance of those systems to pain processing can be defined.

Pain states may be mediated by a number of discrete mechanisms. As reviewed above, these different mechanisms may have different pharmacologies, and different mechanisms may be relevant to different clinical pain states. Accordingly, the ability to target certain human pain states by understanding their mechanisms emphasizes that in screening drug action we must take into account the pain state towards which the agent as a class is being targeted.

Specificity of the Measure: Analgesia Versus Behavioral Dysfunction

High-threshold, potentially tissue-damaging stimuli will evoke a spinally organized reflex or a supraspinally organized escape behavior and signs of discomfort such a vocalization. The spinal reflex activates local spinal circuits leading to a local motor withdrawal. In the intact and unanesthetized animal, such stimuli give rise to an organized response is typically taken to prove that the stimulus has evoked activity in specific ascending spinal and brainstem pathways and that the behavior reflects upon the aversiveness of the information provided by that message transmitted. Drugs or manipulations which prevent the manifestation of that behavior may be considered as analgesics, if they block that behavior, given several considerations.

1. *Block of Motor Function:* Interpretation of a reduction in the behavioral response otherwise induced by a strong stimulus after a drug as an analgesic event requires that the manipulation did not simply alter the ability of the animal to make the response. Appearance of any sign of motor dysfunction must be considered as potentially invalidating the results.
2. *Behavioral Disorganization:* An important limiting consideration of the virtues of supraspinally organized mechanisms in defining the animal parallel of an analgesic is that the drug does not cause a general disruption of organization of behavior (as with a stimulant or a general depressant). For an agent to be classified as an analgesic, other aspects of the animals behavior must be shown to be relatively unimpaired. Thus, agents such as major tranquilizers will block the hot plate licking response, but the animal manifests severe agitation. This dissociation would argue against these agents as analgesics based only on an increase in the response latency and this is consistent with their lack of action in the human pain state.

Factors Influencing Analgesic Activity of a Drug

Mechanism

As reviewed in the discussion of mechanisms, in a given family of tests (such as those for thermal escape: hot plate, tail flick) there is a high similarity in the rank ordering of activity. This concurrence is consistent with the consistency of the mechanisms associated with the several models. On the other hand, across classes of mechanism, different rank ordering of potency can be noted (several examples can be cited): thus on thermal nociceptive measures opiates and α_2 agonists > NMDA antagonist; while in certain neuropathic models such as the Chung model, the ordering of activity is NMDA antagonists/α_2 agonists > opiates. These difference provide presumptive evidence that different mechanisms are in play in the different test types.

Pharmacokinetic Issues

The potency of an agent to induce an effect may generally result in an inability of the drug to gain access to the site of action. Such contributing variables may include rapid metabolism, high protein binding and/or lack of the appropriate diffusion properties, such as high-molecular-weight and low-lipid partition coefficients. Comparisons of potency should ideally be predicated on the effect of the drug at equilibrium. As the kinetics of these agents in vivo is rarely known, it is considered reasonable to default to the measurement made at the time of peak effect after a bolus injection. It is important to consider that in the case of drug interaction studies, as between agonists and antagonists for reversal, or between two proanalgesic agents for assessing the nature of the drug interaction (e.g., additivity versus synergy), the measurements should be at times corresponding to the peak effect of either agent (438).

Pharmacodynamic Issues

The activity of agents which induce their effect by a competitive interaction with a specific membrane site is proportional to the fraction of the receptors occupied (fractional receptor occupancy; FRO). The FRO obeys the law of mass action and, accordingly, is proportional to concentration of drug in the local biophase and the affinity of the drug for the site. We know, however, that the relationship between receptor occupancy and drug effect may vary widely for agents which interact with similar affinities at the same receptor. Thus, as shown in Fig. 9, some agents such as naloxone have no effect, while others, such as buprenorphine, fail to produce a maximum analgesia even at their highest doses, and others produce a maximum effect, even though they may have similar higher binding site affinities (161,427). Because drugs with similar affinities will bind a comparable fraction of the receptors, this difference in maximum achievable effect, even with prolonged delivery, cannot be due to different levels of receptor occupancy. This is

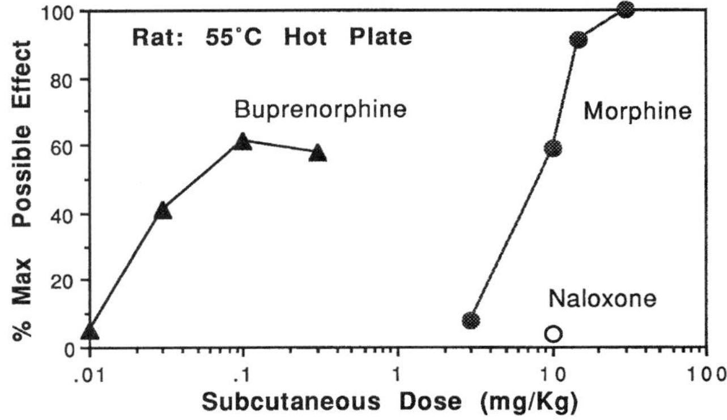

Figure 9. Dose response curves for the effects of subcutaneous naloxone, buprenorphine and morphine in which the effect (expressed as the percentage of the maximum possible effect) is plotted versus drug dose. Note that with this model, buprenorphine is more potent than morphine, but is unable to produce a maximum elevation (100%) of the hot plate response latency.

usually expressed in the following fashion. For agents (A), which bind reversibly with a given site (R), the fraction of receptor occupied (FRO) = $[AR/Rt] = [A]/(k_d + [A])$, where k_d is the dissociation constant of the drug-receptor (AR) complex, and Rt indicates the total number of binding sites. Thus, at a given concentration, two drugs with similar k_d's will, by definition, occupy similar numbers of receptors (329).

This difference in the occupancy-effect relationship results from the property possessed by each agonist called its "efficacy" (329). An agonist (A) interacting with a specific receptor (R) must form complexes (AR) with some fraction of the total receptor population (Rt) to produce a given effect. By definition, an agonist which must occupy a large fraction of the available receptor population to produce a given effect is said to have low efficacy and a small receptor reserve. Thus, if there are fewer functional receptors (i.e., Rt is reduced). This may occur after treatment with an irreversible antagonist (6,260), or, if there is an increase in the number of receptors that must be occupied (i.e., AR is increased), the value of the ratio AR/Rt will approach 1. Should the receptor occupancy (AR) required by an agonist to produce a given effect exceed the available Rt ($AR/Rt > 1$, a logical impossibility), that agonist will become, by definition, a partial agonist (such as buprenorphine). Thus, the dose response curve would become less steep and the curve would plateau at a submaximal level. In contrast, under the same experimental conditions, a second agonist with a higher efficacy, which requires occupancy of only a small fraction of the total receptor population to produce a given effect (i.e., has a larger receptor reserve), will show no change in the maximum achievable drug effect (i.e., AR/Rt remains <1) (189). This characteristic has several important repercussions.

Influence of Drug Efficacy Drug efficacy theoretically impacts on the dose-effect relationship in any case where the ratio (AR/Rt) is altered. Three situations where this happens are stimulus increases, where AR must rise to meet a criterion effect, and those instances where different behaviorally relevant have fractional occupancy requirements and level of tolerance, where Rt is thought to be effectively reduced.

1. The more intense the peripheral, thermal, or mechanical somatic stimulus (120,229,387), or visceral (277,278), the greater the evoked activity in spinal nociceptive neurons, and the greater the dose of opioid required to block the neuronal and behavioral effects of the stimulus (80,141,287,291). This increase in dose requirement associated with more intense stimuli shows the magnitude of the effect of an agonist upon physiological function typically correlates positively with the fraction of the receptors with which the agonist interacts and that the fraction of receptors occupied varies directly with local drug concentrations. If increasing stimulus intensity is modeled simply as an increased release of excitatory neurotransmitters (such as from the primary afferent) and an enhanced depolarization of the projection neurons, and given that there is no change in the number of receptors, the fractional occupancy requirement necessary to produce a given degree of inhibition will rise. If two agents differ in their efficacy, the drug with a higher occupancy requirement (lower efficacy) would display the greater rightward shift/reduction in maximum achievable effect in the dose response curve for any increase in stimulus intensity. These effects have been demonstrated with spinal μ and α_2 agonists (94,333,334). This is further elaborated in Fig. 10.

2. As a corollary of this discussion, suppose that there are two end points evoked by a given stimulus (i.e., a somatomotor and a blood pressure response, both concurrently evoked by a noxious thermal stimulus). The end point requiring the larger receptor occupancy by an agonist to produce a given effect will show the greater rightward shift or a reduction in maximum for the dose response curve (333,334). This paradigm may shed light on the idea that different mu opioids, such as sufentanil and morphine, may be similarly able to manage moderate pain states, but differ in their ability to achieve a maximal analgesic state in the face of an intense afferent drive (e.g., intraoperative stimuli versus postoperative pain management) (94).

3. With regard to tolerance, following exposure to equiactive spinal concentrations of two agonists which differ in efficacy as defined by dose response curve shifts in the presence of irreversible antagonists—opioid: sufentanil > morphine (260); α_2: dexmedetomidine > clonidine (393)—the degree of rightward shift in the intrathecal dose response curves is greatest for the agent with the lowest efficacy. Thus, in animals which are tolerant to either morphine or sufentanil, the degree of cross-tolerance is always greater in a morphine-infused animal and less in a sufentanil-infused animal, whether the animal is tested with morphine or sufentanil (375). These results are consistent with the thesis that for a given degree of down regulation of receptors, agonists which have high-occupancy requirements (few spare receptors) will show the greater shift in their respective dose response curves. Similar results have been shown for α_2-adrenoceptor agonists (393).

BRIEF CONSIDERATIONS OF PRECLINICAL SPINAL SAFETY STUDIES

The use of the spinal route of delivery has long been appreciated as a route of drug access available to the clinician for the routine application of agents under specific circumstances including situations where the drug has a central action and does not cross the blood-brain barrier (as with peptides such as growth factors). The drug passes the blood-brain barrier, but has major peripheral side effects such as myelosupression or renal toxicity at therapeutic doses anticancer/antibacterial/antiviral/antifungal agents; and/or the drug exerts its desired therapeutic end point by a spinal action, as with opiate analgesics. The spinal delivery of the agent may thus be used to diminish the "side effects" of the agent with both acute and chronic application.

An important advance in our understanding of nociceptive processing has been the growing insight that the encoding of high-intensity information and the misencoding of low-intensity stimuli is organized to a significant degree at the spinal level. Such insights have occurred because of the use of the direct spinal route of drug delivery in the unanesthetized and intact animal. Thus, the chronic implantation models using common mammals, including the rat and rabbit (456), dog (15), pig (139), sheep (299), and primate (445) have been contributive in defining the analgesic action of important classes of agents including the opiate and α_2 agonists, and the NMDA antagonists, among others. This approach has proven useful for the long-term management of pain with opiates (99,294,364) and α_2 agonists (108,110), and for the management of spasticity with baclofen (65,250).

An important question relates to the safety of novel agents delivered by the spinal route. High concentrations of agents applied into the CSF or into the epidural space exposes local neural tissue to atypical levels of agent. Although there are few specific examples, it is important to note that one of the few instances of defined toxicity associated with the therapeutic use of spinal agents has been reported with lidocaine. This agent has been used often in bolus spinal intrathecal delivery as 4% solution and has a long history of safety in humans. Under normal circumstances, after such a bolus injection, there is a significant dilution of the injectate. In contrast, the use of small bore intrathecal catheters that preclude barbotage and redistribution (324,326) apparently led to an increased incidence of radiculopathies (324), a finding in concert with preclinical studies of drugs injected near nerves (183,184,311).

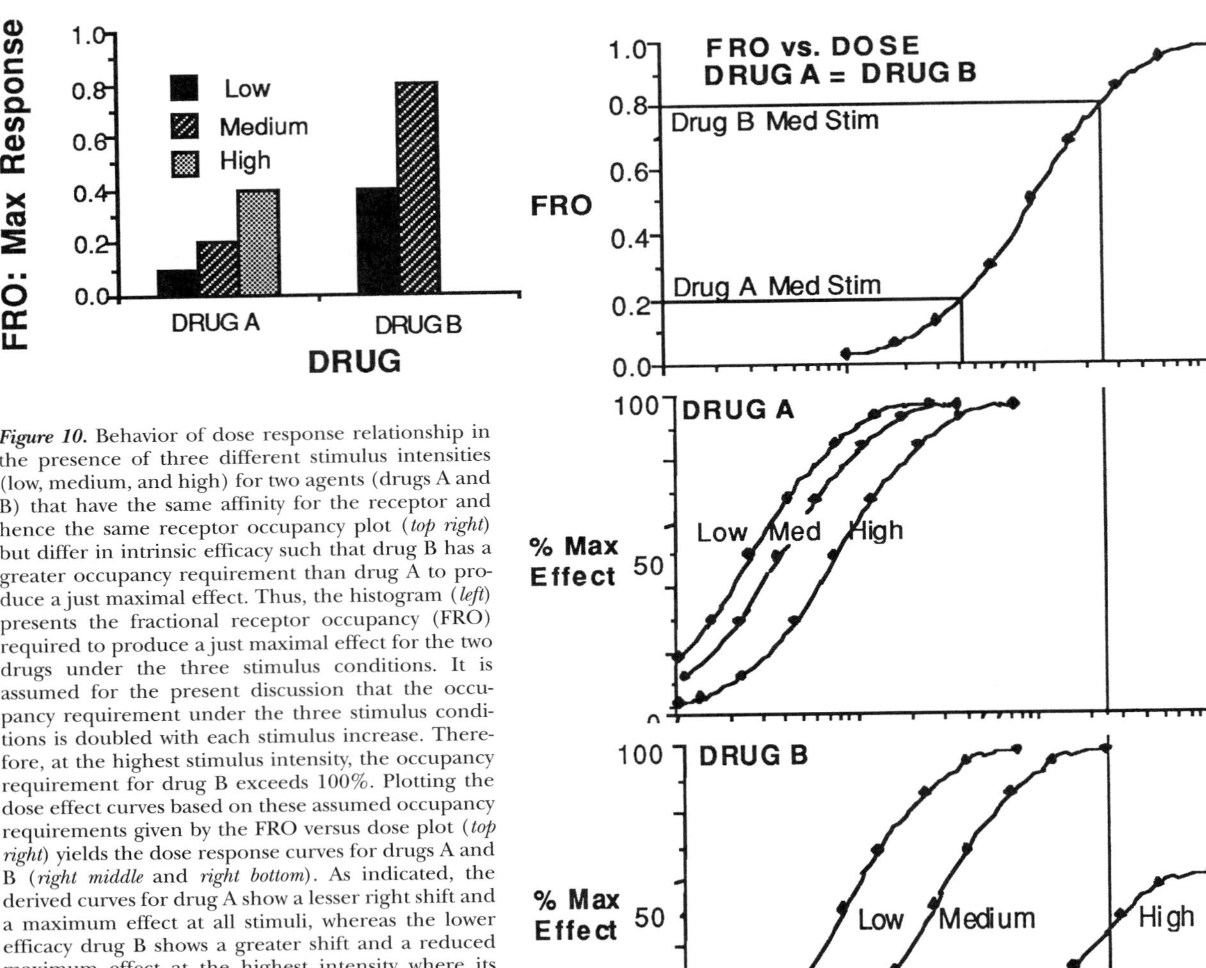

Figure 10. Behavior of dose response relationship in the presence of three different stimulus intensities (low, medium, and high) for two agents (drugs A and B) that have the same affinity for the receptor and hence the same receptor occupancy plot (*top right*) but differ in intrinsic efficacy such that drug B has a greater occupancy requirement than drug A to produce a just maximal effect. Thus, the histogram (*left*) presents the fractional receptor occupancy (FRO) required to produce a just maximal effect for the two drugs under the three stimulus conditions. It is assumed for the present discussion that the occupancy requirement under the three stimulus conditions is doubled with each stimulus increase. Therefore, at the highest stimulus intensity, the occupancy requirement for drug B exceeds 100%. Plotting the dose effect curves based on these assumed occupancy requirements given by the FRO versus dose plot (*top right*) yields the dose response curves for drugs A and B (*right middle* and *right bottom*). As indicated, the derived curves for drug A show a lesser right shift and a maximum effect at all stimuli, whereas the lower efficacy drug B shows a greater shift and a reduced maximum effect at the highest intensity where its FRO requirement exceeds 100%. An example of the analysis is indicated by the *solid lines* for drugs A and B at the medium stimulus. (Reprinted with permission from Dirig DM, Yaksh TL. Intrathecal baclofen and muscimol, but no midazolam, are antinociceptive using the rat-formalin model. *J Pharmacol Exp Ther* 1995;275:219–227.)

Thus, an important message is that the safety of a given agent is dependent upon the parameters of its delivery. No drug can be assumed to be inherently safe when employed at doses or concentrations for which there is no prior experience or safety data. There are two corollaries to this: (a) The issue of the spinal safety of a novel agent, even for one with which there is extensive clinical experience by a nonspinal route, must be considered in targeted preclinical spinal delivery models. (b) The legitimate preclinical safety challenge is to deliver the highest usable dose possible in a small volume (to achieve a high local concentration) or to provide continuous delivery with the highest concentration available (330,331).

Spinal toxicity may be manifested in two areas: (a) effects on physiological function that are secondary to the pharmacology of the agent (as in respiratory depression or urinary retention after spinal opiates and hypotension after α_2 agonists) and (b) effects on tissue morphology or biochemistry that will lead to cell death or permanent dysfunction. In the first case, some of the effects may result not from a spinal action, but from one of kinetic redistribution (as in respiratory depression). In the second case, the change in tissue viability may reflect a direct action of the agent, leading to cell death, due perhaps to excitotoxicity; or may be secondary to changes in tissue perfusion due to vasoconstriction, as with somatostatin (220) or certain nitric oxide synthase inhibitors (462a), or it may result in a direct inflammation of the meninges leading to arachnoiditis and or arteritis, as with certain contrast media (158).

Implementation of a Preclinical Safety Evaluation

It should be stressed that the issues of efficacy and safety are completely dissociable. Accordingly, because a model has the utility for defining the effects of the agent on physiological function, it is not necessarily an indicator of the utility of the model in spinal safety evaluation. In this regard, studies targeted at defining efficacy with acute or chronically delivered agents are not considered adequate for the formal assessment of safety.

The implementation of a preclinical safety evaluation may involve the use of several variants, depending upon the timing of drug delivery and the species. Nevertheless, experience to date suggests several minimum components (443a).

Pharmacology and Physiology of Spinal Drug Action

Studies are required to characterize the behavioral and physiological effects of the agent in routine pharmacological investigations in well-defined animal models. Such investigations might include characterization of the effects of the agent on cardiovascular somatomotor function and general behavior after spinal delivery. The model should provide insights into the mechanisms of the action of the drug and permit assessment of the efficacy of the agent relating to the target action of the agent (as an analgesic, for example).

Spinal Cord Blood Flow

As neural tissue is dependent upon adequate perfusion, it is critical that the local effects of a test agent be shown not to alter the spinal blood flow or its regulation. Thus, such work should consider whether the agent has an effect upon pressure autoregulation, as well as resting flow.

Toxicokinetics

Define the kinetics of the agent after acute or bolus spinal delivery. Ideally, such characterization should include concurrent movement into the intrathecal space (after epidural delivery) and from the spinal space after intrathecal or epidural delivery into the vascular space. If the animal models have been previously characterized with several agents that differ in molecular weight and the kinetics are similar in human studies, the probable relationship between the kinetics in the animal models of a novel agent and the anticipated kinetics in humans can be estimated. Such information can provide some degree of security that the nature of the drug exposure in the animal models will predict the exposure which will be experienced in the human delivery system. If we anticipate that local concentration is a key factor in toxicity, and if the degree of local dilution in humans of a drug with comparable properties exceeds that found in the animal model, then we can assume that the animal spinal canal will be exposed to a concentration profile which is at least equal to, if not exceeding, that observed in humans. Not incidentally, such data will provide justification for the drug delivery paradigm that will be employed in the subsequent safety studies (e.g., continued in bolus; rate of infusion; frequency of bolus injection).

Dose Ranging

Dose ranging studies are required to define the tolerability of the anticipated drug exposure paradigm for the extended period of exposure required in the final phase. These represent "enabling studies" that permit final preparation of the safety study protocol. Several approaches may be employed, including incrementing doses delivered over intervals of several days to weeks, or separate single animal studies in which each animal is exposed to a single dose for the extended period. The incrementing dose model has the advantage of several animals being exposed to the incrementing range. On the other hand, if the early exposure results in tolerance to side effects (as with opiates or α_2 agonists), the dose that can be acutely tolerated by drug tolerant animals will be much higher than that tolerated by drug-naive animals. Initiating the subsequent safety study with the high dose in drug-naive dogs might then lead to an acute crisis.

Safety Study

Safety studies define the effects of chronic spinal drug exposure on tissue morphology and behavioral/physiological function. This component of the drug safety evaluation is the most critical. It is not to be confused with an efficacy study. The essential issue is whether, at defined doses or concentrations and time courses of exposure, an agent exerts any deleterious effects upon spinal cord morphology or function. These studies provide the core of data which enable the investigator to approach the human studies Institutional Review Board (IRB) and the Food and Drug Administration (FDA) to obtain approval to deliver the agent by the tested route in humans under protocol-defined conditions. For agents being developed for commercialization, the safety studies are performed according to regulations outlined in the United State Federal Register (Title 21 Code of Federal Regulations Part 58, Federal Register 22 December 1978 and subsequent amendments effective 12 May 1980, October 1987 and 13 September 1991) and the OECD Principles of Good Laboratory Practice Regulations (OECD, C(81) 30 Final, Annex 2, Effective 1981), as Good Laboratory Practices (GLP) is an essential component for the New Drug Application (NDA). It should be noted that in the course of events, the formal safety evaluation is typically initiated after considerable experience with drug delivery has been accomplished. At this stage, the discovery phase of the drug-systems interaction has been completed. When the safety studies begin, it is anticipated that nothing unexpected relating to the overall characteristics of drug exposure will be observed (see 106,443a).

The above sequence of investigation has in fact governed the formal implementation of several spinally delivered agents. Representative relevant studies reflecting each phase for several such agents are presented in Table 8.

Table 8. SUMMARY OF PRECLINICAL STUDIES UNDERTAKEN TO DEFINE SAFETY OF THREE REPRESENTATIVE DRUGS FOR HUMAN SPINAL DELIVERY

Study phase	Epidural sufentanil	Epidural clonidine	Intrathecal neostigmine
Preclinical pharmacology	Rat/cat (442)	Rat (391,393), sheep (107), pig (136)	Sheep (167), rat (272), sheep (27)
Spinal cord blood flow	?	Sheep (109), pig (136)	Sheep (167)
Preclinical safety	Rat/cat (442), dog (330)	Dog (444), rat (138)	Dog (436)
Kinetics	Dog (383)	Sheep (111), sheep (44), pig (137)	Dog (436)

Preclinical Models of Spinal Toxicity

Preclinical models of spinal toxicity have two elements: (a) the animal preparation, and (b) the dose selection and treatment paradigm. In the animal model, such safety studies targeting spinal intrathecal or epidural drug action typically employ animal models prepared with chronic intrathecal or epidural catheters to unencumbered access to the target space. Several such models will be noted below. With regard to the treatment paradigm, several issues must be considered.

Drug Exposure

First, tissue toxicity must be considered to be a separate issue from characterizing the acute physiological effects of the agent. The tissue safety studies require a degree of extended exposure in animals which are otherwise physiologically competent (e.g., minimally sedated or not significantly hypotensive). Drug dosing for evaluation may thus require lower doses to permit prolonged exposure. This might be referred to as the maximum usable dose (MUD).

Secondly, the drug delivery regimen must be considered as part of the model. In the absence of a specific mechanism, it is anticipated that tissue toxicity will be a function of local concentration and time of exposure. Note that the concentration of drug at the site will vary as a function of injection volume and total dose. Accordingly, a robust preclinical study will employ the MUD dose for some extended period. This suggests a routine chronic infusion model. While this applies for agents which are cleared rapidly, for agents with a relatively longer half-life, continuous infusion may result in a progressive accumulation, which will lead to physiologically intolerable side effects. Such considerations would require a lower total dose. This issue brings into focus the role of drug dose versus the injectate concentration at the site. In the human spinal lidocaine toxicity referred to above, the total dose was typically within accepted limits (as defined by potential cardiotoxicity which might be associated with an inadvertent systemic delivery of the agent). Accordingly, continuous infusion paradigms may lead to the use of lower total doses (to avoid accumulating drug levels that lead, for example, to behavioral depression) and thus preclude the study of higher local concentrations. In this regard, a more robust safety test could involve in fact be a bolus delivery where, for a given total dose, a higher acute exposure concentration may be achieved. Other factors that may define the nature of the delivery paradigm would be the maximum concentration of the available agent (as limited by the solubility of the agent or by the manufactured formulation that will be available for utilization). These comments indicate the importance of having spinal toxicokinetic data available to aid in the definition of the optimal exposure paradigm and to permit rational justification of that paradigm to regulatory authorities.

Animal Models

The implementation of a "new" safety model requires at least a demonstration of the ability of the model to display toxicity, e.g., validation. Given the apparent absence of toxicological signs, an important question would be how sensitive are the test models to displaying toxicity and, given the dose of agent employed, how robustly were the test systems challenged?

Rat The rat has been used extensively in studies where a chronically placed intrathecal catheter was used in defining the toxicity of different agents. The published literature indicates that spinal delivery of a number of agents has been shown to produce both behavioral and histopathologically defined indices of tissue injury. Thus, spinally administered dynorphin (220), somatostatin (125,220,262), ICI 174864 (220), and DPDPE-TFA (440) have been shown to produce significant signs of neuronal damage following a single dose of the respective agent. In contrast, the spinal delivery of multiple intrathecal doses of the following agents were reported to be without an effect on the histological appearance of the rat spinal cord: DADL (bolus) (293), DPDPE HCl (bolus) (440), clonidine, guanafacine (bolus) (138), R-phenylisopropyl adenosine (bolus) (188), sufentanil, alfentanil or morphine (442), ketamine, MK801, dextrorphan (bolus: T. L. Yaksh, D. Quint, and M. Marsala, unpublished observations, 1997), 3-(2-carboxypiperazin-4-yl)propyl-1-phosphonic acid (CPP) and kynurenic acid (199) carbachol (bolus) (388) and droperidol (142). While the studies cited cannot exclude the likelihood that a novel agent deemed safe in that model will not show toxicity later in other paradigms, the positive results observed with even the single dose regimens and the lack of behavioral signs of toxicity with repeated or continued dosing, using a wide variety of agents, provide supportive evidence that the rodent model is able to detect toxicity with some but not all agents. Importantly, agents in which there have been negative signs of toxicity include a wide range of agents that have been given in humans, including clonidine, morphine, alfentanil and sufentanil. Aside from evident morphological changes, the incidence of toxicity following spinal drug delivery frequently appears to correlate with irreversible hindlimb motor dysfunction and this likely provides a clear index of focal neurotoxicity. Thus, following single spinal intrathecal injections, dose-related, irreversible hindlimb dysfunction has been observed with somatostatin (125,220,262), dynorphin A(-(1-17), (2-17), (1-8), (1-7) and (3-8) (45,381), and ICI 174864 (223). These effects are typically associated with a general debilitation of the animal and a variety of changes, such as in the micturition response, suggestive of autonomic dysfunction. In contrast, other spinal agents such as arginine vasopressin may produce reversible weakness but has no effect on neuronal appearance (222). Together, the above comments suggest that multiple bolus dose spinal delivery in the rat can serve as an important index of local drug toxicity.

Dog The dog has been widely used for intrathecal and epidural spinal toxicity testing. To date, a variety of agents have been examined in the dog model, including morphine (28-day intrathecal bolus) (330), sufentanil (28-day intrathecal bolus) (330), alfentanil (28-day intrathecal bolus) (330), bupivacaine (continuous, 3–14 weeks) (48), baclofen (28-day intrathecal continuous infusion) (331), clonidine (28-day epidural continuous infusion) (444), and bupivacaine (201). Typically, based on behavior and physiology, CSF chemistry and systematic light level microscopy, these studies have not shown evidence of histopathology.

Rabbits Intrathecal and epidural safety studies have been accomplished in rabbit models with a variety of compounds, including ketamine (231,232), midazolam (231), local anesthetics (173) and meptazinol (228).

Other Species Pigs (136,138,315) and primates (1,89,100) have been occasionally employed in safety studies of spinally delivered agents with results published in the peer-reviewed literature. Sheep models have been employed for the formal safety investigation of a number compounds, including opiates (68,318), gangliosides (69), and enkephalinase inhibitors (67).

Choice of Species

At the present state of the art there is no a priori indication that one safety model in particular is preferred on the basis of the species. As there is uncertainty as to how concentration and toxicity will scale up to humans, there is a sense that at least one species should be a relatively large animal (such as dog or sheep). At the other end of the scale, the evolving data from rat models has given credence that this model may present an important rational alternative. Determining factors for selection would appear to be related more to the convergence of utility and robustness of the model, expense of the animal (e.g., rat, rabbit, or dog versus primate), maintenance expenses (e.g., rat and dog versus sheep and primate) and, perhaps more importantly, the existence of a body of literature which serves to validate its sensitivity. It is interesting to note that there is a surprisingly small amount of published material on primate spinal toxicology, and at present there are no specific data supporting the validity of this model in predicting spinal drug safety in humans. As the number of classes of agents that are examined and moved to humans grows, the ability of these several models to predict safety will be practically evaluated.

FINAL COMMENTS

In light of the above, it should be emphasized that safety studies must always be considered as indicators and not absolute predictors. The spinal delivery of novel agents in humans should be accomplished after appropriate preclinical safety testing, and even then they should be considered as "canaries in a coal mine." The absence of toxicity may only give us some sense of confidence that within the narrow dose range that was studied, the agent over the time of exposure will not produce an untoward effect. On the other hand, if toxicity is noted in such preclinical studies, it becomes the responsibility of the investigator to define the mechanisms of toxicity and decide whether it is idiopathic to that specific model. To carry the analogy further, a dead canary in a mine may have died of old age, but it behooves us to assess the cause of its demise prior to further advance.

ETHICAL CONSIDERATION IN PRECLINICAL PAIN MODELS

Experimental Method and Advances in Pain Research

Our understanding of the biology of neural function in general and the mechanism of pain processing specifically has advanced in the last 100 years, from the appreciation of the neuron as a discrete unit to a breathtaking appreciation of the richness of the synaptic and membrane function which gives systems constructed from such neurons a complexity and plasticity, appearing short of miraculous. These advances in our understanding of system biology have come by the application of the experimental method to the living organism. Thus, while the observation of "experiments of nature" (e.g., stroke, tumor, trauma, genetic variants) are important sources of information, the nature of the natural model is limited by a process over which there is no control (e.g., variances in the size of the infarct or tumor). In contrast to studies limited to the products of natural intervention, the experimental method induces systematic interventions into a well-defined system and defines casual relationships based on the covariance of intervention with outcome. Once such covariances are established, they may be used to predict unstudied events. This serves to confirm the validity of the hypothesis and to employ the hypothesized relationship as a tool for expanding the knowledge base.

As in other areas of biology, the use of clinical observation and experimental method has given remarkable insights into our understanding of nociception. Such an example is that cited in Chapter 1 regarding the role of the ventrolateral tract. Brown-Sequard, circa 1850, noted contralateral sensory loss in animals after spinal hemisection. Gower, in 1888, observed the behavioral sequelae of a gunshot wound injuring the ventrolateral quadrant of the cervical cord. Spiller later predicted the location of a spinal lesion upon seeing the characteristic contralateral analgesia sparing light touch. Finally, Martin and Beer each systematically undertook such interventions in humans and displayed the characteristics of pain relief. Similar examples, related to virtually every area of understanding regarding pain can be cited, from the actions of opiates to the development of novel drug classes to the role of growth factors. In such cases, insights provided by the application of the experimental method to biologic systems have led to important advances in our understanding of nociceptive processing and the control of the pain state.

Ethical Imperatives in Pain Research

The study of pain mechanisms poses a logical conundrum in that the goal of the investigator is to minimize the stress to which the animal is exposed and at the same time to define the systems which process nociceptive information. At one extreme, the sacrifice of the animal and the study of elements of the system in vitro (e.g., such as isolated nerves, spinal slices or neurons) allows the minimum exposure of the animal to adverse stimulus conditions. At the other extreme, a stimulus associated with tissue injury exposes the animal to a condition which by its nature is not readily escapable. Thus, while the benefits derived from animal research is evidenced by the contents of the clinical literature, the implementation of animals, particularly those in the unanesthetized state, and exposure of those animals to stimulus conditions which lead to nociception place a great moral obligation on the investigator. Selection of in vivo models and their implementation must be governed by several considerations, several of which will be noted below.

Hypothesis-Driven Work

In science in general, but in the area of work with the intact organism in particular, the nature of the study should be driven by organized hypotheses. Such frameworks permit the rational definition of the stimulus conditions, the experimental treatments and permits a systematic definition of the groups to be investigated. Such systematic formulations serve two purposes. First, it provides the framework for the scientific justification of the research methodology and strategy. Second, attention to experimental design permits the formulation of an efficient and powerful study. The goal of the investigator is to assure that the study design is of adequate power to accept or reject the hypotheses in question. While this serves to minimize group size, the goal is to employ groups sizes that provide adequate power to permit hypotheses rejection. Experiments with inadequate power because of group size is in fact wasteful.

Hypotheses-driven work does not exclude the ability to exercise intuition, but it argues that the framework of the intuition involving the animal experiment must be exposed to the same rigorous thinking and considerations that defines group size, model selection and animal treatment.

In Vitro Versus In Vivo Biological Models

Biological models may range from ex vivo to in vivo. It is evident that the issues of pain and suffering in animal research are simplified in the in vitro model. Yet, there is no protocol which can assert a priori that in vitro is superior or inferior to in vivo paradigms. It is the hypothesis and the type of data which is sought that defines the utility of one model over another. To the extent that the hypothesis seeks to define, for example, the pharmacology of a population of dorsal horn terminals, it may be possible that the in vitro model is adequate, if not superior. On the other hand, it has been repeatedly demonstrated that the complexity of the neural organization is such that the collection of systems may possess properties that are not evident from the precise working of each element. Moreover, the definition of the role played by a given system in a particular function such as nociceptive processing may not be determinable a priori. This later statement is true because the "pain state" is the behavioral manifestation of the product of the interaction of multiple systems. Accordingly, the ability to infer the particular contribution of a given system (such as a population of dorsal horn terminals) must be confirmed in the conjoint functioning of the collection of systems. Specifically, as discussed in this chapter, the concept of analgesia is operationally defined by an attenuation of the unconditioned organized response of the animal to an otherwise aversive stimulus. Such information cannot be garnered from an in vitro model or from one which does not involve supraspinal processing (e.g., a spinal reflex). Similarly, interfering changes in motor function induced by a given treatment would preclude the use of this terminology with respect to that treatment. An example relates to the action of morphine at the level of the spinal cord. Thus, single unit studies reveal that opiates and GABA-B agonists will inhibit the firing of dorsal neurons evoked by high-threshold afferents and will inhibit the activation of ventral horn neurons (see Chapters 58 and 62). Whether these spinal agents have an analgesic action, i.e. can selectively alter the response to a noxious stimulus, however, can be defined only in terms of the behavior of the unanesthetized and intact organism. Accordingly, animal studies employing intact, unanesthetized systems demonstrated that spinal morphine produced a selective analgesia and, unexpectedly, no motor weakness (446), whereas the spinal actions of baclofen are characterized by a moderate analgesia, but prominent motor dysfunction (416). Such insights may arise from the effects of such agents on the function of the intact system.

Anesthetic State of the Intact Biological Model

The utilization of an in vivo model may employ an anesthetic state. The anesthetic condition removes the intact system from being exposed to a pain state, in part by the removal of the high order function which otherwise processes that input. The utility of the anesthetized model is clear. Extensive electrophysiological literature has provided considerable insights into the connectivity and pharmacology of afferent pathways (see Chapter 36). Such information is in fact directly parallel to the state of anesthesia that is employed in humans undergoing surgery and accordingly would be deemed predictive of the pharmacology of this not uncommon clinical state. Moreover, the utility of such information generated in the anesthetized animal has proven to possess significant predictive power for system function. The definition of the response properties of dorsal horn and brainstem neurons, and the pharmacology of synapses in these regions, have all been characterized in models that are under planes of anesthesia which would be acceptable to humans undergoing similar interventions (e.g., spinal surgery). It should be emphasized that the presence of anesthesia may provide a false sense of security that there is an adequate "pain-free" state. This can only be assured by the continued monitoring of the preparation. Appropriate attention to the depth of anesthesia (absence of cranial reflexes, stable autonomic function) serves to define a state in which there is an absence of "pain." These considerations are particularly relevant when treatment leading to muscle relaxation is involved as the overt motion associated with the lightening of the anesthetic state would be blocked. Moderate changes in ventilation or gas flow, and alterations in pump or drip rates can lead to unanticipated changes in anesthetic depth. It is inexcusable that a monitoring lapse should occur leaving the animal at risk for such inadvertent changes in anesthetic depth.

While the use of an anesthetized preparation has many advantages from the perspective of removing the animal from a pain state and permitting significant tissue interventions, the anesthetic state does reflect the powerful suppressive action of agents on a number of systems which by definition are relevant to nociceptive processing (66). Moreover, as in the in vitro models, the anesthetized preparation cannot provide the components of behavior which define the pain state, and the role played by these suppressed systems would be absent.

As emphasized in this chapter, there is a growing appreciation that in the postinjury state, there are long-term changes that reflect changes in the phenotype of the system and its organization. This evolving line of hypotheses emphasizes that animal models, necessary to mimic the human state, may require an extended exposure (see below) which could not be managed by use of an extended anesthetic. It should be emphasized that this comment does not represent an approval of the animal being required to endure unnecessary stressful components of the environment. Thus, surgical interventions generate wounds, which by any criteria would be considered discomforting. Such pain components are not considered necessary and must be managed as appropriate.

Stimulus Exposure

It is a tenet of work with the intact organism that the magnitude of such stimuli be limited to the briefest interval and intensity consistent with the explicit goals of the experiments. For acute stimuli, as in thermal escape tests, this exposure may be defined by the unconditioned efforts of the animal to escape the stimulus. Alternately, in the absence of an escape effort, it might be defined by the maximum exposure that does not produce tissue injury. There are models in which tissue injury may be inflicted and the sequelae of that injury is a component of the hypothesis under investigation. In this case, the duration of the exposure must be uniquely defined by the duration necessary for the acquisition of an adequate data set. One example is the formalin test. The animal receives an injection of irritant (formalin) into the paw, resulting in a pain state which persists for an extended interval of several hours. The investigator may be able to conclude, based on systematic observation, that an adequate data set may be obtained in the first 40 or 60 min. Accordingly, at this time the animal should be terminally anesthetized. If, however, the hypothesis suggests that events which transpire in the first 40 min may be manifested by changes at 24 hrs, then the case may be made that in those animals the study should be terminated at that time.

Minimization of the Stimulus Stress Provided by the Experimental Condition

In the preceding comments, the issues addressed reflect on the considerations that lead progressively to biological models which are in an unanesthetized state. It is an important premise that all aspects be managed to minimize any component of the stimulus environment that leads to a pain state that is not a part of the experimental hypothesis. In the most general sense this may be interpreted in terms of attention to the maintenance of the appropriate physiological environment (e.g., food, water, temperature, humidity, clean bedding, quiet environment and gentle handling). Aberrations in these variable can lead to significant variations in the animal's response to the defined experimental stimuli. Rough handling and aggressive restraint serve as experimental elements that will increase the variability of the experimental model (101). It is poor science to ignore such variables. There is little doubt that adequate training of the animal and prior adaptation to the environment will serve to reduce the changes in behavior that occur as a result of adaptation and the stimulation provided by the simple novelty of the test environment.

At a more complex level, the experimental intervention can itself lead to stimulus components that alter the ultimate properties of the biologic systems being studied. Thus, postoperatively, incisions should, where possible, be allowed to heal. It is not uncommon after a brief surgery for rats to display a 10–15% loss in body weight that will be recovered over the next several days. This minimization of stress and nociception that is not required for testing the hypothesis must be considered an essential responsibility of the investigator. The ability of the postinjury pain state, generating persistent afferent input to alter the response characteristics, is a repeated theme in current pain investigations. The contribution of the surgical insult is as much a contribution to the organization of the pain state in the animal model as is anesthetic and perhaps even the intended experimental pain stimulus. Attention to minimizing that input seems crucial. Indeed, such control appears relevant even in the anesthetized preparation. Wind-up and spinal facilitations have been shown to occur in the halothane-anesthetized animal (91). Accordingly, in extensive tissue resection and laminectomy, the afferent drive generated by the preparation is considerable and in the absence of control must represent as much a part of the stimulus milieu as the brief intended activation of the sural nerve.

Responsibility of the Investigator

The scientists who work with animal models have two responsibilities: (1) to undertake hypotheses-driven research that will yield reliable and valid insights into the function of the biological model, and (2) to minimize the nonhypothesis-related stress that may result from the intervention. The first and the second responsibilities provide a potential conflict of interest. Accordingly, each investigator must accept the fact that he /she has a third responsibility and that is to accept oversight from the community of researchers with whom he/she interacts. This oversight may be formal, as in the structure of the institutional animal care and use committees, or informal, as a result of the comments of his / her colleagues. To some, it may seem onerous to have one's judgment questioned, but it is essential. It provides a backdrop against which the virtue of a research endeavor may be independently gauged and a caution to maintain the appropriate treatment of the biological system. It is the minimum price that must be paid for the privilege of undertaking research with the living organism.

REFERENCES

1. Abouleish E, Barmada MA, Nemot EM, Tung A, Winter P. Acute and chronic effects of intrathecal morphine in monkeys. *Br J Anaesth* 1981;53:1027–1032.
2. Abram SE, Winne RP. Intrathecal acetyl cholinesterase inhibitors produce analgesia that is synergistic with morphine and clonidine in rats. *Anesth Analg* 1995;81:501–507.
3. Abram SE, Yaksh TL. Systemic lidocaine blocks nerve injury-induced hyperalgesia and nociceptor-driven spinal sensitization in the rat. *Anesthesiology* 1994;80:383–391.
4. Ackerman WE III. Transient neurologic toxicity after subarachnoid anesthesia with hyperbaric 5% lidocaine. *Anesth Analg* 1993;77: 1306.
5. Adams JU, Geller EB, Adler MW. Receptor selectivity of icv morphine in the rat cold water tail-flick test. *Drug Alcohol Depend* 1994; 35:197–202.
6. Adams JU, Paronis CA, Holtzman SG. Assessment of relative intrinsic activity of mu-opioid analgesics in vivo by using beta-funaltrexamine. *J Pharmacol Exp Ther* 1990;255:1027–1032.
7. Advokat C, Rutherford D. Selective antinociceptive effect of excitatory amino acid antagonists in intact and acute spinal rats. *Pharmacol Biochem Behav* 1995;51:855–860.
8. Ahlgren SC, Levine JD. Mechanical hyperalgesia in streptozotocin-diabetic rats is not sympathetically maintained. *Brain Res* 1993;616: 171–175.
9. Ahlgren SC, White DM, Levine JD. Increased responsiveness of sensory neurons in the saphenous nerve of the streptozotocin-diabetic rat. *J Neurophysiol* 1992;68:2077–2085.
10. Al-Rodhan N, Chipkin R, and Yaksh TL. The antinociceptive effects of SCH-32615, a neutral endopeptidase (enkephalinase) inhibitor, microinjected into the periaqueductal, ventral medulla and amygdala. *Brain Res* 1990;520:123–130.
11. Alhaider AA, Lei SZ, Wilcox GL. Spinal 5-HT3 receptor-mediated antinociception: possible release of GABA. *J Neurosci* 1991;11: 1881–1888.
12. Aloisi AM, Albonetti ME, Carli G. Behavioural effects of different intensities of formalin pain in rats. *Physiol Behav* 1995;58:603–610.
13. Arena, J.M. *Poisoning toxicology, symptoms, treatments.* 4th edn. Springfield, IL: Charles C. Thomas, 1970.
14. Arner S, Meyerson BA. Lack of analgesic effect of opioids on neuropathic and idiopathic forms of pain. *Pain* 1988;33:11–23.
15. Atchison SR, Durant PAC, Yaksh TL. Cardiorespiratory effects and kinetics of intrathecally injected D-Ala2-D-Leu5-enkephalin and morphine in unanesthetized dogs. *Anesthesiology* 1986;65:609–616,.
16. Attal N, Jazat F, Kayser V, Guilbaud G. Further evidence for "pain-related" behaviours in a model of unilateral peripheral mononeuropathy. *Pain* 1990;41:235–251.
17. Backonja M, Arndt G, Gombar KA, Check B, Zimmermann M. Response of chronic neuropathic pain syndromes to ketamine: a preliminary. *Pain* 1994;56:51–7.
18. Barber RP, Vaughn JE, Saito K, McLaughlin BJ, Roberts E. GABAergic terminals are presynaptic to primary afferent terminals in the substantia gelatinosa of the rat spinal cord. *Brain Res* 1978;141: 35–55.
19. Bartolini A, Ghelardini C, Fantetti L, Malcangio M, Malmberg-Aiello P, Giotti A. Role of muscarinic receptor subtypes in central antinociception. *Br J Pharmacol* 1992;105:77–82.
20. Basbaum AI. Distribution of glycine receptor immunoreactivity in the spinal cord of the rat: cystochemical evidence for a differential glycinergic control, of Lamina I and Lamina V neurons. *J Comp Neurol* 1988;278:330–336.
21. Baukrowitz T, Yellen G. Use-dependent blockers and exit rate of the last ion from the multi-ion pore of a K^+ channel. *Science* 1996; 271:653–656.
22. Belfrage M, Sollevi A, Segerdahl M, Sjolund KF, Hansson P. Systemic adenosine infusion alleviates spontaneous and stimulus evoked pain in patients with peripheral neuropathic pain. *Anesth Analg* 1995;81:713–717.
23. Bennett GJ, Xie YK. A peripheral mononeuropathy in rat that produces disorders of pain sensation like those seen in man. *Pain* 1988;33:87–107.
24. Berberich P, Hoheisel U, Mense S. Effects of a carrageenan-induced myositis on the discharge properties of group III and IV muscle receptors in the cat. *J Neurophysiol* 1988;59:1395–1409.
25. Berge OG, Tjolsen A. Tail-flicks, temperatures and latencies: comments on Lichtman et al. *Pain* 1994;57:256–8.
26. Borgbjerg FM, Svensson BA, Frigast C, Gordh T Jr. Histopathology after repeated intrathecal injections of preservative-free ketamine in the rabbit: a light and electron microscopic examination. *Anesth Analg* 1994;79:105–111.
27. Bouaziz H, Tong C, Eisenach JC. Postoperative analgesia from intrathecal neostigmine in sheep. *Anesth Analg* 1995;80: 1140–1144.
28. Bourgoin S, Le Bars D, Artaud F, et al. Effects of kelatorphan and other peptidase inhibitors on the in vitro and in vivo release of methionine-enkephalin-like material from the rat spinal cord. *J Pharmacol Exp Ther* 1986;238:360–366.
29. Braas KS, Newby AL, Wilson VS, Snyder SH. Adenosine containing neurons in the brain localized by immunocytochemistry. *J Neurosci* 1986;6:1952–1961.
30. Brau ME, Nau C, Hempelmann G, Vogel W. Local anesthetics potently block a potential insensitive potassium channel in myelinated nerve. *J Gen Physiol* 1995;105:485–505.
31. Brennum J, Arendt-Nielsen L, Horn A, Secher NH, Jensen TS. Quantitative sensory examination during epidural anaesthesia and analgesia in man: effects of morphine. *Pain* 1993;52:75–83.
32. Brennum J, Dahl JB, Moiniche S, Arendt-Nielsen L. Quantitative sensory examination of epidural anaesthesia and analgesia in man: effects of pre- and post-traumatic morphine on hyperalgesia. *Pain* 1994;59:261–271.
33. Brose W, Pfeifer B, Hassenbusch S, et al. SNX-111 produces analgesia in patients with intractable pain: phase I/II results. Presented at the World Congress of Anesthesiologists, April 1996.
34. Brose WG, Cousins MJ. Subcutaneous lidocaine for treatment of neuropathic cancer pain. *Pain* 1991;45:145–8.
35. Buck SH, Burks TF. The neuropharmacology of capsaicin: review of some recent observations. *Pharmacol Rev* 1986;38:179–226.
36. Burchiel KJ, Ochoa JL. Surgical management of post-traumatic neuropathic pain. *Neurosurg Clin North Am* 1991;2:117–26.
37. Butler SH, Godefroy F, Besson JM, Weil-Fugazza J. A limited arthritic model for chronic pain studies in the rat. *Pain* 1992;48:73–81.
38. Calcutt NA, Jorge MC, Yaksh TL, Chaplan SR. Tactile allodynia and formalin hyperalgesia in streptozotocin-diabetic rats: effects of insulin, aldose reductase inhibition and lidocaine [Abstract]. *Pain* 68: 293–299,1996.
39. Calcutt NA, Li L, Yaksh TL, Malmberg AB. Different effects of two aldose reductase inhibitors on nociception and prostaglandin E. *Eur J Pharmacol* 1995;285:189–97.
40. Calcutt NA, Malmberg AB, Yamamoto T, Yaksh TL. Tolrestat treatment prevents modification of the formalin test model of prolonged pain in hyperglycemic rats *Pain* 1994;58:413–420,.
41. Cambell JN, Raja SN, Meyer RA, Mackinnon SE. Myelinated afferents signal the hyperalgesia associated with nerve injury. Pain *1988*; 32:89–94.
42. Cameron AA, Cliffer KD, Dougherty PM, Willis WD, Carlton SM. Changes in lectin, GAP-43 and neuropeptide staining in the rat superficial dorsal horn following experimental peripheral neuropathy. *Neurosci Lett* 1991;131:249–252.
43. Carlton SM, Westlund KN, Zhang D, Willis WD. GABA-immunoreactive terminals synapse on primate spinothalamic tract cells. *J Comp Neurol* 1992;322:528–537.
44. Castro MI, Eisenach JC. Pharmacokinetics and dynamics of intravenous, intrathecal, and epidural clonidine in sheep. *Anesthesiology* 1989;71:418–25.
45. Caudle RM, Isaac L. Intrathecal dynorphin(1-13) results in an irreversible loss of the tail-flick reflex in rats. *Brain Res* 1987;435:1–6.
46. Chabal C, Russell LC, Burchiel KJ. The effect of intravenous lidocaine, tocainide, and mexiletine on spontaneously active fibers originating in rat sciatic neuromas. *Pain* 1989;38:333–338.
47. Chaplan SR, Bach FW, Shafer SL, Yaksh TL. Prolonged alleviation of tactile allodynia by intravenous lidocaine in neuropathic rats. *Anesthesiology* 1995;83:775–785.

48. Chaplan SR, Calcutt NA, Yaksh, TL. Pharmacology of tactile allodynia in the streptozotocin diabetic rat. *Soc Neurosci Abstr* 1995 21:1172.
49. Chaplan SR, Pogrel JW, Yaksh, TL. Role of voltage-dependant calcium channel subtypes in experimental tactile allodynia. *J Pharmacol Exper Ther* 1994;269:1117–1123.
50. Chaplan SR, Malmberg, AB, Yaksh TL. Efficacy of spinal NMDA receptor antagonism in formalin hyperalgesia and nerve injury evoked allodynia in the rat. *Journal of Pharmacology and Experimental Therapeutics* 1997;280:829–838.
51. Chapman V, Dickenson AH. The effects of sandostatin and somatostatin on nociceptive transmission in the dorsal horn of the rat spinal cord. *Neuropeptides* 1992;23:147–152.
52. Cherny NI, Thaler HT, Friedlander-Klar H, et al. Opioid responsiveness of cancer pain syndromes caused by neuropathic or nociceptive mechanisms: a combined analysis of controlled, single-dose studies. *Neurology* 1994;44:857–861.
53. Chi SI, Levine JD, Basbaum AI. Peripheral and central contributions to the persistent expression of spinal cord fos-like immunoreactivity produced by sciatic nerve transection in the rat. *Brain Res* 1993;617:225–237.
54. Chi SI, Levine JD, Basbaum AI. Effects of injury discharge on the persistent expression of spinal cord fos-like immunoreactivity produced by sciatic nerve transection in the rat. *Brain Res* 1994;617: 220–224.
55. Chipkin RE, Berger JG, Billard W, Iorio LC, Chapman R, Barnett A. Pharmacology of SCH 34826, an orally active enkephalinase inhibitor analgesic. *J Pharmacol Exp Ther* 1988;245:829–838.
56. Chipkin RE, Latranyi MB, Iorio LC, Barnett A. Determination of analgesic drug efficacies by modification of the Randall and Selitto rat yeast paw test. *J Pharmacol Methods* 1983;10:223–229.
57. Choi Y, Yoon YW, Na HS, Kim SH, Chung JM. Behavioral signs of ongoing pain and cold allodynia in a rat model of neuropathic pain. *Pain* 1994;59:369–376.
58. Chrubasik J. Intrathecal somatostatin. *Ann NY Acad Sci* 1988;531: 133–145.
59. Chung JM, Choi Y, Yoon YW, Na HS. Effects of age on behavioral signs of neuropathic pain in an experimental rat model. *Neurosci Lett* 1995;183:54–57.
60. Coda BA, Brown MC, Schaffer R, et al. Pharmacology of epidural fentanyl, alfentanil, and sufentanil in volunteers. *Anesthesiology* 1994;81:1149–1161.
61. Coderre TJ. Potent analgesia induced in rats by combined action at PCP and polyamine recognition sites of the NMDA receptor complex. *Eur J Neurosci* 1993;5:390–393.
62. Coderre TJ, Fundytus ME, McKenna JE, Dalal S, Melzack R. The formalin test: a validation of the weighted-scores method of behavioural pain rating. *Pain* 1993;54:43–50.
63. Coderre TJ, Van Empel I. The utility of excitatory amino acid (EAA) antagonists as analgesic agents. I. Comparison of the antinociceptive activity of various classes of EAA antagonists in mechanical, thermal and chemical nociceptive tests. *Pain* 1994;59:345–352.
64. Coderre TJ, Wall PD. Ankle joint urate arthritis in rats provides a useful tool for the evaluation of analgesic and anti-arthritic agents. *Pharmacol Biochem Behav* 1988;29:461–466.
65. Coffey JR, Cahill D, Steers W, et al. Intrathecal baclofen for intractable spasticity of spinal origin: results of a long-term multicenter study. *J Neurosurg* 1993;78:226–232.
66. Collins JG, Kendig JJ, Mason P. Anesthetic actions within the spinal cord. Contributions to the state of general anestehsia. *Trends Neurosci* 1995;18:549–553.
67. Coombs DW, Colburn RW, DeLeo JA, Hoopes PJ, Rhodes CH, Twitchell BB. Acute toxicology of an enkephalinase inhibitor (SCH 32615) given intrathecally in the ewe. *Anesth Analg* 1993;76: 123–123.
68. Coombs DW, Colburn RW, DeLeo JA, Hoopes PJ, Twitchell BB. Comparative spinal neuropathology of hydromorphone and morphine after 9- and 30-day epidural administration in sheep. *Anesth Analg* 1994;78:674–681.
69. Coombs DW, Colburn RW, McCarthy LE, DeLeo JA, Hoopes PJ, Twitchell BB. Neurotoxicology of chronic infusion of the ganglioside GM1 in the ewe: phase I. intrathecal administration. *Anesth Analg* 1993;77:507–515.
70. Cooper BY, Vierck CJ Jr. Vocalizations as measures of pain in monkeys. *Pain* 1986;26:393–407.
71. Cooper BY, Vierck CJ Jr, Yeomans DC. Selective reduction of second pain sensations by systemic morphine in humans. *Pain* 1986; 24:93–116.
72. Corradetti R, Lo Conte G, Moroni F, Passani MB, Pepeu G. Adenosine decreases aspartate and glutamate release from rat hippocampal slices. *Eur J Pharmacol* 1984;104:19–26.
73. Courteix C, Bardin M, Chantelauze C, Lavarenne J, Eschalier A. Study of the sensitivity of the diabetes-induced pain model in rats to a range of analgesics. *Pain* 1994;57:153–160.
74. Cozanitis DA, Friedmann T, Furst S. Study of the analgesic effects of galanthamine, a cholinesterase inhibitor. *Arch Int Pharmacodyn Ther* 1983;266:229–238.
75. D'Amour FE, Smith DL. A method for determining loss of pain sensation. *J Phamacol Exp Ther* 1941;72:74–79.
76. Dahl JB, Brennum J, Arendt-Nielsen L, Jensen TS, Kehlet H. The effect of pre- versus postinjury infiltration with lidocaine on thermal and mechanical hyperalgesia after heat injury to the skin. *Pain* 1993;53:43–51.
77. Dallel R, Raboisson P, Clavelou P, Saade M, Woda A. Evidence for a peripheral origin of the tonic nociceptive response to subcutaneous formalin. *Pain* 1995;61:11–16.
78. Daval G, Verge D, Basbaum AI, Bouroin S, Hamon M. Autoradiographic evidence of serotonin-1 binding sites on primary afferent fibers in dorsal horn of the rat spinal cord. *Neurosci Lett* 1987;83: 71–81.
79. Davies J, Watkins JC. Role of excitatory amino acids receptors in mono- and polysynaptic excitation in the cat spinal cord. *Exp Brain Res* 1983;49:280–290.
80. Davis RE, Callahan MJ, Dickerson M, Downs DA. Pharmacologic activity of CI-977, a selective kappa opioid agonist, in rhesus monkeys. *J Pharmacol Exp Ther* 1992;261:1044–1049.
81. Daw NW, Stein PS, Fox K. The role of NMDA receptors in information processing. *Annu Rev Neurosci* 1993;16:207–222.
82. DeLander GE, Hopkins CJ. Involvement of A2 adenosine receptors in spinal mechanisms of antinociception. *Eur J Pharmacol* 1987;139: 215–223.
83. DeLeo JA, Coombs DW, Willenbring S, et al. Characterization of a neuropathic pain model: sciatic cryoneurolysis in the rat. *Pain* 1994;56:9–16.
84. Desmeules JA, Kayser V, Weil-Fuggaza J, Bertrand A, Guilbaud G. Influence of the sympathetic nervous system in the development of abnormal pain-related behaviours in a rat model of neuropathic pain. *Neuroscience* 1995;67:941–951.
85. Devoghel JC. Small intrathecal doses of lysine-acetylsalicylate relieve intractable pain in man. *J Intern Med Res* 1983;11:90–1.
86. Devor M, Govrin-Lippmann R, Angelides K. Na^+ channel immunolocalization in peripheral mammalian axons and changes following nerve injury and neuroma formation. *J Neurosci* 1993;13:1976–1992.
87. Devor M, Wall PD, Catalan N. Systemic lidocaine silences ectopic neuroma and DRG discharge without blocking nerve conduction. *Pain*, 1992;48:261–268.
88. Devor M, White DM, Goetzl EJ, Levine JD. Eicosanoids, but not tachykinins, excite C-fiber endings in rat sciatic nerve-end neuromas. *Neuroreport* 1992;3:21–24.
89. Dhiri AK, Sanford J, Wyllie MG. Disposition and pharmacokinetics of meptazinol in the CSF. Studies after intrathecal administration in the non-human primate Erythrocebus patas. *Br J Anaesth* 1987; 59:1140–1146.
90. Dickenson AH, Brewer CM, Hayes NA. Effects of topical baclofen on C fibre-evoked neuronal activity in the rat dorsal horn. *Neuroscience* 1985;14:557–562.
91. Dickenson AH, Sullivan AF. Peripheral origins and central modulation of subcutaneous formalin-induced activity of rat dorsal horn neurones. *Neurosci Lett* 1987;83:207–211.
92. Dickenson AH, Sullivan A, Feeney C, Fournie-Zaluski MC, Roques BP. Evidence that endogenous enkephalins produce delta-opiate receptor mediated neuronal inhibitions in rat dorsal horn. *Neurosci Lett* 1986;72:179–182.
93. Dickenson AH, Sullivan AF, Roques BP. Evidence that endogenous enkephalins and a delta opioid receptor agonist have a common site of action in spinal antinociception. *Eur J Pharmacol* 1988;148: 437–439.
94. Dirig DM, Yaksh TL. Differential right shifts in the dose-response curve for intrathecal morphine and sufentanil as a function of stimulus intensity. *Pain* 1995;62:321–328.
95. Dirig DM, Yaksh TL. Intrathecal baclofen and muscimol, but not midazolam, are antinociceptive using the rat-formalin model. *J Pharmacol Exp Ther* 1995;275:219–227.
96. Doucette R, Theriault E, Diamond J. Regionally selective elimination of cutaneous thermal nociception in rats by neonatal capsaicin. *J Comp Neurol* 1987;261:583–591.

97. Drasner K, Rigler ML, Sessler DI, Stoller ML. Cauda equina syndrome following intended epidural anesthesia. Anesthesiology 1992;77:582–585.
98. Dray A, Dickenson A. Systemic capsaicin and olvanil reduce the acute algogenic and the late inflammatory phase following formalin injection into rodent paw. Pain 1991;47:79–83.
99. Driessen JJ, de Mulder PH, Claessen JJ, Diejen D, Wobbes T. Epidural administration of morphine for control of cancer pain: long-term efficacy and complications. Clin J Pain 1989;5:217–222.
100. Drobeck HP, Mayes BA, Barbolt TA, Fabian RJ, Kimball JP, Slighter RR Jr. Subarachnoid administration of iohexol in cynomolgus monkeys. *Acta Radiol* 1986;27:349–355.
101. Dubner R, Bennett GJ. Spinal and trigeminal mechanisms of nociception. *Annu Rev Neurosci* 1983;6:381–418.
102. Dubner R, Kenshalo DR Jr, Maixner W, Bushnell MC, Oliveras JL. The correlation of monkey medullary dorsal horn neuronal activity and the perceived intensity of noxious heat stimuli. *J Neurophysiol* 1989;62:450–457.
103. Duggan AW, Hope PJ, Lang CW. Microinjection of neuropeptide Y into the superficial dorsal horn reduces stimulus-evoked release of immunoreactive substance P in the anaesthetized car. *Neuroscience* 1991;44:733–740.
104. Dykstra LA. Effects of buprenorphine on shock titration in squirrel monkeys. *J Pharmacol Exp Ther* 1985;235:20–25.
105. Dykstra LA, Woods JH. A tail withdrawal procedure for assessing analgesic activity in rhesus monkeys. *J Pharmacol Methods* 1986;15: 263–269.
106. Eide PK, Jorum E, Stubhaug A, Bremnes J, Breivik H. Relief of post-herpetic neuralgia with the N-methyl-D-aspartic acid receptor antagonist ketamine: a double-blind, cross-over comparison with morphine and placebo. *Pain* 1994;58:347–354.
106a. Eisenach JC. Approval for clinical implementation of spinal agent. *Spinal Drug Delivery*, TL Yaksh, Editor. CRC Press, New York. In press, 1998.
107. Eisenach JC, Dewan DM, Rose JC, Angelo JM. Epidural clonidine produces antinociception, but not hypotension, in sheep. *Anesthesiology* 1987;66:496–501.
108. Eisenach JC, DuPen S, Dubois M, Miguel R, Allin D. Epidural clonidine analgesia for intractable cancer pain. The Epidural Clonidine Study Group. *Pain* 1995;61:391–399.
109. Eisenach JC, Grice SC. Epidural clonidine does not decrease blood pressure or spinal cord blood flow in awake sheep. *Anesthesiology* 1988;68:335–340.
110. Eisenach JC, Rauck RL, Buzzanell C, Lysak SZ. Epidural clonidine analgesia for intractable cancer pain: phase I. *Anesthesiology* 1989; 71:647–652.
111. Eisenach JC, Shafer SL, Bucklin BA, Jackson C, Kallio A. Pharmacokinetics and pharmacodynamics of intraspinal dexmedetomidine in sheep. *Anesthesiology* 1994;80:1349–1359.
112. Eisenberg E, LaCross S, Strassman AM. The effects of the clinically tested NMDA receptor antagonist memantine on carrageenan-induced thermal hyperalgesia in rats. *Eur J Pharmacol* 1994;255:123–129.
113. El-Yassir N, Fleetwood-Walker SM, Mitchell R. Heterogeneous effects of serotonin in the dorsal horn of the rat: the involvement of 5-HT1 receptors subtypes. *Brain Res* 1988;456:147–158.
114. Evans WO. A new technique for the investigation of some analgesic drugs on a reflexive behavior in the rat. *Psychopharmacology* 1961;2:318–325.
115. Fainsinger R, Schoeller T, Bruera E. Methadone in the management of cancer pain: a review. *Pain* 1993;52:137–147.
116. Faull RL, Villiger JW, Dragunow M. Neurotensin receptors in the human spinal cord: a quantitative autoradiographic study. *Neuroscience* 1989;29:603–613.
117. Fleetwood-Walker SM, Hope PJ, Mitchell R, El-Yassir N, Molony V. The influence of opioid receptor subtypes on the processing of nociceptive inputs in the spinal dorsal horn of the cat. *Brain Res* 1988;451:213–226.
118. Fleetwood-Walker SM, Mitchell R, Hope PJ, Molony V, Iggo A. An alpha2 receptor mediates the selective inhibition by noradrenaline of nociceptive responses of identified dorsal horn neurones. *Brain Res* 1995;334:243–254.
119. Fleischmann A, Urca G. Tail-pinch induced analgesia and immobility: altered responses to noxious tail-pinch by prior pinch of the neck. *Brain Res* 1993;601:28–33.
120. Foreman RD, Schmidt RF, Willis WD. Effects of mechanical and chemical stimulation of fine muscle afferents upon primate spinothalamic tract cells. *J Physiol (Lond)* 1979;286:215–231.
121. Fredholm BB, Fastbom J, Lindgren E. Effects of N-ethylmaleimide and forskolin on glutamate release from rat hippocampal slices. Evidence that prejunctional adenosine receptors are linked to N-proteins, but not to adenylate cyclase. *Acta Physiol Scand* 1986;127: 381–386.
122. Frisen J, Risling M, Fried K. Distribution and axonal relations of macrophages in a neuroma. *Neuroscience* 1993;55:1003–1013.
123. Furuyama T, Kiyama H, Sato K, et al. Region-specific expression of subunits of ionotropic glutamate receptors (AMPA-type, KA-type and NMDA receptors) in the rat spinal cord with special reference to nociception. *Brain Res Mol Brain Res* 1993;18:141–151.
124. Gamse R, Holzer P, Lembeck F. Indirect evidence for presynaptic location of opiate receptors in chemosensitive primary sensory neurones. *Naunyn Schmiedbergs Arch Pharmacol* 1979;308:281–285.
125. Gaumann DM, Yaksh TL. Intrathecal somatostatin in rats: antinociception only in the presence of toxic effects. *Anesthesiology* 1988;68:733–742.
126. Gaumann DM, Yaksh TL, Tyce GM. Effects of intrathecal morphine, clonidine, and Midazolam on the Somato-sympathoadrenal reflex response in Halothane-anesthetized cats. *Anesthesiology* 1990;73:425–432.
127. Geiger JD, Labella FS, Nagy JI. Characterization and localization of adenosine receptors in rat spinal cord. *J Neurosci* 1984;4: 2303–2310.
128. Gelgor L, Butkow N, Mitchell D. Effects of systemic non-steroidal anti-inflammatory drugs on nociception during tail ischaemia and on reperfusion hyperalgesia in rats. *Br J Pharmacol* 1992;105: 412–416.
129. Gelgor L, Mitchell D. Modality-specific hypersensitivity of dorsal horn convergent neurones during reperfusion of their receptive fields on the rat's tail. *Pain* 1993;55:305–312.
130. Giamberardino MA, Valente R, De Bigontina P, Iezzi S, Vecchiet L. Effects of spasmolytic and/or non-steroidal anti-inflammatory drugs on muscle hyperalgesia of ureteral origin in rats. *Eur J Pharmacol* 1995;278:97–101.
131. Giamberardino MA, Valente R, de Bigontina P, Vecchiet L. Artificial ureteral calculosis in rats: behavioural characterization of visceral pain episodes and their relationship with referred lumbar muscle hyperalgesia. *Pain* 1995;61:459–469.
132. Gillberg PG, d'Ardy R, Aquilonius SM. Autoradiographic distribution of 3H-acetylcholine binding sites in the cervical spinal cord of man and some other species. *Neurosci Lett* 1988;90:197–202.
133. Gillberg PG, Wiksten B. Effects of spinal cord lesions and rhizotomies on cholinergic and opiate receptor binding sites in rat spinal cord. *Acta Physiol Scand* 1986;126:575–582.
134. Go VLW, Yaksh TL. Release of substance P from the cat spinal cord. *J Physiol* 1987;391:141–167.
135. Gohil K, Bell JR, Ramachandran J, Miljanich GP. Neuroanatomical distribution of receptors for a novel voltage-sensitive calcium-channel antagonist, SNX-230 (omega-conopeptide MVIIC). *Brain Res* 1994;653:258–266.
136. Gordh T Jr, Feuk U, Norlen K. Effect of epidural clonidine on spinal cord blood flow and regional and central hemodynamics in pigs. *Anesth Analg* 1986;65:1312–1318.
137. Gordh T Jr, Hartvig P. Cerebrospinal fluid and plasma concentrations of clonidine in pigs after epidural, intravenous and intramuscular administration. *Upsala J Med Sci* 1986;91:311–315.
138. Gordh T Jr, Post C, Olsson Y. Evaluation of the toxicity of subarachnoid clonidine, guanfacine, and a substance P-antagonist on rat spinal cord and nerve roots: light and electron microscopic observations after chronic intrathecal administration. *Anesth Analg* 1986;65:1303–1311.
139. Gordh T Jr, Wiklund L. A method for reliable and simultaneous cannulation of the epidural and subarachnoid spaces in pigs. A tool for the study of cerebrospinal fluid pharmacokinetics and drug penetration of the dura mater. *Upsala J Med Sci* 1986;91: 111–15.
140. Gotz E, Feuerstein TJ, Lais A, Meyer DK. Effects of gabapentin on release of gamma-aminobutyric acid from siices of rat neostriatum. *Arzneimittelforschung* 1993;43:636–638.
141. Gray WD, Osterberg AC, Scuto TJ. Measurement of the analgesic efficacy and potency of pentazocine by the D'Amour and Smith method. *J Pharmacol Exp Ther* 1970,72:154–162.
142. Grip G, Svensson BA, Gordh T Jr, Post C, Hartvig P. Histopathology and evaluation of potentiation of morphine-induced antinociception by intrathecal droperidol in the rat. *Acta Anaesthesiol Scand* 1992;36:145–152.
143. Grundlach AL, Dodd PR, Grabara-Watson WEJ, et al. Deficits of

spinal cord glycine/strychnine receptors in inherited myoclonius of poll Hereford calves. *Science* 1988;241:1807–1810.

144. Gruner W, Silva LR. Omega-conotoxin sensitivity and presynaptic inhibition of glutamatergic sensory neurotransmission in vitro. *J Neurosci* 1994;14:2800–2808.
145. Gurdal H, Sara Y, Tulunay FC. Effects of calcium channel blockers on formalin-induced nociception and inflammation in rats. *Pharmacology* 1992;44:290–296.
146. Habler HJ, Janig W, Koltzenburg M. Receptive properties of myelinated primary afferents innervating the inflamed urinary bladder of the cat. *J Neurophysiol* 1993;69:395–405.
147. Hammond DL. Inference of pain and its modulation from simple behaviors. In: Chapman CR, Loeser JD, eds. *Issues in pain measurement.* New York: Raven Press, 1989:69–91.
148. Hammond DL, Washington JD. Antagonism of L-baclofen-induced antinociception by CGP 35348 in the spinal cord of the rat. *Eur J Pharmacol* 1993;234:255–262.
149. Hamon M, Gallissot MC, Menard F, Gozlan H, Bourgoin S, Verge D. 5-HT3 receptor binding sites are on capsaicin-sensitive fibres in the rat spinal cord. *Eur J Pharmacol* 1989;164:315–322.
150. Handwerker HO, Kilo S, Reeh PW. Unresponsive afferent nerve fibres in the sural nerve of the rat. *J Physiol* 1991;435:229–242.
151. Handwerker HO, Reeh PW. Pain and inflammation. *Pain Res Clin Manage* 1991;4:59–70.
152. Hao JX, Xu XJ, Aldskogius H, Seiger A, Wiesenfeld-Hallin Z. Photochemically induced transient spinal ischemia induces behavioral hypersensitivity to mechanical and cold stimuli, but not to noxious-heat stimuli, in the rat. *Exp Neurol* 1992;118:187–194.
153. Hao JX, Xu XJ, Wiesenfeld-Hallin Z. Systemic N-nitro-L-arginine-ester (L-NAME), inhibitor of nitric oxide synthase, relieves chronic allodynia-like symptom in rats with spinal cord lesion. *Acta Physiol Scand* 1994;150:457–458.
154. Hao JX, Xu XJ, Yu YX, Seiger A, Wiesenfeld-Hallin Z. Transient spinal cord ischEmia induces temporary hypersensitivity of dorsal horn wide dynamic range neurons to myelinated, but not unmyelinated, fiber input. *J Neurophysiol* 1992;68:384–391.
155. Hao JX, Xu XJ, Yu YX, Seiger A, Wiesenfeld-Hallin Z. Baclofen reverses the hypersensitivity of dorsal horn wide dynamic range neurons to mechanical stimulation after transient spinal cord ischemia; implications for a tonic GABAergic inhibitory control of myelinated fiber input. *J Neurophysiol* 1992;68:392–396.
156. Hao JX, Yu YX, Seiger A, Wiesenfeld-Hallin Z. Systemic tocainide relieves mechanical hypersensitivity and normalizes the responses of hyperexcitable dorsal horn wide-dynamic-range neurons after transient spinal cord ischemia in rats. *Exp Brain Res* 1992d;91: 229–235.
157. Hargreaves K, Dubner R, Brown F, Flores C, Joris J. A new and sensitive method for measuring thermal nociception in cutaneous hyperalgesia. *Pain* 1988;32:77–88.
158. Haughton VM. Intrathecal toxicity of iohexol vs. metrizamide. Survey and current state. *Invest Radiol* 1985;20:S14–S17.
159. Healy PJ. Deficits of spinal cord glycine/strychnine receptors in inherited myoclonius of poll Hereford calves. *Science* 1988;241: 1807–1810.
160. Heapy CG, Jamieson A, Russell NJW. Afferent C-fiber and A-delta activity in models of inflammation. *Br J Pharmacol* 1987;90:164P.
161. Heel RC, Brogden RN, Speight TM, Avery GS. Buprenorphine: a review of its pharmacological properties and therapeutic efficacy. *Drugs* 1979;17:81–110.
162. Hendershot LC, Forsaith, J. Antagonism of the frequency of phenylquinone induced writhing in the mouse by weak analgesics and non analgesics. *J Pharmacol Exp Ther* 1959;125:237–240.
163. Herdegen T, Fiallos-Estrada C, Schmid W, Bravo R, Zimmermann M. The transcription factor CREB, but not immediate-early gene encoded proteins, is expressed in activated microglia of lumbar spinal cord following sciatic nerve transection in the rat. *Neurosci Lett* 1992;;142:57–61.
164. Herdegen T, Fiallos-Estrada CE, Schmid W, Bravo R, Zimmermann M. The transcription factors c-JUN, JUN D and CREB, but not FOS and KROX-24, are differentially regulated in axotomized neurons following transection of rat sciatic nerve. *Mol Brain Res* 1992;14:155–165.
165. Holland LN, Goldstein BD. Changes of substance P-like immunoreactivity in the dorsal horn are associated with the "phasic" behavioral response to a formalin stimulus. *Brain Res* 1990; 537:287–292.
166. Holmgren M, Hedner J, Mellstrand T, Nordberg G, Hedner T. Characterization of the antinociceptive effects of some adenosine analogues in the rat. *Naunyn Schmiedebergs Arch Pharmacol* 1986; 334:290–293.
167. Hood DD, Eisenach JC, Tong C, Tommasi E, Yaksh TL. Cardiorespiratory and spinal cord blood flow effects of intrathecal neostigmine methylsulfate, clonidine, and their combination in sheep *Anesthesiology* 1995;82:428–435.
168. Hood DD, Eisenach JC, Tuttle R. Phase I safety assessment of intrathecal neostigmine methylsulfate in humans. *Anesthesiology* 1995;82:331–343.
169. Hope PJ, Fleetwood-Walker SM, Mitchell R. Distinct antinociceptive actions mediated by different opioid receptors in the region of lamina I and laminae III–V of the dorsal horn of the rat. *Br J Pharmacol* 1990;101:477–483.
170. Hope PJ, Jarrott B, Schaible HG, Clarke RW, Duggan AW. Release and spread of immunoreactive neurokinin A in the cat spinal cord in a model of acute arthritis. *Brain Res* 1990;533:292–299.
171. Howe JR, Yaksh TL, Go VLW. The effect of unilateral dorsal root ganglionectomies or ventral rhizotomies on alpha2-adrenoceptor binding to, and the substance P, enkephalin, and neurotensin content of the cat lumbar spinal cord. *Neuroscience* 1987;21: 385–394.
172. Hua X-Y, Boublik JH, Spicer MA, Rivier JE, Brown MR, Yaksh TL. The antinociceptive effects of spinally administered neuropeptide Y in the rat: systematic studies on structure-activity relationship. *J Pharmacol Exp Ther* 1991;258:243–258.

172a.Hua X-Y, Chen P, Hwang JH, Yaksh TL. Antinuciception induced by civamide, an orally active capsaicin analogue. *Pain.* In press 1997.

173. Hughes PJ, Doherty MM, Charman WN. A rabbit model for the evaluation of epidurally administered local anaesthetic agents. *Anaesth Intensive Care* 1993;21:298–303.
174. Hwang J-H, Yaksh TL. The effect of subarachnoid GABApentin on tactile-evoked allodynia in a surgically induced neuropathic pain model in the rat. *Reg Anesth Analg* 22:249–256,1997.
175. Iacono RP, Boswell MV, Neumann M. Deafferentation pain exacerbated by subarachnoid lidocaine and relieved by subarachnoid morphine. Case report. *Reg Anesth* 1994;19:212–215.
176. Idanpaan-Heikkila JJ, Kalso EA, Seppala T. Antinociceptive actions of dexmedetomidine and the kappa-opioid agonist U-50,488H against noxious thermal, mechanical and inflammatory stimuli. *J Pharmacol Exp Ther* 1994;271:1306–1313.
177. Iwamoto ET, Marion L. Characterization of the antinociception produced by intrathecally administered muscarinic agonists in rats. *J Pharmacol Exp Ther* 1993;266:329–338.
178. Janig W. Systemic and specific autonomic reactions in pain: efferent, afferent an endocrine components. *Eur J Anaesthesiol* 1985;2: 319–346.
179. Janssen PAJ, Niemegeers CJE, Dony JGH. The inhibitory effect of fentanyl and other morphine like analgesics on the warm water induced tail withdrawal reflex in the rat. *Arzneimittelforschung* 1963;13:502–507.
180. Jhamandas K, Yaksh TL, Harty G, Szolcsanyi J, Go VLW. Action of intrathecal capsaicin and its structural analogues on the content and release of spinal substance P: selectivity of action and relationship to analgesia. *Brain Res* 1984;306:215–225.
181. Jinno S, Hua X-Y, Yaksh TL. Nicotine and acetylcholine induce release of calcitonin gene-related peptide from rat trachea. *J Appl Physiol* 1994;76:1651–1656.
182. Jurna I, Heinz G. Differential effects of morphine and opioid analgesics on A and C fibre-evoked activity in ascending axons of the rat spinal cord. *Brain Res* 1979;171:573–576.
183. Kalichman MW. Physiologic mechanisms by which local anesthetics may cause injury to nerve and spinal cord. *Reg Anesth* 1993;18: 448–452.
184. Kalichman MW, Moorhouse DF, Powell HC, Myers RR. Relative neural toxicity of local anesthetics. *J Neuropathol Exp Neurol* 1993; 52:234–240.
185. Kar S, Quirion R. Quantitative autoradiographic localization of [^{125}I]neuropeptide Y receptor binding sites in rat spinal cord and the effects of neonatal capsaicin, dorsal rhizotomy and peripheral axotomy. *Brain Res* 1992;574:333–337.
186. Karlsten R, Gordh T Jr. An A1-selective adenosine agonist abolishes allodynia elicited by vibration and touch after intrathecal injection. *Anesth Analg* 1995;80:844–847.
187. Karlsten R, Gordh T, Post C. Local antinociceptive and hyperalgesic effects in the formalin test after peripheral administration of adenosine analogues in mice. *Pharmacol Toxicol* 1992;70:434–438.
188. Karlsten R, Gordh T Jr, Svensson BA. A neurotoxicologic evalua-

tion of the spinal cord after chronic intrathecal injection of R-phenylisopropyl adenosine (R-PIA) in the rat. *Anesth Analg* 1993; 1:731–736.
189. Kenakin TP. *Pharmacologic analysis of drug receptor interactions.* New York: Raven Press, 1988.
190. Khan IM, Taylor P, Yaksh TL. Stimulatory pathways and sites of action of intrathecally administered nicotinic agents. *J Pharmacol Exp Ther* 1994;271:1550–1557.
191. Khayyat GF, Yu YJ, King RB. Response patterns to noxious and non-noxious stimuli in rostral trigeminal relay nuclei. *Brain Res* 1975;97:47–60.
192. Kim SH, Chung JM. An experimental model for peripheral neuropathy produced by segmental spinal nerve ligation in the rat. *Pain* 1992;50:355–363.
193. Kim SH, Na HS, Sheen K, Chung JM. Effects of sympathectomy on a rat model of peripheral neuropathy. *Pain* 1993;55:85–92.
194. Kishimoto N, Kato J, Suzuki T, Arakawa H, Ogawa S, Suzuki H. A case of RSD with complete disappearance of symptoms following intravenous ketamine infusion combined with stellate ganglion block and continuous epidural bloc. Masui. *Jpn J Anesthesiol* 1995; 44:1680–1684.
195. Kocher L, Anton F, Reeh PW, Handwerker HO. The effect of carrageenan-induced inflammation on the sensitivity of unmyelinated skin nociceptors in the rat. *Pain* 1987;29:363–373.
196. Kocsis JD, Honmou O. Gabapentin increases GABA-induced depolarization in rat neonatal optic nerve. *Neurosci Lett* 1994;169: 181–184.
197. Kolhekar R, Meller ST, Gebhart GF. Characterization of the role of spinal N-methyl-D-aspartate receptors in thermal nociception in the rat. *Neuroscience* 1993;57:385–395.
198. Kristensen JD, Karlsten R, Gordh T, Berge OG. The NMDA antagonist 3-(2-carboxypiperazin-4-yl)propyl-1-phosphonic acid (CPP) has antinociceptive effect after intrathecal injection in the rat. *Pain,* 1994;56:59–67.
199. Kristensen JD, Post C, Gordh T Jr, Svensson BA. Spinal cord morphology and antinociception after chronic intrathecal administration of excitatory amino acid antagonists in the rat. *Pain* 1993; 54:309–316.
200. Kristensen JD, Svensson B, Gordh T Jr. The NMDA-receptor antagonist CPP abolishes neurogenic "wind-up pain" after intrathecal administration in humans. *Pain* 1992;51:249–253.
201. Kroin JS, McCarthy RJ, Penn RD, Kerns JM, Ivankovich AD. The effect of chronic subarachnoid bupivacaine infusion in dogs. *Anesthesiology* 1987;66:737–742.
202. Kuraishi Y, Hirota N, Sugimoto M, Satoh M, Takagi H. Effects of morphine on noxious stimuli-induced release of substance P from rabbit dorsal horn in vivo. *Life Sci* 1983;33:693–696.
203. Laird JMA, Rosa C. Dorsal; horn neuronal responses and nociceptive reflexes evoked by graded distention of the ureter in anesthetized rats: a model of acute visceral pain. *Soc Neruosci Abstr* 1995;21:383.
204. LaMotte RH, Lundberg LE, Torebjork HE. Pain, hyperalgesia and activity in nociceptive C units in humans after intradermal injection of capsaicin. *J Physiol* 1992;448:749–764.
205. LaMotte C, Pert CB, Snyder SH. Opiate receptor binding in primate spinal cord: distribution and changes after dorsal root section. *Brain Res* 1976;112:407–412.
206. Lang E, Novak A, Reeh PW, Handwerker HO. Chemosensitivity of fine afferents from rat skin in vitro. *J Neurophysiol* 1990;63: 887–901.
207. Le Bars D, Guilbaud G, Jurna I, Besson JM. Differential effects of morphine on responses of dorsal horn lamina V type cells elicited by A and C fibre stimulation in the spinal cat. *Brain Res* 1976;115: 518–524.
208. Lee SH, Kayser V, Desmeules J, Guilbaud G. Differential action of morphine and various opioid agonists on thermal allodynia and hyperalgesia in mononeuropathic rats. *Pain* 1994;57: 233–240.
209. Lee Y-W, Chaplan SR, Yaksh TL. Systemic and supraspinal, but not spinal, opiates suppress allodynia in a rat neuropathic pain model. *Neurosci Lett* 1995;199:111–114.
210. Lee Y-W, Yaksh TL. Analysis of drug interaction between intrathecal clonidine and MK-801 in peripheral neuropathic pain rat model. *Anesthesiology* 1995;82:741–748.
211. Lee Y-W, Yaksh TL. Pharmacology of the spinal adenosine receptor which mediates the antallodynic action of intrathecal adenosine agonists. *J Pharmacol Exp Ther* 277:1642–1648.
212. Leighton GE, Rodriguez RE, Hill RG, Hughes J. Kappa-opioid agonists produce antinociception after i.v. and i.c.v. but not intrathecal administration in the rat. *Br J Pharmacol* 1988;93:553–560.
213. Leiphart JW, Dills CV, Zikel OM, Kim DL, Levy RM. A comparison of intrathecally administered narcotic and nonnarcotic analgesics for experimental chronic neuropathic pain. *J Neurosurg* 1995;82: 595–599.
214. Levine JD, Feldmesser M, Tecott L, Gordon NC, Izdebski K. Pain-induced vocalization in the rat and its modification by pharmacological agents. *Brain Res* 1984;296:121–127.
215. Lewis T. Experiments relating to cutaneous hyperalgesia and its spread though somatic fibers. *Clin Sci* 1935;2:373–423.
216. Lichtman AH, Smith FL, Martin BR. Evidence that the antinociceptive tail-flick response is produced independently from changes in either tail-skin temperature or core temperature. *Pain* 1993;55:283–295.
217. Lim RK. Pain. *Annu Rev Physiol* 1970;32:269–288.
218. Liu H, Wang H, Sheng M, Jan LY, Jan YN, Basbaum AI. Evidence for presynaptic N-methyl-D-aspartate autoreceptors in the spinal cord dorsal horn. *Proc Natl Acad Sci USA* 1994;91:8383—8387.
219. Llorens-Cortes C, Gros C, Schwartz JC, Clot AM, Le Bars D. Changes in levels of the tripeptide Tyr-Gly-Gly as an index of enkephalin release in the spinal cord: effects of noxious stimuli and parenterally active peptidase inhibitors. *Peptides* 1989;10:609–614.
220. Long JB. Spinal subarachnoid injection of somatostatin causes neurological deficits and neuronal injury in rats. *Eur J Pharmacol* 1988;149:287–296.
221. Long JB, Martinez-Arizala A, Echevarria EE, Tidwell RE, Holaday JW. Hindlimb paralytic effects of prodynorphin-derived peptides following spinal subarachnoid injection in rats. *Eur J Pharmacol* 1988;153:45–54.
222. Long JB, Martinez-Arizala A, Rigamonti DD, Holaday JW. Hindlimb paralytic effects of arginine vasopressin and related peptides following spinal subarachnoid injection in the rat. *Peptides* 1988;9:1335–1344.
223. Long JB, Petras JM, Holaday JW. Neurologic deficits and neuronal injury in rats resulting from nonopioid actions of the delta opioid receptor antagonist ICI 174864. *J Pharmacol Exp Ther* 1988;244: 1169–1177.
224. Loux JJ, Smith S, Salem H. Comparative analgetic testing of various compounds in mice using writhing techniques. *Arzneimittelforschung* 1978;28:1644–1647.
225. Lund JP, Lamarre Y, Lavigne G, Duquet G. Human jaw reflexes. *Adv Neurol* 1983;39:739–755.
226. Luttinger D. Determination of antinociceptive efficacy of drugs in mice using different water temperatures in a tail-immersion test. *J Pharmacol Methods* 1985;13:351–357.
227. Luttinger D, Ferrari R, Perrone MH, Haubrich DR. Pharmacological analysis of alpha-2 adrenergic mechanisms in nociception and ataxia. *J Pharmacol Exp Ther* 1985;232:883–889.
228. Madsen JB, Jensen FM, Faber T, Bille-Hansen V. Chronic catheterization of the epidural space in rabbits: a model for behavioural and histopathological studies. Examination of meptazinol neurotoxicity. *Acta Anaesthesiol Scand* 1993;37:307–313.
229. Maixner W, Dubner R, Bushnell MC, Kenshalo DR Jr, Oliveras JL. Wide-dynamic-range dorsal horn neurons participate in the encoding process by which monkeys perceive the intensity of noxious heat stimuli. *Brain Res* 1986 374:385–388.
230. Maixner W, Dubner R, Kenshalo DR Jr, Bushnell MC, Oliveras JL. Responses of monkey medullary dorsal horn neurons during the detection of noxious heat stimuli. *J Neurophysiol* 1989;62: 437–449.
231. Malinovsky JM, Cozian A, Lepage JY, Mussini JM, Pinaud M, Souron R. Ketamine and midazolam neurotoxicity in the rabbit. *Anesthesiology* 1991;75:91–97.
232. Malinovsky JM, Lepage JY, Cozian A, Mussini JM, Pinaudt M, Souron R. Is ketamine or its preservative responsible for neurotoxicity in the rabbit? *Anesthesiology* 1993;78:109–115.
233. Malmberg AB, Yaksh TL. Antinociceptive actions of spinal nonsteroidal anti-inflammatory agents on the formalin test in the rat. *J Pharmacol Exp Ther* 1992;263:136–146.
234. Malmberg AB, Yaksh TL. Hyperalgesia mediated by spinal glutamate or substance P receptor blocked by spinal cyclooxygenase inhibition. *Science* 1992;257:1276–1279.
235. Malmberg AB, Yaksh TL. Isobolographic and dose-response analyses of the interaction between intrathecal mu and delta agonists: effects of naltrindole and its benzofuran analog (NTB). *J Pharmacol Exp Ther* 1992;263:264–275.
236. Malmberg AB, Yaksh TL. Spinal nitric oxide synthesis inhibition

blocks NMDA-induced thermal hyperalgesia and produces antinociception in the formalin test in rats. *Pain* 1993;54:291–300.
237. Malmberg AB, Yaksh TL. Pharmacology of the spinal action of ketorolac, morphine, ST-91, U50488H, and L-PIA on the formalin test and an isobolographic analysis of the NSAID interaction. *Anesthesiology* 1993;79:270–281.
238. Malmberg AM, Yaksh TL. Spinal actions of non-steroidal anti-inflammatory drugs: evidence for a central role of prostanoids in nociceptive processing. In: *Progress in pharmacology and clinical pharmacology, vol. 10.* New York: Gustav Fischer Verlag, 1993: 91–110.
239. Malmberg AB, Yaksh TL. Voltage-sensitive calcium channels in spinal nociceptive processing: blockade of N- and P-type channels inhibits formalin-induced nociception. *J Neurosci* 1994;14: 4882–4890.
240. Malmberg AB, Yaksh TL. Effect of continuous intrathecal infusion of omega-conopeptides, N-type calcium-channel blockers, on behavior and antinociception in the formalin and hot-plate tests in rats. *Pain* 1995;60:83–90.
241. Malmberg AB, Yaksh TL. Cyclooxygenase inhibition and the spinal release of prostaglandin E2 and amino acids evoked by paw formalin injection: a microdialysis study in unanesthetized rats. *J Neurosci* 1995;15:2768–2776.
242. Malmberg AB, Yaksh TL, Calcutt NA. Anti-nociceptive effects of the GM1 ganglioside derivative AGF 44 on the formalin test in normal and streptozotocin-diabetic rats. *Neurosci Lett* 1993;161: 45–48.
243. Mao J, Price DD, Hayes RL, Lu J, Mayer DJ. Differential roles of NMDA and non-NMDA receptor activation in induction and maintenance of thermal hyperalgesia in rats with painful peripheral mononeuropathy. *Brain Res* 1992;598:271–278.
244. Mao J, Price DD, Hayes RL, Lu J, Mayer DJ, Frenk H. Intrathecal treatment with dextrorphan or ketamine potently reduces pain-related behaviors in a rat model of peripheral mononeuropathy. *Brain Res* 1993;605:164–168.
245. Marchettini P, Lacerenza M, Marangoni C, Pellegata G, Sotgiu ML, Smirne S. Lidocaine test in neuralgia. *Pain* 1992;48:377–382.
246. Marsala M, Yaksh TL. Transient spinal ischemia in the rat: characterization of behavioral and histopathological consequences as a function of the duration of aortic occlusion. *J Cereb Blood Flow Metab* 1994;14:526–535.
247. Marsala M, Yang L, Lee H, Yaksh, TL. Spinal glutamate release displays a delayed, but persistent elevation after peripheral nerve injury in the rat [Abstract]. Presented at the IASP, Vancouver, 1996.
248. Mathisen LC, Skjelbred P, Skoglund LA, Oye I. Effect of ketamine, an NMDA receptor inhibitor, in acute and chronic orofacial pain. *Pain* 1995;61:215–220.
249. McLachlan EM, Janig W, Devor M, Michaelis M. Peripheral nerve injury triggers noradrenergic sprouting within the dorsal root ganglia. *Nature* 1993;363:543–546.
250. McLean BN. Intrathecal baclofen in severe spasticity. *Br J Hosp Med* 1993;49:262–267.
251. McMahon SB. Neuronal and behavioural consequences of chemical inflammation of rat urinary bladder. *Agents Actions* 1988;25: 231–233.
252. McMahon SB, Abel C. A model for the study of visceral pain states: chronic inflammation of the chronic decerebrate rat urinary bladder by irritant chemicals. *Pain* 1987;28:109–127.
253. McMahon SB, Priestley JV. Peripheral neuropathies and neurotrophic factors: animal models and clinical perspectives. *Curr Opin Neurobiol* 1995;5:616–624.
254. Meller ST, Cummings CP, Traub RJ, Gebhart GF. The role of nitric oxide in the development and maintenance of the hyperalgesia produced by intraplantar injection of carrageenan in the rat. *Neuroscience* 1994;60:367–374.
255. Meller ST, Pechman PS, Gebhart GF, Maves TJ. Nitric oxide mediates the thermal hyperalgesia produced in a model of neuropathic pain in the rat. *Neuroscience* 1992;50:7–10.
256. Mellick GA, Mellicy LB, Mellick LB. Gabapentin in the management of reflex sympathetic dystrophy [letter]. *J Pain Symptom Manage* 1995;10:265–266.
257. Mendell LM, Wall PD. Responses of single dorsal cord cells to peripheral cutaneous unmyelinated fibers. *Nature* 1965;206:97–99.
258. Mercadante S, Lodi F, Sapio M, Calligara M, Serretta R. Long-term ketamine subcutaneous continuous infusion in neuropathic cancer pain. *J Pain Symptom Manage* 1995;10:564–568.
259. Miletic V, Randic M. Neurotensin excites cat spinal neurones located in laminae I–III. *Brain Res* 1979;169:600–604.
260. Mjanger E, Yaksh TL. Characteristics of the dose dependent antagonism by b-funaltrexamine of the antinociceptive effects of intrathecal mu agonists. *J Pharmacol Exp Ther* 1991;258:544–550.
261. Moiniche S, Dahl JB, Kehlet H. Time course of primary and secondary hyperalgesia after heat injury to the skin. *Br J Anaesth* 1994; 71:201–205.
262. Mollenholt P, Post C, Rawal N, Freedman J, Hokfelt T, Paulsson I. Antinociceptive and "neurotoxic" actions of somatostatin in rat spinal cord after intrathecal administration. *Pain* 1988;32:95–105.
263. Mollenholt P, Rawal N, Gordh T Jr, Olsson Y. Intrathecal and epidural somatostatin for patients with cancer. Analgesic effects and postmortem neuropathologic investigations of spinal cord and nerve roots. *Anesthesiology* 1994;81:534–542.
264. Moore PK, Oluyomi AO, Babbedge RC, Wallace P, Hart SL. L-NG-nitro arginine methyl ester exhibits antinociceptive activity in the mouse. *Br J Pharmacol* 1991;102:198–202.
265. Morris BJ, Herz A. Distinct distribution of opioid receptor types in rat lumbar spinal cord. *Naunyn Schmiedebergs Arch Pharmacol* 1987; 336:240–243.
266. Moulin DE, Max MB, Kaiko RF, et al. The analgesic efficacy of intrathecal D-Ala2-D-Leu5-enkephalin in cancer patients with chronic pain. *Pain* 1985;23:213–221.
267. Mushlin BE, Grell R, Cochin J. Studies on tolerance. I. The role of the interval between doses on the development of tolerance to morphine. *J Pharmacol Exp Ther* 1976;196:280–287.
268. Myslinski NR, Randic M. Responses of identified spinal neurones to acetylcholine applied by micro-electrophoresis. *J Physiol* 1977; 269:195–219.
269. Na HS, Leem JW, Chung JM. Abnormalities of mechanoreceptors in a rat model of neuropathic pain: possible involvement in mediating mechanical allodynia. *J Neurophysiol* 1993;70:522–528.
270. Nagaro T, Shimizu C, Inoue H, et al. The efficacy of intravenous lidocaine on various types of neuropathic pain. Masui. *Jpn J Anesthesiol* 1995;44:862–867.
271. Nagasaka H, Awad H, Yaksh TL. Peripheral and spinal actions of opioids in the blockade of the autonomic response evoked by compression of the inflamed knee joint. *Anesthesiology* 1996,85: 808–816.
272. Naguib M, Yaksh TL. Antinociceptive effects of spinal cholinesterase inhibition and isobolographic analysis of the interaction with mu and alpha 2 receptor systems. *Anesthesiology* 1994; 80:1338–1348.
273. Nagy JI, Vincent SR, Staines WA, Fibiger HC, Reisine TD, Yamamura HI. Neurotoxic action of capsaicin on spinal substance P neurons. *Brain Res* 1980;186:435–444.
274. Nasstrom J, Karlsson U, Post C. Antinociceptive actions of different classes of excitatory amino acid receptor antagonists in mice. *Eur J Pharmacol* 1992 212:21–29.
275. Neil A, Attal N, Guilbaud G. Effects of guanethidine on sensitization to natural stimuli and self-mutilating behaviour in rats with a peripheral neuropathy. *Brain Res* 1991;565:237–246.
276. Ness TJ, Gebhart GF. Centrifugal modulation of the rat tail flick reflex evoked by graded noxious heating of the tail. *Brain Res* 1986;386:41–52.
277. Ness TJ, Gebhart GF. Characterization of neuronal responses to noxious visceral and somatic stimuli in the medial lumbosacral spinal cord of the rat. *J Neurophysiol* 1987;57:1867–1892.
278. Ness TJ, Gebhart GF. Quantitative comparison of inhibition of visceral and cutaneous spinal nociceptive transmission from the midbrain and medulla in the rat. *J Neurophysiol* 1987;58:850–865.
279. Ness TJ, Gebhart GF. Characterization of neurons responsive to noxious colorectal distension in the T13-L2 spinal cord of the rat. *J Neurophysiol* 1988;60:1419–1438.
280. Ness TJ, Gebhart GF. Colorectal dissension as a noxious visceral stimulus: physiologic and pharmacologic characterization of pseudaffective reflexes in the rat. *Brain Res* 1988;450:153–169.
281. Ness TJ, Gebhart GF. Visceral pain: a review of experimental studies. *Pain* 1990;41:167–234.
282. Ness TJ, Jones SL, Gebhart GF. Contribution of the site of heating to variability in the latency of the rat tail flick reflex. *Brain Res* 1987;426:169–172.
283. Neugebauer V, Geisslinger G, Rumenapp P, et al. Antinociceptive effects of R(-)- and S(+)-flurbiprofen on rat spinal dorsal horn neurons rendered hyperexcitable by an acute knee joint inflammation. *J Pharmacol Exp Ther* 1995;275:618–628.

284. Neugebauer V, Lucke T, Schaible HG. N-methyl-D-aspartate (NMDA) and non-NMDA receptor antagonists block the hyperexcitability of dorsal horn neurons during development of acute arthritis in rat's knee joint. *J Neurophysiol* 1993;70:1365–1377.
285. Neugebauer V, Weiretter F, Schaible HG. Involvement of substance P and neurokinin-1 receptors in the hyperexcitability of dorsal horn neurons during development of acute arthritis in rat's knee joint. *J Neurophysiol* 1995;73:1574–1583.
286. Nolan A, Livingston A, Waterman A. Antinociceptive actions of intravenous alpha 2-adrenoceptor agonists in sheep. *J Vet Pharmacol Ther* 1987;10:202–209.
287. O'Callaghan JP, Holtzman SG. Quantification of the analgesic activity of narcotic antagonists by a modified hot-plate procedure. *J Pharmacol Exp Ther* 1975;192:497–505.
288. O'Connor TC, Abram SE. Halothane enhances suppression of spinal sensitization by intrathecal morphine in the rat formalin test. *Anesthesiology* 1994;81:1277–1283.
289. Ohkubo T, Shibata M, Takahashi H, Inoki R. Roles of substance P and somatostatin on transmission of nociceptive information induced by formalin in spinal cord. *J Pharmacol Exp Ther* 1990;252: 1261–1268.
290. Okuda K, Nakahama H, Miyakawa H, Shima K. Arthritis induced in cat by sodium urate: a possible animal model for tonic pain. *Pain* 19984;18:287–297.
291. Oliveras JL, Maixner W, Dubner R, et al. The medullary dorsal horn: a target for the expression of opiate effects on the perceived intensity of noxious heat. *J Neurosci* 1986;6:3086–3093.
292. Ono H, Mishima A, Ono S, Fukuda H, Vasko MR. Inhibitory effects of clonidine and tizanidine on release of substance P from slices of rat spinal cord and antagonism by alpha-adrenergic receptor antagonists. *Neuropharmacology* 1991;30:585–589.
293. Onofrio BM, Yaksh TL. Intrathecal delta-receptor ligand produces analgesia in man. *Lancet* 1983;1:1386–1387.
294. Onofrio BM, Yaksh TL. Long-term pain relief produced by intrathecal morphine infusion in 53 patients. *J Neurosurg* 1990;72: 200–209.
295. Oshita S, Yaksh TL, Chipkin R. The antinociceptive effects of intrathecally administered SCH32615, an enkephalinase inhibitor in the rat. *Brain Res* 1990;515:143–148.
296. Otterness IG, Gans DJ. Nonsteroidal anti-inflammatory drugs: an analysis of the relationship between laboratory animal and clinical doses, including species scaling. *J Pharm Sci* 1988;77:790–795.
297. Owens CM, Zhang D, Willis WD. Changes in the response states of primate spinothalamic tract cells caused by mechanical damage of the skin or activation of descending controls. *J Neurophysiol* 1992; 67:1509–1527.
298. Pascual J, del Arco C, Gonzalez AM, Pazos A. Quantitative light microscopic autoradiographic localization of alpha 2-receptors in the human brain. *Brain Res* 1992;585:116–127.
299. Payne R, Madsen J, Harvey RC, Inturrisi CE. A chronic sheep preparation for the study of drug pharmacokinetics in spinal and ventricular CSF. *J Pharmacol Methods* 1986;16:277–296.
300. Pazos A, Cortés R, Palacios JM. Quantitative autoradiographic mapping of serotonin receptors in the rat brain. I & II. Serotonin-2 receptors. *Brain Res* 1985;346:205–249.
300a. Pazos A, Palacios JM. Quantitative autoradiographic mapping of seratonin receptors in the rat brain. I. seratonin-1 receptors. *Brain Research*, 1985;346:205–230.
301. Pelissier T, Paeile C, Soto-Moyano R, Saavedra H, Hernandez A. Analgesia produced by intrathecal administration of the kappa opioid agonist, U-50,488H, on formalin-evoked cutaneous pain in the rat. *Eur J Pharmacol* 1990;190:287–293.
302. Penn RD, Paice JA, Kroin JS. Octreotide: a potent new non-opiate analgesic for intrathecal infusion. *Pain* 1992;49:13–19.
303. Penning J, Yaksh TL. Interaction of intrathecal morphine with bupivacaine and lidocaine in the rat. *Anesthesiology* 1992;77: 1186–1200.
304. Perrot S, Attal N, Ardid D, Guilbaud G. Are mechanical and cold allodynia in mononeuropathic and arthritic rats relieved by systemic treatment with calcitonin or guanethidine? *Pain* 1993;52: 41–47.
305. Persson J, Axelsson G, Hallin RG, Gustafsson LL. Beneficial effects of ketamine in a chronic pain state with allodynia, possibly due to central sensitization. *Pain* 1995;60:217–222.
306. Pert A, Yaksh T. Sites of morphine induced analgesia in the primate brain: relation to pain pathways. *Brain Res* 1974;80:135–140.
307. Picard P, Boucher S, Regoli D, Gitter BD, Howbert JJ, Couture R. Use of non-peptide tachykinin receptor antagonists to substantiate the involvement of NK1 and NK2 receptors in a spinal nociceptive reflex in the rat. *Eur J Pharmacol* 1993;232:255–261.
308. Piercey MF, Schroeder LA. A quantitative analgesic assay in the rabbit based on the response to tooth pulp stimulation. *Arch Int Pharmacodyn Ther* 1980;248:294–304.
309. Portenoy RK. Cancer pain management. *Semin Oncol* 1993;20: 19–35.
310. Portenoy RK. Pharmacologic management of cancer pain. *Semin Oncol* 1995;22:112–120.
311. Powell HC, Kalichman MW, Garrett RS, Myers RR. Selective vulnerability of unmyelinated fiber Schwann cells in nerves exposed to local anesthetics. *Lab Invest* 1988;59:271–280.
312. Price DD, Mao J, Frenk H, Mayer DJ. The N-methyl-D-aspartate receptor antagonist dextromethorphan selectively reduces temporal summation of second pain. *Pain* 1994;59:165–174.
313. Price DD, McHaffie JG. Effects of heterotopic conditioning stimuli on first and second pain: a psychophysical evaluation in humans. *Pain* 1988;34:245–252.
314. Price GW, Kelly JS, Bowery NG. The location of GABAB receptor binding sites in mammalian spinal cord. *Synapse* 1987;1:530–538.
315. Punto L. Lumbar leptomeningeal and radicular reactions after the subarachnoid injection of water-soluble contrast media, meglumine iocarmate (dimer-Xr) and metrizamide (amipaquer). An experimental study in the pig. *Acta Vet Scand Suppl* 1980:1–47.
316. Raja SN, Meyer RA, Campbell JN. Peripheral mechanisms of somatic pain. *Anesthesiology* 1988;68:571–90.
317. Randall LO, Selitto, JJ. A method for measurement of analgesic activity on inflamed tissue. *Arch Int Pharmacodyn Ther* 1957;111: 409–419.
318. Rawal N, Nuutinen L, Raj PP, et al. Behavioral and histopathologic effects following intrathecal administration of butorphanol, sufentanil, and nalbuphine in sheep. *Anesthesiology* 1991;75: 1025–1034.
319. Reis DJ, Fuxe K. Depletion of noradrenaline in brainstem neurons during sham rage behaviour produced by acute brainstem transection in cat. *Brain Res* 1968;7:448–451.
320. Ren K, Hylden JL, Williams GM, Ruda MA, Dubner R. The effects of a non-competitive NMDA receptor antagonist, MK-801, on behavioral hyperalgesia and dorsal horn neuronal activity in rats with unilateral inflammation. *Pain* 1992;50:331–344.
321. Ren K, Williams GM, Hylden JL, Ruda MA, Dubner R. The intrathecal administration of excitatory amino acid receptor antagonists selectively attenuated carrageenan-induced behavioral hyperalgesia in rats. *Eur J Pharmacol* 1992;219:235–243.
322. Rice AS. Topical spinal administration of a nitric oxide synthase inhibitor prevents the hyper-reflexia associated with a rat model of persistent visceral pain. *Neurosci Lett* 1995;187:111–114.
323. Rice AS, McMahon SB. Pre-emptive intrathecal administration of an NMDA receptor antagonist (AP-5) prevents hyper-reflexia in a model of persistent visceral pain. *Pain* 1994;57:335–340.
324. Rigler ML, Drasner K, Krejcie TC, et al. Cauda equina syndrome after continuous spinal anesthesia. *Anesth Analg* 1991;72:275–281.
325. Rock DM, Kelly KM, MacDonald RL. Gabapentin actions on ligand- and voltage-gated responses in cultured rodent neurons. *Epilepsy Res* 1993;16:89–98.
326. Ross BK, Coda B, Heath CH. Local anesthetic distribution in a spinal model: a possible mechanism of neurologic injury after continuous spinal anesthesia. *Reg Anesth* 1992;17:69–77.
327. Rowbotham MC, Reisner-Keller LA, Fields HL. Both intravenous lidocaine and morphine reduce the pain of postherpetic neuralgia. *Neurology* 1991;41:1024–1028.
328. Roza C, Laird JM. Pressor responses to distension of the ureter in anaesthetised rats: characterisation of a model of acute visceral pain. *Neurosci Lett* 1995;198:9–12.
329. Ruffolo RR. Review: important concepts of receptor theory. *J Auton Pharmacol* 1982;2:277–295.
330. Sabbe MB, Grafe MR, Mjanger E, Tiseo PJ, Hill HF, Yaksh TL. Spinal delivery of sufentanil, alfentanil, and morphine in dogs. Physiologic and toxicologic investigations. *Anesthesiology* 1994;81: 899–920.
331. Sabbe MB, Grafe MR, Pfeifer BL, Mirzai THM, Yaksh TL. Toxicology of baclofen continuously infused into the spinal intrathecal space of the dog. *Neurotoxicology* 1993;14:397–410.
332. Sabbe MB, Penning JP, Ozaki GT, Yaksh TL. Spinal and systemic action of the $\alpha 2$ receptor agonist dexmedetomidine in dogs.

Antinociception and carbon dioxide response. *Anesthesiology* 1994; 80:1057–1072.
333. Saeki S, Yaksh TL. Suppression by spinal alpha-2 agonists of motor and autonomic responses evoked by low- and high-intensity thermal stimuli. *J Pharmacol Exp Ther* 1992;260:795–802.
334. Saeki S, Yaksh TL. Suppression of nociceptive responses by spinal mu opioid agonists: effects of stimulus intensity and agonist efficacy. *Anesth Analg* 1993;77:265–274.
335. Sahley TL, Berntson GG. Antinociceptive effects of central and systemic administrations of nicotine in the rat. *Psychopharmacology* 1979;65:279–283.
336. Salter MW, Henry JL. Evidence that adenosine mediates the depression of spinal dorsal horn induced by peripheral vibration in the cat. *Neuroscience* 1987;22:631–650.
337. Samuelsson H, Hedner T. Pain characterization in cancer patients and the analgetic response to epidural morphine. *Pain* 1991;46: 3–8.
338. Samuelsson H, Malmberg F, Eriksson M, Hedner T. Outcomes of epidural morphine treatment in cancer pain: nine years of clinical experience. *J Pain Symptom Manage* 1995;10:105–112.
339. Santicioli P, Del Bianco E, Maggi CA. Adenosine A1 receptors mediate the presynaptic inhibition of calcitonin gene-related peptide release by adenosine in the rat spinal cord. *Eur J Pharmacol* 1993;231:139–142.
340. Santicioli P, Del Bianco E, Tramontana M, Maggi CA. Adenosine inhibits action potential-dependent release of calcitonin gene-related peptide- and substance P-like immunoreactivities from primary afferents in rat spinal cord. *Neurosci Lett* 1992;144:211–214.
341. Saria A, Javorsky F, Humpel C, Gamse R. 5-HT receptor antagonism inhibit sensory neuropeptide release from the rat spinal cord. *Neuroreport* 1990;1:104–106.
342. Sato A, Sato Y, Schmidt RF. Catecholamine secretion and adrenal nerve activity in response to movements of normal and inflamed knee joints in cats. *J Physiol* 1986;375:611–624.
343. Sawynok J, Dickson C. Involvement of GABA in the antinociceptive effect of gamma-acetylenic GABA (GAG), an inhibitor of GABA-transaminase. *Gen Pharmacol* 1983;14:603–607.
344. Sawynok J, Sweeney MI. The role of purines in nociception. *Neuroscience* 1989;32:557–569.
345. Sawynok J, Sweeney MI, White TD. Classification of adenosine receptors mediating antinociception in the rat spinal cord. *Br J Pharmacol* 1986;88:923–930.
346. Schaible HG, Grubb BD. Afferent and spinal mechanisms of joint pain. *Pain* 1993;55:5–54.
347. Schaible HG, Jarrott B, Hope PJ, Duggan AW. Release of immunoreactive substance P in the spinal cord during development of acute arthritis in the knee joint of the cat: a study with antibody microprobes. *Brain Res* 1990;529:214–223.
348. Schaible HG, Schmidt RF. Time course of mechanosensitivity changes in articular afferents during a developing experimental arthritis. *J Neurophysiol* 1988;60:2180–2195.
349. Schmauss C, Yaksh TL. In vivo studies on spinal opiate receptor systems mediating antinociception. II. Pharmacological profiles suggesting a differential association of mu, delta and kappa receptors with visceral chemical and cutaneous thermal stimuli in the rat. *J Pharmacol Exp Ther* 1983;228:1–12.
350. Schneider MC, Hampl KF, Kaufmann M. Transient neurologic toxicity after subarachnoid anesthesia with hyperbaric 5% lidocaine. *Anesth Analg* 1994;79:610.
351. Schneider SP, Perl ER. Selective excitation of neurones in the mammalian spinal dorsal horn by aspartate and glutamate in vitro: correlation with location and excitatory input. *Brain Res* 1985;360:339–343.
352. Seguin L, Le Marouille-Girardon S, Millan MJ. Antinociceptive profiles of non-peptidergic neurokinin1 and neurokinin2 receptor antagonists: a comparison to other classes of antinociceptive agent. *Pain* 1995;61:325–343.
353. Sengupta JN, Gebhart GF. Characterization of mechanosensitive pelvic nerve afferent fibers innervating the colon of the rat. *J Neurophysiol* 1994;71:2046–2060.
354. Serrao JM, Stubbs SC, Goodchild CS, Gent JP. Intrathecal midazolam and fentanyl in the rat: evidence for different spinal antinociceptive effects *Anesthesiology* 1989;70:780–786.
355. Sessle BJ, Hu JW. Raphe-induced suppression of the jaw-opening reflex and single neurons in trigeminal subnucleus oralis, and influence of naloxone and subnucleus caudalis. *Pain* 1981;10:19–36.
356. Sewell RD, Gonzalez JP, Pugh J. Comparison of the relative effects of aspirin, mefenamic acid, dihydrocodeine, dextropropoxyphene and paracetamol on visceral pain, respiratory rate and prostaglandin biosynthesis. *Arch Int Pharmacodyn Ther* 1984;268: 325–334.
357. Sheen K, Chung JM. Signs of neuropathic pain depend on signals from injured nerve fibers in a rat model. *Brain Res* 1993;610: 62–68.
358. Sherman SE, Loomis CW. Morphine insensitive allodynia is produced by intrathecal strychnine in the lightly anesthetized rat. *Pain* 1994;56:17–29.
359. Shir Y, Seltzer Z. A-fibers mediate mechanical hyperesthesia and allodynia and C-fibers mediate thermal hyperalgesia in a new model of causalgia from pain disorders in rats. *Neurosci Lett* 1990; 115:62–67.
360. Shir Y, Seltzer Z. Effects of sympathectomy in a model of causalgiform pain produced by partial sciatic nerve injury in rats. *Pain* 1991;45:309–320.
361. Singer E, Placheta P. Reduction of 3H-muscimol binding sites in rat dorsal spinal cord after neonatal capsaicin treatment. *Brain Res* 1980;202:484–487.
362. Sivilotti LG, Thompson SW, Woolf CJ. Rate of rise of the cumulative depolarization evoked by repetitive stimulation of small-caliber afferents is a predictor of action potential windup in rat spinal neurons in vitro. *J Neurophysiol* 1993;69:1621–1631.
363. Sivilotti LG, Woolf CJ. The contribution of GABAA and glycine receptors to central sensitization: disinhibition and touch-evoked allodynia in the spinal cord. *J Neurophysiol* 1994;72:169–179.
364. Sjoberg M, Appelgren L, Einarsson S, et al. Long-term intrathecal morphine and bupivacaine in "refractory" cancer pain I. Results from the first series of 52 patients. *Acta Anaesth Scand* 1991;35: 30–43.
365. Skingle M, Hayes AG, Tyers MB. Antinociceptive activity of clonidine in the mouse, rat and dog. *Life Sci* 1982;31:1123–1132.
366. Skingle M, Tyers MB. Further studies on opiate receptors that mediate antinoception: tooth pulp stimulation in the dog. *Br J Pharmacol* 1980;70:323–327.
367. Sluka KA, Rees H, Westlund KN, Willis WD. Fiber types contributing to dorsal root reflexes induced by joint inflammation in cats and monkeys. *J Neurophysiol* 1995;74:981–989.
368. Smith GD, Harrison SM, Wiseman J, Elliott PJ, Birch PJ. Pre-emptive administration of clonidine prevents development of hyperalgesia to mechanical stimuli in a model of mononeuropathy in the rat. *Brain Res* 1993;632:16–20.
369. Smith TW, Buchan P, Parsons DN, Wilkinson S. Peripheral antinociceptive effects of N-methyl morphine. *Life Sci* 1982;31: 1205–1208.
370. Smith TW, Follenfant RL, Ferreira SH. Antinociceptive models displaying peripheral opioid activity. International. *J Tissue Reactions* 1985;7:61–67.
371. Snyder R, Hui G, Flugstad P, Viarengo C. More cases of possible neurologic toxicity associated with single subarachnoid injections of 5% hyperbaric lidocaine. *Anesth Analg* 1994;78:411.
372. Sorkin LS, Westlund KN, Sluka KA, Dougherty PM, Willis WD. Neural changes in acute arthritis in monkeys. IV. Time-course of amino acid release into the lumbar dorsal horn. *Brain Res Brain Res Rev* 1992;17:39–50.
373. Sosnowski M, Stevens CW, Yaksh TL. Assessment of the role of A1/A2 adenosine receptors mediating the purine antinociception, motor and autonomic function in the rat spinal cord. *J Pharmacol Exp Ther* 1989;250:915–922.
374. Sosnowski M, Yaksh TL. Role of spinal adenosine receptors in modulating the hyperesthesia produced by spinal glycine receptor antagonism. *Anesth Analg* 1989;69:587–592.
375. Sosnowski M, Yaksh TL. Differential cross-tolerance between intrathecal morphine and sufentanil in the rat. *Anesthesiology* 1990; 73:1141–1147.
376. Stanfa LC, Dickenson AH. Electrophysiological studies on the spinal roles of endogenous opioids in carrageenan inflammation. *Pain* 1994;56:185–191.
377. Stanfa LC, Dickenson AH. Enhanced alpha-2 adrenergic controls and spinal morphine potency in inflammation. *Neuroreport* 1994;5: 469–472.
378. Stanfa LC, Sullivan AF, Dickenson AH. Alterations in neuronal excitability and the potency of spinal mu, delta and kappa opioids after carrageenan-induced inflammation. *Pain* 1992;50: 345–354.
379. Stein C, Millan MJ, Herz A. Unilateral inflammation of the hind-

paw in rats as a model of prolonged noxious stimulation: alterations in behavior and nociceptive thresholds. *Pharmacol Biochem Behav* 1988;31:455–451.

380. Stein C, Millan MJ, Shippenberg TS, Peter K, Herz A. Peripheral opioid receptors mediating antinociception in inflammation. Evidence for involvement of mu, delta and kappa receptors. *J Pharmacol Exp Ther* 1989;248:1269–1275.
381. Stevens CW, Yaksh TL. Dynorphin A and related peptides administered intrathecally in the rat: a search for putative κ opiate receptor activity. *J Pharmacol Exp Ther* 1986;238:833–838.
382. Stevens CW, Yaksh TL. Potency of infused spinal antinociceptive agents is inversely related to magnitude of tolerance after continuous infusion. *J Pharmacol Exp Ther* 1989;250:1–8.
383. Stevens RA, Petty RH, Hill HF, et al. Redistribution of sufentanil to cerebrospinal fluid and systemic circulation after epidural administration in dogs. *Anesth Analg* 1993;76:323–327.
384. Sugimoto T, Bennett GJ, Kajander KC. Transsynaptic degeneration in the superficial dorsal horn after sciatic nerve injury: effects of a chronic constriction injury, transection, and strychnine. *Pain* 1990;42:205–213.
385. Sullivan AF, Dickenson AH, Roques BP. Delta-opioid mediated inhibitions of acute and prolonged noxious-evoked responses in rat dorsal horn neurones. *Br J Pharmacol* 1989;98:1039–1049.
386. Suman-Chauhan N, Webdale L, Hill DR, Woodruff GN. Characterization of [^{3}H]gabapentin binding to a novel site in rat brain: homogenate binding studies. *Eur J of Pharmacol* 1993;244:293–301.
387. Surmeier DJ, Honda CN, Willis WD. Responses of primate spinothalamic neurons to noxious thermal stimulation of glabrous and hairy skin. *J Neurophysiol* 1986;56:328–350.
388. Svensson BA, Sottile A, Gordh T Jr. Studies on the development of tolerance and potential spinal neurotoxicity after chronic intrathecal carbachol-antinociception in the rat. *Acta Anaesthesiol Scand* 1991;35:141.
389. Swenzen GO, Chakrabarti MK, Sapsed-Byrne S, Whitwam JG. Selective depression by alfentanil of group III and IV somatosympathetic reflexes in the dog. *Br J Anaesthes* 1988;61:441–445.
390. Taiwo YO, Coderre TJ, Levine JD. The contribution of training to sensitivity in the nociceptive paw-withdrawal test. *Brain Res* 1989; 487:148–151.
391. Takano Y, Yaksh TL. Relative efficacy of spinal alpha-2 agonists, dexmedetomidine, clonidine and ST-91, determined in vivo by using N-ethoxycarbonyl-2-ethoxy-1,2-dihydroquinoline, an irreversible antagonist. *J Pharmacol Exp Ther* 1991;258:438–446.
392. Takano Y, Yaksh TL. Characterization of the pharmacology of intrathecally administered alpha-2 agonists and antagonists in rats. *J Pharmacol Exper Ther* 1992;261:764–772.
393. Takano Y, Yaksh TL. Chronic spinal infusion of dexmedetomidine, ST-91 and clonidine: spinal alpha 2 adrenoceptor subtypes and intrinsic activity. *J Pharmacol Exp Ther* 1993;264:327–335.
394. Tal M. The threshold for eliciting the jaw opening reflex in rats is not increased by neonatal capsaicin. *Behav Brain Res* 1984;13: 197–200.
395. Tiseo PJ, Adler MW, Liu-Chen LY. Differential release of substance P and somatostatin in the rat spinal cord in response to noxious cold and heat; effect of dynorphin A(1-17). *J Pharmacol Exp Ther* 1990;252:539–545.
396. Todd AJ, McKenzie J. GABA-immunoreactive neurons in the dorsal horn of the spinal cord. *Neuroscience* 1989;31:799–806.
397. Todd AJ, Sullivan AC. Light microscopic study of the coexistence of GABA-Like and glycine-like immunoreactivities in the spinal cord of the rat. *J Comp Neurol* 1990;296:496–505.
398. Todd AJ, Watt C, Spike RC, Sieghart W. Colocalization of GABA, glycine, and their receptors at synapses in the rat spinal cord. *J Neurosci* 1996;16:974–982.
399. Torebjork HE, Lundberg LE, LaMotte RH. Central changes in processing of mechanoreceptive input in capsaicin-induced secondary hyperalgesia in humans. *J Physiol* 1992; 448:765–780.
400. Tsuruoka M, Matsui A, Matsui Y. Quantitative relationship between the stimulus intensity and the response magnitude in the tail flick reflex. *Physiol Behav* 1988;143:79–83.
401. Tyers MB. A classification of opiate receptors that mediate antinociception in animals. *Br J Pharmacol* 1980;69:503–512.
402. Vasko MR, Cartwright S, Ono H. Adenosine agonists do not inhibit the K^+ stimulated release of substance P from rat spinal cord slices. *Soc Neurosci Abstr* 1986;12:799.
403. Vierck CJ, Cooper BY, Franzen O, Ritz LA, Greenspan JD. Behavioral analysis of CNS pathways and transmitter systems involved in conduction and inhibition of pain sensations and reactions in primates. *Prog Psychobiol Physiol Psychol* 1983;10:113–165.
404. Wagner R, DeLeo JA, Coombs DW, Myers RR. Gender differences in autotomy following sciatic cryoneurolysis in the rat. *Physiol Behav*, 1995;58:37–41.
405. Wagner R, DeLeo JA, Heckman HM, Myers RR. Peripheral nerve pathology following sciatic cryoneurolysis: relationship to neuropathic behaviors in the rat. *Exp Neurol* 1995;133:256–264.
406. Wakisaka S, Kajander KC, Bennett GJ. Abnormal skin temperature and abnormal sympathetic vasomotor innervation in an experimental painful peripheral neuropathy. *Pain* 1991;46:299–313.
407. Wall PD, Scadding JW, Tomkiewicz MM. The production and prevention of experimental anaesthesia dolorosa. *Pain* 1984;6: 175–182.
408. Weiss B, Laties VG. Characteristics of aversive thresholds measured by a titration schedule. *J Exp Anal Behav* 1963;6:563–572.
409. Welty DF, Schielke GP, Vartanian MG, Taylor CP. Gabapentin anticonvulsant action in rats: disequilibrium with peak drug concentrations in plasma and brain microdialysate. *Epilepsy Res* 1993;16: 175–181.
410. Wheeler-Aceto H, Cowan A. Standardization of the rat paw formalin test for the evaluation of analgesics. *Psychopharmacology* 1991;104:35-44.
411. Wheeler-Aceto H, Porreca F, Cowan A. The rat paw formalin test: comparison of noxious agents. *Pain* 1990;40:229–238.
412. White WF, Heller AH. Glycine receptor alteration in the mutant mouse spastic. *Nature* 1982;298:655–657.
413. Wikler A. Sites and mechanisms of action of morphine and related drugs in the central nervous system. *Pharmacol Rev* 1950;2: 435–506.
414. Willenbring S, Beauprie IG, DeLeo JA. Sciatic cryoneurolysis in rats: a model of sympathetically independent pain. Part 1: Effects of sympathectomy. *Anesth Analg* 1995;81:544–548.
415. Willenbring S, DeLeo JA, Coombs DW. Differential behavioral outcomes in the sciatic cryoneurolysis model of neuropathic pain in rats. *Pain* 1994;58:135–140.
416. Wilson PR, Yaksh TL. Baclofen is antinociceptive in the spinal intrathecal space of animals. *Eur J Pharmacol* 1978;51:323–330.
417. Woolf CJ. Long term alterations in the excitability of the flexion reflex produced by peripheral tissue injury in the chronic decerebrate rat. *Pain* 1984;18:325–43.
418. Woolf CJ, Shortland P, Coggeshall RE. Peripheral nerve injury triggers central sprouting of myelinated afferents. *Nature* 1992; 355:75–8..
419. Woolfe G, MacDonald AD. The evaluation of the analgesic action of pethidine hydrochloride (Demerol). *J Pharmacol Exp Ther* 1944; 80:300–307.
420. Xu XJ, Hao JX, Aldskogius H, Seiger A, Wiesenfeld-Hallin Z. Chronic pain-related syndrome in rats after ischemic spinal cord lesion: a possible animal model for pain in patients with spinal cord injury. *Pain* 1992;48:279–290.
421. Xu XJ, Hao JX, Seiger A, Arner S, Lindblom U, Wiesenfeld-Hallin Z. Systemic mexiletine relieves chronic allodynialike symptoms in rats with ischemic spinal cord injury. *Anesth Analg* 1992;74: 649–652.
422. Xu XJ, Hao JX, Seiger A, Wiesenfeld-Hallin Z. Systemic excitatory amino acid receptor antagonists of the alpha-amino-3-hydroxy-5-methyl-4-isoxazolepropionic acid (AMPA) receptor and of the N-methyl-D-aspartate (NMDA) receptor relieve mechanical hypersensitivity after transient spinal cord ischemia in rats. *J Pharmacol Exp Ther* 1993;267:140–144.
423. Yaksh TL. Inhibition by etorphine of the discharge of dorsal horn neurons: effects on the neuronal response to both high- and low-threshold sensory input in the decerebrate spinal cat. *Exp Neurol* 1978;60:23–40.
424. Yaksh TL. Opiate receptors for behavioral analgesia resemble those related to the depression of spinal nociceptive neurons. *Science* 1978;199:1231–1233.
425. Yaksh TL. In vivo studies on spinal opiate receptor systems mediating antinociception. I. Mu and delta receptor profiles in the primate. *J Pharmacol Exp Ther* 1983;226:303–316.
426. Yaksh TL. Effects of spinally administered agents on spinal cord blood flow: a need for further studies. *Anesthesiology* 1983;59:1–2.
427. Yaksh TL. Multiple opioid receptor systems in brain and spinal cord. *Eur J Anaesthesiol* 1984;1:171–243.
428. Yaksh TL. Behavioral and autonomic correlates of the tactile evoked allodynia produced by spinal glycine inhibition: effects of

modulatory receptor systems and excitatory amino acid antagonists. *Pain* 1989;37:111–123.
429. Yaksh TL. Studies in animals should precede human use of spinally administered drugs. *Anesthesiology* 1989;70:4–6.
430. Yaksh TL. The spinal actions of opioids. In: Herz A, ed. *Handbook of experimental pharmacology, vol. 104/II.* Berlin: Springer-Verlag, 1993:53–90.
431. Yaksh TL, Chaplan SR, Malmberg AB. Future directions in the pharmacological management of hyperalgesic and allodynic pain states: the NMDA receptor. In: Chiang CN, Finnegan LP, eds. *Medications development for the treatment of pregnant addicts and their infants. NIDA research monograph series no. 149.* Rockville, MD: U.S. Dept. of Health and Human Services, 1995:84–101.
432. Yaksh TL, Chipkin RE. Studies on the effect of SCH-34826 and thiorphan on [Met5]enkephalin levels and release in rat spinal cord. *Eu J Pharmacol* 1989;167:367–373.
433. Yaksh TL, Dirksen R, Harty GJ. Antinociceptive effects of intrathecally injected cholinomimetic drugs in the rat and cat. *Eur J Pharmacol* 1985;117:81–88.
434. Yaksh TL, Elde RP. Factors governing release of methionine enkephalin-like immunoreactivity from mesencephalon and spinal cord of the cat in vivo. *J Neurophysiol* 1981 46:1056–1107.
435. Yaksh TL, Farb D, Leeman S, Jessell T. Intrathecal capsaicin depletes substance P in the rat spinal cord and produces prolonged thermal analgesia. *Science* 1979;206:481–483.
436. Yaksh TL, Grafe MR, Malkmus S, Rathbun ML, Eisenach JC. Studies on the safety of chronically administered intrathecal neostigmine methylsulfate in rats and dogs. *Anesthesiology* 1995;82: 412–427.
437. Yaksh TL, Jage J, Takano Y. Pharmacokinetics and pharmacodynamics of medullar agents. c. The spinal actions of α_2-adrenergic agonists as analgesics. *Baillieres Clin Anaesthesiol* 1993;7: 597–614.
438. Yaksh TL, Malmberg AB. Interaction of spinal modulatory receptor systems. In: Fields HL, Liebeskind JC, eds. *Progress in pain research and management, vol. 1.* Seattle: IASP Press, 1994:151–171.
439. Yaksh TL, Malmberg AB. Central pharmacology of nociceptive transmission. In: Wall P, Melzack R, eds. *Textbook of pain.* 3rd ed. Edinburgh: Churchill Livingstone, 1994:165–200.
440. Yaksh TL, Malmberg AB, Grafe M, Hruby V, Hasseth R. Preclinical safety studies for cyclic [D-penicillamine-2-D-penicillamine 5] enkephalin (DPDPE) a delta opioid analgesic delivered intrathecally. *Fund Appl Toxicol Suppl* 1996;30:24.
441. Yaksh TL, Malmberg AB, Ro S, Schiller P, Goodman M. Characterization of the spinal antinociceptive activity of constrained peptidomimetic opioids. *J Pharmacol Exp Ther* 1995;275:63–72.
442. Yaksh TL, Noueihed RY, Durant PA. Studies of the pharmacology and pathology of intrathecally administered 4-anilinopiperidine analogues and morphine in the rat and cat. *Anesthesiology* 1986;64: 54–66.
443. Yaksh TL, Pogrel JW, Lee YW, Chaplan SR. Reversal of nerve ligation-induced allodynia by spinal alpha-2 adrenoceptor agonists. *J Pharmacol Exp Ther* 1995;272:207–214.
443a. Yaksh TL, Rathbun M, and Dragan J. *Spinal Drug Delivery*, TL Yaksh, Editor. CRC Press, New York. In press, 1998.
444. Yaksh TL, Rathbun ML, Jage J, Mirzai T, Grafe M, Hiles RA. Pharmacology and toxicology of chronically infused epidural clonidine HCl in dogs. *Fund Appl Toxicol* 1994;23:319–335.
445. Yaksh TL, Reddy SVR. Studies in the primate on the analgetic effects associated with intrathecal actions of opiate, a-adrenergic agonists and baclofen. *Anesthesiology* 1981;54:451–467.
446. Yaksh TL, Rudy TA. Analgesia mediated by a direct spinal action of narcotics. *Science* 1976;192:1357–1358.
447. Yaksh TL, Sabbe MB, Lucas D, Mjanger E, Chipkin RE. Effects of [N-(L-(1-Carboxy-2-phenyl) ethyl]-L-phenylalanyl-b-alanine (SCH32615), a neutral endopeptidase (enkephalinase) inhibitor, on levels of enkephalin, encrypted enkephalins and substance P in cerebrospinal fluid and plasma of primates. *J Pharmacol Exper Ther* 1991;256:1033–1041.
448. Yaksh TL, Schmauss C, Micevych PE, Abay EO, Go VLW. Pharmacological studies on the application, disposition and release of neurotensin in the spinal cord. *Annu NY Acad Sci* 1982;400: 228–243.
449. Yaksh TL, Wilson PR. Spinal serotonin terminal system mediates antinociception. *J Pharmacol Exp Ther* 1979;208:446–453.
450. Yamamoto T, Shimoyama N, Mizuguchi T. The effects of morphine, MK-801, an NMDA antagonist, and CP-96,345, an NK1 antagonist, on the hyperesthesia evoked by carageenan injection in the rat paw. *Anesthesiology* 1993;78:124–133.
451. Yamamoto T, Shimoyama N, Mizuguchi T. Effects of FK224, a novel cyclopeptide NK1 and NK2 antagonist, and CP-96,345, a nonpeptide NK1 antagonist, on development and maintenance of thermal hyperesthesia evoked by carrageenan injection in the rat paw. *Anesthesiology* 1993;79:1042–1050.
452. Yamamoto T, Yaksh TL. Stereospecific effects of a nonpeptidic NK1 selective antagonist, CP-96,345: Antinociception in the absence of motor dysfunction. *Life Sci* 1991;49:1955–1963.
453. Yamamoto T, Yaksh TL. Spinal pharmacology of thermal hyperesthesia induced by incomplete ligation of sciatic nerve. I. Opioid and nonopioid receptors. *Anesthesiology* 1991;75:817–826.
454. Yamamoto T, Yaksh TL. Effects of intrathecal capsaicin and an NK-1 antagonist, CP, 96-345, on the thermal hyperalgesia observed following unilateral constriction of the sciatic nerve in the rat. *Pain* 1992;51:329–334.
455. Yamamoto T, Yaksh TL. Spinal pharmacology of thermal hyperesthesia induced by constriction injury of sciatic nerve. Excitatory amino acid antagonists. *Pain* 1992;49:121–128.
456. Yamamoto T, Yaksh TL. Studies on the spinal interaction of morphine and the NMDA antagonist MK-801 on the hyperesthesia observed in a rat model of sciatic mononeuropathy. *Neurosci Lett* 1992;135:67–70.
457. Yamamoto T, Yaksh TL. Comparison of the antinociceptive effects of pre- and posttreatment with intrathecal morphine and MK801, an NMDA antagonist, on the formalin test in the rat. *Anesthesiology* 1992d;77:757–763.
458. Yamamoto T, Yaksh TL. Effects of colchicine applied to the peripheral nerve on the thermal hyperalgesia evoked with chronic nerve constriction. *Pain* 1993;55:227–233.
459. Yanez A, Sabbe MB, Stevens CW, Yaksh TL. Interaction of midazolam and morphine in the spinal cord of the rat. *Neuropharmacology* 1990;29:359–364.
460. Yanez AM, Wallace M, Ho R, Shen D, Yaksh TL. Touch-evoked agitation produced by spinally administered phospholipid emulsion and liposomes in rats. *Anesthesiology* 1995;82:1189–1198.
461. Yang CY, Wu WH, Zbuzek VK. Antinociceptive effect of chronic nicotine and nociceptive effect of its withdrawal measured by hot-plate and tail-flick in rats. *Psychopharmacology* 1992;106: 417–420.
462. Yang L-C, Marsala M, Yaksh TL. Knee joint inflammation in rat: a potential role of spinal PGE2 and NO release in hypersensitivity state. *Anesthesiology* 1995;83:A794.
462a. Yezierski RP, Liu S, Ruenes GL, Busto R, Dietrich WD. Neuronal damage following intraspinal injection of a nitric oxide synthase inhibitor in the rat. *Journal of Cerebral Blood Flow and Metabolism* 1996;16:996–1004.
463. Yokota T, Nishikawa N, Nishikawa Y. Effects of strychnine upon different classes of trigeminal subnucleus caudalis neurons. *Brain Res* 1979;168:430–434.
464. Yoshioka H, Tsuneto S, Kashiwagi T. Pain control with morphine for vertebral metastases and sciatica in advanced cancer patients. *J Palliat Care* 1994;10:10–13.
465. Zanchetti A. Reflex and brain stem inhibition of sham rage behaviour. *Prog Brain Res* 1968;22:195–205.
466. Zarbin MA, Wamsley JK, Kuhar MJ. Glycine receptor: light microscopic autoradiographic localization with [^{3}H]strychnine. *J Neurosci* 1981;1:532–547.
467. Zhang AL, Hao JX, Seiger A, et al. Decreased GABA immunoreactivity in spinal cord dorsal horn neurons after transient spinal cord ischemia in the rat. *Brain Res* 1994;656:187–190.
468. Zieglgansberger W, Bayerl H. The mechanism of inhibition of neuronal activity by opiates in the spinal cord of cat. *Brain Res* 1976;115:111–128.

Anesthesia: Biologic Foundations, edited by
Tony L. Yaksh et al. Lippincott–Raven Publishers,
Philadelphia © 1997.

CHAPTER 41

PSYCHOPHYSICAL MEASUREMENT OF NORMAL AND ABNORMAL PAIN STATES AND ANALGESIA

DONALD D. PRICE

The sensory state produced by a high-intensity mechanical or thermal stimulus applied to the body, or an injury and the changes in the perception of body function after an injury is readily associated by common appreciation and experience with a "pain" state. The development of an understanding of the mechanisms underlying this sensory condition and systematic efforts to modify that state are predicated on the ability to define reliably and without injury the behavioral components induced by such stimulus conditions in verbal (humans) and nonverbal models (infants and animals). The measurement and assessment of physical pain, like that of other sensory modalities, has relied on the application of psychophysical methods and concepts. However, the application of psychophysical methods to the quantitative assessment of pain has a history differing considerably from that of other sensory modalities. Whereas the major psychophysical attributes of most sensory modalities (i.e., vision, audition, somesthesis) have been carefully characterized, those characterizing pain are less well documented. There are at least three reasons why this is so.

1. There has been a fundamental disagreement as to whether pain operates as a sensory modality or as a motivation (55,66).
2. It has been argued that the pain system, unlike that of other sensory systems, operates in a fashion that is limited to dealing with crude discriminative information (e.g., the stimulus is adequate and yields a pain state or it is not adequate and does not yield a pain state) (59,100).
3. Technically, there has been difficulty with the precision with which noxious stimuli activating the various sensory modalities can be controlled and quantified. For example, in visual psychophysics, the ease of quantifying light energy in physical units (e.g., intensity, spectral frequency) and manipulating its parameters (e.g., stimulus shape, contrast and spatial frequency) has facilitated the considerable advances made in understanding the underlying neural mechanisms of vision (52,96). In contrast, quantification and control of the stimuli that produce pain have been far less precise. This is in large part a result of the fact that many such stimuli, by their very nature, are potentially damaging and difficult to present repeatedly with the same effect, whereas others, like electrical stimuli, which are more easily controlled, result in the synchronous activation of an abnormal mix of afferents in a manner that does not resemble the effects produced by "natural" stimuli.

Despite these mitigating factors, efforts to characterize the psychophysical attributes of pain have a long history. One of the early systematic efforts in this century was made by Hardy et al. (33–35). To present a quantifiable and controlled stimuli, they developed a heat lamp, or "dolorimeter," with which they could deliver precise levels of radiant heat. The intensity of the heat stimulus was varied by changing the voltage on the lamp, whereas stimulus area and duration were controlled via an aperture diaphragm and shutter inserted between the lamp and the subject's skin. Questions regarding pain thresholds, adaptation, spatial summation, intensity functions, and discrimination of intensity could thus be addressed in a systematic fashion. With such an approach, they began to evaluate the verbal report of humans so stimulated and thereby characterize the psychophysical components of the human state evoked by such stimuli (34,35). Although reliable and reproducible correlations between the stimulus properties and the pain report were noted, their approach unexpectedly yielded negative, or marginally positive confirmation of the effects of clinically proven analgesics (3,4). From a historical perspective, the consequence of this "failure" to adequately describe what was already known on the basis of clinical experience markedly dampened subsequent enthusiasm for the use of an experimental approach to pain in humans (for reviews, see refs. 26,66).

Within the past two decades, because of an increased insight into the underlying mechanisms of pain and analgesia, there has been a resurgence of interest in psychophysical characterization of pain states. This resurgence has been accompanied by significant methodological and conceptual advances in the use of quantifiable and controllable stimuli in studies of experimental pain. Moreover, in part because of the evolving appreciation of the underlying neurophysiology of substrates associated with pain behavior, there has been a move away from global and complex measures related to the affective dimension of pain (e.g., such as pain tolerance), to direct scaling of the responses evoked by suprathreshold components of stimuli which evoke a pain state. Furthermore, since it has been acknowledged explicitly that pain is comprised of multiple dimensions (i.e., sensory-discriminative and affective-motivational), multiple scales developed for these dimensions have been shown to yield important correlative insights. The incorporation of these methodological and conceptual changes has led to experimental paradigms that directly relate quantifiable suprathreshold stimuli to neural responses and quantifiable human judgments of different aspects of the pain experience.

This chapter discusses the conceptual and methodological advances as they relate to the measurement and assessment of pain, pain mechanisms, and pharmacological treatments for pain. This discussion has four specific objectives: (a) description of approaches to measurement and quantification of the human pain state; (b) characterization of the psychophysical attributes of "normal pain," and consideration of the neural, behavioral, and perceptual consequences of manipulating stimulus intensity and intensity differences, stimulus site, duration, and other spatial and temporal parameters; (c) characterization of psychophysical characteristics associated with the sensory abnormalities of various types of pathophysiological states (e.g., reflex sympathetic dystrophy); and (d) consideration of how various conventional and nonconventional analgesic drugs can differentially influence the sensory-discriminative and affective dimensions of normal and pathophysiological pain processing.

METHODS OF PAIN MEASUREMENT

Overview of Paradigms of Pain Assessment

Measurement of pain, like the measurement of visual acuity or auditory thresholds, depends upon the response of the observer who is subjected to the stimulus. Exposure to a physical stimulus yields a personal experience that is reported by the observer. In a general sense, the assessment of a sensory experience can be accomplished in terms of a comparison to known standards or by an effort to quantify a specific criterion response with a given physical intensity.

Technically, the paradigm may induce a pain state by the application of a physical stimulus or employ a stimulus associated with tissue injury. Practically, to provide a measure of pain intensity, the observer (patient) may be asked to rate the perceived intensity of the recent stimulus on a scale ranging over a continuum from none to some maximum. This rating is implicitly based on some standard. In many instances, the rating is defined on the basis of no pain (0 on the scale) to the worst imaginable pain (10 on the scale). Under those conditions, the patient is in effect being asked to match the current sensory state with that of events that the observer has previously experienced (e.g., match to experience). Alternately, the observer may be asked to match an intensity of the pain experience induced by a well-controlled experimental stimulus with that which results from injury (e.g., match to standard).

In addition to the matching of intensity, the observer/patient who is exposed to a pain stimulus or pain state can be instructed to note and scale different dimensions of their experience. For example, they can be required to observe and judge (by matching to standard or experience) the relative intensity of the sensation, the degree of its "immediate unpleasantness," spatial distribution, and quality (sharp, dull, aching, throbbing). These separate judgments are by no means exclusive to pain and have a long history in the psychophysics of vision, audition, taste, smell, and somatosensory modalities. One can make separate and exquisitely precise judgments of intensity, pitch, timbre, volume, and density of the same sound stimuli as well as their pleasantness or unpleasantness.

The assessment paradigms outlined above implies a sensory continuum in which the magnitude of the degree of pain or some attribute associated with that state can be quantified as a function of stimulus intensity. Such a continuum also implies a point (stimulus intensity) at which the stimulus is not longer judged as painful. As noted initially, though controversial, this underlying principle implies a threshold. Paradigms which assess pain thresholds thus attempt to identify that point on a continuum of increasing stimulus intensity that dichotomously distinguishes a nonpainful from a painful experience. While intuitively useful, thresholds provide no information as to the magnitude of the pain state at stimulus intensities other than at the threshold intensity. By virtue of the way the threshold stimulus is determined (see below), information on the continuum of the stimulus versus response relationship is not obtained. To address this limitation, direct scaling methods of pain assessment have been formalized for pain measurement in both patients and normal volunteer subjects. These methods have utilized two basic approaches (26): rating scale methods in which subjects rate pain intensity on scales with clearly defined numerical limits and intervals or on verbal rating scales whose words directly indicate a rank order; and magnitude scaling procedures in which direct ratings are made on continuous scales of sensation intensity or unpleasantness, without constraints of categories or whole numbers. These sophisticated measuring paradigms have the common advantage of being able to provide relative changes in the stimulus response relationship across stimulus intensities. In the following sections, the methods of pain threshold assessment, simple verbal and numerical magnitude assessments, and magnitude scaling/cross modality matching scaling are briefly summarized.

Pain Threshold Measurement

Pain threshold methods were used by Hardy et al. (35) and Beecher (4) following World War II, but they have since diminished in popularity in pain research and in sensory psychophysics in general. There are two general procedures for obtaining pain threshold: the method of limits and the method of constant stimuli (31). In the former method, the stimulus intensity is increased to a point where the subject responds in the affirmative for each stimulus and then the stimulus is decreased to a point where the subject responds in the negative for each stimulus. The stimulus intensity midway between these two limiting intensities is considered threshold. In the method of constant stimuli, stimulus intensity is increased in steps to a point at which the subject responds in the affirmative 50% of the time when that stimulus is presented (31). In either method, a stimulus intensity is identified that represents the boundary between painful and nonpainful experience.

Given careful and adequate instructions to subjects, pain thresholds are reliable, generalizable across subjects, and simple to obtain. Depending on instructions to subjects, pain thresholds can be obtained separately for sensory discriminative (e.g., pricking pain threshold) or affective (e.g., unpleasantness) dimensions of pain (8,66). However, threshold measures have several drawbacks. As originally noted in the work of Hardy et al., under some experimental conditions, these models are insensitive to effects of clinically proven analgesic drugs for reasons that are still not entirely clear (4,17). Pain threshold measures are unable to directly compare the magnitude of pain states at different stimulus intensities. or to provide a ratio (e.g., one stimulus is perceived as being twice the intensity of another).

Verbal and Numerical Rating Scales

Verbal rating scales (i.e., mild, moderate, severe) and numerical rating scales (i.e., 0–5, 0–10) are often relatively simple and for that reason are very commonly used in clinical assessment of pain and in pain research. Words or numbers on these scales refer only to rank ordering and cannot be used to reflect ratios of magnitude. Such scales are therefore termed ordinal scales. For example, if someone initially rates their pain as 989 and then 969 after a treatment, one can conclude that the pain has reduced in intensity but not that it has reduced by 25%. One variant of an ordinal rating scale is the verbal category scale, the categories of which are designed to imply a rank ordering. The scale designed by Melzack and Torgerson (58) and later included in the McGill Pain Questionnaire (56), has for example, the five categories of "mild, discomforting, distressing, horrible, and excruciating." Other rating scales are simple numerical scales (e.g., 0–5 or 0–10) that are sometimes anchored by verbal descriptors indicative of extremes such as "no pain" and "severe pain." The advantage of ordinal rating scales is their relative simplicity. The most useful attribute of such rating scales is that they can be used to rapidly ascertain whether pain intensity has increased, decreased, or remained the same. These scales are widely used by health care professionals in ascertaining pain and effects of pain treatments. The scales are easily understand and can respond to a 0–5 pain scale, where "5" equals the most "severe pain imaginable" and "0" equals "no pain." Unfortunately, for the purposes of clinical pain assessment, simple verbal numerical rating scales and verbal descriptor scales are widely misused and misinterpreted. Several problems may be noted. Rating scales cannot in principle be used to assess percent pain relief because the numbers on these scales reflect the rank order of pain intensity. Verbal descriptor scales are sensitive to internal response biases of the patients. For example, human observers have a tendency to perseverate in using numbers or words. Thus, if a patient uses the number "5" to rate his or her pain at one time, he or she will have a strong memory for that numerical rating and will tend to use it again despite actual changes in pain intensity. This characteristic is even more likely with verbal descriptor ratings. Stimulus-pain response curves obtained using simple numerical rating scales are different depending on whether most of the stimulus intensities are concentrated toward the low or high end of the pain stimulus intensity range. Thus, the distribution of responses will be skewed and accordingly biased.

Direct Magnitude Scaling Methods

Direct magnitude scaling techniques rely on the capacity of human observers to represent the perceived intensity of one type of sensation by making responses on another physical continuum. For example, patients could adjust a sound intensity or the length of a line to represent perceived intensity of a pain sensation. As there are essentially an infinite number of sound intensities or line lengths that could be used to represent pain intensity, these indices reflect interval or continuous data. Such a scaling method, referred to generically as analog scales, have become extremely popular in pain research and in clinical pain assessment. They have several distinct advantages over other measurement methods (38,73–75,82–85,88,89). Direct scaling techniques represent a continuous variable computation of ratios of the intensity of one pain to another. This then provides information about percent change (71,73,82). Simple numerical scales or verbal descriptor scales, as discussed above, can only measure the rank order of different pain intensities. Patients may use visual analog scaling paradigms in a very consistent manner to rate quite different types of pain, including low back myofascial pain, jaw muscle pain, and even experimental pain (73,74,82). For a particular type of pain, the ratings are very consistent across time and are generalizable across different groups. The visual analog scale can be adapted to separately measure pain sensation intensity and pain unpleasantness or pain related emotional disturbance (71,74,82).

PSYCHOPHYSICAL ATTRIBUTES OF NORMAL PAIN

The properties of the sensation evoked by well-defined physical stimuli have been widely studied. The relationship of the stimulus intensity-sensation relationship may be considered as having a number of specific attributes. These attributes serve to characterize the psychophysical properties of the pain state. These attributes include (a) threshold intensities for the evocation of the pain state, (b) adaptation to the stimulus of a given intensity, (c) the function describing the stimulus intensity-pain magnitude relationship, (d) discriminability of painful stimuli, (e) temporal properties of the sensation evoked by a given stimulus, and (f) spatial characteristics of the sensation evoked by a stimulus. These attributes define the characteristics of the stimulus-sensation relationship and accordingly serve to delimit the operating properties of the underlying anatomical and physiologically defined system. Much of what has been accomplished in defining these response properties have involved thermal stimulation; and, this will serve as a framework for the following discussion. A more extensive review of this topic is provided in ref. 83.

Heat-Induced Thresholds for Pain and Withdrawal Reflexes

Increasing skin temperature will result in reports of warmth and at higher temperatures in reports of pain, with the intensity of the pain report or the vigor of the escape response increasing monotonically as the intensity is raised yet further (1,35). Qualitatively, characteristics of the pain are associated with the report of increasing magnitude with the report of an initial pricking sensation at suprathreshold intensities. Hardy et al. (35) were the first to quantify stimulus parameters that give rise to pain and discover some of its psychophysical attributes. Using controlled radiant heat stimuli applied to darkened skin (to enhance absorption and reduce variability due to reflectance), they demonstrated a significant difference between the characteristics underlying radiant heat-induced pain and judgments of warmth. Unlike warmth thresholds, pain thresholds for radiant heat depend primarily on the absolute temperature of the skin, and very little on the rate with which the skin temperature increases or the size of the body area stimulated (30,33–35). Using threshold methodology, they further determined that the minimal skin temperature at which pain is perceived ranges in humans of 42.7–45.7°C, with the average being 44.5°C. Radiant heat pain thresholds are extremely reliable for any given body area, but vary among different sites on the body. For example, the thresholds for the thigh and lower back are the lowest, averaging 42.6°C and 42.2°C, respectively, and highest for the finger pads and heel, averaging 47.1°C and 53.7°C, respectively (35).

Of considerable importance is the observation that several types of thermally evoked withdrawal reflexes and escape behaviors are initiated in a variety of mammalian species at a skin temperature at or close to 45°C, an intensity that corresponds with the pain threshold determined in humans by Hardy et al. (35). These observations indicate that there may be neural substrates for the various components of pain and pain-related behaviors that are common across all mammals. It is this assumption that common neural mechanisms underlie various pain-related behaviors across species that forms the basis for algesic tests in animals to evaluate the efficacy of analgesic drugs (55). The lack of an effect of clinically efficacious analgesics on pain threshold in humans (3,5) may well have resulted from the contribution of the pricking component of the thermally induced pain state to the assessment of threshold.

Adaptation to Maintained Stimulation

Adaptation, the diminution of perceived sensation with constant stimulus intensity, is a property believed to be characteristic of sensory systems, e.g., vision, audition and non aversive somatic. However, it is a common experience that pain, produced by a maintained high-intensity mechanical or thermal stimulus, persists for as long as one attends to it. This suggests that, unlike other sensory systems, adaptation plays a minimal role in the pain state. Adaptation has, however, not been characterized adequately. This is in part because tissue damage can be a consequence of maintaining a noxious stimulus on the same area of skin. Aside from ethical considerations, tissue damage can change the transduction properties of peripheral terminals (see Chapters 32 and 33).

The hypothesis that adaptation may play a minimal role in pain was first tested in a study by Greene and Hardy in 1958 (30). Trained observers were asked to control the intensity of a radiant heat stimulus such that the observer would continue to perceive the sensation of pricking pain. Rather than increasing the stimulus intensity, as would be predicted if adaptation were taking place, the subjects gradually lowered the stimulus intensity required to maintain the pricking pain. Thus, over 13 min, the average threshold temperature to evoke the pricking sensation decreased modestly from ~45°C to 44°C. These results indicate that at threshold temperatures, adaptation is not a salient characteristic of heat-induced pain, and not incidentally that neural mechanisms exist (i.e., those subserving hyperalgesia) that decrease pain threshold during prolonged nociceptive stimulation.

To assess whether the phenomena of adaptation pertains to supra-threshold temperatures, a combined psychophysical and neurophysiological study employing prolonged repetitive noxious heat stimulation (repetitive immersion of a finger in a water bath at a constant temperature fixed at 45–49°C) showed that a modest adaptation occurred within the first 2 min of repetitive stimulation. However, no additional change in pain ratings occurred during the following 20-min interval (19). At the neurophysiological level in animals, similar results were with regard to the responses of dorsal horn nociceptive neurons engendered by the same stimulus exposures (19).

Other studies using maintained rather than repetitive nociceptive heat stimuli have shown that significant, though incomplete adaptation occurs in the responses of primary nociceptive and spinothalamic tract neurons (5). The partial adaptation of primary afferent and central neurons to maintained nociceptive (45–53°C) stimuli is at odds with psychophysical studies showing minimal adaptation to similar stimuli. This apparent contradiction between the behavior of the whole animal and the activity of primary afferents and some central nociceptive neurons may be explained partly by how nociceptive neurons at successive levels of the nervous system respond to maintained noxious stimuli. As one records the activity of neurons at successively higher levels from the spinal cord to the cerebral cortex, there is a progressive loss of adaptation (39,41–43,102). For example, nociceptive neurons in VPLc of the lateral thalamus adapt more slowly to sustained nociceptive temperatures (i.e., 45–50°C) than do spinothalamic tract neurons (41,43), and nociceptive neurons in SI cortex (particularly those with restricted receptive fields) adapt even more slowly than do VPLc neurons (42). The slow adaptive rate of cortical neurons more nearly approximates that of human perception itself. That mechanisms should exist for overriding peripheral nociceptive adaptation has obvious significance for the degradation of signals that lead to protective escape and avoidance behaviors in the presence of tissue-damaging stimuli would be maladaptive.

Encoding of Intensity and Affect

As noted above, with increasing skin temperature, the sensation progresses from warmth to pain. The pain report evoked by a cutaneous thermal stimulus has been shown repeatedly to follow a positively accelerating power function (19,21,45,66,68, 71,73,83), as illustrated in Fig. 1. The exponent of the power function is consistently greater than 2.0 for pain sensation. Thus, for the data presented in Fig. 1, the function that describe pain sensation intensity have exponents of 2.1 (73). The functions obtained using a visual analogue scale are very consistent across different groups of subjects, including both pain patients and pain-free volunteer groups (Fig. 1). Given the progressive shift from warmth to pain with increasing stimulus thermal intensities, it might be argued that there is a single function that reflects a continuum of sensation. Several lines of evidence in fact does not support this thesis. Consideration of the exponent for temperature versus warmth and pain reveals the latter to be routinely >2.0 and the former <2.0 (0.5–1.6) (94), depending on the stimulus area. The perception of warmth intensity and the threshold for warmth are dependent on the rate of rise of skin temperature, whereas pain threshold and pain intensity are far less influenced by such factors (34,35,52). Differences also exist in spatial summation attributes between pain and warmth (see below). Finally, warmth and pain are processed separately as defined by neurophysiological evidence that separate neuronal populations which process warmth and nociception (36,45,66,102). These clear differences in psychophysical attributes indicate that heat-induced pain cannot be construed as a simple extension of warmth and must be considered a separate sensory dimension.

Regardless of whether radiant heat or contact heat is used as a noxious stimulus, the neural responses of peripheral and central nociceptive neurons follow functions that generally parallel those of human psychophysical magnitude estimations described above, as shown in Fig. 2 (5,23,39,41–43,45–48,66,70, 72,77). The similarity between the nociceptive temperature-pain intensity rating functions (Fig. 1) and nociceptive temperature-neural response functions obtained from electrophysiological experiments is strong evidence that pain intensity information is encoded and transmitted along neural pathways in a relatively straight forward fashion. In other words, there is no radical transformation or distortion of information about intensity at successively higher stages of central neural processing. However, while this principle may be applicable to initial pains evoked by brief nociceptive stimuli, it may be totally inappropriate for others. For, as will be discussed below, there are remarkable temporal transformations that apply to heat-induced "second pain." It is the latter type of pain that is related to central mechanisms underlying inflammatory pain, hyperalgesic states, and pathophysiological pain. These phenomena are not related in a simple and direct manner to impulse frequency in primary nociceptive afferents.

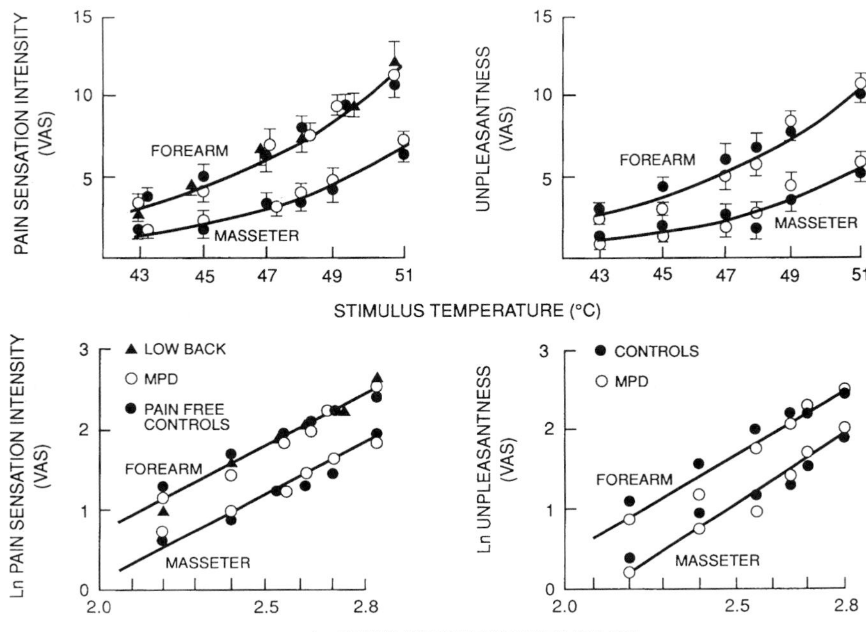

Figure 1. Visual Analogue Scale (VAS) measurements of the relationship between temperature of the skin and the judgment of pain sensation intensity and its unpleasantness. The data were obtained from low back (LB) and myofacial pain dysfunction (MPD), patients as well as pain-free control subjects, and are plotted in linear coordinates in the *upper pair of graphs* and in double logarithmic coordinates in the *lower pair of graphs.* Each *point* on the graphs represents the group average for a given temperature; *vertical lines* through the points represent SEMs (these conventions are followed in subsequent figures). Despite the large difference between the VAS ratings of the intensity of the facial (area over the masseter muscle) and forearm stimuli on the pair of graphs to the left, the exponents (i.e., the slopes) of the functions were identical (2.1). A similar result was obtained for ratings of unpleasantness (*right*) with the slopes equal to 2.4 and 2.7, respectively. (Reprinted, in adapted form, with permission from Price DD, Harkins SW. The combined use of experimental pain and visual analogue scales in providing standardized measurement of clinical pain. *Clin J Pain* 1987;3:1–8.)

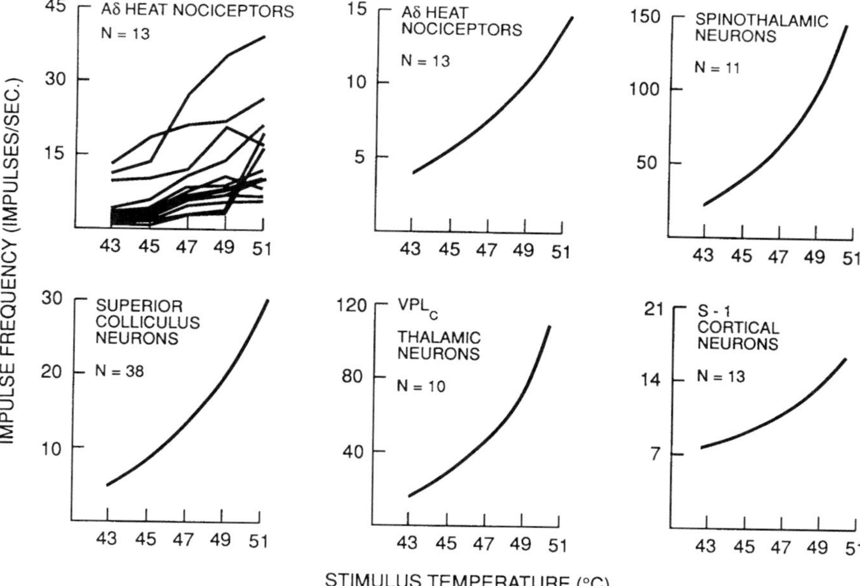

Figure 2. Heat-induced responses in populations of nociceptive neurons at various levels in the nervous system. *Upper left:* The functions of 13 individual A-delta nociceptive neurons are shown (to the right: their population function is shown). Note that regardless of the specific area of the nervous system examined, the stimulus-response relationships for all populations are similar positively accelerating power functions.

A higher exponent for pain affect (2.7) compared with pain sensation (2.1) reflects the fact that unpleasantness ratings are systematically lower than sensory ratings when both dimensions of pain are rated on the same length visual analogue scales (73,74). This has the effect of increasing the slope when plotted in logarithmic coordinates. However, unpleasantness ratings are subject to a good deal of influence by psychological factors. The lower ratings in this case are due to the assurances made to the participants that the stimuli would be brief, would not produce tissue damage, and would remain within tolerable limits. Very different ratings would likely occur if subjects were made anxious about the pain stimuli (68).

Pain Intensity Discriminability

If one can detect the intensity of a noxious stimulus, one must also be able to detect differences in noxious intensities. What is surprising, however, is the sensitivity of this capability. It has been demonstrated that both humans and monkeys can detect temperature shifts of 0.2–0.3°C at nociceptive (>47°C) intensity levels (11,12), as shown in Fig. 3. This discriminative ability is even greater than that found for warmth, which, at 39°C, is 0.3–0.5°C. The ability to detect 0.2–0.3°C within the nociceptive range of 45–51°C is generally consistent with the presence of 21 levels of just-noticeable differences obtained when studying radiant heat-induced pain (35). The psychophysical capacity to discriminate very small difference in stimulus intensity within the range of nociceptive temperatures of 45–51°C is precisely paralleled by a similar discriminative capacity of primary afferent and central nociceptive neurons (10,11,49). Primary C-polymodal nociceptive afferents (87,99), Trigeminothalamic neurons (11), and medial thalamic neurons of primates (10) all have been demonstrated to differentially respond to stimulus intensity differences of 0.2°C within the thermal nociceptive range.

Temporal Characteristics of Heat-Induced Pain

A brief stimulus of 51°C, can evoke two distinct pain sensations called, "first" and "second" pain (65–67,78). First pain is usually a well-localized, sharp, pricking sensation, whereas second pain occurs about 1 s later and is a dull, throbbing, or burning sensation. Second pain is more diffuse and/or less well localized than first pain. Cross-modality matching and visual analogue scaling methods have been used to analyze the curious property of temporal suppression found in first pain and temporal summation found in second pain (78,85). As shown in Fig. 4, the intensities of first and second pain, respectively, decrease and increase throughout a train of nociceptive heat pulses. First pain decreases in intensity whenever the interstim-

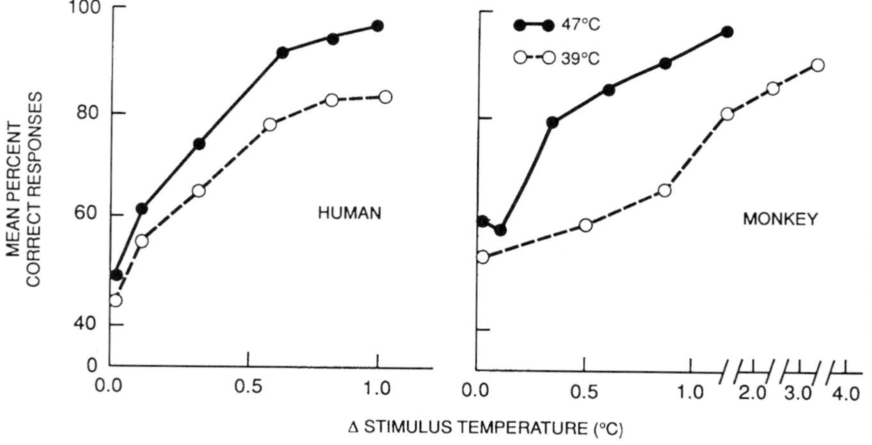

Figure 3. Functions describing the capabilities of human subjects (n = 3) and a monkey to discriminate small changes in temperature in the noxious (47°C, *solid lines*) and innocuous (39°C, *dashed lines*) ranges. Each *point* represents the average of 100 trials. Note that small temperature shifts (0.2–0.3°C) can be discriminated readily in both innocuous and noxious ranges. Corresponding neural data are presented in Fig. 5. (Reprinted, in adapted form, with permission from Bushnell MC, Taylor MB, Duncan GH, Dubner R. Discrimination of innocuous and noxious thermal stimuli applied to the face in human and monkey. *Somatosens Res* 1983;1:199–129.)

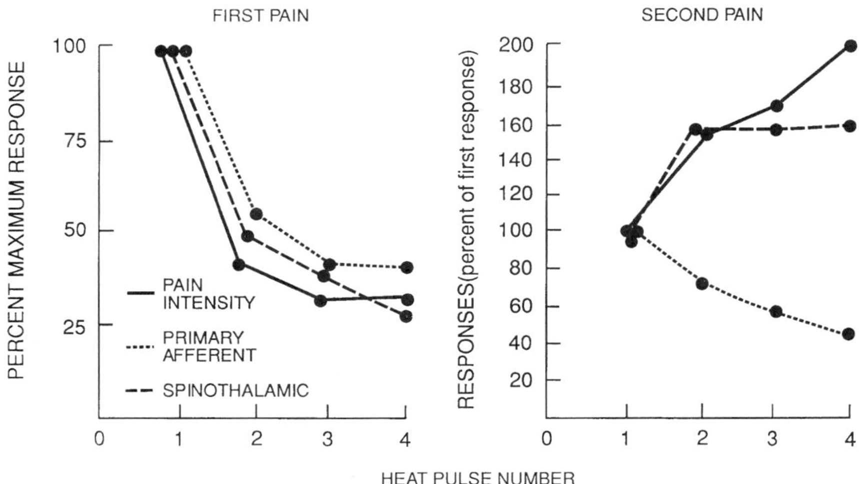

Figure 4. Repetitive heat pulses produce different effects on first and second pain. Repeating a 51°C heat pulse produced a striking decrement in the neural responses of primary afferents and spinothalamic neurons, as well as the judged intensity of first pain (*left*). However, these same stimulus conditions produced very different results for second pain (*right*). In this case, only the long-latency primary afferent activity (associated with second pain) decreased with repetitive stimulation. Long-latency spinothalamic activity and judgments of second pain sensation intensity actually increased in this situation. Apparently, a CNS mechanism exists for amplifying second pain with repetitive noxious stimuli. (Reprinted, in adapted form, with permission from Price DD, Hayes RL, Ruda MA, Dubner R. Spatial and temporal transformations of input to spinothalamic tract neurons and their relation to somatic sensation. *J Neurophysiol* 1978;41:933–947.)

ulus interval is :≤80 s, but only if the same spot on the skin is stimulated repeatedly. Second pain increases in intensity whenever the interstimulus interval is ≤3 s, even when the stimulus moves from spot to spot during the train of heat pulses, and even after total blockade of the peripheral impulses necessary for first pain (78). Thus, the mechanisms for first pain suppression and second pain summation are separate. The former likely is the result of heat-induced suppression of A-delta heat nociceptive afferents and the latter likely is the result of central summation mechanisms activated by C-polymodal nociceptive afferents.

Several observations support these two assertions. When a single 51°C heat pulse is applied to the skin at a distal site such as the hand or foot, a short latency response is evoked in A-delta heat nociceptive primary afferents and in the spinothalamic neurons on which these primary afferents converge (77,78). A longer latency discharge is evoked in C-polymodal primary afferents and in the spinothalamic tract neurons on which these C afferents converge. The characteristics of these neural responses, obtained in monkeys, help to explain psychophysical responses of human subjects to similar heat-pulse stimuli as described below. During a train of heat pulses, the responses of A-delta heat nociceptive primary afferents, the short latency responses of spinothalamic neurons and the sensation of first pain all undergo a progressive reduction over a similar time course (Fig. 4). A parsimonious explanation for this combination of results is that the heat-induced suppression of first pain is the result of the suppression of first order afferents. By contrast, several observations indicate that the slow temporal summation related to second pain is dependent on CNS mechanisms, specifically those within the dorsal horn of the spinal cord (77). The most compelling bit of evidence that responses of first order afferents are not the basis for this summation is the fact that the responses of C-primary nociceptive afferents do not temporally summate in response to trains of heat pulses. In fact, the response of C-fiber afferents undergo progressive suppression similar to that of A-delta heat nociceptive afferents. On the other hand, there is a summation of C-afferent induced responses of spinothalamic tract neurons to repeated heat pulses. This summation has a magnitude and time course that parallel those of second pain. As can be seen in Fig. 4, these summations persist even when the responses of C-polymodal nociceptive afferents become progressively reduced. Finally, summation of long latency responses of spinothalamic tract neurons and second pain occur when electrical shocks are used to activate C afferents, the vast majority of which are C-polymodal nociceptive afferents (64–66). This combination of observations indicates that the neural mechanisms critical for temporal summation of second pain exist at the level of synaptic interactions between C-polymodal nociceptive afferents and spinothalamic tract neurons. These synaptic interactions are now known to involve long-duration excitatory processes related to activation of the NMDA (*N*-methyl-D-aspartate) receptor by the glutamate neurotransmitter and prolonged excitatory neuromodulation by released peptides, such as substance P (for review, see ref. 80; also see Chapters 36 and 60). For example, dextromethorphan, an antitussive and NMDA antagonist, selectively attenuates both C-fiber mediated temporal summation in the dorsal horn and temporal summation of second pain in humans (81).

Spatial Summation

Heat-induced pain has been distinguished from heat-induced warmth in that the latter exhibits considerable spatial summation (40,52,94–96). Summation of warmth takes place generously over large areas of the body surface, and as stimulus area increases, the overall perceived intensity of warmth increases. However, the slope of the stimulus-response function obtained when relating stimulus temperature to perceived warmth (in double-logarithmic coordinates) decreases in magnitude with increasing stimulus area. Therefore, the same change in temperature over a small area has a proportionately greater effect than that same change spread over a larger area. Furthermore, the perceived warmth intensity functions converge at a common point near pain threshold (94).

In contrast to psychophysical studies of warmth, studies of heat-induced pain have only recently concluded that spatial summation exists for pain (19,21,83,84). Earlier studies showed equivocal evidence for spatial summation of pain (18, 30,34,35,40,60). Given its potentially critical role in understanding the neural mechanisms of pain as well as the obvious medical implications of this property of high-intensity stimulation, it is astonishing that direct scaling analyses have been applied to testing spatial summation of pain only within the past several years.

In the three separate studies (19,21,84) that used direct scaling methods, human observers made visual analogue scale ratings for pain sensation intensity and for unpleasantness in response to contact heat-induced pain stimuli over different areas of skin surface. As shown in Fig. 5, considerable spatial summation occurred in both the intensity and unpleasantness dimensions. Although spatial summation was evident throughout a wide range of temperatures, it was far larger at temperatures which exceeded the threshold for pain (47–51°C) than at those near pain threshold (43–46°C) (Fig. 5). The spatial summation of pain was characterized by an upward parallel displacement (left shift) of the stimulus-response function in

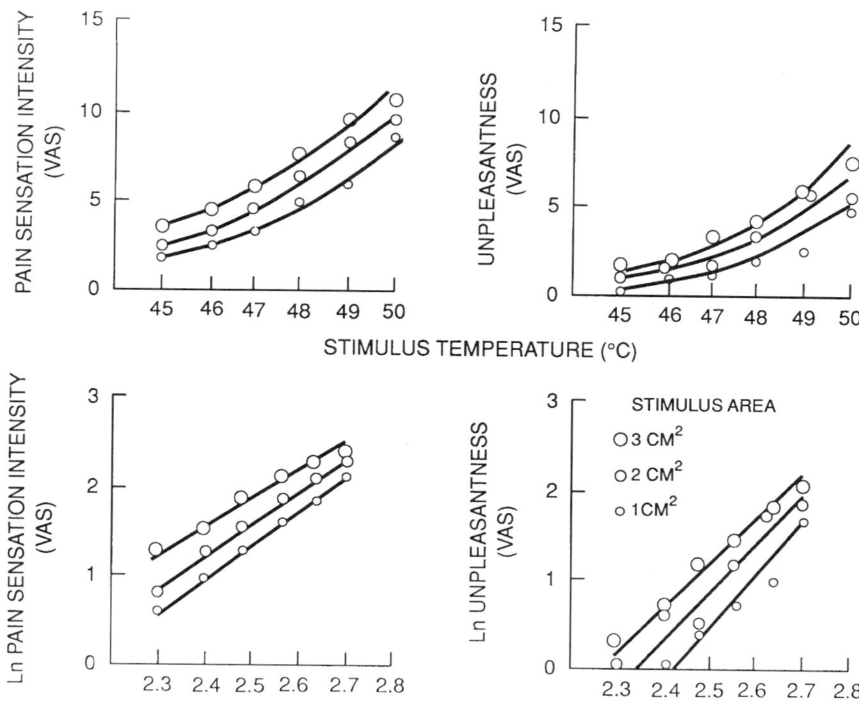

Figure 5. Spatial summation of pain. Nociceptive temperature-VAS-sensory (*left*) and VAS-affective (*right*) functions are plotted here in linear (*top*) and double-logarithmic (*bottom*) coordinates. The sizes of the stimuli (heat probes) are indicated by the *open circles*. The functions are clearly positively accelerating in linear coordinates, and are linear in double-logarithmic coordinates. This demonstrates that spatial summation makes a greater contribution to subjective awareness as the stimulus size increases. (Reprinted, in adapted form, with permission from Price DD, McHaffie JG, Larson MA. Spatial summation of heat-induced pain: influence of stimulus area and spatial separation of stimuli on perceived pain sensation intensity and unpleasantness. *J Neurophysiol* 1989;62:1270–1279.)

double-logarithms coordinates (Fig. 5). A similar parallel displacement in double-logarithmic coordinates is evident when these nociceptive stimuli are delivered to identically sized areas of skin in two regions of the body with different nociceptive thermal sensitivity, the ventral forearm and the facial area over the masseter muscle (73) (Fig. 1). In this instance, the spatial summation is likely to occur as a result of greater density of heat nociceptors in the forearm as compared to the masseter region. The quantitative factors that underlie spatial summation are similar even when different means are used to generate it, e.g., when different sizes of peripheral stimuli are applied, or when the same size stimuli are delivered to regions of different nociceptor density.

The minimal spatial summation observed with stimuli of intensities near pain threshold is consistent with previous studies (30,34) and serves to explain why spatial summation of pain has eluded investigators. The spatial summation property of pain is very different from that of warmth, for which spatial summation occurs maximally near threshold. This difference, in turn, may be related to the fact that the steepest portion of the stimulus-response curve for warmth is near warmth threshold, whereas that for heat-induced pain is well above pain threshold; that is, the function is positively accelerating.

Radiation

A feature of heat-induced pain that is the perceived spread or "radiation" of pain from a stimulus site. While this phenomena may share common mechanisms with summation, it differs technically in that summation reflects the interaction of two or more stimulation incites, whereas for radiation, the region to which pain is referred extends beyond the focal area of a single stimulus. The magnitude of radiation depends upon the magnitude of the local afferent drive originating from the stimulus. Thus, at or near pain threshold, the perceived area of the painful stimulus is confined to the actual area and location of the stimulus itself. However, as the stimulus intensity is elevated above pain threshold, the perceived area of painful sensation extends beyond the boundaries of the actual stimulus. This property was demonstrated in a human psychophysical experiment (77) and is represented in Fig. 6. The 5-s stimuli of randomly varying intensities were applied to the ventral forearm. The incidence of the perceived spread of painful sensations increased from 0 near pain threshold (45°C) to 90% at 51°C. The spread of sensation was not the result of conduction of heat on the skin, since at the highest temperatures used, skin temperatures 2–3 mm from the edge of the thermode were unaltered.

Based on the characteristics of the stimulus which evokes certain pain syndrome, radiation is an attribute believed to be common for many types of clinical pains, including myofascial

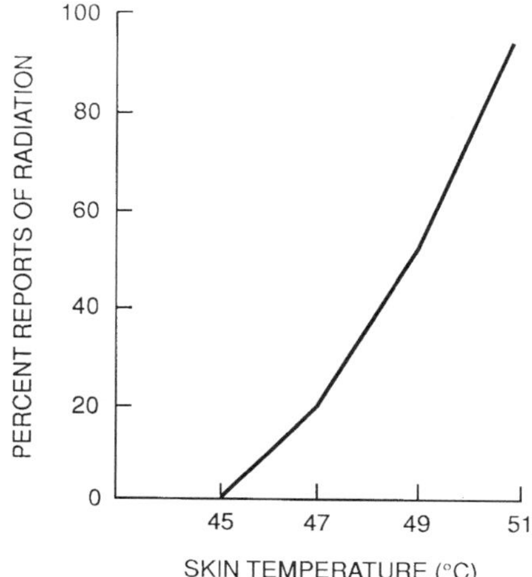

Figure 6. Radiation of pain as a function of skin temperature. As skin temperature increases, the likelihood of reporting radiation of painful sensations increases. (Reprinted, in adapted form, with permission from Price DD, Hayes RL, Ruda MA, Dubner R. Spatial and temporal transformations of input to spinothalamic tract neurons and their relation to somatic sensation. *J Neurophysiol* 1978;41:933–947.)

pain and certain neuropathological pains such as postherpetic neuralgia, trigeminal neuralgia, and causalgia (98). The extent of radiation often covaries with the intensity of the pain itself, remaining confined to a dermatome at low intensities and observed to extend across dermatomes rostral and caudal to the dermatome corresponding to the stimulation site at high intensities.

PSYCHOPHYSICAL ATTRIBUTES OF PATHOPHYSIOLOGICAL PAIN

The psychophysical attributes of pain discussed thus far pertain to those evoked by brief stimuli that are not necessarily damaging and are typically monomodal, e.g., thermal or mechanical and frequently brief in exposure. However, when tissue is injured, as in burns or after surgery (see Chapters 43 and 44), and nerves are damaged (see Chapter 32 and 56), the impact upon function is to induce complex patterns of afferent input and central changes in function . These stimulus conditions will yield pain reports characterized by additional attributes, including "spontaneous" pain, hyperalgesia, and allodynia. Hyperalgesia is a pain state that is reported to be more intense than would otherwise be evoked by a given noxious stimulus. Allodynia is pain evoked by a normally innocuous (nonpainful) stimulus, such as one which otherwise evokes reports of light touch, cooling, or warmth. Both hyperalgesia and allodynia can be thermal or mechanical.

It has been known for >20 years that injury-induced changes can lead to sensitization of the peripheral terminal of primary nociceptive afferent neurons (5,6,14) (see Chapters 30 and 31) and a facilitation of the responsiveness of central nociceptive neurons (6,80,90) (see Chapter 36). These altered stimulus response functions are believed to account for the components of tissue injury-induced hyperalgesia and allodynia.

After nerve injury, significant changes in organization lead to pain reports that appear to be spontaneous (e.g., no evident stimulus) and are characterized by syndromes in which zones of heat hyperalgesia are present (in some patients) and in which larger zones of mechanical hyperalgesia and/or allodynia are present (in most patients)(27,79).

Hyperalgesia and Allodynia

Examples of heat-induced hyperalgesia are shown in Fig. 7, which present data from two patients with unilateral distal extremity injuries and which have been identified by virtue of their positive response to sympathetic block as suffering from reflex sympathetic dystrophy (RSD) patients (79). Assessment of reported pain intensities of stimuli applied to injured regions and homologous contralateral nonpathological zones revealed that the reported intensities of equivalent stimuli of the injured territory exceeded those from the noninjured zone over a wide range of stimulus intensities (43–49°C). However, the difference between injured and noninjured zones was greatest at the lower end of the stimulus range, 43–45°C (Fig. 7). This pattern of increased responsiveness near "normal" threshold for the nerve injured observer is comparable to that obtained for C-polymodal nociceptive afferents and for human ratings of heat-induced pain after heat-induced injury of the skin (14,15). In both heat-induced injury and reflex sympathetic dystrophy, the hyperalgesia is likely to be dynamically maintained by tonic input from primary nociceptive afferents, particularly C-polymodal afferents (27). This tonic input is likely to be related to a "sensitization" of these primary afferents, both in the case of heat injury and in RSD. The sensitization of primary afferents in the latter case, however, appears to lack its usual association with injured skin. Based on the curves presented in Fig. 7, it is also likely that the thermal thresholds for pain were lowered in these two patients, so that heat allodynia was also likely to be present in these patients as well. Cold allodynia also has been shown to be a common characteristic of RSD patients (9,14,15).

Mechanical Hyperalgesia and Allodynia

Two distinct types of mechanical allodynia have been characterized in neuropathic pain patients. The first is termed low-threshold A-beta allodynia based on the presumed role played by A-beta afferents in evoking the pain state (79). Several lines of evidence support the apparent association of A-beta with the initiation of the pain state. The pain state occurs in response to

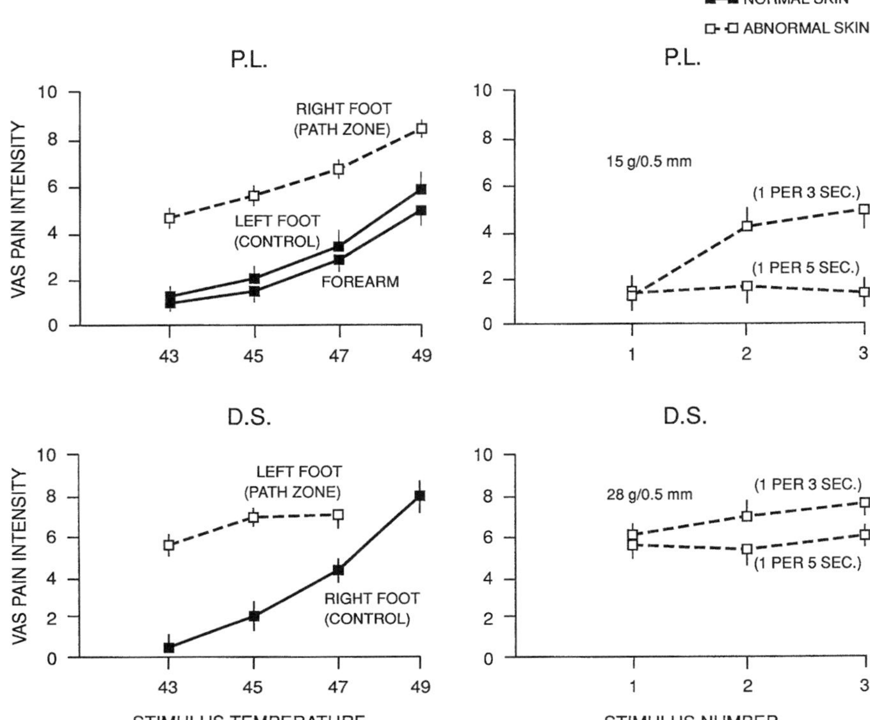

Figure 7. Pain intensity (VAS) ratings of two patients (P.L. and D.S.) who both had heat-induced hyperalgesia (*left graphs*) and temporal summation of mechanical allodynia (*right graphs*) to repeated von Frey filament stimulation. Note that temporal summation occurred with stimuli delivered 1/3 s but not 1/5 s (*right graphs*).

electrical stimulation of the lowest threshold axons in nerves supplying the pathological zone, e.g., large myelinated fibers (14,15,79). It occurs in response to very gentle mechanical stimuli (69). It It is abolished by blockade of the largest, fastest conducting, axons within nerves (27). Adequate stimuli evoke a response with a reaction time consistent with conduction in myelinated afferents (14,15). It is commonly characterized by the fact that moving stimuli or stimulus onset or offset are more painful than static mechanical stimuli (67,69). The other type of mechanical allodynia is characterized by evidence that A-beta afferents do not seem to be involved (see above) and that more intense but normally painless stimuli are required to evoke pain (69). For example, 15–600-g von Frey filament stimuli, which are well above threshold for A-beta primary mechanoreceptive afferents but are rarely painful under normal circumstances, evoke pain when applied to the pathological zones of these patients. This type of mechanical allodynia is termed high threshold, and it well may be mediated by nociceptive afferents that have thresholds below that of normal pain threshold (5).

Pathophysiological Mechanisms of Slow Temporal Summation

Regardless of whether the mechanical allodynia is A-beta or high threshold, it often has characteristics similar to pains normally evoked by unmyelinated C-nociceptive afferents (61, 64–67,69,79). For some RSD patients, slow temporal summation of burning pain occurs when gentle mechanical stimuli or electrical stimulation of A-beta afferents are applied at rates of once per 3 s, as shown in Fig. 8. For other patients, slow temporal summation occurs only with more intense but normally nonpainful mechanical stimuli. Still other patients do not exhibit slow temporal summation with these types of repetitive mechanical stimuli. Both mechanical allodynia and slow temporal summation of allodynia are completely or nearly completely reversed by anesthetic blockade of sympathetic ganglia in those RSD patients tested, indicating that these sensory abnormalities are dynamically maintained by sympathetic efferent activity, presumably activity which induces continuous input over nociceptive afferents. Slow temporal summation of mechanical allodynia, particularly that induced by stimulation of A-beta afferents, is abnormal since such types of stimuli do not evoke pain in pain-free subjects nor in these same pain patients when such stimuli are delivered to homologous contralateral pain-free zones. In fact, A-beta afferent stimulation even at extremely high frequencies does not evoke pain in normal human subjects (66,102). Therefore, A-beta mechanical allodynia and abnormal slow temporal summation of mechanical allodynia may represent an exaggeration and/or abnormal triggering of physiological mechanisms that already exist in normal pain-free individuals. Such mechanisms can be demonstrated in the latter by temporal summation of experimentally induced second pain (Fig. 4), as described earlier. Thus, under some pathological conditions after nerve injury, A-beta input must somehow gain access to and trigger the same NMDA receptor-slow temporal summation mechanism that is normally activated by C-afferent stimulation (see above). In other pathological conditions, sensitized nociceptors themselves are likely to be the direct proximal cause of the slow temporal summation of mechanical allodynia.

Relationships Between Slow Temporal Summation of Allodynia and Spontaneous Pain

Mechanical allodynia and slow temporal summation of allodynia may well be integrally related to the patients ongoing "spontaneous" pain. This relationship could occur if continuous input from A-beta low-threshold afferents (evoked in the normal course of mechanical stimulation from walking, sitting or even contact with clothes) activated slow temporal summation of a type of burning, aching, or throbbing pain that built up slowly and dissipated slowly over time. This possibility was explicitly tested by comparing intensities of ongoing pain between patients who demonstrated slow temporal summation versus those who did not (79). The former had significantly higher intensities of ongoing pain (mean = 7.0 on visual analogue pain scale) than the latter (mean = 4.0 on visual analogue pain scale). Therefore, exaggerated or abnormally triggered mechanisms of slow temporal summation are likely to form at least part of the basis of persistent pain that sometimes follows nerve injury.

PSYCHOPHYSICAL ASSESSMENT OF ANALGESIA PRODUCED BY PHARMACOLOGICAL TREATMENTS

The psychophysical attributes of normal and abnormal pain states and the capacity to measure them offer a potential basis for determining how pharmacological interventions influence different aspects of pain. This section deals with psychophysical assessment of the mechanisms of various types of drugs that influence pain. Only studies in which psychophysical methods and controlled experimental stimuli were used will be discussed. The drugs to be discussed are by no means most of those which are used clinically but are to be considered representative of various pharmacological classes of drugs. Moreover, since present knowledge of many of these classes of drugs is quite limited, particularly in relation to human psychophysical studies, corresponding discussions of some of these drugs will be brief if not absent.

Opiates

The effects of narcotic analgesics on both experimental and clinical pain have been studied extensively in humans. Yet, it has been unclear as to which dimensions of pain experience

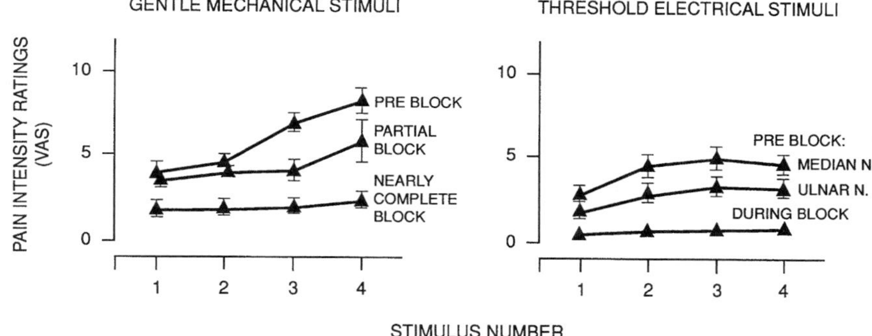

Figure 8. Slow temporal summation of A-beta allodynia in an RSD patient. Pain intensity ratings (VAS) were made by this patient in response to trains of stimuli likely to activate A-beta afferents. These ratings were made before and during successful sympathetic blocks. *Left:* Slow temporal summation of burning pain in response to trains of very gentle mechanical stimuli and its attenuation by sympathetic block. *Right:* Slow temporal summation of pain in response to transcutaneous electrical stimulation of A-beta afferents and its attenuation by sympathetic block. (Based on data presented in ref. 80.)

and which types of pain are most affected (3,4,25). Until the end of the seventies, a prevalent explanation of narcotic analgesia was that opiates reduce the affective-motivational dimension of pain much more than its sensory discriminative dimension (3,4,25). Animal models, however emphasized that opiates by a spinal and supraspinal action could clearly alter the processing of nociceptive afferent traffic (see Chapter 58). This generalization regarding the affective component in humans was largely based on the findings of Beecher (4) that pain thresholds were increased very little by morphine. However, in 1979, Gracely et al. (29) found that fentanyl, a short-acting synthetic opioid, reduced painful sensations but not the unpleasantness associated with suprathreshold tooth pulp stimulation. Subsequent studies that also used direct scaling of experimental pains, including heat pain (75,85) and cold pressor pain (63), have likewise confirmed opiate-induced attenuation of suprathreshold pain sensation intensities. However, that opiate analgesics would reduce only the sensory dimension of pain, as found by Gracely et al. (29), or only unpleasantness components of pain, as found in earlier studies (3,4), is perplexing in view of considerable evidence that opiates inhibit transmission of nociceptive information at the first spinal cord synapse in ascending somatosensory pathways (54,55,101). After all, there is no evidence that sensory or affective components of pain are differentiated at the level of primary nociceptive afferents or at the level of the spinal cord. The observed lack of morphine's effect on pain thresholds in Beecher's studies may have been the result of insensitive or inappropriate measures. In contrast, Gracely et al. (29) explained their observed lack of effect of fentanyl on pain affect on the basis of offsetting dysphoric side effects of opiates in pain-free volunteer subjects, an explanation supported by previous studies (see references in ref. 29).

In an attempt to resolve some of these disparate findings and consequent explanations of mechanisms of narcotic analgesia, Price et al. (85) examined the effects of different doses of morphine on sensory and affective visual analogue scale (VAS) responses to suprathreshold levels of experimentally induced heat pain in an experimental context designed to minimize side effects of morphine. Normal volunteer human subjects, who did not have ongoing clinical pain and were not undergoing medical procedures, lay on hospital beds throughout the experimental session. Different groups of subjects received different doses of morphine sulfate (0.04–0.08 mg/kg) or saline placebo intravenously and on a double blind basis. Morphine reduced both sensory intensity and unpleasantness VAS ratings of graded 5-s nociceptive temperature stimuli (45–51°C) in a dose-dependent manner, as shown in Fig. 9. Although these doses reduced both VAS-sensory and VAS-affective ratings, they did not alter the basic relationship between pain sensation intensity and degree of unpleasantness, because the same regression line derived for the sensory-affective relationship applied to both pre- and postdrug conditions, as shown in Fig. 10. Reductions in pain sensation and unpleasantness were approximately the same. Similar results were obtained in a study of fentanyl's analgesic effects on experimental heat pain and clinical pain (75). Fentanyl produced nearly equal reductions in VAS-sensory and VAS-affective responses to experimental pain (i.e., 45–51°C) but slightly greater reductions in clinical pain VAS-affective as compared to clinical pain VAS-sensory ratings. The combined results of both morphine and fentanyl studies indicate that both sensory and affective dimensions of pain are reduced by morphine and that reductions in unpleasantness can be accounted for mainly by reductions in pain sensation intensity. Additional selective effects on pain affect may result from supraspinal effects of opiates that produce euphoria or sedation and these additional effects may apply more to clinical than to experimental pain (25).

A similar confusion has existed with regard to whether opiates differentially inhibit different types of pain. For example, some investigators have claimed that analgesic effects of opiates are detectable on those forms of experimental pain whose long duration and severity simulate that of clinical pain (3,4,91). Yet several studies have demonstrated analgesic effects of opiates on pains evoked by brief experimental stimuli (29,63,75,85). Other investigators have asserted that opiates reduce diffuse dull pain more than sharp intermittent pain (91) or that opiates inhibit "second" pain (mediated by slow-conducting unmyelinated C afferents) but not "first" pain (mediated by A-delta afferents) (20).

These assertions can be tested in studies in which different types of pains are measured in the same subjects (and in some cases patients) and experimental context. A study that simultaneously compared fentanyl's analgesic effects on clinical low back pain and experimentally induced heat pain (45–51°C/5-s pulses) found that intravenous administration of 0.8 and 1.1 μg/kg fentanyl reduced VAS-sensory ratings of clinical pain and experimental pain by equal extents (75). Thus, the antinociceptive effects of opiates appear similar for very differ-

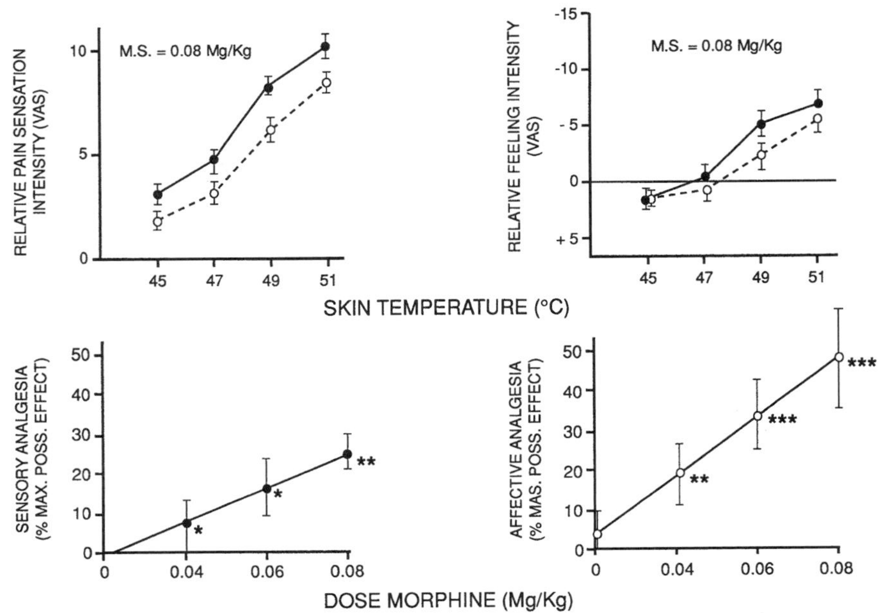

Figure 9. Top: Skin temperature-VAS pain sensory functions (*top left*) and skin temperature-VAS affective functions (*top right*) before and after intravenous injection of 0.08 mg/kg morphine sulfate. *Closed circles* and *solid lines* are based on group mean baseline VAS responses, and *open circles* and *dashed lines* are based on group mean VAS responses after morphine administration. Each *point* is the average of eight subjects, and *vertical bars* are SEMs. *Top right:* The ordinate of the skin temperature-pain affects graph is divided into positive (+) and negative (-) scales, which respectively indicate relative magnitudes of pleasantness and unpleasantness. *Bottom:* Dose response curves for effects of morphine on sensory-intensive (*lower left*) and affective responses (*lower right*) to 45–51°C 5-s temperatures. The degree of analgesia is expressed as average percent of decrease in area under the 45–51°C stimulus-VAS response curve. Paired *t* tests comparing subjects' areas under the stimulus-response curve before and after morphine resulted in p values: *p > 0.05; **p < 0.01; ***p < 0.001.

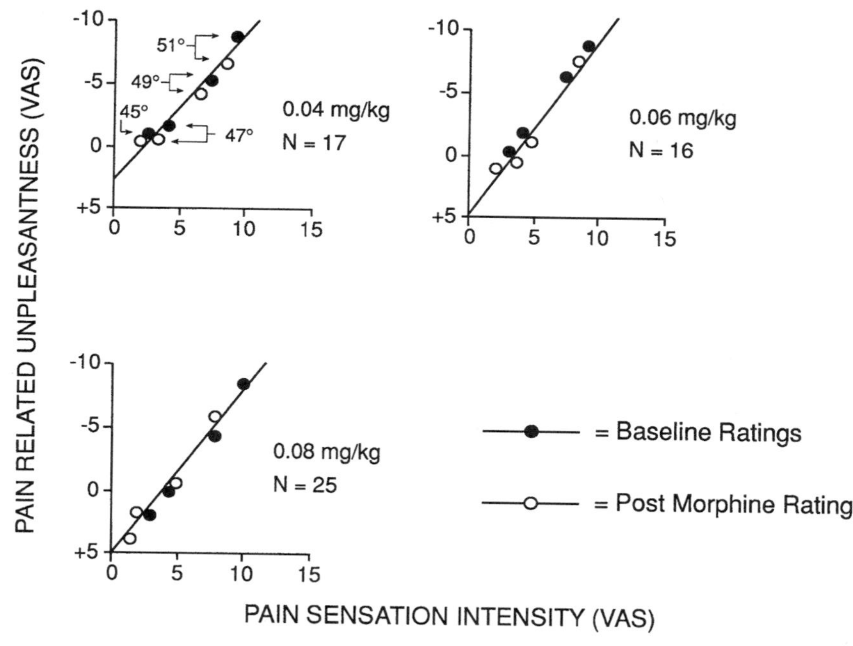

Figure 10. Pain-related unpleasantness plotted as a function of pain sensation intensity for experimentally induced heat pain. The same *regression line* applies to both pre- and postdrug conditions in the case of 0.06 mg/kg (*left*) and 0.08 mg/kg (*right*). Four data *points* obtained for each condition are based on the four temperatures presented (45°C, 47°C, 49°C, 51°C). That the same *regression line* applies to both pre- and postdrug conditions despite reductions in sensory and affective ratings indicates that affect is likely to be reduced as a consequence of reduction in pain sensation.

ent types of pain, such as brief heat pulses to the skin and chronic low back pain.

Nonetheless, there is evidence that pains evoked by different types of primary nociceptive afferents are differentially inhibited by opiate analgesics. Cooper et al. (20) examined effects of intramuscular injections of 5 and 10 mg of morphine on perceived intensities of first and second pains evoked by brief stimuli. They found that regardless of whether electrical, mechanical, or thermal stimulation was used, the initial pains related to impulse conduction in A-delta primary afferents were unaffected by these doses of morphine. In striking contrast, the magnitude of late (second) pain sensations produced by these same types of stimuli was consistently and significantly reduced by doses of 5 or 10 mg of morphine. They concluded that morphine preferentially attenuates the central excitatory effects evoked by impulses in unmyelinated nociceptive afferents (related to second pain). It could be argued, however, that the artificial or highly synchronous nature of the afferent barrage evoked by brief stimuli prevented inhibitory effects of morphine on first pain. A subsequent study (85) using heat pulses generated by a constant contact thermode showed that 0.08 mg/kg morphine (i.v.) produced inhibitory effects on both first and second pain, as shown in Fig. 11, but that morphine also had an especially potent inhibitory effect on the temporal summation of second pain that occurs when heat pulses are delivered at 3-s intervals. Thus, whether morphine reduces second pain by a greater extent than first pain may depend somewhat on temporal parameters of stimulation. Since morphine can inhibit slow temporal summation of second pain, it can prevent the occurrence of intense summated second pain by a greater extent than first or second pain evoked by single stimuli (Fig. 11). It has been suggested above that temporal summation of second pain reflects mechanisms that are related to hyperalgesia and that such summation mechanisms are exaggerated and/or abnormally triggered in pathophysiological pain states. If so, then narcotic analgesics may be especially effective in attenuating such pains before they are allowed to summate over

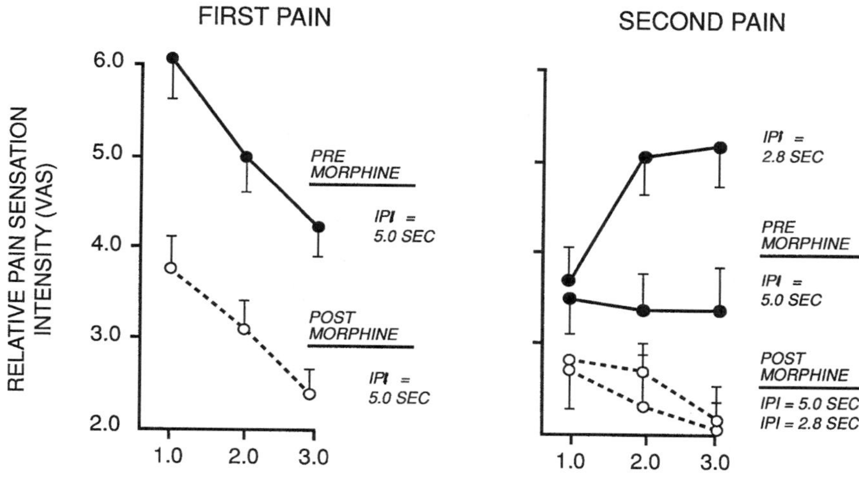

Figure 11. Perceived pain sensation (VAS) magnitudes of first pain (*left*) and second pain (*right*) evoked by trains of three noxious heat pulses 1 h before (*solid lines* and *filled circles*) and 1 h after (*dashed lines* and *open circles*) intravenous administration of morphine sulfate. Each *point* is the group mean of 30 responses obtained from 10 subjects (±1 SE of the estimate). The interstimulus intervals (IPI) of the different trains are indicated at the right of each curve.

time. For example, the administration of opiate analgesics prior to surgery may help prevent the hyperalgesic states that often follow tissue injury.

Finally, the relationship between the intensity of pain and the degree of inhibition of pain by opiates requires some clarification. It would be convenient if a given dose of an opiate inhibited various intensities of pain by the same percentage. One would not have to know much about the pretreatment intensity of pain in order to predict percent relief. Unfortunately, such does not appear to be the case. As shown in Fig. 9, various doses of morphine shift the stimulus-response curves to the right in a parallel manner. A very similar parallel shift occurs with fentanyl (75), electroacupuncture (84), dorsal column stimulation (51), and transcutaneous electrical nerve stimulation (50). In examining these shifts, one can see that various intensities of pain are reduced by a nearly constant numerical extent and not a constant percentage. Thus, for example, 0.08 mg/kg (i.v.) morphine sulfate reduced the pain intensity evoked by 51°C by ~17%, whereas it reduced the pain intensity evoked by 45°C by nearly 50% (Fig. 9). The same dose of an opiate reduces lower-intensity pains by a greater percent than high-intensity pains. This principle is likely to apply to clinical pains, since it has been shown that a given dose of an opiate reduces experimental pain and clinical pain intensity by an internally consistent extent (75). Such a principle may help account for the observation that diffuse low intensity pains are reduced by opiates to a greater extent than are sharp intense pains.

Although some would claim that psychophysical studies of opiate analgesia are clearly limited in that they cannot directly determine how various doses and types of narcotic analgesics will affect clinical pain, the combined and simultaneous analysis of narcotic analgesics on experimental and clinical pain allows for a direct comparison of an opiate analgesicís effect on the different types of pain. Moreover, these psychophysical analyses have advantages in determining the mechanisms of narcotic analgesia and in comparing the relative potencies of various doses and types of analgesic medications and treatments. For example, the morphine dose-response curve shown in Fig. 9 can be used as a reference standard in comparing the analgesic efficacy of various treatments for pain.

Nitrous Oxide

Concentrations of nitrous oxide (N_2O) that are usually below that which produces unconsciousness are commonly used in dentistry and medicine to ameliorate pain and stress. Although analgesic effects of N_2O have been well documented in humans, only recently have well-designed psychophysical studies been carried out that characterize this form of pain control (24,32,86). Based on average responses of groups of human volunteer subjects, it is clear that concentrations of 30–45% of N_2O increase pain thresholds (24,86) or reduce ratings of pain sensation intensity (32).

Of the few attempts to characterize N_2O analgesia through the use of direct scaling techniques, that of Heft et al. (32) is of particular interest because they used the same verbal descriptor scales and a similar experimental design as that used by Gracely et al. (29) to characterize fentanyl analgesia (see above). They compared analgesic effects produced by 33% N_2O and 67% O_2, 100% O2, and air on a double blind basis. Only the N_2O and O_2 combination significantly reduced sensory verbal descriptor ratings but not unpleasantness ratings of graded levels of noxious tooth shocks. These results are very similar to that found for fentanyl, as described earlier, and again it is somewhat perplexing that an analgesic would reduce sensory but not affective responses related to pain. However, a possible reason for this pattern of results can be given that is similar to the one given above for fentanyl. Several studies have shown that N_2O disrupts cognitive performance, including psychomotor performance (86,92). Thus, the cognitive impairment induced by N_2O may be experienced as aversive, a possibility consistent with the observation that five of 19 subjects in one N_2O experiment withdrew within 3–4 min after N_2O administration (86). Thus, the aversive effects of N_2O may offset the reductions in pain unpleasantness that would otherwise occur as a result of the reduction in pain sensation intensity.

Another rather striking characteristic of N_2O analgesia is that acute tolerance rapidly develops in some subjects and not others, rendering the analgesic effects highly variable within and between subjects (86). Ramsey et al. (86) found that six of 14 subjects developed rapid tolerance to analgesic effects of 35–40% N_2O, as assessed by tooth pulp stimulation-evoked pain thresholds. This tolerance occurred over a period of 30–40 min in those subjects who exhibited tolerance but was completely absent in other subjects.

An appreciation of the possible offsetting aversive effects of N_2O and the development of rapid tolerance in some subjects is very important clinically. Future research should be aimed at methods for identifying the subset of individuals who develop tolerance to N_2O analgesia and the problem of rapid tolerance should be recognized amongst those who use N_2O as a clinical analgesic.

Benzodiazepines

Although tranquilizers such as diazepam have been known to reduce the anxiety associated with invasive medical procedures, little explicit investigation has been made with respect to their influence on pain. Using verbal descriptor scaling techniques in combination with cross-modality matching procedures, Gracely et al. (28) demonstrated that 5 mg diazepam (i.v.), a common tranquilizer, significantly reduced affective descriptor responses to painful electrocutaneous shock without altering sensory descriptor responses. The reductions were greatest for low-intensity noxious stimuli. These results can easily be interpreted in terms of reduction in the anxiety associated with experimental pain because diazepam has been well characterized as an anxiety-reducing agent. At least part of the unpleasantness of pain is related to anxiety associated with possible harm to tissue and with other negative consequences. This interpretation is indirectly supported by the fact that other treatments known to reduce anxiety result in a pattern of effects on pain similar to that just described for diazepam. Thus, both saline placebo and other cognitive manipulations have been shown to selectively reduce the affective dimension of pain and to have their largest effects at the low end of the nociceptive stimulus range (26,28,68).

N-Methyl-D-Aspartate Antagonists

Significant recent advances have been made in the understanding of neurotransmitter mechanisms of nociception within the spinal cord, particularly in relationship to central hyperalgesia. As discussed above, hyperalgesic/allodynic mechanisms appear common to neuropathic pain and certain types of inflammatory pain. These mechanisms involve excitotoxic effects of excitatory amino acids, such as glutamate and aspartate, which are synaptically released by primary nociceptive afferents onto second order nociceptive neurons of the spinal cord dorsal horn (6,97) (see Chapters 34 and 36). In brief, the released glutamate and aspartate binds to some postsynaptic receptors that mediate fast excitatory responses and to *N*-methyl-D-aspartate (NMDA) receptors that mediate long-duration depolarization. The long-duration depolarization, initiated by NMDA receptor activation and additionally by released substance P, summates slowly over time. This mechanism is likely to be the basis for slow temporal summation of C-nociceptive afferent-evoked impulse discharges of dorsal horn neurons and is therefore likely to be causally related to slow temporal summation of C-afferent-evoked second pain in normal pain-free individuals as well as slow temporal summation of mechanical allodynia in neuropathic pain patients (80). Slow temporal summation of C-afferent-evoked responses of spinal cord dorsal horn neurons is also likely to provide much of the basis of central hyperalgesia, as has been suggested by Thompson and Woolf (97).

If NMDA receptor mechanisms are involved in summation of second pain as shown by Price et al. (81) and in hyperalgesic states in humans, then some types of normal and pathophysiological pains should be reduced by NMDA antagonists. Although one study has demonstrated inhibitory effects of NMDA antagonists on temporal summation of second pain, other studies have indeed shown that NMDA antagonists effectively reduce both experimental and clinical pains that are likely to involve hyperalgesic states. Maurset et al. (53) compared the analgesic efficacy of 0.3 mg/kg ketamine (which has NMDA antagonist activity) and 0.7 mg/kg pethidine (a synthetic narcotic analgesic) on experimental ischemic pain and postoperative pain after oral surgery. Both types of pain are likely to involve hyperalgesic mechanisms. Naloxone (1.6 mg) or placebo was given 5 min before the analgesic drug. Both ketamine and pethidine were effective against the two types of pain studied. However, naloxone prevented the analgesic effect of pethidine but not that of ketamine. The authors interpreted their results as indicating that ketamine analgesia is mediated by a nonopioid mechanism, possible involving PCP-receptor-mediated blockade of the NMDA-receptor-operated ion channel. In further support of this hypothesis, Klepstad et al. (44) have provided important results showing that S-ketamine (0.10 ± 0.15 mg/kg = effective dose) was approximately four times as potent as R-ketamine (0.50 mg = effective dose) in reducing experimentally induced ischemic pain, in particular its slow increase over time. In this experiment, these isomers of ketamine and saline placebo were administered on a double blind basis. The fourfold difference in analgesic potency was consistent with their relative affinity for PCP (phencyclidine) binding sites. These results support an involvement of NMDA receptors in normal human pain perception.

A role of NMDA receptors in pathophysiological pain was recently supported by Byas-Smith et al. (13) and Park et al. (62) in two complementary studies. The first showed that subanesthetic doses of ketamine were effective in inhibiting the allodynia and spontaneous pain associated with neuropathic pain in chronic pain patients (13). The second showed similar effects of ketamine n allodynia and spontaneous pain after intradermal capsaicin injection, an acute model of pathophysiological pain in humans (62).

CONCLUSIONS

Different dimensions of pain and different mechanisms of pain can be differentially measured in experimental paradigms that use controlled intensities of nociceptive stimuli and in studies in which experimental pain and clinical pain are studied together. Psychophysical studies of normal pain processing have demonstrated the fundamental psychophysical attributes of pain, which include highly reliable pain thresholds, minimal adaptation of pain intensity in the presence of maintained nociceptive stimulation, slow temporal summation of C-afferent-mediated pain but not A-afferent-mediated pain, spatial summation, and radiation of perceived area of pain sensation at suprathreshold levels of nociceptive stimulation.

Pathophysiological mechanisms of pain often represent exaggerations or abnormal triggering of the same mechanisms that are present in normal pain processing. For example, in certain forms of neuropathic pain and in some but not all patients, repetitive input from A-beta afferents appears to trigger the same slow temporal summation mechanism that is triggered in normal individuals by repetitive input from C-polymodal nociceptive afferents. These pathophysiological expressions of pain mechanisms can be identified in individual patients through the use of standardized sensory tests and have important implications for treating various types of pathophysiological pain.

The psychophysical attributes of normal and abnormal pain states and the capacity to measure them provide the basis for determining how pharmacological interventions influence different aspects of pain. This approach has shown that opiates reduce both sensory-discriminative and affective-motivational dimensions of pain and that reduction in the latter is probably a major consequence of reduction in the former. However, opiates such as morphine have a more powerful inhibitory effect on nociceptive mechanisms triggered by C-nociceptive afferents than by A-delta nociceptive afferents, and this differential effect may partly account for clinical impressions that opiates reduce diffuse dull, aching, or burning pains more than brief sharp punctate pains (i.e., pinprick). Benzodiazepines appear to selectively reduce the affective dimension of pain, probably by means of an antianxiety effect. N_2O inhibits the sensory discriminative aspects of pain as well as that of other somatosensory modalities and is characterized by acute tolerance in some patients. Finally, NMDA antagonists show considerable promise as agents that reverse hyperalgesic states that result from nerve injury or inflammation of injured tissue. These effects are beginning to be demonstrated in human psychophysical studies in neuropathic pain patients and in human experimental studies of hyperalgesia.

REFERENCES

1. Adair EE, Stevens JC, Marks LE. Thermally induced pain: the dol scale and the psychophysical power law. *Am J Psychol* 1968;82: 147–164.
2. Barrell JJ, Price DD. The perception of first and second pain as a function of psychological set. *Percept Psychophys* 1975;17:163–166.
3. Beecher HK. Limiting factors in experimental pain. *J Chron Dis* 1956;4.
4. Beecher HK. *Measurement of subjective responses: quantitative effects of drugs.* New York: Oxford University Press, 1959.
5. Beitel RE, Dubner R. Response of unmyelinated (C) polymodal nociceptors to thermal stimuli applied to monkey's face. *J Neurophysiol* 1976;39:116–117.
6. Bennett GJ. Evidence from animal models on the pathogenesis of painful peripheral neuropathy, and its relevance for pharmacotherapy. In: Basbaum AI, Besson JM, eds. *Towards a new pharmacotherapy.* Chichester, U.K.: John Wiley, 1991:365–379.
7. Bennett GJ, Xie YK. A peripheral mononeuropathy in rat that produces disorders of pain sensation like those seen in man. *Pain* 1988;33:87–107.
8. Blitz B, Dinnerstein AJ. Effects of different types of instructions on pain parameters. *J Abnorm Psychol* 1968;73:276–280.
9. Bonica JJ. Causagesia and other reflex sympathetic dystrophies. In: Bonica JJ, ed. *The management of pain.* Philadelphia: Lea & Febiger, 1990:220–256.
10. Bushnell MC, Duncan GH. Sensory and affective aspects of pain perception: is medial thalamus restricted to emotional issues? *Exp Brain Res* 1989;78:415–418.
11. Bushnell MC, Duncan GH, Dubner R, He LF. Activity of trigeminothalamic neurons in medullary dorsal horn of awake monkeys trained in a thermal discrimination task. *J Neurophysiol* 1984;52: 170–187.
12. Bushnell MC, Taylor MB, Duncan GH, Dubner R. Discrimination of innocuous and noxious thermal stimuli applied to the face in human and monkey. *Somatosens Res* 1983;1:119–129.
13. Byas-Smith MG, Max MB, Gracely RH, Bennett GJ. Intravenous ketamine and alfentanyl in patients with chronic causalgic pain and allodynia. In: *Abstracts of the 7th World Congress.* Seattle, Wa: I.A.S.P. Press, 1993:454.
14. Campbell JN, Raja SN, Meyer RA. Painful sequelae of nerve injury. In: Dubner R, Gebhart GF, Bond MR, eds. *Pain research and clinical management.* New York: Elsevier, 1988:135–143.
15. Campbell JN, Raja SN, Meyer RA, MacKinnon SE. Myelinated afferents signal the hyperalgesia associated with nerve injury. *Pain* 1988;32:89–94.

16. Chapman CR, Casey KL, Dubner R, Foley KM, Gracely RH, Reading AE. Pain measurement: an overview. *Pain* 1985;22:1–31.
17. Chapman LF, Dingman HF, Ginzberg SP. Failure of systemic analgesic agents to alter the absolute sensory threshold for the simple detection of pain. *Brain* 1965;88:1011–1022.
18. Chery-Croze S, Duclaux R. Discrimination of painful stimuli in human beings: influence of stimulation area. *J Neurophysiol* 1980; 44:1–10.
19. Coghill RC, Mayer DJ, Price DD. Wide dynamic range but not nociceptive specific neurons encode multidimensional features of prolonged repetitive heat stimuli. *J Neurophysiol* 1993;69: 703–716.
20. Cooper BY, Vierck CJ, Yeomans DC. Selective reduction of second pain sensations by systemic morphine in humans. *Pain* 1986;24: 93–116.
21. Douglass DK, Carstens E, Watkins LR. Spatial summation in human pain perception. *Soc Neurosci Abstr* 1988;13:283.
22. Dubner R, Beitel RE, Brown FJ. A behavioral animal model for the study of pain mechanisms in primates. In: Weisenberg M, Tursky B, eds. *Pain: new perspectives in therapy and research.* New York: Plenum Press, 1976:155–170.
23. Dubner R, Price DD, Beitel RE, Hu JW. Peripheral neural correlates of behavior in monkey and human related to sensory-discriminative aspects of pain. In: Anderson DJ, Matthews B, eds. *Pain in the trigeminal region.* Amsterdam: Elsevier, 1977:57–66.
24. Dworkin SF, Chen ACN, Schubert MM, Clark DW. Analgesic effects of nitrous oxide with controlled painful stimuli. *J Am Dent Assoc* 1983;107:581–585.
25. Gilman AG, Goodman LS, Gilman A. *The pharmacological basis of therapeutics.* New York: Macmillan, 1980.
26. Gracely RH. Psychophysical assessment of human pain. In: Bonica JJ, Liebeskind JC, Albe-Fessard D, eds. *Advances in pain research and therapy.* New York: Raven Press, 1979:805–824.
27. Gracely RH, Lynch SA, Bennett GJ. Painful neuropathy: altered central processing maintained dynamically by peripheral input. *Pain* 1992;51:175–194.
28. Gracely RH, McGrath PA, Dubner R. Validity and sensitivity of ratio scales of sensory and affective verbal pain descriptors: manipulation of affect by diazepam. *Pain* 1978;5:19–29.
29. Gracely RH, McGrath P, Dubner R. Narcotic analgesia: fentanyl reduces the intensity but not the unpleasantness of painful tooth pulp sensations. *Science* 1979;203:1261–1263.
30. Greene LC, Hardy JD. Spatial summation of pain. *J Appl Physiol* 1958;13:457–464.
31. Guilford JP. *Psychometric methods.* New York: McGraw-Hill, 1954.
32. Heft MW, Gracely RH, Dubner R. Nitrous oxide analgesia: a psychological evaluation using verbal descriptor scaling. *J Dent Res* 1984;63:129–132.
33. Hardy JD. Thresholds of pain and reflex contraction as related to noxious stimuli. *J Appl Physiol* 1953;5:225–239.
34. Hardy JD, Wolff HG, Goodell H. Studies on pain. A new method for measuring pain threshold: observations on spatial summation of pain. *J Clin Invest* 1940;19:649–657.
35. Hardy JD, Wolff HG, Goodell H. *Pain sensations and reactions.* Baltimore: Williams and Wilkins, 1952.
36. Hellon RF, Mitchell D. Convergence in a thermal afferent pathway in the rat. *J Physiol (Lond)* 1975;248:359–376.
37. Hoffman DS, Dubner R, Hayes RL, Medlin TP. Neuronal activity in medullary dorsal horn of awake monkeys trained in a thermal discrimination task I: responses to innocuous and noxious thermal stimuli. *J Neurophysiol* 1981;46:409–427.
38. Jensen MP, Karoly P. Self-report scales and procedures for assessing pain in adults. In: Turk DC, Melzack R, eds. *Handbook of pain assessment.* New York: Guilford Press, 1993, 135–151.
39. Kenshalo DR, Anton F, Dubner R. S-1 cortical nociceptive neurons participate in the encoding process by which monkeys perceive the intensity of noxious thermal stimulation. *Brain Res* 1988;454:378–382.
40. Kenshalo DR, Decker T, Hamilton A. Spatial summation on the forehead, forearm, and back produced by radiant and conducted heat. *J Comp Physiol Psychol* 1967;63:510–515.
41. Kenshalo DR Jr, Giesler GJ, Leonard RB, Willis WD. Responses of neurons in primate ventral posterior lateral nucleus to noxious stimuli. *J Neurophysiol* 1980;43:1594–1614.
42. Kenshalo DR Jr, Isensee O. Responses of primate S1 cortical neurons to noxious stimuli. *J Neurophysiol* 1980;50:1479–1496.
43. Kenshalo DR Jr, Leonard RB, Chung JM, Willis WD. Responses of primate spinothalamic neurons to graded and to repeated noxious heat stimuli. *J Neurophysiol* 1979;42:1370–1389.
44. Klepstad P, Maurset A, Moberg ER, Oye I. Evidence of a role for NMDA receptors in pain perception. *Eur J Pharmacol* 1990;187: 513–518.
45. La Motte RH, Campbell JN. Comparison of responses of warm and nociceptive C-fiber afferents in monkey with human judgments of thermal pain. *J Neurophysiol* 1978;41:509–528.
46. Larson MA, McHaffie JG, Stein BE. Response properties of nociceptive and low threshold mechanoreceptive neurons in the hamster superior colliculus. *J Neurosci* 1987;7:547–564.
47. Larson MA, McHaffie JG, Stein BE. Quantitative evaluation of nociceptive neurons in rat trigeminal pars caudalis. *Soc Neurosci Abstr* 1988;14:122.
48. Maixner W, Dubner R, Bushnell MC, Kenshalo DR Jr, Oliveras JL. Wide-dynamic-range dorsal horn neurons participate in the encoding process by which monkeys perceive the intensity of noxious heat stimuli. *Brain Res* 1986;374:385–388.
49. Maixner W, Dubner R, Kenshalo DR Jr, Bushnell MC, Oliveras JL. Responses of monkey medullary dorsal horn neurons during detection of noxious heat stimuli. *J Neurophysiol* 1989;62:437–449.
50. Marchand S, Bushnell MC, Duncan GH. Modulation of heat pain perception by high frequency transcutaneous electrical nerve stimulation (TENS). *Clin J Pain* 1991;7:122–129.
51. Marchand S, Bushnell MC, Duncan GH, Molina-Negro P, Martinez SN The effects of dorsal column stimulation on measures of clinical and experimental pain in man. *Pain* 1991;45:249–257.
52. Marks LW. *Sensory processes. The new psychophysics.* New York: Academic Press, 1974.
53. Maurset A, Skoglund LA, Hustveit O, Oye I. Comparison of ketamine and pethidine in experimental and postoperative pain. *Pain* 1989;36:37–41.
54. Mayer DJ, Price DD. Central nervous system mechanisms of analgesia. *Pain* 1976;2:379–404.
55. Mayer DJ, Price DD. A physiological and psychological analysis of pain: a potential model of motivation. In: Ptaff DW, eds. *The physiological mechanisms of motivation.* New York: Springer-Verlag, 1982: 433–471.
56. Melzack R, Casey KL. Sensory motivational and central control of determinants of pain. In: Kenshalo DR, eds. *The skin senses.* Springfield, IL: Charles C. Thomas, 1968:423–439.
57. Melzack R, Rose G, McGinty D. Skin sensitivity to thermal stimuli. *Exp Neurol* 1962;6:300–314.
58. Melzack R, Torgerson WS. On the language of pain. *Anesthesiology* 1971;34:50–59.
59. Mountcastle VB. Pain and temperature sensibilities. In: Mountcastle VB, eds. *Medical physiology, vol. 1.* 13th ed. Saint Louis: Mosby, 1974:348–381.
60. Murgatroyd D. *Spatial summation of pain for large body areas. Defense Atomic Support Agency report.* Washington, DC: Defense Atomic Support Agency, 1964.
61. Noordenbos W. *Pain.* Amsterdam: Elsevier, 1959.
62. Park KM, Max MB, Robinovitz E, Gracely RH, Bennett GJ. Effects of intravenous ketamine and alfentanil on hyperalgesia induced by intradermal capsaicin. In: *Abstracts of the 7th World Congress.* Seattle, WA: I.A.S.P. Press, 1993:454.
63. Posner J, Telekes A, Crowley D, Phillipson R, Peck AW. Effects of an opioid on cold-induced pain and the CNS in healthy volunteers. *Pain* 1985;23:73–82.
64. Price DD. Characteristics of second pain and flexion reflexes indicative of prolonged central summation. *Exp Neurol* 37:371–391.
65. Price DD. Modulation of first and second pain by peripheral stimulation and by psychological set. In: Bonica JJ, Fessard DA, eds. *Advances in pain research and therapy.* New York: Raven Press, 1976: 427–432.
66. Price DD. *Psychological and neural mechanisms of pain.* New York: Raven Press, 1988.
67. Price DD. Characterizing central mechanisms of pathological pain states by sensory testing and neurophysiological analysis. In: Casey KL, eds. *Pain and central nervous system disease: the central pain syndromes.* New York: Raven Press, 1991:103–115.
68. Price DD, Barrell JJ, Gracely RH. A psychophysical analysis of experiential factors that selectively influence the affective dimension of pain. *Pain* 1980;8:137–149.
69. Price DD, Bennett GJ, Rafii A. Psychophysical observations on patients with neuropathic pain relieved by a sympathetic block. *Pain* 1989;36:209–218.

70. Price DD, Browe AC. Responses of spinal cord neurons to graded noxious and non-noxious stimuli. *Exp Neurol* 1975;48:201–221.
71. Price DD, Bush FM, Long S, Harkins SW. A comparison of pain measurement characteristics of mechanical visual analogue and simple numerical rating scales. *Pain* (in press).
72. Price DD, Dubner R, Hu JW. Trigeminothalamic neurons in nucleus caudalis responsive to tactile, thermal, and nociceptive stimulation of monkey's face. *J Neurophysiol* 1976;39:936–953.
73. Price DD, Harkins SW. The combined use of experimental pain and visual analogue scales in providing standardized measurement of clinical pain. *Clin J Pain* 1987;3:1–8.
74. Price DD, Harkins SW, Baker C. Sensory-affective relationships among different types of clinical and experimental pain. *Pain* 1986;28:297–307.
75. Price DD, Harkins SW, Rafii A, Price C. A simultaneous comparison of fentanyl's analgesic effects on experimental and clinical pain. *Pain* 1986;24:197–203.
76. Price DD, Hayashi H, Dubner R, Ruda MA. Functional relationships between neurons of marginal and substantia gelatinosa layers of primate dorsal horn. *J Neurophysiol* 1979;41:933–947.
77. Price DD, Hayes RL, Ruda MA, Dubner R. Spatial and temporal transformations of input to spinothalamic tract neurons and their relation to somatic sensation. *J Neurophysiol* 1978;41:933–947.
78. Price DD, Hu JW, Dubner R, Gracely RH. Peripheral suppression of first pain and central summation of second pain evoked by noxious heat pulses. *Pain* 1977;3:57–68.
79. Price DD, Long S, Huitt C. Sensory testing of pathophysiological mechanisms of pain in patients with reflex sympathetic dystrophy. *Pain* 1992;49:163–173.
80. Price DD, Mao J, Mayer DJ. Central neural mechanisms of normal and abnormal pain states. In: Fields HL, Liebeskind JC, eds. *Pharmacological approaches to the treatment of chronic pain: new concepts and critical issues.* Seattle, WA: I.A.S.P. Press, 1994:61–84.
81. Price DD, Mao J, Frank H, Mayer, DJ. The N-methyl-D-aspartate receptor antagonist dextromethorphan selectively reduces temporal summation of second pain in man. *Pain* 1994;59:165–174.
82. Price DD, McGrath PA, Rafii A, Buckingham B. The validation of visual analogue scales as ratio scale measures for chronic and experimental pain. *Pain* 1983;17:45–56.
83. Price DD, McHaffie JG, Stein BE. The psychophysical attributes of heat-induced pain and their relationships to neural mechanisms. *J Cogn Neurosci* 1992;4:1–14.
84. Price DD, McHaffie JG, Larson MA. Spatial summation of heat-induced pain: influence of stimulus area and spatial separation of stimuli on perceived pain sensation intensity and unpleasantness. *J Neurophysiol* 1989;62:1270–1279.
85. Price DD, Von der Gruen A, Miller J, Rafii A, Price C. A psychophysical analysis of morphine analgesia. *Pain* 1985;22:261–269.
86. Ramsey DS, Brown AC, Woods SC. Acute tolerance to nitrous oxide in humans. *Pain* 1992;51:367–373.
87. Robinson CJ, Torebjork HE, La Motte R. Psychophysical detection and pain ratings of incremental stimuli: a comparison with nociceptor responses in humans. *Brain Res* 1983;274:87–106.
88. Scott J, Huskisson EC. Graphic representation of pain. *Pain* 1976; 2:175–184.
89. Seymour RA, Simpson JM, Charlton JE, Phillips ME. An evaluation of length and end-phrase of visual analogue scales in dental pain. *Pain* 1985;21:177–186.
90. Simone DA, Baumann TK, Lamotten RH. Dose-dependent pain and mechanical hyperalgesia in humans after intradermal injection of capsaicin. *Pain* 1989;38:99–107.
91. Smith GM, Egbert LD, Markowitz RA, Mosteller F, Beecher HK. An experimental pain method sensitive to morphine in man: the submaximum effort tourniquet technique. *J Pharmacol Exp Ther* 1966;154:324–332.
92. Sonnenschein RR, Jamison R, Loveseth LJ, Cassels WH, Ivy AC. A study on the mechanism of nitrous oxide analgesia. *J Appl Physiol* 1948;1:254–258.
93. Stein BE, Price DD, Gazzaniga MS. Pain perception in a man with total corpus callosum transection. *Pain* 1989;38:51–56.
94. Stevens JC, Marks LE. Spatial summation and the dynamics of warmth sensation. *Percept Psychophys* 1971;9:291–298.
95. Stevens SS. To honor Fechner and repeal his law. *Science* 1961; 133:80–86.
96. Stevens SS. *Psychophysics. Introduction to its perceptual, neural, and social prospects.* New York: John Wiley, 1975.
97. Thompson SWN, Woolf CJ. Primary afferent-evoked prolonged potentials in the spinal cord and their central summation: role of the NMDA receptor. In: Bond MR, Charlton JE, Woolf CJ, eds. *Proceedings of the Vth World Congress on Pain, vol. 4.* Amsterdam: Elsevier, 1990:291–298.
98. Travell JG, Simmons DG. *Myofascial pain and dysfunction: the trigger point manual.* Baltimore: Williams & Wilkins, 1983.
99. Torebjork HE, LaMotte RH, Robinson CJ. Peripheral neural correlates of magnitude of cutaneous pain and hyperalgesia: Simultaneous recordings in humans of sensory judgements of pain and evoked responses in nociceptors with C-fibers. *J Neurophysiol* 1984; 51:325–339.
100. Wall PD. On the relation of injury to pain (The First John J. Bonica Lecture). *Pain* 1976;6:253–264.
101. Watkins LR, Mayer DJ. Organization of endogenous opiate and nonopiate pain control systems. *Science* 1982;216:1185–1192.
102. Willis WD. *The pain system.* Basel: Karger, 1985.
103. Zimmermann M. Neurophysiology of nociception. In: Porter R, ed. *International review of physiology. Neurophysiology II, vol. 10.* Baltimore: University Park Press, 1976:179–221.

Anesthesia: Biologic Foundations, edited by Tony L. Yaksh et al. Lippincott–Raven Publishers, Philadelphia © 1997.

CHAPTER 42

ORGANIZATION OF HORMONAL RESPONSES TO HIGH-THRESHOLD AFFERENT INPUT: AUTONOMIC AND PITUITARY SECRETIONS IN HUMANS

DOROTHEE GAUMANN

It has been long appreciated that tissue injury can lead to a variety of physiological effects that may have unwelcome consequences. Thus, injury in humans and animals can increase heart rate, cardiac inotrophy, and blood pressure and accordingly increase myocardial oxygen consumption (96); diminish gastric motility leading to ileus (46,134); increase catabolic processes (148); depress immune functions (119,142); and produce a hypercoagulable state (39,154). As a whole, these events reflect the syndrome that is the stress response (see Chap. 72).

The mechanisms underlying these effects are multiple. Surgical intervention leads to tissue injury. Tissue injury results in (a) activation of high-threshold afferents; (b) release of a variety of active factors from the site of injury, including a wide variety of cytokines and prostanoids; and (c) the occurrence of ancillary conditions such as hypotension, hemorrhage, hypothermia, hypoglycemia, ischemia, and reperfusion-injury. The principal nonsomatic efferent limbs of these effects are (a) releasing factors from the hypothalamus that act on the pituitary, (b) pituitary hormones that reach the systemic circulation to act on different end organs and endocrine glands, including the adrenal cortex, (c) the sympathetic nervous system, which leads to stimulation of the adrenal medulla with subsequent hormonal responses, and of sympathetic nerves mediating cardiovascular reflexes, and (d) cytokines released from a variety of local and circulating cell systems that exert powerful effects upon hormone release and organ function.

INITIATING STIMULI FOR THE HORMONAL COMPONENT OF THE STRESS RESPONSE

Neurogenic Linkages

After peripheral injury, the neurogenic component leading to the stress response is mediated by small high-threshold primary afferents (121) (see Chapter 39). As reviewed in Chapters 38 and 71, small afferent input can activate spinobulbar projections, which can subsequently activate bulbospinal projections to the intermediolateral cell columns to stimulate preganglionic sympathetic outflow (8,90). Similarly, spinofugal afferent input can reach hypothalamic centers both by direct spinohypothalamic inputs (26) as well as by several spinobulbohypothalamic projections from the medulla (133) and the parabracheal nucleus (11). The excitatory input serves to activate local interneurons, either by a direct excitation or by the release of local factors that attenuate the release of inhibitory factors, such as dopamine. This leads accordingly to pituitary secretion of factors into the systemic circulation. Organizationally, these pathways possess many characteristics that are similar to those which define the encoding of the somatic component of the pain state. As discussed below, manipulations which diminish that input can serve to attenuate the organized stress response.

Circulating Factors

In addition to the afferent drive, tissue injury and inflammation serve to evoke the local release of a variety of active factors such as cytokines, and endotoxins. These circulating factors can exert direct suppressive effects upon vascular permeability, immune function, smooth muscle contractility, and activity in peripheral afferent terminals (see below). In addition, these agents have direct effects upon pituitary and adrenal secretion (34,53,72). Moreover, these factors may additionally serve to upregulate the message and synthesis of the secreted materials (42), serving to amplify the response evoked by the injury stimulus.

In humans, these changes in hormonal secretion play an important role in the postinjury-surgical pain state. In the following sections, the time-dependent nature of the responses that are induced in the postoperative state will be summarized. Several important covariates can influence the particular components of the evoked hormonal response. These include the anesthetic regime and the nature of the stimulus. Thus, in the perioperative period, several distinct stimulus events can be defined: endotracheal intubation, which evokes a nociceptive reflex by mechanical activation of vagal and somatic afferents that innervate the larynx and trachea; and surgical stimulation, secondary to incision and retraction, which, can result in stimulation of somatic and/or visceral afferents (see Chapter 43). As will be reviewed, the magnitude of the response as measured by a variety of physiological and hormonal indices is directly proportional to the degree of tissue trauma, with superficial surgery presenting the weakest and upper abdominal and thoracic surgery the strongest stimulus. During cardiac surgery, the period of cardiopulmonary bypass is a potent stimulator of the endocrine system observed during surgery, probably due to the combination of a variety of highly unphysiologic stimuli such as hypothermia, hypotension, hemodilution, and changes in blood flow characteristics and foreign body responses. Endotracheal extubation and the early postoperative period may be highly stressful, as nociception is no longer suppressed by general anesthesia, and catabolic stressors induced by additional factors, such as shivering, and emotional drives may amplify the endocrine response.

In the following sections, components and organization of the autonomic response observed in the perioperative period are considered.

PITUITARY HORMONES

The pituitary is divided into an anterior (adenohypophysis) and posterior (neurohypophysis) component, connected to the ventral hypothalamus by the infundibulum at the median eminence. Along the infundibulum travels the hypothalamohypophyseal tract. This system arises from magnocellular neurons in the paraventricular/supraoptic nucleus that synthesizes a variety of hormones that are transported along the tract to be released into the capillary net formed by the inferior hypophyseal artery. These cells provide the source of oxytocin and vasopressin. Cells in the anterior pituitary release into the local capillary net. The releasing activity of these anterior cells is governed by releasing factors released by hypothalamic neurons (parvocellular) which make contact with the walls of the long and short portal vessels, forming a hemoneural contact zone. Products secreted from these terminals then are transported by the local portal system which then feeds the anterior pituitary cells. These releasing and inhibitory factors thus control the secretory activity of the neurons in question. The activity of the anterior projecting neurons is governed in part by a variety of local interneurons that release monoamines, particularly dopamine.

Forebrain as well as ascending pathways gain access to the hypothalamus by long monosynaptic pathways (spinohypothalamic) as well as by polysynaptic pathways from the brainstem (122) (see Chapter 12). C-fiber input can thus induce activation of hypothalamo-pituitary secretion. In addition, as noted below, a number of cytokines released secondary to tissue injury can exert a direct effect upon pituitary secretory systems.

Adrenocorticotropin and β-Endorphin

These hormones are secreted in response to hypothalamic corticotropin-releasing factor (CRF). They are derived from a common precursor molecule, pro-opiomelanocortin (POMC), and are released concomitantly following a variety of different stressors (58). Both peptides show a circadian periodicity with peaks in the morning and lowest levels at night.

Adrenocorticotropin (ACTH) stimulates the production of adrenal cortical hormones, mainly cortisol. Basal levels in humans are in the range of 3–17 pmol/L, and the half-life in plasma is ~15 min. During cardiopulmonary resuscitation, levels may rise tenfold as compared to control (88).

β-endorphin belongs to the POMC derived family of endogenous opioids, which have been hypothesized to have broad regulatory or modulating actions on cardiovascular, immunologic, endocrine, and metabolic functions, as well as on pain perception (3). Under clinical stress conditions, however, the importance of circulating β-endorphin is not well defined and an involvement in hormonal, metabolic and cardiovascular changes is not apparent (82). Systemic β-endorphin may partially reflect endorphin activity in the central nervous system, which plays an important role in stress adaptation and analgesia (27). Baseline levels of β-endorphin are in the range of 3–12 pmol/L (30), and plasma half-life is longer than for ACTH, ~45 min (82). During major trauma up to 12-fold increases in β-endorphin have been observed (89). Importantly, a significant fraction of the β-endorphin immunoreactivity is in the acetylated form, which has no activity at an opioid receptor (2).

Increases in ACTH and β-endorphin levels during different types of surgery are presented in Table 1. Both peptides typically display comparable increases rapidly after endotracheal intubation, reach peaks during surgery or in the early postoperative period, remain elevated during the first postoperative hours and are usually back to baseline on the first postoperative day (30,75). As indicated above, the degree of stimulation is the combined result of the extent and severity of surgery, the level of anesthesia and the anesthetics employed.

Prolactin

Secretion of prolactin, which is under the inhibitory control of hypothalamic dopamine, is observed following a variety of stressors. As its main physiologic function is related to lactation, the significance of prolactin in the stress response is uncertain. However, stimulating effects on the cardiovascular and immune system may be of importance (25).

Plasma levels are in the range of 2–10 ng/ml for men and 5–20 ng/ml for women, with highest levels observed during nocturnal sleep. Its plasma half-life is ~20 min. The release of prolactin during nociceptive stimulation, largely depends on the site of stimulation (69). Prolactin secretion, which is independent of growth hormone secretion, is presented in Table 2 during various types of surgery. Prolactin levels rise rapidly following endotracheal intubation, remain elevated during surgery, gradually decreased during the first postoperative

Table 1. ADRENOCORTICOTROPIN (ACTH) AND β-ENDORPHIN RESPONSE TO DIFFERENT TYPES OF SURGERY

Type of surgery	Main anesthetic	Intubation	Surgery	ECC	Extubation	RR 0–1 h	RR 2–6 h	Reference
			ACTH (ratio of baseline)					
Minor orthopedic	Isoflurane/fentanyl	nm	1.4	—	nm	4.3	3.7	1
Gynecologic laparotomy	Halothane/N_2O	nm	7.0	—	nm	nm	5.0	82
Gynecologic laparotomy	N_2O, fentanyl	nm	1.4	—	nm	nm	2.0	82
Cesarian section	Isoflurane/N_2O	3.1	3.1	—	nm	nm	1.7	113
Major abdominal	Fentanyl, N_2O	2.0	5.4	—	nm	4.2	3.7	75
Cholecystectomy	Enflurane/N_2O	nm	17	—	17	16	5.0	13
			β-endorphin (ratio of baseline)					
Minor orthopedic	N_2O/fentanyl	nm	1.9	—	nm	nm	1.1	30
Gynecologic laparotomy	Halothane/N_2O	nm	4.0	—	nm	nm	3.5	82
Gynecologic laparotomy	N_2O/fentanyl	nm	2.0	—	nm	nm	2.4	82
Abdominal hysterectomy	Halothane/N_2O	nm	6.2	—	6.1	6.3	nm	135
Cesarian section	Isoflurane/N_2O	3.2	3.2	—	nm	nm	2.0	113
Major abdominal	Fentanyl/N_2O	2.5	5.0	—	nm	4.0	3.9	75
Cardiac surgery	Fentanyl	nm	1.5	4.0	—	nm	nm	70

Plasma concentrations, expressed as ratio of baseline value, measured before the beginning of anesthesia, at time points: after intubation, during surgery and extracorporal circulation (ECC), after extubation and postoperatively in the recovery room (RR) between 0–1 and 2–6 h.
N_2O, nitrous oxide; nm, not measured.

Table 2. GROWTH HORMONE AND PROLACTIN RESPONSE TO DIFFERENT TYPES OF SURGERY

Type of surgery	Main anesthetic	Intubation	Surgery	ECC	RR 0–1 h	RR 2–6 h	Reference
			Growth hormone (ratio of baseline)				
Minor surgery	Halothane/N_2O	nm	1.4	—	nm	nm	95
Major surgery	Halothane/N_2O	nm	3.6	—	nm	nm	95
Gynecologic laparotomy	Halothane/N_2O	nm	4.8	—	nm	4.0	82
Gynecologic laparotomy	N_2O/fentanyl	nm	1.3	—	nm	1.6	82
Abdominal hysterectomy	Althesin	nm	12.4	—	8.4	4	15
Abdominal hysterectomy	Halothane/N_2O	nm	17	—	23	2	101
Cholecystectomy	Halothane/N_2O	nm	10	—	13	13	36
Cardiac surgery	Sufentanil	0.5	1.2	1.3	1.0	nm	19
Cardiac surgery	Sufentanil	1.0	2.1	nm	nm	9.2	37
			Prolactin (ratio of baseline)				
Appendectomy	Isoflurane/N_2O	nm	5.0	—	nm	nm	85
Minor + major surgery	Halothane/N_2O	nm	3.0	—	nm	nm	95
Abdominal hysterectomy	Isoflurane/N_2O	nm	4.1	—	5.0	5.0	31
Abdominal hysterectomy	Althesin	nm	12	—	8.4	4.0	15
Cardiac surgery	Sufentanil	4.2	4.2	2.0	1.9	nm	19

Plasma concentrations, expressed as ratio of baseline value, measured before the beginning of anesthesia, at time points: after intubation, during surgery and extracorporal circulation (ECC), and postoperatively in the recovery room (RR) between 0–1 and 2–6 h.

N_2O, nitrous oxide; nm, not measured.

hours and are back to baseline on the first postoperative day. As the prolactin secretion may be modulated by a variety of anesthetics in opposing directions, its clinical usefulness as an indicator of the surgical stress response is questionable (13).

Growth Hormone

Release of growth hormone (GH) is under hypothalamic control and influenced by various metabolic parameters, such as glucose and amino acids. Apart from its main function to promote growth, it has several metabolic effects, including (a) increases in protein synthesis, (b) glucose utilization, and (c) lipolysis, which are probably of some importance in the stress response. Basal levels in the adult are <3 ng/ml, and half-life in plasma is 20–30 min. GH is released in response to various stressors, including exercise. Increases in GH levels to surgical trauma are summarized in Table 2. Levels start to rise during the first hour of operation, after reaching a peak intra- or postoperatively, they gradually decline.

Arginine-Vasopressin

Arginine-vasopressin (AVP), or antidiuretic hormone, is formed in hypothalamic nuclei and transported via axons to the posterior lobe of the hypothalamus, where it is stored and from where it is released in response to various stimuli. These stimuli mainly originate from osmo-, baro-, and stretch-receptors, aimed at maintaining blood pressure and volume, as well as plasma osmolarity, within normal limits. But pain and fear also evoke AVP secretion. The main effect of AVP is on the kidney, where it leads to the retention of water. At pharmacological concentrations it has potent vasoconstrictor action by a direct effect on vascular smooth muscle.

Basal levels in the adult are in the range of 1–3 μ/ml; the half-life in plasma is 6–10 min. During surgery, AVP-levels rise gradually within 1 h and remain elevated during the initial postoperative period. Under general anesthesia with fentanyl and N_2O, AVP rose by a factor of 1.6 during orthopedic or gynecologic surgery (23) and by a factor of six during abdominal aortic surgery (112). In this last group, AVP continued to

Table 3. CORTISOL AND ALDOSTERONE RESPONSE TO DIFFERENT TYPES OF SURGERY

Type of surgery	Main anesthetic	Intubation	Surgery	ECC	Extubation	RR 0–1 h	RR 2–6 h	Reference
			Cortisol (ratio of baseline)					
Craniotomy	Isoflurane, N_2O	1.0	1.4	—	1.8	2.6	nm	50
Orthopedic	Isoflurane, fentanyl	nm	1.0	—	nm	2.1	1.7	1
Orthopedic/gynecologic	N_2O, sufentanil	nm	1.3	—	nm	1.6	nm	23
Abdominal hysterectomy	Halothane, N_2O	nm	0.9	—	nm	2.3	3.2	81
Abdominal hysterectomy	Isoflurane, N_2O	nm	4.2	—	—	5.2	5.1	31
Cholecystectomy	Halothane, N_2O	nm	2.5	—	nm	3.3	3.8	36
Cholecystectomy	Enflurane, N_2O	nm	4.0	—	4.5	4.8	4.8	13
Major abdominal	N_2O, fentanyl	0.8	1.7	—	nm	1.9	2.2	75
Major abdominal	Isoflurane, N_2O	0.8	2.3	—	3.0	3.0	nm	4
Cardiac surgery	Sufentanil	nm	0.7	1.0	—	1.1	2.1	37
Cardiac surgery	Sufentanil	1.0	0.8	0.7	—	2.6	nm	19
			Aldosterone (ratio of baseline)					
Craniotomy	Isoflurane, N_2O	0.8	1.7	—	2	2.3	nm	50
Orthopedic	N_2O, fentanyl	nm	1.3	—	nm	nm	0.6	30
Gynecologic laparotomy	Enflurane, N_2O	nm	2.3	—	nm	2.9	3.5	45
Major abdominal	Isoflurane, N_2O	nm	2.8	—	nm	6.4	nm	4

Plasma concentrations of cortisol and aldosterone, expressed as ratio of baseline value, measured before the beginning of anesthesia, at time points: after intubation, during surgery and extracorporal circulation (ECC), after extubation and postoperatively in the recovery room (RR) between 0–1 and 2–6 h.

N_2O, nitrous oxide; nm, not measured.

rise postoperative by a factor of nine, compared to preoperative values. Not only pain, but positive pressure ventilation and hypotension contribute to AVP-secretion during the perioperative period (65,108).

ADRENAL CORTEX

The glucocorticoid, cortisol, is secreted in response to ACTH, exhibiting a similar diurnal rhythm with peaks in the early morning. Cortisol is one of the major stress hormones, necessary for a variety of adaptational functions. It acts on the intermediary metabolism, leading to increased protein catabolism and increased hepatic glucogenesis. It is necessary for the maintenance of blood pressure, has a slight mineralocorticoid effect and depresses immune function.

Plasma levels are in the range of 200–700 nmol/L, and the half-life in plasma is ~80 min. Table 3 presents cortisol levels during different types of surgery and anesthesia. Cortisol levels do not increase immediately following intubation. This is in contrast to the ACTH response (Table 1), probably due to the short time delay between ACTH-release and adrenal cortical stimulation. During surgery, the time course of cortisol levels corresponds closely to ACTH, but increases in ACTH from baseline are usually higher than for cortisol. During the postoperative period, cortisol levels tend to be elevated for a prolonged period, possibly due to stimulating actions of tissue factors (see below) (104).

The mineralocorticoid aldosterone, which plays an important role in sodium and fluid homeostasis, is partially under the control of ACTH. Other regulatory mechanisms include the renin-angiotensin system, which is activated intraoperatively during periods of hypotension (12). Basal aldosterone levels are in the range of 0.1–0.4 nmol/L. During normotensive surgery, increases correspond to those of cortisol (Table 3).

SYMPATHETIC NERVOUS SYSTEM

Activation of the sympathetic nervous system occurs rapidly to a wide variety of stressors, including pain and different forms of shock. This sympathetic reflex response consists of cardiovascular reflexes, mediated via peripheral sympathetic nerves, and of endocrine responses resulting in the release of catecholamines and neuropeptides. Catecholamines are released from the adrenal medulla and postganglionic nerve fibers. Adrenal catecholamine secretion occurs according to the intensity and type of stimulation (83). Epinephrine is the main hormone secreted from the adrenal in humans, but dopamine may also be released during high intensity stimulation (136). Norepinephrine is the major transmitter in postganglionic sympathetic nerve fibers, mediating cardiovascular reflexes. Only a small percentage of it gets access to the blood stream, as its major part is subjected to presynaptic re-uptake or metabolism (100). The half-life of catecholamines in plasma is 1–3 min. Basal levels in unpremedicated healthy patients before induction of anesthesia were 0.36 ng/ml for norepinephrine and 0.07 ng/ml for epinephrine (50).

The importance of the sympatho-adrenal medullary system in maintaining homeostasis in various emergency situations such as pain, hemorrhage or major emotions, has been appreciated since the beginning of this century (21). The different physiologic effects of norepinephrine and epinephrine such as stimulation of the heart, vasodilation in skeletal muscle, vasoconstriction of vessels supplying nonvital organs, bronchodilation, immobilization of the gut, and mobilization of liver glycogen and free fatty acids, contribute to support emergency reactions of the organism (148). Although, the physiologic importance of circulating dopamine is not completely known, it is a component of the physiological stress response, as well as of stress-related disease (136).

Catecholamines

The release of catecholamine induced by different sensory and cardioregulatory stimuli vary widely in humans. Twofold increases occur with changing from the supine to the standing position. Up to 16-fold increases are observed during acute myocardial infarction (64) and up to 20-fold increases in septic shock (9). Hypoglycemia selectively increases epinephrine levels by a factor of 50 (48). A very high degree of sympathetic stimulation occurs during cardiopulmonary resuscitation, where systemic norepinephrine and epinephrine concentrations may rise by a factor of 300 and 30, respectively (150). Marked increases in dopamine have been observe during physical exercise, hypoglycemia and major surgery, where increases may be comparable to norepinephrine.

Table 4 summarizes the catecholamine and cardiovascular response to endotracheal intubation. In all cases, a marked increase in blood pressure and heart rate occurred immediately following intubation. This physiological response contrasts to changes in catecholamines, which usually showed only slight increases. It thus seems that endotracheal intubation may lead to a differential activation of different components of the sympathetic nervous system (128). These data correspond to animal experiments, where high intensity nociceptive stimulation evoked prominent hemodynamic responses, but only marginal increases in catecholamines (52).

Increases in catecholamines during different types of surgery are presented in Table 5. Increases in epinephrine were generally higher than in norepinephrine, indicating a significant involvement of the adrenal medulla. The response of catecholamines to cardiac surgery and during extracorporal circulation are shown in Table 6, where epinephrine levels increase up to 30-fold from baseline. Awakening from anesthesia and the early postoperative period may be more stressful than surgery itself insofar as catecholamine release is concerned. This is shown in Table 7, where increases in catecholamines are often higher than during surgery. Also during this period, increases in epinephrine exceed those of norepinephrine.

Neuropeptides

A variety of neuropeptides have been identified in the sympathetic terminal as well as in the chromaffin cells of the adrenal medulla (60,143). In many instances, these peptides and catecholamine stores are found in the same chromaffin cells.

Neuropeptide Y (NPY) is contained in sympathetic nerve fibers and in the adrenal medulla, from where it may be released together with catecholamines during sympathetic stimulation (22). NPY is a potent vasoconstrictor exerting its effects through a direct vascular action and a potentiation of adrenergic neurotransmission (146). It may further alter cardiac output and regional blood flow distribution and exert chronotropic and inotropic effects on the heart through inhibition of vagal activity (76). It inhibits renin release independently of any hemodynamic effects (28). Resting plasma concentrations of NPY reflect, similarly to norepinephrine, spillover from sympathetic nerve terminals and are in the range of 20–30 pmol/L (141). The half-life of NPY in the circulation at physiological concentrations is ~20 min and is thus considerably longer than that of catecholamines (107).

During sympathetic stimulation, NPY plasma concentrations seem to be a selective marker of postganglionic sympathetic nerve activity, closely correlated to increases in norepinephrine plasma levels (117). NPY concentrations increase by a factor of two during myocardial infarction and by a factor of four during extensive exercise and vaginal delivery (92,144). In cardiac surgery, NPY increases by a factor of two during thoracotomy and of three during cardiopulmonary bypass, whereas norepinephrine increases by a factor of 2.3 and 3.2, respectively (93).

Table 4. SYMPATHETIC STIMULATION FOLLOWING ENDOTRACHEAL INTUBATION

Anesthesia	NE (×BL)	EPI (×BL)	BP (Δ BL, mm Hg)	HR (ΔBL, bpm)	Reference
Fentanyl, thiopental	1	1	+30	+22	49
Thiopental, N_2O	1.2	1	+30	+23	123
Papaveretum, thiopental	1.2	1.2	+23	+26	35
Thiopental	1.2	nm	+30	+30	20
Thiopental, N_2O, enflurane	1.2	1.4	+27	+20	99
Thiopental, N_2O, enflurane	1.3	1	+19	+15	149
Thiopental or propofol	1.3	2	+25	+19	55
Thiopental	1.4	1	+25	+34	86
Thiopental	1.5	4	+13	+30	71
Fentanyl, thiopental, N_2O	1.5	1.6	+30	+17	131

Maximal increase in plasma concentrations of norepinephrine (NE) and epinephrine (EPI), expressed as ratio of baseline value (×BL), and in blood pressure (BP) and heart rate (HR), expressed as change (Δ) from baseline (BL) following endotracheal intubation.
N_2O, nitrous oxide; nm, not measured.

Table 5. CATECHOLAMINE RESPONSE TO DIFFERENT TYPES OF SURGERY

Type of surgery	Main anesthetic	NE (×BL)	EPI (×BL)	DA (×BL)	Reference
Craniotomy	Isoflurane, N_2O	1.2	1.1	nm	50
Minor orthopedic	Isoflurane, fentanyl	1.5	1.2	nm	1
Minor orthopedic	N_2O, fentanyl	2.9	3.3	nm	30
Orthopedic or gynecologic	N_2O, sufentanil	1.0	1.1	1.3	23
Gynecologic laparotomy	Enflurane, N_2O	1.4	3.7	3.3	45
Abdominal hysterectomy	Halothane, N_2O	1.3	2	nm	81
Cholecystectomy	Enflurane, N_2O	2.3	9	nm	13
Abdominal aortic	N_2O, fentanyl	1.7	5	nm	112
Major abdominal	N_2O, fentanyl	2.7	4.5	nm	75

Maximal increase in plasma concentrations of norepinephrine (NE), epinephrine (EPI) and dopamine (DA), expressed as ratio of baseline value (x BL), measured before the beginning of anesthesia.
N_2O, nitrous oxide; nm, not measured.

Table 6. CATECHOLAMINE SECRETION DURING CARDIAC SURGERY

	NE (ratio of BL)		EPI (ratio of BL)		DA (ratio of BL)		
Main anesthetic	Surgery	ECC	Surgery	ECC	Surgery	ECC	Reference
Halothane	1.7	4.0	6.8	30	2.3	10	127
Fentanyl	0.7	4.5	1	24	0.5	14	127
Fentanyl	0.8	3.5	0.7	4.5	1.2	2.6	137
Fentanyl	3.2	6.5	3.5	21	nm	nm	126
Sufentanil	0.7	5.7	0.8	11	1.1	4.8	19
Sufentanil	1	2.5	1	3	nm	nm	37

Maximal increase in plasma concentrations of norepinephrine (NE), epinephrine (EPI) and dopamine (DA), expressed as ratio of baseline value (BL), measured before the beginning of anesthesia, during surgery before extracorporal circulation (ECC) and during ECC.
nm, not measured.

Table 7. CATECHOLAMINE RESPONSE DURING POSTOPERATIVE PERIOD

	Extubation (ratio of baseline)		Postoperative 0–1 h (ratio of baseline)		Postoperative 2–6 h (ratio of baseline)		
Type of surgery	NE	EPI	NE	EPI	NE	EPI	Reference
Craniotomy	1.3	1.2	1.7	1.5	nm	nm	50
Minor orthopedic	1.7	2.2	1.7	2.5	nm	nm	1
Minor orthopedic	nm	nm	0.5	1.0	0.8	1.5	30
Gynecologic laparotomy	nm	nm	0.7	1.0	3.8	1.1	45
Abdominal aortic	nm	nm	2.7	10	2.9	14	112
Major abdominal	nm	nm	3	12	2.6	8	75
Cholecystectomy	2.5	16	4	4	2.5	6.5	13
Major abdominal	2.5	22	3	22	nm	nm	4

Maximal increase in plasma concentrations of norepinephrine (NE) and epinephrine (EPI), expressed as ratio of baseline value, measured before the beginning of anesthesia.
nm, not measured.

Enkephalin

Enkephalins are opioid peptides contained within the adrenal chromaffin cells and released by preganglionic stimulation. Blood pressure depressant effects have been described for enkephalin. These effects are due to an action on pulmonary J-receptors, the heart, vascular smooth muscle, and are mediated by modulation of baro- and chemoreceptor reflexes (68). However, the intravenous injection of methionine (Met)-enkephalin in humans causes a brief increase in blood pressure and heart rate (54). These diverging hemodynamic responses also occur with other opioids and are dependent on factors such as anesthesia, species, dose, site of injection, and cardiovascular status (43). Further actions, mediated by enkephalins, include modulation of adrenal medullary secretion (80) and immune function (110). While enkephalins can interact with central opioid receptors to regulate nociceptive processing, plasma levels of enkephalin generated by stress are unlikely to influence these central receptors due to the peptidic structure of these agents and the presence of the blood-brain barrier. Nevertheless, there are data to suggest that activity in vagal afferents may be induced by peripheral enkephalins and this peripheral action can alter nociceptive transmission (106,114).

Resting plasma concentrations of Met-enkephalin in humans vary between 14 and 140 pg/ml (24). Circadian variations have been reported with lowest levels occurring between 4:00 and 8:00 p.m. (56). The half-life of Met-enkephalin opioid activity in human plasma is 8 min (17).

Intense physical exercise does not lead to constant increases in Met-enkephalin plasma levels (47,103). During migraine episodes, Met-enkephalin concentrations rise by a factor of 10, possibly related to some degree to the underlying pain (102). In patients subjected to abdominal hysterectomy under halothane/N_2O anesthesia, Met-enkephalin concentrations only increase by a factor of two following endotracheal intubation. During surgery and in the postoperative period, these levels rapidly decrease back to baseline, while other stress hormones, ACTH and β–endorphin rise constantly (135). Met-enkephalin, therefore, seems not to be a reliable marker of the sympathetic stress response.

TISSUE-DERIVED STIMULATORS OF THE ENDOCRINE RESPONSE

Stimulating effects on the endocrine response do not only originate from afferent nervous input, but also from active factors that are released from various inflammatory cells and the immune system (14). A large group of polypeptides, the cytokines, which include the interleukins (IL), the tumor necrosis factors (TNF) and the interferons, may modulate the hormonal response to surgical trauma (63) (see Chap. 20). These cytokines have a variety of immunologic, metabolic, hematologic and hormonal functions. Table 8 provides a brief summary of a number of interleukins and their role that have been thus far identified. The magnitude of the contribution of these factors is only now becoming widely understood. They may exert a direct physiological effect by altering smooth muscle function and vascular permeability. In addition, through receptor mediated mechanisms, agents such as TNF and IL-1a can alter the expression of a variety of peptides in secretory systems including the adrenal chromaffin cells (42).

IL-6

IL-6 is a principal cytokine released during routine surgery and is produced in tissue by local fibroblasts, macrophages and endothelial cells. IL-6 baseline levels are in the range of 0–40 pg/ml (31) and the elimination half-life in the circulation is 55 min. In the perioperative period, IL-6 circulating levels correspond to the severity of trauma and reflect tissue damage (32). Increases in IL-6 plasma concentrations precede changes in other interleukins and acute phase proteins. IL-6, like other cytokines, especially IL-1 and TNF-α, stimulates the hypothalamo-pituitary-adrenal axis at the different levels (94). However, during surgery, IL-6 release occurs later than increases in ACTH and cortisol. Therefore, a specific role in the acute endocrine response to surgery is unlikely (101). In the postoperative period, however, IL-6, possibly together with TNF-α, may sustain the cortisol response, as IL-6 and cortisol levels remain elevated during several postoperative days, while ACTH levels rapidly decline to baseline on the first postoperative day (31,104).

Endothelins

Endothelins (ET) are a group of peptides with potent vasoconstrictor properties, which are released from the endothelium in response to anoxia, catecholamines and shear stress. Low levels of endothelin (ET-1: 0.25–5 pg/ml) are normally present in the circulation representing a spillover from the endothelium. Endothelins have a plasma half-life of <2 min (98). Under experimental conditions, endothelins stimulate the hypothalamo-pituitary-adrenal axis (66) and aldosterone (29) and adrenal catecholamine secretion (16). Major surgical

Table 8. SUMMARY OF SEVERAL PRINCIPAL CYTOKINES AND THEIR ACTIONS

IL-1	Induction and facilitation of B and T cells to antigen; activated PLA_2 yielding increase in prostanoids and platelet activating factor; stimulates catabolism resulting in wasting of muscle, bone resorption, and cartilage destruction
IL-2	Stimulates T cells and T-cell cytokines
IL-3	Promotes granulocytes, macrophages and mast cells
IL-4	Stimulates proliferation/maturation of B cells/mast cells; depresses formation of macrophage TNF/IL-1
IL-5	Facilitates proliferation of B cells
IL-6	Promotes proliferation/differentiation of B cells; stimulates production of colony stimulating factors
IL-7	Promotes B cell progenitors
IL-8	Stimulates macrophages; neutrophil chemotactic agent
IL-9	Facilitates mast cells growth
IL-10	Depresses clonal expansion of T cells
Platelet derived growth factors (PDGF)	Stimulates proliferation of fibroblasts, endothelial cells, and fibroblasts
Tumor necrosis factor (TNF-α/β)	Stimulates synthesis of cytokines; activates expression of adhesion molecules; activates fibroblasts, osteoclasts, and chondrocytes

For futher detail, see refs. 5,38,63,111.

stress and vascular injury increase circulating levels of endothelin. During surgery, endothelin concentrations correlate with duration of operation and blood loss. They may increase by a factor of up to two during cardiac procedures and levels remain elevated during the first postoperative days (130). However, as there is no correlation between endothelin concentrations and endocrine or hemodynamic function (61,77), the importance of endothelins as indices of stress is limited.

EFFECTS OF ANESTHETICS UPON THE SURGICAL STRESS RESPONSE

It is appreciated that anesthetics and analgesics serve in a principal capacity to regulate the magnitude of the stress response that is generated by the induction of an injury state. It is commonly appreciated that these agents may have discriminable effects upon the evoked response.

Volatile Anesthetics

In humans, halothane, enflurane, isoflurane inhibit the pain-evoked endocrine and autonomic response by inhibiting noxious afferent input and transmission at various levels of the central nervous system (78,105,120). With regard to the sympathetic reflex response, ganglionic transmission (18), baroreceptor reflexes (125) and catecholamine storage and release mechanisms are inhibited (116,139). The individual components of the autonomic reflex response show different degrees of susceptibility to the suppressant effects of a single volatile anesthetic, and for given anesthetic depths, the different volatiles can vary in their potency to inhibit individual components of this reflex (124,125).

A method of assessing the level of anesthesia, consists in analyzing the hemodynamic and endocrine response to surgery (115). It has been postulated, that the more profound the level of anesthesia, the more suppressed is the sympathetic reflex response. The implementation of this concept is reflected in the notion of MACBAR (minimum alveolar concentration that blocks the adrenergic response) (115) as opposed to MAC, the volatile anesthetic concentration that blocks the somatic response (e.g., limb withdrawal or movement) (40,138) to the stimulus. Typically, MACBAR values for the commonly used anesthetics exceed the MAC values, consistent with the concept that the sensitivity of the autonomic response to both volatile and injectable anesthetics are less than for the somatic responses. Complete suppression of the endocrine and autonomic response to major surgery, with volatile or injectable anesthetics alone is often difficult. A deep level of anesthesia achieved with a volatile will often lead to profound cardiovascular depression, which will itself evoke counterregulatory stimulating sympathetic and endocrine responses, based on autonomic reflexes that are not blocked at the corresponding anesthetic concentrations (12).

Regional Anesthetics

Regional anesthetic blocks will induce a complete block of afferent transmission and accordingly block the sensory message otherwise induced by tissue injury. A variety of clinical studies have emphasized that spinal anesthetics can almost completely block the hormonal signs of stress otherwise evoked by surgical interventions (41,73,118,104). Such results suggest that a principal component of the stress response mediated by an operative intervention reflects upon a neurogenic component. It is clear however, that to the extent that the injury itself leads to the release of circulating levels of active hormones, that the block of afferent input would have little influence on the actions of these secreted factors, e.g., cytokines and endotoxins (see above).

Receptor-Selective Agents

Opioids

Systemic opioids act on specific receptors in brain and spinal cord, which are associated with pathways which regulate nociceptive transmission (151,152) (see Chapter 58). Occupation of these receptors leads to selective inhibition of nociceptive afferent input and thus to mitigation or blockade of nociceptive-evoked autonomic or endocrine responses. Apart from their inhibitory effect on nociception, opioids have, on their own, modulatory effects on various aspects of endocrine function (57,62). A large number of clinical studies have compared the endocrine inhibitory effects of opioids during surgery to other types of general anesthesia. In the majority of studies, the endocrine and autonomic response to surgery were effectively suppressed by opioids given at high doses. However, clinical studies show, that even excessive doses of opioids alone do not completely block the surgical-evoked stress response (67,109). This is likely due to several reasons: (a) Opioids act on specific receptors that may not be effectively coupled to, or be involved in all the pathways activated during surgery; baroreceptor- and hypoglycemia-evoked sympathetic responses seem to be unaffected by opioids (53,140). (b). All components of high-intensity afferent transmission are not uniformly blocked by opiates (91).

α_2-Adrenergic Agonists

Agents such as clonidine act on α_2-adrenergic receptors in brain and spinal cord, which are involved in pain processing and cardiovascular regulation. They exert inhibitory effects on nociceptive processing at the level of the spinal cord (153) (see Chapter 59). The main effect on pain-evoked responses is probably due to inhibitory effects on sympathetic outflow at the level of the brain stem and spinal cord (59,145), leading to a reduction in basal blood pressure, and circulating catecholamine concentrations. However, the spontaneous sympathetic activity is more readily suppressed than stimulation-evoked responses (52). Clonidine, the classical representative of this group, has further inhibitory effects on pituitary ACTH secretion (84), which leads to a reduction in cortisol and aldosterone secretion during surgery (50).

CONCLUSIONS

The endocrine and autonomic response to nociceptive stimulation is complex. During surgery, input of different sensory modalities from different dermatomes evokes responses that cannot be predicted on the basis of the response to a single stimulus alone. Different systems are activated to different degrees and may modify each others responses. Further, stimulation is repeated and long-lasting, probably inducing adaptive mechanisms (10). Tachycardia and hypertension may be detrimental if unrestrained or prolonged, possibly leading to myocardial ischemia and infarction in patients with reduced cardiac function (74,79).

Current anesthesia techniques are aimed at decreasing the stress response to surgery, based on the idea that intraoperative and postoperative mortality and morbidity may be reduced, and postoperative recovery and overall outcome improved (74,147). Spinal neural blockade has been shown, depending on the level of the block and the type of surgery, to be able to completely inhibit surgically evoked stress responses (6,74). Whether certain anesthetics or anesthesia techniques are more beneficial for specific surgical procedures or patients is still subject to discussion. Currently applied anesthetic techniques usually provide sufficient hemodynamic and endocrine stability that severe adverse outcome due to anesthesia is extremely rare (44). However, the endocrine and autonomic response to trauma and pain is only one aspect that contributes to patient outcome. The overall management throughout the perioperative period is decisive in reducing morbidity and mortality (129,132). Nevertheless, there is increasing evidence that adequate control of nociceptive transmission during the postoperative pain period can significantly impact upon myocardial indices of ischemia in the postoperative period. For example it seems probable that regional anesthesia in combination of with systemic or spinal opiates can significantly reduce the incidence of tachycardia in high-risk patients (7,33,87,97).

The mechanisms underlying these positive effects upon perioperative morbidity occurring from a block of the "stress response" are complex. Consider for example one manifestation of the issues underlying the apparent beneficial effect of perioperative pain management on morbidity in high-risk cardiac patients noted in the preceding paragraph. As reviewed above, intraoperative stimuli and the products of tissue injury can activate somatosympathetic reflexes (see Chapter 39), leading to the release of a variety of trophic hormones that can impact upon cardiac function. Regional techniques and opiates have been shown to block the neurogenic components of those reflexes in a manner that is more efficacious than volatile anesthetics alone (at a concentration that alone does not suppress cardiac function). It is important to note in the case of regional anesthetic procedures, particularly those targeted at the thoracic level, that there is not only a block of the afferent innervation, but cardiac afferents and efferent connections as well. It is appreciated that during myocardial ischemia sympathetic afferents are activated (see Chapter 39), which in turn leads to viscero(cardiac) sympathetic reflexes that serve to increase heart rate, decrease coronary blood flow and constrict systemic vascular beds.

Finally, regional anesthetic approaches have been shown to have positive effects on postoperative hypercoaguability. In this regard, these effects of blocking the afferent-evoked stress response would jointly serve to reduce cardiac work, improve supply and demand ratios for the myocardium, and reduce the likelihood of coronary thrombosis secondary to clot formation. This brief summary of one aspect of perioperative stress reflects upon the complexity of the events associated with the results of adequate block of the afferent evoked limb of the perioperative pain response. It is certain that, as further insights are gained into the physiology of these systems, additional complexities of the effects of nociceptive input on system function will be appreciated.

REFERENCES

1. Adams HA, Schmitz CS, Baltes-Götz B. Endocrine Stressreaktion, Kreislauf- und Aufwachverhalten bei totaler intravenöser und Inhalationsanästhesie. *Anaesthesist* 1994;43:730–737.
2. Akil H, Shiomi H, Matthews J. Induction of the intermediate pituitary by stress: synthesis and release of a nonopioid form of beta-endorphin. *Science* 1985;227:424–426.
3. Akil H, Watson SJ, Young E, Lewis ME, Khachturian H, Walker JM. Endogenous opioids: biology and function. *Annu Rev Neurosci* 1984;7:223–255.
4. Amar D, Shamoon H, Frishman WH, Lazar EJ, Salama MD. Effects of labetalol on perioperative stress markers and isoflurane requirements. *Br J Anaesth* 1991;67:296–301.
5. Arai KI, Lee F, Miyajima A, Miyatake S, Arai N, Yokota T. Cytokines: coordinators of immune and inflammatory responses. *Annu Rev Biochem* 1990;59:783–836.
6. Bardram L, Funch-Jensen P, Jensen P, Crawford ME, Kehlet H. Recovery after laparoscopic colonic surgery with epidural analgesia, and early oral nutrition and mobilisation. *Lancet* 1995;345: 763–764.
7. Beattie WS, Buckley DN, Forrest JB. Epidural morphine reduces the risk of postoperative myocardial ischaemia in patients with cardiac risk factors. *Can J Anaesth* 1993;40:532–541.
8. Benarroch EE. The central autonomic network: functional organization, dysfunction, and perspective. *Mayo Clin Proc* 1993;68: 988–1001.
9. Benedict CR, Graham-Smith DG. Plasma noradrenaline and adrenaline concentrations and dopamine-beta-hydroxylase activity in patients with shock due to septicemia, trauma and hemorrhage. *Q J Med* 1978;47:1–20.
10. Bereiter DA, DeMaria EJ, Engeland WC, Gann DS. Endocrine responses to multiple sensory input related to injury. *Adv Exp Med Biol* 1988;245:251–63.
11. Berkley KJ, Scofield SL. Relays from the spinal cord and solitary nucleus through the parabrachial nucleus to the forebrain in the cat. *Brain Res* 1990;529:333–338.
12. Bernard JM, Pinaud M, Macquin-Mavier I, Remi JP, Passuti N. Hypotensive anesthesia with isoflurane and enflurane during total hip replacement: a comparative study of catecholamine and renin angiotensin responses. *Anesth Analg* 1989;69:467–472.
13. Bickel U, Wiegand-Löhnert C, Fleischmann JW, et al. Different modulation of the perioperative stress hormone response under neurolept-anesthesia or enflurane for cholecystectomy. *Horm Metab Res* 1991;23:178–184.
14. Blalock JE. A molecular basis for bidirectional communications between the immune and neuroendocrine systems. *Physiol Rev* 1989;69:1–32.
15. Blunnie WP, McIlroy PDA, Merrett JD, Dundee JW. Cardiovascular and biochemical evidence of stress during major surgery associated with different techniques of anesthesia. *Br J Anaesth* 1983; 55:611–618.
16. Boarder MR, Marriott DB. Endothelin-1 stimulation of noradrenaline and adrenaline release from adrenal chromaffin cells. *Biochem Pharmacol* 1991;41:521–526.
17. Boarder MR, McArdle W. Breakdown of small enkephalin derivatives and adrenal peptide E by human plasma. *Biochem Pharmacol* 1986;35:1043–1047.
18. Bosnjak ZJ, Dujic Z, Roerig DL, Kampine JP. The effects of halothane on acetylcholine release and sympathetic ganglionic transmission. *Anesthesiology* 1988;60:500–506.
19. Bovill JG, Sebel PS, Fiolet JWT, Touber JL, Kok K, Philbin DM. The influence of sufentanil on endocrine and metabolic responses to cardiac surgery. *Anesth Analg* 1983;62:391–397.
20. Bullington J, Mouton S, Rigby J, et al. The effect on age on the sympathetic response to laryngoscopy and tracheal intubation. *Anesth Analg* 1989;68:603–608.
21. Cannon WB. The emergency function of the adrenal medulla in pain and the major emotions. *Am J Physiol* 1914;23:356–372.
22. Chaminade M, Foutz AS, Rossier J. Co-release of enkephalins and precursors with catecholamines from the perfused cat adrenal in situ. *J Physiol (Lond)* 1984;353:157–169.
23. Clark NJ, Meuleman T, Liu WS, Zwanikken P, Pace N, Stanley TH. Comparison of sufentanil-N_2O and fentanyl-N_2O in patients without cardiac disease undergoing general surgery. *Anesthesiology* 1987; 66:130–135.
24. Clement-Jones V, Lowry PJ, Rees LH, Besser GM. Met-enkephalin circulates in human plasma. *Nature* 1980;283:295–297.
25. Clevenger CV, Russel DH, Appasamy PM, Prystowsky MB. Regulation of interleukin 2-derived T-lymphocyte proliferation by prolactin. *Proc Natl Acad Sci USA* 1990;87:6460–6464.
26. Cliffer KD, Burstein R, Giesler GJ Jr. Distributions of spinothalamic, spinohypothalamic, and spinotelencephalic fibers revealed by anterograde transport of PHA-L in rats. *J Neurosci* 1991;11:852–868.
27. Cohen MR, Pickar D, Dubois M, Bunney WE. Stress-induced plasma beta-endorphin immunoreactivity may predict postoperative morphin usage. *Psychiatry Res* 1982;6:7–12.
28. Corder R, Vallotton MB, Lowry PJ, Ramage AG. Neuropeptide Y lowers plasma renin activity in the anaesthetized cat. *Neuropeptides* 1989;14:111–114.
29. Cozza E, Chiou S, Gomez-Sanchez CE. Endothelin-1 potentiation of angiotensin II stimulation of aldosterone production. *Am J Physiol* 1992;R85–R89.
30. Crozier TA, Beck D, Schlaeger M, Wuttke W, Kettler D. Endocrinologic changes following etomidate, midazolam, or methohexital for minor surgery. *Anesthesiology* 1987;66:628–635.
31. Crozier TA, Müller JE, Quittkat D, Sydow M, Wuttke W, Kettler D. Effects of anaesthesia on the cytokine responses to abdominal surgery. *Br J Anaesth* 1994;72:280–285.
32. Cruickshank AM, Fraser WD, Burns HJG, Van Damme J, Shenkin A. Response of serum interleukin-6 in patients undergoing elective surgery of varying intensity. *Clin Sci* 1990;79:161–165.
33. de Leon-Casasola OA, Lema MJ, Karabella D, Harrison P. Postoperative myocardial ischemia: epidural versus intravenous patient-controlled analgesia. A pilot project. *Reg Anesth* 1995;20:105–112.

34. Del Rey A, Besedovsky HO. Metabolic and neuroendocrine effects of pro-inflammatory cytokines. *Eur J Clin Invest* 1992;S1:10–15.
35. Derbyshire DR, Smith G, Achola KJ. Effect of topical lignocaine on the sympathoadrenal responses to tracheal intubation. *Br J Anaesth* 1987;59:300–304.
36. Desborough JP, Edlin SA, Burrin JM, Bloom SR, Morgan M, Hall GM. Hormonal and metabolic responses to cholecystectomy: comparison of extradural somatostatin and diamorphine. *Br J Anaesth* 1989;63:508–515.
37. Desborough JP, Hall GM, Hart GR, Burrin JM, Bloom SR. Hormonal responses to cardiac surgery: effects of sufentanil, somatostatin and ganglion block. *Br J Anaesth* 1990;64:688–695.
38. Dinarello CA. The biological properties of interleukin-1. *Eur Cytokine Netw* 1994;5:517–531.
39. Donadoni R, Baele G, Devulder J, Rolly G. Coagulation and fibrinolytic parameters in patients undergoing total hip replacement: influence of the anaesthesia technique. *Acta Anaesthesiol Scand* 1989;33:588–592.
40. Eger EI II, Saidman LJ, Brandstater B. Minimum alveolar anesthetic concentration: a standard of anesthetic potency. *Anesthesiology* 1965;26:756–763.
41. Engquist A, Brandt MR, Fernandes A, Kehlet H. The blocking effect of epidural analgesia on the adrenocortical and hyperglycemic responses to surgery. *Acta Anaesthesiol Scand* 1977;21: 330–335.
42. Eskay RL, Eiden LE. Interleukin-1 alpha and tumor necrosis factor-alpha differentially regulate enkephalin, vasoactive intestinal polypeptide, neurotensin, and substance P biosynthesis in chromaffin cells. *Endocrinology* 1992;130:2252–2258.
43. Feuerstein G. The opioid system and central cardiovascular control: analysis of controversies. *Peptides* 1985;6:51–56.
44. Forrest JB, Cahalan MK, Rehder K, et al. Multicenter study of general anesthesia: II. Results. *Anesthesiology* 1990;72:262–268.
45. Fragen RJ, Shanks CA, Molteni A, Avram MJ. Effects of etomidate on hormonal responses to surgical stress. *Anesthesiology* 1984;61: 652–656.
46. Furness JB, Costa M. Adynamic ileus, its pathogenesis and treatment. *Med Biol* 1974;52:82–89.
47. Gaillard RC, Bachman M, Rochat T, Egger D, Haller de R, Junod AF. Exercise induced asthma and endogenous opioids. *Thorax* 1986;41:350–354.
48. Garber AJ, Cryer PE, Santiago JV, Haymond MW, Pagliara AS, Kipnis DM. The role of adrenergic mechanisms in the substrate and hormonal response to insulin-induced hypoglycemia in man. *J Clin Invest* 1976;58:7–15.
49. Gaumann DM, Tassonyi E, Fathi F, Griessen M. Effects of topical laryngeal lidocaine on sympathetic response to rigid panendoscopy under general anesthesia. *ORL* 1992;54:49–53.
50. Gaumann DM, Tassonyi E, Rivest RW, Fathi M, Reverdin AF. Cardiovascular and endocrine effects of clonidine premedication in neurosurgical patients. *Can J Anaesth* 1991;38:837–843.
51. Gaumann DM, Yaksh TL. Adrenal and intestinal secretion of catecholamines and neuropeptides during splanchnic artery occlusion shock. *Circ Shock* 1988;26:391–407.
52. Gaumann DM, Yaksh TL, Tyce GM. Effects of intrathecal morphine, clonidine, and midazolam on the somato-sympathetic reflex response in halothane-anesthetized cats. *Anesthesiology* 1990; 73:425–432.
53. Gaumann DM, Yaksh TL, Tyce GM, Lucas DL. Opioids preserve the adrenal medullary response evoked by severe hemorrhage: studies on the adrenal catecholamine and met-enkephalin secretion in halothane anesthetized cats. *Anesthesiology* 1988;68:743–753.
54. Giles T, Sander GE, Rice JC, Quiroz AC. Systemic methionine-enkephalin evokes cardiostimulatory responses in the human. *Peptides* 1987;8:609–612.
55. Gin T, O'Meara ME, Kan AF, Leung RKW, Tan P, Yau G. Plasma catecholamines and neonatal condition after induction of anaesthesia with propofol or thiopentone at cesarean section. *Br J Anaesth* 1993;70:311–316.
56. Govoni S, Salar G, Colombo F, Pasinetti G, Trabucchi M, Mingrino S. Episodic secretion of Met-enkephalin immunoreactive material in human plasma and CSF. *Pharmacol Res Comm* 1986;18:155–159.
57. Grossman A, Rees LH. The neuroendocrinology of opioid peptides. *Br Med Bull* 1983;39:83–88.
58. Guillemin R, Vargo T, Rossier J, et al. Beta-endorphin and adrenocorticotropin are secreted concomitantly by the pituitary. *Science* 1977;197:1367–1369.
59. Guyenet PG, Cabot JB. Inhibition of sympathetic preganglionic neurons by catecholamines and clonidine: mediation by an alpha-adrenergic receptor. *J Neurosci* 1981;1:908–917.
60. Hacker GW, Bishop AE, Terenghi G, et al. Multiple peptide production and presence of general neuroendocrine markers detected in 12 cases of human phaeochromocytoma and in mammalian adrenal glands. *Virchows Arch* 1988;412:399–411.
61. Hähnel J, Mutschler D, Huhn W, et al. Perioperative Endothelin-, ACTH-, und Kortisol-plasma- konzentrationen bei Koronarbypasspatienten. *Anaesthesist* 1994;43:635–641.
62. Hall GM, Lacoumenta S, Hart GR, Burrin JM. Site of action of fentanyl in inhibiting the pituitary-adrenal response to surgery in man. *Br J Anaesth* 1990;65:251–253.
63. Hamblin AS. Cytokines. In: Dale MM, Foreman JC, Fan T-P, eds. *Textbook of immunophamracology.* 3rd ed. Oxford, U.K.: Blackwell Scientific, 1994:179–192.
64. Hart BB, Stanford GG, Ziegler MG, Lake RC, Chernow B. Catecholamines: study of interspecies variation. *Crit Care Med* 1989;17: 1203–1222.
65. Hemmer M, Viquerat CE, Suter PM, Vallotton MB. Urinary antidiuretic hormone excretion during mechanical ventilation and weaning in man. *Anesthesiology* 1980;52:395–400.
66. Hirai M, Miyabo S, Ooya E, et al. Endothelin-3 stimulates the hypothalamic-pituitary-adrenal axis. *Life Sci* 1991;48:2359–2363.
67. Hjortso NC, Christensen NJ, Andersen T, Kehlet H. Effects of the extradural administration of local anaesthetic agents and morphine on the urinary excretion of cortisol, catecholamines and nitrogen following abdominal surgery. *Br J Anaesth* 1985;57:400–406.
68. Holaday JW. Cardiovascular effects of endogenous opiate systems. *Annu Rev Pharmacol Toxicol* 1983;23:541–594.
69. Hotta H, Sato A, Sato Y, et al. Somatic afferent regulation of plasma prolactin in anesthetized rats. *Jpn J Physiol* 1993;43: 501–509.
70. Hynynen M, Lehtinen AM, Salmenperäm M, Fyhrquist F, Takkunen O, Heinonen J. Continuous infusion of fentanyl or alfentanil for coronary aretry surgery. *Br J Anaesth* 1986;58:1260–1266.
71. James MFM, Beer RE, Esser JD. Intravenous magnesium sulfate inhibits catecholamine release associated with tracheal intubation. *Anesth Analg* 1989;68:772–776.
72. Jones TH, Kennedy RL. Cytokines and hypothalamic-pituitary function. *Cytokine* 1993;5:531–538.
73. Kehlet H. Epidural analgesia and the endocrine-metabolic response to surgery. Update and perspectives. *Acta Anaesthesiol Scand* 1984;28:125–127.
74. Kehlet H. Modification of responses to surgery by neural blockade: clinical implications. In: Cousins MJ, Bridenbaugh PO, eds. *Neural blockade in clinical anesthesia and management of pain.* Philadelphia: Lippincott, 1988:145–188.
75. Kho HG, Kloppenborg PWC, Egmond van J. Effects of acupuncture and transcutaneous stimulation analgesia on plasma hormone levels during and after major abdominal surgery. *Eur J Anaesthesiol* 1993;10:197–208.
76. Kilborn MJ, Potter EK, McCloskey DI. Neuromodulation of the cardiac vagus: comparison of neuropeptides Y and related peptides. *Regul Pept* 1985;12:155–161.
77. Knothe CH, Boldt J, Zickmann B, Balesteros M, Dapper F, Hempelmann G. Endothelin plasma levels in old and young patients during open heart surgery: correlations to cardiopulmonary and endocrinology parameters. *J Cardiovasc Pharmacol* 1992; 20:664–670.
78. Kochs E, Treede RD, Schulte am Esch J, Bromm B. Modulation of pain-related somatosensory evoked potentials by general anesthesia. *Anesth Analg* 1990;71:225–230.
79. Kopin IJ, Eisenhofer G, Goldstein D. Sympathoadrenal medullary system and stress. *Adv Exp Med Biol* 1988;245:11–23.
80. Kumakura K, Karoum F, Guidotti A, Costa E. Modulation of nicotinic receptors by opiate receptor agonists in cultured adrenal chromaffin cells. *Nature* 1980;283:489–492.
81. Lacoumenta S, Paterson JL, Burrin J, Causon RC, Brown MJ, Hall GM. Effects of two differing halothane concentrations on the metabolic and endocrine responses to surgery. *Br J Anaesth* 1986; 58:844–850.
82. Lacoumenta S, Yeo TH, Burrin JM, Hall GM. Beta-endorphin infusion to modulate the hormonal and metabolic response to surgery. *Clin Enodcrinol* 1987;26:657–666.
83. LaGamma EF, Adler JE, Black IB. Impulse activity differentially regulates [leu]enkephalin and catecholamine characters in the adrenal medulla. *Science* 1984;224:1102–1104.
84. Lanes R, Herrera A, Palacios A, Moncada G. Decreased secretion

of cortisol and ACTH after oral clonidine administration in normal adults. *Metabolism* 1983;32:568–570.

85. Lanza V, Mercadante S, Latteri MT, Bellanca L. La réponse neuroendocrinienne à l'anesthésie par isoflurane. *Ann Fr Anesth Reanim* 1986;5:120–123.
86. Lavies NG, Meiklejohn BH, May AE, Achola KJ, Fell D. Hypertensive and catecholamine response to tracheal intubation in patients with pregnancy-induced hypertension. *Br J Anaesth* 1989; 63:429–434.
87. Liem TH, Hasenbos MA, Booij LH, Gielen MJ. Coronary artery bypass grafting using two different anesthetic techniques. Part 2: Postoperative outcome. *J Cardiothorac Vasc Anesth* 1992;6:156–161.
88. Lindner KH, Strohmenger HU, Ensinger H, Hetzel WD, Ahnefeld FW, Georgieff M. Stress hormone response during and after cardiopulmonary resuscitation. *Anesthesiology* 1992;77:662–668.
89. Lloyd DA, Teich S, Rowe MI. Serum endorphin levels in injured children. *Surg Gynecol Obstet* 1991;172:449–452.
90. Loewy AD. Forebrain nuclei involved in autonomic control. *Prog Brain Res* 1991;87:253–268.
91. Lund C, Selmar P, Hansen OB, Jensen CM, Kehlet H. Effect of extradural morphine on somatosensory evoked potentials to dermatomal stimulation. *Br J Anaesth* 1987;59:1408–1411.
92. Lundberg JM, Pernow J, Franco-Cereceda A, Rudehill A. Effects of antihypertensive drugs on sympathetic vascular control in relation to neuropeptide Y. *J Cardiovasc Pharmacol* 1987;10:S51–S68.
93. Lundberg JM, Torssell L, Sollevi A, et al. Neuropeptide Y and sympathetic vascular control in man. *Regul Pept* 1985;13:41–52.
94. Lyson K, McCann SM. The effect of interleukin-6 on pituitary hormone release in vivo and in vitro. *Neuroendocrinology* 1991;54: 262–266.
95. Malatinsky J, Vigas M, Jurcovicova J, Jezova D, Garayova S, Minarikova M. The patterns of endocrine response to surgical stress during different types of anesthesia and surgery in man. *Acta Anaesth Belg* 1986;37:23–31.
96. Mangano DT, Browner WS, Hollenberg M, London MJ, Tubau JF, Tateo IM. Association of perioperative myocardial ischemia with cardiac morbidity and mortality in men undergoing noncardiac surgery. The Study of Perioperative Ischemia Research Group. *N Engl J Med* 1990;323:1781–1788.
97. Mangano DT, Siliciano D, Hollenberg M, et al. Postoperative myocardial ischemia. Therapeutic trials using intensive analgesia following surgery. The Study of Perioperative Ischemia (SPI) Research Group. *Anesthesiology* 1992;76:342–353.
98. Masaki T, Yanagisawa M, Goto K. Physiology and pharmacology of endothelins. *Med Res Rev* 1992;12:391–421.
99. Meiklejohn BH, Coley S. Pressor and catecholamine response to nasal intubation of the trachea. *Br J Anaesth* 1989;63:283–286.
100. Merin RG. Pharmacology of the autonomic nervous system. In: Miller RD, ed. *Anesthesia, vol. 2.* New York: Churchill Livingstone, 1986:945–982.
101. Moore CM, Desborough JP, Powell H, Burrin JM, Hall GM. Effects of extradural anesthesia on interleukin-6 and acute phase response to surgery. *Br J Anaesth* 1994;72:272–279.
102. Mosnaim AD, Chevesich J, Wolf ME, Freitag FG, Diamond S. Plasma methionine enkephalin. Increased levels during migraine episodes. *Headache* 1986;26:278–281.
103. Mougin C, Baulay A, Henriet MT, et al. Assessment of plasma opioid peptides, beta-endorphin and met-enkephalin, at the end of an international nordic ski race. *Eur J Appl Physiol* 1987;56:281–286.
104. Naito Y, Tamai S, Shingu K, et al. Responses of plasma adrenocorticotrophic hormone, cortisol and cytokines during and after upper abdominal surgery. *Anesthesiology* 1992;77:426–431.
105. Namiki A, Collins JG, Kitahata LM, Kikuchi H, Homma E, Thalhammer JG. Effects of halothane on spinal neuronal responses to graded noxious heat stimulation in the cat. *Anesthesiology* 1980;53: 475–480.
106. Olson GA, Olson RD, Kastin AJ. Endogenous opiates: 1990. *Peptides* 1991;12:1407–1432.
107. Pernow J, Lundberg JM, Kaijser L. Vasoconstrictor effects in vivo and plasma disappearance rate of neuropeptide Y in man. *Life Sci* 1987;40:47–54.
108. Peters J, Schlaghecke R, Thouet H, Arndt JO. Endogenous vasopressin supports blood pressure and prevents severe hypotension during epidural anesthesia in conscious dogs. *Anesthesiology* 1990; 73:694–702.
109. Philbin DM, Rosow CE, Schneider RC, Koski G, D'Ambra MN. Fentanyl and sufentanil anesthesia revisited: how much is enough? *Anesthesiology* 1990;73:5–11.
110. Plotnikoff NP, Murgo AJ, Miller GC, Corder CN, Faith RE. Enkephalins: immunomodulators. *Fed Proc* 1985;44:118–122.
111. Powrie F, Coffman RL. Cytokine regulation of T-cell function: potential for therapeutic intervention. *Trends Pharmacol Sci* 1993;-14:164–168.
112. Quintin L, Roudot F, Roux C, et al. Effects of clonidine on the circulation and vasoactive hormones after aortic surgery. *Br J Anaesth* 1991;66:108–115.
113. Ramanathan J, Coleman P, Sibai B. Anesthetic modification of hemodynamic and neuroendocrine responses to cesarean delivery in women with severe preeclampsia. *Anesth Analg* 1991;73:772–779.
114. Randich A, Maixner W. (D-Ala2)-Methionine enkephalinamide reflexively induces antinociception by activating vagal afferents. *Pharmacol Biochem Behav* 1984;21:441–448.
115. Roizen MF, Horrigan RW, Frazer BM. Anesthetic doses blocking adrenergic (stress) and cardiovascular responses to incision—MACBAR. *Anesthesiology* 1981;54:390–398.
116. Rorie DK, Hunter LW, Lunn JJ. Halothane decreases the release of neuropeptide Y and 3,4-dihydroxyphenylglycol from superfused segments of the dog pulmonary artery. *Anesthesiology* 1990;73:722–730.
117. Russell AE, Cain MD, Kapoor V, Morris MJ, Chalmers JP. Neuropeptide Y-like immunoreactivity of plasma during hypoglycemia in man. *J Auton Nerv Syst* 1989;26:85–88.
118. Rutberg H, Hakanson E, Anderberg B, Jorfeldt L, Martensson J, Schildt B. Effects of the extradural administration of morphine, or bupivacaine, on the endocrine response to upper abdominal surgery. *Br J Anaesth* 1984;56:233–238.
119. Salo M. Effects of anaesthesia and surgery on the immune response. *Acta Anaesthesiol Scand* 1992;36:201–220.
120. Samso E, Farber NE, Kampine JP, Schmeling WT. The effects of halothane on pressor and depressor responses elicited via the somatosympathetic reflex: a potential antinociceptive action. *Anesth Analg* 1994;79:971–979.
121. Sato A, Sato Y, Schmidt RF. Catecholamine secretion and adrenal nerve activity in response to movements of normal and inflammed knee joints in cats. *J Physiol (Lond)* 1986;375:611–624.
122. Sawchenko PE, Swanson LW. The organization and biochemical specificity of afferent projections to the paraventricular and supraoptic nuclei. *Prog Brain Res* 1983;60:19–29.
123. Scheinin B, Lindgren L, Randell T, Scheinin H, Scheinin M. Dexmedetomidine attenuates sympathoadrenal responses to tracheal intubation and reduces the need for thiopentone and peroperative fentanyl. *Br J Anaesth* 1992;68:126–131.
124. Seagard JL, Elegbe EO, Hopp FA, et al. Effects of isoflurane on the baroreceptor reflex. *Anesthesiology* 1983;59:511–520.
125. Seagard JL, Hopp FA, Donegan JH, Kalbfleisch JH, Kampine JP. Halothane and the carotid sinus reflex. *Anesthesiology* 1982;57: 191–202.
126. Sebel PS, Aun C, Fiolet J, Noonan K, Savege TM, Colvin MP. Endocrinological effects of intrathecal morphine. *Eur J Anaesthesiol* 1985;2:291–296.
127. Sebel PS, Bovill JG, Schellekens APM, Hawker CD. Hormonal responses to high-dose fentanyl anaesthesia. *Br J Anaesth* 1981;53: 941–948.
128. Sellgren J, Pontén J, Wallin BG. Percutaneous recording of muscle nerve sympathetic activity during propofol, nitrous oxide, and isoflurane anesthesia in humans. *Anesthesiology* 1990;73: 20–27.
129. Sharrock NE, Cazan MG, Hargett MJL, Williams-Russo P, Wilson PD. Changes in mortality after total hip and knee arthroplasty over a ten-year period. *Anesth Analg* 1995;80:242–248.
130. Shirakami G, Magaribuchi T, Shingu K, et al. Effects of anesthesia and surgery on plasma endothelin levels. *Anesth Analg* 1995;80: 449–453.
131. Shribman AJ, Smith G, Achola KJ. Cardiovascular and catecholamine responses to laryngoscopy with and without tracheal intubation. *Br J Anaesth* 1987;59:295–299.
132. Slogoff S, Keats AS. Does perioperative myocardial ischemia lead to postoperative myocardial infarction? *Anesthesiology* 1985;62:107–114.
133. Smith DW, Day TA. c-fos expression in hypothalamic neurosecretory and brainstem catecholamine cells following noxious somatic stimuli. *Neuroscience* 1994;58:765–775.
134. Smith J, Kelly KA, Weinshilboum RM. Pathophysiology of postoperative ileus. *Arch Surg* 1977;112:203–209.

135. Smith R, Besser GM, Rees LH. The effect of surgery on plasma beta-endorphin and methionine-enkephalin. *Neurosci Lett* 1985; 55:17–21.
136. Snider ST, Kuchel O. Dopamine: an important neurohormone of the sympathoadrenal system. Significance of increased peripheral dopamine release for the human stress response and hypertension. *Endocrinol Rev* 1983;4:291–309.
137. Stanley TH, Berman L, Green O, Robertson D. Plasma catecholamine and cortisol responses to fentanyl-oxygen anesthesia for coronary-artery operations. *Anesthesiology* 1980;53:250–253.
138. Steffey EP, Eger EI II. Hyperthermia and halothane MAC in the dog. *Anesthesiology* 1974;41:392–396.
139. Sumikawa K, Matsumoko T, Ishizaka N, Nagai H, Amenomori Y, Amamkata Y. Mechanism of the differential effects of halothane on nicotonic and muscarinic-receptor mediated responses of the dog adrenal medulla. *Anesthesiology* 1982;57:444–450.
140. Taborsky GJ, Halter JB, Porte D. Morphine suppresses plasma catecholamine responses to laparotomy but not to 2-deoxyglucose. *Endocrinol Metab* 1982;5:E317–E322.
141. Theodorsson-Norheim E, Hemsén A, Lundberg JM. Radioimmunoassay for neuropeptide Y (NPY): chromatographic characterization of immunoreactivity in plasma and tissue extracts. *Scand J Lab Clin Invest* 1985;45:355–365.
142. Toft P, Svendsen P, Tonnesen E, Rasmussen JW, Christensen NJ. Redistribution of lymphocytes after major surgical stress. *Acta Anaesthesiol Scand* 1993;37:245–249.
143. Toth IE, Hinson JP. Neuropeptides in the adrenal gland: distribution, localization of receptors, and effects on steroid hormone synthesis. *Endocr Res* 1995;21:39–51.
144. Ullman B, Franco-Cereceda A, Hulting J, Lundberg JM, Sollevi A. Elevation of plasma neuropeptide Y-like immunoreactivity and noradrenaline during myocardial ischemia in man. *J Intern Med* 1990;228:583–589.
145. Unnerstall JR, Kopajtic TA, Kuhar MJ. Distribution of alpha$_2$-agonist binding sites in the rat and human central nervous system: analysis of some functional, anatomic correlates of the pharmacologic effects of clonidine and related adrenergic agents. *Brain Res Rev* 1984;7:69–101.
146. Walker P, Grouzmann E, Burnier M, Waeber B. The role of neuropeptide Y in cardiovascular regulation. *Trends Pharmacol Sci* 1991;12:111–115.
147. Wall PD. The prevention of postoperative pain. *Pain* 1988;33: 289–290.
148. Weissmann C. The metabolic response to stress: an overview and update. *Anesthesiology* 1990;73:308–327.
149. Wilson IG, Meiklejohn BH, Smith G. Intravenous lignocaine and sympathoadrenal responses to laryngoscopy and intubation. The effect of varying time of injection. *Anaesthesia* 1991;46:177–180.
150. Wortsman J, Frank S, Cryer PE. Adrenomedullary response to maximal stress in humans. *Am J Med* 1984;77:779–784.
151. Yaksh TL. The spinal actions of opioids. In: Herz A, ed. *Handbook of experimental pharmacology, vol. 104/II.* Berlin: Springer-Verlag, 1993:53–90.
152. Yaksh TL, Al-Rodhan NRF, Jensen, TS. Sites of action of opiates in production of analgesia. In: *Progress in brain research, vol. 77.* Amsterdam: Elsevier Science, 1988:371–394.
153. Yaksh TL, Jage J, Takano Y. Pharmacokinetics and pharmacodynamics of medullar agents. C. The spinal actions of α_2-adrenergic agonists as analgesics. *Baillieres Clin Anaesthesiol* 1993;7:597–614.
154. Ygge J. Changes in blood coagulation and fibrinolysis during the postoperative period. *Am J Surg* 1970;119:225–232.

Anesthesia: Biologic Foundations, edited by
Tony L. Yaksh et al. Lippincott–Raven Publishers,
Philadelphia © 1997.

CHAPTER 43

THE DEVELOPMENT AND RESOLUTION OF POSTINJURY PAIN

THERESE C. O'CONNOR AND STEPHEN E. ABRAM

Prevention and management of acute pain has been the focus of much research over the past 20 years. Despite this, acute postoperative and posttraumatic pain still causes significant suffering and continues to challenge physicians today. No matter how successfully or how skillfully conducted, surgery produces tissue trauma and releases potent mediators of inflammation and pain. Without treatment, sensory input from injured tissue reaches spinal cord neurons and causes subsequent responses to be enhanced. Postoperative pain contributes not only to patient discomfort, but also to longer recovery periods, more complications, and greater use of scarce health care resources. The ability to provide adequate postoperative pain relief by simple and safe methods is presently one of the major challenges for health care providers.

The physiologic risks associated with untreated pain are many and varied and greatest in frail patients with other illnesses such as heart or lung disease, those undergoing major surgical procedures, and the very young or very old. Pain may lead to shallow breathing and cough suppression in an attempt to "splint" the diaphragm. Pain of chest or upper abdominal origin in the spontaneously breathing patient causes a decrease in diaphragmatic function (36) and an increase in abdominal and lower intercostal muscle tone during exhalation (30). This results in decreased vital capacity, tidal volume, functional residual capacity, and alveolar ventilation. Atelectasis may develop with consequent venous admixture and hypoxia. Ability to cough is restricted, resulting in retention of secretions and, eventually, infection. Recovery is slow as chest physiotherapy is difficult and aggravation of pain by deep breathing and coughing limits patient cooperation, further increasing the likelihood of complications. There may be increased work of breathing causing increased oxygen consumption and lactic acid production associated with heightened muscle tone. Also, reflex motor activity associated with pain may result in muscle spasm, which may further increase pain. Skeletal muscle immobilization, venous stasis, and platelet aggregation predispose to deep venous thrombosis and pulmonary embolism.

Pain causes stimulation of the sympathetic nervous system and therefore tachycardia, increased peripheral resistance, hypertension, increased cardiac work load, and myocardial oxygen consumption. The risk of myocardial ischemia or even infarction is therefore increased. Increased sympathetic activity can increase intestinal secretions and smooth muscle sphincter tone, and decrease intestinal motility. Gastric stasis and dilation may occur. Pain can also cause a decrease in motility of the bladder and urethra with consequent difficulty in micturition and retention of urine.

Pain is one of the factors that causes the neuroendocrine and metabolic response to injury. This includes stimulation of the hypothalamus, increased catecholamine and catabolic hormone secretion, including cortisol, adrenocorticotropic hormone (ACTH), antidiuretic hormone (ADH), growth hormone (GH), adenosine 3',5'-cyclic monophosphate (cAMP), glucagon, aldosterone, renin, and angiotensin 11, and a decrease in secretion of anabolic hormones including insulin and testosterone (53) (see Chap. 14). This results in sodium and water retention, hyperglycemia, ketosis and lactic acidosis, and progression to a catabolic state with a negative nitrogen balance.

In the pregnant woman, severe, unrelieved pain during prolonged labor may increase oxygen consumption and maternal acidosis, increase gastrointestinal stasis, inhibit uterine contraction, and decrease uterine blood flow. These factors may pose a serious risk to both mother and fetus (see Chap. 17).

MECHANISMS OF POSTINJURY PAIN STATE

After physical injury to the tissue, the sensations arising from that injury are the result of activity in populations of small afferents that may arise from or are adjacent to the site of injury. Consideration of the complexity of the peri-injury site emphasizes that it is not a trivial issue to initially consider the identity and modality of the stimulus that is generating the afferent message.

Origin of the Postinjury Stimulus

Sensory fibers respond to a range of physical stimuli, including thermal, mechanical (physical distortion), as well as chemical.

Mechanical Distortion

Mechanical distortion of the free nerve ending can arise from the distention of soft tissue and increased parenchymal pressure due to tissue swelling, stretching of bone fascia, or joint deformation (see Chaps. 5 and 20). As reviewed previously, many of the small unmyelinated primary afferents are indeed polymodal and are potentially activated by such mechanical stimuli (see Chap. 4). Different organ systems will likely be differentially subject to mechanical activation. Thus, injury to the tooth or the bone underlying fascia represents confined spaces in which increased volume would be readily transduced into increased distortion of compressible tissue. Alternately, the free nerve ending after organ system injury may be exposed to an otherwise exaggerated degree of distortion, in the face of physiologic ranges of motion. These injuries would include joint injury or the margins of bone fractures.

The mechanical sensitivity of the small afferent terminal can be significantly augmented in the face of a number of inflammatory stimuli. This will be considered further below.

Chemical Products

In the face of injury, inspection of the milieu of the injury reveals the presence of a variety of products that include those produced by damaged tissue, those released by blood vessels, as well as substances released by afferent nerve fibers themselves, by sympathetic fibers, and by various immune cells.

The effects of these substances or inflammatory mediators are to activate or sensitize afferent fibers, effects that are produced by changing membrane ion channels, which are coupled directly via receptors or are regulated through receptor-coupled second messenger systems (see Chap. 6). These second messenger cascades have the ability to alter gene transcription. In this way long-term changes in the biochemistry of sensory neurons are induced, resulting in the expression of new proteins and receptors, and the induction of new enzymes. All of these changes can affect profoundly the characteristics of nociceptors and their ability to transmit pain signals.

Products Released from Primary Afferents Lewis (59) noted that the spread of hyperalgesia following cutaneous tissue injury coincided with the development of a flare or reddening of the skin surrounding the injury. It has long been known that the development of a flare is associated with vasodilatation that is dependent on neural mechanisms, and the spread of hyperalgesia that is dependent on peripheral nerves. Peripheral afferent axons can mediate the spread of hyperalgesia by liberating pain-producing or pain-enhancing substances into the uninjured skin around the injury. Recent evidence suggests that one mediator of neurogenic inflammation is substance P. It may produce its peripheral effects in part by a direct action on adjacent afferents or by indirect processes that would include, for example, degranulation of inflammatory cells.

Lembeck and Gamse (56) have proposed a model for peripheral mechanisms of inflammation and the spread of hyperalgesia. According to this model, tissue damage following injury causes a release of potassium from damaged cells, bradykinin from blood, and histamine from mast cells. Together, these substances stimulate nociceptors and induce the production of prostaglandins. Prostaglandins trigger inflammation and facilitate the activation of nociceptors. The substance most prevalent in vesicles isolated from terminals of small diameter fibers, both centrally and peripherally, is the neuropeptide substance P. Substance P is not the only peptide found in myelinated sensory neurons; over a dozen peptides have been found in primary sensory neurons and may contribute to the development of neurogenic inflammation. The stimulation of nociceptors causes the release of substance P from their nerve terminals, and as the level of stimulation increases, pain signals are generated. When released from peripheral terminals, substance P induces vasodilatation, producing a flare response, as well as causing a further release of histamine from adjacent mast cells (83). The release of further histamine results in the initiation of a repetition of the cycle in adjacent neurons, leading to increasing inflammation and the spread of hyperalgesia to uninjured tissue. The effect of this release of proinflammatory agents is to sensitize adjacent nociceptors (secondary hyperalgesia), resulting in an increase in the spontaneous activity of some nociceptors that can produce membrane depolarization of dorsal horn neurons. Under these conditions, inputs at synapses that were ineffective under normal conditions may be able to generate action potentials after sensitization.

Tissue Products Exposure to severe or prolonged noxious stimulation results in tissue damage. The damage is reflected by a destruction of cells, as well as nerve endings, at the site of injury. For example, potassium (K^+) and adenosine triphosphate (ATP), which are contained in the cells of tissue, are released following injury. The release of K^+ and ATP causes a sensitization of nerve endings and in this way, produces pain sensations. Following tissue injury there is also a local release of serotonin and bradykinin from blood, as well as histamine release from damaged mast cells. Tissue damage is also followed by the production and accumulation of arachidonic acid metabolites in inflammatory perfusate. Prostaglandins, the cyclooxygenase products of arachidonic acid metabolism, cause a sensitization of C-fiber nociceptors. It has been suggested that prostaglandins facilitate inflammation, the sensitization of nociceptors, and hyperalgesia by enhancing the effects of other previously released substances (see Chap. 34).

Evidence is now accumulating that exposure to severe and prolonged noxious stimulation causes a variety of substances to be released following cell damage, while others are synthesized during the events that follow tissue injury (28). They include reactive oxygen species, protons, kinins, prostanoids, ATP, serotonin, and histamine. These substances have a profound qualitative and quantitative impact on the production of inflammation and on afferent fiber activity causing pain sensations (see Chap. 6).

Reactive oxygen species (ROS) include hydrogen peroxide, superoxide, and hydroxyl species, and are normal products of electron transfer reactions, which are important for the regulation of gene transcription activities. Normally, the production of ROS is finely controlled by the antioxidase activity of superoxide dismutase and catalase. During the ischemia that follows the rapid vasoconstriction response upon tissue injury, ROS concentrations decrease to unphysiologically low levels and therefore switch off antioxidant activity. However, tissue reperfusion creates oxidative stress, which leads to the production of a number of factors including gene products encoding enzymes with free radical scavenging (catalase), tissue repair activity (collagenase, stromelysin), as well as the production of cytokines, cell surface receptors, adhesion molecules, and growth factors. Hydrogen peroxide enhances the effects of other inflammatory mediators such as bradykinins and prostaglandins. During inflammation or nerve injury, an inducible form of nitric oxide (NO) occurs, which has an important role in the regulation of an inducible form of cyclooxygenase activity and hence the production of inflammatory prostanoids. In addition, NO may alter the responsiveness of sensory neurons to inflammatory chemicals such as bradykinin (81).

Proton production is increased in inflammation and is likely to be involved in inflammatory hyperalgesia and in the sensation of muscle aching after exercise. Exogenously administered acidic solutions produced a rapid but transient increase in membrane cation activity, as well as a more prolonged permeability increase in sensory neurons. This can give rise to sustained nerve activation as well as an enhanced mechanosensitivity (84).

There is compelling evidence linking bradykinin with the pathologic processes that accompany tissue damage and inflammation, especially the production of pain and hyperalgesia (29). Kinins exert a number of proinflammatory effects including the release of prostanoids, cytokines, and free radicals from a variety of cells. They also stimulate postganglionic sympathetic neurons to affect blood vessel caliber (42). They degranulate mast cells to release histamine as well as other inflammatory mediators and also cause plasma extravasation by contraction of vascular endothelial cells. Kinins are potent algogenic substances and induce pain by directly stimulating nociceptors in skin, joint, and muscle, as well as by sensitizing them to heat and mechanical stimuli.

Prostanoids (prostaglandins, leukotrienes, hydroxy-acids) are among the most important mediators of inflammatory hyperalgesia and are generated from arachidonic acid by cyclooxygenase and lipoxygenase enzyme activity. Prostaglandins sensitize neurons, reducing their activation threshold and enhancing their responses to other stimuli (7).

ATP activates sensory neurons and increases their permeability to cations. Adenosine, formed by the breakdown of ATP, also provokes pain and hyperalgesia (8). This is likely to be due to the production of cAMP and a reduction in potassium ion permeability leading to hyperexcitability of afferent fibers.

Serotonin can cause direct excitation of sensory neurons by increasing sodium permeability. It is released from mast cells and platelets during tissue inflammation or injury. Activation of cAMP-dependent processes appears to be required for 5-HT–induced sensitization (57).

Histamine can be released following mast cell degranulation by a number of inflammatory mediators including substance P, interleukin-1, and nerve growth factor. It can then act on sensory neurons to produce itching at low concentrations and pain at higher concentrations. Indeed, sensory neurons express histamine receptors, and activation of these receptors increases membrane calcium permeability in a variety of sensory neurons, which can provoke the release of sensory neuropeptides, prostaglandins leading to hyperalgesia, and proinflammatory effects (75).

Nerve growth factor (NGF) is thought of as a target factor responsible for the survival and maintenance of the phenotype of specific sets of peripheral and central neurons during development and maturation. Recent evidence suggests that inflammation-induced increases in NGF in the periphery may be the linchpin that connects tissue damage to the accompanying hyperalgesia. It appears that the physiologic role of NGF in sensory neurons is highly dependent on their developmental context (58).

SOMATIC VERSUS VISCERAL PAIN

Somatic Pain

We use the term *pain* to define all sensations that hurt or are unpleasant; however, there are several distinct types of pain. The pain that is elicited when noxious stimuli threaten to damage body tissue is a key part of the body's defense mechanisms, protecting the body from a potentially hostile external environment by initiating behavioral and reflex avoidance tactics. A specific set of primary sensory neurons encode the intensity, duration and quality of noxious stimuli and can locate such stimuli by means of their organized projections to the spinal cord or trigeminal nucleus. This "ouch" pain is therefore an important element of the human nervous system, which, clinically, only needs to be temporarily suppressed or disabled during surgical procedures where tissue damage is deliberately produced. Pain following injury can be considered to have a biologically useful function that is protective to the body. This is achieved by rendering the injured tissue and surrounding area hypersensitive to all stimuli so that contact with external stimulus is avoided. Since the pain is protective in function, it is important to address the question of whether complete elimination of such pain is appropriate or whether it would be more beneficial to reduce it to a level where it can still fulfill a protective function. For example, the comfort of complete pain relief in patients who have undergone abdominal surgery and the advantages of possible earlier mobilization and fewer respiratory complications must be weighed against risks of wound dehiscence because of an excess of movement (92). Profound analgesia may also mask the appreciation of catastrophic occurrences such as nerve compression by an ill-fitting cast or a compartment syndrome.

Somatic pain arises from structures innervated by somatic nerves e.g., skin, muscle, periosteum, synovium. Direct injury causes stimulation of peripheral nociceptors in these structures, thus stimulating pain fibers, which carry the message to the spinal cord and thence to the brain. Because the pain is transmitted via somatic nerves, it is usually easily localized and confined to the distribution of the nerve supplying that structure. Its character is sharp and pain may be intense.

Visceral Pain

The sensibility of some visceral tissue differs profoundly from that of somatically innervated tissue (62). While pain of cutaneous origin is usually focal and well localized, pain of visceral origin is poorly localized in two distinct ways. In some cases visceral pain may be referred to distant structures and in other cases pain is perceived as being deep in the body. This latter type of pain is usually perceived as arising from the midline and may be either anterior or posterior in location. One example is the early pain of appendicitis, initially perceived in the midline. Another example is the pain felt after myocardial infarction. Visceral pain is usually perceived over an area much larger than that of the stimulus, i.e., it is extensive and with diffuse boundaries. It is frequently associated with a sense of nausea and malaise (62). Autonomic and motor reflexes associated with deep pains are often extreme and prolonged.

Much visceral pain is localized to distant structures, a phenomenon known as referred pain. The area to which the pain is referred is usually segmental and superficial, i.e., to muscle, skin, or both, innervated by the same spinal nerves as the affected viscus. A typical example is the pain that develops with nociceptive stimulation of the diaphragm, which is often located to the shoulder tip.

For noxious stimuli applied to cutaneous (or somatic) receptors, increasing the area over which a stimulus acts causes a modest increase in perceived pain, but the threshold for pain is not markedly reduced (73). However, for visceral receptors, unlike skin, spatial summation of stimuli may reduce significantly the effective threshold for pain. For example, for hollow viscera the distending pressures associated with pain may not be tissue damaging, and estimates of the threshold pressures producing pain in a particular viscus often vary markedly. This may explain the failure of localized mechanical stimuli, even frankly damaging ones, to produce pain.

For almost all intrathoracic, intraabdominal, and pelvic viscera, pain perception is a function of visceral afferent (sometimes termed sympathetic afferent) fibers. These neurons accompany sympathetic efferent axons in the sympathetic chain and intraabdominal and intrathoracic plexuses, but most, like other afferent fibers, have their cell bodies in the dorsal root ganglia and synapse with dorsal horn neurons.

High-frequency activation of the visceral afferents in turn activates dorsal horn pain projection neurons, producing pain perceived within cutaneous referral sites. This referred pain is probably the result of viscerosomatic convergence, the phenomenon of a single spinothalamic tract neuron that can be activated by either visceral or somatic stimuli or a combination of the two (see Chap. 12). Another type of convergence, reported by Bahr and colleagues (3), is based on the existence of afferent neurons with two sensory branches, one visceral (sympathetic afferent) and one somatic. It is not possible to locate the site of a painful stimulus to the gut with any accuracy, because stimulation of widely distant sites can give rise to the same referred sensations.

ORIGINS OF POSTOPERATIVE PAIN

A wide range of tissues are injured during surgical trauma. Somatic structures known to contain nociceptors include skin, muscle, fascia, tendons, ligaments, bursae, joints, intervertebral disks, and periosteum. Injury to any such structures may be associated with nociceptor activation. Many of these structures, such as joints and bursae, give rise to painful afferent impulses in response to normally nonpainful stimuli, such as movement or pressure, under conditions of inflammation and injury. Visceral pain may be evoked in the postoperative period by distention of a hollow viscus (gut, ureter), capsular distention of a solid viscus (liver, spleen, kidney), or pleural or peritoneal irritation (pleuritis, hemothorax, pneumothorax, peritonitis, irritation from intraperitoneal gas following laparoscopy). Aside from these specific stimuli leading to small afferent activation, it has been increasingly appreciated that compression, transection, or ischemia of a peripheral nerve in the course of the operation can yield effects with long-term consequences that may be categorized as being neuropathic in character (see Chaps. 20, 23, and 24).

While there are few studies that have investigated which specific tissues provide the source of postoperative pain, a few have provided some indirect information. Local infiltration of skin, muscle, and fascia following inguinal herniorrhaphy provides effective analgesia (27,31). This is not surprising, since there is little cause for visceral pain following this procedure. It seems likely, however, that body wall pain is the primary source of discomfort following major abdominal surgery, since pain ratings are consistently higher during movement or coughing than at rest (19). On the other hand, Joris et al. (49) found that deep, dull, poorly localized pain, which they characterized as visceral, encountered after laparoscopic cholecystectomy, was aggravated by coughing but not by movement. They found that this "visceral" component was more intense than "parietal," or well-localized body wall pain. They also described a third component of shoulder pain that was presumably related to diaphragmatic irritation. Interestingly, none of these pain components was relieved by intraperitoneal bupivacaine, suggesting either that the peritoneum itself is probably not the source of pain or that there was not sufficient anesthetic instilled to relieve such a source of pain.

Synovial inflammation appears to be a substantial component of postoperative pain following arthroscopic surgery, as intraarticular nonsteroidal anti-inflammatory drugs (NSAIDs) have been shown to provide effective analgesia (77).

DURATION OF PAIN AFTER INJURY

There can be a great deal of variability in the duration of pain following injury, since the severity of the injury and the structures traumatized will have a great influence on the resultant injury and healing process. Since the surgical trauma resulting from a given operation is fairly uniform, it would make the most sense to study the severity of postoperative pain over time in order to assess the intensity of acute pain over time. Unfortunately, most studies of postoperative pain are of relatively short duration, since most of these studies are performed by anesthesiologists whose access to postoperative patients is limited to the immediate perioperative period. Discussions of postoperative pain and its management are conspicuously absent in the surgical literature (the authors could not find a single chapter on the topic in surgery texts). However, a few studies have involved assessment of pain scores and analgesic requirements extending beyond the usual 24 to 48 hours.

Near Time Injury Pain States

Studies that provide data regarding severity of postoperative pain over time generally record both pain scores and analgesic utilization. Declining nociception is indicated by reductions in pain scores, decreasing analgesic use, or both.

Most studies that evaluate pain over the initial three postoperative days show modest decrements in pain scores and/or analgesic use during that period. Benzon et al. (5) showed an initial reduction in visual analogue scale (VAS) scores over the initial 12 hours following thoracotomy, with very little subsequent change in the ensuing 2.5 days. Opiate utilization, whether epidural fentanyl or patient-controlled analgesia (PCA) morphine, was unchanged during that period. Delaunay et al. (20) reported low and stable pain scores and a 30% reduction in opioid use through the early portion of the third postoperative day among patients receiving epidural fentanyl following abdominal surgery. Dawson et al. (19) reported a reduction in mean PCA morphine use from 2.5 to 1.6 to 1.3 mg/hr during the initial three days following abdominal surgery. Pain both at rest and with movement remained unchanged over that period. A study assessing the analgesic effects of epidural bupivacaine or morphine showed a 25% reduction in pain scores from the first to the third day with both techniques (32). Duration of pain relief after bolus injections increased more than twofold for bupivacaine and fourfold for morphine during that period of time. Parker et al. (71) were unable to demonstrate any significant reduction in PCA use over the initial 72 hours among patients undergoing abdominal hysterectomy. Modest reductions in dose over the 3-day period were seen for patients who received PCA plus infusion morphine. Similar findings are seen in children. A 3-day study evaluating the efficacy of continuous subcutaneous morphine infusions in children showed a 37% decrease in the infusion rate required to maintain VAS scores of 0 and 1 on a three-point scale (63).

Intermediate-Term Pain States

Only a few studies have assessed acute pain after the initial 3 days. Wasylak et al. (88) assessed patients daily for 5 days following abdominal hysterectomy, and reassessed pain at discharge (on day 5 to 8 for most patients) and at 2-week follow-up. There was a steady decline in morphine use over the first 4 days, whether PCA or IM prn administration was used (Fig. 1). During that interval, vital capacity doubled (Fig. 2) and ambulatory function improved daily. Mean VAS pain scores declined steadily, and remained at about 15 (0–100 scale) at discharge and at 2 weeks postoperatively. There was a similar reduction in Magill Pain Questionnaire scores over time (Fig. 3).

Guinard et al. (41) assessed pain scores and respiratory parameters following thoracotomy in patients receiving either thoracic or lumbar epidural fentanyl or intravenous fentanyl. For all groups, there was a steady reduction in VAS scores at rest and with coughing over the first 48 hours. At the time of discharge pain scores at rest and with coughing were roughly half of the 48-hour scores. Forced expiratory volume in one second (FEV_1) was about 25% of the preoperative control value immediately postoperative, and rose to about 40% of control at 48 hours and to 80% of control at discharge.

Deneuville et al. (23) showed a steady reduction in pain scores over a 5-day period following thoracotomy in patients treated with IM buprenorphine. VAS pain scores (0–10) fell from a mean of 4.5 during the first 8 hours to a mean of 2.0 on day 5. Unfortunately, daily analgesic use was not recorded. FEV_1 was about 30% of preoperative control on the day of surgery, 50% of control on day 5, and 60% of control on day 10.

Dahl et al. (18) assessed pain scores and analgesic use for 7 days in patients receiving epidural morphine plus bupivacaine for the first 48 hours following knee arthroplasty. Systemic analgesic use peaked on the fourth postoperative day and declined by 60% by day 7. There was little pain at rest throughout the study. Mean VAS pain scores (0–100) with movement were 40 on the first postop day, 22 on the fourth day, and 15 on the seventh day.

De Leon-Cassola et al. (22) provide the most extensive profile of postoperative pain over the first 6 days following surgery. They studied a total of over 4000 patients who received a com-

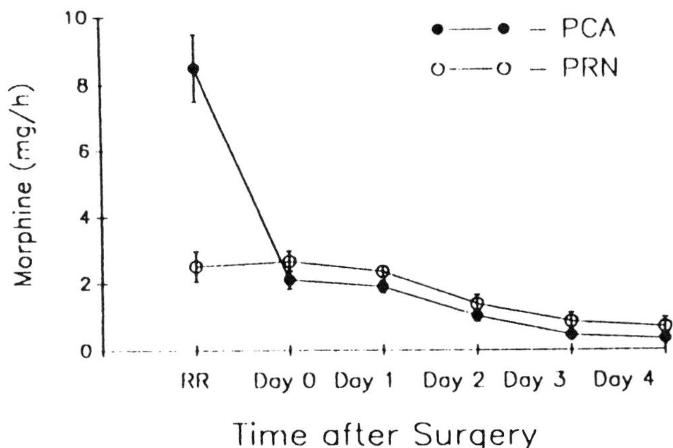

Figure 1. Mean intramuscular and intravenous PCA morphine doses administered to patients following abdominal hysterectomy. RR, recovery room. Day 0 extends from RR discharge to 24:00 hours. (From ref. 88, with permission.)

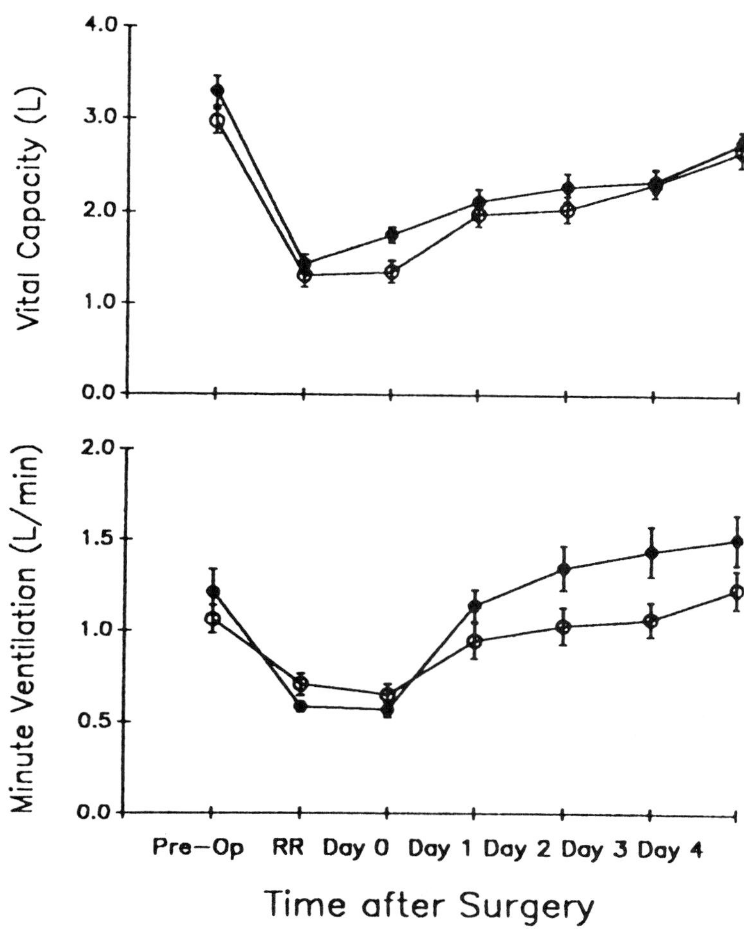

Figure 2. Respiratory function during the postoperative period following abdominal hysterectomy. *Open circles,* IM morphine treatment; *closed circles,* IV PCA morphine treatment. (From ref. 88, with permission.)

bination of epidural morphine and bupivacaine, adjusted to reduce VAS pain scores during cough or movement to <5. Under these circumstances, analgesic use should provide a reasonable measure of pain severity. They reported a mean daily epidural morphine requirement of 14.4 mg on day one, 9.6 mg on day 3, and 6.0 mg on day 6. Supplemental intravenous morphine was required for the first 3 days only . The same group of investigators assessed the postoperative epidural opioid requirements for cancer patients undergoing surgery who were either opioid naive or were receiving opioids chronically prior to surgery (21). They found that the chronic opioid group required about twice the daily epidural morphine dose, needed more intravenous morphine supplementation, and required epidural analgesia for a period nearly three times longer than that required by the opioid-naive group.

Tonsillectomy is associated with considerable postoperative discomfort, particularly with swallowing, and patients are typically unable to resume normal diets for 5 to 7 days (61). Jebeles et al. (46) reported that both constant pain and pain on swallowing remained at a mean VAS score >50 (0–100) for the first 5 postoperative days, and there was still some pain with swallowing after 10 days.

The data reviewed here represent mean scores and analgesic use profiles. Obviously, there is considerable variation in duration of pain among individual patients. Prior opioid use, as mentioned above, is one factor that can influence analgesic use. There are a variety of circumstances that can lead to more severe or prolonged postoperative pain. These include the presence of a preexisting painful disorder, such as cancer, acquired immunodeficiency syndrome (AIDS), chronic pancreatitis, or sickle cell disease. The development of a painful traumatic neuropathy may prolong postoperative pain and analgesic requirements. Intercostal neuralgia is relatively common after lateral thoracotomy. Ilioinguinal and iliohypogastric neuralgias may be encountered following hernia repair, and saphenous neuralgias are occasionally seen after vein harvests for vascular and coronary bypass surgery. Patients with preexisting ischemic pain are likely to develop long-standing postamputation or phantom limb pain following limb amputation. Reflex sympathetic dystrophy occasionally develops following surgery involving the extremities, and may dramatically increase pain and prolong the interval to a low pain state.

CONTRIBUTION OF CENTRAL SENSITIZATION

While it is clear that after peripheral injury there will be a peripherally mediated change in the transducer function of the afferent terminal, it is clear from preclinical work that changes in spinal processing occur that are induced by noxious stimuli during surgery and that these changes may augment the subsequent pain report. There is compelling evidence that acute afferent barrages of high-frequency C-fiber activity associated with tissue trauma or nerve injury will generate changes in spinal sensory processing that leads to a hyperalgesic state (see Chap. 9). Well-characterized human studies using intradermal capsaicin or repetitive electrical stimuli have demonstrated the psychophysical parallels of this central facilitation in humans generated by persistent small afferent stimulation (see Chap. 2). It appears almost certain that this change in postinjury processing accounts for an important component of the postsurgical pain state.

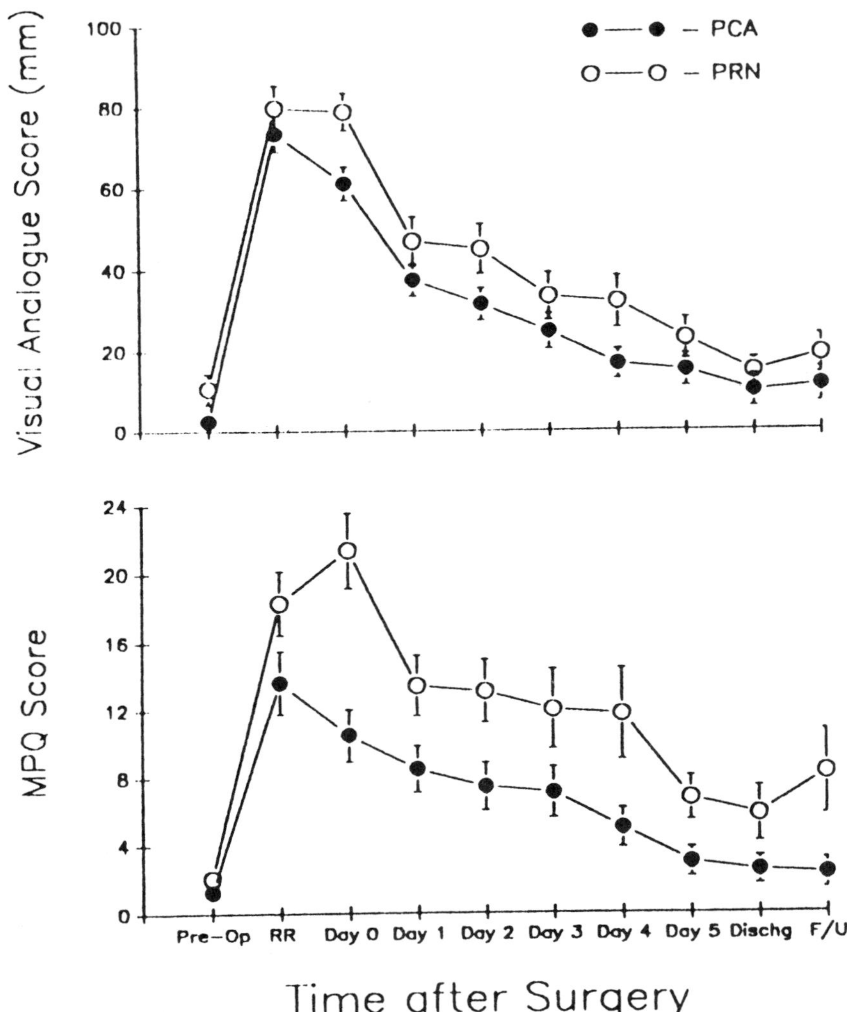

Figure 3. Pain levels reported by patients after abdominal hysterectomy in patients treated with IM or IV PCA morphine as measured by visual analogue or McGill Pain Questionnaire. Discharge was at 5 or 6 days postoperative, and follow-up (F/U) was 2 weeks postoperative. (From ref. 88, with permission.)

Mechanisms

A growing body of evidence suggests that administration of certain analgesic interventions prior to noxious stimulation, termed preemptive analgesia, can inhibit the establishment of spinal sensitization. This has raised the possibility that pain after surgery might be reduced by preventing intraoperative nociceptive impulses from reaching the spinal cord. The significance of this approach lies not only in the obvious benefit of protecting the patient at the time of surgical trauma but also in the possibility that such pretreatment will prevent the development of specific central neural changes that later amplify the peripheral signal and contribute to heightened postoperative pain.

The mechanisms responsible for central sensitization are now well recognized. The intracellular events that give rise to this phenomenon are initiated by the effects of excitatory amino acids on the *N*-methyl-D-aspartate (NMDA) receptor (14), and are prevented by spinal administration of NMDA antagonists (25), by blocking the nociceptive impulses from reaching the spinal cord, and possibly by drugs that limit the release of excitatory amino acids from nerve terminals in the dorsal horn, such as opioids (See Chaps. 9 and 13).

In recent years there has been increasing interest in the possible effects of general anesthetic agents on the processing of nociceptive activity in the spinal cord. Based on convergent lines of data from animal and human studies it seems certain that postinjury hyperalgesia is generated during the anesthetic state because processes set into play by afferent input are poorly blocked with volatile anesthetics at clinically relevant concentrations or by the combinations of anesthetics that are usually used. Studies utilizing single-unit recording techniques demonstrate that sensitization of dorsal horn neurons can be demonstrated in halothane-anesthetized animals (26). Studies of substance P or glutamate release from primary afferents are frequently demonstrated in animals that are anesthetized with volatile anesthetics. There is no reason to suspect that volatile anesthetics will alter either the binding of these transmitters to their respective receptors or the postsynaptic biochemical changes that occur secondary to those receptor activations, such as the increase in intracellular calcium, mediated by NMDA site activation. Animal studies have examined the role of general anesthetics in suppressing spinal sensitization through the use of the formalin test. These studies show that the volatile anesthetics and propofol at best produce only partial suppression of centrally mediated hyperalgesia, and some agents, such as thiopental or combinations of nitrous oxide with volatile agents, produce no suppression at all (70). It is likely, therefore, that noxious stimulation occurring intraoperatively can contribute to the central sensitization that occurs postoperatively.

Preemptive Analgesia

The observation that certain types of afferent input can condition central systems to upregulate the processing of the postinjury message has several important consequences. One that has been of particular import is the concept of "preemptive analgesia." In this scenario, pharmacologic treatment that alters nociceptive processing may be construed as preventing the development of the subsequent postinjury facilitation.

The idea that local anesthetic blocks or spinally administered opioids given before the afferent barrage can diminish the magnitude of the postoperative pain state is supported by animal data (1,14). This effect occurs, however, not because these agents are "analgesics," but because they act to prevent the postsynaptic effects (through a blockade of afferent transmitter release) that yield the facilitated state. Indeed agents such as the NMDA antagonists are not analgesic in the usual sense, but they prevent the development of facilitation by acting postsynaptically to prevent the biochemical events that lead to the facilitated state (see Chap. 9). There is an increasing amount of clinical literature that addresses the issue of the influence of preemptive analgesia on postoperative pain. Much of the literature deals with the effect of local or regional analgesia on postoperative pain ratings and analgesic requirements.

The dental profession recognized the potential value of regional anesthesia in preventing a hyperalgesic state long before the physiologic mechanisms were demonstrated. In 1947 Hutchins and Reynolds (44,78) observed that patients who underwent restorations or extractions under nitrous oxide anesthesia, without block anesthesia, experienced a hyperalgesic state lasting several weeks, characterized by pain referred to the previously stimulated teeth evoked by mechanical stimulation of the nasal epithelium. Patients who had similar procedures performed under block anesthesia failed to exhibit this phenomenon. The authors suggested in a subsequent publication that this was "evidence of a prolonged central excitatory state."

There is substantial evidence from clinical studies that regional anesthetic techniques, instituted prior to incision, are associated with lower pain ratings and analgesic requirements postoperatively. McQuay et al. (64) examined the influence of regional anesthesia on the time to first analgesic request among orthopedic surgical patients. They found that, among patients who received no preoperative opiates, the mean time to first analgesic request was 2 hours for general anesthesia patients versus 8 hours for patients who had regional anesthetics. The difference was significant.

Regional Blocks

The effect of the addition of femoral nerve block to general anesthesia for knee surgery was assessed by Ringrose and Cross (79). Patients who received preincisional femoral block were compared to those who had general anesthesia alone. Patients in the nerve block group required significantly less opioid in the first 24 hours. In a smaller subgroup of patients, they compared analgesic requirements for patients given blocks preoperatively with those blocked at the end of surgery. The group treated before incision used significantly less postoperative analgesic. Parnass et al. (72) examined the effects of general anesthesia versus epidural anesthesia in 260 patients undergoing ambulatory knee arthroscopic surgery. They found that discharge times were shorter, and the incidence of pain and nausea/vomiting was less, in the epidural group. Gottfreosdottir et al. (38) conducted a double-blind prospective clinical investigation to determine whether retrobulbar bupivacaine block had an effect on postoperative pain, nausea, and intra- and postoperative use of analgesics in 32 patients undergoing retinal detachment surgery performed under general anesthesia. Postoperative pain score and nausea were significantly lower in the retrobulbar block group during the first postoperative hours than in the control group, with significantly fewer patients requiring parenteral pain relief during the first 48 hours after surgery. Katz et al. (50), in a study of patients undergoing lower abdominal surgery, compared patients who received preoperative lumbar epidural bupivacaine to patients receiving lumbar epidural bupivacaine 30 min after incision. They found a reduction in postoperative morphine consumption at 24, 48, and 72 hours after surgery of 30%, 25%, and 22%, respectively, in the preoperative bupivacaine group.

On the other hand, several studies comparing pre- versus postoperative regional analgesia have failed to demonstrate a preemptive effect. One randomized, double-blind study (74) examined 36 patients who received a standard general anesthetic for abdominal hysterectomy or myomectomy. They received either 15 ml of bupivacaine 0.5% with adrenaline by lumbar epidural injection 15 min before surgery or the same dose at the end of surgery but before waking. There was no difference in postoperative pain scores between the two groups. Dahl et al. (18) studied 32 patients undergoing total knee arthroplasty who were randomized to receive an identical epidural blockade initiated 30 min before surgical incision or at closure of the surgical wound. They found no significant differences were observed in request for additional opioids, or in pain scores at rest or during mobilization of the operated limb, during or after cessation of the regimen.

Local Infiltration Data

Some randomized studies have confirmed the efficacy of preincisional local infiltration in reducing postoperative pain. The simplest model examines the influence of preincisional local anesthetic infiltration of the surgical field on the severity of postoperative pain. Two of the first studies of this type, published almost simultaneously, compare preoperative to postoperative local anesthetic wound infiltration in patients undergoing inguinal herniorrhaphy under general anesthesia. Both studies were blinded and randomized. Interestingly, the results were quite different. Ejlersen et al. (31) found that patients treated prior to incision requested postoperative analgesia significantly later, despite the expectation that their local anesthetic dissipated sooner. In addition, the preincision-treated patients required fewer postoperative analgesic doses, and a significantly greater percentage of pretreated patients required no postoperative analgesics. Dierking et al. (27) were unable to demonstrate such a relationship between pretreatment and analgesic need. There was no significant difference in time to first analgesic request between pretreated and posttreated patients. Likewise there was no difference with respect to pain scores at rest, during activity, or with coughing at any time during the first 24 hours or at 7 days postoperatively. It is surprising that such similar studies should yield such disparate results. However, the difference in the studies may lie in the choice of intraoperative technique. The Ejlersen study employed thiopentone, nitrous oxide, and a muscle relaxant, but no opiate during surgery, while the patients in the Dierking study received alfentanil prior to the incision. Some animal data suggest that nociceptor-induced spinal sensitization is significantly attenuated by opiate pretreatment, and that preemptive use of alfentanil in both groups may have obscured the potential differences between groups in the Dierking study. This study design factor may also have influenced the results of other subsequent studies.

Jebeles et al. (46) compared preincisional bupivacaine to saline infiltration of the tonsillar bed in patients undergoing tonsillectomy with isoflurane and nitrous oxide. No opiates were given intraoperatively. The study demonstrated significantly lower spontaneous pain for 5 days in the local anesthetic group and significantly less pain with swallowing in the bupivacaine group for as long as 10 days postoperatively.

It is not clear from the local infiltration studies whether the reduction in postoperative analgesic requirements is the result of local effects of the anesthetic on the traumatized tissues, or the result of blocking afferent impulses from reaching the spinal cord. Tverskoy et al. (86) addressed this issue in a study of inguinal herniorrhaphy patients who were randomized to receive general anesthesia, general anesthesia plus preincisional local anesthesia, or spinal anesthesia. Patients received no intraoperative opiates. Patients given spinal anesthesia had a significantly longer interval to first analgesic request, had significantly lower pain scores, and had significantly less pain with mechanical pressure to the wound than patients who had general anesthesia alone. These findings suggest that deafferentation of noxious input indeed plays a role in the attenuation of postoperative pain by preincisional technique. A peripheral tissue effect of the local anesthetic is not ruled out however, since the patients who received local infiltration had significantly less pain with movement or wound pressure and longer latencies to first analgesic requests than the spinal anesthesia patients.

Opioids

There is less clinical evidence for the ability of preincisional opiate administration to block spinal sensitization. In the same study that evaluated the effects of regional anesthesia, McQuay et al. (64) investigated the effects of opioid premedication in patients undergoing orthopedic procedures with general anesthesia. They found that patients who received preoperative narcotics had a significantly longer mean interval to first analgesic request (5 versus 2 hours for the control group). Again, this study is less than ideal, since neither the opioid drug nor the dose was specified, and selection was not randomized. A study by Kiss and Killian (54) also concludes that opioid premedication reduces postoperative analgesic needs. They showed that patients who received 50 mg meperidine intramuscularly preoperatively were less likely to request postoperative analgesics following laminectomy under general anesthesia. Unfortunately, this study also has some major flaws, including the use of different preoperative tranquilizers in the two groups and the administration of fentanyl preincisionally in all patients. Tverskoy et al. (86) investigated whether the induction and maintenance of anesthesia with the use of fentanyl reduced postoperative pain and wound hyperalgesia beyond the period when these effects can be explained by the direct analgesic action of these drugs. They found that the intensity of pain to suprathreshold pressure on the wound was decreased in the fentanyl group compared to controls. However, there was no statistically significant change in spontaneous incisional or movement-associated pain compared with the control group. The results suggest that fentanyl preemptively decreases wound hyperalgesia. On the other hand, Collis et al. (15) found no significant difference in postoperative morphine requirements or cutaneous sensitivity between a group receiving a large opioid premedication and one that received a small premed.

Katz et al. (51) evaluated the ability of preincisional epidural fentanyl to modify postthoracotomy pain. They administered 4 μg fentanyl in 20 ml saline in the lumbar epidural space either just before or just after incision and rib retraction. The group that received epidural fentanyl prior to incision exhibited significantly lower pain scores at 6 hours postoperatively and had lower postoperative morphine consumption between 12 and 24 hours postoperatively. Values for pain ratings and morphine use were not significantly different at any other times. The relatively minor benefits observed with preoperative use of fentanyl may be related to the lumbar, as opposed to the thoracic, level of administration. Also administration of the epidural fentanyl after only 15 min of surgical trauma in the postincisional group may have reduced the apparent magnitude of the preemptive analgesic effect.

Cyclooxygenase Inhibitors

Central prostanoids have been implicated in producing a facilitated state both centrally and peripherally (see Chap. 34). Evidence for a preemptive analgesic effect from NSAIDs is not particularly convincing. Murphy and Medley (67) compared preoperative indomethacin with postoperative administration for pain relief following elective thoracic surgery. They found no significant difference between groups in terms of pain ratings, opioid requirement, or in the incidence of adverse effects. Similarly, Fletcher et al. (35) compared preincisional with postincisional intravenous ketorolac on postoperative pain and analgesic consumption using a randomized, double-blind, placebo-controlled design in patients undergoing total hip replacement. They demonstrated some benefit of preoperative ketorolac, but only in the immediate postoperative period, i.e., during the first 6 hours postoperatively.

CHRONIC POSTINJURY PAIN

Relatively rarely, a pathologic state of chronic pain may develop that can involve more or less permanent changes in the central nervous system, persisting long after the original injury has healed. There has been much interest recently in the involvement of spinal cord synaptic plasticity in hyperalgesia and allodynia of chronic pain syndromes. The fact that evidence of hyperesthesia can persist for weeks after a noxious stimulus in the absence of preoperative analgesic use leads one to speculate that afferent blockade prior to onset of the noxious input might prevent the development of certain chronic pain states.

Damage to peripheral tissue and injury to nerves typically produces persistent pain and hyperalgesia. However, there are significant differences in the underlying peripheral mechanisms of nociceptive and neuropathic pain. Damage to cutaneous or deep (muscle, joint, or viscera) tissue is typically associated with peripheral inflammation, while injury to nerves often leads to pathologic peripheral nerve processes, including neural degeneration, neuroma formation, and the generation of spontaneous neural inputs. It is generally accepted that the nociceptive pain produced by tissue injury is significantly influenced by inflammatory changes, while neuropathic pain is influenced by pathologic alterations in peripheral nerve function. Evidence suggests that although nociceptive and neuropathic pain depend on separate peripheral mechanisms, they are both significantly influenced by changes in CNS function.

Phantom Limb Pain

There are a variety of clinical problems that may develop following amputation that have some similarities whether the amputation involved physical loss of a limb or body organ, or avulsion of the nerve plexus supplying the limb resulting in total deafferentation. Experience of a sensation of the intact limb being present, which can involve all sensory modalities, including movement, is commonly experienced by amputees. This is the classical phantom limb. The sensation may not necessarily be unpleasant, although this may perhaps depend on the condition of the limb prior to amputation.

Pain experienced in a limb at the time of, or shortly before, amputation frequently persists in the phantom limb. This type of phantom limb pain, characterized by the persistence or recurrence of a pain, prior to amputation is typically experienced in the same location in the limb and has the same character as the pain that was present preamputation (65). Pain "memories" that have been demonstrated include painful diabetic ulcers, gangrene, corns, blisters, ingrown toenails, cuts, and deep injury (52). These pains and sensations are frequently felt so vividly that the patient may find it difficult to believe that the limb has been removed, and many patients are embarrassed to admit the presence of phantom sensations, and are relieved when it is explained that this is common.

If pain is experienced at or near time of amputation, there is a high probability that it will persist in the phantom limb (47,52). Reports of pain memories in phantom limbs appear to be less common when there has been a discontinuity, or a pain-free interval, between the experience of pain and the amputation (52). This is consistent with the observation that the relief of preamputation pain by continuous epidural block for 3 days prior to amputation decreases the incidence of phantom limb pain compared to patients undergoing epidural anesthesia induced just prior to surgery. The difference in incidence of phantom limb pain was still evident 6 months later (2). Another study (45) compared the incidence of phantom pain in patients who received epidural analgesia begun 24 to 48 hours preoperatively to patients given general anesthesia. The epidural group experienced lower incidence of phantom pain at 7 days, 6 months, and 1 year postoperatively.

Other possible associated factors in the development of phantom pain include a trend for severe pains to be represented with a greater frequency than mild pains, and facilitation of reactivation of the pain memory by the integration of multimodal inputs established prior to amputation. These associated visual, tactile, and motor components that had accompanied the original pain include such visual elements as that of a discolored and festering diabetic ulcer, and the foul smell of putrid diabetic ulcers and gangrene (52).

Pain also persists in patients with deafferentation that does not involve amputation. Deafferentation with a relatively intact limb is most vividly illustrated in the brachial plexus avulsion injury (48,76). The paralyzed and anesthetic arm is a focus of severe phantom pain, often of a crushing nature. Patients with spinal cord injuries may also experience pain in the anesthetic deafferented region (6,16). Examples of this type of pain include a patient who continued to feel the pain of an ingrown toenail after a complete spinal cord transection (68), as well as seven patients with partial peripheral nerve injury and subsequent pain who underwent complete nerve and graft or ligation but redeveloped pain of the same character and in the same area as the pain they had experienced prior to nerve resection (69).

Some postamputation pains arise in the stump. This may be due to localized stump trauma from poorly fitting prostheses, bone spurs, or neuroma formation. The pain often presents as acutely tender areas on the stump. Tactile stimulation of these areas may give rise to stabbing or electric shock–like pains, sometimes accompanied by clonic movements of the stump. This type of pain is of peripheral origin, whereas phantom limb pain is probably of a central deafferentation type and is associated with reduced inhibitory stimuli from the limb.

Neuropathic Pain

Nerve injury leads to pathologic changes, including nerve degeneration, neuroma formation, and the generation of spontaneous neural inputs. While the immediate effects of injury on nerve transmission are generally understood, it is often forgotten that secondary changes occur with release of chemicals from nerves, from damaged cells, and as a result of the release of enzyme products. There is also a tertiary phase of nerve injury, with invasion of the injured area by fibroblasts and phagocytes. Damaged nerves and capillaries "sprout" and infiltrate the injured area. The sprouting nerves include sensory, sympathetic, and motor nerve fibers (43).

Under optimal conditions one of these regenerating sprouts reaches peripheral target tissue. Growth then stops, peripheral receptor function is restored and excess sprouts are culled. When forward growth is prevented, terminal end bulbs persist and sprouts either turn back on themselves or form a tangled mass. This structure is a "neuroma." Many studies (10,11,39,66,82,90) have found that a neuroma is a major site of ectopic discharge especially in mechanosensitive "hot spots" clustered in the 3 mm closest to the nerve end. While locally applied corticosteroids have been shown to prevent development of ectopic discharge and to suppress ongoing discharge in established neuromas in animal models, there is little clinical data establishing a role for steroids in the perioperative period (24).

In addition to spontaneous activity arising at the site of nerve injury, it is likely that central mechanisms play a substantial role in the development of postoperative neuropathic pain. There is considerable evidence that spinally mediated hyperalgesia may be triggered by afferent discharges originating from the site of nerve injury. One example of such evidence is the ability of NMDA antagonists to reduce the hyperalgesic effect of chronic sciatic nerve ligation injury in rats (93).

Neuropathic pain is occasionally encountered after inguinal hernia repair. It characterized by allodynia and burning, dysesthetic pain that persists or recurs along the incision scar. Injury to the ilioinguinal, iliohypogastric, or genitofemoral nerves is thought to be the most likely cause of this troublesome condition. Postthoracotomy neuralgia is seen fairly often, and produces a similar type of pain along the thoracotomy scar, most likely the result of stretching, injury, or transection of an intercostal nerve. Saphenous neuralgia may occur after saphenous nerve harvest for coronary bypass or peripheral vascular vein grafts.

Reflex Sympathetic Dystrophy

Reflex sympathetic dystrophy (RSD) is occasionally triggered by surgical trauma, particularly procedures involving the palmar aspect of the hand or the plantar aspect of the foot. The syndrome (also known as sympathetically maintained pain and complex regional pain syndrome type I) typically consists of burning pain in the extremity, allodynia, autonomic dysfunction (vasodilation or vasoconstriction, hyperhydrosis), edema, joint dysfunction, and muscle weakness and/or tremor. Late manifestations consist of dystrophic skin changes, bone demineralization, and muscle atrophy. The syndrome is likely the result of both central and peripheral mechanisms. Sensitization of spinal neurons responsive to noxious stimulation is a likely component of the pathologic process. In addition, there is evidence for sensitization of peripheral mechanoreceptors, leading to a situation of heightened afferent input in response to nonnoxious stimulation, plus supernormal activation of spinothalamic and other pain projection pathways, leading to allodynia, burning, and dysesthesias (80). In addition, there may be central dysregulation of autonomic function in patients with RSD. Evidence for alterations in sympathetic regulatory function following injury was provided by Blumberg and Janig (9), who demonstrated loss of the normal reciprocity between skin and muscle vasoconstrictors following peripheral nerve lesions in cats. Skin vasoconstrictors are normally under the influence of hypothalamic centers. They are normally involved in thermoregulation, and tend to be inhibited by stimuli that activate muscle vasoconstrictors, which are under medullary control. Following peroneal nerve lesions, skin vasoconstrictors begin to respond like muscle vasoconstrictors and appear to be under medullary control.

There are few published data on the incidence of RSD after surgery. Since the incidence of this condition is very low compared to the incidence of postamputation pain, it would be difficult to study the effect of different anesthetic techniques on the development of RSD. However, regional anesthetic techniques initiated preoperatively and continued into the postoperative period are often utilized for patients with a history of RSD, particularly when surgery involves a previously affected limb.

ETHNIC AND GENDER DIFFERENCES

Numerous workers have concluded that sociodemographic parameters influence the perception and communication of pain as well as its treatment. Reports of pain severity have been found to vary with ethnic and cultural background, as well as age, gender, education, and socioeconomic class (4,91). A few comparisons between ethnic groups on the severity of acute postoperative or obstetric pain have also been reported. Using a VAS to rate pain, Western women were found to rate the pain of delivery as less severe than Middle Eastern women (89). Faucett et al. (33) compared self-reported postoperative dental pain among four ethnic groups: Asian, African-American, European, and Latino. The subjects of European descent reported significantly less severe pain than those of African-American or Latino descent, and less pain than those of Asian descent also, although this did not reach significance. In another study, however, women of African-American, Anglo-Saxon, Irish, Italian, and Jewish heritage did not vary in their reports of episiotomy pain (34).

Specific conclusions from a large body of literature about ethnic differences in pain severity are difficult to make, however, because of variations in the ethnicities and clinical disorders investigated and possible confounding factors such as gender and varying degrees of integration between ethnic groups. Faucett et al.'s (33) study did examine covariates such as age, gender, education, and generation and found that regardless of ethnic group, men reported less severe pain than women. This difference is also reported in other studies (87,91). The multidisciplinary nature of pain has led investigators to hypothesize that factors such as control, beliefs about pain and pain behavior, and anxiety may contribute to reports of pain severity. Ethnic or gender differences in terms of these psychological factors may influence pain self-reporting, and sociocultural influences on reporting pain are also likely differ between groups (17).

Laboratory comparisons of pain threshold and tolerance have the advantage of control over the application, intensity, duration, and nature of the painful stimulus. Studies of ethnic differences in experimental pain have included a wide variety of stimuli such as mechanical pressure, radiant heat, electrical stimulation, and cold pressor pain. Although results from these studies have been mixed, Northern European or Caucasian groups were more often reported to have higher pain tolerance than other racial or ethnic groups (13,55,87,91).

Differences may exist between ethnic groups in the potency of the endogenous pain-modulating system. Pharmacologic differences have been demonstrated between ethnic groups for substances with known effects on pain such as prostaglandins (85), alcohol (12), beta-blockers (37), caffeine (40), and psychotropic medications (60). While differences in the rate of metabolism of opioids or local anesthetics have not yet, to our knowledge, been investigated, such differences if they exist, could contribute to differences in pain appreciation between ethnic groups. Further investigation into this subject, with more rigorous methodologic consistency, is required.

CONCLUSIONS

Our expanding understanding of the mechanisms involved in the generation of postinjury pain are bound to stimulate new interventions that will diminish the severity of postoperative and posttraumatic pain and reduce their physiologic consequences. While some new interventions will probably require neuraxial drug administration, there are clear advantages to the development of systemically administered pharmacologic agents with specificity toward those mechanisms responsible for adverse effects of tissue injury. There is a substantial need to develop techniques that affect peripheral tissue mechanisms, neuropathic conditions, and changes in central nervous system sensory processing. Identification of individuals at risk for the development of severe or prolonged pain is another worthwhile goal. The transfer of knowledge of the basic mechanisms already accumulated into the clinical realm should go a long way toward reversing the adverse consequences of tissue injury.

REFERENCES

1. Abram SE, Yaksh TL. Morphine but not inhalation anesthesia blocks post-injury facilitation: the role of preemptive suppression of afferent transmission. *Anesthesiology* 1993;78:713–721.
2. Bach S, Noreng MF, Tjellden NU. Phantom limb pain in amputees during the first 12 months following limb amputation, after preoperative epidural blockade. *Pain* 1988;33:297–301.
3. Bahr R, Blumberg H, Janig W. Do dichotomizing afferent fibers exist which supply visceral organs as well as somatic structures? *Neurosci Lett* 1981;24:25.
4. Bates MS, Edwards WT, Anderson KO. Ethnocultural influences on variation in chronic pain perception. *Pain* 1993;52:101–112.
5. Benzon HT, Wong HK, Belavic AM, et al. A randomized double-blind comparison of epidural fentanyl infusion versus patient-controlled analgesia with morphine for postthoracotomy pain. *Anesth Analg* 1993;76:316–322.
6. Berger M, Gerstenbrand F. Phantom illusions in spinal cord lesions. In: Siegfried J, Zimmerman M, eds. *Phantom and stump pain.* Berlin: Springer, 1981;66–73.
7. Birell GJ, McQueen DS, Iggo A, Colman RA, Grubb BD. PGI2-induced activation and sensitization of articular mechanoreceptors. *Neurosci Letts* 1991;124:5–8.
8. Bleehan T, Keele CA. Observations on the algogenic actions of adenosine compounds on the human blister base preparation. *Pain* 1977;3:367–377.
9. Blumberg H, Janig W. Changes in vasoconstrictor neurons supplying cat hindlimb following chronic nerve lesions: a model for studying mechanisms of reflex sympathetic dystrophy? *J Auton Nerve Syst* 1983;7:399–418.
10. Blumberg H, Janig W. Discharge pattern of afferent fibers from a neuroma. *Pain* 1984:20;335–353.
11. Burchiel KJ. Effects of electrical and mechanical stimulation on two foci of spontaneous activity which develop in primary afferent neurons after peripheral axotomy. *Pain* 1984:18;249–265.
12. Chan AW. Racial differences in alcohol sensitivity. *Alcohol* 21: 93–104.
13. Chapman W, Jones C. Variations in cutaneous and visceral pain sensitivity in normal subjects. *J Clin Invest* 1944;23:81–91.
14. Coderre TJ, Melzack R. The contribution of excitatory amino acids to central sensitization and persistent nociception after formalin-induced tissue injury. *J Neurosci* 1992;12:3665–3670.
15. Collis R, Brandner B, Bromley LM, Woolf CJ. Is there any clinical advantage of increasing the pre-emptive dose of morphine or combining pre-incisional with postoperative morphine administration? *Br J Anaesth* 1995;74:396–399.
16. Conomy JP. Disorders of the body image after spinal cord injury. *Neurology* 1973;23:842–850.
17. Craig K. Social disclosure, coactive peer companions. and social modelling determinants of pain communications. *Can J Behav Sci/Rev Can Sci Comp* 1978;10:91–103.
18. Dahl JB, Daugaard JJ, Rasmussen B. Immediate and prolonged effects of pre- versus postoperative epidural analgesia with bupivacaine and morphine on pain at rest and during mobilisation after total knee arthroplasty. *Acta Anaesth Scand* 1994;38:557–561.
19. Dawson PJ, Libreri FC, Jones DJ, et al. The efficacy of adding a continuous intravenous morphine infusion to patient-controlled analgesia (PCA) in abdominal surgery. *Anaesth Intens Care* 1995;23: 453–458.
20. Delaunay L, Leppert C, Dechaubry V, et al. Epidural clonidine decreases postoperative requirements for epidural fentanyl. *Reg Anesth* 1993;18:176–180.
21. de Leon-Casasola OA, Myers DP, Donaparthi S, et al. A comparison of postoperative epidural analgesia between patients with chronic cancer taking high doses of oral opioids versus opioid-naive patients. *Anesth Analg* 1993;76:302–307.
22. de Leon-Casasola OA, Parker B, Lema MJ, et al. Postoperative epidural bupivacaine-morphine therapy. Anesthesiology 1994;81:368–375.
23. Deneuville M, Bissier A, Regnard JF, et al. Continuous intercostal analgesia with 0.5% bupivacaine after thoracotomy: a randomized study.
24. Devor M, Govrin-Lippmann, Raber P. Corticosteroids suppress ectopic neural discharge originating in experimental neuromas. *Pain* 1985;22:127–137.
25. Dickenson AH and Sullivan AF. Evidence for a role of the NMDA receptor in the frequency dependent potentiation of deep rat dor-

sal horn nociceptive neurones following C fibre stimulation. *Neuropharmacology* 1987;26:1235–1238.
26. Dickenson AH, Sullivan AF. Subcutaneous formalin-induced activity of dorsal horn neurones in rat: differential response to an intrathecal opiate administered pre or post formalin. *Pain* 1987;30:349–360.
27. Dierking GW, Dahl JB, Kanstrup K, et al. Effect of pre- vs postoperative inguinal field block on postoperative pain after herniorrhaphy. *Br J Anaesth* 1992;68:344–348.
28. Dray A. Inflammatory mediators of pain. *Br J Anaesth* 1995;75: 125–131.
29. Dray A, Perkins M. Bradykinin and inflammatory pain. *TINS* 1993;16:99–104.
30. Duggan J, Drummond GB. Activity of lower intercostal and abdominal muscle after surgery in humans. *Anesth Analg* 1987:55;852.
31. Ejlersen E, Andersen HB, Eliasen K, et al. A comparison between preincisional and postincisional lidocaine infiltration and postoperative pain. *Anesth Analg* 1992;74:495–8.
32. El-Baz NMI, Faber LP, Jensik RJ. Continuous epidural infusion of morphine for treatment of pain after thoracic surgery.
33. Faucett J, Gordon N, Levine J. Differences in postoperative pain severity among four ethnic groups. *J Pain Symptom Manage* 1994;9: 383–389.
34. Flannery RB, Sos J, McGovern P. Ethnicity as a factor in the expression of pain. *Psychosomatics* 1981;22:39–50.
35. Fletcher D, Zetlaoui P, Monin M, Bombart M, Samii K. Influence of timing on the analgesic effect of intravenous ketorolac after orthopedic surgery. *Pain* 1995;61:291–297
36. Ford GT, Whitelaw WA, Rosenal TW, et al. Diaphragmatic function after upper abdominal surgery in humans. *Am Rev Respir Dis* 1983: 127;431.
37. Freis ED. Antihypertensive agents. In: Kalow W, ed. *Ethnic differences in reactions of drugs and xenobiotics.* New York: Alan R. Liss, 1986.
38. Gottfreosdottir MS, Gislason I, Stefansson E, et al. Effects of retrobulbar bupivacaine on post-operative pain and nausea in retinal detachment surgery. *Acta Ophthalmol* 1993;71:544–547.
39. Govrin-Lippmann R, Devor M Ongoing activity in severed nerves: source and variation with time. *Brain Res* 1978:159;406–410.
40. Grant DM, Tang BK, Kalow W. Variability in caffeine metabolism. *Clin Pharmacol Ther* 1983;33:591–602.
41. Guinard J-P, Mavrocordatos P, Chiolero R and Carpenter RL. A randomized comparison of intravenous versus lumbar and thoracic epidural fentanyl for analgesia after thoracotomy. *Anesthesiology* 1992;77:1108–1115.
42. Hall JM, Geppeti P. Kinins and kinin receptors in the nervous system. *Neurochem Int* 1995;56:17–26.
43. Horch KW, Lisney SJW. On the number and nature of regenerating myelinated axons after lesions of cutaneous nerves in the cat. *J Physiol (Lond)* 1981:313;287–299.
44. Hutchins HC, Reynolds OE. Experimental investigation of the referred pain of aerodontalgia. *J Dent Res* 1947;26:3–8.
45. Jahangiri M, Bradley JWP, Jayatunga AP, et al. Prevention of phantom limb pain after major lower limb amputation by epidural infusion of diamorphine, clonidine and bupivacaine. *Ann R Coll Surg Engl* 1994;76:324–326.
46. Jebeles JA, Reilly JS, Gutierrez JF, et al. The effect of pre-incisional infiltration of tonsils with bupivacaine on the pain following tonsillectomy under general anesthesia. *Pain* 1991;47:305–308.
47. Jensen TS, Krebs B, Nielsen J, Rasmussen P. Immediate and long-term phantom pain in amputees. incidence, clinical characteristics and relationship to pre-amputation pain. *Pain* 1985;21:267–278.
48. Jensen TS, Rasmussen P. Phantom pain and related phenomena after amputation. In: Wall PD, Melzack R, eds. *Textbook of pain,* 2nd ed. Edinburgh: Churchill Livingstone, 1989;508–521.
49. Joris J, Thiry E, Paris P, et al. Pain after laparoscopic cholecystectomy: characteristics and effect of intraperitoneal bupivacaine. *Anesth Analg* 1995;81:379–384.
50. Katz J, Clairoux M, Kavanagh BP. Pre-emptive lumbar epidural anaesthesia reduces postoperative pain and patient-controlled morphine consumption after lower abdominal surgery. *Pain* 1995;59:395–403.
51. Katz J, Kavanagh BP, Sandler AN, et al. Preemptive analgesia. Clinical evidence of neuroplasticity contributing to postoperative pain. *Anesthesiology* 1992;77:439–446.
52. Katz J, Melzack R. Pain "memories" in phantom limbs: review and clinical observations. *Pain* 1990;43:319–336.
53. Kehlet H. Pain relief and modification of the stress response. In: Cousins MJ, Philips GD, eds. *Acute pain management.* New York: Churchill Livingstone, 1986;49.
54. Kiss IA, Killian M. Does opiate premedication influence postoperative analgesia? A prospective study. *Pain* 1992;48:157–158.
55. Knox VJ, Shum K, McLaughlin DM. Response to cold pressor pain and to acupuncture analgesia in oriental and occidental patients. *Pain* 1977;4:49–57.
56. Lembeck F, Gamse R. Substance P in peripheral sensory processes. In: Porter R, O'Connor M, eds. *Substance P in the nervous system.* Ciba Foundation Symposium 91. London: Pitman, 1982;85.
57. Levine JD, Fields HL, Basbaum AI. Peptides and the primary afferent nociceptor. *J Neurosci* 1993;13:2273–2286.
58. Lewin GR, Mendell LM. Nerve growth factor and nociception. *TINS* 1993;16:353–359.
59. Lewis T. The nocifensor system of nerves and its reactions. *Br Med J* 1937;491:194–431.
60. Lin KM, Poland RE, Smith MW, Strickland TL, Mendoza R. Pharmacokinetic and other related factors affecting psychotropic responses in Asians. *Psychopharmacol Bull* 1991;27:427–439.
61. MacGregor FB, Albert DM, Bhattacharyya AB. Post-operative morbidity following pediatric tonsillectomy; a comparison of bipolar diathermy dissection and blunt dissection. *Int J Pediatr Otorhinolaryngol* 1995;31:1–6.
62. McMahon SB, Dmitrieva N, Koltzenburg. Visceral pain. *Br J Anaesth* 1995;75:132–144.
63. McNicol R. Postoperative analgesia in children using continuous S.C. morphine. *Br J Anaesth* 1993;71:752–756.
64. McQuay HJ, Carroll D, Moore RA. Postoperative orthopedic pain—the effect of opiate premedication and local anesthetic blocks. *Pain* 1988;33:291–295.
65. Melzack R. Phantom limb pain: implications for treatment of pathologic pain. *Anesthesiology* 1971;35:409–419.
66. Meyer RA, Raja SN, Cambell JN, Mackinnon SE, Dellon AL. Neural activity originating from a neuroma in the baboon. *Brain Res* 1985:325;255–260.
67. Murphy DF, Medley C, Preoperative indomethacin for pain relief after thoracotomy: comparison with postoperative indomethacin. *Br J Anaesth* 1993;70:298–300.
68. Nathan PW. Pain traces left in the central nervous system. In: Keele CA, Smith R, eds. *The assessment of pain in man and animals.* Edinburgh: Livingstone, 1962;129–134.
69. Noordenbos W, Wall PD. Implications of the failure of nerve resection and graft to cure chronic pain produced by nerve lesions. *J Neurol Neurosurg Psychiatry* 1981;44:1068–1073.
70. O'Connor TC, Abram S. Inhibition of nociception-induced spinal sensitization by anesthetic agents. *Anesthesiology* 1995;82:259–266.
71. Parker RK, Holtman B, White PF. Patient-controlled analgesia: does a concurrent opioid infusion improve pain management after surgery? *JAMA* 1991;266:1947–1952.
72. Parnass SM, McCarthy RJ, Bach BR, et al. Beneficial impact of epidural anesthesia on recovery after outpatient arthroscopy. *Arthroscopy* 1993;9:91–95.
73. Price DD, McHaffe J, Larson M. Spatial summation of heat induced pain: influence of stimulus area and spatial separation of stimuli on perceived sensation intensity and unpleasantness. *J Neurophysiol* 1989;62:1270.
74. Pryle BJ, Vanner RG, Enriquez N, et al. Can pre-emptive lumbar epidural blockade reduce postoperative pain following lower abdominal surgery? *Anaesthesia* 1993;48:120–123.
75. Rang HP, Bevan SJ, Dray A. Nociceptive peripheral neurons: cellular properties. In: Wall PD, Melzack R, eds. *Textbook of pain.* Edinburgh: Churchill Livingstone, 1994;57–58.
76. Reisner H. Phantom sensations (phantom arm) in plexus paralysis. In: Siegfried J, Zimmerman M, eds. *Phantom and stump pain.* Berlin: Springer, 1981;62–65.
77. Reuben SS, Connelly NR. Postoperative analgesia for outpatient arthroscopic knee surgery with intraarticular bupivacaine and ketorolac. *Anesth Analg* 1995;80:1154–1157.
78. Reynolds OE, Hutchins HC. Reduction of central hyper-irritability following block anesthesia of peripheral nerve. *Am J Physiol* 1948; 152:658–662.
79. Ringrose NH, Cross MJ. Femoral nerve block in knee joint surgery. *Am J Sports Med* 1984;12:398–402.
80. Roberts WJ. A hypothesis on the physiological basis for causalgia and related pains. *Pain* 1986;24:297–311.
81. Rueff C, Patel IA, Urban L, Dray A. Regulation of bradykinin sensitivity in peripheral sensory fibres of the rat by nitric oxide and cyclic GMP. *Neuropharmacology* 1994;33:1139–1145.
82. Scadding JW Development of ongoing activity, mechanosensitivity,

and adrenalin sensitivity in severed peripheral nerve axons. *Exp Neurol* 1981:73;345–364.
83. Sosnowski M, Lebrun P, Fodderie L. Receptors, Neuropathways and mechanisms. *Anesth Clin North Am* 1992;10:211–228.
84. Steen KH, Reeh PW, Anton F, Handwerker HO. Protons selectively induce lasting excitation and sensitization to mechanical stimuli of nociceptors in rat skin, in vitro. *J Neurosci* 1992;12:86–95.
85. Stein M, O'Malley K, Kilfeather S. Ethnic differences in cyclic AMP accumulation: effect on alpha 2-, beta 2-, and prostanoid receptor responses. *Clin Pharmacol Ther* 1990;47:360–365.
86. Tverskoy M., Cozacov C., Ayache M., et al. Postoperative pain after inguinal herniorrhaphy with different types of anesthesia. *Anesth Analg* 1990;70:29–35.
87. Walsh N, Schoenfield L, Ramamurthy S, Hoffman J. Normative model for cold pressor test. *Am J Phys Med Rehabil* 1989;68:6–11.
88. Wasylak TJ, Abbott FV, English MJM, et al. Reduction of postoperative morbidity following patient-controlled morphine. *Can J Anaesth* 1990;37:726–731.
89. Weisenberg M, Caspi Z. Cultural and educational influences on pain of childbirth. *J Pain Symptom Manage* 1989;4:13–19.
90. Wiezenfeld Z, Lindblom U. Behavioural and electrophysiological effects of various types of peripheral nerve lesions in the rat: a comparison of possible models for chronic pain. *Pain* 1980:8;285–298.
91. Woodrow KM, Friedman GD, Siegelaub AB, Collen MF. Pain tolerance; differences according to age, sex and race. *Psychosom Med* 1972;34:548–556.
92. Woolf CJ, Chong M-S Preemptive analgesia—treating post-operative pain by preventing the establishment of central sensitization. *Anesth Analg* 1993;77:1–18.
93. Yamamoto T, Yaksh TL. Studies on the spinal interaction of morphine and the NMDA antagonist MK801 on the hyperalgesia observed in a rat model of sciatic mononeuropathy. *Neurosci Lett* 1992;135:67–70.

Anesthesia: Biologic Foundations, edited by Tony L. Yaksh et al. Lippincott–Raven Publishers, Philadelphia © 1997.

CHAPTER 44

BURN PAIN

BRENDAN S. SILBERT, PATRICIA F. OSGOOD, AND DANIEL B. CARR

Encouraging recent data from the National Center for Health Statistics documents a moderate decline over the past 20 years in medical care requirements due to burns and other fire-related injuries such as smoke inhalation (9). Despite this favorable trend, the latest estimates in the 1990s still exceed 5,500 annual deaths in the United States from fire and burn-related causes, a figure fivefold greater than annual deaths from air travel or all forms of machinery-related injuries. Over one million Americans per year seek medical care for burns, of whom 23,000 are admitted to specialized burn centers and nearly 30,000 others are admitted to acute care hospitals (9). The demographics of burn injury remain strikingly similar to those described by the young physician Jacob Bigelow in the first issue of *The New England Journal of Medicine*: "Very dangerous cases often occur in children, whose clothes are accidentally kindled; in intoxicated persons...and in those exposed to conflagrations, or by explosions of...inflammable gases" (7).

Bigelow further observed, "The distressing effects of these injuries, when they exist in an extensive degree, are exceeded by few diseases" and described the pain as "of a peculiar kind, resembling that from the continued application of fire to the part." He also noted, "The peculiar appearance of a burnt surface has commonly been supposed to require a peculiar treatment" and surveyed the "different and opposite modes of (burn) treatment, whose apparent success or failure at different times has occasioned considerable disputes regarding their apparent efficacy." His early, controlled experiments—probably the first in America, if not the world—to examine the comparative efficacy of then-current regimens employed rabbits with bilateral ear scald burns in which each ear was treated according to a different regimen. He even mentioned topical application of opioid ("laudanum") to the inflamed area as a treatment recommended by a Mr. Kentish, but unfortunately he did not test this approach experimentally.

Given this interest in understanding burn pathophysiology and analgesia at the dawn of American medicine, the limited degree to which subsequent preclinical advances in understanding the pathophysiology of burn injury have improved patients' quality of life is disappointing. In contrast to other clinically common forms of nociceptive stimuli, burns are associated with tissue destruction and local liberation of inflammatory mediators (35). Burns that exceed 15% of total body surface area (BSA) provoke systemic hormonal responses (107) and are frequently associated with potentially devastating multisystem impairment (35). While patient survival has improved markedly due to early excision and grafting (11) in conjunction with sophisticated intensive care (34,140), comparatively little attention has been given to pain control. Nevertheless, therapeutic procedures such as sequential skin excision and grafting, and repeated dressing changes impose a constant barrage of acute painful stimuli that may continue for weeks, months, or even years. To contemporary society, "burn injury and death represent a significant if not catastrophic social problem....Serious burns are one of the most costly and medically intensive injuries that can occur to a person" (135). To the individual, "Burns are a truly overwhelming personal catastrophe. They cause extreme and prolonged pain, and too frequently result in profound disfigurement. The lives of those injured and the lives of their families are disrupted, often for months, or even years" (135). Few would question the value of psychological support to deal not only with pain but also with the high prevalence of depressive and posttraumatic stress syndromes in such circumstances (75), but there is still today "a great...discrepancy between the reported emotional needs of patients and services provided" in the United States and Canada (62). Thus, the problem of burn pain urgently needs the collaborative efforts of preclinical scientists and health care providers to elucidate the basic mechanisms of pain after tissue burn, to apply this knowledge to improve analgesic therapies, and finally to deliver these to the bedside.

THERMAL NOCICEPTION

The initial quantitation of stimulus parameters that give rise to pain in human subjects was accomplished by Hardy and colleagues (54) in 1940. They employed sequentially increasing radiant heat directed onto the skin to determine a subject's pain threshold, and found that this threshold was extremely reliable for any specific area yet differed as much as 5°C between different locations on the body (54,55). Subsequent refinement of quantitative sensory testing has led to the widespread use of contact thermal testing, in which a probe that may be heated or cooled precisely is applied in contact with the skin (85). For both methods of assessing pain perception in relation to skin temperature, in a variety of mammalian species withdrawal behaviors and escape reflexes as well as (in humans) pain reports are elicited as skin temperatures rise above 45°C (117) or, with contact methods, below 10°C (Fig. 1). From 35°C to 45°C, warmth is perceived as a separate sensory dimension mediated through separate neuronal sensory populations and pathways distinct from those mediating painful heat above 45°C (117). As temperature is increased progressively above 45°C, the magnitudes of pain-related

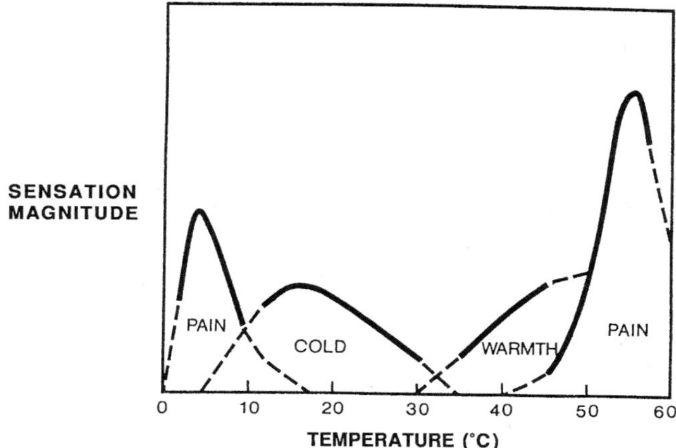

Figure 1. Diagrammatic illustration of sensations evoked by stimulation in different physiologic ranges of temperature (abscissa) versus arbitrary sensation magnitude (ordinate). The *curves* are estimates based on established neurophysiologic data; *thick lines* indicate the normally prevalent type of perception; *hatched lines* indicate borderline rages with overlapping perceptions or subperceptual activation of respective receptor types. (From ref. 85.)

behaviors in animals or pain intensity reports in humans follow a positively accelerating power function (117) (Fig. 2). A similar, positively accelerating response of discharge frequency as a function of rising temperature above 45°C has been demonstrated in electrophysiologic measurements of peripheral and central nociceptive neurons (Fig. 3), strongly suggesting that heat-induced "pain intensity information is encoded and transmitted in neural pathways in a relatively straightforward fashion" (117).

A brief stimulus of 51°C evokes two distinct pain sensations in humans. "First pain" occurs immediately and is well localized, sharp, and pricking. "Second pain" follows about a second later, is less well localized, and is described as dull, throbbing, or burning. Repetitive brief heat "pulses" of 51°C produce consistent decreases in subsequent neural "first pain" responses of primary afferents and spinothalamic neurons in primates, and correspondingly parallel decreases in intensity reports of "first pain" in humans (118). Interestingly, the same repetitive stimulus produced very different responses of "second pain" (Fig. 4). While long-latency afferent responses decrease, long-latency spinothalamic activity and perceived pain intensity both increase with repetitive stimulation. This disparity between first-pain suppression and second-pain summation has been suggested by Price (117) to result from heat-induced suppression of Aδ heat nociceptive afferents, and central summation in pathways activated by C-polymodal nociceptive afferents. Meyer and Campbell (97), however, directly studied the responses of C and A nociceptive afferents to thermal stimuli before and after a 30-second, 53°C burn to the glabrous skin of the hand in monkeys, and compared these to subjective responses in human volunteers. Meyer and Campbell reached the conclusion that C fibers code thermal pain intensity near threshold 43° to 48°C, and that A fibers code for pain associated with prolonged temperatures above this range and for hyperalgesia shortly after burn. It is possible that distinct mechanisms and neurotransmitters may mediate hyperalgesia arising after noxious thermal stimulation versus other forms of noxious stimuli (e.g., mechanical or chemical). Meller (94) has reviewed the evidence that different excitatory amino acids and different signal transduction pathways (see Chap. 36) mediate different forms of nociception-induced hyperalgesia (Fig. 5). Henry and Radhakrishnan (60), however, contend that while processing of different nociceptive inputs may be mediated by different mechanisms, central hyperexcitability provoked by such inputs relies on overlapping, similar mechanisms.

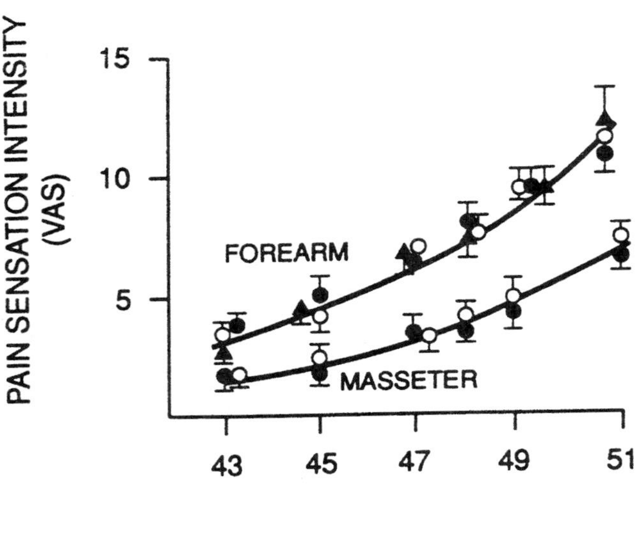

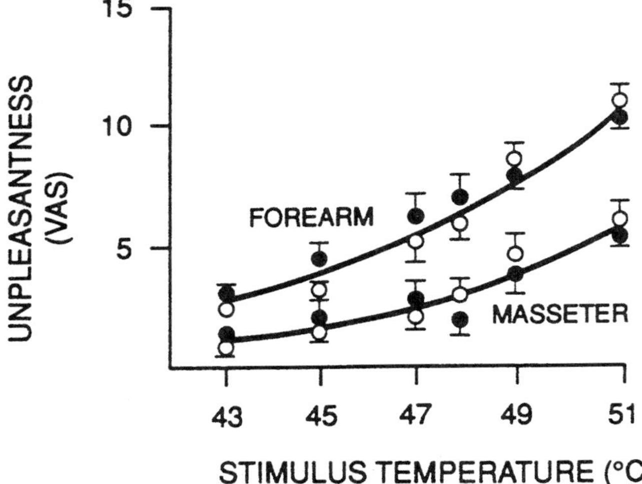

Figure 2. Visual analogue scale (VAS) measurements of the relation between skin temperature and the judgment of pain sensation intensity and unpleasantness. The data were obtained from patients with lower back pain (▲) and myofascial pain dysfunction (MPD) (○) as well as from pain-free control subjects (●) and are plotted in linear coordinates. Each point on the graphs represents the group average for a given temperature; *vertical lines* through the points represent standard errors of the mean (these conventions are followed in subsequent Figures). Despite the large difference between the VAS ratings of the intensity of the facial (area over the masseter muscle) and forearm stimuli on the pair of curves on the *top,* the exponents of the functions were identical (2.1). A similar result was obtained for ratings of unpleasantness *(bottom).* (From ref. 117.)

Two findings—radiation and spatial summation—from human psychophysical studies of heat-induced pain may have mechanisms in common with those identified in preclinical studies of summation of second pain. *Radiation* refers to the perceived spread of pain from the stimulus site; *spatial summation* means that pain intensity and unpleasantness induced by a constant, suprathreshold temperature are both greater as the stimulus is applied over a greater area of skin (Fig. 6). Both phenomena have parallels in the clinical symptoms described by patients with pain well after their acute thermal injury (see below).

EXPERIMENTAL BURN PAIN IN VOLUNTEERS

Burn depth and extent are obvious determinants of pain and clinical outcome after thermal injury (7,11,34,35,49). However, the relationship between burn depth, area, and clinical pain can be complex and inconstant, even in a single patient during a single hospitalization (2). Physiologic and nociceptive responses to tissue burn evolve through distinct phases that involve different mediators, mechanisms, and pathways (15). Therapies such as excision and grafting, or frequent serial dressing changes, that allow present-day patients to survive burns uniformly fatal in prior years, produce substantial pain for long after the burn trauma itself. To these factors are added the tolerance that universally develops when burn patients are started on continuous opioid infusions; the additional pain burden associated with operations to release scarred, contracted tissue or to reconstruct disfiguring injuries; and finally the challenge of mobilization and functional rehabilitation. Unraveling such complexity will no doubt take years. However, some experimental data in volunteers, and limited clinical observations in patients allow us to piece together an overview of the key features of different stages in the natural history of burn pain.

First-degree burns, in which the skin is reddened but not moist, blistered, or swollen, are usually considered minor

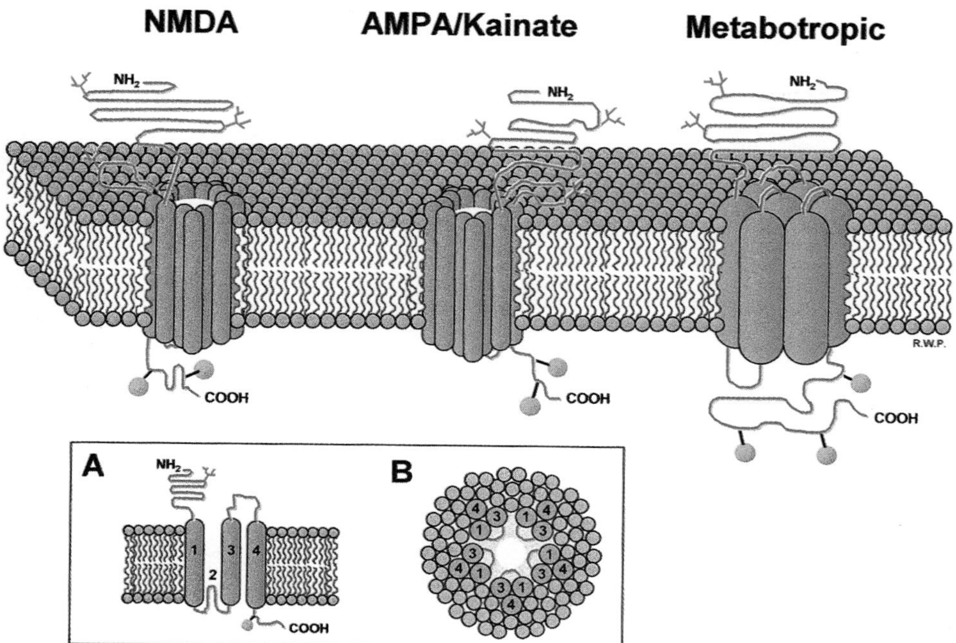

Color Plate 1. Proposed models of the subunit structure of the NMDA *(left)*, AMPA/kainate *(center)*, and metabotropic *(right)* glutamate receptors. Membrane-spanning domains are shown in *blue*, and other regions in *dark green*. Extracellular cites may be glycosylated, as indicated by the branched structures in *red*, and intracellular sites may be phosphorylated, as indicated by the *orange* spheres. In the models shown, NMDA and AMPA/kainate receptor subunits have three membrane-spanning domains (designated 1,3,4) and a loop (designated 2) that enters but does not traverse the palne of the membrane (**Inset**, A). NMDA and AMPA/kainate receptor-ion channels consist of groups of five subunits arranged around a central pore (shown in cross-section in **Inset**, B). Metabotropic receptors are linked to intracellular second messenger systems and have seven membrane-spanning domains. Extracellular and intracellular domains of NMDA and AMPA/kainate receptors are shown on only one subunit for clarity. *(See Figure 15-1.)*

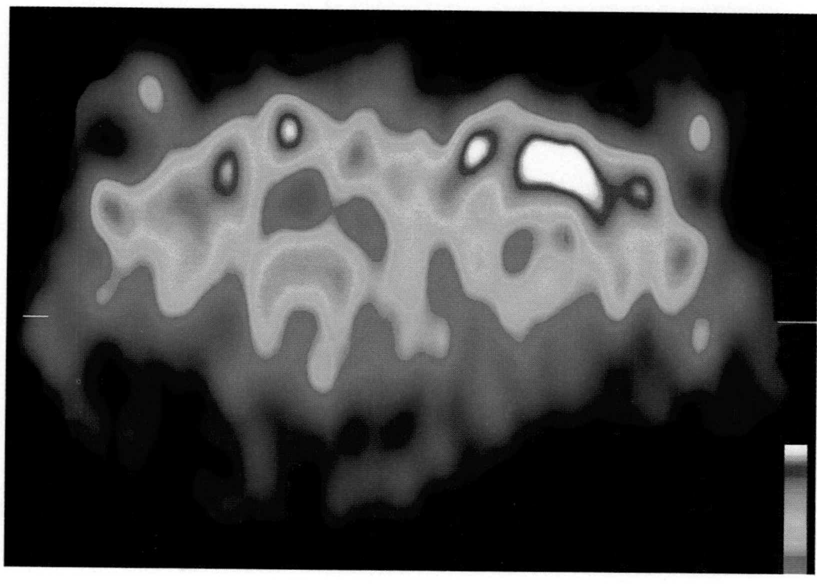

Color Plate 2. A representative surface=coil ^{19}F image showing detailed distribution of sevoflurane in a rat brain. *(See Figure 23-6.)*

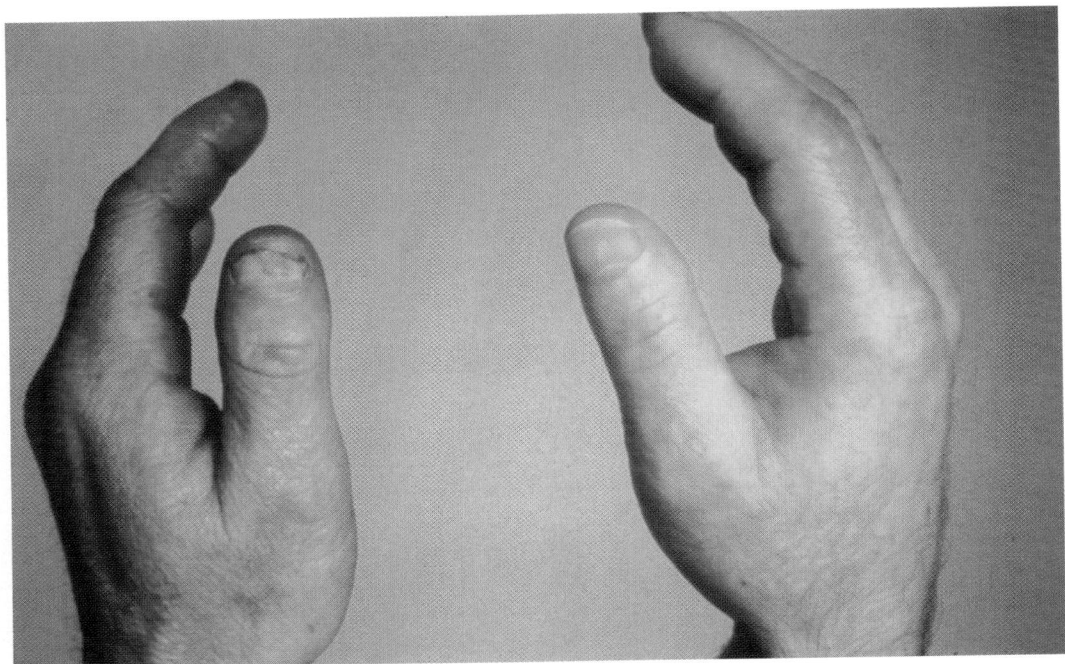

Color Plate 3. Acute stage RSD. In this case, the patient suffered a right wrtist sprain 6 weeks earlier. Note the edema, discoloration of the afflicted extremity, and the glossiness of the skin. The uninjured hand shows the normal wear and tear of a construction worker. At this time, the patient displayed a prominent tactile allodynia and a spontaneious burning dysethesia that encompassed the hand and forearm. A blockade of sympathetic function at this time by a stellate ganglion block resulted in a transient (3 days) reversal of the evident syndrome and the hyperpathia. *(See Figure 56-1.)*

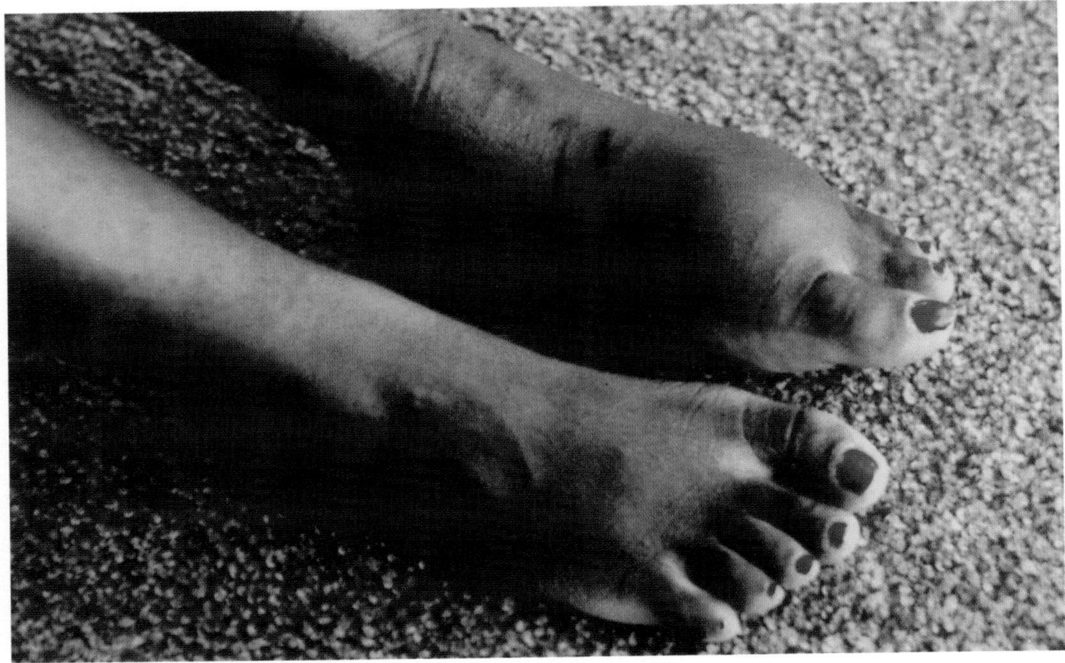

Color Plate 4. Dystrophic stage of RSD in the left foot. In this case, the patient sufffered blunt trauma to the dorsum of the foot 6 months earlier. Particularly noteworthy is the evident edema, muscle wasting of the ankle, and changes in hair growth in the afflicted limb. *(See Figure 56-2A.)*

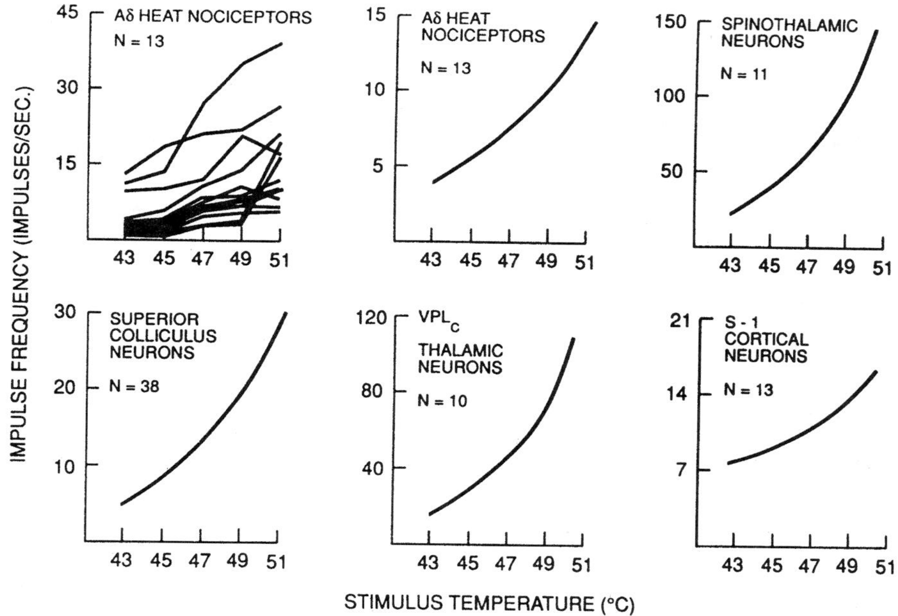

Figure 3. Heat-induced responses in populations of nociceptive neurons at various levels in the nervous system. *Upper left* and *center:* The functions of 13 individual Aδ heat nociceptive neurons (their population function is to the *right*). Note that regardless of the specific area of the nervous system examined, the stimulus-response relations for all populations are similar positively accelerating power functions. (From ref. 117.)

(34,49,140). Bigelow (7) advised, "In slight burns where no vesications have taken place, and where resolution appears practicable, we should resort to cold applications, either of water or of spirit; since in this way the most speedy relief is generally given to the pain, and likewise, as in other inflammations, resolution is accelerated." This advice, while eminently sensible, applies only to first-aid treatment and not to the more serious second- and third-degree burns for which patients are hospitalized. Shortly after the end of these more serious burn injuries (well before most patients reach the hospital or even the ambulance) the skin and underlying tissue are no longer hot, and a clinical priority is to avoid hypothermia due to heat loss and fluid evaporation from injured skin. Yet in each instance of burn trauma, the initial interval of hyperthermia resulting in skin and soft tissue temperatures into the 50°C range and higher no doubt produce noxious stimuli as described in the introductory synopsis of thermal hyperalgesia. These stimuli are fully capable of eliciting the first and second pains that produce central sensitization in experiments outlined above. Moiniche et al. (100) studied the time course of primary (i.e., within the injured area) and secondary hyperalgesia (i.e., in surrounding undamaged tissue) after 5 minutes of a 49°C, 15 by 25 mm first-degree burn of the medial calf in eight healthy volunteers. After this brief stimulus, pain thresholds inside the injured area assessed by heat or pressure fell significantly and stayed low for nearly 2 days. The area of secondary hyperalgesia to pinprick remained enlarged for over a day, and was negatively correlated with the decline in heat pain detection threshold within the injured area (Fig. 7). These findings, consistent with original observations by Hardy and colleagues (55), support the concept that secondary hyperalgesia (a central process) is sustained by primary hyperalgesia and indicate that the time course of both phenomena can last 300-fold longer than the mild thermal stimulus that triggers them. The same group, using the same model, found that the effects of skin infiltration with lidocaine shortly before burn were absent within 2 hours, suggesting that short-lived afferent blockade was ineffective in overriding persistent primary hyperalgesia (30). More recently, also in the same model but giving a larger dose of subcutaneous lidocaine prior to burn injury, they achieved over 7 hours of local anesthesia (111). This more prolonged, preemptive nerve block produced a significant reduction in the area of secondary hyperalgesia evident at least 12 hours postburn (Fig. 8), suggesting that "reduced central hyperexcitability (due to afferent local anesthetic blockade) may contribute to the attenuation of primary hyperalgesia observed."

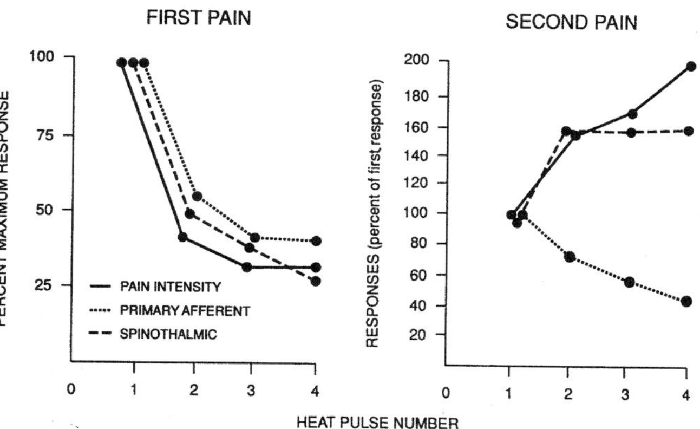

Figure 4. Repetitive heat pulses produce different effects on first and second pain. Repeating a 51°C heat pulse produced a striking decrement in the neural responses of primary afferents and spinothalamic neurons, as well as the judged intensity of first pain *(left)*. Yet these same stimulus conditions produced very different results for second pain *(right)*. In this case only the long-latency primary afferent activity (associated with second pain) decreased with repetitive stimulation. Long-latency spinothalamic activity and judgments of second pain sensation intensity actually increased in this situation. Apparently, a central nervous system mechanism exists for amplifying second pain with repetitive noxious stimuli. (Adapted from ref. 117.)

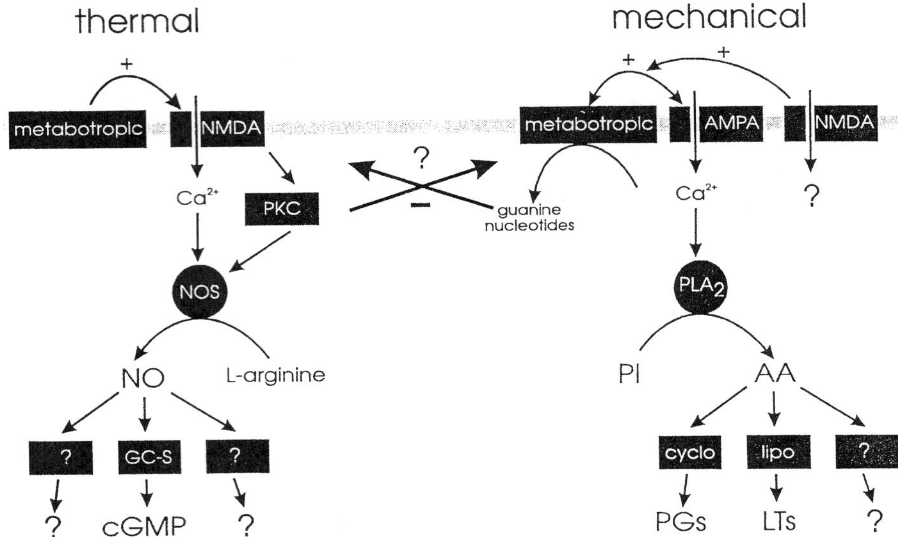

Figure 5. Proposed general scheme of receptor-mediated and intracellular cascade of events resulting in thermal and mechanical hyperalgesia, and the potential interactions between the systems responsible for thermal and mechanical hyperalgesia that might possibly exist in a single neuron. (Adapted from ref. 94.)

PATTERNS OF CLINICAL BURN PAIN

Volunteer studies in which preemptive interventions are evaluated can be most helpful in understanding the clinical biology of burn pain, but are not replicable in the clinical setting in which initial injuries are more severe and completed minutes to hours before medical care commences. As a practical matter, patients with extensive burn trauma often are disoriented, require prompt resuscitation and intensive care to sustain life in the face of multisystem injury, and often receive immediate general anesthesia to secure the airway and conduct trauma surgery such as release of edematous skin and excision of necrotic tissue. In this setting, self-report of pain intensity is not available, and parameters such as pulse rate or blood pressure that are sometimes used as weak surrogates for self-report cannot be relied upon as markers of nociception. The authors are aware of no studies that explore whether there are different long-term outcomes after applying different analgesic regimens during the resuscitative phase. However, about one-third of those patients with severe burns who do not require general anesthesia for early resuscitation report minimal to moderate pain shortly after their injury (22,25). In light of the clear preclinical and experimental human evidence that even a brief period of moderate skin heating produces prolonged central hyperalgesia, the conventional explanation for the absence of early pain in such patients (e.g., "the nerve endings are burned off") seems oversimplified. Instead, preclinical studies in animal models (see below) indicate that immediate postburn analgesia observed in a substantial fraction of survivors reflects active neural and humoral mechanisms of stress-induced analgesia. The authors' observation (137) of an inverse correlation between plasma β-endorphin levels and mean pain scores during burn dressing changes (Fig. 9) provides evidence for one humoral mechanism.

In light of the obvious difficulties in conducting clinical studies in the resuscitative phase of burn treatment, the majority of pain assessments and analgesic trials in the postburn setting begin after resuscitation, during subacute, in-hospital care that involves frequent serial dressing changes and periodic operations for skin excision, grafting, or reconstructive plastic surgery. Undertreatment of pain is widespread but especially likely in those who are unable to advocate for themselves because they are critically ill, intubated, and/or very young (108). Although pain can be relatively mild at rest, therapeutic procedures may cause unbearable pain (113). Visual analogue scale ratings of pain intensity on a 0 to 10 scale, and associated behaviors in relation to burn dressing changes in a group of children and young adults aged from 8 to 17 (mean ± SD = 14 ± 2.5) were observed by the authors (137) and are presented in Table 1.

A later study by the authors (2) evaluated 118 observations of pain during burn dressing changes in 48 patients between the ages of 7 and 17 (mean ± SD = 13.6 ± 2.5). This later study confirmed earlier observations that peak pain intensity occurred during the burn dressing change, and found a clear positive correlation between the percentage of body surface area burned and the mean pain score during burn dressing change. Opioid therapy had less effect on pain intensity in patients with more extensive burns, consistent with the development of opioid tolerance prior to the period when they were studied, an opioid-resistant and presumably neuropathic origin of pain ("phantom skin") in such patients, or both. Importantly, we observed a significant positive correlation between the percentage of body surface area with third-degree (full-thickness) burn and the mean pain score during burn dressing change (Fig. 10). In other words, despite the widely espoused clinical dictum that "third-degree burns don't hurt" the reality is that they *do* hurt, and that larger third-degree burns hurt more. This unexpected finding may be accounted for by the current clinical practice of excising necrotic or dying tissue until viable tissue is reached, thereby causing intact nerves to be divided and injured, and/or that the rim of viable yet damaged tissue containing sensitized nociceptors within areas of first- and second-degree burns is more extensive in patients with larger areas of third-degree burn.

Additional clinical evidence for a neuropathic component of postburn pain comes from pilot observations by Choiniere and colleagues (24), who contacted 104 adult patients from 1 to 7 years after discharge from a burn treatment center and conducted a formal interview to ascertain pain symptom prevalence. Eighty-two percent reported paresthesias or similar sensations such as tingling, stiffness, cold sensations, or numbness, and 35% complained of pain in the scarred tissue. This report also noted earlier anecdotal references to chronic pain or paresthesias in healed burns. More recently, a survey study of members of the Phoenix Society for Burn Survivors by the

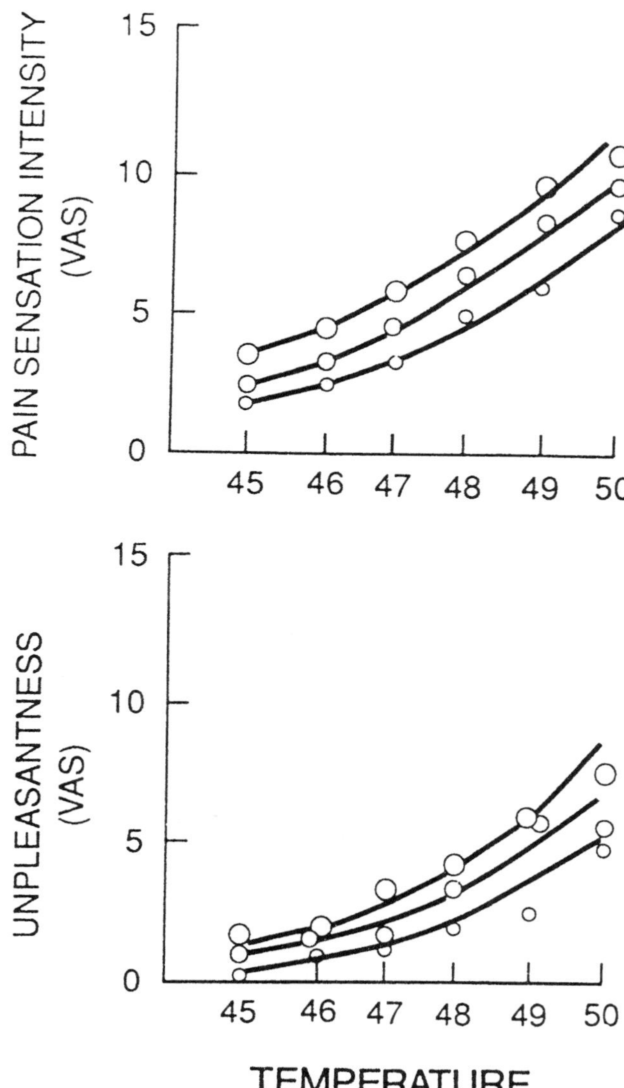

Figure 6. Spatial summation of pain. Nociceptive temperature—VAS-sensory *(top)* and VAS-affective *(bottom)* functions are plotted here in linear coordinates. The sizes of the stimuli (heat probes) are indicated by the *unfilled circles.* The functions are clearly positively accelerating in linear coordinates and are linear in double-logarithmic coordinates, demonstrating that spatial summation makes a greater contribution to subjective awareness as the stimulus size increases. (Adapted from ref. 117.)

authors confirmed these findings of persistent, ongoing pain long after burn injury in 231 adult respondents (31).

In summary, as Freund and Marvin (49), Choiniere (22), and others (15) have emphasized, the pain intensity reported by patients after tissue burn varies tremendously and can even fluctuate markedly in a single patient, depending on that patient's level of activity and intercurrent procedures. After first-degree burns, pain intensity is normally mild to moderate, yet as Kehlet's group has shown, hyperalgesia can persist for days. Even second- or third-degree burns that occur quickly must involve an interval of progressive heating of the skin and underlying tissues. Hence it is likely that even before the point of irreversible thermal tissue injury (e.g., protein denaturation and neurolysis), central sensitization occurs and makes the task of providing analgesia a challenging one. With frank tissue destruction, as in second- or third-degree burns, the sensitizing stimulus is followed by prolonged inflammation and ongoing pain-producing clinical interventions such as excision and graft-

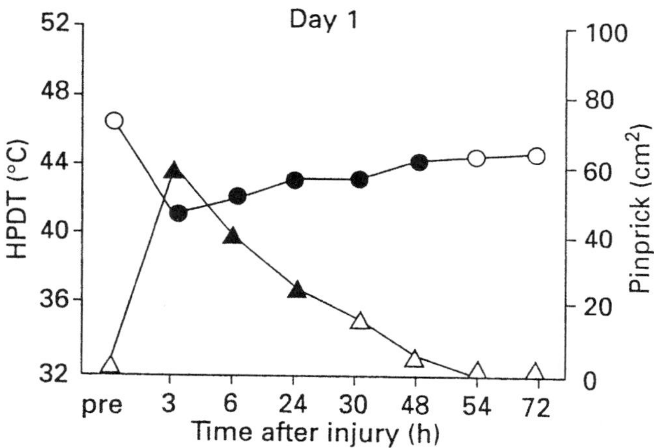

Figure 7. Relationship between heat pain detection thresholds (HPDT) (the least temperature perceived as painful) inside the injury (●) and area of hyperalgesia to pinprick outside the injury (Pinprick) (▲) on two examination days after thermal injury (median values; $n = 8$). *Open symbols:* baseline (pre-) values and values not significantly different from baseline. *Closed symbols:* values significantly different from baseline (p <.05 with Bonferroni's correction). (Adapted from ref. 100.)

ing, or dressing changes. Later, sprouting of abnormal nerve buds occurs at the regenerating margin of injured tissue. These insults taken together combine to amplify and prolong pain, resulting in, as Choiniere (22) has reviewed, a prevalent impression among published clinical reports that pain threshold decreases and pain intensity increases during serial burn dressing changes. In this fashion, the clinical observation of prolonged, severe pain after tissue burn is reminiscent of postherpetic neuralgia after acute herpes zoster (142), except that in the case of zoster, clinical care does not involve further traumatizing or manipulating the injured site. A hypothetical picture of the natural history of pain intensity versus time, as a function of the degree and extent of initial burn injury, is shown in Fig. 11. Indeed, a puzzle of clinical pain after severe burn injury (as after acute herpes zoster) is why pain resolves at all in the 30% to 50% of postburn patients who recover without chronic pain. Much preclinical work has been done on understanding the transition from acute to chronic pain, and some work sheds light on the relevant biology of burn injury itself. As a preface to describing current and future therapeutic approaches to the

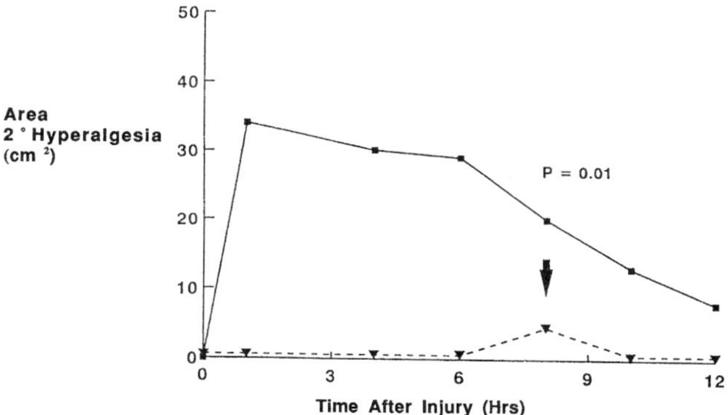

Figure 8. Area of secondary hyperalgesia to pinprick (von Frey, 175 mN). Presented values are medians for the 14 subjects with sufficient blocks lasting less than 12 hours. *Dotted line,* legs with block; *full-drawn line,* unblocked legs. The *arrow* indicates the median return of cold sensation. Time 0 hours indicates observation before thermal injury. P value represents difference between legs after resolution of the nerve block. (Adapted from ref. 111.)

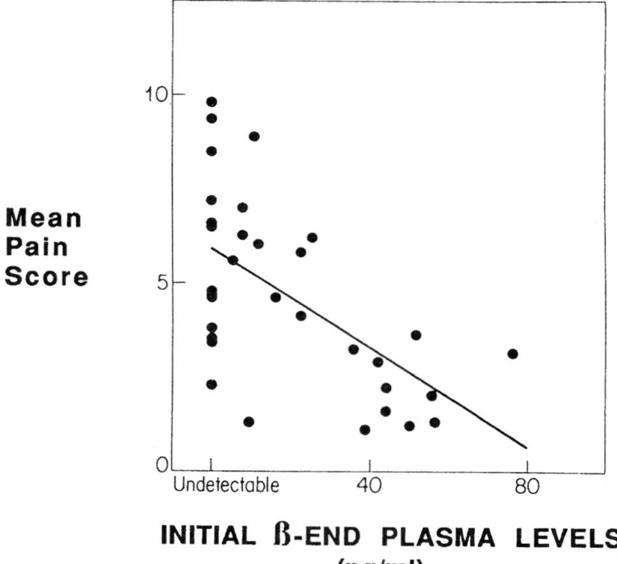

Figure 9. The relationship of the initial [before analgesic and burn dressing change (BDC)] β-endorphin plasma immunoactivity and mean pain score for the time of BDC; scores obtained at intervals of 1 min or less throughout the BDC (r = -.60, p <.001, n = 33). (Adapted from ref. 137.)

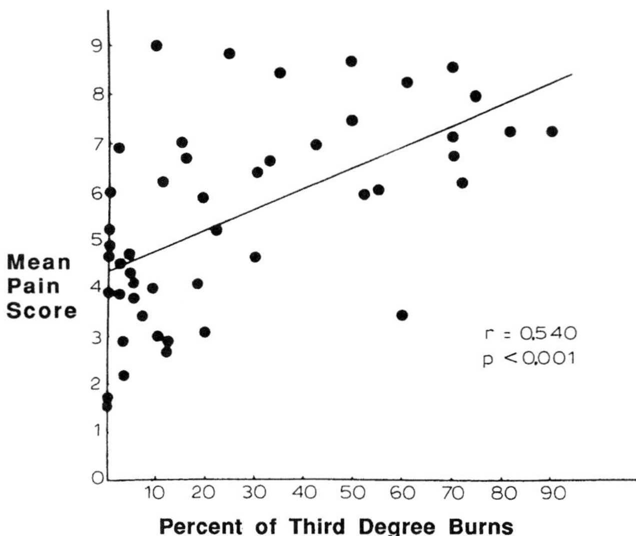

Figure 10. The relationship between third-degree burns and mean pain scores during BDC. Each point represents an average of the mean pain scores for each subject (number of subjects = 48; BDC = 118). As the percent of third-degree burn area increases, mean pain scores also increase. (Adapted from ref. 2.)

therapy of pain after tissue injury, it will be helpful to survey this literature.

BURN-INDUCED HYPERALGESIA

Burn pain follows the physical destruction of tissue by flame, scald, electricity, radiation, or chemical agents. The immediate first and second pains at the time of the initial injury are due to the activation of thermal nociceptors (see above) that will be destroyed along with other tissue as temperatures rise and persist. After the initial insult, when the temperature of the injured tissue has returned to normal, pain persists as the result of high-frequency afferent discharges from damaged yet viable nerve endings (1,35). Nerve endings that are completely destroyed become silent until they begin to regenerate (36,37).

Burn-induced nociceptor sensitization, nerve injury, destruction and regeneration, and soft tissue scarring evolve against a background of an intense local inflammatory response (99) and a series of profound systemic metabolic adaptations (17,33). Thermal injury severe enough to cause a second- or third-degree burn lyses cells and liberates virtually every mediator identified within the "sensitizing soup" that activates or awakens peripheral nociceptors (125,149). These mediators of chemical hyperalgesia include potassium, bradykinin, tachykinins such as substance P, prostaglandins, leukotrienes, interleukins, catecholamines, serotonin, histamine, and other excitatory amino acids. The unique sequence of insults caused by thermal injury—first thermal hyperalgesia, then chemical

Table 1. PAIN SCORES ASSOCIATED WITH VARIOUS PROCEDURES AND BEHAVIORS[a]

	Pain score (± S.D.)	No. of observations
Procedure		
Removal of outer layer of bandage	1.5 ± 1.31	25
Removal of innermost layer of bandage	8.6 ± 1.78	28
Debridement	6.9 ± 2.84	111
Silver nitrate poured on wound or bandage	4.1 ± 3.03	16
Salve applied to burn injury	3.2 ± 3.16	27
Behavior		
Sleepy	1.1 ± 1.46	7
Eating or drinking	1.4 ± 1.65	10
Talking (conversation)	3.5 ± 2.16	11
"It hurts"	7.3 ± 2.25	15
Shouting, yelling	8.3 ± 2.15	26
Moaning or crying	8.3 ± 1.53	36
Expletives	9.1 ± 1.64	8
Screaming	10.0 ± 0	14

[a]Procedures and behaviors during BDC documented in the observer's records are presented with the mean pain scores occurring at the time of these events.

From ref. 137.

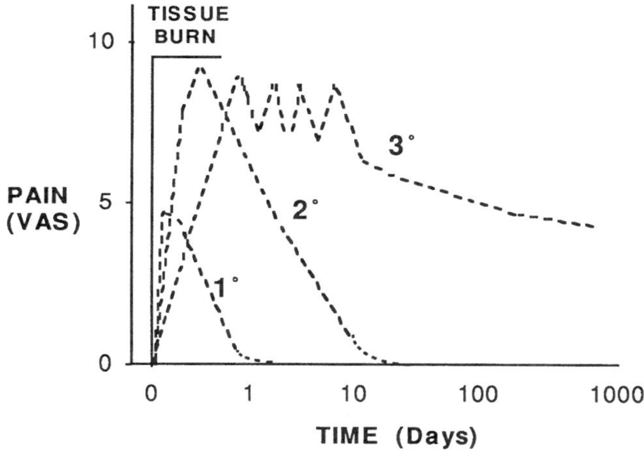

Figure 11. Hypothetical course of pain intensity as a function of time (log-scale) after tissue burn that produces 1°, 2°, or 3° injury. Note fluctuation of pain during clinical care (e.g., excision, grafting, dressing changes, mobilization) of 3° burn.

hyperaglesia, then care-driven tissue trauma, then scarring and distortion—precludes any model of burn injury other than burn itself from simulating accurately the cascade of in vivo events triggered by this form of trauma. The uniqueness and complexity of burn pain, and the absence of convincing in vitro models for its study, are especially clear when one considers that serious burns provoke acute, stress-induced analgesia (8,107,141) and later, a massive outpouring of antiinflammatory adrenal corticosteroids (5,63). Nonetheless, in view of the limited experimental literature on preclinical and clinical burns, and the vast amount learned to date on fundamental properties of nociceptive neurons (122) and their responses to inflammation (83), some degree of extrapolation from results obtained in nonburn models [e.g., of sepsis (61a) or inflammatory pain] is justifiable.

In the periphery at the site of tissue burn, the "soup" of inflammatory mediators sensitizes already-active thermal nociceptors (see Chap. 31). Commonly in severe trauma, other injuries occur along with the burn so mechanical nociception (e.g., due to crush injury) may also contribute to postburn sensitization. Chemical excitation and sensitization of peripheral sensory neurons occurs through two major receptor types. Type I receptors are directly linked to ion channels; these may be activated, for example, by serotonin (via the 5-HT_3 receptor), adenosine triphosphate discharged from damaged cells, and glutamate (via the peripheral kainic acid receptor) (122). Type II receptors are coupled to intracellular G proteins that may either be inhibitory or excitatory. Examples of excitatory receptors identified on peripheral nociceptive neurons are B_2 receptors for bradykinin (58,134), neurokinin 1 and 2 receptors for substance P, the H_1 receptor for histamine, and receptors for eicosanoids and catecholamines (see Chap. 3). The latter two classes of compounds are known, through experiments relying upon cyclooxygenase inhibition (45) or sympathectomy (65), respectively, to mediate wound healing and scar formation after third-degree burn. Little is known concerning the specific value of blocking either pathway as a means to enhance analgesia after third-degree burn. Recent studies of experimental first-degree burn in normal volunteers found no antinociceptive or anti-inflammatory benefit from topically applied glucocorticoid (112) or nonsteroidal anti-inflammatory drug (101). A third receptor family (type III), linked to tyrosine kinase, mediates the actions of growth factors such as nerve growth factor (NGF) upon sensory neurons. Paralleling the pattern of the knowledge gap on type II receptors in nociception, investigation of growth factors' roles in burn wound healing has far outpaced work on their influence on postburn pain and analgesia—despite a burgeoning literature on the importance of growth factors in analgesia in nonburn models.

Of all the neuropeptides, substance P has a uniquely well-documented role in peripheral and central excitation by noxious stimuli (86), including thermal injury. Substance P is cosynthesized from a common precursor along with neurokinins A and B in the dorsal root ganglion (76), from which it is transported both centrally to the dorsal horn of the spinal cord and peripherally to nerve terminals in tissues. Substance P is colocalized with calcitonin gene-related peptide in small sensory neurons that project to the skin. Scald injury leads to an increase in substance P content in dog paw lymph, caused by local release from peripheral branches of primary sensory neurons (68). Noxious heating of the skin releases immunoreactive substance P and neurokinin A in the substantia gelatinosa of the cat (44). This central increase of substance P occurs within 3 hours of formalin-induced inflammation (104) but the corresponding time course following thermal injury has not yet been determined. Substance P released in the periphery can induce contraction of endothelial cells and extravasation of plasma, prime mast cells for degranulation by other agents such as histamine, and stimulate nitric oxide synthesis to produce vasodilation.

Observations on the peripheral algesic actions of substance P—and its functional antagonists, the endogenous opioid peptides (82,103)—have greatly expanded our perspective on nociception from a process confined within the nervous system to one in which endogenous mediators produce analgesic and algesic effects by actions on immune as well as neural mechanisms (16,124). Unraveling the many origins and actions of neuropeptides such as endogenous opioids and their targets is still not complete, but evidence accumulated during the past decade strongly suggests that immune responses at the site of tissue inflammation are modulated by endogenous opioids (132). Shortly after radioimmunoassays for the endogenous opioids became available, it became clear that β-endorphin is derived from a common precursor to adrenocorticotropic hormone (ACTH). Initially, during the late 1970s and early 1980s, findings of elevated plasma levels of β-endorphin during classical stress paradigms (14,50) were interpreted as simply an extension of the well-known phenomenon of pituitary-adrenal activation by stress and at best only indirect evidence concerning analgesia, which was conceptualized as a central nervous system process. However, by the mid-1980s clues emerged that endotoxin exposure caused rises in plasma β-endorphin levels disproportionately high in relation to the mild hypotension that resulted (51), and that the origin of ACTH and β-endorphin during lipopolysaccharide exposure was not the pituitary but instead white blood cells (52,53).

The above suggestions of endorphin-mediated bidirectional communication between immune and nervous systems helped to explain scattered observations of correlations between perceived pain intensity and plasma β-endorphin levels in diverse clinical settings such as burn injury (137), after oral (56) or general (115) surgery, or during transcutaneous electrical nerve stimulation (TENS) therapy (46). The pace of observations that in aggregate blurred the distinction between nociceptive and immune responses quickened. Hargreaves and colleagues (57) demonstrated that analgesia produced by corticotropin-releasing hormone depended on the release of pituitary β-endorphin into the circulation, acting presumably upon peripheral sites. Herz, Stein, and colleagues (120,133) found that white cells at the site of experimental inflammation injury synthesize β-endorphin, which serves as an immunomodulator. Smith and Blalock (130,145) and others (87,138) observed that white cells can activate the pituitary-adrenal axis either by secreting cytokines such as interleukin-1 that stimulate hypothalamic corticotropin-releasing hormone to evoke pituitary ACTH release, or by secreting ACTH to stimulate the adrenal cortex directly. The authors have reported that a small, peripheral burn injury (too small to provoke a systemic pituitary-adrenal response) is accompanied in the rat by a rise in wound fluid levels of β-endorphin and corticosterone as sampled from a subcutaneous chamber (18). This intrachamber rise occurs despite stable plasma levels of both hormones, and even occurs when plasma levels of β-endorphin decline as a result of preburn systemic administration of either morphine or fentanyl. These results are consistent with local production of β-endorphin (Fig. 12) and corticosterone during the local inflammatory response beneath the cutaneous burn, production that is not suppressed by systemic opioid. They may also reflect burn-induced increases in vascular permeability that allow transport of β-endorphin or corticosterone from plasma into the chamber. Additional evidence for corticotropin-releasing hormone-like bioactivity arising from the site of peripheral tissue burn comes from our observation of a pituitary-adrenal response detected after burn in rats with prior pituitary-to-kidney autotransplant, i.e., without brain-pituitary connections (12). Thus, while the experimental data in the burn model is incomplete compared to the thorough descriptions of other experimental models of inflammation, it is consistent with them and indicates local, nonclassically regulated production of hormones first described in the pituitary-adrenal axis. Given β-endorphin's importance as both a cytokine and a neuropeptide (59), the likelihood that local opioid production influences local substance P release and/or actions, and the known function of substance P as a trophic factor in wound healing and nerve regeneration (143), further investigation of the regulation and long-term effects of local opioid action after thermal trauma is warranted.

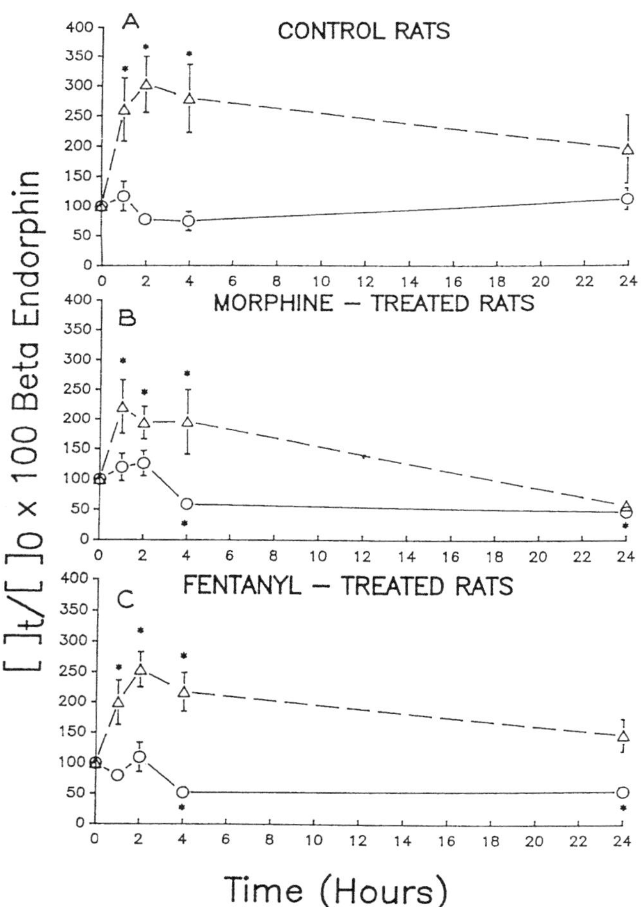

Figure 12. β-Endorphin levels in wound fluid (*triangles,* "chamber" and plasma; *circles,* "blood") samples in rats after unilateral thermal injury of 3% to 5% total body surface area and **(A)** no other drug treatment; **(B)** pretreatment with intravenous morphine, 4 mg/kg; or **(C)** pretreatment with intravenous fentanyl 0.02 mg/kg and repeat of this dose each hour for 4 hours. (Adapted from ref. 17.)

The key role that spinal nociceptive processing and reorganization play in acute and chronic sequelae of trauma is covered in detail by other authors in earlier chapters of this section (see Chaps. 7, 11, and 13) and will not be repeated here. However, since Coderre and Melzack (27) presented evidence over a decade ago for a central mechanism in sensitization after acute thermal injury, and subsequently identified roles for substance P and glutamate in this process (28), it appears appropriate to describe spinal responses to burn injury if only to summarize the little that is known about these burn-induced central changes and the many knowledge gaps to be closed.

The early-immediate proto-oncogene c-*fos* is rapidly expressed in postsynaptic dorsal horn neurons following afferent nociceptive stimuli including heating (64). Fos, the protein product of c-*fos*, after combining with Jun (the protein product of c-*jun*) to form a dimer, binds to the nuclear regulatory site AP-1, which is involved in transcription of many genes in many tissues, including enkephalins and dynorphin within the spinal cord (43). The presence of Ca^{2+} is essential for the transcriptional activation of the c-*fos* proto-oncogene (102). The entry of Ca^{2+} follows activation of the *N*-methyl-D-aspartate (NMDA) receptor Mg^{2+}-gated Ca^{2+} channel or voltage-gated Ca^{2+} channels controlled by other receptors. Although c-*fos* is a nonspecific index of cellular depolarization rather than a specific marker of nociceptive activity, there is good evidence that *c-fos* participates in regulation of opioid gene expression at the spinal level (61). Not surprisingly, thermal stimulation increases c-*fos*–labeled cells in the ventral-most laminae (84) where we have previously described burn-induced increases in enkephalin messenger RNA (mRNA) (see below). Noxious chemical and mechanical stimuli also evoke c-*fos* expression followed by enkephalin and then dynorphin expression in dorsal horn (42,123). Morphine pretreatment in advance of a noxious stimulus produces dose-dependent inhibition of c-*fos* expression (116). Chronic administration of morphine has also been shown to decrease levels of preproenkephalin gene expression (139).

Molecular techniques allow tracking of the early responses to thermal injury. The mRNA encoding for the enkephalins increases after unilateral limb burn both ipsi- and contralaterally in laminae I and II of the dorsal horn of the spinal cord innervating the area of cutaneous burns (127). Such increases are detectable 4 hours postburn using in situ hybridization. Both the number of cells expressing the gene and the number of grains per neuron are increased. We have performed preliminary studies (data unpublished) that suggest the mRNA encoding for dynorphin is also increased at 4 hours postburn. The increases in mRNA expression for the precursors to enkephalins and dynorphin seen several hours after acute thermal injury are consistent with those evident in nonburn models of experimental inflammation (66,98), in which the distinctive time courses of each response have been characterized in greater detail, and the several hour duration of stress-induced, naltrexone-reversible analgesia induced by acute burn in the rat (107). It would be an oversimplification, however, to say that dynorphin or enkephalin expression in dorsal horn are determinants of stress-induced analgesia, since they are more likely to be markers rather than causes of descending modulatory control (47,92).

Relatively little direct information is available concerning the specific neurochemical changes that subserve long-term changes of sensitization and reorganization in spinal cord ("plasticity") after acute burn. The combination of tissue inflammation, peripheral nerve injury, serial skin excision, grafting, and dressing changes, scarring, and analgesic treat-

Table 2. STATE-DEPENDENT PROCESSING IN THE DORSAL HORN STATES—CLINICAL SYNDROMES

Mode	Name	Syndrome
1	Control state	Physiologic sensitivity
2	Suppressed state	Hyposensitivity
3	Sensitized state	Postinjury hypersensitivity Inflammatory pain Peripheral neuropathic pain
4	Reorganized state	Peripheral neuropathic pain Central neuropathic pain

Adapted from ref. 147.

ment defy simple analysis. It is of note that the rat model used by Woolf (146) to demonstrate central sensitization within the spinal cord used a thermal injury as the nociceptive stimulus. This sensitization is manifested by prolonged excitability of dorsal horn cells and expansion of their receptive fields (93). Woolf (147) has described the dorsal horn as capable of operating in four modes, the transition between modes being governed by incoming sensory input. These modes, termed "control, suppressed, sensitized, and reorganized" (Table 2) are well-suited to the natural history of burn pain. Similarly, his schematic models of the sensitized and reorganized states provide plausible frameworks for understanding how the peripheral injuries present after burn give rise to the clinical syndromes of acute analgesia, subacute hyperalgesia, and chronic pain (Fig. 13).

Persistent input from peripheral nociceptors plays a pivotal role in the shift from mode 2 to mode 3. In fact, increased responses and lower thresholds are observed in C-fiber mechanical and thermal nociceptors following heat injury in monkeys, which correspond to the development of hyperalgesia observed in human subjects (77). While both A- and C-fiber mechanoheat nociceptors contribute to hyperalgesia following heat injury, C-fiber mechanoheat nociceptors contribute more following mild heat injuries while the reverse is true for more intense injuries (78). Structural reorganization of the dorsal horn and aberrant sensory processing are characteristic of mode 4, in which neuropathic pain arises from central as well as peripheral sites.

Biochemical events within cells of the dorsal horn that become sensitized and reorganized as a result of ongoing C fiber input are well described but relatively little work has been done to confirm their involvement in postburn pain. Intrathecal administration of substance P or neurokinin A produce hyperalgesia similar to that produced by thermal injury; this hyperalgesia is reversed by treatment with a substance P antagonist (28). There is strong evidence that other neuropeptides identified within C fibers (calcitonin gene-related peptides, vasoactive intestinal peptide, cholecystokinin) also provoke central hyperalgesia after thermal injury, as do the excitatory amino acids aspartate and glutamate (26). Selective activation of the excitatory, ionotropic glutamate receptor by intrathecal administration of NMDA mimics the hyperalgesia that follows tissue burn; this hyperalgesic response is reversed with an NMDA antagonist (28). In contrast, the analgesic effect of endogenous glutamate release in the periaqueductal gray of mice during stress contributes to analgesia (126). Reinforcing interactions between distinct neuropeptide algesic transmitters such as substance P and calcitonin gene-related peptide, and between excitatory amino acids and neuropeptides such as substance P and glutamate, take place within the dorsal horn (131,148). Ninety percent of C fibers that contain substance P also contain glutamate (96). Indeed, co-release of substance P and glutamate to activate simultaneously the NK-1 and NMDA receptors, respectively, appears necessary to induce postsynaptic depolarization sufficiently prolonged to overcome the basal, voltage-dependent magnesium block of the NMDA receptor, as glutamate by itself is unable to do so (41,119). Antagonists at several sites on the NMDA receptor complex are under active investigation for use in reversing sensitized dorsal horn neurons back to their basal, "mode 1" state (73). The analgesic/anesthetic ketamine, long applied in clinical burn care (see below) because of its sympathomimetic and respiratory-sparing effects (15,22,38,49,73,91,140,144) is now recognized to block the calcium channel of the NMDA

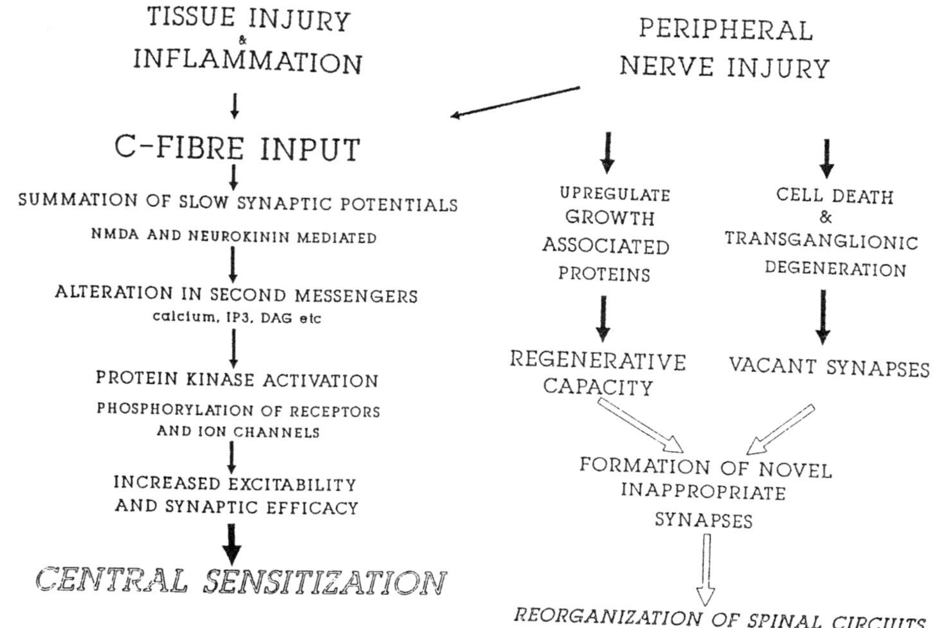

Figure 13. Inflammation and injury of tissue, combined with peripheral nerve injury, together yield cascades of intra- and trans-cellular responses that produce central sensitization and reorganization of spinal circuits. (Adapted from ref. 147.)

receptor complex (38), and in preclinical models (39) prevents or reverses the temporal summation of C-fiber afferent impulses (Fig. 14). MK-801, which acts on the same (phencyclidine-binding) site within the calcium channel as ketamine, blocks the development of thermal hyperalgesia in a rat model of ligation-induced neuropathic pain (32).

As reviewed previously (see Chaps. 34 and 36), concurrent binding of glutamate to NMDA and non-NMDA (e.g., AMPA) receptors, substance P to the NK-1 receptor, and glycine to its receptor adjoining the NMDA receptor, gives rise to sustained postsynaptic depolarization and an influx of calcium and sodium (38,119). The inrush of calcium into the postsynaptic neuron causes activation of nitric oxide synthase (NOS) and protein kinase C (PKC), along with translocation of the latter enzyme from cytosol to cell membrane. PKC phosphorylates multiple proteins, and thereby contributes to long-term changes in neuronal function and structure (e.g., dendritic sprouting) induced by persistent nociception. Coderre and colleagues (29) have shown the importance of PKC for the persistent hyperalgesia produced by a thermal stimulus to the hindpaw of rats. Calcium-induced NOS activation to generate NO also plays an important role in nociceptive processing (95). Intriguingly, both PKC and NO are involved not only in the generation of dorsal horn sensitization and hyperalgesia, but also in the development of morphine tolerance (4). Physiologic adaptations in dorsal horn neurons that occur in common during both processes include NMDA receptor activation, calcium influx, and the activation of PKC and NOS. For example, rats made tolerant to morphine develop thermal hyperalgesia (88), and rats subject to an experimental ligation mononeuropathy have a diminished antinociceptive response to morphine (89). PKC in dorsal horn, activated either during morphine tolerance or hyperalgesia, phosphorylates the NMDA calcium channel and reduces magnesium-dependent channel blockade, thereby augmenting NMDA receptor activity and postsynaptic excitation (20). Further, in vitro data show that PKC, activated either as a result of morphine tolerance or persistent nociception, can facilitate desensitization of μ-opiate receptor coupling to the potassium channel (21). The actions of intracellular NO resemble those of PKC but are accomplished via somewhat different pathways such as cyclic guanosine monophosphate (cGMP)-dependent protein kinases (95). Acute morphine antinociception is enhanced (121) and the development of morphine tolerance impeded (74) by concurrent administration of a NOS inhibitor, results that echo the beneficial analgesic effects of blockade of PKC translocation by GM1 ganglioside (29). As referred to above, the typical burn involves a combination of noxious and destructive, yet brief tissue heating, and subsequent inflammation, peripheral nerve injury, scarring, and therapy such as serial skin excisions, grafts, and dressing changes—all accompanied by frequent or continuous opioid therapy. While there has been regrettably little direct study in burn models, it is plausible that at virtually every step in the patient's course cellular mechanisms of hyperalgesia surveyed herein are likely to be active.

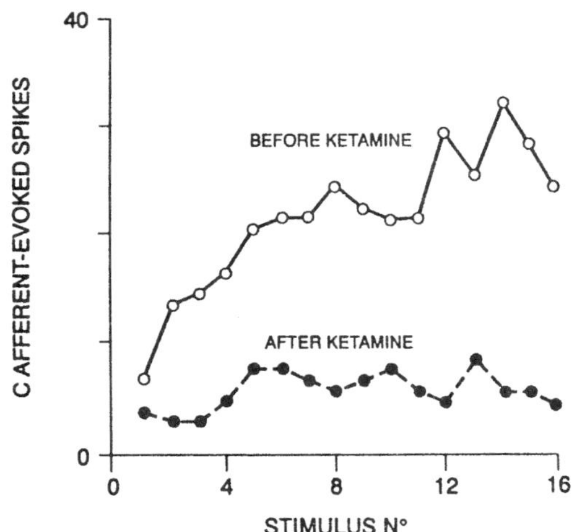

Figure 14. Slow temporal summation of C-afferent-induced impulse discharges is potently reduced by ketamine (2 mg/kg), an NMDA antagonist. The number of impulses discharged per C-afferent volley by a wide dynamic range (WDR) neuron is plotted during a train of repetitive electrical nerve stimuli at C-afferent strength before and after systemic administration of ketamine. (Based on data presented in ref. 39. Adapted from ref. 119.)

POSTBURN ANALGESICS: ENDOGENOUS, EXOGENOUS, AND THEIR INTERACTION

It is the authors' experience that many patients with postburn pain rapidly develop opioid tolerance and hence suffer moderate to severe pain (especially during burn dressing changes) despite continuously escalating opioid bolus doses or increasing rates of continuous opioid infusion (2,15,108,137). This scenario is particularly common among patients for whom specialized consultation for postburn pain control is requested. From the above survey of postburn hyperalgesia, and its newly appreciated links to opioid tolerance, this unfortunate course of events might be predicted and, possibly in the near future, averted through agents designed to block peripheral nociceptive afferent input, central glutamate release, and/or activation of the NMDA receptor, PKC, NOS, or a combination of these actions. Because the focus of this section is on mechanisms underlying clinical pain states rather than their comprehensive clinical assessment and management, we will not cover nonpharmacologic modes of pain relief. However, we emphasize that for burn survivors and clinicians alike, these approaches (which include distraction, relaxation, visualization, and other cognitive-behavioral methods) are valuable adjuncts to pharmacotherapy and merit wide application in daily clinical practice (14,22,49,108).

Pharmacotherapy for burn pain during the initial period of hospital therapy relies widely on μ opioids, chiefly morphine but occasionally fentanyl, for the opioid tolerant patient who requires extremely high opioid doses. In the several hours after acute thermal injury in the rat, opioids with preferential binding to μ (morphine), κ (U50,488H), or both μ and δ [biphalin (128)] receptors all show enhanced potency in prolonging tail flick latency in the rat after intravenous administration (129). Similar immediate postburn enhancement of potency in the tail flick latency assay after intravenous administration was found by the authors for the morphine metabolite, morphine-6-glucuronide (80). Interestingly, intrathecally administered morphine or morphine-6-glucuronide had lower potency (morphine) or a trend to lower potency (morphine-6-glucuronide) when tested in the same postburn interval (79,80). One possible explanation for the divergence between increased systemic analgesic potency and decreased intrathecal potency is a putative peripheral site of opioid action in the immediate postburn interval. Hargreaves and colleagues, for example, found that injection of low doses of opioids at the site of peripheral inflammation produced analgesia even though the same doses were ineffective when given outside the inflamed area (126). Stein and coworkers (120, 132,133) among others have produced, as surveyed earlier, a variety of preclinical and clinical data that strongly support the concept of peripheral opioid effects. Such observations raise the possibility that peripherally active opioids might have therapeutic value when applied to the site of the burn—an idea that clearly antedates Bigelow's (7) review in the early

19th century but that still has not been tested! A major limitation in the design of the authors' studies that explored postburn shifts of opioid potency was their failure to measure burn wound pain per se, for example by pressure or heat testing at the burn site itself; clearly the latter needs to be accomplished.

Opioids of the κ category, such as nalbuphine or butorphanol, have received increasing attention in the clinical realm because of their theoretical ceiling effect on respiratory depression—a major concern when using μ opioids. They may also be as or more effective than morphine in counteracting inflammatory pain (33). Since the clinically available κ agonists are also μ antagonists, one must be careful not to give an opioid of the former class to a patient who has already been receiving drugs of the latter class lest one precipitate withdrawal. Nalbuphine appears as effective as morphine for the pain of debridement (81). To evaluate preclinically the effects of morphine and butorphanol at a time when the acute burn had subsided and hence to simulate their use when burn dressing changes would have commenced, we determined the potency of both drugs systemically administered to rats 2 days after thermal injury (106). The median effective dose (ED_{50}) of morphine was unchanged in both tail flick and tail pinch (71) assays, while the potency of butorphanol increased in both assays 2 days after burn. Combination of a fixed dose (0.5 mg/kg) morphine plus graded doses of butorphanol led to a flat dose-response curve for tail flick latency in burned rats, and a dose-response curve similar to that of butorphanol alone for tail pinch latency in burned rats. Here, too, as with the authors' earlier animal studies on opioid potency in the early postburn period, the use of standard antinociceptive testing rather than wound-specific pain assessment limits the clinical generalizability of these results.

Administration of opioids during the acute postburn interval is not contraindicated but requires care (14). The acutely hypovolemic patient is at risk of hypotension and respiratory depression. Altered pharmacokinetics and, as described above, pharmacodynamics, of analgesics following thermal injury are but a special case of widely documented changes in drug disposition, action, and metabolism in that setting following acute burn change the handling of analgesic drugs (91). These changes may be unpredictable. Shortened distribution and elimination half-lives may require larger doses to achieve the same therapeutic result. Others have found morphine elimination to be similar in burned and nonburned patients (average 27% total body surface area) (114), while we have found an increased morphine clearance and decreased elimination half-life with increasing total body surface area burned up to 80%, beyond which clearance decreases toward control levels (105). When morphine is used, particularly over prolonged periods, the glucuronide metabolites play an active role in analgesia (79,80). Individual adjustment of dose and frequency, with careful titration to analgesic requirements and side effects is necessary. As a rule, intravenous doses of opioids by either bolus or infusion are used. Opioids may be given in a variety of routes (3) and protocols. To overcome large inter- and intrapatient variability in analgesic requirements, patient-controlled analgesia has been employed with favorable results, particularly during burn dressing changes (23,72). The apparent advantage of patient-controlled opioid delivery during burn dressing change may reflect not simply improved pharmacologic titration, but also an enhancement of patient control during this painful procedure; nondrug interventions to encourage patients to actively participate in their care have also produced favorable results (6,70). Indeed, a recent counterintuitive observation that pain and anxiety during burn care in a center that routinely gave patients no opioids were equally well controlled as in one that routinely gave opioids suggests the immense importance that behavioral approaches may have (48), as well as the great room for improvement in pharmacotherapy routinely offered to patients.

Such improvement in bedside pharmacotherapy need not wait for the availability of the drugs of tomorrow. Apart from the anxiolytic anticonvulsants presently available and widely used in acute care as well as cancer pain control, local anesthetics offer another relatively safe, attractive therapeutic option for postburn pain control. The relatively short half-life of lidocaine allows it to be infused during a dressing change and then discontinued and rapidly cleared after. Jonsson and colleagues (67) have reported encouraging results for this approach in a burn pain population. Given recent interest in extending earlier clinical reports of benefit from systemically administered local anesthetics in neuropathic pain states (19,136), this avenue appears promising for further preclinical and clinical study in relation to postburn pain. For the moment, a safe middle ground, supported by clinical trial data (10,49,109), is to employ topical local anesthetic at skin sites subject to invasive, painful procedures such as graft harvesting or dressing changes. Unfortunately, the therapeutic approach normally used to deliver regional anesthesia for relief of acute or cancer pain (i.e., via chronic indwelling epidural or plexus catheters) is severely limited in the postburn setting owing to the practical problems of catheter placement through or adjoining burned tissue and sterile maintenance in burn patients, who are at great risk for bacteremia and infection (7,11,32,34,35,107).

Other than opioids, local anesthetics, and ketamine (which as described above has now been recognized after decades of use to have possible specific advantages in treating postburn hyperalgesia) no other agent in current clinical use for burn pain control has been specifically developed to match the unique analgesic needs of this population. Nonsteroidals have a role for first-degree burns, but not on a routine basis for more serious injury as they can interfere with coagulation and increase the likelihood of gastrointestinal blood loss—two issues that loom large in routine care of the patient with a major burn. Indeed, general inhalational anesthesia (or, more recently, infusion anesthesia with propofol) is widely used not only for operative procedures but also for dressing changes simply because other current analgesic measures so often prove inadequate (49,108). Given the severe metabolic and multisystem insult that burns pose for many patients (40), any approach to analgesia must be accomplished in the "gentlest" physiologic fashion. In providing inhalational anesthesia to the burned patient, for example, great care must be taken to minimize the use of nitrous oxide, since repeated exposure has the potential for bone marrow depression in patients and operating room staff (110).

Choiniere (22) has written, "Clinical studies must be conducted to evaluate critically the efficacy of the available interventions [for postburn pain] and to develop more clear-cut guidelines for their application, according to the burn severity, age group, attitudes and coping abilities of the patients....The search for the best means of providing and maintaining optimal analgesia in burn patients presents a challenge for both researchers and clinicians alike." To these needs must be added the recognition on the part of the public that burn pain can, and must, be treated. The traditional undertreatment of burn pain—particularly in children—is a well documented, reprehensible state of affairs (113). In this era of rising patient awareness and empowerment, it is inevitable that patients and their families will increasingly question, even challenge, whether all that can be done has been done to improve quality of life by aggressively controlling pain, as is now possible for cancer and in other serious illness. Their doctors and nurses, those who fashion the policies these health care providers must follow, and researchers devising more effective forms of therapy for the still unmet needs in burn pain control must join together to face this challenge.

ACKNOWLEDGMENTS

We are indebted to Stanislaw Szyfelbein, M.D., the Director of Anesthesiology at the Shriners Burns Institute, Boston, for his vision and commitment to the analgesic needs of burned children, that led him to initiate "Project Pain" and recruit the authors to help advance its cause. We also thank Drs. John Remensnyder and Richard J. Kitz, the respective chiefs of the Shriners Burns Unit and the Department of Anesthesia, Massachusetts General Hospital, under whose enlightened leadership this collaborative project flourished. Alan Jeffrey Breslau, founder and Executive Director of the Phoenix Society for Burn Survivors, provided access to its membership during the survey of their chronic pain, and inspiration in many other ways. Support for many of the studies described herein, and the preparation of this manuscript, was provided by the Armington Fund and the Richard Saltonstall Charitable Foundation.

REFERENCES

1. Anand KJS, Carr DB. The neuroanatomy, neurophysiology, and neurochemistry of pain, stress and analgesia in newborns and children. *Pediatr Clin North Am* 1989;36:795–822.
2. Atchison NE, Osgood PF, Carr DB, Szyfelbein SK. Pain during burn dressing change in children: relationship to burn area, depth and analgesic regimens. *Pain* 1991;47:41–45.
3. Atchison NE, Szyfelbein SK, Osgood PF, Kazianis A, Wolf JH, Grandy RP. MS Contin: time released pain relief for burn patients. *J Pain Symptom Manage* 1991;6:144–156.
4. Basbaum AI. Insights into the development of morphine tolerance. *Pain* 1995;61:349–352.
5. Batstone GF, Hinks L, Whitefoot R, Bloom S, Laing JE. Hormonal changes after thermal injury. *Burns* 1976;2:27–225.
6. Beales JG. Factors influencing the expectation of pain among patients in a children's burn unit. *Burns* 1983;9:187–192.
7. Bigelow J. Observations and experiments on the treatment of injuries occasioned by fire and related substances. *N Engl J Med* 1812;1:52–64.
8. Bodnar RJ, Kelly DD, Brutus M, Glusman M. Stress-induced analgesia: neuronal and humoral determinants. *Neurosci Biobehav Rev* 1980;4:87–100.
9. Brigham PA, McLoughlin E. Burn incidence and medical care use in the United States: estimates, trends, and data sources. *J Burn Care Rehabil* 1996;17:95–107.
10. Brofeldt BT, Cornwell P, Doherty D, Batra K, Gunther RA. topical lidocaine in the treatment of partial-thickness burns. *J Burn Care Rehabil* 1989;10:63–68.
11. Caldwell FT Jr, Wallace BH, Cone JB. Sequential excision and grafting of the burn injuries of 1507 patients treated between 1967 and 1986: end results and the determinants of death. *J Burn Care Rehabil* 1996;17:137–146.
12. Carr DB, Ballantyne JC, Osgood PF, Kemp JW, Szyfelbein SK. Pituitary-adrenal stress response in the absence of brain-pituitary connections. *Anesth Analg* 1989;69:197–201
13. Carr DB, Bergland RM, Hamilton A, et al. Endotoxin-stimulated opioid peptide secretion: two secretory pools and feedback control in vivo. *Science* 1982;217:845–848.
14. Carr DB, Jacox AK, Chapman CR, et al. *Acute pain management: operative or medical procedures and trauma (clinical practice guideline).* Rockville, MD: Agency for Health Care Policy and Research, U.S. Department of Health & Human Services, 1992.
15. Carr DB, Osgood PF, Szyfelbein SK. Treatment of pain in acutely burned children, In: Schechter NL, Berde CB, Yaster M, eds. *Pain in infants, children and adolescents.* Baltimore: Williams & Wilkins, 1993;495–504.
16. Carr DJJ, Blalock JE. Neuropeptide hormones and receptors common to the immune and neuroendocrine systems: bidirectional pathway of intersystem communication. In: Ader R, Cohen N, Felten DL, eds. *Psychoneuroimmunology.* New York: Academic Press, 1991;573–588.
17. Cepeda MS, Carr DB. The neuroendocrine response to postoperative pain. In: Ferrante FM, VadeBoncouer T, eds. *Postoperative pain management.* New York: Churchill Livingstone, 1993;79–106.
18. Cepeda MS, Lipkowski AW, Langlade A, Osgood PF, Erlich PH, Hargreaves K, Szyfelbein SK, Carr DB. Local increases of subcutaneous β-endorphin immunoactivity at the site of thermal injury. *Immunopharmacology* 1993;25:205–213.
19. Chaplan SR, Bach FW, Shafer SL, Yaksh TL. Prolonged alleviation of tactile allodynia by intravenous lidocaine in rats. *Anesthesiology* 1995;83:775–785.
20. Chen L, Huang LYM. Protein kinase C reduces Mg^{++} block of NMDA-receptor channels as a mechanism of modulation. *Nature* 1992;356:521–523.
21. Chen Y, Yu L. Differential regulation by cAMP-dependent protein kinase C of the mu opioid receptor coupling to a G protein activated K channel. *J Biol Chem* 1994;269:7839–7842.
22. Choiniere M. The pain of burns. In: Wall PD, Melzack R, eds. *Textbook of pain,* 3rd ed. New York: Churchill Livingstone, 1994;523–537.
23. Choiniere M, Grenier R, Paquette C. Patient-controlled analgesia: a double blind study in burn patients. *Anaesthesia* 1992;47:467–472.
24. Choiniere M, Melzack R, Papillon J. Pain and paresthesia in patients with healed burns: an exploratory study. *J Pain Symptom Manage* 1991;6:437–444.
25. Choiniere M, Melzack R, Rondeau J, Girard N, Paquin M. The pain of burns: characteristics and correlates. *J Trauma* 1989;282: 1531–1539.
26. Coderre TJ, Katz J, Vaccarino AL, Melzack R. Contribution of central neuroplasticity to pathological pain. *Pain* 1993;52:259–285.
27. Coderre T, Melzack R. Increased pain sensitivity following heat injury involves a central mechanism. *Behav Brain Res* 1985;15: 259–262.
28. Coderre TJ, Melzack R. Central neural mediators of secondary hyperalgesia following heat injury to rats: neuropeptides and excitatory amino acids. *Neurosci Lett* 1991;131:71–74.
29. Coderre TJ, Yashpal K, Pitcher GM, Quirion R. Anatomical and pharmacological evidence for a contribution of protein kinase C to persistent nociception and hyperalgesia after noxious chemical and thermal stimulation. In: Gebhart GF, Hammond DL, Jensen TS, eds. *Proceedings of the 7th World Congress on Pain.* Seattle: IASP Press, 1994;373–384.
30. Dahl JB, Brennum J, Arendt-Nielsen L, Jensen TS, Kehlet H. The effect of pre- versus postinjury infiltration with lidocaine on thermal and mechanical hyperalgesia after heat injury to the skin. *Pain* 1993;53:43–51.
31. Dauber A, Carr DB, Breslau AJ. Burn survivors' pain experiences: a questionnaire-based survey. 7th World Congress on Pain, Paris, 1993.
32. Davar G, Hama A, Deykin A, Vos B, Maciewicz R. MK-801 blocks the development of thermal hyperalgesia in a rat model of experimental painful neuropathy. *Brain Res* 1991;553:327– 330.
33. Davies JWL, ed. *Physiological responses to burning injury.* New York: Academic Press, 1982.
34. Deitch EA. The management of burns. *N Engl J Med* 1990;323: 1249–1253.
35. Demling RH. Burns. *N Engl J Med* 1985;313:1389–1398.
36. Demling RH. Pathophysiological changes after cutaneous burns and approach to initial resuscitation. In: Martyn JAJ, ed. *Acute management of the burned patient.* Philadelphia: WB Saunders, 1990;12–24.
37. Devor M. The pathophysiology of damaged peripheral nerves. In: Wall PD, Melzack R, eds. *Textbook of pain,* 3rd ed. New York: Churchill Livingstone, 1994;79–100.
38. Dickenson AH. NMDA receptor antagonists as analgesics. In: Fields HL, Liebeskind JC, eds. *Pharmacological approaches to the treatment of chronic pain: new concepts and critical issues. Progress in Pain Research and Management,* vol 1. Seattle: IASP Press, 1994;173–187.
39. Dickenson AH, Sullivan AF. Evidence for a role of the NMDA receptor in the frequency dependent potentiation of deep rat dorsal horn nociceptive neurons following C-fiber stimulation. *Neuropharmacology* 1987;26:1235–1238.
40. Dolecek R, Brizio-Molteni L, Molteni A, Traber D, eds. *Endocrinology of thermal trauma.* Philadelphia: Lea & Febiger, 1990.
41. Dougherty PM, Willis WD. Enhancement of spinothalamic neuron responses to chemical and mechanical stimuli following combined micro-iontophoretic application of N-methyl-D-aspartic acid and substance P. *Pain* 1991;47:85–93.
42. Draisci G, Iadorola MJ. Temporal analysis of increases in c-fos, preprodynorphin and preproenkephalin mRNAs in rat spinal cord. *Mol Brain Res* 1989;6:31–37.
43. Dubner R, Ruda MA. Activity-dependent neuronal plasticity following tissue injury and inflammation. *Trends Neurosci* 1992;15: 96–103.

44. Duggan AW, Morton CR, Zhao ZQ, Hendry IA. Noxious heating of the skin releases immunoreactive substance P in the substantia gelatinosa of the cat: a study with antibody microprobes. *Brain Res* 1987;403:345–349.
45. Ehrlich HP. Antiinflammatory drugs in the vascular response to burn injury. *J Trauma* 1984;24:311–318.
46. Facchinetti F, Sandrini G, Petralgia F. Concomitant increase in nociceptive flexion reflex threshold and plasma opioids following transcutaneous nerve stimulation. *Pain* 1984;19:295–303.
47. Fields HL, Basbaum AI. Central nervous system mechanisms of pain modulation. In: Wall PD, Melzack R, eds. *Textbook of pain,* 3rd ed. New York: Churchill Livingstone, 1994;243–257.
48. Foertsch CE, O'Hara MW, Kealey GP, Foster LD, Schumacher EA. A quasi-experimental, dual-center study of morphine efficacy in patients with burns. *J Burn Care Rehabil* 1995;16:118–126.
49. Freund PR, Marvin JA. Postburn pain. In: Bonica JJ, ed. *The management of pain,* 2nd ed. Philadelphia: Lea & Febiger, 1990;481–489.
50. Guillemin R, Vargo T, Rossier J, et al. Beta-endorphin and adrenocorticotropin are secreted concomitantly by the pituitary gland. *Science* 1977;197:1367–1369.
51. Hamilton AJ, Carr DB, LaRovere JM, Black P McL. Endotoxic shock elicits greater endorphin secretion than hemorrhage. *Circ Shock* 1986;19:47–54.
52. Harbour DV, Smith EM, Blalock JE. Splenic lymphocyte production of an endorphin during endotoxic shock. *Brain Behav Immun* 1987:1:123–133.
53. Harbour-McMenamin D, Smith EM, Blalock JE. Bacterial lipopolysaccharide induction of leukocyte-derived corticotropin and endorphins. *Infect Immun* 1985;48:813–817.
54. Hardy JD, Wolff HG, Goodell H. Studies on pain. A new method for measuring pain threshold: observations on spatial summation of pain. *J Clin Invest* 1940; 19: 649–657.
55. Hardy JD, Wolff HG, Goodell H. *Pain sensations and reactions.* Baltimore: Williams & Wilkins, 1952.
56. Hargreaves K, Dionne R, Mueller G. Plasma β-endorphin-like immunoreactivity, pain and anxiety following administration of placebo in oral surgery in patients. *J Dent Res* 1983;62:1170–1173.
57. Hargreaves KM, Christopher MF, Dionne RA, Mueller GP. The role of pituitary β-endorphin in mediating corticotropin-releasing factor-induced antinociception. *Am J Physiol* 1990;258:E235–E242.
58. Hargreaves KM, Troullos ES, Dionne RA, Schmidt EA, Schafer SC, Joris JL. Bradykinin is released during acute and chronic inflammation: therapeutic implications.
59. Heijnen CJ, Kavelaars A, Ballieux RE. Beta-endorphin: cytokine and neuropeptide. *Immunol Rev* 1991;119:41–63.
60. Henry JL, Radhakrishnan V. Hyperalgesia following noxious thermal, mechanical, or chemical stimulation involves overlapping spinal mechanisms and interactive participation of excitatory amino acids and neuropeptides. *APS J* 1994;3:249–256.
61. Herdegren T, Leah JD, Walker T, Bassler B, Zimmerman M. Activated neurones in CNS pathways detected via early gene protein products. *Pain* 1990;suppl 5:SS97.
61a. Holaday JW, Neugebauer E, Carr DB. Meta². An analysis of meta-analyses of mediators in septic shock. In: Neugebauer EA, Holaday JW, eds. *Handbook of mediators in septic shock.* Boca Raton, FL: CRC Press; 1993;523–534.
62. Holaday M, Yarbrough A. Results of a hospital survey to determine the extent and type of psychologic services offered to patients with severe burns. *J Burn Care Rehab* 1996;17:280–284.
63. Hume DM, Nelson DH, Miller DV. Blood and urinary 17-hydroxycorticosteroids in patients with severe burns. *Ann Surg* 1956;143: 316–329.
64. Hunt SP, Pini A, Evan G. Induction of c-*fos*-like protein in spinal cord neurones following sensory stimulation. *Nature* 1987;240: 1328–1331.
65. Hunt TK. Basic principles of wound healing. *J Trauma* 190;30: S122–S128.
66. Iadarola MJ, Douglass J, Civelli O, Naranjo JR. Differential activation of spinal cord dynorphin and enkephalin neurons during hyperalgesia: evidence using cDNA hybridization. *Brain Res* 1988; 455:205–212.
67. Jonsson A, Cassuto J, Hanson B. Inhibition of burn pain by intravenous lignocaine infusion. *Lancet* 1990;338:151–152.
68. Jonsson C, Brodin E, Dalsgaard C, Haegerstrand A. Release of substance P-like immunoreactivity in dog paw after scalding injury. *Acta Physiol Scand* 1986;126:21–24.
69. Joris JL, Dubner R, Hargreaves KM. Opioid analgesia at peripheral sites: a target for opioids released during stress and inflammation. *Anesth Analg* 1987;66:1277–1281.
70. Kavanagh CT, Lasoff E, Eide Y, et al. Learned helplessness and the pediatric burn patient: dressing change behavior and serum cortisol and β-endorphin. *Adv Pediatr* 1991;38:335–363.
71. Kemp JW, Osgood PF, Kazianis A, Atchison NE, Carr DB, Szyfelbein SK. Tail pinch latency test: conditioned vocalization improves reliability without producing opioid mediated stress analgesia. *Pharmacologist* 1988;30:108–118.
72. Kinsella J, Glavin R, Reid WH. Patient-controlled analgesia for burn patients: a preliminary report. *Burns* 1988;14:500–503.
73. Klepstad P, Maurset A, Moberg ER, Oye I. Evidence of a role for NMDA receptors in pain perception. *Eur J Pharmacol* 1990;187: 513–518.
74. Kolesnikov YA, Pick CG, Cisweska G, Pasternak GW. Blockade of tolerance to morphine but not K opioids by a nitric oxide synthase inhibitor. *Proc Natl Acad USA* 1993;90:5162– 5166.
75. Konigova R. The psychological problems of burned patients: the Rudy Hermans lecture 1991. *Burns* 1992;18:189–199.
76. Krause JE, Chirgwin JM, Carter JS, Xu ZS, Hershey AD. Three rat preproenkephalin mRNAs encode neuropeptides substance P and neurokinin A. *Proc Natl Acad Sci USA* 1987;84:881–885.
77. La Motte RH, Thalhammer JG, Robinson CJ. Peripheral neural correlates of magnitude of cutaneous pain and hyperalgesia: a comparison of neural events in monkey with sensory judgements in human. *J Neurophysiol* 1983;50:1–26.
78. La Motte RH, Thalhammer JG, Torebjork HE, Robinson CJ. Peripheral neural mechanisms of cutaneous hyperalgesia following mild heat injury. *J Neurosci* 1982;2:765–781.
79. Langlade A. Effets analgesiques compares de la morphine et de la morphine-6- glucuronide lors d'une douleur aigue experimentale: la brulure. [Doctoral thesis], University of Paris, 1994.
80. Langlade A, Carr DB, Serrie A, Silbert BS, Syzfelbein SK, Lipkowski AW. Enhanced potency of intravenous, but not intrathecal, morphine and morphine-6-glucuronide after burn trauma. *Life Sci* 1994;54:1699–1709.
81. Lee JJ, Marvin JA, Heimbach DM. Effectiveness of nalbuphine for relief of burn pain. *J Burn Care Rehabil* 1989;10:241–246.
82. Lembeck F. Donnerer J. Opioid control of the function of primary afferent substance P fibres. *Eur J Pharmacol* 1985;114:241–246.
83. Levine J, Taiwo Y. Inflammatory pain. In: Wall PD, Melzack R, eds. *Textbook of pain,* 3rd ed. New York: Churchill Livingstone, 1994; 45–56; *Clin Pharmacol Ther* 1988;44:613–621.
84. Lima D, Esteves F, Coimbra A. c-*fos* Activation by noxious input of spinal neurons projecting to the nucleus of the tractus solitarius in the rat. In: Gebhart GF, Hammond DL, Jensen TS, eds. *Proceedings of the 7th World Congress on Pain.* Seattle: IASP Press, 1994; 423–434.
85. Lindblom U. Analysis of abnormal touch, pain and temperature sensation in patients. In: Boivie J, Hansson P, Lindblom U, eds. *Touch, temperature and pain in health and disease: mechanisms and assessments.* Seattle: IASP Press, 1994;63–84.
86. Lipkowski AW, Carr DB. Neuropeptides: peptide and nonpeptide analogs. In: Gutte B, ed. *Peptides: synthesis, structures and applications.* New York: Academic Press, 1995;287–320.
87. Lumpkin MD. The regulation of ACTH secretion by interleukin-1. *Science* 1987;238:452–454.
88. Mao J, Price DD, Mayer DJ. Thermal hyperalgesia in association with the development of morphine tolerance in rats: roles of excitatory amino acid receptors and protein kinase C. *J Neurosci* 1994; 14:2301–2312.
89. Mao J, Price DD, Mayer DJ. Experimental mononeuropathy reduces the antinociceptive effects of morphine: implications for the common intracellular mechanisms involved in morphine tolerance and pain. *Pain* 1995;61:353–364.
90. Martyn JAJ. Ketamine pharmacology and therapeutics. *J Burn Care Rehabil* 1987;8:146–148.
91. Martyn JAJ. Clinical pharmacology and therapeutics in burns. In: Martyn JAJ, ed. *Acute management of the burn patient.* Philadelphia: WB Saunders, 1990;180–200.
92. Mayer DJ, Manning BH. The role of opioid peptides in environmentally-induced analgesia. In: Tseng LF, ed. *The pharmacology of opioid peptides.* Langhorn, PA: Harwood, 1995;345–395.
93. McMahon SB, Wall PD. Receptive fields of rat lamina I projection cells move to incorporate a nearby region of injury. *Pain* 1984;19: 235–247.
94. Meller ST. Thermal and mechanical hyperalgesia: a distinct role

for different excitatory amino acid receptors and signal transduction pathways? *APS J* 1994;3:215–231
95. Meller ST, Gebhart GF. Nitric oxide (NO) and nociceptive processing in the spinal cord. *Pain* 1993;52:127–136.
96. Merighi A, Polak JM, Theodosis DT. Ultrastructural visualisation of glutamate and aspartate immunoreactivities in the rat dorsal horn, with special reference to the co-localisation of glutamate, substance P and calcitonin gene-related peptide. *Neuroscience* 1991;4067–4090.
97. Meyer RA, Campbell JN. Myelinated nociceptive afferents account for the hyperalgesia that follows a burn to the hand. *Science* 1981; 213:1527–1530.
98. Millan MJ, Czlonkowski A, Morris B, et al. Inflammation of the hind limb as a model of unilateral, localized pain: influence on multiple opioid systems in the spinal cord of the rat. *Pain* 1988;35: 299–312.
99. Miller SE, Miller CL, Trunkey DD. The immune consequences of trauma. *Surg Clin North Am* 1982;62:167–183.
100. Moiniche S, Dahl JB, Kehlet H. Time course of primary and secondary hyperalgesia after heat injury to the skin. *Br J Anaesth* 1993; 71:201–205.
101. Moiniche S, Pedersen JL, Kehlet H. Topical ketorolac has no antinociceptive or anti-inflammatory effect in thermal injury. *Burns* 1994;20:483–486.
102. Morgan JI and Curran T. Role of ion flux in the control of c-fos expression. *Nature* 1986;322:552–555.
103. Mudge AW, Leeman SE, Fischbach GD. Enkephalin inhibits release of substance P from sensory neurons in culture and decreases action potential duration. *Proc Natl Acad Sci USA* 1979; 76:526–530.
104. Noguchi K, Morita Y, Kiyama H, Sato M, Ono K, Tohyama M. Preproenkephalin gene expression in the rat spinal cord after noxious stimuli. *Mol Brain Res* 1989;5:227–234.
105. Osgood PF, Atchison NE, Carr DB, Szyfelbein SK. Morphine pharmacokinetics in children following acute burns and after recovery from burns. In: Bond ME, Charlton JE, Woolf CJ, eds. *Proceedings of the VIth World Congress on Pain.* New York: Elsevier Science, 1991; 175–180.
106. Osgood PF, Kazianis A, Kemp JW, Atchison NE, Carr DB, Szfelbein SK. Dose effects of morphine and butorphanol alone and in combination after burn injury in the rat. *J Burn Care Rehabil* 1995;16: 394–399.
107. Osgood PF, Murphy JL, Carr DB, Szyfelbein SK. Increases in plasma β-endorphin and rat tail flick latency in the rat following burn injury. *Life Sci* 1987;40:547–554.
108. Osgood PF, Szyfelbein SK. Management of burn pain in children. *Pediatr Clin North Am* 1989;36:1001–1013.
109. Owen TD, Dye D. The value of topical lignocaine gel in pain relief on skin graft donor sites. *Br J Plastic Surg* 1990;43:480–482.
110. Parbrook GD. Leucopenic effects of prolonged nitrous oxide treatment. *Br J Anaesth* 1967;39:119–127.
111. Pedersen JL, Crawford ME, Dahl JB, Brennum J, Kehlet H. Effect of preemptive nerve block on inflammation and hyperalgesia after human thermal injury. *Anesthesiology* 1996;84:1020–1026.
112. Pedersen JL, Moiniche S, Kehlet H. Topical glucocorticoid has no antinociceptive or anti-inflammatory effect in thermal injury. *Br J Anesth* 1994;72:379–382.
113. Perry S, Heidrich G. Management of pain during debridement: a survey of U.S. pain units. *Pain* 1982;13:267–280.
114. Perry S, Inturrisi CE. Analgesia and morphine disposition in burn patients. *J Burn Care Rehabil* 1983;4:276–279.
115. Pickar D, Cohen M, Dubois M. The relationship of plasma cortisol and β-endorphin immunoreactivity to surgical stress and postoperative analgesic requirement. *Gen Hosp Psychiatry* 1983;5:93–98.
116. Presley RW, Menetrey D, Levine JD, Basbaum AI. Systemic morphine suppresses noxious stimulus-evoked Fos protein-like immunoreactivity in the rat spinal cord. *J Neurosci* 1990;10:323– 335.
117. Price DD. Psychophysical measurement of normal and abnormal pain processing. In: Boivie J, Hansson P, Lindblom U, eds. *Touch, temperature and pain in health and disease: mechanisms and assessments.* Seattle: IASP Press, 1994;3–25.
118. Price DD, Hu JW, Dubner R, Gracely RH. Peripheral suppression of first pain and central summation of second pain evoked by noxious heat pulses. *Pain* 1977;3:57–68.
119. Price DD, Mao J, Mayer DJ. Central neural mechanisms of normal and abnormal pain states. In: Fields HL, Liebeskind JC, eds. *Pharmacological approaches to the treatment of chronic pain: new concepts and critical issues. Progress in Pain Research and Management,* vol 1. Seattle: IASP Press, 1994;61–84.
120. Przewlocki R, Hassan AHS, Lason W, Epplen C, Herz A, Stein C. Gene expression and localization of opioid peptides in immune cells of inflamed tissue: functional role in antinociception. *Neuroscience* 1992;48:491–500.
121. Przewlocki R, Machelska H, Przewlocka B. Inhibition of nitric oxide synthase enhances morphine antinociception in the rat spinal cord. *Life Sci* 1993;53:1–5.
122. Rang HP, Bevan S, Dray A. Nociceptive peripheral neurons: cellular properties. In: Wall PD, Melzack R, eds. *Textbook of pain,* 3rd ed. New York: Churchill Livingstone, 1994;57– 78.
123. Ruda MA, Iadorola MJ, Cohen LV, Young WS. In situ hybridization histochemistry and immunohistochemistry reveal an increase in spinal dynorphin biosynthesis in a rat model of inflammation and hyperalgesia. *Proc Natl Acad Sci USA* 1988;85:622–626.
124. Sanders VM. The role of opioid peptides in immune function. In: Tseng LF, ed. *The pharmacology of opioid peptides.* Langhorn, PA: Harwood, 1995;411–23.
125. Schmidt RF, Schaible H-G, Messlinger K, Heppelmann B, Hanesch U, Pawlak M. Silent and active nociceptors: structure, functions, and clinical implications. In: Gebhart GF, Hammond DL, Jensen TS, eds. *Proceedings of the 7th World Congress on Pain.* Seattle: IASP Press, 1994:213–250.
126. Siegfried B, Nunes de Souza RL. NMDA receptor blockade in the periaqueductal grey prevents stress induced analgesia in attacked mice. *Eur J Pharmacol* 1989;168:239–242.
127. Silbert BS, Crosby G, Chaar M, Marota JJA, Lipkowski AW, Cepeda MS, Osgood PF, Carr DB. Thermal injury alters opioid gene expression in rat spinal cord. *Pain* 1990;5:S122.
128. Silbert BS, Lipkowski AW, Cepeda SM, Szfelbein SK, Osgood PF, Carr DB. Analgesic activity of a novel bivalent opioid compared to morphine via different routes of administration. *Agents Actions* 1991;33:382–387.
129. Silbert BS, Lipkowski AW, Cepeda MS, Syzfelbein SK, Osgood PF, Carr DB. Enhanced potency of receptor-selective opioids after acute burn injury. *Anesth Analg* 1991;73:427–433.
130. Smith EM, Blalock JE. Human lymphocyte production of corticotropin and endorphn-like substances: association with leukocyte interferon. *Proc Natl Acad Sci USA* 1981;78;7530–7534.
131. Smullin DH, Skilling SR, Larson AA. Interaction between substance P, calcitonin gene related product, taurine and excitatory amino acids in the spinal cord. *Pain* 1990;42:93–101.
132. Stein C. Peripheral mechanisms of opioid analgesia. *Anesth Analg* 1993;76:182–191.
133. Stein C, Hassan AH, Przewlocki R, Gramsch, Peter K, Herz A. Opioids from immunocytes interact with receptors of sensory nerves to inhibit nociception in inflammation. *Proc Natl Acad Sci USA* 1990;867:5935–5939.
134. Steranka LR, Manning DC, DeHaas CJ, et al. Bradykinin as a pain mediator: receptors are localized to sensory neurons and antagonists have analgesic actions. *Proc Natl Acad Sci USA* 1988;85: 3245–3249.
135. Stouffer DJ. *Journeys through hell: stories of burn survivors' reconstruction of self and identity.* Lanham, MD: Rowman & Littlefield, 1995.
136. Strichartz G. Protracted relief of experimental neuropathic pain by systemic local anesthetics: how, where and when. *Anesthesiology* 1995;83:654–655.
137. Szyfelbein SK, Osgood PF, Carr DB. The assessment of pain and plasm β-endorphin immunoreactivity in burned children. *Pain* 1985;22:173–182.
138. Uehara A, Gottschall PE, Dahl RR, Arimura A. Interleukin-1 stimulates ACTH release by an indirect action which requires endogenous corticotropin-releasing factor. *Endocrinology* 1987; 121:1580–1583.
139. Uhl GR, Ryan JP, Schwartz JP. Morphine alters gene expression. *Brain Res* 1988;459:391–397.
140. Vassallo SA, Martyn JAJ. Pathophysiology and anesthetic management of burn injury. *Semin Anesth* 1989;8:275–284.
141. Watkins LR, Mayer DJ. Organization of endogenous opiate and nonopiate pain control systems. *Science* 1982;216:1185–1192.
142. Watson CPN, ed. *Herpes zoster and postherpetic neuralgia.* Pain research and clinical management, vol 8. New York: Elsevier, 1993.

143. Weihe E, Nohr A, Muller SD, Buchler M, Friess H, Zentel H-J. The tachykinin neuroimmune connection in inflammatory pain. *Ann NY Acad Sci* 1991;632:283–295.
144. Wilson GR, Tomlinson P. Pain relief in burns—how we do it. *Burns* 1988;14:331–332.
145. Woloski BMNRJ, Smith EM, Meyer WJ, Fuller GM, Blalock JE. Corticotropin-releasing activity of monokines. *Science* 1985;230: 1035–1037.
146. Woolf CJ. Evidence for the central component of post-injury pain hypersensitivity. *Nature* 1983;306:686–688.
147. Woolf CJ. The dorsal horn: state-dependent sensory processing and the generation of pain. In: Wall PD, Melzack R, eds. *Textbook of pain,* 3rd ed. New York: Churchill Livingstone, 1994;101–112.
148. Yaksh TL, Malmberg AB. Interaction of spinal modulatory receptor systems. In: Fields HL, Liebeskind JC, eds. *Pharmacological approaches to the treatment of chronic pain: new concepts and critical issues. Progress in Pain Research and Management,* vol 1. Seattle: IASP Press, 1994;151–171.
149. Youn Y, LaLonde C, Demling R. The role of mediators in response to thermal injury. *World J Surg* 1992;16:30–36.

Anesthesia: Biologic Foundations, edited by Tony L. Yaksh et al. Lippincott–Raven Publishers, Philadelphia © 1997.

CHAPTER 45

PAIN MECHANISMS ASSOCIATED WITH LABOR AND DELIVERY

JOHN S. McDONALD

HISTORICAL PERSPECTIVE

Parturition represents an important stimulus that activates physiologic pathways that can lead to a pain state. Surprisingly, however, there have been many inaccurate and confusing notions about the nature of the pain of parturition that persist to the present day. In 1844 Lee (47) noted that labor was a "painless process." In the early 1900s Behan (7) stated in his book, a classic at that time, that childbirth was a painless process like menstruation. Further, he noted that the incidence of pain reports appeared to occur with advancement of cultures, as labor pain was allegedly nonexistent in women of primitive cultures. In the 1930s Dick-Read (25) supported this thesis. This individual was an evangelist who spent much of his time condemning pharmacologic pain relief methods and supported only "natural childbirth." The modern psychoprophylaxis method now popular in some parts of the United States grew from a modification of the natural childbirth method of Dick-Read. Psychoprophylaxis was also popular in the then Soviet Union and was practiced throughout Europe as "Lamaze," a French modification (45). The claim of painless childbirth is now a well-accepted cultural myth supported by naive sociologic surveys, although studies have disputed its existence (29,30,39,49,50).

One of the great pioneers of obstetric anesthesia development in the United States, Dr. John J. Bonica, had records on some 2700 parturients that confirmed 65% had moderate to severe pain in labor (75). Much of that work came from personal observation or interviews and was not standardized. However, subsequent systematic epidemiologic work using the McGill Pain Questionnaire essentially confirmed the magnitude of the problem. Melzack (53) determined that about 65% to 68% of primiparas and multiparas rated their labor pain as severe or very severe in nature. Of significance, 23% of primiparas and 11% of multiparas rated their pain as "horrible." Thus, the current belief is that the pain of labor is not only real, but also severe in the degree of pain experienced.

The above comments emphasizing the importance of the physiologic substrate associated with the birth process are not to be construed as suggesting that emotional constructs do not influence the pain state associated with delivery. Ample supporting data emphasize that intervening variables such as emotional, psychological, and motivational factors can enhance the reported intensity of the pain experience (20,27,31,44,51,52, 54–56,62,64,75).

Historically, thinking such as that outlined above suggested that childbirth was painless, as well as the societal and philosophical influences on the obligation to suffer without complaint, paradoxically recognizing the discomfort of parturition, has frequently served to resist the implementation of changes even when medical advances helped in making labor less painful. The practice of using anesthesia during the 19th century is thus characterized by acrimonious debate as to the virtue relieving women of the suffering attendant to delivery. The acceptance by Queen Victoria of anesthesia for delivery was an important factor in influencing the social acceptability of interventions meant to reduce birth pain.

Although significant inroads have been made in the United States, well-meaning proponents of "natural childbirth" and "psychoprophylaxis" have tried to help in areas that do not have an adequate health care team to care for parturient women. Even today there are some people who are not cognizant of the wide margin of safety that now exists and the degree of comfort that can be provided by use of the modern continuous delivery of low concentrations of several pharmacologic approaches and, perhaps most importantly, the advantages that accrue to mother and newborn. Unfortunately, misconceptions exist among the public, including some physicians, nurses, midwives, and other health professionals, about the remarkable effectiveness of this methodology. Currently, many centers are developing an impressive body of evidence that suggests the appropriate management of obstetric pain may in fact reduce maternal and perinatal morbidity. This advantage applies not only in high-risk pregnancies, but in normal, low-risk pregnancies as well.

This chapter discusses the pain associated with normal labor and delivery in an effort to enhance understanding of the complexity of the mechanisms of the pain of parturition.

BEHAVIORAL AND PHYSIOLOGIC COROLLARIES OF LABOR PAIN

There is little doubt that there are adequate physical stimuli that can initiate and sustain a pain state during the birthing experience and that many of the physiologic and biochemical corollaries of the pain state accompany the birthing experience (e.g., the sympathoadrenal secretory responses, the cardiovascular correlates).

Behavioral Corollaries of Labor Pain

There are three stages of labor (first, second, and delivery) corresponding to the positioning of the fetus in the birth canal, the state of uterine activity, and the degree of dilation of the cervix. Each state has a unique dermatomal distribution of referred discomfort and reported intensity. The distribution and progression of this pain state is presented in Fig. 1.

Phase 1

The first phase in its initial presentation reflects a circumferential band that encompasses the T11/T12 dermatome. The sensation is typically described as an "ache." As labor progresses to a cervical dilatation of about 3 to 4 cm, the intensity of the referred pain increases, the pain descriptors transition to "sharp" and "cramping," and the referred pain distribution expands to include the T10 and L1 dermatome. Labor is characterized by a specific type of repetitive pain that is found nowhere else in nature. It starts with small stimuli of intrauterine pressures only 25 to 35 mm Hg and short durations of only 20 to 30 seconds and gradually increases in both intensity and duration until intrauterine pressures are generated up to 50 to 75 mm Hg in late labor with long durations reaching nearly 35 to 60 seconds. Furthermore, and very important,

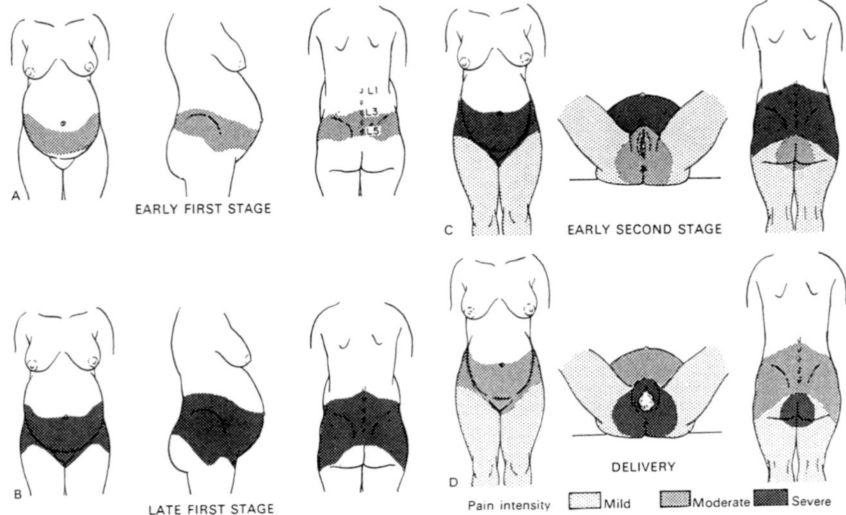

Figure 1. The intensity and distribution of parturition pain during the various phases of labor and delivery. **A:** In the early first stage the pain is referred to the T11 and T12 dermatomes. **B:** In the late first stage, however, the severe pain is also referred to the T10 and L1 dermatomes. **C:** In the early second stage uterine contractions remain intense and produce severe pain in the T10 to L1 dermatomes. At the same time the presenting part exerts pressure on pelvic structures and thus causes moderate pain in the very low back and perineum, and often produces mild pain in the thighs and legs. **D**: Intensity and distribution of pain during the latter phase of the second stage and during actual delivery. The perineal component is the primary cause of pain, whereas uterine contractions produce moderate pain. (From ref. 11a.)

these stimuli are often separated by only 1 to 2 minutes of relaxation periods.

All patients have varying responses to this early labor stimulus, but in general, women cope reasonably well if they are psychologically prepared and emotionally stable at the onset of labor through about 3 to 4 cm. After that there tends to be a general distribution of patients into the poor, fair, and good tolerance of the progressive increasing intensity of pain as the patient continues on through increasing levels of dilatation. One dramatic phenomenon that is associated with the first stage in all labors is the sudden increase in the level of pain with rupture of the fetal membranes and spillage of the amniotic fluid. Once this occurs many patients discover that contractions become almost intolerable without some "rescue" type of analgesia.

Phase 2

As the cervix reaches a state of maximum dilation, the pain state results in a severe pain report in the T10/L1 dermatome. There is also the report of pain in the low back and a mild pain state reported in the thighs and legs and the perineal region (S1-S2).

Delivery

Principal pain referral is to the perineal region (S1/S2) and a mild referral to the thighs and the T10-L1 dermatomes.

Physiologic Corollaries of Labor Pain

In the absence of appropriate anesthetic or analgesic regimens, a variety of biochemical and physiologic changes in the mother and parturient are noted. These changes are almost certainly driven by the sensory message evoked by the birthing process, that is, they represent the symptomatology of a significant pain state.

Release of Stress Hormones

During the delivery process, significant increases in the levels of adrenal (catecholamines, corticosteroids) (63,77,90) and pituitary [β-endorphin; adrenocorticotropic (ACTH)] (28,33,73) hormones are observed in humans and in animal models, with concentrations being typically elevated from approximately two- to sixfold during active labor and the peak concentrations being observed at delivery. Importantly, these changes are typically blocked by appropriate regional techniques (see Chaps. 42 and 72).

Cardiovascular Parameters

The significant mass and metabolic component added by the fetus alters the physiology of the maternal circulation. Such changes include increased blood volume and hemodilution (e.g., as blood volume increases without an increase in red cells). The mass presented by the fetus also represents an important component, because of the additional metabolic burden necessitating increased cardiac output, and as a reflection of the potential mechanical compression of the large veins that can reduce cardiac return by compression of the inferior vena cava and other pelvic veins. During parturition, there is a significant increase in cardiac output up to 50% of prelabor measures. In addition, there are associated increases in blood pressure and cardiac output during uterine contractions that are reported as painful. Such pain states can also evoke enhanced respiratory effort and an induced alkalosis (16,58).

It should be stressed that these physiologic and biochemical corollaries to the birth process have consequences not only for the mother but also for the fetus. In primate studies, noxious stimuli resulted in fetal bradycardia and a fall in oxygenation (59,60). Moreover, not surprisingly, given the large levels of circulating vasoactive hormones in conjunction with the respiratory alkalosis, there can be a decrease in umbilical and uterine blood flow (61,77) and an associated deleterious effect on fetal cardiovascular function (46,60). Such burdens may have modest effects on maternal-fetal function in uncomplicated deliveries, but may have untoward consequences in the face of predisposing maternal limitations (e.g., heart disease, preeclampsia or diabetes (16).

Stages of Labor Pain

Stage 1

Stage 1, or the first stage of labor, begins with the onset of regular contractions that lead to a progressive dilatation of the lower uterine segment and the cervix. The first stage ends with complete dilatation of the cervix.

Much of the emphasis on the mechanism of the pain associated with this first stage of labor relates to the actual dilatation of the cervix, dilatation of the lower uterine segment, and distention, with stretching and even tears of the involved tissues.

The role of uterine contractions or any muscular ischemia that may occur is not clear. The cyclic contraction of the uterus provides results in isometric conditions transmitted by the fetus against the cervix. It is thought that the distention of the hollow smooth muscle of the bowel is responsible for "typical" visceral pain (see Chap. 39), and that the same mechanism is operative at the cervix. Nevertheless, Braxton Hicks contractions result in significant elevations in uterine pressure, do not cause pain, and by definition do not dilate the cervix, but can result in a cervical thinning that ultimately decreases the length of labor (see Chap. 46 for additional discussion of the role of uterine contraction in generating pain states).

Other possibilities for pain production during the first stage include (a) the compression of nerves by uterine musculature, (b) uterine musculature ischemia during pressure peaks at each contraction because the reservoir blood leaves the uterus during these times, (c) cervical contractions during sympathetic stimulation periods after stresses, and (d) uterine contractions acting against a closed cervix.

Stage 2

At complete dilatation of the cervix, there is a lessening of nociceptive input from the dilated cervix, but the uterine contractions continue, often against very effective and stringent resistive forces. The pain in the second stage comes from continued distention of the lower vaginal track and fresh dilatation of the vaginal outlet, including muscular tension and tearing during the final descent of the fetus through the birth canal. It must be noted that the second stage of labor may last less than 1 hour, but 1, 2, or even 3 hours in duration is not unusual. During this interval there is descent of the fetus until the fetal head begins to negate the mid-pelvis at the level of the ischeal tuberosity. The eventual passage of the fetal head through the mid-pelvis results in distention and stretching of the tissues of the mid- and lower vagina, distention of the outlet, and eventual dilatation to make way for passage of the fetal head, shoulders, and body. As will be considered below, these latter anatomic changes are accomplished with maximum stimulation via the nociceptive pathways by way of the pudendal nerves to dorsal root ganglia located at the S2-4 levels. There is also a significant sensory spillover to other adjacent pathways via the lower sacrum, perianal, and even upper thigh regions.

Some women find that with complete dilatation, it hurts too much to push against the strong tension of the perineal muscles until some type of analgesia is administered, such as an epidural with sacral distribution or, preferably, a caudal that provides analgesia yet allows the mother motor capability so that she can adequately push. Alternatively, reflecting on the distribution of this afferent innervation that is relevant during stage 2, pudendal blocks can be efficacious (see below).

MECHANISMS OF LABOR PAIN

Innervation of the Birth Canal

There are five main components of the birth canal: (a) the body of the uterus, (b) the lower uterine segments, (c) the cervix, (d) the vaginal wall, and (5) the vulva (perineal). This innervation is summarized in Fig. 2 of Chap. 46. Selective blocks and anatomical tracing of the afferent innervation have demonstrated their respective afferent innervation.

Body of Uterus/Lower Uterine Segments

This structure is innervated by afferents with cell bodies in the dorsal root ganglia of the T10-T12 and L1 segments. These afferents travel with the sympathetic afferents that form the pelvic and cervical plexi. They then pass though the pelvic plexus (inferior, medial, and superior), hypogastric to the lumbar sympathetic chain, and then to the thoracic sympathetic chain. Here they exit by the rami communicantes of the respective lower thoracic and upper lumbar roots. Retrograde transport studies in the cat have shown that the majority of dorsal root ganglion cells innervating the uterine horn are located in lumbar ganglia. In contrast, dorsal root ganglion innervating the cervix are located in sacral ganglia (42) (see below).

Cervix

The lower uterine segments and the cervix are innervated by similar populations of afferents that travel though the sympathetic plexi. Classical reports as early as 1893 (36) and 1949 (24) had argued that the cervix and lower uterine segments were innervated by pelvic nerve afferents (nervi erigentes). Studies by Bonica (11) using regional blocks in human have instead pointed to the likelihood that cervical innervation travels with the innervation of the uterus and not by the sacral plexus. On the other hand, single-unit recording has emphasized that uterine and cervical stimulation can activate pelvic nerve afferents (8).

Perineal Region

Innervation of the perineal region passes to the S2-S4 roots and thence to the spinal dorsal horn by the pudendal nerve.

While the above discussion relates to the role of afferents that travel with the sympathetic efferent (hypogastric), the role of the fibers traveling with the pelvic nerves is less clear. Labeling studies and single-unit recording in rats have suggested that the innervation may be more complex than is commonly thought. Thus, receptive fields of hypogastric afferents are largely found on the uterine horns, ligaments, and cervix. In contrast, receptive fields for afferents traveling in the pelvic nerve are found on the cervix, fornix, and the vagina (8).

Bilateral section of the T13-L2 roots, through which hypogastric afferents pass, eliminated the response to uterine distention in L1 and L6 cells (see below). Conversely, bilateral section of the L6-S2 roots, through which pelvic afferents pass, had no effect on neuronal activity evoked by uterine distention, but section of both sets of roots eliminated responses to cervix stimulation in L6 spinal neurons (89). Using retrograde tract tracing techniques in the cat, it was observed that 70% to 80% of the axons from the uterine-cervix appear to pass through the pelvic nerve and the remainder through the pudendal nerve, while innervation of the uterine horns was believed to be largely in the sympathetic nerves (41).

Fiber Types

Consistent with other systems associated with visceral innervation, the principal fiber types of which the innervation of the uterus and cervix are composed are Aδ (small myelinated) and C (unmyelinated) axons.

Recording from uterine innervation has demonstrated large populations that are clearly activated by mechanical distention and by local tissue ischemia (7a). Not surprisingly, given the character of the sensory afferents, the close intraarterial injection or topical application of a variety of algesic substances, including KCl, serotonin, and bradykinin, can induce a significant increase in unit activity (7a,38). Hypogastric nerve afferents were activated by relatively intense levels of uterine distention (74). In the pelvic nerve, fibers with mechanoreceptive fields were typically slowly adapting. The axons with receptive fields in the uterus and cervix were also slowly adapting mechanoreceptors and these axons were sensitized by hypoxia (8). Pelvic nerve fibers were markedly more sensitive to uterine and cervical mechanostimulation than hypogastric nerve fibers. Similarly, pelvic nerve fibers were more likely to respond to chemical stimuli than hypogastric nerve fibers. These results suggest that afferent fibers in the pelvic and hypogastric nerves subserve different functions (9,10). Based on the effective stimulus, hypogastric fibers seem more closely allied with the pain state during parturition. In short, based on the effective stimuli, it appears that (a) the input from the uterus to the spinal cord is principally by way of the hypogastric nerve; (b) input from the cervix is by way of both the pelvic and hypogastric nerves; and (c) consistent with effects of peripheral blockade (see above), pelvic innervation appears to play a relatively minimal role in the early phases of labor pain.

Transmitter Content

By the criterion of capsaicin sensitivity, it has been shown that pelvic innervation of the uterus and cervix contain a variety of peptide transmitters, including calcitonin gene-related peptide (CGRP), galanin and the tachykinins, substance P, neurokinin A, and vasoactive intestinal polypeptide (17,65–67). As commonly observed in somatic afferents, a number of these peptides have been observed to be co-contained in subpopulations of these afferents. For example, this has been shown with CGRP and galanin (67). In retrogradely marked dorsal root ganglion cells in the cat, a variety of peptides were observed including CGRP, cholecystokinin (CCK), leucine-enkephalin (LENK), somatostatin, substance P, and vasoactive intestinal polypeptide (VIP). In order of frequency of positive immunoreactivity, the incidence of peptides in uterine projecting sacral DRG cells was VIP (71%), CGRP (42%), substance P (18%), and CCK and LENK (13%). In lumbar dorsal root ganglia, the incidence was CGRP (51%), VIP (34%), substance P (28%), LENK (17%), and CCK (13%) (41). These results suggest that the uterine cervix receives a prominent VIP- and CGRP-containing afferent innervation. The percentage of neurons containing VIP is considerably greater than that observed in afferent pathways to other pelvic organs. In addition to the peptides, afferent axons in the pelvic plexus have been shown to display reduced nicotinamide adenine dinucleotide phosphate (NADPH)-positive staining, indicating that they likely can synthesize and release nitric oxide (68,76).

It should be noted that this diversity of afferent transmitters found to innervate the pelvic viscera is important in the context that such local terminals are able to mediate a local release of the terminal contents into the target organ. Such antidromic afferent activity has been well characterized to play an important role in a variety of somatic and cutaneous systems (see Chaps. 31 and 33). Current evidence argues that such release may also alter local blood flow and smooth muscle tone in the pelvic viscera (72). The presence of NADPH-positive (a marker for nitric oxide synthase) afferent terminals supports the likelihood that a local release of nitric oxide (NO) may play a role in the local smooth muscle tone, and that the inhibitory effects of CGRP on stimulated uterine contraction may be mediated by local NO release (76).

Central Projections

Spinal Cord

Cervix Single-unit recording in dorsal horn neurons revealed units activated by cervical stimulation, distributed in the ventral portions of the dorsal horn in T13-L1 and throughout the dorsal horn in L6-S2 (9,10). These cells had extensive visceral-somatic convergence. Thus, such neurons in T13-L1 typically displayed large bilateral receptive fields extending to the perineum and hind limbs and were typically activated by colonic distention. Neurons in L6-S2 receiving cervical-uterine input had cutaneous receptive fields in the same regions as those in T13-L1, but these fields were smaller and had cutaneous receptive fields limited to the perineum (10).

Uterus Stimulation of the uterine horns revealed cells activated in T13-L1 and relatively fewer in L4 to S2. Importantly, complex interactions have been reported in spinal neuronal populations. Thus, as noted, few L6-S2 neurons were excited by uterine distention, but a significant proportion was inhibited (10). Retrograde transport studies have shown that the majority (70–80%) of afferent input to the uterine cervix passes through the pelvic nerve and the remainder through the pudendal nerve, whereas afferent input to the uterine horn appears to travel in sympathetic nerves. The most prominent labeling is present in Lissauer's tract and in lamina I and outer lamina II on the lateral edge of the dorsal horn, while some axons may continue through lamina V into the dorsal gray commissure (42).

Supraspinal Projections

As anticipated from the organization of visceral afferents, outflow from dorsal horn excitation travels via the ventral lateral pathways (see Chaps. 35 and 37) to the brain stem and thalamus. Distention of the uterine horn or vaginal canal and superfusion of the uterus with prostaglandin (PG)$F_{2\alpha}$ and bradykinin (BK) resulted in vigorous activation of the somatic responsive cells lying in the ventrobasal complex (see Chap. 37). Importantly, this activity was similar to that which would otherwise induce escape behavior in the unanesthetized rat (34). Electrophysiologic mapping studies have shown that projections to the thalamus from pelvic nerve input were found principally in the posterolateral nucleus (VPLp) and to a lesser extent in the dorsal, lateral, and medial aspects of the posterior complex directly adjacent to VPLp. The region surrounding the middle and caudal part of the ventral posterolateral nucleus (VPL) received a stronger input from the pelvic nerve than that around the rostral pole of VPL (18). Many of these thalamic cells had an anticipated viscerosomatic convergence and were activated by low-threshold mechanical stimuli that were located primarily in the lower back, the thigh, and, to a lesser extent, the hindpaw.

It has long been suspected that pelvic organ input might play an important role in the hormonal correlates associated with the ongoing parturition process. Vaginocervical stimulation, which occurs during mating or parturition, is believed to stimulate a number of neuroendocrine responses including the secretion of oxytocin, prolactin, and luteinizing hormone (43,50a). In parturient rats, excitation of afferent traffic was investigated by examining for the appearance of the immediate early gene *c-fos* (50a). In that work, a large increase was observed in the brain stem neurons in both the nucleus of the tractus solitarius and in the ventrolateral medulla, as well as more rostrally in the medial preoptic nucleus, the anteroventral periventricular region, and the hypothalamic supraoptic nucleus. This suggests that these brain stem sites may form part of the afferent pathway from the uterus and cervix to the preoptic area and the hypothalamus (50a). Electrophysiologic studies have shown that uterine horn distention excited neurons in the hypothalamic paraventricular nucleus (PVN), although, interestingly, probing of the cervix had no effect. Stimulation of the hypogastric and pelvic nerves excited 55% and 30% of the neurons tested, respectively (4). Such observation emphasizes that pelvic or uterine input can exert a potent excitatory effect on these hypothalamic neurons associated with trophic and secretory functions.

Parturition-Induced Afferent Processing

While it is clear that parturition will evoke activity in ascending systems and this is able to induce a well-defined pain state corresponding to the segmental distribution of the afferent input, it is also appreciated that such processing at the spinal level is able to evoke a certain degree of regulation of afferent drive. Thus, as noted above, uterine distention evoked activity in L6 neurons, whereas cervical input induced inhibition in a significant percentage of these cells (9,10). This inhibition appeared to be mediated by input through the pelvic nerve. In T13/L1, populations of neurons were excited by uterine distention and a percentage were inhibited by cervical pressure. Importantly, spinal section at T10 increased the incidence of neurons excited by uterine stimulation and decreased the inhibitory responses to cervix stimulation (89). Such data suggest that the evoked output of dorsal horn neurons otherwise excited by uterine input may be modulated by a spinobulbospinal loop driven by input, in this case from the cervix. Such brain stem loops have been shown to be activated by high-intensity somatic (87) and visceral cervical distention (81) and are thought to play an important role in regulating spinal afferent processing (5). Such regulation may have implications in some aspects of the response generated during parturition. Thus, there are studies indicating that nociceptive thresholds, as measured by acute stimuli, are elevated during pregnancy in rats and these effects are blocked by section of the hypogastric nerve (32). In humans, the literature suggesting that labor increases the pain threshold is controversial.

MANAGEMENT OF PARTURITION PAIN

Earlier methods of pain relief centered on use of a variety of inhalation or parenteral drug delivery protocols to produce an analgesic state. Such approaches typically involved the use of N_2O or methoxyflurane mixtures delivered as required (16) or the incremental use of parenteral opioid (16). Such approaches can produce moderately effective relief, but are potentially accompanied by depression of respiration between pain, delayed gastric emptying, and, more importantly, a tendency to produce moderate depression in the fetus that may persist from minutes to hours after delivery.

Regional Anesthetic Approaches

The appreciation of the innervation of the phases of labor emphasizes that the pain associated with parturition may be effectively approached by blocking afferent innervation using regional nerve blocks at the level of the peripheral nerve, at the level of the dural sac, or by a combination of the approaches. The virtue of these approaches has been yet extended by the systematic application of "continuous" procedures.

There are several advantages accruing from regional protocols using local anesthetics: (a) complete blockade of the afferent message and complete pain relief; (b) little or no systemic effects yielding maternal or neonatal depression; and (c) the mother is able to remain alert, which serves to minimize the chances of aspiration (16). There are several disadvantages of the regional approach: (a) sympathetic blockade can result from the use of spinal regional techniques and can lead to hypotension; (b) complete block of the efferent limb of the innervation of the perineal musculature may interfere with the mechanisms of internal rotation, leading to an increased incidence of unusual fetal presentations; (c) blockade of the afferent limb may reduce the urge of the patient to bear down and accordingly prolong the second stage of the delivery; and (d) such spinal procedures may be contraindicated for patients with coagulopathies (23,78).

Peripheral Nerve Blocks

Consistent with the innervation of the pelvic viscera and uterus, paracervical blockade provides disruption of the innervation of the cervix and the uterus, serving to effectively block the pain associated with the first stage of delivery. The pudendal blockade results in prevention of the input associated with the perineal pain.

Spinal Blocks

There are approaches that are extradural (caudal or epidural) and intradural (spinal). The caudal approach entails the placement of a catheter through the sacrum to the S1/L5 vertebrae and the delivery of a sufficient volume of anesthetic to achieve a block to T10-T12. With the use of lower concentrations of anesthetics, e.g., 0.25% bupivacaine, it is impossible to provide adequate relief of phase 1 labor pain with a somewhat reduced risk of hypotension and motor blockade. As labor progresses and rotation has occurred, the density of the block can be increased to provide anesthesia for the second phase (16).

The epidural approach is widely employed. It involves the placement of the epidural catheter at or around L5 and the delivery of adequate volumes to achieve a sufficiently dense block to extend from T10 to S5. An important variant on this approach is to place a single catheter at the level of the T12 vertebra and a second catheter with its tip at the level of the S3 vertebra. The differential blockade achieved by the respective catheters serves to target those dermatomes that are responsible for stage 1 and stage 2 delivery, respectively. The ability to localize the block has the advantages of (a) reducing the total dose required (thereby reducing the likelihood of systemic toxicity to either mother or fetus), (b) minimizing the hypotension, and (c) reducing the blockade of motor function and retaining the ability to bear down through the use of the abdominal musculature.

Delivery of the drug extends from T10 to the S5 spinal segments. While the approach has several advantages including the small volume of anesthetic required, it also induces a potent sympathetic blockade, is potentially associated with significant hypotension and with lower limb paralysis, and can be accompanied by a postdural puncture headache. The hypotension can be attenuated by prior volume loading of the patient while the headaches are minimized with small-gauge needles (16).

Use of Spinal Receptor Selective Agents

The use of spinal anesthetics has been an effective tool in minimizing pain of parturition. There is, however, a growing application that afferent transmission at the spinal level may be altered by an action of several receptor selective agents within the spinal canal. At present the most widely used alternative to local anesthetics are opiates. The use of intrathecal or epidural morphine (79), fentanyl, or sufentanil has typically been reported to produce adequate relief of first-stage labor pain, but the effects on second-stage labor pain are less assured (70). In more recent studies, higher doses of intrathecal agents such as sufentanil have been reported to be effective in second-stage labor. Based on the pharmacology of visceral afferents, it seems reasonable that spinal opiates should be adequate for such small afferent intervention (see Chap. 58). Meperidine has been reported to be effective in late-stage labor (37). It should be noted that at the concentrations typically employed, meperidine may also possess a significant local anesthetic action (85) and this may account in part for its reported activity.

Advantages of Adequate Pain Relief During Parturition

Appropriate management of pain associated with parturition has a number of positive effects. Data in the last few years have supported the fact that this analgesic method reduces catecholamines, β-endorphins, ACTH, and cortisol releases as a result of a nonpainful labor due to the selective effects of the epidural (1,19,40,61,73,77,90). Further meritorious effects of epidural analgesia include a reduction in the usual marked ele-

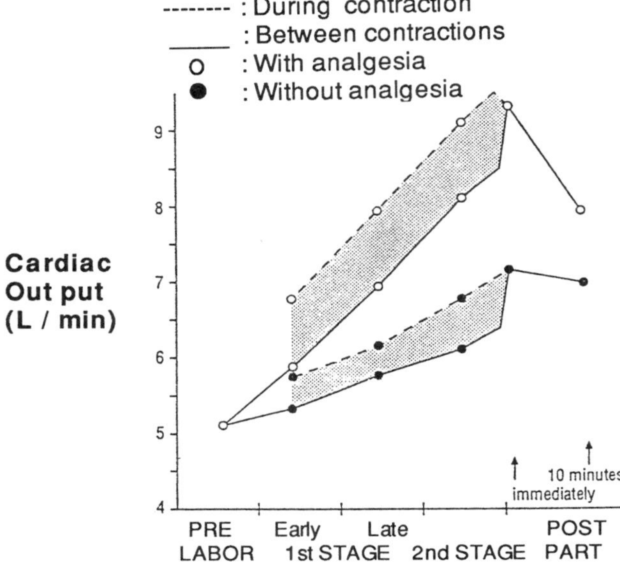

Figure 2. Cardiac outputs in two groups of patients. One group without analgesia that shows progressive increases at both contraction times and between contractions, and the other group with epidural analgesia at the same time periods. Note the smaller increases in cardiac outputs at all comparative levels of labor. Thus, the effective increase in cardiac work is much reduced by the epidural regional analgesia method.

vations in the systolic and diastolic blood pressures and a reduction in the left ventricular work attendant to delivery. This helps to protect those mothers who may have borderline cardiovascular efficiency due to either previous disease or a more recent diagnosis of pregnancy-induced hypertension, essential hypertension, or pulmonary disease processes (3,35,48).

Figure 2 displays the beneficial effect of epidural analgesia in reducing cardiac outputs as already described. This author commonly used a combination of the lumbar epidural for labor in cardiac risk patients, including several patients with mitral stenosis and a few with pulmonary hypertension with minimal dosages of dilute local anesthetic for first-stage pain relief, and then converted to a caudal epidural, with extremely dilute concentrations of local anesthetic for late second stage and delivery with forceps over a sensory denervated perineum with a generous episiotomy. This type of combined epidural placement and activation during the two different stages resulted in a completely pain-free first and second stage and allowed a controlled forceps delivery by the obstetrician; it also was accomplished with essentially no changes in either heart rate or blood pressure during both of the aforementioned stages.

It would appear that the epidural anesthetic is an appropriate anesthetic method for labor and delivery especially in view of both the analgesic impact and the decrease in impact of the pain-induced sympathetic hyperactivity that eliminates that portion of the increase in cardiac output and blood pressure caused by pain. Past clinical studies show the effectiveness of the labor epidural in reduction of the increase in cardiac output, cardiac work, and blood pressure in parturients with heart disease, pregnancy-induced hypertension (preeclampsia), and pulmonary hypertension (15,80).

PSYCHOLOGICAL ASPECTS

Effect of Psychology on Labor and Pain Interpretation

In the past few years clinical research has stressed the importance of psychological aspects of labor and the impact of the pain experience (21,22,57,71). There are several psychodynamic mechanisms including anxiety, attention, and motivation that will be discussed. There is little question that the dynamics of anxiety, anticipation of the possibility of pain, the appreciation of the unknown aspect of the intensity and type of pain, and certain ethnic factorials have significant impact on the final pain experience itself. The final expression or reaction to pain is referred to as pain behavior. This behavior has been distilled down to a numerical index as of recent times that confounds the complexity of the issue of this behavior to a degree that some have wondered if it does more bad to confuse the response to a pain stimulus than it does good in regard to standardization of pain.

Anxiety is perhaps one of the most significant factors that enhance the pain response to noxious stimulation (21,22). At the same time, reduction of anxiety and methods to reduce emotional stress associated with noxious experiences also help to increase one's tolerance of such an experience and thus reduces the overall pain experience. Attention is another factor that can block the response to pain due to a noxious experience, and battlefield injury is always quoted as one of the most demonstrative of attention blocking of pain responses, i.e., an injury will not be manifested immediately on the field as painful because of the intense attention needed by the individual at the time. Motivation is another psychodynamic mechanism that has influence on the physiologic behavior (6,71). Such motivation when sufficiently strong may result in remarkable behavior of a Herculean nature, and there are many stories that corroborate such a phenomenon. It is suggested that certain of these psychodynamic mechanisms inhibit transmission of pain signals at the level of the dorsal root ganglion or even in enhancement of inhibitory pathways. On the other hand, it is also likely that when interpreted to enhance the pain experience, these mechanisms speed and facilitate noxious signal transfer.

Effect of Labor and the Pain Interpretation on the Patient

The most common impact of labor and delivery on the patient is the well-known postpartum depression. This has been variously blamed on hormonal fluctuations and other physiologic phenomena in the few days postdelivery. This is usually short lived and reversible with merely a little sincere understanding. On the other hand, the memory and experience of severe labor pain has produced serious long-term maladjustments and bad effects in regard to mental health and well-being. Some have also impacted negatively on the mother-baby bonding and have eventually caused disruption of normal maternal feelings, undue fear of childbirth, and negative thoughts about sexual relationships (53,54,62,69,86). These negative impacts also occurred in natural childbirth situations without the benefit of analgesia. Both Stewart (83) and Melzack et al. (55) pointed out examples of failed achievements in natural childbirth classes that resulted in feeling of failure as mothers and depression and loss of interest in sex after delivery. Finally, some husbands of such women had guilt feelings and their potency was affected, to the extent that they had to undergo psychotherapy to counteract such effects.

CONCLUSIONS

The organization of labor pain may be summarized as follows. Step 1 in the first stage of labor is caused by an active uterine contraction. This in turn stimulates the dilatation of the cervix, which elicits pain sensations in the paracervical nerves known as the inferior hypogastric plexus. These fibers find their way to the spinal cord with entry levels at T10-T12 and L-1. In the second stage of labor, pain is caused by distention and dilatation of the perineum as the head negotiates the vaginal outlet. This stimulates pain fiber branches of the pudendal nerve. These fibers synapse at the S2-4 cord levels.

The rise of increasingly sophisticated regional anesthetic procedures have led to increased efforts to provide patients with an interruption of the nociceptive input due to cervical dilatation, pelvic tissue pressure, and stretching. Many notable anesthesiologists and others have paved the way for a better understanding and designed the concept of regional pain relief to offer the parturient a pleasant and respectable labor and delivery. A few of these early giants, but by no means a complete list, would include Cleland, Hingson, and Bonica. All three of these physicians had a common thread in their dedication and commitment to obstetric anesthesiology. This thread was a deep compassion for suffering. Cleland took time from his busy schedule as a surgical resident to study and work out the pain pathways of labor. He published his epoch work in 1938 that, with one small exception, was identical to what was summarized above. He did this because he heard nightly from his call room the cries of agony of laboring women that pierced his mind and stimulated him to develop his research project. I was fortunate enough to experience his genius on several occasions during my early training period in Oregon.

Hingson had an enormous dedication to helping mankind in all types of suffering. He set up worldwide organizations to immunize hundreds of thousands of patients all over the globe and is given credit for eradicating smallpox as a threat to humans. He went about his work in the labor and delivery area with the zeal and voracity of a Southern Baptist minister who was everywhere, trying to come up with solutions for better methods of pain relief and better methods that would maintain respectability and enjoyment for the mother during the birth process. I was fortunate enough to witness such commitment firsthand on several of my visits to Dr. Hingson's center.

Bonica personally witnessed the near death of his beloved wife, Emma, during delivery of their firstborn daughter. As the leader in anesthesiology in the great Northwest, he decided to better prepare anesthesiologists to take improved care of laboring mothers. I was most fortunate to be trained by Dr. Bonica in the specialty of anesthesiology, after I completed my obstetrics and gynecology residency. The women of today enjoy the fruits of the labors of such men as these, plus the many after them who have carried on and still carry on the search for better and safer methods of pain relief. They all emphasized the need for a cross-education of the obstetrician and anesthesiologist, providing a thorough understanding of the many complex aspects of the pain of childbirth.

REFERENCES

1. Abboud TK, Artal R, Henriksen EH, Earl S, Kammula RK. Effects of spinal anesthesia on maternal circulating catecholamines. *Am J Obstet Gynecol* 1982;142Z:252–4.
2. Abboud TK, Sarkis F, Hung TT, Khoo SS, Varakian L, Henriksen E, Noueihed R, Goebelsmann U. Effects of epidural anesthesia during labor on maternal plasma beta-endorphin levels. *Anesthesiology* 1983;59:1–5.
3. Adams JQ, Alexander AM. Alterations in cardiovascular physiology during labor. *Obstet Gynecol* 1958;12:542.
4. Akaishi T, Robbins A, Sakuma Y, Sato Y. Neural inputs from the uterus to the paraventricular magnocellular neurons in the rat. *Neurosci Lett* 1988;84(1):57–62.
5. Basbaum AI, Fields HL. Endogenous pain control systems: brain stem spinal pathways and endorphin circuitry. *Annu Rev Neurosci* 1984;7:309.
6. Beecher HK. *Measurement of subjective responses.* New York, Oxford University Press, 1959.
7. Behan RJ. *Pain.* New York: Appleton, 1914.

7a. Berkley KJ, Robbins A, Sato Y. Afferent fibers supplying the uterus in the rat. *J Neurophysiol* 1988;59:142–163.

8. Berkley KJ, Hotta H, Robbins A, Sato Y. Functional properties of afferent fibers supplying reproductive and other pelvic organs in pelvic nerve of female rat. *J Neurophysiol* 1990;63:256–272.
9. Berkley KJ, Hubscher CH, Wall PD. Neuronal responses to stimulation of the cervix, uterus, colon, and skin in the rat spinal cord. *J Neurophysiol* 1993;69:545– 556.
10. Berkley KJ, Robbins A, Sato Y. Functional differences between afferent fibers in the hypogastric and pelvic nerves innervating female reproductive organs in the rat. *J Neurophysiol* 1993;69: 533–544.
11. Bonica JJ. *Principles and practice of obstetric analgesia and anesthesia,* vol 1 and 2. Philadelphia: FA Davis, 1969.

11a. Bonica JJ. *Obstetric analgesia and anesthesia,* 2nd ed. Seattle: University of Washington Press, 1980;46–47.

12. Bonica JJ. Presidential address. In: Bonica JJ, Lindblom U, Iggo A, eds. *Advances in pain research and therapy,* vol 5. New York: Raven Press, 1983.
13. Bonica JJ. Mechanisms and pathways of parturition pain. In: Genazxzani AR, Nappi G, Facchinetti F, Martingnoni E, eds. *Pain and reproduction.* Casterton Holl, Carnfort: Parthenon, 1988; 182–191.
14. Bonica JJ. Anatomic and physiologic basis of nociception and pain. In: Bonica JJ, ed. *The management of pain,* 2nd ed. Philadelphia: Lea & Febiger, 1990;28–94.
15. Bonica JJ, McDonald JS. *Principles and practice of obstetric analgesia and anesthesia.* 2nd ed. Baltimore: Williams & Wilkins, 1995.
16. Bonica JJ, Ueland K. Heart disease. In: Bonica JJ, ed. *Principles and practice of obstetric analgesia and anesthesia,* vol 2. Philadelphia: FA Davis, 1969;941–977.
17. Brauer MM, Lincoln J, Sarner S, Blundell D, Milner P, Passaro M, Burnstock G. Maturational changes in sympathetic and sensory innervation of the rat uterus: effects of neonatal capsaicin treatment. *Int J Dev Neurosci* 1994;12:157–171.
18. Bruggemann J, Vahle-Hinz C, Kniffki KD. Projections from the pelvic nerve to the periphery of the cat's thalamic ventral posterolateral nucleus and adjacent regions of the posterior complex. *J Neurophysiol* 1994;72(5):2237–2245.
19. Buchan PC. Emotional stress in childbirth and its modification by variations in obstetric management—epidural analgesia and stress in labor. *Acta Obstet Gynecol Scand* 1980;59:319.
20. Bundsen P. Subjectiva resultat av smartlindring under forlossning-En enkatundersoknine. *Lakartidningen* 1975;3:139.
21. Chapman CR. Psychological factors in postoperative pain and their treatment. In: Smith G, Covino B, eds. *Acute pain,* vol 1. London: Butterworths International Medical Review, 1985.
22. Chapman CR, Turner JAP. Psychologic and psychosocial aspects of acute pain. In: Bonica JJ, ed. *The management of pain,* 2nd ed. Philadelphia: Lea & Febiger, 1990;122–132.
23. Chestnut DH, Vandewalker GE, Owen CI, Bates JN, Choi WW. The influence of continuous epidural bupivacaine analgesia on the second stage of labor and method of delivery in nulliparous women. *Anesthesiology* 1987;66:774–780.
24. Cleland JGP. Continuous peridural and caudal analgesia in obstetrics. *Curr Res Anesth Analg* 1949;28:61.
25. Dick-Read GP. *Childbirth without fear.* New York: Harper, 1953.
26. Dubner R, Bennett G. Spinal and trigeminal mechanisms of nociception. *Annu Rev Neurosci* 1983;6:281.
27. Eustace TD. Cognitive, attitudinal, and socioeconomic factors influencing parents' choice of childbirth procedure. *Dissertation Abstr Int* 1978;39:1474B.
28. Fettes I, Fox J, Kuzniak S, Shime J, Gare D. Plasma levels of immunoreactive beta-endorphin and adrenocorticotropic hormone during labor and delivery. *Obstet Gynecol* 1984;64:359–362.
29. Ford CS. *A comparative study of human reproduction.* Yale University Publications in Anthropology. New Haven: Yale University Press, 1945.
30. Freedman LZ, Ferguson VS. The question of "painless childbirth" in primitive cultures. *Am J Orthopsychiatry* 1950;20:363.
31. Fridh G, Kopare T, Gaston-Johansson F, Norvell KT. Factors associated with more intense labor pain. *Res Nurs Health* 1988;11: 117–124.
32. Gintzler AR, Peters LC, Komisaruk BR. Attenuation of pregnancy-induced analgesia by hypogastric neurectomy in rats. *Brain Res* 1983;277:186–188.
33. Goebelsmann U, Abboud TK, Hoffman DI, Hung TT. Beta-endorphin in pregnancy. *Eur J Obstet Gynecol Reprod Biol* 1984;17: 77–89.
34. Guilbaud G, Berkley KJ, Benoist JM, Gautron M. Responses of neurons in thalamic ventrobasal complex of rats to graded dis-

tension of uterus and vagina and to uterine suprafusion with bradykinin and prostaglandin F2 alpha. *Brain Res* 1993;614(1-2): 285–290.

35. Hansen JM and Ueland K. The influence of caudal analgesia on cardiovascular dynamics during normal labor and delivery. *Acta Anaesthesiol Scand* 1966;23(suppl 10):449.
36. Head H. On disturbances of sensation with special reference to the pain of visceral disease. *Brain* 1893;16:1.
37. Honet JE, Arkoosh VA, Norris MC, Huffnagle HJ, Silverman NS, Leighton BL. Comparison among intrathecal fentanyl, meperidine, and sufentanil for labor analgesia. *Anesth Analg* 1992;75: 734–739.
38. Hong SK, Han HC, Yoon YW, Chung JM. Response properties of hypogastric afferent fibers supplying the uterus in the cat. *Brain Res* 1993;622(1-2):215–225.
39. Jochelson W. *The Yukaghir and the Youkaghirized Tungus*: Vol XIII of the Memoirs of American Museum of Natural History which constitutes at the same time Vol. IX, Part I, of the Jesup North Pacific expedition. New York and Leiden: American Museum of Natural History, 1910.
40. Joupplila R, Hollmen A. The effect of segmental epidural analgesia on maternal and foetal acid-base balance, lactate, serum potassium and creatine phosphokinase during labour. *Acta Anaesthesiol Scand* 1976;20:259.
41. Kawatani M, de Groat WC. A large proportion of afferent neurons innervating the uterine cervix of the cat contain VIP and other neuropeptides. *Cell Tissue Res* 1991;266(1):191–196.
42. Kawatani M, Takeshige C, de Groat WC. Central distribution of afferent pathways from the uterus of the cat. *J Comp Neurol* 1990; 302(2):294–304.
43. Keverne EB, Kendrick KM. Maternal behaviour in sheep and its neuroendocrine regulation. *Acta Paediatr Suppl* 1994;397:47–56.
44. Kohen N. "Natural" childbirth among the Kankanaly-Igorot. *Bull NY Acad Med* 1986;62:768.
45. Lamaze F. *Qu'est-ce que l'accouchement sans douleur par la methode psychoprophylactique? Ses principes, sa realisation, se resultats.* Paris: Savouret Connaitre, 1956.
46. Lederman RP, Lederman E, Work BA Jr, McCann DS. The relationship of maternal anxiety, plasma catecholamines, and plasma cortisol to progress in labor. *Am J Obstet Gynecol* 1978:132:495–500.
47. Lee R. *Lecture on the theory and practice of midwifery.* Philadelphia: Barrington and Hosswell, 1844.
48. Lees MM, Scott DB, Kerr MG. Haemodynamic changes associated with labour. *Br J Obstet Gynaecol* 1970;77:29.
49. Lefebvre L, Carli G. Parturition pain in non-human primates: pain and auditory concealment. *Pain* 1985;21:315.
50. Levy-Strauss C. *Sorciers et psychanalyse.* Geneva: LeCourier de l'Unecso, 1956;808–810.

50a. Luckman SM. Fos expression within regions of the preoptic area, hypothalamus and brain stem during pregnancy and parturition. *Brain Res* 1995;669(1):115–124.

51. Lundh W. Modraundervisning. Forlossningstraning eller foraldrakunskap? [Ph.D. Dissertation], Pedagogiska Institutionen. Stockholm Universitet, 1974.
52. Marx JL. Dysmenorrhea: basic research leads to a rational therapy. *Science* 1979;205:175.
53. Melzack R. The myth of painless childbirth. The John J. Bonica Lecture. *Pain* 1984;19:321 .
54. Melzack R, Taenzer P, Feldman P, Kinch RA. Labour is still painful after prepared childbirth training. *Can Med Assoc J* 1981; 125:357–363.
55. Melzack R, Kinch R, Dobkin P, Lebrun M, Taenzer P. Severity of labour pain: influence of physical as well as psychologic variables. *Can Med Assoc J* 1984;130:579–584.
56. Melzack R, Schaffelberg D. Low-back pain during labor. *Am J Obstet Gynecol* 1987;156:901.
57. Merskey H, Spear FG. *Pain:* psychological and psychiatric aspects. London: Baillière, Tindall and Cassell, 1967.
58. Miller FC. Hyperventilation during labor. *Am J Obstet Gynecol* 1974;120:489.
59. Morishima HO, Pedersen H, Finster M. Effects of pain on mother, labour and fetus. In: Marx GF, Bassell GM, eds. *Obstetric analgesia and anaesthesia.* Amsterdam: Elsevier North Holland, 1980;197–210.
60. Morishima HO, Pedersen H, Finster M. The influence of maternal psychological stress on the fetus. *Am J Obstet Gynecol* 1978;134:286.
61. Motoyama EK, Rivard G, Acheson F, Cook CD. The effect of changes in maternal pH and P-CO2 on the P-O2 of fetal lambs. *Anesthesiology* 1967;28:891–903.
62. Nettelbladt P, Fagerstrom CF. Uddenberg N. The significance of reported childbirth pain. *J Psychol Res* 1976;20:215.
63. Neumark J, Hammerle AF, Biegelmayer C. Effects of epidural analgesia on plasma catecholamines and cortisol in parturition. *Acta Anaesthesiol Scand* 1985;29:555.
64. Norr KL, Block CR, Charles A, Meyering S, Meyers E. Explaining pain and enjoyment in childbirth. *J Health Soc Behav* 1977;18: 260–275.
65. Papka RE. Some nerve endings in the rat pelvic paracervical autonomic ganglia and varicosities in the uterus contain calcitonin gene-related peptide and originate from dorsal root ganglia. *Neuroscience* 1990; 39:459–470.
66. Papka RE, McNeill DL. Light- and electron-microscopic study of synaptic connections in the paracervical ganglion of the female rat: special reference to calcitonin gene-related peptide, galanin- and tachykinin (substance P and neurokinin A)-immunoreactive nerve fibers and terminals. *Cell Tissue Res* 1993;271:417–428.
67. Papka RE, McNeill DL. Coexistence of calcitonin gene-related peptide and galanin immunoreactivity in female rat pelvic and lumbosacral dorsal root ganglia. *Peptides* 1992;13:761–767.
68. Papka RE, McNeill DL, Thompson D, Schmidt HH. Nitric oxide nerves in the uterus are parasympathetic, sensory, and contain neuropeptides. *Cell Tissue Res* 1995;279(2):339–349.
69. Pearson JF, Davies P. The effect of continuous lumbar epidural analgesia upon fetal acid- base status during the first stage of labour. *Br J Obstet Gynaecol* 1974;81:971.
70. Phillips G. Continuous infusion epidural analgesia and labor: the effect of adding sufentanil to 0.125% bupivacaine. *Anesth Analg* 1988;87:462–465.
71. Pilowsky I. Abnormal illness behavior and sociocultural aspects of pain. In: Kosterlitz HW, Terenius LY, eds. *Pain and society.* Weinheim: Verlag Chemie, 1980;445–460.
72. Pinter E, Szolcsanyi J. Plasma extravasation in the skin and pelvic organs evoked by antidromic stimulation of the lumbosacral dorsal roots of the rat. *Neuroscience* 1995; 68(2):603–614.
73. Raisanen I, Paatero H, Salminen K, Laatikainen T. Beta-endorphin in maternal and umbilical cord plasma at elective cesarean section and in spontaneous labor. *Obstet Gynecol* 1986;67:384–387.
74. Robbins A, Sato Y, Hotta H, Berkley KJ. Responses of hypogastric nerve afferent fibers to uterine distension in estrous or metestrous rats. *Neurosci Lett* 1990;110(1-2):82–85.
75. Scott-Palmer J, Skevington SM. Pain during childbirth and menstruation: a study of locus of control. *J Psychosom Res* 1981;25:151.
76. Shew RL, Papka RE, McNeill DL, Yee JA. NADPH-diaphorase-positive nerves and the role of nitric oxide in CGRP relaxation of uterine contraction. *Peptides* 1993;14(3):637–641.
77. Shnider SM, Abboud TK, Artal R, Henriksen EH, Stefani SJ, Levinson G. Maternal catecholamines decrease during labor after lumbar epidural anesthesia. *Am J Obstet Gynecol* 1983;147:13–15.
78. Sibai BM, Taslimi MM, El-Nazer A, Amon E, et al. Maternal-perinatal outcome associated with the syndrome of hemolysis, elevated liver enzymes and low platelets in sever preeclampsia-eclampsia. *Am J Obstet Gynecol* 1986;155:501.
79. Skerman JH, Thompson BA, Goldstein MT, Jacobs MA, et al. Combined continuous epidural fentanyl and bupivacaine in labor: a randomized study. *Anesthesiology* 1985;63:A450.
80. Sorensen MB, Korshin JD, Fernandes A, Secher O. The use of epidural analgesia for delivery in a patient with pulmonary hypertension. *Acta Anaesthesiol Scand* 1982;26:180–182.
81. Steinman JL, Komisaruk BR, Yaksh TL, Tyce GM. Spinal cord monamines mediate the antinociceptive effects of vaginal stimulation in rats. *Pain* 1983;16:155–166.
82. Sternbach RA. *The psychology of pain.* New York: Raven Press, 1978.
83. Stewart DE. Psychiatric symptoms following attempted natural childbirth. *Can Med Assoc J* 1982;127:713.
84. Sullivan KA, Traurig HH, Papka RE. Ontogeny of neurotransmitter systems in the paracervical ganglion and uterine cervix of the rat. *Anat Rec* 1994;240(3):377–386.
85. Swayze CR, Skerman JH, Walker EB, Sholte FG. Efficacy of subarachnoid meperidine for labor analgesia. *Reg Anesth* 1991;16: 309–313.
86. Thalme B, Belfrage P, Raabe N. Lumbar epidural analgesia in labour. *Acta Obstet Gynaecol Scand* 1974;53:27.

87. Tyce GM, Yaksh TL. Monoamine release from cat spinal cord by somatic stimuli: an intrinsic modulatory system. *J Physiol (Lond)* 1981;314:513–529.
88. Wall PD, Hubscher CH, Berkley KJ. Intraspinal modulation of neuronal responses to uterine and cervix stimulation in rat L1 and L6 dorsal horn. *Brain Res* 1993;622(1-2):71–78.
90. Westgren M, Lindahl SGE, Norden NEP Maternal and fetal endocrine stress response at vaginal delivery with and without an epidural block. *J Perinat Med* 1986;14:235.
91. Woolf CJ. Long-term alterations in the excitability of the flection reflex produced by peripheral tissue injury in the chronic decerebrate rat. *Pain* 1984;18:325.
92. Woolf CJ. Recent advances in the pathophysiology of acute pain. *Br J Anaesth* 1989;63:139.

Anesthesia: Biologic Foundations, edited by Tony L. Yaksh et al. Lippincott–Raven Publishers, Philadelphia © 1997.

CHAPTER 46

DYSMENORRHEA

ANDREA RAPKIN, NATALIA LUZINA RASGON, AND KAREN J. BERKLEY

Dysmenorrhea, a Greek term meaning painful menstruation, has been the subject of investigation since the time of Hippocrates (50,131). Dysmenorrhea has commonly been subclassified as primary or secondary. Primary dysmenorrhea is menstrual pain that begins and persists with menstrual flow and occurs in the absence of underlying pelvic pathology, whereas secondary dysmenorrhea is menstrual pain accompanied by organic pelvic pathology (e.g., adenomyosis, endometriosis, polyps, myomas, intrauterine devices, pelvic infection, cervical stenosis) (50,131).

It seems certain that primary dysmenorrheic episodes reflect the activation of pelvic afferent innervation that lead to a pain state. The effective stimulus leading to such activation is not clear, but several components appear relevant: (a) an intense intrauterine pressure can be exerted by the contractile myometrium (12,122,142); (b) local hormonal factors can influence afferent terminal excitability (e.g., eicosanoid and hormonal); (c) changes in CNS processing that alter the encoding of the afferent message; and (d) behavioral (affective-motivational) components defining the context of the stimulus environment. As will be discussed below, although considerable emphasis is typically placed on myometrial contractility, it is very likely that these several factors all significantly contribute, in an interactive fashion, to the etiology of dysmenorrhea.

MYOMETRIAL CONTRACTILITY ASSOCIATED WITH DYSMENORRHEA

Contractile Parameters

Intrauterine pressure can be monitored in women with a transcervical intrauterine microballoon-tipped catheter (123) or with a catheter top microtransducer system (144). Various parameters are then calculated: (a) Active pressure, measured in mm Hg, is the average amplitude of pressure cycles (contractions). (b) Resting pressure, measured in mm Hg, is the average increase of pressure (tonus) from a baseline value when the uterus is relaxed between contractions. (c) Frequency is the number of contractions in a given unit of time. (d) Velocity, measured in mm Hg/s, is the rate of the change of pressure during contractions. The overall severity of the associated pain state may then be evaluated in relation to these parameters (5,123).

Uterine activity in dysmenorrheic patients as compared with controls is characterized by high resting pressure, high active pressure, and high frequency of contractions (123), with the contractions typically displaying a high velocity (5). That these increased parameters are important in the etiology of dysmenorrhea is supported by the fact that treatment regimens that reduce the contractions are considered effective in reducing dysmenorrhea. For example, nonsteroidal anti-inflammatory drugs (NSAIDs) such as nimesulide, mefenamic acid, and ibuprofen lower fundal resting pressure and/or decrease contraction frequency and concomitantly reduce dysmenorrhea (121,142,150). Similarly, uterine contractions evoked by prostaglandins, by estrogen, and by vasopressin as well as spontaneous activity in isolated human myometrium are associated with calcium influx in vitro and in vivo (7,54,61). Calcium channel blocking agents such as nifedipine concomitantly reduce contractile activity and dysmenorrhea (28,62).

Uterine Hypoxia

Each of these increased myometrial contractile parameters results in a decreased uterine blood flow. It can therefore be postulated that dysmenorrhea is secondary to uterine hypoxia. At least six lines of evidence support this hypothesis: (a) Pressure measured within the uterus during dysmenorrheic menstrual cramping often vastly exceeds the perfusion pressure (4). (b) Simultaneous measurements of intrauterine pressure and arterial blood flow demonstrate the blood flow decreases during uterine contractions and that pain is greatest at the time of this diminished flow (4). (c) Congestive dysmenorrhea is a common feature among women with "pelvic congestion," a condition that comprises dilated pelvic veins and vascular stasis and therefore results in poor blood flow and hypoxemia of pelvic organs including the uterus (11,12). (d) There are a greater number of gap junctions between the smooth muscle cells of the myometrium in patients with severe dysmenorrhea (67). Gap junctions between adjacent smooth muscle cells facilitate propagation of contractions over the uterus (33,64). A greater number of gap junctions would therefore promote decreased blood flow over larger areas of the uterus during each intense contraction. (e) In animal studies, psychophysical experiments have shown that rats will attempt to escape from distention of their uterine horn only when the distention produces obvious uterus ischemia and the uterine pressure exceeds the rat's mean blood pressure (21,25). (f) It is argued that the reduction of resting pressure and contraction frequency by NSAIDs produces a reduction in pain because the decreased myometrial activity results in an improvement of blood flow (150).

LOCAL HORMONAL FACTORS

Eicosanoids

The main pathogenic mechanism that has been associated with the development of dysmenorrhea is the hyperproduction of eicosanoids (8,16,47). Such high concentrations appear to result from an increased production by the endometrium rather than from an altered metabolic degradation (51).

The term "eicosanoid" is the collective name for unsaturated lipids derived from arachidonic acid or similar polyunsaturated fatty acid precursors, via the cyclooxygenase or lipoxygenase metabolic pathways. This group of substances includes prostaglandins, thromboxanes, leukotrienes, lipoxins, and various hydroxy- and hydroperoxy-fatty acids. Although prostaglandins are thought to be the main eicosanoids involved in dysmenorrhea, some evidence exists as well for leukotrienes (112).

Prostanoids

Prostaglandins are formed by a series of enzymatic reactions on phospholipids liberated from the cell membrane. The lysosomal enzyme phospholipase A2 hydrolyzes these phospholipids into arachidonic acid that is then converted by the cyclooxygenase into the cyclic endoperoxides PGG_2 and PGH_2. Subsequent reduction and isomerization of the latter leads to the formation of PGE_2 and $PGF_{2\alpha}$ (Fig. 1).

Prostaglandin synthesis is possible only under conditions of sufficient amounts of precursor such as arachidonic acid. Free

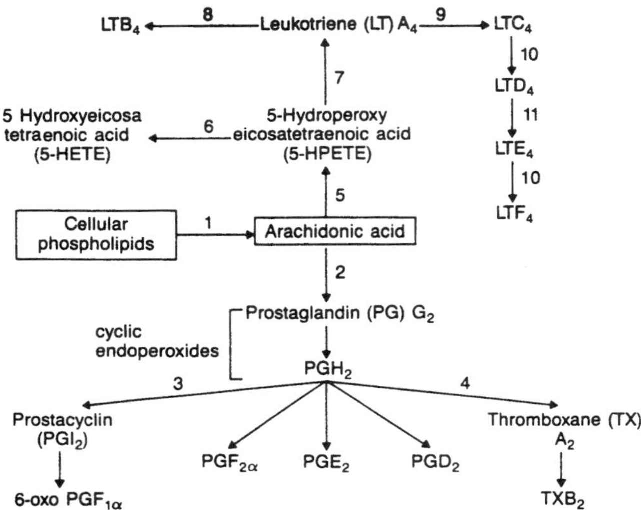

Figure 1. Prostaglandin and leukotriene products of arachidonic acid. *(1)* Phospholipase A_2 (inhibited by phospholipase inhibitor whose synthesis is stimulated by corticosteroids). *(2)* Cyclooxygenase (inhibited by NSAID and BW-755C). *(3)* Prostacyclin synthetase. *(4)* Thromboxane synthetase. *(5)* 5-Lipoxygenase (inhibited by BW-755C). *(6)* Glutathione peroxidase. *(7)* Dehydrogenase. *(8)* Leukotriene A_4 epoxide hydrolase. *(9)* Glutathione transferase. *(10)* Glutamyl transferase. *(11)* Cysteinylglycine dipeptidase. (Reprinted with permission from Chaudhuri G. Physiologic aspects of prostaglandins and leukotrienes. *Semin Reprod Endocrinol* 1985;3:219–230.)

arachidonic acid is rapidly converted into prostaglandins or lipids. The level of activity of the enzyme phospholipase depends on the amount of free intracellular calcium ions. Thus, the amount of prostaglandin synthesis can be controlled by calcium transport (38,107).

The suggestion that prostaglandins are involved in the pathogenesis of primary dysmenorrhea is supported by several observations: (a) Administration of $PGF_{2\alpha}$ and PGE_2 produce pain similar to dysmenorrheic pain (93,132). (b) The clinical symptoms of primary dysmenorrhea are similar to those induced by the administration of $PGF_{2\alpha}$ and PGE_2 for the induction of labor (16). (c) The increased production of prostaglandins by the endometrium during luteal and menstrual phases of the cycle is consistent with the occurrence of primary dysmenorrhea mainly in ovulatory cycles (16, 49). (d) The concentrations of $PGF_{2\alpha}$ and PGE_2 in the endometrium and menstrual fluid and $PGF_{2\alpha}$ metabolic 15-keto-13, 14-dihydro $PGF_{2\alpha}$ in plasma of dysmenorrheic women are significantly higher than in controls (94). (e) Inhibitors of prostaglandin synthesis are very effective in the treatment of dysmenorrhea (16,150). (f) Prostaglandins (and estrogens) provoke the formation of gap junctions while agents blocking prostaglandins may prevent their formation (150). (g) Free radicals are products of lipid peroxidation which is an intermediate step in prostaglandin synthesis. There is a significant elevation of the free fatty acid precursors and end products of lipid peroxidation (Schiff bases) in patients with dysmenorrhea as compared to controls (96). Antioxidants impede lipid peroxidation, thus stabilize membranes, reduce prostaglandin synthesis and can therefore potentially alleviate menstrual pain (96).

The involvement of prostaglandins in primary dysmenorrhea is also supported by studies on arginine vasopressin. Akerlund et al. (5) showed an increased secretion of endogenous vasopressin after osmotic stimulation (intravenous infusion of hypertonic saline). Several reports describe the interaction of vasopressin with prostaglandins. Vasopressin infusion has been found to increase the plasma concentration of $PGF_{2\alpha}$ metabolite in dysmenorrhea (147). Furthermore, the plasma levels of vasopressin remain elevated in patients whose dysmenorrhea is successfully controlled by prostaglandin synthetase inhibitors, suggesting that vasopressin acts by stimulating prostaglandin synthesis (148). Other findings, however, suggest that the vasopressin also must have direct effects on the myometrium (16).

In the above comments, the role of prostaglandins in altering myometrial contractile parameters and producing hypoxia are considered to be the intervening mechanism accounting for their role in dysmenorrhea (94,118,143). However, at least three additional mechanisms are also likely, as pain can be evoked by prostaglandins without an increase in uterine contraction (64).

First, considerable data suggest that prostaglandins may act to stimulate and sensitize uterine afferent nerve endings directly, as prostaglandins have been shown to do in other tissues (119, 137). Such sensitization could result in the evocation of activity in uterine afferent fibers by uterine conditions that normally do not affect activity in hypogastric nerve afferent axons, but do so in conditions in which the uterus has been irritated (19,25). Prostaglandins may sensitize the uterus to actions by other agents. For example, in vitro, PGE has been shown to sensitize the guinea pig uterus to the contractile effects of vasopressin, oxytocin, histamine and electrical stimulation (157).

Second, prostacyclins can cause spasm of the uterine artery (122), which may thus be the source of pain rather than the uterus itself.

Third, prostaglandins could act at the level of the CNS in the spinal cord. Continued activity in uterine afferent fibers during repetitive episodes of menstrual pain could lead to increased excitability of spinal cord neurons and elevated arachidonic acid levels (99) (see Chapter 36). As such, NSAIDs may act at the spinal cord level as well as peripherally in women with dysmenorrhea.

Leukotrienes

Recent experimental data suggest that leukotrienes might be alternative pathogenic factors in dysmenorrhea. Up to 30% of patients with primary dysmenorrhea do not respond to prostaglandin inhibiting agents and some cases could be due to excess leukotrienes (64,127). As with prostaglandins, there is evidence that leukotrienes can act by stimulating uterine contractions (95) or by affecting sensory nerve endings directly (100) or possibly by the other mechanisms listed above.

Studies in vivo and in vitro have shown that LTC_4 and LTD_4, at concentrations similar to those of PGE_2 and $PGF_{2\alpha}$, elicit uterine contractions similar to those elicited by the prostaglandins (35,154). Specific LTC_4-binding sites have recently been demonstrated in uterine tissues of nonpregnant women, especially in luminal epithelial cells of the endometrium, stromal cells, circular and elongated myometrial smooth muscle and arteriolar smooth muscle. This suggests that LTC_4 might regulate contractility of the uterine tissues, either through a direct action or via an increase in local prostaglandin and thromboxane production (40), or both. LTB_4, on the other hand, is a potent chemotactic factor that also induces hyperalgesia and enhances vascular permeability (32,90). Vascular reperfusion subsequent to hypoxia would generate oxygen-free radicals, which in turn might stimulate the cyclooxygenase pathway (114,138).

Platelet Activating Factor

Platelet activating factor is a lipid derivative with a broad range of biological activities. It originates from membrane phospholipids, which, after detachment of a fatty acid due to the action of phospholipase A2, are transformed into lysoplatelet activating factor, which is then converted into platelet activating factor. Besides facilitating platelet activation, it mediates many processes of inflammation and induces the contraction of intestinal and bronchial smooth muscle (34). It is also able to stimulate the contraction of human myometrial strips in vivo in a concentration-dependent manner (111). Considerable data exist indicating that platelet activating factor probably acts via interaction with specific uterine receptors to modulate prostaglandin and possibly leukotriene synthesis (10,143). Of importance, therefore, is that, like leukotrienes, platelet activating factor might play significant pathogenic roles in dysmenorrheic women unresponsive to antiprostaglandin drugs (102).

Endocrinological Factors

Effects Upon Uterine Function

An imbalance of ovarian hormones may be a part of the etiology of dysmenorrhea. It has been postulated that estrogen priming followed by exposure to progesterone is necessary to cause primary dysmenorrhea, and therefore the latter can be seen only in ovulatory cycles (8,50). Increased luteal phase estrogen levels have been described in women with dysmenorrhea (96,148,163).

Ovarian hormonal involvement in dysmenorrhea is likely to be indirect by means of their influences peripherally on prostaglandin synthesis and myometrial contractility (3,76,84, 158). Estrogens can stimulate synthesis and/or release of $PGF_{2\alpha}$ (148) and vasopressin (1,63,64) as well as increase spontaneous uterine activity. Treatment with oral contraceptives, especially those that are gestagen-dominated, change the balance of ovarian hormones to a progesterone-dominated environment. Falling progesterone levels cause lysosomes in endometrial cells to release phospholipase. These hydrolyze phospholipids to generate arachidonic acid. In contrast, high progesterone levels stabilize the lysosomes (49). Thus, a progesterone-dominated cycle in women is associated with decreased uterine activity. In one study, oral contraceptive administration resulted in decreased frequency and amplitude of spontaneous uterine contractions and reduced sensitivity to exogenous $PGF_{2\alpha}$ (55). In nondysmenorrheic women, subendometrial contractions decrease in frequency, amplitude and percentage during the luteal phase (97) as progesterone levels increase.

In rats, the pattern of uterine contractions is altered considerably during the proestrus stage of their estrous cycle (46,52) when progesterone levels have increased following estrogen increases (65) as well as during pseudopregnancy (46,101). These changes consist mostly of a reduction in frequency (contractions become much less regular) and direction, and the changes are prevented by administration of RU486, a progesterone antagonist (46). Rats are much less likely during proestrus and pseudopregnancy (when progesterone levels are high), to attempt to escape uterine distention stimuli (22).

Other peripheral effects of ovarian hormones that might be related to dysmenorrhea are progesterone's effects on the binding of calcium in cell structures that result in decreases in the influx of free calcium through its channels (88). Additionally, progesterone has been shown to diminish the uterine effects of vasopressin (88). And, finally, the sensitivity of uterine afferent fibers in rats to uterine stimulation changes as a function of the estrous cycle, suggesting ovarian hormones could influence activity in afferent fibers relatively directly (128).

An imbalance of ovarian hormones could also be important in the etiology of dysmenorrhea by means of their influences on neurons within the CNS, both on autonomic and motor output systems and on sensory systems (134).

CNS-Processing Influence on Hormone Release

A likely etiological factor in dysmenorrhea may involve influences on the reproductive tract arising from the CNS (113, 149). Numerous studies in animals have demonstrated that disconnection of the reproductive tract from the CNS by means of peripheral neurectomies can affect reproductive events. For example, in rats, pelvic neurectomies produce dystocia (74,115). Similarly, studies have also shown that output through the hypogastric and pelvic nerves can influence uterine contractility (136) as well as uterine blood flow (129). Furthermore, this output is likely to be influenced by neural systems descending from the brainstem and forebrain, particularly the hypothalamus (43,77,91,135). Thus, alterations in central neural systems associated with the reproductive tract have the potential for producing dysmenorrhea by influencing neural output to the uterus and other pelvic organs that could then affect any of the variables discussed in the previous sections. Two of many examples of potentially influential CNS alterations include those that might occur in endogenous opioid neurochemistry and γ-aminobutyric acid (GABA) action.

Endogenous Opioids Endogenous opioid (EOP) systems play an important role in hypothalamic-pituitary ovarian function (27). Opioid peptides are participants in the coordination and control of the menstrual cycle (27). Estradiol and progesterone increase β-endorphin concentrations during the luteal phase of the menstrual cycle and this is followed by a rapid fall of opioid peptides at menstruation (27). This situation suggests a complex mechanism for triggering dysmenorrhea, in which abnormalities in opioid systems, such as those that might occur under stress, could affect (a) central neural influences on ovarian hormonal homeostasis that would alter myometrial contractility and eicosanoid production and/or (b) hypothalamic-descending influences on spinal autonomic output to the uterus. Currently, there is no direct evidence supporting the opioid involvement in the pain of dysmenorrhea. However various studies have demonstrated that dysmenorrhea responds therapeutically to elevation of endogenous opioid peptides. There is a well-described response to placebo in dysmenorrheic patients (57). Additionally, it has been shown in vitro and in vivo that α-tocopherol can stimulate synthesis and secretion of EOPs, particularly β-endorphins, significantly above the level noted with placebo administration (96). In patients with primary dysmenorrhea, administration of α-tocopherol, and not placebo, at the height of the pain attack caused an elevation of β-endorphin immunoreactivity in venous blood and decrease of PGE2 concentration both in venous and menstrual blood (85). In a controlled study, treatment of dysmenorrheic patients with α-tocopherol during three consecutive menstrual cycles alleviated pain in significant number of women. Administration of naloxone on the first day of their relatively pain-free menstruation triggered an immediate onset of menstrual cramps. Naloxone-induced pain in these patients is likely to be due to a blockade of opioid receptors and, thus, impeded opioid regulation of pain perception (86).

GABA The inhibitory neurotransmitter GABA is closely associated with endogenous steroidal hormone release (44,98) and this association has wide ranging implications for the etiology of a number of pathological conditions. In addition, GABAergic neurons are components of circuits within both the spinal cord and brain that include neuronal membrane receptors for ovarian steroids (117). Furthermore, ovarian steroids can directly modulate GABAergic receptors (103). Thus, hormonal imbalances have the potential of altering GABAergic mechanisms in many parts of the nervous system. Within the hypothalamus, imbalances could affect systems that descend to influence autonomic circuitry within the spinal cord controlling output to the uterus. Within the spinal cord, hormonal effects of GABAergic mechanisms most certainly include circuits in the dorsal horn associated with nociception (see below). Although autoradiographic binding and immunohistochemical studies indicate minimal GABA involvement within intermediolateral column spinal autonomic circuitry, GABA is certainly an important agent within spinal autonomic circuitry surrounding the central canal (lamina X) and peripherally within autonomic ganglia themselves (75,152).

NEURAL MECHANISMS OF DYSMENORRHEA: BEYOND THE UTERUS

The previous sections in this chapter have dealt with events that occur within potential sources of dysmenorrhea located in the periphery (e.g., the uterus) and modulation of these peripheral events by eicosanoid, hormonal, behavioral, and neural efferent (output) factors. The experience of dysmenorrheic pain, however, like that of any conscious sensation, requires processing of afferent sensory information by the nervous system.

Innervation of the Uterus

The female pelvic visceral reproductive organs are innervated mainly by two nerves—the hypogastric and the pelvic (erigentes) nerves. Pelvic somatic structures are innervated by the pudendal nerves. Although the hypogastric and pelvic nerves are autonomic nerves whose efferent functions are assumed, a large proportion of the fibers in these nerves is afferent to the spinal cord (80,113,149). As described in considerable detail by Bonica (29,30), hypogastric afferent fibers travel by way of the uterine and cervical plexuses, passing through the pelvic (inferior hypogastric) and middle hypogastric plexuses and finally through the superior hypogastric (presacral nerve) and aortic plexuses to enter the lumbar and lower thoracic sympathetic chain and arrive at the spinal cord via posterior roots of the T10, T11, T12, and L1 spinal nerves. Pelvic nerve fibers travel by way of the pelvic (inferior hypogastric) and pudendal plexuses to arrive at the spinal cord through posterior roots of the S2, S3, and S4 spinal nerves. This is summarized in Fig. 2.

Extensive analyses of pain control by discrete blocks with local anesthetics in women undergoing labor by Bonica et al. (30) demonstrated that pain in the first and second stages of labor was alleviated by various discrete blocks that interfered with fibers traveling in the hypogastric nerve. Additional blocks interfering with input from the pelvic and pudendal nerves were not necessary until later in the second and third stages of labor.

These results indicated that fibers conveying information about the intense events that occur mostly in the uterus and cervix during the first stages of labor travel to the spinal cord by way of the hypogastric nerve and not by way of the pelvic or pudendal nerves. These latter nerves would instead convey information about intense events that occur mostly in the vaginal canal and perineum during the second stage. This topographic innervation pattern is supported by studies in rats that demonstrate that unmyelinated afferent fibers in the hypogastric nerve convey information mainly about intense stimuli occurring in the uterus and cervix, whereas unmyelinated afferent fibers in the pelvic nerve convey information about both gentle and intense stimuli occurring in the cervix and vaginal canal (17,18,20,22,116).

In accord with these results, earlier clinical studies showed that hypogastric (presacral) neurectomies can alleviate intractable dysmenorrhea in women (41,45,66). In addition, such neurectomies can eliminate escape responses to uterine distention stimuli in rats (21). It is important to note, however, that in both humans and rats hypogastric neurectomies can be ineffective or only temporarily effective (21,151). Similarly, it is well known that parous status influences dysmenorrhea—i.e., that intensity of dysmenorrhea is reduced in parous women. One hypothesis is that this reduction is due to the adrenergic nerve terminal degeneration and uterine neurotransmitter loss that occurs during pregnancy and is only partially restored after pregnancy (140). However, recent studies in the rat have shown that this apparent loss produces no obvious changes in the terminations of these fibers in the spinal cord (125). In addition, the uterus becomes hyperinnervated

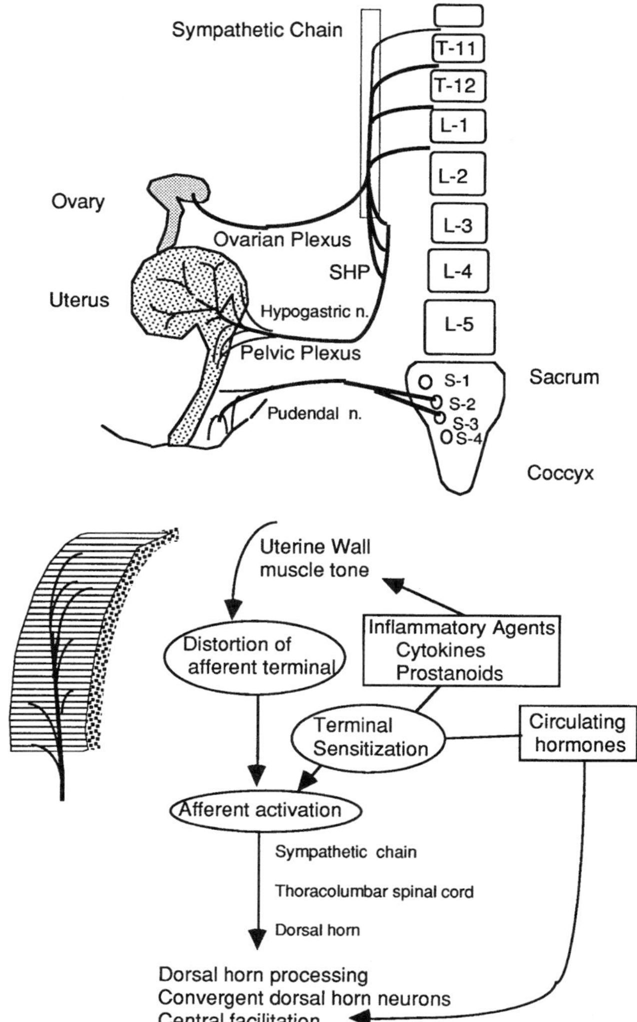

Figure 2. *Top:* Organization showing the principal afferent innervation of the uterus being provided by the hypogastric nerve traveling through the pelvic plexus and the superior hypogastric plexus (SHP) to join the sympathetic chain to innervate the T11/12 and L1-2 segments of the spinal cord; e.g., these afferents have their ganglion cells in the respective dorsal roots. The pudendal nerve originating form the S2-S3/S4 roots provide the somatic afferent innervation for the non visceral pelvic tissues. The ovary receives afferent innervation via the ovarian plexus and projects though the sympathetic chain. *Bottom:* Contributing components that may lead to a dysmenorrheic pain state. Uterine afferent out flow may develop from a combination of changes in uterine muscle tone and the elaboration of prosensitizing factors (such as cytokines and prostanoids, as well as circulating hormones. This out flow provides excitatory input into the spinal cord where it is processed as other visceral input (see Chapter 12). In addition, there is reason to speculate that circulating factors accompanying the menstrual cycle may exert a central facilitatory influence.

immediately postpartum (72). Together, these results suggest that mechanisms for pain of supposed uterine origin involves consideration of other factors in addition to the uterus' peripheral afferent innervation, such as CNS mechanisms (see below).

Central Projections of Pelvic Afferent Input

Unfortunately, very little is known about how information arising from the uterus is processed within the CNS. Recent studies in rats have shown, however, that a distention stimulation of the uterus can activate a surprisingly large percentage of neurons located in many somatovisceral sensory regions; i.e., in the dorsal horn of the caudal spinal cord (T13-S-2) (24), in the dorsal column nuclei (78), in the solitary nucleus (79), and in and near the ventroposterolateral nucleus of the thalamus (26). Electrical stimulation of the uterus has also been shown to activate neurons in the thalamus and primary somatic sensory areas of cortex in the rat and cat (13).

With the exception of the solitary nucleus, most of the CNS neurons responsive to uterine stimulation in these studies were additionally responsive to stimulation of somatic structures located both within and outside the dermatomes supplied by the spinal nerves through which the uterine afferents travel to the spinal cord (mainly T13, L1, and L2 in the rat). Convergence from other visceral organs (e.g., colon) was also observed. Further studies in the spinal cord indicated extensive spread of this information through many segments and considerable intersegmental intraspinal modulation of that information (153). For example, uterine stimulation activated neurons in the dorsal horn of the L6/S1 segment (as well as T13/L1 segments) and this L6/S1 activation was prevented by hypogastric neurectomies or transection of the spinal cord between L2 and L6. Further studies in the thalamus indicated that neurons responsive to uterine and somatic stimulation could also be activated by application of prostaglandins ($PGF_{2\alpha}$) and bradykinin to the uterus (70). While this application evoked giant uterine contractions, the neural response was not necessarily a result of these contractions, particularly those produced by bradykinin.

Taken together, these results indicate (a) that information about intense uterine stimulation has access to a large population of neurons in somatosensory and visceral regions throughout the CNS; (b) that this information is subject to considerable modulation by information converging from other somatic and visceral body structures; and (c) that the neuronal activity provoked by intense mechanical uterine stimulation (i.e., balloon distention) is not always clearly associated with other abnormal uterine events, such as strong contractions. It would be premature at this stage to attempt to use these facts for proposing any detailed CNS mechanisms for dysmenorrhea. However, it is evident from these facts that several components provide substrates for processing such information.

BEHAVIORAL FACTORS

Some authors have suggested that women with dysmenorrhea have lower pain tolerance. Procacci et al. (120) noted lowered-pain thresholds during the luteal phase with a subsequent steady rise that reached a peak towards the end of menstruation. In a study by Hapidou and DeCatanzaro (73), almost identical results were obtained using two different pain induction techniques. Women with dysmenorrhea reported less pain during the follicular phase compared with the luteal phase during a cold pressor task, a finding not present in controls (73). However, other studies have shown no differences between dysmenorrheic and nondysmenorrheic women using a variety of measures of somatic pain sensitivity including pain threshold and pain tolerance, self-reported estimates of pain and affective and physiological changes during the course of an ischemic pain procedure (2,6).

A biopsychosocial model of primary dysmenorrhea includes environmental and behavioral factors that may alter the severity of menstrual discomfort (108). Emotional distress and stress exacerbate dysmenorrhea (69,92,108). The response to stress ultimately involves liberation of endogenous opioid peptides (104,133) that affect CNS function as described above. In addition, opioid peptides can mobilize calcium from intracellular storage sites (82,150) or affect calcium channels (83) and increased intracellular calcium can result in muscle spasm, ischemia, and pain.

ORGANIZING PRINCIPLES FOR PAIN IN THE DYSMENORRHEIC STATE

The etiology of dysmenorrhea, like that of many other clinical persistent pain conditions is multifactorial. In any case, it seems probable that the syndrome reflects the activation of afferent processing through central substrates. Accordingly, several issues are relevant: (a) What is the effective stimulus? (b) What are the essential conditions under which such stimuli evoke a pain state? (c) What are the central pathways relevant to this input? The two major categories of etiological factors are those occurring in the periphery and those within the CNS. Figure 2 provides a summary of this organization.

Peripheral Mechanisms

The most logical source for episodes of dysmenorrheic pain comprises events occurring within the uterus itself that become transduced into afferent traffic that travels to the spinal cord by hypogastric and pelvic nerves. These nerves, like many visceral afferents can be shown to be mechanosensitive and to respond to changes in the local chemical environment. Such events clearly include intense contractile myometrial activities that give rise to hypoxic conditions. Thus, (a) the mechanical pressure, (b) the chemical sequelae of hypoxia, e.g., increased extracellular K or an increase in H^+ ion concentrations, or (c) locally acting hormones (e.g., prostanoids, kinins or cytokines) can activate unmyelinated afferents (see Chapter 6). Importantly many of these chemical products can interact to both activate and to sensitize the afferent terminal through receptor-mediated mechanisms. Under such conditions, afferents that are typically activated only by extreme mechanical or chemical stimuli can become activated by relatively mild stimulus conditions. Although all of the details of this scenario have not been applied to the present syndrome, it appears likely that some components of this substrate could activate uterine afferent fibers in such a fashion that information would be processed within the CNS in a manner that could provoke pain state. The existence of mechanisms that serve to sensitize the afferent terminal may provide a peripheral explanation as to why even intense uterine pressures or contractions are not invariably associated with dysmenorrhea or uterine pain. In the absence of a peripheral sensitization, uterine afferents may not be adequately activated by such mechanical stimuli. Also included would be unknown mechanisms that modify uterine innervation either by (a) affecting the sensitivity of afferent fibers so that myometrial conditions that normally do not activate uterine afferent fibers would do so or by (b) changing uterine innervation patterns in other ways (such as those occurring during pregnancy and immediately postpartum).

CNS Mechanisms

Facilitated Processing

The experience of dysmenorrhea requires central processing of afferent information that originates from the uterus. Dysmenorrhea could result simply from the initiation of neural activity in parts of the CNS thought to serve some role in pain by provocative peripheral pelvic stimuli. Detailed mechanisms for such activation are not yet understood, but intense uterine stimuli can indeed increase neural activity in relevant CNS structures. There is a growing appreciation that in somatic afferents, repetitive afferent input can induce a state of facilitated processing at the level of the spinal cord (see Chapter 36). It is likely that mechanisms that regulate certain components of somatic and visceral afferent processing in general will also apply specifically to the organization of the response in dysmenorrhea. Thus, given the scenario of paroxysmal uterine wall contractions depolarizing afferent terminals that have been sensitized by a variety of inflammatory products, it seems reasonable that central facilitatory processes will be brought into play.

Referred Pain

An important feature of dysmenorrheic pain along with its deeply-localized cramping aches is its "referral" to somatic cutaneous and muscle tissues in the perineum, upper thighs and back. Such referred pains are considered to reflect a central convergence of somatic and visceral input onto common projections neurons (36,105) (see Chapter 39). With respect to the uterus, one good example is labor pain. During labor, somatic regions to which pain is referred progress from the T10-11 dermatomes into the L2-S3 dermatomes as parturition progresses into the second stage (see Chapter 17). Presumably, this is the mechanism for the referred somatic pains of dysmenorrhea; i.e., their provocation originates in uterine tissue. On the other hand, such provocation can occur in the other direction. For example, the extreme painful crises evoked by the passage of kidney stones through the ureter can be reelicited in patients long after the disease has resolved simply by gently stimulating muscles or subcutaneous tissue in the region of referral (68). In women with chronic pelvic pain, tender points in the lower abdominal wall can often be found (11,141). This "referral hyperalgesia" is thought to be due to long-lasting central sensitizations that were produced by prior pathological or intense events (106). The existence of these long-lasting sensitization mechanisms indicates that even certain cases of dysmenorrhea thought to be primary (i.e., without underlying peripheral organic pathology) could be virtually entirely of CNS origin. Rather than being due to sensitization of peripheral structures, dysmenorrheic pains could arise in part from CNS activity brought about by certain environmental and hormonal conditions that would be impotent in individuals without previous central-sensitizing history.

An additional variable that may be considered relates to the complicated interaction between the sex hormones that are cyclically secreted and their potential central actions. One example can be cited pertaining to such interactions. It is appreciated that the state of facilitated processing the spinal cord is mediated in part by the release of glutamate and the subsequent activation of NMDA receptor sites (160) (see Chapter 36). Recent work has demonstrated that in pyramidal cells spine and synapse density fluctuate with ovarian steroid levels across the estrous cycle and the delivery of estradiol will mimic that increase (155). This appears to be a use dependent phenomena as the change in hippocampal dendritic spine density is dependent upon NMDA receptor activation (161). This enhanced spinal surface and receptors correlates with enhanced glutamatergic activity in hippocampus. Thus, estrogen pretreatment has no effect on hippocampal membrane properties, but increases glutamatergic synaptic excitability, inducing repetitive firing (159). These models though not strictly related to pain processing, provide support for the assertion that these cyclical hormones can transiently alter neurotransmission through certain receptor systems. Importantly, as noted, at the spinal cord level these receptor systems have a pronounced influence upon the gain of the afferent transmission system activated by small afferent input.

THERAPEUTIC APPROACHES

NSAIDs

The main stay of treatment for dysmenorrhea is the use of NSAIDs (14,64). This emphasizes the likely role played by prostanoids in the syndrome. It should be stressed, however, that while uterine or plasma prostanoids are elevated in dysmenorrhea (47) and uterine smooth muscle is significantly impacted by prostaglandins (see above), it is not clear that the uterine muscle is the principal site of NSAID action. Thus, measurement of "uterine contractility" in dysmenorrheic patients receiving NSAIDS revealed that contractile strength as well as pattern was unaltered although significant pain relief was noted (124). These observations thus suggest that additional mechanisms may be involved in the effects of the NSAIDs. Such additional mechanisms may include effects not related to cyclooxygenase inhibition or to alternate sites other than smooth muscle in the uterus or even the smooth muscle itself. As reviewed elsewhere (see Chapter 34), most NSAIDs have complex mechanisms of action. For example, meclofenamic acid is not only a potent inhibitor of cyclooxygenase, but will in addition will inhibit the formation of 5-HETE and LTB_4 from human neutrophils and will antagonize the direct effect of certain prostanoids on several peripheral tissues (42). Alternately, as noted above, repetitive afferent input will produce a central state of facilitation that is mediated in part by the release of prostanoids at the spinal level (see Chapter 61). Such facilitated states in animal models have been shown to be attenuated by spinal cyclooxygenase inhibition (99) (see Chapter 40).

Oral Contraceptives

An additional therapy for dysmenorrhea has been oral contraceptives. These medications have long been known to have some efficacy in the treatment of the primary syndrome (110). Such treatment may serve to reduce uterine contractions and may alter a number of corollary variables. Thus, after initiation of such treatments, uterine contractions were reduced, and plasma levels of vasopressin and prostaglandins were reduced. Given the dissociation of circulating prostaglandins and uterine contraction, the pain relief and uterine activity may be complexly associated, but discriminable events (56).

CONCLUSION

A number of factors appear to have the potential of mediating the pain state of primary dysmenorrhea. Studies focused on the peripheral tissue emphasize the likelihood that mechanical stimuli resulting from uterine tone may contribute, but alone cannot account for the pain syndrome. In addition, it appears likely that the local chemical milieu, including a variety of cytokines (such as prostaglandins and hormones), serve to sensitize the peripheral nerve endings of the visceral afferents. In addition, there are central connections that may exacerbate the syndrome by altering the hormonal milieu. As well, there is the central encoding system whereby the information generated by the contractions of the smooth muscle and its adjoining connective tissues is processed. The periodicity of the pain state suggests that the correlated changes in secretion is an important component. The observation that a variety of hormones can in fact evoke a peripheral change in afferent sensitivity and the growing body of knowledge suggesting that circulating hormones can also have effects upon central excitability may reflect an important step in our appreciation of the organization of this syndrome.

REFERENCES

1. Abel MH, Baird DT. The effect of 17-B oestradiol and progesterone on prostaglandin production by human endometrium maintained in organ culture. *Endocrinology* 1980;106:1599–1605.
2. Aberger EW, Denney DR, Hutchings DF. Pain sensitivity and coping strategies among dysmenorrheic women: much ado about nothing. *Behav Res Ther* 1983;21:119–27.
3. Ahumada HH, Valles De Bourges V, Imares Ayala. Variations in serum fluid and lipoproteins throughout the menstrual cycle. *Fertil Steril* 1985;44:88–94.
4. Akerlund M, Andersson KE, Ingemarsson I. Effects of terbutaline on myometrial activity, uterine activity, uterine blood flow and lower abdominal pain in women with primary dysmenorrhea. *Br J Obstet Gynecol* 1976;83:673–678.

5. Akerlund M, Stromberg P, Forsling ML. Primary dysmenorrhea and vasopressin. *Br J Obstet Gynecol* 1979;86:484–487.
6. Amodei N, Nelson-Greay RO. Reactions of dysmenorrheic and non-dysmenorrheic women to experimentally induced pain throughout the menstrual cycle. *J Behav Med* 1990;12:373–385.
7. Andersson K, Ulmsten U. Effects of nifedipine on myometrial activity and lower abdominal pain in women with primary dysmenorrhea. *Br J Obstet Gynecol* 1978:142–148.
8. Avant RF. Dysmenorrhea. *Prim Care* 1988;15:549–559.
9. Backon J. Mechanism of analgesic effect of clonidine in the treatment of dysmenorrhea. *Med Hypotheses* 1991;36:223–224.
10. Battye KM, O'Neill C, Evans G. Evidence of platelet-activating factor suppresses uterine oxytocin-induced 13, 14-dihydro- 15-keto-prostaglandin F2α release and phosphatidylinositol hydrolysis in the ewe. *Biol Reprod* 1992;47:213–219.
11. Beard RW, Highman JW, Pearce S, Reginal PW. Diagnosis of pelvic varicosities in women with chronic pelvic pain. *Lancet* 1984;2: 946–949.
12. Beard RW, Gangar K, Pearce S. Chronic gynaecological pain. In: Wall PD, Melzack R, eds. *Textbook of pain.* Edinburgh: Churchill Livingstone, 1994:597–614.
13. Befort JJ, Albe-Fessard D. Zones de projections thalamiques et corticales de líuterus chez le chat et le rat. *J Physiol Paris* 1966;58:204.
14. Benassi L, Bertani D, Avanzini A. An attempt at real prophylaxis of primary dysmenorrhea: comparison between meclofenamate sodium and naproxen sodium. *Clin Exp Obstet Gynecol* 1993;20: 102–107.
15. Benedek G, Szikazai M. Potentiation of thermoregulatory and analgesic effects of morphine by calcium antagonists. *Pharmacol Res* 1984;16:1009–1018.
16. Benedetto C. Eicosanoids in primary dysmenorrhea, endometriosis and menstrual migraine. *Gynecol Endocrinol* 1989;3:71–94.
17. Berkley KJ, Robbins A, Sato Y. Uterine afferent fibers in the rat. In: Schmidt RF, Shaible HG, Vahle-Hinz C, eds. *Fine afferent nerve fibers and pain.* Weinheim, Germany: Vch Verlagsgesellschaft, 1987: 127–136.
18. Berkley KJ, Robbins A, Sato Y. Afferent fibers supplying the uterus in the rat. *J Neurophysiol* 1988;59:142–163.
19. Berkley KJ, Robbins A, Sato Y. Sensory input from contractions of the uterus in the rat. *Soc Neurosci Abstr* 1988;14:727.
20. Berkley KJ, Hotta H, Robbins A, Sato Y. Functional properties of afferent fibers supplying reproductive and other pelvic organs in pelvic nerve of female rat. *J Neurophysiol* 1990;63:256–272.
21. Berkley KJ, Scofield S, Wood E. Uterine pain: the role of ischemia and the hypogastric nerve. *Soc Neurosci Abstr* 1990;16:416.
22. Berkley KJ. Changes in uterine compliance and escape responses to uterine distention as a function of estrous stage in the awake rat. *J Auton Nerv Syst* 1993;43:61.
23. Berkley KJ, Robbins A, Sato Y. Functional differences between afferent fibers in the hypogastric and pelvic nerves innervating female reproductive organs in the rat. *J Neurophysiol* 1993;69: 533–544.
24. Berkley KJ. Communications from the uterus (and other tissues). In: Besson JM, Guilbaud G, eds. *Pharmacological aspects of the peripheral neurons involved in nociception.* Amsterdam: Elsevier, 1993:39–47.
25. Berkley KJ, Hubscher CH, Wall PD. Neuronal responses to stimulation of the cervix, uterus and colon in the rat spinal cord. *J Neurophysiol* 1993;69:545–556.
26. Berkley KJ, Guilbaud G, Benoist JM, Gautron M. Responses of neurons stimulation of uterus, cervix, vagina, colon and skin. *J Neurophysiol* 1993;69:557–568.
27. Bicknell RJ. Endogenous opioid peptides and hypothalamic neuroendocrine neurones. *J Endocrinol* 1985;107:437–446.
28. Bolton TB. Mechanism of action of transmitters and other substances on smooth muscle. *Physiol Rev* 1979;59:606.
29. Bonica JJ, Mcdonald JS. The pain of childbirth. In: Bonica JJ, ed. *The management of pain.* 2nd ed. Philadelphia: Lea & Febiger, 1990: 1313–1343.
30. Bonica JJ. Labour pain. In: Wall PD, Melzack R, eds. *Textbook of pain.* Edinburgh: Churchill Livingstone, 1994:615–641.
31. Bray MA, Cunningham FM, Ford-Hutchinson AW, Smith MJH. Leukotriene B4: a mediator of vascular permeability. *Br J Pharmacol* 1981;72:483.
32. Bray MA. The pharmacology and pathophysiology of leukotriene B_4. *Br Med Bull* 1983;39:249–254.
33. Burghardt RC, Fletcher WH. Physiological roles of gap junctional communication in reproduction. In: Carsten ME, Miller JD, eds. *Uterine function: molecular and cellular aspects.* New York: Plenum Press, 1990:277–313.
34. Camussi G, Brentjens J, Bussolino F, Tetta C. Role of platelet activating factor in immunopathological reactions. *Adv Inflamm Res* 1986;11:97.
35. Carracher R, Hahn DW, Ritchie DM, Mcguire JL. Involvement of lipoxygenase products in myometrial contractions. *Prostaglandins* 1983;26:23.
36. In: Casey KL, ed. *Pain and central nervous system disease: the central pain syndromes.* New York: Raven Press, 1991.
37. Chan WY, Dawood MY. Prostaglandin levels in menstrual fluid of non-dysmenorrheic and of dysmenorrheic subjects with and without oral contraceptive or ibuprofen therapy. *Adv Prostaglandin Thromboxane Leukot Res* 1980;8:1443–1447.
38. Chance B, Sides H, Boveris A. Hyperoxide metabolism in mammalian organs. *Physiol Rev* 1979;59:527–589.
39. Chaudhuri G. Physiologic aspects of prostaglandins and leukotrienes. *Semin Reprod Endocrinol* 1981;3:219–230.
40. Chegini N, Rao CHV. The presence of leucotriene C4- and prostacyclin-binding sites in non-pregnant uterine tissue. *J Clin Endocrinol Metab* 1988;58:813.
41. Colcock BP. Presacral neurectomy for the relief of severe primary dysmenorrhea. *Surg Clin Am* 1941;21:855–864.
42. Conroy MC, Randinitis EJ, Turner JL. Pharmacology, pharmacokinetics, and therapeutic use of meclofenamate sodium. *Clin J Pain* 1991;1:S44–S48.
43. Corodimas KP, Morrell JI. Estradiol-concentratin forebrain and midbrain neurons project directly to the medulla. *J Comp Neurol* 1990;291:609–620.
44. Costa E, Paul SM. *Neurosteroids and brain function. Fidia Research Foundation symposium series, vol. 8.* New York: Thieme Medical, 1991.
45. Cotte G. Resection of the presacral nerve in the treatment of obstinate dysmenorrhea. *Am J Obstet Gynecol* 1937;33:1034–1040.
46. Crane LH, Martin L. Effects of the progesterone antagonist ru486 on myometrial activity in vivo in early pregnant and pseudopregnant rats. *Reprod Fertil Dev* 1992;4:161–166.
47. Creatsas G, Deligeoroglou E, Zachari A, et al. Prostaglandins: PGF2α, PGE2, 6-keto-PGF1α and TXB2 serum levels in dysmenorrheic adolescents before, during and after treatment with oral contraceptives. *Eur J Obstet Gynecol Reprod Biol* 1990;36:292–298.
48. Dawood MY. Dysmenorrhea. *J Reprod Med* 1985;30:154–166.
49. Dawood MY. Current concepts in the etiology and treatment of primary dysmenorrhea. *Acta Obstet Gynecol Scand Suppl* 1986;138: 7–10.
50. Dawood MY. Dysmenorrhea and prostaglandins: pharmacological and therapeutical considerations. *Drugs* 1987;22:42–56.
51. Dawood MY. Nonsteroidal anti-inflammatory drugs and changing attitudes toward dysmenorrhea. *Am J Med* 1988;5A:23–29.
52. Downing SJ, Porter DG, Redstone CD. Myometrial activity in rats during the oestrous cycle and pseudopregnancy: interaction of oestradiol and progesterone. *J Physiol* 1981;317:425–433.
53. Drugs for Dysmenorrhea. *Med Lett Drugs Ther* 1979;21:81–84.
54. Ducsay CA. Calcium channels: role in myometrial contractility and pharmacological applications of calcium entry blockers. In: Carsten ME, Miller JD, eds. *Uterine function: molecular and cellular aspects.* New York: Plenum Press, 1990:169–194.
55. Ekstrom P, Juchnicka E, Laudanski T, Akerlund M. Effect of an oral contraceptive in primary dysmenorrheaóchanges in uterine activity and reactivity to agonists. *Contraception* 1989;40:39–47.
56. Ekstrom P, Akerlund M, Forsling M, Kindahl H, Laudanski T, Mrugacz G. Stimulation of vasopressin release in women with primary dysmenorrhoea and after oral contraceptive treatment—effect on uterine contractility. *Br J Obstet Gynaecol* 1992;99:680–684.
57. Fedele L, Marchini M, Acaia B, Garagiola U, Tiengo M. Dynamics and significance of placebo response in primary dysmenorrhea. *Pain* 1989;36:43–47.
58. Feine JS, Bushnell MC, Miron D, Duncan GH. Sex differences in the perception of noxious heat stimuli. *Pain* 1991;44:255–262.
59. Ferreira SH. Site of analgesic action of aspirin-like drugs and opioids. In: Beers RE, Basset EG, eds. *Mechanism of pain and analgesic compounds.* New York: Raven Press, 1979:P309.
60. Forman A, Andersson KE, Ulmsten U. Combined effects of diflunisal and nifedipine on uterine contractility in dysmenorrheic patients. *Adv Prostaglandin* 1982;23:237–246.
61. Forman A, Andersson KE, Persson CG, Ulmsten U. Relaxant effects of nifedipine on isolated human myometrium. *Acta Pharmacol Toxicol* 1979;45:81.

62. Forman A, Ulmsten U, Anderson KE. Aspects of inhibition of myometrial hyperactivity in primary dysmenorrhea. *Acta Obstet Gynecol Scand Suppl* 1983;113:71–76.
63. Forsling ML, Stromberg P, Akerlund M. Effect of ovarian steroids on vasopressin secretion. *J Endocrinol* 1982;95:147–151.
64. Fraser IS. Prostaglandins, prostaglandin inhibitors and their roles in gynaecological disorders. *Baillieres Clin Obstet Gynecol* 1992;6: 829–852.
65. Freeman ME. The nonpregnant uterus as an endocrine organ. *News Physiol Sci* 1988;3:31–32.
66. Garcia CR, David SS. Pelvic endometriosis: infertility and pelvic pain. *Am J Obstet Gynecol* 1977;129:740–747.
67. Garfield RE, Hayashi RH. Presence of gap junctions in the myometrium of women during various stages of menstruation. *Am J Obstet Gynecol* 1980;138:569.
68. Giamberardino MA, Valente R, Vecchiet L. Muscular hyperalgesia of renal/ureteral origin. In: Vecchiet L, Albe-Fessard D, Lindblom U, Giamberardino MA, eds. *New trends in referred pain and hyperalgesia. Pain research and clinical management, vol. 7.* Amsterdam: Elsevier, 1993.
69. Gomibuchi H, Taketani Y, Doi M, Yoshida K, Mizukawa H, Kaneko M, Kohda K, Takei T, Kimura Y, Liang SG. Is personality involved in the expression of dysmenorrhea in patients with endometriosis? *Am J Obstet Gynecol* 1993;169:723–725.
70. Guilbaud G, Berkley JJ, Benoist JM, Gautron M. Responses of neurons in thalamic ventrobasal complex of rats to graded distention of uterus and vagina to uterine suprafusion with bradykinin and prostaglandin F2α. *Brain Res* 1993;614:285–290.
71. Gulyaeva NG, Luzina NL, Levshina IP, Kryzhanovskii GN. Stage of inhibition of lipid peroxidation during stress. *Bull Exp Biol Med* 1988;106:1684–1688.
72. Haase EB, Schramm LP. Postpartum hyperinnervation in the uterus of the rat. *Soc Neurosci Abstr* 1993;19:508.
73. Hapidou EG, De Catanzaro D. Sensitivity to cold pressor pain in dysmenorrheic and non-dysmenorrheic women as a function of menstrual cycle phase. *Pain* 1988;34:277–283.
74. Higuchi T, Uchide K, Honda K, Negoro H. Pelvic neurectomy abolishes the fetus expulsion reflex and induces dystocia in the rat. *Exp Neurol* 1987;96:443–455.
75. Hills JM, Jessen KR. Transmission: g-aminobutyric acid (Gaba), 5-hydroxytryptamine (5-Ht) and dopamine. In: Burnstock G, Hoyale CHV, eds. *Autonomic neuroeffector mechanisms.* Chur, Switzerland: Harwood Academic, 1992:465–507.
76. Hockel M, Holzer PA, Brockerhoff P. Determination of long-chain nonesterified fatty acid in sera of young women in different phases of the menstrual cycle. Application of a new gas chromatographic microliter method. *Gynecol Obstet Invest* 1983;16: 51–58.
77. Holstege G. Some anatomical observations on the projections from the hypothalamus to brainstem and spinal cord: an hrp and autoradiographic tracing study in the cat. *J Comp Neurol* 1987; 260:90–126.
78. Hubscher CH, Berkley KJ. Neuronal responses to stimulation of uterus, cervix and vaginal canal in the rat gracile nucleus. *Soc Neurosci Abstr* 1992;18:494.
79. Hubscher CH, Berkley KJ. Neuronal responses to stimulation of uterus, cervix, vaginal canal and colon in the rat solitary nucleus. *Soc Neurosci Abstr* 1993;19:514.
80. Hulsebosch CE, Coggeshall RE. An analysis of the axon populations in the nerves to the pelvic viscera in the rat. *J Comp Neurol* 1982;211:1–10.
81. Hunskaar S, Fasmer Ole Bernt, Hole Kjell. Acetylsalicylic acid, paracetamol and morphine inhibit behavioral responses to intrathecally administered substance P or capsaicin. *Life Sci* 1985;37:1835–1841.
82. Kamaswamy S, Rajasekaran M, Bapha JS. Role of calcium in prolactin analgesia. *Arch Int Pharmacodyn Ther* 1986;28:356–360.
83. Kavaliers M. Calcium channel blockers inhibit the antagonistic effects of phe-met-arg-phe-amide (fmrfamide) on morphine and stress-induced analgesia in mice. *Brain Res* 1987;415:380–384.
84. Kelly RW, Lumsden MA, Abel M, Baird DT. The relationship between menstrual blood loss and prostaglandin production in human: evidence for increased availability of arachidonic acid in women suffering from menorrhagia. *Prostaglandins Leukot Essent Fatty Acids* 1984;16:69–78.
85. Kryzhanowsky GN, Bakuleva LP, Luzina NL, Vinogradov VA, Yarigin KN, Kubatiev AA. Endogenous opioid system in α-tocopherol analgesic effect with special reference to dysmenorrhea. *Bull Exp Biol Med* 1988;2:148–149.
86. Kryzhanovsky GN, Luzina NL, Yarygin KN. Alpha-tocoperhol induced activation of the endogenous opioid system. *Bull Exp Biol Med* 1989;566–567.
87. Laatikainen TJ. Corticoptropin-releasing hormone and opioid peptides in reproduction and stress. *Ann Med* 1991;23:489–496.
88. Lalos O, Joelsson I. Effect of an oral contraceptive on uterine tonicity in women with primary dysmenorrhea. *Acta Obstet Gynecol Scand* 1981;60:229–232.
87. Leadem CA, Kalra SF. Reversal of beta-endorphin-induced blockade of ovulation and luteinizing hormone surge with prostaglandin E2. *Endocrinology* 1985;117:684–689.
90. Levine JD, Lau W, Kwait G, Goetzel EJ. Leucrotriene B4 produces hyperalgesia that is dependent on polymorphonuclear leucocytes. *Science* 1984;225:743.
91. Loewy AD, Spyer KM, eds. *Central regulation of autonomic functions.* Oxford: Oxford University Press, 1990.
92. Logue CM, Moos RH. Perimenstrual symptoms: prevalence and risk factors. *Psychosom Med* 1986;48:388–414.
93. Lundstrom V. The myometrial response of intrauterine administration of PGF2α and PGE2 in dysmenorrheic women. *Acta Obstet Gynecol Scand* 1977;56:167–172.
94. Lundstrom V, Green K. Endogenous levels of prostaglandin $F_2\alpha$ and its main metabolites in plasma and endometrium of normal and dysmenorrheic women. *Am J Obstet Gynecol* 1978;130:640–646.
95. Lundstrom V. The uterus. In: Bygdeman M, Berger GS, Keith LG, eds. *Prostaglandins and their inhibitors in clinical obstetrics and gynecology.* 1st ed. Lancaster, U.K.: MTP Press, 1986:59.
96. Luzina Nl. *Antioxidants in the treatment of dysmenorrhea.* Moscow, 1988:1–129.
97. Lyons EA, Ballard G, Taylor PJ, Levi CS, Zheng XH, Kredenstser JV. Characterization of subendometrial myometrial contractions throughout the menstrual cycle in normal fertile women. *Fertil Steril* 1991;55:771–774.
98. Majewska MD. Neurosteroids: endogenous bimodal modulators of the $GABA_a$ receptor. Mechanism of action and physiological significance. *Prog Neurobiol* 1992;38:379–395.
99. Malmberg AB, Yaksh TL. Antinociceptive actions of spinal nonsteroidal anti-inflammatory agents on the formalin test in the rat. *J Pharmacol Exp Ther* 1992;263:136–263.
100. Martin HA. Leukotrine B_4 induced decrease in mechanical and thermal thresholds of C-fiber mechanonociceptros in rat hairy skin. *Brain Res* 1990;509:273–279.
101. Martin L, Crane LH. In vivo myometrial activity in the rat during the oestrous cycle: studies with a novel technique of video laparoscopy. *Reprod Fertil Dev* 1991;3:185–199.
102. Massobrio M, Benedetto C, Rosi A, Marozio L, Nigam S. Eicosanoids and platelet activating factor dysmenorrhea. In: Genazzani AR, Nappi G, Faccinetti F, Martignoni E, eds. *Pain and reproduction.* Carnforth, U.K.: Parthenon, 1988:63.
103. Mccarthy MM, Coirini H, Schumacher M, Pfaff DW, Mcewen BS, Schwartz-Giblin S. Ovarian steroid modulation of [^{3}H]muscimol binding in the spinal cord of the rat. *Brain Res* 1991;556:321–323.
104. McCubbin JA. Stress and endogenous opioids. Behavioral and circulatory interactions. *Biol Psychiatry* 1993;35:91–122.
105. McMahon SB, Wall PD. Physiological evidence of brancing of peripheral unmyelinated sensory afferent fibers in the rat. *J Comp Neurol* 1987;261:130–136.
106. McMahon SB, Lewin GR, Wall PD. Central hyperexcitability triggered by noxious inputs. *Curr Opin Neurobiol* 1993;3:602–610.
107. Mehta JL. Influence of calcium-channel blockers on platelet function and arachidonic acid metabolism. *Am J Cardiol* 1985;55: 158b–164b.
108. Metheny WP, Smith RP. The relationship among exercise, stress and primary dysmenorrhea. *J Behav Med* 1989;12:569–586.
109. Miller R. How do opiates act? *Trends Neurosci* 1984;7:184–185.
110. Mishell Dr Jr. Noncontraceptive benefits of oral contraceptives. *J Reprod Med* 1993;38:1021–1029.
111. Montucchio G, Massobrio M, Alloatti GET. In vitro oxytocic activity of platelet activating factor on human myometrium. In: Samuelsson B, Paoletti R, Ramwell PW, eds. *Advances in prostaglandin, tromboxane, and leucrotriene research.* New York: Raven Press, 1987:1129.
112. Omini C, Daffonchio L, Paoletti R. Eicosanoids and pain. In: Genazzani AR, Nappi G, Facchinetti F, Martignoni E, eds. *Pain and reproduction.* Carnforth, U.K.: Parthenon, 1988:49–51.

113. Papka RE, Traurig HH. Autonomic efferent and visceral sensory innveration of the female reproductive system: special reference to neurochemical markers in nerves and ganglionic connections. In: Maggi CA, ed. *Nervous control of the urogential system.* Chur, Switzerland: Harwood Academic, 1993:423–466.
114. Parantainen J, Vapaatalo H, Hokkanen E. Clinical aspects of prostaglandins and leucrotrienes in migraine. *Cephalgia* 1986;6:95.
115. Peeters G, De Vos N, Houvenaghel A. Elimination of the fergusion reflex by section of the pelvic nerves in the lactating goat. *J Endocrinol* 1971;49:125–130.
116. Peters LC, Kristal MB, Komisaruk B. Sensory innervation of the external and internal genitalia of the female rat. *Brain Res* 1987; 408:199–204.
117. Pfaff D, Keiner M. Atlas of estradiol-concentrating cells in the central nervous system of the female rat. *J Comp Neurol* 1973;151: 121–158.
118. Pickles VR, Hall WJ, Best FA, Smith GN. Prostaglandins in endometrium and menstrual fluid from normal and dysmenorrheic subjects. *J Obstet Gyencol Br Common Wlth* 1965;72:185–192.
119. Pitchford S, Levine JD. Prostaglandins sensitize nociceptors in cell culture. *Neurosci Lett* 1991;132:105–108.
120. Procacci P, Zoppi M, Maresca M, Romano S. Studies of pain threshold in man. In: Green JR, Thompson RA, eds. *Advances in neurology.* New York: Raven Press, 1974.
121. Pulkkinen MO, Csapo AL. The effect of ibuprofen on the intrauterine pressure and menstrual pain of dysmenorrheic patients. *Prostaglandins* 1978;15:1055–1062.
122. Pulkkinen MO. Prostaglandins and the non-pregnant uterus. The pathophysiology of dysmenorrhea. *Acta Obstet Gynecol Scand Suppl* 1983;113:63–67.
123. Pulkkinen MO. Alterations in intrauterine pressure, menstrual fluid prostaglandin F Levels, and pain dysmenorrheic women treated with nimesulide. *J Clin Pharmacol* 1987;27:65–69.
124. Pulkkinen M, Monti T, Macchiocchi A. Analysis of uterine contractility after administration of the non-steroidal antiinflammatory drug nimesulide. *Acta Obstet Gynecol Scand* 1992;71:181–185.
125. Rai P, Lamotte CC. Neuropeptide immunoreactivity in the thoracic and sacral dorsal horn of pregnant rats. *Soc Neurosci Abstr* 1993;19:514.
126. Ramaswamy S, Rajasekaran M, Bapha JS. Role of calcium in prolactin analgesia. *Arch Int Pharmacodyn Ther* 1986;283:56–60.
127. Rees M. Dysmenorrhea. *Br J Obstet Gynecol* 1988;95:833.
128. Robbins A, Sato Y, Hotta H, Berkley KJ. Responses of hypogastric nerve afferent fibers to uterine distension in estrous or metestrous rats. *Neurosci Lett* 1990;110:82–85.
129. Robbins A, Sato Y. Cardiovascular changes in response to uterine stimulation. *J Autonom Nerv Sys* 1991;33:55–64.
130. Robbins A, Berkley KJ, Sato Y. Estrous cycle variation of afferent fibers supplying reproductive organs in the female rat. *Brain Res* 1992;596:353–356.
131. Rosenwaks Z, Seegar-Jones G. Menstrual pain, its origin and pathogenesis. *J Reprod Med* 1980;25:207–212.
132. Roth-Brandel U, Bygdeman M, Wiqvist N. Effect of intravenous administration of prostaglandin E1 and F2α on the contractility of the non-pregnant human uterus in vivo. *Acta Obstet Gynecol Scand* 1970;49:19–25.
133. Rushen J, Schwarze N, Ludewig J, Foxcroft G. Opioid modulation of the effects of repeated stress on acth, cortisol, prolactin and growth hormone in pigs. *Physiol Behav* 1993;53:973–978.
134. Sakamoto Y, Suga S, Sakuma Y. Estrogen-sensitive neurons in the female rat ventral tegmental area: a dual route for the hormone action. *J Neurophysiol* 1993;70:1469–1475.
135. Saper CB, Loewy AD, Swanson RE. Direct hypothalamic autonomic connections. *Brain Res* 1976;117:305–312.
136. Sato Y, Hayaski RH, Garfield RE. Mechanical responses of the rat uterus, cervix, and bladder to stimulation of hypogastric and pelvic nerves in vivo. *Biol Reprod* 1989;40:209–219.
137. Schepelmann K, Messlinger K, Schaible HG, Schmidt RF. Inflammatory mediators and nociception in the joint: excitation and sensitization of slowly conducting afferent fibers of catís knee by prostaglandin I_2. *Neuroscience* 1992;50:237–247.
138. Setty BN, Ganley C, Stuart MJ. Effects of changes in oxygen tension on vascular and platelet hydroxy acid metabolites. II. Hypoxia increases 15-hydroxyeicosatetraenoic acid, a proangiogenic metabolites. *Pediatrics* 1985;75:911.
139. Shigeru O, Hironaka A. Hyperalgesic action in mice of intracerebroventriculary administered arachidonic acid PGE2, PGF2α and PGD2 effects of analgetic drugs on hyperalgesia. *J Pharmacobiol Dyn* 1986;9:902–908.
140. Sjoberg NO. Dysmenorrhea and uterine neurotransmitters. *Acta Obstet Gynecol Scand Suppl* 1979;87:57–59.
141. Slocumb JC. Neurological factors in chronic pelvic pain: trigger points and the abdominal pelvic pain syndrome. *Am J Obstet Gynecol* 1984;149:536–543.
142. Smith RP, Powell JR. Intrauterine pressure changes during dysmenorrhea therapy. *Am J Obstet Gynecol* 1982;143:286–289.
143. Smith K, Kelly RW. Effect of platelet-activating factor on the release of PGF2α and PGE2 by separated cells of human endometrium. *J Reprod Fertil* 1988;82:271–276.
144. Smith RP. Pressure-velocity analysis of uterine muscle during spontaneous dysmenorrheic contractions in vivo. *Am J Obstet Gynecol* 1989;160:1400–1405.
145. Smith RP, Heltzel JA. Interrelation of analgesia and uterine activity in women with primary dysmenorrhea. A preliminary report. *J Reprod Med* 1991;36:260–264.
146. Stromberg P, Forsling ML. Primary dysmenorrhea and vasopressin. *Br J Obstet Gynecol* 1979;86:484–487.
147. Stromberg P, Akerlund M, Forsling ML, Kindahl H. Involvement of prostaglandins in vasopressin stimulation of the human uterus. *Br J Obstet Gynecol* 1983;90:332–337.
148. Stromberg P, Akerlund M, Forsling ML, Granstrom E, Kindahl H. Vasopressin and prostaglandins in premenstrual pain and dysmenorrhea. *Acta Obstet Gynecol Scand* 1984;63:533–538.
149. Traurig HH, Papka R. Autonomic efferent and visceral sensory innervation of the female reproductive system: special reference to the functional roles of nerves in reproductive organs. In: Maggi CA, ed. *Nervous control of the urogenital system.* Chur, Switzerland: Harwood Academic, 1993:103–141.
150. Ulmsten U. Uterine activity and blood flow in normal and dysmenorrheic women. In: Dawood MY, Mcguire JL, Demers LM, eds. *Premenstrual syndrome and dysmenorrhea.* Baltimore: Urban and Schwarzenberg, 1985:103–124.
151. Vercellini P, Fedele L, Bianchi S, Candiani GB. Pelvic denervation for chronic pain associated with endometriosis: fact or fancy? *Am J Obstet Gynecol* 1991;165:745–749.
152. Waldvogel HJ, Faull RLM, Jansen KLR, et al. Gaba, Gaba receptors and benzodiazepine receptors in the human spinal cord: an autoradiographic and immunohistochemical study at the light and electron microscopic levels. *Neuroscience* 1990;39:361–385.
153. Wall PD, Hubscher CH, Berkley KJ. Intraspinal modulation of neuronal responses to uterine and cervix stimulation in rat L1 and L6 dorsal horn. *Brain Res* 1993;622:71–78.
154. Weichman BM, Tucker SS. Contraction of guinea pig uterus by synthetic leucotrienes. *Prostaglandins* 1982;24:245.
155. Weiland NG. Estradiol selectively regulates agonist binding sites on the N-methyl-D-aspartate receptor complex in the Ca1 region of the hippocampus. *Endocrinology* 1992;131:662–668.
156. Whittle G, Slade P, Ronalds C. Social support in women reporting dysmenorrhea. *J Psychosom Med* 1987;31:1079–1084.
157. Williams TJ. Interactions between prostaglandins, leukotrienes and other mediators of inflammation. *Br Med Bull* 1983;39: 239–242.
158. Witter FR, Di Blasi NC. Effect of steroid hormones on arachidonic acid metabolites of endothelial cells. *Obstet Gynecol* 1984;63:747–751.
159. Wong M, Moss RL. Long-term and short-term electrophysiological effects of estrogen on the synaptic properties of hippocampal Ca1 neurons. *J Neurosci* 1992;12:3217–3225.
160. Woolf CJ, Thompson SW. The induction and maintenance of central sensitization is dependent on N-methyl-D-aspartic acid receptor activation; implications for the treatment of post-injury pain hypersensitivity states. *Pain* 1991;44:293–299.
161. Woolley CS, Mcewen BS. Estradiol regulates hippocampal dendritic spine density via an N-methyl-D-aspartate receptor-dependent mechanism. *J Neurosci* 1994;14:7680–7687.
162. Woods NF. Relationship of socialization and stress to perimenopausal symptoms, disability and menstrual attitudes. *Nurs Res* 1985;34:145–149.
163. Ylkorkala O, Puolakka J, Kaupilla A. Serum gonadotropins, prolactin and ovarian steroids in primary dysmenorrhea. *Br J Obstet Gynecol* 1979;86:648.

Anesthesia: Biologic Foundations, edited by Tony L. Yaksh et al. Lippincott–Raven Publishers, Philadelphia © 1997.

CHAPTER 47

OROFACIAL INFLAMMATION AND PAIN

KENNETH M. HARGREAVES, JAMES Q. SWIFT, SHARON M. GORDON, AND RAYMOND A. DIONNE

The management of acute orofacial pain is, in many ways, the management of inflammation in tissue that is innervated by the trigeminal nerve distribution. The classical signs of inflammation, namely, pain, edema, local increased temperature, redness, and loss of function (Fig. 1), occur following procedures such as surgical extractions of impacted teeth (78). This has led to the general recognition of the utility of the surgical extraction of third molars as a clinical model for evaluating physiologic mechanisms of inflammatory pain and their pharmacologic modulation (31), as well as evaluating novel and prototypic analgesics (9).

MECHANISMS OF ACUTE OROFACIAL PAIN

Acute pain is usually caused by either noxious stimuli of an intensity sufficient to produce tissue damage, or the release of inflammatory mediators that stimulate receptors located on terminal endings of nociceptive afferent nerve fibers. These fibers are distributed throughout the body and are prevalent in trigeminal nerves innervating tooth pulp, oral mucosa, periapical tissue, bone, and muscle. As described in Chaps. 31 and 32, there are two major classes of nociceptors: the C and the Aδ nerve fibers. In tooth pulp, there are at least three to eight times more unmyelinated C fibers as compared to Aδ fibers (44,80). Activation of dental pulp nerves, by either thermal, mechanical, chemical, or electrical (e.g., electrical dental pulp tester) stimuli, results in a nearly pure sensation of pain (3).

Pulpal C-Fiber Afferents

The C-fibers are unmyelinated nerve fibers with a relatively slow conduction velocity; they respond to chemical, thermal, and mechanical stimuli. The C fibers likely mediate the delayed (or "second") sensation of pain, which is generally described as

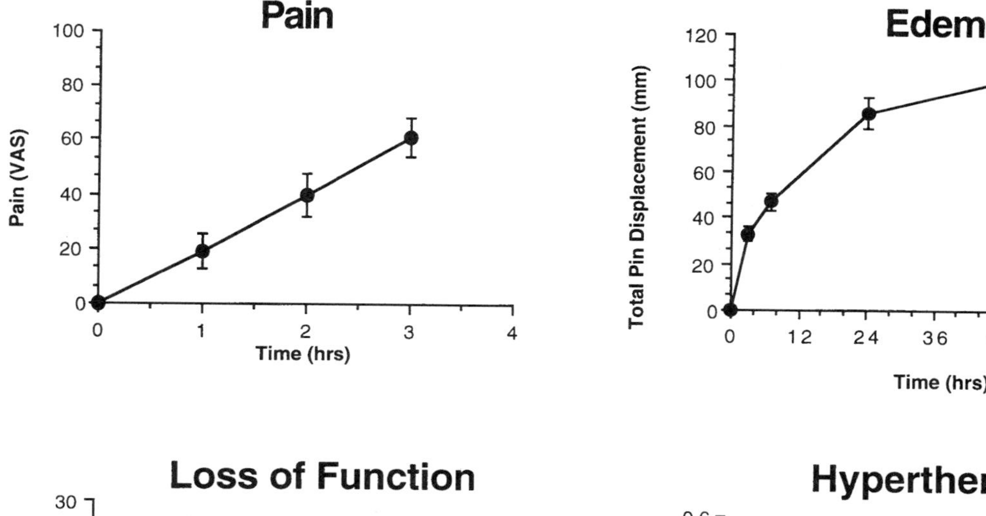

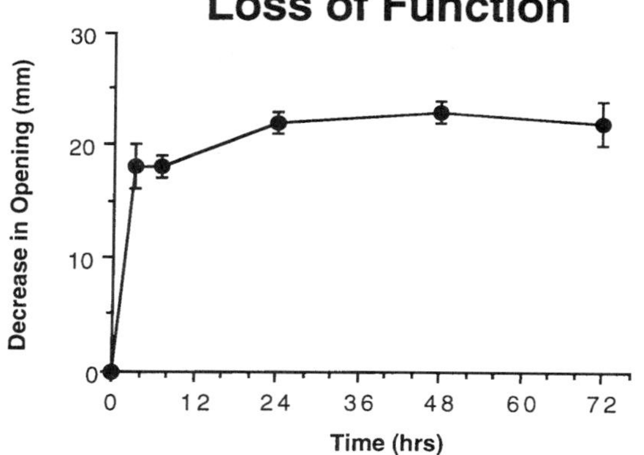

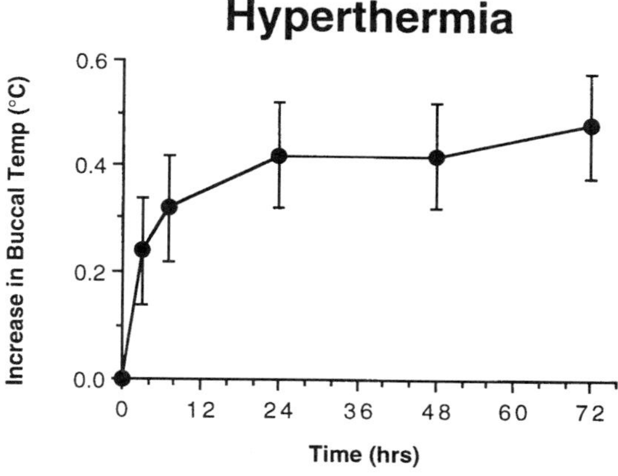

Figure 1. Composite figure illustrating the time-response curves for development of the classic signs of inflammation in the oral surgery clinical pain model. Four of the five signs of inflammation (pain, edema, hyperthermia, and loss of function [erythema was not measured]) were collected in 24 patients after the surgical removal of impacted third molars. (Data collated and redrawn from ref. 78.)

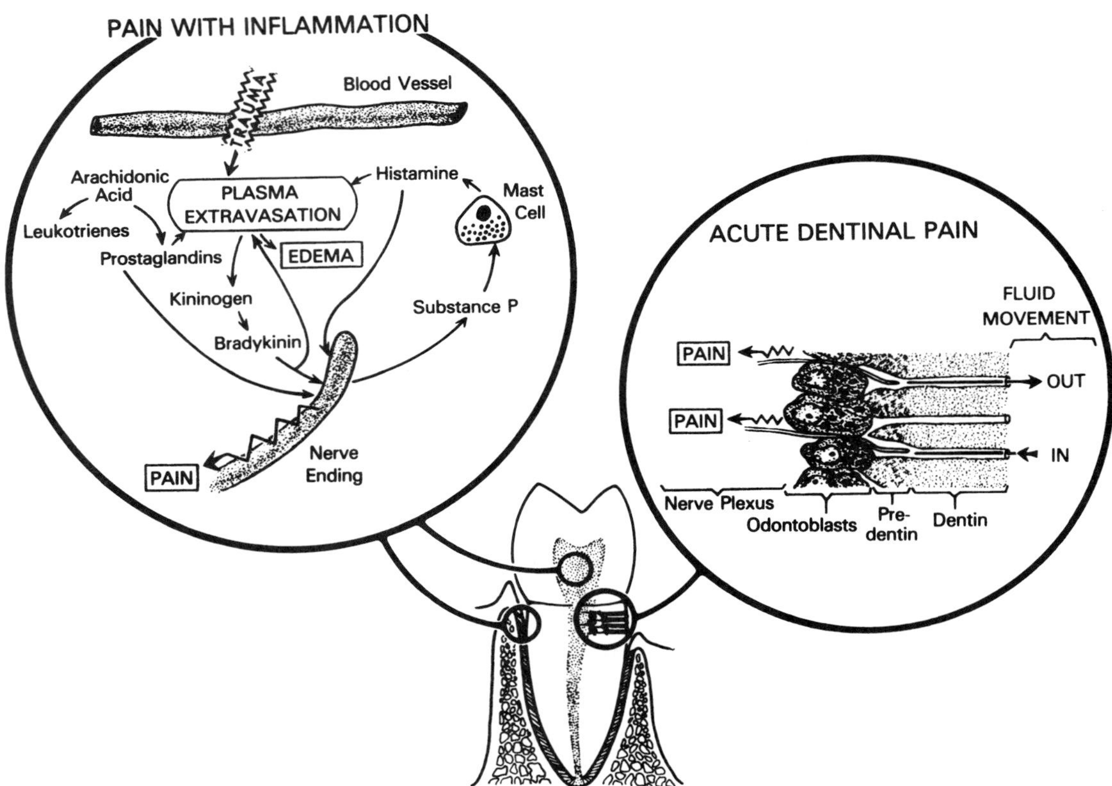

Figure 2. Schematic diagram of two mechanisms for the peripheral stimulation of nociceptive (pain-detecting) nerve fibers in the orofacial region. **Insert:** Acute dentinal pain: According to the hydrodynamic theory, stimuli that cause fluid movement in exposed dentinal tubules results in the stimulation of nociceptive nerve fibers. **Insert:** Pain with inflammation: Trauma activates a cascade resulting in the synthesis or release of prostaglandins, bradykinin, substance P, and histamine (as well as other mediators not shown). The interrelationships of these inflammatory mediators form a positive feedback loop allowing inflammation to persist far beyond cessation of the dental procedure. (From ref. 35a.)

having a throbbing, aching or burning perceptual quality (17,82) (see Chap. 41). In tooth pulp, many C fibers are reported to innervate the pulpal stroma, including blood vessels (Fig. 2). Pulpal C fibers are thought to have a predominant role for encoding inflammatory pain arising from dental pulp. This hypothesis is supported by the distribution of C fibers in dental pulp, their responsiveness to inflammatory mediators (55,64), and the perceptual qualities (e.g., dull, aching pain) of pain associated with pulpitis.

Pulpal Aδ-Fiber Afferents

The second major group of nociceptive fibers are the A fibers. The Aδ nerve fibers are lightly myelinated fibers with a relatively fast conduction velocity. These fibers are generally responsive to noxious mechanical stimuli, with limited responsiveness to chemical or thermal stimuli. They have been proposed to mediate the initial (or "first") sensation of pain, which has a sharp, stabbing, or bright perceptual quality (17) (see Chap. 41). In tooth pulp, many Aδ fibers are reported to innervate the dentinal tubules (6). The innervation pattern of dentinal tubules is presented in Fig. 2. The frequency of dentinal tubule innervation varies according to its location within the pulp, and ranges from a relatively high level of innervation in tubules beneath pulp horns (e.g., >40% innervated), to a low level of innervation in tubules near the root apex (e.g., <0.5%). Many Aδ fibers can be stimulated by mechanical movement of fluid through dentinal tubules (62–64), and are thought to contribute to dentinal hypersensitivity pain.

Interestingly, large-diameter, rapidly conducting, Aβ fibers have been reported in dental pulp, and also respond to stimuli that evoke dentinal sensitivity in humans (63). The innervation of dentinal tubules with these myelinated fibers is consistent with the sharp, stabbing qualities of pain associated with dentinal hypersensitivity.

A generally accepted hypothesis for the transduction of dentinal pain is fluid movement within dentinal tubules. For example, the ability of substances to produce dentinal pain after application to exposed dentinal tubules is directly related to their osmotic strength (2). A common clinical example is the pain following application of a candy onto a tooth with exposed tubules; the high osmolar sucrose solution can activate Aδ fibers innervating dentinal tubules (63,64). Therapeutic approaches for managing dentinal pain include interventions that occlude dentinal tubules, thereby reducing fluid movement. A more complete review of dentinal hypersensitivity is available (2,32,80).

Central Projections of Orofacial Afferents

Following activation, the A, δ, and C fibers from the orofacial region transmit nociceptive signals primarily via trigeminal nerves to the trigeminal nuclei in the brainstem. The trigeminal nerves are divided into three principal components—anteromedially, the ophthalmic; posterolaterally, the mandibular; and in an intermediate position, the maxillary branch. The cell bodies of these axons are in the ganglion of the fifth nerve (the gasserian ganglion). The central distribution enters the brain stem through the portio major, although a small percentage (20%) may additionally travel through the motor root (portio minor) (85), a possible parallel to the so-called ventral root afferents that have been observed in spinal cord (see

Chap. 35). In addition, noxious information from additional regions from orofacial regions is conveyed by other cranial nerves (17,18.51,75).

Although several studies implicate the trigeminal nucleus caudalis as a primary site for processing orofacial nociceptive input involved in perception, it should be noted that trigeminal nociceptors terminate in other nuclei as well (11,17, 22,51,56,69,75,86). Interruption of these signals, by the use of long-acting local anesthetics, evokes profound postoperative analgesia (13).

PERIPHERAL RESPONSES TO OROFACIAL INFLAMMATION

In contrast to a transient pain-producing stimulus (e.g., venipuncture, etc.), pain associated with inflammation is often characterized by a prolonged period of hyperalgesia. This is due in part to the sustained actions of peripheral inflammatory mediators that are thought to interact in the development of a local positive-feedback cycle (Fig. 2) and to plastic changes in the CNS ("central hyperalgesia") (see Chaps. 36 and 40).

Release of Active Factors from Injured Pulpal Tissues

In the periphery, tissue trauma or inflammation initiates the local positive feedback cycle by activating the synthesis of prostaglandins and evoking the release of bradykinin from its blood-borne precursor, kininogen, and of histamine from mast cells. Since prostaglandins, bradykinin, and histamine all increase either the permeability or dilatation of local blood vessels, they act synergistically to increase plasma extravasation (Fig. 2) (see Chap. 33). It is this accumulation of extravasated fluid into tissue spaces that produces the clinical sign of edema. In addition, plasma extravasation replenishes these short-lived local mediators by providing a fresh supply of kininogen, prostaglandins (activated by bradykinin), histamine, and other mediators. The continued synthesis or release of these inflammatory mediators, the process of nociceptor sensitization, and persistent changes in the CNS may contribute to the prolonged duration of inflammatory pain.

It is important to note that while many of these products may indeed induce a pain report or state, little is known regarding (a) the actual tissue concentration of these chemical mediators during inflammation and pain; (b) how the pain state covaries with their respective levels; and (c) how pharmacologic manipulations actually alter their local levels. Such information has made it difficult to assess to what extent such agents are involved in mediating pain due to different types of orofacial inflammation.

To address these issues, we have developed a microdialysis method that permits collection of inflammatory mediators in awake dental pain patients, who can simultaneously provide verbal pain reports (29,71–74,77). Following a standard surgical extraction of impacted mandibular third molars, a sterile microdialysis probe is implanted into the surgical wound. Dialysate samples are collected for up to 8 hours after surgery, and later analyzed for the inflammatory mediator of interest. Advantages of the microdialysis method include (a) exclusion of peptidases and precursors at the tissue level, (b) quantitative recoveries of inflammatory mediators, and (c) minimal disruption of the inflamed tissue (i.e., saline is not being pumped into the tissue).

These clinical studies have used microdialysis probes to collect immunoreactive bradykinin (iBK), prostaglandin E_2 (iPGE$_2$), leukotriene B_4 (iLTB$_4$), substance P (iSP), and other mediators present in inflamed peripheral tissue. These inflammatory mediators were selected due to their known proinflammatory actions. The oral surgery model was selected for these studies since it is a well-recognized clinical model of surgically induced pain and inflammation, which easily permits the temporary implantation of microdialysis probes into awake patients who can simultaneously provide pain reports.

The time-course studies indicate that immunoreactive prostaglandin E_2 (iPGE$_2$), bradykinin (iBK), leukotriene B_4 (iLTB$_4$), and substance P (iSP) are all detectable in tissue dialysates collected from the extraction sites of awake patients after surgical removal of impacted third molars (29,71–74,77). The data presented in Table 1 illustrate typical values for the time of peak release and corresponding peak concentrations of these mediators. Importantly, the peak concentrations of all four of these mediators are greater than the K_d values for binding of the mediators to their respective receptors (the K_d value is the concentration of the mediator that binds to 50% of its receptors). This comparison suggests that all of these mediators are present at physiologically relevant concentrations, and that they may contribute to the development of acute dental pain and inflammation.

Corresponding pharmacologic studies have evaluated the effects of nonsteroidal anti-inflammatory drugs (NSAIDs) and systemic steroid treatment on tissue levels of inflammatory mediators in oral surgery patients. As compared to placebo-treated patients, administration of either flurbiprofen, ibuprofen, or methylprednisolone significantly reduces tissue levels of iBK, iPGE$_2$, and iSP (29,71–74,77). The results of a double-blind comparison of systemic methylprednisolone (125 mg) to placebo for altering postsurgical tissue levels of iBK is presented in Fig. 3. Interestingly, a single preoperative injection of methylprednisolone produced a substantial and prolonged reduction in tissue levels of iBK (29). Methylprednisolone also reduces tissue levels of mediators such as iPGE$_2$ and iSP, supporting the clinical efficacy of glucocorticoids (71).

Table 1. PEAK TISSUE LEVELS OF SELECTED INFLAMMATORY MEDIATORS AS MEASURED BY MICRODIALYSIS PROBES IMPLANTED INTO MODELS OF OROFACIAL INFLAMMATION

	Clinical studies		Animal studies	
Mediator	Oral surgery	Perio. surgery	Control TMJ	Inflamed TMJ
iPGE$_2$	5–7 nmol/L	261 μmol/L	0.2 nmol/L	1–2 nmol/L
iBradykinin	12–20 nmol/L	NM	0.04 nmol/L	0.2 nmol/L
iSubstance P	1 nmol/L	NM	NM	NM
iLTB4	2–4 nmol/L	0.6 nmol/L	NM	NM

Immunoreactive levels of these mediators were determined by RIA or ELISA. Tissue dialysates were collected using microdialysis probes implanted into awake postsurgical oral surgery patients (n = 15–50), periodical surgery patients (n = 9), and anesthetized rabbits with inflamed TMJs (n = 21). The TMJ in the anesthetized rabbits was inflamed with local injection of carrageenan.

LTB4, leukotriene B4; NM, not measured; TMJ, temporomandibular joint.

Data from refs. 29, 65, 71, 73, 74, and 77.

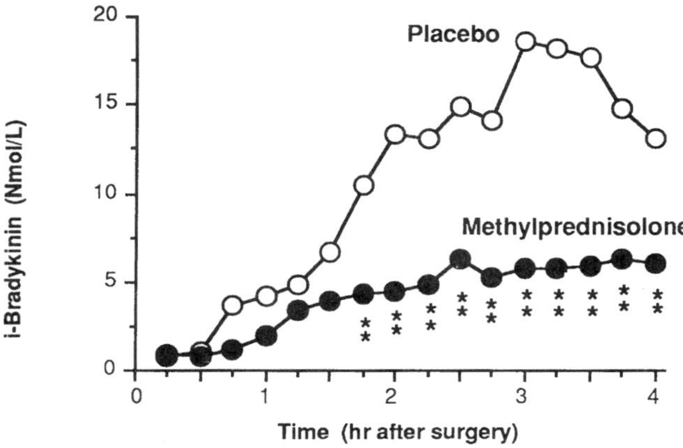

Figure 3. Effect of pretreatment with methylprednisolone (125 mg iv, 2 hr before surgery) or placebo on tissue levels of immunoreactive bradykinin in 36 oral surgery patients. Tissue levels of immunoreactive bradykinin were collected by microdialysis probes implanted into the extraction site and measured by a radioimmunoassay. $^{**}p<.01$. (Modified from ref. 29.)

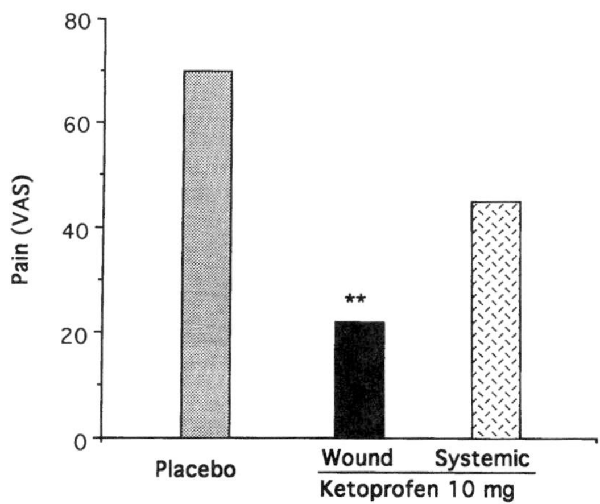

Figure 4. Comparison of the analgesic effects of 10 mg ketoprofen administered directly to mandibular third molar extraction sites ("wound"), in comparison to the same dose of the drug orally ingested ("systemic") or to a placebo using a double-dummy, double-blind experimental design. $^{**}p<.01$ by ANOVA. (Data modified from ref. 15.)

Collectively, these microdialysis studies provide a biochemically based approach for (a) identifying inflammatory mediators released in peripheral tissue of orofacial pain subjects; (b) determining their pharmacologic regulation; and (c) evaluating their interactions and contributions to the development of pain and inflammation. We are currently extending this method to clinical cases of surgery performed on chronically inflamed tissue (e.g., periodontal tissue, temporomandibular joint space; see Table 1). Thus, these findings (Table 1) indicate that the inflammatory response in chronically inflamed tissue is even greater than that observed in the oral surgery model (65). This difference in tissue response may be related to the presence of chronic inflammatory cells that are already in place in tissues selected for periapical or periodontal surgeries.

Demonstration of substantial levels of inflammatory mediators in surgical wounds has led to potentially novel therapeutic studies. For example, tissue levels of immunoreactive PGE_2 peak at early time points in the low nmol/L concentrations (Table 1), suggesting that arachidonic acid metabolites may play a major role in peripheral sensitization of nociceptors. Moreover, NSAIDs are particularly effective analgesics in the oral surgery model (10,14), although they produce systemic side effects such as dyspepsia. Accordingly, peripheral administration of an NSAID directly into a surgical wound may produce profound analgesia at doses that produce little, if any, systemic adverse effects due to less exposure at target organs for toxicity.

This hypothesis was tested in oral surgery patients by comparing the analgesic response of ketoprofen 10 mg gel following local wound administration to oral ingestion of the ketoprofen gel (16,25). The results indicate that local administration of low dose of an NSAID directly into surgical wounds produces significantly greater analgesia than the same dose of the drug administered systemically (Fig. 4) while producing lower plasma drug levels (15). These results indicate that local drug delivery systems may have utility for increasing the therapeutic index of analgesic, anti-inflammatory, or even antibiotic drugs. Further, these and other studies (61,67) suggest that NSAID analgesia in humans may be mediated predominantly by peripheral mechanisms. Collectively, these findings are more consistent with the classic Vane hypothesis of peripheral NSAID action than with the recent suggestion that NSAID analgesia is mediated primarily by spinal cord mechanisms (58). Interestingly, in other studies, it was shown that topical ketorolac had no effect upon inflammation or pain reports in experimental burn patients (60) (see Chap. 61), suggesting that different peripheral injuries may indeed possess distinct pharmacologic profiles.

Release of Peptides from Pulpal Afferents

In addition to the activation and sensitization of certain nociceptors, another effect of inflammatory mediators is to modulate the release of neuropeptides stored in the peripheral nociceptive nerve ending (Fig. 2). The cell body of the primary afferent nerve fiber synthesizes the neuropeptides substance P and calcitonin gene-related peptide (CGRP) (as well as other substances) that are transported both to the CNS and to the periphery. These neuropeptides are highly concentrated in peripheral tissue such as dental pulp and periapical tissue. These neuropeptides are released during activation of certain afferent fibers (e.g., nociceptors) and engage physiologic targets associated with the development of neurogenic inflammation.

Peptide Release

Electrical or chemical stimulation of peripheral pulpal nerves is a sufficient stimulus for these fibers to release iSP and iCGRP from the tooth pulp (28,37,66). Importantly, this peripheral release is a general phenomenon, not limited to the tooth pulp, and has been shown to occur as well in the skin (59), knee joint (84), trachea (41), heart (20, Lundberg, 1992), and lung (54) (see Chap. 33).

Dental pulp is an ideal model tissue for investigations into terminal peptide release since it contains large numbers of small afferent terminals, high concentrations of neuropeptides, and the predominant sensation following stimulation of pulp is pain (see above). These anatomical and physical characteristics indicate that this tissue permits evaluation of a relatively rich supply of nociceptors. Thus, in vitro pulp tissue is removed from freshly extracted bovine mandibular incisors, sectioned, and loaded into superfusion chambers. In this model, several points have been demonstrated (19,28,42,43):

1. Depolarizing concentrations of potassium (e.g., 50 mM) evokes the release of iCGRP from the pulp.
2. Capsaicin (an agent that stimulates populations of C fibers; see Chap. 6) evokes release of iCGRP.
3. The release of iCGRP is calcium dependent, reflecting the general property that peptide release from the central and peripheral terminal of the primary afferent requires calcium for the secretory process.

4. The immunoreactivity CGRP measured in the perfusate co-elutes with authentic CGRP when passed over separative columns.

It is important to note that the presence of active factors may stimulate release of neuropeptides from the afferent terminal. However, in the face of a persistent inflammation, additional processes may be brought into play, including an upregulation in transmitter availability. Thus, the peripheral tissue content of immunoreactive substance P (iSP) and CGRP (iCGRP) is substantially altered during inflammation (4,5,26,45,46). In general, mild-to-moderate forms of injury evoke a substantial increase in tissue content of iSP and iCGRP (4,5). For example, pulpal levels of these neuropeptides increase more than twofold by 7 days after pulpal exposure (Fig. 5). In contrast, more severe forms of injury produce tissue necrosis with a decrease in pulpal neuropeptide content.

Factors Regulating Release of Peptides from the Pulpal Afferent

In contrast to the relative wealth of studies detailing the proinflammatory pharmacology of peripheral neuropeptides and their responses to pulpal inflammation, there is a relative lack of studies on the mechanisms regulating peripheral neuropeptide secretion. As detailed in the above section, it is likely that this is an important area of research since these peptides can modulate inflammation and healing, and undergo dynamic responses in tissue content in response to inflammation. Accordingly, drugs that alter secretion of neuropeptides may have clinically important anti-inflammatory, analgesic, or healing properties.

In addition to mediators that stimulate neuropeptide release, a number of drugs inhibit release. Figure 6 presents the results of a study evaluating the effects of lidocaine and epinephrine on suppressing the evoked release of iCGRP from dental pulp. Both lidocaine and epinephrine significantly inhibit potassium-evoked release of iCGRP from pulp. At these concentrations, the combination of the two drugs does not provide additional inhibitory effects. Demonstration that lidocaine inhibits neuron activity supports the validity of the pulp superfusion method. Interestingly, epinephrine produces nearly the same magnitude of inhibition as lidocaine (Fig. 6). Additional studies indicate that other adrenergic agonists such as norepinephrine (at nmol/L concentrations), clonidine (an α_2-receptor agonist), and salbutamol (a β-receptor agonist) have potent actions for inhibiting the capsaicin-evoked release of iCGRP (19). This raises the possibility that the enhanced efficacy observed with the vasoconstrictor-containing local anesthetic drugs may be due not only to vasoconstriction, but also to an inhibitory action of adrenergic agonists on certain primary afferent fibers. If subsequent research supports this hypothesis, then it is possible that adrenergic agents other than epinephrine or levonordefrin may provide superior local anesthetic adjuncts for control of peripheral hyperalgesia.

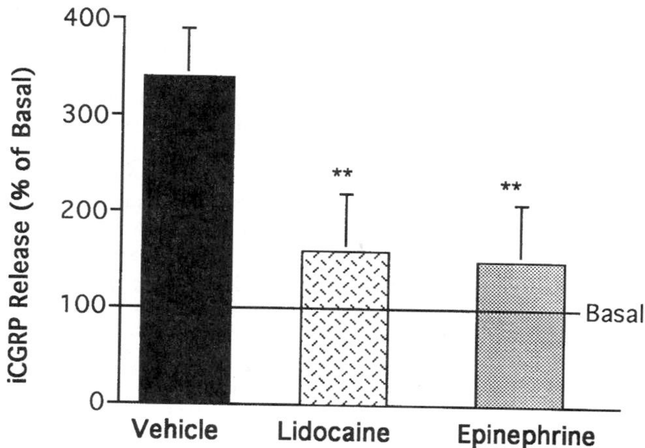

Figure 6. Effect of pretreatment with vehicle, lidocaine (20 mg/ml solution), or epinephrine (10 μg/ml) on altering potassium-evoked release of iCGRP from dental pulp. Chambers (n = 6–10) were pretreated with one of the three treatments, and then exposed to a depolarizing concentration of potassium. *Horizontal line* depicts basal release rates. **p<.01 versus vehicle control group. (Modified from ref. 19.)

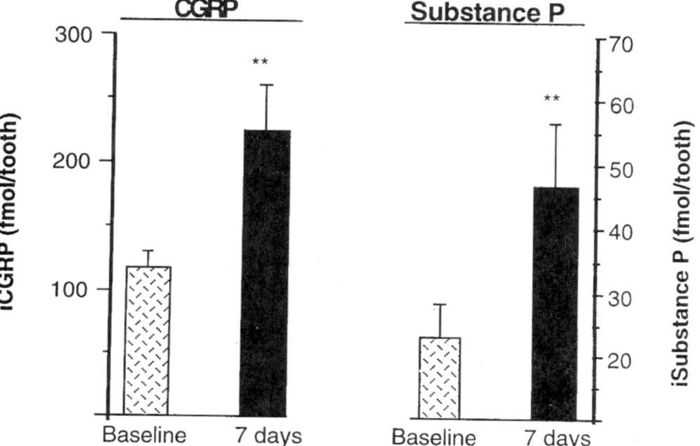

Figure 5. Effect of pulpal exposure on pulpal levels of immunoreactive CGRP *(left)* and substance P *(right).* Rats were anesthetized with halothane, mandibular molars were either left untreated *(speckled bars)* or exposed with a 33 $^1/_2$ burr *(filled bars).* Pulp was collected 7 days later, extracted and measured for immunoreactive CGRP and substance P by radioimmunoassays (RIAs). Error bars = S.E.M.; N = 8–10/group. ** = p<.01 versus corresponding control. (Data modified from ref. 4.).

Role of Peripheral Peptide Release

Peripheral neuropeptides may modulate inflammation by altering the release or metabolism of inflammatory mediators. Neuropeptides, such as substance P, act with other inflammatory mediators to stimulate the release of histamine, PGE_2, collagenase, interleukin-1, interleukin-6, and tumor necrosis factor (49,52,53). Additional studies indicate that these neuropeptides, and possibly additional factors of primary afferent fiber origin, are critical for the resolution of inflammation and the initiation of successful healing. (7,36,47). For example, it has been shown that denervation of the inferior alveolar nerve substantially increases the magnitude of pulpal necrosis following pulp exposure (5). Destruction of small sensory afferents with capsaicin has been shown to slow wound healing (21,68). Collectively, these studies indicate that certain primary afferent fibers not only detect and signal the occurrence of tissue damage, they also respond to the development of tissue inflammation and healing.

CENTRAL PROCESSES INITIATED BY OROFACIAL PAIN

Role of Endogenous Regulatory Systems Activated by Trigeminal Input

Considerable work has led to the appreciation that nociceptive input evoked by small afferent activity can reflexively evoke increases in the activity in regulatory pathways (1). Such pathways have included bulbospinal pathways that release noradrenaline and serotonin (81), and brain stem and spinal systems that release endogenous opiates such as met-enkephalin from the brainstem and spinal cord (83). The organization of various aspects of these pathways have been provided elsewhere in this volume (bulbospinal systems, see Chap. 38; spinal modulatory systems, see Chaps. 34 and 36).

Several studies have used the oral surgery model to evaluate the role of an endogenous opioid analgesic system activated in patients experiencing acute stress (30,50). These studies have used naloxone as an intervention, interpreting naloxone-enhanced pain as evidence for activation of endogenous opioid analgesic system(s). In general, these studies indicate that an endogenous opioid analgesic system is active in unsedated patients during surgery and at later time points during the development of acute postoperative pain. For example, the i.v. injection of naloxone 10 mg more than doubles the perception of intraoperative pain as compared to placebo-treated patients (Fig. 7).

Acute injury leads to a coordinated neuroendocrine stress response. Several studies have measured markers of the pituitary-adrenal and sympathoadrenal axes in patients undergoing oral surgery (12,23,27,30,34,79). The results indicate that oral surgery and acute postoperative pain constitute physiologically relevant stimuli for evoking secretion of immunoreactive β-endorphin (27,30). Circulating levels of immunoreactive β-endorphin increase in placebo-treated patients during oral surgery and after loss of local anesthesia; levels are also increased in a compensatory fashion during naloxone-induced hyperalgesia (Fig. 7). These observations may be clinically relevant since oral surgery patients pretreated with low doses of dexamethasone have lower levels of circulating β-endorphin and significantly greater levels of postoperative pain as compared to patients treated with placebo (27). Moreover, administration of corticotropin releasing factor (CRF) to postoperative patients stimulates secretion of immunoreactive β-endorphin and significantly reduce postoperative pain in patients following extraction of impacted third molars (34). The existence of a peripheral site of action for opiate-induced analgesia provides a potential target for circulating opioid peptides (33) (see Chap. 58).

Role of Endogenous Facilitation

Acute orofacial inflammation is often associated with hyperalgesia. Hyperalgesia is characterized by the presence of spontaneous pain, a decreased pain threshold, and an increased magnitude of perceived pain for a given stimulus (82). Indeed, clinical testing for the presence of hyperalgesia can be used as a diagnostic criterion in the field of endodontics (35).

The origins of this hyperalgesia in orofacial pain likely arises from two components: (a) activation and sensitization of peripheral nociceptors, and (b) development of a facilitated state of processing in the central nervous system (CNS).

Peripheral Components of Hyperalgesia

The peripheral factors have been outlined above. Pulpal inflammation and injury lead to the elaboration of active factors that can served to increase plasma extravasation and sensitize/activate free nerve endings. The reports of pain following tooth percussion is actually the evaluation of a reduced threshold to mechanical stimuli. The "throbbing" pain of pulpitis may be due to the mechanical nociceptive threshold of sensitized pulpal C fibers reduced to the extent that the arterial pressure wave of a heartbeat is sufficient to activate pulpal nociceptors since these units can depolarize in synchrony with the heart rate during pulpal inflammation (64).

Central Components of Hyperalgesia

As reviewed elsewhere (see Chap. 36), it is widely appreciated that repetitive small afferent input can induce a state of prominent facilitation such that after such conditioning, a modest input can generate a prominent output, and the receptive fields of such neurons are enlarged. Such processes also hold for the trigeminal system. For example, neurons in the nucleus caudalis exhibit a substantial increase in staining for immunoreactive *c-fos* following inflammation of dental pulp or the maxillary sinus (8,70). Additional studies have determined prolonged changes in activity of neurons of the trigeminal nuclei following induction of peripheral orofacial inflammation (38,69,86) or deafferentation of tooth pulp (39,48). These central changes, together with inflammation-induced changes in peripheral neuron activity (40,87), likely contribute to the development of orofacial pain and hyperalgesia. Indeed, clinical psychophysical studies on orofacial pain patients is consistent with plasticity changes leading to altered central neuronal processing of noxious stimuli (57,76).

An important implication of the afferent-evoked facilitation has been the ability to reduce the postinjury pain state by reducing the initiating afferent barrage. This process is referred to as "preemptive" analgesia (see Chaps. 36 and 43). This hypothesis proposes that blockade of nociceptive afferent input should inhibit the development of central hyperalgesia, leading to reduced postoperative pain. Recently, this hypothesis has been tested in the oral surgery model. The utility of this clinical model

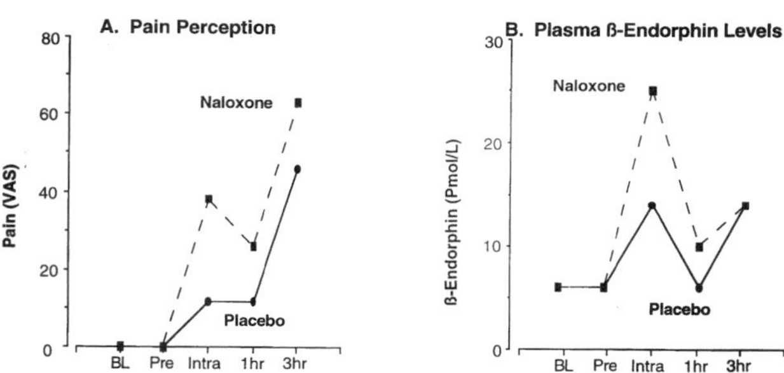

Figure 7. Evaluation of stress responses to surgical extractions of third molars in awake, unsedated patients. Pain was measured by a visual analogue scale (VAS) and circulating levels of immunoreactive β-endorphin were collected at a baseline session 1 week prior to surgery (BL), and on the day of surgery at preoperative (Pre), and intraoperative (Intra) time points, and at 1 and 3 hours after completion of surgery. All patients (n = 24) were injected with a local anesthetic prior to surgery and then injected on a double-blind basis with either naloxone (10 mg iv) or placebo (saline) 5 min into surgery. β-endorphin levels were measured by RIA. (Modified from ref. 30.)

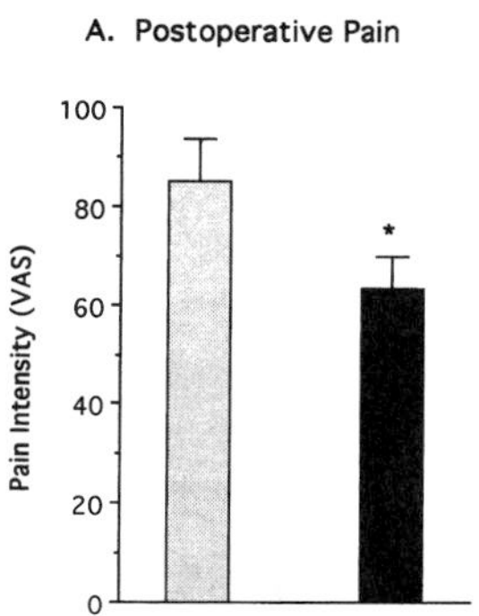

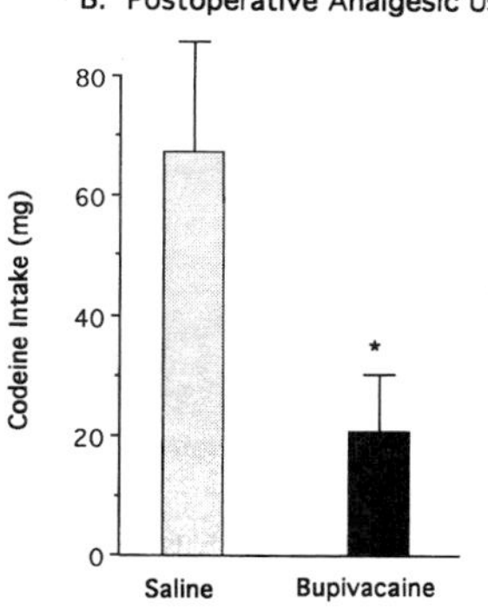

Figure 8. Evaluation of the efficacy of preemptive analgesia on the development of postsurgical pain intensity and the intake of a codeine analgesic. Patients (n = 44) underwent general anesthesia with propofol and were then given inferior alveolar nerve block injections of either 0.5% bupivacaine (with 1:200,000 epinephrine) or saline (with 1:200,000 epinephrine). Surgical extractions of third molars was completed, and pain *(left panel)* and codeine intake *(right panel)* were measured at 48 hours after surgery. *p<.05 versus saline vehicle. (Modified from ref. 24.).

for testing the preemptive hypothesis is based on the fact that patients have no preexisting pain. In this study, 48 patients underwent general anesthesia and were then given a peripheral anesthetic nerve block using either bupivacaine with 1:200,000 epinephrine, or a vehicle control consisting of saline with 1:200,000 epinephrine (24). Following the nerve block, the mandibular third molars were surgically extracted. Patient reports of pain and consumption of analgesics were monitored at 48 and 72 hours after the surgery, times that far exceed the duration of bupivacaine anesthesia. The results (Fig. 8) indicate that blockade of sensory input during and immediately after oral surgery reduced both postoperative pain and consumption of analgesics long after the anesthetic effects have dissipated. These results provide support for the hypothesis that peripheral afferent neuronal barrage during tissue injury and acute inflammation produces central nervous system hyperexcitability that contributes to increased postoperative pain.

CONCLUSIONS

Basic and clinical studies of orofacial pain have contributed to our understanding of pharmacologic regulation of inflammatory mediator release, activation of peripheral sensory neurons, and central changes including neuroendocrine stress responses and the development of hyperalgesia. Since the oral surgery model has been shown to be predictive of other inflammatory pain models, it is likely that continued research will lead to increased knowledge of the pharmacologic and physiologic mechanisms of inflammatory pain.

ACKNOWLEDGMENT

This work is supported in part by NIDR grants R29DE09860, R01DE11277, K16DE0027, and P30DE09737. We wish to acknowledge the excellent technical support of Heidi Geier, Jennelle Durnett-Richardson, Pat Kane, and Julie Heller in these projects, and the superb dental student research projects conducted by Mark Engelstad, Karen Reese, and Susan Buck of the University of Minnesota.

REFERENCES

1. Basbaum AI, Fields HL. Endogenous pain control systems: brainstem spinal pathways and endorphin circuitry. *Annu Rev Neurosci* 1984;7:309–38.
2. Brannstrom M: The hydrodynamic theory of dentinal pain: sensation in preparations, caries and the dentinal crack syndrome. *J Endodon* 1986;12:453–457.
3. Brown AC, Beeler WJ, Kloka AC, Fields RW. Spatial summation of pre-pain and pain in human teeth. *Pain* 1985;21:1–16.
4. Buck S, Reese K, Cane P, Hargreaves KM. Pulpal exposure induces changes in levels of peripheral neuropeptides. *J Dent Res* 1994;73: 314.
5. Byers M, Taylor P, Khayat B, Kimberly C. Effects of injury and inflammation on pulpal and periapical nerves. *J Endodon* 1990;16: 78–84.
6. Byers M: Dental sensory receptors. *Int Rev Neurobiol* 1984;25:39–94.
7. Byers MR, Taylor PE. Effect of sensory denervation on the response of rat molar pulp to exposure injury. *J Dent Res* 1993;72:613–8.
8. Byers MR. Dynamic plasticity of dental sensory nerve structure and cytochemistry. *Arch Oral Biol* 1994;39(suppl):13S–21S.
9. Cooper SA, Beaver WT. A model to evaluate mild analgesics in oral surgery outpatients. *Clin Pharmacol Ther* 1976;20:241–250.
10. Cooper SA: New peripherally-acting oral analgesic agents. *Annu Rev Pharmacol Toxicol* 1983;23:617–647.
11. Dallel R, Raboisson P, Woda A, Sessle BJ. Properties of nociceptive and non-nociceptive neurons in trigeminal subnucleus oralis of the rat. *Brain Res* 1990;521:95–106.
12. Dionne R, Goldstein D, Wirdzek P. Effects of diazepam premedication and epinephrine-containing local anesthetic on cardiovascular and plasma catecholamine responses to oral surgery. *Anesth* 1984;63:640–646.
13. Dionne R: Suppression of dental pain by the preoperative administration of flurbiprofen *Am J Med* 1986;80:41–49.
14. Dionne RA, Gordon S. Nonsteroidal anti-inflammatory drugs for acute pain control. *Dent Clin North Am* 1994;8:645–667.
15. Dionne RA, Gordon SM, Rowan JS. Pharmacokinetic comparison of peripherally versus orally administered ketoprofen gel. *J Dent Res* 1995;74:420.
16. Dionne RA, Tahara MA, Rowan JS. Peripheral administration of low dose ketoprofen is analgesic in the oral surgery model. *7th World Congress on Pain,* 1993.
17. Dubner R, Bennett G: Spinal and trigeminal mechanisms of nociception. *Annu Rev Neurosci* 1983;6:381–418.
18. Dubner R, Kenshalo DR, Maixner W, Bushnell MC, Oliveras. The correlation of monkey medullary dorsal horn neuronal activity and the perceived intensity of noxious heat. *J Neurophysiol* 1989;62: 450–457.
19. Engelstad M, Garry M, Jackson D, Geier H, Hargreaves KM. Adrenergic inhibition of iCGRP release from capsaicin-sensitive fibers in dental pulp. *Abstr Soc Neurosci* 1992;18:690.
20. Franco-Cereceda A, Lundberg JM. Capsazepine inhibits low pH- and lactic acid-evoked release of calcitonin gene-related peptide from sensory nerves in guinea-pig heart. European Journal of Pharmacology 1992;22:183–4.
21. Gallar J, Pozo MA, Rebollo I, Belmonte C. Effects of capsaicin on corneal wound healing. *Invest Ophthalmol Vis Sci* 1990;31: 1968–74.
22. Gobel, S, Falls W, Hockfield S. The division of the dorsal and ventral horns of the mammalian caudal medulla into eight layers using anatomical criteria. In: Anderson D, Matthews B, eds. *Pain in the trigeminal region.* Amsterdam: Elsevier Science, 1977;443–453.
23. Goldstein D, Dionne R, Sweet J, Gracely R, Brewer B, Gregg R, Keiser H. Circulatory, plasma catecholamine, cortisol, lipid, and psychological responses to a real-life stress (third molar extraction): effects of diazepam sedation and of inclusion of epinephrine with the local anesthetic. *Psychosom Med* 1982;44:259–272.
24. Gordon SM, Dionne RA, Brahim J, Dubner R. Blockade of peripheral neuronal barrage reduces post-operative pain. *J Dent Res* 1995; 74:178.
25. Gordon SM, Tahara MA, Rowan JS, Dionne RA, Dubner R. Comparative analgesic efficacy of peripherally versus orally administered ketoprofen gel. *J Dent Res* 1994;73:438.
26. Grutzner E, Garry M, Hargreaves KM. Effect of injury on pulpal levels of immunoreactive substance P and CGRP *J Endodon* 1992; 18:553–557.
27. Hargreaves K, Schmidt E, Mueller G, Dionne R. Dexamethasone alters plasma levels of beta-endorphin and post-operative pain. *Clin Pharmacol Ther* 1987;42:601–607.
28. Hargreaves KM, Bowles WR, Garry G. An in vitro method to evaluate regulation of neuropeptide release from dental pulp *J Endodon* 1992;18:597–600.
29. Hargreaves KM, Costello A. Glucocorticoids suppress release of immunoreactive bradykinin from inflamed tissue as evaluated by microdialysis probes. *Clin Pharmacol Ther* 1990;48:168–178.
30. Hargreaves KM, Dionne R, Goldstein D, Mueller G, Dubner R. Naloxone, fentanyl and diazepam modify plasma beta-endorphin levels during surgery. *Clin Pharmacol Ther* 1986;40:165–171.
31. Hargreaves KM, Dionne R. Evaluating endogenous mediators of pain and analgesia in clinical studies. In: Max M, Portenoy R, Laska E, eds. *The design of analgesic clinical trials.* New York: Raven Press, 1990;579–598.
32. Hargreaves KM, Dubner R. Mechanisms of pain and analgesia. In: Dionne R, Phero J, eds. *Management of pain and anxiety in dental practice.* New York: Elsevier Science, 1992;18–40.
33. Hargreaves KM, Joris J. The peripheral analgesic effects of opioids. *J Am Pain Soc* 1993;2:51–59.
34. Hargreaves KM, Mueller G, Dubner R, Goldstein D, Dionne R. Corticotropin releasing factor (CRF) produces analgesia in humans and rats. *Brain Res* 1987b;422:154–157.
35. Hargreaves KM, Swift JQ, Roszkowski MT, Bowles WR, Garry MG, Jackson DL: Pharmacology of peripheral neuropeptide and inflammatory mediator release. *Oral Surg Oral Med Oral Path* 1994; 78:503–510.
35a. Hargreaves KM, Troullos E, Dionne RA. Pharmacologic rationale for the treatment of acute pain. *Dental Clin North Am* 1987;31:675– 694.
36. Heden P, Jernbeck J, Kjartansson J, Samuelson U. Increased skin flap survival and arterial dilation by calcitonin gene-related peptide. *Scand J Plast Reconstr Surg* 1989;23:11–16.

37. Heyeraas KJ, Kim S, Raab WH, Byers MR, Liu M. Effect of electrical tooth stimulation on blood flow, interstitial fluid pressure and substance P and CGRP-immunoreactive nerve fibers in the low compliant cat dental pulp. *Microvascular Res* 1994;47:329–343.
38. Hu JW, Sessle BJ, Raboisson P, Dallel R, Woda A. Stimulation of craniofacial muscle afferents induces prolonged facilitory effects in trigeminal nociceptive brain-stem neurons. *Pain* 1992;48:53–60.
39. Hu JW, Sharav Y, Sessle BJ. Effects of one- or two-stage deafferentation of mandibular and maxillary tooth pulps on the functional properties of trigeminal brainstem neurons. *Brain Res* 1990; 516:271–279.
40. Hu JW, Yu XM, Vernon H, Sessle BJ. Excitatory effects on neck and jaw muscle activity of inflammatory irritant applied to cervical paraspinal tissues. *Pain* 1993;55:243–250.
41. Hua X-Y, Jinno S, Back SM, Tam EK, Yaksh TL. Multiple mechanisms for the effects of capsaicin, bradykinin and nicotine on CGRP release from tracheal afferent nerves: role of prostaglandins, sympathetic nerves and mast cells. *Neuropharmacology* 1994;33:1147–1154.
42. Jackson D, Aanonsen L, Durnett-Richardson J, Geier H, Hargreaves KM. An evaluation of the effects of excitatory amino acids in bovine dental pulp. *Abstr Soc Neurosci* 1993;19:966.
43. Jackson D, Garry M, Engelstad M, Geier H, Hargreaves KM. Evaluation of iCGRP secretion from dental pulp in response to inflammatory mediators. *Abstr Soc Neurosci* 1992;18:689.
44. Johnson D, Harshbarger J, Rymer H. Quantitative assessment of neural development in human premolars. *Anat Rec* 1983;205: 421–429.
45. Khayat B, Byers M. Responses of nerve fibers to pulpal inflammation and periapical lesions in rat molars demonstrated by calcitonin gene-related peptide immunocytochemistry. *J Endodon* 1988;14:577–587.
46. Kimberly C, Byers M. Inflammation of rat molar pulp and periodontium causes increased calcitonin gene related peptide and axonal sprouting. *Anat Rec* 1988;222:289–300.
47. Kjartannson J, Dalsgaard C. Calcitonin gene-related peptide increases survival of a musculocutaneous critical flap in the rat *Eur J Pharmacol* 1987;42:355–358.
48. Kwan CL, Hu JW, Sessle BJ. Effects of tooth pulp deafferentation on brainstem neurons of the rat trigeminal subnucleus oralis. *Somatosens Motor Res* 1993;10:115–131.
49. Lembeck F, Holzer P. Substance P as a neurogenic mediator of antidromic vasodilation and neurogenic plasma extravasation. *Arch Pharmacol* 1979;310:175–183.
50. Levine J, Gordon N, Fields, H. The mechanism of placebo analgesia. *Lancet* 1978;2:654–657.
51. Light AR. *The initial processing of pain and its descending control: spinal and trigeminal systems.* Basel: Karger, 1992.
52. Lotz M, Carson D, Vaughan J. Substance P activation of rheumatoid synoviocytes: neural pathway in pathogenesis of arthritis. *Science* 1987;235:893–895.
53. Lotz M, Vaughan J, Carson D. Effect of neuropeptides on production of inflammatory cytokines by human monocytes. *Science* 1988;241:1218–1221.
54. Lou YP, Karlsson JA, Franco-Cereceda A, Lundberg JM. Selectivity of ruthenium red in inhibiting bronchoconstriction and CGRP release induced by afferent C-fibre activation in the guinea-pig lung. *Acta Physiol Scand* 1991;142:191–9.
55. Madison S, Whitels, EA, Suarez-Roca H, Maixner W. Sensitizing effects of leukotriene B4 on intradental primary afferents. *Pain* 1992;49:99–104.
56. Maixner W, Dubner R, Kenshalo DR, Bushnell MC, Oliveras JL. Responses of monkey medullary dorsal horn neurons during the detection of noxious heat stimuli. *J Neurophysiol* 1989;62:437–439.
57. Maixner W, Fillingim R, Booker D, Sigurdsson A. Sensitivity of patients with painful temporomandibular disorders to experimentally evoked pain. *Pain* 1995;63:341–352.
58. Malmberg A, Yaksh T. Antinociceptive actions of spinal nonsteroidal agents on the formalin test in the rat. *J Pharmacol Exp Ther* 1992;263:136–146.
59. Mirzai THM, Yaksh TL. Studies on the release of CGRP into the skin blister base. In: Besson JM, Guilbaud G, Ollat H, eds. *Peripheral neurons in nociception:* physio-pharmacological aspects. Paris: John Libbey Eurotext, 1994;125–136.
60. Moiniche S, Pedersen JL, Kehlet H. Topical ketorolac has no Antinociceptive or anti-inflammatory effect in thermal injury. *Burns* 1994;20:483–486.
61. Moore UJ, Seymour RA, Rawlins MD. The efficacy of locally applied aspirin and acetaminophen in postoperative pain after third molar surgery. *Clin Pharmacol Ther* 1992;52:292–296.
62. Narhi M. Activation of dental pulp nerves of the cat and the dog with hydrostatic pressure. *Proc Finn Dent Soc* 1978;74(suppl V):1–64.
63. Narhi M, Jyvasjarv E, Virtanen A, Huopaniemi T, Ngassapa D, Hirvonen T: Role of intradental A and C type nerve fibers in dental pain mechanisms. *Proc Finn Dent Soc* 1992;88:(suppl 1):507–516.
64. Narhi M: The characteristics of intradental sensory units and their responses to stimulation. *J Dent Res* 1985;64:564–571.
65. O'Brien T, Wolff L, Roszkowski M, Hargreaves KM. Tissue levels of PGE2, LTB4 and pain after periodontal surgery. *J Dent Res* 1994; 73:379.
66. Olgart L, Gazelius B, Brodin E, Nilsson G. Release of substance P-like immunoreactivity from the dental pulp. *Acta Physiol Scand* 1977;101:510–512.
67. Penniston SG, Hargreaves KM. Evaluation of periapical injection of ketorolac for management of endodontic pain. *J Endodontics* 1996;22:55–59.
68. Peskar BM, Lambrecht N, Stroff T, Respondek M, Muller KM. Functional ablation of sensory neurons impairs healing of acute gastric mucosal damage in rats. *Dig Dis Sci* 1995;40:2460–2464.
69. Raboisson P, Dallel R, Clavelou P, Sessle BJ, Woda A. Effects of subcutaneous formalin on the activity of trigeminal brain stem nociceptive neurones in the rat. *J Neurophysiol* 1995;73:496–505.
70. Roche AK, Kajander KC. Evaluation of fos labeling in the rabbit brain following induction of sinusitis. *Abstr Soc Neurosci* 1995;21: 893.
71. Roszkowski M, Swift JQ, Hargreaves KM. Local tissue release of immunoreactive substance P, bradykinin, PGE2 and LTB4 in a model of surgically-induced inflammation. *Abstr Soc Neurosci* 1993; 19:521.
72. Roszkowski M, Swift JQ, Hargreaves KM. Effects of ibuprofen on iPGE2, iLTB4, iBradykinin and iSubstance P in surgery patients. *J Dent Res* 1994;73:190.
73. Roszkowski MT, Swift JQ, Hargreaves KM. Corticosteroids attenuate the local release of immunoreactive substance P following third molar surgery. *J Dent Res* 1993;72:186.
74. Roszkowski MT, Swift JQ, Hargreaves KM. Prostaglandin E2 tissue levels increase following third molar extraction. *J Dent Res* 1992;71: 178.
75. Sessle B. Neurophysiology of orofacial pain. *Dent Clin North Am* 1987;31:595–614.
76. Sigurdsson A, Maixner W. Effects of experimental and clinical noxious counterirritants on pain perception. *Pain* 1994;57:265– 275.
77. Swift JQ, Garry MG, Roszkowski M, Hargreaves KM. Effect of flurbiprofen on tissue levels of immunoreactive bradykinin and acute post-operative pain. *J Oral Maxillofac Surg* 1993;51:112–116.
78. Troullos E, Hargreaves KM, Butler D, Dionne R. Comparison of non-steroidal anti-inflammatory drugs, flurbiprofen and ibuprofen, to methylprednisolone for suppression of post-operative pain and edema. *J Oral Maxillofac Surg* 1990;48:945–952.
79. Troullos E, Hargreaves KM, Goldstein D, Stull R, Dionne R. Epinephrine suppresses stress-induced increases in plasma immunoreactive β-endorphin in humans. *J Clin Endocrinol Metab* 1989;69: 546–551.
80. Trowbridge H. Review of dental pain—histology and physiology. *J Endodon* 1986;12:445–452.
81. Tyce GM, Yaksh TL. Monoamine release from cat spinal cord by somatic stimuli: an intrinsic modulatory system. *J Physiol (Lond)* 1981;314:513–529.
82. Willis W. *The pain system.* Basel: Karger, 1985.
83. Yaksh TL, Elde RP. Factors governing release of methionine enkephalin-like immunoreactivity from mesencephalon and spinal cord of the cat *in vivo. J Neurophysiol* 1981;46:1056–1075.
84. Yaksh TL. Substance P release from knee joint afferent terminals: modulation by opioids. *Brain Res* 1988;458:319–324.
85. Young RF. Unmyelinated fibers in the trigeminal motor root. Possible relationship to the results of trigeminal rhizotomy. *J Neurosurg* 1972;35:87–95.
86. Yu XM, Sessle BJ, Hu JW. Differential effects of cutaneous and deep application of inflammatory irritant on mechanoreceptive field properties of trigeminal brain stem nociceptive neurons. *J Neurophysiol* 1993;70:1704–1707.
87. Yu XM, Sessle BJ, Vernon M, Hu JW. Effects of inflammatory irritant application to the rat temporomandibular joint on jaw and neck muscle activity. *Pain* 1995;60:143–149.

Anesthesia: Biologic Foundations, edited by Tony L. Yaksh et al. Lippincott–Raven Publishers, Philadelphia © 1997.

CHAPTER 48

CANCER PAIN: PATHOPHYSIOLOGY AND SYNDROMES

KATHRYN J. ELLIOTT AND RUSSELL K. PORTENOY

In the cancer population, chronic or recurrent pain is experienced by more than one-third of patients in active therapy and more than two-thirds of those with advanced disease (22,90). Cancer pain often results from specific patterns of injury to somatic, visceral, or nervous system structures. The origin of this injury may be the disease itself, any of a variety of treatments (e.g., radiation) used to combat the disease, or some factor unrelated to the disease or its treatment.

As reviewed in earlier chapters, there are multiple mechanisms by which afferent information is encoded to produce a message associated with noxious events. These mechanisms reflect the role of multiple systems that involve many distinct transmitter and receptor classes. Diverse therapeutic approaches may be proposed to regulate these varied mechanisms. Cancer pain rarely reflects a single injury, and the multiplicity of processes involved in each patient underscores the potential utility of multiple therapeutic approaches. The specific clinical strategy is based on accurate diagnosis derived from knowledge of the common pain syndromes that result from cancer and its therapy (22,78,93).

GENERAL CLASSIFICATIONS OF CANCER PAIN STATES

Syndrome

Classification of cancer pain can be approached through description of detailed pain syndromes unique to the cancer population. These syndromes are usually a direct result of the neoplasm or an antineoplastic therapy. Thus, surveys of cancer patients referred to the Memorial Sloan Kettering Cancer Center (MSKCC) Pain Service show that 77–80% of inpatients have pain due to tumor, 15–19% have pain as a result of cancer therapy, and 3–5% have pain that is unrelated to cancer or its therapy (90,187). Among outpatients, almost two-thirds of the pain problems result from direct tumor involvement and one quarter results from cancer therapy (93).

Cancer pain syndromes can be acute or chronic. Acute pain, which is defined by a recent onset and a course that is anticipated to be brief, is extremely common in the cancer population. In contrast to chronic pain syndromes, acute pain syndromes usually result from therapeutic or diagnostic interventions (Table 1). There has been little effort to define acute pain syndromes (45), and the following descriptions focus on the more problematic chronic pains (Table 2).

Inferred Pathophysiology

A classification of cancer pain can be developed according to inferred pain mechanisms. Based on phenomenology and associated findings on examination, radiography, and electrodiagnostic studies, pain syndromes can be categorized into those that are believed to be sustained predominantly by processes related to normal nociception (e.g., initiated by the activation of small, primary afferents that are activated by relatively high-intensity stimuli) and those that are sustained predominantly by neuropathic mechanisms. So-called nociceptive pains, which are presumed to relate in some manner to ongoing tissue injury, may be divided into those associated with damage to somatic structures (somatic pain: e.g., skin, muscle, bone) and those associated with damage or to distention of visceral structures (visceral pain). Neuropathic pains are presumed to be sustained by aberrant somatosensory processing that is induced in either the peripheral or central nervous system by injury to neural tissue (see Chapters 5 and 28).

Somatic pain is the most prevalent type of pain in the cancer population. The origin of this somatic stimulus typically results from direct tumor invasion of soft tissue and bone. Somatic pain is usually readily localized to specific body regions. The pain is usually a familiar aching, throbbing, or stabbing, and there is usually focal tenderness. As reviewed previously, protracted input from small afferents activated by focal injury can yield extended regions of secondary hyperalgesia and tactile allodynia, or tenderness (see Chapter 2).

Visceral pain results from obstruction, infiltration, or compression of viscera. Obstruction of hollow viscus yields pain that is poorly localized, intermittent, and readily compared in character to states generated by abdominal cramps. Injury to or inflammation of organ capsules (e.g., such as kidney or liver), mesentery, or related connective tissue often produces an aching or throbbing pain. The visceral pains may be well localized to a specific cutaneous site (e.g., referred pain) and may

Table 1. ACUTE CANCER PAIN SYNDROMES

- Acute pain associated with diagnostic and therapeutic interventions
  - Acute pain associated with diagnostic interventions
    - Lumbar puncture headache
    - Bone marrow biopsy
    - Lumbar puncture
  - Acute postoperative pain
  - Acute pain caused by other therapeutic interventions
    - Pleurodesis
    - Tumor embolization
  - Acute pain associated with analgesic techniques
    - Spinal opioid hyperalgesia syndrome
- Acute pain associated with anticancer therapies
  - Acute pain associated with chemotherapy infusion techniques
    - Intravenous infusion pain
    - Hepatic artery infusion pain
    - Intraperitoneal chemotherapy abdominal pain
  - Acute pain associated with chemotherapy toxicity
    - Mucositis
    - Painful peripheral neuropathy
    - Diffuse bone pain from transretinoic acid or colony stimulating factors
  - Acute pain associated with hormonal therapy
    - Luteinizing hormone releasing factor tumor flare in prostate cancer
    - Hormone-induced acute pain flare in breast cancer
  - Acute pain associated with radiation therapy
    - Oropharyngeal mucositis
    - Acute radiation enteritis and proctocolitis
  - Acute pain associated with infection

Table 2. CHRONIC CANCER PAIN SYNDROMES

- Tumor-related pain syndromes
  - Bone pain
    - Multifocal or generalized bone pain
    - Vertebral syndromes
    - Atlantoaxial destruction and odontoid fractures
    - C7-T1 syndrome
    - T12-L1 syndrome
    - Sacral syndrome
    - Back pain and epidural compression
    - Pain syndromes of the bony pelvis and hip
  - Headache and facial pain
    - Intracerebral tumor
    - Leptomeningeal metastases
    - Base of skull metastases
  - Tumor involvement of the peripheral nervous system
    - Tumor-related radiculopathy
    - Cervical plexopathy
    - Brachial plexopathy
    - Malignant lumbosacral plexopathy
    - Tumor-related mononeuropathy
    - Paraneoplastic painful peripheral neuropathy
  - Pain syndromes of the viscera and miscellaneous tumor-related syndromes
    - Hepatic distention syndrome
    - Midline retroperitoneal syndrome
  - Paraneoplastic nociceptive pain syndromes
    - Tumor-related gynecomastia
- Chronic pain syndromes associated with cancer therapy
  - Postchemotherapy pain syndromes
    - Chronic painful peripheral neuropathy
    - Avascular necrosis of femoral or humeral head
  - Chronic pain associated with hormonal therapy
    - Gynecomastia with hormonal therapy for prostate cancer
  - Chronic postsurgical pain syndromes
    - Postmastectomy pain syndrome
    - Postradical neck dissection
    - Postthoracotomy pain
    - Phantom pain syndromes
    - Stump pain
  - Chronic postradiation pain syndromes
    - Plexopathies
    - Chronic radiation myelopathy

produce cutaneous hyperesthesia, e.g., a local nocifensor tenderness (52). Pain referral patterns may be explained in part by the common segmental origins of nerves that innervate migrating autonomic viscera and nerves that innervate dermatomes. The neural basis for this referral may be viscerosomatic convergence onto wide dynamic range (WDR) spinal neurons (276).

Cancer-related neuropathic pain most often results from tumor compression or infiltration of peripheral nerves or nerve roots. In a recent survey of cancer inpatients referred to the Pain Service at MSKCC, 30% of the pain diagnoses were neurological (108). Neuropathic pain is highly variable. It may be characterized by spontaneous burning or other abnormal, "unfamiliar" sensations. Aside from the spontaneous ongoing components of the dysesthetic state, evoked sensations include allodynia (pain to a normally nonnoxious stimulus) and hyperalgesia (exaggerated pain response to an otherwise noxious stimulus). These pain states often have dynamic components such that touching or rubbing may lead to a larger area of referred pain (see Chapters 2 and 9). There may or may not be motor, sensory, or autonomic dysfunction in the distribution of the involved nerve.

The widespread acceptance of this classification by clinicians reflects the common distinctions observed clinically among pain syndromes that result from injury to somatic, visceral, or neural tissues, respectively. Although the pain mechanisms (nociceptive versus neuropathic) inferred to exist on the basis of patient characteristics cannot be confirmed in every case, the classification has proven to be useful in both the evaluation of patients with cancer pain syndromes and therapeutic decision making. Although classification according to inferred pain mechanisms has had limited scientific validation and probably represents a gross simplification of very complex pathophysiologic events, it is nonetheless a heuristic starting point for elucidation of underlying pain mechanisms and communication between clinicians and neurobiologists.

The above discussion depicts the components that may be associated with pain states that evolve as a result of cancer or its treatment. In the following sections, pain syndromes will be considered from a functional and mechanistic perspective. As will be noted, many of the syndromes reflect a complex composite of several inferred pathophysiologies.

SOMATIC PAIN SYNDROMES

Tumor invasion of soft tissue, skin, and bone will generate a progressive nociception. Reduction of bulk by surgical excision, radiation, or chemotherapeutic interventions will frequently reduce the reported pain state (see below).

Soft Tissue

Tumor involvement in soft tissue results in a pain state believed to be mediated in part by the activation of small somatic afferents. Such afferents largely travel with the somatic innervation. In contrast, the innervation of the viscera travels with the sympathetic or parasympathetic components (see Chapters 12 and 17).

Activity in primary afferents is known to be closely associated with a pain state (see Chapter 2). Such activation can be generated by (a) mechanical compression of soft tissue or by distention of nonextensible or noncompressible elements (e.g., fascia), as occurs with increasing tumor bulk; (b) tumor-mediated release of inflammatory mediators; or (c) iatrogenic injury produced by surgery or other interventions.

Pain syndromes related to tumor bulk likely involve chronic compression of pain-sensitive structures. If the compression involves an afferent axon, this can lead to a nerve injury syndrome, either due to the physical distortion of the axon or to nerve ischemia (see Chapter 3). In either case, a neuropathic condition can result (see below). If the compression impinges upon the terminal, mechanoreceptive afferents may be activated. Small polymodal C-fiber afferents are activated by mechanical stimuli and the presence of inflammatory products (see below) can enhance that response (see Chapters 6). Many tumors are known to be secretors of a variety of peptides (substance P, vasoactive intestinal peptide, somatostatin), amines (serotonin, histamine) and cytokines (67,126,146), and any or all of these may be involved in the activation of primary afferents. Moreover, the increased vascularity and leakiness around tumor margins, which is perhaps secondary to the release of local products, such as substance P (increases local vascular permeability) or peritumoral inflammation, lead to the increased presence of inflammatory cells. Such conditions can also result in the local release of a variety of cytokines, prostanoids and kinins (e.g., bradykinin). As reviewed in Chapters 6, such agents are also able to stimulate and sensitize afferent nerve endings.

Bone

Invasion of bone by primary neoplasms or metastases is a common cause of cancer pain. Bone lesions can usually be identified by plain radiography or skeletal scintigraphy (119). Skeletal scintigraphy is more sensitive than plain radiography; 35–50% of lesions detected by scintigraphy are not detected on plain radiographs (119) and scintigraphy often detects lesions months earlier than radiographs (128). Scintigraphy may be falsely negative, however, particularly in a region of previously irradiated bony metastases (143).

Evolving bone lesions, as evidenced by scintigraphy, may or may not be correlated with increasing pain states. Once a lesion is painful, however, radiation or chemotherapeutic interventions that halt the tumors growth are frequently associated with a diminishing pain report. Local radiotherapy is usually effective for single sites of metastasis (214). With widely disseminated cancer, hemibody irradiation (155,225), or systemic strontium-89 (209,214) can be palliative. Patients with multifocal bone pain have also found relief from a variety of adjuvant drugs (e.g., corticosteroids, bisphosphonates, or calcitonin), many of which probably exert their effect through symptomatic alterations of the processes leading to bone erosion.

Bone pain may also be caused by treatment effects. Shoulder pain exacerbated by movement of the joint may be seen due to osteonecrosis of the head of the humerus, a complication of corticosteroid therapy or radiation therapy. Similarly, necrosis of the femoral head, which has been associated with both short-term (85) and long-term corticosteroid administration (81), may present with localized hip pain radiating to the knee. Knee pain alone is an uncommon presentation of this lesion. Regardless of the site, avascular necrosis is characterized by pain that precedes radiologic changes by a prolonged period. Bone scintigraphy and MRI are more sensitive than radiography early in the disease course. Pain and joint immobility may severely compromise ambulation and may require joint replacement (189).

The origin of pain secondary to tumor invasion of bone is not well understood. Bone structures are, however, highly innervated. Fascia and periosteum are highly vascular and innervated by small axons with extensive axonal ramifications containing substance P and calcitonin gene-related peptide (125,132). These peptides are markers for small, typically high-threshold, primary afferents (see Chapter 7). It is likely that the lytic processes associated with bony erosion result in (a) alterations in structural integrity and stress on the nerve endings or expansion of the fascia, resulting in a mechanical stimulus; and (b) the release of active factors that serve to activate free nerve endings that are found in bone and fascia (15). Bone invasion thus causes activation of nociceptors in periosteum and endosteum (68), a process that may be additionally mediated by osteoclast function (96,97) and by the lytic processes associated with tumor and the resulting inflammation.

Vertebral Metastasis

The spine is the most common site of bone metastasis, particularly in populations with breast, lung, prostate, and kidney tumors (119). These tumors may metastasize to the vertebral column through an extensive system of venous anastomoses, which connect venous drainage from breast, lung, prostate, or pelvic malignancies to Batson's vertebral venous plexus (14,210). Most patients have multiple silent foci of bone metastases at the time they present with localized pain (24). Back pain due to vertebral metastases is an extremely common clinical problem.

The vertebrae and associated epidural structures (dura, disc, facets) are widely innervated by small, peptide-containing afferents (1,2), which are distributed in a segmentally organized fashion (235). Such afferents likely serve to transduce the mechanical and chemical processes that are associated with tumor invasion of the vertebral bodies and canal.

Growth of tumor within the spine can result in a chronic root compression, with consequences on nerve function as outlined above. In addition to nerve compression secondary to tumor invasion, dorsal root ganglia may also be an important site of impulse generation in the presence of a local tumor. At L4 and L5 nerve roots, for example, the ganglia are primarily intraforaminal, and at S1, they are principally intraspinal (147); such proximally placed ganglia may be prone to damage by spinal neoplasm. Importantly, dorsal root ganglion cells show considerable sensitivity to both local chemical stimuli through coupled receptors on the cell body (229,275), as well as mechanical compression (131). Chronic nerve compression or even distal axon injury can cause the ganglion cell to become a spontaneous generator of action potentials (29). Compression of nerve can induce increased intraganglionic pressure (224), an event that can also lead to increased spontaneous discharges. Accordingly, a number of mechanisms exist whereby tumor compression and the release of local active factors secondary to the tumor presence can activate populations of small primary afferents.

When back pain occurs, it mandates a careful clinical assessment designed to characterize the underlying structural lesion. As outlined above, considerable data indicate that bone is significantly innervated. Back pain may also signal tumor invasion of the epidural space, which can activate afferents innervating the periosteum and fascia.

Epidural compression of the spinal cord or cauda equina is a serious complication of vertebral metastasis, the outcome of which is improved by early diagnosis followed by effective therapy (usually radiation and sometimes surgery or chemotherapy). When plain radiographs demonstrate a >50% collapse of the vertebral body, there is an 87% likelihood of associated epidural extension; the probability of epidural extension is 31% with damage limited to pedicle erosion and 7% with tumor confined to the vertebral body (110). If the symptoms suggest epidural extension (e.g., "crescendo" pain or radicular pain), neurological signs indicate damage to nerve roots or spinal cord, or plain radiography demonstrates a suspicious lesion, then definitive imaging of the epidural space is justified. Magnetic resonance imaging (MRI) is the preferred method to evaluate the epidural space and the extent of bony and soft tissue disease (19,264).

There are many discrete pain syndromes related to vertebral metastases. A description of these syndromes clarifies the importance of clinical assessment in defining the underlying structural abnormalities associated with pains inferred to be due to somatic nociception.

1. *Odontoid Fracture:* Fracture of the odontoid due to tumor invasion of the C2 vertebrae presents with progressive neck pain, which is exacerbated by flexion of the neck and radiates over the posterior aspect of the vertex. Fractures of the odontoid process may result in secondary subluxation associated with spinal cord or brain stem compression. In such cases, progressive pain is followed by neurologic signs of sensory, motor, and autonomic dysfunction (245).

2. *C7-T1 Vertebral Body Metastases:* Metastases to the C7-T1 vertebral bodies present with pain that may localize to the adjacent paraspinal areas or be referred inferiorly to the interscapular region. There may be radiation of dull aching pain into one or both shoulders. Nerve root compression may result in radicular pain in the arm and hand. With paravertebral sympathetic chain involvement, a Horner's syndrome can develop (143).

3. *L1 Metastases:* Pain in the mid-back aggravated by sitting or lying and relieved by standing is the presentation of metastatic involvement of the L1 vertebral body. This may evolve into band-like radicular pain radiating anteriorly or to both paraspinal lumbosacral regions, or even referred solely to the sacroiliac joint or superior iliac crest.

4. *Sacral Metastases:* Metastases to the sacrum, which are most common in patients with pelvic malignancies, present with low back or coccygeal pain exacerbated by lying or sitting and relieved by walking. Patients with progressive sacral metastases may also develop a neuropathic pain syndrome from involvement of the adjacent sacral plexus.

Base of Skull Metastases

Base of skull metastases commonly present with face or head pain and various cranial nerve palsies (18). Tumors that commonly metastasize to the base of skull include breast, lung and prostate carcinoma (112,215). Base of skull invasion may also occur from local extension of nasopharyngeal tumors (183) or perineural spread of tumors originating in the head and neck (50). Base of skull metastases are difficult to diagnose with plain radiographs and require MRI or CT scan imaging. Early diagnosis and subsequent treatment of metastases with radiation therapy is most likely to result in improvement in neurological function and pain relief (257).

1. *Orbital Syndrome:* Neoplastic invasion of the orbit can produce continuous progressive orbital and supraorbital pain. Blurred vision is followed by diplopia, and examination may reveal external ophthalmoplegia and proptosis with sensory loss in the first division of the trigeminal nerve.
2. *Parasellar Syndrome:* The parasellar syndrome presents as unilateral supraorbital or frontal headache and diplopia without proptosis. There may be associated oculomotor paresis or papilledema present on examination.
3. *Middle Fossa Syndrome:* Most patients with the middle fossa syndrome present with paresthesias or sensory loss in the second or third division of the trigeminal nerve. Patients usually have a dull ache in the cheek or jaw. Some develop pain similar to trigeminal neuralgia without trigger points. Sensory symptoms in the trigeminal distribution precede the development of masseter and pterygoid weakness.
4. *Jugular Foramen Syndrome:* The presenting symptoms of the jugular foramen syndrome include hoarseness and dysphagia. Glossopharyngeal neuralgia and unilateral pain behind the ear may be the presenting complaints, with weakness of the palate, vocal cords, trapezius, sternocleidomastoid, and tongue. Cranial nerve XII impairment may occur if the hypoglossal canal is also involved, and a Horner's syndrome (ptosis, miosis, and anhidrosis) may be observed if the sympathetic chain is involved adjacent to the jugular foramen.
5. *Occipital Condyle Syndrome:* Tumor invasion of the occipital condyle may produce severe unilateral occipital pain, which is exacerbated by neck flexion and associated with neck stiffness and occipital tenderness (112). A 12th nerve paresis may accompany the pain.
6. *Clivus Metastases:* A destructive lesion of the clivus may produce vertex headache exacerbated by neck flexion. Pareses of lower cranial nerves may occur as the lesion progresses.
7. *Sphenoid Sinus Metastases:* Sphenoid sinus metastases often present with bifrontal headache radiating to the temples. There may also be intermittent retro-orbital pain associated with nasal congestion and diplopia. Examination can reveal unilateral or bilateral sixth nerve paresis.

VISCERAL PAIN SYNDROMES

Obstruction, infiltration or compression of visceral structures, including hollow viscus and supporting connective tissues, produce an extremely diverse group of pain syndromes that are together categorized as visceral nociceptive. As reviewed previously (see Chapter 12), visceral organ systems are innervated by two populations of afferents: (a) "sympathetic" afferents: axons which travel with the sympathetics and the cell bodies of which are in the dorsal root ganglia; and (b) vagal afferents, cell bodies of which are in the nodose ganglia and the axons of which travel with the vagus. These visceral afferents are typically small, slowly conducting and activated by a variety of chemical stimuli and/or mechanical stimuli, associated with distention of the smooth muscle or capsule. As with somatic afferents these axons show significant sensitization with local inflammation (see Chapters 6 and 18). Sympathetic afferents project within the dorsal horn in a somatotopic fashion and synapse with dorsal horn neurons that receive convergent input from somatic afferents (see Chapter 12). This convergence is believed to account for the referred pain states generated by visceral injury for the local nocifensor tenderness that is associated with the visceral injury (175).

The effective stimulus that evokes activity in these systems is likely similar to those outlined above in somatic pain states. Thus, visceral afferents are typically defined in terms of their mechanical sensitivity and chemosensitivity (16,140,191,231). Although mild distention of a hollow viscus is not adequate to produce a pain state, extreme distention or the presence of inflammation can yield clearly defined pain states.

Two common visceral pain states are illustrative of these processes.

Liver Metastases

The liver is involved by tumor in one third of all cancer patients, and in one half of patients with primaries of the biliary system, breast, lung, and stomach (135,232). In addition to pain, patients may experience malaise, heaviness in the right upper abdomen, weight loss, and hepatomegaly (232), usually without jaundice. There may be only mild abnormalities of conjugated bilirubin, transaminase, and alkaline phosphatase.

The pain in such patients likely occurs as a result of injury to nociceptors that invest the hepatic capsule or nearby structures, including the inferior surface of the diaphragm or the chest wall. The pain caused by capsular injury is usually localized to the right upper abdomen and steady and aching in character. It may be associated with tenderness to palpation and cutaneous hyperesthesia (52).

Sensory nerve terminals have been identified in the parenchyma with particular densities around the local vasculature (196). Numerous peptide-containing axons have been observed (86). Vagal innervation of the liver is well known, but it is not known whether this innervation accounts for regulatory feedback for homeostasis (194) or for nociception. Electrophysiological studies have shown that neuronal outflow from the liver, traveling in the splanchnic distribution is activated by a variety of agents, such as bradykinin (164).

Referred pain from involvement of the liver capsule may be experienced in the subscapular region, right flank, lower paraspinal back or right shoulder. The latter referred site is associated with diaphragmatic irritation (232). In this regard, mechanical stimulation of the hepatic vein, the hepatic parenchyma as well as the inferior vena cava will result in the activation of axons traveling in the phrenic nerve and C5 nerve root (152). These results suggest that inflammatory products and expansive processes in the liver may activate a variety of small afferents that reach the spinal cord by at least two routes.

Pancreatic Carcinoma

The incidence of adenocarcinoma of the pancreas has increased threefold during the past 30 years (272). This tumor is now the fourth cause of cancer death in the United States (130). Pancreatic cancer is associated with a triad of pain, cachexia and depression. Pain is present in ~80% of patients prior to death (130), most of whom experience epigastric pain or epigastric pain that radiates to the mid-back. The pain is characteristically relieved by forward flexion and exacerbated by spinal extension. Patients may also develop localized right upper abdominal pain if there is biliary tract obstruction, and a more diffuse and intermittent upper abdominal pain if there is pancreatic duct obstruction (130).

Pain is thought to result from activation of primary afferent nerves that innervate the damaged gland or increase firing during intermittent obstruction of the pancreatic duct or biliary duct; activation of nociceptors that invest surrounding blood vessels and connective tissue may also be involved. Changes in nerve morphology have been observed in chronic pancreatitis and such changes may lead to alterations in the discharge properties of these innervating afferents (20). These afferents travel with the sympathetic innervation of the gland passing through the celiac plexus and entering the spinal cord with the splanchnic nerves. The efficacy of celiac plexus blocks is support for the role played by these projections (227). Back pain may be referred from somatic injury to the posterior abdomen wall produced by the tumor or retroperitoneal lymphadenopathy (34,263), or from tumor involvement of the bowel, kidney, ureter, uterus, or rectum (52). These pains may thus resemble spinal disease (124).

NEUROPATHIC PAIN SYNDROMES

The cancer-related neuropathic pain syndromes comprise disorders due to tumor infiltration or compression of nerve, ganglion cells or roots (if within the vertebral canal, as outlined above), or due to the remote effects of malignancy on peripheral nerves (78). Axonal injury, which results in focal demyelination and neuroma formation, most likely contributes to the development of the abnormal sensations associated with neuropathic pain. These abnormal sensations include nonpainful paresthesias (abnormal sensations) and dysesthesias. The dysesthesias are often reported as spontaneous burning or stabbing, which may be associated with allodynia, hyperpathia, or hyperalgesia (182). Some patients develop neuropathic pain states that are relatively refractory to routine therapeutic maneuvers, including opioid administration (5).

Pain can also result from other neural processes, such as enhanced nociception due to sympathetic efferent activity, which has been shown to sensitize peripheral nociceptors in the setting of nerve injury (230), or abnormal impulse formation (30,39) in damaged sensory afferents (see Chapter 5).

General Mechanisms

When tumor invades peripheral nerve or compresses peripheral nerve, pain can result, in part, from sensitization of peripheral sensory receptors, especially mechanoreceptors and nociceptors, or from the local tissue inflammatory response to the tumor (33,49,150,166) (Table 3). Experimentally, it has been demonstrated that chronic nerve compression will lead to (a) development of local axon injury sites that develop spontaneous afferent activity and cross talk between populations of axons (63); (b) appearance of spontaneous activity in the dorsal root ganglion cells of the injured nerve (131); (c) appearance of sympathetic sprouting at the peripheral injury site and in the dorsal root ganglion of the injured axon and development of an excitation by sympathetic input into the injury site and the dorsal root ganglion (177); and (d) sprouting of the central terminals of the Ab axon from lamina III and deeper, up into lamina I and II (266). These complex events are reviewed in detail in Chapters 13 and 28. Together, these processes induced by peripheral nerve injury, can lead to a state in which sympathetic outflow can increase afferent input at several sites and low-threshold mechanoreceptor afferents can yield activity in circuitry that was originally activated by small typically high-threshold afferent input. Moreover, it appears probable that this enhanced spontaneous input may cause a central state of sensitization, whereby the persistent abnormal impulses from peripheral receptors (49,230) and primary afferents (258) changes the neuronal properties (267) and receptive fields (13,32,133) of central neurons in the pain pathways. This central sensitization may combine with the development of a relative imbalance in presynaptic (219), postsynaptic (69,95,243) or descending inhibition (247) that exacerbates hyperexcitable central neurons (212,249) and may sustain the neuropathic pain (see Chapters 13 and 28).

These hyperexcitable neurons may also develop at higher levels of the nervous system. Studies with positron emission tomography, for example, suggest that pain may be associated with a more widespread activation of brain structures, including bilateral thalamus and cingulate gyrus (127,248), than occurs normally following a noxious stimulus (51) (see Chapter 10). This more extensive increase in both blood flow and glucose metabolism in bilateral structures related to nociceptive pathways may reflect the rostral spread of central sensitization, which could underlie the development of some chronic pain states (Table 2).

Table 3. MECHANISMS OF NEUROPATHIC PAIN

Sensitization of peripheral receptors
- Adrenergic activation
- Neurogenic inflammation with activation
- Changes in receptor thresholds
- Expansion of receptor fields

Ectopic activity in primary afferents
- Demyelination-induced exposure of Na^{2+} channels
- Aberrant coupling of efferent sympathetics and sensory afferents

Neuroma formation
- Accumulation of Na^{2+} channels
- Axonal cross-excitation

Ectopic activity in the dorsal root ganglia
- Noradrenergic sprouting in DRG
- Activity-dependent cross-excitation

Central sensitization of spinal cord (dorsal horn) neurons
- Increasing action potential response with repetitive stimuli
- Lowering of response thresholds of wide dynamic range neurons
- Spontaneous activity of dorsal horn projection neurons
- Expansion of receptive fields.

Central sensitization of more rostral CNS sensory/pain pathways

Neuropathic Syndromes Associated with Peripheral Nerves

Painful Cranial Mononeuropathies, Including Neuralgias

Facial pain, with or without headache, results from tumor infiltration or compression of nerves in the head and neck. Some of the syndromes present with focal lancinating head pain. This subtype of neuropathic pain, which has been termed lancinating neuralgia, may be related to discrete neoplastic lesions.

Glossopharyngeal neuralgia, which may be associated with syncope and hypotension, has been reported in patients with leptomeningeal metastases (238), the jugular foramen syndrome (see below) (112), and head and neck malignancy (167,220,202). Severe pain in the neck or temporal region with retro-auricular or mastoid radiation, may be the prodrome to a syncopal episode.

Pain that mimics classic trigeminal neuralgia can occur with middle and posterior fossa tumors (28). Up to 10% of patients with classical trigeminal neuralgia harbor an unrecognized CNS tumor and tend to have a younger age at presentation than patients with idiopathic trigeminal neuralgia (44). Brief, lancinating pains in the absence of trigger points can also occur with leptomeningeal metastases (58,161).

Continuous facial pain due to trigeminal nerve damage also occurs in patients with base of skull metastases (28) and those with perineural spread of tumor from cutaneous or head and neck malignancies (11,80). Twenty-five percent of patients with squamous carcinoma of the head and neck will have evidence of perineural invasion by tumor at the time of surgical resection (35), and perineural spread of tumor is present in 88% of patients with squamous carcinoma of the head and neck at autopsy (35). The pain in these patients often occurs in conjunction with incomplete peripheral facial nerve involvement (25,50).

Unilateral facial pain may also occur with tumor infiltration of the lung apex and tumor irritation of the intrathoracic vagal nerve. The pain may be centered around the eye, cheek or ear, and is presumed to result from the convergence of vagal afferents and somatosensory afferents in the trigeminal tract and nucleus (17,255).

Intercostal Neuropathy

The most common example of compression and infiltration of the peripheral nerve is intercostal nerve entrapment that occurs as a result of metastatic involvement of a rib (93). Intercostal neuropathy commonly results in burning pain and dysesthesia in a region of dermatomal sensory loss. Such intercostal nerve syndromes show some correspondence to iatrogenic lesions as noted in postthoracotomy syndromes (see Chapter 24).

Painful Peripheral Neuropathy

Painful peripheral neuropathy has diverse causes in the cancer population: multiple vitamin deficiencies; metabolic derangements due to renal dysfunction, hepatic dysfunction, or diabetes; neurotoxic effects of chemotherapy (37,184,273); direct tumor invasion (122); and paraneoplastic syndromes (4) may all result in painful peripheral neuropathy. Although the paraneoplastic syndromes are rare causes, they may herald an occult malignancy and are important to recognize (122). Their course is usually independent of the primary tumor (211), with the exception of the painful neuropathies associated with multiple myeloma, which can respond to primary antineoplastic therapy (12,56,178,211).

The syndrome of paraneoplastic dorsal root ganglionopathy may present with pain, tingling paresthesias, and burning distal dysesthesias. These symptoms are associated with marked impairment of joint position sense, pseudoatheotosis of the hands, sensory ataxia, and loss of deep tendon reflexes (211). The disorder results from an autoimmune, inflammatory infiltration of dorsal root ganglion; lesions of the spinal cord, brain stem, or limbic lobe may also be present (4). It is most often associated with small cell carcinoma of the lung, but may occasionally be seen in patients with other malignancies, such as breast, ovary or colon carcinoma (4). ANNA-1 seropositivity ("anti-Hu") indicates a paraneoplastic etiology. This finding should be followed by a search for an occult cancer, usually small cell lung cancer. The tumor may present many years after the development of symptoms (40).

A painful sensorimotor neuropathy may also occur as a paraneoplastic syndrome (56,259). This lesion has a variable presentation, which ranges from distal extremity sensory loss with painful dysesthesias to extensive distal weakness and wasting. There is rarely a Guillain-Barré syndrome (206).

Painful dysesthesias, paresthesias, restless legs and hyperpathia associated with mild weakness, sensory loss or autonomic dysfunction may follow treatment with neurotoxic chemotherapy. The mechanisms responsible for the pain in these disorders are unknown. Treatment with vincristine may result in severe pain associated with marked impairment of fine finger movements, loss of two-point discrimination and vibratory sensation, and selective weakness of the distal hand and feet extensors (especially finger extensors) (57). Cisplatin therapy usually produces a sensory neuropathy with cramps, sensory paresthesias in the extremities, and large fiber sensory loss (251). Pain is unusual in this neuropathy. Cisplatin neuropathy is related to the cumulative dose received by the patient (184), and off-therapy deterioration may continue for months after cisplatin withdrawal (234). Paclitaxel, a newer antineoplastic agent with activity against ovarian, breast, lung, and head and neck malignancies, also induces a painful sensory or sensorimotor peripheral neuropathy (221). Patients with peripheral neuropathy prior to paclitaxel therapy (for example, related to nutrition, diabetes, alcohol, or chemotherapy) are prone to developing a severe neuropathy. Rarely, proximal motor weakness and autonomic dysfunction can also occur.

Cervical, Brachial, and Lumbosacral Plexopathy

Tumor infiltration of the cervical, brachial, or lumbosacral plexus causes pain in the neck, arm, or leg, respectively. Symptoms and signs mimic multiple peripheral nerve or nerve root involvement.

Cervical Plexopathy The cutaneous branches of the cervical plexus emerge into the posterior triangle of the neck. These nerves may be injured by tumor, cervical trauma, or infection (27). This injury may produce cervical pain in the preauricular and postauricular areas and over the anterior shoulder and neck (240). Sensory afferent fibers from the cervical plexus enter the spinal tract of the trigeminal along with the sensory afferents from cranial nerves V, VII, IX, and X. Consequently, there is much overlap of the pain referral patterns in the head and neck (26). A Horner's syndrome may be present if the superior cervical ganglion is involved.

Postradical Neck Dissection Syndrome Radical neck dissection may result in a postsurgical neuropathic pain syndrome as a result of damage to the cutaneous branches of the cervical plexus. These patients also often develop poor posture due to the loss of supporting muscles around the shoulder capsule, which may result in a "droopy shoulder syndrome" (246) and subsequent brachial plexus stretch or suprascapular nerve entrapment (31).

Malignant Brachial Plexopathy Malignant brachial plexopathy occurs most commonly in patients with metastatic breast carcinoma and those with lung carcinoma that arises from the superior sulcus of the lung apex (Pancoast syndrome) (173). Pain in the shoulder girdle, elbow, and medial hand is often the initial presentation of malignant brachial plexopathy (92). In a series of patients with Pancoast tumor treated at MSKCC, the median duration of time from the onset of symptoms to correct diagnosis was eight months (173). The pain is followed weeks to months later by progressive weakness, sensory loss, dysesthesias, and hyperpathia in the C7, C8, and T1 segmental distribution, often with an associated depression in the triceps reflex. This pattern of findings suggests predominant involvement of the lower plexus. Brachial plexopathy may also develop from extension of tumor from supraclavicular lymph nodes. This may produce an upper plexopathy with proximal shoulder pain and predominant C5 and C6 segmental involvement (92).

One half of all patients with Pancoast tumor will develop epidural extension. This complication is often heralded by a progressive brachial panplexopathy (143), a Horner's syndrome, or the development of crescendo pain (Fig. 1). These findings suggest proximal extension and require further imaging studies to assess for epidural spinal cord compression (89,151). Arm pain exacerbated with neck maneuvers and associated with segmental reflex loss or motor weakness (222), with or without evidence of a myelopathy and autonomic dysfunction, also suggests radiculopathy due to epidural tumor and requires radiographic examination of the epidural space. Patients with recurrent pain after definitive treatment most often have local recurrence of their tumor.

Other Causes of Brachial Plexopathy Not all arm pain in the cancer patient is due to direct tumor infiltration. The acute onset of pain in the shoulder and arm followed by progressive weakness in the shoulder girdle may be the presentation of idiopathic brachial plexopathy (252). Idiopathic brachial plexopathy can be differentiated from a malignant plexopathy with the appropriate imaging studies and the improvement in the neurological abnormalities over time. Intraarterial administration of chemotherapy, which may result in an acute painful brachial plexopathy, may produce irreversible deficits (228).

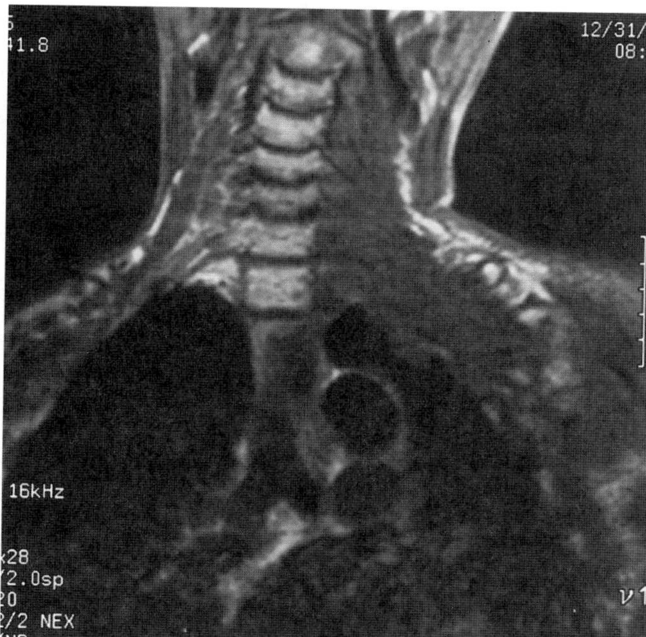

Figure 1. A patient with breast carcinoma and a left brachial plexopathy who developed escalating pain. MRI reveals tumor extending proximally to involve the cervical paraspinal muscles adjacent to the cervical vertebral bodies.

Trauma to the brachial plexus can occur during catheter placement or positioning (117,157).

An acute ischemic brachial plexopathy, often associated with subclavian occlusion, may follow radiation therapy (99). A reversible brachial plexopathy resembling acute brachial plexitis may also occur during the course of mantle radiation therapy in patients with Hodgkin's disease (170) or may follow supervoltage radiation therapy in 1% of patients with breast carcinoma (226).

Radiation-induced fibrosis of the brachial plexus does not usually present with severe pain, but with slowly progressive weakness and sensory loss predominantly affecting the upper plexus. Pain is present in only 18% of patients at presentation (90). Radiation skin changes, lymphedema, the absence of a tumor mass on imaging of the brachial plexus, and the presence of myokymic discharges on electromyographic (EMG) studies (84,118,160) support the diagnosis of radiation plexopathy. However, definitive diagnosis may require surgical exploration.

Malignant Lumbosacral Plexopathy Tumor invasion of the lumbar plexus can produce progressive lower abdominal, buttock or leg pain (205), followed by sensory loss and weakness in varying patterns. The differential diagnosis is often lengthy; for example, meningeal disease may also present with multiple radicular leg pains, and bony metastases to the hip may also result in referred pain in the knee (114).

Pain is the most frequent initial symptom of malignant lumbosacral plexopathy, and develops in most patients during the course of the disease (54,78,102). Pain may be the only symptom in one-quarter of patients, and a very small proportion present with pain associated with local autonomic involvement (54,83,102). Perineal sensory loss and sphincter impairment, hydronephrosis, leg edema and palpable tenderness, or a rectal mass may also be present in some patients (136).

Other Causes of Lumbosacral Plexopathy Regional iliac administration of intra-arterial chemotherapy may result in a lumbosacral plexopathy or mononeuropathy. The acute onset of pain, weakness, and paresthesias follows the infusion, possibly due to small vessel damage and plexus infarction (38).

Radiation fibrosis of the lumbosacral plexus may occur 1–30 years following radiation therapy. Similar to radiation-induced fibrosis of the brachial plexus, pain is uncommon and severe pain is rare. The lesion is associated with slowly progressive unilateral or bilateral leg weakness, numbness, and paresthesias (3,250). Both intracavitary radium pelvic implants used for therapy of gynecological malignancy and intraoperative irradiation are associated risk factors (100,107,148).

Other causes of painful plexopathy include an idiopathic, presumably inflammatory, lesion (23,82); plexus infarction from diabetes or vasculitis; and compression due to an iliopsoas hemorrhage, a large abdominal aneurysm/dissection (98), or from a psoas abscess. In addition, malignant peripheral nerve tumors and second primary tumors may occur in a previously irradiated area, such as lumbosacral plexus. This lesion may occur following radiation to any plexus or nerve, and may present years following radiation therapy (70,94,253). Patients with neurofibromatosis are at increased risk and surgical exploration may be required for definitive diagnosis in patients with progressive pain and a mass in the affected plexus.

Spinal Neuropathic Syndromes

Epidural Spinal Cord and Cauda Equina Compression

Back pain exacerbated by recumbency, cough, sneeze, or strain and associated with focal vertebral tenderness may be the only symptom of epidural tumor. Back pain usually precedes neurological signs of epidural spinal cord or cauda equina compression (ESCC) by weeks to months. ESCC is the second most common neurologic complication of cancer (203), occurring in 10% of patients (210). ESCC may be the presentation of the underlying malignancy, especially in patients with lymphoma (195). In up to 10% of patients, back pain may be the only symptom despite high-grade epidural disease (113). Most patients develop ESCC (210) through adjacent tumor spread from vertebral metastases. Patients with lymphoma, however, may develop ESCC without vertebral body metastases, as the lymphoma reaches the epidural space via spread through the intervertebral foramina.

The pain of ESCC is focal, radicular, or referred (195). The focal pain, which results from tumor involvement of the vertebral periosteum, is dull, localized and often exacerbated by palpation and recumbency. The radicular pain results from compression of nerve roots. It is typically unilateral when lumbar (222) or cervical, and bilateral when thoracic (222) in the latter case, it is often described as a tight band across the abdomen or chest. As discussed previously, referred unilateral or bilateral sacroiliac or iliac crest pain may occur with L1 vertebral compression (241), and referred mid-scapular or shoulder pain may be seen with C7-T1 vertebral compression with epidural disease. So-called "funicular pain" is a referred pain that is typically dysesthetic and experienced below the site of spinal cord compression. It is thought to result from compression of the sensory tracts in the spinal cord (195).

Following a period of progressive pain, the patient with untreated ESCC will develop weakness, sensory loss, autonomic dysfunction, and reflex abnormalities (195). The weakness will be segmental in distribution if there is a predominantly radicular involvement from nerve root compression, or pyramidal in distribution if the spinal cord is affected (241). Sensory symptoms and signs may be segmental or nondermatomal. There may be ascending paresthesias culminating in a sensory level or marked loss of all sensation below a dermatomal level in a paraplegic patient. The sensory level may correspond to the level of the epidural tumor or may develop many segments caudal to the level of the epidural tumor. Bladder and bowel dysfunction usually occurs late in the course of ESCC, unless tumor compresses the conus medullaris (241). Conus medullaris compression can rapidly progress, with the development of symmetrical perineal pain, symmetrical sacral (saddle) sensory loss, and paraplegia. A small number of patients develop ESCC with progressive ataxia from early compression of the spinocerebellar tracts (195,210).

The neurological outcome in patients with epidural spinal cord compression is directly related to level of function at the time of treatment (101,121,222,237,274). Consequently, early diagnosis is essential. As discussed previously, the decision to undertake definitive imaging of the epidural space is based on the symptoms and signs, and the results of imaging studies. Algorithms have been described to assist in this management (207,218). Ten percent of patients have multiple levels of ESCC on their initial evaluation, and the entire spine should usually be imaged (113).

The treatment of ESCC includes corticosteroids, radiation therapy, chemotherapy and surgery. Neurosurgical therapy of ESCC is considered in patients with ESCC due to an unknown primary and in patients who have relapsed after radiation therapy, have spinal instability (or bone fragments compressing the spinal cord) (119), or develop progressive neurological impairment during radiation therapy (119,210,244). Some patients with high-grade lesions from radioresistant tumors are also considered for surgery. The prompt use of radiotherapy is usually sufficient treatment for the pain and neurological deficits, even when the tumor is relatively radioresistant (105,123).

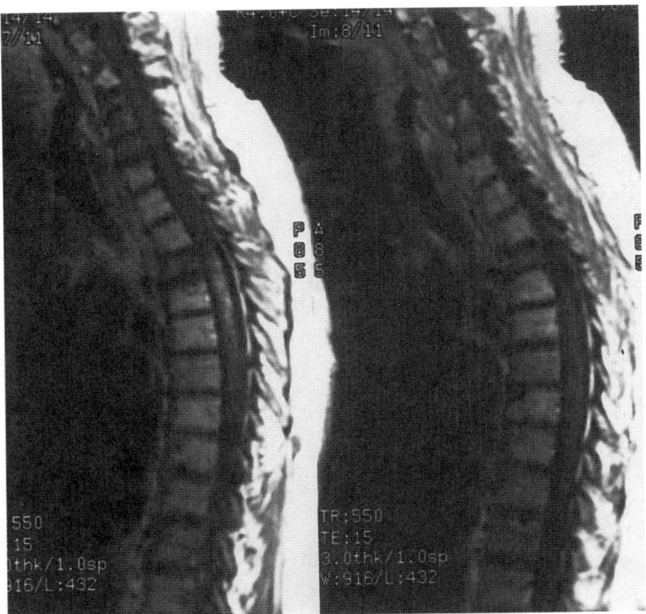

Figure 2. A woman with breast carcinoma who developed myelopathy and leg pain 6 months following irradiation for epidural spinal cord compression. MRI suggests a swollen spinal cord and spinal necrosis compatible with progressive radiation myelopathy.

Other Spinal Cord Syndromes

Reagan et al. (217) described four spinal cord syndromes associated with radiation: (a) a transient syndrome characterized by paresthesias that resolves spontaneously; (b) a progressive syndrome, which may be preceded by paresthesias and is characterized by progressive weakness, autonomic dysfunction and sensory loss; (c) a rare syndrome of acute paraplegia or quadriplegia, which presumably results from spinal cord infarction related to radiation-induced changes in blood vessels; and (d) a rare syndrome of lower motor neuron disease with atrophy, loss of deep tendon reflexes, fasciculation, and weakness in upper or lower extremities, which presumably results from radiation-induced anterior horn cell damage. All but the last of these syndromes can be associated with neuropathic pain, which originates from root or cord pathology (172).

Progressive radiation-induced myelopathy may stabilize or progress to a Brown-Sequard syndrome (spinal cord hemisection) (141) or a transverse myelopathy, with complete paralysis (21,260). A refractory central pain syndrome may develop. Rapid fractionation schedules and large dose per fraction, total dose, treatment time, and length of spinal cord irradiated (>10 cm) are predisposing risk factors (159,163,207,260). Three-fourths of reported cases of progressive radiation-induced thoracic myelopathy occur within the first 18 months after completion of radiotherapy (159) and the majority of patients present within 6 months to 2 years of radiation therapy (Fig. 2).

Treatment of radiation myelopathy is symptomatic. The anticoagulants heparin and warfarin may have a role in slowing progression, at least for a time (105).

Epidural lipomatosis is a rare complication of corticosteroid therapy and may present with back pain and rapidly evolving epidural spinal cord compression, which may mimic epidural abscess (88,115,145). The lesion can also present as a painful lumbar radiculopathy (88). Patients develop back pain, radicular pain, weakness, numbness, and dysesthesias (88). Patients may develop this syndrome after only a short course of corticosteroids or even with use of a steroid inhaler (88).

Spinal cord ischemia (from tumor compression of the spinal radicular arteries), meningeal metastases, epidural hematoma or abscess, subluxation of the spine from pathological spinal fracture, or a central herniated disc may also mimic ESCC from tumor and produce a spinal cord syndrome (36). Management varies greatly and accurate diagnosis is extremely important.

Meningeal Metastases

Pain is present in about one half of patients with meningeal metastases. Back pain, radicular pain, multiple root and cranial nerve symptoms, and headache may occur in any combination (106,199). A cauda equina syndrome occurs in 30% of these patients (261).

Evaluation of the cerebrospinal fluid (CSF) for cell count, protein, glucose, and malignant cells is needed to establish the diagnosis of meningeal metastases. Imaging studies, particularly contrast-enhanced MRI also may be useful in diagnosis (42,111). CSF flow studies (41), CSF flow cytometry (48), and tumor marker studies such as CEA, LDH isoenzymes, β_2 microglobulin, or glucosephosphate isomerase may assist diagnosis and evaluation of therapeutic response (48,193,254).

Other Neuropathic Pains in Cancer Patients

Postmastectomy Syndrome

Burning dysesthesias in the arm and anterior chest wall may be the presentation of the postmastectomy syndrome (265). This syndrome results from damage to the intercostobrachial nerve, a cutaneous branch of the second and third intercostal nerves that innervates the axilla and upper medial and posterior arm (6). The presence of this syndrome is not associated with recurrent disease (109). There may be a trigger point in the scar. The postmastectomy syndrome is believed to be due to the formation of a neuroma at the end of a severed nerve (256).

Postthoracotomy Syndrome

Thoracotomy may result in a postsurgical neuropathic pain syndrome due to transection of the intercostal nerves. This syndrome is characterized by segmental thoracic sensory loss, dysesthesias, and hyperalgesia. New or progressive thoracic pain following cancer surgery is usually due to recurrent neoplasm (144,173).

Phantom Limb and Stump Pain

Phantom limb pain is a chronic neuropathic pain perceived in an absent body part. There are wide variations in the reported incidence of phantom limb pain (233). A prospective study of patients without cancer found a 59% prevalence at 2 two years, with persistent late phantom pain significantly more frequent in patients with coexistent stump pain (142).

Stump pain is due to neuroma formation in the region of the amputation. It is present in 10–25% of patients who undergo amputation and is often associated with a palpable neuroma. Stump pain may be worsened by inadequate local blood supply, infection (especially osteomyelitis), or poorly fitting prosthesis. In the cancer population, recurrent disease must be considered when either phantom pain or stump pain recurs or progresses.

Therapy for established phantom limb pain has been generally unsatisfactory. Postsurgical phantom limb pain has been reported to be minimized with preoperative epidural blockade using an opioid/anesthetic combination (10) or opioid/anesthetic plus spinal clonidine (139). Successful treatment of early phantom pain has been reported with a calcitonin (137). Recently, three patients with established phantom limb pain obtained analgesia with parenteral infusion of the *N*-methyl-D aspartate receptor antagonist, ketamine hydrochloride (239). These data suggest that prevention of central sensitization by any of by a variety of methods, or the use of an NMDA receptor antagonist to attenuate central sensitization after it occurs, may be effective approaches for this syndrome.

Herpetic and Postherpetic Neuralgia

Patients with cancer have an increased incidence of herpes zoster infection. The dermatomal herpetic eruption often occurs in a region of tumor pathology or in a previous radiation port. Immunocompromised patients with a hematological malignancy who develop acute herpes zoster have an increased risk of developing disseminated herpetic infection (223), herpes zoster myelitis (61), or other diverse neurological complications of zoster (76).

Acute herpetic neuralgia may develop for a prolonged period prior to rash eruption ("preherpetic neuralgia") (103) or may be seen in the absence of a rash in conjunction with a variety of neurological complications, including facial paresis, myelitis, aseptic meningitis, encephalitis, or radiculopathy (71,73,120,176,186). This widening spectrum of 9zoster sine herpete9 (72,162) complicates the clinical diagnosis and may require detailed diagnostic evaluation, including imaging studies, CSF studies, and specific immunological tests for herpes zoster, including the use of polymerase chain reaction to examine the CSF for VZV DNA (104).

The management of acute herpetic neuralgia in the cancer population relies on prompt antiviral therapy in adequate dosages (262) and management of pain with a combination of analgesics and/or local nerve blocks if required. Corticosteroids are not used in the management of acute herpetic neuralgia in patients with cancer. The management of postherpetic neuralgia may be difficult. Therapeutic options are needed for patients who develop refractory pain. These options could potentially include CNS specific calcium channel blockers and/or *N*-methyl-D-aspartate receptor antagonists. In a recent controlled study, eight patients with established postherpetic neuralgia were administered saline, morphine or the NMDA receptor antagonist, ketamine. Following intravenous administration of ketamine 0.15mg/kg, patients developed significant relief of pain, and significant decrease in "wind-up pain" produced with repetitive pricking of the affected skin region with a von Frey filament (74).

GENERAL CONSIDERATION OF MECHANISMS IN CANCER PAIN MANAGEMENT

As reviewed above, the presentation of pain in a cancer patient typically reflects a composite of syndromes that may involve initiating mechanisms which reflect protracted afferent input originating from somatic and visceral organ systems and an altered organization of afferent encoding secondary to nerve injury. Accordingly, it is reasonable to consider the utility of multiple interventions in cancer pain management.

Agents Altering Somatic Afferent Input

In many cases, the tumor or the sequelae of treatment has resulted in the activation of systems that employ small afferent populations. As reviewed elsewhere (see Chapter 4), many pain states evoked by tissue injury, tissue compression, or the elaboration of inflammatory products are mediated by the excitatory input generated by small primary afferents. Elimination of that input will constitute an important variable in controlling the pain state. Thus, reduction of the stimulus (e.g., elimination of the tumor, reduction of tumor bulk) will minimize this component of the pain state. Blocking the input pathways with local anesthetics or severing the relevant afferent pathway can also be effective.

Within the central neuraxis, the modulation of afferent transmission can be achieved by a variety of drugs, the most important of which are the opioids (91). As reviewed elsewhere (see Chapters 30 and 31), opioids may exert powerful modulatory effect upon small afferent input at the spinal and supraspinal levels. At the spinal levels, the effects are demonstrably selective for small afferent input. To the extent that a pain state depends upon the afferent input mediated by small afferents, opioids will, in principle, regulate that input. In addition, opioids can have positive effects on mood (138) and, accordingly, can lessen suffering.

To the extent that a pain state is dependent upon processing systems that are independent of small afferent input, as in many neuropathic states wherein large afferents are believed to be essential, it might be anticipated that opioids would have correspondingly less efficacy. Indeed, it does appear that in some human (179) and animal (270) neuropathic pain states, opioids are less effective. It should be stressed, however, that all post–nerve injury states are not the same and in humans (134,165), as well as animal models (7,53), the underlying mechanisms may involve an opioid sensitive component.

Other drug classes are known to alter afferent transmission at the spinal level in humans but at present are not commercially available or are not practical. Drugs in this category include delta opioid agonists (188,200) (see Chapter 30), α_2 agonists (75) (for clonidine, see Chapter 32), and the cholinesterase inhibitor neostigmine (129).

Agents Altering Facilitated States of Somatic Afferent Processing

As reviewed above, injury, such as that produced by a tumor, may induce spontaneous activity in nociceptive pathways and a state of central sensitization. Evidence has pointed to the role of prostaglandins in both central and peripheral components of this action (see Chapter 34). The efficacy of NSAIDS in cancer pain, and particularly that associated with bony metastasis, is well appreciated and likely reflects the role of prostaglandins in nociceptive processing and the local release of prostanoids secondary to the lytic processes associated with tumor invasion (see Chapter 6). NSAIDs are instituted at the first step of the World Health Organization (WHO) ladder (91), and are utilized, with other agents, throughout the course of cancer therapy.

As emphasized above and in Chapters 9 and 13, insights into the role of central facilitory processes has led to the appreciation of the role played by a number of other receptors systems, notably those for glutamate. Thus, one promising group of experimental drugs known to attenuate central sensitization is the subclass of excitatory amino acid (EAA) receptor antagonists, the *N*-methyl-D-aspartate (NMDA) receptor antagonists (267). NMDA receptor antagonists have demonstrated efficacy in a variety of experimental pain models (55,77,79,171,271) (see Chapter 13). Favorable reports have suggested efficacy in patients with postoperative pain (174) and mixed cancer pain and neuropathic pain (74,153,201,239). For example, the antitussive dextromethorphan is an NMDA receptor antagonist (46,47,87,192) that can attenuate the "wind-up" phenomenon (66) and nociceptive behavior in animals (77,79). A psychophysical correlate of wind-up in humans has also been reduced by dextromethorphan (213). Extensive work remains to assure the safety and efficacy of these new therapies for neuropathic pain. Safety remains a particular concern with drugs that have unique modes of action. For example, neuropathological evaluation following large doses of both competitive and noncompetitive NMDA receptor antagonists in the adult rat revealed neuronal vacuolation in the cingulate cortex, retrosplenial cortex, and other neuronal regions suggestive of a neurotoxic effect from excessive NMDA receptor blockade (197,198; but see ref. 8).

Future efforts will likely target the actions of these and other similarly active classes of agents.

Agents That Alter Neuropathic Components of the Cancer Pain State

As reviewed above, the etiology and characteristics of the pain may lead to the conclusion that it is neuropathic, or related to changes in processing secondary to nerve injury. On the basis of current understanding of mechanisms that may be involved in this type of pain, particularly as it concerns the role of large afferents, it is not surprising that this pain may not display the same sensitivity to "analgesics" as does the somatic component. Thus, it may be speculated that the failure of opioids to induce pain relief may reflect, in part, the degree to which the pain state is not mediated by small afferents. The unique pharmacology of post–nerve injury pain suggests the value of several other interventions.

First, preclinical studies have shown that the glutamate receptors may be relevant to maintaining the allodynia that characterizes many neuropathic pains. As noted above, preliminary data with NMDA receptor antagonists have pointed to the possible efficacy of such interventions. Obviously, these new drugs have to be carefully studied in controlled clinical trials to determine their efficacy in neuropathic cancer pain.

Second, it has been shown that nerve compression and injury will lead to spontaneous afferent traffic, and this may be due in part to an accumulation of sodium channels in the injured axon (62). As reviewed in Chapters 27 and 36, intravenous local anesthetics such as lidocaine have been shown to have efficacy in managing at least some components of the neuropathic state in humans (154) and animals (43). These sodium channels, presumably the source of the ectopic activity, can also be blocked by the use of selected adjuvant agents with membrane-stabilizing properties, such as carbamazepine (30,39,64). New agents that prevent or reverse these central nervous system changes will likely serve to enhance the management of cancer-related neuropathic pain refractory to opioid drugs (65,66,116, 158,180).

Third, as noted, after experimental nerve injury, a linkage between sympathetic outflow and afferent excitation develops. The mechanism underlying the sympathetically maintained pain state have been reviewed in detail elsewhere (see Chapters 28). At least some component of the neuropathic cancer pain state may be sustained by such experimentally produced mechanisms. Spinal α_2 agonists, such as clonidine, have been reported to exert potent effects upon neuropathic states induced by nerve injury in animals (270) or in late stage cancer patients showing significant refractoriness to opioids (216).

Combination Drug Approaches to Cancer Pain Management

The afferent component of cancer pain is likely composed to varying degrees of somatic input arising from small afferents, facilitated states generated by the repetitive afferent input, and by a number of mechanisms that alter the encoding process such that input generated by large afferents generates responses associated with noxious input. The optimal approach to the management of such a complex state must involve multiple families of agents. It is clear that well considered polypharmacy can improve the well-being of patients. Two examples are widely appreciated.

1. The combination of NSAIDs and opioids is encouraged by the WHO (see above). While such synergy may reflect the role of repetitive small afferent input, and the peripheral and central role of prostanoids in augmenting the response to a C-fiber stimulus, extensive clinical experience supports their combined use and efficacy for cancer pain. Preclinical studies have confirmed the powerful interaction observed clinically between prostaglandins inhibitors and opioids (269).

2. Cancer pain states that are ineffectively managed by even high doses of opioids alone can show considerable relief when a local anesthetic is combined with reduced doses of opioid (60,181,236). The mechanism of this response is not known. Animal studies have shown a powerful synergy between opioids and ineffective doses of local anesthetics and it has been speculated that the combination serves to reduce the dorsal horn small afferent input and transmitter release (204).

Preclinical studies have similarly shown other interactions to be synergistic, but their clinical relevance has not been demonstrated. These include opioids and α_2 agonists (185), μ and δ agonists (269), and cholinesterase inhibitors and opioids (190).

Consideration of Side Effects in Cancer Pain Management

Although considerable relief can be achieved for the cancer pain patient with aggressive use of several modalities, care must be taken because of the potential for additional side effects. Several examples include the direct side effects of a drug (e.g., NSAIDs) (see Chapter 34), the accumulation of metabolites that have undesirable side effects (e.g., as with normeperidine), or the appearance of side effects because high doses are used.

With regard to the latter case, the development of the spinal hyperalgesic syndrome below the level of an intraspinal opioid infusion is a striking example. This pain syndrome, which may be associated with hyperalgesia/allodynia, painful muscle spasms, and myoclonus, is a poorly recognized complication of intraspinal opioid administration (59,149,242). In a retrospective review, 13% of patients receiving intraspinal opioids for management of cancer pain developed this complication (149), which was strongly associated with dosage of intraspinal opioid and with the presence of either a plexopathy or a spinal cord lesion. In this retrospective review, it was unclear whether the presence of neuropathic injury was the sole risk factor, or whether escalating neuropathic pain induced the clinicians to deliver large dosages of intraspinal opioids. Careful clinical evaluation is needed to differentiate this pain syndrome from alternative causes of pain.

The hyperalgesia syndrome closely resembles strychnine toxicity and may result from an imbalance in inhibitory spinal circuitry, possibly induced by presynaptic opioid blockade of the spinal inhibitory surround. Nonopioid excitatory effects have been ascribed to one of the principal metabolites of morphine (morphine-3-glucuronide) (268). Both animal data and clinical experience suggest that benzodiazepines (by increasing inhibition and possibly through their anticonvulsant action), in conjunction with lowering or discontinuing the intraspinal opioid, will rapidly reverse the syndrome. The spinal hyperalgesia syndrome should be considered a pain emergency (59,149). Continuation of high dosages of intraspinal opioids may result in generalization of the syndrome (149). Spinal imaging should be considered in the patient without known risk factors given the association with spinal cord pathology.

CONCLUSION

Cancer pain may be viewed as a model for the evaluation of the diverse pathophysiologies that may be responsible for chronic pain. It is now widely recognized that a comprehensive assessment of cancer-related pain may allow the clinician to infer the pathophysiology of the pain and identify the pain syndrome. This information can help define the status of the underlying disease and clarify the options for both primary therapy and analgesic techniques.

Although the clinical understanding of pain mechanisms will undoubtedly evolve as more becomes known about nociceptive and neuropathic processes, a simple categorization of syndromes into those that are predominantly nociceptive and those that are predominantly neuropathic has proved useful in developing strategies for evaluation and treatment. Similarly, efforts to define the characteristics of pain syndromes continue, but there is already a strong emphasis on syndrome recognition as a means to improve diagnostic acumen. The syndromes and inferred pathophysiologies described previously illustrate the usefulness of this information in conceptualizing the spectrum of pain problems that present in cancer patients. Importantly, as insights into the pharmacology of these several pain states evolve, the appreciation of such multiplicity will likely result in the more appropriate management of these complex conditions.

Although the emphasis of this chapter has been on the physiological components of the effects produced by tumor, it is clear that pain is, in part, defined by the "response bias" of the patient. The affective and motivational component of cancer pain and the accompanying suffering can have a devastating impact on the function and well-being of the patient. This aspect of patient care is as important as the diagnosis of underlying mechanisms and other pathophysiologic concerns. In addition to other aspects of care, future developments in the utilization of drug classes that alter mood in a positive fashion (269) may play a major role in the management of this suffering component.

ACKNOWLEDGMENT

K.J.E. is supported, in part, by a grant from the Varicella Zoster Virus (VZV) Foundation, and by NIDA Grant DA 00255.

REFERENCES

1. Ahmed M, Bjurholm A, Kreicbergs A, Schultzberg M. Neuropeptide Y, tyrosine hydroxylase and vasoactive intestinal polypeptide-immunoreactive nerve fibers in the vertebral bodies, discs, dura mater, and spinal ligaments of the rat lumbar spine. *Spine* 1993;18:268–273.
2. Ahmed M, Bjurholm A, Kreicbergs A, Schultzberg M. Sensory and autonomic innervation of the facet joint in the rat lumbar spine. *Spine* 1993;18:2121–2126.
3. Aho KA, Sainio K. Late irradiation-induced lesions of the lumbosacral plexus. *Neurology* 1983;33:953–955.
4. Anderson NE, Cunningham JM, Posner JB. Autoimmune pathogenesis of paraneoplastic neurologic syndromes. *Crit Rev Neurobiol* 1987;3:245–299.
5. Arner S, Meyerson BA. Lack of analgesic effect of opioids on neuropathic and idiopathic forms of pain. *Pain* 1988;33:11–23.
6. Assa J. The intercostobrachial nerve in radical mastectomy. *J Surg Oncol* 1974;6:123–126.
7. Attal N, Chen YL, Kayser V, Guilbaud G. Behavioural evidence that systemic morphine may modulate a phasic pain-related behaviour in a rat model of peripheral mononeuropathy. *Pain* 1991;47:65–70.
8. Auer RN, Coulter KC. The nature and time course of neuronal vacuolation induced by the *N*-methyl-D-aspartate antagonist, MK801. *Acta Neuropathol* 1994;87:1–7.
9. Bach F, Agerlin N, Sorenson JB, et al. Metastatic spinal cord compression secondary to lung cancer. *J Clin Oncol* 1992;10:1781–1787.
10. Bach S, Noreng MF, Tjellden NU. Phantom limb pain in amputees during the first 12 months following limb amputation, after preoperative lumbar epidural blockade. *Pain* 1988;33:297–301.
11. Ballantyne AJ, McCarten AB, Ibanez ML. The extension of cancer of the head and neck through peripheral nerves. *Am J Surg* 1963; 106:651–667.
12. Bardwick PA, Zvaifler NJ, Gill GN, et al. Plasma cell dyscrasia with polyneuropathy, organomegaly, endocrinopathy, M protein, and skin changes: the poems syndrome. *Medicine* 1980;59:311–322.
13. Basbaum AI, Wall PD. Chronic changes in the response of cells in adults cat dorsal horn following partial deafferentation. The appearance of responding cells in a previously nonresponsive region. *Brain Res* 1976;116:181–204.
14. Batson OV. The vertebral vein system. Caldwell Lecture 1956. *AJR* 1957;78:195–212.
15. Bennett A. The role of biochemical mediators in peripheral nociception and bone pain. *Cancer Surv* 1988;7:55–67.
16. Berkley KJ, Hubscher CH, Wall PD. Neuronal responses to stimulation of the cervix, uterus, colon, and skin in the rat spinal cord. *J Neurophysiol* 1993;69:545–556
17. Bindoff LA, Haseltine D. Unilateral facial pain in patients with lung cancer: a referred pain via the vagus? *Lancet* 1988;1:812–815.
18. Bingas B. Tumors of the base of the skull. In: Vinken PJ, Bruyn GW, eds. *Handbook of clinical neurology, vol. 17.* Amsterdam: Elsevier, 1974:136–233.
19. Blatt I, Goldhammer Y. Deterioration after lumbar puncture below spinal block. *J Neurosurg* 1988;69:313–314.
20. Bockman DE, Buchler M, Malfertheiner P, Beger HG. Analysis of nerves in chronic pancreatitis. *Gastroenterology* 1988;94:1459–1469.
21. Boden G. Radiation myelitis of the cervical spinal cord. *Br J Radiol* 1948;21:464–469.
22. Bonica JJ. *The management of pain, vol. 1.* 2nd ed. Philadelphia: Lea & Febiger, 1990:400–460.
23. Bradley WG, Chad D, Verghese JP, et al. Painful lumbosacral plexopathy with elevated erythrocyte sedimentation rate: a treatable inflammatory syndrome. *Ann Neurol* 1984;15:457–464.
24. Brady LW, Croll MN. The role of bone scanning in the cancer patient. *Skeletal Radiol* 1979;3:217–222.
25. Brazis PW, Vogler JB, Shaw KE. The "numb cheek-limp lower lid" syndrome. *Neurology* 1991;41:327–328.
26. Brodal A. *Neurological anatomy.* Oxford: Oxford University Press, 1981:527–530.
27. Bruera E, MacDonald RN. Intractable pain in patients with advanced head and neck tumors: a possible role of local infections. *Cancer Treat Rep* 1986;70:691–692.
28. Bullitt E, Tew JM, Boyd J, et al. Intracranial tumors in patients with facial pain. *J Neurosurg* 1986;64:865–871.
29. Burchiel KJ. Spontaneous impulse generation in normal and denervated dorsal root ganglia: sensitivity to alpha-adrenergic stimulation and hypoxia. *Exp Neurol* 1984;85:257–272.
30. Burchiel KJ. Carbamazepine inhibits spontaneous activity in experimental neuromas. *Exp Neurol* 1988;102:249–253.
31. Callahan JD, Scully TB, Shapiro SA, et al. Suprascapular nerve entrapment. A series of 27 cases. *J Neurosurg* 1991;74:893–896.
32. Cameron AA, Pover CM, Willis WD, et al. Evidence that fine primary afferent axons innervate a wider territory in the superficial dorsal horn following peripheral axotomy. *Brain Res* 1992;575:151–154.
33. Campbell JN, Raja SN, Meyer R, et al. Myelinated afferents signal the hyperalgesia associated with nerve injury. *Pain* 1988;32:89–94.

34. Cantwell BMJ, Mannis KA, Harris AL. Back pain—a presentation of metastatic testicular germ cell tumors. *Lancet* 1987:262–264.
35. Carter RL, Pittam MR, Tanner NSB. Pain and dysphagia in patients with squamous carcinomas of the head and neck: the role of perineural spread. *J R Soc Med* 1982;75:598–606.
36. Case Records of the Massachusetts General Hospital (Case 16—1992). *N Engl J Med* 1992;326:1070–1076.
37. Casey EB, Jellife AM, LeQuesne PM, et al. Vincristine neuropathy: clinical and electrophysiological observations. *Brain* 1973;96:69–86.
38. Castellanos AM, Glass JP, Yung KA. Regional nerve injury after intraarterial chemotherapy. *Neurology* 1987;37:834–837.
39. Chabal C, Russell LC, Burchiel KJ. The effect of intravenous lidocaine tocainide, and mexiletine on spontaneously active fibers originating in rat sciatic neuromas. *Pain* 1989;38:333–338.
40. Chalk CH, Lennon VA, Stevens JC, Windebank AJ. Seronegativity for type 1 antineuronal nuclear antibodies ("anti-Hu") in subacute sensory neuronopathy patients without cancer. *Neurology* 1993;43:2209–2211.
41. Chamberlain MC, Corey-Bloom J. Leptomeningeal metastases: indium DTPA CSF flow studies. *Neurology* 1991;41:1765–1769.
42. Chamberlain MC, Sandy AD, Press GA. Leptomeningeal metastases: a comparison of gadolinium-enhanced MR and contrast-enhanced CT of the brain. *Neurology* 1990;40:435–438.
43. Chaplan SR, Bach FW, Shafer SL, Yaksh TL. Systemic lidocaine alleviates mechanical allodynia in rats with experimental neuropathy. *Anesthesiology* 1993;79:A910.
44. Cheng TMW, Cascino TL, Onofrio BM. Comprehensive study of diagnosis and treatment of trigeminal neuralgia secondary to tumors. *Neurology* 1993;43:2298–2302.
45. Cherny NI, Portenoy RK. Cancer pain: principles of assessment and syndromes. In: Wall PD, Melzack R, eds. *Textbook of pain.* 3rd ed. Edinburgh: Churchill Livingston, 1994:787–824.
46. Choi DW. Dextrorphan and dextromethorphan attenuate glutamate neurotoxicity. *Brain Res* 1987;403:333–336.
47. Church J, Lodge D, Berry SC. Differential effects of dextrorphan and levorphanol on the excitation of rat spinal neurons by amino acids. *Eur J Pharmacol* 1985;111:185–190.
48. Cibas ES, Malkin MG, Posner JB, et al. Detection of DNA abnormalities by flow cytometry in cells from cerebrospinal fluid. *Am J Clin Pathol* 1987;88:570–577.
49. Cline MA, Ochoa J, Torebjork HE. Chronic hyperalgesia and skin warming caused by sensitive C nociceptors. *Brain* 1989;112:621–647.
50. Clouston PD, Sharpe DM, Corbett AJ, et al. Perineural spread of cutaneous head and neck cancer. Its orbital and central neurologic complications. *Arch Neurol* 1990;47:73–77.
51. Coghill RC, Talbot JD, Evans AC, et al. Distributed processing of pain and vibration by the human brain. *J Neurosci* 1994;14:4095–4108.
52. Cope Z. *The early diagnosis of the acute abdomen.* London: Oxford University Press, 1957:1–58.
53. Courteix C, Bardin M, Chantelauze C, Lavarenne J, Eschalier A. Study of the sensitivity of the diabetes-induced pain model in rats to a range of analgesics. *Pain* 1994;57:153–160.
54. Dalmau J, Graus F, Marco M. "Hot and dry foot" as initial manifestation of neoplastic lumbosacral plexopathy. *Neurology* 1989;39:871–872.
55. Davar G, Marma A, Deykin A, Vos B, Maciewicz R. MK-801 blocks the development of thermal hyperalgesia in a rat model of experimental painful neuropathy. *Brain Res* 1991;553:327–330.
56. Davis D. Myeloma neuropathy. *Arch Neurol* 1972;27:507–511.
57. DeAngelis LM, Gnecco C, Taylor L, et al. Evolution of neuropathy and myopathy during intensive vincristine/corticosteroid chemotherapy for non-Hodgkin's lymphoma. *Cancer* 1991;67:2241–2246.
58. DeAngelis LM, Payne R. Lymphomatous meningitis presenting as atypical cluster headache. *Pain* 1987;30:211–216.
59. DeConno F, Caraceni A, Martini C, et al. Hyperalgesia and myoclonus with intrathecal infusion of high-dose morphine. *Pain* 1991;47:337–339.
60. de Leon-Casasola OA, Lema MJ. Epidural bupivacaine/sufentanil therapy for postoperative pain control in patients tolerant to opioid and unresponsive to epidural bupivacaine/morphine. *Anesthesiology* 1994;80:303–309.
61. Devinsky O, Cho E-S, Petitio CK, et al. Herpes zoster myelitis. *Brain* 1991;114:1181–1196.
62. Devor M, Govrin-Lippmann R, Angelides K. Na^+ channel immunolocalization in peripheral mammalian axons and changes following nerve injury and neuroma formation. *J Neurosci* 1993;13:1976–1992.
63. Devor M, Wall PD. Cross-excitation in dorsal root ganglia of nerve-injured and intact rats. *J Neurophysiol* 1990;64:1733–1746.
64. Devor M, Wall PD, Catalan N. Systemic lidocaine silences ectopic neuroma and DRG discharge without blocking nerve conduction. *Pain* 1992;48;261–268.
65. Dickenson AH, Sullivan AF. Evidence for a role of the NMDA receptor in the frequency dependent potentiation of rat dorsal horn nociceptive neurones following C fibre stimulation. *Neuropharmacology* 1987;26:1235–1238.
66. Dickenson AH, Sullivan AF, Stanfa LC, McQuay HJ. Dextromethorphan and levorphanol on dorsal horn nociceptive neurones in the rat. *Neuropharmacology* 1991;30:1303–1308.
67. Di Sant'Agnese PA, Cockett AT. The prostatic endocrine-paracrine neuroendocrine) regulatory system and neuroendocrine differentiation in prostatic carcinoma: a review and future directions in basic research. *J Urol* 1994;152:1927–1931.
68. Dray A, Wood JN. Nonopioid molecular signaling mechanisms involved in nociception and antinociception. In: Basbaum A-I, Besson J-M, eds. *Towards a new pharmacotherapy of pain.* New York: John Wiley, 1991:21–34.
69. Dubner R. Neuronal plasticity in the spinal and medullary dorsal horns: a possible role in central pain mechanisms. In: Casey KL, ed. *Pain and central nervous system disease: the central pain syndromes.* New York: Raven Press, 1991:143–155.
70. Ducatman BS, Scheithauer BW, Piepgras DG, et al. Malignant peripheral nerve sheath tumors. A clinicopathological study of 120 cases. *Cancer* 1986;57:2006–2021.
71. Dueland AN, Devlin M, Martin JR, et al. Fatal varicella-zoster virus meningoradiculitis without skin involvement. *Ann Neurol* 1991;29:569–572.
72. Easton HG. Zoster sine herpete causing acute trigeminal neuralgia. *Lancet* 1970;2:1065–1066
73. Echevarria JM, Martinez-Martin P, Tellez A, et al. Aseptic meningitis due to varicella-zoster virus: serum antibody levels and local synthesis of specific IgG, IgM and IgA. *J Infect Dis* 1987;155:959–967.
74. Eide PK, Jorum E, Stubhaug A, et al. Relief of post-herpetic neuralgia with the N-methyl-D-aspartic acid receptor antagonist ketamine: a double-blind, cross-over comparison with morphine and placebo. *Pain* 1994;58:347–354.
75. Eisenach JC, Rauck RL, Buzzanell C, Lysak SZ. Epidural clonidine analgesia for intractable cancer pain: phase I. *Anesthesiology* 1989;71:647–652.
76. Elliott KJ. Other neurological complications of herpes zoster and their management. *Ann Neurol* 1994;35:557–561.
77. Elliott KJ, Brodsky M, Hynansky A, Foley KM, Inturrisi CE. Dextromethorphan suppresses both formalin-induced nociceptive behavior and formalin-induced increase in CNS c-fos mRNA. *Pain* (in press).
78. Elliott K, Foley KM. Neurologic pain syndromes in patients with cancer. *Neurol Clin* 1989;7:333–360.
79. Elliott KJ, Hynansky A, Foley KM, Inturrisi CE. Dextromethorphan is antinociceptive in the mouse formalin test [Abstract]. *Proc Am Pain Soc* 1993.
80. Eng CT, Vasconez LO. Facial pain due to perineural invasion by basal cell carcinoma. *Ann Plast Surg* 1984;12:374–377.
81. Engel IA, Straus DJ, Lacher M, et al. Osteonecrosis in patients with malignant lymphoma: a review of 25 cases. *Cancer* 1981;48:1245–1250.
82. Evans BA, Stevens JC, Dyck PJ. Lumbosacral plexus neuropathy. *Neurology* 1981;31:1327–1330.
83. Evans RJ, Watson CPN. Lumbosacral plexopathy in cancer patients. *Neurology* 1985;35:1392–1393.
84. Fardin P, Lelli S, Negrin P, et al. Radiation-induced brachial plexopathy: clinical and electromyographical (EMG) considerations in 13 cases. *Electromyogr Clin Neurophysiol* 1990;30:277–282.
85. Fast A, Alon M, Weiss S, et al. Avascular necrosis of bone following short term dexamethasone therapy for brain edema. *J Neurosurg* 1984;61:983–985.
86. Feher E, Fodor M, Feher J. Ultrastructural localization of somatostatin- and substance P-immunoreactive nerve fibers in the feline liver. *Gastroenterology* 1992;102:287–294.
87. Ferkany JW, Borosky BJ, Lesser RP, et al. Dextromethorphan for treatment of complex partial seizures. *Neurology* 1990;40:547–549.

88. Fessler RG, Johnson DL, Brown FD, Erickson RK, Reid SA, Kranzler L. Epidural lipomatosis in steroid-treated patients. *Spine* 1992; 17:183–188.
89. Fishman EK, Campbell JN, Kuhlman JE, et al. Multiplanar CT evaluation of brachial plexopathy in breast cancer. *J Comput Assist Tomogr* 1991;15:790–795.
90. Foley KM. Pain syndromes in patients with cancer. In: Bonica JJ, Ventafridda V, eds. *Advances in pain research and therapy, vol. 2.* New York: Raven Press, 1979:59–78.
91. Foley KM. The treatment of cancer pain. *N Engl J Med* 1985;313: 84–95.
92. Foley KM. Brachial plexopathy in patients with breast cancer. In: Harris JR, Hellman S, Henderson IC, et al, eds. *Breast diseases.* Philadelphia: JB Lippincott, 1987.
93. Foley, KM. Pain syndromes in patients with cancer. *Med Clin North Am* 1987;71:169–184.
94. Foley KM, Woodruff JM, Ellis FT. Radiation-induced malignant and atypical peripheral nerve sheath tumors. *Ann Neurol* 1980;7: 311–318.
95. Fromm GH, Nakata M, Kondo T. Differential action of amitriptyline on neurons in the trigeminal nucleus. *Neurology* 1991;41: 1932–1936.
96. Galasko CSB. Mechanisms of bone destruction in the development of skeletal metastasis. *Nature* 1976;263:507–508.
97. Galasko CSB, Bennett A. Relationship of bone destruction in skeletal metastases to osteoclast activation and prostaglandins. *Nature* 1976;263:508–510.
98. Garcia-Diaz JdeD, Balseiro J, Calandre L, Bermejo F. Aortic dissection presenting with neurologic sighs. *N Engl J Med* 1988;-1070.
99. Gerard, JM Franck N, Moussa Z, et al. Acute ischemic brachial plexus neuropathy following radiation therapy. *Neurology* 1989;39: 450–451.
100. Giese WL, Kinsella TJ. Radiation injury to peripheral and cranial nerves. In: Gutin PJ, Lebel SA, Sheline, GE, eds. *Radiation injury to the nervous system.* New York: Raven Press, 1991:383–403.
101. Gilbert RW, Kim JH, Posner JB. Epidural spinal cord compression from metastatic tumor. Diagnosis and treatment. *Ann Neurol* 1978; 3:40–51.
102. Gilchrist JM, Moore M. Lumbosacral plexopathy in cancer patients. *Neurology* 1985;35:1392.
103. Gilden DH, Dueland AN, Cohrs R, et al. Preherpetic neuralgia. *Neurology* 1991;41:1215–1218.
104. Gilden DH, Dueland AN, Devlin ME, et al. Varicella-zoster virus reactivation without rash. *J Infect Dis* 1992;166:530–534.
105. Glantz MJ, Burger PC, Friedman AH, et al. Treatment of radiation-induced nervous system injury with heparin and warfarin. *Neurology* 1994;44:2020–2027.
106. Glass JP, Foley KM. Carcinomatous meningitis. In: Harris JR, Hellman S, Henderson IC, et al, eds. *Breast diseases.* Philadelphia: JB Lippincott, 1987:497–505.
107. Glass JP, Pettigrew LC, Maor M, et al. Plexopathy induced by radiation therapy. *Neurology* 1985;35:1261.
108. Gonzales GR, Elliott KJ, Portenoy RK, Foley KM. The impact of a comprehensive evaluation in the management of cancer pain. *Pain* 1991;47:141–144.
109. Granek I, Ashikari R, Foley KM. Post-mastectomy pain syndrome: clinical and anatomical correlates. *Proc Am Soc Clin Oncol* 1984;3: 122.
110. Graus F, Krol G, Foley KM. [Abstract] Early diagnosis of spinal epidural metastasis (SEM): correlation with clinical and radiological findings. *Proc Am Soc Clin Oncol* 1985;4:269.
111. Gray JR, Wallner KE. Reversal of cranial nerve dysfunction with radiation therapy in adults with lymphoma and leukemia. *Int J Radiat Oncol Biol Phys* 1990;19:439–444.
112. Greenberg HS, Deck MDF, Vikram B, et al. Metastasis to the base of the skull: clinical findings in 43 patients. *Neurology* 1981;31:530–537.
113. Greenberg HS, Kim J-H, Posner JB, et al. Epidural spinal cord compression from metastatic tumor: results from a new treatment protocol. *Am Neurol* 1980;8:361–366.
114. Habermann ET, Sachs R, Stern RE, et al. The pathology and treatment of metastatic disease of the femur. *Clin Orthop* 1982;169: 70–82.
115. Haid RW, Kaufman HH, Schichet SS, et al. Epidural lipomatosis simulating an epidural abscess: case report and literature review. *Neurosurgery* 1987;21:744–747.
116. Haley JE, Sullivan AF, Dickenson AH. Evidence for spinal *N*-methyl-D-aspartate receptor involvement in prolonged chemical nociception in the rat. *Brain Res* 1990;518:218–226.
117. Hanson MR, Breuer AC, Furlan AJ, et al. Mechanism and frequency of brachial plexus injury in open-heart surgery: a prospective analysis. *Ann Thorac Surg* 1983;36:675–679.
118. Harper CM, Thomas JE, Cascino TL, et al. Distinction between neoplastic and radiation-induced brachial plexopathy, with emphasis on the role of EMG. *Neurology* 1989;39:502–506.
119. Harrington KD. *Orthopedic management of metastatic bone disease.* Washington: CV Mosby, 1988.
120. Heller HM, Carnevale NT, Steigbigel RT. Varicella zoster virus transverse myelitis without cutaneous rash. *Am J Med* 1990;68: 550–551.
121. Helweg-Larsen S, Rasmusson B, Sorenson PS. Recovery of gait after radiotherapy in paralytic patients with metastatic epidural spinal cord compression. *Neurology* 1990;40:1234–1236.
122. Henson RA, Urich H. *Cancer and the nervous system.* Boston: Blackwell Scientific, 1982:100–119,368–405.
123. Herbert SH, Solin LJ, Rate WR, et al. The effect of palliative radiation therapy on epidural compression due to metastatic malignant melanoma. *Cancer* 1991;67:2472–2476.
124. Hewitt DJ, Foley KM, Neuroimaging of pain. In: Greenberg, JO, ed. *Neuroimaging: a companion to Adam's and Victor's principles of neurology.* New York: McGraw-Hill, 1995:41–82.
125. Hill EL, Elde R. Distribution of CGRP-, VIP-, D beta H-, SP-, and NPY-immunoreactive nerves in the periosteum of the rat. *Cell Tissue Res* 1991;264:469–480.
126. Hoang P, Fiasse R, Van Heuverzwyn R, Sibille C. Role of cytokines in inflammatory bowel disease. *Acta Gastroenterol Belg* 1994;57: 219–223.
127. Hoffman JM, Hanson MW, Coleman RE. Clinical positron emission tomography imaging. *Radiol Clin North Am* 1993;31:939–959.
128. Holder LE. Clinical radionuclide bone imaging. *Radiology* 1990; 176:607–614.
129. Hood DD, Eisenach JC, Tuttle R. Phase I safety assessment of intrathecal neostigmine methylsulfate in humans. *Anesthesiology* 1995;82:331–343.
130. Horton J. Pain in pancreatic cancer. In: Foley KM, Payne RM, eds. *Current therapy of pain.* Philadelphia: Decker, 1989:332–341.
131. Howe JF, Loeser JD, Calvin WH. Mechanosensitivity of dorsal root ganglia and chronically injured axons: a physiological basis for the radicular pain of nerve root compression. *Pain* 1977;3:25–41.
132. Hukkanen M, Konttinen YT, Rees RG, Gibson SJ, Santavirta S, Polak JM. Innervation of bone from healthy and arthritic rats by substance P and calcitonin gene related peptide containing sensory fibers. *J Rheumatol* 1992;19:1252–1259.
133. Hylden JLK, Nahin RL, Taub RJ, et al. Expansion of receptive fields of spinal lamina I projection neurons in rats with unilateral adjuvant-induced inflammation: the contribution of dorsal horn mechanisms. *Pain* 1989;37:229–243.
134. Iacono RP, Boswell MV, Neumann M. Deafferentation pain exacerbated by subarachnoid lidocaine and relieved by subarachnoid morphine. Case report. *Reg Anesth* 1994;19:212–215.
135. Issebacher KJ. Diseases of the liver. In: Petersdorf R, ed. *Harrison's principles of internal medicine.* Philadelphia: JB Lippincott, 1985: 1485–1486.
136. Jaeckle KA, Young DF, Foley KM. The natural history of lumbosacral plexopathy in cancer. *Neurology* 1985;35:8–15.
137. Jaeger H, Maier C. Calcitonin in phantom limb pain: a double blind study. *Pain* 1992;48:21–27.
138. Jaffe JH, Martin WR. Opioid analgesics and antagonists. In: Gilman AG, Goodman LS, Rall TW, Nies AS, Taylor PT, eds. *The pharmacological basis of therapeutics.* New York: Pergamon Press, 1990:485–521.
139. Jahangiri M, Jayatunga AP, Bradley JWP, Dark CH. Prevention of phantom pain after major lower limb amputation by epidural infusion of diamorphine, clonidine and bupivacaine. *Ann R Coll Surg Engl* 1994;76:324–326.
140. Janig W, Koltzenburg M. On the function of spinal primary afferent fibres supplying colon and urinary bladder. *J Auton Nerv Syst* 1990;Suppl:S89–96.
141. Jellinger K, Sturm KW. Delayed radiation myelopathy in man. *J Neurol Sci* 1971;14:389–408.
142. Jensen TS, Krebs B, Nielsen J, et al. Immediate and long-term phantom limb pain in amputees: incidence, clinical characteristics and relationship to pre-amputation limb pain. *Pain* 1985;21: 267–278.

143. Kanner RM, Martini N, Foley KM. Incidence of pain and other clinical manifestations of superior pulmonary sulcus (Pancoast) tumors. In: Bonica JJ, et al. *Advances in pain research and therapy, vol. 4.* New York: Raven Press, 1982:27–39.
144. Kanner RM, Martini N, Foley KM. Nature and incidence of post-thoracotomy pain. *Proc Am Soc Clin Oncol* 1982;1:152.
145. Kaplan JG, Barasch E, Hirschfeld A, et al. Spinal epidural lipomatosis: a serious complication of iatrogenic Cushing's syndrome. *Neurology* 1989;39:1031–1034.
146. Kema IP, de Vries EG, Slooff MJ, Biesma B, Muskiet FA. Serotonin, catecholamines, histamine, and their metabolites in urine, platelets, and tumor tissue of patients with carcinoid tumors. *Clin Chem* 1994;40:86–95.
147. Kikuchi S, Sato K, Konno S, Hasue M. Anatomic and radiographic study of dorsal root ganglia. *Spine* 1994;19:6–11.
148. Kinsella TJ, Sindelar WF, Lack E, et al. Preliminary results of a randomized study of adjuvant radiation therapy in resectable adult retroperitoneal soft tissue sarcomas. *J Clin Oncol* 1988; 6:18–25.
149. Koke M, Bingel U, Seeber S. Complications of spinal opioid therapy: myoclonus, spastic muscle tone and spinal jerking. *Support Care Cancer* 1994;2:249–252.
150. Kocher L, Anton F, Reeh PW, Handwerker, HO. The effect of carrageenan-induced inflammation on the excitability of unmyelinated skin nociceptors on the rat. *Pain* 1987;29:363–373.
151. Kori SH, Foley KM, Posner JB. Brachial plexus lesions in patients with cancer: 100 cases. *Neurology* 1981;31:45–50.
152. Kostreva DR, Pontus SP. Hepatic vein, hepatic parenchymal, and inferior vena caval mechanoreceptors with phrenic afferents. *Am J Physiol* 1993;265:G15–G20.
153. Kristensen, JD, Svensson B, Gordh T Jr. The NMDA receptor antagonist CPP abolishes neurologic "wind-up pain" after intrathecal administration in humans. *Pain* 1992;51:249–253.
154. Kroner K, Krebs B, Skov J, et al. Immediate and long-term phantom breast syndrome after mastectomy: incidence, clinical characteristics and relationship to pre-mastectomy breast pain. *Pain* 1989;36:327–334.
155. Kuban DA, Delbridge T, El-Mahdi AM, Schellhammer PF. Half-body irradiation for treatment of widely metastatic adenocarcinoma of the prostate. *J Urol* 1989;141:572–574.
156. Kune G, Cole R, Bell S. Observations on the relief of pancreatic pain. *Med J Aust* 1975;2:789–791.
157. Kwaan JHM, Rappaport I. Postoperative brachial plexus palsy. A study in the mechanism. *Arch Surg* 1970;101:612–615.
158. Laird JMA, Cervero F. A comparative study of the changes in receptive-field properties of multireceptive and nocireceptive rat dorsal horn neurons following noxious mechanical stimulation. *J Neurophysiol* 1989;62:854–863.
159. Lambert PM. Radiation myelopathy of the thoracic spinal cord in long term survivors treated with radical radiotherapy using conventional fractionation. *Cancer* 1978;41:1751–1760.
160. Lederman RJ, Wilbourn AJ. Brachial plexopathy: Recurrent cancer or radiation? *Neurology* 1984;34:1331–1335.
161. Leon R. Neuritis of the ophthalmic branch of the trigeminal nerve as isolated manifestation of leptomeningeal carcinomatosis. *Ann Neurol* 1990;28:842.
162. Lewis GW. Zoster sine herpete. *Br Med J* 1958;2:418–421.
163. Locksmith JP, Powers WE. Permanent radiation myelopathy. *Am J Roentgenol* 1968;102:916–926.
164. Longhurst JC, Kaufman MP, Ordway GA, Musch TI. Effects of bradykinin and capsaicin on endings of afferent fibers from abdominal visceral organs. *Am J Physiol* 1984;247:R552–R559.
165. Longobardi JJ, Comens R, Jacobs AM. Epidural morphine as an adjuvant to the treatment of pain in a patient with acute inflammatory polyradiculopathy secondary to Guillain-Barre syndrome. *J Foot Surg* 1991;30:267–268.
166. Lotz M, Vaughan JH, Carson DA. Effects of neuropeptides in production of inflammatory cytokines by human monocytes. *Science* 1988;241:1218–1221.
167. MacDonald DR, Strong E, Nielsen S, et al. Syncope from head and neck cancer. *J Neurooncol* 1983;1:257–267.
168. Malmberg AB, Yaksh TL. Isobolographic and dose-response analyses of the interaction between intrathecal mu and delta agonists: effects of naltrindole and its benzofuran analog (NTB). *J Pharmacol Exp Ther* 1992;263:264–275.
169. Malmberg AB, Yaksh TL. Pharmacology of the spinal action of ketorolac, morphine, ST-91, U50488H, and L-PIA on the formalin test and an isobolographic analysis of the NSAID interaction. *Anesthesiology* 1993;79:270–281.
170. Malow BA, Dawson DM. Neuralgic amyotrophy in association with radiation therapy for Hodgkin's disease. *Neurology* 1991;41: 440–441.
171. Mao J, Price DD, Mayer DJ, Lu J, Hayes RL. Intrathecal MK-801 and local nerve anesthesia synergistically reduce nociceptive behaviors in rats with experimental peripheral mononeuropathy. *Brain Res* 1992;576:254–262.
172. Marcus RB Jr, Million RR. The incidence of myelitis after irradiation of the cervical spinal cord. *J Radiat Oncol Biol Phys* 1990;19: 3–8.
173. Martini N. Pain associated with superior sulcus tumor and its management. In: Arbit E, ed. *Management of cancer-related pain.* New York: Futura Press, 1993:425–435.
174. Maurset A, Skoglind LA, Hustueit O, Oye I. Comparison of ketamine and pethidine in experimental and postoperative pain. *Pain* 1989;36:37–41.
175. Mayer EA, Gebhart GF. Basic and clinical aspects of visceral hyperalgesia. *Gastroenterology* 1994;107:271–293.
176. Mayo DR, Booss J. Varicella zoster-associated neurologic disease without skin lesions. *Arch Neurol* 1989;46:313–315.
177. McLachlan EM, Janig W, Devor M, Michaelis M. Peripheral nerve injury triggers noradrenergic sprouting within the dorsal root ganglia. *Nature* 1993; 363:543–546.
178. McLeod JG, Walsh JC, Pollard JD. Neuropathies associated with paraproteinemias and dysproteinemias. In: Dyck PJ, et al, eds. *Peripheral neuropathy, vol. 2.* Philadelphia: WB Saunders, 1984: 1847–1865.
179. McQuay HJ. Pharmacological treatment of neuralgic and neuropathic pain. *Cancer Surv* 1988;7:141–59.
180. Mendell LM. Physiological properties of unmyelinated fiber projection to the spinal cord. *Exp Neurol* 1966;16:316–332.
181. Mercadante S. Intrathecal morphine and bupivacaine in advanced cancer pain patients implanted at home. *J Pain Symptom Manage* 1994;9:201–207.
182. Mersky H, Bogduk N. *Classification of chronic pain: descriptions of chronic pain syndromes and definition of pain terms.* 2nd ed. Seattle: IASP Press, 1994.
183. Miura T, Hirabuki N, Nishiyama K, et al. Computed tomography findings of nasopharyngeal carcinoma with skull base and intracranial involvement. *Cancer* 1990;65:29–37.
184. Mollman JE, Glover DJ, Hogan WM, et al. Cisplatin neuropathy: Risk factors, prognosis, and protection by WR-2721. *Cancer* 1988; 61:2192–2195.
185. Monasky MS, Zinsmeister AR, Stevens CW, Yaksh TL. Interaction of intrathecal morphine and ST-91 on antinociception in the rat: dose-response analysis, antagonism and clearance. *J Pharmacol Exp Ther* 1990;254:383–392.
186. Morgello S, Block GA, Price RW, Petito CK. Varicella-zoster virus leukoencephalitis and cerebral vasculopathy. *Arch Pathol Lab Med* 1988;112:173–177.
187. Moulin DE, Foley KM. A review of a hospital-based pain service. In: Foley KM, Bonica JJ, Ventafridda V, eds. *Advances in pain research and therapy, vol. 16.* New York: Raven Press, 1990:413–427.
188. Moulin DE, Max MB, Kaiko RF, et al. The analgesic efficacy of intrathecal D-Ala^2-D-Leu^5-enkephalin in cancer patients with chronic pain. *Pain* 1985;23:213–221.
189. Murphy RG, Greenberg ML. Osteonecrosis in pediatric patients with acute lymphoblastic leukemia. *Cancer* 1990;65:1717–1721.
190. Naguib M, Yaksh TL. Antinociceptive effects of spinal cholinesterase inhibition and isobolographic analysis of the interaction with μ and α_2 receptor systems. *Anesthesiology* 1994;80: 1338–1348.
191. Ness TJ, Gebhart GF. Visceral pain: a review of experimental studies. *Pain* 1990;41:167–234.
192. Netzer R, Pflimlin P, Trube G. Dextromethorphan blocks *N*-methyl-D-aspartate-induced currents and voltage-operated inward currents in cultured cortical neurons. *Eur J Pharmacol* 1993;238: 209-216.
193. Newton HB, Fleisher M, Schwartz MK, et al. Glucosephosphate isomerase as a CSF marker for leptomeningeal metastasis. *Neurology* 1991;41:395–398.
194. Niijima A, Meguid MM. Parenteral nutrients in rat suppresses hepatic vagal afferent signals from portal vein to hypothalamus. *Surgery* 1994;116:294–301.
195. Obbens EAMT, Posner JB. Systemic cancer involving the spinal

cord. In: Davidoff RA, ed. *Handbook of the spinal cord.* New York: Marcel Dekker, 1987:451–489.

196. Ohata M. Electron microscope study on the innervation of guinea pig liver—proposal of sensory nerve terminals in the hepatic parenchyme. *Arch Histol Jpn Nippon Soshikigaku Kiroku* 1984;47: 149–178.
197. Olney JW, Labruyere J, Price MT. Pathological changes induced in cerebrocortical neurons by phencyclidine and related drugs. *Science* 1989;244:1360–1362.
198. Olney JW, Labruyere J, Wang G, Wozniak DF, Price MT, Sesma MA. NMDA antagonist neurotoxicity: mechanisms and prevention. *Science* 1991;254:1515–1518.
199. Olson ME, Chernik NL, Posner JB. Infiltration of the leptomeninges by systemic cancer: a clinical and pathologic study. *Arch Neurol* 1974;30:122–137.
200. Onofrio BM, Yaksh TL. Intrathecal delta-receptor ligand produces analgesia in man. *Lancet* 1983;1:1386–1387.
201. Oshima E, Tei K, Kayazawa H, Urabe N. Continuous subcutaneous injection of ketamine for cancer pain. *Can J Anaesth* 1990;37: 385–386.
202. Papay FA, Roberts JK, Wegryn TL, et al. Evaluation of syncope from head and neck cancer. *Laryngoscope* 1989;99:382–388.
203. Patchell RA, Posner JB. Neurologic complications of systemic cancer. *Neurol Clin* 1985;3:729–750.
204. Penning J, Yaksh TL. Interaction of intrathecal morphine with bupivacaine and lidocaine in the rat. *Anesthesiology* 1992;77: 1186–1200.
205. Pettigrew LC, Glass JP, Maor M, et al. Diagnosis and treatment of lumbosacral plexopathies in patients with cancer. *Arch Neurol* 1984;41:1282–1285.
206. Phanthumchinda K, Intragumtornchai T, Kasantikul V. Guillain-Barre syndrome and optic neuropathy in acute leukemia. *Neurology* 1988;38:1324–1326.
207. Philips TL, Buschke F. Radiation tolerance of the thoracic spinal cord. *Am J Roentgenol* 1969;105:659–664
208. Portenoy RK, Lipton RB, Foley KM. Back pain in the cancer patient: an algorithm for evaluation and management. *Neurology* 1987;37:134–138.
209. Porter AT, McEwan AJB, Powe JE, et al. Results of a randomized phase-III trial to evaluate the efficacy of strontium-89 adjuvant to local field external beam irradiation in the management of endocrine resistant metastatic prostate cancer. *Int J Radiat Oncol Biol Phys* 1993;25:805–813.
210. Posner JB. Back pain and epidural spinal cord compression. *Med Clin North Am* 1987;71:185–205.
211. Posner JB. Paraneoplastic syndromes involving the nervous system. In: Aminoff MJ, ed. *Neurology and general medicine.* New York: Churchill Livingstone, 1989:341–364.
212. Price DD. Characterizing central mechanisms of pathological pain states by sensory testing and neurophysiological analysis. In: Casey KL, ed. *Pain and central nervous system disease: the central pain syndromes.* New York: Raven Press, 1991:65–75.
213. Price DD, Mao J, Frenk H, Mayer DJ. The N-methyl-D-aspartate receptor antagonist dextromethorphan selectively reduces temporal summation of second pain in man. *Pain* 1994;59:165–174.
214. Quilty PM, Kirk D, Bolger JJ, et al. A comparison of the palliative effects of strontium-89 and external beam radiotherapy in metastatic prostate cancer. *Radiother Oncol* 1994;31:33–40.
215. Ransom DT, Dinapoli RP, Richardson RL. Cranial nerve lesions due to base of the skull metastases in prostate carcinoma. *Cancer* 190;65:586–589.
216. Rauck RL, Eisenach JC, Jackson K, et al. Epidural clonidine treatment for refractory reflex sympathetic dystrophy. *Anesthesiology* 1993;79:1163–1169.
217. Reagan TJ, Thomas JE, Colby MY Jr. Chronic progressive radiation myelopathy. Its clinical aspects and differential diagnosis. *JAMA* 1968;203:106–110.
218. Redmond J, Friedl KE, Cornett P, et al. Clinical usefulness of an algorithm for early diagnosis of spinal metastatic disease. *J Clin Oncol* 1988;6:154–157.
219. Roberts MHT, Rees H. Denervation supersensitivity in the central nervous system: possible relation to central pain syndromes. In: Casey KL, ed. *Pain and central nervous system disease: the central pain syndromes.* New York: Raven Press, 1991:219–231.
220. Rothstein SG, Jacobs JB, Reede DL. Carotid sinus hypersensitivity secondary to parapharyngeal space carcinoma. *Head Neck Surg* 1987;9:332–335.
221. Rowinsky EK, Eisenhauer EA, Chaudhry V, Arbuck SG, Donehower RC. Clinical toxicities encountered with paclitaxel (Taxol). *Semin Oncol* 1993;20:1–15.
222. Ruff RL, Lanska DJ. Epidural metastases in prospectively evaluated veterans with cancer and back pain. *Cancer* 1989;63: 2234–2241.
223. Rusthoven JJ, Ahlgren P, Elakim T, et al. Risk factors for varicella zoster disseminated infection among adult cancer patients with localized zoster. *Cancer* 1988;62:1641–1646.
224. Rydevik BL, Myers RR, Powell HC. Pressure increase in the dorsal root ganglion following mechanical compression. Closed compartment syndrome in nerve roots. *Spine* 1989;14:574–576.
225. Salazar OM, Rubin P, Hendrickson FR, et al. Single-dose half-body irradiation for palliation of multiple bone metastases from solid tumors. Final radiation therapy oncology group report. *Cancer* 1986;58:29–36.
226. Salner AL, Botnick LE, Herzog AG, et al. Reversible brachial plexopathy following primary radiation therapy for breast cancer. *Cancer Treat Rep* 1981;65:797–802.
227. Saltzburg D, Foley KM. Management of pain in pancreatic cancer. *Surg Clin North Am* 1989;69:629–649.
228. Samuels BL, Kahn CE, Messersmith RN, et al. Brachial plexopathy after intraarterial cisplatin. *J Clin Oncol* 1988;6:1204.
229. Sato K, Kiyama H, Park HT, Tohyama M. AMPA, KA and NMDA receptors are expressed in the rat DRG neurones. *Neuroreport* 1993;4:1263–1265.
230. Sato J, Perl ER. Adrenergic excitation of cutaneous pain receptors induced by peripheral nerve injury. *Science* 1991;251:1608–1610.
231. Sengupta JN, Gebhart GF. Characterization of mechanosensitive pelvic nerve afferent fibers innervating the colon of the rat. *J Neurophysiol* 1994;71:2046–2060.
232. Sherlock S. *Diseases of the liver and biliary tract.* 6th ed. Boston: Blackwell Scientific, 1981.
233. Sherman RA, Sherman CJ, Parker L. Chronic phantom and stump pain among American veterans: results of a survey. *Pain* 1984;18: 83–95.
234. Siegal T, Haim N. Cisplatin-induced peripheral neuropathy: frequent off-therapy deterioration, demyelinating syndromes and muscle cramps. *Cancer* 1990;66:1117–1123.
235. Simmons JW Jr, Ricketson R, McMillin JN. Painful lumbosacral sensory distribution patterns: embryogenesis to adulthood. *Orthop Rev* 1993;22:1110–1118.
236. Sjoberg M, Nitescu P, Appelgren L, Curelaru I. Long-term intrathecal morphine and bupivacaine in patients with refractory cancer pain. Results from a morphine:bupivacaine dose regimen of 0.5:4.75 mg/ml. *Anesthesiology* 1994;80:284–297.
237. Sorenson S, Borgesen SE, Rohde K, et al. Metastatic epidural spinal cord compression. Results of treatment and survival. *Cancer* 1990;65:1502–1508.
238. Sozzi G, Marotta P, Piatti L. Vagoglossopharyngeal neuralgia with syncope in the course of carcinomatous meningitis. *Ital J Neurol Sci* 1987;8:271–276.
239. Stannard CF, Porter GE. Ketamine hydrochloride in the treatment of phantom limb pain. *Pain* 54 1993:227–230.
240. Stewart JD. *Focal peripheral neuropathies.* New York: Elsevier, 1987: 76–84.
241. Stillman M, Foley KM. Breast cancer and epidural spinal cord compression: diagnostic and therapeutic strategies. In: Harris JR, Hellman S, Henderson IC, et al., eds. *Breast diseases.* Philadelphia: JB Lippincott, 1987:488–497.
242. Stillman MJ, Moulin DE, Foley KM. Paradoxical pain following high–dose spinal morphine. *Pain* 1987;S4:5389.
243. Sugimoto T, Bennet GJ, Kajander KC. Transynaptic degeneration in the superficial dorsal horn after sciatic nerve injury: effects of a chronic constriction injury, transection, and strychnine. *Pain* 1990;42:205–213.
244. Sundaresan N, DiGiancinto GV, Hughes JEO. Surgical treatment of spinal metastases. *Clin Neurosurg* 1986;33:503–522.
245. Sundaresan N, Galicich JH, Lane JM, Greenberg HJ. Treatment of odontoid fractures in cancer patients. *J Neurosurg* 1981;54:187–192.
246. Swift TR, Nichols FT. The droopy shoulder syndrome. *Neurology* 1984;34:212–215.
247. Talbot JD, Duncan GH, Bushnell MC. Effects of diffuse noxious inhibitory controls (DNICs) on the sensory-discriminative dimension of pain perception. *Pain* 1989;36:231–238.
248. Talbot JD, Marrett S, Evans AC, et al. Multiple representations of pain in human cerebral cortex. *Science* 1991;251:1355–1358.

249. Tasker RR. Deafferentation. In: Wall PD, Melzack R, eds. *Textbook of pain.* New York: Churchill Livingstone, 1984:119–132.
250. Thomas JE, Cascino TL, Earle JD. Differential diagnosis between radiation and tumor plexopathy of the pelvis. *Neurology* 1985;35: 1–7.
251. Thompson SW, Davis LE, Kornfeld M, et al. Cisplatin neuropathy. Clinical, electrophysiologic, morphologic and toxicologic studies. *Cancer* 1984;54:1269–1275.
252. Tsairis P, Dyck PJ, Mulder DW. Natural history of brachial plexus neuropathy: Report on 99 patients. *Arch Neurol* 1972;27:109–117.
253. Tucker MA, Coleman CN, Cox RS, et al. Risk of second cancers after treatment for Hodgkin's disease. *N Engl J Med* 1988;318:76–81.
254. Twijnstra A, Nooyen WJ, vanZanten AP, et al. Cerebrospinal fluid carcinoembryonic antigen in patients with metastatic and non-metastatic neurological diseases. *Arch Neurol* 1986;43:269–272.
255. van Moll BJM, Vecht CJ. Referred pain to the fact by chest tumors. *Pain Clinic* 1994;7:35–38.
256. Vecht CJ, van de Brand HJ, Wajer OJM, et al. Post-axillary dissection pain in breast cancer due to a lesion of the intercostobrachial nerve. *Pain* 1989;38:171–176.
257. Vikram B, Chu FCH. Radiation therapy for metastases to the base of the skull. *Radiology* 1979;130;465–468.
258. Wall PD, Gutnick M. Ongoing activity in peripheral nerves: the physiology and pharmacology of impulses originating from a neuroma. *Exp Neurol* 1974;43:580–593.
259. Walsh, JC. The neuropathy of multiple myeloma. An electrophysiological and histological study. *Arch Neurol* 1971;25:404–414.
260. Wara WM, Philips TL Sheline GE, Schwade JG. Radiation tolerance of the spinal cord. *Cancer* 1975;35:1558–1562.
261. Wasserstrom WR, Glass JP, Posner JB. Diagnosis and treatment of leptomeningeal metastases from solid tumors: experience with 90 patients. *Cancer* 1982;49:759–772.
262. Whitley RJ, Straus SE. Therapy for varicella-zoster virus infections: where do we stand? *Infect Dis Clin Prac* 1993;2:100–108.
263. Woll PJ, Rankin EM. Persistent back pain due to malignant lymphadenopathy. *Am Rheum Dis* 1987;46:681–683.
264. Wong MC, Krol G, Rosenblum MK. Occult epidural chloroma complicated by acute paraplegia following lumbar puncture. *Ann Neurol* 1992;31:110–112.
265. Wood KM. Intercostobrachial nerve entrapment syndrome. *South Med J* 1978;71:662–663.
266. Woolf CJ, Shortland P, Coggeshall RE. Peripheral nerve injury triggers central sprouting of myelinated afferents. *Nature* 1992; 355:75–78.
267. Woolf CJ, Thompson SWN. The induction and maintenance of central sensitization is dependent on N-methyl-D-aspartic acid receptroactivation; implications for the treatment of post-injury hypersensitivity states. *Pain* 1991;44:293–299.
268. Yaksh TL, Harty GJ. Pharmacology of the allodynia in rats evoked by high-dose intrathecal morphine. *J Pharmacol Exp Ther* 1988;244: 501–507.
269. Yaksh TL, Malmberg AB. Central pharmacology of nociceptive transmission. In: Wall P, Melzack R, eds. *Textbook of pain.* Rev. ed. Edinburgh: Churchill Livingstone, 1994:165–200.
270. Yaksh TL, Pogrel JW, Lee YW, Chaplan SR. Reversal of nerve ligation-induced allodynia by spinal alpha-2 adrenoceptor agonists. *J Pharmacol Exp Ther* 1995;272:207–214.
271. Yamamoto T, Yaksh TL. Spinal pharmacology of thermal hyperesthesia induced by constriction injury of sciatic nerve: excitatory amino acid antagonists. *Pain* 1992;49:121–128.
272. Yang R, Leichman L, Ralls PW, et al. Carcinoma of the exocrine pancreas. In: Valenzuela JE, Reber HA, Ribet A, eds. *Medical and surgical diseases of the pancreas.* New York: Igaku-Shoin, 1991:155–178.
273. Young DF, Posner JB. Nervous system toxicity of the chemotherapeutic agents. In: Vinken PJ, Bruyn GW, eds. *Handbook of clinical neurology, vol. 39.* Amsterdam: Elsevier, 1980:91–129.
274. Young RF, Post EM, King GA. Treatment of spinal epidural metastases. Randomized prospective comparison of laminectomy and radiotherapy. *J Neurosurg* 1980;53:741–748.
275. Zhang X, Bao L, Xu ZQ, et al. Localization of neuropeptide Y Y1 receptors in the rat nervous system with special reference to somatic receptors on small dorsal root ganglion neurons. *Proc Natl Acad Sci USA* 1994;91:11738–11742.
276. Zimmerman M. Central nervous system mechanisms modulating pain-related information: do they become deficient after lesions of the peripheral or central nervous system? In: Casey KL, ed. *Pain and the central nervous system disease: the central pain syndromes.* New York: Raven Press, 1991:183–199.

Anesthesia: Biologic Foundations, edited by Tony L. Yaksh et al. Lippincott–Raven Publishers, Philadelphia © 1997.

CHAPTER 49

MECHANISMS OF PAIN IN ARTHRITIS

MARTIN K. LOTZ

Joint pain is the major subjective symptom of arthritis. It reflects the development of afferent traffic in small, lightly myelinated or unmyelinated afferents that innervate the synovial space. As will be noted below, under normal circumstances, normal joint movement leads to minimal afferent activity, and it is only when the joint is moved through an extreme range that a report of pain is obtained (see Chap. 31). From the point of view of arthritic pain, we will concern ourselves in the present chapter in the review of mechanisms whereby the arthritic condition leads to abnormal afferent traffic and a persistent pain state that is enhanced by otherwise normal movement of the joint.

A major distinction for the purpose of the present discussion is between osteoarthritis as a joint condition not primarily triggered by inflammatory cell-mediated connective tissue destruction and associated with a relatively mild degree of synovial inflammation, and the so-called inflammatory arthropathies, which include rheumatoid arthritis, seronegative arthropathies, and crystal-induced arthritis.

Osteoarthritis is associated with a secondary joint inflammation of varying intensity. Other mechanisms that can additionally contribute to joint pain in osteoarthritis are (a) changes in blood flow in subchondral bone, (b) activation of nerve fibers in the periosteum during bone resorption and (c) by osteophytes, and (d) inflammation of ligaments and distention of the joint capsule by an increased synovial fluid volume. Periarticular tenderness, muscle spasms, and the perception of joint stiffness are frequent components of the arthritic pain syndrome.

Synovitis is the primary triggering mechanism of joint pain in inflammatory arthropathies. Joint inflammation is typically associated with the production of chemical mediators that serve (a) to stimulate otherwise quiescent articular afferents leading to afferent traffic and (b) to sensitize sensory afferent terminals in the joint such that modest and otherwise innocuous joint movement will activate afferents which were originally activated only by the most extreme joint rotation, e.g., "silent nociceptors" (87). This peripheral input is processed at spinal and central levels and triggers pain behavior. Important advances over the past 5 years in our understanding of the central organization of the input generated by an inflamed joint has emphasized that this ongoing small afferent input will lead to prominent changes in central processing that facilitates spinofugal outflow, resulting in a hyperalgesic state with a distinct pharmacology (10,86) (see Chap. 36). This review will discuss the current understanding of mechanisms by which products of synovial inflammation induce joint pain. Mechanisms of antirheumatic therapy will be evaluated as an alternative source of insight into pathways leading to the experience of joint pain (Table 1).

SENSORY INNERVATION OF THE JOINTS

Normal Joint Innervation

Cutaneous afferents and branches of adjacent muscle afferents innervate the joints (26). Sensory innervation extends into joint capsule, ligaments, subchondral bone, periosteum, and synovium. Cartilage is aneural (101). Unmyelinated C fibers (group IV) sensory nerve fibers containing neuropeptides such as calcitonin gene-related peptide (CGRP) and substance P (SP) are present in the synovial lining and sublining tissue and in the vascularized peripheral parts of the joint menisci. Furthermore, periosteum, bone marrow, and the epiphyseal growth plates are innervated, whereas innervation of the diaphyseal and metaphyseal bone is more sparse (41). Normal synovial tissue is richly innervated with both sensory and sympathetic nerves (34). Sympathetic fibers are exclusively located around blood vessels. Mast cells and afferent nerve terminals are frequently observed in all parts of the normal synovium, and densities of mast cells appear to be greatest at sites proximal to the nerve terminals (40). Electrophysiological studies have typically demonstrated that within the range of normal joint movement there is little afferent traffic. Intense deformation or inflammation-induced expansion within the joint (see below) will evoke activity in the group III (A delta) fibers (13,87).

Innervation in Inflamed Joints

Urate crystals (1), carrageenan (74,96), and endotoxin (35) injected into the synovial joint evoke an acute local inflammation, whereas the intradermal injection of killed bacteria suspended in Freund's adjuvant results in a more widespread disease, a chronic polyarthritis (27). A marked sensitivity to modest movement of the stimulation of the affected joint or a hyperalgesia is observed in animals so treated. These animal models display considerable similarities to the human state, with evident increases in joint volume and radiographic signs consistent with a chronic joint inflammation (27). Such models have been widely used for the investigation of the biochemical and behavioral changes associated with chronic joint inflammation (47).

Several changes in synovial innervation have been documented as a result of chronic inflammation. Inflamed synovium from adjuvant arthritic rats shows an absence of SP and CGRP nerves in heavily infiltrated villous synovial tissue, whereas healthy synovial tissue and noninflammatory areas were innervated by SP and CGRP nerves close to normal synovial tissue resident cells (47). With the lower density of nerve fibers in arthritic synovium, there is also a decrease or absence of nerve-associated mast cells (40). A similar loss in nerve fibers is seen in human rheumatoid arthritis synovium (79), which shows an innervation similar to that seen in normal human synovium in the deep tissue layers but an absence of fibers immunoreactive for SP in the more superficial layer. In addition, immunostaining of neuropeptides in the deep tissue is weaker in the arthritic synovium than in normal controls (64).

Table 1. MECHANISMS AND INDUCERS OF JOINT PAIN

Chemical inducers: prostaglandins, kinins, purines, cytokines
Impaired subchondral blood flow
Osteophytes
Increased synovial fluid volume

These findings suggest that neuropeptides are depleted from the nerves. Alternatively, formation of new nerve fibers may occur at a slower rate than proliferation of rheumatoid synovium. Nerve fibers may also be destroyed by locally produced proteolytic enzymes and various reactive oxygen species in the vicinity of inflammatory cells. Collectively, these findings raise the possibility that the discrepancy between the prominent synovial thickening and the relatively low degree of tenderness in some patients with chronic arthritis may at least be in part be due to changes in the density of sensory fibers.

CHEMICAL MEDIATORS OF JOINT PAIN AND INFLAMMATION

As part of the inflammatory process in the synovium, cellular and humoral mediators are produced that maintain the chronic synovitis and cause cartilage degradation (33). These mediators can be distinguished into products of humoral inflammatory systems such as kinins and anaphylatoxins or as products of activated leukocytes and connective tissue cells such as cytokines and arachidonic acid metabolites (see Chaps. 8 and 20). All of these different mediators are integrated into a network where they modulate the production and effects of each other (56), thereby contributing directly or indirectly to the effect upon afferent terminals leading to the generation of joint pain (Fig. 1). This discussion will address mediators that are known to directly affect the sensory nerve terminals, and review regulatory interactions that are relevant to the maintenance of joint pain and inflammation. We will focus on prostaglandins, kinins, cytokines, and purines as they are not only involved with the pathogenesis of joint inflammation and pain but are also the target of established and experimental antirheumatic therapy (Table 2). Additional commentary on the pharmacology of the peripheral afferent terminal is presented in Chapter 33.

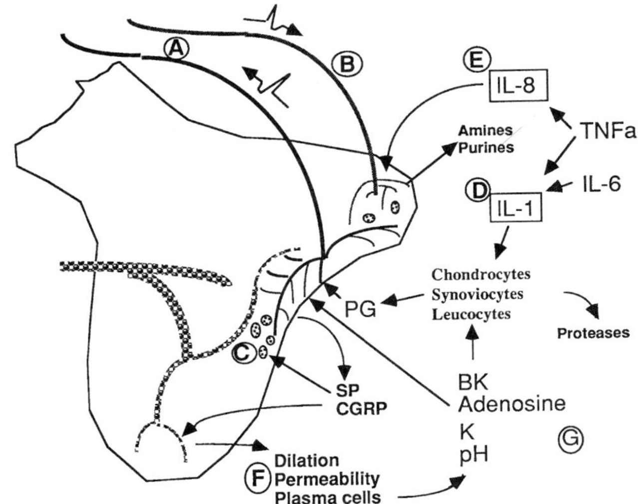

Figure 1. Schematic of several key aspects of the inflammatory milieu of the joint that leads to an afferent barrage in otherwise silent joint afferents. **(A)** Aδ/C fibers, some of which contain SP and CGRP in releasible fractions, innervate synovium, and underlying bone. **(B)** Sympathetic innervation to blood vessels terminate in the synovial space. **(C)** Primary afferents terminate. These afferents lie proximal to capillaries and display typically high levels of mast cells in adjoining tissue. **(D)** In the inflammatory state, a variety of cytokines are released. IL-1 has been shown to produce a proinflammtory reaction by stimulating a variety of local bone cells to release proteases, which exert lytic processes in the synovial capsule, and to evoke the release of prostaglandins. Prostaglandins are known to exert potent stimulatory and sensitizing effects upon joint afferents. **(E)** IL-8 formation appears to exert an excitatory (proalgogenic) effect which requires functional sympathetic terminals and acts through a β-adrenoceptor. **(F)** Activation of periperal afferent terminals leads to the release of SP and CGRP. Importantly, the release may occur as a result of local depolarization of the terminal, or by antidromic invasion of axon collaterals (e.g., antidromic activity). These agents serve (a) to degranulate local mast cells, releasing active products such as histamine and proteases, and (b) to induce capillary vasodilatation and increased capillary permeability (leakiness). These plasma products then contribute to the increased synovial volume and the cytokine/plasma cell content of the synovial space. **(G)** Active products that appear in the synovial space secondary to injury include kinins such as bradykinin, adenosine, and increased extracellular potassium and hydrogen ion concentration. These products can either indirectly (as with bradykinin) or directly (as with adenosine, K, or pH) stimulate small afferent terminals.

Prostanoids and Kinins

The role of prostaglandins (PG) in the induction of pain behavior is well documented, and some of the mechanisms have been clarified. Local application of prostanoids facilitates the evoked activity of C-fiber afferents and generates pain behavior. PG synthesis increases in response to inflammatory tissue injury and inhibition of local cyclooxygenases is associated with analgesic effects. PGI_2 and PGE_2 when applied intraarterially close to the joint causes an excitatory effect, a sensitization to passive movements of the joint (95) and also potentiates bradykinin-induced hyperalgesia (100). PGE_2 has qualitatively similar effects as PGI_2 but excites and sensitizes a lower proportion of articular afferents. Thus, PGI_2 and PGE_2 increase the sensitivity to mechanical as well as to chemical stimulation. It may be an inflammatory mediator that is important for inflammation-evoked activity in slowly conducting afferents and participate in the development of arthritic hyperalgesia and pain (88). This and other evidence suggests that PGE_2 and PGI_2 are the main hyperalgesic metabolites of the cyclooxygenase pathway of arachidonic acid (95). The hyperalgesic effects are the result of a direct action on the primary afferent and attenuated by guanosine 5′-O-(2-thiodiphosphate), suggesting that they are mediated by stimulatory G proteins (2) (see Chap. 4).

Multiple cell types and stimuli contribute to the production of prostaglandins in the arthritic joint. Synoviocytes, chondrocytes, and infiltrating leukocytes produce PG in response to immune complexes, anaphylatoxins, cytokines, neuropeptides, and kinins. PG levels are increased in arthritic synovial fluid and correlate with the severity of inflammation and response to therapy. A role of kinins in the pathogenesis of arthritis has been postulated, but there is only very limited information directly addressing this. Bradykinin (BK) causes a dose-dependent pain response that is mediated by the activation of B2 receptors and reduced by indomethacin or NG-nitroarginine, and abolished by methylene blue. This suggests that BK action depends on the release of prostaglandins and nitric oxide or a related compound and includes the activation of guanylate cyclase that appears to be involved in primary afferent excitation (15).

Table 2. EFFECTS OF CHEMICAL MEDIATORS FOUND IN THE SYNOVIAL SPACE

Mediator	Effect
IL-1	Stimulates peripheral PG synthesis; has central antinociceptive effects
IL-8	Induces hyperalgesia mediated by the sympathetic nervous system and PG independent
IL-6	Activates the IL-1/prostaglandin pathway
TNF-α	Activates both IL-1 and IL-8 pathways
Adenosine	Peripheral hyperalgesia, central antinociceptive effects

In addition to the inhibition of PG synthesis at peripheral sites of inflammation, it has been shown that the ongoing afferent barrage with which such peripheral inflammatory states are associated will evoke a spinal secretion of prostanoids, and this central action can induce a central facilitation of subsequent afferent processing (63). It has been shown that the facilitated spinal state generated by such repetitive input can be diminished by the spinal action of nonsteroidal antiinflammatory drugs (NSAIDs) that will inhibit the synthesis and release of spinal prostaglandins (63) and prevent SP- or glutamate-induced hyperalgesia by inhibiting PG synthesis at the spinal level (62). This mechanism is consistent with the ability of intrathecal glutamate to induce prostaglandin release from spinal cord (91). It thus appears that the analgesic effect of NSAIDs acting as cyclooxygenase inhibitors cannot be exclusively attributed to their inhibitory effects on the synthesis of peripherally formed prostaglandins and that at least some of these compounds also have antinociceptive effects (for further discussion, see Chaps. 36 and 61).

An important observation has been the appreciation that, with chronic stimulation and the activation of certain cells by cytokines released by inflammation (see below), there can be a time-dependent upregulation of cyclooxygenase. Importantly, the inducible form is relevant for two reasons: (a) It increases the ability of the inflamed systems to enhance prostaglandin secretion. (b) The inducible form appears to have a pharmacology that differs from that of the constituitive form (75) (for further discussion, see Chap. 61).

Purines

Adenosine is known to cause pain when injected intravenously or intraarterially (16). There is also evidence of hyperalgesia to mechanical and heat stimuli at the injection site (primary hyperalgesia) but no evidence of mechanical hyperalgesia in the cutaneous area surrounding the injected site (secondary hyperalgesia) (78). It has been speculated that the adjuvant activity of caffeine, an adenosine receptor antagonist, may be mediated in part by the blockade of such a peripheral action of adenosine (85).

While adenosine receptor systems may exert a proalgogenic role in inflammation, adenosine receptor agonist, such as NECA (5′-N-ethylcarboxamidoadenosine) and PIA (N6-phenylisopropyladenosine) or inhibitors of adenosine metabolism possess antinociceptive effects after peripheral and intrathecal administration in animals (43,44,83). There is evidence for the release of spinal adenosine as a result of activity in small diameter capsaicin-sensitive primary afferents in the spinal cord. In view of the antinociceptive actions of adenosine analogs, there has been some interest in the possibility of developing adenosine analogs as analgesic agents. Adenosine triphosphate (ATP) may be a sensory neurotransmitter released from nonnociceptive large diameter primary afferent neurons. The subsequent extracellular conversion of released ATP to adenosine may produce suppression of the transmission of noxious sensory information through small diameter primary afferent fibers (84).

Currently, adenosine kinase inhibitors and adenosine analogs (2-chloro-deoxyadenosine, 2cda) are in clinical trials or under development as novel antiinflammatory agents in the treatment of arthritis, and it will conceptually be of interest to dissociate the effects of these systemic interventions on pain and inflammation.

Cytokines

Cytokines represent a principal mediator system in the pathogenesis of synovial inflammation and cartilage degradation (33). IL-1 and tumor necrosis factor (TNF) are the cytokines held primarily responsible for the production of extracellular matrix-degrading proteases. The role of these cytokines in arthritis has been demonstrated in a multitude of experimental approaches and they are the target for the development of new antirheumatic therapies (55).

Most of the proinflammatory cytokines have hyperalgesic activities in the periphery which appear to be principally mediated by two pharmacologically distinguishable cascades: (a) the IL-1/prostaglandin pathway or (b) the IL-8/sympathetic terminal-mediated pathway (see Chap. 20).

1. *IL-1 Cascade:* IL-1 is a potent peripheral hyperalgesic agent (23). The hyperalgesic effects of IL-1 and prostaglandins appear related but are not identical. IL-1 induces a dose-dependent increase in the sensitivity of rat paws to mechanical stimulation following intraplantar injection. PGE_2 enhances the sensitivity of the skin to both mechanical pressure and thermal stimuli, but IL-1 enhances only sensitivity to pressure. This suggests that IL-1 sensitizes pressure-sensitive but not temperature-sensitive sensory neurons, through a prostaglandin-independent mechanism. Furthermore, hyperalgesia induced by IL-1, but not PGE_2, is inhibited by melanocyte-stimulating hormone, which also antagonizes IL-1 effects in other systems (11,24,37).
2. *IL-8 Cascade:* IL-8 evokes a hyperalgesia that is attenuated by β-adrenoceptor (atenolol) and dopamine receptor (SCH 23390) antagonists and the adrenergic neuron-blocking agent guanethidine. This suggests an intervening role mediated through activity in peripheral sympathetic terminals. IL-8–induced hyperalgesia is not attenuated by the cyclooxygenase inhibitor indomethacin. In contrast, IL-1–evoked hyperalgesia is attenuated by indomethacin but is not altered by changes in sympathetic terminal function. IL-8 was the first endogenous mediator to be identified as evoking hyperalgesia by a prostaglandin-independent mechanism involving the sympathetic nervous system. Because IL-8 is released by activated macrophages and endothelial cells, it may be a humoral link between tissue injury and sympathetic involvement in the postinflammation hyperalgesic state (18).

Other cytokines appear to act through one or both of these two cascades. Thus, IL-6 activates the IL-1/prostaglandin hyperalgesic pathway but not the IL-8/sympathetic-mediated hyperalgesic pathway. TNF activates both pathways. After carrageenin injection into the skin or joint, the hyperalgesia is attenuated by atenolol and by an anti-IL-8 serum. The effects of indomethacin and anti-IL-8 serum are additive, and this combination abolishes carrageenin-evoked hyperalgesia. Thus, in an arthritic joint, it is likely that both mechanisms are activated, and this is at least in part related to cytokine interactions. Antiserum neutralizing endogenous TNF abolishes the response to carrageenin, whereas antisera neutralizing endogenous IL-1β, IL-6, and IL-8 each only partially inhibits the response. TNF thus has an early and crucial role in the development of inflammatory hyperalgesia.

It is important to note that the formation of these several cytokines bring into play a number of mechanisms which involve not only a direct effect upon the inflammatory process or the activation of sensory afferents. These agents also serve to alter the constituitive make up of the products that are secreted by the inflammatory process. Thus, IL-1 is a potent stimulus of PG synthesis in resident mesenchymal cells and infiltrating leukocytes and this may be primarily related to its effects on transcription of the inducible prostaglandin synthase/cyclooxygenase-2 (75). IL-1 is also one of the most potent inducers of IL-8 and IL-6 synthesis in synoviocytes and chondrocytes (29,30,59). During the inflammatory process in the joint, this cytokine directly activates the IL-1/prostaglandin pathway and indirectly activates the IL-8/sympathetic-mediated hyperalgesic pathway.

A central role of cytokines in the regulation of pain behavior has only recently been investigated. After central administration, IL-1 and TNF *increased* pain thresholds in the rat. The analgesic effect of TNF was completely antagonized by anti-IL-1 antibodies. Moreover, the cyclooxygenase inhibitor indomethacin did not antagonize the increase of nociceptive thresholds induced by either cytokine(7). Corticotrophin releasing factor (CRF) induces an analgesic effect that, as observed with the two cytokines, is not reversible by naloxone. A similar observation was made in humans and experimental animals after exposure to stressful conditions suggesting that the two cytokines share with corticotrophin releasing hormone some characteristics of stress mediators (6). As IL-1 is a stimulus of CRF release from the hypothalamus, it was possible that CRF is involved in the antinociception induced by IL-1. Experiments with CRF antagonists suggested that the antinociception induced by IL-1 is mediated, at least in part, by the peripheral action of CRF (46).

Neuropeptides

Neuropeptides not only function in their classical role as signaling molecules between neurons but are also involved in bidirectional interactions with joint tissue cells and leukocytes. Neuropeptides are thus not only modulators of pain but also affect intraarticular inflammatory responses. Furthermore, neuropeptides are not only the product of neurons but can also originate from connective tissue cells and leukocytes.

Primary Afferent Peptides

Neuropeptides, contained within sensory nerve terminals in the synovium, have been detected in synovial fluids (SF) from arthritis patients (Table 3). Synovial fluid SP levels exceeded plasma levels in most types of arthritis and were elevated in rheumatoid arthritis (RA), osteoarthritis (OA), Reiter's syndrome, and posttrauma patients (66). Higher levels of SP-like immunoreactivity (SPLI) were found in the SF of patients with RA compared with OA (67,71). Conversely, SPLI content in synovial tissue was higher in OA than in RA, suggesting that there is an active secretory process of SPLI into the SF in RA, thus depleting SPLI stores in the synovium (71). Levels of CGRP II and VIP-like immunoreactivity in synovial fluid were also higher in RA than in OA (36). Plasma levels did not show a difference between OA and RA (36,67).

The extracellular movement of afferent neuropeptides from the peripheral afferent terminal represents a well-defined neurotransmitter event (see Chap. 6). Activation of a small afferent terminal by a physical (mechanical) or pharmacological (e.g., a cytokine) stimulus yields a local terminal depolarization that either directly or indirectly by antidromic invasion of an axon collateral will open local voltage-sensitive Ca channels and result in the local release of the content of the local afferent terminal. In normal tissue, antidromic stimulation of the articular nerve leads to an increase in SP release into synovial perfusates (102). During experimentally induced acute monoarthritis in rats SP-, NKA-, CGRP-, and NPY-LI in synovial fluid occurred in both knees after injections with the proinflammatory substances only into the right joints (8). Similar release has been observed in a variety of tissues (38,54). Importantly, the release of these afferent neuropeptides has been shown to be regulated by a variety of pharmacological events. Thus, by an action upon the peripheral terminal, opiates can serve to diminish the antidromically evoked release of SP from the knee joint.

Table 3. ORIGIN AND EFFECTS OF NEUROPEPTIDES IN SYNOVIAL FLUID

Neuropeptide	Origin	Effects on pain inflammation
Substance P	C-fibers	- -
Eosinophils CGRP	C-fibers	- -
VIP	C-fibers	-
Enkephalins	monocytes	- - / -
Lymphocytes		
Chondrocytes		
Synoviocytes		

Nonafferent Peptides

Several neuropeptides found in arthritic synovial fluid are not only produced by neurons but also by inflammatory cells derived from bone marrow and resident connective tissue cells (Table 3). An example of this is the demonstration of the extraneuronal production of enkephalins. Activated monocytes and lymphocytes express the preproenkephalin gene and monocytes secrete completely processed enkephalins (48). Enkephalin immunoreactivity can be detected in synovial fluids from arthritis patients. This originates from several intraarticular cell sources. Human articular chondrocytes express the preproenkephalin gene and secrete met-enkephalin (97). Enkephalin immunoreactivity is also present in rheumatoid synovium and produced by cultured synoviocytes. The regulatory control of enkephalin production in these joint tissue cells is of interest since it is inhibited by IL-1 and increased by TGF-β, which is a cytokine that also antagonizes the proinflammatory effects of IL-1. The importance of the appearance of the enkephalins in the extracellular space during inflammation is emphasized by work that has demonstrated (a) the presence of opioid receptors on sensory nerve endings and (b) that opioids acting upon specific opioid receptor subtypes have no effect upon normal sensory function, but will reduce the hyperalgesia associated with the inflammatory state (75,92–94) (see Chap. 30) for additional discussion) and (c) reduce the spontaneous discharge in afferents innervating inflamed tissues (3,82). Although the mechanisms of this opioid receptor influence of the facilitated state of the afferent innervating inflamed tissue is not known, the biological relevance of this system is suggested by the upregulation of opioid peptide synthesis in leukocytes and joint tissue cells during inflammation.

Regulation of Neuropeptide Levels in Synovial Fluid

The biologic activity of neuropeptides in synovial fluid is regulated by their enzymatic degradation. The SP peptidases, neutral endopeptidase (NEP) (3.4.24.11), and angiotensin-converting enzyme (ACE) are significantly increased in plasma and synovial fluid of patients with RA when compared to patients with OA and healthy controls (67). Normal human synovium failed to show any immunoreactivity for NEP. In the disease groups, there was intense staining of cells surrounding blood vessels, data consistent with the hypothesis that a proportion of synovial fibroblasts are the major source of this enzyme in the arthritic joint (65). Changes in the cerebrospinal fluid levels of these peptidases have also been detected during experimentally induced arthritis. NEP and dynorphin-converting enzyme (DCE) were significantly lowered in the acute phase of collagen II–induced arthritis. Based on these adaptive changes, a functional role of these enzymes in processing pain-related neuropeptides has therefore been suggested (80).

THE ROLE OF PRIMARY SENSORY NEURONS IN INFLAMMATION

Two points should be stressed. First, as reviewed above, inflammation yields a pain state that is mediated by an excitation of small afferent terminals. Second, this release results in an increase in the local extracellular levels of these peptides which permit them to exert a variety of local effects.

Effects of Afferent Neuropeptides

SP has been shown to (a) activate lymphocytes (70); (b) stimulate in monocytes the production PGE and of cytokines such as IL-1, TNF, and IL-6 (60); (c) increase in fibroblasts the expression of extracellular matrix degrading proteases (58); (d) represent a stimulus for the continued production of IL-1 and other cytokines; and (e) exert a direct smooth muscle relaxant effect and increase capillary permeability (61).

The cascade involving the neuropeptides is extremely complex, and interaction occurs at multiple points between elements of the cascade. Three examples will be cited for illustration of the types of potential interactions.

1. Intraarticular injection of IL-1 or TNF in rabbit knees increases the number of leukocytes in the joint fluid and enhances cartilage degradation. Both cytokines also increase SP levels in the joint fluid. Treatment with indomethacin or dexamethasone reduced leukocyte counts, and PGE_2 and SP concentrations but not IL-1–induced proteoglycan loss (76). Elevated SP and PGE_2 in the joint may thus amplify or sustain an initial receptor-mediated inflammatory response to IL-1 (77).
2. Kinins belong to the group of inflammatory mediators that stimulate SP release. In a blister model in the rat footpad, perfusion of bradykinin elicited both vasodilatation and plasma extravasation. In rats pretreated as neonates with capsaicin to destroy primary sensory afferents, the inflammatory response to bradykinin was significantly smaller. Nitric oxide (NO), a potent endothelial cell-derived vasorelaxation factor, was suggested as an additional intermediate since the selective inhibitor of NO synthase, NG-nitro-L-arginine, attenuated the inflammatory response to bradykinin in control rats with a further decrease in the response in capsaicin-pretreated rats (45). Vasodilatation and plasma extravasation induced by application of SP were reduced by an inhibitor of nitric oxide formation(39).
3. The interactions between SP and other neuropeptides can be additive, synergistic, or antagonistic. Vasoactive intestinal peptide (VIP) has qualitatively opposing effects to SP in the regulation of inflammation and smooth muscle contraction. The interaction with CGRP, which is usually localized and coreleased with SP, is additive or synergistic. Perfusion of capsaicin through the knee joint of the rat increased plasma extravasation transiently. Perfusion of SP or CGRP, jointly released by acute capsaicin administration, evoked an increase in plasma extravasation that was greater and of longer duration than that produced by capsaicin (28).

Contribution of SP to Pathogenesis of Arthritis

The role of SP to the evolution of the arthritic state has been studied in various experimental models, most commonly in the adjuvant-induced arthritis in rats. A neurogenic component has been demonstrated for different models of acute joint inflammation and is mediated through sensory afferent or sympathetic efferent nerve fibers. In adjuvant-induced arthritis in rats, joints more densely innervated with SP fibers developed more severe joint destruction and infusion of SP increased severity (53). Intraarticular injection of SP in rat knee joints results in a pronounced inflammatory response. However, prior intraarticular injection of capsaicin, a neurotoxin that can selectively desensitize, deplete, and abolish (with neonatal treatment) populations of SP-containing primary afferents (22), will significantly attenuate the arthritic response (49,51). Similarly, pretreatment of rat knees with a SP receptor antagonist almost completely inhibited the inflammatory response to carrageenan, providing further support for a role of SP in acute joint inflammation (50). Blocking SP effects at the peripheral site of inflammation has the potential to have beneficial effects in controlling joint inflammation (57,99).

ADAPTIVE CHANGES IN NEUROPEPTIDE SYNTHESIS IN ARTHRITIS

Fluctuations in the intensity of pain reported by arthritis patients are not always correlated with quantitatively similar changes in the extent of synovial inflammation. These differences are the possible consequence of adaptive changes in peptide or receptor synthesis by neurons in the spinal circuitry. Aside from the relatively acute (minutes to hours) changes in spinal processing associated with the ongoing small afferent input (see Chapter 9), there is increasing evidence that persistent (days) activity in small afferents will lead to alterations in the amount of message and the subsequent increase in the expression of prohormones and receptors in both the central and peripheral terminals.

Central Terminals

Following the initiation of adjuvant-induced monoarthritis, the expression of genes encoding the prohormones of SP and CGRP are increased in the dorsal root ganglia innervating the affected joint. This effect is relatively specific in that mRNA encoding vasoactive intestinal polypeptide (VIP) is not induced. These increases occur around the time of onset of acute inflammation (8 h) and persist until chronic arthritis develops after 14 days (20,31). This increased message is accompanied by an increase in prohormone, and SP and CGRP immunoreactivity by as much as 50% is also seen in the dorsal root ganglia and horn in arthritic rats (14,32,42,73). This is consistent with marked increases in gene expression of β-preprotachykinin and α-CGRP mRNAs. Similar changes have been observed during adjuvant-induced paw inflammation.

The tissue level of immunoreactive Met-enkephalin-Arg^6-Gly^7-Leu^8, a peptide derived from proenkephalin, and proenkephalin messenger RNA and prodynorphin messenger RNA levels increases after adjuvant inoculation and remains enhanced until day 14 (81). In polyarthritic rats, in which all four limbs showed swelling, inflammation, and hyperalgesia, a pronounced elevation is seen in the level of mRNA-encoding prodynorphin (proenkephalin B) in the lumbosacral spinal cord. In addition, the levels of immunoreactive dynorphin A1-17, a primary gene product of this precursor, are greatly increased. In polyarthritic rats, fibers and varicosities are much more intensely stained throughout the cord, particularly in laminae I/II, IV, and V and dorsolateral to the central canal. Monolaterally inflamed rats injected in the right hindpaw showed pathological changes only in this limb. Correspondingly, in unilateral inflammation, an elevation in immunoreactive dynorphin was seen exclusively in the ipsilateral dorsal horn. A pronounced intensification of the immunohistochemical staining of these neurons is seen in chronic arthritis. These findings demonstrate an enhancement in the functional activity of spinal cord-localized dynorphin neurons in the response to chronic arthritic inflammation (98). The μ-, δ-, and κ-opioid binding sites in the superficial layers (laminae I–II) of the lumbar and cervical enlargements of the spinal cord are complexly changed over time postadjuvant injection (5).

Peripheral Afferent Terminal

In addition to the increase in prohormones and receptors in the central terminal, there is little doubt that persistent afferent terminal inflammation will lead to an increased presence of the several hormones at the peripheral terminal. The axonal transport of both SP and CGRP towards the inflamed paw, as determined after sciatic nerve ligation, is increased. Nerve growth factor content is increased in the sciatic nerve of the inflamed paw and may have a regulatory function in the stimulation of sensory neuropeptide synthesis during prolonged inflammatory processes (21).

This information from experimentally induced arthritis thus suggests that quantitative and qualitative changes in neuropeptide gene expression and biosynthesis occur in response to the persistent input generated by acute and chronic inflammation. These findings open new perspectives for the understanding of pain regulation and therapeutic interventions in arthritis patients.

PSYCHOLOGICAL EFFECTS UPON PAIN

Pain as a neurophysiologic phenomenon is triggered by chemical or mechanical activation of nerve fibers in the joint and transmission of the peripheral signals to the brain. Pain as a subjective experience and clinical symptom is also a manifestation of the individual patient's history and an integration and interpretation of the peripheral stimulus in the context of the patient's psychological structure.

Pain behavior is profoundly modulated by psychological variables, and this has implications for the assessment and management of arthritis patients. Psychological variables characteristic for arthritis patients that are preexisting in the premorbid personality (prior to the onset of the arthritis) may contribute to the onset of the actual inflammatory disease process and determine the patients' strategies to cope with pain and disability. Antidepressants are a useful adjunct to the pharmacologic management of patients with arthritis, and their efficacy is usually manifested by a reported reduction in the pain-related disability associated with arthritis. These medications are not thought to affect peripheral components of the pain response but alter the patient's affective status (see Chapter 37).

MECHANISMS OF ACTION OF ANTIRHEUMATIC DRUGS

The local activity of joint inflammation using the degree of joint swelling as a clinical measure appears to correlate with biochemical markers in the synovial fluid such as IL-6, neopterin, and PG, as well as with leukocyte counts (72). However, neither clinical nor biochemical markers of inflammation correlate as well with the severity of joint pain in patients with chronic arthritis. Patients who are on stable pharmacologic regimens and have no significant detectable change in biochemical markers or joint swelling may report substantial variations in joint pain. Conversely, certain effective antirheumatic drugs such as methotrexate (MTX), which are not known to directly modulate pain generation, do profoundly reduce pain much sooner than joint swelling or biochemical markers of inflammation decrease. Some of these discrepancies may be explained by psychological effects on pain thresholds. Alternatively, as yet uncharacterized mediator systems or mechanisms of drug action may be involved. Here, we will contrast information on the mechanism of antirheumatic drugs with the current understanding of joint pain modulation (Table 4).

The management of rheumatoid arthritis (RA) involves the use of various classes of therapeutic agents to induce symptomatic relief and reduce disease activity. Aspirin and nonsteroidal antiinflammatory drugs are used as "first-line" therapy to reduce joint pain and swelling. For reduction or inhibition or the underlying disease process "second-line" or disease-modifying antiinflammatory rheumatic drugs such as antimalarials, gold salts, D-penicillamine, sulfasalazine, azathioprine, and MTX are being used. Randomized placebo-controlled trials have demonstrated the efficacy of these compounds in RA. Improvement in standard parameters of disease activity, including the number of painful and swollen joints, duration of morning stiffness, and erythrocyte sedimentation rate has been noted with these second-line drugs.

Table 4. SUMMARY OF ANALGETIC MECHANISMS OF ANTIRHEUMATIC DRUGS

Drug	Action
Salicylates	Central and peripheral antiinflammatory effects; inhibition of cyclooxygenase
NASIDs	Inhibit PG synthesis peripherally and in spinal cord
Glucocorticoids	Inhibit expression of proinflammatory mediator genes (cytokines, inducible cyclooxygenase, inducible nitric oxide synthase
MTX	Increases adenosine release

Pharmacologic treatment of patients with OA is exclusively directed at pain management, and presently no drugs are available for modification of the disease process. One study specifically compared antiinflammatory doses and analgesic doses of the nonsteroidal drug ibuprofen with acetaminophen as a pure analgesic in the treatment of patients with osteoarthritis of the knee (9). All three regimens resulted in similar improvement in pain scores, suggesting that at least for this study population synovial inflammation may not have been the primary triggering mechanism for joint pain.

Capsaicin

Topical capsaicin has been suggested for temporary relief of neuralgia following episodes of herpes zoster infections and in the treatment of diabetic neuropathy. Clinical investigations of topical capsaicin include trials in chronic pain syndromes such as postherpetic neuralgia, postmastectomy neuroma, reflex sympathetic dystrophy syndrome, diabetic neuropathy, psoriasis, hemodialysis-associated itching, and vulvar vestibulitis (77). In a double-blind-randomized study, 70 patients with osteoarthritis and 31 with rheumatoid arthritis received capsaicin or placebo for 4 weeks. Significantly more relief of pain was reported by the capsaicin-treated patients than the placebo patients (45). These findings suggest that topical capsaicin is a potentially useful drug for the treatment of painful OA of the hands (68).

Glucocorticoids/NSAIDS

The delineation of the role of TNF, IL-1, IL-6, and IL-8 in the development of inflammatory hyperalgesia, taken together with the finding that the production of these cytokines as well as that of the inducible cyclooxygenase are inhibited by steroidal antiinflammatory drugs, provides a mechanism of action for these drugs in the treatment of inflammatory hyperalgesia (19). Glucocorticoids may also influence pain and mood control via central effects on enkephalin neurons especially in the basal ganglia (mood) and on all β-endorphin (β-END) neurons of the arcuate nucleus, while most of the dynorphin neurons are not directly controlled by GC (12).

As reviewed above, there is strong evidence supporting both a central and peripheral role of agents that act as cyclooxygenase inhibitors in controlling the pain associated with the arthritic joint. The classic consideration of the utilization of these agents has been predicated (as their name implies) on the ability of these agents to reduce the inflammatory state. Such a reduction in inflammation was believed to be an important if not essential component of their efficacy in arthritis. However, as reviewed elsewhere (see Chapter 61), significant dissociation can be demonstrated for drugs in this class with respect to their efficacy as analgesics and their ability to reduce inflammatory signs (69). It seems certain that reduction in inflammatory signs cannot alone account for the significant activity of these agents.

MTX

Methotrexate has become the most popular second line antirheumatic drug. It equals gold and is better than azathioprine when examining radiographic erosions (25). Dihydrofolate reductase is the drug's target enzyme. However, based on the fact that folate supplementation of MTX-treated rheumatoid arthritis patients reduces toxicity without altering efficacy suggests that inhibition of this enzyme is not complete and not essential for efficacy at therapeutic doses. Several lines of evidence now suggest that one of the major mechanisms of MTX action is modulation of purine metabolism. Polyglutamates of MTX are direct inhibitors of thymidylate synthase and folate-dependent enzymes of purine biosynthesis, and the efficacy of MTX may involve blockade of these pathways. Blockage of aminoimidazole carboxamide ribotide transformylase, the folate-dependent enzyme responsible for the insertion of carbon 2 into the purine ring, produces an immunosuppression mediated by secondary inhibition of adenosine deaminase and S-adenosyl homocystein hydrolase by aminoimidazolecarboxamide metabolites (4). One hypothesis on the effect of MTX on adenosine release is that, by inhibition of 5-aminoimidazole-4-carboxamide ribonucleotide (AICAR) transformylase, MTX induces the accumulation of AICAR, the nucleoside precursor of which (5-aminoimidazole-4-carboxamide ribonucleoside, also referred to as acadesine) has previously been shown to cause adenosine release from ischemic cardiac tissue.

MTX significantly increases adenosine release by fibroblasts and by endothelial cells. MTX treatment inhibits neutrophil adherence by enhancing adenosine release from fibroblasts since digestion of extracellular adenosine by added adenosine deaminase completely abrogated the effect of MTX on neutrophil adherence. Acadesine also promotes adenosine release from and inhibits neutrophil adherence to connective tissue cells. The observation that the antiinflammatory actions of MTX are due to the capacity of MTX to induce adenosine release may form the basis for the development of an additional class of antiinflammatory drugs (17). Because purine biosynthesis is a fundamental process in cellular homeostasis, blocking this pathway may also be responsible for the MTX-induced decrease in leukotriene production (52) and IL-1 (89) and IL-8 (90) expression.

Clinically, MTX causes a significant reduction in joint pain and stiffness. The differential effects of purines on nociception at the peripheral and central levels raise the interesting possibility that the MTX effect on pain may be predominantly an effect related to increased levels of adenosine in the spinal cord and the CNS and that the increased levels in the inflamed joints are effective in reducing inflammation by interfering with the extravasation of leukocytes but for unknown reasons do not trigger increased pain.

CONCLUSION

Joint pain and inflammation are closely associated. Synovial inflammation is augmented by and generates chemical stimuli that can interact with primary afferent terminals innervating the inflamed region. However, it is important to recognize that, in addition to inflammation, other disturbances of joint homeostasis due to cartilage loss can cause pain. In osteoarthritis, the most common joint disease, these other mechanisms are more important. This is evidenced by the lower efficacy of antiinflammatory agents in controlling pain in osteoarthritis as compared to rheumatoid arthritis and the finding of similar efficacy of NSAIDs that differ in their antiinflammatory activity but are similar as analgesics in osteoarthritis.

A substantial amount of information suggests that, in arthritis, inflammation and pain are not only causally related but are both the product of a network of chemical mediator interactions. Products of the inflammatory process such as prostaglandins and cytokines that originate from infiltrating leukocytes as well as resident connective tissue cells are in different ways involved in the induction of pain. Conversely, so-called neuropeptides bind to specific receptors on inflammatory and connective tissue cells and modulate their secretory and proliferative activity. Most inflammatory arthropathies are chronic processes, and in addition to the acute signals provided by chemical inducers of pain, adaptive changes occur via alterations in neuropeptide gene and receptor expression. Careful evaluation of arthritis patients often reveals a lack of correlation between changes in the intensity of pain and inflammation. The experience of joint pain is the result of central processing of a chemical or mechanical activation of the sensory fibers in the joint. Central processing integrates the patient's affective history and current status and is a target for pharmacologic pain modulation.

Evaluation of the mechanisms of action of antirheumatic therapy in part reveals rather plausible interactions where the improvement in joint pain is readily explained by the inhibition of inflammatory mediator production. NSAIDs inhibit PG production peripherally and at the spinal cord level. Glucocorticoids inhibit the production of proinflammatory cytokines, inducible cyclooxygenase, and inducible nitric oxide synthase in arthritic joints. MTX, the most commonly used remittive therapy in rheumatoid arthritis, raises interesting contradictions. Its antiinflammatory effects are ascribed to a stimulation of adenosine release. Purines have nociceptive activities in the periphery. However, when administered centrally, they are antinociceptive. Central effects of MTX are unknown.

As much as pain and inflammation are integrated in their peripheral pathogenesis and central processing of peripheral pain signals is recognized as an important component in forming pain behavior, central processing may modulate peripheral inflammation. The antiinflammatory effects of centrally administered salicylates represent an intriguing phenomenon to elucidate central interactions of mediators and mechanisms that govern pain and inflammation.

REFERENCES

1. Agudelo CA, Schumacher HR, Phelps P. Effect of exercise on urate crystal-induced inflammation in canine joints. *Arthritis Rheum* 1972;15:609–616.
2. Ahlgren SC, Levine JD. Mechanical hyperalgesia in streptozotocin-diabetic rats. *Neuroscience* 1993;52:1049–1055.
3. Andreev N, Urban L, Dary A. Opioids suppress spontaneous activity of polymodal nociceptors in rat paw skin induced by ultraviolet irradiation. *Neuroscience* 1994;58:793–798.
4. Baggott JE, Morgan SL, Ha TS, Alarcon GS, Koopman WJ, Krumdieck CL. Antifolates in rheumatoid arthritis: a hypothetical mechanism of action. *Clin Exp Rheumatol* 1993;11:S101–S105.
5. Besse D, Weil-Fugazza J, Lombard MC, Butler SH, Besson JM. Monoarthritis induces complex changes in μ-, δ- and κ-opioid binding sites in the superficial dorsal horn of the rat spinal cord. *Eur J Pharmacol* 1992;223:123–131.
6. Bianchi M, Sacerdote P, Locatelli L, Mantegazza P, Panerai AE. Corticotropin releasing hormone, interleukin-1α, and tumor necrosis factor-α share characteristics of stress mediators. *Brain Res* 1991;546:139–142.
7. Bianchi M, Sacerdote P, Ricciardi-Castagnoli P, Mantegazza P, Panerai AE. Central effects of tumor necrosis factor α and interleukin-1α on nociceptive thresholds and spontaneous locomotor activity. *Neurosci Lett* 1992;148:76–80.
8. Bileviciute I, Lundeberg T, Ekblom A, Theodorsson E. Bilateral changes of substance P-, neurokinin A-, calcitonin gene-related peptide- and neuropeptide Y-like immunoreactivity in rat knee joint synovial fluid during acute monoarthritis. *Neurosci Lett* 1993;153:37–40.
9. Bradley JD, Brandt KD, Katz BP, Kalasinski LA, Ryan SI. Comparison of an antiinflammatory dose of ibuprofen, an analgesic dose of ibuprofen, and acetaminophen in the treatment of patients with osteoarthritis of the knee. *N Engl J Med* 1991;325:87–91.

10. Brick JE, Brick JF. Neurologic manifestations of rheumatologic disease. *Neurol Clin* 1989;7:629–639.
11. Cannon JG, Tatro JB, Reichlin S, Dinarello CA. Alpha melanocyte stimulating hormone inhibits immunostimulatory and inflammatory actions of interleukin 1. *J Immunol* 1986;137:2232–2236.
12. Cintra A, Fuxe K, Solfrini V, et al. Central peptidergic neurons as targets for glucocorticoid action. Evidence for the presence of glucocorticoid receptor immunoreactivity in various types of classes of peptidergic neurons. *J Steroid Biochem Mol Biol* 1991;40:93–103.
13. Clark FJ. Information signaled by sensory fibers in medial articular nerve. *J Neurophysiol* 1975;38:1464–1472.
14. Collin E, Mantelet S, Frechilla D, et al.Increased in vivo release of calcitonin gene–related peptide-like material from the spinal cord in arthritic rats. *Pain* 1993;54:203–211.
15. Corrado AP, Ballejo G. Is guanylate cyclase activation through the release of nitric oxide or a related compound involved in bradykinin-induced perivascular primary afferent excitation? *Agents Actions Suppl* 1992;36:238–250.
16. Crea F, Gaspardone A, Kaski JC, Davies G, Maseri A. Relation between stimulation site of cardiac afferent nerves by adenosine and distribution of cardiac pain: results of a study in patients with stable angina. *J Am Coll Cardiol* 1992;20:1498–1502.
17. Cronstein BN, Eberle MA, Gruber HE, Levin RI. Methotrexate inhibits neutrophil function by stimulating adenosine release from connective tissue cells. *Proc Natl Acad Sci USA* 1991;88:2441–2445.
18. Cunha FQ, Lorenzetti BB, Poole S, Ferreira SH. Interleukin-8 as a mediator of sympathetic pain. *Br J Pharmacol* 1991;104:765–767.
19. Cunha FQ, Poole S, Lorenzetti BB, Ferreira SH. The pivotal role of tumour necrosis factor a in the development of inflammatory hyperalgesia. *Br J Pharmacol* 1992;107:660–664.
20. Donaldson LF, Harmar AJ, McQueen DS, Seckl JR. Increased expression of preprotachykinin, calcitonin gene–related peptide, but not vasoactive intestinal peptide messenger RNA in dorsal root ganglia during the development of adjuvant monoarthritis in the rat. *Brain Res Mol Brain Res* 1992;16:143–149.
21. Donnerer J, Schuligoi R, Stein C. Increased content and transport of substance P and calcitonin gene–related peptide in sensory nerves innervating inflamed tissue: evidence for a regulatory function of nerve growth factor in vivo. *Neuroscience* 1992;49:693–698.
22. Dray A. Mechanism of action of capsaicin-like molecules on sensory neurons. *Life Sci* 1992;51:1759–1765.
23. Ferreira SH, Lorenzetti BB, Bristow AF, Poole S. Interleukin-1b as à potent hyperalgesic agent antagonized by a tripeptide analogue. *Nature* 1988;334:698–700.
24. Follenfant RL, Nakamura-Craig M, Henderson B, Higgs GA. Inhibition by neuropeptides of interleukin-1β–induced, prostaglandin-independent hyperalgesia. *Br J Pharmacol* 1989;98:41–43.
25. Furst DE. Methotrexate: new mechanisms and old toxicities. *Agents Actions Suppl* 1993;44:131–137.
26. Gardner E. The distribution and termination of nerves in the knee joint of the cat. *J Comp Neurol* 1944;80:32.
27. Gouret C, Mocquet G, Raynaud G. Use of Freundís adjuvant arthritis test in anti-inflammatory drug screening in the rat: value of animal selection and preparation at the breeding center. *Lab Anim Sci* 1976;26:281–287.
28. Green PG, Basbaum AI, Levine JD. Sensory neuropeptide interactions in the production of plasma extravasation in the rat. *Neuroscience* 1992;50:745–749.
29. Guerne PA, Carson DA, Lotz M. IL-6 production by human articular chondrocytes. Modulation of its synthesis by cytokines, growth factors, and hormones in vitro. *J Immunol* 1990;144:499–505.
30. Guerne PA, Zuraw BL, Vaughan JH, Carson DA, Lotz M. Synovium as a source of interleukin 6 in vitro. Contribution to local and systemic manifestations of arthritis. *J Clin Invest* 1989;83:585–592.
31. Hanesch U, Pfrommer U, Grubb BD, Heppelmann B, Schaible HG. The proportion of CGRP-immunoreactive and SP-mRNA containing dorsal root ganglion cells is increased by a unilateral inflammation of the ankle joint of the rat. *Regul Pept* 1993;46: 202–203.
32. Hanesch U, Pfrommer U, Grubb BD, Schaible HG. Acute and chronic phases of unilateral inflammation in ratís ankle are associated with an increase in the proportion of calcitonin gene–related peptide-immunoreactive dorsal root ganglion cells. *Eur J Neurosci* 1993;5:154–161.
33. Harris ED Jr. Rheumatoid arthritis. Pathophysiology and implications for therapy. *N Engl J Med* 1990;322:1277–1289.
34. Heppelmann B, Schaible HG. Origin of sympathetic innervation of the knee joint in the cat: a retrograde tracing study with horseradish peroxidase. *Neurosci Lett* 1990;108:71–75.
35. Herman AG, Moncada S. Proceedings: release of prostaglandins and incapacitation after injection of endotoxin in the knee joint of the dog. *Br J Pharmacol* 1975;53:465.
36. Hernanz A, De Miguel E, Romera N, Perez-Ayala C, Gijon J, Arnalich F. Calcitonin gene–related peptide II, substance P and vasoactive intestinal peptide in plasma and synovial fluid from patients with inflammatory joint disease. *Br J Rheumatol* 1993;32: 31–35.
37. Holdeman M, Lipton JM. Antipyretic activity of a potent α-MSH analog. *Peptides* 1985;6:273–275.
38. Hua XY. Tachykinins and calcitonin gene related peptide in relation to peripheral functions of capsaicin-sensitive sensory neurons. *Acta Physiol Scand Suppl* 1986;551:1–45.
39. Hughes SR, Williams TJ, Brain SD. Evidence that endogenous nitric oxide modulates oedema formation induced by substance P. *Eur J Pharmacol* 1990;191:481–484.
40. Hukkanen M, Gronblad M, Rees R, et al. Regional distribution of mast cells and peptide containing nerves in normal and adjuvant arthritic rat synovium. *J Rheumatol* 1991;18:177–183.
41. Hukkanen M, Konttinen YT, Rees RG, Santavirta S, Terenghi G, Polak JM. Distribution of nerve endings and sensory neuropeptides in rat synovium, meniscus and bone. *Int J Tissue React* 1992;14:1–10.
42. Kar S, Gibson SJ, Polak JM. Origins and projections of peptide-immunoreactive nerves in the male rat genitofemoral nerve. *Brain Res* 1990;512:229–237.
43. Karlsten R, Gordh T, Post C. Local antinociceptive and hyperalgesic effects in the formalin test after peripheral administration of adenosine analogues in mice. *Pharmacol Toxicol* 1992;70:434–438.
44. Keil GJ, DeLander GE. Spinally-mediated antinociception is induced in mice by an adenosine kinase-, but not by an adenosine deaminase-, inhibitor. *Life Sci* 1992;51:PL171–PL176.
45. Khalil Z, Helme RD. The quantitative contribution of nitric oxide and sensory nerves to bradykinin-induced inflammation in rat skin microvasculature. *Brain Res* 1992;589:102–108.
46. Kita A, Imano K, Nakamura H. Involvement of corticotropin-releasing factor in the antinociception produced by interleukin-1 in mice. *Eur J Pharmacol* 1993;237:317–322.
47. Konttinen YT, Hukkanen M, Segerberg M, et al. Relationship between neuropeptide immunoreactive nerves and inflammatory cells in adjuvant arthritic rats. *Scand J Rheumatol* 1992;21:55–59.
48. Kuis W, Villiger PM, Leser HG, Lotz M. Differential processing of proenkephalin-A by human peripheral blood monocytes and T lymphocytes. *J Clin Invest* 1991;88:817–824.
49. Lam FY, Ferrell WR. Inhibition of carrageenan induced inflammation in the rat knee joint by substance P antagonist. *Ann Rheum Dis* 1989;48:928–932.
50. Lam FY, Ferrell WR. Capsaicin suppresses substance P–induced joint inflammation in the rat. *Neurosci Lett* 1989;105:155–158.
51. Lam FY, Ferrell WR. Neurogenic component of different models of acute inflammation in the rat knee joint. *Ann Rheum Dis* 1991;50:747–751.
52. Leroux JL, Damon M, Chavis C, Crastes de Paulet A, Blotman F. Effects of a single dose of methotrexate on 5- and 12-lipoxygenase products in patients with rheumatoid arthritis. *J Rheumatol* 1992; 19:863–866.
53. Levine JD, Clark R, Devor M, Helms C, Moskowitz MA, Basbaum AI. Intraneuronal substance P contributes to the severity of experimental arthritis. *Science* 1984;226:547–549.
54. Levine JD, Grubb BD. Afferent and spinal mechanisms of joint pain. *J Neurosci* 1993;13:2273–2286.
55. Lotz M. Prospects of immunotherapy in rheumatoid arthritis. *Rev Rhum Engl Ed* 1993;60:3–9.
56. Lotz M. Cytokines and their receptors. In: Koopman W, ed. *Arthritis and Allied Conditions, 13th ed.* Baltimore: Williams and Wilkins, 1997:439–478.
57. Lotz M. Experimental models of arthritis: identification of substance P as a therapeutic agent and use of capsaicin to manage joint pain and inflammation. *Semin Arthritis Rheum* 1994.
58. Lotz M, Carson DA, Vaughan JH. Substance P activation of rheumatoid synoviocytes: neural pathway in pathogenesis of arthritis. *Science* 1987;235:893–895.
59. Lotz M, Terkeltaub R, Villiger PM. Cartilage and joint inflammation. Regulation of IL-8 expression by human articular chondrocytes. *J Immunol* 1992;148:466–473.

60. Lotz M, Vaughan JH, Carson DA. Effect of neuropeptides on production of inflammatory cytokines by human monocytes. *Science* 1988;241:1218–1221.
61. Louis SM, Jamieson A, Russell NJ, Dockray GJ. The role of substance P and calcitonin gene related peptide in neurogenic plasma extravasation and vasodilatation in the rat. *Neuroscience* 1989;32:581–586.
62. Malmberg AB, Yaksh TL. Hyperalgesia mediated by spinal glutamate or substance P receptor blocked by spinal cyclooxygenase inhibition. *Science* 1992;257:1276–1279.
63. Malmberg AB, Yaksh TL. Cyclooxygenase inhibition and the spinal release of prostaglandin E2 and amino acids evoked by paw formalin injection: a microdialysis study in unanesthetized rats. *J Neuroscience* 1995;15:2768–2776.
64. Mapp PI, Kidd BL, Gibson SJ, et al. Substance P-, calcitonin gene–related peptide- and C-flanking peptide of neuropeptide Y-immunoreactive fibres are present in normal synovium but depleted in patients with rheumatoid arthritis. *J Neuroscience* 1995; 15:2768–2776.
65. Mapp PI, Walsh DA, Kidd BL, Cruwys SC, Polak JM, Blake DR. Localization of the enzyme neutral endopeptidase to the human synovium. *J Rheumatol* 1992;19:1838–1844.
66. Marshall KW, Chiu B, Inman RD. Substance P and arthritis: analysis of plasma and synovial fluid levels. *Arthritis Rheum* 1990;33:87–90.
67. Matucci-Cerinic M, Lombardi A, Leoncini G, et al. Neutral endopeptidase (3.4.24.11) in plasma and synovial fluid of patients with rheumatoid arthritis. A marker of disease activity or a regulator of pain and inflammation? *Rheumatol Int* 1993;13:1–4.
68. McCarthy GM, McCarty DJ. Effect of topical capsaicin in the therapy of painful osteoarthritis of the hands. *J Rheumatol* 1992;19: 604–607.
69. McCormack K, Brune K. Dissociation between the antinociceptive and anti-inflammatory effects of the nonsteroidal anti-inflammatory drugs. A survey of their analgesic efficacy. *Drugs* 1991;41: 533–547.
70. McGillis JP, Mitsuhashi M, Payan DG. Immunomodulation by tachykinin neuropeptides. *Ann NY Acad Sci* 1990;594:85–94.
71. Menkes CJ, Renoux M, Laoussadi S, Mauborgne A, Bruxelle J, Cesselin F. Substance P levels in the synovium and synovial fluid from patients with rheumatoid arthritis and osteoarthritis. *J Rheumatol* 1993;20:714–717.
72. Miltenburg AM, van Laar JM, de Kuiper R, Daha MR, Breedveld FC. Interleukin-6 activity in paired samples of synovial fluid. Correlation of synovial fluid interleukin-6 levels with clinical and laboratory parameters of inflammation. *Br J Rheumatol* 1991; 30: 186–189.
73. Minami M, Kuraishi Y, Kawamura M, et al. Enhancement of preprotachykinin A gene expression by adjuvant-induced inflammation in the rat spinal cord: possible involvement of substance P–containing spinal neurons in nociception. *Neurosci Lett* 1989;98:105–110.
74. Moncada S, Ferreira SH, Vane JR. Inhibition of prostaglandin biosynthesis as the mechanism of analgesia of aspirin-like drugs in the dog knee joint. *Eur J Pharmacol* 1975;31:250–260.
75. Nagasaka H, Awad H, Yaksh TL. Peripheral and spinal actions of opioids in the blockade of the autonomic response evoked by compression of the inflamed knee joint. *Anaesthesiology* 1996; 85: 808–816.
76. O'Byrne EM, Blancuzzi V, Wilson D, et al. Effects of indomethacin, triamcinolone, and dexamethasone on recombinant human interleukin-1–induced substance P and prostaglandin E2 levels in rabbit knee joints. *Agents Actions* 1991;34:46–48.
77. O'Byrne EM, Blancuzzi V, Wilson DE, Wong M, Jeng AY. Elevated substance P and accelerated cartilage degradation in rabbit knees injected with interleukin-1 and tumor necrosis factor. *Arthritis Rheum* 1990;33:1023–1028.
78. Pappagallo M, Gaspardone A, Tomai F, Iamele M, Crea F, Gioffre PA. Analgesic effect of bamiphylline on pain induced by intradermal injection of adenosine. *Pain* 1993;53:199–204.
79. Pereira da Silva JA, Carmo-Fonseca M. Peptide containing nerves in human synovium: immunohistochemical evidence for decreased innervation in rheumatoid arthritis. *J Rheumatol* 1990; 17:1592–1599.
80. Persson S, Post C, Holmdahl R, Nyberg F. Decreased neuropeptide-converting enzyme activities in cerebrospinal fluid during acute but not chronic phases of collagen induced arthritis in rats. *Brain Res* 1992;581:273–282.
81. Przewlocka B, Lason W, Przewlocki R. Time-dependent changes in the activity of opioid systems in the spinal cord of monoarthritic ratsóa release and in situ hybridization study. *Neuroscience* 1992;46: 209–216.
82. Russell NJ, Schaible HG, Schmidt RF. Opiates inhibit the discharges of fine afferent units from inflamed knee joint of the cat. *Neurosci Lett* 1987;76:107–112.
83. Sabetkasai M, Zarrindast MR. Antinociception: interaction between adenosine and GABA systems. *Arch Int Pharmacodyn Ther* 1993;322:14–22.
84. Sawynok J, Sweeney MI. The role of purines in nociception. *Neuroscience* 1989;32:557–569.
85. Sawynok J, Yaksh TL. Caffeine as an analgesic adjuvant: a review of pharmacology and mechanisms of action. *Pharmacol Rev* 1993; 43:45–85.
86. Schaible HG, Grubb BD. Afferent and spinal mechanisms of joint pain. *Pain* 1993;55:5–54.
87. Schaible HG, Schmidt RF. Time course of mechanosensitivity changes in articular afferents during a developing experimental arthritis. *J Neurophysiol* 1988;60:2180–2195.
88. Schepelmann K, Messlinger K, Schaible HG, Schmidt RF. Inflammatory mediators and nociception in the joint: excitation and sensitization of slowly conducting afferent fibers of catís knee by prostaglandin I2. *Neuroscience* 1992;50:237–247.
89. Segal R, Mozes E, Yaron M, Tartakovsky B. The effects of methotrexate on the production and activity of interleukin-1. *Arthritis Rheum* 1989;32:370–377.
90. Seitz M, Dewald B, Ceska M, Gerber N, Baggiolini M. Interleukin-8 in inflammatory rheumatic diseases: synovial fluid levels, relation to rheumatoid factors, production by mononuclear cells, and effects of gold sodium thiomalate and methotrexate. *Rheumatol Int* 1992;12:159–164.
91. Sorkin LS. NDMA evokes an L-NAME sensitive spinal release of glutamate and citrullin. *Neuroreport* 1993;4:479–482.
92. Stein C, Comisel K, Haimerl E, et al. Analgesic effect of intraarticular morphine after arthroscopic knee surgery. *N Engl J Med* 1991;325:1123–1126.
93. Stein C, Gramsch C, Herz A. Intrinsic mechanisms of antinociception in inflammation: local opioid receptors and β-endorphin. *J Neurosci* 1990;10:1292–1298.
94. Stein C, Hassan AH, Przewlocki R, Gramsch C, Peter K, Herz A. Opioids from immunocytes interact with receptors on sensory nerves to inhibit nociception in inflammation. *Proc Natl Acad Sci USA* 1990;87:5935–5939.
95. Taiwo YO, Levine JD. Effects of cyclooxygenase products of arachidonic acid metabolism on cutaneous nociceptive threshold in the rat. *Brain Res* 1990;537:372–374.
96. Van Arman CG, Nuss GW, Risley EA. Interactions of aspirin, indomethacin and other drugs in adjuvant-induced arthritis in the rat. *J Pharmacol Exp Ther* 1973;187:400–414.
97. Villiger PM, Lotz M. Expression of prepro-enkephalin in human articular chondrocytes is linked to cell proliferation. *EMBO J* 1992; 11:135–143.
98. Weihe E, Millan MJ, Hollt V, Nohr D, Herz A. Induction of the gene encoding pro-dynorphin by experimentally induced arthritis enhances staining for dynorphin in the spinal cord of rats. *Neuroscience* 1989;31:77–95.
99. Weisman MH, Hagaman C, Lotz M, Yaksh TL. Preliminary findings on the role of synovial fluid neuropeptide suppression by topical capsaicin in rheumatoid arthritis. *Semin Arthritis Rheum* 1994.
100. Whelan CJ, Head SA, Poll CT, Coleman RA. Prostaglandin (PG) modulation of bradykinin-induced hyperalgesia and oedema in the guinea-pig paw–effects of PGD2, PGE2 and PGI2. *Agents Actions Suppl* 1991;32:107–111.
101. Wyke B. The neurology of joints: a review of general principles. *Clin Rheum Dis* 1981;7:223–239.
102. Yaksh TL. Substance P release from knee joint afferent terminals: modulation by opioids. *Brain Res* 1988;458:319–324.

Anesthesia: Biologic Foundations, edited by Tony L. Yaksh et al. Lippincott–Raven Publishers, Philadelphia © 1997.

CHAPTER 50

PAIN IN ACQUIRED IMMUNE DEFICIENCY SYNDROME

CLAUDIA L. SOMMER AND ROBERT R. MYERS

With AIDS having emerged as a rapidly spreading, fatal disease in the early 1980s, the focus of clinical concern was on issues of acute medical management rather than the management of pain. However, reports on abdominal pain in patients with AIDS were first published in 1983, primarily as an aid in elucidating the differential diagnosis of intraabdominal opportunistic infections and "true" acute abdomen (4,12,73, 155). Case reports of AIDS patients with painful conditions like peripheral neuropathies (187,122) and polyradiculopathies (37,57,138), or conditions causing headache like toxoplasmosis or cryptococcal meningitis (30,223), followed during the first decade of patient management in the northern hemisphere. The first systematic reports on prevalence and management of pain in patients with AIDS were by Schofferman (176) and Lebovits (117) in the late 1980s, and other series have followed (3,77,115,126,131,142,185). An awareness of the pertinence of pain to this syndrome is now widely appreciated and documented in nursing journals in articles stressing the importance of adequate pain control in AIDS patients (31,116,177).

There is not a definitive pain syndrome in AIDS. As in cancer, pain arises from a spectrum of diseases affecting all organ systems. As will be reviewed below, the predominant mechanisms of pain in AIDS are those associated with inflammatory pain, tumor pain, and neuropathic pain. Pain in AIDS, like in any other syndrome, may point to the underlying disease, and treatment directed at the cause may be possible. However, the involvement of the immune system in AIDS complicates the treatment of disease and limits some forms of therapy. Painful neuropathic states may arise from the antiviral therapy itself. Treatment of the underlying disease may be lengthy, and symptomatic pain treatment may be necessary during that time. Furthermore, pain is more prevalent in the later stages of AIDS (176,185), when therapy of the underlying disease is rarely possible. AIDS pain is then comparable to terminal cancer pain, and it is at this point that aggressive palliative treatment is mandatory.

PREVALENCE OF PAIN IN AIDS

According to published studies, the prevalence of pain in AIDS varies from 54% to 61% in hospital inpatients and hospice patients (117,118,176) and from 54% to 80% in outpatients (49,131,185). In terminally ill patients, rates as high as 94% have been reported (145). In general, the prevalence of pain appears to increase with disease progression. Singer et al. (185) found an association between the number of new pains in AIDS patients and low-CD4 cell counts. Among the reported pains, abdominal and oropharyngeal pain are common. Other frequent complaints include headache, neuropathic, chest, and musculoskeletal pain (117,176,185). Inadequate pain control in AIDS patients and a lack of awareness by physicians of the problem have been criticized (3,118,131) since sufficient pain relief can often be achieved even in advanced stages with appropriate medication (3,49). These common pain referrals will be considered in the following sections.

CLINICAL PRESENTATION

Abdominal Pain

In a series of 458 nonselected consecutive AIDS patients, severe abdominal pain was observed in 15% (147). In this series, the predominant site of pain together with other key symptoms had a high-diagnostic value in <50% of the patients.

Abdominal pain in patients with AIDS has received much attention, since it frequently gives rise to problems of diagnosis and management (12,102,155,182,199,212,218). With treatment of the first AIDS patients, it became clear that AIDS presented with an unusual spectrum of intraabdominal pathology (155). Whereas guidelines for the diagnosis of most types of abdominal pain are generally well established, different rules apply for patients with AIDS, since common diseases may present in a different way and unusual diseases are frequent.

Localizing signs are often misleading due to the contributions of immunosuppression, cachexia, and prior antibiotic therapy. In a series of 235 patients with AIDS, Barone et al. (12) found 12% who had undergone evaluation for abdominal pain. The causes were infectious diarrhea (12 patients), ileus or organomegaly (eight patients), Kaposi sarcoma (three patients), Meckel's diverticulum, perforated duodenal ulcer, Burkitt's lymphoma, and duodenitis. In a series of 160 AIDS patients referred for gastrointestinal investigation, Edwards et al. (55) reported 20% of them to suffer from abdominal pain. Infections with cryptosporidium, shigella, salmonella, campylobacter, and cytomegalovirus (CMV) were often associated with abdominal cramps. Seventy-five percent of the patients with CMV ileitis and colitis improved with alimentary rest and Ganciclovir.

Occurrence of severe abdominal pain has been typically associated with reduced survival. The indication for emergency laparotomy is limited. Although mortality is higher than in the general population, morbidity is more common after emergency operations. In some studies, surgical interventions have been shown to reduce overall morbidity and mortality in AIDS patients with symptoms of an acute abdomen (48). Whitney et al. (212) recently found a perioperative mortality of 12% and 26% major complications in a series of 63 emergency laparotomies for appendicitis, visceral perforation or obstruction, peritonitis, or hemorrhage. Davidson et al. (43), from their experience with 28 AIDS patients who underwent emergency laparotomy, recommend early intervention in CMV toxic megacolon, whereas less benefit is to be expected from surgery in patients with abdominal pain from atypical mycobacterial infection or lymphoma. Elective surgery has been successfully used for palliation of cytomegalovirus enterocolitis, with complete or partial improvement of lower abdominal pain, diarrhea, and fever (189). The differentiation between AIDS-related causes and non-AIDS-related causes is useful, as was shown in a report on appendicitis in 28 AIDS patients, where only 30% of the patients had normal appendices and an AIDS-related pathology, and no perioperative deaths occurred (213). In addition, a wide variety of causes of abdominal pain in AIDS patients has been described: gastric carcinoma (99), pancreatitis, which may also due to antiretroviral treatment (220), cholangitis and cholangiopathy (22,32,46,50,63,215), histoplasmosis of the colon (11), gastrointestinal cryptosporidiosis (4), strongyloides infection (136), aseptic peritonitis, bacillary angiomatosis (90), and toxic shock (145).

Treatment in most of these conditions must be directed at the underlying cause, i.e., antibiotic or surgical. Adjuvant symptomatic treatment includes measures usually taken for abdominal pain such as antispasmodics, nonopioid and opioid analgesics, and sufficient palliation in the case of untreatable disease.

Oral Cavity and Esophageal Pain

Oral and esophageal pain is a major problem in AIDS patients. Lebovits (117) found oral cavity pain in 11% of their series of AIDS patients. Odynophagia may be the presenting symptom of newly seroconverted patients. A typical presentation is the combination of palatal and esophageal ulcers with a maculopapular rash. One third of AIDS patients have esophageal symptoms of dysphagia and odynophagia in the course of the disease (35). In advanced disease, odynophagia leads to substantial loss in quality of life, may hinder food uptake, and further deteriorate the often already compromised nutritional status of the patient (105).

Retroviruses have been detected by electronmicroscopy in biopsy specimens from such patients (159). Oropharyngeal candidiasis, which occurs in up to 75% of HIV-seropositive patients, is, although frequently asymptomatic, the most common cause of oral cavity pain (145). Other causes of oral cavity pain are oral ulcerations by herpes simplex virus, which are often combined with perioral lesions, cytomegalovirus, Epstein-Barr virus, mycobacterial infections, cryptococci, or histoplasmosis. Several AIDS-associated diseases presenting with oral pain have been described as the presenting symptom in AIDS: painful gingivitis (168), osteomyelitis of the jaw (54), and nasopharynx-carcinoma (89). Oral hairy leukoplakia may be painful, but the pain responds to surgical excision and acyclovir therapy (91). Bacterial infections cause necrotizing gingivitis as well as dental abscesses and are associated with pain and tooth loss.

Another condition associated with oral cavity pain is recurrent aphtous stomatitis (98). The differential diagnoses include herpes simplex infection and Wegener's granulomatosis, which have to be excluded by viral cultures and histologic studies. Seventy percent of patients with aphtous ulcers suffer from the idiopathic type (143). These aphtous ulcers are divided into two types, minor and major aphtous ulcers. In the more common "minor" form, aphtous ulcers last typically for 7–14 days, are limited to the superficial layers of the mucosa, and heal without scarring (28). Ten percent of the ulcers present as the major type (periadenitis mucosa necrotica recurrens). Major ulcers are larger, may persist for as long as 30 days, involve the deeper muscular layer, and can cause severe pain, dysphagia, and facial edema. They often remain unresponsive to treatment and scar upon healing (28). Major aphtous ulcers seem to be increased in AIDS patients as compared with the general population (84).

Symptomatic relief can be obtained with topical application of viscous lidocaine or other local anesthetics. Systemic therapy with colchicine, dapsone, or nonsteroidal anti-inflammatory drugs (NSAIDs) has anecdotally been reported to be beneficial (143). Steroid therapy appears to be efficient in most patients for pain control and to promote healing of the ulcers (9,10,51). Thalidomide has been used as an alternative in patients who were unresponsive to steroids. In two patients with severe recurrent aphtous stomatitis described by Nicolau and West (143), thalidomide led to rapid ulcer resolution and pain alleviation. Immunomodulation by decreasing tumor necrosis factor production in macrophages (172,191) may be one mechanism of action of thalidomide. Obviously, due to its teratogenic potential, thalidomide should not be used in women of childbearing age. Whether thalidomide may diminish deterioration in AIDS-related neuropathies has not been conclusively shown (87).

Kaposi's sarcoma in the oral mucosa and oropharynx may rarely cause oral pain. Radiation yields good functional and cosmetic results as well as relief from pain (145,209).

Esophageal candidiasis and its resultant ulcerations are responsible for a large number of the cases of odynophagia, varying between 25% and 79% in different series (21,35,58,127,162,203). Fluconazole or a combination of amphotericin B and flucytosine allow efficient treatment (26). Other etiologies of esophagitis include other fungal infections like *Torulopsis glabrata* (201) and *Histoplasma capsulatum* (64). Esophagitis can also be caused by mycobacteria (80, 47), herpes simplex (203) or Eppstein-Barr virus (106), cytomegalovirus, and HIV itself (21,159). A distinct entity of idiopathic esophageal ulcers that are very painful and difficult to treat has been described (9,10, 51,71,110,121,149,196). Kotler et al. (109) describe a follow-up on 12 patients with severe odynophagia, weight loss, and chest pain, in whom large undermined esophageal ulcers with acute inflammation were found. No evidence of the infectious agents known to frequently cause esophageal ulcers were found, neither was evidence of a tumor, although evidence of HIV was detected locally in all ulcers. Whether HIV expression in the cells occurs as the cause of, or as a response to, esophageal inflammation is unclear. The authors suggest that HIV is reactivated from by cytokines or inflammatory mediators in this condition, since the number of staining cells detected by in situ hybridization and by immunohistochemistry was too low to allow the conclusion that HIV itself causes the inflammation. Pain in this condition is disabling and sometimes refractory to parenteral opiates. In addition to odynophagea, spontaneous substernal pain and severe, prolonged postprandial pain are part of the condition, as well as occasionally midline back pain.

Corticosteroids administered orally, intravenously, or by intralesional injection relieved the symptoms and promoted ulcer healing. After intralesional therapy, pain decreased within hours of the procedure, and after oral and intravenous application within 36–48 h. Pain recurred 7–10 days after intralesional injections. On repeat injections, prolonged responses were observed. Oral steroids were able to provide long-term relief, and could be tapered and discontinued in two thirds of the patients. Symptomatic recurrence occurred if therapy was discontinued too early. Otherwise, ulcer healing could be documented endoscopically in five patients. Five of the 12 patients developed new infectious diseases in temporal relationship with the steroid therapy, implying a possible causative role by deteriorating the patient's immune status. For symptomatic treatment, a combination of antacids and topical analgesics has been advocated (145). Gehanno et al. (72) report a series of 12 HIV seropositive patients with pharyngeal pain of unknown origin not relieved by analgesics. In these patients, thalidomide proved to be the only effective means of healing the ulcers and of suppressing pain. Esophageal ulceration has also been reported after zidovudine treatment (56).

Anorectal Pain

Anorectal pain is a common complaint in AIDS patients and is frequently caused by ulcerative and infectious processes. In a study of 340 homosexual and bisexual men with AIDS, 34% of the patients had anorectal disease (210). Conditions associated with pain were perirectal abscesses, cytomegalovirus proctitis, fissures, and herpes simplex infection. About half of the patients required surgical treatment. The complication rate with surgery was high such that conservative treatment was recommended (12,210). In 74 HIV seropositive patients, ulcerative anal disease was treated by sphincterotomy, debridement, antiviral therapy, or intralesional steroid therapy (205). Significant pain relief was achieved in most and healing in about half of the patients. Goldberg et al. (78) report a series of 163 HIV seropositive patients, 47 of whom had clinical evidence of an infectious process. Seventy-nine percent of these patients complained of anorectal pain. On examination, perianal tenderness, condylomata, ulcers, and anal fissures were found. Evidence of an infectious agent was found in 68% of the patients. Organisms frequently identified were herpes simplex, cytomegalovirus, *Neisseria gonorrhoeae,* and chlamydia. Medical or surgical treatment or a combination of both improved or resolved symptoms in 69% of the patients. Wilcox and Schwartz (213) describe a syndrome with idiopathic anorectal ulceration in AIDS patients, where etiology remains undetermined despite an extensive search for a pathogen. Therapy is symptomatic, with NSAIDs often effective in achieving pain control (150).

A rarer cause of rectal pain are malignant squamous tumors of the anus, which present with bleeding, pain, pruritus, and discharge. Proctologic examination reveals an ulcerated lesion, proliferative or infiltrating, with the diagnosis confirmed by biopsy (125, 197). Local excision and radiation therapy allow palliation.

Chest Pain

Chest pain is highly prevalent in AIDS patients. In 134 hospital patients, the chest was the most frequent pain location (22%) (117). This was assumed to be due to the high prevalence of *Pneumocystis carinii* pneumonia in their population (57%). Retrosternal burning on deep inspiration is characteristic of *Pneumocystis carinii* pneumonia. The acute onset of pleuritic chest pain may indicate pneumothorax due to *Pneumocystis carinii* pneumonia (13). Other pulmonary infections may equally be associated with pain, as has been reported for various types of bacterial pneumonia (33), pneumonia caused by mycobacterium tuberculosis and atypical mycobacteria (150), necrotizing pneumonitis (202), pulmonary actinomycosis (108), aspergillosis (45,107), *Pneumocystis carinii* combined with *Cryptococcus neoformans* infection (2), cytomegalovirus infection (127), and non-Hodgkin's-lymphoma (154). Radcliffe et al. (160) report a case of rheumatic fever manifesting as chest pain. Esophageal diseases may also manifest with chest pain, although the additional symptoms of odynophagia and dysphagia usually lead to the correct diagnosis (see above). Herpes zoster radiculitis is another cause of chest pain that is usually easy to diagnose (see below). An aneurysm of the thoracic aorta due to giant cell mesaortitis caused acute, severe chest pain (20). Among the differential diagnoses were Marfan's syndrome, vasculitis due to tuberculosis or syphilis or HIV, or rheumatologic diseases.

In most cases, treatment of the underlying conditions giving rise to chest pain either by antibiosis or by surgery will also abolish pain. During the treatment phase, NSAIDs and TENS, or opiates may be necessary to give pain relief (124).

Arthritic Pain

Whether there is an association between rheumatic diseases and AIDS is a matter of debate (190). A number of syndromes with painful arthritides and arthralgias have been described that may be partially overlapping. Statistically, the manifestation of some rheumatologic diseases is slightly increased as compared to the general population. In a review of the literature between 1981 and 1988, Kaye (103) found Reiter's syndrome and reactive arthritis to be the most common rheumatologic manifestations of AIDS, with psoriasis, myositis, and Sicca syndrome also being prominent. A prospective study with a series of 121 stage IV patients (166) reported rheumatologic diseases in 25% of the population. Buskila et al. (29) found rheumatologic symptoms in 34 of 52 patients, mild arthralgia included. In a series of 101 patients, involvement of the musculoskeletal system was observed in 72% (16). A prospective study of persistent arthralgia was carried out on 331 consecutive female inpatients in Rwanda, and arthralgia turned out to be a strong predictor of an HIV infection. Persistent arthralgia was present in 7% of the HIV seropositive patients and only in 0.8% of the HIV seronegative patients (173). Comparing the data of 556 AIDS patients with other studies composed primarily of homosexual men, it was concluded that the type of rheumatic complaint is more related to the risk factors than to HIV itself (141).

Although rheumatic manifestations are clearly not limited to an AIDS-affiliated etiology, such inflammatory states observed in AIDS patients appear to encompass a different spectrum than in the general population and are known to be associated with severe pain (169). Reiter's syndrome is encountered frequently, and in some patients, precipitating bacterial infections, e.g., by shigella, yersinia, and campylobacter, have been implicated. In the majority of cases, however, no specific infection could be identified (104). Preexisting psoriasis and psoriatic arthritis have been found to be exacerbated in AIDS patients (101) and may be associated with the immunodeficiency. The arthritis is often more severe than usual and is typically refractory to conventional therapy. In most patients, depletion of circulating $CD4^+$ lymphocytes is present by the time that arthritis is detected, but only limited data on synovial immunopathology are available. Occasionally, a rheumatic disease may be the initial presentation of AIDS. Thus, Arend et al. (6) describe a patient with general malaise, pain in several joints and muscles, lymphadenopathy, livedo reticularis, an elevated sedimentation rate, mild pancytopenia, a positive ANF, anticardiolipin antibodies, and circulating immune complexes. A syndrome of severe intermittent oligoarthralgia without evidence of synovitis, which lasted 2–24 h, has been referred to as an HIV-associated painful articular syndrome (16). In a series of 123 AIDS patients referred to rheumatologists, acute peripheral nonerosive arthritis without evidence of an infective agent other than the HIV virus and with a definite inflammatory infiltrate on synovial biopsy was the most prominent diagnosis (167). This arthritis usually persisted until death. In this series, 18 patients had nonspecific spinal pain, five had noninflammatory arthropathy, and 20 had arthralgias and myalgias of unknown cause. In a few patients, infectious joint disease was discovered (*Staphylococcus aureus, Neisseria gonorrhoeae,* tuberculosis, and others) and successfully treated with antibiotics. AIDS-associated arthritis is an extremely painful condition. Rynes (169) described four patients with this syndrome, which is oligoarthritic, most frequently affecting the knees and ankles. The joints are swollen, erythematous, and very tender. Movement may be impeded by pain. In spite of the clinical appearance of an inflammatory arthritis, synovial fluid analysis and histologic studies in these patients were surprisingly unremarkable.

HIV virus has been identified in synovial fluid (211), but the etiology of AIDS-associated arthritis has not yet been established. Treatment with intraarticular application of steroids and NSAIDs has been reported to bring prompt pain relief (169), and spontaneous resolution is possible. In contrast, in inflammatory arthritis of undetermined type, characterized by inflammatory synovial fluid and unusually severe symptoms affecting the knees and sometimes also upper extremity joints, as in the patients described by Rowe et al. (167), the symptoms were resistant to NSAIDs and persistent functional limitation caused by severe pain and stiffness resulted (65). A syndrome of incapacitating arthralgias without any evidence of synovitis has also been described, which often made opioid treatment necessary (169). An active factor which served to sensitize nerve endings but did not lead to an inflammatory state is one possible source of this aberrant pain state (see Chapters 3 and 6).

Other pain conditions hard to treat include bursitis and myalgias. The latter pose a diagnostic problem, because myositis may be difficult to detect in AIDS patients due to the unreliability of laboratory parameters. Rynes (169) states that a common characteristic of the AIDS-associated rheumatic diseases is severe pain in the lower extremities, regardless of whether the pain is generated from joints, muscles, or bursae. Why pain is so severe as compared with non-AIDS patients with similar arthritides is unknown. Subclinical neuropathy or aberrant response of the CNS due to HIV infection have been suggested (169) (see below). Standard treatment includes oral analgesics, NSAIDs, and intraarticular corticosteroids. Oral or parenteral administration of high-dose corticosteroids is considered controversial because of the potential risk of facilitating opportunistic infections by additional immunosuppression (see below).

Myalgia

Myalgia can be caused by myopathy or myositis, and it may also be an accompanying symptom of rheumatic diseases primarily attacking the joints (see Chapter 27) or of other infectious diseases. Myalgia has been described in 56% of patients with acute seroconversion to HIV (200). Polymyositis is the most common myopathy in AIDS (42). It may occur at any stage of the HIV infection, often early and sometimes as the presenting symptom. The symptoms are proximal muscle weakness and pain with serum studies revealing an elevated creatine kinase. Muscle biopsy shows inflammatory infiltrates with phagocytosis and fiber necrosis (40). The pathogenesis is unknown, although direct viral infection of muscle cells has been proposed (103). There is, however, no evidence of virus in muscle itself, since only surrounding inflammatory cells were immunoreactive with HIV in immunohistochemistry (40). In another type of myopathy associated with proximal weakness and myalgia, prominent clinical and electrodiagnostic features contrast with modest findings on muscle biopsy. In this condition, only a few scattered necrotic fibers can be found without evidence of inflammation (112,183,194). Younger et al. (222) describe a case of recurrent myoglobinuria and myalgia in a HIV seropositive patient, who was asymptomatic between episodes and had no clinical evidence of AIDS. In this patient's biopsy, muscle fiber necrosis was present without inflammation. Pyomyositis, caused by *Staphylococcus aureus* or by *Mycobacterium avis*, characterized by localized muscle pain, swelling and tenderness, has been reported in AIDS patients (19,216,217).

Drugs in the treatment of AIDS, especially AZT, have been associated with the development of myalgia and myositis, including a necrotizing noninflammatory myopathy (18,81, 128,163). In AZT-induced myopathy, inflammatory infiltrates may be found. Differentiation from true inflammatory myopathies may be difficult (34,41). Muscle biopsy in AZT myopathy may show ragged red fibers, and, indeed, mitochondrial dysfunction has been identified as the cause of this disorder (7,134). However, most patients with AIDS and myopathy, including those taking AZT, are supposed to have HIV-related rather then AZT-related disease (184).

The inflammatory myopathy (polymyositis) may improve with immunomodulating treatment such as plasmapheresis, intravenous immunoglobulins, or steroids (184). Dalakas et al. (42) report that immunosuppressive treatment of polymyositis brings improvement in ~50% of patients, although the success of treatment varies in other studies. Whether there is an increased risk of opportunistic infections with immunosuppression is not yet clear; however, the symptoms of pyomyositis respond well to steroids, as in non-AIDS patients (113). The treatment for AZT-myopathy is cessation of the drug. Reduction of the dosage has not been shown to be of benefit (34).

Headache

In AIDS patients, headaches encompass a large number of differential diagnoses, from relatively benign conditions, including tension headache, migraine, and sinus infections, to serious diseases like HIV encephalitis and atypical aseptic meningitis, opportunistic infections, and neoplasms of the CNS. Headache was the most frequent complaint in the longitudinal study on painful symptoms in ambulatory HIV-infected men by Singer et al. (185), and its prevalence increased with duration of the disease. In a survey of hospitalized patients with AIDS, headache was the second most frequent complaint after chest pain (117). In another study of 100 hospitalized patients (142), headache was the fourth major cause of pain. HIV encephalitis and atypical aseptic meningitis may cause headache (145). Encephalopathy presents with poor concentration, mental slowing, lack of coordination, and disturbance of gait. Dementia progresses with advance of the disease; survival after the onset of dementia averages ~6 months (25,130). HIV infection has been shown in cerebral macrophages, lymphocytes, and microglial cells (135,207). It is proposed that immune activation in the CNS leads to excessive production of cytokines and toxic products that damage the neuronal cells, which have not otherwise been affected (25).

Atypical aseptic meningitis is characterized by headache and meningism without evidence of an infectious agent in the CSF. It may be part of the acute febrile illness accompanying the acquisition of the virus (94), or it may occur as chronic meningitis later in the course of the infection (95). Frequently, headache indicates opportunistic infection. Sinusitis headache is experienced as dull pressure (142). Cryptococcal meningitis, one of the most commonly encountered opportunistic infections, presents with slowly progressive symptoms of headache, neck stiffness and fever. Cerebral toxoplasmosis may present with headache, however, focal neurologic symptoms or seizures may occur first, depending on the location of the toxoplasmoma (123). Computed cerebral tomography (CCT) reveals typical ring-enhancing lesions, although the lesions may be difficult to differentiate from cerebral lymphoma or other tumors. Antitoxoplasmal therapy, which is often used as a trial to confirm the diagnosis, brings clinical improvement and diminution of the lesions seen in CCT. If a toxoplasma abscess is located in the thalamic region, it can give rise to classical contralateral thalamic pain. The typical syndrome of paresthesias, deep aching pain and hypersensitivity to touch on the contralateral arm and leg has been described (79).

Other cerebral infections leading to headache are cytomegalovirus infection, herpes simplex and herpes zoster infection, and progressive multifocal leukencephalopathy (PML) induced by a papovavirus (145). Frequently encountered neoplasms include primary cerebral lymphoma and metastatic systemic lymphoma. Intracranial Kaposi sarcoma has also been described. Symptoms are those of increased intracranial pressure like headache, nausea and vomiting, seizures or focal neurological deficits. AZT treatment induces headache in nearly 16% of the ambulatory patients studied by Singer (185). None of their patients discontinued the drug due to headaches, and in most cases, AZT-related headache subsided over time (153,185).

Treatment of AIDS-related headache is often directed at the underlying process. Symptomatic and adjuvant treatment of pain includes aminacetophen, NSAIDs, tricyclic antidepressants (such as amitryptiline) and opiates. Biofeedback and relaxation techniques may be of value in tension headache (124,150). Several mechanisms underlying headache have been reviewed elsewhere (see Chapter 25).

Peripheral neuropathy pain

Syndromes

Several types of neuropathy are typically seen in patients with AIDS including symmetric predominantly sensory painful neuropathy, CMV neuropathy and polyradiculopathy. Other types of neuropathy that occur in AIDS do not differ clinically from those seen in the general population, e.g., Guillain-Barré syndrome and mononeuropathies due to vasculitis.

Sensory Neuropathies The most frequently encountered type of peripheral neuropathy in AIDS is painful predominantly sensory neuropathy, which has been found to occur in 10–30% of patients (36,122,148,187). Cornblath and McArthur (39) evaluated 40 patients with HIV infection and neuropathy, 26 of whom had predominantly sensory neuropathy. Most of these patients had AIDS for >4 months; only six patients had AIDS-related complex (ARC). The prognosis is very bad for such patients, and many die within 6 months of the onset of neuropathy. The most common complaint in this population is pain in the soles. Patients are observed to walk on their heels to avoid pressure on their feet, and some cannot wear normal shoes (38). Pain is described as burning or as intense pins and needles, involving the soles and the dorsum of the feet (70). Light touch or contact with bed sheets increases the pain. Most complaints are symmetrical and limited to the feet. Even when symptoms progress, no spreading of symptoms above the ankle is observed. Symptoms of autonomic failure, like impotence or urinary symptoms, may be present (70). Clinical signs of neuropathy, like absent or reduced ankle jerks and elevated pain or vibration thresholds, are usually present. Although weakness is rare, electrophysiology often reveals involvement of both the sensory and the motor system.

Axonal atrophy has been found to be the morphological correlate in painful, as opposed to nonpainful neuropathy in AIDS (68), and a possible link between axonal atrophy and the generation of pain has been assumed (68,181,198). Occasionally, segmental demyelination has been reported (119). In their ultrastructural study of twelve sural nerves from AIDS patients with sensory or sensorimotor neuropathy, Mezin et al. (133) also describe axonal atrophy, however, in this study no data on the painfulness of the neuropathy are given.

Mononeuritis multiplex occurs in all stages of the HIV infection, but if it occurs in AIDS, it indicates a poor prognosis (113). Pain is not an obligatory symptom. The term "mononeuritis multiplex" is descriptive indicating dysfunction of multiple peripheral nerves, and different etiologies may underlie the condition. It is often due to vasculitis (36,70,74,112,170), or to CMV infection (82,171) and sometimes to lymphoma (70).

A different type of neuropathy which may also be associated with pain and paresthesias is cytomegalovirus neuropathy, in which there is electron microscopic evidence of CMV in macrophages, endoneurial fibroblasts and endothelial cells (171). The patients develop a rapidly progressive, multifocal sensorimotor neuropathy late in the course of AIDS. Histologically the neuropathy is characterized by multifocal necrotic endoneurial lesions which look like multiple endoneurial microabscesses. Treatment with ganciclovir may be of benefit. Robert et al. (164) describe a patient with a sensorimotor neuropathy which started with painful burning dysesthesias and rapidly progressed to generalized weakness with fasciculations. CMV inclusions were prominent in endothelial cells of small epineurial and epimysial cells in this patient.

Spinal and Root Pathologies Lumbosacral polyradiculopathy due to invasion of the nerve roots by CMV occurs in about 1% of patients with AIDS (14,88). It presents with low back pain, often associated with radicular or perianal radiation. A progressive areflexic paraplegia leading to flaccid paraparesis evolves over 1–6 weeks (69). Pathologic changes are multiple foci of inflammatory infiltrates in the cauda equina and lumbosacral roots, associated with destruction of axons and myelin. Prognosis is very poor and death often occurs within weeks of onset. Ganciclovir or the combination of ganciclovir and foscarnet were of benefit in some patients when given early (67,83,137).

Selective gracile tract degeneration has been reported, with the suggestion of a direct retroviral infection of the lumbosacral dorsal root ganglion cells with subsequent proximal to distal axonal degeneration (161). Although direct infection with HIV has been proposed, improvement with AZT has rarely been seen (38,219). An association with concurrent CMV infection has been observed in 80% of the 25 patients reported by Fuller et al. (70). Indeed, a dorsal root ganglionitis due to CMV has been described (27,164). Evidence of CMV infection has also been found in autopsies of patients who died with peripheral neuropathy (82). Thus, CMV infection with proximal nerve root dysfunction may contribute to the pathogenesis of axonal neuropathy. Symptomatic treatment with tricyclic antidepressants, anticonvulsants, or topical capsaicin has been used, as would be the routine in the non-HIV population. According to Penfold and Clark (150), mexiletine, like in diabetic neuropathy (44), provided considerable improvement in the treatment of pain, paresthesias and dysaesthesias.

Inflammatory Demyelinating Peripheral Neuropathies In inflammatory demyelinating peripheral neuropathies, which occur with seroconversion, ARC, and less frequently with AIDS, pain is not a prominent symptom, but there may be painful paresthesias (25,75,148). As in Guillain-Barré syndrome or in chronic inflammatory demyelinating neuropathy (CIDP), the pathogenesis is supposed to be autoimmune (148). The course may be benign with remission, or with relapse and remissions; corticosteroids and plasmapheresis have been used as treatment (37).

Herpes Zoster Herpes zoster may cause a predominantly sensory, painful neuropathy (see Chapter 27). Herpes viruslike particles have been shown in the axoplasmic matrix of myelinated fibers in patients with sensory neuropathies (61). Herpes zoster radiculitis is more frequent and causes the typical dermatomal pain. In the thoracic segments, it causes severe chest pain (117). Herpes zoster may affect up to one fourth of HIV-infected patients (113). In a survey of 112 homosexual men, herpes zoster was found to be a predictor of AIDS (132). Severity of zoster and degree of pain were indicators of poor outcome. Treatment, in addition to antiviral treatment with aciclovir, consists of NSAIDs in the acute phase, and carbamazepin, tricyclic antidepressants, or local capsaicin for postherpetic neuralgia.

Origin of Neuropathic Changes

The complexity of the peripheral neuropathic changes outlined above suggest that there are diverse mechanisms that account for these syndromes. Chapters 3 and 5 in this volume review a number of the general components associated with changes in axonal integrity and function secondary to injury and neurotoxicity. In addition to the direct peripheral changes that may occur as a result of a variety of pathologies (e.g., AIDS virus, CMV infection, herpes zoster), these changes in nerve function and integrity may well lead a variety of reactive central changes within the dorsal horn, including loss of interneurons and alterations in the expression of transmitters and receptors (see Chapters 3, 5, and 28). Such changes have been shown to result in spontaneous activity in primary afferents, dorsal root ganglia, and aberrant dorsal horn activity (see Chapters 5 and 28). The role of central changes due to a direct CNS involvement in spinal cord and at higher centers on pain states is as yet poorly understood. A number of general mechanisms may, however, be particularly relevant to the AIDS neuropathology.

Vascular Changes Vascular abnormalities which might lead to a decrease in tissue oxygenation have been observed in other types of neuropathy (53,156,157,178,192,195,206), including an animal model of painful neuropathy (191) (see Chapter 3). Mezin et al. (133) describe the presence of endoneurial vascular abnormalities consisting of basement membrane thickening, endothelial necrosis, and capillary remnants. Axonal atrophy and endoneurial capillary thickening may thus play a role in the development of a painful neuropathic syndrome.

Local Cytokine Elaboration A dysregulation of endoneurial macrophages resulting in excessive production of tumor necrosis factor (TNF) and other interleukins has been proposed to be involved in the pathogenesis of this neuropathy (85,139) (see Chapter 3). TNF has previously been shown to be involved in the pathogenesis of inflammatory and neuropathic pain (62,191). Gp120, the coat protein of HIV, binds to the dorsal root ganglia and may damage the peripheral nerve (5). Interestingly, neuropathy is very rare in children with AIDS, an observation that again may shed light on the pathogenesis of this neuropathy. Dalakas and Pezeshkpour (41) found tubuloreticular profiles in the endothelial cells of an AIDS patient with painful sensory neuropathy. Since these structures have been associated with interferon production (86), the authors speculate on a neurotoxic component in the pathogenesis of the neuropathy. Therapeutically, tricyclic antidepressants, anticonvulsants, NSAIDs, and opioids have been used with varying success (38). The symptoms are unresponsive to steroids or plasmapheresis, which is an argument against an autoimmune pathogenesis.

Drug-Induced Neuropathies A variety of chemotherapeutic agents used in cancer (see Chapter 20) and aids have been shown to induce neuropathology. The antiviral agents ddI (2′3′-dideoxyinosine) and ddC (2′3′-dideoxycytidine) have both been shown to produce painful neuropathy. In a phase I trial of ddI (111), eight of 37 patients developed the neuropathy and, with ddC (221), 10 of 20 patients. The neuropathies are dose-related and reversible. Combination of both drugs appears to exacerbate the neuropathy (120). Since AZT (3′-azido-3′-deoxythymidine) produces different side effects, mostly bone marrow suppression, a regime of AZT alternating with ddC has been proposed (23,186). In a study by Berger et al. (15), all patients with high doses of ddC (>0.03 mg/kg every 4 h) developed painful neuropathy with a mean onset of 7.7 weeks. Treatment with lower doses produced a similar neuropathy, although of milder severity and later onset. Except for the time course, the neuropathy was very similar to AIDS-related painful peripheral neuropathy. Indeed, ddC has been implicated as an axonal toxin (52). The neuropathy begins to resolve 3–5 weeks after discontinuation of the drug. The mechanisms of many of these neuropathologies are in fact poorly understood and represent a rich area of future investigation.

Total Body Pain and Skin Pain

Total body pain and skin pain are observed in terminally ill AIDS patients (140,176). The syndrome has been described as diffuse overwhelming distress (140). Attention to the psychological needs of the patient at this stage is very important. Pressure sore pain adds to generalized skin pain in emaciated patients. Lesions of Kaposi sarcoma contribute to skin pain. Good nursing care and adequate choice of beds and mattresses are essential. NSAIDs may be of benefit. Pain from pressure sores may be relieved by topical treatment (100). Opiates should be administered until pain control is achieved.

Pain in Children

Pain is more difficult to assess in young children than in adults, but there is little doubt that children with AIDS can suffer significant pain. While there are no exact data on the incidence of pain in children with AIDS, a study of >300 children with HIV infection reported a high incidence of acute and chronic pain due to the disease itself and to invasive medical procedures (146).

If symptoms or signs of typical painful conditions are present, like candida esophagitis or diarrhea, it is easier to estimate the extent of pain. Otherwise, behavioral disorders of the children must be assessed as symptomatic of pain. These may be crying crises, or sudden crying without apparent causes, catatonic appearance, or cachexia and retiration (204). Pain due to gastrointestinal and neurological manifestation seems to be frequent, while pain due to rheumatologic manifestations appears less frequent than in adults (146,180).

The problems in pain management are inability to assess pain in the young children, frequent parental denial of the disease and thus the child's pain, and strong family resistance to the use of narcotics due to negative experiences with drug abuse (208). In the case series of 300 children with HIV, it was judged that only one third of the children received adequate pain control. Special care protocols and a multidisciplinary approach that included support of parents has been shown to be successful (208). Therapeutic strategies using chronic intravenous lines to reduce pain caused by intermittent procedures has been useful (60).

Iatrogenic Sources of Pain

The induction of painful neuropathy by ddC and ddI has been discussed above. Other pain syndromes due to medication have been reported, like diarrhea and abdominal pain in a patient receiving ketoconazole (92), painful peripheral neuropathy and stomatitis with ddC, and diarrhea and abdominal pain with ddI (1). Right upper quadrant pain occurred in patients receiving interleukin-2 4–5 days after starting infusion, with gallbladder wall-thickening being present on sonography (158). Symptoms resolved after interleukin-2 infusion was reduced or stopped, but recurred on reinstallation of treatment. Painful esophageal ulcer has been reported after AZT treatment in three patients (55). Chemically induced pain has been connected anecdotally with several other agents, like interferon-alpha (175) and anti-CD 16 antibody (193). Severe medication-induced pain may thus prevent the administration of agents directed against HIV or the opportunistic infections.

SYMPTOMATIC MANAGEMENT

There is general consensus that pain management in AIDS should include treating the underlying disease (opportunistic infection, neoplasm) as far as possible by surgery, antibiotic, antifungal, or antiviral agents. This should, however, not delay symptomatic treatment. During and following the initiation of causative treatment, the same measures should be used that are employed in the treatment of cancer pain (117,150). Patients often rely on pain as the indicator of the severity and progression of their disease.

Inadequate treatment of pain in AIDS has been criticized (131,145). The reasons on the patient's side may be limited capacity to communicate the pain due to an organic mental disorder, and on the physician's side by lack of knowledge of common pain syndromes and their treatment, by focus on treatment of underlying diseases only, by fear of the adverse effects of pain-relieving drugs like further immunosuppression or respiratory depression, and by fear of uncontrolled reaction of drug addicts. Hoyt et al. (97) compared the perception of pain by chemically dependent and not dependent patients with AIDS, since previous studies had found a lower tolerance in dependent subjects than in control subjects for experimentally induced pain (93,129). They found no difference between the groups. Pain relief was achieved for 62% of patients in the chemically dependent group and for 52% of patients in the nondependent group. In the study of Anand et al. (3), adequate pain control could be achieved equally in substance abusers and nonsubstance abusers after consultation with the pain control service, using around-the-clock opioid analgesia adjusted daily as necessary.

Mild to moderate pain may be treated with NSAIDs or acetaminophen on a fixed schedule. If this does not yield sufficient pain control, a weak opioid like codeine or dextropropoxyphene should be added. If pain still persists, the weak opioid should be substituted by a strong opioid such as morphine. The dose should be increased stepwise until either pain control is achieved or adverse effects prevent further increase (145). Slow-release morphine was found useful in seriously ill, not hospitalized AIDS patients, often until the time of death (49). Subcutaneous application was used as an alternative for those not able to swallow.

As in cancer pain, some pains are not responsive to opioids. Among these are pain from neuropathies, some headaches, visceral pain and pressure sore pain (145). Tricyclic antidepressants can be useful in neuropathic pain, and may have to be added to regular analgesic therapy. In one study (142), drug users were found not to respond well to the sole use of tricyclic antidepressants for neuropathic pain such that the addition of weak opiates was required. Opiates can be given at night to reduce daytime drowsiness. In this way, they may also improve sleep and mood. TENS and acupuncture may be used as adjuvant measures or for otherwise not controllable neuropathic pain. Special measures, like intraarticular steroid injections, nerve blocks or trigger point injections may be used according to the diagnosis. Nonpharmacological forms of treatment include biofeedback, relaxation training, hypnosis, and psychotherapeutic and cognitive behavioral techniques (24,145,150). The value of pain clinics and ambulatory pain services has been demonstrated (3,142,185).

The treating physician needs to be vigilant for adverse drug effects. Opioids lead to constipation, and unless the patient suffers from diarrhea due to gastrointestinal infection, laxatives are required. Morphine and NSAIDs competitively inhibit AZT glucuronidation, which may lead to AZT toxicity depending on the dose of AZT administered (163). In cell culture, opioids have been shown to promote HIV replication in human mononuclear cells (151,152), and there are indications of immune modulation by opioids in HIV-negative drug users (144). There is, however, no evidence so far that these consequences of opioid use have practical implications in pain treatment of AIDS patients, though there is at present little systematic data. In patients on methadone maintenance therapy, a normalization of the alterations of cellular immunity induced by diamorphin (heroin) has been shown (144).

The indication for systemic steroids, which may be useful in the treatment of inflammatory neuropathies, myopathies or in arthropathies, has to be strictly posed due to their additional immunosuppressive effects. While some groups found a good response to steroid therapy with no adverse effects (59,174), others reported progression of Kaposi sarcoma or exacerbation of opportunistic infections (17,40,76,114,179). Other immunosuppressants like methotrexate and azathioprine have been associated with the progression of immunodeficiency. In addition, HIV patients may not benefit from them, as they probably require an intact CD4-cell network for their pharmacological action (145).

Because of CNS involvement in most AIDS patients, it has been suggested that centrally acting analgesics might further deteriorate mental function, although there is no evidence of such an effect. Hypomania was observed in one AIDS patient receiving amitriptyline for neuropathic pain (96). In general, AIDS patients seem to be more susceptible to the anticholinergic effects of tricyclic antidepressants (8), yet new antidepressants, which have fewer anticholinergic side effects, are often less efficacious in pain control. Alternately, as reviewed elsewhere, tricyclic antidepressant may also serve as NMDA antagonists and the effects of the classes of agent on AIDS-related pain states is unknown.

Ultimately, the utility of various pharmacological therapies will reflect upon the underlying etiology for the pain state. As reviewed in this chapter, it is clear that AIDS syndromes can induce pain states that, like cancer, cross the spectra of mechanisms from insults that reflect tissue injury (as in frank tissue lesions) to chronic inflammatory states as in the arthralgias and arthrides to complex neuropathic components. To the extent that different classes influence one or more of these underlying component mechanisms, it can be predicted that they will have a correlated efficacy. Thus, in the face of a predominant neuropathic component, opiates may be less efficacious, whereas therapeutic approaches such as the so-called membrane stabilizers (e.g., carbamzapine) or systematic local anesthetics may prove particularly effective (see Chapters 28 and 36). Short of curing the underlying disease entity, advances in our understanding of the mechanisms for these several pain states will likely lead to advances in our ability to manage the pain states associated with AIDS and its related syndromes.

REFERENCES

1. Abrams DI, Goldman AI, Launer C, et al. A comparative trial of didanosine or zalcitabine after treatment with zidovudine in patients with human immunodeficiency virus infection. *N Engl J Med* 1994;330:657–662.
2. Albrecht H, Stellbrink HJ, Fenske S, Koperski K, Greten H. Doppelinfektion der Lunge durch *Pneumocystis carinii* und *Cryptococcus neoformans* bei einem AIDS-Patienten. *Pneumologie* 1993;47:640–642.
3. Anand A, Carmosino L, Glatt AE. Evaluation of recalcitrant pain in HIV-infected hospitalized patients. *J Acquir Immune Defic Syndr Hum Retrovirol* 1994;7:52–56.
4. Andreani T, Modigliani R, leCharpentier Y, et al. Acquired immunodeficiency with intestinal cryptosporidiosis: possible transmission by Haitian whole blood. *Lancet* 1983;1:1187–1191.
5. Apostolski S, McAlarney T, Quattrini A, et al. The gp120 glycoprotein of human imunodefieciency virus type 1 binds to sensory ganglion neurons. *Ann Neurol* 1993;34:855–863.
6. Arend SM, Westedt ML, Hogewind BL. Een reumatisch ziekteheeld als eerste uiting von een HIV-infectie. *Ned Tijdschr Geneesk* 1992;136:584–586.
7. Arnaudo E, Dalakas M, Shanske S, Moraes CT, DiMauro S, Schon EA. Depletion of muscular mitochondrial DNA in AIDS patients with zidovudine-induced myopathy. *Lancet* 1991;1:508–510.
8. Ayuso JL. Use of psychotropic drugs in patients with HIV infection. *Drugs* 1994;47:599–610.
9. Bach MC, Howell DA, Valenti AJ, Smith TJ, Winslow DL. Aphthous ulceration of the gastrointestinal tract in patients with the acquired immunodeficiency syndrome (AIDS). *Ann Intern Med* 1990;112:465–466.
10. Bach MC, Valent AJ, Howell DA, Smith TJ. Odynophagia from aphtous ulcers of the pharynx and esophagus in the acquired immunodeficiency syndrome (AIDS). *Ann Intern Med* 1988;109:338–339.
11. Balthazar EJ, Megibow AJ, Barry M, Opulencia JF. Histoplasmosis of the colon in patients with AIDS: imaging findings in four cases. *Am J Roentgenol* 1993;161:585–587.
12. Barone JE, Gingold BS, Arvanitis ML, Nealon Jr TF. Abdominal pain in patients with acquired immune deficiency syndrome. *Ann Surg* 1986;204:619–623.
13. Battegay M, Greminger P, Luthy R. Pneumothorax als Komplikation einer *Pneumocystis carinii* Pneumonie. *Dtsch Med Wochenschr* 1989;114:1562–1565.
14. Behar R, Wiley C, McCutchan JA. Cytomegalovirus polyradiculopathy in acquired immune deficiency syndrome. *Neurology* 1987;37:557–561.
15. Berger AR, Arezzo JC, Schaumburg HH, et al. 2′,38-dideoxycytidine (ddC) toxic neuropathy: a study of 52 patients. *Neurology* 1993;43:358–362.
16. Berman A, Espinoza LR, Diaz JD, et al. Rheumatic manifestations of human immunodeficiency virus infection. *Am J Med* 1988;85:59–64.
17. Bernstein B, Flomenberg P, Letzer D. Disseminated cryptococcal disease complicating steroid therapy for *Pneumocystis carinii* pneumonia in a patient with AIDS. *South Med J* 1994;87:537–538.
18. Bessen LJ, Greene JB, Louie E, Sietzman P, Weinberg H. Severe polymyositis-like syndrome associated with zidovudine therapy of AIDS and ARC. *N Engl J Med* 1988;318:708.
19. Blumberg HM, Stephens DS. Pyomyositis and human immunodeficiency virus infection. *South Med J* 1990;83:1092–1095.
20. Boggian K, Leu HJ, Schneider J, Turina M, Oertle D. True aneurysm of the ascending aorta in HIV disease [German]. *Schweiz Med Wochenschr* 1994;124:2083–2087.
21. Bonacini M, Young T, Laine L. The causes of esophageal symptoms in human immunodeficiency virus infection. *Arch Intern Med* 1991;151:1567–1572.

22. Bouche H, Housset C, Dumont JL, et al. AIDS-related cholangitis: diagnostic features and course in 15 patients. *J Hepatol* 1993;17: 34–39.
23. Bozzette SA, Richman DD. Salvage therapy for zidovudine-intolerant HIV-infected patients with alternating and intermittent regimens of zidovudine and dideoxycytidine. *Am J Med* 1990;88: 24S–26S.
24. Breitbart W. Psychiatric aspects of pain and HIV disease. *Focus* 1990;5:1–2.
25. Brew BJ. The clinical spectrum and pathogenesis of HIV encephalopathy, myelopathy, and peripheral neuropathy. *Curr Opin Neurol* 1994;7:209–216.
26. Brockmeyer NH, Hantschke D, Olbricht T, Hengge UA, Goos M. Vergleichende Untersuchung zur Therapy der Candida-Oesophagitis bei HIV-1-infizierten Patienten mit Fluconazol oder Amphotericin B und Flucytosin. *Mycoses* 1991;34:83–86.
27. Budzilovich GN, Avitabile A, Niedt G, Aleksie SN, Rosenblum MK. Polyradiculopathy and sensory ganglionitis due to cytomegalovirus in acquired immune deficiency syndrome (AIDS). *Prog AIDS Pathol* 1989;1:143–157.
28. Burns RA, Davis WJ. Recurrent aphtous stomatitis. *Am Fam Physician* 1985;32:99–104.
29. Buskila D, Gladman DD, Langevitz P, Bookman AA, Fanning M, Salit IE. Rheumatologic manifestations of infection with the human immunodeficiency virus (HIV). *Clin Exp Rheumatol* 1990;8: 567–573.
30. Carne C. ABC of AIDS: neurological manifestations. *BMJ* 1987; 294:1399–1401.
31. Carr G, Neild J, MacDonald V, Meadows J. Nursing beliefs and pain management. *Nurs Standard* 1991;5:54–56.
32. Cello JP. Acquired immunodeficiency syndrome cholangiopathy: spectrum of disease. *Am J Med* 1989;86:539–546.
33. Chaisson RE. Bacterial pneumonia in patients with human immunodeficiency virus infection. *Semin Respir Infect* 1989;4: 133–138.
34. Chalmers AC, Greco CM, Miller RG. Prognosis in AZT myopathy. *Neurology* 1991;41:1181–1184.
35. Conolly GM, Hawkins D, Harcourt-Webster JN, Parsons PA, Husain OAN, Gazzard BG. Oesophageal symptoms, their causes, treatment and prognosis in patients with the acquired immunodeficiency syndrome. *Gut* 1989;30:1033–1039.
36. Cornblath DR. Treatment of the neuromuscular complications of human immunodefieciency virus infection. *Ann Neurol* 1988;23: S88–S91.
37. Cornblath DR, McArthur JC. Predominantly sensory neuropathy in patients with AIDS and AIDS-related complex. *Neurology* 1988; 38:794–796.
38. Cornblath DR, McArthur JC, Griffin JW. The spectrum of peripheral neuropathies in HTLV-III infection. *Muscle Nerve* 1986;9:76.
39. Cornblath DR, McArthur JC, Kennedy GE, Witte AS, Griffin JW. Inflammatory demyelinating peripheral neuropathies associated with human T-lymphotrophic virus type III infection. *Ann Neurol* 1987;21:32–40.
40. Dalakas MC, Illa I, Pezeshkpour GH, Laukaitis JP, Cohen B, Griffin JL. Mitochondrial myopathy caused by long term zidovudine therapy. *N Engl J Med* 1990;332:1098–1105.
41. Dalakas MC, Pezeshkpour GH. Neuromuscular diseases associated with human immunodeficiency virus infection. *Ann Neurol* 1988; 23:S38–S48.
42. Dalakas MC, Pezeshkpour GH, Gravell M, Sever JL. Polymyositis associated with AIDS retrovirus. *JAMA* 1986;256:2381–2383.
43. Davidson T, Allen-Mersh TG, Miles AJ, et al. Emergency laparotomy in patients with AIDS. *Br J Surg* 1991;78:924–926.
44. Dejgård A, Petersen P, Kastrup J. Mexiletine for treatment of chronic painful diabetic neuropathy. *Lancet* 1988;1:9–11.
45. Denning DW, Follansbee SE, Scolaro M, Norris S, Edelstein H, Stevens DA. Pulmonary aspergillosis in the acquired immunodeficiency syndrome. *N Engl J Med* 1991;324:654–662.
46. DeRodriguez CV, Fuhrer J, Lake-Bakaar G. Cytomegalovirus colitis in patients with acquired immunodeficiency syndrome. *J R Soc Med* 1994;87:203–205.
47. DeSilva R, Stoopack PM, Raufman JP. Esophageal fistulas associated with mycobacterial infection in patients at risk for AIDS. *Radiology* 1990;175:449–453.
48. Deziel DJ, Hyser MJ, Doolas A, Bine SD, Blaauw BB, Kessler HA. Major abdominal operations in acquired immunodeficiency syndrome. *Am Surg* 1990;56:455–450.
49. Dixon P, Higginson I. AIDS and cancer pain treated with slow release morphine. *Postgrad Med J* 1991;67:S92–S94.
50. Dowsett JF, Miller R, Davidson R, et al. Sclerosing cholangitis in acquired immunodeficiency syndrome. Case reports and review of the literature. *Scand J Gastroenterol* 1988;23:1267–1274.
51. Dretler RH, Rausher DB. Giant esophageal ulcer healed with steroid therapy in an AIDS patient. *Rev Infect Dis* 1989;11:768–769.
52. Dubinsky RM, Yarchoan R, Dalakas M, Broder S. Reversible axonal neuropathy from the treatment of AIDS and related disorders with 2′,3′-dideoxycytidine (ddC). *Muscle Nerve* 1989;12: 856–860.
53. Dyck PJ, Hansen S, Karnes J. Capillary number and percentage closed in human diabetic sural nerve. *Proc Natl Acad Sci USA* 1985; 82:2513–2517.
54. Edelstein H, Chirurgi VA, Hybarger CP. Osteomyelitis of the jaw in patients infected with the human immunodeficiency virus. *South Med J* 1993;86:1215–1218.
55. Edwards P, Turner J, Gold J, Cooper DA. Esophageas ulceration induced by zidovudine. *Ann Intern Med* 1990;112:65–66.
56. Edwards P, Wodak A, Cooper DA, Thompson IL, Penny R. The gastrontestinal manifestations of AIDS. *Aust NZ J Med* 1990;20: 141–148.
57. Eidelberg D, Sotrel A, Vogel H, et al. Progressive polyradiculopathy in acquired immune deficiency syndrome. *Neurology* 1986;36: 912–916.
58. Eisner MS, Smith PD. Etiology of odynophagia and dysphagia inpatients wtihthe acquired immunodeficiency syndrome (AIDS). *Gastroenterology* 1990;98:A446.
59. Espinoza LR, Aguilar JL, Berman A. Drug selection for rheumatic manifestations of aquired immunodeficiency syndrome. *Am J Med* 1988;85:895–896.
60. Fahrenheim E, Wintergerst U, Belohradsky BH. Minderung von Schmerzerlebnissen chronisch kranker Kinder bei intermittierender Infusionstherapie. *Monatsschr Kinderheilkd* 1993;141:330–332.
61. Ferrari S, Bonetti B, Monaco S, et al. AIDS associated predominantly sensory neuropathy. The role of herpes viruses. *Acta Neurol (Napoli)* 1990;12:75–78.
62. Ferreira S, Lorenzetti B, Pool S. Bradykinin initiates cytokine-mediated inflammatory hyperalgesia. *Br J Pharmacol* 1993;110: 1227–1231.
63. Forbes A, Blanshard C, Gazzard B. Natural history of AIDS related sclerosing cholangitis: a study of 20 cases. *Gut* 1993;34:116–121.
64. Forsmark CE, Wilcox CM, Daragh TM, Cello JP. Disseminated histoplasmosis in AIDS: and unusual case of esophageal involvement and gastrointestinal bleeding. *Gastrointest Endosc* 1990;36: 604–605.
65. Forster SM, Seifert MH, Keat AC, et al. Inflammatory joint disease and human immunodefieciency virus infection. *Br J Med* 1988; 296:1625.
66. Fuller GN. Cytomegalovirus and the peripheral nervous system in AIDS. *J Acquir Immune Defic Syndr Hum Retroviral* 1992;5:S33–S36.
67. Fuller GN, Gill SK, Guiloff RJ, et al. Ganciclovir for lumbosacral polyradiculopathy in AIDS [Letter]. *Lancet* 1990;1:48–49.
68. Fuller GN, Jacobs JM, Guiloff RJ. Association of painful peripheral neuropathy in aids with cytomegalovirus infection. *Lancet* 1989;2: 937–941.
69. Fuller GN, Jacobs JM, Guiloff RJ. Axonal atrophy in the painful peripheral neuropathy in AIDS. *Acta Neuropathol* 1990;81:198–203.
70. Fuller GN, Jacobs JM, Guiloff RJ. Nature and incidence of peripheral nerve syndromes in HIV infection. *J Neurol Neurosurg Psychiatry* 1993;56:372–381.
71. Gaylor RE, Stone EG, Glaser RL, Singleton KB, Crespo JH. Chronic esophageal ulcers in an AIDS patient. *Gastrointest Endosc* 1986;32:370–371.
72. Gehanno P, Barry B, Depondt J, et al. Syndromes hyperalgiques bucco-pharynges observes au cours du SIDA. *Ann Otolaryngol Chir Cervicofac* 1990;107:311–313.
73. Gerstein HC, Fanning MM, Read SE, Shepherd FA, Glynn MF. AIDS in a patient with hemophilia receiving mainly cryoprecipitate. *Can Med Assoc J* 1984; 131:45–47.
74. Gherardi R, Lebargy F, Gaulard P, Mhiri C, Bernaudin JF, Gray F. Necrotizing vasculitis and HIV replication in peripheral nerves. *N Engl J Med* 1989;321:685–686.
75. Gibbels E, Diederich N. Human imunodeficiency virus (HIV)-related chronic relapsing inflammatory demyelinating polyneuropathy with multifocal unusual onion bulbs in sural nerve biopsy. *Acta Neuropathol* 1988;75:529–534.

76. Gill PS, Loureiro C, Bernstein-Singer M, Rarick MU, Sattler F, Levine AM. Clinical effect of glucocorticoids on Kaposi sarcoma related to the acquired immunodeficiency syndrome (AIDS). *Ann Intern Med* 1989;110:937–940.
77. Glare P. Pain in patients with advanced AIDS. *Annu Conf Australas Soc HIV Med* 1993;5:60.
78. Goldberg GS, Orkin BA, Smith LE. Microbiology of human immunodeficiency virus anorectal disease. *Dis Colon Rectum* 1994; 37:439–444.
79. Gonzales GR, Herskovitz S, Rosenblum M, et al. Central pain from cerebral abscess: thalamic syndrome in AIDS patients with toxoplasmosis. *Neurology* 1992;42:1107–1109.
80. Goodman P, Pinero SS, Rance RM, Mansell PWA, Uribe-Botero G. Mycobacterial oesophagitis in AIDS. *Gastrointest Radiol* 1989;14: 103–105.
81. Gorard DA, Henry K, Guiloff RJ. Necrotizing myopathy and zidovudine. *Lancet* 1988;1:1050.
82. Grafe MR, Wiley CA. Spinal cord and peripheral nerve pathology in AIDS: the role of cytomegalovirus and human immunodeficiency virus. *Ann Neurol* 1989;25:561–566.
83. Gravelau P, Perol R, Chapman A. Regression of cauda equina syndrome in AIDS patient being treated with ganciclovir [Letter]. *Lancet* 1989;1:511–512.
84. Greenspan JS, Greenspan D, Winkler JR. Diagnosis and management of the oral manifestations of HIV infection and AIDS. *Infect Dis Clin North Am* 1988;2:373–385.
85. Griffin JW, Wesselingh SL, Griffin DE, Glass JD, McArthur JC. Peripheral nerve disorders in HIV infection, similarities and contrasts with CNS disorders. In: Price QW, Perry SW, eds. *HIV, AIDS and the brain.* New York: Raven Press, 1994:159–182.
86. Grimley PM, Kang Y-H, Frederick W, et al. Interferon-related leucocyte inclusions in acquired immune deficiency syndrome: localization in T cells. *Am J Clin Pathol* 1984;81:147.
87. Guiloff RJ, Fuller GN, Roberts A, et al. Nature, incidence and prognosis of neurological involvement in the acquired immunodeficiency syndrome in central London. *Postgrad Med J* 1988;64: 919–925.
88. Günzler V. Thalidomide in human immunodeficiency virus (HIV) patients. *Drug Safety* 1992;7:116–134.
89. Hald J, Larsen PL. Nasopharyngeal carcinoma in an HIV-positive patient causing severe morbidity and early death. *J Laryngol Otol* 1993;107:149–150.
90. Haught WH, Steinbach J, Zander DS, Wingo CS. Case report: bacillary angiomatosis with massive visceral lymphadenopathy. *Am J Med Sci* 1993;306:236–240.
91. Herbst JS, Morgan J, Raab-Traub N, Resnick L. Comparison of the efficacy of surgery and acyclovir therapy in oral hairy leukoplakia. *J Am Acad Dermatol* 1989;21:753–756.
92. Hernandez-Sampelayo T. Fluconazole versus ketoconazole in the treatment of oropharyngeal candidiasis in HIV-infected children. Multicentre Study Group. *Eur J Clin Microbiol Infect Dis* 1994;13: 340–344.
93. Ho A, Dole U. Pain perception in drug-free and in methadone-maintained human ex-addicts. *Soc Exp Biol Med* 1979;162:392–395.
94. Ho DD, Rota TR, Schooley RT, et al. Isolation of HTLV-III from cerebrospinal fluid and neural tissues of patients with neurologic syndromes related to AIDS. *N Engl J Med* 1985;313:1493–1497.
95. Hollander H, Stringari S. Human immunodeficiency virus associated meningitis: clinical course and correlations. *Am J Med* 1987; 83:813.
96. Holmes VF, Fricchione GL. Hypomania in an AIDS patient receiving amitriptyline for neuropathic pain. *Neurology* 1989;39:305.
97. Hoyt MJ, Nokes K, Newshan G, Staats JA, Thorn M. The effect of chemical dependency on pain perception in persons with AIDS. *J Assoc Nurses AIDS Care* 1994;5:33–38.
98. Hutton KP, Rogers RS. Recurrent aphtous stomatitis. *Dermatol Clin* 1987;5:761–768.
99. Ishikawa M, Suzuki S, Akudo Y, Toyota T, et al. An autopsy case of AIDS with hemophilia A who died of DIC and gastrointestinal bleeding associated with gastric carcinoma (signet ring cell carcinoma) [Japanese]. *Rinsho Ketsueki* 1994;35:886–891.
100. Jepson BA. Relieving the pain of pressure sores. *Lancet* 1992; 1:503–504.
101. Johnson TM, Duvic M, Rapini RP, Rios A. AIDS exacerbates psoriasis. *N Engl J Med* 1985;313:1415.
102. Katz MH, French DM. AIDS and the acute abdomen. *Emerg Med Clin Am* 1989;7:575–589.
103. Kaye BR. Rheumatologic manifestations of infection with human immunodeficiency virus (HIV). *Ann Intern Med* 1989;111:158–167.
104. Keat A, Rowe I. Reiter's syndrome and associated arthritides. *Rheum Dis Clin North Am* 1991;17:25–42.
105. Keithley JK, Kohn CL. Managing nutritional problems in people with AIDS. *Oncol Nurs Forum* 1990;17:23–27.
106. Kitchen VS, Helbert M, Francis ND, et al. Epstein-Barr virus associated oesophageal ulcers in AIDS. *Gut* 1990;31:1223–1225.
107. Klapholz A, Salomon N, Perlman DC, Talavera W. Aspergillosis in the acquired immunodeficiency syndrome. *Chest* 1991;100: 1614–1618.
108. Klapholz A, Talavera W, Rorat E, Salsitz E, Widrow C. Pulmonary actinomycosis in a patient with HIV infection. *Mt Sinai J Med* 1989; 56:300–303.
109. Kotler DP, Reka S, Orenstein JM, Fox CH. Chronic idiopathic esophageal ulceration in the acquired immunodeficiency syndrome. *J Clin Gastroenterol* 1992;15:284–290.
110. Kumar A, Posner G, Colby S, Nicholas A. Giant esophageal ulcers in AIDS-related complex. *Gastrointest Endosc* 1988;34:153–154.
111. Lambert JS, Seidlin M, Reichman RC, et al. 2′,3′-Dideoxyinosine (ddI) in patients with the acquired immunodeficiency syndrome or AIDS-related complex. A phase I trial. *N Engl J Med* 1990;322: 1333–40.
112. Lange DJ. AAEM minimonograph 41: neuromuscular diseases associated with HIV-1 infection. *Muscle Nerve* 1994;17:16–30.
113. Lange DJ, Britton CB, Younger DS, Hays AP. The neuromuscular manifestations of human immunodeficiency virus infections. *Arch Neurol* 1988;45:1084–1088.
114. Langtry JA, Copeman PW. Late secondary syphilis altered by systemic corticosteroids in a human immunodeficiency virus antibody postitive man. *J R Soc Med* 1990;83:49.
115. Larue F, Brasseur L, Musseault P, Demeulemeester R, Bonifassi L, Bez G. Pain and H.I.V. infection. A French national survey. *Int Conf AIDS* 1993;9:74.
116. Laskin MEA. Pain management in the patients with AIDS. *J Adv Med Surg Nurs* 1988;1:37–43.
117. Lebovits AH, Lefkowitz M, McCarthy D, et al. The prevalence and management of pain in patients with AIDS: a review of 134 cases. *Clin J Pain* 1989;5:245–248.
118. Lebovits AH, Smith G, Maignan M, Lefkowitz M. Pain in hospitalized patients with AIDS: analgesic and psychotropic medications. *Clin J Pain* 1994;101:156–161.
119. Leger JM, Bouche P, Bolgert F, et al. The spectrum of polyneuropathies in patients infected with HIV. *J Neurol Neurosurg Psychiatry* 1989;52:1369–1374.
120. LeLacheur S, Simon GL. Exacerbation of dideoxycytidine-induced neuropathy with dideoxycytidine. *J AIDS* 1991;4:538–539.
121. Levine MS, Loercher G, Katzka DA, Herlinger H, Rubesin SE, Laufe I. Giant, human immunodeficiency virus–related ulcers in the esophagus. *Radiology* 1991;180:323–326.
122. Levy RM, Bredesen DE, Rosenblum ML. Neurological manifestations of the acquired immune deficiency syndrome (AIDS): experience at UCSF and review of the literature. *J Neurosurg* 1985;62: 475–495.
123. Levy RM, Bredesen DE, Rosenblum ML. Opportunistic central nervous system pathology in patients with AIDS. *Ann Neurol* 1988; 23:S7–S12.
124. Lewis MS, Warfield CA. Management of pain in AIDS. *Hosp Pract* 1990;25:51–54.
125. Lorenz HP, Wilson W, Leigh B, Crombleholme T, Schecter W. Squamous cell carcinoma of the anus and HIV infection. *Dis Colon Rectum* 1991;34:336–8.
126. Loveless M, Bell L, Coodley G. Pain associated with HIV disease and its complications. *Int Conf AIDS* 1993;9:74.
127. Lucente FE, Meiteles LZ, Pincus RL. Bronchoesophageal manifestations of acquired immunodeficiency syndrome. *Ann Otol Rhinol Laryngol* 1988;97:530–533.
128. Manji H, Harrison MJ, Round JM, et al. Muscle disease, HIV and zidovudine: the spectrum of muscle disease in HIV-infected individuals treated with zidovudine. *J Neurol* 1993;240:479–488.
129. Martin J, Ingles J. Pain tolerance and narcotic addiction. *Br J Soc Clin Psychol* 1965;4:224–229.
130. McArthur JC, Hoover DR, Bacellar MA, et al. Dementia in AIDS patients: incidence and risk factors. *Neurology* 1993;43: 2245–2252.
131. McCormack JP, Li R, Zarowny D, Singer J. Inadequate treatment of pain in amulatory HIV patients. *Clin J Pain* 1993;9:279–283.

132. Melbye W, Grossman RJ, Goedert JJ, Eyster ME, Biggar RJ. Risk of aids after herpes zoster. *Lancet* 1987;1:728–731.
133. Mezin P, Brion J-P, Vermont J, Micoud M, Stoebner P. Ultrastructural changes associated with peripheral neuropathy in HIV/AIDS. *Ultrastruct Pathol* 1991;15:593–602.
134. Mhiri C, Baudrimont M, Bonne G, et al. Zidovudine myopathy: a distinctive disorder associated with mitochondrial dysfunction. *Ann Neurol* 1991;29:606–614.
135. Michaels J, Price RW, Rosenblum MK. Microglia in the giant cell encephalitis of acquired immune deficiency syndrome: proliferation, infection and fusion. *Acta Neuropathol* 1988;76:373–379.
136. Miller RG, Storey JR, Greco CM. Ganciclovir in the treatment of progressive AIDS-related polyradiculopathy. *Neurology* 1990;40: 569–574.
137. Miller SE. Helminthic infections in the acquired immunodeficiency syndrome. *J Electron Microsc Tech* 1988; 8:133–135.
138. Mishra BB, Sommers W, Koski CL, Greenstein JI. Acute inflammatory demyelinating polyneuropathy in the acquired immune deficiency syndrome. *Ann Neurol* 1985;18:131–132.
139. Monte SMDL, Gabuzda DH, Ho DD, et al. Peripheral neuropathy in the acquired immunodeficiency syndrome. *Ann Neurol* 1988;23: 485–492.
140. Moss V. Palliative care in advanced HIV disease: presentation, problems and palliation. *AIDS* 1990;4:S235–S242.
141. Munoz-Fernandez S, Cardenal A, Balsa A, et al. Rheumatic manifestations in 556 patients with human immunodeficiency virus infection. *Semin Arthritis Rheum* 1991; 21:30–9.
142. Newshan GT, Wainapel SF. Pain characteristics and their management in persons with AIDS. *J Assoc Nurses AIDS Care* 1993;4:53–59.
143. Nicolau D, West TE. Thalidomide: treatment of severe recurrent aphthous stomatitis in patients with AIDS. *DICP* 1990;24: 1054–1056.
144. Novick DM, Ochshorn M, Ghali V, et al. Natural killer cell activity and lymphocyte subsets in parenteral heroin abusers and long-term methadone maintenance patients. *J Pharmacol Exp Ther* 1989; 250:606–610.
145. O'Neill WM, Sherrard JS. Pain in human immunodeficiency virus disease: a review. *Pain* 1993;54:3–14.
146. Oleske J, Czarniecki L, Boland M. Pain in children with HIV infection. *Int Conf AIDS* 1993;9:74.
147. Parente F, Cernuschi M, Antinori S, et al. Severe abdominal pain in patients with AIDS: frequency, clinical aspects, causes, and outcome. *Scand J Gastroenterol* 1994;29:511–515.
148. Parry GJ. Peripheral neuropathies associated with human immunodeficiency. *Ann Neurol* 1988;23:S49–S53.
149. Pedro-Botet J, Miralles R, Sauleda J, Rubies-Prat J. Idiopathic ulcer of the esophagus in the AIDS syndrome: a potential life threatening complication. *Gastrointest Endosc* 1986;32:84–87.
150. Penfold J, Clark AJM. Pain syndromes in HIV infection. *Can J Anaesth* 1992;39:724–730.
151. Peterson PK, Gekker G, Chao CC, Schut R, Molitor TW, Balfour Jr HH. Cocaine potentiates HIV-1 replication in human peripheral blood mononuclear cell cocultures. *J Immunol* 1991;146:81–84.
152. Peterson PK, Sharp BM, Gekker G, Portoghese PS, Sannerud K, Balfour Jr HH. Morphine promotes the growth of HIV-1 in human peripheral blood mononuclear cell cocultures. *AIDS* 1990; 4:869–873.
153. Pinching AJ, Helbert M, Peddle B, et al. Clinical experience with zidovudine for patients with acquired immune deficiency syndrome and acquired immune deficiency syndrome-related complex. *J Infect* 1989;18:33–40.
154. Polish LB, Cohn DL, Ryder JW, Myers AM, O'Brien RF. Pulmonary non-Hodgkin's lymphoma in AIDS. *Chest* 1989;96: 1321–1326.
155. Potter DA, Danforth DN Jr, Macher AM, Longo DL, Stewart L, Masur H. Evaluation of abdominal pain in the AIDS patient. *Ann Surg* 1984;199:332–339.
156. Powell FC, Spooner KM, Shawker TH, et al. Symptomatic interleukin-2–induced cholecystopathy in patients with HIV infection. *AJR* 1994;163:11–21.
157. Powell H, Myers R, Lampert P. Changes in Schwann cells and vessels in lead neuropathy. *Am J Pathol* 1982;109:193–205.
158. Powell H, Rosoff J, Myers R. Microangiopathy in human diabetic neuropathy. *Acta Neuropathol* 1985;68:295–305.
159. Rabeneck L, Popovic M, Gartner S, et al. Acute HIV infection presenting with painful swallowing and esophageal ulcers. *JAMA* 1990;263:2318–2322.
160. Radcliffe KW, McLean KA, Benbow AG. Acute rheumatic fever in human immunodeficiency virus infection. *J Infect* 1991;22: 187–189.
161. Rance NE, McArthur JC, Cornblath DR, Landstrom DL, Griffin JW, Price DL. Gracile tract degeneration in patients with sensory neuropathy and AIDS. *Neurology* 1988;38:265–271.
162. Raufman JP. Odynophagea and dysphagia in AIDS. *Gastroenterol Clin North Am* 1988;17:599–614.
163. Richman DD, Fischl MA, Grieco MH, et al. The toxicity of azidothymidine (AZT) in the treatment of patients with AIDS and AIDS-related comples. *N Engl J Med* 1987;317:192–197.
164. Robert MH, Geraghty JJ, Miles SA, Cornford ME, Vinters HV. Severe neuropathy in a patient with acquired immune deficiency syndrome (AIDS). *Acta Neuropathol* 1989;79:255–261.
165. Rhodes RH, Ward JM, Cowan RP, Moore PT. Immunohistochemical localization of human immunodeficiency viral antigens in formalin-fixed spinal cords with AIDS myelopathy. *Clin Neuropathol* 1989;8:22–27.
166. Rogeaux O, Fassin D, Gentilini M. Etude de la prevalence des manifestations rhumatologiques au cours de l'infection par le virus de l'immunodeficience humaine. *Ann Med Interne (Paris)* 1993;144:443–448.
167. Rowe IF, Forster SM, Seifert MH, et al. Rheumatological lesions in individuals with human immunodeficiency virus. *Q J Med* 1989; 272:1167–1184.
168. Rowland RW, Escobar MR, Friedman RB, Kaplowitz LG. Painful gingivitis may be an early sign of infection with the human immunodeficiency virus. *Clin Infect Dis* 1993;16:233–236.
169. Rynes RI. Painful rheumatic syndromes associated with human immunodeficiency virus infection. *Rheum Dis Clin North Am* 1991; 17:79–87.
170. Said G, Lacroix C, Andriev JN, et al. Necrotizing arteritis in patients with inflammatory neuropathy and human immunodeficiency virus (HIV-III) infection. *Neurology* 1987;37:139–146.
171. Said G, Lacroix C, Chemouilli P, et al. Cytomegalovirus neuropathy in acquired immunodeficiency syndrome: a clinical and pathological study. *Ann Neurol* 1991;29:139–146.
172. Sampaio EP, Sarno EN, Galilly R, Cohn ZA, Kaplan G. Thalidomide selectively inhibits tumor necrosis factor alpha production by stimulated human monocytes. *J Exp Med* 1991;173:699–703.
173. Saraux A, Taelman H, Clerinx J, et al. Persistent arthralgia and its association with HIV infection in Rwanda. *J Acquir Immune Defic Syndr Hum Retrovirol* 1994;7:158–62.
174. Saulsbury FT, Bringelsen KA, Normansell DE. Effect of prednisone on human immunodeficiency virus infection. *South Med J* 1991;84:431–435.
175. Schiff RD, Headley Jr RN, Self S, Garvin AJ, Stuart RK. Treatment of peripheral T-cell lymphoma (PTCL) with recombinant alpha-interferon (RINF-ALPHA). *Proc Annu Meet Am Soc Clin Oncol* 1989; 8:A1042.
176. Schofferman J. Pain: diagnosis and management in the palliative care of AIDS. *J Palliat Care* 1988;4:46–49.
177. Scholz MJ. Don't overlook pain in AIDS patients. *RN* 1993;56:89.
178. Schröder JM. Proliferation of epineurial capillaries and smooth muscle cells in angiopathic peripheral neuropathy. *Acta Neuropathol* 1986;72:29–37.
179. Schulhafer EP, Grossman ME, Fagin G, Bell KE. Steroid-induced Kaposi's sarcoma in a patient with pre-AIDS. *Am J Med* 1987;82: 313–317.
180. Schuval SJ, Bonagura VR, Ilowite NT. Rheumatologic manifestations of pediatric human immunodeficiency virus infection. *J Rheumatol* 1993;20:1578–1582.
181. Sharma AK, Britland ST, Young RJ, et al. Morphological abnormalities in the sural nerve of patients with and without clincal syndromes of diabetic neuropathy. In: Ward J, Goto Y, eds. *Diabetic neuropathy.* New York: John Wiley, 1990:29–45.
182. Sievert W, Brooy JTL. HIV-related gastrointestinal disease. *Med J Aust* 1993;158:175–178.
183. Simpson DM. Neuromuscular complications of human immunodeficiency virus infection. *Semin Neurol* 1992;12:34–42.
184. Simpson DM, Bender AN. Human immunodeficiency virus-associated myopathy: analysis of 11 patients. *Ann Neurol* 1988;24: 79–84.
185. Singer EJ, Zorilla C, Fahy-Chandon B, Chi S, Syndulko K, Tourtellotte WW. Painful symptoms reported by ambulatory HIV-infected men in a longitudinal study. *Pain* 1993;54:15–19.
186. Skowron G, Merigan TC. Alternating and intermittent regimens

of zidovudine (3′-azido-3′-deoxythymidine) and dideoxycytidine (2′,3′-dideoxycytidine)in the treatment of patients with acquired immunodeficiency syndrome (AIDS) and AIDS-related complex. *Am J Med* 1990;88:20S–23S.
187. Snider WD, Simpson DM, Nielson S, Gold JWM, Metroka CE, Posner JB. Neurological complications of the acquired immune deficiency syndrome: analysis of 50 patients. *Ann Neurol* 1983;14: 403–418.
188. So YT, Holtzman DM, Abrams DI, Olney RK. Peripheral neuropathy associated with acquired immunodeficiency syndrome. 1988; 45:945–948.
189. Soderlund C, Bratt GA, Engstrom L, et al. Surgical treatment of cytomegalovirus enterocolitis in severe human immunodeficiency virus infection. Report of eight cases. *Dis Colon Rectum* 1994;37: 63–72.
190. Solinger AM, Hess EV. Rheumatic diseases and AIDS—is the association real? *J Rheumatol* 1993;20:678–683.
191. Sommer C, Myers RR. Inhibition of TNF by thalidomide abolishes an early phase of thermal hyperalgesia in neuropathic rats. *J Neurol* 1994; 241:S36.
192. Sommer C, Schroder JM. Immune mediated neuropathy and myopathy in post streptococcal disease: electron microscopical, morphometrical, and immunohistochemical studies. *Clin Neuropathol* 1992;11:77–86.
193. Soubrane C, Visonneau S, Khayat D, et al. Study of biological and immunological events associated with infusions of monoclonal anti-CD 16 antibody (3G8) in HIV-infected thrombocytopenic patients. *Proc Annu Meet Am Assoc Cancer Res* 1990;31:A1233.
194. Stern R, Gold J, Dicarlo EF. Myopathy complicating the acquired immune deficiency syndrome. *Muscle Nerve* 1987;10:318–322.
195. Stoebner P, Mezin P, Vila A, Grosse R, Kopp N, Paramelle B. Microangiopathy of endoneurial vessels in hypoxemic chronic obstructive pulmonary disease. *Acta Neuropathol* 1989;78:388–395.
196. Strohlein S, Posner G, Colby S, Nicholas A. Giant esophageal ulcers in patients with AIDS-related complex. *Dysphagia* 1986;1:84–87.
197. Suduca P. Malignant epidermoid tumors of the anus. Etiopathogenesis and clinical aspects. *Ann Gastroenterol Hepatol (Paris)* 1994; 30:189–191.
198. Thomas PK. Vascular factors in the causation of diabetic neuropathy. *Trends Neurosci* 1987;10:6–8.
199. Thuluvath PJ, Connolly GM, Forbes A, Gazzard BG. Abdominal pain in HIV infection. *Q J Med* 1991;78:275–285.
200. Tindall B, Barke S, Donovan B, et al. Characterization of the acute clinical illness associated with human immunodeficiency virus infection. *Arch Intern Med* 1988;148:945–949.
201. Tom W, Aaron JS. Esophageal ulcers caused by torulopsis glabrata in a patient with acquired immune deficiency syndrome. *Am J Gastroenterol* 1987;82:766–768.
202. Torre D, Sampietro C, Fiori GP, Luzzaro F. Necrotizing pneumonitis and empyema caused by *Streptococcus cremoris* from milk. *Scand J Infect Dis* 1990;22:221–222.
203. Varsky CG, Yahni VD, Freire MC, et al. Patologia esofagica en pacientes con virus de SIDA. Etiologia y diagnostico. *Acta Gastroenterol Latinoam* 1991;21:67–83.
204. Veber F, Halpern-Weil F, Blanche S, Griscelli C. Pain and HIV infection in children. *J Pain Symptom Manage* 1989;4:S5.
205. Viamonte M, Dailey TH, Gottesman L. Ulcerative disease of the anorectum in the HIV+ patient. *Dis Colon Rectum* 1993;36:801–805.
206. Vital C, Deminiere C, Lagueny A, et al. Peripheral neuropathy with essential mixed cryoglobulinemia: biopsies from 5 cases. *Acta Neuropathol* 1988;75:605–610.
207. Watkins BA, Dorn HH, Kelly WB, et al. Specific tropism of HIV-1 for microglial cells in primary human brain cultures. *Science* 1990; 249:549–553.
208. Weil-Halpern F, Debre M, Griscelli C. Efficacy of pluridisciplinary approach to the best care of severe pain in AIDS children. *Int Conf AIDS* 1993;9:534.
209. Westermann VA, Muller RP, Adler M, Bendick C, Rasokat H. Strahlentherapie epidemischer Kaposi-Sarkome bei AIDS-Patienten. *Strahlenther Onkol* 1990;166:705–709.
210. Wexner SD, Smithy WB, Milsom JW, Dailey TH. The surgical management of anorectal diseases in AIDS and pre-AIDS patients. *Dis Colon Rectum* 1986;29:719–723.
211. Whitney TM, Brunel W, Russell TR, Bossart KJ, Schecter WP. Emergent abdominal surgery in AIDS: experience in San Francisco. *Am J Surg* 1994;168:239–243.
212. Whitney TM, Macho JR, Russell TR, Bossart KJ, Heer FW, Schecter WP. Appendicitis in acquired immunodeficiency syndrome. *Am J Surg* 1992;164:467–470.
213. Wilcox CM, Schwartz DA. Idiopathic anorectal ulceration in patients with human immunodeficiency virus infection. *Am J Gastroenterol* 1994;89:599–604.
214. Wind P, Chevallier JM, Jones D, Frileux P, Cugnenc PH. Cholecystectomy for cholecystitis in patients with acquired immune deficiency syndrome. *Am J Surg* 1994;168:244–2466.
215. Withrington RH, Cornes P, Harris JWR, et al. Isolation of human immunodeficiency virus from synovial fluid of a patient with reactive arthritis. *BMJ* 1987;294:484.
216. Wolf RF, Sprenger HG, Mooyaart EL, Tamsma JT, Kengen RA, Weits J. Nontropical pyomyositis as a cause of subacute, multifocal myalgia in the acquired immunodeficiency syndrome. *Arthritis Rheum* 1990;33:1728–1732.
217. Wrzolek MA, Chandrakant R, Kozlowski PB, Sher JH. Muscle and nerve involvement in AIDS patient with disseminated mycobacterium avium intracellulare infection. *Muscle Nerve* 1989;March: 247–249.
218. Wyatt SH, Fishman EK. The acute abdomen in individuals with AIDS. *Radiol Clin North Am* 1994;32:1023–1043.
219. Yarchoan R, Browers P, Spitzer AR, et al. Response of human-immunodeficiency-virus-associated neurological disease to 3′-azido-3′-deoxythymidine. *Lancet* 1987;1:132–135.
220. Yarchoan R, Mitsuya H, Pluda JM, et al. The National Cancer Institute phase I study of 2′,3′-dideoxyinosine administration in adults with AIDS or AIDS-related complex: analysis of activity and toxicity profiles. *Rev Infect Dis* 1990;12 Suppl 5:S522–33.
221. Yarchoan R, Perno CF, Thomas RV, et al. Phase I studies of 2′,3′-dideoxycytidine in severe human immunodeficiency virus infection as a single agent and alternating with zidovudine (AZT). *Lancet* 1988;1:76–81.
222. Younger DS, Hays AP, Uncini A, Lange DJ, Lovelace RE, DiMauro S. Recurrent myoglobinuria and HIV seropositivity; incidental or pathogenic association? *Muscle Nerve* 1989;10:842–843.
223. Zuger A, Louie E, Holzman R, Simberkoff M, Rahal J. Cryptococcal disease in patients with acquired immuno-deficiency syndrome. Diagnostic features and outcome of treatment. *Ann Intern Med* 1986;104:234–240.

Anesthesia: Biologic Foundations, edited by
Tony L. Yaksh et al. Lippincott–Raven Publishers,
Philadelphia © 1997.

CHAPTER 51

POSTTHORACOTOMY PAIN

MARK S. WALLACE

In the immediate postoperative period after thoracic surgery, severe pain may be reported in 70% of the patient population (1). The majority of these patients will have a complete resolution of the pain within days, as in other postoperative pain states (see Chapter 15). A significant number of patients will, however, experience long-term postthoracotomy pain. Reports on the incidence of chronic postthoracotomy pain at 6 months have ranged from 26% to 67% (33,64,66,72,79). Of the patients with persistent pain, 9–66% will require medical intervention, and many will be refractory to therapy (33,66,72,79).

Although the causes of postthoracotomy pain are usually identifiable, treatment can be difficult. The most common causes fall into the categories of peripheral nerve injury, scar pain, myofascial pain, and tumor recurrence. In general, thoracotomy patients are a relatively homogenous group. Accordingly, they may serve as a model for investigating chronic pain from peripheral nerve injuries.

This chapter discusses the etiology of postthoracotomy pain, the underlying mechanisms, and responses to therapy based on these underlying mechanisms.

ETIOLOGY AND PATHOPHYSIOLOGY

Causes of postthoracotomy pain fall into five major categories: (a) peripheral nerve injury, (b) scar pain, (c) myofascial pain, (d) tumor recurrence, and (e) herpes zoster infection (Table 1). Each of these mechanisms will be discussed below.

Peripheral Nerve Injury

Humans

Because of their location in the intercostal space, intercostal nerves are susceptible to surgical trauma (see Figs. 2 and 3 in Chapter 52). Rib retraction can partially damage the nerve, and a misplaced suture can cause a chronic nerve compression, resulting in pain associated with a wide range of sensory deficits. Rib resection transects the nerve and leads by definition to deafferentation (loss of sensory input). All such interventions can lead to intercostal neuralgias, but rib resection appears to have a higher incidence (59,60). Overall, the incidence of postthoracotomy neuralgia ranges from 1% to 15% (30,32,59,60,66). Surgical techniques using rib retraction cause a 1–8% incidence (30,32,59,60,66), and the incidence of neuralgias with rib resection approaches 10–15% (59,60)

The pain resulting from intercostal nerve damage appears no different from the neuropathic syndrome typically associated with a peripheral nerve injury (Table 2). The pain is felt in the region of sensory deficit (if present), and there may be a delay of weeks to months between the thoracotomy and onset of the pain. The pain is described as dysesthetic and burning with a superimposed shooting component, which appears episodically and persists for seconds to minutes. Frequently, allodynia, a painful sensation evoked by a low-threshold mechanical stimulus, can be demonstrated in the painful area (Fig. 1) (44).

Animal Models

The mechanisms of the post nerve injury pain state has been widely investigated in animal models. Complete deafferentation of a limb will result in self-mutilation (autotomy) of the limb, as animals with a pharmacologically induced functional deafferentation using chronic perineural lidocaine infusion will ignore the limb (12,27). These findings suggest that autotomy is a behavior in response to some state secondary to the lesion rather than a response to a simple nonpainful sensory deafferentation. In rats, deafferentation can result in the progressive development of spontaneous activity in lamina V dorsal horn cells, corresponding to the denervated segment, which project supraspinally. This hyperactivity begins as early as 6 h after section and may be evident for weeks. As these cell systems are believed to play a role in nociceptive traffic (see Chapter 35), this activity could account for the developing sensation driving the autotomy behavior (75). More recently, models of nerve injury have been developed involving chronic compression of sciatic nerve (Bennett model) (15), partial ligation of the sciatic nerve (105), and ligation of the L5/6 nerve roots (Chung model) (67). These manipulations lead to a well-defined thermal hyperalgesia and tactile allodynia, respectively (see Chapters 32 and 40).

Both peripheral and central mechanisms have been proposed to explain the pain associated with peripheral nerve injury.

Peripheral Mechanisms Peripheral mechanisms have focused on the development of spontaneous activity in the injured axon. Nerve transection leads to Wallerian degeneration of the distal segment while the proximal end will attempt regeneration (see Chapter 30). This regeneration results in axonal sprouts which collectively form neuromas (see Chapter 5). Unlike the normal, uninjured axon, these neuroma display (a) spontaneous activity, (b) mechanosensitivity, and (c) chemical sensitivity to norepinephrine, thus developing an excitatory response to sympathetic stimulation (see Chapter 28) (11,39,63,101). The afferent activity in these sprouts peak at 1–7 weeks after the lesions, which may explain the delay in developing neuropathic pain (64).

Partial nerve injuries associated with a chronic compression may result from rib retraction, misplaced sutures, and scar tis-

Table 1. ETIOLOGIES OF POSTTHORACOTOMY PAIN

Peripheral nerve injury
Scar pain
Myofascial pain
Tumor recurrence
Herpes zoster infection

Table 2. CLINICAL FEATURES OF A POST NERVE INJURY PAIN STATE

Reported pain in the absence of a detectable tissue injury or damaging process
Existence of a definable injury to nerve integrity
Dysesthetic sensation referred to region of nerve injury
Allodynia
Episodic paryoxysmal shooting or stabbing pain
Pain in the region of sensory deficit
Delay in onset after initial injury

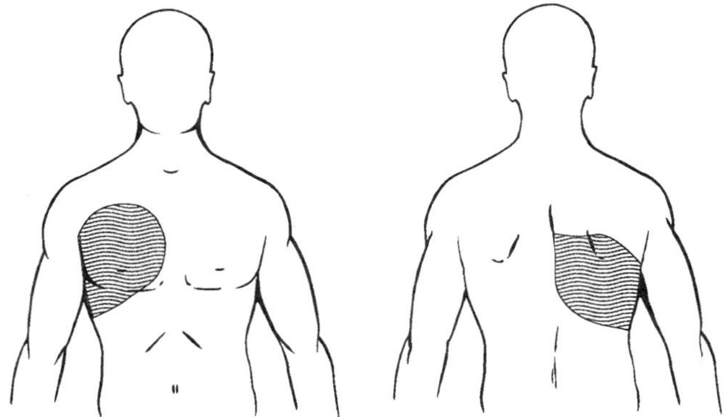

Figure 1. Typical pain distribution in a patient suffering from postthoracotomy pain. The pain usually occurs around the incision and occurs secondary to injury to the intercostal nerve. For explanation of other causes, see text.

sue. Because acute nerve compression usually results in transient afferent activity and no prolonged effect on nerve function, it is unlikely that acute nerve compression from rib retraction (in the absence of nerve injury) contributes to postthoracotomy pain (61). However, such focal injuries to nerves can lead to small regions of demyelination. These demyelinated patches can generate ectopic impulses (19). Partial section of nerves can theoretically give rise to microneuromas, which possess the same properties of large neuromas (121).

In addition to spontaneous activity in the sprouts, the damaged axon may develop a secondary site of spontaneous activity and mechanosensitivity at the cell bodies in the dorsal root ganglion (61,115). The spontaneous generator of nerve activity could thus be from either of these three peripheral sites.

In the cases of the several regions, the source of the spontaneous activity is not certain, but several lines of investigation have pointed to the increase in sodium channels in the terminals of the injured axon and the increase in sensitivity to locally released products such as epinephrine (39).

Animal studies have demonstrated that injury to peripheral nerves spares the unmyelinated C fibers (see Chapter 30) (45,46). Examination of nerves with chronic compression reveals loss of large and small myelinated axons with a relative preservation of small unmyelinated axons (6,49,65,91). The significance of this has been demonstrated with selective block of small myelinated axons, which transmit the sharp first pain after noxious stimuli. This block results in an enhanced and prolonged second pain transmitted by the small unmyelinated axons (93). It appears that myelinated primary afferents, including Aδ and Aβ fibers, inhibit pain transmission neurons in the dorsal horn that are activated by unmyelinated fibers (44). This is the basis of the gate control theory set forth by Melzack and Wall (83). Although it appears that this loss of large fiber afferent input contributes to the pain of chronic nerve compression, treatment of these nerves with capsaicin, a neurotoxin which selectively destroys unmyelinated fibers, has no effect upon the pain state (125).

Central Mechanisms After peripheral nerve injury, a variety of events occur that may lead to the spontaneous pain and hyperpathia characterizing the postthoracotomy pain state. As reviewed in Chapter 56, nerve injury leads to (a) central spouting of large afferents in the dorsal horn from the deeper laminae into the substantia gelatinosa, a region typically innervated by C fibers; (b) loss of dorsal horn neurons, which may mediate a local modulation over large afferent-evoked excitation; and (c) sympathetic innervation of the injured neuroma and the dorsal root ganglion cell. Such a functional reorganization would serve to mediate an underlying allodynia. In addition, the spontaneous activity in the injured afferent originating from the neuroma and/or the dorsal root ganglion cell of the injured axon will result in a conditioning barrage on to dorsal horn neurons. Such protracted afferent input has been shown to be associated with the release of excitatory amino acids and the generation of a facilitated state mediated by spinal NMDA receptors (see Chapter 60). *N*-methyl-D-aspartate (NMDA) receptor activity is known to generate a state of facilitated processing at the spinal level, which leads to an exaggerated response to low- and high-threshold afferent input (115). In animal models of neuropathic pain, such glutamate receptor activation will lead to a state of allodynia and hyperalgesia (see Chapters 9 and 33). The possibility that the postthoracotomy hyperpathia results in part from the ongoing activity, secondary to the nerve injury, driving central systems, raises the likelihood that such a neuropathic state may be ameliorated by at least transient blocks of the injury site. Such loss of hyperpathia after a focal block of an injury has been demonstrated in the human (55). A detailed discussion of these mechanisms is beyond the scope of this chapter but is reviewed elsewhere (see Chapter 56).

Scar Pain

Pain within the postthoracotomy scar can cause significant discomfort to the patient. The incidence of postthoracotomy scar pain is unknown, but the incidence after mastectomy has been estimated to be 23–35% (70). Usually, patients with painful scars present with trigger points rather than diffuse pain in the entire scar. These trigger points are most likely the result of microcompression of small nerves or microneuromas that develop within the scar (14,35). Histologic examination of scar tissue has revealed numerous demyelinated axons and neuromas (47). Thus, the pathophysiology of these microcompressions and microneuromas follow the discussion presented earlier in this chapter. Continuous burning and aching pain extending beyond the immediate area of the scar are most likely due to an intercostal nerve injury.

Although unusual, some patients may complain of constant itchiness and pain in the scar. Nara (86) demonstrated that patients with this complaint had elevated levels of histamine and serotonin within the scar tissue. Shiga (104) reported that histidine contents (which is a measure of histamine levels) increased more in areas of scar contracture than in areas without contracture. Histamine is released from mast cells, and serotonin is released from platelets secondary to tissue trauma. Both substances have been demonstrated to stimulate peripheral nociceptors (see Chapter 33) (7,71).

Myofascial Pain

Myofascial pain is among the more frequent causes of severe disabling pain. This syndrome is reviewed in Chapter 29. Postthoracotomy patients may suffer from this syndrome. There are several possible mechanisms leading to myofascial pain in this group of patients. The intercostal neuralgia and scar pain previously described may be exacerbated by movement; therefore, the patient will limit movement. It has been demonstrated that sedentary patients are more likely to develop myofascial pain than patients who exercise regularly (106,107). Limitation of movement in these patients may contribute to myofascial pain. Cailliet (20) proposed that trigger points are caused by the presence of blood and extracellular material that are not reabsorbed after soft tissue damage. This results in adhesions, which limit the gliding action of muscles, resulting in tension and spasms (20). Prolonged tension and spasm within the muscle can cause muscle fatigue and local ischemia, which stimulates the release of algogenic agents such as histamine, kinins, and prostaglandins (127). These algogenic substance may stimulate further pain and spasm leading to a vicious cycle.

Due to their location, the intercostal and serratus anterior muscles are likely to be damaged during a thoracotomy. Other muscles that may be damaged include the pectoralis major and minor, latissmus dorsi, levator scapulae, and teres major and minor (89). Indeed, the serratus anterior muscle is likely to be involved in postthoracotomy pain as it has been demonstrated that blockade of the long thoracic nerve (which supplies this muscle) relieves the pain in some patients (97). Also, denervation of a muscle may lead to denervation hypersensitivity. This can lead to a supersensitivity of the muscle to biochemical agents and nerve impulses (3,23,56,113). Gunn (58) claims that trigger points may develop in muscles as a result of this denervation hypersenstivity.

Tumor Recurrence

Postthoracotomy pain may also be the result of direct tumor invasion. Tumor invasion of the bone is the most common cause of pain from metastatic disease followed by tumor compression or infiltration of peripheral nerves or plexuses (see Chapter 20) (48). Bronchial carcinoma may metastasize to the chest wall and involve the ribs and intercostal nerves. The pain of rib metastasis can be confused with postthoracotomy pain as described above. The pain associated with recurrence may, however, be initially constant and aching without the hyperpathia associated with peripheral nerve damage. Possible mechanisms for the pain from rib metastasis include (a) release of algogenic substances (prostaglandins, bradykinin, substance P, histamine) from the damaged bone tissue, which stimulates the nerve endings of the endosteum, (b) stretching of the periosteum by increasing tumor size, (c) fractures, and (d) tumor compression and invasion of the intercostal nerves leading to a neuropathic component (see Chapter 48) (90,102).

Fractured ribs may result in an acute mechanical compression of the intercostal nerve resulting in a sharp neuralgic pain radiating into the distribution of the injured nerve. Increased tumor size may lead to a compression neuropathy and the eventual infiltration of the nerve will lead to total destruction and the development of the deafferentation pain. Therefore, initially the pain is caused by peripheral mechanisms but soon progresses to central mechanisms (14).

Superior pulmonary sulcus tumors may compress or infiltrate the lower brachial plexus resulting in Pancoast's syndrome. This syndrome produces pain in the shoulder, scapula, and posterior aspect of the arm and elbow. The mechanism behind the pain of this syndrome is similar to peripheral nerve injury, although a significant number of these patients will develop classic causalgia of the upper extremity (14).

Acute Herpes Zoster and Postherpetic Neuralgia

A miscellaneous cause of postthoracotomy pain is from acute herpes zoster and postherpetic neuralgia. This syndrome has been reviewed in Chapter 55. Because the infection commonly occurs over the site of tumor involvement or at previous radiation therapy sites, this complication may be more common in patients with thoracotomies for lung cancer (21). Also, the infection most commonly occurs in the mid thoracic dermatomes, which also corresponds to the thoracotomy incision (119).

The mechanisms underlying the pain of acute herpes zoster and postherpetic neuralgia are poorly understood. Theories on the mechanism of acute herpes zoster include sensitization of the affected mechanoreceptors by sympathetic hyperactivity or other chemical mediators such as substance P (see Chapter 55). Sympathetic blockade has been widely reported to relieve the pain of acute herpes zoster although its effect in postherpetic neuralgia is much less dramatic (29). In acute herpes zoster, inflammation has been demonstrated in the dorsal horn as well as the dorsal root ganglion and peripheral nerve, therefore the pain may involve both peripheral and central mechanism (52). The mechanisms underlying the pain of postherpetic neuralgia probably follows that of a peripheral nerve injury as loss of large nerve fibers has been described (5).

PHARMACOLOGY OF THE POSTTHORACOTOMY PAIN STATE

Once the underlying etiology of the postthoracotomy pain is determined, an understanding of the basic mechanisms behind the etiology is essential to a well-directed treatment plan. This section will consider various treatment modalities used in postthoracotomy pain as well as discuss the proposed mechanism of treatment success or failure. Table 3 presents the various treatment modalities used in postthoracotomy pain. The clinician needs to characterize the pain and examine the patient to determine what therapy is indicated. As outlined in the beginning of this chapter, patients with postthoracotomy pain present with pain characterized by one or more of three pain quality categories: (a) dysesthetic, burning pain with allodynia; (b) neuralgic pain characterized by intermittent sharp, shooting or lancinating pain; and (c) deep, diffuse, poorly localized pain.

Dysesthetic, Burning Pain With Allodynia

Sympathetic Blockade

In postthoracotomy pain patients who complain of dysesthesia, allodynia, and burning pain, it needs to be determined if the pain is sympathetically mediated. As discussed in the above pathophysiology section, damaged peripheral nerves form axonal sprouts and occasionally neuromas which may be activated by catecholamines. A phentolamine challenge is a simple procedure which will determine if the pain possesses component driven by sympathetically derived products (96). A phentolamine challenge is preferred over neural blockade for several reasons. First, the local anesthetic administered for the block may be absorbed and provide pain relief by another mechanism (see below). Second, somatic blockade does not provide information on the mechanism of the pain as both somatic and sympathetic fibers are blocked. Third, due to the technical difficulty of sympathetic blocks, false negatives are common. Once it is determined if the pain is sympathetically mediated, several approaches can be taken.

If the pain is sympathetically mediated, a trial of sympathetic blockade in conjunction with the tricyclic antidepressants (see below) may be tried. This sympathetic blockade can be achieved by either intercostal or thoracic sympathetic block. There is much controversy over the value of repeated sympathetic blockade in the treatment of sympathetically mediated pain. In the treatment of causalgia, some authors claim complete and lasting pain relief with single or repeated sympathetic block, whereas others state sympathetic blocks rarely, if ever, provide permanent relief. The discrepancy between these groups probably lies in the difference in the interval between

Table 3. SUMMARY OF TREATMENT MODALITIES FOR POSTTHORACOTOMY PAIN

Pharmacologic: tricyclic antidepressants, anticonvulsants, systemic local anesthetics, NSAIDs, opioids
Neural blockade: paravertebral, intercostal, epidural, trigger point injections, scar infiltration
Neurostimulation: transcutaneous electrical nerve stimulation, dorsal column nerve stimulation
Neuroablation: cryoanalgesia, chemical neurolysis, dorsal root entry zone lesions

onset of the pain and initiation of block therapy (17). As discussed in the pathophysiology of intercostal nerve injury, initially the pain arises from peripheral mechanisms which may be more likely to respond to sympathetic blockade. However once central changes have occurred, long-lasting relief from sympathetic blockade may be less likely. In this author's opinion, sympathetic blockade performed early can be very helpful. Sympathetic blockade alone in the late phase of postthoracotomy pain is rarely helpful; however, in conjunction with other therapeutic modalities such as physical therapy and the tricyclics, it can be of great value. The mechanism behind sympathetic neural blockade is a decrease in sympathetic outflow thus decrease release of norepinephrine from sympathetic nerve terminals. Thus, there is less norepinephrine available to stimulate the sensitized nerve endings or neuromas (98,100).

Oral adrenolytic drugs may also be useful in providing pain relief in these patients. Prazosin and phenoxybenzamine have effectively relieved the pain of causalgia therefore it is reasonable to assume these agents would be beneficial in postthoracotomy pain that is sympathetically mediated (1,53). Whereas sympathetic neural blockade decreases norepinephrine release, the oral adrenolytic agents block the α_1 receptors, which have been implicated in mediating sympathetic pain (34).

It is conceivable to say that α_2 agonists should provide pain relief in these patients by a similar mechanism of sympathetic neural blockade. α_2 receptors will reduce release from sympathetic terminals. Accordingly, it has been demonstrated in humans that topical clonidine relieves the hyperalgesia in patients with sympathetically maintained pain (34). Animal studies have demonstrated that spinal α_2 agonists suppress neuropathic pain in animals. (94,95,123). The mechanism of this spinal action of spinal α_2 agonists is not clear, but it may reflect upon the sympatholytic activity of these agents observed after spinal delivery (see Chapter 59).

Tricyclic Antidepressants

The tricyclic antidepressants have been proven useful in a variety of neuropathic pain syndromes, especially when the pain has a prominent dysesthetic or burning quality (18). Although patients suffering from postthoracotomy pain may be depressed secondary to their pain, the tricyclics seem to have analgesic properties independent of their antidepressant properties (117,118). Furthermore, the analgesia from the tricyclics occur at a lower dose required for the antidepressant effect (54,117). The analgesic actions of the tricyclic antidepressants is discussed in Chapter 64. Current thinking suggests that the basis of the analgesia seen with tricyclic antidepressants may relate to (a) inhibition of uptake of norepinephrine and serotonin into nerve terminals of the central nervous system and/or (b) blockade of the NMDA receptor (see Chapter 64). Brain stem serotonergic and noradrenergic neurons project to the spinal dorsal horn, where they modulate incoming nociceptive transmission. Thus, the tricyclics may stimulate these brain stem neurons to block incoming pain impulses into the spinal dorsal horn (42). This action may, however, appear paradoxical given that it is presumed that in some patients the syndrome may be driven by an enhanced noradrenergic terminal activity, a mechanism that would be facilitated by agents that block catecholamine reuptake. The NMDA receptor antagonists are known to block the generation of a facilitated state of processing and are effective in post nerve injury animal models (see Chapter 60).

Systemic Local Anesthetics

A logical step in the differential treatment of this subtype of postthoracotomy pain is a trial of systemic local anesthetics, such as lidocaine. Long-term therapy is best accomplished with the orally active agent mexiletine. Long-term mexiletine therapy is not without risk, and it is reasonable before embarking on such treatment, to attempt identification of those patents who would benefit from mexiletine. A lidocaine challenge is a simple test used to determine if the pain is sensitive to sodium channel blockers. This test is performed by infusing 5 mg/kg of lidocaine i.v. over a 30-min interval (4). End points to infusion are a 50% reduction in pain or unacceptable side effects such as tinnitus, dizziness, nausea, or muscle twitching. These signs precede seizure activity and infusion should be discontinued if observed to be present. Wallace et al. (116) demonstrated a reduction in the allodynic area of a patient with postthoracotomy pain who received an intravenous lidocaine infusion (Fig. 2). The antihyperpathic effect of lidocaine has been supported in animal studies, which show selective suppression of A-delta and C-fiber nociceptors (37,111,121). There have also been reports of prolonged analgesia after a single dose of intravenous lidocaine in patients with neuropathic pain (67,37,92). There are also reports of the same phenomenon after single peripheral local anesthetic blocks (2,68). The mechanism behind this phenomenon is poorly understood. As noted above, after nerve injury there appears to be an increase in spontaneous neural activity in the neuroma and dorsal root ganglia of the injured axons. This spontaneous activity is blocked by lidocaine in concentrations which do not alter axonal conduction (see Chapter 63) (40). Mexiletine, a sodium channel blocker in the same class of medications as lidocaine, is available in an oral preparation and has been used to treat chronic neuropathic pain states (25,36,108,110). The mechanism of mexiletine and lidocaine analgesia is most likely by stabilizing nerve membranes and reducing or impairing the spontaneous activity in damaged small myelinated axons. If it is determined that the pain is sensitive to lidocaine, mexiletine can be initiated and the dose gradually increased up to a maximum dose of 10 mg/kg or until pain relief achieved (108).

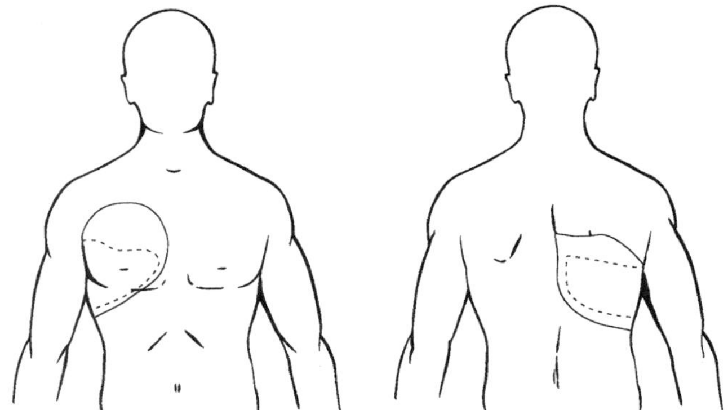

Figure 2. Representation of the decrease in mechanical allodynia in a patient with postthoracotomy pain who received an intravenous lidocaine infusion. The *solid line* represents the mechanical allodynia distribution prior to the lidocaine infusion. The *dotted line* represents the mechanical allodynia after completion of the lidocaine infusion. (Reprinted with permission from Wallace MS, Dyck JB, Rossi SS, Yaksh TL. Computer-controlled lidocaine infusion for the evaluation of neuropathic pain after peripheral nerve injury. *Pain*, 1996;66:69–77.)

Phenothiazines

The use of phenothiazines alone in chronic pain is controversial although they are used frequently in combination with opioids for chronic pain. There is evidence in animal studies that dopaminergic systems are involved in pain modulation (73,126). The phenothiazines have been reported to be effective in the treatment of a variety of peripheral neuropathies including diabetic neuropathy and postherpetic neuralgia (41,58,78,88). Therefore, it seems a reasonable approach to try this class of drugs if other treatments fail in these patients.

Opiates/NSAIDs

In general, the opioids and nonsteroidal anti-inflammatory drugs (NSAIDs) are not very effective in treating pain that is dysesthetic and allodynic in nature. The dysesthesia and allodynia observed in these patients are thought to be mediated through large myelinated afferents that activate sensitized nociceptors within the central nervous system (22). This phenomenon explains the low-efficacy of the opioids in peripheral nerve injury pain. The opioids are thought to act presynaptically to inhibit the release of substance P from unmyelinated fibers in the dorsal horn (see Chapter 58) (26). They do not inhibit input of the large myelinated afferents and therefore cannot affect the allodynia mediated by these fibers. However, opioids also act on supraspinal receptors which activate descending inhibitory control on nociception primarily through the noradrenergic and serotonergic systems (122). This mechanism of action may explain some efficacy of opiates in postthoracotomy pain states.

Through the cyclooxygenase system, tissue damage and inflammation results in the release of prostaglandins which activate or sensitize unmyelinated fibers but not large and small myelinated fibers (16,49). However, dysesthesias and allodynia usually persist long after the inflammation has subsided. Therefore, NSAIDs become less effective because the unmyelinated fibers become less important in mediating the pain in these patients.

Stimulation Modalities

A more conservative approach to this subtype of postthoracotomy pain is transcutaneous electrical nerve stimulation (TENS). Several studies have reported this technique to be the most successful after peripheral nerve injury (13,76,77,84). One study specifically stated that peripheral nerve injury pain that is sympathetically mediated responds the best to TENS (13). This gives further support to determining if the postthoracotomy pain is sympathetically mediated. Although the mechanism of TENS analgesia is poorly understood, high-frequency and low-intensity stimulation is thought to exert its analgesia through selective activation of large myelinated afferents which inhibit dorsal horn pain transmission (83,120). In contrast, high-intensity and low-frequency stimulation produces analgesia that is prolonged and naloxone reversible (120). Thus, the latter technique most likely stimulates both large and small myelinated afferents. As mentioned earlier, injury to the intercostal nerve may result in loss of large and small myelinated afferents thus loss of the inhibitory control these fibers exert. By stimulating the remaining large myelinated afferents, analgesia is provided.

Other Approaches

If the more conservative approaches described above fails, it may be necessary to consider more invasive procedures. Dorsal column stimulation (DCS) has gained widespread acceptance as a pain relieving technique since its introduction by Shealy in 1967 (103). The burning dysesthetic pain of postthoracotomy patients is fairly localized therefore should be amenable to DCS. DCS has proved efficacious in deafferentation pain of peripheral origin and postherpetic neuralgia (80,99). The mechanism behind DCS is similar to TENS. However, instead of stimulating large myelinated primary afferents directly, large myelinated afferents of the dorsal columns are stimulated and antidromically activate large myelinated primary afferent terminals in the dorsal horn (15). Animal studies have demonstrated that DCS segmentally inhibits wide dynamic range neurons (120).

Peripheral and central neurolysis should be reserved for patients with a short life expectancy because of the risk of neuralgia from this procedure (30). Cryoablation of the intercostal nerve has been the most frequent method of neurolysis for postthoractomy pain, however, long-term pain relief has not been demonstrated (31,32,74). Dorsal root entry zone (DREZ) lesions have been reported effective for deafferentation pain following peripheral nerve injury but due to the invasiveness of this procedure, it should be one of last resort (50,51). The success of this procedure seems to be greatest with nerve root avulsions and spinal cord injury. Lower success rates have been found after more peripheral nerve injury such as postherpetic neuralgia. Avulsion rhizotomies and spinal cord injuries are associated with spontaneous activity of second-order neurons within the dorsal horn, whereas peripheral lesions cause spontaneous activity of the peripheral nerve and dorsal root ganglion (44). DREZ lesions are directed at the hyperexcitable second order neurons thus explaining the higher success in more central nerve lesions (87). Therefore, DREZ lesions are less likely to be of any benefit in this group of pain patients.

Consideration of the use of neurolytic procedures should always be tempered by the appreciation what a nerve lesion can do to central organization. Thus, there is now literature that suggests that cryoneurolysis may itself generate a neuropathic state (38).

Intermittent Sharp, Shooting, or Lancinating Pain

An important component of the postthoracotomy pathology is the behavioral syndrome in which pain described as flashing, shooting, and stabbing are reported. This syndrome may be spontaneous or elicited by stimulating a trigger point. As discussed earlier in this chapter, nerve damage can lead to ectopic impulses from demyelinated segments, neuronal sprouts and near the dorsal root ganglion. It is hypothesized that this component underlies the lancinating sensations.

Anticonvulsants

With the discovery that the anticonvulsants successfully treat trigeminal neuralgia, this class of drug has found a place in the treatment of neuropathic pain with a "shooting" component (10). Swerdlow and colleagues determined that lancinating pain could be treated with a number of anticonvulsant drugs including phenytoin, carbamazepine, clonazepam and valproic acid (109). Carbamazepine has become the anticonvulsant of choice with phenytoin following a close second. The mechanism behind the pain relief of the anticonvulsants is thought to be similar to the local anesthetics. Phenytoin and carbamazepine block voltage-sensitive sodium channels, which probably explains their pain relief in this class of patients. Carbamazepine causes the greatest inhibition (24).

The increased use of mexiletine for neuropathic pain, has led to the replacement of the anticonvulsants as first line therapy. If the shooting pain can be elicited, an intravenous lidocaine challenge can be performed as described above. If positive, mexiletine therapy can be started. If the pain cannot be elicited, a lidocaine challenge is not possible, however mexiletine therapy can be started empirically. The mechanism of mexiletine pain relief is believed to be through sodium channel blockade and membrane stabilization as described above. This membrane stabilization inhibits the spontaneous activity of the damaged nerve fiber. The new anticonvulsant, gabapentin, may replace the older anticonvulsants and mexiletine because of the extremely low side effect profile (85). This new agent has been reported to be effective in the treatment of reflex sympathetic dystrophy (81,82). The exact mechanism of gabapentin is unknown. Although it has a GABA-like structure, it does not appear to act on the GABA receptor (112).

Deep, Dull, Diffuse, Poorly Localized Pain

Postthoracotomy pain is sometimes described as dull, diffuse and poorly localized. This pain description is consistent with nociceptive pain which is somatic in origin and is more likely to result in a referred pain. Underlying causes of this type of pain include myofascial pain or soft tissue/bone pain from tumor recurrence. The order of sensitivity of deep structures of the thorax are as follows (under normal conditions): periosteum has the lowest threshold, followed by ligaments, fibrous structures of the joints, tendons, fasciae, and muscles. If these tissues are damaged or if inflammation is present, the stimulus thresholds required to elicit pain reports are lowered (62). Any of these structures may be the cause of pain, however, the treatment is essentially the same regardless of the etiology.

NSAIDs and Opioids

The NSAIDs and opioids can be quite effective in managing postthoracotomy pain of somatic origin. Tissue damage and inflammation result in the release of prostaglandins which activate or sensitize unmyelinated fibers. The breakdown of arachidonic acid to prostaglandins is mediated by the cyclooxygenase enzyme. The NSAIDs inhibit cyclooxygenase, which explains there effectiveness in this type of pain (see Chapter 61) (16,56).

Whereas the opioids are quite ineffective in peripheral nerve injury, they can be very effective in pain of somatic origin. Tissue damage and inflammation not only result in the release of prostaglandins but also other algogenic substances such as potassium, serotonin, bradykinin, histamine, leukotrienes, and substance P. All of these substances either activate or sensitize small unmyelinated fibers (44). It is clear that deep somatic pain is primarily mediated by small unmyelinated afferent. Since the opioids act presynaptically to inhibit the release of substance P from unmyelinated fibers in the dorsal horn, they are effective analgesics in postthoracotomy pain of somatic origin (26). The above discussion explains the common practice of combining opioids with NSAIDs.

Trigger Point Injections

If the postthoracotomy pain is myofascial in origin, discrete trigger points can usually be identified in the muscles of the thorax distant from the site of nerve injury. Referred pain is secondary to the trigger points and treatment should be directed to the latter. As discussed earlier, myofascial pain is believed to reflect a somatic reflex cycle which can be interrupted. This can be accomplished by trigger point injections with local anesthetic or spraying the skin overlying the trigger point with a vapor coolant. These treatments are rarely of benefit when done alone and it is necessary to combine this treatment with stretching of the affected muscle (114). If the myofascial pain is determined to be located in the serratus anterior muscle, blockade of the long thoracic nerve has been demonstrated to relieve the spasm (97). Intercostal nerve blocks may also be performed to relieve spasms of the intercostal muscles.

It seems clear that postthoracotomy pain of somatic origin is the result of peripheral mechanisms and less likely to have central processing abnormalities. Therefore, this type of pain is more likely to benefit from peripheral or central neurolysis. If these patients fail more conservative therapy such as the NSAIDS and systemic opioids and they have a short life span, then neurolysis may be considered. If their life expectancy is long, then a more conservative therapy may involve implantable devices for stimulation or drug delivery. The basic principles behind opioid therapy discussed above also apply for intraspinal opioid therapy.

CONCLUSIONS

Postthoracotomy pain may be typified by several distinct sensory components: (a) dysesthetic, burning pain with allodynia; (b) neuralgic pain characterized by intermittent sharp, shooting or lancinating pain; and/or (c) deep, diffuse, poorly localized pain. Consideration of the state suggests several underlying etiologies; however, intercostal nerve injury is the most common cause. Such nerve injuries give rise to well-defined changes in peripheral and central processing components. Based on these mechanisms, it can be anticipated that different treatment modalities may be most effective against specific components of the postthoracotomy pain state.

REFERENCES

1. Abram SE, Lightfoot RW. Treatment of long-standing causalgia with prazosin. *Reg Anesth* 1981;6:79–81.
2. Arner S, Lindblom U, Meyerson BA, Molander C. Prolonged relief of nerualgia after regional anesthetic blocks. A call for further experimental and systematic clinical studies. *Pain* 1990;43: 287–297.
3. Axelsson J, Thesleff S. A study of supersensitivity in denervated mammalian skeletal muscle. *J Physiol* 1959;174:178.
4. Bach FW, Jensen TS, Kastrup J, Stigsby B, Dejgard A. The effect of intravenous lidocaine on nociceptive processing in diabetic neuropathy. *Pain* 1990;40:29–34.
5. Barrett AP. Herpes zoster virus infection: a clinicopathologic review and case reports. *Aust Dental J* 1990;35:328–332.
6. Basbaum AI, Gautro M, Jazat F, et al. The spectrum of fiber loss in a model of neuropathic pain in the rat: an electron microscopic study. *Pain* 1991;47:359–367.
7. Beck PW, Handwerker HO. Bradykinin and serotonin effects on various types of cutaneous nerve fibers. *Pflugers Arch* 1974;347: 209–222.
8. Benedetti C, Bonica JJ, Bellucci G. Pathophysiology and therapy of postoperative pain: a review. In: Benedetti C, Chapman CR, Moricca G, eds. *Advances in pain research and therapy, vol. 7.* New York: Raven Press, 1984:373–407.
9. Bennett GJ, Xie YK. A peripheral mononeuropathy in rat that produces disorders of pain sensation like those seen in man. *Pain* 1988;33:87–107.
10. Bergouignan M. Successful cure of essential facial neuralgias by sodium diphenylhydantoinate. *Rev Laryngol Otol Rhinol (Bord)* 1942;63:34–41.
11. Blumberg H, Janig W. Discharge pattern of afferent fibers from a neuroma. *Pain* 1984;20:335–353.
12. Blumenkopf B, Lipman JJ. Studies in autotomy: its pathophysiology and usefulness as a model of chronic pain. *Pain* 1991;45: 203–209.
13. Bohm E. Transcutaneous electrical nerve stimulation in chronic pain after peripheral nerve injury. *Acta Neurochir (Wien)* 1978;40: 277–285.
14. Bonica JJ, Buckley FP. Regional analgesia with local anesthetics. In: Bonica JJ, ed. *The management of pain.* 2nd ed. Philadelphia: Lea & Febiger, 1990:1883–1966.
15. Bonica JJ, Yaksh T, Liebeskind JC, Pecknick RN, Depaulis A. Biochemistry and modulation of nociception and pain. In: Bonica JJ, ed. *The management of pain.* 2nd ed. Philadelphia: Lea & Febiger, 1990:95–121.
16. Bonica JJ. Anatomic and physiologic basis of nociception and pain. In: Bonica JJ, ed. *The management of pain.* 2nd ed. Philadelphia: Lea & Febiger, 1990:28–94.
17. Bonica JJ. Causalgia and other reflex sympathetic dystrophies. In: Bonica JJ, ed. *The management of pain.* 2nd ed. Philadelphia: Lea & Febiger, 1990:220–243.
18. Bruera E, Ripamonti C. Adjuvants to opioid analgesics. In: Patt RB, ed. *Cancer pain.* 1st ed. Philadelphia: Lippincott, 1993: 143–159.
19. Burchiel KJ. Abnormal impulse generation in focally demyelinated trigeminal roots. *J Neurosurg* 1980;53:674–683.
20. Caillet R. *Soft tissue pain and disability.* Philadelphia: Davis, 1977.
21. Campa JA, Payne R. Pain syndromes due to cancer treatment. In: Patt RB, ed. *Cancer pain.* 1st ed. Philadelphia: Lippincott, 1993: 41–56.
22. Campbell JN, Raja SN, Meyer RA, et al. Myelinated afferents signal the hyper algesia associated with nerve injury. Pain 1988;32:89–94.
23. Cannon WB, Rosenblueth A. *The supersensitivity of denervated structures.* New York: Macmillan, 1949.
24. Ragsdale OS, McPhee JC, Sheuer T, Catterall WA. Common molecular determinants of local anesthetic antiarrhythmic and anti-

convulsant block of voltage-gated Na^+ channels. *Cres Nat Acad Sci USA* 1993;93:9270–9275.
25. Chabal C, Jacobson L, Mariano A, Chaney E, Britell CW. The use of oral mexiletine for the treatment of pain after peripheral nerve injury. *Anesthesiology* 1992;76:513–517.
26. Chang HM, Berde CB, Holz GG, Steward GF, Kream RM. Sufentanil, morphine, met-enkephalin, and kappa-agonist (U-50, 488H) inhibit substance P release from primary sensory neurons: a model for presynaptic spinal opioid actions. *Anesthesiology* 1989; 70:672–677.
27. Coderre TJ, Grimes RW, Melzack R. Deafferentation and chronic pain in animals: an evaluation of evidence suggesting autotomy is related to pain. *Pain* 1986;26:61–84.
28. Coderre TJ, Katz J, Vaccarino AL, Melzack R. Contribution of central neuroplasticity to pathological pain: review of clinical and experimental evidence. *Pain* 1993;52:259–285.
29. Colding A. The effect of regional sympathetic blocks in the treatment of herpes zoster: a survey of 300 cases. *Acta Anaesthesiol Scand* 1969;13:133–141.
30. Conacher ID, Locke T, Hilton C. Neuralgia after cryoanalgesia for thoracotomy. *Lancet* 1986;1:277.
31. Conacher ID. Percutaneous cryotherapy for post-thoracotomy nerualgia. *Pain* 1986;25:227–228.
32. Conacher ID. Therapists and therapies for post-thoracotomy neuralgia. *Pain* 1992;48:409–412.
33. Dajczman E, Gordon A, Kreisman H, Wolkove N. Long-term posthoracotomy pain. *Chest* 1991;99:270–274.
34. Davis KD, Treede RD, Raja SN, Meyer RA, Campbell JN. Topical application of clonidine relieves hyperalgesia in patients with sympathetically maintained pain. *Pain* 1991;47:309–317.
35. Defalque RJ, Bromley JJ. Poststernotomy neuralgia: a new pain syndrome. *Anesth Analg* 1989;69:81–82.
36. Dejgard A, Petersen P, Kastrup J. Mexiletine for treatment of chronic painful diabetic neuropathy. *Lancet* 1988;2:9.
37. deJong RH, Nace RA. Nerve impulse conduction during intravenous lidocaine injection. *Anesthesiology* 1968;29:22–28.
38. DeLeo JA, Coombs DW, Willenbring S, et al. Characterization of a neuropathic pain model: sciatic cryoneurolysis in the rat. *Pain* 1994;56:9–16.
39. Devor M. Neuropathic pain and injured nerve: peripheral mechanisms. *Br Med Bull* 1990;47:619–630.
40. Devor M, Lomazov P, Matzner O. Sodium channel accumulation in injured axons as a substrate for neuropathic pain. *Prog Pain Res Manage* 1994;3:207–230.
41. Farber GA, Burks JW. Chlorprothixene therapy for herpes zoster neuralgia. *South Med J* 1974;67:808–812.
42. Fields HL. Central nervous system mechanisms for control of pain transmission. In: Fields HL, ed. *Pain.* New York: McGraw-Hill, 1987:99–131.
43. Fields HL. Painful dysfunction of the nervous system. In: Fields HL, ed. *Pain.* New York: McGraw-Hill, 1987:133–169.
44. Fields HL. The peripheral pain sensory system. In: Fields HL, ed. *Pain.* New York: McGraw-Hill, 1987:13–40.
45. Fink BR, Cairns AM. A bioenergetic basis of peripheral nerve fiber dissociation. *Pain* 1982;12:307–317.
46. Fink BR, Cairns AM. Differential tolerance of mammalian myelinated and unmyelinated nerve fibers to oxygen lack. *Reg Anesth* 198;7:2–6.
47. Finnesson BE. *Diagnosis and management of pain syndromes.* Philadelphia: WB Saunders, 1962:233–235.
48. Flower RJ, Moncada S, Vane JR. Analgesic-antipyretics and anti-inflammatory agents; drugs employed in the treatment of gout. In: Goodman, Gilman, Rall, Murad, eds. *The pharmacologic basis of therapuetics.* 1985:674–715.
49. Fowler TJ, Ochoa J. Unmyelinated fibres in normal and compressed peripheral nerves of the baboon: a quantitative electron microscopic study. *Neuropathol Appl Neurobiol* 1975;1:247–265.
50. Friedman AH, Bullitt E. Dorsal root entry zone lesions in the treatment of pain following brachial plexus avulsions, spinal cord injury and herpes zoster. *Appl Neurophysiol* 1988;51:164–169.
51. Friedman AH, Nashold BS. Dorsal root entry zone lesions for the treatment of postherpetic neuralgia. *Neurosurgery* 1984;15: 969–970.
52. Galer BS, Portenoy RK. Acute herpetic and postherpetic neuralgia: clinical features and management. *Mt Sinai J Med* 1991;58: 257–266.
53. Ghostine SY et al. Phenoxybenzamine in the treatment of causalgia: Report of 40 cases. *J Neurosurg* 1984;60:1263.
54. Glassman AH, Perel JM, Shostak M, Kantor SJ, Fleiss Jl. Clinical implications of imipramine plasma levels for depressive illness. *Arch Gen Psychiatry* 1977;34:197–204.
55. Gracely RH, Lynch SA, Bennett GJ. Painful neuropathy: altered central processing maintained dynamically by peripheral input. *Pain* 1992;51:175–194.
56. Gunn CC. Causalgia and denervation supersensitivity. *Am J Acupuncture* 1979;7:317.
57. Gunn CC. Prespondylosis and some pain syndromes following denervation supersensitivity. *Spine* 1980;5:185.
58. Hallett M, Tandon D, Berardelli A. Treatment of peripheral neuropathies. *J Neurol Neurosurg Psychiatry* 1985;48:1193–1207.
59. Hansen JL. Intercostal nerualgia following thoraco-abdominal surgery. *Acta Chir Scand Suppl* 1973;433:180–182.
60. Hansen JL. Thoracotomi og intercostalneuralgi. *Nord Med* 1951; 46:1710.
61. Howe JF, Loeser JD, Calvin WH. Mechanosensitivity of dorsal root ganglia and chronically injured axons: a physiological basis for the radicular pain of nerve root compression. *Pain* 1977;3: 25–41.
62. Inman VT, Saunders JBdeCM. Referred pain from skeletal structures. *J Nerv Ment Dis* 1944;99:660.
63. Janig W, Kollmann W. The involvement of the sympathetic nervous system in pain. *Arzneimmittelforschung* 34:1066–1073, 1984.
64. Janig W. Pathophysiology of nerve following mechanical injury. In: Dubner R, Gebhart GF, Bond MR, eds. *Proceedings of the 5th World Congress on Pain.* Amsterdam: Elsevier Science, 1988:80–86.
65. Jefferson D, Eames RA. Subclinical entrapment of the lateral femoral cutaneous nerve: an autopsy study. *Muscle Nerve* 1979;2: 145–154.
66. Kalso E, Perttunen K, Kaasinen S. Pain after thoracic surgery. *Acta Anaesthesiol Scand* 1992;36:96–100.
67. Kim SH, Chung JM. Sympathectomy alleviates mechanical allodynia in an experimental animal model for neuropathy in the rat. *Neurosci Lett* 1991;134:131–134.
68. Kirvela O, Antila H. Thoracic paravertebral block in chronic postoperative pain. *Reg Anesth* 1992;17:348–350.
69. Knner RM, Martini N, Foley KM. Nature and incidence of postthoracotomy pain. *Proc Am Soc Clin Oncol* 1982;1:152.
70. Kroner K, Knudsen UB, Lundby L, Hvid H. Long-term phantom breast syndrome after mastectomy. *Clin J Pain* 1992;8:346–350.
71. Lembeck F. Sir Thoma Lewis's nocifensor system, histamine and substance-P-containing primary afferent nerves. *Trends Neurosci* 1983;6:106–108.
72. Lerut T, Coosemans W, Christiaens R, Gruwez JA. The Belsey Mark IV antireflux procedure: indications and long-term results. *Acta Gastroenterol Belg* 1990;LIII:585–590.
73. Lindvall O, Bjorklund A, Skagerberg G. Dopamine-containing neurons in the spinal cord: anatomy and some functional aspects. *Ann Neurol* 1983;14:255–260.
74. Lloyd JW, Barnard JDW, Glynn CJ. Cryoanalgesia. A new approach to pain relief. *Lancet* 1976;2:932–933.
75. Lombard MC, Larabi Y. Electrophysiological study of cervical dorsal horn cells in partially deafferented rats. *Adv Pain Res Ther* 1983; 5:147–154.
76. Long DM. Electrical stimulation of the nervous system for pain control. *Electroencephalogr Clin Neurophysiol Suppl* 1978;34:343–348.
77. Long DM. Uses of percutaneous electical stimulation of the nervous system. *Med Prog Technol* 1977;5:47–50.
78. Maciewicz R, Bouchoms A, Martin JB. Drug therapy of neuropathic pain. *Clin J Pain* 1985;1:39–49.
79. Matsunaga M, Dan K, Manabe FY, Hara F. Residual pain of 90 thoracotomy patients with malignancy and non-malignancy. *Pain* 1990;5:S148.
80. Meglio M, Cioni B, Prezioso A, Talamonti G. Spinal cord stimulation in the treatment of postherpetic pain. *Acta Neurochir Suppl* 1989;46:65–66.
81. Mellick GA, Mellick LB. Gabapentin in the management of reflex sympathetic dystrophy [Letter]. *J Pain Symptom Manage* 1995;13:96.
82. Mellick LB, Mellick GA. Successful treatment of reflex sympathetic dystrophy with gabapentin [Letter]. *Am J Emerg Med* 1995;13:96.
83. Melzack R, Wall PD. Pain mechanisms: a new theory. *Science* 1965; 150:971–978.
84. Melzack R. Prolonged relief of pain by brief, intense transcutaneous somatic stimulation. *Pain* 1975;1:357–373.
85. Murdoch LA. Gabapentin—a novel anticonvulsant. *Axone* 1994;16: 56.

86. Nara T. Histamine and 5-hydroxytryptamine in human scar tissue. *Ann Plastic Surg* 1985;14:244–247.
87. Nashold BS, Alexander E. Neurosurgical treatment of chronic pain. In: Tollison CD, ed. *Handbook of chronic pain managment.* Baltimore: Williams & Wilkins, 1989:125–135.
88. Nathan PW. Chloroprothixene (Taractan) in post-herpetic neuralgia and other severe chronic pain. *Pain* 1978;5:367–371.
89. Nguyen H, Nguyen HV. The two key muscles in thoracotomy for excision of the lung. The latissmus dorsi and the levator scapulae muscles. *J Chir (Paris)* 1986;123:626–634.
90. Nielsen OS, Munro AJ, Tannock IF. Bone metastases: pathophysiology and management policy. *J Clin Oncol* 1991;9:509–524.
91. Ochoa J, Noordenbos W. Pathology and disordered sensation in local nerve lesions: an attempt at correlation. *Adv Pain Res Ther* 1979;3:67–90.
92. Petersen P, Kastrup J. Dercum's disease (adiposis dolorosa). Treatment of the severe pain with intravenous lidocaine. *Pain* 1987;28: 77–80.
93. Price DC, Hu JW, Dubner R, Gracely RH. Peripheral suppression of first pain and central summation of second pain evoked by noxious heat pulses. *Pain* 1977;3:57–68.
94. Puke MJ, Wiesenfeld-Hallin Z. The differential effects of morphine and the alpha 2-adrenoreceptor agonists clonidine and exmedetomidine on the prevention and treatment of experimental neuropathic pain. *Anesth Analg* 1993;77:104–109.
95. Puke MJ, Xu XJ, Wiesenfeld-Hallin Z. Intrathecal administration of clonidine suppresses autotomy, a behavioral sign of chronic pain in rats after sciatic nerve section. *Neurosci Lett* 1991;133:199–202.
96. Raja SN, Treede RD, Davis KD, Campbell JN. Systemic alphaadrenergic blockade with phentolamine: a diagnostic test for sympathetically maintained pain. *Anesthesiology* 1991;74:691–698.
97. Ramamurthy S, Hickey R, Maytorena A, Hoffman J, Kalantri A. Long thoracic nerve block. *Anesth Analg* 1990;71:197–199.
98. Roberts, WA, Elardo SM. Sympathetic activation of A-delta nociceptors. *Somatosens Res* 1985;3:33–44.
99. Sanchez-Ledesma MJ, Garcia-March G, Diaz-Cascajo P, Gomez-Moreta J, Broseta J. Spinal cord stimulation in deafferentation pain. *Sterotact Funct Neurosurg* 1989;53:40–45.
100. Sanjue H, Jun Z. Sympathetic facilitation of sustained discharges of polymodal nociceptors. *Pain* 1989;38:85–90.
101. Scadding JW. Development of ongoing activity, mechanosensitivity and adrenaline sensitivity in severed peripheral nerve axons. *Exp Neurol* 1981;73:345–364.
102. Scher HI, Yagoda A. Bone metastases: pathogenesis, treatment, and rationale for use of resorption inhibitors. *Am J Med* 1987;82: 6–28.
103. Shealy CN, Taslitz N, Mortimer J, Becker DP. Electrical inhibition of pain: experimental evaluation. Anesth Analg 1967;46:299–305.
104. Shiga J. Histidine in the human skin scars. *J Plast Reconstr Surg (Jpn)* 1976;19:288.
105. Shir Y, Seltzer Z. A-fibers mediate mechanical hyperesthesia and allodynia and C-fibers mediate thermal hyperalgesia in a new model of causalgiform pain disorders in rats. *Neurosci Lett* 1990; 115:62–67.
106. Simons DG. Muscle pain syndromes, part II. *Am J Phys Med* 1976; 55:15.
107. Simons DG. Muscle pain syndromes, part I. *Am J Phys Med* 1975; 54:289.
108. Stracke H, Meyer UE, Schumacher HE, Federlin K. Mexiletine in the treatment of diabetic neuropathy. *Diabetes Care* 1992;15: 1550–1555.
109. Swerdlow M, Cundill JG. Anticonvulsant drugs used in the treatment of lancinating pain. A comparison. *Anaesthesia* 1981;36: 1129–1132.
110. Tanelian DL, Brose WG. Neuropathic pain can be relieved by drugs that are use-dependent sodium channel blockers: lidocaine, carbamazepine, and mexiletine. *Anesthesiology* 1991;74: 949–951.
111. Tanelian DL, Maclver MB. Analgesic concentrations of lidocaine suppress tonic A-delta and C fiber discharges produced by acute injury. *Anesthesiology* 1991;74:934–936.
112. Taylor CP. Gabapentin: mechanism of action. In: Levy RH, Mattson RH, Meldrum BS, eds. *Antiepileptic drugs.* New York: Raven Press, 1995:829–841.
113. Tower SS. The reaction of muscle to denervation. *Physiol Rev* 1939; 19:1.
114. Travell JG, Simons DG. *Myofascial pain and dysfunction: the trigger point manual.* Baltimore: Williams & Wilkins, 1983.
115. Wall PD, Devor M. Sensory afferent impulses originate from dorsal root ganglia as well as from the periphery in normal and nerve injured rats. *Pain* 1983;17:321–339.
116. Wallace MS, Dyck JB, Rossi SS, Yaksh TL. Computer-controlled lidocaine infusion for the evaluation of neuropathic pain after peripheral nerve injury. *Pain* 1996;66:69–77.
117. Watson CP, Evans RJ, Reed K, Merskey H, Goldsmith L, Warsh J. Amitriptlyine versus placebo in postherpetic neuralgia. *Neurology* 1982;32:671–673.
118. Watson CPN, Evans RJ. A comparative trial of amitriptyline and zimelidine in post-herpetic neuralgia. *Pain* 1985;23:387–394.
119. Watson CPN. Postherpetic neuralgia. *Neurol Clin* 1989;7:231–248.
120. Willis WD. Modulation of primate spinothalamic tract dicharges. In: Kruger L, Liebeskind JC, eds. *Advances in pain research and therapy. Vol. 6.* New York: Raven Press, 1984:217–240.
121. Woolf CJ, Wiesenfeld-Hallin Z. The systemic administration of local anaesthetics produces a selective depression of C-afferent fibre evoked activity in the spinal cord. *Pain* 1985;23:361–374.
122. Yaksh TL, Al-Rodham NRF, Jensen TS. Sites of action of opiates in production of analgesia. In: *Progress in brain research, vol. 77.* New York: Elsevier Science, 1988:371–394.
123. Yaksh TL, Pogrel JW, Lee YW, Chaplan SR. Reversal of nerve ligation-induced allodynia by spinal alpha-2 adrenoceptor agonists. *J Pharmacol Exp Ther* 1995;272:207–214.
124. Yaksh TL. The spinal pharmacology of facilitation of afferent processing evoked by high threshold afferent input of the postinjury pain state. *Curr Opin Neurol Neurosurg* 1993;6:250–256.
125. Yamamoto T, Yaksh TL. Effects of intrathecal capsaicin and an NK-1 antagonist on the thermal hyperalgesia observed following unilateral constriction of the sciatic nerve in the rat. *Pain* 1992;51: 329–334.
126. Yehuda S, Youdim MB. The increased opiate action of beta-endorphin in iron-deficient rats: the possible involvement of dopamine. *Eur J Pharmacol* 1984;104:245–251.
127. Zimmerman M. Peripheral and central nervous mechanisms of nociception, pain and pain therapy: facts and hypotheses. In: Bonica JJ, Liebeskind JC, Albe-Fessard DG, eds. *Advances in pain research and therapy, vol. 3.* New York: Raven Press, 1979:3–32.

Anesthesia: Biologic Foundations, edited by Tony L. Yaksh et al. Lippincott–Raven Publishers, Philadelphia © 1997.

CHAPTER 52

BREAST PAIN

ANNE M. WALLACE, MAREK K. DOBKE, AND MARK S. WALLACE

Surgical intervention into a soft tissue may lead to unavoidable injury to muscle and fat masses, the development of scar tissues, local reactions to foreign bodies (as may be employed in reconstruction), and lesions of sensory afferents that traverse or terminate in the surgical region. These occurrences are characteristics of most surgical procedures, but apply with particular clarity to interventions involving the breast. Whether for reconstruction or for more aggressive interventions related to removing tumor in cancer therapy, there are documented insults to structure and innervation. In addition, the treatment for malignancy may involve chemotherapy, known to induce peripheral neuropathies, and the use of radiation. Such radiation, while targeted at the tumor, may often unavoidably injure the underlying brachial plexus, leading to an additional neuropathy (see Chapter 48). In spite of this degree of intervention, it has not been widely appreciated that pain may be a sequelae of these treatments. Typically, the concern with tumor reoccurrence has left the problems related to the pain resulting from these interventions largely unappreciated. Importantly, because of the target area of the surgery, there is often a misconception that the syndrome is essentially the same as that described loosely as postthoracotomy pain. Although certain components of the two pain states overlap, they in fact reflect quite distinct syndromes (see Chapter 51). The present chapter will therefore consider the incidence, etiology, and underlying mechanisms that may account for the postmastectomy pain state. In addition, the breast after surgery may undergo reconstruction, and this in itself may yield discrete pain states. Finally, the breast is a complex tissue having secretory function and displays marked hormonal sensitivity. It is subject, in the absence of malignancy, to apparently symptomatic conditions that can be reported as painful (e.g., mastalgia). This state will also be considered.

ETIOLOGY

One in eight women will develop breast cancer. In the absence of metastasis, a small percentage (~6%) of these women will present with breast pain as a primary complaint (145). In the face of frank metastasis to bone and soft tissue, the incidence of pain in the site of metastasis is virtually 100%. Of these women diagnosed with cancer, ~60% will be treated with mastectomy as a curative procedure, with or without surgical reconstruction (1). Although cure of disease is of overriding importance, some of these women, once surgically treated, are left with an ill-defined postmastectomy and postreconstruction pain syndrome. Four to 14% of women suffer postmastectomy pain (4,45,55,134,136), although it may be as high as 31% (121,132). This suggests that there is a large population of women who will suffer significant pain secondary to the treatment of breast cancer; in a population of 250 million, ~500,000 to 2.5 million women, conservatively, may be so afflicted.

The onset of postmastectomy pain ranges from 2 weeks to 6 months. Moreover, 23–100% report abnormal sensation in the axilla and medial aspect of the arm (36,71,102,127,129). The pain described ranges from mild to intractable and disabling. In its most florid presentation, the pain was frequently persistent and characterized in those so afflicted with several components: (a) a general burning, aching sensation referred to the tissue region underlying the mastectomy in the axilla, medial upper arm, and/or chest; (b) paroxysmal episodes of shooting and lancinating pain. In addition, following mastectomy, 10–64% of women will report phantom breast sensations with the majority of women noticing the phantom breast within 1 week (2,71,74,75). Of these women reporting phantom breast sensations, 80% are painful (65).

The nature of the pain state described above results in a significant impairment in the ability to perform of daily occupational activities. These numbers represent many women whose quality of life is notably impaired, despite adequate treatment of their breast cancer.

INNERVATION OF THE BREAST

The innervation of the breast and surrounding tissue is intricate in its association with the brachial plexus (120). As indicated in Fig. 1, the long thoracic nerve arises from the roots of C5, C6, and C7 and innervates the serratus anterior muscle. The thoracodorsal nerve from C6 innervates the latissimus dorsi muscle. Injury to either of these nerves may occur due to vigorous traction during modified radical mastectomy, even though they are routinely spare (38,86). The innervation of the pectoralis major and minor muscles is via the lateral and medial pectoral nerves, respectively, though there is some variability over which nerve innervates which muscle. These nerves arise as roots from the lateral (C5,6,7) and medial (C8,T1) cords of the brachial plexus.

Innervation of the skin of the breast comes from the third though the sixth intercostal nerves (Fig. 2). The anterior end of these nerves turn superficially as the anterior cutaneous nerves and, passing through the sternal intercostal space, penetrate the muscle and divide into short medial cutaneous branches. These branches go to the midline of the body, whereas longer lateral branches extend to the nipple line. These branches essentially innervate the medial half of the breast and are as such called the medial mammary branches (Fig. 3). Each intercostal nerve after the second also gives off a lateral cutaneous nerve. The well-described intercostobrachial nerve is the equivalent branch of the second intercostal nerve (136) (Fig. 2).

The lateral branches divide into anterior and posterior branches to further innervate the rest of the breast (Fig. 3). Although it is routinely thought that the anterior branch of the fourth lateral cutaneous nerve is the single nerve to the nipple (39), there is a great deal of variation as to where the medial and lateral branches unite. It is therefore not possible to always predict whether the innervation of the nipple and areola comes from the medial or lateral mammary nerves, or is shared by both (27,42,94,128). Again, these are important factors when considering breast-sparing surgery where the nipple is maintained.

PATHOGENESIS

Postmastectomy pain is a complex problem that likely has a number of contributing causes. The syndrome has long been thought to have a significant psychological component. The patient must recover from a type of ablative surgery, with all its

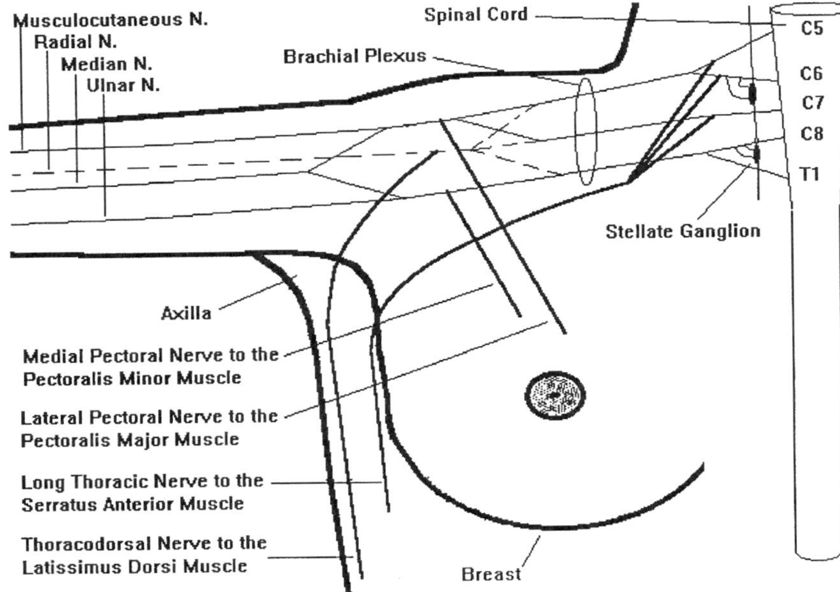

Figure 1. Origin of innervation of the musculture around the breast. The medial and lateral pectoral nerves arise from the medial and lateral cord of the brachial plexus, respectively, and course to their respective muscles (pectoralis minor and major). The long thoracic nerve arises from the C5–C7 roots and courses through the medial axilla and down the lateral chest wall to innervate the serratus anterior muscle. The thoracodorsal nerve arises from the posterior cord of the brachial plexus and courses in the posterior aspect of the axilla and down the posteriolateral chest wall to innervate the latissimus dorsi muscle. All of these nerves carry postganglionic sympathetic fibers originating from the stellate and middle cervical ganglion. Damage to these nerves during mastectomy may result in neuropathic pain. Also note the close relationship of the breast and axilla to the brachial plexus. Radiation to the breast and axilla may damage the nerves described here as well as the brachial plexus.

sequelae, suffer a major impact upon body image, and at the same time muster the emotional and psychological resources to fight against cancer. Accordingly, the underlying physiological component to the pain state may be overlooked in the thinking that much of its cause is psychological. In order to enhance the knowledge of postmastectomy pain (and that caused, or exacerbated, by reconstruction), a basic understanding of its origin must be obtained. The sources of the pain associated with breast surgery and secondary to cancer may arise from a number of sources. These sources may be broadly divided into states secondary to tissue injury or nerve injury.

Somatic Pain: Tissue Injury

An obvious acute source of pain arises from the common problems associated with tissue injury, secondary to the surgical procedure. After recovery from the surgery, pain associated with a somatic origin may arise as a result of tumor recurrence. Tumor invasion of the ribs causes well-known bone pain.

Mechanisms of the pain from rib metastasis include (a) release of algogenic substances (prostaglandins, bradykinin, substance P, histamine) from the damaged bone tissue that stimulate the nerve endings of the endosteum, (b) stretching of the periosteum by increasing tumor size, and (c) fracture (see Chapter 48) (14,100,114).

Neuropathic Pain

The verbal descriptors employed in a significant proportion of the postmastectomy pain patient (including lancinating and shooting) bear significant similarity to those employed by patients suffering from pain secondary to evident nerve injury (see Chapter 56). This, along with the effects of surgery, radiation, and chemotherapy, strongly support a role for nerve

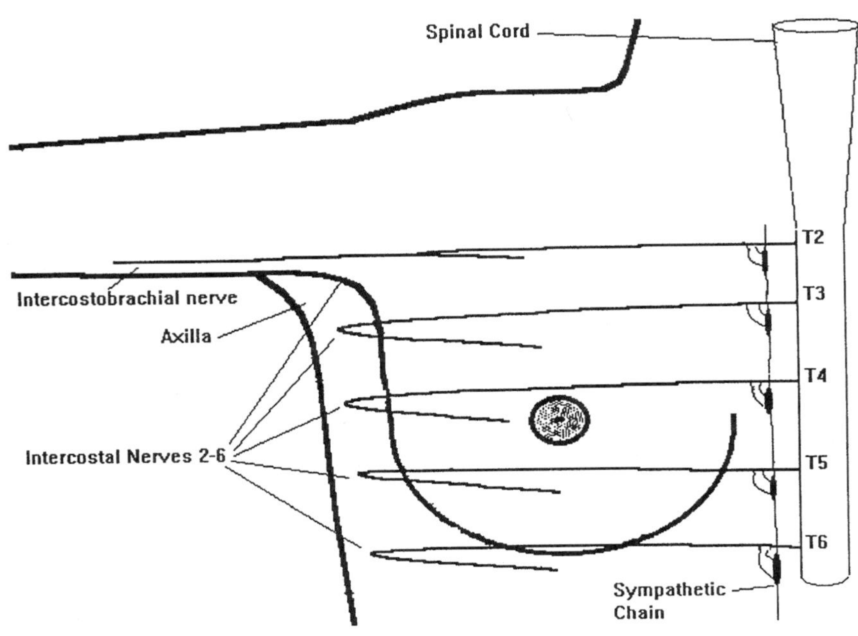

Figure 2. Cutaneous and glandular innervation of the breast and axilla. The innervation of the breast arises from intercostal nerves 3–6. The innervation of the nipple is from the fourth intercostal nerve. The intercostobrachial nerve arises from the second intercostal nerve and courses through the superficial axilla to innervate the axilla and skin of the upper inner arm. All of these nerves may be injured during mastectomy, which may lead to neuropathic pain.

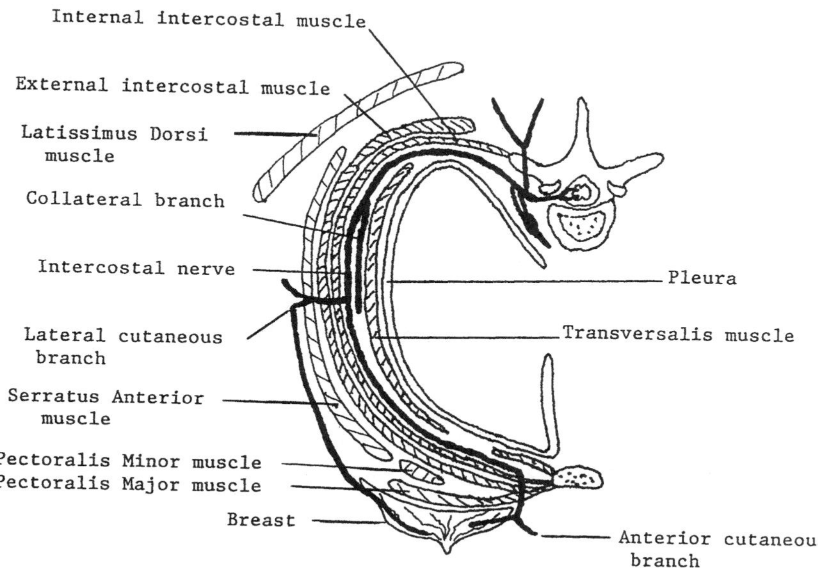

Figure 3. Nerves and muscles of the thoracic wall. The thickness of the intercostal muscles is exaggerated. The breast receives innervation from the lateral cutaneous and anterior cutaneous branch of the intercostal nerves 3–6.

injury in the postmastectomy pain state. The following sections will consider the innervation of the breast and chest wall and the injury perpetrated on that innervation by therapy and cancer invasion.

Nerve Damage

Surgical Injury Aside from frank section of nerves that innervate the lesioned region, several nerves typically undergo mechanical injury in breast surgery. The innervation of the pectoralis muscles via the lateral and medial pectoral nerves may be injured during mastectomy (due to traction or scarring), despite sparing adjacent muscle or fascia (95).

The intercostobrachial nerve has been reportedly injured in 80–100% of mastectomy patients undergoing axillary dissection and has been described as the cause of the axillary and upper arm pain from which these women suffer (36,71,102, 129).

Nonsurgical Injury. Several nonsurgical causes of nerve injury also exist. Radiation after surgical therapy may enhance or cause a pain syndrome. Severity and time of onset is proportional to total dose in animal and humans (70,103,130). Importantly, many of these effects may appear with considerable delay after even low-dose radiation (51,103). As indicated in Fig. 1, the radiation exposure to the axilla essentially encompasses not only the local innervation, but the cords of the bracheal plexus. Electron microscopic examination of the sciatic nerve 12 months after radiation showed a significant decrease in nerve fiber density, with loss being particularly prominent in the central portion of the nerve, primarily in the large fiber populations. In addition, an increase in microtubule and neurofilament density was observed. These changes are consistent with (but do not prove) that radiation may result in a nerve injury due in part to damage to the microvascular supply of the peripheral nerve with subsequent ischemia (3, 6,73, 79). In other work, it has been shown that radiation leading to necrosis will also induce increases in the local presence of a variety of cytokines, including TNF-α and interleukin-6 (76). As reviewed else where, these factors can play an important role in the initiation of degenerative nerve processes (see Chapter 30).

Chemotherapy commonly used for breast cancer, such as the taxols (35,59), the vinca alkaloids (53) and a variety of combination protocols employing several agents, including *cis*-platnin and methotrexate (105,119), are commonly appreciated to induce neuropathic states. Such neuropathies are frequently characterized by a stocking and glove syndrome common to systemic chemical peripheral neurotoxicity. Importantly, there appears to be an enhancement of the neuropathic effects of radiation and chemotherapy (101). The mechanisms of these neurotoxicities are multiple, but likely reflect upon the ability of many of these agents to influence microtubules and neurofilaments and accordingly alter axon transport.

Fibrosis of the surrounding connective tissue will result in local constrictive and compressive forces, which can lead to secondary nerve injury (13).

Finally, metastasis can lead to space-occupying masses that can lead to a chronic nerve compression syndrome. Such compression can alter vascular perfusion and increase endoneurial pressure leading to loss of nerve function (see Chapter 30). This may progress to total nerve tissue destruction and may involve the brachial plexus.

Mechanisms Underlying the Neuropathic Pain State.

Preclinical studies have provided a number of insights into the systems that may be altered in the face of nerve injury. Details of such alterations have been reviewed else where in this volume (see Chapters 36, 40, and 56). As an overview, following peripheral nerve ligation or section, several events occur, signaling long-term changes in peripheral and central processing. Several classes of events can be noted.

1. Persistent small afferent fiber activity originates after an interval of days to weeks from the lesioned site (neuroma) and from the dorsal root ganglion (DRG) of the injured nerve (9,131).

2. The sprouted terminals display a characteristic growth cone that possesses transduction properties that were not possessed by the original axon. These include significant mechanical and chemical sensitivity. Thus, these sprouted endings may have sensitivity to a number of humoral factors, such as prostaglandins, catecholamines, and cytokines (31). In addition, it is known that these regenerating terminals have significant densities of various ion channels, notably those for sodium (32). Increased ionic conductance may result in the increase in spontaneous activity that develops in a sprouting axon.

3. Prominent changes in the morphology of the DRG cells is observed. Recent data, for example, has indicated that following peripheral lesion there is a hyperinnervation of the type A ganglion cells by postganglionic sympathetic terminals to form basketlike structures around large-diameter axo-

tomized sensory neurons and leading to a coupling such that sympathetic stimulation can activate such neurons (88). In addition, at this time, there is the development of a cross talk between A and C fibers in the ganglion (33).

4. Lesions of the sensory nerve have been shown to result in sprouting of large (presumably low-threshold) primary afferents from their normal site of termination in Rexed lamina III and deeper into the lamina II of the substantial gelatinosa, a region that normally receives all of the C-fiber input (140).

5. Prominent morphological changes have been identified in the spinal dorsal horn ipsilateral to the ligation. The mechanism of these changes is not clear, but the possibility of persistent changes secondary to the chronic afferent barrage or to a change in factors transported from the lesioned site seem likely. Transsynaptic changes signal significant changes in dorsal horn function (23,37).

6. Repetitive small afferent input (as generated from injured tissue, cross talk between injured axons or spontaneous activity in neuromas or ganglion cells) will lead to a state of central facilitation. Considerable data indicates that such protracted states induces its activity by the release of excitatory amino acids and peptides (see Chapters 7 and 8). The postsynaptic action of these products leads to the subsequent release of a variety of products, including those originating from cyclooxygenase and nitric oxide synthase. Such agents have been shown to enhance the response of dorsal horn neurons to otherwise modest input, e.g., hyperalgesia and allodyia (23,37).

Hypothesized mechanisms for postmastectomy pain may be extrapolated from knowledge of other peripheral nerve injuries and the preclinical models in part outlined above. Animal studies on peripheral nerve transection report deafferentation as a cause of pain (10,22,83). Deafferentation, or complete loss of sensory input, causes high-frequency discharge of dorsal horn cells (lamina V) corresponding to the denervated segment. Discharge begins at ~6 h and can last for weeks. Nociceptive input from the damaged peripheral nerves induces sensitization of the dorsal horn cells such that low-threshold tactile stimuli, acting through large myelinated afferents, may mediate allodynia (painful response to a nonpainful stimuli) (143). This sensitization appears to result from the release of neuropeptides and excitatory amino acids in the dorsal horn which work through second messenger systems to induce long-term CNS changes (23,37,143).

Peripheral pain mechanisms may also be used to explain the initiating pathophysiology of neuropathic postmastectomy pain. Focal injuries to nerves can lead to short patches of demyelination which generate ectopic foci (16); painful neuroma or microneuroma formation may occur (31,66,113,145). Both primary and secondary spontaneous activity with increased mechanosensitivity in the axonal sprouts (67) or increased mechanosensitivity near the cell bodies of the dorsal root ganglia has been shown (61,131). Finally, chronic nerve compression as a result of ischemia, scarring, radiation fibrosis or lymphedema may result in loss of large and small myelinated fibers with relative preservation of small unmyelinated fibers resulting in loss of inhibitory inputs into the dorsal horn cells (7,44). Again, these mechanisms have not been described for postmastectomy pain, but are extrapolated from other peripheral nerve injury literature.

As noted above, a significant proportion of women report a phantom breast state after resection. Phantom limb is a well-described phenomenon that occurs almost universally following amputation (69). This could be explained by the fact that breasts, in contrast to limbs, do not mediate kinesthetic sensory impulses, which, together with kinetic and exteroceptive sensations, constitute the phantom-related phenomenon (69,116). Another explanation of the relatively low incidence of phantom breast syndrome could be that the somatosensory cortical area that represents the breast is relatively small (137). Because the nipple has the richest nerve supply, phantoms are most related to this area. If premastectomy pain is present, there is a higher incidence of phantom breast pain (74).

The role of the central components related to reorganization of central processing and the role of central facilitation in postmastectomy pain states remains to be essentially defined. Advances in this area will occur with the systematic assessment of the pharmacology of the postmastectomy pain state. Nevertheless, the clear behavioral components suggesting a prominent neuropathic component and the clear parallels with other nerve injury conditions strongly support the hypothesis that such nerve injury and the changes induced both peripherally and centrally may account mechanistically for the observed pain report. Accordingly, although there is surprisingly little systematic work with this pain conditions, these mechanisms offer a number of therapeutic alternatives.

Postreconstruction Pain

Chronic pain after breast reconstruction is yet another area of breast cancer therapy that is poorly described. The incidence of pain followed by reconstruction with breast implants may be as high as 47% (132). Breast reconstruction can be accomplished immediately after mastectomy or may be delayed for any length of time. Reconstruction methods include autologous tissue, most commonly the transverse rectus abdominus myocutaneous (TRAM) flap or the latissimus dorsi flap. Very commonly used also is tissue expansion followed by placement of a permanent breast implant. Pain associated with tissue expansion may be an ischemic effect on nerves, causing long-term nerve damage (117), or may be due to direct damage to nerves during surgical dissection (77). The pectoral nerves may be directly injured at the time of tissue expander placement for breast reconstruction because the devices are purposefully placed under the muscle. Also the thoracodorsal nerve may be injured upon elevation of the latissimus for coverage of a tissue expander. Chronic pain with permanent implants may be due to scar tissue around the implant (capsule), chronically compressing the peripheral nerves (68). Implants may produce myofascial pain in the pectoralis major minor or serratus anterior muscles (62). Observations of the implant capsule pocket reveal several findings: sensation to touch is barely present and only appreciated if forceful; sensation to mechanical deformation is present but vague and poorly localized; thermoreceptors are functional; and the capsule can be cut painlessly but stretching is perceived as pain (64). No histochemical or biological studies have been performed directly on the scar capsule to determine more precisely the neuronal anatomy. At present, the pain mechanism appears to be compressive.

The incidence of chronic pain after autologous tissue reconstruction is unknown but seems to be low. Flap reinnervation, however, is significantly altered and presents a quality of life issue to the reconstructed patient (60,72,78). The TRAM breast reconstruction has been shown to recover sensation progressively in the postoperative period, but the perception of vibration and pressure is in general significantly poorer than in the normal female (80,118). It is, however, a difficult issue to study because normal breast sensibility is variable (128). The intercostal nerves that enter the rectus abdominus muscle are routinely thought to be predominantly motor, and thus the contractions that result from pedicled TRAM flaps are avoided by direct attempts to ligate these nerves. In fact, 30% of the nerves are sensory-containing afferents from muscle spindles (118) and are capable of either enhancing sensation to the flap, if spared, or being a source of chronic pain, if injured. In addition, the TRAM flap has been shown to recover sensibility better than the latissimus dorsi flap with breast implant (80). This is probably due to the increased number of sensory end organs in the transferred rectus versus latissimus muscles. The issue of sensibility in postmastectomy flaps and reconstruction flaps is an important one; clinically, decreased or abnormal sensations may be as bothersome as pain; scientifically, an understanding of reinnervation lends a basis to the understanding of pain formation.

Mastalgia

Mastalgia (from Latin), or mastodynia (from Greek), is defined as pain in the breast. It is a prevalent, distressing symptom, occurring in all age groups. However, defining the true incidence of mastalgia is problematic since almost every female gives a history of at least some incidence of breast pain. Multiplicity of breast pain states, hormonal characteristics, and lack of consistent correlation between histological characteristics of mammary gland tissue and patient's complaints create empiric clinical management. Patients with normal histology of breast tissue may present with mastalgia. On the other hand, pain may be a presenting symptom of such pathology as inflammatory or malignancy states (139). Absence of animal models for mastalgia research create difficulties in developing an understanding of the problem as well as difficulties in developing effective therapeutic interventions.

Two main patterns of breast pain has been distinguished: cyclical and noncyclical. In general practice, two thirds of the patients will complain of cyclical mastalgia (139). Cyclical breast pain may affect young women before the age of 20; however, in most, the pain starts in the third decade and rarely after the age of 50 (106,139). In the context of normal breast development, benign breast disorders leading to mastalgia are considered to be an aberration of normal cyclical changes within the breasts of women during reproductive years (63). Half of the patients describe their pain as a bilateral "heaviness or fullness." Patients with a component of nonpuerperal mastitis (duct ectasia) and hyperprolactinemia more frequently experience sharp pain in the form of stabbing and cutting (104,106). The majority of patients report no diurnal variation of the pain (106).

In patients with cyclical mastalgia, the pain is usually exacerbated or occurs during the premenstrual period. Prolactin and/or aldosterone excess, increased estrogen/progesterone ratio, progesterone allergy, prostaglandin excess, vitamin deficiency, hypoglycemia, and psychosomatic factors have all been implicated in the pathogenesis of this type of pain (97). The effectiveness of reassurance, reduction of stress, reduction in intake of salt, methylxanthines (e.g., caffeine), animal fats, dairy products, and vitamin B6 supplementation is evidence that the etiology of cyclical mastalgia is multifactorial (54,97). However, research on the possible role of gammalinolenic acid and other essential fatty acids in the treatment of mastalgia as well as anecdotal reports on the importance of diet in the etiology of breast pain points towards abnormal lipid metabolism as the underlying cause of the problem at the breast cell level (49,54). Primrose oil, which is traditionally used for the treatment of mastalgia, is a rich natural source of gammalinolenic acid and seems to regulate circulating and cellular profiles of essential fatty acids, eicosanoids, and cholesterol transportation (49).

Prolactin appears to be pivotal in producing changes in breast physiology that lead to pain. It is a polypeptide secreted by the anterior pituitary and is normally inhibited by dopamine (prolactin inhibiting factor), which is secreted by the hypothalamus. Breast pain associated with inflammatory changes (duct ectasia) and nonpuerperal mastitis may be a symptom of hyperprolactinemia. The term neurogenic hyperprolactinemia has been introduced describing hyperprolactinemia due to breast stimulation, injury, and inflammation which leads to pain. Breast surgery or herpes zoster of the breast or chest wall may also lead to increased prolactin levels and the above clinical picture (104). Therefore, prolactin may not only be important in the pathophysiology of cyclical but also noncyclical mastalgia.

TREATMENT

Whereas postmastectomy and postreconstruction pain result from peripheral nerve injury, mastalgia involves mechanisms at the breast cellular level and peripheral nerve terminals. The treatment of these two types of pain are different.

Postmastectomy Pain

If peripheral nerve injury is considered as the etiology of the breast pain, it is reasonable to hypothesize that the pain may have a sympathetically mediated component. Damaged peripheral nerves form axonal sprouts and occasionally neuromas which may be activated by norepinephrine. An intravenous phentolamine challenge is a simple procedure that will determine if the pain is sympathetically mediated (108). Because of the complex innervation of the breast, isolated sympathetic blockade may prove difficult and further supports a phentolamine challenge as the initial treatment to avoid a false negative. Once the determination of sympathetically mediated pain is diagnosed, several approaches may be taken.

Tricyclic Antidepressants

The tricyclic antidepressants have been proven useful in a variety of neuropathic pain syndromes, especially when the pain has a prominent dysesthetic or burning quality (15). Although patients suffering from postmastectomy pain may be depressed secondary to the pain and the fact that they are facing cancer, the tricyclics seem to have analgesic properties independent of their antidepressant properties (133,135). Furthermore, the analgesia from the tricyclics occur at a lower dose than required for the antidepressant effect (52,133). The inhibition of the uptake of norepinephrine and serotonin into nerve terminals of the CNS forms the basis of the analgesia seen with tricyclic antidepressants. Brain stem serotonergic and noradrenergic neurons project to the spinal dorsal horn, where they modulate incoming nociceptive transmission. Thus, the tricyclics may stimulate these brain stem neurons to block incoming pain impulses into the spinal dorsal horn (43). Recent studies have suggested that at least some of the tricyclic antidepressants may function as antagonists of the *N*-methyl-D-asparate receptor (NMDA) (see Chapter 64). NMDA receptor antagonists have been described in preclinical and limited clinical models as being effective in certain neuropathic pain states. A trial of sympathetic or somatic blockade in conjunction with the tricyclic antidepressants may be tried. These neural blockades can be achieved by intercostal nerve blocks, thoracic sympathetic block, stellate ganglion block (if a high enough volume is used to reach the thoracic sympathetic chain) or epidural blockade. There is much controversy over the value of repeated neural blockade in the treatment of sympathetically mediated pain. Though controversial, sympathetic or neural blockade performed early in the course of the pain may be helpful. Many women with postmastectomy pain develop frozen shoulders. At the least, early intervention provides pain relief necessary for aggressive physical therapy to be employed. If pain relief can be achieved with neural blockade, then this should always be pursued in conjunction with a physical therapy program. The neural blockade performed early will thus not only enhance physical therapy but *may* also prevent central changes that may occur in the dorsal horn as a result of the pain.

α-Adrenoceptor Agents

There are few systematic studies on the use of adrenoceptor agonists or antagonists on the postmastectomy pain state. However, the mechanism behind sympathetic and somatic blockade is a decrease in sympathetic outflow thus decrease release of active factors from sympathetic nerve terminals, which can otherwise stimulate sensitized nerve endings, neuromas, or dorsal root ganglion cells (89,110,112). It is conceivable that spinal α_2 agonists, because of their sympatholytic action on preganglionic neurons (40,50) could provide pain relief in these patients by a similar mechanism. Studies have demonstrated that spinal α_2 agonists suppress neuropathic pain in animals (107,144) and RSD in humans (109). It has also been demonstrated in humans that topical clonidine relieves the hyperalgesia in patients with sympathetically maintained pain (28). This is believed to reflect a presynaptic effect of clonidine in the sympathetic terminals in the vicinity of the site of application.

While neural blockade and α_2 agonists reduce peripheral catecholamine release, the available oral adrenolytic agents block the α_1 receptors, which have been implicated in mediating sympathetic pain (28). Prazosin and phenoxybenzamine have effectively relieved the pain of causalgia; therefore, it is reasonable to assume these agents would be beneficial in postmastectomy pain.

Systemic Local Anesthetics

A logical step is a trial of systemic local anesthetics. Long-term therapy is best accomplished with mexiletine because lidocaine is not active following oral administration. Long-term mexiletine therapy is not without risk, and it is reasonable before embarking on such treatment, to attempt identification of those patients who would benefit from mexiletine. A lidocaine challenge is a simple test used to determine if the pain is sensitive to sodium channel blockers. This test is performed by infusing up to 5 mg/kg of lidocaine i.v. over 30–45 min (5). End points to infusion are a 50% reduction in pain or unacceptable side effects such as tinnitus, dizziness, nausea, or muscle twitching. These signs prelude seizure activity and should be watched for and the infusion discontinued if present.

The effects of lidocaine on afferent processing are complex (see Chapter 63). In brief, preclinical studies have shown that in order of decreasing sensitivity (higher plasma levels), lidocaine will block spontaneous activity in neuroma; block spontaneous activity in ganglion of injured axon; block spinal activity evoked by protracted C-fiber discharge (central facilitation); block activity evoked in C fiber by local tissue injury; and block conduction in uninjured axon (30,34,125,141). Mexiletine, a sodium channel blocker in the same class of medications as lidocaine, is available in an oral preparation and has been used to treat chronic neuropathic pain states (20,29,122,124). As noted above, lidocaine i.v. does not seem to suppress C-fiber activity because limb ischemic pain, which selectively blocks large and small myelinated fibers, is not relieved by lidocaine (11,111). If the pain is sensitive to lidocaine, mexiletine can be started and the dose gradually increased until pain relief is achieved up to a maximum dose of 10 mg/kg (122).

Anticonvulsants

With the discovery that the anticonvulsants successfully treat trigeminal neuralgia, this class of drug has found a place in the treatment of neuropathic pain with a shooting component (8). Swerdlow and Cundill (123) determined that lancinating pain could be treated with a number of anticonvulsant drugs, including phenytoin, carbamazepine, clonazepam, and valproic acid. Carbamazepine has become the anticonvulsant of choice, with phenytoin following a close second. However, the new anticonvulsant, gabapentin, may replace the older anticonvulsants because of the extremely low side effect profile (96). This new agent has been reported to be effective in the treatment of reflex sympathetic dystrophy (90,91). The mechanism behind the pain relief of the anticonvulsants are thought to be similar to the local anesthetics. Phenytoin and carbamazepine block voltage-sensitive sodium channels which probably explains their pain relief in this class of patients. Carbamazepine causes the greatest inhibition (19). The exact mechanism of gabapentin is unknown. Although it has a GABA-like structure, it does not appear act on the GABA receptor (126).

Phenothiazines

The use of phenothiazines alone in chronic pain is controversial although they are used frequently in combination with opioids for chronic pain. There is evidence in animal studies that dopaminergic systems are involved in pain modulation (80,146). The phenothiazines have been reported to be effective in the treatment of a variety of peripheral neuropathies, including diabetic neuropathy and postherpetic neuralgia (41,56,87,99). Therefore, it seems a reasonable approach to try this class of drugs if other treatments fail.

Opioids and NSAIDs

In general, the opioids and nonsteroidal antiinflammatory drugs (NSAIDs) are not very effective in treating pain secondary to nerve injury. The dysesthesia and allodynia observed in postmastectomy pain is thought to be mediated through large myelinated afferents that activate sensitized nociceptors within the CNS (18). This phenomenon explains the low-efficacy of the opioids in peripheral nerve injury pain. The opioids are thought to act presynaptically to inhibit the release of substance P from unmyelinated fibers in the dorsal horn (21). They do not inhibit input of the large myelinated afferents therefore cannot affect the allodynia mediated by these fibers. However, the opioids also act on supraspinal receptors that activate descending inhibitory control on nociception (142). This mechanism of action may provide some pain relief in these patients.

Through the cyclooxygenase system, tissue damage and inflammation results in the release of prostaglandins that activate or sensitize high-threshold unmyelinated fibers (46,100). Repetitive small afferent activation can lead to the release of prostanoids from the spinal cord, where they are believed to facilitate central nociceptive processing leading to a concurrent spinally mediated facilitation (see Chapter 9). However, dysesthesias and allodynia usually persists long after the inflammation has subsided. Therefore, NSAIDs may become less effective because the unmyelinated fibers become less important in modulating the pain in these patients.

Whereas the opioids and NSAIDs are ineffective in peripheral nerve injury, they can be very effective in pain originating from tissue damage and inflammation such as rib infiltration of tumor and rib fracture.

Nerve Stimulation

A conservative approach to postmastectomy pain is transcutaneous electrical nerve stimulation (TENS). Several studies have reported this technique to be the most successful after peripheral nerve injury (12,84,85,93). One study specifically stated that peripheral nerve injury pain, which is sympathetically mediated, responds the best to TENS (12). Although the mechanism of TENS analgesia is poorly understood, high-frequency and low-intensity stimulation is thought to exert its analgesia through selective activation of large myelinated afferents which inhibit dorsal horn pain transmission (92,138). In contrast, high-intensity and low-frequency stimulation produces analgesia that is prolonged and naloxone reversible (138). Thus, the latter technique most likely stimulates both large and small myelinated afferents. As mentioned earlier, injury to the intercostobrachial nerve may result in loss of large and small myelinated afferents, thus loss of the inhibitory control these fibers exert. By stimulating the remaining large myelinated afferents, analgesia may be provided. On the other hand, the issue of allodynia mediated by large afferents after nerve injury suggests the mechanism of the disorder and/or the therapy are inadequately understood.

Neurolysis

Peripheral and central neurolysis should be reserved for patients with a short life expectancy because of the high risk of neuralgia from this procedure (24). Cryoablation of the second or third intercostal nerve may be used and has been demonstrated effective in the management of postthoracotomy pain (25,26,82). Dorsal root entry zone lesions have been reported effective for deafferentation pain following peripheral nerve injury, but due to the invasiveness of this procedure, it should be one of last resort (47,48). The success of this procedure seems greatest with nerve root avulsions and spinal cord injury. Lower success rates have been found after more peripheral nerve injury. Avulsion rhizotomies and spinal cord injuries are associated with spontaneous activity of second-order neurons within the dorsal horn whereas peripheral lesions cause spontaneous activity of the peripheral nerve and dorsal root ganglion (44). DREZ lesions are directed at the hyperexcitable second order neurons, thus explaining the higher success in more central nerve lesions (98). Therefore, DREZ lesions are less likely to be of any benefit in this group of pain patients.

Mastalgia

Agents which improve mastalgia have effects at different levels of the hypothalamic-pituitary-ovarian-breast axis (54). Bromocriptine, effective in the treatment of cyclical, premenopausal mastalgia, acts primarily as a dopaminergic agonist decreasing prolactin release (54). Several other, "hormonally active" agents such as danazol (androgen) or tamoxifen (nonsteroidal antiestrogen) or finally reduction of dietary fat lead to decreased prolactin activity at the breast tissue level (54).

Hypothalamic gonadotropin releasing hormone (GnRH) agonists, specifically the luteinizing-releasing hormone agonist goserelin, reversibly induces suppression of pituitary gonadotrophins and have been used in patients with recurrent and refractory mastalgia (57). Although positive response rates have been reported as high as 97%, the effect of prolonged hypoestrogenism on bone metabolism in healthy premenopausal women is a major concern (58).

CONCLUSIONS

This chapter emphasizes the complexity of the pain state that arises from the management of pain syndromes that arise from surgical intervention into the breast. The multiple effects arising from tissue and nerve injury induced by the surgery, the changes in nerve function secondary to radiation and chemotherapy, and the lytic properties of the tumor mass itself all combine to yield a complex pain state. Given the major changes in systems function induced by such interventions, it is little surprise that this condition is characterized by a high incidence of pain complaint. It is perhaps all the more remarkable that relatively few studies have targeted this systems. Accordingly, there are few definitive studies to which one can point as indicating a systematic assessment of one therapeutic appropriate over an other. In large part, we suspect that the failure to recognize the postmastectomy pain state as having both neuropathic and somatic pain components may account for the relative variability that does arise in the extant literature. On the positive side, the major insights that have arisen from our growing understanding of mechanism give promise that this pervasive pain state can be managed with increasing efficiency and success.

REFERENCES

1. ACS (American Cancer Society). *Cancer facts and figures.* Atlanta: American Cancer Society, 1992.
2. Aitken DR, Minton JP. Complications associated with mastectomy. *Surg Clin North Am* 1983;63:1331–1352.
3. Ampil FL. Radiotherapy for carcinomatous brachial plexopathy. *Cancer* 1985;56:2185–2188.
4. Assa J. The intercostobrachial nerve in radical mastectomy. *J Surg Oncol* 1974;6:123–126.
5. Bach FW, Jensen TS, Kastrup J, Stigsby B, Dejgard A. The effect of intravenous lidocaine on nociceptive processing in diabetic neuropathy. *Pain* 1990;40:29–34.
6. Bagley FH, Walsh JW, Cady B, Salzman FA, Oberfield RA, Pazianos AG. Carcinomatous versus radiation-induced brachial plexus neuropathy in breast cancer. *Cancer* 1978;41:2154–2157.
7. Basbaum AI, Gautro M, Jazat F, et al. The spectrum of fiber loss in a model of neuropathic pain in the rat: an electron microscopic study. *Pain* 1991;47:359–367.
8. Bergouignan M. Successful cure of essential facial neuralgias by sodium diphenylhydantoinate. *Rev Laryngol Otol Rhinol (Bord)* 1942;63:34–41.
9. Blumberg H, Janig W. Discharge pattern of afferent fibers from a neuroma. *Pain* 1984;20:335–353.
10. Blumenkopf B, Lipman JJ. Studies in autotomy: its pathophysiology and usefulness as a model of chronic pain. *Pain* 1991;45: 203–209.
11. Boas RA, Covino BG, Shahnarian A. Analgesic responses to IV lignocaine. *Br J Anaesth* 1982;54:501–505.
12. Bohm E. Transcutaneous electrical nerve stimulation in chronic pain after peripheral nerve injury. *Acta Neurochir* 1978;40:277–285.
13. Bonica JJ, Buckley FP. Cancer pain. In: Bonica JJ, ed. *The management of pain.* 2nd ed. Philadelphia: Lea & Febiger, 1990:400–460.
14. Bonica JJ. Anatomic and physiologic basis of nociception and pain. In: Bonica JJ, ed. *The management of pain.* 2nd ed. Philadelphia: Lea & Febiger, 1990:28–94.
15. Bruera E, Ripamonti C. Adjuvants to opioid analgesics. In: Patt RB, ed. *Cancer pain.* 1st ed. Philadelphia: Lippincott, 1993:143–159.
16. Burchiel KJ. Abnormal impulse generation in focally demyelinated trigeminal roots. *J Neurosurg* 1980;53:674–683.
17. Campbell JN, Raja SN, Meyer RA, et al. Myelinated afferents signal the hyperalgesia associated with nerve injury. *Pain* 1988;32: 89–94.
19. Ragsdale OS, McPhee JC, Scheuer T, Catterall WA. Common molecular determinants of local anesthetic antiarrhythmic and anticonvulsant block of voltage-gated Na^+ channels. *Proc Nat Acad Sci USA* 1996;93:9270–9275.
20. Chabal C, Jacobson L, Mariano A, Chaney E, Britell CW. The use of oral mexiletine for the treatment of pain after peripheral nerve injury. *Anesthesiology* 1992;76:513–517.
21. Chang HM, Berde CB, Holz GG, Steward GF, Kream RM. Sufentanil, morphine, met-enkephalin, and kappa-agonists (U-50, 488H) inhibit substance P release from primary sensory neurons: a model for presynaptic spinal opioid actions. *Anesthesiology* 1989; 70:672–677.
22. Coderre TJ, Grimes RW, Melzack R. Deafferentation and chronic pain in animals: an evaluation of evidence suggesting autotomy is related to pain. *Pain* 1986;26:61–84.
23. Coderre TJ, Katz J, Vaccarino AL, Melzack R. Contribution of central neuroplasticity to pathological pain: review of clinical and experimental evidence. *Pain* 1993;52:259–285.
24. Conacher ID, Locke T, Hilton C. Neuralgias after cryoanalgesia for thoracotomy. *Lancet* 1986;1:277.
25. Conacher ID. Percutaneous cryotherapy for post-thoracotomy neuralgia. *Pain* 1986;25:227–228.
26. Conacher ID. Therapists and therapies for post-thoracotomy neuralgias. *Pain* 1992;48:409–412.
27. Cowie AT. Overview of the mammary gland. *J Invest Dermatol* 1974; 63:2–9.
28. Davis KD, Treede RD, Raja SN, Meyer RA, Campbell JN. Topical application of clonidine relieves hyperalgesia in patients with sympathetically maintained pain. *Pain* 1991;47:309–317.
29. Dejgard A, Petersen P, Kastrup J. Mexiletine for treatment of chronic painful neuropathy. *Lancet* 1988;2:9.
30. deJong RH, Nace RA. Nerve impulse conduction during intravenous lidocaine injection. *Anesthesiology* 1968;29:22–28.
31. Devor M. Neuropathic pain and injured nerve: peripheral mechanisms. *Br Med Bull* 1990;47:619–630.
32. Devor M, Govrin-Lippmann R, Angelides K. Na^+ channel immunolocalization in peripheral mammalian axons and changes following nerve injury and neuroma formation. *J Neurosci* 1993;13: 1976–1992.
33. Devor M, Wall PD. Cross-excitation in dorsal root ganglia of nerve-injured and intact rats. *J Neurophys* 1990;64:1733–1746.

34. Devor M Wall PD, Catalan N. Systemic lidocaine silences ectopic neuroma and DRG discharge without blocking nerve conduction. *Pain* 1992;48:261–268.
35. Dieras V, Marty M, Tubiana N, et al. Phase II randomized study of paclitaxel versus mitomycin in advanced breast cancer. *Semin Oncol* 1995;22:33–39.
36. Downing R, Windsor CWO. Disturbance of sensation after mastectomy. *BMJ* 1984;288:1650.
37. Dubner R, Basbaum AI. Spinal dorsal horn plasticity following tissue or nerve injury. In: Wall PD, Melzack R, eds. *Textbook of pain.* London: Churchill Livingstone, 1993:225–242.
38. Duncan MA, Lotze MT, Gerber LH, Rosenberg SA. Incidence, recovery, and management of serratus anterior muscle palsy after axillary node dissection. *Phys Ther* 1983;63:1243–1247.
39. Edwards EA. Surgical anatomy of the breast. In: Goldwyn RM, ed. *Plastic and reconstructive surgery of the breast.* Boston: Little Brown, 1976;37–57.
40. Eisenach JC, Chuanyao T. Site of hemodynamic effects of intrathecal α_2-adrenergic agonists. *Anesthesiology* 1991;74:766–771.
41. Farber GA, Burks JW. Chlorprothixene therapy for herpes zoster neuralgia. *South Med J* 1974;67:808–812.
42. Farina MA, Newby BG, Lani HM. Innervation of the nipple-areola complex. *Plast Reconstr Surg* 1980;66:497–501.
43. Fields HL. Central nervous system mechanisms for control of pain transmission. In: Fields HL, ed. *Pain.* New York: McGraw-Hill, 1987:99–131.
44. Fields HL. Painful dysfunction of the nervous system. In: Fields HL, ed. *Pain.* New York: McGraw-Hill, 1987:133–169.
45. Foley KM. Pain syndromes in patients with cancer. *Med Clin North Am* 1978;71:177–178.
46. Fowler TJ, Ochoa J. Unmyelinated fibres in normal and compressed peripheral nerves of the baboon: a quantitative electron microscopic study. *Neuropathol Appl Neurobiol* 1975;1:247–265.
47. Friedman AH, Bullitt E. Dorsal root entry zone lesions in the treatment of pain following brachial plexus avulsions, spinal cord injury and herpes zoster. *Appl Neurophysiol* 1988;51:164–169.
48. Friedman AH, Nashold BS. Dorsal root entry zone lesions for the treatment of postherpetic neuralgia. *Neurosurgery* 1984;15:969–970.
49. Gateley CA. Gammalinolenic acid: possible modes of action in the treatment of mastalgia. *Breast* 1993;2:67–69.
50. Gaumann DM, Yaksh TL, Tyce GM. Effects of intrathecal morphine, clonidine, and midazolam on the somato-sympathoadrenal reflex response in halothane-anesthetized cats. *Anesthesiology* 1990; 73:425–432.
51. Gillette EL, Mahler PA, Powers BE, Gillette SM, Vujaskovic Z. Late radiation injury to muscle and peripheral nerves. *Int J Radiat Oncol Biol Phys* 1995;31:1309–1318.
52. Glassman AH, Perel JM, Shostak M, Kantor SJ, Fleiss JL. Clinical implications of imipramine plasma levels for depressive illness. *Arch Gen Psychiatry* 1977;34:197–204.
53. Goa KL; Faulds D. Vinorelbine. A review of its pharmacological properties and clinical use in cancer chemotherapy. *Drugs Aging* 1994;5:200–234.
54. Goodwin PJ, Neelan W, Boyd NF. Cyclical mastopathy: a critical review of therapy. *Br J Surg* 1988;75:837–844.
55. Granek I, Ashikari R, Foley KM. The postmastectomy pain syndrome: clinical and anatomical correlates. *Proc ASCO* 1984;3:122.
56. Hallett M, Tandon D, Berardelli A. Treatment of peripheral neuropathies. *J Neurol Neurosurg Psychiatry* 1985;48:1193–1207.
57. Hamed H, Chanday WA, Caletti W, Fentiman IS. LHRH analogue for treatment of recurrent and refractory mastalgia. *Ann R Coll Surg* 1990;72:221–224.
58. Hamed H, Fogelman I, Smith P, Gregory W, Fentiman IS. Effect of a GnRH analogue on bone mass in premenopausal patients with mastalgia. *Breast* 1993;2:75–82.
59. Holmes FA, Valero V, Walters RS, et al. The M. D. Anderson Cancer Center experience with Taxol in metastatic breast cancer. *Monogr Natl Cancer Inst* 1993;15:161–169.
60. Hoppenreijs TJ, Freihofer HP, Brouns JJ, Buraset I, Manni JJ. Sensibility and cutaneous reinnervation of pectoralis major myocutaneous island flaps. A preliminary clinical report. *J Craniomaxillofac Surg* 1990;18:237–242.
61. Howe JF, Loeser JD, Calvin WH. Mechanosensitivity of dorsal root ganglia and chronically injured axons: a physiological basis for the radicular pain of nerve root compression. *Pain* 1977;3:25–41.
62. Huang TT. Breast and subscapular pain following submuscular placement of breast prostheses. *Plast Reconstr Surg* 1990;86: 275–280.
63. Hughes LE, Mansel RE, Webster DJT. Aberrations of normal development and involution (ANDI): a new perspective on pathogenesis of and nomenclature of benign breast disorders. *Lancet* 1987;3:1316–1319.
64. Jabaley ME, Das SK. Late breast pain following reconstruction with polyurethrane-covered implants. *Plast Reconstr Surg* 1986;78: 390–395.
65. Jamison K, Wellisch DK, Katz RI, Pasnav RO. Phantome breast syndrome. *Arch Surg* 1979;114:93–95.
66. Janig W, Kollman W. The involvement of the sympathetic nervous system in pain. *Arzneimittelforschung* 1984;34:1066–1073.
67. Janig W. Pathophysiology of nerve following mechanical injury. In: Dubner R, Gebhart GF, Bond MR, eds. *Proceedings of the 5th World Congress on Pain.* Amsterdam: Elsevier Science, 1988:80–86.
68. Janson RA. Implant arm: axillary compression from breast prostheses. *Plast Reconstr Surg* 1985;75:420–422.
69. Jensen TS, Rasmussen P. Amputation. In: Wall PD, Melzack R, eds. *Textbook of pain.* Edinburgh: Churchill Livingstone, 1984:402–412.
70. Johnstone PA, DeLuca AM, Bacher JD, et al. Clinical toxicity of peripheral nerve to intraoperative radiotherapy in a canine model. *Int J Radiat Oncol Biol Phys* 1995;32:1031–1034.
71. Karydas I, Fentiman IS, Habib F, Hayward JL. Sensory changes after treatment of operable breast cancer. *Breast Cancer Res Treat* 1986;8:55–59.
72. Katsantonis GP. Neurotization of pectoralis major myocutaneous flap by the hypoglossal nerve in tongue reconstruction: clinical and experimental observations. *Laryngoscope* 1988;98:1313–1323.
73. Kori SH, Foley KM, Posner JB. Brachial plexus lesions in patients with cancer: 100 cases. *Neurology* 1981;31:45–50.
74. Kroner K, Knudsen UB, Lundby L, Hvid H. Long-term phantom breast syndrome after mastectomy. *Clin J Pain* 1992;8:346–350.
75. Kroner K, Krebs B, Skov J, Jorgensen HS. Immediate and long-term phantom breast syndrome after mastectomy: incidence, clinical characteristics and relationship to pre-mastectomy breast pain. *Pain* 1989;36:327–334.
76. Kureshi SA, Hofman FM, Schneider JH, Chin LS, Apuzzo ML, Hinton DR. Cytokine expression in radiation-induced delayed cerebral injury. *Neurosurgery* 1994;35:822–830.
77. Laban E, Kon M. Lesion of the long thoracic nerve during transaxillary breast augmentation: an unusual complication. *Ann Plast Surg* 1990;24:445–446.
78. Lahteenmaki T, Waris T, Asko-Seljavaara S, Sundell B. Recovery of sensation in free flaps. *Scand J Plast Reconstr Surg Hand Surg* 1989; 23:217–222.
79. Ledrman RJ, Wilbourn AJ. Brachial plexopathy: recurrent cancer or radiation? *Neurology* 1984;34:1331–1335.
80. Lehman C, Gumener R, Montandon D. Sensibility and cutaneous reinnervation after breast reconstruction with musculocutaneous flaps. *Ann Plast Surg* 1991;26:325–327.
81. Lindvall O, Bjorklund A, Skagerberg G. Dopamine-containing neurons in the spinal cord: anatomy and some functional aspects. *Ann Neurol* 1983;14:255–260.
82. Lloyd JW, Barnard JDW, Glynn CJ. Cryoanalgesia. A new approach to pain relief. *Lancet* 1976;2:932–933.
83. Lomabard MC, Larabi Y. Electrophysiological study of cervical dorsal horn cells in partially deafferented rats. *Adv Pain Res Ther* 1983;5:147–154.
84. Long DM. Electrical stimulation of the nervous system for pain control. *Electroencephalogr Clin Neurophysiol Suppl* 1978;34:343–348.
85. Long DM. Uses of percutaneous electrical stimulation of the nervous system. *Med Prog Technol* 1977;5:47–50.
86. Lotze MT, Duncan MA, Gerber LH, et al. Early versus delayed shoulder motion following axillary dissection. *Ann Surg* 1981;193: 288–295.
87. Maciewicz R, Bouchoms A, Martin JB. Drug therapy for neuropathic pain. *Clin J Pain* 1985;1:39–49.
88. McLachlan EM, Janig W, et al. Peripheral nerve injury triggers noradrenergic sprouting within dorsal root ganglia. *Nature* 1993; 363:543–546.
89. McLachlan EM, Janig W, Devor M, Michaelis M. Peripheral nerve injury triggers noradrenergic sprouting within the dorsal root ganglia. *Nature* 1993;363:543–546.
90. Mellick GA, Mellick LB. Gabapentin in the management of reflex sympathetic dystrophy [Letter]. *J Pain Symptom Manage* 1995;10: 265–266.

91. Mellick LB, Mellick GA. Successful treatment of reflex sympathetic dystrophy with gabapentin [Letter]. *Am J Emerg Med* 1995; 13:96.
92. Melzack R, Wall PD. Pain mechanisms: a new theory. *Science* 1965; 150:971–978.
93. Melzack R. Prolonged relief of pain by brief, intense transcutaneous somatic stimulation. *Pain* 1975;1:357–373.
94. Montaga W. Histology and cytochemistry of human skin. XXXV. The nipple and areola. *Br J Dermatol* 1970;83:2–13.
95. Moosman DA. Anatomy of the pectoral nerves and their preservation in modified radical mastectomy. *Am J Surg* 1980;139:883.
96. Murdoch LA. Gabapentin—a novel anticonvulsant. *Axone* 1994; 16:56.
97. Nachtigali RD. Femala reproductive disorders. In: Fitzgerald PA, ed. *Handbook of clinical endocrinology*. Chicago: Jones Medical, 1986: 289–336.
98. Nashold BS, Alexander E. Neurosurgical treatment of chronic pain. In: Tollison CD, ed. *Handbook of chronic pain management*. Baltimore: Williams & Wilkins, 1989:125–135.
99. Nathan PW. Chloroprothixene (Taractan) in post-herpetic neuralgia and other severe chronic pain. *Pain* 1978;5:367–371.
100. Nielsen OS, Munro AJ, Tannock IF. Bone metastases: pathophysiology and management policy. *J Clin Oncol* 1991;9:509–524.
101. Olsen NK, Pfeiffer P, Mondrup K, Rose C. Radiation-induced brachial plexus neuropathy in breast cancer patients. *Acta Oncol* 1990;29:885–890.
102. Paredes JP, Puente JL, Potel J. Variation in sensitivity after sectioning the intercostobrachial nerve. *Am J Surg* 1990;160:525–528.
103. Parsons JT, Bova FJ, Fitzgerald CR, Mendenhall WM, Million RR. Radiation optic neuropathy after megavoltage external-beam irradiation: analysis of time-dose factors. *Int J Radiat Oncol Biol Phys* 1994;30:755–763.
104. Peters F, Sehuth W. Hyperprolactinemia and non-puerperal mastitis (duct ectasia). *JAMA* 1989;261:1618–1620.
105. Powles TJ, Jones AL, Judson IR, Hardy JR, Ashley SE. A randomised trial comparing combination chemotherapy using mitomycin C, mitozantrone and methotrexate (3M) with vincristine, anthracycline and cyclophosphamide (VAC) in advanced breast cancer. *Br J Cancer* 1991;64:406–410.
106. Preece PE, Hughes LE, Mansel RE, Baum M, Button PM, Gravelle IM. Clinical syndromes of mastalgia. *Lancet* 1976;670–673.
107. Puke MJ, Xu XJ, Wiesenfeld-Hallin Z. Intrathecal administration of clonidine suppresses autotomy, a behavioral sign of chronic pain in rats after sciatic nerve section. *Neurosci Lett* 1991;133: 199–202.
108. Raja SN, Treede RD, Davis KD, Campbell JN. Systemic alpha-adrenergic blockade with phentolamine: a diagnostic test for sympathetically maintained pain. *Anesthesiology* 1991;74:691–698.
109. Rauck RL, Eisenach JC, Jackson K, et al. Epidural clonidine treatment for refractory reflex sympathetic dystrophy. *Anesthesiology* 1993;79:1163–1169.
110. Roberts WA, Elardo SM. Sympathetic activation of A-delta nociceptors. *Somatosens Res* 1985;3:33–44.
111. Rowlingson JC, DiFazio CA, Foster J, Carron H. Lidocaine as an analgesic for experimental pain. *Anesthesiology* 1980;52:20–22.
112. Sanjue H, Jun Z. Sympathetic facilitation of sustained discharge of polymodal nociceptors. *Pain* 1989;38:85–90.
113. Scadding JW. Development of ongoing activity, mechanosensitivity and adrenaline sensitivity in severed peripheral nerve axons. *Exp Neurol* 1981;73:345–364.
114. Scher HI, Yagoda A. Bone metastases: pathogenesis, treatment, and rationale for use of resorption inhibitors. *Am J Med* 1987;82: 6–28.
115. Seltzer MH. The significance of breast complaints as correlated with age and breast cancer. *Am Surg* 1992;58:413–417.
116. Simmel ML. A study of phantoms after amputation of the breast. *Neuropsykologica* 1966;4:331–350.
117. Sinow JD, Cunningham BL. Intraluminal lidocaine for analgesia after tissue expansion: a double-blind prospective trial in breast reconstruction. *Ann Plast Surg* 1992;28:320–325.
118. Slezak S, McGibbon B, Dellon AL. The sensational transverse rectus abdominus musculocutaneous (TRAM) flap: return of sensibility after TRAM breast reconstruction. *Ann Plast Surg* 1992;28: 210–217.
119. Somlo G, Doroshow JH, Forman SJ, et al. High-dose cisplatin, etoposide, and cyclophosphamide with autologous stem cell reinfusion in patients with responsive metastatic or high-risk primary breast cancer. *Cancer* 1994;73:125–134.
120. Southwick HW, Slaughter DP, Humphrey LT. Anatomy and physiology of the breast and axilla. In: Southwick HW, ed. *Surgery of the breast*. Chicago: Yearbook, 1968:15–21.
121. Stevens PE, Dibble SL, Miaskowski C. Prevalence, characteristics, and impact of postmastectomy pain syndrome: an investigation of women's experiences. *Pain* 1995;61:61–68.
122. Stracke H, Meyer UE, Schumacher HE, Federlin K. Mexiletine in the treatment of diabetic neuropathy. *Diabetes Care* 1992;15: 1550–1555.
123. Swerdlow M, Cundill JG. Anticonvulsant drugs used in the treatment of lancinating pain. A comparison. *Anaesthesia* 1981;36: 1129–1132.
124. Tanelian DL, Brose WG. Neuropathic pain can be relieved by drugs that are use-dependent sodium channel blockers: lidocaine, carbamazepine, and mexiletine. *Anesthesiology* 1991;74:949–951.
125. Tanelian DL, Maclver MB. Analgesic concentrations of lidocaine suppress tonic A-delta and C fiber discharges produced by acute injury. *Anesthesiology* 1991;74:934–936.
126. Taylor CP. Gabapentin: mechanism of action. In: Levy RH, Mattson RH, Meldrum BS, eds. *Antiepileptic drugs*. New York: Raven Press, 1995:829–841.
127. Temple WJ, Ketcham AS. Preservation of the intercostobrachial nerve during axillary dissection for breast cancer. *Am J Surg* 1985; 150:585–588.
128. Terzis JK, Vincent MP, Wilkins LM, Rutledge K, Deane LM. Breast sensibility: a neurophysiological appraisal in the normal breast. *Ann Plastic Surg* 1987;19:318–322.
129. Vecht CJ, Van de Brand HJ, Wajer OJM. Post-axillary dissection pain in breast cancer due to a lesion of the intercostobrachial nerve. *Pain* 1989;38:171–176.
130. Vujaskovic Z, Gillette SM, Powers BE, Thurmond DN, Gillette EL, Colacchio TA. Ultrastructural morphometric analysis of peripheral nerves after intraoperative irradiation. *Int J Radiat Biol* 1995; 68:71–76.
131. Wall PD, Devor M. Sensory afferent impulses originate from dorsal root ganglia as well as from the periphery in normal and nerve injured rats. *Pain* 1983;17:321–339.
132. Wallace MS, Wallace AM, Lee J, Dobke MK. Pain after breast surgery: A survey of 282 women. *Pain* 1996;66:195–205.
133. Watson CP, Evans RJ, Reed K, Merskey H, Goldsmith L, Warsh J. Amitriptyline versus placebo in postherpetic neuralgia. *Neurology* 1982;32:671–673.
134. Watson CPN, Evans RJ, Watt VR. The post-mastectomy pain syndrome and the effect of topical capsaicin. *Pain* 1989;38:177–186.
135. Watson CPN, Evans RJ. A comparative trial of amitriptyline and zimelidine in postherpetic neuralgia. *Pain* 1985;23:387–394.
136. Watson CPN, Evans RJ. Intractable pain with breast cancer. *Can Med Assoc J* 1982;126:263–266.
137. Weinstein S, Vetter RJ, Sersen EA. Phantoms following breast amputation. *Neuropsykologica* 1970;8:185–197.
138. Willis WD. Modulation of primate spinothalamic tract discharges. In: Kruger L, Liebeskind JC, eds. *Advances in pain research and therapy. Vol. 6*. New York: Raven Press, 1984:217–240.
139. Wisbey JR, Kumar S, Mansel RE, Preece PE, Pye JK, Hughes LE. Natural history of breast pain. *Lancet* 1983;672–674.
140. Woolf CJ, Shortland P. Peripheral nerve injury triggers central sprouting of myelinated afferents. *Nature* 1992;355:75–78.
141. Woolf CJ, Wiesenfeld-Hallin Z. The systemic administration of local anaesthetics produces a selective depression of C-afferent fibre evoked activity in the spinal cord. *Pain* 1985;23:361–374.
142. Yaksh TL, Al-Rodham NRF, Jensen TS. Sites of action of opiates in production of analgesia. In: *Progress in brain research, vol. 77*. New York: Elsevier Science, 1988:371–394.
143. Yaksh TL, Malmberg AB. Central pharmacology of nociceptive transmission. In: Wall P, Melzack R, eds. *Textbook of Pain*. 3rd ed. Edinburgh: Churchill Livingstone, 1994:165–200.
144. Yaksh TL, Pogrel JW, Lee YW, Chaplan SR. Reversal of nerve ligation-induced allodynia by spinal alpha-2 adrenoceptor agonists. *J Pharmacol Exp Ther* 1995;272:207–214.
145. Yaksh TL. New horizons in our understanding of the spinal physiology and pharmacology of pain processing. *Semin Oncol* 1993;20:6–18.
146. Yehuda S, Youdim MB. The increased opiate action of beta-endorphin in iron-deficient rats: the possible involvement of dopamine. *Eur J Pharmacol* 1984;104:245–251.

Anesthesia: Biologic Foundations, edited by Tony L. Yaksh et al. Lippincott–Raven Publishers, Philadelphia © 1997.

CHAPTER 53

TRIGEMINAL ORGANIZATION WITH SPECIAL REFERENCE TO THE TRIGEMINOVASCULAR SYSTEM AND CRANIAL PAIN

GEOFFREY M. BOVE AND MICHAEL A. MOSKOWITZ

The trigeminal nerve, a mixed cranial nerve containing both sensory and motor components, transmits sensory information from the face, cornea, oral cavity, teeth, and meninges. It acts as a sentry to the organism, providing critical information about food texture, liquid character, and inspired air quality. Though the nerve carries most sensory modalities in its various axon types, one of its primary functions is to signal actual or impending damage to innervated structures (nociception), causing the sensation of pain and hopefully leading to an appropriate evasive behavior. Three major divisions innervate contiguous skin areas. Unlike spinal dermatomes, these divisions have very little peripheral overlap (160). The facial skin and oral mucosa are among the most densely innervated tissues in the body, allowing high tactile discrimination and sensory feedback (179). Although the nerve has a lower percentage of unmyelinated fibers compared to spinal nerves (50% versus 80%) (100,147,187), corneal branches are the most densely unmyelinated in the body (150,189). Trigeminal branches often run very close to the cutaneous or mucosal surfaces, making them susceptible to injury; this is reflected in a high incidence of both pathology and pain from tissues such as paranasal sinuses, teeth, and periodontium (61). The meninges, innervated primarily by the trigeminal nerve and considered an important source of head pain (121,184), may share similar properties given that 5–15% of the population suffers from migraine headache (107).

This chapter will concentrate on the role of unmyelinated and thinly myelinated trigeminal nerve fibers, which transmit nociception (impulses that may lead to pain) and participate in axon reflexes, releasing neuropeptides at their distal terminals. The trigeminal intracranial innervation, called the trigeminovascular system (121), provides an interesting example that is relevant to other tissues innervated by the trigeminal nerve, and is relevant to several pain states, including migraine headache.

ANATOMY OF THE TRIGEMINAL SYSTEM

Peripheral Nerve

The trigeminal nerve contains three major branches, the ophthalmic, maxillary, and mandibular nerves, all of which transmit general sensory and nociceptive impulses. In brief, the ophthalmic nerve (V_1) innervates the skin from the upper eyelids to the vertex, the conjunctiva of the upper lid, the cornea, the mucosal tissue of the sinuses, and the anterior cranial fossa. The maxillary nerve (V_2) innervates the skin of the middle third of the face, the palate, maxillary teeth and supporting structures, nasal mucosa, and the dura of the middle cranial fossa. The mandibular nerve (V_3) innervates the skin overlying the mandible, the temporomandibular joint, the external ear, the lower teeth and supporting structures, and the dura corresponding to the distribution of the middle meningeal artery (Table 1). Besides the sensory fibers, the mandibular nerve conveys motor fibers to the muscles of mastication. There is no autonomic component to the trigeminal nerve, though parasympathetic and sympathetic fibers join various trigeminal branches in their peripheral course.

Central to the ganglion, the trigeminal splits into sensory (portia major) and motor (portia minor) divisions. As visceral efferent fibers are not thought to course in the motor root, the observation that ~20% of the axons are unmyelinated may be similar to the anatomy of the lumbar and sacral spinal cord, where afferent fibers pass with the ventral roots (188). This presence of afferents in the motor root may explain in part the preservation of tactile sensitivity and facial pain following trigeminal rhizotomy (80).

Trigeminal Ganglion

The sensory fibers from the three divisions converge on the trigeminal ganglion (also called the semilunar or Gasserian ganglion) where their pseudounipolar neurons are housed. This arrangement is similar to spinal nerves, which have their cell bodies located outside the central nervous system in the dorsal root ganglia. In the trigeminal ganglion, the neurons are arranged somatotopically and according to their division (32,92,93). Thus, the cell bodies of V_1 are located anteromedially, those of V_3 are located posterolaterally, and the cell bodies of V_2 are located between them. Fibers of proprioception pass through the ganglion to their cell bodies located in the mesencephalic trigeminal nucleus, the only nucleus in the central nervous system that contains primary afferent neurons (83).

Examination of the cell bodies within the trigeminal systems reveal them to be composed of large (type A) and small (type B) ganglion cells. As in the spinal sensory ganglia, the small ganglion cells contain a variety of peptides including substance P and calcitonin gene-related peptide. This will be discussed further below.

Central Organization of the Trigeminal Roots

From the ganglion, trigeminal afferent fibers travel in the trigeminal root to enter the brain stem venterolaterally at the level of the rostral pons (100). During this short course, the fibers separate according to size and intermingle with fibers from other divisions (62). At the pontine entry zone, the fine myelinated and unmyelinated fibers coalesce to form the deep ventral division (60,173). This is similar to spinal primary afferent fibers, which merge to take a ventrolateral position in the dorsal root before entering the spinal dorsal horn (105,106). The trigeminal fibers then descend in the medial brain stem to terminate below obex in the substantia gelatinosa of the trigeminal nucleus caudalis, extending to and merging with the upper cervical spinal cord (39,135,175).

Table 1. SUMMARY OF TRIGEMINAL AFFERENT DIVISIONS

Division	Projection sites: Extracranial structures	Projection sites: Intracranial structures
Opthalmic	Skin between the upper eyelids and the vertex, the conjunctiva of the upper lid, the cornea, the frontal, sphenoid, and ethmoid sinus mucosa.	Dura of the anterior cranial fossa and vault, including the upper tentorium cerebelli and falx cerebri.
Maxillary	Skin of the middle one-third of the face from the lower eyelid to the upper lip, palate, maxillary teeth, and nasal mucosa.	Dura of the middle cranial fossa.
Mandibular	Skin overlying the mandible, the auricle, the external auditory meatus and anterior exterior part of the tympanic membrane, the lower teeth and supporting structure, and temporomandibular joint.	Dura corresponding to the distribution of the middle meningeal artery.

It should be noted here, however, that the nucleus caudalis also receives afferent input from the upper cervical dorsal roots and the facial, glossopharyngeal, and vagus nerves (60,160, 182). Importantly, as with the spinal segments, there is significant collateralization of the roots as they enter the dorsal root entry zone, and these collaterals from a given segmental level may gain access to neurons in distal segments. Such extrasegmental projections provide an adequate substrate for somatotopic convergence that may underlie unusual pain referral patterns that do not reflect known peripheral nerve distributions. It is no wonder that painful syndromes of the head and neck present with such diversity.

The brain stem trigeminal projections are divided into a main sensory nucleus and a spinal nucleus that extends caudally to the upper cervical spinal cord. Anatomically, the spinal nucleus presents rostrocaudally in three subdivisions: nucleus oralis, nucleus interpolaris, and nucleus caudalis (135). The somatotopic arrangement present in the trigeminal ganglion is reflected in the descending trigeminal tract and in the main sensory and spinal nuclei (92)

Large afferent fibers bifurcate within the brain stem, yielding ascending and descending branches that terminate in the main sensory and spinal nuclei (68). Physiologic studies are consistent with the anatomic evidence for widespread termination of trigeminal afferents within the several trigeminal brainstem subdivisions. Neurons activated by low-intensity mechanical stimuli are found within the main sensory nucleus and nuclei oralis, interpolaris, and caudalis (94,96). Neurons responsive to thermal or noxious stimuli have been reported in the nucleus caudalis (33,38,41,145). Significantly, trigeminal neurons can be driven by input from spinal afferent collaterals and other cranial nerves. Stimulation as far caudally as the C2 root produces an excitation of neurons receiving trigeminal input (95). Such widespread convergence points to the likelihood that unusual pain syndromes (as are seen in atypical facial neuralgias) might reflect the contribution of these collateral projections. The role of the nucleus caudalis in pain is supported by the observation that trigeminal tractotomy at the level of the medullary obex relieves ipsilateral facial pain with preservation of touch (164). Studies with neurons in the nucleus caudalis indicate two principal classes that have response properties similar to those found in spinal cord (145). Neurons in the marginal layer of nucleus caudalis (lamina I) are typically "nociceptive specific." The receptive fields of these neurons are predominantly ipsilateral and small in size. The second group of neurons, called "wide dynamic range," are situated ventrally in the magnocellular portion of the nucleus caudalis. These neurons receive convergent input from large and small diameter primary afferents, which are activated by light touch, hair movement, vibration, and noxious stimuli (110,161).

Trigeminofugal Projections

Retrograde tract recordings have shown that the ventrobasal thalamus receives largely contralateral projections from the entire trigeminal sensory complex, with the possible exception of the nucleus oralis of the spinal nucleus (51). Neurons in the superficial laminae project strongly to the submedius and ventroposterior and posterior nuclear regions of the thalamus. Neurons in the deeper laminae are distributed primarily the zona incerta and posterior hypothalamus (78). Neurons in the nucleus caudalis responsive to noxious or innocuous stimuli, or both, project to more rostral levels within the trigeminal complex and also to the ventroposterior thalamus (145,172).

Neurons of the main sensory nucleus and nucleus oralis can be activated by electrical stimulation of the nucleus caudalis. Activation of the nucleus caudalis by topical strychnine (a glycine receptor antagonist) potentiates the response of main sensory and nucleus caudalis neurons to both noxious and innocuous stimuli. Conversely, cold block of the nucleus caudalis decreases the responses of neurons in the nucleus oralis and main sensory nucleus to peripheral stimulation. Consistent with these observations, electrical stimulation or strychnine on the nucleus caudalis has been reported to hyperpolarize the preterminal endings of primary afferent neurons in the nucleus oralis (96,159). Thus, neurons of the nucleus caudalis may activate primary afferent terminals synapsing on neurons in the more rostral sensory trigeminal nuclei.

For details of the organization of the trigeminal nuclear complex and trigeminal afferent pathways in the central nervous system, the reader is referred elsewhere (39,59,60,135,160) (see Chapter 47).

TRIGEMINAL SYSTEM AND EXTRACRANIAL PAIN

Trigeminal Afferent Processing Evoked by Small Afferent Input

The rich innervation of the skin, nasal, and buccal structures facilitates the transduction of mechanical and thermal stimuli as well as the effects of tissue injury to these structures. The anatomical and neurochemical organization of the primary afferents and the trigeminal medullary dorsal horn displays significant homology to the noncranial somatosensory system. Accordingly, the principles underlying trigeminal nociceptive processing are remarkably similar to those defined for other somatic nociceptive processing. Predictably, noxious mechanical and thermal stimuli applied to the regions innervated by the trigeminal nerve will result in discharges of primary afferent nociceptors and also in trigeminal nuclear areas.

Chemical stimuli secondary to inflammation are known to play an important role in extracranial pain states, and their effects have been well documented for cornea and tooth pulp (see Chapters 32 and 47). This input is subject to regulation by a pharmacology comparable to that discussed for spinal afferent input. Accordingly, these systems display a well-defined central facilitation (24,64). The small afferent-evoked excitation of trigeminal projection neurons is subject to modulation like neurons of the dorsal horn (25) (see Chapter 38). Thus, facial and mandibular nociceptive reflexes and the neuronal response to noxious facial stimuli are suppressed by opioids and α_2 agonists (28,134,171).

Facial neuralgias often present with unusual somatotopic distributions that encompass multiple, often noncontiguous dermatomes. Convergence of afferent input from the upper shoulders, neck, scalp, and face provides a theoretical substrate for these apparently anomalous referred pain states. This convergence may also provide an afferent-evoked reflex substrate for otherwise unanticipated manifestations associated with altered muscle tone, such as those observed in fibromyalgia and myofascial pain syndromes (see Chapter 57).

Trigeminal Afferent Processing Evoked by Large Afferent Input

Innocuous stimuli activates larger diameter afferent fibers, and does not normally lead to pain. Under certain conditions, however, innocuous stimuli can generate a well-defined pain state (allodynia). Such conditions have been described for many cranial nerves, including the trigeminal (see below), facial (26), glossopharyngeal (152), and vagus (170). These neuralgias can be subdivided into two broad classes: typical and atypical. Typical neuralgias are defined as those having a distribution consistent with one of the cranial nerves or a combination of its branches. The sensory spectrum of atypical neuralgias varies widely and characteristically does not follow known innervation patterns. As noted above, significant convergence on medullary and upper cervical afferent projections clearly provides a substrate for at least some components of such anomalous pain states.

Current thinking regarding trigeminal neuralgia (tic douloureux) provides an opportunity to study some aspects of the underlying organization of the trigeminal system. Typically triggered by an innocuous tactile stimulus on the face, its sensations are reported as resembling electric shock, or as stabbing or shooting pain. These symptoms occur intermittently, from every few seconds to once per day. The incidence increases after 50 years and is somewhat more common in women (49). The mechanisms underlying the apparently aberrant processing are not certain, but probably reflect both peripheral and central factors.

Compression, distortion, or stretching of the trigeminal nerve by adjacent arteries or be slow-growing tumors are considered associated with an increased likelihood for trigeminal neuralgia (50). As reviewed in Chapters 32 and 56, chronic nerve compression can lead to focal demyelination, which can result in the generation of abnormal impulses at the injury site as well as in the ganglion cells of the injured axons (75,177), and trophic changes may lead to crosstalk between the injured axons and dorsal root ganglion cells (48,177). Direct stimulation may also activate nociceptors intrinsic to the nerve sheath, as has been described recently for peripheral nerves (11).

However, it seems unlikely that simple compression can account for the syndrome. Mechanical pressure on a nerve manifests as sensory, reflex, and motor changes, but not pain (76,139). Slowly growing tumors more commonly yield sensory deficits (17). Trigeminal neuralgia is not considered to be opiate sensitive, arguing against a simple activation of small afferent pathways. On the other hand, activation of large afferents also fails to account for the pain state since simple high-frequency stimulation of trigeminal afferents does not ordinarily lead to a report of pain (115).

There is little doubt that peripheral nerve injury can induce transynaptic changes in the substantia gelatinosa, indicating local alterations in synaptic and neuronal morphology (85,168). Early pharmacological studies (96,186) have emphasized that the transient antagonism of medullary dorsal horn glycine receptors will induce signs of a potent allodynia and a facilitation of the discharge evoked in trigeminal wide dynamic range neurons by low-threshold afferents. This observation has spinal cord parallels (163,185). Although current data do not indicate that trigeminal neuralgia is associated with a loss of activity in dorsal horn GABA or glycinergic sites, modest changes in these inhibitory amino acid functions may be promising directions of investigation.

TRIGEMINAL SYSTEM AND INTRACRANIAL PAIN

Clinical observations support the contention that intracranial pain from migraine, tumor growth, and other sources are mediated by the trigeminal nerve. A common referent for such central pain states is the generic term "headache." It is not the purpose of this section to review in detail the many manifestations of such syndromes (132,158). However, there are several broad categories that indicate the range of mechanisms involved in pain referred to the head, including tension headaches and migraine. Clinically, it is important to note that these conditions rarely exist in a pure form.

Chronic tension headaches have several criteria, including a perception of pressing/tightening (nonpulsating quality of mild to moderate intensity), bilateral localization, and lack of aggravation by physical exertion (22). As poorly understood as they are common, tension headaches are often attributed to increased activity in pericranial or nuchal musculature, and tenderness of pericranial myofascial tissue has been reported (82). Nevertheless, a significant proportion of such patients display normal EMG activity (141).

Migraine is a complex of syndromes that may or may not appear with a prodromal auditory or visual sensation (aura). The pain of migraine is typically moderate to severe, pulsating, unilateral, and aggravated by physical exertion. It is often accompanied by nausea, vomiting, and/or photophobia (22). Common migraine with aura has been the subject of extensive investigation, and a number of components of the pathophysiology of the attack appear evident. These include a local oligemia in the cortical regions associated with the aura (e.g., visual cortex for a visual aura) that spreads over the interval of the attack to other cortical regions (47,131), and the appearance of a DC shift (spreading depression) that moves as the symptoms of the migraine evolve (6).

Although mechanisms underlying these clinical syndromes will be discussed further below, it is important to emphasize that their etiology implies activity in the trigeminal afferent system. Thus, trigeminal rhizotomy abolishes the headache associated with histamine infusion. (140). Rhizotomy (69,133,138), alcohol injection (67,137), and bulbar tractotomy (133) reportedly provide relief of migraine headache, but only when the ophthalmic nerve is rendered analgesic. During cerebral embolism, pain may be referred to the ophthalmic and maxillary dermatomes (3,45).

Clinical studies have demonstrated the pain sensitivities of various intracranial structures during mechanical and electrical stimulation in conscious humans (138,148,183). Noxious stimulation of dural arteries and sinuses, the arteries of Willis' circle, and parts of the dura caused pain but no other perception. The most sensitive structures were the blood vessels, and traction was the most noxious stimulus. In general, the dura covering the base of the skull was much more sensitive than that covering the superior cerebrum and cerebellum. The pial arteries and veins were insensitive except at their origins, where traction and electrical stimulation caused an aching pain, accompanied by nausea.

Other structures stimulated, including brain parenchyma, pia, choroid, and the ventricular system, were not pain sensitive (148). However, the findings of insensitivity must be interpreted with caution because the investigators may have not provided an appropriate stimulus. Not all nociceptive fibers are mechanosensitive (119), and some may be chemospecific (146). Also, electrical stimulation must be very close to the transductive mechanism or axon to evoke an action potential.

Innervation of the Intracranial Meninges and Vasculature

Anatomical and immunochemical techniques have demonstrated that the trigeminal nerve provides the principal afferent pathway from the meninges and intracranial blood vessels (1,2,44,114,138,165), referred to as the trigeminovascular system. In humans, afferent meningeal fibers originate from all trigeminal divisions as well as the vagus and upper three cervical nerves (1,44,77,87,89,97,113,114,154,165). As reviewed above, the trigeminal nerve innervates supratentorial structures, including the dura of the anterior and middle cranial fossae. In laboratory animals, a branch of the ethmoidal nerve provides the primary innervation of these structures. The circle of Willis is also innervated primarily by the trigeminal nerve, though the caudal portion also receives sensory fibers from the upper cervical nerves (1,154).

Histological studies have shown that the pattern and density of innervation of the intracranial blood vessels and meningeal connective tissues are similar to those of their extracranial counterparts (54,88,120). The large blood vessels, especially those of the rostral circle of Willis, have a very dense innervation, which becomes less dense with smaller vessel caliber (129,174). The meninges contain a more sparse innervation, and the majority of fibers are associated with arteries (40,88,120). Experiments using retrograde axonal transport of horseradish peroxidase and wheat germ agglutinin have confirmed that these fibers originate from the trigeminal nerve. When placed on various intracranial arteries the transported substance labels trigeminal ganglion cells (113,114). Further evidence for the importance of the trigeminal nerve comes from studies examining early immediate gene upregulation after noxious stimulation. Intracranial application of capsaicin or autologous blood causes an upregulation of the c-*fos* gene in the substantia gelatinosa of the trigeminal nucleus and upper cervical spinal cord, and can be revealed by immunohistochemistry (30,31,86,127,128).

The presence of referred pain with migraine raises the possibility that trigeminovascular axons branch and/or afferent inputs from other tissues converge within the trigeminal nucleus caudalis. Individual trigeminovascular axons do branch widely at their peripheral targets, and may supply more than one major artery (Fig. 1) (10,116). This type of branching has been observed for many other tissues (4,11,23,117,156) and may contribute to the poor spatial resolution of pain reported by migraine patients, but is not likely to cause referred pain (118). Though there are reports of axonal branching close to the sensory ganglia (5,143), this is considered to be rare (37,70), and does not occur with trigeminovascular neurons (10,116). Convergent input does occur, but in the second order neurons of the nucleus caudalis (166,167), also consistent with features of other tissues (9,55,142,144,157). Hence, pain referral from within the cranium is likely to occur thorough central mechanisms, referred to as the "convergence-projection" theory of Ruch (151). The nucleus caudalis receives input from tissues of the head and neck (84,136,182), suggesting that pathologies of these other tissues can mimic or result in intracranial pain, and vice versa (Fig. 1). Though supported anatomically and clinically (169,176), details of this convergence and its consequences have yet to be demonstrated.

Trigeminovascular Neurochemistry

The neuropeptides substance P (SP) and calcitonin gene-related peptide (CGRP) are colocalized in secretory vesicles (53,63,120,180), and are released from nociceptors both at the site of stimulation and via an antidromic mechanism (Fig. 2) (for review, see ref. 181). SP release promotes vascular relax-

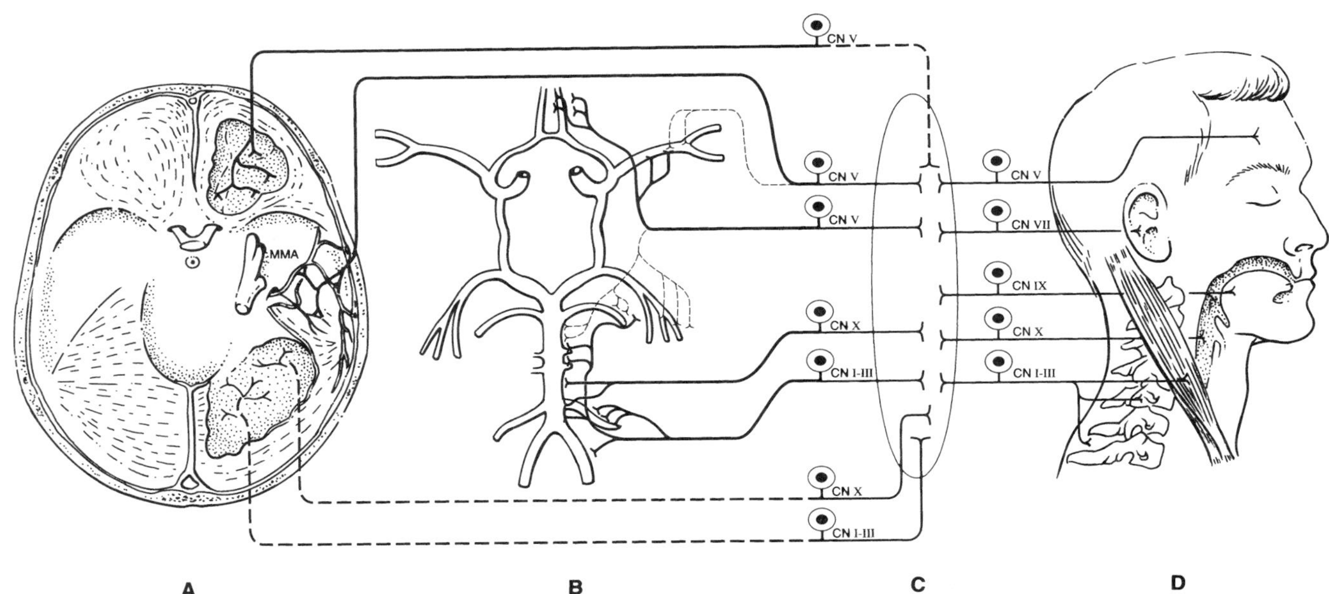

Figure 1. Sources of sensory input to the trigeminal nucleus. *Left:* The circle of Willis and dura mater are innervated by the trigeminal (CN 5), vagus (CN 10), and upper cervical (C1–3) nerves. *Right:* Tissues innervated by the trigeminal, facial (CN 7), glossopharyngeal (CN 9), vagus, and upper cervical nerves. These nerves project to the nucleus caudalis. MMA, middle meningeal artery.

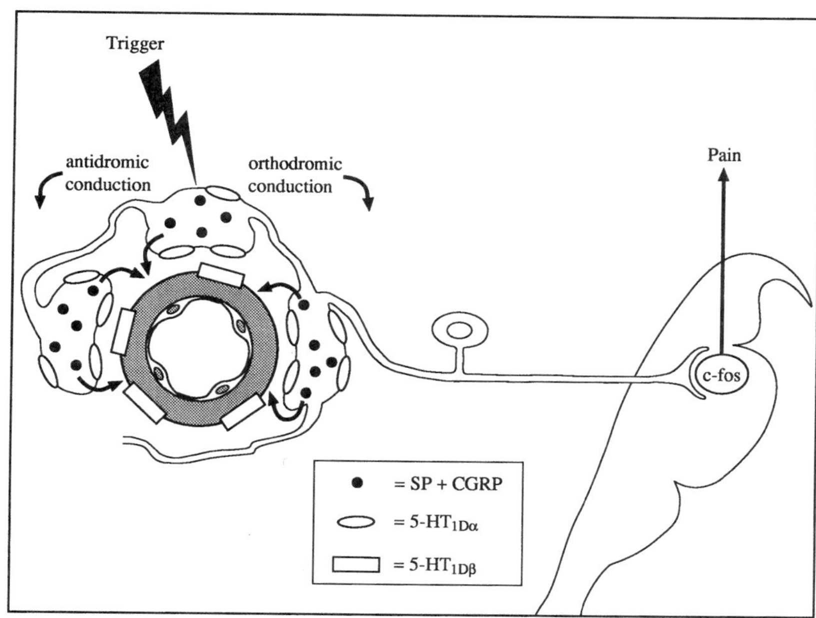

Figure 2. Trigeminovascular neurovascular junction. After triggering, antidromic and orthodromic conduction causes the primary afferent fiber to release substance P (SP) and calcitonin gene-related peptide (CGRP), leading to increased vascular dimension and permeability. The afferent impulses activate *c-fos* in the nucleus caudalis and may lead to pain. 5-HT_{1D} receptor subtypes are distributed on the nerve terminals and blood vessel.

ation, enhances permeability (27,43,91), and may sensitize nociceptors to mechanical stimulation (7,126). CGRP is a potent vasodilator (13,14) and also inhibits SP degradation (103), potentiating its action (130). SP and CGRP have been identified in primary afferent neurons innervating most tissues (99,102,162), including trigeminal neuronal axons innervating mammalian pia-arachnoid (including pial arteries) (108,109), cerebral arteries (129,174), and dura mater (40,88,120). These substances are located in small caliber nerve fibers both associated and unassociated with blood vessels, and do not have differentiated terminals (40,43,120).

SP and CGRP, as well as neurokinin A (NKA), are released by an axon reflex mechanism, causing vasodilation and plasma extravasation. This process, termed neurogenic inflammation (NI), was first described by Bayliss (8) and later referred to as the nocifensive system by Lewis (104). NI appears to be an adaptive mechanism, promoting increased local metabolism in response to damage in the area of innervation. However, NI may be maladaptive in certain settings, and is being implicated as a component of chronic diseases such as migraine, arthritis, and asthma. It has been described in many different tissues [for review, see Holzer (73)]. NI is produced experimentally by electrical stimulation of C-fiber polymodal nociceptors or by administration of noxious substances, such as capsaicin (52,79, 90,155). Though depolarization of peripheral trigeminal axons isolated from their roots and central connections is sufficient for inducing NI (27), in the intact organism it is likely that NI occurs in concert with the release of substances from autonomic sources via reflex mechanisms (57). It must be stressed that the vasodilatation of NI has not been linked to the pain accompanying migraine or other painful symptoms.

Markowitz et al. (111) developed a model using electrical stimulation of the trigeminal ganglion or capsaicin administration to induce dural NI. When labeled plasma proteins are administered following trigeminal nerve stimulation, leakage into the surrounding tissue can be measured. The model is relevant to migraine, since the stimulation induces changes in CGRP levels in the cranial blood of animals (18) that are comparable to those in human migraneurs during their headache phase (57). Also, the dosages and time course of drugs required to treat headaches and block NI are similar (20,153). For recent reviews of NI in migraine, the reader is referred to Moskowitz (123,124) and Edvinsson and Goadsby (42).

Electrophysiology of Trigeminovascular Nociceptors

Many electrophysiological properties of primary afferent nociceptors from cutaneous, visceral, and deep somatic tissues have been elucidated (23,117,146,156). The electrophysiological properties of trigeminovascular nociceptors have remained obscure, probably due to technical problems related to their inaccessibility. We have collected single unit data from nociceptors with mechanically sensitive receptive fields on dura (12). These nociceptors have properties similar to those innervating deep somatic tissues (11). Extracellular recordings from second order neurons of the nucleus caudalis have revealed wide dynamic range and nociceptive-specific neurons responding to electrical, mechanical, and bradykinin stimulation of dural blood vessels (34,35,166,167). The majority of these neurons also had cutaneous or corneal receptive fields. Most recently, nucleus caudalis neurons have been recorded that respond to noxious stimulation of face or cornea and also respond to superfusion of the subarachnoid space with a low pH solution containing inflammatory mediators (41). These studies emphasize that the intracranial blood vessels are a potential source of nociception.

Specialized Receptors of the Trigeminovascular System

Though ergot alkaloids have been used for decades to treat migraine headaches, their mechanism of action was unknown. Recent studies have shown that ergot alkaloids and sumatriptan, both of which can abort migraine, have in common their high affinity for 5-HT_{1D} receptors (36,125). These receptors are found on intracranial and a few extracranial blood vessels (29, 66) where they cause contraction (29,65), and on dural trigeminovascular afferents, where they are inhibitory (21,112). Because ergot alkaloids and sumatriptan cause constriction of intracranial blood vessels (66), and because there have been reports of vasodilation associated with migraine [reviewed by Moskowitz (122)], this mechanism has been proposed as mediating the anti-migraine effects. However, there is significant experimental evidence that ergot alkaloids and sumatriptan function through 5-HT_{1D} receptors located on trigeminovascular nerve fibers (Fig. 2). First, these drugs block NI following electrical stimulation of the trigeminal ganglion or intravenous capsaicin administration (20,21,112); however, plasma extravasation induced by exogenous SP or NKA is not affected (153). Second, plasma CGRP in the rat superior sagittal sinus (18) and the human jugular vein (56,58) decreases after administration of sumatriptan and ergot alkaloids. Third, markers of the inflammatory response (e.g., platelet aggregation, mast cell degranulation, and the formation of endothelial microvilli, vacuoles, and vesicles) are also reduced by these agents (19). Fourth, expression of *c-fos* in the trigeminal nucleus in response to intracisternal irritants, a mechanism dependent on nociceptor activity, is reduced by the drugs (31,128).

When one considers that ergot alkaloids and sumatriptan block NI in the dura but not in extracranial tissues (20), the above findings are consistent with a 5-HT_{1D} receptor subtype specific to the trigeminovascular system. Molecular biological techniques have demonstrated that the 5-HT_{1D} receptor family consists of at least two related receptors encoded by different genes, termed $5\text{-HT}_{1D\alpha}$ and $5\text{-HT}_{1D\beta}$ (178). Human and guinea pig trigeminal ganglia express the $5\text{-HT}_{1D\alpha}$, but not the $5\text{-HT}_{1D\beta}$, mRNA (149). However, specific binding sites were not found on the ganglion's neurons (15), suggesting that the receptor proteins are transported primarily to the trigeminovascular fibers. Importantly, the $5\text{-HT}_{1D\beta}$ receptor is selectively expressed by pial vascular smooth muscle (66). The receptor specificity opens the potential to develop receptor-selective medications that do not cause undesired vasoconstrictive side effects.

Gamma-aminobutyric acid (GABA) receptors have also been implicated in trigeminovascular pharmacology. Sodium valproate, a GABA transaminase inhibitor and glutamic acid decarboxylase activator, has been shown to be effective in the prophylactic and acute treatment of migraine (71,72,81,98). Sodium valproate and the GABA_A agonist muscimol decrease dural plasma extravasation caused by SP or trigeminal stimulation by bicuculline-sensitive mechanisms (101). In rats neonatally treated with capsaicin, which significantly decreases unmyelinated and thinly myelinated nerve fibers (16,46,74), similar effects were observed, suggesting that GABA_A receptors are not located on capsaicin-sensitive primary afferents. Removal of the sphenopalatine ganglion abolishes the effect of valproate or muscimol on dural plasma extravasation, suggesting that GABA_A receptors are on intracranial parasympathetic fibers (V. Limmroth, unpublished data, 1996). These data support an indirect mediation of the trigeminovascular system by GABA_A agonists, and provide a novel target for new antimigraine drugs.

Recent studies demonstrated that α_2-adreno-, histamine H3, and somatostatin receptor agonists reduce dural neurogenic inflammation. Though implicating these receptors as modulators of intracranial pain, their relationships to clinical migraine are unclear. As for GABA_A, these receptors may provide interesting targets for drug development.

Activation of the trigeminovascular system is necessary for the perception of most intracranial pain. Besides transmitting nociception, the trigeminovascular fibers perform an efferent function, releasing neuropeptides that mediate neurogenic inflammation. Drugs effective in migraine block neurogenic inflammation and nociceptive impulses through interactions with specific receptors expressed on trigeminal nerve fibers. Anatomical studies suggest that pain referral patterns accompanying migraine are likely to occur through convergence in the trigeminal nucleus. Because the trigeminovascular innervation shares many of these features with other parts of the trigeminal system, it serves as a good example of trigeminal organization.

Acknowledgment: M.A.M. is the recipient of the Bristol-Myers Unrestricted Award in Neuroscience. G.M.B. is supported by F32-ARO8239-03. We thank Drs. Volker Limmroth and Christian Waeber for their helpful comments on this chapter.

REFERENCES

1. Arbab MAR, Wiklund L, Svengaard NA. Origin and distribution of cerebral vascular innervation from superior cervical, trigeminal and spinal ganglia with retrograde and anterograde WGA-Hrp tracing in the rat. *Neuroscience* 1986;19:695–708.
2. Arnold F. *Icones nervorum capitis.* Heidelberg: J. C. B. Mohr, 1860.
3. Auerbach S. Headache in cerebral embolitic disease. *Stroke* 1981; 12:367–369.
4. Bahns E, Ernsberger U, Jänig W, Nelke A. Discharge properties of mechanosensitive afferents supplying the retroperitoneal space. *Pflugers Arch* 1986;407:519–525.
5. Bahr R, Blumberg H, Jänig W. Do dichotomizing afferent fibers exist which supply visceral organs as well as somatic structures? A contribution to the problem of referred pain. *Neurosci Lett* 1981; 24:25–28.
6. Barkley GL, Tepley N, Nagel-Leiby S, Moran JE, Simkins RT, Welch KM. Magnetoencephalographic studies of migraine. *Headache* 1990;30:428–434.
7. Basbaum AI, Levine JD. The contribution of the nervous system to inflammation and inflammatory disease. *Can J Physiol Pharmacol* 1991;69:647–651.
8. Bayliss WM. On the origin of the spinal cord of the vaso-dilator fibers of the hind-limb, and on the nature of these fibers. *J Physiol (Lond)* 1900;26:173.
9. Berkley KJ, Hubscher CH, Wall PD. Neuronal responses to stimulation of the cervix, uterus, colon, and skin in the rat spinal cord. *J Neurophysiol* 1993;69:545–556.
10. Borges LF, Moskowitz MA. Do intracranial and extracranial trigeminal afferents represent divergent axon collaterals? *Neuroscience Lett* 1983;35:265–270.
11. Bove GM, Light AR. Unmyelinated nociceptors of rat paraspinal tissues. *J Neurophysiol* 1995;73:1752–1762.
12. Bove GM, Moskowitz MA. Primary afferent neurons innervating guinea pig dura. *J Neurophysiology* 1997;77:299–308.
13. Brain SD, Tippins JR, Morris HR, MacIntyre I, Williams TJ. Potent vasodilator activity of calcitonin gene-related peptide in human skin. *J Invest Dermatol* 1986;87:533–536.
14. Brain SD, Williams TJ, Tippins JR, Morris HR, MacIntyre I. Calcitonin gene-related peptide is a potent vasodilator. *Nature* 1985; 313:54–56.
15. Bruinvels AT, Landwehrmeyer B, Moskowitz MA, Hoyer D. Evidence for the presence of $5\text{-HT}_{1\beta}$ receptor messenger RNA in neurons of the rat trigeminal ganglia. *Eur J Pharmacol* 1992;227: 357–359.
16. Buck SH, Burks TF. The neuropharmacology of capsaicin: review of some recent observations. *Pharmacol Rev* 1986;38:179–226.
17. Bullitt E, Tew JM, Boyd J. Intracranial tumors in patients with facial pain. *J Neurosurg* 1986;64:865–871.
18. Buzzi MG, Carter WB, Shimizu T, Heath H, Moskowitz MA. Dihydroergotamine and sumatriptan attenuate levels of CGRP in plasma in rat superior saggital sinus during electrical stimulation of the trigeminal ganglion. *Neuropharmacology* 1991;30:1193–1200.
19. Buzzi MG, Dimitriadou V, Theoharides T, Moskowitz MA. 5-Hydroxytryptamine receptor agonists for the abortative treatment of vascular headaches blocks mast cell, endothelial, and platelet activation within the rat dura mater after trigeminal stimulation. *Brain Res* 1992;583:137–149.
20. Buzzi MG, Moskowitz MA. The antimigraine drug, sumatriptan (GR43175), selectively blocks neurogenic plasma extravasation from blood vessels in dura mater. *Br J Pharmacol* 1990;99:202–206.
21. Buzzi MG, Moskowitz MA, Peroutka SJ, Byun B. Further characterization of the specific 5-HT receptor which mediates blockade of neurogenic plasma extravasation in rat dura mater. *Br J Pharmacol* 1991;103:1421–1428.
22. Cephalalgia. Classification of and diagnostic criteria for headache disorders, cranial neuralgia, and facial pain. *Cephalalgia* 1988; 8:3–96.
23. Cervero F. Sensory innervation of the viscera: peripheral basis of visceral pain. *Physiol Rev* 1994;74:95–138.
24. Chen L, Huang LY. Protein kinase C reduces Mg^{2+} block of NMDA-receptor channels as a mechanism of modulation. *Nature* 1992;356:521–523.
25. Chiang CY, Hu JW, Dostrovsky JO, Sessle BJ. Changes in mechanoreceptive field properties of trigeminal somatosensory brainstem neurons induced by stimulation of nucleus raphe magnus in cats. *Brain Res* 1989;485:371–381.

26. Clark LP, Taylor AS. Tic douloreaux of the nervus intermedius. *JAMA* 1942;119:255.
27. Couture R, Cuello AC. Studies on the trigeminal antidromic vasodilatation and plasma extravasation in the rat. *J Physiol (Lond)* 1984;346:273–285.
28. Curtis AL, Marwah J. Evidence for alpha adrenoceptor modulation of the nociceptive jaw-opening reflex in rats and rabbits. *J Pharm Exp Ther* 1986;238:576–579.
29. Cushing DJ, Baez M, Kursar JD, Schenk K, Cohen ML. Serotonin-induced contraction in canine coronary artery and saphenous vein: role of a 5-HT_{1D}-like receptor. *Life Sci* 1994;54:1671–1680.
30. Cutrer FM, Moussaoui S, Garret C, Moskowitz MA. The non-peptide neurokinin-1 antagonist, RPR 100893, decreases c-fos expression in trigeminal nucleus caudalis following noxious chemical meningeal stimulation. *Neuroscience* 1995;64:741–750.
31. Cutrer FM, Schoenfeld D, Limmroth V, Panahian N, Moskowitz MA. Suppression by the sumatriptan analogue, CP-122,228 of c-fos immunoreactivity in trigeminal nucleus caudalis induced by intracisternal capsaicin. *Br J Pharmacol* 1995;114:987–992.
32. Darian-Smith I, Mutton P, Proctor R. Functional organization of the tactile cutaneous afferents within the semilunar ganglion and trigeminal spinal tract of the cat. *J Neurophysiol* 1965;28:682–694.
33. Davis KD, Dostrovsky JO. Activation of trigeminal brain-stem nociceptive neurons by dural artery stimulation. *Pain* 1986;25:395–401.
34. Davis KD, Dostrovsky JO. Responses of feline trigeminal spinal tract nucleus neurons to stimulation of the middle meningeal artery and saggital sinus. *J Neurophysiol* 1988;59:648–666.
35. Davis KD, Dostrovsky JO. Cerebrovascular application of bradykinin excites central sensory neurons. *Brain Res* 1988;446: 401–406.
36. Delganis AV, Peroutka SJ. 5-Hydroxytriptamine-1D receptor agonism predicts antimigraine efficacy. *Headache* 1991;31:228.
37. Devor M, Wall PD, McMahon SB. Dichotomizing somatic nerve fibers exist in rats but they are rare. *Neurosci Lett* 1984;49:187–192.
38. Dickenson AH, Hellon RF, Taylor DLM. Facial thermal input to the trigeminal spinal nucleus of rabbits and rats. *J Comp Neurol* 1979; 185:203–210.
39. Dubner R, Gobel S, Price DD. Peripheral and central trigeminal "pain" pathways. In: Bonica JJ, Albe-Fessard D, eds. *Advances in pain research and therapy.* New York: Raven Press, 1976:137–148.
40. Düring M, Bauersachs M, Böhmer B, Veh RW, Andres KH. Neuropeptide Y- and substance P-like immunoreactive nerve fibers in the rat dura meter encephali. *Anat Embryol* 1990;182:363–373.
41. Ebersberger A, Ringkamp M, Reeh PW, Handwerker HO. Perfusion of the meninges of the rat and recording in the brainstem: an electrophysiological model for headache? In: Olesen J, Moskowitz MA, eds. *Experimental headache models in animals and man.* New York: Raven Press, 1995:217–232.
42. Edvinsson L, Goadsby PJ. Neuropeptides in migraine and cluster headache. *Cephalalgia* 1994;14:320–327.
43. Edvinsson L, McCulloch J, Uddmann R. Substance P: immunohistological localization and effect upon feline pial arteries in vitro and in situ. *J Physiol* 1981;318:251–258.
44. Feindel W, Penfield W, McNaughton F. The tentorial nerves and localization of intracranial pain. *Neurology* 1960;10:555–563.
45. Fisher CM. Clinical syndromes in cerebral arterial occlusion. In: Fields W, ed. *Pathogenesis and treatment of cerebrovascular disease.* Springfield, IL: Charles C. Thomas, 1961:123–164.
46. Fitzgerald M. Capsaicin and sensory neurones—a review. *Pain* 1983;15:109–130.
47. Friberg L, Olesen J, Lassen NA, Olsen TS, Karle A. Cerebral oxygen extraction, oxygen consumption, and regional cerebral blood flow during the aura phase of migraine. *Stroke* 1994;25:974–979.
48. Fried K, Govrin-Lippmann R, Devor M. Close apposition among neighboring axonal endings in a neuroma. *J Neurocytol* 1993;22(8): 663–681.
49. Fromm GH. Pathophysiology of trigeminal neuralgia. In: Fromm GH, Sessle B, eds. *Trigeminal neuralgia.* Boston: Butterworth, 1991: 105–130.
50. Fromm GH, Terrence CF, Maroon JC. Trigeminal neuralgia. Current concepts regarding etiology and pathogenesis. *Arch Neurol* 1984;41:1204–1207.
51. Fukushima T, Kerr FWL. Organization of trigeminothalamic tracts and other thalamic afferent systems of the brainstem in the rat: presence of gelatinosa neurons with thalamic connections. *J Comp Neurol* 1979;183:169–184.
52. Gamse R, Holzer P, Lembeck F. Decrease of substance P in primary afferent neurones and impairment of neurogenic plasma extravasation by capsaicin. *Br J Pharmacol* 1980;68:207–213.
53. Gibbins IL, Furness JB, Costa M, MacIntyre I, Hillyard CJ, Girgis S. Co-localization of calcitonin gene-related peptide-like immunoreactivity with substance P in cutaneous, vascular and visceral sensory neurons of guinea pigs. *Neurosci Lett* 1985;57:125–130.
54. Gibbins IL, Morris JL, Furness JB, Costa M. Innervation of systemic blood vessels. In: Burnstock G, Griffith SG, eds. *Nonadrenergic innervation of blood vessels, vol. II.* Boca Raton, FL: CRC Press, 1988:1–36.
55. Gillette RG, Kramis RC, Roberts WJ. Characterization of spinal somatosensory neurons having receptive fields in lumbar tissues of cats. *Pain* 1993;54:85–98.
56. Goadsby PJ, Edvinsson L. Sumatriptan reverses the changes in calcitonin gene related peptide seen in the headache phase of migraine. *Cephalalgia* 1991;11:3–4.
57. Goadsby PJ, Edvinsson L. The trigeminovascular system and migraine: studies characterizing cerebrovascular and neuropeptide changes seen in humans and cats. *Ann Neurol* 1993;33:48–56.
58. Goadsby PJ, Edvinsson L, Ekman R. Release of vasoactive peptides in the extracerebral circulation of humans and the cat during activation of the trigeminovascular system. *Ann Neurol* 1988; 23:193–196.
59. Gobel S. Principles of organization in the substantia gelatinosa layer of the spinal trigeminal nucleus. In: Bonica JJ, Albe-Fessard D, eds. *Advances in pain research and therapy.* New York: Raven Press, 1976:165–170.
60. Gobel S, Purvis MB. Anatomical studies of the organization of the spinal V nucleus: the deep bundles and the spinal V tract. *Brain Res* 1972;48:27–44.
61. Gregg JM. Neurological disorders of the maxillofacial region. In: Kruger GO, ed. *Textbook of oral and maxillofacial surgery.* St. Louis: CV Mosby, 1979:666–710.
62. Gudmundsson K, Rhoton AL Jr, Rushton JG. Detailed anatomy of the intracranial portion of the trigeminal nerve. *J Neurosurg* 1971;35:592.
63. Gulbenkian S, Merighi A, Wharton J, Varndell IM, Polak JM. Ultrastructural evidence for the coexistence of calcitonin gene-related peptide and substance P in secretory vesicles of peripheral nerves in the guinea pig. *J Neurocytol* 1986;15:535–542.
64. Hamba M, Hisamitsu H, Muro M. Wind-up of tooth pulp-evoked responses and its suppression in rat trigeminal caudalis neurons. *Brain Res Bull* 1992;29:883–889.
65. Hamel E, Bouchard D. Contractile 5-HT_1 receptors in human isolated pail arterioles: correlation with 5-HT_{1D} binding sites. *Br J Pharmacol* 1991;102:227–233.
66. Hamel E, Fan E, Linville D, Ting V, Villemure J-G, Chia L-S. Expression of mRNA for the serotonin -hydroxytriptamine-1D-receptor subtype in human and bovine cerebral arteries. *Mol Pharmacol* 1993;44:242–246.
67. Harris W. Alcohol injection of the gasserian ganglion for migrainous neuralgia. *Lancet* 1940;2:481–482.
68. Hayashi H. Distribution of vibrissae afferent fiber collaterals in the trigeminal nuclei as revealed by intra-axonal injection of horseradish peroxidase. *Brain Res* 1980;183:442–446.
69. Haynes WG. Surgical treatment of intractable unilateral cephalgia. *JAMA* 1948;136:538–541.
70. Häbler H-J, Jänig W, Koltzenburg M. Dichotomizing unmyelinated afferents supplying pelvic viscera and perineum are rare in the sacral segments of the cat. *Neurosci Lett* 1988;94:119–124.
71. Hering R, Kuritzky A. Sodium valproate in the prophylactic treatment of migraine: a double-blind study versus placebo. *Cephalalgia* 1992;12:81–84.
72. Hering R, Steiner TJ. Sodium valproate in the treatment of acute migraine attacks. In: *Abstracts of the 6th International Headache Conference.* 1993.
73. Holzer P. Local effector functions of capsaicin-sensitive sensory nerve endings: involvement of tachykinins, calcitonin gene-related peptide and other neuropeptides. *Neuroscience* 1988;24: 739–768.
74. Holzer P. Capsaicin: cellular targets, mechanisms of action, and selectivity for thin sensory neurons. *Pharmacol Rev* 1995;43: 143–201.
75. Howe JF, Calvin WH, Loeser JD. impulses reflected from dorsal root ganglia and from focal nerve injuries. *Brain Res* 1976;116: 139–144.
76. Howe JF, Loeser JD, Calvin WH. Mechanosensitivity of dorsal root ganglia and chronically injured axons: a physiological basis

for the radicular pain of nerve root compression. *Pain* 1977;3: 25–41.
77. Imamura J, Saunders MC, Keller JT. Projections of cervical nerves to the rat medulla. *Neurosci Lett* 1986;70:46–51.
78. Iwata K, Kenshalo DR, Dubner R, Nahin RL. Diencephalic projections from the superficial and deep laminae of the medullary dorsal horn in the rat. *J Comp Neurol* 1992;321:404–420.
79. Jancso N, Janscó-Gábor A, Szolcsányi J. Direct evidence for neurogenic inflammation and its prevention by denervation and by pretreatment with capsaicin. *Br J Pharmacol Chemother* 1967;31: 138–151.
80. Jannetta PJ, Rand RW. Transtentorial retrogasserian rhizotomy in trigeminal neuralgia. In: Rand RW, ed. *Microsurgery*. St. Louis: Mosby, 1969:156–169.
81. Jensen R, Brinck T, Oleson J. Sodium valproate has a prophylactic effect in migraine without aura: a triple-blinded, placebo controlled crossover study. *Neurology* 1994;44:647–651.
82. Jensen R, Rasmussen BK, Pedersen B, Olesen J. Muscle tenderness and pressure pain thresholds in headache. A population study. *Pain* 1993;52:193–199.
83. Johnson R. The radix mesencephalica trigemini. *J Comp Neurol* 1909;19:593.
84. Kanaka R, Schaible HG, Schmidt RF. Activation of fine articular afferent units by bradykinin. *Brain Res* 1985;327:81–90.
85. Kapadia SE, LaMotte CC. Deafferentation-induced alterations in the rat dorsal horn: I. comparison of peripheral nerve injury vs. rhizotomy effects on presynaptic, postsynaptic, and glial processes. *J Comp Neurol* 1987;266:183–187.
86. Kaube H, Keay KA, Hoskin KL, Bandler R, Goadsby PJ. Stimulation of the superior saggital sinus in the cat evokes c-fos expression in the caudal medulla and upper cervical spinal cord. *Cephalalgia* 1993;13:S118.
87. Keller JT, Beduk A, Saunders MC. Origin of fibers innervating the basilar artery of the cat. *Neurosci Lett* 1985;58:263–268.
88. Keller JT, Marfurt CF. Peptidergic and seratoninergic innervation of the rat dura mater. *J Comp Neurol* 1991;309:515–534.
89. Keller JT, Saunders MC, Beduk A, Jollis JG. Innervation of the posterior fossa dura of the cat. *Brain Res Bull* 1985;14:97–102.
90. Kenins P. Identification of the unmyelinated sensory nerves which evoke plasma extravasation in response to antidromic stimulation. *Neurosci Lett* 1981;25:137–141.
91. Kenins P, Hurley JV, Bell C. The role of substance P in the axon reflex in the rat. *Br J Dermatol* 1984;111:551–559.
92. Kerr FWL. The divisional organization of afferent fibers of the trigeminal nerve. *Brain* 1963;86:721–732.
93. Kerr FWL. Somatotopic organization of the trigeminal ganglion neurones. *Arch Neurol* 1964;11:593–602.
94. Kerr FWL, Kruger L, Schwassmann HO, Stern R. Somatotopic organizaton of mechanoreceptor units in the trigeminal complex of the macaque. *J Comp Neurol* 1968;34:127–144.
95. Kerr FWL, Olafson RA. Trigeminal and cervical volleys, convergence on single units in the spinal gray at C-1 and C-2. *Arch Neurol* 1961;5:171–178.
96. Khayyat GF, Yu YJ, King RB. Response patterns to noxious and nonnoxious stimuli in rostral trigeminal relay nuclei. *Brain Res* 1975; 97:47–60.
97. Kimmel DL. Innervation of the spinal dura mater and dura mater of the posterior cranial fossa. *Neurology* 1961;11:800–809.
98. Kozubski W, Sokolowski P. Sodium valproate vs. ergot derivatives in acute treatment of migraine attacks. In: *Abstracts of the 10th Migraine Trust International Symposium*. London, 1994.
99. Kruger L, Silverman JD, Mantyh PW, Sternini C, Brecha NC. Peripheral patterns of calcitonin-gene-related peptide general somatic sensory innervation: cutaneous and deep terminations. *J Comp Neurol* 1989;280:291–302.
100. Kruger L, Young RF. Specialized features of the trigeminal nerve and its central connections. In: Samii M, Jannetta PJ, eds. *The cranial nerves*. New York: Springer, 1981:273–301.
101. Lee WS, Limmroth V, Ayata C, et al. Peripheral GABAA receptor mediated effects of sodium valproate on dural plasma extravasation to substance P and trigeminal stimulation. *Br J Pharmacol* 1995; 116:1661–1667.
102. Lee Y, Takami K, Kawai Y, et al. Distribution of calcitonin gene-related peptide in the rat peripheral nervous system with reference to its coexistence with substance P. *Neuroscience* 1985;15:1227–1237.
103. LeGreves P, Nyberg F, Terenius L, Hökfelt T. Calcitonin gene-related peptide is a potent inhibitor of substance P degradation. *Eur J Pharmacol* 1985;115:309–311.
104. Lewis T. The nocifensor system of nerves and its reactions. *BMJ* 1937;1:431–435,491–494.
105. Light AR, Perl ER. Reexamination of the dorsal root projection to the spinal dorsal horn including observations on the differential termination of coarse and fine fibers. *J Comp Neurol* 1979;186: 117–131.
106. Light AR, Perl ER. Spinal termination of functionally identified primary afferent neurons with slowly conducting myelinated fibers. *J Comp Neurol* 1979;186:133–150.
107. Linet MS, Stewart WF. The epidemiology of migraine headache. In: Blau JN, ed. *Migraine: clinical, therapeutic, conceptual and research aspects*. London: Chapman and Hall, 1987:451–477.
108. Liu-Chen L-Y, Mayberg MR, Moskowitz MA. Immunohistochemical evdence for a substance P–containing trigeminovascular pathway to pial arteries in cats. *Brain Res* 1983;268:162–166.
109. Liu-Chen LY, Han DH, Moskowitz MA. Pia arachnoid contains substance P originating from trigeminal neurons. *Neuroscience* 1983; 9:803–808.
110. Maixner W, Dubner R, Kenshalo DRJ, Bushnell MC, Oliveras JL. Responses of monkey medullary dorsal horn neurons during the detection of noxious heat stimuli. *J Neurophysiol* 1989;62:437–449.
111. Markowitz S, Saito K, Moskowitz MA. Neuorgenically mediated leakage of plasma protein occurs from blood vessels in dura mater but not brain. *J Neurosci* 1987;7:4129–4136.
112. Matsubara T, Moskowitz MA, Byun B. CP-93,129, a potent and selective 5-$HT_{1\beta}$ receptor agonist blocks neurogenic plasma extravasation within rat but not guinea pig dura mater. *Br J Pharmacol* 1991;104:3–4.
113. Mayberg M, Langer RS, Zervas NT, Moskowitz MA. Perivascular meningeal projections from cat trigeminal ganglia: possible pathway for vascular headaches in man. *Science* 1981;213:228–230.
114. Mayberg MR, Zervas NT, Moskowitz MA. Trigeminal projections to supratentorial pial and dural blood vessels in cats demonstrated by horseradish peroxidase histochemistry. *J Comp Neurol* 1984;223:46–56.
115. McGrath PA, Gracely RH, Dubner R, Heft MW. Non-pain and pain sensations evoked by tooth pulp stimulation. *Pain* 1983;15:377–388.
116. McMahon MS, Norregaard TV, Beyerl BD, Borges LF, Moskowitz MA. Trigeminal afferents to cerebral arteries and forehead are not divergent axon collaterals in cat. *Neurosci Lett* 1985;60:63–68.
117. Mense S. Nociception from skeletal muscle in relation to clinical pain. *APS Journal* 1993;54:241–289.
118. Mense S. Referral of muscle pain: new aspects. *APS J* 1994;3:1–9.
119. Meyer RA, Davis KD, Cohen RH, Treede R-D, Campbell JN. Mechanically insensitive afferents (MIAs) in cutaneous nerves of monkey. *Brain Res* 1991;561:252–261.
120. Messlinger K, Hanesch U, Baumgärtel M, Trost B, Schmidt RF. Innervation of the dura mater encephali of cat and rat: ultrastructure and calcitonin gene-related peptide-like and substance P-like immunoreactivity. *Anat Embryol* 1993;188:219–273.
121. Moskowitz MA. The neurobiology of vascular head pain. *Ann Neurol* 1984;16:157–168.
122. Moskowitz MA. Neurogenic versus vascular mechanisms of sumaptrin and ergot alkaloids in migraine. *Trends Pharmacol Sci* 1992;13: 307–311.
123. Moskowitz MA. Neurogenic inflammation in the pathophysiology and treatment of migraine. *Neurology* 1993;43:S16–S20.
124. Moskowitz MA. Drug mechanisms in acute migraine. In: Gebhart GF, Hammond DL, Jensen TS, eds. *Progress in pain research and management*. Seattle: IASP Press, 1994:755–764.
125. Moskowitz MA, Waeber C. The 5-HT_{1D} receptor subtype and migraine headache. In: Municio AM, Miras-Portugal MT, eds. *Cell transduction, second messengers, and protein phosphorylation in health and disease*. New York: Plenum Press, 1994:199–204.
126. Nakamura Craig M, Gill BK. Effect of neurokinin A, substance P and calcitonin gene related peptide in peripheral hyperalgesia in the rat paw. *Neurosci Lett* 1991;124:49–51.
127. Nozaki K, Boccalini P, Moskowitz MA. Expression of c-fos immunoreactivity in brainstem after meningeal irritation by blood in the subarachnoid space. *Neuroscience* 1992;49:669–680.
128. Nozaki K, Moskowitz MA, Boccalini P. CP-93,129, sumatriptan, dihydroergotamine block c-*fos* expression within rat trigeminal nucleus caudalis caused by chemical stimulation of the meninges. *Br J Pharmacol* 1992;106:409–415.
129. Nozaki K, Uemura Y, Okamoto S, Kikuchi H, Mizuno N. Origins and distribution of cerebrovascular nerve fibers showing calcitonin gene-related peptide-like immunoreactivity in the major cerebral artery of the dog. *J Comp Neurol* 1990;297:219–226.

130. Oku R, Satoh M, Fujii N, Otaka A, Yajima H, Takagi H. Calcitonin gene-related peptide promotes mechanical nociception by potentiating release of substance P from the spinal dorsal horn in rats. *Brain Res* 1987;403:350–354.
131. Oleson J. Cerebral blood flow in migraine with aura. *Pathol Biol* 1992;40:318–324.
132. Oleson J, Bonica JJ. Headache. In: Bonica JJ, ed. *The management of pain.* Philadelphia: Lea & Fibiger, 1990:687–726.
133. Olivecrona H. Notes on the surgical treatment of migraine. *Acta Med Scand* 1947;196:229–238.
134. Oliveras JL, Maixner W, Dubner R, et al. The medullary dorsal horn: a target for the expression of opiate effects on the perceived intensity of noxious heat. *J Neurosci* 1986;6:3086–3093.
135. Olszewski J. On the anatomical and functional organization of the spinal trigeminal nucleus. *J Comp Neurol* 1950;92:401–413.
136. Ohlen A, Lindbom L, Staines W, et al. Substance P and calcitonin gene-related peptide: immunohistochemical localisation and microvascular effects in rabbit skeletal muscle. *Naunyn Schmiedebergs Arch Pharmacol* 1987;336:87–93.
137. Penfield W. Operative treatment of migraine and observations on the mechanism of vascular pain. *Trans Am Acad Opthamol Otolaryngol* 1932;37:67.
138. Penfield W, McNaughton F. Dural headache and innervation of the dura mater. *Arch Neurol Psychiatry* 1940;44:43–75.
139. Perl ER. Mode of action of nociceptors. In: Hirsch C, Zotterman Y, eds. *Cervical pain.* Oxford: Pergamon Press, 1972:157–164.
140. Pickering GW. Observations on the mechanism of headache produced by histamine. *Clin Sci* 1933;1:77–101.
141. Pickoff H. Is the muscular model of headache still viable? A review of conflicting data. *Headache* 1984;24:186–198.
142. Pierau FK, Fellmer G, Taylor DC. Somato-visceral convergence in cat dorsal root ganglion neurones demonstrated by double-labelling with fluorescent tracers. *Brain Res* 1984;321:63–70.
143. Pierau FK, Taylor DCM, Abel W, Friedrich B. Dichotomizing peripheral fibers revealed by intracellular recording from rat sensory neurones. *Neurosci Lett* 1982;31:123–128.
144. Pomeranz B, Wall PD, Weber WV. Cord cells responding to fine myelinated afferents from viscera, muscle, and skin. *J Physiol (Lond)* 1968;199:511–532.
145. Price DD, Dubner R, Hu JW. Trigeminothalamic neurons in nucleus caudalis responsive to tactile, thermal, and nociceptive stimulation of monkey's face. *J Neurophysiol* 1976;39:936–953.
146. Raja SN, Meyer RA, Campbell JN. Peripheral mechanisms of somatic pain. *Anesthesiology* 1988;68:571–590.
147. Ranson SW. Cutaneous sensory fibers and sensory conduction. *Arch Neurol Psychiatry* 1931;26:1122–1144.
148. Ray BS, Wolff HG. Experimental studies on headache. *Arch Surg* 1940;41:813–856.
149. Rebeck GW, Maynard KI, Hyman BT, Moskowitz MA. Selective 5-HT_{1D} alpha serotonin receptor gene expression in trigeminal ganglia: Implications for antimigraine drug development. *Proc Natl Acad Sci USA* 1994;91:3666–3669.
150. Rozsa AJ, Beuerman RW. Density and organization of free nerve endings in the corneal epithelium of the rabbit. *Pain* 1982;14:105–120.
151. Ruch TC. Visceral sensation and referred pain. In: Fulton JF, ed. *Howell's textbook of physiology.* 15th ed. Philadelphia: WB Saunders, 1946:385–401.
152. Rushton JG, Stevens JC, Miller RH. Glossopharyngeal (vagoglossopharyngeal) neuralgia: a study of 217 cases. *Arch Neurol* 1981;38:201–205.
153. Saito K, Markowitz S, Moskowitz MA. Ergot alkaloids block neurogenic extravasation in dura mater: proposed action in vascular headaches. *Ann Neurol* 1988;24:732–737.
154. Saito K, Moskowitz MA. Contributions from the upper cervical dorsal roots and trigeminal ganglia to the feline circle of Willis. *Stroke* 1989;20:524–526.
155. Saria A, Gamse R, Petermann J, Fischer JA, Theodorsson-Norheim E, Lundberg JM. Simultaneous release of several tachykinins and calcitonin gene related peptide from rat spinal cord slices. *Neurosci Lett* 1986;63:310–314.
156. Schaible HG, Grubb BD. Afferent and spinal mechanisms of joint pain. *Pain* 1993;55:5–54.
157. Schaible HG, Schmidt RF, Willis WD. Convergent inputs from articular, cutaneous and muscle receptors onto ascending tract cells in the cat spinal cord. *Exp Brain Res* 1987;66:479–488.
158. Schoenen J, Noordhout AM. Headache. In: Melzack R, Wall P, eds. *Textbook of pain.* London: Churchill Livingstone, 1994:495–521.
159. Scibetta BJ, King RB. Hyperpolarizing influence of trigeminal nucleus caudalis on primary afferent preterminals in trigeminal nucleus oralis. *J Neurophysiol* 1969;32:229–238.
160. Selby G. Diseases of the fifth cranial nerve. In: Dyck PJ, ed. *Peripheral neuropathy.* Philadelphia: WB Saunders, 1984:1224–1265.
161. Sessle BJ, Hu JW, Amano N, Zhong G. Convergence of cutaneous, tooth pulp, visceral, neck and muscle afferents onto nociceptive and non-nociceptive neurones in trigeminal subnucleus caudalis (medularry dorsal horn) and its implications for referred pain. *Pain* 1986;27:219–235.
162. Silverman JD, Kruger L. Calcitonin-gene-related-peptide-immunoreactive innervation of the rat head with emphasis on specialized sensory structures. *J Comp Neurol* 1989;280:303–330.
163. Sivilotti L, Woolf CJ. The contribution of GABAA and glycine receptors to central sensitization: disinhibition and touch-evoked allodynia in the spinal cord. *J Neurophysiol* 1994;72:169–179.
164. Sjoqvist O. Studies on pain conduction of the trigeminal nerve. *Acta Psychiatr Neurol Scand* 1938;17:1–139.
165. Steiger HJ, Tew JM, Keller JT. The sensory representation of the dura mater in the trigeminal ganglion of the cat. *Neurosci Lett* 1982;31:231–236.
166. Strassman A, Mason P, Moskowitz MA, Maciewitz R. Response of brainstem trigeminal neurons to electrical stimulation of the dura. *Brain Res* 1986;379:242–250.
167. Strassman AM, Potrebic S, Maciewicz RJ. Anatomical properties of brainstem trigeminal neurons that respond to electrical stimulation of dural blood vessels. *J Comp Neurol* 1994;346:349–365.
168. Sugimoto T, Bennett GJ, Kajander KC. Strychnine-enhanced transsynaptic degeneration of dorsal horn neurons in rats with an experimental painful peripheral neuropathy. *Neurosci Lett* 1989;98:139–143.
169. Taylor JR, Finch P. Acute injury of the neck: anatomical and pathological basis of pain. *Ann Acad Med Singapore* 1993;22:187–192.
170. Tew JM. Treatment of pain of glossopharyngeal and vagus nerves by percutaneous neurolysis. In: Youmanns J, ed. *Neurological surgery.* Philadelphia: WB Saunders, 1982:3609–3612.
171. Thomas DA, Anton F, Kenshalo DRJ, Williams GM, Dubner R. Noradrenergic and opiod systems interact to alter the detection of noxious thermal stimuli and facial scratching in monkeys. *Pain* 1993;55:63–70.
172. Tiwari RK, King RB. Fiber projections from trigeminal nucleus caudalis in primate (squirrel monkey and baboon). *J Comp Neurol* 1974;158:191–206.
173. Torvik A. Afferent connections to the sensory trigeminal nuclei, the nucleus of the trigeminal tract. *J Comp Neurol* 1956;106:51–141.
174. Tsai SH, Tew JM, McLean JH, Shipley MT. Cerebral arterial innervation by nerve fibers containing calcitonin gene-related peptide (CGRP): I. Distribution and origin of CGRP perivascular innervation in the rat. *J Comp Neurol* 1988;271:435–444.
175. Uhl GR, Walther D, Nishimori T, Buzzi MG, Moskowitz MA. Jun B, c-jun, jun D and c-fos mRNAs in nucleus caudalis neurons: rapid selective enhancement by afferent stimulation. *Brain Res Mol Brain Res* 1991;11:133–141.
176. Vernon H, Steiman I, Hagino C. Cervicogenic dysfunction in muscle contraction headache and migraine: a descriptive study. *J Manip Physiol Ther* 1992;15:418–429.
177. Wall PD, Devor M. Sensory afferent impulses originate from dorsal root ganglia as well as from the periphery in normal and nerve injured rats. *Pain* 1983;17:321–339.
178. Weinshank RL, Zgombick JM, Macchi MJ, Branchek TA, Hartig PR. Human seratonin 1D receptor is encoded by a subfamily of wo distinct genes: 5-$HT_{1D\alpha}$ and 5-$HT_{1D\beta}$. *Proc Natl Acad Sci USA* 1992;89:3630–3634.
179. Weinstein S. Intensive and extensive aspects of tactile sensitivity as a function of body part, sex and laterality. In: Kenshalo D, ed. *The skin senses.* Springfield, IL: Charles C. Thomas, 1968:195–219.
180. Wharton J, Gulbenkian S, Bloom SR, Polak JM. The capsaicin sensitive (afferent) innervation of the guinea pig cardiovascular system contains both calcitonin gene-related peptide (CGRP) and substance P (SP). *Neurosci Lett* 1985;S22:S86.
181. White WJ, Field KJ. Anesthesia and surgery of laboratory animals. *Vet Clin North Am Small Anim Pract* 1987;17:989–1017.
182. Wilson-Pauwels L, Akesson EJ, Stewart PA. *Cranial nerves.* Toronto: B.C. Decker, 1988.
183. Wirth FP Jr, Van Buren M. Referral of pain from dural stimulation in man. *J Neurosurg* 1971;34:630–642.
184. Wolff HG. *Headache and other head pain.* New York: Oxford University Press, 1972.

185. Yaksh TL. Behavioral and autonomic correlates of the tactile evoked allodynia produced by spinal glycine inhibition: effects of modulatory receptor systems and excitatory amino acid antagonists. *Pain* 1989;37:111–123.
186. Yokota T, Nishikawa N, Nishikawa Y. Effects of strychnine upon different classes of trigeminal subnucleus caudalis neurons. *Brain Res* 1979;168:430–434.
187. Young RF. Fiber spectrum of the trigeminal sensory root of the frog, cat and man determined by electron microscopy. In: Anderson DJ, Matthews B, eds. *Pain in the trigeminal region.* New York: Elsevier, 1977:137–147.
188. Young RF. Unmyelinated fibers in the trigeminal motor root. Possible relationship to the results of trigeminal rhizotomy. *J Neurosurg* 1978;49:538–543.
189. Zander E, Weddell G. Observations on the innervation of the cornea. *J Anat* 1951;85:68–99.

Anesthesia: Biologic Foundations, edited by
Tony L. Yaksh et al. Lippincott–Raven Publishers,
Philadelphia © 1997.

CHAPTER 54

DIABETIC NEUROPATHY

RAYAZ A. MALIK AND NIGEL A. CALCUTT

Long-term changes in neural function following changes in the ability to mobilize blood glucose have been long appreciated. Indeed, we consider diabetes to be the most frequent cause of peripheral neuropathy in the Western world. In the present chapter, we consider the presentation and the hypothesized etiology of the disorder.

CLINICAL PRESENTATION OF DIABETIC NEUROPATHY

Diabetes is a commonly occurring metabolic disorder that may be broadly divided into insulin-dependent (type 1) or insulin-independent (type 2) syndromes. There are a variety of complications associated with both types of diabetes including retinopathy, micro- and macroangiopathy, nephropathy, and neuropathy. Diabetic neuropathy may typically present as either a diffuse symmetric polyneuropathy or as a focal or multifocal neuropathy. Abnormal sensations, including pain, are described in all types of diabetic neuropathy, and pain often represents the major clinical complaint (91).

DIFFUSE SYMMETRIC POLYNEUROPATHY

Pain is a common symptom in patients with diffuse distal sensory polyneuropathy and occurs most frequently in the feet and legs. The pain is characterized by a deep-seated aching with superimposed lancinating stabs or burning sensations which are particularly troublesome at night. The onset of pain is insidious and, once established, is often irreversible (141).

A transient, probably metabolic, neuropathy often referred to as hyperglycemic neuropathy, can occur in either newly diagnosed insulin-dependent diabetic patients with a period of unrecognized and significant hyperglycemia or in diabetic patients with poor metabolic control (126). This form is characterized by superficial sensory symptoms, principally paresthesiae with occasional dysaesthesia, along with a modest reduction in nerve conduction velocity and resistance to ischaemic conduction failure. All of these symptoms generally resolve after establishment of normoglycemia.

The converse of hyperglycemic neuropathy is insulin neuritis, an acute and severe painful neuropathy that develops after institution of strict glycemic control following a period of poor glycemic control (63). A similar condition has been reported in young diabetic girls with weight loss due to anorexia nervosa (118). Both of these conditions appear similar to the syndrome of "diabetic cachexia" (45), which also exhibits an acute painful neuropathy.

A distinct and extremely troublesome variant termed acute painful neuropathy has been described in a small group of male diabetic patients (5). This condition was associated with precipitous weight loss and presented with severe lancinating pain in the feet and cutaneous hyperalgesia with nocturnal exacerbation. Though highly unpleasant, there was only a relatively mild neuropathy as indicated by preservation of motor function, occasional loss of ankle jerks, and dissociated sensory loss. Quantitative sensory testing demonstrated a principally small-fiber neuropathy with loss of thermal perception and preservation of vibration sense. The outlook for this neuropathy is good as the symptoms resolved in all but one patient over ~6 months following improved glycemic control and weight gain and did so without any residual neurological deficits.

A group of young insulin-dependent diabetic patients have recently been described who developed a severe early onset polyneuropathy characterized by distal paresthesiae and, in one case, dysesthesiae over the anterior trunk (105). All patients had severe symptoms indicating autonomic involvement and quantitative testing confirmed a severe peripheral and autonomic neuropathy. Clinical examination showed dissociated sensory loss and a predominantly small-fiber deficit producing an impairment of pain and temperature sensation with relative preservation of large fiber function in the form of normal touch, vibration and position sense.

FOCAL AND MULTIFOCAL NEUROPATHY

These neuropathies generally occur in older diabetic patients and, though particularly troublesome with regard to painful symptoms, have a good outlook with almost complete recovery over ~12 months (6). Focal lesions that affect limb nerves may be associated with pain in the nerve distribution or may produce painful symptoms attributed to the carpal and cubital tunnel syndromes and meralgia paresthetica involving the median, ulnar and lateral cutaneous nerve of the thigh respectively. Oculomotor nerve palsy usually presents with pain behind and above the eye, which precedes ptosis and diplopia by several days (7,144). Deficits reach their nadir within 2–3 days, persist for several weeks and gradually resolve over 3–5 months. Proximal motor neuropathy, formerly known as diabetic amyotrophy, can be extremely painful in the thigh, buttocks, and perineum, with severe nocturnal exacerbation (50). This syndrome is associated with asymmetric loss of the patellar reflex, neurogenic atrophy, and subsequent wasting of the thigh. Generally, the patient makes a slow recovery over 12–15 months with complete remission of painful symptoms, although some neurological disability remained in nearly half of patients studied (104).

Truncal mononeuropathy presents with an acute onset of a girdlelike pain radiating around the chest or abdomen which is described as a deep, aching, or boring pain but may also be jabbing, burning, or tearing with nocturnal exacerbation and significant weight loss (63). This is accompanied by hyperpathia and hyperesthesia to pinprick over the affected area with occasional focal paralysis of the abdominal wall (10) and denervation of paraspinous muscles. The prognosis is generally good with recovery from painful symptoms usually occurring within a few months, although in a few cases it may take as long as 2 years.

POTENTIAL MECHANISMS

Although the precise etiology of pain in human diabetic neuropathy is unclear, both peripheral and central mechanisms are assumed to play an important role. The potential contribution of changes in the peripheral nerves have been most widely studied, largely due to the incomplete accessibility and understanding of the pathophysiology of pain in the central nervous system.

Abnormal Plasma Glucose

Diabetes is characterized by aberrant glucose regulation, and it has been suggested that glucose levels per se may influence nociception. Both diabetic and nondiabetic patients infused with glucose develop a lower-stimulus threshold and tolerance of pain when compared to nondiabetic normoglycemic patients (95). However, others were unable to confirm the observation that acute hyperglycemia influences the heat pain threshold in diabetic patients and painful episodes in these patients were not associated with elevated blood sugar levels (27). Hypoglycemia can also produce painful symptoms and the neuropathy associated with an insulinoma is painful (126). Thus, wide fluctuations in the glycemic state of poorly controlled diabetics may expose nerves to both hypo- and hyperglycemic episodes capable of inducing pain. An abnormal lowering of the nociceptive threshold, thereby evoking pain in response to normal physicochemical stimulation, may also be the basis of chronic hyperalgesia in some of the focal neuropathies (130). Nevertheless, simple changes in glucose levels do not appear to be solely responsible for many of the characteristics of painful diabetic neuropathy.

Axonal Atrophy, Degeneration, and Regeneration

The pathology of diabetic neuropathy involves segmental demyelination, axonal atrophy and a progressive fiber degeneration with the subsequent appearance of clusters of regenerating fibers. All of these abnormalities have the potential to be involved in the generation of pain, although the current understanding of the contribution of each is limited.

Atrophy

Reduced axonal calibre may initiate changes in the temporal patterning of impulses, thereby altering normal sensation and producing pain sensations. One study has reported an association between axonal atrophy and pain in neuropathic diabetics (14), but this is balanced by two other studies that failed to demonstrate axonal atrophy in biopsies from patients with painful diabetic neuropathy (77,120).

Degeneration

Axonal degeneration may contribute to the generation of pain in diabetics (43) as degeneration arising from physical nerve injury is associated with a variety of other neuropathic pain states (see Chapters 55 and 56). However, two recent studies comparing diabetic patients with and without painful neuropathy failed to find a relationship between active fiber degeneration and painful neuropathy (14,77).

Regeneration

Ectopic impulse generation from regenerating small myelinated and unmyelinated axons has been proposed as a mechanism of pain generation in neuroma after sciatic nerve section in rats (see Chapter 32). Sural nerve biopsies from a range of painful neuropathies demonstrate damage principally to the Aδ and C fibers, whereas those neuropathies with large fiber damage do not generally manifest pain (125). Brown et al. (16) assessed sural nerve morphometry in three diabetic patients with an acute painful neuropathy and reported a significant degree of small-fiber regeneration in the form of unmyelinated fiber sprouts. From this data they proposed that painful diabetic neuropathy was a small-fiber neuropathy with the pain sensations arising from ectopic discharges emanating from regenerating unmyelinated fibers. The report of regenerative clusters in the sural nerve of a young female who developed an acute painful neuropathy following continuous subcutaneous insulin therapy was consistent with this proposal (78). The hypothesis was extended by the suggestion that more effective fiber regeneration may initiate pain in patients with painful sensory neuropathy (14,15), and a study of proximal nerve from patients with proximal motor neuropathy demonstrated more regenerative activity in those patients with more severe symptoms (104). A mechanism by which regeneration may be associated with ectopic activity is suggested by the observation of a correlation between plasma noradrenaline levels and the severity of pain in patients with diabetic neuropathy (131). Regenerating nociceptive afferents may develop ectopic adrenergic sensitivity which, in the presence of raised levels of neurotransmitter released locally by damaged sympathetic axons, could potentially produce pain somewhat analogous to reflex sympathetic dystrophy (see Chapter 28). However, the association between regenerative activity and pain is not clear, and a number of studies have reported that unmyelinated fiber regeneration is a characteristic of both painful and painless diabetic neuropathy and that there appears to be no relationship between the degree of regeneration of both myelinated and unmyelinated sural nerve fibers and pain (14,15,77,79).

It is clear that there is no simple association between the physiologic, biochemical, and structural abnormalities of nerves of diabetic patients and the presence and type of pain experienced. Human studies are obviously limited by practical and ethical considerations, and investigators have turned to animal models of diabetes in order to investigate potential mechanisms.

PRECLINICAL MODELS OF DIABETES MELLITUS

Spontaneous hyperglycemia, arising from insulin deficiency or resistance, has been noted in many species and is a not infrequently reported disorder of aging domestic pets such as dogs and cats. Because of the need for large numbers of genetically homogeneous animals, rodents are most commonly used in experimental studies. The commercially available BB Wistar rat and NOD mouse provide models of spontaneously developing type 1 (insulin-deficient) diabetes, while there are also a number of rodent colonies that model spontaneous type 2 (insulin-independent) diabetes, such as the Zucker rat, the db/db mouse, and the ob/ob mouse. However, the majority of experimental studies have been performed using animals where diabetes is induced by surgical, dietary, or chemical means. Rodents are more frequently used to investigate the complications arising from hyperglycemia. The sand rat (*Psammomys obesus*) develops an obese diabetes when changed from a natural diet of low-calorific plants to a standard laboratory diet, and feeding normal rats and mice diets containing 20–40% galactose is used to selectively increase hexose sugar metabolism in the absence of insulin deficiency or increased blood glucose levels. Chemically induced diabetes is the most widely used animal model of type 1 diabetes. The injection of either streptozotocin or alloxan causes a rapid and selective destruction of the β cells of the pancreas, leading to insulin deficiency and profound hyperglycemia with blood glucose levels in the 20–40 mmol/L range. Such animals may survive for a period of weeks to months, particularly if supplemented with insulin to modulate the severity of hyperglycemia and protect muscle from extreme wasting.

There are a number of important caveats that must precede consideration of the sensory abnormalities present in diabetic animals. Most obviously, it is not possible to directly determine perception of pain in animals and investigators are restricted to the use of physiological indicators and behavioural responses as measurement end points. The animal models of diabetes available are also limited in their representation of the complications associated with human diabetes, particularly with regard to diabetic neuropathy. No fiber loss or overt pathology has been reported in the sciatic nerves of diabetic rodents

(110), which contrasts with the marked fiber degeneration that often accompanies sensory loss in neuropathic diabetic patients described above. However, this may be considered of benefit to experimental studies as degeneration of sensory fibers may be excluded from the potential mechanisms that underlie abnormalities of sensory function. The absence of marked pathologic changes in peripheral nerves of diabetic rats is likely to be due to the relatively short life span of such animals (1–2 years maximum with insulin therapy) compared to the many years that a patient may be diabetic before developing neuropathy. Thus, the studies performed in diabetic animals should be viewed as representing aspects of relatively acute and severe diabetes.

The majority of studies in humans and animals have focused on the sciatic nerve, which contains a mixed population of motor and sensory fibers. At present, there is little evidence to suggest that the widely reported and studied disorders of peripheral nerves, including reduced mean axonal calibre, accumulation of the polyol pathway metabolites sorbitol and fructose, myo-inositol depletion, reduced Na^+-K^+ ATPase activity and nerve ischaemia (129; and for review, see ref. 126) are selective for populations of sensory or motor axons. A number of disorders are, however, likely to have particular impact on sensory function.

Nerve Structure

A recent study has shown myelin-splitting in the spinal roots of long-term diabetic rats, which was qualitatively more notable in the dorsal versus the ventral roots (121). More subtle structural disorders are also present in sensory neurons within weeks of the onset of diabetes in rats. These include reduced neuronal cell volume in the dorsal root ganglion (DRG) that is associated with a decreased mean axonal calibre in the sciatic nerve (60,112). Axonal atrophy is presumed to arise from deficits in the slow axonal transport of cytoskeletal elements (90), reduced mRNA for cytoskeletal proteins in sensory cell bodies (94), and possibly also the impairment of amino acid uptake by cell bodies in the DRG (127). Functional sensory nerve regeneration (44) after crush injury is impaired by diabetes and is accompanied by attenuated DRG cell body responses such as in the injury-induced induction of ornithine decarboxylase (89) and VIP (21).

Sensory Neurotransmitters

Changes in nerve structural proteins are accompanied by reduced levels of the sensory neuropeptides substance P and calcitonin gene-related peptide (CGRP) in the DRG and sciatic nerve (23,40,101,135). It is well established that nerve growth factor (NGF) regulates synthesis of these neuropeptides (76). Consequently, studies demonstrating reduced retrograde axonal transport of NGF (61), reduced NGF mRNA and protein in the peripheral target organs and nerves of diabetic rats (46,47,59) and that NGF treatment of diabetic rats restores nerve neuropeptide levels (39) suggest that deficient neurotrophic support of sensory nerves may underlie the reduced neuropeptide levels. Reduced peripheral axonal transport of neuropeptides from the DRG may contribute to the impaired flare and weal response in skin (49) although reports of a concurrent increase in skin substance P content (49,117,135) may also indicate impaired neurotransmitter release. The central axonal transport of sensory neuropeptide from the DRG that would be involved in spinal nociceptive processing have not yet been studied, nor have the in vivo release properties of any neurotransmitters and modulators. However, there have been reports that K^+-evoked release of substance P from spinal cord slices of diabetic rats in vitro is enhanced rather than decreased (70), along with an increase in substance P binding sites (69). Whether any of the above contribute to the functional sensory disorders present in diabetic animals remains to be established.

Electrophysiology

The detection of reduced motor and sensory nerve conduction velocities within weeks of the onset of chemically induced diabetes (93) has underpinned the use of rodents to model diabetic neuropathy because similar disorders are often present in newly diagnosed diabetic patients (133) and may be predictive for the future onset of more overt neuropathy (42). In patients, aggressive insulin therapy rapidly restores conduction velocities to near normal (133), indicating a metabolic origin and the same is true in diabetic rats (54). The precise etiology of the disorder is not yet understood although the efficacy of inhibitors of the glucose-metabolizing enzyme aldose reductase in preventing or reversing nerve conduction deficits in diabetic rodents without altering plasma insulin or glucose levels implicates exaggerated flux through this enzyme and subsequent parts of the polyol pathway (129). Recent studies have also shown that levels of the Schwann cell–derived neurotrophic factor CNTF are reduced in the sciatic nerve of both diabetic and galactose-fed rats (22) and that ciliary neuronotrophic factor (CNTF) treatment prevents reduced sensory but not motor nerve conduction velocity in galactose-fed rats (92). However, as the deficit rarely exceeds a 10–15% decline in sensory nerve conduction velocity it is unlikely to contribute to other disorders of sensory function that may be equated to pain states.

As discussed above and elsewhere in this volume, ectopic discharges from primary afferents undergoing degeneration and regeneration may contribute to some of the painful symptoms of diabetic patients (16) (see Chapter 56). It is not easy to test this hypothesis in animals studies as the sciatic nerves of diabetic rodents show no obvious fiber degeneration or regeneration (110) and an initial report of increased spontaneous activity in C fibers of diabetic rats (17) has not been confirmed (2, 103). Single fiber studies in streptozocin-diabetic rats have demonstrated that while C fibers show no evidence of spontaneous activity or changes in the thresholds for thermal or mechanical stimulation, there is an enhanced afterdischarge following a sustained mechanical stimulus and increased firing following a sustained suprathreshold mechanical stimulus (2). Diabetic rats also had proportionately fewer thermally and mechanically insensitive C fibers than controls and more C fibers that responded to cold. In contrast, the only parameter of Aδ fibers that was altered by diabetes was a reduction in mechanical threshold and no changes were noted in the properties of Aβ fibers. Interestingly, while both nerves of diabetic patients (119) and animals (109) show a resistance to ischaemic conduction blockade, the sensory nerves are less likely to recover (108), indicating a greater susceptibility to ischaemic injury.

Nociceptive Thresholds

Acute, High-Threshold Stimuli

Diabetic patients may develop an increase in thermal perception and thermal pain perception thresholds in the presence (or absence) of a painful neuropathy (9). The equivalent studies in animals are those that have measured the response (licking or removing the afflicted limb) time to acute high-threshold thermal stimuli that incorporate a supraspinal component, such as the hot plate test. The literature is somewhat equivocal about the effect of diabetes on the hot plate responses of rats and mice, with reports of increased response times (3,8,20,29,51) being balanced by others showing no change (99,100) or a decrease (48). Where the tail flick test has been used to measure spinal nociceptive reflexes, diabetic rats are widely (34,73,74) but not always (4) reported to show reduced response times, whereas diabetic mice may exhibit reduced (99), increased (75) or unchanged response times (71,113).

The responses to high-threshold mechanical stimuli, as measured by the paw pressure (Randall-Selitto) and tail pinch tests have also been studied in diabetic rodents. There is general agreement that threshold values to the paw pressure test are reduced in both insulin-deficient and insulin-replete diabetic rats (1,33–35,136), with one exception (3). Reduced response times have also been reported to the tail pinch test in both diabetic rats (64, 69)and mice (66–68,71), although there is a report of an increased response time to tail pinch in diabetic mice (75). It is suggested that these behavioural indices of mechanical hyperalgesia may be related to the altered electrophysiologic properties of C and Aδ fibers in diabetic rats (2). However, it should be noted that the response thresholds in paw pressure tests are of the order of 100–400 g and that pinch tests also apply extreme mechanical force so that the relevance of these tests to painful neuropathy in diabetic patients is questionable.

Acute, Low-Threshold Stimuli

Concurrent with thermal hyperalgesia, 2–4 weeks of streptozotocin diabetes induces a thermal allodynia with rats responding to tail flick tests at temperatures (10°C and 42°C) that did not elicit a response in controls (34). Diabetic rats do not exhibit notable touch-evoked allodynia over their body or head. However, in tests using graded von Frey hairs to apply low-level (1–15 g force) mechanical pressure to the dorsal hindpaw (28), diabetic rats developed an allodynia that could be prevented or reversed by restoring normoglycemia by insulin treatment (18). Whether this corresponds to the touch-evoked allodynia that occurs in the hands and feet of some neuropathic diabetic patients remains to be established.

Prolonged Nociceptive Stimuli

The pain sensations described by neuropathic diabetic patients are often prolonged or continuous and vary from superficial paraesthesiae to deeper nerve and muscular pain (see above). However, the traditional tests of nociception are based on a short-lasting stimulus, often of high intensity, and exclude examination of stimulus-induced modulatory mechanisms that may occur in both the peripheral and central nervous systems. It is therefore also of interest to study the response to a prolonged nociceptive stimulus in diabetic animals in order to detect possible differences in modulatory mechanisms that could contribute to the prolonged or continuous pain experienced by some diabetic patients.

A commonly employed model of a prolonged nociceptive stimulus is the formalin test (41,97). The subcutaneous injection of a dilute formalin solution evokes a behavioural syndrome that may be divided into a transient flinching of the injected paw over the first 1–2 min after injection (phase 1), a period of quiescence (Q phase) during the following 20 min and then a second (phase 2) prominent and protracted phase of flinching. The first phase results from the acute activation of afferent Aβ, Aδ, and C fibers, whereas the second phase is believed to include peripheral inflammation and the prolonged activation of Aδ and C fibers together with increased sensitivity of spinal cord neurons (37,57,98) (see Chapter 9). Pharmacologic studies have suggested that there is amplification of the nociceptive input at the spinal level, involving glutaminergic *N*-methyl-D-aspartate (NMDA) and peptidergic neurokinin (NK-1) receptor activation (137,138), cyclooxygenase-mediated prostaglandin E_2 release (80,82) and nitric oxide production (81) (see Chapter 36). However, the response remains dependent on primary afferent activity (30, 38). Changes in behavioural responses to the formalin test have been reported in both diabetic rats and mice (34,65,83). In streptozocin-diabetic rats, an increased frequency of flinching of the formalin-injected paw is particularly notable during the normally silent Q phase (19,20,83). Whether this represents exaggerated and prolonged primary afferent activity, as noted after mechanical stimulation (2), changes in postsynaptic characteristics (69), impediments of descending inhibitory systems that may suppress activity during the Q phase (85) or other supraspinal mechanisms is not yet clear.

Experimental Therapies in Preclinical Models

A major goal of the study of pain mechanisms in animals is to enable assessment of potential therapeutic agents and a number of studies have attempted to normalize the aberrant nociceptive responses reported in diabetic rodents.

Glycemic Control

Insulin treatments that restore normoglycemia or attenuate hyperglycemia prevent abnormalities in the hot plate (regarding increased response time in streptozocin-diabetic rats, see ref. 29) and tail flick (regarding reduced response time in streptozocin, alloxan, and BB Wistar diabetic rats, see refs. 73 and 74) tests. Intensive insulin treatment from the onset of diabetes also prevents touch-evoked allodynia and increased activity during the Q phase of the formalin test in streptozocin-diabetic rats (18). This indicates that the above disorders are not likely to be due to neurotoxic actions of the diabetogenic agents. Moreover, insulin deficiency per se is unlikely to be the sole cause, as similar disorders are found in animal models of diabetes where insulin levels are normal or exaggerated (regarding reduced response thresholds to paw pressure tests in the sand rat and galactose-fed rat and increased formalin-induced flinching in the galactose-fed rat, see refs. 20 and 136). Thus, it is probable that most disorders of nociception found in diabetic animals are due to hyperglycemia or its consequences. Some studies have suggested that transient hyperglycemia is able to increase the response time to certain nociceptive tests (3,73,74), as has been reported in nondiabetic humans (95). Interestingly, the antinociceptive actions of opioids are suppressed by increased glucose levels (29,99,100,113). However, reduced response times take 7–21 days of diabetes to develop to the tail flick and paw pressure tests (1,34), and the reduced response time to the tail flick test is not amenable to acute normalization of blood glucose levels in streptozocin-diabetic rats after prolonged diabetes (74). These data suggest that prolonged hyperglycemia or its sequelae produces distinct effects on nociception.

Aldose Reductase Inhibitors

Exaggerated flux through aldose reductase, the first enzyme of the polyol pathway, has been associated with many of the biochemical, functional and structural disorders present in peripheral nerves of diabetic animals (129). The galactose-fed rat is used to produce increased blood and tissue levels of a hexose sugar in the absence of insulin deficiency or increased blood glucose levels and also selectively models increased flux through aldose reductase alone. This is because dulcitol, the product of galactose metabolism by aldose reductase, is not further metabolized by the polyol pathway. Galactose-fed rats exhibit a reduced response threshold during the paw pressure test (136) and increased response frequency during the Q phase of the formalin test (20). Moreover, aldose reductase inhibitors, which did not affect the formalin test in control rats or hyperglycemia in diabetic rats, suppressed the exaggerated flinching during the Q phase of the formalin test in streptozocin-diabetic rats (19,20) providing a further link between flux through the polyol pathway and altered nociception in diabetic rats.

Other Pharmacological Agents

A variety of other compounds, which may not necessarily be directed at the mechanisms underlying altered nociception in diabetic rodents but nevertheless could provide therapeutic effects, have recently been investigated. Gangliosides reverse increased flinching during the Q phase in diabetic rats, but also suppress phases 1 and 2 in both control and streptozocin-diabetic rats, suggesting a mechanism not specific to the diabetes-induced disorder (83). Treating diabetic rats with NGF reduced the elevated tail flick response time in diabetic rats, although the potential effect of NGF on response times in control rats was not reported and could confound interpretation of this finding (4). Reduced response thresholds in the paw pressure test were shifted towards normal by RP-67580 (NK_1 receptor antagonist), tricyclic antidepressants, lidocaine, and morphine, although the latter required greater doses than in controls (33,35). A similar effect was achieved by manipulating cAMP levels in the paw skin by intradermal injection of an adenylate cyclase inhibitor or phosphodiesterase, which degrades cAMP (1). Thus, while caution is required in equating particular nociceptive disorders in diabetic animals to the pain syndromes experienced by diabetic patients, animal models of diabetes are now becoming a potentially useful tool in the evaluation of the efficacy of therapeutic agents in treating sensory disorders.

CLINICAL TREATMENT

The treatment of pain in diabetic neuropathy should ideally entail a detailed assessment of the underlying lesions followed by an appropriately tailored therapy. Initially, other possible causes of neuropathy such as alcohol, vitamin B_{12} deficiency, or use of drugs, which may cause neuropathy, should be carefully excluded. Metabolic control should be optimized gradually and analgesics such as nonsteroidal antiinflammatory agents may be tried, although these are often ineffective. In the absence of remission, the array of therapeutic options discussed in greater detail below should be employed while narcotic analgesics are not helpful and should be avoided. An important point to remember when considering clinical trial data is the strong placebo response, which can occur in up to 60% of patients, particularly in clinical trials using intravenous infusions.

Glycemic Control

Improved glycemic control is clearly of great benefit in preventing the progression of diabetic neuropathy (124). Pain in patients with acute proximal neuropathy and acute painful neuropathy associated with weight loss both respond well to improved glycemic control, and the use of continuous subcutaneous insulin infusion has also been shown to benefit patients with severe painful neuropathy (11). However, one should be cautious in improving glycemic control too rapidly in previously poorly controlled patients due to the risk of developing insulin neuritis (63).

Tricyclic Antidepressants

These are currently the most effective drugs in the treatment of mild to moderate painful neuropathy (96) (see Chapter 64). Controlled clinical trials have demonstrated that antidepressant drugs are effective in the relief of painful neuropathy in patients with both normal and depressed moods (86). Interestingly, the primary mode of action does not appear to be through relief of depression alone, as the onset of action is faster than would be expected and the dosage required to relieve pain is much lower than necessary to relieve depression. Furthermore, the therapeutic efficacy for the relief of painful neuropathy is achieved irrespective of the presence of depression (134). Alleviation, rather than abolition, of pain is achieved presumably by inhibiting reuptake of noradrenaline at synapses in central descending pain control systems, although a peripheral antinociceptive effect has also been proposed (87). Side effects of these compounds include the anticholinergic effects of a dry mouth, urinary retention, postural hypotension, impotence, and cardiac arrhythmias, all of which are particularly troublesome in elderly patients and should therefore be carefully monitored. Amitryptylline and imipramine are the two most commonly used agents of this group. Desipramine has less anticholinergic side effects, produces less sedation but relieves pain equally as effectively as amitryptylline (88). Mianserin is a nontricyclic antidepressant that showed benefit in an early trial (139), but a more recent controlled trial failed to find any efficacy (116). This may be related to the lack of inhibitory effect on noradrenaline reuptake exhibited by this compound. Mianserin also has a greater predilection for the development of allergic blood disorders such as agranulocytosis and aplastic anaemia and is therefore not widely used. Initially, there was a vogue to combine the tricyclic antidepressants with a phenothiazine. However, in view of the unproven efficacy and the risk of developing tardive dyskinesia, this is not currently practiced. It should also be noted that, although tricyclic antidepressants may relieve painful symptoms of diabetic neuropathy, they probably do not address the underlying etiology or impede the progression of neuropathy.

Selective Serotonin Reuptake Inhibitors

Both paroxitene (115) and citalopram (114) have been shown to relieve sensory symptoms, although fluoxitene relieved pain only in patients with depression (88). The mechanism of action is presumed to be potentiation of the action of 5-hydroxytryptamine by inhibiting uptake. These compounds have fewer antimuscarinic effects and are less sedative than the tricyclic antidepressants and also display lower cardiotoxicity.

Anticonvulsants and Antiarrythmics

Phenytoin has been shown to benefit patients with painful neuropathy in some (26) but not all (107) studies. Carbamazepine is also effective and, as it is only a weak sedative, may be used during the day providing an advantage over the more efficacious but also more sedative tricyclic antidepressants (102). Side effects include dizziness, gastrointestinal disturbances, abnormal liver function, and ataxia. It has been suggested that, as these compounds affect sodium conductance, they decrease ectopic discharges by stabilising peripheral neuronal membranes. Antiarrythmics such as intravenous lignocaine and oral mexilitine may also reduce nerve fiber spontaneous activity and mechanoreceptor sensitivity and have been shown to be effective in treating a range of painful neuropathies including diabetic truncal neuropathy (72) and severe distal painful neuropathy (36) (see Chapter 63).

Aldose Reductase Inhibitors

This class of compounds prevent excessive flux of glucose through the polyol pathway and target a potential mechanism underlying diabetic neuropathy. They have proved extremely successful in preventing and reversing biochemical and functional disorders in the peripheral nerves of diabetic animals (129) and prevented hyperalgesia in the rat formalin test (19,20). It is suggested that aldose reductase inhibitors may prevent progression of diabetic neuropathy and perhaps even reverse established neuropathy but their benefit to diabetic patients remains unproven (84). An early open-label study (62) and a short-term placebo-controlled study (140) with the aldose reductase inhibitor Sorbinil demonstrated qualitative reduction of painful symptoms. Studies with a more potent inhibitor, the first a double-blind study (12) and the second a withdrawal study (106) have also demonstrated benefit to patients with painful neuropathy, although the former reported improvement in paresthesiae rather than pain. Recent studies show promising evidence of efficacy against both spontaneous pain and sensory loss (52,132).

Gangliosides

Gangliosides are glycosphingolipids of particular abundance in membranes of nervous tissue that have been considered as potential therapeutic agents for diabetic and other neuropathies based upon their neuronotrophic and neuritogenic properties (13). Antinociceptive actions are reported in animal models of neuropathic and formalin-induced hyperalgesia (56,83). Although their clinical use has been questioned in an unresolved debate regarding possible associations between ganglioside treatment and Guillain-Barré syndrome (53), limited effects in alleviating diabetic pain have been noted (55).

Capsaicin

Topically applied capsaicin has been shown to relieve the painful symptoms of diabetic neuropathy (24,25). Capsaicin may cause the release and ultimate depletion of substance P from sensory nerve terminals, thereby reducing nociceptor function (see Chapter 33).

Vasoactive Substances

Vascular abnormalities probably play an important role in the pathogenesis of diabetic neuropathy (123) and may also regulate pain, prompting studies exploring the use of vasoactive substances in the treatment of painful diabetic neuropathy. At present, the benefits of a wide range of drugs influencing physiologic systems from haemorheology to vascular supply are divided. Pentoxifylline and cyclandelate, agents that improve the rheological properties of blood, were ineffective in patients with painful diabetic neuropathy (31,32,58). However, Iloprost a prostacyclin analogue and potential peripheral vasodilator demonstrated considerable relief from painful symptoms (111) while a significant improvement in painful symptoms occurred following intravenous and subsequent oral administration of the antioxidant α–lipoic acid (142).

Transdermal (143), but not oral clonidine (31) has also been shown to benefit patients with painful diabetic neuropathy. At low dose, clonidine is an agonist of postsynaptic α_2-adrenoceptors in the brain, thereby suppressing sympathetic outflow. At higher doses, which may well be achieved locally by transdermal administration, it activates peripheral α_2-adrenoceptors on the adrenergic nerve endings, mediating negative-feedback suppression of noradrenaline release, thus presenting a possible mechanism for pain relief (see Chapter 32). Such topical application has been advantageous in neuropathic states that are believed to be sympathetically dependent (see Chapter 56).

Physical Measures

Transcutaneous electrical nerve stimulation has been recommended (128) but was not found to be effective in painful diabetic neuropathy (5). A recent double-blind study employing a spinal cord stimulator has shown considerable relief of pain in diabetic patients with severe painful neuropathy (122).

CONCLUSIONS

Although progress has been made in characterizing diabetic neuropathy, there is no current unifying hypothesis describing the etiology of the disorder. Painful neuropathy occurs in a significant proportion of diabetic patients and is both debilitating and notoriously difficult to treat. The inconsistent and varied presentation of pain symptoms provides further challenges for those that would develop therapeutic interventions selectively targeted at preventing or treating pain. Good glycemic control is clearly the most desirable therapy, but practical and social constraints often preclude long-term maintenance of strict euglycemia by many diabetics. Clinical and experimental studies have described several disorders, including exaggerated glucose metabolism, endoneurial hypoxia, fiber degeneration, and regeneration, which are all potential contributors to pain. The growing appreciation that long-term changes in afferent function can evoke reactive changes in the neuron such as increased expression of neurotransmitters, channels, and receptors may suggest that such changes are also a component of this chronic pain state. Future studies may be directed towards achieving insight into how the neurochemistry of afferents is influenced by the biochemical and structural disorders present in diabetic nerve. That linkage will provide an important tool in developing selective therapeutic agents with which to treat this very prevalent pain condition.

REFERENCES

1. Ahlgren SC, Levine JD. Mechanical hyperalgesia in streptozocin-diabetic rats. *Neuroscience* 1993;52:1049–1055.
2. Ahlgren SC, White DM, Levine JD. Increased responsiveness of sensory neurons in the saphenous nerve of the streptozocin-diabetic rat. *J Neurophysiol* 1992;68:2077–2085.
3. Akunne HC, Soliman KF. The role of opioid receptors in diabetes and hyperglycemia-induced changes in pain threshold in the rat. *Psychopharmacology* 1987;93:167–172.
4. Apfel SC, Arezzo JC, Brownlee M, Federoff H, Kessler JA. Nerve growth factor administration protects against experimental diabetic sensory neuropathy. *Brain Res* 1994;634:7–12.
5. Archer AG, Watkins PJ, Thomas PK, Sharma AK, Payan J. The natural history of acute painful neuropathy in diabetes mellitus. *J Neurol Neurosurg Psychiatry* 1983;46:491–499.
6. Asbury AK. Focal and Multifocal neuropathies of diabetes. In: Dyck PJ, Thomas PK, Asbury AK, Winegrad AI, Porte D. eds. *Diabetic neuropathy.* Philadelphia: Saunders, 1987:45–55.
7. Asbury AK, Aldridge H, Hershberg R, Fisher CM. Oculomotor palsy in diabetes mellitus: a clinico-pathological study. *Brain* 1970; 93:555–566.
8. Bansinath M, Ramabadran K, Turndorf H, Puig MM. Effect of yohimbine on nociceptive threshold in normoglycemic and streptozocin-treated hyperglycemic mice. *Pharmacol Biochem Behav* 1989;33:459–463.
9. Benbow SJ, Chan AW, Bowsher D, MacFarlane IA, Williams G. A prospective study of painful symptoms, small-fibre function and peripheral vascular disease in chronic painful diabetic neuropathy. *Diabetic Med* 1994;11:17–21.
10. Boulton AJM, Angus E, Ayyar DR, Weiss R. Diabetic thoracic polyradiculopathy presenting as abdominal swelling. *BMJ* 1984; 289:798–799.
11. Boulton AJM, Drury F, Clarke B, Ward JD. Continuous subcutaneous insulin infusion in the management of painful diabetic neuropathy. *Diabetes Care* 1982;5:386–390.
12. Boulton AJM, Levin S, Comstock J. A multicentre trial of the aldose-reductase inhibitor, Tolrestat, in patients with symptomatic diabetic neuropathy. *Diabetologia* 1990;33:431–437.
13. Bradley WG. Critical review of gangliosides and thyrotropin-releasing hormone in peripheral neuromuscular diseases. *Muscle Nerve* 1990;13:833–842.
14. Britland ST, Young RJ, Sharma AK, Clarke BF. Association of painful and painless diabetic polyneuropathy with different patterns of nerve fibre degeneration and regeneration. *Diabetes* 1990; 39:898–908.
15. Britland ST, Young RJ, Sharma AK, Clarke BF. Acute and remitting painful diabetic polyneuropathy: a comparison of peripheral nerve fibre pathology. *Pain* 1992;498:361–370.
16. Brown MJ, Martin JR, Asbury AK. Painful diabetic neuropathy: a morphometric study. *Arch Neurol* 1976;33:164–171.

17. Burchiel KJ, Russell LC, Lee RP, Sima AA. Spontaneous activity of primary afferent neurons in diabetic BB/Wistar rats. A possible mechanism of chronic diabetic neuropathic pain. *Diabetes* 1985; 34:1210–1213.
18. Calcutt NA, Jorge MC, Chaplan SC. Tactile allodynia in diabetic rats: effects of insulin and systemic lidocaine. *Diabetologia* 1995;38: A234.
19. Calcutt NA, Li L, Yaksh TL, Malmberg AB. Different effects of two aldose reductase inhibitors on nociception and prostaglandin E. *Eur J Pharmacol* 1995;285:189–197.
20. Calcutt NA, Malmberg AB, Yamamoto T, Yaksh TL. Tolrestat treatment prevents modification of the formalin test model of prolonged pain in hyperglycemic rats. *Pain* 1994;58:413–420.
21. Calcutt NA, Mizisin AP, Yaksh TL. Impaired induction of vasoactive intestinal polypeptide after sciatic nerve injury in the streptozocin-diabetic rat. *J Neurol Sci* 1993;119:154–161.
22. Calcutt NA, Muir D, Powell HC, Mizisin AP. Reduced ciliary neuronotrophic factor-like activity in nerves from diabetic or galactose-fed rats. *Brain Res* 1992;575:320–324.
23. Calcutt NA, Tomlinson DR, Willars GB, Keen P. Axonal transport of substance P-like immunoreactivity in ganglioside-treated diabetic rats. *J Neurol Sci* 1990;96:283–291.
24. Capsaicin Study Group. Treatment of painful diabetic neuropathy with topical capsaicin. A multicentre, double-blind, vehicle controlled study. *Arch Intern Med* 1991;151:2225–2229.
25. Capsaicin Study Group. Effect of treatment with capsaicin on daily activities of patients with painful diabetic neuropathy. *Diabetes Care* 1992;15:159–165.
26. Chadda VS, Mathur MS. Double-blind study on the effects of diphenylhydantoin sodium on diabetic neuropathy. *J Assoc Phys India* 1978;26:403–408.
27. Chan AW, MacFarland IA, Bowsher DR, Wells JCD. Does acute hyperglycaemia influence heat pain threshold? *J Neurosurg* 1988; 57:688–690.
28. Chaplan SR, Bach FW, Pogrel JW, Chung JM, Yaksh TL. Quantitative assessment of tactile allodynia in the rat paw. *J Neurosci Methods* 1994;53:55–63.
29. Chu PC, Lin MT, Shian LR, Leu SY. Alterations in physiologic functions and in brain monoamine content in streptozocin-diabetic rats. *Diabetes* 1986;35:481–485.
30. Coderre TJ, Vaccarino AL, Melzack R. Central nervous system plasticity in the tonic pain response to subcutaneous formalin injection. *Brain Res* 1990;535:155–158.
31. Cohen KL, Lucibello FE, Chomiak M. Lack of effect of clonidine and pentoxifylline in short-term therapy of diabetic peripheral neuropathy. *Diabetes Care* 1990;13:1074–1077.
32. Cohen SM, Mathews T. Pentoxifylline in the treatment of distal diabetic neuropathy. *Angiology* 1991;42:741–746.
33. Courteix C, Bardin M, Chantelauze C, Lavarenne J, Eschalier A. Study of the sensitivity of the diabetes-induced pain model in rats to a range of analgesics. *Pain* 1994;57:153–160.
34. Courteix C, Eschalier A, Lavarenne J. Streptozocin-induced diabetic rats: behavioural evidence for a model of chronic pain. *Pain* 1993;53:81–88.
35. Courteix C, Lavarenne J, Eschalier A. RP-67580, a specific tachykinin NK1 receptor antagonist, relieves chronic hyperalgesia in diabetic rats. *Eur J Pharmacol* 1993;241:267–270.
36. Dejgard A, Peterson P Kastrup J. Mexilitine for treatment of chronic painful diabetic neuropathy. *Lancet* 1988;1:9–11.
37. Dickenson AH, Sullivan AF. Subcutaneous formalin-induced activity of dorsal horn neurones in the rat: differential response to an intrathecal opiate administered pre or post formalin. *Pain* 1987; 30:349–360.
38. Dickenson AH, Sullivan AF. Peripheral origins and central modulation of subcutaneous formalin-induced activity of rat dorsal horn neurones. *Neurosci Lett* 1987;83:207–211.
39. Diemel LT, Brewster WJ, Fernyhough P, Tomlinson DR. Expression of neuropeptides in experimental diabetes; effects of treatment with nerve growth factor or brain-derived neurotrophic factor. *Mol Brain Res* 1994;21:171–175.
40. Diemel, LT, Stevens E, Willars GB, Tomlinson DR. Depletion of substance P and calcitonin gene-related peptide in sciatic nerve of rats with experimental diabetes; effects of insulin and aldose reductase inhibition. *Neurosci Lett* 1992;137:253–256.
41. Dubuisson D, Dennis SG. The formalin test: a quantitative study of the analgesic effects of morphine, meperidine, and brain stem stimulation in rats and cats. *Pain* 1977;4:161–174.
42. Dyck PJ, Karnes JL, Daube J, O'Brien P, Service FJ. Clinical and neuropathological criteria for the diagnosis and staging of polyneuropathy. *Brain* 1985;108:861–880.
43. Dyck PJ, Lambert EH, O'Brien PC. Pain in peripheral neuropathy related to rate and kind of fibre degeneration. *Neurology* 1976;26: 466–471.
44. Ekstrom PAR, Tomlinson DR. Impaired nerve regeneration in streptozocin-diabetic rats. Effects of treatment with an aldose reductase inhibitor. *J Neurol Sci* 1989;93:231–237.
45. Ellenberg M. Diabetic neuropathic cachexia. *Diabetes* 1974;23: 418–423.
46. Fernyhough P, Diemel LT, Brewster WJ, Tomlinson DR. Deficits in sciatic nerve neuropeptide content coincide with a reduction in target tissue nerve growth factor messenger RNA in streptozocin-diabetic rats: effects of insulin treatment. *Neuroscience* 1994;62: 337–344.
47. Fernyhough P, Diemel LT, Brewster WJ, Tomlinson DR. Altered neurotrophin mRNA levels in peripheral nerve and skeletal muscle of experimentally diabetic rats. *J Neurochem* 1995;64: 1231–1237.
48. Forman LJ, Estilow S, Lewis M, Vasilenko P. Streptozocin diabetes alters immunoreactive beta-endorphin levels and pain perception after 8 wk in female rats. *Diabetes* 1986;35:1309–1313.
49. Gamse R, Jancso G. Reduced neurogenic inflammation in streptozocin-diabetic rats due to microvascular changes but not to substance P depletion. *Eur J Pharmacol* 1985;118:175–180.
50. Garland HT. Diabetic amyotrophy. *BMJ* 1955;2:1287–1290.
51. Ginawi OT. Morphine analgesia in normal and alloxanized mice. *Arch Int Pharmacodynam Ther* 1992;318:13–20.
52. Goto Y, Hotta N, Shigeta Y, Sakamoto N, Kikkawa R. Effects of an aldose reductase inhibitor, epalrestat, on diabetic neuropathy. Clinical benefit and indication for the drug assessed from the results of a placebo-controlled double-blind study. *Biomed Pharmacother* 1995;49:269–277.
53. Granieri E, Casetta I, Govoni V, Tola MR, Paolino E, Rocca WA. Ganglioside therapy and Guillain-Barré syndrome: a historical cohort fails to demonstrate an association. *Neuroepidemiology* 1991; 10:161–169.
54. Greene DA, De Jesus PV Jr, Winegrad AI. Effects of insulin and dietary myoinositol on impaired peripheral motor nerve conduction velocity in acute streptozocin diabetes. *J Clin Invest* 1975;55: 1326–1336.
55. Hallet M, Flood T, Slater N, Dambrosia J. Trial of ganglioside therapy for diabetic neuropathy. *Muscle Nerve* 1987;10:822–825.
56. Hayes RL, Mao J, Price DD, et al. Pretreatment with gangliosides reduces abnormal nociceptive responses associated with a rodent peripheral mononeuropathy. *Pain* 1992;48:391–396.
57. Heapy CG, Jamieson A, Russell NJW. Afferent C-fibre and A-delta activity in models of inflammation. *Br J Pharmacol* 1987;90:164P.
58. Heimans JJ, Drukarch B, Matthaei I, et al. Cyclandalate in diabetic neuropathy. A double-blind placebo-controlled, randomized, crossover study. *Acta Neurol Scand* 1991;84:483–486.
59. Hellweg R, Hartung H-D. Endogenous levels of NGF are altered in experimental diabetes mellitus: a possible role for NGF in the pathogenesis of diabetic neuropathy. *J Neurosci Res* 1990;26: 258–267.
60. Jakobsen J. Axonal dwindling in early experimental diabetes. I. A study of cross sectioned nerves. *Diabetologia* 1976;12:539–546.
61. Jakobsen J, Brimijoin S, Skau K, Sidenius P, Wells D. Retrograde axonal transport of transmitter enzymes, fucose-labelled protein and nerve growth factor in streptozocin-diabetic rats. *Diabetes* 1981;30:797–803.
62. Jaspan J, Masell R, Herold K, Bartkus C. Treatment of severely painful diabetic neuropathy with an aldose reductase inhibitor: relief of pain and improved somatic and autonomic nerve function. *Lancet* 1983;2:758–762.
63. Jordan WR. Neuritic manifestations in diabetes mellitus. *Arch Intern Med* 1936;57:307.
64. Kamei J, Aoki T, Kasuya Y. Periaqueductal gray matter stimulation-produced analgesia in diabetic rats. *Neurosci Lett* 1992a;142: 13–16.
65. Kamei J, Hitosugi H, Kasuya Y. Formalin-induced nociceptive responses in diabetic mice. *Neurosci Lett* 1993;149:161–164.
66. Kamei J, Hitosugi H, Kawashima N, Aoki T, Ohhashi Y, Kasuya Y. Antinociceptive effect of mexiletine in diabetic mice. *Res Commun Chem Pathol Pharmacol* 1992;77:245–248.
67. Kamei J, Kawashima N, Kasuya Y. Role of spleen or spleen prod-

ucts in the deficiency in morphine-induced analgesia in diabetic mice. *Brain Res* 1992;576:139–142.
68. Kamei J, Kawashima N, Ohhashi Y, Kasuya Y. Effects of diabetes on stress-induced analgesia in mice. *Brain Res* 1992d;580:180–184.
69. Kamei J, Ogawa M, Kasuya Y. Development of supersensitivity to substance P in the spinal cord of the streptozocin-induced diabetic rats. *Pharmacol Biochem Behav* 1990;35:473–475.
70. Kamei J, Ogawa Y, Ohhashi Y, Kasuya Y. Alterations in the potassium-evoked release of substance P from the spinal cord of streptozocin-induced diabetic rats in vitro. *Gen Pharmacol* 1991a;22:1093–1096.
71. Kamei J, Ohhashi Y, Aoki T, Kasuya Y. Streptozocin-induced diabetes in mice reduces the nociceptive threshold, as recognized after application of noxious mechanical stimuli but not of thermal stimuli. *Pharmacol Biochem Behav* 1991;39:541–544.
72. Kastrup J, Petersen P, Dejgard A. Treatment of chronic painful diabetic neuropathy with intravenous lidocaine infusion. *BMJ* 1986;292:173.
73. Lee JH, McCarty R. Glycemic control of pain threshold in diabetic and control rats. *Physiol Behav* 1990;47:225–230.
74. Lee JH, McCarty R. Pain threshold in diabetic rats: effects of good versus poor diabetic control. *Pain* 1992;50:231–236.
76. Levine AS, Morley JE, Wilcox G, Brown DM, Handwerger BS. Tail pinch behavior and analgesia in diabetic mice. *Physiol Behav* 1982;28:39–43.
76. Lindsay RM, Harmar AJ. Nerve growth factor regulates expression of neuropeptide genes in adult sensory neurons. *Nature* 1989;337:362–364.
77. Llewelyn JG, Gilbey SG, Thomas PK, King RHM, Muddle JR, Watkins PJ. Sural nerve morphometry in diabetic autonomic and painful sensory neuropathy. *Brain* 1991;114:867–892.
78. Llewelyn JG, Thomas PK, Fonesca V, King RHM, Dandona P. Acute painful diabetic neuropathy precipitated by strict glycaemic control. *Acta Neuropathol* 1986;72:157–163.
79. Malik RA, Tesfaye S, Veves A, Ward JD, Boulton AJM. Sural nerve fibre pathology with progression of human diabetic neuropathy. *Diabetologia* 1994;37:A79–304.
80. Malmberg AB, Yaksh TL. Antinociceptive actions of spinal nonsteroidal anti-inflammatory agents on the formalin test in the rat. *J Pharmacol Exp Ther* 1992;263:136–146.
81. Malmberg AB, Yaksh TL. Spinal nitric oxide synthesis inhibition blocks NMDA-induced thermal hyperalgesia and produces antinociception in the formalin test in rats. *Pain* 1993;54:291–300.
82. Malmberg AB, Yaksh, TL. Cyclooxygenase inhibition and the spinal release of prostaglandin E_2 and amino acids evoked by paw formalin injection: A microdialysis study in unanesthetized rats. *J Neurosci* 1995;15:2768–2776.
83. Malmberg AB, Yaksh TL, Calcutt NA. Anti-nociceptive effects of the GM1 ganglioside derivative AGF 44 on the formalin test in normal and streptozocin-diabetic rats. *Neurosci Lett* 1993;161:45–48.
84. Masson EA, Boulton AJM. Aldose reductase inhibitors in the treatment of diabetic neuropathy: a review of the rationale and clinical evidence. *Drugs* 1990;39:190–202.
85. Matthies BK, Franklin KB. Formalin pain is expressed in decerebrate rats but not attenuated by morphine. *Pain* 1992;51:199–206.
86. Max MB, Culnane M, Schafer SC. Amitryptyline relieves diabetic neuropathy pain in patients with normal or depressed moods. *Neurology* 1987;37:589–596.
87. Max MB, Kishore-Kumar R, Schafer FC, et al. Efficacy of desipramine in painful diabetic neuropathy. *Pain* 1991;45:3–9.
88. Max MB, Lynch SA, Muir J, Shoaf SE, Smoller B, Dubner R. Effects of desipramine, amitryptyline and fluoxetine on pain in diabetic neuropathy. *N Engl J Med* 1992;326:1250–1256.
89. McLean WG, Chapman JE, Cullum NA. Impaired induction of ornithine decarboxylase activity following nerve crush in the streptozocin-diabetic rat. *Diabetologia* 1987;30:963–965.
90. Medori R, Autilio-Gambetti L, Monaco S, Gambetti P. Experimental diabetic neuropathy: impairment of slow transport with changes in axon cross-sectional area. *Proc Natl Acad Sci USA* 1985;82:7716–7720.
91. Melton LJ III, Dyck PJ. Clinical features of the diabetic neuropathies. In: Dyck PJ, Thomas PK, Asbury AK, Winegrad AI, Porte D. eds. *Diabetic neuropathy.* Philadelphia: WB Saunders, 1987:27–35.
92. Mizisin AP, Bache M, DiStefano P, Lindsay RM, Calcutt NA. Effects of BDNF or CNTF treatment on galactose neuropathy. *Soc Neurosci Abs* 1995;21:1535.
93. Moore SA, Peterson RG, Felten DL, O'Connor BL. A quantitative comparison of motor and sensory conduction velocities in short- and long-term streptozocin- and alloxan-diabetic rats. *J Neurol Sci* 1980;48:133–152.
94. Mohiuddin L, Fernyhough P, Tomlinson DR. Reduced levels of mRNA encoding endoskeletal and growth-associated proteins in sensory ganglia in experimental diabetes. *Diabetes* 1995;44:25–30.
95. Morley GK, Mooradian AD, Levine AL, Morley JE. Mechanisms of pain in diabetic peripheral neuropathy: effects of glucose on pain perception in humans. *Am J Med* 1984;77:79–86.
96. Pfiefer MA, Ross DR, Schrager JP, et al. A highly successful and novel model for treatment of chronic painful diabetic peripheral neuropathy. *Diabetes Care* 1993;16:1103–1115.
97. Porro CA, Cavazzuti M. Spatial and temporal aspects of spinal cord and brainstem activation in the formalin pain model. *Prog Neurobiol* 1993;41:565–607.
98. Puig S, Sorkin LS. Subcutaneous formalin evoked activity in single fibers of rat sural nerve. *Soc Neurosci Abstr* 1994;20:319.
99. Ramabadran K, Bansinath M, Turndorf H, Puig MM. The hyperalgesic effect of naloxone is attenuated in streptozocin-diabetic mice. *Psychopharmacology* 1989;97:169–174.
100. Raz I, Hasdai D, Seltzer Z, Melmed RN. Effect of hyperglycemia on pain perception and on efficacy of morphine analgesia in rats. *Diabetes* 1988;37:1253–1259.
101. Robinson JP, Willars GB, Tomlinson DR, Keen P. Axonal transport and tissue contents of substance P in rats with long-term streptozocin-diabetes. Effects of the aldose reductase inhibitor "statil." *Brain Res* 1987;426:339–348.
102. Rull JA, Quibrera R, Gonzales-Milan H, Castehada OL. Symptomatic treatment of peripheral diabetic neuropathy with carbamazepine (Tegrotol): a double-blind cross-over study. *Diabetologia* 1969;5:215–218.
103. Russell LC, Burchiel KJ. Abnormal activity in diabetic rat saphenous nerve. *Diabetes* 1993;42:814–819.
104. Said G, Goulon-Goeau C, Lacroix C, Moulonguet A. Nerve biopsy findings in different patterns of proximal diabetic neuropathy. *Ann Neurol* 1994;35:559–569.
105. Said G, Goulon-Goeau C, Slama G, Tchobroutsky G. Severe early onset polyneuropathy in insulin-dependent diabetes mellitus. *N Engl J Med* 1992;326:1257–1263.
106. Santiago JV, Sonksen PH, Boulton AJM, et al. Withdrawal of the aldose reductase inhibitor Tolrestat in patients with diabetic neuropathy: effect on nerve function. *J Diabetes Complications* 1993;7:170–178.
107. Saudek CD, Werns S, Reidenberg MM. Phenytoin in the treatment of diabetic symmetrical polyneuropathy. *Clin Pharmacol Ther* 1977;22:196–199.
108. Schneider U, Nees S, Grafe P. Differences in sensitivity to hyperglycemic hypoxia of isolated rat sensory and motor nerve fibers. *Ann Neurol* 1992;31:605–610.
109. Seneviratne KN, Peiris OA. The effects of hypoxia on the excitability of the isolated peripheral nerves of alloxan-diabetic rats. *J Neurol Neurosurg Psych* 1969;32:462–469.
110. Sharma AK, Thomas PK. Peripheral nerve structure and function in experimental diabetes. *J Neurol Sci* 1974;23:1–15.
111. Shindo H, Tanata M, Aida K, Onaya T. Clinical efficacy of a stable prostacyclin analogue, Iloprost, in diabetic neuropathy. *Prostaglandins* 1991;41:85–96.
112. Sidenius P, Jakobsen J. Reduced perikaryal volume of lower motor and primary sensory neurons in early experimental diabetes. *Diabetes* 1980;29:182–186.
113. Simon GS, Dewey WL. Narcotics and diabetes. I. The effect of streptozocin-induced diabetes on the antinociceptive potency of morphine. *J Pharmacol Exp Ther* 1981;218:318–324.
114. Sindrup SH, Bjerre U, Dejgaard A, Brosen K, Aaes-Jorgensen T, Gram LF. The selective serotonin reuptake inhibitor Citalopram relieves the symptoms of diabetic neuropathy. *Clin Pharmacol Ther* 1992;52:547–552.
115. Sindrup SH, Grodum E, Gram LF, Beck-Nielsen H. Concentration response relationship in Paroxetine treatment of diabetic neuropathy symptoms: a patient blinded dose-escalation study. *Ther Drug Monit* 1991;13:408–414.
116. Sindrup SH, Tuxen C, Gram LF, Skjold T, Brosen K, Beck-Nielsen H. Lack of effect of Mianserin on the symptoms of diabetic neuropathy. *Eur J Clin Pharmocol* 1992;43:251–255.
117. Smith WJ, Diemel LT, Leach RM, Tomlinson DR. Central hypoxaemia in rats provokes neurological defects similar to those seen

in experimental diabetes mellitus: evidence for a partial role of endoneurial hypoxia in diabetic neuropathy. *Neuroscience* 1991;45:255–259.

118. Steele JM, Young RJ, Lloyd GG, Clarke BF. Clinically apparent eating disorders in young diabetic women: associations with painful neuropathy and other complications. *BMJ* 1987;294:859–866.
119. Steiness IB. Vibratory perception in diabetics during arrested blood flow to the limb. *Acta Med Scand* 1959;163:195–205.
120. Sugimura K, Dyck PJ. Sural nerve myelin thickness and axis cylinder calibre in human diabetes. *Neurology* 1981;31:1087–1091.
121. Tamura E, Parry G. Severe radicular pathology in rats with long-standing diabetes. *J Neurol Sci* 1995;127:29–35.
122. Tesfaye S, Watt J, Benbow SJ, Pang KA, Miles J, Macfarlane IA. Electrical spinal-cord stimulation for painful diabetic peripheral neuropathy. *Lancet* 1996;348:1698–1701.
123. Tesfaye S, Malik RA, Ward JD. Vascular factors in diabetic neuropathy. *Diabetologia* 1994;37:847–854.
124. The Diabetes Control and Complications Trial Research Group. The effects of intensive treatment of diabetes on the development and progression of long-term complications in insulin-dependent diabetes mellitus. *N Engl J Med* 1993;329:977–986.
125. Thomas PK. The anatomical substratum of pain: evidence derived from morphometric studies of peripheral nerve. *Can J Neurol Sci* 1974;1:92–97.
126. Thomas PK, Tomlinson DR. Diabetic and hypoglycaemic neuropathy. In: Dyck PJ, Thomas PK, Griffin JW, Low PA, Poduslo JF, eds. *Peripheral neuropathy.* 3rd ed. Philadelphia: WB Saunders, 1993:1219–1250.
127. Thomas PK, Wright DW, Tzebelikos E. Amino acid uptake by dorsal root ganglia from streptozocin-diabetic rats. *J Neurol Neurosurg Psych* 1984;47:912–916.
128. Thorsteinsson G. Management of painful diabetic neuropathy. *JAMA* 1977;238:2697–2702.
129. Tomlinson DR. Aldose reductase inhibitors and the complications of diabetes mellitus. *Diabetic Med* 1993;10:214–230.
130. Torebjork HE, La Motte RH, Robinson CJ. Peripheral nerve correlates of magnitude of cutaneous pain and hyperalgesia: simultaneous recordings of human sensory judgements of pain and evoked responses in nociceptor C fibres. *J Neurophysiol* 1984;51:325–339.
131. Tsigos C, Reed P, White A, Young RJ. Plasma epinephrine and norepinephrine in painful and painless diabetic polyneuropathy. *Diabetes* 1990;39:A498.
132. Uchida K, Kigoshi T, Nakano S, Ishii T, Kitazawa M, Morimoto S. Effect of 24 weeks of treatment with epalrestat, an aldose reductase inhibitor, on peripheral neuropathy in patients with non-insulin-dependent diabetes mellitus. *Clin Ther* 1995;17:460–466.
133. Ward JD, Barnes CG, Fisher DJ, Jessop JD, Baker RW. Improvement in nerve conduction following treatment in newly diagnosed diabetics. *Lancet* 1971;1:428–430.
134. Ward JD, Hanssen KF, Krans HMJ, Tesfaye S. Treatment of diabetic neuropathy. *Diabetes Nutr Metab* 1994;7:369–379.
135. Willars GB, Calcutt NA, Compton AM, Tomlinson DR, Keen P. Substance P levels in peripheral nerve, skin, atrial myocardium and gastrointestinal tract of rats with long-term diabetes mellitus. Effects of aldose reductase inhibition. *J Neurol Sci* 1989;91:153–164.
136. Wuarin-Bierman L, Zahnd GR, Kaufmann F, Burcklen L, Adler J. Hyperalgesia in spontaneous and experimental animal models of diabetic neuropathy. *Diabetologia* 1987;30:653–658.
137. Yamamoto T, Yaksh TL. Stereospecific effects of a nonpeptidic NK1 selective antagonist, CP-96,345: antinociception in the absence of motor dysfunction. *Life Sci* 1991;49:1955–1963.
138. Yamamoto T, Yaksh TL. Comparison of the antinociceptive effects of pre- and post treatment with intrathecal morphine and MK801, an NMDA antagonist, on the formalin test in the rat. *Anesthesiology* 1992;77:757–63.
139. Young RJ, Clarke BF. Pain relief in diabetic neuropathy: the effectiveness of Imipramine and related drugs. *Diabetic Medicine* 1985;2:363–366.
140. Young RJ, Ewing DJ, Clarke BF. A controlled clinical trial of sorbinil, an aldose reductase inhibitor, in chronic painful diabetic neuropathy. *Diabetes* 1983;32:938–942.
141. Young RJ, Zhou YQ, Rodrigues E, Prescott RJ, Ewing DJ, Clarke BF. Variable relationship between peripheral somatic and autonomic neuropathy in patients with different syndromes of diabetic polyneuropathy. *Diabetes* 1986;35:192–197.
142. Ziegler D, Hanefeld M, Ruhnau KJ, et al. Treatment of symptomatic diabetic peripheral neuropathy with the antioxidant alpha-lipoic acid. A 3 week randomised controlled trial (personal communication, 1995).
143. Ziegler D, Lynch SA, Muir J, Benjamin J, Max B. Transdermal clonidine versus placebo in painful diabetic neuropathy. *Pain* 1992;43:403–408.
144. Zorilla E, Kozak GP. Opthalmoplegia in diabetes mellitus. *Ann Intern Med* 1967;67:968–974.

Anesthesia: Biologic Foundations, edited by
Tony L. Yaksh et al. Lippincott–Raven Publishers,
Philadelphia © 1997.

CHAPTER 55

HERPES ZOSTER AND POSTHERPETIC NEURALGIA

MICHAEL C. ROWBOTHAM AND KIRK TAYLOR

Herpes zoster (HZ), a disease of the primary afferent system, is one of the most common of all neurological disorders (42,61). Clues to the neural basis of zoster appeared in the literature early in the 19th century. Bright noted the peripheral nervelike territorial spread in 1831; von Barensprung related the cutaneous eruption to necrosis in the corresponding dorsal root ganglion in 1862; and Head and Campbell correlated clinical features of the acute eruption with postmortem changes in a series of cases to construct dermatomal maps of the human body in 1900 (1,46). Lewis and Marvin (64) hypothesized in 1927 that "the virus causing the mischief in the root ganglion spreads along the sensory tract to the skin, there setting up a distinct inflammatory change," but quickly discarded the theory as too inconsistent with the data available at the time. In 1965, Hope-Simpson (52) expanded on earlier theories that zoster represented reactivation of latent varicella zoster virus (VZV) by proposing that the virus was initially introduced during childhood varicella but kept in a latent state by the immune system. Using restriction endonuclease analysis, Straus et al. (103) finally proved reactivation of latent virus as the origin of zoster by showing in 1984 that virus isolates during varicella and zoster outbreaks are identical. Cellular immunity prevents reactivation; whether this is by keeping the virus in a latent state or by preventing viral spread to the periphery is not yet clear (104). Cell-mediated immunity specifically to VZV declines with age, especially after the age of 60 (5,45).

Once reactivated, virus produced in dorsal root ganglion cells undergoes transport along involved peripheral nerve to the skin to produce the characteristic vesicular rash (104). Infectious virus and its antigens are present in neurons, nerve-associated satellite cells, peripheral nerves, and the skin. Inflammation is intense within the dorsal root ganglion and peripheral nerve of the involved spinal (or trigeminal) segment, portions of the skin served by that ganglion, and occasionally extending rostral into the spinal cord even beyond the dorsal horn (5,28,46,104,115). Most of the complications of HZ are related to the destructive intensity of the inflammation, including cranial nerve palsies, eye destruction, and myelitis (52,86,89). The acute pain of HZ is almost certainly the result of inflammation and destruction of the involved dorsal root ganglia and nerves, the nervi nervorum located in the protective sheaths of the involved nerves, and peripheral tissues (6). This combination of inflammation, tissue destruction, and nerve irritation and destruction produces a very severe pain with prominent burning, itching, dysesthesias, and extreme pain from any skin contact (13,52,86). Although HZ is nonpainful in a small minority, many patients describe the pain of acute HZ as the most severe pain they have ever experienced. Most patients with postherpetic neuralgia (PHN) describe the pain of acute HZ as the most severe phase.

These subjects related to etiology and clinical presentation will be expanded in the following sections.

TERMINOLOGY AND EPIDEMIOLOGY OF ZOSTER AND POSTHERPETIC NEURALGIA

Terminology

The pain accompanying HZ was recognized by the early Greeks. The Greek term "herpes," meaning "something that creeps," was used to designate chronic cutaneous diseases. The unilateral, creeping, erythematous rash is well described by pairing herpes with the Greek term for the belt a warrior used to secure his armor, "zoster." The common designation of "shingles" is derived from the Latin word cingere, "to gird." Zona, a term commonly used in Europe for zoster, refers to the characteristic unilateral restricted area affected. Probably the most colorful and descriptive phrase for zoster was penned in 1979 by an anonymous writer as "a belt of roses from hell" (1).

There have been several terms proposed for pain that outlasts the acute zoster outbreak. The simplest is to consider all pain beginning with zoster to be zoster-associated pain (ZAP). Besides the unfortunate acronym, this term also suggests that the mechanism of the acute pain is the same as the mechanism of the chronic pain. Because the majority of patients with acute zoster recover without lasting pain or other sequelae, it is semantically useful to differentiate chronic pain following zoster from acute zoster pain (23,52). The terms postzoster neuralgia (PZN) and postherpetic neuralgia (PHN) are equivalent. The most conservative definition of PHN would be pain in the affected region lasting longer than 3 or 6 months after crusting of the skin lesions, as patients with pain at 6 months are likely to continue to have pain ≥1 years postzoster. However, most clinicians and many clinical trials have used 1 month after crusting of the skin lesions to define the start of PHN (86).

Incidence

In healthy persons under the age of 20, the incidence of zoster is 0.42–0.74 cases per 1,000 person-years (43,89). The elderly are at greatly increased risk not only for developing HZ, with an incidence of 4.5–10.1 cases per 1,000 person-years (13,42,52,89). Overall, ~15% of people who have had varicella develop zoster. Of those surviving to the age of 80, roughly a third will have had an episode of zoster. The risk of developing a second attack of zoster appears to be as great as the first attack (52,76). Immune system compromise is associated with a greatly increased risk of developing zoster (37,38). Adult cancer patients have a rate that is 6.2 per 1,000 person-years (100). Children with leukemia have a rate that may be >100-fold higher than their healthy peers (43,45). HIV-infected persons also have a much higher risk of zoster (37).

Chronic PHN occurs in ~10–15% of all HZ patients. The elderly are at greatly increased risk not only for developing HZ, but also for PHN following HZ (13,23,52,89). Less than

4% of children develop PHN after zoster. Zoster at the age of 60 has an incidence of PHN of 47% and, by the age of 80, up to 80% will develop PHN. In an unfortunate minority, PHN persists for years or even a lifetime. Again the elderly are at disproportionately high risk for PHN pain lasting >1 year. Precise figures on the prevalence of PHN are not available, but extrapolation from published population-based studies indicates ~180,000 persons suffer from PHN in the United States (13,23,52,61,89).

PREHERPETIC NEURALGIA, ZOSTER SINE HERPETE, AND SUBCLINICAL ZOSTER

Preherpetic Manifestation

In elderly patients presenting with acute and severe chest or abdominal pain that cannot be explained, incipient zoster is high on the differential diagnosis list. Although it is common for patients to describe pain, itching, and paresthesias for 2–4 days before the first lesions become apparent, Gilden et al. (39) have described a group of patients with pain preceding zoster by up to 100 days and even longer. The pathophysiologic basis of such long-lasting preherpetic neuralgia is not certain. Because the disorder begins with virus reactivation in dorsal root ganglion neurons, one may speculate that pain would begin as soon as tissue inflammation or destruction occurs. The preherpetic pain would be experienced as arising within the skin or deeper tissues because of the dorsal root ganglion origin of the disturbance. Perhaps the reactivation is able to be kept in check for a prolonged period by the immune system before viral transport finally progresses all the way to the skin to produce the characteristic lesions.

Acute Zoster Without Rash

Lewis described several cases of what he felt was acute zoster without the rash, or "zoster sine herpete," in 1958 (63). He suggested that zoster could be the cause of a number of syndromes that were otherwise unexplained, including unilateral segmental pain with or without visceral disturbances, painful unilateral muscle paresis, ophthalmic disturbances with eyeball or ocular muscle involvement, and otalgia with palsies or taste loss. In 1970, Easton (27) demonstrated a 16-fold antibody titer rise in his own case of VZV-induced trigeminal pain. Subsequent case reports suggest VZV is an uncommon, but now well-documented, cause of isolated neurologic disorders. In immunocompetent patients with diverse disorders, including transverse myelitis, cranial or peripheral polyneuritis, aseptic meningitis, and encephalitis, VZV has been documented as the cause by either VZV isolation, intrathecal VZV antibody production, high VZV titers in blood or cerebrospinal fluid, and diagnostic titer rises (29,47,73). Recently, Gilden et al. (41) used VZV DNA extraction from cerebrospinal fluid to support a viral etiology in two otherwise healthy men with radicular pain lasting 5–8 months.

Subclinical Zoster

Subclinical zoster can also occur. Luby et al. observed fluctuations in VZV antibody titers in the absence of symptoms in renal transplant patients in 1977 (68). Ljungman et al. (65) observed 102 patients before and after bone marrow transplantation; 36% developed clinical zoster and another 26% had subclinical reactivation based on either a fourfold or greater rise in VZV antibody titers or development of a positive lymphocyte transformation response. The phenomenon was proven by Wilson et al. (117), who used the polymerase chain reaction to demonstrate viremia in 19% of 37 bone marrow transplant patients who had no symptoms of zoster (117).

PREDICTORS OF PHN DEVELOPMENT

It is not clear why only a minority of patients develop PHN when the great majority have significant pain during acute zoster. Several factors may be relevant.

1. *Immune competency:* In general, immune system competence does not seem to be a factor (3,37,38,100).
2. *Location:* Location of the rash on the face (especially when the eye is involved) nearly doubles the risk of developing PHN. When established, the facial pain seems to last longer than in other locations (52). Curiously, lumbar and sacral PHN were of the shortest duration in the Hope-Simpson's series (52).
3. *Antibody titer:* Severe skin lesions and a large rise in VZV antibody titers are markers of a more severe outbreak and also increase the risk of PHN (48).
4. *Severity of acute pain and personality:* Severe acute herpetic pain seems to predispose a patient to suffer from PHN, but the explanation could be varying degrees of personality factors, more severe outbreak, etc. In a large retrospective study, Engberg et al. (31) studied whether psychosocial stress influenced the course of zoster and the development of PHN. Although mood alteration due to continuing pain could have influenced their recollections, patients experiencing psychosocial stress at the time of the zoster outbreak had more severe zoster pain and continued to view their habits and activities as changed negatively due to PHN.
5. *Sensory threshold changes:* Nurmikko et al. (80) carried out detailed sensory examinations in 31 patients at 4–28 days into acute zoster. As a group, the acute zoster patients had an elevated threshold for vibration detection and difficulty detecting innocuous temperature changes in the warm to cool range within the affected dermatome. Heat pain thresholds were not elevated in the 12 subjects tested because four subjects were sufficiently hyperalgesic to balance the remaining eight hypoalgesic subjects. At the 3-month reevaluation, seven patients had PHN. A stepwise logistic regression analysis revealed thermal threshold asymmetry to predict development of PHN. Whether the thermal threshold asymmetry is a specific marker because it indicates deafferentation is necessary for development of PHN or is only a marker that a severe outbreak occurred because demonstrable injury to the primary afferent system was present is an important question for future study.

FACTORS PREVENTING THE DEVELOPMENT OF PHN

Nerve Blocks

Anecdotal reports, totaling thousands of patients, have been used to argue both for and against nerve blocks early in the course of HZ to prevent PHN (15,19,35,48,50,91,106,118,123). As nerve blocks during the acute HZ phase can be dramatically effective in reducing pain, and there is an association between severity of acute herpetic pain and development of PHN, the approach has merit. The debate on this topic remains clouded by two issues.

First, there are no properly controlled studies of adequate size to test the hypothesis. Proof that PHN can be prevented by use of repetitive nerve blocks early in the course of zoster, and the risk:benefit ratio of this approach, can only be gained through a study with random assignment to either nerve block or conservative pain control methods. Because pain will resolve in the great majority of cases by 3 months postzoster, matching for duration of HZ outbreak at study entry, age, location of HZ, sensory abnormalities (including thermal sensory testing), and severity of HZ pain will be critically important. Tenicela et al. (106) attempted a double-blind, crossover study of sympathetic blocks, but their sample size of 20 was far too small to overcome the effect of the natural history of the disorder. A study sample in the hundreds would be necessary; it seems unlikely such a study will be carried out soon.

Second, the debate has placed an excessive emphasis on the role of the sympathetic nervous system. In many studies, the local anesthetic epidural and stellate ganglion blocks most commonly used are both referred to as sympathetic blocks (15,19,48,50,106,118,123). For example, in Winnie and Hartwell's (118) study of prevention of PHN by sympathetic blocks, approximately half the patients were treated via the epidural route. Both C-nociceptor primary afferents and sympathetic efferents are unmyelinated fibers and both are affected by epidural blocks. Furthermore, electrophysiologic studies do not support an association between fiber size and concentration dependence (36). The strongest case for a sympathetic nervous system component to acute zoster pain is the relief of trigeminal zoster pain by stellate ganglion block. In addition, primary afferent nociceptors are known to develop a response to local release of norepinephrine (NE) after nerve injury and increased numbers of α receptors are synthesized (25,85,108). However, even local anesthetic blocks of the stellate ganglion for cranial pain are not completely selective for the sympathetic nervous system. Systemic lidocaine has been shown to block nerve injury-induced hyperalgesia and nociceptor-driven spinal sensitization in animal models (2). In humans, systemically administered local anesthetics relieve a variety of pains, including zoster and PHN pain, and vascular uptake from the region of the stellate ganglion is so rapid that peak venous blood levels occur within five minutes (95,101,122). Regional sympathetic blocks for neck, arm, and leg involvement by zoster carry the possibility of pain relief by spread to nearby sensory nerves, especially when larger volumes are used (22). Controlled studies of alternative techniques for blocking the actions of the sympathetic nervous system, such as intravenous phentolamine, have not been reported.

There is a strong emphasis on beginning nerve blocks as soon as possible after the onset of zoster in order to have the best chance of preventing PHN (15,19,48,50,106,118). The natural history of the disorder makes this claim difficult to evaluate. As pain with acute zoster may be transient, with each passing day after zoster onset the total available pool of nerve block candidates shrinks as pain spontaneously remits in some. Therefore, by 3 weeks after zoster onset, those destined to develop PHN occupy a much greater percentage of the total pool than at 1 week after zoster onset. The nerve block technique used may not be critical as peripheral nerve blocks (including intercostal blocks), epidural administration of local anesthetic and narcotic, and even very low-risk and simple techniques such as skin infiltration with local anesthetic may relieve pain (91). It is clear from all studies that once PHN is established, the likelihood that nerve blocks will permanently relieve pain falls dramatically (15,19,118).

Antiviral/Steroid Medication

There is agreement among published trials that acyclovir at the onset of HZ reduces pain in the short term (5). Although a metanalysis of four acyclovir trials claimed a 42% reduction in PHN, most large trials indicate acyclovir to have little effect on the likelihood of developing long-lasting postherpetic pain (5,18,53,74,119,120). Studies of two newer antivirals, famciclovir and valacyclovir, provide encouraging data by showing faster rates of pain resolution when compared to placebo or acyclovir (7,107).

There have been five trials of steroids for prevention of PHN (32,88,116,120). Two early studies showed benefit in reducing the incidence of PHN (88). Later studies, including comparisons of steroids plus acyclovir indicates steroids reduce early pain without a definite impact on long-term pain (32,116,120). Administering steroids plus local anesthetic by the epidural route is a frequent clinical practice; how this compares with a tapering course of oral steroids is unknown.

PATHOPHYSIOLOGY OF POSTHERPETIC PAIN

Viral Replication

It has been proposed that persistent low-level virus replication could be responsible for some cases of PHN. Viewed this way, unilateral segmental pain would be related to VZV replication in four ways: (a) preherpetic neuralgia, in which pain is present but the virus has not yet reached the skin to produce the characteristic rash; (b) acute zoster, in which viral replication and transport has extended from dorsal root ganglion neurons to affected skin; (c) zoster sine herpete, in which viral replication occurs but rash never appears; and (d) postherpetic neuralgia, in which viral replication and transport for a limited period of time affects the skin, but pain persists because viral replication never completely ceases. However, in only a few cases has persistent viral replication been demonstrated in immunocompetent patients with PHN, making it speculative that a significant proportion of PHN cases could be accounted for in this way (40). In the very limited pathological data published in the 20th century are a few examples of inflammatory cell infiltrates present 100 days and longer in otherwise uncomplicated cases of PHN (115). This suggests that prolonged inflammation is associated with some cases of postherpetic pain. Whether or not the inflammation is related to persistent viral expression in these cases is completely unknown. Anecdotally, treatment of chronic PHN patients with acyclovir does not appear to provide much benefit, although this treatment modality has not been subjected to a controlled trial.

Neuropathic Pain State

The most widely accepted view is that PHN is a neuropathic pain, resulting from damage to or abnormal functioning of the nervous system (79,86). Postmortem studies have shown that in nearly every case, only one dorsal root ganglion and its connections are affected (115). During acute zoster, inflammation and destruction of the neural apparatus extends from the dorsal root to the skin (5,6,28,46,52,86,89,104). In the chronic state, nerve cell loss in the dorsal root ganglion, fibrosis of the dorsal root, peripheral nerve and skin, and thinly myelinated axons consistent with remyelination have been reported (24,46,78,112,115). Postmortem studies by Watson et al. (115) have shown that the dorsal horn of the spinal cord may be atrophic in chronic PHN.

Patients with PHN collectively describe three components to their discomfort: (a) a constant, deep, aching, "bruised," or burning sensation, (b) a spontaneous, recurrent, neuralgic, shooting or electric shocklike pain, and (c) an allodynic, superficial, sharp, radiating, burning, tender, dysesthetic or "itch"-like sensation evoked by wearing clothing, very light touch, or gentle pressure on the skin (94,112). The mechanism(s) behind each of these complaints is not certain.

Noordenbos (79) reported that patients who did not develop PHN after zoster had no sensory deficits on clinical examination, but patients who developed PHN had sensory deficits. Noordenbos noted the presence of allodynia, including the production of pain by stimuli at the threshold for detection. He felt, based in part on pathological study of intercostal nerves by light microscopy, that zoster produced preferential loss of large diameter myelinated sensory fibers in some patients and that the pain was due to the loss of the normal inhibitory function of these fibers on CNS pain transmission neurons. Unfortunately, his methods could not distinguish between large diameter fibers attempting to regenerate and unmyelinated C-fibers. Following Noordenbos' seminal work, many workers have believed that the pain of PHN is due to deafferentation and central reorganization (10,81,82,115).

Nurmikko and Bowsher (81) compared 42 patients presenting for treatment of PHN with a group of 20 patients who had previously been seen for therapy of acute zoster but had not developed PHN. Consistent with Noordenbos's and Watson and colleagues' reports, they found that there were significant sensory deficits in the area of pain in the PHN patients, but examination of the area of the herpetic outbreak in 90% of the patients who had not developed PHN revealed normal sensation (79,112). In the PHN patients, the group means for all sensory modalities tested (warm, cold, and heat pain thresholds; tactile, pinprick, two-point discrimination, and vibration thresholds) were abnormal compared to the unaffected mirror image area. Allodynia to gently brushing the skin was present in 87% of their sample of PHN patients. Nurmikko and Bowsher postulated that the allodynia was a result of central reorganization consequent to deafferentation such that second order pain transmission neurons became capable of responding to A-beta low-threshold mechanoreceptors. Bowsher (10) later concluded in a review paper that the degree of pain in PHN is determined by the extent of loss of unmyelinated and small myelinated primary afferent function and is due to changes in the spinal cord resulting from deafferentation.

Based on a study of 10 patients with PHN and allodynia on examination compared to three patients who did not experience PHN after zoster and 10 healthy controls, Baron and Saguer (4) concluded that C-nociceptors were not involved in the signaling and maintenance of allodynia. Skin temperature, skin resistance, resting blood flow, and thermally evoked blood flow was the same in PHN skin and contralateral uninvolved skin. The flare reaction to iontophoresed histamine was significantly impaired in allodynic PHN skin, and little pain or itch was provoked. The severity of the defect in flare response was strongly correlated with the severity of spontaneous pain complaint, which they felt supported central deafferentation as the major mechanism for the pain. Although iontophoresis of histamine does stimulate a C-fiber–mediated axon flare response, this is an indirect measure of C-nociceptor function, and corroborating evidence in the form of detailed baseline sensory findings was not provided. Jancso et al. (55) previously reported defects in the flare response to capsaicin in both PHN and zoster. LeVasseur et al. (62) reported defects in the flare response to capsaicin in PHN skin compared to control sites distant from the area, but found no correlation of pain and capsaicin induced flare response.

Rowbotham and Fields (94) reported their analysis of the sensory features of PHN in 1989, based on a clinical study of 12 patients with PHN. Although the area of greatest sensory loss and scarring was generally included in the area of maximum pain, the most severe pain correlated best with the area of most severe allodynia. Areas of severe allodynia often had minor or no clinical sensory deficit. Areas of perceived abnormal sensation (including allodynia) sometimes extended far beyond the borders of visible scarring and beyond the borders of the original rash (Fig. 1). Using an infrared device for determining skin temperature that does not require skin contact, it was reported that allodynic skin was sometimes asymmetrically warm, and that extensively deafferented areas without allodynia were sometimes asymmetrically cool. Infiltrating the most severely allodynic skin with dilute lidocaine frequently produced a dramatic reduction in pain severity. The findings suggested that afferent input was critical for maintaining PHN pain in most cases and that abnormal C-nociceptor activity arising in fibers that were still functionally connected to their peripheral and central targets could account for the sensory and thermographic findings and the response to local anesthetic skin infiltration.

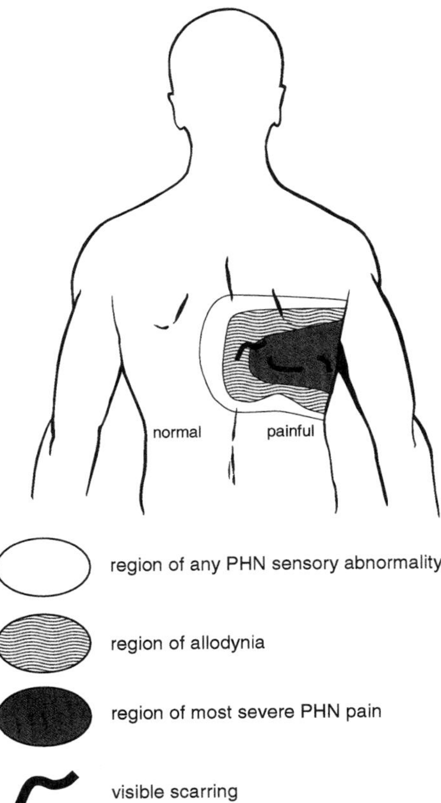

Figure 1. Topography of PHN pain and sensory disturbances. The size of the different regions varies from <50 cm^2 to well over 1,000 cm^2. In exceptional cases, the region of nonpainful sensory disturbance and allodynia may extend far beyond the borders of visible scarring or the original rash, and may even extend a short distance across the midline. Scarring is most often included in the patient-defined area of greatest pain.

Multiple Mechanism

More than one pain mechanism may thus be necessary to account for the continuing pain of PHN (34). A subset of patients have severe sensory deficits, little or no allodynia, and little or no pain relief from peripheral neural blockade (94). In such patients, the precise mechanism of such pain is obscure, but is possibly related to enduring changes in the CNS induced by deafferentation (6,67,121). In contrast, patients with prominent allodynia may have important pain generators located in the skin. As primary afferents of all types, including nociceptors, are damaged during acute zoster, there is a source for increased primary afferent activity via ectopic impulse generation, as has been demonstrated in both animal models of experimental nerve injury and humans with peripheral nerve injury (14,25,60,108). The intensely painful stimulus of acute HZ could produce sensitization of spinal cord neurons maintained by continuing input from damaged C-nociceptors in the area of pain. Instead of rewiring in the dorsal horn of the spinal cord to produce pain from innocuous mechanoreceptor stimulation, the mechanism of allodynia in some PHN patients could thus be analogous to areas of secondary hyperalgesia observed after experimental capsaicin injection (60,121). In this situation, continuing C-nociceptor input is required to maintain pain and allodynia as cuff block of A-beta fibers blocks allodynia but not pain, while C-fiber block eliminates both allodynia and ongoing burning pain. It is interesting to note that to the degree that opiates have efficacy at low doses in PHN (see below), it differs in principle from other forms of neuropathy where opiates may show relatively less activity (see Chapter 56). Given that opiates are able most efficiently to alter C-fiber transmission (see Chapter 58), such efficacy would point to a syndrome in part mediated though a C-fiber-driven linkage.

THERAPY OF POSTHERPETIC NEURALGIA

The essence of established PHN is the chronicity of the pain and its resistance to therapy (86). The devastating impact of PHN on a patient's life should never be underestimated. Patients over the age of 65 nearly always know one or more people who have recovered uneventfully from zoster and so blame themselves for the continuing pain. After a time, many patients are afraid to "burden" their friends and relatives with any discussion of their continuing pain. Social isolation, depression, and even suicide occur with sufficient frequency to make PHN one of the more significant health problems of the elderly.

The only therapy proven effective for PHN in multiple- and independent-controlled studies are the tricyclic antidepressants (58,70,72,86,109,110,112,113). Beyond that, the number of options with any proof of efficacy is quite limited. Opioids and anticonvulsant or antiarrhythmic medications may be of substantial benefit in selected patients, although they have not yet been proven of long-term benefit in prospective, controlled trials (83,87,95,97,112). Transcutaneous electrical nerve stimulation (TENS) presents almost no risks and is occasionally of benefit (86). Topical medications containing capsaicin, local anesthetics, or aspirin-like compounds hold significant promise (96). Patients with PHN in the C4 to T4 dermatomes (affecting the shoulder) and L1 to S2 dermatomes (hip and knee) may develop limitation of joint movement due to pain and can benefit from physical therapy.

Patients refractory to widely accepted interventions should be referred to a pain management center, preferably a multidisciplinary treatment program, that is experienced in managing difficult cases of PHN. This is particularly important if more invasive therapies are being considered, such as intrathecal opioid infusion pumps, spinal cord stimulation, deep brain stimulation, surgical destructive lesions, and neurolytic nerve blocks. Psychological intervention, including education about pain physiology, can address depression, concern over chronic fatigue, and perceived global loss of ability to function at the preillness level. Counseling, combined with biofeedback or relaxation therapies, can occasionally be very helpful.

Antidepressants

The tricyclic antidepressants amitriptyline and desipramine have been established to be effective in well-designed, controlled clinical trials (58,70,109,110,113) (see Chapter 64). Antidepressants remain the oral medication treatment of first choice for PHN. Major published trials are listed in Table 1.

Although desipramine appears to have fewer side effects than amitriptyline, all tricyclic antidepressants have unpleasant and potentially dangerous adverse effects, including altered cardiac conduction, orthostatic hypotension, dry mouth, constipation, urinary retention, confusion and memory impairment, and seizures (16,44). Alternatives exist, such as serotonin (5HT)–specific reuptake inhibitors (SSRI) antidepressants like fluoxetine, sertraline, paroxetine, and trazodone, and mixed 5HT-NE antidepressants such as maprotiline, nefazodone, and venlafaxine. Compared to the newer antidepressants, tricyclic antidepressants present greater hazards in patients who may intentionally or accidentally take an overdose. *All* antidepressants have the potential for significant side effects, however. Fluoxetine alters serum levels of some other drugs and may cause troublesome nausea, diarrhea, anxiety, tremor, insomnia, symptomatic hyponatremia, and suicidal ideation, but is essentially free of changes in cardiac conduction and blood pressure. Trazodone may be sedating, cause significant orthostatic hypotension, and can cause priapism in men. Maprotiline has a higher incidence of seizures than other antidepressants. Venlafaxine may produce hypertension.

At present, the mechanism of antidepressant analgesia is incompletely understood. One obvious possibility is that they act within the CNS by enhancing neurotransmission at biogenic amine links of the well-described brain stem to dorsal horn nociceptive modulating system (33) (see Chapters 38 and 58). 5HT and NE projections have been demonstrated between brain stem nuclei implicated in nociceptive modulation as well as from these nuclei to the dorsal horn. The action of either or both transmitters may be critical to the function of this endogenous system. Nearly all antidepressants have been shown to have analgesic activity in a variety of animal pain models (54) (see Chapter 64). More recently, many of the tricyclic antidepressants have been shown to have antagonist activity at the *N*-methyl-D-asparate (NMDA) receptor site (see Chapter 64). Such receptor antagonisms is known to have potent effect upon a number of neuropathic (allodynia) as well as facilitated pain states that are C-fiber driven (see Chapter 64). It remains to be determined if differences in the characteristics of analgesic activity between the different antidepressants relate to their differences in effects on biogenic amine systems, but the studies reported to date with fluoxetine and zimelidine indicate lower analgesic activity for 5HT-selective drugs (71,110). However, a trial of the relatively selective noradrenergic drug maprotiline also showed it was not as effective as amitriptyline (113).

Differences among antidepressants in binding to neurotransmitter receptors of human brain and rat brain synaptosomes that may explain the clinical side effect profiles of these drugs (90). α-Adrenergic receptor blockade is associated with orthostatic hypotension, histamine receptor effects with sedation and possibly weight gain, acetylcholine receptor effects with constipation, dry mouth, blurred vision, nightmares, confusional states, and impaired memory. Amitriptyline affects a

Table 1. SUMMARY OF CLINICAL TRIALS WITH TRICYCLIC ANTIDEPRESSANTS AND POST HERPETIC NEURALGIA

Source	Drugs	n	Controlled?	Benefit?
Woodforde et al. (1965)	Amitriptyline	14	No	
Watson et al. (109)	Amitriptyline	24	Yes	Yes
Max et al. (70)	Amitriptyline, lorazepam	58	Yes	Amitriptyline only
Watson and Evans (110)	Amitriptyline, zimelidine	15	Yes	Amitriptyline only
Kishore-Kumar et al. (58)	Desipramine	26	Yes	Yes
Watson et al. (111)	Various	208	No	
Watson et al. (113)	Amitriptyline, maprotiline	35	Yes	Both effective

large number of neurotransmitter systems; 5HT, NE, and dopamine reuptake are inhibited, and histamine H1, acetylcholine, and α_1- and α_2-adrenergic receptor antagonism is significant. Relative to amitriptyline, desipramine only weakly affects histamine and α_1 and α_2 receptors, and is less potent at blocking acetylcholine receptors, but potently blocks NE reuptake. Fluoxetine is a potent and selective inhibitor of 5HT reuptake. Relative to both amitriptyline and desipramine, fluoxetine has almost no effect on histamine H1, muscarinic acetylcholine, and α_1 and α_2 receptors, but potently blocks 5HT reuptake. Studies that have examined the relationship between dose or blood level and clinical analgesic response have produced conflicting results (58,69–72,109,110,113).

A common misconception among patients is that antidepressants are of no value in treating pain unless associated with depression because their pain-reducing effect is only a by-product of mood elevation. The animal literature is unequivocal regarding a direct analgesic action of antidepressants (54). In addition, studies by Max et al. (69) using amitriptyline clearly show that pain relief is independent of the presence or absence of depression. The analgesic effects of antidepressants are variably expressed. Some patients report they feel better and tolerate their discomfort more easily, but the underlying pain is unchanged. Others note significant qualitative changes in their pain pattern, such as the cessation of lancinating pain and allodynia (58). In a fortunate few, the pain and dysesthesias disappear altogether. Overall, controlled studies show that the majority of PHN patients treated with tricyclic antidepressants report at least partial pain relief, with continued pain or return of pain during treatment periods with placebo (72) (see Chapter 64).

Unfortunately, in clinical practice the results are not as good (112). Elderly patients with PHN who already have other significant health problems, especially cognitive impairment, are particularly difficult to treat with antidepressants. To increase the likelihood of successful completion of the medication trial, it is very important that the patient understand the side effects appear immediately and the benefits may be subtle at first and slow to develop. Commitment to giving the medication a fair chance is crucial. Unless the patient's medical condition indicates otherwise, the literature supports starting with a tricyclic antidepressant, particularly desipramine or amitriptyline. Start with a dose low enough that the patient is very likely to tolerate it initially and then slowly increase the dose every 3–5 days. Continue to increase the dose until pain relief occurs, intolerable side effects develop, or blood levels well into the therapeutic range are documented. An adequate trial would be 2 weeks at a minimum of 75 mg/day of a tricyclic antidepressant or, better yet, 2 weeks at a dose that produces blood levels in the antidepressant range. If the trial fails to relieve pain or is not tolerated, a trial of an alternate antidepressant is warranted, either another tricyclic, an SSRI, or one of the newer mixed 5HT-NE reuptake blocking antidepressants. However, when the first agent fails to relieve PHN pain, the response rate to subsequent antidepressant trials is uncertain.

Opioids

One obvious approach is to use opioid analgesics, and there is ample anecdotal evidence that many patients achieve satisfactory long-term control of their pain without untoward effects (83,87,95,97,112). A placebo-controlled study showed intravenous morphine reduced the pain of PHN (95). Although longer term controlled trials have not been completed, Pappagallo et al. have recently reported excellent results after 6 months of treatment in 16 of 20 consecutive cases using slow-release morphine or oxycodone (83). In individual patients, opioids may succeed even when multiple trials of antidepressants have failed; in others, opioids may provide equivalent relief with fewer side effects (97,112).

Other Oral Medications

Despite the prominence and severity of the pain in PHN, there are few controlled trials of other therapeutic agents. A variety of other medications have been tried, including anticonvulsants such as carbamazepine and valproate, neuroleptics such as chlorprothixene and phenothiazines, and histamine receptor blockers such as cimetidine (86). None have been proven effective compared to placebo and can not be recommended until a thorough trial of antidepressants has been completed. Although i.v. lidocaine has been shown in a controlled trial to relieve PHN pain, prospective controlled trials of the oral congener, mexiletine, have not been reported (95). Anticonvulsants have been anecdotally recommended especially for lancinating, electric shocklike pains in PHN, but antidepressants are also effective for this subtype of PHN pain (58,70). Recently released anticonvulsants such as gabapentin have a favorable side effect profile, but have not been studied in large scale, open-label, or controlled studies. Benzodiazepines are used with some frequency in clinical practice, even though the study by Max et al. (70) showed lorazepam ineffective compared to amitriptyline. Phenothiazines present particular problems with side effects in the elderly and have little to recomment them as monotherapy or combined with an antidepressant. NMDA blocking agents, such as ketamine, have been reported to reduce PHN pain when given intravenously, and orally in one case report, but their role in long-term management of this condition remains to be determined (30,49).

Topical Agents

Because the disease begins with a skin rash that leads to scarring and hypersensitive skin, therapy directed at cutaneous nerves is logical. Three types of topically applied medications have been intensively studied in recent years; capsaicin, local anesthetic preparations, and aspirin and nonsteroidal antiinflammatory drugs (NSAIDs) (96).

Although the original outbreak of HZ may be extensive, most PHN patients have only limited areas of affected skin that they feel is the source of their pain (79,94,112). Only a modest amount of an effective preparation would then need to be applied to produce pain relief. Unlike antidepressants, topical therapies have few systemic side effects. Nearly all patients are potential candidates for topical therapy, and for some there are no other practical alternatives. It seems logical, though unproven, that patients with prominent superficial pain and allodynia would be more likely to respond to topicals than those with deep pain and no allodynia. Published trials of topical agents for PHN are listed in Table 2.

Capsaicin

Capsaicin-containing preparations have received much attention in recent years. Capsaicin selectively stimulates and then blocks unmyelinated primary afferents with eventual depletion of substance P and other peptide transmitters from nociceptive primary afferents (51) (see Chapter 33). These afferents release the same transmitter both peripherally (where they help promote neurogenic inflammation) and at their CNS termination in the dorsal horn (see Chapter 30). Repeated application of capsaicin on normal skin produces a sensory deficit to thermal stimuli, loss of flare response from intradermal histamine, and other changes expected from depletion of peptide transmitters.

Several studies of topical capsaicin for PHN have been carried out, with mixed results (7,9,11,17,26,84,111,112,114). Controversy has surrounded clinical trials of capsaicin because blinding such studies is nearly impossible as a high percentage of patients report significant warmth or a burning sensation on application (17). When all the PHN patients could recognize

Table 2. SUMMARY OF CLINICAL TRIALS WITH TOPICAL AGENTS AND POSTHERPETIC NEURALGIA

Source	Agent	n	Duration	Controlled?	Benefit?
Watson et al. (111)	Capsaicin 0.025%	33	4 weeks	No	
Bernstein et al. (7)	Capsaicin 0.075%	32	6 weeks	Yes	Yes
Drake et al. (26)	Capsaicin 0.025%	30	3 weeks	Yes	No
Bjerring et al. (9)	Capsaicin 0.1%	8	8 weeks	No	
Peikert et al. (84)	Capsaicin 0.025%	39	8 weeks	No	
Bruxelle et al. (11)	Capsaicin 0.030%	59	4 weeks	Yes	Yes
Watson et al. (114)	Capsaicin 0.075%	143	6 weeks	Yes	Yes
Rowbotham and Fields (93)	Lidocaine gel 10%	11	Single session	No	
Kissin et al. (59)	Lidocaine in glycerin	6	Variable	No	
Stow et al. (102)	Lidocaine-prilocaine 5% cream	12	Single session	No	
Riopelle et al. (92)	Lidocaine 9% in petrolatum	22	Single session	No	
Rowbotham et al. (98)	Lidocaine gel 5%	39	Single session	Yes	Yes
Rowbotham et al. (99)	Lidocaine patch 5%	35	Single session	Yes	Yes
King (57)	Aspirin/chloroform	42	Variable	No	
DeBenedittis et al. (20)	Aspirin/diethyl ether	10	Variable	No	
DeBenedittis et al. (21)	Aspirin/diethyl ether	17	Variable	No	
	Aspirin, diclofenac, indomethacin	7	Single session	Yes	Yes
Kassirer (56)	Aspirin in moisturizing lotion	4	Variable	No	
McQuay et al. (75)	Benzydamine cream	23	Variable	Yes	No

capsaicin effects, Bjerring et al. (9) abandoned use of blinding and placebo controls in their study of capsaicin-induced sensory changes using argon laser stimuli. Although 5 of their 8 patients reported pain relief during the 5-week trial, none were still using the cream in open-label follow-up 1 month later. Even at the 0.025% concentration, 66–79% of patients have reported burning with application in the uncontrolled studies of Peikert (84), Watson (111), and their colleagues. Drake et al.'s (26) controlled study of 30 patients using a 0.025% concentration showed no benefit compared to placebo. Two controlled studies showed benefit using 0.030% and 0.075% concentrations in a total of 91 subjects (7,11). Significant differences from placebo appear after ≥4 weeks of therapy and subjects are instructed to apply the compound ≥4 times per day. In Peikert et al.'s uncontrolled study of 39 patients, although 19/39 reported improvement, only 33% continued to use the drug at follow-up (84). The largest double-blind, vehicle-controlled study is that of Watson et al. (114), who reported efficacy in a group of 143 patients using the 0.075% cream. By the end of the 6-week study, 39% reported pain relief with capsaicin compared to 11% with vehicle. The magnitude of the pain reduction was not large, only a 15% reduction from baseline. In addition to the 6-week blinded trial, 77 subjects were followed for up to 2 years and experienced stable or improved pain relief in more than 80% of the cases.

Local Anesthetic

Local anesthetic preparations in five different vehicles have been reported effective for PHN, two of which have shown efficacy in double-blind, vehicle-controlled studies (59,92,93,98, 99,102). In one, 39 subjects treated with 5% lidocaine in a gel vehicle using a three-session crossover design that included application on the contralateral, mirror-image skin as an additional control, showed both efficacy and a local site of action (98). In the other, efficacy was shown in 35 patients using lidocaine 5% in a soft, self-adherent patch compared with both vehicle and no-treatment controls (99). Stow et al. (102) reported relief using 5% lidocaine-prilocaine cream (EMLA). Although Kissin et al. (59) reported a small number of patients whose PHN pain was temporarily relieved by lidocaine in a liquid base containing mostly isopropyl alcohol, this is not a suitable vehicle for chronic use. Riopelle et al. (92) recently reported 9% lidocaine in a petrolatum vehicle to be effective for acute zoster pain. Placebo-controlled, longer-term efficacy studies have not been reported for any local anesthetic preparations.

Antiinflammatory Agents

There has been significant interest in topical application of aspirin and antiinflammatory medications mixed in chloroform or diethyl ether (20,21,57,96). The solution is daubed onto the painful skin. As the solvent evaporates, the active drug is left behind to penetrate to cutaneous nerve endings. In a recent uncontrolled study, King reported excellent results in both acute herpetic pain and PHN in 42 consecutive patients treated this way (57). Similar to King's method, De Benedittis et al. reported benefit from the use of 750–1,500 mg of acetylsalicylic acid crushed to a fine powder and mixed into 20–30 ml of diethyl ether in 25 patients with either acute zoster or PHN (20). In a follow-up study, his group reported that both acute herpetic pain and PHN were relieved with daily use of aspirin in diethyl ether (21). Single session comparative studies of aspirin, diclofenac, and indomethacin have shown benefit compared to placebo (21). Morimoto et al. (77) reported that both indomethacin (in self-adherent poultice form) and a chloroform-aspirin combination were effective, but the poultice was much easier to use. Kassirer et al. (56) reported anecdotally that aspirin in a cream base was also effective. The only negative study is that of McQuay et al. (75), who carried out a carefully designed, multiple-dose, placebo-controlled crossover study of benzydamine in 23 patients.

Theoretical advantages of local anesthetic preparations and aspirin/NSAID preparations over capsaicin would be efficacy with the first few applications, a lower incidence of burning sensations, and possibly a lower frequency of application. All three types of topicals presumably share modulation of cutaneous sensory fiber function, especially that of small diameter nerve fibers, as their mechanism of action (96). No studies directly comparing the different types of topical therapies have been reported.

INVASIVE THERAPIES

Neurolysis

Although local anesthetic nerve blocks are highly effective in the very short term (hours to days), and particularly useful in the initial weeks and months after the onset of HZ, all authors agree they are of limited benefit as long-term therapy for established PHN (15,19,35,48,50,91,106,118,123). Neurolytic nerve blocks, nerve sectioning, and other ablative procedures are occasionally proposed as treatment, but have little proof of efficacy. With the exception of reports on DREZ (dorsal root entry zone) lesions and mesencephalic tractotomy, the majority of the literature on surgical ablative therapies is more than a decade old, predating the widespread use of antidepressants and topical therapies (12,66). The number of cases treated with any particular procedure has been small.

Neuostimulation

Neuromodulatory procedures such as deep brain stimulation appears to be effective in some patients. Although they are very expensive and require considerable ongoing care, implanted opioid pumps and spinal stimulators offer the advantage of a trial period before permanent implantation. Long-term benefits of pumps and stimulators for PHN patients in relation to other available therapies remains uncertain.

REFRACTORY PHN

Unfortunately, some patients with PHN continue to have intolerable pain despite multiple antidepressant trials, anticonvulsant and antiarrhythmic trials, a variety of opioids, and several different topical agents. TENS units, physical therapy, and psychological intervention does not alleviate their suffering. Direct local anesthetic nerve block may transiently and partially reduce pain in such cases. In some patients, even trials of high-dose intravenous opioids, i.v. ketamine, and continuous epidural local anesthetic plus narcotic for several days fails to relieve pain. Should these patients be offered more invasive therapies? The case of trigeminal PHN reported by Sugar and Bucy in 1951 (105) is especially instructive as a spectacular failure. Their patient continued to report pain despite treatment that included alcohol injection into the supraorbital nerve, division of the sensory root, alcohol injection into the trigeminal ganglion, stellate ganglion block, electroconvulsive therapy, extirpation of the contralateral then ipsilateral sensory cortex, and finally, prefrontal lobotomy. With the increasing use of antidepressants, opioids, and topical therapies, the number of cases of truly refractory PHN is hopefully diminishing. Without a prospective series of cases treated surgically after very carefully documented trials of more conservative approaches, it is impossible to know if surgical responders would have also responded to noninvasive therapy.

FUTURE RESEARCH

PHN is a painful disorder uniquely suited for clinical research. Much can be learned about the mechanisms and management of neuropathic pain in general from well-designed studies of patients with PHN. PHN is common, typically strikes otherwise healthy persons in a relatively restricted age distribution, is unilateral, and, in one nerve root territory, has a clearly defined onset and relatively consistent symptomatology.

There remain a large number of questions in search of answers:

1. Many authors have documented nerve damage from the skin through the peripheral nerve apparatus to the dorsal root, but recent postmortem studies by Watson et al. (115) have shown that the dorsal horn of the spinal cord may be significantly atrophied in chronic PHN, as well. This raises the issue as to whether CNS changes alter the response to therapy, making PHN more like chronic spinal cord injury pains that rarely respond to treatment.
2. Finally, if it is possible to predict, based on pain profile, sensory testing, or response to i.v. pharmacological challenges, which therapy would offer the most long-term benefit for a particular PHN patient.
3. The role played by the extent and severity of sensory disturbance in the ongoing symptomatology and response to therapy must be systematically defined.
4. Definition of opioid dosing and the long-term efficacy of such clinical treatment has not been defined with respect to tolerance and/or dependence.
5. Characterization in a systematic fashion of topical agent actions is necessary. Such agents would appear to offer the most appropriate therapeutic ratio by having the most moderate side effects in patients where baseline cognitive impairment is an issue.

REFERENCES

1. Abraham N, Murray J. The belt of roses from hell: historical aspects of herpes zoster and post-herpetic neuralgia. In: Watson CPN, ed. *Herpes zoster and postherpetic neuralgia.* Amsterdam: Elsevier Science, 1993:1–6.
2. Abram SE, Yaksh TL. Systemic lidocaine blocks nerve injury-induced hyperalgesia and nociceptor-driven spinal sensitization in the rat. *Anesthesiology* 1994;80:383–391.
3. Balfour HH. Varicella zoster virus infections in immunocompromised hosts. A review of the natural history and management. *Am J Med* 1988;85:68–73.
4. Baron R, Saguer M. Postherpetic neuralgia: are C-nociceptors involved in signalling and maintenance of tactile allodynia? *Brain* 1993;116:1477–1496.
5. Bean B, Deamant C, Aeppli D. Acute zoster: course, complications and treatment in the immunocompetent host. In: Watson CPN, ed. *Herpes zoster and postherpetic neuralgia.* Amsterdam: Elsevier Science, 1993:37–58.
6. Bennett GJ. Hypotheses on the pathogenesis of herpes zoster-associated pain. *Ann Neurol* 1994;35:S38–S41.
7. Bernstein JE, Korman NJ, Bickers DR, et al. Topical capsaicin treatment of chronic postherpetic neuralgia. *J Am Acad Dermatol* 1989;21:265–270.
8. Beutner KR, Friedman DJ, Forszpaniak C, Anderson PL, Wood MJ. Improved therapy for herpes zoster in immunocompetent adults: valacyclovir HCL compared with acyclovir. *Antimicrob Agents Chemother* (in press).
9. Bjerring P, Arendt-Nielsen L, Soderberg U. Argon laser induced cutaneous sensory and pain thresholds in post-herpetic neuralgia: quantitative modulation by topical capsaicin. *Acta Dermatol Venereol* 1990;70:121–125.
10. Bowsher D. Sensory change in postherpetic neuralgia. In: Watson CPN, ed. *Herpes zoster and postherpetic neuralgia.* Amsterdam: Elsevier Science, 1993:97–108.
11. Bruxelle J, Luu M, Kong-a-Siou D. Randomized double-blind study of topical capsaicin for treatment of post-herpetic neuralgia. In: *Congress Abstracts, 7th World Congress on Pain.* Seattle: IASP Publications, 1993:187.
12. Burchiel KJ. Deafferentation syndromes and dorsal root entry zone lesions. In: Fields HL, ed. *Pain syndromes in neurology.* London: Butterworths, 1990:201–222.
13. Burgoon C, Burgoon J, Baldridge G. The natural history of herpes zoster. *JAMA* 1957;164:265–269.
14. Coderre TJ, Katz J, Vaccarino AL, Melzack R. Contribution of central neuroplasticity to pathological pain: review of clinical and experimental evidence. *Pain* 1993;52:259–285.
15. Colding A. Treatment of pain: organization of a Pain clinic: treatment of acute herpes zoster. *Proc R Soc Med* 1971;66:541–543.
16. Cookson J. Side-effects of antidepressants. *Br J Psychiatry* 1993;20:20–24.
17. Cotton P. Compliance problems, placebo effect cloud trials of topical analgesic. *JAMA* 1990;264:13–14.
18. Crooks RJ, Jones DA, Fiddian A. Zoster-associated chronic pain: an overview of clinical trials with acyclovir. *Scand J Infect* 1991;80:62–68.
19. Dan K, Higa K, Noda B. Nerve block for herpetic pain. In: Fields HL, Cervero F, Dubner R, eds. *Advances in pain research and therapy, vol. 9.* New York: Raven Press, 1985:831–838.
20. DeBenedittis G, Lorenzetti A, Besana F. A new topical treatment for acute herpetic neuralgia and postherpetic neuralgia. *Pain* 1990;S5:S57.
21. DeBenedittis G, Besana F, Lorenzetti A. A new topical treatment for acute herpetic neuralgia and postherpetic neuralgia: the

aspirin/diethyl ether mixture. An open-label study plus a double-blind controlled clinical trial. *Pain* 1992;48:383–390.
22. Dellemijn PLI, Fields HL, Allen RR, McKay WR, Rowbotham MC. The interpretation of Pain relief and sensory changes following sympathetic blockade. *Brain* 1994;117:1475–1487.
23. DeMoragas J, Kierland R. The outcome of patients with herpes zoster. *Arch Dermatol* 1957;75:193–196.
24. Denny-Brown D, Adams R, Fitzgerald P. Pathologic features of herpes zoster: a note on geniculate herpes. *Arch Neurol Psychiatr* 1944;51:216–231.
25. Devor M, Rappaport ZH. Pain and the pathophysiology of damaged nerve. In: Fields HL, ed. *Pain syndromes in neurology.* London: Butterworths, 1990:47–84.
26. Drake HF, Harries AJ, Gamester RE, et al. Randomised double-blind study of topical capsaicin for treatment of post-herpetic neuralgia [Abstract]. *Pain* 1990;S5:S58.
27. Easton HG. Zoster sine herpete causing acute trigeminal neuralgia. *Lancet* 1970;2:1065–1066.
28. Ebert M. Histologic changes in sensory nerves of the skin in herpes zoster. *Arch Dermatol* 1949;60:641–648.
29. Echevarria JM, Martinez-Martin P, Tellez A, et al. Aseptic meningitis due to varicella-zoster virus: serum antibody levels and local synthesis of specific IgG, IgM, and IgA. *J Infect Dis* 1987;155: 959–967.
30. Eide PK, Jorum E, Stubhaug A, Bremnes J, Breivik H. Relief of post-herpetic neuralgia with the N-methyl-D-aspartic acid receptor antagonist ketamine: a double-blind, cross-over comparison with morphine and placebo. *Pain* 1994;58:347–354.
31. Engberg IB, Grondahl GB, Thibom K. Patients' experiences of herpes zoster and postherpetic neuralgia. *J Adv Nurs* 1995;21: 427–433.
32. Esmann V, Kroon S, Peterslund NA, et al. Prednisolone does not prevent post-herpetic neuralgia. *Lancet* 1987;2:126–129.
33. Fields HL, Heinricher MM, Mason P. Neurotransmitters in nociceptive modulatory circuits. *Annu Rev Neurosci* 1991;14:219–245.
34. Fields HL, Rowbotham MC. Multiple mechanisms of neuropathic pain: a clinical perspective. In: Gebhart GF, Hammond DL, Jensen TS, eds. *Proceedings of the 7th World Congress on Pain, Progress in Pain Research and Management, vol. 2.* Seattle: IASP Press, 1994:437–454.
35. Fine PG. Nerve blocks, herpes zoster, and postherpetic neuralgia. In: Watson CPN, ed. *Herpes zoster and postherpetic neuralgia.* Amsterdam: Elsevier, 1993:173–183.
36. Fink B, Cairns A. Lack of size-related differential sensitivity to equilibrium conduction block among mammalian myelinated axons exposed to lidocaine. *Anesth Analg* 1987;66:948.
37. Freidman-Kein AE, Lafleur FL, Gendler E, et al. Herpes zoster: a possible early clinical sign for development of acquired immunodeficiency syndrome. *J Am Acad Dermatol* 1986;14:1023–1028.
38. Gershon A. Zoster in immunosuppressed patients. In: Watson CPN, ed. *Herpes zoster and postherpetic neuralgia.* Amsterdam: Elsevier, 1993:73–86.
39. Gilden DH, Dueland AN, Cohrs R, et al. Preherpetic neuralgia. *Neurology* 1991;41:1215–1218.
40. Gilden DH. Herpes zoster with postherpetic neuralgia—persisting pain and frustration. *N Engl J Med* 1994;330:932–934.
41. Gilden DH, Wright RR, Schneck SA, Gwaltney JM Jr, Mahalingam R. Zoster sine herpete, a clinical variant. *Ann Neurol* 1994;35: 530–533.
42. Glynn C, Crockford G, Gavaghan D, Cardno P, Price D, Miller J. Epidemiology of shingles. *Proc R Soc Med* 1990;83:617–619.
43. Guess HA, Broughton DD, Melton LJ, Kurland LT. Epidemiology of herpes zoster in children and adolescents: a population-based study. *Pediatrics* 1985;76:512–517.
44. Halper JP, Mann JJ. Cardiovascular effects of antidepressant medications. *Br J Psychiatry* 1988;153:87–98.
45. Hardy I, Gershon AA, Steinberg SP, LaRuss P. The incidence of zoster after immunization with live attenuated varicella vaccine. *N Engl J Med* 1991;325:1545–1550.
46. Head H, Campbell A. The pathology of herpes zoster and its bearing on sensory localization. *Brain* 1900;23:353–523.
47. Heller HM, Carnevale NT, Steigbigel RT. Varicella zoster virus transverse myelitis without cutaneous rash. *Am J Med* 1990;88: 550–551.
48. Higa K, Dan K, Manabe H, Noda B. Factors influencing the duration of treatment of acute herpetic Pain with sympathetic nerve block: importance of severity of herpes zoster assessed by the maximum antibody titers to varicella-zoster virus in otherwise healthy patients. *Pain* 1988;32:147–157.
49. Hoffmann V, Coppejans H, Vercauteren M, Adriaensen H. Successful treatment of postherpetic neuralgia with oral ketamine. *Clin J Pain* 1994;10:240–242.
50. Hogan QH. The sympathetic nervous system in post-herpetic neuralgia. *Reg Anesth* 1993;18:271–273.
51. Holzer P. Local effector functions of capsaicin-sensitive sensory nerve endings: involvement of tachykinins, calcitonin gene-related peptide and other neuropeptides. *Neuroscience* 1988;24: 739–768.
52. Hope-Simpson R. The nature of herpes zoster: a long-term study and a new hypothesis. *Proc R Soc Lond B Biol Sci* 1965;58:9–20.
53. Huff JC, Bean B, Balfour HH Jr, et al. Therapy of herpes zoster with oral acyclovir. *Am J Med* 1988;85:84–89.
54. Hwang AS, Wilcox GL. Analgesic properties of intrathecally administered heterocyclic antidepressants. *Pain* 1987;28:343–355.
55. Jancso G, Husz S, Simon N. Impairment of axon reflex vasodilatation after herpes zoster. *Clin Exp Dermatol* 1983;8:27–31.
56. Kassirer MR. King and Robert, concerning the management of pain associated with herpes zoster and of post-herpetic neuralgia. *Pain* 1988;35:368–369.
57. King RB. Topical aspirin in chloroform and the relief of pain due to herpes zoster and postherpetic neuralgia. *Arch Neurol* 1993;50: 1046–1053.
58. Kishore-Kumar R, Max MB, Schafer SC, et al. Desipramine relieves post-herpetic neuralgia. *Clin Pharmacol Ther* 1990;47:305–312.
59. Kissin I, McDanal J, Xavier AV. Topical lidocaine for relief of superficial pain in postherpetic neuralgia. *Neurology* 1989;39: 1132–1113.
60. Koltzenburg M, Torebjork HE, Wahren LK. Nociceptor modulated central sensitization causes mechanical hyperalgesia in acute chemogenic and chronic neuropathic pain. *Brain* 1994;117: 579–591.
61. Kurtzke JF. Neuroepidemiology. *Ann Neurol* 1984;16:265–277.
62. LeVasseur SA, Gibson SJ, Helme RD. The measurement of capsaicin-sensitive sensory nerve fiber function in elderly patients with pain. *Pain* 1990;41:19–25.
63. Lewis GW. Zoster sine herpete. *BMJ* 1958;2:418–419.
64. Lewis T, Marvin HM. Observations relating to vasodilatation arising from antidromic impulses, to herpes zoster and trophic effects. *Heart* 1927;14:27–47.
65. Ljungman P, Lonnqvist B, Gahrton G, Ringden O, Sundqvist V-A, Wahren B. Clinical and subclinical reactivations of varicella-zoster virus in immunocompromised patients. *J Infect Dis* 1986;153: 840–847.
66. Loeser JD. Surgery for postherpetic neuralgia. In: Watson CPN, ed. *Herpes zoster and postherpetic neuralgia.* Amsterdam: Elsevier, 1993:221–238.
67. Lombard MC, Larabi Y. Electrophysiological study of cervical dorsal horn cells in partially deafferented rats. In: Bonica JJ, Lindblom U, Iggo A, eds. *Advances in pain research and therapy, vol. 5.* New York: Raven Press, 1983:147–154.
68. Luby J, Ramirez-Ronda C, Rinner S, Hull A, Vergne-Marini P. A longitudinal study of varicella zoster virus in renal transplant recipients. *J Infect Dis* 1977;135:659–663.
69. Max MB, Culnane M, Schafer SC, et al. Amitriptyline relieves diabetic neuropathy pain in patients with normal or depressed mood. *Neurology* 1987;37:589–596.
70. Max M, Schafer S, Culnane M, et al. Amitriptyline, but not lorazepam, relieves postherpetic neuralgia. *Neurology* 1988;38:1427–1432.
71. Max MB, Lynch SA, Muir J, et al. Effects of desipramine, amitriptyline, and fluoxetine on pain in diabetic neuropathy. *N Engl J Med* 1992;326:1250–1256.
72. Max MB. Treatment of post-herpetic neuralgia: antidepressants. *Ann Neurol* 1994;35:S50–S53.
73. Mayo Dr, Boos J. Varicella zoster-associated neurologic disease without skin lesions. *Arch Neurol* 1989;46:313–315.
74. McKendrick MW, McGill JI, Wood MJ. Lack of effect of acyclovir on postherpetic neuralgia. *BMJ* 1989;298:431.
75. McQuay HJ, Carroll D, Moxon A, et al. Benzydamine cream for the treatment of post-herpetic neuralgia: minimum duration of treatment periods in a cross-over trial. *Pain* 1990;40:131–135.
76. Molin L. Aspects of the natural history of herpes zoster. *Acta Dermatol Venereol* 1969;49:569–583.
77. Morimoto M, Inamori K, Hyodo M. The effect of indomethacin stupe for post-herpetic neuralgia—particularly in comparison with chloroform-aspirin solution [Abstract]. *Pain* 1990;S5:S59.
78. Muller S, Winkelmann R. Cutaneous nerve changes in zoster. *J Invest Dermatol* 1969;52:71–77.

79. Noordenbos W. *Pain.* Amsterdam: Elsevier Science, 1959.
80. Nurmikko TJ, Räsänen A, Häkkinen V. Clinical and neurophysiological observations on acute herpes zoster. *Clin J Pain* 1990;6:284–290.
81. Nurmikko T, Bowsher D. Somatosensory findings in postherpetic neuralgia. *J Neurol Neurosurg Psychiatry* 1990;53:135–141.
82. Nurmikko T. Sensory dysfunction in postherpetic neuralgia. In: Boivie J, Hansson P, Lindblom U, eds. *Touch, temperature, and pain health and disease: mechanisms and assessments. Progress in pain research and management, vol. 3.* Seattle: IASP Press, 1994:133–141.
83. Pappagallo M, Campbell JN. Chronic opioid therapy as alternative treatment for post-herpetic neuralgia. *Ann Neurol* 1994;35:S54–S56.
84. Peikert A, Hentrich M, Ochs G. Topical 0.025% capsaicin in chronic post-herpetic neuralgia: efficacy, predictors of response and long-term course. *J Neurol* 1991;238:452–456.
85. Perl ER. Causalgia and reflex sympathetic dystrophy revisited. In: Boivie J, Hansson P, Lindblom U, eds. *Touch, temperature, and pain health and disease. Progress in pain research and management, vol. 3.* Seattle: IASP Press, 1994:231–248.
86. Portenoy R, Duma C, Foley K. Acute herpetic and postherpetic neuralgia: clinical review and current management. *Ann Neurol* 1986;20:651–664.
87. Portenoy R, Foley K. Chronic use of opioid analgesics in non-malignant pain: report of 38 cases. *Pain* 1986;25:171–186.
88. Post BT, Philbrick JT. Prevention of postherpetic neuralgia by corticosteroids. In: Watson CPN, ed. *Herpes zoster and postherpetic neuralgia.* Amsterdam: Elsevier, 1993:159–172.
89. Ragozzino M, Melton L, Kurland L, et al. Population based study of herpes zoster and its sequelae. *Medicine* 1982;61:310–316.
90. Richelson E. Antidepressants and brain neurochemistry. *Mayo Clin Proc* 1990;65:1227–1236.
91. Riopelle JM, Naraghi M, Grush K. Chronic neuralgia incidence following local anesthetic therapy for herpes zoster. *Arch Dermatol* 1984;120:747–750.
92. Riopelle J, Lopez-Anaya A, Cork RC, et al. Treatment of the cutaneous pain of acute herpes zoster with 9% lidocaine (base) in petrolatum/paraffin ointment. *J Am Acad Dermatol* 1994;30:757–767.
93. Rowbotham M, Fields H. Topical lidocaine reduces pain in postherpetic neuralgia. *Pain* 1989;38:297–302.
94. Rowbotham MC, Fields HL. Post-herpetic neuralgia: the relation of Pain complaint, sensory disturbance, and skin temperature. *Pain* 1989;39:129–144.
95. Rowbotham MC, Reisner LA, Fields HL. Both intravenous lidocaine and morphine reduce the Pain of post-herpetic neuralgia. *Neurology* 1991;41:1024–1028.
96. Rowbotham MC. Topical agents for post-herpetic neuralgia. In: Watson CPN, ed. *Herpes zoster and postherpetic neuralgia.* Amsterdam: Elsevier, 1993:185–203.
97. Rowbotham MC. Managing post-herpetic neuralgia with opioids and local anesthetics. *Ann Neurol* 1994;35S:S46–S49.
98. Rowbotham MC, Davies PS, Fields HL. Topical lidocaine gel relieves postherpetic neuralgia. *Ann Neurol* 1995;37:246–253.
99. Rowbotham MC, Davies PS, Verkempinck C, Galer BS. Lidocaine patch: double-blind controlled study of a new treatment method for post-herpetic neuralgia. *Pain* (press).
100. Rusthoven JJ, Ahlgren P, Elhakim T, et al. Varicella-zoster infection in adult cancer patients. *Arch Intern Med* 1988;148:1561–1566.
101. Shanbrom E. Treatment of herpetic pain and postherpetic neuralgia with intravenous procaine. *JAMA* 1961;176:1041–1043.
102. Stow PJ, Glynn CJ, Minor B. EMLA cream in the treatment of postherpetic neuralgia: efficacy and pharmacokinetic profile. *Pain* 1989;39:301–305.
103. Straus SE, Smith HA, Ruyechen WT, Henderson DK, Blaese RM, Hay J. Endonuclease analysis of viral DNA from varicella and subsequent zoster infections in the same patient. *N Engl J Med* 1984;311:1362–1364.
104. Straus S. Varicella-zoster virus infections: biology, natural history, treatment, and prevention. *Ann Int Med* 1988;108:221–237.
105. Sugar O, Bucy P. Postherpetic trigeminal neuralgia. *Arch Neurol Psychiatry* 1951;65:131–145.
106. Tenicela R, Lovasik D, Eaglestein W. Treatment of herpes zoster with sympathetic blocks. *Clin J Pain* 1985;1:63–67.
107. Tyring S, Barbarash RA, Nahlik JE, et al. Famciclovir for the treatment of acute herpes zoster: effects on acute disease and postherpetic neuralgia. *Ann Intern Med* (in press).
108. Wall PD, Gutnick M. Ongoing activity in peripheral nerves: the physiology and pharmacology of impulses originating from a neuroma. *Exp Neurol* 1974;43:580–593.
109. Watson C, Evans R, Reed K, et al. Amitriptyline vs placebo in postherpetic neuralgia. *Neurology* 1982;32:671–673.
110. Watson CPN, Evans RJ. A comparative trial of amitriptyline and zimelidine in postherpetic neuralgia. *Pain* 1985;23:387–394.
111. Watson C, Evans R, Watt V. Postherpetic neuralgia and topical capsaicin. *Pain* 1988;33:333–340.
112. Watson CPN, Evans RJ, Watt VR, Birkett N. Post-herpetic neuralgia: 208 cases. *Pain* 1988;35:289–297.
113. Watson CPN, Chipman M, Reed K, Evans RJ, Birkett N. Amitriptyline versus maprotiline in postherpetic neuralgia: a randomized, double-blind, crossover trial. *Pain* 1992;48:29–36.
114. Watson CPN, Tyler KL, Bickers DR, Millikan LE, Smith S, Coleman E. A randomized vehicle-controlled trial of topical capsaicin in the treatment of postherpetic neuralgia. *Clin Ther* 1993;15:510–526.
115. Watson CPN, Deck JH. The neuropathology of herpes zoster with particular reference to postherpetic neuralgia and its pathogenesis. In: Watson CPN, ed. *Herpes zoster and postherpetic neuralgia.* Amsterdam: Elsevier, 1993:139–158.
116. Whitley RJ, Weiss H, Gnann J, et al. The efficacy of steroid and acyclovir therapy of herpes zoster in the elderly. *J Invest Med* 1995;43:A114.
117. Wilson A, Sharp M, Koropchak C, Ting S, Arvin A. Subclinical varicella-zoster virus viremia, herpes zoster, and T lymphocyte immunity to varicella-zoster viral antigens after bone marrow transplantation. *J Infect Dis* 1992;165:119–126.
118. Winnie AP, Hartwell PW. Relationship between time of treatment of acute herpes zoster with sympathetic blockade and prevention of post-herpetic neuralgia: clinical support for a new theory of the mechanism by which sympathetic blockade provides therapeutic benefit. *Reg Anesth* 1993;18:277–282.
119. Wood MJ, Ogan PH, McKendrick MW, et al. Efficacy of oral acyclovir treatment of acute herpes zoster. *Am J Med* 1988;85:79–83.
120. Wood MJ, Johnson RW, McKendrick MW, Taylor J, Mandal BK, Crooks J. A randomized trial of acyclovir for 7 days or 21 days with and without prednisolone for treatment of acute herpes zoster *N Engl J Med* 1994;330:896–900.
121. Woolf CJ, Shortland P, Coggeshall RE. Peripheral nerve injury triggers central sprouting of myelinated afferents. *Nature* 1992;355:75–78.
122. Wulf H, Maier C, Schele HA, Wabbel W. Plasma concentration of bupivacaine after stellate ganlion blockade. *Anesth Analg* 1991;72:546–8.
123. Yanagida H, Suwa K, Corssen G. No prophylactic effect of early sympathetic blockade on postherpetic neuralgia. *Anesthesiology* 1987;66:73–76.

Anesthesia: Biologic Foundations, edited by Tony L. Yaksh et al. Lippincott–Raven Publishers, Philadelphia © 1997.

CHAPTER 56

CAUSALGIA/REFLEX SYMPATHETIC DYSTROPHY

PAMELA A. PIERCE AND WILLIAM G. BROSE

The clinical pain syndrome that can accompany peripheral nerve injuries had been mentioned only sporadically in the medical literature prior to 1864. However, in that year, Silas Weir Mitchell and his colleagues (113) produced the classic description of the post–nerve injury pain state in a publication entitled "Gunshot Wounds and Other Injuries of Nerves." Mitchell, a physician during the American Civil War, described a burning pain usually present in the hands or feet of soldiers with peripheral nerves that had been injured, typically by the low-velocity impact of the miniball. In these patients, a hyperesthetic state existed in the affected limb, such that the "rattling of a newspaper, a breath of air, . . . or the shock of the feet in walking" would give rise to an increase in pain. The only relief from the burning sensation seemed to be obtained by soaking the affected limb in water. Mitchell introduced the term *causalgia* from the Greek words *kausos* (heat) and *algos* (pain) to refer to the clinical entity he had reported. Since that time alternate terms have appeared in the literature as a further understanding of the pathophysiology of the disease developed (46). *Sudeck's atrophy,* described in 1900, refers to the bony absorption present in advanced stages of the disease. Other terms include *traumatic angiospasm, posttraumatic osteoporosis, minor causalgia, shoulder-hand syndrome, acute atrophy of bone, osteodystrophy, peripheral acute trophoneurosis, traumatic vasospasm, postinfarctional sclerodactyly, reflex neurovascular dystrophy, reflex dystrophy of the extremities,* and *reflex algodystrophy* (89). Recent additions to this confusing nomenclature include *sympathetically maintained pain syndrome* and *complex regional pain syndrome.*

Rene Leriche (98), a French surgeon was perhaps the first to suggest a link between the sympathetic nervous system and causalgia. He promoted sympathectomy for the treatment of causalgia, reasoning that therapeutic response indicated a mechanistic link. The term *reflex sympathetic dystrophy* (RSD) is credited to Evans in 1947, emphasizing the role of the sympathetic nervous system in the disorder. The majority of medical discourse on the subject of RSD has linked increased sympathetic outflow to the evaluation and maintenance of the disease. The clinical and basic observations provided here indicate that this explanation is at least incomplete. RSD has become an extensively used term to refer to the syndrome of chronic burning pain in an extremity and associated dystrophic tissue changes, including bone atrophy, in which blockade of sympathetic function is believed to reduce the observed pain state. Whereas RSD has many etiologies, the term *causalgia* has been reserved for the specific cases of RSD associated with specific identifiable nerve injury. The link drawn between the sympathetic nervous system and RSD as well as the similarity on clinical presentation of many patients with RSD or causalgia has led to the more recent promotion of the term *sympathetically maintained pain* (SMP). These additional changes in nomenclature further suggest the concept that dysfunction of the sympathetic nervous system may be causally related to the clinical syndrome. This causal link appears to be true in only some cases or at some times in the course of disease. Attempts to further describe the heterogeneous group of patients presenting with signs and symptoms of RSD have led to the even more recent terminology of complex regional pain syndrome (CRPS) (156). Given the continued publication of myriad opinions regarding RSD and the poorly defined etiology and pathogenesis in these patients, the promotion of yet further classification should be anticipated for some time.

DEFINITIONS AND EPIDEMIOLOGY

Causalgia

Causalgia is defined as "burning pain, allodynia, and hyperpathia, usually in the hand or foot, after partial injury of a nerve or one of its major branches" (International Association for the Study of Pain [IASP] taxonomy [112]). Allodynia refers to pain due to a stimulus that does not normally provoke pain, whereas hyperpathia is a pain syndrome characterized by increased reaction to a stimulus, especially a repetitive stimulus, as well as an increased threshold (see Chaps. 2 and 13). Essential features of causalgia are a burning pain and cutaneous hypersensitivity with signs of sympathetic hyperactivity in the portion of limb innervated by partially injured nerve.

Various reports have placed the incidence of causalgia after major nerve injury between 2% and 3% (135). A review of the literature indicates the majority of causalgia occurs with trauma to the median nerve, the sciatic nerve and its branches, and the brachial plexus (16). The higher incidence of causalgia in median and sciatic nerve distributions may reflect the fact that the majority of sympathetic fibers to the upper and lower extremities are carried in these nerves. Since the clinical presentation and course of causalgia is virtually identical to RSD, these diseases are discussed together in the Clinical Manifestations section and referred to as RSD.

Reflex Sympathetic Dystrophy

The IASP defines RSD as a "continuous pain in a portion of an extremity after trauma which may include fracture but does not involve a major nerve, associated with sympathetic hyperactivity." The pain is described as "burning, continuous, exacerbated by movement, cutaneous stimulation, or stress." The common clinical component to the syndrome as defined is the alteration of one or more elements of the pain state with an intervention that lowers the release of sympathetic transmitter from the distal sympathetic terminals in the afflicted limb. Such blockade may be achieved by surgical removal, anesthetic block, terminal depletion (as with guanethedine), or postsynaptic blockade (as with phentolamine).

Although numerous causative agents have been reported in the development of RSD, accidental trauma is the most common cause (16). The trauma is usually mild in nature and the severity of the RSD symptoms does not frequently correlate with the evident degree of injury. The trauma can often involve a minor fracture or sprain injury, or a crush or traumatic amputation injury usually of the hand, wrist, foot, or ankle. Iatrogenic trauma to extremities such as surgery, amputation of digits or limbs, poor cast fitting, etc. have also been reported to cause RSD in a number of cases (68).

In addition to traumatic injury, neurologic diseases such as stroke, cervical disk disease, diabetic neuropathy, and multiple sclerosis have been related to the onset of an RSD syndrome (16). The presence of RSD in the hand and upper extremity of patients recovering from myocardial infarction has also been reported in a significant number of patients (139,157). Although many factors have been associated with the development of RSD, a large percentage of cases (25%) present with no definable precipitating event (55). Psychological testing shows approximately one-third of patients with RSD score abnormally; however, no single psychological disorder can be consistently identified (126,159). Moreover, it should be emphasized that is unclear whether emotional or psychological disturbances predisposes to the development of RSD or rather develop as a consequence of the unrelenting symptoms of the disease.

Patients developing RSD usually range in age from 20 to 60 years (159,164); however, a small number of cases of RSD have been reported in children (12,61). In both children and adults, there is a female preponderance of approximately 2:1 to 3:1.

Although the incidence of RSD following limb injuries is probably significantly less than 1%, this small fraction reflects a significant number of cases, given the frequency of mild extremity trauma such as sprains, crush injuries, and minor fractures. Whereas the published literature supports the above view, alternative proposals could be described. The spectrum of signs and symptoms reported by patients and described by physicians could lead one to speculate that mild self-limiting physiologic changes of RSD occur commonly following injury but because of their transient nature they are not reported. While the prevalence of this syndrome is widely accepted, it is not universal. As emphasized above, (a) specific injuries do not reliably lead to the disorder, (b) patients may appear with the diagnosis in spite of an absence of definable injury, and (c) there is a lack of a reliable definition of time course of the evolution of the pathology; accordingly, treatment that appears to alter the manifestation of the syndrome may reflect upon the natural history of the untreated disease. These points have led Ochoa (119) to challenge the definition of RSD as a disease or even a definable syndrome. In the last instance, differential efficacy of even multiple blocks has led to a query regarding the actual role played by the sympathetic nerve terminals in a post–nerve injury syndrome (165,166).

CLINICAL MANIFESTATIONS

The clinical presentation of RSD/causalgia is often described in terms of grades and stages. Intensity of symptoms/signs can be divided into grade 1 (severe), grade 2 (moderate), and grade 3 (mild), while the clinical course is identified in stages: acute, dystrophic, and atrophic (13,16,17). Although there is considerable variation, it is the clinical impression that the course of the RSD syndrome progresses through three stages, each typically lasting approximately 3 to 6 months (16,17,151).

Grade 1 RSD presents with acute onset of severe burning pain that is constant in nature, and hyperalgesia and hyperesthesia that are exacerbated by minimal physical or emotional disturbances. Marked hypersympathetic tone is evident by severe vasomotor and sudomotor instability.

Grade 2 RSD presents with a dull, aching, diffuse pain, described as throbbing, which has developed more insidiously than grade 1 RSD. Only mild signs of increased sympathetic outflow are present.

Grade 3 is a mild form of RSD that is often overlooked by clinicians but that results in increased intensity and duration of pain than otherwise would be expected in the affected extremity.

Acute Stage

The initial signs and symptoms of RSD develop within days or up to 3 to 4 weeks following injury. The acute stage of RSD consists of (a) burning pain not localized to a dermatome or nerve distribution that usually starts in the distal part of an extremity, (b) abnormal cutaneous sensitivity, (c) reduced function, (d) general appearance of the limb, and (e) changes in sympathetic tone. An example of such an acute stage is shown in Fig. 1.

Hyperalgesia and hyperpathia are frequently present to such a degree that the patient guards the affected extremity with extreme caution against the slightest physical disturbance, as Silas Weir Mitchell and colleagues described in 1864.

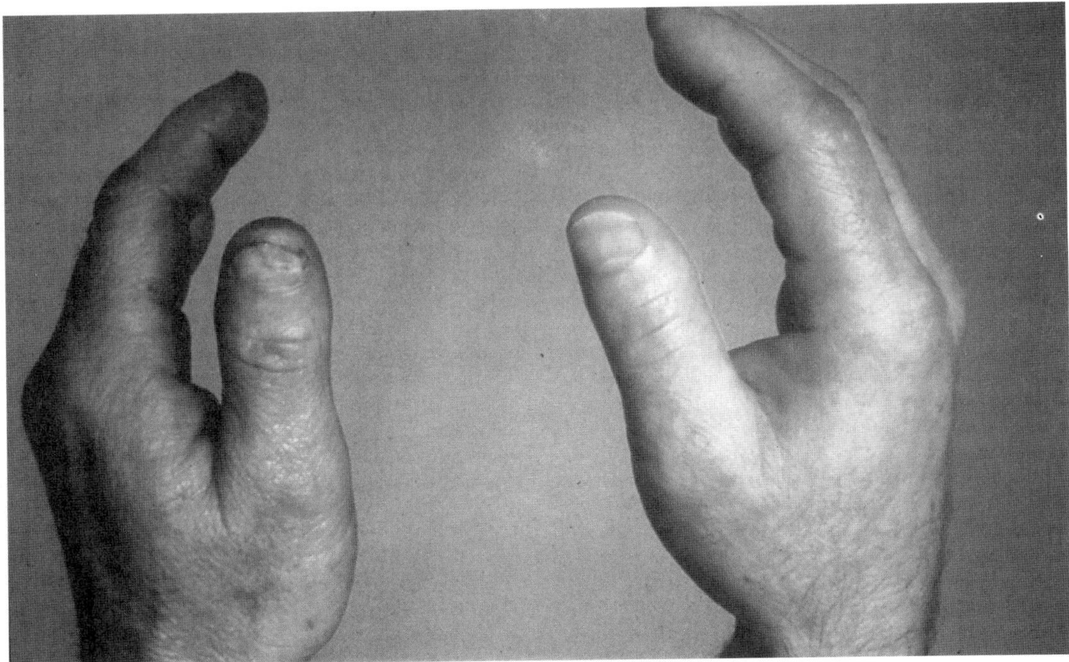

Figure 1. Acute stage RSD. In this case, the patient suffered a right wrist sprain 6 weeks earlier. Note the edema, discoloration of the afflicted extremity, and the glossiness of the skin. The uninjured hand shows the normal wear and tear of a construction worker. At this time, the patient displayed a prominent tactile allodynia and a spontaneous burning dysesthesia that encompassed the hand and forearm. A blockade of sympathetic function at this time by a stellate ganglion block resulted in a transient (3 days) reversal of the evident syndrome and the hyperpathia *(See colorplate 30.)*

After the onset of the reported pain state, a decreased range of motion of the joints of the afflicted limb is observed and an evident muscle spasm is noted.

The general appearance of the limb is altered such that the limb often appears edematous and the skin is dry, 2° to 4°C warmer than the contralateral limb and mildly erythematous, reflecting vasodilatation within the limb.

Toward the end of the acute stage, signs of increased sympathetic tone develop in the affected limb, such as hyperhidrosis, decreased limb temperature (as compared to simultaneous measures made of the contralateral limb), and cold intolerance, reflecting vasoconstriction. Nails and hair show increased growth and hair is coarser.

If treatment is initiated during this stage of the disease process, a large percentage of patients will show at least a transient resolution of their symptoms. Left untreated, however, the disease process often continues on to the second stage within 1 to 3 months.

Dystrophic Stage

The second or dystrophic stage of RSD consists of continued signs of increased sympathetic tone in the affected limb, and pain that continues to be burning in nature with hyperesthesia and hyperpathia present. During the dystrophic stage the pain can either intensify or lessen relative to the acute stage. This

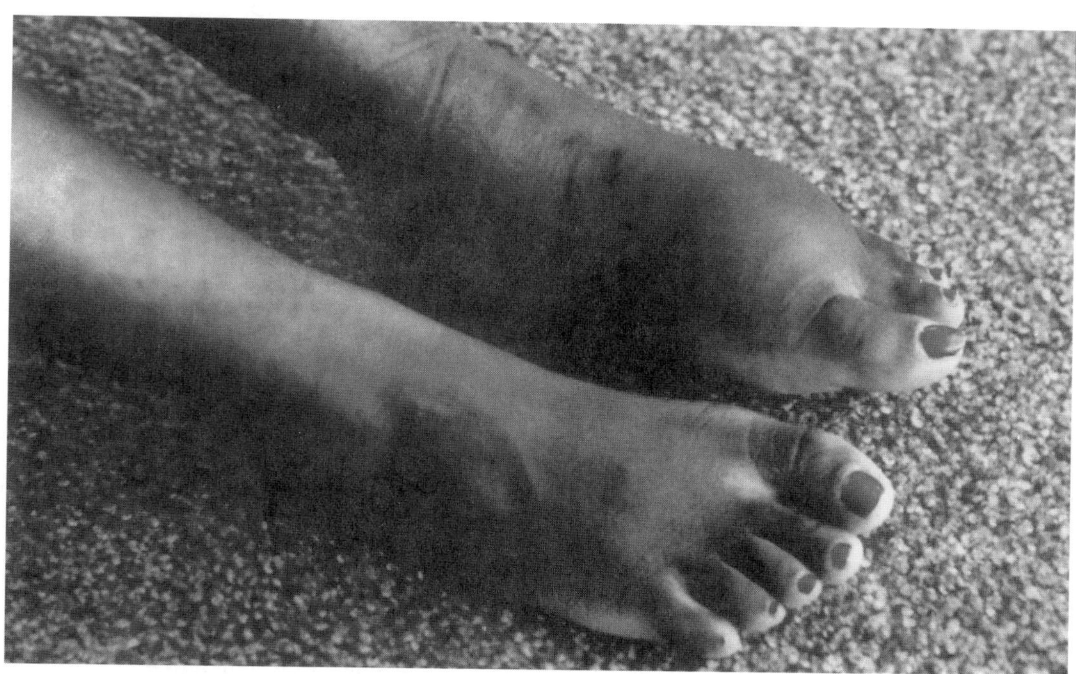

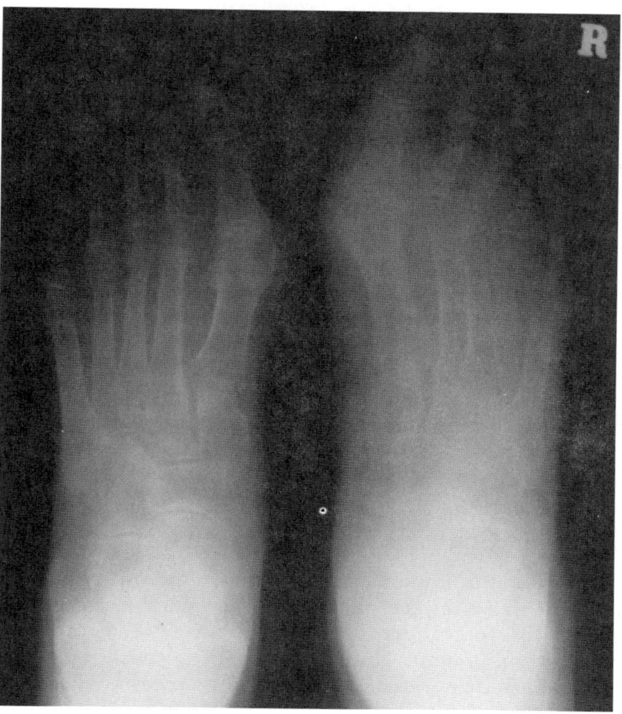

Figure 2. **(A)** Dystrophic stage of RSD in the left foot. In this case, the patient suffered blunt trauma to the dorsum of the foot 6 months earlier. Particularly noteworthy is the evident edema, muscle wasting of the ankle, and changes in hair growth in the afflicted limb. *(See colorplate 4.)* **(B)** X-ray reveals the significant dimineralization of the left (injured) foot. At the time of the photograph, the patient reported a severe burning dysesthesia. At approximately 3 months after injury, a lumbar sympathetic block was effective in inducing a transient pain relief. A lumbar surgical sympathectomy was performed. The symptoms, however, returned after 1 month and subsequent local anesthetic sympathectomies were not effective. At the time of the photograph, the patient was receiving significant pain relief from subcutaneous lidocaine infusion using an ambulatory pump.

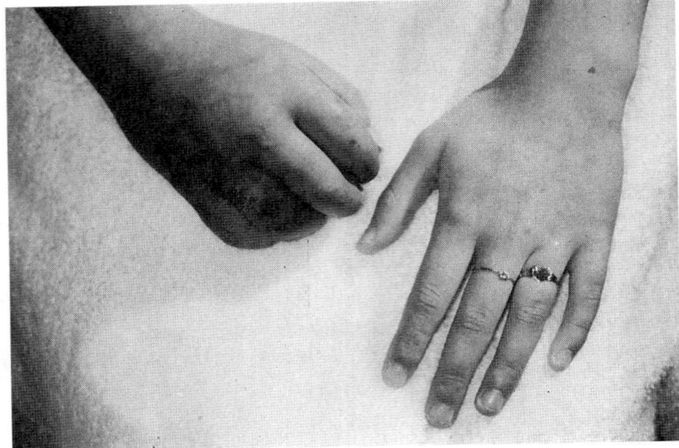

Figure 3. A later-stage dystrophic RSD. This photograph was taken at 10 months after a hyperextension injury to the left hand. Evident are the muscle wasting, changes in hair growth edema, discoloration, and contractures of the afflicted extremity. Multiple sympathetic blocks resulted in pain relief that persisted for up to 1 to 2 weeks, but the syndrome continued to progress.

stage is also marked by (a) the development of muscle wasting; (b) decreased hair growth and thinning of hair and brittle nails, as shown in Fig. 2; and (c) radiographic changes. Isolated subperiosteal, endosteal, or intracortical bone resorption can be detected on plain radiographs as well as bony erosions (Fig. 3) (55). It is at this stage that many cases of RSD are diagnosed, frequently after the patient has seen numerous physicians and other diagnoses have been excluded. Extensive treatment consisting of sympathetic blockade and physical therapy can reverse the disease process but are not always successful late in the dystrophic stage. Therapeutic approaches to RSD are discussed later in this chapter.

Atrophic Stage

As RSD progresses beyond 6 months, patients enter the third or atrophic stage, with skin and tissue changes that are essentially irreversible. Although pain can be severe at this stage, it is often diminished to a significant degree. The atrophic changes consist of (a) a smooth, glossy appearance to the skin; (b) digits appear thin and tapered; (c) atrophy of subcutaneous tissues and muscle wasting; (d) pale, cool, and dry extremity; (e) nails remain brittle with hypertrichosis; (f) flexion contractures are present; (g) distal extremity joints have markedly decreased range of motion; and (h) radiography changes consist of a more diffuse osteoporosis than during the dystrophic stage and reveals markedly widened medullary space and thinned cortex. Juxtaarticular bone erosions are frequently present (55).

Although the atrophied extremity at this stage is essentially nonfunctional, aggressive therapy may increase range of motion and decrease pain in the limb.

Differential Diagnosis

Since causalgia/RSD is a clinical diagnosis based on a constellation of symptoms and signs that can be consistent with other disease processes, the diagnosis becomes one of exclusion. This often results in a time delay between onset of symptoms and effective therapy, at which point the disease may be refractory to treatment. As a result of this delay and refractoriness to treatment, these later-stage patients often constitute a significant percentage of cases seen in pain management clinics. Although RSD remains a difficult disease to manage clinically, many inroads are being made into the understanding of the disease process, thereby possibly leading to more efficacious therapies. The following sections review basic pain mechanisms and current theories relating to the pathophysiology of RSD.

PSYCHOPHYSICS OF THE CAUSALGIC/RSD PAIN STATE

The psychophysics of the post–nerve injury pain state has been reviewed in previous chapters (see Chaps. 40 and 41). In brief, however, it should be noted that the sensory state associated with the post–nerve injury condition is characterized by (a) a spontaneous component (e.g., burning dysesthesia), and (b) a hyperpathia reflected by an exaggerated response to an otherwise noxious stimulus. In each case, it can be demonstrated that these components may be routinely manifested in the post–nerve injury pain state, without further intervention, e.g., static manifestation. In addition, both the dysesthesia and hyperpathia may display *dynamic* components that evolve as a result of provocative exposure of the patient to conditioning stimuli.

Static Components of the Sensory Condition

Aside from the spontaneous burning sensations, detailed investigations have emphasized that multiple elements can be variously identified that reflect a hyperalgesia to heating and particularly cooling and a prominent tactile allodynia (122,127; see Chap. 2). While these hyperpathias may have different time courses, and show differences between patients in terms of their relative prominence, they are principally distributed in the injured extremity.

Psychophysical studies for the tactile allodynia, using differential nerve block with local anesthetics and limb compression have uniformly emphasized that the sensation is mediated by the activation low-threshold, rapidly conducting, and presumably large primary afferents (Aβ fibers) (23,63,100). These mechanosensitive fibers signal vibratory sense, light touch, and position sense in normal skin, but not painful stimuli. The production of pain by Aβ stimulation indicates that central neurons have altered the processing of Aβ input from the periphery. Lindblom and Verrillo (100) studied 11 patients with peripheral neuralgia after trauma and found that nonnoxious mechanical stimuli produced pain with reaction time measurements too short to allow conduction in C fibers. Campbell and colleagues (23) performed sensory testing in 17 patients with hyperalgesia after nerve injury and found that differential ischemic block and differential local anesthetic block abolished pain at a time when tactile sensation was eliminated but C-fiber–mediated temperature sensation was intact. Furthermore, reaction time measurements were performed that indicated that myelinated afferents, possibly Aβ fibers, conducted the signals interpreted as painful by the patient. Bennett's team (63) studied four patients with RSD and similarly found that mechanoallodynia was mediated by Aβ low-threshold afferents using differential ischemic block and reaction time measurements. Interestingly, they also found that local anesthetic block of the initial region of trauma abolished allodynia and spontaneous pain over the entire limb, indicating that the altered central processing of Aβ stimulation is maintained by ongoing peripheral input and that the central process can revert to normal if the peripheral input is abolished.

Dynamic Components of the Sensory Condition

In addition to the static components of the psychophysics of the post–nerve injury pain state, considerable information emphasizes that these pain states can have a prominent dynamic component. Thus, light repetitive touching of a primary area of dysesthesia can lead to large areas of altered sensory function, such as allodynia that extends ipsilateral to distal dermatomes (90; see Chap. 41). Specific examination of mechanical hyperalgesia using ischemia-induced nerve block has indicated that the dynamic component was mediated by A fibers, whereas the static hyperalgesia disappeared when the small, likely unmyelinated afferents were blocked (122,129). The observation that local anesthetic block of a local neuroma may, for the duration of the block, reverse a more broadly distributed dysesthesia hyperalgesia strongly suggests that afferent traffic associated with focal nerve injury is particularly responsible for supporting the pain states. This finding suggests that a dynamic process may be responsible for a major component of the post–nerve injury pain state (63).

BASIC MECHANISMS OF CAUSALGIA/RSD

While there are numerous proposed etiologies underlying the development of RSD, the basic unifying theme relates to some degree of nerve damage. For instance, direct nerve trauma in the case of causalgia, minor nerve damage in bone fractures, sprains and crush injuries, and neurologic disease in patients with stroke and multiple sclerosis may result in RSD. To understand the pathophysiology behind the development of RSD, we must consider the possible interplay between peripheral afferent sensory neurons, dorsal horn neurons, higher-order pain-processing midbrain and cortical neurons, and the sympathetic nervous system. Although much knowledge has accumulated over the past few decades regarding the neurotransmission of pain signals in both normal and chronic disease states, many questions remain unanswered. The potential mechanisms involved in the pathogenesis of RSD will be presented separately for both the peripheral and central nervous systems. It is likely that these processes overlap in RSD and cannot be considered as distinct mechanisms.

Peripheral Mechanisms

Local Role of Peripheral Afferent Terminals

The classic response to tissue injury is the local appearance of erythema, edema, and hyperalgesia. This constellation of symptoms is essentially the same as those present in the initial stages of RSD. A significant factor in the development of local symptoms after tissue damage appears to be the release of neuropeptides from nociceptive C-fiber afferent terminals, referred to as neurogenic inflammation or axon reflex (20,99,106; see Chap. 33). In addition to functioning as afferent conducting axons for nociceptive signaling, C fibers behave as neuroeffector cells, releasing neuropeptides such as substance P (SP), neurokinin A, and calcitonin gene-related peptide (CGRP) from their peripheral terminals (124,125,169; see Chap. 33). Direct injection of neuropeptides found in C-fiber terminals into human skin causes a wheal and flare reaction (51). Inflammatory responses to antidromic stimulation of C fibers (81) can be blocked by SP antagonists (96,114) or pretreatment with capsaicin, which depletes peptide transmitters from C-fiber terminals (53,76). Other neuropeptides, such as vasoactive intestinal polypeptide (VIP), somatostatin, and galanin have been localized to C-fiber neurons and also produce wheal and flare reactions when injected into human skin (4,67).

SP has been the most extensively studied neuropeptide in the peripheral nervous system. SP is a potent vasodilator and produces plasma extravasation with resulting edema formation (97). Furthermore, SP triggers the release from mast cells of inflammatory mediators, such as histamine, 5-hydroxytryptamine (5-HT), platelet-activating factor (PAF), and leukotrienes (48,73,82). These compounds may play a role in the sensitization of nociceptive afferents to painful stimuli (30) and produce vasodilation and plasma extravasation (14,118). In addition to stimulating mast cell release, SP modulates immunologic activity by enhancing phagocytosis (8), inducing release of cytokines from monocytes (85,104), and increasing immunoglobulin production (155).

CGRP is also released from the peripheral terminal of stimulated nociceptive afferent terminals and may play a role in edema formation present in limbs affected by RSD. CGRP is a potent vasodilator (19), and potentiates tissue edema produced by agents such as SP, histamine, bradykinin, and platelet-activating factor (18). Other neuropeptides, neurokinins A and B, have both been shown to produce plasma extravasation (74); however, only neurokinin A appears to be present in the periphery (115). In addition to the release of proinflammatory mediators, other neuropeptides present in C-fiber terminals such as somatostatin and galanin have been shown to inhibit capsaicin-induced plasma extravasation, thereby possibly exerting negative feedback control of neurogenic inflammation (65).

In patients with RSD, nerve damage may produce excessive antidromic stimulation of C fibers, releasing neuropeptides that result in vasodilation, edema secondary to plasma extravasation, and release of mast cell mediators that produce sensitization of the C-fiber terminals and resulting hyperalgesia. Using animal models of chronic pain states, such as adjuvant-induced monoarthritis in rats, studies show increased synthesis and transport to the periphery of neuropeptides in nociceptive neurons (42,153). In man, neuropeptide levels in synovial fluid from chronically inflamed joints are elevated (93). It is likely that neurogenic inflammation plays at least an initial role in the pathogenesis of RSD, specifically the production of erythema, edema, and hyperalgesia.

Injured Primary Afferent Terminals

Under normal circumstances, the peripheral sensory afferent shows minimal spontaneous activity. The axon itself, unlike the terminal region where normal transduction may occur, is essentially insensitive to the chemical products of injury and does not respond to graded mechanical stimuli. In contrast, it is now appreciated that after nerve injury, axons will initially undergo retrograde chromatolysis and then initiate sprouting. In the absence of contact with the target organ, these sprouts will form organized structures that are called neuromas (37; see Chaps. 30 and 32). These neuromas endow the primary afferent with properties not normally present in the intact axon.

Spontaneous Activity Over intervals after nerve injury ranging from days to weeks, neuromas have been found to generate spontaneous ectopic discharges (see Chap. 32). This spontaneous activity may arise from altered electrical properties that stem from the insertion of a variety of ion channels into the neuroma membrane. While such has been identified for sodium (108), it is likely, though as yet unidentified, that a variety of channels including those for calcium and potassium may also be influenced. It is important to note that insofar as sodium channels are concerned systemic administration of lidocaine in concentrations less than required for inhibition of axonal nerve conduction will block the spontaneous activity in these neuromas (40,171).

In addition to the spontaneous generator represented by the neuroma, it has been shown that spontaneous activity may also arise independently from the ganglion cell of the injured axon (38). Like the activity in the neuroma, the activity in the DRG cell is also inhibited by low concentrations of sodium channel blockers (40) .

This spontaneous afferent activity could account for at least a component of the spontaneous dysesthetic pain state and, as will be noted below, such spontaneous activity can alter nociceptive processing in the spinal cord.

Transduction of Mechanical Activity Unlike uninjured axons, neuromas display the ability to transduce graded mechanical stimuli (37; see Chap. 32).

Chemosensitivity Neuromas display the presence of coupled excitatory receptor systems. Thus, topical application of a variety of chemicals has been shown to evoke activity originating from the neuroma, including adrenergic agonists and prostanoids (41,87). Stimulation of sympathetic efferents and administration of systemic norepinephrine increase ectopic discharge from neuromas, an effect that is blocked by α-adrenergic antagonists (39,87).

Ephaptic Linkages in the Neuroma Ephaptic linkages may develop between sympathetic efferents or somatomotor axons and sensory afferents. Within the neuroma, immature, unmyelinated axon sprouts exist in close apposition to such terminals (37,50,147). Such ephaptic linkages also appear to develop in the dorsal root ganglion cells of the injured axons. Thus, it is possible to envision how cross talk can evolve between otherwise isolated axon populations. Importantly such cross talk has been shown to occur between large and small afferents (3).

The appearance of spontaneous activity in the sensory afferent and the development of unusual transduction properties provide mechanisms by which a "spontaneous" sensory event may occur in the absence of an evident stimulus. Moreover, as will be reviewed below, such spontaneous activity can serve to evoke an alteration in afferent processing that can itself lead to a hyperpathic state in which otherwise innocuous stimuli may serve to generate a pain state (see Chaps. 36 and 40).

Sympathetic Efferents

Although the classic symptoms of RSD, such as vasomotor instability and hyperhidrosis, usually occur late in the acute stage of the disease, suggesting increased sympathetic tone to the affected limb, there is evidence that postganglionic sympathetic terminals may be involved in the pathogenesis of RSD much earlier in the disease process. Several animal models of post–nerve injury hyperalgesia and allodynia exist that involve partial nerve injury to peripheral or spinal nerves (11,83,148). In all three models, signs of hyperalgesia and allodynia rapidly develop in the affected limb, which are relieved to a large extent by sympathectomy (7,84,152; see Chap. 40). Likewise, as indicated by the differential diagnosis, in certain classes of patients after peripheral nerve injury, hyperalgesia and pain can be at least temporarily alleviated by pharmacologic or surgical sympathectomy (102).

An important question is, how are sympathetic nerves involved in producing or maintaining painful conditions? Sympathetic stimulation is known *not* to excite nociceptors in normal skin (149). In damaged nerves, however, both electrical stimulation of postganglionic sympathetics or close arterial injection of norepinephrine produces excitation of C-fiber nociceptors, an effect that appears to be mediated by α-adrenergic receptors (143). The increased sensitivity of partially injured nerves to adrenergic agonists may be secondary to an increase in nociceptor terminal α receptors. Studies on patients with RSD report a decrease in pain with use of systemic α-adrenergic antagonists (6,132). A small trial of transdermal application of the α_2-agonist clonidine produced a reduction of hyperalgesia only at the site of application (35). The authors suggest a local inhibition of norepinephrine release by α_2 receptors located preterminally on the sympathetic efferents may decrease postsynaptic activation of α-adrenergic receptors, perhaps on sensory nerve terminals.

Electrical and chemical sympathetic stimulation has also been shown to contribute to neurogenic inflammation and vascular permeability (31,101). These effects do not appear to be mediated by norepinephrine since this amine has been shown to actually decrease plasma extravasation and edema formation (31,123). Rather, additional substances present in sympathetic terminals, such as prostaglandin E_2 and adenosine triphosphate (ATP) (21,94) may be involved. Prostaglandin E_2 significantly potentiates plasma extravasation produced by bradykinin, histamine, and leukotriene B_4 (94,161,173). ATP has also been shown to produce PE (25,31). Neuropeptide Y (NPY) is present in sympathetic terminals and is released upon stimulation (105,158). NPY does not cause plasma extravasation (31) but acts as a potent vasoconstrictor, perhaps contributing with norepinephrine to the decreased skin temperature and pallor observed in the dystrophic stage of RSD.

Patients with RSD often develop periods of erythema and edema alternating with periods of coolness and pallor of their affected extremity (16). It is possible that neurogenic inflammation and plasma extravasation compete with vasoconstrictive properties of sympathetic efferents, causing these swings in regulation of cutaneous vascular tone. Furthermore, the presence of livedo reticularis in RSD suggests that this counterbalance of vascular regulation may vary significantly between local regions (146).

Although patients often present with signs of increased sympathetic tone to the affected extremity, the study by Drummond and colleagues (43) actually noted a decrease in sympathetic neurotransmitters and metabolites in limbs affected with RSD. This suggests the possibility that while the products of sympathetic terminal activity may indeed have impact on the transduction properties of injured (spouting) sensory afferents, it is not necessarily the sympathetic terminals innervating the peripheral injury site that are responsible. Two possible alternative mechanisms exist for altering peripheral sympathetic tone:

1. The adrenal medulla is activated in a parallel fashion to sympathetic outflow through the splanchnic innervation (see Chap. 14). If there is a specific change in the sensitivity of the peripheral, injured, afferent terminal, then the secretion of adrenal medullary products could indeed contribute to that terminal activation.
2. An alternative to the activation of the afferent pathway by sympathetic terminals from the injury site relates to the observation by McLachlan and colleagues (110) that following peripheral nerve injury in the rat, sympathetic postganglionic perivascular axons sprout onto sensory neuron cell bodies in the dorsal root ganglia of lesioned nerves. Importantly, this sprouting was observed bilaterally, although it was largely limited to the segment of injury. Stimulation of segmental preganglionic outflow produced activation of the sensory afferent neurons, which was antagonized by phentolamine. This finding is suggestive of a mechanism for sympathetically maintained pain after peripheral nerve injury, since altered central mechanisms can produce nociception from stimulation of peripheral large Aβ fibers (see following section on Central Mechanisms).

It is likely that in patients with RSD, a combination of the above peripheral mechanisms and additional as yet undefined mechanisms underlie the clinical syndrome. As noted, patients who develop RSD/causalgia following peripheral injury commonly present with spontaneous pain at rest, increased sensitivity to mechanical stimulation, and a reduction of pain levels with sympathetic blockade (16,102). Furthermore, as reviewed in previous sections, peripheral nerve injury initiates processes influencing central nervous system signaling, leading to a complex feedback interaction between peripheral and central pain transmission pathways. Current theories regarding spinal cord and higher-order sensory neurons and their role in RSD are discussed in the following section.

Central Mechanisms

While peripheral injury that involves nerve may result in changes in local terminal function, which alters the transduction process that can account for the post–nerve injury hyperalgesia, several components suggest that the process may additionally involve a higher level of organization: (a) hyperalgesia and allodynia, initially localized to the site of injury, such as a crush to the hand or a severe ankle sprain, often spreads to involve the entire limb; (b) the syndrome starts a unilateral phenomenon and spreads to involve contralateral body surface; and (c) a dynamic component of the post–nerve injury pain state entails conditioning input that appears to drive a facilitated response (e.g., hyperalgesia and allodynia). This section considers several mechanisms that support an altered central processing in the post–nerve injury pain states (for further discussion see Chap. 40).

Spinal Cord Dorsal Horn Neurons

Ample data suggest that the processing of afferent input into the dorsal horn may be altered by dynamic elements such as produced by persistent afferent input (as occurs after peripheral nerve injury) and by central changes in connectivity that may occur secondary to sprouting or dorsal horn cell death.

Facilitated Processing The involvement of multiple dermatomes that display properties of hyperalgesia after peripheral injury is believed to be secondary to increased cutaneous receptive fields and decreased thresholds of spinal cord neurons. For example, Cook et al. (32) demonstrated that electrical stimulation of peripheral C-fiber afferents in the hind limb of the rat produces an increase in the size of cutaneous receptive fields and a decrease in the mechanical threshold of both lumbar nociceptive-specific (NS) and wide dynamic range (WDR) dorsal horn neurons (see Chap. 8). Electrical stimulation at strengths that only activate large myelinated afferents had no effect. NS neurons are usually located in the superficial lamina (Rexed layers I and II) of the dorsal horn and respond under normal circumstances only to noxious stimulation (91), whereas WDR neurons are located deeper in the dorsal horn in Rexed layers IV and V and respond to both low-threshold input from large myelinated afferents and noxious inputs from C-fiber afferents (128). Expanded receptive fields of NS and/or WDR neurons have also been demonstrated after sciatic nerve transection in the cat (69), chemical irritation with mustard oil in the rat (175), and adjuvant-induced hind limb inflammation in the rat (70), in which case the increased receptive fields and decreased mechanical thresholds correlated with the occurrence of hyperalgesia to thermal stimuli. Electrophysiologic studies of dorsal root ganglion neurons with A-δ or C-fiber conduction velocities indicate that peripheral nociceptors do not demonstrate increased cutaneous receptive fields after peripheral injury, further supporting a role of altered central processes (70).

The receptive field size of a dorsal horn neuron depends in part on the projection of the peripheral projection of the afferent that can induce excitation in that neuron. As reviewed previously (Chap. 9), afferent collaterals from a given segmental input can induce excitation with decreasing probability at segments that are increasingly distant from the level of afferent entry. Processes that serve to increase the excitability of this distant afferent input can be appreciated to increase the size of the receptive field of the neuron in question. Two processes may play a role in the increased receptive field size and decreased threshold of dorsal horn neurons to mechanical stimulation after peripheral injury: (a) induction of a facilitated state by persistent small afferent drive, and (b) alteration in dorsal horn processing secondary to changes evoked by afferent nerve injury.

1. Prolonged depolarization due to C-fiber neurotransmitters: Neurotransmitters known to be present in C-fiber afferents terminals in the dorsal horn, such as substance P, CGRP, and glutamate (28,36; see Chap. 34), have been shown to produce slow depolarizing potentials that are long-lasting and can summate (116,140,163). Excitatory postsynaptic potentials that are normally ineffective in activating dorsal horn neurons would then become suprathreshold after neuronal membranes have been previously depolarized from C-fiber neurotransmitter release after injury. As evidence, prior electrical stimulation of C-fiber afferents, but not large myelinated afferents, produces increased mechanosensitive receptive field size and decreased threshold of rat dorsal horn neurons (32). The facilitated activation of WDR neurons as a result of high-frequency stimulation involving C-fiber afferent activity has been termed "wind-up" (111). Both the wind-up effect in WDR neurons and the expansion of receptive field size of dorsal horn neurons after C-fiber afferent stimulation are inhibited by antagonists to a subclass of glutamate receptors, *N*-methyl-D-aspartate (NMDA) receptors (34,178).
2. Loss of inhibitory inputs onto dorsal horn neurons: There is accumulating information that after peripheral nerve injury a variety of events may transpire at the site of injury (see Chap. 3), leading to changes in growth factor release and transport that may in turn lead to changes in dorsal horn morphology and function (79,160). Following sciatic nerve constriction, dorsal root ganglion neurons display increased firing frequency and small dark-staining neurons appear in spinal laminae I to III, showing signs of transsynaptic degeneration and exaggerated behavior that is enhanced by spinal administration of inhibitory neurotransmitter antagonists (160,183). There is evidence that dynorphin upregulation in the spinal cord after injury may increase dorsal horn neuron depolarization by glutamate via NMDA receptors, enhancing the "excitotoxic" potential of excitatory amino acids on the small inhibitory interneurons (24). Importantly, after nerve injury, application of axon transport blockers has been shown to attenuate the behavioral hyperalgesia associated with such injury (184). Alternatively, loss of dorsal horn inhibitory interneurons has been hypothesized to be due to excessive release of excitatory amino acids, such as glutamate, from sensory neurons following injury, leading to excessive depolarization via NMDA receptors and subsequently death of interneurons (44).

Loss of inhibitory interneurons or their postsynaptic action within the dorsal horn of the spinal cord can apparently lead to increased receptive field size and decreased threshold of dorsal horn neurons, which in turn would produce peripheral hyperalgesia. For example, spinal administration of inhibitory neurotransmitter antagonists produces allodynia in rodents (180) and produces expansion of dorsal horn receptive fields (107, 185).

Role of Large Afferents As reviewed above, it seems certain, based on human observations, that the initiation of certain components of the post–nerve injury hyperpathia results from the activation of large, low-threshold primary afferents (Aβ). The central mechanisms underlying the ability of Aβ mechanoreceptors to signal the perception of pain is an area of active research. Several mechanisms present themselves:

1. Enhanced excitability of dorsal horn neurons: WDR neurons receive input from both mechanoreceptors and nociceptors. It is possible that during injury, the initial barrage of C-fiber afferent activity onto WDR neurons produces wind-up, which then causes these cells to fire in a pattern that is perceived as painful after Aβ stimulation. Sensory testing in RSD patients has shown that the presence of slow temporal summation of mechanical allodynia, similar to the wind-up phenomenon, is closely correlated with the degree of RSD pain (129).
2. Altered central projections: Under normal circumstances, large myelinated (Aβ) afferents project into

Rexed lamina III and deeper. Small afferent tend to project into lamina I and II (see Chap. 35). Following peripheral nerve injury, the central terminals of myelinated afferents have been demonstrated to sprout into laminae II of the spinal cord, a region consisting mostly of NS neurons. (177). In the presence of this synaptic reorganization, stimulation of Aβ fibers could produce excitation of NS neurons and be perceived as painful.

3. Altered afferent transmitter release: A third possible mechanism underlying mechanoallodynia is alterations in spinal cord neurochemical content that occur in the dorsal horn after peripheral injury. Increased levels of certain peptides, such as dynorphin and vasoactive intestinal polypeptide (71,150), and decreased levels of other peptides, such as SP and CGRP (22,167) and stimulation of growth proteins (176), occur in the dorsal horn after peripheral injury in animal models (see Chap. 32).

Preganglionic Sympathetic Neurons

Central mechanisms may also play a role in altering sympathetic nervous system function in RSD. The normal reflex sympathetic activity observed with stimulation of peripheral sensory afferent fibers is an inhibition of sympathetic cutaneous vasoconstrictor neurons and excitation of sympathetic muscle vasoconstrictor neurons. This differential effect is observed both in preganglionic sympathetic cell bodies within the intermediolateral column of the spinal cord (57) and postganglionic sympathetic axons (15). Following chronic peripheral nerve lesions of the hindlimb, however, the reflex pattern of sympathetic cutaneous vasoconstrictor neurons in both lesioned nerves and an intact nerve changed to that of muscle vasoconstrictor neurons. In this model, noxious stimulation no longer inhibits cutaneous vasoconstrictor neurons within days following nerve lesions, suggesting that this alteration in reflex patterns may account for the blood flow abnormalities observed following injury in such diseases as RSD or causalgia (77). It is possible that an absolute increase in sympathetic outflow is not responsible for the symptoms observed in RSD, consistent with the results found by Drummond et al. (43) and Bennett's team (170) showing a decrease in sympathetic neurotransmitters and metabolites in RSD-affected limbs in both humans and an animal model of RSD. Similarly, the studies by Janig (77) would suggest that differential control at the spinal cord level between cutaneous and muscle sympathetic neurons, rather than an overall increase in sympathetic activity, may be responsible for vasomotor instability observed in RSD.

Spinal Cord Ventral Horn Neurons

Altered central mechanisms present in the ventral horn of the spinal cord may account for some of the motor disturbances seen in the later stages of RSD, such as weakness, muscle spasm, and increased reflexes (145). Similar to the effects of C-fiber activation on dorsal horn neurons, nociceptive afferent activation produces slow depolarizing potentials in ventral horn neurons (86,163) that can summate and outlast the initial stimulus. Application of an SP antagonist and capsaicin have been shown to inhibit these C-fiber–induced depolarizations in rat ventral horn neurons (2). Furthermore, intrathecally administered SP and CGRP facilitate the nociceptive flexor withdrawal reflex in rats (174). Other nociceptor neurotransmitters, such as glutamate, may be involved in sensitization of motor neurons, since NMDA receptors have been shown to mediate depolarization of motor neurons by C-fiber afferents (163). This nociceptive sensitization of motor neurons within the spinal cord is yet another example of possible central processes involved in the pathogenesis of RSD.

Descending Brain Stem Neurons

In addition to sensory afferent input, the spinal cord also receives descending input from brain stem nuclei on to the dorsal and ventral horn and preganglionic sympathetic neurons (see Chap. 11). This bulbospinal input may display alterations in chronic pain states such as RSD. Stimulation of brain stem serotonergic neurons within the raphe nuclei and intrathecally administered serotonin both produce antinociception (138). Serotonin applied on preganglionic sympathetic neurons within the spinal cord produces both excitatory and inhibitory effects (57). Similarly, brain stem noradrenergic neurons located in the locus coeruleus project to the spinal cord (130), and electrical stimulation of these neurons produces antinociception as evidenced by an inhibition of the nociceptive tail-flick withdrawal reflex—an action mediated by α_2-adrenoreceptors in the lumbar spinal cord (78). Furthermore, intrathecally applied noradrenergic antagonists produce hyperalgesia in rats with a pharmacology suggestive of an effect mediated via α_2-

Table 1. SUMMARY OF POST–NERVE INJURY EVENTS CORRELATING WITH EVOLUTION OF PAIN STATE

Peripheral nerve injury	Spontaneous pain behavior Allodynia/Hyperalgesia
Acute post-injury (seconds to minutes)	
Injury discharge	Release of afferent transmitters and activation of dorsal horn neurons
Delayed post-injury (days to weeks)	
Nerve injury—retrograde chromatolysis	Local macrophages—release of local actors (IL-1) Schwann cells—growth factor (NGF) Axon transport of active factors to DRG Increased DRG synthesis receptors/channels
Afferent sprouting	Aβ afferent innervation into lamina II of dorsal horn
Development of ephaptic linkages in DRG /Neuroma	Cross talk between A and C afferents
Insertion of receptors and channels in neuroma	Development of (a) spontaneous activity, (b) chemical sensitivity (adrenergic and prostaglandins), and (c) mechanical sensitivity
Increased spontaneous activity in afferents	Increased spinal release of excitatory amino acids Increased NMDA receptor activity Facilitated processing and hyperalgesia/allodynia Enhanced expression of immediate early genes
Sprouting of sympathetics into neuroma and DRG and increased chemosensitivity	Coupling of excitability of DRG and neuroma to sympathetic efferent activity
Transport of central factors/loss of tropic factors; increased aberrant input	Loss of dorsal horn inhibitory interneurons—allodynia/hyperpathia

See Chap. 13 and (181).

adrenoreceptors (141). The role of descending monoaminergic neurons in nociceptive processing and sympathetic neuronal activity in patients with RSD is not known at present.

Summary of Post–Nerve Injury Mechanism

In the preceding discussion, a number of interrelated mechanisms have been considered that may account for the several components of the post–nerve injury pain state. These multiple variables are summarized in Table 1. It should be stressed that the concept is that the post–nerve injury state represents a cascade that evolves over time as a result of diverse influences. The events outlined below typically represent the changes that have been identified in the preclinical models. It is not clear at present which ones (if not all) actually occur in the human state, and, if they do occur, what their distribution is across cases. This is an important future development in our understanding of the neurobiology of these post–nerve injury conditions.

CURRENT THERAPIES FOR RSD/CAUSALGIA

In a complex and chronic pain syndrome such as RSD there is no doubt that numerous alterations in nociceptive signal processing develop during the onset of the syndrome to account for the pronounced allodynia, hyperalgesia, and signs of sympathetic dysregulation. Possible peripheral and central mechanisms have been presented that may play a role in the pathogenesis of RSD, yet to date very little progress has been made in the treatment of this frustrating condition. This section discusses the current therapeutic approaches to the treatment of RSD.

A number of problems make the treatment of RSD/causalgia difficult. The initial difficulty is correctly diagnosing the condition. Despite causalgia and RSD being identified as specific entities for many years, many physicians are not aware of the presenting symptoms and do not entertain the diagnosis of RSD until the condition has progressed to later stages, at which point the condition appears more refractory to treatment. More recent publication of signs and symptoms of RSD and the formation of RSD support groups including the Reflex Sympathetic Dystrophy Syndrome Association (RSDSA) has significantly changed awareness of the disease. Throughout the first 120 years since Silas Weir Mitchell's description, those orthopedists, psychiatrists, neurologists, and anesthesiologists who treated these patients attempted to educate the general medical community about this syndrome in hopes of altering the natural history of the disease. The lack of clear etiology and pathogenesis, however, prevented RSD from being accepted by the general medical community. The evolution of the patient advocacy movement in the 1980s and 1990s, however, has promoted widespread public education about these signs and symptoms, thereby driving physician exposure and rapidly changing the frequency of the diagnosis being applied. Besrza's initial estimates published in 1990 suggest that less than 1% of all injuries will develop RSD. However, recent publication in the lay press and paraprofessional literature suggests the incidence of RSD diagnosis is rapidly increasing likely beyond the 1% mark (119,134). While some authors would point to the evolution of work environments creating repetitive strain/cumulative trauma as being the cause, one must also consider the impact of this on diagnosis and incorrect classification. The imprecise mechanistic understanding for this disease as described previously is a recognized failure of the conventional biomedical model in RSD/causalgia. The opposing forces have created a growing conflict in pain medicine where new models integrating the biomedical and psychosocial aspects of health and disease can be promoted. The pain state has led to trophic changes that may reflect in part a disuse syndrome (e.g., stiffened joints, demineralization, and muscle wasting). Clinical symptoms of burning pain, history of a proximal injury, and the presence of intermittent vasomotor sudomotor and pilomotor signs form a very heterogeneous group of patients to be diagnosed as RSD. There is no consensus regarding biologic markers of the disease and in fact there is frank argument among writers regarding this dilemma (120). Furthermore, the most commonly prescribed pain medications, nonsteroidal anti-inflammatory agents and opioids, do not have established clinical efficacy in this disease. Although numerous treatments have been tested in the past, the mainstay of therapy for RSD is sympathetic blockade.

Sympathetic Blockade

Since the initial use of sympathectomy for relief of causalgia pain in the First World War, this has remained the primary therapy in many post–nerve injury pain syndromes (16). The dramatic relief obtained with sympathetic blockade in many patients with RSD reinforces the hypothesized role of the sympathetic nervous system in the pathophysiology of RSD. However, to simply identify RSD as a disease of sympathetic hyperactivity is incomplete. As noted previously, the levels of products released from the systemic circulation do not indicate that the hyperactivity is simply due to an exaggerated sympathetic overflow. This suggests, mechanistically, that peripheral release may be normal, but that either the site of release or the receptor coupling at the afferents has been exaggerated.

To facilitate the review of clinical information, a brief review of normal sympathetic efferent neurotransmission is in order. Sympathetic efferent responses are thought to arise from stimulation of several brainstem nuclei, including medullary raphe nuclei that in turn communicate with sympathetic primary efferent cell bodies in the intermediolateral cell column within the spinal cord from T1 through L2 (see Chaps. 38,71). These primary cell bodies give rise to the preganglionic fibers that constitute the gray rami communicans. These fibers are joined by visceral afferent fibers to make up the paravertebral sympathetic ganglion that extends from the C2-4 vertebral level to the lumbosacral plexus and pelvic plexus (by way of the hypogastric plexus). The preganglionic sympathetic efferents terminate in ganglia making up the various autonomic plexi, and release norepinephrine as a primary neurotransmitter.

It should be further stressed that while the postganglionic neurons are largely thought of in terms of their ability to secrete catecholamines, sympathetic terminal activation releases catecholamines, NPY, prostaglandins, and ATP (see Chaps. 42,71). Of equal importance, the peripheral terminals of the sympathetics are subject to significant control by local receptors on their terminals. Thus, the peripheral terminals of these sympathetic nerves also have α_2 and 5-HT1 receptors on the preganglionic terminal that can locally inhibit transmitter release.

A number of approaches have been employed to reduce sympathetic influence. It is important to appreciate that while the end results of different interventions may in fact lead to a sympathectomy, the nature of the sympathectomy may differ in terms of the components of the sympathetic nervous system that are affected and the profile of sympathetic terminal release. As reviewed above, it is increasingly reasonable to speculate that the syndrome of RSD may involve a composite of mechanisms ranging from spontaneous activity at the peripheral nerve ending of the sprouting axon, to a conditioning of the spinal processing system, to the development of sensitivity at the sprouts, to sympathetic products, to the changes in the innervation of the dorsal root ganglion. Different interventions lead to prominent differences in which of the specific components of this scenario are affected. Some components of interventions targeted at reducing sympathetic activity are presented in Table 2.

Table 2. SUMMARY OF EFFECTS OF SEVERAL MANIPULATIONS ON COMPONENTS OF THE SYMPATHETIC-SOMATOSENSORY INTERACTION

Treatment	Regional block of sympathetic efferent	Regional block of afferent terminal activity/input	Block of sympathetic terminals at DRG of injured axon	Block of adrenal secretion/ α-receptor–mediated activity
Surgical or chemical denervation of sympathetic chain	Yes	No/Yes	Yes	No
Sympathetic ganglion block	Yes	No/Yes	Yes	No
IV local anesthetic	No	Yes (spontaneous act)	Yes/No	No
IV phentolamine	Yes/No	No	Yes	Yes
Spinal local anesthetic	Yes	Yes/No	Yes	Yes
Spinal clonidine	Yes/No	Yes	Yes	Yes
IV regional sympathetic depletors (guanethedine; bretylium)	Yes	No	No	No
Topical phentolamine	Yes	No	No	No

Therapeutic Interventions

Spinal Anesthesia

The epidural or intrathecal delivery of local anesthetics can produce a powerful anesthesia. At blocking doses that reduce blood pressure, antagonism of the hyperalgesia and dysesthetic pain state can be observed in patients with RSD (33,92); however, this therapy as a long-term treatment is not practical. It is not possible because of the overlap in effects to discriminate clearly between the possible effects on afferent input and the loss of sympathetic outflow.

The spinal delivery of α_2-agonists has been shown to produce a powerful reduction in the allodynia in preclinical models (182) and in the RSD pain state in cancer patients (133). This effect has been hypothesized to reflect an inhibitory influence of the α_2 receptors on the preganglionic neurons (182). Such inhibition has been demonstrated (45). Interestingly, the spinal action of opiates is typically unaccompanied by an effect on blood pressure, emphasizing their lack of influence on ganglionic sympathetic outflow. It has been suggested that this difference between spinal α_2-agonists and opiate agonists accounts for their different efficacy in treating RSD pain states (182).

Regional Sympathetic Ganglionic Blockade

Local anesthetic blockade of selective sympathetic ganglia, e.g., stellate ganglion, lumbar sympathetic, or celiac plexus blocks, have been employed for achieving a local sympathetic denervation of the sympathetic outflow to the respective body region. Pain relief from these blocks has typically been considered to be diagnostic of a sympathetically maintained pain state. Such blocks, often repeated as a series, serve to reduce the spontaneous dysesthesia and reverse the hyperalgesia (16, 172). It should be noted that to the extent that an afferent population travels with the sympathetics (e.g., the presumed innervation of blood vessel and visceral organs), these axons would also be blocked by the local anesthetic. Often permanent chemical or surgical sympathetic denervation is performed if repeated sympathetic blockade with local anesthesia provides only temporary pain relief.

Systemic IV Local Anesthetics

It has been demonstrated that IV local anesthetics in concentrations that do not inhibit axonal conduction (e.g., 1 to 2 μg/ml) can be employed to diminish the post–nerve injury pain state (26,41,162). It is important to note that the spontaneous activity of the sprouted terminal and the dorsal root ganglion cell is particularly sensitive to modest plasma levels of lidocaine (see Chap. 63). Given the probable role of spontaneous activity in altering the processing of spinal sensory input (see above), this ability to block spontaneous activity might serve to reduce the facilitated processing (see Chap. 40). A recent study demonstrated that peripheral nerve injury pain states are more likely to respond to intravenous lidocaine infusions than pain resulting from central nervous system injury, and that 66% of RSD patients had "partial" or "excellent" pain relief from the lidocaine infusion (52). Because of the minimal effects on blood pressure, it is not likely that this treatment approach is mediated by an action on the sympathetic terminal. However, this has not as yet been systematically studied.

IV Regional Depleting Agents

Agents such as bretylium, reserpine, and guanethidine are known to deplete sympathetic terminal stores. Intravenous regional administration of such agents has been employed and has been shown to produce a reversal of the spontaneous dysesthesia and hyperalgesias observed in the post-injury pain state (49,66,109). This approach leads to a local inactivation of sympathetic terminals and leaves transmitter release from adrenals and other parts of the afferent system (e.g., the DRG) unaltered.

IV α Blockers

Adrenergic blocking agents, most commonly α-adrenergic antagonists, have been reported to be effective in relieving RSD pain after systemic administration (5,56,132; but see 165,166). Side effects, specifically orthostatic hypotension, are significant with this systemic therapy. The use of intravenous phentolamine, an α-adrenergic antagonist, has been suggested as a test to determine if pain is sympathetically maintained (5,132).

Topical α Active Agents

Transdermally applied clonidine, an α_2-agonist, has been reported to be effective after local activity achieved under a skin patch, presumably through the inhibition of norepinephrine release by a preterminal action on sympathetic terminals (35).

Summary of Expected Consequences of Several Sympatholytic Approaches

Although some patients with RSD and some animal models of peripheral nerve injury display decreased pain and hyperalgesia with α-adrenergic blockade (39,87,143), the role of the sympathetic nervous system in RSD may extend beyond the release of norepinephrine by sympathetic efferents. For example, other mediators involved in neurogenic inflammation and plasma extravasation, such as prostaglandins and ATP, are released by sympathetics, and the postsynaptic actions of these agents would not be blocked by phentolamine. Therefore, the lack of efficacy of phentolamine in patients with RSD does not necessarily indicate that their pain is not sympathetically maintained.

It is clear from the above that the several interventions that may be anticipated to alter sympathetic function will necessarily have distinct effects, based on their anatomic locus of action. To summarize, we may rationally consider the following:

1. Spinal: Local anesthetics or α_2-agonists such as clonidine diminish the excitability of all preganglionic cells or block preganglionic transmission.
2. Surgical sympathectomy serves to block outflow by interdicting the efferent pathways. The regions blocked depend on the pathways cut, e.g., lumbar versus cervical chain, unilateral versus bilateral. Such interventions likely lead to a denervation of the ganglion and the neuroma, but do not necessarily prevent the release of circulating products from the adrenal medulla. Note that circulating factors can induce adrenal secretion (see Chap. 42). Thus, sympathectomy will not necessarily preclude the release of sympathetic hormones from that source.
3. IV drugs provide a whole body effect. Phentolamine thus serves to block adrenergic receptors that are believed to be postsynaptic to the sympathetic terminal on the primary afferent sprout and in the ganglion.
4. The IV local anesthetic is believed to exert a direct effect on the spontaneously active sprout, though not the sympathetics themselves.
5. Regional blockade produces a local terminal inactivation by depleting the sympathetic terminal of its contents. A regional procedure does not affect release from other sympathetic systems (such as the adrenal) nor would it influence the sympathetic terminals that reach the respective dorsal root ganglion or the effluent from the adrenals.

Alternative Therapies

Diverse classes of agents have been tested in RSD patients. Such classes include corticosteroids (58), β-adrenergic blockers (168), α-adrenergic blockers (56), calcium channel blockers (131), and calcitonin (60). Most clinical reports of novel RSD therapies consist of small patient populations and are often open-label in design. Moreover, significant side effects have been observed with these agents in clinical practice.

Corticosteroids

High-dose corticosteroids may provide some degree of relief from the symptoms of RSD (58,89), possibly by inhibiting prostaglandin release from sympathetic efferents and thereby decreasing plasma extravasation and C-fiber sensitization. However, the significant side effects of this therapy are well known.

Calcium Channel Blockers

A study of the calcium channel blocker nifedipine showed some success in decreasing RSD pain; however, the sample size was small and the study was open-label (131). In addition, normotensive patients can develop orthostatic hypotension and headaches from this therapy. The possible efficacy of calcium channel blocker treatment may result from the ability of these agents to relax smooth muscle and increase peripheral blood flow, thereby antagonizing the vasoconstrictor effects of norepinephrine in the affected limb. Development of selective vasodilating agents without significant effects on systemic blood pressure may prove useful in the therapy of RSD.

Calcitonin

Recently, a study of intranasal calcitonin in RSD patients was performed that was double-blinded and randomized, but suggested only limited efficacy in a subset of RSD patients (60). Of interest, intravenous calcitonin has recently been shown to significantly reduce phantom limb pain (75). Furthermore, studies suggest that the antinociceptive actions of calcitonin may be mediated via serotonergic mechanisms (29,144). Additional studies on the role of calcitonin in chronic pain states, such as RSD, and the possible actions of this agent on serotonergic neurotransmission are needed.

Opioids

The pain of RSD and causalgia is often reported to be refractory to systemic opioids. Bolus epidural morphine was reported to be without significant effect on post–nerve injury pain patients (5). However, continuous intrathecal morphine administration for refractory RSD has been reported to be effective both for the pain and edema associated with RSD in the small number of patients studied (62,146).

Local anesthetic block of the stellate ganglion is commonly effective for upper-extremity RSD pain; however, morphine injected around the stellate ganglion in patients with upper-extremity RSD has been shown to have no effect on RSD pain (59). Peripheral C-fiber afferent terminals are thought to contain μ-opioid receptors, since μ receptor-selective agonists inhibit C-fiber–mediated plasma extravasation (10,65) and block substance P release (179).

The modest effect of opiates in such causalgic pain states may reflect upon the role played by large primary afferents in the allodynic components of the pain state and the absence of opiate receptors on those classes of afferents (see Chap. 58). In other studies examining the spontaneous activity observed in dorsal horn neurons in rats after brachial plexus lesions, it was found that opiates had effects only at considerably higher systemic doses (103). The effectiveness of continuous intrathecal morphine may result from a modest degree of inhibition by intrathecal morphine of sympathetic activation within the spinal cord (80). It should be noted that to the degree that small afferent input drives some component of the hyperpathia or dysesthesia, spinal morphine should alter that component. Such systematic screening of patients for such sensitivity of different components of the respective post–nerve injury pain state appears warranted.

NMDA Receptor Antagonists

There is increasing evidence that post–nerve injury pain states in preclinical models may be mediated in part by an increase in spinal glutamatergic activity at the NMDA class of receptors (182; see Chap. 13). There is limited work suggesting that NMDA antagonists can alter facilitated processing in human pain states. In the post–nerve injury pain patients, a case report using an intrathecally delivered NMDA antagonist has shown that a dynamic component of a dysesthetic pain state is indeed diminished (90; see Chap. 60).

Other Agents

As reviewed in Chap. 13, preclinical studies have provided significant insights into the pharmacology of the preclinical neuropathic state. Thus, as reviewed in that chapter, a variety of promising directions have been identified, such as the utilization of N-channel blockers (27) and adenosine A_1 agonists (95,154). Continued developments in these fields may be expected to contribute to the development of additional mechanisms and accordingly more efficacious avenues of therapeutic intervention.

Adjunctive Therapy

The combination of regional sympathetic blockade followed by aggressive active and passive range-of-motion physical therapy is considered to be the first line of therapy for RSD (16). Again, early diagnosis and correct treatment are essential in halting the progression of this condition. Transcutaneous electrical nerve stimulation (TENS) has been reported to be effective in relieving the pain of RSD in some patients (136), yet aggravates the pain in others (1). A number of studies using small patient populations have reported moderate success with spinal cord stimulators (9,137,142). The mechanisms underlying the efficacy of this therapy is unclear, but may be related to altered nociceptive input to higher brain centers and/or an effect on peripheral sympathetic activity (117). It is also important to emphasize psychological therapies in the treatment of RSD/causalgia in order to obtain a multidisciplinary approach to these often debilitating disease states. Ochoa (121) has recently questioned the role of the sympathetic nervous system in RSD and states that "the inescapable conclusion is that an overall majority of patients qualifying for the . . . diagnoses of RSD . . . carry a distinct, potentially treatable, neuropsychiatric cerebral disorder."

FUTURE DIRECTIONS

Although RSD and causalgia are not common entities, they are frequently encountered in chronic pain clinics because of the progressive and unrelenting nature of the condition and the ineffectiveness of commonly used analgesics. Recent advances in our understanding of the peripheral generation and transmission of nociceptive signaling, mechanisms of tissue inflammation, and central sensory processing will lead to improved therapies for many chronic pain conditions. The role of the sympathetic nervous system in chronic pain and inflammation is also an area of intense research effort, and therapeutic advances should be especially applicable to the treatment of RSD and causalgia.

In basic science research the observation of two different responses to an identical intervention suggests the existence of different underlying mechanisms to account for the variation in response. Currently, RSD/causalgia are grouped together based on similar symptoms and findings that are recognized as consistent with the syndrome. Although it is obviously compelling to group these patients together in this way, so that study of unifying characteristics can be proposed, review of the clinical literature and the day-to-day management of several hundred patients with RSD suggests the mechanism may differ between patients. Whether the different mechanisms coexist coincidentally or causally is unknown. Whether peripheral mechanisms explain early findings while central mechanisms account for later changes is at present merely speculation. If such dynamic evolution of mechanisms for different grades, stages, or clinical features does exist, the impact of genetic code or environment (including medical intervention) on the rate of evolution would need to be considered.

To anticipate answers to all of the above questions from basic science research would be a mistake. The limitation of changing clinical practice, based on observations from a petri dish are clear to most clinicians and researchers alike. However, the value of extremely careful and controlled behavioral animal studies must also be carefully considered because of species differences and limitations of experimental models. Many of the remaining important questions must be answered through appropriately designed clinical research with clearly defined clinical outcome measurements.

Finally, while the present discussions focused largely on frank injury to the nerve generated by section or compression, the findings in such investigations likely have implications for a diversity of pain states. One example that is clearly relevant is that associated with metastatic disease, where aside from chronic tumor compression of nerve, interventions such as surgery, radiation, and chemotherapy can indeed induce nerve injury. It seems intuitive that such pain states may well possess a greater fraction of neuropathic mechanisms than commonly considered (see Chaps. 48 and 51,52). Similarly, in the case of syndromes such as diabetic neuropathy (see Chap. 54) or AIDS (see Chap. 22), the disease process itself leads to alterations in nerve structure and function. Such changes also likely lead to components that will in time be appreciated for their common effect on neuronal systems that lead to the aberrant encoding of sensory information.

REFERENCES

1. Abrams SE. Increased sympathetic tone associated with transcutaneous electrical stimulation. *Anesthesiology* 1976;45:575–577.
2. Akagi H, Konishi S, Otsuka M, Yanagisawa M. The role of substance P as a neurotransmitter in the reflexes of slow time courses in the neonatal rat spinal cord. *Br J Pharmacol* 1985;84(3):663–673.
3. Amir R, Devor M. Axonal cross-excitation in nerve-end neuromas: comparison of A- and C-fibers. *J Neurophysiol* 1992;68:1160–1166.
4. Anand P, Bloom SR, McGregor GP. Topical capsaicin pretreatment inhibits axon reflex vasodilatation caused by somatostatin and vasoactive intestinal polypeptide in human skin. *Br J Pharmacol* 1983;78:665–669.
5. Arner S. Intravenous phentolamine test: diagnostic and prognostic use in reflex sympathetic dystrophy. *Pain* 1991;46:17–22.
6. Arner S, Meyerson BA. Lack of analgesic effect of opioids on neuropathic and idiopathic form of pain. *Pain* 1988;33:11–23.
7. Attatal N, Jazat F, Kayser V, Guilbaud G. Further evidence for "pain-related" behaviours in a model of unilateral peripheral mononeuropathy. *Pain* 1990;41:235–251.
8. Bar SZ, Goldman R, Stabinsky Y, Gottlieb P, Fridkin M, Teichberg VI, Blumberg S. Enhancement of phagocytosis—a newly found activity of substance P residing in its N-terminal tetrapeptide sequence. *Biochem Biophys Res Commun* 1980;94:1445–1451.
9. Barolat G, Schwartzman R, Woo R. Epidural spinal cord stimulation in the management of reflex sympathetic dystrophy. *Stereotact Functional Neurosurg* 1989;53:29–39.
10. Bartho L, Sebok B, Szolcsanyi J. Indirect evidence for the inhibition of enteric substance P neurones by opiate agonists but not by capsaicin. *Eur J Pharmacol* 1982;77:273–279.
11. Bennett GJ, Xie YK. A peripheral mononeuropathy in rat that produces disorders of pain sensation like those seen in man. *Pain* 33: 87–107.
12. Bernstein BH, Singsen BH, Kent JT, Kornreich H, King K, Hicks R, Hanson V. Reflex neurovascular dystrophy in childhood. *J Pediatr* 1978;93:211–215.
13. Betcher AM, Casten DF. Reflex sympathetic dystrophy. *Anesthesiology* 1955;16:994–1000.
14. Bignold LP, Lykke AW. Time courses and refractoriness of enhanced vascular permeability induced by histamine, serotonin and bradykinin in synovialis of the rat. *Experientia* 1979;35: 1645–1647.
15. Blumberg H, Janig W. Reflex patterns in postganglionic vasoconstrictor neurons following chronic nerve lesions. *J Auton Nerv Syst* 1985;14:157–189.
16. Bonica JJ. Causalgia and other reflex sympathetic dystrophies. In: *The management of pain.* Philadelphia: Lea & Febiger, 1990; 240–243.
17. Bonica JJ. Causalgia and other reflex sympathetic dystrophies. *Postgrad Med* 1973;53:143–148.
18. Brain SD, Williams TJ. Inflammatory oedema induced by synergism between calcitonin gene-related peptide (CGRP) and mediators of increased vascular permeability. *Br J Pharmacol* 1985;86: 855–860.
19. Brain SD, Williams TJ, Tippins JR, Morris HR, MacIntyre I. Calcitonin gene-related peptide is a potent vasodilator. *Nature* 1985; 313:54–56.
20. Bruce AN. Vasodilator axon reflexes. *Q J Exp Physiol* 1913;6: 339–354.
21. Burnstock G, Sneddon P. Evidence for ATP and noradrenaline as cotransmitters in sympathetic nerves. *Clin Sci* 1986;68:89–92.
22. Cameron AA, Cliffer KD, Dougherty PM, Willis WD, Carlton SM. Changes in lectin, GAP-43 and neuropeptide staining in the rat superficial dorsal horn following experimental peripheral neuropathy. *Neurosci Lett* 1991;131(2):249–252.
23. Campbell JN, Raja SN, Meyer RA, Mackinnon SE. Myelinated afferents signal the hyperalgesia associated with nerve injury. *Pain* 1988;32(1):89–94.
24. Caudle RM, Isaac L. Influence of dynorphin (1-13) on spinal reflexes in the rat. *J Pharmacol Exp Ther* 1988;246(2):508–513.

25. Chahl LA. Interactions of substance P with putative mediators of inflammation and ATP. *Eur J Pharmacol* 1977;44:45–49.
26. Chaplan SR, Bach FW, Shafer SL, Yaksh TL. Prolonged alleviation of tactile allodynia by intravenous lidocaine in neuropathic rats. *Anesthesiology* 1995;83:775–785.
27. Chaplan SR, Pogrel JW, Yaksh TL. Role of voltage-dependent calcium channel subtypes in experimental tactile allodynia. *J Pharmacol Exp Ther* 1994;269:1117–1123.
28. Chung K, Lee WT, Carlton SM. The effects of dorsal rhizotomy and spinal cord isolation on calcitonin gene-related peptide-labeled terminals in the rat lumbar dorsal horn. *Neurosci Lett* 1988;90(1-2):27–32.
29. Clementi G, Prato A, Conforto G, Scapagnini U. Role of serotonin in the analgesic activity of calcitonin. *Eur J Pharmacol* 1984;98(3-4):449–451.
30. Cline MA, Ochoa J, Torebjork HE. Chronic hyperalgesia and skin warming caused by sensitized C nociceptors. *Brain* 1989; 621–647.
31. Coderre TJ, Basbaum AI, Levine JD. Neural control of vascular permeability: Interactions between primary afferents, mast cells, and sympathetic efferents. *J Neurophysiol* 1989;62:48–58.
32. Cook AJ, Woolf CJ, Wall PD, McMahon SB. Dynamic receptive field plasticity in rat spinal cord dorsal horn following C-primary afferent input. *Nature* 1987;325(7000):151–153.
33. Cooper DE, DeLee JC, Ramamurthy S. Reflex sympathetic dystrophy of the knee. Treatment using continuous epidural anesthesia. *J Bone Joint Surg [Am]* 1989;71:365–369.
34. Davies SN, Lodge D. Evidence for involvement in N-methylaspartate receptors in wind-up of class 2 neurones in the dorsal horn of the rat. *Brain Res* 1987;424(2):402–406.
35. Davis KD, Treede RD, Raja SN, Meyer RA, Campbell JN. Topical application of clonidine relieves hyperalgesia in patients with sympathetically maintained pain. *Pain* 1991;47:309–317.
36. De Biasi S, Rustioni A. Glutamate and substance P coexist in primary afferent terminals in the superficial laminae of spinal cord. *Proc Natl Acad Sci USA* 1988;85(20):7820–7824.
37. Devor M, Bernstein JJ. Abnormal impulse generation in neuromas: electrophysiology and ultrastructure. In: Culp WJ, Ochoa J, eds. *Abnormal nerves and muscles as impulse generators.* New York: Oxford University Press, 363–380.
38. Devor M, Govrin-Lippmann R, Angelides K. Na+ channel immunolocalization in peripheral mammalian axons and changes following nerve injury and neuroma formation. *J Neurosci* 1993; 13(5):1976–1992.
39. Devor M, Janig W. Activation of myelinated afferents ending in a neuroma by stimulation of the sympathetic supply in the rat. *Neurosci Lett* 1981;24:43–47.
40. Devor M, Wall PD, Catalan N. Systemic lidocaine silences ectopic neuroma and DRG discharge without blocking nerve conduction. *Pain* 1992;48:261–268.
41. Devor M, White DM, Goetzl EJ, Levine JD. Eicosanoids, but not tachykinins, excite C-fiber endings in rat sciatic nerve-end neuromas. *Neuroreport* 1992;3(1):21–24.
42. Donnerer J, Schuligoi R, Stein C. Increased content and transport of substance P and calcitonin gene-related peptide in sensory nerves innervating inflamed tissue: evidence for a regulatory function of nerve growth factor in-vivo. *Neuroscience* 1992;49: 693–698.
43. Drummond PD, Finch PM, Smythe GA. Reflex sympathetic dystrophy: the significance of differing plasma catecholamine concentrations in affected and unaffected limbs. *Brain* 1991;114(pt 5):2025–2036.
44. Dubner R, Max MB. Painful peripheral neuropathies: mechanisms and treatment. In: Besson JM, ed. *Serotonin and pain.* Amsterdam: Elsevier Science, 327–338.
45. Eisenach JC, Chuanyao T. Site of hemodynamic effects of intrathecal α2-adrenergic agonists. *Anesthesiology* 1991;74:766–771.
46. Escobar PL. Reflex sympathetic dystrophy. *Orthop Rev* 1986; 15(10):646–651.
47. Evans JA. Reflex sympathetic dystrophy. *Surg Gynecol Obstet* 1946; 82:36.
48. Fewtrell CM, Foreman JC, Jordan CC, Oehme P, Renner H, Stewart JM. The effects of substance P on histamine and 5-hydroxytryptamine release in the rat. *J Physiol (Lond)* 1982;330:393–411.
49. Ford SR, Forrest WH Jr, Eltherington L. The treatment of reflex sympathetic dystrophy with intravenous regional bretylium. *Anesthesiology* 1988;68:137–140.
50. Fried K, Govrin-Lippmann R, Devor M. Close apposition among neighbouring axonal endings in a neuroma. *J Neurocytol* 1993;22: 663–681.
51. Fuller RW, Conradson TB, Dixon CM, Crossman DC, Barnes PJ. Sensory neuropeptide effects in human skin. *Br J Pharmacol* 1987; 92:781–788.
52. Galer BS, Miller KV, Rowbotham MC. Response to intravenous lidocaine infusion differs based on clinical diagnosis and site of nervous system injury. *Neurology* 1993;43:1233–1235.
53. Gamse R, Holzer P, Lembeck F. Decrease of substance P in primary afferent neurones and impairment of neurogenic plasma extravasation by capsaicin. *Br J Pharmacol* 1980;68:207–213.
54. Garret C. Distribution of neurokinin B in rat spinal cord and peripheral tissues: comparison with neurokinin A and substance P and effects of neonatal capsaicin treatment. *Neuroscience* 1992;48: 969–978.
55. Genant HK, Kozin F, Bekerman C, McCarty DJ, Sims J. The reflex sympathetic dystrophy syndrome. A comprehensive analysis using fine-detail radiography, photon absorptiometry, and bone and joint scintigraphy. *Radiology* 1975;117:21–32.
56. Ghostine SY, Comair YG, Turner DM, Kassell NF, Azar CG. Phenoxybenzamine in the treatment of causalgia. Report of 40 cases. *J Neurosurg* 1984;60:1263–1268.
57. Gilbey MP, Stein RD. Characteristics of sympathetic preganglionic neurones in the lumbar spinal cord of the rat. *J Physiol* 1991;432: 427–443.
58. Glick EN. Reflex dystrophy (algoneurodystrophy): results of treatment by corticosteroids. *Rheumatol Phys Med* 1973;12:84–88.
59. Glynn C, Casale R. Morphine injected around the stellate ganglion does not modulate the sympathetic nervous system nor does it provide pain relief. *Pain* 1993;53(1):33–37.
60. Gobelet C, Walburger M, Meier JL. The effect of adding calcitonin to physical treatment on reflex sympathetic dystrophy. *Pain* 1992;48:171–175.
61. Goldsmith DP, Vivino FB, Eichenfield AH, Athreya BH, Heyman S. Nuclear imaging and clinical features of childhood reflex neurovascular dystrophy: comparison with adults. *Arthritis Rheum* 1989;32:480–485.
62. Goodman RR, Brisman R. Treatment of lower extremity reflex sympathetic dystrophy with continuous intrathecal morphine infusion. *Appl Neurophysiol* 1987;50:425–426.
63. Gracely RH, Lynch SA, Bennett GJ. Painful neuropathy: altered central processing maintained dynamically by peripheral input. *Pain* 1992;51:175–194.
64. Green PG, Basbaum AI, Levine JD. Sensory neuropeptide interactions in the production of plasma extravasation in the rat. *Neuroscience* 1992;50:745–749.
65. Green PG, Levine JD. Delta- and kappa-opioid agonists inhibit plasma extravasation induced by bradykinin in the knee joint of the rat. *Neuroscience* 1992;49(1):129–133.
66. Hannington-Kiff JG. Intravenous regional sympathetic block with guanethidine. *Lancet* 1974;1(875):1019–1020.
67. Hokfelt T, Elde R, Johansson O, Luft R, Nilsson G, Arimura A. Immunohistochemical evidence for separate populations of somatostatin-containing and substance P-containing primary afferent neurons in the rat. *Neuroscience* 1976;1:131–136.
68. Horowitz SH. Iatrogenic causalgia: classification, clinical findings and legal ramifications. *Arch Neurol* 1984;41:821–826.
69. Hylden JL, Nahin RL, Dubner R. Altered responses of nociceptive cat lamina I spinal dorasal horn neurons after chronic sciatic neuroma formation. *Brain Res* 1987;411(2):341–350.
70. Hylden JL, Nahin RL, Traub RJ, Dubner R. Expansion of receptive fields of spinal lamina I projection neurons in rats with unilateral adjuvant-induced inflammation: the contribution of dorsal horn mechanisms. *Pain* 1989;37:229–243.
71. Iadarola MJ, Brady LS, Draisci G, Dubner R. Enhancement of dynorphin gene expression in spinal cord following experimental inflammation: stimulus specificity, behavioral parameters and opioid receptor binding. *Pain* 1988;35:313–326.
72. Issues and opinions, letters and responses regarding Ochoa editorial. *Muscle Nerve* 1995;18:452–462.
73. Iwamoto I, Tomoe S, Tomioka H, Yoshida S. Leukotriene B4 mediates substance P-induced granulocyte infiltration into mouse skin. Comparison with antigen-induced granulocyte infiltration. *J Immunol* 1993;151:2116–2123.
74. Jacques L, Couture R, Drapeau G, Regoli D. Capillary permeability induced by intravenous neurokinins. Receptor characterization and mechanism of action. *Naunyn Schmiedebergs Arch Pharmacol* 1989;340:170–179.

75. Jaeger H, Maier C. Calcitonin in phantom limb pain: a double-blind study. *Pain* 1992;43:21–27.
76. Jancso N, Jancso-Gabor A, Szolcsanyi J. Direct evidence for neurogenic inflammation and its prevention by denervation and by pretreatment with capsaicin. *Br J Pharmacol* 1967;32:32–41.
77. Janig W. The sympathetic nervous system in pain. *Eur J Anesthesiol* 1995;10(S): 53–60.
78. Jones SL. Descending noradrenergic influences on pain. *Prog Brain Res* 1991;88:381–394.
79. Kapadia SE; LaMotte CC. Deafferentation-induced alterations in the rat dorsal horn: I. Comparison of peripheral nerve injury vs. rhizotomy effects on presynaptic, postsynaptic, and glial processes. *J Comp Neurol* 1987;266:183–197.
80. Karoum F, Commissiong J, Wyatt RJ. Effects of morphine on norepinephrine turnover in various functional regions of rat spinal cord. *Biochem Pharmacol* 1982;31:3141–3143.
81. Kenins P. Identification of the unmyelinated sensory nerves which evoke plasma extravasation in response to antidromic stimulation. *Neurosci Lett* 1981;25:137–141.
82. Kiernan JA. The involvement of mast cells in vasodilatation due to axon reflexes in injured skin. *Q J Exp Physiol Cogn Med Sci* 1972;57: 311–317.
83. Kim SH, Chung JM. An experimental model for peripheral neuropathy produced by segmental spinal nerve ligation in the rat. *Pain* 1992;50:355–363.
84. Kim SH, Chung JM. Sympathectomy alleviates mechanical allodynia in an experimental animal model for neuropathy in the rat. *Neurosci Lett* 1991;134:131–134.
85. Kimball ES, Persico FJ, Vaught JL. Substance P, neurokinin A, and neurokinin B induce generation of IL-1-like activity in P388D1 cells. Possible relevance to arthritic disease. *J Immunol* 1988;141: 356–409.
86. King AE, Thompson SW, Woolf CJ. Characterization of the cutaneous input to the ventral horn in vitro using the isolated spinal cord-hind limb preparation. *J Neurosci Methods* 1990;35: 39–46.
87. Korenman EM, Devor M. Ectopic adrenergic sensitivity in damaged peripheral nerve axons in the rat. *Exp Neurol* 1981;72:63–81.
88. Korin F, McCarty DJ, Sims J and Genant H. The reflex sympathetic dystrophy syndrome 1. Clinical and histologic studies: evidence for bilaterality, response to corticosteroids and articular involvement. *Am J Med* 1976;60:321–331.
89. Kozin F, Ryan LM, Carerra GF, Soin JS, Wortmann RL. The reflex sympathetic dystrophy syndrome (RSDS). III. Scintigraphic studies, further evidence for the therapeutic efficacy of systemic corticosteroids, and proposed diagnostic criteria. *Am J Med* 1981;70(1): 23–30.
90. Kristensen JD, Svensson B, Gordh T Jr. The NMDA-receptor antagonist CPP abolishes neurogenic "wind-up pain" after intrathecal administration in humans. *Pain* 1992;51:249–253.
91. Kumazawa T, Perl ER. Excitation of marginal and substantia gelatinosa neurons in the primate spinal cord: indications of their place in dorsal horn functional organization. *J Comp Neurol* 1978; 177:417–434.
92. Ladd AL, DeHaven KE, Thanik J, Patt RB, Feuerstein M. Reflex sympathetic imbalance. Response to epidural blockade. *Am J Sports Med* 1989;17:660–667.
93. Larsson J, Ekblom A, Henriksson K, Lundeberg T, Theodorsson E. Immunoreactive tachykinins, calcitonin gene-related peptide and neuropeptide Y in human synovial fluid from inflamed knee joints. *Neurosci Lett* 1989;100:326–330.
94. Lee A, Coderre TJ, Basbaum AI, Levine JD. Sympathetic neuron factors involved in bradykinin-induced plasma extravasation in the rat. *Brain Res* 1991;557:146–148.
95. Lee YW, Yaksh TL. Pharmacology of the spinal adenosine receptor which mediates the antiallodynic effect of intrathecal adenosine agonists. *J Pharmacol Exp Ther* 1996;277.
96. Lembeck F, Donnerer J, Bartho L. Inhibition of neurogenic vasodilation and plama extravasation by substance P antagonists, somatostatin and [D-Met2, Pro5] enkephalinamide. *Eur J Pharmacol* 1982;85:171–176.
97. Lembeck F, Holzer P. Substance P as neurogenic mediator of antidromic vasodilation and neurogenic plasma extravasation. *Naunyn Schmiedebergs Arch Pharmacol* 1979;310:175–183.
98. Leriche R. De la causalgie envisagee come une nevrite du sympathique et son traitement per la denudation et l'excision des plexus nerveux periarteriels. *Presse Med* 1916;24:153.
99. Levine JD, Moskowitz MA, Basbaum AI. The contribution of neurogenic inflammation in experimental arthritis. *J Immunol* 1985; 843S–847S.
100. Lindblom U, Verrillo RT. Sensory functions in chronic neuralgia. *J Neurol Neurosurg Psychiatry* 1979;42(5):422–435.
101. Linde B, Chisolm G, Rosell S. The influence of sympathetic activity and histamine on the blood-tissue exchange of solutes in canine adipose tissue. *Acta Physiol Scand* 1974;92:145–155.
102. Loh L, Nathan PW. Painful peripheral states and sympathetic blocks. *J Neurol Neurosurg Psychiatry* 1978;41:664–671.
103. Lombard MC, Besson JM. Attempts to gauge the relative importance of pre- and postsynaptic effects of morphine on the transmission of noxious messages in the dorsal horn of the rat spinal cord. *Pain* 1989;37:335–345.
104. Lotz M, Vaughan JH, Carson DA. Effect of neuropeptides on production of inflammatory cytokines by human monocytes. *Science* 1988;241:1218–1221.
105. Lundberg JM, Martinsson A, Hemsen A, Theodorsson NE, Svedenhag J, Ekblom B, Hjemdahl P. Co-release of neuropeptide Y and catecholamines during physical exercise in man. *Biochem Biophys Res Commun* 1985;133:30–36.
106. Maggi CA, Meli A. The sensory-efferent function of capsaicin-sensitive sensory neurons. *Gen Pharmacol* 1988;19:1–43.
107. Markus H, Pomeranz B. Saphenous has weak ineffective synapses in sciatic territory of rat spinal cord: electrical stimulation of the saphenous or application of drugs reveal these somatotopically inappropriate synapses. *Brain Res* 1987;416:315–321.
108. Matzner O, Devor M. Hyperexcitability at sites of nerve injury depends on voltage-sensitive Na+ channels. *J Neurophysiol* 1994;72: 349–359.
109. McKain CW, Urban BJ, Goldner JL. The effects of intravenous regional guanethidine and reserpine. A controlled study. *J Bone Joint Surg* 1983;65:808–811.
110. McLachlan EM, Janig W, Devor M, Michaelis M. Peripheral nerve injury triggers noradrenergic sprouting within dorsal root ganglia. *Nature* 1993;363:543–546.
111. Mendell LM. Physiological properties of unmyelinated fiber projection to the spinal cord. *Exp Neurol* 1966;16:316–332.
112. Merskey H. Classification of chronic pain: description of chronic pain syndromes and definitions of pain terms. *Pain* 1986;3(suppl): S215–S211.
113. Mitchell SW, Moorehouse GR, Keen WW. *Gunshot wounds and other injuries of nerves.* Philadelphia: JB Lippincott, 1864.
114. Morton CR, Chahl LA. Pharmacology of the neurogenic oedema response to electrical stimulation of the saphenous nerve in the rat. *Naunyn Schmiedebergs Arch Pharmacol* 1980;314:271–276.
115. Moussaoui SM, Le Prado N, Bonici B, Faucher DC, Cuine F, Laduron PM, Garret C. Distribution of neurokinin B in rat spinal cord and peripheral tissues: comparison with neurokinin A and substance P and effects of neonatal capsaicin treatment. *Neuroscience* 1992;48:969–978.
116. Murase K, Randic M. Actions of substance P on rat spinal dorsal horn neurones. *J Physiol* 1984;346:203–217.
117. Naver H, Augustinsson LE, Elam M. The vasodilating effect of spinal dorsal column stimulation is mediated by sympathetic nerves. *Clin Auton Res* 1992;2(1):41–45.
118. Northover AM, Northover BJ. The effects of histamine, 5-hydroxytryptamine and bradykinin on rat mesenteric blood vessels. *J Pathol* 1969;98:265–275.
119. Ochoa J. Reflex sympathetic dystrophy (RSD): a tragic error in medical science. *Hypocrates' Lantern* 1995;3(2):1–6.
120. Ochoa JL. Essence, investigation, and management of "neuropathis" pains: hopes from acknowledgement of chaos. [Editorial]. *Muscle Nerve* 1993;16:991–1008.
121. Ochoa JL. Reflex sympathetic dystrophy: a disease of medical understanding. *Clin J Pain* 1992;8:363–366.
122. Ochoa JL, Yarnitsky D. The triple cold syndrome. Cold hyperalgesia, cold hypoaesthesia and cold skin in peripheral nerve disease. *Brain* 1994;117(pt 1):185–197.
123. O'Duffy G, Chahl LA. Effect of catecholamines on oedema induced by inflammatory agents in the rat. *Eur J Pharmacol* 1979; 57:377–386.
124. Olgart L, Gazelious B, Brodin E, Nilsson G. Release of substance P-like immunoreactivity from the dental pulp. *Acta Physiol Scand* 1977;101:510–512.
125. Pernow B. Role of tachykinins in neurogenic inflammation. *J Immunol* 1985;812S–815S.

126. Poplawski ZJ, Wiley AM, Murray JF. Post-traumatic dystrophy of the extremities. *J Bone Joint Surg [Am]* 1983;65:642–655.
127. Price DD, Bush FM, Long S, Harkins SW. A comparison of pain measurement characteristics of mechanical visual analogue and simple numerical rating scales. *Pain* 1994;56:217–226.
128. Price DD, Dubner R. Neurons that subserve the sensory-discriminative aspects of pain. *Pain* 1977;3:307–338.
129. Price DD, Long S, Huitt C. Sensory testing of pathophysiological mechanisms of pain in patients with reflex sympathetic dystropy. *Pain* 1992;49(2):163–173.
130. Proudfit HK, Clark FM. The projections of locus coeruleus neurons to the spinal cord. *Prog Brain Res* 1991;88:123–141.
131. Prough DS, McLeskey CH, Poehling GG, Koman LA, Weeks DB, Whitworth T, Semble EL. Efficacy of oral nifedipine in the treatment of reflex sympathetic dystrophy. *Anesthesiology* 1985;62(6): 769–769.
132. Raja SN, Treede RD, Davis KD, Campbell JN. Systemic alpha-adrenergic blockade with phentolamine: a diagnostic test for sympathetically maintained pain. *Anesthesiology* 1991;74:691–698.
133. Rauck RL, Eisenach JC, Jackson K, Young LD. et al. Epidural clonidine treatment for refractory reflex sympathetic dystrophy. *Anesthesiology* 193;79:1163–1169.
134. Reflex Sympathetic Dystrophy Syndrome Association of America. *RSDSA Review* 1995(winter).
135. Richards RL. Causalgia—a centennial review. *Arch Neurol* 1967;16: 339–350.
136. Richlin DM, Carron H, Rowlingson JC, Sussman MD, Baugher WH, Goldner RD. Reflex sympathetic dystrophy: successful treatment by transcutaneous nerve stimulation. *J Pediatr* 1978;93: 84–86.
137. Robaina FJ, Rodriguez JL, de Vera JA, Martin MA. Transcutaneous electrical nerve stimulation and spinal cord stimulation for pain relief in reflex sympathetic dystrophy. *Stereotact Functional Neurosurg* 1989;52:53–62.
138. Roberts MH. 5-Hydroxytryptamine and antinociception. *Neuropharmacology* 1984;23:1529–1536.
139. Russek HI. Shoulder-hand syndrome following myocardial infarction. *Med Clin North Am* 1958;42:1555–1561.
140. Ryu PD, Gerber G, Murase K, Randic M. Actions of calcitonin gene-related peptide on rat spinal dorsal horn neurons. *Brain Res* 1988;441:357–361.
141. Sagen J, Proudfit HK. Effect of intrathecally administered noradrenergic antagonists on nociception in the rat. *Brain Res* 1984; 310:295–301.
142. Sanchez-Ledesma MJ, Garcia-March G, Diaz-Cascajo P, Gomez-Moreta J, Broseta J. Spinal cord stimulation in deafferentation pain. *Stereotact Functional Neurosurg* 1989;53:40–45.
143. Sato J, Perl ER. Adrenergic excitation of cutaneous pain receptors induced by peripheral nerve injury. *Science* 1991;251:1608–1610.
144. Satoh M, Akaike A, Nakazawa T, Takagi H. Evidence for involvement of separate mechanisms in the production of analgesia by electrical stimulation of the nucleus reticularis paragigantocellularis and nucleus reticularis paragigantocellularis and nucleus raphe in the rat. *Brain Res* 1980;194:525–529.
145. Schwartzman RJ. Reflex sympathetic dystrophy and causalgia. *Neurol Clin* 1992;10:953–973.
146. Schwartzman RJ, Kerrigan J. The movement disorder of reflex sympathetic dystrophy. *Neurology* 1990;40:57–61.
147. Seltzer Z, Devor M. Ephaptic transmission in chronically damaged peripheral nerves. *Neurology* 1979;29:1061–1064.
148. Seltzer Z, Dubner R, Shir Y. A novel behavioral model of neuropathic pain disorders produced in rats by partial sciatic nerve injury. *Pain* 1990;43:205–218.
149. Shea VK, Perl ER. Failure of sympathetic stimulation to affect responsiveness of rabbit polymodal nociceptors. *J Neurophysiol* 1985;54:513–519.
150. Shehab SA, Atkinson ME. Vasoactive intestinal polypeptide increases in areas of the dorsal horn of the spinal cord from which other neuropeptides are depleted following peripheral axotomy. *Exp Brain Res* 1986;62:422–430.
151. Shelton RM; Lewis CW. Reflex sympathetic dystrophy: a review. *J Am Acad Dermatol* 1990;22:513–520.
152. Shir Y, Seltzer Z. A-fibers mediate mechanical hyperesthesia and allodynia and C-fibers mediate thermal hyperalgesia in a new model of causalgiform pain disorders in rats. *Neurosci Lett* 1990; 115:62–67.
153. Smith GD, Harmar AJ, McQueen DS, Seckl JR. Increase in substance P and CGRP, but not somatostatin content of innervating dorsal root ganglia in adjuvant monoarthritis in the rat. *Neurosci Lett* 1992;137:257–260.
154. Sosnowski M, Yaksh TL. Role of spinal adenosine receptors in modulating the hyperesthesia produced by spinal glycine receptor antagonism. *Anesth Analg* 1989;69:587–592.
155. Stanisz AM, Befus D, Bienenstock J. Differential effects of vasoactive intestinal peptide, substance P, and somatostatin on immunoglobulin synthesis and proliferations by lymphocytes from Peyer's patches, mesenteric lymph nodes, and spleen. *J Immunol* 1986;136:152–156.
156. Stanton Hicks MW, Hessenbusch S, Haddox JD, Boas R, Wilson P. Reflex sympathetic dystrophy: changing concepts and taxonomy. *Pain* 1995;63:127–133.
157. Steinbrocker O, Spitzer N, Friedman HH. The shoulder-hand syndrome in reflex dystrophy of the upper extremity. *Ann Intern Med* 1948;29:22–29.
158. Stjarne L, Lundeberg JM, Astrand P. Neuropeptide Y—a cotransmitter with noradrenaline and adrenosine 5'-triphosphate in the sympathetic nerves of the mouse vas deferens? A biochemical, physiological and electropharmacological study. *Neuroscience* 1986; 18:151–166.
159. Subbarao J, Stillwell GK. Reflex sympathetic dystrophy syndrome of the upper extremity: analysis of total outcome of management of 125 cases. *Arch Phys Med Rehabil* 1981;62:549–554.
160. Sugimoto T, Bennett GJ, Kajander KC. Strychnine-enhanced transsynaptic degeneration of dorsal horn neurons in rats with an experimental painful peripheral neuropathy. *Neurosci Lett* 1989; 98:139–143.
161. Svensjo E. Bradykinin and prostaglandin E1, E2, and F2 alpha-induced macromolecular leakage in the hamster cheek pouch. *Prostaglandins Med* 1:397–410.
162. Tanelian DL, MacIver MB. Analgesic concentrations of lidocaine suppress tonic A-delta and C fiber discharges produced by acute injury. *Anesthesiology* 1991;74:934–936.
163. Thompson SW, Gerber G, Sililotti LG, Woolf CJ. Long duration ventral root potentials in the neonatal rat spinal cord in vitro; the effects of ionotropic and metabotropic excitatory amino acid receptor antagonists. *Brain Res* 1992;595:87–97.
164. Tietjen R. Reflex sympathetic dystrophy of the knee. *Clin Orthop Rel Res* 1986;209:234–243.
165. Verdugo RJ, Campero M, Ochoa JL. Phentolamine sympathetic block in painful polyneuropathies. II. Further questioning of the concept of "sympathetically maintained pain." *Neurology* 1994;44: 1010–1014.
166. Verdugo RJ, Ochoa JL. "Sympathetically maintained pain." I. Phentolamine block questions the concept. *Neurology* 1994;44: 1003–1010.
167. Villar MJ, Cortes R, Theodorsson E, Wiesenfeld-Hallin Z, Schalling M, Fahrenkrug J, Emson PC, Hokfelt T. Neuropeptide expression in rat dorsal root ganglion cells and spinal cord after peripheral nerve injury with special reference to galanin. *Neuroscience* 1989;33:587–604.
168. Visitsunthorn U, Prete P. Reflex sympathetic dystrophy of the lower extremity: a complication of herpes zoster with dramatic response to propranolol. *West J Med* 1981;135:62–66.
169. Wahlestedt C, Beding B, Ekman R, Oksala O, Stjernschantz J, Hakanson R. Calcitonin gene-related peptide in the eye: release by sensory nerve stimulation and effects associated with neurogenic inflammation. *Regul Pept* 1986;16:107–115.
170. Wakisaka S, Kajander KC, Bennett GJ. Abnormal skin temperature and abnormal sympathetic vasomotor innervation in an experimental painful peripheral neuropathy. *Pain* 1991;46: 299–313.
171. Wall PD, Gutnick M. Ongoing activity in peripheral nerves: the physiology and pharmacology of impulses originating from a neuroma. *Exp Neurol* 1974;43:580–593.
172. Wang JK, Johnson KA, Ilstrup DM. Sympathetic blocks for reflex sympathetic dystrophy. *Pain* 1985;23:13–17.
173. Wedmore CV, Williams TJ. Control of vascular permeability by polymorphonuclear leukocytes in inflammation. *Nature* 1981;289: 646–650.
174. Woolf C, Weisenfeld-Hallin Z. Substance P and calcitonin gene-related peptide synergistically modulate the gain of the nociceptive flexor withdrawal reflex in the rat. *Neurosci Lett* 1986;66: 226–230.
175. Woolf CJ, King AE. Dynamic alterations in the cutaneous

mechanoreceptive fields of dorsal horn neurons in the rat spinal cord. *J Neurosci* 1990;10:2717–2726.

176. Woolf CJ, Reynolds ML, Molander C, O'Brien C, Lindsay RM, Benowitz LI. The growth-associated protein GAP-43 appears in dorsal root ganglion cells and in the dorsal horn of the rat spinal cord following peripheral nerve injury. *Neuroscience* 1990;34: 465–478.
177. Woolf CJ, Shortland P, Coggeshall RE. Peripheral nerve injury triggers central sprouting of myelinated afferents. *Nature* 1992; 355:75–78.
178. Woolf CJ, Thompson SW. The induction and maintenance of central sensitization is dependent on N-methyl-D-aspartic acid receptor activation: implications for the treatment of post-injury pain hypersensitivity states. *Pain* 1991;44:293–299.
179. Yaksh TL. Substance P release from knee joint afferent terminals: modulation by opioids. *Brain Res* 1988;458:319–324.
180. Yaksh TL. Behavioral and autonomic correlates of the tactile evoked allodynia produced by spinal glycine inhibition: effects of modulatory receptor systems and excitatory amino acid antagonists. *Pain* 1989;37:111–123.
181. Yaksh TL. Neurologic mechanisms of pain. In: Cousins MJ, Bridenbaugh PO, eds. *Neural blockade. Clinical anesthesia and management of pain,* 2nd ed. Philadelphia: JB Lippincott, 1996, in press.
182. Yaksh TL, Pogrel JW, Lee YW, Chaplan SR. Reversal of nerve ligation-induced allodynia by spinal alpha-2 adrenoceptor agonists. *J Pharmacol Exp Ther* 1995;272: 207–214.
183. Yamamoto T, Yaksh TL. Effects of intrathecal strychnine and bicuculline on nerve compression-induced thermal hyperalgesia and selective antagonism by MK-801. *Pain* 1993;54:79–84.
184. Yamamoto T, Yaksh TL. Effects of colchicine applied to the peripheral nerve on the thermal hyperalgesia evoked with chronic nerve constriction. *Pain* 1993;55:227–233.
185. Yokota T, Nishikawa Y. Action of picrotoxin upon trigeminal subnucleus caudalis neurons in the monkey. *Brain Res* 1979;171: 369–373.

Anesthesia: Biologic Foundations, edited by Tony L. Yaksh et al. Lippincott–Raven Publishers, Philadelphia © 1997.

CHAPTER 57

FIBROMYALGIA

FREDERICK WOLFE

Fibromyalgia is a clinical syndrome that may be defined operationally as (a) referral of pain complaints to large areas of the body; (b) decreased pain threshold, as identified by the presence of many tender points; and (c) the presence of a number of characteristic symptoms. The constellation of commonly associated symptoms may include sleep disturbance, fatigue, psychological problems, headaches, and an irritable bowel syndrome. Additional observed components believed associated with the syndrome are listed in Table 1. The diagnosis and the syndrome is controversial for three reasons:

1. Populations studies have suggested that pain threshold as well as key fibromyalgia symptoms are typically distributed in the population (57,259), and that the formal diagnosis of a fibromyalgia syndrome based on an arbitrary cutoff point (for example, 11 tender points versus 10 tender points, see below) is misleading (57, 259).
2. The strong associations with various measures of psychological dysfunction (see below) have suggested that the syndrome largely reflects the manifestation of psychological factors.
3. Some have averred that fibromyalgia is merely a form of a chronic pain that happens to be associated with decreased pain threshold, but is otherwise not different from other chronic pain syndromes (185).

This chapter considers this diagnosis and these issues.

Table 1. PREVALENCE OF PAIN AND SYMPTOMS IN THE 1990 ACR STUDY OF CRITERIA FOR THE CLASSIFICATION OF FIBROMYALGIA (248)

Criterion	% Positive	Classification accuracy
Pain symptoms		
Pain posterior thorax	72.3	73.9
15+ painful sites	55.6	70.6
Neck pain	85.3	67.5
Low back pain	78.8	66.6
Widespread pain	97.6	65.9
Symptoms		
Sleep disturbance	74.6	73.8
"Pain all over"	67.0	73.6
Fatigue	81.4	71.7
Morning stiffness >15 minutes	77.0	67.2
Paresthesias	62.8	63.6
Anxiety	47.8	62.9
Headache	52.8	62.3
Prior depression	31.5	58.0
Irritable bowel syndrome	29.6	57.1
Sicca symptoms	35.8	55.4
Urinary urgency	26.3	54.2
Dysmenorrhea history	40.6	53.4
Raynaud's phenomenon	16.7	51.6
Modulating factors		
Noise	24.0	68.5
Cold	79.3	66.6
Poor sleep	76.0	65.2
Anxiety	69.0	63.7
Humidity	59.6	63.6
Stress	63.0	60.4
Fatigue	76.7	60.3
Weather change	66.1	60.3
Warmth	78.0	50.8

Modified from ref. 248, with permission.

NOMENCLATURE

Classifications

Fibromyalgia is said to be of a primary, secondary, concomitant, or traumatic nature. *Primary fibromyalgia* is defined when no other disease is present that could explain the symptoms or cause the fibromyalgia. In *secondary fibromyalgia* another condition is believed to cause the reported symptoms comprising the fibromyalgia diagnosis. In *concomitant fibromyalgia* another disorder is present but no causal relationship is implied. These definitions are unsatisfactory since it is not known what causes fibromyalgia and how other diseases may interact with the syndrome. *Posttraumatic fibromyalgia* is terminology that is sometimes applied when the syndrome is noted following an injury (252). The term is used in a descriptive rather than a causal way because the tissue relationship between trauma and fibromyalgia is not well understood.

Two different logical processes led to the evolution of this terminology. First, in order to study fibromyalgia, other disorders whose symptoms and physical findings might overlap with fibromyalgia needed to be excluded. Historically, this dichotomy reinforced the notion that fibromyalgia was primarily a disorder of young women—essentially by restricting the condition to the young who did not have other diseases. The second logical process assumed that fibromyalgia could be caused by illnesses such as hypothyroidism, sleep apnea, or rheumatoid arthritis. This assessment was typically based on case reports or small clinical series. These causal links remain largely unsubstantiated, and while the term *secondary fibromyalgia* is still used, it is synonymous with *concomitant fibromyalgia.* In 1990 the American College of Rheumatology criteria for the classification of fibromyalgia abolished the distinction between primary and secondary or concomitant fibromyalgia at the level of diagnosis "because no differences between the various putative classifications could be found in symptoms or diagnostic criteria sensitivity or specificity" (248). The significance of a unified fibromyalgia diagnosis is that fibromyalgia is not a disorder of exclusion, but one that describes a constellation of rheumatic and nonrheumatic conditions.

Tender Points Versus Trigger Points

An important issue in the fibromyalgia syndrome is the question of the sensitivity of the patient to an external stimulus. Under these conditions it may be found that in addition to the spontaneous pain report, the patient will display small areas where a pressure stimulus yields an apparently exaggerated report of discomfort. These areas may be referred to as "tender" points. Such an observation bears operational similarity to the concept of a "trigger" point, but is believed to reflect different phenomena. Often different authors appear to use these phrases interchangeably.

In the present discussion, tender points are areas in muscles, tendon, fat pads, or over bone where the pain threshold to palpation is ordinarily reduced. Many such areas exist in the body (148,208). For use in the diagnosis of fibromyalgia, small groups of particularly sensitive tender points have been identified. Although a number of groupings or maps have been proposed, the map most commonly in use is that proposed by Wolfe et al. (248) in their paper, "The 1990 American College of Rheumatology Criteria for the Classification of Fibromyalgia" (Fig. 1 and Table 2). The concept of tender points carries with it no causal or pathogenic mechanism; tender points are just tender areas regardless of what other characteristics they may have. To identify a positive tender point, a fixed force (usually about 4 kg/mm^2)is applied to the area. A positive tender point is one in which the patient states that the palpation is painful. Most persons in the general population have few or no tender points (57,260). In general, fibromyalgia tenderness, as evidenced by a high count of tender points, is a manifestation of the decreased pain threshold of the syndrome.

Trigger points, as defined in the case of myofascial pain syndromes, are believed to reflect a very local aberration, typically in a muscle mass at which a focal mechanical stimulus may evoke a pain report, predictably referred to a larger region of tissue.

Mechanistically, the tender point is believed to reflect a general decrease in the pain threshold. This will be discussed further below. In contrast, the trigger point may reflect an abnormal afferent connectivity that evokes a pain state in an observer that may otherwise have "normal" pain thresholds. Thus, one hypothesis has suggested the role of muscle spindles and sympathetically activated intrafusal contractions. (121a, 166a). It is is unclear at this time whether these two phenomena indeed reflect discriminable mechanisms. It is clear that should these two mechanisms exist, the phrases *trigger point* and *tender point* should not be used interchangeably. There is, however, nothing within these two constructs that prevent a tender point from also being a trigger point, or, stated another way, fibromyalgia and the myofascial pain syndrome can coexist.

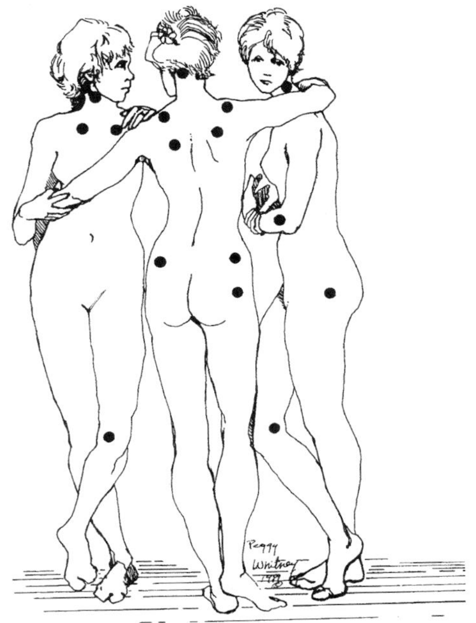

Figure 1. The 18 tender point sites of the 1990 American College of Rheumatology (ACR) criteria for the classification of fibromyalgia (248). Eleven of 18 tender points satisfies the tenderness criterion.

Table 2. THE 1990 AMERICAN COLLEGE OF RHEUMATOLOGY CRITERIA FOR THE CLASSIFICATION OF FIBROMYALGIA (248)

1. History of widespread pain
   Definition: Pain is considered widespread when all of the following are present: pain in the left side of the body, pain in the right side of the body, pain above the waist, and pain below the waist. In addition, axial skeletal pain (cervical spine or anterior chest or thoracic spine or low back) must be present. In this definition shoulder and buttock pain is considered as pain for each involved side. "Low back" pain is considered lower segment pain.
2. Pain in 11 of 18 tender point sites on digital palpation.
   Definition: Pain, on digital palpation, must be present in at least 11 of the following 18 tender point sites:
   Occiput: bilateral, at the suboccipital muscle insertions.
   Low cervical: bilateral, at the anterior aspects of the intertransverse spaces at C5-C7.
   Trapezius: bilateral, at the midpoint of the upper border.
   Supraspinatus: bilateral, at origins, above the scapula spine near the medial border.
   2nd rib: bilateral, at the second costochondral junctions. Just lateral to the junctions on upper surfaces.
   Lateral epicondyle: bilateral, 2 cm distal to the epicondyles.
   Gluteal: bilateral, in upper outer quadrants of buttocks in anterior fold of muscle.
   Greater trochanter: bilateral, posterior to the trochanteric prominence.
   Knees: bilateral, at the medial fat pad proximal to the joint line.
   Digital palpation should be performed with an approximate force of 4 kg.
   For a tender point to be considered "positive" the subject must state that the palpation was painful. "Tender" is not to be considered painful.

For classification purposes patients will be said to have fibromyalgia if both criteria 1 and 2 are satisfied. Widespread pain must have been present for at least 3 months. The presence of a second clinical disorder does not exclude the diagnosis of fibromyalgia. (From ref. 248, with permission.)

Definite fibromyalgia: All of the characteristic fibromyalgia features.

Probable fibromyalgia: Two of the three characteristic fibromyalgia features.

Possible fibromyalgia: One of the three characteristic fibromyalgia features and two of the three indeterminate fibromyalgia features.

EPIDEMIOLOGY

Prevalence

The prevalence of fibromyalgia was noted to be 5.7% (38) in general medical clinics and 2.1% in family practice settings (108). In rheumatology clinics, fibromyalgia prevalence was higher, 12% (254) to 20% (271) of new patients. The agreement regarding diagnostic criteria (248) and the comparability of older criteria (271) has led to useful estimates of prevalence in the community. The only North American study noted the prevalence to be 0.5% and 3.7% in men and women, respectively, and 2.0% for both sexes combined (260). European prevalence estimates have been as high as 10.5% (85). A recent, well-designed study from the United Kingdom did not report specific prevalence, but prevalence can be calculated to be over 4% for both sexes combined (57). Overall, adult prevalence (both sexes) is about 2% to 3% when all studies are considered (182,187,260). Wolfe and colleagues (260) noted that the prevalence of fibromyalgia increases with age (Fig. 2), a result germane to our understudying of possible pathogenesis. Prevalence in children is based on a small (nonpopulation) sample, yielding results for boys of 3.9%, girls of 8.8%, and both sexes of 6.2% (34).

A number of problems exist in the determination of prevalence of fibromyalgia. Recent data suggest that the degree of

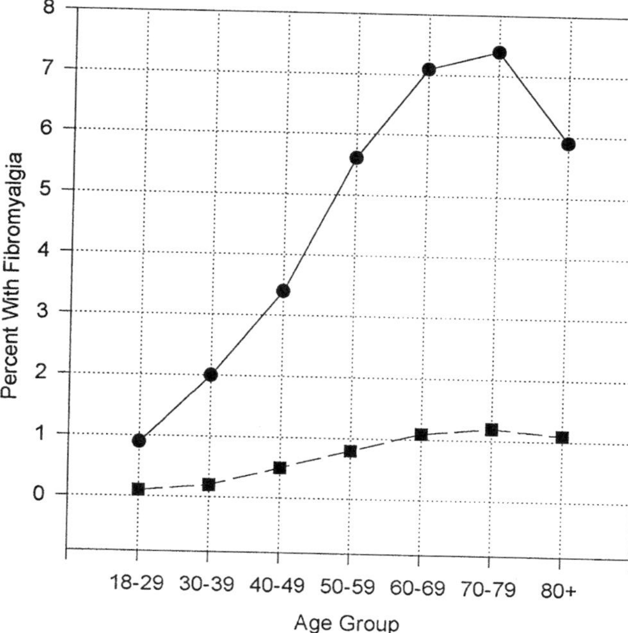

Figure 2. Age- and sex-specific prevalence of fibromyalgia in the Wichita population for persons aged 18 and above. Circles are women, squares men (260).

tenderness found in fibromyalgia represents about the 95th percentile of tenderness in the population (259), and that tenderness is distributed almost normally in the population. Figure 3 demonstrates a probability distribution curve for the general populations for dolorimetry scores and tender point counts. Data such as these suggest that classification of one individual with 11 tender points as having fibromyalgia and another with only 9 or 10 tender points may represent an artificial division (57,259). In addition, because different examiners may exert different force during the examination, prevalence estimates can vary as a function of interobserver difference, and it is probable that some of the differences in population estimates is based on this phenomenon.

Sex Distribution

Fibromyalgia is most common in women (85% to 90% or greater), both in the clinic and in the community, and female predominance (67%) also has been observed in children by Buskila and colleagues (34).

DIAGNOSIS AND DIAGNOSTIC METHODOLOGIES

Fibromyalgia is diagnosed clinically when widespread pain, decreased pain threshold to palpation, and characteristic symptoms are all present together. Because there are many symptoms occurring in tandem with decreased thresholds, fibromyalgia has been characterized as a disorder of pain modulation (170,209,212,263), pain amplification, (212,214) and as the "irritable everything" syndrome (214). We conceptualize fibromyalgia as a syndrome in which the threshold for all stimuli appears to be decreased and/or that stimuli appear to be amplified in their effect.

Pain

At a clinical level, mildly noxious stimuli are perceived as more intense and often as severe pain (Fig. 4). The distribution(s) of the pain referral are broad and more generalized. Common regions for rheumatic pain such as low back, cervical spine, knees, and hands are often involved first, and the pain is often severe. Figure 5 displays pain drawings from four patients with fibromyalgia. The figure emphasizes the characteristic distribution of fibromyalgia pain: widespread, axial, radiating, and joint associated. The extent of the pain is often surprising and in and of itself may suggest the diagnosis. Similarly, more severe pain than might be expected almost anywhere, but particularly in peripheral joints, suggests fibromyalgia.

Pain Threshold

Tender Point Assessment

Another manifestation of the generally decreased pain threshold is the presence of tenderness (tender points) at specific anatomic locations. Figure 1 presents the 18 tender point sites used by the 1990 American College of Rheumatology (ACR) Criteria for the Classification of Fibromyalgia (248). As noted above, tender point sites represent specific areas of muscle, tendon, and fat pads that are much more tender to palpation than surrounding sites. Many maps of tender point sites have been presented (38,89,208,220,248,271). In fibromyalgia patients, pain is elicited by palpating the tender point site with approximately 4 kg of force. Palpation is usually performed using the second and third fingers or the thumb, and often

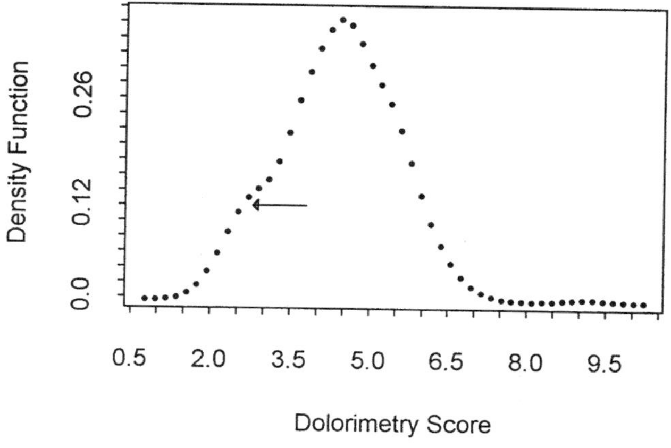

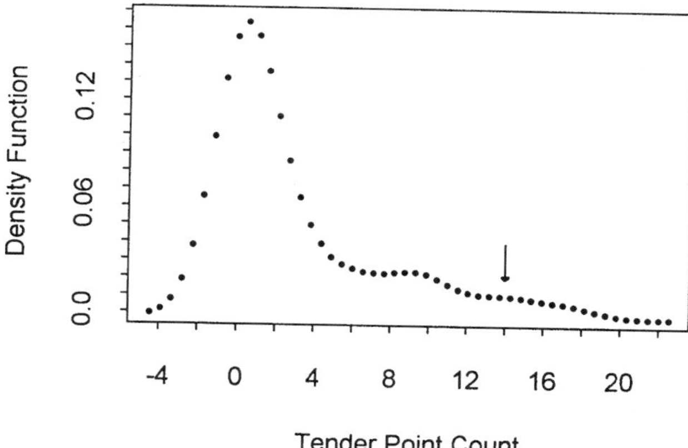

Figure 3. Probability distributions for dolorimetry scores (*left*) and tender point counts (*right*) from a general population sample of mean age of 54.1 years. *Arrows* show median dolorimetry score and tender point count for persons with fibromyalgia.

Total Body Pain (Pain Threshold = 0)

Total Pain Score = 276

Stimulus Intensity

Number of Potentially Painful Stimuli

No Fibromyalgia (Pain Threshold = 6)

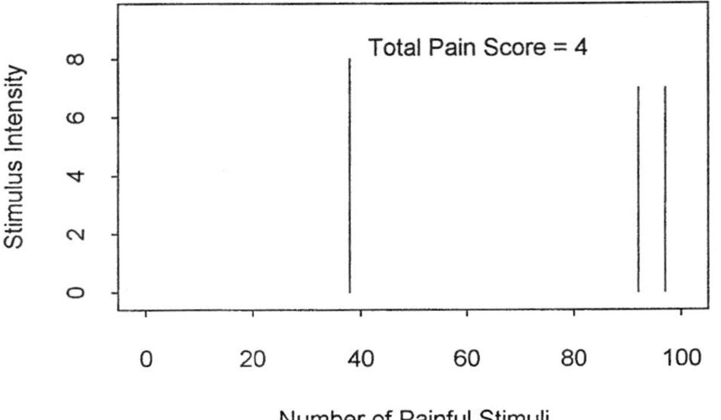

Mild Fibromyalgia (Pain Threshold = 4)

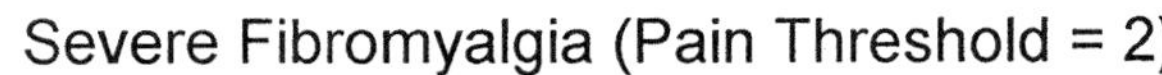

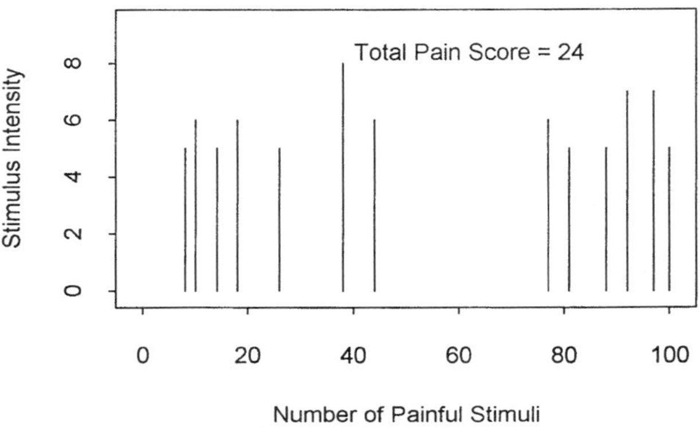

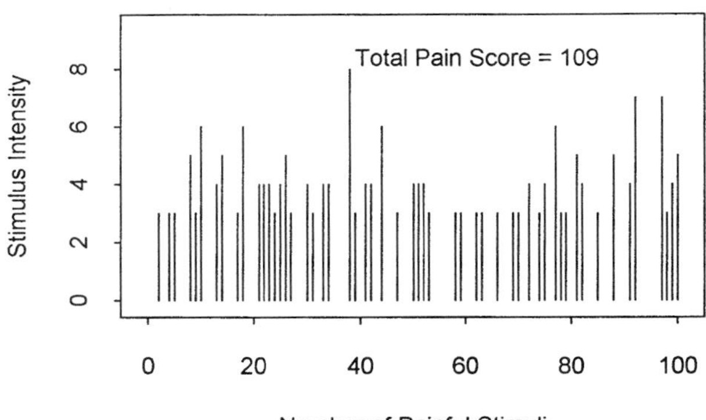

Figure 4. A model of pain and pain thresholds in fibromyalgia. Lines represent 100 potentially painful and nonpainful stimuli occurring over an arbitrary period indicated. Stimuli are indicated on the x-axis. Intensity of stimuli are indicated by the height of the vertical lines (y-axis). A total pain score is determined by summing the "heights" above pain threshold over all the stimuli. In the *upper left panel* all stimuli are treated as "painful." Lines on the figure indicate arbitrary pain thresholds of 6, 4, and 2. The figure on the *upper right* displays "painful stimuli" and pain score for a person without fibromyalgia, while the *lower* figures display hypothetical diagrams for those with mild and severe fibromyalgia. Thus, persons with fibromyalgia, having a decreased pain threshold, will experience more pain and more severe pain.

with a rolling motion. Practically, one can learn how much pressure to apply by palpating "normal" individuals. The amount of force that does not elicit tenderness in a nonfibromyalgia patient (just below the pressure pain threshold) is the correct pressure to use. Smaller, thinner, less muscled individuals are more sensitive to pressure. Thus, the comparison group for training purposes is those with similar physiques.

Verbal Scaling

Attempts have been made to quantify the tender point. Yunus and colleagues (271) introduced the concept of "severe" tenderness ("Ouch!, that really hurts") as a diagnostic criterion in 1981. Russell et al. (197,248) proposed a categoric scoring for tenderness: no pain = 0; mild pain (complaint of pain without grimace, flinch, or withdrawal) = 1; moderate pain (complaint of pain plus grimace or flinch) = 2; severe pain (complaint of pain plus marked flinch or withdrawal) = 3; and unbearable pain (patient withdraws without palpation) = 4. In the ACR method, the method generally used, the patient is asked if the examination "hurt" or was "painful" at each site examined. A positive tender point is one in which the patient states that the examination caused pain. Tender point sites are ordinarily tender, and patients frequently reply when asked about pain, "It's tender." To have a reliable method, the "tenderness" descriptor should not be accepted as reflecting a pain state per se (248) and the patient should be explicitly asked whether the examination caused "pain." It is the patient's response that defines the painfulness of the stimulus rather than the examiner's interpretation.

The use of quantitative measures has several goals. First, it may identify those with "severe" or "important" tenderness, thereby recognizing that fibromyalgia is a disorder of severe pain and tenderness. In addition, it might help to exclude patients who indicated that they have (mild) pain wherever palpated, even at sites that are almost never tender. An additional goal in measuring tenderness is in the quantification of any improvement. Total myalgic scores or the Tender Point Index are methods that have been used to assess the effects of treatment (39,42,45,54,65,105,165,195,201). The problems with measured tenderness is that while it has good intraobserver reliability, the interobserver is less impressive. Using Russell's method, the ACR criteria study (248) noted that counts of tender points based on the presence of any tenderness (pain = 1) were significantly better than tender point scores or tender point counts using moderate or severe tenderness (pain = 2 or 3) in identifying subjects with a diagnosis of fibromyalgia (248). The differences noted were primarily a result of increasing interobserver variability.

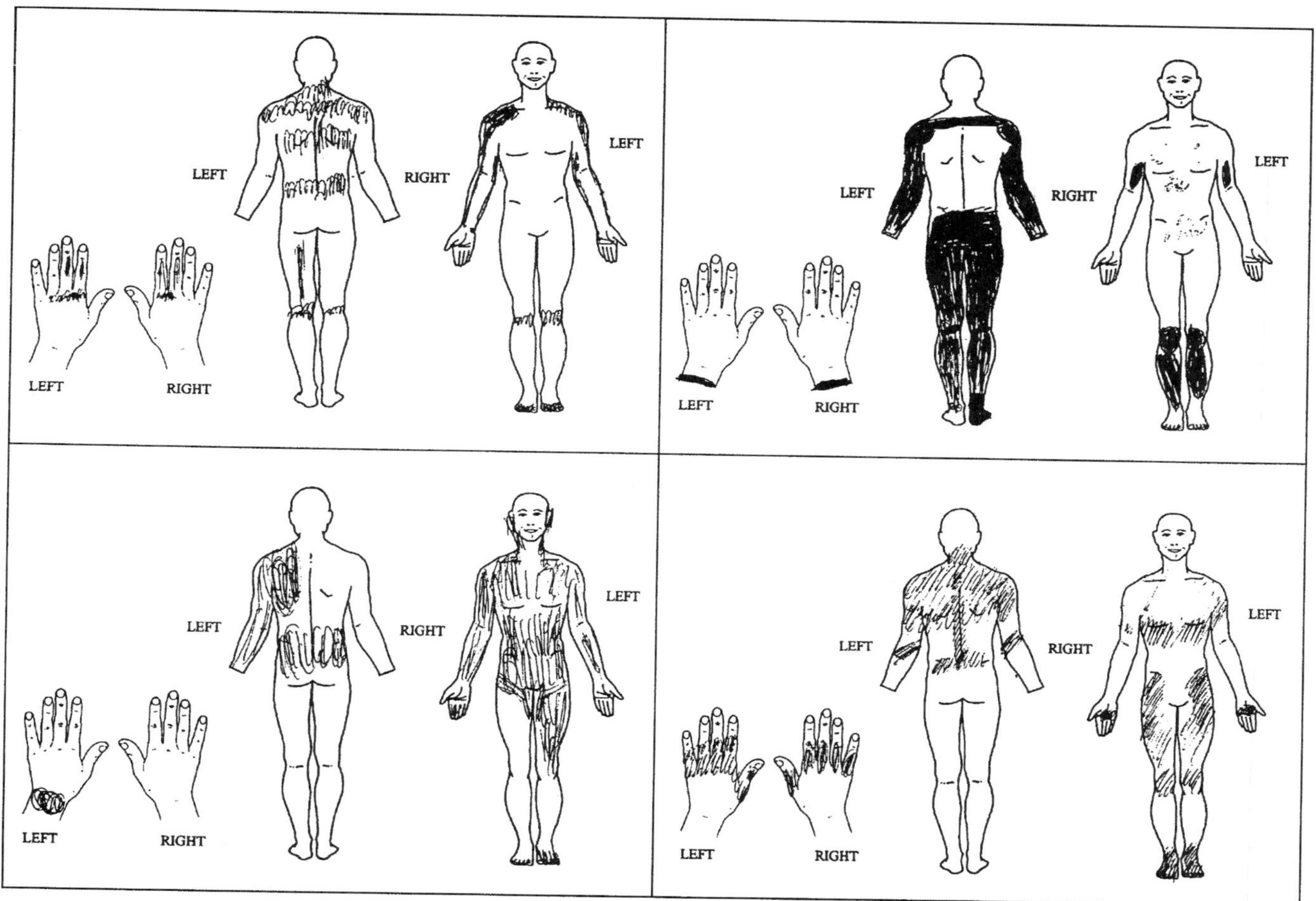

Figure 5. Pain drawings from four patients with fibromyalgia emphasizing the characteristic distribution of fibromyalgia pain: widespread, axial, radiating, and joint associated. (From ref. 251.)

Tenderness can be quantified somewhat more objectively by the use of pressure algometers, or dolorimeters. Two instruments in common use are the Chatillon dolorimeter (Chatillon Instruments, Long Island City, NY) and the Fischer algometer (78,81). Algometers remove the variability of the palpating force during digital examination as well as the need to interpret the patient's response. A positive response evoked by a stimulus equal to or less than 4 kg/1.77 Cm^2 has been used as the threshold for a positive tender point (56,218,219,248). Dolorimetry, however, is frequently less useful for diagnosis than digital palpation (248). Reanalysis of data from the ACR criteria study (248) indicated that 73% of fibromyalgia patients were identified by dolorimetry as opposed to 90% by manual palpation, with an overall accuracy of 73% for dolorimetry and 84% for palpation. Among the reasons for the poorer performance of dolorimetry is that it is an inherently more difficult and inaccurate technique, as the tactile clues necessary to locate palpation site are missing and that the rolling motion of manual palpation may elicit tenderness not noted by direct focal compression.

How many tender points should be examined and found positive to permit a positive diagnosis of fibromyalgia has been a matter of controversy (220,247,248,271). The ACR criteria (Table 2) required 11 of 18 (61%). Previous studies (using the mild or greater criterion for tenderness) examined as many as 25 sites (19) and as few as 14 (220) and the percentage of points-positive required for diagnosis has ranged from 86% (220) to 46% (148). Complicating the issue of what is the correct number and percent positive is whether symptom criteria should also be used in diagnosis, as in the older Yunus criteria (271), and whether the comparison or control group represents other patients with pain or "normals." Lautenschläger and associates (148) found 11 of 24 (46%) yielded the best sensitivity when compared with normal volunteers. When the comparison groups were other rheumatic disease patients, 11 of 18 (61%) was the best cutoff point (248). Thus, whether one uses the 18 tender points recommended by the ACR or other maps, about 60% of tender point should be positive to satisfy the tender point criterion.

Other Symptomatology

Symptoms associated with the diagnosis of fibromyalgia have been extensively studied (12,15,38,52,64,237,257,271). The sensitivity and specificity of the various symptom and symptom combinations in fibromyalgia and rheumatic disease control patients are reported in Table 1 (248). Sleep disturbance, fatigue, and morning stiffness are present in from 75% to 81% of patients, while "pain all over," paresthesia, headache, and anxiety occur in 49% to 67% of patients (248). Symptom criteria and the pattern of pain may allow identification of persons with fibromyalgia. But symptom criteria alone will have an unacceptable false-positive rate, particularly in those with other rheumatic conditions, as indicated in Table 1. In the 1990 ACR classification criteria study, the addition of symptom criteria to the tender point count and the presence of widespread pain did not improve criteria sensitivity and specificity (248).

THE CLINICAL SYNDROME

Onset

Childhood Fibromyalgia

Few studies of fibromyalgia in childhood have been performed (7,34,36,51,158,210,235,236,268), although there is a general recognition of its existence. Childhood and adult fibromyalgia were found to be similar characteristics in one study of 33 patients presenting at age 17 or under (268). Children, however, reported more subjective swelling and aggravation of symptoms by activity then did adults, while in areas where arthritis occurs in adults (low back and hand, for example) symptoms were less common. Anxiety was reported in 70% and depression in 55%. General fatigue (91%), chronic headaches (54%), and irritable bowel syndrome (27%) were also noted. In another report from a rheumatology clinic, almost 17% of pediatric patients had fibromyalgia (51). Preliminary, limited data are available on the prognosis of childhood fibromyalgia. Of 15 children satisfying the tender point criterion for fibromyalgia in an epidemiologic study (34), only 27% satisfied criteria at follow-up 30 months later, and pain thresholds as measured by dolorimetry increased substantially (35).

Adult Fibromyalgia

Fibromyalgia occurring in adults can be divided into several patterns: childhood onset of symptoms, gradual onset of symptoms in adult life, fibromyalgia in association with repeated differing musculoskeletal problems, fibromyalgia following trauma (249), and fibromyalgia following apparent viral infection. Only recently have these patterns been studied (31).

1. Childhood onset: Patients presenting as young and middle-aged adults often describe a lifelong history of mild musculoskeletal complaints, usually beginning in adolescence, often with articular pain (knees). They appear to have difficulty with athletic activities in school. Later they seem to have repeated minor musculoskeletal problems. In addition, this group may have irritable bowel syndrome and migraine headaches also develop within this period of life. Yunus et al. reported 15% (264) to 28% (271) with childhood onset.
2. Gradual onset: This state reflects the simplest condition in the adult in which there is a gradual onset of slowly increasing pain, emerging in an otherwise healthy individual (246).
3. Postsurgical or viral onset: Usually occurring in a generally previously healthy individual, this state is characterized by a rapid onset of symptoms following an viral or flu-like syndrome. Depending on the sample and the specific question asked, this type of onset has been reported by patients in 6% (152), 18% (246), 22% (31), and 55% (28) of the examined population.
4. Chronic musculoskeletal pain onset: Two subgroups are identified. In the first, fibromyalgia develops as a concomitant of other musculoskeletal problems, particularly osteoarthritic complaints of the axial skeleton and peripheral joints. Patients complain more than would be expected about their "arthritic" problems and about more arthritic problems than are expected. Presentation is usually in the later middle-aged or the elderly. In the second subgroup, fibromyalgia is diagnosed in a background of major musculoskeletal medical complaints and multiple surgical interventions, and is associated with marked pain behavior. Individual frequently have long surgical and medical histories, significant anxiety, and aspects of somatization disorders (48,142). Often one problem follows the next over many years. When fibromyalgia is diagnosed it is not clear if an onset date can be determined.
5. Posttraumatic fibromyalgia: Following injury, regional pain patterns with symptoms suggestive of a fibromyalgic symptoms may appear, usually in a unilateral shoulder girdle region. The pain then spreads to envelop the entire arm. Gradually, one by one, all of the other limbs may become involved. This pattern also has been described in the workplace setting (153,155,252). Even where fibromyalgia is clearly present it can coexist with a myofascial pain syndrome, and one can often find areas corresponding to definitions of trigger points, areas that are much more tender than the other fibromyalgia tender point regions, and that were at the original site of complaint. The link between trauma and fibromyalgia on a pathophysiologic basis is often very tenuous, and requires further investigation (106,107,154,216). Percentages of studies reporting trauma as an initiating event have varied from 15% (152) to 42% (31).

Clinical Presentations: Diagnosis and Differential Diagnosis

Fibromyalgia is frequently misdiagnosed, either as rheumatoid arthritis or osteoarthritis (271). Patients may present with articular symptoms that emphasize peripheral joint pain, often at the knees, shoulders, hands, and wrists (189). Inflammatory rheumatic disorders may be considered instead of fibromyalgia because of the complaint of swelling; patients report the mild soft tissue swelling that accompanies fibromyalgia as articular swelling. Similarly, osteoarthritic enlargement may also be reported as swelling. Arthralgic presentations may be a result of pain amplification in mildly osteoarthritic joints, or be contributed to by soft tissue swelling and its associated mild periarticular pressure increase. Entrapment neuropathies may be considered when paresthesias predominate, often with associated pain (207,246). Surgical treatment is a common concomitant. Mild soft tissue swelling and amplification of central mechanisms for paresthesia may be among the mechanism for this presentation. Systemic lupus erythematosus is not infrequently suggested by the generalized symptomatology when a positive antinuclear antibody is identified by laboratory testing. A small percentage of patients have definite features of a connective tissue disorder, but do not appear to develop such a disorder during long-term follow-up (64). General pain amplification and predominance of axial skeletal complaints often lead to consideration of compressive nerve root and disk syndromes. The prevalence of axial skeletal surgery is high among those with the syndrome (48). Childhood fibromyalgia may be misdiagnosed as juvenile or adult rheumatoid arthritis for reasons similar to those in adults: joint pain and reported swelling.

The chronic fatigue syndrome (CFS) shares many features in common with fibromyalgia. The main difference at a clinical level is the predominance of the incapacitating nature of the fatigue in CFS and the predominance of pain in fibromyalgia. Most studies have noted significant diagnostic overlap (27,94, 99,171), although this has not been observed universally (176, 261). Differences in the proportion of patients satisfying one as opposed to two diagnoses may relate to the selection practices of tertiary fibromyalgia and chronic fatigue syndrome referral clinics, where patients with most characteristic features are referred, compared to community practice where selection is less common.

Clinical Symptoms

Fatigue

Fatigue is among the most common of symptoms of fibromyalgia, being noted in 77% of patients in the ACR study (248). In a general population survey approximately 66% of subjects with fibromyalgia complained of fatigue (260). Campbell et al.'s (38) suggestion that fatigue be qualified by the definition of (usually or often) being "too tired during the day to do what I want to do" adds an appropriate method of assessment. Visual analogue and other scales recently developed may add additional reliable ways of assessment (29,253).

Sleep Disturbance

Moldofsky et al. (172) originally described the sleep disturbance of fibromyalgia in terms of *alpha delta intrusion* observable in EEGs during sleep studies. "Awaking unrefreshed" is the construct that has been adopted as the most effective way of ascertaining the clinical complaint (38,257). Sleep disturbance has been an obligatory or semi-obligatory criterion for fibromyalgia diagnosis in earlier criteria sets (220,271). In the ACR study 74.6% reported the symptom (248), while in the community approximately 74% had the symptom (260).

Morning Stiffness

Stiffness is a predominant symptom in all studies, ranging from 75% (93,152,248,254) to 100% (38) of cases. In the community, stiffness occurred at a rate of approximately 76% (260).

Irritable Bowel Syndrome

Irritable bowel syndrome (IBS) has been reported in 34% to 53% of studies (38,93,254,270,271) including 35.7% in the ACR criteria study (248). Using a validated self-administered questionnaire, Triadafilopoulus et al. (225) reported altered bowel function in 73%; and 64% reported abdominal pain. The prevalence of IBS is dependent on referral pattern, definition of IBS, and the assiduousness of the examiner.

Irritable Bladder Syndrome

This symptom has not been widely studied in fibromyalgia (237). It may manifest itself as reports of frequent urinary tract infections or as urinary urgency. Urgency was found in 26.3% of fibromyalgia patients as compared with 15.5% of controls in the ACR criteria study (248).

Headache

Chronic headache, either as migraine (271) or other headache, has been reported in 44% to 58% of patients with fibromyalgia (15,38,93,248,254,270,271). Headache may begin in adolescence in many patients whose pain first begins in that period of life.

Paresthesia

Paresthesias were among the most common finding in the ACR study (62%) (248). It has been noted by others at rates varying from 26% (271) to 71% (15). In the community, paresthesias were reported by approximately 63% (260).

Psychological Abnormality

Psychological factors have been intensively studied in fibromyalgia. This interest has been fueled by the common clinical observation of increased psychological abnormality in those with fibromyalgia compared with other patients, an observation supported by a large number of studies of studies (2,4,10,26,69,72,100,110,122,123,140,147,150,151,179,198,202, 229,230,234,245,260). In the face of such observations it is often easy to forget that many, perhaps most, patients with fibromyalgia are psychologically normal (20). Even so, fibromyalgia patients differ from those with other rheumatic diseases. Hawley and Wolfe (110) noted that 48.6% and 29.3% of unselected clinic fibromyalgia patients ($N = 543$) had AIMS depression scores at levels of possible (AIMS depression score of 3.0) and probable (AIMS depression score of 4.0) clinical depression, respectively, compared with 34.5% and 19.1% of all other clinic patients ($N = 5610$). Thus, depression, variously defined, is 10% to 15% more common in those with fibromyalgia. Corollary observations from a study of marital status in rheumatic disease provide additional insight into fibromyalgia; divorce rates were higher among fibromyalgia patients (10.1%) compared with all other rheumatic conditions (6.6%) (112).

A few studies have not found evidence of psychological abnormality in fibromyalgia when compared to other rheumatic disease and general medical patients (1,26,52), or have suggested a history of past major depression and increased family depression but not current psychiatric diagnosis (92,123). The prevalence of psychological abnormalities among fibromyalgia patients for anxiety (4,123,124,245), depression (3,4,110,179,192,245), somatization or emphasis bodily concerns including hypochondriasis (26,142,150,192, 202), coping (230), daily hassles (59,230), and history of major depression (3,92,123,124) has been widely noted. Psychopathology has been hypothesized using the Minnesota Multiphasic Personality Inventory (MMPI) data [both not adjusting (25,184,115) and adjusting for somatic or disease related items] (150), and in studies of the Symptom Check List-90-r (SCL-90-r) scales (4,142), and the Basic Personality Inventory (BPI) (202). Wolfe et al. (260) studied fibromyalgia in the general population. They noted that fibromyalgia occurred more frequently in those with high scores for anxiety, depression, general (psychological) severity (SCL-90), and increased divorce rates. These data then extend to the general population observations made in the clinic.

Physical Findings Other Than Measurements of Pain Threshold

Swelling

Patients frequently complain of swelling, often in characteristic locations—around the elbows, in the hands, and in the medial aspect of the knees. This was originally called "subjective swelling" (271). While *subjective* tended to mean both not observed by physicians and not present, it has become clear that such swelling does exist. Patients can point out tightness of their wristwatch band, and the loss of the skin lines over the metacarpophalangeal (MCP) joints (observable by physicians). Swelling is nonarticular, and often improves during the course of the day. It is possible that such swelling is related to complaints of carpal tunnel symptoms among fibromyalgia patients. The complaint of swelling is important in diagnosis since it may be misinterpreted as joint swelling rather than soft tissue swelling. In the community study of fibromyalgia, approximately 71% reported joint swelling, although such swelling was not observed by the study investigators (260).

Neurogenic Inflammation

Reactive hyperemia was described as a clinical sign early in the description of fibromyalgia (6,220). Quantification of the presence of erythema in the skin following mechanical (palpation) or chemical (capsaicin) stimulation was demonstrated by Littlejohn et al., who showed increased erythema in those with fibromyalgia compared with controls (156) and normals (101). While common, this finding during routine clinical examination does not have sufficient specificity to be used for diagnosis since it is seen (in lesser proportion) in others with rheumatic diseases (248). When carefully quantitated it accurately classified 74.5% of patients compared with normal controls (101).

Tissue Compliance

Tissue compliance (79,80) is significantly lower in patients with fibromyalgia, and has good diagnostic specificity (101).

Skin Fold Tenderness

Grasping the upper border of the trapezius and rolling it between the fingers produces complaints of pain in many persons with fibromyalgia. Originally suggested by Smythe and Moldofsky (220) as a characteristic physical finding, this assessment of tenderness at the trapezius was found to have a diagnostic accuracy of 71.2% in the ACR criteria study (248). When applied to the thoracic region, however, sensitivity was 96.6% and diagnostic accuracy 92.5% against normal controls (101). Skin fold tenderness is another measure of pain threshold.

The investigation of tissue compliance, reactive hyperemia, and thoracic skin fold tenderness was pioneered by Granges and Littlejohn (101). Although not yet investigated in subjects with other rheumatic conditions, available data suggest these additional physical signs might be reliable and useful in diagnosis.

Laboratory Studies

Routine laboratory studies are generally normal in fibromyalgia unless an addition disorder is present that is associated with laboratory abnormalities. A small subset of fibromyalgia patients (20.5%) who had features suggestive of a connective tissue disorder, including Raynaud's phenomenon (30.5%), sicca syndrome (14%), low C3 (17%), immunoglobulin G (IgG) deposition at the dermal epidermal junction (14%), and positive antinuclear antibodies (23%) was identified by Dinerman et al. (64). No identifiable connective tissue disorder was noted on long-term follow-up, leaving the meaning of these observations unclear. Ledingham et al. (152) noted antinuclear antibodies (ANA) and rheumatoid factor positivity in 18% and 14%, respectively. The results of Ledingham et al. and Dinerman et al. might have been the result of referral bias, specifically the tendency to refer for evaluation those patients with abnormal laboratory studies and unexplained symptoms.

A series of antibody-related findings have been reported. Antibodies to serotonin receptor have been reported recently in fibromyalgia (143). Two studies noted deposition of IgG at the dermal epidermal junction (43,44), while another found IgG attachment to collagen bundles but not at the dermal-epidermal junction (71). Antistriated muscle antibodies and anti-smooth muscles antibodies (but not other autoantibodies) were found in 40% to 55% of fibromyalgia patients but not in controls in a single study (130). But other reports found no evidence of increases in antibodies (13), and all additional reviews have failed to find increases in the various autoantibodies. In addition, sophisticated studies of cytokines and immune regulation in fibromyalgia have disclosed no abnormalities (238).

Course and Outcome

The outcome of fibromyalgia is unclear because adequate methods have not been developed to assess the specific fibromyalgic element in a setting where other chronic disorders also cause pain. For example, in fibromyalgia in patients with chronic low back problems, questionnaires that assess presence or severity of pain will always be abnormal even if fibromyalgia is no longer present. A second problem concerns the weight that should be given to specific fibromyalgic symptoms. It is not clear, for example, whether pain threshold should be thought of as an important outcome measure. Clinical observations suggest that even in patients who are clearly better, pain threshold may remain unchanged. Understanding of the actual outcome of fibromyalgia is likely to require the identification of fibromyalgia subsets based on severity, psychological factors, and age. Thus, an additional problem with understanding the outcome of fibromyalgia is that most available data concern patients with disease of long duration who have been referred to specialty clinics, while it is clear that improvement generally occurs in a wide spectrum of chronic pain patients (58,241). Using data that are available, fibromyalgia appears to be a chronic, rather unchanging disorder that rarely ends in remission. (15,48,74,111,115,152). In one study from a referral clinic (152), 4 years after initial examination 97% still had symptoms, and 85% fulfilled diagnostic criteria and had significant self-reported functional abnormalities on the Health Assessment Questionnaire (HAQ) (86). Fibromyalgia related to trauma also is reported as chronic as well as severe (102).

Functional Disability

Self-reported functional problems have been noted frequently. Using the Stanford Health Assessment Questionnaire (HAQ) (86), significantly abnormal scores averaging approximately 1.00 (0–3 scale) were found in the United States (109) and the United Kingdom. (152). A correlation of $r = -.61$ between HAQ scores and ability to perform work tasks was noted in the United States (49).

Work Disability

Work disability and compensation is related to country and social system. In two reports from one center in the United States, 6.3% (48) and 9.3% (49) reported being disabled, while 5.7% were receiving disability payments, 30.4% reported having to change jobs because of their illness, and 17% retired because of fibromyalgia (49). In another center 22% reported being disabled, and 33% changed jobs because of the illness (162). A preliminary study of 620 patients from several centers indicated that 14.9% had received disability payments. Of these patients 8.8% received payments from the federal government (Social Security Disability) (47). After an average of 7 years of fibromyalgia, 55% of Swedish patients were unable to do necessary household tasks and 24% were receiving disability pensions (15).

Pathophysiology

The definition of the pathophysiology associated with fibromyalgia is complicated by the lack of an absolute diagnosis. Accordingly, one may only hypothesize the relevance of several potential substrates (21,164,188). Focusing on the central issue of an exaggerated pain response evoked by a firm compression of large expanses of muscle and soft tissue, one might presume that an important physiologic component is an exaggerated afferent evoked response. Several possibilities can be considered speculative.

Anomalous Processing of Afferent Information

Sensitized Peripheral Afferents A component could arise from a facilitated response on the part of a sensitized high-threshold afferent. Such sensitization could occur as a result of systemic factors that lead to afferent sensitization. As reviewed, a variety of circulating cytokines have the ability to induce spontaneous activity and sensitization by a direct action on the terminal (see Chap. 6) and in the dorsal root ganglion cells of small afferents (see Chap. 3). To the extent that the diagnosis reflects a wide distribution of the "tender" regions, a circulating factor that exerts a broad influence on the neuraxis represents an inviting hypothesis. Peripheral manifestation of neurogenic inflammation as manifested by reactive hyperemia have also been demonstrated (101,113,156). This suggests a hyperactive peripheral sensory terminal. A variety of mechanisms have been suggested to contribute to such peripheral end organ mechanisms, including immune components, deconditioning of the musculature, altered secretion of circulating hormones (such as somatomedin C), which may influence local afferent transduction (14,23,159,169,173,193).

Sympathetic Contributions It is appreciated that in the face of nerve injury there can be an induced sprouting of sympathetic terminals into the vicinity of sensory afferent and their ganglion cells, and these projections can result in an excitatory coupling (see Chap. 28). It has in fact been reported that sympathetic blockade can abolish or reduce tender points (11,18). Many of the secondary manifestations of the syndrome appear to be related to autonomic system activity including dry eyes and mouth, irritable bowel syndrome, paresthesias, soft tissue swelling, and peripheral temperature changes. Autonomic features, as with the neuroendocrine abnormalities cited below, might be secondary concomitants of other manifestations of the syndrome rather than being intrinsic to the syndrome itself.

Changes in Central Processing Preclinical studies have provided insights into several central mechanisms that would support a generalized tenderness, or hyperalgesia. Thus, small afferent input can induce central states of facilitation that are mediated by well-defined afferent transmitter systems such as those for substance P and glutamate (see Chap. 7). Substance P in the CNS, although not in plasma (190), appears to be higher in those with fibromyalgia than in normals or in those with other pain problems (194,196,232). Such input can activate spinal systems that can yield a facilitated processing of the afferent traffic (5,37,50; see Chap. 9). Such spinal systems may include the local action of cyclooxygenase and nitric oxide synthase systems releasing prostaglandins and nitric oxide, respectively (see Chap. 34). In addition, there is ample data to suggest that bulbospinal pathways can also serve to inhibit nociceptive processing. Accordingly, a withdrawal of that inhibition might lead to a general hyperalgesia (9). On the other hand, it is now appreciated that bulbospinal input may serve to facilitate the processing of afferent traffic leading to a hyperalgesia (see Chap. 11). In addition to these transmitter-mediated changes in function, it is currently appreciated that long-term changes in afferent traffic can induce significant changes in the connectivity and the efficacy of local circuitry, such as is associated with an increase in transmitter synthesis, coupled receptors, and ion channels (66–68) (see Chaps. 7 and 9). These observations are in accord with considerations of a central changes resulting in facilitated processing (188, 263).

The relationship between axial skeletal pain and bladder symptoms (irritable bladder syndrome) (237) as well as symptoms of abdominal pain (136) might be associated with increases in receptive fields and spatial summation of nociception, representing a "referred pain" syndrome (see Chap. 12).

Behavioral/Psychological Contributions

As noted, there are important corollaries with fibromyalgia diagnoses and the psychological state of the patient. Arguably, pain may induce altered psychological status and depression. It is widely appreciated that such changes contribute to the behavioral manifestation of the patient (123,126,203,213). Genetic, gender, and aging changes have also been established (123, 177,221). The clinical corollary of such a model is that central as well as peripheral processing mechanisms may cause or exacerbate the syndrome. The high lifetime history (and family history) of major depression has led to a suggestion that a constitutional predisposition to develop the syndrome exists, perhaps on a biochemical basis, particularly in view of the apparent link between serotonin and depression and fibromyalgia (122). Whether or not the psychological state of the patient can be considered the primary component, the psychological and, in the larger sense, the psychosocial clearly represent exacerbating factors. This view draws support from patient statements (181), clinical associations between psychological manifestations and pain, and, inferentially, from the numerous studies showing more psychological distress and abnormality among those with fibromyalgia than with other conditions.

Other generalized measures of CNS dysfunction have been described, including abnormal cortisol diurnal response (166, 194), increased prolactin levels (76,135), abnormal response to thyroid-stimulating hormone (41,174,244), low levels of serotonin or its metabolites centrally and in the CNS (119,120,196), and abnormal central levels of amino acids (193,265).

Exacerbating Factors

Fibromyalgia is exacerbated by a number of factors, including sleep disturbance (4,126; see below) muscle pain and abnormality, and psychological and physical stress. In some instances these exacerbating factors have been seen to be the primary cause or explanation for the syndrome. The importance of muscle in fibromyalgia and the suggestion that fibromyalgia is primarily a disorder of muscle abnormality has had strong support in Scandinavia (8,11,14,16,17,60,61,116, 117,127,128,131–133,157,272), and in the United States by Bennett and coworkers (21–23,137), but this has been challenged by others (70,138,206,266,267). The central role for muscle derives from two propositions: (a) that most pain and dysfunction in fibromyalgia comes directly from muscle abnormality, and (b) that muscle abnormality causes pain and dysfunction and is also the major nociceptive force in the syndrome. Support for the hypotheses comes from biopsy studies, studies of muscle energy metabolism, nuclear magnetic resonance (NMR) studies, and from reports showing clinical functional abnormalities (8,11,14,16,17,60,61,116,117,127,128, 131–133,157,272). Biopsy abnormalities have been criticized as being nonspecific and artifactual, or might be the result of confusion between myofascial pain syndromes and local muscle disorders and fibromyalgia. In addition, a number of studies of energy metabolism have found no significant abnormality (205,206,242). Fibromyalgia has been noted to develop following interleukin-2 therapy for malignancy (239).

MANAGEMENT OF FIBROMYALGIA

The complex interaction of pain, fatigue, sleep problems, concomitant conditions, psychosocial factors, and demographic factors suggests that treatment requires more than just piecemeal efforts or simple drug or physical interventions to improve fibromyalgia. Although it is traditional to consider fibromyalgia to be one entity, patients differ significantly in pain severity, psychological difficulty, disease duration, and concomitant conditions, and they have different prognoses. A number of treatment failures might have been the result of the inclusion of those with long-term, recalcitrant, and psychologically associated fibromyalgia, as opposed to those with shorter duration of symptoms and less severe problems. While pain, and its psychological, social, and societal consequences represent the major problems in fibromyalgia, exacerbating factors are areas for useful intervention. As noted above, however, individual fibromyalgia patients differ, and not all factors are present (in equal amounts) in each patient. Treatment should be individualized (161).

Sleep Disturbance

There is little doubt that sleep disturbances exacerbate symptoms of fibromyalgia (4,15,152,230,248,264,271). For their presumed ability to alter sleep patterns, a series of agents have been used in the treatment of the disorder, most commonly including amitriptyline, cyclobenzaprine, other tricyclics, combined anxiolytic-antidepressants, and specific hypnotics (24,26, 33,42,45,64,88,91,95,103,134,163,186,191,195,200,201,231).

Amitriptyline is the most commonly used agent, and has been shown to be better than placebo in several short-term trials (42,95,134,201). Efficacy, however, is limited. Short-term improvement in pain scores of 26% to 32% was noted in the most positive study (95). Cyclobenzaprine, which differs from amitriptyline by a only single double bond, appears to be slightly less effective (24,186,191,200). Long-term results do not show the same degree of efficacy. Only about a third of patients starting such therapy will continue it for as long as a year, and symptoms do not improve and actually begin to reverse toward pretreatment levels a few weeks after beginning therapy (40,42). A report of a controlled 208-patient, 6-month trial of amitriptyline, cyclobenzaprine, and placebo indicated no benefit for either active drug beyond the first few weeks of therapy (39,40). Anecdotal case reports have provided data indicating that only a third of patients can recognize benefit from the amitriptyline (134). Although the hypothesized mechanism of benefit for tricyclics is through their effect on the putative non-REM sleep abnormality (220), at least one study has shown that cyclobenzaprine does not alter stage IV sleep in patients with fibromyalgia (191). Aprazolam, an agent with effects on anxiety and depression in the doses employed, appears to have marginal benefit in the syndrome in one study (195) and no benefit in another (145). Thus, the role of tricyclics in fibromyalgia treatment is controversial. One possible reason for the failure of these agents in clinical trials is that sleep disturbance is only one, and often not the major, exacerbating factor for most patients with the syndrome. For those patients for whom sleep is the predominant problem, tricyclics and similar agents may prove useful, but if they are not they should be discontinued. Fibromyalgia patients are sensitive to or even intolerant of usual doses of tricyclics. Small doses (e.g., 10 to 25 mg of amitriptyline) just before sleep are more easily tolerated. The hazard of using tricyclics in persons with longstanding complex problems, of which sleep is only one, is that the drug is almost always insufficient in and of itself. Few patients are cured with tricyclics, and their prescription alone may continue a failing pattern of therapy consisting of one drug after another drug, rather than a potentially more comprehensive and effective approach.

Mechanical Stimuli

Persistent nociceptive stimuli may exacerbate fibromyalgia (211,213,215,216). Stress on the cervical and lumbar spine through abnormal work and sleep postures has been suggested as exacerbating the syndrome (211,213,215,216). Smythe (211,213,215,216) has suggested, however, that the tender points in the cervical spine are responding to local irritation, and that the cervical complex, as well as similar areas in the lumbar spine, may be responsible for the radiation and maintenance of pain. This hypothesis has not been tested formally, but an observational study by Smythe (217) demonstrated a reduction in tender points by the use of a specially designed cervical pillow. Anecdotally, such simple interventions appear to be helpful and are inexpensive and nontoxic. Changes in the workplace and home include using chairs of the correct height and support, cervical support pillows, firm mattresses, and avoidance of work in positions that call for repeated hypertension of the neck and abnormal lumbar postures. These suggestions have long been prominent and useful in physical medicine, and should provide inexpensive and useful benefit in fibromyalgia.

Myofascial Pain

Myofascial trigger points are an area of controversy as to their definition and pathologic significance (250). While trigger points are found in many normal, noncomplaining individuals, in persons with fibromyalgia a lowered-pain threshold may lead to a perceived intensification of trigger point pain to levels above pain threshold, or even to an intensification of clinically painful trigger points. Still another role for trigger points might be through their contribution to the total nociceptive load, and it is possible that amelioration might be beneficial. The treatment of trigger points in fibromyalgia has not been studied, and there is little evidence that such treatments (209), including injection, spraying with cold spray, and stretching, or other modalities provide more than symptomatic relief. Anecdotally, some patients with discrete areas of severe local tenderness may be improved following injection. It is important to treat concomitant problems of patients with fibromyalgia, for not all pain is from fibromyalgia, but all pain contributes to the problem of fibromyalgia. But cautions are in order. Just as routine prescription of drug can be harmful, so can routine injections. Injection therapy when used more than infrequently may be counterproductive. There is no evidence that multiple simultaneous injections of tender areas in patients are beneficial, and considerable theoretical and practical reasons suggest that such treatments not be employed.

Treatment of Other Musculoskeletal Disorders

Population data as well as clinical data suggest that most persons with fibromyalgia are above age 50. As such, they can be expected to have other musculoskeletal conditions. Treatment of concomitant conditions may improve fibromyalgia symptoms. In patients with inflammatory arthritis who are treated with corticosteroids during a flare-up, marked reductions in tender point counts and pain scores can be observed (256). Nonsteroidal antiinflammatory drugs (NSAIDs) can be of value in some patients with osteoarthritis and with degenerative disorders of the axial skeleton. NSAID therapy in uncomplicated (primary) fibromyalgia has not been shown to be of benefit in several controlled trials (95,195,269), but might be expected to be useful in concomitant fibromyalgia.

Exercise

Controlled trials have shown aerobic exercise programs to be of benefit in fibromyalgia (96,125,165,168). In the most important study of exercise, McCain et al. (165) studied 42 patients with fibromyalgia who were randomized to receive either a program of stretching exercises or a program of aerobic exercises consisting of indoor bicycle riding during 20 weeks of closely supervised training. Cardiovascular fitness improved in the aerobic group, but not in those undergoing stretching. Pain threshold scores improved in the aerobic group, as did patient and physician global assessment scores. Pain scores improved too, although the improvement was not statistically significant. While this study demonstrated the benefit of aerobic exercise, the extent of the benefit was small and did not extend to all subjects. Both group improved in psychological status, as measured by the SCL-90-r.

Exercise programs are attractive for a number of reasons beyond improvement in physical capacity, reasons that include self-motivation and goal setting. Exercise is frequently suggested by clinicians, and attempts to incorporate exercise into treatment programs have been widespread. But even in strong, well-staffed treatment programs with well-motivated patients that incorporate exercise, few patients achieve goals of aerobic fitness set for them (40). Often overall improvement in fibromyalgia in those participating in exercise program is almost of an equal degree in those meeting as well as those not meeting aerobic fitness goals (40,165,168). Thus, it is possible that some benefit from these programs is derived from participation in the program and some benefit from success in the program.

It is common for patients with fibromyalgia to have physical therapy prescribed. But there are no data to suggest benefit, nor reason to believe that such programs should be effective. In fact, one small study in Sweden (32) failed to show benefit for physical therapy combined with self-management education. Even among well-motivated patients who make a full and earnest effort at aerobic exercise, some find that it leads to increased pain and are unable to proceed or to make progress. An unusual susceptibility to muscle microtrauma by ordinary activities has been suggested by Bennett (21), and this might be one mechanism for increased pain. Increased pain might be related to mechanical factors involving the lumbar spine in a manner similar to that seen in spinal stances, or through stimulation of nociceptors at arthritic lower extremity joints. The reasons for exacerbation by exercise have not been studied. In spite of this, exercise increases health, a sense of well-being, endurance, and psychological well-being, and should be recommended for whatever benefit can accrue.

Psychological Interventions

Although psychological abnormalities and clinical depression have been reported frequently in those with fibromyalgia, there have been few specific and controlled trials of pharmacotherapy or psychotherapies in the syndrome. Studies in the last few years, however, have attempted to evaluate the effectiveness of specific treatments (62,83,97,98,139,233). A variety of interventions with psychological content have been used (32,55,62,77,83,97,98,105,139,144,167,175,180,183,228,233, 236).Cognitive behavioral and restructuring is among the most commonly used psychological intervention, and preliminary reports are encouraging (62,83,97,98,139,175,236). Other interventions have included hypnosis (105), biofeedback (75, 87,118), and various group psychoeducational interventions including stress reduction and relaxation programs (30,62,97, 183), self-management educational programs (32,73,141), and pain schools or clinics (146).

It is difficult to measure the success of these interventions individually, for they are combined often with other treatments (e.g., pharmacotherapy or exercise in a setting of a pain management clinic (see below)) (30,62,97,121).

Pain

One study of data from five centers noted that 36% of fibromyalgia patients were receiving analgesics. Narcotic usage was limited. In general, over-the-counter analgesic therapy with aspirin, acetaminophen, and ibuprofen was commonly employed (47). There is a general sense that opiates should not be employed in this primary syndrome. Even so, this recommendation has not been studied, and a trial of narcotics in this and other benign pain syndromes is overdue.

NSAID therapy has been studied widely, and it is among the interventions aimed specifically at pain. However, these agents have not been found to be of benefit in controlled trials (95,195,269). NSAID use is common in the clinic, however, reflecting either an efficacy not noticed in controlled trials or continued prescription by physicians in lieu of an acceptable alternative (47).

Other Treatment Interventions

A number of other therapies have not been shown to be effective. Prednisone is not effective in the treatment of fibromyalgia (53), nor is somatostatin (258). Other pharmacologic therapies with marginal or uncertain benefit include fluoxetine (55,77,90,255), serotonin receptor (S2) blockers (222), 5-hydroxy-L-tryptophan (46,184), muscle relaxants (231). and S-adenyslmethionine (129,224).

Nonpharmacologic therapies have included biofeedback (75), electroacupuncture (63), acupuncture (63,149), hot and cold treatments (199), homeopathic treatment (25,82), transcutaneous electrical stimulation (TENS) therapy (104), and various methods of support (e.g.. cervical pillows) for correction of mechanical stress especially in the cervical area (214, 243), and general support and reassurance that fibromyalgia is not a progressive disabling disease (114,243,262).

Comprehensive Treatment Programs

The general inefficacy of usual treatments for those with severe fibromyalgia has led to the management of fibromyalgia using concepts and techniques developed in pain management clinics (84,167). These techniques require prolonged interventions that may last from weeks (175) to months (30). Many disciplines may be involved, including psychologists, psychiatrists, physical and occupational therapists, nurses, exercise therapists, exercise physiologists, rheumatologists, social workers, and vocational counselors, and the treatments can be very expensive. Techniques may include relaxation training, electromyogram (EMG) biofeedback, cognitive restructuring, aerobic and stretching exercise, biomechanics training, pacing, and family education. It is difficult to evaluate such programs because it is almost impossible to develop adequate controls and because selection processes, compliance, and dropouts influence results (226), and long-term follow-up is rarely reported (227). In addition, the milieu in which treatment is administered may be more important than the treatment itself (223).

Results of such therapies have been variable. A comprehensive 3-week program yielded improvements in psychological measures including a 47% reduction in depression, a 26% reduction in trait anxiety, and a 30% reduction in pain at the study conclusion for those completing the program (175). Preliminary positive reports of have come from a number of centers (30,62,96,97,144). Adding physiotherapy to self management was not more effective than self-management over a 6-week period (32). What the effective agent is in such programs is unclear, but it may be the program rather than specific components of the program, including exercise.

Data from other sources suggest that pain management programs can be helpful (160,178,240), but it may be that the improvement is generic rather than fibromyalgia specific. Uncontrolled, the value of such programs is at present unproven in fibromyalgia. Reduction in medical costs as a consequence of participating in a comprehensive pain management clinic for a spectrum of pain disorders has been demonstrated (240). Long-term follow-up studies will be required to place these therapies in prospective in fibromyalgia. Perhaps most important in the treatment programs for fibromyalgia will be the identification of subsets of patients who are and who are not capable of response. Not all patients need drugs or exercise, although all can benefit from engagement, explanation, encouragement (204), and understanding. For many patients the pharmacologic or nonpharmacologic interventions listed above will be sufficient.

REFERENCES

1. Ahles TA, Khan SA, Yunus MB, et al. Psychiatric status of patients with primary fibromyalgia, patients with rheumatoid arthritis, and subjects without pain—a blind comparison of DSM-III diagnoses. *Am J Psychiatry* 1991;148:1721–1726.
2. Ahles TA, Yunus MB, Riley SD, et al. Psychological factors associated with primary fibromyalgia syndrome. *Arthritis Rheum* 1984;27: 1101–1106.
3. Alfici S, Sigal M, Landau M. Primary fibromyalgia syndrome—a variant of depressive disorder? *Psychother Psychosom* 1989;51: 156–161.
4. Anch AM, Lue FA, MacLean AW, Moldofsky H. Sleep physiology and psychological aspects of the fibrositis (fibromyalgia) syndrome. *Can J Psychol* 1991;45:179–184.
5. Arroyo JF, Cohen ML. Unusual responses to electrocutaneous stimulation in refractory cervicobrachial pain—clues to a neuropathic pathogenesis. *Clin Exp Rheumatol* 1992;10:475–482.
6. Astrand PO. Exercise physiology and its role in disease prevention and in rehabilitation. *Arch Phys Med Rehabil* 1987;68:305–309.
7. Balague F, Nordin M. Back pain in children and teenagers. *Baillieres Clin Rheumatol* 1992;6:575–593.
8. Bartels EM, Danneskiold-Samsoe B. Histological abnormalities in muscle from patients with certain types of fibrositis. *Lancet* 1986;1: 755–757.
9. Basbaum AI, Fields HL. Endogenous pain control systems: brainstem spinal pathways and endorphin circuitry. *Annu Rev Neurosci* 1984;7:309–338.
10. Baumstark KE, Buckelew SP, Sher KJ, et al. Pain behavior predictors among fibromyalgia patients. *Pain* 1993;55:339–346.
11. Bäckman E, Bengtsson A, Bengtsson M, et al. Skeletal muscle function in primary fibromyalgia. Effect of regional sympathetic blockade with guanethidine. *Acta Neurol Scand* 1988;77:187–191.

12. Becirovic E, Matanovic B, Kapor M, Rajin G. (Treatment of clinical manifestations of extra-articular rheumatism using electrophoresis with thiomucase.) *Med Arh* 1982;36:209–212.
13. Bengtsson A, Ernerudh J, Vrethem M, Skogh T. Absence of autoantibodies in primary fibromyalgia. *J Rheumatol* 1990;17:1682–1683.
14. Bengtsson A, Henriksson KG. The muscle in fibromyalgia—a review of Swedish studies. *J Rheumatol Suppl* 1989;19:144–149.
15. Bengtsson A, Henriksson KG, Jorfeldt L, et al. Primary fibromyalgia. A clinical and laboratory study of 55 patients. *Scand J Rheumatol* 1986;15:340–347.
16. Bengtsson A, Henriksson KG, Larsson J. Reduced high-energy phosphate levels in the painful muscles of patients with primary fibromyalgia. *Arthritis Rheum* 1986;29:817–821.
17. Bengtsson A, Henriksson KG, Larsson J. Muscle biopsy in primary fibromyalgia. Light-microscopical and histochemical findings. *Scand J Rheumatol* 1986;15:1–6.
18. Bengtsson M, Bengtsson A, Jorfeldt L. Diagnostic epidural opioid blockade in primary fibromyalgia at rest and during exercise. *Pain* 1989;39:171–180.
19. Bennett RM. Fibrositis: misnomer for a common rheumatic disorder. *West J Med* 1981;134:405–413.
20. Bennett RM. Personal communication, 1987.
21. Bennett RM. Beyond fibromyalgia: ideas on etiology and treatment. *J Rheumatol Suppl* 1989;19:185–191.
22. Bennett RM, Clark SR, Goldberg L, et al. Aerobic fitness in patients with fibrositis: a controlled study of respiratory gas exchange and ^{133}xenon clearance from exercising muscle. *Arthritis Rheum* 1989;32:454–460.
23. Bennett RM, Clark SR, Campbell SM, Burckhardt CS. Low levels of somatomedin C in patients with the fibromyalgia syndrome—a possible link between sleep and muscle pain. *Arthritis Rheum* 1992;35:1113–1116.
24. Bennett RM, Gatter RA, Campbell SM, et al. A comparison of cyclobenzaprine and placebo in the management of fibrositis: a double-blind controlled study. *Arthritis Rheum* 1988;31:1535–1542.
25. Berry H. Homeopathic treatment and fibrositis (letter). *BMJ* 1989;299:858
26. Birnie DJ, Knipping AA, van Rijswijk MH, et al. Psychological aspects of fibromyalgia compared with chronic and nonchronic pain. *J Rheumatol* 1991;18:1845–1848.
27. Buchwald D, Garrity D. Comparison of patients with chronic fatigue syndrome. fibromyalgia, and multiple chemical sensitivities. *Arch Intern Med* 1994;154:2049–2053.
28. Buchwald D, Goldenberg DL, Sullivan JL, Komaroff AL. The "chronic, active Epstein-Barr virus infection" syndrome and primary fibromyalgia. *Arthritis Rheum* 1987;30:1132–1136.
29. Burckhardt CS, Clark SR, Bennett RM. The fibromyalgia impact questionnaire—development and validation. *J Rheumatol* 1991;18:728–733.
30. Burckhardt CS, Clark SR, Campbell SM, et al. Multidisciplinary treatment of fibromyalgia. *Scand J Rheumatol Suppl* 1992;21:51 (abstr).
31. Burckhardt CS, Clark SR, Campbell SM, et al. The onset of fibromyalgia: an analysis of early symptoms and initiating events. *Arthritis Rheum* 1992;53:S241(abstr).
32. Burckhardt CS, Mannerkorpi K, Bjelle A. A randomized, controlled clinical trial of education and physical for women with fibromyalgia (FMS). *Arthritis Care Res* 1992;5:S17(abstr).
33. Bush C, Ditto B, Feuerstein M. A controlled evaluation of paraspinal EMG biofeedback in the treatment of chronic low back pain. *Health Psychol* 1985;4:307–321.
34. Buskila D, Press J, Gedalia A, et al. Assessment of nonarticular tenderness and prevalence of fibromyalgia in children. *J Rheumatol* 1993;20:368–370.
35. Buskila D, Gedalia A, Neumann L, et al. Fibromyalgia in children: an outcome study. *J Rheumatol* 1995;22:525–528.
36. Calabro JJ. Fibromyalgia (fibrositis) in children. *Am J Med* 1986;81:57–59.
37. Callaghan M, Sternbach RA, Nyquist JK, Timmermans G. Changes in somatic sensitivity during transcutaneous electrical analgesia. *Pain* 1978;5:115–127.
38. Campbell SM, Clark S, Tindall EA, et al. Clinical characteristics of fibrositis. I. A "blinded," controlled study of symptoms and tender points. *Arthritis Rheum* 1983;26:817–824.
39. Carette S, Bell M, Reynolds J, et al. A controlled trial of amitriptyline (AM), cyclobenzaprine (CY) and placebo (P) in fibromyalgia. *Arthritis Rheum* 1992;35:S112(abstr).
40. Carette S, Bell MJ, Reynolds WJ, et al. Comparison of amitriptyline, cyclobenzaprine, and placebo in the treatment of fibromyalgia—a randomized, double-blind clinical trial. *Arthritis Rheum* 1994;37:32–40.
41. Carette S, Lefrancois L. Fibrositis and primary hypothyroidism. *J Rheumatol* 1988;15:1418–1421.
42. Carette S, McCain GA, Bell DA, Fam AG. Evaluation of amitriptyline in primary fibrositis. A double-blind, placebo-controlled study. *Arthritis Rheum* 1986;29:655–659.
43. Caro XJ. Immunofluorescent studies of skin in primary fibrositis syndrome. *Am J Med* 1986;81:43–49.
44. Caro XJ, Wolfe F. Johnston WH, Smith AL. A controlled and blinded study of immunoreactant deposition at the dermal-epidermal junction of patients with primary fibrositis syndrome. *J Rheumatol* 1986;13:1086–1092.
45. Caruso I, Sarzi Puttini PC, Boccassini L, et al. Double-blind study of dothiepin versus placebo in the treatment of primary fibromyalgia syndrome. *J Int Med Res* 1987;15:154–159.
46. Caruso I, Sarzi Puttini P, Cazzola M, Azzolini V. Double-blind study of 5-hydroxytryptophan versus placebo in the treatment of primary fibromyalgia syndrome. *J Int Med Res* 1990;18:201–209.
47. Cathey MA, Wolfe F, Roberts FK, et al. Demographic, work disability, service utilization and treatment characteristics of 620 fibromyalgia patients in rheumatologic practice. *Arthritis Rheum* 1990;33:S10(abstr).
48. Cathey MA, Wolfe F, Kleinheksel SM, Hawley DJ. Socioeconomic impact of fibrositis. A study of 81 patients with primary fibrositis. *Am J Med* 1986;81:78–84.
49. Cathey MA, Wolfe F, Kleinheksel SM, et al. Functional ability and work status in patients with fibromyalgia. *Arthritis Care Res* 1988;1:85–98.
50. Cervero F, Laird JMA, Pozo MA. Selective changes of receptive field properties of spinal nociceptive neurones induced by noxious visceral stimulation in the cat. *Pain* 1992;51:335–342.
51. Cicuttini F, Littlejohn GO. Female adolescent rheumatological presentations: the importance of chronic pain syndromes. *Aust Paediatr J* 1989;25:21–24.
52. Clark S, Campbell SM, Forehand ME, et al. Clinical characteristics of fibrositis. II. A "blinded," controlled study using standard psychological tests. *Arthritis Rheum* 1985;28:132–137.
53. Clark S, Tindall E, Bennett RM. A double blind crossover trial of prednisone versus placebo in the treatment of fibrositis. *J Rheumatol* 1985;12:980–983.
54. Clark SR, Burckhardt CS, Campbell SM, et al. Pain behavior and treatment outcomes in fibromyalgia patients. *Arthritis Rheum* 1992;35:S350(abstr).
55. Cortet B, Houvenagel E, Forzy G, et al. Evaluation of the effectiveness of a serotonin-agonist (fluoxetin hydrochloride)—an open study in patients with fibromyalgia. *Rev Rhum Mal Osteoartic* 1992;59:497–500.
56. Cott A, Parkinson W, Bell MJ, et al. Interrater reliability of the tender point criterion for fibromyalgia. *J Rheumatol* 1992;19:1955–1959.
57. Croft P, Schollum J, Silman A. Population study of tender point counts and pain as evidence of fibromyalgia. *Br Med J* 1994;309:696–699.
58. Crook J, Weir R, Tunks E. An epidemiological follow-up survey of persistent pain sufferers in a group family practice and specialty pain clinic. *Pain* 1989;36:49–61.
59. Dailey PA, Bishop GD, Russell IJ, Fletcher EM. Psychological stress and the fibrositis/fibromyalgia syndrome. *J Rheumatol* 1990;17:1380–1385.
60. Danneskiold-Samsoe B, Christiansen E, Bach Andersen R. Myofascial pain and the role of myoglobin. *Scand J Rheumatol* 1986;15:174–178.
61. Danneskiold-Samsoe B, Christiansen E, Lund B, Andersen RB. Regional muscle tension and pain (fibrositis): effect of massage on myoglobin in plasma. *Scand J Rehabil Med* 1982;15:17–20.
62. de Voogd JN, Knipping AA, De Blecourt ACE, van Rijswijk MH. Treatment of fibromyalgia syndrome wtih psycho-motor therapy and marital counseling. *J Muscle Pain* 1993;1:273–281.
63. Deluze C, Bosia L, Zirbs A, et al. Electroacupuncture in fibromyalgia—results of a controlled trial. *Br Med J* 1992;305:1249–1252.
64. Dinerman H, Goldenberg DL, Felson DT. A prospective evaluation of 118 patients with the fibromyalgia syndrome: prevalence of Raynaud's phenomenon, sicca symptoms, ANA, low complement, and Ig deposition at the dermal-epidermal junction. *J Rheumatol* 1986;13:368–373.

65. Drewes AM, Andreasen A. Jennum P, Nielsen KD. Zopiclone in the treatment of sleep abnormalities in fibromyalgia. *Scand J Rheumatol* 1991;20:288–293.
66. Dubner R, Basbaum AI. Spinal dorsal horn plasticity following tissue or nerve injury. In: Wall PD, Melzack R, eds. *Text Book of Pain*. London: Churchill Livingstone, 1993;225–242.
67. Dubner R. Neuronal plasticity and pain following peripheral tissue inflammation or nerve injury. In: Bond MR, Charlton JE, Woolf CJ, eds. *Proceedings of the Vth World Congress on Pain*. New York: Elsevier Science, 1991;263–276.
68. Dubner R. Hyperalgesia and expanded receptive fields. *Pain* 1992; 48:3–4.
69. Egle UT, Rudolf ML, Hoffmann SO, et al. (Personality markers, defense behavior and illness concept in patients with primary fibromyalgia.) *Z Rheumatol* 1989;48:73–78.
70. Elam M. Johansson G, Wallin BG. Do patients with primary fibromyalgia have an altered muscle sympathetic nerve activity. *Pain* 1992;48:371–375.
71. Enestrom S, Bengtsson A, Lindstrom F, Johan K. Attachment of IgG to dermal extracellular matrix in patients with fibromyalgia. *Clin Exp Rheumatol* 1990;8:127–135.
72. Ercolani M, Trombini G, Chattat R, et al. Fibromyalgic syndrome: depression and abnormal illness behavior multicenter investigation—multicenter investigation. *Psychother Psychosom* 1994;61: 178–186.
73. Evenson M, Anderle-Johnson D. Learned helplessness and self-efficacy in fibromyalgia: a team approach. *Arthritis Care Res* 1992; 5:S13(abstr).
74. Felson DT, Goldenberg DL. The natural history of fibromyalgia. *Arthritis Rheum* 1986;29:1522–1526.
75. Ferraccioli GF, Ghirelli L, Scita F, et al. EMG-biofeedback training in fibromyalgia syndrome. *J Rheumatol* 1987;14:820–825.
76. Ferraccioli GF, Cavalieri F, Salaffi F, et al. Neuroendocrinologic findings in primary fibromyalgia (soft tissue chronic pain syndrome) and in other chronic rheumatic conditions (rheumatoid arthritis, low back pain). *J Rheumatol* 1990;17:869–873.
77. Finestone DH, Ober SK. Fluoxetine and fibromyalgia (letter). *JAMA* 1990;264:2869–2870.
78. Fischer AA. Pressure threshold meter: its use for quantification of tender spots. *Arch Phys Med Rehabil* 1986;67:836–838.
79. Fischer AA. Muscle tone in normal persons measured by tissue compliance. *JONOMAS* 1987;8:227–233.
80. Fischer AA. Tissue compliance meter for objective, quantitative documentation of soft tissue consistency and pathology. *Arch Phys Med Rehabil* 1987;68:122–125.
81. Fischer AA. Pressure algometry over normal muscles. Standard values, validity and reproducibility of pressure threshold. *Pain* 1987;30:115–126.
82. Fisher P, Greenwood A, Huskisson EC, et al. Effect of homeopathic treatment on fibrositis (primary fibromyalgia) (see comments). *BMJ* 1989;299:365–366.
83. Flor H, Birbaumer N. Comparison of the efficacy of electromyographic biofeedback, cognitive-behavioral therapy, and conservative medical interventions in the treatment of chronic musculoskeletal pain. *J Consult Clin Psychol* 1993;61:653–658.
84. Flor H, Turk DC, Rudy TE. Relationship of pain impact and significant other reinforcement of pain behaviors: the mediating role of gender, marital status and marital satisfaction. *Pain* 1989;38:45–50.
85. Forseth KO, Gran JT. The prevalence of fibromyalgia among women aged 20–49 years in Arendal, Norway. *Scand J Rheumatol* 1992;21:74–78.
86. Fries JF, Spitz PW, Kraines RG. Measurement of patient outcome in arthritis. *Arthritis Rheum* 1980;23:137–145.
87. Fritz G, Fehmi L. Primary fibrositis: a skeletal muscle disroder treated with biofeedback-assisted attention training. *Biofeed Self Regul* 1983;8:332–333(abstr).
88. Gambert SR, Gartgwaite TL, Pontzer CH, et al. Running elevates plasma B-Endorphin Immunoreactivity and ACTH in untrained human subjects. *Proc Soc Exp Biol Med* 1981;168:1–4.
89. Garvey TA, Marks MR, Wiesel SW. A prospective, randomized, double-blind evaluation of trigger-point injection therapy for low-back pain. *Spine* 1989;14:962–964.
90. Geller SA. Treatment of fibrositis with fluoxetine hydrochloride (Prozac). *Am J Med* 1989;87:594–595.
91. Gerster JC, Suter P, Daehler M. Maprotiline in primary fibrositis syndrome—a double blind controlled study. In: Muller W, ed. *Generalisierte Tendomyopathie (Fibromyalgie)*. Darmstadt: Steinkopff Verlag, 1991;279–282.
92. Goldenberg DL. Psychologic studies in fibrositis. *Am J Med* 1986; 81:67–70.
93. Goldenberg DL. Fibromyalgia syndrome. An emerging but controversial condition. *JAMA* 1987;257:2782–2787.
94. Goldenberg DL. Fibromyalgia, chronic fatigue syndrome, and myofascial pain syndrome. *Curr Opin Rheumatol* 1991;3:247–258.
95. Goldenberg DL, Felson DT, Dinerman H. A randomized, controlled trial of amitriptyline and naproxen in the treatment of patients with fibromyalgia. *Arthritis Rheum* 1986;29:1371–1377.
96. Goldenberg DL, Kaplan KH, Nadeau MG. The impact of cognitive-behavioral therapy (CBT) on fibromyalgia. *Arthritis Rheum* 1991;34:S190(abstr).
97. Goldenberg DL, Kaplan KH, Nadeau MG. A prospective study of stress reduction, relaxation response (SRRR) therapy in fibromyalgia. *J Muscle Pain* 1994;2:53–56.
98. Goldenberg DL, Kaplan KH, Nadeau MG, et al. A controlled study of a stress-reduction, cognitive-behavioral treatment program in fibromyalgia. *J Muscle Pain* 1994;2:67–66.
99. Goldenberg DL, Simms RW, Geiger A, Komaroff AL. High frequency of fibromyalgia in patients with chronic fatigue seen in a primary care practice. *Arthritis Rheum* 1990;33:381–387.
100. Goodnick PJ, Sandoval R. Psychotropic treatment of chronic fatigue syndrome and related disorders. *J Clin Psychiatry* 1993;54: 13–20.
101. Granges G, Littlejohn GO. A comparative study of clinical signs in fibromyalgia/fibrositis syndrome, healthy and exercising subjects. *J Rheumatol* 1993;20:344–351.
102. Greenfield S, Fitzcharles MA, Esdaile JM. Reactive fibromyalgia syndrome. *Arthritis Rheum* 1992;35:678–681.
103. Gronblad M, Nykanen J, Konttinen Y, et al. Effect of zopiclone on sleep quality, morning stiffness, widespread tenderness and pain and general discomfort in primary fibromyalgia patients—a double-blind randomized trial. *Clin Rheumatol* 1993;12: 186–191.
104. Guven Z, Ozaras N, Kayhan O, et al. The effect of different TENS modalities on pain in fibromyalgia syndrome. *Scand J Rheumatol Suppl* 1992;21:49(abstr).
105. Haanen HCM, Hoenderdos HTW, Van Romunde LKJ, et al. Controlled trial of hypnotherapy in the treatment of refractory fibromyalgia. *J Rheumatol* 1991;18:72–75.
106. Hadler NM. Work-related disorders of the upper extremity part I: cumulative trauma disorders—a critical review. *Occup Prob Med Pract* 1989;4:1–8.
107. Hadler NM. When is an 'idiopathic' rheumatic disease a personal injury? *Occup Prob Med Pract* 1991;6(1):1–8.
108. Hartz A, Kirchdoerfer E. Undetected fibrositis in primary care practice. *J Fam Pract* 1987;25:365–369.
109. Hawley DJ, Wolfe F. Pain, disability, and pain/disability relationships in seven rheumatic disorders: a study of 1522 patients. *J Rheumatol* 1991;18:1552–1557.
110. Hawley DJ, Wolfe F. Depression is not more common in rheumatoid arthritis: a 10 year longitudinal study of 6,608 rheumatic disease patients. *J Rheumatol* 1993;20:2025–2031.
111. Hawley DJ, Wolfe F, Cathey MA. Pain, functional disability, and psychological status: a 12-month study of severity in fibromyalgia. *J Rheumatol* 1988;15:1551–1556.
112. Hawley DJ, Wolfe F, Cathey MA, Roberts FK. Marital status in rheumatoid arthritis and other rheumatic disorders: a study of 7,293 patients. *J Rheumatol* 1991;18:654–660.
113. Helme RD, Littlejohn GO, Weinstein C. Neurogenic flare responses in chronic rheumatic pain syndromes. *Clin Exp Neurol* 1987;23:91–94.
114. Hench PK, Mitler MM. Fibromyalgia. 2. Management guidelines and research findings. *Postgrad Med* 1986;80:57–64, 69.
115. Henriksson C, Gundmark I, Bengtsson A, Ek AC. Living with fibromyalgia—consequences for everyday life. *Clin J Pain* 1992;8: 138–144.
116. Henriksson KG. Muscle pain in neuromuscular disorders and primary fibromyalgia. *Eur J Appl Physiol* 1988;57:348–352.
117. Henriksson KG. Muscle pain in neuromuscular disorders and primary fibromyalgia. *Neurologija* 1989;38:213–221.
118. Hester G, Grant AE, Russell IJ. Psychological evaluation and behavioral treatment of patients with fibrositis. *Arthritis Rheum* 1982;25:S148(abstr).
119. Houvenagel E, Forzy G, Leloire O, et al. (Cerebrospinal fluid monoamines in primary fibromyalgia.) *Rev Rhum Mal Osteoartic* 1990;57:21–23.
120. Houvenagel E, Forzy G, Cortet B, Vincent G. 5-Hydroxy indol

acetic acid in cerebrospinal fluid in fibromyalgia. *Arthritis Rheum* 1990;33:S55
121. Hoydalsmo O. Johannsen I, Harstad H, et al. Effects of multidisciplinary training programmme in fibromyalgia. *Scand J Rheumatol Suppl* 21 1992;21:51(abstr).
121a. Hubbard DR. Berkoff GM. Myofascial trigger points show spontaneous needle EMG activity. *Spine* 1993;18(13):1803–1807.
122. Hudson JI, Goldenberg DL, Pope HG, et al. Comorbidity of fibromyalgia with medical and psychiatric disorders. *Am J Med* 1992;92:363–367.
123. Hudson JI, Hudson MS, Pliner LF, et al. Fibromyalgia and major affective disorder: a controlled phenomenology and family history study. *Am J Psychiatry* 1985;142:441–446.
124. Hudson JI, Pliner LF, Hudson MS, et al. The dexamethasone suppression test in fibrositis. *Biol Psychiatry* 1984;19:1489–1493.
125. Isomeri R, Mikkelsson M, Latikka P. Effects of amitriptyline and cardiovascular fitness training on the pain of fibromyalgia patients. *Scand J Rheumatol Suppl* 1992;21:47(abstr).
126. Jacks DA. Fibromyalgia (letter). *NZ Med J* 1981;94:237
127. Jacobsen S, Bartels EM, Danneskiold-Samsoe B. Single cell morphology of muscle in patients with chronic muscle pain. *Scand J Rheumatol* 1991;20:336–343.
128. Jacobsen S, Danneskiold-Samsoe B. Inter-relations between clinical parameters and muscle function in patients with primary fibromyalgia. *Clin Exp Rheumatol* 1989;7:493–498.
129. Jacobsen S, Danneskiold-Samsoe B, Andersen RB. Oral S-adenosylmethionine in primary fibromyalgia-double-blind clinical evaluation. *Scand J Rheumatol* 1991;20:294–302.
130. Jacobsen S, H:yer-Madsen M, Danneskiold-Samsoe B, Wiik A. Screening for autoantibodies in patients with primary fibromyalgia syndrome and a matched control group. *APMIS* 1990;98: 655–658.
131. Jacobsen S, Holm B. Muscle strength and endurance compared to aerobic capacity in primary fibromyalgia syndrome. *Clin Exp Rheumatol* 1992;10:419–420.
132. Jacobsen S, Jensen LT, Foldager M, Danneskiold-Samsoe B. Primary fibromyalgia: clinical parameters in relation to serum procollagen type III aminoterminal peptide. *Br J Rheumatol* 1990;29: 174–177.
133. Jacobsen S, Wildschiodtz G, Danneskiold-Samsoe B. Isokinetic and isometric muscle strength combined with transcutaneous electrical muscle stimulation in primary fibromyalgia syndrome. *J Rheumatol* 1991;18:1390–1393.
134. Jaeschke R, Adachi JD, Guyatt G, et al. Clinical usefulness of amitriptyline in fibromyalgia: the results of 23 N-of-1 randomized controlled trials. *J Rheumatol* 1991;18:447–451.
135. Jara LJ, Gomez-Sanchez C, Espinoza LR. Prolactin in primary fibromyalgia and rheumatoid arthritis. *J Rheumatol* 1991;18: 480–481.
136. Jorgensen LS, Fossgreen J. Back pain and spinal pathology in patients with functional upper arm abdominal pain. *Scand J Gastroenterol* 1990;45:1234–1241.
137. Jubrias SA, Bennett RM, Klug GA. Increased incidence of a resonance in the phosphodiester region of P-31 nuclear magnetic resonance spectra in the skeletal muscle of fibromyalgia patients. *Arthritis Rheum* 1994;37:801–807.
138. Kalyan Raman UP, Kalyan Raman K, Yunus MB, Masi AT. Muscle pathology in primary fibromyalgia syndrome: a light microscopic, histochemical and ultrastructural study. *J Rheumatol* 1984;11: 808–813.
139. Kaplan KH, Goldenberg DL, Galvin-Nadeau M. The impact of a meditation-based stress reduction program on fibromyalgia. *Gen Hosp Psychiatry* 1993;15:284–289.
140. Kellgren JH, Samuel EP. The sensitivity and innervation of the articular muscle. *J Bone Joint Surg* 1950;32:84–91.
141. Kelly J, Fransen J, Devonshire R. Fibromyalgia self-help class. *Arthritis Care Res* 1992;5:S13(Abstract)
142. Kirmayer LJ, Robbins JM, Kapusta MA. Somatization and depression in fibromyalgia syndrome. *Am J Psychiatry* 1988;145:950–954.
143. Klein R, Berg PA. A comparative study on antibodies to nucleoli and 5-hydroxytryptamine in patients with fibromyalgia syndrome and tryptophan-induced eosinophilia-myalgia syndrome. *Clin Invest* 1994;72:541–549.
144. Kogstad O, Hintringer F, Jonsson YM. Patients with fibromyalgia in pain school. *J Muscle Pain* 1993;1:261–265.
145. Krag NJ, Norregaard J, Larsen JK, Danneskiold-Samsoe B. A blinded, controlled evaluation of anxiety and depressive symptoms in patients with fibromyalgia, as measured by standardized psychometric interview scales. *Acta Psychiatr Scand* 1994;89: 370–375.
146. Kramer JS, Yelin EH, Epstein WV. Social and economic impacts of four musculoskeletal conditions. *Arthritis Rheum* 1983;26:901–907.
147. Kravitz HM, Katz R, Kot E, et al. Biochemical clues to a fibromyalgia-depression link: imipramine binding in patients with fibromyalgia or depression and in healthy controls. *J Rheumatol* 1992;19:1428–1432.
148. Lautenschläger J, Bruckle W, Seglias J, Müller W. Lokalisierte druckschmerzen in der diagnose der generalisierten tendomyopathie (fibromyalgie). *Z Rheumatol* 1989;48:132–138.
149. Lautenschläger J, Schnorrenberger CC, Müller W. Akupunktur bei generalisierter tendomyopathie (fibromyalgie-syndrom). *Dtsch Zschr Akup* 1989;32:122–128(abstr).
150. Leavitt F, Katz RS. Is the MMPI invalid for assessing psychological disturbance in pain related organic conditions. *J Rheumatol* 1989; 16:521–526.
151. Leavitt F, Katz RS, Golden HE, et al. Comparison of pain properties in fibromyalgia patients and rheumatoid arthritis patients. *Arthritis Rheum* 1986;29:775–781.
152. Ledingham J, Doherty S, Doherty M. Primary fibromyalgia syndrome—an outcome study. *Br J Rheumatol* 1993;32:139–142.
153. Littlejohn GO. Repetitive strain syndrome: an Australian experience (editorial). *J Rheumatol* 1986;13:1004–1006.
154. Littlejohn GO. Medicolegal aspects of fibrositis syndrome. *J Rheumatol Suppl* 1989;19:169–173.
155. Littlejohn GO. Fibrositis/fibromyalgia syndrome in the workplace. *Rheum Dis Clin North Am* 1989;15:45–60.
156. Littlejohn GO, Weinstein C, Helme RD. Increased neurogenic inflammation in fibrositis syndrome. *J Rheumatol* 1987;14: 1022–1025.
157. Lund N, Bengtsson A, Thorborg P. Muscle tissue oxygen pressure in primary fibromyalgia. *Scand J Rheumatol* 1986;15:165–173.
158. Malleson PN, Almatar M, Petty RE. Idiopathic musculoskeletal pain syndromes in children. *J Rheumatol* 1992;19:1786–1789.
159. Martin M, Remy J, Daburon F. In vitro growth potential of fibroblasts isolated from pigs with radiation-induced fibrosis. *Int J Radiat Biol* 1986;49:821–828.
160. Maruta T, Swanson DW, McHardy MJ. Three year follow-up of patients with chronic pain who were treated in a multidisciplinary pain management center. *Pain* 1990;41:47–53.
161. Masi AT. Management of fibromyalgia syndrome: a person-centered approach. *J Musculo Med* 1994;11:27–37.
162. Mason JH, Simms RW, Goldenberg DL, Meenan RF. The impact of fibromyalgia on work: a comparison with RA. *Arthritis Rheum* 1989;32:S197(abstr).
163. Matthews DA, Manu P, Lane TJ. Evaluation and management of patients with chronic fatigue. *Am J Med Sci* 1991;302:269–277.
164. McCain GA. Nonmedicinal treatments in primary fibromyalgia. *Rheum Dis Clin North Am* 1989;15:73–90.
165. McCain GA, Bell DA, Mai FM, Halliday PD. A controlled study of the effects of a supervised cardiovascular fitness training program on the manifestations of fibromyalgia. *Arthritis Rheum* 1988;31: 1135–1141.
166. McCain GA, Tilbe KS. Diurnal hormone variation in fibromyalgia syndrome: a comparison with rheumatoid arthritis. *J Rheumatol Suppl* 1989;19:154–157.
166a. McNulty WH, Gevirtz RN, Hubbard DR, Berkoff GM. Needle electromyographic evaluation of trigger point response to a psychological stressor. *Psychophysiology* 1994;31:313–316.
167. Melvin JL. Fibromyalgia. In: Melvin JL, ed. *Rheumatic disease in the adult and child: occupational therapy and rehabilitation*, vol 3. Philadelphia: F.A. Davis, 1988;62–74.
168. Mengshoel AM, Komnaes HB, Forre O. The effects of 20 weeks of physical fitness training in female patients with fibromyalgia. *Clin Exp Rheumatol* 1992;10:345–349.
169. Miller MH, Littlejohn GO. Jones BW, Strand H. Clinical comparison of cultured human epithelial cells and rat liver as substrates for the fluorescent antinuclear antibody test. *J Rheumatol* 1985;12: 265–269.
170. Moldofsky H. Rheumatic pain modulation syndrome: the interrelationships between sleep, central nervous system serotonin, and pain. *Adv Neurol* 1982;33:51–57.
171. Moldofsky H. Fibromyalgia, sleep disorder and chronic fatigue syndrome. In: Block GR, Whelan J, eds. *Chronic fatigue syndrome.* Chichester: J. Wiley, 1993;262–279.

172. Moldofsky H, Scarisbrick P, England R, Smythe HA. Musculoskeletal symptoms and non-REM sleep disturbance in patients with "fibrositis syndrome" and healthy subjects. *Psychosom Med* 1975;37:341–351.
173. Moldofsky H, Warsh JJ. Plasma tryptophan and musculoskeletal pain in non-articular rheumatism ("fibrositis syndrome"). *Pain* 1978;5:65–71.
174. Neeck G, Riedel W. Thyroid function in patients with fibromyalgia syndrome. *J Rheumatol* 1992;19:1120–1122.
175. Nielson WR, Walker C, McCain GA. Cognitive behavioral treatment of fibromyalgia syndrome—preliminary findings. *J Rheumatol* 1992;19:98–103.
176. Norregaard J, Bulow PM, Prescott E, et al. A four-year follow-up study in fibromyalgia. Relationship to chronic fatigue syndrome. *Scand J Rheumatol* 1993;22:35–38.
177. Pellegrino MJ, Waylonis GW, Sommer A. Familial occurrence of primary fibromyalgia. *Arch Phys Med Rehabil* 1989;70:61–63.
178. Peters. J.L, Large, R.G. A randomised control trial evaluating in- and outpatient pain management programmes. *Pain* 1990;41: 283–293.
179. Piergiacomi G, Blasetti P, Berti C, et al. Personality pattern in rheumatoid arthritis and fibromyalgic syndrome. Psychological investigation. *Z Rheumatol* 1989;48:288–293.
180. Pilowsky I, Barrow CG. A controlled study of psychotherapy and amitriptyline used individually and in combination in the treatment of chronic intractable, 'psychogenic' pain. *Pain* 1990;40: 3–19.
181. Potts MK, Silverman SL. The importance of aspects of treatment for fibromyalgia (fibrositis). Differences between patient and physician views. *Arthritis Care Res* 1990;3:11–18.
182. Prescott E, Kjoller M. Jacobsen S, et al. Fibromyalgia in the adult Danish population: I. Prevalence study. *Scand J Rheumatol* 1993;22: 233–237.
183. Probst J-Y, Monsch A. Gruppen and Schmerzbewaltigung bei der generalisierten tendomyopathie (GTM). In: Muller W, ed. *Generalisierte Tendomyopathie (fibromyalgie).* Darmstadt: Steinkopff Verlag, 1991;351–354.
184. Puttini PS, Caruso I. Primary fibromyalgia syndrome and 5-hydroxy-L-tryptophan—a 90-day open study. *J Int Med Res* 1992;20: 182–189.
185. Quimby LG, Block SR, Gratwick GM. Fibromyalgia: generalized pain intolerance and manifold symptom reporting. *J Rheumatol* 1988;15:1264–1270.
186. Quimby LG, Gratwick GM, Whitney CD, Block SR. A randomized trial of cyclobenzaprine for the treatment of fibromyalgia. *J Rheumatol Suppl* 1989;19:140–143.
187. Raspe HH, Baumgartner C, Wolfe F. The prevalence of fibromyalgia in a rural German community: how much difference do different criteria make? *Arthritis Rheum* 1993;36(suppl 9):S48.
188. Reilly PA, Littlejohn GO. Fibrositis/fibromyalgia syndrome: the key to the puzzle of chronic pain (Editorial). *Med J Aust* 1990;152: 226–227.
189. Reilly PA, Littlejohn GO. Peripheral arthralgic presentation of fibrositis/fibromyalgia syndrome. *J Rheumatol* 1992;19:281–283.
190. Reynolds WJ, Chiu B, Inman RD. Plasma substance P levels in fibrositis. *J Rheumatol* 1988;15:1802–1803.
191. Reynolds WJ, Moldofsky H, Saskin P, Lue FA. The effects of cyclobenzaprine on sleep physiology and symptoms in patients with fibromyalgia. *J Rheumatol* 1991;18:452–454.
192. Robbins JM, Kirmayer LJ, Kapusta MA. Illness worry and disability in fibromyalgia syndrome. *Int J Psychiatry Med* 1990;20:49–63.
193. Russell IJ. Neurohormonal aspects of the fibromyalgia syndrome. *Rheum Dis Clin North Am* 1989;15:149–168.
194. Russell IJ, Orr MD, Littman B, et al. Elevated cerebrospinal fluid levels of substance P in patients with the fibromyalgia syndrome. *Arthritis Rheum* 1994;37:1593–1601.
195. Russell IJ, Fletcher EM, Michalek JE, et al. Treatment of primary fibrositis/fibromyalgia syndrome with ibuprofen and alprazolam—a double-blind, placebo-controlled study. *Arthritis Rheum* 1991;34:552–560.
196. Russell IJ, Vaeroy H. Javors M, Nyberg F. Cerebrospinal fluid biogenic amine metabolites in fibromyalgia/fibrositis syndrome and rheumatoid arthritis. *Arthritis Rheum* 1992;35:550–556.
197. Russell IJ, Vipraio GA, Morgan WW, Bowden CL. Is there a metabolic basis for the fibrositis syndrome? *Am J Med* 1986;81:50–54.
198. Samborski W, Stratz T, Kretzmann WM, et al. (Comparative studies of the incidence of vegetative and functional disorders in backache and generalized tendomyopathies.) *Z Rheumatol* 1991;50: 378–381.
199. Samborski W, Stratz T, Sobieska M, et al. (Intraindividual comparison of whole body cold therapy and warm treatment with hot packs in generalized tendomyopathy.) *Z Rheumatol* 1992;51:25–30.
200. Santandrea S, Montrone F, Sarziputtini P, et al. A double-blind crossover study of 2 cyclobenzaprine regimens in primary fibromyalgia syndrome. *J Int Med Res* 1993;21:74–80.
201. Scudds RA, McCain GA, Rollman GB, Harth M. Improvements in pain responsiveness in patients with fibrositis after successful treatment with amitriptyline. *J Rheumatol Suppl* 1989;16:98–103.
202. Scudds RA, Rollman GB, Harth M, McCain GA. Pain perception and personality measures as discriminators in the classification of fibrositis. *J Rheumatol* 1987;14:563–569.
203. Sharpe M, Peveler R, Mayou R. Invited review: the psychological treatment of patients with functional somatic symptoms—a practical guide. *J Psychosom Res* 1992;36:515–529.
204. Silman AJ. ME/fibromyalgia symposium. *Br J Rheumatol* 1992;31: 130–131.
205. Simms RW, Roy S, Hrovat M, et al. Fibromyalgia syndrome (FMS) is not associated with abnormalities in muscle energy metabolism. *Scand J Rheumatol Suppl* 1992;21:19(abstr).
206. Simms RW, Roy SH, Hrovat M, et al. Lack of association between fibromyalgia syndrome and abnormalities in muscle energy metabolism. *Arthritis Rheum* 1994;37:794–800.
207. Simms RW, Goldenberg DL. Symptoms mimicking neurologic disorders in fibromyalgia syndrome. *J Rheumatol* 1988;15:1271–1273.
208. Simms RW, Goldenberg DL, Felson DT, Mason JH. Tenderness in 75 anatomic sites. Distinguishing fibromyalgia patients from controls. *Arthritis Rheum* 1988;31:182–187.
209. Simons DG, Travell JG. Myofascial origins of low back pain. *Postgrad Med* 1983;73:66–108.
210. Singsen B. Research advances in pediatric rheumatic diseases: of mice, stress, and data sets. *J Pediatr* 1986;384–386.
211. Smythe H. Links between fibromyalgia and myofascial pain syndromes. *J Rheumatol* 1992;19:842–843.
212. Smythe HA. Fibrositis as a disorder of pain modulation. *Clin Rheum Dis* 1979;5:823–832.
213. Smythe HA. Nonarticular rheumatism and psychogenic musculoskeletal syndromes. In: McCarty DJ, ed. *Arthritis and allied conditions.* Philadelphia: Lea and Febiger, 1985;1083–1094.
214. Smythe HA. "Fibrositis" and other diffuse musculoskeletal syndromes. In: Kelley WN, Harris ED Jr, Ruddy S, Sledge CB, eds. *Textbook of rheumatology,* vol 2. Philadelphia: WB Saunders, 1985; 481–489.
215. Smythe HA. Referred pain and tender points. *Am J Med* 1986;81: 90–92.
216. Smythe HA. The "repetitive strain injury syndrome" is referred pain from the neck. *J Rheumatol* 1988;15:1604–1608.
217. Smythe HA. The C6-7 syndrome—clinical features and treatment response. *J Rheumatol* 1994;21:1520–1526.
218. Smythe HA, Buskila D, Urowitz S, Langevitz P. Control and "fibrositic" tenderness: comparison of two dolorimeters. *J Rheumatol* 1992;19:768–771.
219. Smythe HA, Gladman A, Dagenais P, et al. Relation between fibrositic and control site tenderness—effects of dolorimeter scale length and footplate size. *J Rheumatol* 1992;19:284–289.
220. Smythe HA, Moldofsky H. Two contributions to understanding of the "fibrositis" syndrome. *Bull Rheum Dis* 1977;28:928–931.
221. Stormorken H, Brosstad F. Fibromyalgia—family clustering and sensory urgency with early onset indicate genetic predisposition and thus a true disease. *Scand J Rheumatol* 1992;21:207
222. Stratz T, Mennet P, Benn HP, Müller W. Blockade of S2 receptors—a new approach to therapy of primary fibromyalgia syndrome. *Z Rheumatol* 1991;50:21–22.
223. Talo S, Rytokoski U, Puukka P. Patient classification, a key to evaluate pain treatment: a psychological study in chronic low back pain patients. *Spine* 1992;17:998–1011.
224. Tavoni A, Vitali C, Bombardieri S, Pasero G. Evaluation of S-adenosylmethionine in primary fibromyalgia. A double-blind crossover study. *Am J Med* 1987;83:107–110.
225. Triadafilopoulos G, Simms RW, Goldenberg DL. Bowel dysfunction in fibromyalgia syndrome. *Dig Dis Sci* 1991;36:59–64.
226. Turk DC, Rudy TE. Neglected factors in chronic pain treatment outcome studies—referral patterns, failure to enter treatment, and attrition. *Pain* 1990;43:7–25.
227. Turk DC, Rudy TE. Neglected topics in the treatment of chronic

pain patients—relapse, noncompliance, and adherence enhancement—review article. *Pain* 1991;44:5–28.
228. Tyber MA. Lithium carbonate augmentation therapy in fibromyalgia. *Can Med Assoc J* 1990;143:902–904.
229. Urrows S, Affleck G, Tennen H, Higgins P. Unique clinical and psychological correlates of fibromyalgia tender points and joint tenderness in rheumatoid arthritis. *Arthritis Rheum* 1994;37: 1513–1520.
230. Uveges JM, Parker JC, Smarr KL, et al. Psychological symptoms in primary fibromyalgia syndrome: relationship to pain, life stress, and sleep disturbance. *Arthritis Rheum* 1990;33:1279–1283.
231. Vaeroy H, Abrahamsen A, Frre O, Kass E. Treatment of fibromyalgia (fibrositis syndrome): a parallel double blind trial with carisoprodol, paracetamol and caffeine (Somadril comp) versus placebo. *Clin Rheumatol* 1989;8:245–250.
232. Vaeroy H, Helle R, Frre O, et al. Elevated CSF levels of substance P and high incidence of Raynaud phenomenon in patients with fibromyalgia: new features for diagnosis. *Pain* 1988;32:21–26.
233. Vandvik IH, Forseth KO. A bio-psychosocial evaluation of ten adolescents with fibromyalgia. *Acta Paediatr* 1994;83:766–771.
234. Vanhoudenhove B, Vasquez G, Neerinckx E. Tender points or tender patients—the value of the psychiatric in-depth interview for assessing and understanding psychopathological aspects of fibromyalgia. *Clin Rheumatol* 1994;13:470–474.
235. Varni JW, Bernstein BH. Evaluation and management of pain in children with rheumatic diseases. *Rheum Dis Clin North Am* 1991; 17:985–1000.
236. Walco GA, Ilowite NT. Cognitive-behavioral intervention for juvenile primary fibromyalgia syndrome. *J Rheumatol* 1992;19: 1617–1619.
237. Wallace DJ. Genitourinary manifestations of fibrositis: an increased association with the female urethral syndrome. *J Rheumatol* 1990;17:238–239.
238. Wallace DJ, Bowman RL, Wormsley SB, Peter JB. Cytokines and immune regulation in patients with fibrositis (letter) (published erratum appears in Arthritis Rheum 1989;32(12):1607). *Arthritis Rheum* 1989;32:1334–1335.
239. Wallace DJ, Margolin K, Waller P. Fibromyalgia and interleukin-2 therapy for malignancy (letter). *Ann Intern Med* 1988;108:909.
240. Weir R, Browne GB, Tunks E, et al. A profile of users of specialty pain clinic services—predictors of use and cost estimates. *J Clin Epidemiol* 1992;45:1399–1415.
241. Whitney CW, Vonkorff M. Regression to the mean in treated versus untreated chronic pain. *Pain* 1992;50:281–285.
242. Wigers SH, Aasly J. 31 Phosphorus magnetic resonance spectroscopy of leg muscle of patients with fibromyalgia. *Scand J Rheumatol Suppl* 1992;21:26(abstr).
243. Wilke WS, Corbo DD. Fibrositis/fibromyalgia: causes and treatment. *Compr Ther* 1989;15:47–54.
244. Wilke WS, Sheeler LR, Makarowski WS. Hypothyroidism with presenting symptoms of fibrositis. *J Rheumatol* 1981;8:626–631.
245. Wolfe F, Cathey MA, Kleinheksel SM, et al. Psychological status in primary fibrositis and fibrositis associated with rheumatoid arthritis. *J Rheumatol* 1984;11:500–506.
246. Wolfe F. The clinical syndrome of fibrositis. *Am J Med* 1986;81: 7–14.
247. Wolfe F. Development of criteria for the diagnosis of fibrositis. *Am J Med* 1986;81:99–104.
248. Wolfe F, Smythe HA, Yunus MB, et al. The American College of Rheumatology 1990 Criteria for the Classification of Fibromyalgia: Report of the Multicenter Criteria Committee. *Arthritis Rheum* 1990;33:160–172.
249. Wolfe F. Fibromyalgia. In: Bellamy N, ed. *Prognosis in the rheumatic diseases.* Dordrecht: Kluwer Academic, 1991;321–332.
250. Wolfe F, Simons DG, Fricton JR, et al. The fibromyalgia and myofascial pain syndromes—a preliminary study of tender points and trigger points in persons with fibromyalgia, myofascial pain syndrome and no disease. *J Rheumatol* 1992;19:944–951.
251. Wolfe F. Fibromyalgia and problems in classification of musculoskeletal disorders. In: Vaeroy H, Merskey H, eds. *Progress in fibromyalgia and myofascial pain.* Amsterdam: Elsevier Science, 1993;217–235.
252. Wolfe F. Post-traumatic fibromyalgia: a case report narrated by the patient. *Arthritis Care Res* 1994;7:161–165.
253. Wolfe F. Data collection and utilization: a methodology for clinical practice and clinical research. In: Wolfe F, Pincus T, eds. *Rheumatoid arthritis:* pathogenesis, *assessment, outcome, and treatment.* New York: Marcel Dekker, 1994;463–514.
254. Wolfe F, Cathey MA. Prevalence of primary and secondary fibrositis. *J Rheumatol* 1983;10:965–968.
255. Wolfe F, Cathey MA, Hawley DJ. A double-blind placebo controlled trial of fluoxetine in fibromyalgia. *Scand J Rheumatol* 1994; 23:255–259.
256. Wolfe F, Cathey MA, Kleinheksel SM. Fibrositis (fibromyalgia) in rheumatoid arthritis. *J Rheumatol* 1984;11:814–818.
257. Wolfe F, Hawley DJ, Cathey MA, et al. Fibrositis: symptom frequency and criteria for diagnosis. An evaluation of 291 rheumatic disease patients and 58 normal individuals. *J Rheumatol* 1985;12:1159–1163.
258. Wolfe F, Mullis M, Cathey MA. A double blind placebo controlled trial of somatostatin in fibromyalgia. *Arthritis Rheum* 1991;34: S188(abstr).
259. Wolfe F, Ross K, Anderson J, Russell IJ. Aspects of fibromyalgia in the general population: sex, pain threshold, and fibromyalgia symptoms. *J Rheumatol* 1995;22:151–156.
260. Wolfe F, Ross K, Anderson J, et al. The prevalence and characteristics of fibromyalgia in the general population. *Arthritis Rheum* 1995;38:19–28.
261. Wysenbeek AJ, Shapira Y, Leibovici L. Primary fibromyalgia and the chronic fatigue syndrome. *Rheumatol Int* 1991;10:227–229.
262. Yunus MB. Diagnosis, etiology, and management of fibromyalgia syndrome: an update. *Compr Ther* 1988;14:8–20.
263. Yunus MB. Towards a model of pathophysiology of fibromyalgia—aberrant central pain mechanisms with peripheral modulation. *J Rheumatol* 1992;19:846–850.
264. Yunus MB, Ahles TA, Aldag JC, Masi AT. Relationship of clinical features with psychological status in primary fibromyalgia. *Arthritis Rheum* 1991;34:15–21.
265. Yunus MB, Dailey JW, Aldag JC, et al. Plasma tryptophan and other amino acids in primary fibromyalgia—a controlled study. *J Rheumatol* 1992;19:90–94.
266. Yunus MB, Kalyan Raman UP, Kalyan Raman K, Masi AT. Pathologic changes in muscle in primary fibromyalgia syndrome. *Am J Med* 1986;81:38–42.
267. Yunus MB, Kalyan-Raman UP, Masi AT, Aldag JC. Electron microscopic studies of muscle biopsy in primary fibromyalgia syndrome: a controlled and blinded study. *J Rheumatol* 1989;16:97–101.
268. Yunus MB, Masi AT. Juvenile primary fibromyalgia syndrome. A clinical study of thirty-three patients and matched normal controls. *Arthritis Rheum* 1985;28:138–145.
269. Yunus MB, Masi AT, Aldag JC. Short term effects of ibuprofen in primary fibromyalgia syndrome: a double blind, placebo controlled trial (published erratum appears in *J Rheumatol* 1989; 16(6):855). *J Rheumatol* 1989;16:527–532.
270. Yunus MB, Masi AT, Aldag JC. A controlled study of primary fibromyalgia syndrome: clinical features and association with other functional syndromes. *J Rheumatol Suppl* 1989;19:62–71.
271. Yunus MB, Masi AT, Calabro JJ, et al. Primary fibromyalgia (fibrositis): clinical study of 50 patients with matched normal controls. *Semin Arthritis Rheum* 1981;11:151–171.
272. Zidar J, Blackman E, Bengtsson A, Henriksson KG. Quantitative EMG and muscle tension in painful muscles in fibromyalgia. *Pain* 1990;40:249–254.

Anesthesia: Biologic Foundations, edited by
Tony L. Yaksh et al. Lippincott–Raven Publishers,
Philadelphia © 1997.

CHAPTER 58

PHARMACOLOGY AND MECHANISMS OF OPIOID ANALGESIC ACTIVITY

TONY L. YAKSH

Among the remedies which it has pleased almighty God to give to man to relieve his sufferings, none is so universal and efficacious as opium.

Sydenham, 1680

The potent effects of opiates in altering animal or human responses to strong and potentially tissue-damaging stimulus has been long appreciated, as suggested by the quotation attributed to Sydenham. The potency of the effect and the specificity of the action is indicative of a highly organized substrate that regulates the processing of and response to nociceptive information. This chapter reviews some of the mechanisms by which this family of agents exerts its actions as defined by preclinical investigations. The use of opiates in humans to manage pain is pervasive and references can be found in the chapters related to the specific pain states.

OPIOID RECEPTORS

Subtypes

At present, agents classified as opioids are believed to exert their effect by a specific interaction with one or more subclasses of three opiate receptors, designated as μ, δ, and κ. Early in vivo pharmacologic work provided the initial definition of the profile of actions that became associated with the definition of the three principal receptor types. Thus, work by Martin and colleagues (91) in spinally transected dogs led to the classification of agents that were acting at μ and κ sites. The subsequent work by Kosterlitz's team (83) using in vitro smooth muscle bioassays with the newly discovered enkephalin peptides led to the designation of the δ receptor subclass. The profile of this activity is summarized in Table 1.

Receptor isolation and cloning have been accomplished for the μ (28,29,152), δ (71), and κ (29,80,92) receptor classes. Some characteristics of these receptors are presented in Table 2. Studies on the characteristics of these cloned receptors expressed in heterologous cell lines have indicated that (a) they possess an agonist structure activity relationship that resembles those defined in in vivo and ex situ bioassays, (b) they are negatively coupled through G_i proteins to adenylate cyclase, and (c) they display seven transmembrane spanning regions. In general, these receptors show considerable structural homology with each other and to other G-protein–coupled receptors, such as for vasopressin, somatostatin, and substance P, which display the seven transmembrane spanning regions. Characteristically, they display sequences that are highly conserved in regions spanning the transmembrane domain and the intracellular loops (160).

A number of subclasses of the principal categories of receptors have been postulated based on their differential pharmacology: μ_1 and μ_2 (107), δ_1 and δ_2 (66), and k_{1-4} (107), with the characteristics of these subtype receptors continuing to evolve as new agents are developed. It is important to note that in many cases the clones have not yet demonstrated multiple types. However, the possibility of systematic changes in receptor protein structure by posttranslational processing cannot be discounted. Moreover, the separation of subclasses within the subtypes has frequently depended on a limited structure activity relationship. Thus, for example, the separation of μ_1 and μ_2 has been almost exclusively based on the ability of noncompetitive antagonists (such as naloxonazine) to antagonize one or another effect of an opioid agonist (analgesia is reversed, respiratory depression is not [107]). In the case of the μ subclasses, no selective agonists have been described thus far. In contrast, in the case of the δ subclasses, selective competitive agonists (δ_1: DPDPE; δ_2: deltorphin) have been identified and a distinctive antagonist activity profile has been obtained for both sites (δ_1: 7-brenzylidenenaltrexone: δ_2: naltriben) (54,66,144).

In this review, the primary classifications will be emphasized.

Membrane Action

Agonist occupancy of opioid receptors typically leads to several events that serve to inhibit the activation of the neuron. μ and δ agonists have been shown to depress adenosine 3′,5′-cyclic monophosphate (cAMP) formation. μ, δ (198), and on occasion κ (52) receptors can induce a membrane hyperpolarization through the activation of an inwardly rectifying K^+ channel. This effect of the μ receptor is mediated by the activation of membrane G_o proteins, while the δ effects are mediated by $G_{i/o}$ proteins of a different nature (27). In addition to the hyperpolarization induced by μ and δ agonist receptor occupancy, there is a concurrent inhibition of the opening of voltage-sensitive Ca^{2+} channels (67,110), which will subsequently depress the terminal release of neurotransmitters from the cell. These joint actions lead to a powerful, receptor-mediated inhibition that is typically observed with opiates. κ Receptors appear to be distinctly coupled and have been shown to depress Ca^{2+} conductance in neurons. While the principal effect of the μ receptor appears mediated through an inhibitory effect, several lines of work have suggested that, under certain conditions the μ receptors may couple through G_s protein and exert a stimulatory effect (130). The significance of this action is less certain, however, than for the inhibitory effect, which appears to be broadly noted.

SITES OF OPIATE ANTINOCICEPTIVE ACTION

The systemic delivery of an opioid produces a selective alteration in the animal's response to a strong and otherwise aversive thermal or mechanical stimulus. This antinociceptive effect is characterized by a structure activity relationship and antagonistic profile indicative of an action mediated by an opioid receptor. The essential issue is where are such receptors located? The methodologic approach to such an issue is to deliver the agent to specific sites in the organism and to define the effect and the pharmacology of the action if there is an effect after local exposure.

For central delivery, such work has involved the placement of microinjection guide cannulae stereotaxically into specific brain sites and affixing them to the skull. Through the chronic guide,

Abbreviations are presented on last page.

Table 1. OPIOID RECEPTOR SUMMARY

Receptor	Bioassay	Agonists	Antagonists
μ	Guinea pig ileum	Morphine, sufentanil, meperidine, DAMGO	Naloxone, naltrexone,β-funaltrexamine
δ	Mouse vas deferens	DPDPE, DADLE, deltorphin, DSLET	Naloxone, DALCE, BNTX,[1] naltrindole
κ	Rabbit vas deferens	Butorphanol, bremazocine, spiradoline	Naloxone, Nor-BNI

See refs. 66 and 171.

a smaller injection cannula is inserted to deliver small volumes of injectate (0.2 to 0.5 μl). In the spinal cord, this local delivery has entailed the placement of a spinal catheter into the intrathecal or epidural spaces (186,187). In each case, the important issue has been to assess the effects of a local drug on the nociceptive behavior of the intact and unanesthetized animal.

Brain (Supraspinal) Sites

Mapping of brain sites in animals prepared with microinjection cannulae has shown that opioid receptors associated with systems that modulate the animals pain behavior are found in several surprisingly restricted brain regions. Table 3 summarizes several of the sites of action that have been identified. The schematic localization of these sites is presented in Fig. 1. The best characterized of these sites so identified is the mesencephalic periaqueductal gray (PAG). Microinjections of morphine into this region block nociceptive responses in the unanesthetized rat, rabbit, cat, dog, and primate (see below). This local effect serves to block not only spinally mediated reflexes such as the tail flick, but supraspinally organized responses such as in the formalin test (88), hot plate test (Fig. 2), or using shock titration (192). This effect on a spinal reflex of a supraspinally injected agent emphasizes the possible activation of bulbospinal projections, which will be discussed below. Importantly, these effects are reversed by low doses of naloxone given either systemically or into the microinjection site.

Mesencephalic Periaqueductal Gray

Tsou and Jiang (157) discovered in 1963 that the local action of morphine in the periventricular gray would block thermally evoked hind limb reflexes, and this was subsequently verified in a variety of species, including the rat (129,192), mouse (31), cat (103), dog (163), and primate (108,109). Within the PAG, a somatotopic organization has been reported for opiate action (68,192). As indicated in Table 2, based on the relative activity of several receptor agonists and antagonists, the effects appear to be mediated by μ but not δ or κ (177). Binding studies focusing on the PAG have identified a single high-affinity μ site for which δ and κ agonists have low affinity and that is coupled to a G protein (38,39).

Mesencephalic Reticular Formation

Bilateral injections of opiates into the mesencephalic reticular formation significantly increase escape latency with only modest effects on spinal reflexes (53). The pharmacology of this system is thought to implicate a μ site.

Medulla

Two distributions of opiate-sensitive sites have been identified within the caudal medulla: (a) medial sites overlapping the nucleus raphe (65), and (b) lateral sites coinciding with the nucleus gigantocellularis (65,127). The pharmacology of these systems suggests both μ and δ sites exist within the caudal medulla (65).

Substantia Nigra

Bilateral microinjection of opioids into the substantia nigra evokes an increase in the tail flick and hot plate response latencies in rats without evidence of significant motor impairment or change in the response to nonnoxious stimuli (12,13). Examination of the agonist and antagonist pharmacology of the nigra action reveals the role of μ, but not δ or κ, receptors (11).

Nucleus Accumbens/Ventral Forebrain

Microinjections of opiates into the ventral forebrain, notably the nucleus accumbens, preoptic, and arcuate nuclei, block spinal nociceptive reflexes (85,155). Tseng and Wang (155) observed that in the preoptic and arcuate regions, β-endorphin and morphine yielded a dose-dependent, naloxone-reversible increase in tail flick latencies. In the nucleus accumbens, β-endorphin, but not morphine, displays significant activity, suggesting two receptors (155).

Within the ventral forebrain microinjections of μ, δ, and κ agonists into the region referred to as the area tempestas has been shown to attenuate thermal nociception.

Amygdala

Morphine given into the basolateral amygdala increased escape latencies but not spinal reflex latencies (117,192). The pharmacology of the amygdala has not been characterized, but μ opioid agonists are active (117,177,192).

Thalamus and Cortex

Several microinjection mapping studies of opiate action have failed to observe activity following thalamic or cortical injections (108,192), but others (112) reported that microinjection of morphine into the anterior pretectal region of the rat, but not adjacent nuclei, resulted in an inhibition of the tail flick.

Supraspinal Mechanisms of Opiate Antinociception

The multiplicity of opiate sites guarantees that the role of systems with which the opiate receptors are coupled varies in the

Table 2. SUMMARY OF STRUCTURAL CHARACTERISTICS OF CLONED OPIATE RECEPTORS

Characteristics	μ	δ	κ
Gene family	Seven transmembrane spanning loops G_i protein coupled	Seven transmembrane spanning loops G_i protein coupled	Seven transmembrane spanning loops G_i protein coupled
mRNA size	10–16 kb	4.5 kb	5.2 kb
Glycosylation sites	5	2	2
No. of amino acids	398	372	380

Table 3. SUMMARY OF CHARACTERISTICS OF ACTIONS OF OPIATES GIVEN INTO VARIOUS SITES IN THE UNANESTHETIZED RAT

Microinjection sites	Antinociceptive action		Pharmacology	Reference
	Reflex	Escape		
Forebrain/diencephalon				
Amygdala (corticomedial)	0	++	μ?	118,192
N. accumbens	+		μ?	155
Mesencephalon				
Periaqueductal gray	+++	+++	$\mu >> \delta = \kappa = 0$	65,124,131
Mesencephalic reticular formation	++	++	μ?	54
Substantia nigra	++	++	$\mu >> \delta = \kappa = 0$	13
Lower brainstem				
Medial medulla	++	++	$\mu = \delta > \kappa = 0$	18,65
Spinal cord	+++	+++	$\mu = \delta > \kappa > 0$	35,87,128,183
Peripheral site[a]	+++		$\mu = \kappa > \delta = 0$	97,135

Reflex: tail flick/ jaw jerk; Escape: Hot plate/paw pressure.
Relative activity: +++ > ++ >+ > 0.
[a]Inflamed knee joint or foot pad.

way they alter nociceptive processing. Accordingly, it is unlikely that all of the mechanisms whereby opiates act within the brain to alter nociceptive transmission are identical. A brief overview of several classes of mechanisms, particularly as they pertain to the periaqueductal gray, are provided below and presented schematically in Fig. 3.

Descending Control

Mu and δ opiates acting in the brain stem inhibit spinal nociceptive reflexes, reduce the spinal neuronal activity evoked by noxious stimuli, and alter supraspinally organized pain behavior. As discussed in detail elsewhere (180), bulbospinal pathways exert a powerful regulatory influence over spinal cord afferent processing. These effects are in accord with studies in which (a) activation of bulbospinal pathways that contain noradrenaline or 5-HT inhibits spinal nociceptive activity (47,48); (b) enhancement of spinal monoamine receptor activity by local delivery of α_2/5-HT agonists inhibits spinal activity (32, 115,148,191); (c) microinjection of opiates into brain stem sites increases the spinal release or turnover of 5-HT and/or noradrenaline (147,190); and (d) intrathecal injection of α_2 or serotonergic antagonists reverses the effects of brain stem opiates on spinal reflexes and analgesia (3,26). These observations emphasize that the actions of opiate agonists in the PAG are associated with an increase in spinofugal outflow and this influence can regulate spinal nociceptive processing.

The mechanisms that cause the increased activity in bulbospinal pathways are of particular organizational interest,

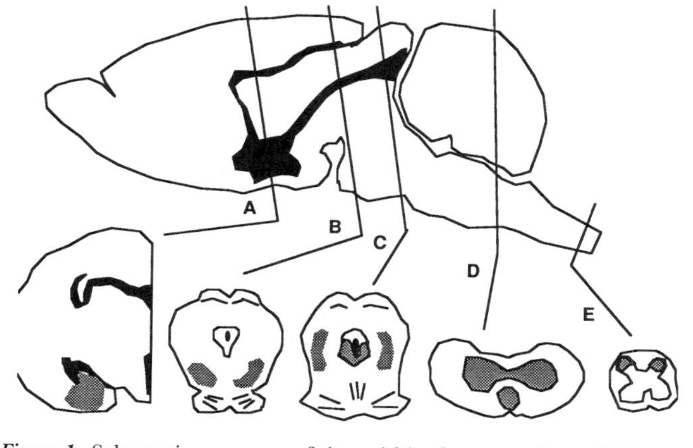

Figure 1. Schematic summary of sites within the neuraxis at which opiate injections result in a prominent increase in the nociceptive threshold. The approximate planes of section at which the coronal sections are taken are indicated. *Darkened regions* indicate the cerebral aqueductal location. The *light shading* indicates the active regions. **A:** Diencephalic—active regions within the basolateral amygdala. **B:** Mesencephalic—active sites within the substantia nigra. **C:** Mesencephalic—lateral regions are the mesencephalic reticular formation; medial region is the periaqueductal gray. **D:** Medulla—site indicates the rostral ventral medulla with the midline suture corresponding to the raphe magnus. **E:** Spino/medullary—active regions refer to the substantia gelatinosa in the spinal and medullary dorsal horn. See text for additional discussion.

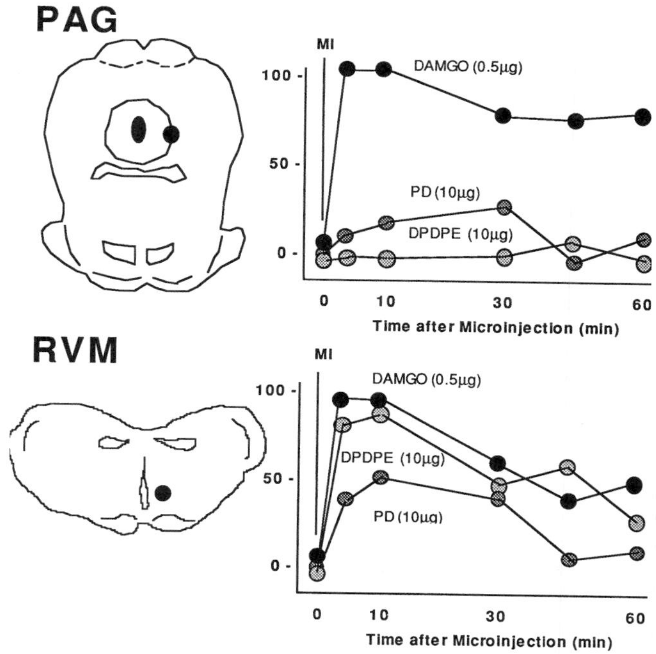

Figure 2. Percent of the maximum possible effect for escape from the 52.5°C hot plate, plotted as a function of time after the injection of a µ agonist (DAMGO: 0.5 µg), a δ agonist (D-Pen[2]-D-Pen[5]-enkephalin [DPDPE]: 10 µg), or a κ agonist (PD117302: 10µg) into the periaqueductal gray (PAG) *(top)* or the rostroventral medulla (RVM) *(bottom)* at the sites indicated in the adjacent histologic representation. Each site received the three injections at 3- to 5-day intervals. Injections were made in a volume of 0.3 µl.

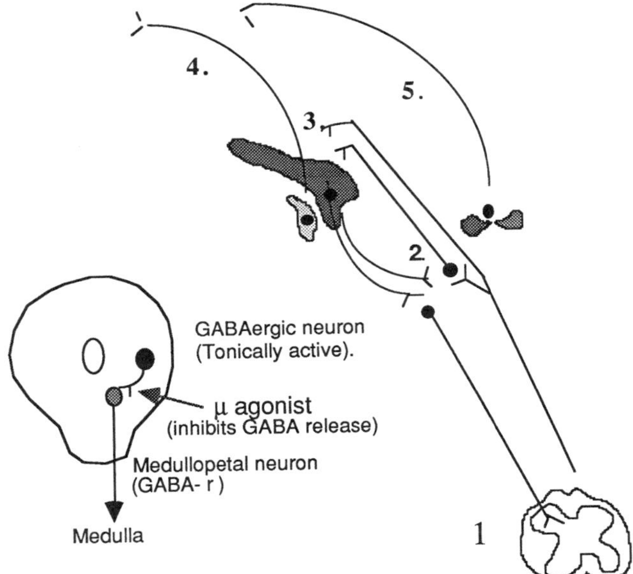

Figure 3. **Left:** Schematic of organization of opiate action within the periaqueductal gray. In this schema, μ opiate actions block the release of GABA from tonically active systems that otherwise regulate the projections to the medulla, leading to an activation of PAG outflow. **Right:** The overall organization of the several mechanisms whereby PAG injections of opiate agonist can alter nociceptive processing are presented in the adjacent schematic. The following mechanisms are hypothesized: (1) PAG projection to the medulla that serves to activate bulbospinal projections releasing serotonin and/or noradrenaline at the spinal level. (2) PAG outflow to the medulla, where local inhibitory interaction results in an inhibition of ascending medullary projections to higher centers. (3) Opiate binding within the PAG may be preterminal on the ascending spinofugal projection. This preterminal action would inhibit input into the medullary core and mesencephalic core. (4/5) Outflow from the PAG can serve to act to modulate excitability of dorsal raphe (4) and locus coeruleus (5) from which ascending serotonergic and noradrenergic projections originate to project to limbic/forebrain. See text for other considerations.

given the membrane inhibitory effects of the μ opioids. Current thinking emphasizes that the outflow of the periaqueductal gray is under modulatory control by GABAergic neurons (Fig. 3). Thus, the local opiates inhibit activity in this population of tonically active neurons, and this inhibition would permit the drive of excitation. Opiates have been shown to diminish a tonic GABA release from the PAG (116), while $GABA_A$ antagonists enhance the activity of local neurons.

Brain stem-Brain stem Inhibition of Afferent Traffic

Spinomedullary and spinal mesencephalic projections are thought to play a role in the generation of the message evoked by high-threshold stimuli. Stimulation within the periaqueductal gray can inhibit nucleus reticulo-gigantocellularis neurons (93). Fields and colleagues (41) have shown powerful mesencephalic influences upon medullary cell populations. Given the role played by the medullary system in the ascending pain traffic, it seems probable that some of these cells may represent projection neurons that contribute to the rostral movement of nociceptive information.

Direct Inhibition of Brain stem Afferent Traffic

Many regions in which opioids exert their effects, such as within the mesencephalon and medulla, receive significant input from direct spinobulbar projections or collaterals of spinodiencephalic projections. Cervical hemisection results in a reduction in opiates in medulla PAG and the mesencephalic reticular formation ipsilateral to the hemisection (113). This suggests that opiate binding may be presynaptic on spinofugal terminals, and that locally administered opiates might alter nociceptive processing through reduction of the excitation otherwise evoked by the spinofugal projections.

Forebrain Mechanism Modulating the Response

Ample evidence suggests that opiates may interact with brain stem mechanisms to alter input by a variety of direct and indirect systems. The behavioral sequelae of systemic appear to reflect a change in the affective component of the response to the strong pain stimulus. Numerous *rostral* projections arise from the dorsal raphe nucleus (5-HT) and the locus coeruleus (noradrenaline) that connect the periaqueductal gray matter with forebrain systems that are known to influence motivational and affective components of behavior, including the n. accumbens, amygdala, and lateral thalamus (85,86). The locus coeruleus has ample projections into the limbic forebrain and thalamus (2). Both monoaminergic systems are strongly implicated in emotionality and in the maintenance of conscious arousal. Lesions of raphe dorsalis diminish the effects of morphine (123), and depletion of serotonin has been classically known to produce a high level of irritability in rats (151).

Considerable data suggest that the periaqueductal gray matter may represent an important nexus for higher level organization in which components of "fear" and "anxiety" may be regulated as part of a loop that involves the limbic forebrain and other rostral structures (8,9).

Spinal Action

Behavioral Effects

Intrathecal administration of opioids reliably attenuates the response of the animal to a variety of unconditioned somatic and visceral stimuli that otherwise evoke an organized escape behavior in a variety of species, including the mouse (64), rat (186), rabbit (186), guinea pig (L. Crone, unpublished observations), cat (159,167), dog (122), and primate (macaque) (170,177,185). The antinociceptive end points in which spinal opiates have been shown to be effective are presented in Table 4.

Pharmacology

The pharmacology of spinal opioids has been examined extensively from the perspective of agonist structure activity relationships, antagonist structure activity relationships, and antagonist potency. In general, in the tests outlined above, spinal opioids produce a monotonic dose- dependent increase in the response latency (tail flick, hot plate, skin twitch), the magnitude of the response (writhing, number of paw licks, change in blood pressure), and the threshold for escape (paw pressure, shock titration) (see above for references). Based on the consideration of the available data, several points regarding the pharmacology of spinal opiates may be summarized:

1. The structure activity relationship of these opioids over a range of two to three orders of magnitude is similar for the end points and across species.
2. The rank order of potency in producing a block of spinal reflexes after intrathecal delivery correlates with the potency of agents on the guinea pig ileum and on the mouse vas deferens (184), suggesting a role for the μ and δ receptors in virtually all end points, except certain neuropathic pain models (see Table 3). The κ-preferring agonists studied thus far typically have lower apparent efficacy (128).
3. Intrathecal opioids are subject to a competitive antagonism by naloxone. For agents classified as μ-preferring agonists (morphine, sufentanil, DAME), the pA_2 (dose required to double the median effective dose [ED_{50}] of the agonist) is similar across all tests examined (writhing, hot plate, and tail flick) in the rat and across

Table 4. MODELS OF NOCICEPTION IN WHICH SPINAL OPIATES HAVE BEEN EXAMINED

General stimulus	Animal	Specific model	Reference
Acute thermal stimuli	Rat	Hot plate (52.5°)/tail flick	188
	Rat	Tail dip evoked hypertension and tachycardia	96
	Dog/cat	Skin twitch	122,159,167
	Primate	Thermal escape	101; also this chapter
Acute mechanical	Rat	Paw pressure	146
	Rat	Tail clamp/pinch	73
Acute visceral	Rat	Colonic distention	98
Acute electrical shock	Rat	Tail shock/vocalization	150,188
	Primate	Shock titration	170
Acute chemical stimuli	Rat	Writhing	128
	Rat	Intradermal formalin	193
Chronic neurogenic	Rat	Autonomy-neurectomy	164
	Rat	Chronic nerve compression (Bennett model)	194
	Rat	Root ligation (Chung model—inactive)	78
Fictive pain stimuli generated by intrathecal drug treatment	Rat	Intrathecal strychnine (inactive)	174

species (rat and primate) and is about 0.1 times the dose required to antagonize agonists classified as δ and κ (182). Receptor-preferring antagonists block the agonists for the respective receptors. Thus, δ-preferring opioids (DPDPE, DADL) but not μ-preferring opioids (morphine, DAMGO), have been shown to be reversed by naltrindole (187). The pharmacology of these effects appear to be similar across a number of species, including rat (54,87,143,144) and primate (170,178, 185; Fig. 4).

Based on the above overview, a case can be made that in the spinal cord of infrahuman species, there are at least three distinguishable subpopulations of opioid receptors that, according to the homology of their agonist and antagonist structure activity profiles, resemble the subclassifications designated as μ, δ, and κ.

Mechanisms of Spinal Opiate Action

Initial studies demonstrated that opiates applied by iontophoresis (25,43) or systemically in spinally transected animals

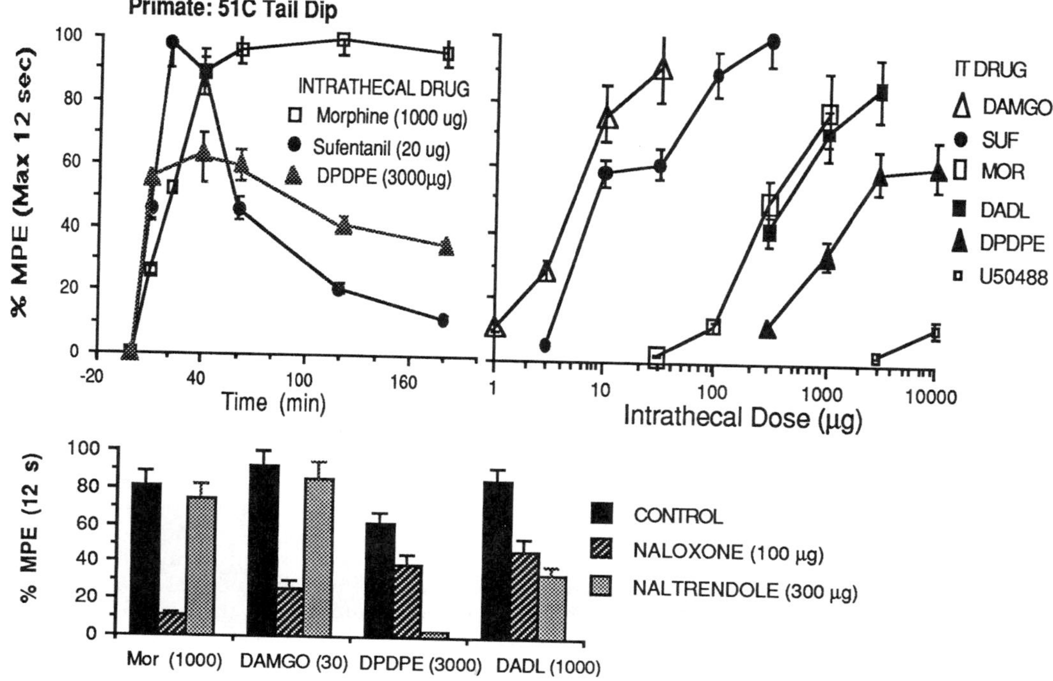

Figure 4. **Top left:** Time effect curve for the effects of intrathecal μ (morphine, sufentanil) and δ (DPDPE) agonists on the response latency to withdraw the tail of the cynomologous primate from a 51°C waterbath. Each line presents the mean and SEM of four experiments. **Top right:** Intrathecal dose effect curve for intrathecal μ (DAMGO; SUF; MOR), δ (DADL; DPDPE), or κ (U50488) agonists. **Bottom:** Reversal of the effects of intrathecal morphine (1000 μg), DAMGO (30 μg), DPDPE (3000 μg), and DADL (1000 μg) after pretreatment with intrathecal saline (control), naloxone (100 μg), or naltrindole (300 μg). *$p<.05$ as compared to control.

(77,166,167) would inhibit selectively the discharge of spinal dorsal horn neurons activated by small (high-threshold) but not large (low-threshold) afferents. Fleetwood-Walker and colleagues (43) examined the pharmacology of the inhibition of dorsal horn neurons by iontophoretically applying receptor preferring agonists for the μ (DAMGO), δ (DPDPE), and κ (U50488). In lamina I, with nociceptive specific neurons or with multireceptive (WDR) neurons, μ and δ agonists exerted a suppressive effect on the nociceptive component; κ agonists had no effect. In laminae II to V, μ and δ agonists were with minimal effect, while κ agonists caused a selective inhibition of the nociceptive component. Recording-evoked activity in lamina II neurons in spinal cord slices revealed that μ (DAMGO) and δ_1 (DPDPE) agonists produced a dose-dependent reduction in the excitatory postsynaptic potentials. In contrast, the δ_2 agonists (D-Ala^2-Glu^4-deltorphin) had less than a 50% effect at the highest dose examined.

Receptor autoradiography with opiate ligands has revealed a number of important characteristics of spinal opiate binding. Binding was limited for the most part to the upper laminae of Rexed, particularly in the substantia gelatinosa (20,51,94), the region in which small afferents show their principal termination. The proportions of the μ, δ and κ opioid binding sites, assessed by autoradiography in laminae I and II, were found to be approximately 70%, 20%, and 10%, respectively. Dorsal rhizotomies result in a significant reduction in dorsal horn binding, suggesting that the binding corresponding to μ, δ, and κ sites were all reduced by 50% to 75% in the dorsal horn ipsilateral to the lesions, and that a significant proportion of all three binding sites was associated with the degenerating primary afferents (15,16). This association was consistent with the observation that opiate binding was found in the dorsal root ganglia (40). This organization suggested that opiates might thus exert a portion of their activity by a presynaptic effect on primary afferents and a postsynaptic effect on dorsal horn projection neurons. Confirmation of the presynaptic action was provided by the observation that opiates in vitro and in vivo would reduce the release of primary afferent peptide transmitters such as substance P (SP) that were contained in small primary afferents. Thus, morphine, DAMGO, DPDPE, and DADL, but not U50488 (1,50,62,179), would block SP and/or CGRP release in vivo.

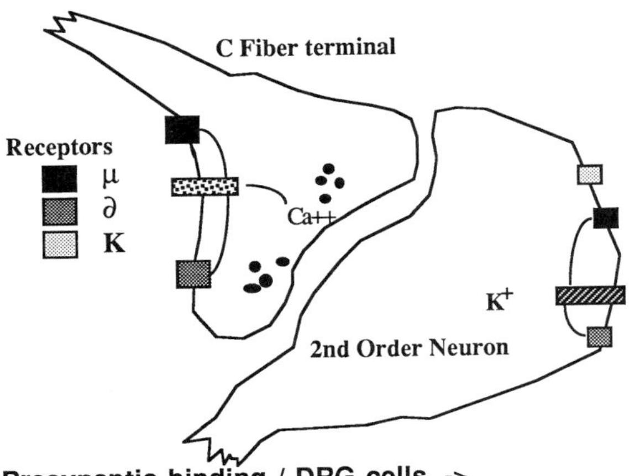

Figure 5. Schematic presents a summary of the anticipated organization of opiate receptors in the dorsal horn regulating nociceptive processing. As indicated, μ/δ and κ binding is high in the dorsal horn, particularly in the region associated with the termination of small unmyelinated afferents (C fibers). A significant proportion of these sites are located on the terminals of the small afferent, as suggested by the loss of such binding after rhizotomy. In addition, there is a postafferent terminal localization of these sites that are apparently coupled through the G_i protein to κ channels, leading to a hyperpolarization of the neuron. Occupancy of the presynaptic μ and δ sites reduces the release of SP and/or CGRP in part by an inhibition of the opening of voltage-sensitive calcium channels. See text for further discussion.

A postsynaptic action was demonstrated by the ability of opiates to block the excitation of dorsal horn neurons evoked by glutamate, presumably reflecting a direct activation of the dorsal horn neuron (199). The presynaptic action corresponded to the ability of opiates to prevent the opening of voltage-sensitive Ca^{2+} channels, thereby preventing release. The activation of potassium channels leading to a hyperpolarization was consistent with the direct postsynaptic inhibition. The joint ability of μ and δ opiates to reduce the release of excitatory neurotransmitters from C fibers as well as decrease the excitability of dorsal horn neurons is believed to account for the powerful and selective effect on spinal nociceptive processing (Fig. 5).

Peripheral Nerves

Behavioral Effects

It has been a principal tenet of opiate analgesia that these agents are centrally acting. Direct application of opiates to the peripheral nerve can in fact produce a local anesthetic-like action at high concentrations, but this is not naloxone reversible and is believed to reflect a "nonspecific" action (49). Moreover, in pain models using normal animals, it can be demonstrated that if the agent does not readily penetrate the brain, its opiate actions are limited.

Alternately, studies employing the direct injection of these agents into peripheral sites have demonstrated that under conditions of inflammation where there is a "hyperalgesia," the local action of opiates can have a normalizing effect on the exaggerated thresholds. This has been demonstrated by the response to mechanical stimulation of inflamed paw (135) or inflamed knee joints (97). As indicated in Fig. 6, examination of the pharmacology of this articular action has emphasized the likely role of μ and κ, but perhaps less importantly δ sites (96,135).

Mechanisms of Peripheral Action

While the opiate "binding" sites are transported in the peripheral sensory axon (74), there is no evidence that these sites are coupled to mechanisms governing the excitability of the membrane. Thus, high doses of agents such as sufentanil can block the compound action potential, but this is not naloxone reversible and is thought to reflect a "local anesthetic" action of the lipid-soluble agent (49). It has been shown that opiate receptors exist on the distant peripheral terminals of C fibers and that agonist occupancy of these sites can block the antidromic release of C-fiber transmitters (e.g., SP) (173).

The models in which peripheral opiates appear to work are those that possess a significant degree of inflammation and are characterized by a hyperalgesic component. This raises the possibility that these peripheral actions normalize a process leading to an increased sensitivity to the local stimulus environment, but does not alter normal transduction. Previous work has indeed demonstrated that local opiates in the knee joint (119) and in the skin (3) can reduce the firing of spontaneously active afferents observed when these tissues are inflamed. The mechanisms of the antihyperalgesic effects of opiates applied to the inflamed regions (such as the knee joint) are unexplained. It is possible, for example, that opiates may act on inflammatory cells that are present and releasing cytokines and on products that activate or sensitize the nerve terminal (136).

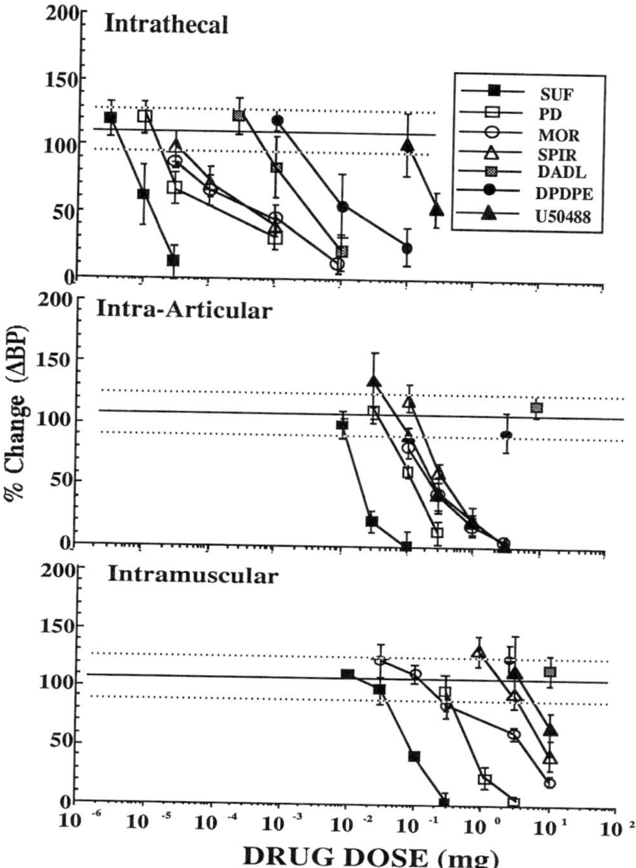

Figure 6. The dose response of the suppressive effects of maximum suppression of the evoked change in blood pressure (expressed as the mean ± SEM of the compression evoked change in blood pressure) after injection intrathecally *(top)*, intraarticularly (IA) *(middle)*, and intramuscularly (IM) *(bottom)* of SUF, PD, MOR, SPIR, DADL, DPDPE and U-50,488H. Each point presents the mean ± SEM of four to eight rats. Because the IA injection alone of the vehicle produced an augmentation response, all IM drug injections were given concurrently with an IA injection of saline. The *horizontal lines* indicate the mean *(solid)* ± SEM *(dotted lines)* for rats receiving IA saline and no other drug at time zero.

Interactions Between Opiate Modulatory Systems

As outlined above, opioids with an action limited to several sites, notably the spinal cord and brain stem, produce a powerful alteration in nociceptive processing. After systemic delivery, the net result reflects the contribution of the interactive component resulting from the concurrent action of the sites. Ample evidence indicates that the effects of concurrent opiate receptor occupancy result in a powerful functional facilitation. Several specific instances are outlined.

Brain stem–Spinal Cord

It was observed early on that (a) both spinal and supraspinal sites can support a maximum analgesic effect and (b) delivery of an opioid antagonist into the cerebral ventricles (156,162) or into the lumbar intrathecal space (188) can produce a complete antagonism of the effects of a systemic opioid agonist. This led to the speculation that the interaction between the spinal and supraspinal sites was synergistic (184). This hypothesis was substantiated by the observation that concurrent spinal and supraspinal administration of morphine (intracerebroventricularly) would lead to a prominent synergy, as indicated by hyperbolic isobolograms (197). Similar results have been observed in mice (118) (see ref. 149 for discussion of analysis of synergic interactions).

Supraspinal–Supraspinal

As noted above, in the brain multiple sites exist that possess opioid receptors through which an agonist can exert an antinociceptive effect. Co-microinjection of opiates into the periaqueductal gray and locus coeruleus (19) resulted in a synergic interaction, while co-injection into the periaqueductal gray and nucleus reticularis gigantocellularis (166) displayed only an additive relationship.

Spinal Cord–Spinal Cord

Several opiate system interactions are believed to exist within the spinal cord. First, as discussed in the section on spinal opiates, there is strong reason to conclude that the potent antinociceptive effects observed with spinally delivered opiate agonists reflects upon a concurrent interaction preterminally on the primary afferent and postterminally on second-order neurons. That concurrent effect results in a reduction in the magnitude of the stimulus provided by the afferent input through a reduction in the release of afferent transmitters and concurrently serving to reduce the excitability of the second-order neuron by its hyperpolarization. Hypothetically, it is this concurrent action that leads to a significant therapeutic ratio. Thus, in lieu of the effect on input, the concentrations required to block activation of dorsal horn projection neurons might be equivalent to those that would also influence motor neuron excitability.

Consistent with the powerful nonlinear interaction between spinal and supraspinal opiates, and given the considered role of bulbospinal systems in mediating some of the supraspinal actions of opiates, it has been shown that the concurrent spinal delivery of α_2 and μ, as well as α_2 and δ opioid agonists, yields a potent synergistic interaction. Importantly, nonlinear interactions have been also been reported between μ and δ agonists (180,181).

SIMILARITY OF OPIATE MECHANISMS IN HUMAN AND ANIMAL MODELS

Site of Action

Supraspinal

In humans it is not feasible to routinely assess the site of action within the brain where opiates may act to alter nociceptive transmission. However, intracerebroventricular opioids have been employed in humans for pain relief in cancer patients (75,76,79,81). An important characteristic of this action is that the time of onset is relatively rapid for even the water-soluble agent morphine. Gamma scans of human brain after injection of I-123–morphine have shown that the agent, even one hour after injection, remains close to the ventricular lumen (145). This distribution is consistent with the slow permeation of the water-soluble agent from the ventricular lumen (59). Given the rate of diffusion for such a drug and the size of the human brain, it seems reasonable to hypothesize that the site of opiate action in the human must lie close to the ventricular lumen. In this regard, the preclinical studies in species such as the primate have emphasized the importance of the periaqueductal sites. Such a site of action would in fact lie in close proximity to the ventricles and permit a relatively rapid access of a slowly moving drug from the ventricular lumen. While an extensive activity relationship has not been achieved with human intracerebroventricular delivery, morphine and β-endorphin have been delivered and β-endorphin appears to show a greater activity (45), a finding consistent with its greater molar potency in vitro (171).

Spinal

There is extensive literature indicating that opiates delivered spinally can induce a powerful analgesia in humans. The pharmacology of this action has been widely studied and it appears certain that μ, δ, and, to a lesser degree, κ agonists are effective after intrathecal or epidural delivery (172). The effects of spinal opiates are reversed by low doses of systemic naloxone (23,102,114). Importantly, for spinally delivered agents modulating acute nociception in animal models such as the rodent, the hot plate test reveals an ordering of activity that closely resembles that observed in humans for controlling clinical pain states. This similarity is indicated by the close regression observed when the approximate relative ordering of activity observed in rats and after spinal delivery in humans is plotted (Fig. 7).

Peripheral Actions

The findings regarding opiates injected in the periphery in preclinical models led to clinical work showing that injection of morphine into the knee joint of humans after knee surgery (58,70,134) had a potent antihyperalgesic effect. The appropriate controls emphasize that the effects are indeed mediated by a local action and not by a CNS redistribution. These results are in close accord with the observation reported in the animal models of hyperalgesia induced by peripheral inflammation. There are to date no pharmacologic profiles assessed. However, the efficacy noted in the rat models of κ agonists provides support for this as an important future consideration.

Human Clinical Pain States and Opiate Activity

Stimulus Modality

The mechanisms of opiate action have been widely studied. Accordingly, the ability of such agents to alter a particular human pain state is in a sense a diagnosis of some of the mechanisms that may underlie the human clinical pain condition. As reviewed in Table 4, opiates have been shown to have efficacy in a variety of preclinical models, notably those that employ high-intensity, potentially tissue-damaging stimuli that work through the activation of small afferents (see Chap. 40). This action corresponds to the anticipated mechanisms underlying the human postinjury (operative/trauma) pain state and likely reflects upon the importance of this afferent substrate in those circumstances (see Chaps. 41,43).

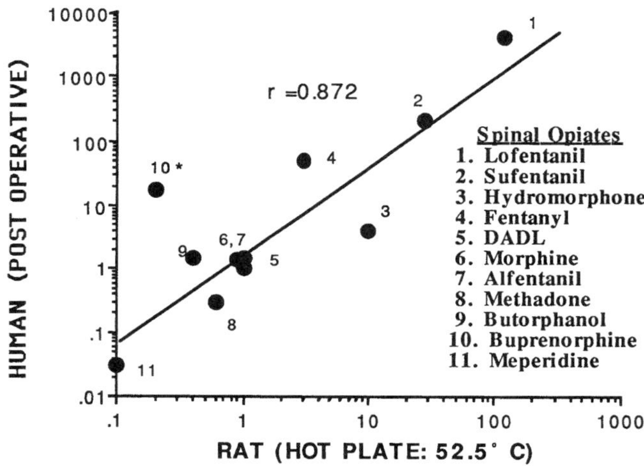

Figure 7. The relative ordering of activity for clinically effective doses of spinal opiates in the postoperative pain state expressed relative to the activity of morphine (e.g., morphine = 1) in humans is plotted versus the ordering of activity relative to morphine after spinal delivery in the rat model on the 52°C hot plate test. * Indicates that buprenorphine on the hot plate is a partial agonist. (Data from ref. 172.)

In contrast to their well-defined efficacy in states associated with small afferent activation, in preclinical models spinal opiates have only modest effects in several models associated with allodynia, either induced by intrathecal strychnine or after nerve injury (Chung model) (Table 4). The mechanism underlying this lack of spinal efficacy has been speculated to be the result of the lack of a role of small afferents in that syndrome (see Chap. 40). Two points should be emphasized with regard to opiates and neuropathic syndromes. First, while some preclinical models of neuropathic pain are indeed refractory (as in the intrathecal strychnine model and the Chung model), the Bennett model of thermal hyperalgesia is readily reversed by spinal opiates. Thus, there are preclinical neuropathic states that are in fact readily affected by opiates. Second, even models that are refractory to spinal opiates appear to be influenced by supraspinal actions (78). The reason for this supraspinal action is not certain, but may represent either the activation of a descending pathway that influences the processing or a supraspinal effect upon the "affective" component of the pain state. The important point is that based on the preclinical models, we would anticipate that at least some components of human neuropathic pain may indeed be relatively refractory while others are relatively sensitive. Epidural morphine has been indicated as being relatively ineffective in treating populations of post–nerve injury pain patients (6). But this observation is controversial. At present, there appear to be no a priori reasons to conclude that all post–nerve injury pain patients will be constituted by a homogeneous mix of mechanisms. Systematic examination of post–nerve injury pain states often reveals composite static and dynamic symptoms involving various component modalities, e.g., extreme sensitivity to touch, pressure, heat, and cold (100,195,196). There are surprisingly few data at present defining the relative opioid sensitivity to these characteristics (see Chap. 41). It seems certain, however, that in populations of neuropathic patients, there are distinct differences in opioid sensitivity (44,111). Accordingly, it is important to know that neuropathic pain conditions likely possess multiple underlying mechanisms, some that are modulated by opioid receptors and some that are not. Thus, for example, the allodynic components were induced by spontaneous activity in a population of C fibers, leading to a state of central facilitation (see Chap. 36), and that allodynic state might be efficaciously regulated by opiate agonists.

Two examples of the complexity associated with the prediction of opiate efficacy in clinical pain states involving nerve injury is seen in the syndromes of postherpetic neuralgia and cancer. In postherpetic neuralgia, the tactile component of the disorder, pain evoked by repeatedly pricking the affected skin area, may be aggravated by systemic morphine (37,105). Cancer pain states may be typically constituted of a number of components: tumor mass, release of active factors that sensitize and stimulate small afferents, compression of the nerve, and iatrogenic events, such as severing of the nerve, radiation, or chemotherapy, that lead to nerve damage (see Chap. 48). Systematic studies on the utilization of opiates in cancer have typically yielded positive results, with a fraction of the population displaying components of their pain state that were relatively refractory to opioid action (5,30,46,55,56). It is important to stress that in practice the definition of opiate sensitivity must be considered to be a relative concept with the continuum being defined by the intensity of the stimulus (i.e., intense stimuli being more insensitive to opiates than high-intensity stimuli) and substrate (spinal outflow driven by a C-fiber input being more sensitive to opiates than an output driven by a low-threshold input).

Pharmacodynamics of Human Opiate Action

The action of opiate agonists is defined by the receptor on which the agonist acts, the affinity of the agent for the receptor, and the efficacy of the agent once it occupies that receptor. The previous discussions have emphasized the role played by the opiate receptor in regulating afferent processing. An important component of evaluating drug action is the efficacy of the analgesic agent. As the concentration of the drug at the receptor is elevated, the number of occupied receptors increases. The efficacy of the agonist is defined in terms of the magnitude of drug effect produced by a given level of occupancy. An agent that produces a full effect by occupying a small fraction of the available receptors is said to have greater efficacy than one that produces a lesser effect for the same fraction of receptor occupancy. Agents that have affinity but no efficacy are antagonists. The methods for determining efficacy, typically by the use of irreversible antagonists, are reviewed in Chap. 40. Examples of opiate agonists, ranked in order of their efficacy, are sufentanil > morphine > buprenorphine > naloxone (which has no efficacy). It is important to note that efficacy is not predicted by potency. Buprenorphine doses are typically in the range of μg/kg, whereas morphine doses may be in the mg/kg range (see Chap. 40, Appendix 1). Preclinical pharmacology has shown that for a μ opioid agonist, efficacy may impact in two areas: (a) the magnitude of dose increases in the face of stimulus increases, and (b) the degree of cross-tolerance. The possible relevance of these preclinical characteristics to human models will be briefly considered. For further discussion of the analyses, see Chap. 40.

Dose-Response Shifts with Increased Stimulus Intensity

Increasing the intensity of the stimulus leads to a right shift in the dose-response curve, reflecting the increased occupancy requirement necessary to produce a criterion level of response suppression (e.g., adequate analgesia). Preclinical work has shown that for a given stimulus increase, the degree of right shift is less for an agent with low-receptor occupancy requirements (e.g., a high-efficacy agonist, such as sufentanil) than for an agent with high-occupancy requirements (e.g., a lower-efficacy agonist such as morphine). It is suggested that this phenomenon has its parallels in humans. For analgesia, the necessary doses of sufentanil and morphine are typically in the range of 1 μg/kg and 50 μg/kg, respectively (7,89,90,104,121). In contrast, for the extreme conditions associated with the intraoperative environment, sufentanil doses in the range of 20 μg/kg are reported; for morphine, doses as high as 3 to 6 mg/kg have been reported to be necessary to produce similar control over the autonomic response (4,22,84,126). Calculation of these ratios suggests that from mild or moderate to severe pain, the dose of sufentanil is increased by a factor of 20, while for morphine the increase is 60 to 180. Such results, while less precise than those obtained in the preclinical model, indicate parallel pharmacodynamic properties of the human clinical pain state and those predicted from the preclinical behavior of these opiate agonists.

Plateau Effect in Analgesic Action

It is appreciated that certain classes of agents are highly efficacious in managing mild pain states (e.g., codeine and buprenorphine). Nevertheless, with stronger stimuli such agents may be insufficient. This loss of clinical efficacy may indicate that such agents, often classified as partial agonists, have an affinity for the receptor, but a limited receptor efficacy. Accordingly, in the World Health Organization (165) guidelines (the WHO ladder), it is recognized that these agents may be highly appropriate for managing the mild to moderate components of the pain. On the other hand, as the pain intensity rises, these agents, even at very high doses, may be ineffective. Moreover, as these agents may have efficacy at the receptor, they will compete with other agents that also interact with that site, such as morphine. In this regard, it is emphasized that as the pain state rises, it is appropriate to move to a higher efficacy agonist and remove the one with the lower efficacy.

Analgesic Tolerance

Preclinical studies have uniformly emphasized that continued systemic, intracerebral, or spinal exposure to an opiate agonist over a period of days yields a progressive reduction in the effect produced by a fixed dose of that agent and increases the dose required to produce a given analgesic effect (e.g., shift the dose effect curve to the right) (175). Systematic studies have indicated that the dose effect curve is similar to a curve for irreversible antagonists, e.g., the right shift is accompanied by a decreasing maximum (119,120,138,140). Given the stability of the model, the invariant nature of the pain stimulus, and the stability of drug dosing, this incrementation in dose is believed to reflect a "pharmacologic tolerance." The mechanism of this phenomenon is not appreciated, although it has been long studied. Pharmacologic tolerance does not appear to correlate to the significant change in the number of receptors, although there may be a reduction in the efficiency of the G protein coupling for agents acting through receptors that are so coupled (as are the μ/κ/δ sites) (99,107). The tolerance has been shown to have two pharmacologic properties: (a) there appears to be little cross-tolerance between agents that act at separate receptors (e.g., μ versus δ [120,141]; μ versus α_2 [138,185]); and (b) there is an asymmetric cross-tolerance between agents that act at the same receptor, but differ in intrinsic activity (106,133; see Chap. 40).

In human cancer patients, incrementation of dose has been observed to be a widely varying phenomenon that, unlike the animal model, may occur over an extended period of months to years (44,46). In many instances (a) the incrementation in doses may be increased by escalating tumor growth or psychological stress, (b) there may be no change for extended periods, and (c) there may be a reduction in analgesic utilization concurrent with reduction in tumor by interventional therapies (46). These observations do not indicate that humans do not display tolerance. Houde and colleagues (63) demonstrated a right shift in the dose-response curves with exposure in cancer patients. In well-controlled studies, bone marrow transplant patients displayed a rapid incrementation in doses (60,61). In postoperative pain patients, the doses of epidural morphine required to produce postoperative relief was significantly elevated in patients with chronic opiate exposure (34).

Further evidence that pharmacologic tolerance occurs in humans has properties similar to that observed in animals is further suggested by observations suggesting a lack of cross-tolerance between agents that act at distinct receptors, or an asymmetric cross-tolerance between agents that differ in efficacy. Thus, though limited in scope, the δ opioid agonist D-Ala[2]-D-Leu-[5]-enkephalin was observed to have a potent action after spinal delivery in cancer patients who were tolerant to morphine (95). With regard to asymmetric cross-tolerance, it has been shown that in chronic cancer pain patients who were on high doses of systemic morphine and who underwent surgery for tumor resection, postoperative management of pain showed poor responses to elevated doses of epidural morphine. In contrast, sufentanil was observed to be considerably more efficacious (33).

Complexity of Opioid Drug Action

In the preceding sections, the focus has been on the ability of certain structurally related classes of agents to produce a particular alteration in nociceptive processing. The common pharmacology of these agents causes them to be defined as opioid in character. On the other hand, it should be remembered that each agent is a molecule with a variety of effects not necessarily mediated at an opiate site. Thus, the ability of morphine to induce histamine release (10) and the local anesthetic effects of meperidine (69) are not related to an opiate action. Accordingly, we should not be surprised that specific molecules may possess additional properties. One such interesting area has been the observation that methadone and ketobemedine may be noncompetitive antagonists at the *N*-methyl-D-aspartate (NMDA) receptor (36,72). This property may be of importance given the role played by the NMDA receptor in certain neuropathic pain states (see Chaps. 40 and 60) and in regulating the development of opiate tolerance (153,154). It is important in this regard to note that clinical experience in chronic pain management has often shown that pain states that are not managed by one opiate agonist (such as morphine) may benefit from trials with an alternate agonist (such as methadone) (46). Some of this benefit may arise from different pharmacokinetics and idiosyncratic differences between patients. Alternately, it may reflect upon a particular property of the drug either by its relative efficacy at an opiate receptor or, as in this case, because of a property peculiar to the particular structure of the agent.

The message that must be drawn from these closing observations is that the pain state is complex, and even drugs with which we have great experience may possess novel properties. In view of the system complexities, the guidelines for the administration of such agents in managing pain must always be individual dose titration and the selection of the agent with attention to the magnitude and nature of the clinical pain syndrome.

CONCLUSIONS

This overview of opioid receptor activity raises a number of important issues that have relevance to the understanding of pain and pain processing.

1. The ability of opiates to produce a powerful effect on the organized response of the animal to a strong and potentially tissue damaging stimulus reflects first upon the action mediated by a specific family of receptors.
2. The antinociceptive effects associated with such receptor occupancy reflects the coupling of these receptors to specific neuronal systems that are part of a circuitry that either regulates the excitability of a neuronal pathway (as in the bulbospinal projections that control spinal activity) or serves to directly impede the release of a transmitter link (as in the prevention of the release of a neurotransmitter from the primary afferent or by hyperpolarizing the projection neuron).
3. The complexity of each of these systems alone is amplified by the appreciation that the organized processing is impacted at many levels by even a locally acting agent (as in the PAG or in the spinal cord where a single site reflects multiple effects). Importantly, in many cases it appears certain that the concurrent involvement of the separate components yields a physiologic or biochemical consequence that is greater than additive (e.g., synergistic). The synergy permits significant effects on function at levels of receptor occupancy at which other systems (e.g., respiratory or autonomic) are not sufficiently affected to produce a physiologically relevant action. These mechanisms and their synergistic interactions likely affect the way opiates exert a relatively potent, yet selective, effect on nociceptive processing.
4. Our appreciation of the actions of the opiate systems provides important insights into the mechanisms by which antinociceptive information is processed. Thus, the characteristics of the antinociception are defined by the systems with which the opiates interact. For neuropathic pain, it might be speculated that in pain states in which the afferent drive is mediated by low-threshold myelinated afferents (as in allodynia), the agent may be relatively less effective than in a pain state mediated by input from small afferents (with which opiate receptors are believed to be associated in the spinal cord).
5. Finally, while the data for the action of these agents in humans are relatively less exhaustive than for the preclinical models, there is a prominent compatibility across species when site of action, pharmacology, and pharmacodynamic properties are considered. Thus, there is little doubt that in humans, as in the animal model, it is possible to demonstrate comparable supraspinal, spinal, and peripheral actions. This similarity in pharmacology and function provides validating support for the conclusion that animal models reveal mechanisms of processing that are present in the human.

REFERENCES

1. Aimone LD, Yaksh TL. Opioid modulation of capsaicin-evoked release of substance P from rat spinal cord in vivo. *Peptides* 1989;10:1127–1131.
2. Amaral DG, Sinnamon HM. The locus ceruleus: neurobiology of a central noradrenergic nucleus. *Prog Neurobiol* 1977;9:147–196.
3. Andreev N, Urban L, Dray A. Opioids suppress spontaneous activity of polymodal nociceptors in rat paw skin induced by ultraviolet irradiation. *Neuroscience* 1994;58:793–798.
4. Arens JF, Benbow BP, Ochsner JL, Theard R. Morphine anesthesia for aortocoronary bypass procedures. *Anesth Analg* 1972;52:901–909.
5. Arner S, Arner B. Differential effects of epidural morphine in the treatment of cancer-related pain. *Acta Anaesth Scand* 1985;29:32–36.
6. Arner S, Meyerson BA. Lack of analgesic effect of opioids on neuropathic and idiopathic forms of pain. *Pain* 1988;33:11–23.
7. Bailey PL, Streisand JB, East KA, East TD, Isern S, Hansen TW, Posthuma EF, Rozendaal FW, Pace NL, Stanley TH. Differences in magnitude and duration of opioid-induced respiratory depression and analgesia with fentanyl and sufentanil. *Anesth Analg* 1990;70:8–15.
8. Bandler R, Carrive P, Zhang SP. Integration of somatic and autonomic reactions within the midbrain periaqueductal grey, viscerotopic, somatotopic and functional organization. *Prog Brain Res* 1991;87:269–305.
9. Bandler R, McCulloch T, McDougall A, Prineas S, Dampney R. Midbrain neural mechanisms mediating emotional behaviour. *Int J Neurol* 1985;19:40–58.
10. Barke KE, Hough LB. Opiates, mast cells and histamine release. *Life Sci* 1993;53(18):1391–1399.
11. Baumeister AA. The effects of bilateral intranigral microinjection of selective opioid agonists on behavioral responses to noxious thermal stimuli. *Brain Res* 1991;557:136–145.
12. Baumeister AA, Hawkins MF, Anticich TG, Moore LL, Higgins TD, Vaughn A, Chatellier MO. Bilateral intranigral microinjection of morphine and opioid peptides produces antinociception in rats. *Brain Res* 1987;411:183–186.
13. Baumeister AA, Nagy M, Hebert G, Hawkins MF, Vaughn A, Chatellier MO. Further studies of the effects of intranigral morphine on behavioral responses to noxious stimuli. *Brain Res* 1990;525:115–125.
14. Behbehani MM, Jiang MR, Chandler SD, Ennis M. The effect of GABA and its antagonists on midbrain periaqueductal gray neurons in the rat. *Pain* 1990;40(2):195–204.
15. Besse D, Lombard M-C, Zajac J-M, Roques BP, Besson J-M. Pre- and postsynaptic location of mu, delta and kappa opioid receptors in the superficial layers of the dorsal horn of the rat spinal cord. In: *International Narcotics Research Conference (INRC)*. New York: Alan R. Liss, 1990;182.
16. Besse D, Lombard MC, Besson JM. Autoradiographic distribution of mu, delta and kappa opioid binding sites in the superficial dorsal horn, over the rostrocaudal axis of the rat spinal cord. *Brain Res* 1991;548(1-2):287–291.
17. Besse D, Lombard MC, Zajac JM, Roques BP, Besson JM. Pre- and postsynaptic distribution of mu, delta and kappa opioid receptors in the superficial layers of the cervical dorsal horn of the rat spinal cord. *Brain Res* 1990;521(1-2):15–22.
18. Bodnar RJ, Williams CL, Lee SJ, Pasternak GW. Role of mu 1-opiate receptors in supraspinal opiate analgesia: a microinjection study. *Brain Res* 1988;447:25–34.
19. Bodnar R, Paul D, Pasternak GW. Synergistic analgesic interac-

tions between the periaqueductal gray and the locus coeruleus. *Brain Res* 1991;558:224–230.

20. Bouchenafa O, Livingston A. Distribution of immunoreactive met-enkephalin and autoradiographic [3H]DAGO and [^{3}H]DPDPE in the spinal cord of sheep. *Advances in the Biosciences*, 1989,75:289.
21. Bourgoin S, Benoliel JJ, Collin E, Mauborgne A, Pohl M, Hamon M, Cesselin F. Opioidergic control of the spinal release of neuropeptides. Possible significance for the analgesic effects of opioids. *Fundam Clin Pharmacol* 1994;8(4):307–321.
22. Bovill JG, Warren PJ, Schuller JL, vanWezel HB, Hoeneveld MH. Comparison of fentanyl, sufentanil, and alfentanil anesthesia in patients undergoing valvular heart surgery. *Anesth Analg* 1984;63: 1081–1086.
23. Bromage PR, Camporesi E, Leslie J. Epidural narcotics in volunteers: sensitivity to pain and to carbon dioxide. *Pain* 1980;9: 145–160.
24. Cahill CM, White TD, Sawynok J. Spinal opioid receptors and adenosine release: neurochemical and behavioral characterization of opioid subtypes. *J Pharmacol Exp Ther* 1995;275(1):84–93.
25. Calvillo O, Henry JL, Neuman RS. Effects of morphine and naloxone on dorsal horn neurones in the cat. *Can J Physiol Pharmacol* 1974;52:1207–1211.
26. Camarata PJ, Yaksh TL. Characterization of the spinal adrenergic receptors mediating the spinal effects produced by the microinjection of morphine into the periaqueductal gray. *Brain Res* 1985; 336:133–142.
27. Carter BD, Medzihradsky F. Go mediates the coupling of the mu opioid receptor to adenylyl cyclase in cloned neural cells and brain. *Proc Natl Acad Sci USA* 1993;90(9):4062–4066.
28. Chen Y, Mestek A, Liu J, Hurley JA, Yu L. Molecular cloning and functional expression of a mu-opioid receptor from rat brain. *Mol Pharmacol* 1993;44:8–12.
29. Chen Y, Mestek A, Liu J, Yu L. Molecular cloning of a rat kappa opioid receptor reveals sequence similarities to the mu and delta opioid receptors. *Biochemic J* 1993;295:625–628.
30. Cherny NI, Thaler HT, Friedlander-Klar H, Lapin J, Foley KM, Houde R, Portenoy RK. Opioid responsiveness of cancer pain syndromes caused by neuropathic or nociceptive mechanisms: a combined analysis of controlled, single-dose studies. *Neurology* 1994; 44(5):857–861.
31. Criswell HD. Analgesia and hyperreactivity following morphine microinjections into mouse brain. *Pharmacol Biochem Behav* 1976; 4:23–26.
32. Danzebrink RM, Gebhart GF. Evidence that spinal 5-HT$_1$, 5-HT$_2$ and 5-HT$_3$ receptor subtypes modulate responses to noxious colorectal distention in the rat. *Brain Res* 1991;538:64–75.
33. de Leon-Casasola OA, Lema MJ. Epidural bupivacaine/sufentanil therapy for postoperative pain control in patients tolerant to opioid and unresponsive to epidural bupivacaine/morphine. *Anesthesiology* 1994;80(2):303–309.
34. de Leon-Casasola OA, Myers DP, Donaparthi S, Bacon DR, Peppriell J, Rempel J, Lema MJ. A comparison of postoperative epidural analgesia between patients with chronic cancer taking high doses of oral opioids versus opioid-naive patients. *Anesth Analg* 1993;76(2):302–307.
35. Drower EJ, Stapelfeld A, Rafferty MF, de Costa BR, Rice KC, Hammond DL. Selective antagonism by naltrindole of the antinociceptive effects of the delta opioid agonist cyclic[D-penicillamine2-D-penicillamine5] enkephalin in the rat. *J Pharmacol Exp Ther* 1991;259:725–731.
36. Ebert B, Andersen S, Krogsgaard-Larsen P. Ketobemidone, methadone and pethidine are non-competitive N-methyl-D-aspartate (NMDA) antagonists in the rat cortex and spinal cord. *Neurosci Lett* 1995;187(3):165–168.
37. Eide PK, Jorum E, Stubhaug A, Bremnes J, Breivik H. Relief of post-herpetic neuralgia with the N-methyl-D-aspartic acid receptor antagonist ketamine: a double-blind, cross-over comparison with morphine and placebo. *Pain* 1994;58(3):347–354.
38. Fedynyshyn JP, Kwiat G, Lee N. Characterization of high affinity opioid binding sites in rat periaqueductal gray P2 membrane. *Eur J Pharmacol* 1989;159:83–88.
39. Fedynyshyn JP, Lee NM. Mu type opioid receptors in rat periaqueductal gray-enriched P2 membrane are coupled to G-protein-mediated inhibition of adenylyl cyclase. *FEBS Lett* 1989;253:23–27.
40. Fields HL, Heinricher MM, Mason P. Neurotransmitters in nociceptive modulatory circuits. *Annu Rev Neurosci* 1991;14:219–245.
41. Fields HL, Emson PC, Leigh BK, Gilbert RFT, Iverses LL. Multiple opiate receptor sites on primary afferent fibres. *Nature (Lond)* 1980;284:351–353.
42. Fleetwood-Walker SM, Hope PJ, Mitchell R, El-Yassir N, Molony V. The influence of opioid receptor subtypes on the processing of nociceptive inputs in the spinal dorsal horn of the cat. *Brain Res* 1988;451:213–226.
43. Fleetwood-Walker S M, Mitchell R, Hope P J, El-Yassir N, Molony V, Bladon CM. The involvement of neurokinin receptor subtypes in somatosensory processing in the superficial dorsal horn of the cat. *Brain Res* 1990;519:169–182.
44. Foley KM. Misconceptions and controversies regarding the use of opioids in cancer pain. *Anti-Cancer Drugs* 1995;suppl 3:4–13.
45. Foley KM, Kourides IA, Inturrisi CE, Kaiko RF, Zaroulis CG, Posner JB, Houde RW, Li CH. Beta-endorphin: analgesic and hormonal effects in humans. *Proc Natl Acad Sci USA* 1979;76: 5377–5381.
46. Foley KM. The role of opioid analgesics in neuropathic pain. In: Besson JM, Guilbaud G, ed. *Lesions of the primary afferent fibers as a tool for the study of clinical pain.* Amsterdam: Elsevier Science, 1991;277–292.
47. Gebhart GF, Jones SL. Effects of morphine given in the brain stem on the activity of dorsal horn nociceptive neurons. *Prog Brain Res* 1988;77:229–243.
48. Gebhart GF, Sandkuhler J, Thalhammer J, Zimmerman M. Inhibition in spinal cord of nociceptive information by electrical stimulation and morphine microinjections at identical sites in midbrain of the cat. *J Neurophysiol* 1984;51:75–89.
49. Gissen AJ, Gugino LD, Datta S, Miller J, Covino BG. Effects of fentanyl and sufentanil on peripheral mammalian nerves. *Anesth Analg* 1987;66:1272–1276.
50. Go VL, Yaksh TL. Release of substance P from the cat spinal cord. *J Physiol* 1987;391:141–167.
51. Gouardères C, Cros J, Quirion R. Autoradiographic localization of μ, δ and κ opioid receptor binding sites in rat and guinea pig spinal cord. *Neuropeptides* 1985;5:331–342.
52. Grudt TJ, Williams JT. Kappa-opioid receptors also increase potassium conductance. *Proc Natl Acad Sci USA* 1993;90(23): 11429–11432.
53. Haiger HJ, Spring DD. A comparison of the analgesic and behavioral effects of [D-Ala^2] met-enkephalinamide and morphine in the mesencephalic reticular formation of rats. *Life Sci* 1978;23: 1229–1240.
54. Hammond DL, Stewart PE, Littell L. Antinociception and delta-1 opioid receptors in the rat spinal cord: studies with intrathecal 7-benzylidenenaltrexone. *J Pharmacol Exp Ther* 1995;274(3):1317–1324.
55. Hanks GW. Pain management in cancer patients. *Therapie* 1992; 47(6):489–493.
56. Hanks GW, Justins DM. Cancer pain: management. *Lancet* 1992; 339(8800):1031–1036.
57. Harada Y, Nishioka K, Kitahata LM, Nakatani K, Collins JG. Contrasting actions of intrathecal U50,488H, morphine, or [D-Pen2, D-Pen5] enkephalin or intravenous U50,488H on the visceromotor response to colorectal distension in the rat. *Anesthesiology* 1995; 83(2):336–343.
58. Haynes TK, Appadurai IR, Power I, Rosen M, Grant A. Intra-articular morphine and bupivacaine analgesia after arthroscopic knee surgery. *Anaesthesia* 1994;49:54–56.
59. Herz, A and Tescehmacher, H. Activities and sites of antinociceptive action of morphine-like analgesics and kinetics of redistribution following intravenous, intracerebral and intraventricular application. *Adv Drug Res* 1971;6:79–119.
60. Hill HF, Coda BA, Mackie AM, Iverson K. Patient-controlled analgesic infusions: alfentanil versus morphine. *Pain* 1992;49(3): 301–310.
61. Hill HF, Mackie AM, Coda BA, Iverson K, Chapman CR. Patient-controlled analgesic administration. A comparison of steady-state morphine infusions with bolus doses. *Cancer* 1991;67(4):873–882.
62. Hirota N, Kuraishi Y, Hino Y, Sato Y, Satoh M, Takagi H. Met-enkephalin and morphine but not dynorphin inhibit the noxious stimuli-induced release of substance P from rabbit dorsal horn in situ. *Neuropharmacology* 1985;24:567–570.
63. Houde RW, Wallenstein SL, Beaver WT. Evaluation of analgesics in patients with cancer pain. In: Lasagna L, ed. *Clinical pharmacology international encyclopedia of pharmacology and therapeutics,* vol 1. Oxford: Pergamon Press, 1966;59–97.
64. Hylden JLK, Wilcox GL. Pharmacological, characterization of sub-

stance P induced nociception in mice: modulation by opioid and noradrenergic agonists at the spinal level. *J Pharmacol Exp Ther* 1983;226:398–404.

65. Jensen TS, Yaksh TL. Comparison of the antinociceptive action of mu and delta opioid receptor ligands in the periaqueductal gray matter, medial and paramedial ventral medulla in the rat as studied by the microinjection technique. *Brain Res* 1986;372:301–312.
66. Jiang Q, Takemori AE, Sultana M, Portoghese PS, Bowen WD, Mosberg HI, Porreca F. Differential antagonism of opioid delta antinociception by [D-ala2,Leu5,Cys6]-enkephalin and naltrindole 5′-isothiocyanate: evidence for delta receptor subtypes. *J Pharmacol Exp Ther* 1991;257:1069–1075.
67. Kaneko S, Fukuda K, Yada N, Akaike A, Mori Y, Satoh M. Ca2+ channel inhibition by kappa opioid receptors expressed in *Xenopus* oocytes. *Neuroreport* 1994;5(18):2506–2508.
68. Kasman GS, Rosenfeld JP. Opiate microinjections into midbrain do not affect the aversiveness of caudal trigeminal stimulation but produce somatotopically organized peripheral hypoalgesia. *Brain Res* 1986;383:271–278.
69. Kaya K, Babacan A, Beyazova M, Bolukbasi N, Akcabay M, Karadenizli Y. Effects of perineural opioids on nerve conduction of N. suralis in man. *Acta Neurol Scand* 1992;85(5):337–339.
70. Khoury GF, Chen ACN, Garland DE, Stein C. Intra-articular morphine, bupivacaine, and morphine/bupivacaine for pain control after Knee videoarthroscopy. *Anesthesiology* 1992;77:263–266.
71. Kieffer BL, Befort K, Gaveriaux-Ruff C, Hirth CG. The delta-opioid receptor: isolation of a cDNA by expression cloning and pharmacological characterization. *Proc Natl Acad Sci USA* 1992;89: 12048–12052.
72. Krug M, Matthies R, Wagner M, Brodemann R. Non-opioid antitussives and methadone differentially influence hippocampal long-term potentiation in freely moving rats. *Eur J Pharmacol* 1993; 231(3):355–361.
73. Kuraishi Y, Hirota N, Satoh M, Takagi H. Antinociceptive effects of intrathecal opioids, noradrenaline and serotonin in rats: mechanical and thermal algesic tests. *Brain Res* 1985;326:168–171.
74. Laduron PM. Axonal transport of opiate receptors in capsaicin-sensitive neurones. *Brain Res* 1984;294:157–160.
75. Lazorthes Y. Intracerebroventricular administration of morphine for control of irreducible cancer pain. *Ann NY Acad Sci* 1988;531: 123–132.
76. Lazorthes Y, Verdie JC, Caute B, Maranhao R, Tafani M. Intracerebroventricular morphinotherapy for control of chronic cancer pain. *Prog Brain Res* 1988;77:395–405.
77. Le Bars D, Menétrey D, Conseiller C, Besson JM. Depressive effects of morphine upon lamina V cells activities in the dorsal horn of the spinal cat. *Brain Res* 1975;98:261–277.
78. Lee YW, Chaplan SR, Yaksh TL. Systemic and supraspinal, but not spinal, opiates suppress allodynia in a rat neuropathic pain model. *Neurosci Lett* 1995;199(2):111–114.
79. Lenzi A, Galli G, Gandolfini M, Marini G. Intraventricular morphine in paraneoplastic painful syndrome of the cervicofacial region: experience in thirty-eight cases. *Neurosurgery* 1985;17:6–11.
80. Li S, Zhu J, Chen C, Chen YW, Deriel JK, Ashby B, Liu-Chen LY. Molecular cloning and expression of a rat kappa opioid receptor. *Biochem J* 1993;295(pt 3):629–633.
81. Lobato RD, Madrid JL, Fatela LV, Sarabia R, Rivas JJ, Gozalo A. Intraventricular morphine for intractable cancer pain: rationale, methods, clinical results. *Acta Anaesthesiol Scand Suppl* 1987;85: 68–74.
82. Lombard MC, Besson JM. Attempts to gauge the relative importance of pre- and postsynaptic effects of morphine upon the transmission of noxious messages in dorsal horn of the rat spinal cord. *Pain* 1989;37:335–345.
83. Lord JA, Waterfield AA, Hughes J, Kosterlitz HW. Endogenous opioid peptides: multiple agonists and receptors. *Nature* 1977;267: 495–499.
84. Lowenstein E, Hallowell P, Levine FH, Daggett WM, Austen WG, Laver MB. Cardiovascular response to large doses of intravenous morphine in man. *N Engl J Med* 1969;281:1389–1393.
85. Ma QP, Han JS. Neurochemical and morphological evidence of an antinociceptive neural pathway from nucleus raphe dorsalis to nucleus accumbens in the rabbit. *Brain Res Bull* 1992;28:931–936.
86. Ma QP, Yin GF, Ai MK, Han JS. Serotonergic projections from the nucleus raphe dorsalis to the amygdala in the rat. *Neurosci Lett* 1991;134:21–24.
87. Malmberg AB, Yaksh TL. Isobolographic and dose response analyses of the interaction between intrathecal mu and delta agonists: Effects of naltrindole and its benzofuran analog NTB. *J Pharmacol Exp Ther* 1992;263:264–275.
88. Manning BH, Morgan MJ, Franklin KB. Morphine analgesia in the formalin test: evidence for forebrain and midbrain sites of action. *Neuroscience* 1994;63:289–294.
89. Marshall BE, Wollman H. General anesthetics. In: Gilman AG, Goodman LS, Rall TW, Murad F, eds. *Goodman and Gilman's the pharmacological basis of therapeutics.* New York: Macmillan, 1985; 276–301.
90. Marshall H, Popreus C, McMillan I, McPherson SG, Nimmo WS. Relief of pain by infusion of morphine after operation. Does tolerance develop? *Br Med J* 1985;291:19–21.
91. Martin WR, Eades CG, Thompson WO, Thompson JA, Flanary HG. Morphine physical dependence in the dog. *J Pharmacol Exp Ther* 1974;189:759–771.
92. Meng F, Xie GX, Thompson RC, Mansour A, Goldstein A, Watson SJ, Akil H. Cloning and pharmacological characterization of a rat kappa opioid receptor. *Proc Natl Acad Sci USA* 1993;90:9954–9958.
93. Mohrland S, Gebhart G. Effects of focal electrical stimulation and morphine microinjection in the periaqueductal gray of the rat mesencephalon on neuronal activity in the medullary reticular formation. *Brain Res* 1980;201:23–37.
94. Morris BJ, Herz A. Distinct distribution of opioid receptor types in rat lumbar spinal cord. *Naunyn Schmiedebergs Arch Pharmacol* 1987; 336:240–243.
95. Moulin DE, Max MB, Kaiko RF, Inturrisi CE, Maggard J, Yaksh TL, Foley KM. The analgesic efficacy of intrathecal D-Ala^2-D-Leu^5-enkephalin in cancer patients with chronic pain. *Pain* 1985;23: 213–221.
96. Nagasaka H, Yaksh TL. Effects of intrathecal μ, δ, and κ agonists on thermally evoked cardiovascular and nociceptive reflexes in halothane-anesthetized rats. *Anesth Analg* 1995;80:437–443.
97. Nagasaka H, Awad H, Yaksh TL. Peripheral and spinal actions of opioids in the blockade of the autonomic response evoked by compression of the inflamed knee joint. *Anesthesiology* 1996,85:808,816.
98. Ness TJ, Gebhart GF. Differential effects of morphine and clonidine on visceral and cutaneous spinal nociceptive transmission in the rat. *J Neurophysiol* 1989;62:220–230.
99. Nestler EJ. Cellular responses to chronic treatment with drugs of abuse. *Crit Rev Neurobiol* 1993;7(1):23–39.
100. Ochoa JL, Yarnitsky D. Mechanical hyperalgesias in neuropathic pain patients: dynamic and static subtypes. *Ann Neurol* 1993;33(5): 465–472.
101. Oliveras J-L, Maixner W, Dubner R, Bushnell MC, Duncan G, Thomas DA, Bates R. Dorsal horn opiate administration attenuates the perceived intensity of noxious heat stimulation in behaving monkey. *Brain Res* 1986;371:368–371.
102. Onofrio BM, Yaksh TL. Intrathecal delta-receptor ligand produces analgesia in man [letter]. *Lancet* 1983;1(8338):1386–1387.
103. Ossipov MH, Goldstein FJ, Malseed RT. Feline analgesia following central administration of opioids. *Neuropharmacology* 1984;23: 925–929.
104. Owens H, Reekie RM, Clements JA, Watson R, Nimmo WS. Analgesia from morphine and ketamine. A comparison of infusions of morphine and ketamine for post operative analgesia. *Anaesthesia* 1987;42:1051–1056.
105. Pappagallo M, Campbell JN. Chronic opioid therapy as alternative treatment for post-herpetic neuralgia. *Ann Neurol* 1994;35(suppl): S54–56.
106. Paronis CA, Holtzman SG. Development of tolerance to the analgesic activity of mu agonists after continuous infusion of morphine, meperidine or fentanyl in rats. *J Pharmacol Exp Ther* 1992; 262(1):1–9.
107. Pasternak GW. Pharmacological mechanisms of opioid. *Clin Neuropharmacol* 1993;16:1–18.
108. Pert A, Yaksh TL. Sites of morphine induced analgesia in the primate brain: relation to pain pathways. *Brain Res* 1974;80: 135–140.
109. Pert A, Yaksh TL. Localization of the antinociceptive action of morphine in primate brain. *Pharmacol Biochem Behav* 1975;3: 133–138.
110. Piros ET, Prather PL, Loh HH, Law PY, Evans CJ, Hales TG. Ca2+ channel and adenylyl cyclase modulation by cloned mu-opioid receptors in GH3 cells. *Mol Pharmacol* 1995;47(5):1041–1049.
111. Portenoy RK, Foley KM, Inturrisi CE. The nature of opioid responsiveness and its implications for neuropathic pain: new hypotheses derived from studies of opioid infusion. *Pain* 1990;43(3):273–286.

112. Prado WA. Antinociceptive effect of agonists microinjected into the anterior pretectal nucleus of the rat. *Brain Res* 1989;493: 145–154.
113. Ramberg DA, Yaksh TL. Effects of cervical spinal hemisection of dihydromorphine binding in brain stem and spinal cord in cat. *Brain Res* 1989;483:61–67.
114. Rawal N, Mollefors K, Axelsson K, Lingardh G, Widman B. An experimental study of urodynamic effects of epidural morphine and of naloxone reversal. *Anesth Analg* 1983;62:641–647.
115. Reddy SVR, Maderdrut JL, Yaksh TL. Spinal cord pharmacology of adrenergic agonist-mediated antinociception. *J Pharmacol Exp Ther* 1980;213:525–533.
116. Renno WM, Mullett MA, Beitz AJ. Systemic morphine reduces GABA release in the lateral but not the medial portion of the midbrain periaqueductal gray of the rat. *Brain Res* 1992;594(2): 221–232.
117. Roerig SC, Fujimoto JM. Multiplicative interaction between intrathecally and intracerebroventricularly administered mu opioid agonists but limited interactions between delta and kappa agonists for antinociception in mice. *J Pharmacol Exp Ther* 1989;249: 762–768.
118. Rodgers RJ. Elevation of aversive threshold in rats by intraamygdaloid injection of morphine sulfate. *Pharmacol Biochem Behav* 1977;6:385–390.
119. Russell NJW, Schaible H-G, Schmidt RF. Opiates inhibit the discharges of fine afferent units from inflamed knee joint of the cat. *Neurosci Lett* 1987;76:107–112.
120. Russell RD, Leslie JB, Su YF, Watkins WD, Chang KJ. Continuous intrathecal opioid analgesia: tolerance and cross-tolerance of mu and delta spinal opioid receptors. *J Pharmacol Exp Ther* 1987; 240(1):150–158.
121. Rutter PC, Murphy F, Dudley HAF. Morphine controlled trial of different methods of administration for post operative pain relief. *Br Med J* 1980;1:12–13.
122. Sabbe MB, Grafe MR, Mjanger E, Tiseo PJ, Hill HF, Yaksh TL. Spinal delivery of sufentanil, alfentanil and morphine in dogs. Physiologic and toxicologic investigations. *Anesthesiology* 1994;81: 899–920.
123. Samanin R, Gumulka W, Valzelli L. Reduced effect of morphine in midbrain raphe lesioned rats. *Eur J Pharmacol* 1970;10:339.
124. Sanchez-Blazquez P, Garzon J. Evaluation of delta receptor mediation of supraspinal opioid analgesia by in vivo protection against the beta-funaltrexamine antagonist effect. *Eur J Pharmacol* 1989; 159:9–23.
125. Sandouk P, Serrie A, Urtizberea M, Debray M, Got P, Scherrmann JM. Morphine pharmacokinetics and pain assessment after intracerebroventricular administration in patients with terminal cancer. *Clin Pharmacol Ther* 1991;49:442–448.
126. Sanford TJ, Smith NT, Dec-Silver H, Harrison WK. A comparison of morphine, fentanyl, and sufentanil anesthesia for cardiac surgery: induction, emergence, and extubation. *Anesth Analg* 1986;65:259–266.
127. Satoh M, Oku R, Akaike A. Analgesia produced by microinjection of L-glutamate into the rostral ventromedial bulbar nuclei of the rat and its inhibition by intrathecal a-adrenergic blocking agents. *Brain Res* 1983;261:361–364.
128. Schmauss C, Yaksh TL. In vivo studies on spinal opiate receptor systems mediating antinociception. II. Pharmacological profiles suggesting a differential association of mu, delta and kappa receptors with visceral chemical and cutaneous thermal stimuli in the rat. *J Pharmacol Exp Ther* 1984;228:1–12.
129. Sharpe LG, Garnett JE, Cicero TJ. Analgesia and hyperreactivity produced by intracranial microinjections of morphine into the periaqueductal gray matter of the rat. *Behav Biol* 1974;11:303–313.
130. Shen K-F, Crain SM. Dual opioid modulation of the action potential duration of mouse dorsal root ganglion neurons in culture. *Brain Res* 1989;491:227–242.
131. Smith DJ, Perrotti JM, Crisp T, Cabral ME, Long JT, Scalzitti JM. The mu opiate receptor is responsible for descending pain inhibition originating in the periaqueductal gray region of the rat brain. *Eur J Pharmacol* 1988;156:47–54.
132. Sosnowski M, Stevens CW, Yaksh TL. Assessment of the role of A1/A2 adenosine receptors mediating the purine antinociception, motor and autonomic function in the rat spinal cord. J Pharmacol Exp Ther 1989;250:915–922.
133. Sosnowski M, Yaksh TL. Differential cross-tolerance between intrathecal morphine and sufentanil in the rat. *Anesthesiology* 1990; 73:1141–1147.
134. Stein C, Comisel K, Haimerl E, Yassouridis A, Lehrberger K, Herz A, Peter K. Analgesic effect of intra-articular morphine after arthroscopic knee surgery. *N Engl J Med* 1991;325:1123–1126.
135. Stein C, Millan MJ, Shippenberg TS, Peter K, Herz A. Peripheral opioid receptors mediating antinociception in inflammation. Evidence for involvement of mu, delta and kappa receptors. *J Pharmacol Exp Ther* 1989;248:1269–1275.
136. Stein CS. Peripheral mechanism of opioid analgesia. *Anesth Analg* 1993;76:182–191.
137. Stevens CW, Lacey CB, Miller KE, Elde RP, Seybold VS. Biochemical characterization and regional quantification of mu, delta and kappa opioid binding sites in rat spinal cord. *Brain Res* 1991; 550(1):77–85.
138. Stevens CW, Monasky MS, Yaksh TL. Spinal infusion of opiate and alpha-2 agonists in rats: tolerance and cross-tolerance studies. *J Pharmacol Exp Ther* 1988;244:63–70.
139. Stevens CW, Seybold VS. Changes of opioid binding density in the rat spinal cord following unilateral dorsal rhizotomy. *Brain Res* 1995;687(1-2):53–62.
140. Stevens CW, Yaksh TL. Studies of morphine and D-ala^2-D-leu^5-enkephalin (DADLE) cross-tolerance after continuous intrathecal infusion in the rat. *Anesthesiology* 1992;76:596–603.
141. Stevens CW, Yaksh TL. Potency of infused spinal antinociceptive agents is inversely related to magnitude of tolerance after continuous infusion. *J Pharmacol Exp Ther* 1989;250:1–8.
142. Stewart PE, Hammond DL. Evidence for delta opioid receptor subtypes in rat spinal cord: studies with intrathecal naltriben, cyclic[D-Pen2,D-Pen5] enkephalin and [D-Ala2,Glu4]deltorphin. *J Pharmacol Exp Ther* 1993;266(2):820–828.
143. Stewart PE, Hammond DL. Activation of spinal delta-1 or delta-2 opioid receptors reduces carrageenan-induced hyperalgesia in the rat. *J Pharmacol Exp Ther* 1994;268(2):701–708.
144. Stewart PE, Holper EM, Hammond DL. Delta antagonist and kappa agonist activity of Naltriben: evidence for differential kappa interaction with the delta 1 and delta 2 opioid receptor subtypes. *Life Sci* 1994;55(4):PL79–84.
145. Tafani JA, Lazorthes Y, Danet B, Verdie JC, Esquerre JP, Simon J, Guiraud R. Human brain and spinal cord scan after intracerebroventricular administration of iodine-123 morphine. *Int J Radiat Appl Instrument (Part B, Nucl Med Biol)* 1989;16:505–509.
146. Taiwo YO, Coderre TJ, Levine JD. The contribution of training to sensitivity in the nociceptive pain-withdrawal test. *Brain Research*, 1989, 487:148–51.
147. Takagi H, Shiomi H, Kuraishi Y, Fukui K, Ueda H. Pain and the bulbospinal noradrenergic system: Pain-induced increase in normetanephrine content in the spinal cord and its modification by morphine. *Eur J Pharmacol* 1979;54:99–107.
148. Takano Y, Yaksh TL. Characterization of the pharmacology of intrathecally administered alpha-2 agonists and antagonists in rats. *J Pharmacol Exp Ther* 1992;261:764–772.
149. Tallarida RJ, Porreca F, Cowan A. Statistical analysis of drug-drug and site-site interactions with isobolograms. *Life Sci* 1989;45: 947–961.
150. Tang AH, Schoenfeld MJ. Comparison of subcutaneous and spinal subarachnoid injections of morphine and naloxone of analgesic tests in the rat. *Eur J Pharmacol* 1978;52:215–223.
151. Tenen SS. Antagonism of the analgesic effect of morphine and other drugs by p-chlorophenylalanine, a serotonin depletor. *Psychopharmacology* 1968;12:278.
152. Thompson RC, Mansour A, Akil H, Watson SJ. Cloning and pharmacological characterization of a rat mu opioid receptor. *Neuron* 1993;11(5):903–913.
153. Tiseo PJ, Cheng J, Pasternak GW, Inturrisi CE. Modulation of morphine tolerance by the competitive N-methyl-D-aspartate receptor antagonist LY274614: assessment of opioid receptor changes. *J Pharmacol Exp Ther* 1994;268(1):195–201.
154. Trujillo KA, Akil H. Inhibition of opiate tolerance by non-competitive N-methyl-D-aspartate receptor antagonists. *Brain Res* 1994; 633(1-2):178–188.
155. Tseng LF, Wang Q. Forebrain sites differentially sensitive to beta-endorphin and morphine for analgesia and release of Met-enkephalin in the pentobarbital-anesthetized rat. *J Pharmacol Exp Ther* 1992;261:1028–1036.
156. Tsou K. Antagonism of morphine analgesia by the intracerebral microinjection of nalorphine. *Acta Physiol Sinica* 1963;26: 332–337.
157. Tsou K, Jang CS. Studies on the site of analgesic action of morphine by intracerebral microinjection. *Sci Sin* 1964;13:1099–1109.

158. Tung AS, Yaksh TL. *In vivo* evidence for multiple opiate receptors mediating analgesia in the rat spinal cord. *Brain Res* 1982;247:75–83.
159. Tung AS, Yaksh TL. The antinociceptive effects of epidural opiates in the cat: studies on the pharmacology and the effects of lipophilicity in spinal analgesia. *Pain* 1982;12:343–356.
160. Uhl GR, Childers S, Pasternak G. An opiate-receptor gene family reunion. *Trends Neurosci* 1994;17:89–93.
161. Vasko MR, Cartwright S, Ono H. Adenosine agonists do not inhibit the K+ stimulated release of substance P from rat spinal cord slices. *Soc Neurosci Abstr* 1986;12:799.
162. Vigouret J, Tesechemacher H, Albus K, Herz A. Differentiation between spinal and supraspinal sites of action of morphine when inhibiting the hind limb flexor reflex in rabbits. *Neuropharmacology* 1973;12:111–121.
163. Wettstein JG, Kamerling SG, Martin WR. Effects of microinjections of opioids into and electrical stimulation (ES) of the canine periaqueductal gray (PAG) on electrogenesis (EEG), heart rate (HR), pupil diameter PD), behavior and analgesia. *Neurosci Abstr* 1982;8:229
164. Wiesenfeld-Hallin Z. The effects of intrathecal morphine and naltrexone on autotomy in sciatic nerve sectioned rats. *Pain* 1984; 18:267–278.
165. World Health Organization. *Cancer pain relief and palliative caare.* Geneva: World Health Organization, 1990.
166. Xia LY, Huang KH, Rosenfeld JP.Behavioral and trigeminal neuronal effects of rat brain stem-nanoinjected opiates. *Physiol Behav* 1992;52:65–73.
167. Yaksh TL. Analgetic actions of intrathecal opiates in cat and primate. *Brain Res* 1978;153:205–210.
168. Yaksh TL. Inhibition of etorphine of the discharge of dorsal horn neurons: Effects upon the neuronal response to the both high- and low-threshold sensory input in the decerebrate spinal cat. *Exp Neurol* 1978;60:23–40.
169. Yaksh TL. Direct evidence that spinal serotonin and noradrenaline terminals mediate the spinal antinociceptive effects of morphine in the periaqueductal gray. *Brain Res* 1979;160:180–185.
170. Yaksh TL. *In vivo* studies on spinal opiate receptor systems mediating antinociception. I. Mu and delta receptor profiles in the primate. *J Pharmacol Exp Ther* 1983;226:303–316.
171. Yaksh TL. Multiple opioid receptor systems in brain and spinal cord. *Eur J Anaesthesiol* 1984;1:171–243.
172. Yaksh TL. Spinal opiates: a review of their effect on spinal function with emphasis on pain processing. *Acta Anaesthesiol Scand* 1987;31:25–37.
173. Yaksh TL. Substance P release from knee joint afferent terminals: modulation by opioids. *Brain Res* 1988;458:319–324.
174. Yaksh TL. Behavioral and autonomic correlates of the tactile evoked allodynia produced by spinal glycine inhibition: effects of modulatory receptor systems and excitatory amino acid antagonists. *Pain* 1989;37:111–123.
175. Yaksh TL. Tolerance: factors involved in changes in the dose-effect relationship with chronic drug exposure. In: Basbaum AI, Besson L-M, eds. *Towards a new pharmacotherapy of pain.* Dahlem Workshop Reports. John Wiley, New York 1991;157–179.
176. Yaksh TL. The spinal action of opioids. In: Herz A, ed. *Handbook of experimental pharmacology.* Berlin: Springer-Verlag, 1993;53–90.
177. Yaksh TL, Al-Rodhan NRF, Jensen TS. Sites of action of opiates in production of analgesia. Progress in Brain Research 1988, 77:371–394.
178. Yaksh TL, Gross KE, Li CH. Studies on the intrathecal effect of b-endorphin in primate. *Brain Res* 1982;241:261–269.
179. Yaksh TL, Jessell TM, Gamse R, Mudge AW, Leeman SE. Intrathecal morphine inhibits substance P release from mammalian spinal cord *in vivo. Nature* 1980;286:155–156.
180. Yaksh TL, Malmberg AB. Central pharmacology of nociceptive transmission. In: Wall P, Melzack R, eds. *Textbook of pain,* 3rd ed. Edinburgh, UK: Churchill Livingstone, 1994;165–200.
181. Yaksh TL, Malmberg AB. Interaction of spinal modulatory receptor systems. In: Fields HL, Liebeskind JC, eds. *Progress in pain research and management,* vol 1. Seattle: IASP Press, 1994;151–171.
182. Yaksh TL, Noueihed R. The physiology and pharmacology of spinal opiates. *Annu Rev Pharmacol* Toxicol 1985;25:433–462.
183. Yaksh T, Noueihed RY, Durant PAC. Studies of the pharmacology and pathology of intrathecally administered 4-anilinopiperidine analogues and morphine in rat and cat. *Anesthesiology* 1986;64: 54–66.
184. Yaksh TL, Pogrel JW, Lee YW, Chaplan SR. Reversal of nerve ligation-induced allodynia by spinal alpha-2 adrenoceptor agonists. *J Pharmacol Exp Ther* 1995;272:207–214.
185. Yaksh TL, Reddy SVR. Studies in the primate on the analgetic effects associated with intrathecal actions of opiates, a-adrenergic agonists and baclofen. *Anesthesiology* 1981;54:451–467.
186. Yaksh TL, Rudy TA. Analgesia mediated by a direct spinal action of narcotics. *Science* 1976;192:1357–1358.
187. Yaksh TL, Rudy TA. Chronic catheterization of the spinal subarachnoid space. *Physiol Behav* 1976;17:1031–1036.
188. Yaksh TL, Rudy TA. Studies on the direct spinal action of narcotics in the production of analgesia in the rat. *J Pharmacol Exp Ther* 1977;202:411–428.
189. Yaksh TL, Rudy TA. Narcotic analgesics: CNS sites and mechanisms of action as revealed by intracerebral injection techniques. *Pain* 1978;4:299–359.
190. Yaksh TL, Tyce GM. Microinjection of morphine into the periaqueductal gray evokes the release of serotonin from spinal cord. *Brain Res* 1979;171:176–181.
191. Yaksh TL, Wilson PR. Spinal serotonin terminal system mediates antinociception. *J Pharmacol Exp Ther* 1979;208:446–453.
192. Yaksh TL, Yeung JC, Rudy TA. Systematic examination in the rat of brain sites sensitive to the direct application of morphine: Observation of differential effect within the periaqueductal gray. *Brain Res* 1976;114:83–103.
193. Yamamoto T, Yaksh TL. Comparison of the antinociceptive effects of pre- and posttreatment with intrathecal morphine and MK801, an NMDA antagonist, on the formalin test in the rat. *Anesthesiology* 1992;77:757–763.
194. Yamamoto T, Yaksh TL. Spinal pharmacology of thermal hyperesthesia induced by incomplete ligation of sciatic nerve. I. Opioid and nonopioid receptors. *Anesthesiology* 1991;75:817–826.
195. Yarnitsky D, Ochoa JL. Release of cold-induced burning pain by block of cold-specific afferent input. *Brain* 1990;113(pt 4): 893–902.
196. Yarnitsky D, Ochoa JL. Differential effect of compression-ischaemia block on warm sensation and heat-induced pain. *Brain* 1991;114(pt 2):907–913.
197. Yeung JC, Rudy TA. Multiplicative interaction between narcotic agonism expressed at spinal and supraspinal sites of antinociceptive action as revealed by concurrent intrathecal and intracerebroventricular injections of morphine. *J Pharmacol Exp Ther* 1980; 215:633–642.
198. Yoshimura M, North RA. Substantia gelatinosa neurones in vitro hyperpolarised by enkephalin. *Nature (Lond)* 1983;305:529–530.
199. Zieglgänsberger W, Bayerl H. The mechanism of inhibition of neuronal activity by opiates in the spinal cord of cat. *Brain Res* 1976;115:111–128.

Abbreviations. 5-HT: 5 hydroxytryptamine; BNTX: 7-benzylidenenaltrexone; cAMP: cyclic adenosine monophosphate; CGRP: calcitonin gene related peptide; CNS: central nervous system; DADL: D-Ala2-D-Leu5-enkephalin; DALCE: [D-Ala2,Leu5,Cys6] enkephalin; DAME: [D-Ala2, Met5] enkephalin amide; DAMGO: [D-Ala2,NMePhe4,Gly-ol5]enkephalin; DPDPE: [D-Pen2,D-Pen5]enkephalin; DSLET: [D-Ser2,Leu5,Thr6]enkephalin; GABA: gama amino butyric acid; IA: Intra-articularly; IM: Intramuscular; MOR: Morphine; mRNA: messenger RNA; NMDA: n-methyl-d-asparate; nor-BNI: norbinaltorphimine; PAG: periaqueductal gray; PD; PD117302: (trans-N-methyl-N-[2-(1 pyrrolidinyl)cyclohexyl]benzo[b]thiophene-4 acetamide); SEM: standard error of the mean; sP: substance P; SPIR: Spiradoline; SUF: sufentanil; U50488:trans-3,4-dichloro-N-methyl-N-[2-(1-pyrrolidinyl)-cyclohexyl] benzeneacetamide; UPHIT: 1S,2S-trans-2-isothiocyanato-4,5-dichloro-N methyl-N-[2-(1-pyrrolidinyl)cyclohexyl]-benzeneacetamide

Anesthesia: Biologic Foundations, edited by
Tony L. Yaksh et al. Lippincott–Raven Publishers,
Philadelphia © 1997.

CHAPTER 59

ANALGESIC DRUG CLASSES IN THE MANAGEMENT OF CLINICAL PAIN: α_2-AGONISTS

JAMES C. EISENACH

α_2-Adrenoreceptors are present at peripheral, spinal, and supraspinal sites, and α_2-adrenergic mechanisms serve to modulate a wide variety of behavioral and physiologic functions including pain transmission, the state of arousal, and autonomic outflow. Table 1 lists a number of common α_2-agonists and -antagonists.

After the classic work of Ahlquist in the 1940s separating the α- and β-adrenoceptor classes, work in the middle 1970s emphasized the likelihood that there were two subclasses of α receptors, α_1 and α_2. Based on receptor isolation, pharmacologic profiles, and receptor cloning, it is now appreciated that there are likely a minimum of three or four subtypes of α_2-receptors (10). The role played by these subtypes are at present not certain, although several lines of data suggest the possibility that subtypes may be associated with several actions of α_2-adrenoceptor agonists (10). This chapter does not consider possible α_2-receptor subtype affiliation because of the absence, at present, of appropriately selective subtype selective agents.

MECHANISMS

Analgesic Actions

Early studies indicated that the spinal delivery of adrenaline extract would result in a powerful antinociceptive action in animal models (79). Studies by Swedish investigators demonstrated that catecholamine precursors would inhibit spinal nociceptive reflexes by the release of catecholamines from bulbospinal terminals (3). Subsequent investigations revealed that electrical stimulation in the brain stem or the microinjection of opiates into the periaqueductal gray would yield a powerful analgesia that was found to be mediated by the activation of these pathways. Evidence supporting that contention was the observation that the effects of supraspinal manipulation were associated with (a) the spinal release of noradrenaline, (b) antagonism of the behavior effect by the spinal delivery of noradrenergic antagonists (11,81) (see Chap. 40), and (c) by the observation that the spinal delivery of adrenergic agonists mimicked the antinociceptive effect (68). These pharmacodynamic studies indicated that the spinal actions were mediated by an α_2-adrenergic receptor. Preclinical studies emphasized that these spinal antinociceptive actions could be observed across species including mouse (42), rat (68), dog (70,83), sheep (21,51), and primate (84). These antinociceptive effects have been observed on a wide variety of nociceptive models involving acute nociceptive (68), facilitated states of nociceptive processing (53), visceral pain models (17), and neuropathic pain models (80,82,85) (see Chap. 40).

Table 1. SUMMARY OF α_2 PREFERRING AGENTS

Agents	α_2/α_1 ratio	Comments
Agonists		
Clonidine	>100:1	Considerable human use
Detomidine	>1000:1	Racemic mixture; veterinary use
Dexmedetomidine	>1000:1	Active isomer of detomidine
Xylazine	>100:1	Veterinary sedative
Guanfacine	>100:1	Longer systemic half-life
Guanabenz	>100:1	
Antagonists		
Phenoxybenzamine		Noncompetitive α blocker
Phentolamine		Competitive α blocker
Yohimbine	>100:1	Competitive α_2 blocker
Raulwolfscine	>100:1	Competitive α_2 blocker

The mechanisms of these effects are believed to be associated with a spinal modulation of small afferent transmission at sites pre- and postsynaptic to the small primary afferent. This thinking is based on (a) the location of α_2 binding in the dorsal horn, in the vicinity of C-fiber terminals, and by the incomplete loss of α_2 binding with rhizotomy (40); (b) the ability of α_2-agonists to reduce the release of C-fiber neurotransmitters (9,62,75); and (c) the ability of α_2-agonists to hyperpolarize dorsal horn neurons, presumably by an increase in potassium conductance though a G_i-coupled protein (59).

Sedation

In addition to the analgesic action, α_2-agonists given systemically are known to produce sedation. This sedation is associated with prominent EEG synchronization. The mechanisms of this effect are poorly understood, but intracranial drug delivery studies have suggested that this effect may be mediated in part by an action within the brain stem, possibly upon α_2-receptors within the locus coeruleus (20,55).

Autonomic Outflow

α_2-Agonists have powerful hypotensive effect in animals and humans. The initial organization of the α_2-receptor was believed to be preterminal on sympathetic efferents and as such could reduce sympathetic outflow by blocking local terminal release. Early work demonstrated that α_2-preferring agonists would induce a centrally mediated hypotensive action. The early investigations pointed to a supraspinal action that was believed to reflect upon a suppression of activity in brain stem neurons (39). This depression led to a reduction in bulbospinal-mediated excitation of spinal preganglionic neurons located in the intermediolateral cell column. Other work demonstrated that spinal adrenergic agonists would reduce splanchnic nerve outflow (52) and adrenal secretion (31). It has been subsequently confirmed that α_2-agonists can reduce sympathetic outflow by a direct action at the spinal level on preganglionic outflow (29).

SYSTEMIC ADMINISTRATION OF α_2-AGONISTS

Analgesia has not been commented upon in the larger literature concerning the oral administration of α_2-adrenergic agonists (clonidine, guanfacine, guanabenz) for hypertension. Nonetheless,there is some evidence that acute systemic administration of α_2-adrenergic agonists can cause clinically meaningful pain relief and can exert a MAC-sparing effect (see below). The sites of action for pain relief after systemic administration have not specifically been investigated.

Postoperative Pain

This pain state represents most commonly a mixture of somatic and visceral nociception with a poorly defined component of hyperalgesia. Acute systemic administration (oral, intramuscular, intravenous) of the α_2-adrenergic agonists clonidine and dexmedetomidine causes analgesia in postoperative patients and volunteers (43,64). Although there are conflicting reports , the preponderance of data suggest that minor, short-lasting, or incomplete analgesia is achieved when α_2-adrenergic agonists are administered by these routes. In addition, analgesia following systemically administered α_2-adrenergic agonists is frequently accompanied by bothersome side effects, including sedation, hypotension, and dry mouth.

Table 2 presents several selected clinical studies that highlight clinical experience with systemic α_2-adrenergic agonists for postoperative pain (6,19,71). Segal et al. (71) administered oral followed by transdermal clonidine to maintain plasma clonidine concentrations in the targeted therapeutic range for treatment of hypertension (1 to 2 ng/ml) in a group of patients receiving general anesthesia for abdominal surgery. Compared to the placebo control, postoperative morphine use was reduced by 40% to 50% in those receiving clonidine, indicating an analgesic effect. Pain scores were identical in the two groups.

Whether these types of studies demonstrate analgesia from clonidine per se is difficult to determine for several reasons. Clonidine may interfere with alfentanil elimination, and plasma concentrations of this opioid were greater in those receiving clonidine than placebo in the Segal et al. (71) study. As noted, α_2-adrenergic agonists have sedative/anesthetic effects and reduce the MAC of volatile anesthetics and opioids (1,32). It is conceivable that, despite attempts at anesthetic titration, anesthesia was more profound in patients receiving clonidine than in those receiving placebo, which could have led to a "preemptive" effect to reduce postoperative analgesic requirements. Other studies of similar design have been unable to duplicate these findings.

The situation is not much clearer when these drugs are administered IV in the acute postoperative, rather than intraoperative period. Both clonidine and dexmedetomidine have been administered IV in the recovery room for postoperative pain. Dexmedetomidine demonstrates a minor degree of analgesia compared to standard analgesics (Fig. 1), and is accompanied by sedation and bradycardia (2). Similarly, clonidine, 300 μg, did not affect patient-controlled analgesia (PCA) meperidine usage compared to placebo when administered following cholecystectomy (74). The duration of analgesia is relatively brief (<2 hr) with either clonidine or dexmedetomidine, necessitating repeat bolus or continuous infusion for sustained analgesia. In most cases, clonidine or dexmedetomidine have not been administered as the sole analgesic, but as a supplement to opioids or nonsteroidal antiinflammatory drugs (NSAIDs).

Bolus IV administration of clonidine or dexmedetomidine is unlikely to be routinely employed for postoperative analgesia because of the rapid onset of intense sedation, hypotension, and bradycardia. As exemplified by dexmedetomidine, doses causing complete analgesia also exhibit a high incidence of significant hemodynamic side effects (bradycardia, hypotension) (2). Whether continuous IV infusion or sustained release preparations will have an ancillary role for postoperative pain control is not certain.

One approach that holds promise is the combination of opioid and α_2-adrenergic agonist IV PCA solutions. For example, Bernard and colleagues (5) demonstrated similar analgesia from an IV fentanyl/clonidine infusion after spinal surgery to that from intrathecal morphine, although at the price of more sedation.

Neuropathic Pain

Systemic administration of α_2-adrenergic agonists for chronic pain is largely restricted to those with neuropathic pain, and few controlled studies have been performed. For example, transdermal clonidine provides minimal analgesia in patients with diabetic neuropathy (86), and oral clonidine is similar to codeine in the treatment of postherpetic neuralgia (54). Some clinicians claim efficacy and commonly employ oral or transdermal clonidine for patients with chronic neuropathic pain, but many do not. The quality of studies within this indication is not such that definitive conclusions can be drawn. Carroll et al. (12) compared epidural to IV clonidine in a group of chronic pain patients with an unspecified character of pain. They observed minor effects of clonidine by either route, and concluded that routine use of clonidine in this patient population was not likely to be helpful.

α_2-Agonists cause sympatholysis by both peripheral and central actions, and it is perhaps by this action that clonidine demonstrates some efficacy in the treatment of sympathetically maintained pain. Whereas the beneficial effect of oral clonidine is uncertain, Raja's team (18) has clearly demonstrated that transdermal clonidine yields analgesia in an area surrounding the patch in patients with sympathetically maintained pain. Since they have also demonstrated that subcutaneous norepinephrine exacerbates pain in these individuals, they hypothesize that local application of clonidine causes analgesia by presynaptic inhibition of norepinephrine release from sympathetic nerves onto afferent terminals. The usefulness of topically applied α_2-adrenergic agonists is currently limited by the restricted area of analgesia immediately surrounding the patch and side effects from systemic absorption, although there is one case report of efficacy beyond the patch border (48).

Visceral Pain

Whereas systemically administered α_2-adrenergic agonists exhibit activity in a variety of animal models of visceral pain, there are no clinical trials of these agents for visceral pain syndromes. Intravenous clonidine reduces myocardial infarct size in patients admitted with evolving myocardial infarction (87), but whether this effect is due to sympatholysis, decreased heart rate, and decreased myocardial oxygen utilization or to pain relief is unknown, as pain and its relief were not reported. Intravenous clonidine has been used in the treatment of hypertensive emergencies in preeclamptic

Table 2. SYSTEMIC CLONIDINE FOR POSTOPERATIVE ANALGESIA

Surgery	Route	Placebo	Analgesia	Reference
Abdominal	Oral—transdermal	Yes	↓PCA morphine use by 40–50%	71
Spinal	IV	Yes	↓Morphine use by 50%	6
Abdominal	IV	Yes	↓Morphine use by 25%	19

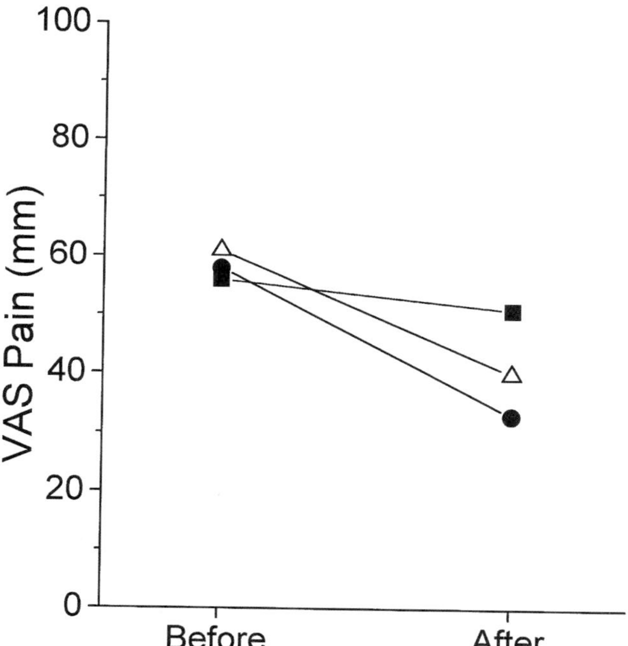

Figure 1. Postoperative pain before and after intravenous administration of diclofenac *(filled square)*, oxycodone *(filled circle)*, or dexmedetomidine *(open triangle)*. (Data from ref. 2.)

women during labor (44), but effects on perception of pain, if any, were not reported.

INTRASPINAL (EPIDURAL/SPINAL) ADMINISTRATION OF α_2-AGONIST

The above discussion suggests a limited clinical role of intravenous α_2-adrenergic agonists for pain relief, since they are relatively weak analgesics and are accompanied by a high incidence of bothersome side effects. In contrast, the majority of clinical studies with intraspinal administration suggests α_2-adrenergic agonists can produce near-complete analgesia alone and interact in a useful manner with other intraspinal analgesics. Preclinical safety studies indicated that spinal clonidine has no deleterious effects upon spinal cord blood flow in pigs and sheep (25,36), and systematic long-term intrathecal exposure in rats (37) or chronic epidural infusion in dogs (83) is without histopathologic consequence.

Postoperative Pain

Epidural clonidine causes dose-dependent analgesia in postoperative patients, as determined by pain report, duration of complete analgesia, and reduction in supplemental morphine use (Fig. 2). There has been some confusion regarding epidural clonidine analgesia in this group, due to differing definitions of pain relief and different dosages used and definition of adequate analgesia. For example, a small dose (150 µg) of clonidine causes brief analgesia compared to placebo, defined as a 50% reduction in visual analogue scale (VAS) pain report (7), but the same dose has no effect compared to placebo defined as IV PCA meperidine use following thoracotomy (35). In contrast, larger doses (400 to 800 µg) cause complete analgesia for several hours and, compared to placebo, reduce IV PCA morphine use after cesarean section (26,41,56).

A recent pharmacokinetic-pharmacodynamic study in volunteers helps to explain some of these disparate clinical reports. In that study (22) epidural clonidine, 700 µg, was injected as a single bolus, the cerebrospinal fluid (CSF) was sampled via an indwelling spinal catheter, and the pain report to a noxious cold stimulus was measured. Clonidine caused analgesia that was closely correlated with simultaneous clonidine concentration in CSF, with an EC_{95} of 130 ng/ml (Fig. 3). From the CSF pharmacokinetics observed in that study, one can calculate the time from epidural bolus injection until CSF clonidine decreases below this EC_{95}, and there is a close correlation between this time and the observed time of complete analgesia following different doses of epidural clonidine in clinical studies (Fig. 3).

Epidural clonidine analgesia is brief in comparison to morphine, necessitating continuous infusion for sustained analgesia. A variety of studies have examined clonidine infusion rates of 10 to 40 µg/hr following surgery, and demonstrates rate-dependent reduction in supplemental IV PCA morphine use, from 15% to 20% reduction after 10 µg/hr to >60% reduction after 40 µg/hr (41,56). Compared to placebo, these 24- to 48-hr infusions do not cause sedation, respiratory depression, or clinically significant hypotension and bradycardia.

Systematic preclinical studies with spinally delivered α_2-adrenergic agonists have shown that the analgesic effects produced by these agents may be enhanced synergistically in the presence of other spinal analgesics and anesthetics (see ref. 81a for review). Such drug interactions have been the subject of several investigations in patients with postoperative pain. Clonidine intensifies and prolongs sensory anesthesia and analgesia from spinal and epidural injection of local anesthetics (58,66).

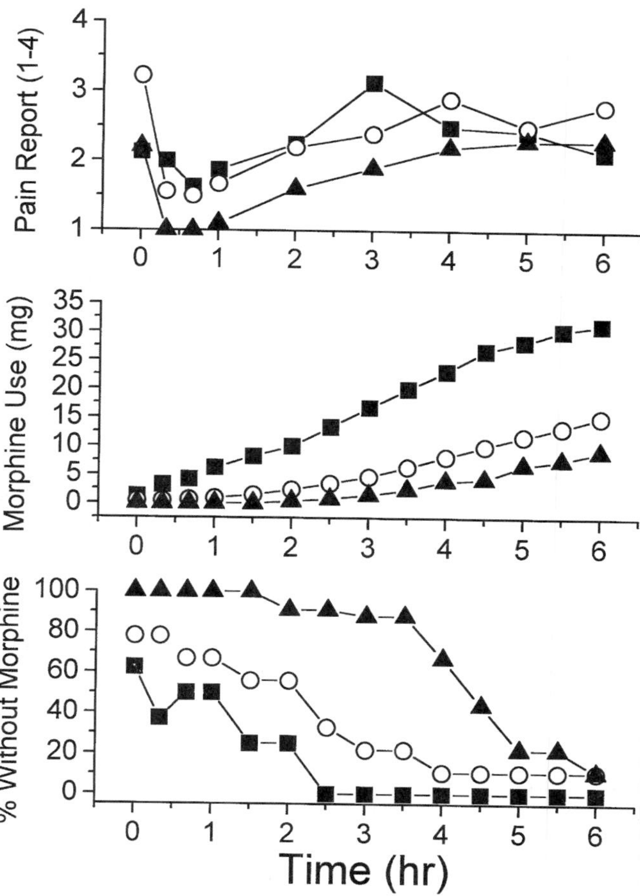

Figure 2. Pain report, cumulative IV PCA morphine rescue use, and percent of patients not requesting morphine over time after epidural bolus injection in an open-label trial of clonidine, 100–300 µg *(filled square)*, 400–600 µg *(open circle)*, or 700–900 µg *(filled triangle)*. (Data from ref. 26.)

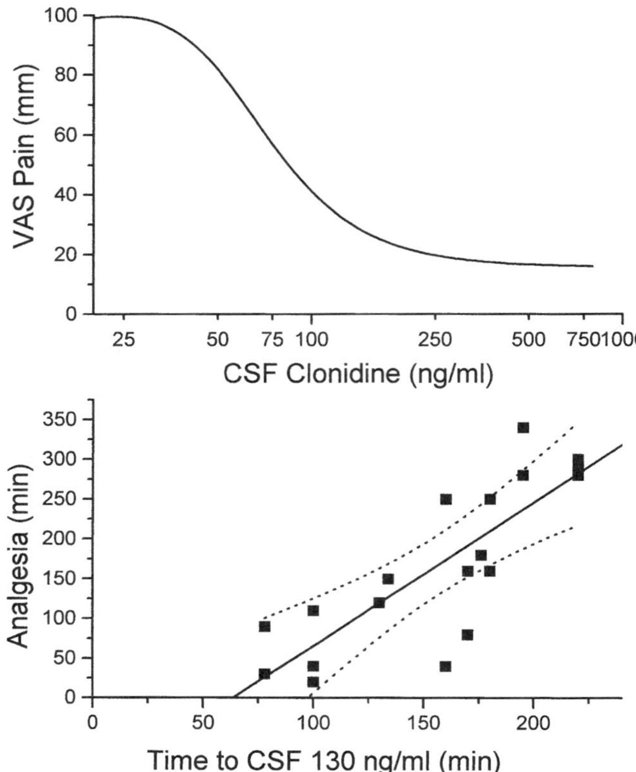

Figure 3. Relationship between experimental pain and lumbar CSF clonidine concentration **(upper panel)**, and between clinical report of duration of complete analgesia and calculated time until reduction in CSF clonidine to the EC_{95} for experimental pain **(lower panel)**. The *upper curve* is a sigmoid fit of experimental data and the *lower curve* is fit by linear regression with 95% confidence intervals. (Data from ref. 22.)

For example, clonidine, 150 µg, increases by over 100% the duration of anesthesia from bupivacaine, 50 mg epidurally or 5 mg intrathecally (49). In addition to this prolongation, clonidine also intensifies local anesthetic blocks as seen by diminished perception of tourniquet pain when it is added to spinal bupivacaine in patients undergoing lower extremity orthopedic procedures (8).

The mechanisms by which clonidine enhances local anesthetic-induced analgesia is unclear. It may represent an interaction between synaptic/Na^+ channel blockade by local anesthetics and/or receptor stimulation by α_2-adrenergic agonists in the spinal cord. Alternatively, the observation that clonidine enhances both motor and sensory block from intraspinal local anesthetics suggests that clonidine may alter disposition of the local anesthetics by local vasoconstriction or some other mechanism.

In contrast to the positive interaction between clonidine and other local anesthetics, 2-chloroprocaine inhibits clonidine analgesia (41). This is similar to the inhibition of spinal opioid analgesia in humans by 2-chloroprocaine (28), and the long duration of this effect suggests an interaction with a 2-chloroprocaine metabolite or additive in that solution (ethyleneglycotetraacetic acid [EGTA]) rather than with 2-chloroprocaine itself. Regardless of mechanism, clonidine's efficacy is diminished after epidural 2-chloroprocaine, and these agents should probably be separated by at least 6 hours.

The interaction between epidural clonidine and opioids has been the focus of several clinical studies. The results with morphine are conflicting, likely reflecting the unique time course of that opioid. For example, in rats, which exhibit a similar time course of analgesia from spinal clonidine or morphine alone, these drugs exhibit synergy when combined (63). In contrast, addition of clonidine to morphine has no effect on the intensity or duration of morphine analgesia following a single injection (78). This is not surprising, since clonidine's duration of action (<5 hr) would be unlikely to affect the long-acting (>18 hr) morphine alone. When clonidine is administered by continuous epidural infusion with morphine postoperatively, an enhancement is observed (57). This is due perhaps to sustained effect of clonidine by continuous infusion and hence sustained interaction with the action of morphine.

Clonidine has been combined with fentanyl epidurally in several studies in postoperative patients. In contrast to morphine, fentanyl has a relatively brief duration of action that is similar to clonidine's and one would therefore be more likely to observe an interaction from their contribution. For example, addition of clonidine 150 µg/hr to fentanyl 100 µg prolongs the duration of fentanyl twofold, from approximately 2 hours to nearly 5 hours (69). This is not due to altered disposition of fentanyl, as addition of clonidine has no effect on plasma fentanyl pharmacokinetics.

Analgesics can interact in an additive or supra-additive (synergistic) manner. The latter is of particular clinical interest, as the dose of each component can be dramatically decreased, thereby decreasing the incidence of side effects. The simplest and most reliable method of distinguishing additive from synergistic interactions is isobolographic analysis (76). In this design, a dose response for analgesia is obtained for each drug alone and a fixed-ratio combination of the two together. Using this approach, profound synergy has been observed in animals between intraspinal α_2-adrenergic agonists and opioids (63). Compared to each drug alone, in combination as little as 5% of each drug is needed to get the same degree of analgesia.

Only one clinical study has employed isobolographic analysis to determine the type of interaction between epidural opioids and α_2-adrenergic agonists. In that study (23), the dose of

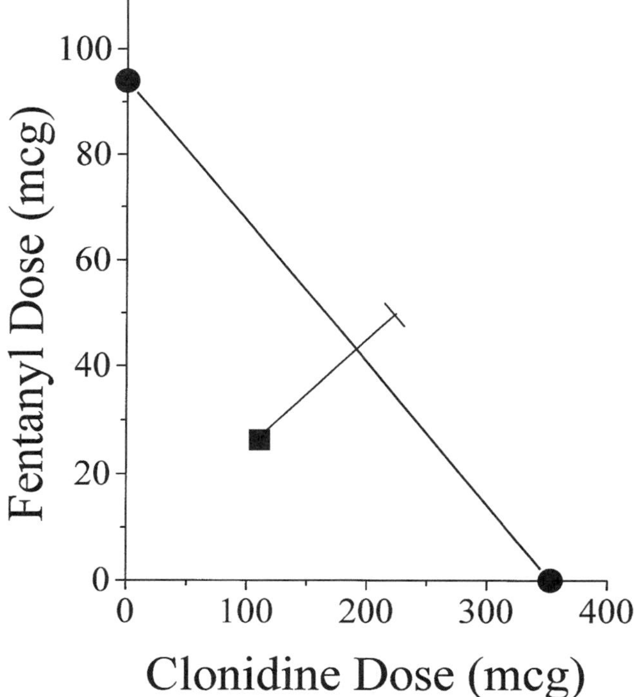

Figure 4. Isobologram at the ED_{50} level describing the interaction between epidural fentanyl *(ordinate)* and epidural clonidine *(abscissa)* in women with post–cesarean section pain. The interaction point lies within the synergistic area of the isobologram, but the 95% confidence limits overlap the line of additivity. Therefore, an additive interaction is not excluded. (Data from ref. 23.)

epidural fentanyl required to provide effective analgesia in 50% of women after cesarean section was 94 μg, while that of clonidine was 350 μg. These values are in keeping with previous studies of fentanyl and the above review of epidural clonidine. The combination dose producing this degree of effect (30 μg fentanyl plus 100 μg clonidine), although less than 60% of what one would predict from an additive interaction, did not differ significantly from additivity (Fig. 4). Nonetheless, less drug is required when these are combined; there was some suggestion of improved efficacy with the combination, and minimal side effects were observed.

As important as the degree of interaction between α_2-adrenergic agonists and opioids for analgesia is their interaction in causing side effects. Common to both types of drugs is dose-dependent sedation, yet their combination does not cause more, and may cause less, sedation than each drug alone, presumably because of the reduced dose of each component. Also, respiratory depression is the most common dangerous side effect of intraspinal opioids, and there has been some suggestion that epidural clonidine may cause mild respiratory depression (4,30). However, combination of α_2-adrenergic agonists and opioids by systemic administration does not alter the degree of respiratory depression from opioid alone in animals and humans. Whereas this has not been formally examined after intraspinal administration, there have been no reports of severe respiratory depression following combined injection of clonidine and an opioid.

Neuropathic Pain

The first report of epidural clonidine use in humans was for chronic pain with a neuropathic component, where it demonstrated efficacy (77). Several anecdotal or uncontrolled series followed, generally demonstrating efficacy even in patients in whom opioids were ineffective (33,34,77). Clinically, neuropathic pain may be relatively "opioid insensitive," requiring larger doses of opioids than nonneuropathic pain. Animal models of neuropathic pain have been developed, some of which are opioid insensitive, and in each case where they have been examined, α_2-adrenergic agonists have shown efficacy (see Chap. 40). For example, lumbosacral spinal dorsal root ligation (as described by Chung) yields a unilateral hyperalgesic state that is sensitive to sympathetic block, and has been considered a reasonably good model of sympathetically maintained neuropathic pain (46). Behavioral hyperalgesia in this model is exquisitely sensitive to spinally administered α_2-adrenergic agonists.

Another animal model of neuropathic pain highlights the difference between opioids and α_2-adrenergic agonists. In that model, which involves peripheral nerve section leading to autotomy, morphine is more effective than clonidine intrathecally as a "preemptive" measure (65). That is, pretreatment with morphine is more effective than clonidine in diminishing autotomy following the insult. In contrast, intrathecal clonidine's apparent potency increases significantly after the insult, when hyperalgesia is present. These results led the authors to conclude that intrathecal injection of opioids may be more effective than α_2-adrenergic agonists in prevention of this neuropathic pain, but that α_2-adrenergic agonists may be preferred in the treatment of established hyperalgesic pain.

Epidural and intrathecal clonidine have been reported to have benefit in the treatment of neuropathic nonmalignant pain. For example, Glynn et al. (34) observed sustained and effective analgesia following a relatively small dose (150 μg) of epidural clonidine in patients with spinal cord injury and chronic pain. Similar results have been obtained in other studies, suggesting that, as in the animal model, lower doses of clonidine are required in the treatment of neuropathic pain than in the treatment of acute, somatic pain. In a blinded comparison between epidural morphine and clonidine in patients with chronic, nonmalignant pain, at least one drug was effective in nearly all of the patients, although some patients received relief from only one of the two drugs (33).

Another likely patient population to receive benefit from intraspinal α_2-adrenergic agonists is the post–nerve injury pain patients, in whom a component of the pain is maintained by sympathetic activity. As previously discussed, topical clonidine relieves allodynia in a small area surrounding its application, presumably by inhibition of norepinephrine release from peripheral sympathetic nerve endings, but it is limited in use by the restricted site of analgesia and by systemic side effects. IV or oral clonidine have not been demonstrated to be effective in patients with sympathetically maintained pain. In contrast, epidural administration of clonidine does produce effective analgesia in these patients.

Rauck et al. (67) utilized a double-blind, placebo-controlled design to test the efficacy of epidural clonidine, 300 and 700 μg by bolus, in patients with long-standing, intractable reflex sympathetic dystrophy. Clonidine, but not saline, decreased pain report. Although the two clonidine doses did not differ in degree of analgesia, sedation was greater following the 700 μg dose. A majority of patients then entered an open-label, chronic infusion trial, in which they received epidural clonidine, 10 to 50 μg/hr titrated to pain relief for 2 to 12 weeks. Clonidine was well tolerated, without evidence of clinically significant sedation or hypotension, and produced sustained reductions in pain report during infusion.

This report raises several questions regarding the utility of epidural clonidine in sympathetically maintained pain. Whether intraspinal α_2-adrenergic agonists would have advantages over local anesthetic sympathetic block in the initial treatment of reflex sympathetic dystrophy has not been explored. Similarly, whether continuous infusion of epidural clonidine in patients with long-standing reflex sympathetic dystrophy would improve limb function as well as relieve pain has not been tested. Finally, although it is conceivable that clonidine could cause analgesia by sympatholysis via systemic redistribution, initial results of a blinded, crossover trial comparing oral to epidural clonidine in patients with reflex sympathetic dystrophy demonstrate analgesia only with epidural administration (Rauck, personal communication).

The mechanisms by which intraspinal α_2-adrenergic agonists produce analgesia in sympathetically maintained pain may include three sites of action. In the spinal cord dorsal horn, α_2-adrenergic agonists inhibit excitatory neurotransmitter release from noxious stimulation as well as hyperpolarize dorsal horn neurons that receive nociceptive input (60). In the spinal cord intermediolateral cell column, α_2-adrenergic agonists decrease sympathetic outflow (38). Finally, in the periphery, α_2-adrenergic agonists diminish norepinephrine release from sympathetic terminals (47), which can excite damaged sensory afferents. In all three instances, to the degree that the pain state was maintained by sympathetic activity, the local effects of the α_2-agonists would impede that activation.

Visceral Pain

In animals, intraspinally administered α_2-adrenergic agonists inhibit behavioral, neurochemical, or neurophysiologic effects following noxious visceral stimuli, including colorectal or duodenal distention (17). Clinically, the only application of an intraspinal α_2-adrenergic agonists for treatment of visceral pain has been the use of epidural clonidine for labor analgesia. Two types of studies have been performed. In the first, epidural clonidine (50 to 100 μg) has been added to the local anesthetic, bupivacaine, and has been demonstrated to intensify and prolong the effect of a subanalgesic dose of bupivacaine (50,61). In the second, intrathecal clonidine alone (100 to 200 μg) has been administered, resulting in rapid onset, near-complete analgesia lasting 1 to 3 hours (13). In both types of studies, clonidine has produced dose-dependent, mild sedation and mild reductions in maternal blood pressure, without significant fetal or neonatal effects.

Protracted Utilization of Spinal α_2-Agonists

Protracted pain states typically present a dilemma for pain management. Several lines of research have focused on the relatively long-term administration of spinal clonidine. In nonmalignant states, much of the literature regarding the use of epidural clonidine is anecdotal or individual case reports, and caution should be exercised in its interpretation. As discussed, Carroll et al. (12) examined, using a double-blind protocol, analgesia from epidural clonidine in a group of patients with chronic pain who had previously claimed benefit from this therapy in an open-label trial. In the blinded study, neither epidural nor IV administration of clonidine caused analgesia. Additional studies utilizing a double-blind, placebo-controlled design are needed to establish the usefulness of intraspinal α_2-adrenergic agonists in this patient population.

Intraspinal clonidine has been examined in the treatment of cancer pain in patients who have failed intraspinal opioid therapy. For example, Coombs et al. (16) reported effective analgesia and reduction in opioid use in a woman with severe cancer pain that had become poorly responsive to intrathecal opioids. They further reported a series of such patients, all studied in an open-label manner, and observed sustained analgesia from continuous intrathecal clonidine infusion, accompanied by sedation and decreased blood pressure, but no evidence of neurotoxicity (14–16). Similarly, we observed in an open-label, dose-ranging study, dose-dependent analgesia from epidural clonidine in cancer patients with severe pain despite receiving hundreds of milligrams of epidural morphine per day (27). As with intrathecal administration, bolus epidural clonidine was associated with sedation and decreased blood pressure. Many, although not all, of these cancer patients had pain that was primarily neuropathic in nature.

Recently, a double-blind, placebo-controlled trial of epidural clonidine for intractable cancer pain has been completed (24). In this study, 85 patients with severe cancer pain not responding to large doses of epidural morphine were randomized to receive epidural clonidine by continuous infusion, 30 µg/hr, or an equivalent volume of saline, for 2 weeks. Epidural morphine rescue was provided by a PCA device, and success was defined as a reduction in pain or in morphine use, with the other variable not increasing. In that study, efficacy of epidural clonidine was dependent on the nature of the patients' pain. Approximately 40% of the patients had pain of the somatic type, and clonidine was no more effective than saline in these patients. In contrast, the success rate of epidural clonidine in the remaining patients, all of whom had neuropathic pain, was 56%, significantly higher than the 5% success rate in the placebo-treated group. Significant hypotension from clonidine was only observed in two of these severely ill cancer patients, and sedation with continuous infusion did not differ between clonidine- and placebo-treated patients. These results suggest epidural clonidine is well tolerated and effective in cancer patients with neuropathic pain who fail opioid therapy, and are supported by a variety of laboratory studies. As previously discussed, intraspinally administered α_2-adrenergic agonists are effective in animal models of neuropathic pain.

An additional consideration regarding the long-term use of α_2-agonists is the minimal cross-tolerance that has been reported between opioids and α_2-agonists in preclinical models (45,72,73). Thus, in the human model one would expect that if tolerance to opioids had occurred in some of these patients, clonidine would remain effective. This is corroborated by analgesic efficacy of epidural clonidine, 30 µg/hr, in cancer patients receiving large doses of opioid, since this clonidine dose is not larger than that required in postoperative, opioid-naive patients. For this reason, some authors have recommended the use of intraspinal clonidine to provide a "drug holiday" in patients tolerant to opioids, allowing recovery from tolerance and return to opioids in the future if necessary.

CONCLUSIONS

The systemic administration of α_2-adrenergic agonists can produce a significant MAC-sparing action in animals and humans. This MAC-sparing action likely reflects the combined sedative and antinociceptive action of the agent exerting a concurrent spinal and supraspinal action. Accordingly, it is clear that with the pharmacologic actions of the α_2-agonists that are currently available, the systemic route of delivery is not able to produce a meaningful selective analgesia. The exception to this comment may be the localized effect surrounding the site of topically applied agonist in patients with sympathetically maintained pain. In contrast, epidural or intrathecal administration of α_2-adrenergic agonists causes clear, dose-dependent analgesia in postoperative patients and patients with neuropathic and visceral (laboring women) pain components. Side effects, primarily sedation and hypotension, will limit the use of this therapy to combination with local anesthetics or opioids or to settings where unique efficacy has been demonstrated, e.g., neuropathic pain, opioid tolerance, reflex sympathetic dystrophy.

ACKNOWLEDGMENTS

This work was supported by grants GM35523 and GM48085 from the National Institutes of Health.

REFERENCES

1. Aho M, Lehtinen A-M, Erkola O, Kallio A, Korttila K. The effect of intravenously administered dexmedetomidine on perioperative hemodynamics and isoflurane requirements in patients undergoing abdominal hysterectomy. *Anesthesiology* 1991;74:997–1002.
2. Aho MS, Erkola OA, Scheinin H, Lehtinen A-M, Korttila KT. Effect of intravenously administered dexmedetomidine on pain after laparoscopic tubal ligation. *Anesth Analg* 1991;73:112–118.
3. Anden NE, Jukes MGM, Lundberg A. The effect of dopa on the spinal cord. 2. A pharmacological analysis. *Acta Physiol Scand* 1966; 67:387–397.
4. Bailey PL, Sperry RJ, Johnson GK, Eldredge SJ, East KA, East TD, Pace NL, Stanley TH. Respiratory effects of clonidine alone and combined with morphine, in humans. *Anesthesiology* 1991;74: 43–48.
5. Bernard J-M, Hommeril J-L, Legendre M-P, Passuti N, Pinaud M. Spinal or systemic analgesia after extensive spinal surgery: Comparison between intrathecal morphine and intravenous fentanyl plus clonidine. *J Clin Anesth* 1993;5:231–236.
6. Bernard J-M, Hommeril J-L, Passuti N, Pinaud M. Postoperative analgesia by intravenous clonidine. *Anesthesiology* 1991;75:577–582.
7. Bonnet F, Boico O, Rostaing S, Saada M, Loriferne J-F, Touboul C, Abhay K, Ghignone M. Postoperative analgesia with extradural clonidine. *Br J Anaesth* 1989;63:465–469.
8. Bonnet F, Diallo A, Saada M, Belon M, Guilbaud M, Boico O. Prevention of tourniquet pain by spinal isobaric bupivacaine with clonidine. *Br J Anaesth* 1989;63:93–96.
9. Bourgoin S, Pohl M, Mauborgne A, Benoliel JJ, Collin E, Hamon M, Cesselin F. Monoaminergic control of the release of calcitonin gene-related peptide- and substance P-like materials from rat spinal cord slices. *Neuropharmacology* 1993;32:633–640.
10. Bylund DB. Subtypes of α_2-adrenoceptors: pharmacological and molecular biological evidence converge. *TIPS* 1988;9:356–361.
11. Camarata PJ, Yaksh TL. Characterization of the spinal adrenergic receptors mediating the spinal effects produced by the microinjec-

tion of morphine into the periaqueductal gray. *Brain Res* 1985;336:133–142.
12. Carroll D, Jadad A, King V, Wiffen P, Glynn C, McQuay H. Single-dose, randomized, double-blind, double-dummy cross-over comparison of extradural and i.v. clonidine in chronic pain. *Br J Anaesth* 1993;71:665–669.
13. Chiari A, Berger R, Lorber C, Gosch M, Klimscha W. Intrathecal sufentanil and clonidine for obstetric analgesia. *Anesthesiology* 1994; 81:A1141(abstr).
14. Coombs DW, Saunders R, Gaylor M, LaChance D, Jensen L. Clinical trial of intrathecal clonidine for cancer pain. *Reg Anaesth* 1984; 9:28(abstr).
15. Coombs DW, Saunders RL, Fratkin JD, Jensen LE, Murphy CA. Continuous intrathecal hydromorphone and clonidine for intractable cancer pain. *J Neurosurg* 1986;64:890–894.
16. Coombs DW, Saunders RL, LaChance D, Savage S, Ragnarsson TS, Jensen LE. Intrathecal morphine tolerance: Use of intrathecal clonidine, DADLE, and intraventricular morphine. *Anesthesiology* 1985;62:357–363.
17. Danzebrink RM, Gebhart GF. Antinociceptive effects of intrathecal adrenoceptor agonists in a rat model of visceral nociception. *J Pharmacol Exp Ther* 1990;253:698–705.
18. Davis KD, Treede RD, Raja SN, Meyer RA, Campbell JN. Topical application of clonidine relieves hyperalgesia in patients with sympathetically maintained pain. *Pain* 1991;47:309–317.
19. De Kock MF, Pichon G, Scholtes J-L. Intraoperative clonidine enhances postoperative morphine patient-controlled analgesia. *Can J Anaesth* 1992;39:537–544.
20. De Sarro GB, Bagetta G, Ascioti C, Libri V, Nistico G. Microinfusion of clonidine and yohimbine into locus coeruleus alters EEG power spectrum: effects of aging and reversal by phosphatidylserine. *Br J Pharmacol* 1988;95:1278–1286.
21. Detweiler DJ, Eisenach JC, Tong C, Jackson C. A cholinergic interaction in *alpha*$_2$ adrenoceptor-mediated antinociception in sheep. *J Pharmacol Exp Ther* 1993;265:536–542.
22. Eisenach J, Detweiler D, Hood D. Hemodynamic and analgesic actions of epidurally administered clonidine. *Anesthesiology* 1993;78: 277–287.
23. Eisenach JC, D'Angelo R, Taylor C, Hood DD. An isobolographic study of epidural clonidine and fentanyl after cesarean section. *Anesth Analg* 1994;79:285–290.
24. Eisenach JC, DuPen S, Dubois M, Miguel R, Allin D, and Epidural Clonidine Study Group. Epidural clonidine analgesia for intractable cancer pain. *Pain* 1995;61:391–399.
25. Eisenach JC Grice SC. Epidural clonidine does not decrease blood pressure or spinal cord blood flow in awake sheep. *Anesthesiology* 1988;68:335–340.
26. Eisenach JC, Lysak SZ, Viscomi CM. Epidural clonidine analgesia following surgery: Phase I. *Anesthesiology* 1989;71:640–646.
27. Eisenach JC, Rauck RL, Buzzanell C, Lysak SZ. Epidural clonidine analgesia for intractable cancer pain: Phase I. *Anesthesiology* 1989; 71:647–652.
28. Eisenach JC, Schlairet TJ, Dobson CE, II, Hood DH. Effect of prior anesthetic solution on epidural morphine analgesia. *Anesth Analg* 1991;73:119–123.
29. Eisenach JC, Tong C. Site of hemodynamic effects of intrathecal α_2-adrenergic agonists. *Anesthesiology* 1991;74:766–771.
30. Furst SR, Weinger MB. Dexmedetomidine, a selective α_2-agonist, does not potentiate the cardiorespiratory depression of alfentanil in the rat. *Anesthesiology* 1990;72:882–888.
31. Gaumann DM, Yaksh TL, Tyce GM. Effects of intrathecal morphine, clonidine, and midazolam on the somato-sympathoadrenal reflex response in halothane-anesthetized cats. *Anesthesiology* 1990; 73:425–432.
32. Ghignone M, Quintin L, Duke PC, Kehler CH, Calvillo O. Effects of Clonidine on narcotic requirements and hemodynamic response during induction of fentanyl anesthesia and endotracheal intubation. *Anesthesiology* 1986;64:36–42.
33. Glynn C, Dawson D, Sanders R. A double-blind comparison between epidural morphine and epidural clonidine in patients with chronic non-cancer pain. *Pain* 1988;34:123–128.
34. Glynn CJ, Teddy PJ, Jamous MA, Moore RA, Lloyd JW. Role of spinal noradrenergic system in transmission of pain in patients with spinal cord injury. *Lancet* 1986;ii:1249–1250.
35. Gordh T Jr. Epidural clonidine for treatment of postoperative pain after thoracotomy. A double-blind placebo-controlled study. *Acta Anaesth Scand* 1988;32:702–709.
36. Gordh T Jr, Feuk U, Norlen K. Effect of epidural clonidine on spinal cord blood flow and regional and central hemodynamics in pigs. *Anesth Analg* 1986;65:1312–1318.
37. Gordh T Jr, Post C, Olsson Y. Evaluation of the toxicity of subarachnoid clonidine, guanfacine, and a substance P-antagonist on rat spinal cord and nerve roots: Light and electron microscopic observations after chronic intrathecal administration. *Anesth Analg* 1986;65:1303–1311.
38. Guyenet PG, Cabot JB. Inhibition of sympathetic preganglionic neurons by catecholamines and clonidine: Mediation by an a-adrenergic receptor. *J Neurosci* 1981;1:908–917.
39. Head GA. Central monoamine neurons and cardiovascular control. *Kidney Int* 1992;37:S8–13.
40. Howe JR, Yaksh TL, Go VLW. The effect of unilateral dorsal root ganglionectomies or ventral rhizotomies on α_2-adrenoceptor binding to, and the substance p, enkephalin, and neurotensin content of, the cat lumbar spinal cord. *Neuroscience* 1987;21:385–394.
41. Huntoon M, Eisenach JC, Boese P. Epidural clonidine after cesarean section: appropriate dose and effect of prior local anesthetic. *Anesthesiology* 1992;76:187–193.
42. Hylden J, Wilcox GL. Pharmacological characterization of substance P induced nociception in the mouse. Modulation by opioid and adrenergic agonists at the spinal level. *J Pharmacol Exp Ther* 1983;226:398–404.
43. Jaakola M-L, Salonen M, Lehtinen R, Scheinin H. The analgesic action of dexmedetomidine—a novel α_2-adrenoceptor agonist—in healthy volunteers. *Pain* 1991;46:281–285.
44. Johnston CI, Aickin DR. The control of high blood pressure during labour with clonidine ("Catapres"). *Med J Aust* 1971;2:132–135.
45. Kalso EA, Sullivan AF, McQuay HJ, Dickenson AH, Roques BP. Cross-tolerance between *mu* opioid and *alpha*-2 adrenergic receptors, but not between *mu* and *delta* opioid receptors in the spinal cord of the rat. *J Pharmacol Exp Ther* 1993;265:551–558.
46. Kim SH, Chung JM. Sympathectomy alleviates mechanical allodynia in an experimental animal model for neuropathy in the rat. *Neurosci Lett* 1991;134:131–134.
47. Kiowski W, Hulthen UL, Ritz R, Buhler FR. Prejunctional α2-adrenoceptors and norepinephrine release in the forearm of normal humans. *J Cardiovasc Pharmacol* 1985;7(suppl 6):S144–S148.
48. Kirkpatrick AF, Derasari M, Glodek JA, Piazza PA. Postherpetic neuralgia: a possible application for topical clonidine. *Anesthesiology* 1992;76:1065–1066.
49. Klimscha W, Chiari A, Krafft P, Plattner O, Taslimi R, Mayer N, Weinstabl C, Schneider B, Zimpfer M. Hemodynamic and analgesic effects of clonidine added repetitively to continuous epidural and spinal blocks. *Anesth Analg* 1995;80:322–327.
50. Le Polain B, De Kock M, Scholtes JL, Van Lierde M. Clonidine combined with sufentanil and bupivacaine with adrenaline for obstetric analgesia. *Br J Anaesth* 1993;71:657–660.
51. Ley S, Waterman A, Livingston A. The influence of chronic pain on the analgesic effects of alpha2-adrenoceptor agonist, xylazine, in sheep. *J Vet Pharmacol Ther* 1991;14:141–144.
52. LoPachin RM, Rudy TA. The effects of intrathecal sympathomimetic agents on neural activity in the lumbar sympathetic chain of rats. *Brain Res* 1981;224:195–198.
53. Malmberg AB, Yaksh TL. Pharmacology of the spinal action of ketorolac, morphine, ST-91, U50488H, and L-PIA on the formalin test and an isobolographic analysis of the NSAID interaction. *Anesthesiology* 1993;79:270–281.
54. Max MB, Schafer SC, Culnane M, Dubner R, Gracely RH. Association of pain relief with drug side effects in postherpetic neuralgia: A single-dose study of clonidine, codeine, ibuprofen, and placebo. *Clin Pharmacol Ther* 1988;43:363–371.
55. Maze M, Tranquilli W. Alpha-2 adrenoceptor agonists: Defining the role in clinical anesthesia. *Anesthesiology* 1991;74:581–605.
56. Mendez R, Eisenach JC, Kashtan K. Epidural clonidine analgesia after cesarean section. *Anesthesiology* 1990;73:848–852.
57. Motsch J, Gräber E, Ludwig K. Addition of clonidine enhances postoperative analgesia from epidural morphine: A double-blind study. *Anesthesiology* 1990;73:1067–1073.
58. Nishikawa T, Dohi S. Clinical evaluation of clonidine added to lidocaine solution for epidural anesthesia. *Anesthesiology* 1990;73: 853–859.
59. North RA, Williams JT, Suprenant A, Christie MJ. Mu and delta opioid receptors belong to a family of receptors that are coupled to potassium channels. *Proc Natl Acad Sci USA* 1987;84:5487–5491.
60. North RA, Yoshimura M. The actions of noradrenaline on neu-

rones of the rat substantia gelatinosa in vitro. *J Physiol* 1984;349: 43–55.
61. O'Meara ME, Gin T. Comparison of 0.125% bupivacaine with 0.125% bupivacaine and clonidine as extradural analgesia in the first stage of labour. *Br J Anaesth* 1993;71:651–656.
62. Ono H, Mishima A, Ono S, Fukuda H, Vasko MR. Inhibitory effects of clonidine and tizanidine on release of substance P from slices of rat spinal cord and antagonism by α-adrenergic receptor antagonists. *Neuropharmacology* 1991;30:585–589.
63. Ossipov MH, Harris S, Lloyd P, Messineo E. An isobolographic analysis of the antinociceptive effect of systemically and intrathecally administered combinations of clonidine and opiates. *J Pharmacol Exp Ther* 1990;255:1107–1116.
64. Porchet HC, Piletta P, Dayer P. Objective assessment of clonidine analgesia in man and influence of naloxone. *Life Sci* 1990;46: 991–998.
65. Puke MJC, Wiesenfeld-Hallin Z. The differential effects of morphine and the α_2-adrenoceptor agonists clonidine and dexmedetomidine on the prevention and treatment of experimental neuropathic pain. *Anesth Analg* 1993;77:104–109.
66. Racle JP, Benkhadra A, Poy JY, Bleizal B. Prolongation of isobaric bupivacaine spinal anesthesia with epinephrine and clonidine for hip surgery in the elderly. *Anesth Analg* 1987;66:442–446.
67. Rauck RL, Eisenach JC, Jackson K, Young LD, Southern J. Epidural clonidine treatment for refractory reflex sympathetic dystrophy. *Anesthesiology* 1993;79:1163–1169.
68. Reddy SVR, Maderdrut JL, Yaksh TL. Spinal cord pharmacology of adrenergic agonist-mediated antinociception. *J Pharmacol Exp Ther* 1980;213:525–533.
69. Rostaing S, Bonnet F, Levron JC, Vodinh J, Pluskwa F, Saada M. Effect of epidural clonidine on analgesia and pharmacokinetics of epidural fentanyl in postoperative patients. *Anesthesiology* 1991; 75:420–425.
70. Sabbe MB, Penning JP, Ozaki GT, Yaksh TL. Spinal and systemic action of the α_2 receptor agonist dexmedetomidine in dogs: antinociception and carbon dioxide response. *Anesthesiology* 1994; 80:1057–1072.
71. Segal IS, Jarvis DJ, Duncan SR, White PF, Maze M. Clinical efficacy of oral-transdermal clonidine combinations during the perioperative period. *Anesthesiology* 1991;74:220–225.
72. Solomon RE, Gebhart GF. Intrathecal morphine and clonidine: antinociceptive tolerance and cross-tolerance and effects on blood pressure. *J Pharmacol Exp Ther* 1988;245:444–454.
73. Stevens CW, Monasky MS, Yaksh TL. Spinal infusion of opiate and α_2-agonists in rats: tolerance and cross-tolerance studies. *J Pharmacol Exp Ther* 1988;244:63–70.
74. Striebel WH, Koenigs DI, Krämer JA. Intravenous clonidine fails to reduce postoperative meperidine requirements. *J Clin Anesth* 1993;5:221–225.
75. Takano M, Takano Y, Yaksh TL. Release of calcitonin gene-related peptide (CGRP), substance P (SP), and vasoactive intestinal polypeptide (VIP) from rat spinal cord: modulation by α_2 agonists. *Peptides* 1993;14:371–378.
76. Tallarida RJ, Porreca F, Cowan A. Statistical analysis of drug-drug and site-site interactions with isobolograms. *Life Sci* 1989;45: 947–961.
77. Tamsen A, Gordh T. Epidural clonidine produces analgesia (letter). *Lancet* 1984;2:231–232.
78. van Essen EJ, Bovill JG, Ploeger EJ. Extradural clonidine does not potentiate analgesia produced by extradural morphine after meniscectomy. *Br J Anaesth* 1991;66:237–241.
79. Weber HU. Anaesthesia durch adrenalin. *Verh Dtsch Ges Inn Med* 1904;21:616–619.
80. Xu XJ, Hao JX, Aldskogius H, Seiger A, Weisenfeldt-Hallin Z. Chronic pain-related syndrome in rats after ischemic spinal cord injury. A possible animal model for pain in patients with spinal cord injury. *Pain* 1992;48:279–290.
81. Yaksh TL. Direct evidence that spinal serotonin and noradrenaline terminals mediate the spinal antinociceptive effects of morphine in the periaqueductal gray. *Brain Res* 1979;160:180–185.
81a. Yaksh TL, Malmberg AB. Interaction of spinal modulatory receptor systems. In: Fields HL, Liebeskind JC, eds. *Progress in pain research and management*, vol 1. Seattle: IASP Press, 1994;151–171.
82. Yaksh TL, Pogrel JW, Lee YW, Chaplan SR. Reversal of nerve ligation-induced allodynia by spinal *alpha*-2 adrenoceptor agonists. *J Pharmacol Exp Ther* 1995;272:207–214.
83. Yaksh TL, Rathbun M, Jage J, Mirzai T, Grafe M, Hiles RA. Pharmacology and toxicology of chronically infused epidural clonidine HCl in dogs. *Fundam Appl Toxicol* 1994;23:319–335.
84. Yaksh TL, Reddy SVR. Studies in the primate on the analgetic effects associated with intrathecal actions of opiates, alpha adrenergic agonists and baclofen. *Anesthesiology* 1981;54:451–467.
85. Yamamoto T, Yaksh TL. Spinal pharmacology of thermal hyperesthesia induced by incomplete ligation of sciatic nerve: I. Opioid and nonopioid receptors. *Anesthesiology* 1991;75:817–826.
86. Zeigler D, Lynch SA, Muir J, Benjamin J, Max MB. Transdermal clonidine versus placebo in painful diabetic neuropathy. *Pain* 1992;48:403–408.
87. Zochowski RJ, Lada W. Intravenous clonidine treatment in acute myocardial infarction (with comparison to a nitroglycerin-treated and control group). *J Cardiovasc Pharmacol* 1986;8(suppl 3): S41–S45.

Anesthesia: Biologic Foundations, edited by
Tony L. Yaksh et al. Lippincott–Raven Publishers,
Philadelphia © 1997.

CHAPTER 60

MODULATION OF NMDA RECEPTOR FUNCTION FOR PAIN TREATMENT

JENS D. KRISTENSEN AND TORSTEN GORDH

The last decade of pain research has given new insights into the physiology and pathophysiology of pain. An important issue has been the recognition of the dynamic nature of nociceptive transmission. Electrophysiologic and behavioral studies carried out in preclinical (see Chaps. 36 and 40) and clinical (see Chap. 41) models have provided detailed characterization of time- and stimulus-dependent alterations in the encoding of somatosensory information. Pharmacologic investigations have provided insights into the transmitter and receptor mechanisms that are responsible for this altered processing. As reviewed previously (see Chaps. 9 and 13), current thinking has emphasized that an important component of these changes is the role played by the glutamate receptor of the *N*-methyl-D-aspartate (NMDA) subtype. Our knowledge of the NMDA receptor's role in pain processing derives primarily from basic scientific studies. From these experimental investigations it has been convincingly documented that the NMDA receptor complex is involved in the transmission and modulation of nociceptive information at the spinal cord level (101). Drugs that interfere with NMDA receptor function may constitute new classes of pharmaceuticals for the future treatment of pain.

Excitatory amino acids (EAA) play an important role in systems mediating the central nervous effects evoked by afferent input. Their release from both afferents and interneurons at the spinal level as well as their role in mediating at least a component of the supraspinal excitation induced by ascending afferent traffic has been well documented (33) (see Chap. 37). EAAs that are released into the extracellular space gain access to several specific classes of receptors, including sites designated as NMDA receptors and several non-NMDA receptors, α-amino-3-hydroxy-5-methyl-4-isoxazole propionic acid (AMPA), and the metabotrophic glutamate receptor (mGlu) (Fig. 1) (see Chap. 17). The specific role of these receptors is not fully known. It is believed that AMPA and mGlu have a general effect by inducing short excitatory postsynaptic potentials, whereas the NMDA receptor amplifies and prolongs the response to depolarization. The EAAs and their corresponding receptors are widely distributed throughout the central nerve system, at both the spinal and the supraspinal level.

NEURONAL PLASTICITY, THE NMDA RECEPTOR, AND PAIN

Neuronal plasticity is the ability of the central nervous system to modify its structure and function in response to evolution, experience, or injury. Hyperexcitability of the dorsal horn neurons may be referred to as an activity-dependent form of neuronal plasticity. There is now substantial evidence that these changes are caused by intracellular events evoked by agonist occupancy of the NMDA receptor.

A theoretical sequence of events has been proposed (18,99). Stimulation of afferent C fibers results in the release of EAAs and neuropeptides, such as substance P and calcitonin gene-related peptide (CGRP) (101a). As reviewed in Chap. 34, the EAAs induce fast excitatory postsynaptic potentials via AMPA and mGlu receptors, whereas the neuropeptides produce slow synaptic potentials. If the stimulation is intense, these slow potentials may summate to produce a cumulative depolarization that can overrule the voltage-dependent Mg^{2+} block of the NMDA receptor, and hence result in amplification of the depolarization caused by the influx of calcium ions. The role of mGlu receptor may be to enhance the NMDA receptor activity. Glutamate binding to mGlu receptor will lead to activation of protein kinase C, which is believed to catalyze the phosphorylation of subunits of the NMDA receptor, resulting in enhanced NMDA receptor-mediated Ca^{2+} entry (83). This NMDA receptor-mediated increase in intracellular calcium initiates a cas-

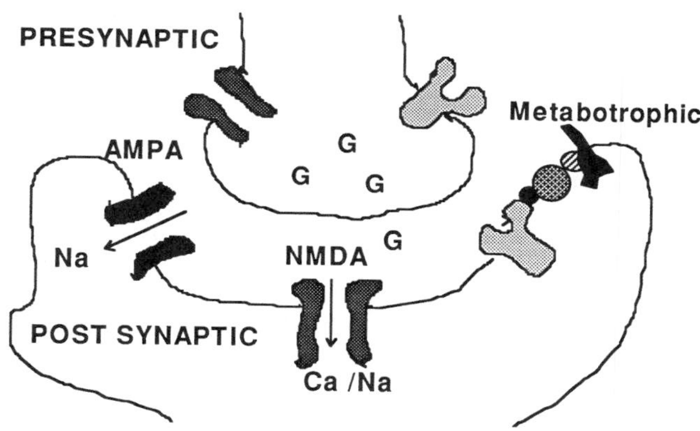

GLUTAMATE RECEPTORS

	METABOTROPHIC	IONOTROPHIC: NMDA	IONOTROPHIC: AMPA
Agonists	Glutamate LAP4 Quisqualate	Glutamate NMDA	Glutamate AMPA Kainate
Antagonist	L-AP3	MK801 CPP Memantine Dextrophan Ketamine 7 Chlorokynureic acid (glycine site) Ilfenprodil (polyamine site)	CNQX

Figure 1. Excitatory amino acid sites. The metabotrophic receptors, when activated by the release of glutamate (G), result in an activation of a number of effector systems leading to increases in phospholipase A_2, C, and D, decreases in adenylate cyclase, and a reduction in N-type Ca^{2+} channel activity. These receptors have been identified pre- and postterminally. The ionotrophic receptors are characterized by the ionophore and the respective agonists: *N*-methyl-D-aspartate (NMDA) and α-amino-3-hydroxy-5-methyl-isoxazole (AMPA). NMDA sites are Ca^{2+} and Na^{2+} ionophores while the non-NMDA sites largely pass smaller cations. Representative agonists and antagonists at these several sites are listed in the above table. NMDA sites have been identified both pre- and postterminally. Thus, in the face of glutamate release, a presynaptic facilitation may be induced by an action at an NMDA site to increase glutamate release or depress its release by an interaction with a metabotrophic receptor.

cade of intracellular events, responsible for the development of neuronal plasticity, i.e., changes in the function or structure of the nerve cell. Thus, while neuropeptides and EAA acting at the non-NMDA receptors lower the threshold for neuron activation, the NMDA receptor activation amplifies and prolongs the response to depolarization.

Implications for Clinical Pain and its Treatment

A possible clinical correlate to this hyperexcitability of the dorsal horn neurons may be such states of hyperexcitability as allodynia and secondary hyperalgesia that may occur in acute nociceptive pain, e.g., postoperative pain. As the postinjury pain state is characterized by a persistent discharge of small afferents, and given that such discharge can induce a facilitated state in animals (see Chap. 40) and humans (see Chap. 41), it is likely that hyperexcitability is an important constituent of acute and postoperative pain (100). Accordingly, pharmacologic intervention through antagonism of the NMDA receptor is a theoretical possibility, in combination with drugs that reduce afferent input to the spinal cord (such as local anesthetics or opiates; see Chap. 58). This effect of NMDA antagonism likely accounts for the popular appreciation among anesthesiologists that ketamine, an agent with affinity for the NMDA site, has, in addition to its dissociative anesthetic effects, analgesic properties in the perioperative or trauma state (12,12a; see below). However, the clinical situation of acute and postoperative pain is relatively easy to handle with currently available pharmacologic agents, such as local anesthetics, nonsteroidal antiinflammatory drugs (NSAIDs), and opioids.

In contrast, patients suffering from neuropathic pain can describe types of pain sensations that are refractory to conventional pain treatment, and it is for these patients that the need for new treatment strategies is most urgent. Research into the role of NMDA receptors in nociceptive perception has provided valuable knowledge about the pathophysiology underlying neuropathic pain, and raised the idea that intervention in the NMDA receptor function may represent a new pharmacologic tool for its treatment. Neuropathic pain states are often followed by signs of spinal cord hyperexcitability, such as persistent pain, hyperpathia, spread of pain outside the territory of the injured nerve, and aftersensation. Excessive and/or long-lasting activity in nociceptive afferents may by different forms of synaptic plasticity that result in neuronal dysfunction and even neurotoxicity, thus implying a contribution of the NMDA receptor system to the development of the abnormal sensations experienced in chronic pain (18). Activation of the NMDA receptor triggers the expression of gene transcription factors such as c-*fos* and related immediate-early genes that can produce long-term changes in the synaptic function, lasting for a few hours to up to several months. Loss of inhibitory neurons may result as excessive depolarization induces neurotoxicity, either from high concentrations of EAA (80) or by the action of, for example, dynorphin (9). These mechanisms may cause permanent changes in nociceptive processing, hence leading to chronic pain states characterized by anomalous sensory properties.

NMDA RECEPTOR

The complexity of the NMDA receptor is highlighted by the presence of at least nine pharmacologically distinct binding sites by which the receptor activity can be regulated (22,58,75,76). These are (a) the NMDA recognition site, (b) a glycine or coactivator binding site, (c) a magnesium binding site within the channel, (d) a phencyclidine site within the channel, (e) an inhibitory divalent action site that can bind Zn^{2+}, (f) a phosphorylation site where protein kinase C and adenosine 3′,5′-cyclic monophosphate (cAMP)-dependent protein kinase can modulate the channel function, (g) a redox site, (h) an arachidonic acid site, and (i) a polyamine site (Fig. 2). Furthermore, molecular cloning of the genes for the NMDA receptor as well as for other EAA receptors has revealed that each receptor comprises a number of subunits, and the variability in the way these subunits combine may represent a molecular basis for functional diversity of the receptors (87).

The NMDA receptor channel complex is further characterized by being both ligand and voltage dependent. At resting membrane potential the channel is blocked in a voltage-dependent manner by binding of Mg^{2+} inside the ion channel (53,68). This block can be removed if the membrane potential is increased by activity at other EAA receptors or by a neuropeptide, such as substance P or CGRP. Ligand stimulation at the NMDA recognition site will then allow an influx of Ca^{2+}, together with Na^{+} (46). This NMDA-mediated influx of Ca^{2+} may initiate a cascade of intracellular biochemical events related to the main physiologic effects of NMDA receptor activation (14):

1. The increase in intracellular Ca^{2+} initiates the expression of proto-oncogenes (e.g., c-*fos*) (90), which are vital in controlling cell differentiation and development. These immediate-early genes encode proteins that act as transcription factors by binding to the DNA or to DNA-binding proteins in the promoter region of

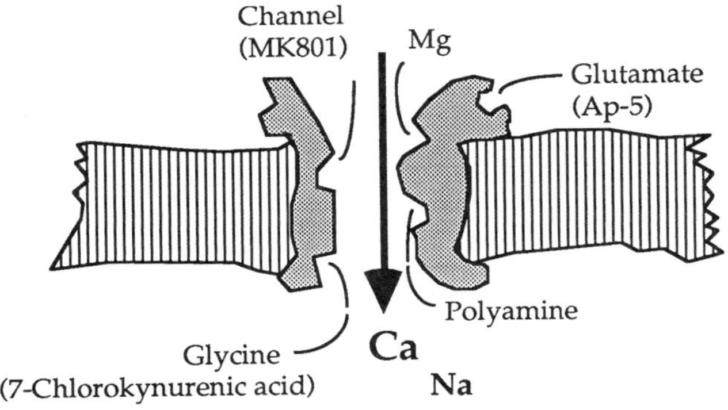

Figure 2. NMDA receptor function. At first, the complexity of the NMDA receptor and its associated ion channel may appear somewhat daunting, but knowledge of the system not only explains how and why the NMDA receptor becomes active but provides the means of interrupting it. The channel associated with the NMDA receptor is blocked by normal resting physiologic levels of magnesium, and so no change in excitability of the neurons possessing NMDA receptors can occur until this is removed. The magnesium block is only removed by a shift in the membrane voltage toward depolarization. Thus, the binding of glutamate to the receptor alone is insufficient to activate the channel. The receptor channel complex is unique because of this dual requirement—the channel is gated by both ligand binding, glutamate on the receptor to the receptor, and by the membrane voltage. An added degree of complexity is that glycine is a required coagonist with glutamate for activation of the receptor, acting at a strychnine-insensitive site closely associated with the NMDA receptor. Thus, for the NMDA receptor channel to operate, certain particular conditions need to be met: the release and binding of glycine and glutamate together with a non–NMDA-induced depolarization to remove the magnesium. C-fiber stimulation induces the release of glutamate but also with excitatory peptides, and the latter may provide the required depolarization to remove the block. Another possibility is that excitatory amino acids activate AMPA receptors on the cell, depolarize the membrane, and so allow the NMDA receptor to operate. The net result is that the NMDA receptor-channel complex is not a participant in "normal" synaptic transmission due to the unique ligand gating (the binding of glutamate to the receptor) and voltage gating (the magnesium block having to be removed) of the system before the channel can operate. However, when the correct conditions are achieved, the complex will suddenly become activated and add a powerful depolarizing or excitatory drive to spinal afferent processing.

the target genes (60). It has been suggested that c-*fos* is involved in the transcriptional control of genes coding for neurotransmitters such as enkephalin and dynorphin (62).

2. Increased intracellular Ca^{2+} leads to the activation of phospholipase C activity. This serves to catalyze the hydrolysis of polyphosphatidylinositol to inositol triphosphate (IP_3) and diacylglycerol. Whereas IP_3 stimulates the release of intracellular stores of Ca^{2+}, thus producing a positive feedback, diacylglycerol stimulates both transcription and activation of protein kinase C (89). Protein kinase C (PKC) is believed to activate and enhance synaptic transmission by stimulation of transduction and release of neurotransmitters (66), and by reducing the voltage-dependent Mg^{2+} block at the NMDA receptor channel (10).
3. Increased intracellular Ca^{2+} results in the activation of neuronal phospholipase A_2, which induces release of arachidonic acid. Arachidonic acid has been shown to stimulate the release of CGRP (25). In addition, arachidonate serves additionally as a substrate for cyclooxygenase, and spinal prostanoids have been shown to be released by persistent afferent input and to enhance spinal glutamate release (48).
4. Intracellular Ca stimulates synthesis and release of nitric oxide (NO) (23). NO is released from intracellular L-arginine residues by a Ca^{2+}-dependent NO synthase and regulates the synthesis of cyclic guanosine monophosphate (cGMP). The NMDA receptor is probably the most potent EAA receptor in the activation of NO synthase (36). It has been suggested that NO acts as a retrograde secondary messenger by stimulating the presynaptic neuron, hence increasing its excitability (4). Antagonism of both the NMDA receptor and NO-synthase seems to attenuate analgesic tolerance to some opioids (21a). Spinal NO synthase inhibitors have been shown to diminish the facilitated state induced by NMDA receptor activation and by persistent afferent input (47a).

By these several discrete mechanisms, the spinal NMDA receptor complex constitutes a system that can lead to a variety of synaptic activities, differing according to their magnitude and duration, as well as the history of their activation.

Clearly, the NMDA receptor does not function as a simple on-off switch. Several unique properties constitute mechanisms by which the NMDA receptor function can be regulated, thus giving the NMDA receptor a central role for modulation of not only afferent nociceptive input, but also the function and structure of the entire synapse. Such properties include (a) the numerous mutually differing binding sites at the NMDA receptor; (b) the existence of NMDA receptor subunits with variable configuration; (c) variability in the combination of NMDA receptor subunits, depending on anatomic location in the central nervous system; (d) interference from other neurotransmitters acting both on non-NMDA receptors, such as AMPA and mGlu, and on other receptors, such as neuropeptide receptors and intrinsic inhibitory receptors; and (e) the possibility of initiating both positive and negative feedback circuits (e.g., by activating an inhibition).

Modulation of NMDA Receptor-Mediated Effects

There are three different ways to modulate NMDA receptor function: (a) inhibition of glutamate release or increasing uptake from the presynaptic site, (b) blocking of the NMDA receptor, and (c) blocking of the effect resulting from NMDA receptor activation.

Presynaptic Inhibition of Production or Release of Glutamate

A straightforward approach to intervening with the activation of the NMDA receptor and to preventing the initiation of the cascade that it can trigger is to prevent the release of EAA and neuropeptides from the primary afferent. The obvious clinical correlate to this is to prevent afferent signaling to the spinal cord, e.g., by using local and regional anesthetic techniques as well as potent systemic analgesics. The concept of preemptive analgesia, i.e., to administer analgesics before the stimulus occurs, was reactualized by Woolf (99), and its importance is generally acknowledged (56,100). The difficulty experienced in most clinical studies in providing evidence of the benefit of timing, i.e., to administer analgesia before or after starting surgery (15,74), may have been due in part to an adequate preoperative basic analgesia. The dynamic of the plastic changes induced by acute pain has been elegantly demonstrated by Torebjørk and colleagues (92), who showed that secondary hyperalgesia following capsaisin injection can only temporary be avoided by coadministration of a local anesthetic. The secondary hyperalgesia will show up as soon as the effect of the local anesthetic has disappeared. This suggests that acute pain must be treated continuously in order to avoid central sensitization.

Specific pharmacologic treatment can reduce presynaptic glutamate release. It has been suggested that stimulation of the adenosine A1 receptor situated at the presynaptic end terminal inhibits glutamate release in experimental studies (86). When adenosine was given intravenously to volunteers, it was found to alleviate ischemic tornique pain (84), and recently intrathecal administration of the adenosine analogue R-PIA was shown to reduce allodynia in a patient with neuropathic pain (35).

Recently, a new class of drugs has been introduced that is claimed to inhibit presynaptic glutamate release. One of these, lamotrigine, is introduced as a new antiepileptic drug, acting by inhibition of glutamate release through use-dependent blockade of voltage-sensitive sodium channels and stabilization of neuronal membranes (42). The clinical role of this class of drugs for the treatment of pain has not yet been established. Experimentally, systemic lamotrigine raised the pain threshold in a rat model of hyperalgesia (64). According to clinical trials for antiepileptic therapy in over 4,000 patients, lamotrigine appears to be relatively safe from a toxicologic point of view (95). A possible serious side effect of lamotrigine is toxic epidermal necrolysis (946).

Antagonizing the NMDA Receptor Sites

There are several ways to block the effect of released glutamate at the NMDA receptor complex, but much research remains to be accomplished on this issue before the potentials of blocking each of the different receptor sites can be mapped. NMDA receptor antagonists, acting at the transmitter recognition site, the polyamine site, the glycine site, and at the ion channel, have been tested in clinical trials for the treatment of epilepsy and stroke (44). The variety of ways for the NMDA receptor to regulate nociceptive processing implies that there may also be several ways to inhibit its functioning, thus encouraging the development of new drugs having specific functional effects at the NMDA receptor complex.

Glutamate Site

There are several potent, competitive antagonists acting at the glutamate binding site that are of interest for clinical use. Most of these are introduced for the treatment of stroke and other kinds of ischemic neuronal injury, e.g., *cis*-4-phosphonomethyl-2-piperidine carboxylic acid (CGS19755), and D-3-(2-carboxypiperazin-4-yl)-1-propenyl-1-phosphonic acid (CPPene). These drugs may also be valuable for the treatment of pain. The major drawback of these drugs is their psychotomimetic side effects that can result from systemic administration. As NMDA receptors are widely distributed in the central nervous system and involved in a large number of neuronal processes, the competitive property of these blockers probably makes it difficult to achieve a therapeutic drug concentration at the target organ with high-glutamate concentration without interfering with other NMDA receptor mediated activities, where the concentration of glutamate may be within the normal physiologic range. To avoid supraspinal effects, spinal administration may be the only route by which to administer competitive NMDA receptor antagonists to conscious patients. However, gene cloning of NMDA receptors has revealed differences in the configuration of the receptor complex, depending on the location in the central nervous system (61). This may lead to second- or third-generation antagonists that are active on spinal, but not supraspinal, NMDA receptors.

Channel Blockers

Repetitive, high-frequency synaptic activity that produces prolonged depolarization of the cell membrane to levels above -50 mV can reduce the Mg^{2+} blocking of the channel, hence allowing Ca^{2+} to enter the cell when the NMDA receptor is activated by recognition site agonists. Pharmacologic blocking of the Ca^{2+} channel is use dependent, i.e., the channel must be open before the blockers can enter the channel. Even unblocking of the channel is agonist dependent, suggesting that the blockers can become trapped in the channel. Theoretically, this type of NMDA antagonists ought to have the advantage of being most effective at sites with high NMDA receptor activity.

The dissociative anesthetic ketamine represent the NMDA antagonist that has been most extensively used to test the influence of NMDA receptors in pain transmission in humans. This topic will be discussed later in this chapter. Other clinically available channel blockers are dextrorphan, dextromethorphan, and memantine, all weak channel blockers with low affinity for the phencyclidine (PCP) site and short duration of action.

Felbamate is an antiepileptic drug, the mechanism of action of which is unknown. In whole-cell voltage clamp recordings from cultured rat hippocampal neurons, clinically relevant concentrations of felbamate (0.1 to 3 mM) inhibited NMDA responses and potentiated γ-aminobutyric acid (GABA) responses (79). Single-channel recordings indicated that the effect on NMDA responses occurred via a channel-blocking mechanism, although it has also been suggested that felbamate is active at the glycine site (54). Felbamate is the first anticonvulsant drug with dual action on both excitatory (NMDA) and inhibitory (GABA) brain mechanisms.

Glycine Site

The glycine site is a modulator site at the NMDA receptor complex present in the same protein subunit as the NMDA recognition site (63). Occupancy at the glycine site is an absolute prerequisite for NMDA receptor activation, and the role of the glycine site seems to be modulation of the NMDA-mediated synaptic response (52). Thus, the release of glutamate from the primary afferent mediates the synaptic transmission, whereas changes in extracellular glycine modulate the NMDA receptor's role in the transmission. Cloning of NMDA receptor subunits suggests the existence of subtypes with differentiated affinity for glycine (41,61).

Kynurenic acid is experimentally the best-studied glycine site antagonist, although its affinity for the site is low. It is nonselective, being similarly potent at NMDA and non-NMDA receptors (71). Newer antagonists, such as L687414, are more selective and potent at the glycine site. L687414 is effective in experimental studies on stroke and convulsion in doses that do not produce vacuolization of neurons or alterations in brain glucose metabolism (28).

Polyamine Site

The polyamine site is an intracellular binding site that can modulate the affinity of other agonists and antagonists. The modulatory effect seems complex and dependent on residual activity at the other binding sites (69). Spermidine and spermine, which are agonists to the polyamine site, enhance binding of MK-801 and glycine to the NMDA receptor. In the formalin test in rats, a synergistic effect was found of the combined administration of the channel blocker MK-801 and spermine, whereas the polyamine site antagonist ifenprodil failed to produce any analgesic effects (13). Ifenprodil and its analogue SL 82.0715 exert a dose-dependent, but incomplete, inhibition of the NMDA receptor by antagonist action at the polyamine site (8). More information is needed on the role of the polyamine site in regulation of the NMDA receptor.

Antagonizing the Effects of NMDA Receptor Activation

A third possibility is to intervene in the secondary events that result from activation of the NMDA receptor complex. As reviewed above, NMDA receptor activation initiates a cascade of events that leads to a facilitated state. In this regard, it has been suggested that NSAIDs and acetaminophen are effective at the spinal level (7,34,47,47a), probably by interacting with the synthesis of prostaglandins or NO. NO seems to play a central role in the secondary events that result from activation of the NMDA receptor (47a,57). NO is catalyzed by the enzyme NO synthase (NOS). This enzyme converts arginine into free NO and citrulline. Only certain types of neurons contain NOS. In the spinal cord, NOS-like immunoreactivity has been identified in the dorsal horn and around the central canal, loci important for sensory processing. NOS is a calmodulin-sensitive enzyme. The binding of Ca^{2+}/calmodulin complexes to the enzyme results in activation of catalytic activity. It is through the generation of NO that several neurotransmitters, including glutamate, acetylcholine, substance P, histamine, and bradykinin, are thought to activate guanylyl cyclase and increase cellular concentrations of cGMP in the CNS. Thus, neurotransmitters that increase intracellular calcium levels could be expected to stimulate guanylyl cyclase activity in neurons containing NOS (59).

NMDA activation enhances NO synthesis from arginine, implicating NO as an important mediator of NMDA effects, such as nociception and neurotoxicity. This also implies that antagonism of NO production could have antinociceptive effects, especially in pain states with signs of central sensitization, hypothetically produced by NMDA receptor activation. Some structural analogues to arginine function as NOS antagonists, and block the production of NO. Experimentally, it has been shown that intrathecal administration of the NOS by L-NG-monomethylarginine (L-NMMA) produces a dose-dependent antihyperalgesic effect (30,47a), suggesting a theoretically new mechanism to induce spinal analgesia.

Protein kinase C activity seems to play a central in the events resulting from NMDA receptor activation (5). Inhibitors of PKC, of which staurosporin is one of the most potent, inhibit ischemic neuronal damage, and may also be a tool for the study of PKC's role in nociceptive transmission. However, clinical inhibition of PKC is probably not feasible, as PKC plays a crucial role in signal transduction for the activation of many cellular functions and even for the control of cell proliferation.

Interaction with Other Receptor Systems

Although the NMDA receptor may have a fundamental part to play in the development of pathologic pain, it should be remembered that pain processing results from the integrated action of a number of receptor systems. Experimental studies on interaction have shown synergistic effects from the combination of NMDA antagonists acting at different sites in the NMDA receptor complex (13) or by the combination of NMDA antagonism with substances acting on other receptor systems, such as μopioids.

Of particular importance is the recent observations that concurrent NMDA receptor antagonism can attenuate the tolerance development otherwise observed after chronic exposure to μ opioid (19,21a,92a) or α_2-adrenergic agonists (19a). Reports that tolerance to μ opioids can be attenuated by NOS inhibitors (38) suggest the likelihood that a cascade of events initiated by NMDA receptor occupancy may be necessary for the appearance of such downregulation. Hence, polypharmacy may be a future key to achieving effective long-term pain control.

CLINICAL EXPERIENCES WITH NMDA ANTAGONISTS

Ketamine

It is mainly from studies using ketamine that we have obtained information regarding the role of NMDA receptors in humans. Ketamine is a dissociative anesthetic agent that binds to the phencyclidine site of the NMDA receptor-gated calcium channel and inhibits the NMDA receptor noncompetitively (1,45,102). Of the two enantiomers, the affinity of S-ketamine for the PCP site is about four times as high as that of R-ketamine (37). Ketamine also interacts with the μ- and nonopioid σ-binding site but at a lower affinity than that for the PCP site (37). Ketamine in high doses, resulting in plasma concentrations of about 1 μg/ml, produces a dissociative anesthesia. When comparing the effects of ketamine in vivo with its receptor affinities obtained from in vitro studies, a positive correlation was observed between the analgesic effect and binding to the PCP site of the NMDA receptor (37). Some 50% NMDA receptor occupancy corresponded to anesthetic levels of S-ketamine, whereas a 20% to 30% receptor occupancy was related to analgesia (103).

Studies in Volunteers

Sadove et al. (82) found that 0.44 mg/kg of ketamine raised the pain threshold in a human model, using electrical ear algesimetry. They describe mild side effects of a predominantly pleasant nature, but warn of the temptation to abuse it due to the description of a pleasant psychic experience from the volunteers. Pharmacokinetic studies in a human model of ischemic pain have shown that an analgesic effect can be achieved with low doses of ketamine, viz. 0.25 mg/kg IV and 0.5 mg/kg IM, producing plasma concentrations of about 100 ng/ml and 150 ng/ml, respectively (12,26). Maurset et al. (51) studied the mechanism of action of low-dose ketamine. They showed analgesic properties of ketamine that were independent of opioid receptors in patients with postoperative pain as well as in human volunteers subjected to an ischemic pain model. They also describe a correlation between the inhibition constant for the PCP receptor and analgesic potency of the two enantiomers S- and R-ketamine, suggesting that the analgesic effect of low-dose ketamine is due, at least in part, to binding to the PCP site of the NMDA receptor (37).

Using S-[N-methyl-11C] ketamine as a tracer in combination with "cold" S-ketamine in positron emission tomography (PET) technique, a direct relationship was shown between specific S-ketamine binding in human CNS and its analgesic and psychopharmacologic effects (29). In this study it was also shown that the analgesic effect on ischemic tornique pain could be reduced in a dose-dependent manner, without affecting warm and cold thresholds or heat and cold pain, measured with the Marstock Thermotest. Furthermore, it was found that, even at the lowest dose of 0.1 mg/kg S-ketamine, the analgesic effect was accompanied by cognitive disturbances, such as changes in hearing and visual functions, altered body image, and feeling of unreality and insobriety.

These studies demonstrate an analgesic effect of low-dose ketamine in ischemic pain, in doses where "normal" physiologic pain transmission seems unaffected. It is also quite evident that this analgesic effect cannot be separated from disturbances in cognitive functions, such as hearing, vision, and mood.

Postoperative Pain

The analgesic effect of low-dose ketamine has been demonstrated in several studies, using clinical postoperative pain as a model. Postoperative pain includes acute nociceptive pain with peripheral and central sensitization, resulting in, for example, NMDA-mediated secondary hyperalgesia.

Intramuscular low-dose ketamine (1 mg/kg) was as good as meperidine (1 mg/kg) for postoperative pain treatment after cholecystectomy in 42 patients (27) or thoracic surgery in 30 patients (16). In both studies, the psychotomimetic side effect of ketamine was claimed to be low and insignificantly different from that found after meperidine.

Following major abdominal surgery in 40 patients requiring postoperative ventilator treatment, benzodiazepines were administered in combination with either placebo or low-dose ketamine in a bolus of 30 mg followed by a continuous infusion (about 0.8 μg/kg/h) for 8 hours. Opioids were given as a supplement. Ketamine reduced the need for opioids and only 4 of 20 ketamine-treated patients were given a total of five supplementary opioid doses, compared with 13 of 20 patients in the placebo group, who received a total of 30 doses of opioid (33a). Diazepam 5 mg was given every fourth hour during ventilator treatment and only mild psychotomimetic side effects were observed, with no difference between the ketamine and placebo groups.

Postoperative continuous infusion of ketamine in a dose of about 0.36 mg/kg/h together with midazolam (about 0.075 mg/kg/h) was given to asthmatic patients following hysterectomy. This afforded the same pain relief as 1.5 mg/kg meperidine administered as a bolus every 4 hours. Some 84% of the patients treated with ketamine would accept the same analgesic procedure for future operations, as compared with 72% in the meperidine-treated patients (32).

In some studies, ketamine has been used to explore the importance of preemptive analgesia. Roytblat et al. (81) showed, in a surprisingly small number of patients (11 ketamine and 11 placebo), that a low dose of ketamine (0.15 mg/kg) given as a bolus after induction of anesthesia, but before surgical stimulation, in patients undergoing open cholecystectomy significantly reduced the postoperative patient-controlled need for opioids compared with placebo-treated patients (48.7 ± 1.25 mg morphine in the ketamine group and 29.5 ±5.2 mg in the placebo group during the 24 hours following surgery). The analgesic part of the anesthesia consisted of fentanyl 5 μg/kg, isoflurane, and nitrous oxide. In another study of patients undergoing hysterectomy (93), the analgesic part of the anesthesia consisted of isoflurane + fentanyl, isoflurane + ketamine, or isoflurane only (nine patients in each group). The results suggested a preemptive effect of fentanyl and ketamine on wound hyperalgesia when measured 24 and 48 hours after surgery, whereas postoperative meperidine consumption, spontaneous pain, and movement-associated pain in the fentanyl and ketamine groups did not differ from that in the patients receiving isoflurane only. However, when ketamine at a rate of 5, 10, or 20 mg/h was added to continuous infusions of 1 mg/h of morphine in elderly patients after upper abdominal surgery, no beneficial effects on postoperative pain were evident (19b). A higher dose of ketamine resulted in an increased incidence of postoperative dreaming.

On the whole, low-dose ketamine seems to be effective for the treatment of postoperative pain. Some studies also indicate a preemptive effect. The difference in the frequency of side effects between healthy volunteers and postoperative patients is probably due to the coadministration of benzodiazepines, which were used in the majority of the postoperative studies. An important advantage of ketamine is that it produces less respiratory depression and sedation than opioids (16,27,32,33a).

Neuropathic Pain

Neuropathic pain results from functional abnormalities caused by injury or disease in the peripheral and central nervous system, and is often associated with sensory dysfunctions that can be characterized as quantitative (e.g., hyperalgesia), qualitative (e.g., allodynia), spatial (e.g., spread of pain outside the territory of the injured nerve), or temporal (e.g., aftersensation lasting for minutes to hours). Normally these pain sensations respond rather poorly to conventional treatment, and the need for new pharmacologic tools for effective pain treatment is obvious. Theoretically, it is within the pathologic pain states represented by neuropathic pain that the NMDA receptor is believed to play an important role.

The difficulty of performing controlled and randomized studies in patients with neuropathic pain is evident from the few studies that have been published on the issue. In a double-blind, crossover study in eight patients suffering from postherpetic neuralgia of a mean duration of 3.8 years, the effect of intravenous administration of ketamine was compared with that of morphine and placebo (20). Ketamine, given in a dose of 0.15 mg/kg, gave pain relief and inhibited wind-up–like pain in contrast to the effect of morphine in a dose of 0.075 mg/kg. Both ketamine and morphine reduced allodynia. Furthermore, ketamine normalized abnormal heat pain sensation in four of the eight patients. However, all eight patients experienced more pronounced side effects following ketamine than after morphine. Another patient with 6-week-old postherpetic neuralgia was successfully treated with ketamine (31). Pain relief was obtained by continuous subcutaneous infusion of 0.5 mg/kg/h, as well as by oral administration of between 400 and 1000 mg/day. No side effects were reported.

Stannard and Porter (88) successfully treated three patients suffering from phantom limb pain by continuous systemic administration of low-dose ketamine (0.125 to 0.2 mg/kg/h). Prior to the treatment, all patients had phantom pain for several years. Side effects were mild in one patient, whereas another became agitated and frightened. However, two of the three patients could continue with the treatment.

In a double-blind and placebo-controlled study, low-dose IV ketamine (0.25 mg/kg) gave significant but brief pain relief in five of six patients with neuropathic pain characterized by hyperexcitability phenomenon and afterdischarge (3). Despite the small dose, psychotomimetic side effects were reported by all the patients who experienced pain relief. Continuous infusion of ketamine (about 0.8 mg/kg/h) together with benzodiazepine was tested in one patient but could not be maintained due to side effects, whereas single-bolus doses were well tolerated. Mankowitz et al. (49) treated seven patients with intractable pain in the back, lower abdomen, and legs in an open study of epidural ketamine in a dose of 4 mg. All patients experienced relief lasting from 30 min to 6 hours.

Persson et al. (72) described a case report of a 17-year-old girl with an opioid-resistant allodynia due to a long-standing superficial wound for whom IV ketamine in doses between 0.2 and 0.5 mg/kg in combination with 1 to 2 mg midazolam could allow painless dressing of the wound. Furthermore, repeated treatment with midazolam and ketamine in the same doses two to four times a day for several months depressed both allodynia and pathologic heat-pain thresholds. Although spontaneous remission might have been involved, this observation could also be indicative of a ketamine-induced reversal of central sensitization. No side effects were reported.

Whereas these studies suggest that ketamine can alleviate different types of neuropathic pain, the profile of the psychomimetic side effects indicates the limitation of its clinical use. However, more controlled clinical studies are needed in order to establish the clinical value of long-term ketamine treatment.

Side Effects from Subanesthetic Doses of Ketamine

It was recognized early that ketamine, even in low doses, produced psychotomimetic effects (17), and this property is a major drawback to its use for clinical pain treatment. Ketamine is related to phencyclidine (PCP, or Sernyl), which was initially developed for anesthetic use, but the unavoidable occurrence of serious psychotomimetic side effects led to its abandonment. Ketamine seems to produce similar side effects, though less pronounced and of shorter duration. Dizziness, a floating sensation, visual distortions, illusions, nightmares, amnesia, alteration of the form and content of thought, and altered bodily and environmental perception are some of the side effects accompanying ketamine, even in low doses (40), and these side effects are correlated to binding of ketamine in the CNS (29).

Competitive NMDA Receptor Antagonist: CPP

We have previously published a report on the clinical use of a competitive NMDA receptor antagonist (39). The patient suffered from a severe neuropathic pain condition, caused by a nerve injury (Fig. 3). Her pain syndrome had the following four characteristics: (a) at rest she suffered from a continuous deep pain sensation mediolaterally on her left thigh, i.e., matching the innervation area of the anterior cutaneous branches of the femoral nerve; (b) low-threshold and brief mechanical or thermal stimulation of her left thigh in the territory of the injured nerve caused an immediate, severe pain sensation (allodynia), followed by (c) a pronounced increase in the basic pain level lasting from minutes to hours after termination of the stimulation (afterdischarge, wind-up), which (d) evoked pain sensation spread beyond the territory of the injured nerve, extending downward to the foot and upward to the left side of the abdomen and thorax up to the level of Th_2. This pain, which embraced most of the left side of the body,

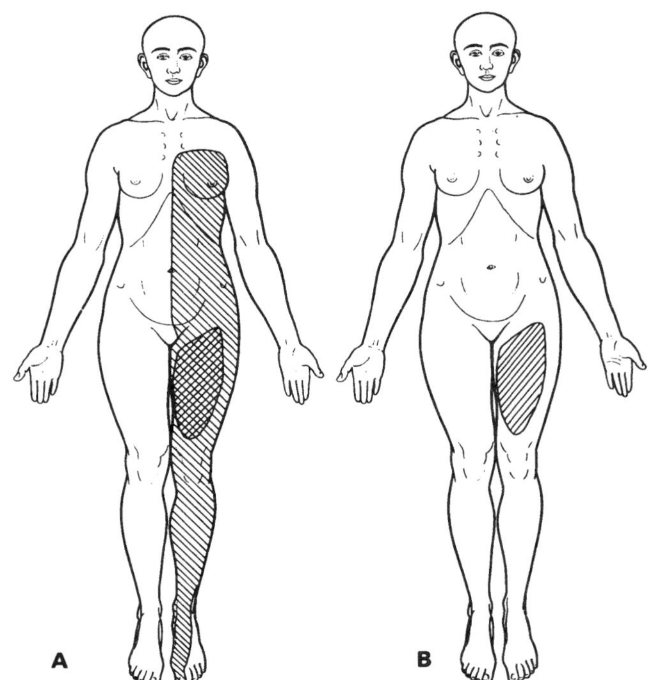

Figure 3. Sensory changes in a woman suffering from a neuropathic state before and after the intrathecal injection of the competitive NMDA receptor antagonist CPP. (From ref. 39.)

lasted from minutes to hours. Her main problem was sleeplessness due to pain triggered by movements and mechanical stimulation of her leg during the night. The condition frequently caused the patient to become totally exhausted, requiring hospitalization and deep sedation with benzodiazepine for a day or two to allow her to obtain some rest. Intrathecal administration of 90 mg hyperbaric 5% lidocaine produced an apparent sensory and motor block extending from Th_{10} to S_5, although the continuous deep pain persisted unchanged. The allodynia to mechanical and thermal stimulation, as well as the afterdischarge and spread of pain, was markedly alleviated, but none of the components was completely abolished.

After intrathecal injection of 200 nmol 3-(2-carboxypiperazine-4-yl)propyl-1-phosphonic acid (CPP), afterdischarge and the spread of pain beyond the territory of the injured nerve were completely abolished following brief, low-threshold, mechanical, and thermal stimulation. The immediate allodynia and the continuous deep pain sensation were still present with the same severity as before the injection of CPP, but these pain sensations were now strictly limited to the territory of the injured nerve (Fig. 3).

The normal sensory and motor function was not affected at all by spinal NMDA receptor inhibition. The patient could walk and experienced normal sensations to nociceptive stimulation. The thermal sensory and pain thresholds were unchanged, when compared with pre-CPP values, over both the affected and the unaffected skin areas. No changes were observed in the response to low- and high-threshold mechanical stimulation, proprioception, or sensitivity to vibration. No changes could be observed in motor function, coordination, and reflexes, and the patient could micturate normally. Heart rate and blood pressure were unaffected. About 4 hours after the administration of CPP, the patient developed a long-lasting state of anxiety, uneasiness, and hyperacusis, similar to the side effects that can be produced by ketamine.

An important finding in this human study was that normal sensory and motor functions appeared to be completely unaffected by intrathecal CPP. Hence, only pathologic pain, i.e., pain sensations resulting from spinal cord hyperexcitability due to neuronal plasticity, was affected. This is consistent with the results of several experimental studies in neuropathic pain models where NMDA antagonists could alleviate hyperalgesia without affecting latency to noxious stimulation in normal tissue (77,101,101b). This stands in contrast to the effects of opioids, which in the clinical situation are effective in the treatment of nociceptive pain, whereas they are often ineffective against neuropathic pain with hyperpathia (2). This characteristic of NMDA receptor antagonists, viz. their capacity to dampen hyperexcitability of the spinal cord without affecting normal sensory transmission, is of fundamental importance to its potential clinical use. It implies the possibility of avoiding the drawbacks associated with other spinal analgesics, such as motor dysfunction (following local anesthetics) resulting in immobilization, and reduced sensibility (following both local anesthetics and morphine). Sensibility fulfills an important physiologic function in warning of potential tissue damage. Furthermore, the finding supports the organization proposed by Woolf (99) that pain can be divided into two distinct and qualitatively different categories: physiologic pain caused by transient non–tissue-injurious noxious stimuli, and pathologic pain caused by peripheral and central sensitization of the somatosensory system following tissue injury. The study suggests that parts of hyperpathia can be reduced by means of CPP in the clinical situation of neuropathic pain, although the profile of potential side effects needs to be further explored.

Dextrorphan

Dextrorphan is the primary metabolite of the antitussive drug dextromethorphan, which is well tolerated by humans. Experimental studies have shown that dextrorphan has antagonistic properties at the channel site of the NMDA receptor (11). In experimental studies on neuropathic pain, dextrorphan has shown antinociceptive effects (50,91). In volunteers, dextrorphan reduced temporal summation of electrical and thermally evoked second pain, without affecting the amplitude of the first pain (73). However, McQuay et al. (55) was unable to demonstrate any beneficial effect of dextromethorphan in a heterogeneous group of 21 patients suffering from neuropathic pain.

Memantine

Memantine (1-amino-3,5-dimethyl-adamantane) is an analogue of amantadine, which is used clinically for the treatment of Parkinson's disease (97). In vitro studies have shown that memantine is an open-channel NMDA blocker with rapid blocking and unblocking rates and with stronger voltage than use dependency (10,70). However, its affinity for the NMDA receptor is lower than that of ketamine. As shown by extracellular recording from spinal cord neurons, memantine reduced the neurons' responses to noxious but not to innocuous pressure on the knee in normal rats, whereas in rats with acute arthritis memantine reduced the responses to both noxious and innocuous pressure (65). In experimental thermal hyperalgesia induced by injecting carrageenan, memantine in doses without motor effect reduced the hyperalgesia when given before (but not after) the carrageenan injection. No clinical studies on memantine for the treatment of pain has been reported.

Other Clinically Available Drugs that May Act via NMDA Receptors

Tricyclic Antidepressants

Antidepressants have been one of the few agents available for pharmacologic treatment of neurogenic pain (28). There is evidence that their antinociceptive effect may be due, at least in part, to interaction with the NMDA receptor function (see Chap. 37). Tricyclic antidepressants block the induction of long-term potentiation by inhibitory action on NMDA receptors (96). The mechanism of action is not known, but chronic (14 daily injections) treatment of mice with the prototypic tricyclic antidepressant imipramine significantly alters ligand binding to the NMDA receptor complex (67). This effect may be due to blocking of the $Ca2^{+}$ channel (85) or interference with the zinc site (78). Intrathecal amitryptyline behaves in preclinical models as do NMDA antagonists (21).

Antiepileptic Drugs

It is suggested that the NMDA receptor is involved in generating many types of seizures, and epilepsy represents a disease in which antagonists to the NMDA receptor may prove useful as a therapeutic agent (98). There is also evidence that some of the well-known antiepileptics act by interfering with the NMDA receptor function. In vitro studies have shown that valproic acid depresses NMDA-induced depolarization in the presence of both non-NMDA antagonists and GABA antagonists (24). This suggests that valproic acid has an action that interferes with the NMDA receptor function. The new antiepileptic drugs felbamate and lamotrigine, which have been mentioned earlier, are also claimed to interact with NMDA receptor function.

NSAIDs

Earlier, NSAIDs were believed to exert their action in the periphery, but there is now substantial evidence to suggest a central action (94). Microdialysis technique in unanesthetized rats has shown that formalin injection in the paw triggers the release of glutamate and prostaglandin E_2 (PGE_2), which could be restricted by pretreatment with intraperitoneal or intrathecal S-ibuprofen (48). Intrathecal (IT) administration of NSAIDs reduces experimental hyperalgesia elicited by IT administration of NMDA or substance P (47). These studies suggest that the spinal prostanoid system is involved in nociception and that NSAIDs exert an antinociceptive effect by a spinal action, involving NMDA receptor function. In a rat model, where intrathecal administration of NMDA produced characteristic pain-related behavior, pretreatment with acetaminophen or NSAIDs had an inhibitory effect, and this antinociceptive action could be reversed by administering L-arginine (6,7). Furthermore, NMDA- (but not kainate-) induced *c-fos* messenger RNA (mRNA) expression could be abolished by indomethacin in vitro (43). These studies suggest that the antinociceptive effects of NSAIDs include a central component related to NMDA receptor-induced activation of the NO system. As altered gene expression is believed to play an important part in the development of neuronal plasticity and central sensitization, these studies suggest a new and more active role of NSAIDs in clinical pain treatment.

FUTURE DIRECTIONS

The weight of the preclinical and the few clinical studies clearly supports a fundamental role of the NMDA receptor system in clinical pain states involving pathologic pain, such as that observed after tissue injury (postoperative/ trauma) and/or nerve injury (neurogenic pain). If the result can be confirmed in controlled clinical studies, modulation of NMDA receptor function may constitute an important new principle for clinical pain treatment, and several new options for pharmacologic intervention will be open. It is for patients suffering from chronic pain that the need for new treatment strategies is most urgent. The development of an effective pharmacologic treatment for these patients would represent a fundamental breakthrough in clinical pain treatment. The use of ketamine for the treatment of neuropathic pain is inspiring and useful in order to study what kind of chronic pain may benefit from NMDA receptor blockade, although ketamine probably cannot be used as a therapeutic on a larger scale. The major concern is the psychotomimetic side effect produced by drugs that interfere with the NMDA receptor complex. As the NMDA receptor is widely distributed in the central nervous system, and is involved in a number of neuronal processes, it is difficult to use this class of drugs systemically. Other routes of administration, e.g., spinal, may circumvent the problem, though in so doing will limit its clinical use. Molecular cloning of the genes for the NMDA receptor as well as for other EAA receptors has revealed that the receptors consist of a number of subunits, and the variability in the way these subunits combine may represent a molecular basis for functional diversity of the receptors (87), and hence a way to identify antagonists acting specifically on receptors involved in pain processing. Furthermore, the role of the different modulatory sites at the NMDA receptor has not yet been explored, and the development of drugs exerting a specific action on these sites may also be a way to separate therapeutic effects from side effects. Finally, even though each of these potential approaches per se may not be sufficient to reveal pain, it is possible that synergistic effects can be obtained by their combination or when combined with drugs acting at other receptor systems involved in pain transmission.

The last 10 years of research in the functioning of the NMDA receptor complex and its role in modulating and transmitting nociceptive information has indeed expanded our knowledge of pain physiology and pathophysiology, as well as shown the need for further research on the issue. The future challenge is to apply this new knowledge to the development of novel treatment strategies for pain treatment.

ACKNOWLEDGMENTS

This work is supported by the Swedish Medical Research Council, grant no. 9077, and the Lions Fund for Cancer Research.

REFERENCES

1. Anis NA, Berry SC, Burton NR, Lodge D. The dissociative anesthetics ketamine and phencyclidine selectively reduce excitation of central mammalian neurones by N-methylaspartate. *Br J Pharmacol* 1983;79:565–575.
2. Arnér S, Meyerson BA. Lack of analgesic effect of opioids on neuropathic and idiopathic forms of pain. *Pain* 1988;33:11–23.
3. Backonja M, Arndt G, Gombar KA, Check B, Zimmermann M. Response of chronic neuropathic pain syndromes to ketamine: a preliminary study. *Pain* 1994;56:51–57.
4. Baringa M. Is nitric oxide the "retrograde messenger"? *Science* 1991;254:1296–1297.
5. Ben-Ari Y, Aniksztejn L, Bregestovski P. Protein kinase C modulation of NMDA currents: an important link for LTP induction. *TINS* 1992;15:333–339.
6. Björkman R. Central antinociceptive effects of non-steroidal anti-inflammatory drugs and paracetamol. *Acta Anaesthesiol Scand* 1995; 39(suppl):1–44.
7. Björkman R, Hallman KM, Hedner J, Hedner T, Henning M. Acetaminophen blocks spinal hyperalgesia induced by NMDA and substance P. *Pain* 1994;57:259–265.
8. Carter C, Rivy JP, Scatton B. Ifenprodil and SL 82.0715 are antagonists at the polyamine site of the N-methyl-D-aspartate (NMDA) receptor. *Eur J Pharmacol* 1989;164:611–612.
9. Caudle RM, Isaac L. A novel interaction between dynorphin(1-13) and an N-methyl-D-aspartate site. *Brain Res* 1988;443:329–332.
10. Chen L, Huang LYM. Protein kinase C reduces Mg_{2+} block of NMDA-receptor channels as a mechanism of modulation. *Nature* 1992;356:521–523.
11. Choi DW, Peters S, Viseskul V. Dextrorphan and levorphanol selectively block N-methyl-D-aspartate receptor-mediated neurotoxicity on cortical neurons. *J Pharmacol Exp Ther* 1987;242:713–720.
12. Clausen L, Sinclair DM, Van Hasselt CH. Intravenous ketamine for postoperative analgesia. *South Afr Med J* 1975;49:1437–1440.
12a. Clements JA, Nimmo WS. Pharmacokinetics and analgesic effects of ketamine in man. *Br J Anaesth* 1981;53:27–30.
13. Coderre TJ. Potent analgesia induced in rats by combined action at PCP and polyamine recognition sites of the NMDA receptor complex. *Eur J Neurosci* 1993;5:390–393.
14. Cotman CW, Monaghan DT, Ganong AH. Excitatory amino acid neurotransmission: NMDA receptors and Hebb-type synaptic plasticity. *Annu Rev Neurosci* 1988;11:61–80.
15. Dahl JB, Hansen BL, Hjortsø N-C, Erichsen CJ, Møiniche S, Kehlet H. Influence of timing on the effect of continuous extradural analgesia with bupivacaine and morphine after major abdominal surgery. *Br J Anaesth* 1992;69:4–8.
16. Dich NJ, Svendsen LB, Berthelsen P. Intramuscular low-dose ketamine versus pethidine for postoperative pain treatment after thoracic surgery. *Acta Anaesthesiol Scand* 1992;36:583–587.
17. Domino EF, Chodoff P, Corssen G. Pharmacologic effects of CI-581, a new dissociative anesthetic, in man. *Clin Pharmacol Ther* 1965;6:279–291.
18. Dubner R, Ruda MA. Activity-dependent neuronal plasticity following tissue injury and inflammation. *Trends Neurosci* 1992;15:96–103.
19. Dunbar SA, Yaksh TL. Intrathecal MK801 attenuates intrathecal morphine tolerance and withdrawal in the rat. *Anesthesiology* 1994; 81:A838.
19a. Dunbar SA, Buerkle H, Yaksh TL. Spinal infusion of NMDA antagonist MK801 attenuates spinal tolerance to the alpha2 agonist ST91 in the rat. *Anesth Analg* 1996;in press.
19b. Edwards ND, Fletcher A, Cole JR, Peacock JE. Combined infusions of morphine and ketamine for postoperative pain in elderly patients. *Anaesthesia* 1993;48:124–127.
20. Eide PK, Jørum E, Stubhaug A, Bremnes J, Breivik H. Relief of post-herpetic neuralgia with the N-methyl-D-aspartic acid receptor antagonist ketamine: a double-blind, cross-over comparison with morphine and placebo. *Pain* 1994;58:347–354.
21. Eisenach JC, Gebhart GF. Intrathecal amitriptyline acts as an N-methyl-D-aspartate receptor antagonist in the presence of inflammatory hyperalgesia in rats. *Anesthesiology* 1995;83:1046–1054.

21a. Elliott K, Minami N, Kolesnikov YA, Pasternak GW. The NMDA receptor antagonists, LY274614 and MK-801, and the nitric oxide synthase inhibitor, NG-nitro-L-arginine, attenuate analgesic tolerance to the mu-opioid morphine but not to kappa opioids. *Pain* 1994;56:69–75.
22. Fagg GE, Massieu L. Excitatory amino acid receptor subtypes. In: Meldrum BS, eds. *Excitatory amino acid antagonists.* Oxford: Blackwell Scientific, 1991;39–63.
23. Garthwaite J, Garthwaite G, Palmer RM, Moncada S. NMDA receptor activation induces nitric oxide synthesis from arginine in brain slices. *Eur J Pharmacol* 1989;172:413–416.
24. Gean PW, Huang CC, Hung CR, Tsai JJ. Valproic acid suppresses the synaptic response mediated by the NMDA receptors in rat amygdalar slices. *Brain Res Bull* 1994;33:333–336.
25. Geppetti P, DelBianco E, Tramontana M, Vigano M, Folco GC, Maggi CA, Manzini S, et al. Arachidonic acid and bradykinin share a common pathway to release neuropeptide from capsaicin-sensitive sensory nerve fibers of the guinea pig heart. *J Pharmacol Exp Ther* 1991;259:759–765.
26. Grant IS, Nimmo WS, Clements JA. Pharmacokinetics and analgesic effects of i.m. and oral ketamine. *Br J Anaesth* 1981;53: 805–810.
27. Hagelin A, Lundberg D. Ketamine for postoperative analgesia after upper abdominal surgery. *Clin Ther* 1981;4:229–233.
28. Hargreaves RJ, Rigby M, Smith D, Hill RG. Lack of effect of L-687,414 ((+)-cis-4-methyl-HA-966), an NMDA receptor antagonist acting at the glycine site, on cerebral glucose metabolism and cortical neuronal morphology. *Br J Pharmacol* 1993;110:36–42.
29. Hartvig P, Valtysson J, Lindner CJ, Kristensen JD, Karlsten R, Gustafsson L, Persson J , et al. CNS effects of subdissociative doses of (S)-ketamine are related to plasma and brain concentrations measured with positron emission tomography in healthy volunteers. *Clin Pharmacol Ther* 1995;58:165–173.
30. Hedner T, Qian-Ling G, Hedner J, Samuelsson H. Involvement of nitric oxide (NO) in nociceptive processing in the rat (abstract). Scandinavian Association for the Study of Pain, 1991, 15th Annual Meeting.
31. Hoffmann V, Coppejans H, Vercauteren M, Adriaensen H. Successful treatment of postherpetic neuralgia with oral ketamine. *Clin J Pain* 1994;10:240–242.
32. Jahangir SM, Islam F, Aziz L. Ketamine infusion for postoperative analgesia in asthmatics: a comparison with intermittent meperidine. *Anesth Analg* 1993;76:45–49.
33. Jensen TS, Yaksh TL. Brainstem excitatory amino acid receptors in nociception: Microinjection mapping and pharmacological characterization of glutamate-sensitive sites in the brainstem associated with algogenic behavior. *Neuroscience* 1992;46:535–547.
33a. Joachimsson P-O, Hedstrand U, Eklund A. Low-dose ketamine infusion for analgesia during postoperative ventilator treatment. *Acta Anaesthesiol Scand* 1986;30:697–702.
34. Jurna I, Spohrer B, Bock R. Intrathecal injection of acetylsalicylic acid, salicylic acid and indomethacin depress C fibre evoked activity in the rat thalamus and spinal cord. *Pain* 1992;49:249–256.
35. Karlsten R, Gordh T. An A1-selective adenosine agonist abolishes allodynia elicited be vibration and touch after intrathecal injection. *Anesth Analg* 1995;80:844–847.
36. Kiedrowski L, Costa E, Wroblewski JT. Glutamate receptor agonists stimulate nitric oxide synthetase in primary cultures of cerebellar granule cells. *J Neurochem* 1992;58:335–341.
37. Klepstad P, Maurset A, Moberg ER, Oye I. Evidence of a role for NMDA receptors in pain perception. *Eur J Pharmacol* 1990;187: 513–518.
38. Kolesnikov YA, Pick CG, Pasternak GW. NG-nitro-L-arginine prevents morphine tolerance. *Eur J Pharmacol* 1992;221:399–400.
39. Kristensen JD, Svensson B, Gordh TJ. The NMDA-receptor antagonist CPP abolishes neurogenic 'wind-up pain' after intrathecal administration in humans. *Pain* 1992;51:249–253.
40. Krystal JH, Karper LP, Seibyl JP, Freeman GK, Delaney R, Bremner JD, Heninger GR, et al. Subanesthetic effects of the noncompetitive NMDA antagonist, ketamine, in humans. Psychotomimetic, perceptual, cognitive, and neuroendocrine responses. *Arch Gen Psychiatry* 1994;51:199–214.
41. Kutsuwada T, Kashiwabuchi N, Mori H, Sakimura K, Kushiya E, Araki K, Meguro H, et al. Molecular diversity of the NMDA receptor channel [see comments]. *Nature* 1992;358:36–41.
42. Leach MJ, Marden CM, Miller AA. Pharmacological studies of lamotrigine, a novel potential antiepileptic drug: II. Neurochemical studies on the mechanism of action. *Epilepsia* 1986;27:490–497.
43. Lerea LS, McNamara JO. Ionotropic glutamate receptor subtypes activate c-fos transcription by distinct calcium-requiring intracellular signaling pathways. *Neuron* 1993;10:31–41.
44. Lipton SA. Prospects for clinically tolerated NMDA antagonists: open-channel blockers and alternative redox states of nitric oxide. *Trends Neurosci* 1993;12:527–532.
45. Lodge D, Johnson KM. Noncompetitive excitatory amino acid receptor antagonists. *Trends Pharmacol Sci* 1990;11:81–86.
46. MacDermott AB, Mayer ML, Westbrook GL, Smith SJ, Barker JL. NMDA-receptor activation increases cytoplasmic calcium concentration in cultured spinal cord neurones [published erratum appears in *Nature* 1986;321(6073):888]. *Nature* 1986;321:519–522.
47. Malmberg AB, Yaksh TL. Hyperalgesia mediated by spinal glutamate or SP receptor blocked by spinal cyclooxygenase inhibition. *Science* 1992;257:1276–1279.
47a. Malmberg AB, and Yaksh TL. Spinal nitric oxide synthesis inhibition blocks NMDA-induced thermal hyperalgesia and produces antinociception in the formalin test in rats. *Pain* 1993;54:291–300.
48. Malmberg AB, Yaksh TL. Cyclooxygenase inhibition and the spinal release of prostaglandin E_2 and amino acids evoked by paw formalin injection: a microdialysis study in anesthetized rats. *J Neurosci* 1995;15:2768–2776.
49. Mankowitz E, Brock-Utne JG, Cosnett JE, Green-Thompson R. Epidural ketamine. *S Afr Med J* 1982;61:441–442.
50. Mao J, Price DD, Hayes RL, Lu J, Mayer DJ, Frenk H. Intrathecal treatment with dextrorphan or ketamine potently reduces pain-related behaviors in a rat model of peripheral mononeuropathy. *Brain Res* 1993;605:164–168.
51. Maurset A, Skoglund LA, Hustveit O, Oye I. Comparison of ketamine and pethidine in experimental and postoperative pain. *Pain* 1989;36:37–41.
52. Mayer ML, Vyklicky LJ, Clements J. Regulation of NMDA receptor desensitization in mouse hippocampal neurons by glycine. *Nature* 1989;338:425–427.
53. Mayer ML, Westbrook GL, Guthrie PB. Voltage-dependent block by Mg^{2+} of NMDA responses in spinal cord neurones. *Nature* 1984; 309:261–263.
54. McCabe RT, Wasterlain GG, Kucharczyk N, Sofia RD, Vogel JR. Evidence for anticonvulsant and neuroprotectant action of felbamate mediated by strychnine-insensitive glycine receptors. *J Pharmacol Exp Ther* 1993;264:1248–1252.
55. McQuay HJ, Carroll D, Jadad AR, Glynn CJ, Jack T, More RA, Wiffen PJ. Dextromethorphan for the treatment of neuropathic pain: a double-blind randomised controlled crossover trial with integral n-of-1 design. *Pain* 1994;59:127–133.
56. McQuay HJ, Dickenson AH. Implications of nervous system plasticity for pain management. *Anaesthesia* 1990;45:110–102.
57. Meller ST, Gebhart GF. Nitric oxide (NO) and nociceptive processing in the spinal cord. *Pain* 1993;52:127–136.
58. Miller B, Sarantis M, Traynelis SF, Attwell D. Potentiation of NMDA receptor currents by arachidonic acid. *Nature* 1992;355: 722–725.
59. Mocanda S, Palmer RJM, Higgs EA. Nitric oxide: physiology, pathophysiology and pharmacology. *Pharmacol Rev* 1991;43: 109–142.
60. Monaghan DT, Bridges RJ, Cotman CW. The excitatory amino acid receptors: Their classes, pharmacology, and distinct properties in the function of the central nervous system. *Annu Rev Pharmacol Toxicol* 1989;29:365–402.
61. Monyer H, Sprengel R, Schoepfer R, Herb A, Higuchi M, Lomeli H, Burnashev N, et al. Heteromeric NMDA receptors: molecular and functional distinction of subtypes. *Science* 1992;256:1217–1221.
62. Morgan JI, Curran T. Stimulus transcription coupling in neurons: role of cellular immediate-early genes. *Trends Neurosci* 1989;12: 459–462.
63. Moriyoshi K, Masu M, Ishii T, Shigemoto R, Mizuno N, Nakanishi S. Molecular cloning and characterization of the rat NMDA receptor [see comments]. *Nature* 1991;354:31–37.
64. Nakamura-Craig M, Follenfant RL. Lamotrigine and analogs: a new treatment for chronic pain? In: Gebhart GF, Hammond DL, Jensen TS, eds. *Proceedings of the 7th World Congress on Pain.* Seattle: IASP Press, 1994;725–730.
65. Neugebauer V, Kornhuber J, Lucke T, Schaible HG. The clinically available NMDA receptor antagonist memantine is antinociceptive on rat spinal neurones. *Neuroreport* 1993;4:1259–1262.
66. Nishizuka Y. Studies and perspectives of protein kinase C. *Science* 1986;233:305–312.
67. Nowak G, Trullas R, Layer RT, Skolnick P, Paul IA. Adaptive

changes in the N-methyl-D-aspartate receptor complex after chronic treatment with imipramine and 1-aminocyclopropanecarboxylic acid. *J Pharmacol Exp Ther* 1993;265:1380–1386.

68. Nowak L, Bregestovski P, Ascher P, Herbet A, Prochiantz A. Magnesium gates glutamate-activated channels in mouse central neurones. *Nature* 1984;307:462–465.
69. Oblin A, Schoemaker H. Complex allosteric modulation of the binding of the NMDA receptor antagonist [3H]CGP39653. *Eur J Pharmacol* 1994;266:103–106.
70. Parsons CG, Gruner R, Rozental J, Millar J, Lodge D. Patch clamp studies on the kinetics and selectivity of N-methyl-D-aspartate receptor antagonism by memantine (1-amino-3,5-dimethyladamantan). *Neuropharmacology* 1993;32:1337–1350.
71. Perkins MN, Stone TW. Action of kynurenic acid and quinolinic acid in the rat hippocampus in vivo. *Exp Neurol* 1985;88:570–579.
72. Persson J, Axelsson G, Hallin RG, Gustafsson LL. Beneficial effects of ketamine in a chronic pain state with allodynia, possibly due to central sensitization. *Pain* 1995;60:217–222.
73. Price DD, Mao J, Frenk H, Mayer DJ. The N-methyl-D-aspartate receptor antagonist dextromethorphan selectively reduces temporal summation of second pain in man. *Pain* 1994;59:165–174.
74. Pryle BJ, Vanner RG, Enriquez N, Reynolds F. Can pre-emptive lumbar epidural blockade reduce postoperative pain following lower abdominal surgery. *Anesthesia* 1993;48:120–123.
75. Ransom RW, Stec NL. Cooperative modulation of [3H]MK-801 binding to the N-methyl-D-aspartate receptor-ion channel complex by L-glutamate, glycine, and polyamines. *J Neurochem* 1988;51:830–836.
76. Raymond LA, Blackstone CD, Huganir RL. Phosphorylation and modulation of recombinant GluR6 glutamate receptors by cAMP-dependent protein kinase. *Nature* 1993;361:637–641.
77. Ren K, Hylden JLK, Williams GM, Ruda MA, Dubner R. The effect of a non-competitive NMDA receptor antagonist, MK-801, on behavioral hyperalgesia and dorsal horn neuronal activity in rats with unilateral inflammation. *Pain* 1992;50:331–344.
78. Reynolds IJ, Miller RJ. Tricyclic antidepressants block N-methyl-D-aspartate receptors: similarities to the action of zinc. *Br J Pharmacol* 1988;95:95–102.
79. Rho JM, Donevan SD, Rogawski MA. Mechanism of action of the anticonvulsant felbamate: opposing effects on N-methyl-D-aspartate and gamma-aminobutyric acidA receptors. *Ann Neurol* 1994;35:229–234.
80. Rothman SM, Olney JW. Glutamate and the pathophysiology of hypoxic-ischemic brain damage. *Ann Neurol* 1986;19:105–111.
81. Roytblat L, Korotkoruchko A, Katz J, Glazer M, Greemberg L, Fisher A. Postoperative pain: the effect of low-dose ketamine in addition to general anesthesia. *Anesth Analg* 1993;77:1161–1165.
82. Sadove MS, Shulman M, Hatano S, Fevold N. Analgesic effects of ketamine administered in subdissociative doses. *Anesth Analg* 1971;50:452–457.
83. Scoepp DD, Conn PJ. Metabotropic glutamate receptors in brain function and pathology. *Trends Pharmacol Sci* 1993;14:13–20.
84. Segerdahl M, Ekblom A, Sollevi A. The influence of adenosine, ketamine, and morphine on experimentally induced ischemic pain in healthy volunteers. *Anesth Analg* 1994;79:787–791.
85. Sernagor E, Kuhn D, Vyklicky LJ, Mayer ML. Open channel block of NMDA receptor responses evoked by tricyclic antidepressants. *Neuron* 1989;2:1221–1227.
86. Sosnowski M, Yaksh TL. Role of spinal adenosine receptors in modulating the hyperesthesia produced by spinal glycine receptor antagonism. *Anesth Analg* 1989;69:587–592.
87. Sprengel R, Seeburg PH. The unique properties of glutamate receptor channels. *FEBS Lett* 1993;325:90–94.
88. Stannard CF, Porter GE. Ketamine hydrochloride in the treatment of phantom limb pain. *Pain* 1993;54:227–230.
89. Sugiyama H, Ito I, Hirono C. A new type of glutamate receptor linked to inositol phospholipid metabolism. *Nature* 1987;325:531–533.
90. Szekely AM, Barbaccia ML, Alho H, Costa E. In primary cultures of cerebellar granule cells the activation of N-methyl-D-aspartate-sensitive glutamate receptors induces c-fos mRNA expression. *Mol Pharmacol* 1989;35:401–408.
91. Tal M, Bennett GJ. Dextrorphan relieves neuropathic heat-evoked hyperalgesia in the rat. *Neurosci Lett* 1993;151:107–10.
92. Torebjørk E. Nociceptor modulation of central sensitization to tactile stimuli. In: Bovie J, Hansson P, Lindblom U, eds. *Touch, temperature, and pain in health and disease.* Seattle: IASP Press, 1994.
92a. Trujillo KA, Akil H Inhibition of morphine tolerance and dependance by the NMDA receptor antagonist MK-801. *Science* 1991;251:85–87.
93. Tverskoy M, Oz Y, Isakson A, Finger J, Bradley EJ, Kissin I. Preemptive effect of fentanyl and ketamine on postoperative pain and wound hyperalgesia [see comments]. *Anesth Analg* 1994;78:205–209.
94. Urquhart E. Central analgesic activity of non-steroidal anti-inflammatory drugs in animal and human pain models. *Semin Arthritis Rheum* 1993;23:198–205.
94b. Wadelius M, Karlsson T, Wadelius C, Rane A: Lamotrigine and toxic epidermal necrolysis. *The Lancet* 1996;348:1041.
95. Vajda FJE. New anticonvulsants. *Curr Opin Neurol Neurosurg* 1992;5:519–525.
96. Watanabe Y, Saito H, Abe K. Tricyclic antidepressants block NMDA receptor-mediated synaptic responses and induction of long-term potentiation in rat hippocampal slices. *Neuropharmacology* 1993;32:479–486.
97. Wesemann W, Sturm G, Fünfgeld EW. Distribution and metabolism of the potential anti-Parkinson drug memantine in the human. *J Neural Transm* 1980;16(suppl):143–148.
98. Wilson WA, Stasheff S, Swartzwelder S, Clark S, Anderson WW, Lewis D. The NMDA receptor in epilepsy. In: Watkins JC, Collingridge GL, eds. *The NMDA receptor.* Oxford: Oxford University Press, 1990;167–176.
99. Woolf CJ. Recent advances in the pathophysiology of acute pain. *Br J Anaesth* 1989;63:139–146.
100. Woolf CJ. Central mechanisms of acute pain. In: Bond MR, Charlton JE, Woolf CJ, eds. *Pain research and clinical management, vol. 4, Proc. VI World Congress on Pain.* Amsterdam: Elsevier Science, 1991;25–34.
101. Yaksh TL, Chaplan SR, Malmberg AB. Future directions in the pharmacological management of hyperalgesic and allodynic pain states: the NMDA receptor. In: Chiang CN, Finnegan LP, eds. *Medications development for the treatment of pregnant addicts and their infants.* NIDA Research Monograph Series #149. Rockville, MD: US Dept. of Health and Human Services, 1995.
101a. Yaksh TL, Malmberg AB. Central pharmacology of nociceptive transmission. In: Wall P, Melzack R, eds. *Textbook of Pain,* 3rd ed. Edinburgh, UK: Churchill Livingstone, 1994;165–200.
101b. Yamamoto T, Yaksh TL. Spinal pharmacology of thermal hyperesthesia induced by constriction injury of sciatic nerve. Excitatory amino acid antagonists. *Pain* 1992;49:121–128.
102. Yamamura T, Harada K, Okamura A, Kemmotsu O. Is the site of action of ketamine anesthesia the N-methyl-D-aspartate receptor? *Anesthesiology* 1990;72:704–10.
103. Øye I, Paulsen O, Mauerset A. Effects of ketamine on sensory perception: evidence for a role of N-methyl-D-aspartate receptors. *J Pharmacol Exp Ther* 1991;260:1209–1213.

Anesthesia: Biologic Foundations, edited by Tony L. Yaksh et al. Lippincott–Raven Publishers, Philadelphia © 1997.

CHAPTER 61

ANTIPYRETIC-ANALGESIC DRUGS

KAY BRUNE AND TONY L. YAKSH

ANTIPYRETIC ANALGESICS

After tissue injury, there is the appearance of repetitive activity in small primary afferent neurons that are otherwise silent (see Chap. 3). Moreover, because of the changes in the chemical milieu around the afferent terminal, there is an increase in the sensitivity of the terminal to otherwise subthreshold stimuli. The appearance of spontaneous afferent activity and facilitated responding has been shown to alter central processing at both the spinal and supraspinal level (see Chaps. 36 and 40). Behaviorally, the spontaneous activity and the facilitated processing lead to a condition in which a continuing pain state is reported and otherwise subthreshold stimuli are found to evoke pain, that is, this situation reflects a state of hyperalgesia. Early research revealed that different classes of agents known to be antifebrile would also yield an attenuation of the hyperalgesic components, that is, they would serve to normalize the pain threshold. Such effects were observed to occur without remarkable changes in consciousness or perception. Although these agents varied considerably in structure, they were considered to form a therapeutically useful class of agents that was designated, because of the agents' common actions, as antipyretic analgesics (54). Because many members of this functional class display antiinflammatory properties but are clearly acting by mechanism other than those employed by steroids, these agents are often referred to as a nonsteroidal antiinflammatory agents (NSAIDs). While this is a common acronym many of these agents have actually only modest antiinflammatory actions.

In any case, these characteristics typically serve to differentiate these drugs from opioids, which, beside their analgesic actions, also have sedative and euphoric effects. The terms used in the literature, such as *nonopioid analgesics* and *weak analgesics,* are misnomers, because they imply that they have only a modest effect upon pain processing. As will be noted, there are a variety of pain states in which these agents have proven to be extraordinarily efficacious, e.g., in rheumatic diseases, cancer, and in posttraumatic injury.

While the diverse chemical structures indicate the likelihood of diverse actions, a common factor that links the physiologic actions of these agents is their ability to antagonize the synthesis of prostaglandins. This insight had the dual consequence of providing a unifying hypothesis for the actions of the agents and for underlining the powerful role played by these lipidic acids in the inflammatory state and in central neurotransmission processes.

HISTORY

The Roman and Greek military field physicians were using extracts from the willow and poplar for the treatment of painful injuries and rheumatic complaints, probably arthrosis (Dioscorides of Anazarbos, a 1st century A.D. botanist and physician). According to numerous traditions, such extracts were used for similar indications in the Middle Ages (100). Hildegard von Bingen, for example, describes in her herbal books the use of willow bark and leaves for treating pain, inflammation, and fever (12th century). The Reverend E. Stone became famous through a letter to the Royal Society of Medicine in 1763, in which he communicated that such an extract relieved his gouty pains. He presumed that the willow, which was known to grow on marshy areas, had absorbed the healing power of the swamp and thus could mediate a therapeutic action. The first clear description of the principles of action of willow extract is from Piria in Italy in 1838, after the Frenchman Leroux in 1829 identified salicin in plant extracts as the first precursor of salicylic acid. Kolbe, in Germany, finally succeeded in establishing a synthetic method to produce salicylic acid in 1874. von Heyden, one of Kolbe's pupils, built the first industrial facility to produce salicylic acid near Dresden in 1877. Stricker, in Berlin, introduced salicylic acid to the therapy of the rheumatic diseases in 1876. His paper appeared two months before similar data from MacLagan were published in the Lancet. The chemist Hoffmann (1897) synthesized acetylsalicylic acid (ASA) from salicylic acid on an industrial scale because his father was a rheumatic patient who had been taking between 10 and 15 g of salicylate in powder form and had found the acetylated product to be more acceptable. In the 1950s phenylbutazone, which served as an acidic partner in a water-soluble complex with aminophenazone, was recognized as the most active known antiinflammatory drug. The systematic search for antiinflammatory drugs using animal experiments led in the 1960s, 1970s, and 1980s to preparation of numerous antiinflammatory analgesic acids such as indomethacin, ibuprofen, diclofenac, naproxen, and piroxicam, to name only the most important in the sequence of their discovery.

Phenazone, a nonacidic agent, was discovered and synthesized more or less accidentally in Erlangen, Germany. The later Nobel Prize winner Emil Fischer had developed methods to synthesize ring structures containing nitrogen using phenylhydrazine. His pupil Knorr tried to produce chinolin by these techniques in order to obtain a synthetic antipyretic drug. The pharmacologic studies of his agents, carried out by the pharmacologist Filehne also in Erlangen, showed that some methyl-substituted ring structures possess antipyretic activity. One of the most successful products of synthesis was phenazone, named antipyrine by Knorr and Filehne. It was the first purely synthetic drug in the world. Its introduction as an antipyretic and later also as an analgesic drug led to the discovery of phenazone derivatives, that are still used every year in ton quantities.

Finally, acetanilid, the predecessor of paracetamol, was discovered in Strasbourg by the clinicians Cahn and Hepp through an error of their supplying pharmacy. They had ordered naphthalene as a therapy against worms. They received acetanilid instead. The worms survived. The patient, however, presented with decreasing fever. Acetanilid was introduced as antifebrin, but was later replaced by phenacetin, a better-tolerated derivative, and finally by paracetamol (acetaminophen), which is believed to be safer.

CLASSIFICATION OF ANTIPYRETIC ANALGESICS

While a large number of agents have been synthesized that fall into the functional class of antipyretic analgesics, they may be largely subdivided into several principal subgroups. On the one hand, there are a series of acidic agents that derive primarily from salicylic and acetylsalicylic acids. They possess in common some presumably essential physicochemical properties, including lipophilic-hydrophilic polarity, a pKa between 3 and 6 and a very high protein binding in human and animal organisms (Table 1). To this group belong, from the chemical point of view, salicylates, arylacetic acids, arylpropionic acids, fenamates, and different keto-enolic acids including the oxicams and phenylbutazone.

A second group consists of nonacidic derivatives of phenazone including prodrugs such as metamizol (dipyrone). This group has different physicochemical characteristics, e.g., its representatives are neutral or moderately alkaline, bind only in limited proportion to plasma proteins, and do not have hydrophilic-lypophilic polarity (Table 2). A third group consists to date of only one drug, paracetamol (acetaminophen), an almost neutral substance with limited polarity and protein binding (Table 2).

Important for the therapy of pain is the classification into acids on the one hand and nonacidic compounds on the other, because the acidic antipyretic analgesics show clear antiinflammatory effects at therapeutic doses, while the nonacidic agents exert only analgesic effects at such doses. A possible explanation for these differences is presented in the following sections.

NOCICEPTOR SENSITIZATION BY PROSTANOIDS

In the early 1960s, it was appreciated that cellular injury could give rise to the elaboration of lipidic acids that was syn-

Table 1. ACIDIC ANTIPYRETIC ANALGESICS (= ANTI-INFLAMMATORY ANTIPYRETIC ANALGESICS, NSAIDS): CHEMICAL CLASSES, STRUCTURES, PHYSICO-CHEMICAL AND PHARMACOLOGICAL DATA, THERAPEUTIC DOSAGE

Chemical class Monosubstance (subclass)	Structure	pK_a	Plasma protein binding	$t_{1/2}$[a]	t_{max}[b]	bioavailability	Daily Oraldosage in adults
Salicylates							
Acetylsalicylic acid		3,5	50–70%	~0,25 h	~0,25 h	50–70%	1–4 g
Salicylic acid (active metabolite)		2,9	80–95% dose dependent	2,5–4,5 h dose dependent	0,5–2 h	80–100%	—
Diflunisal	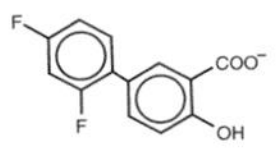	3,3	98–99,9% dose dependent	9–13 h dose dependent	2–3 h	80–100%	1 g
Arylacetic acids							
Indomethacin (Indolacetate)	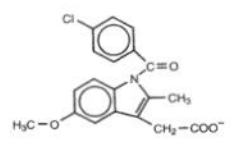	4,3	90–99%	2–3 h (~11 h) very variable EHC[c]	1–2 h	~100%	50–150 mg
Diclofenac (Fenac-class)	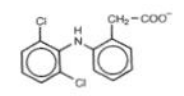	3,9	99,7%	1–2 h	1–12 h very variable	30–80% first pass	50–150 mg
Arylpropionic acids (Profen-class)							
Ibuprofen	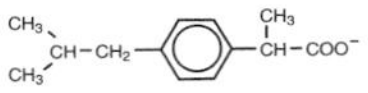	4,6	99,5%	1,5–2,5 h	0,5–2 h	80–100%	0,6–2,4 g
Ketoprofen	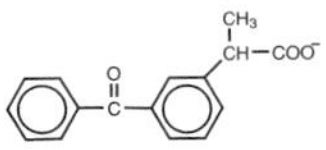	5,3	99,2%	1,5–2,5 h (~8 h)	1–2 h	~100%	150–200 mg
Naproxen	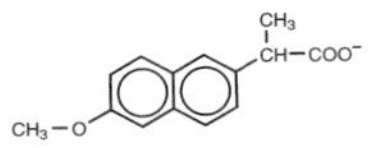	4,1	99,7%	13–15 h	2–4 h	90–100%	0,5–1 g
Flurbiprofen	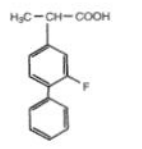	4,2	>99%	2,5–4 h (-8 h)	1,5–3 h	no data	150–200 mg
Keto-enol acids							
Piroxicam (Oxicam)	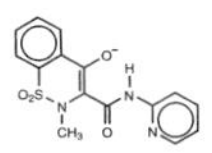	5,9	99,3%	14–160 h (~50 h) very variable EHC[c]	~2 h 2. Peak: 4–8 h	~100%	20 mg initially: 40 mg
Azapropazone	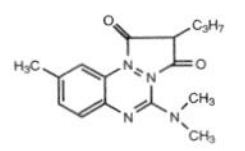	6,5	90–99%	9–17 h	4–6 h	80–95%	0,6–1,2 g
Phenylbutazone (Pyrazolidindione)	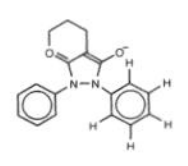	4,8	96–99%	24–96 h (~75 h) very variable ECH[c]	2–5 h	80–100%	0,2 g initially: 0.4 g

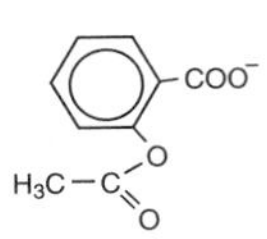

[a]Terminal half-life of elimination.
[b]Time to reach maximum plasma concentration after oral administration.
[c]EHC, enterohepatic circulation.

Table 2. NONACIDIC ANALGESICS: CHEMICAL CLASSES, STRUCTURES, PHARMACOKINETIC DATA, THERAPEUTIC DOSAGE

Chemical class Monosubstance	Structure	Plasma protein binding	$t_{½}$[a]	t_{max}[b]	Oral bioavailability	Daily dosage in adults
Aniline derivatives						
Paracetamol (acetaminophen)	NHCOCH₃ / OH	5–50% dose dependent	1,5–2,5 h	0,5–1,5 h	70–100% dose dependent	1–4 g
Pyrazolinone[c]						
Phenazone (antipyrine)		<10%	11–12 h	0,5—2 h	~100% dose dependent	1–4 g
Propyphenazone (isopropylantipyrine)		~10%	1–2,5 h	0,5–1,5 h	~100% dose dependent	1–4 g
Metamizole-Na (dipyrone-Na)[d]		<20%	—	—	—	1–4 g
4-MAP[e]		58%	2–4 h	1–2 h	~100%	—
4-AP[f] (active metabolites)		48%	4—5,5 h			—

[a]Terminal half-life of elimination.
[b]Time to reach maximum plasma concentration after oral administration.
[c]Terms like pyrazole and, incorrectly, pyrazolone are also in use.
[d]Noraminopyrinemethanosulfonate-Na.
[e]4-MAP, 4-methylaminophenazone.
[f]4-AP, 4-aminophenazone.

thesized in the presence of molecular oxygen. Early chemistry emphasized, on the basis of structure and bioassay, that these lipidic acids constituted a large and functionally diverse family (Fig. 1). An important observation was that essential to their formation was a membrane-bound intracellular enzyme that was necessary for the insertion of the oxygen in to the structure. This enzyme was referred to as cyclooxygenase (105).

At the end of the 1960s, Vane (121) and Smith and Willis (110) demonstrated that ASA and other analgesic acids (but not salicylic acid) acted as potent inhibitors of the synthesis of the lipidic acid products prostaglandins by a competitive and noncompetitive interaction with the membrane-bound cyclooxygenase (121–123). Given the elevated levels of prostaglandins in inflamed tissues, and the ability of prostanoids to produce marked sensitization, it was concluded that inhibition of the inhibition of prostaglandin synthesis was the principal mechanism of NSAID/antipyretic analgesic drug action. The structure of the cyclooxygenase is a large globular protein, with the active site, a heme-like structure, being located at the bottom of a deep channel that is able to accept the long folded structure of the lipidic acid precursors (95). At present it is believed that the cyclooxygenase inhibitors act by preventing access of the lipidic acid to the active site.

In recent work, it has been shown that cyclooxygenase may exist as two isozymes, a constitutive form that is typically present (COX1) and an inducible form (COX2) that has been shown to appear after cellular activation of cytosolic protein kinase (45,90,133). Thus, after the induction of inflammation, there is an appearance of message for COX2 within an hour while COX2 protein will appear by several hours. Importantly, studies on the relative potency of various cyclooxygenase inhibitors have shown that the majority of the clinically useful NSAIDs have little or no selectivity for either isozyme, or at best a modest preference for COX1 (77,81). Recent work with more selective agents has indicated that both COX1 and COX2 may have an important role in regulating central and peripheral mechanisms of hyperalgesia. Importantly, as will be discussed below, at present it appears that many of the undesirable effects, such as gastric erosion are mediated by the COX1 isozyme. However, studies with COX2 knockout mice indicate that they appear to have significant kidney injury, a finding consistent with the importance of prostaglandins in renal function (see below).

It has been shown that the antiinflammatory acids, on the basis of their high protein binding and their acidic character, readily leave the blood in inflamed tissue and are sequestered therein. Here they reach particularly high-intracellular concentrations (15,17,98). Consequently they inhibit prostaglandin synthesis first of all in inflamed tissue, and thereby reduce pain and other prostaglandin-mediated or -enhanced symptoms of inflammation. While the antipyretic analgesics appear to have as a common action the ability to antagonize the production of prostaglandins, it should be emphasized that these structurally diverse agents can exert a variety of additional effects. On the basis of their local high concentrations in inflamed tissue, they are also able to interact with other processes that might alter the local excitability of the local nerve endings and curb numerous other processes. Among these many effects are activation of complement, histamine release, enhanced leukocyte invasion, and others (for review see 14). In many cases, these actions may be idiopathic for the specific agent.

MECHANISMS OF ACTION

The functional characteristics of the actions of the antipyretic analgesics and their potential effects upon inflammatory processes, mediated in part by the inhibition of cyclooxygenase, have provided presumptive insights into the mechanisms of action of this structurally heterogeneous family of agents.

Peripheral Site of Action

Systematic experiments showed that the acidic antipyretic analgesics typically produced measurable, but varying degrees of, inhibition of inflammatory and antinociceptive reactions in animal models (87). Early work emphasized that the animal models in which such agents could be shown to have measurable activity frequently possessed an inflammatory component, e.g., the pressure threshold test in the inflamed paw (89,114).

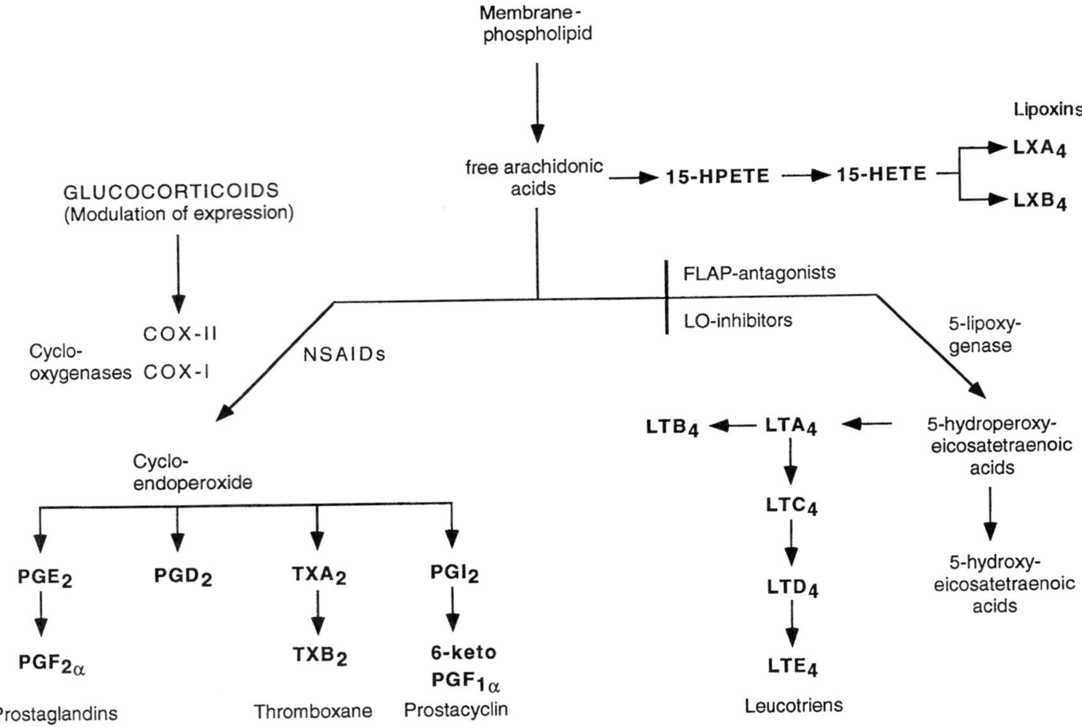

Figure 1. Eicosanoid biosynthesis; pharmacologic means of interference. As a consequence of injury to the cell by an inflammatory stimulus, free arachidonic acid is released from membrane phospholipids. The cyclooxygenases and the lipoxygenases are the key enzymes mediating the formation of prostaglandins (PGs), prostacyclin, thromboxane (TX), and leukotrienes (LTs) (together termed eicosanoids). PG synthesis is blocked by NSAIDs (inhibition of cyclooxygenases). The glucocorticoids modulate the expression of cyclooxygenases and lipoxygenases and thereby influence eicosanoid formation in several organs. By exclusively inhibiting cyclooxygenases (NSAID), there is a facilitation of the 5-lipoxygenase pathway resulting in an increase of LT synthesis. This cascade of reactions can be inhibited by FLAP (5-lipoxygenase-activating peptide) antagonists and by FLAP inhibitors. Both groups of drugs are currently under clinical evaluation. Moreover, by means of other lipoxygenases, hydroxyacids can be formed that can be further metabolized to lipoxins (LX). The biologic significance of lipoxins has not been clearly defined (HETE: hydroxyeicosatetraenoic acid; HPETE: hydroperoxyeicosa tetraenoic acid).

Such observations strongly suggested an important peripheral component. Early cross-perfusion studies in dogs by Lim (67) indicated that ASA had a peripheral action in blocking the acute algogenic behavior evoked by local delivery of bradykinin, while opiates had a central action. This association between local inflammation and the apparent actions of the antipyretic analgesics was consistent with the early appreciation that injury would lead to the release of active factors that would evoke pain when applied to the human blister base or parenterally in animals. This affiliation was emphasized by their additional designation as NSAIDs. Current work has continued to emphasize the mechanistic importance of a peripheral action. Thus, a major component of pain originates after tissue injury. Such tissue injury leads to a pain state through the stimulation of nociceptive C fibers, which terminate in the vicinity of the injury site (12,107; see Chap. 33). These nociceptors are typically believed to terminate in so-called free nerve endings. Studies defining the transduction characteristics of these free nerve endings have shown them to possess several characteristics: (a) A given afferent terminal may be activated by a variety of high intensity mechanical and thermal stimuli, as well as by a number of endogenous and exogenous chemical products. Hence, they are called polymodal nociceptors (107). (b) The frequency of the discharge will be enhanced as a function of stimulus intensity or chemical concentration. (c) Most of the C-polymodal nociceptors have little if any spontaneous activity, and large fractions of the afferents show little if any activity even under extremes of stimulus conditions. These afferents have been called "silent nociceptors" (see Chap. 33). Such silent nociceptors may display a remarkable increase in sensitivity after tissue injury. This increase in sensitivity is mediated by the release of active factors, secondary to the local tissue injury.

In the peri-injury milieu, prostaglandins are formed and released (9,36,37,50,52,118,130). Direct application of these lipidic acids can indeed stimulate and sensitize peripheral afferent terminals. However, in addition, to the prostanoids, as reviewed in Chap. 6, a variety of other products are released into the extravascular-extracellular milieu, such as protons, potassium, bradykinin, histamine, serotonin, and a variety of cytokines. These agents have also been shown to stimulate and sensitize primary afferent terminals. Importantly, the excitatory effect of several of these products (such as bradykinin) but not others (such as protons or potassium) appears to be in large part by the local release and action of prostanoids (53). This pervasive role played by prostanoids as an intermediary emphasizes that their inhibition removes a significant component of the postinjury products that act on the local afferent terminal (see Chaps. 36 and 40). Given the importance of discharge frequency in these C fibers for encoding the intensity of the afferent message, the ability of local factors to evoke spontaneous activity and to increase the sensitivity of the terminals to peripheral stimuli can be seen as exceedingly relevant to the magni-

Table 3. SITE OF ACTION AND EFFECT OF ANTIPYRETIC ANALGESICS

Monosubstance group	Main site of action for analgesia (additional sites of action)	Actions			
		Analgesic	Antipyretic	Anti-inflammatory	Spasmolytic
Acetylsalicylic acid NSAID *acidic*	Nociceptor (dorsal spinal cord)	Good	Good	Good	Limited in therapeutic dose [a]
Paracetamol Aniline derivative *nonacidic*	Dorsal spinal cord (nociceptor, brain)	Weak	Good	None in therapeutic-dose	None in therapeutic dose
Metamizol Pyrazole derivative *nonacidic*	Dorsal spinal cord (nonciceptor, brain)	Strong	Strong	Limited in therapeutic-dose	Confirmed

[a]NSAIDs act through inhibition of prostaglandin synthesis which causes relaxation of smooth muscles.

tude of the pain sensation. This model indicates in addition that these agents will have minimum effects on "normal" pain thresholds, where prostaglandins synthesis are not believed to play a role.

The correlation between drug action and the role of the attenuation of the peripheral inflammatory state provides an appropriate explanation for the historically appreciated efficacy of these agents in a variety of painful inflammatory states, such as arthritis. Yet, it was clear early that such an affiliation could not alone provide a unique mechanism of the actions of these agents as a group. Thus, it was appreciated that there was a clear dissociation between the analgesic actions of the agents and their antiinflammatory efficacy (75) (Tables 3, 4, and 5). The nonacidic antipyretic analgesics only modestly inhibit prostaglandin synthesis in inflamed tissues, and this is probably the reason they do not have an antiinflammatory effect. At similar dosage phenazone and paracetamol had only very weak (phenazone) or no activity (paracetamol) (15,18,64,121). How they mediate their analgesic effects remains at present somewhat hypothetical. Research in humans (40) illustrated a comparable spectrum of action of these drugs and confirmed the clinical experience of rheumatologists who considered the antiinflammatory acids (e.g., salicylates) as "antirheumatics," in that they reduce inflammatory signs and produce a reduction in the pain state, while agents such as phenazone and paracetamol have analgesic effects, but little effect upon inflammation.

Central Action

While it is clear that the antipyretic analgesics can exert an action on inflammation, early behavioral analyses have indicated a central analgesic effect of these drugs (13) as well. Recently, it has been demonstrated in humans and animals that electrophysiologic responses or reflexes evoked by electrical stimulation of small afferent input can be attenuated by these agents in animal models. Thus, systemically administered antipyretic analgesics suppress activity in thalamic neurons that are evoked by electrical stimulation of small primary afferents (4,21,48,57). Electrical stimulation directly activates primary afferents and thus obviates the likelihood that these agents are acting peripherally to alter facilitated transduction. Some evidence suggests that the efficacy of systemic paracetamol may depend on intact bulbospinal serotonergic pathways (117). Central effects have been similarly disclosed in humans (96, 127).

Intrathecal injection of NSAIDs at doses that are inactive after systemic administration attenuates the behavioral response to certain types of noxious stimuli, such as in models of protracted nociception (e.g., in inflammation), and diminishes spinal facilitated processing (71,72,132). A likely spinal action is supported in humans by the observations that spinal delivery of lysine acetylsalicylate was effective in late stage cancer patients (27,28,94).

The spinal effects of these antipyretic analgesics suggest that under the appropriate circumstances cyclooxygenase products may be formed and released from local systems and that they might augment the processing of nociceptive stimuli. Previous work has indeed demonstrated that repetitive small afferent input can, through the activation of spinal *N*-methyl-D-aspartate (NMDA) receptors, increase the spinal release of prostanoids (73,74,111,112). This effect is presumably mediated by an increase in phospholipase activity secondary to increased extracellular calcium. Such activation of small afferents and the spinal injection of NMDA can indeed induce a spinally mediated hyperalgesia that is attenuated by the spinal delivery of NMDA antagonists and, importantly, by spinal cyclooxygenase inhibitors (71,72). In addition, systemically administered antipyretic analgesics can in fact exert a central effect on prostaglandins release. It has been shown that parenterally delivered agents can produce a dose-dependent suppression of

Table 4. ANTIPYRETIC ANALGESIC DOSES (MG/KG BODY WEIGHT) NECESSARY FOR ACHIEVING ANALGESIC RESPONSE AND ANTI-INFLAMMATORY EFFECTS IN ANIMAL EXPERIMENTS; FOR COMPARISON, THE MINIMAL ANALGESIC DOSES (MG/KG BODY WEIGHT) USED CLINICALLY

	Acetylsalicylic acid	Indomethacin	Paracetamol	Metamizole
		Dosage in mg/kg		
Pain model: stretch spasm	~150	inactive till 2	inactive till 240	~50
Pain model: edema pain	~50	1–2	inactive till 100	inactive till 400
Inflammation model: edema inhibition	~90	~2,5	inactive till 150	inactive till 150
Clinical analgesia: minimum dose	~7	<1	~7	~5

Modified after Brune K, Müller N., Kobal G.: Methoden zur experimentellen Erfassung analgetischer Wirkungen. In: Burger O.K., Grosdanoff P., Henschler D., Kraupp O., Schnieders B. eds. (Hrsg.): *Aktuelle Probleme der Biomedizin*. Berlin, New York: de Gruyter, 1986.

Table 5. ACIDIC ANTIPYRETIC ANALGESICS (ACIDIC ANTI-INFLAMMATORY ANALGESICS, NSAIDS): INHIBITION OF PROSTAGLANDIN SYNTHESIS (IN VITRO INHIBITORY POTENCY ON CYCLOOXYGENASE, IC50-VALUE)

	Terminal half-life			
Potency: IC_{50} (-log mol/L)	**Very long: >> 24 h**	**Long: 12–18 h**	**Middle: 4–12 h**	**Short 1–4 h**
Very strong: 8–9				Indomethacin, flurbiprofen
Strong: 7–8			Tornoxicam, ketorolac	Diclofenac, ketoprofen
Intermediate: 6–7	Piroxicam, tenoxicain	Naproxen		
Weak: 3–6	Phenylbutazon	Diflunisal	Azapropazone	Ibuprofen, aspirin

evoked prostanoid release from spinal cord (74). Nonacidic antipyretic analgesics readily cross into the central nervous system (CNS) (Fig. 2), and there reduce prostanoid synthesis (Fig. 2). Since the acidic antiinflammatory analgesics also pass into the central nervous system, although more slowly, it is understandable why these agents mediate some analgesic effects in the spinal cord in addition to their clear antipyretic action in the hypothalamus.

Support for a supraspinal action of NSAIDs is also provided by the observation that intracerebroventricular delivery of several NSAIDs produce antinociception in several animal models, including the mechanical threshold with the inflamed paw (38,99), the rat hot plate (25), and the writhing response (6) and the hyperalgesic response in arthritic rats (91). Further, central injection of ketoprofen has been shown to diminish activity evoked in thalamic neurons in arthritic rats (11). Microinjection mapping studies have indicated activity in the periaqueductal gray matter, ventromedial thalamus, medial preoptic area, and the nucleus raphe magnus (7).

Finally, it should be stressed that, as in the periphery, antipyretic analgesics may have a variety of actions on mechanisms that can alter neurotransmission, by mechanisms other than an action on cyclooxygenase. Among these actions are direct effects upon G protein, hydrolysis of phosphoinositides, and interactions with the several components of the glutamate receptor (76).

CLINICAL UTILITY OF ANTIPYRETIC ANALGESICS

General Properties

The antipyretic analgesics have revealed considerable efficacy in a wide spectrum of clinical conditions in which pain is a prominent component (Table 6). Importantly, the efficacy of these agents indirectly reveals the pervasive role played by prostanoids in these various human pain conditions. This section briefly reviews the efficacy of these agents in several selected pain states.

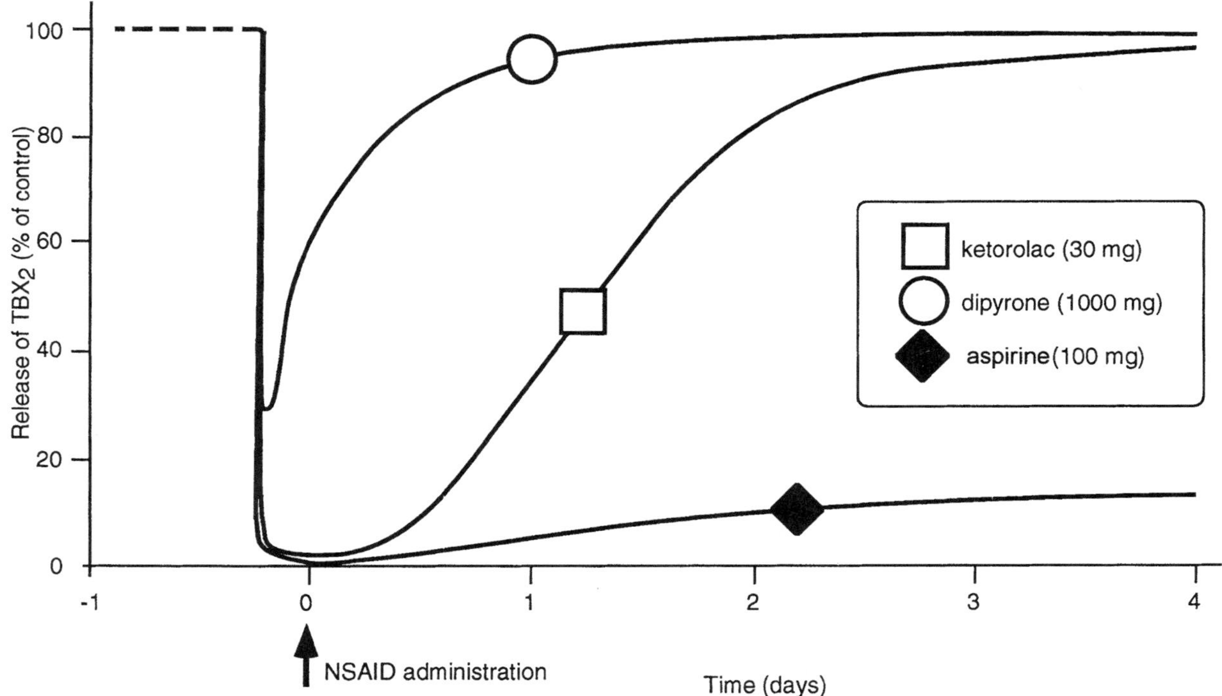

Figure 2. The influence of different NSAIDs on thrombocyte aggregation presented as inhibition of thromboxane-B_2 (TXB_2-release). Acetylsalicylic acid (aspirin) (400 mg po), leads to an intense and prolonged (many days) inhibition of thrombocyte aggregation, consequent to irreversible enzyme inhibition (acetylation of the thrombocyte cyclooxygenase). Ketorolac-trometamol (30 mg I.M.) reversibly inhibits thrombocyte aggregation for almost 2 days. Metamizole-sodium (1000 mg I.M.), has only a limited effect, which disappears after one day.

Table 6. INDICATIONS FOR ANTIPYRETIC ANALGESICS

Indications	**Acidic antipyretic analgesics (anti-inflammatory antipyretic analgesics, NSAIDs)**[a]		
Acute and chronic pain, produced by inflammation of different etiology	**High dose** **Arylacetic acids** **Arylpropionic acids** **Keto-enolic acids**	**Middle dose** **Arylacetic acids** **Arylpropionic acids** **Keto-enolic acids**	**Low dose** **Salicylates** **Arylpropionic acids**
Arthritis: chronic polyarthritis (rheumatoid arthritis) ankylosing spondilytis (Morbus Bechterew) acute gout (gout attack)	diclofenac, indomethacin ibuprofen piroxicam, (phenylbutazone)[b]	diclofenac, indomethacin ibuprofen piroxicam, (phenylbutazone)[b]	no
Cancer pain (e.g. bone metastasis)	indomethacin[c], diclofenac[c] ibuprofen[c] piroxicam[c]	indomethacin[c], diclofenac[c] ibuprofen[c] piroxicam[c]	acetylsalicylic acid ibuprofen[c]
Active arthrosis (acute pain-inflammatory episodes)	no	diclofenac, indomethacin ibuprofen piroxicam	ibuprofen, ketoprofen
Miofascial pain syndromes (antipyretic analgesics are often prescribed but of limited value)	no	diclofenac ibuprofen piroxicam	ibuprofen, ketoprofen
Posttraumatic pain, swelling	no	indomethacin, diclofenac ibuprofen	acetylsalicylic acid ibuprofen
Postoperative pain, swelling[d]	no	indomethacin, diclofenac ibuprofen	azapropazone ibuprofen
Temporary pain with inflammatory components:			
Dysmenorrhoea	no	no	ibuprofen, ketoprofen, naproxen
Headache, migraine, tooth pain	no	no	acetylsalicylic acid, ibuprofen
Fever and limb pain associated with viral infections	no	no	acetylsalicylic acid, ibuprofen

Indications	**Nonacidic anti-inflammatory analgesics**	
Pain and fever	**Pyrazolinone**	**Aniline**
Spastic pain (colics)	metamizole	no
Conditions associated with high fever	metamizole[c], propyphenazone	no
Acute and chronic intense pain	metamizole[e], propyphenazone	no
Cancer pain	metamizole[c], propyphenazone[c]	paracetamol[c]
Headache, migraine	metamizole[c], propyphenazone,	paracetamol[f]
General disturbances associated with viral infections (fever and limb pain in influenza infections)	propyphenazone, phenazone	paracetamol

[a]Dosage range of NSAIDs and example of monosubstances (but note dosage prescribed for each agent).
[b]Indicated only in gout attacks.
[c]Compare the sequence staged scheme of WHO for cancer pain.
[d]Blood coagulation and renal function must be normal.
[e]If other analgesics and antipyretics are contraindicated, e.g. gastro-duodenal ulcer, blood coagulation disturbances, asthma.
[f]In particular patients.

It should be noted that the rational therapeutic utilization of this family of agents is dependent on several characteristics that are reflective of their mode of actions and their pharmacokinetic behaviors in the human body:

1. The maximum achievable effects are theoretically limited by the extent to which the pain state is mediated by prostaglandins. If there is a prominent component of the state that is not mediated by the prostanoid, then to that degree the actions of the antipyretic analgesics will be limited. Thus, theoretically, if there is maximum suppression of the cyclooxygenase, it is not clear that supramaximal systemic doses provide any advantage. Given the likely central actions of the agent, it is possible that recommended dosing will not achieve maximum central cyclooxygenase inhibition. There is, however, little systematic data on this issue. In any case, because the highest usable systemic dose in humans is defined by side effects (see below), it is not possible to define a clear plateau effect in the clinical literature.
2. Maximum dosing regimens are typically governed by the tolerable side effects of the agent. These side effects are typically dependent on dose and duration of administration (as with GI bleeding). Idiosyncratic characteristics of the patient may contribute as well. Accordingly, careful attention to dosing must be the rule in long-term delivery because of the side-effect profile of the several agents (see below) and the chronicity of administration. In this regard, these agents have widely varying kinetics with distinctive half-lives (see Table 7). Because of the possibility of dose cumulation, appropriate dosing intervals should be given and closely attended to. Although there exists no clear correlation between the plasma half-life of elimination and the duration of action of these drugs, for chronic and intense inflammatory pain drugs with a sufficiently high

potency and slow rate of elimination such as the oxicams may be used with advantage (Table 6). Naturally, the higher risk of damage to the gastrointestinal tract and the kidneys must be taken into account. For acute pain that occurs regularly, e.g., at noon in some patients with osteoarthrosis, antiinflammatory acids that are safe and have a rapid onset of absorption, but are also eliminated rapidly, such as ibuprofen or diclofenac, can be selected.

3. It is clear that different agents may exert different effects upon inflammatory processes. Accordingly, analgesic effects may not uniformly correlate with changes in inflammatory signs, e.g., reduction in joint volume in arthritics.
4. Because several clinically useful antipyretic analgesics likely exert their actions by a common mechanism, e.g., inhibition of cyclooxygenase, there is no rationale to administer them in combination. On the other hand, aside from potentially harmful drug interaction (see below), the implementation of antipyretic analgesic therapy may yield its most effective therapeutic advantage in combinations with other families of agents, e.g., opiates. Under certain conditions, powerful synergies have been noted in systematic experimental studies (70,131). Different classes of analgesics should not, however, be combined routinely under clinical conditions because (a) enhanced effects are not always seen and (b) the incidence of side effects may be increased.

Postoperative Pain

After surgical interventions, there is an interval in which there is a protracted pain state requiring intervention (see Chaps. 40 and 43). Early investigations demonstrated that postoperative narcotic requirement could be significantly reduced by the use of antipyretic analgesics (62). The literature has in fact emphasized the efficacy of this family of functionally allied agents. Current work has typically demonstrated a reduction in the postoperative pain state as measured by visual analogue scales or by the indirect method of establishing reductions in the time to first analgesic request or total narcotic consumption during the postoperative interval (22,82). Such efficacy has been demonstrated after thoracotomy (3,92,101), abdominal and gynecologic surgeries (23), a variety of orthopedic interventions including hip arthroplasty (19,26), and abdominal surgery (20,44). This effective treatment applies cyclooxygenase inhibitors in a very vulnerable period of the patient's treatment. Consequently, an increased risk of ulcer formation and kidney failure appears plausible (2,10,24).

Cancer Pain

As reviewed in Chap. 48, "cancer pain" typically reflects a syndrome with a complex etiology involving a variety of causally related events including (a) soft tissue injury or mechanical distortion (tumor expansion in viscera; bone/fascia); (b) lytic processes (as in tumor erosion of the bone or skin); (c) release of neurohumors that directly or indirectly activate small afferents, as in amine precursor uptake and decarboxylation (APUD)-derived tumors; and (d) nerve injury secondary to tumor compression, activation of immune processes, or iatrogenic events such as nerve section for tumor removal, as in postmastectomy pain or radiation injury. Based on the presumed mechanisms of action, it is clear that a number of inflammatory components of the cancer pain states should prove to be particularly sensitive to the actions of the antipyretic analgesics and indeed this is the case. This has led to the widely appreciated World Health Organization (WHO) ladder sequence, in which the antipyretic analgesics are the first line of implementation and that with progressive incrementation in the pain state their use is supplemented by the addition of narcotics (39,115). A number of systematic trials have confirmed the efficacy of these agents. Thus, in double-blinded, within-patient randomized trials, these agents were highly effective in pain relief from the visceral and somatic sites and were relatively well tolerated (68,79,124,125). The potent effect upon the pain secondary to bony invasion clearly reflects upon the important role of the prostaglandins in mediating the pain secondary to the lytic processes of tumor invasion. While there is little systematic data, the failure of these agents in managing all of the components of the pain state reflects not upon their intrinsic weakness, but upon the limited role played by prostanoids in the pain secondary to other C-fiber stimulation processes and in particular to neuropathic mechanisms. The combined use of the antipyretic analgesics with opioids provides a strong tool for cancer pain management. Not only do the opiates provide an additional intervention in the input related to small afferent input, but the mood-altering aspects of opiates provide an additional component to the well-being of the suffering patient.

Arthritis

As reviewed in Chap. 48, arthritis presents a chronic disorder leading to the loss of joint control and crippling. This process is accompanied by chronic pain and joint inflammation. As noted, a frequent component of the synovial fluid is elevated levels of prostanoids. Such local actions can induce spontaneous activity in small joint afferents and increase their sensitivity to modest joint movement (107; see Chap. 33). It is thus mechanistically conceivable that the antipyretic analgesics would have a significant impact on the pain of arthritis. Extensive trials with a wide variety of antipyretic analgesics have been accomplished. Such studies have largely emphasized repeatedly the efficacy of such a therapeutic approach (46). Consumption of agents such as aspirin may range from the occasional two to four 325-mg tablets to literally several grams per day for extended periods in arthritics (46,55,59,97). Importantly, the classic efficacy of these agents in this state has been construed as support for the concept that they serve to diminish the inflammatory state. However, as reviewed in detail, the analgesic activity of these agents often appears to be independent of their ability to reduce inflammatory signs (75).

Low Back Pain

Low back pain may originate from a variety of possible sources. To the extent that the phenomenon is mediated in part by an inflammatory process that influences the terminal sensitivity of the small primary afferents, it would appear reasonable that the antipyretic analgesic agents would possess ameliorating effects upon the pain state. While there are surprisingly few systematic studies in this regard, it has been argued that a significant percentage of the low back pain syndrome could be managed by the appropriate use of analgesics, particularly the antipyretic analgesics at least during the first 2 weeks after onset (35).

Neuropathic Pain States

As reviewed in Chaps. 40 and 56, a number of mechanisms are believed to underlie the pain state that is initiated by nerve injury. It is typically considered that antipyretic analgesic actions are not efficacious in this pain state. However, there are few published systematic studies. As reviewed in Chap. 30, the peri–nerve injury environment is characterized by the release of factors that can initiate inflammatory responses. There is considerable evidence that sprouting terminals may develop particular chemosensitivity. The eicosanoids prostaglandin I_2

(PGI_2) and 8(R),15(S)-dihydroxyicosatetraenoic acid (8(R), 15(S)-diHETE) both excite C fibers in the chronic neuromas of rat sciatic nerve but not A fibers (31). Also, in the post–nerve injury state, neuromas and the dorsal root ganglion cells of the injured axons can develop spontaneous activity (29,30; see Chap. 32). In such conditions, it is possible that this continued afferent activity may induce a state of central facilitation that has some component that is mediated by the spinal synthesis and release of prostaglandins (see Chap. 36). Accordingly, it is possible that at least some, though clearly not all, components of neuropathic pain states may be influenced temporarily by this class of agents.

Burn

Mild burns (first degree), e.g., sunburn, yield an erythema and ample evidence of local inflammation. Such inflammation is accompanied by a cutaneous sensitization (84; see Chaps. 31 and 41). Under these circumstances, the antipyretic analgesics are effective in preclinical models. (129). Progressively more severe burns result in an exacerbation of the injury state, and these conditions are associated with evident increases in the secretion of cytokines, kinins and prostanoids (50a; see Chap. 44).

The ongoing activity in these afferents generated by the release of active factors can then lead to a central state of facilitation (see Chap. 36). It is generally presumed that these NSAIDs may exert their effect upon these tissue injury states generated by burns at the site of injury. Interestingly, in experimental burn studies in humans, neither an NSAID (ketorolac) nor a glucocorticoid actually had any antiinflammatory or, more importantly, any antinociceptive effect upon postburn hyperalgesia (83,93). This argues for a potential central action of these agents and raises the possibility that under certain conditions the peripheral afferent message is not mediated by a cyclooxygenase mechanism.

Clinically, systematic utilization of cyclooxygenase inhibitors in the burn injury state where there may be considerable capillary injury and leakage may be rendered problematic because of the effects of these agents upon platelet aggregation and clotting. Nevertheless, studies with the antipyretic analgesics have emphasized that this is not a major clinical concern if antipyretic analgesics other than ASA are used (e.g., ASA irreversibly blocks the platelet aggregation for days) (Fig. 2).

Fibromyalgia/Myositis

States of muscle pain with diagnosed trigger points are referred to as a fibromyalgia or a myositis. As reviewed in Chap. 29, there is considerable controversy as to the origin of these pain conditions. Antipyretic analgesics are widely employed in these pain states, although with limited success (41).

Systemic Infections (Common Cold; Influenza)

There is a widespread utilization of antipyretic analgesics for the pyrexia and aches and pain (algogenic and hyperalgesia) that are associated with a systemic (viral) infection. It is generally considered that the antipyretic effect is largely mediated by an inhibition of cyclooxygenase activity. Thus, intracerebral microinjection studies have emphasized a probable central action of the febrile actions within the hypothalamus, mediated in part by the local synthesis, release, and action of prostanoids (85,113,128). The central injection of NSAIDs into this region can have an antipyrogenic effect.

The origin of the general systemic effects of infections leading to a proalgesic state may be reasonably speculated to result from changes in circulating cytokines that derive secondary to immune reactivity of circulating and resident cells such as leukocytes and macrophages (49,61). Thus, for example, systemic endotoxin has been demonstrated to increase circulating levels of tumor necrosis factor-α (TNF-α) (80). Such cytokines would likely serve to initiate a cascade that would readily lead to activity in and sensitization of peripheral afferents. Thus, the delivery of a variety of systemic agents such as interleukin-1 (IL-1) or TNF-α can result in the firing of local small afferents and hyperalgesia (42; Linda Sorkin, unpublished observation). Although not specifically examined, it further appears likely that these multiple cytokines could exert a potent synergy in such stimulation and sensitization, as they do in other systems, for example in shock, where the resulting state has a strong cyclooxygenase-sensitive component (33). The efficacy of systemic cyclooxygenase inhibition in the clinical state associated with systemic infection suggests an important role for prostaglandins. Whether this action is mediated by a central action (as discussed above) or relates to an inhibition of the release of circulating prostanoids is not known.

ADVERSE EFFECTS OF ANTIPYRETIC ANALGESICS

The principal adverse effects associated with the actions of antipyretic analgesics relate to their primary effect upon prostaglandin synthesis (Fig. 1). Table 7 is a compilation of the typical actions of prostaglandins and the effects that may be seen after persistent inhibition of prostaglandins synthesis. This table reveals that prostaglandins are not only mediators of pain and inflammation in injured tissues, but also are constantly released and, as tissue hormones, regulate local blood circulation, production of mucus and of hydrochloric acid in the stomach, and many other cellular and organ functions. Moreover, the toxicity of these agents is clearly dependent on the local concentration. As mentioned previously, the acidic antiinflammatory analgesics are not distributed uniformly in the organism, and they particularly inhibit prostaglandins synthesis in organ systems in which they reach high concentrations. These drugs reach particularly high local concentrations in two situations: (a) where the capillary bed is open and both the free and bound drug can leave the blood circulation, and (b) in areas of the body where acidic extracellular pH values dominate. Such conditions prevail in inflamed tissue and under normal conditions in the lining of the upper gastrointestinal tract, the liver, bone marrow, and the kidneys. Consequently, it is not surprising that occasionally all acidic antipyretic analgesics may produce unwanted effects through inhibition of prostanoid synthesis (see Fig. 2) . Erosions, ulceration, and bleeding in the gastrointestinal tract, inhibition of thrombocyte function, and functional impairment of liver cells and kidneys are, to varying degrees, the typical side effects of all antiinflammatory acids (Table 8). Moreover, these agents may lead to an increase in leukotriene synthesis, particularly in patients with preimpaired mucosal tissues, such as occurs in chronic obstructive lung diseases (asthma and related conditions) in which there is infiltration of the tissue with inflammatory cells. Consequently, pseudoallergic asthma and hay fever–like reactions are frequent. Rarely, the reaction may be generalized and include the whole circulation. Shock reactions can then occur (8). Table 8 summarizes the most important adverse effects of antiinflammatory acids.

Several factors increase the likelihood of side effects. First, the risk is exacerbated in the case of preimpaired organ systems, such as occurs in asthmatic patients and in patients with gastrointestinal ulcers, in partial renal failure, and in disturbances of normal blood clotting. Second, environmental

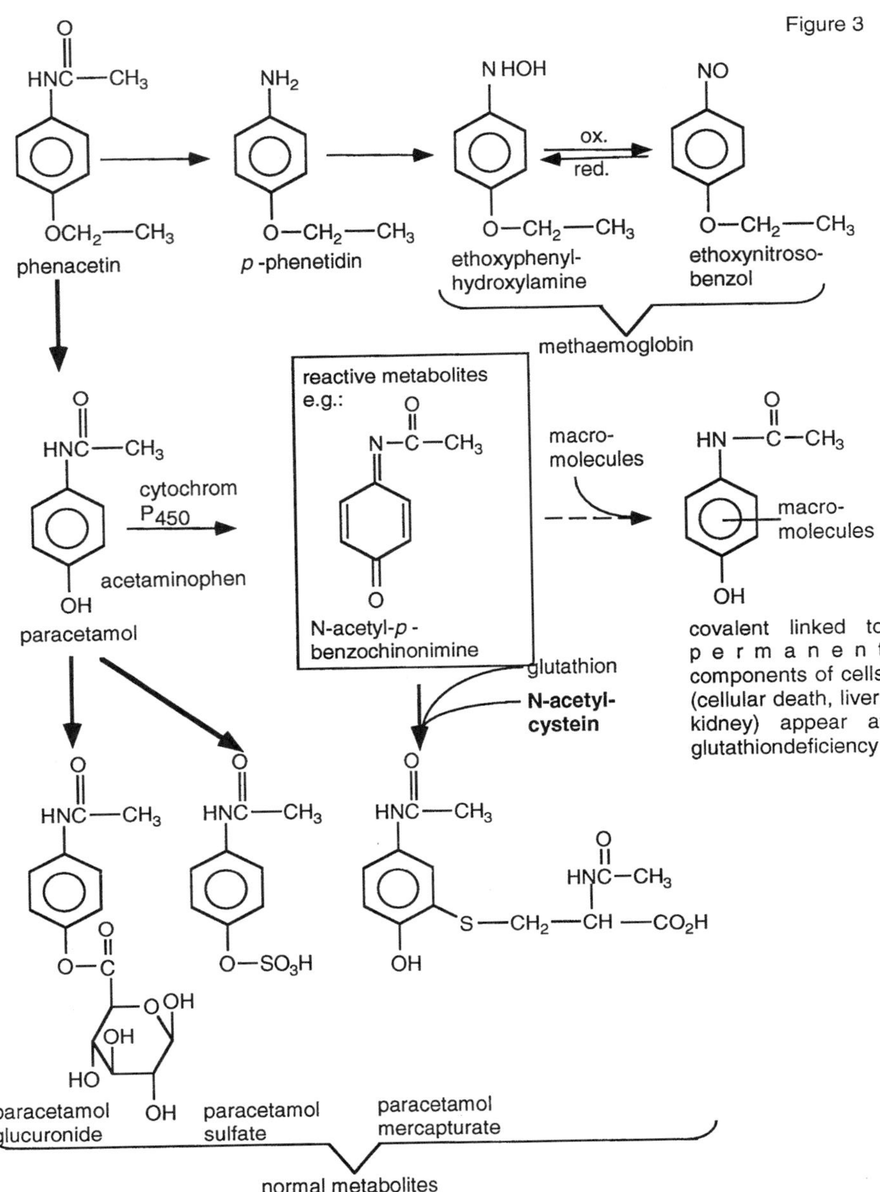

Figure 3. Metabolism of paracetamol (acetaminophen) and phenacetin. The conjugative steps of the metabolism of paracetamol are saturable. If the conjugating systems are overloaded, e.g., following administration of over 10 g of the drug, detoxification of the reactive intermediate (chinone-imine) through SH donators may also be exhausted. Then the chinone-imine binds to the cellular macromolecules, e.g., DNA in the liver resulting in cell death.

stressors may contribute to risk liability. Thus, operative stress increases the vulnerability of the gastrointestinal tract mucosa, and reduced renal perfusion or function may lead to a greater likelihood of renal injury.

At first it may be surprising that the incidence of these adverse effects is not the same for all NSAIDs (43,47,51,60,63, 65,88,102,103,106). An explanation for drug-specific undesired actions may derive from some additional drug-specific characteristics that may lead to interactions with certain "mediators." The structural similarity of indomethacin to serotonin, for example, could be responsible for the high incidence of central nervous system disorders such as vertigo, headache, and nausea. The high incidence of epileptiform seizures in patients following fenamate overdosage is group specific (120). The molecular basis for this remains unclear.

Of greatest significance with regard to antipyretic analgesic inflammatory activity appears to be the local concentration of the drug in the gastrointestinal tract, blood, liver, and kidneys during drug absorption, distribution, and excretion. If absorption already begins in the stomach, as is the case for aspirin, then injuries to the gastric mucosa will be more frequent, as compared to modern, more lipophilic agents that are absorbed distal to the stomach. The high rate of enterohepatic circulation seen with piroxicam, phenylbutazone, and indomethacin may be a reason for the gastrointestinal bleeding frequently observed with these agents. Sali-

Table 7. SUMMARY OF THE MOST IMPORTANT BIOLOGICAL ACTIONS OF PROSTAGLANDINS (PGS), THROMBOXANE (TX) AND LEUKOTRIENES (LTS) [a]

Organ/System	PG/TX/LT	Action	Effect of acidic anti-inflammatory analgesics
Central nervous system	PG	amplified pain transmission and processing in dorsal spinal cord	pain inhibition at spinal level
		induction of fever	fever lowering
Nociceptor	PG	increasing sensitivity (hyperalgesia)	normalization of increased sensitivity
Kidney	PG	increasing renal blood flow, diuresis	water and electrolyte retention
Smooth muscles			
Blood vessels	PG	vasodilatation	inhibition of inflammation closing of the Ductus arteriosus Botalli
	TX, (PG) [b]	vasoconstriction	shock (very rare)
Bronchi	PG	broncial relaxation	asthma-like (pseudoallergic) attacks (increased LT-synthesis)
	TX, LT, (PG)[b]	bronchial constriction	
Bowel	PG	contraction, (relaxation)	diarrhoea (irritation of the mucosa)
Uterus	PG	contraction of the corpus (gravidity) relaxation of the cervix	premature birth
Exocrine glands			
Bronchi	LT	increased secretion of viscuos mucous	asthma-like (pseudoallergic) attacks
Stomach	PG	reduced acid secretion and increased secretion of mucous and HCO_3	gastro-duodenal ulcer
Bowel	PG	increased secretion of mucous, water and electrolytes	intestinal ulcer
Blood	PG	inhibition of thrombocyte aggregation	blood coagulation disturbances (only in pre-impaired coagulation)
	TX	increased thrombocyte aggregation	thromboembolic prophylaxis
	LT	increased microvascular permeability, plasma exudation	shock probably also by means of increased LT-synthesis
Immune system	LT	chemotaxis of polymorphonuclear leukocytes, eosinophiles, and monocytes increased functions of polymorphonuclear and neutrophile leukocytes (multiple studies do not yet offer a single interpretation of these complex interactions)	small
	PG	(multiple studies do not yet offer a single interpretation of these complex interactions)	small

[a]This list offers a very simplified review and is by far complete. Differential actions of the individual prostaglandins (prostacyclin I = I PGI, PGE, PGF, PGD) or leukotrienes (LTB, LTC, LTD) are not discussed.
[b]No typical action for prostaglandins in general, produced only by one representative of this class.

cylate and ibuprofen do not recirculate in humans and are correspondingly relatively harmless to the lower sections of the gastrointestinal tract (108). A similar situation also applies to the kidneys. Impaired renal function causes increased prostaglandin production in the renal cortex, which is required to maintain sufficient blood circulation in the renal medulla. If this prostaglandin production is chronically inhibited, as is the case for potent inhibitors of prostaglandin synthesis with slow excretion rates (see Table 7), the incidence of functional and morphologically irreversible renal injuries will be more frequent and threatening as compared to drugs that are weak inhibitors and are rapidly eliminated.

Analogous to the different distribution profiles of nonacidic antipyretic analgesics is the profile of their side effects (16). In particular, they typically lack some of the toxic actions on the gastrointestinal tract and kidneys of the antiinflammatory acids. The inhibition of blood coagulation by metamizol is limited and temporary, except when very large doses are administered (Fig.2). Pseudoallergic reactions have been described only for high doses of metamizol and propyphenazone (16). These reactions are facilitated by parenteral administration. Like all other drugs, phenazone and its derivatives may also on occasion trigger genuine allergic reactions including agranulocytosis (116). Very rare skin reactions are observed in connection with the intensive use of all antipyretic analgesics. They may be slightly more frequent when eliminated slowly (half-life >1 to 2 days), e.g., phenylbutazone.

On the basis of its metabolism to a known reactive oxidation product (Fig. 3), paracetamol may lead to life-threatening liver cell injury following overdose or if administered to subjects with liver disease (1,69,104). If timely diagnosis of overdosage is made, lethal liver injury may be prevented by administration of N-acetylcysteine in the first 12 hours, because paracetamol (chinone-imine) is detoxified by means of the thiol (SH-) group.

Modern medicine sometimes enthusiastically practices polypharmacy. Drug interactions are thus likely, but fortunately life-threatening drug interactions are rare. The antipyretic analgesics discussed here present with a wide spectrum of drug interactions. Both groups, acidic and nonacidic analgesics, show both pharmacodynamic and pharmacokinetic interactions. The most relevant drug interactions for therapy are summarized in Table 9. In particular, the older, antiinflammatory acids with high-protein binding and lower-potency e.g., acetylsalicylic acid and phenylbutazone, present with a list of drug interactions on the basis of their high albumin binding and consequently interactions at protein binding sites. The release of vitamin K antagonists or oral antidiabet-

Table 8. IMPORTANT UNWANTED DRUG ACTIONS (UDAS) OF THE ANTIPYRETIC ANALGESICS AND THEIR INCIDENCE

	UDA (I = incidence)									Toxicity			
	Often I>1:100	Occasionally/rarely 1:100>I>1:1.000				Exceptions I<1:10.000				Acute overdosage			Chronic
Acidic antipyretic analgesics (NSAIDs)													
Salicylates													
acetylsalicylic acid	G_f	A	C	G_u	K	B				B	G_u	C_c	K(?)
salicylic acids	?	?				?				?	?	C_u	K(?)
diflunisal	G_f	A	G_u	K		B	C	L		?	?	C	K(?)
Arylacetic acids													
indomethacin	G_f	A	G_u	K	C	B				?	G_u	C	K(?) B
diclofenac	G_f	A	G_u	K	L	B	C			?	?	C	K(?) B
Arylpropionic acids													
ibuprofen	G_f	A	G_u	K		B	C	L		B(?)	G_u	C	K(?)
ketoprofen	G_f	A	G_u	K		B	C	L		B(?)	G_u(?)	C	K(?)
naproxen	G_f	A	G_u	K		B	C	L		B(?)	G_u	C	K(?)
flurbiprofen	G_f	A	G_u	K		B	C	L		B(?)	G_u	C	K(?)
Keto-enol acids													
piroxicam	G_f(G_u)	A	G_u	K		B	C	L		B(?)	G_u	C_c	K
azapropazone	G_f(G_u)	A	G_u	K		B	C	L		B(?)	G_u	C_c	K
phenylbutazone	G_f(G_u)	A	G_u	K		B	C	L		B	G_u	C_c	K B
Nonacidic antipyretic analgesics													
Anilines													
paracetamol		A				B	C	L	K(?)	B(?)	K,L	C	L K(?)
Pyrazolinone													
phenazone		A				B	C				L(?)	C	
propyphenazone		A				B	C					C	
metamizole		A				B	L					C	

Abbreviations:
A: allergic reactions.
B: blood and bone marrow impairments.
C: central nervous system disturbances, reversible.
C_c: coma and death reported.
G_f: gastrointestinal impairment, functional or mild.
G_u:gastrointestinal impairment, ulcer, bleedings.
K: renal impairment.
L: liver impairment.
?: no interpretable data available.

ics from albumin binding sites may augment inhibition of blood clotting or may lead to acute hypoglycemia. The inhibitory effect on blood coagulation (acetylation of thrombocyte cyclooxygenases inhibits the thrombocyte aggregation for many days) makes it impossible to use ASA in conditions involving reduced blood clotting (see above). All other drug interactions are more important (inhibition of diuretic activity, increasing the effect of lithium, of hyperkalemia in reduced renal function, and of angiotensin-converting enzyme [ACE]-inhibitor dosage) or less important (inhibition of absorption or acceleration of elimination by other antiinflammatory acids or antacids).

The recent characterization of cyclooxygenase isozymes and early pharmacologic studies characterizing their action have recently provided preliminary observations that at least some of these side effects may be mediated by the constitutive form of the enzyme (e.g., COX1). This seems to be particularly true of the gastrointestinal effects. The clinical relevance of such separations remain to be determined, but it provides some suggestion that further developments of more selective agents with fewer side effects may yet be in the offing.

CONCLUSIONS

The long history of use of the antipyretic analgesics and the development of an understanding of their mechanisms of action have paralleled our growing recognition of the mechanisms of nociceptive transmissions and the peripheral and central role of cyclooxygenase products in neurotransmission in general, and nociceptive processing in particular. The roles of prostanoids as facilitatory agents for afferent sensitivity in the periphery and afferent-evoked excitation in the spinal cord are important concepts providing the mechanism for their potent antihyperalgesic actions. The efficacy of these agents in severe pain states, such as in the postoperative patient or the cancer patient suffering form bone metastases, is consistent with the mechanisms that have been developed in the preclinical models. The recent insights showing that the COX enzyme can undergo a distinct upregulation in the face of continued tissue injury or afferent input and the observation that this isozyme may have a unique pharmacology indicate that further therapeutically relevant developments can be expected.

Table 9. IMPORTANT DRUG INTERACTIONS OF ANTIPYRETIC ANALGESICS

Antipyretic analgesics	A:	(Modified) action	Mechanisms involved	Comments
Other drugs	**B:**	**(Modified) action**	**Mechanisms involved**	
Acidic antipyretic analgesics (anti-inflammatory antipyretic analgesics, NSAIDs)[a]				
Acids	A:	analgesic effect↑	renal clearance↓	
Antacids	A:	analgesic effect↓	renal clearance↑ or absorption↓	
Aldosterone antagonists	B:	diuretic effect↓	natriuresis↓	
Antidiabetics (oral)	B:	hypoglycemic effect↑	plasma protein binding↓ or elimination↓	*salicylate and ibuprofen salicylate and phenylbutazone especially during treatment with tolbutamide*
Antihypertensives	B:	antihypertensive effect↓	Na^+-and H_2O-retention↑	*NSAIDs except salicylates*
Anticoagulants (oral)	A:	thrombocyte aggregation↓	thromboxan synthesis↓	
	B:	hypothrombinic effect↑ (coumarin plasma concentration↑ free fraction)	plasma protein binding↓ or metabolism↓	*high risk with salicylate and phenylburazone low risk with indomethacin diclofenac and piroxicam monitoring of prothromobin time*
b-receptor blocker	B:	antihypertensive effect↓	Na^+-and H_2O-retention↑ (PG-synthesis↓)	*indomethacin and naproxen*
Corticosteroids	A/B:	ulcerogenic effect↑	additional	*gastroprotection*
Digitoxin	B:	plasma concentration↓	metabolism↑ (enzyme induction)	*phenylbutazone*
Digoxin	B:	plasma concentration↑	?	*indomethacin, diclofenac and ibuprofen clinical relevance?*
Diuretics	A:	analgetic effect↓	renal clearance↑	*indomethacin plasma level >>*
	B:	diuretic effect↓ antihypertensive effect↓	Na^+- and H_2O-retention↑ (PG-synthesis↓)	
K^+-savings diuretics	B:	hyperkalemia	K^+-retention	*monitoring of potassium plasma concentration*
Lithium	B:	toxicity↑ plasma concentration –	renal clearance↓	*dosage adjusment monitoring of lithium plasma concentration*
Methotrexat	B:	toxicity↑ plasma concentration↑	renal clearance↓ resp. plasma protein binding↓	*dosis adjustment ketoprofen contraindicated*
Phenytoin	B:	plasma concentration↑	plasma protein binding↓	*salicylates, ibuprofen, and piraxicam clinical relevance?*
Uricosurics	A:	analgesic effect↑	renal clearance↓	*indomethacin plasma concentration*
	B:	uricosuric effect↓	renal clearance↑ or plasma protein binding>>	
Nonacidic anti-inflammatory analgetics				
Paracetamol				
Anticonvulsants Barbiturates Rifampicin	A:	liver toxicity↑	toxic metabolite↑ (enzyme induction)	*avoid combinations*
Chloramphenicol	B:	toxicity↑	half-life↑	
Anticoagulants (oral)	B:	hypothrombinemic effect↑	?	*monitoring of prothrombin time*
Phenazone[b]				
Anticonvulsants Barbiturates	A:	duration of action↓ analgetic effect↓	metabolism↑ (enzyme induction)	
Cimetidine			elimination↓	
Disulfiram b-receptors blocker	A:	accumulation risk↑		
Warfarin	B:	hypothrombinemic effect↑		*monitoring prothrombin time*

[a]Drug interactions of antipyretic analgesics are summarized here. In spite of a considerably homogenous spectrum of drug interactions, one must pay attention to the particular monosubstances (see comments below), above all the differences are between salicylates and the common NSAIDs. Especially for phenylbutazone (and other butazones) a variety of interactions with other drugs has been demonstrated (because of its many interactions, only an incomplete list is given).

[b]For other pyrazolinone (metamizole and propyphenazone) dangerous drug interactions have not been described.

Abbreviations: ↑ = increasing, ↓ = decreasing

REFERENCES

1. Agnelli G, Cosmi B. Antipyretic analgesics. In: Dukes MNG, Aronson JK, eds. *Side effects of drugs,* annual 15. Amsterdam/London/New York/Tokyo: Elsevier, 1991;85–91.
2. Aitken HA, Burns JW, McArdle CS, Kenny GN. Effects of ketorolac trometamol on renal function. *Br J Anaesth* 1992;68(5):481–485.
3. Anderson SK, al Shaikh BA. Diclofenac in combination with opiate infusion after joint replacement surgery. *Anaesth Intensive Care* 1991;19(4):535–538.
4. Attal N, Kayser V, Eschalier A, et al. Behavioural and electrophysiological evidence for an analgesic effect of a non-steroidal anti-inflammatory agent, sodium diclofenac. *Pain* 31988;5:341–348.
5. Benet LZ, Williams RL. Design and optimization of dosage regiments; pharmacokinetic data. In: Goodman Gilan A, Rall TW, Nies AS, Taylor P, eds. *The pharmacological basis of therapeutics,* 8th ed. New York: Pergamon Press, 1990;1650–1735.
6. Björkman R, Hedner J, Hedner T, et al. Central naloxone-reversible antinociception by diclofenac in the rat. *Naunyn Schmiedebergs Arch Pharmacol* 1990;342:171–176.
7. Björkman RL, Hedner T, Hallman KM, et al. Localization of the central antinociceptive effects of diclofenac in the rat. *Brain Res* 1992;590:66–73.
8. Bochner BS, Lichtenstein LM. Anaphylaxis. *N Engl J Med* 1991;324:1785–1790.
9. Bombardieri S, Cattani P, Ciabattoni G, Di Munno O, Pasero G, Patrono C, Pinca E, Pugliese F. The synovial prostaglandin system in chronic inflammatory arthritis: differential effects of steroidal and nonsteroidal anti-inflammatory drugs. *Br J Pharmacol* 1981;73(4):893–901.
10. Boras-Uber LA, Brackett NC Jr. Ketorolac-induced acute renal failure. *Am J Med* 1992;92(4):450–452.
11. Braga PC. Ketoprofen: i.c.v. injection and electrophysiological aspects of antinociceptive effect. *Eur J Pharmacol* 1990;184:273–280.
12. Brune K. Spinal cord effects of antipyretic analgesics. *Drugs* 1994;47(suppl 5):21–27.
13. Brune K, Bucher K, Walz D. The avian microcrystal arthritis ll. Central versus peripheral effects of sodium salicylate, acetaminophen und colchicine. *Agents Actions* 1974;4:27–33.
14. Brune K, Glatt Markus, Graf P. Mechanisms of action of anti-inflammatory drugs. *Gen Pharmacol* 1976;7:27–33.
15. Brune K, Lanz R. Pharmacokinetics of non-steroidal anti-inflammatory drugs. In: Bonta IL, Bray MA, Parnham MJ, eds. *Handbook of inflammation,* vol 5. Amsterdam: Elsevier Science, 1985;413–449.
16. Brune K, McCormack K. The over-the-counter use of nonsteroidal anti-inflammatory drugs and other antipyretic analgesics. In: Lewis AJ, Furst DE, eds. *Nonsteroidal anti-inflammatory drugs: mechanisms and clinical uses,* 2nd ed. New York: Marcel Dekker, 1994;97–126.
17. Brune K, Rainsford KD, Schweitzer A. Biodistribution of mild analgesics. *Br J Clin Pharmacol* 1980;10(suppl 2):279–284.
18. Brune K, Rainsford KD, Wagner K, Peskar BA. Inhibition by anti-inflammatory drugs of prostaglandin production in cultured macrophages—factors influencing the apparent drug effects. Arch Pharmacol 1981;315:269–276.
19. Buchanan JM, Baldasera J, Poole PH, Halshaw J, Dallard JK. Postoperative pain relief; a new approach: narcotics compared with non-steroidal anti-inflammatory drugs. *Ann R Coll Surg Engl* 1988;70:332–335.
20. Burns JW, Aitken HA, Bullingham RE, McArdle CS, Kenny GN. Double-blind comparison of the morphine sparing effect of continuous and intermittent i.m. administration of ketorolac. *Br J Anaesth* 1991;67(3):235–238.
21. Carlsson K-H, Monzel W, Jurna I. Depression by morphine and the non-opioid analgesic agents, metamizol (dipyrone), acetylsalicylate, and paracetamol of activity in rat thalamus neurones evoked by electrical stimulation of nociceptive afferents. *Pain* 1988;32:313–326.
22. Cashman J, McAnulty G. Nonsteroidal anti-inflammatory drugs in perisurgical pain management. Mechanisms of action and rationale for optimum use. *Drugs* 1995;49:51–70.
23. Cataldo PA, Senagore AJ, Kilbride MJ. Ketorolac and patient controlled analgesia in the treatment of postoperative pain. *Surg Gynecol Obstet* 1993;176(5):435–438.
24. Committee on Safety of Medicines. Ketorolac: new restrictions on dose and duration of treatment. *Curr Probl Pharmacovigilance* 1993;19:5–6.
25. de Beaurepaire R, Suaudeau C, Chait A, et al. Anatomical mapping of brain sites involved in the antinociceptive effects of ketoprofen. *Brain Res* 1990;536:201–206.
26. DeAndrade JR, Maslanka M, Maneatis T, Bynum L, Burchmore M. The use of ketorolac in the management of postoperative pain. *Orthopedics* 1994;7(2):157–166.
27. Devoghel JC. Intrathecal injection of lysine-acetylsalicylate in man with intractable cancer pain. In: Jurna I, Yaksh TL, eds. *Progress in pharmacology and clinical pharmacology,* vol 10. Stuttgart, New York: Gustav Fischers Verlag, 1993;111–118.
28. Devoghel JC. Small intrathecal doses of lysine-acetylsalicylate relieve intractable pain in man. *J Int Med Res* 1983;11:90–91.
29. Devor M, Wall PD, Catalan N. Systemic lidocaine silences ectopic neuroma and DRG discharge without blocking nerve conduction. *Pain* 1992;48(2):261–268.
30. Devor M, Wall PD. Cross-excitation in dorsal root ganglia of nerve-injured and intact rats. *J Neurophysiol* 1990;64(6):1733–1746.
31. Devor M, White DM, Goetzl EJ, Levine JD. Eicosanoids, but not tachykinins, excite C-fiber endings in rat sciatic nerve-end neuromas. *Neuroreport* 1992;3(1):21–24.
32. Dinarello CA. Biology of interleukin 1. *FASEB J* 1988;2:108–115.
33. Dinarello CA, Okusawa S, Gelfand JA. Interleukin-1 induces a shock-like state in rabbits: synergism with tumor necrosis factor and the effect of cyclooxygenase inhibition. *Prog Clin Biol Res* 1989;286:243–263.
34. Dinchuk JE, Car BD, Focht RJ, Johnston JJ, Jaffee BD, Covington MB, Contel NR, Eng VM, Collins RJ, Czerniak PM, et al. Renal abnormalities and an altered inflammatory response in mice lacking cyclooxygenase II. *Nature* 1995;378(6555):406–409.
35. DiPalma JR, DiGregorio GJ. Management of low back pain by analgesics and adjuvant drugs. *Mt Sinai J Med* 1991;58(2):101–108.
36. Dromgoole SH, Furst DE, Desiraju RK, Nayak RK, Kerschenbaum MA, Paulus HE. Tolmetin kinetics and synovial fluid prostaglandin E levels in rheumatoid arthritis. *Clin Pharmacol Ther* 1982;32:371–377.
37. Egg D, Gunther R, Herold M, Kerschbaumer F. Prostaglandins E2 and F2 alpha concentrations in the synovial fluid in rheumatoid and traumatic knee joint diseases. *Z Rheumatol* 1980;39(5-6):170–17
38. Ferreira SH. Prostaglandins: peripheral and central analgesia. In: Bonica LL, ed. *Advances in pain research and therapy.* New York: Raven Press, 1983;627–634.
39. Foley KM. The treatment of cancer pain. *N Engl J Med* 1985;313:84–95.
40. Forster C, Magerl W, Beck W, Geiβlinger G, Gall T, Brune K, Handwerker HO. Differential effects of dipyrone, ibuprofen, and paracetamol on experimentally induced pain in man. *Agents Actions* 1992;35:112–121.
41. Fricton JR, Awad EA, eds. Myofascial pain and fibromyalgia. *Adv Pain Res Ther* 1990;17.
42. Fukuoka H, Kawatani M, Hisamitsu T, Takeshige C. Cutaneous hyperalgesia induced by peripheral injection of interleukin-1 beta in the rat. *Brain Res* 1994;657(1-2):133–140.
43. Gabriel SE, Jaakkimainen L, Bombardier C. Risk for serious gastrointestinal complications related to use of nonsteroidal anti-inflammatory drugs. A meta-analysis. *Ann Intern Med* 1991;115:787–796.
44. Gillies GW, Kenny GN, Bullingham RE, McArdle CS. The morphine sparing effect of ketorolac tromethamine. A study of a new, parenteral non-steroidal anti-inflammatory agent after abdominal surgery. *Anaesthesia* 1987;42(7):727–731.
45. Goppelt-Struebe M. Regulation of prostaglandin endoperoxide synthase (cyclooxygenase) isozyme expression. *Prostaglandins Leukot Essent Fatty Acids* 1995;52(4):213–222.
46. Gotzsche PC. Review of dose-response studies of NSAIDs in rheumatoid arthritis. *Dan Med Bull* 1989;36:395–399.
47. Griffin MR, Piper JM, Daugherty JR, Snowden M, Ray WA. Nonsteroidal anti-inflammatory drug use and increased risk for peptic ulcer disease in elderly persons. *Ann Intern Med* 1991;114:257–263.
48. Groppetti A, Braga PC, Biella G, et al. Effect of aspirin on serotonin and metenkephalin in brain: correlation with the antinociceptive activity of the drug. *Neuropharmacology* 1988;27:499–505.
49. Hajjar DP, Pomerantz KB. Signal transduction in atherosclerosis: integration of cytokines and the eicosanoid network. *FASEB J* 1992;6(11):2933–2941.

50. Harms BA, Bodai BI, Smith M, Gunther R, Flynn J, Demling RH.Prostaglandin release and altered microvascular integrity after burn injury. *J Surg Res* 1981;31(4):274–280.

50a. Heideman M, Bengetsson A. The immunologic response to thermal injury. *World J Surg* 1992;16;53–56.

51. Henry D, Dobson A, Turner C. Variability in the risk of major gastrointestinal complications from nonaspirin anti-inflammatory drugs. *Gastroenterology* 1993;105:1078–1088.

52. Herndon DN, Abston S, Stein MD. Increased thromboxane B2 levels in the plasma of burned and septic burned patients. *Surg Gynecol Obstet* 1984;159(3):210–213.

53. Hua XY, Jinno S, Back SM, Tam EK, Yaksh TL. Multiple mechanisms for the effects of capsaicin, bradykinin and nicotine on CGRP release from tracheal afferent nerves: role of prostaglandins, sympathetic nerves and mast cells. *Neuropharmacology* 1994;33(10):1147–1154.

54. Insel PA. Analgesic-antipyretics and anti-inflammatory agents; Drugs employed in the treatment of rheumatoid arthritis and gout. In: Gilman AG, Rall TW, Nies AS, Taylor P, eds. *Goodman and Gilman's the pharmacological basis of therapeutics,* 8th ed. New York: Macmillan, 1990;640.

55. Jacobs J, Keyserling JA, Britton M, et al. The total cost of care and the use of pharmaceuticals in the management of rheumatoid arthritis: the Medi-Cal program. *J Clin Epidemiol* 1988;41:215–223.

56. Jänig W. Experimental approach to reflex sympathetic dystrophy and related syndromes. *Pain* 1991;46:241–245.

57. Jurna I, Brune K. Central effects of the non-steroid anti-inflammatory agents, indomethacin, ibuprofen and diclofenac, determined in C fibre-evoked activity in single neurones of the rat thalamus. *Pain* 1990;4:71–80.

58. Jurna I, Yaksh TL. *Central mechanisms for analgesia by acetylsalicylic acid and (functionally) related compounds.* Jena-New York: Gustav Fischer Verlag Stuttgart, 1993.

59. Kantor TG. Current modalities in arthritic diseases. *Am J Med* 1987;83:2–5.

60. Kaufman D.W, Kelly JP, Sheehan JE, Laszlo A, Wiholm BE, Alfredsson L, Koff RS, Shapiro S. Nonsteroidal anti-inflammatory drug use in relation to major upper gastrointestinal bleeding. *Clin Pharmacol Ther* 1993;53:485–493.

61. Kelley J. Cytokines of the lung. *Am Rev Respir Dis* 1990;141(3): 765–788.

62. Kweekel-de Vries WJ, Spierdijk J, Mattie H, Hermans JM. A new soluble acetylsalicylic acid derivative in the treatment of postoperative pain. *Br J Anaesth* 1974;46:133–135.

63. Langman MJS, Weil J, Wainwright P, Lawson DH, Rawlins MD, Logan RFA, Murphy M, Vessey MP, Colin-Jones DG. Risks of bleeding peptic ulcer associated with individual non-steroidal anti-inflammatory drugs. *Lancet* 1994;343:1075–1078.

64. Lanz R, Polster P, Brune K.. Antipyretic analgesics inhibit prostaglandin release from astrocytes and macrophages similarly. *Eur J Pharmacol* 1986;130:105–109.

65. Laporte JR, CarnÈ X, Vidal X, Moreno V, Juan J. Upper gastrointestinal bleeding in relation to previous use of analgesics and nonsteroidal anti-inflammatory drugs. *Lancet* 1991;337:85–89.

66. Levy M, Flusser D, Zylber-Katz E, Granit L. Plasma kinetics of dipyrone metabolites in rapid and slow acetylators. *Eur J Clin Pharmacol* 1984;27:453–458.

67. Lim RKS. Pain. *Annu Rev Physiol* 1970;32:269–288.

68. Lomen PL, Samal BA, Lamborn KR, Sattler LP, Crampton SL. Flurbiprofen for the treatment of bone pain in patients with metastatic breast cancer. *Am J Med* 1986;80:83–87.

69. Maddrey WC. Hepatic effects of acetaminophen enhances toxicity in alcoholics. *J Clin Gastroenterol* 1987;9:180–185.

70. Malmberg AB, Yaksh TL. Pharmacology of the spinal action of ketorolac, morphine, ST-91, U50488H, and L-PIA on the formalin test and an isobolographic analysis of the NSAID interaction. *Anesthesiology* 1993;79:270–281.

71. Malmberg AB, Yaksh TL. Antinociception produced by spinal delivery of the S and R enantiomers of flurbiprofen in the formalin test. *Eur J Pharmacol* 1994;256:205–209.

72. Malmberg AB, Yaksh TL. Antinociceptive actions of spinal nonsteroidal anti-inflammatory agents on the formalin test in the rat. *J Pharmacol Exp Ther* 1992;263:136–146.

73. Malmberg AB, Yaksh TL. Capsaicin-evoked prostaglandin E2 release in spinal cord slices: relative effect of cyclooxygenase inhibitors. *Eur J Pharmacol* 1995;in press.

74. Malmberg AB, Yaksh TL. Cyclooxygenase inhibition and the spinal release of prostaglandin E2 and amino acids evoked by paw formalin injection: A microdialysis study in unanesthetized rats. *J Neurosci* 1995;in press.

75. McCormack K, Brune K. Dissociation between the antinociceptive and anti-inflammatory effects of the nonsteroidal anti-inflammatory drugs. A survey of their analgesic efficacy. *Drugs* 1991;41: 533–547.

76. McCormack K. Non-steroidal anti-inflammatory drugs and spinal nociceptive processing. *Pain* 1994;59(1):9–43.

77. Meade EA, Smith WL, DeWitt DL. Differential inhibition of prostaglandin endoperoxide synthase (cyclooxygenase) isoenzymes by aspirin and other non-steroidal anti-inflammatory drugs. *J Biol Chem* 1993;268:6610–6614.

78. Meller ST, Gebhart GF. Nitric oxide (NO) and nociceptive processing in the spinal cord. *Pain* 1993;52:127–136.

79. Mercadante S. Celiac plexus block versus analgesics in pancreatic cancer pain. *Pain* 1993;52:187–192.

80. Michie HR, Manogue KR, Spriggs DR, Revhaug A, O'Dwyer S, Dinarello CA, Cerami A, Wolff SM, Wilmore DW. Detection of circulating tumor necrosis factor after endotoxin administration. *N Engl J Med* 1988;318(23):1481–1486.

81. Mitchel JA, Akarasereenont P, Thiemermann C, et al. Selectivity of nonsteroidal antiinflammatory drugs as inhibitors of constitutive and inducible cyclooxygenase. *Proc Natl Acad Sci USA* 1994;90: 11693–11697.

82. Moote C. Efficacy of nonsteroidal anti-inflammatory drugs in the management of postoperative pain. *Drugs* 1992;44(suppl 5): 14–29.

83. Moiniche S, Pedersen JL, Kehlet H. Topical ketorolac has no antinociceptive or anti-inflammatory effect in thermal injury. *Burns* 1994;20(6):483–486.

84. Moiniche S, Dahl JB, Kehlet H. Time course of primary and secondary hyperalgesia after heat injury to the skin. *Br J Anaesth* 1993; 71(2):201–205.

85. Myers RD, Rudy TA, Yaksh TL. Effect in the rhesus monkey of salicylate on centrally-induced endotoxin fevers. *Neuropharmacology* 1971;10:775–778.

86. Neugebauer V, Schaible HG. Evidence for a central component in the sensitization of spinal neurons with oint input during the development of acute arthritis in cat's knee. *J Neurophysiol* 1990;64: 299–311.

87. Neugebauer V, Schaible HG, He X, Lücke T, Gründling P, Schmidt RF, Electrophysiological evidence for a spinal antinociceptive action of dipyrone. *Agents Actions* 1994;41:62–70.

88. Nobili A, Mosconi P, Franzosi MG, Tognoni G. Non-steroidal anti-inflammatory drugs and upper gastrointestinal bleeding, a post-marketing surveillance case-control study, Pharmacoepidemiol. *Drug Saf* 1992;1:65–72.

89. O'Callaghan JP, Holtzman SG. Quantification of the analgesic activity of narcotic antagonists by a modified hot-plate procedure. *J Pharmacol Exp Ther* 1975;192:497–505.

90. O'Neill GP, Hutchinson AW. Expression of mRNA for cyclooxygenase-1 and cyclooxygenase-2 in human tissues. *FEBS Lett* 1993;330: 156–165.

91. Okuyama S, Aihara H. The mode of action of analgesic drugs in adjuvant arthritic rats as an experimental model of chronic inflammatory pain: possible central analgesic action of acidic nonsteroidal anti-inflammatory drugs. *Jpn J Pharmacol* 1994;35:95–103.

92. Pavy T, Medley C, Murphy DF. Effect of indomethacin on pain relief after thoracotomy. *Br J Anaesthesia* 1990;65(5):624–627.

93. Pedersen JL, Moiniche S, Kehlet H. Topical glucocorticoid has no antinociceptive or anti-inflammatory effect in thermal injury. *Br J Anaesth* 1994;72(4):379–382.

94. Pellerin M, Hardy F, Abergel A, et al. Doleur chronique rebelle des cancereux. Interet de l'injection intrarachidienne d'acetylsalicylate de lysine. Soixante observations. *Presse Med* 1987;16: 1465–1468.

95. Picot D, Loll PJ, Garavito RM. The x-ray crystal structure of the membrane protein prostaglandin H2 synthase-1. *Nature* 1994; 367(6460):243–249.

96. Piletta P, Porchet HC, Dayer P. Central analgesic effect of acetaminophen but not of aspirin. *Clin Pharmacol Ther* 1991;49: 350–354.

97. Preston SJ, Arnold MH, Beller EM, et al. Comparative analgesic and antiinflammatory properties of sodium salicylate and acetylsalicylic acid (aspirin) in rheumatoid arthritis. *Br J Clin Pharmacol* 1989;27:607–611.

98. Rainsford KD, Schweitzer A, Brune K. Autoradiographic and biochemical observations on the distribution of non-steroid anti-inflammatory drugs. *Arch Int Pharmacodyn Ther* 1981;250:180–194.
99. Rampin O, Harrewyn JM, Albe-Fessard D. Effect antalgique de l'administration centrale du ketoprofene chez le rat. *Rev Rhum Mal Osteoartic* 1988;55:779–780.
100. Rey R. *History of pain* (Wallace LE, Cadden JA, Cadden SW, trans.) Paris: Editions La Decouverte, 1993;1–409.
101. Rhodes M, Conacher I, Morritt G, Hilton C. Nonsteroidal antiinflammatory drugs for postthoracotomy pain. A prospective controlled trial after lateral thoracotomy. *J Thorac Cardiovasc Surg* 1992;103(1):17–20.
102. Rodriguez LAG, Walker AM, Gutthann SP. Nonsteroidal antiinflammatory drugs and gastrointestinal hospitalizations in saskatchewan: a cohort study, *Epidemiology* 1992;3:337–342.
103. Rodriguez LAG. Risk of upper gastrointestinal bleeding and perforation associated with individual non-steroidal anti-inflammatory drugs. *Lancet* 1994;343:769–772.
104. Rumac BH. Acetaminophen overdose in children and adolescents. *Pediatr Clin North Am* 1986;33:691–701.
105. Samuelsson B. Bisynthesis of prostaglandins. *Fed Proc* 1972;31: 1442–1460.
106. Savage RL, Moller PW, Ballantyne CL, Wells JE. Variation in the risk of peptic ulcer complications with nonsteroidal antiinflammatory drug therapy. Arthritis Rheum 1993;36:84–90.
107. Schaible H-G, Grubb BD. Afferent and spinal mechanisms of joint pain. *Pain* 1993;55:5–54.
108. Schneider HT, Nuernberg B, Dietzel K, Brune K. Biliary elimination of non-steroidal anti-inflammatory drugs in patients. *Br J Clin Pharmacol* 1990;29:127–131.
109. Shimada SG, Otterness IG, Stitt JT. A study of the mechanism of action of the mild analgesic dipyrone. *Agents Actions* 1994;41: 188–192.
110. Smith JB, Willis AL. Aspirin selectively inhibits prostaglandins production in platelets. *Nature* 1971;321:235–237.
111. Sorkin LS. Intrathecal ketorolac blocks NMDA-evoked spinal release of prostaglandin E2 and thromboxane B2. *Anesthesiology* 1993;79:A909.
112. Sorkin LS. Release of amino acids and PGE2 into the spinal cord of lightly anesthetized rats during development of an experimental arthritis: enhancement of C-fiber evoked release. *Soc Neurosci Abst* 1992;18:429.10.
113. Stitt JT. Differential sensitivity in the sites of fever production by prostaglandin E1 within the hypothalamus of the rat. *J Physiol* 1991;432:99–110.
114. Taber RI. Predictive value of analgesic assays in mice and rats. *Adv Biochem Psychopharmacol* 1973;8:191–211.
115. Takeda F. WHO cancer pain relief programme. *Pain Res Clin Manage* 1991;4:467–474.
116. The international agranulocytosis and aplastic anemia study. Risks of agranulocytosis and aplastic anemia. A first report of their relation to drug use with special reference to analgesics. *JAMA* 1986; 256:1749–1757.
117. Tjolsen A, Lund A, Hole K. Antinociceptive effect of paracetamol in rats is partly dependent on spinal serotonergic systems. *Eur J Pharmacol* 1991;193(2):193–201.
118. Tokunaga M, Ohuchi K, Yoshizawa S, Tsurufuji S, Rikimaru A, Wakamatsu E. Change of prostaglandin E level in joint fluids after treatment with flurbiprofen in patients with rheumatoid arthritis and osteoarthritis. *Ann Rheum Dis* 1981;40(5):462–465.
119. Travers AF. A fatality after antipyrine administration. *Clin Pharmacol Ther* 1991;49:695–696.
120. Vale JA, Meredith TJ. Acute poisoning due to non-steroidal anti-inflammatory drugs - clinical features and management. *Med Toxicol* 1986;1:12–31.
121. Vane J. Inhibition of prostaglandin synthesis as a mechanism of action for aspirin-like drugs. Nature New Biol 1971;231:232–237.
122. Vane J. The evolution of non-steroidal anti-inflammatory drugs and their mechanisms of action. *Drugs* 1987;33(suppl 1):18–27.
123. Vane J. Towards a better aspirin. *Nature* 1994;367:215–216.
124. Ventafridda V, De Conno F, Panerai AE, Maresca V, Monza GC, Ripamonti C. Non-steroidal anti-inflammatory drugs as the first step in cancer pain therapy: double-blind, within-patient study comparing nine drugs. *J Int Med Res* 1990;18:21–29.
125. Ventafridda V, Toscani F, Tamburini M, Corli O, Gallucci M, Gottlieb A, Speranza R, De Conno F. Sodium naproxen versus sodium diclofenac in cancer pain control. *Arzneimittelforschung* 1990; 40(10):1132–1134.
126. Vlahov V, Badian M, Verho M, Bacracheva N. Pharmacokinetics of metamizol metabolites in healthy subjects after a single oral dose of metamizol dosium. *Eur J Clin Pharmacol* 1990;38:61–65.
127. Willer JC, De Broucker T, Bussel B, et al. Central analgesic effect of ketoprofen in humans: electrophysiological evidence for a supraspinal mechanism in a double-blind and cross-over study. *Pain* 1989;38:1–7.
128. Williams JW, Rudy TA, Yaksh TL, Viswanathan CT. An extensive exploration of the rat brain for sites mediating prostaglandin-induced hyperthermia. *Brain Res* 1977;120(2):251–262.
129. Winder CV, Wax J, Burr V, Been M, Rosiere CE. A study of pharmacological influences on ultraviolet erythema in guinea pigs. *Arch Int Pharmacodyn* 1958;116:261–292.
130. Wittenberg RH, Willburger RE, Kleemeyer KS, Peskar BA. In vitro release of prostaglandins and leukotrienes from synovial tissue, cartilage, and bone i n degenerative joint diseases. Arthritis Rheum 1993;36(10):1441–1450.
131. Yaksh TL, and Malmberg AB. Interaction of spinal modulatory receptor systems. In: Fields HL, Liebeskind JC, eds. *Progress in pain research and management,* vol 1. Seattle: IASP Press, 1994;151–171.
132. Yaksh TL. Central and peripheral mechanisms for the analgesic action of acetylsalicylic acid. In: Barett HJM, Hirsh J, Mustard JF, eds. *Acetylsalicylic acid:* new uses for an old drug. New York: Raven Press, 1982;137–151.
133. Yamagata K, Andreasson KI, Kaufmann WE, et al. Expression of a mitogen-inducible cyclooxygenase in brain neurons: regulation by synaptic activity and glucocorticoids. *Neuron* 1993, 11:371–386.

Anesthesia: Biologic Foundations, edited by Tony L. Yaksh et al. Lippincott–Raven Publishers, Philadelphia © 1997.

CHAPTER 62

GABAERGIC DRUGS AND THE CLINICAL MANAGEMENT OF PAIN

DONNA L. HAMMOND AND BRENT A. GRAHAM

Anesthesiologists use a wide variety of agents that mimic or enhance the actions of γ-aminobutyric acid (GABA) in the central nervous system. These agents include inhalational anesthetics (e.g., halothane, isoflurane), barbiturate anesthetics (e.g., thiopental, pentobarbital), and benzodiazepine receptor agonists or antagonists (e.g., diazepam, midazolam, flumazenil). Other clinically used drugs that mimic or enhance the actions of GABA include baclofen for the treatment of spasticity, barbiturate sedatives and anticonvulsants (e.g., phenobarbital), and gabapentin for the treatment of seizures. The development of such a large number of drugs having diverse pharmacologic activities and clinical utilities is not surprising when one considers (a) the widespread distribution of GABA within the central nervous system, (b) its preeminent role as an inhibitory neurotransmitter, and (c) the complexity of its receptors. What is surprising, however, is the limited clinical utility of GABAergic drugs for the treatment of pain. This chapter briefly reviews the pharmacology of GABA receptors, discusses the large body of evidence obtained in laboratory animals that suggests GABAergic agents should be effective analgesics for the treatment of acute or neuropathic pain, and contrasts these studies with the results of clinical investigations that indicate that such agents are of limited utility and efficacy in the treatment of pain. In addition, it highlights questions that may warrant further clinical investigation.

INTRODUCTION TO GABA AND ITS RECEPTORS

An inhibitory amino acid neurotransmitter, GABA is widely distributed throughout the brain and spinal cord and is considered to be the preeminent inhibitory neurotransmitter in the central nervous system (14,78,105). Its actions and the characteristics of the receptors at which it acts have been reviewed in depth both in this volume and elsewhere (9–12,14, 28,53,70,80,105). For this reason, only a brief overview will be provided.

The existence of at least two types of the GABA receptor, $GABA_A$ and $GABA_B$, is now well established (11,28,70,80,105). The $GABA_A$ receptor is classically defined as the bicuculline-sensitive, baclofen-insensitive site at which GABA acts. Prototypic agonists for the $GABA_A$ receptor include isoguvacine, muscimol, and THIP (4,5,6,7-tetrahydroisoxazolo-[5,4-c]pyridin-3-ol). Antagonists for this receptor include bicuculline and picrotoxin. The $GABA_B$ receptor is defined as the bicuculline-insensitive, baclofen-sensitive site at which GABA acts. The prototypic agonist for the $GABA_B$ receptor is baclofen (Lioresal). Several antagonists of the $GABA_B$ receptor are now available, including phaclofen, 2-OH-saclofen, and CGP35348. More recently, the existence of a third subtype of the GABA receptor, termed the $GABA_C$ receptor, has been proposed (26,52,61,116). It is currently defined as the baclofen-insensitive, bicuculline-insensitive site at which GABA acts and appears to be localized nearly exclusively to the retina. Preferential agonists for this receptor include *trans*- and *cis*-4-aminocrotonic acid. These receptors are summarized in Table 1.

The $GABA_A$ receptor is actually a complex of binding sites for GABA, barbiturate anesthetics and anticonvulsants, steroid anesthetics, convulsant agents, and benzodiazepine receptor agonists, inverse agonists, and antagonists (14,70,105) (see Chap. 16). The $GABA_A$ receptor complex is comprised of five subunits (α, β, γ, δ, or ρ) that form the walls of a ligand-gated ion channel permeable to Cl^- (14,69,99). Multiple isoforms of each of these subunits have been identified. The results of expression studies indicate that the pharmacologic profile of the $GABA_A$ receptor complex (i.e., its affinity for GABA and other $GABA_A$ receptor ligands, as well as the efficacy of these ligands and other modulatory agents) is dependent on the composition and stoichiometry of the various subunits (14,28,69,76,99,115). Activation of the $GABA_A$ receptor results in an increase in Cl^- conductance and hyperpolarization of the neuron (9). This GABA- induced increase in Cl^- flux is augmented in the presence of low concentrations of benzodiazepine receptor agonists or barbiturates, which bind to the adjacent modulatory sites of the complex. However, at high concentrations, these same agents appear to interact directly with the channel to increase Cl^- flux (40,53).

Unlike the $GABA_A$ receptor, the $GABA_B$ receptor is a G-protein–coupled receptor. The actions of GABA at this receptor are mediated by inhibitory G proteins. Activation of the $GABA_B$ receptor results either in an increase in K^+ conductance, which causes hyperpolarization of the neuron, or a decrease in Ca^{2+} influx, which decreases neurotransmitter release (10,11,80). The former effect is a predominantly postsynaptic event, whereas the latter is a predominantly presynaptic effect. Either event results in an inhibition of neural transmission.

$GABA_B$ RECEPTOR LIGANDS AND ANALGESIA: POTENTIAL INSIGHTS FROM ANIMAL STUDIES

A large number of studies have examined the antinociceptive potency and efficacy of the prototypic $GABA_B$ receptor agonist baclofen in the laboratory mouse, rat, or primate using different measures of nociception. Collectively, the results of these studies provide strong evidence that $GABA_B$ receptor agonists are effective analgesics. For example, systemic administration of baclofen to the mouse or rat produces dose-dependent antinociception in the writhing, tail flick, and hot plate tests (22, 49,51,63,95,113), as well as in the shock titration test in the primate (49,51). These effects occur at doses below those at which flaccidity is observed, although the therapeutic index is admittedly small. Later investigations identified the spinal cord as an important site in the central nervous system at which baclofen acts to produce antinociception. Intrathecal administration of baclofen produces a dose-dependent antinociception in the tail flick and hot plate tests in the mouse and the rat (4,42,43, 50,114), and increases the titration threshold for noxious electrical stimuli in the primate (118). The finding that acute transection of the spinal cord significantly decreases the antinociceptive effect of systemically administered baclofen suggests that a supraspinal site, or an interaction of spinal and supraspinal

Table 1. CHARACTERISTICS OF THREE TYPES OF GABA RECEPTOR

	Bicuculline	Baclofen	Agonist	Antagonist
$GABA_A$	Sensitive	Insensitive	Isoguvacine Muscimol THIP[a]	Bicuculline Picrotoxin
$GABA_B$	Insensitive	Sensitive	Baclofen	Phaclofen 2-OH-saclofen CGP35348[b]
$GABA_C$	Insensitive	Insensitive	TACA[c] CACA[d]	Unknown

[a]4,5,6,7-tetrahydroisoxazolo-[4,5-c]pyridin-3-ol.
[b]3-amino-propyl(diethoxymethyl)phosphinic acid.
[c]*trans*-4-aminocrotonic acid.
[d]*cis*-4-aminocrotonic acid.

sites, is also important. Indeed, microinjection of baclofen at supraspinal sites including the lateral ventricles, periaqueductal gray, and the ventromedial medulla produces antinociception, although the effect is modest in magnitude (64,65,109). Intrathecal administration of the $GABA_B$ receptor antagonist CGP35348 antagonizes the antinociceptive effect of subcutaneously administered baclofen to a greater extent than does microinjection of the same dose at sites in the ventromedial medulla of the rat (110). Thus, the antinociceptive effects of systemically administered baclofen appear to be mediated predominantly by $GABA_B$ receptors in the spinal cord. Additional evidence for the importance of GABA and spinal $GABA_B$ receptors in the production of antinociception is provided by the finding that intrathecal administration of two different $GABA_B$ receptor antagonists, phaclofen or CGP35348, antagonizes the antinociception produced by activation of the endogenous pain modulatory pathways that originate in the ventromedial medulla (74).

Until very recently, the majority of studies of baclofen's antinociceptive effects used conventional measures of acute nociception such as the tail flick or hot plate test. More recent studies have assessed its efficacy using models of inflammatory or neuropathic pain. For example, intrathecal (IT) administration of baclofen produces a dose-dependent suppression of the behavioral response to subcutaneous (sc) injection of formalin in the hind paw of the rat (25). The recent development of several animal models of neuropathic pain, including loose ligation or partial transection of the sciatic nerve (7,96), ligation of the L5-L6 spinal nerve (54), or focal ischemia of the spinal cord (44,46), has afforded new opportunities to study the mechanisms responsible for this difficult-to-treat entity and to identify new pharmacologic therapies. The results of these investigations suggest that a loss of GABA may contribute to the development of allodynia (a syndrome in which application of a nonpainful stimulus evokes pain) and chronic pain. For example, transection of the sciatic nerve results in a modest decrease in the number of GABA-immunoreactive neurons in the spinal cord (15). In normal rats, antagonism of spinal $GABA_B$ receptors by intrathecal injection of high doses of CGP35348 produces allodynia to innocuous mechanical stimuli that is similar to that produced by focal ischemia of the spinal cord (45). Subcutaneous administration of baclofen, a $GABA_B$ receptor agonist, suppresses the behavioral allodynia and hypersensitivity of dorsal horn neurons to innocuous mechanical stimuli that develop after spinal cord ischemia in the rat (44,46). Finally, sc or IT administration of baclofen reverses the thermal or mechanical hyperalgesia induced by loose ligation of the sciatic nerve in the rat (101,119). Collectively, these findings suggest that $GABA_B$ receptor agonists may be efficacious in the treatment of neuropathic pain and that deficits in GABA and in $GABA_B$ receptor function may contribute to or be responsible for neuropathic pain.

GABA$_B$ RECEPTOR LIGANDS AND ANALGESIA: CLINICAL STUDIES AND EXPERIENCE

The results of the studies conducted in laboratory animals of the antinociceptive effects of baclofen are consistent and substantive, and would appear to predict that this and other $GABA_B$ receptor agonists should be effective analgesics in humans. However, these findings contrast markedly with the results of clinical investigations of baclofen. Few studies of baclofen's efficacy against acute pain have been conducted, and the results of these are not in agreement. In a double-blind study of postoperative dental pain with sufficient sensitivity to detect the antinociceptive effects of 650 mg of acetaminophen, 20 mg p.o. of racemic baclofen did not differ from placebo (108). This dose of baclofen is estimated to provide plasma levels of ~0.4 (μg/ml, well within the range at which spasticity is alleviated (58,108). By comparison, in a double-blind, placebo-controlled study of its efficacy against pain induced by dilation and clamping of the cervix, IV administration of 0.3 mg/kg or 0.6 mg/kg racemic baclofen significantly increased the diameter to which the cervix could be dilated without the need for local anesthetic (19). Also, in a study of acute low back pain, 30 to 80 mg/day of baclofen was concluded to be significantly better than placebo in reducing lumbar pain and tenderness (23). Baclofen's interaction with opioid analgesics for the treatment of acute perioperative pain has also been examined. In a study of acute uterine pain, coadministration of 0.3 mg/kg IV baclofen with an analgesic dose of fentanyl did not produce any greater analgesia than did 0.3 mg/kg IV baclofen alone (19). In another study, patients scheduled for transsphenoidal hypophysectomy were pretreated with either saline, 0.6 mg/kg IM baclofen for 5 days, or a bolus injection of 0.6 mg/kg IV baclofen. Perioperative analgesia was provided by IV injection of fentanyl. In patients receiving baclofen, the interval between doses of fentanyl was significantly longer, and less fentanyl was required for perioperative pain control than in patients receiving saline (84).

The doses of baclofen administered in these clinical studies were within the range that alleviated spasticity resulting from spinal injury or multiple sclerosis, and that produced dose-limiting side effects in a significant portion of the population (e.g., nausea, heaviness of the limbs, sedation). Yet, despite administration of purportedly effective doses, these limited studies do not provide impressive evidence of baclofen's efficacy in the management of acute pain or of the existence of a satisfactory separation between the analgesic dose and the dose at which limiting side effects occur (i.e., a suitable therapeutic index). However, in hindsight, it is important to note these early investigations were conducted with the racemic mixture of baclofen, which was the only form available at that time. The racemic mixture of baclofen is not nearly as well tolerated as is the active isomer, L-baclofen (31). Furthermore, the D-isomer of baclofen can antagonize the antinociceptive effects of the L-isomer (94). Its presence in the racemic mixture would be expected to limit analgesic efficacy of the drug. Thus, it is possible that the analgesic efficacy of baclofen was obscured in early studies because of the inability to administer higher doses and the presence of the D-isomer in the racemic mixture. However, perhaps more important than the issue of isomers is the route of administration. In these early studies, baclofen was administered either by oral, intramuscular, or intravenous routes. Its efficacy by the intrathecal route of administration was not examined. However, studies conducted in the late 1980s indicated that intrathecally administered baclofen effectively managed the spasticity resulting from spinal cord injury or multiple sclerosis. Moreover, intrathecally administered baclofen was better tolerated than systemically administered baclofen (17,62,85,86). Although systemically administered baclofen is not currently indicated for the management of acute pain, these retrospective observations raise the intriguing possibility that effective management of acute pain could be achieved by intrathecal administration of the L-isomer of baclofen.

More consistent findings have been made with respect to baclofen's efficacy in trigeminal neuralgia. Fromm and Terrence (31) conducted a series of double-blind, placebo-controlled crossover trials of baclofen, as well as open trials of baclofen in typical and atypical trigeminal neuralgia. In an initial open trial with racemic baclofen, 12 patients with typical trigeminal neuralgia refractory to carbamazepine treatment were administered 60 to 80 mg/day of racemic baclofen. Baclofen decreased the frequency and severity of the paroxysmal attacks in 6 of the 12 patients. In four of the six remaining patients, relief was provided by the addition of previously ineffective doses of carbamazepine. In another group of ten patients, the addition of baclofen to either carbamazepine or phenytoin therapy decreased the frequency and severity of attacks in seven of the patients (32). Similar findings were reported by others (5,102). Fromm and colleagues (33) later extended these initial findings to a single crossover, double-blind study in ten patients and to a larger open trial of 50 patients in which 40 to 80 mg/day p.o. baclofen significantly reduced or prevented the paroxysmal attacks of trigeminal neuralgia (33). In a final study, these same investigators reported that the L-isomer of baclofen was better tolerated by patients and produced fewer dose-limiting side effects than did the racemic mixture. Although Fromm and colleagues concluded that baclofen was not effective in the treatment of atypical facial pain (33), there is a case report that atypical facial pain resulting from ectasia of the basilar artery was effectively treated by 40 mg p.o. baclofen (72).

In neuropathic pain conditions other than trigeminal neuralgia, the efficacy of baclofen is not as clear-cut. In an open trial, Terrence et al. (107) reported that 44 mg/day p.o. baclofen was effective in treating facial postherpetic neuralgia, but not spinal postherpetic neuralgia or the burning dysesthesia of diabetic neuropathy. However, an open trial of 1 mg/kg/day p.o. baclofen and a case report of two patients receiving 20 mg/day of baclofen reported that baclofen alleviated the pain associated with diabetic neuropathy (3,102). Finally, two reports suggest that intrathecally administered baclofen may relieve central pain. In an open trial of five patients suffering from unilateral allodynia or dysesthetic pain of the upper and lower extremities after focal cerebral stroke in the pons, thalamus, or corona radiata, intrathecal administration of 50 to 150 μg of baclofen provided relief within one hour in four patients (104). In a double-blind, placebo-controlled study of pain in patients with spinal spasticity resulting from spinal cord injury or multiple sclerosis, intrathecal administration of 50 μg of baclofen suppressed the spontaneous and allodynic dysesthetic pain, as well as spasm-related pain (48). Collectively, these studies suggest that baclofen is an effective treatment for trigeminal neuralgia in patients refractory to carbamazepine and that under certain conditions it may also be an effective treatment for central or neuropathic pain. Further controlled studies of its efficacy in the treatment of central and neuropathic pain appear to be warranted, particularly those in which the more active L-isomer is administered by the intrathecal route.

$GABA_A$ RECEPTOR LIGANDS AND ANALGESIA: INSIGHTS FROM ANIMAL STUDIES

Numerous investigators have examined the antinociceptive efficacy of prototypic $GABA_A$ receptor agonists such as isoguvacine, muscimol, or THIP in the laboratory animal. Systemic administration of muscimol or THIP produces antinociception in the hot plate, tail flick, or writhing tests in the mouse or the rat (39,49,51,81,95,113) and the shock titration test in the primate (8,49,51). However, the therapeutic indices of THIP (i.e., antinociceptive dose/sedative dose) and of muscimol (i.e., antinociceptive dose/lethal dose) are very small (51,113). Furthermore, despite THIP's affinity for the $GABA_A$ receptor, in many of these studies its antinociceptive effects are not antagonized by subconvulsant doses of bicuculline or picrotoxin, suggesting an action at a bicuculline-insensitive $GABA_A$ receptor (perhaps the now-recognized $GABA_C$ receptor?). Systemic administration of γ-vinyl GABA, an irreversible inhibitor of GABA transaminase that increases the levels of GABA in the central nervous system, also produces antinociception in some of these tests (13,95).

The antinociception produced by systemic administration of $GABA_A$ receptor agonists is likely to be mediated by an action at both supraspinal and spinal $GABA_A$ receptors. A spinal site of action is supported by several lines of evidence. Intrathecal administration of prototypic $GABA_A$ agonists such as muscimol, THIP, or isoguvacine produces modest antinociception in the mouse and the rat (1,42,73,89,112). Intrathecal administration of benzodiazepine receptor agonists such as diazepam or midazolam, which enhance the actions of GABA at the $GABA_A$ receptor, also produce antinociception in the rat, rabbit, or dog (21,29,36,82,88,98). Conversely, intrathecal administration of $GABA_A$ receptor antagonists such as bicuculline or picrotoxin produces allodynia and hyperalgesia (89,117) and increases the reactivity of spinal cord dorsal horn neurons to innocuous stimuli (100). Finally, intrathecal administration of $GABA_A$ receptor antagonists attenuates, whereas intrathecal administration of benzodiazepine receptor agonists enhances, the antinociception produced by activation of the endogenous pain modulatory pathways that originate in the ventromedial medulla (73) and periaqueductal gray (66).

In contrast to spinal $GABA_A$ receptors, activation of supraspinal $GABA_A$ receptors enhances sensitivity to noxious stimuli. Microinjection of $GABA_A$ receptor agonists such as muscimol or THIP at sites in the nucleus raphe magnus or periaqueductal gray produces hyperalgesia (24,27,47), whereas microinjection of the $GABA_A$ receptor antagonist bicuculline at these sites or intracisternally produces antinociception (27,47,79,112). These findings suggest that the brain stem neurons from which the endogenous pain modulatory pathways originate are subject to a tonic, inhibitory input from GABAergic neurons. Antagonism of this inhibitory input disinhibits (i.e., activates) this important bulbospinal pathway for the production of antinociception. Conversely, activation of these receptors results in inhibition of this pathway and the production of hyperalgesia. The lack of or only modest antinociceptive activity of systemically administered benzodiazepines or barbiturates (see below) may therefore reflect the opposing action of GABA at supraspinal and spinal $GABA_A$ receptors (Table 2). Moreover, the ability of systemically administered barbiturates and benzodiazepines to antagonize the analgesic effects of opiates (antianalgesic activity) (55,56,83,91) may reflect a preferential enhancement of GABA at supraspinal $GABA_A$ receptors (i.e., hyperalgesia) (18,71,91,122), as opposed to spinal $GABA_A$ receptors (i.e., analgesia).

Table 2. OPPOSING ACTIONS OF $GABA_A$ RECEPTOR LIGANDS ADMINISTERED AT SUPRASPINAL AND SPINAL SITES

Site of injection	$GABA_A$ agonist	$GABA_A$ antagonist
Spinal	Antinociception	Allodynia Hyperalgesia
Supraspinal	Hyperalgesia	Antinociception

As with the $GABA_B$ receptor ligands, most studies of the role of $GABA_A$ receptor ligands in the production of antinociception have used conventional measures of acute nociception. It is only recently that its role in chronic and neuropathic pain conditions has been examined, and with conflicting results. In the formalin test, intrathecal injection of muscimol produces a bicuculline-reversible suppression of the pain behaviors evoked by injection of formalin in the hind paw of the rat (25). However, the effects of intrathecally administered benzodiazepine receptor agonists are controversial. Intrathecal injection of 30 μg of midazolam does not significantly suppress formalin-induced pain behaviors evoked by sc injection of formalin in the hind paw even at a high dose of 30 μg (25), but intrathecal injection of 15 to 30 μg of midazolam at the cervical level suppresses the pain behaviors induced by injection of formalin in the muzzle of the rat (2). Finally, systemic administration of 0.5 to 5 mg/kg of diazepam greatly increases the pain behaviors during the normally quiescent period between phase 1 and phase 2 of the formalin response (30). The bases for these discrepancies is unclear, although the pronociceptive effects of systemically administered diazepam may reflect preferential enhancement of supraspinal $GABA_A$ receptors and inhibition of the descending inhibitory pathways originating in the medulla. With respect to neuropathic pain, systemic administration of muscimol or THIP does not alleviate the tactile allodynia and enhanced responsiveness of dorsal horn neurons to innocuous tactile stimuli produced by spinal cord ischemia (46; Z. Wiesenfeld-Hallin, personal communication). However, in a model of neuropathic pain induced by loose ligation of the sciatic nerve in the rat, the resultant thermal hyperalgesia is alleviated by intrathecal administration of the $GABA_A$ receptor agonist muscimol (119) and enhanced by pretreatment with a $GABA_A$ receptor antagonist (120). These latter findings suggests that an action of GABA at $GABA_A$ receptors in the spinal cord may play a protective role and that agents that either directly activate or that enhance the actions of GABA at $GABA_A$ receptors in the spinal cord may be effective in the treatment of certain types of neuropathic pain.

$GABA_A$ RECEPTOR LIGANDS AND ANALGESIA: HUMAN STUDIES AND EXPERIENCE

Although no $GABA_A$ receptor agonists are currently available for the treatment of pain in humans, at least one such agent has undergone clinical evaluation in the past. Intramuscular administration of 10 or 20 mg of THIP (Gaboxadol) increased the detection threshold and tolerance threshold for painful electrical stimulation of tooth pulp as compared to placebo. In an open trial of THIP in patients with chronic pain of malignant origin, intramuscular administration of 10 to 25 mg of THIP reduced the pain intensity (57). However, at these therapeutic doses patients in both studies reported significant side effects including sedation, dizziness, and blurred vision (57,67). Although these side effects precluded further development of this particular $GABA_A$ receptor agonist, its efficacy in acute pain suggests that $GABA_A$ receptor agonists with a greater therapeutic index may represent a plausible and novel therapeutic approach to pain management.

As discussed previously, an alternate approach to activation of $GABA_A$ receptors is the administration of benzodiazepine receptor agonists. At low concentrations these agents do not directly activate the receptor, but rather enhance the actions of endogenous GABA (40,53). The majority of studies of the effects of systemically administered diazepam or midazolam concluded that these benzodiazepine receptor agonists did not reduce either the sensory or affective components of cold-pressor–induced pain (103,121), tourniquet-induced pain (20, 103), thermal pain (16,41), or pain induced by electrical stimulation of tooth pulp (38), although the tolerance threshold for tourniquet-induced pain was reportedly increased (16). This universal finding is not surprising when one considers that systemically administered benzodiazepines are likely to enhance the actions of GABA at both spinal and supraspinal $GABA_A$ receptors having opposing actions on nociception (Table 2). Indeed, in a pilot study of acute postoperative pain in which the action of midazolam was restricted to the spinal cord by intrathecal administration, it effectively reduced somatic, but not visceral, pain (35). In a later, double-blind study of chronic low back pain, intrathecal administration of 2 mg of midazolam reduced visual analogue and verbal report scores of the intensity of the pain, as well as the scores on the short-form McGill Pain Questionnaire for the sensory and affective components of low back pain for a period of at least 2 weeks. The magnitude of pain relief produced by midazolam was comparable to that produced by epidural administration of 80 mg of methylprednisolone. Furthermore, one-third to one-half of midazolam-treated patients were able to reduce their concomitant intake of pain medication in the 2-month follow-up period (97). This finding is consistent with the antinociceptive effects of $GABA_A$ receptor agonists in the spinal cord.

NOVEL COMPOUNDS BASED ON GABA

Recently, several anticonvulsants were developed that stimulate or simulate the actions of GABA in the central nervous system and that cross the blood-brain barrier (87,93). For example, gabapentin (Neurontin) is a structural analogue of GABA that readily crosses the blood-brain barrier, but whose mechanism of antiepileptic action is still unknown (34,93,106). Although it has no affinity for or direct action at GABA receptors (90), it appears to increase the concentration of GABA by enhancing its release or synthesis (37,59,68). It also inhibits the transport of neutral L-amino acids in the brain (106,111). Although gabapentin did not produce antinociception in acute models in the mouse or the rat (6), current data suggest that this agent can reduce neuropathic pain states in animal models by a spinal action, and this effect was not reversed by intrathecal $GABA_A$ or $GABA_B$ receptor antagonists (50a). Moreover, a case study reported that gabapentin reduced pain in five of five patients suffering from reflex sympathetic dystrophy (75). Clearly, further investigations of its efficacy in reflex sympathetic dystrophy and other neuropathic pain conditions will need to be made under more controlled, stringent conditions. However, it is intriguing that intravenous administration of 10 to 60 mg/kg of gabapentin in the cat decreased neuronal excitability in the trigeminal nucleus in a manner similar to that of carbamazepine and baclofen (60). This latter finding suggests that clinical trials of gabapentin in trigeminal neuralgia may also be warranted.

Finally, another new anticonvulsant, γ-vinyl GABA (vigabatrin), may also bear further investigation in the management of acute and neuropathic pain. An irreversible inhibitor of GABA transaminase, vigabatrin increases the concentration of GABA in the central nervous system and is well tolerated at therapeutic doses (92). Both compounds may mimic or enhance the actions of GABA at $GABA_A$ and $GABA_B$ receptors and consequently possess analgesic efficacy in acute or chronic, neuropathic pain. It will be of particular interest to establish the efficacy of these agents after intrathecal or epidural administration in man, as the evidence for an antinociceptive action of GABA at spinal $GABA_A$ and $GABA_B$ receptors is perhaps the most convincing.

CONCLUSIONS

Studies conducted in the laboratory animal predict that drugs that activate or mimic the action of GABA at either $GABA_A$ or $GABA_B$ receptors, particularly in the spinal cord, are effective analgesics for the treatment of acute and neuropathic pain. However, the corresponding clinical experience is by no means as persuasive or as impressive as the preclinical literature would predict. At present, relatively little is known about the analgesic effects of these agents in the clinical setting, and past findings may be confounded by the choice of drug with which to test the hypothesis and by the use of a systemic route of administration. A review of the clinical literature provides hints that this class of pharmacologic agent may be efficacious and that further studies of the role of these agents may be warranted. Examples of questions that may be addressed by future studies include (1) Is L-baclofen efficacious and well tolerated for the management of acute pain, neuropathic pain, or central pain when administered by the intrathecal route? (2) Are $GABA_A$ receptor agonists and benzodiazepine receptor agonists effective analgesics for the management of acute pain and neuropathic pain when administered intrathecally? (3) Are the new GABA-based anticonvulsants effective in the treatment of neuropathic or central pain, and under what conditions?

ACKNOWLEDGMENTS

This work was supported by Public Health Service Grant DE11423 to D.L.H.

REFERENCES

1. Aanonsen LM, Wilcox GL. Muscimol, gamma-aminobutyric $acid_A$ receptors and excitatory amino acids in the mouse spinal cord. *J Pharmacol Exp Ther* 1989;248:1034–1038.
2. Aigouy L, Fondras JC, Pajot J, Schoeffler P, Woda A. Intrathecal midazolam versus intrathecal morphine in orofacial nociception: An experimental study in rats. *Neurosci Lett* 1992;139:97–99.
3. Anghinah R, Oliveira ASB, Gabbai AA. Effect of baclofen on pain in diabetic neuropathy. *Muscle Nerve* 1994;17:958–959.
4. Aran S, Hammond DL. Antagonism of baclofen-induced antinociception by intrathecal administration of phaclofen or 2-hydroxysaclofen, but not delta-aminovaleric acid in the rat. *J Pharmacol Exp Ther* 1991;257:360–368.
5. Baker KA, Taylor JW, Lilly GE. Treatment of trigeminal neuralgia: Use of baclofen in combination with carbamazepine. *Clin Pharm* 1985;4:93–96.
6. Bartoszyk GD, Meyerson N, Reimann W, Satzinger G, von Hodenberg A. Gabapentin. In: Meldrum BS, Porter RJ, eds. *Current problems in epilepsy.* London: John Libbey, 1986;147–163.
7. Bennett GJ, Xie YK. A peripheral mononeuropathy in rat that produces disorders of pain sensation like those seen in man. *Pain* 1988;33:87–107.
8. Bloss JL, Hammond DL. Shock titration in the rhesus monkey: Effects of opiate and non-opiate analgesics. *J Pharmacol Exp Ther* 1985;235:423–430.
9. Bormann J. Electrophysiology of $GABA_A$ and $GABA_B$ receptor subtypes. *Trends Neurosci* 1988;11:112–116.
10. Bowery NG. $GABA_B$ receptors: past, present and future. In: Bowery NG, Bittiger H, Olpe HR, eds. *$GABA_B$ receptors in mammalian function.* Chicester: John Wiley, 1990;3–28.
11. Bowery NG. $GABA_B$ Receptor Pharmacology. *Annu Rev Pharmacol Toxicol* 1993;33:109–147.
12. Bowery, NG Pratt, GD. $GABA_B$ receptors as targets for drug action. *Arzneimittelforschung* 1992;42:215–223.
13. Buckett WR. Irreversible inhibitors of GABA transaminase induce antinociceptive effects and potentiate morphine. *Neuropharmacology* 1980;19:715–722.
14. Burt DR, Kamatchi GL. $GABA_A$ receptor subtypes: from pharmacology to molecular biology. *FASEB J* 1991;5:2916–2923.
15. Castro-Lopes JM, Tavares I, Coimbra A. GABA decreases in the spinal cord dorsal horn after peripheral neurectomy. *Brain Res* 1993;620:287–291.
16. Chapman CR, Feather BW. Effects of diazepam on human pain tolerance and pain sensitivity. *Psychosom Med* 1973;35:330–340.
17. Coffey RJ, Cahill D, Steers W, et al. Intrathecal baclofen for intractable spasticity of spinal origin: results of a long-term multicenter study. *J Neurosurg* 1993;78:226–232.
18. Collins JG, Ren K, Saito Y, Iwasaki H, Tang J. Plasticity of some spinal dorsal horn neurons as revealed by pentobarbital-induced disinhibition. *Brain Res* 1990;525:189–197.
19. Corli O, Roma G, Bacchini M, et al. Double-blind placebo-controlled trial of baclofen, alone and in combination, in patients undergoing voluntary abortion. *Clin Ther* 1984;6:800–807.
20. Coulthard P, Rood JP. An investigation of the effect of midazolam on the pain experience. *Br J Oral Maxillofac Surg* 1992;30:248–251.
21. Crawford ME, Jensen FM, Toftdahl DB, Madsen JB. Direct spinal effect of intrathecal and extradural midazolam on visceral noxious stimulation in rabbits. *Br J Anaesth* 1993;70:642–646.
22. Cutting DA, Jordan CC. Alternative approaches to analgesia: baclofen as a model compound. *Br J Pharmacol* 1975;54:171–179.
23. Dapas F, Hartman SF, Martinez L, et al. Baclofen for the treatment of acute low-back syndrome: a double-blind comparison with placebo. *Spine* 1985;10:345–349.
24. Depaulis A, Morgan MM, Liebeskind JC. GABAergic modulation of the analgesic effect of morphine microinjected in the ventral periaqueductal grey matter of the rat. *Brain Res* 1987;436:223–228.
25. Dirig DM, Yaksh TL. Intrathecal baclofen and muscimol, but not midazolam are antinociceptive in the rat-formalin model. *J Pharmacol Exp Ther* 1995;275:219–227.
26. Djamgoz MBA. Diversity of GABA receptors in the vertebrate outer retina. *Trends Neurosci* 1995;18:118–120.
27. Drower EJ, Hammond, DL. GABAergic modulation of nociceptive threshold: effects of THIP and bicuculline microinjected in the ventral medulla of the rat. *Brain Res* 1988;450:316–324.
28. Dunn SMJ, Bateson AN, Martin IL. Molecular neurobiology of the $GABA_A$ receptor. *Int Rev Neurobiol* 1994;36:51–96.
29. Edwards M, Serrao JM, Gent JP, Goodchild CS. On the mechanism by which midazolam causes spinally mediated analgesia. *Anesthesiology* 1990;73:273–277.
30. Franklin KBJ, Abbott FV. Pentobarbital, diazepam, and ethanol abolish the interphase diminution of pain in the formalin test: evidence for pain modulation by $GABA_A$ receptors. *Pharmacol Biochem Behav* 1993;46:661–666.
31. Fromm GH, Terrence CF. Comparison of L-baclofen and racemic baclofen in trigeminal neuralgia. *Neurology* 1987;37:1725–1728.
32. Fromm GH, Terrence CF, Chattha AS. Treatment of face pain. *Trans Am Neurol Assoc* 1980;105:486–488.
33. Fromm GH, Terrence CF, Chattha AS. Baclofen in the treatment of trigeminal neuralgia: double-blind study and long-term follow-up. *Ann Neurol* 1984;15:240–244.
34. Goa KL, Sorkin EM. Gabapentin. A review of its pharmacological properties and clinical potential in epilepsy. *Drug* 1993;46: 409–427.
35. Goodchild CS, Noble J. The effects of intrathecal midazolam on sympathetic nervous system reflexes in man—a pilot study. *Br J Clin Pharmacol* 1987;23:273–285.
36. Goodchild CS, Serrao JM. Intrathecal midazolam in the rat: Evidence for spinally mediated analgesia. *Br J Anaesth* 1987;59: 1563–1570.
37. Gotz E, Feuerstein TJ, Lais A, Meyer DK. Effects of gabapentin on release of gamma-aminobutyric acid from slices of rat neostriatum. *Arzneimittelforschung* 1993;43:636–638.
38. Gracely RH, Dubner R, McGrath PA. Fentanyl reduces the intensity of painful tooth pulp sensations: Controlling for detection of active drugs. *Anesth Analg* 1982;61:751–755.
39. Grognet A, Hertz F, DeFeudis FV. Comparison of the antinociceptive actions of THIP and morphine. *Pharmacol Res Comm* 1982; 14:993–999.
40. Haefly W, Polc P. Physiology of GABA enhancement by benzodiazepines and barbiturates. In: Olsen RW, eds. *Benzodiazepine/GABA receptors and chloride channels.* New York: Alan R. Liss, 1986; 97–133.
41. Hall GM, Whitman JG, Morgan M. Effect of diazepam on experimentally induced pain thresholds. *Br J Anaesth* 1974;46:50–53.
42. Hammond DL, Drower EJ. Effects of intrathecally administered THIP, baclofen and muscimol on nociceptive threshold. *Eur J Pharmacol* 1984;103:121–125.
43. Hammond DL, Washington JD. Antagonism of L-Baclofen-induced antinociception by CGP 35,348 in the spinal cord of the rat. *Eur J Pharmacol* 1993;234:255–262.
44. Hao J-X, Xu X-J, Aldskogius H, Seiger Å, Wiesenfeld-Hallin Z. Allodynia-like effect in rat after ischemic spinal cord injury photochemically induced by laser irradiation. *Pain* 1991;45:175–185.
45. Hao J-X, Xu X-J, Wiesenfeld-Hallin Z. Intrathecal-aminobutyric $acid_B$ ($GABA_B$) receptor antagonist CGP 35348 induces hypersen-

sitivity to mechanical stimuli in the rat. *Neurosci Lett* 1994;182: 299–302.
46. Hao J-X, Xu X-J, Yu Y-X, Seiger Å, Wiesenfeld-Hallin Z. Baclofen reverses the hypersensitivity of dorsal horn wide dynamic range neurons to mechanical stimulation after transient spinal cord ischemia: Implications for a tonic GABAergic inhibitory control of myelinated fiber input. *J Neurophysiol* 1992;68:392–396.
47. Heinricher MM, Kaplan HJ. GABA-mediated inhibition in rostral ventromedial medulla: role in nociceptive modulation in the lightly anesthetized rat. *Pain* 1991;47:105–113.
48. Herman RM, D'Luzansky SC, Ippolito R. Intrathecal baclofen suppresses central pain in patients with spinal lesions. A pilot study. *Clin J Pain* 1992;8:338–345.
49. Hill RC, Maurer R, Buescher H-H, Roemer D. Analgesic properties of the GABA-mimetic THIP. *Eur J Pharmacol* 1981;69:221–224.
50. Hwang AS, Wilcox GL. Baclofen, γ-Aminobutyric acid$_B$ receptors and substance P in the mouse spinal cord. *J Pharmacol Exp Ther* 1989;248:1026–1033.
50a. Hwang JH and Yaksh TL. The effect of intrathecal gabapentin on tactile-evoked allodynia in a surgically induced neuropathic pain model in the rat. *Reg Anesth* 1996;in press.
51. Hynes MD, Leander JD, Frederickson RCA, Ho PPK, Johnson DW, Archer RA. Evaluation of THIP in standard tests of analgesic activity: occurrence of antinociception and hyperalgesia. *Drug Devel Res* 1984;4:405–419.
52. Johnston GAR. Multiplicity of GABA receptors. In: Olsen RW, Venter JC, eds. *Benzodiazepine/GABA receptors and chloride channels.* New York: Alan R. Liss, 1986;57–71.
53. Kerr DIB, Ong J. GABA agonists and antagonists. *Med Res Rev* 1992;12:593–636.
54. Kim SH, Chung JM. An experimental model for peripheral neuropathy produced by segmental spinal nerve ligation in the rat. *Pain* 1992;50:355–363.
55. Kissin I, Brown P, Bradley E Jr. Morphine and fentanyl anesthetic interactions with diazepam: Relative antagonism in rats. *Anesth Analg* 1990;71:236–241.
56. Kitahata LM, Saberski L. Are barbiturates hyperalgesic? *Anesthesiology* 1992;77:1059–1061.
57. Kjaer M, Nielsen H. The analgesic effect of the GABA-agonist THIP in patients with chronic pain of malignant origin. A phase-1-2 study. *Br J Clin Pharmacol* 1983;16:477–485.
58. Knutsson E, Lindblom U, Märtensson A. Plasma and cerebrospinal fluid levels of baclofen (Lioresal) at optimal therapeutic responses in spastic paresis. *J Neurol Sci* 1974;23:473–484.
59. Kocsis JD, Honmou O. Gabapentin increases GABA-induced depolarization in rat neonatal optic nerve. *Neurosci Lett* 1994;169: 181–184.
60. Kondo T, Fromm GH, Schmidt B. Comparison of gabapentin with other antiepileptic and GABAergic drugs. *Epilepsy Res* 1991;8: 226–231.
61. Kusama T, Spivak CE, Whiting P, Dawson VL, Schaeffer JC, Uhl GR. Pharmacology of GABA ρ1 and GABA A/B receptors expressed in *Xenopus* oocytes and COS cells. *Br J Pharmacol* 1993; 109:200–206.
62. Lazorthes Y, Sallerin-Caute B, Verdie J, Bastide R, Carillo J. Chronic intrathecal baclofen administration for control of severe spasticity. *J Neurosurg* 1990;72:393–402.
63. Levy RA, Proudfit HK. The analgesic action of baclofen [β-(4-chlorophenyl)-γ-aminobutyric acid]. *J Pharmacol Exp Ther* 1977; 202:437–445.
64. Levy RA, Proudfit HK. Analgesia produced by microinjection of baclofen and morphine at brain stem sites. *Eur J Pharmacol* 1979; 57:43–55.
65. Liebman JM, Pastor G. Antinociceptive effects of baclofen and muscimol upon intraventricular administration. *Eur J Pharmacol* 1980;61:225–230.
66. Lin Q, Peng Y, Willis WD. Glycine and GABA$_A$ antagonists reduce the inhibition of primate spinothalamic tract neurons produced by stimulation in periaqueductal gray. *Brain Res* 1994;654: 286–302.
67. Lindeburg T, Folsgard S, Sillesen H, Jacobsen E, Kehlet H. Analgesic, respiratory and endocrine responses in normal man to THIP, a GABA-agonist. *Acta Anesthesiol Scand* 1983;27:10–12.
68. Löscher W, Honack D, Taylor CP. Gabapentin increases aminooxyacetic acid-induced GABA accumulation in several regions of rat brain. *Neurosci Lett* 1991;128:150–154.
69. Lüddens H, Wisden W. Function and pharmacology of multiple GABA$_A$ receptor subunits. *Trends Pharmacol Sci* 1991;12:49–51.
70. MacDonald RL, Olsen RW. GABA$_A$ receptor channels. *Annu Rev Neurosci* 1994;17:569–602.
71. Mantegazza P, Parenti M, Tammiso R, Vita P, Zambotti F, Zonta N. Modification of the antinociceptive effect of morphine by centrally administered diazepam and midazolam. *Br J Pharmacol* 1982; 75:569–572.
72. Martins IP, Ferro JM. Atypical facial pain, ectasia of the basilar artery, and baclofen: a case report. *Headache* 1989;29:581–583.
73. McGowan MK, Hammond DL. Antinociception produced by microinjection of L-glutamate into the ventromedial medulla of the rat: mediation by spinal GABA$_A$ receptors. *Brain Res* 1993;620: 86–96.
74. McGowan MK, Hammond DL. Intrathecal GABA$_B$ antagonists attenuate the antinociception produced by microinjection of L-glutamate into the ventromedial medulla of the rat. *Brain Res* 1993;607:39–46.
75. Mellick LB, Mellick GA. Successful treatment of reflex sympathetic dystrophy with gabapentin. *Am J Emerg Med* 1995;13:96.
76. Mertens S, Benke D, Mohler H. GABA$_A$ receptor populations with novel subunit combinations and drug binding profiles identified in brain by α_5- and δ-subunit-specific immunopurification. *J Biol Chem* 1993;268:5965–5973.
77. Milligan G, Bond AR, Lee M. Inverse agonism: pharmacological curiosity or potential therapeutic strategy. *Trends Pharmacol Sci* 1995;16:10–13.
78. Mody I, DeKoninck Y, Otis TS, Soltesz I. Bridging the cleft at GABA synapses in the brain. *Trends Neurosci* 1994;17:
79. Moreau JL, Fields HL. Evidence for GABA involvement in midbrain control of medullary neurons that modulate nociceptive transmission. *Brain Res* 1986;397:37–46.
80. Mott DD, Lewis DV. The pharmacology and function of central GABA$_B$ receptors. *Int Rev Neurobiol* 1994;36:97–223.
81. Murray TF, McGill W, Cheney DL. A comparison of the analgesic activities of 4,5,6,7-tetrahydroisoxazolo[5,4-c]pyridin-3-ol (THIP) and 6-chloro-2[1-piperazinyll]pyrazine (MK212). *Eur J Pharmacol* 1983;90:179–184.
82. Niv D, Whitwam JG, Loh L. Depression of nociceptive sympathetic reflexes by the intrathecal administration of midazolam. *Br J Anaesth* 1983;55:541–547.
83. Ossipov MH, Gebhart GF. Light pentobarbital anesthesia diminishes the antinociceptive potency of morphine administered intracranially but not intrathecally in the rat. *Eur J Pharmacol* 1984; 97:137–140.
84. Panerai AE, Massei R, De Silva E, Sacerdote P, Monza G, Mantagazza P. Baclofen prolongs the analgesic effect of fentanyl in man. *Br J Anaesth* 1985;57:954–955.
85. Penn RD. Intrathecal baclofen for spasticity of spinal origin: seven years of experience. *J Neurosurg* 1992;77:236–240.
86. Penn RD, Savoy SM, Corcos D, et al. Intrathecal baclofen for severe spinal spasticity. *N Engl J Med* 1989;320:1517–1521.
87. Perucca E. The clinical pharmacology of the new antiepileptic drugs. *Pharmacol Res* 1993;28:89–196.
88. Pomeranz B, Nguyen P. Intrathecal diazepam suppresses nociceptive reflexes and potentiates electroacupuncture effects in pentobarbital-anesthetized rats. *Neurosci Lett* 1987;77:316–320.
89. Roberts LA, Beyer C, Komisaruk BR. Nociceptive responses to altered GABAergic activity at the spinal cord. *Life Sci* 1986;39: 1667–1674.
90. Rock DM, Kelly KM, MacDonald RL. Gabapentin actions on ligand- and voltage-gated responses in cultured rodent neurons. *Epilepsy Res* 1993;16:89–98.
91. Rosland JH, Hole K. 1,4-Benzodiazepines antagonize opiate-induced antinociception in mice. *Anesth Analg* 1990;71:242–248.
92. Sabers A, Gram L. Pharmacology of vigabatrin. *Pharmacol Toxicol* 1992;70:237–243.
93. Satzinger G. Antiepileptics from gamma-aminobutyric acid. *Arzneimittelforschung* 1994;44:261–266.
94. Sawynok J, Dickson C. D-Baclofen is an antagonist at baclofen receptors mediating antinociception in the spinal cord. *Pharmacology* 1985;31:248–259.
95. Sawynok J, LaBella FS. On the involvement of GABA in the analgesia produced by baclofen, muscimol and morphine. *Neuropharmacology* 1982;21:397–403.
96. Seltzer W, Dubner R, Shir Y. A novel behavioral model of neuro-

pathic pain disorders produced in rats by partial sciatic nerve injury. *Pain* 1990;43:205–218.

97. Serrao JM, Marks RL, Morley SJ, Goodchild CS. Intrathecal midazolam for the treatment of chronic mechanical low back pain: a controlled comparison with epidural steroid in a pilot study. *Pain* 1992;48:5–12.
98. Serrao JM, Stubbs SC, Goodchild CS, Gent JP. Intrathecal midazolam and fentanyl in the rat: Evidence for different spinal antinociceptive effects. *Anesthesiology* 1989;70:780–786.
99. Sieghart W. $GABA_A$ receptors: ligand-gated Cl^- ion channels modulated by multiple drug-binding sites. *Trends Pharmacol Sci* 1992; 13:446–450.
100. Sivilotti L, Woolf CJ. The contribution of $GABA_A$ and glycine receptors to central sensitization: Disinhibition and touch-evoked allodynia in the spinal cord. *J Neurophysiol* 1994;72:169–179.
101. Smith GD, Harrison SM, Birch PJ, Elliott PJ, Malcangio M, Bowery NG. Increased sensitivity to the antinociceptive activity of (±)baclofen in an animal model of chronic neuropathic pain, but not chronic inflammatory hyperalgesia. *Neuropharmacology* 1994; 33:1103–1108.
102. Steardo L, Leo A, Marano E. Efficacy of baclofen in trigeminal neuralgia and some other painful conditions. *Eur Neurol* 1984;23: 51–55.
103. Stern JA, Brown M, Ulett GA, Sletten I. A comparison of hypnosis, acupuncture, morphine, valium, aspirin and placebo in the management of experimentally induced pain. *Ann NY Acad Sci* 1977; 296:175–193.
104. Taira T, Tanikawa T, Kawamura H, Iseki H, Takakura K. Spinal intrathecal baclofen suppresses central pain after a stroke. *J Neurol Neurosurg Psychiatry* 1994;57:381–382.
105. Tanelian DL, Kosek P, Mody I, MacIver B. The role of the $GABA_A$ receptor/chloride channel complex in anesthesia. *Anesthesiology* 1993;78:757–776.
106. Taylor CP. Emerging new perspectives on the mechanism of action of gabapentin. *Neurology* 1994;44 (Suppl. 5):S10–16.
107. Terrence CF, Fromm GH, Tenicela R. Baclofen as an analgesic in chronic peripheral nerve disease. *Eur Neurol* 1985;24:380–385.
108. Terrence CF, Potter DM, Fromm GH. Is baclofen an analgesic? *Clin Neuropharmacol* 1983;6:241–145.
109. Thomas DA, McGowan MK, Hammond DL. Microinjection of baclofen in the ventromedial medulla of the rat produces antinociception or hyperalgesia. *J Pharmacol Exp Ther* 1995;275:274–284.
110. Thomas DA, Navarrete I, Graham BA, McGowan MK, Hammond DL. Contribution of spinal and brain stem sites to the antinociception produced by the systemic administration of baclofen. *Neurosci Abstr* 1995;21:
111. Thurlow RJ, Brown JP, Gee NS, Hill DR, Woodruff GN. [^{3}H]gabapentin may label a system-L-like neutral amino acid carrier in brain. *Eur J Pharmacol* 1993;247:341–345.
112. Ueda H, Ge M, Satoh M, Takagi H. Subconvulsive doses of intracisternal bicuculline methiodide, a $GABA_A$ receptor antagonist, produce potent analgesia as measured in the tail pinch test in mice. *Eur J Pharmacol* 1987;136:129–131.
113. Vaught JL, Pelley K, Costa LG, Setler P, Enna SJ. A comparison of the antinociceptive responses to the GABA-receptor agonists THIP and baclofen. *Neuropharmacology* 1985;24:211–216.
114. Wilson PR, Yaksh TL. Baclofen is antinociceptive in the spinal intrathecal space of animals. *Eur J Pharmacol* 1978;51:323–330.
115. Wisden W, Laurie DJ, Monyer H, Seeburg PH. The distribution of 13 $GABA_A$ receptor subunit mRNAs in the rat brain. I. Telencephalon, diencephalon, mesencephalon. *J Neurosci* 1992;12: 1040–1062.
116. Woodward RM, Polenzani L, Miledi R. Characterization of bicuculline/baclofen-insensitive γ-aminobutyric acid receptors expressed in *Xenopus* oocytes. I. Effects of Cl^- channel inhibitors. *Mol Pharmacol* 1992;42:165–173.
117. Yaksh TL. Behavioral and autonomic correlates of the tactile evoked allodynia produced by spinal glycine inhibition: effects of modulatory receptor systems and excitatory amino acid antagonists. *Pain* 1989;37:111–123.
118. Yaksh TL, Reddy SVR. Studies in the primate on the analgetic effects associated with intrathecal actions of opiate, alpha-adrenergic agonists and baclofen. *Anesthesiology* 1981;54:451–467.
119. Yamamoto T, Yaksh TL. Spinal pharmacology of thermal hyperesthesia induced by incomplete ligation of sciatic nerve. *Anesthesiology* 1991;75:817–826.
120. Yamamoto T, Yaksh TL. Effects of intrathecal strychnine and bicuculline on nerve compression-induced thermal hyperalgesia and selective antagonism by MK-801. *Pain* 1993;54:79–84.
121. Zacny JP, Coalson D, Young C, et al. A dose-response study of the effects of intravenous midazolam on cold pressor-induced pain. *Anesth Analg* 1995;80:521–525.
122. Zambotti F, Zonta N, Tammiso R, Ferrario P, Hafner B, Mantegazza P. Reversal of the effect of centrally administered diazepam on morphine antinociception by specific (Ro 15-1788 and Ro 15-3505) and non-specific (bicuculline and caffeine) benzodiazepine antagonists. *Naunyn Schmiedebergs Arch Pharmacol* 1986;333:43–46.

Anesthesia: Biologic Foundations, edited by
Tony L. Yaksh et al. Lippincott–Raven Publishers,
Philadelphia © 1997.

CHAPTER 63

SYSTEMIC USE OF LOCAL ANESTHETICS IN PAIN STATES

SANDRA R. CHAPLAN, FLEMMING W. BACH,
AND TONY L. YAKSH

The topical/regional use of local anesthesia with cocaine was well established prior to the turn of the century. Procaine and lidocaine, first synthesized in 1904 and 1948, respectively, were the next drugs with recognized local anesthetic properties to be developed (16,74). Reports of general anesthetic properties of intravenously infused local anesthetics date back to the 1940s, with demonstrations that these agents could be used to augment the anesthetic effects of nitrous oxide (41). Analgesic effects of these compounds in various pain states in unanesthetized patients were recognized early in the World War II era and documented in a number of anecdotal series (12,50,80,87; see 49 for review). Particular interest in these reports resides in the contention that such treatment provides specific analgesia for pain states presenting special management difficulties and in which opiates are found to be of limited benefit (27,50,96). The impact of these observations may have been lessened by similar anecdotal accounts claiming highly nonspecific benefits to general health and well-being from the IV infusion of local anesthetics (3). In the ensuing decades, both procaine and lidocaine have continued to enjoy clinical popularity, albeit declining, as systemically administered anesthetic adjuncts (14,30); lidocaine appears to have an anesthetic-sparing property that plateaus at approximately 40% at a plasma level between 1 and 2 μg/ml, after which increasing plasma levels do not provide additional benefit (56) and toxicity may be evident.

In the past decade, interest in the use of systemic local anesthetics has been strongly renewed by clinical trials demonstrating utility in specific neuropathic pain states. More recently, growing appreciation of the differences in the pharmacology and electrophysiology of facilitated pain states, and availability of accepted animal models of neuropathic pain produced by nerve injury, have permitted more rigorous investigations of differential effects on pain states. This chapter summarizes what is currently known regarding clinical effects, laboratory investigations, and mechanisms of action of analgesic, and more importantly, antihyperalgesic effects of systemically delivered local anesthetics.

ACUTE PAIN: CONTROLLED STUDIES

Clinical Trials

The earliest controlled trials on the effects of procaine (4 mg/kg IV administered) (68) and lidocaine (1 g IV administered) (7) demonstrated positive analgesic effects on postoperative pain. Two recent double-blind randomized controlled studies on postoperative pain, both yielding similar blood concentrations of lidocaine, resulted in conflicting conclusions, one finding decreases in both visual analogue scale (VAS) scores and opioid consumption (23), and the other finding no effect on either VAS scores or stress hormones in patients immediately after abdominal hysterectomy (13). Postoperative myalgias induced by intraoperative succinylcholine administration were alleviated by IV lidocaine (52). Acute migraine pain was not alleviated by a low dose of IV lidocaine—1 mg/kg (91). The two studies examining local anesthetic infusions in burn patients have been in agreement: pain was reduced by procaine infusion in patients suffering from burns (50). Similarly, a recent study has documented relief of burn pain from IV lidocaine infusion (60).

Experimental Pain Stimuli

Several recent controlled studies have been performed using experimental acute pain models (Table 1). These studies confirm that lidocaine at concentrations below 3 μg/ml is not a general analgesic. Of note, Boas et al. (15) are perhaps responsible for the first systematic observation that the effects of local anesthetics may be divergent in pain states of different origins, as reported in their investigation studying the simultaneous effect of IV lidocaine on experimental acute ischemic pain induced by the tourniquet technique and on preexisting neuropathic pain in the same subjects. At blood lidocaine concentrations above 3 μg/ml both kinds of pain were reduced, whereas only the neuropathic pain was reduced at lower concentrations, leading to the suggestion that there is a mild general analgesic effect of lidocaine at blood concentrations above 3 μg/ml, and that neuropathic pain may be selectively reduced at lower concentrations. In one of the few clinical studies to examine both analgesic actions and mechanisms, Bach et al. (5) found that lidocaine increased the threshold at which the nociceptive flexion reflex was elicited, a withdrawal reflex that is mainly spinally organized. These data suggest that intrinsic spinal nociceptive circuits are sensitive to systemic lidocaine, and are supported by several clinical studies documenting a depressant effect of systemically administered lidocaine on somatosensory-evoked potentials recorded intraoperatively (95) or in awake patients (66).

CHRONIC PAIN

Uncontrolled Studies

A retrospective series describes the effect of lidocaine at a dose of 1 to 5 mg/kg on 182 cases of various chronic pain states (42). In this heterogeneous patient population, 83 (46%) responded favorably to treatment. Most responders were patients with radicular low back pain and peripheral nerve lesions. Patients with mechanical back pain, myofascial syndromes, phantom limb pain, and postherpetic neuralgia were poor responders. Another retrospective study (48) focused solely on neuropathic pain and reported a high number of responders (87%) when the painful condition was related to a primary lesion of the peripheral nervous system, whereas primary CNS lesions showed lower-response rates (31%). Idiopathic pain conditions and reflex sympathetic dystrophy showed poor response rates.

Controlled Studies

Pain resulting from peripheral nerve injury or polyneuropathy seems most consistently sensitive to local anesthetics. Con-

Table 1. ANALGESIC EFFECT OF SYSTEMIC LOCAL ANESTHETICS: CONTROLLED STUDIES

	Pain syndrome	*N*	Treatment	Design	Concentration	Effect parameters	Result	Reference
Acute pain Experimental	Healthy volunteers	14	Lidocaine	RCDBX	1–3 μg/ml	Tourniquet pain threshold Tourniquet pain tolerance	NS NS	Rowlingson
	Healthy volunteers	11	Bupivacaine	RCDBX	0.1–1.8 μg/ml	Tourniquet pain threshold Tourniquet pain tolerance	NS NS	Friedman
	Diabetic/healthy volunteers	8	Lidocaine 5 mg/kg	RCDBX		Heat pain threshold Cold pain threshold	NS NS	Bach
	Diabetic/healthy volunteers	3	Lidocaine 5 mg/kg	RCDBX		Nociceptive flexion reflex threshold	Threshold ↑	Bach
	Healthy volunteers	10	Lidocaine 3.7 mg/kg	RCDBX	2 μg/ml	Laser pain detection Laser pain tolerance	NS NS	Nielsen
Clinical	Migraine	25	Lidocaine 1 mg/kg	RCDB		VAS	NS	Reutens
	Postoperative pain	20	Lidocaine 2 mg/min	RCDB	1–2 μg/ml	VAS	Pain ↓, opioid use ↓	Cassuto
	Postoperative pain	18	Lidocaine 2 mg/kg/h	RCDB	1.5–2 μg/ml	VAS, stress hormones	NS	Birch
	Postoperative pain	40	Procaine 4–6.5 mg/kg	OC		Pain and comfort report	Pain ↓, comfort ↑	Keats et al.
	Postoperative pain	302	Lidocaine 1 g	OC		Pain report	Pain ↓	Bartlett
Chronic pain Nociceptive	Cancer bone pain	10	Lidocaine 5 mg/kg	RCDBX		VAS	NS	Sjøgren
Neuropathic	Diabetic neuropathy	15	Lidocaine 5 mg/kg	RCDBX	1.7–6.5 μg/ml	VAS/symptom score	Pain ↓	Kastrup
	Diabetic neuropathy	16	Mexiletine 10 mg/kg/d	RCDBX	3.4 μmol/L	VAS/symptom score	Pain ↓	Dejgaard
	Peripheral nerve injury	11	Mexiletine 750 mg/d	RCDBX		VAS	Pain ↓	Chabal
	Postherpetic neuralgia	19	Lidocaine 5 mg/kg	RCDBX	1–4.8 μg/ml	VAS	Pain ↓	Rowbotham
	Central pain	8	Lidocaine 1 mg/kg	CSB		Verbal rating scale	Pain ↓	Backonja
	Neuropathy: cancer/treatment	10	Lidocaine 5 mg/kg	RCDBX		Allodynia VAS	NS	Ellemann
	Diabetic neuropathy	95	Mexiletine 225–675 mg/d	RCDB		VAS, McGill	NS	Stracke
	Malignant plexopathy	10	Lidocaine 5 mg/kg	RCDBX		VAS	NS	Bruera
	Trigeminal neuralgia	12	Tocainide 20 mg/d	RCDBX	29 μmol/L	VAS	Comparable to carbamazepine	Lindström

R, randomized; C, controlled; DB, double blind; SB, single blind; X, crossover; O, open trial.

trolled studies on effects of systemic local anesthetics on chronic pain are systematically presented in Table 1. Only a single-controlled study has been performed in chronic nociceptive pain, with a negative finding (98). As can be seen by scanning the table, the results however are generally more uniformly positive for neuropathic pain conditions, but, as can also be appreciated, there are conflicting results from well-controlled studies.

There may be several explanations for these discrepancies. Differing treatment paradigms may account for lack of accord in observations: studies employing low doses, or shorter infusion durations producing lower peak plasma concentrations, may be predisposed toward negative results. Documentation of treatment effect is a difficult matter: many chronic pain patients, in addition to having pain in more than one location, may be experiencing localized pain involving more than one mechanism, and it may be unrealizable to precisely define which pain is quantified. Some authors have employed neuropathy symptom scores instead of simple subjective pain scales to attempt to overcome this problem (31,67). Severity of pretreatment pain may influence responses to intervention. Lidocaine is extensively protein-bound in the bloodstream, primarily to α_1-acid glycoprotein, yet lidocaine plasma concentrations are ordinarily reported as total drug (protein-bound plus free drug). This carrier protein, α_1-acid glycoprotein, is an acute-phase reactant, and may be elevated in inflammatory states as well as malignancies; other disease states may result in plasma protein deficiencies. Thus, actual free drug concentrations may be much lower than suspected from total drug measurements in, for example, cancer patients, and the opposite may obtain in patients with marked protein losses or hepatic synthetic abilities. Pain diagnoses as grouped according to current taxonomic understanding may also conceal significant heterogeneity related to the time course, severity, or other factors modifying the underlying disorder. Thus, a large study on patients with diabetic neuropathy revealed no significant overall effect of mexiletine, an orally bioavailable lidocaine analogue, evaluated on a VAS scale or a McGill scale. However, certain subgroups categorized according to types and course of complaints showed clear effect on both scales (104). Finally, studies may have included patients with significant confounding effects due to previous treatments.

Few data are available on the dose-response relationships between lidocaine and pain alleviation. In humans, as in animals, 90% of circulating lidocaine is metabolized in the liver; some metabolites, such as monoethylglycinexylidide (MEGX) and glycinexylidide (GX), possess pharmacologic activity (17). The oral bioavailability of lidocaine is low, due to extensive first-pass metabolism. After an IV injection, an initial redistribution phase with a half-life ($t_{1/2}$) of 5 min is followed by a final elimination phase with $t_{1/2}$ of 1.5 to 2 hours (55). Most studies reporting effects of systemic lidocaine administered 5 mg/kg over 30 to 60 minutes. From the data in Table 1 it might be concluded that a blood lidocaine concentration above 1.5 to 2 μg/ml is required to demonstrate effects. However, in the studies assembled, blood samples were collected at various time points relative to infusions. A recent study examined the dose and concentration effects on VAS reports during infusions of lidocaine in 13 patients; the median effective dose (ED_{50}) of lidocaine was 372 mg, in good accord with the common practice mentioned above (47). At these lidocaine levels side effects are common but harmless, limited to light-headedness, a sense of intoxication, and perioral paresthesias. Apart from dysarthria and, rarely, nystagmus, neurologic signs are not seen.

Most of the studies discussed to this point deal with short-lasting effects of lidocaine, barely outlasting the infusion. An intriguing aspect of this subject, however, is the reports of pain-relieving effects lasting from several days to up to 2 to 3 weeks (5,6,42,67,89). While it is relatively easy to hypothesize a mechanism related to well-known acute effects on excitable membranes to explain short-term pain relief by systemic local anesthetics, it is more difficult to speculate regarding a mechanism to explain sustained analgesia. This topic will be discussed in more detail in the following section, since the bulk of studies on the subject are performed in animals.

PRECLINICAL MODELS AND LOCAL ANESTHETIC ACTION

Preclinical studies addressing the analgesic effects of systemically administered local anesthetics are most rationally considered in terms of the several discrete models employed. As reviewed in Chap. 40, some preclinical models provide corollaries to acute painful stimuli, analogous to acute postinjury or experimental pain in humans. Others employ stimuli with more sustained characteristics, resolving over a period of many minutes or several hours, which resemble post–tissue injury pain states with persistent nociceptive activity. A third class of preclinical models induces a mono- or polyneuropathy by either surgical or metabolic means, thus generating behaviors suggestive of neuropathic conditions. In the following sections, the action of systemic local anesthetics are considered in the context of these three principal categories of pain states.

Acute Nociceptive Stimulation

Acute noxious stimuli against which the effect of systemic local anesthetics have been measured in both behavioral and electrophysiologic studies include:

Thermal stimuli: measured as tail flick to heat, time-to-escape behavior on the hot plate, or paw withdrawal to a selective thermal probe application (54).

Noninjurious mechanical stimuli: paw pressure or pinch device, measuring vocalization or withdrawal attempts to a deep mechanical stimulus (105).

Acute mechanical injury to primary afferent terminals: as in the explanted corneal abrasion model (106).

Acute responses to noxious chemical stimuli: as in the paw flinch/licking responses in the formalin test (39,108).

In the formalin test, two phases of flinching activity have been reliably described and correlated with respective phases of increased peripheral nerve and dorsal horn neuronal activity. The first phase (0–5 min) is interpreted to reflect reactions to an acute noxious stimulus, and is usually followed by a brief quiescent phase (5–10 min) during which behavior is reduced. The second, tonic phase (10–60 min) is discussed below; further details of these models are presented in Chap. 40.

It should be stressed that the available data on the actions of intravenous local anesthetics are limited and distributed across several models and species. Comparisons of the studies are additionally hindered by the use for the most part of dose responses rather than blood level data, since volumes of distribution differ substantially among species, and doses are not comparable across species.

Actions of Local Anesthetics in Models of Acute Pain

Parenteral delivery of local anesthetics has revealed mixed results (Table 2). At doses not associated with side effects, lidocaine and bupivacaine caused no significant changes in hot plate escape latency (110); analgesia was seen, however, with the lidocaine analogue tocainide. Lidocaine had no significant effect on the first phase of the rat formalin paw test at plasma concentrations in the range of 3 to 6 μg/ml or on the thermal withdrawal latencies of normal rat paws (contralateral to nerve-ligated extremities) at plasma levels of 1 μg/ml (1). Vocalization thresholds of normal rats to paw compression was significantly elevated by IV lidocaine doses of 1 to 9 mg/kg for a period of 6 hours (28). Bartolini et al. (8) found analgesic properties of subcutaneous (s.c.) bupivacaine, lidocaine, and procaine in the mouse hot plate test and the rat tail flick test, which were reversed by pretreatment with atropine, leading these investigators to advance an analgesic mechanism involving presynaptic muscarinic acetylcholinergic receptor enhancement. To date no further studies have explored this hypothesis.

Acute physiologic preparations have shown lidocaine to have depressant effects on firing of second-order neurons. These effects are sustained for many minutes (even hours) after acute administration. Dose-related suppression of neurons in rexed lamina V to high-threshold mechanical and noxious thermal stimuli, lasting up to 50 minutes after bolus delivery, is seen in decerebrate cats (3 to 10 μg/ml) (38). In comparison, activity evoked in primary afferent neurons by electrical stimulation of the tooth pulp (an area selectively innervated by nociceptive C fibers) was not blocked by intravenous lidocaine at any sublethal dose, although blockade was possible with the noncompetitive sodium channel blocker tetrodotoxin (51). Thus, a higher degree of sodium channel blockade may be required to block peripheral nerve activity, particularly if evoked by a synchronous volley as with an intense electrical stimulus.

Persistent Postinjury Pain States

The second phase of paw flinching/licking (10–60 min) of the formalin test is considered a model of reactions to tonic rather than acute noxious stimulation, and has been shown to reflect facilitation of neural activity at the spinal cord level, with recruitment of *N*-methyl-D-aspartate (NMDA)-type glutamate receptor activity (53). Similarly, cutaneous mustard oil application generates a sustained nociceptive response based on prolonged and selective C-fiber stimulation (59,112). The visceral writhing test evaluates responses to activation of unmyelinated visceral afferents by intraperitoneal (i.p.) chemical irritants (88). As reviewed in Chap. 36, these models are believed to reflect a cascade of events initiated by the persistent small afferent input. This cascade involves activation of spinal glutamate receptor subtypes. Accordingly, it is possible to pharmacologically reconstitute "chronic" or facilitated spinal cord transmission by the use of iontophoresed glutamatergic excitatory amino acids. Thus, NMDA application produces augmented wide dynamic range neuronal (WDR) firing (firing similar to that produced by intensive C-fiber intensity afferent stimulation—windup) (36,37,53), and NMDA antagonism reverses windup and windup-like facilitation. Sustained central activity is demonstrable after the application of NMDA-type glutamate agonists (37), which leads not only to electrophysiologic facilitation of neuronal responses but also to the behavioral manifestation of tactile allodynia (4) and thermal hyperalgesia (76).

Table 2. ACUTE NOCICEPTION STUDIES

Model	Drug	Effect	Reference
Behavioral			
Hot plate (rat)	Lidocaine 20 mg/kg i.p.	No analgesia	110
	Tocainide 100 mg/kg i.p.	Dose-related analgesia	
	Bupivacaine 12.5 mg/kg i.p.	No analgesia	
Formalin (rat), 1st phase	Lido 10 mg/kg i.v.	No analgesia	1
Formalin (mouse), 1st phase	Mexiletine 30 mg/kg i.p.	Reduced phase 1	63
Paw pressure (rat)	Lidocaine 1–9 mg/kg i.v.	Dose-related suppression of vocalization	28
Hot plate (mouse)	Procaine, to 50 mg/kg s.c.	Dose-related analgesia, all agents, both tests	8
Tail flick (rat)	Bupivacaine, to 25 mg/kg s.c.		
	Lidocaine, to 30 mg/kg s.c.		
Electrophysiologic			
Trigeminal nucleus (cat) tooth pulp stimulation	Lidocaine 15–30 mg/kg i.v.	No effect	51
	Tetrodotoxin 2–8? μ/kg i.v.	Blocked response	
Dorsal horn (rat), thermal paw stimulation	Lidocaine 5–10 mg/kg i.v.	Dose-related WDR firing suppression	38
Dorsal horn (rat) thermal/mechanical paw stimulation	Lidocaine 5 mg/kg i.a.	Both agents: reduction or abolition of WDR response	112
	Tocainide, 50 mg/kg i.a.		
Dorsal horn, (rat) thermal/mechanical paw stimulation	Lidocaine 3–4 mg/kg i.v.	Suppression of WDR firing	101
In vitro			
Corneal abrasion (rabbit)	Lidocaine 10–60 μM, bath	Dose-related decreased primary afferent firing	106

Actions of Local Anesthetics in Models of Tonic Pain

Investigations using tonic stimuli (Table 3), such as the formalin test phase 2 or mustard oil, have yielded uniformly positive results on afferent responses (1,63). The single study to examine behavioral responses to a noxious visceral stimulus (8) also revealed positive results. Woolf and Wiesenfeld-Hallin (112) showed that the reduction by lidocaine or tocainide of sural nerve reflexes elicited by selective C-fiber stimulation was sustained over 30 minutes, and was more significant than the suppression of other noxious responses. A companion study showed that this response was not due to axonal or terminal blockade, since axonal conduction was unaffected, as was neurogenic extravasation into the paw; they concluded that the action was on polysynaptic C-fiber–evoked responses (112). While in vitro work has shown that lidocaine can suppress the spontaneous firing of injured primary afferent terminals, this effect was observed only at free lidocaine concentrations of around 5 μg/ml; this concentration of free drug is not obtained clinically due to the sequestering effect of extensive plasma protein binding (see above). The foregoing studies suggest a pronounced effect on C-fiber–evoked responses, since the formalin test is largely sustained by ongoing low-level C-fiber discharge, and visceral nociception is mediated by small unmyelinated fibers.

The specific interaction of local anesthetics with neurotransmitter systems has been explored in behavioral as well as electrophysiologic in vivo and ex vivo preparations. Kamei et al. (63) have shown decreased agitation in the mouse after lidocaine pretreatment to subsequent intrathecal (IT) substance P (SP) as well as somatostatin. Bach et al. (4) have shown decreased agitation and tactile allodynia due to IT NMDA application after IV lidocaine pretreatment in the rat. These studies provide important behavioral parallels to the electrophysiologic studies, also showing decreased WDR responses to iontophoretic glutamate after IV lidocaine pretreatment (but not iontophoretic lidocaine), but not after IV bupivacaine. Interestingly, Biella and colleagues (10,11) observed augmented responses after IV lidocaine with iontophoretic NMDA, but decreased responses to iontophoretic quisqualate and strychnine, suggesting an action on either non–NMDA-type glutamatergic receptors or glycinergic sites. In vitro investigations of the neurotransmitter basis for suppression of responses have shown both inhibition of K^+-evoked SP release from diabetic mouse spinal cord (64) and reduction of the NMDA-evoked component of C-fiber slow ventral root potentials in neonatal rat spinal cord (81). Both these studies find these effects at free drug bath concentrations exceeding those targeted clinically (range, 40 to 60 μM). Other investigators have shown decreased binding of SP to spinal cord (73); the dose range is somewhat higher than IV levels and more compatible with levels achieved by iontophoresis. Lidocaine, procaine, and cocaine, but not tetrodotoxin, block the formation of long-term potentiation (LTP) in the hippocampus by a mechanism that may involve inhibition of Ca^{2+}/calmodulin-dependent protein kinase II (99). The formation of facilitated pain responses in the spinal cord is thought to be analogous to hippocampal LTP mechanisms.

Neuropathic Pain States

Given the clinical observations that local anesthetics may be unusually efficacious in painful neuropathies, a number of studies have attempted to replicate this in the laboratory, using behavioral, electrophysiologic, and other criteria (see Chap. 13). The effects of systemic local anesthetics have been investigated in several models of chronic neuropathic pain in the rat (Table 4).

Peripheral Nerve Injury Models

Two chronic nerve compression models have been investigated using intravenous/intraperitoneal local anesthetics, one devised by Bennett and Xie (9) calling for four loose ligatures around the distal sciatic nerve, and the other by Kim and Chung (70) calling for tight selective ligation of spinal nerves L5 and L6. In addition, a model of neuroma formation after nerve transection has provided for study of abnormal discharge patterns from neuromas and dorsal root ganglions (DRG) (24,34). Following trauma to a peripheral nerve, substantial functional alterations occur in both the baseline and the evoked electrical activity of both the peripheral and central nervous systems. Sustained, low-level ectopic spontaneous activ-

Table 3. TONIC MODELS OF NOCICEPTION

Model	Drug	Effect	Reference
Behavioral			
Formalin (rat), phase 2	Lidocaine 10 mg/kg	Reduced phase 2	1
Formalin (mouse) phase 2	Mexiletine 30 mg/kg	Reduced phase 2	63
Writhing, acetic acid (mouse)	Procaine, to 50 mg/kg s.c. Bupivacaine, to 25 mg/kg s.c. Lidocaine, to 30 mg/kg s.c.	Dose-related analgesia, all agents, all three tests	8
Awake IT application SP, SST, (diabetic/mouse)	Mexiletine 30 mg/kg, i.p.	Decreased nociception	63
Awake IT application NMDA (rat)	Lidocaine (2 μg/ml) plasma	Suppression of allodynia	4
Correlate			
Neurogenic extravasation (raw paw)	Lidocaine 5 mg/kg i.a. Tocainide 50 mg/kg i.a.	No blockade	112
Electrophysiologic			
Rat dorsal horn, mustard oil	Lidocaine 5 mg/kg i.a. Tocainide 50 mg/kg i.a.	Suppression of sural nerve reflex	112
Rat dorsal horn, glutamate	Lidocaine 3–4 mg/kg i.v.	Inhibition of excitation	10
Rat dorsal horn/NMDA	Lidocaine 3–4 mg/kg i.v.	Potentiation of WDR firing	10
Quisqualate		Suppression of WDR firing	
Strychnine		Suppression	
In vitro			
NMDA-evoked C-fiber activity	Lidocaine 40–60 μM	Reduction and slowing	81
K^+-evoked SP release, sp cord slice diabetic mouse	Mexiletine 10^{-5}M	Inhibition	64
Formation of LTP, hippocampal slice	Lidocaine Procaine Cocaine TTX	Blockade Blockade Blockade No blockade	99

ity originates at the site of neuroma formation in large peripheral axons (24) as well as in DRG cells (62) and dorsal horn neurons that project supraspinally (75,86). These changes in electrical activity are associated with peripheral and central changes including alterations in receptor expression (94,113), second messenger function (77,78), and possibly altered balance of inhibitory/excitatory neurotransmitters (115; see Chap. 56).

Diabetes

Paw hyperalgesia results from streptozocin-induced diabetes (28,29). The precise pathophysiology of nerve injury is not known; several hypotheses have been advanced to explain this form of neuropathic pain, including overactivity of the aldose reductase pathway leading to polyol metabolite accumulation, nerve ischemia, altered trophic factor balance, neuronal loss, substance P level alterations, and other neurotransmitter alterations (for review see Chap. 54). This model shows increased sensitivity to mechanical paw pressure, controversial responses to thermal stimuli, and increased responses to the formalin test.

Spinal Cord Ischemia

A unique model of spinal cord injury generated by controlled spinal cord ischemia resulted in allodynia-like reactions to segmental fur brushing, with vocalization (114). The histopathology of this particular model, generated by targeted irradiation, has not been reported; however, the injury is reportedly confined to the spinal cord, thus creating a selective lesion at this level of the neuraxis.

Actions of Local Anesthetics in Models of Neuropathic Pain States

In painful neuropathy models reported to date, systemically administered lidocaine suppresses well-described hyperalgesic responses to thermal stimuli, tactile allodynia to light mechanical stimuli, and mechanical hyperalgesia to deep pressure stimuli. In two models of nerve compression, paw withdrawal thresholds to heat and light touch are restored toward normal by nontoxic doses of lidocaine IV (1,25) (Fig. 1). It has recently been shown that this effect is duplicated neither by regional application of lidocaine on the nerve constriction site, nor by IT application of doses of lidocaine sufficient to cause brief spinal anesthesia. Bupivacaine, however, appears to be inactive in two models (11,26). A recent study has shown extended prophylaxis of the onset of thermal hyperalgesia in the Bennett rat model, a single preligation dose having an effect for 3 weeks or more (100).

In the model of ischemic spinal cord injury, Xu et al. (114) have shown that mexiletine, 15 to 30 mg/kg i.p. (as well as to some extent tocainide, but not morphine, clonidine, carbamazepine, baclofen muscimol, or guanethidine), suppresses vocalization to segmental fur brushing for over 120 minutes. This model, as well as the Chung tight ligation model, is noteworthy in this respect as representing two models wherein local anesthetics are specifically antihyperalgesic, but opiates have decreased effectiveness (72).

In diabetic rats, lowered thresholds for paw withdrawal to pressure are normalized by IV lidocaine, with a duration of bolus effect of >8 hours (Fig. 2). Similarly, systemic lidocaine markedly normalizes tactile allodynia to von Frey hairs in diabetic rats for an extended period (20). The neuropathic models in general are remarkable for reports of extended antihyperalgesia, in some instances outlasting likely kinetics of the drug or possible metabolites (25).

Effect of Local Anesthetics on Post–Nerve Injury Neuronal Activity

A number of studies have examined the effects of lidocaine on peripheral and dorsal horn electrical activity. Lidocaine, mexiletine, and tocainide cause transient suppression of spontaneous activity in ectopic generator foci in the injured peripheral nerve in a dose-dependent manner (24). The concentration of lidocaine required to suppress abnormal electrical activity appears to

Table 4. NEUROPATHIC MODELS

Model	Drug	Effect	Reference
Behavioral			
Spinal cord ischemia (rat)	Mexiletine 15–30 mg/kg	Suppression of allodynia	114
Tail pinch (diabetic mouse)	Mexiletine 10, 30 mg/kg	Decreased response	64
	Lidocaine 30 mg/kg	No effect	
Bennett nerve compression	Lidocaine 0.6–6.6 mg i.v.	Increased thermal latency	1
Chung nerve compression	Plasma [lidocaine] 1–2 μg/ml	Prolonged suppression of allodynia; no effect	Chaplan et al. 1994
	Plasma [bupivacaine] <4 μg/ml		
Diabetic neuropathy (rat)	Lidocaine 1–9 mg/kg i.v.	Increased paw pressure threshold	28
Bennett compression (rat)	6–8 mg/kg i.v.	Prevention of development of thermal hyperalgesia × 3 weeks	100
Diabetic neuropathy (rat)	Lidocaine 60 mg/kg, i.p.	Suppression of paw allodynia	20
Electrophysiologic			
Bennett compression (rat)	Lidocaine 3–4 mg/kg	Decreased spontaneous WDR hyperactivity	102
Sciatic neuroma (rat)	Lidocaine		35
	ED_{50} 6 mg/kg	Neuroma firing suppression	
	ED_{50} 1 mg/kg	DRG firing suppression	
Bennett compression (rat)	Lidocaine 4 mg/kg	Inhibition of DRG, dorsal horn neurons	Sotgiu 1994
Sciatic neuroma (rat)	Lidocaine Mexiletine Tocainide	Suppression of automaticity	Chabal and Jacobson 1989

decrease moving centrally from neuroma to dorsal root ganglion to spinal cord: the lidocaine ED_{50} for discharge suppression in neuroma has been reported to be 6 mg/kg, whereas that for the dorsal root ganglion is 1 mg/kg (35), and Sotgiu et al. (101,102) reported that while intravenous lidocaine 4 mg/kg selectively suppresses both increased activity in dorsal root ganglion and second-order neurons ipsilateral to chronic nerve compression, the onset is significantly shorter and the duration of effect significantly longer in spinal cord.

MECHANISMS OF ACTIVITY

Kinetic Considerations of the Systemic Route

The most common implementation of local anesthetics is by topical or regional application. Such application of relatively high concentrations of drug directly in the vicinity of the axon induces conduction blockade by preventing the propagation of action potentials across a critical length of nerve. The possibility of selective blockade of one type of axon versus another appears difficult to support under these circumstances, since a steep concentration gradient obtains between the interior and exterior of the nerve bundle, and it is likely that an adequate concentration to provide selective blockade of fibers in the nerve interior will block all axons on the outside. On the other hand, intravenously delivered agents are distributed by the vascular tree first to inner and then to outer areas of the nerve bundle, initially reversing but likely ultimately reducing the gradient (58), since with continuous intravenous delivery of agent it is probable that pseudo–steady states in the nerve are proportional to plasma concentrations. Thus, some consideration of possibilities of selective blockade of more vulnerable axon types or locations has particular merit in the case of intravenous delivery.

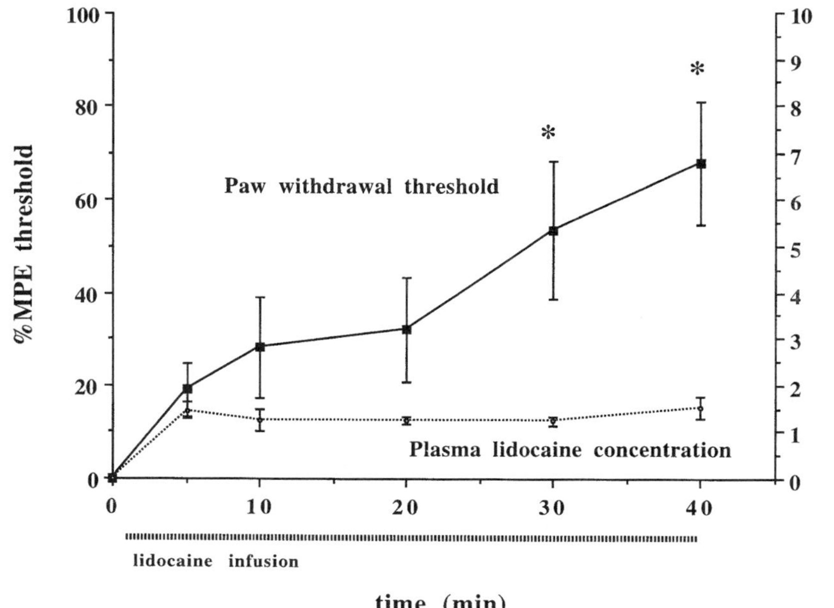

Figure 1. Effect of IV lidocaine on tactile allodynia: Chung neuropathy model. Illustration of pseudo–steady state plasma concentrations of lidocaine (mean 1.34 ± 0.07 μg/ml) concurrent with significant increases in paw withdrawal thresholds to von Frey hairs, seen beginning 30 minutes after attaining targeted plasma lidocaine levels ($p < .001$, repeated measures ANOVA). X-axis: time; left y-axis: paw withdrawal thresholds expressed as percent of maximum possible drug effect; right y-axis: plasma lidocaine levels, μg/ml (25).

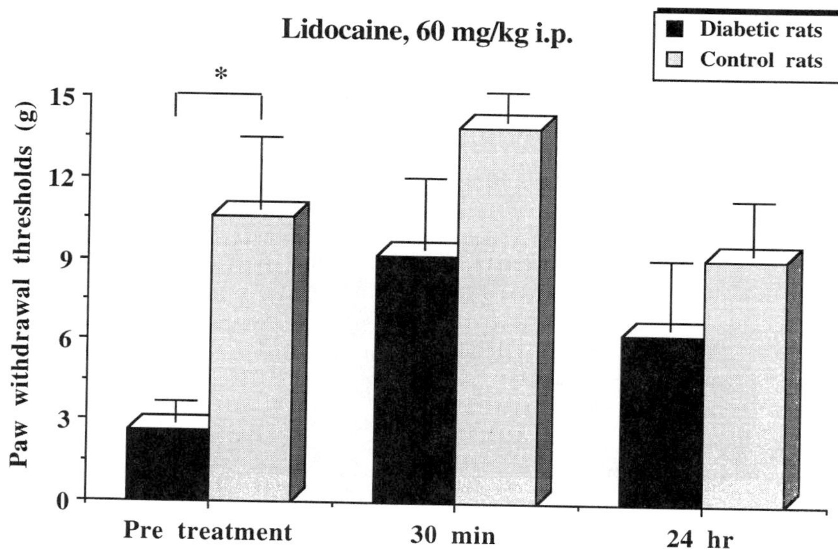

Figure 2. Effect of lidocaine on tactile allodynia and diabetic neuropathy. Streptozotocin diabetic rats have significantly lower mean paw withdrawal thresholds to von Frey hairs than control rats (*p =.03, unpaired t-test) prior to lidocaine treatment. After i.p. lidocaine treatment, thresholds are no longer significantly different, an effect that persists at least 24 hours (20). X-axis: paw withdrawal thresholds (g).

Effects upon Peripheral Transduction of the Physical Stimulus: Role of Voltage-Dependent Sodium Channels in Post–Nerve Injury States

Reversible sodium channel blockade is the major described pharmacologic property of the local anesthetics (for review see 19). Lidocaine and procaine have similar use-dependent properties, also somewhat similar to anticonvulsants (43). It is possible that this action of lidocaine may be augmented in excitable tissues after injury, in a way that remains to be elucidated. For example, after injury, the expression of different isoforms of both acetylcholine receptors and sodium channels at the neuromuscular junction (109,111) leads to a distinct pharmacology of the postinjury state. Functionally differing subpopulations of sodium channels have already been well described within the normal dorsal root ganglia of both invertebrates and vertebrates (21,84). Channels associated with the smaller dorsal root ganglion cells, which likely give rise to small unmyelinated fibers (C fibers), display the particular characteristic of use-dependent blockade with lidocaine (93). Although the role of C fibers per se has been questioned in both the induction and maintenance of tactile allodynia (22,90,97), it is speculated that under conditions of injury the altered characteristics of sodium channels in a changed environment could perhaps render them subject to exaggerated use-dependent blockade by lidocaine. Markedly increased density of sodium channels proximal to a peripheral nerve ligation in the fish Apteronotus and in human neurons has been demonstrated in immunohistochemical observations (33). In the injured myelinated peripheral nerve of the rat, randomization of channels over the axon as well as clustering at the axon tip replaces the normal clustering at the nodes of Ranvier (32,44,46). There is evidence that numbers of sodium channels increase due to de novo manufacture after in vivo demyelination with doxorubicin (45). Membrane functional characteristics are hypothetically altered in that the density of channels, in a mathematical model, leads to increased channel opening probability (79). Actual channel subtype, or proportion of subtypes, may be altered over the time course of injury/repair (92). Such changes may explain the appearance of spontaneous activity in primary afferents (see Chap. 5), and may also provide the basis for altered susceptibility to systemic local anesthetics. It should be borne in mind, however, that, where examined, the concentrations of lidocaine required to silence these peripheral sites are relatively elevated compared to effective concentrations at central nervous system sites (see above).

Sympatholytic Effects

Clinical pain syndromes have been functionally divided into two important categories: those that are responsive to sympatholysis and those that are not (2). The role of local anesthetic infusion should thus be considered with regard to effects on the sympathetic nervous system. One of the results of preferential use-dependent blockade of small unmyelinated C fibers or their respective somata could hypothetically be blockade of fibers or cell bodies of sympathetic neurons. Tabatabai and Booth have shown that the sympathetic ganglia are particularly sensitive to prolonged local anesthetic blockade. As described above, systemically administered lidocaine does not block neurogenic extravasation, leading to the conclusion that axons are unaffected by this treatment (112). Evidence from animal studies points to an effect that is independent of sympathetic suppression, since intravenous lidocaine has been shown to be antihyperalgesic in a model that is not responsive to sympathectomy (9) as well as one that is responsive to sympatholysis by several means (69,71). While some reduction in sympathetic activity has been documented as an effect of intravenous lidocaine (40), this appears to be a minor consequence of lidocaine-evoked hypertension/tachycardia with reflex sympathetic attenuation. Most studies show no significant or minimal effects of systemically administered lidocaine on sympathetic efferent activity in nonpain models (i.e., models in which relief of pain is not a possible indirect reason for decreased catecholamine secretion) (57,82,83,116).

Non–Sodium Channel Mechanisms of Action

Several lines of evidence suggest that non–sodium channel mechanisms of analgesia are plausible explanations for the antihyperalgesic actions of systemically administered local anesthetics. The contrasting effects of some local anesthetics suggest that there is a range of efficacies against hyperalgesia that perhaps does not correlate with local anesthetic efficacy/potency. Biella et al. (11) showed that WDR suppression was achieved by systemic lidocaine, but not by iontophoresed lidocaine and not by intravenous bupivacaine. They suggested that biotransformation of systemic lidocaine might be a prerequisite for the relevant activity, and proposed on the basis of iontophoretic excitatory substance studies that a glycinergic action was the most consistent mechanism for the putative lidocaine metabolite. Butterworth and Cole (18) have also suggested that a metabolite of procaine, diethylaminoethanol, reduces excitability of hippocampal pyramidal cells without abolishing action potentials. Others have shown blockade of other receptor systems, as above: NMDA receptors, SP receptors, and acetylcholine receptors. Smith et al. (99) propose an intracellular site of action for the LTP inhibition of cocaine, possibly interfering with calmodulin, thus indirectly suggesting that other local anesthetics may have a similar action. Several additional reports have suggested that lidocaine has second messenger blocking effects (61,65,85,103,107); however, the concentrations employed in those studies in general far exceed the physiologic range, rendering their applicability difficult to evaluate.

REFERENCES

1. Abram SE, Yaksh TL. Systemic lidocaine blocks nerve injury-induced hyperalgesia and nociceptor-driven spinal sensitization in the rat. *Anesthesiology* 1994;80:383–391.
2. Arnér S. Intravenous phentolamine test: diagnostic and prognostic use in reflex sympathetic dystrophy. *Pain* 1991;46:17–22.
3. Aslan A. A new method for the prophylaxis and treatment of aging with Novocain-eutrophic and rejuvenating effects. *Therapiewoche* 1956;7:14–17.
4. Bach FW, Chaplan SR, Yaksh TL. Studies on the spinal pharmacology of a new model of allodynia. *Ann Neurol* 1994;36:288A.
5. Bach FW, Jensen TS, Kastrup J, Stigsby B, Dejgård A. The effect of intravenous lidocaine on nociceptive processing in diabetic neuropathy. *Pain* 1990;40:29–34.
6. Backonja M, Gombar KA. Response of central pain syndromes to intravenous lidocaine. *J Pain Symptom Manage* 1992;7:172–178.
7. Bartlett EE, Hutaserani O. Xylocaine for the relief of postoperative pain. *Anesth Analg* 1961;40:296–304.
8. Bartolini A, Galli A, Ghelardini C, et al. Antinociception induced by systemic administration of local anaesthetics depends on a central cholinergic mechanism. *Br J Pharmacol* 1987;92:711–721.
9. Bennett GJ, Xie Y-K. A peripheral mononeuropathy in rat that produces disorders of pain sensation like those seen in man. *Pain* 1988;33:87–107.
10. Biella G, Lacerenza M, Marchettini P, Sotgiu ML. Diverse modulation by systemic lidocaine of iontophoretic NMDA and quisqualic acid induced excitations on rat dorsal horn neurons. *Neurosci Lett* 1993;157:207–210.
11. Biella G, Sotgiu ML. Central effects of systemic lidocaine mediated by glycine spinal receptors: an iontophoretic study in the rat spinal cord. *Brain Res* 1992;603:201–206.
12. Bigelow N, Harrison I. General analgesic effects of procaine. *JPET* 1944;81:368–373.
13. Birch K, Jorgensen J, Chraemmer-Jorgensen B, Kehlet H. Effect of i.v. lignocaine on pain and the endocrine metabolic responses after surgery. *Br J Anaesth* 1987;59:721–724.
14. Blancato LS, Peng AT, Alonsabe D. Intravenous lidocaine. Adjunct to general anesthesia for endoscopy. *N Y State J Med* 1970;70: 1659–1660.
15. Boas R, Covino B, Shahnarian A. Analgesic responses to IV lignocaine. *Br J Anaesth* 1982;54:501.
16. Braun H. über einige neuer örtliche Anaesthetica (Stovain, Alypin, Novocain). *Dtsch Klin Wochenschr* 1905;31:1667.
17. Burney RG, DiFazio CA, Peach MJ, Petrie KA, Silvester MJ. Antiarrhythmic effects of lidocaine metabolites. *Am Heart J* 1974;88: 765–769.
18. Butterworth JF, Cole LR. Low concentrations of procaine and diethylaminoethanol reduce the excitability but not the action potential amplitude of hippocampal pyramidal cells. *Anesth Analg* 1990;71:404–410.
19. Butterworth JF, Strichartz GR. Molecular mechanisms of local anesthesia: a review. *Anesthesiology* 1990;72:711–734.
20. Calcutt NA, Jorge MC, Yaksh TL, Chaplan SR. Tactile allodynia and formalin hyperalgesia in streptozotocin-diabetic rats: effects of insulin, aldose reductase inhibition, and lidocaine. *Pain* 1996; 68:293–299.
21. Campbell DT. Large and small vertebrate sensory neurons express different Na and K channel subtypes. *Proc Natl Acad Sci USA* 1992; 89:9569–9573.
22. Campbell JN, Raja SN, Meyer RA, Mackinnon SE. Myelinated afferents signal the hyperalgesia associated with nerve injury. *Pain* 1988;32:89–95.
23. Cassuto J, Wallin G, Hogstrom S, Faxen A, Rimback G. Inhibition of postoperative pain by continuous low-dose intravenous infusion of lidocaine. *Anesth Analg* 1985;64:971–974.
24. Chabal C, Russell LC, Burchiel KJ. The effect of intravenous lidocaine, tocainide, and mexiletine on spontaneously active fibers originating in rat sciatic neuromas. *Pain* 1989;38:333–338.
25. Chaplan SR, Bach FW, Shafer SL, Yaksh TL. Prolonged alleviation of tactile allodynia by intravenous lidocaine in neuropathic rats. *Anesthesiology* 1995;83:775–785.
26. Chaplan SR, Bach FW, Yaksh TL. A lidocaine metabolite has superior anti-allodynia activity in a rat neuropathy model. American Pain Society 14th Annual Scientific Meeting, 1995, no. 95795.
27. Collins EB. The use of intravenous procaine infusion in the treatment of postherpetic neuralgia. *Med J Aust* 1969;2:27–28.
28. Courteix C, Bardin M, Chantelauze C, Lavarenne J, Eschalier A. Study of the sensitivity of the diabetes-induced pain model in rats to a range of analgesics. *Pain* 1994;57:153–160.
29. Courteix C, Eschalier A, Lavarenne J. Streptozocin-induced diabetic rats: behavioural evidence for a model of chronic pain. *Pain* 1993;53:81–88.
30. de Clive-Lowe SG, Desmond J, North J. Intravenous lignocaine anaesthesia. *Anaesthesia* 1958;13:139–146.
31. Dejgård A, Petersen P, Kastrup J. Mexiletine for treatment of chronic painful diabetic neuropathy. *Lancet* 1988;1:9–11.
32. Devor M, Govrin-Lippmann R, Angelides K. Na+ channel immunolocalization in peripheral mammalian axons and changes following nerve injury and neuroma formation. *J Neurosci* 1993;13: 1976–1992.
33. Devor M, Keller CH, Deerinck TJ, Levinson SR, Ellisman MH. Na+ channel accumulation on axolemma of afferent endings in nerve end neuromas in Apteronotus. *Neurosci Lett* 1989;102:149–154.
34. Devor M, Keller CH, Ellisman MH. Spontaneous discharge of afferents in a neuroma reflects original receptor tuning. *Brain Res* 1990;517:245–250.
35. Devor M, Wall PD, Catalan N. Systemic lidocaine silences ectopic neuroma and DRG discharge without blocking nerve conduction. *Pain* 1992;48:261–268.
36. Dickenson AH. A cure for wind up - NMDA receptor antagonists as potential analgesics. *Trends Pharmacol Sci* 1990;11:307–309.
37. Dickenson AH, Sullivan AF. Evidence for involvement of N-methyl-D-aspartate receptors in 'wind-up' of class 2 neurones in the dorsal horn of the rat. *Brain Res* 1987;424:402–406.
38. Dohi S, Kitahata LM, Toyooka H, Ohtani M, Namiki A, Taub A. An analgesic action of intravenously administered lidocaine on dorsal-horn neurons responding to noxious thermal stimulation. *Anesthesiology* 1979;51:123–126.
39. Dubuisson D, Dennis SG. The formalin test: a quantitative study of the analgesic effects of morphine, meperidine, and brain stem stimulation in rats and cats. *Pain* 1977;4:161–174.
40. Ebert TJ, Mohanty PK, Kampine JP. Lidocaine attenuates efferent sympathetic responses to stress in humans. *J Cardiothorac Vasc Anesth* 1991;5:437–443.
41. Edmonds GW, Comer WH, Kennedy JD, Taylor IB. Intravenous use of procaine in general anesthesia. *JAMA* 1949;141:761–765.
42. Edwards WT, Habib F, Burney RG, Begin G. Intravenous lidocaine in the management of various chronic pain states: a review of 211 cases. *Reg Anesth* 1985;10:1–6.
43. Elliott P. Action of antiepileptic and anaesthetic drugs on Na- and Ca-spikes in mammalian non-myelinated axons. *Eur J Pharmacol* 1990;175:155–163.
44. England JD, Gamboni F, Ferguson MA, Levinson SR. Sodium channels accumulate at the tips of injured axons. *Muscle Nerve* 1994;17:593–598.
45. England JD, Gamboni F, Levinson SR. Increased numbers of sodium channels form along demyelinated axons. *Brain Res* 1991; 548:334–337.
46. England JD, Gamboni F, Levinson SR, Finger TE. Changed distribution of sodium channels along demyelinated axons. *Proc Natl Acad Sci USA* 1990;87:6777–6780.
47. Ferrante FM, Paggioli J, Cherukuri S, Arthur GR. The analgesic response to intravenous lidocaine in the treatment of neuropathic pain. *Anesth Analg* 1996; 82:91–97.
48. Galer BS, Miller KV, Rowbotham MC. Response to intravenous lidocaine infusion differs based on clinical diagnosis and site of nervous system injury. *Neurology* 1993;43:1233–1235.
49. Glazer S, Portenoy RK. Systemic local anesthetics in pain control. *J Pain Symptom Manage* 1991;6:30–39.

50. Gordon RA. Intravenous novocaine for analgesia in burns. *Can Med Assoc J* 1943;49:478–481.
51. Haegerstam G. Effect of i.v. administration of lignocaine and tetrodotoxin on sensory units in the tooth of the cat. *Br J Anaesth* 1979;51:487–491.
52. Haldia KN, Chatterji S, Kackar SN. Intravenous lignocaine for prevention of muscle pain after succinylcholine. *Anesth Analg* 1973; 52:849–852.
53. Haley JE, Sullivan AF, Dickenson AH. Evidence for spinal N-methyl-D-aspartate receptor involvement in prolonged chemical nociception in the rat. *Brain Res* 1990;518:218–226.
54. Hargreaves K, Dubner R, Brown F, Flores C, Joris J. A new and sensitive method for measuring thermal nociception in cutaneous hyperalgesia. *Pain* 1988;32:77–88.
55. Hayes AHJ. Intravenous infusion of lidocaine in the control of ventricular arrhythmias. In: Scott DB, Julian DG, eds. *Lidocaine in the treatment of ventricular arrhythmias.* Edinburgh and London: E. & S. Livingstone, 1971;189.
56. Himes RS, DiFazio CA, Burney RG. Effects of lidocaine on the anesthetic requirements for nitrous oxide and halothane. *Anesthesiology* 1977;47:437–440.
57. Hogan QH, Stadnicka A, Stekiel TA, Bosnjak ZJ, Kampine JP. Effects of epidural and systemic lidocaine on sympathetic activity and mesenteric circulation in rabbits. *Anesthesiology* 1993;79: 1250–1260.
58. Holmes CM. Intravenous regional blockade. In: Cousins MJ, Bridenbaugh PO, eds. *Neural blockade in clinical anesthesia and management of pain,* 2nd ed. Philadelphia: JB Lippincott, 1988.
59. Jancso G, Kiraly E, Jancso-Gabor A. Direct evidence for an axonal site of action of capsaicin. *Naunyn Schmiedebergs Arch Pharmacol* 1980;313:91–94.
60. Jönsson A, Cassuto J, Hanson B. Inhibition of burn pain by intravenous lignocaine infusion. *Lancet* 1991;338:151–152.
61. Kai T, Nishimura J, Kobayashi S, Takahashi S, Yoshitake J, Kanaide H. Effects of lidocaine on intracellular Ca^{2+} and tension in airway smooth muscle. *Anesthesiology* 1993;78:954–965.
62. Kajander KC, Wakisaka S, Bennett GJ. Spontaneous discharge originates in the dorsal root ganglion at the onset of a painful peripheral neuropathy in the rat. *Neurosci Lett* 1992;138:225–228.
63. Kamei J, Hitosugi H, Kasuya Y. Effects of mexiletine on formalin-induced nociceptive responses in mice. *Res Commun Chem Pathol Pharmacol* 1993;80:153–162.
64. Kamei J, Hitosugi H, Kawashima N, Aoki T, Ohhashi Y, Kasuya Y. Antinociceptive effect of mexiletine in diabetic mice. *Res Commun Chem Pathol Pharmacol* 1992;77:245–248.
65. Kanbara T, Tomoda MK, Sato EF, Ueda W, Manabe M. Lidocaine inhibits priming and protein tyrosine phosphorylation of human peripheral neutrophils. *Biochem Pharmacol* 1993;45:1593–1598.
66. Kasaba T, Nonoue T, Yanagidani T, Maeda M, Kosaka Y. [Effects of intravenous lidocaine administration on median nerve somatosensory evoked potentials.] *Masui* 1991;40:713–716.
67. Kastrup J, Petersen P, Dejgård A, Angelo HR, Hilsted J. Intravenous lidocaine infusion—a new treatment of chronic painful diabetic neuropathy? *Pain* 1987;28:69–75.
68. Keats AS, D'Alessandro GL, Beecher HK. A controlled study of pain relief by intravenous procaine. *JAMA* 1951;147:1761–1763.
69. Kim SH, Chung JM. Sympathectomy alleviates mechanical allodynia in an experimental animal model for neuropathy in the rat. *Neurosci Lett* 1991;134:131–134.
70. Kim SH, Chung JM. An experimental model for peripheral neuropathy produced by segmental spinal nerve ligation in the rat. *Pain* 1992;50:355–363.
71. Kim SH, Na HS, Sheen K, Chung JM. Effects of sympathectomy on a rat model of peripheral neuropathy. *Pain* 1993;55:85–92.
72. Lee YW, Chaplan SR, Yaksh TL. Systemic and supraspinal, but not spinal, opiates suppress allodynia in a rat neuropathic pain model. *Neurosci Lett* 1995;186:1–4.
73. Li YM, Wingrove DE, Too HP, et al. Local anesthetics inhibit substance P binding and evoked increases in intracellular Ca^{2+}. *Anesthesiology* 1995;82:166–173.
74. Löfgren N. *Studies on local anesthetics. Xylocaine: a new synthetic drug. Inaugural dissertation.* Stockholm: Hoeggstroms, 1948.
75. Lombard MC, Besson JM. Attempts to gauge the relative importance of pre- and postsynaptic effects of morphine on the transmission of noxious mesages in the dorsal horn of the rat spinal cord. *Pain* 1989;37:335–345.
76. Malmberg AB, Yaksh TL. Hyperalgesia mediated by spinal glutamate or substance-P receptor blocked by spinal cyclooxygenase inhibition. *Science* 1992;257:1276–1279.
77. Mao J, Mayer DJ, Hayes RL, Price DD. Spatial patterns of increased spinal cord membrane-bound protein kinase-C and their relation to increases in C-14-2-deoxyglucose metabolic activity in rats with painful peripheral mononeuropathy. *J Neurophysiol* 1993;70:470–481.
78. Mao JR, Price DD, Mayer DJ, Hayes RL. Pain-related increases in spinal cord membrane-bound protein kinase-C following peripheral nerve injury. *Brain Res* 1992;588:144–149.
79. Matzner O, Devor M. Na+ conductance and the threshold for repetitive neuronal firing. *Brain Res* 1992;597:92–98.
80. Morton R, Spitzer K, Steinbrocker O. Intravenous procaine as an analgesic and therapeutic procedure in painful, chronic neuromusculoskeletal disorders. *Anesthesiology* 1949;10:629–633.
81. Nagy I, Woolf CJ. Lignocaine selectively reduces C fibre-evoked neuronal activity in rat spinal cord in vitro by decreasing N-methyl-D-aspartate and neurokinin receptor-mediated post-synaptic depolarizations; implications for development of novel centrally acting analgesics. *Pain* 1996;64:59–70.
82. Nishikawa K, Fukuda T, Yukioka H, Fujimori M. Effects of intravenous administration of local anesthetics on the renal sympathetic nerve activity during nitrous oxide and nitrous oxide-halothane anesthesia in the cat. *Acta Anaesthesiol Scand* 1990;34: 231–236.
83. Nishikawa K, Terai T, Morimoto O, Yukioka H, Fujimori M. Effects of intravenous lidocaine on cardiac sympathetic nerve activity and A-V conduction in halothane-anesthetized cats. *Acta Anaesthesiol Scand* 1994;38:115–120.
84. Omri G, Meiri H. Characterization of sodium currents in mammalian sensory neurons cultured in serum-free defined medium with and without nerve growth factor. *J Membr Biol* 1990;115: 13–29.
85. Onozuka M, Watanabe K, Imai S, Nagasaki S, Yamamoto T. Lidocaine suppresses the sodium current in Euhadra neurons which is mediated by cAMP-dependent protein phosphorylation. *Brain Res* 1993;628:335–339.
86. Paleček J, Dougherty PM, Kim SH, et al. Responses of spinothalamic tract neurons to mechanical and thermal stimuli in an experimental model of peripheral neuropathy in primates. *J Neurophysiol* 1992;68:1951–1966.
87. Papper EM, Brodie BB, Lief PA, Rovenstine EA. Studies on the pharmacological properties of procaine and di-ethyl-amino-ethanol. *NY J Med* 1948;48:1711–1714.
88. Pearl J, Harris LS. Inhibition of writhing by narcotic antagonists. *J Pharmacol Exp Ther* 1966;154:319–323.
89. Petersen P, Kastrup J. Dercum's disease (adiposis dolorosa). Treatment of the severe pain with intravenous lidocaine. *Pain* 1987;28: 77–80.
90. Price DP, Bennett GJ, Rafii A. Psychophysical observations on patients with neuropathic pain relieved by a sympathetic block. *Pain* 1989;36:273–288.
91. Reutens DC, Fatovich DM, Stewartwynne E, Prentice DA. Is intravenous lidocaine clinically effective in acute migraine. *Cephalalgia* 1991;11:245–247.
92. Rizzo MA, Waxman SG, Kocsis JD. Differential properties of voltage-dependent Na+ channels following axotomy in cutaneous afferent DRG neurons of adult rat. *Soc Neurosci Abs* 1995;21:715.9.
93. Roy ML, Narahashi T. Differential properties of tetrodotoxin-sensitive and tetrodotoxin-resistant sodium channels in rat dorsal root ganglion neurons. *J Neurosci* 1992;12:2104–2111.
94. Sato J, Perl ER. Adrenergic excitation of cutaneous pain receptors induced by peripheral nerve injury. *Science* 1991;251:1608–1610.
95. Schubert A, Licina MG, Glaze GM, Paranandi L. Systemic lidocaine and human somatosensory-evoked potentials during sufentanil-isoflurane anaesthesia. *Can J Anaesth* 1992;39:569–575.
96. Shanbrom E. Treatment of herpetic pain and postherpetic neuralgia with intravenous procaine. *JAMA* 1961;176:1041–1043.
97. Shir Y, Seltzer Z. A-fibers mediate mechanical hyperesthesia and allodynia and C-fibers mediate thermal hyperalgesia in a new model of causalgiform pain disorders in rats. *Neurosci Lett* 1990; 115:62–67.
98. Sjøgren P, Banning A-M, Hebsgaard K, Petersen P, Gefke K. Intravenøs lidokain i behandlingen af kroniske smerter forårsaget af knoglemetastaser. *Ugeskr Læger* 1989;151:2144–2146.
99. Smith DA, Browning M, Dunwiddie TV. Cocaine inhibits hippocampal long-term potentiation. *Brain Res* 1993;608:259–265.

100. Sotgiu ML, Castagna A, Lacerenza M, Marchettini P. Pre-injury lidocaine treatment prevents thermal hyperalgesia and cutaneous thermal abnormalities in a rat model of peripheral neuropathy. *Pain* 1995;61:3–10.
101. Sotgiu ML, Lacerenza M, Marchettini P. Selective inhibition by systemic lidocaine of noxious evoked activity in rat dorsal horn neurons. *Neuroreport* 1991;2:425–428.
102. Sotgiu ML, Lacerenza M, Marchettini P. Effect of systemic lidocaine on dorsal horn neuron hyperactivity following chronic peripheral nerve injury in rats. *Somatosens Mot Res* 1992;9: 227–233.
103. Spedding M, Berg C. Antagonism of Ca2+ induced contractions of K+-depolarized smooth muscle by local anesthetics. *Eur J Pharmacol* 1985;108:143–150.
104. Stracke H, Meyer U, Schumacher HE, Federlin K. Mexiletine in the treatment of diabetic neuropathy. *Diabetes Care* 1992;15: 1550–1555.
105. Takesue EI, Schaefer W, Jukniewicz E. Modification of the Randall-Selitto analgesic apparatus. *J Pharm Pharmacol* 1969;21: 788–789.
106. Tanelian DL, Maclver MB. Analgesic concentrations of lidocaine suppress tonic A-delta and C-fiber discharges produced by acute injury. *Anesthesiology* 1991;74:934–936.
107. Tomoda MK, Tsuchiya M, Ueda W, Hirakawa M, Utsumi K. Lidocaine inhibits stimulation-coupled responses of neutrophils and protein kinase C activity. *Physiol Chem Phys & Med NMR* 1990;22: 199–210.
108. Wheeler-Aceto H, Porreca F, Cowan A. The rat paw formalin test: comparison of noxious agents. *Pain* 1990;40:229–238.
109. White MM, Chen LQ, Kleinfield R, Kallen RG, Barchi RL. SkM2, a Na+ channel cDNA clone from denervated skeletal muscle, encodes a tetrodotoxin-insensitive Na+ channel. *Mol Pharmacol* 1991;39:604–608.
110. Wiesenfeld-Hallin Z, Lindblom U. The effect of systemic tocainide, lidocaine, and bupivacaine on nociception in the rat. *Pain* 1985; 23:357–360.
111. Witzemann V, Barg B, Nishikawa Y, Sakmann B, Numa S. Differential regulation of muscle acetylcholine receptor gamma- and epsilon-subunit mRNAs. *FEBS Lett* 1987;223:104–112.
112. Woolf CJ, Wiesenfeld-Hallin Z. The systemic administration of local anesthetics produces a selective depression of C-afferent fibre evoked activity in the spinal cord. *Pain* 1985;23:361–374.
113. Xie YK, Xiao WH, Li HQ. The relationship between new ion channels and ectopic discharges from a region of nerve injury. *Sci China B* 1993;36:68–74.
114. Xu XJ, Hao JX, Seiger A, Arnér S, Lindblom U, Wiesenfeld-Hallin Z. Systemic mexiletine relieves chronic allodynia-like symptoms in rats with ischemic spinal cord injury. *Anesth Analg* 1992;74:649–652.
115. Yaksh T. Behavioral and autonomic correlates of the tactile evoked allodynia produced by spinal glycine inhibition: effects of modulatory receptor systems and excitatory amino acid antagonists. *Pain* 1989;37:111–123.
116. Yoneda I. [Effect of intravenous lidocaine infusion on arterial baroreflex]. *Masui* 1993;42:652–663.

Anesthesia: Biologic Foundations, edited by Tony L. Yaksh et al. Lippincott–Raven Publishers, Philadelphia © 1997.

CHAPTER 64

ANTIDEPRESSANTS AS ANALGESICS

S. H. SINDRUP

The first tricyclic antidepressant, imipramine, was introduced in the treatment of depression more than 35 years ago (70). A few years later, the first report on the analgesic effect of this drug appeared (99). Subsequently, numerous observations on the analgesic effect of tricyclic antidepressants have been published. Their beneficial effect in various chronic pain conditions are now well documented in double-blind, placebo-controlled, clinical trials (82), and, as will be reviewed below, experimental studies in humans and animals have indicated an acute pain relieving effect. The efficacy of these tricyclic agents in managing pain states thus appears to be beyond dispute. In recent years other types of antidepressants have been studied as well.

Antidepressants have mainly been used in the treatment of chronic, neuropathic pain states. Pain in such conditions is considered to respond poorly or not at all to mild analgesics [aspirin, nonsteroidal anti-inflammatory drugs (NSAIDs)], and opioids are less likely to result in a good response than in nociceptive pain (92) (see Chaps. 58 and 67). The pain relief obtained with antidepressants is usually partial, and troublesome side effects are frequent. Such characteristics may present as important problems in patients that require long-term treatment. However, the lack of effective and well-tolerated alternative treatments continues to justify their use in neuropathic pain.

An important consideration relates to the functional mechanisms whereby these agents influence pain behavior. Their potent actions in attenuating indices of depression and the known role played by depression in pain, particularly that of a chronic nature, has made the effects of this family of agents on nociception difficult to elucidate. This chapter reviews the current clinical evidence for the analgesic effect of antidepressants, discusses the mechanism of action, and considers clinically relevant pharmacokinetics.

ACTION OF ANTIDEPRESSANT DRUGS IN HUMAN PAIN STATES

Antidepressants have been widely tried in a range of clinical pain conditions. This chapter focuses on studies with a randomized, double-blind, and placebo-controlled design. Such studies represent the only valid source of documentation, since pain is subjective and heavily influenced by placebo effects. The use of antidepressants in psychogenic pain disorders, i.e., pain disorders in which no organic disease can be detected, are not considered here. An overview of studies on antidepressants in chronic, organic pain conditions is given in Table 1.

Chronic Painful Diabetic Neuropathy

Tricyclic antidepressants were introduced in the treatment of chronic, painful, diabetic neuropathy about 15 years ago on the basis of uncontrolled, clinical observations (31,47). Subsequently, the benefits of the tricyclic antidepressants imipramine, desipramine, amitriptyline, nortriptyline, and clomipramine have been confirmed in double-blind, placebo-controlled trials, most of them with a crossover design (53,71,85,86,122,125,134). The effect has only been questioned in one study, composed of only six patients with amitriptyline against placebo (95). The studies showing a positive effect were composed of 9 to 59 patients and differed in rating of symptoms. In some studies only pain was rated, whereas in others ratings also included paresthesia, dysesthesia, and sleep disturbances. Defining a positive response to these tricyclic drugs in terms of at least "moderate relief," there is typically a responder frequency from 50% to 90% for imipramine, clomipramine, and amitriptyline, and from 45% to 60% for desipramine. As a rule, only up to 30% of the patients are totally relieved of symptoms on a tricyclic drug. In some studies, a combination of a tricyclic antidepressant and a neuroleptic drug (fluphenazine) was used (53,95), but this combination is apparently not necessary since tricyclic antidepressants sufficed in the other studies (71,85,86,122,125,134). Care should be taken in the interpretation of such interaction studies because the plasma concentration of tricyclic antidepressants can be elevated secondary to a reduced metabolism associated with concomitant neuroleptic treatment (56).

Mianserin is a nontricyclic antidepressant. This agent showed no effect on the symptoms of chronic, painful, diabetic neuropathy in a trial that also included imipramine (127). However, the effect of imipramine in that study was considerably weaker than in other similar studies. It can therefore not be excluded that mianserin may have a minor pain-relieving effect in this condition.

More recently introduced antidepressants are the selective serotonin reuptake inhibitors. Two drugs from this class, paroxetine and citalopram, have been shown to relieve diabetic neuropathy symptoms, but apparently with a lower efficacy than the tricyclics (117,123). These findings are contrasted by the apparent lack of effect of fluoxetine (87), which is a selective serotonin reuptake inhibitor.

Acute painful diabetic neuropathy is a distinct disease entity differing from the chronic painful diabetic neuropathy, by having an acute onset of symptoms and showing remission within a year (4,15). All of the studies discussed above were performed in patients with chronic painful neuropathy. A small trial with six patients with acute painful diabetic neuropathy showed a significantly better pain relief from imipramine than from placebo (150). The results obtained in patients with chronic symptoms may thus be considered to reflect upon the effects observed with the acute disease.

Postherpetic Neuralgia

A beneficial effect of tricyclic antidepressants in postherpetic neuralgia is well established. Amitriptyline and desipramine have in controlled trials shown a better effect than placebo (69,88,142). In an open, controlled study, clomipramine in combination with carbamazepine had a better effect than transcutaneous electric nerve stimulation (49). The responder frequency (as discussed above) ranged from 47% to 66% in the studies on amitriptyline and desipramine.

Other Peripheral Neuropathies

A few randomized, double-blind studies included mixed patient groups with peripheral neuropathy of different origin.

Table 1. OVERVIEW OF DOUBLE-BLIND, CONTROLLED, CLINICAL TRIALS OF ANTIDEPRESSANTS IN DIFFERENT PAIN CONDITIONS

	Results indicating an effect of antidepressants		Results indicating no effect of antidepressants	
Pain condition	**Drug**	**Reference**	**Drug**	**Reference**
Diabetic neuropathy	Imipramine/amitriptyline	Turkington et al. 1980 (134)	Amitriptyline	Mendel et al. 1986 (95)
	Imipramine	Kvinesdal et al. 1984 (71)	Mianserin	[a]Sindrup et al. 1992 (127)
	Nortriptyline	Gomez-Perez et al. 1985 (53)	Fluoxetine	Max et al. 1992 (87)
	Amitriptyline	Max et al. 1987 (85)		
	Imipramine	Sindrup et al. 1989 (122)		
	Imipramine, paroxetine	[a]Sindrup et al. 1990 (123)		
	Clomipramine, desipramine	[b]Sindrup et al. 1990 (125)		
	Desipramine	Max et al. 1991 (86)		
	Imipramine	[a]Sindrup et al. 1992 (127)		
	Citalopram	[b]Sindrup et al. 1992 (117)		
	Amitriptyline, desipramine	Max et al. 1992 (87)		
Postherpetic neuralgia	Amitriptyline	Watson et al. 1982(142)		
	Amitriptyline	Max et al. 1988 (88)		
	Desipramine	Kishore-Kumar et al. 1990 (69)		
Peripheral neuropathy of different etiology	Clomipramine	Langohr et al. 1982 (74)		
	Clomipramine,nortriptyline	Panerai et al. 1990 (98)		
Central pain	Amitriptyline	Leijon et al. 1989 (76)	Trazodone	Davidoff et al. 1987 (30)
Atypical facial pain	Phenalzine	Lascelles 1966 (75)		
	Amitriptyline	Sharav et al. 1987 (116)		
Migraine (prophylaxis)	Amitriptyline	Gomersall et al. 1973 (52)	Clomipramine	[a]Langohr et al. 1985 (73)
	Amitriptyline	Couch et al. 1979 (27)		
	Amitriptyline	Ziegler et al. 1987 (152)		
Chronic tension headache	Amitriptyline	Lance et al. 1964 (72)		
	Amitriptyline	[b]Diamond et al. 1971 (35)		
	Maprotiline	Fogelholm et al. 1983 (43)		
Arthritis	Imipramine	McDonald Scott 1969 (90)	Amitriptyline	Ganvir et al. 1980 (48)
	Imipramine	Gringas 1976 (58)	Clomipramine	Grace et al. 1985 (55)
	Amitriptyline	Frank et al. 1988 (44)	Desipramine, trazodone	Frank et al. 1988 (44)
Chronic low back pain			Imipramine	Jenkins et al. 1976 (65)
			Imipramine	[c]Alcoff et al. 1982 (1)
			Amitriptyline	Pheasant et al. 1983 (102)
"Mixed patients"	Amitriptyline	Zitman et al. 1990 (155)		
	Amitriptyline	[b]McQuay et al. 1992 (93)		

For details, please refer to the text and individual references.
[a]High dropout rate on clomipramine may have influenced the results.
[b]Significant effect of low dose (10–60 mg/day) but higher dose (25–150 mg/day) not different from placebo.
[c]Pain severity showed borderline significant effect on imipramine ($p < .058$).

Clomipramine had a significantly better effect than aspirin in patients with mostly mononeuropathy from trauma, surgical procedures, or infections (74), and both clomipramine and nortriptyline were shown to relieve pain in a group of patients with pain following limb amputation, phantom stump pain, postherpetic neuropathy, or posttraumatic nerve lesions (98). It should be noted that the title of the latter publication incorrectly states that the target patients suffered from central pain, although the study only included patients with peripheral neuropathic pain.

Central Poststroke Pain and Miscellaneous Neurogenic Pain States

Amitriptyline has been shown to be superior to both placebo and carbamazepine in a well-designed study on patients with central poststroke pain (76). In that study, it was also found that the pain relief from carbamazepine was not significantly different from placebo. The responder frequency on amitriptyline was 67%.

In a randomized, double-blind, placebo-controlled trial with a parallel-group design in patients with dysesthetic pain in traumatic myelopathy, the selective serotonin reuptake inhibitor trazodone was found to be ineffective (30), but the sample size (9 + 9 patients) was rather small for a parallel-group design. In atypical facial pain (a central pain syndrome?), controlled studies have shown that both a monoamine oxidase (MAO) inhibitor (phenelzine) and amitriptyline were better than placebo (75,116). There is no evidence of an effect of antidepressants in trigeminal neuralgia.

Migraine and Tension Headache

Migraine prophylaxis with amitriptyline is well documented in adequately controlled trials (27,52,152). The tricyclic drug clomipramine was ineffective in a controlled study (73), but there was a high dropout rate during clomipramine treatment. In the study of Gomersall and Stuart (52), the patients had fewer attacks on amitriptyline than on placebo, whereas in the study of Couch and Hassanein (27) 55% improved on amitriptyline as compared to 34% on placebo. In the study of Gomersall and Stuart, the treatment was maintained for up to 6 months, and it was clearly suggested that the effect is maintained in the long term. In general, these drugs will not be drugs of first choice for migraine prophylaxis although the study of Ziegler et al. (152) found amitriptyline equally effective with propranolol. In a recent paper (153), it was reported that a better response on amitriptyline was associated with female gender, headache of short duration, and high frequency of attacks.

Studies of tricyclic antidepressants in chronic tension headache are almost uniformly positive (35,48,72), but this disease entity may actually have a psychogenic origin, and in the studies quoted all or at least a majority of the patients were rated to be depressed. The study of Diamond and Baltes (35) revealed that a low dose of amitriptyline (10 to 60 mg/day) was effective, whereas a higher dose (25 to 150 mg/day) was not significantly different from placebo.

Other Chronic Pain Conditions

In arthritis, some studies favor imipramine (58,90) and amitriptyline (44), while others do not find amitriptyline (48) and clomipramine (55) different from placebo. Further, the study of Frank et al. (44) included desipramine and trazodone and the effect of these drugs could not be distinguished from placebo.

There is no solid evidence of an effect of tricyclic antidepressants in chronic low back pain patients (1,65,102). This patient group may also be very heterogeneous since the pain in many patients may have a psychogenic origin, but one of the studies came out with a borderline significant effect of imipramine (1).

Mixed Patient Groups and Influence of Pain Characteristics

In an excellent study, it has been shown that a very low dose of amitriptyline (25 mg/day) relieves pain in a mixed group of patients with chronic nonmalignant pain (93). The patient group also comprised back pain patients, who are considered to be relatively unresponsive to antidepressants (see above), and there was no measurable changes in mood scores. In a later study, it was found that the effect could be increased by increasing amitriptyline doses to 50 or 75 mg/day (91). A modest effect in a mixed group of patients has also been reported by others (155). These data and general considerations lead one to focus more on pain characteristics (type of pain) than on the disease process underlying the development of pain symptoms. In clinical practice, it is often held that antidepressants are especially useful in the treatment of steady pain of dysesthetic and burning character. It is obvious from the overview presented above that the analgesic efficacy of antidepressants are best documented in neuropathic pain in which these pain types are generally more frequent than in nociceptive pain. Only a fraction of the antidepressant studies quoted above included a description of the patients' pain symptoms (69,76,85,87,88,123, 125,134,142) and even fewer indicated which pain types are alleviated by antidepressants. Further, many patients in these trials experienced several types of pain. However, it can be concluded from studies in both diabetic neuropathy (85,123,125) and postherpetic neuralgia (88) that tricyclic antidepressants relieve both steady (burning, aching, etc.) and brief or lancinating pain. Therefore, the clinical preference for carbamazepine in the control of lancinating pain and antidepressants in steady pain does not appear to be justified from these data.

PHARMACODYNAMIC PROFILE OF ANTIDEPRESSANT DRUGS

Numerous studies, mainly employing receptor binding techniques, have clarified the pharmacodynamic profile of different antidepressants. The pharmacodynamics of antidepressants described below form the background on which their hypothesized mechanism of action in pain treatment will be considered. This chapter considers several prototypical antidepressants that have been used in pain treatment, and a summary of their action is given in Table 2.

Tricyclic Antidepressants

The tricyclic structure has led to the development of a wide variety of agents with powerful pharmacologic effects on various components of neurotransmission. It is probable that the mechanisms of action will reflect upon the potential membrane effects these agents can exert.

Monoamine Uptake

Tricyclic antidepressants are associated with an important presynaptic blockade of the uptake process for monoamines such as serotonin (5-HT) and noradrenaline (NA) (19,20). Tricyclic agents with antidepressant actions, such as imipramine, amitriptyline, and clomipramine, are potent inhibitors of 5-HT

Table 2. PHARMACODYNAMIC PROFILE OF DIFFERENT ANTIDEPRESSANTS

	Reuptake inhibition		Receptor blockade				
	Serotonin	Noradrenaline	α-Adrenergic[a]	H_1- histaminergic	Muscarinic cholinergic	Opioid receptor interaction	Quinidine-like effect
Classical TCAs							
Imipramine	+	+[b]	+	+	+	+	+
Clomipramine	+	+[b]	+	+	+	+	?
Amitriptyline	+	+[b]	+	+	+	+	+
Desipramine	-	+	(+)	(+)	(+)	+	+
Nortriptyline	-	+	+	(+)	+	+	+
Selective serotonin reuptake inhibitors							
Paroxetine	+	-	-	-	(+)	?	-
Citalopram	+	-	-	-	-	?	-
Fluoxetine	+	-	-	-	-	(+)	-
Tetracyclic antidepressant							
Mianserin	-[c]	(+)	+	+	-	(+)	-

TCAs, Tricyclic antidepressants.
[a]α_1- and α_2-adrenergic receptor interaction not differentiated.
[b]Effect mainly through metabolites, i.e., desipramine, desmethylclomipramine, and nortriptyline, respectively.
[c]Mianserin appears to be antiserotonergic.
The pharmacodynamic profiles are as interpreted from references given in text.

reuptake, whereas they do not have a corresponding effect upon NA reuptake (59). However, their major metabolites (i.e., desipramine, nortriptyline, and desmethylclomipramine, respectively) are relatively potent NA reuptake inhibitors (59). Therefore, in a clinical setting, imipramine, amitriptyline, and clomipramine must be considered as balanced inhibitors of 5-HT and NA reuptake. The metabolites desipramine and nortriptyline are themselves used as drugs, i.e., tricyclic antidepressants, which are relatively selective NA reuptake inhibitors. Doxepine and maprotiline are relatively potent noradrenaline reuptake inhibitors from this drug class (59,109); they are similar to desipramine.

Receptor Blockade

The tricyclic compounds display a number of direct receptor interactions. Thus, the tricyclic compounds block (a) α_1-and α_2-adrenergic, (b) H_1-histaminergic, and (c) muscarinic cholinergic receptors, although with distinct interdrug patterns and potencies (59). All tricyclics bind at opiate receptors, but the affinity for those receptors is very modest (13,59,64).

Recent studies indicate that tricyclic antidepressants bind at the *N*-methyl-D-aspartate (NMDA) subtype of the glutamate receptor (108) and block NMDA-mediated synaptic activity (139). These drugs can, as do NMDA receptor antagonists, provide protection against NMDA-induced toxicity (18,89) and have a preclinical antihyperalgesic profile similar to NMDA antagonists (see below). Importantly, these actions at the NMDA receptor occur at concentrations comparable to those required to block monoamine reuptake.

Most of tricyclic antidepressants exert a "quinidine-like" effect on the heart, i.e., they prolong the duration of the QRS complex and to a lesser degree also the QT interval due to a membrane stabilizing effect (40,42,50,136,137). For quinidine, this effect on the heart is paralleled by a local blocking effect on peripheral nerves (67), but it is not known if this is also the case for the tricyclic antidepressants.

Besides these immediate receptor and nonreceptor effects, it has also been suggested that long-term treatment with tricyclic antidepressants upregulate 5-HT_{1A}-receptors and downregulate 5-HT_2-receptors (38,78).

Selective Serotonin Reuptake Inhibitors

Recent efforts in drug development have led to the development of antidepressants that are selective inhibitors of serotonin reuptake. Examples of this drug class are fluoxetine, paroxetine, and citalopram. These drugs block the reuptake of serotonin, but are without effect on noradrenaline reuptake (63,129,133). Further, selective serotonin reuptake inhibitors have no or very weak postsynaptic blocking effects (63,129,133) and do not induce quinidine-like effects on the electrocardiogram (37,42,79). Fluoxetine has a lower affinity to opiate receptors than the tricyclic antidepressants (13), whereas the possible interaction of the other drugs from this class with opiate receptors has not been studied. Trazodone is a selective, though less potent, inhibitor of serotonin reuptake (109) and is likewise without anticholinergic and antihistaminergic effects (110) but displays serotonin receptor antagonism (129). It has a lower affinity for opiate receptors than the tricyclics (64).

Other Antidepressants

Mianserin is a tetracyclic antidepressant with a pharmacodynamic profile quite different from the tricyclics (8,59,130). It is not an inhibitor of serotonin reuptake and may actually block postsynaptic serotonergic receptors. As a noradrenaline reuptake inhibitor, it is much weaker than the tricyclic antidepressants, but does cause some excessive noradrenaline release, probably by blocking presynaptic α_2-adrenergic receptors. The affinity of mianserin for the opiate receptor is also lower than that of the tricyclics (13), and it has no quinidine-like effect on the heart (101).

Monoamine oxidase inhibitors interfere with the degradation of serotonin and noradrenaline, and their action may therefore be somehow similar to tricyclic antidepressants with a balanced reuptake inhibition of serotonin and noradrenaline.

MECHANISM OF ACTION OF ANTIDEPRESSANTS IN PAIN TREATMENT

The exact mechanism of action of antidepressants in the treatment of depression is not known, and this is also the case for the use of antidepressants in pain treatment. However, recent studies in pain treatment have increased our knowledge on this issue considerably.

Antidepressant Versus Analgesic Effect

Depressed patients often complain of pain (138). Conversely, it is recognized that in some patients pain masks a genuinely depressed state (77). The common appreciation that pain may consist of a "sensory-discriminative" and an "affective motivational" component (94) emphasizes that agents that by their pharmacology can alter this emotional component can have a distinct ameliorating impact on the pain state (21,22). Thus, it could be suggested that the pain-diminishing effect of the antidepressants may be closely linked to the antidepressant effect of the drugs. Several lines of evidence, however, may be marshaled to indicate that the analgesic effects are likely not uniquely defined in terms of either the antidepressant effect or a simple change in afferent transmission:

1. Effects in pain patients not suffering from depression. The first controlled trial on antidepressants in painful diabetic neuropathy indicated pain relief through the antidepressant effect (134), since it was found that nearly all the patients had a substantial degree of depression and that pain relief was followed by relief of depressive symptoms. However, more recent studies have shown that amitriptyline, imipramine, and desipramine relieve diabetic neuropathy symptoms in patients with both normal and depressed mood (85,86,123). Similar findings have been reported for antidepressants used in the treatment of postherpetic neuralgia (69,88), central poststroke pain (76), arthritis (44), and migraine (27,152).
2. Time of onset of drug effect. Studies have indicated that the full effect of these agents as analgesics in diabetic neuropathy is achieved much faster (within 1 week) (123, 125) (Fig. 1) than the antidepressant actions assessed in melancholic depression (gradually over 3 to 8 weeks). If one takes into account the initial small dose and short dose titration period used in many studies, a similar, comparatively more rapid onset in analgesia than in altered depression scores has been reported in other neuropathic states (74,76,98). Also in the mixed patient group studied by McQuay et al. (91,92) a similar pattern was observed (Fig. 2). Some studies describe an increasing effect over 6 weeks (69,85,87,88), but this discrepancy can to some extent be explained by a 3-week-dose titration period.
3. Relative dose dependency of analgesia and antidepressant action. It has generally been found that lower doses or plasma concentrations of the tricyclic antidepressants are required to obtain pain relief than that required to obtain an antidepressant effect. With respect to plasma concentrations, this has been most extensively studied for imipramine in diabetic neuropathy. In a fixed dose study (71), it was found that patients with notable improvement on imipramine had higher plasma concentrations of imipramine plus desipramine than patients

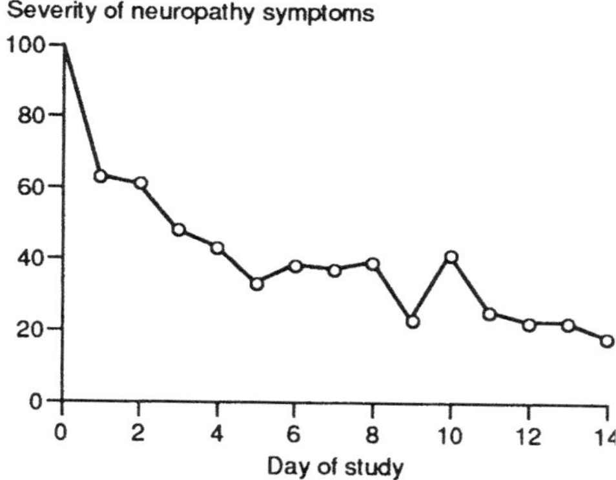

Figure 1. Daily neuropathy symptoms given as percent of the severity observed during placebo or drug-free baseline by day of study in patients treated with imipramine for chronic painful diabetic neuropathy. Median value indicated (○). (Data from ref. 123.)

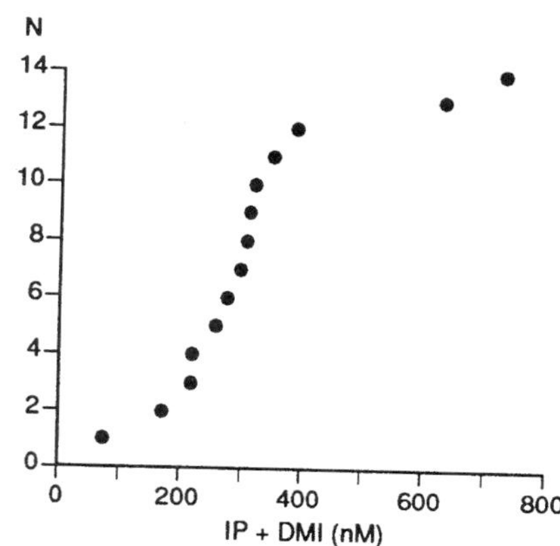

Figure 3. Cumulated numbers of patients (●) experiencing more than 95% of maximal response by plasma concentration of imipramine (IP) plus its active metabolite desipramine (DMI) during an imipramine dose-titration study in patients with chronic painful diabetic neuropathy. (Data from ref. 118.)

with no therapeutic effect. The lower effective level appeared to be around 400 nM. This level was later further supported in a dose titration study, since plasma drug levels above 400 nM were required obtain an individual maximal response in the majority of patients (124) (Fig. 3). The lower effective plasma concentration of imipramine plus desipramine in the treatment of depression is about 700 nM (107). Further, in postherpetic neuralgia (142), lower effective plasma levels of amitriptyline and its active metabolite nortriptyline than in the treatment of depression (154) have been found. However, identical effective plasma concentrations for treatment of pain and depressive conditions have been indicated in other studies on amitriptyline (85,88). The recent finding of efficacy of an extremely low dose of amitriptyline (25 mg) in chronic pain patients (93) supports the former view.

4. Acute antinociceptive effects of tricyclic agents. An "analgesic" effect of antidepressants is also suggested from experimental human (16,26,104) and animal (13,32,64,106) studies in which the models are not believed to possess a "depressive" component. In these studies, it has been shown that various antidepressants have an acute antinociceptive effect, since they increased thresholds to painful stimuli. Animal studies show that systemic or spinally delivered tricyclic agents augment the effects of opiates and prevent the development of facilitated pain states (such as in the formalin test, see below).

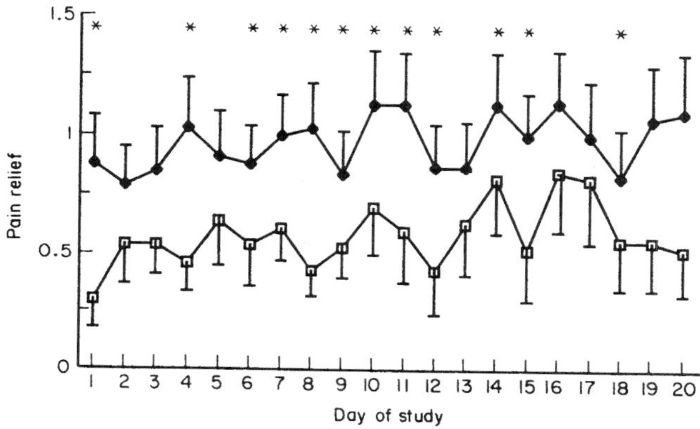

Figure 2. Mean (SEM) daily pain relief scores by day of study for amitriptyline 25 mg/day (■) and for placebo (□) in a mixed group of patients with chronic pain. (From ref. 93, with permission).

The many indications that antidepressants have a genuine analgesic effect not depending on their effect on depression does not preclude that the basic mechanisms of action in pain and depression may be related.

Potential Mechanisms

Nearly all the pharmacodynamic actions of tricyclic antidepressants can be shown to have potential effects on systems that process nociceptive information.

Monoamine Uptake Blockade

Monoamine systems not only play an important role in regulating the afferent traffic, but also serve to influence the emotionality of the animal. Importantly, if the effects of the tricyclic antidepressant molecule is mediated by an enhanced release of either 5-HT or noradrenaline, its actions in that model should display the appropriate antagonist receptor pharmacology.

At the spinal level, the activation of serotonergic (128,147) and α_2-adrenoceptors (146) produces a powerful modulation of spinal nociceptive processing. Serotonin and noradrenaline arising from the respective bulbospinal projections can by an action upon specific spinal receptors modulate small afferent evoked excitation (23,41,97,103,105,111,148). Given that small afferent input will evoke spinal release of 5-HT and noradrenaline (135), factors increasing the extracellular levels of these monoamines at the spinal level would enhance spinal receptor occupancy and induce an enhanced modulation of spinal input, resulting in antinociception (62). The activation of such bulbospinal pathways is reviewed in detail elsewhere (see Chaps. 11 and 30).

At the supraspinal levels, forebrain monoamine projections arising from brainstem nuclei go to a variety of limbic structures that are known to play an important role in regulating the animal's emotionality (6,7,45). Thus, the raphe dorsalis provides 5-HT projections to rostral sites, including the n. accumbens, amygdala, and lateral thalamus (80,81,144). Similarly, the locus coeruleus has strong noradrenergic projections into the limbic forebrain and thalamus (3,144). 5-HT and noradrenergic systems are implicated in the manifestation emotionality and maintenance of consciousness. Depletion of serotonin by treatment with p-chlorphenylalanine, for example, has been classically known to produce rats that were particularly irritable (131). Thus, while the nature of the interaction between the activity generated by small afferent input and the forebrain systems receiving monoamine input is at present uncharacterized, such systems may play an important role in the affective motivational component that contributes to pain behavior (33,46). Enhancing the terminal activity of these catecholamine systems by blocking reuptake might thus reasonably provide an important point of action for the uptake blocking properties of the tricyclic compounds.

NMDA Antagonist Activity

The affinity of the tricyclic compounds for the NMDA receptor has led to the speculation that these agents may serve in that capacity. Current thinking has indicated that spinal NMDA receptors may serve to induce a state of facilitated afferent processing (see Chaps. 36 and 60). Two forms of facilitated processing may be briefly considered as relevant to the potential actions of tricyclic agents at an NMDA-like receptor. First, repetitive small afferent input will yield a facilitated response of dorsal horn neurons (96), and this facilitation is believed to be correlated with the behavioral parallel of hyperalgesia (146). Ample data emphasize that the small afferent evoked facilitation can be diminished by the spinal delivery of NMDA antagonists (36). The intrathecal delivery of NMDA induces a thermal hyperalgesia, and this hyperalgesia is reversed by NMDA antagonist (83). In recent work, it has been shown that the hyperalgesia is also reversed by intrathecal amitryptiline (38a) (Fig. 4). In behavioral models involving a chronic injury or inflammation, such as the inflamed knee joint or after the injection of formalin into the paw, NMDA antagonists by a spinal action can diminish the hyperalgesic component (24,149). The spinal delivery of tricyclic antidepressants has in fact also been shown to reduce phase 2 (the facilitated component) but not phase 1 (the acute nociceptive component) of the formalin test (Fig. 4). Similarly, after peripheral cutaneous inflammation, the associated thermal hyperalgesic component is reduced by intrathecal amitryptiline (38a). Second, rodent models of nerve injury such as the Bennett model and the Chung model yield neuropathic states of thermal hyperalgesia and tactile allodynia, respectively (see Chap. 30). The spinal delivery of NMDA antagonists has been shown to diminish the hyperalgesic components (146). In recent work, the spinal delivery of amitriptyline has in fact been shown to reduce the hyperalgesic state in the two models of thermal hyperalgesia and tactile allodynia (Fig. 4). As reviewed in Chap. 40, it has been suggested that NMDA-antagonists may relieve neurogenic pain in humans (54) and inhibits central temporal summation in the nociceptive system (5). This body of experimental evidence in humans and animals is consistent with the clinical profile of activity of the tricyclic agents reviewed below.

Opioid Receptor Activity

Several animal experiments have focused on the opioid receptor interaction as the central mechanism of tricyclics in pain treatment (13,32,64,106) and found that the antinociceptive effect is partially reversed by naloxone. However, this does not prove a direct link between opioid receptor interaction and antinociception, since opioid neurons could be secondarily stimulated by nonopioid neurons. Furthermore, the apparent low efficacy of opioids in neuropathic pain (93) and a relatively low affinity of antidepressants for the opioid receptor (13,59,64) speaks against this as the mechanism of action.

Other Receptors/Mechanisms

It has been suggested (150) that tricyclics relieve diabetic neuropathy by blockade of highly sensitive α-adrenergic receptors on sprouts from diseased peripheral nerves. These receptors can otherwise be endogenously stimulated by noradrenaline released by sympathetic nerve discharge (34,114,115). Also, blockade of α_2-adrenergic receptors in some regions of the CNS may cause antinociception (105). Antinociception from antihistamines and thus H1-receptor blockade, has been indicated in humans in both experimental and clinical settings (14,113).

The possible quinidine-like effects on peripheral nerves may be expected to cause a local analgesic effect (67).

There is no evidence of an antinociceptive effect of blockade of muscarinic cholinergic receptors; on the contrary, stimulation of these receptors may have such an effect (61).

Clinical Correlates

The antinociceptive mechanism of antidepressants has been most extensively studied in diabetic neuropathy. The importance of noradrenaline reuptake inhibition is indicated by studies showing a beneficial effect of the relatively selective noradrenaline inhibitors desipramine (86,87,125) and nortriptyline (53). The latest study of Max et al. (87) even indicated that desipramine was equally effective with amitriptyline. Likewise, some studies have shown a pain relieving effect of the selective serotonin reuptake inhibitors paroxetine and citalopram (117,123), whereas fluoxetine has been reported to be without effect (87). However, the involvement of serotonergic mechanisms is indirectly indicated by the lack of effect of

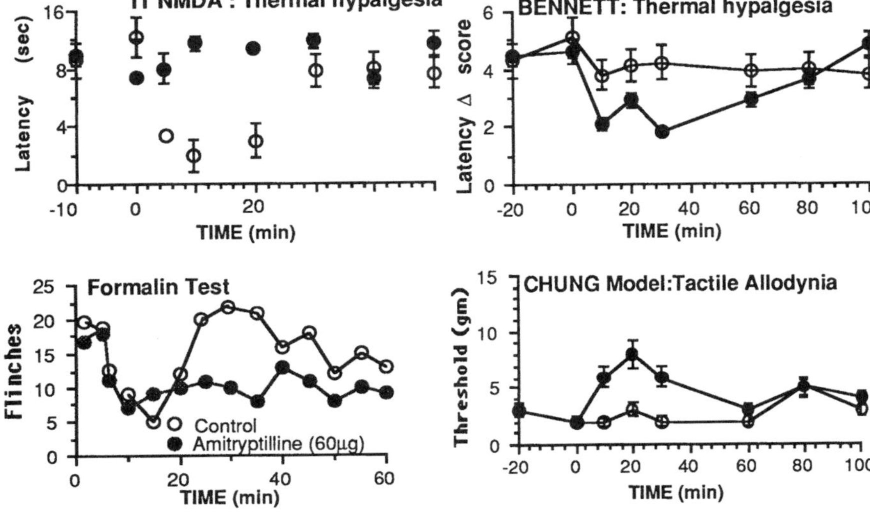

Figure 4. Top left: The effects of intrathecal (IT) amitriptyline (60 μg) or control (saline) on the thermal hyperalgesia induced by the IT delivery of NMDA (1 μg). *Bottom left:* Flinching of the hind paw after injection of formalin into the left hand paw. *Top right:* Thermal latency in a Bennett model of nerve ligation yielding a thermal hyperalgesia (9), expressed as difference in score between latency of nonlesioned and lesioned paw; smaller number is normal. Tactile escape thresholds in the Chung model of nerve ligation yielding a tactile allodynia; increased threshold is normal (68). *Bottom right:* As indicated, intrathecal amitriptyline reversed the tactile allodynia and thermal hyperalgesia induced by nerve injury or by the spinal delivery of NMDA, and attenuated the second, but not the first, phase of flinching induced in the formalin test. (From Yaksh and Spath, unpublished observations.)

mianserin (127), which may be directly antiserotonergic (cf. above). The comparative efficacy of drugs with the full range of pharmacologic actions of tricyclics as represented by clomipramine, and more selective compounds desipramine (noradrenergic) and paroxetine/citalopram (serotonergic) is shown in Fig. 5. The apparent lower efficacy of the selective serotonin reuptake inhibitors than of clomipramine may be attributed both to the lack of noradrenaline reuptake inhibition and to the fact that these compounds are without postsynaptic and quinidine-like effects (cf. above). The possible lower efficacy of desipramine, in contrast, seems mainly to be attributed to the lack of serotonin reuptake effect of this drug, since it does possess postsynaptic and quinidine-like effects.

Studies in other conditions have also focused on reuptake inhibition of serotonin and noradrenaline. The noradrenergic drug desipramine relieves postherpetic neuralgia (69), but other studies have shown that tricyclics with the full range of pharmacologic actions are more efficient than the noradrenergic compounds in this condition (141) and in a mixed group of patients with peripheral neuropathy (98). Selective serotonin reuptake inhibitors have been disappointing in postherpetic neuralgia (140) and posttraumatic myelopathy (30), but appeared to be effective in a mixed patient group (66). In the study on myelopathy, trazodone was used and it should be remembered that this compound to some extent is antiserotonergic along with its selective effect on serotonin reuptake.

Taken together, these studies seem to indicate that both reuptake inhibition of noradrenaline and serotonin are important for the effect of tricyclic antidepressants in pain treatment. However, it cannot be excluded that the receptor blockade (such as for the NMDA receptor) and the quinidine-like actions add to the efficacy. Therefore, from the point of view of efficacy, the older tricyclics with the full range of actions should be preferred as drugs of first choice. Consideration of contraindications and side effects may require that the more selective compounds are tried in spite of their apparent lower efficacy (cf. Section 6.0).

The upregulation of 5-HT_{1A}-receptors by chronic treatment with the tricyclics has not achieved much attention. This effect may explain why some studies show that the antinociceptive effect slightly increases after several weeks of treatment on the same dose (69,85–88). A maximal effect of the other pharmacologic actions has supposedly been achieved for some time. These considerations suggest a biphasic effect-time profile of tricyclic antidepressants in pain treatment.

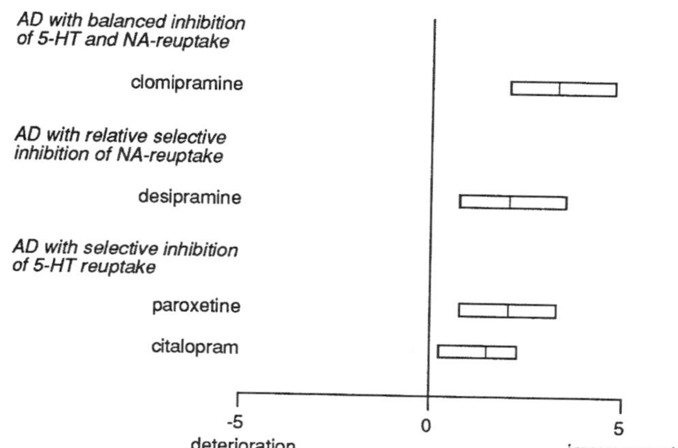

Figure 5. Median *(vertical line)* with 95% confidence interval *(box)* for the difference in neuropathy score between antidepressant (AD) and placebo in patients with chronic painful diabetic neuropathy. Antidepressants grouped according to their potential for inhibiting serotonin (5-HT) and noradrenaline (NA) reuptake. (Data from refs. 117, 123, 125.)

PHARMACOKINETICS AND DOSING

Pharmacokinetics of Antidepressants

A pronounced interindividual variation in pharmacokinetics is a common feature of the tricyclic antidepressants. A 30-fold variation in steady-state plasma concentrations on identical doses has been reported for imipramine (107), and variations on this order or lower are found, e.g., amitriptyline, desipramine, nortriptyline, and clomipramine (11,28,29,60, 112). The metabolism of these drugs to a large extent depends on the sparteine/debrisoquine oxygenase (CYP2D6) (17), the source of the sparteine/debrisoquine oxidation polymorphism. The extremes of the pharmacokinetic variation of these drugs are therefore made up by poor metabolizers of sparteine devoid of hepatic CYP2D6 (151) and fast extensive metabolizers with high activity of the enzyme. Population studies have shown that 7% of whites are poor metabolizers of sparteine (2), and that the poor metabolizes phenotype is inherited as an autosomal, recessive trait (39). The pharmacokinetics of the selective serotonin reuptake inhibitors is also characterized by some interindividual variations (10,28,29) that to some extent depend on the sparteine oxidation polymorphism (118,121).

Another feature of the pharmacokinetics of some of the antidepressants, e.g., imipramine, desipramine, paroxetine, fluoxetine, and probably also clomipramine, is dose-dependent kinetics (10,25,28,119,120,124,125), i.e., there is not a linear relationship between dose and plasma concentrations. Therefore, dose increments may cause nonproportionally higher increments in drug levels.

Dosing

As discussed earlier, lower effective plasma levels of tricyclic antidepressants have been indicated for pain treatment than for the treatment of depression, e.g., the effective level of imipramine plus desipramine in diabetic neuropathy is probably 300 to 500 nM. However, the therapeutic index is still quite low since the toxic level is probably around 1500 to 2000 nM (100). The combination of low therapeutic index and the pronounced interindividual pharmacokinetic variation makes standard dosing inappropriate, since a standard dose of 100 mg imipramine results in toxic concentrations in some patients and subtherapeutic levels in others (124). As the effect probably reaches a maximum within a week, it seems feasible to titrate the dose on the basis of therapeutic response. However, it should be remembered that these drugs are effective in at most 70% of patients, and the effect is modest in the majority of these patients. A few measurements of plasma drug concentrations should be performed in order to avoid toxicity and be able to increase doses that produce subtherapeutic plasma levels. It seems justified to recommend that drug level for each drug be kept well below the upper limit of the therapeutic interval for treatment of depression. Dose adjustment according to side effects to achieve an optimal effect is not generally recommended, since some side effects, e.g., dry mouth, occur at subtherapeutic concentrations (12,51,57,132). It can be speculated that such a dosing policy may have resulted in an underestimation of the efficacy of tricyclic antidepressants in some of the trials referred to above.

Plasma concentration effect relations are not so clear-cut for selective serotonin reuptake inhibitors in diabetic neuropathy (117,123,126), and since these drugs are widely nontoxic, it is probably not necessary to carry out therapeutic drug monitoring of their use.

A therapeutic window for amitriptyline in postherpetic neuralgia has been suggested (143), and as mentioned higher doses of amitriptyline appeared to be ineffective in tension headache in a study showing an effect on lower doses (35).

However, no other studies have indicated such a relationship for either amitriptyline or other antidepressants.

SIDE EFFECTS

The side effects of tricyclic antidepressants are probably mainly a result of blockade of muscarinic, cholinergic, histaminergic, and α-adrenergic receptors. The most common side effects are dry mouth, blurred vision (accommodation), problems with micturition, fatigue, dizziness, and orthostatic hypotension. It may be possible in patients with special problems to choose an antidepressant with less pronounced effect on the pertinent receptor. For orthostatic hypotension, it has been shown that nortriptyline produces significantly fewer reactions of this type than imipramine (132).

The tricyclics also have a negative inotropic effect on the heart and influence the heart in a quinidine-like way (112a). The use of these drugs therefore may be problematic or directly contraindicated in patients with some cardiac diseases. Also, the main toxicity of tricyclics in overdose are related to their cardiac effects.

The selective serotonin reuptake inhibitors are somewhat better tolerated (28,29,123) with respect to the trivial side effect and because they probably do not influence cardiac function. However, these drugs do cause some side effects, notably fatigue, nausea, and gastric upset.

The monoamine oxidase inhibitors may give rise to sleep disturbances, anxiety, and confusion. The main problem with these drugs are potential interactions with other drugs and foods, but this is less problematic with the newer reversible, selective monoamine oxidase A inhibitors. However, these have not been tried in pain treatment.

CONCLUSION AND PERSPECTIVES

During the past decade tricyclic antidepressants have become a mainstay in the treatment of different chronic neuropathic pain conditions, and they have also gained a minor role as adjunctive treatment in other chronic pain conditions. The mechanism of action of these drugs may be related to their ability to inhibit presynaptic reuptake of serotonin and noradrenaline, but other pharmacologic actions of these drugs, such as their ability to block the NMDA receptor, may also play a role. It is important to be aware of the great pharmacokinetic variability that is so characteristic of these drugs. This implies that special attention must be paid to the dosage regimen. An important issue remains in the general sense as to whether these agents as a family serve to induce their ameliorating effect on the pain state through an effect on the emotional component (e.g., as antidepressants) or in terms of an effect on afferent processing. The current body of data provides support for both general mechanisms. Future studies in human and animal experimental models should serve to illuminate the relative contribution of these several roles.

Other antidepressants, such as monoamine oxidase inhibitors and selective serotonin reuptake inhibitors, may in the future turn out to be interesting alternative drugs, but they have been tried in relatively few controlled studies. The selective serotonin reuptake inhibitors are important because they are better tolerated than the tricyclic antidepressants.

The antidepressants usually provide only partial pain relief, but this may be acceptable, since antidepressants are most often used in conditions where other treatments fail. However, the search for new drugs is warranted, especially for the treatment of neuropathic pain. This search may be inspired by the results from the trials of antidepressants reviewed in this chapter combined with knowledge of the pharmacodynamic effects (e.g., receptor interaction profile) of the different antidepressants.

REFERENCES

1. Alcoff J, Jones E, Rust P, Newman R. Controlled trial of imipramine for chronic low back pain. *J Fam Pract* 1982;14: 841–846.
2. Alván G, Bechtel P, Iselius L, Gundert-Remy U. Hydroxylation polymorphisms of debrisoquine and mephenytoin in European populations. *Eur J Clin Pharmacol* 1990;39:533–537.
3. Amaral DG, Sinnamon HM. The locus coereuleus: neurobiology of a central noradrenergic nucleus. *Prog Neurobiol* 1977;9: 147–196.
4. Archer AG, Watkins PJ, Thomas PK, Sharma AK, Payan J. The natural history of acute painful neuropathy in diabetes mellitus. *J Neurol Neurosurg Psychiatry* 1983;46:491–499.
5. Arendt-Nielsen L, Petersen-Felix S, Fischer M, Bak P, Bjerring P, Zbinden AM. The effect of NMDA-antagonist (Ketamine) on single and repeated nociceptive stimuli—a double-blind, placebo-controlled experimental human study. *Anesth Analg* 1995;81: 63–68.
6. Bandler R, Carrive P, Zhang SP. Integration of somatic and autonomic reactions within the midbrain periaqueductal grey, viscerotopic, somatotopic and functional organization. *Prog Brain Res* 1991;87:269–305.
7. Bandler R, McCulloch T, McDougall A, Prineas S, Dampney R Midbrain neural mechanisms mediating emotional behavior. *Int J Neurol* 1985;19:40–58.
8. Baumann PA, Maître L. Blockade of presynaptic α-receptors and of amine uptake in the rat brain by the antidepressant mianserine. *Naunyn Schmiedeberg Arch Pharmacol* 1977;300:31–37.
9. Bennett GJ, Xie YK. A peripheral mononeuropathy in rat that produces disorders of pain sensation like those seen in man. *Pain* 1988;33:87–107.
10. Bergstrom RF, Lemberger L, Farid NA, Wolen RL. Clinical pharmacology and pharmacokinetics of fluoxetine: a review. *Br J Psychiatry* 1988;153(suppl 3):47–50.
11. Bertilsson L, Aberg-Wistedt A. The debrisoquine hydroxylation test predicts steady-state plasma levels of desipramine. *Br J Clin Pharmacol* 1983;15:388–390.
12. Bertram U, Kragh-Sørensen P, Rafaelsen OJ, Larsen NE. Saliva secretion following long-term antidepressant treatment with nortriptyline controlled by plasma levels. *Scand J Dent Res* 1979;87: 58–64.
13. Biegon A, Samuel D. Interaction of tricyclic antidepressants with opiate receptors. *Biochem Pharmacol* 1980;29:460–462.
14. Bjerring P. Effect of antihistamines on argon laser-induced cutaneous sensory and pain thresholds and on histamine-induced wheal and flare. *Skin Pharmacol* 1989;2:210–216.
15. Boulton AJM, Armstrong WD, Scarpello JHB, Ward JD. The natural history of painful diabetic neuropathy—a 4-year study. *Postgrad Med J* 1983;59:556–559.
16. Bromm B, Meier W, Scharein E. Imipramine reduces experimental pain. *Pain* 1986;25:245–257.
17. Brøsen K, Gram LF. Clinical significance of the sparteine/debrisoquine oxidation polymorphism. *Eur J Clin Pharmacol* 1989;36: 537–547.
18. Cai Z, McCaslin PP. Amitriptyline, desipramine, cyproheptadine and carbamazepine, in concentrations used therapeutically, reduce kainate- and N-methyl-D-aspartate-induced intracellular Ca^+ levels in neuronal cultures. *Eur J Pharmacol* 1992;219:53–57.
19. Carlsson A, Corrodi H, Fuxe K, Hökfelt T. Effect of antidepressant drugs on the depletion of intraneuronal brain 5-hydroxytryptamine stores caused by 4-methyl-ethyl-meta-tyramine. *Eur J Pharmacol* 1969;5:357–366.
20. Carlsson A, Corrodi H, Fuxe K, Hökfelt T. Effect of some antidepressant drugs on the depletion of intraneuronal brain catecholamine stores caused by 4,32dimethyl-meta-tyramine. *Eur J Pharmacol* 1969;5:367–373.
21. Chapman CR. Psychological aspects of postoperative pain control. *Acta Anesthesiol Belg* 1992;43:41–52.
22. Chapman CR, Gavrin J. Suffering and its relationship to pain. *J Palliat Care* 1993;9:5–13.
23. Chitour D, Dickenson AH, Le Bars D. Pharmacological evidence for the involvement of serotonergic mechanisms in diffuse noxious inhibitory controls (DNIC). *Brain Res* 1982;236:329–337.
24. Coderre TJ, Melzack R. The contribution of excitatory amino acids to central sensitization and persistent nociception after formalin-induced tissue injury. *J Neurosci* 1992;12:3665–3670.

25. Cooke RG, Warsh JJ, Stancer HC, Reed KL, Persad E. The non-linear kinetics of desipramine and 2-hydroxydesipramine in plasma. *Clin Pharmacol Ther* 1984;36:343–349.
26. Coquoz D, Porchet HC, Dayer P. Effet analgésique central d'anti-dépresseurs à mode d'action distinct: désipramine, fluvoxamine et moclobémide. *Schweiz Med Wschr* 1991;121:1843–1845.
27. Couch JR, Hassanein RS. Amitriptyline in migraine prophylaxis. *Arch Neurol* 1979;36:695–699.
28. Danish University Antidepressant Group (DUAG). Citalopram: clinical effect profile in comparison with clomipramine. A controlled multicenter study. *Psychopharmacology* 1986;90:131–138.
29. Danish University Antidepressant Group (DUAG). Paroxetine: a selective serotonin reuptake inhibitor showing better tolerance, but weaker antidepressant effect than clomipramine in a controlled multicenter study. *J Affective Disord* 1990;18:289–299.
30. Davidoff G, Guarracini M, Roth E, Sliwa J, Yarkony G. Trazodone hydrochloride in the treatment of dysesthesic pain in traumatic myelopathy: a randomized, double-blind, placebo-controlled study. *Pain* 1987;29:151–161.
31. Davis JL, Lewis SB, Gerich JE, Kaplan RA, Schultz TA, Wallin JD. Peripheral diabetic neuropathy treated with amitriptyline and fluphenazine. *JAMA* 1977;238:2291–2292.
32. De Felipe M, de Ceballos ML, Fuentes JA. Hypoalgesia induced by antidepressants in mice: a case for opioids and serotonin. *Eur J Pharmacol* 1986;193–199.
33. Derryberry D, Tucker DM. Neural mechanisms of emotion. *J Consult Clin Psychol* 1992;60:329–38.
34. Devor M. Nerve pathophysiology and mechanisms of pain in causalgia. *J Auton Nerv Syst* 1983;7:371–384.
35. Diamond S, Baltes BJ. Chronic tension headache—treated with amitriptyline—a double-blind study. *Headache* 1971;1(11): 110–116.
36. Dickenson AH, Sullivan AF. Evidence for a role of the NMDA receptor in the frequency dependent potentiation of deep rat dorsal horn nociceptive neurones following C fibre stimulation. *Neuropharmacology* 1987;26:1235–1238.
37. Edwards JG, Goldie A, Papayanni-Papasthatis S. Effect of paroxetine on the electro-cardiogram. *Psychopharmacol* 1989;97:96–98.
38. Eide PK, Hole K. The role of 5-hydroxytryptamine (5-HT) receptor subtypes and plasticity in the 5-HT systems in the regulation of nociceptive sensitivity. *Cephalalgia* 1993;13:75–85.
38a. Eisenach JC, Gebhart GF. Intrathecal amitriptyline acts as an N-methyl-D-aspartate antagonist in the presence of inflammatory hyperalgesia in rats. *Anesthesiology* 1995;83:1046–54.
39. Evans DAP, Mahgoub A, Sloan TP, Idle JR, Smith RL. A family and population study of the genetic polymorphism of debrisoquine oxidation in a white British population. *J Med Genet* 1980;17: 102–105.
40. Faravelli C, Brat A, Marchetti G, Franchi F, Padeletti L, Michelucci A, Pastorino A. Cardiac effects of clomipramine treatment. ECG and left ventricular systolic time intervals. *Neuropsychobiology* 1983;9: 113–118.
41. Fields HL, Basbaum AI. Endogenous pain control mechanisms. In: Wall PD, Melzach R, eds. *Textbook of pain.* London: Churchill Livingstone, 1984;142–152.
42. Fisch C. Effect of fluoxetine on the electrocardiogram. *J Clin Psychiatry* 1985;46:42–44.
43. Fogelholm R, Murros K. Maprotiline in chronic tension headache: a double-blind cross-over study. *Headache* 1985;25: 273–275.
44. Frank RG, Kashani JH, Parker JC, Beck NC, Brownlee-Duffeck M, Elliot TR, Haut AE, Atwood C, Smith E, Kay DR. Antidepressant analgesia in rheumatoid arthritis. *J Rheumatol* 1988;15:1632–1638.
45. Franklin KBJ.Analgesia and the neural substrate of reward. *Neurosci Biobehav Rev* 1989;13:149–154.
46. Frysztak RJ; Neafsey EJ. The effect of medial frontal cortex lesions on cardiovascular conditioned emotional responses in the rat. *Brain Res* 1994;643:181–193.
47. Gade GN, Hofeldt FD, Treece GL. Diabetic neuropathic cachexia. Beneficial response to combination therapy with amitriptyline and fluphenazine. *JAMA* 1980;243:1160–1161.
48. Ganvir P, Beaumont G, Seldrup J. A comparative trial of clomipramine and placebo as adjunctive therapy in arthralgia. *J Int Med Res* 1980;8(suppl 3):60–66.
49. Gerson GR, Jones RB, Luscombe DK. Studies on the concomitant use of carbamazepine and clomipramine for the relief of post-herpetic neuralgia. *Postgrad Med J* 1977;53:104–109.
50. Giardina E-GV, Bigger JT, Glassman AH, Perel JM, Kantor SJ. The electrocardiographic and anti arrhythmic effects of imipramine hydrochloride at therapeutic plasma concentrations. *Circulation* 1979;60:1045–1052.
51. Glassman AH, Carino JS, Roose SP. Adverse effects of tricyclic antidepressants: focus on the elderly. In: Usdin E, Åsberg M, Bertilsson L, Sjöqvist F, eds. *Frontiers in biochemical and pharmacological research in depression.* New York: Raven Press, 1984;391–398.
52. Gomersall JD, Stuart A. Amitriptyline in migraine prophylaxis. Changes in pattern of attacks during a controlled clinical trial. *J Neurol Neurosurg Psychiatry* 1973;36:684–690.
53. Gomez-Perez FJ, Rull JA, Dies H, Rodriguez-Rivera JG, Gonzales-Barranco J, Lozano-Casteñeda O. Nortriptyline and fluphenazine in the symptomatic treatment of diabetic neuropathy. A double-blind cross-over study. *Pain* 1985;23:395–400.
54. Gordh T, Kristensen JD. The NMDA-receptor antagonist CPP abolishes neurogenic "wind-up pain" after intrathecal administration in humans. *Reg Anesth* 1992;17(suppl 3):82.
55. Grace EM, Bellamy N, Kassam Y, Buchanan WW. Controlled, double-blind randomized trial of amitriptyline in relieving articular pain and tenderness with rheumatoid arthritis. *Curr Med Res Opin* 1985;9:426–429.
56. Gram LF, Fredricson Overø K. Drug interaction: inhibitory effect of neuroleptics on metabolism of tricyclic antidepressants in man. *Br Med J* 1972;1:463–465.
57. Gram LF, Kragh-Sørensen P, Kristensen CB, Møller M, Pedersen OL, Thayssen P. Plasma level monitoring of antidepressants: theoretical basis and clinical application. In: Usdin E, Åsberg M, Bertilsson L, Sjöqvist F, eds. *Frontiers in biochemical and pharmacological research in depression.* New York: Raven Press, 1984;399–411.
58. Gringas M. A clinical trial of tofranil in rheumatic pain in general practice. *J Int Med Res* 1976;4(suppl 2):41–49.
59. Hall H, Ögren S-O. Effects of antidepressant drugs on different receptors in the brain. *Eur J Pharmacol* 1981;70:393–407.
60. Hammer W, Sjöqvist F. Plasma levels of monomethylated tricyclic antidepressants during treatment with imipramine-like compounds. *Life Sci* 1967;6:1895–1903.
61. Hartvig P, Gillberg PG, Gordh T, Post C. Cholinergic mechanisms in pain and analgesia. *Trend Pharmacol Sci* 1989;Dec. suppl:75–79.
62. Hwang AS, Wilcox GL. Analgesic properties of intrathecally administered heterocyclic antidepressants. *Pain* 1987;28: 343–355.
63. Hyttel J. Neurochemical characterization of a new potent serotonin reuptake inhibitor: Lu 10-171. *Psychopharmacology* 1977;51: 225–233.
64. Isenberg KE, Cicero TJ. Possible involvement of opiate receptors in the pharmacological profiles of antidepressant compounds. *Eur J Pharmacol* 1984;103:57–63.
65. Jenkins DG, Ebbutt AF, Evans CD. Tofranil in the treatment of low back pain. *J Int Med Res* 1976;4:28–40.
66. Johansson F, von Knorring L. A double-blind controlled study of a serotonin uptake inhibitor (zimelidine) versus placebo in chronic pain patients. *Pain* 1979;1(7):69–78.
67. Juan H. Inhibition of the algesic effect of bradykinin and acetylcholine by mepacrine. *Naunyn Schmiedebergs Arch Pharmacol* 1977; 301:23–27.
68. Kim SH, Chung JM. An experimental model for peripheral neuropathy produced by segmental spinal nerve ligation in the rat. *Pain* 1992;50:355–363.
69. Kishore-Kumar R, Max MB, Schafer SC, Gaughan AM, Smoler B, Gracely RH, Dubner R. Desipramine relieves postherpetic neuralgia. *Clin Pharmacol Ther* 1990;47:305–312.
70. Kuhn R. Treatment of depressive states with imipramine hydrochloride. *Am J Psychiatry* 1958;115:459–464.
71. Kvinesdal B, Molin J, Frøland A, Gram LF. Imipramine treatment of painful diabetic neuropathy. *JAMA* 1984;251:1727–1730.
72. Lance JW, Curran DA. Treatment of chronic tension headache. *Lancet* 1964;1:1236–1239.
73. Langohr HD, Gerber WD, Koletzki E, Mayer K, Schroth G. Clomipramine and metoprolol in migraine prophylaxis—a double-blind crossover study. *Headache* 1985;25:107–113.
74. Langohr HD, Stöhr M, Petruch F. An open and double-blind cross-over study on the efficacy of clomipramine (Anafranil) in patients with painful mono- and polyneuropathies. *Eur Neurol* 1982;21:309–317.
75. Lascelles RG. Atypical facial pain and depression. *Br J Psychiatry* 1966;112:651–659.

76. Leijon G, Boivie J. Central post-stroke pain—a controlled trial of amitriptyline and carbamazepine. *Pain* 1989;36:27–36.
77. Lopez Ibor JJ. Masked depression. *Br J Psychiatry* 1972;120: 245–258.
78. Lund A, Mjellem-Joly N, Hole K. Desipramine administered chronically, influences 5-hydroxytryptamine$_{1A}$-receptors, as measured by behavioral tests and receptor binding in rats. *Neuropharmacology* 1992;31:25–32.
79. Lyby K, Elsborg L, Høpfner Petersen HE, Skovlund E. Long-term safety of citalopram. *Psychopharmacol* 1988;96(suppl):S268.
80. Ma QP, Han JS. Neurochemical and morphological evidence of an antinociceptive neural pathway from nucleus raphe dorsalis to nucleus accumbens in the rabbit. *Brain Res Bull* 1992;28: 931–936.
81. Ma QP, Yin GF, Ai MK, Han JS. Serotonergic projections from the nucleus raphe dorsalis to the amygdala in the rat. *Neurosci Lett* 1991;134:21–24.
82. Magni G. The use of antidepressants in the treatment of chronic pain. *Drugs* 1991;42:730–748.
83. Malmberg AB, Yaksh TL. Hyperalgesia mediated by spinal glutamate or substance P receptor blocked by spinal cyclooxygenase inhibition. *Science* 1992;257:1276–1279.
84. Marshall JB, Forker AD. Cardiovascular effects of tricyclic antidepressant drugs: therapeutic usage, overdose, and management of complications. *Am Heart J* 1982;103:401–414.
85. Max MB, Culnane M, Schafer SC, Gracely RH, Walther DJ, Smoller B, Dubner R. Amitriptyline relieves diabetic neuropathy pain in patients with normal or depressed mood. *Neurology* 1987;37:589–596.
86. Max MB, Kishore-Kumar R, Schafer SC, Meister B, Gracely RH, Smoller B, Dubner R. Efficacy of desipramine in painful diabetic neuropathy: a placebo-controlled trial. *Pain* 1991;45:3–9.
87. Max MB, Lynch SA, Muir J, Shoaf SE, Smoller B, Dubner R. Effects of desipramine, amitriptyline, and fluoxetine on pain in diabetic neuropathy. *N Engl J Med* 1992;326:1250–1256.
88. Max MB, Schafer SC, Culnane M, Smoller B, Dubner R, Gracely RH. Amitriptyline, but not lorazepam, relieves postherpetic neuralgia. *Neurology* 1988;38:1427–1432.
89. McCaslin PP, Yu XZ, Ho IK, Smith TG. Amitriptyline prevents N-methyl-D-aspartate (NMDA)-induced toxicity, does not prevent NMDA-induced elevations of extracellular glutamate, but augments kainate-induced elevations of glutamate. *J Neurochem* 1992;59:401–405.
90. McDonald Scott WA. The relief of pain with an antidepressant in arthritis. *Practitioner* 1969;202:802–807.
91. McQuay HJ, Carroll D, Glynn CJ. Dose-response for analgesic effect of amitriptyline in chronic pain. *Anaesthesia* 1993;48: 281–285.
92. McQuay HJ, Jadad AR, Carroll D, Faura C, Glynn CJ, Moore RA, Liu Y. Opioid sensitivity of chronic pain: a patient-controlled analgesia method. *Anaesthesia* 1992;47:757–767.
93. McQuay HJ, Carroll D, Glynn CJ. Low dose amitriptyline in the treatment of chronic pain. *Anaesthesia* 1992;47:646–652.
94. Melzack R, Casey KL. Sensory, motivational, and central control determinants of pain: a new conceptual model. In: Kenshalo D, ed. *The skin senses.* Springfield, IL; Charles C. Thomas, 1968; 423–443.
95. Mendel CM, Klein RF, Chappell DA, Dere WH, Gertz BJ, Karam JH, Lavin TN, Grunfeld C. A trial of amitriptyline and fluphenazine in the treatment of painful diabetic neuropathy. *JAMA* 1986;255:637–639.
96. Mendell LM, Wall PD. Responses of single dorsal cord cells to peripheral cutaneous unmyelinated fibers. *Nature* 1965;206: 97–99.
97. Mohrland JS, Gebhart GF. Effect of selective destruction of serotonergic neurons in nucleus raphe magnus on morphine-induced antinociception. *Life Sci* 1980;27:2627–2632.
98. Panerai AE, Monza G, Movilia P, Bianchi M, Francucci BM, Tiengo M. A randomized, within-patient, cross-over, placebo-controlled trial on the efficacy and tolerability of the tricyclic antidepressants chlorimipramine and nortriptyline in central pain. *Acta Neurol Scand* 1990;82:34–38.
99. Paoli F, Darcourt G, Corsa P. Note préliminaire sur l'action de l'imipramine dans les états douloureux. *Rev Neurol* 1960;2: 503–504.
100. Pedersen OL, Gram LF, Kristensen CB, Møller M, Thayssen P, Bjerre M, Kragh-Sørensen P, Klitgaard NA, Sindrup E, Hole P, Brinkløv M. Overdosage of antidepressants: clinical and pharmacokinetic aspects. *Eur J Clin Pharmacol* 1982;23:513–521.
101. Peet M, Tienari P, Jaskari MO. A comparison of the cardiac effects of mianserin and amitriptyline in man. *Pharmacopsychiatry* 1977;10: 309–312.
102. Pheasant H, Bursk A, Goldfarb J, Azen SP, Weiss JN, Borelli L. Amitriptyline and chronic low-back pain. A randomized double-blind crossover study. *Spine* 1983;8:552–557.
103. Post C, Minor BG, Davies M, Archer T. Analgesia induced by 5-hydroxytryptamine receptor agonists is blocked or reversed by noradrenaline-depletion in rats. *Brain Res* 1986;363:18–27.
104. Poulsen L, Arendt-Nielsen L, Brosen K, Gram LF, Sindrup SH. The hypoalgesic effect of imipramine in different human experimental pain models. *Pain* 1995;60:287–293.
105. Proudfit HK. Pharmacologic evidence for the modulation of nociception by noradrenergic neurons. In: Fields HL, Besson J-M, eds. *Progress in brain research.* Amsterdam: Elsevier Scientific, 1988;77: 357–370.
106. Reichenberg K, Gaillard-Plaza G, Montastruc JL. Influence of naloxone on the antinociceptive effects of some antidepressant drugs. *Arch Int Pharmacodyn* 1985;275:78–85.
107. Reisby N, Gram LF, Bech P, Nagy A, Petersen GO, Ortmann J, Ibsen I, Dencker SJ, Jacobsen O, Krautwald O, Søndergård I, Christiansen J. Imipramine: clinical effects and pharmacokinetic variability. *Psychopharmacology* 1977;54:263–272.
108. Reynolds, IJ, Miller, RJ. Tricyclic antidepressants block N-methyl-D-aspartate receptors: similarities to the action of zinc. *Br J Pharmacol* 1988;95:95–102.
109. Richelson E, Pfenning M. Blockade by antidepressants and related compounds of biogenic amine uptake into rat brain synaptosomes: most antidepressants selectively block norepinephrine uptake. *Eur J Pharmacol* 1984;104:277–286.
110. Richelson E. Antidepressants: effects on histaminic and muscarinic receptors. In: Gram LF, Usdin E, Dahl SG, Kragh-Sørensen P, Sjöqvist F, Morselli PL, eds. *Clinical pharmacology in psychiatry. Bridging the experimental therapeutic gap.* London and Basingstoke: Macmillan, 1983;288–300.
111. Roberts MHT. 5-hydroxytryptamine and antinociception. *Neuropharmacology* 1984;23:1529–1536.
112. Rollins DE, Alván G, Bertilsson L, Gilette JK, Mellström B, Sjöqvist F, Träskman L. Interindividual differences in amitriptyline demethylation. *Clin Pharmacol Ther* 1980;1(28):121–129.
112a. Roos JC. Cardiac effects of antidepressant drugs. A comparison of the tricyclic antidepressants and fluvoxamine. *Br J Clin Pharmacol* 1983;3(suppl 15);439–445.
113. Rumore MM, Schlichting DA. Clinical efficacy of antihistaminics as analgesics. *Pain* 1986;25:7–22.
114. Sanjue H, Jun Z. Sympathetic facilitation of sustained discharges of polymodal nociceptors. *Pain* 1989;38:85–90.
115. Sato J, Perl ER. Adrenergic excitation of cutaneous pain receptors induced by peripheral nerve injury. *Science* 1991;251:1608–1611.
116. Sharav Y, Singer E, Schmidt E, Dionne RA, Dubner R. The analgesic effect of amitriptyline on chronic facial pain. *Pain* 1987;31: 199–209.
117. Sindrup SH, Bjerre U, Dejgaard A, Brøsen K, Aaes-Jørgensen T, Gram LF. The selective serotonin reuptake inhibitor citalopram relieves the symptoms of diabetic neuropathy. *Clin Pharmacol Ther* 1992;52:547–552.
118. Sindrup SH, Brøsen K, Gram LF, Hallas J, Skjelbo E, Allen A, Allen GD, Cooper SM, Mellows G, Tasker TCG, Zussmann BD. The relationship between paroxetine and the sparteine oxidation polymorphism. *Clin Pharmacol Ther* 1992;51:278–287.
119. Sindrup SH, Brøsen K, Gram LF. Nonlinear kinetics of imipramine in low and medium plasma level ranges. *Ther Drug Monit* 1990;12:445–449.
120. Sindrup SH, Brøsen K, Gram LF. Pharmacokinetics of the selective serotonin reuptake inhibitor paroxetine: non-linearity and relation to the sparteine oxidation polymorphism. *Clin Pharmacol Ther* 1992;51:288–295.
121. Sindrup SH, Brøsen K, Hansen MGJ, Aaes-Jørgensen T, Overø KF, Gram LF. Pharmacokinetics of citalopram in relation to the sparteine and the mephenytoin oxidation polymorphisms. *Ther Drug Monit* 1993;15:11–17.
122. Sindrup SH, Ejlertsen B, Frøland A, Sindrup EH, Brøsen K, Gram LF. Imipramine treatment in diabetic neuropathy: relief of subjective symptoms without changes in peripheral and autonomic nerve function. *Eur J Clin Pharmacol* 1989;37:151–153.

123. Sindrup SH, Gram LF, Brøsen K, Eshøj O, Mogense EF. The selective serotonin reuptake inhibitor paroxetine is effective in the treatment of diabetic neuropathy symptoms. *Pain* 1990;42: 135–144.
124. Sindrup SH, Gram LF, Skjold T, Frøland A, Beck-Nielsen H. Concentration-response relationship in imipramine treatment of diabetic neuropathy symptoms. *Clin Pharmacol Ther* 1990;47: 509–515.
125. Sindrup SH, Gram LF, Skjold T, Grodum E, Brøsen K, Bech-Nielsen H. Clomipramine vs. desipramine in the treatment of diabetic neuropathy symptoms. A double-blind cross-over study. *Br J Clin Pharmacol* 1990;30:683–691.
126. Sindrup SH, Grodum E, Gram LF, Beck-Nielsen H. Concentration-response relationship in paroxetine treatment of diabetic neuropathy symptoms: a patient-blinded dose-escalation study. *Ther Drug Monit* 1991;13:408–414.
127. Sindrup SH, Tuxen C, Gram LF, Grodum E, Skjold T, Beck-Nielsen H. Lack of effect of mianserin on the symptoms of diabetic neuropathy. *Eur J Clin Pharmacol* 1992;43:251–255.
128. Solomon R E, Gebhart G F 1988 Mechanisms of effects of intrathecal serotonin on nociception and blood pressure in rats. *J Pharmacol Exp Ther* 1988;245:905–912.
129. Stark P, Fuller RW, Wong DT. The pharmacologic profile of fluoxetine. *J Clin Psychiatry* 1985;46:7–13.
130. Starke K, Göthert M, Kilbinger H. Modulation of neurotransmitter release by presynaptic autoreceptors. *Physiol Rev* 1989;69: 864–989.
131. Tenen SS. Antagonism of the analgesic effect of morphine and other drugs by p-chlorophenylalanine, a serotonin depletor. *Psychopharmacology* 1968;12:278–85.
132. Thayssen P, Bjerre M, Kragh-Sørensen P, Møller M, Petersen OL, Kristensen CB, Gram LF. Cardiovascular effects of imipramine and nortriptyline in elderly patients. *Psychopharmacology* 1981;74: 360–364.
133. Thomas DR, Nelson DR, Johnson AM. Biochemical effects of the antidepressant paroxetine, a specific 5-hydroxytryptamine uptake inhibitor. *Psychopharmacology* 1987;93:193–200.
134. Turkington RW. Depression masquerading as diabetic neuropathy. *JAMA* 1980;243:1147–1150.
135. Tyce GM, Yaksh TL. Monoamine release from cat spinal cord by somatic stimuli: an intrinsic modulatory system. *J Physiol (Lond)* 1981;314:513–529.
136. Veith RC, Friedel RO, Bloom V, Bielski R. Electrocardiogram changes and plasma desipramine levels during treatment of depression. *Clin Pharmacol Ther* 1980;27:796–802.
137. Vohra J, Burrows G, Hunt D, Sloman G. The effect of toxic and therapeutic doses of tricyclic antidepressant drugs on intracardiac conduction. *Eur J Cardiol* 1975;3:219–227.
138. von Knorring L, Perris C, Eisemann M, Eriksson U, Perris H. Pain as a symptom in depressive disorders. I. Relationship to diagnostic subgroup and depressive symptomatology. *Pain* 1983;15: 19–26.
139. Watanabe Y, Saito H, Yamawaki, S. Antidepressants block NMDA receptor-mediated synaptic responses and induction of long term potentiation in rat hippocampal slices. *Neuropharmacology* 1993; 32:479–486.
140. Watson CPN, Evans RJ. A comparative trial of amitriptyline and zimelidine in post-herpetic neuralgia. *Pain* 1985;23:387–394.
141. Watson CPN, Chipman M, Reed K, Evans RJ, Birkett N. Amitriptyline versus maprotiline in postherpetic neuralgia: a randomized, double-blind, crossover trial. *Pain* 1992;48:29–36.
142. Watson CPN, Evans RJ, Reed K, Merskey H, Goldsmith L, Warsh J. Amitriptyline versus placebo in postherpetic neuralgia. *Neurology* 1982;32:671–673.
143. Watson CPN. Therapeutic window for amitriptyline analgesia. *Can Med Assoc J* 1984;130:105–106.
144. Westlund K N, Sorkin L S, Ferrington DG, Carlton SM, Willcockson HH, Willis WD 1990 Serotoninergic and noradrenergic projections to the ventral posterolateral nucleus of the monkey thalamus. *J Comp Neurol* 1990;295:197–207.
145. Yaksh TL, Jage J, Takano Y. Pharmacokinetics and pharmacodynamics of medullar agents. c. The spinal actions of α_2-adrenergic agonists as analgesics. In: Aitkenhead AR, Benad G, Brown BR, et al., eds. *Baillière's clinical anesthesiology*, vol 7, no. 3. London: Baillière Tindall, 1993;597–614.
146. Yaksh TL. The spinal pharmacology of facilitation of afferent processing evoked by high-threshold afferent input of the post injury pain state. *Curr Opin Neurol Neurosurg* 1993;6:250–256.
147. Yaksh TL, Wilson PR. Spinal serotonin terminal system mediates antinociception. *J Pharmacol Exp Ther* 1979;208:446–453.
148. Yaksh TL. Direct evidence that spinal serotonin and noradrenaline terminals mediate the spinal antinociceptive effects of morphine in the periaqueductal gray. *Brain Res* 1979;160:180–185.
149. Yamamoto T, Yaksh TL. Spinal pharmacology of thermal hyperesthesia induced by constriction injury of sciatic nerve. Excitatory amino acid antagonists. *Pain* 1992;121–128.
150. Young RJ, Clarke BF. Pain relief in diabetic neuropathy: the effectiveness of imipramine and related drugs. *Diabetic Med* 1985;2: 363–366.
151. Zanger UM, Vilbois F, Hardwick JP, Meyer UA. Absence of hepatic cytochrome P450bufl causes genetically deficient debrisoquine oxidation in man. *Biochemistry* 1988;27:5447–5454.
152. Ziegler DK, Hurwitz A, Hassanein RS, Kodanaz HA, Preskorn SH, Mason J. Migraine prophylaxis. A comparison of propranolol and amitriptyline. *Arch Neurol* 1987;44:486–489.
153. Ziegler DK, Hurwitz A, Preskorn S, Hassanein R, Seim J. Propranolol and amitriptyline in prophylaxis of migraine. *Arch Neurol* 1993;50:825–830.
154. Ziegler VE, Co BT, Taylor JR, Clayton PJ, Biggs JT. Amitriptyline plasma levels and therapeutic response. *Clin Pharmacol Ther* 1976; 19:795–801.
155. Zitman FG, Linssen ACG, Edelbroek PM, Stijnen T. Low dose amitriptyline in chronic pain: the gain is modest. *Pain* 1990;42: 35–42.

C

THE CARDIO-VASCULAR SYSTEM

Anesthesia: Biologic Foundations, edited by Tony L. Yaksh et al. Lippincott–Raven Publishers, Philadelphia © 1997.

CHAPTER 65

CARDIAC ELECTROPHYSIOLOGY

ZELJKO J. BOSNJAK AND CARL LYNCH III

NORMAL IMPULSE CONDUCTION WITHIN THE HEART

The electrical behavior of the heart with its intrinsic, continuous, rhythmic activity has been the source of wonder and speculation for years. Recent application of microelectrophysiologic techniques combined with molecular biologic isolation of channels has considerably broadened our understanding of cardiac electrophysiology; however, the variable and sometimes conflicting data obtained from different species and tissues, under varying conditions and temperatures, remain to be completely integrated into a comprehensive model that has consistent predictive value. Nonetheless, the considerable information is yielding useful concepts to guide physiologic and pharmacologic intervention. Although anesthetics can alter myocardial electrophysiologic behavior, the intrinsic stability of the system is well maintained.

The ionic currents and membrane permeability changes responsible for generation and conduction of the action potential (AP) in cardiac tissue are similar to those in nerves. The fast depolarization is due to a sudden massive inward movement of positive charges, primarily Na^+ with some Ca^{2+}, while repolarization is due to the net outward movement of positive charges, primarily K^+. Unlike nerve APs, which resemble a sudden spike, most cardiac APs can be divided in five phases, with a sustained plateau between depolarization and repolarization (Fig. 1): phase 0—rapid depolarization, phase 1—initial rapid repolarization, phase 2—plateau, phase 3—final rapid repolarization, and phase 4—electrical diastole. During phase 4 the resting conductance for K^+ is substantial, yet there is little current since the resting membrane potential (RMP) is near the equilibrium potential for K^+ (E_K: -85 to -95 mV). During the plateau there is a large electrochemical gradient driving K^+ out of the cell, but the reduced permeability permits only a small outward current. Nevertheless, it more than neutralizes ongoing inward current, resulting in a small net outward current that is responsible for the low rate of repolarization of the plateau.

Cable Considerations

The most important membrane factors for cardiac impulse propagation (conduction) are active membrane generator properties and passive membrane properties (140). The generator, or current source, is the inward current (mostly Na^+) flowing down its electrochemical gradient during phase 0 of the AP, which depends on the number of available channels and Na^+ electrochemical gradient. This inward current provides the source of the energy needed for conduction, providing the positive changes required to discharge the membrane by neutralizing the excess negative charges that maintain RMP. However, the ions also can flow out through the adjacent membrane that is not yet excited. Because this passive membrane can contain (by its electrical capacitance) or conduct current introduced by the source, it is considered the sink. The interaction of the source with the sink determines the characteristics of conduction and whether electrotonic effects (local, nonpropagated) or successful impulse propagation will result following excitation of adjacent cells. The rate of rise of the AP, velocity of cardiac AP propagation, and AP overshoot or amplitude and duration all provide a measure of the ability of the current source to saturate current sink. When excitation proceeds from adjacent fast response fibers with high resting membrane potentials, the large entering current causes a profound depolarization (large AP amplitude) that is likely to result in successful impulse propagation. In contrast, excitation from adjacent slow response fibers (or depressed fast response fibers) is more likely to result in only electrotonic effects. Fast response fibers have a high safety factor (excess of activation current over that required to produce successful propagation), whereas slow or depressed fast response fibers have a low safety factor of conduction.

A cable analysis has been found useful for describing properties of the sink of cardiac tissue (140). For instance, a biologic cable (e.g., strands of Purkinje fibers) consists of a low-resistance intracellular core that is surrounded by insulation (sarcolemma) of relative low conductance (high resistance), immersed in a low-resistance solution (extracellular fluid). When membrane conductance is low (i.e., resistance is high), less incoming current leaks out through the membrane and depolarization (discharge from the membrane) occurs more rapidly and farther down the length of the fiber. The cable properties also depend on the ability of the current to flow along the fiber. The larger diameter fibers with low longitudinal resistances, such as Purkinje fibers, conduct far better than smaller diameter muscle cells. Since myocardial tissue consists of multicellular strands, the rate of depolarization and conductance also depends on the electrophysiologic connections between cells (gap junctions). There are, however, recognized limitations to cable analysis of cardiac conduction (140). Varying structural complexities of cardiac cells, including number of low-resistance gap junctions (168) and variations in fiber geometry (165), must play an important role in determining the speed of impulse propagation. For example, continuous cable theory would not predict a dependence of velocity of conduction on the direction of conduction, as has been shown by several investigators (403,430,431).

Nevertheless, numerous previous studies have estimated the role of the active component (phase 0 inward current, largely Na^+) of cardiac conduction based on cable considerations. For example, maximal rate of rise of phase 0 of the AP (dV/dt_{max} phase 0) is sometimes considered a measure of conduction velocity and peak inward current (i_{ionic}), based on the assumption that i_{ionic} is defined by: $i_{ionic} = dV/dt_{max} \bullet c_m$, where c_m is the fiber capacity per unit length. Although the linear strands of normal Purkinje fibers belie their complex architecture (197), it is surprising that an approximate proportional relationship is usually seen between dV/dt_{max} phase 0 and conduction velocity as predicted by cable theory. Although this relation even exists as an approximation in other cardiac muscle tissues of yet more complicated architecture (140), there are limitations. For example, the amplitude of dV/dt_{max} phase 0 as a measure of peak Na current (I_{Na}) has recently been shown to be highly sensitive to membrane conductance. When membrane resistance was decreased by increasing external K^+ even when membrane potential was fixed, dV/dt_{max} was depressed. Even though peak I_{Na} was unchanged, because more depolar-

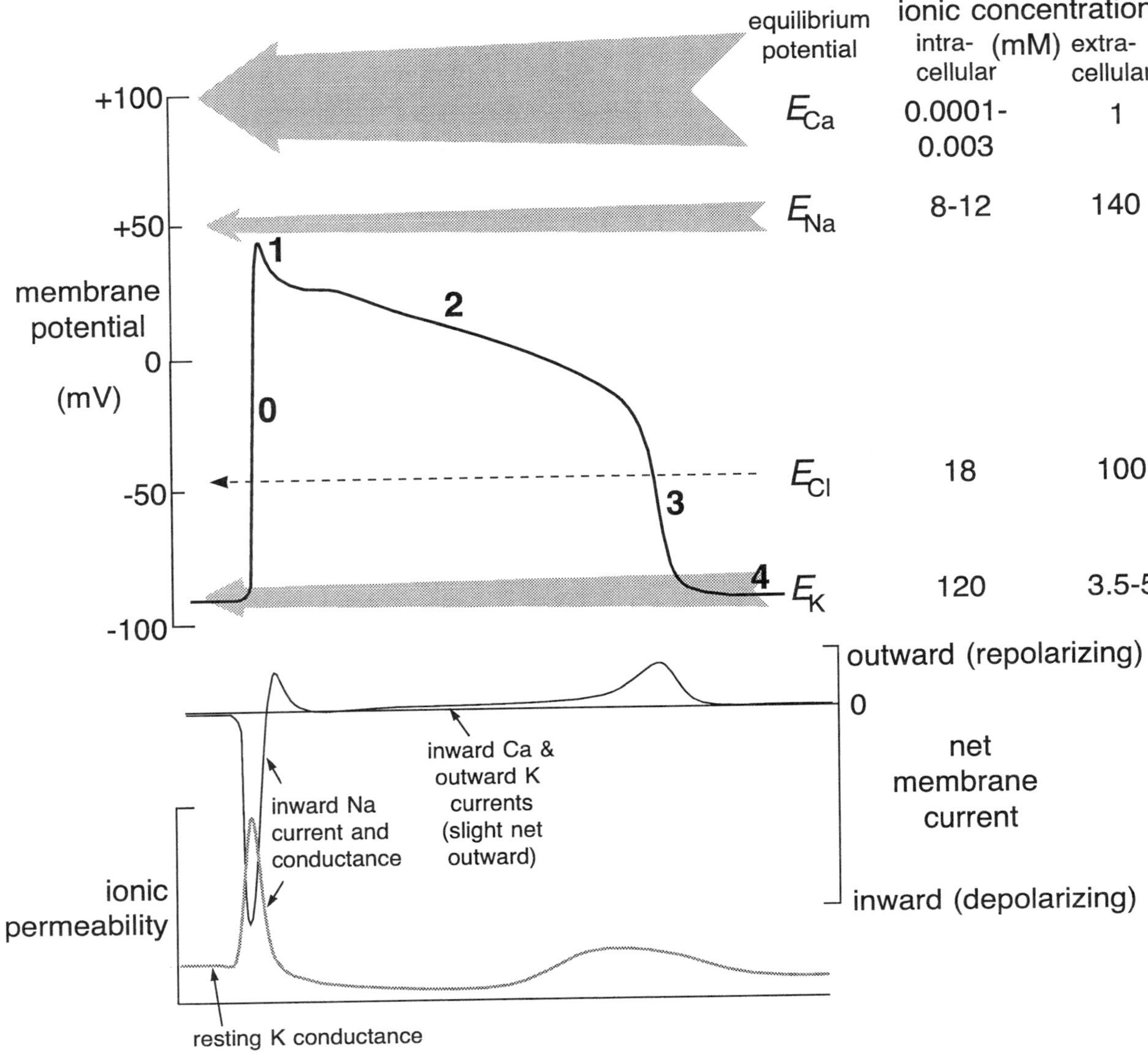

Figure 1. Schematic representation of the cardiac action potential (AP) and the concurrent net membrane ionic current and permeability changes in the cell membrane that are responsible. The net membrane current is that present when the individual parallel or opposed ionic currents are summed and it is approximated by dV/dt, the rate of change of the membrane potential. The *arrows* indicate the range of ionic equilibrium potentials (E_{ion}) for K^+, Na^+, Ca^{2+}, and Cl^- gradients. E_{ion} was calculated according to the Nernst equation at 37°C: $E_{ion} = (62mV/n)(\log[ion]_o/[ion]_i)$ where n is the charge on the ion and subscripts i and o designate intra- and extracellular (outside); 62 mV is calculated from RT/F × ln 10 (to convert from natural logarithms to $\log_{10}$); R = 8.314 volt/coulomb/K/mole, a Faraday (F) = 96,493 coulombs/mole of charge, and T = 310K at 37°C. Intracellular concentrations are those based on estimates using intracellular ion selective electrodes (83,285,342); values may vary depending on the tissue (33). The phases of the AP are indicated: rapid initial upstroke (0), initial depolarization (1), plateau (2), late repolarization (3), diastole (4).

izing current leaked from the fiber, the rate of depolarization was decreased (505). In fast response fibers, inward current (I_{Na}) and conduction velocity are not linearly related (417). This nonlinear relationship appears more likely in slow response settings where the inward current is a much lower density I_{Ca}, dV/dt_{max} phase 0 is far smaller, and conduction velocity is much slower, even though dV/dt_{max} is proportional to I_{Ca} (247).

Inward Currents

The rapid depolarization observed in muscle and Purkinje fibers depends primarily on Na^+ current and secondarily upon Ca^{2+} current.

Sodium Current

It is of critical importance to cardiac muscle function that there are sufficient number of available Na channels so that a large depolarizing current can spread very rapidly to adjacent cells and tissue, rapidly conducting APs throughout the cardiac muscle. This is accomplished by the abundance of these channels in the sarcolemma of cardiac tissues, especially in the Purkinje system, where the density is estimated to be as high as 24 to 60 per μm^2 of membrane (141). Atrial and ventricular muscle probably have far lower densities of 4 to 8 channels per μm^2 (141), or about 20,000 to 40,000 based on the surface area of the average myocyte (158,212). The major factor determining the availability of Na channels is the membrane voltage. Because normal cardiac muscle membrane potential (V_m) is between -80 to -90 mV, it is within 15 to 25 mV of threshold potential at which sufficient Na channels open so that the entering Na^+ causes a regenerative depolarization. Although the channels activate with a time constant of less than 1 msec, most of them also inactivate rapidly at negative membrane potentials. Negative to -80 mV, a large fraction of Na channels are not inactivated (Fig. 2); rapid depolarization positive to -70 mV results in a regenerative opening and an AP. When the potential is positive to -65 mV, more than 75% of the channels are inactivated, and there are usually too few available to open and generate the large inward current required to propagate AP. In the region from -65 to -80 mV, 35% to 65% of the channels may be available, which may be enough for an abnormally slow conducted AP.

Changes in the extracellular K^+ ($[K^+]_o$) will alter the resting potential of the cardiac cells, which alters the density of available (noninactivated) Na channels responsible for the conduction the AP in Purkinje fibers and muscle. When myocardial cells are partially depolarized, as occurs with hyperkalemia, fewer channels are available and conduction is impaired (Fig. 2). This is readily apparent clinically as the widened QRS complex representing slowed conduction through the ventricle. This voltage-inactivating effect of increased $[K^+]_o$ is employed clinically in the application of cardioplegia solutions, where 20 to 30 mM K^+ depolarize the heart to -50 to -35 mV. In this potential range almost all Na channels will be inactivated and normal APs cannot occur, resulting in plegia ("paralysis") of the heart. This potential, however, is above the mechanical threshold, that is, Ca^{2+} is not released from the sarcoplasmic reticulum (SR) to activate contractions, so that energy is not consumed generating tension.

The Na channel protein conformation responds to the local electrical field across the membrane, which will differ somewhat from the actual membrane potential, since the local membrane field includes the surface charges present at each membrane-aqueous interface. The extracellular surface charge is typically negative, in part created by negatively charged phospholipids or acidic amino acids on the external channel surface, and it reduces the membrane field that maintains Na channels in their activatible state. These negative membrane surface charges are in part neutralized by cations in the extracellular media, especially by divalent cations (Ca^{2+} or Mg^{2+}). When the membrane potential is decreased by hyperkalemia, part of the local membrane field can be restored by increasing the neutralization of the negative surface charge by increasing the extracellular concentration of Ca^{2+} or Mg^{2+}. When a greater membrane field is restored, fewer Na channels will be inactivated at any given measurable membrane potential (108), shifting the apparent voltage dependence of the Na channels to more positive potentials (Fig. 2). This phenomenon accounts for the improved conduction observed when Ca^{2+} or Mg^{2+} is administered during the hyperkalemic states (270). This beneficial action of extracellular divalent cations in shifting Na channel voltage dependence, may be attenuated by a voltage-dependent Na channel blockade by divalent ions that is prominent at high concentrations (≥5 mM) (416).

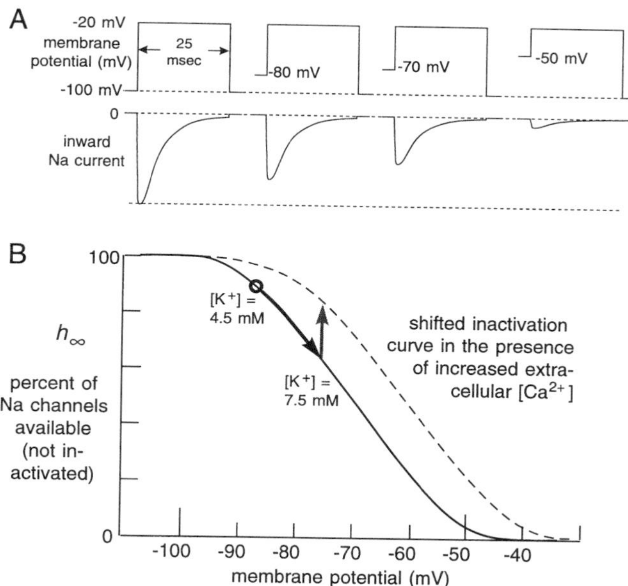

Figure 2. **A:** Typical Na^+ currents from cardiac myocytes elicited from various resting potentials. With more positive resting potentials less Na^+ current is present because fewer channels are available. **B:** The steady-state inactivation of the Na channel. The *solid curve* indicates the usual fraction of Na channels available opening as a function of resting membrane potential from which repolarization occurred. With depolarization, such as that due to hyperkalemia (indicated by *arrow*), fewer channels will be available and conduction will be slowed (increased K^+ conductance may also contribute). At any given membrane potential, increased extracellular Ca^{2+} makes more Na channels available for activation *(dashed inactivation curve)* that will tend to restore conduction. These actions are consistent with neutralization of the membrane surface charge that influences Na channel gating.

A very small fraction of cardiac Na channels appear not to inactivate rapidly, providing sustained current even during the plateau of the AP (22,167). This subpopulation of channels provides a small "window current" that persists for the duration of depolarization and contributes to the plateau phase of the Purkinje fiber AP (22,86). A distinctive feature of cardiac Na channels, as opposed to the distinct isoforms present in brain, is their relative insensitivity to tetrodotoxin and greater sensitivity to local anesthetic blockade, possibly due to a second binding site (6). One of the actions of pure Na channel blocking agents (and certain local anesthetics) is to decrease the plateau duration, presumably by blocking the Na channel "window" current that persists in the plateau (469), although this effect is modest in ventricular muscle.

Calcium Currents

The slow inward current of cardiac tissue has been clearly defined as the influx through channels selective for divalent cations (Ca^{2+}, and also Ba^{2+} and Sr^{2+}). While there are at least two types of Ca channels in heart, the L-type ($I_{Ca,L}$, long-lasting, high threshold, low-voltage-activating positive to -40 mV) channel is by far the most common and important myocardial Ca channel (28,54,202,355,391). Through this channel flows the Ca^{2+} current that maintains the internal Ca^{2+} stores necessary for contractions. It is modulated by β-adrenergic stimulation (238,526), and is also the channel sensitive to the commonly used "calcium antagonists," the 1,4-dihydropyridines (DHPs, e.g., nifedipine), the phenylalkylamines (e.g., verapamil), and the benzothiazepines (e.g., diltiazem) (287). With a basic structure similar to the Na channel, the major pore-forming α_1-subunit of the cardiac L-type Ca channel was first cloned from and expressed for rabbit (336). The comparable human α_1-subunit (designated hHT-1) consists of 2,180 amino acids and is 92.8% identical to the rabbit channel, although variations between species in the intracellular N-terminus of the protein and in the number of potential phosphorylation sites are present (413). The cardiac L-type channel a_1 subunit (now designated a_{1C}) is closely related to α_1 the skeletal muscle DHP receptor (α_{1S} subunit), which gates Ca^{2+} release in skeletal muscle, and to a distinct L-type channel present in endocrine tissue (α_{1D}). The a_1 subunit usually has three associated subunits (α_2, β, γ) at least some of which appear to modulate ionic conductance (76). Also like the Na channel, asymmetric membrane charge movements are detectable with applied voltage changes ("gating charge") and appear to reflect voltage-induced molecular rearrangements of the Ca channel voltage sensor, which open the channel and permit Ca^{2+} flux (36,136).

L-type channel activation and inactivation appear to reflect multiple processes, and one of the major modulators seems to be Ca^{2+} itself, particularly the $[Ca^{2+}]$ present at the internal pore mouth. Although there is a component of voltage-dependent inactivation of L-type channels as seen in the Na channels, the major mechanism that stops influx through the channel at the plateau potentials (~0 mV) appears to be a rise in $[Ca^{2+}]_i$ (170), probably the Ca^{2+} that accumulates at the interior channel mouth (30,525). Curiously, L-type channels show a distinct frequency-dependent facilitation that requires Ca^{2+} entry (524,537). Increase in intracellular Ca^{2+} by photolysis also appears to enhance currents by increasing the number of activated channels (30). Although other factors may contribute (30), a convincing case can be made for Ca^{2+} binding to calmodulin and activating the multifunctional Ca^{2+}-calmodulin–dependent protein kinase (CaMKII), which phosphorylates a site on or near the Ca^{2+} channel (524). This phosphorylation results in slower inactivation of current and faster recovery from inactivation, both actions being consistent with an increased negative charge on the inner membrane surface. Clustering of Ca channels may influence the accumulation of local $[Ca^{2+}]_i$, and thus the regional variation in density of Ca channels may also play a modulatory role, enhancing facilitation (101). Because the voltage dependence of activation and inactivation overlaps, that is, there are membrane potentials at which a fraction of channels will be open but not inactivated (typically about 10% of channels at ~-10mV), ongoing L-type "window" current can flow during the AP plateau (421). The slowly inactivating channels will pass increasing current as repolarization occurs during the AP plateau, which can actually lead to increasing $I_{Ca,L}$ during this time (Fig. 3).

One class of the Ca channel modulators, dihydropyridines, binds to particular site on the cardiac Ca channel, and depending on the exact drug structure, they may either inhibit channel opening or shift the channel to a long opening mode (Bay K 8644) (402). Specific drug effects are also dependent on the membrane potential, which can markedly influence channel structure and function (402). For example, partial depolarization, as occurs in cardiac muscle with hyperkalemia or ischemia, markedly increases the binding of and inhibition by nifedipine. This behavior may explain the particular benefit of these agents in primarily depressing vascular smooth muscle or benefiting ischemia. This potential-dependent binding represents variation of the modulated receptor hypothesis first proposed for the local anesthetics binding by Na channels (200,208). In contrast, the frequency-dependent binding of verapamil is similar to the frequency-dependent block of Na channels by the local anesthetics (122,287,325). The binding to the DHPs also modulates the binding of the phenylalkylamines or benzothiazepines by altering their distinctly different sites on the molecule (see "Calcium Channels," Chap. X). As with decreased $[Ca^{2+}]_o$, blockade of the Ca channel has variable effects on the AP. In Purkinje fibers, although the AP plateau may be depressed, the AP duration may be enhanced (248). This effect may be related to Ca^{2+}-dependent control of repolarizing K^+ and Cl^- currents.

The transient Ca channel (T-type, low threshold, activating when the membrane potential becomes positive to -65 mV) identified as $I_{Ca,T}$ has been identified in number of tissues (34,129,171,202,341,355,512). In contrast to the L-type channel, it inactivates far more rapidly (Figs. 3 and 4). While it accounts for only 10% of I_{Ca} ventricular and atrial tissue (355,512), it may account for as much as 40% of current in Purkinje fibers (129,202,463), in which it may contribute to the pacemaker depolarization as in sinoatrial tissue. While $I_{Ca,T}$ appears to contribute to the latter half of the SA nodal depolarization, and its blockade (by 40 μM Ni^{2+}) can slow spontaneous nodal firing, $I_{Ca,L}$ appears to contribute the majority of depolarizing current in nodal cells (116,171).

The Ca channels are not only a site for pharmacologic intervention by specific Ca^{2+} entry blockers, it is also clear that these channels are susceptible to inhibition by volatile anesthetics

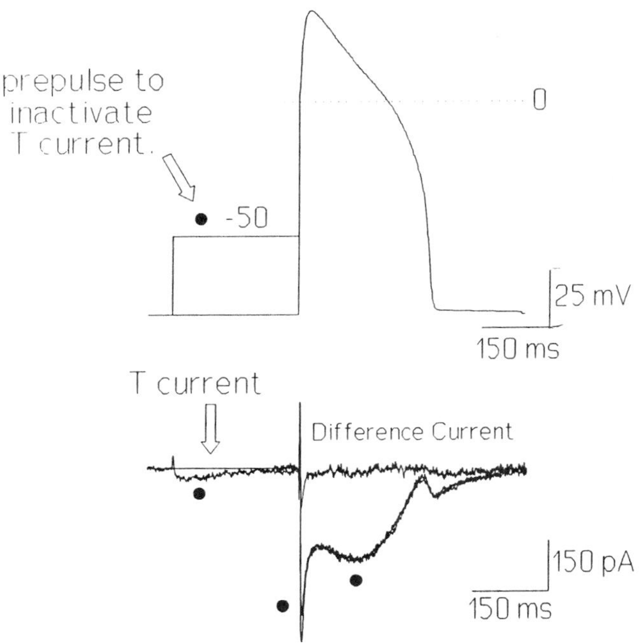

Figure 3. Inward Ca^{2+} currents in a guinea pig myocyte elicited in response to a voltage-clamped depolarization shaped like an action potential. When the AP voltage profile was preceded by a depolarization from the holding potential of -90 mV to -50 mV, the T-type Ca channels were inactivated. The small, rapid "difference current" is the T-type component of the inward Ca^{2+} current with depolarization from -90 mV. Note the L-type current has a rapidly inactivating component and a sustained component, which actually increases during repolarization due to the increasing driving force ($V_m = E_{Ca}$). (Figure courtesy of J.J. Pancrazio.)

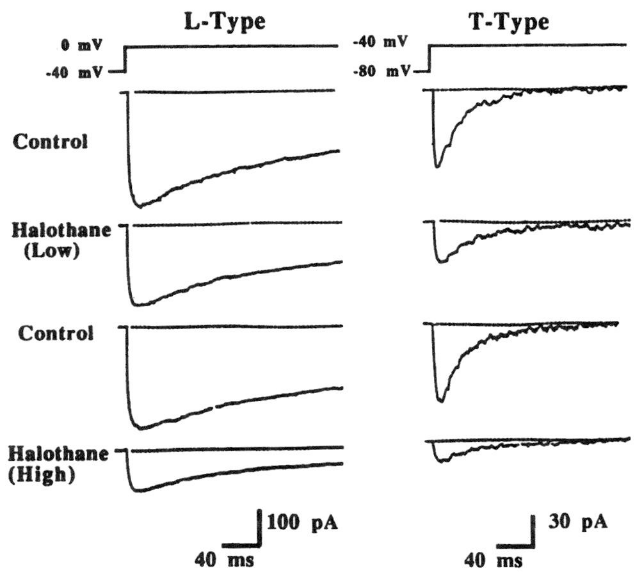

Figure 4. Concentration-dependent effects of halothane on L- and T-type calcium currents in a single canine cardiac Purkinje cell. L-type current was elicited by depolarizing the cell from -40 to 0 mV *(left)*. T-type current was elicited by depolarizing the cell from -80 to -40 mV *(right)*. Exposure of the cell to 0.7% (low) and 1.5% (high) concentrations of halothane depressed both L- and T-type currents in a dose-dependent and reversible manner. (From ref. 129, with permission.)

(Fig. 4). Since the initial suggestion that halothane depresses Ca^{2+} currents (307), it has become clear that the volatile anesthetics specifically depress Ca^{2+} currents of myocardial tissue (44,54,129,215,348,449,450). The exact mechanism of this action remains to be elucidated, although an enhanced rate of inactivation and a greater effect on the noninactivating component appear to contribute (365). In addition to the volatile anesthetics, thiopental and thiamylal have also been clearly demonstrated to decrease I_{Ca} in myocardial tissues (215,364). Likewise, the ketamine can decrease I_{Ca} in myocardial tissue (126). In addition to these anesthetics, citrate ion at concentrations present during rapid blood infusion is capable of decreasing myocardial I_{Ca}, an effect that is separate from its Ca^{2+} chelating action (41).

Potassium Channels and Currents

A number of K channels are responsible for maintaining the resting conductance as well as providing the primary neutralizing ionic efflux to counteract the inward Na^+ and Ca^{2+} currents (Table 1). The K^+ efflux occurs at various points in the cardiac AP cycle by ion passage through a wide variety different K channels, representing at least two different ion channel superfamilies (137,205,271,273,337,445). These channels are responsible not only for the pattern of repolarization in various regions of the heart, but also for modulating excitability via the resting membrane conductance (G_m) and refractory periods. While the similarities and differences that exist among species must be defined, the large number of different channels clearly represents distinct receptors with the potential for specific pharmacologic intervention. The various ion channels present in myocardial tissue are summarized in Table 1.

Inwardly Rectifying K Channels

The rate and character (AP duration) of cardiac impulse conduction are modulated by the resting K^+ conductance (G_K). When G_K is increased, incoming current from adjacent cells and via the membrane "leak" out through the K channels and depolarization is slowed (505). This membrane conductance appears to be due to expression of channel proteins from a family of inwardly rectifying (IR) K channels, of which 12 have been identified by molecular biologic methods (271). The membrane channels are composed from subunits that possess only two α-helical membrane spanning regions, with a connecting extracellular region that lines the pore (see "Potassium Channels," Chap. X). Combinations of different subunits (heteromultimers) may be very important in determining the channel behavior responsible for the various currents (271).

The Inward Rectifier (G_{K1})

Anomalous and Rectifying Behavior The resting potassium conductance of myocardium (G_{K1}) is responsible for maintaining the resting potential at its equilibrium potential. However, G_{K1} has two peculiar and very important characteristics that are primarily responsible for membrane electrical behavior of the heart. First, the channel conductance is pro-

Table 1. CARDIAC ION CHANNELS

Channel	Symbol	Activation	Inactivation	Pharmacologic modulators
Sodium ("fast")	I_{NA}	Very fast	Fast, except for a "slow" fraction that reopens	Local anesthetics and phenytoin (use-dependent), tetrodotoxin (weak)
Calcium ("slow")				
L-type (or HVA, high-voltage activated)	$I_{Ca,L}$	Fast	Slow, large Ca^{2+}-dependent component	Dihydropyridines, benzothiazepines, phenylalkylamines, Cd^{2+}
T-type	$I_{Ca,T}$	Fast	Moderate	Amiloride, tetramethrin, Ni^{2+}, Cd^{2+}
Potassium, inwardly rectifying				
Inward rectifier	I_{K1} (IRK)	Instantaneous	Mg^{2+} and polyamine block of outward current	Cs^+, Ba^{2+} (100 μM), thiopental, zero K^+
G protein activated	$I_{K(ACh,Ado)}$ (GIRK)	Open when activated	Mg^{2+} block of outward current	
ATP (-inactivated)	$I_{K(ATP)}$	Open when activated	Mg^{2+} block of outward current	Sulfonylureas, amiodarone, quinidine; activators: benzopyrans, cyanoguanidines, nicotinamides, diazoxide, minoxidil
Potassium, voltage-activated				
Plateau or background	$I_{K,p}$	Very rapid	None?	Ba^{2+}(1 mM)
Transient outward (early outward)	I_{to1}	Fast	Moderate	4-AP (1 mM), bupivacaine, quinidine
	$I_{K(Ca)}$, $I_{to2?}$	Fast	Moderate	4-AP (10 mM), tedisamil
Delayed current (delayed rectifier)	$I_{K,r}$	Moderate	None	Quinidine (HK2)
	I_{RAK},I_{HK2}	Very rapid	Slight	d-sotalol, dofetilide, E4031, quinidine, UK-68,798, 1mM La^{3+}
	$I_{K,s}$	Slow	None	Indapamide, clofilium, quinidine, amiodarone
Potassium, other				
Na-activated	$I_{K(Na)}$	Open when active		
Fatty-acid activated	$I_{K,AA}$,$I_{K,PC}$	Open when active		
Pacemaker	If	Slow	Slow	1–2mMCs^+
Chloride				
Transient outward	$I_{Cl(Ca)}$,$I_{to2?}$	Fast	Fast	SITS, DIDS
CFTR	$I_{Cl,cAMP}$	Open when active	None	DNDS
Stretch-activated				SITS, DNDS, anthracene-9-carboxylic acid

CFTR, cystic fibrosis transmembrane regulator; DIDS, 4,4′-dithiocyanatostilbene; DNDS, 4,4′-dinitrostilbene-2,2′-disulfonic acid; SITS, 4-acetomido-4′-isothiocyanatostilbene-2,2′-disulfonic acid; TEA^+, tetraethylammonium ion.

portional to the square root of $[K^+]_o$ (398). For instance, when $[K^+]_o$ is greater, ions can pass more rapidly through the channel, but when $[K^+]_o$ is low, ion flux is reduced. This peculiar behavior may have two benefits: (a) K^+ loss may be reduced when $[K^+]_o$ is low; and (b) when $[K^+]_o$ is higher and the Na pump is activated, the negative current generated (three Na^+ are pumped out for two K^+ pumped in) will not profoundly hyperpolarize the cell, or thereby alter its behavior (201). One consequence of this behavior is the dependence on $[K^+]_o$ of myocardial V_m, which is shown in Fig. 5A. The agreement with the predicted Nernst potential for K^+ (E_K) is excellent until $[K^+]_o$ becomes very low (<2.5 mM), where the cell fails to hyperpolarize further. When the $[K^+]_o$ gets very low, G_{K1} virtually shuts down, and even very slight Na^+ leaks prevent further hyperpolarization or may even depolarize the cell, which occurs in ≥1 mM $[K^+]_o$ (419). Consequently, with extreme hypokalemia, even though the E_K is very negative, arrhythmias may become common because there is little K^+ conductance to stabilize the membrane. Because the ability to pass current increases with $[K^+]_o$, even against a larger concentration gradient, this behavior of G_{K1} has been called "anomalous."

Second, many ion channels pass ions equally well in either direction, according to the potential applied and transmembrane ion concentrations. While G_{K1} readily permits external K^+ to enter from outside the cell, with increasingly positive (>10–20 mV) electrical gradients applied inside the cell (such as an action potential), less K^+ can leave the cell—the channel acts as a diode or rectifier, hence the name inward rectifier. This effect is shown in the relation of current to voltage (the "I-V curve") in Fig. 5B. After the cell becomes positive to -65 to 70 mV, the greater positive potentials actually cause less current to flow (the "negative conductance" region). When channels are excised from the cell, they lose their rectifying behavior, leading to the suggestion that the rectification is due to an intracellular blocking particle that occludes the channel. A likely candidate for the blocking species is intracellular Mg^{2+}, which has been found to block outward K^+ current (224,315,317,475). Although Na^+ has been shown to possess blocking properties, a more modest modulatory role is present physiologically (316). Another candidate for the intrinsic rectifying factor is cytoplasmic polyamines (spermidine, putrescine, spermine) that can demonstrate a clear voltage-dependent block of outward current (297). Whatever the physiologic blocker may be, this rectifying action has a very important result. While conductance is well maintained around E_K, when cardiac muscle is depolarized to the plateau potential (0 to +25 mV) by entry of Na^+ and Ca^{2+}, K^+ cannot escape from the cell to eliminate the positive charge. If this channel was not blocked by Mg^{2+} to prevent outward K^+ flux, K^+ would rapidly leave the cell and repolarize it, so that the plateau would be small or nonexistent. This failure to elim-

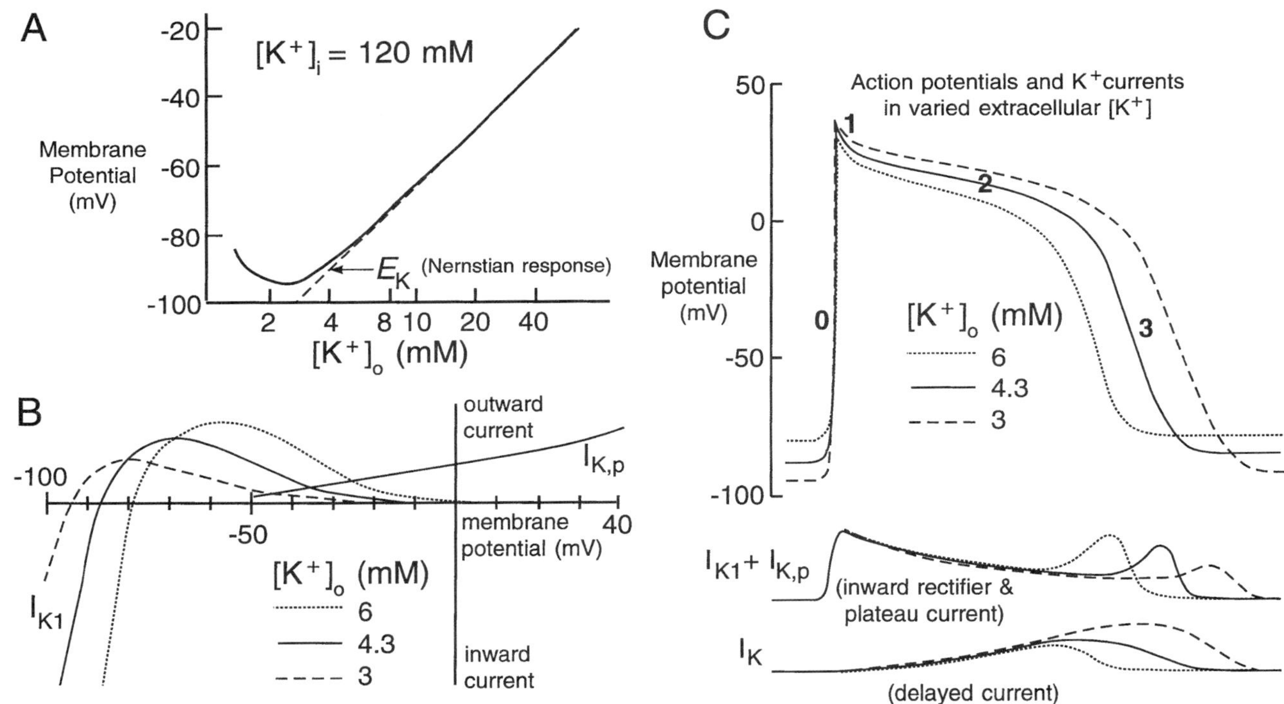

Figure 5. Electrophysiologic effects of the inward rectifier (G_{K1}). **A:** The calculated Nernst equilibrium potential for K^+ (E_K) and the membrane potential (V_m) recorded in myocardial tissue are shown. The intracellular K^+ ($[K^+]_i$) is based on measurements in Purkinje fibers and ventricular muscle (83,285,342). Due to the dependence of the resting potassium conductance (G_{K1}, inward rectifier) on extracellular K^+ ($[K^+]_o$), as $[K^+]_o$ declines the membrane potential deviates increasingly from the E_K as G_{K1} decreases. At very low $[K^+]_o$ cell may actually depolarize (33). **B:** The current voltage (I-V) relation of G_{K1}. When increased potassium is present externally, there is a shift toward depolarizing potential; however, the conductance increases so a greater depolarizing current will be required to decrease the membrane potential. With decreased $[K^+]_o$, the lower conductance means that less current will generate a larger depolarization. The outward current observed with positive potentials appears to be due to a separate plateau or background conductance ($I_{K,p}$) (24). **C:** Effects of varied $[K^+]_o$ on the action potential configuration. As the delayed current is activated, with increased $[K^+]_o$, G_{K1} is enhanced so that outward currents through it result in an earlier repolarization and termination of the plateau. The opposite effect is observed in low $[K^+]_o$ when G_{K1} is reduced, and the delayed current must contribute more outward current, which requires a longer period of time-dependent activation. In either case, a component of repolarizing outward current is present because of $I_{K,p}$ that is relatively insensitive to $[K^+]_o$. Inward currents are not shown. For a discussion and mathematical description, respectively, see Surawicz (441) and Luo and Rudy (301). (From ref. 304, with permission.)

inate K^+ down its electrochemical gradient potentiates the depolarization caused by entering Na^+, and is also in large part responsible for maintaining the plateau.

EFFECTS OF ALTERED EXTRACELLULAR $[K^+]_o$ In the presence of low $[K^+]_o$ (2.5 mM), conductance (G_{K1}) is low (membrane resistance is high) so only a modest amount of current (flowing from adjacent tissue) leads to a large depolarization from the resting potential (-95 mV) to near the AP threshold (-70 mV). In contrast, when $[K^+]_o$ is high, the membrane conductance is high (membrane resistance is low) because of the inherent behavior G_{K1}, so that positive charges (as K^+) escape from the cell more rapidly. Although the membrane is more depolarized so that it is closer to the action potential threshold, the cell is unlikely to be more excitable because current will more readily pass through the membrane and therefore not depolarize it. While a smaller depolarization is required to get to threshold (-65 mV) from the resting potential (-75 mV), even more current (either from adjacent tissue or from an electrode) may be necessary to depolarize the cell compared to that when $[K^+]_o$ is low. A major effect of hyperkalemia is slowed conduction, due to the need for increased depolarizing current to reach threshold, and a decrease in AP duration as more outward K^+ current causes loss of depolarizing charge from the cells. When external K^+ is moderately low (2–3.5 mM) and the cells are more hyperpolarized, more Na channels are available, which results in improved AP conduction. Although a greater depolarization is required, the G_{K1} is decreased so that any current (from adjacent cells, or cell damage) causes more depolarization toward threshold. The result may be a greater excitability and a tendency for extra membrane depolarizations (ectopy).

The behavior and $[K^+]_o$-dependence of G_{K1} also profoundly influence repolarization. Once the repolarization process has been initiated by the delayed current (I_K, see below) and V_m becomes negative to -30 mV, G_{K1} increases progressively, permitting an increase in K^+ efflux and enhancing the rate of repolarization. In fact, G_{K1} is the major repolarizing current during the later half of repolarization (301). Consequently, increases or decreases in conductance with hyper- or hypokalemia, respectively, will decrease or increase AP duration as indicated in Fig. 5C (301). Likewise, specific blockade of G_{K1} by 50 to 100 μM Ba^{2+} (158) or by certain barbiturates (e.g., thiopental [364]) will prolong the AP duration by extending the later phase. In contrast, the volatile anesthetics cause a modest decrease (364; Bosnjak et al., *unpublished data*) that does not appear to dramatically alter AP duration.

In addition to G_{K1}, the resting K conductance is strongly modulated by at least two additional major K conductances with IR properties. These channels are normally inactive, but when activated they can contribute to stabilizing the membrane potential as well as to speeding repolarization. Ongoing experiments are beginning to define the molecular character of the channels responsible (271).

Protein-G Linked K Channels (GIRK) Neurotransmitter regulation of cardiac membrane conductance is mediated in part by activation of a separate rectifying K channel via the ubiquitous protein-G membrane signaling system. Muscarinic agonists, as well as a variety of other agents, have been found to activate inwardly rectifying K^+ current via a pertussis toxin–sensitive G protein leading to cellular hyperpolarization (73). Thus, the function of the pertussis toxin–sensitive G_i protein is not limited to inhibition of adenylyl cyclase, but includes ion channel gating. The gated channel (termed $I_{K(ACh)}$) depends on the intracellular guanosine triphosphate (GTP) concentration (371). The GTP dependence was confirmed by the use of GTP analogues, and can be persistently activated by hydrolysis-resistant GTP analogues present at the intracellular surface (62) such as guanosine 5'-0-(3-thiotriphosphate) (GTP-γ-S), which irreversibly binds to G proteins. If G_i protein binds GDP, it will inactivate. Guanosine 5'-0-(2-thiodiphosphate) (GDP-β-S) is an analogue that retains the G_i in the inactive form, and intracellular injection of this analogue blocks the acetylcholine (ACh) effect on the K^+ current (62). G_i links not only the atrial myocardial cell muscarinic (M2) receptor, but also the A1 adenosine receptor, as well as the platelet activating factor receptor for activation of $I_{K(ACh)}$ (hence $I_{K(ACh, Ado)}$) (38,379). Activation of $I_{K,ACh}$ is also possible in single channel experiments on isolated patches in the presence of hydrolysis-resistant GTP, even after pertussis toxin uncouples the channel from the ACh receptor. In the classic description of the G protein–linked cascades, receptor activation leads to dissociation of the $G_{\beta\gamma}$ subunit from the G_α subunit with the binding of GTP, which frees the G_α subunit to act on a membrane effector (77,82). It has recently been shown, however, that it is the availability of the $G_{\beta\gamma}$ subunit that is responsible for activating $I_{K(ACh, Ado)}$ (506).

The exact definition of the structural similarity of $I_{K(ACh, Ado)}$ to G_{K1} came with the molecular biologic isolation of the genetic material for this G protein–linked IR channel (now termed GIRK) and the demonstration of a structure most consistent with the two-transmembrane domains (95,273). However, the isolated expressed channel showed behavior distinct from the native channel. Recently, Krapivinsky and coworkers (271) have isolated another similar channel protein (termed CIR) and provided evidence that the $I_{K(ACh, Ado)}$ channel is really a heteromultimer of GIRK and CIR. This CIR/GIRK1 channel shows G protein–gated behavior and other characteristics of the native channel.

The ATP-Regulated K^+ Channel, $I_{K(ATP)}$ When adenosine triphosphate (ATP) is reduced in cardiac muscle cells, a K^+ channel is activated as described first by Noma (359). This channel is distinct from G_{K1}, having higher conductance (462), and has been reported in vascular smooth muscle, brain, skeletal muscle, kidney, and pancreatic β-cells (169), although the properties of the channels in different tissues appear variable (100). Like I_{K1} and $I_{K(ACh, Ado)}$, $I_{K(ATP)}$ also has some inwardly rectifying characteristics that appear to be mediated in part by Mg^{2+}. The channel is sensitive to $[H^+]$ and is also activated by decreases in pH (234,269).

A prominent feature of this channel is its regulation by a variety of drugs. It is blocked or inhibited by a variety of sulfonylurea derivatives (e.g., glyburide, glibenclamide, tolbutamide) (40,139). A wide variety of compounds including benzopyrans (e.g., cromakalin, lemakalin), cyanoguanidines (e.g., pinacidil), nicotinamide (e.g., nicorandil), as well as diazoxide and minoxidil are known to activate these channels (507). In addition, the potential for initiating myocardial protection with these compounds has been emphasized (127,169).

When the channel is activated in the presence of intracellular ATP-depletion such as that caused by ischemia or hypoxia (40,245,461), this current it postulated to play a protective role by abbreviating the AP, decreasing Ca^{2+} entry, and reducing further ATP depletion. Although hypoxia or ischemia does not reduce ATP to levels low enough to activate a majority of channels (<100 μM ATP) (359), the activity of only a very small fraction (<1%) may be sufficient to enhance K^+ efflux (502). Furthermore, ATP may be compartmentalized, being at a lower concentration near the membrane surface (63,186). In this setting, the sodium pump may be inhibited and K^+ efflux via K_{ATP} channels will accumulate outside the cell, causing some depolarization. Blockade of K_{ATP} channels by glibenclamide increases heart infarct size in a rabbit model in the absence of preconditioning, but blockade did not prevent the beneficial effect of preconditioning (454). The effect of K_{ATP} channel openers is also equivocal (482). The role that such channels may play in arrhythmias and the effects of their activation and blockade remain to be fully defined.

The identification of this channel as being a member of the IR K channel family was based on its cloning and sequencing (termed RNKATP) (8) and similarity to an ATP-regulated channel cloned from the kidney (205). However, the CIR K channel previously noted is virtually identical to RNKATP, leading to speculation that a combination RNKATP/CIR, with some additional channel protein (which binds sulfonylureas) and possibly another subunit, is required for true expression of the $I_{K(ATP)}$ channel. The possibility that RNKATP/CIR may combine with another protein and exhibit more complex behavior has been suggested with the demonstration that $G_{i\alpha}$ may modulate the behavior of $I_{K(ATP)}$ (261).

Voltage-Activated K⁺ Currents

The voltage-activated K channels typically represent that superfamily in which the subunits have six transmembrane domains, and demonstrate variable rates of activation and inactivation. However, additional types may also be present.

The Background (or Plateau) K⁺ Current Single-channel studies have clearly demonstrated that G_{K1} turns off completely with depolarization (as shown in Fig. 5B) in the presence of physiologic intracellular Mg^{2+} (224,315,317,475), and will therefore be unavailable to provide any countercurrent to the calcium current and Na^+ current during the AP plateau. Yet an outward current (as shown in Fig. 5B) is evident on whole cell recordings even at positive potentials (398). This current has been observed in isolation and termed the background or plateau current ($I_{K,p}$) (24). This background conductance is blocked by only 1 mM Ba^{2+}, but is unaffected by low or zero $[K^+]_o$, which inactivates G_{K1}. This small amplitude current activates very rapidly on depolarization (527) and can provide a small amount of outward current, which will contribute toward repolarization of the action potential during the plateau (24).

In addition, in rat atrium a very rapidly activating, noninactivating current has been documented (I_{RAK}) that is sensitive to the organic cation 4-aminopyridine (4-AP) (59) and is probably responsible for the very fast repolarization observed in tissue from this species. The channel has also been cloned and expressed, showing great similarity to a neuronal rat K^+ channel BK2 (369). The kinetic behavior and conductance are very similar to a quinidine-sensitive K channel cloned from human atrium (HK2) (133,427,428) as well as a channel observed in canine ventricular epicardium (233).

Delayed K⁺ Current Subtypes The cardiac tissue displays a time- and voltage-dependent K^+ current that is responsible for repolarizing cells (324). Since its activation was slow (324), and because this channel was thought to pass outward current, as opposed to the inward rectification of G_{K1}, this repolarizing current has been frequently termed the delayed rectifier (also delayed current). Initially labeled I_{x1} in studies by Noble and Tsien (357,358) the current (conductance) is typically indicated as simply I_K (G_K) (327). This delayed current plays a critical role in initiating phase 3 of repolarization, but because of the dependence of G_{K1} on $[K^+]_o$, the influence of G_K on repolarization varies with $[K^+]_o$. As indicated in Fig. 5, when $[K^+]_o$ is low G_K plays a more dominant role, while in higher $[K^+]_o$, G_{K1} contributes more to repolarization.

A number of studies have shown that the delayed K^+ current is kinetically complex, sometimes showing fast and sometimes slow components of activation (163,327,358). Two distinct components have been identified. In guinea pig myocytes, a rapidly activating, inwardly rectifying current can be specifically blocked by certain class III antiarrhythmic agents (d-sotalol, E-4031, dofetilide) as well as by 1 µM La^{3+}, which has been designated $I_{K,r}$ (241,400,401). This current is similar in kinetics to an I_K present in the atrial node (420), and recently identified in rabbit ventricular myocytes, where an E-4031–sensitive $I_{K,r}$ appears to be the only delayed current present (481). When $I_{K,r}$ is blocked, the plateau of the AP is significantly prolonged, although the phase 3 repolarization rate is largely unaltered (401,481). Following blockade of $I_{K,r}$, a nonrectifying delayed current that activates more slowly remains ($I_{K,s}$).

$I_{K,r}$ has distinct behavior in that while it begins to slowly activate when $V_m \geq -40$ mV, it appears to rapidly inactivate when depolarizations exceed 0 mV (401). This results in effective rectifying behavior, so that repolarizing current is smaller early in the plateau phase ($V_m \sim +20$ mV) and increases later in the plateau (V_m <-10 mV), accelerating repolarization. Recently, a gene candidate for this current has been identified in humans as closely related to the *ether-a-go-go* K channel (eag) first identified in *Drosophila* (499) and subsequently described in human hippocampus (500). This human *ether-a-go-go* gene (HERG) is strongly expressed in human heart (93) and when expressed in *Xenopus* oocytes it demonstrates electrophysiologic behavior very similar to that observed for $I_{K,r}$ (92). Unlike $I_{K,r}$, however, methanesulfonanilides do not appear to block HERG, a process that may involve an additional subunit. Mutations in this gene appear to account for familial based long QT syndromes that are associated with *torsades de pointes* ventricular arrhythmias and sudden death (93).

The Slow Delayed Current The kinetically slower I_K channel ($I_{K,s}$) activity appears to be modulated by a number of pathways including intracellular Ca^{2+} (455,456), the adenosine 3',5'-cyclic monophosphate (cAMP)-dependent protein kinase (PKA) (492,493), as well as protein kinase C (456–458,493). Although increased $[Ca^{2+}]_i$ is not required for I_K, it is capable of enhancing the current. Unlike most voltage-activated K channels, I_{Ks} may represent a peculiar exception. Molecular biologic studies suggest that the channel may be composed of very small subunit structures of only 103 amino acids and be identical to the MinK channel. The current is blocked by indapamide (466). This current also appears to be markedly decreased by the volatile anesthetics, particularly halothane (364; Bosnjak et al., *unpublished data*); however, the decreased AP duration typically observed with halothane (303,449) suggests that I_{Ks} has a modest contribution in repolarization or there is an even greater depression of the depolarizing currents.

The Transient Outward Currents, I_{to}, and Early Repolarization Additional K^+ outward currents that are variably present in different cardiac tissues are the transient outward currents (I_{to}, also early outward, I_{eo}) (85,237,423,424). These rapidly activating and inactivating currents markedly alter or abbreviate the AP configuration in various cardiac myocytes, influencing excitability and contractility. The identification as K^+ currents is strongly suggested by their blockade or inhibition by 4-AP (120,159,254,274,293) and internal quaternary ammonium ions (246). The current appears in both Ca^{2+}-dependent (71,120,222,423) and -independent forms (158,159,498), the latter having many features in common with the neuronal transient K^+ current I_A (158,159). Such a current from human heart has recently been cloned and expressed (372), and seems to be the primary voltage-dependent K^+ current in human myocardium (477,504). During the course of development, the expression of I_{to} increases in human atrium, being present more often and more prominent in adult tissue than in neonates (91).

In the pacemaker tissue of the sinoatrial (SA) node, a transient current has been documented that contributes to repolarizations; however, it differs from other I_{to} in being somewhat less selective for K^+ (351). Several transient outward currents have been documented in atrial muscle from a variety of tissues, the most prominent in the Ca^{2+}-independent form that is largely responsible for the dramatically abbreviated plateau of the atrial AP (78,128). Variation within the atrial muscle, with more I_{to} present in the epicardium than in the endocardium, has also been described (498). The role and requirement of the Ca^{2+}-dependent I_{to} ($I_{K,Ca}$) is unclear.

One of the prominent features of the Purkinje fiber AP is the phase 1 "notch" indicated in Fig. 1. In contrast to atrial muscle in which the repolarization process initiated I_{to} persists and results a shortened AP duration, in Purkinje fibers the AP plateau is restored for an extended period, in part due to the decreased G_{K1} (163). Although there is certainty of an I_{to} in

Purkinje fibers, its exact character seems to be species dependent. In cow and calf Purkinje fibers, a Ca^{2+}-activated current is clearly demonstrable that has a very high single channel conductance (71,423), while in the sheep conduction system I_{to} appears to be Ca^{2+}-independent (71,85). These differences emphasize that pharmacologic intervention toward a single K^+ current will require species specific data.

The presence of I_{to} in *ventricular cells* varies with species, being the major repolarizing current in rat (120,237), but absent in guinea pig (458). Although a 4-AP–sensitive current has been demonstrable in ventricular myocytes (274), it has become evident more recently that there is differential transmural distribution. Approaching the epicardial surface, cells have shorter APs and a phase 1 "notch" not observed in endocardial cells (144,160,258), but are similar to those of Purkinje fibers that possess I_{to}. Although the similar orientation of the R and T vectors on the ECG required a briefer epicardial versus endocardial AP duration, the cellular basis for this phenomenon was documented only when the presence of a prominent I_{to} was found in epicardial, but not in endocardial, canine ventricular cells (293). Application of 4-AP eliminates the phase 1 "notch" in the epicardial AP and increases AP duration, but has minimal effect on endocardial AP duration. In addition to explaining the ECG T-wave direction, these currents may be altered with various myocardial disease states, with diminished I_{to} observed in myocytes derived from failing human ventricle (347), a canine peri-infarction zone (298), or hypertrophied rat ventricle (460).

The Chloride Currents

Cl^- currents are thought to play a modest role in cardiac electrophysiologic behavior in the absence of most hormonal stimuli. However, it has become evident that a variety of Cl^- channels also exist in cardiac tissue that can assume a prominent role under certain conditions. It is important to recognize that the Nerst equilibrium potential for Cl^- (E_{Cl}) is -45 to -65 mV (211), so that influx of Cl^- through specific anion channels may contribute a repolarizing current when the V_m is positive to E_{Cl}, while efflux of Cl^- when V_m is negative to E_{Cl} will represent a depolarizing current. These channels are usually blocked by a variety of negatively charged aromatic organic acids (2).

The Ca^{2+}-Activated Cl^- Current As already noted, a repolarizing current is partly responsible for initial repolarization (phase 1) of the AP. While a distinct K^+ current (I_{to1}) clearly plays a role, the initial descriptions of the outward current (the "initial outward" or "positive dynamic" current) in cardiac Purkinje fibers showed sensitivity to external Cl^-, suggesting it might be a Cl channel (119,142). Some of the confusion regarding this current has resolved with the recognition that both K and Cl channels probably contribute. This Cl^- current appears to be activated by Ca^{2+} released from sarcoplasmic reticulum (SR) stores, since inhibition of Ca^{2+} release from the SR by depletion with caffeine or ryanodine slows the phase 1 repolarization (2,535,536). This inactivating Cl^- current, now designated $I_{Cl(Ca)}$ as well as I_{to2}, has been found in a variety of myocardial tissue, including atrial cells and ventricular myocytes isolated from the epicardium and myocardial regions (534). Recent experiments selectively inhibiting $I_{to1}(K^+)$ and I_{to2} (Cl^-) suggest that at physiologic heart rates the latter is the dominant current responsible for the initial repolarization, at least in atrial tissue (497). This Ca^{2+}-dependent control component permits the increased contractile state of the myocardium, associated with an increase in rate and increased intracellular Ca^{2+}, to increase channel opening, which will then accelerate repolarization and decrease AP duration. The decreased AP duration will then cause earlier relaxation and a longer diastolic interval, permitting more appropriate cardiac metabolic balance. However, when Ca^{2+} is released from overloaded SR stores, activation of $I_{Cl(Ca)}$ may generate a depolarizing potential in cells at RMP (534).

The Cystic Fibrosis Transmembrane Regulator While there is normally no resting Cl^- conductance in cardiac tissue, a channel has clearly been defined that is activated by β-adrenergic stimulation (25,123,183,184,443) via phosphorylation by protein kinase A (cAMP controlled). The channel appears to be similar in many characteristics to the Cl channel that has been identified as the defective gene in cystic fibrosis (cystic fibrosis transmembrane regulator, CFTR) (2), and is a member of the ATP binding cassette (ABC) family of proteins that include a variety of membrane transporters. As with other members of this class, this channel also appears to require binding of a nucleotide triphosphate, typically ATP, although it is unclear if ATP is hydrolyzed in the transport cycle (412). This channel is insignificant in sinoatrial and atrial cells, and is more prominent in epicardial than endocardial ventricular cells (443). Activation of this channel by β-adrenoceptor activation results in depolarizing current that may actually cause depletion of intracellular Cl^- (349), and can contribute to AP abbreviation as well (211).

Other Cl Channels In addition, a Cl^- current has been noted in guinea pig ventricular myocytes activated by protein kinase C. However, this channel appears to have characteristics distinct from the PKA activated CFTR. Another Cl^- channel activated by stretch (172) or swelling (429) has been documented in atrial myocytes, but its role is unclear.

Coordination of Membrane Currents During Normal Cardiac Conduction

The phases of the cardiac AP can now be examined in greater detail, better defining the roles of the various currents (Fig. 6).

Resting Membrane Potential (Phase 4) The cardiac transmembrane potential during the electrical quiescence, i.e., resting membrane potential (RMP), varies among cardiac cell types, along with other AP characteristics and conduction velocities (432). Potassium is the major ion determining the RMP because during phase 4, as noted, the cell membrane is quite permeable to K^+, but relatively impermeable to other ions. While providing very stable electrical behavior, the K^+ gradient is maintained at considerable energetic expense (5–10% of myocardial O_2) by the "Na pump," or Na^+-K^+ adenosine triphosphatase (ATPase) of the sarcolemma. This protein uses energy supplied by the hydrolysis of an ATP to transport Na^+ out of the myocytes and K^+ into the myocytes and maintain respectively low and high intracellular levels. Since three Na^+ are pumped out of the cell for two K^+ pumped into the cell for each ATP consumed (425,452), the Na^+-K^+ ATPase is electrogenic (i.e., it generates a net outward current) and tends to make the cell RMP more negative. Depending on the activity transmembrane potential and Na^+ and Ca^{2+} concentrations inside and outside the cell, a non-ATP consuming Na-Ca exchanger can reversibly transport Ca^{2+} or Na^+ into or out of cells (64,281,283). During rest it exchanges three entering Na^+ as it eliminates one Ca^{2+} in one cycle, and generates a net inward (depolarizing) current. In parallel with the Na-Ca exchanger, an ATP-dependent Ca^{2+} transport system also exists in the cardiac sarcolemma (74); however, it is probably responsible for elimination of only a small fraction of Ca^{2+} (277). Consequently, the Na pump not only eliminates the Na^+ that enters via Na channels during the phase 0 depolarization, it also removes from the cell the Na^+ that enters via the Na-Ca exchanger to Ca^{2+}. While the charge entry via the Na-Ca exchanger neutralizes to a small extent the outward Na pump current, the Na pump generates a modest hyperpolarization of cardiac tissue, which probably results in a modest influx of K^+ via G_{K1}. When the Na pump has a higher baseline activity, as seen with hyperthyroidism, the increased outward current is sufficient to slightly decrease AP duration on ventricular myocytes (117).

Because they lack or have a decreased G_{K1}, pacemaker cells and Purkinje fibers, respectively, do not have stable RMP.

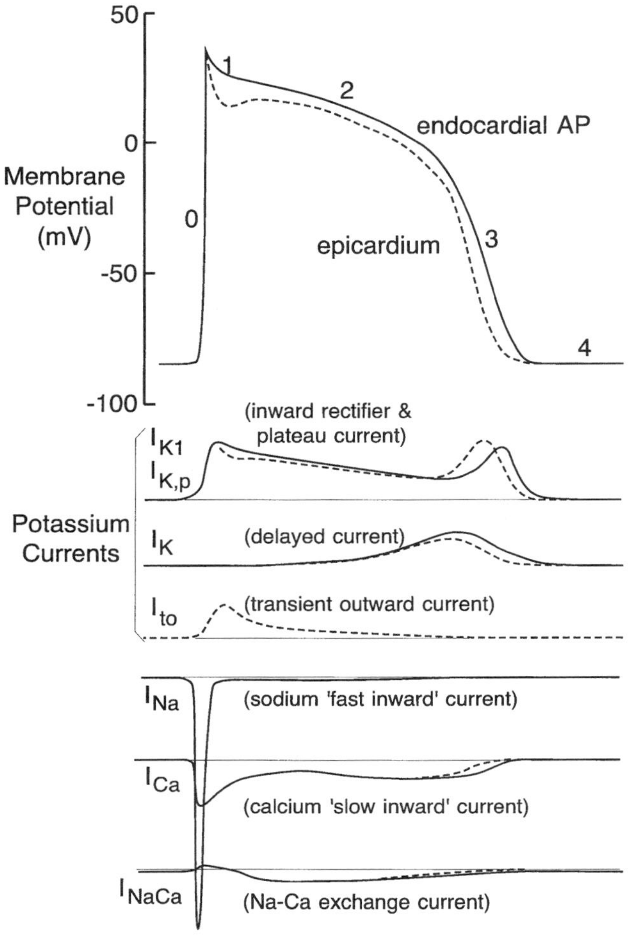

Figure 6. The five distinct phases of the action potential are the result of several inward currents (sodium, I_{Na}; calcium, $I_{Ca,L}$ and $I_{Ca,T}$; Na-Ca exchange, $I_{Na/Ca}$), and outward currents carried mostly by potassium (delayed rectifier, I_K; inward rectifier, I_{K1}; and transient outward, I_{to}). Not included in the figure is outward current due to the Na^+/K^+ ATPase, as well as chloride current and a variety of other K^+ currents, e.g., $I_{K(ACh)}$, $I_{K(ATP)}$, $I_{K(Ado)}$, activated under particular conditions (sympathetic stimulation, ischemia).

Instead they depolarize slowly during diastole, phase 4 (or diastole) depolarization, which causes the automaticity of the heart.

AP Upstroke—Depolarization (Phase 0) The depolarizing stimulus must be of sufficient strength to reduce the level of transmembrane potential to threshold. This is about -65 mV in normal Purkinje fibers. Once threshold has been achieved, an "all-or-none" action AP response occurs. This AP will propagate to excite other cardiac tissue. Smaller depolarizing stimuli, ones that do not bring the cell to threshold, result in nonpropagated, electrotonic effects. The ionic basis for the upstroke of the AP depends on the fiber type. In fast response fibers, namely atrial and ventricular muscle or Purkinje fibers with high (more negative) RMP, rapid AP upstroke velocities (V_{max} phase 0), and distinct overshoots, the AP upstroke is due to the rapid influx of Na^+ through Na channels. The Na current lasts only 1 to 2 msec in most fast response fibers. The Ca^{2+} channels, especially the T-type, actually activate rather quickly (<5 msec); however, it is the massive depolarization generated by I_{Na} that is ultimately responsible for the rapidity of phase 0. In slow response fibers, namely SA node and AV node cells with low (less negative) maximum diastolic potential, reduced V_{max} phase 0, and little or no overshoot, depolarization during phase 0 is largely dependent on the slow inward current carried predominantly by Ca^{2+}.

AP Repolarization and Plateau (Phases 1–3) A number of currents contribute to AP repolarization phases 1 and 3 and to the AP plateau, phase 2 (Fig. 6). The inactivation of the Na current and the Ca current (especially T-type), combined with the transient outward K and Cl currents (I_{to}), produce the net efflux of charge that is responsible for early rapid repolarization (phase 1) from about +40 to near +20 mV. In cells lacking I_{to}, such as guinea pig ventricular myocytes, the AP lacks a phase 1, but rather begins with a gradual repolarizing plateau (212). The effect of I_{to} in ventricular tissue is shown in Fig. 5, where the presence of the early outward current in the epicardium leads to the phase 1 "notch" and contributes to a decrease in AP duration. Also contributing to repolarization may be briefly "reversed" flux through the Na-Ca exchanger (45); with the rapid Na^+ influx, the rise in $[Na^+]$ near the membrane before there is substantial Ca^{2+} entry or release should reverse the driving force of the exchanger so that one Ca^{2+} will enter as the Na^+ are expelled, resulting in a net outward (repolarizing) current. This "reversal" flow may be only very brief, but still sufficient to contribute Ca^{2+} influx and outward current.

During the AP plateau phase, when membrane conductance for all ions is reduced, a variety of currents contribute small components. Particularly in proximal Purkinje fibers with prominent plateaus, however, a small Na "window" current contributes to the AP plateau (86). The Na "window" current might be explained by the existence of two different Na channel populations, or two different modes of operation of the same Na channel (531). Although most Na channels are inactivated, a few continue in a sustained opening mode at around 0 mV (Na window current), while inward L-type Ca currents also contribute. While IR K (G_{K1}) channels are blocked, the plateau K current ($I_{K,p}$) provides an ongoing, counterbalancing efflux of charge. At this point in the plateau, the Na-Ca exchanger may also help to maintain the plateau by generating a net inward charge (three Na^+ in for one Ca^{2+} out) (121). Nonetheless, the gradual depolarization of phase 2 means that the outward current is slightly greater. The outward (delayed) rectifying K^+ current (I_K) and inward (anomalous) rectifying K^+ currents (I_{K1}) are responsible for final rapid repolarization (phase 3). The gradual activation of I_K, and persistence of any I_{to}, along with time-dependent and voltage-dependent inactivation of the I_{Ca}, also contribute to the early phase 3 repolarization. However, as V_m becomes negative to -30 or -40 nV, G_{KI} begins to conduct increasing outward current, especially with higher $[K^+]_o$, and is responsible for accelerating the repolarization at the end of the AP.

During the cardiac AP plateau, fibers cannot be reexcited regardless of stimulus strength; that is, they are absolutely refractory (140). The principal reason for absolute refractoriness is that the vast majority of Na channels are inactivated during the AP plateau and are thus unable to generate current for an AP upstroke. Repolarization must occur before the Na channels can open. In fast response fibers, restoration of the normal resting membrane potential is usually sufficient for full recovery of excitation, as depicted in Fig. 7. Between the end of the absolute refractory period and full recovery of excitation, the fibers are relatively refractory. During the relative refractory period, the stimulus required for excitation is larger than normal, and the resulting AP is either too small to propagate or it will propagate more slowly than normal. In slow response or depressed fast response fibers, the relative refractory period may extend several hundred milliseconds beyond full repolarization.

Other K^+ currents involved in repolarization that may operate under special circumstances include (a) Ca-activated K^+ current, which accelerates repolarization in the Ca-overloaded heart; (b) Na-activated K^+ current, which may promote repolarization in Na-overloaded heart; (c) ATP-sensitive K^+ current,

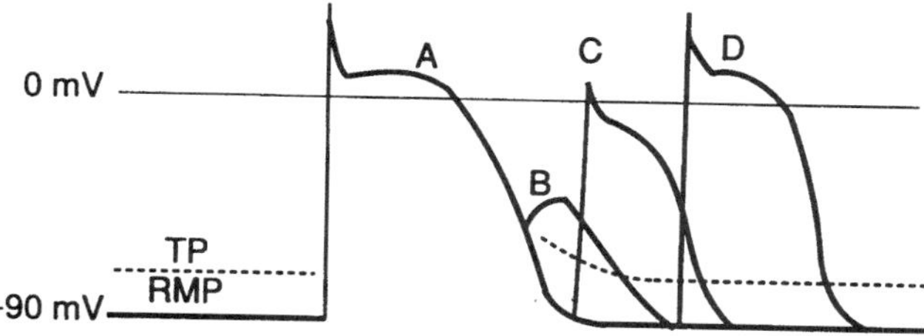

Figure 7. Schematic representation of quiescent Purkinje fiber action potential (AP). TP, threshold potential *(dashed line).* Note that TP is higher for stimuli applied during final rapid repolarization (AP phase 3). RMP, resting membrane potential. Stimuli during the absolute refractory period (A) fail to produce any response. Stimulus occurring early during the relative refractory period (B) will produce only local, nonpropagated (electrotonic) responses. During the latter part of the B, stimulus C will produce a propagated AP, although it will conduct slowly due to its smaller rate of rise and amplitude. Stimulus D at the end of the relative refractory period will produce a normal AP, one that conducts normally due to its normal rate of rise and amplitude. (From ref. 12, with permission.)

normally inhibited by ATP, but that opens up with depletion of energy stores; (d) acetylcholine-activated K^+ current, which activates in response to vagal stimulation and hyperpolarizes resting cardiac cells; and (e) arachidonic acid–activated K^+ current, which is activated by arachidonic acid and other fatty acids, especially at low pH (253). Concerning K repolarization currents, as the transmembrane potential becomes more negative during the latter phases of repolarization, K^+ conductance (as the result of K^+ current) increases. Inward-going rectification enhances the outward movement of K^+ during repolarization, thereby accelerating repolarization by further increasing K^+ conductance. This regenerative increase in K^+ conductance partly explains the all-or-none repolarization. Therefore, toward the end of the AP plateau, a large repolarizing current will result in full repolarization to normal resting membrane or maximum diastolic potential levels.

Initiation and Conduction of the Heart Beat

Initiation of the Cardiac AP—The Pacemaker Potential

While the previously noted channels can provide a mechanism for propagation of an AP once initiated, the intact heart has the important property of spontaneous, regular activity in the absence of neural input. This pacemaking property is due to the presence of specific regions of small tissue that have a spontaneous depolarization during rest; these generate an AP that is propagated through the atrium and then through the ventricle. The sequence of depolarization is normally initiated by a specialized region of tissue in the sinoatrial (SA) node. Although difficult to identify grossly, this small group of microscopically distinct cells have few mitochondria, no sarcoplasmic reticulum (SR) or organized myofibrils, and have been termed round cells (46). When not undergoing an action potential (AP) the cells undergo a very gradual depolarization from ~-60 mV (the maximum diastolic potential at the end of repolarization) at a rate of 20 to 100 mV/sec (Fig. 8). This process is the diastolic depolarization (DD), or pacemaker potential. The prominent DD of SA and atrioventricular (AV) nodes is due to a complex combination of changing ionic permeabilities. Critical to the intrinsic repetitive firing of the pattern of pacemaker tissue is the absence and presence of distinct ionic conductances. In contrast to the ventricular and atrial muscle, the pacemaking tissues of the heart have virtually no detectable resting G_{K1} conductance to fix the resting membrane potential (RMP) near E_K (221), so the RMP is much more able to "float." The term *maximum diastolic potential* instead of RMP refers to the maximum level of transmembrane potential attained during diastole in automatic fibers. Thus, very modest ionic currents can depolarize these tissues, while the activation of K channels will tend to hold RMP closer to E_K, and shunt depolarizing current.

The Pacemaker Current, I_f Although DD was initially defined as an inactivating K^+ current (I_{K2}) (190,357), subsequent studies clearly demonstrated that the depolarization is due to an inward current (109,110,112,320,321). The current was found to be an ionic pathway activated by membrane potentials negative to -40 to -50 mV and sensitive to changes in both $[Na^+]_o$ and $[K^+]_o$. The channel is relatively nonspecific, permitting both depolarizing Na^+ influx as well as K^+ efflux. However, near diastolic potentials in nodal tissue (-50 to -60 mV), the channel permits a depolarizing inward current (mostly Na^+ influx). The channel is inhibited and enhanced by muscarinic (112) and adrenergic receptor activation (113), respectively, thereby modulating heart rate. The molecular character of this channel remains to be defined.

While the role and necessity of a depolarizing inward current has been emphasized (111), and while it may play a primary role, the ionic flux through the delayed K and Ca channels also plays a role in regulating diastolic depolarization. The deactivation of the delayed current (I_K, probably the slow component) and the activation of Ca^{2+} currents appear to contribute. When 40 µM Ni^{2+} is applied to block $I_{Ca,T}$, the latter half of the DD is remarkably prolonged, suggesting that $I_{Ca,T}$, in addition to I_f, contributes depolarizing current to the diastolic depolarization (171). When an internal membrane potential of ~-50 mV is reached, the depolarization rate increases to 1 to 2 V/sec, creating a slowly depolarizing AP. Although Na channels may be present in SA node (298), they are inactivated by the low resting potential and slow DD, and never observed physiologically. Since the $I_{Ca,L}$ is not activated negative to -40 mV, it appears to generate the inward current for phase 0 of the SA and atrioventricular (AV) nodal AP, but not to DD (171,179). Figure 8 shows schematically the currents that appear to account for the cyclic nature of the cardiac pacemaker.

In the SA and AV nodes, the combined kinetics of K channel inactivation and I_f activation are able to depolarize these cells to the activation threshold potential of Ca channels in a relatively short interval (300–900 msec, depending on species, development, autonomic nervous system input, and temperature). In contrast, the His-Purkinje system possesses less G_{K1} than is present in ventricular muscle (163), but has a sufficient amount to achieve a far more negative RMP. Spontaneous depolarizations occur at a much slower rate than observed in the nodal tissue, but eventually reach the Na channel threshold, eliciting a fast, rapidly conducted AP. Pacemaker currents can be observed in ventricular tissue (523), but due to the sustained high level of G_{K1} such currents probably have modest physiologic significance, with spontaneous pacemaking rarely present.

It is of interest, however, that the Rasmusson et al. (380) model successfully simulates pacemaker behavior in normal frog sinus venosus cells, which lack I_f. These investigators combined measurements of I_K and I_{Ca} with estimates of background currents, Na-K pump currents, Na-Ca exchange currents, and intracellular buffering systems for Ca^{2+}. The key conclusions of this model are the following: (a) Pacemaking does not result from one current, but rather from the interaction of I_K background currents, the intracellular Ca^{2+} concentration, and the absence of I_{K1}. (b) The Na-Ca exchange of inward current immediately after repolarization is small because of intracellular Ca^{2+} buffering, and it declines as the intracellular concentration of Ca^{2+} is reduced by the Na-Ca exchanger. The Na-K pump current is time-invariant and small. These currents cannot generate the pacemaker potential, but they are large enough to influence it. (c) Accumulation and/or depletion of ions just beneath or just outside the surface membrane play no

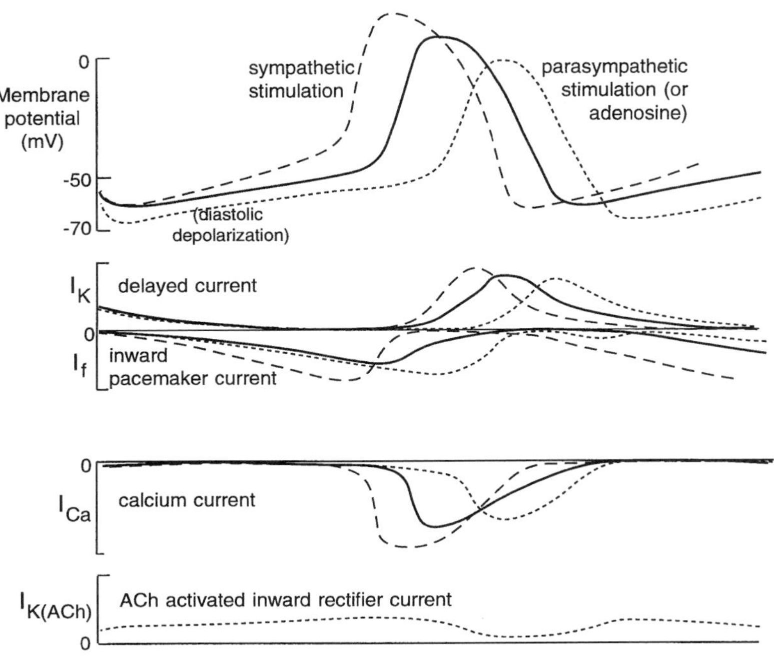

Figure 8. The currents responsible for pacemaker potentials in the sinoatrial (and also the atrioventricular) node. As indicated in the *center panel,* the diastolic depolarization (DD) is the result of the turn off of the delayed K^+ current (I_K), as well as the hyperpolarization-induced activation of the inward pacemaker current (I_f) (221). The decline in the potassium conductance combined with the inward current result in the gradual depolarization until the action potential threshold is approached and Ca channels open. The I_{Ca} probably represents T-type channels initially activated during the latter half of the DD with the L-type channels providing the major current responsible for the AP upstroke (171). In the presence of β-adrenergic stimulation the I_f is enhanced as are the L-type calcium currents. The activated pacemaker current results in a rapid diastolic depolarization; the enhanced $I_{Ca,L}$ results in a larger and faster phase zero of the AP. This latter effect may result in faster conduction of the action potential through the nodal tissue. In the presence of muscarinic stimulation, the pacemaker potential is depressed while an inward rectifier current ($I_{K(ACh)}$) is stimulated by the acetylcholine (also by adenosine). This channel tends to maintain the cells in a hyperpolarized condition, decreasing the rate of diastolic depolarization by requiring a larger pacemaker current. Furthermore, the pacemaker current itself appears to be depressed by muscarinic stimulation (112). (From ref. 304, with permission.)

significant role in the pacemaker process. While the Rasmusson et al. (380) sinus venosus mode lacks I_f, known to be present in many mammalian SA node cells, the model results would have been the same if I_f were included, provided its voltage-dependent activation was very small at the voltage range of the SA node pacemaker potential (32). It would only contribute if the SA node cells were hyperpolarized by activation of other K channel currents, such as might occur with vagal stimulation, e.g., $I_{K,ACh}$ (32).

The Conduction of the Cardiac AP Through the Heart

The action potential configurations in the various regions of the heart and their temporal relationship are shown in Fig. 9.

The Sinoatrial (SA) Node The slow AP present in SA nodal tissue has been noted previously. This nodal slow AP invades the zone of surrounding cells, which have more myofibrils and appear microscopically more as muscle (46). These cells also spontaneously depolarize, but not as rapidly. As the cells become more muscle-like in character, they have a more negative resting potential, more active Na channels, and therefore a more rapid AP depolarization. Occasionally, islands of cells near the SA node may take over as dominant pacemaker with a slightly faster diastolic depolarization.

Atrial Muscle Once the depolarization reaches atrial muscle, which has a -85 to -90 mV resting potential, the AP spreads rapidly, with a particularly rapid conduction pathway (Bachman's bundle) toward the left atrium. In comparison to ventricular muscle, the atrial AP duration is considerably shorter, with a less prominent plateau, consistent with its far briefer contraction. However, the short AP duration in atrial tissue permits another action potential to occur much sooner, so that relatively high rates are achievable (i.e., atrial flutter). It is noteworthy that in rabbit (158), guinea pig (212), and human (477) atrial tissue the resting conductance is lower, but also less rectifying at depolarized potentials than in ventricular tissue. Consequently, during the plateau more repolarizing current can escape from atrial cells to abbreviate the AP. The greater outward current at depolarized potentials may represent a persisting low level of activity of $I_{K(ACh)}$, prominent in atrial tissue but less rectifying than G_{K1}. In addition, the atrial cells have a prominent I_{to} that contributes to the initial repolarization (158,212,477),

Atrioventricular (AV) Node When the AP reaches the borders of the atrial muscle, the AP stops at the nonconducting fibrous tissue that forms the annulus for each atrioventricular valve. At a junction of the atrial-ventricular septa, the arriving atrial AP passes through a transitional zone of cells (A-N zone), smaller than the normal atrial cells and separated from them by fibrous tissue. The AP is markedly slowed as it transits the compact or N region of the node, composed of round cells similar anatomically and physiologically to the SA node cells (328). Located on the superior right ventricular edge of the ventricular septum, the AV node is similar to the SA node, except for having a slower rate of diastolic depolarization. The AP conduction velocity then increases as it travels through a second transitional zone (N-H region) to the bundle of His, from which it is embryologically distinct (229). By virtue of its slow diastolic depolarization, it is a backup system of impulse initiation, in case the SA node or atrial conduction fails. The delay between the atria and ventricular contraction permits better augmentation of ventricular filling. The node is also a frequency gate, so that if the atria flutter (~300 bpm) or fibrillate, the ventricle will not be driven at a rate incompatible with effective pump function (328). This AV node represents the only electrical continuity and means of conduction between the atria and ventricles, except for individuals who have abnormal direct conduction pathways between the atria and ventricles (Wolff-Parkinson-White and Lown-Ganong-Levine syndromes).

The Bundle of His and Purkinje Network Uniform initiation of contraction of all the ventricular myocytes is achieved by specialized myocytes that form large-diameter (50–80 μm) fibers with very sparse myofibrils or sarcoplasmic reticulum. The APs of this system are characterized by the most rapid rate of depolarization (400–800 V/sec) in the heart. The bundle of His, which has sufficiently high current density that it generates a discrete voltage signal, is a specialized group of large conducting fibers that emanates from the AV node and that divides into a right ventricular branch, an anterior left ventricular branch, and a large posterior left ventricular branch. Each branch forms a network of Purkinje fibers that spreads over the inner surface of the heart, rapidly carrying depolarization to the entire endothelial surface. These large diameter fibers have a conduction velocity of ~4 m/sec that permits the rapid conduction of the AP from the AV node to the endocardial surface

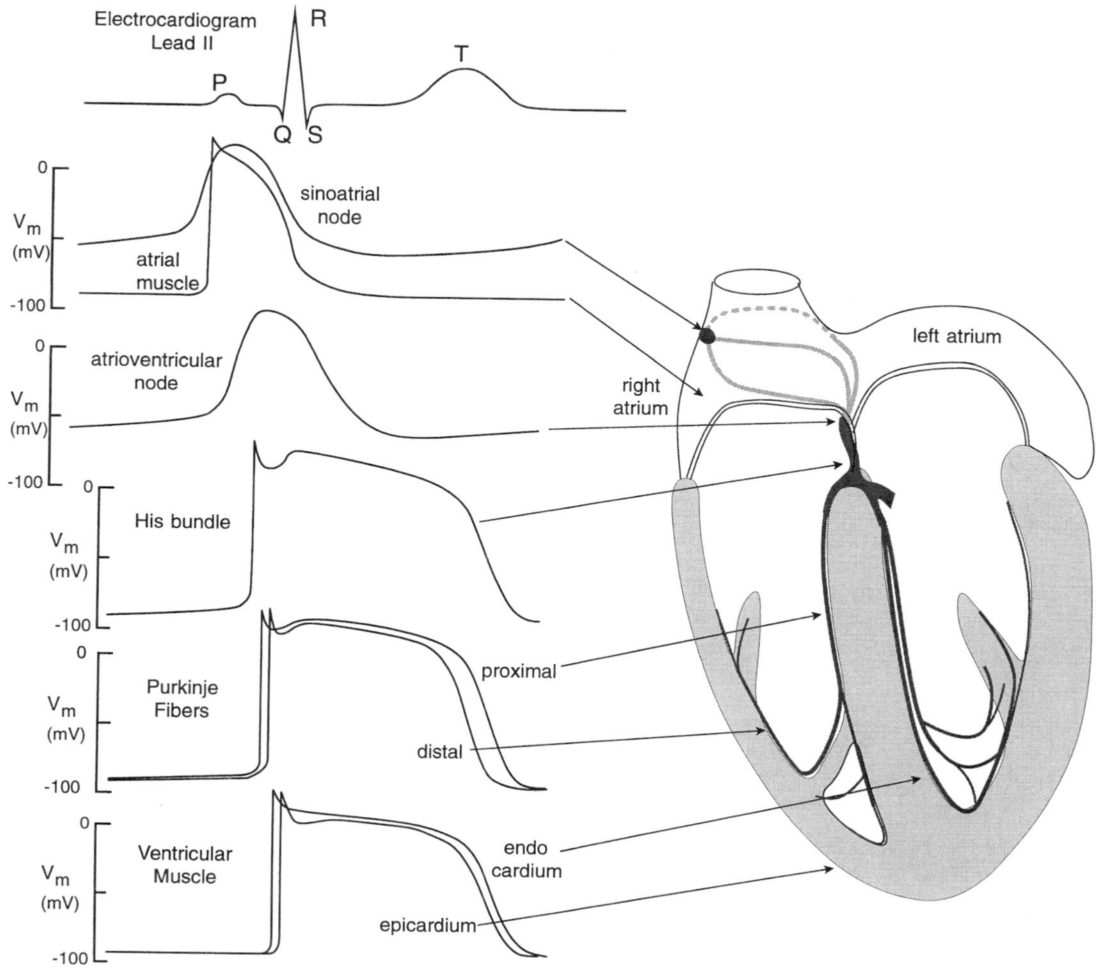

Figure 9. Conduction of the depolarization through the heart. The action potential configurations in the various regions of the heart and their temporal relationship are shown.

of the ventricular muscle in ~30 msec. The APs in the Purkinje system are also the longest in the heart, and the proximal (nearest the His bundle) are depolarized for a substantially longer time (40–80 msec) than those distal fibers that form electrical junctions with the myocardium (Fig. 9; see Fig. 14). Consequently, the cardiac impulses cannot go retrograde under normal conditions, protecting the heart from many erratic and premature beats that might be initiated in the distal regions. These fibers also have a very slow diastolic depolarization, which can provide pacemaking capability if the SA and AV nodes fail, although the rates are very slow (10–20 bpm).

The depolarization of the ventricular wall occurs in 80 to 100 msec, generating significant current that is detected as QRS complex of the electrocardiogram. This wave of depolarization is normally oriented in endocardial-epicardial direction and is transmitted by the extracellular fluid to all parts of the body. During the plateau of the AP, virtually no current is flowing, and there is relative electrical silence. Considerable heterogeneity has been reported for AP durations at various locations in the ventricular wall (294), and such heterogeneity has been suggested as a substrate for arrhythmogenesis (258,294). Epicardial APs are shorter than those in the endocardium; they repolarize slightly before and more uniformly than those in the endocardium (144), and as a consequence the wave of repolarization that sweeps from the epicardium to the endocardium also causes a positive deflection of the electrocardiogram (Fig. 9).

The decreased AP duration in the epicardium results from the presence of a greater and/or more rapidly activated K conductance. Canine epicardial myocytes show a more prominent component of I_{Ks} than epicardial cells, which may account for the difference (162). However, I_{Ks} has not been demonstrated in human myocardium (477), and endo- versus epicardial differences in I_{to} may have far greater relevance (132,293,294). A similar high density of I_{to} has recently been reported in subepicardial versus subendocardial cells from human ventricle, with the subepicardial cells also having more favorable recovery kinetics (504).

Modulation of Cardiac Action Potentials and Conduction

Rate-Dependent Effects

Alterations in Ca^{2+} entry via the Ca channel and the amount of Ca^{2+} released from intracellular stores appear to have complex effects upon cardiac APs, which are related in large part to the secondary effects of altered intracellular Ca^{2+} ($[Ca^{2+}]_i$) modulation of other ion channels and cell functions. When Ca^{2+} entry was altered by varying extracellular Ca^{2+} ($[Ca^{2+}]_o$), the increased $[Ca^{2+}]_o$ resulted in increased AP plateau and shortened duration, while decreased $[Ca^{2+}]_o$ resulted in a decreased AP plateau and increased AP duration (248,469). Part of the Ca^{2+}-dependent effect to enhance delayed K^+ current appears to be modulated by calmodulin-mediated activation in a process not involving phosphorylation (356). The more prominent effect may be mediated by Ca^{2+}-activated Cl^- and/or K^+ transient outward currents.

G Protein–Linked Receptor-Mediated Effects

Cardiac conduction is modulated by various ligands acting through receptors and pathways. The vast majority of receptors in the heart and peripheral cardiovascular system that modulate their function belong to a family of receptors whose actions are mediated by activation of the guanine nucleotide binding proteins, or G proteins. After activation by these specific receptors, G proteins activate (or inhibit) a variety of ion channels or second-messenger generating enzymes (43,207,305). When ligands (norepinephrine, histamine, etc.) bind in the cleft of these receptors, a conformational change occurs on the intracellular surface of the receptor that promotes dissociation of the heterotrimeric G protein complex. Guanosine diphosphate (GDP) and the tightly coupled βγ subunit dissociate away from the α subunit, which is then free to bind guanosine triphosphate (GTP). The GTP-bound α subunit forms an activating complex that then regulates the membrane effector systems (198), at least until the GTP is hydrolyzed. The βγ subunit also appears to play an important signaling role, either by direct interaction with membrane constituents directly or by binding to and inactivating α subunits (217,227,506).

Cyclic AMP–Dependent, Kinase (PKA)-Mediated Effects The most widely studied G protein signal pathway, which is highly relevant to cardiac conduction, is the regulation of adenylyl cyclase (AC) that produces the second messenger cAMP. In addition to the profound modulating effect of the catecholamines via the β-adrenergic receptor (β-AR), histamine (via H_2 receptor), ATP (via P_2 purinergic), and glucagon mediate their primary actions by activating G_s, the stimulatory G protein, which activates AC, increases intracellular [cAMP], and has the various actions mediated by PKA.

Phosphorylation of the L-type Ca channel alters its gating behavior, changing its behavior to a new "mode" in which the open intervals are more sustained, so that a greater number of Ca^{2+} ions may enter the cell (326). $I_{Ca,L}$ is markedly increased as indicated in Fig. 10. In addition, $I_{Ca,L}$ activates at more negative V_m, enhancing channel opening with depolarization (35,238). A similar effect appears to be present for Na channels (360), although a parallel shift of inactivation to more negative voltages can result in a decreased I_{Na} in certain settings (411).

In addition to enhancing Ca and Na channels, a number of channels appear to be activated by PKA. A profound action occurs in pacemaking tissue in which I_f is increased, increasing the rate of diastolic depolarization, and leading to the increased heart rate typical of b-adrenergic activation (see Fig. 8). The enhanced $I_{Ca,L}$ results in a larger and faster phase 0 of the nodal APs, which will result in faster conduction of the action potential through the nodal tissue. The delayed K current (492), as well as the transient outward current (I_{to}) (350), are both enhanced by phosphorylation, which will serve to abbreviate the AP, an important electrophysiologic effect that ensures that the contractile state is not prolonged. In addition, the CFTR Cl^- conductance is also activated, which will also have a repolarizing action on the plateau, but a depolarizing effect during diastole that may contribute to automaticity. While the increased inward Ca^{2+} and Na^+ may enhance conduction, the repolarizing currents predominate during the plateau so that AP duration is not increased or even decreases. These effects are summarized in Fig. 11.

Other intracellular effects of PKA activation will enhance intracellular Ca^{2+} accumulation by the SR and Ca^{2+} cycling. Following phosphorylation, phospholamban no longer provides a brake on the SR Ca pump so that Ca^{2+} can be accumulated at a far greater rate (257). The combination of increased Ca^{2+} entry and SR accumulation means a far greater amount of Ca^{2+} will

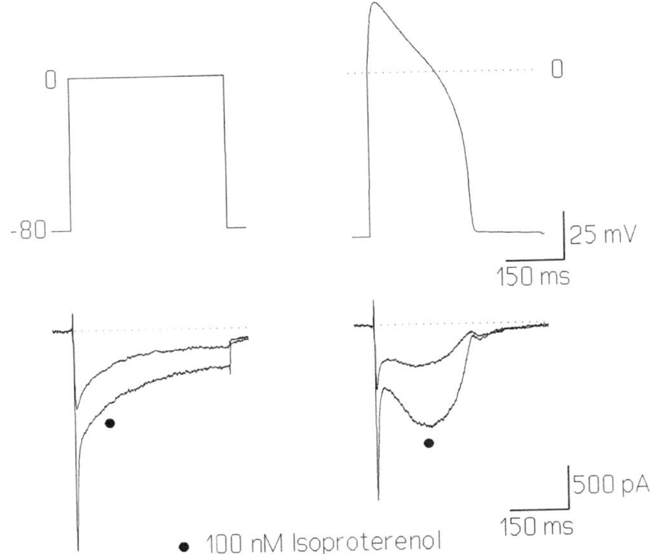

Figure 65-10. Enhancement of Ca^{2+} currents by β-adrenergic stimulation with isoproterenol. Ca^{2+} currents in guinea pig myocytes were elicited in response by voltage-clamped depolarizations of either square wave or cardiac AP wave form. Note the enhancement of the rapidly inactivating and slowly inactivating component. Such activation may particularly enhance the late current observed during the AP depolarization. The Na^+ and K^+ currents were blocked by the inclusion of tetrodotoxin and Cs^+, respectively, in the perfusate (Figure courtesy of J. J. Pancrazio.)

be accumulated with each beat. This effect may be even further increased by effects on the cardiac CaRC, whose function is enhanced by PKA phosphorylation (444). While such changes primarily relate to inotropic action, the increased intracellular Ca^{2+} can lead to overloading and oscillatory release of Ca^{2+}, which can activate depolarizing currents.

The β-adrenergic receptors (β-AR) in the myocardium are both the $β_1$-AR and $β_2$-AR subtypes. $β_2$-AR appears to be present in both pacemaker tissues and myocytes, and are activated by isoproterenol and specific agonists such as Zinterol (513), but not by norepinephrine. The effects noted above apply to the actions of $β_1$-AR stimulation, but not to $β_2$-AR. $β_2$-AR activation does not appear to decrease myofibril Ca^{2+} sensitivity or markedly increase SR Ca^{2+}. It does enhance I_{Ca}, but the effect is distinct from that of b_1-AR stimulation (513). These differential actions may depend on different pools of AC or compartmentalized cAMP, and may have potentially important therapeutic implications. $β_2$-AR activation is not as arrhythmogenic as $β_1$-AR stimulation, nor does it shorten the contraction.

The AC-inhibitory G protein G_i is activated in myocardial tissue by acetylcholine (ACh, M_2 muscarinic receptors [29]) or adenosine (A_1-adenosine receptors (422)) as indicated in Fig. 12. Such G_i activation can strongly inhibit AC and thereby reverse the effect of β-AR stimulation, so that cAMP levels and the physiologic functions return toward nonstimulated levels (49). In human myocardium adenosine appears to be more efficiently coupled than ACh in this inhibitory regulatory pathway (49). The inhibitory actions appear to be mediated at least in part by release of βγ subunits from $Gα_i$, which then bind $Gα_s$, resulting in the loss AC activation (227). Within cardiac tissue, this action is most obvious in the pacemaker tissues. These tissues appear to possess a very high resting adenylyl cyclase activity resulting in a high activity of I_f and $I_{Ca,L}$ even in the absence of β-AR stimulation. Consequently, muscarinic and A_1 purinergic stimulation by adenosine will depress I_f and $I_{Ca,L}$ (112,370), slowing the diastolic depolarization and AP conduction veloc-

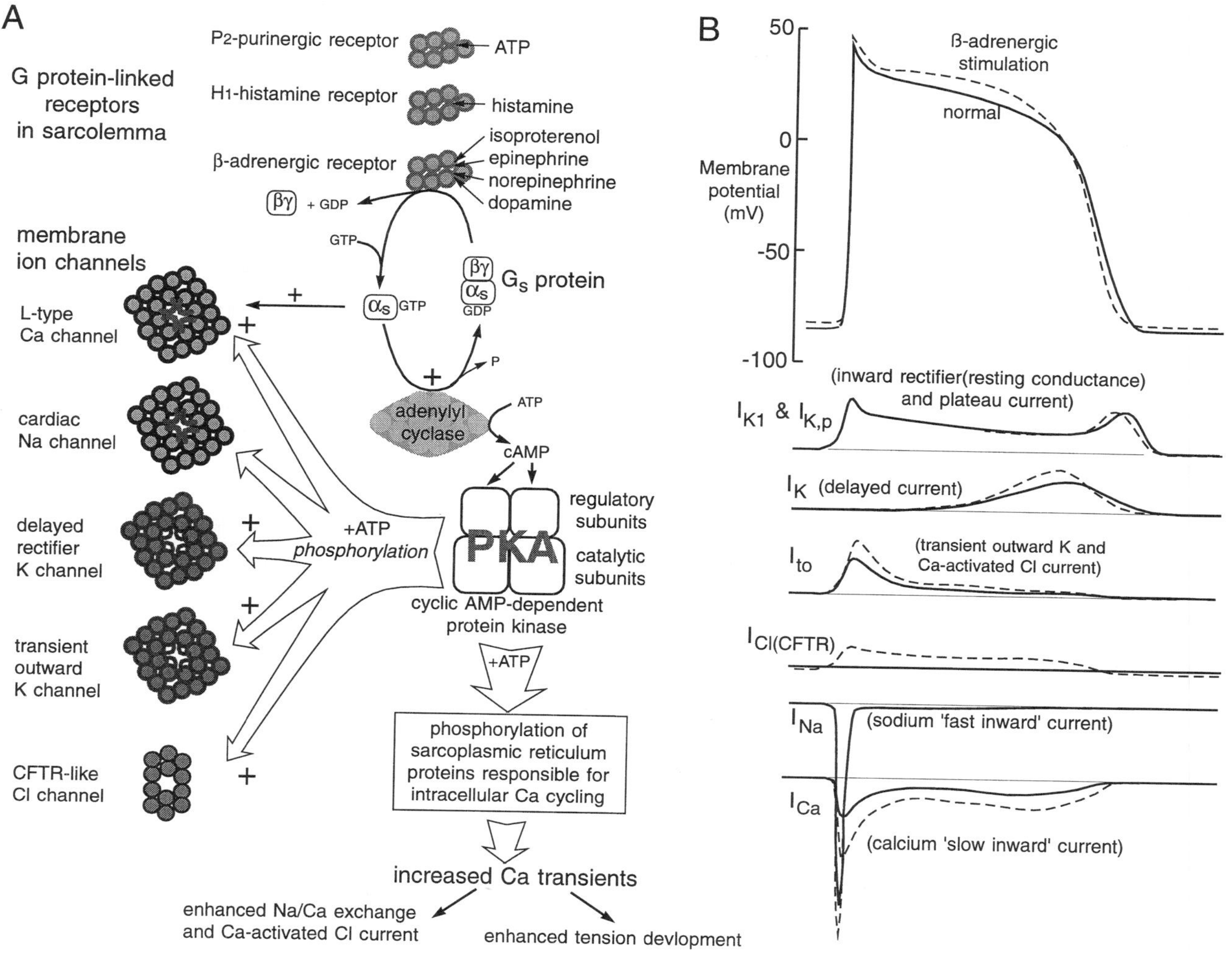

Figure 11. Cardiac ion channel modulation via phosphorylation by cAMP-dependent protein kinase (PKA). **A:** PKA-modulated pathways as viewed from the membrane surface. Ligand binding in the cleft of the transmembrane heptahelical β-adrenergic, H_2 histamine, or P_2 purinergic receptors catalyzes conversion of the G_s complex into its βγ and α_s subunits. The α_s subunit binds GTP and stimulates production of cAMP via adenylyl cyclase (AC), which converts intracellular ATP into cAMP. When cAMP binds to the regulatory component of PKA, the catalytic component is liberated and free to phosphorylate a number of membrane channel proteins. The phosphorylated channels are more active, showing a higher opening probability at a given membrane potential. Activated α_s may also directly gate Ca channels in the heart without involvement of cAMP, although this is probably a minor effect. *Shaded objects* represent transmembrane proteins; *open objects* are intracellular processes. **B:** Changes in membrane currents and the cardiac AP, induced by PKA (and direct α_s) enhancement of ion channel function.

ity. While the isoproterenol enhancement of I_{Ca} in ventricular myocytes can be reversed by adenosine (223), in the absence of β-adrenoceptor stimulation the effect of adenosine or ACh on I_{Ca} and shortening is modest (58,223). Nevertheless, adenosine may cause an ongoing tonic inhibition of the β-AR/AC interaction that increases the dose requirement for β-AR ligands (65). The β-adrenergic responsiveness declines with age, exhibiting evidence of decreased cAMP production and decreased phosphorylation of the various proteins involved (235), an effect that may be mediated in part by enhanced adenosine in the aged heart (115). An important component of modulation of $I_{Ca,L}$ appears to involve nitric oxide as well (see below).

Direct G-Protein–Mediated Effects The most important of the directly modulated cardiac ion currents is $I_{K(ACh,Ado)}$. As noted, ligand binding to M_2 muscarinic or A_1 adenosine receptors activates G_i, releasing βγ, which then opens the $K_{ACh,Ado}$ channel, subsequently causing the cells to be hyperpolarized and less excitable due to the increase in resting K^+ conductance (Fig. 12). The result is a profound decrease in the rate of diastolic depolarization of pacemaker tissue and a slowing of heart rate (see Fig. 8) (39). While ACh release by vagal stimulation can decrease the rate of automaticity or AV nodal conduction, increased tissue adenosine also plays a prominent role in activating $I_{K(ACh, Ado)}$. Adenosine that is generated secondary to ischemia, particularly in regions supplied by the posterior descending coronary artery, can cause complete heart block by its action at the AV node. Exogenously administered adenosine can be employed therapeutically to block AV conduction that is too rapid, or to block reentry loops that utilize the SA or AV node by hyperpolarizing the tissue (114). Because of the direct G_i coupling that does not require inhibition of AC or a decline in cAMP, $I_{K(ACh)}$ can exert its action very rapidly (≤ 1 sec) to depress diastolic depolarization and slow heart rate. Following an initial stimulation by ACh, a second stimulation potentiates the K^+ current induced by a second stimulus (496). The increased current appears to be mediated by glibenclamide-sensitive ATP-inhibited K chan-

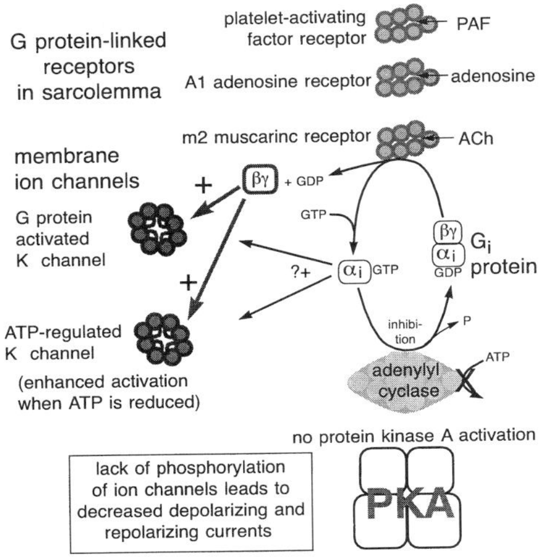

Figure 12. The G_i protein-modulated pathways as viewed from the membrane surface. Ligand binding to the transmembrane heptahelical M_2 muscarinic, α_1-adrenergic, or A_1 adenosine receptor has multiple actions. When agonist binds in the cleft of these G protein–linked receptors, the activated receptor catalyzes the dissociation of the G_i α_i-$\beta\gamma$ protein complex. The $\beta\gamma$ subunit then directly activates inwardly rectifying K channels in myocardial membranes. The α_i subunit binds GTP and interacts with adenylyl cyclase (AC) to inhibit its activity, opposing activation by α_s-GTP subunits (see Fig. 11). This inhibition is terminated by the GTPase activity of the AC-activated α_i subunit, breaking down GTP to GDP and allowing the inactive α_i-GDP to reassociate with the $\beta\gamma$ subunit. Although Gα-GTP may activate the K channel, the activation of $K_{(ACh, Ado)}$ by the freed, dissociated $\beta\gamma$ subunit may be the major activator of this channel, leading to increased K^+ conductance that stabilizes the resting membrane potential and hyperpolarizes pacemaking tissue. *Shaded objects* represent transmembrane proteins.

nels, by a process that is dependent on Ca^{2+} release from the SR and activation of protein kinase C (495). Thus, while ACh directly activates $I_{K(ACh,Ado)}$, it may also indirectly enhance ATP-sensitive K channels.

While $I_{K(ACh,Ado)}$ is present in human ventricular myocytes, its activation by ACh is far more modest than in the atrial myocytes and it makes a modest contribution to total K conductance (267). However, its activation can shorten AP duration, which may in turn inhibit contractility by decreasing Ca^{2+} entry (58). In contrast, adenosine binding to A_1 receptors represents a major influence in ventricular tissue, decreasing AP duration via $I_{K(ACh,Ado)}$ as well as inhibiting AC.

In addition, G_s activation appears to directly increase Ca channel currents (519,520). However, the importance and relevance of this action to physiologic function is unclear (182). Direct activation by β_2-AR might explain observed behavior that differs from that seen with β_1 activation. Likewise, stimulation of P_2-purinergic receptors appears to enhance opening of L-type channels via a pathway involving a G_s pathway exclusive of cAMP production (405).

Protein Kinase C–Mediated Effects Another major G protein pathway involves the activation of the phospholipases, enzymes that metabolize phospholipid components of the cell membranes (426,435). The primary enzymes of interest in myocardium are phospholipase C (PLC) types, which are also activated by a G protein, specifically G_q. PLC cleaves the phosphoester linkage of diphosphoinositide to produce the phosphated sugar, inositol trisphosphate (IP_3), leaving a glycerol with two fatty acids (diacylglycerol, DAG) in the plasmalemma. The protein kinase C (PKC) class of enzymes are then activated by the combined actions of Ca^{2+} and DAG. In addition to effects on the Na/H antiport, PKC also has other important actions on ion channels. PKC activation appears to blunt the stimulation by I_{Ca} of β-AR stimulation (528). A documented PKC action also involves delayed K current enhancement (457,493) which mediates the decrease in the AP duration observed with β_1-adrenoceptor stimulation (458). PKC has also been demonstrated to decrease L-type Ca channel currents in some systems, although its contribution remains to be defined (57). Another major action of PKC is activation of the Na/H antiport so that H^+ is eliminated from the cell, which results in a more alkaline intracellular milieu (153,451), increasing intracellular pH from 7.1 to 7.3. While intracellular alkalinization seems beneficial, it occurs at the expense of increased Na^+ entry, which can have profound implications for regulation of intracellular [Ca^{2+}] by Na-Ca exchange.

Effects of the Autonomic Nervous System

The behavior of the sympathetic and parasympathetic effects cannot be simply considered as being counterbalancing forces on myocardial conduction and contraction that are centrally integrated. Both their anatomic proximity in the cardiac plexi and their physiologic and pharmacologic behavior indicate that the sympathetic and sympathetic nerves continuously modulate each other.

Parasympathetic Effects The effects of vagally released ACh are profound decreases in heart rate, mediated via $I_{K(ACh,Ado)}$ and possibly $I_{K(ATP)}$, as well as by the inhibition of AC and the subsequent PKA cascades, as described previously. In addition to its cellular actions, it is important to recognize that a major effect of vagal outflow is the influence that ACh exerts on sympathetic tone by presynaptic inhibition of norepinephrine release (476,514).

Sympathetic Stimulation The actions of catecholamines in the ventricles are different in the conduction system and myocardium and include effects mediated by activation of both α- and β-adrenergic receptors. Sympathetic stimulation can also decrease vagal outflow also via the release of neuropeptide Y (NPY) (515). While vagal depression of sympathetics is usually dominant over sympathetic depression of vagal tone, sustained NPY release prior to vagal stimulation has a more profound vagolytic effect.(514)

β-Adrenergic Effects Norepinephrine and epinephrine, acting at β-ARs, have little effect on conduction at constant heart rate in Purkinje fibers either in vivo or in vitro, except perhaps to improve conduction in depressed fibers (206,491). Conduction across the Purkinje muscle junctions and in the myocardium is rapidly enhanced by β-AR receptor activation due to phosphorylation of intracellular proteins by cAMP-dependent protein kinases and increased gap junctional conductance (69,103,104,479). β-AR activation and cAMP-dependent phosphorylation may also modulate peak inward Na^+ current, and potentially conduction, in a voltage-dependent fashion (318,411). The β-adrenergic effects of catecholamines shortening action potential duration (APD) in Purkinje and myocardial fibers are associated with increases of inward Ca^{2+} current, as well as marked increases in outward K^+ currents (I_K and I_{to}) and Cl^- currents shortening APD (25,149). The β-mediated reduction in refractory period due to APD shortening may contribute to arrhythmogenesis, particularly in the ischemic heart. In the myocardium, the β-AR mediated decrease of APD and effective refractory period may be antagonized by acetylcholine or vagal stimulation (27,312).

α-Adrenergic Effects Catecholamines acting at α-AR are not known to modulate Purkinje fiber conduction velocity, except in the presence of halothane (385). One preliminary report suggests that high concentrations of phenylephrine may produce cell-to-cell uncoupling between paired myocytes (68), although a-adrenergic effects on myocardial conduction velocity have not been reported. However, α-AR stimulation under certain conditions augments the prominent $I_{Ca,T}$ in Purkinje fibers (463). In contrast to β-AR stimulation, α-AR activation increases APD in Purkinje fibers at constant pacing rate (164), and α-adrenergic agonists (phenylephrine) prolong refractory periods, an effect not seen in the myocardium (311). α-Adrenergic prolongation of Purkinje fiber APD is thought to involve inhibition of outward K^+ currents (286). In ventricular myocytes, α-AR activation appears to inhibit the background G_{K1} via a pertussis toxin–sensitive pathway (131). In general, the responses to α-adrenergic stimulation on action potential duration are generally opposite to those elicited by β-receptor stimulation (164).

Cyclic GMP and Nitric Oxide-Dependent Effects

Although not as prominent on the cAMP/AC system, cyclic GMP is a modulatory second messenger pathway present in myocardium. Cyclic GMP production can be initiated by either of two main routes: (a) binding of natriuretic peptides (atrial, brain) to their membrane-bound receptors, whose intracellular domains possess guanylyl cyclase activity; or (b) binding of nitric oxide (NO) to soluble guanylyl cyclase. Cyclic GMP can activate or inhibit phosphodiesterases (PDE), thereby altering [cAMP]- and PKA-mediated actions. In low concentrations, cGMP appears to augment the stimulatory action of cAMP by inhibition of a cGMP-sensitive PDE (334,361). At higher cGMP concentrations, cAMP-enhanced I_{Ca} is decreased by activation of guanylyl cyclase. This latter effect appears mediated by cGMP-dependent protein kinase in mammalian ventricular myocytes (361,490), while in rabbit SA nodal cells the action appears to be mediated by a cGMP-activated PDE (178), similar to the action seen in amphibian atrium (334). Nitric oxide, either produced by endothelium, myocytes themselves, or from sodium nitroprusside, consistently decreases myocardial contractions (60), an action likely to be mediated by the cGMP-mediated actions on I_{Ca}.

The NO-guanylyl cyclase pathway also plays a critical role in the muscarinic actions of ACh in inhibiting $I_{Ca,L}$, since the action is blocked by inhibitors of nitric oxide synthase (NOS) and duplicated by the NO donor SIN-1 (177). In pacemaker cells, the inhibitory action of M_2 receptor activation was completely absent when cAMP-specific phosphodiesterase (cGMP-activated) was inhibited by IBMX (178). Consequently, direct inhibition of adenylyl cyclase by G_i plays a minimal role in decreasing cAMP-enhanced $I_{Ca,L}$. Of note, the direct action of ACh via G_i in stimulating $I_{K(ACh,Ado)}$ is not altered by the same interventions (178).

ABNORMAL CONDUCTION AND AUTOMATICITY IN THE HEART

Abnormal cardiac electrophysiologic phenomena include uneven prolongation of conduction and refractoriness with the depressed fast response, abnormal automaticity, early or delayed afterpotentials with triggering, and reentrant excitation. These abnormal mechanisms may result when normal electrophysiologic processes are acutely disrupted by the effects of disease or altered physiologic states including autonomic, metabolic or electrolyte imbalance, adverse drug effects, myocardial ischemia or hypoxia, alteration in pH, and hypothermia. In addition, chronic disease processes such as hypertension or coronary insufficiency can result in hypertrophy, fibrosis and scarring, and cardiomyopathic changes in the myocytes.

Altered Normal Automaticity

The pacemaker with the highest rate is normally found in the SA node. However, the pacemaker discharge can also occur from ectopic sites of latent or subsidiary pacemakers. Latent pacemakers can be found at sites of subsidiary atrial pacemakers inferior to the SA node, along the sulcus terminalis, at more remote ectopic atrial sites (e.g., Bachman's bundle, coronary sinus), the atrioventricular valve rings, the AV node margins, and the His-Purkinje system. Spontaneous phase 4 depolarization in latent pacemaker cells is normally prevented from reaching threshold potential due to overdrive suppression of automaticity by the more rapidly firing SA node (259,531). Ectopic pacemakers may be manifested through default of the primary pacemaker with latent pacemaker escape, or through usurpation by latent pacemakers. With default and escape, SA node discharge slows sufficiently or there is conduction block somewhere between the SA node and ectopic pacemaker, thereby permitting latent pacemaker escape at an appropriate rate for that pacemaker. With usurpation, the discharge rate of the late pacemaker is inappropriately enhanced relative to the SA node rate, so that it usurps control of the heart for one or more beats. Pacemaker default, escape and usurpation are manifestations of altered normal automaticity (161,531). Altered normal automaticity means that although the ionic mechanisms for automaticity in the affected fibers remain unchanged, the kinetics or magnitude of the currents responsible for automaticity are altered.

Abnormal Automaticity

As compared to altered normal automaticity, abnormal automaticity is due to an ionic mechanism that is substantially different from that for normal automaticity in the same fiber type (e.g., Purkinje fibers), or it occurs in fibers that do not normally exhibit automaticity (e.g., atrial and ventricular muscle) (161,531). Depolarization of Purkinje, atrial, or ventricular muscle by disease or other interventions can accelerate existing spontaneous activity or induce abnormal automaticity in previously quiescent fibers (102,125). Abnormal automaticity has been found in Purkinje fibers removed from dogs subjected to myocardial infarction, in rat myocardium damaged by epinephrine, in human atrial samples, and in ventricular myocardium from patients having aneurysectomies or endocardial resection for recurrent ventricular tachyarrhythmias (531). The ionic mechanism(s) for abnormal automaticity have not been firmly established and probably vary depending on the fiber type, amount of membrane depolarization, and on the intervention or condition that initiated automaticity. That the slow inward current (I_{Ca}) might be involved was suggested by experiments in which verapamil, but not lidocaine, suppressed automaticity in partially depolarized Purkinje fibers (125).

Afterdepolarizations and Triggered Activity

An abnormal form of impulse initiation that is critically dependent on preceding afterdepolarizations has been termed triggered activity (90,509). This activity is separate and distinct from automaticity, which results from spontaneous diastolic depolarization caused by the pacemaker current. Afterdepolarizations are oscillations in the transmembrane potential that follow the upstroke of an action potential (AP). Afterpotentials with or without sustained (triggered) rhythmic activity may occur at virtually any level of transmembrane potential (509). For instance, afterpotentials may occur early, i.e., during repolarization of the AP (early afterdepolarizations, EAD), or they may be delayed until after repolarization is complete (delayed afterdepolarization, DAD) and the prior RMP has been reestablished. DADs frequently are preceded by early afterhyperpolarizations. When EAD or DAD are large enough to achieve threshold potential for activation of a regenerative inward current, the resulting APs are referred to as triggered. If these perpetuate themselves, the process is referred to as triggered sustained rhythmic activity, as opposed to automatic sustained rhythmic activity. The key characteristic of automatic rhythms that distinguishes them from triggered rhythmic activity is that they can arise in the absence of any prior electrical activity (509).

Early Afterdepolarizations

EADs occur in the late plateau of the AP or during phase 3 repolarization (509). Under certain conditions, EAD can lead to "second upstrokes" (90,94) and a propagated AP. The second AP occurring during repolarization is triggered in the sense that it is evoked by an EAD, which in turn was induced by a prior AP. The second AP may be followed by other APs, all arising near membrane potentials characteristic of the plateau phase. Such sustained rhythmic activity may continue for a variable number of beats, but terminates when repolarization returns the V_m to more negative level.

Since the membrane conductance during the plateau is relatively low, small increases in inward current or decreases in outward are sufficient to cause depolarizations. EADs typically arise with interventions or drugs that reduce the K^+ conductances, delay repolarization, and increase the AP duration. For example, the large ionic radius cation Cs^+ blocks G_{K1} and activates EADs, an effect enhanced by decreased $[K^+]_o$ (94), which also decreases G_{K1}. Blockade of G_{K1} by Ba^{2+} can also be used to generate EADs and triggered activity (442). Delay of repolarization or its clinical equivalent, prolongation of the QT interval of the ECG, are also observed with class IA and III antiarrhythmic drugs, such as quinidine (290) and almokalant, respectively (72,290,511). The long QT syndrome can occur spontaneously in families and is associated with syncope, seizures, and sudden death due to ventricular arrhythmias, typically the peculiar undulating torsades de pointes rhythm (414). Recently, a number of different mutations in the human K channel equivalent to the delayed current $I_{K,r}$ (HERG) have been described that are associated with long QT syndrome in a variety of families (93). Since repolarizing current through $I_{K,r}$ as well as I_{K1} are increasingly enhanced by $[K^+]_o$, elevations in $[K^+]_o$ may be useful to enhance K^+ conductance and prevent EADs.

Under most circumstances, the inward current responsible for the EAP during the AP plateau and early during phase 3 is unlikely to be normal cardiac Na channels, since most Na channels are inactivated. Instead, L-type Ca^{2+} "window" current probably plays an important role in generating the EAD, particularly when enhanced by sympathetic stimulation (232,530). As the depolarization begins to invade previously repolarized regions of muscle, progressively more current can flow through reactivated Na channels and permit an AP to be triggered throughout the tissue. However, a mutation of the cardiac Na channel has recently been associated with a mutation in the cardiac Ca channel that results in a deletion in the region of channel thought to be associated with inactivation (494). Presumably, failure of the channel to inactivate may result in a persisting inward current that prolongs the AP and can initiate an EAD.

Finally, EADs show a cycle length (heart rate) dependence; that is, EAD amplitude and the likelihood of triggered activity increases at lower heart rates (509) and is suppressed by the overdrive hyperpolarization resulting from rapid rates (94). The increased inward current generated by the Na pump in eliminating the greater Na^+ load due to higher beating rates is apparently sufficient to make up for the relative lack of inward current due to absence or inhibition of repolarizing K^+ currents. The greater $[Ca^{2+}]_i$ seen at high rates may also enhance repolarizing currents (I_{to2}, $I_{Cl(Ca)}$, I_K) and prevent the low K^+ conductance state that serves as a substrate for EAD.

Delayed or Late Afterdepolarizations

Delayed (DADs) or late (LADs) afterdepolarizations are repolarizations that occur after the AP has fully repolarized, and may or may not reach the threshold for activation of a propagated AP and triggered ectopic beats. DADs have been observed in Purkinje fibers and in atrial and ventricular muscle (509). DADs themselves arise from an inward current that is distinct from the pacemaker currents discussed earlier, which is termed the transient inward current (284). The common feature of those settings in which DADs occur is circumstances that promote loading (or rather overloading) of SR intracellular Ca^{2+} stores (509). Digitalis and cardiac glycoside toxicity are well-known causes of DAD and triggered activity, first studied in detail in isolated cardiac tissues over 20 years ago (98,135,185). More recently, endogenous digitalis-like substances have been shown to induce DAD and triggered activity (256), the most notable being palmitoyl-L-carnitine (418). Cardiac glycosides cause DAD by inhibition of the Na pump, which leads to accumulation of intracellular Na^+ and reduction of the Na^+ gradient. The reduced driving force for Na^+ entry across the sarcolemma in turn diminishes Ca^{2+} extrusion from the cell by the Na-Ca exchanger. Catecholamines may also cause the necessary increase in intracellular Ca^{2+} for DAD to occur (384,509), by increasing $I_{Ca,L}$ and SR uptake of Ca^{2+}.

The transient inward current, also called an "internal oscillator" (464), then results from a sudden elevation in myoplasmic Ca^{2+} produced by the oscillatory release of Ca^{2+} from the overloaded sarcoplasmic reticulum, possibly due to Ca-induced Ca release (130,509). Evidence exists for at least three pathways by which the late release of Ca^{2+} can induce the transient depolarizing inward current: (a) increased myoplasmic Ca^{2+} activates an inward cation channel, whereby Na^+ entry down its concentration gradient depolarizes the cell; (b) increased myoplasmic Ca^{2+} gives rise to inward current through electrogenic Ca-Na exchange, the elimination of each Ca^{2+} resulting in three Na^+ entering with one net change (509); and (c) Ca^{2+} may activate $I_{Cl(Ca)}$, which can depolarize the cell toward E_{Cl} (40 mV). Such depolarizations have been observed in the absence of a functional Na-Ca exchanger (534). In contrast to EADs, DADs increase in amplitude with increased heart rate or prematurity of the prior impulses (508,509) due to increased Ca^{2+} entry associated with these interventions. In all these settings, the cell compensates by accumulating the excess Ca^{2+} in the SR. The ability of the DAD to reach threshold and trigger and AP appears to be augmented by reduced $[K^+]$, which decreases G_{K1} and enhances the depolarization caused by the transient inward current (157).

The arrhythmias seen with reperfusion of the myocardium seem to be initiated in the subendocardium, at the border of the reperfused zone. The overload of ischemic cells with Ca^{2+} upon reperfusion, in addition to enhanced catecholamine release, would be very likely to contribute to loading of Ca^{2+} stores and the initiation of LADs, leading to triggered arrhythmias. The mechanism does not appear to involve reentry in all cases, since there is no continuous activation between the preceding sinus beat and the subsequent ventricular tachycardia (VT). VT is maintained by both reentry and nonreentry (373).

During ischemia and the resulting acidosis, the increased intracellular H^+ is removed from the cell by the Na^+/H^+ antiport, increasing Na^+ entry and raising $[Na^+]_i$ (352,446). The decreased Na^+ gradient then results in less Ca^{2+} elimination and increased cellular dysfunction (173,410,446). Upon reperfusion, Ca^{2+} overload may also be exacerbated. Blockade of the antiport (causing worse acidosis) or blockade of other Na^+ by other routes actually proved beneficial (410,483). While there does not appear to be an increased I_{Na} (329), reduction of Na^+ entry can improve myocardial recovery (483) and prevent ventricular fibrillation (352,518). The Na^+ overload can then interfere with Ca^{2+} elimination, and worsen Ca^{2+} overload upon reperfusion (173,446). α_1-AR stimulation, which enhances the activity of Na^+/H^+ antiport, worsens reperfusion arrhythmias, and this effect can be blocked by inhibition of the antiport (517).

Loss of Membrane Potential

One of the common mechanisms underlying abnormal electrophysiologic processes is loss of membrane potential (LMP) in fast response fibers. With reduced Na^+ channel availability at depolarized levels of RMP, fewer Na^+ channels can be activated (Figs. 2 and 7). Thus, less Na^+ current is generated and conduction is slowed. AP upstroke velocity (V_{max} phase 0), overshoot, and amplitude are reduced and may approximate values measured in slow response fibers. LMP also affects AP repolarization, and may extend AP duration. Refractoriness in fast response cells with LMP may lag behind recovery of RMP, similar to slow response tissue. Finally, fast response cells with LMP are distinguished from cells found in transitional zones between working myocardium and the SA or AV nodes (532). Purkinje fibers with LMP are termed depressed fast response fibers. Because the pathophysiologic processes responsible for LMP are likely to be nonuniform, there is likely to be heterogeneous depression of the fast response (155,531). Therefore, depending on Na^+ channel availability, conduction velocities may be only somewhat reduced from those reported for fast response fibers, or more similar to those for slow response fibers. Similarly, there may be uneven prolongation of refractoriness. Thus, conduction of the depressed fast response fibers creates conditions that are favorable for reentrant excitation. LMP in fast response fibers may also contribute to early or delayed afterpotentials and triggering, or to abnormal forms of automaticity (155).

A primary mechanism causing loss of RMP is hyperkalemia, which can be readily induced in the myocardial interstitium by ischemia. While decreased activity of the Na^+/K^+-ATPase reduces reaccumulation of K^+ into myocytes, interstitial myocardial $[K^+]$ can rise rapidly during ischemia (e.g., 0.68 mM/minute), an effect that is in part due to activation of $I_{K,ATP}$ as cellular energy stores are depleted (502). The decreases in AP duration and amplitude and decreases in conduction velocity both in vivo and in vitro can be duplicated by infusion of elevated $[K^+]_o$ solution (145,415). Such partial depolarization as slowed conduction serves as a substrate for reentry and arrhythmias (see below).

Reentrant Excitation

During the normal heart beat, the propagating AP is extinguished after sequential activation of the atria and ventricles, either because it is surrounded by refractory tissue that has just been excited or because it encounters the inexcitable tissue (230). Reentrant excitation occurs when a propagating AP somehow persists to reexcite nonrefractory atrial or ventricular tissue (also termed reentry, circus movement, reciprocal beat, echo beat, or reciprocating tachycardia) (230,531). The basic criteria for ascribing an arrhythmia to reentry were first formulated by Mines (339,340) and are summarized as follows (11,230). First, an area of unidirectional block of conduction must be shown. Second, the reentry pathway must be defined; that is, movement of the excitatory wavefront should be observed to progress through the pathway, to return to its point of origin, and then again to follow the same pathway. Third, to rule out a focal origin (i.e., automatic, triggered), one must be able to terminate reentry by interrupting the circuit at some point. Two basic requirements for the initiation of reentrant arrhythmias are unidirectional block and slow conduction, and there are a number of different forms of reentry that have been described.

Unidirectional Block

Where there is rapid propagation of an impulse through tissue in which regional differences in the duration of refractory periods exist, propagation may fail in regions with the longest refractory periods (230). These regions will be available for reexcitation, provided that the appropriate conditions exist for the impulse to return to the site of former block. This reexcitation is unlikely in normal working myocardium, because even at fast heart rates there is substantial time during diastole when excitability is normal. However, the circumstances are more favorable during propagation of premature impulses, which may arise spontaneously or be induced by premature electrical stimulation. Reentry induced by premature beats is facilitated because refractory periods are shorter at short cycle lengths. Therefore, the pathways over which the impulse must propagate to return to the site of unidirectional block are shortened as well. In normal ventricular tissue it is difficult to produce sufficient nonuniformity with premature stimulation for unidirectional block (230), but by changing local temperature it is possible to produce the necessary increase in dispersion of refractoriness for reentry (275).

A site for unidirectional block could be present at the point where a thin bundle of cells inserts into a large muscle mass such as the Purkinje fiber–ventricular muscle junction (PFMJ) (230). While unidirectional block at the PFMJ has not been confirmed for normal fibers, the antegrade conduction delay at the PFMJ may be longer than the retrograde delay (319). However, with experimental interventions that inactivate Na^+ channels, antegrade block may occur while retrograde conduction is possible (i.e., unidirectional block) (333). Subsequent studies have shown that the PFMJ is better represented by a three-dimensional model of overlying two-dimensional sheets rather than a strand of terminal Purkinje fibers inserting into a three-dimensional ventricular muscle mass (480). Reasons for unidirectional block between Purkinje and ventricular muscle layers include differences in the excitability of the two layers, differences in thickness of the two layers, and increased coupling resistance at sites showing unidirectional block (240). Furthermore, sites where the cross-sectional area of interconnected cells suddenly increases may be sites for unidirectional block (230). An example is the junction of accessory pathways with ventricular muscle in patients with ventricular preexcitation (Wolff-Parkinson-White syndrome) (230). Experimental studies have shown that geometrical factors (e.g., fiber branching sites, junctions of separate muscle bundles) are an important cause for unidirectional block and reentry in cardiac tissue with uniform membrane properties (430,431). Finally, the way myocardial cells are connected to each other influences conduction velocity, with conduction velocity in the transverse direction about one-third that in the longitudinal direction (230,430).

Slow Conduction

One of the conditions required for reentry is sufficient delay of the propagating impulse in an alternate pathway to allow tissue proximal to the site of unidirectional block to recover from refractoriness (230). Therefore, reentry would be facilitated by conduction that was slower than normal. In fast response fibers, the speed of conduction is largely dependent on the magnitude of Na inward current during phase 0 of the AP. The magnitude of the Na inward current depends on the fraction of open Na channels, in turn determined by the level of membrane potential at which the AP is initiated and the time following initiation of the previous AP upstroke. Because time is needed for Na channels to recover from inactivation, the amplitude and upstroke velocities of premature APs initiated during repolarization are reduced and conduction velocity is low (Figs. 2 and 7). Reentry may occur during propagation of a premature AP in a region with different AP durations because of unidirectional block and slow conduction. Reentry may also occur in fibers with persistent low levels of membrane potential. At levels between -60 and -70 mV, about one-half the Na channels are inactivated (150). Recovery from inactivation after such an AP is prolonged, and may extend beyond full repolarization (156). Furthermore, reentry may occur in partially depolarized fast response fibers, even with normally propagated responses, when local differences in membrane potential give rise to areas of slow conduction intermingled with areas of conduction block. Finally, coupling resistance between adjacent cells is another factor that may affect the speed of conduction (230). As coupling resistance increases, conduction velocity decreases. Increased intracellular Ca^{2+} and acidosis are two factors that may increase coupling resistance (230).

Loss of RMP, as observed with increased $[K^+]$ as occurs with myocardial ischemia or hypoxia, is frequently responsible for slowed conduction. In settings of acute ischemia, such depolarization facilitates reentry and is the likely cause of arrhythmias (231,415). In the absence of reperfusion, the arrhythmias associated with ischemia per se do not appear to be mediated by Ca^{2+} overload and DAD triggering (278).

Reentry with an Anatomic Obstacle

Over 80 years ago Mines (339) proposed the simplest model of reentry in cardiac tissue, which involves a fixed anatomic obstacle. An important feature of this model of reentry was the existence of an excitable gap. The excitable gap implies that impulses originating outside the reentry circuit can penetrate the circuit and influence the reentrant rhythm (230). However, because normal pacemakers of the heart are usually overdriven during reentrant tachycardia, impulses used to penetrate the reentry circuit and terminate tachycardia must be supplied by external electrical stimuli or mechanical stimulation. There are several variations on reentry involving a fixed anatomic obstacle. Some investigators used alternating current or rapid atrial pacing to induce circus movement (atrial flutter) around the orifices of the vena cavae in dogs (291), but the question remained whether naturally occurring obstacles in the atria were large enough for sustained reentry to occur. It was further suggested that anisotropic conduction in the atria would remove the need for a large anatomic obstacle (368). It was believed that specialized intranodal pathways, with faster conduction velocities than surrounding atrial tissue, could form the loops necessary for reentry (368). It is now generally accepted that the anatomically discrete, intranodal, or interatrial conducting pathways are nonexistent. Nevertheless, preferential atrial conduction may occur because of geometric fiber arrangements within the atrial myocardium or differing electrophysiologic properties among fibers (9). Furthermore, the way myocardial cells are coupled influences conduction, with conduction faster in the direction of fiber orientation (230,430). This also could provide the anisotropy required for reentry (230). It has been postulated that the combination of an anatomic obstacle with an adjacent area of depressed conduction would facilitate reentry (5). Finally, changes in electrophysiologic properties may reduce the size of anatomic obstacle for reentry (230).

Reentry without an Anatomic Obstacle

Allessie and coworkers (3) induced circus movement tachycardia in small pieces of isolated left atria from rabbit hearts by a properly timed premature stimulus. In this preparation, no anatomic obstacles are present, and the reentrant circuit is completely defined by the electrophysiologic properties of the tissue involved. After the initial studies of Spach and coworkers (430,431) showing that anisotropic properties of cardiac muscle per se could provide the spatial nonuniformity required for reentry, a number of studies performed on reentry in a variety of cardiac tissues and models (230) described the characteristics of anisotropic reentry. Anisotropic reentry is functional in the sense that no gross anatomic obstacle is present. However, in contrast to the leading circle model, anisotropic reentry is characterized by the presence of a distinct excitable gap. The excitable gap is produced by changes in propagated AP duration at pivotal points within the reentry circuit (230) so that certain tissues may be excitable when nearby tissues are depolarized and can provide sufficient depolarizing current to activate an AP. When such temporal dispersion in AP duration and refractory period is produced experimentally in ventricular tissue, tachycardia can be induced by an appropriate single stimulation (275). Since hypoxia or ischemia results in AP shortening (245,461), regions of myocardium may be repolarized at times when other areas may remain depolarized (393). In hypertrophied myocardium, there is greater dispersion of refractory periods and greater vulnerability to ventricular fibrillation (268). When such dispersion is reduced by inhibition of K channels, ventricular vulnerability is reduced, while verapamil, which does not alter dispersion, does not reduce vulnerability.

Finally, reflection is a form of reentry occurring in a one-dimensional structure, where the impulse is conducted to and fro over the same pathway (230,394). The important result of studies such as these is that impulse propagation across a small (1–2 mm) segment of inexcitable tissue is discontinuous and can result in delays of one to several hundred milliseconds, the time required for proximal cells to recover their excitability and be available for reexcitation (230). Such a situation may exist in hearts with regional ischemia, where local inhomogeneities may give rise to conditions similar to those used in experimental models(199).

Because of the slow conduction and prolonged refractoriness, the SA and AV nodes are both natural sites for reentry. However, it has not been possible to produce sustained SA node reentry tachycardia in experimental models, although it has been possible to demonstrate circus movement (i.e., echo beats) (4). Nonetheless, there is clinical evidence that some clinical paroxysmal supraventricular tachycardias (PSVT) are due to SA node reentry. It is possible that with pathophysiologic alterations, the chances for sustained SA node reentry are enhanced (230). The AV node may be involved in reentry tachycardia in two ways. One requires participation of other tissues (i.e., the AV node is one part of a larger pathway); the other does not (230). In patients with ventricular preexcitation syndrome (Wolff-Parkinson-White syndrome), a type of PSVT, termed AV reciprocating tachycardia, is initiated by a properly timed atrial or ventricular premature beat that is blocked in one of the two AV connections (i.e., the AV node or accessory pathway). With AV reciprocating tachycardia, the reentrant pathway includes the atrium, AV node, ventricular specialized conducting system and myocardium, and accessory pathways. Reentry responsible for PSVT may also be confined to the AV node (331).

Reentry is probably the cause for many tachyarrhythmias, including both atrial and ventricular forms. However, it is difficult under in vivo experimental conditions or in humans to prove unequivocally that reentry exists. In intact heart or humans, a host of confounding variables could affect the in vitro mechanisms for reentry discussed above (230,531). Criteria that may be used to show that a particular tachyarrhythmia is due to reentry include the initiation or termination of tachycardia by pacing or extrastimulation, the demonstration of electrical activity spanning diastole, fixed coupling, and entrainment and resetting of tachycardia (531).

ANESTHETIC EFFECTS ON NORMAL AND ABNORMAL CONDUCTION

Local Anesthetic Actions

Following systemic absorption, excessive concentrations of local anesthetics are depressant to the cardiovascular system.

The primary site of action is the myocardium, but most produce arteriolar vasodilatation as well. Direct cardiovascular effects are usually apparent only after central nervous system toxicity, but this may not be the case with bupivacaine and etidocaine. The cardiac electrophysiologic actions of local anesthetics are most pronounced in fast response fibers such as atrial and ventricular muscle and Purkinje fibers, the cells with their action potential upstrokes largely dependent on the Na channel.

The dose of bupivacaine necessary to cause cardiovascular collapse in the sheep in the presence of hypoxia and acidosis was about half that required for lidocaine (345). Additionally, the mean dose of bupivacaine causing vascular collapse was significantly lower in pregnant versus nonpregnant ewes (345). In normocarbic cats, subconvulsant doses of bupivacaine produced a nodal and ventricular arrhythmias, whereas convulsant doses of lidocaine did not (99). Cardiac toxicity with bupivacaine in dogs included increased atrial conduction time and AV nodal refractoriness, decreased left ventricular contractility, ventricular tachyarrhythmias, and electromechanical dissociation (209). In isolated rat hearts, bupivacaine was more potent than lidocaine in decreasing the atrial rate and delaying atrioventricular conduction (262). In isolated guinea pig hearts bupivacaine was six to ten times more potent than lidocaine in decreasing heart rate, contractility, and myocardial oxygen consumption (447). In in vitro studies acidosis and hypoxia enhance the bradycardic effects of bupivacaine more than lidocaine (53,396,436). Additionally, hypercapnic acidosis and hypoxia slowed SA node rate in the neonatal and adult guinea pig hearts, the effect of which was additive to that produced by lidocaine and bupivacaine (53). However neither hypoxia nor acidosis alone appear sufficient to alter local anesthetic–induced depression (436). Finally, combined hypoxia and acidosis cause a greater effect in sinus rate in neonatal compared to adult guinea pig hearts.

The cardiovascular effects of equipotent doses of lidocaine and bupivacaine were examined for neural blockade following intravascular injection into chronically instrumented sheep (266). While animals convulsed with both drugs, serious arrhythmias were seen only with bupivacaine and transient S-T changes or sinus tachycardia with lidocaine. In a subsequent study, also in sheep, bupivacaine cardiotoxicity was enhanced by hypercarbia, acidosis, and hypoxia (392). Thus, evidence from both in vitro and in vivo animal studies suggest that hypoxia and acidosis, which could result from CNS and circulatory depression with bupivacaine, would increase the likelihood of serious arrhythmias following inadvertent intravascular injection of bupivacaine.

Many of the arrhythmic effects of bupivacaine and lidocaine can be explained by the modulated receptor hypothesis (79,80). According to this hypothesis, different local anesthetics block Na channels by binding to a common receptor site. bupivacaine and possibly lidocaine may also exert a weak Ca channel blocking action based on their ability to depress myocardial slow action potentials (88,208,302). Drug affinity for the Na channel receptor site is determined by the state of the channel, which could be resting, open, or inactivated. Rate constants defining association and dissociation of a drug from its receptors are different for each channel state and different drugs. In ventricular myocytes Na channels are blocked by local anesthetics in the open and inactivated states; the resting state displays the least affinity for local anesthetics (79). Lidocaine, a smaller and less lipid soluble molecule than bupivacaine, rapidly blocks Na channels in both open and inactivated states. Lidocaine, compared to bupivacaine, binds more loosely and exhibits less block of the Na channels at faster heart rates (use dependence). Bupivacaine has also been shown to block Na channels in the inactivated state much more avidly than lidocaine and has a low affinity for open and rested Na channels (80). Because bupivacaine is so tightly bound to inactivated Na channels, the half-life for recovery from block during the resting state is much longer. Consequently, at intermediate heart rates, Na channel block by bupivacaine can accumulate. This could explain the greater occurrence of cardiac conduction and rhythm disturbances with bupivacaine at doses that produce comparable neurotoxic symptoms to lidocaine.

The cardiac electrophysiologic effects of bupivacaine and lidocaine that might contribute to reentrant arrhythmias were investigated in a rabbit Purkinje fiber ventricular muscle preparation (344). High concentrations of bupivacaine but not lidocaine reduced maximum diastolic potential in Purkinje fibers, but not in ventricular muscle. Both bupivacaine and lidocaine reduced action potential upstroke velocity and amplitude in Purkinje and ventricular muscle fibers, but reductions were greater with bupivacaine. Both drugs produced comparable shortening of action potential duration and increases in effective refractory period–action potential duration ratio. However, while Purkinje fiber to ventricular muscle (P-M) conduction time was increased by both local anesthetics, bupivacaine produced P-M block in 90 to 100% of the preparations, while P-M block occurred in only one preparation with lidocaine. Finally, recovery of excitability and return to control values for P-M conduction time with bupivacaine took four to eight times longer than with lidocaine. These alterations in electrical properties of Purkinje and ventricular muscle fibers were interpreted by the authors as conducive to reentrant ventricular arrhythmias. Indeed, its prolonged Na channels blockade is similar to class IC arrhythmias, known to induce wide QRS complex ventricular tachycardias (290).

While attention has focused on the Na channel blocking properties, bupivacaine also blocks I_{to} (75). Such blockade of a K^+ current may contribute to prolongation and dispersion of AP durations through the ventricular wall and increase the risk of ventricular tachycardia. The arrhythmias seen with bupivacaine toxicity have sometimes been torsades de pointes (250), seen with type IA antiarrhythmias such as quinidine (290), which has also been shown to depress I_{to} as well as other K channels (521). Consequently, the proarrhythmic action of bupivacaine may represent a combined type IA and IC antiarrhythmic toxicity.

The management of cardiac toxicity following massive doses of bupivacaine were evaluated by Kasten and Martin (249,250). It was shown that bretylium was effective against inducible ventricular tachycardia in bupivacaine-treated dogs. Furthermore, the cardiovascular collapse following bupivacaine occurred either as sustained ventricular tachycardia or, more commonly, bradycardia with electromechanical dissociation. All animals could be resuscitated with bretylium or epinephrine and atropine. While the doses of epinephrine and atropine used by Kasten and Martin (249) for resuscitation were much greater than those recommended for cardiopulmonary resuscitation (84), one report suggests that higher than recommended doses of epinephrine may be effective for some resuscitations (265).

While most of the attempts to treat bupivacaine cardiac toxicity have been varied and controversial (243,250,251,276,314) and not very successful, they have focused on the role of Na channels to explain suppression of cardiac action potential conduction. Agents that alter the duration of the plateau phase of the cardiac action potential may affect the toxicity of the bupivacaine because bupivacaine-induced block of cardiac Na channels develops mostly during the action potential plateau when Na channels are inactivated (80), an effect potentiated by the I_{to} blockade. Shortening of action potential duration and hyperpolarization of resting membrane potential have been suggested as potentially effective approaches in the treatment of bupivacaine-induced cardiac toxicity (80). These mechanisms may be responsible for the partial reversal of bupivacaine-induced AV block observed in a study using pinacidil and bimakalim (48). Because bupivacaine-induced block of cardiac Na channels develops primarily during the action potential plateau when Na channels are in an inactive state, these K_{ATP} channel openers could reduce the Na channel block due to bupivacaine by attenuating the plateau phase of action potential in the AV conduction system. The K_{ATP} channel openers could also be effective if they hyperpolarize AV nodal cells.

The attenuating effects of the K_{ATP} channel openers on bupivacaine-induced AV conduction block were reversed completely by glibenclamide, a specific blocker of ATP-dependent K channels (139). This indicates that the major mechanism of action of these compounds is through ATP-sensitive K channels. The presence of this specific K channel in AV nodal cells has also been confirmed (242). It remains to be determined whether any beneficial effects of clinically safe concentrations of K_{ATP} channel openers can be used to treat bupivacaine-induced cardiac toxicity in vivo. Because bupivacaine and other K_{ATP} channel openers individually produce cardiac depression and coronary vasodilation, treatment of bupivacaine-induced cardiac toxicity with K_{ATP} channel openers, although improving AV conduction, might worsen cardiac depression and cause excessive coronary vasodilation.

The central neurogenic action of local anesthetics may also contribute to the local anesthetic cardiotoxicity (196,453). The investigators have injected saline and local anesthetics bupivacaine, lidocaine, and procaine at approximately equipotent neural blocking doses into the right lateral cerebral ventricle of chronically instrumented cats (196). Additional cats were given intravenous bupivacaine to determine whether electrocardiographic ECG changes following intracerebroventricular (ICV) infusion of bupivacaine were due to a direct cardiac action following systemic absorption. No arrhythmias (sinus tachycardia excluded) were observed after the ICV infusion of saline or bupivacaine. One of six (lidocaine), five of seven (procaine), and 10 of 10 cats (bupivacaine) developed ventricular arrhythmias following ICV infusion. It was speculated that the similarity between these CNS effects of local anesthetics and digitalis and suggested that a common neuroexcitatory mechanism could involve central adrenergic stimulation (196). The concomitant cardiovascular and CNS toxicity with bupivacaine or lidocaine were also considered (453). Equimolar amounts of either drug were injected into one of three discrete medullary vasomotor centers in adult chloral hydrate–anesthetized rats. At any of these areas both local anesthetics produce bradycardia and hypotension. In addition, when they were injected at the nucleus tractus solitarius, ventricular arrhythmias were observed in 55% of animals. In all animals with lidocaine, arrhythmias spontaneously reverted to sinus rhythm. With bupivacaine, arrhythmias reverted to sinus rhythms in half of the animals but were fatal in others. Several explanations were offered for these findings. First, the modulated receptor hypothesis explains both cardiovascular and CNS toxicity with local anesthetics. Second convulsions with the local anesthetics might alter blood-brain barrier permeability and enhance their uptake into cardiovascular regulatory centers. Third, the antiarrhythmic action of lidocaine might oppose centrally stimulated arrhythmias due to lidocaine toxicity. Fourth, greater accumulation of bupivacaine in the brain during convulsions might explain the nearly simultaneous CNS and cardiovascular toxicity.

GENERAL ANESTHETIC EFFECTS ON NORMAL AND ABNORMAL CONDUCTION

Supraventricular Impulse Initiation and Conduction

Inhalational anesthetics halothane, enflurane, and isoflurane were shown to directly depress SA nodal automaticity (Fig. 13) in a manner antagonized by increasing extracellular Ca^{2+} (51). These actions are consistent with anesthetic depression of T- and L-type Ca^{2+} currents in Purkinje and ventricular myocytes (54,129), although no studies have directly examined anesthetic effects on the pacemaker current (I_f) underlying automatic phase 4 diastolic depolarization in SA nodal or Purkinje fibers. Similar slowing of the primary SA pacemaker is observed during anesthesia relative to conscious controls in the presence of pharmacologic autonomic blockade (14). The direct actions of halothane on the action potentials of atrial muscle fibers (189,204) include depression of the plateau and

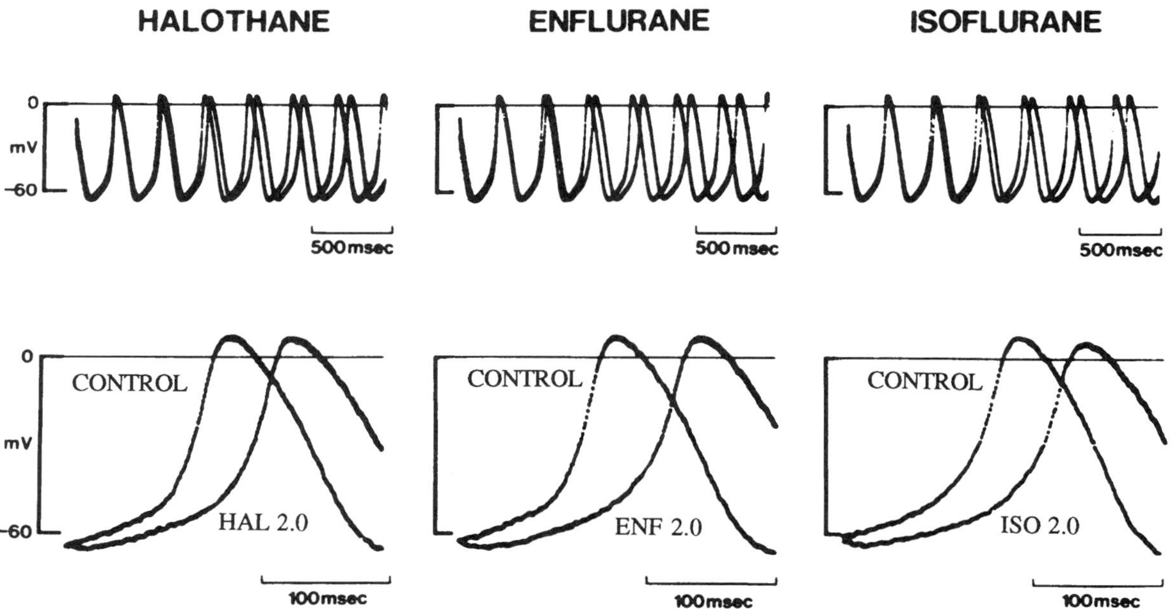

Figure 13. The effects of halothane, enflurane, and isoflurane on the action potentials of spontaneously active fibers in the guinea pig SA nodal region. The action potential tracings of the control and after 5 minutes of the exposure to anesthetics (2 MAC) are superimposed at two different speeds and magnifications. (From ref. 51, with permission.)

slight prolongation of terminal repolarization, while those of enflurane and isoflurane have not been reported. The effects of halothane, enflurane, and isoflurane anesthesia on specialized atrial and AV nodal refractory periods and AV nodal conduction time are influenced substantially by indirect changes in autonomic activity, are highly dependent on the specific model employed (paced or spontaneous), and suggest potential modest direct anesthetic effect increasing refractoriness and AV conduction delay that may be masked in vivo by other adrenergic- and reflex-mediated effects (12,19–21). No study has directly examined anesthetic actions on the action potential characteristics of AV nodal cells.

Depression of SA nodal automaticity by inhalational anesthetics in combination with changes in cardiac autonomic activity may be related to the emergence of subsidiary pacemaker function and atrial arrhythmias in patients without known heart disease. Normally the intrinsically more rapid rate of automatic phase 4 depolarization of the primary SA nodal pacemaker fibers maintains "dominance" over other potential sites of automaticity (atrial, AV junctional, and ventricular Purkinje fibers exhibiting spontaneous phase 4 diastolic depolarization) by a mechanism known as "overdrive inhibition" (478). The consequence of more frequent depolarization of subsidiary pacemakers by the SA node is an increased Na^+ influx and K^+ efflux per unit of time. This produces relative activation of the electrogenic Na^+-K^+ pump and outward hyperpolarizing current that increases the maximum diastolic potential (more negative) and reduces the slope of phase 4 depolarization of subsidiary automatic fibers. On cessation of overdrive Na^+ influx decreases, intracellular Na^+ falls, pump current decreases, and the membrane potential during the pause gradually returns toward threshold with resumption of spontaneous activity at a low rate that gradually increases to the rate present before overdrive. Thus, anesthetic depression of SA nodal automaticity, assuming less depression of automaticity or greater anesthetic inhibition of hyperpolarization by the Na^+-K^+ pump mechanism (377) in other portions of the conduction system, may permit escape of subsidiary pacemakers from SA nodal dominance.

Some early studies of myocardial sensitization by anesthetics to the arrhythmogenic effects of epinephrine (387,465) noted the occurrence of abnormal supraventricular foci in atrial and ECG recordings just prior to onset of ventricular arrhythmias. Atlee and Malkinson (16) characterized these shifts of activity (subsidiary atrial or wandering pacemaker, atrial ectopy, AV dissociation) as arrhythmias of "development" and demonstrated that they occur at lower doses of epinephrine than ventricular arrhythmias both with the more "sensitizing" agent halothane as well as with enflurane and isoflurane (17). In superfused atrial preparations, halothane, enflurane, and isoflurane produce a noncompetitive rightward shift in the positive chronotropic response of the SA node to epinephrine and isoproterenol (437). In addition, in atrial preparations perfused through the SA nodal artery, low concentrations of both epinephrine and norepinephrine, either with or without halothane, frequently shift the site of earliest activation to subsidiary atrial pacemaker locations along the sulcus terminalis (374). These studies, suggesting that catecholamines may augment automaticity of subsidiary atrial pacemakers more so than the SA node, were also performed in a chronically instrumented dog model (485,510). The results of these studies indicate that halothane and enflurane, but not isoflurane, "sensitize" the heart to atrial arrhythmias compared to awake control responses, increasing the degree or severity of shifts to subsidiary sites, including the His bundle, for a given epinephrine dose. In addition, they suggest that baroreceptor mediated vagal inhibition of the SA node contributes to such shifts in the conscious state and at lower compared to higher halothane concentrations.

The role of atrial arrhythmia development as a harbinger or contributor to generation of more severe arrhythmias (ventricular ectopy, bigeminy, and ventricular tachycardia) with anesthetics and catecholamines is unknown. Simultaneous β-adrenergic-mediated effects of catecholamines on AV conduction may include abbreviation of AV nodal conduction time at rapid atrial rates and shortening of the AV nodal functional refractory period, the minimum coupling interval or most premature response conducted to the His bundle (134,330,343). These actions of epinephrine during anesthesia may potentially result in conduction of irregularly coupled supraventricular activity through the AV node and the His-Purkinje system to the myocardium earlier during the relative refractory period than would be expected without adrenergic facilitation of AV conduction. Moe et al. (343) observed in pentobarbital anesthetized dogs that actions of epinephrine on AV nodal refractoriness and conduction of premature atrial responses could produce aberrant ventricular conduction at rapid pacing rates in animals that usually only exhibit functional bundle branch block at low pacing rates. The importance of this "filtering" function of the AV node in preventing premature excitation of the ventricles during the vulnerable period is exemplified in certain animal models (neonatal goats, pigs) lacking normal AV nodal conduction delays that exhibit ventricular tachycardia or fibrillation induced by premature atrial stimuli (378).

Halothane and enflurane were shown to cause similar, dose-dependent prolongation of atrioventricular (AV) nodal conduction time and refractoriness (18–20), but atrial refractoriness appears less affected by increasing halothane (19,20). Other investigators found no effect of increasing isoflurane on AV nodal conduction time (47). The effects of halothane, enflurane, and isoflurane were examined on supraventricular conduction and refractoriness in chronically instrumented dogs (13). Compared to awake animals, AV nodal conduction time is prolonged in anesthetized dogs by about 20% with 1.6 minimal alveolar concentrations of enflurane and halothane. The prolongation was less, however, with isoflurane (12). While no data exist for anesthetic effects on specialized cardiac conduction and refractoriness in humans, animal studies suggest that none of the contemporary inhalation anesthetics are likely to be a cause for second- or third-degree AV block in the absence of intrinsic conduction system disease or drugs that prolong AV conduction time. Furthermore, anesthetic effects on functional properties of the AV node in the clinical setting are likely to be affected by autonomic compensatory mechanisms, while those on the ventricular conduction and refractoriness are less likely to be so affected (87).

Ventricular Impulse Initiation and Conduction

Early studies have shown that halothane depresses automaticity in pacemakers of the ventricular specialized conducting system (Purkinje fibers) (296,386). Recently, the effects of halothane, enflurane, and isoflurane on automaticity and recovery of automaticity from overdrive suppression were determined in canine Purkinje fibers derived from normal hearts (280). It was concluded that all three volatile anesthetics at clinically relevant concentrations increased the rate of automaticity of normal Purkinje fibers exposed to epinephrine, and that this increase is explained by enhanced phase 4 depolarization. In addition, recovery of automaticity from overdrive suppression is enhanced by enflurane but is little affected by halothane and isoflurane.

Halothane was shown to produce larger decreases of Purkinje fiber action potential duration (APD) as compared to ventricular fiber APD, a reduction of the rate of phase 0 depolarization (V_{max}) at higher concentrations in both tissues, and prolongation of conduction times in Purkinje fibers (189). These actions of halothane have subsequently been confirmed both in vitro and in vivo. Compared to conscious controls, halothane, enflurane, and isoflurane slightly (5–10%) and similarly prolong ventricular conduction intervals measured utilizing His bundle recordings with little added depression at high compared to lower concentrations (10,12,14,18,19,474). The prolongation of conduction intervals was not shown to be rate dependent (15,474). In Purkinje fibers the depression of conduction velocity by high concentrations of halothane may be related to reduction of the peak inward Na^+ current (66,216). Additional actions increasing longitudinal resistance (188) and depressing cell-to-cell coupling at cardiac gap junctions (70,353,449) may contribute to more marked depression of conduction at Purkinje fiber–muscle junctions (147), sites of intrinsically poor cell coupling (239,381). In contrast to Purkinje fibers, a similar study of conduction in ventricular muscle fibers (362) indicated that halothane and enflurane depress conduction velocity with less influence on V_{max}, again suggesting an important anesthetic influence on cell-to-cell coupling that could potentially affect anisotropic propagation in cardiac muscle, the variation of conduction velocity with the direction of propagation.

At constant heart rate, APD and refractory periods are longer in certain regions of the His-Purkinje system (the false tendons) than in the endocardium, longer in the endocardium than epicardium, and longer in the epicardium at the apex than at the base of the heart (Figs. 6 and 9) (23,67,176, 332,343). The refractory periods of the bundle branches shorten more than those of the myocardium at higher steady-state rate (176), and both Purkinje and myocardial fibers exhibit alternans of APD (alternating short and long durations that are damped over time) at rapid stimulation rates and after abrupt changes in rate before reaching steady-state values (397,448). In addition, at high compared to low steady-state rates there is decreased dispersion of myocardial refractory periods (174,393), a major determinant of vulnerability fibrillation during the relative refractory period (175). Finally, the refractoriness of the myocardium can also be influenced importantly by mechanical factors such as volume loading and dilation, which can heterogeneously shorten refractory periods and increase vulnerability to induction of arrhythmias (383). Therefore, the significance of anesthetic shortening of refractory periods in ventricular tissues and their potential relationship to the occurrence of reentry may involve complex indirect as well as direct effects of anesthesia on heart rate, cardiac autonomic efferent activity, and hemodynamic changes that may not be readily assessed in vitro.

At constant stimulation rate, volatile anesthetics decrease Purkinje fiber APD in the false tendons more so than in apical fibers exhibiting shorter APD, and at equianesthetic concentrations the actions of enflurane and isoflurane decrease false tendon fiber APD more so than halothane, as shown in Fig. 14 (375). Although the actions of enflurane and isoflurane on refractoriness in the His-Purkinje system in vivo have not been determined, halothane was found to decrease refractoriness in the bundle branches at high compared to lower concentrations and more so at low- than high-paced rate (474). Myocardial fibers are less sensitive than Purkinje fibers to anesthetic effects on refractory characteristics (189) and the comparative effects of volatile anesthetics on the APD of myocardial fibers are not well established. It was reported (189) that 2% halothane decreased APD and the effective refractory period of sheep myocardial fibers, while other investigators (307) have noted shortening of APD with 3% halothane in the guinea pig. Enflurane at high concentrations (3%) decreases APD (306), while isoflurane increases APD in guinea pig papillary muscles (303). No studies have systematically examined actions of volatile anesthetics on myocardial repolarization in the normal heart in vivo compared to the awake control state. It was observed that following cardiac denervation in dogs, chloroform added to basal pentobarbital anesthesia prolongs the duration and increases the dispersion of myocardial refractory periods (175). Denniss et al. (105) reported that 2% halothane increased myocardial effective refractory periods relative to awake control values, without change of QT intervals or vulnerability to induction of tachyarrhythmias by programmed stimulation techniques. Similar refractory period prolongation by halothane was observed in the nonischemic zone of animals with chronic infarction and is a major mechanism responsible for reduction of the inducibility of ventricular tachycardia in this model (105,107,151,213). Recent studies clearly indicate that halothane, isoflurane, and enflurane have an important direct effects on myocardial repolarization as manifested by prolongation of the QT or QT_c intervals in animal models following pharmacologic autonomic nervous system blockade, and similar actions have been reported in human studies during anesthesia (389,408). The mechanism underlying anesthetic actions on the uniformity of myocardial repolarization, reflected by the QT interval, is not known but may involve changes in activation time due to slowing of conduction in the Purkinje system and myocardium as well as potential differ-

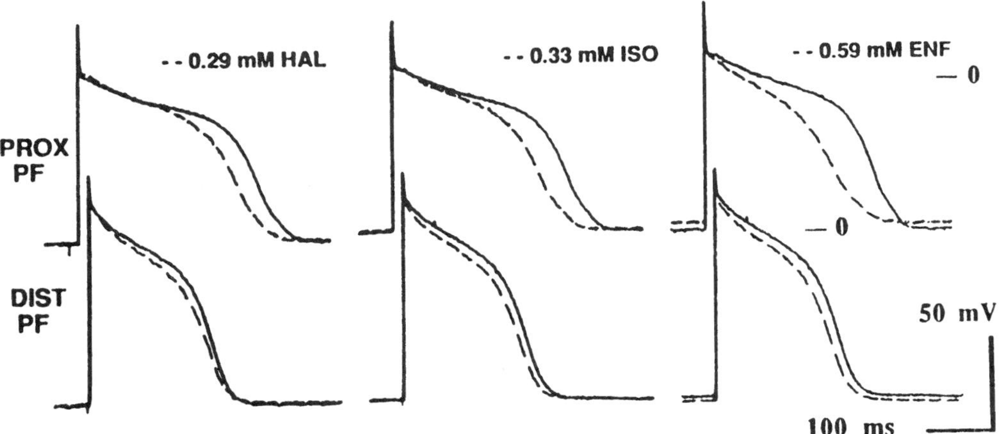

Figure 14. Simultaneously recorded single proximal (PROX.) and distal (DIST.) Purkinje fiber action potentials from the dog under control conditions *(solid tracings)* and after exposure *(dashed tracings)* to halothane (HAL), isoflurane (ISO), and enflurane (ENF). Each anesthetic produces a larger decrease of proximal than distal fiber action potential duration. (From ref. 375, with permission.)

ences of anesthetic actions on repolarization of myocardial fibers in different regions of the heart.

Anesthetic-Catecholamine Interaction

Despite the many studies over the years of the possible mechanisms underlying this adverse interaction, the cellular electrophysiologic basis for the occurrence of cardiac arrhythmias in association with endogenously released or exogenously administered catecholamines during inhalational anesthesia remains unclear (55).

The ability of some anesthetics to reduce the dose of epinephrine required to induce ventricular arrhythmias (363), which is usually measured as an infusion rate or product of rate time duration, is a classic example of an adverse drug interaction. The electrophysiologic basis for this phenomenon, referred to as sensitization, as well as the mechanisms generating the arrhythmias, remains unknown. Although the arrhythmogenic dose of epinephrine (ADE) in the conscious canine model is about 35 μg/kg, and about 5 μg/kg during 1.25 minimum alveolar concentration (MAC) halothane anesthesia (236), the corresponding arrhythmogenic plasma concentrations (APC) of epinephrine with threshold doses in the awake control state have not been reported. Doses and APC of epinephrine in neurally intact ventilated dogs with different types of anesthesia have been reported (193–195,438). These studies indicate that the epinephrine required to produce this particular arrhythmia end point (≥4 PVC/15 sec) varies over about a 10- to 20-fold range with different anesthetics. Other reports indicate that the range of doses producing different types of arrhythmias, e.g., atrial arrhythmias versus PVCs versus ventricular bigeminy, tachycardia or fibrillation, is also reduced with more sensitizing agents (16,17), although the APC of epinephrine for different types of arrhythmias has not been reported.

It was reported that the phenomenon of sensitization to the arrhythmogenic effects of catecholamines occurs at remarkably low anesthetic concentrations. For instance, it was shown that relative to a nonsensitizing etomidate basal anesthetic (335), halothane produces a dose-related fourfold reduction of APC of epinephrine at halothane concentrations of 0 to 0.5 vol%, with little or no additional reduction at higher concentrations (194). The same group reported about an eightfold reduction of APC by thiopental (195), again relative to basal etomidate anesthesia, at plasma thiopental concentrations up to about 50 μg/ml, a concentration estimated to be equivalent to about 1 MAC of inhalational anesthesia. These studies suggest that (a) the direct electrophysiologic actions of volatile anesthetics on cardiac tissues, including their actions on transmembrane potentials and ionic currents, automaticity, and conduction that generally occur at concentrations ≥0.5 MAC, may be less important in the phenomenon of sensitization than neural influences at low anesthetic concentrations; and (b) that direct anesthetic effects may only influence the underlying mechanisms generating arrhythmias at higher concentrations. Recent reports that the central α_2-agonist dexmedetomidine and the imidazoline α_2-antagonist atipamezole, agents that alter the balance of central vagosympathetic outflow, substantially (two- to threefold) increase and decrease, respectively, the APC of epinephrine during halothane anesthesia (191,192). These studies strongly suggest that reflex-mediated changes in cardiac autonomic efferent activity have an important influence on the arrhythmic doses of epinephrine during anesthesia, and probably in the awake control state as well.

The role of blood pressure and heart rate was examined in thiopental-halothane anesthetized, vagotomized dogs; it was found that either increasing atrial pacing rate or elevation of blood pressure by aortic occlusion consistently induced bigeminy with fixed coupling intervals during subthreshold infusions of epinephrine (529). In addition, increasing atrial pacing rate could both induce and "overdrive" the arrhythmia at higher rate, suggesting a reentrant mechanism rather than a triggered arrhythmia, and sustained bigeminy could be converted to sinus rhythm by stimulation of the right vagus nerve during atrial pacing. However, other studies in neurally intact halothane-anesthetized dogs (without thiopental) suggest no pressure dependence, based on the observation that artificially reducing the blood pressure response with nitroprusside does not elevate the arrhythmogenic dose of epinephrine (323). However, other investigators found that elevating blood pressure with angiotensin II largely substitutes for the pressure elevation due to phenylephrine in the production of arrhythmias by isoproterenol with halothane (193). In this study, rapid atrial pacing did not substitute for the presence of isoproterenol in production of arrhythmias by phenylephrine, suggesting that increased rate may not play an important role in the halothane-epinephrine interaction.

The relative contribution of cardiac β_1- and α_1-adrenergic receptor activation on the ADE during halothane anesthesia was reported by Maze and Smith (323). The threshold dose was elevated 13-fold by the α_1-antagonist prazocin but only an estimated fivefold by β_1-adrenergic blockade with metoprolol. Subsequent studies by the same group (433) demonstrated a strong correlation between the individual ADE during halothane anesthesia and responsiveness to the pressor effects of phenylephrine, but no correlation between ADE and responsiveness to the positive chronotropic effects of isoproterenol. In addition, α_1-adrenergic blockade (droperidol or doxazosin) produced dose-related elevation of the ADE with halothane, strongly suggesting an important contribution of cardiac α_1-adrenergic receptor activation to induction of halothane-epinephrine arrhythmias (322). Furthermore, it was suggested that full expression of catecholamine-induced arrhythmias during halothane anesthesia requires activation of both α_1- and β-adrenergic receptors in the heart and that the adrenergic mechanism involves a synergistic interaction between both receptors as assessed by simultaneous administration of the agonists phenylephrine and isoproterenol (193).

Some of the recent efforts have been directed toward examining the possible role of abnormal conduction in the Purkinje system with halothane and catecholamines (486). This role was suggested by earlier findings that halothane slows conduction and shortens refractory periods in the conduction system (474) and that α- and β-adrenergic effects of sympathetic efferent activity produce nonuniform refractory period changes in the conduction system in vivo (473). In addition, one older report of Reynolds and Chiz (385) indicated that an a-adrenergic effect of epinephrine (4.5 mM) potentiated the modest slowing of conduction produced by halothane in Purkinje fibers. The interaction of catecholamines and anesthetics on Purkinje fiber conduction is readily examined in vitro by measuring the conduction time between action potentials recorded from false tendon fibers several millimeters apart in a fast-flow low-volume tissue chamber (486). Epinephrine did not significantly influence conduction velocity, while halothane alone produces slight (<3%) slowing and a decrease of action potential duration relative to drug free control. However epinephrine with halothane produces marked transient depression of conduction (-17%) without significant reduction of the rate of phase 0 depolarization (V_{max}), a major determinant of conduction velocity. Compared to halothane, smaller depression of conduction is observed with isoflurane, and with norepinephrine in the presence of either halothane or isoflurane, although again to a lesser degree than with epinephrine. Figure 15 shows the effect of changing the order of administration of high doses of halothane and epinephrine on conduction velocity. Epinephrine alone induces minimal biphasic changes of conduction velocity, while halothane added with continued epinephrine exposure decreased velocity to about 1.8 m/s from a control of 2.1 m/s. However, the usual clinical order of administration produced markedly different effects. Halothane alone decreased the velocity to about 1.9 m/s, while epinephrine added in the presence of halothane transiently decreases conduction velocity to about 1.3 m/s within 3 to 5 min, with return to 1.7 m/s by 20 min in the presence of both anesthetic and catecholamine. Thus, this negative dromotropic interaction is characterized by (a) depression of conduction velocity with the combination of epinephrine and halothane, regardless of order, to a steady-state value (about 1.75 m/s at 40 min) that differs from the additive effects of either epinephrine (minimal) or halothane (moderate) alone; and (b) substantially greater transient depression of conduction when the catecholamine is administered to fibers previously exposed to the anesthetic. The time course of this interaction suggests two competing processes: one rapid and transiently slowing conduction within a few minutes, similar to the time of onset of halothane-epinephrine arrhythmias in vivo, and the other gradually returning conduction velocity to more normal values over 10 to 15 minutes despite continued exposure to both agents. In addition, the marked decrease and gradual increase of velocity due to epinephrine after halothane appears similar to the small negative and positive changes of conduction velocity produced by epinephrine alone. This observation suggests that the negative dromotropic interaction may represent an amplification of a "normal" effect of high epinephrine doses, rather than potentiation by epinephrine of the modest slowing of conduction produced by halothane.

The latest in vitro results indicate that the depression of conduction is not attenuated by either β_1- (metoprolol) or β_1- and β_2- (propranolol) adrenergic receptor blockade, that the responses are completely attenuated by the α_1 antagonist prazocin, and that similar slowing of conduction occurs with the α_1-agonist phenylephrine but not with the α_2-agonist clonidine (487). Figure 16 illustrates the responses of the nadir of conduction velocity slowing (open circles) with epinephrine at high halothane concentration (0.7 mM, about 3 MAC). The depression of conduction velocity by epinephrine is dose related and produces about a 20% depression (to 1.7 m/s), relative to halothane alone (1.9 m/s), at a concentration of epinephrine (0.2 mM) comparable to arrhythmogenic plasma concentrations in vivo. This action is attenuated by the α_1-subtype antagonist WB4101 more so than by CEC (472), indicating that the modulation of conduction by epinephrine with halothane involves activation of the same α_1-WB4101–sensitive adrenoceptor as that which has been reported to increase Purkinje fiber APD and automaticity. Under steady-state conditions (at 150 bpm), the degree of conduction slowing in the false tendons is only modest (-5% relative to halothane) with 0.2 mM epinephrine and 1.7 MAC halothane, and conduction block does not occur even at unphysiologic concentrations of epinephrine (5 mM) and halothane (2.75%). It appears that the a_1-mediated negative dromotropic effect of epinephrine would not contribute to arrhythmias in the absence of anesthetics and that it may produce only minimal depression of conduction in combination with subanesthetic (0.5%) sensitizing concentrations of halothane. On the other hand, this action at higher epinephrine and halothane concentrations, by delaying endocardial activation by impulses descending through different parts of the His-Purkinje system, may contribute to increased disparity of repolarization times in the conduction system and myocardium and thereby potentially facilitate abnormal conduction and generation of reentrant ventricular tachycardia or fibrillation by single premature ventricular impulses.

The mechanisms by which halothane and activation of the α_1-WB4101-sensitive adrenergic receptor depress conduction are not known but may involve a combination of actions on active (largely peak Na^+ current) and passive (membrane capacitance, intracellular and gap junctional resistance) membrane properties that determine conduction velocity. Because the depression of conduction occurs without large changes in V_{max}, modulation of cell-to-cell coupling may be involved (147). Actions of halothane that could contribute to slowing of conduction include inhibition of inward Na^+ currents (66,216), increased membrane capacitance and longitudinal resistance (188), and reduction of gap junctional conductance (70,449). In addition, it is possible that indirect anesthetic actions on second messengers levels, reducing cAMP and increasing cGMP (203,488,489) in combination with adrenergic effects, may affect Na^+ channel activity (411) or modulate gap junctional conductance and cell-to-cell coupling (69,104).

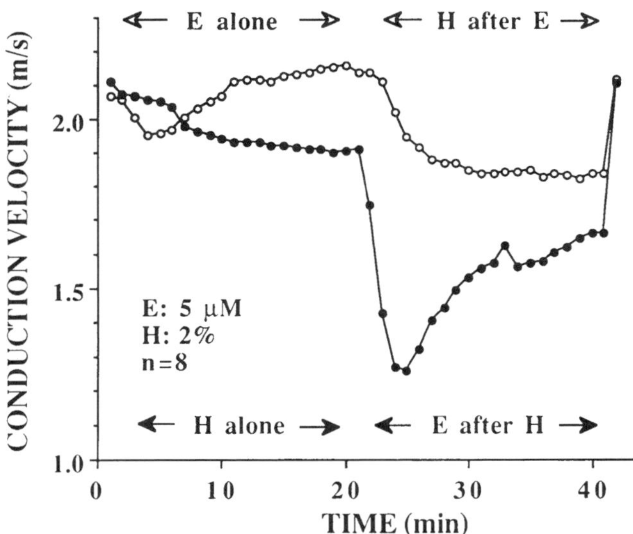

Figure 15. Changes of canine Purkinje fiber conduction velocity in one group of preparations after the addition of epinephrine (E) alone, followed by halothane (H) in the presence of E, compared to H alone and E in the presence of H. Standard deviations were omitted for clarity. Differences of mean conduction velocity between times of > 0.08 m/s were significant at p <.05. (From ref. 467, with permission.)

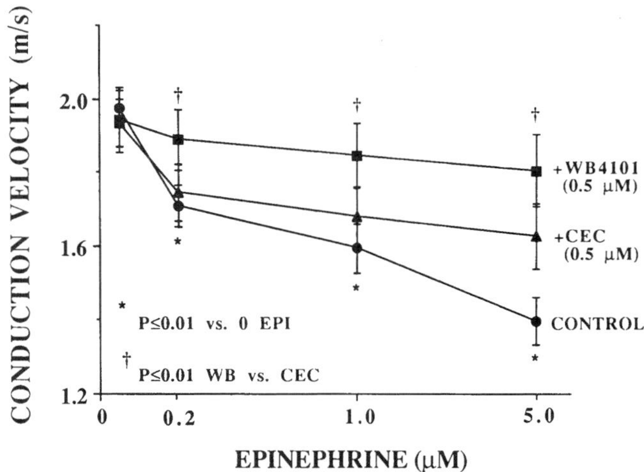

Figure 16. Average peak depressions of canine Purkinje fiber conduction velocity at 2–5 min of epinephrine (EPI) administration in the presence of high halothane (0.7 mM or 3 MAC). The Krebs' solution contained 0.2 μM propranolol. The responses of 12 preparations are compared to control (0 EPI). Thereafter, two groups of six preparations each were treated with the α_1-subtype receptor blockers chloroethylclonidine (CEC) and WB4101 and the dose response curves to EPI were repeated. (From ref. 467, with permission.)

At present, there is no evidence that the signal transduction pathway activated by the α_1-WB4101–sensitive subtype receptor, resulting in generation of IP_3 and DAG, is involved in modulation of Na^+ channel activity or cell-to-cell coupling. However, one preliminary report indicates that high concentrations of phenylephrine (10 mM) can depress coupling between pairs of rat myocytes (68). Therefore, it is possible that a synergistic interaction between the effects of WB4101-sensitive α_1-adrenergic receptor activation and volatile anesthetics on cell-to-cell coupling, both in the His-Purkinje system and myocardium, may be responsible for the negative dromotropic effects of catecholamines in combination with volatile anesthetics.

Myocardial Ischemia and Infarction

Ischemia and infarction are likely to initiate the reentry type of ventricular arrhythmias, while those with reperfusion may be triggered (56,231). The actions of different anesthetics on reentry are sometimes studied in Purkinje fibers derived from 24-hour-old infarcted canine hearts (468). Ischemic fibers from this model exhibit abnormal electrophysiologic characteristics conducive to reentry, including loss of membrane potential, reduced AP amplitude and upstroke velocity, and prolonged AP duration (56,148). All contemporary volatile anesthetics (but isoflurane the most) increase the disparity between repolarization times of ischemic and nonischemic Purkinje fibers, as well as increase the conduction time of premature impulses into the infarcted zone, changes favorable to reentry (471). Concerning the induction of reentry with halothane and isoflurane, halothane increases both the incidence and range of premature intervals inducing reentry, while isoflurane only shortens premature coupling intervals for reentry (470). In contrast, under in vivo conditions and several days to weeks following infarction, halothane suppresses the induction of reentrant ventricular tachycardia (107,151). This difference may in part reflect the effects of normalization of the abnormal AP characteristics in Purkinje fibers 2 to 3 days after infarction (231). Also, the substrate that supports reentry in chronic infarction models may be less dependent on depressed fiber AP characteristics as compared to differences in specific fiber geometry (231). Finally, recent studies suggest that reentry in chronic in vivo models may involve the leading circle mechanism in fibers that exhibit marked directional differences of conduction velocity and cell-to-cell coupling (503).

Although the mechanisms underlying myocardial cell injury following reperfusion of ischemic myocardium are multifactorial and poorly understood, excess Ca^{2+} influx and intracellular accumulation appear important to the development of arrhythmias (56). Intracellular Ca^{2+} may increase for several reasons: (a) increased sarcolemmal permeability to Ca^{2+}, (b) enhanced release of intracellular Ca^{2+}, (c) decreased capacity of sarcoplasmic reticulum for binding Ca^{2+}, and (d) impaired Na^+-Ca^{2+} exchange. Regardless of cause, increased intracellular Ca^{2+} may facilitate arrhythmias due to abnormal mechanisms for automaticity or triggered activity. While none of the contemporary volatile anesthetics opposed abnormal automaticity in fibers from infarcted hearts, all did oppose triggered activity from delayed afterdepolarizations (DAD), with enflurane most potent (Fig. 17) (280). The contemporary anesthetics might oppose DAD-induced triggering by decreasing intracellular Ca^{2+} availability through inhibition of the slow-inward current or by affecting Ca^{2+} release from the sarcoplasmic reticulum (56). Finally, antifibrillatory effects of all the contemporary inhalation anesthetics have been demonstrated in a canine acute coronary artery occlusion-reperfusion model (272).

Role of Calcium

A number of electrophysiologic actions of volatile anesthetics on cardiac tissues have been related to depression of transsarcolemmal ionic currents, particularly the inward Ca^{2+} current present during the plateau phase following depolarization (54,129,215,306,307,449) but also the Na^+ current responsible for depolarization (66,216), as well as the various outward K^+ currents during repolarization (439,440). Anesthetic inhibition of Ca^{2+} currents, which serve as the trigger for release of intracellular Ca^{2+} sequestered in the sarcoplasmic reticulum, and reduction of Ca^{2+} stored in the SR (252) are well established as largely responsible for anesthetic-induced contractile depression (395) and may similarly underlie important antiarrhythmic actions on abnormal automatic activity associated with intracellular Ca^{2+} "overload." Cellular Ca^{2+} homeostasis (478) may be disturbed by excessive loading related to increased rate, producing increased Ca^{2+} influx per unit of time, and increased inward Ca^{2+} current resulting from catecholamine exposure. In addition, Ca^{2+} overload may also be produced by diminished extrusion of Ca^{2+}, secondary to depression of the energy dependent electrogenic Na^+-K^+ pump, and by accumulation of intracellular Na^+ ions and reduced exchange of intracellular Ca^{2+} for extracellular Na^+, as occurs in digitalis toxicity and ischemia. Abnormal oscillatory Ca^{2+} release from the overloaded SR in early diastole produces aftercontractions, the transient inward current and afterdepolarizations that increase in amplitude with increased stimulation rate and may initiate bursts of triggered activity. Early studies demonstrated anesthetic inhibition of isoproterenol stimulated slow action potential responses, largely carried by Ca^{2+} ions, in K^+ depolarized papillary muscle preparations (306,307). Subsequent studies utilizing voltage clamp techniques in single ventricular and Purkinje fibers have shown similar depression of Ca^{2+} channel currents by equianesthetic concentrations of halothane, enflurane, and isoflurane (54,129). These actions are associated with dose-related reductions (except isoflurane) of the peak intracellular Ca^{2+} transient associated with the Ca^{2+} influx and SR Ca^{2+} release accompanying contraction (50,52), which suggest that anesthetic actions would be expected to oppose or reduce Ca^{2+} overload.

The actions of volatile anesthetics depressing inward Ca^{2+} currents may underlie important antiarrhythmic actions on triggered activity due to delayed afterdepolarizations (DADs) in several different experimental models including digitalis intoxication, catecholamine stimulation, and ischemia.

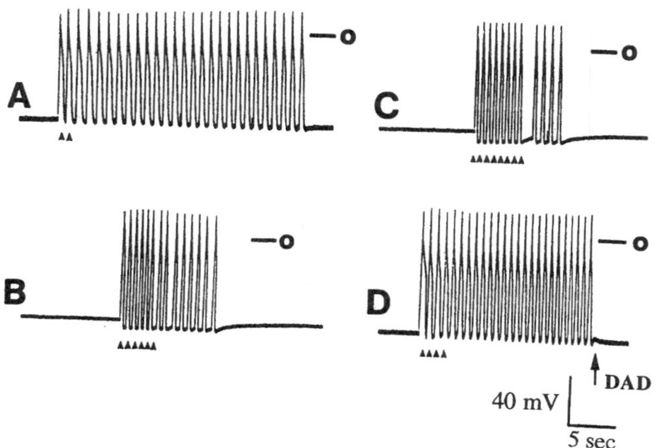

Figure 17. Representative tracings of Purkinje fiber action potentials from 24-hour infarcted canine heart illustrating the effects of anesthetics on triggered activity. **A:** Rhythmic activity is triggered by two driven beats *(arrows)* in the absence of anesthetics. **B:** With 1.5% halothane, six driven beats are required for a short train of rhythmic activity. **C:** With 3.5% enflurane, triggered activity requires eight driven beats. **D:** With 2% isoflurane, triggered activity requires four driven beats and is followed by a delayed afterdepolarization (DAD) *(large arrow)*. (From ref. 280, with permission.)

Reynolds and Horne (388), Morrow and coworkers (296,346), and Gallagher and coworkers (151,152) have demonstrated antagonism by halothane of ventricular tachyarrhythmias due to digitalis toxicity in vivo. Enflurane and isoflurane may have similar antiarrhythmic actions (226). Gallagher et al. (152) examined the actions of halothane on ouabain-intoxicated Purkinje fibers exhibiting typical afterdepolarization-triggered arrhythmias potentiated by increasing extracellular Ca^{2+} and stimulation rate. Halothane reduced the amplitude of DADs in a manner antagonized by increasing Ca^{2+}, but it did not inhibit the ventricular tachycardia resulting from EADs induced by Cs^+. Freeman and Li (146) similarly demonstrated antiarrhythmic actions of halothane on the amplitude of DADs, the accompanying abnormal intracellular Ca^{2+} transients and triggered responses induced by isoproterenol in enzymatically dispersed canine myocytes. Monitoring cell length of single stimulated rat myocytes, Zuckerman and Wheeler (533) reported inhibition by halothane of spontaneous interbeat waves and late aftercontractions due to isoproterenol and norepinephrine, as well as early aftercontractions induced by these agonists or phenylephrine. The inhibition by halothane of these types of sympathomimetic-induced arrhythmogenic responses is probably due to reduction of the inward Ca^{2+} current, the cellular Ca^{2+} load, and secondary processes of abnormal SR Ca^{2+} release. Halothane and isoflurane have also been shown to depress triggered afterdepolarizations induced by epinephrine in human atrial fibers obtained at the time of cardiac surgery (299). Subendocardial Purkinje fibers that survive overlying the ischemic region of 24-hour-old infarcted canine hearts are well known to exhibit triggered arrhythmias due to DADs that are potentiated by increasing drive rate, elevated extracellular Ca^{2+}, and catecholamines (124). Turner et al. (468) have shown that halothane reduces the rate of spontaneous arrhythmias originating in the ischemic region of infarcted hearts, and that halothane and enflurane, but not isoflurane, increase the number of drive stimuli required to induce triggered activity in ischemic fibers, as shown in Fig. 17 (280). None of the anesthetics tested decreased the rate of slow (40–50 bpm) sustained automaticity of Purkinje fibers derived from infarctions. In vivo studies of spontaneous ventricular tachycardia in dogs 24 hours following experimental infarction demonstrate that halothane anesthesia tends to reduce the overall heart rate and markedly decreases the percentage of ventricular ectopic beats (97% to 35%) relative to the conscious control state (151). This substantial antiarrhythmic action in ischemia could in part reflect direct anesthetic inhibition of abnormal automaticity as well as indirect anesthetic effects reducing cardiac sympathetic efferent activity (310,407) and plasma catecholamine concentrations (390).

While a number of in vitro studies have examined anesthetic actions on normal automaticity in ventricular tissues, less is known about their actions on automaticity in vivo. Reynolds et al. (386) observed depression of spontaneous phase 4 diastolic depolarization by halothane in Purkinje fibers both with and without epinephrine, although in our laboratory, halothane, isoflurane, and particularly enflurane were found to modestly increase spontaneous rate (from about 30 to <60 bpm) in Purkinje fibers previously exposed to high (2, 15 μM) epinephrine concentrations (279). The actions of enflurane, and to a lesser extent halothane and isoflurane, were associated with shortened recovery time following overdrive, consistent with a previous report (377) that enflurane may directly increase Purkinje fiber automaticity by an action suppressing the normal mechanism of overdrive inhibition. Other investigators have examined the effects of halothane on the emergence of ventricular pacemakers utilizing supramaximal vagal stimulation to produce complete heart block (296). Relative to basal pentobarbital anesthesia, halothane prolonged the escape time and slowed the rate of idioventricular pacemakers. However, assessment of anesthetic effects on the automaticity of ventricular escape pacemakers may be complicated by cholinergic effects depressing automaticity in the proximal bundle branches (26), and probably adrenergically mediated enhancement of automaticity due to baroreflex activation during AV block. No studies have examined direct anesthetic actions on idioventricular pacemaker function following experimental complete heart block or phenomena such as "overdrive excitation" of ventricular pacemaker activity during norepinephrine infusions, which may represent induction of triggered activity, reported to occur with acute AV block in pentobarbital anesthetized animals (478).

In summary, concerning the arrhythmic potential of the contemporary volatile anesthetics, one can suggest the following. First, any of these agents appears conducive to bradycardia and AV conduction disturbances. This would be due to their direct depressant action on the slow response (SA and AV nodes) or depressed fast response (atrial or ventricular muscle, Purkinje fibers). Second, in depressed fibers (e.g., with myocardial ischemia/infarction), halothane (and likely both enflurane and isoflurane) is conducive to reentrant excitation (increased temporal dispersion of refractoriness). In contrast, halothane (and likely enflurane and possibly isoflurane) is expected to oppose abnormal automaticity and DAD-triggered sustained rhythmic activity. The latter effect might explain halothane's effectiveness against ouabain-induced ventricular arrhythmias (152). Third, there are no data for anesthetic effects on early afterdepolarization (EAD) or EAD-induced triggered automaticity. The latter may be the mechanism for *torsades de pointes* tachycardia in patients with idiopathic or acquired long QT syndrome (180). One should note that halothane, enflurane, and isoflurane prolong the QTc interval (QT interval corrected for heart rate) independent of changes in autonomic tone in chronically instrumented dogs (389).

Intravenous Anesthetics and Adjuncts

Barbiturates and Hypnotics

A number of different barbiturates including thiopental and methohexital have been found to inhibit transsarcolemmal influx of Ca^{2+} (97,143,214,215,263,364). While thiopental has little effect on RMP and AP amplitude in ventricular tissue (143), it decreases the height of the AP plateau and the rate of depolarization during phase 0 (143) yet increases AP duration (143,214,367). While at very high concentrations of thiopental severely depresses AP amplitude, increases AP duration, and ultimately abolishes APs (255), at lower concentrations it induces spontaneous activity in rabbit papillary muscle (264), an effect influenced by intracellular Ca^{2+} stores. This action is similar to that mechanism responsible for delayed afterpotentials, which can be induced by thiopental (309). Consequently, in addition to depression of I_{Ca}, these effects of thiopental appear to be mediated by a decrease in K^+ permeability, specifically blockade of G_{K1}. Such inhibition of the inward rectifier will prolong AP duration and enhance membrane excitability (366). If barbiturates such as thiopental and thiamylal (37) decrease resting G_K and potentiate DADs, it may also explain their ability to potentiate epinephrine-induced ventricular arrhythmias with cyclopropane (308), halothane (16,195), enflurane, and isoflurane (17). Although propofol does not show the prolongation of AP duration observed with thiopental (367), it also lowers the threshold for ventricular arrhythmias caused epinephrine injection in dogs (244). In contrast, etomidate does not appear to alter arrhythmia induction by epinephrine (195).

Opiates and Other Agents

An opioid fentanyl is thought to reduce heart rate via a central mechanism that leads to decreased sympathetic and increased vagal efferent tone (96). In animals, about 90% of the bradycardia seen with fentanyl use resulted from enhanced vagal activity, and 10% from decreased sympathetic efferent tone (382). In this respect, fentanyl is similar to other opiates, except meperidine, that can cause tachycardia (138). Tachycardia with meperidine may be related to its structural similarity to atropine or to reflex-caused increase in heart rate with hypotension. The centrally mediated increase in vagal tone produced by fentanyl can be reversed by naloxone, which implicates the involvement of central opiate receptors as mediators for this effect (7). Premedication with atropine is expected to reduce bradycardia with any of the opiates. In addition to indirect actions, fentanyl directly reduces SA node rate, potentiates the action of ACh, and may inhibit acetylcholinesterase activity (295).

Similar to fentanyl, morphine may also have direct negative chronotropic (SA node) and dromotropic (AV node) actions (106). These actions may in part explain reduced vulnerability to ventricular fibrillation with morphine (106). In addition to direct effects, it was demonstrated that endogenous endorphins can attenuate β-adrenergic stimulation and possibly contribute to reduced ventricular arrhythmias (282). Based on similar actions to morphine, a reduced incidence of ventricular arrhythmias following tracheal intubation in adults and children given fentanyl (292) may be due to fentanyl's central vagal actions, or to attenuation of sympathetic effects.

Like thiopental, ketamine has multiple direct effects on various cardiac ionic currents, as well as indirect actions mediated via stimulatory effects on the autonomic nervous system. By blocking the reuptake of monoamines such norepinephrine (300,399), the electrophysiologic effects of sympathetic stimulation may be evident. These actions will combine with ketamine's direct depressant effects on Ca^{2+} and K^+ currents. By depressing I_{to}, ketamine can prolong the duration of APs in which I_{to} accelerates repolarization, which in turn increases the duration of Ca^{2+} entry (126). Inhibition of the resting K^+ conductance (G_{K1}) and delayed current may also contribute to AP prolongation (126). In contrast, I_{Ca} is directly depressed by ketamine on the compensating actions on (31,126). In intact animals ketamine appears to decrease epinephrine-induced arrhythmias, an effect attributed to an increased refractory period (118) and possibly mediated by actions on the K^+ conductances. Ketamine also reduced digitalis-induced arrhythmias (225).

Droperidol, which may be used in fixed combination with fentanyl, has in vitro electrophysiologic properties similar to quinidine and procainamide (187). Droperidol prevents epinephrine-halothane–induced ventricular tachycardia and ventricular fibrillation following coronary artery ligation in cats (42). Finally, droperidol with fentanyl increases both antegrade and retrograde refractoriness in the accessory pathway of patients with Wolff-Parkinson-White syndrome (166).

Neuromuscular Blocking Agents

Succinylcholine A number of different arrhythmias can be associated with the use of succinylcholine (SCh), and they are attributed to its direct or indirect actions, or other factors (e.g., airway manipulation under light anesthesia). The mechanism for bradycardia and arrhythmias with SCh (1,181) is not established. Bradycardia after a single dose of SCh most likely results from stimulation of cardiac muscarinic receptors, which are most prominent in the SA and AV nodes. SCh also stimulates presynaptic nicotinic receptors, thereby causing the release of norepinephrine. The net effect could be a small and variable increase or decrease in heart rate (354). Other drugs used during the course of anesthesia could alter or intensify the action of SCh (218,220). Enhanced vagal activity is also likely involved in bradydysrhythmia following repeat doses of SCh (1,61,89). While Schoenstadt and Whitcher (409) have suggested that choline produced by hydrolysis of the initial dose of SCh "sensitized" the heart to repeated doses of SCh, in a more recent study repeated doses of SCh produced only an increase in heart rate (516). Concerning a mechanism for bradycardia and arrhythmias with repeat doses of SCh, Nigrovic (354) has suggested that activation by SCh of presynaptic nicotinic receptors causes the release of norepinephrine. Activation of these as well as postsynaptic muscarinic receptors following a single dose of SCh results in opposing actions, with little effect on heart rate. With a repeat dose of SCh, cardiac muscarinic receptors would be stimulated but presynaptic receptors would remain desensitized, resulting in bradycardia or asystole.

Lack of periodic neuronal activation of skeletal muscle causes a proliferation of extrajunctional nicotinic ACh receptors (313). When patients experience prolonged nondepolarizing neuromuscular blockade, widespread lower motor neuron dysfunction (spinal cord injury or disease), or widespread upper motor neuron dysfunction (closed-head injury, stroke) that results in disuse or immobilization of a large skeletal muscle mass, the activation of AChRs by SCh administration will release a large amount of K^+. In addition, extensive burns or trauma as well as severe infection can also cause massive K^+ efflux from muscle upon exposure to SCh, although it is less clear that it is primarily due to increased AChR under these settings. In any case, if K^+ release spills over from the extracellular fluid so that the increased serum K^+ is of sufficient magnitude, severe ventricular arrhythmias will occur (459). Such an increase in serum $[K^+]$ results in depolarization of myocardium with associated slowed conduction (widened QRS), which may eventually result in reentrant ventricular tachycardia. If severe enough, coordinated ventricular activity will cease and result in irregular slow depolarizations (ventricular fibrillation). If circulation can be maintained, muscle will take up the lost K^+, reducing serum $[K^+]$ and cardiac conduction can be restored.

Nondepolarizing Relaxants Strong arrhythmic associations are not evident for any of the nondepolarizing muscle relaxants (NDMRs). All are competitive antagonists at postjunctional cholinergic receptors at the motor end-plate. Although these receptors have certain features in common with nicotinic receptors located in autonomic ganglia, they are not identical (501). Thus, it should not be surprising that NDMRs, which vary in potency as neuromuscular blockers, also vary in potency as ganglionic blockers. In addition to ganglionic blockade, potentially adverse cardiovascular effects may result from block of cardiac muscarinic receptors or drug-induced release of histamine (404). An increase in heart rate with gallamine or pancuronium likely involves block of the cardiac muscarinic receptors (210,288), but there may be a direct blocking action on the vagus itself (289). The latter was not thought to be a ganglionic blocking action or blockade of axonal conduction, but rather an affect at the pre- or postganglionic nerve terminal (289). These vagolytic actions of gallamine and pancuronium should also facilitate AV nodal conduction, which has been confirmed for pancuronium in dogs anesthetized with halothane (154). Normally, vagal impulses also attenuate sympathetic outflow presynaptically, decreasing the release of norepinephrine (476,514). Blockade of presynaptic muscarinic receptors on sympathetic nerve endings by pancuronium and gallamine (484) will also contribute to increased sympathetic activation of the heart observed with these agents (404).

Direct cardiac electrophysiologic effects of pancuronium have been examined in vitro (228). Recordings were made from quiescent and spontaneously active papillary muscle fibers during superfusion with pancuronium alone, or with epinephrine, verapamil, or propranolol. Pancuronium prolonged AP duration and increased resting potential, AP magnitude, and the rate of rise of phase 0 of the AP. These effects are consistent with the nonspecific effects of pancuronium on the Na^+, Ca^{2+}, and K^+ currents, but their physiologic significance is uncertain (228). Additionally, pancuronium induced automaticity in 12% of fibers. With epinephrine, normal or abnormal forms of automaticity were induced in 80% of fibers. In three driven fibers with a reduced level of membrane potential, there were DAD and what appear to be triggered AP. Abnormal automaticity and DAD could be abolished with verapamil, but not consistently with propranolol. Jacobs et al. (228) speculated that these findings might explain certain clinical instances of AV nodal tachycardia and ventricular arrhythmias with pancuronium. Considering these findings, it is somewhat interesting to note that pancuronium has been reported not to affect the dose of epinephrine for ventricular arrhythmias with halothane (406).

Several clinical reports indicate that vecuronium, particularly with large doses of opiates or reflex vagal stimulation, may be associated with severe bradycardia and even asystole (81,260,338, 376,434,522). In patients about to undergo coronary artery surgery, Inoue et al. (219) found that the combination of etomidate, vecuronium, and a small dose of fentanyl led to the greatest reduction in heart rate. When thiopental was substituted for etomidate, the reduction in heart rate was significantly less. Bradycardia responded to atropine, but often after a short period of AV junctional rhythm (219).

REFERENCES

1. Abdul-Rasool IH, Sears DH, Katz RL. The effect of a second dose of succinylcholine on cardiac rate and rhythm following induction of anesthesia with etomidate or midazolam. *Anesthesiology* 1987;67: 795–797.
2. Ackerman MJ, Clapham DE. Cardiac chloride channels. *Trends Cardiovasc Med* 1993;3:23–28.
3. Allessie MA, Bonke FI, Schopman FJ. Circus movement in rabbit atrial muscle as a mechanism of tachycardia. III. The "leading circle" concept: a new model of circus movement in cardiac tissue without the involvement of an anatomical obstacle. *Circ Res* 1977; 41:9–18.
4. Allessie MA, Bonke FIM. Direct demonstration of sinus node reentry in the rabbit heart. *Circ Res* 1979;44:557–568.
5. Allessie MA, Lammers WJ, Bonke IM, Hollen J. Intra-atrial reentry as a mechanism for atrial flutter induced by acetylcholine and rapid pacing in the dog. *Circulation* 1984;70:123–135.
6. Alpert LA, Fozzard HA, Hanck DA, Makielski JC. Is there a second external lidocaine binding site on mammalian cardiac cells. *Am J Physiol* 1989;257:H79–H84.
7. Arndt JO, Mikat M, Parasher C. Fentanyl's analgesic, respiratory, and cardiovascular actions in relation to dose and plasma concentrations in unanesthetized dogs. *Anesthesiology* 1984;61:355–361.
8. Ashford MLJ, Bond CT, Blair TA, Adelman JP. Cloning and functional expression of a rat heart K_{ATP} channel. *Nature* 1994;370: 456–459.
9. Atlee JL III. Normal electrical activity of the heart. In: *Perioperative cardiac dysrhythmias.* Chicago: Year Book Medical, 1990;14–56.
10. Atlee JL III, Alexander SC. Halothane effects on conductivity of the AV node and His-Purkinje system in the dog. *Anesth Analg* 1977;56:378–386.
11. Atlee JL III, Bosnjak ZJ. Mechanisms for cardiac dysrhythmias during anesthesia. *Anesthesiology* 1990;72:347–374.
12. Atlee JL III, Brownlee Sw, Burstrom RE. Conscious-state comparisons of the effects of inhalation anesthetics on specialized atrioventricular conduction times in dogs. *Anesthesiology* 1986;64: 703–710.
13. Atlee JL III, Dayer AM, Houge JC. Chronic recording from the His bundle of the awake dog. *Basic Res Cardiol* 1984;79:627–638.
14. Atlee JL III, Hamann SR, Brownlee SW, Kreigh C. Conscious state comparisons of the effects of the inhalation anesthetics and diltiazem, nifedipine, or verapamil on specialized atrioventricular conduction times in spontaneously beating dog hearts. *Anesthesiology* 1988;68:519–528.
15. Atlee JL III, Homer LD, Tobey RE. Diphenylhydantoin and lidocaine modification of A-V conduction in halothane-anesthetized dogs. *Anesthesiology* 1975;43:49–56.
16. Atlee JL III, Malkinson CE. Potentiation by thiopental of halothane — epinephrine-induced arrhythmias in dogs. *Anesthesiology* 1982;57:285–288.
17. Atlee JL III, Roberts FL. Thiopental and epinephrine-induced dysrhythmias in dogs anesthetized with enflurane or isoflurane. *Anesth Analg* 1986;65:437–443.
18. Atlee JL III, Rusy BF. Halothane depression of A-V conduction studied by electrograms of the bundle of His in dogs. *Anesthesiology* 1972;36:112–118.
19. Atlee JL III, Rusy BF. Atrioventricular conduction times and atrioventricular nodal conductivity during enflurane anesthesia in dogs. *Anesthesiology* 1977;47:498–503.
20. Atlee JL III, Rusy BF, Kreul JF. Supraventricular excitability in dogs during anesthesia with halothane and enflurane. *Anesthesiology* 1978;49:407–413.
21. Atlee JL III, Yeager TS. Electrophysiologic assessment of the effects of enflurane, halothane and isoflurane on properties affecting supraventricular re-entry in chronically instrumented dogs. *Anesthesiology* 1989;71:941–952.
22. Attwell D, Cohen I, Eisner D, Ohba M, Ojeda C. The steady state TTX sensitive ("window") sodium current in cardiac Purkinje fibers. *Pflugers Arch* 1979;379:147–152.
23. Autenrieth G, Surawicz B, Kuo CS. Sequence of repolarization on the ventricular surface in the dog. *Am Heart J* 1975;89:463–69.
24. Backx PH, Marban E. Background potassium current active during the plateau of the action potential in guinea pig ventricular myocytes. *Circ Res* 1993;72:890–900.
25. Bahinski A, Nairn AC, Greengard P, Gadsby DC. Chloride conductance regulated by cyclic AMP-dependent protein kinase in cardiac myocytes. *Nature* 1989;340:718–721.
26. Bailey JC, Greenspan K, Elizari MV, Anderson GJ, Fisch C. Effects of acetylcholine on automaticity and conduction in the proximal portion of the His-Purkinje specialized conduction system of the dog. *Circ Res* 1972;30:210–216.
27. Bailey JC, Watanabe AM, Besch HR, Lathrop DA. Acetylcholine antagonism of the electrophysiological effects of isoproterenol on canine cardiac Purkinje fibers. *Circ Res* 1979;44:378–383.
28. Balke CW, Rose WC, Marban E, Wier WG. Macroscopic and unitary properties of physiological ion flux through T-type Ca^{2+} channels in guinea-pig heart cells. *J Physiol* 1992;456:247–266.
29. Barnard EA. Separating receptor subtypes from their shadows. *Nature* 1988;335:301–302.
30. Bates SE, Gurney AM. Ca^{2+}-dependent block and potentiation of L-type calcium current in guinea-pig ventricular myocytes. *J Physiol* 1993;466:345–365.
31. Baum VC, Tecson ME. Ketamine inhibits transsarcolemmal calcium entry in guinea pig myocardium: direct evidence by single cell voltage clamp. *Anesth Analg* 1991;73:804–807.
32. Baumgarten CM, Fozzard HA. Cardiac resting and pacemaker potentials. In: Fozzard HA, Haber E, Jennings RB, Katz AM, Morgan HE, eds. *The heart and cardiovascular system—scientific foundations.* New York: Raven Press, 1991;963–1001.
33. Baumgarten CM, Singer DH, Fozzard HA. Intra- and extracellular potassium activities, acetylcholine and resting potential in guinea pig atria. *Circ Res* 1984;54:65–73.
34. Bean BP. Two kinds of calcium channels in canine atrial cells: differences in kinetics, selectivity, and pharmacology. *J Gen Physiol* 1985;86:1–31.
35. Bean BP, Nowycky MC, Tsien RW. β-Adrenergic modulation of calcium channels in frog ventricular heart cells. *Nature* 1984;307: 371–375.
36. Bean BP, Rios E. Nonlinear charge movement in mammalian cardiac ventricular cells. *J Gen Physiol* 1989;94:65–93.
37. Bednarski RM, Majors LJ, Atlee JL. Potentiation by thiamylal and thiopental of halothane-epinephrine induced ventricular arrhythmias in dogs. *Am J Vet Res* 1985;46:1829–1831.
38. Belardinelli L, Isenberg G. Isolated atrial myocytes: adenosine and acetylcholine increase potassium conductance. *Am J Physiol* 1983; 224:H734–H737.
39. Belardinelli L, Linden J, Berne RM. The cardiac effects of adenosine. *Prog Cardiovasc Dis* 1989;32:73–97.
40. Benndorf K, Bollman G, Friedrich M, Hirche H. Anoxia induces time-independent K^+ current through K_{ATP} channels in isolated guinea-pig heart. *J Physiol* 1992;454:339–357.
41. Bers DM, Hryshko LV, Harrison SM, Dawson DD. Citrate decreases contraction and Ca current in cardiac muscle independent of its buffering action. *Am J Physiol* 1991;260:C900–C909.
42. Bertolo L, Novakovic L, Penna M. Antiarrhythmic effects of droperidol. *Anesthesiology* 1972;37:529–535.
43. Birnbaumer L. G Proteins in signal transduction. *Annu Rev Pharmacol Toxicol* 1990;30:675–705.
44. Blanck TJJ, Runge S, Stevenson RL. Halothane decreases calcium channel antagonist binding to cardiac membranes. *Anesth Analg* 1988;67:1032–1035.
45. Blaustein MP. Sodium/calcium exchange and the control of contractility in cardiac muscle and vascular smooth muscle. *J Cardiovasc Pharmacol* 1988;12(suppl 5):S56–S68.

46. Bleeker WK, McKaay AJC, Masson-Pevot M, Bouman LN, Becker AE. The functional and morphological organization of the rabbit sinus node. *Circ Res* 1980;46:11–22.
47. Blitt CD, Raessler KL, Wightman MA, Groves BM, Wall CL, Geha DG. Atrioventricular conduction in dogs during anesthesia with isoflurane. *Anesthesiology* 1979;50:210–212.
48. Boban M, Stowe DF, Gross GJ, Pieper GM, Kampine JP, Bosnjak ZJ. Potassium channel openers attenuate atrioventricular block by bupivacaine in isolated hearts. *Anesth Analg* 1993;76:1259–1265.
49. Böhm M, Gierschik P, Schwinger RHG, Uhlmann R, Erdmann E. Coupling of M-cholinoceptors and A_1 adenosine receptors in human myocardium. *Am J Physiol* 1994;266:H1951–H1958.
50. Bosnjak ZJ, Aggarwal A, Turner LA, Kampine JM, Kampine JP. Differential effects of halothane, enflurane, and isoflurane and papillary muscle tension in guinea pigs. *Anesthesiology* 1992;76:123–131.
51. Bosnjak ZJ, Kampine JP. Effects of halothane, enflurane and isoflurane on the SA node. *Anesthesiology* 1983;58:314–321.
52. Bosnjak ZJ, Kampine JP. Effects of halothane on transmembrane potentials, Ca^{++} transients, and papillary muscle tension. *Am J Physiol* 1986;251:H374–H381.
53. Bosnjak ZJ, Stowe DF, Kampine JP. Comparison of lidocaine and bupivacaine depression of sinoatrial nodal activity during hypoxia and acidosis in adult and neonatal guinea pigs. *Anesth Analg* 1986; 65:911–917.
54. Bosnjak ZJ, Supan FD, Rusch NJ. The effects of halothane, enflurane and isoflurane on calcium currents in isolated canine ventricular cells. *Anesthesiology* 1991;74:340–345.
55. Bosnjak ZJ, Turner LA. Halothane, catecholamines, and cardiac conduction: anything new? *Anesth Analg* 1991;72:1–4.
56. Bosnjak ZJ, Warltier DC. New aspects of cardiac electrophysiology and function: effects of inhalational anesthetics. In: Conzen P, Peter K, eds. *Baillière's clinical anaesthesiology*, vol 7. London: Baillière-Tindal, 1993.
57. Boutjdir M, Restivo M, Wei Y, El-Sherif N. α_1- β-Adrenergic interactions on L-type calcium current in cardiac myocytes. *Pflugers Arch* 1992;421:397–399.
58. Boyett MR, Kirby MS, Orchard CH, Roberts A. The negative inotropic effect of acetylcholine on ferret ventricular myocardium. *J Physiol* 1988;404:613–635.
59. Boyle WA, Nerbonne JM. A novel type of depolarization-activated K^+ current in isolated adult rat atrial myocytes. *Am J Physiol* 1991; 29:H1236–H1247.
60. Brady AJB, Warren JB, Poole-Wilson PA, Williams TJ, Harding SE. Nitric oxide attenuates cardiac myocyte contraction. *Am J Physiol* 1993;265:H176–H182.
61. Brandt MR, Viby-Mogensen J. Halothane anesthesia and suxamethonium. *Acta Anaesthesiol Scand* 1978;67 (Suppl):76–83.
62. Breitwieser GE, Szabo G. Mechanism of muscarinic receptor-induced K^+ channel activation as revealed by hydrolysis-resistant GTP analogues. *J Gen Physiol* 1988;91:469–493.
63. Bricknell OL, Opie LH. Effects of substrate on tissue metabolic changes in the isolated rat heart during underperfusion and on release of lactate dehydrogenase and arrhythmias during reperfusion. *Circ Res* 1978;43:102–115.
64. Bridge JHB, Smolley JR, Spitzer KW. The relationship between charge movements associated with I_{Ca} and $I_{Na\text{-}Ca}$ in cardiac myocytes. *Science* 1990;248:376–378.
65. Brown LA, Humphrey SM, Harding SE. The anti-adrenergic effect of adenosine and its blockade by pertussis toxin: a comparative study in myocytes isolated from guinea-pig, rat and failing human hearts. *Br J Pharmacol* 1990;101:484–488.
66. Buljubasic N, Berci V, Supan DF, et al. Depression of the Na^+ current by halothane and isoflurane in the rabbit Purkinje fiber. *Anesthesiology* 1993;79:A392.
67. Burgess MJ, Green LS, Millar K. The sequence of normal ventricular recovery. *Am Heart J* 1972;84:660–669.
68. Burt JM, Spray DC. Adrenergic control of gap junction conductance in cardiac myocytes. *Circulation* 1988;78 (Suppl II):99–113.
69. Burt JM, Spray DC. Inotropic agents modulate gap junctional conductance between cardiac myocytes. *Am J Physiol* 1988;254: H1206–H1210.
70. Burt JM, Spray DC. Volatile anesthetics block intercellular communication between neonatal rat myocardial cells. *Circ Res* 1989; 65:829–837.
71. Callewaert G, Vereecke J, Carmeliet E. Existence of calcium-dependent potassium channel in the membrane of cow cardiac Purkinje fibres. *Pflugers Arch* 1986;406:424–426.
72. Carlsson L, Abrahamsson C, Andersson B, Duker G, Schiller-Linhardt G. Proarrhythmic effects of the class III agent almokalant: importance of infusion rate, QT dispersion, and early afterdepolarisations. *Cardiovasc Res* 1993;27:2186–2193.
73. Carmeliet E, Mubagwa K. Characterization of the acetylcholine-induced potassium current in rabbit cardiac Purkinje fibres. *J Physiol* 1985;371:219–237.
74. Caroni P, Carafoli E. An ATP-dependent Ca^{2+} pumping system in dog heart sarcolemma. *Nature* 1980;283:765–767.
75. Castle NA. Bupivacaine inhibits the transient outward K^+ current but not the inward rectifier in rat ventricular myocytes. *J Pharmacol Exp Ther* 1990;255:1038–1046.
76. Catterall WA, Scheuer T, West JW, et al. Structure and modulation of voltage-gated sodium channels. In: Spooner PM, Brown AM, Catterall WA, Kaczorowski GJ, Strauss HC, eds. *Ion channels in the cardiovascular system.* Armonk, NY: Futura, 1994;317–340.
77. Cerbai E, Klöckner U, Isenberg G. The α subunit of the GTP binding protein activates muscarinic potassium channels of the atrium. *Science* 1988;240:1782–1783.
78. Clark RB, Giles WR, Imaizumi Y. Properties of the transient outward currents in rabbit atrial cells. *J Physiol* 1988;405:147–168.
79. Clarkson CW, Hondeghem LM. Evidence for a specific receptor site for lidocaine, quinidine, and bupivacaine associated with cardiac sodium channels in guinea pig ventricular myocardium. *Circ Res* 1985;56:496–506.
80. Clarkson CW, Hondeghem LM. Mechanisms for bupivacaine depression of cardiac conduction: fast block of sodium channels during the action potential with slow recovery from block during diastole. *Anesthesiology* 1985;62:396–405.
81. Clayton D. Asystole associated with vecuronium (Letter). *Br J Anaesth* 1986;58:937–938.
82. Codina J, Yatani A, Grenet D, Brown AM, Birmbaumer L. The α subunit of GTP binding protein G_k opens atrial potassium channels. *Science* 1987;236:442–445.
83. Cohen CJ, Fozzard HA, Sheu SS. Increase in intracellular sodium activity during stimulation in mammalian cardiac muscle. *Circ Res* 1982;50:651–662.
84. Committee. Standards and guidelines for cardiopulmonary resuscitation (CPR) and emergency cardiac care (ECC). *JAMA* 1986; 255:2905–2989.
85. Coraboeuf E, Carmeliet E. Existence of two transient outward currents in sheep Purkinje fibres. *Pflugers Arch* 1982;392:352–359.
86. Coraboeuf E, Deroubaix E, Colombe A. Effect of tetrodotoxin on the action potentials of the conducting system in the dog heart. *Am J Physiol* 1979;236:H561–H567.
87. Corr PB, Yamada KA, Witkowski FX. Mechanisms controlling cardiac autonomic function and their relation to arrhythmogenesis. In: Fozzard HA, Haber E, Jennings RB, Katz AM, Morgan HE, eds. *The heart and cardiovascular system.* New York: Raven Press, 1986; 1343–1403.
88. Coyle DE, Sperelakis N. Bupivacaine and lidocaine blockade of calcium-mediated slow action potentials in guinea pig ventricular muscle. *J Pharmacol Exp Ther* 1987;242:1001–1005.
89. Cozanitis DA, Dundee JW, Khan MM. Comparative study of atropine and glycopyrrolate and suxamethonium-induced changes in cardiac rate and rhythm. *Br J Anaesth* 1980;52:291–293.
90. Cranefield DF. Action potentials, after potentials and arrhythmias. *Circ Res* 1977;41:415–423.
91. Crumb WJ Jr, Pigott JD, Clarkson CW. Comparison of I_{to} in young and adult human atrial myocytes: evidence for developmental changes. *Am J Physiol* 1995;268:H1335–H1342.
92. Curran ME, Splawski I, Timothy KW, Vincent GM, Green ED, Keating MT. A mechanistic link between an inherited and an acquired cardiac arrhythmia: *HERG* encodes the I_{Kr} potassium channel. *Cell* 1995;81:299–307.
93. Curran ME, Splawski I, Timothy KW, Vincent GM, Green ED, Keating MT. A molecular basis for cardiac arrhythmia: *HERG* mutations cause long QT syndrome. *Cell* 1995;80:795–803.
94. Damiano BP, Rosen MR. Effects of pacing on triggered activity induced by early afterdepolarizations. *Circulation* 1984;69:1013–1025.
95. Dascal N, Schreibmayer W, Lim NF, et al. Atrial G protein-activated K^+ channel: expression cloning and molecular properties. *Proc Natl Acad Sci USA* 1993;90:10235–10239.
96. Daskalopoulos N, Laubie M, Schmitt H. Localization of the central sympatho-inhibitory effects of a narcotic analgesic agent, fentanyl in cats. *Eur J Pharmacol* 1975;33:91–97.

97. Davies AO, McCans DR. Effects of barbiturate anesthetics and ketamine on the force-frequency relation of cardiac muscle. *Eur J Pharmacol* 1979;59:65–73.
98. Davis LD. Effects of changes in cycle length on diastolic depolarization produced by ouabain in canine Purkinje fibers. *Circ Res* 1973;32:206–214.
99. de Jong RH, Ronfeld RA, DeRosa RA. Cardiovascular effects of convulsant and supraconvulsant doses of amide local anesthetics. *Anesth Analg* 1982;61:3–9.
100. de Weille JR. Modulation of ATP sensitive potassium channels. *Cardiovasc Res* 1992;26:1017–1020.
101. DeFelice LJ. Molecular and biophysical view of the Ca channel: a hypothesis regarding oligomeric structure, channel clustering, and macroscopic current. *J Memb Biol* 1993;133:191–202.
102. Delmar M, Jalife J. Low Bα-induced pacemaker current in well-polarized cat papillary muscle. *Am J Physiol* 1987;252:H258–H268.
103. DeMello WC. Modulation of junctional permeability. *Fed Proc* 1984;43:L2692–L2996.
104. DeMello WC. Effects of isoproterenol and 3-isobutyl-1-methylxanthine on junctional conductance in heart cell pairs. *Biochim Biophys Acta* 1989;1012:291–298.
105. Denniss AR, Richards DA, Taylor AT, Uther JB. Halothane anesthesia reduces inducibility of ventricular tachyarrhythmias in chronic canine myocardial infarction. *Basic Res Cardiol* 1989;84:5–12.
106. DeSilva RA, Verrier RL, Lown B. Protective effect of vagotonic action of morphine sulfate on ventricular vulnerability. *Cardiovasc Res* 1978;12:167–172.
107. Deutsch N, Hantler CB, Tait AR, Uprichard A, Schork MA, Knight PR. Suppression of ventricular arrhythmias by volatile anesthetics in a canine model of chronic myocardial infarction. *Anesthesiology* 1990;72:1012–1021.
108. Dichtl A, Vierling W. Inhibition by magnesium of calcium inward current in heart ventricular muscle. *Eur J Pharmacol* 1991;204:243–248.
109. DiFrancesco D. A new interpretation of the pace-maker current in calf Purkinje fibres. *J Physiol* 1981;314:359–376.
110. DiFrancesco D. A study of the ionic nature of the pace-maker current in calf Purkinje fibres. *J Physiol* 1981;314:377–393.
111. DiFrancesco D. Pacemaker mechanisms in cardiac tissue. *Annu Rev Physiol* 1993;55:455–472.
112. DiFrancesco D, Ducouret P, Robinson RB. Muscarinic modulation of cardiac rate at low acetylcholine concentrations. *Science* 1989;243:669–671.
113. DiFrancesco D, Ferroni D, Mazzanti A, Tromba C. Properties of the hyperpolarizing-activated current (i_f) in cells isolated from the rabbit sino-atrial node. *J Physiol* 1986;377:61–88.
114. DiMarc JP, Miles W, Akhtar M, et al. Adenosine for paroxysmal supraventricular tachycardia: dose ranging and comparison with verapmil in placebo-controlled, multicellular trials. *Ann Intern Med* 1990;113:104–110.
115. Dobson JG, Fenton RA. Adenosine inhibition of β-adrenergic induced responses in aged hearts. *Am J Physiol* 1993;265:H494–H503.
116. Doerr T, Denger R, Trautwein W. Calcium currents in single SA nodal cells of the rabbit heart studied with action potential clamp. *Pflügers Arch* 1989;413:599—603.
117. Doohan MM, Hool LC, Rasmussen HH. Thyroid status and Na^+-K^+ pump current, intracellular sodium, and action potential duration in rabbit heart. *Am J Physiol* 1995;268:H1838–H1846.
118. Dowdy EG, Kaya K. Studies of the mechanism of cardiovascular responses to CI-581. *Anesthesiology* 1968;29:931–943.
119. Dudel J, Peper K, Rüdel R, Trautwein W. The dynamic chloride component of membrane current in cardiac Purkinje fibers. *Pflugers Arch* 1967;295:197–212.
120. Dukes ID, Morad M. The transient K^+ current in rat ventricular myocytes: evaluation of its Ca^{2+} and Na^+ dependence. *J Physiol* 1991;435:395–420.
121. Egan TM, Noble D, Noble SJ, Powell T, Spindler AJ, Twist VW. Sodium-calcium exchange during the action potential in guinea-pig ventricular cells. *J Physiol* 1989;411:639–661.
122. Ehara T, Kaufmann R. The voltage and time-dependent effects of (-) verapamil on the slow inward current in isolated cat ventricular myocardium. *J Pharmacol Exp Ther* 1978;207:49–55.
123. Ehara T, Matsuura H. Single-channel study of the cyclic AMP-regulated chloride current in guinea-pig ventricular myocytes. *J Physiol* 1993;464:307–320.
124. El-Sherif N, Gough WB, Zeiler RH, Mehra R. Triggered ventricular rhythms in 1-day-old myocardial infarction in the dog. *Circ Res* 1983;52:566–579.
125. Elharrar V, Zipes DP. Voltage modulation of automaticity in cardiac Purkinje fibers. In: Zipes DP, Bailey JC, Elharrar V, eds. *The slow inward current and cardiac arrhythmias.* The Hague: Martinus Nijhoff, 1980;357–373.
126. Endou M, Hattori Y, Nakaya H, Gotoh Y, Kanno M. Electrophysiological mechanisms responsible for inotropic responses to ketamine in guinea pig and rat myocardium. *Anesthesiology* 1992;76:409–418.
127. Escande D, Cavero I. K^+ channel openers and 'natural' cardioprotection. *Trends Pharmacol Sci* 1992;13:269–271.
128. Escande D, Coulombe A, Faivre J-F, Deroubaix E, Corabeouf E. Two types of transient outward currents in adult human atrial cells. *Am J Physiol* 1987;249:H142–H148.
129. Eskinder H, Rusch NJ, Supan FD, Kampine JP, Bosnjak ZJ. The effects of volatile anesthetics on L-type and T-type calcium channel currents in canine Purkinje cells. *Anesthesiology* 1991;74:919–926.
130. Fabiato A. Calcium-induced release of calcium from the cardiac sarcoplasmic reticulum. *Am J Physiol* 1983;245:C1–C14.
131. Fedida D, Braun AP, Giles WR. Alpha 1–adrenoceptors reduce background K^+ current in rabbit ventricular myocytes. *J Physiol* 1991;441:673–684.
132. Fedida D, Giles WR. Regional variations in action potentials and transient outward current in myocytes isolated from rabbit left ventricle. *J Physiol* 1991;442:191–209.
133. Fedida D, Wible B, Wang Z, et al. Identity of a novel delayed rectifier current from human heart with a cloned K^+ channel current. *Circ Res* 1993;73:210–216.
134. Ferrier GR, Dresel PE. Relationship of the functional refractory period to conduction in the atrioventricular node. *Circ Res* 1974;35:204–214.
135. Ferrier GR, Saunders JH, Mendez C. A cellular mechanism for the generation of ventricular arrhythmias by acetylstrophanthidin. *Circ Res* 1973;32:600–609.
136. Field AC, Hill C, Lamb GD. Asymmetric charge movement and calcium currents in ventricular myocytes of neonatal rat. *J Physiol* 1988;406:277–297.
137. Folander K, Smith JS, Antanavage J, Bennett C, Stein RB. Cloning and expression of the delayed-rectifier I_{sK} channel from neonatal rat heart and diethylstilbestrol-primed rat uterus. *Proc Natl Acad Sci USA* 1990;87:2975–2979.
138. Foldes FF, Shiffman HP, Kronfeld PP. The use of fentanyl, meperidine, or alphaprodine for neuroleptanesthesia. *Anesthesiology* 1970;33:35–42.
139. Fosset M, De Weille JR, Green RD, Schmid-Antomarchi H, Lazdunski M. Anti-diabetic sulfonylureas control action potential properties in heart cells via high affinity receptors that are linked to ATP-dependent K^+ channels. *J Biol Chem* 1988;263:7933–7936.
140. Fozzard HA, Arnsdorf MF. Cardiac electrophysiology. In: Fozzard HM, Haber E, Jennings RB, eds. *The heart and cardiovascular system.* New York: Raven Press, 1991;63–98.
141. Fozzard HA, Hanck DA. Sodium channels. In: Fozzard HA, Haber E, Jennings RB, Katz AM, Morgan HE, eds. *The heart and cardiovascular system—scientific foundations.* New York: Raven Press, 1991;1091–1119.
142. Fozzard HA, Hiraoka M. The positive dynamic current and its inactivation properties in cardiac Purkinje fibres. *J Physiol* 1973;234:569–586.
143. Frankl WS, Poole-Wilson PA. Effects of thiopental on tension development, action potential, and exchange of calcium and potassium in rabbit ventricular myocardium. *J Cardiovasc Pharmacol* 1981;3:554–565.
144. Franz MR, Bargheer K, Rafflenbeul W, Haverich A, Lichtlen PR. Monophasic action potential mapping in human subjects with normal electrocardiograms: direct evidence for the genesis of the T wave. *Circulation* 1987;75:379–386.
145. Franz MR, Flaherty JT, Platia EV, Bulkley BH, Weisfeldt ML. Localization of regional myocardial ischemia by recording of monophasic action potentials. *Circulation* 1984;69:593–604.
146. Freeman LC, Li Q. Effects of halothane on delayed afterdepolarizations and calcium transients in dog ventricular myocytes exposed to isoproterenol. *Anesthesiology* 1991;74:146–154.
147. Freeman LC, Muir WW III. Effects of halothane on impulse propagation in Purkinje fibers and at Purkinje-muscle junctions: relationship of V_{max} to conduction velocity. *Anesth Analg* 1991;72:5–10.

148. Friedman PL, Stewart JR, Wit AL. Spontaneous and induced cardiac arrhythmias in subendocardial Purkinje fibers surviving extensive myocardial infarction in dogs. *Circ Res* 1973;33:617–625.
149. Gadsby DC. Effects of beta-adrenergic catecholamines on membrane currents in cardiac cells. In: Rosen MR, Janse MJ, Wit AL, eds. *Cardiac electrophysiology: a textbook.* Mount Kisco, NY: Futura, 1990;857–876.
150. Gadsby DC, Witt AL. Electrophysiologic characteristics of cardiac cells and the genesis of cardiac arrhythmias. In: Wilkersen RG, ed. *Cardiac pharmacology.* New York: Academic Press, 1981;229–241.
151. Gallagher JD. The effects of halothane on ventricular tachycardia in intact dogs. *Anesthesiology* 1991;75:866–875.
152. Gallagher JD, Bianchi JJ, Gessman LJ. Halothane antagonizes ouabain toxicity in isolated canine Purkinje fibers. *Anesthesiology* 1989;71:695–703.
153. Gambassi G, Spurgeon HA, Lakatta EG, Blank PS, Capogrossi MC. Different effects of α- and β-adrenergic stimulation on cytosolic pH and myofilament responsiveness to Ca^{2+} in cardiac myocytes. *Circ Res* 1992;71:870–882.
154. Geha DG, Rozelle BC, Raessler KL, Groves BM, Wightman MA, Blitt CD. Pancuronium bromide enhances atrioventricular conduction in halothane anesthetized dogs. *Anesthesiology* 1977;46:342–345.
155. Gettes LS, Cascio WE. Effects of acute ischemia on cardiac electrophysiology. In: Fozzard HA, Haber E, Jennings RB, eds. *The heart and cardiovascular system: scientific foundations.* New York: Raven Press, 1991;2021–2054.
156. Gettes LS, Reuter H. Slow recovery from inactivation of inward currents in mammalian myocardial fibres. *J Physiol* 1974;240: 703–724.
157. Gilat E, Nordin CW, Aronson RS. The role of reduced potassium conductance in generating triggered activity in guinea-pig ventricular muscle. *J Mol Cell Cardiol* 1990;22:619–928.
158. Giles WR, Imaizumi Y. Comparison of potassium currents in rabbit atrial and ventricular cells. *J Physiol* 1988;405:123–145.
159. Giles WR, Van Ginneken ACG. A transient outward current in isolated cells from the crista terminalis of rabbit heart. *J Physiol* 1985; 368:243–264.
160. Gilmour RF Jr, Zipes DP. Different electrophysiological responses of canine endocardium and epicardium to combined hyperkalemia, hypoxia, and acidosis. *Circ Res* 1980;46:814–825.
161. Gilmour RF Jr, Zipes DP. Abnormal automaticity and related phenomena. In: Fozzard HA, Haber E, Jennings RB, eds. *The heart and cardiovascular system.* New York: Raven Press, 1986;1239–1257.
162. Gintant GA. Regional differences in I_K density in canine left ventricle: role of $I_{K,s}$ in electrical heterogeneity. *Am J Physiol* 1995;268: H604–H613.
163. Gintant GA, Datyner NB, Cohen IS. Gating of delayed rectification in acutely isolated canine cardiac Purkinje myocytes. *Biophys J* 1985;48:1059–1069.
164. Giotti A, Ledda F, Mannaioni PF. Effects of noradrenaline and isoprenaline, in combination with alpha- and beta-receptor blocking substances, on the action potential of cardiac Purkinje fibres. *J Physiol* 1973;229:99–113.
165. Goldstein SS, Rall W. Changes in action potential shape and velocity for changing core conductor geometry. *Biophys J* 1974;14: 731–757.
166. Gomez-Arnau J, Marquez-Montes J, Avello F. Fentanyl and droperidol effects on refractoriness of the accessory pathway in the Wolff-Parkinson-White syndrome. *Anesthesiology* 1983;58: 307–313.
167. Grant AO, Starmer CF. Mechanisms of closure of cardiac sodium channels in rabbit ventricular myocytes: single-channel analysis. *Circ Res* 1987;60:897–913.
168. Gros D, Jongsma HJ. The cardiac connection. *News Physiol Sci* 1991;6:34–40.
169. Gross GJ, Auchampach JA. Role of ATP dependent potassium channels in myocardial ischaemia. *Cardiovasc Res* 1992;26: 1011–1016.
170. Hadley RW, Hume JR. An intrinsic potential-dependent inactivation mechanism associated with calcium channels in guinea-pig myocytes. *J Physiol* 1987;389:205–222.
171. Hagiwara N, Irisawa H, Kameyama M. Contribution of two types of calcium currents to the pacemaker potentials of rabbit sinoatrial node cells. *J Physiol* 1988;395:233–253.
172. Hagiwara N, Masuda H, Shoda M, Irisawa H. Stretch-activated anion currents of rabbit cardiac myocytes. *J Physiol* 1992;456: 285–302.
173. Haigney MCP, Miyata H, Lakatta EG, Stern MD, Silverman HS. Dependence of hypoxic cellular calcium loading on Na^+-Ca^{2+} exchange. *Circ Res* 1992;71:547–557.
174. Han J, Millet D, Chizzonitti B, Moe GK. Temporal dispersion of recovery of excitability in atrium and ventricle as a function of heart rate. *Am Heart J* 1966;71:481–487.
175. Han J, Moe GK. Nonuniform recovery of excitability in ventricular muscle. *Circ Res* 1964;14:44–60.
176. Han J, Moe GK. Cumulation effects of cycle length on refractory periods of cardiac tissues. *Am J Physiol* 1969;217:106–109.
177. Han X, Shimoni Y, Giles WR. An obligatory role for nitric oxide in autonomic control of mammalian heart rate. *J Physiol* 1994;476: 309–314.
178. Han X, Shimoni Y, Giles WR. A cellular mechanism for nitric oxide-mediated cholinergic control of mammalian heart rate. *J Gen Physiol* 1995;106:45–65.
179. Hancox JC, Levi AJ. L-type calcium current in rod- and spindle-shaped myocytes isolated from rabbit atrioventricular node. *Am J Physiol* 1994;267:H1670–H1680.
180. Hanich RF, Levine JH, Spear JF. Autonomic modulation of ventricular arrhythmias in cesium chloride-induced long QT syndrome. *Circulation* 1988;77:1149–1161.
181. Hannallah RS, Oh TH, McGill WA, Epstein BS. Changes in heart rate and rhythm after intramuscular succinylcholine with or without atropine in anesthetized children. *Anesth Analg* 1986;65: 1329–1332.
182. Hartzell HC, Fischmeister R. Direct regulation of cardiac Ca^{2+}channels by G proteins: neither proven nor necessary? *Trends Pharmacol Sci* 1992;13:380–385.
183. Harvey RD, Clark CD, Hume JR. Chloride current in mammalian cardiac myocytes - Novel mechanism for autonomic regulation of action potential duration and resting membrane potential. *J Gen Physiol* 1990;95:1077–1102.
184. Harvey RD, Hume JR. Autonomic regulation of a chloride current in heart. *Science* 1989;244:983–985.
185. Hashimoto K, Moe GK. Transient depolarization induced by acetylstrophanthidin in specialized tissue of dog atrium and ventricle. *Circ Res* 1973;32:618–624.
186. Hasin Y, Barry WH. Myocardial metabolic inhibition and membrane potential, contraction, and potassium uptake. *Am J Physiol* 1984;247:H322–H329.
187. Hauswirth O. Effects of droperidol on sheep Purkinje fibers. *Naunyn Schmiedebergs Arch Pharmacol* 1968;261:133–142.
188. Hauswirth O. The influence of halothane on the electrical properties of cardiac Purkinje fibers. *J Physiol* 1968;201:42P-43P.
189. Hauswirth O. Effects of halothane on single atrial ventricular and Purkinje fibers. *Circ Res* 1969;24:745–750.
190. Hauswirth O, Noble D, Tsien RW. Separation of the pace-maker and plateau components of delayed rectification in cardiac Purkinje fibres. *J Physiol* 1972;225:211–235.
191. Hayashi Y, Kambayashi T, Maze M. Role of imidazoline-preferring receptors in the genesis of epinephrine-induced arrhythmias in halothane-anesthetized dogs. *Anesthesiology* 1993;78:524–530.
192. Hayashi Y, Sumikawa K, Maze M. Dexmetomidine prevents epinephrine-induced arrhythmias through stimulation of central α_2 adrenoceptors in halothane-anesthetized dogs. *Anesthesiology* 1991; 75:113–117.
193. Hayashi Y, Sumikawa K, Tashiro C, Yoshiya I. Synergistic interaction of $alpha_1$- and beta-adrenoceptor agonists on induction arrhythmias during halothane anesthesia in dogs. *Anesthesiology* 1988;68:902–907.
194. Hayashi Y, Sumikawa K, Yamatodani A, Kamibayashi T, Kuro M, Yoshiya I. Myocardial epinephrine sensitization with subanesthetic concentrations of halothane in dogs. *Anesthesiology* 1991;74: 134–137.
195. Hayashi Y, Sumikawa K, Yamatodani A, Tashiro C, Wada H, Yoshiya I. Myocardial sensitization by thiopental to arrhythmogenic action of epinephrine in dogs. *Anesthesiology* 1989;71: 929–935.
196. Heavner JE. Cardiac dysrhythmias induced by infusion of local anesthetics into the lateral cerebral ventricle of cats. *Anesth Analg* 1986;65:133–138.
197. Hellam DC, Studt JW. A core-conductor model of the cardiac Purkinje fibre based on structural analysis. *J Physiol* 1974;243:637–660.
198. Hepler JR, Gilman AG. G proteins. *Trends Biochem Sci* 1992;17: 383–387.
199. Hill JL, Gettes LS. Effect of acute coronary artery occlusion on

local myocardial extracellular K^+ activity in swine. *Circulation* 1980; 61:768–778.

200. Hille B. Local anesthetics: hydrophilic and hydrophobic pathways for the drug-receptor interactions. *J Gen Physiol* 1977;69:497–515.
201. Hille B. *Ionic channels of excitable membranes*, 2nd ed. Sunderland, MA: Sinauer Associates, 1992.
202. Hirano Y, Fozzard HA, January CT. Characteristics of L- and T-type Ca^{2+} currents in canine cardiac Purkinje fibers. *Am J Physiol* 1989; 256:H1478–H1492.
203. Hirota K, Ito Y, Kuze S, Momose Y. Effects of halothane an electrophysiologic properties and cyclic adenosine 3',5' -monophosphate content in isolated guinea pig hearts. *Anesth Analg* 1992;74: 564–569.
204. Hirota K, Momose Y, Takeda R, Nakanishi S, Ito Y. Prolongation of the action potential and reduction of the delayed outward K^+ current by halothane in single frog atrial cells. *Eur J Pharmacol* 1986; 126:293–295.
205. Ho K, Nichols CG, Lederer WJ, et al. Cloning and expression of an inwardly rectifying ATP-regulated potassium channel. *Nature* 1993;362:31–38.
206. Hoffman BF, Singer DH. Appraisal of the effects of catecholamines on cardiac electrical activity. *Ann N Y Acad Sci* 1967;139:914–939.
207. Holmer SR, Homcy CJ. G proteins in the heart: a redundant and diverse transmembrane signaling network. *Circulation* 1991;84: 1891–1902.
208. Hondeghem LM, Katzung BG. Time- and voltage-dependent interactions of antiarrhythmic drugs with cardiac sodium channels. *Biochim Biophys Acta* 1977;472:373–398.
209. Hotvedt R, Refsum H, Helgesen KG. Cardiac electrophysiologic and hemodynamic effects related to plasma levels of bupivacaine in the dog. *Anesth Analg* 1985;64:388–394.
210. Hughes R, Chapple DJ. Effects of non-depolarizing neuromuscular blocking agents on peripheral autonomic mechanisms in cats. *Br J Anaesth* 1976;48:59–68.
211. Hume JR, Levesque PC, Hart PJ, Tsung SS, Chapman T, Horowitz B. Molecular physiology of cAMP-dependent chloride channels in heart. In: Spooner PM, Brown AM, Catterall WA, Kaczorowski GJ, Strauss HC, eds. *Ion channels in the cardiovascular system.* Armonk, NY: Futura, 1994;169–184.
212. Hume JR, Uehara A. Ionic basis of the different action potential configurations of single guinea-pig atrial and ventricular myocytes. *J Physiol* 1985;368:525–544.
213. Hunt GB, Ross DL. Comparison of effects of three anesthetic agents on induction of ventricular tachycardia in a canine model of myocardial infarction. *Circulation* 1988;78:221–226.
214. Ikemoto Y. Reduction by thiopental of the slow-channel-mediated action potential of canine papillary muscle. *Pflugers Arch* 1977;372: 285–286.
215. Ikemoto Y, Yatani A, Arimura H, Yoshitake J. Reduction of the slow inward current of isolated rat ventricular cells by thiamylal and halothane. *Acta Anaesthesiol Scand* 1985;29:583–586.
216. Ikemoto Y, Yatani A, Imoto Y, Arimura H. Reduction in the myocardial sodium current by halothane and thiamylal. *Jpn J Physiol* 1986; 36:107–121.
217. Iñiguez-Lluhi J, Kleuss C, Gilman AG. The importance of G-protein βγ subunits. *Trends Cell Biol* 1993;3:230–236.
218. Inoue K, Arndt JO. Efferent vagal discharge and heart rate in response to methohexitone, althesin, ketamine, and etomidate in cats. *Br J Anaesth* 1982;54:1105–1115.
219. Inoue K, El-Banayosy A, Stolarski L, Reichelt W. Vecuronium-induced bradycardia following induction of anaesthesia with etomidate or thiopentone, with or without fentanyl. *Br J Anaesth* 1988; 60:10–17.
220. Inoue K, Reichelt W. Asystole and bradycardia in adult patients after a single dose of suxamethonium. *Acta Anaesthesiol Scand* 1986; 30:571–573.
221. Irisawa H, Brown HF, Giles W. Cardiac pacemaking in the sinoatrial node. *Physiol Rev* 1993;73:197–227.
222. Isenberg G. Cardiac Purkinje fibers. $[Ca^{++}]_i$ controls the potassium permeability via the conductance components G_{K1} and G_{KL}. *Pflugers Arch* 1977;371:77–85.
223. Isenberg G, Belardinelli L. Ionic basic for the antagonism between adenosine and isoproterenol on isolated mammalian ventricular myocytes. *Circ Res* 1984;55:309–325.
224. Ishihara K, Mitsuiye T, Noma A, Takano M. The Mg^{2+} block and intrinsic gating underlying inward rectification of the K^+ current in guinea-pig cardiac myocytes. *J Physiol* 1989;419:297–320.
225. Ivankovich AD, El-Etr AA, Janeczko GF, Maronic JP. The effects of ketamine and of Innovar anesthesia on digitalis tolerance in the dog. *Anesth Analg* 1975;54:106–111.
226. Ivankovich AD, Miletich DJ, Grossman RK. The effects of enflurane, isoflurane, fluroxene, methoxyflurane and diethyl-ether anesthesia on oubian tolerance in the dog. *Anesth Analg* 1976;55: 360–365.
227. Iyengar R. Molecular and functional diversity of mammalian Gs-stimulated adenylyl cyclases. *FASEB J* 1993;7:768–775.
228. Jacobs HK, Lim S, Salem MR, Rao TLK, Mathru M, Smith BD. Cardiac electrophysiologic effects of pancuronium. *Anesth Analg* 1985; 64:693–699.
229. James TN. Cardiac conduction system: fetal and postnatal development. *Am J Cardiol* 1970;6:1083–1095.
230. Janse MJ. Re-entrant arrhythmias. In: Fozzard HA, Haber E, Jennings RB, eds. *The heart and cardiovascular system: scientific foundations.* New York: Raven Press, 1991;2055–2094.
231. Janse MJ, Wit AL. Electrophysiological mechanisms of ventricular arrhythmias resulting from myocardial ischemia and infarction. *Physiol Rev* 1989;69:1049–1169.
232. January CT, Riddle JM. Early afterdepolarizations: mechanism of induction and block. A role for L-type Ca^{2+} current. *Circ Res* 1989; 64:977–990.
233. Jeck CD, Boyden PA. Age-related appearance of outward currents may contribute to developmental differences in ventricular repolarization. *Circ Res* 1992;71:1390–1403.
234. Jiang C, Mochizuki S, Poole-Wilson PA, Harding SE, MacLeod KT. Effect of lemakalim on action potentials, intracellular calcium, and contraction in guinea pig and human cardiac myocytes. *Cardiovasc Res* 1994;28:851–857.
235. Jiang M, Moffat M, Narayanan N. Age-related alterations in the phosphorylation of sarcoplasmic reticulum and myofibrillar proteins and diminished contractile response to isoproterenol in intact rat ventricle. *Circ Res* 1993;72:102–111.
236. Joas TA, Stevens WC. Composition of the arrhythmic doses of epinephrine during forane, halothane and enflurane anesthesia in dogs. *Anesthesiology* 1971;35:48–53.
237. Josephson IR, Sanchez-Chapula J, Brown AM. Early outward current in rat single ventricular cells. *Circ Res* 1983;54:157–162.
238. Josephson IR, Sperelakis N. Phosphorylation shifts the time-dependence of cardiac Ca^{++} channel gating currents. *Biophys J* 1991;60:491–497.
239. Joyner RW, Overholt ED. Effects of octanol on canine subendocardial Purkinje-to-ventricular transmission. *Am J Physiol* 1985;249: H1228–H1231.
240. Joyner RW, Overholt ED, Ramza B, Veenstra RD. Propagation through electrically coupled cells: two inhomogeneously coupled cardiac tissue layers. *Am J Physiol* 1984;247:H596–H609.
241. Jurkiewicz NK, Sanguinetti MC. Rate-dependent prolongation of cardiac action potentials by a methanesulfonanilide class III antiarrhythmic agent. *Circ Res* 1993;72:75–83.
242. Kakei M. Adenosine-5'-triphosphate-sensitive single potassium channel in the atrioventricular node cell of the rabbit heart. *J Physiol* 1984;352:265–284.
243. Kambam JR, Kinney WW, Matsuda F, Wright W, Holaday DA. Epinephrine and phenylephrine increase cardiorespiratory toxicity of intravenously administered bupivacaine in rats. *Anesth Analg* 1990;70:543–545.
244. Kamibayashi T, Hayashi Y, Sumikawa K, Yamatodani A, Kawabata K, Yoshiya I. Enhancement by propofol of epinephrine-induced arrhythmias in dogs. *Anesthesiology* 1991;75:1035–1040.
245. Kardesch M, Hogencamp CE, Bing RJ. The effect of complete ischemia on the intracellular electrical activity of the whole mammalian heart. *Circ Res* 1958;6:715–720.
246. Kass RS, Scheuer T, Malloy KJ. Block of outward current in cardiac Purkinje fibres by injection of quaternary ammonium ions. *J Gen Physiol* 1982;79:1041–1063.
247. Kass RS, Seigelbaum SA, Tsien RW. Three-microelectrode voltage clamp experiments in calf cardiac Purkinje fibres: Is slow inward current adequately measured? *J Physiol* 1979;290:201–225.
248. Kass RS, Tsien RW. Control of action potential duration by calcium ions in cardiac Purkinje fibers. *J Gen Physiol* 1976;67: 599–617.
249. Kasten G, Martin S. Successful cardiovascular resuscitation after massive intravenous bupivacaine overdosage in anesthetized dogs. *Anesth Analg* 1985;64:491–497.
250. Kasten GW, Martin ST. Bupivacaine cardiovascular toxicity: com-

parison of treatment with bretylium and lidocaine. *Anesth Analg* 1985;64:911–916.
251. Kasten GW, Martin ST. Comparison of resuscitation of sheep and dogs after bupivacaine-induced cardiovascular collapse. *Anesth Analg* 1986;65:1029–1032.
252. Katsuoka M, Kobayashi K, Ohnishi T. Volatile anesthetics decrease calcium content of isolated myocytes. *Anesthesiology* 1989;70:954–960.
253. Katz AM. Cardiac Ion Channels. *New Engl J Med* 1993;328:1244–1251.
254. Kenyon JL, Gibbons TW. 4-Aminopyridine and the early outward current of sheep cardiac Purkinje fibres. *J Gen Physiol* 1979;73:139–157.
255. Kiba T. Effects of thiopental and pentobarbital sodium on the transmembrane potentials of the rabbit's atria in special reference to interaction with catecholamine. *Jpn J Pharmacol* 1966;16:168–179.
256. Kieval RS, Bulter VPJ, Derguini F. Cellular electrophysiologic effects of vertebrate digitalis-like substances. *J Am Coll Cardiol* 1988;11:637–643.
257. Kim HW, Steenart NAE, Ferguson DG, Kranias EG. Functional reconstitution of the cardiac sarcoplasmic reticulum Ca^{2+}-ATPase with phospholamban in phospholipid vesicles. *J Biol Chem* 1990;265:1702–1709.
258. Kimura S, Bassett AL, Kohya T, Kozlovskis PL, Myerburg RJ. Simultaneous recording of action potentials from endocardium and epicardium during ischemia in the isolated cat ventricle: relation of temporal electrophysiologic heterogeneities to arrhythmias. *Circulation* 1986;74:401–409.
259. Kirchhof CJ, Bonke FI, Allessie M. Evidence for the presence of electrotonic depression of pacemakers in the rabbit atrioventricular node: the effects of uncoupling from the surrounding myocardium. *Basic Res Cardiol* 1988;83:190–201.
260. Kirkwood I, Duckworth RA. An unusual case of sinus arrest. *Br J Anaesth* 1983;55:1273.
261. Kirsch GE, Codina J, Birnbaumer L, Brown AM. Coupling of ATP-sensitive K^+ channels to A_1 receptors by G proteins in rat ventricular myocytes. *Am J Physiol* 1990;28:H820–H826.
262. Komai H, Rusy BF. Effects of bupivacaine and lidocaine on AV conduction in the isolated rat heart. *Anesthesiology* 1981;55:281–285.
263. Komai H, Rusy BF. Differences in the myocardial depressant action of thiopental and halothane. *Anesth Analg* 1984;63:313–318.
264. Komai H, Rusy BF. Calcium and thiopental-induced spontaneous activity in rabbit papillary muscle. *J Mol Cell Cardiol* 1986;18:73–79.
265. Koscove EM, Paradis NA. Successful resuscitation from cardiac arrest using high-dose epinephrine therapy. *JAMA* 1988;259:3031–3034.
266. Kotelko DM, Schnider SM, Dailey PA, et al. Bupivacaine-induced cardiac arrhythmias in sheep. *Anesthesiology* 1984;60:10–18.
267. Koumi S-I, Wasserstrom JA. Acetylcholine-sensitive muscarinic K^+ channels in mammalian ventricular myocytes. *Am J Physiol* 1994;266:H1812–H1821.
268. Kowey PR, Friehling TD, Sewter J, et al. Electrophysiological effects of left ventricular hypertrophy: effect of calcium and potassium channel blockade. *Circ Res* 1991;83:2067–2075.
269. Koyano T, Kakei M, Nakashima H, Yoshinaga M, Matsuoka T, Tanaka H. ATP-regulated K^+ channels are modulated by intracellular H^+ in guinea-pig ventricular cells. *J Physiol* 1993;463:747–766.
270. Kraft LF, Katholi RE, Woods WT, James TN. Attenuation by magnesium of the electrophysiologic effects of hyperkalemia on human and canine heart cells. *Am J Cardiol* 1980;45:1191–1195.
271. Krapivinsky G, Gordon EA, Wickman K, Velimirovic B, Krapivinsky L, Clapham DE. The G-protein-gated atrial K^+ channel I_{KACh} is a heteromultimer of two inwardly rectifying K^+ channel proteins. *Nature* 1995;374:135–141.
272. Kroll DA, Knight PR. Antifibrillatory effects of volatile anesthetics in acute occlusion/reperfusion arrhythmias. *Anesthesiology* 1984;61:657–661.
273. Kubo Y, Baldwin TJ, Jan YN, Jan LY. Primary structure and functional expression of a mouse inward rectifier potassium channel. *Nature* 1993;362:127–133.
274. Kukushkin NI, Gainullin RZ, Sosunov EA. Transient outward current and rate dependence of action potential duration in rabbit cardiac ventricular muscle. *Pflugers Arch* 1983;399:87–92.
275. Kuo C-S, Munakata K, Reddy CP, Surawicz B. Characteristics and possible mechanism of ventricular arrhythmia dependent on the dispersion of action potential durations. *Circulation* 1983;67:1356–1367.
276. Lacombe P, Blaise G, Hollmann C, Tanguay M, Loulmet D. Isoproterenol corrects the effects of bupivacaine on the electrophysiologic properties of the isolated rabbit heart. *Anesth Analg* 1991;72:70–74.
277. Langer GA. Calcium and the heart: exchange at the tissue, cell, and organelle levels. *FASEB J* 1992;6:893–902.
278. Lappi MD, Billman GE. Effect of ryanodine on ventricular fibrillation induced by myocardial ischaemia. *Cardiovasc Res* 1993;27:2152–2159.
279. Laszlo A, Polic S, Kampine JP, Turner LA, Atlee JL, Bosnjak ZJ. Anesthetics and automaticity in latent pacemaker fibers. I. Effects of halothane, enflurane and isoflurane on automaticity and recovery of automaticity from overdrive suppression in Purkinje fibers derived from canine hearts. *Anesthesiology* 1991;75:98–105.
280. Laszlo A, Polic S, Kampine JP, Turner LA, Atlee JL III, Bosnjak ZJ. Halothane, enflurane and isoflurane on abnormal automaticity and triggered rhythmic activity of Purkinje fibers from 24–hour-old infarcted canine hearts. *Anesthesiology* 1991;75:847–853.
281. LeBlanc N, Hume JR. Sodium current-induced release of calcium from cardiac sarcoplasmic reticulum. *Science* 1990;248:372–376.
282. Lechner RB, Gurll NJ, Reynolds DG. Intracoronary naloxone in hemorrhagic shock: dose-dependent stereospecific effects. *Am J Physiol* 1985;249:H272–H277.
283. Lederer WJ, Niggli E, Hadley RW. Sodium-calcium exchange in excitable cells: fuzzy space. *Science* 1991;248:371–372.
284. Lederer WJ, Tsien RW. Transient inward current underlying arrhythmogenic effects of cardiotonic steroids in Purkinje fibers. *J Physiol* 1976;263:73–100.
285. Lee CO, Fozzard HA. Membrane permeability during low potassium depolarization in sheep cardiac Purkinje fibers. *Am J Physiol* 1979;237:C156–C165.
286. Lee JH, Steinburg SF, Rosen MR. A WB4101–sensitive alpha-a adrenergic receptor subtype modulates repolarization in canine Purkinje fibers. *J Pharmacol Exp Ther* 1991;258:681–687.
287. Lee KS, Tsien RW. Mechanism of calcium channel blockade by verapamil, D600, diltiazem and nitrendipine in single dialysed heart cells. *Nature* 1983;302:790–794.
288. Lee Son S, Waud BE. Potencies of neuromuscular blocking agents at the receptors of the atrial pacemaker and the motor endplate of the guinea pig. *Anesthesiology* 1977;47:34–36.
289. Lee Son S, Waud DR. A vagolytic action of neuromuscular blocking agents at the pacemaker of the isolated guinea pig atrium. *Anesthesiology* 1978;48:191–194.
290. Levine JH, Morganroth J, Kadish AH. Mechanisms and risk factors for proarrhythmia with type Ia compared with Ic antiarrhythmic drug therapy. *Circulation* 1989;80:1063–1069.
291. Lewis T, Feil HS, Stroud WD. Observations upon flutter and fibrillation. II. The nature of auricular flutter. *Heart* 1920;7:191–346.
292. Lindgren L, Saarnivaara L, Klemola U-M. Protection of fentanyl against cardiac dysrhythmias during induction of anaesthesia. *Eur J Anaesth* 1987;4:229–233.
293. Litovsky SH, Antzelevitch C. Transient outward current prominent in canine ventricular epicardium but not endocardium. *Circ Res* 1988;62:116–126.
294. Liu D-W, Gintant GA, Antzelevitch C. Ionic bases for electrophysiological distinctions among epicardial, midmyocardial, and endocardial myocytes from the free wall of the canine left ventricle. *Circ Res* 1993;72:671–687.
295. Loeb JM, Lichtenthal PR, de Tarnowsky JM. Parasympathomimetic effects of fentanyl on the canine sinus node. *J Auton Nerv Syst* 1984;11:91–94.
296. Logic JR, Morrow DH. The effect of halothane on ventricular automaticity. *Anesthesiology* 1972;36:107–111.
297. Lopatin AN, Makhina EN, Nichols CG. Potassium channel block by cytoplasmic polyamines as the mechanism of intrinsic rectification. *Nature* 1994;372:366–369.
298. Lue W-M, Boyden PA. Abnormal electrical properties of myocytes from chronically infarcted canine heart: alterations in Vmax and the transient outward current. *Circulation* 1992;85:1175–1188.
299. Luk H-N, Lin C-I, Wei J, Chang C-L. Depressant effects of isoflurane and halothane on isolated human atrial fibers. *Anesthesiology* 1988;69:667–676.
300. Lundy PM, Gverzdys S, Frew R. Ketamine: evidence of tissue-spe-

cific inhibition of neuronal and extraneuronal catecholamine uptake processes. *Can J Physiol Pharmacol* 1985;63:298–303.

301. Luo C, Rudy Y. A model of the ventricular cardiac action potential: depolarization, repolarization, and their interaction. *Circ Res* 1991;68:1501–1526.
302. Lynch C III. Depression of myocardial contractility in vitro by bupivacaine, etidocaine, and lidocaine. *Anesth Analg* 1986;65: 551–559.
303. Lynch C III. Differential depression of myocardial contractility by halothane and isoflurane *in vitro*. *Anesthesiology* 1986;64:620–631.
304. Lynch C III. Cellular electrophysiology of the heart. In: Lynch C III, ed. *Clinical cardiac electrophysiology: perioperative considerations.* Philadelphia: JB Lippincott, 1994;1–52.
305. Lynch C III, Jaeger JM. The G protein cell signalling system. In: Lake C, ed. Advances in anesthesia 11. Chicago: Mosby-Year Book, 1994;65–112.
306. Lynch C III, Vogel S, Pratila MG, Sperelakis N. Enflurane depression of myocardial slow action potentials. *J Pharmacol Exp Ther* 1982;222:405–409.
307. Lynch C III, Vogel S, Sperelakis N. Halothane depression of myocardial slow action potentials. *Anesthesiology* 1981;55:360–368.
308. MacCannell KL, Dresel PE. Potentiation by thiopental of cyclopropane-adrenaline cardiac arrhythmias. *Can J Physiol Pharmacol* 1964;42:627–639.
309. Mantelli L, Manzini S, Mugelli A, Ledda F. The influence of some cardiodepressant drugs on the histamine-induced restoration of contractility in potassium-depolarized heart preparations. *Arch Int Pharmacodyn* 1981;254:99–108.
310. Martins JB. Autonomic control of ventricular tachycardia: sympathetic neural influence on spontaneous tachycardia 24 hours after coronary occlusion. *Circulation* 1985;72:933–942.
311. Martins JB, Wendt DJ. α-Adrenergic effects on relative refractory period in Purkinje system of intact canine left ventricle. *Am J Physiol* 1989;257:H1156–H1164.
312. Martins JB, Zipes DP. Effects of sympathetic and vagal nerves on recovery properties of the endocardium and epicardium of the canine left ventricle. *Circ Res* 1980;46:100–110.
313. Martyn JAJ, White DA, Gronert GA, Jaffe RS, Ward JM. Up-and-down regulation of skeletal muscle acetylcholine receptors. *Anesthesiology* 1992;76:822–843.
314. Matsuda F, Kinney WW, Wright W, Kambam R. Nicardipine reduces the cardiorespiratory toxicity of intravenously administered bupivacaine in rats. *Can J Anaesth* 1990;37:920–923.
315. Matsuda H. Magnesium gating of the inwardly rectifying K^+ channel. *Annu Rev Physiol* 1991;53:289–298.
316. Matsuda H. Effects of internal and external Na^+ ions on inwardly rectifying K^+ channels in guinea-pig ventricular cells. *J Physiol* 1993;460:311–326.
317. Matsuda H, Saigusa A, Irisawa H. Ohmic conductance through the inwardly rectifying K channel and blocking by internal Mg^{2+}. *Nature* 1987;325:156–159.
318. Matsuda JJ, Lee H, Shibata EF. Enhancement of rabbit cardiac sodium channels by β-adrenergic stimulation. *Circ Res* 1992;70: 199–207.
319. Matsuda K, Kamiyama A, Hoshi T. Configuration of the transmembrane potential of the Purkinje-ventricular fiber junction and its analysis. In: Sano T, Mizuhira J, Matsuda K, eds. *Electrophysiology and ultrastructure of the heart.* New York: Grune & Stratton, 1967;177–188.
320. Maylie J, Morad M. Ionic currents responsible for the generation of pace-maker current in the rabbit sino-atrial node. *J Physiol* 1984; 355:215–235.
321. Maylie J, Morad M, Weiss J. A study of pace-maker potential in rabbit sino-atrial node: measurement of potassium activity under voltage-clamp conditions. *J Physiol* 1981;311:161–178.
322. Maze M, Hayward E, Gaba DM. Alpha$_1$-adrenergic blockade raises epinephrine-arrhythmia threshold in halothane-anesthetized dogs in a dose-dependent fashion. *Anesthesiology* 1985;63:611–615.
323. Maze M, Smith CM. Identification of receptor mechanism mediating epinephrine-induced arrhythmias during halothane anesthesia. *Anesthesiology* 1983;59:322–326.
324. McAllister RE, Noble D. The time and voltage dependence of the slow outward current in cardiac Purkinje fibres. *J Physiol* 1966;186: 632–662.
325. McDonald TF, Pelzer D. Cat ventricular muscle treated with D600: characteristics of calcium channel block and unblock. *J Physiol* 1984;352:217–241.
326. McDonald TF, Pelzer S, Trautwein W, Pelzer DJ. Regulation and modulation of calcium channels in cardiac, skeletal, and smooth muscle cells. *Physiol Rev* 1994;74:365–507.
327. McDonald TF, Trautwein W. The potassium current underlying delayed rectification in cat ventricular muscle. *J Physiol* 1978;274: 217–246.
328. Meijler F, Anse MJ. Morphology and electrophysiology of the mammalian atrioventricular node. *Physiol Rev* 1988;68:608–649.
329. Mejía-Alvarez R, Marban E. Mechanism of the increase in intracellular sodium during metabolic inhibition - direct evidence against mediation by voltage-dependent sodium channels. *J Mol Cell Cardiol* 1992;24:1307–1320.
330. Mendez C, Han J, Moe GK. A comparison of the effects of epinephrine and vagal stimulation upon the refractory periods of the A-V node and the bundle of His. *Naunyn Schmiedebergs Arch Pharmacol* 1964;248:99–116.
331. Mendez C, Moe GK. Demonstration of a dual A-V nodal conduction system in the isolated rabbit heart. *Circ Res* 1966;19:378–393.
332. Mendez C, Mueller WJ, Merideth J, Mow GK. Interaction of transmembrane potentials in canine Purkinje fibers and at Purkinje fiber-muscle junctions. *Circ Res* 1969;24:361–372.
333. Mendez C, Mueller WJ, Urguiaga X. Propagation of impulses across the Purkinje fiber-muscle junctions in the dog heart. *Circ Res* 1970;26:135–150.
334. Méry P-F, Pavoine C, Belhassen L, Pecker F, Fischmeister R. Nitric oxide regulates cardiac Ca^{2+} current. Involvement of cGMP-inhibited and cGMP-stimulated phosphodiesterases through guanylyl cyclase activation. *J Biol Chem* 1993;268:26286–26295.
335. Metz S, Maze M. Halothane concentration does not alter the threshold for epinephrine-induced arrhythmias in dogs. *Anesthesiology* 1985;62:470–474.
336. Mikami A, Imoto K, Tanabe T, et al. Primary structure and functional expression of the cardiac dihydropyridine-sensitive calcium channel. *Nature* 1989;340:230–233.
337. Miller C. 1990: Annus mirabilis of potassium channels. *Science* 1991;252:1092–1096.
338. Milligan KR, Beers HT. Vecuronium-associated cardiac arrest (letter). *Anaesthesia* 1985;40:385.
339. Mines GR. On dynamic equilibrium in the heart. *J Physiol* 1913;46: 349–382.
340. Mines GR. On circulating excitations in heart muscle and their possible relation to tachycardia and fibrillation. *Trans R Soc Canada* 1914;IV:43–52.
341. Mitra R, Morad M. Two types of Ca^{2+} in guinea pig ventricular myocytes. *Proc Natl Acad Sci USA* 1986;83:5340–5344.
342. Miura DS, Hoffman BF, Rosen MR. The effect of extracellular potassium on the intracellular potassium ion activity and transmembrane potential of beating canine cardiac Purkinje fibers. *J Gen Physiol* 1977;69:463–474.
343. Moe GK, Mendez C, Han J. Aberrant A-V impulse program propagation in the dog heart: a study of functional bundle branch block. *Circ Res* 1965;16:261–286.
344. Moller RA, Covino BG. Cardiac electrophysiologic effects of lidocaine and bupivacaine. *Anesth Analg* 1988;67:107–114.
345. Morishima HO, Pedersen H, Finster M, et al. Bupivacaine toxicity in pregnant and nonpregnant ewes. *Anesthesiology* 1985;63:134–139.
346. Morrow DH, Townley NT. Anesthesia and digitalis toxicity: an experimental study. *Anesth Analg* 1964;43:510–519.
347. Nabauer M, Beuckelmann D, Erdmann E. Characteristics of transient outward current in human ventricular myocytes from patients with terminal heart failure. *Circ Res* 1993;73:386–394.
348. Nakao S, Hirat H, Kagawa Y. Effects of volatile anesthetics on cardiac calcium channels. *Acta Anaesthesiol Scand* 1989;33:326–330.
349. Nakaya H, Hattori Y, Tohse N, Shida S, Kanno M. Beta-adrenoceptor-mediated depolarization of the resting membrane in guinea-pig papillary muscles: changes in intracellular Na^+, K^+ and Cl^- activities. *Pflugers Arch* 1990;417:185–193.
350. Nakayama T, Fozzard HA. Adrenergic modulation of the transient outward current in isolated canine Purkinje cells. *Circ Res* 1988;62: 162–172.
351. Nakayama T, Irisawa H. Transient outward current carried by potassium and sodium in quiescent atrioventricular node cells of rabbit. *Circ Res* 1985;57:65–73.
352. Neubauer S, Newell JB, Ingwall JS. Metabolic consequences and predictability of ventricular fibrillation in hypoxia: a ^{31}P- and ^{23}Na-magnetic resonance study of the isolated rat heart. *Circulation* 1992;86:302–310.

353. Niggli E, Rüdisüli A, Maurer P, Weingart R. Effects of general anesthetics on current flow across membranes in guinea pig myocytes. *Am J Physiol* 1989;256:C273–C281.
354. Nigrovic V. Succinylcholine, cholinoceptors, and catecholamines: proposed mechanism of early adverse haemodynamic reactions. *Can Anaesth Soc J* 1984;31:382–394.
355. Nilius B, Hess P, Lansman JB, Tsien RW. A novel type of cardiac calcium channel in ventricular cells. *Nature* 1985;316:443–446.
356. Nitta J, Furukawa T, Marumo F, Sawanobori T, Hiraoka M. Subcellular mechanism for Ca^{2+}-dependent enhancement of delayed rectifier K^+ current in isolated membrane patches of guinea pig ventricular myocytes. *Circ Res* 1994;74:96–104.
357. Noble D, Tsien RW. The kinetics and rectifier properties of the slow potassium current in cardiac Purkinje fibres. *J Physiol* 1968; 195:185–214.
358. Noble D, Tsien RW. Outward membrane currents activated in the plateau range of potentials in cardiac Purkinje fibres. *J Physiol* 1969;200:205–231.
359. Noma A. ATP-regulated K^+ channels in cardiac muscle. *Nature* 1983;305:147–148.
360. Ono K, Fozzard HA, Hanck DA. Mechanism of cAMP-dependent modulation of cardiac sodium channel current kinetics. *Circ Res* 1993;72:807–815.
361. Ono K, Trautwein W. Potentiation by cyclic GMP of β-adrenergic effect on Ca^{2+} current in guinea-pig ventricular cells. *J Physiol* 1991;443:387–404.
362. Ozsaki S, Nakaya H, Gotoh Y, Azuma M, Kemmotsu O, Kanno M. Effects of halothane and enflurane on conduction velocity and maximum rate of action potential upstroke in guinea pig papillary muscles. *Anesth Analg* 1989;68:219–225.
363. Pace NL, Ohmura A, Wong KC. Epinephrine-induced arrhythmias: effects of exogenous prostaglandins and prostaglandin synthesis inhibition during halothane-O_2 anesthesia in the dog. *Anesth Analg* 1979;58:401–404.
364. Pancrazio JJ, Frazer MJ, Lynch C III. Barbiturate anesthetics depress the resting K^+ conductance of myocardium. *J Pharmacol Exp Ther* 1993;265:358–365.
365. Pancrazio JJ, Lynch C III. Effect of volatile anesthetics on cardiac calcium current kinetics. *Biophys J* 1994;66:A95.
366. Pancrazio JJ, Park WK, Lynch C III. Effects of enflurane on voltage-gated membrane currents of bovine adrenal chromaffin cells. *Neurosci Lett* 1992;146:147–151.
367. Park WK, Lynch C III. Propofol and thiopental depression of myocardial contractility—a comparative study of mechanical and electrophysiologic effects in isolated guinea pig ventricular muscle. *Anesth Analg* 1992;74:395–405.
368. Pastelin G, Mendez R, Moe GK. Participation of atrial specialized conduction pathways in atrial flutter. *Circ Res* 1978;42:386–393.
369. Paulmichl MP, Nasmith P, Hellmiss R, et al. Cloning and expression of a rat cardiac delayed rectifier potassium channel. *Proc Natl Acad Sci USA* 1991;88:7892–7895.
370. Petit-Jacques J, Bescond J, Bois P, Lenfant J. Particular sensitivity of the mammalian heart sinus node cells. *News Physiol Sci* 1994;9: 77–79.
371. Pfaffinger PJ, Martin JM, Hunter DD, Nathanson NM, Hille B. GTP-binding proteins couple cardiac muscarinic receptors to a K^+ channel. *Nature* 1985;317:536–538.
372. Po S, Snyders DJ, Baker R, Tamkun MM, Bennett PB. Functional expression of an inactivating potassium channel cloned from human heart. *Circ Res* 1992;71:732–736.
373. Pogwizd SM, Corr PB. Electrophysiologic mechanisms underlying arrhythmias due to reperfusion of ischemic myocardium. *Circulation* 1987;76:404–426.
374. Polic S, Atlee JL, Laszlo A, Kampine JP, Bosnjak ZJ. Anesthetics and automaticity in latent pacemaker fibers. II. Effects of halothane and epinephrine or norepinephrine on automaticity of dominant and subsidiary atrial pacemakers in the canine heart. *Anesthesiology* 1991;75:298–304.
375. Polic S, Bosnjak ZJ, Marijic J, Hoffman RG, Kampine JP, Turner LA. Actions of halothane, isoflurane and enflurane on the regional action potential characteristics of canine Purkinje fibers. *Anesth Analg* 1991;73:603–611.
376. Pollok AJP. Cardiac arrest immediately after vecuronium. *Br J Anaesth* 1986;58:936–937.
377. Pratila M, Vogel S, Sperelakis N. Inhibition by enflurane and methoxyflurane of postdrive hyperpolarization in canine Purkinje fibers. *J Pharmacol Exp Ther* 1984;229:603–607.
378. Preston JB, McFadden S, Moe GK. Atrioventricular transmission in young mammals. *Am J Physiol* 1959;197:236–240.
379. Ramos-Franco J, Lo CF, Breitwieser GE. Platelet-activating factor receptor-dependent activation of the muscarinic K^+ current in bullfrog atrial myocytes. *Circ Res* 1993;72:786–794.
380. Rasmusson RL, Clark JW, Giles WR. A mathematical model of a bullfrog cardiac pacemaker cell. *Am J Physiol* 1990;259: H352–H369.
381. Rawling DA, Joyner RW, Overholt ED. Variations in the functional electrical coupling between the subendocardial Purkinje and ventricular layers of the canine left ventricle. *Circ Res* 1985;57: 252–261.
382. Reitan JA, Stengert KB, Wymore ML, Martucci RW. Central vagal control of fentanyl-induced bradycardia during halothane anesthesia. *Anesth Analg* 1978;57:31–36.
383. Reiter MJ, Synhorst DP, Mann DE. Electrophysiological effects of acute ventricular dilation in the isolated rabbit heart. *Circ Res* 1988;62:554–562.
384. Reuter H, Scholz H. A study of the ion selectivity and the kinetic properties of the calcium dependent slow inward current in mammalian cardiac muscle. *J Physiol* 1977;264:17–47.
385. Reynolds AK, Chiz JF. Epinephrine-potential slowing of conductance in Purkinje fibers. *Res Commun Chem Pathol Pharmacol* 1974; 9:633–645.
386. Reynolds AK, Chiz JF, Pasquet AF. Halothane and methoxyflurane —a comparison of their effects on cardiac pacemaker fibers. *Anesthesiology* 1970;33:602–610.
387. Reynolds AK, Chiz JF, Tanikella TK. On the mechanism of coupling in adrenalin-induced bigeminy in sensitized hearts. *Can J Physiol Pharmacol* 1975;53:1158–1171.
388. Reynolds AK, Horne ML. Studies on the cardiotoxicity of oubain. *Can J Physiol Pharmacol* 1969;47:165–170.
389. Riley DC, Schmeling WT, Al-Wathiqui MH, Kampine JP, Warltier DC. Prolongation of the QT interval by volatile anesthetics in chronically instrumented dogs. *Anesth Analg* 1988;67:741–749.
390. Roizen MF, Moss J, Henry DP, Kopin IJ. Effects of halothane on plasma catecholamines. *Anesthesiology* 1974;41:432–439.
391. Rose WC, Balke CW, Wier WG, Marban E. Macroscopic and unitary properties of physiological ion flux through L-type Ca^{2+} channels in guinea-pig heart cells. *J Physiol* 1992;456:267–284.
392. Rosen MA, Thigpen JW, Schnider SM, Foutz SE, Levinson G, Koike M. Bupivacaine-induced cardiotoxicity in hypoxic and acidotic sheep. *Anesth Analg* 1985;64:1089–1096.
393. Rosenbaum DS, Kaplan DT, Kanai A, et al. Repolarization inhomogeneities in ventricular myocardium change dynamically with abrupt cycle length shortening. *Circulation* 1991;84:1333–1345.
394. Rozanski GJ, Jalife J, Moe GK. Reflected reentry in nonhomogeneous ventricular muscle as a mechanism of cardiac arrhythmias. *Circulation* 1984;69:163–173.
395. Rusy BF, Komai H. Anesthetic depression of myocardial contractility: a review of possible mechanisms. *Anesthesiology* 1987;67: 745–766.
396. Sage DJ, Feldman HS, Arthur R, et al. Influence of lidocaine and bupivacaine on isolated guinea pig atria in the presence of acidosis and hypoxia. *Anesth Analg* 1984;63:1–7.
397. Saitoh H, Bailey JC, Surawicz B. Alterations of action potential duration after abrupt shortening of cycle length: differences between dog Purkinje and ventricular fibers. *Circ Res* 1988;62: 1027–1040.
398. Sakmann B, Trube G. Conductance properties of single inwardly rectifying potassium channels in ventricular cells from guinea-pig heart. *J Physiol* 1984;347:641–657.
399. Salt PJ, Barnes PK, Beswick FJ. Inhibition of neuronal and extraneuronal uptake of noradrenaline by ketamine in the isolated perfused rat heart. *Br J Anaesth* 1979;51:835–838.
400. Sanguinetti MC, Jurkiewicz NK. Lanthanum blocks a specific component of I_K and screens membrane surface charge in cardiac cells. *Am J Physiol* 1990;28:H1881–H1889.
401. Sanguinetti MC, Jurkiewicz NK. Two components of cardiac delayed rectifier K^+ current: differential sensitivity to block by class III antiarrhythmic agents. *J Gen Physiol* 1990;96:195–215.
402. Sanguinetti MC, Kass RS. Voltage-dependent block of calcium channel current in the calf cardiac Purkinje fiber by dihydropyridine calcium channel antagonists. *Circ Res* 1984;55:336–348.
403. Sano T, Takayama N, Shimamoto T. Directional difference of conduction velocity in cardiac ventricular syncytium studied by microelectrodes. *Circ Res* 1959;7:262–267.

404. Savarese JJ, Lowenstein E. The name of the game: no anesthesia by cook book. *Anesthesiology* 1985;62:703–705.
405. Scamps F, Nilius B, Alvarez J, Vassort G. Modulation of L-type Ca channel activity by P_2-purinergic agonist in cardiac cells. *Pflugers Arch* 1993;422:465–471.
406. Schick LM, Chapin JC, Munson ES, Kushins LG. Pancuronium, d-tubocurarine, and epinephrine-induced arrhythmias during halothane anesthesia in dogs. *Anesthesiology* 1980;52:207–209.
407. Schmeling WT, Bosnjak ZJ, Kampine JP. Anesthesia and the autonomic nervous system. *Semin Anesth* 1990;9:223–231.
408. Schmeling WT, Warltier DC, McDonald DJ, Madsen KE, Atlee JL, Kampine JP. Prolongation of the QT interval by enflurane, isoflurane, and halothane in humans. *Anesth Analg* 1991;72:137–144.
409. Schoenstadt DA, Whitcher CE. Observations on the mechanism of succinylcholine-induced cardiac arrhythmias. *Anesthesiology* 1963; 24:358–362.
410. Scholz W, Albus U, Linz W, Martorana P, Lang HJ, Schölkens BA. Effects of Na^+/H^+ exchange inhibitors in cardiac ischemia. *J Mol Cell Cardiol* 1992;24:731–740.
411. Schubert B, Vandongen AM, Kirsch GE, Brown AM. Inhibition of cardiac Na^+ currents by isoproterenol. *Am J Physiol* 1990;258: H977–H982.
412. Schultz BD, Venglarik CJ, Bridges RJ, Frizzell RA. Regulation of CFTR Cl^- channel gating by ADP and ATP analogues. *J Gen Physiol* 1995;105:329–362.
413. Schultz D, Mikala G, Yatani A, et al. Cloning, chromosomal localization, and functional expression of the α_1 subunit of the L-type voltage-dependent calcium channel from normal human heart. *Proc Natl Acad Sci USA* 1993;90:6228–6232.
414. Schwartz PJ, Periti M, Malliani A. The long QT syndrome. *Am Heart J* 1975;109:378–390.
415. Senges J, Mizutani T, Pelzer D, Brachman J, Sonnhof U, Kübler W. Effect of hypoxia on the sinoatrial node, atrium and atrioventricular node in the rabbit heart. *Circ Res* 1979;44:856–863.
416. Sheets MF, Hanck DA. Mechanisms of extracellular divalent and trivalent cation block of the sodium current in canine cardiac Purkinje cells. *J Physiol* 1992;454:299–320.
417. Sheets MF, Hanck DA, Fozzard HA. Nonlinear relationship between V_{max} and I_{Na} in canine cardiac Purkinje cells. *Circ Res* 1988;63:386–398.
418. Shen J-B, Pappano AJ. Palmitoyl-carnitine acts like ouabain on voltage, current, and contraction in guinea pig ventricular cells. *Am J Physiol* 1995;268:H1027–H1036.
419. Sheu S-S, Korth M, Lathrup DA, Fozzard HA. Intra- and extra-cellular K^+ and Na^+ activities and resting membrane potential in sheep cardiac Purkinje strands. *Circ Res* 1980;47:692–700.
420. Shibasaki T. Conductance and kinetics of delayed rectifier potassium channels in nodal cells of the rabbit heart. *J Physiol* 1987;387: 227–250.
421. Shorofsky SR, January CT. L- and T-type Ca^{2+} channels in canine cardiac Purkinje cells. Single-channel demonstration of L-type Ca^{2+} window current. *Circ Res* 1992;70:456–464.
422. Shryock J, Song Y, Wang D, Baker SP, Olsson RA, Belardinelli L. Selective α_2-Adenosine receptor agonists do not alter action potential duration, twitch shortening, or cAMP accumulation in guninea pig, rat, or rabbit isolated ventricular myocytes. *Circ Res* 1993;72:194–205.
423. Siegelbaum SA, Tsien RW, Kass RS. Role of intracellular calcium in the transient outward current of calf Purkinje fibres. *J Physiol* 1977;269:611–613.
424. Siegelbaum SA, Tsien RW, Kass RS. Calcium-activated outward current in calf Purkinje fibres. *J Physiol* 1980;299:485–506.
425. Skou JC. The Na-K pump. *News Physiol Sci* 1992;7:95–100.
426. Smrcka AV, Hepler JR, Brown KO, Sternweiss PC. Regulation of polyphosphoinositide-specific phospholipase C activity by purified G_q. *Science* 1991;251:804–807.
427. Snyders DJ, Knoth KM, Robards SL, Tamkun MM. Time-, state- and voltage-dependent block by quinidine of a cloned human cardiac channel. *Mol Pharmacol* 1992;41:332–339.
428. Snyders DJ, Tamkun MM, Bennett PB. A rapidly activating and slowly inactivating potassium channel cloned from human heart: functional analysis after stable mammalian cell culture expression. *J Gen Physiol* 1993;101:513–543.
429. Sorota S. Swelling-induced chloride-sensitive current in canine atrial cells revealed by whole-cell patch clamp. *Circ Res* 1992;70: 679–687.
430. Spach MS, Miller WT III, Dolber PC. The discontinuous nature of propagation in normal canine cardiac muscle. Evidence for recurrent discontinuities of intracellular resistance that affect membrane currents. *Circ Res* 1981;48:39–54.
431. Spach MS, Miller WT III, Dolber PC. The functional role of structural complexities in the propagation of depolarization in the atrium of a dog. Cardiac conduction disturbances due to discontinuities of effective axial resistivity. *Circ Res* 1982;50:175–191.
432. Sperelakis N. Origin of the cardiac resting potential. In: Berne RM, ed. *Handbook of physiology section 2: the cardiovascular system,* vol 1 (the heart). Bethesda: American Physiological Society, 1979;187–267.
433. Spiss CK, Maze M, Smith CM. Alpha-adrenergic responsiveness correlates with epinephrine dose for arrhythmias during halothane anesthesia in dogs. *Anesth Analg* 1984;63:297–300.
434. Starr NJ, Sethna DH, Estafanous F, Bowman FO Jr, Gersony WM. Bradycardia and asystole following rapid administration of sufentanil and vecuronium. *Anesthesiology* 1986;64:521–523.
435. Sternweis PC, Smrcka AV. Regulation of phospholipase C by G proteins. *Trends Biochem Sci* 1992;17:502–506.
436. Stowe DF, Bosnjak ZJ, Kampine JP. Effect of hypoxia on adult and neonatal pacemaker rates. *Obstet Gynecol* 1985;66:649–656.
437. Stowe DF, Dujic Z, Bosnjak ZJ, Kalbfleisch JH, Kampine JP. Volatile anesthetics attenuate sympathomimetic actions on the guinea pig SA node. *Anesthesiology* 1988;68:887–894.
438. Sumikawa K, Ishizaka N, Suzaki M. Arrhythmogenic plasma levels of epinephrine during halothane, enflurane and pentobarbital anesthesia in the dog. *Anesthesiology* 1983;58:322–325.
439. Sunnergren KP, Fairman RP, deBlois GG, Glauser FL. Effects of protamine, heparinase, and hyaluronidase on endothelial permeability and surface charge. *J Appl Physiol* 1987;63:1987–1992.
440. Supan DF, Eskinder H, Buljubasic N, Kampine JP, Bosnjak ZJ. Effects of inhalational anesthetics on K^+ current in canine cardiac Purkinje cells (abstract). *FASEB J* 1991;5:A1742.
441. Surawicz B. Role of potassium channels in cycle length dependent regulation of action potential duration in mammalian cardiac Purkinje and ventricular muscle fibres. *Cardiovasc Res* 1992; 26:1021–1029.
442. Takanaka C, Singh BN. Barium-induced nondriven action potentials as a model of triggered potentials from early afterdepolarizations: significance of slow channel activity and differing effects of quinidine and amiodarone. *J Am Coll Cardiol* 1990;15: 213–221.
443. Takano M, Noma A. Distribution of the isoprenaline-induced chloride current in rabbit heart. *Pflugers Arch* 1992;420:223–226.
444. Takasago T, Imagawa T, Shigekawa M. Phosphorylation of the cardiac ryanodine receptor by cAMP-dependent kinase. *J Biochem (Tokyo)* 1989;106:872–877.
445. Tamkun MM, Knoth KM, Walbridge JA, Kroemer H, Roden DM, Glover DM. Molecular cloning and characterization of two voltage-gated K^+ channel CDNAs from human ventricle. *FASEB J* 1991;5:331–337.
446. Tani M, Neely JR. Role of intracellular Na^+ in Ca^{2+} overload and depressed recovery of ventricular function of reperfused ischemic rat hearts: possible involvement of H^+-Na^+ and Na^+-Ca^{2+} exchange. *Circ Res* 1989;65:1045–1056.
447. Tanz RD, Heskett T, Loehning RW, Fairfax CA. Comparative cardiotoxicity of bupivacaine and lidocaine in the isolated perfused mammalian heart. *Anesth Analg* 1984;63:549–556.
448. Tchou PJ, Lehmann MH, Dongas J. Effect of sudden rate acceleration on the human His-Purkinje system: adaptation of refractoriness in a dampened oscillatory pattern. *Circulation* 1986;73: 920–929.
449. Terrar DA, Victory JGG. Effects of halothane on membrane currents associated with contraction in single myocytes isolated from guinea-pig ventricle. *Br J Pharmacol* 1988;94:500–508.
450. Terrar DA, Victory JGG. Isoflurane depresses membrane currents associated with contractions in myocytes isolated from guinea-pig ventricle. *Anesthesiology* 1988;69:742–749.
451. Terzic A, Pucéat M, Clément O, Scamps F, Vassort G. α_1-Adrenergic effects on intracellular pH and calcium and on myofilaments in single rat cardiac cells. *J Physiol* 1992;447:275–292.
452. Thomas RC. Electrogenic sodium pump in nerve and muscle cells. *Physiol Rev* 1972;52:563–594.
453. Thomas RD, Behbehani MM, Coyle DE, Denson DD. Cardiovascular toxicity of local anesthetics: an alternative hypothesis. *Anesth Analg* 1986;65:444–450.
454. Thornton JD, Thornton CS, Sterling DL, Downey JM. Blockade

of ATP-sensitive potassium channels increases infarct size but does not prevent preconditioning in rabbit hearts. *Circ Res* 1993; 72:44–49.

455. Tohse N. Calcium-sensitive delayed rectifier potassium current n guinea pig ventricular cells. *Am J Physiol* 1990;27:H1200–H1207.
456. Tohse N, Kameyama M, Irisawa H. Intracellular Ca^{2+} and protein kinase C modulate K^+ current in guinea pig heart cells. *Am J Physiol* 1987;22:H1321–H1324.
457. Tohse N, Kameyama M, Sekiguchi K, Shearman MS, Kanno M. Protein kinase C activation enhances the delayed rectifier potassium current in guinea-pig heart cells. *J Mol Cell Cardiol* 1990;22: 725–734.
458. Tohse N, Nakaya H, Kanno M. α_1-Adrenoceptor stimulation enhances the delayed rectifier K^+ current of guinea pig ventricular cells through the activation of protein kinase C. *Circ Res* 1992;71:1441–1446.
459. Tolmie JD, Joyce TH, Mitchell GD. Succinylcholine danger in the burned patient. *Anesthesiology* 1967;28:467–470.
460. Tomita F, Bassett AL, Myerburg RJ, Kimura S. Diminished transient outward currents in rat hypertrophied ventricular myocytes. *Circ Res* 1994;75:296–303.
461. Trautwein W, Gottstein U, Dudel J. Der Aktionsstrom der Myokardfaser im Sauerstoffmangel. *Pflugers Arch* 1954;260:40–60.
462. Trube G, Hescheler J. Inward-rectifying channels in isolated patches of the heart cell membrane: ATP-dependence and comparison with cell-attached patches. *Pflugers Arch* 1984;401:178–184.
463. Tseng GN, Boyden PA. Multiple types of Ca^{2+} currents in single canine Purkinje cells. *Circ Res* 1989;65:1735–1750.
464. Tsien RW, Kass RS, Weingart R. Cellular and subcellular mechanisms of cardiac pacemaker oscillations. *J Exp Biol* 1979;81: 205–215.
465. Tucker WK, Rackstein AD, Munson ES. Comparison of arrhythmic doses of adrenaline, metaraminal, ephedrine and phenylephrine during isoflurane and halothane anaesthesia in dogs. *Br J Anaesth* 1974;46:392–396.
466. Turgeon J, Daleau P, Bennett PB, Wiggins SS, Selby L, Roden DM. Block of the I_{Ks}, the slow component of the delayed rectifier K^+ current, by the diuretic agent indapamide in guinea pig myocytes. *Circ Res* 1994;75:879–886.
467. Turner LA, Bosnjak ZJ. Autonomic and anesthetic modulation of cardiac conduction and arrhythmias. In: Lynch C III, ed. *Clinical cardiac electrophysiology: perioperative considerations.* Philadelphia: JB Lippincott, 1994;53–84.
468. Turner LA, Bosnjak ZJ, Kampine JP. Actions of halothane on the electrical activity of Purkinje fibers derived from normal and infarcted canine hearts. *Anesthesiology* 1987;67:619–629.
469. Turner LA, Marijic J, Kampine JP, Bosnjak ZJ. A comparison of the effects of halothane and tetrodotoxin on the regional repolarization characteristics of canine Purkinje fibers. *Anesthesiology* 1990; 73:1158–1168.
470. Turner LA, Polic S, Hoffmann RG, Kampine JP, Bosnjak ZJ. Action of halothane and isoflurane on Purkinje fibers in the infarcted canine heart: conduction, regional refractoriness and reentry. *Anesth Analg* 1993;76:1387–1400.
471. Turner LA, Polic S, Hoffmann RG, Kampine JP, Bosnjak ZJ. Actions of volatile anesthetics on ischemic and nonischemic Purkinje fibers in the infarcted canine heart: regional action potential characteristics. *Anesth Analg* 1993;76:726–733.
472. Turner LA, Vodanovic S, Kampine JP, Bosnjak ZJ. WB4101 sensitive α_1-adrenergic depression of conduction in canine Purkinje fibers exposed to halothane (abstract). *FASEB J* 1993;7:A96.
473. Turner LA, Zuperku EJ, Bosnjak ZJ, Kampine JP. Autonomic modulation of refractoriness in canine specialized His-Purkinje system. *Am J Physiol* 1985;248:R515–R523.
474. Turner LA, Zuperku EJ, Purtock RV, Kampine JP. *In vivo* changes in canine ventricular cardiac conduction during halothane anesthesia. *Anesth Analg* 1980;59:327–334.
475. Vandenberg CA. Inward rectification of a potassium channel in cardiac ventricular cells depends on internal magnesium ions. *Proc Natl Acad Sci USA* 1987;84:2560–2564.
476. Vanhoutte PM, Levy MN. Prejunctional cholinergic modulation of neurotransmission in the cardiovascular system. *Am J Physiol* 1980; 238:H275–H281.
477. Varró A, Nánási PP, Lathrop DA. Potassium currents in isolated human atrial and ventricular cardiocytes. *Acta Physiol Scand* 1993; 149:133–142.
478. Vassalle M. Overdrive suppression and overdrive excitation. In: Rosen MR, Janse MJ, Wit AL, eds. *Cardiac electrophysiology: a textbook.* 175–189. Mount Kisco: Futura, 1990;
479. Veenstra RD. Physiological modulation of cardiac gap junction channels. *J Cardiovasc Electrophysiol* 1991;2:168–89.
480. Veenstra RD, Joyner RW, Rawling DA. Purkinje and ventricular activation sequences of canine papillary muscle: effects of quinidine and calcium on Purkinje-ventricular conduction delay. *Circ Res* 1984;54:500–515.
481. Veldkamp MW, Ginneken ACGV, Bouman LN. Single delayed rectifier channels in the membrane of rabbit ventricular myocytes. *Circ Res* 1993;72:865–878.
482. Venkatesh N, Stuart JS, Lamp ST, Alexander LD, Weiss JN. Activation of ATP-sensitive K^+ channels by chromakalim: effects on cellular K^+ loss and cardiac function in ischemic and reperfused mammalian ventricle. *Circ Res* 1992;71:1324–1333.
483. Ver Donck L, Borgers M, Verdonck F. Inhibition of sodium and calcium overload pathology in the myocardium: a new cytoprotective principle. *Cardiovasc Res* 1993;27:349–357.
484. Vercruysse P, Bossuyt P, Hanegreefs G, Verbeuren TJ, Vanhoutte PM. Gallamine and pancuronium inhibit pre-junctional and post-junctional muscarinic receptors in canine saphenous veins. *J Pharmacol Exp Ther* 1979;209:225–230.
485. Vicenzi MN, Woehlck HJ, Bosnjak ZJ, Atlee JL III. Anesthetics and automaticity of dominant and latent pacemakers in chronically instrumented dogs. II. Effects of enflurane and isoflurane during exposure to epinephrine with and without muscarinic blockade. *Anesthesiology* 1993;79:1316–1323.
486. Vodanovic S, Turner LA, Hoffmann RG, Kampine JP, Bosnjak ZJ. Transient negative dromotropic effects of catecholamines on Purkinje fibers exposed to halothane and isoflurane. *Anesth Analg* 1993;592–597.
487. Vodanovic S, Turner LA, Kampine JP, Bosnjak ZJ. α_1-Mediated transient negative dromotropic effect in canine Purkinje fibers exposed to halothane (abstract). *FASEB J* 1993;7:A96.
488. Vulliemoz Y. Volatile anesthetics and second messengers in cardiac tissue. In: Wheeler DW, Blanck TJJ, eds. *Mechanisms of anesthetic action in muscle. Advances in experimental medicine and biology 301.* New York: Plenum Press, 1991;169–180.
489. Vulliemoz Y, Verosky M, Triner L. Effect of halothane on myocardial cyclic AMP and cyclic GMP content of mice. *J Pharmacol Exp Ther* 1986;236:181–186.
490. Wahler GM, Dollinger SJ. Nitric oxide donor SIN-1 inhibits mammalian cardiac calcium current through cGMP-dependent protein kinase. *Am J Physiol* 1995;268:C45–C54.
491. Wallace AG, Sarnoff SJ. Effects of cardiac sympathetic nerve stimulation on conduction in the heart. *Circ Res* 1964;14:86–92.
492. Walsh KB, Begenisich TB, Kass RS. β-Adrenergic modulation in the heart: independent regulation of K and Ca channels. *Pflugers Arch* 1988;411:232–234.
493. Walsh KB, Kass RS. Regulation of a heart potassium channel by protein kinase A and C. *Science* 1988;242:67–69.
494. Wang Q, Shen J, Splawski I, et al. *SCN5A* mutations associated with an inherited cardiac arrhythmia, long QT syndrome. *Cell* 1995;80:805–811.
495. Wang YG, Lipsius SL. Acetylcholine activates a glibenclamide-sensitive K^+ current in cat atrial myocytes. *Am J Physiol* 1995;268: H1322–H1334.
496. Wang YG, Lipsius SL. Acetylcholine potentiates acetylcholine-induced increases in K^+ current in cat atrial myocytes. *Am J Physiol* 1995;268:H1313–H1321.
497. Wang Z, Fermini B, Feng J, Nattel S. Role of chloride currents in repolarizing rabbit atrial myocytes. *Am J Physiol* 1995;268: H1992–H2002.
498. Wang Z, Fermini B, Nattel S. Repolarization differences between guinea pig atrial endocardium and epicardium: evidence for a role of I_{to}. *Am J Physiol* 1991;260:H1501–H1506.
499. Warmke J, Drysdale R, Ganetzky B. A distinct potassium channel polypeptide encoded by the *Drosophila eag locus. Science* 1991;252: 1560–1562.
500. Warmke JW, Ganetzky B. A family of potassium channel genes related to eag in Drosophila and mammals. *Proc Natl Acad Sci USA* 1994;91:3438–3442.
501. Weiner N, Taylor P. Drugs acting at synaptic and neuroeffector junctional sites. In: Gilman AG, Goodman LS, Rall TW, Murad F, eds. *The pharmacological basis of therapeutics.* New York: Macmillan, 1985;66–99.
502. Weiss JN, Vankatesh, N., Lamp, S.T. ATP-sensitive K^+ channels

and cellular K^+ loss in hypoxic and ischaemic mammalian ventricle. *J Physiol* 1992;447:649–673.

503. Weiss JN, Nademanee K, Stevenson WG, Singh B. Ventricular arrhythmias in ischemic heart disease. *Ann Intern Med* 1991;114: 784–797.
504. Wettwer E, Amos GJ, Posival H, Ravens U. Transient outward current in human ventricular myocytes of subepicardial and subendocardial origin. *Circ Res* 1994;75:473–482.
505. Whalley DW, Wendt DJ, Starmer CF, Rudy Y, Grant AO. Voltage-independent effects of extracellular K^+ on the Na^+ current and phase 0 of the action potential in isolated cardiac myocytes. *Circ Res* 1994;75:491–502.
506. Wickman KD, Iniguez-Lluhl JA, Davenport PA, et al. Recombinant G-protein $\beta\gamma$-subunits activate the muscarinic-gated atrial potassium channel. *Nature* 1994;368:255–257.
507. Wilde AAM, Janse MJ. Electrophysiological effects of ATP sensitive potassium channel modulation: implications for arrhythmogenesis. *Cardiovasc Res* 1994;28:16–24.
508. Wit AL, Cranefield PF. Triggered and automatic activity in the canine coronary sinus. *Circ Res* 1977;41:435–445.
509. Wit AL, Rosen MR. Afterdepolarizations and triggered activity. In: Fozzard HA, Haber E, Jennings RB, Katz AM, Morgan HE, eds. *The heart and cardiovascular system: scientific foundations.* New York: Raven Press, 1991;2113–2163.
510. Woehlck HJ, Vicenzi MN, Bosnjak ZJ, Atlee JL III. Anesthetics and automaticity of dominant and latent pacemakers in chronically instrumented dogs. I. Methodology, conscious state, and halothane anesthesia: comparison with and without muscarinic blockade during exposure to epinephrine. *Anesthesiology* 1993;79:1304–1315.
511. Woosley RL. Antiarrhythmic drugs. *Annu Rev Pharmacol Toxicol* 1991;31:427–455.
512. Wu J, Lipsius SL. Effects of extracellular Mg^{2+} on T- and L-type Ca^{2+} currents in single atrial myocytes. *Am J Physiol* 1990;259: H1842–H1850.
513. Xiao P-P, Lakatta EG. β_1-Adrenoceptor stimulation and β_2-adrenoceptor stimulation differ in their effects on contraction, cytosolic Ca^{2+}, and Ca^{2+} current in single rat ventricular cells. *Circ Res* 1993;73:286–300.
514. Yang T, Levy MN. Sequence of excitation as a factor in sympathetic-parasympathetic interactions in the heart. *Circ Res* 1992;71:898–905.
515. Yang T, Levy MN. Effects of intense antecedent sympathetic stimulation on sympathetic neurotransmission in the heart. *Circ Res* 1993;72:137–144.
516. Yasuda I, Hirano T, Amaha K, Fudeta H, Obara S. Chronotropic effects of succinylcholine and succinylmonocholine on the sinoatrial node. *Anesthesiology* 1982;57:289–292.
517. Yasutake M, Avkiran M. Exacerbation of reperfusion arrhythmias by α_1 adrenergic stimulation: a potential role for receptor mediated activation of sarcolemmal sodium-hydrogen exchange. *Cardiovasc Res* 1995;29:222–230.
518. Yasutake M, Ibuki C, Hearse DJ, Avkiran M. Na^+/H^+ exchange and reperfusion arrhythmias: protection by intercoronary infusion of a novel inhibitor. *Am J Physiol* 1994;267:H2430–H2440.
519. Yatani A, Brown AM. Rapid b-adrenergic modulation of cardiac calcium channel currents by a fast G protein pathway. *Science* 1989;245:71–74.
520. Yatani A, Codina J, Imoto Y, Reeves JP, Birnbaumer L, Brown AM. A G protein directly regulates mammalian cardiac calcium channels. *Science* 1987;238:1288–1292.
521. Yatani A, Wakamori M, Mikala G, Bahinski A. Block of transient outward-type cloned cardiac K^+ channel currents by quinidine. *Circ Res* 1993;73:351–359.
522. Yeaton P, Teba L. Sinus node exit block following administration of vecuronium. *Anesthesiology* 1988;68:177–178.
523. Yu H, Chang F, Cohen IS. Pacemaker current exists in ventricular myocytes. *Circ Res* 1993;72:232–236.
524. Yuan W, Bers DM. Ca-dependent facilitation of cardiac Ca current is due to Ca-calmodulin-dependent protein kinase. *Am J Physiol* 1994;267:H982–H993.
525. Yue DT, Backx PH, Imredy JP. Calcium-sensitive inactivation in the gating of single calcium channels. *Science* 1990;250: 1735–1738.
526. Yue DT, Herzig S, Marban E. β-Adrenergic stimulation of calcium channels occurs by potentiation of high-activity gating modes. *Proc Natl Acad Sci USA* 1990;87:753–757.
527. Yue DT, Marban E. A novel cardiac potassium channel that is active and conductive at depolarized potentials. *Pflugers Arch* 1988;413:127–133.
528. Zheng J-S, Christie A, Levy M, Scarpa A. Ca^{2+} mobilization by extracellular ATP in rat cardiac myocytes: regulation by protein kinase C and A. *Am J Physiol* 1992;263:C933–C940.
529. Zink J, Sasyniuk BI, Dresel PE. Halothane-epinephrine-induced cardiac arrhythmias and the role of heart rate. *Anesthesiology* 1975; 43:548–555.
530. Zipes DP. The long QT interval syndrome: a rosetta stone for sympathetic related ventricular tachyarrhythmias. *Circulation* 1991; 84:1414–1419.
531. Zipes DP. Genesis of cardiac arrhythmias: electrophysiological considerations. In: Braunwald E, ed. *Heart Disease.* Philadelphia: WB Saunders, 1992;588–627.
532. Zipes DP, Miyazaki T. The autonomic nervous system and the heart: basis for understanding interactions and effects on arrhythmia development. In: Zipes DP, Jalife J, eds. *Cardiac electrophysiology: from cell to bedside.* Philadelphia: WB Saunders, 1990.
533. Zuckerman R, Wheeler D. Effect of halothane on arrhythmogenic responses induced by sympathomimetic agents in single rat heart cells. *Anesth Analg* 1991;72:596–603.
534. Zygmunt AC. Intracellular calcium activates a chloride current in canine ventricular myocytes. *Am J Physiol* 1994;267:H1984–H1995.
535. Zygmunt AC, Gibbons WR. Calcium-activated chloride current in rabbit ventricular myocytes. *Circ Res* 1991;68:424–437.
536. Zygmunt AC, Gibbons WR. Properties of the calcium-activated chloride current in heart. *J Gen Physiol* 1992;99:391–414.
537. Zygmunt AC, Maylie J. Stimulation-dependent facilitation of the high threshold calcium current in guinea-pig ventricular myocytes. *J Physiol* 1990;428:653–671.

Anesthesia: Biologic Foundations, edited by Tony L. Yaksh et al. Lippincott–Raven Publishers, Philadelphia © 1997.

CHAPTER 66

MYOCARDIAL EXCITATION-CONTRACTION COUPLING

CARL LYNCH III

Excitation-contraction (EC) coupling is the mechanism by which depolarization of the cellular membrane activates contraction. The critical aspects of the process involve carefully regulated changes in the concentration of myoplasmic Ca^{2+} ($[Ca^{2+}]_i$) that surrounds the contractile proteins (actin and myosin) and controls their interaction, and that in turn determines myocyte shortening and force development. The primary control of $[Ca^{2+}]_i$ is achieved via an intracellular compartment, the sarcoplasmic reticulum (SR), from which Ca^{2+} can be rapidly released and into which it is rapidly reaccumulated. The entry and efflux of extracellular Ca^{2+} across the surface membrane is responsible for triggering the release from Ca^{2+} stores as well as maintaining the quantity of Ca^{2+} in the SR. The Ca^{2+} fluxes are mediated via a variety of channels, exchangers, and pumps that are distributed in a highly regimented manner within the external and intracellular membranes, and that are likewise exquisitely structured around the contractile proteins. In addition, the sensitivity of the myofibrils to Ca^{2+} is a finely modulated and cooperative response that also determines the amount of tension developed.

Since both skeletal and cardiac muscle have a highly organized striated structure, skeletal muscle has served as a model for cardiac tissue. While the two share many common features, there are a number of major differences in their basic biochemical and physiologic characteristics that serve their different functional roles. In contrast to skeletal muscle, in which the strength of contraction is controlled by the number of fibers activated by motor neurons, cardiac muscle is an electrical syncytium in which *all* cells are stimulated to contract under normal conditions. The strength of cardiac contractions is instead controlled by the degree of contractile activation, which is determined by the amount of activator Ca^{2+} and the length of the initial degree of myofilament overlap. The varied tension generation that is seen with changes in cardiac volume (Starling's [472] law of the heart) or rate of beating (positive frequency staircase) results from two intrinsic characteristics of the myocardium: (a) variation in the myofibril Ca^{2+} sensitivity, and (b) alteration in the amount of activator Ca^{2+}. The steep length-dependence of force generation by myocardium and the variable store of releasable Ca^{2+} activated by entering Ca^{2+} represent two major features in which cardiac differs from skeletal muscle. During the sustained cardiac action potential (AP), the voltage-dependent entry of Ca^{2+} and Na^+ and their interaction via the Na^+-Ca^{2+} exchange also mean that electrophysiologic behavior and EC coupling are highly integrated, interdependent functions. In addition to functional constraints determined by the fine subcellular structure, the Ca^{2+} fluxes, as well as the responses by actin and myosin, are tightly modulated by regulation of the activity of the various enzymes and transport proteins. A variety of extrinsic factors, such as inotropic stimulation or ischemia, also modulate their effects by alterations in these intrinsic determinants of cardiac contractility.

STRUCTURE OF THE CARDIAC MYOCYTE

Unlike skeletal muscle, which is composed of long, multinucleated fibers, atrial and ventricular muscle in mammals is composed of individual myocytes (mono- or binucleate). These cells are typically 80 to 150 μm in length with elliptical cross sections of 5 to 15 × 20 to 30 μm (Fig. 1A) and are composed of numerous bundles of contractile protein myofibrils (158). The central bundles of myofibrils may extend the length of the cell, terminating at each end. More superficial myofibrils may terminate along the length of the fiber, resulting in squared-off indentations where junctions are formed with adjacent myocytes. The myocytes are arranged longitudinally and attached at various end-to-end, end-to-side, and side-to-side connections, resulting in interconnected strands. As a consequence, the average cardiac myocyte is electrically coupled and mechanically tethered, at least in part, to about seven other myocytes (470). Myocytes are coupled at intercalated disks, a complex interdigitation of membrane structures that maintain mechanical integrity via cytoskeletal membrane proteins such as vinculin and permit electrical continuity via transmembrane ion channels called connexons (or gap junctions) (36,159, 297). Connexons in the heart are formed from six monomers of connexin 42 (42 kd molecular weight), a member of a large family of gap junction-forming proteins. Two of the large homohexameric connexon hemichannels present in the membrane of adjacent cells become juxtaposed end to end to form a highly conductive channel between cells. Previous work employing isolated myocytes has suggested that one effect of volatile anesthetics is to depress coupling between myocytes, particularly at higher anesthetic concentrations (85,305). If individual myocytes become electrically isolated, they will shorten and contribute to cardiac contraction; however, it is not known whether such cell uncoupling occurs either in intact tissue or clinically.

The sarcomere is the basic functional unit of contraction responsible for the striations typical of both skeletal and cardiac muscle. This unit is a 2.0 to 2.5 μm wide cross section of fiber, extending between two Z lines. Extending longitudinally along the axis of the fiber and centered between the Z lines are hexagonally packed myosin filaments (1.55 μm long). These filaments interdigitate with and overlap the hexagonally packed but thinner actin filaments (1.15 μm long) arising from each Z line (Fig. 1B). The ends of the actin filaments from adjacent sarcomeres meet and combine with a variety of cytoskeletal proteins (α-actinin, talin, integrin) and anchor fibers at the Z line. The surface membrane is linked to the Z line by the structural protein vinculin. In addition, stretching between the Z lines and running parallel to the actin and myosin filaments are long protein strands, which are composed of a very high molecular weight polypeptide called titin (316). The actin and myosin filaments are also separated into bundles 0.5 to 1 μm in diameter (myofibrils), each containing 300 to 1000 filaments of each type (Fig. 1B). In addition, microtubules (tubulin) and longitudinally oriented intermediate filaments (primarily desmin) are also present in myocytes, partitioning them into quasi-compartments to prevent disruption of the complex internal architecture. These structural cellular components also increase the passive stiffness of the cardiac myocytes, at least in comparison with skeletal muscle (156).

The surface membrane (plasmalemma or sarcolemma) of the myocytes is a typical lipid bilayer containing the various

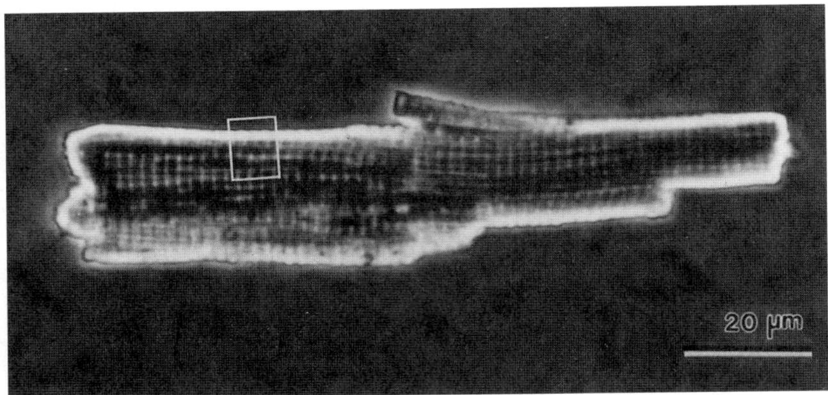

A

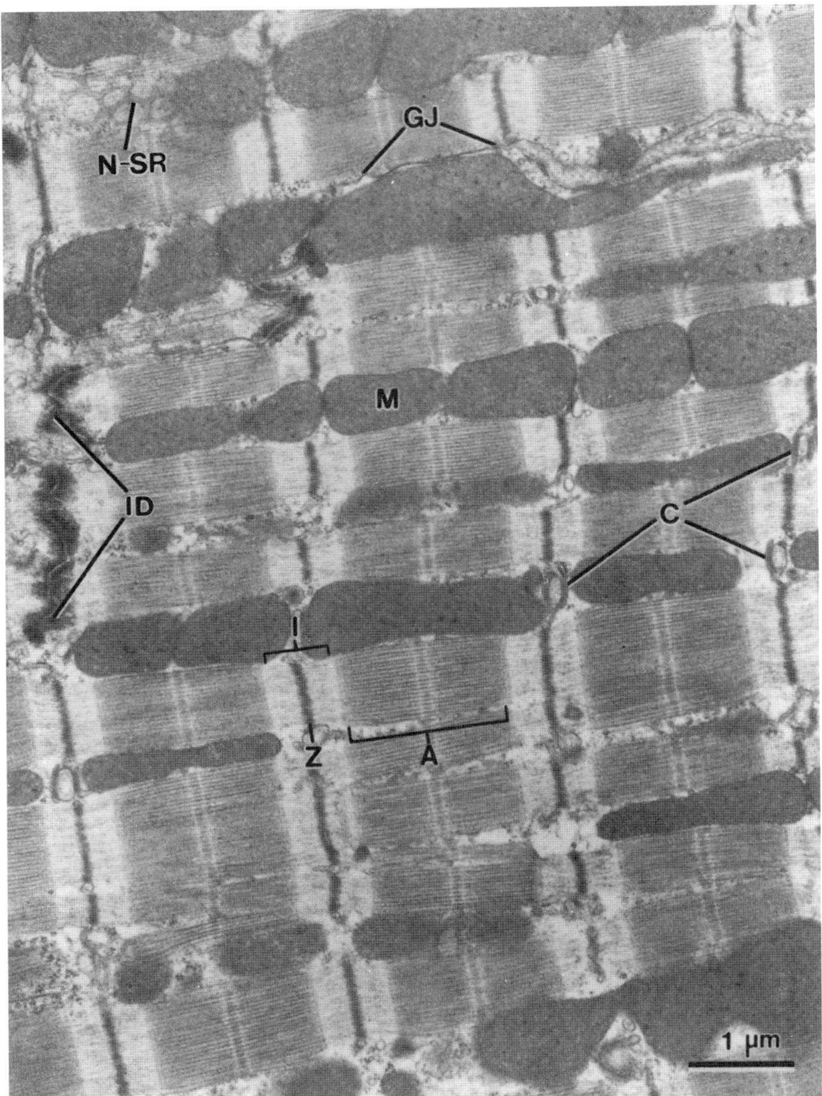

B

Figure 1. **A:** Phase contrast light micrograph of enzymatically isolated rat ventricular myocardial cell. Periodic banding pattern of myofibrils is due to the sarcomeric striations. The uneven contour of the cell is the result of myofibrils of shorter overall lengths teminating at the regions that form junctions with other myocytes along the length of the cell. **B:** Transmission electron micrograph of a longitudinal thin section through rat ventricular myocardial cells, the area shown being equivalent in size and orientation to the *white square* in A. The bulk of each cell is occupied by the myofibrils, oriented along the long axis of each cell and exhibiting the characteristic banding pattern formed by the A bands (where actin and myosin filaments overlap), I bands (consisting primarily of actin filaments), and Z lines (composed in large part of α-actinin) that bisect each I band. At the end of myofibrils, a collection of specialized junctions (the intercalated disks [ID]) connect adjacent cells at the position Z lines would occupy. Mitochondria (M) are arranged either in rows among the myofibrils or in clusters beneath the cell membrane, where they frequently closely appose gap junctions (GJ), an example of which appears as a *thin dark line* at this magnification. The internal membrane system of the sarcoplasmic reticulum (SR) appears in the form of tubular retes (network SR: N-SR) on the surfaces of myofibrils. Continuous with the network SR are specialized flattened saccules of junctional SR (see Fig. 7), which are apposed either to the surface sarcolemma or its tubular extensions, the transverse tubules, to form complexes known as couplings (C), which frequently are located at the levels of the Z lines. (Electron and photomicrograph kindly provided by Michael Forbes.)

receptors, transport proteins, and structural components. A cylindrical sheath enclosing the cell contents and structural proteins, the sarcolemma may be removed (chemically or mechanically) without disturbing the organized structure of sarcomeres, which can continue to function so long as they are bathed in solutions appropriate for the intracellular milieu. However, the plasmalemma and the closely adherent extracellular mucopolysaccharide basement membrane have a complex structure. At each Z line the sarcolemma forms tubular invaginations (0.1 µm diameter) called transverse tubules, or T tubules, which form a network across the ventricular myocyte. In contrast to the much narrower (0.01 to 0.02 µm diameter) T tubules of skeletal muscle fibers in which the basement membrane is absent, the basement membrane extends into and lines the T tubules of cardiac myocytes. T tubules are critical in carrying the surface depolarization and Ca^{2+} entry to the interior of the myocyte to initiate myofibrillar activation. The greater volume and basement membrane of the cardiac myocyte T tubule may be important as a Ca^{2+} store, whereas Ca^{2+} entry from T tubules is not required to activate internal Ca^{2+} release in skeletal muscle fibers. T tubules are frequently not seen in small diameter atrial myocytes (158).

Each of the 10 to 70 myofibrils seen in the cross section of a myocyte is surrounded by a membranous network, the sarcoplasmic reticulum (SR), the lumen of which contains a high concentration of Ca^{2+} (Fig. 1B). At the Z line the network of SR is juxtaposed to the T tubules. The SR membrane that faces the T tubules contains an array of highly specialized, very large homotetrameric protein complexes, the Ca release channels. These are responsible for controlling the release of Ca^{2+}, which activates tension development. This junctional SR is also characterized by a larger lumen that contains calsequestrin, a protein that binds Ca^{2+} with a low affinity and provides an extra "sink" of releasable Ca^{2+}. In addition to couplings with the T tubules, the SR occasionally forms junctions with the surface membrane, another location where Ca^{2+} release may be activated. The functional structure here is similar to that usually found in smooth muscle. In addition, free SR vesicles, or corbular SR, may be found in mammalian myocytes (158).

Because of the continuous high rate of energy consumption by the myocardium, myocytes require a large number of mitochondria. A very high density of adenosine triphosphate (ATP)-producing organelles is obviously critical in a continuously active tissue like the heart, in contrast with most types of skeletal muscle. Myocardial mitochondria frequently occupy 30% to 40% of cell volume, depending on the species, and are organized in rows between the separate myofibrils. This architecture provides a short diffusion distance between the sites of ATP production and utilization by the SR and myofibrils, and it may represent a partial diffusion barrier to other intracellular substances (139).

In the heart, the interconnected strands of myocytes are enmeshed in a thin network of collagen fibers (perimysium) and gathered into small interconnecting bundles, which are also sheathed in connective tissue. While mechanical continuity within the myocytes is generated by the cytoskeletal proteins (talin, α-actinin, integrin, dystrophin, and titin), tissue-level structural organization and generation of macroscopic force by the heart is due to the extracellular basal lamina and microfibrils (endomysium or struts), which connect the sarcolemma and basal lamina to the collagen matrix surrounding cell bundles (536). These endomysial fibers provide lateral cell-to-cell structural continuity and are attached to the perimysium. Collagen fibers serve as the major structural protein of the interstitium and provide the scaffolding for the myocytes and blood vessels. A large population of fibroblasts is responsible for the synthesis of the collagen, of which approximately 85% is type I and 11% is type III, constituting predominantly the thick and thin fibers, respectively. The endomysial tethers appear to contain both collagen types (536). The connective tissue and collagen present in the extracellular space is 2% to 6% of muscle dry weight, far greater than in skeletal muscle. While there do not appear to be any passive, noncontractile elements in series with the myocytes (87), this extracellular matrix provides an important elastic component parallel to the contractile cellular elements, which can generate considerable passive tension when myocardium is stretched. This interstitial framework thereby contributes considerably to the diastolic properties of the myocardium. The collagen fibers, endomysial mesh, and struts that attach to the sarcolemma at the Z line of myocytes protect them from being overstretched and maintain the unloaded geometry of the LV (341). However, this collagen matrix is also responsible for remodeling of the myocardium when subjected to hypertrophic stimuli (hypertension, hyperthyroidism) or injury (536). Even in the absence of permanent myocyte injury such as stunning, degradation of structural collagen can occur (574).

MYOFILAMENT FORCE GENERATION

A well-recognized feature of cardiac behavior is the length-dependence of its contractility, which is expressed in its more integrated form by Starling's law of the heart: "Within physiological limits the larger the volume of the heart, the greater the energy of its contraction and the amount of chemical change at each contraction" (440,472). Such length-dependent contractile behavior, which is far steeper than that observed in skeletal muscle, results in faster relaxation and greater efficiency in intact myocardium and is based on the distinct biochemical features of cardiac contractile machinery. While contractile force is determined in part by the quantity of Ca^{2+} released to the myofibrils, the myofibrils themselves have a variable Ca^{2+} sensitivity that depends on the length of, and tension generated within, the myocyte sarcomeres.

The Myofilaments

Most of the details of the myofilament interactions that actually generate tension in striated muscle have been defined from studies in skeletal muscle and isolated myofibrillar proteins. The concept of force generation by myosin cross-bridges between the myosin and actin filaments (242,243) and the accompanying biochemical cycle in which ATP is hydrolyzed (329) are widely accepted, and considerable detail is now available regarding these processes.

Actin Filaments

The actin monomer, composed of 375 amino acids, shows very little variation among species and serves as the molecular basis for an array of cytoskeletal activities in a wide variety of cells. Each actin monomer is composed of two side-by-side peanut-shaped domains and has dimensions of approximately 5.5 × 5.5 × 3.5 nm. Binding sites for a divalent cation (Ca^{2+}, Mg^{2+}) and an adenosine nucleotide (ATP or adenosine diphosphate [ADP]) are located between domains, and these are critical cofactors (540). Occupation of the binding sites is apparently necessary for the conformational structure of the monomer to form the 9 to 10 nm diameter filaments (F-actin), the helical polymer composed of two intertwined strands of actin monomers (Fig. 2A). The monomers are held together by strong noncovalent interactions, primarily between the inner "large" domains (363,451).

The outer "small" domain of each actin monomer forms the lateral component of F-actin filament that possesses the major binding sites for myosin. Acidic amino acids on the outermost edge form an initial site for interaction with a loop of myosin that is rich in basic lysine residues. This initial actin-myosin interaction is a weak electrostatic interaction that is sensitive to solutions of high ionic strength, and may account for nonspecific interactions between actin and myosin (229). In addition to the "weak" electrostatic interaction, higher affinity binding sites for myosin that employ multiple amino acid residues are located on each actin monomer. These sites are closer to the central axis of the filament (230,258,451), partially in the grooves formed by the two intertwined helical actin strands (Fig. 2B).

In the grooves of an actin filament lie elongated coiled-coil, α-helical dimers of tropomyosin (144). Each such dimer overlaps and controls the availability of seven actin monomers (~40 nm) (68) and also has an associated troponin complex. The troponin complex, composed of an inhibitory (TnI), a Ca^{2+} binding (TnC), and a tropomyosin-binding (TnT) subunit, regulates the position of the tropomyosin dimer within the groove and thereby determines whether the high-affinity myosin binding sites are accessible (144). TnC is a dumbbell-

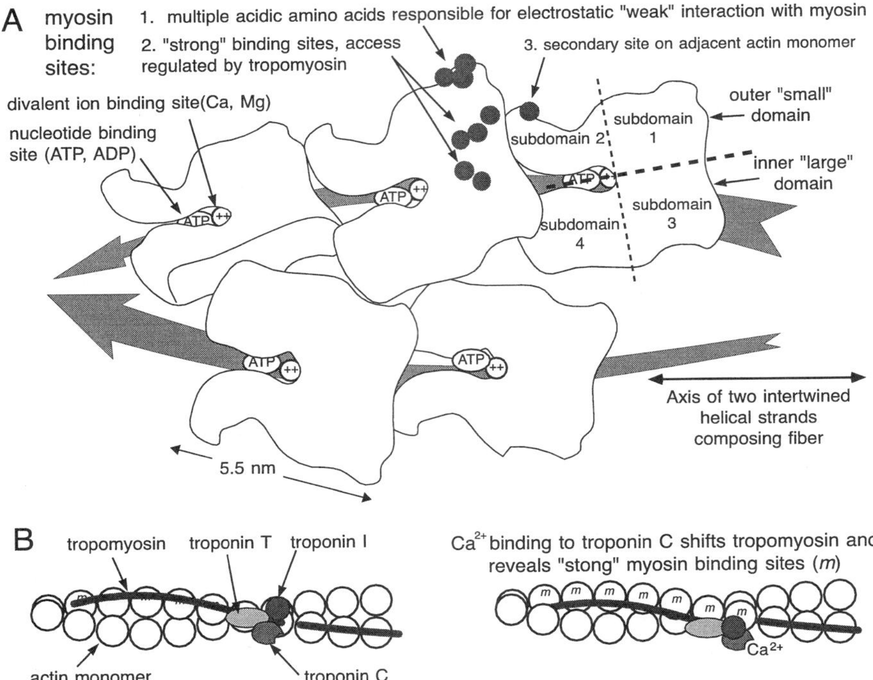

Figure 2. **A:** Basic shape, structure, and arrangement of actin individual monomers (approximately 55 x 55 x 35 nm) as arranged to form an actin filament. Each monomer has been subdivided into four indicated subdomains. The amino and carboxy terminae of the amino acid sequence both reside in subdomain 1 of the outer domain, which is a major binding site for myosin. **B:** Schematic of the Ca^{2+}-activated "switch" of the troponin-tropomyosin complex on actin. When Ca^{2+} binds to troponin C (TnC), the attraction for the inhibitory subunit troponin I (TnI) is increased. When TnT is moved into closer apposition with TnC, the tropomyosin strand rotates further into the tropomyosin groove, revealing the myosin binding site (*m*) on actin. Recent molecular models suggest that myosin may actually bind to sites on two adjacent monomers (425).

shaped molecule, with two Ca^{2+} binding sites at each end. The binding sites are the "EF hand" Ca^{2+} binding sites observed on calmodulin, parvalbumin, myosin light chains, and a variety of Ca^{2+} binding proteins. Sites III and IV at the COOH-terminal end bind either Ca^{2+} or Mg^{2+}, usually the latter under physiologic conditions, and are not involved in the molecule's regulatory function. In skeletal muscle, sites I and II near the NH_2-terminus bind Ca^{2+} (421), while in cardiac troponin, amino acid substitutions at site I have eliminated its Ca^{2+} binding, so only a single site has regulatory control. At rest (during diastole), when the myoplasmic Ca^{2+} concentration ($[Ca^{2+}]_i$) is approximately 80 to 100 nM (~0.1 μM) and no Ca^{2+} is bound to the TnC regulatory Ca^{2+} site, the Tn complex stabilizes the position of the tropomyosin molecule so that higher affinity sites for myosin attachment are occluded. However, TnT appears to play an important role in keeping the TnC-TnI bound to tropomyosin-actin complex, as well as distributing the effect of the tropomyosin along the length of the actin filament over seven actin monomers (144).

When $[Ca^{2+}]_i$ rises to the 0.5 to 2 μM, Ca^{2+} binding to TnC is postulated to reveal a hydrophobic surface on the NH_2 terminus (216) that results in stronger coupling of the TnI to TnC (534) and uncoupling TnI from actin (420,498). This rearrangement of the Tn complex results in a conformational shift of tropomyosin in the actin filament to a position deeper in the groove and closer to the central axis of the fiber, thereby revealing the sites on actin to which the myosin head groups can bind strongly (Fig. 2B). By binding to TnC, this activator Ca^{2+} acts like a switch to turn on actin-myosin interaction. The protein-protein interaction between actin and troponin-tropomyosin complex is bidirectional. If a myosin is bound to an actin monomer of a filament so that the tropomyosin-troponin complex is shifted to a noninhibitory position, TnC has a higher Ca^{2+} affinity (68,168).

Myosin

Each cardiac myosin is a 520-kd protein comprised of two heavy chains (MHC), each chain being either an α or β isoform composed of 1939 amino acids. Each chain contains a globular head domain (subfragment 1, S1), a tightly coiled rod (coiled-coil) section (S2), and a light meromyosin (LMM), as well as a two associated light chains and C protein. The LMM of two individual myosin proteins form an elongated straight segment, and it is these segments that aggregate to form the myosin (thick) filaments, with the head groups facing outward to bind to actin (Fig. 3A). It is the flexion or rotation of the 19-nm-long head group after binding to an actin monomer that generates the tension along the axis of the myosin and actin filaments, and the total force generated within the muscle is proportional to the total number of head groups actively cycling. The 16 to 18 kd myosin light chains, essential (ELC, LC1) and regulatory (RLC, LC2), bind in the narrower "neck" region the S1 subunit of the molecule, where the two head groups join to form the coiled coil.

Each of the two S1 head groups of a myosin appear to operate independently. In addition to careful biochemical studies, detailed structural studies of the myosin S1 have now permitted a far more detailed picture of the tension generating cycle (Fig. 3B) (107,157,425). A long α-helical strand within the myosin S1 stretches from the ATP binding site, near the actin binding region, through the narrow neck region to the point where it joins the S2 and LMM segments. A flexible "hinge" region halfway along the length of the S1 segment is important for generating the conformational change associated with tension generation. In the absence of ATP the myosin is firmly attached to actin (a rigor complex) and the S1 head group is in a more extended state. In a multistep process, ATP binds to its "pocket" on S1 and opens a cleft across the actin binding region, which make dissociation of myosin from actin energetically favorable (107,157). Actin and myosin may remain weakly associated via electrostatic interactions that permit far greater mobility. During or after hydrolysis of ATP, the S1 appears to undergo a bend at the hinge region that "cocks" the myosin for a subsequent "power stroke." The rebinding of myosin to actin is also a multistep process. "Weak" initial electrostatic binding can occur while ATP is bound and may initiate ATP hydrolysis, but ATP hydrolysis favors isomerization to a "strong" binding by myosin to sites on actin deeper within the filament groove. One of the strong interactions of myosin with actin is between helix-loop-helix regions of exposed hydrophobic amino acids and

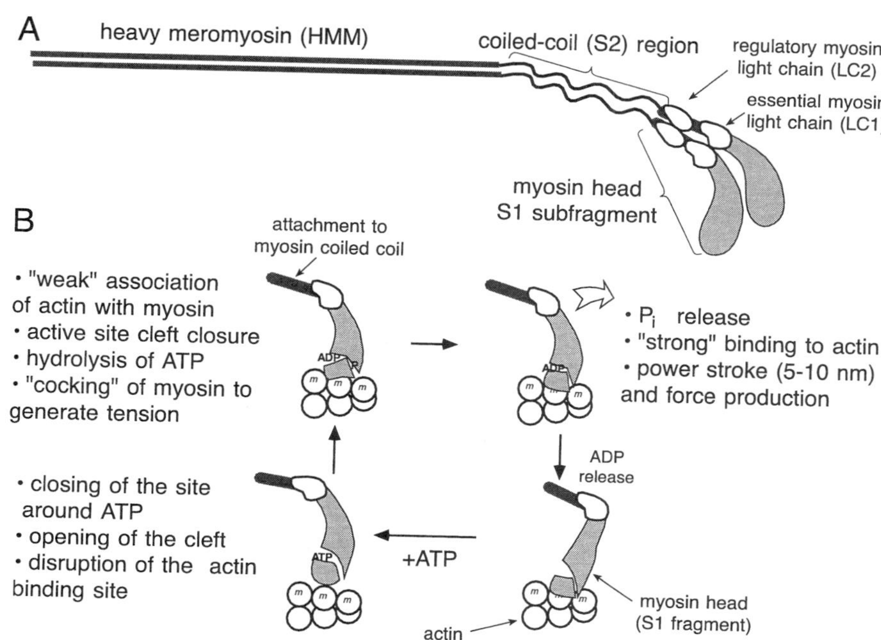

Figure 3. **A:** Basic structure of the myosin molecules (two heavy chains and two pairs of light chains) that combine to form a single myosin hexamer, which in turn combine to form the thick filaments of striated muscle. **B:** Schematic of the cycle of the myosin head (S1) in force generation. Dissociation of myosin's strong binding actin requires the binding of ATP to a cleft site on the myosin head near its actin binding site. Weak electrostatic association of myosin and actin may persist. Closure of the site is accompanied by myosin assuming a "cocked" position that can generate tension upon binding to actin, and hydrolysis of ATP. Subsequently there is strong binding of myosin to sites on actin, followed by release of P_i, which then permits the "power stroke" and force production. The cleft opens permitting ADP to dissociate, but leaves myosin tightly bound to actin. (Based on the model of Rayment et al. [425] and Cooke [107].)

charged residues, regions that showing considerable conservation among species and stereospecificity of binding. Another region of strong binding involves a pair of proline residues on actin that interact with a conserved arginine residue on a loop of myosin (451), mutation of which is associated with a form of familial hypertrophic cardiomyopathy (177). The resulting myosin–ADP–P_i complex in the strongly bound state then releases the free inorganic phosphate (P_i). The release of P_i allows closure of cleft on the binding site; there is rapid release of ADP and straightening of the myosin head while bound to actin filaments—constituting the conformational change that generates the power stroke and force development (511).

While the free energy for the power stroke is ultimately derived from ATP hydrolysis, the hydrolysis occurs while the actin and myosin are only weakly bound, and a large conformational change in the nucleotide binding pocket does not occur with the power stroke. Instead, the energy for the power stroke conformational change may arise from the formation of the strong bond between actin and myosin. The tighter association markedly reduces the exposure of a highly hydrophobic region, which should liberate considerable free energy (107). While myosin binds primarily to subdomain 1 of actin (Fig. 2A), it also appears to interact with the adjacent actin monomer in the smaller subdomain 2. An important component of the process is the ELC (LC1) located near the hinge region of S1, the presence of which appears to be critical in regulating the power stroke (157).

The cycle begins again when ATP binds to myosin and provides the energy for release from actin. If other myosin head groups are generating tension and shortening has occurred, the myosin can bind to an actin monomer further along the filament, with each power stroke accounting for 10 nm in length (411). If no shortening has occurred and tropomyosin has not occluded the active site on actin, the myosin may rebind in the same location to continue tension generation (while other myosin S1s are cycling). In intact skeletal muscle, however, mechanical evidence suggests that the myosin head will bind more than once to actin sites and undergo a number of power strokes per ATP hydrolyzed (324). The number of power strokes per ATP may be determined by load, with multiple strokes at high loads but single power strokes when the applied force is high (565). This conclusion is also consistent with energetic considerations and may result from steric considerations imposed by intact myofibrils and the activation of multiple myosin head groups.

In smooth muscle, the RLC (LC2) plays a prominent role in maintaining myosin adenosine triphosphatase (ATPase) activity and RLC phosphorylation controls the actin-myosin interaction, but its role in modulation of cardiac force development is less well defined (325). However, the combination of the ELC (LC2) and C protein appears to increase the actin-activated ATPase activity (343). Two closely related MHC isoforms exist (α and β) that differ in the rate at which they cycle through actin binding, ATP binding, and ATP hydrolysis. The isoforms can combine as different forms of myosin termed fast (V_1, αα), medium (V_2, αβ), and slow (V_3, ββ) forms of myosin (351,402) based on their ATPase activity. The latter form predominates in adult cardiac tissue. In animal models, V_1 and V_2 isoforms are expressed in neonatal animals, or in hyperthyroidism (320), but their importance in human myocardium has not been demonstrated.

The cross-bridge cycling rate is also modulated by the products of the reaction. Since P_i is a product of the actin-myosin reaction sequence, rises in [P_i] would be expected to inhibit both ATPase activity and force generation by simple mass action. However, the depression of force generation is more profound than predicted and proportionally greater than the decrease in ATPase activity (i.e., the muscle is less efficient) (131). This effect has been attributed to decrease in free energy release available from ATP hydrolysis when [P_i] is increased (131). H^+ is also a by-product of the cycling of the S1 head group, seen even with the "weak" initial interaction and perhaps reflecting underlying conformational changes. Decreased pH also reduces force development but has little effect on ATPase activity, demonstrating a divorce between ATP hydrolysis and force. Whatever the mechanisms, since P_i and H^+ both accumulate markedly during ischemia, the resulting decrease in force generation and efficiency may be profound. Pharmacologically, 2,3-butanedione monoxime (BDM) has been recognized as a potent inhibitor of force development in both cardiac and skeletal muscle due to its decreasing effect on the myosin cycling rate. This compound directly decreases tension by stabilizing the myosin head group in the unattached or weakly bound ADP·P-bound state (215). By stabilizing this state, fewer ATPs are hydrolyzed and fewer head groups are able to attach to actin to generate force (14).

In addition to movement of myosin along the actin filament, the helical nature of the actin filament may result in its right-hand rotation. The elastic energy of the twist will be stored in the filament lattice, and the transfer of torque along the filament may be sufficient to transform the lattice structure of the Z line in which they are anchored (388). This alteration in cellular or F-actin geometry may also contribute to the force dependence of Ca^{2+}-binding by TnC.

FORCE- AND LENGTH-DEPENDENT CONTRACTILE ACTIVATION

Our understanding of the actin-myosin interaction has been largely derived from skeletal muscle, and it appears to apply to cardiac muscle. However, skeletal and cardiac muscle have marked distinctions. Force development in skeletal muscle is maximal at 2.0 to 2.5 μm sarcomere length, but decreases at sarcomere lengths >2.5 μM where actin-myosin filament overlap begins to decrease. In cardiac muscle, such lengthening of sarcomeres in intact muscle is virtually impossible because of the extensive connective tissue that surrounds the myocytes and fibers (536). Of greater physiologic relevance is the force development with shortening. In skeletal muscle, force decreases only gradually with shorter sarcomere lengths <1.8 μm, but in myocardium the relationship of active force vs length has a far steeper slope. At 80% of optimal length (sarcomere length: 1.7 μm), skeletal muscle generates 80% to 85% of maximum force, while cardiac muscle achieves only 10% to 15% of maximum force (168). When the cardiac sarcomeres are contracted and short (≤1.8 μm) there is very modest active force development for a given $[Ca^{2+}]_i$, yet small amounts of stretch result in far greater active force development (see Fig. 6A,B) (256,257,500).

Substantial evidence exists that the apparent affinity of TnC for Ca^{2+} decreases with sarcomere length. In "skinned" cardiac ventricular trabeculae in which all Ca^{2+} regulatory processes have been eliminated, sarcomere length and force as well as the surrounding $[Ca^{2+}]$ can be carefully controlled (217,223, 224). When sarcomeres are shorter, a higher $[Ca^{2+}]$ is required to achieve the same relative force (percent of maximum at the given length) (217). Examined in an opposite way, when the sarcomere length or force is increased, there is an increase in the amount of Ca^{2+} bound to TnC at longer sarcomere lengths (223). Contrary to expectation, the TnC Ca^{2+} affinity and amount of Ca^{2+} binding appears to be reduced when there is the greatest overlap and interaction of actin and myosin (Fig. 4) (4,168,217,223,224,264). When the same $[Ca^{2+}]_i$ is present in the myoplasm, more myofibrils appear activated and more force is generated when cardiac myocytes are stretched (217,264). Further work documents that this behavior arises from the myofibrils and is not an artifact due to length-dependent effects on the SR or peculiar to skinned muscle fibers (438). Evidence points to force rather than sarcomere length per se as the sensor that influences Ca^{2+} sensitivity. When vanadate ion (V_i) is present in the myofibrillar milieu, a myosin–ADP–V_i complex is formed that does not interact with actin, and the result is a marked reduction in binding of Ca^{2+} to the regulatory site on TnC regardless of the sarcomere length of the myofibrils (533). Prior experiments also suggest that the effect is not dependent on length per se, but rather on the degree of interaction between the filaments (4,438).

The greater force/length sensitivity of myocardium has been attributed to the cardiac TnC isoform, since this effect is reduced or not seen when skeletal muscle TnC is substituted for cardiac TnC (13,187). However, this effect has not been observed in some experiments (373), nor is it apparent with slow skeletal muscle fibers expressing cardiac TnC (533). An alterative (or additional) explanation has been suggested involving the cellular geometry (168). Since cardiac myocytes have a constant volume, at a greater length the diameter will be reduced and myofilaments will come closer together, which should permit greater interaction of myosin heads with actin. When short fibers are subjected to a modest degree of osmotic compression, the result is an increase in force development as well as increased Ca^{2+} sensitivity and binding (168). Such behavior, in which less Ca^{2+} is required to bind to TnC when force-generating myosin head groups are attached to actin, can be further explained if tropomyosin is forced to stay in its non-inhibiting position once a strong interaction is formed by

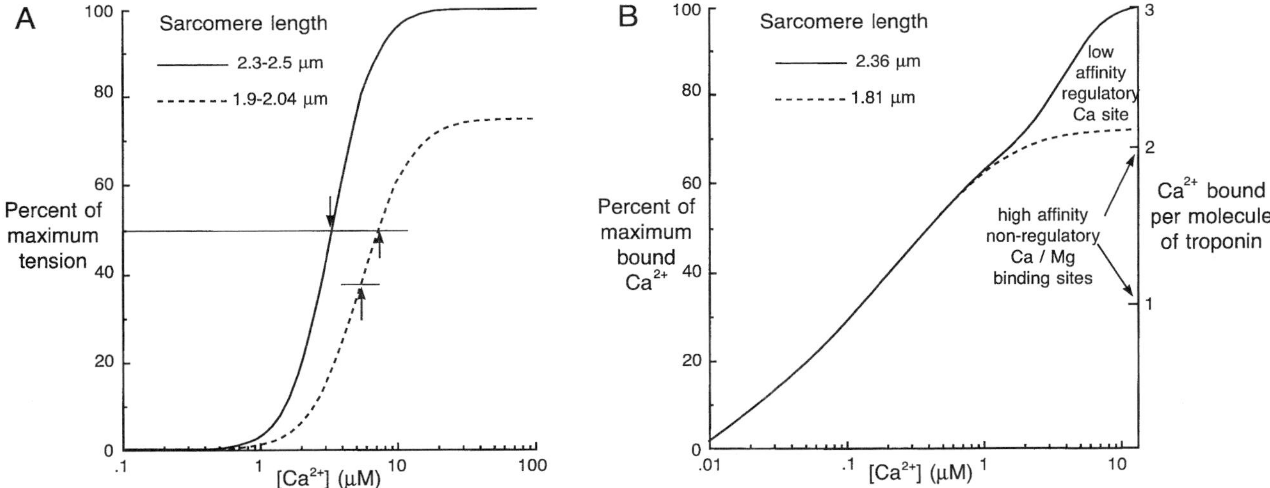

Figure 4. Length- (force-) dependent alteration in Ca^{2+} sensitivity and affinity of myofibrils. **A:** Length-dependent shift in Ca^{2+} sensitivity of tension development in chemically permeabilized rat ventricular trabeculae. Note the decreased maximum tension and Ca^{2+} sensitivity at the shorter sarcomere length, so that <20% instead of 50% of maximum tension is observed with 3.0 μM Ca^{2+}. At the shorter length 4.9 μM Ca^{2+} is required to obtain 50% activation;to obtain the same tension as at the longer length, $[Ca^{2+}]$ would have to be increased to ~8 μM. (Data from ref. 217.) **B:** Length-dependent enhancement of Ca^{2+} binding by troponin C in permeabilized bovine ventricular fiber bundles determined by a double isotope technique. Two Ca^{2+} bind to nonregulatory sites at $[Ca^{2+}]$ below 1 μM. Ca^{2+} binding to the regulatory site is modulated by fiber length so that at the shorter length, less Ca^{2+} is bound to the regulatory site. (Data from ref. 224.)

myosin on actin. Although the binding of Ca^{2+} to TnC has a higher affinity, the binding is no longer required to permit myosin to strongly interact with actin. If Ca^{2+} diffuses off from TnC (in spite of the greater affinity), it becomes available to bind to another TnC and activate other regions of the actin filament. If the same or another myosin head rapidly binds to actin, keeping the tropomysin-complex in the noninhibiting position deeper in the actin groove, then an extra cycle(s) of tension generation by myosin can occur, extending the effectiveness of the Ca^{2+} activation. Since more myosin-actin interaction is possible when myocyte diameter is smaller and myofilaments are more closely opposed (longer length, higher osmolarity), force-dependent binding could result. Such cooperative interaction between TnC-mediated Ca^{2+} activation and myosin binding to actin can be used to effectively model cardiac mechanics (298).

Shortening Deactivation

Whatever the mechanism, the force dependence of myofibril activation also has an important corollary with regard to relaxation: the shorter the muscle length, the more rapidly relaxation occurs. This phenomenon is called length- (or load-) dependent relaxation, or shortening deactivation. Because TnC Ca^{2+} affinity is decreased when a muscle shortens more (when tension is lower and fewer myosins are strongly bound to actin), a muscle allowed to shorten relaxes sooner (81,82,412). As suggested by studies using aequorin (3,235,293) and confirmed by fura-2 $[Ca^{2+}]_i$ measurements (15), the rate of decline of Ca^{2+} transients is altered by varying the length and tension development of the myocardium. The decreased Ca^{2+} affinity of TnC that occurs due to shortening results in a detectably higher cytoplasmic $[Ca^{2+}]_i$ since Ca^{2+} diffuses off of TnC into the myoplasm (235). With quick release of tension, there is a transient increase in $[Ca^{2+}]_i$ caused by the lower affinity (Fig. 5) (122). Presumably, when shortening occurs instead of force development, fewer myosin cross-bridges on actin will permit more tropomyosin-troponin complexes to return to their inhibitory position, in which TnC's affinity for Ca^{2+} is decreased. The result of shortening is the transient elevation in $[Ca^{2+}]_i$ as Ca^{2+} is released from TnC. If there is no shortening, $[Ca^{2+}]_i$ ultimately declines more slowly since equilibration between TnC and SR uptake takes longer. When shortening does occur, the duration of contractile activity is briefer and the relaxation rate is somewhat more dependent on SR uptake of Ca^{2+}, since the rapid release requires more rapid reaccumulation of Ca^{2+}.

Mechanics

The cooperativity between myosin-actin interaction and TnC Ca^{2+} binding yields an extremely steep length dependence of active force generation at shorter sarcomere lengths, while the extensive envelopment of extracellular matrix and collagen fibers causes a dramatic rise in force at longer lengths. The result is that force development by myocardium has a very steep, virtually linear length dependence (Fig. 6A) (256,257, 500). When a cardiac muscle is activated, either exclusive force development (isometric shortening or isovolumic contraction) or shortening (unloaded isotonic shortening) can be arranged experimentally, or some combination of force development and shortening (Fig. 6B). If instead of force development, shortening occurs from a longer sarcomere length because a greater number of myosin units are active due to the cooperative interaction with TnC Ca^{2+} affinity, a longer muscle will shorten more against a given resisting force within a given time. When the steep length dependence of cardiac contractility is expressed as muscle shortening instead of force development, the result is the classic observation of greater shortening at greater velocity, as clearly delineated by Sonnenblick (471) in isolated muscle (Fig. 6C). As noted above, when shortening

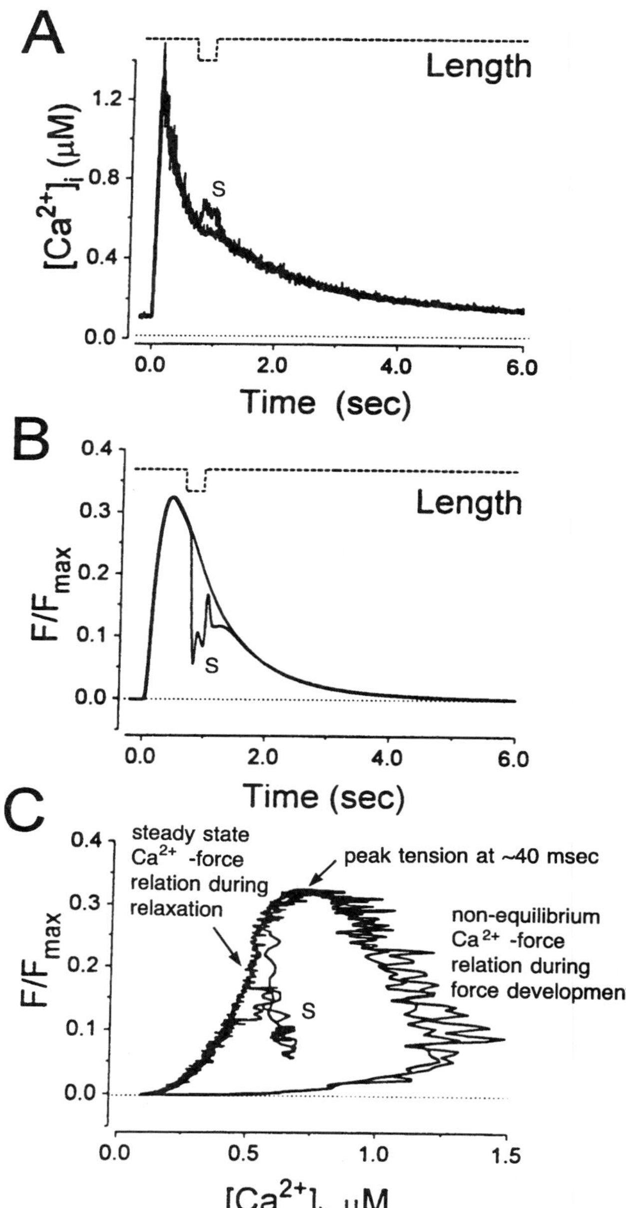

Figure 5. Alterations in myoplasmic Ca^{2+} ($[Ca^{2+}]_i$) responsible for force development (F) where F_{max} was the maximal force observed in tetanized muscle in 6.0 mM Ca^{2+}. $[Ca^{2+}]_i$ was calculated from the ratio of Ca^{2+}-free and Ca^{2+}-bound fura-2 dye, which had been injected iontophoretically into rat trabeculae. When a sudden shortening (quick release) of the muscle was made at the indicated time, force declined with a coincident increase in $[Ca^{2+}]_i$ observed upon release (indicated by *S*), with subsequent reuptake of Ca^{2+} when lengthening was reimposed. The change in $[Ca^{2+}]_i$ appears to represent alteration in the affinity in troponin C with length change. The plot of $[Ca^{2+}]_i$ versus F/Fmax shows the transient excess of Ca^{2+} during development of force, and the steady-state relation observed during the declining muscle relaxation phase. During the brief shortening, a transient relative excess of Ca^{2+} occurred (S). (From ref. 122, with permission.)

occurs, the duration of contractile activity is decreased (shortening deactivation); regardless of the initial length, if shortening begins at a lower force, duration of contractile activation will be decreased.

Since the change in TnC Ca^{2+} affinity occurs within a single cardiac cycle, the mechanical consequences of this effect can

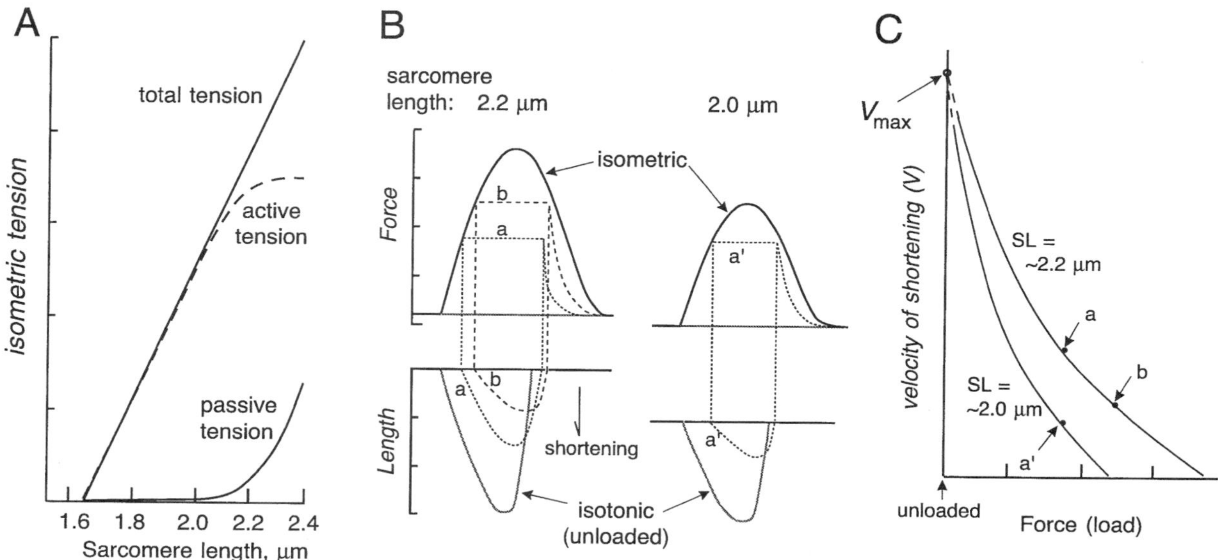

Figure 6. The interaction of initial length and preload on force development and velocity of shortening. **A:** Dependence of active and passive force on muscle length. The difference between the total and passive tension is the active developed tension *(dotted line)*. **B:** Simultaneous tracings of tension and length from a typical papillary muscle experiment. The *left panel* shows the response at 2.2 μm sarcomere length, while the *right panel* shows the response at the shorter length 2.0 μm sarcomere length. Once any given force is attained, shortening is a linear function of the initial length. At the shorter length, the muscle can attain less maximum tension (as plotted in A), and also shortens less rapidly. The maximum velocity of shortening is the initial slope of the length tracing and is plotted in **C,** according to the analysis first described by Sonnenblick (471).

also be observed physiologically in cardiac muscle in which there is some combination of force and shortening. This effect has important implications with regard to ventricular function, energy consumption, and perfusion. For any given initial length or resting force, the muscle shortens less rapidly and not as far as the afterload is increased, that is, more cross-bridges cycle to generate greater force, but do not cause the myofibrils to shorten as much. When there is great resistance to ejection and high intraventricular pressures, there is less shortening deactivation and relaxation is retarded (84). It follows that systole and ATP consumption by greater cycling of myosin will be prolonged, while diastole will be shortened. When there is considerable shortening and ventricular ejection and less force is thereby developed, Ca^{2+} diffuses more readily off of TnC than when systole is abbreviated. Such length dependence of relaxation is a clear demonstration of myocardial economy, since ATP would be consumed needlessly if myosin continued to cycle once shortening and ejection of blood had occurred. Conversely, against a higher afterload, a more sustained contraction will be important to eject blood.

Consequently, end-systolic length and tension will strongly influence the rate of relaxation. This effect may explain the apparent dependence of oxygen consumption on cardiac diastolic wall stress. Since during diastole the myocardium is relaxed (Ca^{2+} is accumulated and myofibrils are not interacting), it is difficult to reconcile how this state could influence myocardial energy use. It seems likely that lower diastolic wall stress (and smaller diameter) will result in a decreased myofibrillar Ca^{2+} sensitivity. If there is the same degree of shortening during the subsequent systole to a smaller end systolic diameter, Ca^{2+} will diffuse off of TnC more rapidly with a shorter duration of tension development and less energy consumption. This phenomenon may also explain in part the interesting and seemingly contradictory result that dogs whose hearts are depressed by volatile anesthetics have improved diastolic relaxation when extracellular Ca^{2+} is increased, which also increases systolic shortening (403).

The myofilament sensitivity to Ca^{2+} and the resulting degree of activation are also modulated by receptor-mediated systems that control TnI subunit phosphorylation as noted below. While the myofibrils are the primary cellular system responsive to cell dimension or tension, the SR also shows length-dependent behavior. SR Ca^{2+} stores increase following an increase in length (5). As opposed to the instantaneous effect caused by length-dependence of TnC and Ca^{2+}, the length-dependent SR effect develops over a number of contractions and appears to account for a more modest component (15–25%) of the positive inotropic effect. The phenomenon is not limited to isolated muscle, but is readily demonstrable in intact animals (313).

Passive Force Development

The other component that sharply defines the myocardial length-force relationship is the passive behavior mediated by the passive intracellular stress-strain relation and the extracellular connective tissue. Below sarcomere lengths of 2.2 μm, the intrinsic myofibrillar stress-strain relation generated by the polypeptide titin is largely responsible for the very modest increase in force caused by stretching myocardium (316). At longer sarcomere lengths, extracellular collagen fibrils become stretched in intact cardiac muscle, which prevents the muscle from being passively stretched beyond that point where total tension declines (257,316,500). This passive length-force component increases steeply at the muscle length at which active tension development levels off. The contribution of the passive components is evident, for example, when the collagen strands that surround myocytes are enzymatically digested, shifting the passive tension curve to the right (341). The combination of the steep active length-force relation at short sarcomere lengths due to cardiac TnC with the steep passive length-force relation at long sarcomere lengths results in a total length-force relation that is virtually linear over the functional range (Fig. 6A). This linear combination of active and passive components extends to three dimensions in the intact ventricle and provides a simple quantitative description of the heart, particularly when applied to ventricular function and pressure-volume relations.

REGULATION OF INTRACELLULAR Ca^{2+}

In addition to modulation of the degree of myofibrillar activation by length and force, the other major determinant of myocardial contractility is the regulation of the amount of Ca^{2+} made available to activate each beat of the heart. When $[Ca^{2+}]_i$ is increased and binds to TnC, myosin cross-bridges will be formed, thereby generating more tension. With normal action potentials (APs), a distinct Ca^{2+} transient can be measured by either aequorin or spectrofluorometric dyes (indo-1, fura-2) (136,174,319,399,547,550). This increase in $[Ca^{2+}]_i$ peaks in about 20 msec, with the peak force (or shortening) occurring during the falling phase of $[Ca^{2+}]_i$ (see Fig. 5). The changing $[Ca^{2+}]_i$ results from the transient Ca^{2+} excess in the myoplasm until it binds to TnC, with subsequent redistribution from TnC into the SR during relaxation.

The amount and source of activator Ca^{2+} in the myoplasm surrounding the myofibrils in mammalian hearts is determined by an intermixture and cycling of two Ca^{2+} sources: a small amount of Ca^{2+} entering from extracellular milieu, and a far greater amount of Ca^{2+} released from the sarcoplasmic reticulum (SR) pool. Upon depolarization, Ca^{2+} enters the cell through the surface membrane, which triggers release of a far greater amount of Ca^{2+} from the SR store into the myoplasm. Since the extracellular milieu and SR lumen have a free Ca^{2+} concentration of ~1 mM, versus a myoplasmic $[Ca^{2+}]$ surrounding the myofibrils at rest of 0.1 μM, Ca^{2+} flows passively from either source down an enormous concentration (and electrical) gradient. After Ca^{2+} binds to the myofibrils to activate contraction, relaxation ensues as Ca^{2+} is removed from the myoplasm into the SR and out of the myoplasm. In either case, transport against the large concentration gradients requires expenditure of energy. The amount of activator Ca^{2+} that arises from the extracellular space versus the SR lumen varies according to such factors as age, species, heart rate, and temperature, all of which frequently differ in experimental studies.

Ca^{2+} Fluxes Activating Contraction

Most of the Ca^{2+} that enters the myocyte during the AP depolarization is insufficient to bind to and activate a significant number of the myofibrils to generate relevant physiologic force (37). However, this entry serves two critical purposes that are not required in skeletal muscle. First, Ca^{2+} entering at the T tubule near junctional SR is required for activation of release from the SR (142). Second, since Ca^{2+} leaks from the SR during the diastolic interval of the myocardium (46,299), the Ca^{2+} entry replenishes the SR store. At regular, steady-state beating, the same amount of Ca^{2+} that enters via the cell membrane during the AP must subsequently be eliminated, but the Ca^{2+} cycled by this pathway is modest (typically 5% to 20% of activator Ca^{2+}) compared to the amount that is alternately released and taken up by the SR.

Ca Release from the Sarcoplasmic Reticulum (SR)

As first noted by A.V. Hill (219) almost five decades ago, in order for contractile activation and relaxation to proceed rapidly, the distance over which Ca^{2+} must diffuse from its entry site into the myoplasm to TnC must be very short. The SR membrane networks that envelop each of the <1 μm diameter myofibrils (see Fig. 1B) provide multiple sites for release and uptake of Ca^{2+} and ensure short diffusion distances for Ca^{2+}, providing the required speed for activation and relaxation. A single depolarization activates release of a substantial fraction (~50%) of Ca^{2+} stored in the junctional SR of myocardium, as assessed by either caffeine-induced release (26) or electron-probe microanalysis (370,538). Adult myocardial cells have an extensive SR network, but certain species such as rat rely more exclusively on the SR than do species such as rabbit (27). Fetal mammalian myocardium as well as neonatal myocardium from certain species is similar to frog heart in having a far less developed SR structure and function, so that immature myocardium relies far more on extracellular Ca^{2+} entry by both the voltage-gated Ca channels (VGCC) and Na^+-Ca^{2+} exchanger to mediate contractions (9,31). However, the atrium of human neonates appears to possess a releasable intracellular Ca^{2+} store (208).

The Ca Release Channel Activation of myofibrils by Ca^{2+} requires not only proximity of an adequate quantity of Ca^{2+} but also a mechanism for rapid efflux. The Ca release channels of the Ca^{2+} stored in the SR permit a large fraction to rapidly (10 to 20 msec) diffuse out of the SR lumen and into the myoplasm. Each Ca release channel (CaRC) is a homotetramer, composed of four monomers arranged with a rosette or quatrefoil symmetry (108,353,524). Each monomer has transmembrane domains that extend to the SR lumen and a very large N-terminus region that occupies cytoplasmic space between the SR membrane and the T-tubular membrane. These cytoplasmic portions of the CaRC are sufficiently large that they are seen in micrographs as the electron-dense "foot" structures that form a bridge between the adjacent membranes (Fig. 7A); they also contain an internal channel (524) as well as the various binding sites for Ca^{2+}, ryanodine, ATP, anthraquinones, and other drugs that regulate the opening of this channel (108,353). When the channel opens the plant alkaloid ryanodine binds tightly, causing the channel to remain open but with a conductance less than half of the control value. By blocking the CaRCs open, ryanodine causes loss of Ca^{2+} from the SR, resulting in marked depression of cardiac contractions. The intense binding of ryanodine has provided the name *ryanodine receptor* for this protein, as well as permitted its isolation and ultimately its cloning. One of three CaRC isoforms isolated by molecular genetic techniques (108,196,344,353,359,400,576), the cardiac isoform is designated RYR2 (for ryanodine receptor). It is also present in the brain. When incorporated into artificial bilayers, these channels have a very single high channel conductance, capable of permitting a high rate of Ca^{2+} efflux from the SR lumen. Ca^{2+} selectivity arises from a tighter binding of the ion as it passes through the channel. Monovalent ions pass through more rapidly, and the pore is of sufficient magnitude to permit small sugar molecules to pass (108).

Although it appears that the SR Ca^{2+} efflux is initially into the junctional space between the SR and T tubules, the Ca^{2+} presumably diffuses rapidly into the surrounding myoplasm. Since each myofibril is of typically less than 1 μm in diameter and each half sarcomere is less than 1.2 μm long, the distance over which Ca^{2+} must diffuse from the junctional SR to TnC on the actin filaments is very short, so that the time dependence of this process is minimal.

Ca^{2+}-Induced Ca^{2+} Release For over a decade it has been evident that in contrast to skeletal muscle, in which removal of extracellular Ca^{2+} permits ongoing release of internal Ca^{2+} (8,184), entry of extracellular Ca^{2+} is required to activate release from the SR for cardiac tissue (141–143). In skeletal muscle a specialized, truncated L-type Ca channel subunit ($\alpha 1_S$) located in the T tubules is directly coupled to the skeletal muscle CaRC (RYR1) (108,353). Although Ca^{2+} can activate RYR1 channel opening, voltage-induced conformational changes in $\alpha 1_S$ are transmitted to the CaRC to open RYR1 and to permit Ca^{2+} efflux from the SR into the myoplasm (495). In cardiac tissue, the L-type channel ($\alpha 1_C$ subunit) does not possess the structure to activate CaRCs (174,175); instead this I_{Ca} acts as "trigger Ca^{2+}" to activate opening of the cardiac CaRC (RYR2). The Ca^{2+} that enters L-type Ca channel (or via the Na^+-Ca^{2+} exchanger) is sufficient by itself to activate only a small fraction of myofibrils. Instead the primary function of $I_{Ca,L}$ is to bind to Ca^{2+} receptors

A

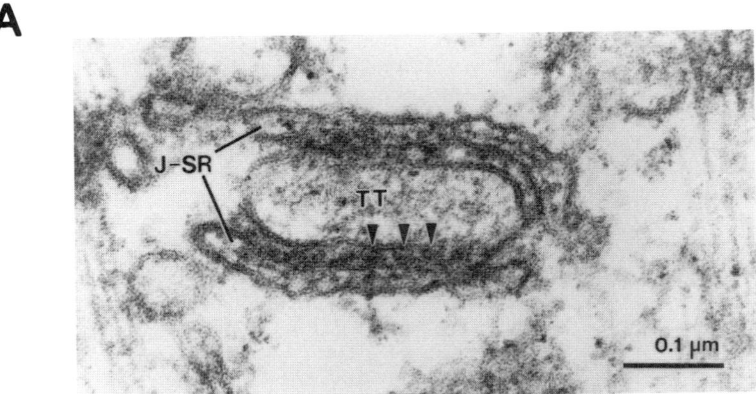

B1

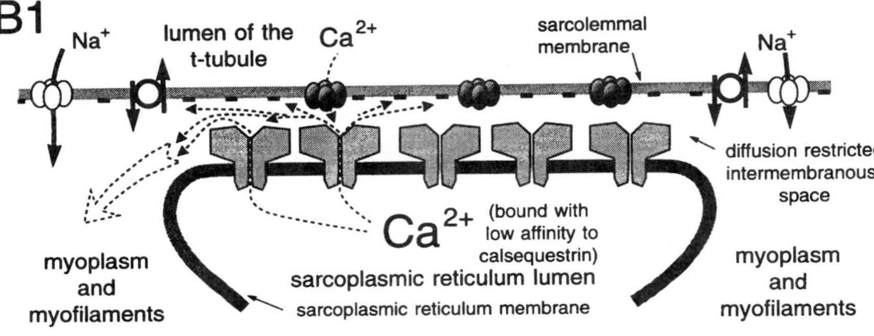

B2

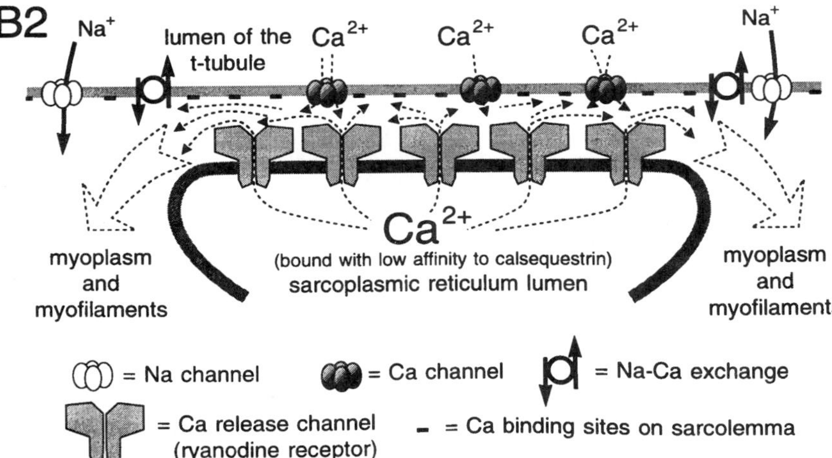

Figure 7. Coupling between the T tubule and sarcoplasmic reticulum (SR) of a cardiac myocyte. **A:** High magnification electron micrograph of a myocardial coupling in a rat ventricular cell. The internal membrane component is the junctional SR (J-SR), characteristically flattened and containing dense granular material within the lumen (in part calsequestrin). In the cleft between junctional SR and a transverse tubule (TT) there appear periodically spaced opaque structures known as "SR feet" or "junctional processes" (indicated by *arrowheads*), which are the Ca release channels (CaRC, ryanodine receptors) that open to release sequestered Ca^{2+} from the SR lumen. **B:** Cardiac tissue demonstrates a graded release of Ca^{2+} from the SR store, in spite of the fact that the Ca release channels (Ca RC) are Ca^{2+}-activated. This effect may in part be explained by the diffusion restricted space created by the junctional cleft between the cytoplasmic faces of the T tubule and JSR membranes, indicated schematically. **B1:** With small depolarizations or partial Ca^{2+} channel blockade, some CaRCs are activated. However, because of the low-affinity binding sites on the sarcolemma or prolonged exposure to Ca^{2+}, the Ca^{2+} released from the CaRC is not sufficient to activate all surrounding CaRCs. **B2:** With more profound Ca^{2+} entry into the intermembranous space, most or all of the CaRCs will be activated, resulting in complete release of SR Ca^{2+}. Calculations suggest that in this space $[Ca^{2+}]$ may rise to 100–500 μM (413,476). (Electron micrograph kindly provided by Michael Forbes. From ref. 335, with permission.)

on the CaRC to activate opening and release of the SR Ca^{2+}, a process termed Ca^{2+}-induced Ca^{2+} release (CICR) (142). The Ca^{2+} release activated by the trigger Ca^{2+} depends on a number variables. When extracellular Ca^{2+} is reduced ≤0.5 mM, the resulting SR release Ca^{2+} transient is decreased disproportionately, as if trigger Ca^{2+} ($I_{Ca,L}$) may have been incompletely triggered from the SR store (161). In addition to the amount of entering Ca^{2+}, the quantity of the SR Ca^{2+} store also modulates the amount of activated release, or the "gain" on the SR release mechanism (252). For a given influx of trigger Ca^{2+}, the amount of Ca^{2+} released from the SR will be greater in the SR is more replete (252). During a normal twitch, at least half of the Ca^{2+} present in the SR (as assessed by caffeine activated release) is released (26), which may represent 60% to 75% of the physiologically releasable store.

Much of the behavior of the CaRC and CIRC has been determined from studies in which cardiac CaRC behavior has been examined in bilayers. When exposed to an activating $[Ca^{2+}]$, the probability of channel opening (P_o) increases (10). When exposed to a sustained rise in Ca^{2+}, the cardiac CaRC channel adapts and P_o decreases so that channel is closed (191). A further increase in $[Ca^{2+}]$ once again induces opening, to which the channel again adapts with a decreased P_o.

While the CIRC from the SR, activated by Ca^{2+} entry via L-type voltage-gated Ca channels, is now well established (99,387), a question exists as to type of control. If Ca^{2+} entry stimulates Ca^{2+} release, one would anticipate a positive feedback loop. That is, once Ca^{2+} flux from a CaRC was initiated, all CaRCs in the vicinity would be activated (387,477). This process would result in a release of all of the SR Ca^{2+} store. However, there instead appears to be finely graded release, with the quantity of Ca^{2+} released dependent on the amount of entering Ca^{2+} (549). While the adaptation and decreased CaRC channel activity seen with ongoing Ca^{2+} exposure may contribute to the limitation on positive feedback, such adaptation may be to slow to provide a complete explanation. Ultrastructural features of membrane systems may also be important. Between the T tubule, where Ca^{2+} enters, and the apposed junctional sarcoplasmic reticulum (JSR) membrane containing CaRC there is diffusion-restricted or "fuzzy" space (300,307,387), which may be critical in regulation of CIRC and the graded release that occurs with Ca^{2+} entry (Fig. 7). An appropriately graded response can be provided by local control models that depend on Ca^{2+} gradients in the neighborhood of a channel: a "calcium synapse" in which Ca^{2+} entry through an L-type channel activates a single CaRC, and a "cluster bomb" model in which a small group of CaRC can be activated together (476,477). While there currently is no definite answer, these models can at least demonstrate the graded behavior seen experimentally when local domains of Ca^{2+} are permitted. Low-affinity sites on the sarcolemmal membrane and Na^+-Ca^{2+} exchange may be critical to buffering Ca^{2+} release (413,419), muting the response of nearby CaRCs, and preventing an "all-or-nothing" Ca^{2+} release. A purely descriptive model has also been proposed by Callewaert (86). While massive activation of release occurs during each beat caused by the depolarization-induced Ca^{2+} entry, in quiescent cells the spontaneous opening of a single CaRC may result in a localized "spark" of Ca^{2+} (93) that does not go on to cause a regenerative release of a large quantity of Ca^{2+}.

The CaRC has a very high single channel conductance (about 10x greater than the L-type Ca channel) so that the stored Ca^{2+} can rapidly leave. To prevent this rapid efflux of positive ions from generating a high negative charge within the SR lumen, which retards further efflux, high-conductance K channels are also present in the SR membrane. Countermovement of K^+ into the SR presumably prevents large membrane potentials from being generated in the SR (354,510).

Ca Release Channel Modulation and Drug Effects The cardiac CaRC also appears to be more readily phosphorylated than the skeletal muscle isoform by protein kinase A (adenosine 3',5'-cyclic monophosphate [cAMP]-dependent) and Ca^{2+}-calmodulin–dependent kinases (483). Such phosphorylation provides an additional modulatory mechanism that is associated with increased channel opening (556). It may also explain how perfusion of hearts with decreased or increased extracellular Ca^{2+} (0.2 to 5.6 mM) caused a subsequent down- or upregulation of CaRC Ca^{2+} flux, respectively, that was maintained when SR was subsequently isolated (1).

A variety of drugs also may play modulatory roles. The best example is the effect of caffeine, which in pharmacologic concentrations (1 to 25 mM) is widely used to "empty" Ca^{2+} stores from various tissues, a process mediated by opening of the CaRC (468). More clinically relevant are the anthroquinone antineoplastic drugs that induce CaRC opening (60,414), a process that may contribute to the cardiomyopathy associated with these agents. The immunosuppressant drug FK506 binds to a specific protein (FKBP) that is closely associated with the CaRC, although its physiologic function is unclear (253).

Calsequestrin Another important constituent of the SR is the 45-kd protein calsequestrin, which binds up to 40 Ca^{2+} per molecule and is about half-saturated at ~500 μM Ca^{2+} (364,455). Of the 391 amino acids that compose the cardiac isoform of this protein, 109 are negatively charged to provide the multiple binding sites for Ca^{2+} (455). Such low-affinity binding reduces the effective $[Ca^{2+}]$ within the SR lumen from 1 to 5 mM to about 0.1 to 0.5 μM, so that the gradient against which the SR Ca^{2+} ATPase has to pump is considerably reduced, yet at the same time permits rapid mobilization and efflux from the SR when the CaRC is open. In addition to calsequestrin, a protein called triadin has been identified in skeletal junctional SR that may coordinate release between the CaRC and calsequestrin (164,244,274); however, its possible role in cardiac muscle activity remains undefined.

Entry of Extracellular Ca^{2+}

The two major pathways for Ca^{2+} entry from the extracellular milieu are the L-type Ca channel and the Na/Ca exchanger, although the latter protein plays an even more prominent role in Ca^{2+} elimination from the cell. Because of the regular entry of Ca^{2+} with each beat via these pathways, the SR can stay continually charged with Ca^{2+}. For each individual beat, the primary function of these influx pathways is to provide the trigger Ca^{2+} to activate the CaRCs.

Voltage-Gated Ca Channels Two types of VGCCs are present in myocardium, the T type (transient) and L type (long-lasting). While the former plays a role in pacemaking (192) and assumes a considerable fraction (~40%) of I_{Ca} in Purkinje fibers (220), these channels are very modest in ventricular tissue and appear to play little role in excitation-contraction coupling. The dihydropyridine-sensitive L-type channels are the major source of the entering Ca^{2+} current ($I_{Ca,L}$) into the myocyte. These channels are activated when the membrane is depolarized positive to -40 mV, which requires more than a 40 mV depolarization from the resting potential under most circumstances. The Na channel is responsible for the rapid and large depolarization required to open these channels, and under normal conditions $I_{Ca,L}$ cannot sustain a propagated AP.

A major modulator of L-type VGCC activity appears to be Ca^{2+} itself. During the course of a single AP, the $I_{Ca,L}$ inactivates more rapidly when Ca^{2+} is the conducted ion. A counteracting effect is that an increased concentration of local Ca^{2+}, perhaps accumulating near the inner pore mouth with rapid (physiologic) stimulation rates, appears to enhance the channel activity (29,116). Enhancement of channel opening in this setting may be due to channel phosphorylation by the calmodulin-sensitive kinase (CaM kinase II) (570). Phosphorylation is also frequently mediated by cAMP-dependent protein kinase (PKA) (activated most notably by the β-adrenoceptor), causing the much greater $I_{Ca,L}$ and Ca^{2+} entry observed with b-adrenergic stimulation (426). This phosphorylation shifts L-type VGCC into a mode in which channel openings are more frequent and sustained (572). In this setting of enhanced $I_{Ca,L}$, even if Na channels are inactivated by partial depolarization, propagated "slow" APs can be achieved because there is sufficient inward Ca^{2+} current to result in a regenerative AP. As one might anticipate, the Ca^{2+} released from the SR appears to enhance Ca^{2+}-dependent inactivation (252,309).

The Na^+-Ca^{2+} Exchanger The Na^+-Ca^{2+} exchanger (NCE) of the myocardium is a 108-kd, 970 amino acid protein present in the plasmalemma and possessing a large cytoplasmic domain located between the sixth and seventh of twelve postulated transmembrane domains (386). Unlike the ion ATPases ("pumps"), the exchanger does not consume ATP, but rather employs the potential energy in the Na^+ gradient to translocate Ca^{2+} against its gradient in a process that is reversible (71,376). Critical to its behavior is the fact that the exchanger is electrogenic, that is, 3 Na^+ exchange for 1 Ca^{2+}. Thus there is a net transfer of 1 charge *into* the cell, for 1 Ca^{2+} moved *out* of the cell; the Ca^{2+} flux is measurable as a current (I_{NaCa}) in the opposite direction (110). Furthermore, the membrane potential can greatly alter the amplitude of the Ca^{2+} flux, as well as its direction. The membrane potential at which the Ca^{2+} flux reverses ($E_{rev,Na\text{-}Ca}$) is given by: $E_{rev,Na\text{-}Ca} = 3 \cdot E_{Na} - 2 \cdot E_{Ca}$, where E_{Na} and E_{Ca} are the Na^+ and Ca^{2+} equilibrium potentials defined by the Nerst equation (269). For example, 3 Na^+ enter the cell down their 10- to 15-fold gradient (E_{Na} ~+60 mV) through the exchanger and are able to move 1 Ca^{2+} against its 10,000-fold gradient (E_{Ca} ~+120 mV) when the membrane potential is negative to −60 mV. Since the normal resting potential is <−80 mV, this can occur during rest. With a sufficient electrochemical gradient Ca^{2+} can cause Na^+ to be translocated against its normal gradient (i.e., out of the cell), such as during the peak of an AP when the membrane potential goes to +40 mV. The exchanger reverses direction and mediates Ca^{2+} entry and Na^+ efflux (and a net outward I_{NaCa}), augmenting entry via the L-type Ca channel. Such I_{NaCa}-mediated entry declines sharply after Ca^{2+} release and entry has raised $[Ca^{2+}]_i$ to ~1 μM and made $E_{rev,Na\text{-}Ca} > 0$ mV, near the plateau of the AP (53). Since during the AP plateau membrane potential is near $E_{rev,Na\text{-}Ca}$, increases in $[Na^+]_i$ may cause decreases in the amount of Ca^{2+} elimination, or even cause persisting Ca^{2+} entry (200,504). Since exchange is electrogenic, $I_{Na\text{-}Ca}$ exchange current may also modulate AP duration, increasing it during periods of Ca^{2+} elimination.

Ca^{2+} entry via the exchanger is clearly sufficient to the activate Ca^{2+} release from the SR (306,310,312), and it may also serve to load the SR stores (393). Ca^{2+} entry during the later phases of the AP may load the SR for the subsequent AP (504). While a large Na^+ gradient is required to eliminate Ca^{2+} during diastole, too large a gradient may prevent Ca^{2+} entry by this pathway during the peak of the AP (311). Calculations suggest that the exchanger could contribute as much as 65% of the entering Ca^{2+} that triggers release from the SR (311), but there is disagreement as to whether such reversed Ca^{2+} flow into the myocyte has physiologic relevance (99,310), particularly with regard to activating Ca^{2+} release from the SR (318,458).

The NCE appears to modulate the Ca^{2+} content of a small compartment of the cell, localized near the membrane. Langer and coworkers (301,419) have postulated that a large fraction of the Ca^{2+} that the NCE regulates is bound to anionic phospholipids of the sarcolemmal inner leaflet. The compartment is also responsive to the amount of Ca^{2+} present in the junctional SR and may correspond to the "cleft" present between sarcolemma and JSR (see Fig. 7B), which is in equilibrium with the Ca^{2+} on the JSR. Such a model may be attractive if the Na^+ that enters during an AP accumulates in a "fuzzy" subsarcolemmal space (307), decreasing its gradient, and thereby inducing greater exchanger-mediated Ca^{2+} entry while the cell is depolarized during the AP plateau.

The role of the NCE appears to assume greater importance in the neonates of species such as rabbit in which the SR is underdeveloped and intracellular Ca^{2+} stores are limited (9). In neonatal rabbit myocytes, the exchanger plays a predominant role, and Ca^{2+} entry via this path is far more important than that via L-type VGCC (541). The NCE may also play an important role in rate-dependent changes in contractility (200).

Ca^{2+} Removal and Relaxation

Critical to relaxation within mammalian heart is the ability to decrease the $[Ca^{2+}]_i$ well below the threshold at which it activates contraction, usually to <0.10 μM. While rapid relaxation first depends on Ca^{2+} diffusion off of TnC, a force-dependent process as noted above, it subsequently requires the rapid accumulation into the SR by the Ca^{2+}-ATPase (Ca pump). The other processes available for removing Ca^{2+} from the myoplasm (Na^+-Ca^{2+} exchange, sarcolemmal Ca^{2+} pump activity, mitochondrial Ca^{2+}) are simply too slow to permit the rapid relaxation seen in the normally working heart (28,47).

Ca^{2+} Uptake by the SR

Ca^{2+} accumulation into the SR is accomplished by the the cardiac isoform of the sarcoplasmic/endoplasmic reticulum Ca^{2+}-ATPase (SERCA2), which is responsible for reaccumulating all of the released Ca^{2+} back into the SR lumen (186). SERCA2 is a 105-kd protein composed of 997 amino acids, which is the isoform expressed in slow skeletal muscle (65,66). As typical of membrane transport proteins, this protein has hydrophobic intramembranous helices that bind and translocate ions, while the bulk of the protein is located in the myoplasmic domains, including the ATP binding and modulatory regions. One ATP is hydrolyzed to transfer two Ca^{2+} into the SR lumen (coupling ratio of 2) (206,342). This efficiency is greater than that of either the plasma membrane Ca^{2+}-ATPase (PMCA) or the combined action of the Na pump and Na/Ca exchanger. The SERCAs are specifically inhibited by the terpenoid drug thapsigargin (266), which completely eliminates the twitch response in isolated myocytes by preventing uptake of Ca^{2+} into SR, resulting in its depletion (241,251). Curiously, the effect of either thapsigargin or cyclopiazonic acid, another SERCA inhibitor, is far more limited in intact muscle (30).

During a normal contraction, Ca^{2+} binds to TnC after its release from the SR. Ca^{2+} will dissociate from TnC and can either rebind, continuing to activate myosin-actin interactions, or bind to the higher affinity Ca^{2+} binding sites on the SERCA. Due to the dense distribution of the ATPase on the longitudinal (or network) SR that surrounds the length of the myofibrils, and because it has a higher affinity for Ca^{2+} (K_M = 0.18 μM) than TnC (K_M = 0.5 μM) (18), Ca^{2+} will be increasingly bound to the high-affinity ATPase Ca^{2+} binding sites. Ca^{2+} is then translocated into the SR lumen and diffuses off of the now low-affinity Ca^{2+} sites, becoming unavailable for the rest of that contraction. From its location in the longitudinal SR, Ca^{2+} diffuses to the JSR, which contains the CaRCs and from which it is released. The strategic location and ability of the SR to rapidly accumulate Ca^{2+} is evident when the SR stores have been depleted during rest. If the SR Ca^{2+}-ATPase is inhibited by thapsigargin, rest contractions are enhanced because a fraction of entering Ca^{2+} is normally taken up by the SR is now available to bind to TnC to activate force development (26).

In rat myocytes the amount of Ca^{2+} taken up into the SR Ca^{2+} appears to be related to level of resting $[Ca^{2+}]_i$. When entry of Ca^{2+} into the cell was enhanced by either an increase in extracellular $[Ca^{2+}]$ or stimulation rate, there was an increase in diastolic $[Ca^{2+}]_i$, an increase in the systolic Ca^{2+} transient mediated by SR release, and enhanced shortening (161). In fact, there was a relatively linear relation between diastolic and peak systolic $[Ca^{2+}]_i$, representing the amount of stored Ca^{2+}.

The primary means by which cardiac Ca^{2+}-ATPase activity is modulated occurs by regulation of the number active ATPase molecules. In addition to SERCA2, an important accompanying membrane protein is phospholamban, a 52 amino acid peptide with a single transmembrane domain that typically exists as a homopentamer (169,466). In its unphosphorylated state, phospholamban binds to and inhibits SERCA2, thereby reducing the rate of Ca^{2+} accumulation into the SR. When the protein kinases become activated and phosphorylate phospholamban, its inhibitory action on Ca^{2+}-ATPase ceases (268).

While the majority of ATP consumption in the working heart is by myosin ATPase, both theoretical considerations as well as experimental studies suggest that "activation energy" for myocardial contractions accounts for ~25% of energy consumption (441). Such activation energy is that which is related to cycling of activator Ca^{2+} through the SR. Since SR Ca^{2+} efflux is a passive process, the energy consumption is related ATP use by the SR Ca pump when it accumulates Ca^{2+} into the SR.

Removal of Ca^{2+} from the Myocyte

The decline in activator Ca^{2+} from the SR is primarily achieved by reuptake into the SR, which released the bulk of the activator Ca^{2+}. Nevertheless, the quantity of Ca^{2+} that enters with each beat during steady-state beating (via Ca channels and the Na/Ca exchanger) must be eliminated from the myocyte to prevent overloading the SR with Ca^{2+}.

The Na^+-Ca^{2+} Exchanger The system primarily responsible for removal of Ca from the cell is the Na^+-Ca^{2+} exchanger (42,72). When the Na^+ gradient is reduced or eliminated, contractions are markedly enhanced, since the $[Na^+]$ gradient driving Ca^{2+} elimination is inadequate (314,559). Obviously, the Na^+ gradient that is maintained by the Na^+,K^+-ATPase (Na pump) is critical to eliminating Ca^{2+}. The Na pump is also electrogenic, normally pumping 3 Na^+ out and 2 K^+ into the cell, employing energy derived from ATP hydrolysis (234). Although there is no direct link between the exchanger and the Na pump, their interaction via the $[Na^+]_i$ makes it seem as if 1 ATP is consumed to "pump" 1 Ca^{2+} out and 2 K^+ in, with no net charge movement. The Na pump is also required to eliminate the Na^+ that enters via Na channels, which represents an additional energy burden. The capacity of the Na^+-Ca^{2+} exchange can only reduce the Ca^{2+} transient at a rate that is three to four times slower than the SR Ca pump (40). However, during diastole it is of sufficient magnitude to be able to eliminate the smaller quantity of Ca^{2+} that entered the cell, 7–25% of the amount released and taken up by the SR. When rest is prolonged, the exchanger appears capable of mediating the loss of Ca^{2+} from the SR store, which can eventually result in total depletion of the SR (27,41,47). The contribution of the Na^+-Ca^{2+} exchanger to Ca^{2+} removal from the myoplasm does vary among species, being far smaller in rat (7%) where SERCA activity accounts for 92% of the $[Ca^{2+}]_i$ reduction. In rabbit, SERCA-mediated uptake into the SR still accounts for the majority of the $[Ca^{2+}]_i$ reduction (70%), but the Na^+-Ca^{2+} exchanger accounts for 28% of the reduction (27). Since these experiments were performed in insulated myocytes at 22°C and at stimulation rates far lower than physiologic, the contribution of SERCA to relaxation may be somewhat greater under physiologic conditions. Nevertheless, the predominant role of the SR in mediating relaxation, with a significant fraction of elimination via the Na^+-Ca^{2+} exchange activity (greater in the rabbit), is consistent with the physiologic behavior of intact tissue (37,460). In human myocardium, the distribution of Ca^{2+} fluxes upon relaxation may be somewhere between rat and rabbit.

Relevant to such discussion is the distribution of the Na^+-Ca^{2+} exchanger. This structure appears to be located throughout the sarcolemma (265), although its density appears to be somewhat higher in the T tubules when tested with monoclonal antibodies (162). As such it may be located strategically to eliminate Ca^{2+} as it is slowly lost from junctional SR, particularly since the junctional cleft represents a diffusion-restricted space (see Fig. 7) (300). In fact, the cytoplasmic Ca^{2+} binding (K_D) of the Na^+-Ca^{2+} exchanger is only 0.6 μM (365), which would be inadequate to rapidly reduce myoplasmic Ca^{2+} to the typical resting levels of 0.1 μM. The presence of release at a diffusion-restricted site such as the junctional cleft and other subsarcolemmal sites would permit a locally elevated Ca^{2+} concentration at which the exchanger could work.

The Plasma Membrane Ca^{2+}-ATPase (PMCA) In addition to the Na^+-Ca^{2+} exchange, Ca^{2+} can also be eliminated from the myocyte via a Ca^{2+} ATPase (Ca pump) located in the surface plasma membrane (PMCA). These proteins are particularly important in tissues such as erythrocytes that contain no Na^+-Ca^{2+} exchanger. The basic conformational structure is similar to the Ca pump of the SR, but differences include a lower apparent coupling ratio (1 Ca:1 ATP) and distinctly different modulatory pathways. PMCAs contain a specific binding site for Ca^{2+}-calmodulin, which is a prominent regulatory mechanism (532). In addition, acidic phospholipids can enhance the turnover rate of the pump, as can phosphorylation by protein kinases (532). Although present in the cardiac plasmalemma, the PMCA has a low capacity and does not contribute substantially to myoplasmic Ca^{2+} removal under normal settings (299,300). Since on any cardiac beat <10% of the Ca^{2+} increase is due to Ca^{2+} influx, and since >90% and possibly all of entering Ca^{2+} is eliminated by the Na^+-Ca^{2+} exchanger (72,110), it is likely that <1% of activator Ca^{2+} is eliminated by this pathway (25,27). By itself the PMCA requires at least 30 times longer than the SERCA to reduce $[Ca^{2+}]$ to relaxation levels (28).

Continuous Ca^{2+} Circulation and Rate Dependence

In skeletal muscle that remains inactive, there is little change in its ability to generate tension with a depolarization since the internal SR store of Ca^{2+} that activates myofibrils is present after long periods of rest. This behavior is in sharp contrast to contractions of myocardium of most mammalian species, which show an exponential decline in contractile force with rest (isolated intact rat myocardium is an important exception). Unlike skeletal muscle, in which the SR tightly retains Ca^{2+}, the cardiac SR Ca^{2+} is in far more active exchange with the extracellular milieu. The inverse phenomenon is the classically described positive force-frequency relation (staircase, or treppe) (275), also observed in human myocardium (150,152,203,415).

Effects of Rest

During inactivity, Ca^{2+} is eliminated from cardiac SR Ca^{2+}, a process that occurs without any apparent increase in resting myoplasmic $[Ca^{2+}]$ or tension development (39,41,47). Perhaps mediated by such events as the spontaneous "sparks" of Ca^{2+} release from the SR in the absence of depolarization (93), the incrementally released Ca^{2+} is gradually eliminated by the Na^+-Ca^{2+} exchanger. With sustained (>5 min) rest, Ca^{2+} is eliminated from the SR so that the resulting "rested state" contraction is minuscule compared to those at normal rates, and the SR is depleted of Ca^{2+} (Fig. 8, *left panels*) (539). After prolonged rest, it may require 20 to 100 beats for the normally releasable SR store of Ca^{2+} to be replenished and show an unchanging contraction at any given rate. The importance of the exchanger is evidenced by the fact that in low external Na^+, the rest contraction is not depressed but enhanced (331,456) and the SR store remains replete with Ca^{2+} (38). The importance of the Na^+ gradient is also exemplified by study of rat heart, in which contractions after rest are sustained or increased in amplitude. Rat heart has a higher intracellular $[Na^+]$ of ~13 mM (versus ~7 mM in rabbit), and the smaller Na^+ gradient favors Ca^{2+} entry rather than elimination during rest (460). Therefore, the SR pool stays filled with Ca^{2+}, an effect seen with low extracellular Na^+ in other species (44). In view of the increased $[Na^+]_i$, the observation that rat heart relies more on sarcolemmal Ca^{2+}-ATPase for Ca^{2+} elimination is not surprising (383).

Rate-Dependent Alteration in Contractility

An obvious example of intrinsic variation of Ca^{2+} stores occurs with variation in heart rate. At physiologic rates, the bulk (90% to 95%) of activator Ca^{2+} is derived from loaded SR stores, although the small amount entering from outside is responsible for inducing Ca^{2+} release and contributing 5% to 10% of Ca^{2+} for myofibrillar activation. As indicated schematically in Fig. 8 (*right panels*), these two sources of Ca^{2+} are apparently intermingled. Relaxation occurs as 90% to 95% of Ca^{2+} is reaccumulated in the SR, and 5% to 10% of the Ca^{2+} (equal to the amount that entered) is eliminated from the cell by the Na^+-Ca^{2+} exchanger before depolarization stimulates the next beat. As the heart rate slows, with more time for the Ca^{2+} to "leak" from the SR and then be eliminated from the myocyte, the contractions are smaller and the entering Ca^{2+} now represents a higher fraction (perhaps 10% to 20%) of activator Ca^{2+}. In contrast, the positive inotropic effect of increased heart rate has been recognized for over a century as the "treppe" or staircase—specifically, the positive force-frequency relation observed in almost all mammalian species. The major exception is isolated rat myocardium, which may be an artifact of the preparation, since it is not observed in isolated rat ventricular myocytes (161). The simplest view of the phenomenon assumes that in the diastolic period between depolarization there is less time for Ca^{2+} to leak out of the SR and be eliminated from the cell; consequently, more Ca^{2+} is available for release to stimulate each subsequent contraction.

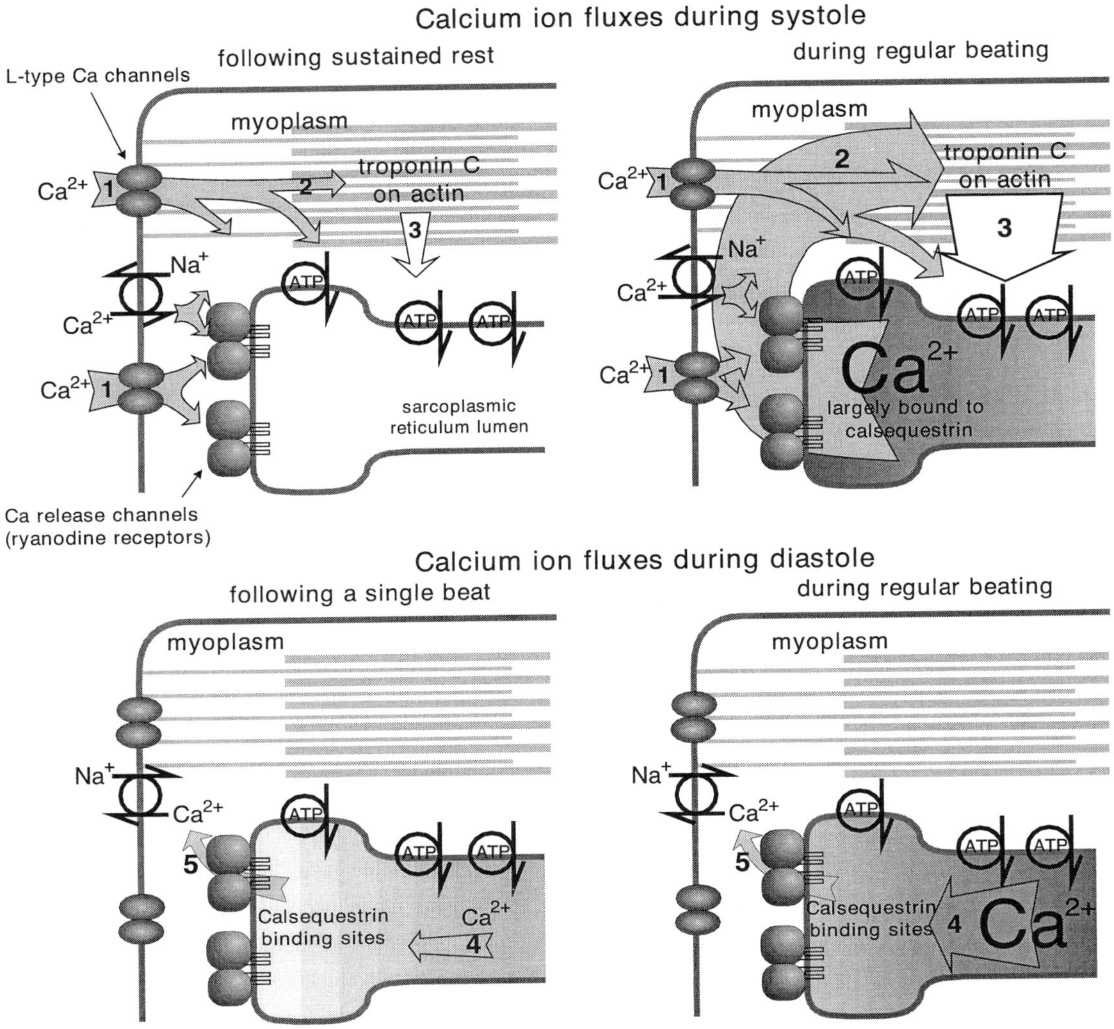

Figure 8. Schematic of Ca^{2+} cycling by the myocardium during systole *(upper panels)* and diastole *(lower panels)*, and which differs between regular beating *(right panels)* and following sustained rest *(left panels)*. Upon depolarization, Ca^{2+} enters via L-type Ca channels and also via the Na^+-Ca^{2+} exchanger to initiate systole (step 1). When the sarcoplasmic reticulum (SR) store is filled *(upper right)*, the action of entering Ca^{2+} is to activate the Ca release channels of the junctional SR (JSR) to activate release of Ca^{2+}, which is the predominant activator Ca^{2+} that binds to troponin C to permit actin-myosin interaction (step 2). Following rest, the SR is depleted of Ca^{2+}, so a significant fraction of Ca^{2+} is taken up into the SR. In either case, only a small fraction of entering Ca^{2+} may actually reach the myofibrils. Following tension development, Ca^{2+} diffuses off of troponin C and binds to the higher-affinity binding sites on the Ca-ATPase (Ca pump) located on the longitudinal (or network) SR and that then transports it to the SR lumen (step 3). During diastole, Ca^{2+} moves toward the junctional SR lumen (step 4) and the Ca^{2+} that "leaks" from the SR is slowly eliminated from the myocyte by the Na-Ca exchange (step 5). If diastole is not prolonged, the bulk of the Ca^{2+} is still present in the junctional SR lumen and available for release with the subsequent depolarization. As rest is prolonged the SR is increasingly depleted of its Ca^{2+} store. If the SR is empty, a number of cycles of Ca^{2+} entry are required to load it.

A small fraction of the cardiac cycle (50 to 200 msec) may be required to transfer Ca^{2+} from the LSR to the JSR, so that at very high heart rates with short diastolic intervals, not all of the SR pool of Ca^{2+} is at a release site. When a premature beat occurs, the contraction may be reduced because Ca^{2+} is not yet in a releasable JSR location. However, during the subsequent pause there is time for accumulation in the JSR release site of an enhanced Ca^{2+}, including that from the extra beat; then there is a marked potentiation of the next beat (postextrasystolic potentiation) (571). With very high heart rates, the continued Ca^{2+} entry of each AP with reduced time between contractions for Ca^{2+} elimination can result in SR Ca^{2+} overload.

Alteration in [Na⁺]ᵢ The decreased time between depolarizations at greater heart rates also reduces the time available for elimination of Na^+ from the cell. Increases in stimulation rate result in an increase in myoplasmic Na^+ (typically indicated as intracellular ionic activity, a^i_{Na}), observed both in Purkinje fibers (62,101) and in ventricular tissue (101,529). In fact, the relation between contractile force and a^i_{Na} is relatively linear (201). The increased a^i_{Na} caused by the increased heart rate shifts the Na/Ca exchanger reversal potential, which can be detected as an increase in outward current in voltage clamped myocytes (200). This increased current represents more Ca^{2+} entry via this exchanger pathway during the initial phase of the AP plateau, while the gradient for Ca^{2+} elimination will be slightly reduced. Such increased outward current may contribute to the shorter AP duration observed at higher stimulation rates (200).

Calmodulin and Ca²⁺-Dependent Phosphorylation The increase in Ca^{2+} that mediates the rate dependence of tension development is not only the result of altered time for elimination and altered balance between entry and elimination via the exchanger. It is now clear that increased frequency of depolarizations and accompanying Ca^{2+} entry also directly alters a variety of the Ca^{2+} regulating pathways. The function of the various ion channels and enzymes can be modulated via phosphorylation by a multifunction Ca-calmodulin (CaM)-dependent kinase (CaM kinase II), which is activated when Ca^{2+} combines with calmodulin to form an activating complex. Control of the various Ca^{2+} pathways by this enzyme remains to be fully elucidated, yet it appears to explain a variety of processes seen with increased heart rate as well as with increased extracellular Ca^{2+} (562). One action of CaMK II may be phosphorylation of L-type Ca channels, facilitating Ca^{2+} entry. When CaMK II is inhibited, the Ca^{2+} entry dependent increase in $I_{Ca,L}$ is markedly reduced (570). Increases in stimulation rate or extracellular Ca^{2+} (and hence peak and mean $[Ca^{2+}]_i$) appear to increase not only $I_{Ca,L}$, but more importantly the SR Ca^{2+}-ATPase responsible for accumulation and SR Ca^{2+} uptake (563). The effect of phosphorylation by CaMK II appears to be an increase in the turnover rate (V_{max}) of the enzyme (347). In fact, rapid pacing results in a persisting enhancement of Ca^{2+}-ATPase and the CaRC (1). Although its physiologic significance remains to be delineated, the cardiac CaRC has a site for phosphorylation not present in the skeletal muscle CaRC, which when phosphorylated by CaM kinase II activates the channel (556). Consequently, in response to an increase in heart rate and the resulting increase in average myoplasmic Ca^{2+}, CaMK II represents a sensitive effector that increases the Ca^{2+} cycling within the myocardium, which in turn can partly account for the positive frequency staircase seen in many species. Such a Ca^{2+}-dependent phosphorylation system is an intrinsic pathway to enhance the contractility of the heart with increases in rate.

Since the phosphorylation of these enzyme systems results in greater Ca^{2+} cycling, each beat will consume more energy to permit Ca^{2+} SR uptake and elimination from the cell, while the greater number of activated myofibrils will also increase ATP consumption. Consequently, the increased oxygen consumption increase associated with an increased heart rate will be due not only to increased beats per unit time, but also to slightly greater energy consumption per beat.

Additional Effects on Ca^{2+} Stores

As noted previously, $E_{rev,NaCa}$ becomes much more positive after Ca^{2+} release, with calculated values of +10 to +40 mV (53,134), which are in the range of the AP plateau. When the voltage is clamped near these potentials, there is no longer a decline in measured Ca^{2+} transients caused by Na^+-Ca^{2+} exchange (21,110). Both $[Ca^{2+}]_i$ (and consequently $E_{rev,NaCa}$) and AP plateau decline together (53,134). While the Na^+-Ca^{2+} exchange current (I_{NaCa}) can influence AP duration, modest alteration in AP plateau amplitude and duration may alter the time during which Ca^{2+} enters through the exchanger, before Ca^{2+} elimination begins. With a very positive AP plateau of extended duration (as when repolarizing K^+ currents are inhibited) the period of exchanger Ca^{2+} influx may be extended. Conversely, when the AP plateau is short and more negative (as when K^+ conductances are increased), more Ca^{2+} can be eliminated by the exchanger. Since the exchanger competes to a certain extent with the SR Ca^{2+}-ATPase for Ca^{2+}, when Ca^{2+} removal begins later (as in the former case) more Ca^{2+} will accumulated in the SR and contractility will be greater. In the latter case, when the exchanger eliminates more Ca^{2+}, contractility will be reduced. However, since the Ca^{2+} influx corresponds to outward I_{NaCa} this process is self-correcting: larger, longer APs increase outward I_{NaCa} (and Ca influx), which decreases amplitude and duration.

Pharmacologic blockade of Ca^{2+} channels can also decrease cardiac contractility. This effect is both direct and indirect. By decreasing the amount of triggering Ca^{2+}, the activation of Ca^{2+} release may be reduced; however, it is unknown whether there may be a substantial excess of Ca^{2+} normally entering to activate release of the much greater SR store. Initially with Ca^{2+} channel blockade and decreased Ca^{2+} entry, Ca^{2+} elimination via the surface membrane will exceed Ca^{2+} entry, resulting in a gradual reduction in the SR Ca^{2+} store and reduced contractility.

The Role of the Mitochondria

In addition to synthesizing ATP by employing a proton gradient across the inner and outer membranes, mitochondria also carefully regulate Ca^{2+} via a Ca^{2+}-H^+ exchanger and Ca^{2+} uniport pathways (188). Na^+-Ca^{2+} antiport is also present and responsible for elimination of Ca^2 from the mitochondria. The rate of Ca^{2+} uptake has been shown to be too slow to contribute to Ca^{2+} regulation within a contractile cycle (367,446). When the physiologic pathways for decreasing myoplasmic Ca^{2+} are inhibited by eliminating $[Na^+]_o$ to inhibit Na^+/Ca^{2+}, the Ca^{2+} released into the myoplasm by caffeine will be assimilated by the mitochondria over a time course of 10 seconds (24,28), a process 50- to 100-fold slower than the normal Ca^{2+} accumulation into the SR. This Ca^{2+} will redistribute to the SR once Ca^{2+} reuptake is restored (by caffeine removal). When $[Na^+]_i$ is partially depleted, initial Ca^{2+} reuptake is enhanced and subsequent redistribution from the mitochondria, mediated by the mitochondrial Na^+-Ca^{2+} antiport, is delayed.

During hypoxia or ischemia, the loss of the proton gradient may result in Ca^{2+} loading of mitochondria. Sustained Ca^{2+} overload leads to mitochondrial swelling, and ultimately to disruption. However, in contrast to pathologic conditions, the increased "average" myoplasmic $[Ca^{2+}]$ that occurs with increased heart rate of β-adrenergic activation may have important physiologic functions. Under such settings, gradual uptake of Ca^{2+} over time may result in a modest increase in mitochondrial $[Ca^{2+}]$ (198,367,558), which can in turn enhance the activity of intramitochondrial dehydrogenases and lead to an appropriate increase in ATP synthesis (77).

EXTRINSIC MODULATION OF CONTRACTILITY

The major mechanism by which the autonomic nervous system as well as other hormones and transmitters influence cardiac function is an alteration in the function of the various ion transport pathways in cardiac membranes. While any resulting change in heart rate may in and of itself alter contractile function (see above), activation of the various pathways exerts a strong, direct modulating effect on the amount of activator Ca^{2+} and also acts on myofibrillar Ca^{2+} sensitivity and function. The changes in $[Ca^{2+}]_i$ can in turn influence membrane potential via Na^+-Ca^{2+} exchange and certain ion currents. Activation of various processes is appropriately coordinated, so that if the duration of tension development is shortened by enhanced relaxation, the AP duration will also be decreased. The primary processes and pathways that modulate cardiac function are listed in Table 1.

G Protein–Linked Receptor-Mediated Effects

The vast majority of receptors in the heart and peripheral cardiovascular system that modulate function belong to a family of membrane proteins whose actions are mediated by activation of the guanine nucleotide-binding proteins, or G proteins. These molecules act as highly specialized intracellular messengers. After they are activated by specific receptors, they in turn activate (or inhibit) a variety of cell effector pathways such as ion channels or second-messenger generating enzymes (48,228,338). The G protein–linked receptors are distinctive in having seven transmembrane α-helical segments, which create a central cleft (not a channel) on the extracellular surface.

Table 1. PATHWAYS AND MECHANISMS OF EXTRINSIC MODULATION OF CARDIAC CONTRACTILITY

Ligand	Membrane Receptor	Pathway	Cellular effect	Action
PG I_2 (prostacyclin)	IP		↑ Delayed I_K, I_{to}, and Cl conductance	↓ AP duration → sl ↓ Ca^{2+} entry
Serotonin	5-HT_2	→G_s protein	↑ Myosin turnover rate	↑ Contractility
Glucagon	Glucagon	↑ Adenylyl cyclase	↑ I_{Ca} (?direct G_s effect	↑↑ Ca^{2+} entry
Histamine	H_2 histamine	↑ cAMP	↑ CaRC activity	SR Ca^{2+} release
epinephrine, NE, isoproterenol, dopamine	β_1 adrenergic, β_2 adrenergic	↑ Protein kinase A activity Phosphorylation	↓ Phospholamban (Plm) inhibition of SR Ca ATPase →	↑ SR Ca^{2+} uptake → ↑↑ Ca^{2+}cycling through the SR,
			TnC Ca^{2+} affinity (via TnI phosphorylation)	faster relaxation
		→ $G_?$ protein	↓ Transient inward & other K currents	↑ AP duration → ↑ Ca^{2+}
NE, epinephrine	α_1 adrenergic	→ G_q protein ↑ phospholipase C	↑ Na^+,K^+ ATPase activity →	decrease in Ca^{2+} accumulation
Angiotensin II	Angiotensin II	activity → ↑ IP_3	↑ Na^+/H^+ exchange	↑ pH → ↑ Ca^{2+}
Endothelin	Endothelin	and ↑ diacylglycerol ↑ protein kinase C		sensitivity of myofilaments
			?? ↑ CaRC activity and ?? ↓ Plm inhibition	?? ↑ SR Ca^{2+} uptake and release
Adenosine, ?ATP	A1 purinergic	G_i protein ↓ Adenylyl cyclase	$I_{K(Ado,ACh)}$ Effects opposite to those seen	↓ AP duration → ↓ Ca^{2+}
Acetylcholine	M2 muscarinic → ↑ Guanylyl	↓ cAMP production ↑ cGMP → PDE activation	with adenylyl cyclase activation ↓I_{Ca} (?)	↓ Ca^{2+} entry
NO (from endothelium)	cyclase (myoplasmic "soluble") activation	→ ↓ cAMP	Certain effects opposite to those seen with ↑ cAMP	
Atrial natriuretic factors	Receptor/→ guanylyl cyclase ("particulate")	↑ cGMP → PDE activation → ↓ cAMP	Activation of Na/K/Cl ion cotransporter	? altered cell volume

AP, action potential; CaRC, Ca^{2+} release channel; IP_3, inositol 1,4,5–trisphosphate; NE, norepinephrine; NO, nitric oxide; PDE, phosphodiesterase; SR, sarcoplasmic reticulum, Tn, tropinin.
Adapted from ref. 335.

When ligands (norepinephrine, histamine, etc.) bind in the cleft of these receptors, a conformational change occurs on the intracellular surface of the receptor that promotes dissociation of the heterotrimeric G protein complex. Guanosine diphosphate (GDP) and the tightly coupled $\beta\gamma$ subunit dissociate away from the α subunit, which is then free to bind GTP. The GTP-bound α subunit forms an activating complex that then regulates the membrane effector systems (211), at least until the GTP is hydrolyzed. The $\beta\gamma$ subunit also appears to play an important signaling role, either by direct interaction with membrane constituents or by binding to and inactivating the a subunits (97,247,250).

Cyclic AMP–Dependent Protein Kinase Actions

The most widely studied G protein signal pathway, which is highly relevant to the cardiovascular system, is the regulation of adenylyl cyclase (AC). This produces the second messenger cAMP. By binding to their specific receptors in the myocardium, catecholamines (via the β-adrenoceptors, β_1-AR, β_2-AR) (454), histamine (via the H_2 receptor) (352), prostacyclin (via the IP receptor) (6), serotonin (via the 5-HT_4 receptor) (401), and glucagon mediate their primary actions by activating G_s, the stimulatory G protein, which in turn activates AC. The increased intracellular [cAMP] then activates the cAMP-dependent protein kinase (PKA), thus phosphorylating a variety of proteins that leads to the increase in contractility and heart rate. These PKA-mediated effects are shown schematically in Fig. 9 and discussed below.

Myofibrils Phosphorylation of TnI decreases the affinity of TnC for Ca^{2+} (433), an effect that will decrease actin-myosin interaction and contractility unless Ca^{2+} has been increased. However, the other actions of PKA noted below serve to markedly enhance the depolarization-induced increase in myoplasmic Ca^{2+}, which more than offsets the decreased Ca^{2+} affinity of TnC for Ca^{2+} so that contractility is ultimately enhanced (136). Consequently, the prominent effect of the decreased Ca^{2+} affinity is to cause more rapid dissociation of Ca^{2+} from TnC, permitting relaxation to occur more quickly. Within the context of a higher heart rate (see below) this decreased contractile duration is critical to permitting an adequate diastolic period for coronary flow and ventricular filling. In addition to these actions, β-AR activation appears to have an independent effect to increase the rate of myosin cross-bridge turnover, an action that will also serve to increase tension development (226). Finally, the C-protein molecule located on myosin is also phosphorylated in the presence of β-AR stimulation (176,289), possibly contributing to this positive inotropic action by increasing the rate of myosin cross-bridge turnover or cycling(226,231,439).

Ca^{2+} Cycling The major mechanism by which β-AR stimulation increases contractile force is by an increase in the amount of Ca^{2+} cycled, resulting in a marked increase in the measurable Ca^{2+} transient, which is proportionally far greater than the increase in force development (136). When compared to increased force elicited by elevated extracellular [Ca^{2+}], the Ca^{2+} transient seen with β-AR activation is far greater (Fig. 10A). Such enhanced Ca^{2+} cycling results from PKA-mediated phosphorylation of (a) the L-type Ca channel, (b) phospholamban, and (c) the Ca release channel. Phosphorylation of the L-type Ca channel alters its gating behavior, changing to a new "mode" in which the open intervals are more sustained so that a greater number of Ca^{2+} ions may enter the cell (350). Although the increase in $[Ca^{2+}]_i$ can contribute to Ca^{2+}-mediated inactivation of the channel, the net effect is still a marked increase in the peak current and total Ca^{2+} influx. However, entering Ca^{2+} is not the primary regulator of activation; phosphorylation of SR proteins appears to be more critical in increasing myocardial Ca^{2+} (459). When the inhibition of the

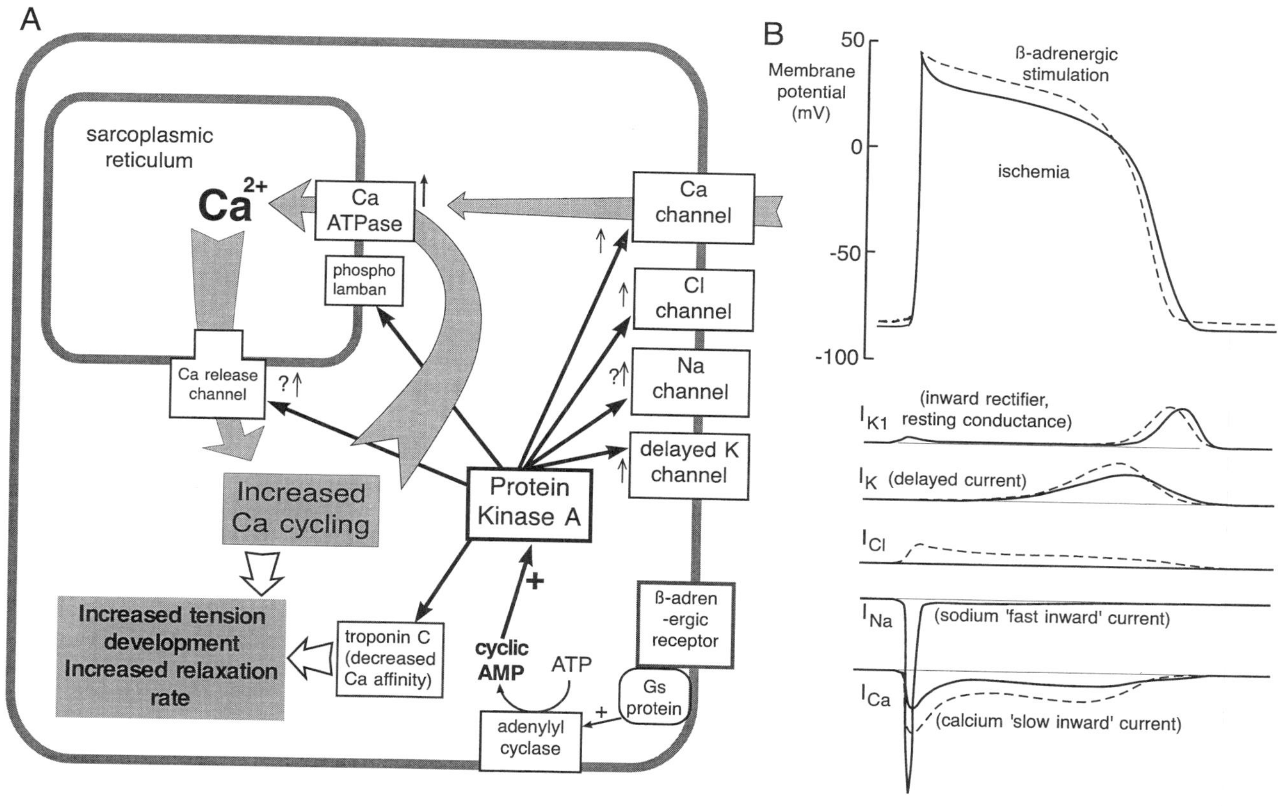

Figure 9. Sites of cellular action of β-adrenergic stimulation and protein kinase A activation that increase force development **(A)**, with the accompanying changes in the cardiac action potential and ionic currents **(B)**. While phosphorylation of troponin C (TnC) decreases Ca^{2+} affinity, the increase in the amount of cycled Ca^{2+} is more than sufficient to overcome the lower affinity, so that more TnC subunits bind Ca^{2+}, resulting in greater myofibrillar activation and peak force. However, the lower TnC Ca^{2+} affinity and greater Ca^{2+}-ATPase activity in the sarcoplasmic reticulum permit faster relaxation. Similar PKA-mediated effects can also be observed with histamine, prostacyclin, serotonin, and glucagon stimulation, or with phosphodiesterase inhibition, which prevents cyclic breakdown of cyclic AMP.

SR Ca pump by phospholamban is prevented, either by injection of specific antibody (459) or by ablation of the gene so that the protein is not expressed(328), the result is increased myocardial contractility and loss of inotropic response to β-AR stimulation. Following phosphorylation, phospholamban no longer provides a brake on the SR Ca pump, so Ca^{2+} can be accumulated at a far greater rate (268). This increased rate has been attributed to an increase in the turnover rate (V_{max}) of the ATPase of well over twofold (18); in addition, a decrease in Ca^{2+} binding affinity has also been reported when phospholamban assumes an inhibitory (nonphosphorylated) form (347). Certainly the combination of increased Ca^{2+} entry and SR accumulation means a far greater amount of accumulated Ca^{2+}. The greater amount of SR Ca^{2+} also appears to be released at an enhanced rate following phosphorylation of the cardiac CaRC (or a closely associated protein) by PKA, whose function is also enhanced (494,568). Following phosphorylation, sensitivity to baseline Ca^{2+} is decreased, but the response to a given incremental increase in $[Ca^{2+}]$ is an increased initial channel opening followed by faster adaptation (decay of activity) compared to the nonphosphorylated state (515). Such greater peak of CaRC activity and faster adaptation, so that the channel may be more rapidly available for subsequent activity, are features present in β-adrenergically treated muscle.

While the increased amount of Ca^{2+} cycling overcomes the decreased troponin complex Ca^{2+} sensitivity to cause the positive inotropic effect, these processes are not uniformly activated by β-AR stimulation of PKA. In isolated myocardium, the Ca^{2+} transient amplitude and kinetics (due to SR Ca^{2+} release) and the peak force are enhanced by the lowest isoproterenol concentrations (1 nM), but 5 to 10 nM isoproterenol is required to enhance relaxation, consistent with decreased TnC Ca^{2+} sensitivity (396).

In addition to enhancing Ca^{2+} entry and release, PKA appears to activate a number of other channels. In pacemaking tissue, the pacemaker current (I_f) is increased, which increases the rate of diastolic depolarization and leads to the increased heart rate typical of β-adrenergic activation. As previously noted, increased rate by itself has positive inotropic actions. PKA phosphorylation also increases in the delayed K current (526), the transient outward (I_{to}) current (382), and a Cl^- conductance, all of which will tend to abbreviate the AP and ensure that the contractile state is not overly prolonged. Although the decrease in AP duration will slightly abbreviate the duration of the Ca^{2+} current, the net effect of β-AR stimulation will be an increased Ca^{2+} influx because of the great increase in open L-type Ca channels. Although the greater amount of entering Ca^{2+} contributes in greater SR loading, over a sustained period the greater Ca^{2+} influx must be balanced by greater Ca^{2+} efflux. The greater efflux is mediated via the Na^+-Ca^{2+} exchanger, which obligates greater Na^+ entry and its elimination via the Na^+-K^+ ATPase.

The β-ARs (β-AR) in the myocardium are both the $β_1$-AR and $β_2$-AR subtypes. $β_2$-AR is present on both pacemaker tissues and myocytes and is not activated by norepinephrine, but by isoproterenol and specific agonists such as Zinterol (560). The

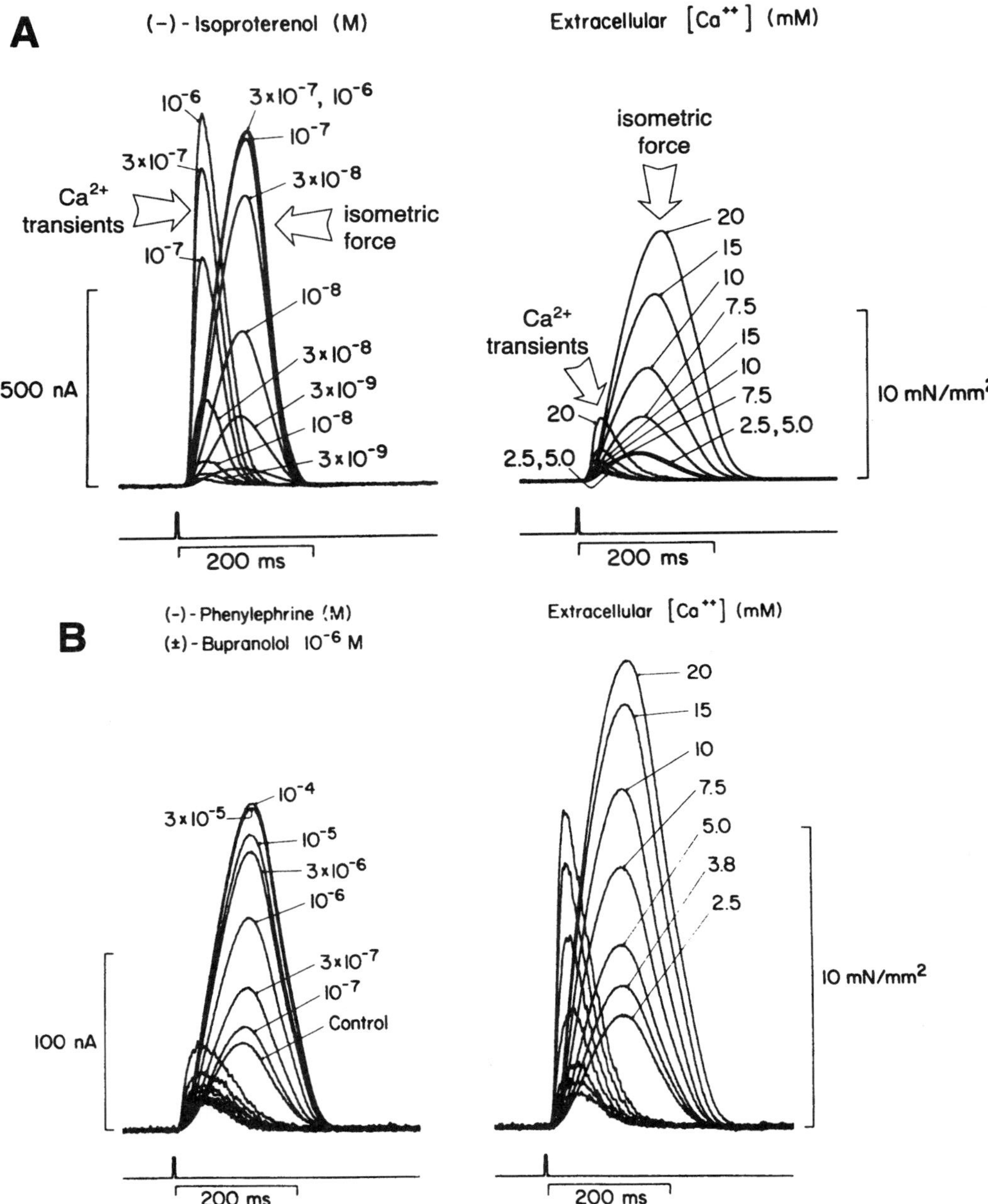

Figure 10. Alteration in the myocardial Ca^{2+} transient (sharply peaking initial tracings) and the accompanying tension caused by β-adrenergic stimulation with isoproterenol versus α-adrenergic stimulation by phenylephrine. **A:** Effects of various concentrations of (-)-isoproterenol *(left panel)* or extracellular Ca^{2+} *(right panel)* on isometric contractions and accompanying aequorin light signals monitoring intracellular Ca^{2+}. Responses are those observed in isolated rabbit papillary muscle at a temperature of 37.5°C with a stimulation interval of 1 sec. Responses were averaged from 128 contractions to improve the signal-to-noise ratio. **B:** Effects of various concentrations of (-)-phenylephrine *(left panel)* and of increased extracellular Ca^{2+} *(right panel)* on aequorin signals and isometric contractions. Conditions are identical to those employed in A, but in a different muscle. (±)-bupranol (10^{-6} M) was present during the phenylephrine study to prevent β-adrenergic stimulation. Note the far greater increase in the Ca^{2+} transient observed with β-adrenergic stimulation compared to α_1-adrenergic stimulation. Greater maximal force of shorter duration could ultimately be achieved with β-adrenergic stimulation. (From ref. 136, with permission.)

effects noted above apply primarily to the actions of β_1-AR stimulation, but are not usually attributed to β_2-AR. β_2-AR activation does not appear to decrease myofibril Ca^{2+} sensitivity, nor does it markedly increase SR Ca^{2+} uptake or increase the rate of relaxation and abbreviate contractions, effects associated with disinibition of Ca-ATPase by β_1-AR stimulation. Whereas β_2-AR activation enhances I_{Ca}, the effect is distinct from that of β_1-AR stimulation, demonstrating less inactivation of current, which may contribute to AP prolongation (560). β_2-AR activation is not as arrhythmogenic as β_1-AR stimulation, probably because it does not induce profound SR Ca^{2+} loading, which can result in oscillatory release of Ca^{2+}, delayed afterdepolarizations, and ectopic beats. These different actions may depend on different locations of AC or compartmentalized cAMP, and may have potentially important therapeutic implications. The differential actions do not appear so profound in failing human myocytes, however, and low epinephrine concentrations appear to mediate their actions via β_2-AR activation (117).

While G_s activation also appears to directly increase Ca channel currents (566,567), the importance and relevance of this action to physiologic function is unclear (202). Direct activation by β_2-ARs might explain observed behavior that differs from that seen with β_1-AR activation (560). Likewise, stimulation of P_2-purinergic receptors appears to enhance opening of L-type channels via a pathway involving a G_s pathway exclusive of cAMP production (445).

Cyclic AMP Regulation by Phosphodiesterase In addition to regulation of [cAMP] (and PKA protein phosphorylation) by regulation of AC-mediated cAMP synthesis, there is also hydrolytic breakdown of cAMP by alterations in phosphodiesterase activity. A variety of cAMP-phosphodiesterase enzymes exist whose activity can be modulated by intracellular constituents (151,155). Inhibition of cAMP hydrolysis by inhibitors of varying specificity (methylxanthenes such as theophylline and caffeine; bipyridines such as amrinone and milrinone) can be employed to increase cAMP, with its consequent increase in contractile function. Certain phosphodiesterases and phosphatases are also regulated by intracellular messengers (e.g., cyclic GMP), which provide an additional modulatory system on cAMP and the PKA phosphorylation (94,155,348).

Inhibition of Adenylyl Cyclase When myocardial tissue is activated by acetylcholine (ACh, via M_2 muscarinic cholinoceptors [22]) or adenosine (via A_1-adenosine receptors (464)) there is activation of the AC-inhibitory G protein, G_i. Such G_i activation can strongly inhibit AC and decrease cAMP levels toward nonstimulated levels (54), thereby reversing the positive inotropic effects of β-AR stimulation, an "antiadrenergic" effect (63,232, 248). The inhibitory actions appear to be mediated at least in part by release of βγ subunits from $G\alpha_i$, which then bind $G\alpha_s$, resulting in the loss of AC activation (250). In the absence of β-AR stimulation, the effect of adenosine or ACh on I_{Ca} in ventricular muscle is modest (63,248). Vagal stimulation has a far more modest effect on ventricular contractility because the nerves primarily release ACh on sympathetic nerve endings, presynaptically decreasing release (323). Consequently, vagal stimulation causes a more profound decrease in contractility that is enhanced by sympathetic stimulation. In human myocardium, adenosine actions mediated by A_1-receptors appear to be more efficiently coupled than ACh in this inhibitory regulatory pathway (54). Adenosine release secondary to ischemia may activate G_i and inhibit AC, thereby decreasing contractility.

In addition to effects mediated by alteration in AC activity, ligand binding to M_2 muscarinic or A_1 adenosine receptors activates G_i, which then directly activates an inwardly rectifying cardiac K^+ conductance ($I_{K(ACh)}$, $I_{K(Ado)}$, or $I_{K(ACh,Ado)}$) (35,63,521, 528). These increases in the resting K^+ conductance will slow diastolic depolarization in pacemaker tissues and decrease heart rate, indirectly altering contractile behavior. $I_{K(ACh,Ado)}$ is also present in human ventricular myocytes, but it is largely inactive under normal circumstances and makes only a modest contribution to total K^+ conductance (287). However, even in the absence of β-AR stimulation, a depressant effect on ventricular function may be present when ACh is directly applied to the myocardium (63), mediated via M_2 receptors present on ventricular myocytes. Although a modest reduction in peak Ca^{2+} current may be present, the increased $I_{K(ACh,Ado)}$ markedly decreases AP duration, which decreases the duration of Ca^{2+} influx (63). The abbreviated AP duration reduces total Ca^{2+} current so that the ongoing Na^+-Ca^{2+} exchange leads to a net loss of Ca^{2+} from SR stores and contractility decreases significantly.

Effect of Phospholipase C Activation

Another major G protein pathway involves the activation of the phospholipases, enzymes that metabolize phospholipid components of the cell membranes (469,478). When activated by a G protein (as shown in Fig. 11), specifically by G_q (and possibly G_i), phospholipase C (PLC) cleaves the phosphoester linkage of diphosphoinositide to produce the phosphated sugar, inositol 1,4,5-trisphosphate (IP_3), and leaves a glycerol with two fatty acids (diacylglycerol [DAG]) in the plasmalemma. Each of these agents can then act as a second messenger. The activity of PLC can also be enhanced by Ca^{2+}, with activity increasing when [Ca^{2+}] increases above resting cellular levels (0.1 μM) (428).

Protein Kinase C and [H]$_i$ Effects The protein kinase C (PKC) class of over 11 enzymes is dependent on the presence of certain phospholipids such as DAG, although a number of lipophilic tumor promoters (the phorbol esters) are widely used experimentally to activate these enzymes. A major subgroup of this kinase class is activated by the presence of Ca^{2+}. In its cytoplasmic state PKC has an autoinhibitory portion that binds to and inhibits the active site, but in the presence of Ca^{2+} and DAG in the membrane bilayer the enzyme binds to the plasmalemma with a resulting conformational change that reveals the active site (Fig. 11A) (443). In cellular homogenates the enzyme can phosphorylate a variety of the molecules activated by PKA, including phospholamban and TnC (249,375,389). However, PKC also has other important actions. PKC may mediate the α_1-adrenergic activation of the Na^+/H^+ antiport so that H^+ is eliminated from the cell, resulting in a more alkaline intracellular milieu (173,505). PKC also has important actions on ion channels. After an initial increase in activity of L-type Ca channels, PKC activation with phorbol esters decreases their opening (294), and increased PKC activity appears to blunt the stimulation of I_{Ca} by β-AR stimulation (575) and decrease L-type Ca channel currents (61). In addition, PKC can activate the delayed K^+ current in myocytes.

IP_3 Effects IP_3 binds to and activates Ca^{2+} flux through a specific intracellular receptor. The IP_3 receptor is a homotetrameric protein, smaller in size (2,749 amino acids per monomer) yet similar in structure to the CaRC (171). When IP_3 in the myoplasm is increased and binds to this receptor, the protein behaves as a Ca^{2+} channel that releases Ca^{2+} from intracellular sarcoplasmic/endoplasmic reticulum stores. This receptor-activated channel is prominent in smooth muscle and in neuronal, endocrine, and hepatic cells (154). Several recent investigations suggest that inositol trisphosphate (IP_3) promotes Ca^{2+} release from cardiac SR (17,124,391), and that this IP_3-induced Ca^{2+} release is enhanced in hypertrophic myocardium (262). However, the IP_3 receptor has a very restricted distribution in the myocardium, being located near the intercalated disks (267), and its physiologic role in the release of Ca^{2+} in this location or in cardiac tissue in general is unclear.

α_1-Adrenergic Effects

The potential importance of possible PKC-mediated actions is exemplified by the positive inotropic action of α_1-adrenoceptor (α_1-AR) stimulation. Phenylephrine (PE), as well as norepinephrine in the presence of β-AR blockade, causes an increase in both atrial and ventricular contractility that is associated with an increase in AP duration (140,147), effects demonstrable in human ventricular myocardium (80,452). Following a transient decrease in shortening (variable with species), isolated myocytes showed increased shortening, which correlated with increased intracellular alkalinity and presumed increased myofibrillar Ca^{2+} sensitivity (140,146). In contrast to β-AR effects, the positive inotropic actions of α_1-AR stimulation in papillary muscles appear with a proportionally smaller increases in the [Ca^{2+}]$_i$ transient than in developed force (136) (Fig. 10B). While contractile and pH effects of α_1-AR were prevented by blockade of the Na^+/H^+ antiport with amiloride derivatives, in skinned fibers the inotropic effect of PE was not prevented by such agents, suggesting some direct phosphorylation of myofilaments (146,505).

In addition to the effects on myofibrillar sensitivity, α_1-AR stimulation also increases the amplitude of the Ca^{2+} transient,

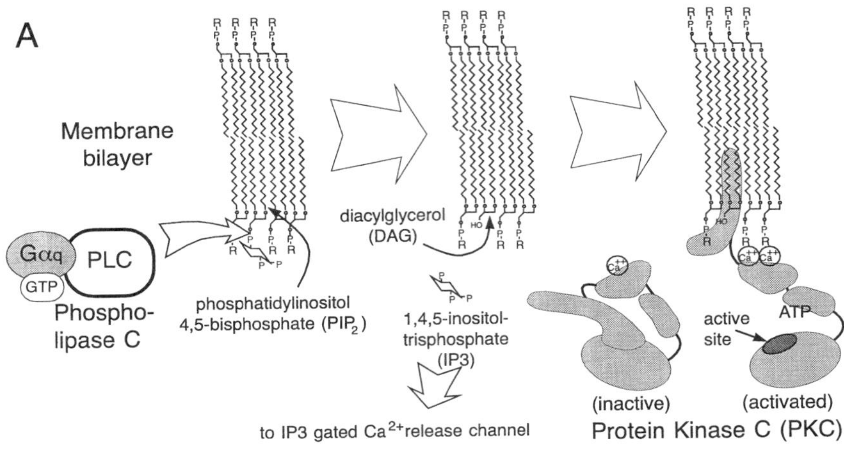

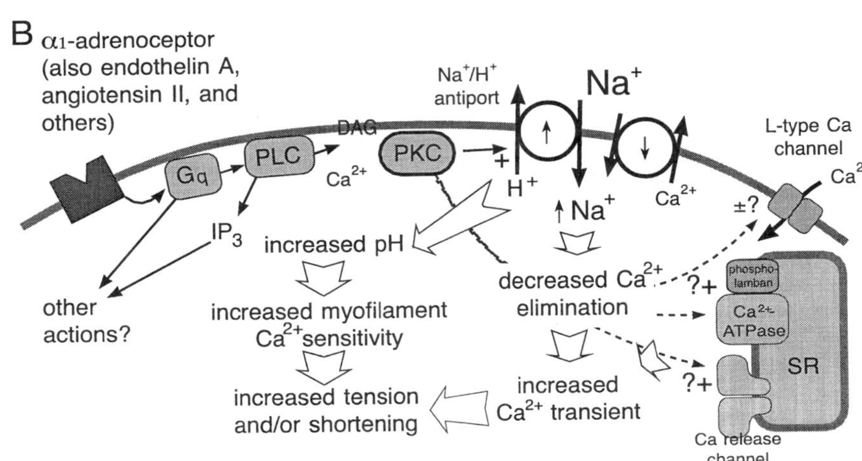

Figure 11. Phospholipase C (PLC) and protein kinase C (PKC) cellular activation pathways. **A:** Proposed membrane molecular pathway for PLC production of diacylglycerol (DAG) and inositol 1,4,5–trisphosphate (IP_3). Activation of PKC appears to involve movement of an autoinhibitory pseudosubstrate region of the molecule to reveal the active site, which occurs when there is intimate association of PKC with the membrane, as well as a requirement for Ca^{2+} (for many PKC subtypes). **B:** Proposed mechanisms of the positive inotropic effects of α_1-adrenergic stimulation (and other G_q-linked receptors) and PKC activation on cardiac myocytes. PKC causes activation of the Na^+/H^+-antiport, which in turn increases myofilament Ca^{2+} sensitivity, while SR uptake and release may possibly be enhanced. In addition, via a pathway separate from PKC, K channel inhibition causes shorter action potentials with a less positive plateau, resulting in less Ca^{2+} current and less Ca^{2+} elimination via the Na-Ca exchanger (not shown).

although the effect is far more modest than that seen with β-AR stimulation (136,394). The mechanism for the increased Ca^{2+} transient is somewhat obscure. As previously noted, α_1-AR and PKC activation do not cause a marked increase in $I_{Ca,L}$. Likewise, while activated exogenous PKC can mediate phosphorylation of phospholamban (249,375) and CaRC (108), which could enhance SR uptake and Ca^{2+} release (132), proteins located in the SR membrane do not appear to be influenced by activation of native PKC in the surface membrane. Certain studies suggest that the positive inotropic actions of α_1-AR stimulation does not involve PKC (138). A more likely explanation involves a probable G protein–mediated inhibition of variety of K^+ currents. Although enhancement of delayed K^+ currents by PKC has been demonstrated (509,527), the predominant action of α_1-AR stimulation is a prominent inhibition of the transient outwardly (145,147) and inwardly rectifying K^+ current. This inhibition results in an AP with a prolonged and more positive plateau (80,140), which thereby provides a longer period for $I_{Ca,L}$. In addition, because the Na^+-Ca^{2+} exchange is very sensitive to membrane potential and $[Na^+]_i$, the greater and longer depolarization will result in slower rate of Ca^{2+} elimination and a greater compensatory uptake into the SR. These combined effects may account for the significant increase in the Ca^{2+} transient seen with α_1-AR stimulation. These effects are the opposite of those observed with ACh and adenosine, which shorten the AP results in marked negative inotropy even though peak I_{Ca} shows little change (63).

In spite of the increased Ca^{2+}-ATPase activity, the α_1-AR enhanced contractions do not show the enhanced relaxation and shorter duration as seen with β_1-AR stimulation (136), probably because of the greater Ca^{2+} sensitivity. Because the tension may in fact be prolonged, in the intact organ this effect may result in a decreased diastolic interval, potentially decreasing the time for coronary perfusion. The myocardial inotropic effect of an α_1-agonist alone is surprising; however, the decrease in cardiac output due to increased vascular resistance may mask its inotropic action. Such positive α_1-AR inotropic effects have been documented using methoxamine in human volunteers (111).

The α_1-ARs have been cloned and divided into four subtypes, α_{1a} to α_{1d} (218). The α_{1a}-AR is blocked by WB4011 and seems to mediate its actions via PLC activation, with subsequent activation of PKC. The α_{1b}-subtype, defined by its sensitivity to chloroethylclonidine (CEC), appears to mediate its action at least in part by increasing the activity of the Na^+,K^+-ATPase (555), a pathway that also appears to involve PLC activation (304). The Na^+,K^+-ATPase activation may account for the decrease in ventricular contractility observed initially with α_1-adrenergic stimulation by phenylephrine (140). Such enhancement of Na^+ elimination should ultimately maintain a larger Na^+ gradient, which will enhance elimination of Ca^{2+} from the cell.

Distinct from the action of the pure β-AR agonist isoproterenol, which shortens the duration of contractions, are the effects of combined β-AR and α_1-AR activation seen with epinephrine and especially with norepinephrine, the major natural sympathetic agonist of the heart. The marked decrease in myofibril Ca^{2+} sensitivity seen with pure β_1-AR stimulation is far less than with mixed β- and α_1-AR activation, and the duration of contractions shows less reduction (136). Certain aspects of the combined β- and α_1-AR stimulation may be viewed a complementary; for example, the enhanced Na^+,K^+-ATPase and

Na^+ gradient provides a mechanism for removal of the increased Ca^{2+} entry via L-type channels. Recent evidence suggests that α_1-AR stimulation and increased PKC activity can modulate the β-AR stimulated PKA phosphorylation, which regulates actin-myosin activity (348).

Endocardial Endothelium, Nitric Oxide, and Cyclic GMP

In addition to forming the lining of the blood vessels, endothelial cells also line the chambers of the heart, lying directly on the basal membrane and connective tissue that surrounds the endocardial myocytes. Although not as dramatic as the vascular endothelial actions on smooth muscle, this endocardial endothelium (EE) does modulate myocardial function (114). Both a negative inotropic effect (myocardial relaxant factor [MRF]) and a stimulatory contractile effect (myocardial contractile factor [MCF]) are demonstrable. The depressant action is relatively modest, is evidenced primarily by an earlier onset of relaxation, and appears to be mediated by nitric oxide (NO) (64,114,185). The action can be blocked by inhibition of NO synthase and can be duplicated by sodium nitroprusside (SNP) (64,185). Since there is typically improvement in cardiac output due to decreased vascular resistance with SNP administration in whole animal experiments or clinical settings, the modest myocardial depressant effect of SNP is probably masked. In fact, in isolating ejecting hearts, peak LV pressure and LV-dP/dt were unchanged by SNP, although it induced premature ventricular relaxation (185).

The typically modest effect of NO and SNP appears to be mediated by activation of a cytoplasmic guanylyl cyclase (94). Both NO (generated by the NO donor SIN-1) and cyclic GMP (cGMP) have been shown to modulate $I_{Ca,L}$. The effect of low concentrations of NO is an enhancement of $I_{Ca,L}$, mediated by an inhibition of a cGMP-sensitive phosphodiesterase (PDE), leading to a increase in cAMP (358,398) and greater activation of PKA. At higher cGMP concentrations, cAMP-enhanced $I_{Ca,L}$ is decreased, an effect mediated by cGMP-dependent protein kinase in mammalian ventricular myocytes (398,525).

The effects of NO, however, are not restricted to the endothelium. The actions of NO and activation of guanylyl cyclase have also been implicated in the actions of muscarinically mediated inhibition of contractions and counteraction against adrenergic activation (19,398,525). This effect can be demonstrated in isolated myocytes, which constitutively express an endothelial cell form of NO synthase (ecNOS, or NOS III) (20). When NO synthesis in inhibited or NO is prevented from acting, the action of muscarinic agents to reverse the adrenergic enhancement $I_{Ca,L}$ are not observed (20,197,525), although NOS inhibition has no effect on the enhancement of $I_{K(ACh)}$ (197). It is unclear whether the antiadrenergic effect of adenosine is similarly mediated by an NO pathway.

Endothelin

The MCF derived from EE is likely to be an endothelin, a stimulatory vasoconstricting peptide secreted by the endothelium that has been shown to have positive inotropic effects on ventricular myocytes (276) and papillary muscles (508). As with α_1-agonists, endothelin receptors appear to activate the G_q-PLC-PKC cascade resulting in intracellular alkalization (276). This in turn increases myofilament Ca^{2+} sensitivity (530), which is sufficient to reverse the effects of an imposed acidosis (531). As with α_1-AR stimulation, there does not appear to be a significant enhancement of $I_{Ca,L}$, whereas effects on the SR may play an important role (508). The threshold concentration for the positive inotropy of endothelin is ~0.3 nM, which is about 10 times greater than required for activation of vascular smooth muscle (368). In rat heart trabeculae, experiments with the specific endothelin A inhibitor BQ-123 suggest that baseline endothelin release contributes to maintenance of contractility, but this effect may be less prominent in other species (349).

Other Hormonal Effects

Angiotensin

The sequential action of renin (released by the glomerulosa cells of the kidney) and angiotensin converting enzyme (ACE, present on the endothelial cell membrane) on angiotensinogen produces angiotensin II (AII), which in addition to its effects on the vasculature also influences the myocardium. Binding to the G protein–linked AT1 receptor activates the PLC pathway outlined above, with a positive cardiac inotropic effect similar to that of the α_1-agonists in which relaxation is not accelerated (371). In the hypertrophied left ventricle of the rat the IP_3-enhanced release of Ca^{2+}, possibly combined with an enhanced myofibrillar Ca^{2+} affinity, may contribute to impaired relaxation (371). In addition, increased intracellular Ca^{2+} loading may occur secondary to enhanced Na channel function and Na^+ entry (369). While these effects lead to an augmented contractile state, they may also delay relaxation and result in the impaired filling seen in pressure-overload hypertrophy. This may be especially true in the presence of concomitant myocardial ischemia (129). Additional major actions of AII appear to include longer term modulation, involving regulation of cardiac protein synthesis and contributing to myocardial hypertrophy (514). Since these actions can be inhibited by pretreatment with an angiotensin converting enzyme (ACE) inhibitor, they provide an important avenue of treatment for patients with diastolic heart failure beyond the traditional use of these drugs as peripheral vasodilators.

Atrial Natriuretic Peptides (ANP)

The heart not only secretes atrial natriuretic peptide from the atria, it also has receptors that respond to such hormones. Unlike the vast array of G protein–linked receptors, the ANP receptors respond with enzymatic activity when binding ligand and generate cyclic GMP when activated. Unlike the soluble guanylyl cyclases that respond to NO, these receptors are termed "particulate" guanylyl cyclase. The actions of cGMP have been noted, although it is unclear whether the cGMP produced by ANP receptors or stimulated by NO are produced and have their actions in the same cell compartments. One effect of ANP-activated cGMP is related to regulation of cell volume and involves the activation of $Na^+/K^+/2Cl^-$ cotransporter, which is in part responsible for control of myocyte volume (100).

Thyroid Hormone

Thyroid hormone has profound metabolic consequences in a variety of tissues. The primary alterations in the myocardium are usually attributed to the effects triiodothyronine (T_3) involved alterations in nuclear synthetic machinery. Such changes involve alteration in myosin isozyme from V_3 toward the faster V_1(320) and greater expression of β-ARs (121,554). These processes contribute dramatically to enhancing tension development. However, in addition to these chronic actions that require time for protein synthesis, T_3 has also been found to have apparently direct actions in a variety of cellular processes that can cause an immediate increase in inotropy. T_3 has direct effects on mitochondrial respiratory rate that do not require protein synthesis (474,475), which may involve enhanced function of adenine nucleotide translocase (128). Mitochondria from hypothyroid rats rapidly respond to T_3 with an increase in ATP production and oxygen consumption (474). T_3 also enhances function of the sarcolemmal Ca^{2+}-ATPase and the Na^+-K^+ ATPase. T_3 enhancement of the Na pump results in a decrease in $[Na^+]_i$ (123), an effect that may be offset in the beating heart by the direct action of T_3 in increasing I_{Na} (127). Enhanced Na^+ entry may increase sarcolemmal Ca^{2+} cycling by increasing the influx and efflux mediated by Na^+-Ca^{2+} exchange. These direct effects may be important in the myocardial dysfunction following cardiopulmonary bypass (CPB), since a significant decline in T_3 is associated with CPB (69) and dopamine administration (516). Myocardial depression following CPB can be relieved by T_3 administration (392).

MYOCARDIAL CONTRACTILE DYSFUNCTION

Decreased contractile function of the myocardium may be either transient, or permanent, depending on the nature of the insult and the cellular response. Transient deterioration in function may arise from a variety of reversible causes, while the dysfunction seen with myocardial failure may also have a reversible component.

Effects of Ischemia and Hypoxia

With the loss of delivery of oxygen and/or nutrients to the myocardial cells, the ATP stores are rapidly depleted and the tissue subsequently undergoes a specific sequence of mechanical and electrophysiologic events (75,88,103,315) (Fig. 12). Within ten minutes of onset the tension development is reduced by >60%, with an accompanying rise in resting tension (ischemic contracture) as $[Ca^{2+}]_i$ rises. The contracture is reduced, but not eliminated, by rest or reduced temperature during the hypoxia (315). In this setting, peak tension and the rate of relaxation are slowed due to impaired SR Ca^{2+} reuptake (492), and since less Ca^{2+} is accumulated less is available for release to generate subsequent twitches. Also contributing to the decreased SR release may be a relatively less sensitive response of the CaRC; in studies employing photo-released Ca^{2+}, the cardiac CaRC adapts to higher Ca^{2+} by decreasing Ca^{2+} efflux; the CaRC remains closed until a substantial step increase in Ca^{2+} again activates opening (191).

In isolated cells, hypoxia is associated with a rise of $[Ca^{2+}]_i$ to ~200 μM and recovery with reoxygenation, while cells that do not recover show a much greater increase to ~400 μM in both the cytosol and mitochondria (366). The SR appears to play an important role in postanoxic Ca^{2+} regulation on reoxygenation (366,465). However, global ischemia is associated with the depressed SR function that persists following reoxygenation (113,259). This may be secondary to Ca^{2+}-ATPase dysfunction (259) as well as to inappropriate opening of the SR Ca release channel in certain cases (113). Decreased Ca^{2+} responsiveness of the myofibrils also appears to contribute to the decreased contractility (194).

Simultaneous with deterioration of mechanical function, the AP duration is markedly reduced and the cell typically depolarizes by 10 to 20 mV (75,103). This effect is associated with a decreased rate of depolarization, an increase in the resting conductance, and a decreased slow inward current (522). The increase in conductance is due to the activation of a specific K channel that is inactivated by ATP, the K_{ATP} channel (390), and blocked by the sulfonylurea drugs (115,133). This K_{ATP} channel appears structurally related to the inward rectifier (G_{K1}) with each subunit having only two transmembrane segments (221). The K_{ATP} channel also inwardly rectifies due to Mg^{2+} blockade, albeit to a lesser extent than the G_{K1} (233,345). The channel becomes active when ATP is depleted with ongoing ischemia/hypoxia, resulting in increased K^+ conductance with less depolarization and decreased AP duration, an effect that appears to be more prominent in epicardial cells (172). This K_{ATP} channel activation accounts for the ST segment elevation seen during myocardial ischemia (290) and the increased K^+ efflux and extracellular accumulation seen during hypoxia or ischemia (537). When $I_{K(ATP)}$ is activated by aprikalim (11) or pinacidil (103) prior to an ischemic insult, the postischemic mechanical dysfunction is reduced. This effect may be mediated in part via coronary vessel effects (see below), but the decreased AP duration due to $I_{K(ATP)}$ combined with the intracellular acidosis (523) will decrease the duration and intensity of I_{Ca}, thus decreasing the rate of Ca^{2+} entry. The sulfonylurea drug glybenclamide is a specific blocker of the K_{ATP} channel that attenuates the decrease in AP duration observed during

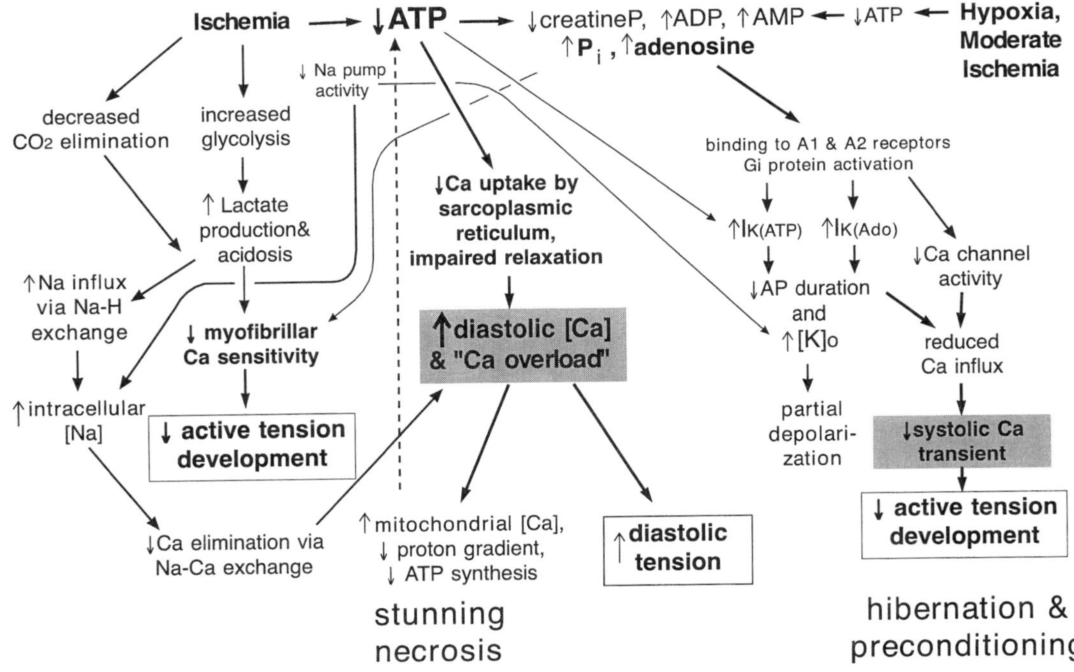

Figure 12. Effects of ischemia on energy substrates, H^+, and Ca^{2+} regulation resulting in a myocardial depressant effects. Depending on the extent and duration of hypoxia or ischemia, effects may vary from transient actions (preconditioning) to more sustained stunning, or if ongoing may result in permanent tissue necrosis.

ischemia and worsens the postischemic dysfunction. In addition, sustained (≥1 hr) ischemia is associated with a decrease in G_s protein and its activation of adenylyl cyclase by β-ARs, an effect that will also decrease the response to β-AR stimulation (491). During reperfusion, the affinity of β-ARs shows a compensatory increase in the previously ischemic region (519).

A by-product of ischemia is the ultimate breakdown of ATP to adenosine, which has a critical regulatory role not only in coronary flow (see below), but also on myocyte function. Activation of by adenosine of A_1 receptors will enhance $I_{K(Ado,ACh)}$ channel activation and thereby abbreviate the AP. Furthermore, the K_{ATP} channel is also modulated by $G\alpha_i$, and its activation by ATP deficiency appears to be enhanced by the presence of A_1 activation (270). The decreased action potential duration may be beneficial in decreasing metabolic demand by decreasing the duration of Ca^{2+} entry and the resulting Ca^{2+} overload, although the greater dispersion of action potential duration may have a potential proarrhythmic effect (551). In addition, adenosine will have dramatic effects on the pacemaker rate via activation of $I_{K(Ado,ACh)}$ channels, which will hyperpolarize nodal tissue and depress diastolic depolarization.

Acidosis

The acidosis that accompanies ischemia contributes to mechanical dysfunction by decreasing myofilament responsiveness to Ca^{2+} (194), as well as by a decrease in I_{Ca} (166,272,273,523). The decreased Ca^{2+} entry and myofilament activation will both serve to decrease ATP consumption. During ischemia and the resulting acidosis, the increased intracellular H^+ is removed from the cell by the Na^+/H^+ antiport (or exchange), causing increased Na^+ entry with an associated rise in $[Na^+]_i$ (384,496). Na^+ entry is also necessary to eliminate the excessive intracellular Ca^{2+} (193,450,496). However, Na^+-Ca^{2+} exchange is steeply dependent on $[Na^+]_i$ (548) so that maintenance of the normal $[Na^+]_i$ of 7 to 10 mM is critical for proper control of intracellular Ca^{2+}. While metabolic inhibition does not appear to increase I_{Na} (355), reduction of Na^+ entry can improve myocardial recovery (520) and prevent ventricular fibrillation (384). The decreased Na^+ gradient that results from H^+ elimination results in greater Ca^{2+} accumulation and increased cellular dysfunction. Blockade of the antiport (causing a greater degree of acidosis) as well as blockade of Na^+ entry by other routes proves beneficial (450,520), improving mechanical recovery from ischemia or anoxia. The Na^+ overload resulting from H^+ elimination from the cell also worsens Ca^{2+} overload upon reperfusion (193,496). When anoxic myocytes in acidic medium are reoxygenated at pH 7.4, inhibition of the antiport and prevention of excessive Na^+ loading protects myocytes from hypercontracture and Ca^{2+} oscillations (295). When metabolic inhibition was imposed upon myocytes, $[Na^+]_i$ was increased threefold, an effect caused by suppressed extrusion by the Na pump as well as by function of the Na^+/H^+ antiport (444). While Ca^{2+} elimination by the Na^+-Ca^{2+} exchanger was reduced by the energy depletion and the increased $[Na^+]$, the contracture seemed to result more from depletion than from the Ca^{2+} overload.

A corollary of the Na^+/H^+ antiport-induced Ca^{2+} overload is that extracellular acidosis, by decreasing the H^+ gradient for efflux, should reduce the antiport-induced influx Na^+ and resulting rise in $[Ca^{2+}]_i$. Indeed, in isolated rat trabeculae subjected to ATP depletion, reduction of extracellular pH from 7.4 to 6.2 decreased the rise in $[Ca^{2+}]_i$ and enhanced recovery of contractility upon restoration of metabolic function (517). Nevertheless, the presence of the added buffering capacity of blood does ameliorate the internal acidification and delay ischemic contractures (564). Application of extracellular acidosis in the absence of ischemia or hypoxia clearly has a myocardial depressant effect associated with decreased I_{Ca}, but the effect is relatively modest above pH 7.1 (166). The intracellular acidification that results from an elevation of CO_2 shows partial recovery mediated by the Na/H^+ antiport (96). While a decrease in myocardial sensitivity to catecholamine stimulation is frequently suggested, the magnitude of this effect above 7.0 is poorly described. In isolated tissue at pH 6.8 there is a decrease in catecholamine sensitivity; however, the maximal increase in contractility is not depressed (506).

Reperfusion and Stunning

When tissue that has been totally ischemic is reperfused, a number of additional processes take place to further degrade myocyte function and viability. Upon restoration of flow, mitochondria may be sufficiently functional to permit restoration of Ca^{2+} regulation or, depending on the duration of the insult, there may be further deterioration and worsening of the Ca^{2+} overload, ultimately causing cell death (366,416). A factor contributing to the progression of injury is production of oxygen free radicals upon reintroduction of oxygenated blood (56,291). Xanthine dehydrogenase may be converted to xanthine oxidase in the presence of elevated cytosolic Ca^{2+}. This enzyme may produce oxygen free radicals, employing the purine derived from adenosine as added substrate. Of greater importance may be free radicals generated by polymorphonuclear leukocytes, which are activated upon reentry into the previously ischemic vasculature (291). Free radicals will injure not only the myocardium but its vasculature as well, so that perfusion may be further degraded. Oxidative stress and peroxidation of membrane lipids may destroy membrane integrity so that ionic gradients are no longer be maintained and unregulated Ca^{2+} entry is further increased (381), a process that may occur in endothelial cells and myocytes as well. While cells have the capability to scavenge free radicals via reduced glutathione (GSH) and glutathione peroxidase, that capacity may be exceeded. Oxidative stress evidenced by decreases in GSH has been observed in human hearts following cardiopulmonary bypass (153).

Free radical formation may also contribute to loss of Ca^{2+} regulation, since oxidating agents cause the Ca release channel to be activated (227,417). This may permit further leak of accumulated Ca^{2+} into the myoplasm, where it can cause further energy expenditure (either by mitochondrial uptake, elimination from the cell, or activation of myofibrils). The sequence of Ca^{2+} overload leading to free radical formation may continue, possibly degrading membrane integrity and causing further Ca^{2+}overload, which clearly leads to cell death.

If an episode of ischemia is not sufficient to result in cell death, the myocardium undergoes a period of recovery during which it is "stunned," exhibiting markedly depressed contractility (67). The scenario of events that leads to this depressed function has been summarized as a gradual uncontrolled rise in cytoplasmic Ca^{2+} during ischemia, a transient worsening of Ca^{2+} overload upon reperfusion, and a persistent but ultimately reversible decrease in myofibrillar Ca^{2+} sensitivity (292). Because Ca^{2+} regulation is largely restored, the contractile deficit appears to be caused by an alteration in the myofibrillar Ca^{2+} sensitivity. This has been demonstrated recently in permeabilized segments of stunned and normal porcine myocardium in which a significant decrease in Ca^{2+} sensitivity was observed in myocardial biopsies (pCa shifted from 5.88 to 5.69, with no change in maximal tension) (225). Similar changes were not seen, however, in stunned rat heart (120).

Preconditioning

If myocardium is subjected to a brief (~5 min) episode of ischemia, the myocardium is "preconditioned," that is, it tolerates subsequent episodes of ischemia for a more sustained period before cell death occurs (302,380). The protective effect includes improved recovery of contractile function following an ischemic insult and reperfusion, as well as protecting the heart against ischemic arrhythmias (409). Preconditioning lasts for a relatively brief period (<1 hr), although a more long-term effect may be present (409). The process seems to require the activity of adenosine, which appears not only to activate $K_{ACh,Ado}$, but also to modulate the function of K_{ATP} channels (270). Blockade of adenosine receptors appears to largely block the protection elicited by preconditioning (302,409), while enhancement of adenosine tissue levels with acadesine extends the duration of the preconditioning effect (513). In addition, catecholamines (512) and bradykinin (183) also appear to induce preconditioning via α_1 and β_2 receptors, respectively. In all cases, the process appears to involve activation of protein kinase C, since its inhibition can prevent the protection normally observed following brief ischemia (183,321,409,512,569), but the exact processes activated or inhibited by PKC in this setting remain to be completely defined. Support for the notion that the rise in cytoplasmic Ca^{2+} is the initiating cause for stunning (or at least strongly associated with it) (292) comes from the observation that preconditioning partially inhibits the ischemic rise in cytoplasmic Ca^{2+} and attenuates the contractile dysfunction of stunning (473). The rise in cytoplasmic Na^+ is decreased, suggesting that it may contribute to the development of the Ca^{2+} overload as noted previously.

Myocardial Failure

Ongoing contractile failure of the heart may be due to destruction or loss of contractile tissue, perpetual dyscoordinated contraction, alteration in ventricular architecture, or decreased contractile activity of the individual myocytes themselves (317). While scarring and fibrotic changes may impair contractile efficiency of the ventricle, studies in isolated myocytes from failing hearts suggest that their ability to contract in response to maximal Ca^{2+} stimulation is not impaired (160,195,199,453), that is, the cellular systems to activate contractions are intact and maximal responsiveness of the myofibrils to Ca^{2+} is not changed. Instead, two major functional defects have been defined in myocytes from failing hearts. The first appears to be a prolongation of the Ca^{2+} transient and impaired isometric relaxation (189,360,372), changes that are also demonstrable in experimental hypertrophy (190). These changes would appear to be explained by decreased SERCA2 messenger RNA (mRNA) (356) and lower SERCA2 protein levels (205), which would result in a decrease in the maximum Ca^{2+} reuptake rate. These changes are of sufficient magnitude to be associated with a decrease in the tension-independent heat production since there is less ATP breakdown when less Ca^{2+} is actively transported (204). In failing myocardium, a decrease in Ca release channel mRNA is also reported (73), as well as a reduction in L-type Ca channel density measured with $[^3H]$nitrendipine (178). In contrast to SERCA, mRNA for the Na/Ca exchanger is increased in failed human myocardium (484), a response that would be an appropriate compensatory response by the myocyte to reduce the cellular Ca^{2+} load. Consequently, a decrease in the proteins responsible for Ca^{2+} cycling contributes to the contractile defect.

A second major consequence of heart failure is the loss of responsiveness to β-adrenergic stimulation mediated by AC activation (74,199). Decreased β-adrenergic sensitivity is demonstrable in both atrial and ventricular cells isolated from failing hearts (78,199) as well as in intact tissue (160,453), which results in decreased cAMP synthesis in response to β-adrenergic stimulation (151,179). A decrease in the density of β-adrenoceptors is reported by autoradiographic methods (74,178). Patients with cardiac failure typically exhibit excessive plasma concentrations of norepinephrine (102,507), and β-adrenergic desensitization is also present in myocardium that has been subjected to continuous, excessive adrenergic stimulation (254). This continuous stimulation apparently results in increased levels of the inhibitory G protein, G_i, which are observed in failing myocardial tissues (149,385). This "antiadrenergic" effect of G_i activation, which inhibits AC and causes decreased [cAMP], markedly reduces the normal sympathetic responsiveness of the heart and contributes to cardiac failure (78,79,167).

Both the decrease in SERCA proteins and loss of adrenergic responsiveness, which can markedly enhance SR Ca^{2+} uptake, would be expected to markedly alter contractile behavior. Since Ca^{2+} uptake into the SR contributes to the normal positive force-frequency relation, it is not surprising that the normal positive frequency staircase is absent in dilated cardiomyopathy, an effect observable both in vitro (152,415) and in clinical settings (150,203).

Anesthetic Actions on Subcellular Pathways

Alteration in cardiac contractile function by anesthetics is a common phenomenon, although actions have not always been separated from effects on the vasculature in general, nor from effects on sympathetic outflow to the heart, which can dramatically influence myocardial performance. Studies on isolated myocardium and myocytes have permitted identification of distinct effects of anesthetic agents, which need to be understood within the context of entire cardiovascular control and function. Effects of a variety of inhalational anesthetics on various cell processes are discussed below and summarized in Table 2.

Inhalational Anesthetics

The volatile anesthetics have long been known to depress myocardial contractility in a dose-dependent fashion (76,424). This depression is most prominent with isometric contractions, and is slightly less profound when shortening is examined (181,236). With regard to presently used clinical anesthetics, at equi-anesthetic concentrations the amount of depression caused by halothane or enflurane appears to be greater than that seen with isoflurane (119,236,238,331,480,482). These agents alter a number of specific mechanisms of cardiac EC coupling in an agent-specific fashion (436). As determined by various investigators, when the activating $[Ca^{2+}]_i$ is controlled volatile anesthetics directly depress tension development of isolated cardiac myofibrils (214,379,485,486,488), as well as decreasing myofibrillar ATPase activity (357,410). At relevant clinical levels, however, these actions are modest and do not account for the greater contractile depression seen in intact myocardial tissue to 50% to 60% of control. In chemically skinned myofibrils, 2 MAC anesthetics typically cause only a 10% to 15% depression of maximal force, although a loss of myofibrillar Ca^{2+} sensitivity and a decrease in maximal force of 27% to 28% is reported for isoflurane and halothane in human skinned cardiac fibers at 20°C (499). In these preparations devoid of intact membrane systems, increase in stiffness/force has been interpreted as a decrease in the number of cross-bridges as well as decreased force per cross-bridge (378). High anesthetic concentations and reduced temperature (17°C) may reduce cross-bridge cycling rate (213). However, when intact cardiac muscle is stimulated by Ba^{2+}, cross-bridge kinetics are unaltered by anesthetics (461) and their effects can be duplicated by decreasing Ca^{2+} availability with nifedipine (95). The importance of myocyte membrane systems in mediating the action of anesthetics has been further emphasized by experiments in which varied membrane disruption techniques were employed (214).

When the negative inotropic effects of anesthetics are compared as force development (isometric) versus shortening (isotonic), anesthetics typically depress force development rather more than the maximum velocity of shortening (181,236,263,462,463,490). However, when contractile depression is produced by a decrease in external $[Ca^{2+}]$ ($[Ca^{2+}]_o$), the pattern of greater depression of isometric versus isotonic contractions is the same as that caused by anesthetics (236)

Table 2. EFFECTS OF INHALATIONAL ANESTHETIC ON SITES OF MYOCARDIAL EXCITATION-CONTRACTION COUPLING

Volatile anesthetic	Ca channel effects	Ca release channel and SR Ca stores	Relaxation (Ca reuptake)	Na-Ca exchange	Contractile proteins
Halothane	Moderate depression	Moderate depletion due to CaRC activation	Slight Ca-ATPase activation	Modest-moderate inhibition	Slightly decreased Ca^{2+} sensitivity
Enflurane	Moderate depression	Moderate depletion due to CaRC activation, cooling-induced, and late release depressed	Ca-ATPase activation	Strong inhibition	Slightly decreased Ca^{2+} sensitivity
Isoflurane	Modest-moderate depression	No CaRC activation, possible modest depletion due to nonspecific leak; cooling-induced and late release depressed	± Effect	Moderate inhibition	Decreased sensitivity at higher concentration
Nitrous oxide	? Modest depression	No apparent effect	No effect		Minimal depression

The effects noted are in relative terms (modest, 10–20%; moderate, 30–50%; strong, > 50%) and are noted for 1 to 2 MAC for the volatile anesthetic. Summarized from various sources including Baum (31–34), Blanck (51,52,92,95,461), Bosnjak (57–59), Haworth (209,210), Housmans (16,90,91,236,237,240), Komai and Rusy (119,278–281,283,284,435–437), Lynch (165,303,331,333,337), Murat (377–379), Ohnishi (260,261,395), Su (485,487,488), Terrar (493,501–503), Wheeler (542–545), and others. AP, action potential.

(Fig. 13). The anesthetics also cause some acceleration of isotonic and isometric relaxation that may indicate a possible decrease in affinity of TnC for Ca^{2+} (236,240), although no direct alteration in TnC Ca^{2+} affinity by halothane has been reported (49). Studies in which intracellular Ca^{2+} transients are recorded suggest that isoflurane may, however, decrease Ca^{2+} sensitivity, especially at higher concentrations (57). When anesthetic effects are examined at differing muscle lengths, including shorter lengths at which TnC Ca^{2+} affinity is decreased, the relative decrease in force development is unchanged (16). As with the effect on the kinetics of shortening and force development, the effect is similar to that seen with reduction of $[Ca^{2+}]_o$, suggesting that alteration is myofibrillar Ca^{2+} responsiveness contributes modestly to anesthetics' negative inotropic action. In summary, while alteration in the actin-myosin interaction by anesthetics probably contributes to contractile depression, it accounts for only 20% to 30% of the observed effect.

The greater contribution to myocardial depression appears with alteration of Ca^{2+} handling by the myocardium (418) and depression of the Ca^{2+} transient that activates the myofibrils (57,58). The important role of Ca^{2+} was suggested by early studies demonstrating the ability of increased $[Ca^{2+}]_o$ to overcome the depressant action of anesthetics (422,423), although this is a relatively nonspecific effect. Intracellular Ca^{2+} transients and the resulting tension demonstrate a clear anesthetic depression of transient amplitude (Fig. 14) (57,58,434), suggesting effects are primarily related to altered activator Ca^{2+} (although at higher isoflurane concentrations this may be less true) (57). One of the major effects of the volatile anesthetics clearly is depression of I_{Ca}, both via L- and T-type channels (59,246,332, 340,501,502), although it is uncertain whether the degree of depression by halothane and isoflurane is similar at equi-anesthetic doses (59,331,407). Depressant actions on I_{Ca} have also been reported for enflurane (59,339) and sevoflurane (207). Biochemical studies also demonstrate the ability of anesthetics to alter the L-type Ca channel conformation as assessed by binding of nitrendipine (^{3}HNTP) (50,126,308,449) or a phenylalkylamine analogue (D600) (222). Halothane appears to be the most potent in regard to its ability to inhibit ^{3}HNTP binding to cardiac sarcolemmal Ca channels as well as in decreasing affinity for ^{3}HNTP (126). Since I_{Ca} in part triggers SR Ca^{2+} release, this action may contribute to decreasing Ca^{2+} released by the SR.

The volatile anesthetics have specific and direct effects on SR function, with evidence from a variety of experiments in whole tissue or isolated cells demonstrating an apparent decrease in

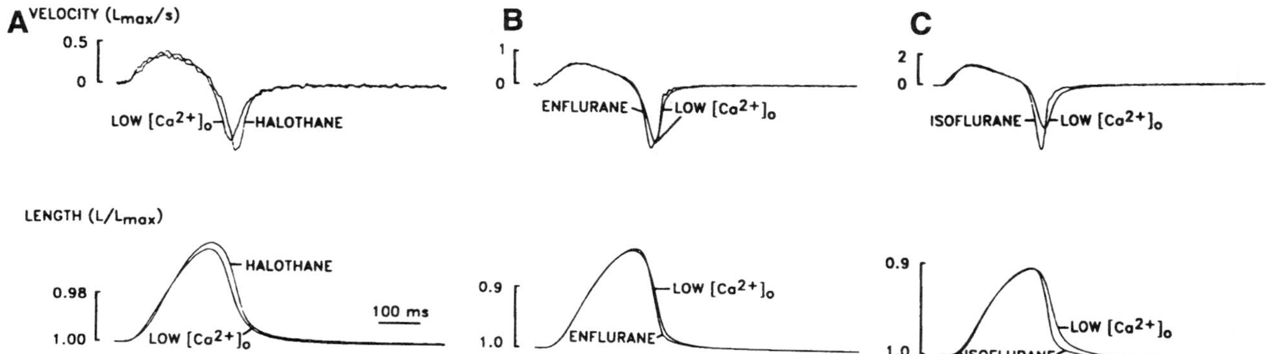

Figure 13. Effects of volatile anesthetics on cardiac myofibrillar mechanics. Shortening responses (shown as upward deflections) of preloaded isotonic twitches in three different muscles. In each case, the muscle was exposed to approximately 1 MAC anesthetic and allowed to recover, and then exposed to a decreased Ca^{2+} concentration, which caused a similar decrease in shortening. **A:** The responses are shown for 1% halothane and 0.38 μM Ca^{2+}. B: 2% Isoflurane and 0.45 μM Ca^{2+}; and 1.5% isoflurane and 0.9 μM Ca^{2+}. Note the similar pattern of shortening under the decreased inotropic conditions caused by the aesthetics for low Ca^{2+}. (From ref. 236, with permission.)

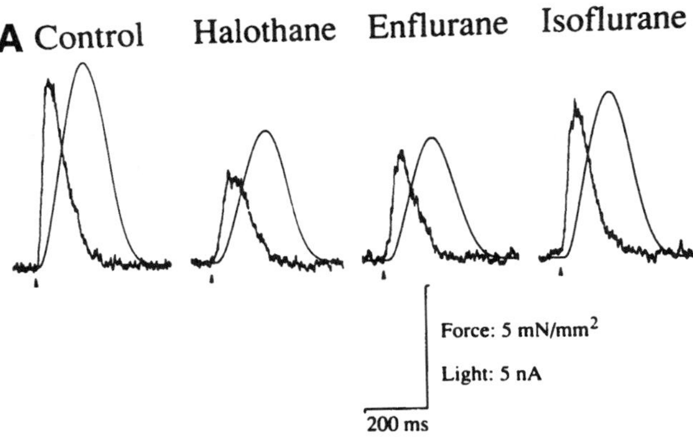

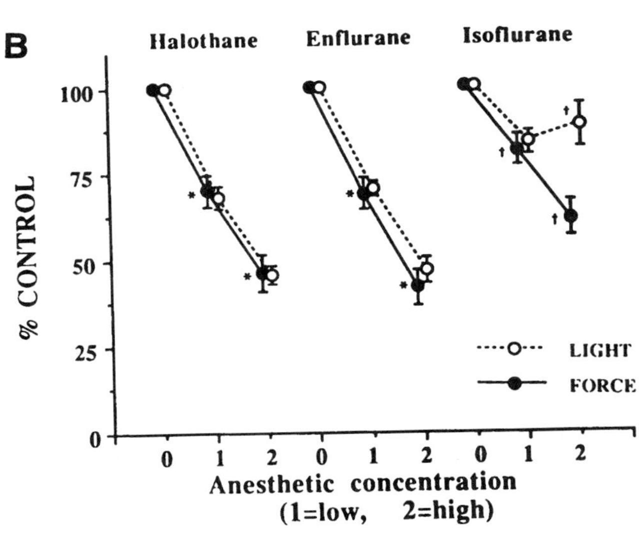

Figure 14. Alteration in the myocardial Ca^{2+} transient (sharply peaking initial tracings) and the accompanying force caused various anesthetic agents. **A:** Effects of approximately 1.2 MAC concentrations of anesthetics (1.1% halothane, 2.2% enflurane, 1.6% isoflurane) on isometric contractions and on the aequorin light signal in response to Ca^{2+}, recorded from single isolated guinea pig papillary muscles. Muscles had been injected with small amounts of aequorin to determine intracellular Ca^{2+} concentrations, and responses shown are those that accompany 1 Hz pacing (indicated at the *arrowhead)* at 30°C. **B:** Average effects of halothane, enflurane, or isoflurane at approximately 0.8 MAC (1 = low) and 1.2 MAC (2 = high). ******p* <.05 versus 0 (no anesthetic control); †*p* <.05 isoflurane versus other anesthetics at the same concentrations (*n* = 13). (From ref. 57, with permission.)

SR retention of Ca^{2+} (260,261,279,281–284,331,487,542–545), which is clearly evident in isolated SR vesicles (92,165). Applications of halothane (212,260,261,543–545,553) and enflurane (260,261,543,552) have been reported to activate release of Ca^{2+} from SR stores, while the effect is far less prominent or not evident with isoflurane (543,552). Sudden application of solution equilibrated with halothane or enflurane can actually cause transiently enhanced twitch force or shortening with a subsequent rapid decline in contractility (261,326,340,545), which is consistent with transiently augmented release of SR Ca^{2+}. This effect is not observed with isoflurane (326). The action of the volatile anesthetics is strikingly similar to the actions of caffeine to activate release of SR Ca^{2+} (260), and like the Ca^{2+} releasing action of caffeine, halothane-activated SR Ca^{2+} release causes the appearance of large conductance channels (not seen with isoflurane) (406).

The combined action of anesthetics in reducing I_{Ca} and the releasable store of Ca^{2+} can account in large measure for the observed decrease in Ca^{2+} transients. Isoflurane's depression of Ca^{2+} transients as well as force is less than that caused by equianesthetic concentrations of enflurane and halothane (57). This smaller action of isoflurane is consistent with the fact that a considerably higher concentration of isoflurane is required to activate SR release of Ca^{2+} (260). Halothane, unlike isoflurane, specifically activates cardiac CaRCs as determined by ryanodine binding (337) or single-channel bilayer recordings (104). By opening such channels during rest, the SR Ca^{2+} store will be depleted as if there is decreased uptake of Ca^{2+}, as suggested for halothane (but less so for isoflurane) by earlier skinned fiber studies (485,487). Combined with halothane's depressant action on I_{Ca}, its SR Ca^{2+} depletion may also account for the protective action of halothane against ischemia/reperfusion insults (322), although protection of sarcolemmal L-type Ca channels can also be demonstrated (125). Enflurane also appears to enhance CaRC channel opening in isolated bilayer studies (104), consistent with intact myocyte studies documenting SR depletion (543,552), although its alteration of ryanodine binding appears distinct from that of halothane (337). In addition, a nonspecific "leak" from isolated cardiac SR vesicles is identifiable, although its significance in situ is unclear (92,165). While greater Ca^{2+} depletion by halothane may account in part for its greater myocardial depressant action compared to isoflurane, in frog ventricle, which has a poorly developed SR, isoflurane is still less depressant than halothane (336).

Volatile anesthetic effects might also be caused by altered SERCA activity, which could influence the SR accumulation of Ca^{2+}. Although halothane was originally reported to depress ATPase activity (296), at physiologic pH the effects of clinically relevant concentrations (≤2 MAC) are modest (51,52,92,361). Although some depression of Ca^{2+} uptake by halothane was suggested based on the altered rate of decline of Ca^{2+} transients (57), the reduced Ca^{2+} release in and of itself will influence rate of decline of the Ca^{2+} transient (43). Mild stimulatory effects of halothane may be due to its increase in Ca^{2+} efflux via CaRC, while enflurane may have a more direct stimulatory action (361).

A more prominent volatile anesthetic action may be the depression of the $Na^{+}Ca^{2+}$ exchange current with actions that may be as great as those on the Ca^{2+} current (33,209,210). In view of the prominent role of the exchanger in Ca^{2+} entry and elimination in certain species and particularly in neonatal or fetal animals, such actions may prove to be very important. Isolated neonatal myocardium is about 2 to 2.5 times more sensitive than adult tissue to the depressant effects of halothane and isoflurane (31), although sensitivity somewhat closer to that of adult tissue has been noted by others (288). Although neonatal myocardium is has less functional SR (which is depleted far less by isoflurane than by halothane), isoflurane is less depressant than halothane. Both anesthetics decreased AP plateau amplitude, which could reflect decreased inward Ca^{2+} current (31).

Although isoflurane does not appear to open CaRC, isoflurane and enflurane both inhibit a late component of tension made prominent by β-adrenergic stimulation (331,333), depressed by local anesthetics (330,334), and apparently mediated by a form of SR Ca^{2+} release (334). Curiously, isoflurane and enflurane, but not halothane, inhibit release of Ca^{2+} from the SR that is mediated by rapid cooling (278) (Lynch, *unpublished results*). Although this process was thought to involve opening of CaRC (45,467), other pathways appear responsible for the Ca^{2+} release (148), and it may be these that are sensitive to the halogenated ether anesthetics and perhaps also responsible for the late-peak force. Nevertheless, these effects further emphasize the differing effects among the volatile agents on cardiac SR Ca^{2+} handling.

As noted, the positive frequency staircase depends on accumulation of Ca^{2+} in the SR. Since isoflurane has less effect on the SR Ca^{2+} release function, the positive staircase is better maintained and isoflurane causes fractionally less contractile depression at physiologic rates (331,362,557) or in settings in which SR release is maximized, such as potentiated state contractions (119,280,283). However, the frequency dependence of contractile depression of the isoflurane, enflurane, or halothane is not replicated either by ryanodine, reduced $[Ca^{2+}]_o$, or blockade of Ca^{2+} entry by nifedipine (at 30 or 37°C), suggesting that all of these agents alter several aspects of Ca^{2+} handling (362).

In addition to direct actions, the volatile agents may also influence the extrinsic modulators of contractility. The "sensitization" by halothane to catecholamines, which may generate dysrhythmias, may also enhance contractility under certain circumstances (55). This action may be mediated by enhanced β-AR coupling, or more likely by interference with M_2-cholinoceptors (448) that can depress contractile function (63). Since in failing myocardium there is an apparent excess inhibition of AC by the action of the inhibitory G protein (G_i) (78), interference by halothane with G_i (448) may be the mechanism by which it actually has a positive inotropic action and restores the positive force-frequency relationship in failing myocardium (447). While this effect is most obvious is cardiac failure, it may also have a dramatic action when high resting vagal tone is present.

Nitrous Oxide The effects of nitrous oxide in depressing myocardial contractility have long been recognized (182,423, 424). In studies of isolated myocardial tissue, perfusion solutions equilibrated with less than 95% oxygen often cause a depression in contractility due simply to the failure to deliver adequate oxygen (303,481). Consequently, the degree of contractile depression caused by nitrous oxide has occasionally been difficult to separate from that due to suboptimal delivery of oxygen. In studies in which 45% to 50% nitrous oxide (~0.5 MAC) was administered to preparations, developed force is typically decreased by 15% to 20% compared to equivalent substitution of N_2 (90,303). Similar to the behavior of the other agents, shortening is less affected than is force (90). The magnitude of the contractile depression is similar to an equi-anesthetic concentration of halothane (303), although in perfused whole hearts the depressant effect of nitrous oxide may be difficult to distinguish from that caused by the mildest degree of hypoxia (481). When combined with either halothane or isoflurane, nitrous oxide appears to have an additive effect (303). In whole animals and in the clinical setting, the myocardial depression may be offset by increased sympathetic stimulation (130,170) and release of norepinephrine (135), so depressant effects may not be evident. Studies with aequorin-loaded myocardium (91) as well as studies in skinned cardiac fibers (489) show little or no effect of nitrous oxide in depressing myofibrillar responsiveness to Ca^{2+}. Nitrous oxide decreases the transient of activator Ca^{2+} observed in isolated myocardium, but there appears to be little depression of Ca^{2+} uptake or release by the SR (489), leading some investigators to suggest that its depressant effect is mediated primarily by a decrease in transsarcolemmal Ca^{2+} influx (91).

Intravenous Anesthetics

Of the intravenous anesthetics, hypnotics, and analgesics, thiopental and the short-acting barbiturates appear to cause the greatest degree of direct myocardial depression in isolated tissues at clinical concentrations. Thiopental causes a dose-dependent depression of contractility (12,163,239,374,408, 424) whose major mechanism probably involves the depression of $I_{Ca,L}$ (245,405). Although thiopental does not appear to alter Ca^{2+} uptake by the SR, some effect on SR handling of Ca^{2+} may be present (279,408) with an apparent inhibition of the Ca^{2+} release pathway (285). This SR effect may be modest compared the effect mediated by depression of transsarcolemmal Ca^{2+} influx (239). Thiopental's depression of Ca channels may be counterbalanced in part by its ability to prolong the cardiac AP by inhibiting the resting K^+ conductance (405,408).

The effects of ketamine on the myocardium are complex, arising from both indirect and direct actions. In intact animals (479) and in human studies (546), ketamine causes cardiovascular stimulation due to its stimulatory effects on the autonomic nervous system. These effects may be explained by ketamine's blockade of monoamine reuptake, which includes norepinephrine in adrenergic nerves (327,442). However, ketamine has direct positive (2,23,105,430) as well as direct negative (112,180,435) inotropic effects in studies conducted in vitro. While there is impaired neuronal reuptake of catecholamines that may be observed even in vitro (105), ketamine's small positive inotropic effect may result from increased calcium influx (23,430). This is probably an indirect action that results from cardiac AP prolongation secondary to blockade of K^+ conductances (I_{to} and G_{K1}) (137). Also contributing may be a decreased rate of relaxation (404,430), which may be caused by decreased of Ca^{2+} uptake by the SR. In contrast, a negative inotropic effect may predominate due to the direct depression of Ca^{2+} entry (435) in response to inhibition of I_{Ca} (32,137). In patients with impaired function of the sympathetic nervous system, these latter effects may become dominant and lead to acute cardiovascular decompensation (535). Possible impairment of SR Ca^{2+} accumulation may contribute effects at supraclinical levels (100 μM) (430).

Propofol at free concentrations of ≥10 μM depresses the myocardial contractions (12,106,374,408,429); however, this free drug concentration is unlikely to be observed clinically because of propofol's >97% protein binding (457). High serum binding may explain why with blood perfused preparations, no depressant effect was seen with up to 1000 μM propofol (374). While some modest alteration in SR function at high concentrations may be present (408,429), much of the action of propofol appears related to inhibition of transsarcolemmal Ca^{2+} influx, an effect that is compatible with an observed depression of $I_{Ca,L}$ (397,493). Propofol has no apparent action on myofibrillar Ca^{2+} sensitivity (106).

With regard to other intravenous anesthetics, depressant actions on the myocardium are far less prominent, particularly at clinical concentrations. Etomidate has little (271) or no (431,432) effect, although its propylene glycol vehicle did appear decrease relaxation rate, an effect attributed to mildly depressed SR function. While alfentanil (573) and midazolam (427) can be myocardial depressants in isolated tissue, the concentations required to cause depression are well beyond free serum levels with anesthetic doses. Subcellular sites of action of various intravenous anesthetics are listed in Table 3.

Specific depression of L-type channel I_{Ca} has been seen with stimulation of opiate receptors by leu-enkaphalin (561), although the mechanism is unclear. Whether the synthetic narcotics (fentanyl and its congeners) depress I_{Ca} significantly at clinical concentrations and whether they do so by an opiate receptor or another mechanism remain to be determined.

Local Anesthetics

The most notable pharmacologic action of the local anesthetics is their ability to block Na channels. Based on the role that $[Na^+]_i$ can play in modulating contractility via the Na^+/Ca^{2+} exchanger (200), it is not surprising that the local anesthetics may influence cardiac contractility. If Na channels are inhibited by local anesthetics, the decrease in Na^+ entry will result in a lower $[Na^+]_i$, maintaining a larger $[Na^+]$ gradient so that Ca^{2+} elimination via the Na^+/Ca^{2+} will be better maintained. SR Ca^{2+} stores will be less augmented and smaller contractions will result. Blockade of Na channels with tetrodotoxin (TTX) is well characterized to decrease contractile force (118,200,334,518). Since the local anesthetics typically exhibit frequency-dependent or use-dependent blockade of Na channels (98,330), one might anticipate that contractile depression would be greater at high stimulation rates. However, the relative depression of contractility by the local anesthetics actually decreases with increas-

Table 3. EFFECTS OF INTRAVENOUS ANESTHETICS ON SITES OF MYOCARDIAL EXCITATION-CONTRACTION COUPLING

Intravenous anesthetic	Ca channel effects	SR Ca stores	Relaxation (Ca reuptake)	Na-Ca exchange	Contractile proteins
Thiopental	Moderate inhibition; AP prolongation	? decreased release	None observed	?	?
Etomidate	None apparent	None apparent	None apparent	?	?increased cross-bridge kinetics
Ketamine	Modest depression	None apparent	Slightly impaired at veryhigh dose	?	None apparent
Propofol	Modest depression	None apparent	? Slightly impaired uptake	?	None apparent
Opiates	? Modest depression	? None apparent	? None apparent	?	None apparent

Summarized from various sources including Housmans (106,239,286,346), Komai and Rusy (277,281,282), Park (408), Riou (429–431), and others (32,34,493). AP, action potential.

ing rate of beating (330,334). Furthermore, when compared to the effects of TTX, the effects of local anesthetics on contractions differ in character (334) and add to the contractile depression caused by TTX (118). Such additional effects implicate additional cellular pathways. Although local anesthetics have been reported to have no effects on Ca channel mediated ("slow") APs (70), a variety of studies have documented a mild depressant effect of local anesthetics upon Ca^{2+} currents or Ca^{+} channel–mediated action potentials. However, these effects are relatively modest at relevant clinical concentrations (89,109,255,330) and do not resemble the changes seen with Ca^{2+} entry blockade (334). Local anesthetics have been shown to depress Ca^{2+} from skeletal muscle sarcoplasmic reticulum (7), but the required concentration usually is at least an order of magnitude greater than that required for depression of myocardial contractions. Local anesthetics do appear to depress a late component of contraction seen in isoproterenol-stimulated muscles (330,334), which are also depressed by isoflurane and enflurane (333). The potency with which local anesthetics cause contractile depression appears related to their lipid solubility. Among the amide drugs, bupivacaine and etidocaine are 5 to 10 times more potent than lidocaine, depending on the tissue and technique of investigation (83,118,330,497).

ACKNOWLEDGMENTS

The author thanks Michael S. Forbes, Ph.D., for providing the micrographs, and Anna Hall Evans for editorial assistance. Research funding for the author was provided by NIH grant R01 GM34411.

REFERENCES

1. Abdelmeguid AE, Feher JJ. Effect of perfusate [Ca^{2+}] on cardiac sarcoplasmic Ca^{2+} release channel in isolated hearts. *Circ Res* 1992; 71:1049–1058.
2. Adams HR, Parker JL, Mathew BP. The influence of ketamine on inotropic and chronotropic responsiveness of heart muscle. *J Pharmacol Exp Ther* 1977;201:171–183.
3. Allen DG, Eisner DA, Pirolo JS, Smith GL. The relationship between intracellular calcium concentration and contraction in calcium-overloaded ferret papillary muscles. *J Physiol* 1985;364: 169–182.
4. Allen DG, Kentish JC. Calcium concentration in the myoplasm of skinned ferret ventricular muscle following changes in muscle length. *J Physiol* 1988;407:489–503.
5. Allen DG, Kurihara S. The effects of muscle length on intracellular calcium transients in mammalian cardiac muscle. *J Physiol* 1982;327:79–94.
6. Alloatti G, Serazzi L, Levi EC. Prostaglandin I_2 (PGI_2) enhances calcium current in guinea-pig ventricular heart cells. *J Mol Cell Cardiol* 1991;23:851–860.
7. Almers W, Best PM. Effects of tetracaine on displacement currents and contraction of frog skeletal muscle. *J Physiol* 1979;262: 583–611.
8. Armstrong CM, Bezanilla FM, Horowicz P. Twitches in the presence of ethylene-glycol-bis(β-amino-ethyl ether)-*N,N'*-tetraacetic acid. *Biochim Biophys Acta* 1972;267:605–608.
9. Artman M, Ichikawa H, Avkiran M, Coetzee WA. Na^+/Ca^{2+} exchange current density in cardiac myocytes from rabbits and guinea pigs during postnatal development. *Am J Physiol* 1995;268: H1714–H1722.
10. Ashley RH, Williams AJ. Divalent cation activation and inhibition of single calcium release channels from sheep cardiac sarcoplasmic reticulum. *J Gen Physiol* 1990;95:981–1005.
11. Auchampach JA, Maruyama M, Cavero I, Gross GJ. Pharmacological evidence for a role of ATP-dependent potassium channels in myocardial stunning. *Circulation* 1992;86:311–319.
12. Azari DM, Cork RC. Comparative myocardial depressive effects of propofol and thiopental. *Anesth Analg* 1993;77:324–329.
13. Babu A, Sonnenblick E, Gulati J. Molecular basis for the influence of muscle length on myocardial performance. *Science* 1988;240: 74–76.
14. Backx PH, Gao W-D, Azan-Backx MD, Marban E. Mechanism of force inhibition by 2,3-butanedione monoxime in rat cardiac muscle: roles of $[Ca^{2+}]_i$ and cross-bridge kinetics. *J Physiol* 1994;476: 487–500.
15. Backx PH, ter Keurs HEDJ. Fluorescent properties of rat trabeculae microinjected with fura-2 salt. *Am J Physiol* 1993;264: H1098–H1110.
16. Baele P, Housmans PR. The effects of halothane, enflurane, and isoflurane on the length-tension relation of the isolated ventricular papillary muscle of the ferret. *Anesthesiology* 1991;74:281–291.
17. Baker KM, Aceto JA. Characterization of avian angiotensin II cardiac receptors: coupling to mechanical activity and phosphoinositide metabolism. *J Mol Cell Cardiol* 1989;21:375–382.
18. Balke CW, Egan TM, Wier WG. Processes that remove calcium from the cytoplasm during excitation-contraction coupling in intact rat heart cells. *J Physiol* 1994;474:447–462.
19. Balligand J-L, Kelly RA, Marsden PA, Smith TW, Michel T. Control of cardiac muscle cell function by an endogenous nitric oxide signaling system. *Proc Natl Acad Sci USA* 1993;90:347–351.
20. Balligand J-L, Kobzik L, Han X, et al. Nitric oxide-dependent parasympathetic signalling is due to activation of constitutive endothelial (Type III) nitric oxide synthase in cardiac myocytes. *J Biol Chem* 1995;270:14582–14586.
21. Barcenas-Ruiz L, Beukelmann DJ, Wier WG. Sodium-calcium exchange in heart: membrane currents and changes in $[Ca^{2+}]_i$. *Science* 1987;238:1720–1722.
22. Barnard EA. Separating receptor subtypes from their shadows. *Nature* 1988;335:301–302.
23. Barrigon S, De Miguel B, Tamargo J, Tejerina T. The mechanism of the positive inotropic action of ketamine on isolated atria of the rat. *Br J Pharmacol* 1982;76:85–93.
24. Bassani JWM, Bassani RA, Bers DM. Ca^{2+} cycling between sarcoplasmic reticulum and mitochondria in rabbit cardiac myocytes. *J Physiol* 1993;460:603–621.
25. Bassani JWM, Bassani RA, Bers DM. Mitochondrial and sarcolem-

mal Ca^{2+} transport reduce $[Ca^{2+}]_i$ during caffeine contractures in rabbit cardiac myocytes. *J Physiol* 1993;453:591–608.
26. Bassani JWM, Bassani RA, Bers DM. Twitch-dependent SR Ca accumulation and release in rabbit ventricular myocytes. *Am J Physiol* 1993;265:C533–540.
27. Bassani JWM, Bassani RA, Bers DM. Relaxation in rabbit and rat cardiac cells: species-dependent differences in cellular mechanisms. *J Physiol* 1994;476:279–293.
28. Bassani RA, Bassani JWM, Bers DM. Mitochondrial and sarcolemmal Ca^{2+} transport reduce Ca^{2+}during caffeine contractures in rabbit cardiac myocytes. *J Physiol* 1992;453:591–608.
29. Bates SE, Gurney AM. Ca^{2+}-dependent block and potentiation of L-type calcium current in guinea-pig ventricular myocytes. *J Physiol* 1993;466:345–365.
30. Baudet S, Shaoulian R, Bers DM. Effects of thapsigargin and cyclopiazonic acid on twitch force and sarcoplasmic reticulum Ca^{2+} content of rabbit ventricular muscle. *Circ Res* 1993;73:813–819.
31. Baum VC, Klitzner TS. Excitation-contraction coupling in neonatal myocardium: effects of halothane and isoflurane. *Dev Pharmacol Ther* 1991;16:99–107.
32. Baum VC, Tecson ME. Ketamine inhibits transsarcolemmal calcium entry in guinea pig myocardium: direct evidence by single cell voltage clamp. *Anesth Analg* 1991;73:804–807.
33. Baum VC, Wetzel GT. Sodium-calcium exchange in neonatal myocardium: reversible inhibition by halothane. *Anesth Analg* 1994;78:1105–1109.
34. Baum VC, Wetzel GT, Klitzner TS. Effects of halothane and ketamine on activation and inactivation of myocardial calcium current. *J Cardiovasc Pharmacol* 1994;23:799–805.
35. Belardinelli L, Isenberg G. Isolated atrial myocytes: adenosine and acetylcholine increase potassium conductance. *Am J Physiol* 1983; 244:H734–H737.
36. Bennett MVL, Verselis VK. Biophysics of gap junctions. *Semin Cell Biol* 1992;3:29–47.
37. Bers DM. Ca influx and sarcoplasmic reticulum Ca release in cardiac muscle activation during postrest recovery. *Am J Physiol* 1985; 248:H366–H381.
38. Bers DM. Ryanodine and the calcium content of cardiac SR assessed by caffeine and rapid cooling contractures. *Am J Physiol* 1987;253:C408–C415.
39. Bers DM. Rapid cooling contractures in cardiac muscle reflect SR Ca depletion and refilling (abstract). *Biophys J* 1988;53:435a.
40. Bers DM. SR Ca-pump and sarcolemmal Na-Ca exchange in relaxation of cardiac muscle with and without ryanodine. *Biophys J* 1988; 53:436a.
41. Bers DM. SR Ca loading in cardiac muscle preparations based on rapid-cooling contractures. *Am J Physiol* 1989;256:C109–C120.
42. Bers DM, Bassani JWM, Bassani RA. Competition and redistribution among calcium transport systems in rabbit cardiac myocytes. *Cardiovasc Res* 1993;27:1772–1777.
43. Bers DM, Berlin JR. Kinetics of $[Ca]_i$ decline in cardiac myocytes depend on peak $[Ca]_i$. *Am J Physiol* 1995;268:C271–C277.
44. Bers DM, Bridge JHB. Relaxation of rabbit ventricular muscle by Na-Ca exchange and sarcoplasmic reticulum calcium pump - ryanodine and voltage sensitivity. *Circ Res* 1989;65:334–342.
45. Bers DM, Bridge JHB, Spitzer KW. Intracellular Ca^{2+} transients during rapid cooling contractures in guinea-pig ventricular myocytes. *J Physiol* 1989;417:537–553.
46. Bers DM, Christensen DM. Functional interconversion of rest decay and ryanodine effects in rabbit and rat ventricle depends on Na/Ca exchange. *J Mol Cell Cardiol* 1990;22:715–723.
47. Bers DM, Lederer WJ, Berlin JR. Intracellular Ca transients in rat cardiac myocytes: role of Na-Ca exchange in excitation-contraction coupling. *Am J Physiol* 1990;258:C944–C954.
48. Birnbaumer L. G Proteins in signal transduction. *Annu Rev Pharmacol Toxicol* 1990;30:675–705.
49. Blanck TJJ, Chiancone E, Salviati G, et al. Halothane does not alter Ca^{2+} affinity of troponin C. *Anesthesiology* 1992;76:100–105.
50. Blanck TJJ, Runge S, Stevenson RL. Halothane decreases calcium channel antagonist binding to cardiac membranes. *Anesth Analg* 1988;67:1032–1035.
51. Blanck TJJ, Thompson M. Calcium transport by cardiac sarcoplasmic reticulum: modulation of halothane action by substrate concentration and pH. *Anesth Analg* 1981;60:390–394.
52. Blanck TJJ, Thompson M. Enflurane and isoflurane stimulate calcium transport by cardiac sarcoplasmic reticulum. *Anesth Analg* 1982;61:142–145.
53. Blaustein MP. Sodium/calcium exchange and the control of contractility in cardiac muscle and vascular smooth muscle. *J Cardiovasc Pharmacol* 1988;12(Suppl. 5):S56–S68.
54. Böhm M, Gierschik P, Schwinger RHG, Uhlmann R, Erdmann E. Coupling of M-cholinoceptors and A_1 adenosine receptors in human myocardium. *Am J Physiol* 1994;266:H1951–H1958.
55. Böhm M, Schmidt U, Schwinger RHG, Böhm S, Erdmann E. Effects of halothane on b-adrenoceptors and M-cholinoceptors in human myocardium: radioligand binding and functional studies. *J Cardiovasc Pharmacol* 1993;21:296–304.
56. Bolli R, Patel BS, Jeroudi MO, Lai EK, McCay PB. Demonstration of free radical generation in "stunned" myocardium of intact dogs with the use of the spin trap a-phenyl N-tert-butyl nitrone. *J Clin Invest* 1988;82:476–485.
57. Bosnjak ZJ, Aggarwal A, Turner LA, Kampine JM, Kampine JP. Differential effects of halothane, enflurane, and isoflurane on Ca^{2+} transients and papillary muscle tension in guinea pigs. *Anesthesiology* 1992;76:123–131.
58. Bosnjak ZJ, Kampine JP. Effects of halothane on transmembrane potentials, Ca^{++} transients, and papillary muscle tension. *Am J Physiol* 1986;251:H374–H381.
59. Bosnjak ZJ, Supan FD, Rusch NJ. The effects of halothane, enflurane and isoflurane on calcium currents in isolated canine ventricular cells. *Anesthesiology* 1991;74:340–345.
60. Boucek RJ, Jr., Buck SH, Scott F, et al. Anthracycline-induced tension in permeabilized cardiac fibers: evidence for the activation of the calcium release channel of sarcoplasmic reticulum. *J Mol Cell Cardiol* 1993;25:249–259.
61. Boutjdir M, Restivo M, Wei Y, El-Sherif N. α_1- β-Adrenergic interactions on L-type calcium current in cardiac myocytes. *Pflugers Arch* 1992;421:397–399.
62. Boyett MR, Hart G, Levi AJ. Factors affecting intracellular sodium during repetitive activity in isolated sheep Purkinje fibers. *J Physiol* 1987;384:405–429.
63. Boyett MR, Kirby MS, Orchard CH, Roberts A. The negative inotropic effect of acetylcholine on ferret ventricular myocardium. *J Physiol* 1988;404:613–635.
64. Brady AJB, Warren JB, Poole-Wilson PA, Williams TJ, Harding SE. Nitric oxide attenuates cardiac myocyte contraction. *Am J Physiol* 1993;265:H176–H182.
65. Brandl CJ, de Leon S, Martin DR, MacLennan DH. Adult forms of the Ca^{2+}-ATPase of the sarcoplasmic reticulum. *J Biol Chem* 1987; 262:3768–3774.
66. Brandl CJ, Green NM, Korczak B, MacLennan DH. Two Ca^{2+}-ATPase genes: homologies and mechanistic implication of deduced amino acid sequences. *Cell* 1986;44:597–607.
67. Braunwald E, Kloner RA. The stunned myocardium: prolonged, postischemic ventricular dysfunction. *Circulation* 1982;66: 1146–1149.
68. Bremel RD, Weber A. Cooperation within actin filamentin vertebrate skeletal muscle. *Nature New Biol* 1972;238:97–101.
69. Bremner W, Taylor K, Baird S. Hypothalamo-pituitary-thyroid axis function during cardiopulmonary bypass. *J Thorac Cardiovasc Surg* 1978;75:392–399.
70. Brennan FJ, Cranefield PF, Wit AL. Effects of lidocaine on slow responses and depressed fast response action potentials of canine cardiac Purkinje fibers. *J Pharmacol Exp Ther* 1978;204:312–324.
71. Bridge JHB, Bassingthwaighte JB. Uphill sodium transport driven by an inward calcium gradient in heart muscle. *Science* 1983;219: 178–180.
72. Bridge JHB, Smolley JR, Spitzer KW. The relationship between charge movements associated with I_{Ca} and $I_{Na\text{-}Ca}$ in cardiac myocytes. *Science* 1990;248:376–378.
73. Brillantes AM, Allen P, Takahashi T, Izumo S, Marks AR. Differences in cardiac calcium release channel (ryanodine receptor) expression in myocardium from patients with end-stage heart failure caused by ischemic versus dilated cardiomyopathy. *Circ Res* 1992;71:18–26.
74. Bristow MR, Ginsburg R, Minobe W, et al. Decreased catecholamine sensitivity and beta-adrenergic receptor density in failing human hearts. *N Engl J Med* 1982;307:205–211.
75. Brooks WW, Struckow B, Bing OHL. Myocardial hypoxia and reoxygenation: electrophysiologic and mechanical correlates. *Am J Physiol* 1974;226:523–527.
76. Brown BR, Crout JR. A comparative study of the effects of five general anesthetics on myocardial contractility: isometric conditions. *Anesthesiology* 1971;34:236–245.

77. Brown GC. Control of respiration and ATP synthesis in mammalian mitochondria and cells. *Biochem J* 1992;284:1–13.
78. Brown LA, Harding SE. The effect of pertussis toxin on b-adrenoceptor responses in isolated cardiac myocytes from noradrenaline-treated guinea-pigs and patients with cardiac failure. *Br J Pharmacol* 1992;106:115–122.
79. Brown LA, Humphrey SM, Harding SE. The anti-adrenergic effect of adenosine and its blockade by pertussus toxin: a comparative study in myocytes isolated from guinea-pig, rat and failing human hearts. *Br J Pharmacol* 1990;101:484–488.
80. Brückner R, Meyer W, Mügge A, Schmitz W, Scholz H. α-Adrenoceptor-mediated positive inotropic effect of phenylephrine in isolated human ventricular myocardium. *Eur J Pharmacol* 1984;99: 345–347.
81. Brutsaert DL, De Clerck NM, Goethals MA, Housmans PR. Relaxation of ventricular cardiac muscle. *J Physiol* 1978;283:469–480.
82. Brutsaert DL, Housmans PR, Goethals MA. Dual control of relaxation: its role in the ventricular function in the mammalian heart. *Circ Res* 1980;47:637–652.
83. Buffington CW. The magnitude and duration of direct myocardial depression following intracoronary local anesthetics: a comparison of lidocaine and bupivacaine. *Anesthesiology* 1989;70: 280–287.
84. Burkhoff D, de Tombe PP, Hunter WC. Impact of ejection on magnitude and time course of ventricular pressure-generating capacity. *Am J Physiol* 1993;265:H899–H909.
85. Burt JM, Spray DC. Volatile anesthetics block intercellular communication between neonatal rat myocardial cells. *Circ Res* 1989; 65:829–837.
86. Callewaert G. Excitation-contraction coupling in mammalian cardiac cells. *Cardiovasc Res* 1992;26:923–932.
87. Campbell KB, Kirkpatrick RD, Tobias AH, Taheri H, Shroff SG. Series coupled non-contractile elements are functionally unimportant in the isolated heart. *Cardiovasc Res* 1994;28:242–251.
88. Carmeliet E. Cardiac transmembrane potentials and metabolism. *Circ Res* 1978;42:577–587.
89. Carmeliet E, Morad M, Heyden GVd, Vereecke J. Electrophysiological effects of tetracaine in single guinea-pig ventricular myocytes. *J Physiol* 1986;376:143–161.
90. Carton EG, Housmans PR. Role of transsarcolemmal Ca^{2+} entry in the negative inotropic effect of nitrous oxide in isolated ferret myocardium. *Anesth Analg* 1992;74:575–579.
91. Carton EG, Wanek LA, Housmans PR. Effects of nitrous oxide on contractility, relaxation and the intracellular calcium transient of isolated mammalian ventricular myocardium. *J Pharmacol Exp Ther* 1991;257:843–849.
92. Casella ES, Suite DA, Fisher YI, Blanck TJJ. The effect of volatile anesthetics on the pH dependence of calcium uptake by cardiac sarcoplasmic reticulum. *Anesthesiology* 1987;67:386–390.
93. Cheng H, Lederer WJ, Cannell MB. Calcium sparks: Elementary events underlying excitation-contraction coupling in heart muscle. *Science* 1993;262:740–744.
94. Chinkers M, Garbers D. Signal transduction by guanylyl cyclases. *Annu Rev Biochem* 1991;60:553–575.
95. Chung OY, Blanck TJJ, Berman MR. Depression of myocardial force and stiffness without change in crossbridge kinetics: Effects of volatile anesthetics reproduced by nifedipine. *Anesthesiology* 1989;71:444–448.
96. Cingolani H, Koretsune Y, Marban E. Recovery of contractility and pH_i during respiratory acidosis in ferret hearts: role of Na^+-H^+ exchange. *Am J Physiol* 1990;259:H843–H848.
97. Clapham DE, Neer EJ. New roles for G-protein βγ-dimers in transmembrane signalling. *Nature* 1993;365:403–406.
98. Clarkson CW, Hondeghem LM. Mechanisms for bupivacaine depression of cardiac conduction: Fast block of sodium channels during the action potential with slow recovery from block during diastole. *Anesthesiology* 1985;62:396–405.
99. Cleemann L, Morad M. Role of Ca^{2+} channel in cardiac excitation-contraction coupling in the rat: evidence from Ca^{2+} transients and contraction. *J Physiol* 1991;432:283–312.
100. Clemo HF, Feher JJ, Baumgarten CM. Modulation of rabbit ventricular cell volume and $Na^+/K^+/2Cl^-$ cotransport by cGMP and atrial natriuretic factor. *J Gen Physiol* 1992;100:89–114.
101. Cohen CJ, Fozzard HA, Sheu SS. Increase in intracellular sodium activity during stimulation in mammalian cardiac muscle. *Circ Res* 1982;50:651–662.
102. Cohn JN, Levine TB, Olivari MT, et al. Plasma norepinephrine as a guide to prognosis in patients with chronic congestive heart failure. *N Engl J Med* 1984;311:819–823.
103. Cole W, McPherson CD, Sontag D. ATP-regulated K^+ channels protect the myocardium against ischemia/reperfusion damage. *Circ Res* 1991;69:571–581.
104. Connelly TJ, Coronado R. Activation of the Ca^{2+} release channel of cardiac sarcoplasmic reticulum by volatile anesthetics. *Anesthesiology* 1994;81:459–469.
105. Cook DJ, Carton EG, Housman PR. Mechanisms of the positive inotropic effect of ketamine in isolated ferret ventricular papillary muscle. *Anesthesiology* 1991;74:880–888.
106. Cook DJ, Housmans PR. Mechanism of the negative inotropic effect of propofol in isolated ferret ventricular myocardium. *Anesthesiology* 1994;80:859–871.
107. Cooke R. The actomyosin engine. *FASEB J* 1995;9:636–642.
108. Coronado R, Morrissette M, Sukhareva M, Vaughn DM. Structure and function of ryanodine receptors. *Am J Physiol* 1994;266: C1485–C1504.
109. Coyle DE, Sperelakis N. Bupivacaine and lidocaine blockade of calcium-mediated slow action potentials in guinea pig ventricular muscle. *J Pharmacol Exp Ther* 1987;242:1001–1005.
110. Crespo LM, Grantham CJ, Cannell MB. Kinetics, stoichiometry and role for the Na-Ca exchange mechanism is isolated cardiac myocytes. *Nature* 1990;345:618–621.
111. Curiel R, Pérez-González J, Brito N, et al. Positive inotropic effects mediated by a_1 adrenoceptors in intact human subjects. *J Cardiovasc Pharmacol* 1989;14:603–615.
112. Davies AO, McCans DR. Effects of barbiturate anesthetics and ketamine on the force-frequency relation of cardiac muscle. *Eur J Pharmacol* 1979;59:65–73.
113. Davis MD, Lebolt W, Feher JJ. Reversibility of the effects of normothermic global ischemia on the ryanodine-sensitive and ryanodine-insensitive calcium uptake of cardiac sarcoplasmic reticulum. *Circ Res* 1992;70:163–171.
114. De Hert SG, Gillebert TC, Andries LJ, Brutseart DL. Role of the endocardial endothelium in the regulation of myocardial function. Physiologic and pathophysiologic implications. *Anesthesiology* 1993;79:1354–1366.
115. de Weille JR. Modulation of ATP sensitive potassium channels. *Cardiovasc Res* 1992;26:1017–1020.
116. DeFelice LJ. Molecular and biophysical view of the Ca channel: A hypothesis regarding oligomeric structure, channel clustering, and macroscopic current. *J Membr Biol* 1993;133:191–202.
117. del Monte F, Kaumann AJ, Poole-Wilson PA, Wynne DG, Pepper J, Harding SE. Coexistence of functioning β_1- and β_2-adrenoceptors in single myocytes from human ventricle. *Circulation* 1993;88: 854–863.
118. Desai SP, Marsh JD, Allen PD. Contractility effects of local anesthetics in the presence of sodium channel blockade. *Reg Anesth* 1989;14:58–62.
119. DeTraglia MC, Komai H, Rusy BF. Differential effects of inhalational anesthetics on myocardial potentiated-state contractions *in vitro*. *Anesthesiology* 1988;68:534–540.
120. Dietrich DLL, van Leeuwen GR, Stienen GJM, Elzinga G. Stunning does not change the relation between calcium and force in skinned rat trabeculae. *J Mol Cell Cardiol* 1993;25:541–549.
121. Disatnik MH, Shainberg A. Regulation of beta-adrenoceptors by thyroid hormone and amiodarone in rat myocardial cells in culture. *Biochem Pharmacol* 1991;41:1039–1044.
122. Dobrunz LE, Backx PH, Yue DT. Steady-state $[Ca^{2+}]_i$-force relationship in intact twitching cardiac muscle: direct evidence for modulation by isoproterenol and EMD 53998. *Biophys J* 1995;69: 189–201.
123. Doohan MM, Hool LC, Rasmussen HH. Thyroid status and Na^+-K^+ pump current, intracellular sodium, and action potential duration in rabbit heart. *Am J Physiol* 1995;268:H1838–H1846.
124. Dösemeci A, Dhallan RS, Cohen NM, Lederer WJ, Rogers TB. Phorbol ester increases calcium current and simulates the effects of angiotensin II on cultured neonatal rat heart myocytes. *Circ Res* 1988;62:347–357.
125. Drenger B, Ginosar Y, Chandra M, Reches A, Gozal Y. Halothane modifies ischemia-associated injury to the voltage-sensitive calcium channels in canine heart sarcolemma. *Anesthesiology* 1994;81: 221–228.
126. Drenger B, Quigg M, Blanck TJJ. Volatile anesthetics depress calcium channel blocker binding to bovine cardiac sarcolemma. *Anesthesiology* 1991;74:155–165.

127. Dudley J, S C, Baumgarten CM. Bursting of cardiac sodium channels after acute exposure to 3,5,3'-triiodo-L-thyronine. *Circ Res* 1993;73:301–313.
128. Dyke CM, Yeh T Jr, Lehman JD, et al. Triiodothyronine-enhanced left ventricular function after ischemic injury. *Ann Thorac Surg* 1991;52:14–19.
129. Eberli FR, Apstein CS, Ngoy S, Lorell BH. Exacerbation of left ventricular ischemic diastolic dysfunction by pressure-overload hypertrophy: modification by specific inhibition of cardiac angiotensin converting enzyme. *Circ Res* 1992;70:931–943.
130. Ebert TJ, Kampine JP. Nitrous oxide augments sympathetic outflow: Direct evidence from human peroneal recordings. *Anesth Analg* 1989;69:
131. Ebus JP, Stienen GJM, Elzinga G. Influence of phosphate and pH on myofibrillar ATPase activity and force in skinned cardiac trabeculae from rat. *J Physiol* 1994;476:501–516.
132. Edes I, Kranias E. Phospholamban and troponin I are substrates for protein kinase C in vitro but not in intact beating guinea pig hearts. *Circ Res* 1990;67:394–400.
133. Edwards G, Weston AH. The pharmacology of ATP-sensitive potassium channels. *Annu Rev Pharmacol Toxicol* 1993;33:597–637.
134. Egan TM, Noble D, Noble SJ, Powell T, Spindler AJ, Twist VW. Sodium-calcium exchange during the action potential in guinea-pig ventricular cells. *J Physiol* 1989;411:639–661.
135. Eisele JH, Smith NT. Cardiovascular effects of 40 percent nitrous oxide in man. *Anesth Analg* 1972;31:250–260.
136. Endoh M, Blinks JM. Actions of sympathomimetic amines on the Ca^{2+} transients and contractions of rabbit myocardium: reciprocal changes in myofibrillar responsiveness to Ca^{2+} mediated through α- and β-receptors. *Circ Res* 1988;62:247–265.
137. Endou M, Hattori Y, Nakaya H, Gotoh Y, Kanno M. Electrophysiological mechanisms responsible for inotropic responses to ketamine in guinea pig and rat myocardium. *Anesthesiology* 1992;76: 409–418.
138. Endou M, Hattori Y, Tohse N, Kanno M. Protein kinase C is not involved in alpha$_1$-adrenoceptor mediated positive inotropic effect. *Am J Physiol* 1991;260:H27–H36.
139. Engel J, Fechner M, Sowerby AJ, Finch SAE, Stier A. Anisotropic propagation of Ca^{2+} waves in isolated cardiomyocytes. *Biophys J* 1994;66:1756–1762.
140. Ertl R, Jahnel U, Nawrath H, Carmeliet E, Vereecke J. Differential electrophysiologic and inotropic effects of phenylephrine in atrial and ventricular heart muscle preparations from rats. *Naunyn Schmiedebergs Arch Pharmacol* 1992;344:574–581.
141. Fabiato A. Calcium release in skinned cardiac cells: variations with species, tissues, and development. *Fed Proc* 1982;41:2238–2244.
142. Fabiato A. Calcium-induced release of calcium from the cardiac sarcoplasmic reticulum. *Am J Physiol* 1983;245:C1–C14.
143. Fabiato A, Fabiato F. Contraction induced by a calcium-triggered release of calcium from the sarcoplasmic reticulum of single skinned cardiac cells. *J Physiol (Lond)* 1975;249:469–495.
144. Farah CS, Reinach FC. The troponin complex and regulation of muscle contraction. *FASEB J* 1995;9:755–767.
145. Fedida D, Bouchard RA. Mechanisms for the positive inotropic effect of α_1-adrenoceptor stimulation in rat cardiac myocytes. *Circ Res* 1992;71:673–688.
146. Fedida D, Braun AP, Giles WR. α_1-Adrenoceptors in myocardium: functional aspects and transmembrane signalling mechanisms. *Physiol Rev* 1993;73:469–487.
147. Fedida D, Shimoni Y, Giles WR. α-Adrenergic modulation of the transient outward current in rabbit atrial myocytes. *J Physiol* 1990; 423:257–277.
148. Feher JJ, Rebeyka IM. Cooling and pH jump-induced calcium release from isolated cardiac sarcoplasmic reticulum. *Am J Physiol* 1994;267:H962–H969.
149. Feldman AM, Cates AE, Veazey WB, et al. Increase of the 40,000-mol wt pertussis toxin substrate (G protein) in the failing human heart. *J Clin Invest* 1988;82:189–197.
150. Feldman MD, Alderman JD, Aroesty JM, et al. Depression of systolic and diastolic myocardial reserve during atrial pacing tachycardia in patients with dilated cardiomyopathy. *J Clin Invest* 1988; 82:1661–1669.
151. Feldman MD, Copelas L, Gwathmey JK, et al. Deficient production of cyclic AMP: pharmacologic evidence of an important cause of contractile dysfunction in patients with end-stage heart failure. *Circulation* 1987;75:331–339.
152. Feldman MD, Gwathmey JK, Phillips P, Schoen FJ, Morgan JP. Reversal of the force-frequency relationship in working myocardium from patients with end-stage heart failure. *J Appl Cardiol* 1988; 3:272–283.
153. Ferrari R, Alfieri O, Curello S, et al. Occurrence of oxidative stress during reperfusion of the human heart. *Circulation* 1990;81: 201–211.
154. Ferris C, Snyder S. Inositol 1,4,5–trisphosphate-activated calcium channels. *Annu Rev Physiol* 1992;54:469–488.
155. Fischmeister R, Hartzell HC. Regulation of calcium current by low-K_m cyclic AMP phosphodiesterases in cardiac cells. *Am Soc Pharmacol Exp Ther* 1990;38:426–433.
156. Fish D, Orenstein J, Bloom S. Passive stiffness of isolated cardiac and skeletal myocytes in the hamster. *Circ Res* 1984;54:267–276.
157. Fisher AJ, Smith CA, Thoden J, et al. Structural studies of the myosin:nucleotide complex: a revised model for the molecular basis of muscle contraction. *Biophys J* 1995;68:19s-28s.
158. Forbes MS, Sperelakis N. Ultrastructure of mammalian cardiac muscle. In: Sperelakis N, ed. *Physiology and pathophysiology of the heart.* Boston: Martinus Nijhoff, 1984;3–42.
159. Forbes MS, Sperelakis N. Intercalated discs of mammalian heart: a review of structure and function. *Tissue Cell* 1985;17:605–648.
160. Fowler MB, Laser JA, Hopkins GL, Minobe W, Bristow MR. Assessment of the β-adrenergic receptor pathway in the intact failing human heart: progressive receptor down-regulation and subsensitivity to agonist response. *Circulation* 1986;74:1290–1302.
161. Frampton JE, Orchard CH, Boyett MR. Diastolic, systolic and sarcoplasmic reticulum [Ca^{2+}] during inotropic interventions in isolated rat myocytes. *J Physiol* 1991;437:351–375.
162. Frank JS, Mottino G, Reid D, Molday RR, Philipson KD. Distribution of the Na-Ca exchange protein in mammalian cardiac myocytes: an immunofluorescence and immunocolloidal gold-labelling study. *J Cell Biol* 1992;117:337–345.
163. Frankl WS, Poole-Wilson PA. Effects of thiopental on tension development, action potential, and exchange of calcium and potassium in rabbit ventricular myocardium. *J Cardiovasc Pharmacol* 1981;3:554–565.
164. Franzini-Armstrong C, Kenney LJ, Varriano-Marston E. The structure of calsequestrin in triads of vertebrate skeletal muscle: a deep-etch study. *J Cell Biol* 1987;105:49–56.
165. Frazer MJ, Lynch C III. Halothane and isoflurane effects on Ca^{2+} fluxes of isolated myocardial sarcoplasmic reticulum. *Anesthesiology* 1992;77:316–323.
166. Fry CH, Poole-Wilson PA. Effects of acid-base changes on excitation-contraction coupling in guinea-pig and rabbit cardiac ventricular muscle. *J Physiol* 1981;313:141–160.
167. Fu L-X, Feng Q-P, Liang Q-M, et al. Hypersensitivity of Gi protein mediated muscarinic receptor adenylyl cyclase in chronic ischaemic heart failure in the rat. *Cardiovasc Res* 1993;27:2065–2070.
168. Fuchs F. Mechanical modulation of the Ca^{2+} regulatory protein complex in cardiac muscle. *News Physiol Sci* 1995;10:6–11.
169. Fujii J, Ueno A, Kitano K, Tanaka S, Kadoma M, Tada M. Complete complementary DNA-derived amino acid sequence of canine cardiac phospholamban. *J Clin Invest* 1987;79:301–304.
170. Fukanaga AF, Epstein RM. Sympathetic excitation during nitrous oxide-halothane anesthesia in the cat. *Anesthesiology* 1973;39: 23–36.
171. Furuichi T, Yoshikawa S, Miyawaki A, Kentaroh W, Maeda N, Mikoshiba K. Primary structure and functional expression of the inositol 1,4,5–triposphate-binding protein P_{400}. *Nature* 1989;342: 32–38.
172. Furukawa T, Kimura S, Furukawa N, Bassett AL, Myerburg RJ. Role of cardiac ATP-regulated potassium channels in differential responses of endocardial and epicardial cells to ischemia. *Circ Res* 1991;68:1693–1702.
173. Gambassi G, Spurgeon HA, Lakatta EG, Blank PS, Capogrossi MC. Different effects of α- and β-adrenergic stimulation on cytosolic pH and myofilament responsiveness to Ca^{2+} in cardiac myocytes. *Circ Res* 1992;71:870–882.
174. García J, Beam KG. Measurement of calcium transients and slow calcium current in myotubes. *J Gen Physiol* 1994;103:107–123.
175. García J, Tanabe T, Beam KG. Relationship of calcium transients to calcium currents and charge movements in myotubes expressing skeletal and cardiac dihydropyridine receptors. *J Gen Physiol* 1994;103:125–147.
176. Garvey J, Kranias E, Solaro R. Phosphorylation of C-protein, troponin I and phospholamban in isolated rabbit hearts. *Biochem J* 1988;249:709–714.

177. Geisterfer-Lowrance AAT, Kass S, Tanigawa G, et al. A molecular basis for familial hypertrophic cardiomyopathy: a β cardiac myosin heavy chain gene missense mutation. *Cell* 1990;62:999–1006.
178. Gengo PJ, Sabbah HN, Steffen RP, et al. Myocardial beta adrenoceptor and voltage sensitive calcium channel changes in a canine model of chronic heart failure. *J Mol Cell Cardiol* 1992;24: 1361–1369.
179. Ginsburg R, Bristow MR, Billingham ME, Stinson EB, Schroeder JS, Harrison DC. Study of the normal and failing isolated human heart: decreased response of failing heart to isoproterenol. *Am Heart J* 1983;3:272–283.
180. Goldberg AH, Keane PW, Phear PC. Effects of ketamine on contractile performance and excitability of isolated heart muscle. *J Pharmacol Exp Ther* 1970;175:388–394.
181. Goldberg AH, Phear WPC. Alterations in mechanical properties of heart muscle produced by halothane. *J Pharmacol Exp Ther* 1968; 162:101–108.
182. Goldberg AH, Sohn YZ, Phear WPC. Direct myocardial effects of nitrous oxide. *Anesthesiology* 1972;37:373–380.
183. Goto M, Liu Y, Yang X-M, Ardell JL, Cohen MV, Downey JM. Role of bradykinin in protection of ischemic preconditioning in rabbit hearts. *Circ Res* 1995;77:611–621.
184. Graf F, Schatzmann HH. Some effects of removal of external calcium on pig striated muscle. *J Physiol* 1984;349:1–13.
185. Grocott-Mason R, Fort S, Lewis M, Shah A. Myocardial relaxant effect of exogenous nitrous oxide in isolated ejecting hearts. *Am J Physiol* 1994;266:H1699–H1705.
186. Grover AK, Khan I. Calcium pump isoforms: diversity, selectivity and plasticity. *Cell Calcium* 1992;13:9–17.
187. Gulati J, Sonnenblick E, Babu A. The role of troponin C in the length dependence of Ca^{2+}-sensitive force of mammalian skeletal and cardiac muscle fibers. *J Physiol* 1990;444:305–324.
188. Gunter TE, Pfeiffer DL. Mechanisms by which mitochondria transport calcium. *Am J Physiol* 1990;258:C755–C786.
189. Gwathmey JK, Copelas L, Mackinnon R, et al. Abnormal intracellular calcium handling in myocardium from patients with end-stage heart failure. *Circ Res* 1987;61:70–76.
190. Gwathmey JK, P MJ. Altered calcium handling in experimental pressure overload hypertrophy in the ferret. *Circ Res* 1985;57: 836–843.
191. Györke S, Fill M. Ryanodine receptor adaptation: control mechanism of Ca^{2+}-induced Ca^{2+} release in heart. *Science* 1993;260: 807–809.
192. Hagiwara N, Irisawa H, Kameyama M. Contribution of two types of calcium currents to the pacemaker potentials of rabbit sino-atrial node cells. *J Physiol* 1988;395:233–253.
193. Haigney MCP, Miyata H, Lakatta EG, Stern MD, Silverman HS. Dependence of hypoxic cellular calcium loading on Na^+-Ca^{2+} exchange. *Circ Res* 1992;71:547–557.
194. Hajjar R, Gwathmey J. Direct evidence of changes in myofilament responsiveness to Ca^{2+} during hypoxia and reoxygenation in myocardium. *Am J Physiol* 1990;259:H784–H795.
195. Hajjar RJ, Grossman W, Gwathmey JK. Responsiveness of the myofilaments to Ca^{2+} in human heart failure—implications for Ca^{2+} and force regulation. *Basic Res Cardiol* 1992;87:143–159.
196. Hakamata Y, Nakai J, Takeshima H, Imoto K. Primary structure and distribution of a novel ryanodine receptor/calcium release channel from rabbit brain. *FEBS Lett* 1992;312:229–235.
197. Han X, Shimoni Y, Giles WR. A cellular mechanism for nitric oxide-mediated cholinergic control of mammalian heart rate. *J Gen Physiol* 1995;106:45–65.
198. Hansford RG, Hogue B, Prokopczuk A, Wasilewska E, Lewartowski B. Activation of pyruvate dehydrogenase by electrical stimulation, and low-Na^+ perfusion of guinea pig heart. *Biochim Biophys Acta* 1990;1018:282–286.
199. Harding SE, Jones SM, O'Gara P, del Monte F, Vescovo G, Poole-Wilson PA. Isolated ventricular myocytes from failing and non-failing human heart;the relation of age and clinical status of patients to isoproterenol response. *J Mol Cell Cardiol* 1992;24: 549–564.
200. Harrison SM, Boyett MR. The role of the Na^+-Ca^{2+} exchanger in the rate dependent increase in contraction in guinea-pig ventricular myocytes. *J Physiol* 1995;482:555–566.
201. Harrison SM, McCall E, Boyett MR. The relationship between contraction and intracellular sodium in rat and guinea-pig ventricular myocytes. *J Physiol* 1992;449:517–550.
202. Hartzell HC, Fischmeister R. Direct regulation of cardiac Ca^{2+} channels by G proteins: neither proven nor necessary? *Trends Pharmacol Sci* 1992;13:380–385.
203. Hasenfuss G, Holubarsch C, Hermann H-P, Astheimer K, Pieske B, Just H. Influence of the force-frequency relation on haemodynamics and left ventricular function in patients with non-failing hearts and in patients with dilated cardiomyopathy. *Eur Heart J* 1994;15:164–170.
204. Hasenfuss G, Mulieri LA, Holubarsch C, Pieske B, Just H, Alpert NR. Energetics of calcium cycling in nonfailing and failing human myocardium. *Basic Res Cardiol* 1992;87:81–92.
205. Hasenfuss G, Reinecke H, Studer R, et al. Relation between myocardial function and expression of sarcoplasmic reticulum Ca^{2+}-ATPase in failing and nonfailing human myocardium. *Circ Res* 1994;75:434–442.
206. Hasselbach W, Oetlicker H. Energetics and electrogenicity of the sarcoplasmic reticulum calcium pump. *Annu Rev Physiol* 1983;43: 325–339.
207. Hatakeyama N, Momose Y, Ito Y. Effects of sevoflurane on contractile responses and electrophysiologic properties in canine single cardiac myocytes. *Anesthesiology* 1995;82:559–565.
208. Hatem SN, Sweeten T, Vetter V, Morad M. Evidence for presence of Ca^{2+} channel-gated Ca^{2+} stores in neonatal human atrial myocytes. *Am J Physiol* 1995;268:H1195–1201.
209. Haworth RA, Goknur AB. Inhibition of sodium/calcium exchange and calcium channels of heart cells by volatile anesthetics. *Anesthesiology* 1995;82:1255–1265.
210. Haworth RA, Goknur AB, Berkoff HA. Inhibition of Na-Ca exchange by general anesthetics. *Circ Res* 1989;65:1021–1028.
211. Hepler JR, Gilman AG. G proteins. *Trends Biochem Sci* 1992;17: 383–387.
212. Herland JS, Julian FJ, Stephenson DG. Halothane increases Ca^{2+} efflux via Ca^{2+} channels of sarcoplasmic reticulum in chemically skinned rat myocardium. *J Physiol* 1990;426:1–18.
213. Herland JS, Julian FJ, Stephenson DG. Unloaded shortening velocity of skinned rat myocardium: effects of volatile anesthetics. *Am J Physiol* 1990;259:H1118–H1125.
214. Herland JS, Julian FJ, Stephenson DG. Effects of halothane, enflurane, and isoflurane on skinned rat myocardium activated by Ca^{2+}. *Am J Physiol* 1993;264:H224–H232.
215. Herrman C, Wray J, Travers F, Barman T. Effect of 2,3–butanedione monoxime on myosin and myofibrillar ATPases. An example of an uncompetitive uncoupler. *Biochemistry* 1992;31:12227–12232.
216. Herzberg OH, Moult J, James MNG. A model for the Ca2+-induced conformational transition of troponin C: a trigger for muscle contraction. *J Biol Chem* 1986;261:2638–2644.
217. Hibberd MG, Jewell BR. Calcium- and length-dependent force production in rat ventricular muscle. *J Physiol* 1982;329:527–540.
218. Hieble JP, Bylund DB, Clarke DE, et al. Intentional union of pharmacology X. Recommendation for nomenclature of α_1-adrenoceptors: consensus update. *Pharmacol Rev* 1995;47:267–270.
219. Hill AV. On the time required for diffusion and its relation to processes in muscle. *Proc R Soc Lond B* 1948;135:446–453.
220. Hirano Y, Fozzard HA, January CT. Characteristics of L- and T-type Ca^{2+} currents in canine cardiac Purkinje fibers. *Am J Physiol* 1989; 256:H1478–H1492.
221. Ho K, Nichols CG, Lederer WJ, et al. Cloning and expression of an inwardly rectifying ATP-regulated potassium channel. *Nature* 1993;362:31–38.
222. Hoehner P, Quigg M, Blanck T. Halothane depresses D600 binding to bovine heart sarcolemma. *Anesthesiology* 1991;75:1019–1024.
223. Hofmann P, Fuchs F. Evidence for a force-dependent component of calcium binding to cardiac troponin C. *Am J Physiol* 1987;22: C541–C546.
224. Hofmann PA, Fuchs F. Bound calcium and force development in skinned cardiac muscle bundles: effect of sarcomere length. *J Mol Cell Cardiol* 1988;20:667–677.
225. Hofmann PA, Miller WP, Moss RL. Altered calcium sensitivity of isometric tension in myocyte-sized preparations of porcine postischemic stunned myocardium. *Circ Res* 1993;72:50–56.
226. Hoh J, Rossmanith G, Kwan L, Hamilton A. Adrenaline increases the rate of cycling of crossbridges in rat cardiac muscle as measured by pseudo-random binary noise-modulated perturbation analysis. *Circ Res* 1988;62:452–461.
227. Holmberg SRM, Cumming DVE, Kusama Y, et al. Reactive oxygen species modify the structure and function of the cardiac sarcoplasmic reticulum calcium-release channel. *Cardioscience* 1991;2:19–25.

228. Holmer SR, Homcy CJ. G proteins in the heart: a redundant and diverse transmembrane signaling network. *Circulation* 1991;84:1891–1902.
229. Holmes KC. The actomyosin interaction and its control by tropomyosin. *Biophys J* 1995;68:2s-7s.
230. Holmes KC, Popp D, Gebhard W, Kabsch W. Atomic model of the actin filament. *Nature* 1990;347:44–47.
231. Hongo K, Tanaka E, Kurihara S. Alterations in contractile properties and Ca2+ transients by b-and muscarinic receptor stimulation in ferret myocardium. *J Physiol* 1993;461:167–184.
232. Hopwood AM, Harding SE, Harris P. Pertussis toxin reduces the antiadrenergic effect of 2–chloroadenosine on papillary muscle and the direct negative inotropic effect of 2–chloroadenosine on atrium. *Eur J Pharmacol* 1987;141:423–428.
233. Horie M, Irisawa H, Noma A. Voltage-dependent magnesium blockade of adenosine-triphosphate-sensitive potassium channel in single guinea-pig ventricular cells. *J Physiol* 1987;287:251–272.
234. Horisberger J-D, Lemas V, Kraehenbuhl J-P, Rossier B. Structure-function relationship of Na,K-ATPase. *Annu Rev Physiol* 1991;53:565–584.
235. Housmans PD, Lee NKM, Blinks JR. Active shortening retards the decline of the intracellular calcium transient in mammalian heart muscle. *Science* 1983;221:159–161.
236. Housmans PE. Negative inotropy of halogenated anesthetics in ferret ventricular myocardium. *Am J Physiol* 1990;259:H827–H834.
237. Housmans PE, Murat I. Comparative effects of halothane, enflurane, and isoflurane at equipotent anesthetic concentrations on isolated ventricular myocardium of the ferret. I. Contractility. *Anesthesiology* 1988;69:451–463.
238. Housmans PR. Mechanisms of negative inotropy of halothane, enflurane and isoflurane in isolated mammalian ventricular muscle. *Adv Exp Med Biol* 1991;301:199–204.
239. Housmans PR, Kudsioglu ST, Bingham J. Mechanism of the negative inotropic effect of thiopental in isolated ferret ventricular myocardium. *Anesthesiology* 1995;82:436–450.
240. Housmans PR, Murat I. Comparative effects of halothane, enflurane, and isoflurane at equipotent anesthetic concentrations on isolated ventricular myocardium of the ferret. II. Relaxation. *Anesthesiology* 1988;69:464–471.
241. Hove-Madsen L, Bers DM. Sarcoplasmic reticulum Ca^{2+} uptake and thapsigargin sensitivity in permeabilized rabbit and rat ventricular myocytes. *Circ Res* 1993;73:820–828.
242. Huxley AF, Simmons RM. Proposed mechanism of force generation in striated muscle. *Nature* 1971;233:533–538.
243. Huxley HE. The mechanism of muscular contraction. *Science* 1969;164:1356–1366.
244. Ikemoto N, Ronjat M, Mészáros L, Koshita M. Postulated role of calsequestrin in the regulation of calcium release from sarcoplasmic reticulum. *Biochemistry* 1989;28:6764–6771.
245. Ikemoto Y. Reduction by thiopental of the slow-channel-mediated action potential of canine papillary muscle. *Pflugers Arch* 1977;372:285–286.
246. Ikemoto Y, Yatani A, Arimura H, Yoshitake J. Reduction of the slow inward current of isolated rat ventricular cells by thiamylal and halothane. *Acta Anaesthesiol Scand* 1985;29:583–586.
247. Iñiguez-Lluhi J, Kleuss C, Gilman AG. The importance of G-protein βγ subunits. *Trends Cell Biol* 1993;3:230–236.
248. Isenberg G, Belardinelli L. Ionic basic for the antagonism between adenosine and isoproterenol on isolated mammalian ventricular myocytes. *Circ Res* 1984;55:309–325.
249. Iwasa Y, Hosey MM. Phosphorylation of cardiac sarcolemma proteins by the calcium activated phospholipid-dependent kinase. *J Biol Chem* 1984;259:534–540.
250. Iyengar R. Molecular and functional diversity of mammalian Gs-stimulated adenylyl cyclases. *FASEB J* 1993;7:768–775.
251. Janczewski AM, Lakatta EG. Thapsigargin inhibits Ca^{2+} uptake, and Ca^{2+} depletes sarcoplasmic reticulum in intact cardiac myocytes. *Am J Physiol* 1993;265:H517–H522.
252. Janczewski AM, Spurgeon HA, Stern MD, Lakatta EG. Effects of sarcoplasmic reticulum Ca^{2+} load on the gain function of Ca^{2+} release by Ca^{2+} current in cardiac cells (Rapid Communication). *Am J Physiol* 1995;268:H916–H920.
253. Jayaraman T, Brillantes A, Timerman A, et al. FK506 binding protein associated with the calcium release channel (ryanodine receptor). *J Biol Chem* 1992;267:9474–9477.
254. Jones SM, Hunt NA, del Monte F, Harding SE. Contraction of cardiac myocytes from noradrenaline-treated rats in response to isoprenaline, forskolin and dibutyryl cAMP. *Eur J Pharmacol* 1990;191:129–140.
255. Josephson I, Sperelakis N. Local anesthetic blockade of Ca^{2+}-mediated action potentials in cardiac muscle. *Eur J Pharmacol* 1976;40:201–208.
256. Julian FJ, Sollins MR. Sarcomere length-tension relations in living rat papillary muscle. *Circ Res* 1975;37:299–308.
257. Julian FJ, Sollins MR, Moss RL. Absence of a plateau in length-tension relationship of rabbit papillary muscle when internal shortening is prevented. *Nature* 1976;260:340–342.
258. Kabsch W, Mannherz HG, Suck D, Pai EF, Homes KC. Atomic structure of the actin:DNase I complex. *Nature* 1990;347:37–44.
259. Kaplan P, Hendrikx M, Mattheussen M, Mubagwa K, Flameng W. Effect of ischemia and reperfusion on sarcoplasmic reticulum calcium uptake. *Circ Res* 1992;71:1123–1130.
260. Katsuoka M, Kobayashi K, Ohnishi T. Volatile anesthetics decrease calcium content of isolated myocytes. *Anesthesiology* 1989;70:954–960.
261. Katsuoka M, Ohnishi ST. Inhalation anaesthetics decrease calcium content of cardiac sarcoplasmic reticulum. *Br J Anaesth* 1989;62:669–673.
262. Kawaguchi H, Shoki M, Sano H, et al. Phospholipid metabolism in cardiomyopathic hamster heart cells. *Circ Res* 1991;69:1015–1021.
263. Kemmotsu O, Hashimoto Y, Shimosato S. Inotropic effects of isoflurane on mechanics of contraction in isolated cat papillary muscles from normal and failing hearts. *Anesthesiology* 1973;39:470–477.
264. Kentish JC, ter Keurs HEDJ, Ricciardi L, Bucx JJJ, Noble MIM. Comparison between the sarcomere length-force relations of intact and skinned trabeculae from rat right ventricle: influence of calcium concentrations on these relations. *Circ Res* 1986;58:755–768.
265. Kieval R, Bloch R, Lindenmayer G, Ambesi A, Lederer W. Immunofluorescence localization of the Na^+-Ca^{2+} exchanger in heart cells. *Am J Physiol* 1992;163:C545–C550.
266. Kijima Y, Ogunbunmi E, Fleischer S. Drug action of thapsigargin on the $Ca2^+$ pump protein of sarcoplasmic reticulum. *J Biol Chem* 1991;266:22912–22918.
267. Kijima Y, Saito A, Jetton TL, Magnuson MA, Fleischer S. Different intracellular localization of inositol 1,4,5–triphosphate and ryanodine receptors in cardiomyocytes. *J Biol Chem* 1993;268:3499–3506.
268. Kim HW, Steenart NAE, Ferguson DG, Kranias EG. Functional reconstitution of the cardiac sarcoplasmic reticulum Ca^{2+}-ATPase with phospholamban in phospholipid vesicles. *J Biol Chem* 1990;265:1702–1709.
269. Kimura J, Akinori A, Irisawa H. Na-Ca exchange current in mammalian heart cells. *Nature* 1986;319:596–597.
270. Kirsch GE, Codina J, Birnbaumer L, Brown AM. Coupling of ATP-sensitive K^+ channels to A_1 receptors by G proteins in rat ventricular myocytes. *Am J Physiol* 1990;28:H820–H826.
271. Kissin I, Motomura S, Aultman DF, Reves JG. Inotropic and anesthetic potencies of etomidate and thiopental in dogs. *Anesth Analg* 1983;62:961–965.
272. Klöckner U, Isenberg G. Calcium channel current of vascular smooth muscle cells: extracellular protons modulate gating and single channel conductance. *J Gen Physiol* 1994;103:665–678.
273. Klöckner U, Isenberg G. Intracellular pH modulates the availability of vascular L-type Ca^{2+} channels. *J Gen Physiol* 1994;103:647–663.
274. Knudson CM, Stang KK, Jorgensen AO, Campbell KP. Biochemical characterization and ultrastructural localization of a major junctional sarcoplasmic reticulum glycoprotein (triadin). *J Biol Chem* 1993;268:12637–12645.
275. Koch-Weser J, Blinks JR. The influence of the interval between beats on myocardial contractility. *Pharmacol Rev* 1963;15:601–652.
276. Kohmoto O, Ikenouchi H, Hirata Y, Momomura S-I, Serizawa T, Barry WH. Variable effects of endothelin-1 on $[Ca^{2+}]_i$ transients, pH_i, and contraction in ventricular myocytes. *Am J Physiol* 1993;265:H793–H800.
277. Komai H, DeWitt DE, Rusy BF. Negative inotropic effects of etomidate in rabbit papillary muscle. *Anesth Analg* 1984;64:400–404.
278. Komai H, Redon D, Rusy BF. Effects of isoflurane and halothane on rapid cooling contractures in myocardial tissue. *Am J Physiol* 1989;257:H1804–H1811.
279. Komai H, Redon D, Rusy BF. Effects of thiopental and halothane

on spontaneous contractile activity induced in isolated ventricular muscles of the rabbit. *Acta Anaesthesiol Scand* 1991;35:373–379.
280. Komai H, Rusy BF. Effect of halothane on rested-state and potentiated state contraction in rabbit papillary muscle relationship to negative inotropic effect. *Anesth Analg* 1982;61:403–409.
281. Komai H, Rusy BF. Differences in the myocardial depressant action of thiopental and halothane. *Anesth Analg* 1984;63:313–318.
282. Komai H, Rusy BF. Calcium and thiopental-induced spontaneous activity in rabbit papillary muscle. *J Mol Cell Cardiol* 1986;18:73–79.
283. Komai H, Rusy BF. Negative inotropic effects of isoflurane and halothane in rabbit papillary muscles. *Anesth Analg* 1987;66:29–33.
284. Komai H, Rusy BF. Direct effect of halothane and isoflurane on the function of the sarcoplasmic reticulum in intact rabbit atria. *Anesthesiology* 1990;72:694–698.
285. Komai H, Rusy BF. Effect of thiopental on Ca^{2+} release from sarcoplasmic reticulum in intact myocardium. *Anesthesiology* 1994;81:946–952.
286. Kongsayreepong S, Cook DJ, Housmans PR. Mechanism of the direct, negative inotropic effect of ketamine in isolated ferret and frog ventricular myocardium. *Anesthesiology* 1993;79:313–322.
287. Koumi S-I, Wasserstrom JA. Acetylcholine-sensitive muscarinic K^+ channels in mammalian ventricular myocytes. *Am J Physiol* 1994;266:H1812–H1821.
288. Krane EJ, Su JY. Comparison of the effects of halothane on skinned myocardial fibers from newborn and adult rabbit. I. Effects on contractile proteins. *Anesthesiology* 1989;70:76–81.
289. Kranias EG, Garvey JL, Srivastava RD, Solaro RJ. Phosphorylation and functional modifications of sarcoplasmic reticulum and myofibrils in isolated rabbit hearts stimulated with isoprenaline. *Biochem J* 1985;226:113–121.
290. Kubota I, Yamaki M, Shibata T, Ikeno E, Hosoya Y, Tomoike H. Role of ATP-sensitive K+ channel on ECG ST segment elevation during a bout of myocardial ischemia: a study on epicardial mapping in dogs. *Circulation* 1993;88:1845–1851.
291. Kukreja RC, Hess ML. The oxygen free radical system: from equations through membrane-protein interactions to cardiovascular injury and protection. *Cardiovasc Res* 1992;26:641–655.
292. Kusuoka H, Marban E. Cellular mechanisms of myocardial stunning. *Annu Rev Physiol* 1992;54:243–256.
293. Lab MJ, Allen DG, Orchard CH. The effects of shortening on myoplasmic calcium concentration and on the action potential in mammalian ventricular muscle. *Circ Res* 1984;55:825–829.
294. Lacerda AE, Rampe D, Brown AM. Effects of protein kinase C activators on cardiac Ca^{2+} channels. *Nature* 1988;335:249–251.
295. Ladilov YV, Siegmund B, Piper HM. Protection of reoxygenated cardiomyocytes against hypercontracture by inhibition of Na^+/H^+ exchange. *Am J Physiol* 1995;268:H1531–H1539.
296. Lain RF, Hess ML, Gertz EW, Briggs FN. Calcium uptake activity of canine myocardial sarcoplasmic reticulum in the presence of anesthetic agents. *Circ Res* 1968;23:597–604.
297. Lal R, Arnsdorf MF. Voltage-dependent gating and single-channel conductance of adult mammalian atrial gap junctions. *Circ Res* 1992;71:737–743.
298. Landesberg A, Sideman S. Mechanical regulation of cardiac muscle by coupling calcium kinetics with cross-bridge cycling: a dynamic model. *Am J Physiol* 1994;267:H779–H795.
299. Langer GA. Calcium and the heart: exchange at the tissue, cell, and organelle levels. *FASEB J* 1992;6:893–902.
300. Langer GA, Peskoff A, Post JA. How does the Na^+-Ca^{2+} exchanger working the intact cardiac cells? *J Mol Cell Cardiol* 1993;25:637–639.
301. Langer GA, Wang SY, Rich TL. Localization of the Na/Ca exchange-dependent Ca compartment in cultured neonatal rat cells. *Am J Physiol* 1995;268:C119–C126.
302. Lawson C, Downey J. Preconditioning: state of the art myocardial protection. *Cardiovasc Res* 1993;27:542–550.
303. Lawson D, Frazer MJ, Lynch C III. Nitrous oxide effects on isolated myocardium: a reexamination *in vitro*. *Anesthesiology* 1990;73:930–943.
304. Lazou A, Fuller SJ, Bogoyevitch MA, Orfali KA, Sugden PH. Characterization of stimulation of phosphoinositide hydrolysis by α_1-adrenergic agonists in adult rat hearts. *Am J Physiol* 1994;267:H970–H978.
305. Lazrak A, Peres A, Giovannardi S, Peracchia C. Ca-mediated and independent effects of arachidonic acid on gap junctions and Ca-independent effects of oleic acid and halothane. *Biophys J* 1994;67:1052–1059.
306. LeBlanc N, Hume JR. Sodium current-induced release of calcium from cardiac sarcoplasmic reticulum. *Science* 1990;248:372–376.
307. Lederer WJ, Niggli E, Hadley RW. Sodium-calcium exchange in excitable cells: fuzzy space. *Science* 1990;248:371–372.
308. Lee DL, Zhang J, Blanck TJJ. The effects of halothane on voltage-dependent calcium channels in isolated Langenforff-perfused rat heart. *Anesthesiology* 1994;81:1212–1219.
309. Lee KS, Marban E, Tsien RW. Inactivation of calcium channels in mammalian heart cells: joint dependence on membrane potential and intracellular calcium. *J Physiol* 1985;364:395–411.
310. Levesque PC, Leblanc N, Hume JR. Release of calcium from guinea pig cardiac sarcoplasmic reticulum by sodium-calcium exchange. *Cardiovasc Res* 1994;28:370–378.
311. Levi AJ, Brooksby P, Hancox JC. One hump or two? The triggering of calcium release from the sarcoplasmic reticulum and the voltage dependence of contraction in mammalian cardiac muscle. *Cardiovasc Res* 1993;27:1743–1757.
312. Levi AJ, Spitzer KW, Kohmoto O, Bridge JHB. Depolarization-induced Ca entry via Na-Ca exchange triggers SR release in guinea pig cardiac myocytes. *Am J Physiol* 1994;266:H1422–1433.
313. Lew WYW. Mechanisms of volume-induced increase in left ventricular contractility. *Am J Physiol* 1993;265:H1778–H1786.
314. Lewartowski B, Wolska BM, Zdanowski K. The effects of blocking Na-Ca exchange at intervals throughout the physiological contraction-relaxation cycle of single cardiac myocyte. *J Mol Cell Cardiol* 1992;24:967–976.
315. Lewis MJ, Grey AC, Henderson AH. Determinants of hypoxic contracture in isolated heart muscle preparations. *Cardiovasc Res* 1979;13:86–94.
316. Linke WA, Popov VI, Pollack GH. Passive and active tension in single cardiac myofibrils. *Biophys J* 1994;67:782–792.
317. Linzbach AJ. Heart failure from the point of view of quantitative anatomy. *Am J Cardiol* 1960;5:370–380.
318. Lipp P, Niggli E. Sodium current-induced calcium signals in isolated guinea-pig ventricular myocytes. *J Physiol* 1994;474:439–446.
319. Lipp P, Pott L, Callewaert G, Carmeliet E. Calcium transients caused by calcium entry are influenced by the sarcoplasmic reticulum in guinea-pig atrial myocytes. *J Physiol* 1992;454:321–338.
320. Litten RZ, Martin BJ, Low RB, Alpert NR. Altered myosin isozyme patterns from pressure-overloaded and thyrotoxic hypertrophied rabbit hearts. *Circ Res* 1982;50:856–864.
321. Liu Y, Ytrehus K, Downey J. Evidence that translocation of protein kinase C is a key event during ischemic preconditioning of rabbit myocardium. *J Mol Cell Cardiol* 1994;26:661–668.
322. Lochner A, Harper IS, Salie R, Genade S, Coetzee AR. Halothane protects the isolated rat myocardium against excessive total intracellular calcium and structural damage during ischemia and reperfusion. *Anesth Analg* 1994;79:226–233.
323. Löffelholz K, Pappano AJ. The parasympathetic neuroeffector junction of the heart. *Pharmacol Rev* 1985;37:1–24.
324. Lombardi V, Piazzesi G, Linari M. Rapid regeneration of the actin-myosin power stroke in contracting muscle. *Nature* 1992;355:638–641.
325. Lowry S, Trybus KM. Role of skeletal and smooth muscle myosin light chains. *Biophys J* 1995;68:120s-127s.
326. Luk HN, Lin CI, Chang CL, Lee AR. Differential inotropic effects of halothane and isoflurane in dog ventricular tissues. *Eur J Pharmacol* 1987;136:409–413.
327. Lundy PM, Gverzdys S, Frew R. Ketamine: evidence of tissue-specific inhibition of neuronal and extraneuronal catecholamine uptake processes. *Can J Physiol Pharmacol* 1985;63:298–303.
328. Luo W, Grupp IL, Harrer J, et al. Targeted ablation of the phospholamban gene is associated with markedly enhanced myocardial contractility and loss of β-agonist stimulation. *Circ Res* 1994;75:401–409.
329. Lymn RW, Taylor EW. Mechanism of adenosine triphosphate hydrolysis by actomyosin. *Biochemistry* 1971;10:4617–4624.
330. Lynch C III. Depression of myocardial contractility in vitro by bupivacaine, etidocaine, and lidocaine. *Anesth Analg* 1986;65:551–559.
331. Lynch C III. Differential depression of myocardial contractility by halothane and isoflurane *in vitro*. *Anesthesiology* 1986;64:620–631.
332. Lynch C III. Effects of halothane and isoflurane on isolated human ventricular myocardium. *Anesthesiology* 1988;68:429–432.
333. Lynch C III. Differential depression of myocardial contractility by volatile anesthetics *in vitro*: comparison with uncouplers of excitation-contraction coupling. *J Cardiovasc Pharmacol* 1990;15:655–665.

334. Lynch C III. Pharmacological evidence for two types of myocardial sarcoplasmic reticulum Ca^{2+} release. *Am J Physiol* 1991; 260:H785–H795.
335. Lynch C III. The biochemical and cellular basis of myocardial contractility. In: Warltier DC, ed. *Ventricular function.* Baltimore: Williams & Wilkins, 1995;1–67.
336. Lynch C III, Frazer MJ. Depressant effects of volatile anesthetics upon rat and amphibian ventricular myocardium: Insights into mechanisms of action. *Anesthesiology* 1989;70:511–522.
337. Lynch C III, Frazer MJ. Anesthetic alteration of ryanodine binding by cardiac calcium release channels. *Biochim Biophys Acta* 1994;1194:109–117.
338. Lynch C III, Jaeger JM. The G protein cell signalling system. In: Lake C, ed. *Advances in anesthesia,* vol 11. Chicago: Mosby-Year Book, 1994;65–112.
339. Lynch C III, Vogel S, Pratila MG, Sperelakis N. Enflurane depression of myocardial slow action potentials. *J Pharmacol Exp Ther* 1982;222:405–409.
340. Lynch C III, Vogel S, Sperelakis N. Halothane depression of myocardial slow action potentials. *Anesthesiology* 1981;55:360–368.
341. MacKenna D, Omens J, A M, Covell J. Contribution of collagen matrix to passive left ventricular mechanics in isolated rat hearts. *Am J Physiol* 1994;266:H1007–H1018.
342. MacLennan DH. Molecular tools to elucidate problems in exitation-contraction coupling. *Biophys J* 1990;58:1355–1365.
343. Margossian SS. Reversible dissociation of dog cardiac myosin regulatory light chain 2 and its influence on ATP hydrolysis. *J Biol Chem* 1985;260:13747–13754.
344. Marks AR, Tempst P, Hwang KS, et al. Molecular cloning and characterization of the ryanodine receptor/junctional channel complex cDNA from skeletal muscle sarcoplasmic reticulum. *Proc Natl Acad Sci USA* 1989;86:8683–8687.
345. Matsuda H. Magnesium gating of the inwardly rectifying K^+ channel. *Annu Rev Physiol* 1991;53:289–298.
346. Mattheussen M, Housmans PR. Mechanism of the direct, negative inotropic effect of etomidate in isolated ferret ventricular myocardium. *Anesthesiology* 1993;79:1284–1295.
347. Mattiazzi A, Hove-Madsen L, Bers D. Protein kinase inhibitors reduce SR Ca transport in permeabilized cardiac myocytes. *Am J Physiol* 1994;36:
348. McClellan G, Weisberg A, Winegrad S. cAMP can raise or lower cardiac actomyosin ATPase activity depending on α-adrenergic activity. *Am J Physiol* 1994;36:H431–H442.
349. McClellan G, Weisberg A, Winegrad S. Endothelin regulation of cardiac contractility in the absence of added endothelin. *Am J Physiol* 1995;268:H1621–H1627.
350. McDonald TF, Pelzer S, Trautwein W, Pelzer DJ. Regulation and modulation of calcium channels in cardiac, skeletal, and smooth muscle cells. *Physiol Rev* 1994;74:365–507.
351. McNally EM, Kraft R, Bravo-Zehnder M, Taylor DA, Leinwand LA. Full-length rat alpha and beta cardiac myosin heavy chain sequences: comparisons suggest a molecular basis for functional differences. *J Mol Biol* 1989;210:665–671.
352. McNeill JH, Muschek LD. Histamine effects on cardiac contractility, phosphorylase and adenyl cyclase. *J Mol Cell Cardiol* 1972;4:611–624.
353. McPherson PS, Campbell KP. The ryanodine receptor/Ca^{2+} release channel. *J Biol Chem* 1993;268:13765–13768.
354. Meissner G, McKinley D. Permeability of canine cardiac sarcoplasmic reticulum vesicles to K^+, Na^+, H^+, and Cl^-. *J Biol Chem* 1982;257:7704–7711.
355. Mejía-Alvarez R, Marban E. Mechanism of the increase in intracellular sodium during metabolic inhibition—direct evidence against mediation by voltage-dependent sodium channels. *J Mol Cell Cardiol* 1992;24:1307–1320.
356. Mercadier J-J, Lompré AM, Duc P, et al. Altered sarcoplasmic reticulum Ca^{2+}-ATPase gene expression in the human ventricle during end-stage heart failure. *J Clin Invest* 1990;85:305–309.
357. Merin RG, Kumazawa T, Honig CR. Reversible interaction between halothane and Ca2+ on cardiac actomyosin adenosine triphosphatase. *J Pharmacol Exp Ther* 1974;190:1–14.
358. Méry P-F, Pavoine C, Belhassen L, Pecker F, Fischmeister R. Nitric oxide regulates cardiac Ca^{2+} current. Involvement of cGMP-inhibited and cGMP-stimulated phosphodiesterases through guanylyl cyclase activation. *J Biol Chem* 1993;268:26286–26295.
359. Mészáros LG, Volpe P. Caffeine- and ryanodine-sensitive Ca^{2+} stores of canine cerebrum and cerebellum neurons. *Am J Physiol* 1991;261:C1048–C1054.
360. Meuse AJ, Perreault CL, Morgan JP. Pathophysiology of cardiac hypertrophy and failure of human working myocardium—abnormalities in calcium handling. *Basic Res Cardiol* 1992;87:223–233.
361. Miao N, Frazer MJ, Lynch C III. Anesthetic actions on Ca^{2+} uptake and Ca-ATPase activity of cardiac sarcoplasmic reticulum. In: Bosnjak ZJ, Kampine JP, eds. *Anesthesia and cardiovascular disease.* Advances in Pharmacology, vol 31. San Diego: Academic Press, 1994;145–165.
362. Miao N, Lynch C III. Effect of temperature on volatile anesthetic depression of myocardial contractions. *Anesth Analg* 1993;76: 366–371.
363. Milligan R, Whittaker M, Safer D. Molecular structure of F-actin and location of surface binding sites. *Nature* 1990;348:217–221.
364. Mitchell RD, Simmerman HKB, Jones LR. Ca^{2+} binding effects on protein conformation and protein interactions of canine cardiac calsequestrin. *J Biol Chem* 1988;263:1376–1381.
365. Miura Y, Kimura J. Sodium-calcium exchange current. Dependence on internal Ca and Na and competitive binding of external Na and Ca. *J Gen Physiol* 1989;93:1129–1145.
366. Miyata H, Lakatta EG, Stern MD, Silverman HS. Relation of mitochondrial and cytosolic free calcium to cardiac myocyte recovery after exposure to anoxia. *Circ Res* 1992;71:605–613.
367. Miyata H, Silverman HS, Sollott SJ, Lakatta EG, Stern MD, Hansford RG. Measurement of mitochondrial free Ca^{2+} concentration in living single rat cardiac myocytes. *Am J Physiol* 1991;261: H1123–H1134.
368. Moody CJ, Dashwood MR, Sykes RM, et al. Functional and autoradiographic evidence for endothelin 1 receptors on human and rat cardiac myocytes. *Circ Res* 1990;67:764–769.
369. Moorman JR, Kirsch GE, Lacerda AE, Brown AM. Angiotensin II modulates cardiac Na+ channels in neonatal rat. *Circ Res* 1989;65: 1804–1809.
370. Moravec CS, Bond M. Calcium is released from the junctional sarcoplasmic reticulum during cardiac muscle contraction. *Am J Physiol* 1991;260:H989–H997.
371. Moravec CS, Schluchter MD, Paranandi L, et al. Inotropic effects of angiotensin II on human cardiac muscle in vitro. *Circulation* 1990;82:1990.
372. Morgan JP. Abnormal intracellular modulation of calcium as a major cause of cardiac contractile dysfunction. *N Engl J Med* 1991; 325:625–632.
373. Moss R, Nwoye L, Greaser M. Substitution of cardiac troponin C into rabbit muscle does not alter the length dependence of Ca2+ sensitivity of tension. *J Physiol* 1991;440:273–289.
374. Mouren S, Baron J-F, Albo C, Szekely B, Arthaud M, Viars P. Effects of propofol and thiopental on coronary blood flow and myocardial performance in an isolated rabbit heart. *Anesthesiology* 1994;80:634–641.
375. Movsesian MA, Nishikawa M, Adelstein RS. Phosphorylation of phospholamban by calcium-activated, phospholipid-dependent protein kinase. *J Biol Chem* 1984;259:8029–8032.
376. Mullins LJ. The generation of electric currents in cardiac fibers by Na/Ca exchange. *Am J Physiol* 1979;236:C103–C110.
377. Murat I, Hoerter J, Ventura-Clapier R. Developmental changes in effects of halothane and isoflurane on contractile properties of rabbit cardiac skinned fibers. *Anesthesiology* 1990;73:137–145.
378. Murat I, Lechene P, Ventura-Clapier R. Effects of volatile anesthetics on mechanical properties of rat cardiac skinned fibers. *Anesthesiology* 1990;73:73–81.
379. Murat I, Ventura-Clapier R, Vassort G. Halothane, enflurane, and isoflurane decrease calcium sensitivity and maximal force in detergent-treated rat cardiac fibers. *Anesthesiology* 1988;69: 892–899.
380. Murry CE, Jennings RB, Reimer KA. Preconditioning with ischemia: a delay of lethal cell injury in ischemic myocardium. *Circulation* 1986;74:1124–1136.
381. Nakaya H, Tohse N, Kanno M. Electrophysiological derangements induced by lipid peroxidation in cardiac tissue. *Am J Physiol* 1987; 253:H1089–H1097.
382. Nakayama T, Fozzard HA. Adrenergic modulation of the transient outward current in isolated canine Purkinje cells. *Circ Res* 1988;62: 162–172.
383. Negretti N, O'Neill SC, Eisner DA. The relative contributions of different intracellular and sarcolemmal systems to relaxation in rat ventricular myocytes. *Cardiovasc Res* 1993;27:1826–1830.
384. Neubauer S, Newell JB, Ingwall JS. Metabolic consequences and predictability of ventricular fibrillation in hypoxia: a ^{31}P- and ^{23}Na-

magnetic resonance study of the isolated rat heart. *Circulation* 1992;86:302–310.

385. Neumann J, Schmitz W, Scholz H, von Meyerinck D, Doring V, Kalmar P. Increase in myocardial G proteins in heart failure. *Lancet* 1988;ii:936–937.
386. Nicoll DA, Longoni S, Philipson KD. Molecular cloning and functional expression of the cardiac sarcolemmal Na^+-Ca^{2+} exchanger. *Science* 1990;250:562–565.
387. Niggli E, Lederer WJ. Voltage-independent calcium release in heart muscle. *Science* 1990;250:565–568.
388. Nishizaka T, Yagi T, Tanaka Y, Ishiwata S. Right-handed rotation of an actin filament in an *in vitro* motile system. *Nature* 1993;361: 269–71.
389. Noland TA, Jr., Kuo JF. Protein kinase C phosphorylation of cardiac troponin I and troponin T inhibits Ca^{2+}-stimulated MgATPase activity in reconstituted actomyosin and isolated myofibrils, and decreases actin-myosin interactions. *J Mol Cell Cardiol* 1993; 25:53–65.
390. Noma A. ATP-regulated K^+ channels in cardiac muscle. *Nature* 1983;305:147–148.
391. Nosek TM, Williams MF, Zeigler ST, Godt RE. Inositol triphosphate enhances calcium release in skinned cardiac and skeletal muscle. *Am J Physiol* 1986;250:C807–C811.
392. Novitsky D, Human PA, Cooper DKC. Inotropic effect of triiodothyronine following myocardial ischemia and cardiopulmonary bypass: An experimental study in pigs. *Ann Thorac Surg* 1988;45:500–505.
393. Nuss HB, Houser SR. Sodium-calcium exchange-mediated contractions in feline ventricular myocytes. *Am J Physiol* 1992;263: H1161–H1169.
394. O'Rourke B, Reibel DK, Thomas AP. α-Adrenergic modification of the Ca^{2+} transient and contraction in single rat cardiomyocytes. *J Mol Cell Cardiol* 1992;24:809–820.
395. Ohnishi T, Pressman GS, Price HL. A possible mechanism of anesthetic-induced myocardial depression. *Biochem Biophys Res Commun* 1974;57:316–322.
396. Okazaki O, Suda N, Hongo K, Konishi M, Kurihara S. Modulation of Ca^{2+} transients and contractile properties by β-adrenoceptor stimulation in ferret ventricular muscles. *J Physiol* 1990;423: 221–240.
397. Olcese R, Usai C, Maestrone E, Nobile M. The general anesthetic propofol inhibits transmembrane calcium current in chick sensory neurons. *Anesth Analg* 1994;78:955–960.
398. Ono K, Trautwein W. Potentiation by cyclic GMP of β-adrenergic effect on Ca^{2+} current in guinea-pig ventricular cells. *J Physiol* 1991;443:387–404.
399. Orchard CH, Lakatta EG. Intracellular calcium transients and developed tension in rat heart muscle. *J Gen Physiol* 1985;86: 637–651.
400. Otsu K, Willard HF, Khanna VK, Zorzato F, Green NM, MacLennan DH. Molecular cloning of cDNA encoding of the Ca^{2+} release channel (ryanodine receptor) of rabbit cardiac muscle sarcoplasmic reticulum. *J Biol Chem* 1990;265:13472–13483.
401. Ouadid H, Seguin J, Dumuis A, Bockaert J, Nargeot J. Serotonin increases calcium current in human atrial myocytes via the newly described 5–hydroxytryptamine$_4$ receptors. *Mol Pharmacol* 1992; 41:346–351.
402. Pagani E, Julian F. Rabbit papillary muscle myosic isozymes and the velocity of muscle shortening. *Circ Res* 1984;54:586–594.
403. Pagel PS, Kampine JP, Schmeling WT, Warltier DC. Reversal of volatile anesthetic-induced depression of myocardial contractility by extracellular calcium also enhances left ventricular diastolic function. *Anesthesiology* 1993;78:141–154.
404. Pagel PS, Schmeling WT, Kampine JP, Warltier DC. Alteration of canine left ventricular diastolic function by intravenous anesthetics in vivo. Ketamine and propofol. *Anesthesiology* 1992;76: 419–425.
405. Pancrazio JJ, Frazer MJ, Lynch C, III. Barbiturate anesthetics depress the resting K^+ conductance of myocardium. *J Pharmacol Exp Ther* 1993;265:358–365.
406. Pancrazio JJ, Lynch C, III. Differential anesthetic-induced opening of calcium-dependent large conductance channels in isolated ventricular myocytes. *Pflugers Arch* 1994;429:134–136.
407. Pancrazio JJ, Lynch C, III. Effect of volatile anesthetics on cardiac calcium current kinetics. *Biophys J* 1994;66:A95.
408. Park WK, Lynch C, III. Propofol and thiopental depression of myocardial contractility—a comparative study of mechanical and electrophysiologic effects in isolated guinea pig ventricular muscle. *Anesth Analg* 1992;74:395–405.
409. Parratt JR. Protection of the heart by preconditioning: mechanisms and possibilities for pharmacologic exploitation. *Trends Pharmacol Sci* 1994;15:19–25.
410. Pask HT, England PJ, Prys-Roberts C. Effects of volatile inhalational anesthetic agents on isolated bovine cardiac myofibrillar ATPase. *J Mol Cell Cardiol* 1981;13:293–301.
411. Pate E, White H, Cooke R. Determination of the myosin step size from mechanical and kinetic data. *Proc Natl Acad Sci USA* 1993;90: 2451–2455.
412. Pery-man N, Chemla D, Coirault C, Suard I, Riou B, Lecarpentier Y. A comparison of cyclopiazonic acid and ryanodine effects on cardiac muscle relaxation. *Am J Physiol* 1993;265:H1364–H1372.
413. Peskoff A, Post JA, Langer GA. Sarcolemmal calcium binding sites in heart: II. Mathematical model for diffusion of calcium release from the sarcoplasmic reticulum into the diadic region. *J Membr Biol* 1992;129:59–69.
414. Pessah IN, Durie EM, Schiedt MJ, Zimanyi I. Anthraquinone-sensitized Ca^{2+} release channel from rat cardiac sarcoplasmic reticulum: possible receptor-mediated mechanism of doxorubicin cardiomyopathy. *Mol Pharmacol* 1990;37:503–514.
415. Pieske B, Hasenfuss G, Holubarsch C, Schwinger R, Bohm M, Just H. Alterations of the force-frequency relationship in the failing human heart depend on the underlying cardiac disease. *Basic Res Cardiol* 1992;87:213–221.
416. Piper H, Noll T, Siegmund B. Mitochondrial function in the oxygen depleted and reoxygenated myocardial cell. *Cardiovasc Res* 1994;28:1–15.
417. Poole-Wilson P, Holmberg S, Williams A. A possible molecular mechanism for 'stunning' of the myocardium. *Eur Heart J* 1991;12 Suppl F:25–29.
418. Porsius AJ, van Zwieten PA. Influence of halothane on calcium movements in isolated heart muscle and in isolated plasma membranes. *Arch Int Pharmacodyn* 1975;218:29–39.
419. Post JA, Langer GA. Sarcolemmal calcium binding sites in heart: I. Molecular origin in "gas dissected" sarcolemma. *J Membr Biol* 1992;129:49–57.
420. Potter JD, Gergely J. Troponin, tropomyosin, and actin interactions in the Ca^{2+} regulation of muscle contraction. *Biochemistry* 1974;13:2697–2703.
421. Potter JD, Gergely J. The calcium and magnesium binding sites on troponin and their role in the regulation of myofibrillar ATPase. *J Biol Chem* 1975;250:4628–4633.
422. Price HL. Calcium reverses myocardial depression caused by halothane: site of action. *Anesthesiology* 1974;41:576–579.
423. Price HL. Myocardial depression by nitrous oxide and its reversal by Ca^{++}. *Anesthesiology* 1976;44:211–215.
424. Price HL, Helrich M. The effect of cyclopropane, diethyl ether, nitrous oxide, thiopental, and hydrogen ion concentration on the myocardial function of the dog heart-lung preparation. *J Pharmacol Exp Ther* 1955;115:206–216.
425. Rayment I, Holden HM, Whittaker M, et al. Structure of the actin-myosin complex and implications for muscle contraction. *Science* 1993;261:58–65.
426. Reuter H, Scholz H. The regulation of the calcium conductance of cardiac muscle by adrenaline. *J Physiol* 1977;264:49–62.
427. Reves JG, Kissin I, Fournier SE. Negative inotropic effects of midazolam. *Anesthesiology* 1984;60:517–518.
428. Rhee SG, Kim H, Suh P-G, Choi WC. Multiple forms of phosphoinositide-specific phospholipase C and different modes of activation. *Biochem Soc Trans* 1991;19:337–341.
429. Riou B, Besse S, Lecarpentier Y, Viars P. *In vitro* effects of propofol on rat myocardium. *Anesthesiology* 1992;76:609–616.
430. Riou B, Lecarpentier Y, Chemla D, Viars P. Inotropic effect of ketamine on rat cardiac papillary muscle. *Anesthesiology* 1989;71: 116–125.
431. Riou B, Lecarpentier Y, Chemla D, Viars P. *In vitro* effects of etomidate on intrinsic myocardial contractility in rat. *Anesthesiology* 1990;72:330–340.
432. Riou B, Lecarpentier Y, Viars P. Effects of etomidate on the cardiac papillary muscle of normal hamsters and those with cardiomyopathy. *Anesthesiology* 1993;78:83–90.
433. Robertson S, Johnson J, Holroyde M, Kranias E, Potter J, Solaro R. The effect of troponin I phosphorylation on the Ca2+-binding properties of the Ca2+-regulatory site of bovine cardiac troponin. *J Biol Chem* 1982;257:260–263.

434. Robinson M, Harrison SM, Winlow W, Hopkins PM, Boyett MR. The effect of halothane on intracellular calcium and contraction in ventricular cells from rat hearts. *J Physiol* 1993;473:110P.
435. Rusy BF, Amuzu JK, Bosscher HA, Redon D, Komai H. Negative inotropic effect of ketamine in rabbit ventricular muscle. *Anesth Analg* 1990;71:275–278.
436. Rusy BF, Komai H. Anesthetic depression of myocardial contractility: a review of possible mechanisms. *Anesthesiology* 1987;67: 745–766.
437. Rusy BF, Thomas-King PY, King GP, Komai H. Effects of propofol on the contractile state of isolated rabbit papillary rabbit muscles under various stimulation conditions. *Anesthesiology* 1990;73:A559.
438. Saeki Y, Kurihara S, Hongo K, Tanaka E. Alterations in intracellular calcium and tension of activated ferret papillary muscle in response to step length changes. *J Physiol* 1993;463:291–306.
439. Saeki Y, Shiozawa K, Yanagisawa K, Shibata T. Adrenaline increases the rate of cross-bridge cycling in rat cardiac muscle. *J Mol Cell Cardiol* 1990;22:453–460.
440. Sagawa K, Maughan L, Suga H, Sunagawa K. *Cardiac contraction and the pressure-volume relationship.* New York: Oxford University Press, 1988.
441. Sagawa K, Maughan L, Suga H, Sunagawa K. Energetics of the Heart. In: *Cardiac contraction and the pressure-volume relationship.* New York: Oxford University Press, 1988;171–231.
442. Salt PJ, Barnes PK, Beswick FJ. Inhibition of neuronal and extraneuronal uptake of noradrenaline by ketamine in the isolated perfused rat heart. *Br J Anaesth* 1979;51:835–838.
443. Sando JJ, Maurer MC, Bolen EJ, Grisham CM. Role of cofactors in protein kinase C activation. *Cell Signal* 1992;4:595–609.
444. Satoh H, Hayashi H, Katoh H, Terada H, Kobayashi A. Na^+/H^+ and Na^+/Ca^{2+} exchange in regulation of $[Na^+]_i$ and $[Ca^{2+}]_i$ during metabolic inhibition. *Am J Physiol* 1995;268:H1239–H1248.
445. Scamps F, Nilius B, Alvarez J, Vassort G. Modulation of L-type Ca channel activity by P_2-purinergic agonist in cardiac cells. *Pflugers Arch* 1993;422:465–471.
446. Scarpa A, Graziotti P. Mechanisms for intracellular calcium regulation in heart. I. Stopped-flow measurements of Ca uptake by cardiac mitochondria. *J Gen Physiol* 1973;62:756–772.
447. Schmidt U, Schwinger RHG, Böhm M. Halothane restores the altered force-frequency relationship in failing human myocardium. *Anesthesiology* 1995;82:1456–1462.
448. Schmidt U, Schwinger RHG, Böhm M. Interaction of halothane with inhibitory G-proteins in the human myocardium. *Anesthesiology* 1995;83:353–360.
449. Schmidt U, Schwinger RHG, Böhm S, et al. Evidence for an interaction of halothane with the L-type Ca^{2+} channel in human myocardium. *Anesthesiology* 1993;79:332–339.
450. Scholz W, Albus U, Linz W, Martorana P, Lang HJ, Schölkens BA. Effects of Na^+/H^+ exchange inhibitors in cardiac ischemia. *J Mol Cell Cardiol* 1992;24:731–740.
451. Schröder RR, Manstein DJ, Jahn W, et al. Three-dimensional atomic model of F-actin decorated with *Dictyostelium* myosin S1. *Nature* 1993;364:171–174.
452. Schümann HJ, Wagner J, Knorr A, Reidemeister JC, Sadony V, Schramm G. Demonstration in human atrial preparations of α-adrenoceptors mediating positive inotropic effects. *Naunyn Schmiedebergs Arch Pharmacol* 1978;302:333–338.
453. Schwinger RH, Böhm M, Erdmann E. Evidence against spare or uncoupled beta-adrenoceptors in the human. *Am Heart J* 1990; 119:899–904.
454. Schwinn DA, Caron MG, Lefkowitz RJ. The beta-adrenergic receptor as a model for molecular structure-function relationships in G-protein-coupled receptors. In: Fozzard HA, ed. *The heart and cardiovascular system.* New York: Raven Press, 1991;
455. Scott BT, Simmerman HKB, Collins JH, Nadal-Ginard B, Jones LR. Complete amino acid sequence of canine cardiac calsequestrin deduced by cDNA cloning. *J Biol Chem* 1988;263:8958–8964.
456. Seibel K, Karema E, Takeya K, Reiter M. Effects of noradrenaline on an early and late component of the myocardial contraction. *Naunyn Schmiedebergs Arch Pharmacol* 1978;305:65–74.
457. Servin F, Desmonts JM, Haberer JP, Cockshott ID, Plummer GF, Farinotti R. Pharmacokinetics and protein binding of propofol in patients with cirrhosis. *Anesthesiology* 1988;69:887–891.
458. Sham JSK, Cleeman L, Morad M. Gating of the cardiac Ca^{2+} release channel: the role of Na^+ current and Na^+-Ca^{2+} exchange. *Science* 1992;255:850–853.
459. Sham JSK, Jones LR, Morad M. Phospholamban mediates the β-adrenergic-enhanced Ca^{2+} uptake in mammalian ventricular myocytes. *Am J Physiol* 1991;261:H1344–H1349.
460. Shattock MJ, Bers DM. Rat vs. rabbit ventricle: Ca flux and intracellular Na assessed by ion-selective microelectrodes. *Am J Physiol* 1989;256:C813–C822.
461. Shibata T, Blanck TJJ, Sagawa K, Hunter WC. Effect of volatile anesthetics on dynamic stiffness of cardiac muscle in Ba^{2+} contracture. *Anesthesiology* 1989;67:496–502.
462. Shimosato S, Sugai N, Etsten BE. The effect of methoxyflurane on the inotropic state of the myocardium. *Anesthesiology* 1969;30: 506–512.
463. Shimosato S, Sugai N, Iwatsuki N, Etsten BE. The effect of Ethrane on cardiac muscle mechanics. *Anesthesiology* 1969;30:513–518.
464. Shryock J, Song Y, Wang D, Baker SP, Olsson RA, Belardinelli L. Selective α_2-adenosine receptor agonists do not alter action potential duration, twitch shortening, or cAMP accumulation in guinea pig, rat, or rabbit isolated ventricular myocytes. *Circ Res* 1993;72:194–205.
465. Siegmund B, Zude R, Piper HM. Recovery of anoxic-reoxygenated cardiomyocytes from severe Ca^{2+} overload. *Am J Physiol* 1992;263: H1262–H1269.
466. Simmerman HKB, Collins JH, Theibert JL, Wegener AD, Jones LR. Sequence analysis of phospholamban. *J Biol Chem* 1986; 261:13333–13341.
467. Sitsapesan R, Montgomery RAP, MacLeod KT, Williams AJ. Sheep cardiac sarcoplasmic reticulum calcium-release channels: modulation of conductance and gating by temperature. *J Physiol* 1991; 434:469–488.
468. Sitsapesan R, Williams AJ. Mechanisms of caffeine activation of single calcium-release channels of sheep cardiac sarcoplasmic reticulum. *J Physiol* 1990;423:425–439.
469. Smrcka AV, Hepler JR, Brown KO, Sternweiss PC. Regulation of polyphosphoinositide-specific phospholipase C activity by purified G_q. *Science* 1991;251:804–807.
470. Sommer JR, Jennings RB. Ultrastructure of cardiac muscle. In: Fozzard HA, Haber E, Jennings RB, Katz AM, Morgan HE, eds. *The heart and cardiovascular system—scientific foundations.* New York: Raven Press, 1991;3–50.
471. Sonnenblick EH. Determinants of active state in heart muscle; force, velocity, instantaneous muscle length, time. *Fed Proc* 1964; 24:1396–1409.
472. Starling EH. *The Linacre lecture of the law of the heart.* London: Longmans Green, 1918.
473. Steenbergen C, Perlman ME, London RE, Murphy E. Mechanism of preconditioning - ionic alterations. *Circ Res* 1993;72:112–125.
474. Sterling K, Brenner MA, Sakurada T. Rapid effect of triiodothyronine on the mitochondrial pathway in rat liver in vivo. *Science* 1980;210:340–342.
475. Sterling K, Lazarus JH, Milch PO, Sakurada T, Brenner MA. Mitochondrial thyroid hormone receptor: localization and physiological significance. *Science* 1978;201:1126–1129.
476. Stern MD. Theory of excitation-contraction coupling in cardiac muscle. *Biophys J* 1992;63:497–517.
477. Stern MD, Lakatta EG. Excitation-contraction coupling in the heart: the state of the question. *FASEB J* 1992;6:3092–3100.
478. Sternweis PC, Smrcka AV. Regulation of phospholipase C by G proteins. *Trends Biochem Sci* 1992;17:502–506.
479. Stirt JA, Berger JM, Roe SD, Ricker SM, Sullivan SF. Cardiovascular effects of ketamine following administration of aminophylline in dogs. *Anesth Analg* 1982;61:685–688.
480. Stowe DF, Marijic J, Bosnjak ZJ, Kampine JP. Direct comparative effects of halothane, enflurane, and isoflurane on oxygen supply and demand in isolated hearts. *Anesthesiology* 1991;74:1087–1095.
481. Stowe DF, Monroe S, Marijic J, Rooney RT, Bosnjak ZJ, Kampine JP. Effects of nitrous oxide on contractile function and metabolism of the isolated heart. *Anesthesiology* 1990;73:1220–1226.
482. Stowe DF, Monroe SM, Marijic J, Bosnjak ZJ, Kampine JP. Comparison of halothane, enflurane, and isoflurane with nitrous oxide on contractility and oxygen supply. *Anesthesiology* 1991;75: 1062–1074.
483. Strand MA, Louis CF, Mickelson JR. Phosphorylation of the porcine skeletal and cardiac muscle sarcoplasmic reticulum ryanodine receptor. *Biochim Biophys Acta* 1993;1175:319–326.
484. Studer R, Reinecke H, Bilger J, et al. Gene expression of the cardiac Na^+-Ca^{2+} exchanger in end-stage human heart failure. *Circ Res* 1994;75:443–453.

485. Su JY, Bell JG. Intracellular mechanism of action of isoflurane and halothane on striated muscle of the rabbit. *Anesth Analg* 1986;65: 457–462.
486. Su JY, Kerrick WGL. Effects of halothane on Ca2+-activated tension development in mechanically disrupted rabbit myocardial fibers. *Pflugers Arch* 1978;375:111–117.
487. Su JY, Kerrick WGL. Effects of halothane on caffeine-induced tension transients in functionally skinned myocardial fibers. *Pflugers Arch* 1979;380:29–34.
488. Su JY, Kerrick WGL. Effects of enflurane on functionally skinned myocardial fibers from rabbits. *Anesthesiology* 1980;52:385–389.
489. Su JY, Kerrick WGL, Hill SA. Effects of diethyl ether and nitrous oxide on functionally skinned myocardial cells of rabbits. *Anesth Analg* 1984;63:451–455.
490. Sugai N, Shimasato S, Etsten BE. Effect of halothane on force-velocity relations and dynamic stiffness of isolated heart muscle. *Anesthesiology* 1968;29:267–274.
491. Susanni EE, Manders WT, Vatner DE, Vatner SF, Homcy CJ. One hour of myocardial ischemia decreases the activity of the stimulatory guanine-nucleotide regulatory protein G_s. *Circ Res* 1989;65: 1145–1150.
492. Sys SU, Housmans PR, Van Ocken ER, Brutsaert DL. Mechanisms of hypoxia-induced decrease of load dependence of relaxation in cat papillary muscle. *Pflugers Arch* 1984;401:368–373.
493. Takahashi H, Puttick RM, Terrar DA. The effects of propofol and enflurane on single calcium channel currents of guinea-pig isolated ventricular myocytes. *Br J Pharmacol* 1994;111:1147–1153.
494. Takasago T, Imagawa T, Shigekawa M. Phosphorylation of the cardiac ryanodine receptor by cAMP-dependent kinase. *J Biochem (Tokyo)* 1989;106:872–877.
495. Tanabe T, Beam KG, Adams BA, Niidome T, Numa S. Regions of the skeletal muscle dihydropyridine receptor critical for excitation-contraction coupling. *Nature* 1990;346:567–569.
496. Tani M, Neely JR. Role of intracellular Na^+ in Ca^{2+} overload and depressed recovery of ventricular function of reperfused ischemic rat hearts: possible involvement of H^+-Na^+ and Na^+-Ca^{2+} exchange. *Circ Res* 1989;65:1045–1056.
497. Tanz RD, Heskett T, Loehning RW, Fairfax CA. Comparative cardiotoxicity of bupivacaine and lidocaine in the isolated perfused mammalian heart. *Anesth Analg* 1984;63:549–556.
498. Tao T, Gong BJ, Leavis P. Calcium-induced movement of troponin-I relative to actin in skeletal muscle thin filaments. *Science* 1990;247:1339–1341.
499. Tavernier BM, Adnet PJ, Imbenotte M, et al. Halothane and isoflurane decrease calcium sensitivity and maximal force in human skinned cardiac fibers. *Anesthesiology* 1994;80:625–633.
500. ter Keurs HEDJ, Rijnsburger WH, van Heuningen R, Nagelsmit MJ. Tension development and sarcomere length in rat cardiac trabeculae. Evidence of length dependent activation. *Circ Res* 1980;46:703–714.
501. Terrar DA, Victory JGG. Effects of halothane on membrane currents associated with contraction in single myocytes isolated from guinea-pig ventricle. *Br J Pharmacol* 1988;94:500–508.
502. Terrar DA, Victory JGG. Isoflurane depresses membrane currents associated with contractions in myocytes isolated from guinea-pig ventricle. *Anesthesiology* 1988;69:742–749.
503. Terrar DA, Victory JGG. Influence of halothane on contraction at positive membrane potentials in single cells isolated from guinea-pig ventricular muscle. *J Exp Physiol* 1989;74:141–151.
504. Terrar DA, White E. Mechanisms and significance of calcium entry at positive membrane potentials in guinea-pig ventricular muscle cells. *J Exp Physiol* 1989;74:121–139.
505. Terzic A, Pucéat M, Clément O, Scamps F, Vassort G. α_1-Adrenergic effects on intracellular pH and calcium and on myofilaments in single rat cardiac cells. *J Physiol* 1992;447:275–292.
506. Than H, Orchard CH. The effect of acidosis and hypoxia on the response of cardiac muscle isolated from ferret hearts to noradrenaline. *J Physiol* 1991;435:98P.
507. Thomas JA, Marks BH. Plasma norepinephrine in congestive heart failure. *Am J Cardiol* 1978;41:233–243.
508. Tohse N, Hattori Y, Nakaya H, Endou M, Kanno M. Inability of endothelin to increase Ca^{2+} current in guinea-pig heart cells. *Br J Pharmacol* 1990;99:437–438.
509. Tohse N, Kameyama M, Sekiguchi K, Shearman MS, Kanno M. Protein kinase C activation enhances the delayed rectifier potassium current in guinea-pig heart cells. *J Mol Cell Cardiol* 1990;22: 725–734.
510. Tomlins B, Williams AJ. Solubilisation and reconstitution of the rabbit skeletal muscle sarcoplasmic reticulum K^+ channel into liposomes suitable for patch clamp studies. *Pflugers Arch* 1986; 407:341–347.
511. Trayer IP. Molecular motors: coming soon-the movie. *Science* 1993;Nature:101–103.
512. Tsuchida A, Liu Y, Liu GS, Cohen MV, Dowmeny JM. α_1-Adrenergic agonists precondition rabbit ischemic myocardium independent of adenosine by direct activation of protein kinase C. *Circ Res* 1994;75:576–585.
513. Tsuchida A, Yang X-M, Burckhartt B, Mullane KM, Cohen MV, Downey JM. Acadesine extends the window of protection afforded by ischemic preconditioning. *Cardiovasc Res* 1994;28:379–383.
514. Unger T, Gohlke P. Coverting enzyme inhibitors in cardiovascular therapy: current status and future potential. *Cardiovasc Res* 1994;28:146–158.
515. Valdivia HH, Kaplan JH, Ellis-Davies GHR, Lederer WJ. Rapid adaptation of cardiac ryanodine receptors: modulation by Mg^{2+} and phosphorylation. *Science* 1995;267:1997–2000.
516. Van den Berghe G, de Zegher F, Lauwers P. Dopamine and the sick euthyroid syndrome in critical illness. *Clin Endo* 1994;41: 731–737.
517. Van Hardeveld C, Schouten VJA, Muller A, van der Meulen ET, Elzinga G. Exposure of energy-depleted rat trabeculae to low pH improves contractile recovery: role of calcium. *Am J Physiol* 1995; 268:H1510–H1520.
518. Vassalle M, Bhattacharyya M. Local anesthetics and the role of sodium in the force development by canine ventricular muscle and Purkinje fibers. *Circ Res* 1980;47:666–674.
519. Vatner D, Kiuchi K, Manders W, Vatner S. Effects of coronary arterial reperfusion on β-adrenergic receptor-adenylyl cyclase coupling. *Am J Physiol* 1993;264:H196–H204.
520. Ver Donck L, Borgers M, Verdonck F. Inhibition of sodium and calcium overload pathology in the myocardium: a new cytoprotective principle. *Cardiovasc Res* 1993;27:349–357.
521. Visentin S, Wu S-N, Belardinelli L. Adenosine-induced changes in atrial action potential: contribution of Ca and K currents. *Am J Physiol* 1990;258:H1070–H1078.
522. Vleugels A, Vereeke J, Carmeliet E. Ionic currents during hypoxia in voltage-clamped cat ventricular muscle. *Circ Res* 1980; 47:501–508.
523. Vogel S, Sperelakis N. Blockade of myocardial slow inward current at low pH. *Am J Physiol* 1977;233:C99–C103.
524. Wagenknecht T, Grassucci R, Frank J, Saito A, Inui M, Fleischer S. Three-dimensional architecture of the calcium channel/foot structure of sarcoplasmic reticulum. *Nature* 1989;338:167–170.
525. Wahler GM, Dollinger SJ. Nitric oxide donor SIN-1 inhibits mammalian cardiac calcium current through cGMP-dependent protein kinase. *Am J Physiol* 1995;268:C45–C54.
526. Walsh KB, Begenisich TB, Kass RS. β-Adrenergic modulation in the heart: independent regulation of K and Ca channels. *Pflugers Arch* 1988;411:232–234.
527. Walsh KB, Kass RS. Regulation of a heart potassium channel by protein kinase A and C. *Science* 1988;242:67–69.
528. Wang D, Belardinelli L. Mechanism of the negative inotropic effect of adenosine in guinea pig atrial myocytes. *Am J Physiol* 1994;267:H2420–H2429.
529. Wang DY, Chae SW, Gong QY, Lee CO. Role of a^i_{Na} the positive force-frequency staircase in guinea-pig pappillary muscle. *Am J Physiol* 1988;255:C798–C807.
530. Wang J, Morgan JP. Endothelin reverses the effects of acidosis on the intracellular Ca^{2+} transient and contractility in ferret myocardium. *Circ Res* 1992;71:631–639.
531. Wang J, Paik G, Morgan JP. Endothelin 1 enhances myofilament Ca^{2+} responsiveness in aequorin-loaded ferret myocardium. *Circ Res* 1991;69:582–589.
532. Wang K, Villalobo A, Roufogalis B. The plasma membrane calcium pump: a multiregulated transporter. *Trends Cell Biol* 1992;2: 46–51.
533. Wang Y-P, Fuchs F. Length, force, and Ca^{2+}-troponin C affinity in cardiac and slow skeletal muscle. *Am J Physiol* 1994;266: C1077–C1082.
534. Wang Z, Gergely J, Tao T. Characterization of the Ca^{2+}-triggered conformational transition in troponin C. *Proc Natl Acad Sci USA* 1992;89:11814–11817.
535. Waxman K, Shoemaker WC, Lippman M. Cardiovascular effects of anesthetic induction with ketamine. *Anesth Analg* 1980;59:355–358.

536. Weber KT. Cardiac interstitium in health and disease: the fibrillar collagen network. *J Am Coll Cardiol* 1989;13:1637–1652.
537. Weiss JN, Vankatesh, N., Lamp, S.T. ATP-sensitive K+ channels and cellular K+ loss in hypoxic and ischaemic mammalian ventricle. *J Physiol* 1992;447:649–673.
538. Wendt-Gallitelli MF, Isenberg G. Total and free myoplasmic calcium during a contraction cycle: x-ray microanalysis in guinea-pig ventricular myocytes. *J Physiol* 1991;435:349–372.
539. Wendt-Gallitelli MF, Jacob R. Rhythm-dependent role of different calcium stores in cardiac muscle: x-ray microanalysis. *J Mol Cell Cardiol* 1982;14:487–492.
540. Wertman K, Drubin D. Actin constitution: guaranteeing the right to assemble. *Science* 1992;258:750–60.
541. Wetzel GT, Chen F, Klitzner TS. Na^+/Ca^{2+} exchange and cell contraction in isolated neonatal and adult rabbit cardiac myocytes. *Am J Physiol* 1995;268:H1723–H1733.
542. Wheeler DM, Katz A, Rice RT. Effects of volatile anesthetics on cardiac sarcoplasmic reticulum as determined in intact cells. In: Blanck TJJ, Wheeler DM, eds. *Mechanisms of anesthetic action in skeletal, cardiac and smooth muscle.* New York: Plenum Press, 1991; 143–154.
543. Wheeler DM, Katz A, Rice RT, Hansford RG. Volatile anesthetic effects on sarcoplasmic reticulum Ca content and sarcolemmal Ca flux in isolated rat cardiac cell suspensions. *Anesthesiology* 1994;80: 372–382.
544. Wheeler DM, Rice RT, Hansford RG, Lakatta EG. The effect of halothane on the free intracellular calcium concentration of isolated rat heart cells. *Anesthesiology* 1988;69:578–583.
545. Wheeler DM, Rice RT, Lakatta EG. The action of halothane on spontaneous contractile waves and stimulated contractions in isolated rat and dog heart cells. *Anesthesiology* 1990;72:911–920.
546. White PF. Ketamine update: its clinical uses in anesthesia. *Semin Anesth* 1988;7:113–126.
547. Wier WG. Calcium transients during excitation-contraction coupling in mammalian heart: aequorin signals of canine Purkinje fibers. *Science* 1980;207:1085–1087.
548. Wier WG. Cytoplasmic $[Ca^{2+}]$ in mammalian ventricle: dynamic control by cellular processes. *Annu Rev Physiol* 1990;52:467–485.
549. Wier WG, Egan TM, Lopez-Lopez JR, Balke CW. Local control of excitation-contraction coupling in rat heart cells. *J Physiol* 1994; 474:463–471.
550. Wier WG, Yue DT. Intracellular calcium transients underlying the short-term force-interval relationship in ferret ventricular myocardium. *J Physiol* 1986;376:507–530.
551. Wilde AAM, Janse MJ. Electrophysiological effects of ATP sensitive potassium channel modulation: implications for arrhythmogenesis. *Cardiovasc Res* 1994;28:16–24.
552. Wilde DW, Davidson BA, Smith MD, Knight PR. Effects of isoflurane and enflurane on intracellular Ca^{2+} mobilization in isolated cardiac myocytes. *Anesthesiology* 1993;79:73–82.
553. Wilde DW, Knight PR, Sheth N, Williams BA. Halothane alters control of intracellular Ca^{2+} mobilization in single rat ventricular myocytes. *Anesthesiology* 1991;75:1075–1086.
554. Williams TL, Lefkowitz RJ. Thyroid hormone regulation of β-adrenergic receptors number. *J Biol Chem* 1977;252:2787–2789.
555. Williamson AP, Kennedy RH, Seifen E, Lindemann JP, Stimers JR. α_{1b}-Adrenoceptor-mediated stimulation of Na-K pump current in adult rat ventricular myocytes. *Am J Physiol* 1993;264: H1315–H1318.
556. Witcher DR, Kovacs RJ, Schulman H, Cefali DC, Jones LR. Unique phosphorylation site on the cardiac ryanodine receptor regulates calcium channel activity. *J Biol Chem* 1991;266: 11114–11152.
557. Wolf WJ, Neal MB, Matthew BP, Bee DE. Comparison of the in vitro myocardial depressant effects of isoflurane and halothane anesthesia. *Anesthesiology* 1988;69:660–666.
558. Wolska BM, Lewartowski B. Calcium in the *in situ* mitochondria of rested and stimulated myocardium. *J Mol Cell Cardiol* 1991;23: 217–226.
559. Wolska BM, Lewartowski B. The role of sarcoplasmic reticulum and Na-Ca exchange in the Ca^{2+} extrusion from the resting myocytes of guinea-pig heart: comparison with rat. *J Mol Cell Cardiol* 1993;25:75–91.
560. Xiao P-P, Lakatta EG. β_1-Adrenoceptor stimulation and β_2-adrenoceptor stimulation differ in their effects on contraction, cytosolic Ca^{2+}, and Ca^{2+} current in single rat ventricular cells. *Circ Res* 1993;73:286–300.
561. Xiao R-P, Spurgeon HA, Capogrossi MC, Lakatta EG. Stimulation of opioid receptors on cardiac ventricular myocytes reduces L type Ca^{2+} channel current. *J Mol Cell Cardiol* 1993;25:661–666.
562. Xiao RP, Cheng HP, Lederer WJ, Suzuki T, Lakatta EG. Dual regulation of Ca^{2+}/calmodulin-dependent kinase-II activity by membrane voltage and by calcium influx. *Proc Natl Acad Sci USA* 1994; 91:9659–9663.
563. Xu A, Hawkins C, Narayanan N. Phosphorylation and activation of the Ca^{2+} -pumping ATPase of cardiac sarcoplasmic reticulum by Ca^{2+}/calmodulin-dependent protein kinase. *J Biol Chem* 1993; 268:8394–8397.
564. Yan G-X, Kléber AG. Changes in extracellular and intracellular pH in ischemic rabbit papillary muscle. *Circ Res* 1992;71:460–470.
565. Yanagida T, Ishijima A. Forces and steps generated by single myosin molecules. *Biophys J* 1985;68:312s-320s.
566. Yatani A, Brown AM. Rapid β-adrenergic modulation of cardiac calcium channel currents by a fast G protein pathway. *Science* 1989;245:71–74.
567. Yatani A, Codina J, Imoto Y, Reeves JP, Birnbaumer L, Brown AM. A G protein directly regulates mammalian cardiac calcium channels. *Science* 1987;238:1288–1292.
568. Yoshida A, Takahashi M, Imagawa T, Shigekawa M, Takisawa H, Nakamura T. Phosphorylation of ryanodine receptors during β-adrenergic stimulation. *J Biochem (Tokyo)* 1992;111:186–190.
569. Ytrehus K, Liu Y, Downey J. Preconditioning protects ischemic rabbit heart by protein kinase C activation. *Am J Physiol* 1994;266: H1145–H1152.
570. Yuan W, Bers DM. Ca-dependent facilitation of cardiac Ca current is due to Ca-calmodulin-dependent protein kinase. *Am J Physiol* 1994;267:H982–H993.
571. Yue DT, Burkhoff D, Franz MR, Hunter WC, Sagawa K. Postextrasystolic potentiation of the isolated canine left ventricle. *Circ Res* 1985;56:340–350.
572. Yue DT, Herzig S, Marban E. β-Adrenergic stimulation of calcium channels occurs by potentiation of high-activity gating modes. *Proc Natl Acad Sci USA* 1990;87:753–757.
573. Zhang C-C, Su J, Calkins D. Effects of alfentanil on isolated cardiac tissues of the rabbit. *Anesth Analg* 1990;71:268–74.
574. Zhao M, Zhang H, Robinson TF, Factor SM, Sonnenblick EH, Eng C. Profound structural alterations of the extracellular collagen matrix in postischemic dysfunctional ("stunned") but viable myocardium. *J Am Coll Cardiol* 1987;10:1322–1334.
575. Zheng J-S, Christie A, Levy M, Scarpa A. Ca^{2+} mobilization by extracellular ATP in rat cardiac myocytes: regulation by protein kinase C and A. *Am J Physiol* 1992;263:C933–C940.
576. Zorzato F, Fujii J, Otsu K, et al. Molecular cloning of cDNA encoding human and rabbit forms of the Ca^{2+} release channel (ryanodine receptor) of skeletal muscle sarcoplasmic reticulum. *J Biol Chem* 1990;265:2244–2256.

Anesthesia: Biologic Foundations, edited by Tony L. Yaksh et al. Lippincott–Raven Publishers, Philadelphia © 1997.

CHAPTER 67

MECHANICAL FUNCTION OF THE LEFT VENTRICLE

PAUL S. PAGEL AND DAVID C. WARLTIER

Characterization of left ventricular function in the normal and diseased heart has traditionally centered on events that occur during systole. Within this framework, heart failure has been previously defined as the inability of the heart to generate sufficient output to meet the requirements of cellular metabolism. During the past two decades, however, it has become clear that the heart serves dual roles, propelling blood into the high pressure arterial vasculature during systole and collecting blood from the low pressure venous circulation during diastole. This duality has rendered definitions of congestive heart failure based solely on systolic dysfunction inadequate. Failure may result not only from impaired contractile performance resulting in passive obstruction to flow in the systemic or pulmonary venous circulation but also from diastolic dysfunction secondary to increased resistance to ventricular inflow and filling. In fact, clinical signs and symptoms of congestive heart failure may occur because of primary abnormalities in diastolic mechanics in the absence of or preceding significant derangement of systolic function (129,278,565). Comprehensive knowledge of left ventricular function during both systole and diastole creates a foundation for fundamental understanding of normal cardiac physiology and forms the basis for insight into pathophysiologic mechanisms and pharmacologic management of the failing heart. In this chapter, the term *ventricle* refers to the left ventricle unless otherwise specified.

FUNCTIONAL ANATOMY OF THE LEFT VENTRICLE

The complex architecture of the left ventricle allows this pump to efficiently propel blood into the high pressure arterial vasculature. The mitral and aortic valve annuli, the root of the aortic trunk, and the dense, fibrous connective tissue that connects these structures, including the central fibrous body and the left and right fibrous trigones, form the skeletal base of the left ventricle, located at its superior aspect. This cartilaginous skeleton supports the delicate, translucent, and macroscopically avascular mitral and aortic valves, resists the dilating forces of chamber pressure and blood flow, and provides an insertion site for superficial subepicardial muscle fibers (208,499). However, the majority of the left ventricular muscle mass arises as branches from surrounding myocardium and does not originate from the fibrous skeletal base of the heart (208), consistent with the embryologic origin of the heart as an expanded arterial blood vessel (280).

The mitral and aortic valves are remarkably durable structures that facilitate the unidirectional flow of blood through the left ventricle. The mitral valve has two leaflets or cusps (anterior and posterior) that act as passive flaps. Retrograde blood flow toward the valve during isovolumetric contraction and ejection expands the valve leaflets and forces them into direct apposition. The cusps are thickened slightly at the line of apposition and may also contain small fenestrations near the commissure. The mitral valve leaflets are tethered to the distal ventricular wall by thin fibrous threads, termed the chordae tendinae, which originate from the anterior and posterior papillary muscles and insert into the free margins of the corresponding mitral valve leaflets. The papillary muscles are outpouchings of anterior and posteroinferior subendocardial muscle that tighten the chordae tendinae and prevent inversion of the mitral valve and regurgitation of blood into the left atrium during left ventricular systole (312, 500). Clearly, papillary muscle ischemia or infarction may severely compromise the functional integrity of the mitral valve. The mitral valve annulus contracts slightly during systole via a sphincter like effect of the surrounding subepicardial musculature that decreases the cross-sectional area of the orifice and aids in valve closure (452). The aortic valve consists of three symmetric leaflets, the right (adjacent to the ostium of the right coronary artery), the left (adjacent to the ostium of the left main coronary artery), and the posterior (noncoronary) leaflets (4). These cusps open passively under the force of ventricular ejection to almost the entire cross-sectional area of the aortic valve annulus. Dilatations of the aortic root, termed the sinuses of Valsalva, are located immediately behind each cusp and prevent them from adhering to the aortic wall by establishing eddy currents of blood flow during ejection (561). These eddy currents in the sinuses of Valsalva also contribute to closure of the aortic valve leaflets at the termination of ejection (577).

The majority of the blood flow to the left ventricle occurs in diastole when aortic pressure exceeds the intracavitary pressure within this chamber and establishes a positive pressure gradient in each coronary artery. All three major coronary arteries contribute to the blood supply of the left ventricle and, therefore, coronary artery stenosis or occlusion may result in a predictable pattern of left ventricular injury based on their known distribution of supply. The left anterior descending coronary artery and its branches supply the medial half of the anterior left ventricular wall, the apex, and the anterior two-thirds of the ventricular septum. The left circumflex coronary artery and its branches supply the anterior and posterior aspects of the lateral wall. The right coronary artery and its distal branches supply the medial portions of the posterior wall and the posterior one-third of the ventricular septum. Anastomoses between the distal regions of the coronary arteries also exist that may provide an alternative route of blood flow to myocardium distal to a severe coronary artery stenosis or complete occlusion (499).

Contrary to historical anatomic reports dating back to Vesalius and Harvey (231), there are no distinct bands or dividing septa in ventricular muscle that can be defined by unwinding dissection techniques (358,366,497,498). Instead, the left ventricular wall is a thick, fiber-wound continuum of interconnecting muscle fibers (587) characterized by well-ordered, differential alterations in fiber angle from the endocardium surface to epicardium (588). These myocardial fiber angles are maintained in a relatively constant spatial orientation despite changes in wall thickness that occur during the cardiac cycle. Subendocardial and subepicardial muscle fibers follow perpendicular, oblique, helical trajectories from the base to the apex with a reversal of the orientation of these interdigitating sheets occurring at the midaxis of the left ventricle resembling a flattened figure of eight (625), or perhaps more poetically, a raked turban (208). Contraction of these oblique subepicardial and subendocardial fibers causes shortening of the ventricular chamber along its longitudinal axis. In contrast, fibers of the midmyocardium are arranged in a primarily circumferential pattern around the diameter of the left ventricular cavity. Thus, contraction of the left ventricle reduces both the basal-apical length and the diameter of the chamber.

The walls of the left ventricle are thickest near the base and become progressively thin toward the apex. This decline in ventricular wall thickness occurs because reductions in midmyocardial circumferential fibers occur with confluence of the endocardial and epicardial layers at the apex. The ventricular septum is composed of the subendocardial muscle layers of the left and right ventricles and the midmyocardial circumferential fibers from the corresponding layer of the left ventricular free wall (208). Thus, the septum consists of structural elements that are primarily derived from the left ventricle and, not surprisingly, this region of ventricular myocardium contributes to a reduction in left ventricular chamber diameter during contraction. As observed in the ventricular free wall, the septum thickness decreases progressively toward the apex as the circumferential midmyocardial layer diminishes. In contrast to the apical free wall that is composed of subendocardial and subepicardial muscle fibers, however, the apical septum consists of the subendocardial layers of the right and left ventricles (208). Irregular ridges of subendocardium, termed trabeculae carnae, occur on the interior surface of the left ventricle and are typically observed in apical regions. The physiologic function of the trabeculae carnae is unknown. A layer of endocardial endothelium covers the subendocardial muscle on the surface of the left ventricular cavity and recent evidence suggests that this endocardial endothelium may play an important role in the control of myocardial performance in the intact heart (119).

During left ventricular contraction, the apex and ventricular septum remain relatively fixed in three-dimensional space within the mediastinum, while the lateral and posterior walls of the left ventricle shift anteriorly and to the right. These movements displace the longitudinal axis of the ventricular cavity from a line through the mitral valve in diastole to an orientation parallel to the ascending aorta during systole. This relative reorientation of the left ventricular longitudinal axis during the cardiac cycle may promote more effective diastolic filling and enhanced ejection (561). The left ventricular base also descends toward the apex during systole. This caudal movement of the heart results from subendocardial and subepicardial fiber shortening and from mechanical recoil that balances the force of expulsion of blood into the aorta. These gross cardiac movements are facilitated by the smooth visceral and parietal pericardium and the lubrication provided by the 30 to 50 ml of clear or straw-colored pericardial fluid that is normally contained in this serosal structure (499). Diseases of pericardium may affect the cyclical movement of the heart and may have important diastolic functional consequences (see below).

THE LAW OF LAPLACE

The contractile behavior of linear cardiac muscle preparations in vitro must be related to three-dimensional global left ventricular function in vivo in order to examine the ability of the intact heart to collect and propel blood. Although individual cardiac contractile elements develop tension and shorten during contraction and release tension and lengthen during relaxation, the heart as an organ generates pressure and causes ejection of a volume of blood. Changes in muscle tension and length must be transformed into changes in pressure and volume in the intact heart (189). The relationship between myocyte length and ventricular volume can be easily described if the left ventricle is modeled as a simple, pressurized, spherical shell (582). In a sphere, volume (V) is proportional to the cube of the radius (r):

$$V = F(4,3)\ \pi\ r^3$$

Volume is also related to the third power of the length around the ventricular cavity because circumference is equal to $2\pi r$. An ellipsoidal model of ventricular architecture defines three axes corresponding to the anterior-posterior diameter (D_{AP}), the lateral diameter (D_L), and the maximal long axis length (L_M). Ventricular volume is related to each of these dimensions by the formula:

$$V = F(\pi,6)\ D_{AP} \cdot D_L \cdot L_M$$

This technique of measuring left ventricular volume more closely approximates the actual ventricular geometry and has been extensively validated in experimental (95,96,346) and clinical settings (59,68,234).

The relationship between wall stress (tension exerted over a cross-sectional area) and pressure within the ventricle is complex. Three assumptions permit derivation of the law of Laplace, which relates wall stress to pressure and ventricular geometry (189). First, the left ventricular sphere is assumed to have a uniform wall thickness, h, and an internal radius, r. Second, the stress (σ) through the thickness of the ventricular wall is considered to be constant because the wall itself is assumed to be thin. Lastly, the ventricle is assumed to be at rest (i.e., static equilibrium exists for this model). Development of tension in each ventricular myocyte leads to increases in global wall stress during contraction of the ventricle and is translated into pressure within the ventricular cavity. Pressure is a distending force exerted at right angles to the ventricular walls, whereas wall stress is a shear force exerted around the circumference of the ventricle (189). Bisecting the ventricular sphere into two equal halves exposes the internal forces within the ventricular cavity (Fig. 1). The ventricular pressure (p) within the sphere times the internal wall cross-sectional area, πr^2, represents the total force tending to repel the upper and lower hemispheres. The two hemispheres are held together by the total force in the ventricular wall that is equal to the wall stress times the cross-sectional wall area. The two forces must balance such that

$$p\pi r^2 = \sigma[\pi\ (r + h)^2 - \pi r^2]$$

This equation can be algebraically simplified to

$$pr = \sigma\ h\ (2 + h/r)$$

Because the ventricular wall is thin, the ratio of thickness to the internal radius (h/r) must be much smaller than 2 and this term can be neglected. Thus,

$$\sigma = pr\ /2h$$

The law of Laplace for a thin-walled sphere relates the pressure in the left ventricle and its geometry to wall stress. The wall stress in this simple spherical model increases linearly with increases in internal pressure and radius and decreases as the wall becomes thicker. Although the ratio of wall thickness to radius (h/r) is approximately 0.4 at end diastole in the normal

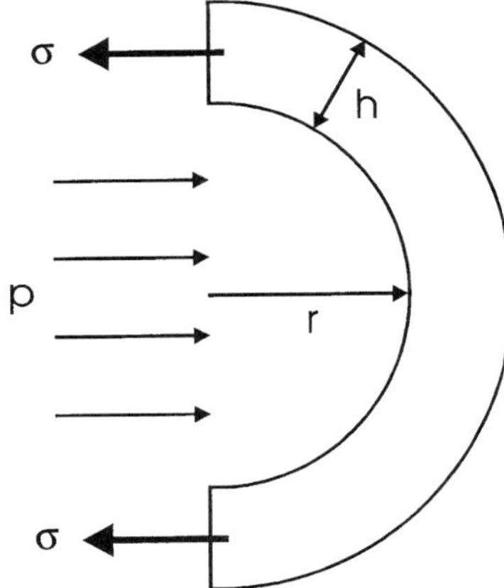

Figure 1. Opposing forces in a theoretical ventricular sphere. Ventricular pressure (p) tends to force the ventricle apart, whereas wall stress (σ) opposes this action. Ventricular radius = r; wall thickness = h. (From ref. 189, with permission.)

heart (524), the simple model of the law of Laplace defined above for a thin-walled sphere provides a useful approximation of relative changes in left ventricular wall stress (162). For example, dilatation of the ventricle (increases in cavity radius) leads directly to an increase in wall stress as well as increases in tension on each muscle fiber within the ventricular wall. Similarly, increases in ventricular pressure result in direct increases in wall stress. The increases in wall stress resulting from dilatation and/or hypertension are directly translated into increases in myocardial oxygen demand because the energy requirements of the myofilaments are greater in order to develop enhanced tension. In contrast, an increase in wall thickness (h) reduces wall stress and tension developed by individual muscle fibers. Thus, ventricular hypertrophy reduces the load on each muscle fiber and decreases wall stress according to the law of Laplace. Ellipsoidal models of ventricular geometry require more complex formulations of the law of Laplace (216,641) and are often corrected with actual dimensions measured by echocardiography (51).

Wall stress is not uniformly distributed across the thickness of the left ventricle in the intact heart (393). Wall stress is highest near the inner surface of the cavity, decreases across the thickness of the ventricular wall, and is lowest at the epicardial surface. These regional differences in wall stress became especially important in ventricular hypertrophy (212,216). Because subendocardial regions of the left ventricle develop higher stress than epicardial regions, the subendocardium is more susceptible to the detrimental consequences of rapid increases in interventricular pressure associated with chronic pressure overload states aortic stenosis or malignant hypertension. Higher wall stress and concomitant increases in oxygen demand also make the subendocardium more susceptible to ischemia. The combination of enhanced myocardial oxygen demand associated with increases in wall stress and decreases in compensatory oxygen supply associated with coronary artery stenosis may lead to the relatively common occurrence of subendocardial myocardial infarction despite the absence of total coronary artery occlusion.

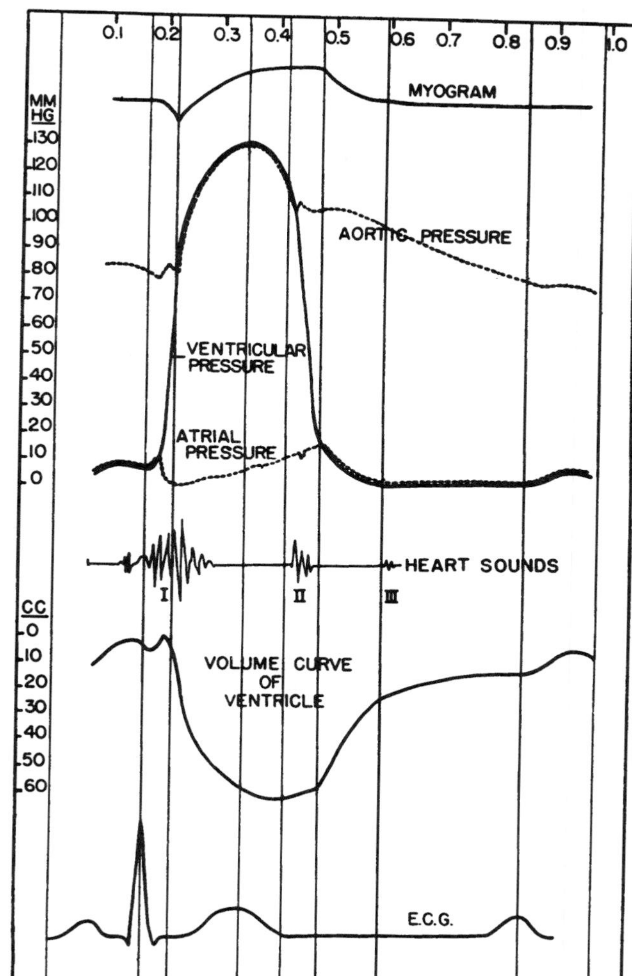

Figure 2. The cardiac cycle. Left ventricular pressure, aortic pressure, and left atrial pressure are correlated with ventricular volume, heart sounds, venous pulse, and the electrocardiogram. (From ref. 660, with permission.)

THE CARDIAC CYCLE

The left ventricular cardiac cycle initially depicted by Carl J. Wiggers (661) (Fig. 2) is composed of a combination of mechanical, electrical, and valvular events. At a sinus rate of 75 beats per minute, the complete cycle for filling and emptying takes approximately 800 msec. The contractile period of the left ventricle (systole) begins with the initial rise of ventricular pressure and closure of the mitral valve following ventricular depolarization (QRS complex). During systole when left ventricular pressure exceeds that in the aorta, there is an opening of the aortic valve and ejection of blood. Systole ends with closure of the aortic valve. Closure of the aortic valve also begins the period of diastole during which ventricular relaxation and filling occur. During normal sinus rhythm, systole and diastole compose approximately one-third and two-thirds of the cardiac cycle, respectively. At higher rates, significant reductions occur primarily in the time spent in diastole.

Under normal conditions, the atrial pressure waveform is composed of three major deflections (Fig. 2). After the P-wave of atrial depolarization is recorded electrocardiographically, the atria contract causing an "a" wave that occurs late in diastole. With initiation of systole, ventricular contraction causes a pressure wave to be transmitted in a retrograde fashion through the atrioventricular valve resulting in an increase in atrial pressure (atrial "c" wave). In the final portion of systole and continuing into early diastole, as venous blood returns from the periphery, atrial filling proceeds. The atrioventricular valve remains closed, and there is a slow increase in atrial pressure that results in the atrial "v" wave.

Ventricular systole is subdivided into a number of components. Isovolumetric contraction occurs between closure of the mitral valve and opening of the aortic valve, and little change in ventricular volume occurs during this period. However, the global geometry of the ventricle changes during isovolumetric contraction. The overall ellipsoidal shape of the ventricle at end diastole is transformed into a more spherical configuration because decreases in the longitudinal axis length occur concomitant with increases in wall thickness (64,523). The rate of upstroke of the ventricular pressure waveform becomes maximal during this time and is often used to estimate myocardial contractility in vivo (left ventricular peak positive dP/dt_{max}; see below). After opening of the aortic valve, a period of rapid ejection occurs. About two-thirds of the ventricular volume is emptied into the aorta during the period of rapid ejection. Ejection slows as ventricular and aortic pressures equalize and when aortic pressure exceeds left ventricular pressure, the aortic valve closes. Thus, the majority of ventricular volume is delivered to the aorta during the first third of ejection and the volume of blood propelled by the ventricle declines precipitously thereafter until the end of systole. The normal end-diastolic left ventricular volume (EDV) is approximately 120 ml and end-systolic volume (ESV) is 40 ml. Thus, normal stroke volume (SV) is about 80 ml and ejection fraction [(EDV – ESV)·100/EDV] is approximately 67% (159).

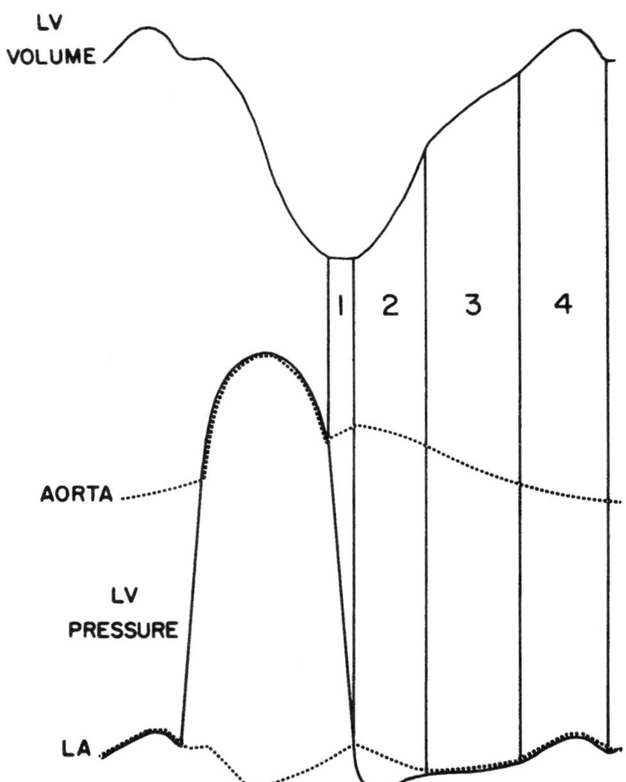

Figure 3. Left ventricular (LV) volume and pressure and aortic and left atrial (LA) pressure during the various phases of diastole: (1) isovolumetric relaxation, (2) rapid ventricular filling, (3) diastasis (slow ventricular filling), (4) atrial systole. (From ref. 458, with permission.)

Diastole is traditionally divided into four phases: isovolumetric relaxation, rapid ventricular filling, diastasis (slow ventricular filling), and atrial systole (Fig. 3). Isovolumetric relaxation begins with closure of the aortic valve and ends with opening of the mitral valve. During this phase, the ventricle is a closed chamber in which no change in volume (in the absence of mitral or aortic valve disease) occurs while intraventricular pressure abruptly decreases in an exponential fashion. Factors that influence the rate of isovolumetric pressure decline may later affect rapid ventricular filling upon opening of the mitral valve, but no actual filling occurs during isovolumetric relaxation (70–72).

The mitral valve opens when ventricular pressure falls below atrial pressure, and the next phase of diastole, rapid ventricular filling, begins. Ventricular pressure continues to decline despite opening early filling because there is continued myocardial relaxation and recoil of myocardial elastic components. These factors contribute to the creation of a pressure gradient between the atrium and ventricle. The rate of decrease of ventricular pressure and the level of atrial pressure when the mitral valve opens defines the extent of the pressure gradient between these chambers (98,258). After the mitral valve opens, the pressure gradient between the atrium and the ventricle depends on the pressures in these respective chambers at any instant in time. The rapid ventricular filling phase of diastole accounts for as much as 80% of the total stroke volume ejected during the next systole. The increase in ventricular volume occurs, to a large degree, while ventricular pressure continues to decrease (Fig. 3, early period of phase 2), emphasizing that relaxation and recoil of elastic elements compressed during the preceding systole continue after the mitral valve opens (111,290,515,516). Ventricular pressure will actually decline to a subatmospheric value if flow across the mitral valve is experimentally obstructed (627,673), implying that the ventricle will fill by a suction mechanism even if atrial pressure is zero (111,290,515,594,604,627,673). Recoil of myocardial elastic components probably produces this ventricular suction mechanism (416). The rapid ventricular filling phase ends with equilibration of atrial and ventricular pressures.

Ventricular filling slows during the middle of diastole (diastasis) because the pressures in the atrium and ventricle are nearly identical. A small amount of blood from pulmonary venous return occurring during this time period (289) adds to the total diastolic filling (usually less than 5%) of the ventricle. Diastasis may become shortened or completely disappear during tachycardia, but this has little effect on overall ventricular filling.

Atrial systole is the final phase of diastole. Contraction of the atrium elevates atrial pressure and increases the positive pressure gradient across the mitral valve, forcing blood into the ventricle. Minimal retrograde flow into pulmonary veins occurs because of the peristaltic-like configuration of atrial contraction and the unique anatomy of the pulmonary venous-atrial junction (341). Atrial systole normally accounts for 15% to 25% of total diastolic filling and the subsequent ventricular stroke volume. However, in pathologic states that decrease ventricular compliance or delay isovolumetric relaxation, atrial "kick" may become critical to maintain an adequate stroke volume because early to mid-diastolic filling is impaired (399,476,510). Loss of atrial contraction following the onset of atrial fibrillation can produce dramatic hemodynamic compromise in patients with early diastolic filling abnormalities, such as those that occur in advanced aortic stenosis or hypertrophic cardiomyopathy.

LEFT VENTRICULAR PRESSURE-VOLUME AND DIMENSION DIAGRAMS

When continuous left ventricular pressure and volume from the Wiggers diagram are plotted simultaneously, a phase space

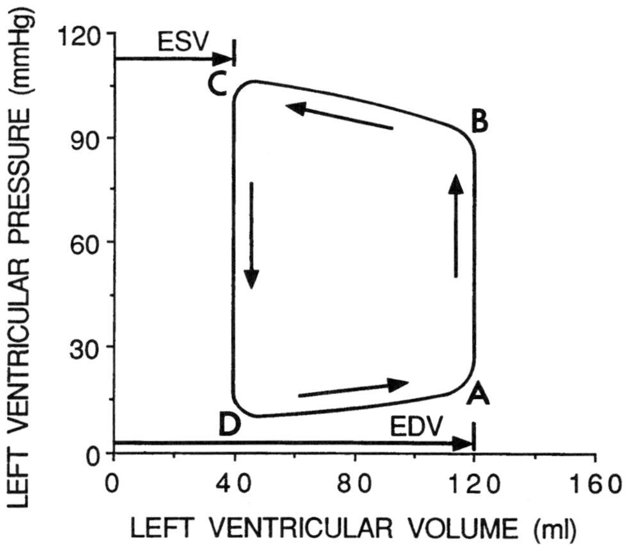

Figure 4. Schematic left ventricular pressure-volume diagram. The cardiac cycle proceeds in a counterclockwise direction *(arrows)*. **A:** End-diastole. **B:** Aortic valve opening. **C:** Aortic valve closure. **D:** Mitral valve opening. Segments AB, BC, CD, and DA represent isovolumetric contraction, ventricular ejection, isovolumetric relaxation, and diastolic filling, respectively. End-diastolic volume (EDV) and end-systolic volume (ESV) can be identified as the *lower right* (point A) and *upper left* (point C) corners of the diagram allowing rapid calculation of stroke volume and ejection fraction. The area of the loop represents stroke work. (From ref. 427, with permission.)

diagram is generated that can be used to analyze systolic and diastolic ventricular function during the cardiac cycle (Fig. 4). Although this technique was first described by Frank (168) in 1898, description of ventricular mechanical performance using pressure-volume diagrams was only popularized much later by Suga and Sagawa (519,601,602). Changes in ventricular pressure with respect to volume occur in a counterclockwise fashion over time. The cardiac cycle begins at end diastole (point A, Fig. 4). An abrupt increase in ventricular pressure with little change in ventricular volume occurs during isovolumetric contraction. Opening of the aortic valve takes place when pressure within the ventricle exceeds that in the aorta (point B, Fig. 4) and systolic ejection begins. Ventricular volume decreases rapidly especially during the first third of this phase as blood is ejected into the aorta. The aortic valve closes at end ejection when ventricular pressure declines below aortic pressure (point C, Fig. 4). A rapid decrease in ventricular pressure with little change in volume (isovolumetric relaxation) then occurs. The mitral valve opens when ventricular pressure is reduced below left atrial pressure (point D, Fig. 4), initiating ventricular diastolic filling. The ventricular pressure-volume loop is completed as large increases in ventricular volume occur with minimal increases in pressure during rapid ventricular filling, diastasis, and atrial systole (see below).

Ventricular pressure-volume diagrams offer several advantages over simple time plots of individual pressure and volume waveforms for the analysis of hemodynamic data. End-diastolic volume (EDV) and end-systolic volume (ESV) can be identified as the lower right (point A) and upper left (point C) corners of the diagram, respectively, allowing rapid calculation of stroke volume (EDV–ESV) and ejection fraction [(EDV–ESV)·100/EDV]. The area of the loop mathematically defines stroke work for each cardiac cycle examined:

$$SW = \int P \cdot dV$$

where SW = stroke work, P = ventricular pressure, and dV = time-dependent changes in ventricular volume.

A series of pressure-volume diagrams of consecutive cardiac cycles can be generated by transient alterations in preload or afterload using mechanical (e.g., vena caval or aortic constriction, respectively) or pharmacologic (e.g., sodium nitroprusside or phenylephrine infusions, respectively) techniques (Fig. 5). This nested set of loops allows calculation of indices of myocardial contractility such as the end-systolic pressure-volume relationship (519) (ESPVR) and the stroke work versus end-diastolic volume relation [a linear Frank-Starling analogue termed "preload recruitable stroke work"(196)]. This family of loops also provides an estimate of diastolic ventricular compliance by the end-diastolic pressure-volume relationship (EDPVR). The two pressure-volume relationships in systole and diastole also define the limits of the work diagram of the ventricle. Although the pressure-volume relationships are determined by the intrinsic properties of the ventricle [systolic (inotropic) and diastolic mechanical (lusitropic) states], the relative positions of the end-diastolic and end-systolic points that lie along these lines for each cardiac cycle are established primarily by venous return and arterial vascular tone (preload and afterload) (275). This unifying connection between the systemic circulation and the inherent properties of the ventricle emphasizes that analysis of overall cardiovascular performance in vivo cannot consider either of these entities entirely independently (273).

The schematic ventricular pressure-volume diagram also provides a useful illustration of basic hemodynamic alterations observed during systolic and diastolic dysfunction as causes for congestive heart failure (214) (Fig. 6). Depression of the normal end-systolic pressure-volume relationship (ESPVR), indicating a decrease in intrinsic myocardial contractility, is distinctive of pure systolic dysfunction (top panel, Fig. 6) and is

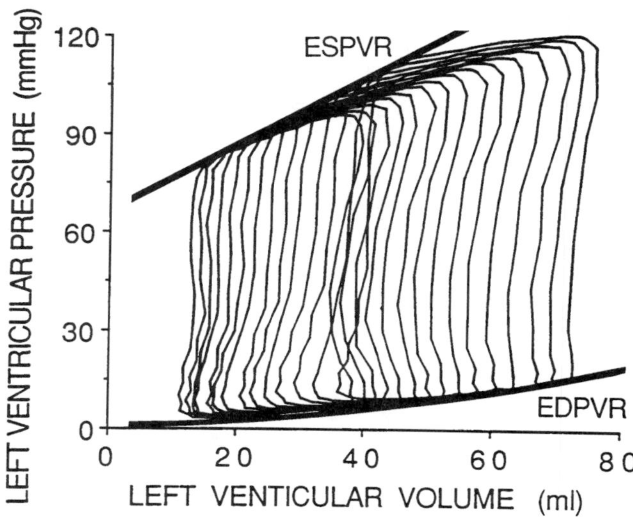

Figure 5. A series of left ventricular pressure-volume loops (representing 14 consecutive cardiac cycles) generated by abrupt occlusion of the inferior vena cava in a conscious dog. The slope of the end-systolic pressure-volume relationship (ESPVR), an index of myocardial contractility, can be calculated by linear regression analysis of the end-systolic pressure and end-systolic volume of each beat. Increases or decreases in the slope of the ESPVR indicate enhanced or depressed contractility, respectively. The end-diastolic pressure-volume relation (EDPVR), an index of diastolic function, can be determined using the end-diastolic pressure and corresponding end-diastolic volume for each cardiac cycle fitted to an exponential relationship (see text). Increases or decreases in ventricular compliance are characterized by depression or elevation of the EDPVR, respectively. (From ref. 427, with permission.)

accompanied by a compensatory ventricular dilatation occurring along a normal end-diastolic pressure-volume relation (EDPVR). Under these circumstances, stroke volume and cardiac output are relatively preserved but compensatory responses maintaining these variables occur at the cost of ventricular dilatation and increased diastolic pressure. Pure diastolic dysfunction is characterized by an increase in resistance to ventricular inflow during a decrease in ventricular compliance (diastolic pressure is higher at any given volume) with relative maintenance of the ESPVR (middle panel, Fig. 6). Stroke volume and cardiac output may be preserved, but because EDPVR is elevated, this occurs at the expense of increased filling pressures. Heart failure may also be manifested by simultaneous systolic and diastolic dysfunction (bottom panel, Fig. 6) with corresponding depression of ESPVR (decrease in contractile state) and elevation of EDPVR (decrease in chamber compliance). Stroke volume and cardiac output may be severely reduced under such conditions because available compensatory mechanisms (e.g., movements along the ESPVR and EDPVR) are limited.

The ventricular pressure-volume relationship can be extrapolated to a single region or dimension within the ventricle and analogous ventricular pressure-regional dimension relationships can be determined (13,163,165,267,268,322,363). Ultrasonic piezoelectric transducers placed within the left ventricular wall can be used experimentally to measure changes in myocardial segment length (163,165,267,268) or midaxis diameter (363) of the ventricular cavity during the cardiac cycle. These ultrasonic transducers can also be placed on the epicardial and endocardial surfaces of the ventricle to measure continuous changes in myocardial wall thickness (13,322). The time for ultrasound to be transmitted between a pair of transducers is directly propor-

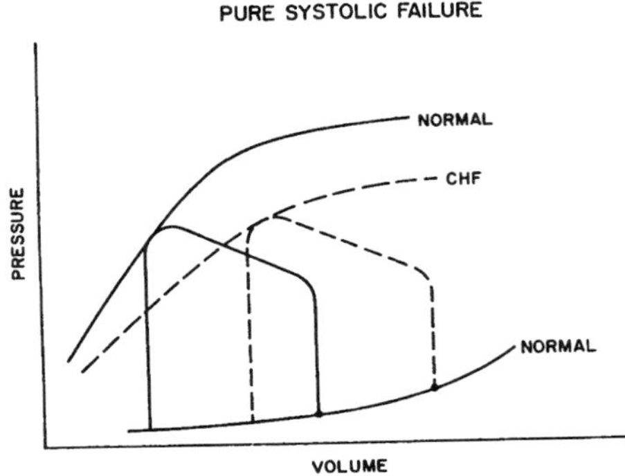

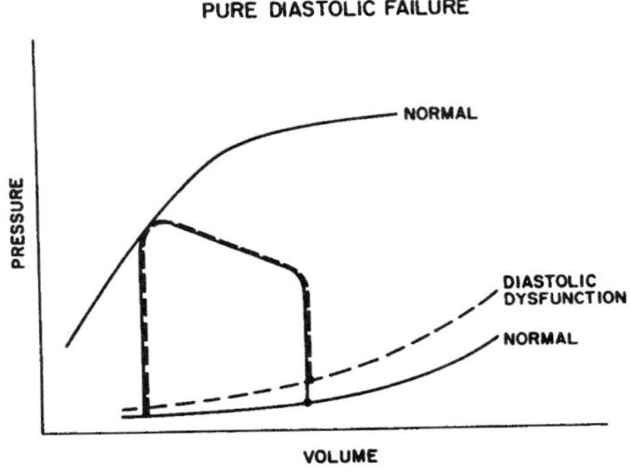

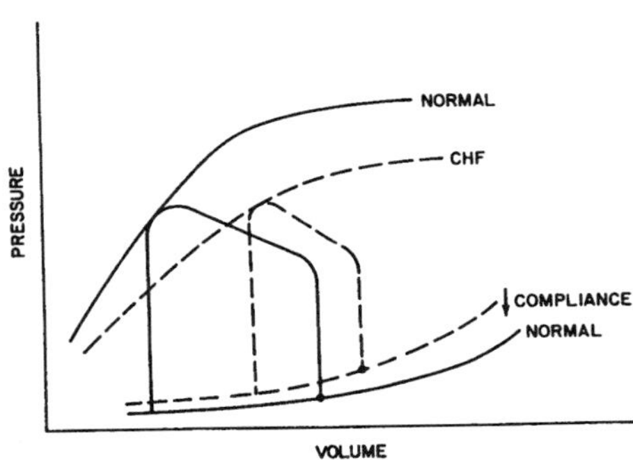

Figure 6. Schematic diagram of left ventricular pressure-volume relationships as derived from loops in pure systolic heart failure *(top panel)*, pure diastolic heart failure *(middle panel)*, and mixed systolic and diastolic failure *(lower panel)*. *Solid lines* represent pressure-volume data from normal hearts and *dashed lines* represent data from hearts in failure. Note the depression of the ESPVR when congestive heart failure (CHF) is due to pure systolic failure compared to maintenance of ESPVR during diastolic dysfunction (characterized by an upward shift of the EDPVR). (From ref. 214, with permission.)

tional to the length between the transducers. Segment length or midaxis diameter normally increases during diastole and shortens during systole, similarly to changes in continuous ventricular volume (Fig. 7). In contrast, myocardial wall thickness decreases in diastole and increases during systole. Abrupt decreases in preload or increases in afterload using mechanical or pharmacologic interventions can be used to generate a series of diagrams for measurement of end-systolic and end-diastolic pressure–segment length, pressure–wall thickness, or pressure—midaxis diameter relationships.

Deformity of the normal shape of the pressure-volume diagram may indicate global ischemia-induced myocardial dysfunction. More commonly, however, there may be only small changes manifested by the global ventricular pressure-volume diagram because myocardial ischemia is a regional phenomenon. In contrast, the pressure-ischemic segment length diagram may be dramatically altered (132,163). Severe ischemia may cause collapse of the loop, indicative of lack of effective stroke work in the region measured (Fig. 8). The pressure–segment length diagram tilts to the right during mild myocardial ischemia. The pressure-length diagram from a moderately ischemic zone can be divided into three regions corresponding to an area of postsystolic shortening (indicating that the ischemic segment cannot contribute to overall left ventricular function because shortening occurs after the end of ejection), systolic lengthening (indicating that paroxysmal aneurysmal bulging of the ischemic region during systole is occurring

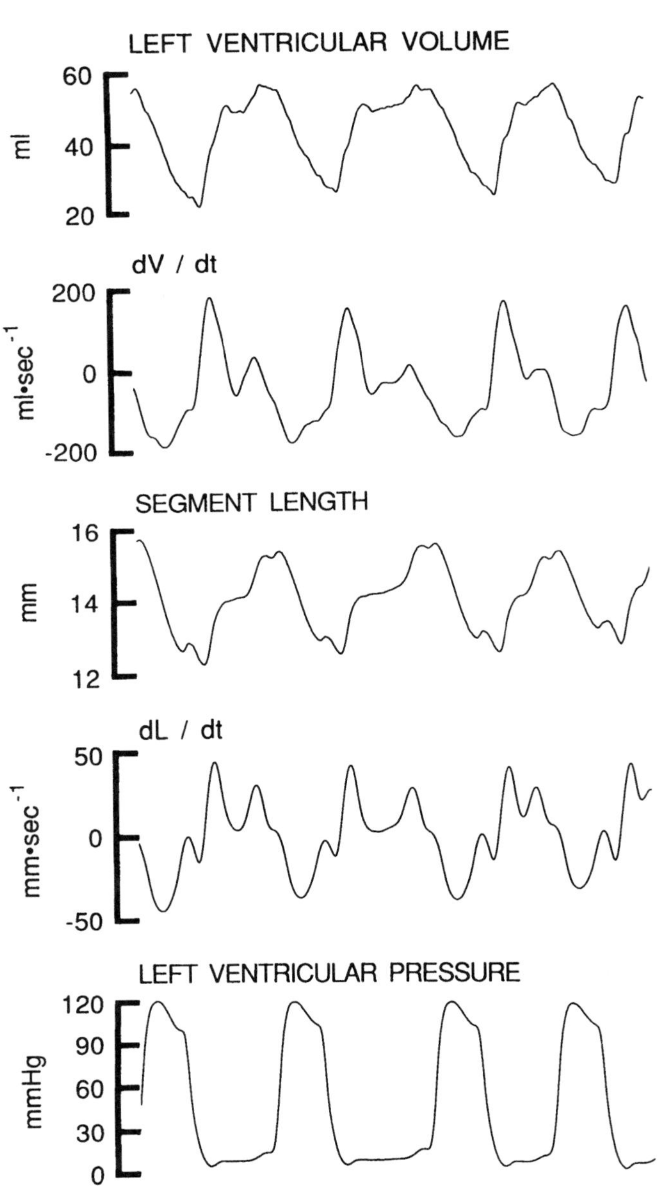

Figure 7. Continuous left ventricular volume, rate of change of volume (dV/dt), segment length, rate of change of segment length (dL/dt), and left ventricular pressure waveforms in a conscious dog. Early diastolic filling can be quantified by the peak filling rate (dV/dt or dL/dt) or a variety of related parameters (see text). (From ref. 427, with permission.)

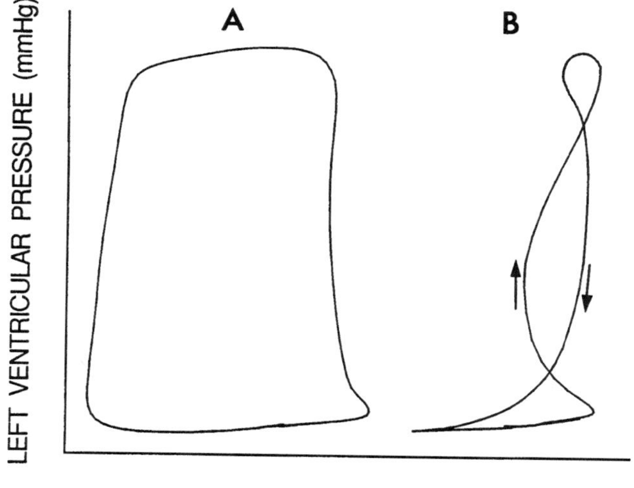

Figure 8. Left ventricular pressure-segment length loops from a conscious dog under control conditions (**A**) and during ischemia (**B**). The *arrows* indicate the direction of movement around the ischemic loop during the cardiac cycle. Ischemia produces passive systolic lengthening, postsystolic shortening, and lack of effective regional stroke work resulting in marked deformity of the loop. (From ref. 427, with permission.)

because of tethering to surrounding normally contracting areas), and an area between that contributes to overall ventricular stroke work (Fig. 9). Use of these parameters has recently been advocated for the quantitation of the intensity of regional myocardial ischemia (518).

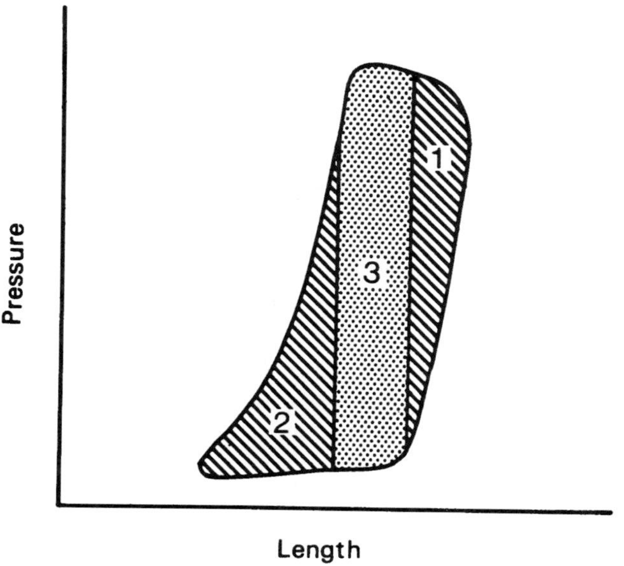

Figure 9. During mild ischemia, the left ventricular pressure-segment length diagram tilts to the right indicating systolic lengthening (region 1) and postsystolic shortening (region 2). The actual work that contributes to pump function (*shaded area;* 3) represents only a fraction of the total loop area. Areas of systolic lengthening or postsystolic shortening do not contribute to pump function. (From ref. 163, with permission.)

EVALUATION OF MYOCARDIAL CONTRACTILITY IN THE INTACT HEART

Although changes in myocardial contractility can be easily characterized in isolated cardiac muscle preparations where rigid control of loading conditions is possible, reliable quantitation of changes in intrinsic contractile state has proven to be an elusive task in vivo. This goal remains important because the ability to accurately measure contractility would allow reliable evaluation of pharmacologic interventions and pathophysiologic processes that alter global ventricular performance. Several fundamental difficulties have contributed to the complexity of this problem and have stimulated considerable research over the past two decades. While a strict definition of preload in terms of instantaneous one-dimensional myofibrillar length is intuitively useful, the dynamic, three-dimensional changes in left ventricular geometry during the cardiac cycle make such a definition of preload of limited practical utility in the intact heart. Similarly, comprehensive definition and quantitative measurement of afterload in vivo does not parallel the concept of afterload in isolated cardiac muscle in either clarity or simplicity. In addition, while myocardial contractility can be purely defined in isolated papillary muscle preparations, all indices of contractile state in vivo developed to date, including those derived from ventricular pressure-volume diagrams, have some degree of dependence on heart rate and loading conditions (273). Thus, the underlying principles used to investigate the physiology of isolated cardiac muscle are not entirely applicable to the study of global cardiac performance. Evaluation of myocardial contractility in vivo must consider not only the intrinsic contractile properties of the myocardium itself but also the impact of changes in heart rate and systemic and pulmonary hemodynamics that may alter preload and afterload.

Quantitation and Regulation of Preload

Preload can be defined as the volume of blood contained within the left ventricular cavity at end diastole in the intact heart. This volume establishes the passive stretch on each myofibril of the ventricle immediately prior to electrical initiation of isovolumetric contraction (572) and is directly related to end-diastolic wall stress. While this definition is intuitively clear, the actual real-time measurement of continuous ventricular volume during the cardiac cycle and the precise characterization of end-diastolic volume over several consecutive beats poses a persistent and difficult problem (74). Ventricular volume can be experimentally assessed using ultrasonic sonomicrometers implanted in a three-dimensional orthogonal array in the subendocardium of the ventricle (74,348,509). Mathematical models of ventricular volume, which make various simplifying assumptions about the geometric architecture of the ventricle, can then be applied to changes in the measurement of these regional dimensions, resulting in continuous estimation of ventricular volume. More recently, the conductance method of measuring left ventricular volume has been advocated (6,17,78,348). This technique involves placement of a multielectrode catheter within the left ventricular cavity to establish multiple electrical current fields and measure time-varying voltage potentials within the chamber (16). Intraventricular conductance is derived from these voltage gradients and left ventricular volume can be estimated. This technique is especially attractive because it can provide a continuous volume signal after percutaneous placement of the catheter without extensive surgical intervention. This method allows sophisticated assessment of left ventricular function in experimental settings in closed-chest animals and in the cardiac catheterization laboratory in humans (74,215,272).

Correlation between conductance catheter measurements of ventricular volume and those derived from dimensional assessment with sonomicrometry is good (6,40) although some controversy remains concerning the relative correlation of these two techniques with more conventional methods of assessing ventricular volume such as Doppler echocardiography or biplane cineangiography (74). Orthogonal three-dimensional crystal arrays and conductance catheter techniques of measurement of continuous ventricular volume offer the advantage that end-diastolic volume can be easily measured in a series of cardiac cycles without the poststudy analysis required in angiographic and echocardiographic methods. Ventricular volume waveforms generated by dimensional assessment or conductance also allow an analysis of a variety of indices of left ventricular systolic and diastolic function derived from ventricular pressure-volume diagrams (see below).

Left ventricular end-diastolic volume is typically not quantitatively measured, and other estimates of ventricular preload are used in the clinical setting. Left ventricular end-diastolic pressure can be determined invasively in the cardiac catheterization laboratory or during cardiac surgery by advancing a fluid-filled or pressure transducer-tipped catheter from the aorta across the aortic valve or through the left atrium across the mitral valve into the ventricular chamber. Left ventricular end-diastolic pressure is related to end-diastolic volume on the basis of the nonlinear end-diastolic pressure-volume relationship (1) (EDPVR; see above). Ventricular end-diastolic pressure, however, only indirectly indicates the degree of end-diastolic volume and may be a poor reflection of volume because of alterations in ventricular compliance produced by declines in contractility or by diastolic dysfunction (1).

With the exception of real-time assessment of end-diastolic dimension using two-dimensional transesophageal echocardiography (2D TEE), the clinical anesthesiologist usually must rely on estimates of left ventricular filling that result from measurements further "upstream" from the ventricle. Left atrial pressure, pulmonary capillary occlusion (wedge) pressure, pulmonary artery diastolic pressure, and right atrial pressure have all been used to estimate left ventricular preload. These indirect indicators of left ventricular end-diastolic volume are influenced by the functional integrity of the structures that separate the specific measurement location from the left ventricle. For example, correlation between right atrial and left ventricular end-diastolic pressure assumes that the fluid column between these chambers has not been influenced by airway pressure during respiration, right ventricular or pulmonary vascular pathology, left atrial dysfunction, or structural abnormalities of the mitral valve (Fig. 10). The complex relationship between these structures may be intact in a healthy patient, but this may not be the case in patients with significant cardiorespiratory pathology who may require accurate monitoring of left ventricular filling to optimize cardiac performance. The correlation between left ventricular end diastolic volume, pulmonary artery occlusion pressure, and right atrial pressure is poor in patients with compromised pump function (226,614), making measurement of "upstream" pressures of limited clinical utility in the assessment of ventricular preload. In the remainder of

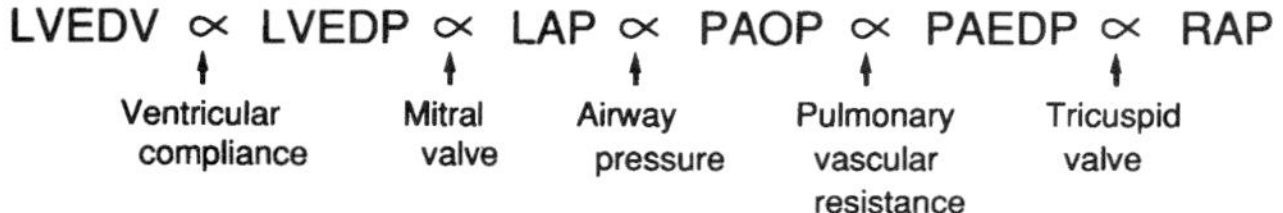

Figure 10. Summary of factors that alter estimates of left ventricular end-diastolic volume "upstream" from the ventricle. LVEDP, left ventricular end-diastolic pressure; LAP, left atrial pressure; PAOP, pulmonary artery occlusion pressure; PAEDP, pulmonary artery end-diastolic pressure; RAP, right atrial pressure. (From ref. 23, with permission.)

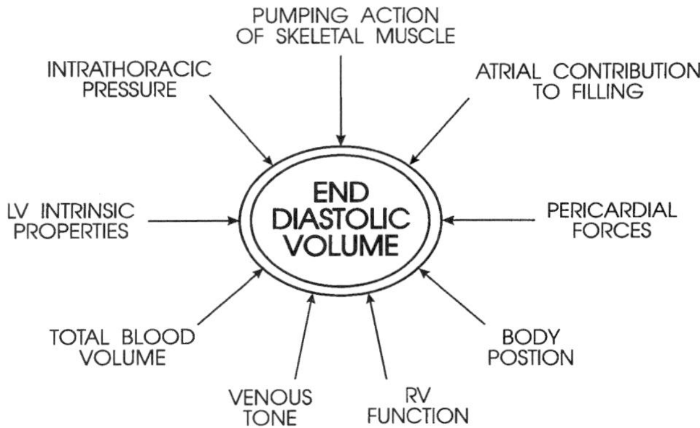

Figure 11. Major influences determining preload in the intact cardiovascular system. (Adapted from ref. 64, with permission.)

this chapter, the term *preload* refers to end-diastolic volume unless otherwise noted.

The return of blood from the low pressure, high compliance venous circulation, and the distribution and absolute quantity of total blood volume combined with the functional integrity of the atrium and the diastolic filling characteristics of the ventricle determine the end-diastolic volume for each cardiac cycle in the intact heart (Fig. 11). Left ventricular stroke volume in vivo is directly related to venous return [Starling's law of the heart (449)] and acute changes in cardiac output are primarily determined by alterations in the return of venous blood from the peripheral circulation. The level of inotropic state plays an important role in the systolic performance of the failing heart, but sole changes in contractile state have little effect on overall cardiac output in the normal left ventricle (58). However, large variations in cardiac output occur in both the normal and diseased heart when venous return is acutely altered by rapid changes in total blood volume, body position, intrathoracic pressure, or venous tone (553). Cardiac output can be relatively maintained in the normal heart if gradual or small changes in these variables (e.g., a decrease in total blood volume of less than 15% to 20%) occur because of compensatory sympathetic nervous system activation. In contrast, concomitant declines in autonomic responsiveness via desensitization and downregulation of cardiac β_1-adrenoceptors may render the failing heart more susceptible to alterations in these determinants of venous return (65,635).

Left ventricular end-diastolic volume is also dependent on the distribution of blood volume between intra- and extrathoracic compartments (64). Gravity-induced pooling of blood in dependent regions occurs with changes in body position. For example, assumption of the supine position from a standing posture increases intrathoracic blood volume and ventricular preload. The cyclical extravascular contraction and relaxation of antigravity muscles in the lower extremities in combination with the venous valvular system helps to maintain adequate venous return in the standing position (553). The artificial application of pressure to the legs, e.g., military antishock trousers (MAST), augments ventricular filling by increasing the ratio of intra- to extrathoracic blood volume. During normal respiration, negative intrathoracic pressure contributes to enhanced venous return to the heart during inspiration. In contrast, positive-pressure ventilation reverses the normal gradient for venous return to the thorax, impeding ventricular filling and decreasing cardiac output. Venoconstriction resulting from elevated sympathetic nervous system tone directly increases venous return. Conversely, venodilators (e.g., nitroglycerin) decrease return of blood to the heart, resulting in a direct decline in end-diastolic volume. Mediastinal and myocardial etiologies of impaired ventricular filling are discussed in detail below.

Quantitation and Regulation of Afterload

The concept of afterload in isolated cardiac muscle preparations is intuitively clear and easily quantitated, but the definition and precise measurement of afterload in the intact, beating heart is complex even under controlled experimental conditions. Impedance to left ventricular outflow by the arterial vasculature provides the qualitative intellectual framework for the concept of afterload in vivo. Several approaches have been advocated in previous attempts to quantitate afterload. The first viewpoint defines an afterload variable through which the left ventricle is coupled to the arterial vasculature (64). In this model, afterload is defined as left ventricular end-systolic wall stress, a calculated parameter that incorporates not only the ventricular pressure and geometric components of the law of Laplace but also the physical characteristics of the arterial system into which the heart propels blood (205,651). Left ventricular volume decreases with simultaneous increases in ventricular pressure and wall thickness during ejection. These changes produce ventricular wall stress that reaches a maximum during the first phase of ventricular ejection (Fig. 12) and decreases thereafter because increases in wall thickness and decreases in chamber size occur despite continued increases in ventricular pressure during the remainder of ejection (49,52,205).

Changes in continuous left ventricular systolic wall stress have several important physiologic consequences. Peak left ventricular systolic wall stress appears to be a principal stimulus of left ventricular hypertrophy in chronic pressure-overload states such as essential hypertension and aortic stenosis (48,216,651). The integral of left ventricular wall stress over time during systole is a major determinant of myocardial oxygen demand (650) (in addition to heart rate, preload, and inotropic state). End-systolic wall stress can also be combined with indices of ventricular emptying to quantitate changes in myocardial contractility (49,104). Finally, left ventricular end-systolic wall stress defines the force that ultimately limits fiber shortening at end ejection and determines the degree of ventricular emptying for a given contractile state. Thus, left ventricular end-systolic wall stress represents the maximal isometric value of instantaneous myocardial force at end ejection for a given chamber size, thickness, and pressure and incorporates both internal cardiac forces and those external to the heart (the arterial system) that oppose it (49,89,104,505,651). The use of left ventricular end-systolic wall stress as a quantitative index of afterload is complicated by geometric assumptions of ventricular shape, the nonlinear distribution of forces from the subendocardium and epicardium, and the nonuniformity of wall thickness (393,523), problems that become especially relevant in the study of pathologic states such as regional myocardial ischemia and postinfarction ventricular remodeling. Several left ventricular wall stress equations have been developed based on radial (σ_r), meridional (σ_m) (216), and circumferential dimensions (σ_c) (394), and controversy continues to exist concerning the application and assumptions presented in each formulation (484).

Another important experimental model describing afterload defined by the interaction between the arterial vascular system and the left ventricle was proposed by Sunagawa et al. (606,607). These investigators used the slope of the end-systolic pressure-volume relation (E_{es}) to define chamber elastance (the ratio of changes in pressure to changes in volume) and argued that the arterial system could be considered to be a second elastic chamber described by effective arterial elastance (E_a) calculated as the slope of the end-systolic aortic pressure-stroke volume relation:

$$P_s = E_a \cdot SV$$

where P_s = end-systolic aortic pressure and SV = stroke volume (Fig. 13). In this framework, the relationship between E_{es} and E_a defined the stroke volume that could be transferred between the ventricle and the arterial system (left ventricular output). This interaction between ventricular and arterial elastance has been used to determine left ventricular pump function under a variety of loading and inotropic conditions in experimental preparations (76,344,413,414,607) and in humans (575). The

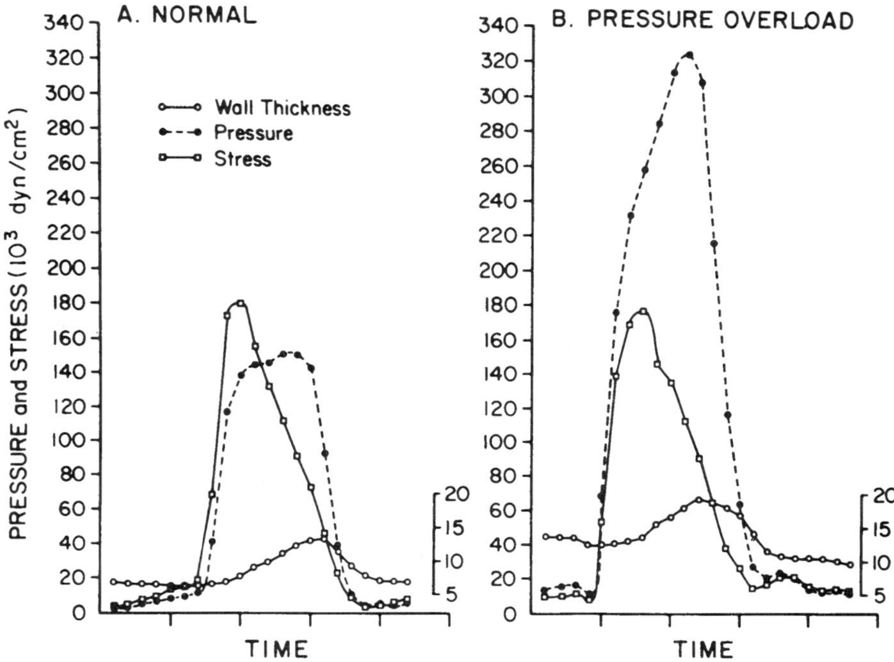

Figure 12. Changes in left ventricular pressure *(solid dots)*, wall thickness *(open dots)*, and wall stress *(open squares)* during the cardiac cycle in the normal **(A)** and pressure-overloaded **(B)** left ventricle. Wall stress peaks during early ejection and declines throughout the remainder of ejection. In the pressure-overloaded ventricle, dramatic increases in ventricular systolic pressure occur, but compensatory increases in wall thickness maintain wall stress in the normal range and configuration. (From ref. 216, with permission.)

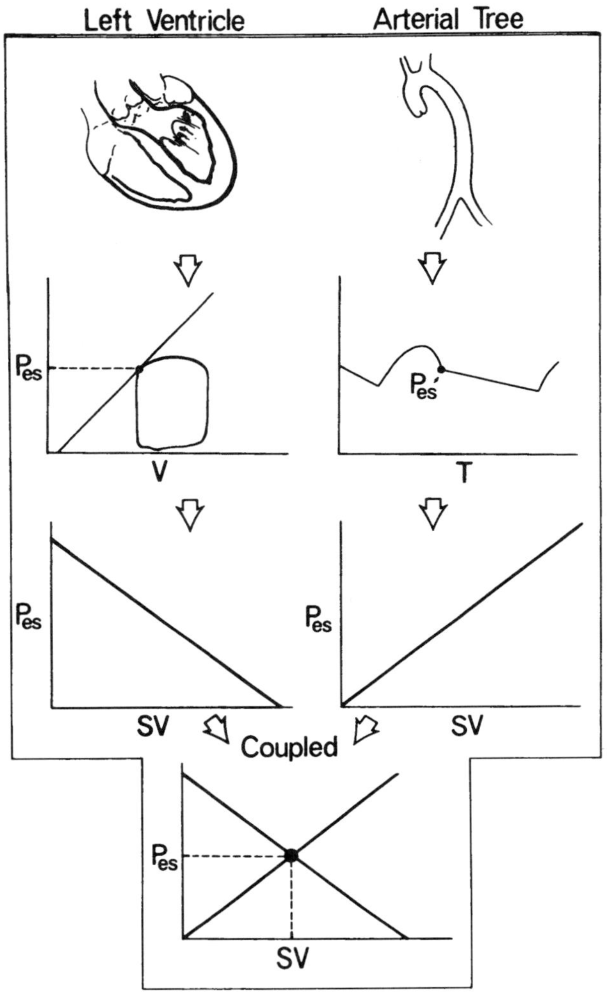

Figure 13. Coupling of the left ventricle to the arterial vasculature in the model of Sunagawa et al. The ventricular system *(left panels)* and the arterial system *(right panels)* are characterized by the relationship between end-systolic pressure (P_{es}) to stroke volume (SV). The intersection of these relations *(bottom panel)* denotes the stroke volume resulting from the coupling of the two systems. (From ref. 520, with permission.)

maximal stroke work performed by the left ventricle can also be assessed using this model, occurring when E_{es} and E_a are optimally balanced (606,607). Myocardial efficiency (the ratio of left ventricular stroke work to myocardial oxygen consumption) can also be calculated (see below), reaching its maximum when the ratio of E_{es} to E_a is approximately 2.0 (76).

A second major approach to the examination of afterload delineates forces purely external to the left ventricle that oppose ejection of a viscous fluid (blood) into a viscoelastic arterial system (391). Arterial input impedance is a dynamic characteristic of the arterial system and is defined by the ratio of arterial pressure to arterial blood flow measured at the aortic root. Arterial input impedance incorporates the pulsatile nature of aortic blood flow independent of left ventricular performance. Calculation of aortic input impedance, however, is very difficult even in highly controlled experimental settings and requires simultaneous and high-fidelity measurement of aortic pressure and blood flow (391). These waveforms are then subjected to Fourier series analysis to generate an arterial input impedance spectrum characterized by modulus and phase curves that are dependent on heart rate and the frequency of reflected waves from the peripheral circulation (Fig. 14). In this context, the arterial input impedance spectrum depends not only on the physical properties (viscoelasticity and vessel diameter) of the artery and the blood (viscosity and density) that determine "characteristic" impedance, but also on the reflected pressure and flow waves generated by more distal parts of the arterial tree that produce frequency-dependent oscillations of local impedance around the characteristic impedance (391). Aortic and pulmonary input impedances have been quantified using this technique in both normal and pathologic states (390,392,447).

The magnitude of arterial input impedance depends primarily on peripheral resistance and can be reasonably approximated with arterial resistance, an index of afterload that assumes a steady state rather than a pulsatile aortic flow (286). Arterial resistance is calculated as a single quotient of aortic pressure and flow, in contrast to aortic input impedance, which results in a time-dependent spectrum of variable resistance to ventricular ejection that incorporates arterial capacitance. This assumption forms the basis for the use of calculated systemic vascular resistance (SVR) to define left ventricular afterload in the clinical setting:

$$SVR = (MAP - RAP) \cdot 80/CO$$

where MAP = mean arterial pressure, RAP = right atrial pressure, CO = cardiac output (aortic flow), and 80 is a factor converting $mmHg \cdot min^{-1} \cdot L^{-1}$ to $dynes \cdot sec \cdot cm^{-5}$. Systemic vascular resistance calculations parallel left ventricular afterload assessment using end-systolic wall stress in a majority of experimental conditions of varying load; however, systemic vascular resistance may underestimate the magnitude of changes in resistance to left ventricular outflow (315).

Another approach in the characterization of left ventricular afterload examines changes in the magnitude (252) and morphology (281,424) of the arterial blood pressure waveform at different sites in the arterial vasculature during the cardiac cycle. In young volunteers, pulse pressure increases from the central aorta to distal peripheral arteries, and peak pressure is reached relatively early in systole in all arteries consistent with observed changes in ventricular wall stress (281). In contrast, older patients with hypertension or cardiomyopathy may manifest increases in proximal aortic characteristic impedance that are enhanced by pressure waves returning from the peripheral arterial tree (increases in local impedance), causing augmentation of arterial pressure later during systole (281,550). This persistent elevation of late systolic blood pressure may depress left ventricular function due to enhanced end-systolic wall stress (123). These findings indicate that not only the magnitude but also the phasic character of the systolic arterial pressure waveform plays an important role in the determination of left ventricular afterload.

Other investigators have studied left ventricular afterload by examining the systolic ejection gradients between the ventricle and proximal aorta using high-fidelity catheterization techniques (445,446) or, more recently, Doppler echocardiography (257). Ejection gradients have two major components consisting of the rate of left ventricular ejection (known as the "Bernoulli" gradient) and the acceleration of blood in the proximal aorta during early systole (known as the "impulse" or "local acceleration" gradient) (446). In normal individuals, the ventricular ejection gradient (flow from ventricle to aorta) peaks during early systole and remains positive throughout the vast majority of systole. In contrast, patients with congestive cardiomyopathy may demonstrate a smaller magnitude of positive pressure gradient between the left ventricle and the aorta. The gradient also declines more rapidly than in normal individuals (Fig. 15), remaining positive for shorter fractions of systole, indicating greater resistance to left ventricular outflow (257). Increases in ejection gradients may also represent augmentation of ventricular afterload resulting from structural abnormalities of the left ventricle independent of peripheral vascular resistance or arterial blood pressure. This occurs when blood is

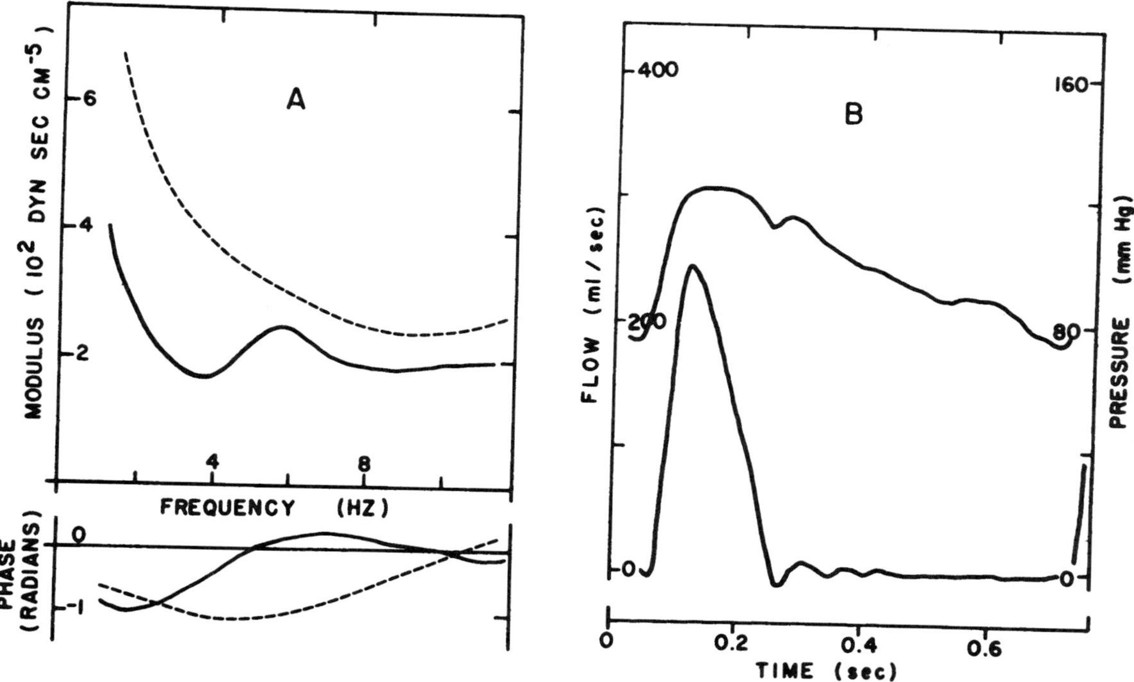

Figure 14. Aortic impedance spectrum in a conscious dog at rest *(solid line; left panel)* and under the conditions of increased stiffness of the aortic wall *(dashed line; left panel)*. The negative phase angle *(left panel, bottom)* in the abnormal dog *(dashed line)* indicates that developed aortic pressure lags behind aortic blood flow. Typical aortic blood flow and aortic blood pressure waveforms during the cardiac cycle in the canine ascending aorta are depicted in the *right panel*. (From ref. 391, with permission.)

rapidly ejected from an enlarged ventricle through a normal-sized aortic annulus in aortic regurgitation (termed "ventriculoannular disproportion") or when the ventricular septum produces resistance to outflow in hypertrophic cardiomyopathy (termed left ventricular "cavity obliteration") (447,674).

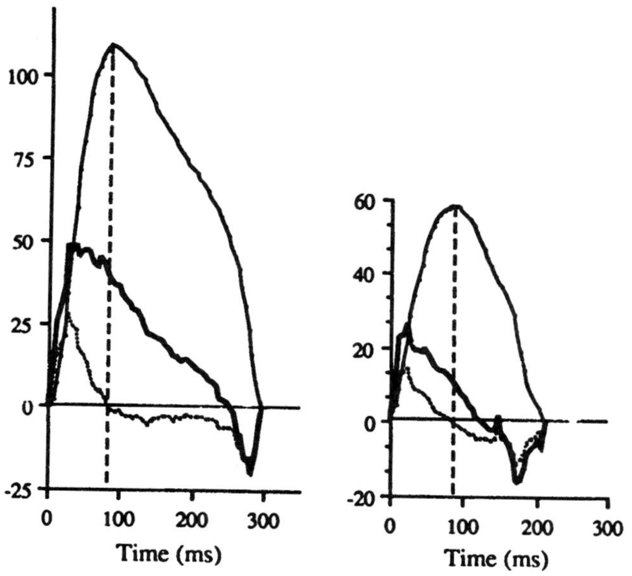

Figure 15. Echocardiographically derived tracings of left ventricular outflow velocity *(solid fine line)*, local acceleration *(dotted fine line)*, and ejection force *(solid thick line)* in a normal patient *(left panel)* and a patient with dilated cardiomyopathy *(right panel)*. At peak velocity *(vertical dashed line)*, the ejection force has decreased below 50% of its peak value in the patient with dilated cardiomyopathy *(right panel)* but remains nearly 90% of its peak value in the normal patient *(left panel)*. (From ref. 257, with permission.)

In summary, afterload is a complex interaction of four fundamental components in the intact cardiovascular system: (a) the pressure generated by, and the geometry of, the left ventricle, intrinsic cardiac factors governing end-systolic wall stress via the law of Laplace; (b) the physical characteristics of the arterial system, defined by the viscoelasticity and size of arterial vessels; (c) the volume and physical properties of the blood contained within the arterial circulation, determined by blood rheology, viscosity, and density; and (d) the total peripheral resistance of the arterial vasculature, characterized by the degree of arteriolar tone. Acute increases in afterload are usually well tolerated in the presence of normal cardiac function, but can result in deterioration of ventricular performance in the failing heart. Neurohumoral compensation for decreased myocardial contractility (e.g., increased sympathetic tone) and structural abnormalities in vascular architecture (e.g., atherosclerosis) cause increases in impedance to left ventricular ejection and further declines in cardiac output. Compensatory ventricular hypertrophy is an important adaptive process to chronic elevations in afterload that decreases end-systolic wall stress and may transiently improve systolic contractile function but also increases the risk of myocardial ischemia and may produce diastolic dysfunction (see below). The primary objective of the pharmacologic or surgical management of chronically elevated afterload focuses on reduction of the inciting stress.

Preload and Afterload in the Left Ventricular Pressure-Volume Diagram

Examination of changes in the schematic left ventricular pressure-volume diagram provides a useful illustration of the theoretical physiologic consequences of alterations in preload and afterload. Increases in preload (represented by end-diastolic volume) are reflected by expansion of the pressure-volume diagram to the right along the end-diastolic pressure-volume curve (EDPVR), with concomitant increases in stroke volume and stroke work (the area inscribed by the pressure-volume dia-

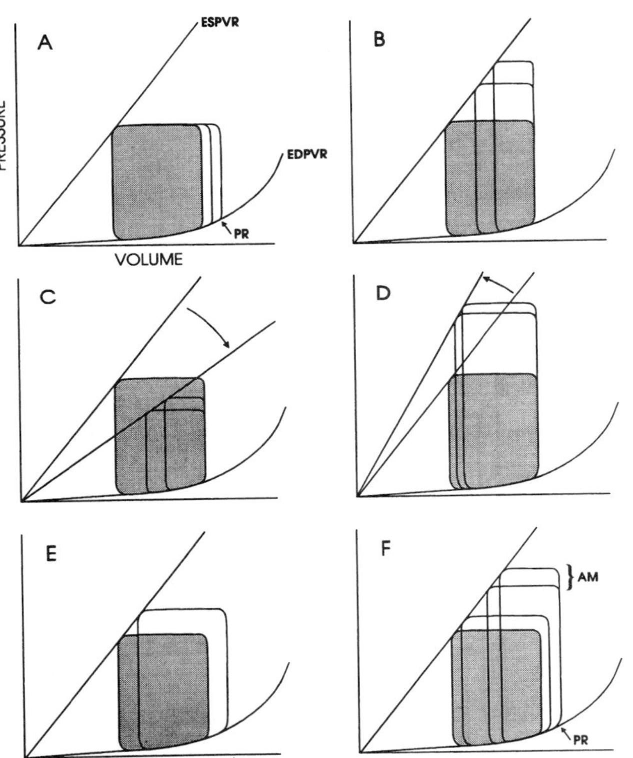

Figure 16. Schematic illustrations depicting the effects of theoretical changes in preload **(A)** and afterload **(B)** in the ventricular pressure-volume model. Changes in preload are identified by movement of the loop along the end-diastolic pressure volume relation line (EDPVR) without change in the intersection with the end-systolic pressure volume relation (ESPVR). Expansion of preload is limited by the distensibility of the ventricle and the physiologic limit at which increases in end-diastolic volume no longer result in increases in stroke volume as identified as preload reserve (PR, panel A). Pure increases in afterload result in an increase in left ventricular pressure and a concomitant decrease in stroke volume (panel B). A decrease in contractility (decrease in ESPVR slope) exacerbates the declines in stroke volume associated with increases in afterload **(C)**. In contrast, increase in contractility allows relative maintenance of stroke volume with progressive increases in afterload **(D)**. Increases in afterload result in compensatory increases in preload, thereby maintaining stroke volume near normal **(E)**. When preload reserve is exhausted during compensation, afterload mismatch occurs and increases in left ventricular systolic pressure are accompanied by dramatic declines in stroke volume **(F)**.

gram), assuming that intrinsic myocardial contractility (slope of the ESPVR) and afterload remain constant (Fig. 16A). The magnitude by which stroke volume and work increase is dependent on the initial location of the end-diastolic volume on the EDPVR. While dramatic increases in stroke volume and work result from a given increase of EDV on the flat portion of the EDPVR, the exponential nature of the EDPVR dictates that smaller increases in stroke volume and work will occur at higher values of EDV because of a continuously steeper rise of the curve. Expansion of preload is ultimately limited by the distensibility of the ventricle, and the amount by which preload can be expanded before reaching this physiologic limit is termed "preload reserve" (64).

The effects of pure changes in afterload can also be predicted by pressure-volume diagram analysis. Assuming that preload and contractile state remain constant, a pure increase in ventricular afterload (e.g., administration of an α_1-adrenergic receptor agonist or mechanical aortic constriction) results in an increase in left ventricular pressure and a concomitant decrease in stroke volume (Fig. 16B). This reduction in stroke volume precipitated by increased impedance to left ventricular outflow is especially marked when myocardial contractility is depressed (e.g., during global myocardial ischemia; Fig. 16C). In contrast, when contractile state is augmented (e.g., administration of a β_1-adrenergic receptor agonist), increases in afterload result in increases in left ventricular pressure with little change in effective stroke volume (Fig. 16D). These observations provide a rationale for the administration of arterial vasodilators (e.g., sodium nitroprusside) in patients with compromised left ventricular systolic function because forward flow is augmented by decreases in left ventricular afterload and occurs concomitant with increases in stroke volume.

In the intact heart, changes in preload and afterload do not occur independently. An abrupt increase in afterload initially results in a slight decrease in stroke volume that is followed in subsequent cardiac cycles by a compensatory increase in preload that effectively normalizes stroke volume (Fig. 16E). Preload reserve limits increases in preload that occur in response to increases in afterload. When preload reserve is exhausted, "afterload mismatch" occurs and increases in left ventricular systolic pressure are accompanied by dramatic declines in stroke volume (Fig. 16F). Clinically, afterload mismatch resulting from limited preload reserve can occur in pressure-overload disease processes such as aortic stenosis, aortic coarctation, and hypertensive cardiomyopathy.

Indices of Contractility Derived from Pressure-Volume Diagrams

End-Systolic Pressure-Volume Relations

Advances in the technology of measurement of continuous ventricular volume in the early 1970s allowed an intense and fruitful reexamination of the relationship between ventricular pressure and volume initially described in the classic work by Frank (168). Suga, Sagawa, and their collaborators (601,602) proposed that the relationship between instantaneous pressure and volume in the isolated left ventricle could be described on the basis of a model of time-varying elastance and that alterations in this relationship provided a relatively load-independent measure of myocardial contractility. During systole, ventricular pressure increases with corresponding declines in volume, resulting in time-dependent increases in the calculated elastance. The maximum value of elastance (E_{max}) occurs at end systole, usually corresponding to the upper left hand corner of the pressure-volume diagram (Fig. 17). Ventricular pressure decreases with concomitant increases in volume during diastole, defining minimum elastance at end diastole.

Suga and Sagawa (601,602) demonstrated that the relationship between ventricular pressure-volume points was linear throughout the cardiac cycle such that

$$E(t) = P(t)/[V(t)-V_0(t)]$$

where $E(t)$ = time-varying elastance, $P(t)$ and $V(t)$ = time-dependent changes in ventricular pressure and volume, respectively, and $V_0(t)$ = time-related changes in unstressed volume (ventricular volume at 0 mm Hg of pressure). These investigators also showed that each E_{max} of a series of pressure-volume diagrams derived from cardiac cycles obtained at various loads, but at constant inotropic and lusitropic states reached the same straight line, determining the end-systolic pressure-volume relationship (ESPVR; Fig. 5). The slope of the ESPVR[1] (desig-

[1]In the isolated heart, E_{max} and E_{es} are nearly identical. However, distinction between them becomes important if large changes in afterload occur during the generation of the ESPVR in vivo. Enhanced afterload delays the timing of ejection and the occurrence of maximal elastance for each beat. This delay in end systole results in a deviation of E_{max} away from the upper left-hand corner of the pressure-volume diagram. Analogously, rapid declines in afterload during systole (e.g., arteriovenous fistula) hasten the occurrence of end systole.

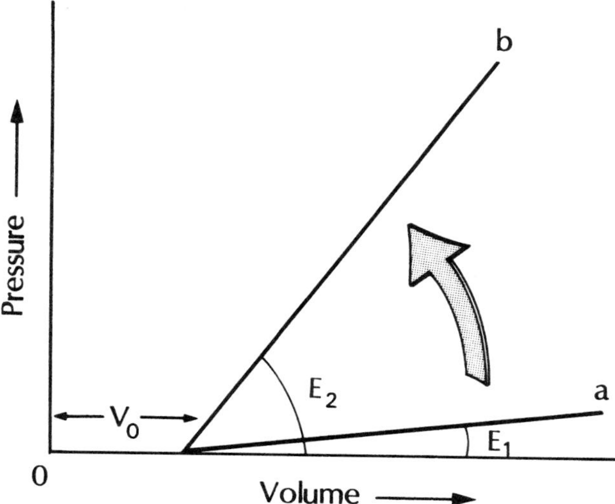

Figure 17. Time-varying elastance in the left ventricular pressure-volume diagram. The end-diastolic pressure-volume relationship *(line a)* is defined by a slope (E_1) and a volume intercept (V_0). When the ventricle contracts, elastance (the ratio of pressure to volume) increases gradually with time *(arrow)*, eventually reaching a maximum *(line b)* with a slope E_2 at end-systole, corresponding to maximal elastance (E_{max}). (From ref. 520, with permission.)

nated as E_{es}) quantitatively defined the inotropic state of the left ventricle, was relatively independent of changes in preload, and incorporated afterload via analysis at end systole (see above). Increases and decreases in intrinsic myocardial contractility were defined by increases and decreases in E_{es}, respectively (Fig. 18). Subsequent investigations demonstrated that in addition to changes in E_{es}, changes in contractility could also be manifested by changes in the unstressed volume (V_0), that is, the left ventricular volume at zero intraventricular pressure (519) (Fig. 19). This observation has been incorporated into a method of assessing contractility using both E_{es} and V_0 (114). Analogous derivation of the end-diastolic pressure-volume relationship (EDPVR; lower right-hand corner of each pressure-volume loop) from a series of differentially loaded cardiac cycles provides a useful framework for the analysis of diastolic mechanical properties (Fig. 5). Importantly, for any set of systolic and diastolic characteristics (ESPVR and EDPVR), contraction, relaxation, and filling of the intact heart is constrained to the boundaries of these relationships (272).

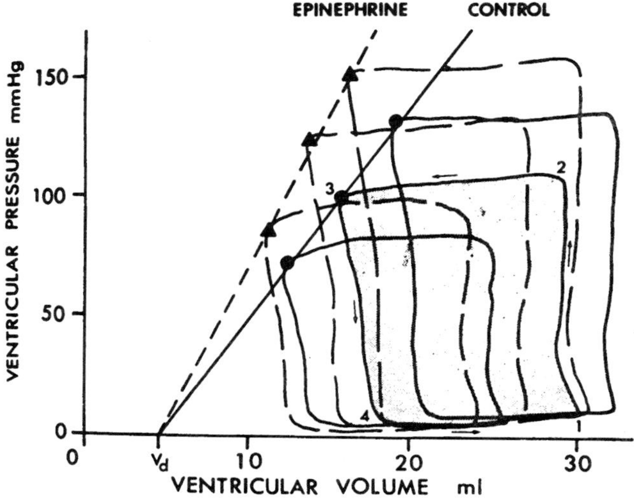

Figure 18. Left ventricular pressure-volume loops and corresponding end-systolic pressure-volume relationships in an isolated heart during control conditions *(circles)* and during an epinephrine infusion *(triangles)*. (From ref. 602, with permission.)

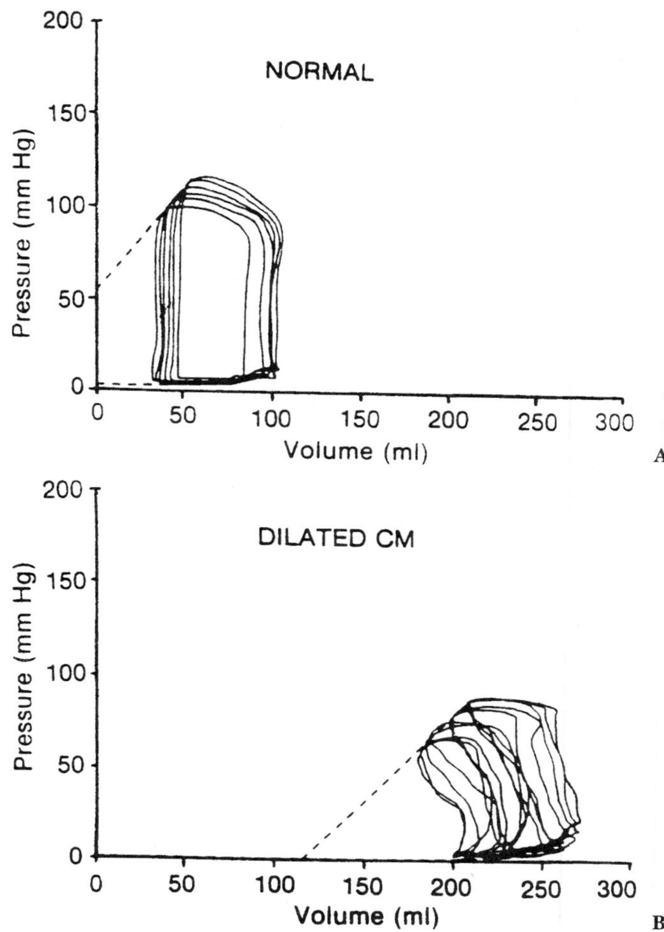

Figure 19. Left ventricular pressure-volume diagrams in a normal patient **(A)** demonstrating a moderately steep ESPVR (high contractility) and a relatively flat EDPVR (high compliance). In contrast, a patient with dilated cardiomyopathy (CM) **(B)** has a flattened ESPVR consistent with declines in contractility as well as a steepened EDPVR indicating decreases in ventricular compliance. The volume intercept is shifted to the right in the patient with dilated cardiomyopathy (B) indicating increased operating volumes. (From ref. 269, with permis-

The ventricular pressure-volume analyses developed by Sagawa et al. (519,601,602) have provided excellent models not only for the assessment of changes in intrinsic myocardial contractility relatively well separated from ventricular loading conditions but also for the analysis of inherent diastolic mechanical properties (519), ventriculoarterial coupling (606,607), and the energetics of the heart (597,598). Applications of the ESPVR and pressure-dimension relationships (13,163,165,267,268,322,363) (e.g., segment length, midaxis diameter, and wall thickness) to the invasive study of systolic function in both experimental animals and humans have been made under a wide variety of pathologic states and pharmacologic interventions, enhancing understanding of cardiac mechanics (520). Noninvasive assessment systolic function with the ESPVR has also been described (to varying degrees of success) using radionuclide ventriculography or two-dimensional echocardiography to assess ventricular volume (259,361). Recently, several limitations to the use of E_{es} as an index of contractile state have been suggested including potential afterload-dependence of the ESPVR (171,630), significant variability in the measurement of E_{es} (345), dependence of E_{es} on autonomic nervous system tone (573), nonlinearity of the ESPVR in the intact heart (77,171,271,345,573,630), dependence of ESPVR on chamber size and shape (28,227), possible dependence of the time-varying elastance model on ejection-mediated alterations in ventricular pressure-generating capacity (75), and potential interaction of the ESPVR with diastolic mechanical properties (678). Despite these potential limitations, the ESPVR provides an excellent framework for the assessment of changes in intrinsic myocardial contractility in both experimental and clinical settings. The reader should consult the superlative textbook on the end-systolic pressure-volume relation by Sagawa et al. (520) for an exhaustive examination of this landmark concept in cardiac physiology.

The dP/dt_{max}–End-Diastolic Volume Relation

Isovolumetric indices of myocardial contractility such as left ventricular peak positive dP/dt are sensitive indicators of inotropic state and are largely independent of afterload (if measured before opening of the aortic valve), but these parameters are substantially influenced by changes in left ventricular preload (375,454,470). Because the left ventricle can be modeled with time-varying elastance (601,602), it can be easily shown (342) that dP/dt_{max} and left ventricular end-diastolic volume are linearly related:

$$dP/dt_{max} = dE/dt_{max} \cdot (EDV - V_0)$$

where dE/dt_{max} = the slope of the relation (peak rate of increase of elastance), EDV = end-diastolic volume (the volume at which dP/dt_{max} occurs during isovolumetric contraction), and V_0 = the volume intercept of the relation. The dP/dt_{max} – EDV relation has been shown to quantitate alterations in contractility in the normal and regionally ischemic left ventricle (342,349). The dP/dt_{max} – EDV relation can be mathematically correlated with the slope of the ESPVR (E_{es}) (342), and interventions that shift the ESPVR without altering E_{es} also shift the volume intercept of the dP/dt_{max} - EDV without changing its slope as well (272). Like the ESPVR, the dP/dt_{max} – EDV relation also displays curvilinearity at higher operating volumes and contractile states, a finding that has been predicted by isolated cardiac muscle mechanics (420).

Preload Recruitable Stroke Work

Another index of myocardial contractility that can be derived from a series of left ventricular pressure-volume loops obtained by transient alteration of loading conditions was developed from reexamination of traditional ventricular function curves using contemporary methodology. Early studies by Frank (167) and Starling (449) related the energy generated by ventricular contraction (e.g., ventricular pressure or cardiac output) to indirect measures of cardiac muscle fiber length (e.g., end-diastolic, pulmonary capillary occlusion or right atrial pressure). This work was extended by Sarnoff and Berglund (526), who used a series of ventricular function curves relating stroke work to filling pressures to describe changes in global myocardial performance. Increases in contractility were indicated by movement of the function curve upward and/or to the left, consistent with the ability of the ventricle to perform greater stroke work at a similar level of preload. Unfortunately, function curves obtained in this manner were nonlinear, difficult to quantify, and used indices of preload (filling pressures) that merely indirectly evaluated end-diastolic volume. Subsequently, Glower et al. (196) used three-dimensional orthogonal sonomicrometry to measure continuous ventricular volume and demonstrated that the relationship between ventricular stroke work and end-diastole volume was linear:

$$SW = M_{sw} \cdot (EDV - V_{sw})$$

where SW = stroke work (calculated by ventricular pressure-volume area for each cardiac cycle), EDV = end-diastolic volume,

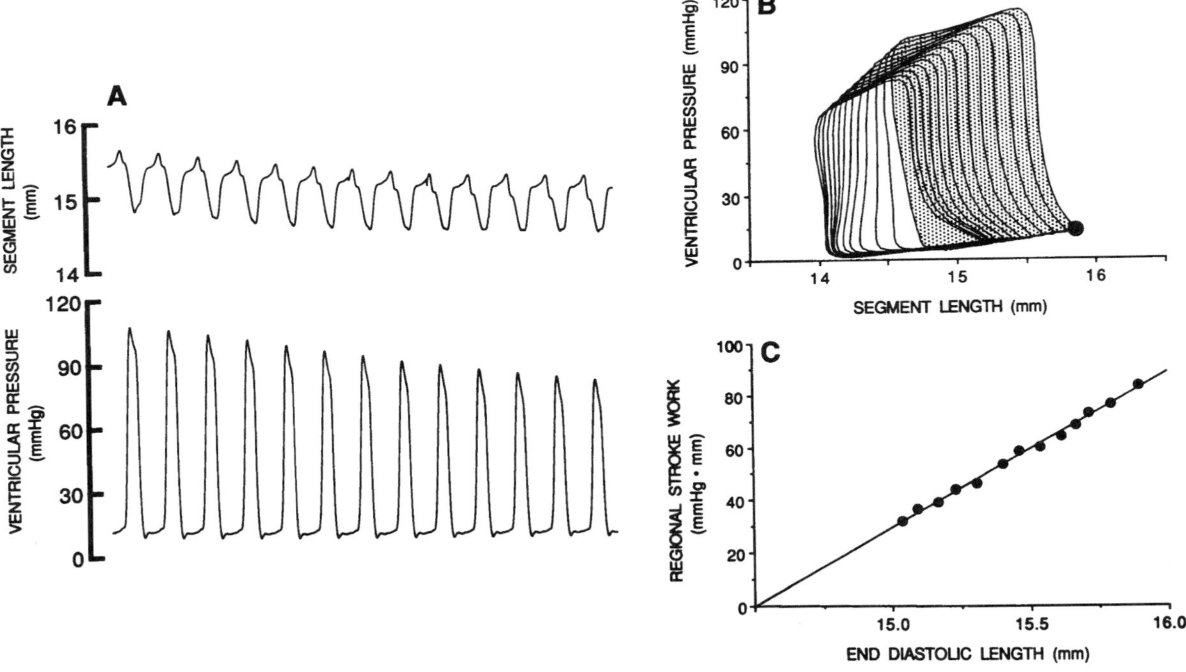

Figure 20. Continuous left ventricular pressure and segment length wave forms **(A)** and resultant pressure-length loops **(B)** in a chronically instrumented dog. Pressure-length diagrams were generated by abrupt occlusion of the inferior vena cava resulting in decreases in ventricular pressure for 13 cardiac cycles. The area of each loop *(shaded area)*, calculated by electronic integration and corresponding to regional stroke work, was plotted against the corresponding end-diastolic segment length *(solid circle)* for each loop (B). A linear regression analysis was then used to define the relationship between regional stroke work and end-diastolic length **(C)**. (From ref. 439, with permission.)

and M_{sw} and V_{sw} = the slope and volume intercept of the relation. This relationship was termed "preload recruitable stroke work" (196) (PRSW) and confirmed a hypothesis proposed by Sarnoff and Berglund (526) three decades earlier. A similar linear relationship between stroke work and one-dimensional segment length (Fig. 20) was also demonstrated by Glower et al. (196). Using these techniques, increases or decreases in intrinsic myocardial contractility were quantitated by appropriate changes in M_{sw}.

PRSW can be calculated using the same pressure-volume diagrams used to assess the ESPVR, and it offers several advantages over the ESPVR. The PRSW relationship is highly linear over a wide variety of loading conditions and contractile states (196, 345), in contrast to the ESPVR, which may be curvilinear under certain conditions in vivo (77,171,271,345,573,630). While the ESPVR may demonstrate a significant degree of afterload sensitivity (171,630), PRSW has been shown to be relatively independent of this variable in a wide physiologic range (196). This occurs despite the potential for the PRSW relation to demonstrate sensitivity to changes in afterload because stroke work must be zero with no load and at infinite load. By integrating data from the entire cardiac cycle (instead of relying on data obtained at an instantaneous definition of end systole), PRSW may also be more reproducible and less variable than the ESPVR while maintaining better linearity and quantitative sensitivity to changes in contractile state at lower ranges of arterial blood pressure than the ESPVR (345). However, integration of data from the entire cardiac cycle also implies that PRSW cannot strictly separate systolic events from diastolic alterations (272). This may be especially important in the setting of profound diastolic dysfunction resulting from myocardial ischemia or ventricular hypertrophy. In addition, partial collapse of the pressure-volume diagram during regional myocardial ischemia (163,518) makes calculation of PRSW technically more difficult than the ESPVR, although an alternative method has been developed that simplifies this process (195). PRSW has been successfully applied as a contractile index under a variety of pathologic conditions as well as under the influence of volatile (430,434) and intravenous anesthetics (435,441).

Other Indices of Myocardial Contractility

Isovolumetric Contraction

High-fidelity, invasive measurement of continuous left ventricular pressure is required to calculate the maximum rate of increase of pressure (dP/dt_{max}), the most commonly used index of global intrinsic inotropic state derived during the isovolumetric phase of ventricular contraction (see Fig. 28). Although changes in dP/dt_{max} are very sensitive to acute alterations in contractile state (375), dP/dt_{max} is less useful when attempting to establish an absolute baseline level of contractility in vivo (454), in contrast to ejection-phase indices such as ejection fraction. Left ventricular dP/dt_{max} is probably most useful in the qualitative assessment of directional changes in contractility produced by acute interventions rather than absolute quantitative evaluation. Left ventricular dP/dt_{max} is considered to be essentially independent of afterload because the peak rate of rise of ventricular pressure usually occurs before the opening of the aortic valve (470). However, dP/dt_{max} is influenced by changes in preload, and alterations in dP/dt_{max} during increases in contractility may be indistinguishable from those induced by variations in preload occurring concurrently (375,470). In addition, dP/dt_{max} may also be influenced by total muscle mass, ventricular chamber size, and abnormalities of the mitral or aortic valves (277). Because dP/dt_{max} is a measure of global systolic function, regional ventricular wall dysfunction caused by myocardial ischemia or infarction of even moderate size may not be sensitively detected. Compensatory increases in contractility (via a Starling mechanism or increases in sympathetic tone) in the nonischemic zones or remodeling hypertrophy in noninfarcted regions may attenuate any potential decrease in dP/dt_{max}. The rate of increase of ventricular pressure at a fixed developed pressure [e.g., dP/dt at 50 mm Hg ventricular pressure (dP/dt_{50})] and the ratio of dP/dt to developed pressure (dP/dt/P), have also been proposed as useful indices of contractility. While these measures of contractility may be less influenced by preload as compared to dP/dt_{max} (376,470), both dP/dt_{50} and dP/dt/P provide little additional information concerning contractile state. A recently developed method incorporates changes in preload into a relation between dP/dt_{max} and end-diastolic volume (342) (see above).

Ejection Phase Indices of Contractility

The most commonly measured index of global myocardial contractility is the ratio of stroke volume to end-diastolic volume or ejection fraction (EF):

$$EF = (EDV - ESV)/EDV$$

Ejection fraction can be calculated using a variety of noninvasive techniques including ventricular cineangiography, echocardiography, and radionuclide ventriculography. A closely related parameter, fractional shortening, can also be determined with these methods as the ratio of end-systolic volume to end-diastolic volume. Assessment of regional derivatives (e.g., using ventricular mid-axis diameter, wall thickness, or segment length) of ejection fraction or fractional shortening are also commonly used in both experimental and clinical settings to evaluate changes in contractile performance.

Ejection fraction averages 67% ± 8% (mean ± SD) in normal patients (159). In the presence of normal mitral and aortic valve function, ejection fraction and fractional shortening are only slighted affected by moderate changes in preload (419). Both variables decrease linearly with increases in afterload and also vary inversely with heart rate, and thus are relatively insensitive indices of contractile function. Ejection fraction and fractional shortening are global measures of cardiac function that may not adequately reflect inconsistencies in regional contraction produced by myocardial ischemia. In addition, ejection fraction and fractional shortening can be misleading in the presence of mitral or aortic valvular pathology, chamber dilatation, or ventricular hypertrophy (47,48,87,130,531,667,668).

The mean velocity of circumferential fiber shortening (V_{cfs}) also provides information about the contractile properties of the intact heart during ejection. This index can be measured using a variety of invasive and noninvasive techniques, including echocardiography using a mid-axis view, and is calculated with the following formula:

$$V_{cfs} = (EED - ESD)/(EED * ET)$$

where EED and ESD = end-distolic and end-systolic diameter, respectively, and ET = ejection time. V_{cfs} may be more sensitive to changes in inotropic state than ejection fraction because velocity, rather than magnitude, of shortening is assessed. V_{cfs} also varies directly with heart rate and inversely with changes in afterload; however, V_{cfs} remains relatively independent of changes in preload because reflex changes in afterload mirror acute alterations in preload, thereby normalizing V_{cfs} in the intact heart (470,471).

Force-Velocity Curves In Vivo

Methods for correcting the inherent heart rate and afterload dependency of ejection-phase indices of contractility in vivo have been suggested that are based on the force-velocity relationship described in isolated papillary muscle preparations. Noninvasive determinations (typically using M-mode or two-dimensional echocardiography and a blood pressure cuff) of left ventricular end-systolic wall stress [circumferential (σ_c) or meridional (σ_m) wall stress, see above] as an index of afterload are combined with heart rate-corrected indices of ventricular ejection such as frac-

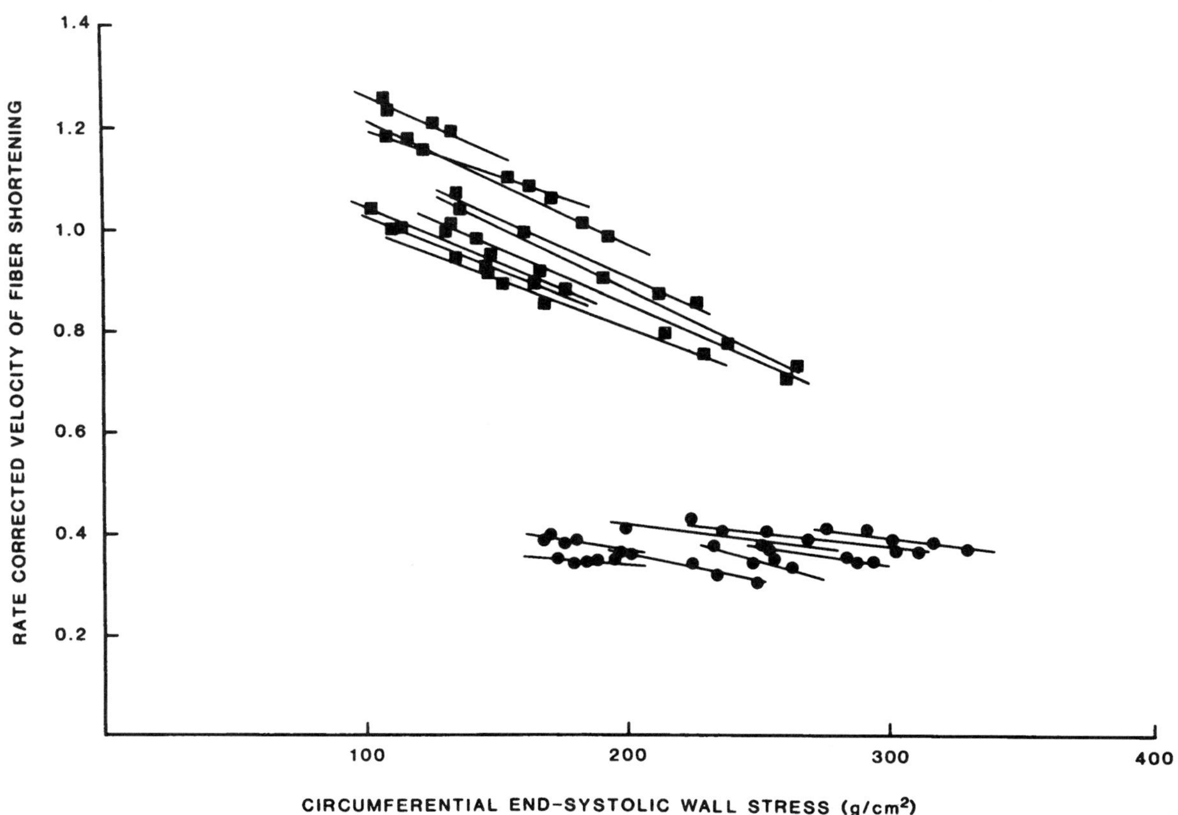

Figure 21. Relationship between the heart rate–corrected velocity of fiber shortening and circumferential end-systolic wall stress in normal patients *(solid squares)* and in patients with congestive heart failure *(solid circles).* (Adapted from ref. 51, with permission.)

tional shortening or V_{cfs}, providing indices of contractility that incorporate afterload and are preload independent over a reasonable physiologic range (48,104). An end-systolic wall stress-V_{cfs} curve (analogous to a force-velocity relation in vitro) can be generated with a pharmacologic intervention that produces an acute change in afterload (e.g., administration of phenylephrine). Changes in this relation accurately reflect acute alterations in myocardial contractility (Fig. 21) and have been used clinically to define basal levels of both enhanced and depressed inotropic state in patients with hypertensive (104,272) and dilated cardiomyopathies (50,104,130,668), respectively. The end-systolic wall stress-V_{cfs} relation has also been employed to ascertain the relative contractile viability of hypertrophic remodeling in cardiomyopathic conditions (48). Recently, the ventricular end-systolic wall stress rate-corrected V_{cfs} relation was used to characterize the relative myocardial depression produced by enflurane and a new volatile anesthetic, sevoflurane, in human volunteers (292).

Ventricular Power Indices of Contractility

Ejection-phase measures of the rate of left ventricular work [power (the product of ventricular pressure and aortic blood flow)] including maximal ventricular power (PWR_{max}) and the rate of power rise are known to be very sensitive to changes in myocardial contractility (511,560,578,579). These indices were intensively studied in the late 1960s but were shown to be highly influenced by left ventricular preload and were technically difficult to derive. Recently, however, improvements in the noninvasive measurement of variables required to calculate power has stimulated reexploration of these techniques (83,281,282,580). Kass and Beyar (270) demonstrated that the quotient of PWR_{max} and the square of end-diastolic volume (PWR_{max}/EDV^2) sensitively reflected changes in inotropic state while maintaining preload and afterload independence when measured invasively. PWR_{max}/EDV^2 can be easily calculated from data obtained in a single cardiac cycle (in contrast to relations derived from a series of left ventricular pressure-volume diagrams), incorporates preload changes, and is highly correlated with the slope of the end-systolic pressure-volume relation (519) (E_{es}) and the dP/dt_{max}-EDV relation (342), two well-established indices of contractility in vivo. Similarly, a regional power quotient using segment length (PWR_{max}/EDL^2) has also been shown to correlate well with the slope of the regional preload recruitable stroke work relation (see below) and has been used to quantitate myocardial depression induced by volatile anesthetics (438). Accurate noninvasive estimation of aortic blood flow, ventricular dimension, and central aortic pressure using Doppler echocardiography combined with tonometry allows measurement of changes in inotropic state using PWR_{max}/EDV^2 in patients (543). Although more study is required to characterize the sensitivity, applicability, and functional limitations of PWR_{max}/EDV^2, this index displays several promising features that have been absent from other measures of contractile state including single cardiac cycle derivation, consistent load independence, and the potential for relatively uncomplicated noninvasive assessment.

REGULATION OF MYOCARDIAL CONTRACTILITY IN VIVO

The regulation of myocardial contractility in the intact heart is complex (Fig. 22). Several intrinsic and extrinsic compensatory mechanisms allow the heart to maintain overall performance when contractile function is reduced by disease states (e.g., myocardial ischemia) or pharmacologic agents (e.g., volatile anesthetics) or when abnormal pressure or volume loads are acutely or chronically imposed. The Frank-Starling

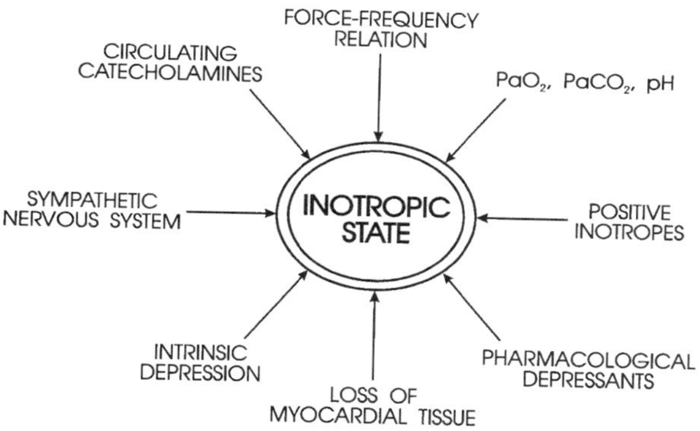

Figure 22. Major influences on intrinsic inotropic state in the intact cardiovascular system. (Adapted from ref. 64, with permission.)

law represents the most important adaptation by which inherent global systolic function can be enhanced. Increased end-diastolic volume optimizes sarcomere length (311) and actin-myosin overlap (203) and augments the sensitivity of the contractile apparatus to calcium (2,287), effects that are directly translated into an increase in contractility. Potentiation of ventricular preload occurs in response to venoconstriction and increases in intravascular volume by renal sodium and water retention resulting from sympathetic nervous system stimulation (134,166,239,305), renin-angiotensin-aldosterone axis activation (18,135,485), enhanced release of vasopressin from the posterior pituitary gland (491,542), and modulation of other vasoactive substances including prostaglandins (328,379,679) and atrial natriuretic peptide (12,663).

Another intrinsic adaptive mechanism by which myocardial contractile state can be self-regulated in vivo is the "force-frequency" relation as described in isolated cardiac muscle preparations in vitro. Contractility increases in direct response to increases in heart rate within a wide physiologic range independent of changes in ventricular loading conditions (64), an effect known as the Bowditch staircase or "treppe." This phenomenon was first demonstrated in isolated myocardium and has also been observed in the isolated (378) and intact heart (172). A longer than normal delay between beats (e.g., precipitated by marked bradycardia or a conduction abnormality) or a pause following a ventricular extrasystole (e.g., a premature ventricular contraction) will also be followed by a stronger contraction in vivo. This phenomenon, termed the interval-strength effect, is an intrinsic property of cardiac muscle and is probably due to a time-induced alteration in calcium availability in the myocyte modulated via enhanced calcium channel opening (659,676). In the intact heart, the interval strength effect is amplified by the additional mechanical actions of increases in diastolic filling time and volume.

Although the "force-frequency" effect plays an important role in the physiologic matching of cardiac output to venous return in the intact heart during exercise (238,459), tachycardia has little effect on overall cardiac performance under normal conditions (639). In contrast, rate-dependent positive inotropic effects are especially important in dilated, failing myocardium. In this condition, enhanced venous return and passive congestion resulting from intravascular volume expansion, augmented venous tone, and primary depression of contractile function can be compensated by increases in rate despite concomitant decreases in diastolic filling time (64,401). Similarly, tachycardia-related increases in myocardial contractility also help to maintain cardiac output in pathologic conditions that limit the extent of ventricular filling (571) (e.g., pericardial tamponade). Contractility becomes reduced at extremely rapid heart rates (greater than 175 beats per minute) associated with pacing or tachyarrhythmias. Very rapid heart rates also limit the extent to which cardiac output can be enhanced because decreases in diastolic duration and filling also occur (400).

Ventricular hypertrophy is a compensatory response to chronically imposed stress resulting from excessive pressure or volume loading conditions (216). Hypertrophy enhances systolic function by augmenting total myocardial contractile mass via increases in the size and/or number of sarcomeres in each myocyte. The increase in contractile performance allows the ventricle to maintain adequate pump function and decrease wall stress in the presence of abnormal elevations in load. However, ventricular hypertrophic processes also simultaneously produce several detrimental effects (see below), including decreases in the intrinsic contractile function of individual myocytes, increases in global myocardial oxygen demand, abnormalities in the transmural distribution of coronary blood flow, and impairment of diastolic function that may ultimately contribute to cardiac decompensation and failure.

Stimulation of the sympathetic nervous system results in the release of norepinephrine from synaptic terminals located on the heart and the peripheral vasculature (115,675). Norepinephrine causes direct positive chronotropic, inotropic, and lusitropic effects mediated via cardiac β_1-adrenoceptors and the intracellular second messenger, cyclic adenosine monophosphate (cAMP) (637), as well as effects in the myocardium mediated via α_1-adrenoceptors that also increase contractility (148). Norepinephrine-induced α_1-adrenergic veno- and vasoconstriction of capacitance and resistance vessels increases venous return to the heart and arterial perfusion pressure to vital organs, respectively (637). Although increases in preload resulting from enhanced venous tone improve cardiac performance by the Frank-Starling mechanism, peripheral arterial vasoconstriction also directly increases impedance to ventricular outflow, an effect that may worsen myocardial function, especially in the setting of heart failure. Activation of presynaptic α_2-adrenoceptors by norepinephrine modulates the central and peripheral actions of this catecholamine by augmenting its reuptake into nerve terminals (200,237). Increases in central sympathetic tone also result in the release of epinephrine from the adrenal medulla (314). Epinephrine also stimulates cardiac β_1-adrenoceptors, enhancing heart rate, contractility, and diastolic relaxation. Activation of β_2-adrenoceptors presynaptically may augment release of norepinephrine (56). The hormonal effects of epinephrine occur more slowly than the neural actions produced by norepinephrine (314) and may represent an important homeostatic mechanism during chronic disease states associated with heart failure (232). A persistent elevation in sympathetic tone or circulating catecholamines associated with depressed myocardial contractility (97, 103,232) may lead to the downregulation of cardiac β_1-adrenoceptors (65,635), decreasing the responsiveness of the failing heart to inotropic and lusitropic augmentation.

The parasympathetic nervous system acts to counterbalance the actions of the sympathetic nervous system in the regulation of myocardial contractility in the intact heart (332,333). Increases in efferent vagal tone and release of acetylcholine result in negative chronotropic and dromotropic effects on the sinoatrial (SA) and atrioventricular (AV) nodes and the electrical conduction pathways, respectively (330). Acetylcholine-induced depression of contractile function also occurs to some degree with increases in parasympathetic outflow via vagal innervation of myocardium (330). Under normal conditions, parasympathetic activity far exceeds sympathetic activity (638, 640). Further increases in parasympathetic tone may occur in response to sympathetic activation, directly attenuating the positive inotropic effects produced by sympathetic stimulation, a process known as "accelerated antagonism" (331–333). In contrast, withdrawal of parasympathetic tone may accompany sympathetic stimulation during exercise or heart failure, an effect that reverses the relative importance of these determinants of overall autonomic nervous system function (637). This decline in parasympathetic control may result in a more vigorous cardiac response to catecholamines derived from stimulation of the sympathoadrenal axis.

MYOCARDIAL ENERGETICS IN THE LEFT VENTRICULAR PRESSURE-VOLUME FRAMEWORK

The total mechanical energy of the heart generated during the cardiac cycle has been characterized using a model based on the left ventricular pressure-volume diagram and the corresponding end-systolic and end-diastolic pressure-volume relations that establish its boundaries in pressure-volume phase space. Suga defined total mechanical energy as the sum of kinetic energy expended during systole (e.g., pressure-volume or stroke work) and potential energy that remains in the chamber wall at end systole (e.g., compressed myocardial series elastic elements) using the total area under the ESPVR line and the systolic component of the pressure-volume diagram above the EDPVR (590). The area outlined by these boundaries was denoted as total systolic pressure-volume area (PVA; Fig. 23) (591). The potential energy stored in the myocardium at end systole was defined as the triangular area between the ESPVR and the EDPVR to the left of the stroke work trajectory. This elastic potential energy has units identical to pressure-volume work (1 mm Hg · mm = $1.333 \cdot 10^{-4}$ joules) and has been presumed to be converted into heat during relaxation and ventricular filling (591,596).

Because total cardiac mechanical energy is equivalent to myocardial oxygen consumption (MVO_2) during aerobic metabolism, Suga et al. (597,599) also proposed that PVA should directly reflect MVO_2. These investigators demonstrated a highly linear correlation ($r \geq .95$) between PVA and measured MVO_2 in the isolated heart under a variety of loading conditions and heart rates: $MVO_2 = A \cdot PVA + D$, where A = slope of the relation and D = the MVO_2 at zero PVA (595,598). The area beneath the MVO_2-PVA line represents the sum of mechanical energy, basal metabolism, and the energy of excitation-contraction coupling (Fig. 24). Increases in myocardial contractility (E_{max}) produced by exogenous positive inotropes including calcium and epinephrine or decreases in contractile state resulting from propranolol or verapamil caused parallel upward or downward shifts in the MVO_2-PVA relation, respectively (79,593,599,600). During alterations in contractile state, the MVO_2-PVA relation was mathematically rewritten as $MVO_2 = A \cdot PVA + B \cdot E_{max} + C$, where B = the sensitivity of the MVO_2-PVA relation to E_{max} and C = basal metabolism (596,600). Within this theoretical framework, increases in MVO_2 associated with enhanced contractility occurred at constant PVA and resulted from proportional increases in the energy of excitation-contraction coupling (Fig. 24). However, the contribution of mechanical energy to total MVO_2 remained constant during changes in intrinsic inotropic state, indicating that the actual biochemical conversion of adenosine triphosphate (ATP) into mechanical energy in the myofilaments is unaffected by contractile state (520). Alterations in the relative magnitude of kinetic and potential energy may also occur during diastolic dysfunction via changes in the slope of the pressure-volume compliance curve (EDPVR); however, measured MVO_2 does not vary under these circumstances if PVA remains constant (596). These findings support the hypothesis that PVA alone, but not the individual kinetic and potential energy elements of PVA, is correlated with MVO_2 (592). The relative load independence of the MVO_2-PVA relation also provided convincing indirect evidence that conventionally used calculated indices of myocardial oxygen consumption, including pressure-time and wall stress-time integrals, were incapable of completely describing alterations in MVO_2 (595,598). MVO_2 has recently been shown to be primarily related to systolic PVA in humans (633), confirming previous evidence obtained in the isolated heart.

The relationship between MVO_2 and PVA also forms the basis for an elegant description of the mechanical efficiency of the heart. Efficiency is traditionally defined as the ratio of useful energy output to total energy input. Using this definition, car-

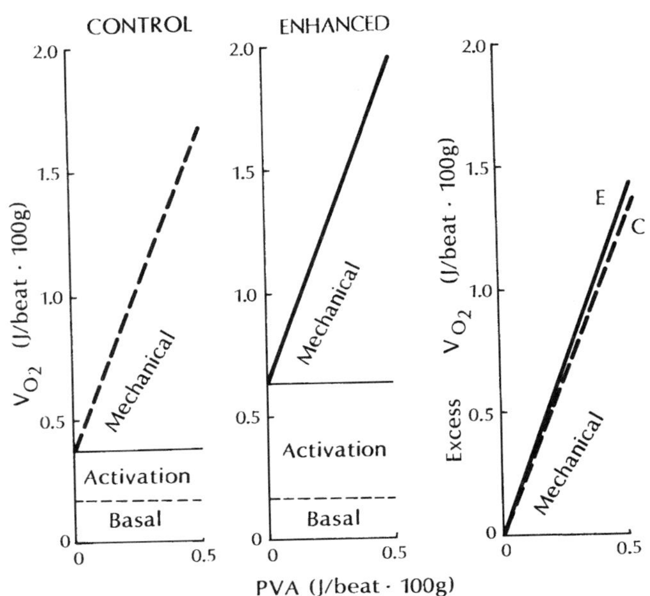

Figure 24. Three myocardial oxygen consumption (VO_2) components for basal metabolism, excitation-contraction coupling, and mechanical contraction control *(left panel)* and enhanced inotropic state *(middle panel)*. The *solid diagonal lines* represent the VO_2-pressure-volume area (PVA) relation observed in each condition. Note that during the infusion of epinephrine *(middle panel)*, the VO_2 component for excitation-contraction coupling activation is markedly increased, causing a parallel upward shift of the VO_2-PVA relation. In the *right panel*, excess VO_2 (total VO_2 minus unloaded VO_2) is plotted against PVA under control conditions (C) or during enhancement of contractile state (E). The two *solid diagonal lines* are transcribed from the *left* and *middle panels* and indicate that the mechanical component of VO_2 is unaffected by contractile state. (From ref. 520, with permission.)

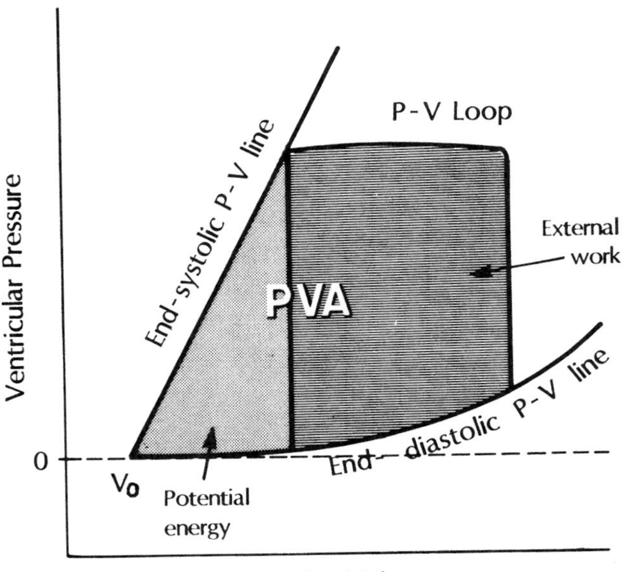

Figure 23. Systolic pressure-volume area (PVA) determined by external work and end-systolic elastic potential energy. (From ref. 520, with permission.)

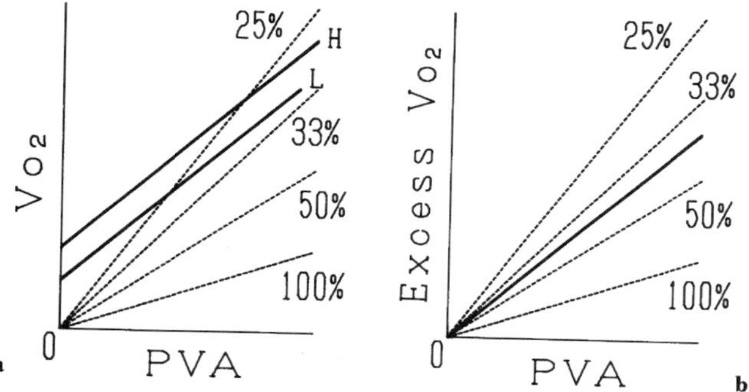

Figure 25. The relation between total myocardial oxygen consumption (VO_2) and systolic pressure-volume area (PVA) and a family of isoefficiency lines (25%, 33%, 50%, and 100%). Two VO_2-PVA relations at low (L) and high (H) contractility are depicted in **a**. The relation between excess VO_2 and PVA and a family of isoefficiency lines is illustrated in **b**. The two excess VO_2-PVA relations during low and high inotropic state are superimposable (see Fig. 24). These data indicate that the efficiency of mechanical activation of the contractile apparatus is approximately 40% and is unaffected by contractile state (see text). (From ref. 592, with permission.)

diac mechanical efficiency is characterized by the quotient of external mechanical work performed by the heart (e.g., stroke work) and total energy supplied to and used by the heart (187,527,600). Because PVA describes total mechanical energy expenditure under aerobic metabolic conditions, myocardial conversion efficiency was defined as the ratio of PVA to MVO_2 and formally characterized the efficiency of the conversion of total energy input to total mechanical energy output (600,603). In addition, because the mechanical contribution of total MVO_2 exceeds basal and excitation-contraction metabolic requirements (Fig. 25), the quotient of PVA and this mechanical component of MVO_2 (termed "excess" MVO_2) was used to define myofibrillar efficiency and described the efficiency of energy

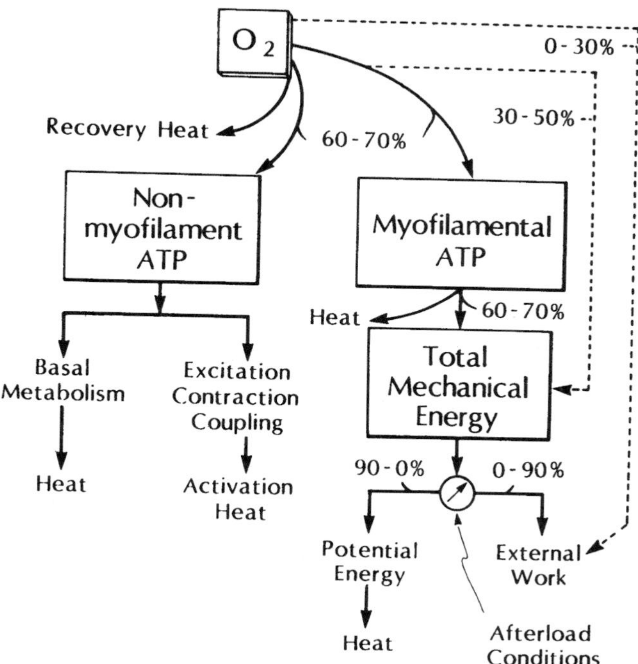

Figure 26. Schematic illustration depicting the transfer of energy from oxygen supply to basal metabolism, excitation contraction coupling, external work, and end-systolic elastic potential energy. The percentages represent the approximate efficiency of each conversion process (see text). (From ref. 520, with permission.)

conversion from the MVO_2 component used for activity of the contractile proteins into the total mechanical energy output. PVA/MVO_2 and PVA/excess MVO_2 ratios are typically examined in relation to superimposed isoefficiency lines and are calculated as the inverse of the slope coefficient ($1/A$) of the MVO_2/PVA slope relation that indicates the relationship between PVA and total or excess MVO_2 at specified efficiencies (Fig. 25). Myocardial conversion efficiency (PVA/MVO_2) varies with PVA and E_{max} (599). In contrast, myofibrillar efficiency (PVA/excess MVO_2) is independent of myocardial contractility because chemomechanical energy transfer at the myofilaments (e.g., the activity of actomyosin ATPase) is unaffected by inotropic state.

Myofibrillar efficiency averages between 30% and 40% in the normal heart. The functional efficiency of the contractile proteins depends on the chemical efficiency of aerobic ATP production by oxidative phosphorylation and the conversion of this high-energy phosphate to mechanical kinetic and potential energy (PVA). The efficiency of ATP formation from O_2 supplied to the cardiac myocyte has been shown to be approximately 65% (188). The efficiency of energy transduction from ATP to PVA must also be about 65% because the product of the efficiencies of ATP production from O_2 and the transfer of this energy to the contractile apparatus must be equal to the myofibrillar efficiency (Fig. 26). These calculations also suggest that the efficiency of energy conversion of ATP to PVA during contraction is relatively constant and occurs independent of changes in contractile state and ventricular loading conditions (592).

LEFT VENTRICULAR FUNCTION DURING DIASTOLE

Invasive Evaluation of Diastolic Function

Isovolumetric Relaxation

Invasive and high-fidelity measurement of ventricular pressure is required to accurately measure changes in isovolumetric relaxation. The rate of decrease of isovolumetric pressure is commonly assessed with the minimum value of the first derivative of ventricular pressure with respect to time ($-dP/dt_{min}$) or a time constant (τ) of isovolumetric left ventricular pressure decline (656). Peak $-dP/dt_{min}$ is a relatively unreliable measure of global relaxation because this index is dependent on developed ventricular pressure, and the rate of pressure decline is measured at only a single time point when using this technique (335,653). The decrease in ventricular pressure from $-dP/dt_{min}$ to the opening of the mitral valve follows a monoexponential time course. The rate of pressure decrease between these points can be determined from a simple mathematical expression:

$$P = A \cdot e^{-t/\tau}$$

where P = ventricular pressure, A = ventricular pressure at $-dP/dt_{min}$, t = time after $-dP/dt_{min}$, and τ = rate of relaxation (msec). A delay in relaxation is reflected by an increase in τ (Fig. 27) that can occur in disease processes such as myocardial ischemia (10,90,251,381,403,537), ventricular hypertrophy (142,319,450,541), and dilated cardiomyopathy (156), or as a result of the action of negative inotropes, such as potent inhalational anesthetics (133,250,432). τ is reduced by an enhanced rate of relaxation that can occur during an increase in heart rate, sympathetic nerve stimulation, or circulating catecholamines. Alterations in the rate of ventricular pressure reduction produced by positive or negative inotropes or by pathologic processes may exist with or without concomitant effects on systolic performance, indicating that nonuniformity between systolic and diastolic events can occur (142,319,450).

The time constant of isovolumetric relaxation is probably dependent on ventricular loading conditions, particularly afterload, although this conclusion remains somewhat controversial (71,178,180,189,266,444,473,576,621,634,677). Certainly in isolated muscle it is evident that greater shortening induces faster

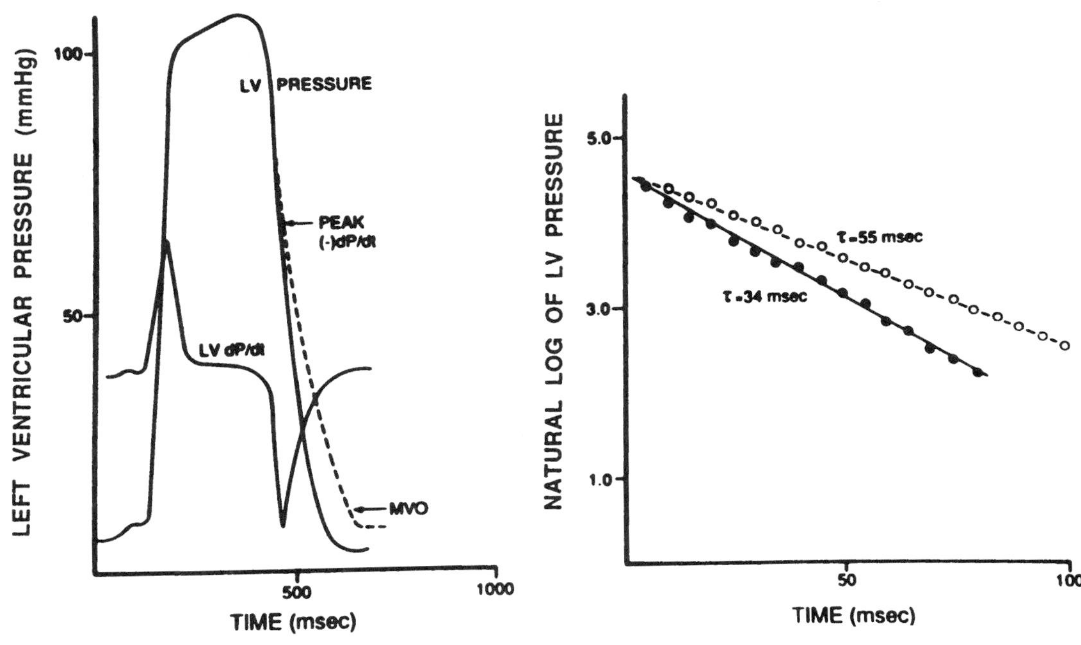

Figure 27. Calculation of the time constant of left ventricular (LV) isovolumetric relaxation (τ). Normal *(solid line)* and delayed *(dashed line)* rates of LV pressure decline are represented in the *left panel.* Plots of the natural logarithm of LV pressure against time and the corresponding time constant of isovolumetric relaxation for normal *(solid circles)* and delayed relaxation *(open circles)* are illustrated in the *right panel.* MVO, mitral valve opening. (From ref. 558, with permission.)

relaxation, an effect that appears to be mediated by length-dependent alterations in Ca^{2+} binding by troponin C (70,247, 287). Because afterload influences the duration of ejection and ventricular muscle shortening (75), afterload will be expected to alter relaxation rate (189). Thus, interpretation of changes in τ as an index of intrinsic myocardial relaxation should be made when loading conditions are held relatively constant (558). There has also been debate as to which portion of the left ventricular pressure curve should be used and whether a zero pressure asymptote should be assumed in the calculation of τ. Methods of evaluating isovolumetric relaxation by allowing ventricular pressure to decay to a natural asymptote rather than being mathematically constrained to fall to zero (as dictated by the equation above) have been proposed (473,621). Nevertheless, τ derived using a zero pressure asymptote has proven to be clinically and experimentally acceptable in describing isovolumetric relaxation as long as acute changes in pericardial pressure do not occur (673).

Early Diastolic Filling

Continuous measurement of ventricular volume or dimension is required for calculation of invasive indices characterizing early diastolic filling. This phase of diastole can be assessed using several techniques including peak filling rate [calculated as the first derivative of the volume-time curve, dV/dt (Fig. 7)], the peak velocity of early diastolic filling, the velocity-time integral (area under the dV/dt curve), the percentage of total diastolic filling time occupied by rapid ventricular filling, and measurements of time intervals between diastolic events such as the time from end systole to peak filling. Peak filling rates and analogous parameters derived from dimensional (e.g., segment length) approximations may be dependent on the region of the ventricle examined (336). The accuracy with which these variables describe early ventricular filling also depends on geometric assumptions used to estimate ventricular volume or cardiac dimension (335).

The early diastolic pressure gradient between atrium and ventricle is a primary determinant of the rate of rapid ventricular filling (258). The pressure gradient across the mitral valve may increase with elevations in left atrial pressure or decreases in atrial compliance. Decreases in this gradient occur as a result of delay in isovolumetric relaxation, reduction of left ventricular compliance, or increase in left ventricular viscoelasticity (the property of a material to demonstrate enhanced resistance to stretch when the rate of application of strain increases). Viscoelastic characteristics of the left ventricle are important during rapid ventricular filling and atrial systole, periods when the rate of change of volume (strain rate) is high (462). The early diastolic transmural pressure gradient is also affected by diastolic suction (416,594,604), especially when filling pressures are low.

Chamber Stiffness

Ventricular chamber stiffness is defined as the ratio of change in pressure to unit change in volume (dP/dV). The inverse of stiffness is compliance (dV/dP). The diastolic pressure-volume relation can be represented mathematically using a simple exponential equation:

$$P = A \cdot e^{Kc \cdot V}$$

where P = ventricular pressure, A = ventricular pressure at zero volume, K_c = the modulus of chamber stiffness, and V = ventricular volume. Because the diastolic pressure-volume relation is considered exponential, the relation between dP/dV (the first derivative of pressure with respect to volume) and ventricular pressure is linear. The slope of this relation defines K_c. Simple dimension measurements such as segment length are often used as substitutes for ventricular volume. The pressure-volume relation shifts to the left, and the slope of the dP/dV versus pressure relationship becomes steeper during an increase in chamber stiffness (Fig. 28).

While intuitively useful, a simple monoexponential description of the relationship between ventricular pressure and volume may be physiologically inappropriate for several reasons (395). Pressure-volume data may be better fit with a three-constant exponential equation, allowing for the possibility that the pressure-volume curve passes through zero (395). Chamber stiffness is also influenced by left ventricular volume and mass,

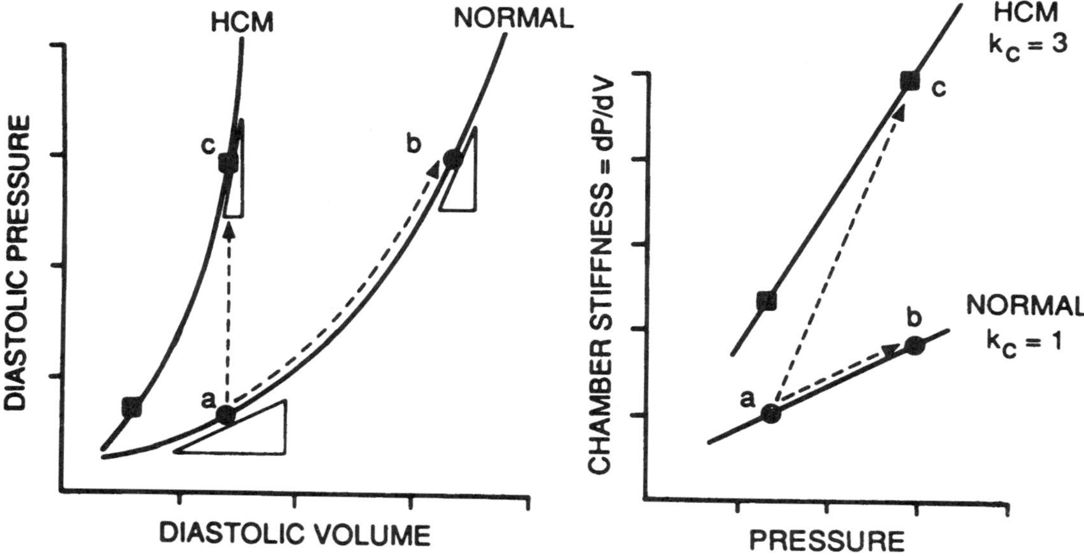

Figure 28. Schematic diagram depicting left ventricular diastolic pressure-volume relations in hypertrophic cardiomyopathy (HCM). The stiffness at any point along a given pressure-volume curve is equal to the slope of the tangent drawn to the curve at that point *(left panel)*. Chamber stiffness changes throughout filling because stiffness is less at smaller volumes (point *a, left panel)* and greater at larger volumes (point *b, left panel)*. The pressure-volume relation in HCM demonstrates a shift to the left and increased diastolic pressure at any given diastolic volume (point *c, left panel)* consistent with increased chamber stiffness. Because the shape of the pressure-volume relation is exponential, the relationship between dP/dV and pressure is linear *(right panel)*. The slope of this relation is termed the modulus of chamber stiffness (K_c). The slope of the dP/dV versus pressure relationship becomes steeper and K_c increases when overall chamber stiffness is increased (HCM, *right panel)*. (From ref. 558, with permission.)

and therefore a comparison of changes in the intrinsic chamber stiffness constant (K_c) between patients, for example, requires normalization for left ventricular wall volume (558). K_c should also be derived from common ranges of left ventricular pressure or normalized so that the range of pressure over which stiffness is calculated is similar between patients or interventions.

Measurements of chamber stiffness do not strictly consider important parallel shifts in the diastolic pressure-volume relationship. A parallel upward shift, for example as produced by an acute increase in pericardial pressure, may make the chamber appear less distensible because the ventricular diastolic pressure would be higher at any given volume (558). Although this parallel upward shift would result in an increase in ventricular diastolic pressure at zero ventricular volume, the slope of the dP/dV versus pressure relation would remain constant, indicating that intrinsic chamber stiffness (K_c) is unaltered. The position of the ventricular pressure-volume curve may ultimately be more important than the actual slope of this relation (192,193) in defining the characteristics of the ventricle, since upward and leftward shifts in the curve, regardless of K_c, imply that a higher pressure is required to distend the ventricle to any given volume.

Myocardial Stiffness

While ventricular chamber stiffness evaluates the ability of the ventricle to passively distend over a range of filling pressures, myocardial stiffness represents the resistance of cardiac muscle to stretching when a stress is applied and, therefore, defines the material properties of myocardium itself (335). Myocardium exhibits properties of an elastic material, developing a resisting force (stress; σ) as muscle length (strain; ε) increases (Hooke's law) during ventricular filling. Forces resisting further increases in muscle length become greater as muscle is stretched, resulting in increased myocardial stiffness. Examination of the ventricular wall stress-strain relationship during diastole allows quantification of myocardial stiffness. Strain is defined as the percent change in volume or muscle length *(L)* from unstressed, equilibrium volume or muscle length *(L_o)*, which is assumed to occur at 0 mm Hg left ventricular pressure. The Lagrangian strain formula is most commonly used to normalize volumes or muscle lengths:

$$\varepsilon = \frac{L - L_o}{L_o}$$

The stress-strain relation is exponential, and stress and strain are typically related by the following equation:

$$\sigma = \alpha(e^{\beta \cdot \varepsilon} - 1)$$

where σ = left ventricular wall stress, ε = Lagrangian strain, α = the coefficient of gain, and β = the modulus of myocardial stiffness. Increases in myocardial stiffness (e.g., as produced by chronic infiltrative processes such as amyloidosis) are indicated by a shift of the stress-strain relationship to the left and an increase in the slope of the linear $d\sigma/d\varepsilon$ versus σ relationship. Comparison of stress-strain data between subjects must be performed under conditions of similar degrees of ventricular wall stress and geometry (395). Chamber stiffness (see above) can also be shown to be directly proportional to myocardial stiffness and inversely related to the ratio of the volume of the ventricular cavity to the volume of the ventricular wall (395).

Ventricular myocardium is not strictly an elastic material but also displays viscoelastic characteristics. Viscoelasticity occurs when forces resisting further deformity are dependent not only on the degree of changes in muscle length but also on the rate at which muscle length is changed. These effects are most apparent during rapid ventricular filling and atrial systole, periods of diastole when the rate of change of ventricular volume is most pronounced. Mathematical descriptions of stress-strain relations incorporating expressions describing instantaneous rate of change of ventricular filling have also been developed that incorporate these viscoelastic effects (462,478):

$$\sigma = \alpha(e^{\beta \cdot \varepsilon} - 1) + \eta \cdot d\varepsilon/dt$$

where η = the viscoelastic constant and $d\varepsilon/dt$ = the rate of change of strain. Although viscous effects may alter ventricular filling to some degree, this is probably of minor importance in the normally functioning heart (417).

Noninvasive Evaluation of Diastolic Function

Doppler Echocardiography

Clinical and experimental noninvasive evaluation of left ventricular filling dynamics can be accomplished using Doppler echocardiographic techniques. Doppler echocardiography measures the velocity of blood flow through the mitral valve by detecting the frequency shift of ultrasound reflected from moving erythrocytes. In transthoracic studies, the ultrasound beam is typically directed from the cardiac apex through the mitral valve, an orientation that is parallel to the direction of diastolic flow. In contrast, when transesophageal echocardiography is used, the ultrasound beam originates from the esophagus and is directed through the mitral valve from the left atrium to the left ventricle. The velocity of flow can be reproducibly measured by Doppler sampling within the mitral valve orifice using these configurations. Total blood flow across the mitral valve is calculated as the product of mitral valve area (assumed to be constant throughout diastole) and the velocity of blood flow (337). Thus, the rate of left ventricular filling is directly proportional to mitral flow velocity measured by the Doppler technique. Doppler recording of blood flow velocity across the mitral valve typically has a biphasic pattern. An early peak of flow velocity (E wave) occurs during rapid early diastolic filling and a late peak of flow velocity (A wave) occurs during atrial systole (Fig. 29). Measurements of flow velocity during diastasis are minimal, consistent with the observation that little ventricular filling occurs during this phase of diastole.

A large number of indices of diastolic function derived from Doppler echocardiography have been proposed (295,296,347, 418). These parameters include the peak heights of the early (E) and late (A) flow velocities, the ratio of peak E to peak A velocity (E/A ratio), the time velocity integrals (TVI) of E and A signals (area under each wave) and ratio of the E and A TVI, the

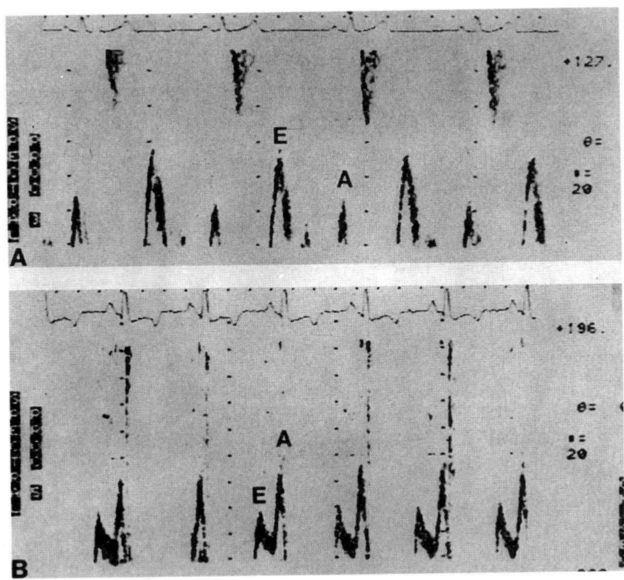

Figure 29. Doppler echocardiographic recordings of mitral blood flow velocity in a normal patient **(A)** and a patient with severe left ventricular (LV) hypertrophy **(B)**. An early peak of blood flow velocity (E wave) occurs during rapid ventricular filling and a late peak of blood flow velocity (A wave) occurs during atrial systole. The E wave is reduced and the A wave is increased in LV hypertrophy, suggesting that the atrial contribution to LV filling is enhanced and early diastolic filling is depressed. (From ref. 347, with permission.)

atrial filling fraction (the ratio of the A wave TVI to the TVI of total mitral inflow), the deceleration time (the interval from peak E wave velocity to zero), and the isovolumetric relaxation time (IVRT; the time from the end of systolic ventricular outflow to mitral valve opening). Doppler assessment of filling dynamics appears to correlate well with angiographic or radionuclide techniques of measuring the rate of ventricular volume change during diastole (174,503,568). Furthermore, the E and A portions of the mitral flow velocity waveform correspond closely to the first derivative of left ventricular volume (dV/dt) or segment length (dL/dt) (Fig. 7) obtained with invasive techniques.

The magnitude and ratio of the early and late peaks of flow velocity are influenced by normal physiologic events (heart rate and rhythm, preload, and atrial inotropic state), aortic or mitral valve disease, right ventricular competence and ventricular septal interaction, and the intrinsic lusitropic (diastolic mechanical) properties of the ventricle itself. Transmitral flow velocities can assume distinctive patterns depending on the nature of diastolic dysfunction. For example, when isovolumetric relaxation is prolonged, the initial pressure gradient between the left atrium and ventricle is reduced, less filling occurs during early diastole, and subsequently, a greater proportion of filling occurs in late diastole during atrial contraction. Thus, abnormal global ventricular relaxation is characterized by a prolongation of the IVRT and deceleration time, the presence of reduced E and simultaneously enhanced A wave velocity, and a low or reversed E/A ratio. These findings have been observed in hypertrophic (373,451,609) or dilated cardiomyopathies (610), during myocardial ischemia or infarction (176,309,398,666), or in the presence of restrictive processes (7) (see Fig. 37). A decrease in ventricular compliance may result in a rapid rise in ventricular diastolic pressure during early diastole, causing a high initial flow velocity signal (E wave). Shortened IVRT and deceleration time and increased E wave velocity are characteristic findings in mitral regurgitation consistent with enhanced isovolumetric relaxation and early ventricular filling. Because the pattern of left ventricular filling is effected by multiple factors, alterations in filling dynamics assessed from Doppler techniques should be interpreted within these potential constraints. Some patients with gross diastolic dysfunction and elevated left ventricular filling pressures may actually demonstrate a normal diastolic filling pattern, a process known as pseudonormalization (7,8,610). Conversely, abnormal patterns of ventricular filling may also be observed in the absence of diastolic pathology (11,19).

The patterns of pulmonary venous blood flow during diastole also provide information about ventricular compliance. Pulmonary venous flow velocity signals can be accurately obtained using pulsed Doppler transesophageal echocardiography (307). The diastolic phase of pulmonary venous blood flow is typically described by an antegrade flow velocity wave (D wave) that begins when the mitral valve opens and a retrograde flow velocity signal observed during atrial contraction, corresponding to the E and A waves of the mitral inflow Doppler signals, respectively (Fig. 30). Examination of patterns of pulmonary blood flow may be especially useful in the presence of ventricular diastolic dysfunction and elevated filling pressures, a clinical setting in which pseudonormalization of mitral inflow velocity waveforms is known to occur (see above). Enhanced retrograde pulmonary venous blood flow may occur before or during atrial systole, strongly implicating the presence of diastolic dysfunction under these circumstances. Doppler pulmonary venous flow velocity signals have been used to evaluate abnormal diastolic function in restrictive and constrictive pericardial diseases, amyloidosis and other infiltrative processes, and cardiac tamponade (307).

Two-Dimensional and M-Mode Echocardiography

Two-dimensional echocardiography allows characterization of left ventricular size, wall motion and thickness, and qualitative analysis of systolic performance (ejection fraction, circum-

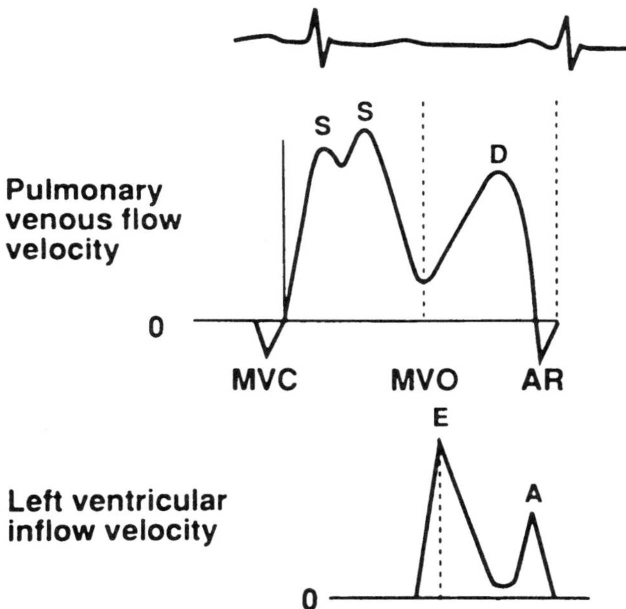

Figure 30. Schematic illustration depicting pulmonary venous flow velocity and the corresponding left ventricular inflow velocity obtained with Doppler echocardiography. During systole, pulmonary venous flow consists of a mono- or biphasic forward flow (S). Diastolic pulmonary venous flow is composed of a single monophasic forward flow (D) and a small retrograde flow associated with atrial contraction (AR), corresponding to the E and A waves of the mitral inflow Doppler signals, respectively. MVC, mitral valve closure; MVO, mitral valve opening. (Adapted from ref. 296, with permission.)

ferential velocity of fiber shortening) as well as definition of abnormalities in valvular structure. This technique also can be used to detect the presence, magnitude, and pathophysiologic consequences (right ventricular diastolic collapse) of pericardial effusions that may adversely affect left ventricular diastolic filling. Two-dimensional echocardiography, however, cannot typically provide further quantitative assessment of diastolic relaxation and filling because of slow sampling rates and poor spatial resolution (347).

In the absence of regional wall motion abnormalities, M-mode echocardiography approximates changes in ventricular volume by using a narrow ultrasound beam combined with rapid sampling to define the sequential position of cardiac structures in time. The rate of change of left ventricular diameter can be used as an index of ventricular filling (628). The rate of ventricular wall thinning can also be measured using M-mode echocardiography, providing another means of quantifying filling dynamics. In general, pulsed Doppler has replaced M-mode echocardiography in the assessment of diastolic function because the latter technique provides only a limited window of detection and may be misleading during asynchrony of ventricular wall motion.

Radionuclide Ventriculography

Recognition of patterns of ventricular filling can be accomplished by radionuclide ventriculography using radiolabeled erythrocytes. The activity of the isotope obtained over the left ventricle (minus background activity) during the diastolic phase of several cardiac cycles is recorded, and the electrocardiogram is used to consistently define end diastole. Relative left ventricular volume (% end-diastolic volume) is approximated by a time-activity curve (Fig. 31). Filling rates during early and late diastole (rapid filling and atrial systole) as well as filling times [such as time to peak filling rate (TPFR)], filling fraction during the first third of diastole ($FF_{1/3}$, an index incorporating rate of relaxation), and relative rapid filling volume can be derived using this technique (42,360,569). Global or regional filling parameters obtained with radionuclide ventriculography require a uniform RR interval in the absence of aortic or mitral valve disease and a high frame acquisition rate with appropriately applied temporal smoothing of raw time-activity data to enhance image resolution and minimize observer bias (558,568).

Factors that Influence Diastolic Function In Vivo

The properties of the left ventricle in diastole contribute to the timing, rate, and extent of ventricular filling. These events are determined by several major factors: the rate and degree of myocardial relaxation, the intrinsic filling properties of the ventricle itself and those imposed by external constraints, and the structure and function of the left atrium, pulmonary venous system, and mitral valve (Fig. 32). Alterations of these diverse structural and mechanical characteristics, while intimately interrelated, may have distinctly different physiologic implications. These factors that influence diastolic performance are summarized in Table 1.

Myocardial Relaxation

Myocyte relaxation depends on the dissociation of Ca^{2+} from troponin C and the active uptake of Ca^{2+} at the subcellular level. The dissociation of contractile elements and recoil of myocardial elastic components compressed during systole lead to global myocardial relaxation. Relaxation is usually complete by the beginning of diastasis under normal circumstances; however, delays in relaxation may dynamically attenuate early diastolic filling and increase the dependence of filling on atrial systole. Prolongation of isovolumetric relaxation may be considered "active elasticity" (214) because the existence of residual cross-bridge formation secondary to lags in energy-dependent deactivation contributes to impaired early filling dynamics. Pathologic processes such as myocardial ischemia (10,369,381,403,537,538) or hypertrophic (319) and congestive cardiomyopathy (219) delay isovolumetric relaxation. It is not surprising that patients with such entities may develop acute diastolic heart failure concomitant with loss of atrial "kick." These disease states may also be associated with incomplete relaxation, an event that occurs as

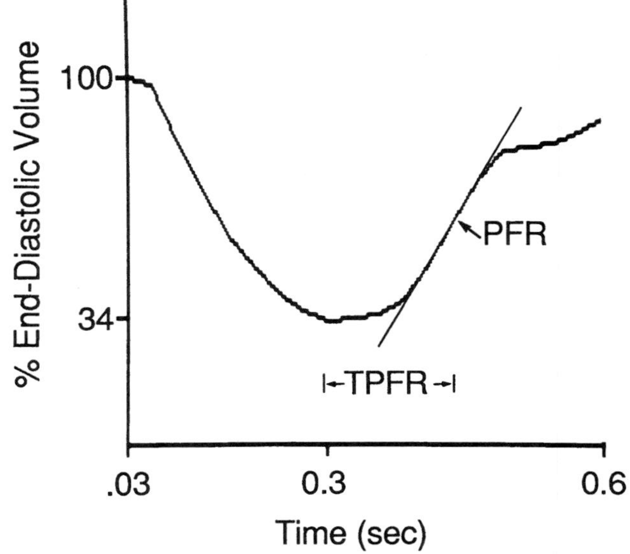

Figure 31. A normal radioactive erythrocyte time-activity curve obtained using radionuclide ventriculography. The maximum filling rate during early diastole (PFR) and the time from minimum left ventricular pressure to peak filling rate (TPFR), indicators of diastolic filling properties, are depicted. (From ref. 347, with permission.)

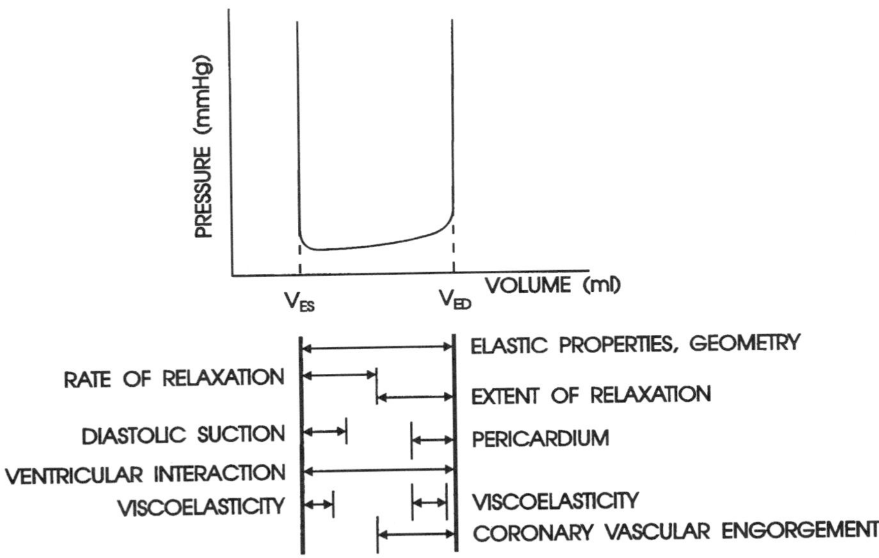

Figure 32. Properties of the left ventricle that contribute to the rate, timing, and extent of ventricular filling. Myocardial elasticity and geometry (size and wall thickness) are important throughout diastole. During early diastole, active relaxation and recoil of elastic energy (diastolic suction) stored in the myocardium during systole determine the atrial-ventricular pressure gradient and early ventricular filling rate. Late in diastole, ventricular interaction and the pericardium become important determinants of filling. Viscoelastic properties of the myocardium are important during rapid ventricular filling and during atrial systole. Coronary vascular engorgement also plays a role in determining the extent of filling in late diastole. V_{ES}, end-systolic volume; V_{ED}, end-diastolic volume. (From ref. 189, with permission.)

a result of residual cross-bridge activation and affects chamber distensibility throughout the entire diastolic phase of the cardiac cycle (Fig. 33A). The concept of incomplete relaxation remains controversial, but upward shifts in the diastolic pressure-volume relation (characteristic of impaired diastolic distensibility) have been observed experimentally in the presence of myocardial ischemia or hypoxia (9). Parallel increases in the pressure-volume relation during diastole have also been observed during exercise (91) or pacing-induced angina (10,25,368,530), consistent with increases in pressure relative to volume throughout diastole (Fig. 33C). Alterations in global ventricular compliance may be at least partially due to incomplete relaxation.

Table 1. DETERMINANTS OF LEFT VENTRICULAR DIASTOLIC FUNCTION

Myocardial relaxation and active elasticity
- End-systolic segment length, greater shortening hastens relaxation
- Residual cross-bridge activation during part or all of diastole
- Slow relaxation, affects early diastolic filling
- Incomplete relaxation, affects compliance throughout diastole

Recoil of elastic elements compressed during systole

Intrinsic ventricular chamber characteristics
- Passive ventricular elasticity (chamber stiffness)
- Ventricular wall thickness (mass)
- Ventricular wall composition (myocardial stiffness)
- Viscoelasticity

Factors extrinsic to the ventricle
- Pericardium
- Right ventricular loading and function
- Turgor of the coronary circulation
- Compression by mediastinal or pulmonary masses
- Pulmonary pathology or positive pressure ventilation

Left atrial structure and function
- Preload
- Wall thickness
- Inotropic state

Pulmonary venous return

Mitral valve competency

Heart rate and rhythm

Prolongation of isovolumetric relaxation may play a role in abnormalities of coronary blood flow (133). Under normal circumstances, 70% to 80% of coronary blood flow to the left ventricle and 90% to 100% of flow to the subendocardium occurs during diastole. Slowing of relaxation because of delays in dissociation of actin-myosin cross-bridges may result in the continued compression of intramyocardial coronary vessels during early diastole when coronary blood flow is usually highest.

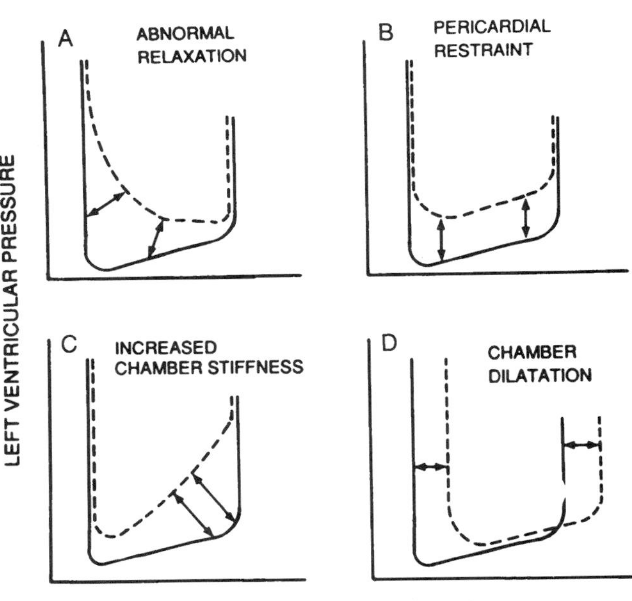

Figure 33. Schematic diagrams illustrating mechanisms responsible for abnormal diastolic function. The normal diastolic ventricular pressure-volume loop is represented by *solid lines.* Abnormal diastolic function resulting from impaired relaxation **(A)**, pericardial restraint **(B)**, increased chamber stiffness **(C)**, chamber dilatation **(D)** are represented by *dashed lines.* (From ref. 558, with permission.)

Decreases in subendocardial flow would be expected to be most prominent during incomplete relaxation because of prolonged elevation of diastolic pressure in the left ventricle. Impairment of coronary perfusion by such a mechanism would further exacerbate preexisting diastolic dysfunction.

Ventricular Filling Characteristics

Ventricular filling is primarily dependent on passive filling properties. Chamber stiffness is determined by several characteristics including the intrinsic properties of the myocardium (myocardial stiffness); the mass, geometry, and composition of the ventricular wall; viscoelastic properties; and extramyocardial impediments to filling. The ventricular pressure-volume relation quantifies the combined effects of these diverse factors (217). For example, alteration of cardiac muscle by edema or chronic infiltrative processes (e.g., amyloidosis or hemachromatosis) or changes in connective tissue composition (e.g., chronic fibrosis) increase intrinsic myocardial stiffness. These properties produce an upward shift of the ventricular pressure-volume curve, indicating that distention of the ventricle at any given volume is accompanied by higher pressures. Disease processes that produce an increase in myocardial wall thickness are also manifested by increases in chamber stiffness, so that higher pressures are necessary to fill the ventricle (Fig. 33C). Viscoelastic effects are exaggerated during rapid ventricular filling and atrial systole and may result in increases in ventricular pressure above the curve predicted by the passive pressure-volume distensibility relationship.

Factors extrinsic to the ventricle also alter filling dynamics. Increases in pericardial pressure (e.g., pericardial effusion, marked biventricular dilatation) or decreases in pericardial compliance (e.g., constrictive pericarditis) restrict filling and produce an upward shift of the pressure-volume relation consistent with the requirement for higher internal pressure in order to distend the ventricle (544) (Fig. 33B). Right ventricular loading also affects left ventricular filling because the right ventricle determines the external pressure exerted on the interventricular septum (57,343,397). External compression of mediastinal structures by surrounding lung tissue can influence ventricular filling. Positive pressure ventilation decreases venous return and compresses the right and left ventricles, thereby impairing filling of these chambers (29,525). Extrinsic compression of the heart by mediastinal or pulmonary masses may also impede left ventricular filling. Lastly, coronary vascular turgor ("erectile effect") may affect the passive ventricular pressure-volume relationship through an increase in stiffness during increases in coronary blood flow (177,647).

The Left Atrium, Pulmonary Venous Circulation, and Mitral Valve

The pressure gradient between the left atrium and ventricle responsible for early diastolic filling is affected not only by the rate and extent of isovolumetric relaxation but also by the left atrial pressure at the time of opening of the mitral valve and the passive properties of both the left atrium and pulmonary venous circulation. Early diastolic filling is potentiated by an increase in left atrial pressure that augments the pressure gradient across the mitral valve (98,258). Pulmonary venous return and left atrial function also play important roles in determining the final stroke volume by affecting filling during diastasis and atrial systole, respectively. Ventricular filling is diminished during mid-diastole because of equilibration of pressures in the atrium and ventricle. Ventricular filling that occurs during this period of diastole is highly influenced by the rate of pulmonary venous return (289).

The force of atrial contraction, the major determinant of filling during late diastole, is affected by atrial preload, wall thickness and configuration, and inotropic state (665). The majority of atrial volume is emptied during rapid ventricular filling when heart rates are slow, implying that little atrial volume remains during later periods of diastole. During sinus tachycardia, diastasis becomes shortened or completely disappears, and atrial systole immediately follows rapid ventricular filling. Atrial contraction preserves cardiac output by rapidly forcing blood into the ventricle during the short time that separates consecutive ventricular systoles under these conditions (190,421). If early diastolic filling is diminished, the left atrium will contain more blood (preload), enhancing the subsequent atrial systole by a Frank-Starling mechanism. Thus, the left atrium can compensate for diminished early filling by providing a booster "kick" of volume at end diastole.

Ventricular filling is not affected by the mitral valve under normal circumstances. However, stenosis of the mitral valve serves as a mechanical obstruction that may limit early diastolic filling. Diastasis cannot occur because atrial and ventricular pressures do not equilibrate, and even filling aided by atrial systole is limited by the obstruction to flow. Mitral stenosis is often accompanied by atrial fibrillation secondary to atrial enlargement, making the atrium useless as a pump and relegating this chamber to the role of a passive conduit.

MECHANICAL CONSEQUENCES OF VENTRICULAR HYPERTROPHY

Prolonged exposure of the ventricle to volume or pressure overload results in myocardial hypertrophy that develops in a pattern specific to the inciting stress (216). Elevated diastolic wall stress and progressive enlargement of left ventricular chamber size are the typical mechanical and structural abnormalities found in eccentric hypertrophy resulting from sustained volume overload (e.g., aortic valvular insufficiency, arteriovenous fistula). Histologically, myocardium exposed to chronic volume overload demonstrates increases in the length and diameter of individual myocytes. Increases in wall stress during systole, concentric ventricular wall thickening, and an increase in the diameter of individual myocytes are the classical features of concentric hypertrophy resulting from long-term pressure overload (e.g., hypertension or aortic stenosis). The precise mechanisms by which these hypertrophic processes are initiated in the myocardial cell are controversial (80,402). Systolic or diastolic wall stress may stimulate sarcomere synthesis in parallel or in series with preexisting contractile units, respectively (216,340) (Fig. 34). Decreases in the ratio of mitochondrial to myofibrillar mass (472) may occur in conjunction with increases in interstitial collagen (5), leading to relative energy depletion, myocyte dysfunction, and initiation of hypertrophic repair. Other degenerative processes in the cardiac cell or hormonal signals may also lead to stimulation of myocardial hypertrophy. Regardless of the specific stimulus, myocardial hypertrophy requires alteration of gene expression via derepression of myocyte DNA, modification of messenger RNA transcription and/or translation, or modulation of posttranslational processing of synthesized proteins (467).

Myocardial hypertrophy is an important compensatory response to both pressure and volume overload that results in partial restoration of wall stress toward normal and improvement of overall cardiac performance. These beneficial effects do not occur without significant adverse physiologic consequences, however. Depression of myocardial contractility often accompanies ventricular hypertrophy associated with chronic pressure overload or cardiomyopathy (109,566). The maximum velocity of shortening (V_{max}), the peak isometric force, and the rate of force development (+dF/dt) of isolated papillary muscles from experimental models of ventricular hypertrophy decrease in the absence of frank heart failure (85,109, 566) (Fig. 35). Depression of intrinsic inotropic state also occurs in hypertrophic myocardium caused by pressure overload in vivo (86,396,567). Primary contractile dysfunction may also be observed late in the natural history of volume-overload hypertrophy, usually in conjunction with overt heart failure

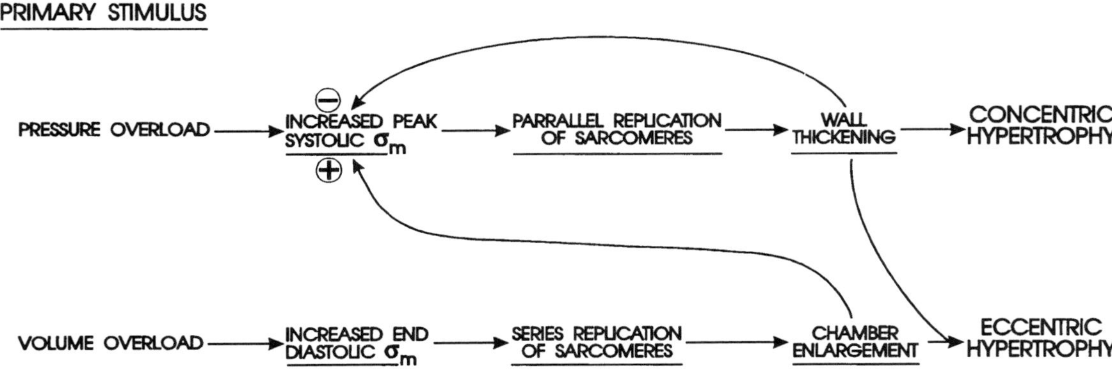

Figure 34. Hypothesis relating wall stress and patterns of ventricular hypertrophy. (From ref. 216, with permission.)

(88,323). The increases in total myocardial mass associated with hypertrophy serve to partially normalize global ventricular performance prior to the onset of failure despite declines in contractile function of individual myocytes (88,396,455,567).

The degree of myocardial depression observed in hypertrophic states is dependent on the time course, severity, and underlying cause of the imposed load (382). Acute imposition of exaggerated pressure or volume load results in early myocardial damage and contractile dysfunction, ventricular dilatation, and initiation of compensatory hypertrophy in conjunction with acute heart failure. Development of hypertrophy in response to a gradually imposed overload or established hypertrophy after an acute event may be associated with relatively normal contractile function (365,382,664). However, persistent elevation of ventricular wall stress resulting from enhanced pressure or volume load places the hypertrophied myocytes at greater risk of early dysfunction and cell death, further increasing the stress on the remaining myocardial cells (60,382). This vicious cycle ultimately leads to overt ventricular decompensation, declines in cardiac output and stroke volume, and congestive heart failure late in the natural history of ventricular hypertrophy. The increase in muscle mass associated with these hypertrophic processes also increases the risk of contractile dysfunction resulting from myocardial ischemia, especially in the presence of concomitant coronary artery disease. Hypertrophy-induced myocardial depression can be reversed in both pressure and volume-overload states by sustained pharmacologic treatment (455) (e.g., antihypertensive agents) or appropriately timed surgical intervention (41,43,45,199,285,517,531, 611) (e.g., aortic or mitral valvuloplasty or replacement).

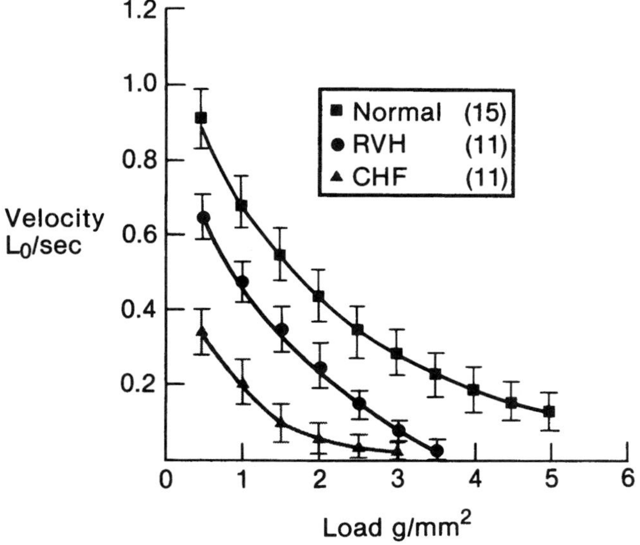

Figure 35. Force-velocity relations in normal cat papillary muscle *(squares)*, right ventricular hypertrophy *(circles)*, and frank congestive heart failure *(triangles)*. (From ref. 567, with permission.)

Myocardial hypertrophy contributes to abnormalities in diastolic function that may further exacerbate overall cardiac performance. End-stage ventricular hypertrophy is associated with marked diastolic dysfunction secondary to prolonged isovolumetric relaxation and reduced diastolic compliance. Decreases in passive diastolic distensibility often occur in myocardial hypertrophy because of alterations in the character and quantity of myocardial collagen (131,151,241,620,649) or because of thickening of the ventricular wall (218). Diastolic dysfunction is also observed in the presence of chronic volume overload (110). Hypertrophied myocardium exhibits enhanced susceptibility to diastolic dysfunction resulting from ischemia (116, 350). Sudden increases in myocardial oxygen demand may result in impaired relaxation and increased resistance to filling in patients with left ventricular hypertrophy resulting from aortic stenosis, despite the presence of a normal coronary vasculature (158,294).

Diastolic function is markedly impaired in hypertrophic cardiomyopathy (asymmetric left ventricular hypertrophy) in the presence or absence of left ventricular outflow tract obstruction during systole. Isovolumetric relaxation may be incomplete and extend throughout diastolic filling (32,350,352). This striking prolongation of isovolumetric relaxation is accompanied by delayed opening of the mitral valve (522) and reduced early ventricular filling (570). An increase in chamber stiffness is also observed in hypertrophic cardiomyopathy (179). This disease process is accompanied by an increased dependence on atrial systole for maintenance of adequate stroke volume and cardiac output (44).

Diastolic dysfunction is a common finding in left ventricular hypertrophy produced by long-standing systemic hypertension (102,372). Decreases in the rate of ventricular filling as evaluated by M-mode echocardiography and increases in isovolumetric relaxation time in the presence of normal systolic function have been correlated with the severity of left ventricular hypertrophy resulting from hypertension (156,256,442). Functional alterations in diastolic filling mechanics appear to develop early in the clinical course of hypertension-induced left ventricular hypertrophy, with systolic decompensation occurring only late in this pathologic process. In fact, low-peak filling rates have been documented in one-third of hypertensive patients with no echocardiographic evidence of left ventricular hypertrophy (559) emphasizing the importance of noninvasive assessment of presence and severity of diastolic dysfunction in this disease.

The cellular mechanisms responsible for myocardial dysfunction in congestive heart failure associated with ventricular hypertrophy have been the subject of multiple recent investigations. Chronic forms of heart failure due to pathologic overloading are associated with a variety of adaptive processes at the tissue, cellular, and subcellular levels (65,274,276,409,482,608). Altered gene regulation and transcription of several myocardial proteins occur in response to long-term overload and as a result of chronic hormonal or paracrine stimulation (261,276, 532,548,574). The structure of the contractile apparatus may be altered by myosin isozyme transformation causing decreased myosin adenosine triphosphatase (ATPase) activity with a consequent decrease in velocity of fiber shortening (362,482).

Transcription of the gene coding for the angiotensin-converting enzyme (ACE) increases fourfold in rat hypertrophied myocardium. Subsequent amplification of production of ACE leads to enhanced conversion of angiotensin I to angiotensin II (532). Increases in circulating angiotensin II levels are associated with pronounced systolic and diastolic dysfunction in the hypertrophied left ventricle of the rat; however, only a portion of the abnormal cardiac performance can be attributed to angiotensin II–induced increases in afterload. Dysfunction can also be attributed to angiotensin II–induced alterations in intracellular Ca^{2+} kinetics via receptor-mediated activation of phospholipase C, leading to the production of diacylglycerol (DAG) and phosphoinositide second messengers (21,22,407) (Fig. 36). While some recent investigations suggest that inositol triphosphate (IP_3) promotes Ca^{2+} release from the sarcoplasmic reticulum (21,128,422) and that this IP_3-induced Ca^{2+} release is enhanced in hypertrophic myocardium (279), DAG activation of protein kinase C may result in the alkalinization of the sarcoplasm and enhanced myofibrillar Ca^{2+} binding. Increased levels of angiotensin II cause elevation of intracellular Ca^{2+} during systole and prolong the Ca^{2+} transient during diastole. This leads to an augmented contractile state but also results in delayed relaxation and impaired filling in pressure-overload hypertrophy, especially in the presence of concomitant myocardial ischemia (136). These actions can be inhibited by pretreatment with an ACE inhibitor, providing an additional explanation for the success of ACE inhibitors in the treatment of patients with diastolic heart failure, beyond the peripheral vasodilating effect of these drugs.

Abnormal handling of intracellular Ca^{2+} has been implicated as a major underlying mechanism for systolic and diastolic dysfunction in patients with end-stage heart failure due to myocardial hypertrophy, especially in the presence of tachycardia (222,223,408). Although acute systolic failure produced by negative inotropic drugs or myocardial ischemia may be associated with decreases in peak Ca^{2+} concentrations available for contractile activation (291,304,320,409,453), myocytes from patients with end-stage diastolic heart failure resulting from hypertrophy demonstrate relatively normal Ca^{2+} kinetics in sys-

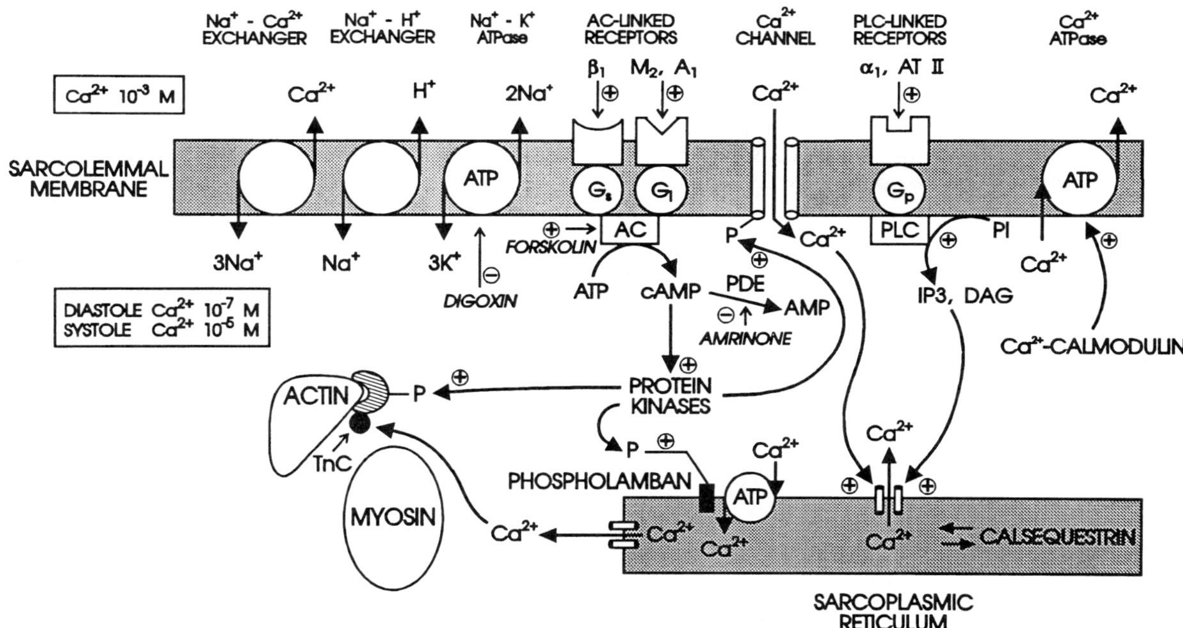

Figure 36. Calcium (Ca^{2+}) homeostasis in the cardiac myocyte. Sarcolemmal membrane depolarization allows influx of Ca^{2+} into the myoplasm through the voltage-dependent Ca^{2+} channel, providing Ca^{2+} for contractile activation and inducing further Ca^{2+} release from stores in the sarcoplasmic reticulum. This process is modulated by adenyl cyclase (AC)- or phospholipase C (PLC)- linked receptors. A β_1-adrenergic agonist combines with its receptor on the sarcolemmal membrane and activates AC via a stimulatory G protein (G_s). This process increases the intracellular concentration of cyclic adenosine monophosphate (cAMP), resulting in activation of protein kinases responsible for phosphorylation of the voltage-dependent Ca^{2+} channel, the regulatory protein of the sarcoplasmic reticular Ca^{2+} ATPase, phospholamban, and the troponin C (TnC) subunit of the tropomyosin-troponin complex. These actions facilitate further Ca^{2+} entry through the Ca^{2+} channel, enhance Ca^{2+} uptake into the sarcoplasmic reticulum by the Ca^{2+}-ATPase, and decrease the affinity of TnC for Ca^{2+}, respectively (see text). Increased cAMP concentrations also result from direct stimulation of AC by forskolin or by inhibition of cAMP degradation by cardiac phosphodiesterase (PDE) blockers such as amrinone. Muscarinic (M_2) or adenosine (A_1) agonists decrease the activity of AC via an inhibitory G protein (G_i), decreasing the intracellular concentration of cAMP. Stimulation of PLC-linked receptors with α_1-adrenergic or angiotensin II agonists activate PLC via a G protein (G_p), splitting the membrane lipid phosphatidyl inositol (PI) into inositol trisphosphate (IP_3) and diacylglycerol (DAG). IP_3 directly stimulates Ca^{2+} release from the sarcoplasmic reticulum. Intracellular Ca^{2+} is also regulated by a Ca^{2+}-ATPase in the sarcolemmal membrane (which is stimulated by Ca^{2+} bound to calmodulin) and by Na^+-Ca^{2+} and Na^+-H^+ exchangers coupled to a Na^+-K^+ ATPase (inhibited by digoxin). (From ref. 428, with permission.)

tole coupled with delays in the clearance of Ca^{2+} from myoplasm during diastole (223). The delay in removal of Ca^{2+} from the contractile apparatus and cytosol contributes to intracellular Ca^{2+} overload in diastole and may result in prolonged isovolumetric relaxation and impaired early ventricular filling. The ATP-dependent Ca^{2+} pump in the sarcoplasmic reticulum is primarily responsible for Ca^{2+} sequestration in the normal myocyte, and abnormal function of this pump occurs in cardiac failure due to myocardial hypertrophy (228,339). Similar dysfunction of the ATP-dependent Ca^{2+} pump takes place during the natural aging process that is associated with diastolic dysfunction (310,359). Depressed expression of transcription of genes coding for the Ca^{2+}-ATPase (383) and the regulatory protein of this enzyme, phospholamban (155), contribute to abnormalities in diastolic Ca^{2+} kinetics and have also been observed in myocytes isolated from some, but not all (410), patients with congestive heart failure (Fig. 36).

A decrease in cyclic adenosine monophosphate (cAMP) production by adenylyl cyclase in myocytes obtained from patients with congestive heart failure has been observed and may play an important role in the development of diastolic dysfunction (157). This second messenger phosphorylates phospholamban, accelerating the uptake of cytosolic Ca^{2+} into the sarcoplasmic reticulum during diastole. Cyclic AMP is also responsible for the phosphorylation of the troponin I subunit of the troponin-tropomyosin complex. This process decreases the affinity of troponin C for Ca^{2+} (274,501,562) and enhances Ca^{2+} dissociation from the regulatory protein. Impaired mitochondrial production of ATP not only decreases the energy available for myocardial contraction and relaxation (276,482) but also decreases intracellular concentrations of cAMP.

Downregulation of β_1-adrenoceptors in the sarcolemma has been described in heart failure (65,635). Decreased β_1-adrenoceptor activation of adenylyl cyclase should result in a reduction of intracellular levels of cAMP. Primary abnormalities in adenylyl cyclase function leading to deficiencies in the production of cAMP may also represent a fundamental defect in cardiac failure (408). Efficiency of production of myocardial cAMP may be impaired secondary to abnormal expression of the excitatory G protein, G_s, which couples a variety of receptor subtypes including β_1-adrenoceptors in the sarcolemmal membrane to adenylyl cyclase in cardiac muscle (Fig. 36). Concentrations of the inhibitory G protein, G_i, are also increased in failing human myocardium (65,154,415). An imbalance in membrane-associated G_i and G_s proteins may be the basis of abnormalities in signal transduction in the cardiac myocyte and contribute to altered Ca^{2+} homeostasis. Inhibition of the degradation of cAMP by pharmacologic blockade of cytosolic phosphodiesterase (e.g., by amrinone or milrinone) or direct activation of adenylate cyclase (e.g., by forskolin) increases intracellular levels of cAMP and acutely improve systolic and diastolic function in both clinical and experimental studies of cardiac failure (65,157,405,457). Enhancement of ventricular function in these studies, however, could equally be related to vasodilation-induced decreases in afterload rather than specific and direct improvement of intrinsic inotropic and lusitropic properties (235). Ca^{2+} homeostasis may be markedly altered in patients with hypertrophic cardiomyopathy, in the presence of normal or hyperdynamic systolic contractility (224). Thus, fundamental abnormalities of Ca^{2+} kinetics in failing myocardium represent a general component of advanced ventricular hypertrophy (Fig. 36).

MECHANICAL CONSEQUENCES OF MYOCARDIAL ISCHEMIA AND INFARCTION

Acute Myocardial Ischemia—Supply Versus Demand

The study of left ventricular function during myocardial ischemia requires specification of the mechanism of the underlying ischemic process. Ischemic episodes resulting from diminished blood supply or increased oxygen demand have different initial functional consequences (9). An abrupt decrease in blood flow as occurs during acute coronary artery occlusion results in a nearly simultaneous systolic contractile dysfunction in the ischemic zone in experimental animals (616,619) and humans (539). Diastolic function, however, is relatively well maintained during the early stages following reduction of coronary blood flow (9,24,66). In contrast, myocardial ischemia produced by tachycardia or exercise in the presence of a coronary artery stenosis is accompanied by striking abnormalities in diastolic function with relative maintenance of systolic function early in the time course of this oxygen demand–related pathologic process (10,90,368,381,403,537).

Acute reduction of coronary blood flow results in a significant decrease in effective segment shortening (hypokinesia) and transmural wall thickening that occur after only a few cardiac

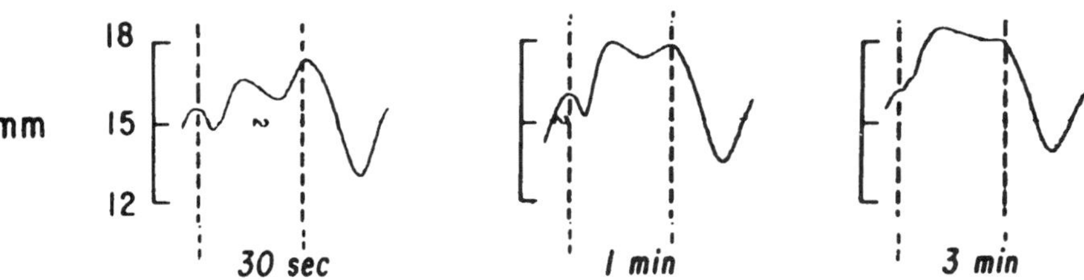

Figure 37. Subendocardial segment length in an ischemic zone before and after coronary artery occlusion (CO) in the anesthetized dog. Note the rapid onset of regional dysfunction with the development of holosystolic expansion within 30 seconds after coronary occlusion. (From ref. 616, with permission.)

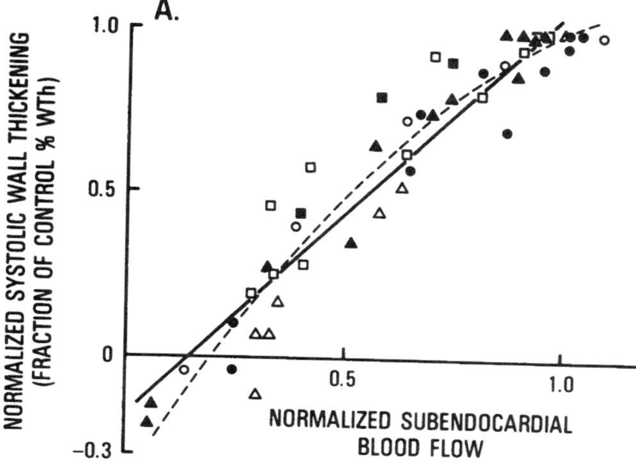

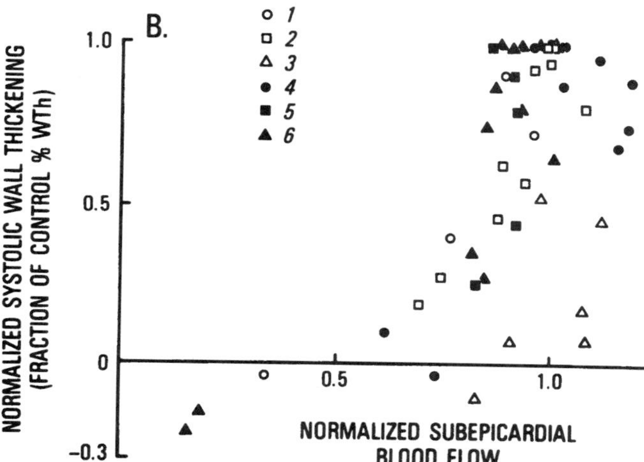

Figure 38. Relationships between myocardial blood flow and regional systolic function in conscious dogs in which brief steady-state levels of reductions of subendocardial **(A)** and subepicardial **(B)** coronary blood flow were produced. Note the high degree of correlation between systolic function and subendocardial blood flow (A). In contrast, no correlation between subepicardial blood flow and function can be derived (B). (From ref. 183, with permission.)

cycles (616). The left ventricular pressure-ischemic segment diagram tilts to the right, indicating development of postsystolic shortening and presystolic lengthening, findings that are consistent with ischemic segment dysfunction and paroxysmal aneurysmal bulging of the ischemic region (dyskinesia), respectively (165,204,334,518) (Fig. 9). Early systolic lengthening occurs within 30 seconds and rapidly becomes holosystolic within one minute of complete coronary artery occlusion (616) (Fig. 37). The ventricular pressure-segment length diagram becomes severely deformed (Fig. 8), collapsing entirely as effective regional stroke work within the ischemic zone declines toward zero (165,518). Hypokinesia of cardiac muscle immediately adjacent (border zone) to the central ischemic region is observed (73,181) concomitant with compensatory increases in wall thickness and shortening of the surrounding normal myocardium (204). These changes in systolic function may be accompanied by ventricular dilatation consistent with thinning and expansion of the acutely ischemic segment and augmented preload and enhanced inotropic state in the remaining functional zones (204,528,616). Wall thinning and lengthening of the ischemic segment occur as tethered normal zones undergo contraction, while the ischemic zone is unable to contract.

Transmural systolic wall thickening in the acutely ischemic zone is determined primarily by subendocardial blood flow and function (182,183). A direct correlation between subendocardial blood flow and transmural wall function (Fig. 38), a "flow-function" relation (507), has been demonstrated in myocardial ischemia resulting from acute coronary artery occlusion (182,183,636) or during exercise in the presence of a graded coronary stenosis (184,185,506). In contrast, poor correlations between subepicardial blood flow and regional wall thickening have been shown in both supply (182,183,636) and demand ischemia (184,185,506). In fact, only dramatic reductions in subepicardial blood flow, which occur with concomitant declines in subendocardial perfusion, result in transmural wall dyskinesia (183). These findings indicate that subendocardial blood flow plays a critical role in determining transmural contractile function (506). This relationship provides the rationale for the detection and quantitative evaluation of the magnitude of latent coronary stenoses by examination of extent and severity of regional wall motion abnormalities during stress induced by exercise (46,321,642), inotropes (26), pacing (367,624), coronary angioplasty (233,669), or surgery (27,327,554) in both experimental and clinical settings.

Regional myocardial ischemia resulting from acute reductions in coronary blood flow produces reversible alterations in diastolic mechanics manifested by prolongation of isovolumetric relaxation (90,369,381), increases in chamber stiffness (25), and a shift to the right of the diastolic compliance curve (a phenomenon termed ischemia-induced diastolic creep) (140) (Fig. 39). Similar findings have been described during exercise-induced ischemia (461,483), and regional differences in compliance have been identified during pacing-induced ischemia in humans (530). These abnormalities in diastolic function can be clinically manifested by the appearance of acute pulmonary edema associated with high left ventricular filling pressures despite relatively normal left ventricular size (126). Declines in

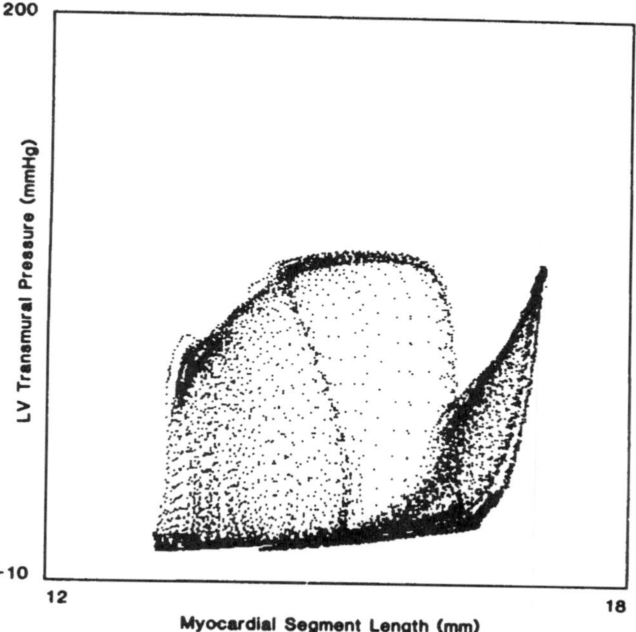

Figure 39. Sequential left ventricular (LV) transmural pressure-segment length diagrams obtained during vena caval occlusion under control conditions *(left loops)* and after acute coronary artery occlusion *(right loops).* Note the shift to the right of the diastolic LV pressure-segment length relation (termed "diastolic creep") that occurs during ischemia. (From ref. 480, with permission.)

peak diastolic filling rates (evaluated using radionuclide techniques) with or without impairment of systolic function have been observed in patients with angiographically documented coronary artery disease (42,389,460). An increase in chamber stiffness (as identified by a steeper diastolic pressure-segment length curve) characterizes ischemic regions, in contrast to normally perfused regions in which compliance is maintained despite increases in both diastolic pressure and segment length. This finding suggests that during ischemia an acute dynamic compensation for regional abnormalities in function occurs in normal zones (318) and may represent a mechanism by which cardiac output can be relatively preserved despite decreases in systolic function in ischemic regions (213).

Although reversal of ischemia-induced diastolic creep has been directly linked to recovery of systolic contractile performance (194), some evidence has suggested that focal diastolic abnormalities are more apparent than abnormalities in systolic function in patients with coronary artery disease (173). Changes in loading conditions or inotropic state produced by pharmacologic interventions have little effect on ventricular compliance in normal myocardium (478,479); however, these modalities significantly alter diastolic mechanics after acute ischemic injury (264) while producing proportionally detrimental actions on systolic performance (480). Alterations in systolic and diastolic function in the presence of myocardial ischemia are intimately related and may result from a common abnormality in myocyte ultrastructure such as overextension of the sarcomere or defective cross-linking of actin and myosin filaments (194,480).

Myocardial ischemia resulting from reduced coronary blood flow or increased oxygen demand is associated with dramatic metabolic consequences that may differ depending on the underlying cause (9). Precipitous declines in aerobic synthesis and intracellular concentrations of ATP and creatine phosphate (CP) occur rapidly (303); however, ATP levels may be relatively spared by selective transfer of high-energy phosphate from CP to adenosine diphosphate (ADP) depending on the severity and duration of coronary blood flow restriction (262,404). In fact, the acute, severe systolic contractile dysfunction associated with diminished blood flow follows a time course that cannot be accounted for solely by decreases in ATP production (404). Lactate produced during anaerobic glycolysis leads to myocyte acidosis (3). Some evidence suggests that the metabolic acidosis and accumulation of inorganic phosphate in combination with myofibrillar stretch and decreases in coronary vascular turgor contribute to the relatively rapid onset of systolic contractile failure while paradoxically maintaining diastolic mechanics (9,24,66). In contrast, altered Ca^{2+} homeostasis appears to play a more important role in the early development of diastolic dysfunction in ischemia caused by increases in oxygen demand (255,351). Increases in left ventricular end-diastolic pressure parallel the intracellular accumulation of Ca^{2+} during diastole in demand ischemia. This response is similar to that observed early during myocyte hypoxia if accumulation of toxic metabolites is prevented by maintenance of coronary perfusion (291).

Myocardial Postischemic, Reperfusion Injury—"Stunned" Myocardium

Reperfusion of myocardium after brief periods of coronary artery occlusion (typically less than 20 min) is associated with delayed recovery of mechanical function during systole and diastole despite return of blood flow to normal levels (236). This reversible postischemic dysfunction, termed "stunned" myocardium (61), may be prolonged but occurs without tissue necrosis (38,39). The duration of myocardial stunning ranges from hours to days and is directly influenced by the extent of coronary collateral perfusion during the occlusion (39). Regional diastolic dysfunction may follow an even more prolonged time course, persisting despite the restoration of systolic function after reperfusion (94). Postischemic, reperfusion injury plays an important role in the natural history of ischemic heart disease because spontaneous reperfusion of ischemic myocardium after thrombosis or coronary vasospasm is known to occur frequently in patients with coronary artery disease. In addition, patients with acute myocardial ischemia often undergo coronary artery reperfusion through interventions, such as thrombolytic therapy, angioplasty, and emergency bypass surgery, in attempts to salvage myocardium at risk for development of infarction. Delayed recovery of myocardial function also occurs in oxygen demand–induced ischemia in the presence of a fixed coronary artery stenosis (243,377,615).

The pathogenesis of stunned myocardium remains unclear despite extensive study (38). Although tissue reperfusion is necessary to preserve myocardial integrity, severe ischemia-induced cellular abnormalities have been implicated in the subsequent development of reperfusion injury (38,39,62,236, 465,652). Intracellular calcium overload (371), depletion of high energy phosphates (118,147,486), production of oxygen-derived free radicals by ischemic myocytes or infiltrating neutrophils (37,149,225,551,680), a reduction in myofilament Ca^{2+} sensitivity (370), and myocyte excitation-contraction uncoupling (306) have all been suggested as contributing etiologies for the contractile dysfunction observed in stunned myocardium. Pharmacologic therapy has focused on modulation of these diverse pathophysiologic abnormalities and a variety of treatment modalities, including calcium channel blocking agents (313,469,613,644), vasodilators (469,547,613,644), β–adrenergic antagonists (297), specific bradycardic agents (210), and free radical scavenging with superoxide dismutase and catalase (211) have all been shown to enhance recovery. More recently, monoclonal antibodies directed against neutrophil-derived cell adhesion molecules (CAMs) have been shown to improve functional recovery after brief myocardial ischemia (551) and heart transplantation (81), respectively. These findings emphasize that neutrophil migration and activation may play a critical role in the development of reperfusion-induced contractile dysfunction (149).

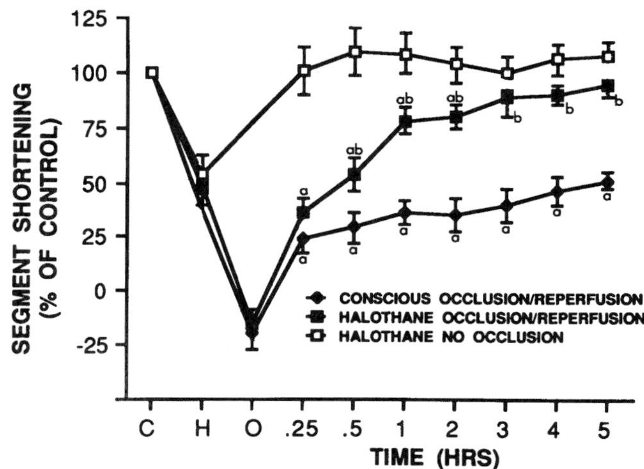

Figure 40. Segment shortening data during coronary artery occlusion (O) and at various times after reperfusion in conscious and halothane-anesthetized dogs. Anesthetized dogs were allowed to emerge from anesthesia after the onset of reperfusion. Comparisons are made at various time intervals to anesthetized dogs allowed to emerge from halothane anesthesia that did not undergo coronary artery occlusion and reperfusion. Recovery of function of stunned myocardium is improved in dogs anesthetized with halothane. Note that the control state (C) indicates awake, unsedated state in each group. (From ref. 643, with permission.)

Volatile anesthetic agents have been shown to improve systolic functional recovery of stunned myocardium when these agents are administered in vivo (643) (Fig. 40) and in vitro (170) before and during, but not after (30), brief periods of myocardial ischemia. These actions presumably result from volatile anesthetic-induced depression of the intracellular Ca^{2+} transient within the myocyte (34,246,513,662) combined with improvement of overall myocardial oxygen supply-demand balance during anesthesia (643). In contrast, recent evidence suggests that nitrous oxide (549) impairs functional recovery of stunned myocardium (see Fig. 49). Nitrous oxide-induced sympathetic nervous system activation (138,504) and imbalances of myocardial oxygen supply and demand represent potential mechanisms by which nitrous oxide further delays contractile recovery of postischemic reperfused myocardium.

Contractile Function After Late Reperfusion and Myocardial Hibernation

Prolonged coronary artery occlusion (e.g.,30 minutes to 3 hours) followed by reperfusion results in severe, persistent contractile dysfunction. Although myocardium within the central ischemic zone may become infarcted, some viable myocardium still remains (191,263), and partial recovery of function eventually occurs over a time course of several weeks (618) (Fig. 41). The duration of coronary occlusion prior to reperfusion and the degree of collateral blood flow during occlusion (502) are the primary determinants of the extent of myocardial necrosis, although reperfusion itself can also cause further tissue injury (298,426). A "wave front" of myocardial cell death spreads from the subendocardium to the subepicardium over time (487,488). Rapid restoration of coronary blood flow decreases myocardial stunning and infarct size and accelerates the process of partial functional repair (317,618). Even late reperfusion is often accompanied by myocardial hypertrophy in border and normal zones as well as in subepicardial myocytes surviving within the central ischemic zone. This compensatory process contributes to improved global and regional ventricular function with ongoing recovery after prolonged coronary artery occlusion and reperfusion (529). The clinical relevance of experimental studies of late reperfusion following coronary artery occlusion cannot be understated. Institution of thrombolytic therapy, coronary angioplasty, or emergent myocardial revascularization in patients within 6 hours of the onset of chest pain directly reduces morbidity and mortality (124,220,221,265,288,423,490,584,657). Late reperfusion may also decrease infarct size, preserve myocardium at risk, and improve overall ventricular function, particularly if interventions are initiated in the first 3 to 4 hours of symptoms (220,481,657).

Chronic myocardial ischemia resulting from continuous, partial reductions in myocardial perfusion produces sustained depression of contractile function without infarction, a phenomenon termed "myocardial hibernation" (63,474). Dysfunction during hibernation may result from the matching of contractile function to the limited energy supply available to each myocyte in the area at risk (377) and may be reversed by relief of the underlying ischemia (475). Myocardial hibernation occurs frequently in humans during prolonged medical management of coronary disease without acute electrocardiographic or clinical evidence of ischemia (63,475). Marked enhancement of ventricular function resulting from reversal of hiberation often occurs after coronary artery bypass surgery (153,370).

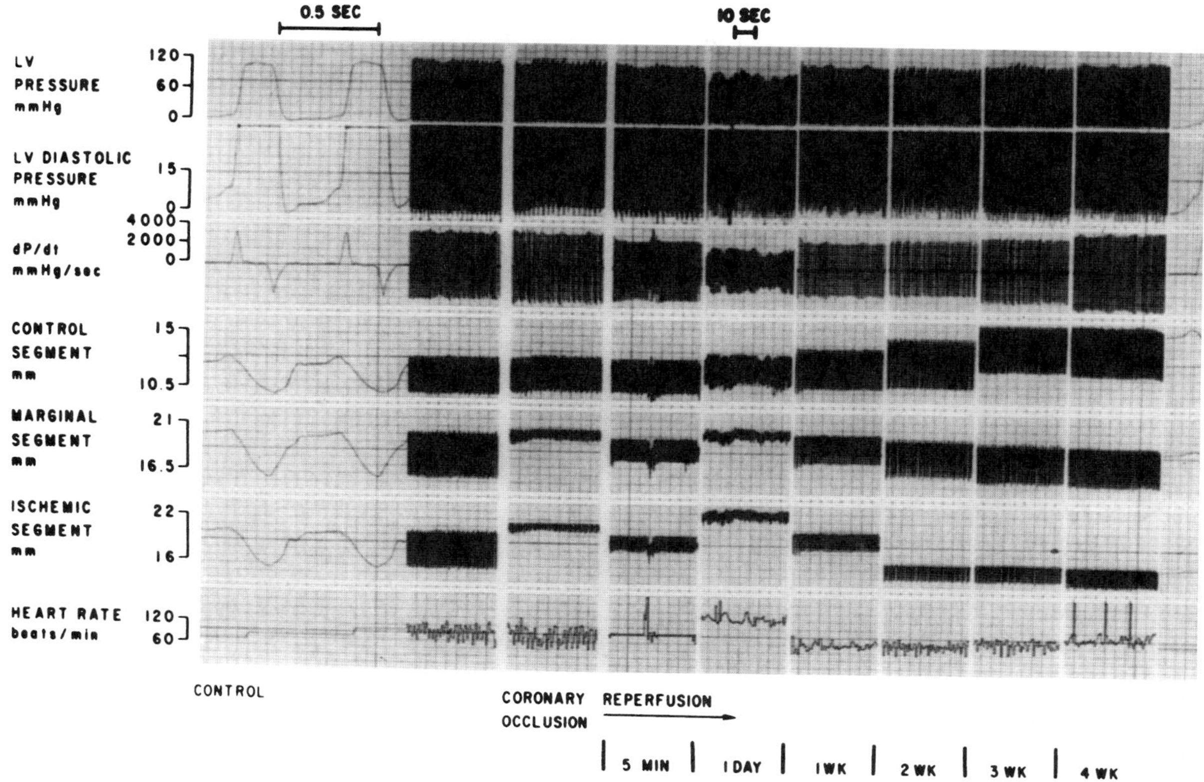

Figure 41. Serial changes in ischemic, marginal, and control segments of left ventricular (LV) myocardium in a conscious dog subjected to 2 hours of coronary artery occlusion followed by reperfusion. Note the gradual recovery of partial function in the ischemic and marginal segments 4 weeks after coronary occlusion. In addition, note the dilatation and enhanced function in the control segment, reflecting hypertrophic adaptation. (From ref. 618, with permis-

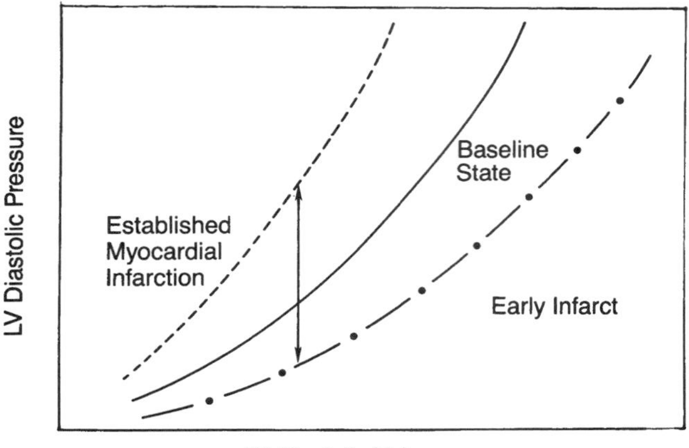

Figure 42. Alterations in diastolic left ventricular (LV) pressure-volume relations occurring early *(dot-dash curve)* and late *(dashed curve)* after myocardial infarction. The pressure-volume relation shifts downward and to the right during early infarction indicating increased ventricular compliance. Upward and leftward shift of the pressure-volume relation (indicating decreased compliance) occurs after an infarction has become established secondary to scar formation and compensatory hypertrophy of noninfarcted myocardium. (From ref. 229, with permission.)

Myocardial Infarction and Ventricular Remodeling

Acute myocardial infarction causes a series of changes in regional and global mechanical function during systole and diastole induced by formation of scar tissue within the infarcted zone and compensatory hypertrophy of remaining viable myocardium in border and unaffected region (496,617). Initially, myocardial infarction results in a rightward shift (increase in compliance) of the diastolic pressure-volume curve (Fig. 42). This increase in ventricular distensibility probably results from thinning and dilatation of the infarcted ventricular segment and loss of coronary turgor (164). Increases in global chamber stiffness, however, are observed within several days following myocardial infarction (244) and can be reduced by early reperfusion (308). Decreases in ventricular distensibility result from scar formation and shrinkage of the infarcted zone as well as adaptive hypertrophy of noninfarcted regions that assume a portion of the function no longer performed by the infarcted zone (380,463,646).

Extensive remodeling of the ventricular architecture results from this segmental hypertrophic process. A combination of pressure- and volume-like overload hypertrophy occurs because noninfarcted myocardium is exposed to increases in both systolic and diastolic wall stress. Late congestive heart failure may develop after extensive myocardial infarction solely as a result of decompensation of regionally hypertrophic myocardium, despite an absence of further ischemic insult (456). Histologically, remodeled myocardium may resemble that observed in patients with end-stage pressure or volume overload (425). An increased susceptibility to ischemia occurring in hypertrophied myocardial segments also exists. Although the underlying etiology of the complex process of ventricular remodeling is incompletely understood, activation of the renin-angiotensin axis and sympathetic nervous system appears to play an important role (339,456).

ANESTHETICS AND VENTRICULAR FUNCTION

Volatile Anesthetics

Modern potent inhalational anesthetics, including halothane, enflurane, and isoflurane, depress myocardial contractile function in the isolated and intact heart. Seminal investigations in the 1960s demonstrated conclusively that halothane produces dose-related depression of force-velocity relations and ventricular function curves in isolated cardiac muscle preparations (198,605) and intact, closed-chest dogs (545), respectively. These findings supported the clinical observations of several investigators who reported halothane-induced circulatory depression in humans (122,141,540,563). Enflurane (546) and isoflurane (283) were also shown to cause dose-dependent decreases in the maximal velocity of shortening (V_{max}), peak developed force, maximal rate of force development (+dF/dt), and work during isotonic contraction in isolated cat papillary muscles. These studies in vitro indicated that enflurane and isoflurane produced direct negative inotropic effects that probably contributed to the cardiovascular depression observed with these agents in vivo (84,581).

Although the contention that volatile anesthetics depress intrinsic inotropic state in vitro was well established by these early studies (283,546,605) controversy remained concerning the relative degree of myocardial depression produced by each of these agents. Early studies of the cardiovascular effects of enflurane in humans suggested that enflurane produced minimal myocardial depression (206,329,374) in direct contrast to halothane (122,141,540). Other investigations, using isovolumetric and ejection-phase measures of contractile function, showed that enflurane and halothane caused very similar negative inotropic effects in dogs (245,387,433), primates (495), and humans (84). These findings were later confirmed using the slope (E_{es}) of the end-systolic pressure–mid-axis diameter relation as a relatively load-independent index of contractile state in chronically instrumented dogs (631). Equi-MAC concentrations of these volatile agents were shown to depress myocardial contractile function to similar degrees in vivo (631).

Studies in humans and experimental animals have suggested a differential depression of contractile function by halothane and isoflurane. Stevens et al. (581) examined the effects of isoflurane on systemic hemodynamics in healthy volunteers and suggested that since little change in cardiac output or the mean rate of ventricular ejection was observed with increasing doses of isoflurane, myocardial function must be relatively preserved as compared to halothane. Nevertheless, dose-dependent declines in stroke volume were observed during isoflurane anesthesia, similar to other volatile anesthetics. Similar findings were reported in surgical patients (207). Tarnow et al. (612) used left ventricular dP/dt to assess contractile state in geriatric patients and found less depression of contractility with isoflurane than halothane. Interpretation of this study, however, was complicated by the presence of baseline intravenous anesthetics and neuromuscular blockade. M-mode transthoracic echocardiography has been used to noninvasively evaluate changes in fractional shortening and the mean velocity of circumferential fiber shortening during equi-MAC halothane or isoflurane in healthy children (670). Myocardial performance was decreased in a dose-dependent fashion when halothane was used but was not significantly altered when isoflurane was administered (670). These studies in humans strongly implied that halothane depresses myocardial contractile function to a greater extent than equi-MAC isoflurane; however, lack of conscious control data, concomitant use of anesthetic adjuvants, differential direct and reflex effects of volatile anesthetics on the systemic circulation, and assessment of changes in contractile state using load-dependent or indirect indicators of ventricular function represented important qualifications in the interpretation of the results of these investigations.

Horan et al. (245), Merin (384), and Pagel et al. (433) used isovolumetric indices of contractility to delineate greater depressant actions of halothane versus isoflurane on myocardial performance in chronically instrumented dogs. Horan et al. showed significant differences in left ventricular dP/dt (40%) and maximum aortic acceleration (32%) when nearly

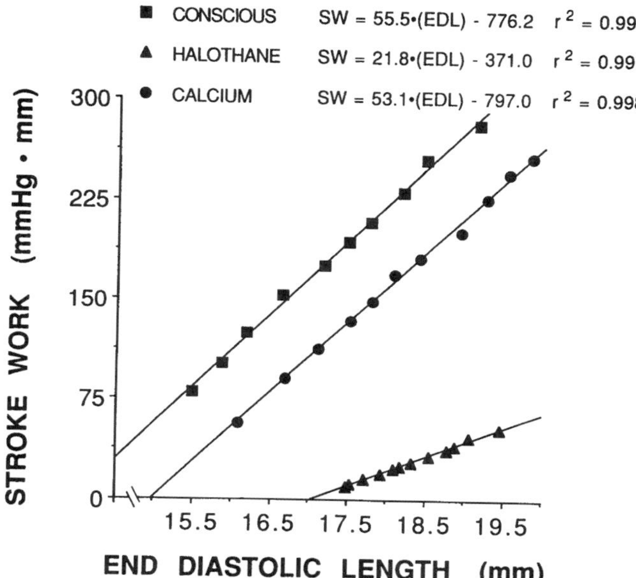

Figure 43. Regional stroke work (SW) versus end-diastolic segment length (EDL) relationship data in the conscious state, during 1.5 MAC halothane and following 5 $mg \cdot kg^{-1} \cdot min^{-1}$ calcium chloride during halothane anesthesia in a chronically instrumented dog. (From ref. 437, with permission.)

equianesthetic-inspired concentrations of halothane (1.0%) and isoflurane (1.2%) were directly compared in the same study. Similar differences in contractile function were inferred in separate investigations by Merin and coworkers (384,388) using nearly identical protocols, although the direct effects of the volatile anesthetics on the systemic circulation or reflex actions mediated through the autonomic nervous system could not be entirely excluded from the analysis. Pagel et al. also demonstrated differences in contractility between isoflurane and halothane in dogs using left ventricular dP/dt_{max} and dP/dt_{50} in the presence and absence of autonomic nervous system function, suggesting that differences in myocardial depression caused by these agents occurred independent of autonomic reflexes.

These investigations (245,384,433) strongly implied a difference between the negative inotropic effects of halothane and isoflurane despite the use of indices of contractile state that are significantly influenced by ventricular loading conditions. The suspected difference in the negative inotropic effects of halothane and isoflurane was later quantified using the slope of the regional preload recruitable stroke work (PRSW) relation and a stroke work analogue of the end-systolic pressure-segment length relationship (ESPLR area) in chronically instrumented dogs with pharmacologic blockade of the autonomic nervous system (430). Isoflurane maintained intrinsic inotropic state an average of 22% higher as compared to equi-MAC inspired concentrations of halothane using these models (430). These results were subsequently confirmed with PRSW using end-tidal anesthetic concentrations in dogs with intact autonomic nervous system function (438), indicating that differential depression of contractility by halothane and isoflurane was probably unrelated to anesthetic-induced differences in underlying autonomic tone. The findings are supported by a growing body of evidence in vitro that also implies a difference in the contractile depression caused by halothane and isoflurane based on differential modulation of intracellular Ca^{2+} homeostasis at several subcellular targets within the cardiac myocyte (33,34,53–55,93, 242,246,248,249,301,357,513,589,662). The negative inotropic actions of volatile anesthetics are exacerbated by hypocalcemia (253), Ca^{2+} channel blocking agents (364,386), or β_1-adrenergic receptor antagonists (364), and can be reversed with administration of exogenous calcium (121,253,437,466) (Fig. 43) or cardiac phosphodiesterase inhibitors (364,429) (Fig. 44).

The cardiovascular effects of desflurane have been the subject of intense recent research. Desflurane produces a systemic and coronary hemodynamic profile that is remarkably similar to that of isoflurane (645). Using isovolumetric and ejection-phase measures of contractility, several investigators (385,433, 654,655) concluded that desflurane and isoflurane also depress myocardial function to nearly equivalent degrees. This contention was supported by Pagel et al. (434), who used the slope of the PRSW relation as an assay of intrinsic inotropic state in chronically instrumented dogs (Fig. 45) and found desflurane and isoflurane to decrease myocardial contractility equally in the presence (436) and absence (434) of autonomic nervous system reflexes. These observations were further supported by Boban et al. (36)in the isolated guinea pig heart.

The cardiovascular effects of another new volatile anesthetic, sevoflurane, have been incompletely studied. Bernard et al. (31) compared the systemic and coronary hemodynamic actions of sevoflurane to those produced by isoflurane in dogs. Using dP/dt_{max} as an index of inotropic state, the investigators

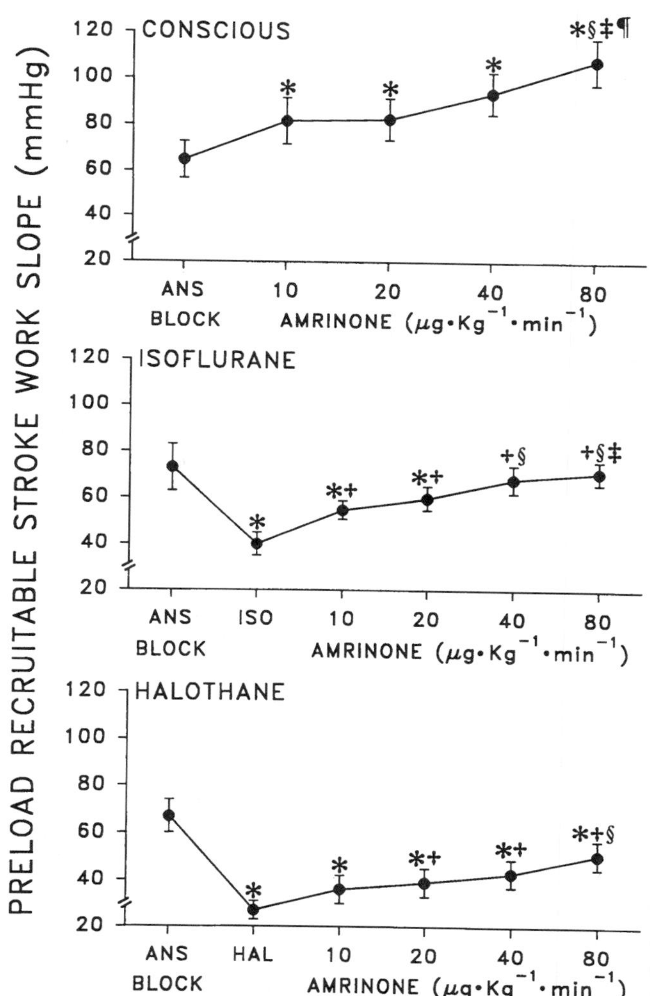

Figure 44. Preload recruitable stroke work slope (M_W) in conscious *(top panel)* and isoflurane (ISO; *middle panel)* or halothane-anesthetized (HAL; *bottom panel)* dogs in the presence of pharmacologic blockade of the autonomic nervous system (ANS block). Note that progressive doses of amrinone increase contractility in the conscious and anesthetized states and partially reverse the negative inotropic effects of halothane and isoflurane. (From ref. 429, with permission.)

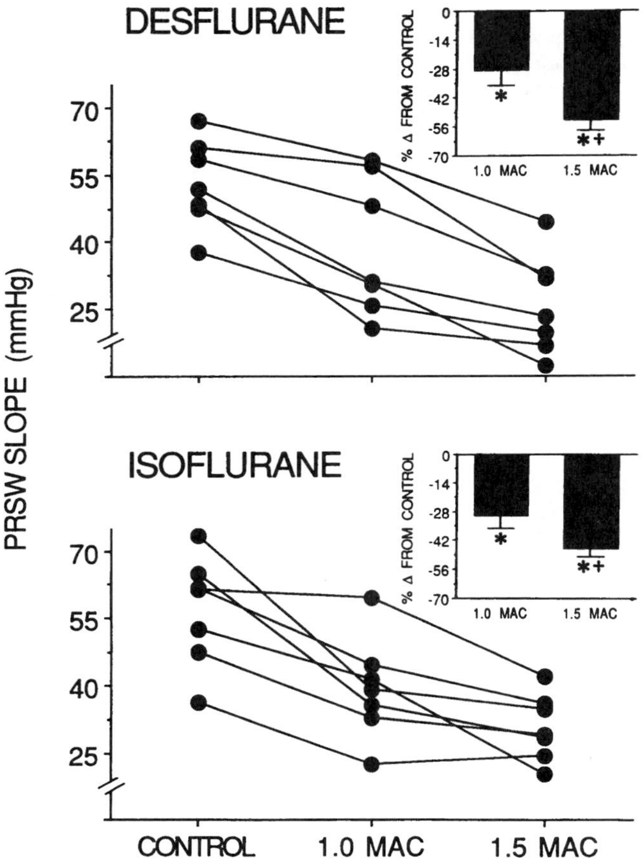

Figure 45. Preload recruitable stroke work (PRSW) slope for eight conscious dogs during control and at 1.0 and 1.5 end-tidal MAC desflurane *(top panel)* and isoflurane *(bottom panel).* Figure insets depict percent changes from control. (From ref. 434, with permission.)

demonstrated that the effect of sevoflurane on myocardial contractile function was indistinguishable from that induced by isoflurane (31). Other reports in humans (175) and experimental animals (15,230,326) have supported these findings and have suggested that sevoflurane may produce less cardiac depression than halothane (15,230,326). A recent study using echocardiography also demonstrated that sevoflurane produces less myocardial depression than equi-MAC concentrations of enflurane in volunteers using the heart rate-corrected velocity of circumferential fiber shortening versus left ventricular end-systolic wall stress relation as an index of contractile state calculated noninvasively (292). Thus, modern volatile anesthetics appear to depress the contractile state in normal ventricular myocardium in the following order: enflurane = halothane > isoflurane = desflurane = sevoflurane.

The effects of isoflurane (283) and enflurane (284) on the mechanics of isolated cat papillary muscle from normal hearts and those with congestive heart failure precipitated by chronic exposure to pressure overload have been compared. Decreases in V_{max} and +dF/dt were observed in both groups in response to isoflurane and enflurane; however, papillary muscles from failing hearts demonstrated significantly greater depression than those from normal hearts. The findings demonstrated that the combined negative inotropic effects of volatile anesthetics and failing myocardium were more pronounced than the actions of isoflurane or enflurane alone (283,284). The investigations also provided important experimental evidence to support the hypothesis that patients with underlying global contractile dysfunction may be more sensitive to the myocardial depressant properties of volatile anesthetics. In experimental models of regional myocardial ischemia (353) or infarction (468), however, declines in contractile function caused by volatile anesthetics were well tolerated and did not precipitate frank systolic dysfunction. These studies implied that the extent of regional ischemia or infarction is an important factor in determining the overall functional consequences imposed by volatile anesthetics. Further study in both experimental and clinical settings of myocardial ischemia, infarction, and hypertrophy are required to provide a more comprehensive understanding of the mechanical interaction between volatile anesthetics and these pathologic states.

The actions of potent inhalational anesthetics on diastolic function in the normal heart have been incompletely studied. Halothane, isoflurane, enflurane, and the new volatile anesthetics, desflurane and sevoflurane, produce dose-related prolongation of isovolumetric relaxation in vivo (Fig. 46) (133,230, 250,432). This delay of isovolumetric relaxation is associated with declines in early ventricular filling (230,429,437), but probably is not of sufficient magnitude to interfere with overall chamber stiffness. The significance of delayed relaxation to early coronary blood flow has also not been thoroughly investigated with volatile anesthetics. Coronary flow is highest during this period

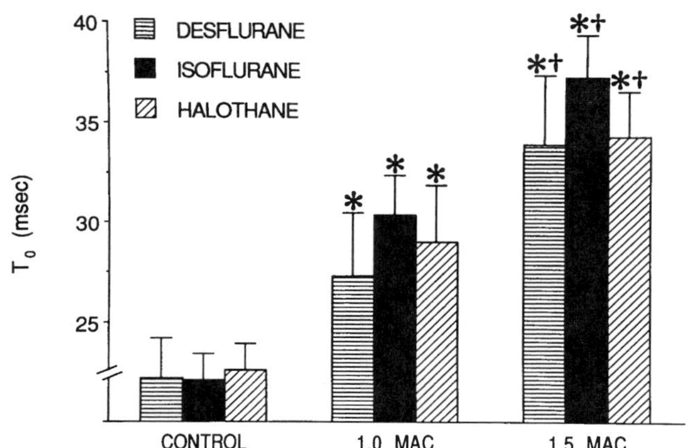

Figure 46. Effects of desflurane, isoflurane, and halothane on the time constant of isovolumetric relaxation calculated using a zero decay assumption (T_0). (From ref. 432, with permission.)

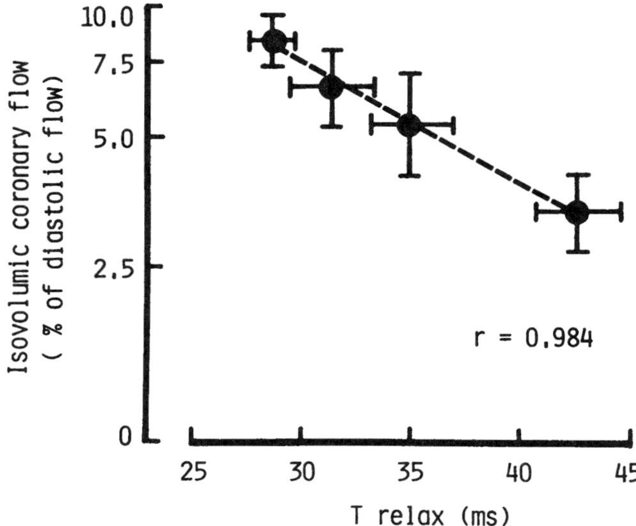

Figure 47. Relationship between the time constant of isovolumetric relaxation (T relax) and isovolumetric coronary blood flow (as expressed as a percentage of total diastolic flow) in halothane-anesthetized, acutely instrumented dogs. (From ref. 133, with permission.)

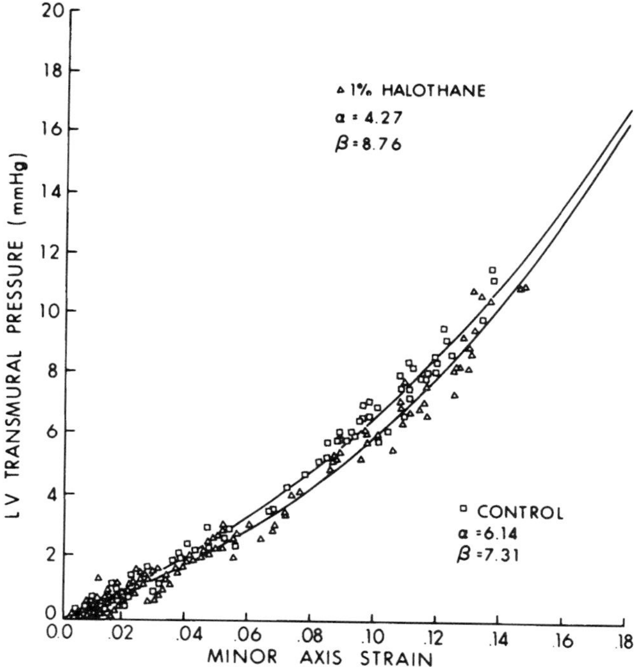

Figure 48. Left ventricular (LV) diastolic transmural pressure-Lagrangian strain relation in a conscious *(squares)* and halothane-anesthetized *(triangles)* dog. The pressure-strain relation qualitatively shifted to the left during halothane anesthesia, but this shift was not statistically significant, indicating that halothane does not produce alterations in intrinsic myocardial stiffness. α, gain; β, modulus of myocardial stiffness. (From ref. 632, with permission.)

of diastole, and an experimental study in dogs has suggested that delays in isovolumetric relaxation lead to impairment of flow (Fig. 47) during halothane anesthesia (133).

Isoflurane, desflurane, and sevoflurane do not alter invasively derived regional myocardial or chamber stiffness (230, 432), indicating that intrinsic ventricular distensibility is unchanged by these agents. Although some indirect evidence suggests that halothane affects diastolic compliance, this conclusion has been disputed by more recent investigations using invasively derived measures of passive ventricular filling. Halothane decreases myocardial compliance in isolated rat left ventricular muscle subjected to paired electrical stimulation in vitro (197). Increases in left ventricular end-diastolic volume as assessed with high-speed, biplane cineradiography are also observed following administration of halothane to dogs (514). Halothane, but not morphine sulfate nor regional major conduction blockade, results in depression of stroke volume at equivalent left ventricular end-diastolic pressures following cardiopulmonary bypass in acutely instrumented swine. The latter finding indirectly suggests a halothane-induced decrease in ventricular compliance (406). In contrast, dynamic stiffness of the series elastic element of myocardium was unaltered by halothane in isolated cat papillary muscle (605). No differences in passive compliance (characterized by a monoexponential pressure-volume relationship) were observed during administration of 1 versus 2 MAC halothane to acutely instrumented, open-chest dogs (209). Halothane (1% to 2%), it has also been found, does not change the end diastolic-minor axis strain relationship (Fig. 48), indicating that halothane does not alter end-diastolic myocardial stiffness (632). Using an end-diastolic pressure-segment length relation normalized with Lagrangian strain in chronically instrumented dogs, halothane, but not isoflurane or desflurane, was nevertheless shown to produce a significant increase in passive regional chamber stiffness calculated using a monoexponential ventricular pressure-segment length relationship (432). This effect was not dose dependent and may have resulted secondary to increases in left ventricular end-diastolic pressure and decreases in systolic contractile performance and heart rate (67). The actions of enflurane on diastolic compliance have yet to be thoroughly characterized. Although volatile anesthetics have been shown to prolong isovolumetric relaxation and impede early ventricular filling in a dose-related fashion, it seems unlikely that these agents, with the possible exception of halothane, affect overall ventricular compliance in vivo. The negative lusitropic properties of potent inhalational anesthetics can be reversed by administration of positive inotropes such as calcium chloride (437) (Fig. 49) or amrinone (Fig. 50) (429). The effects of anesthetic-induced abnormalities in diastolic mechanics in the heart with impaired diastolic performance has yet to be explored in either experimental models or patients with preexisting diastolic dysfunction, and this represents an important goal of

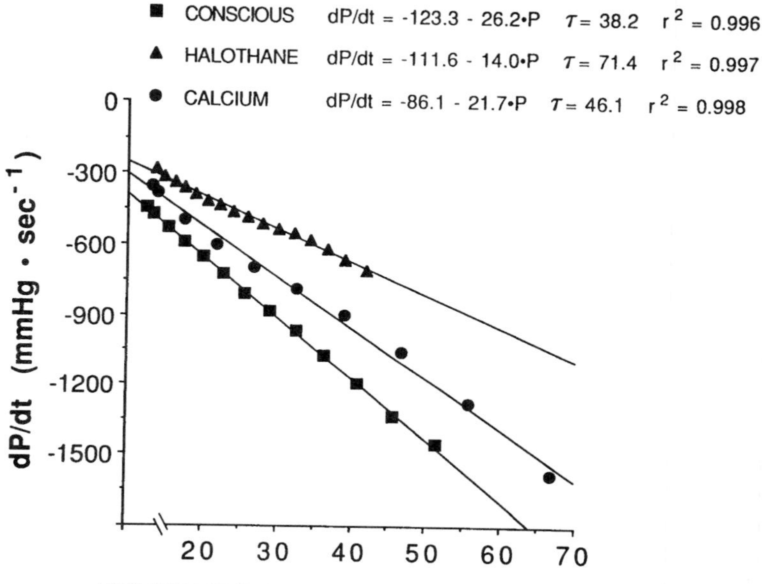

Figure 49. Relationship between left ventricular -dP/dt and pressure used to calculate the time constant of isovolumetric relaxation (τ) in the conscious state, during 1.5 MAC halothane, and during 5 mg·kg^{-1}·min^{-1} $CaCl_2$ in the presence of halothane anesthesia. Note the partial reversal of anesthetic-induced delay in isovolumetric relaxation by $CaCl_2$. (From ref. 437, with permission.)

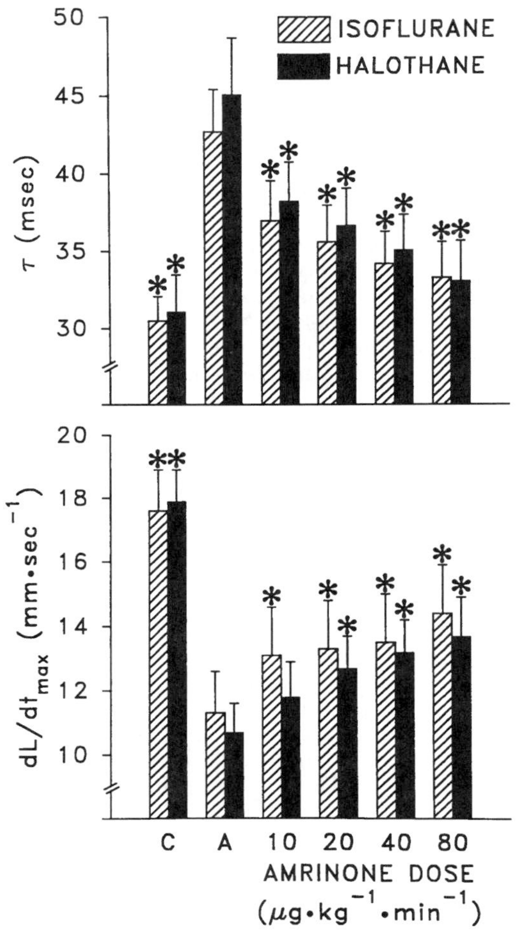

Figure 50. Histograms depicting the effects of intravenous infusions of amrinone on the time constant of isovolumetric relaxation (τ) and maximum segment lengthening velocity (dL/dt_{max}) in conscious (C) and isoflurane *(hatched bars)* or halothane *(solid bars)* anesthetized dogs. *Significantly ($p < 0.05$) different from the anesthetized state (A). (Adapted from ref. 429 with permission.)

future research. It is highly likely that the volatile anesthetics even in low inspired concentrations will exacerbate preexisting diastolic dysfunction and attenuate cardiac performance by negative lusitropic actions independent of effects on systolic function.

Nitrous Oxide

Determination of the effects of nitrous oxide on myocardial contractility in vivo has been a technically difficult task and the obtained results are controversial. Experiments in isolated heart preparations have demonstrated that nitrous oxide causes a direct negative inotropic effect (586). Previous investigations conducted in healthy experimental animals have supported (112,125,146,354,431,622) the contention that nitrous oxide is a direct negative inotrope; however, other studies have failed to verify this conclusion (100,556,632). Conflicting results have also been observed in healthy volunteers (20,127, 145,150,240,338,555,557,671). Evidence that nitrous oxide possesses direct myocardial depressant actions appears to be more uniform in humans with heart disease (144,316,356,583,672) and in experimental models of coronary artery disease in dogs (324,477), but this issue remains unsettled as well (82,552,583).

Several persistent difficulties with previous investigations in vivo have contributed to these contradictory results. First, because nitrous oxide may increase sympathetic nervous system tone (137,138,535), observed changes in contractile function may be influenced by the direct actions of nitrous oxide on the systemic circulation or by reflex effects mediated by the autonomic nervous system (112,557). Second, studies using nitrous oxide alone are difficult to perform and interpret because this gas does not produce total anesthesia at partial pressures less than one atmosphere (145,150,152,338,583,623). Third, protocols examining the effects of nitrous oxide in combination with other volatile anesthetics, opioids, or benzodiazepines are diverse, often difficult to directly compare, and have implied that nitrous oxide may have differential effects on myocardial function depending on the baseline anesthetic (20,100,127,316, 356,555–557,631,671,672). Fourth, the underlying health of the patient or animal population studied appears to influence the obtained results when the effects of nitrous oxide on contractile function are evaluated (143). Lastly, lack of a reliable, load-insensitive measure of myocardial contractility has allowed only qualitative assessment of the effects of nitrous oxide on intrinsic inotropic state in the majority of previous investigations.

The regional PRSW relationship generated from a series of invasively derived left ventricular pressure-segment length diagrams has been used in a recent reexamination of the effects of nitrous oxide on myocardial contractility in autonomically blocked, chronically instrumented dogs anesthetized with isoflurane or sufentanil. The results of this investigation (431) indicated that nitrous oxide produces dose-related depression of myocardial contractile state in the presence of either volatile or opioid-based anesthesia when underlying autonomic nervous system activity is eliminated. The degree of depression of PRSW slope with 70% nitrous oxide was 28% and 41% with sufentanil and isoflurane anesthesia (Fig. 51), respectively, indicating that 70% nitrous oxide decreased myocardial contractility to approx-

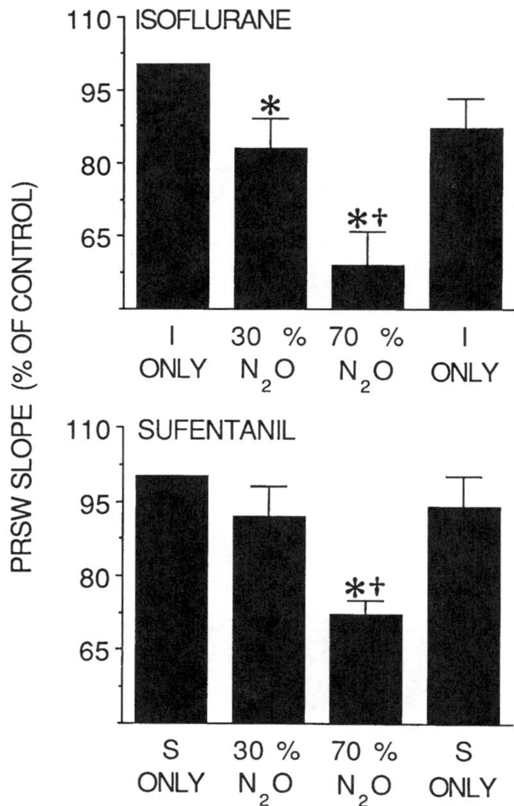

Figure 51. Effects of nitrous oxide (N_2O) on regional preload recruitable stroke work (PRSW) slope in isoflurane (I) or sufentanil (S) anesthetized, chronically instrumented dogs. (Adapted from ref. 431, with permission.)

imately the same extent as 1 MAC isoflurane (430,434). These nitrous oxide–induced myocardial depressant effects may be negated in vivo by concomitant increases in sympathetic tone.

The actions of nitrous oxide on ventricular diastolic function have been incompletely studied in vitro and remain completely uncharacterized in vivo. Carton et al. (92) examined the effects of nitrous oxide on contractility and relaxation in ferret papillary muscle. No changes in the rates of isometric or isotonic relaxation in twitches of equal amplitude were observed in response to nitrous oxide administration. In addition, although modest nitrous oxide–induced increases in maximal lengthening velocity ($-V_{max}$) and maximal rate of decline of force (-dF/dt) were observed, these changes in lusitropic state occurred concomitant with direct decreases in contractile state. Thus, the investigators (92) demonstrated that although nitrous oxide produces direct negative inotropic effects, this anesthetic gas did not modify myocardial relaxation in vitro. Further research is required in order to describe the actions of nitrous oxide on ventricular relaxation, filling, and compliance in the normal and diseased heart.

Intravenous Anesthetics

The effects of intravenous anesthetics, including barbiturates, etomidate, ketamine, and propofol, on systemic hemodynamics and left ventricular systolic function have been extensively studied. Ironically, despite the widespread and long-standing clinical use of barbiturates for anesthetic induction, the actions of these agents on specific indices of systolic and diastolic performance have not been well established. Barbiturates, including thiopental and methohexital, decrease indirect indices of myocardial contractility in vivo (106,160,489,536,564). Thiopental and methohexital have been shown to decrease the slope of a noninvasively derived approximation of the end-systolic pressure-volume relationship (ESPVR) in anesthetized patients (186,325, 411), although the several simplifying assumptions that were used to calculate the ESPVR cloud interpretation of the results and make quantitative assessment of changes in contractility difficult (99). Thiopental decreases ventricular dP/dt_{max} in a dose-related manner in the isolated heart (585) and depresses the tension development and the force-velocity relationship of atrial (14) and ventricular muscle (117,169) in vitro. These actions have been attributed to inhibition of transsarcolemmal Ca^{2+} flux and subsequent declines in availability of intracellular Ca^{2+} for contractile activation (14,35,117,169,254,300). These direct negative inotropic actions combine with barbiturate-induced increases in venous capacitance (139) and transient decreases in central sympathetic nervous system tone to produce the characteristic decreases in mean arterial pressure and cardiac output observed clinically during the administration of these agents (139,161). Further study using relatively load-independent indices of myocardial contractility such as the ESPVR or PRSW derived invasively in experimental animals or humans would provide quantitative insight into the relative effects of barbiturates on systolic ventricular performance. The actions of barbiturates on ventricular diastolic function in vivo have yet to be described; however, barbiturate-induced alterations in intracellular Ca^{2+} homeostasis may have an impact on diastolic performance as well as systolic function.

The hallmark of anesthetic induction with etomidate is remarkable stability of systemic and pulmonary hemodynamics. Investigations in normal patients (113,201,448) and those with cardiovascular disease (105,201,202) have repeatedly demonstrated that etomidate produces little change in hemodynamics. Modest decreases in mean arterial pressure, presumably resulting from declines in central sympathetic nervous system tone, venous return, and peripheral metabolism (464), have been reported with higher doses of etomidate in patients with cardiac disease without apparent negative inotropic effects (201,202). Etomidate has been shown to have little effect on myocardial contractility of isolated normal (493) and cardiomyopathic (494) rat papillary muscle (Fig. 52), presumably by maintaining the availability of intracellular Ca^{2+} for contractile activation in vitro (299). Etomidate also causes little or no myocardial depression in isolated hearts (585) and dogs (69,120,293), as evaluated with isovolumetric and ejection-phase indices of contractility. However, the effects of etomidate on more load-independent measures of contractile state have yet to be established. The actions of etomidate on diastolic function have not been specifically described in vivo.

Induction or maintenance of anesthesia with propofol is associated with significant decreases in systemic arterial pressure (534). Propofol-induced hypotension results from a combination of venous and arterial vasodilation (412,508) and mild direct negative inotropic effects (101,441) (Fig. 53). A growing body of evidence in isolated papillary muscle preparations (14,443) and in dogs (120) and humans (186,325,411) suggests that propofol causes less myocardial depression than equipotent doses of thiopental and methohexital. In chronically instrumented dogs, propofol was found to cause no change in isovolumetric relaxation or regional chamber stiffness even at doses that far exceed the usual clinical range required for anesthesia, indicating that this intravenous anesthetic does not alter diastolic function (440) (Fig. 54). These findings are indirectly supported by two recent investigations in isolated guinea pig ventricular muscle (443) and rat papillary muscle (492). Propofol produces moderate changes in intrinsic myocardial contractility by depressing voltage-dependent transsarcolemmal Ca^{2+} entry and late Ca^{2+} release from sarcoplasmic reticulum (443). In addition, although propofol impairs uptake of Ca^{2+} by the sarcoplasmic reticulum to a small extent, no change in the rate constant of exponential decay of isometric force has been observed in vitro (492). These results are consistent with the hypothesis that propofol does not alter the functional integrity of the sarcoplasmic reticulum with the exception of modest decreases in Ca^{2+} uptake. Thus, although propofol produces some effects on intracellular Ca^{2+} homeostasis during systole and diastole, these perturbations appear to cause only modest derangements in myocardial contractility (441) and no change in lusitropic state.

Since its introduction into clinical practice in 1971, ketamine has been used with widespread success in the induction of anesthesia in certain patients with hemodynamic compromise (658).

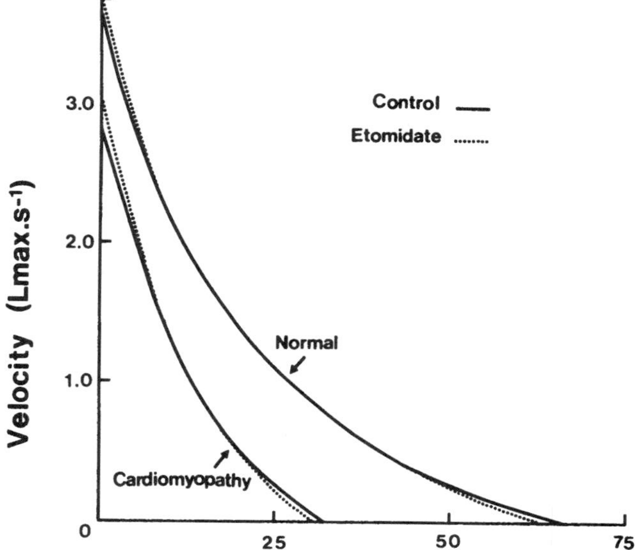

Figure 52. Effects of etomidate (5 mg/ml) on force-velocity relationships of papillary muscles of normal hamsters and those with cardiomyopathy. (From ref. 494, with permission.)

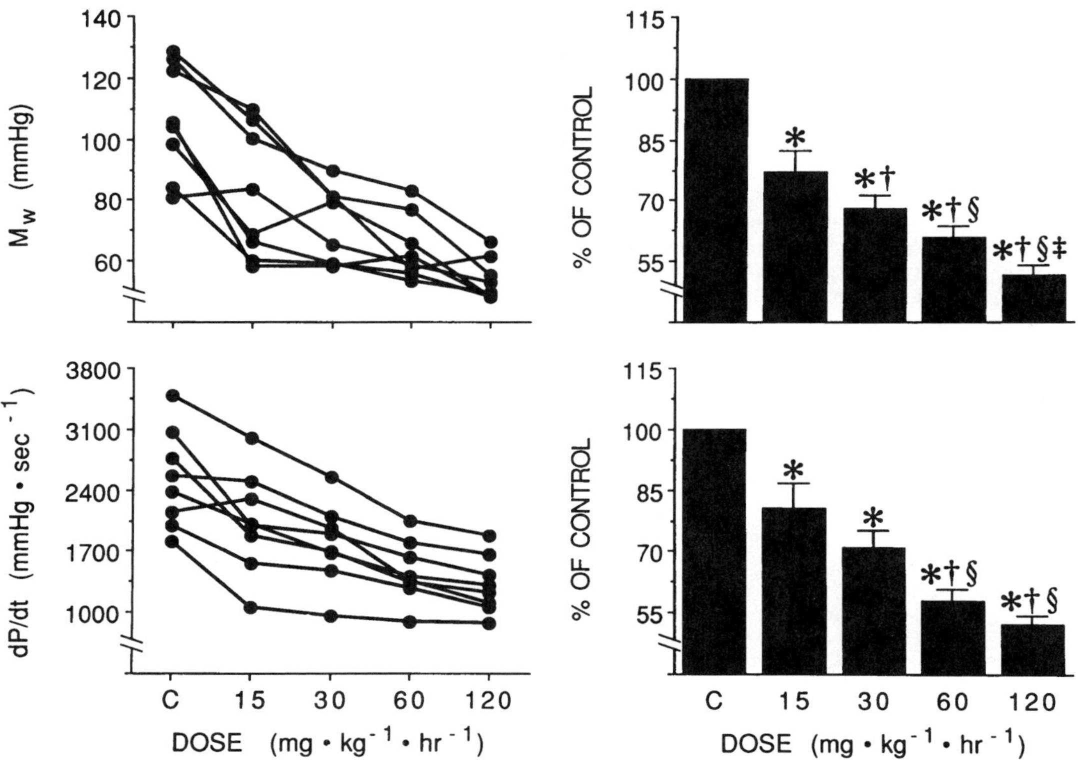

Figure 53. Preload recruitable stroke work slope (M_W; *top left panel)* and left ventricular dP/dt *(bottom left panel)* for each of eight dogs and average data expressed as a percent of control *(top and bottom right panels,* respectively) during control (C) and at various infusions of propofol. (From ref. 441, with permission.)

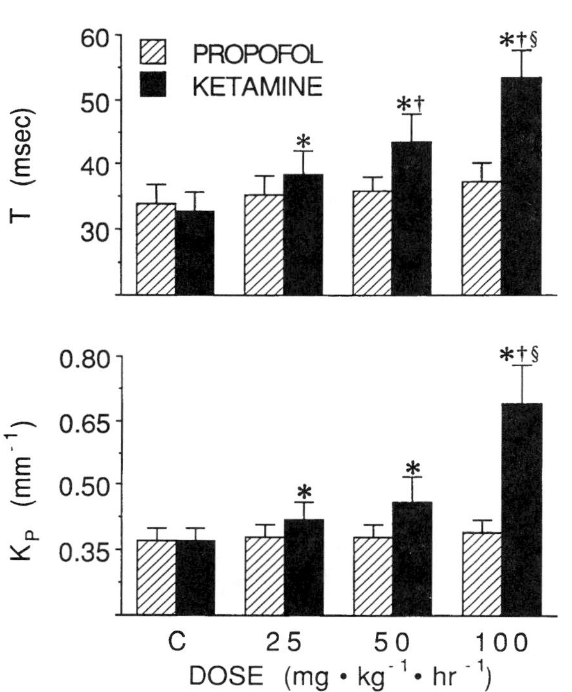

Figure 54. Effects of ketamine and propofol on the time constant of isovolumetric relaxation (T) and regional chamber stiffness (K_P) in chronically instrumented dogs. (From ref. 440, with permission.)

The observation that ketamine can lead to acute hemodynamic decompensation in a subset of critically ill patients with impaired function of the sympathetic nervous system (648) has stimulated exploration of the direct effects of this intravenous anesthetic on cardiovascular function. Ketamine produces dramatic increases in heart rate and arterial pressure in most patients, which can be attributed to the central and peripheral sympathomimetic actions of this drug (658). Ketamine blocks the reuptake of monoamines including norepinephrine in adrenergic nerves, a mechanism of action similar to that of cocaine (355,521). Depletion of catecholamines to the direct vasodilator and myocardial depressant actions of ketamine independent of sympathomimetic effects have been postulated as potential mechanisms of hemodynamic collapse after administration of ketamine in some patients (533,648). The direct effects of ketamine on myocardial contractility in vivo have been difficult to interpret because changes in contractile state are often masked by ketamine-induced increases in sympathetic tone (260,533,626,658). However, ketamine has been shown to produce direct myocardial depressant actions as assessed with the regional PRSW slope in dogs with pharmacologic blockade of the autonomic nervous system (435). This observation is supported by investigations in vitro (107,108,302,512,629) demonstrating ketamine-induced negative inotropic effects when normal adrenergic nerve transmission is impaired. The direct myocardial depression caused by ketamine probably occurs as a result of inhibition of transsarcolemmal Ca^{2+} influx and subsequent decreases in intracellular Ca^{2+} availability without changes in myofibrillar Ca^{2+} sensitivity (302,512). Ketamine also produces diastolic dysfunction in a dose-related manner, prolonging isovolumetric relaxation and increasing regional chamber stiffness (440) (Fig. 54). Thus, cardiovascular collapse observed in the catecholamine-depleted patient during induction of anesthesia with ketamine (656) may be related not only to depression of systolic performance but also to direct alterations in ventricular diastolic function.

ACKNOWLEDGMENTS

The authors extend their appreciation to David Schwabe for technical assistance and to Mimi Mick for her help in the preparation of this chapter.

REFERENCES

1. Alderman EL, Glantz SA. Acute hemodynamic interventions shift the diastolic pressure-volume curve in man. *Circulation* 1976;54: 662–671.
2. Allen DG, Kentish JC. Calcium concentration in the myoplasm of skinned ferret ventricular muscle following changes in muscle length. *J Physiol* 1988;407:489–503.
3. Allen DG, Orchard CH. Myocardial contractile function during ischemia and hypoxia. *Circ Res* 1987;60:153–168.
4. Anderson JE. *Grant's atlas of anatomy*, 7th ed. Baltimore: Williams and Wilkins, 1978.
5. Anversa P, Ricci R, Olivetti G. Quantitative structural analysis of myocardium during physiologic growth and induced cardiac hypertrophy: a review. *J Am Coll Cardiol* 1986;7:1140–1149.
6. Applegate RJ, Cheng CP, Little WC. Simultaneous conductance catheter and dimension assessment of left ventricle volume in the intact animal. *Circulation* 1990;81:638–648.
7. Appleton CP, Hatle LK, Popp RL. Demonstration of restrictive ventricular physiology by Doppler echocardiography. *J Am Coll Cardiol* 1988;11:757–768.
8. Appleton CP, Hatle LK, Popp RL. Relation of transmitral flow velocity patterns to left ventricular diastolic function: new insights from a combined hemodynamic and Doppler echocardiographic study. *J Am Coll Cardiol* 1988;12:426–440.
9. Apstein CS, Grossman W. Opposite initial effects of supply and demand ischemia on left ventricular diastolic compliance: the ischemia-diastolic paradox. *J Mol Cell Cardiol* 1987;19:119–128.
10. Aroesty JM, McKay RG, Heller GV, Royal HD, Als AV, Grossman W. Simultaneous assessment of left ventricular systolic and diastolic dysfunction during pacing-induced ischemia. *Circulation* 1985;71: 889–900.
11. Arora RR, Machac J, Goldman ME, Butler RN, Gorlin R, Horowitz SF. Atrial kinetics and left ventricular diastolic filling in the healthy elderly. *J Am Coll Cardiol* 1987;9:1255–1260.
12. Atarashi K, Mulrow PJ, Franco-Saenz, Shajder R, Rapp J. Inhibition of aldosterone production by an atrial extract. *Science* 1984; 224:992–994.
13. Aversano T, Maughan WL, Hunter WC, Kass D, Becker LC. End-systolic measures of regional ventricular performance. *Circulation* 1986;73:938–950.
14. Azari DM, Cork RC. Comparative myocardial depressive effects of propofol and thiopental. *Anesth Analg* 1993;77:324–329.
15. Azari DM, Cork RC, Conzen P, Vollmar B, Kramer TH. Inotropic effects of sevoflurane compared to isoflurane and halothane (abstract). *Anesthesiology* 1992;77:A628.
16. Baan J, Jong TT, Kerkhof PLM, et al. Continuous stroke volume and cardiac output from intraventricular dimensions obtained with impedance catheter. *Cardiovasc Res* 1981;15:328–334.
17. Baan J, Van der Velde ET, De Bruin HG, et al. Continuous measurement of left ventricular volume in animals and humans by conductance catheter. *Circulation* 1984;70:812–823.
18. Baer PG, McGiff JC. Hormonal systems and renal hemodynamics. *Annu Rev Physiol* 1980;42:589–601.
19. Bahler RC, Vrobel TR, Martin P. The relation of heart rate and shortening fraction to echocardiographic indexes of left ventricular relaxation in normal subjects. *J Am Coll Cardiol* 1983;2:926–933.
20. Bahlman SH, Eger EI, II, Smith NT, et al. The cardiovascular effects of nitrous oxide-halothane in man. *Anesthesiology* 1971;35: 274–285.
21. Baker KM, Aceto JA. Characterization of avian angiotensin II cardiac receptors: coupling to mechanical activity and phosphoinositol metabolism. *J Mol Cell Cardiol* 1989;21:375–382.
22. Baker KM, Singer HA. Identification and characterization of guinea pig angiotensin II ventricular and atrial receptors: coupling to inositol phosphate production. *Circ Res* 1988;62:896–904.
23. Barash PG, Kopriva CJ. Cardiac monitoring. In: Thomas SJ, Kramer JL, eds. *Manual of cardiac anesthesia*. New York: Churchill Livingstone, 1993;23–50.
24. Barry WH. Mechanical dysfunction of the heart during and after ischemia: unraveling the causes. *Circulation* 1990;82:652–654.
25. Barry WH, Brooker JZ, Alderman EL, Harrison DC. Changes in diastolic stiffness and tone of the left ventricle during angina pectoris. *Circulation* 1974;49:255–263.
26. Battler A, Gallagher KP, Froelicher VF, Kumada T, Kemper WS, Ross J Jr. Detection of latent coronary stenosis in conscious dogs: regional functional and electrocardiographic responses to isoprenaline. *Cardiovasc Res* 1980;14:476–481.
27. Beaupre PN, Kremer PF, Cahalan MK, Lurz FW, Schiller NB, Hamilton WK. Intraoperative detection of changes in left ventricular segmental wall motion by transesophageal two-dimensional echocardiography. *Am Heart J* 1984;107:1021–1023.
28. Belcher P, Boerboom LE, Olinger GN. Standardization of end-systolic pressure-volume relation in the dog. *Am J Physiol* 1985;249: H547–H553.
29. Bell RC, Robotham JL, Badke FR, Little WC, Kindred MK. Left ventricular geometry during intermittent positive pressure ventilation in dogs. *J Crit Care* 1987;2:230–244.
30. Belo SE, Mazer CD. Effect of halothane and isoflurane on postischemic "stunned" myocardium in the dog. *Anesthesiology* 1990;73: 1243–1251.
31. Bernard JM, Wouters PF, Doursout MF, Florence B, Chelly JE, Merin RG. Effects of sevoflurane and isoflurane on cardiac and coronary dynamics in chronically instrumented dogs. *Anesthesiology* 1990;72:659–662.
32. Betocchi S, Bonow RO, Bacharach SL, Rosing DR, Maron BJ, Green MV. Isovolumetric relaxation period in hypertrophic cardiomyopathy: assessment by radionuclide angiography. *J Am Coll Cardiol* 1986;7:74–81.
33. Blanck TJJ, Chiancone E, Salvati G, et al. Halothane does not alter Ca^{2+} affinity of troponin C. *Anesthesiology* 1992;76:100–105.
34. Blanck TJJ, Peterson CV, Baroody B, Tegazzin V, Lou J. Halothane, enflurane, and isoflurane stimulate calcium leakage from rabbit sarcoplasmic reticulum. *Anesthesiology* 1992;76:813–821.
35. Blanck TJJ, Stevenson RL. Thiopental does not alter Ca^{2+} uptake by cardiac sarcoplasmic reticulum. *Anesth Analg* 1988;67:346–348.
36. Boban M, Stowe DF, Buljubasic N, Kampine JP, Bosnjak ZJ. Direct comparative effects of isoflurane and desflurane in isolated guinea pig hearts. *Anesthesiology* 1992;76:775–780.
37. Bolli R. Oxygen-derived free radicals and postischemic myocardial dysfunction ("stunned myocardium"). *J Am Coll Cardiol* 1988;12: 239–249.
38. Bolli R. Mechanism of myocardial "stunning." *Circulation* 1990;82: 723–738.
39. Bolli R, Zhu WX, Thornby JI, O'Neill PG, Roberts R. Time course and determinants of recovery of function after reversible ischemia in conscious dogs. *Am J Physiol* 1988;254:H102–H114.
40. Boltwood CM, Appleyard RF, Glantz SA. Left ventricular volume measurement by conductance catheter in intact dogs. Parallel conductance depends on left ventricular size. *Circulation* 1989;80: 1360–1377.
41. Bonchek LI, Olinger GN, Siegel R, Tresch DD, Keelan MH Jr. Left ventricular performance after mitral reconstruction for mitral regurgitation. *J Thorac Cardiovasc Surg* 1984;88:122–127.
42. Bonow RO, Bacharach SL, Green MV, et al. Impaired left ventricular diastolic filling in patients with coronary artery disease: assessment with radionuclide angiography. *Circulation* 1981;64:315–323.
43. Bonow RO, Dodd JT, Maron BJ, et al. Long-term serial changes in left ventricular function and reversal of ventricular dilatation after valve replacement for chronic aortic regurgitation. *Circulation* 1988;78:1108–1120.
44. Bonow RO, Frederick TM, Bacharach SL, et al. Atrial systole and left ventricular filling in hypertrophic cardiomyopathy: effect of verapamil. *Am J Cardiol* 1983;51:1386–1391.
45. Bonow RO, Rosing DR, Kent KM, Epstein SE. Timing of operation for chronic aortic regurgitation. *Am J Cardiol* 1982;50:325–336.
46. Borer JS, Bacharach SL, Green MV, Kent KM, Epstein SE, Johnston GS. Real-time radionuclide cineangiography in the noninvasive evaluation of global and regional left ventricular function at rest and during exercise in patients with coronary-artery disease. *N Engl J Med* 1977;296:839–844.
47. Borow KM. Surgical outcome in chronic aortic regurgitation: a physiologic framework for assessing preoperative predictors. *J Am Coll Cardiol* 1987;10:1165–1170.
48. Borow KM, Colan SD, Neumann A. Altered left ventricular mechanics in patients with valvular aortic stenosis and coarctation of the aorta: effects on systolic performance and late outcome. *Circulation* 1985;72:515–522.
49. Borow KM, Green LH, Grossman W, Braunwald E. Left ventricu-

lar end-systolic stress-shortening and stress-length relations in humans: normal values and sensitivity to inotropic states. *Am J Cardiol* 1982;50:1301–1308.
50. Borow KM, Henderson IC, Neumann A, et al. Assessment of left ventricular contractility in patients receiving doxorubicin. *Ann Intern Med* 1983;99:750–756.
51. Borow KM, Lang RM, Neumann A, Carroll JD, Rajfer SI. Physiologic mechanisms governing hemodynamic responses to positive inotropic therapy in patients with dilated cardiomyopathy. *Circulation* 1988;77:625–637.
52. Borow KM, Neumann A, Lang RM. Milrinone versus dobutamine: contribution of altered myocardial mechanics and augmented inotropic state to improved left ventricular performance. *Circulation* 1986;73(suppl III):153–161.
53. Bosnjak ZB, Kampine JP. Effects of halothane on transmembrane potentials, Ca^{2+} transients, and papillary muscle tension in the cat. *Am J Physiol* 1986;251:H374–H381.
54. Bosnjak ZB, Supan FD, Rusch NJ. The effects of halothane, enflurane, and isoflurane on calcium current in isolated canine ventricular cells. *Anesthesiology* 1991;74:340–345.
55. Bosnjak ZJ, Aggarwal A, Turner LA, Kampine JM, Kampine JP. Differential effects of halothane, enflurane, and isoflurane on Ca^{2+} transients and papillary muscle tension in guinea pigs. *Anesthesiology* 1992;76:123–131.
56. Boudreau G, Peronnet F, De Champlain J, Nadeau R. Presynaptic effect of epinephrine on norepinephrine release from cardiac sympathetic nerves in dogs. *Am J Physiol* 1993;265:H205–H211.
57. Bove AA, Santamore WP. Ventricular interdependence. *Prog Cardiovasc Dis* 1981;23:365–388.
58. Braunwald E. On the difference between the heart's output and its contractile state. *Circulation* 1971;43:171–174.
59. Braunwald E. Assessment of cardiac function. In: Braunwald E, ed. *Heart disease: a textbook of cardiovascular medicine.* Philadelphia: WB Saunders, 1992;419–443.
60. Braunwald E. Pathophysiology of heart failure. In: Braunwald E, ed. *Heart disease: a textbook of cardiovascular medicine.* Philadelphia: WB Saunders, 1992;393–418.
61. Braunwald E, Kloner RA. The stunned myocardium: prolonged, postischemic ventricular dysfunction. *Circulation* 1982;66:1146–1149.
62. Braunwald E, Kloner RA. Myocardial reperfusion: a double-edged sword? *J Clin Invest* 1985;76:1713–1719.
63. Braunwald E, Rutherford JD. Reversible ischemic left ventricular dysfunction: evidence for the "hibernating myocardium". *J Am Coll Cardiol* 1986;8:1467–1470.
64. Braunwald E, Sonnenblick EH, Ross J Jr. Mechanisms of cardiac contraction and relaxation. In: Braunwald E, ed. *Heart disease: a textbook of cardiovascular medicine.* Philadelphia: WB Saunders, 1992;351–392.
65. Bristow MR, Hershberger RE, Port JD, et al. Beta-adrenergic pathways in nonfailing and failing human ventricular myocardium. *Circulation* 1990;82(suppl I):12–25.
66. Bronzwaer JGF, de Bruyne B, Ascoop CAPL, Paulus WJ. Comparative effects of pacing-induced and balloon coronary occlusion ischemia on left ventricular diastolic function in man. *Circulation* 1991;84:211–222.
67. Brower RW, Merin RG. Left ventricular function and compliance in swine during halothane anesthesia. *Anesthesiology* 1979;50:409–415.
68. Brown BG, Bolson EL, Dodge HT. Quantitative contrast angiography for assessment of ventricular performance in heart disease. *J Am Coll Cardiol* 1983;1:73–81.
69. Brussel T, Thiessen JL, Vigfusson G, Lunkenheimer PP, Van Aken H, Lawin P. Hemodynamic and cardiodynamic effects of propofol and etomidate: negative inotropic properties of propofol. *Anesth Analg* 1989;69:35–40.
70. Brutsaert DL, Housmans PR, Goethals MA. Dual control of relaxation. Its role in the ventricular function in the mammalian heart. *Circ Res* 1980;47:637–652.
71. Brutsaert DL, Rademakers FE, Sys SU. Triple control of relaxation: implications in cardiac disease. *Circulation* 1984;69:190–196.
72. Brutsaert DL, Rademakers FE, Sys SU, Gillebert TC, Housmans PR. Analysis of relaxation in the evaluation of ventricular function of the heart. *Prog Cardiovasc Dis* 1985;28:143–163.
73. Buda AJ, Zotz RJ, Gallagher KP. Characterization of the functional border zone around regionally ischemic myocardium using circumferential flow-function maps. *J Am Coll Cardiol* 1986;8:150–158.
74. Burkhoff D. The conductance method of left ventricular volume estimation: methodologic limitations put into perspective. *Circulation* 1990;81:703–706.
75. Burkhoff D, De Tombe PP, Hunter WC. Impact of ejection on magnitude and time course of ventricular pressure-generating capacity. *Am J Physiol* 1993;265:H899–H909.
76. Burkhoff D, Sagawa K. Ventricular efficiency predicted by an analytical model. *Am J Physiol* 1986;250:R1021–R1027.
77. Burkhoff D, Sugiura S, Yue DT, Sagawa K. Contractility-dependent curvilinearity of end-systolic pressure-volume relations. *Am J Physiol* 1987;252:H1218–H1227.
78. Burkhoff D, Van der Velde E, Kass D, Baan J, Maughan WL, Sagawa K. Accuracy of volume measurement by conductance catheter in isolated, ejecting canine hearts. *Circulation* 1985;72:440–447.
79. Burkhoff D, Yue D, Oikawa Y, Franz MR, Schaefer J, Sagawa K. Influence of ventricular contractility on non-work-related myocardial oxygen consumption. *Heart Vessel* 1987;3:66–72.
80. Buttrick P, Malhotra A, Factor S, Greenen D, Leinwand L, Scheuer J. Effect of aging and hypertension on myosin biochemistry and gene expression in the rat heart. *Circ Res* 1991;68:645–652.
81. Byrne JG, Smith WJ, Murphy MP, Couper GS, Appleyard RF, Cohn LH. Complete prevention of myocardial stunning, contracture, low-reflow, and edema after transplantation by blocking neutrophil adhesion molecules during reperfusion. *J Thorac Cardiovasc Surg* 1992;104:1589–1596.
82. Cahalan MK, Prakash O, Rulf ENR, et al. Addition of nitrous oxide to fentanyl anesthesia does not induce myocardial ischemia in patients with ischemic heart disease. *Anesthesiology* 1987;67:925–929.
83. Calafiore P, Stewart WT. Doppler echocardiographic quantitation of volumetric flow rate. *Cardiol Clin* 1990;8:191–202.
84. Calverley RK, Smith NT, Prys-Roberts C, Eger EI II, Jones CW. Cardiovascular effects of enflurane anesthesia during controlled ventilation in man. *Anesth Analg* 1978;57:619–628.
85. Capasso JM, Aronson RS, Sonnenblick EH. Reversible alterations in excitation-contraction coupling during myocardial hypertrophy in rat papillary muscle. *Circ Res* 1982;51:189–195.
86. Capasso JM, Palackal T, Olivetti G, Anversa P. Left ventricular failure induced by long-term hypertension in rats. *Circ Res* 1990;66:1400–1412.
87. Carabello BA, Green LH, Grossman W, Cohn LH, Koster JK, Collins Jr JJ. Hemodynamic determinants of prognosis of aortic valve replacement in critical aortic stenosis and advanced congestive heart failure. *Circulation* 1980;62:42–48.
88. Carabello BA, Nakano K, Corin W, Biederman R, Spann JF Jr. Left ventricular function in experimental volume overload hypertrophy. *Am J Physiol* 1989;256:H974–H981.
89. Carabello BA, Spann JF. The uses and limitations of end-systolic indexes of left ventricular function. *Circulation* 1984;69:1058–1064.
90. Carroll JD, Hess OM, Hirzel HO, Krayenbuehl HP. Exercise-induced ischemia: the influence of altered relaxation on early diastolic pressures. *Circulation* 1983;67:521–528.
91. Carroll JD, Hess OM, Hirzel HO, Turina M, Krayenbuehl HP. Left ventricular systolic and diastolic function in coronary artery disease: effects of revascularization on exercise-induced ischemia. *Circulation* 1985;72:119–129.
92. Carton EG, Wanek LA, Housmans PR. Effects of nitrous oxide on contractility, relaxation and the intracellular calcium transient of isolated mammalian ventricular myocardium. *J Pharmacol Exp Ther* 1991;257:843–849.
93. Casella ES, Suite ND, Fisher YI, Blanck TJ. The effect of volatile anesthetics on the pH dependence of calcium uptake by cardiac sarcoplasmic reticulum. *Anesthesiology* 1987;67:386–390.
94. Charlat ML, O'Neill PG, Hartley CJ, Roberts R, Bolli R. Prolonged abnormalities of left ventricular diastolic wall thinning in the "stunned" myocardium in conscious dogs: time course and relation to systolic function. *J Am Coll Cardiol* 1989;13:185–194.
95. Cheng C-P, Freeman GL, Santamore WP, Constantinescu MS, Little WC. Effect of loading conditions, contractile state, and heart rate on early diastolic left ventricular filling in conscious dogs. *Circ Res* 1990;66:814–823.
96. Cheng CP, Igarashi Y, Little WC. Mechanism of augmented rate of left ventricular filling during exercise. *Circ Res* 1992;70:9–19.
97. Chidsey CA, Harrison DC, Braunwald E. Augmentation of the plasma norepinephrine response to exercise in patients with congestive heart failure. *N Engl J Med* 1962;267:650–654.

98. Choong CY, Abascal VM, Thomas JD, Guerrero JL, McGlew S, Weyman AE. Combined influence of ventricular loading and relaxation on the transmitral flow velocity profile in dogs measured by Doppler echocardiography. *Circulation* 1988;78: 672–683.
99. Coddens J, DeLoof T. End-systolic pressure-volume relationship and arterial elastance: the optimal method to evaluate myocardial contractile effects of anesthetic agents? (Letter). *Anesth Analg* 1992;74:165.
100. Coetzee A, Fourie P, Bollinger C, Badenhorst E, Rebel A, Lombard C. Effect of N_2O on segmental left ventricular function and effective arterial elastance in pigs when added to a halothane-fentanyl-pancuronium anesthetic technique. *Anesth Analg* 1989;69: 313–322.
101. Coetzee A, Fourie P, Coetzee J, et al. Effect of various propofol plasma concentrations on regional myocardial contractility and left ventricular afterload. *Anesth Analg* 1989;69:473–483.
102. Cohen A, Hagan AD, Watkins J, et al. Clinical correlates in hypertensive patients with left ventricular hypertrophy diagnosed with echocardiography. *Am J Cardiol* 1981;47:335–341.
103. Cohn JN, Levine TB, Olivari MT, et al. Plasma norepinephrine as a guide to prognosis in patients with chronic congestive heart failure. *N Engl J Med* 1984;311:819–823.
104. Colan SD, Borow KM, Neumann A. The left ventricular end-systolic wall stress-velocity of fiber shortening relation: a load independent index of myocardial contractility. *J Am Coll Cardiol* 1984; 4:715–724.
105. Colvin MP, Savege TM, Newland PE, et al. Cardiorespiratory changes following induction of anaesthesia with etomidate in patients with cardiac disease. *Br J Anaesth* 1979;51:551–556.
106. Conway CM, Ellis DB. The haemodynamic effects of short acting barbiturates. *Br J Anaesth* 1969;41:534–542.
107. Cook DJ, Carton EG, Housmans PR. Mechanism of the positive inotropic effect of ketamine in isolated ferret ventricular papillary muscle. *Anesthesiology* 1991;74:880–888.
108. Cook DJ, Housmans PR, Rorie DK. Effect of ketamine HCl on norepinephrine disposition in isolated ferret ventricular myocardium. *J Pharmacol Exp Ther* 1992;261:101–107.
109. Cooper G, IV, Tomanek RJ, Ehrhardt JC, Marcus ML. Chronic progressive pressure overload of the cat right ventricle. *Circ Res* 1981;48:488–497.
110. Corin WJ, Murakami T, Monrad ES, Hess OM, Krayenbuehl HP. Left ventricular passive diastolic properties in chronic mitral regurgitation. *Circulation* 1991;83:797–807.
111. Courtois M, Kovacs SJ Jr, Ludbrook PA. Transmitral pressure-flow velocity relation. Importance of regional pressure gradients in the left ventricle during diastole. *Circulation* 1988;78:661–671.
112. Craythorne NW, Darby TD. The cardiovascular effects of nitrous oxide in the dog. *Br J Anaesth* 1965;37:560–565.
113. Criado A, Maseda J, Navarro E, Escarpa A, Avello F. Induction of anaesthesia with etomidate. Haemodynamic study of 36 patients. *Br J Anaesth* 1980;52:803–806.
114. Crottogini AJ, Willshaw P, Barra JG, Armentano R, Cabrera Fischer EI, Pichel RH. Inconsistency of the slope and volume intercept of the end-systolic pressure-volume relationship as individual indexes of inotropic state in dogs: presentation of an index combining both variables. *Circulation* 1987;76:1115–1126.
115. Cryer PE. Physiology and pathophysiology of the human sympathoadrenal neuroendocrine system. *N Engl J Med* 1980;303: 436–444.
116. Cuocolo A, Sax FL, Brush JE, Maron BJ, Bacharach SL, Bonow RO. Left ventricular hypertrophy and impaired diastolic filling in essential hypertension: diastolic mechanisms for systolic dysfunction during exercise. *Circulation* 1990;81:978–986.
117. Davies AE, McCans JL. Effects of barbiturate anesthetics and ketamine on the force-frequency relation of cardiac muscle. *Eur J Pharmacol* 1979;59:65–73.
118. DeBoer LW, Ingwall JS, Kloner RA, Braunwald E. Prolonged derangements of canine purine metabolism after a brief coronary artery occlusion not associated with anatomic evidence of necrosis. *Proc Natl Acad Sci USA* 1980;77:5471–5475.
119. DeHert SG, Gillebert TC, Andries LC, Brutsaert DL. Role of the endocardial endothelium in the regulation of myocardial function: physiologic and pathophysiologic implications. *Anesthesiology* 1993;79:1354–1366.
120. DeHert SG, Vermeyen KM, Adriaensen HF. Influence of thiopental, etomidate, and propofol on regional myocardial function in the normal and acute ischemic heart segment in dogs. *Anesth Analg* 1990;70:600–607.
121. Denlinger JK, Kaplan JA, Lecky JH, Wollman H. Cardiovascular response to calcium administered intravenously to man during halothane anesthesia. *Anesthesiology* 1975;42:390–397.
122. Deutsch S, Linde HW, Dripps RD, Price HL. Circulatory and respiratory actions of halothane in normal man. *Anesthesiology* 1962;23:631–638.
123. Devereux RB. Toward a more complete understanding of left ventricular afterload. *J Am Coll Cardiol* 1991;17:122–124.
124. DeWood MA, Notske RN, Berg R Jr, et al. Medical and surgical management of early Q wave myocardial infarction. I. Effects of surgical reperfusion on survival, recurrent myocardial infarction, sudden death and functional class at 10 or more years of follow-up. *J Am Coll Cardiol* 1989;14:65–77.
125. Diedericks J, Leone BJ, Foex P. Regional differences in left ventricular wall motion in the anesthetized dog. *Anesthesiology* 1989; 70:82–90.
126. Dodek A, Kassebaum DG, Bristow JD. Pulmonary edema in coronary-artery disease without cardiomegaly: paradox of the stiff heart. *N Engl J Med* 1972;286:1347–1350.
127. Dolan WM, Stevens WC, Eger EI, II, et al. The cardiovascular and respiratory effects of isoflurane-nitrous oxide anaesthesia. *Can Anaesth Soc J* 1974;21:557–568.
128. Dosemeci A, Dhallan RS, Cohen NM, Lederer WJ, Rogers TB. Phorbol ester increases calcium current and simulates the effects of angiotensin II in cultured neonatal rat heart myocytes. *Circ Res* 1988;62:347–357.
129. Dougherty AH, Naccarelli GV, Gray EH, Hicks CH, Goldstein RA. Congestive heart failure with normal systolic function. *Am J Cardiol* 1984;54:778–782.
130. Douglas PS, Reichek N, Hackney K, Ioli A, Sutton MG. Contribution of afterload, hypertrophy and geometry to left ventricular ejection fraction in aortic valve stenosis, pure aortic regurgitation and idiopathic dilated cardiomyopathy. *Am J Cardiol* 1987;591398–1404.
131. Douglas PS, Tallant B. Hypertrophy, fibrosis and diastolic dysfunction in early canine experimental hypertension. *J Am Coll Cardiol* 1991;17:530–536.
132. Doyle RL, Foex P, Ryder WA, Jones LA. Difference in ischaemic dysfunction after gradual and abrupt coronary occlusion: effects on isovolumetric relaxation. *Cardiovasc Res* 1987;21:507–514.
133. Doyle RL, Foex P, Ryder WA, Jones LA. Effects of halothane on left ventricular relaxation and early diastolic coronary blood flow in the dog. *Anesthesiology* 1989;70:660–666.
134. Dzau VJ, Hollenberg NK, Williams GH. Neurohormonal mechanisms in heart failure: role in pathogenesis, therapy, and drug tolerance. *Fed Proc* 1983;42:3162–3169.
135. Dzau VJ, Pratt RE. Renin-angiotensin system. In: Fozzard HA, Haber E, Jennings RB, Katz AM, Morgan HE, eds. *The heart and cardiovascular system: scientific foundations.* New York: Raven Press, 1991;1817–1849.
136. Eberli FR, Apstein CS, Ngoy S, Lorell BH. Exacerbation of left ventricular ischemic diastolic dysfunction by pressure-overload hypertrophy: modification by specific inhibition of cardiac angiotensin converting enzyme. *Circ Res* 1992;70:931–943.
137. Ebert TJ. Differential effects of nitrous oxide on baroreflex control of heart rate and peripheral sympathetic nerve activity in humans. *Anesthesiology* 1990;72:16–22.
138. Ebert TJ, Kampine JP. Nitrous oxide augments sympathetic outflow: direct evidence from human peroneal nerve recordings. *Anesth Analg* 1989;69:444–449.
139. Eckstein JW, Hamilton WK, McCammond JM. The effect of thiopental induction on peripheral venous tone. *Anesthesiology* 1961;22:525–528.
140. Edwards CH, II, Rankin JS, McHale PA, Ling D, Anderson RW. Effects of ischemia on left ventricular regional function in the conscious dog. *Am J Physiol* 1981;240:H413–H420.
141. Eger EI, Smith NT, Stoelting RK, Cullen DJ, Kadis DJ, Whitcher CE. Cardiovascular effects of halothane in man. *Anesthesiology* 1970;32:396–409.
142. Eichhorn P, Grimm J, Koch R, Hess O, Carroll J, Krayenbuehl HP. Left ventricular relaxation in patients with left ventricular hypertrophy secondary to aortic valve disease. *Circulation* 1982;65: 1395–1404.
143. Eisele JH. Cardiovascular effects of nitrous oxide. In: Eger EI II, ed. *Nitrous oxide/N_2O.* New York: Elsevier Science, 1985;125–156.
144. Eisele JH, Reitan JA, Massumi RA, Zelis RF, Miller RR. Myocardial

performance and N_2O analgesia in coronary-artery disease. *Anesthesiology* 1976;44:16–20.
145. Eisele JH, Smith NT. Cardiovascular effects of 40 percent nitrous oxide in man. *Anesth Analg* 1972;51:956–963.
146. Eisele JH, Trenchard D, Stubbs J, Guz A. The immediate cardiac depression by anesthetics in conscious dogs. *Br J Anaesth* 1969;41:86–93.
147. Ellis SG, Henschke CI, Sandor T, Wynne J, Braunwald E, Kloner RA. Time course of functional and biochemical recovery of myocardium salvaged by reperfusion. *J Am Coll Cardiol* 1983;1:1047–1055.
148. Endoh M, Blinks JR. Actions of sympathomimetic amines on the Ca^{2+} transients and contractions of rabbit myocardium: peripheral changes in myofibrillar responsiveness to Ca^{2+} mediated through α- and β-adrenoceptors. *Circ Res* 1988;62:247–265.
149. Engler R, Covell JW. Granulocytes cause reperfusion ventricular dysfunction after 15–minute ischemia in the dogs. *Circ Res* 1987;61:20–28.
150. Eriksen S, Johannsen G, Frost N. Effects of nitrous oxide on systolic time intervals. *Acta Anaesthesiol Scand* 1980;24:74–78.
151. Factor SM, Butany J, Sole MJ, Wigle ED, Williams WC, Rojkind M. Pathologic fibrosis and matrix connective tissue in subaortic myocardium of patients with hypertrophic cardiomyopathy. *J Am Coll Cardiol* 1991;17:1343–1351.
152. Falk RB, Jr, Denlinger JK, Nahrwold ML, Todd RA. Acute vasodilation following induction of anesthesia with intravenous diazepam and nitrous oxide. *Anesthesiology* 1978;49:149–150.
153. Fedele FA, Gerwitz H, Capone RJ, Sharaf B, Most AS. Metabolic response to prolonged reduction of myocardial blood flow distal to a severe coronary artery stenosis. *Circulation* 1988;78:729–735.
154. Feldman AM, Cates AE, Veazey WB, et al. Increase of the 40,000–mol wt pertussis toxin substrate (G protein) in the failing human heart. *J Clin Invest* 1988;82:189–197.
155. Feldman AM, Ray PE, Silan CM, Mercer JA, Minobe W, Bristow MR. Selective gene expression in failing human heart: quantification of steady-state levels of messenger RNA in endomyocardial biopsies using the polymerase chain reaction. *Circulation* 1991;83:1866–1872.
156. Feldman MD, Alderman JD, Aroesty JM, et al. Depression of systolic and diastolic myocardial reserve during atrial pacing tachycardia in patients with dilated cardiomyopathy. *J Clin Invest* 1988;82:1661–1669.
157. Feldman MD, Copelas L, Gwathmey JK, et al. Deficient production of cyclic AMP: pharmacologic evidence of an important cause of contractile dysfunction in patients with end-stage heart failure. *Circulation* 1987;75:331–339.
158. Fifer MA, Bourdillon PD, Lorell BH. Altered left ventricular diastolic properties during pacing-induced angina in patients with aortic stenosis. *Circulation* 1986;74:675–683.
159. Fifer MA, Grossman W. Measurement of ventricular volumes, ejection fraction, mass, wall stress, and regional wall motion. In: Grossman W, ed. *Cardiac catheterization, angiography, and intervention.* Philadelphia: Lea & Febiger, 1991;300–318.
160. Fischler M, Dubois C, Brodaty D, et al. Circulatory responses to thiopentone and tracheal intubation in patients with coronary artery disease. *Br J Anaesth* 1985;57:493–496.
161. Flickinger H, Fraimow W, Cathcart RT, Nealon TF Jr. Effect of thiopental induction on cardiac output in man. *Anesth Analg* 1961;40:693–700.
162. Florenzano F, Glantz SA. Left-ventricular mechanical adaptation to chronic aortic regurgitation in intact dogs. *Am J Physiol* 1987;252:H969–H984.
163. Foex P, Francis CM, Cutfield GR, Leone B. The pressure-length loop. *Br J Anaesth* 1988;60(8 suppl 1):65S-71S.
164. Forrester JS, Diamond G, Parmley WW, Swan HJ. Early increase in left ventricular compliance after myocardial infarction. *J Clin Invest* 1972;51:598–603.
165. Forrester JS, Tyberg JV, Wyatt HL, Goldner S, Parmley WW, Swan HJC. Pressure-length loop: a new method for simultaneous measurement of segmental and total cardiac function. *J Appl Physiol* 1974;37:771–775.
166. Francis GS. Neurohormonal mechanisms in congestive heart failure. *Am J Cardiol* 1985;55:15A-21A.
167. Frank O. Zur dynamik des herzmuskels. *Z Biol* 1895;32:370–437.
168. Frank O. Die grundform des arteriellen pulses. *Z Biol* 1898;39:483–526.
169. Frankl WS, Poole-Wilson PA. Effects of thiopental on tension development, action potential, and exchange of calcium and potassium in rabbit ventricular myocardium. *J Cardiovasc Pharmacol* 1981;3:554–565.
170. Freedman BM, Hamm DP, Everson CT, Wechsler AS, Christian CM II. Enflurane enhances postischemic functional recovery in the isolated rat heart. *Anesthesiology* 1985;62:29–33.
171. Freeman GL, Little WC, O'Rourke RA. The effect of vasoactive agents on the left ventricular end-systolic pressure-volume relation in closed chest dogs. *Circulation* 1986;74:1107–1113.
172. Freeman GL, Little WC, O'Rourke RA. Influence of heart rate on left ventricular performance in conscious dogs. *Circ Res* 1987;61:455–464.
173. Freeman ML, Stevens K, Barnes WE, et al. Regional diastolic functional images utilizing time-domain analysis of gated radionuclide ventriculograms. *Am Heart J* 1985;109:890–899.
174. Friedman BJ, Drinkovic N, Miles H, Shih WJ, Mazzoleni A, DeMaria AN. Assessment of left ventricular diastolic function: comparison of Doppler echocardiography and gated blood pool scintigraphy. *J Am Coll Cardiol* 1986;8:
175. Frink EJ Jr, Malan TP, Atlas M, DiNardo JA, Brown BR. Hemodynamic changes during sevoflurane or isoflurane anesthesia in ASA I and ASA II surgical patients (abstract). *Anesthesiology* 1991;75:A156.
176. Fujii J, Yazaki Y, Sawada H, Aizawa T, Watanabe H, Kato K. Noninvasive assessment of left and right ventricular filling in myocardial infarction with a two-dimensional Doppler echocardiographic method. *J Am Coll Cardiol* 1985;5:1155–1160.
177. Gaasch WH, Bing OHL, Franklin A, Rhodes D, Bernard SA, Weintraub RM. The influence of acute alterations in coronary blood flow on left ventricular diastolic compliance and wall thickness. *Eur J Cardiol* 1978;7(Suppl):147–161.
178. Gaasch WH, Carroll JD, Blaustein AS, Bing OHL. Myocardial relaxation: effects of preload on the time course of isovolumetric relaxation. *Circulation* 1986;73:1037–1041.
179. Gaasch WH, Levine HJ, Quinones MA, Alexander JK. Left ventricular compliance: mechanisms and clinical implications. *Am J Cardiol* 1976;38:645–653.
180. Gaasch WL, Blaustein AS, Andrias CW, Donahue RP, Avitall B. Myocardial relaxation: II. Hemodynamic determinants of rate of left ventricular isovolumetric pressure decline. *Am J Physiol* 1980;239:H1–H6.
181. Gallagher KP, Gerren RA, Stirling MC, et al. The distribution of functional impairment across the lateral border of acutely ischemic myocardium. *Circ Res* 1976;58:570–583.
182. Gallagher KP, Kumada T, Koziol JA, McKown MD, Kemper WS, Ross J Jr. Significance of regional wall thickening abnormalities relative to transmural myocardial perfusion in anesthetized dogs. *Circulation* 1980;62:1266–1274.
183. Gallagher KP, Matsuzaki M, Koziol JA, Kemper WS, Ross J Jr. Regional myocardial perfusion and wall thickening during ischemia in conscious dogs. *Am J Physiol* 1984;247:H727–H738.
184. Gallagher KP, Matsuzaki M, Osakada G, Kemper WS, Ross J Jr. Effect of exercise on the relationship between myocardial blood flow and systolic wall thickening in dogs with acute coronary stenosis. *Circ Res* 1983;52:716–729.
185. Gallagher KP, Osakada G, Matsuzaki M, Kemper WS, Ross J Jr. Myocardial blood flow and function with critical coronary stenosis in exercising dogs. *Am J Physiol* 1982;243:H698–H707.
186. Gauss A, Heinrich H, Wilder-Smith OHG. Echocardiographic assessment of the haemodynamic effects of propofol: a comparison with etomidate and thiopentone. *Anaesthesia* 1991;46:99–105.
187. Gibbs CL. Cardiac energetics. *Physiol Rev* 1978;58:175–254.
188. Gibbs CL, Chapman JB. Cardiac mechanics and energetics: chemomechanical transduction in cardiac muscle. *Am J Physiol* 1985;249:H199–H206.
189. Gilbert JC, Glantz SA. Determinants of left ventricular filling and of the diastolic pressure-volume relation. *Circ Res* 1989;64:827–852.
190. Gillam LD, Homma S, Novick SS, Rediker DE, Eagle KA. The influence of heart rate on Doppler mitral inflow patterns (abstract). *Circulation* 1987;76(suppl IV):123.
191. Ginks WR, Sybers HD, Maroko PR, Covell JW, Sobel BE, Ross J Jr. Coronary artery reperfusion. II. Reduction of myocardial infarct size at one week after coronary occlusion. *J Clin Invest* 1972;51:2717–2723.
192. Glantz SA. Computing indices of diastolic stiffness has been counterproductive. *Fed Proc* 1980;39:162–168.

193. Glantz SA, Parmley WW. Factors which affect the diastolic pressure-volume curve. *Circ Res* 1978;42:171–180.
194. Glower DD, Schaper J, Kabas JS, et al. Relation between reversal of diastolic creep and recovery of systolic function after ischemic myocardial injury in dogs. *Circ Res* 1987;60:850–860.
195. Glower DD, Spratt JA, Kabas JS, Davis JW, Rankin JS. Quantification of regional myocardial dysfunction after acute ischemic injury. *Am J Physiol* 1988;255:H85–H93.
196. Glower DD, Spratt JA, Snow ND, et al. Linearity of the Frank-Starling relationship in the intact heart: the concept of preload recruitable stroke work. *Circulation* 1985;71:994–1009.
197. Goldberg AH, Phear WPC. Halothane and paired stimulation: effects on myocardial compliance and contractility. *J Appl Physiol* 1970;28:391–396.
198. Goldberg AH, Ullrick WC. Effects of halothane on isometric contractions of isolated heart muscle. *Anesthesiology* 1967;28: 838–845.
199. Goldman ME, Mora F, Guarino T, Fuster V, Mindich BP. Mitral valvuloplasty is superior to valve replacement for preservation of left ventricular function: an intraoperative two-dimensional echocardiographic study. *J Am Coll Cardiol* 1987;10:568–575.
200. Goldstein DS, Brush Jr JE, Eisenhofer G, Stull R, Esler M. In vivo measurement of neuronal uptake of norepinephrine in the human heart. *Circulation* 1988;78:41–48.
201. Gooding JM, Corssen G. Effect of etomidate on the cardiovascular system. *Anesth Analg* 1977;56:717–719.
202. Gooding JM, Weng JT, Smith RA, Berninger GT, Kirby RR. Cardiovascular and pulmonary responses following etomidate induction of anesthesia in patients with demonstrated cardiac disease. *Anesth Analg* 1979;58:40–41.
203. Gordon AM, Huxley AF, Julian FJ. The variation in isometric tension with sarcomere length in vertebrate muscle fibers. *J Physiol (Lond)* 1966;184:170–192.
204. Goto Y, Igarashi Y, Yamada O, Hiramori K, Suga H. Hyperkinesis without the Frank-Starling mechanism in a nonischemic region of acutely excised canine heart. *Circulation* 1988;77:468–477.
205. Gould KL, Lipscomb K, Hamilton GW, Kennedy JW. Relation of left ventricular shape, function and wall stress in man. *Am J Cardiol* 1974;34:627–634.
206. Graves CL, Downs NH. Cardiovascular and renal effects of enflurane in surgical patients. *Anesth Analg* 1974;53:898–903.
207. Graves CL, McDermott RW, Bidwai A. Cardiovascular effects of isoflurane in surgical patients. *Anesthesiology* 1974;41:486–489.
208. Greenbaum RA, Ho SY, Gibson DG, Becker AE, Anderson RH. Left ventricular fibre architecture in man. *Br Heart J* 1981;45: 248–263.
209. Greene ES, Gerson JI. One versus two MAC halothane anesthesia does not alter the left ventricular diastolic pressure-volume relationship. *Anesthesiology* 1986;64:230–237.
210. Gross GJ, Daemmgen JW. Beneficial effects of two specific bradycardiac agents, AQ-A39 (falipamil) and AQ-AH 208, on reversible myocardial reperfusion damage in anesthetized dogs. *J Pharmacol Exp Ther* 1986;238:422–428.
211. Gross GJ, Farber NE, Hardman HF, Warltier DC. Beneficial actions of superoxide dismutase and catalase in stunned myocardium of dogs. *Am J Physiol* 1986;250:H372–H377.
212. Grossman W. Cardiac hypertrophy: useful adaptation or pathologic process? *Am J Med* 1980;69:576–584.
213. Grossman W. Why is left ventricular diastolic pressure increased during angina pectoris? *J Am Coll Cardiol* 1985;5:607–608.
214. Grossman W. Diastolic dysfunction and congestive heart failure. *Circulation* 1990;81(suppl 3):1–7.
215. Grossman W, Braunwald E, Mann T, McLaurin LP, Green LH. Contractile state of the left ventricle in man as evaluated from end-systolic pressure-volume relations. *Circulation* 1977;56:845–852.
216. Grossman W, Jones D, McLaurin LP. Wall stress and patterns of hypertrophy in the human left ventricle. *J Clin Invest* 1975;56: 56–64.
217. Grossman W, McLaurin LP. Diastolic properties of the left ventricle. *Ann Intern Med* 1976;84:316–326.
218. Grossman W, McLaurin LP, Moos SP, Stefadouros M, Young DT. Wall thickness and diastolic properties of the left ventricle. *Circulation* 1974;49:129–135.
219. Grossman W, McLaurin LP, Rolett EL. Alterations in left ventricular relaxation and diastolic compliance in congestive cardiomyopathy. *Cardiovasc Res* 1979;13:514–522.
220. Group TISAMS. A prospective trial of intravenous streptokinase in acute myocardial infarction (I.S.A.M.): mortality, morbidity, and infarct size at 21 days. *N Engl J Med* 1986;314:1465–1471.
221. Gruppo Italiano per lo Studio della Streptochi-nasi nell'Infarto Miocardico (GISSI). Long-term effects of intravenous thrombolysis in acute myocardial infarction: final report of the GISSI study. *Lancet* 1987;2:871–874.
222. Gwathmey JK, Copelas L, MacKinnon R, et al. Abnormal intracellular calcium handling in myocardium from patients with end-stage heart failure. *Circ Res* 1987;61:70–76.
223. Gwathmey JK, Slawsky MT, Hajjar RJ, Briggs GM, Morgan JP. Role of intracellular calcium handling in force-interval relationships of human ventricular myocardium. *J Clin Invest* 1990;85: 1599–1613.
224. Gwathmey JK, Warren SE, Briggs GM, et al. Diastolic dysfunction in hypertrophic cardiomyopathy: effect on active force generation during systole. *J Clin Invest* 1991;87:1023–1031.
225. Hammond B, Hess ML. The oxygen free radical system: potential mediator of myocardial injury. *J Am Coll Cardiol* 1985;6:215–220.
226. Hansen RM, Viquerat CE, Matthay MA, et al. Poor correlation between pulmonary arterial wedge pressure and left ventricular end-diastolic volume after coronary artery bypass graft surgery. *Anesthesiology* 1986;64:764–770.
227. Hanson DE, Cahill PD, DeCampli WM, et al. Valvular-ventricular interaction: importance of the mitral apparatus in canine left ventricular systolic performance. *Circulation* 1986;73:1310–1320.
228. Harigaya S, Schwartz A. Rate of calcium binding and uptake in normal animal and failing cardiac muscle: membrane vesicles (relaxing system) and mitochondria. *Circ Res* 1969;25:781–794.
229. Harizi RC, Bianco JA, Alpert JS. Diastolic function of the heart in clinical cardiology. *Arch Intern Med* 1988;148:99–109.
230. Harkin CP, Pagel PS, Kersten JR, Hettrick DA, Warltier DC. Direct negative inotropic and lusitropic effects of sevoflurane. *Anesthesiology* 1994;81:156–167.
231. Harvey W. An anatomical disquisition on the motion of the heart and blood in animals (1628). In: Willis FA, Keys TE, eds. *Cardiac classics.* London: Henry Kimpton, 1941;19–79.
232. Hasking GJ, Esler MD, Jennings GL, Burton D, Johns JA, Korner PI. Norepinephrine spillover to plasma in patients with congestive heart failure: evidence of increased overall and cardiorenal sympathetic nervous system activity. *Circulation* 1986;73:615–621.
233. Hauser AM, Gangaharan V, Ramos RG, Gordon S, Timmis GC. Sequence of mechanical, electrocardiographic and clinical effects of repeated coronary occlusion in human beings: echocardiographic observations during coronary angioplasty. *J Am Coll Cardiol* 1985;5:193–197.
234. Hermann HJ. Left ventricular volumes by angiocardiography: comparison of methods and simplification of techniques. *Cardiovasc Res* 1968;2:404–414.
235. Herrmann HC, Ruddy TD, Dec GW, Strauss HW, Boucher CA, Fifer MA. Diastolic function in patients with severe congestive heart failure: comparison of the effects of enoximone and nitroprusside. *Circulation* 1987;75:1214–1221.
236. Heyndrickx GR, Millard RW, McRithchie RJ, Maroko PR, Vatner SF. Regional myocardial function and electrophysiological alterations after brief coronary artery occlusion in conscious dogs. *J Clin Invest* 1975;56:978–985.
237. Heyndrickx GR, Vilaine JP, Moerman EJ, Leusen I. Role of prejunctional alpha$_2$-adrenergic receptors in the regulation of myocardial performance during exercise in conscious dogs. *Circ Res* 1984;54:683–693.
238. Higginbotham MB, Morris KG, Williams RS, McHale PA, Coleman RE, Cobb FR. Regulation of stroke volume during submaximal and maximal upright exercise in normal man. *Circ Res* 1986;58: 281–291.
239. Higgins CB, Vatner SF, Braunwald E. Parasympathetic control of the heart. *Pharmacol Rev* 1973;25:119–155.
240. Hill GE, English JE, Lunn J, et al. Cardiovascular responses to nitrous oxide during light, moderate, and deep halothane anesthesia in man. *Anesth Analg* 1978;57:84–94.
241. Hittinger L, Shannon RP, Bishop SP, Gelpi RJ, Vatner SF. Subendomyocardial exhaustion of blood flow reserve and increased fibrosis in conscious dogs with heart failure. *Circ Res* 1989;65: 971–980.
242. Hoehner PJ, Quigg MC, Blanck TJJ. Halothane depresses D600 binding to bovine heart sarcolemma. *Anesthesiology* 1991;75: 1019–1024.
243. Homans DC, Sublett CE, Dai X-Z, Bache RJ. Persistence of

regional left ventricular dysfunction after exercise-induced myocardial ischemia. *J Clin Invest* 1986;77:66–73.
244. Hood WB Jr, Bianco JA, Kumar R, Whiting RB. Experimental myocardial infarction. IV. Reduction of ventricular compliance in the healing phase. *J Clin Invest* 1970;49:1316–1323.
245. Horan BF, Prys-Roberts C, Roberts JG, Bennett MJ, Foex P. Haemodynamic responses to isoflurane anaesthesia and hypovolaemia in the dog, and their modification by propranolol. *Br J Anaesth* 1977;49:1179–1187.
246. Housmans PR. Negative inotropy of halogenated anesthetics in ferret ventricular myocardium. *Am J Physiol* 1990;259:H827–H834.
247. Housmans PR, Lee NKM, Blinks JR. Active shortening retards the decline of the intracellular calcium transient in mammalian heart muscle. *Science* 1983;221:159–161.
248. Housmans PR, Murat I. Comparative effects of halothane, enflurane, and isoflurane at equipotent anesthetic concentrations on isolated ventricular myocardium of the ferret. I. Contractility. *Anesthesiology* 1988;69:451–463.
249. Housmans PR, Murat I. Comparative effects of halothane, enflurane, and isoflurane at equipotent anesthetic concentrations on isolated ventricular myocardium of the ferret. II. Relaxation. *Anesthesiology* 1988;69:464–471.
250. Humphrey LS, Stinson DC, Humphrey MJ, et al. Volatile anesthetic effects on left ventricular relaxation in swine. *Anesthesiology* 1990;73:731–738.
251. Humphrey LS, Topol EJ, Rosenfeld GI, et al. Immediate enhancement of left ventricular relaxation by coronary artery bypass grafting: intraoperative assessment. *Circulation* 1988;77:886–896.
252. Hunter WC. End-systolic pressure as a balance between opposing effects of ejection. *Circ Res* 1989;64:265–275.
253. Hysing ES, Chelly JE, Jacobson L, Doursout MF, Merin RG. Cardiovascular effects of acute changes in extracellular ionized calcium concentration induced by citrate and $CaCl_2$ infusions in chronically instrumented dogs, conscious and during enflurane, halothane, and isoflurane anesthesia. *Anesthesiology* 1990;72:100–104.
254. Ikemoto Y. Reduction by thiopental of the slow-channel-mediated action potential of canine papillary muscle. *Pflugers Arch* 1977;372:285–286.
255. Ikenouchi H, Kohmoto O, McMillan M, Barry WH. Contributions of $[Ca^{2+}]_i$, $[P_i]_i$, and pH_i to altered diastolic myocyte tone during partial metabolic inhibition. *J Clin Invest* 1991;88:55–61.
256. Inouye I, Massie B, Loge D, et al. Abnormal left ventricular filling: an early finding in mild to moderate systemic hypertension. *Am J Cardiol* 1984;53:120–126.
257. Isaaz K, Pasipoularides A. Noninvasive assessment of intrinsic ventricular load dynamics in dilated cardiomyopathy. *J Am Coll Cardiol* 1991;17:112–121.
258. Ishida Y, Meisner JS, Tsujioka K, et al. Left ventricular filling dynamics: influence of left ventricular relaxation and left atrial pressure. *Circulation* 1986;74:187–196.
259. Iskandrian AS, Hakki AH, Bemis CE, Kane SA, Boston B, Amenta A. Left ventricular end-systolic pressure-volume relation. A combined radionuclide and hemodynamic study. *Am J Cardiol* 1983;51:1057–1061.
260. Ivankovich AD, Miletich DJ, Reimann C, Albrecht RF, Zahed B. Cardiovascular effects of centrally administered ketamine in goats. *Anesth Analg* 1974;53:924–933.
261. Izumo S, Nadal-Ginard B, Mahdavi V. Protooncogene induction and reprogramming of cardiac gene expression produced by pressure overload. *Proc Natl Acad Sci USA* 1988;85:339–343.
262. Jennings RB, Reimer KA, Jill ML, Mayer SE. Total ischemia in dog hearts in vitro: comparison of high energy phosphate production, utilization and depletion, and of adenine nucleotide catabolism in total ischemia in vitro vs. severe ischemia in vivo. *Circ Res* 1981;49:892–900.
263. Jennings RB, Sommers HM, Smyth GA, Flack HA, Linn H. Myocardial necrosis induced by temporary occlusion of a coronary artery in the dog. *Arch Pathol* 1960;70:68–78.
264. Kabas JS, Glower DD, Spratt JA, Snow ND, Rankin JS. Effects of afterload and inotropic state on diastolic properties after ischemic injury (abstract). *Circulation* 1985;72(suppl III):71.
265. Kahn JK, Rutherford BD, McConahay DR, et al. Results of primary coronary angioplasty for acute myocardial infarction in patients with multivessel coronary artery disease. *J Am Coll Cardiol* 1990;16:1089–1096.
266. Karlinger JS, LeWinter MM, Mahler F, Engler R, O'Rourke RA. Pharmacologic and hemodynamic influences on the rate of isovolumetric left ventricular relaxation in the normal conscious dog. *J Clin Invest* 1977;60:511–521.
267. Kaseda S, Tomoike H, Ogata I, Nakamura M. End-systolic pressure-length relations during changes in regional contractile state. *Am J Physiol* 1984;247:H768–H774.
268. Kaseda S, Tomoike H, Ogata I, Nakamura M. End-systolic pressure-volume, pressure-length, and stress-strain relations in canine hearts. *Am J Physiol* 1985;249:H648–H654.
269. Kass DA. Evaluation of left ventricular systolic function. *Heart Failure* 1988;4:198–.
270. Kass DA, Beyar R. Evaluation of contractile state by maximal ventricular power divided by the square of end-diastolic volume. *Circulation* 1991;84:1698–1708.
271. Kass DA, Beyar R, Lankford E, Heard M, Maughan WL, Sagawa K. Influence of contractile state on curvilinearity of *in situ* end-systolic pressure-volume relations. *Circulation* 1989;79:167–178.
272. Kass DA, Maughan WL. From 'Emax' to pressure-volume relations: a broader view. *Circulation* 1988;77:1203–1212.
273. Kass DA, Maughan WL, Guo ZM, Kono A, Sunagawa K, Sagawa K. Comparative influence of load versus inotropic state on indexes of ventricular contractility: experimental and theoretical analysis based on pressure-volume relationships. *Circulation* 1987;76:1422–1436.
274. Katz AM. Cyclic adenosine monophosphate effects on the myocardium: a man who blows hot and cold with one breath. *J Am Coll Cardiol* 1983;2:143–149.
275. Katz AM. Influence of altered inotropy and lusitropy on ventricular pressure-volume loops. *J Am Coll Cardiol* 1988;11:438–445.
276. Katz AM. Cardiomyopathy of overload: a major determinant of prognosis in congestive heart failure. *N Engl J Med* 1990;322:100–110.
277. Katz AM. *Physiology of the heart*, 2nd ed. New York: Raven Press, 1992.
278. Katz AM, Smith VE. Regulation of myocardial function in the normal and diseased heart. Modification by inotropic drugs. *Eur Heart J* 1982;3(suppl D):11–18.
279. Kawaguchi H, Shoki M, Sano H, et al. Phospholipid metabolism in cardiomyopathic hamster heart cells. *Circ Res* 1991;69:1015–1021.
280. Keith A. The functional anatomy of the heart. *Br J Med* 1918;i:361–363.
281. Kelly R, Hayward C, Avolio A, O'Rourke M. Noninvasive determination of age-related changes in the human arterial pulse. *Circulation* 1989;80:1652–1659.
282. Kelly R, Hayward C, Ganis J, Daley J, Avolio A, O'Rourke M. Non-invasive registration of the arterial pressure pulse waveform using high-fidelity applanation tonometry. *J Vasc Med Biol* 1989;1:142–149.
283. Kemmotsu O, Hashimoto Y, Shimosato S. Inotropic effects of isoflurane on mechanics of contraction in isolated cat papillary muscles from normal and failing hearts. *Anesthesiology* 1973;39:470–477.
284. Kemmotsu O, Hashimoto Y, Shimosato S. The effects of fluroxene and enflurane on contractile performance of isolated papillary muscles from failing hearts. *Anesthesiology* 1974;40:252–260.
285. Kennedy JW, Doces J, Stewart DK. Left ventricular function before and following aortic valve replacement. *Circulation* 1977;56:944–950.
286. Kenner T. Some comments on ventricular afterload. *Basic Res Cardiol* 1987;82:209–215.
287. Kentish JC, ter Keurs HEDJ, Ricciardi L, Bucx JJJ, Noble MIM. Comparison between the sarcomere length-force relations of intact and skinned trabeculae from rat right ventricle: influence of calcium concentrations on these relations. *Circ Res* 1986;58:755–768.
288. Kereiakes DJ, Topol EJ, George BS, et al. Favorable and long-term prognosis following coronary artery bypass surgery therapy for myocardial infarction: results of a multicenter trial. *Am Heart J* 1989;118:199–207.
289. Keren G, Meisner JS, Sherez J, Yellin EL, Laniado S. Interrelationship of mid-diastolic mitral valve motion, pulmonary venous flow, and transmitral flow. *Circulation* 1986;74:36–44.
290. Keren G, Sherez J, Megidish R, Levitt B, Laniado S. Pulmonary venous flow pattern — Its relationship to cardiac dynamics. A pulsed Doppler echocardiographic study. *Circulation* 1985;71:1105–1112.
291. Kihara Y, Grossman W, Morgan JP. Direct measurement of

changes in intracellular calcium transients during hypoxia, ischemia, and reperfusion of the intact mammalian heart. *Circ Res* 1989;65:1029–1044.

292. Kikura M, Ikeda K. Comparison of effects of sevoflurane-nitrous oxide and enflurane-nitrous oxide on myocardial contractility in humans. *Anesthesiology* 1993;79:235–243.
293. Kissin I, Motomura S, Aultman DF, Reves JG. Inotropic and anesthetic potencies of etomidate and thiopental in dogs. *Anesth Analg* 1983;62:961–965.
294. Kitzman DW, Higginbotham MB, Cobb FR, Sheikh KH, Sullivan MJ. Exercise intolerance in patients with heart failure anf preserved left ventricular systolic function: failure of the Frank-Starling mechanism. *J Am Coll Cardiol* 1991;17:1065–1072.
295. Klein AL, Cohen GI. Doppler echocardiographic assessment of constrictive pericarditis, cardiac amyloidosis, and cardiac tamponade. *Cleve Clin J Med* 1992;59:278–290.
296. Klein AL, Tajik AJ. Doppler assessment of pulmonary venous flow in healthy subjects and in patients with heart disease. *J Am Soc Echocardiogr* 1991;4:379–392.
297. Kloner RA, Kirshenbaum J, Lange R, Antman EM, Braunwald E. Experimental and clinical observations on the efficacy of esmolol in myocardial ischemia. *Am J Cardiol* 1985;56:40F-48F.
298. Kloner RA, Przyklenk K, Whittaker P. Deleterious effects of oxygen free radicals in ischemia/reperfusion. Resolved and unresolved issues. *Circulation* 1989;80:1115–1127.
299. Komai H, DeWitt DE, Rusy BF. Negative inotropic effects of etomidate in rabbit papillary muscle. *Anesth Analg* 1985;64:400–404.
300. Komai H, Rusy BF. Differences in the myocardial depressant action of thiopental and halothane. *Anesth Analg* 1984;63:313–318.
301. Komai H, Rusy BF. Negative inotropic effects of isoflurane and halothane in rabbit papillary muscles. *Anesth Analg* 1987;66:29–33.
302. Kongsayreepong S, Cook DJ, Housmans PR. Mechanism of the direct, negative inotropic effect of ketamine in isolated ferret and frog ventricular myocardium. *Anesthesiology* 1993;79:313–322.
303. Koretsune Y, Coretti MC, Kusuoka H, Marban E. Mechanism of early ischemic contractile failure: inexcitability, metabolite accumulation, or vascular collapse? *Circ Res* 1991;68:255–262.
304. Koretsune Y, Marban E. Relative roles of Ca^{2+}-dependent and Ca^{2+}-independent mechanisms in hypoxic contractile dysfunction. *Circulation* 1990;82:528–535.
305. Korner PI. Integrative neural cardiovascular control. *Physiol Rev* 1971;51:312–367.
306. Krause SM, Jacobus WE, Becker LC. Alterations in cardiac sarcoplasmic reticulum calcium transport in postischemic "stunned" myocardium. *Circ Res* 1989;65:526–530.
307. Kuecherer HF, Muhiudeen IA, Kusumoto FM, et al. Estimation of mean left atrial pressure from transesophageal pulsed Doppler echocardiography of pulmonary venous blood flow. *Circulation* 1990;82:1127–1139.
308. Kurnik PB, Courtois MR, Ludbrook PA. Diastolic stiffening induced by acute myocardial infarction is reduced by early reperfusion. *J Am Coll Cardiol* 1988;12:1029–1036.
309. Labovitz AJ, Lewen MK, Kern M, Vandormael M, Deligonal U, Kennedy HL. Evaluation of left ventricular systolic and diastolic dysfunction during transient myocardial ischemia produced by angioplasty. *J Am Coll Cardiol* 1987;10:748–755.
310. Lakatta EG. Cardiac muscle changes in senescence. *Annu Rev Physiol* 1987;49:519–531.
311. Lakatta EG. Starling's law of the heart is explained by an intimate interaction of muscle length and myofilament calcium activation. *J Am Coll Cardiol* 1987;10:1157–1164.
312. Lam JHC. Morphology of the human mitral vavle. I. Chordae tendinae: a new classification. *Circulation* 1970;41:449.
313. Lamping KA, Gross GJ. Improved recovery of myocardial segment function following a short coronary occlusion in dogs with nicorandil, a potential new antianginal agent, and nifedipine. *J Cardiovasc Pharmacol* 1985;7:158–166.
314. Landsberg L, Young JB. Catecholamines and the adrenal medulla. In: Wilson JD, Foster DW, eds. *Williams' textbook of endocrinology*. Philadelphia: WB Saunders, 1985;891–965.
315. Lang RM, Borow KM, Neumann A, Janzen D. Systemic vascular resistance: an unreliable index of left ventricular afterload. *Circulation* 1986;74:1114–1123.
316. Lappas DG, Buckley MJ, Laver MB, Daggett WM, Lowenstein E. Left ventricular performance and pulmonary circulation following addition of nitrous oxide to morphine during coronary-artery surgery. *Anesthesiology* 1975;43:61–69.
317. Lavalle M, Cox D, Patrick TA, Vatner SF. Salvage of myocardial function by coronary artery reperfusion 1,2 and 3 hours after occlusion in conscious dogs. *Circ Res* 1983;53:235–247.
318. Lawrence WE, Maughan WL, Kass DA. Mechanism of global functional recovery despite sustained postischemic regional stunning. *Circulation* 1992;85:816–827.
319. Lecarpentier Y, Waldenstrom A, Clergue M, et al. Major alterations in relaxation during cardiac hypertrophy induced by aortic stenosis in guinea pig. *Circ Res* 1987;61:107–116.
320. Lee HC, Mohabir R, Smith N, Franz MR, Clusin WT. Effect of ischemia in calcium-dependent fluorescence transients in rabbit hearts containing indo-1: correlation with monophasic action potentials and contraction. *Circulation* 1988;78:1047–1059.
321. Lee JD, Tajimi T, Guth B, Seitelberger R, Miller M, Ross J Jr. Exercise-induced regional dysfunction with subcritical coronary stenosis. *Circulation* 1986;73:596–605.
322. Lee JD, Tajimi T, Widmann TF, Ross J Jr. Application of end-systolic pressure-volume and pressure-wall thickness relations in conscious dogs. *J Am Coll Cardiol* 1987;9:136–146.
323. Legault F, Rouleau JL, Juneau C, Rose C, Rakusan K. Functional and morphological characteristics of compensated and decompensated cardiac hypertrophy in dogs with chronic infrarenal aorto-caval fistulas. *Circ Res* 1990;66:846–859.
324. Leone BJ, Philbin DM, Lehot JJ, Foex P, Ryder WA. Gradual or abrupt nitrous oxide administration in a canine model of critical coronary stenosis induces regional myocardial dysfunction that is worsened by halothane. *Anesth Analg* 1988;67:814–822.
325. Lepage J-YM, Pinaud ML, Helias JH, Cozian AY, Le Normand Y, Souron RJ. Left ventricular performance during propofol and methohexital anesthesia: isotopic and invasive cardiac monitoring. *Anesth Analg* 1991;73:3–9.
326. Lerman J, Oyston JP, Gallagher TM, Miyasaki K, Volgyesi GA, Burrows FA. The minimum alveolar concentration (MAC) and hemodynamic effects of halothane, isoflurane, and sevoflurane in newborn swine. *Anesthesiology* 1990;73:717–721.
327. Leung JM, O'Kelley B, Browner WS, Tubau J, Hollenberg M, Mangano DT. Prognostic importance of postbypass regional wall-motion abnormalities in patients undergoing coronary artery bypass graft surgery. *Anesthesiology* 1989;71:16–25.
328. Levenson DJ, Simmons Jr CE, Brenner BM. Arachidonic acid metabolism, prostaglandins, and the kidney. *Am J Med* 1982;72: 354–374.
329. Levesque FR, Nanagas V, Shanks C, Shimosato S. Circulatory effects of enflurane in normocarbic human volunteers. *Can Anaesth Soc J* 1974;21:580–585.
330. Levy MN. Parasympathetic control of the heart. In: Randall WC, ed. *Neural regulation of the heart*. New York: Oxford University Press, 1977;95–129.
331. Levy MN. Neural control of the heart: sympathetic-vagal interactions. In: Baan J, Noordergraaf A, Raines J, eds. *Cardiovascular system dynamics*. Cambridge, MA: MIT Press, 1978;365–370.
332. Levy MN, Blattberg B. Effect of vagal stimulation on the overflow of norepinephrine into the coronary sinus during cardiac sympathetic nerve stimulation in the dog. *Circ Res* 1976;38:81–84.
333. Levy MN, Ng M, Martin P, Zieske H. Sympathetic and parasympathetic interactions upon the left ventricle of the dog. *Circ Res* 1966;19:5–10.
334. Lew WYW. Influence of ischemic zone size on nonischemic area function in the canine left ventricle. *Am J Physiol* 1987;252: H990–H997.
335. Lew WYW. Evaluation of left ventricular diastolic function. *Circulation* 1989;79:1393–1397.
336. Lew WYW, LeWinter MM. Regional circumferential lengthening patterns in canine left ventricle. *Am J Physiol* 1983;245:H741–H748.
337. Lewis JF, Kuo LC, Nelson JG, Limacher MC, Quinones MA. Pulsed Doppler echocardiographic determination of stroke volume and cardiac output: clinical validation of two new methods using the apical window. *Circulation* 1984;70:425–431.
338. Lichtenthal P, Philip J, Sloss LJ, Gabel R, Lesch M. Administration of nitrous oxide in normal subjects. Evaluation of systems of gas delivery for their clinical use and hemodynamic effects. *Chest* 1977;72:316–322.
339. Limas CJ, Olivari MT, Goldenberg IF, Levine TB, Benditt DG, Simon A. Calcium uptake by sarcoplasmic reticulum in human dilated cardiomyopathy. *Cardiovasc Res* 1987;21:601–605.
340. Linzbach AJ. Heart failure from the point of view of quantitative anatomy. *Am J Cardiol* 1960;5:370–382.

341. Little RC. Volume pressure relationships of the pulmonary-left heart vascular segment. Evidence for a "valve-like" closure of the pulmonary veins. *Circ Res* 1960;8:594–599.
342. Little WC. The left ventricular dP/dt_{max}-end-diastolic volume relation in closed-chest dogs. *Circ Res* 1985;56:808–815.
343. Little WC, Badke FR, O'Rourke RA. Effect of right ventricular pressure on the end-diastolic left ventricular pressure-volume relationship before and after chronic right ventricular pressure overload in dogs without pericardia. *Circ Res* 1984;54:719–730.
344. Little WC, Cheng CP. Left ventricular-arterial coupling in conscious dogs. *Am J Physiol* 1991;261:H70–H76.
345. Little WC, Cheng CP, Mumma M, Igarashi Y, Vinten-Johansen J, Johnston WE. Comparison of measures of left ventricular contractile performance derived from pressure-volume loops in conscious dogs. *Circulation* 1989;80:1378–1387.
346. Little WC, Cheng CP, Peterson T, Vinten-Johansen J. Response of the left ventricular end-systolic pressure-volume relation in conscious dogs to a wide range of contractile states. *Circulation* 1988; 78:736–745.
347. Little WC, Downes TR. Clinical evaluation of left ventricular diastolic performance. *Prog Cardiovasc Dis* 1990;32:273–290.
348. Little WC, Freeman GL, O'Rourke RA. Simultaneous determination of left ventricular end-systolic pressure-volume and pressure-dimension relationships in closed-chest dogs. *Circulation* 1985;71: 1301–1308.
349. Little WC, Park RC, Freeman GL. Effects of regional ischemia and ventricular pacing on LV dP/dt_{max}-end-diastolic volume relation. *Am J Physiol* 1987;252:H933–H940.
350. Lorell BH, Grossman W. Cardiac hypertrophy: the consequences for diastole. *J Am Coll Cardiol* 1987;9:1189–1193.
351. Lorell BH, Isoyama S, Grice WN, Weinberg EO, Apstein CS. Effects of ouabain and isoproterenol on left ventricular diastolic function during low-flow ischemia in isolated, blood perfused rabbit hearts. *Circ Res* 1988;63:457–467.
352. Lorell BH, Paulus WJ, Grossman W, Wynne J, Cohn PF. Modification of abnormal left ventricular diastolic properties by nifedipine in patients with hypertrophic cardiomyopathy. *Circulation* 1982;65: 499–507.
353. Lowenstein E, Foex P, Francis CM, Davies WL, Yusuf S, Ryder WA. Regional ischemic ventricular dysfunction in myocardium supplied by a narrowed coronary artery with increasing halothane concentration in the dog. *Anesthesiology* 1981;55:349–359.
354. Lundborg RO, Milde JH, Theye RA. Effect of nitrous oxide on myocardial contractility of dogs. *Can Anaesth Soc J* 1966;13: 361–367.
355. Lundy PM, Gverzdys S, Frew R. Ketamine: evidence of tissue specific inhibition of neuronal and extraneuronal catecholamine uptake processes. *Can J Physiol Pharmacol* 1985;63:298–303.
356. Lunn JK, Stanley TH, Eisele J, Webster L, Woodward A. High dose fentanyl anesthesia for coronary artery surgery: plasma fentanyl concentrations and influence of nitrous oxide on cardiovascular responses. *Anesth Analg* 1979;58:390–395.
357. Lynch C III. Differential depression of myocardial contractility by halothane and isoflurane *in vitro*. *Anesthesiology* 1986;64:620–631.
358. MacCullum JB. On the muscular architecture and growth of the ventricles of the heart. *Johns Hopkins Hosp Rep* 1900;9:307–335.
359. Maciel LMZ, Polikar R, Rohrer D, Popovich BK, Dillman WH. Age-induced decreases in the messenger RNA coding for the sarcoplasmic reticulum Ca^{2+}-ATPase of the rat heart. *Circ Res* 1990;67: 230–234.
360. Magorien DJ, Shaffer P, Bush C, et al. Hemodynamic correlates for timing intervals, ejection rate, and filling rate derived from the radionuclide angiographic volume curve. *Am J Cardiol* 1984;53: 567–571.
361. Magorien DJ, Shaffer P, Bush CA, et al. Assessment of left ventricular pressure-volume relations using gated radionuclide angiography, echocardiography, and micromanometer pressure recordings. A new method for serial measurements of systolic and diastolic function in man. *Circulation* 1983;67:844–853.
362. Mahdavi V, Izumo S, Nadal-Ginard B. Developmental and hormonal regulation of sarcomeric myosin heavy chain gene family. *Circ Res* 1987;60:804–814.
363. Mahler F, Covell JW, Ross J Jr. Systolic pressure-diameter relations in the normal conscious dog. *Cardiovasc Res* 1975;9:447–455.
364. Makela VHM, Kapur PA. Amrinone and verapamil-propranolol induced cardiac depression during isoflurane anesthesia in dogs. *Anesthesiology* 1987;66:792–797.
365. Malik AB, Abe T, O'Kane HO, Geha AS. Cardiac performance in ventricular hypertrophy induced by pressure or volume overloading. *J Appl Physiol* 1974;37:867–874.
366. Mall FP. On the muscular architecture of the ventricles of the human heart. *Am J Anat* 1911;11:211–278.
367. Mancini GBJ, Peterson KL, Gregoratos G, Higgins CB. The effects of atrial pacing on global and regional left ventricular function in coronary heart disease assessed by digital intravenous ventriculography. *Am J Cardiol* 1984;53:456–461.
368. Mann T, Brodie BR, Grossman W, McLaurin LP. Effect of angina on the left ventricular diastolic pressure-volume relationship. *Circulation* 1977;55:761–766.
369. Mann T, Goldberg S, Mudge GH Jr, Grossman W. Factors contributing to altered left ventricular diastolic properties during angina pectoris. *Circulation* 1979;59:14–20.
370. Marban E. Myocardial stunning and hibernation: the physiology behind the colloquialisms. *Circulation* 1991;83:681–688.
371. Marban E, Koretsune Y, Coretti M, Chacko VP, Kusuoka H. Calcium and its role in myocardial cell injury during ischemia and reperfusion. *Circulation* 1989;80(suppl 4):17–22.
372. Marcus ML, Mueller TM, Gascho JA, Kerber RE. Effects of cardiac hypertrophy secondary to hypertension on the coronary circulation. *Am J Cardiol* 1979;44:1023–1028.
373. Maron BJ, Spirito P, Green KJ, Wesley YE, Bonow RO, Arce J. Noninvasive assessment of left ventricular diastolic function by pulsed Doppler echocardiography in patients with hypertrophic cardiomyopathy. *J Am Coll Cardiol* 1987;10:733–742.
374. Marshall BE, Cohen PJ, Klingenmaier CH, Neigh JL, Pender JW. Some pulmonary and cardiovascular effects of enflurane (Ethrane) anaesthesia with varying $PaCO_2$ in man. *Br J Anaesth* 1971; 43:996–1002.
375. Mason DT. Usefulness and limitations of the rate of rise of intraventricular pressure (dP/dt) in the evaluation of myocardial contractility in man. *Am J Cardiol* 1969;23:516–527.
376. Mason DT, Braunwald E, Covell JW, Sonnenblick EH, Ross J Jr. Assessment of cardiac contractility: the relation between the rate of pressure rise and ventricular pressure during isovolumetric systole. *Circulation* 1971;44:47–58.
377. Matsuzaki M, Gallagher KP, Kemper WS, White F, Ross J Jr. Sustained regional dysfunction produced by prolonged coronary stenosis: gradual recovery after reperfusion. *Circulation* 1983;68: 170–182.
378. Maughan WL, Sunagawa K, Burkhoff D, Graves WL Jr, Hunter WC, Sagawa K. Effect of heart rate on the canine end-systolic pressure-volume relationship. *Circulation* 1985;72:654–659.
379. McGiff JC, Itskovitz HD. Prostaglandins and the kidney. *Circ Res* 1973;33:479–488.
380. McKay RG, Pfeffer MA, Pasternak RC, et al. Left ventricular remodeling after myocardial infarction: a corollary to infarct expansion. *Circulation* 1986;74:693–702.
381. McLaurin LP, Rollet EL, Grossman W. Impaired left ventricular relaxation during pacing-induced ischemia. *Am J Cardiol* 1973;32: 751–757.
382. Meerson FZ. The myocardium in hyperfunction, hypertrophy, and heart failure. *Circ Res* 1969;25(suppl 2):1–163.
383. Mercadier JJ, Lompre A-M, Duc P, et al. Altered sarcoplasmic reticulum Ca^{2+}-ATPase gene expression in the human ventricle during end-stage heart failure. *J Clin Invest* 1990;85:305–309.
384. Merin RG. Are the myocardial function and metabolic effects of isoflurane really different from those of halothane and enflurane? *Anesthesiology* 1981;55:398–408.
385. Merin RG, Bernard JM, Doursout MF, Cohen M, Chelly JE. Comparison of the effects of isoflurane and desflurane on cardiovascular dynamics and regional blood flow in the chronically instrumented dog. *Anesthesiology* 1991;74:568–574.
386. Merin RG, Chelly JE, Hysing ES, et al. Cardiovascular effects of and interaction between calcium blocking drugs and anesthetics in chronically instrumented dogs. IV. Chronically administered oral verapamil and halothane, enflurane, and isoflurane. *Anesthesiology* 1987;66:140–146.
387. Merin RG, Kumazawa T, Luka NL. Enflurane depresses myocardial function, perfusion, and metabolism in the dog. *Anesthesiology* 1976;45:501–507.
388. Merin RG, Kumazawa T, Luka NL. Myocardial function and metabolism in the conscious dog and during halothane anesthesia. *Anesthesiology* 1976;44:402–415.
389. Miller TR, Goldman KJ, Sampathkumaran KS, Biello DR, Lud-

brook PA, Sobel BE. Analysis of cardiac diastolic function: application in coronary artery disease. *J Nucl Med* 1983;24:2–7.
390. Mills CJ, Gabe IT, Gault JH, et al. Pressure-flow relationships and vascular impedance in man. *Cardiovasc Res* 1970;4:405–417.
391. Milnor WR. Arterial impedance as ventricular afterload. *Circ Res* 1975;36:565–570.
392. Milnor WR, Conti CR, Lewis KB, O'Rourke MF. Pulmonary arterial pulse wave velocity and impedance in man. *Circ Res* 1969; 25:637–649.
393. Mirsky I. Review of various theories for the evaluation of left ventricular wall stresses. In: Mirsky I, Ghista DN, Sandler H, eds. *Cardiac mechanics: physiological, clinical, and mathematical considerations.* New York: John Wiley, 1974;381–409.
394. Mirsky I. Elastic properties of the myocardium: a quantitative approach with physiological and clinical applications. In: Berne RM, ed. *Section 2, the cardiovascular system, volume 1, heart. Handbook of physiology.* Bethesda: American Physiological Society, 1979;501.
395. Mirsky I. Assessment of diastolic function: suggested methods and future considerations. *Circulation* 1984;69:836–841.
396. Mirsky I, Pfeffer JM, Pfeffer MA, Braunwald E. The contractile state as the major determinant in the evolution of left ventricular dysfunction in the spontaneously hypertensive rat. *Circ Res* 1983; 53:767–778.
397. Mirsky I, Rankin JS. The effects of geometry, elasticity, and external pressures on the diastolic pressure-volume and stiffness-strain relations. How important is the pericardium? *Circ Res* 1979;44: 601–611.
398. Mitchell GD, Brunken RC, Schwaiger M, Donohue BC, Krivokapich J, Child JS. Assessment of mitral flow velocity with exercise by an index of stress-induced left ventricular ischemia in coronary artery disease. *Am J Cardiol* 1988;61:536–540.
399. Mitchell JH, Gilmore JP, Sarnoff SJ. The transport function of the atrium. Factors influencing the relation between mean left atrial pressure and left ventricular end diastolic pressure. *Am J Cardiol* 1962;9:237–247.
400. Mitchell JH, Wallace AG, Skinner NS Jr. Intrinsic effects of heart rate on left ventricular performance. *Am J Physiol* 1963;205:41–48.
401. Miyazaki S, Guth BD, Miura T, Indolfi C, Schulz R, Ross J Jr. Changes of left ventricular diastolic function in exercising dogs with and without ischemia. *Circulation* 1990;81:1058–1070.
402. Moalic J-M, Charlemagne D, Mansier P, Chevalier B, Swynghedauw B. Cardiac hypertrophy and failure—A disease of adaptation: modifications in membrane proteins provide a molecular basis for arrhythmogenicity. *Circulation* 1993;87(suppl IV):21–26.
403. Momomura S, Bradley AB, Grossman W. Left ventricular diastolic pressure-segment length relations and end-diastolic distensibility in dogs with coronary stenoses: an angina physiology model. *Circ Res* 1984;55:203–214.
404. Momomura S, Ingwall JS, Parker JA, Sahagian P, Ferguson JJ, Grossman W. The relationships of high energy phosphates, tissue pH, and regional blood flow to diastolic distensibility in the ischemic dog myocardium. *Circ Res* 1985;57:822–835.
405. Monrad ES, McKay RG, Baim DS, et al. Improvement in indexes of diastolic performance in patients with congestive heart failure treated with milrinone. *Circulation* 1984;70:1030–1037.
406. Moores WY, Weiskopf RB, Baysinger M, Utley JR. Effects of halothane and morphine sulfate on myocardial compliance following total cardiopulmonary bypass. *J Thorac Cardiovasc Surg* 1981;81:163–170.
407. Moravec CS, Schluchter MD, Paranandi L, et al. Inotropic effects of angiotensin II in human cardiac muscle in vitro. *Circulation* 1990;82:1973–1984.
408. Morgan JP. Abnormal intracellular modulation of calcium as a major cause of cardiac contractile dysfunction. *New Engl J Med* 1991;325:625–632.
409. Morgan JP, Erny RE, Allen PD, Grossman W, Gwathmey JK. Abnormal intracellular calcium handling, a major cause of systolic and diastolic dysfunction in ventricular myocardium from patients with heart failure. *Circulation* 1990;81(suppl III):21–32.
410. Movsesian MA, Bristow MR, Krall J. Ca^{2+} uptake by cardiac sarcoplasmic reticulum from patients with idiopathic dilated cardiomyopathy. *Circ Res* 1989;65:1141–1144.
411. Mulier JP, Wouters PF, Van Aken H, Vermaut G, Vandermeersch E. Cardiodynamic effects of propofol in comparison with thiopental: assessment with a transesophageal echocardiographic approach. *Anesth Analg* 1991;72:28–35.
412. Muzi M, Berens RA, Kampine JP, Ebert TJ. Venodilation contributes to propofol-mediated hypotension in humans. *Anesth Analg* 1992;74:877–883.
413. Myhre ESP, Johansen A, Bjornstad J, Piene H. The effect of contractility and preload on matching between canine left ventricle and afterload. *Circulation* 1986;73:161–171.
414. Myhre ESP, Johansen A, Piene H. Optimal matching between canine left ventricle and afterload. *Am J Physiol* 1988;254: H1051–1058.
415. Neumann J, Schmitz W, Scholz H, von Meyerinck L, Doring V, Kalmar P. Increase in myocardial G_i-proteins in heart failure. *Lancet* 1988;2:936–937.
416. Nikolic S, Yellin EL, Tamura K, et al. Passive properties of canine left ventricle: diastolic stiffness and restoring forces. *Circ Res* 1988;62:1210–1222.
417. Nikolic SD, Tamura K, Tamura T, Dahm M, Frater RWM, Yellin EL. Diastolic viscous properties of the intact canine left ventricle. *Circ Res* 1990;67:352–359.
418. Nishimura RA, Abel MD, Hatle LK, Tajik AJ. Assessment of diastolic function of the heart: background and current applications of Doppler echocardiography. Part II. Clinical studies. *Mayo Clin Proc* 1989;64:181–204.
419. Nixon JV, Murray RG, Leonard PD, Mitchell JH, Blomqvist CG. Effect of large variations in preload on left ventricular performance characteristic in normal subjects. *Circulation* 1982;65: 698–703.
420. Noda N, Cheng CP, De Tombe PP, Little WC. Curvilinearity of LV end-systolic pressure-volume and dP/dt_{max}-end-diastolic volume relations. *Am J Physiol* 1993;265:H910–H917.
421. Nolan SP, Dixon Jr SH, Fisher RD, Morrow AG. The influence of atrial contraction and mitral valve mechanics on ventricular filling. A study of instantaneous mitral valve flow *in vivo. Am Heart J* 1969;77:784–791.
422. Nosek TM, Williams MF, Zeigler ST, Godt RE. Inositol triphosphate enhances calcium release in skinned cardiac and skeletal muscle. *Am J Physiol* 1986;250:C807–C811.
423. O'Neill W, Timmis GC, Bourdillon PD, et al. A prospective randomized clinical trial of intracoronary streptokinase versus coronary angioplasty for acute myocardial infarction. *N Engl J Med* 1986;314:812–818.
424. O'Rourke M. Arterial stiffness, systolic blood pressure, and logical treatment of arterial hypertension. *Hypertension* 1990;15: 339–347.
425. Olivetti G, Capasso JM, Meggs LG, Sonnenblick E, Anversa P. Cellular basis of chronic ventricular remodeling after myocardial infarction in rats. *Circ Res* 1991;68:856–869.
426. Opie LH. Reperfusion injury and its pharmacologic modification. *Circulation* 1989;80:1049–1062.
427. Pagel PS, Grossman W, Haering JM, Warltier DC. Left ventricular diastolic function in the normal and diseased heart: perspectives for the anesthesiologist. (First of two parts). *Anesthesiology* 1993;79: 836–854.
428. Pagel PS, Grossman W, Haering JM, Warltier DC. Left ventricular diastolic function in the normal and diseased heart: perspectives for the anesthesiologist. (Second of two parts). *Anesthesiology* 1993;79:1104–1120.
429. Pagel PS, Hettrick DA, Warltier DC. Amrinone enhances myocardial contractility and improves left ventricular diastolic function in conscious and anesthetized chronically instrumented dogs. *Anesthesiology* 1993;79:753–765.
430. Pagel PS, Kampine JP, Schmeling WT, Warltier DC. Comparison of end-systolic pressure-length relations and preload recruitable stroke work as indices of myocardial contractility in the conscious and anesthetized, chronically instrumented dog. *Anesthesiology* 1990;73:278–290.
431. Pagel PS, Kampine JP, Schmeling WT, Warltier DC. Effects of nitrous oxide on myocardial contractility as evaluated by the preload recruitable stroke work relationship in chronically instrumented dogs. *Anesthesiology* 1990;73:1148–1157.
432. Pagel PS, Kampine JP, Schmeling WT, Warltier DC. Alteration of left ventricular diastolic function by desflurane, isoflurane, and halothane in the chronically instrumented dog with autonomic nervous system blockade. *Anesthesiology* 1991;74:1103–1114.
433. Pagel PS, Kampine JP, Schmeling WT, Warltier DC. Comparison of the systemic and coronary hemodynamic actions of desflurane, isoflurane, halothane, and enflurane in the chronically instrumented dog. *Anesthesiology* 1991;74:539–551.
434. Pagel PS, Kampine JP, Schmeling WT, Warltier DC. Influence of

volatile anesthetics on myocardial contractility *in vivo*: desflurane versus isoflurane. *Anesthesiology* 1991;74:900–907.
435. Pagel PS, Kampine JP, Schmeling WT, Warltier DC. Ketamine depresses myocardial contractility as evaluated by the preload recruitable stroke work relationship in chronically instrumented dogs with autonomic nervous system blockade. *Anesthesiology* 1992;76:564–572.
436. Pagel PS, Kampine JP, Schmeling WT, Warltier DC. Evaluation of myocardial contractility in the chronically instrumented dog with intact autonomic nervous system function: effects of desflurane and isoflurane. *Acta Anaesthesiol Scand* 1993;37:203–210.
437. Pagel PS, Kampine JP, Schmeling WT, Warltier DC. Reversal of volatile anesthetic-induced depression of myocardial contractility by extracellular calcium also enhances left ventricular diastolic function. *Anesthesiology* 1993;78:141–154.
438. Pagel PS, Nijhawan N, Warltier DC. Quantitation of volatile anesthetic-induced depression of myocardial contractility using a single beat index derived from maximal ventricular power. *J Cardiothorac Vasc Anesth* 1993;7:688–695.
439. Pagel PS, Power MW, Kenny D, Warltier DC. Cocaine depresses myocardial contractility and prolongs isovolumetric relaxation in conscious dogs with partial autonomic nervous system blockade. *J Cardiovasc Pharmacol* 1992;20:25–34.
440. Pagel PS, Schmeling WT, Kampine JP, Warltier DC. Alteration of canine left ventricular diastolic function by intravenous anesthetics in vivo: ketamine and propofol. *Anesthesiology* 1992;76:419–425.
441. Pagel PS, Warltier DC. Negative inotropic effects of propofol as evaluated by the regional preload recruitable stroke work relationship in chronically instrumented dogs. *Anesthesiology* 1993; 78:100–108.
442. Papademetriou V, Gottdiener JS, Fletcher RD, Freis ED. Echocardiographic assessment by computer-assisted analysis of diastolic left ventricular function and hypertrophy in borderline or mild hypertension. *Am J Cardiol* 1985;56:546–550.
443. Park WK, Lynch C III. Propofol and thiopental depression of myocardial contractility: a comparative study of the mechanical and electrophysiologic effects in isolated guinea pig ventricular muscle. *Anesth Analg* 1992;74:395–405.
444. Parmley WW, Sonnenblick EH. Relation between mechanics of contraction and relaxation in mammalian cardiac muscle. *Am J Physiol* 1969;216:1084–1091.
445. Pasipoularides A. Clinical assessment of ventricular ejection dynamics with and without outflow tract obstruction. *J Am Coll Cardiol* 1990;15:859–862.
446. Pasipoularides A, Murgo JP, Miller JW, Craig WE. Nonobstructive left ventricular ejection pressure gradients in man. *Circ Res* 1987; 61:220–227.
447. Patel DJ, DeFreitas FM, Fry DL. Hydraulic input impedance to aorta and pulmonary artery in dogs. *J Appl Physiol* 1963;18:134–140.
448. Patschke D, Bruckner JB, Eberlein JH, Hess W, Tarnow J, Weymar A. Effects of althesin, etomidate and fentanyl on haemodynamics and myocardial oxygen consumption in man. *Can Anaesth Soc J* 1977;24:57–69.
449. Patterson SW, Piper H, Starling E. Regulation of the heart beat. *J Physiol (Lond)* 1914;48:465–513.
450. Paulus WJ, Lorell BH, Craig WE, Wynne J, Murgo JP, Grossman W. Comparison of the effects of nitroprusside and nifedipine on diastolic properties in patients with hypertrophic cardiomyopathy: altered left ventricular loading or improved muscle relaxation? *J Am Coll Cardiol* 1983;2:879–886.
451. Pearson AC, Labovitz AJ, Mrosek D, Williams GA, Kennedy HL. Assessment of diastolic function in normal and hypertrophied hearts: comparison of Doppler echocardiography and M-mode echocardiography. *Am Heart J* 1987;113:1417–1425.
452. Perloff JK, Roberts WC. The mitral apparatus. Functional anatomy of mitral regurgitation. *Circulation* 1972;46:227–.
453. Perreault CL, Meuse AJ, Bentivegna LA, Morgan JP. Abnormal intracellular calcium handling in acute and chronic heart failure: role in systolic and diastolic dysfunction. *Eur Heart J* 1990;11 (suppl C):8–21.
454. Peterson KL, Skloven D, Ludbrook P, Uther JB, Ross J Jr. Comparison of isovolumetric and ejection phase indices of myocardial performance in man. *Circulation* 1974;49:1088–1101.
455. Pfeffer JM, Pfeffer MA, Mirsky I, Braunwald E. Regression of left ventricular hypertrophy and prevention of left ventricular dysfunction by captopril in the spontaneously hypertensive rat. *Proc Natl Acad Sci USA* 1982;79:3310–3314.
456. Pfeffer MA, Braunwald E. Ventricular remodeling after myocardial infarction: experimental observations and clinical implications. *Circulation* 1990;81:1161–1172.
457. Piscione F, Jaski BE, Wenting GJ, Serruys PW. Effect of a single oral dose of milrinone on left ventricular diastolic performance in the failing human heart. *J Am Coll Cardiol* 1987;10:1294–1302.
458. Plotnick GD. Changes in diastolic function - Difficult to measure, harder to interpret. *Am Heart J* 1989;118:637–641.
459. Plotnick GD, Becker LC, Fisher ML, et al. Use of the Frank-Starling mechanism during submaximal versus maximal upright exercise. *Am J Physiol* 1986;251:H1101–H1105.
460. Polak JF, Kemper AJ, Bianco JA, Parisi AF, Tow DE. Resting early peak diastolic filling rate: a sensitive index of myocardial dysfunction in patients with coronary artery disease. *J Nucl Med* 1982;23:471–478.
461. Poliner LR, Farber SH, Glaeser DH, Nylaan L, Verani MS, Roberts R. Alteration of diastolic filling rate during exercise radionuclide angiography: a highly sensitive technique for detection of coronary artery disease. *Circulation* 1984;70:942–950.
462. Pouleur H, Karlinger JS, LeWinter MM, Covell JW. Diastolic viscous properties of the intact canine left ventricle. *Circ Res* 1979;45: 410–419.
463. Pouleur H, Rousseau MF, van Eyll C, Charlier AA. Assessment of regional left ventricular relaxation in patients with coronary artery disease: importance of geometric factors and changes in wall thickness. *Circulation* 1984;69:696–702.
464. Prakash O, Dhasmana M, Verdouw PD, Saxena PR. Cardiovascular effects of etomidate with emphasis on regional myocardial blood flow and performance. *Br J Anaesth* 1981;53:591–599.
465. Preuss KC, Gross GJ, Brooks HL, Warltier DC. Time course of recovery of "stunned" myocardium following variable periods of ischemia in conscious and anesthetized dogs. *Am Heart J* 1987; 114:696–703.
466. Price HL. Calcium reverses myocardial depression caused by halothane: site of action. *Anesthesiology* 1974;41:576–579.
467. Pritzl N, Zak R. Molecular biology of myocardial proteins. *Circulation* 1987;75(suppl I):85–91.
468. Prys-Roberts C, Roberts JG, Foex P, Clarke TN, Bennett MJ, Ryder WA. Interaction of anesthesia, beta-receptor blockade, and blood loss in dogs with induced myocardial infarction. *Anesthesiology* 1976;45:326–329.
469. Przyklenk K, Kloner RA. Effect of verapamil on postischemic "stunned" myocardium: importance of the timing of treatment. *J Am Coll Cardiol* 1988;11:614–623.
470. Quinones MA, Gaasch WH, Alexander JK. Influence of acute changes in preload, afterload, contractile state, and heart rate on ejection and isovolumetric indices of myocardial contractility in man. *Circulation* 1976;53:293–302.
471. Quinones MA, Waggoner AD, Reduto LA, et al. A new, simplified and accurate method for determining ejection fraction with two-dimensional echocardiography. *Circulation* 1981;64:744–753.
472. Rabinowitz M, Zak R. Mitochondria and cardiac hypertrophy. *Circ Res* 1975;36:367–376.
473. Raff GL, Glantz SA. Volume loading slows left ventricular isovolumetric relaxation rate: evidence of load-dependent relaxation in the intact dog. *Circ Res* 1981;48:813–824.
474. Rahimtoola SH. A perspective on the three large multicenter randomized clinical trials of coronary artery bypass surgery for chronic stable angina. *Circulation* 1985;72(suppl 5):123–135.
475. Rahimtoola SH. The hibernating myocardium. *Am Heart J* 1989;117:211–221.
476. Rahimtoola SH, Ehsani A, Sinno MZ, Loeb HS, Rosen KM, Gunnar RM. Left atrial transport function in myocardial infarction. Importance of its booster pump function. *Am J Med* 1975;59: 686–694.
477. Ramsey JG, Arvieux CC, Foex P, et al. Regional and global myocardial function in the dog when nitrous oxide is added to halothane in the presence of critical coronary artery constriction. *Anesth Analg* 1986;65:431–436.
478. Rankin JS, Arentzen CE, McHale PA, Ling D, Anderson RW. Viscoelastic properties of the diastolic left ventricle in the conscious dog. *Circ Res* 1977;41:37–45.
479. Rankin JS, Arentzen CE, Ring WS, Edwards CH, II, McHale PA, Anderson RW. The diastolic mechanical properties of the intact left ventricle. *Fed Proc* 1980;39:141–147.
480. Rankin JS, Gaynor JW, Feneley MP, et al. Diastolic myocardial mechanics and the regulation of cardiac performance. In: Gross-

man W, Lorell BH, eds. *Diastolic relaxation of the heart: basic research and current applications for clinical cardiology.* Boston: Matinus Nijhoff, 1988;111–124.

481. Rankin JS, Newman GE, Muhlbaier LH, Behar VS, Fedor JM, Sabiston DC Jr. The effects of coronary revascularization on left ventricular function in ischemic heart disease. *J Thorac Cardiovasc Surg* 1985;90:818–832.
482. Rappaport L, Swynghedauw B, Mercadier JJ, et al. Physiological adaptation of the heart to pathological overloading. *Fed Proc* 1986;45:2573–2579.
483. Reduto LA, Wickemeyer WJ, Young JB, et al. Left ventricular diastolic performance at rest and during exercise in patients with coronary artery disease. *Circulation* 1981;63:1228–1237.
484. Regen DM. Calculation of left ventricular wall stress. *Circ Res* 1990; 67:245–252.
485. Reid IA, Morris BJ, Ganong WF. The renin-angiotensin system. *Annu Rev Physiol* 1978;40:377–410.
486. Reimer KA, Hill ML, Jennings RB. Prolonged depletion of ATP and of the adenine nucleotide pool due to delayed resynthesis of adenine nucleotides following reversible myocardial ischemic injury in dogs. *J Mol Cell Cardiol* 1981;13:229–239.
487. Reimer KA, Jennings RB. The "wavefront phenomenon" of myocardial ischemic cell death. II. Transmural progression of necrosis within the framework of ischemic bed size (myocardium at risk) and collateral flow. *Lab Invest* 1979;40:633–644.
488. Reimer KA, Lowe JE, Rasmussen MM, Jennings RB. The wavefront phenomenon of ischemic cell death. I. Myocardial infarct size versus duration of coronary occlusion in dogs. *Circulation* 1977;56: 786–794.
489. Reiz S, Balfors E, Friedman A, Haggmark S, Peter T. Effects of thiopentone on cardiac performance, coronary hemodynamics and myocardial oxygen consumption in chronic ischemic heart disease. *Acta Anaesthesiol Scand* 1981;25:103–110.
490. Rentrop R, Blanke H, Karsch KR, Kaiser H, Kostering H, Leitz K. Selective intracoronary thrombolysis in acute myocardial infarction and unstable angina pectoris. *Circulation* 1981;63:307–317.
491. Riegger GAJ, Liebau G, Kochsiek K. Antidiuretic hormone in congestive heart failure. *Am J Med* 1982;72:49–52.
492. Riou B, Besse S, Lecarpentier Y, Viars P. In vitro effects of propofol on rat myocardium. *Anesthesiology* 1992;76:609–616.
493. Riou B, Lecarpentier Y, Chemla D, Viars P. *In vitro* effects of etomidate on intrinsic myocardial contractility in the rat. *Anesthesiology* 1990;72:330–340.
494. Riou B, Lecarpentier Y, Viars P. Effects of etomidate on the cardiac papillary muscle of normal hamsters and those with cardiomyopathy. *Anesthesiology* 1993;78:83–90.
495. Ritzman JR, Erickson HH, Miller ED Jr. Cardiovascular effects of enflurane and halothane on the rhesus monkey. *Anesth Analg* 1976;55:85–91.
496. Roan P, Scales F, Saffer S, Buja LM, Willerson JT. Functional characterization of left ventricular segmental responses during the initial 24 hours and one week after experimental canine myocardial infarction. *J Clin Invest* 1979;64:1074–1088.
497. Robb JS, Robb RC. Abnormal distribution of the superficial muscle bundles in the human heart. *Am Heart J* 1938;15:597–603.
498. Robb JS, Robb RD. The normal heart: anatomy and physiology of the structural units. *Am Heart J* 1942;23:455–467.
499. Robbins SL, Cotran RS. *Pathologic basis of disease.* Philadelphia: WB Saunders, 1979.
500. Roberts WC, Cohen LS. Left ventricular papillary muscles. Description of the normal and a survey of conditions causing them to be abnormal. *Circulation* 1972;46:138–.
501. Robertson SP, Johnson JD, Holroyde MJ, Kranias EG, Potter JD, Solaro RJ. The effect of troponin I phosphorylation on the Ca^{2+}-binding properties of the Ca^{2+}-regulatory site of bovine cardiac troponin. *J Biol Chem* 1982;257:260–263.
502. Rogers WJ, Hood WP Jr, Mantle JA, et al. Return of left ventricular function after reperfusion in patients with myocardial infarction: importance of subtotal stenoses or intact collaterals. *Circulation* 1984;69:338–349.
503. Rokey R, Kuo LC, Zoghbi WA, Limacher MC, Quinones MA. Determination of parameters of left ventricular diastolic filling with pulsed Doppler echocardiography: comparison with cineangiography. *Circulation* 1985;71:543–550.
504. Rorie DK, Tyce GM, Sill JC. Increased norepinephrine release from dog pulmonary artery caused by nitrous oxide. *Anesth Analg* 1986;1986:560–564.
505. Ross J Jr. Applications and limitations of end-systolic measures of ventricular performance. *Fed Proc* 1984;43:2418–2422.
506. Ross J Jr. Mechanisms of regional ischemia and antianginal drug action during exercise. *Prog Cardiovasc Dis* 1989;31:455–466.
507. Ross J Jr. Mechanical consequences of regional myocardial ischemia. In: Fozzard HA, Haber E, Jennings RB, Katz AM, Morgan HE, eds. *The heart and cardiovascular system: scientific foundations.* New York: Raven Press, 1992;1997–2020.
508. Rouby JJ, Andreev A, Leger P, et al. Peripheral vascular effects of thiopental and propofol in humans with artificial hearts. *Anesthesiology* 1991;75:32–42.
509. Rushmer RF, DL F, Ellis RM. Left ventricular dimensions recorded by sonocardiometry. *Circ Res* 1956;4:684–688.
510. Ruskin J, McHale PA, Harley A, Greenfield JC Jr. Pressure-flow studies in man: effect of atrial systole on left ventricular function. *J Clin Invest* 1970;49:472–478.
511. Russell RO Jr, Porter CM, Frimer M, Dodge HT. Left ventricular power in man. *Am Heart J* 1971;81:799–808.
512. Rusy BF, Amuzu JK, Bosscher HA, Redon D, Komai H. Negative inotropic effect of ketamine in rabbit ventricular muscle. *Anesth Analg* 1990;71:275–278.
513. Rusy BF, Komai H. Anesthetic depression of myocardial contractility: a review of possible mechanisms. *Anesthesiology* 1987;67: 745–766.
514. Rusy BF, Moran JE, Vongvises P, et al. The effects of halothane and cyclopropane on left ventricular volume determined by high-speed biplane cineradiography in dogs. *Anesthesiology* 1972;36: 369–373.
515. Sabbah HN, Stein PD. Negative diastolic pressure in the intact canine right ventricle. Evidence of diastolic suction. *Circ Res* 1981; 49:108–113.
516. Sabbah HN, Stein PD. Pressure-diameter relations during early diastole in dogs. Incompatibility with the concept of passive left ventricular filing. *Circ Res* 1981;48:357–365.
517. Safian RD, Warren SE, Berman AD, et al. Improvement in symptoms and left ventricular performance after balloon valvuloplasty in patients with aortic stenosis and depressed left ventricular ejection fraction. *Circulation* 1988;78:1181–1191.
518. Safwat A, Leone BJ, Norris RM, Foex P. Pressure-length loop area: its components analyzed during graded myocardial ischemia. *J Am Coll Cardiol* 1991;17:790–796.
519. Sagawa K. The end-systolic pressure-volume relation of the ventricle: definition, modifications and clinical use. *Circulation* 1981;63: 1223–1227.
520. Sagawa K, Maughan L, Suga H, Sunagawa K. *Cardiac contraction and the pressure-volume relationship.* New York: Oxford University Press, 1988.
521. Salt PJ, Barnes PK, Beswick FJ. Inhibition of neuronal and extraneuronal uptake of noradrenaline by ketamine in the isolated perfused rat heart. *Br J Anaesth* 1979;51:835–838.
522. Sanderson JE, Traill TA, St John Sutton MG, Brown DJ, Gibson DG, Goodwin JF. Left ventricular relaxation and filling in hypertrophic cardiomyopathy: an echocardiographic study. *Br Heart J* 1978;40:596–601.
523. Sandler H, Alderman E. Determination of left ventricular size and shape. *Circ Res* 1974;34:1–8.
524. Sandler H, Dodge HT. Left ventricular tension and stress in man. *Circ Res* 1963;13:91–104.
525. Santamore WP, Bove AA, Heckman JL. Right and left ventricular pressure-volume response to positive end-expiratory pressure. *Am J Physiol* 1984;246:H114–H119.
526. Sarnoff SJ, Berglund E. Ventricular function. I. Starling's law of the heart studied by means of simultaneous right and left ventricular function curves in the dog. *Circulation* 1954;9:706–718.
527. Sarnoff SJ, Braunwald E, Welch GH Jr, Case RB, Stainsby WN, Macruz R. Hemodynamic determinants of oxygen consumption of the heart with special reference to the time-tension index. *Am J Physiol* 1958;192:148–156.
528. Sasayama S, Franklin D, Ross J Jr, Kemper WS, McKown D. Dynamic changes in left ventricular wall thickness and their use in analyzing cardiac function in the conscious dog. *Am J Cardiol* 1976;38:870–879.
529. Sasayama S, Gallagher KP, Kemper WS, Franklin D, Ross J Jr. Regional left ventricular wall thickness early and late after coronary occlusion in the conscious dog. *Am J Physiol* 1981;240: H293–H299.
530. Sasayama S, Nonogi H, Miyazaki S, et al. Changes in diastolic

properties of the regional myocardium during pacing-induced ischemia in human subjects. *J Am Coll Cardiol* 1985;5:599–606.

531. Schuler G, Peterson KL, Johnson A, et al. Temporal response of left ventricular performance to mitral valve surgery. *Circulation* 1979;59:1218–1231.
532. Schunkert H, Dzau VJ, Tang SS, Hirsch AT, Apstein CS, Lorell BH. Increased rat cardiac angiotensin converting enzyme activity and mRNA expression in pressure overload left ventricular hypertrophy: effects on coronary resistance, contractility, and relaxation. *J Clin Invest* 1990;86:1913–1920.
533. Schwartz DA, Horwitz LD. Effects of ketamine on left ventricular performance. *J Pharmacol Exp Ther* 1975;194:410–414.
534. Sebel PS, Lowdon JD. Propofol: a new intravenous anesthetic. *Anesthesiology* 1989;71:260–277.
535. Sellgren J, Ponten J, Wallin BG. Percutaneous recording of muscle nerve sympathetic activity during propofol, nitrous oxide, and isoflurane anesthesia in humans. *Anesthesiology* 1990;73:20–27.
536. Seltzer JL, Gerson JI, Allen FB. Comparison of the cardiovascular effects of bolus v. incremental administration of thiopentone. *Br J Anaesth* 1980;52:527–30.
537. Serizawa T, Carabello BA, Grossman W. Effect of pacing-induced ischemia on left ventricular diastolic pressure-volume relations in dogs with coronary stenoses. *Circ Res* 1980;46:430–439.
538. Serizawa T, Vogel WM, Apstein CS, Grossman W. Comparison of acute alterations in left ventricular relaxation and diastolic chamber stiffness induced by hypoxia and ischemia. Role of myocardial oxygen supply-demand imbalance. *J Clin Invest* 1981;68:91–102.
539. Serruys PW, Wijns W, Van der Brand M, et al. Left ventricular performance, regional blood flow, wall motion, and lactate metabolism during transluminal angioplasty. *Circulation* 1984;70: 25–36.
540. Severinghaus JW, Cullen SC. Depression of myocardium and body oxygen consumption with Fluothane. *Anesthesiology* 1958;19: 165–177.
541. Shapiro LM, McKenna WJ. Left ventricular hypertrophy: relation of structure to diastolic function in hypertension. *Br Heart J* 1984; 51:637–642.
542. Share L. Role of vasopressin in cardiovascular regulation. *Physiol Rev* 1988;68:1248–1284.
543. Sharir T, Van Anden E, Marmor A, Feldman AM, Kass DA. Noninvasive assessment of drug induced load vs inotropic change by maximal ventricular power/EDV^2 in humans (abstract). *Circulation* 1992;86(suppl I):460.
544. Shebetai R. Progress in cardiac tamponade and constrictive pericarditis. In: Yu PN, Goodwin JF, eds. *Progress in cardiology.* Philadelphia: Lea & Febiger, 1986;87–100.
545. Shimosato S, Li TH, Etsten B. Ventricular function during halothane anesthesia in closed chest dog. *Circ Res* 1963;12:63–75.
546. Shimosato S, Sugai N, Iwatsuki N, Etsten BE. The effect of Ethrane on cardiac muscle mechanics. *Anesthesiology* 1969;30:513–518.
547. Shimshak TM, Preuss KC, Gross GJ, Brooks HL, Warltier DC. Recovery of contractile function in post-ischaemic, reperfused myocardium of conscious dogs: influence of nicorandil, a new antianginal agent. *Cardiovasc Res* 1986;20:621–626.
548. Shubeita HE, McDonough PM, Harris AN, et al. Endothelin induction of inositol phospholipid hydrolysis, sarcomere assembly, and cardiac gene expression in ventricular myocytes: a paracrine mechanism for myocardial cell hypertrophy. *J Biol Chem* 1990;265:20555–20562.
549. Siker D, Pagel PS, Pelc LR, Kampine JP, Schmeling WT, Warltier DC. Nitrous oxide impairs functional recovery of stunned myocardium in barbiturate-anesthetized, acutely instrumented dogs. *Anesth Analg* 1992;75:539–548.
550. Simkus GJ, Fitchett DH. Radial arterial pressure measurements may be a poor guide to the beneficial effects of nitroprusside on left ventricular systolic pressure in congestive heart failure. *Am J Cardiol* 1990;66:323–326.
551. Simpson PJ, Todd RF III, Mickelson JK, et al. Sustained limitation of myocardial reperfusion injury by a monoclonal antibody that alters leukocyte function. *Circulation* 1990;81:226–237.
552. Slavik JR, LaMantia KR, Kopriva CJ, Prokop E, Ezekowitz MD, Barash PG. Does nitrous oxide cause regional wall motion abnormalities in patients with coronary artery disease? An evaluation by two-dimensional transesophageal echocardiography. *Anesth Analg* 1988;67:695–700.
553. Smith JJ, Kampine JP. *Circulatory physiology—the essentials,* 3rd ed. Baltimore: Williams & Wilkins, 1990.
554. Smith JS, Cahalan MK, Benefiel DJ, et al. Intraoperative detection of myocardial ischemia in high-risk patients: electrocardiography versus two dimensional transesophageal echocardiography. *Circulation* 1985;72:1015–1021.
555. Smith NT, Calverley RK, Prys-Roberts C, Eger EI II, Jones CW. Impact of nitrous oxide on the circulation during enflurane anesthesia in man. *Anesthesiology* 1978;48:345–349.
556. Smith NT, Corbascio AN. The cardiovascular effects of nitrous oxide during halothane anesthesia in the dog. *Anesthesiology* 1966;27:560–566.
557. Smith NT, Eger EI II, Stoelting RK, Whayne TF, Cullen D, Kadis LB. The cardiovascular and sympathomimetic responses to the addition of nitrous oxide to halothane in man. *Anesthesiology* 1970; 32:410–421.
558. Smith V-E, Zile MR. Relaxation and diastolic properties of the heart. In: Fozzard HA, Haber E, Jennings RB, Katz AM, Morgan HE, eds. *The heart and cardiovascular system: scientific foundations.* New York: Raven Press, 1991;1353–1367.
559. Smith VE, Schulman P, Karimeddini MK, White WB, Meeran MK, Katz AM. Rapid ventricular filling in left ventricular hypertrophy: II. Pathologic hypertrophy. *J Am coll Cardiol* 1985;5:869–874.
560. Snell RE, Luchsinger PC. Determination of the external work and power of the intact left ventricle in intact man. *Am Heart J* 1965; 69:529–537.
561. Sokolow M, McIlroy MB. *Clinical cardiology,* 4th ed. Los Altos, CA: Lange, 1986.
562. Solaro RJ, Moir AJ, Perry SV. Phosphorylation of troponin I and the inotropic effect of adrenaline in the perfused rabbit heart. *Nature* 1976;262:615–617.
563. Sonntag H, Donath U, Hillebrand W, Merin RG, Radke J. Left ventricular function in conscious man and during halothane anesthesia. *Anesthesiology* 1978;48:320–324.
564. Sonntag H, Hellberg K, Schenk HD, et al. Effects of thiopental (Trapanal) on coronary blood flow and myocardial metabolism in man. *Acta Anaesthesiol Scand* 1975;19:69–78.
565. Soufer R, Wohlgelernter D, Vita NA, et al. Intact systolic left ventricular function in clinical congestive heart failure. *Am J Cardiol* 1985;55:1032–1036.
566. Spann JF Jr, Buccino RA, Sonnenblick EH, Braunwald E. Contractile state of cardiac muscle obtained from cats with experimentally produced ventricular hypertrophy and heart failure. *Circ Res* 1967;21:341–354.
567. Spann JF Jr, Covell JW, Eckberg DL, Sonnenblick EH, Ross J Jr, Braunwald E. Contractile performance of the hypertrophied and chronically failing cat ventricle. *Am J Physiol* 1972;223: 1150–1157.
568. Spirito P, Maron BJ. Doppler echocardiography for assessing left ventricular diastolic function. *Ann Intern Med* 1988;109:122–126.
569. Spirito P, Maron BJ, Bonow RO. Noninvasive assessment of left ventricular diastolic function: comparative analysis of Doppler echocardiographic and radionuclide angiographic techniques. *J Am Coll Cardiol* 1986;7:518–526.
570. Spirito P, Maron BJ, Chiarella F, et al. Diastolic abnormalities in patients with hypertrophic cardiomyopathy: relation to magnitude of left ventricular hypertrophy. *Circulation* 1985;72:310–316.
571. Spodick DH. The normal and diseased pericardium: current concepts of pericardial physiology, diagnosis, and treatment. *J Am Coll Cardiol* 1983;1:240–251.
572. Spotnitz HM, Sonnenblick EH, Spiro D. Relation of ultrastructure to function in the intact heart: sarcomere structure relative to pressure volume curves of intact left ventricles of dog and cat. *Circ Res* 1966;18:49–66.
573. Spratt JA, Tyson GS, Glower DD, et al. The end-systolic pressure-volume relationship in conscious dog. *Circulation* 1987;75: 1295–1309.
574. Starksen NF, Simpson PC, Bishopric N, et al. Cardiac myocyte hypertrophy is associated with c-myc protooncogene expression. *Proc Natl Acad Sci USA* 1986;83:8348–8350.
575. Starling MR. Left ventricular-arterial coupling relations in the normal human heart. *Am Heart J* 1993;125:1659–1666.
576. Starling MR, Montgomery DG, Mancini GBJ, Walsh RA. Load independence of the rate of isovolumetric relaxation in man. *Circulation* 1987;76:1274–1281.
577. Stein PD, Munter WA. New functional concept of valvular mechanics in normal and diseased aortic valves. *Circulation* 1971; 44:101–.
578. Stein PD, Sabbah HN. Rate of change of ventricular power: an

indicator of ventricular performance during ejection. *Am Heart J* 1976;91:219–227.
579. Stein PD, Sabbah HN. Ventricular performance measure during ejection: studies in patients of the rate of change of ventricular power. *Am Heart J* 1976;91:599–606.
580. Stein PD, Sabbah HN, Albert DE, Synder JE. Continuous-wave Doppler for noninvasive evaluation of aortic blood velocity and rate of change of velocity: evaluation in dogs. *Med Instrum* 1987;21: 177–182.
581. Stevens WC, Cromwell TH, Halsey MJ, Eger EI II, Shakespeare TF, Bahlman SH. The cardiovascular effects of a new inhalation anesthetic, forane, in human volunteers at constant arterial carbon dioxide tension. *Anesthesiology* 1971;35:8–16.
582. Stillwell GK. The law of Laplace: some clinical applications. *Mayo Clin Proc* 1973;48:863–869.
583. Stoelting RK, Gibbs PS. Hemodynamic effects of morphine and morphine-nitrous oxide in valvular heart disease and coronary-artery disease. *Anesthesiology* 1973;38:45–52.
584. Stone GW, Rutherford BD, McConahay DR, et al. Direct coronary angioplasty in acute myocardial infarction: outcome in patients with single vessel disease. *J Am Coll Cardiol* 1990;15:534–543.
585. Stowe DF, Bosnjak ZJ, Kampine JP. Comparison of etomidate, ketamine, midazolam, propofol, and thiopental on function and metabolism of isolated hearts. *Anesth Analg* 1992;74:547–558.
586. Stowe DF, Monroe SM, Marijic J, Bosnjak ZB, Kampine JP. Comparison of halothane, enflurane, and isoflurane with nitrous oxide on contractility and oxygen supply and demand in isolated hearts. *Anesthesiology* 1991;75:1062–1074.
587. Streeter DD Jr, Bassett DL. An engineering analysis of myocardial fiber orientation in pig's left ventricle in systole. *Anat Rec* 1966; 155:503–511.
588. Streeter DD Jr, Spotnitz HM, Patel DP, Ross J Jr, Sonnenblick EH. Fiber orientation in the canine left ventricle during diastole and systole. *Circ Res* 1969;24:339–347.
589. Su JY, Kerrick WG. Effects of halothane on Ca^{2+}-activated tension development in mechanically disrupted rabbit myocardial fibers. *Pflugers Arch* 1978;375:111–117.
590. Suga H. External mechanical work from relaxing ventricle. *Am J Physiol* 1979;236:H494–H497.
591. Suga H. Total mechanical energy of a ventricle model and cardiac oxygen consumption. *Am J Physiol* 1979;236:H498–H505.
592. Suga H, Futaki S, Goto Y. Energetics of the heart. In: Hori M, Suga H, Baan J, Yellin EL, eds. *Cardiac mechanics and function in the normal and diseased heart.* New York: Springer-Verlag, 1989;157–163.
593. Suga H, Goto Y, Igarashi Y, Yamada O. Ventricular pressure-volume area (PVA) and oxygen consumption under ischemia. In: Yamada K, Katz AM, Toyama J, eds. *Cardiac function under ischemia and hypoxia.* Nagoya, Japan: The University of Nagoya Press, 1986; 315–335.
594. Suga H, Goto Y, Igarashi Y, Yamada O, Nozawa T, Yasamura Y. Ventricular suction under zero source pressure for filling. *Am J Physiol* 1986;251:H47–H55.
595. Suga H, Goto Y, Nozawa T, Yasamura Y, Futaki S, Tanaka N. Force-time integral decreases with ejection despite constant oxygen consumption and pressure-volume area in dog left ventricle. *Circ Res* 1987;60:797–803.
596. Suga H, Goto Y, Yamada O, Igarashi Y. Independence of myocardial oxygen consumption from pressure-volume trajectory during diastole in canine left ventricle. *Circ Res* 1984;55:734–739.
597. Suga H, Hayashi T, Shirahata M. Ventricular systolic pressure-volume area as a predictor of cardiac oxygen consumption. *Am J Physiol* 1981;240:H39–H44.
598. Suga H, Hayashi T, Suehiro S, Hisano R, Shirahata M, Ninomiya I. Equal oxygen consumption rates of isovolumetric and ejecting contractions with equal systolic pressure volume areas in canine left ventricle. *Circ Res* 1981;49:1082–1091.
599. Suga H, Hisano R, Goto Y, Yamada O, Igarashi Y. Effect of positive inotropic agents on the relation between oxygen consumption and systolic pressure-volume area in canine left ventricle. *Circ Res* 1983;53:306–318.
600. Suga H, Igarashi Y, Yamada O, Goto Y. Mechanical efficiency of the left ventricle as a function of preload, afterload, and contractility. *Heart Vessel* 1985;1:3–8.
601. Suga H, Sagawa K. Instantaneous pressure-volume relationships and their ratio in the excised, supported canine left ventricle. *Circ Res* 1974;35:117–126.
602. Suga H, Sagawa K, Shoukas AA. Load-independence of the instantaneous pressure-volume ratio of the canine left ventricle and effects of epinephrine and heart rate on the ratio. *Circ Res* 1973; 32:314–322.
603. Suga H, Yamada O, Goto Y, Igarashi Y, Ishigura H. Constant mechanical efficiency of contractile machinery of canine left ventricle under different loading and inotropic conditions. *Jpn J Physiol* 1984;34:679–689.
604. Suga H, Yasumura Y, Nozawa T, Futaki S, Tanaka N. Pressure-volume relation around zero transmural pressure in excised cross-circulated dog left ventricle. *Circ Res* 1988;63:361–372.
605. Sugai N, Shimosato S, Etsten BE. Effect of halothane on force-velocity relations and dynamic stiffness of isolated heart muscle. *Anesthesiology* 1968;29:267–274.
606. Sunagawa K, Maughan WL, Burkhoff D, Sagawa K. Left ventricular interaction with arterial load studied in isolated canine ventricle. *Am J Physiol* 1983;245:H773–H780.
607. Sunagawa K, Maughan WL, Sagawa K. Optimal arterial resistance for the maximal stroke work studied in isolated canine left ventricle. *Circ Res* 1985;56:586–595.
608. Swynghedauw B. Remodeling of the heart in response to chronic mechanical overload. *Eur Heart J* 1989;10:935–943.
609. Takenaka K, Dabestani A, Gardin JM, et al. Left ventricular filling in hypertrophic cardiomyopathy: a pulsed Doppler echocardiographic study. *J Am Coll Cardiol* 1986;7:1263–1271.
610. Takenaka K, Dabestani A, Gardin JM, et al. Pulsed Doppler echocardiographic study of left ventricular filling in dilated cardiomyopathy. *Am J Cardiol* 1986;58:143–147.
611. Taniguchi K, Nakano S, Kawashima Y, et al. Left ventricular ejection performance, wall stress, and contractile state in aortic regurgitation before and after aortic valve replacement. *Circulation* 1990;82:798–807.
612. Tarnow J, Bruckner JB, Eberlein HJ, Hess W, Patschke D. Haemodynamics and myocardial oxygen consumption during isoflurane (Forane) anaesthesia in geriatric patients. *Br J Anaesth* 1976;48: 669–675.
613. Taylor AL, Golino P, Eckels R, Pastor P, Buja LM, Willerson JT. Differential enhancement of postischemic segmental systolic thickening by diltiazem. *J Am Coll Cardiol* 1990;15:737–747.
614. Teplick RS. Measuring central vascular pressures: a surprisingly complex problem. *Anesthesiology* 1987;67:289–291.
615. Thaulow E, Guth BD, Heusch G, et al. Characteristics of regional myocardial stunning after exercise in dogs with chronic coronary stenosis. *Am J Physiol* 1989;257:H113–H119.
616. Theroux P, Franklin D, Ross J Jr, Kemper WS. Regional myocardial function during acute coronary artery occlusion and its modification by pharmacologic agents in the dog. *Circ Res* 1974;35: 896–908.
617. Theroux P, Ross J Jr, Franklin D, Covell JW, Bloor CM, Sasayama S. Regional myocardial function and dimensions early and late after myocardial infarction in the unanesthetized dog. *Circ Res* 1977;40:158–165.
618. Theroux P, Ross J Jr, Franklin D, Kemper WS, Sasayama S. Coronary arterial reperfusion. III. Early and late effects on regional myocardial function and dimensions in conscious dogs. *Am J Cardiol* 1976;38:599–606.
619. Theroux P, Ross J Jr, Franklin D, Kemper WS, Sasayama S. Regional myocardial function in the conscious dog during acute coronary occlusion and responses to morphine, propranolol, nitroglycerin, and lidocaine. *Circulation* 1976;53:302–314.
620. Thiedemann KU, Holubarsch C, Meduogorac I, Jacob R. Connective tissue content and myocardial stiffness in pressure overload hypertrophy: a combined study of morphologic, morphometric, biochemical and mechanical parameters. *Basic Res Cardiol* 1983;78:140–155.
621. Thompson DS, Waldron CB, Juul SM, et al. Analysis of left ventricular pressure during isovolumetric relaxation in coronary artery disease. *Circulation* 1982;65:690–697.
622. Thorburn J, Smith G, Vance JP, Brown DM. Effect of nitrous oxide on the cardiovascular system and coronary circulation of the dog. *Br J Anaesth* 1979;51:937–942.
623. Thorton JA, Fleming JS, Goldberg AD, Baird D. Cardiovascular effects of 50 percent nitrous oxide and 50 percent oxygen mixture. *Anaesthesia* 1973;28:484–489.
624. Tomoike H, Franklin D, Ross J Jr. Detection of myocardial ischemia by regional dysfunction during and after rapid pacing in conscious dogs. *Circulation* 1978;58:48–56.
625. Torrent-Guasp F. *The cardiac muscle.* Madrid: Fundacin Juan, 1973.

626. Tweed WA, Minuck M, Mymin D. Circulatory response to ketamine anesthesia. *Anesthesiology* 1972;37:613–619.
627. Tyberg JV, Keon WJ, Sonnenblick EH, Urschel CW. Mechanics of ventricular diastole. *Cardiovasc Res* 1970;4:423–428.
628. Upton MT, Gibson DG. The study of left ventricular function from digitized echocardiograms. *Prog Cardiovasc Dis* 1978;20:359–384.
629. Urthaler F, Walker AA, James TN. Comparison of the inotropic action of morphine and ketamine studied in canine cardiac muscle. *J Thorac Cardiovasc Surg* 1976;72:142–149.
630. Van der Velde ET, Burkhoff D, Steendijk P, Karsdon J, Sagawa K, Baan J. Nonlinearity and load sensitivity of end-systolic pressure-volume relation of canine left ventricle in vivo. *Circulation* 1991;83:315–327.
631. Van Trigt P, Christian CC, Fagraeus L, et al. Myocardial depression by anesthetic agents (halothane, enflurane, and nitrous oxide): quantitation based on end-systolic pressure-dimension relations. *Am J Cardiol* 1984;53:243–247.
632. Van Trigt P, Christian CC, Fagraus L, et al. The mechanism of halothane-induced myocardial depression: altered diastolic mechanics versus impaired contractility. *J Thorac Cardiovasc Surg* 1983;85:832–838.
633. Vanoverschelde JLJ, Wijns W, Essamri B, et al. Hemodynamic and mechanical determinants of myocardial O_2 consumption in normal human heart: effects of dobutamine. *Am J Physiol* 1993;265:H1884–H1892.
634. Varma SK, Owen RM, Smucker ML, Feldman MD. Is τ a preload-independent measure of isovolumetric relaxation? *Circulation* 1989;80:1757–1765.
635. Vatner DE, Vatner SF, Fujii AM, Homcy CJ. Loss of high affinity cardiac beta adrenergic receptors in dogs with heart failure. *J Clin Invest* 1985;76:2259–2264.
636. Vatner SF. Correlation between acute reductions in myocardial blood flow and function in conscious dogs. *Circ Res* 1980;47:201–207.
637. Vatner SF. Sympathetic mechanisms regulating myocardial contractility in conscious animals. In: Fozzard HA, Haber E, Jennings RB, Katz AM, Morgan HE, eds. *The heart and cardiovascular system: scientific foundations.* New York: Raven Press, 1991;1709–1728.
638. Vatner SF, Baig H, Manders WT, Ochs H, Pagani M. Effects of propranolol on regional myocardial function, electrograms and blood flow in conscious dogs with myocardial ischemia. *J Clin Invest* 1977;60:353–360.
639. Vatner SF, Braunwald E. Cardiovascular control mechanisms in the conscious state. *N Engl J Med* 1975;293:970–976.
640. Vatner SF, Rutherford JD, Ochs HR. Baroreflex and vagal mechanisms modulating left ventricular contractile responses to sympathomimetic amines in conscious dogs. *Circ Res* 1979;44:195–207.
641. Walker ML Jr, Hawthone EW, Sandler H. Methods for assessing performance for the intact hypertrophied heart. In: Alpert NR, ed. *Cardiac hypertrophy.* New York: Academic Press, 1971;387–405.
642. Wann LS, Faris JV, Childress RH, Dillon JC, Weyman AE, Feizenbaum H. Exercise cross-sectional echocardiography in ischemic heart disease. *Circulation* 1979;60:1300–1308.
643. Warltier DC, Al-Wathiqui MH, Kampine JP, Schmeling WT. Recovery of contractile function of stunned myocardium in chronically instrumented dogs is enhanced by halothane or isoflurane. *Anesthesiology* 1988;69:552–565.
644. Warltier DC, Gross GJ, Brooks HL, Preuss KC. Improvement of postischemic, contractile function by the calcium channel blocking agent nitrendipine in conscious dogs. *J Cardiovasc Pharmacol* 1988;12(suppl 4):S120–S124.
645. Warltier DC, Pagel PS. Cardiovascular and respiratory actions of desflurane: is desflurane different from isoflurane? *Anesth Analg* 1992;75:S17–S31.
646. Warren SE, Royal HD, Markis JE, Grossman W, McKay RG. Time course of left ventricular dilation after myocardial infarction: influence of infarct-related artery and success of coronary thrombolysis. *J Am Coll Cardiol* 1988;11:12–19.
647. Watanabe J, Levine MJ, Bellotto F, Johnson RG, Grossman W. Effects of coronary venous pressure on left ventricular diastolic distensibility. *Circ Res* 1990;67:923–932.
648. Waxman K, Shoemaker WC, Lippmann M. Cardiovascular effects of anesthetic induction with ketamine. *Anesth Analg* 1980;59:355–358.
649. Weber KT, Brilla CG. Pathological hypertrophy and cardiac interstitium. Fibrosis and renin-angiotensin-aldosterone system. *Circulation* 1991;83:1849–1865.
650. Weber KT, Janicki JS. Myocardial oxygen consumption: the role of wall force and shortening. *Am J Physiol* 1977;233:H421–H430.
651. Weber KT, Janicki JS. The dynamics of ventricular contraction: force, length, and shortening. *Fed Proc* 1980;39:188–195.
652. Weisfeldt ML. Reperfusion and reperfusion injury. *Clin Res* 1987;35:13–20.
653. Weisfeldt ML, Scully HE, Frederiksen J, et al. Hemodynamic determinants of maximum negative dP/dt and periods of diastole. *Am J Physiol* 1974;227:613–621.
654. Weiskopf RB, Cahalan MK, Eger EI II, et al. Cardiovascular actions of desflurane in normocarbic volunteers. *Anesth Analg* 1991;73:143–156.
655. Weiskopf RB, Holmes MA, Eger EI II, Johnson BH, Rampil IJ, Brown JG. Cardiovascular effects of I653 in swine. *Anesthesiology* 1988;69:303–309.
656. Weiss JL, Frederiksen JW, Weisfeldt ML. Hemodynamic determinants of the time course of fall in canine left ventricular pressure. *J Clin Invest* 1976;58:751–760.
657. White HD, Norris RM, Brown MA, et al. Effects of intravenous streptokinase on left ventricular function and early survival after acute myocardial infarction. *N Engl J Med* 1987;317:850–855.
658. White PF, Way WL, Trevor AJ. Ketamine — Its pharmacology and therapeutic uses. *Anesthesiology* 1982;56:119–136.
659. Wier W, Yue DT. Intracellular [Ca^{++}] transients underlying the short-term force-interval relationship in ferret ventricular myocardium. *J Physiol (Lond)* 1986;376:507–530.
660. Wiggers CJ. *Circulatory dynamics: physiologic studies.* New York: Grune & Stratton, 1952.
661. Wiggers CJ. The Henry Jackson Memorial Lecture. Dynamics of ventricular contraction under abnormal conditions. *Circulation* 1952;5:321–348.
662. Wilde DW, Knight PR, Sheth N, Williams BA. Halothane alters control of intracellular Ca^{2+} mobilization in single rat ventricular myocytes. *Anesthesiology* 1991;75:1075–1086.
663. Wildey GM, Misono KS, Graham RM. Atrial natriuretic factor: biosynthesis and mechanism of action. In: Fozzard HA, Haber E, Jennings RB, Katz AM, Morgan HE, eds. *The heart and cardiovascular system: scientific foundations.* New York: Raven Press,1991;1777–1796.
664. Williams JF Jr, Potter RD. Normal contractile state of hypertrophied myocardium after pulmonary artery constriction in the cat. *J Clin Invest* 1974;54:1266–1272.
665. Williams JF Jr, Sonnenblick EH, Braunwald E. Determinants of atrial contractile force in the intact heart. *Am J Physiol* 1965;209:1061–1068.
666. Wind BE, Snider AR, Buda AJ, O'Neill WW, Topol EJ, Dilworth LR. Pulsed Doppler assessment of left ventricular diastolic filling in coronary disease before and immediately after coronary angioplasty. *Am J Cardiol* 1987;59:1041–1046.
667. Wisenbaugh T. Does normal pump function belie muscle dysfunction in patients with chronic severe mitral regurgitation? *Circulation* 1988;77:515–525.
668. Wisenbaugh T, Booth D, DeMaria A, Nissen S, Waters J. Relationship of contractile state to ejection performance in patients with chronic aortic valve disease. *Circulation* 1986;73:47–53.
669. Wohlgelernter D, Jaffe CC, Cabin HS, Yeatman LA Jr, Cleman M. Silent ischemia during coronary occlusion produced by balloon inflation: relation to regional myocardial dysfunction. *J Am Coll Cardiol* 1987;10:491–498.
670. Wolf WJ, Neal MB, Peterson MD. The hemodynamic and cardiovascular effects of isoflurane and halothane anesthesia in children. *Anesthesiology* 1986;64:328–333.
671. Wong KC, Martin WE, Hornbein TF, Freund FG, Everett J. The cardiovascular effects of morphine sulfate with oxygen and with nitrous oxide in man. *Anesthesiology* 1973;38:542–549.
672. Wynne J, Mann T, Alpert JS, Green LH, Grossman W. Hemodynamic effects of nitrous oxide administered during cardiac catheterization. *JAMA* 1980;243:1440–1442.
673. Yellin EL, Hori M, Yoran C, Sonnenblick EH, Gabbay S, Frater RW. Left ventricular relaxation in the filling and nonfilling intact canine heart. *Am J Physiol* 1986;250:H620–H629.
674. Yock PG, Hatle L, Popp RL. Patterns and timing of Doppler-detected intracavitary and aortic flow in hypertrophic cardiomyopathy. *J Am Coll Cardiol* 1986;8:1047–1058.
675. Young MA, Hintze TH, Vatner SF. Correlation between cardiac

performance and plasma catecholamine levels in conscious dogs. *Am J Physiol* 1985;248:H82–H88.
676. Yue DT, Burkhoff D, Franz MR, Hunter WC, Sagawa K. Postextrasystolic potentiation of the isolated canine left ventricle: relationship to mechanical restitution. *Circ Res* 1985;56:340–350.
677. Zile MR, Blaustein AS, Gaasch WH. The effect of acute alterations in left ventricular afterload and beta-adrenergic tone on indices of early diastolic filling rate. *Circ Res* 1989;65:406–416.
678. Zile MR, Izzi G, Gaasch WH. Left ventricular diastolic dysfunction limits use of maximum systolic elastance as an index of contractile function. *Circulation* 1991;83:674–680.
679. Zusman RM. Eicosanoids: prostaglandins, thromboxane, and prostacyclin. In: Fozzard HA, Haber E, Jennings RB, Katz AM, Morgan HE, eds. *The heart and cardiovascular system: scientific foundations.* New York: Raven Press, 1991;1797–1815.
680. Zweier JL, Flaherty JT, Weisfeldt ML. Direct measurement of free radical generation following reperfusion of ischemic myocardium. *Proc Natl Acad Sci USA* 1987;84:1404–1407.

Anesthesia: Biologic Foundations, edited by
Tony L. Yaksh et al. Lippincott–Raven Publishers,
Philadelphia © 1997.

CHAPTER 68

THE PERIPHERAL VASCULATURE: CONTROL AND ANESTHETIC ACTIONS

THOMAS A. STEKIEL, WILLIAM J. STEKIEL,
AND ZELJKO J. BOSNJAK

HOMEOSTATIC ROLE OF THE PERIPHERAL CIRCULATION

Delivery, Exchange, and Homeostasis

The primary role of the cardiovascular system is to provide all organ and tissue systems with a volume rate of blood flow commensurate with their metabolic needs and physiologic functions. The right heart provides the motive force (i.e., longitudinal pressure gradient) and volume rate of blood flow through the pulmonary circuit necessary for normal alveolar exchange of respiratory gases and thus for maintenance of their normal arterial and venous concentrations. By simultaneously generating a significantly greater motive force the left heart provides the volume rate of blood flow necessary for nutritional maintenance and function of each organ or tissue system supplied by the systemic circulation. Thus, the peripheral systemic vasculature, together with its numerous integrated intrinsic and extrinsic control mechanisms, constitutes a highly regulated flow distribution system (Fig. 1) (242).

The blood vessels usually included in a functional (i.e., physiologic) definition of the peripheral vasculature are (a) the large and intermediate conduit arteries and veins that convey blood to and from the vascular beds of specific tissues and organ systems in response to the driving pressure generated by the heart; (b) the small arteries and arterioles primarily involved in the regulation of peripheral vascular resistance to blood flow; (c) the smallest diameter vessels (i.e., capillaries) across which the major fraction of transvascular exchange occurs between blood constituents and respective constituents within the surrounding interstitial space (i.e., nutrients, wastes, chemical messengers, water, and heat); (d) the small veins primarily involved in the regulation of the capacity of the systemic vasculature (100,128,188,189,242).

These vessels function synergistically to provide three general modes of support for the functions of specific mammalian tissue and organ systems: (a) delivery of metabolic substrates and removal of metabolic wastes; (b) delivery of humoral factors that can regulate tissue- and organ-specific functions; (c) maintenance of interstitial (and thus intracellular) physical and chemical environments. Regulated physical properties of the interstitial fluid environment include hydrostatic and osmotic pressure (hence interstitial fluid volume) and temperature. Regulated chemical factors in the interstitial environment include concentrations of those ionic and molecular constituents necessary for support of specific parenchymal functions of tissue and organ systems (in addition to metabolic support). The concept of a regulated internal fluid environ-

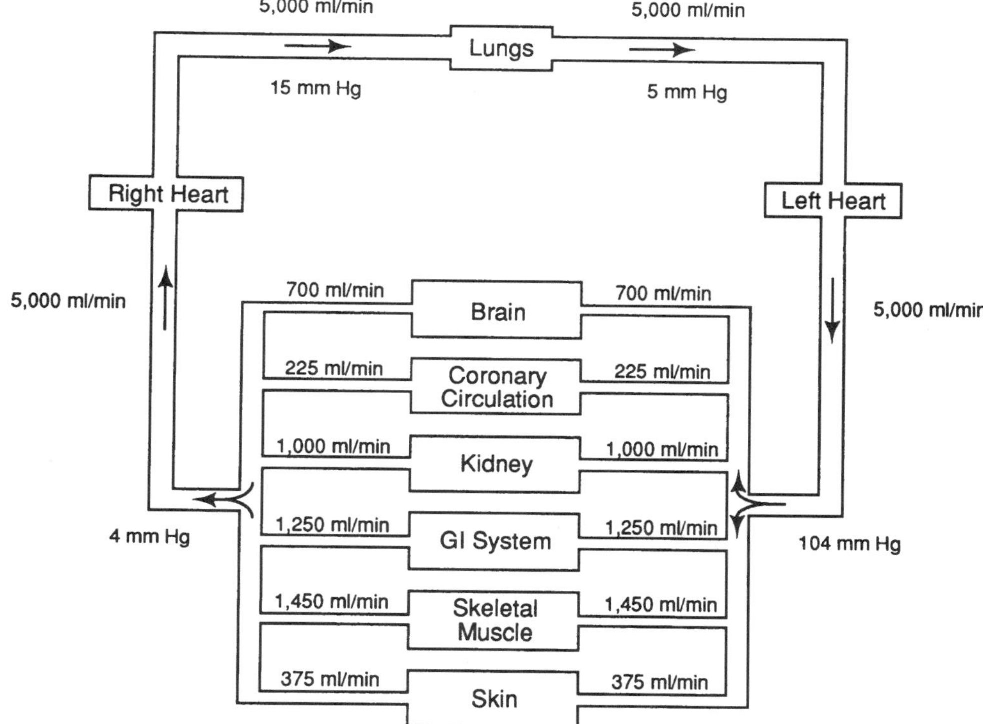

Figure 1. The distribution of resting cardiac output to various organ systems. (From ref. 242, with permission.)

ment (i.e., *milieu intérieur*) was first introduced in the 1850s by the French physiologist Claude Bernard (92). Later this concept was expanded by the American physiologist Walter B. Cannon, who postulated that the internal environment was maintained by the integrated activity of local and reflex control mechanisms. The latter are mediated by the neural, endocrine, and circulatory systems. Cannon introduced the term *homeostasis* to identify such maintenance of a state of uniformity in the body's fluid matrix (34).

STRUCTURAL COMPONENTS OF THE BLOOD VESSEL

Common Structural Characteristics of the Vascular Wall

Tunics and Endothelium

The structural characteristics of the vascular wall as a function of vessel size and location have been described in detail in several excellent reviews (55,120,137,168,197,245,250). The following comparative description summarizes the major structural components present within the walls of blood vessels as a function of their size and location within the peripheral circulation based on the studies described in these reviews. The walls of all blood vessels (including capillaries) have three major anatomical layers (i.e., tunics): the innermost tunica intima, the middle tunica media, and the outermost tunica adventitia (120,168). However, the ratio of the relative thicknesses of these tunics, as well as the content of specific cell and tissue types within each, varies with vessel size, location, and function. For example, the relative thickness of the adventitial and medial (but not the intimal) tunics decreases with distal progression and branching of arterial blood vessels. The intima of all vessels contains a single layer of apposed endothelial cells with their long axes parallel to the direction of blood flow. It also contains a thin basal lamina in most arterial vessels and a subendothelial layer composed largely of collagen and elastin fibrils in the large arteries. The media is primarily composed of smooth muscle cells. However, in the larger vessels it also contains bundles of collagenous fibrils and a network of elastic fibrils. The adventitia is the most variable of the three layers in terms of its thickness and tissue content. In all arteries and most veins it consists of dense fibroelastic tissue without smooth muscle cells. It also contains the *vasa vasorum* (i.e., the small intramural blood vessels providing a nutrient supply to the large systemic vessels with multiple layers of smooth muscle cells within the media) and the sensory and vasomotor innervation when present in the vascular wall (168).

Vessel Types

Large Arteries

The structural (i.e., anatomical) classification of the blood vessels constituting the peripheral vasculature is usually based on the relative content of elastic and muscular tissue located within the adventitial and medial tunics (Fig. 2) (168). Thus, on the arterial side of the circulation, the large-diameter vessels

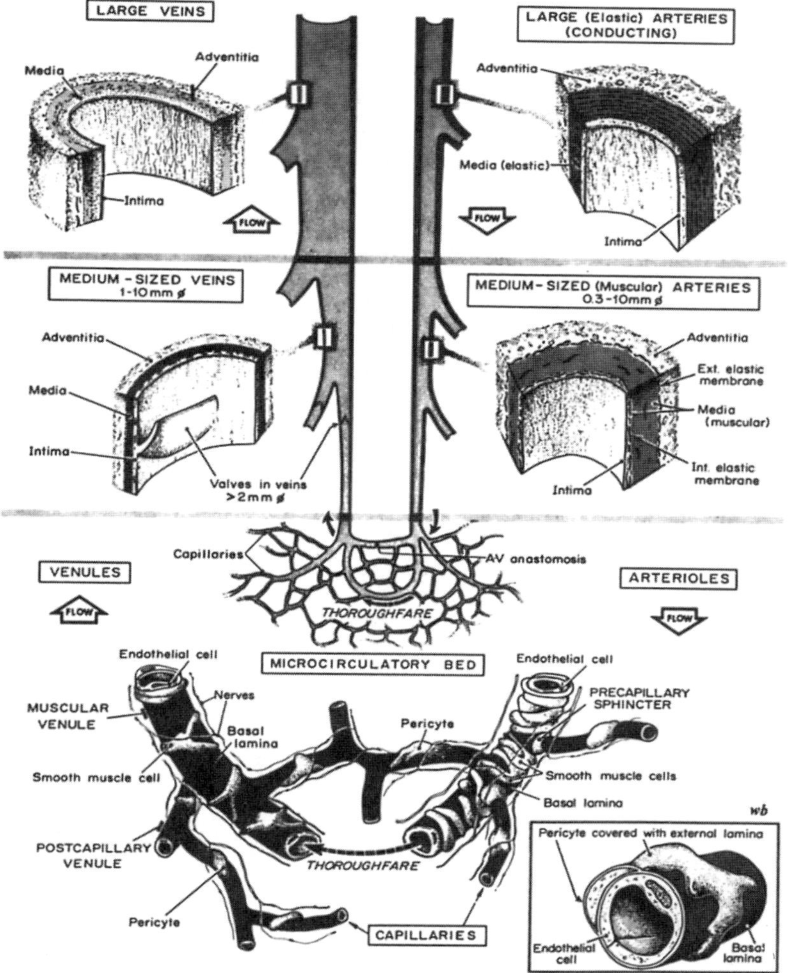

Figure 2. Schematic drawing summarizing major structural characteristics of principal segments of mammalian blood vessels, θ, diameter. (From ref. 168, with permission.)

(e.g., aorta, brachiocephalic trunk, subclavian, carotid, iliac, and pulmonary arteries) are termed *elastic* arteries. They exhibit a relatively thin adventitia. However, they contain multiple fenestrated elastic laminae interspersed among the multiple layers of smooth muscle within the media (Fig. 3) (168). Consequently, they possess a significant distensibility. This vascular parameter, which is a property of the vascular wall per se, is formally defined as the fractional increase in volume of a vascular bed (i.e., relative to its initial volume) per unit increase in transmural pressure. Its value is a function of two components of the vascular wall: (a) passive (i.e., structural), and (b) active (i.e., intrinsic and extrinsic mechanisms that regulate vascular smooth muscle [VSM] tone). Regulation of distensibility is of key hemodynamic importance for maintenance of normal cardiovascular function (see below).

Muscular Arteries

As the large arteries course peripherally, their external and internal diameters become reduced. At the diameter range between 0.3 to 10 mm, they are termed *muscular* arteries because of the increased ratio of smooth muscle to elastic tissue in the media (Fig. 4) (168). Also, the adventitial tunic is wider in these vessels compared to that in elastic arteries. Although some longitudinally oriented elastic fibers are still present in the media, the number of collagenous fibrils is increased significantly. Also, only one distinct fenestrated internal elastic lamina remains to separate the intimal from the medial layer; one less distinct elastic lamina separates the medial from the adventitial layer. The smooth muscle cells within the media are arranged in multiple concentric layers (20 to 25 layers in larger muscular arteries) and are wrapped primarily in a circular orientation around the vessel perpendicular to its long axis. Muscular arteries include such vessels as the facial, brachial, femoral, and celiac arteries.

Small Arteries

With further peripheral progression the diameters of the muscular arteries are further reduced. At a level less than 500 microns (μm), they are termed *small* arteries (137). To clarify terminology at this level of the peripheral vasculature, it is important to note that vessels smaller than 300 μm, visible only by microscopic examination, are defined as components of the *microvascular system.* In turn, the flow of blood through this system is defined as the *microcirculation* (120). The media of the small arteries contains approximately four to six layers of circularly oriented smooth muscle cells. Upon entry into the vascular bed of a particular organ or tissue system (e.g., skeletal muscle), where their diameters range from 150 to 100 μm and the media contains approximately three circular layers of smooth muscle cells, they have been termed *regional feed* arteries (250).

Arterioles

At this peripheral level the vessels branch significantly into smaller vessels termed *arterioles,* where their media contains only two layers of smooth muscle cells (30- to 100-μm diameter range) or one layer in the *terminal arterioles* (25- to 30-μm diameter range) (55,168,197,245). The internal elastic lamina is fragmented and less distinct in the small arteries and absent from most arterioles. The spindle-shaped smooth muscle cells become thinner and very elongated and for the most part each wraps concentrically and almost completely around the vessel perpendicular to its long axis. The arteriolar adventitia is very thin, containing only small bundles of longitudinally arranged collagen fibers (120,168,197).

Capillaries

At the level of the arteriole, the peripheral vasculature undergoes extensive branching in most organs and tissue systems to form vessels with the smallest diameters (4 to 8 μm inner diameter), termed true *capillaries* (120,168,197,245). In addition to their small lumen diameter (approximately the size of the mature erythrocyte), capillaries are distinguished by the structural simplicity of their walls. These consist only of an intima containing a basal lamina, a layer of endothelial cells,

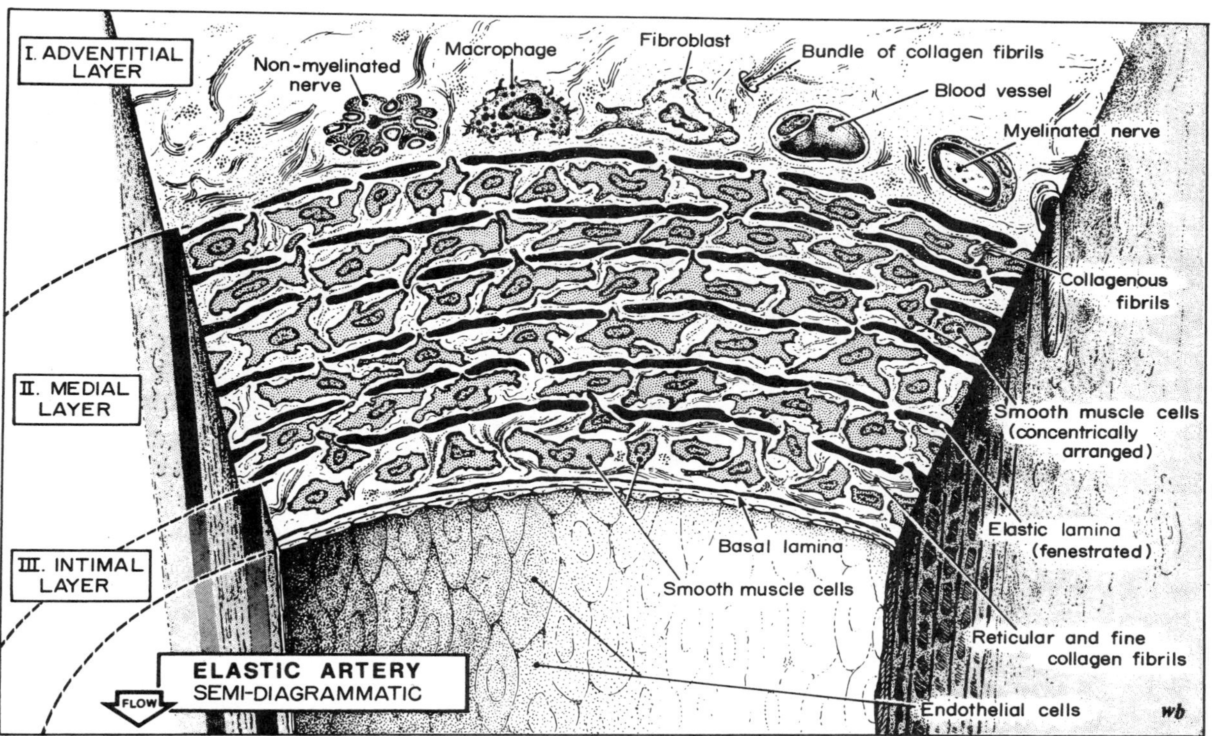

Figure 3. Schematic drawing of major components of the wall of an elastic artery illustrating multiple concentric layers of VSM cells separated by layers of elastic laminae. (From ref. 168, with permission.)

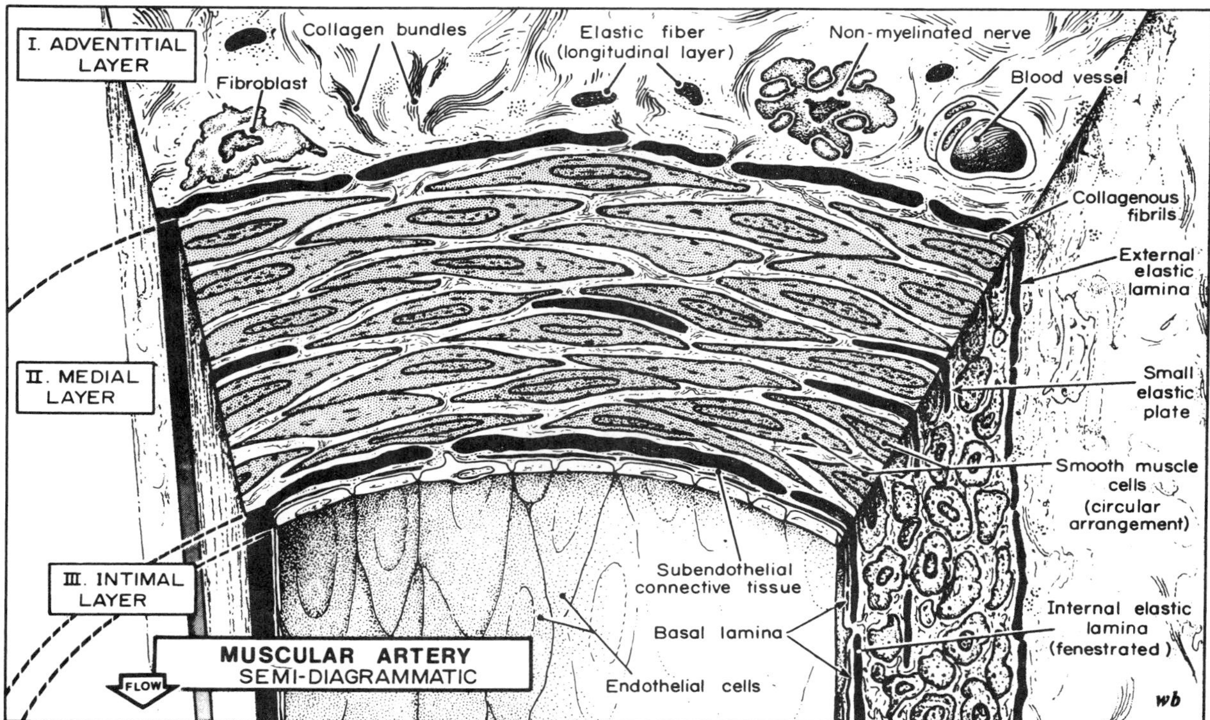

Figure 4. Schematic drawing of the major components of the wall of a muscular artery illustrating multiple layers of smooth muscle cells bordered by an external and internal (but no interspersing) elastic laminae. (From ref. 168, with permission.)

and pericytes (Rouget cells) that surround the endothelial cells at irregular intervals (Fig. 5) (120,168).

Based on the structure of their endothelial cells, capillaries can be subdivided into three categories, namely, continuous, fenestrated, and discontinuous (120,197). The first is the most common, including capillaries supplying skeletal, cardiac, and smooth muscle, and lung and brain (Fig. 5) (197). The basal lamina and endothelium are continuous (i.e., no fenestrations) and the endothelial cells contain plasmalemmal vesicles and transendothelial channels. Fenestrated capillaries (Fig. 6) are most frequently associated with secretory epithelium (e.g., intestine, thyroid gland). They are characterized by endothelial cells with a very thin cytoplasm and a relatively large population of transcellular circular openings (60 to 80 nm) or fenestrae. These span the endothelium without affecting the continuity of the plasma membrane and are usually covered by a thin heparin-proteoglycan–containing diaphragm (197). Discontinuous capillaries (or sinusoids) are found primarily in liver, spleen, and bone marrow (Fig. 7) (120). They are irregular rather than cylindrical in shape with diameters generally larger than that of a single erythrocyte. Their walls are characterized by a discontinuous basal lamina and endothelial cells with open fenestrae or gaps between them that permit large molecules and even blood cells to pass through them (120,197).

Arteriovenous Anastomoses

In addition to capillaries, short, thick-walled, parallel shunt channels (5- to 18-μm diameter) termed *arteriovenous anastomoses (AVAs)* are also present between arterioles and venules in some microvascular beds (e.g., skin of the digits, nailbeds, lips, intestinal mucosa and mesentery, liver, thyroid, erectile tissue, and aortic and carotid bodies) (4,120,197,245). The media of some AVAs contains a significant number of epithelioid cells, which function like smooth muscle cells to regulate volume flow rates through them and consequently the amount of shunting around the capillary network within an organ or tissue system. Of particular functional interest relative to mechanisms regulating blood flow through AVAs is that, like many other vessels in the peripheral circulation, their adventitia contains both myelinated and nonmyelinated nerve fibers. Known local regulators of blood flow through such shunts include local humoral agents presumably released from surrounding parenchymal cells (120).

Postcapillary Venules

The initial efferent vessels that collect blood from the capillaries upon its return to the heart are termed *pericytic postcapillary venules.* They range between 10 and 50 μm in diameter (Fig. 8) (120). The intima of these vessels is composed of thin endothelial cells and surrounding pericytes. Of special interest are the loosely organized endothelial intercellular junctions that represent the weakest endothelial contacts along the entire peripheral vasculature (120,197). These junctions are the preferred sites for extravasation and the diapedesis associated with inflammation due to their particular sensitivity to humoral agents that induce the opening of intercellular junctions (e.g., prostaglandins, histamine, serotonin, and bradykinin). Extravasation of lymphocytes is particularly evident across the wall of postcapillary venules in lymph nodes (197).

Muscular Venules

Progressing more proximally toward the heart, the intima of the postcapillary venules gradually acquires more VSM cells. At the location where these vessels acquire one or two incomplete layers of VSM cells and a sparse innervation compared to arterioles, they are termed *muscular venules* (Fig. 8) (120,168,197). Their intimal endothelial cell layer also becomes more continuous and, as in pericytic venules, the cell membranes contain high-affinity histamine receptors. Of particular functional significance is the evidence for both α and β adrenergic receptors suggesting that these vessels actively participate in the regulation of blood flow and possibly vascular capacitance. Their

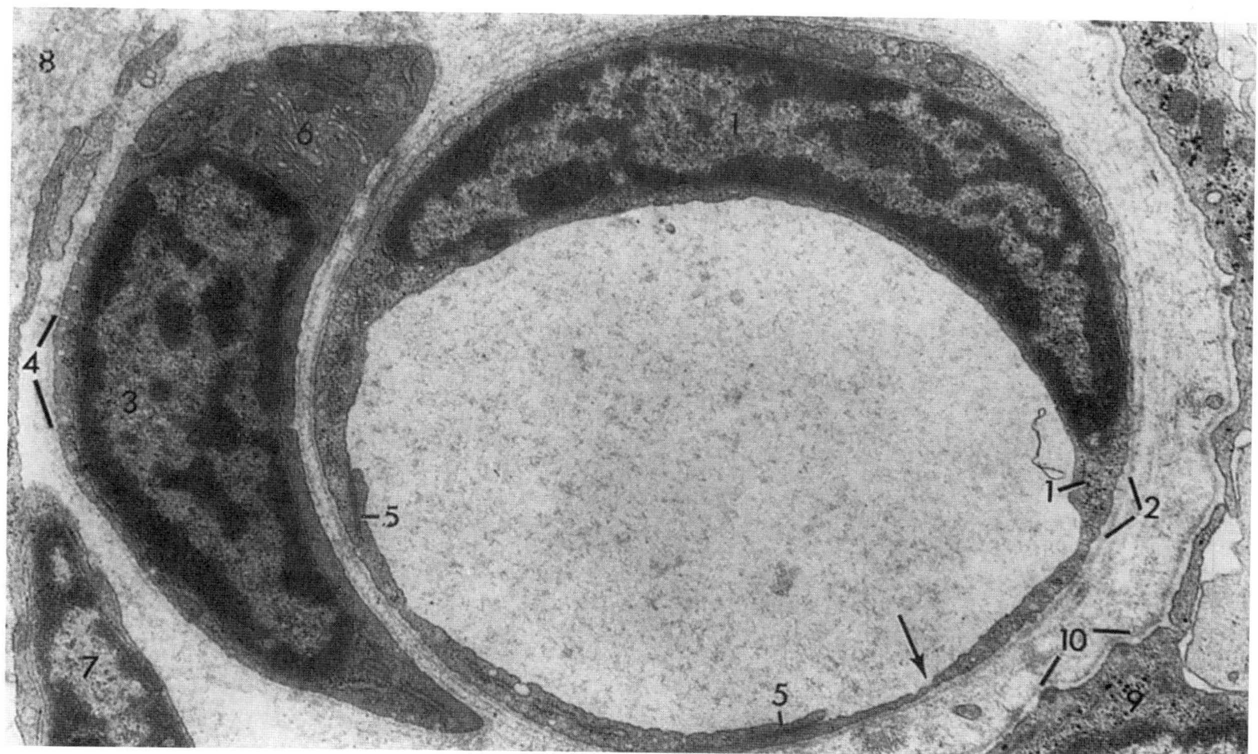

Figure 5. Cross section of the venous end of a 4.5-μm capillary in subepithelial tissue of rat ureter. *Arrow* indicates fenestration. Numbers indicate: (1) endothelial cell; (2) basal lamina; (3) pericyte; (4) external lamina; (5) endothelial cell junctions; (6) Golgi area near nucleus; (7) fibroblast on left lower side of capillary; (8) collagenous fibrils; (9) part of basal cell of transitional epithelium of ureter; (10) subepithelial space between capillary and epithelium of ureter. (From ref. 168, with permission.)

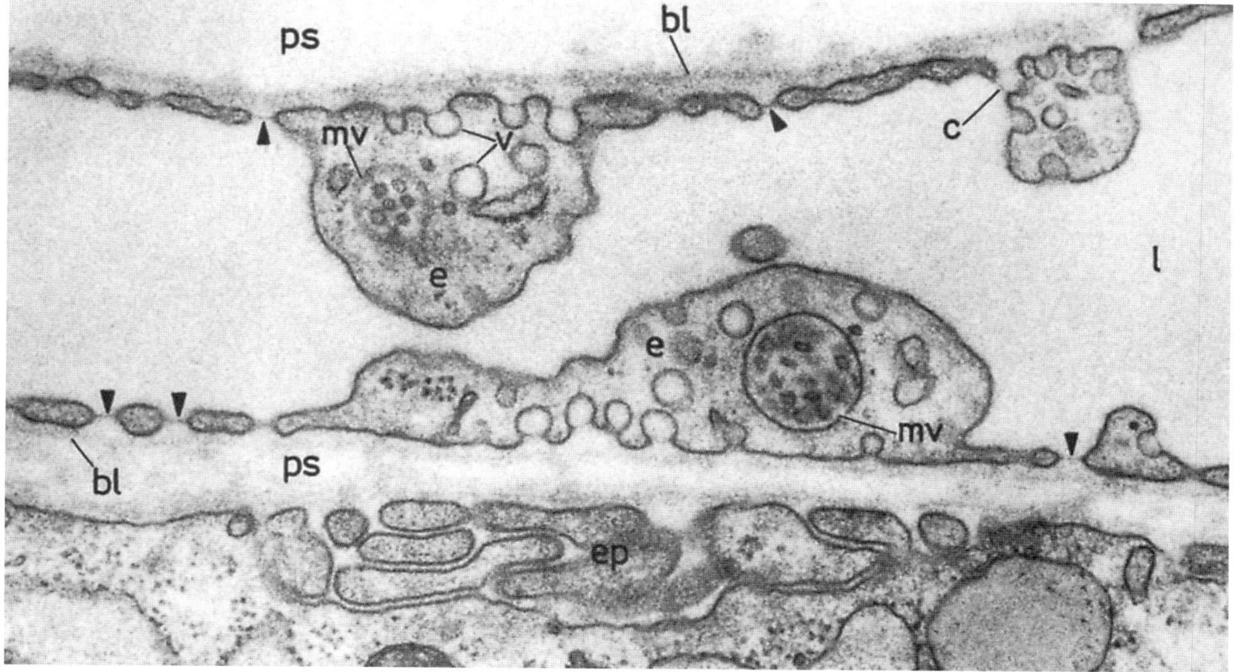

Figure 6. Fenestrated capillary (rat thyroid gland): e, endothelial cells with numerous fenestrae *(arrowheads)* closed by a thin diaphragm; bl, basal lamina; c, single vesicle transendothelial channel; ep, epithelium; l, lumen; mv, multivesicular body; ps, pericapillary space; v, plasmalemmal vesicles. (×40,000). (From ref. 168, with permission.)

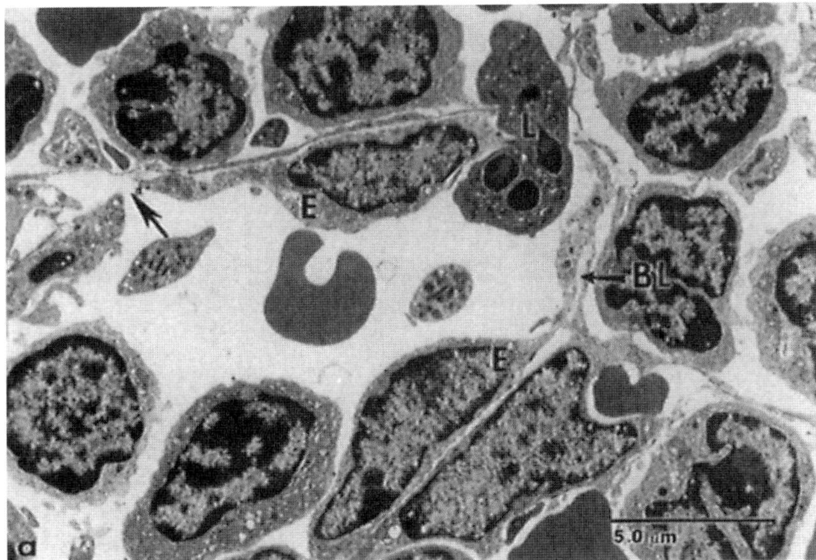

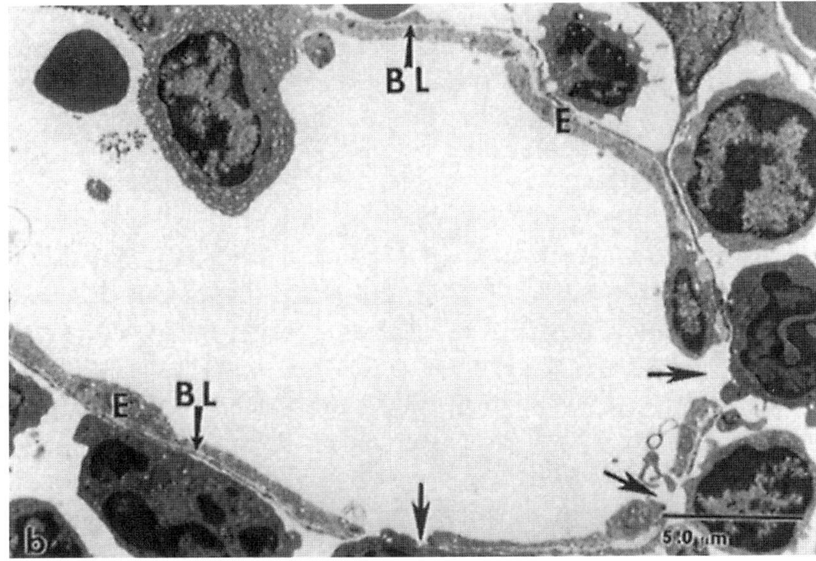

Figure 7. Two discontinuous capillaries (sinusoids) in the spleen (**a** and **b**). Note gaps *(arrows)* between adjacent endothelial cells (E) and the incomplete basal lamina (BL). In **a** note leukocyte (L) in transit through gap between endothelial cells. (From ref. 120, with permission.)

adventitia is thicker than in pericytic venules and in most vascular beds these vessels acquire an increased density of innervation (30,63,120,197).

Veins

The last two general categories of vessels on the venous side of the circulation are the *medium* and *large* veins. Compared to similar categories of vessel on the arterial side of the circulation (and usually in similar locations within a vascular bed), these veins possess relatively thin walls with a sparse content of VSM cells. As in their arterial counterparts, the walls of these vessels are usually described in terms of a tunica intima, tunica media, and tunica adventitia, although the boundaries between these divisions are not very distinct. Hence, bundles of collagenous fibers can be found interspersed among the smooth muscle cells in the medial layer as well as in the adventitial layer. In turn, depending on vessel size and location, VSM cells can be found in any of the three layers (Fig. 9) (168).

Of significant functional importance is the geometric arrangement of the VSM cells relative to the long axis of the vessel. VSM cells course through the venous wall of various veins with a wide variety of pitch angles ranging from 0° (i.e., circularly about the lumen) to 90° (i.e., parallel or longitudinally to the lumen) depending on vessel location and function. Thus, for example, in some vessels in the human, a longitudinal orientation of VSM cells predominates (e.g., veins of the thorax and abdomen), whereas circularly oriented VSM cells occupy more than 50% of the wall in leg veins (168,237). The human portal vein possesses both a strong inner circular and outer longitudinal orientation of VSM cells. In contrast, the long and short intestinal veins have a strong inner circular and weaker outer longitudinal muscle. Rhodin (168) provides an extensive description of the intramural arrangement of VSM cells in small and large veins in various vascular beds. Contraction of the longitudinally arranged VSM cells located within the adventitia contributes to the coordinated maintenance of tone in relatively long segments of veins. Functionally, such contraction, in conjunction with a network of collagen and elastin connective tissue fibers helically interspersed between the VSM cells in both the adventitia and media, contributes greatly to the support and strength of the venous wall. The architectural arrangement of these structural elements leads to the formation of a thin but resilient fibroelastic muscular tube (71), and consequently to the maintenance of vessel patency (70,168,

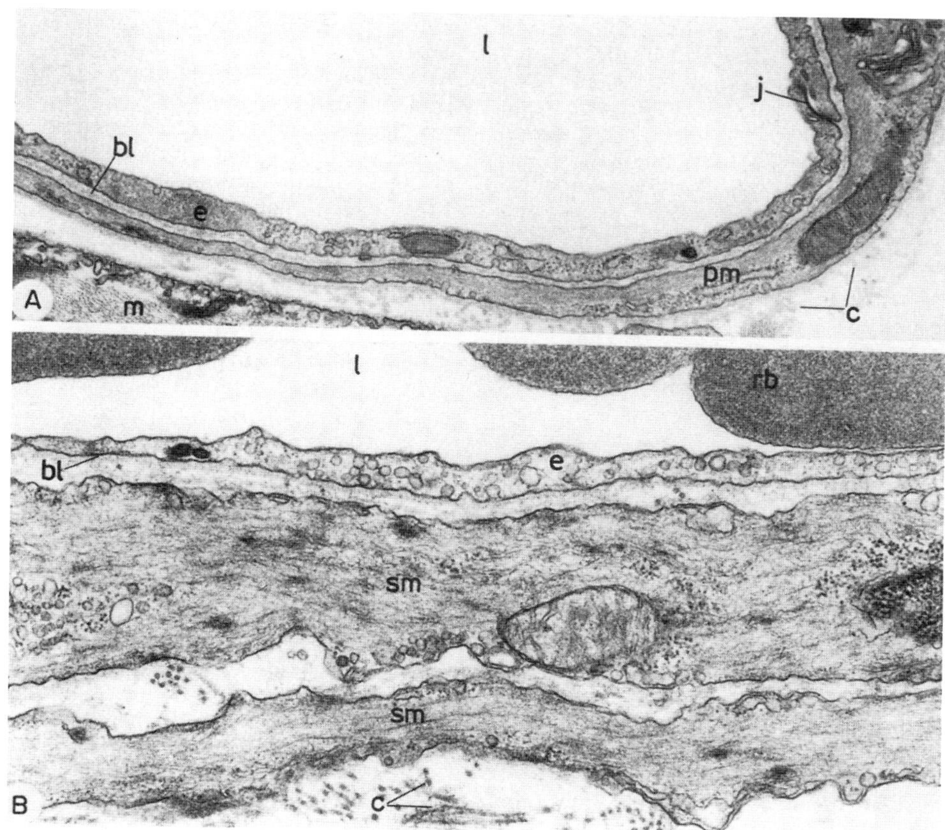

Figure 8. **(A)** Cross-section through a venule (rat diaphragm) at the transition between pericyte and muscular venule (as revealed by structural appearance of cell marked (pm), which possesses characteristics of both pericyte and VSM cell (×27,000). **(B)** Cross-section through a muscular venule (rat diaphragm) (×37,000). Note two smooth muscle cells in media (sm); bl, basal lamina; c, collagen; e, endothelium; j, intercellular junction; l, lumen; m, skeletal muscle fiber; rb, red blood cell. (From ref. 197, with permission.)

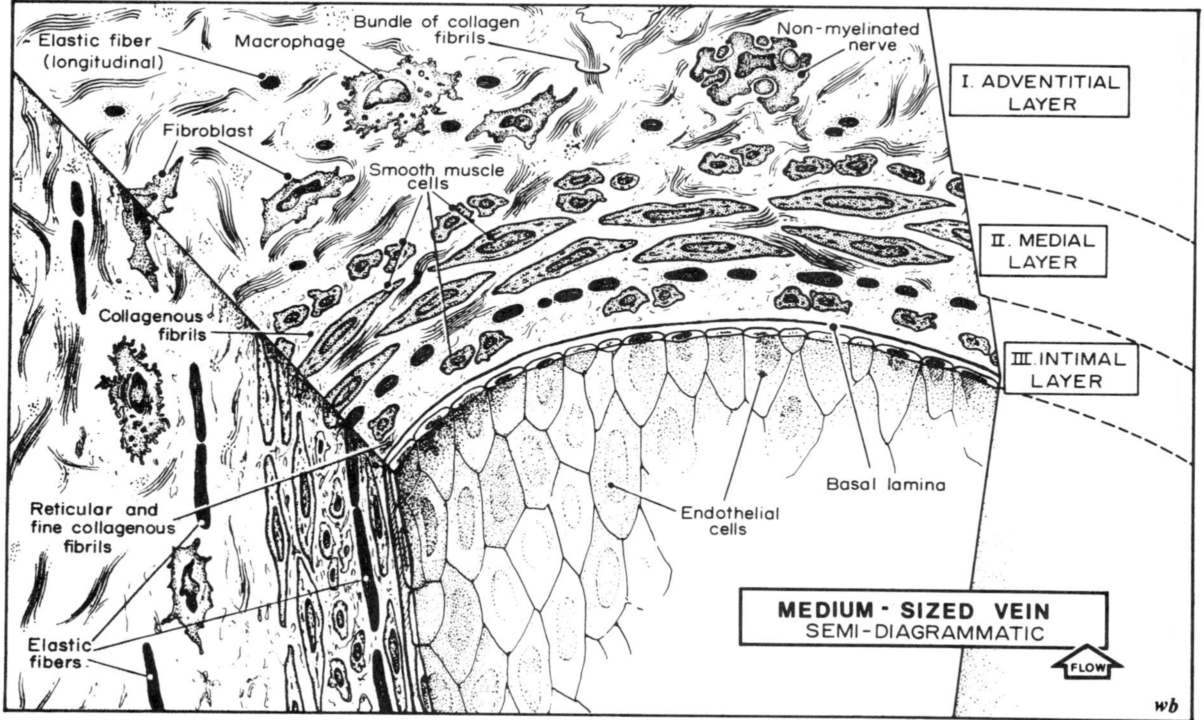

Figure 9. Schematic drawing of the major components of the wall of a medium-sized vein. Note the dispersion of VSM cells in both the medial and intimal layers and their perpendicular and parallel orientation relative to the long axis of the vessel. (From ref. 168, with permission.)

238). This occurs, for example, in long veins of the leg subjected to a continual gravitational stress and in the inferior vena cava subjected to transverse pressure of the viscera (168). As in vessels of similar size and location on the arterial of the circulation, the adventitia of small and large veins also contains two other components that are essential for both the active and passive regulation of venous wall tension. The first is the nutrient vessels of the vascular wall (i.e., the vasa vasorum composed of arterioles, venules, capillaries, and lymph vessels). The second is the innervation within the vascular wall (including both sensory afferents and vasomotor efferents) (30,120,144).

PERIPHERAL MECHANISMS FOR REGULATION OF VASCULAR SMOOTH MUSCLE TONE

Hemodynamic Regulatory Role of Peripheral Vascular Resistance

Fundamental Relationship Between Flow, Driving Pressure, and Resistance to Flow

Hemodynamically, the circulatory system obeys the same basic physical laws of fluid dynamics that govern flow of any fluid driven by a mechanical pump through a single tube or a system of tubes connected in series and in parallel. Interestingly, the concepts leading to the formulation of the hemodynamic application of this law have their origins in three of the most fundamental experimental measurements made in cardiovascular physiology, namely, the estimates of stroke volume made from casts of the ventricular chambers by William Harvey in the 17th century (88), the measurements of both blood pressure and cardiac output by Stephen Hales in the 18th century (82), and the empirical development of the relationship between flow, driving pressure and resistance to flow in small (30 to 140 μm) glass tubes by Jean Poiseuille in the 19th century (152). These and other key historical studies underlying current knowledge of the peripheral circulatory system and its control are succinctly described in an excellent review by Neil (141).

The most widely used equation to express the general relationship between volume rate of flow of blood (Q) (ml/min) through the series and/or parallel-connected vessels in a vascular bed, its hydrostatic driving force, i.e., the pressure difference or driving pressure across the bed ($P_{in} - P_{out}$) (dyne/cm^2), and the total resistance to flow through the bed (R) (peripheral resistance units [PRU] or dyne sec/cm^5) is:

$$Q = (P_{in} - P_{out})/R \quad (1)$$

This equation is analogous to Ohm's law for electrical current (I) (amperes) through a circuit of series and/or parallel-connected wires, electrical driving force, i.e., voltage difference (V_1 - V_2) (volts), and resistance to flow of electrons (R) (ohms). For the condition where flow is approximately steady (i.e., nonpulsatile) and laminar (i.e., nonturbulent), resistance to flow through a single blood vessel is directly proportional to blood viscosity (η), cylindrical vessel geometry ($8/\pi$), and vessel length (L). It is inversely proportional to the fourth power of vessel radius (r^4). This relationship was first established empirically by Poiseuille and later derived theoretically by others (131). Thus, under these conditions:

$$Q = (P_{in} - P_{out})/R = \pi r^4 (P_{in} - P_{out})/8\eta L \quad (2)$$

where

$$R = 8\eta L/\pi r^4 \quad (3)$$

Equations 2 and 3 express Poiseuille's law. These equations indicate that vascular resistance to flow is inversely proportional to the fourth power of internal radius. Thus, under a constant driving pressure the most effective controller of vascular resistance to flow through a single vessel is its internal radius. Since we can assume that each blood vessel segment within a vascular bed obeys Poiseuille's law, the same will be true for total flow through the bed. Thus, it is clear from this equation that flow resistance across a specific vascular bed is regulated primarily by two mechanisms: (a) passive distention or collapse of smaller arterial blood vessels in response to changes in their transmural pressure; (b) active regulation of VSM tone and hence diameter of these vessels by both extrinsic (e.g., neural, humoral, and metabolic) and intrinsic (e.g., myogenic, autocrine, and endothelial) mechanisms.

Poiseuille's law can also be applied to the total systemic circulation with flow defined as cardiac output (CO), driving pressure defined as the difference between mean arterial pressure (MAP) and right atrial pressure (RAP), and resistance to flow defined as total peripheral resistance (TPR):

$$CO = (MAP - RAP)/TPR \quad (4)$$

This equation has been used extensively in experimental and clinical medicine to calculate changes in TPR from direct measurements of CO, arterial pressure, and central venous pressure (assumed to be equal to RAP). The major site of TPR is on the arterial side of the systemic circulation. This is due primarily to a disproportionately large contribution made by the smaller and less distensible arterial vessels and by the inverse proportionality to the fourth power of their radii (Eq. 3). In addition, arterial vessels possess greater levels of VSM tone than veins at the same level of the peripheral circulation. The majority of the peripheral vascular beds of organ systems supplied by the systemic circulation are connected in parallel. Thus:

$$1/TPR = 1/R_1 + 1/R_2 + 1/R_3 + 1/R_n \quad (5)$$

where $R_{1 \to n}$ represent flow resistances of specific vascular beds. From Equation 5 it can be seen that each resistance of a specific vascular bed is larger than TPR and also varies inversely with the number of parallel vessels within the bed. Also, since larger animals have a greater number of vessels connected in parallel in each vascular bed, resistance to flow in specific vascular beds is inversely proportional to animal size. This is illustrated in Table 1 (129).

Physiologic Applications of Poiseuille's Law

Changes in flow resistance across specific vascular beds (calculated from measured total blood flows through them and pressure differences across them) can be used to identify vascular sites and pathologic changes in the mechanisms of control of blood flow that may be involved in various cardiovascular diseases. For example, an increase in calculated resistance across specific vascular beds in the absence of VSM tone provides indirect evidence for a contribution from structural changes (e.g., vessel number density and wall thickness) to the development and /or maintenance of various forms of hypertension (64,136,137,155). In addition, changes of calculated resistance across specific vascular beds in the presence of specific blockers of neural, humoral, endothelial, and intrinsic vascular mechanisms involved in the regulation of VSM tone have helped establish the relative importance of alterations of these regulatory mechanisms in the etiology of various cardiovascular

Table 1. TYPICAL VASCULAR RESISTANCES UNDER BASAL CONDITIONS[a]

Vascular bed	Dog (20 kg)	Man (70 kg)
Pulmonary	320	80
Systemic	4200	1150
Renal (both kidneys)	14,600	5,800
Cerebral	23,400	9,300

[a]Dyn sec/cm^5. (From ref. 129 with permission.)

diseases (e.g., essential hypertension, congestive heart failure, and arteriosclerosis) (64,132,137). Finally, changes in calculated resistance of specific vascular beds have also been used extensively to clarify hemodynamic mechanisms and cardiovascular sites of action of anesthetics (see below).

Physiologic Limitations of Poiseuille's Law

It is important to emphasize that by virtue of the assumptions made in their derivation, the applicability of the above equations for analysis of hemodynamic properties of the cardiovascular system is subject to certain limitations. For example, they are valid only for steady-state or mean values of flow and pressure. Hence, calculated TPR and resistances across specific vascular beds are fair approximations of the ratio of mean pressure difference to mean flow derived from actual pulsatile values. When calculated from pulsatile (i.e., time varying) changes in pressure and flow, this ratio is termed *vascular impedance* and is calculated from an equation requiring knowledge of pulse frequency and vascular distensibility (129).

The requirement for a rigid system is another condition that is not strictly met (thus leading to approximation of calculated variables) when Poiseuille's law is applied to the cardiovascular system. This results in an error in calculated flow resistance that is directly proportional to the compliance of the vascular components within a specific vascular bed. Also, since components of the vascular system possess finite compliances, it must be recognized that changes in vascular resistance are also a function of transmural pressure.

Hemodynamic Regulatory Role of Blood Volume and Vascular Capacity

Mean Circulatory Filling Pressure and Venous Return

In addition to flow resistance, blood volume and vascular capacity are two other closely associated peripheral vascular parameters involved in the regulation of cardiac output and arterial pressure. The effects of these two parameters on these hemodynamic variables are not taken into account in Equation 4 above for circulatory systems composed of rigid tubes. To understand the hemodynamic regulatory role of these two parameters it is necessary first to understand the concept of mean circulatory filling pressure (MCFP), developed by Guyton and colleagues (76,78), and now classically utilized to explain the effect of preload and afterload on cardiac output (9,77).

By definition, MCFP is the equilibrium pressure that is reached throughout the vascular system (before intervention by cardiovascular reflexes or fluid shift through the capillaries) when the pumping action of the heart is temporarily suspended and blood is rapidly transferred from the arterial to the venous side of the circulation. Measurements by Guyton and colleagues (79) indicate that such equilibrium pressure equals 7 mm Hg and is reached within 5 to 7 seconds in the anesthetized dog with a normal blood volume. Since MCFP is a measure of the degree of filling of the circulation, it is directly proportional to intravascular blood volume and inversely proportional to vascular capacity. The latter, in turn, is directly proportional to passive wall compliance and inversely proportional to VSM tone. Conceptually, it is of key importance to understand that MCFP is the average filling pressure throughout the circulatory system. Hence, under normal conditions with the heart pumping and right atrial pressure (RAP) at approximately 0 mm Hg, the driving force (i.e., pressure gradient) for return of blood from the peripheral circulation to the right atrium is proportional to MCFP. In general, venous return (VR) is directly proportional to the difference between MCFP and RAP and inversely proportional to the resistance to venous return (RVR). This relationship can be expressed mathematically in equation form similar to Equation 4 for cardiac output:

$$VR = (MCFP - RAP)/RVR \qquad (6)$$

Experimental evidence in support of Equation 6 has been obtained by Guyton and colleagues (76,78,79).

Under steady-state conditions CO is equal to VR and RAP is close to 0 mm Hg due primarily to the cardiac length-tension response (i.e., Starling's law of the heart) and ventricular volume receptor-initiated reflexes. Consequently, under normal limits of pumping by the heart and under constant peripheral resistance and vascular compliance, CO and MAP are directly proportional to MCFP and thus to blood volume. This relationship is of special significance clinically, since it is part of the rationale for blood infusion to maintain MAP during surgical stress and blood loss.

Equally important is that under normal limits of cardiac performance, MCFP, and thus CO and MAP, are inversely proportional to vascular capacity. Since approximately 70% of the systemic blood volume resides on the highly compliant venous side of the circulation, veins are major regulators of vascular capacity (72,73,80,81,172–175,189–191). Thus, passive (e.g., structural) and active (e.g., VSM tone regulating) mechanisms that modulate venous compliance and hence venous capacity are as important as passive and active mechanisms that regulate peripheral resistance in the maintenance of cardiovascular homeostasis.

Extrinsic Regulation of Peripheral Vascular Tone

Neural Regulation of VSM Contractile Force

Neural, humoral, intrinsic transmural, and endothelial cell mechanisms all contribute to the active regulation of VSM tone in both pre- and postcapillary blood vessels. The classical concept of the peripheral neural mechanism underlying control of VSM tone primarily in the resistance vessels, a theory that prevailed for approximately 50 years, was that an antagonistic action exists between the vasoconstrictor catecholamine, norepinephrine (NE), which is released from the postganglionic sympathetic efferent motoneuron, and the vasodilator, acetylcholine (ACh), released from the postganglionic parasympathetic motoneuron. However, over the past three decades our knowledge of the neuroeffector mechanisms involved in the control of VSM tone in the peripheral vasculature has advanced significantly. Of major importance are the initial seminal studies concerning the structure of the autonomic neuroeffector junction (32) and the concept of cotransmission, i.e., that nerves synthesize, store, and release more than one transmitter at the vascular neuroeffector junction (27,29). The proposed mechanisms of vascular neuromuscular transmission derived from these initial studies have been corroborated and continue to be expanded through additional studies by these investigators and others. The latter are described in several reviews and monographs (28,31,91, 130,142,161,167,188).

Specific functions of sympathetic, parasympathetic, and sensorimotor branches of intrinsic nerves have been identified in particular vascular beds (28,30,31,130,161). A major component of the perivascular nerve plexus is the motor innervation originating in the sympathetic nervous system. Tonic sympathetic neural activity originates in central cardiovascular control centers in the brainstem and in more rostral regions and travels via axons that project to cells in the intermediolateral gray matter in the spinal cord. Neuronal cells in this region send myelinated preganglionic axons to synapse with postganglionic cells within the paravertebral ganglia that form the sympathetic neural chains. Unmyelinated postganglionic axons travel to blood vessels where they form a series of "*en passage*" synapses with VSM fibers. In large vessels these synapses occur at both the adventitial-medial junction and within the media of the vascular wall, whereas in smaller vessels they occur primarily at the adventitial-medial junction. VSM cells within the inner layers of the media (distant from the innervation) are activated

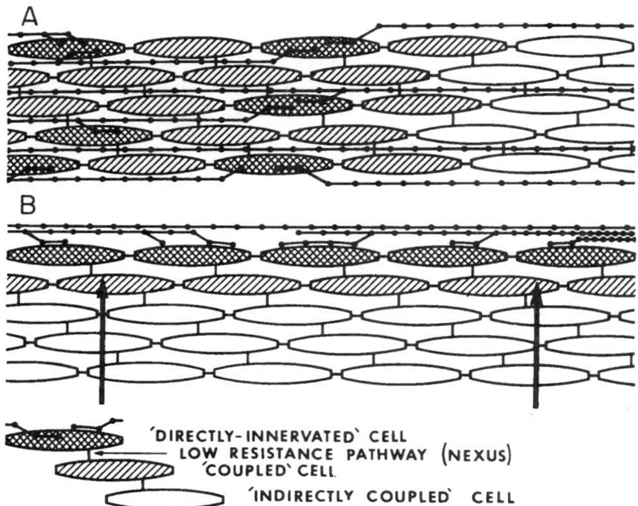

Figure 10. Schematic diagram of **(A)** interspersed innervation among SM cells in visceral organs and VSM fibers in multilayered large arteries; **(B)** innervation primarily in adventitia of small arteries, arterioles, and veins. *Connected dots* represent varicosities in nerves; *arrows,* circulating catecholamines. (From ref. 28, with permission.)

electrically via low-resistance pathways (Fig. 10) (28). In contrast to the sympathetic nervous system, preganglionic fibers of the parasympathetic nervous system originate in cell bodies located in several nuclei within the brainstem and in sacral segments of the spinal cord. These fibers are considerably longer than the postganglionic fibers since the cell bodies of the latter are in ganglia close to or within the tissues that they innervate. In general the distribution of parasympathetic nerves in the cardiovascular system is less extensive than that of sympathetic nerves. When present, it is most prominent in cerebral and genital blood vessels where it exerts a vasodilatory action. However, many blood vessels do not receive any parasympathetic innervation (130,161). The magnitude of the effect of transmitted nerve activity on vascular tone in any particular tissue is a function of the differential distribution of nerve fibers (50). Perivascular nerves exist in both large and small vessels on the arterial side of the circulation extending even to microvessels as small as 20 μm outer diameter (67). On the venous side of the circulation microvessels are not innervated (63).

Each nerve fiber within the perivascular plexus consists of a series of varicosities that contain neurotransmitters stored in discrete intracellular vesicles. Depolarization of the autonomic postganglionic motoneuron leads to opening of voltage-operated "N type" calcium channels in the plasmalemmal membrane and movement of extracellular Ca^{2+} into the nerve fiber cytoplasm (252). The elevated cytoplasmic Ca^{2+} concentration leads to release of vesicles from cytoplasmic binding sites and their movement to active "docking" sites on the intracellular side of the plasmalemmal membrane. Upon docking, neurotransmitter is released from the vesicles that open to the extracellular space between nerve and muscle fiber membranes. The nature of the protein components and biophysical mechanisms involved in the intracellular Ca^{2+}-dependent release and docking of the vesicles and the question concerning the relation between nerve fiber activity and the amount of neurotransmitter released from each vesicle per motor axon action potential is currently a subject of intense investigation (3,5, 102,205,223,235,252).

Released neurotransmitter diffuses passively across the junctional cleft to combine with specific receptors on the VSM cell membrane. Unlike the narrow cleft width between the presynaptic nerve terminal and end plate at the skeletal neuromuscular junction (20 to 40 nm), the width of the cleft at the VSM neuroeffector junction varies between 60 nm and up to 2 μm and is proportional to the diameter of the vessel (11). Also the postjunctional VSM membrane does not have specialized structures opposite the prejunctional varicosities in contrast to the apposition of the end plate to prejunctional membrane active zones in the skeletal neuromuscular junction (31). Depending on the neurotransmitter and the specific VSM receptor activated by it, either an increase or decrease in VSM contractile force (i.e., VSM tone) can be generated in proportion to the respective increase or decrease that occurs in the concentration of intracellular free Ca^{2+} and/or the sensitivity of the VSM myofilaments (146,231).

Neurotransmitters Involved in the Regulation of VSM Contractile Force

The concept that neurons release a single neurotransmitter was considered as doctrine and dominated thinking for approximately 40 years. In a recent review on the functions of cotransmission Kupfermann (107) states that this concept was inferred, but not explicitly stated, by Dale (41) and popularized as "Dale's Principle" by Eccles (52). However, as stated above, beginning with the early studies by Burn and Rand (27) and especially by Burnstock (28,29), evidence in favor of release of two or more bioactive substances from a single neuron continues to accumulate (31,107,161,163). Table 2(31) is a current list of monoamines, purines, amino acids, and polypeptides that are released, along with nitric oxide, from perivascular nerves as either established or putative neurotransmitters.

A general principle that is emerging from studies of the function of these agents is that autonomic nerves possess a "chemical coding." This implies that individual neurons contain a specific combination of transmitter substances, have axons that project to identifiable target sites, and have defined central connections (31,107).

A demonstration of this principle is the cotransmission involving the adrenergic neurotransmitter NE and the purinergic neurotransmitter adenosine triphosphate (ATP), which produce synergistic vasodilation via β-adrenoceptors and P_{2y} purinoreceptors, respectively (39). Also of experimental interest is that the purinergic component responds optimally to short bursts of sympathetic nerve stimulation (1 s or less), whereas the adrenergic component dominates the vasoconstriction during long periods of stimulation (30 s or more)(103). Neuromodulation is another physiologically important function of cotransmitters.

Table 2. ESTABLISHED AND PUTATIVE TRANSMITTERS: PERIVASCULAR NERVES

Noradrenaline (NA)
Acetylcholine (ACh)
Adenosine 5′-triphosphate (ATP)
5-Hydroxytryptamine (5-HT)
Dopamine (DA)
Enkephalin-dynorphin (ENK-DYN)
Vasoactive intestinal polypeptide (VIP)
Peptide histidine isoleucine (PHI)
Substance P (SP)
Gastrin-releasing peptide (GRP)
Somatostatin (SOM)
Neurotensin (NT)
Vasopressin (VP)
Cholecystokinin-gastrin (CCK-GAS)
Neuropeptide Y and pancreatic polypeptide (NPY-PPP)
Galanin (GAL)
Angiotensin (ANG)
Adrenocorticotrophic hormone (ACH)
Calcitonin gene-related peptide (CGRP)
Nitric oxide (NO)

From ref. 31.

This is exemplified by neuropeptide Y (NPY) that is stored and released from sympathetic motor axons. NPY acts presynaptically to reduce release of NE and ATP and postsynaptically to enhance the actions of both of these cotransmitters (31,219).

Parasympathetic perivascular innervation composed of cholinergic vasodilator motor axons has been well established for cerebral and genital organ blood vessels and possibly for small coronary vessels within the heart and within the GI tract, salivary glands, uterus, and pulmonary vascular bed (45,130). However, not all vasodilation is mediated by ACh released from cholinergic motor axons. Another category of perivascular nerves that mediate vasoconstriction or vasodilation is the nonadrenergic noncholinergic (NANC) group of motor axons whose neurotransmitters do not include either NE or ACh. In some organs (e.g., heart) these axons arise from intrinsic ganglia and project to blood vessels within the parenchyma (31). Putative neurotransmitters in the NANC category include vasoactive intestinal polypeptide (VIP) (a known potent vasodilator of many vessels in the sacral region, notably penile vessels) (161), serotonin (vasoconstrictor of coronary vessels) (161), substance P (SP), and calcitonin gene-related peptide (CGRP) (cerebral vasodilator) (53,119), and SP and CGRP (sensorimotor perivascular nerves) (31,69,161).

Nitroxidergic Neurons

Most recently an additional group of NANC neurons that also regulate the vasculature has been identified. These neurons appear to release de novo synthesized nitric oxide (NO) as their neurotransmitter and have been termed *nitroxidergic* neurons by Toda and Okamura (227) and *nitrergic* by Rand et al. (162,164). NO released as neurotransmitter may act at both membrane and intracellular sites to produce VSM relaxation (95). NO is known to hyperpolarize the cell membrane at higher concentrations (162,164). Such hyperpolarization, which may result from activation of potassium (K) channels (110,123), may lead to closure of voltage-dependent VSM plasmalemmal membrane Ca channels. Consequently, intracellular free Ca^{2+} activity ($[Ca^{2+}]_i$) may be reduced below the threshold concentration (approximately 10^{-7} M) necessary for generation of contractile force via actin-myosin bridge formation. Bridge formation results from myosin phosphorylation by myosin light chain kinase, which in turn is activated by an intracellular Ca-calmodulin complex (138) (also see Intrinsic Regulation of Peripheral Vascular Tone, below). NO may also diffuse through the VSM cell membrane and directly activate soluble guanylyl cyclase to produce cyclic guanosine monophosphate (cGMP). Cyclic GMP, in turn, activates a cGMP- dependent protein kinase that causes VSM relaxation by mechanisms as yet not well understood. One is a proposed reduction of intracellular free Ca^{2+} by activation of the Ca pump in the VSM sarcoplasmic reticulum (110), while Ca^{2+} elimination may also be activated by enhanced Na/Ca exchanger activity (65). Another is a proposed reduction in sensitivity of contractile proteins to increases in $[Ca^{2+}]_i$ (121,146,147).

Nitroxidergic neurons similar to those originally described in the CNS (95,204) have now been identified in the mesenteric and other vascular beds (236,248). They coexist with adrenergic nerves and can be identified by a vasodilator response to perivascular nerve stimulation following depletion of norepinephrine neurotransmitter from sympathetic motor axon varicosities by 6-hydroxydopamine and in the presence of cholinergic receptor blockade. As with adrenergic neurons, they are blocked by exogenously applied tetrodotoxin and hexamethonium (225,227). It has been proposed that the function of these neurons is to provide a means to reciprocally balance the vasoconstrictor tone produced by adrenergic neurons in the overall neural regulation of VSM tone. Furthermore, an imbalance in this reciprocal function has been proposed as a possible pathogenesis of certain disease conditions such as hypertension (226). Good evidence now supports the existence of these neurons and they fit well into a hypothetical reciprocal regulatory scheme. However, the relative contribution that they make to the overall regulation of VSM tone (compared with the sympathetic neural input) remains to be demonstrated.

Humoral Regulation of VSM Contractile Force

The net effect of a circulating vasoactive humoral agent (released from a specific endocrine gland or organ or cell system) on VSM tone in a specific vascular bed is dependent on multiple factors. Of key importance are (a) the local intravascular concentration of the humoral agent; (b) the humoral agent's affinity for specific receptors in the VSM cell plasmalemmal membrane; (c) the surface densities of specific receptors activated by the humoral agent in the VSM cell plasmalemmal membrane; and (d) the surface densities of specific ion channels in the VSM plasmalemmal membrane that are opened or closed by the humoral agent when acting either directly or via the receptor and a cascade of membrane-bound and intracellular second messengers.

Adrenal Medullary Catecholamines

The classic example of endocrine regulation of VSM tone is the adrenal medullary release of the catecholamines, NE, and epinephrine (Epi) (77,130). The adrenal medullary chromaffin cells are analogous to the sympathetic postganglionic neurons whose soma are in the paravertebral ganglia. Both release NE upon activation (i.e., depolarization) by ACh neurotransmitter released from respective activated sympathetic preganglionic neurons. However, upon activation, the adrenal medullary chromaffin cells also secrete Epi into the circulation in a concentration ratio averaging 80% Epi to 20% NE (but also dependent on the nature of the stimulus) (77). The NE and Epi released by the adrenal medulla and the NE released as neurotransmitter act in concert as the *sympathoadrenal system*. Circulating Epi is released from the adrenal medulla in response to a wide variety of external and internal physiologic stimuli (e.g., exercise), as well as pathophysiologic stimuli (e.g., hypoxia, emotional stress, hemorrhage, etc.). It produces β–adrenergic receptor-mediated positive chronotropic and inotropic cardiac responses coupled with α-adrenergic receptor-mediated increases and β-adrenergic receptor-mediated decreases in VSM tone in order to maintain adequate driving pressures and perfusion rates to sustain normal function of vital organs. Even a moderate elevation of the plasma level of Epi from a resting plasma level of 30 picograms (pg)/ml to a range of 50 to 100 pg/ml is sufficient to cause a significant increase in heart rate and arterial pressure. Epi thus acts as a cardiovascular-regulating hormone under both physiologic and pathophysiologic conditions (40,130). On the other hand, the normal plasma concentration of NE (200 pg/ml in supine humans) must be elevated approximately sevenfold to produce hemodynamic effects (40,130). This occurs during strenuous exercise or under pathophysiologic conditions such as hemorrhagic hypotension. Thus, humoral NE does not participate significantly in circulatory control under basal conditions (130,195).

Due to the variety of mechanisms involved in the humoral regulation of vasomotor tone, it is not surprising that the net effect of Epi on VSM tone differs in various vascular beds. Since activation of α-adrenergic receptors leads to increased VSM tone, whereas the opposite is true for activation of β-adrenergic receptors, and since Epi exhibits different affinities for α- and β-adrenergic receptors in VSM cell membranes of blood vessels in different vascular beds, its net effect on VSM contractile force results from the algebraic summation of these responses. For example, the arterioles in cutaneous and renal beds constrict, but those in skeletal muscle and the splanchnic bed dilate in response to Epi. Thus, with moderate increases in circulating plasma levels of Epi, total peripheral resistance falls but mean blood pressure rises moderately due to the increase in cardiac output coupled with the attenuating effect of baroreflexes.

The affinity of circulating NE for β-adrenergic receptors is lower than that of Epi, but is equal to that of Epi for α-adrenergic receptors. Consequently, when circulating concentrations of NE are sufficiently elevated (>1500 pg/ml), an elevated TPR, resulting from a generalized vasoconstriction, predominates over an elevated CO. Hence, a rise in mean and systolic pressure results primarily from a rise in diastolic pressure (130) (see also Eq. 4 above).

Renin-Angiotensin System

The vasoactive substances produced by the renin-angiotensin (RA) system in the kidney are considered to be endocrine agents when released into the circulation to modulate VSM tone in nonrenal blood vessels. These substances are classified as *autocrine* agents when modulating tone in intrarenal vessels since, by definition, autocrine control occurs when a substance elaborated by a cell regulates the function of that cell. The renal RA system consists of a set of substrates and enzymes that participate in a cascade of steps to produce the octapeptide angiotensin II (AII), a potent vasoconstrictor, as well as additional smaller peptides exhibiting vasodilator activity (61). The initial report of the existence of this system was made by Tigerstedt and Bergman (224), who demonstrated a hypertensive effect of a saline extract of a rabbit kidney when injected into a second rabbit. The active component in the saline extract of rabbit kidney was named renin and later shown to be an enzyme that catalyzes the formation of a secondary pressor substance (105). The latter was isolated independently from kidney tissue by two groups of investigators (19,149) and eventually given the name *angiotensin*. Classically, it has been established that renin is secreted by the granular cells within the walls of the afferent and efferent arterioles that supply the kidney glomerulus. These cells, together with the contiguous macula densa cells of the thick ascending limb of the nephron tubule and the extraglomerular mesangial cells, form the *juxtaglomerular apparatus*. This apparatus is one component of the tubuloglomerular feedback mechanism that is involved in the autoregulation of renal blood flow and glomerular filtration rate. Such autoregulation is essential for regulation of both extracellular and intravascular volumes and, hence, arterial blood pressure (according to Equations 4 and 6 above). Known stimuli for renal renin release include (a) reduction of extracellular and vascular fluid volumes (via diminished activity of low- and high-pressure volume receptors, consequent reduction of depressor reflex afferent input to the CNS, and consequent increase in renal sympathetic nerve activity to the granular cells); (b) decreases in afferent arteriole perfusion pressure (as occurs in any pathophysiologic state that results in a reduction of arterial blood pressure, e.g., loss of blood volume and/or increase in vascular capacity, cardiac failure); (c) decreased delivery of NaCl to the macula densa (one of the mechanisms involved in the conservation of body Na^+ and maintenance of extracellular and intravascular volumes). Renin cleaves angiotensinogen (a circulating peptide produced by the liver) into a relatively inert 10 amino acid peptide (angiotensin I)(AI). AI, in turn, is cleaved to the 8 amino acid peptide AII in the lung by angiotensin converting enzyme (ACE).

Four major physiologic functions of circulating AII are (a) retention of Na^+ (via stimulation of aldosterone secretion by the glomerulosa cells of the adrenal cortex); (b) vasoconstriction of systemic and renal arterioles to elevate blood pressure; (c) stimulation of antidiuretic hormone (ADH) (vasopressin) secretion from the posterior pituitary and stimulation of the thirst center within the hypothalamus; and (d) enhancement of NaCl reabsorption by the proximal tubule (210). Because of the essential role of these functions in homeostasis, elevated circulating AII also plays an important role in the pathophysiology of a number of cardiovascular and related renal diseases (e.g., hypertension, congestive heart failure, and chronic renal failure) (160,176,177).

The constant quest for new, more specific, drugs for treatment of these diseases has generated much new information about the components of the RA system. In the past few years it has become clear that the RA system is not restricted to the kidney. Local AII-generating systems also exist in brain, adrenal glands, testes, and the arterial wall (21,26,33,47,48,178). Furthermore, information about the multiplicity of renal and related cardiovascular functions of the RA system has continued to expand almost exponentially (160,176,177). Figure 11 is a current schematic representation of the biochemical pathways producing AII and related angiotensin peptides and their interactions with angiotensin subtype receptors (61). New studies have established that AI acts as substrate not only for production of AII, but also for production of the vasodilator heptapeptide *angiotensin-(1-7)* [A-(1-7)] via a family of tissue endopeptidases found in brain, kidney, and vascular endothelium of mammals (61,243). Also, AII itself is the source of two additional biologically active peptides, AIII and AIV. At present, the physiologic functions of these RA components are not

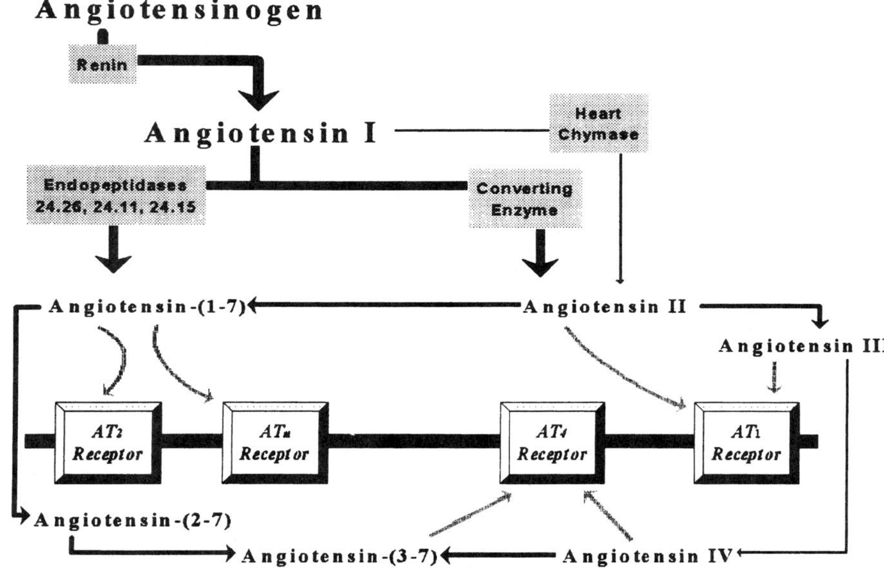

Figure 11. Schematic representation of the biochemical pathways producing biologically active angiotensin peptides and their interactions with angiotensin subtype receptors. (From ref. 61, with permission.)

clear. The autocrine regulation of VSM tone by AII and its vascular receptors in large arteries are described below.

Other Vasoactive Circulating and Local Humoral Agents

Numerous other substances can modulate VSM tone by one or more of three regulatory modes: (a) endocrine regulation (as described above for the catecholamines released from the adrenal medulla and AII synthesized from renin that is released from the kidney); (b) paracrine regulation (defined as regulation by vasoactive substances that are synthesized and released from local nonneural cells adjacent to blood vessels; (c) autocrine regulation (defined as regulation by vasoactive substances synthesized and released from cells within the vascular wall of the vessel itself.

Arginine vasopressin (AVP), also known as *antidiuretic hormone* (ADH), is a nonapeptide that also is an endocrine regulator of VSM tone. This substance, which in high concentrations combines with V_1 receptors on the plasmalemmal membrane to elevate VSM tone, particularly in the coronary and splanchnic vascular beds, is not involved in the maintenance of VSM tone under normal physiologic conditions. However, reductions of blood volume and blood pressure greater than approximately 7% profoundly increase plasma concentrations of vasopressin (e.g., from a resting concentration of <2 pg/ml to 23 pg/ml following a 30% reduction) (169). This plasma increase results from release of vasopressin from pituicytes (neurosecretory terminals of the magnocellular neurons where it is synthesized). The perikarya of these cells lie in the paraventricular (PVN) and supraoptic (SON) nuclei of the anterior hypothalamus. Their terminals lie within the pars nervosa of the neurohypophysis (posterior pituitary). Release of AVP is mediated by both low- and high-pressure baroreflex activation of nerve cells within the brainstem with axons that project to the PVN and SON.

In addition to their function as neurotransmitters and/or cotransmitters, substances such as histamine (a biogenic amine) and serotonin (5-hydroxytryptamine) also act as vasoactive paracrine agents. Histamine, which is released from most cells in vascular beds (including VSM cells) in response to local injury and by antigen-antibody reactions, is a potent dilator of arterioles and venules in the dog, monkey, and human, but a vasoconstrictor in cats and rodents (130). These vascular actions are mediated by H_1 and H_2 receptors on the VSM cell plasmalemmal membrane. Sufficient liberation of histamine also affects the peripheral circulation by increasing venular permeability to plasma proteins, which, in turn, leads to edema, a reduction of plasma volume, and hypotension.

In the peripheral tissues serotonin is synthesized by neurons, the enterochromaffin cell of the gut, and by the pineal gland. In high concentrations it is taken up from the circulation by platelets from which it is later released (130). The vasoaction of this substance is variable depending on animal species, its site of action (i.e., nerve terminal, VSM cell, endothelial cell), blood vessel size, available receptor type, and basal level of VSM tone. Neurally, serotonin is taken up, stored in, and released as a "false transmitter" from sympathetic nerves (101,161). Serotonin can cause vasodilation by inhibiting the release of NE from sympathetic nerve terminals. However, serotonin also vasoconstricts large arteries and veins with varying levels of sensitivity, whereas it vasodilates arterioles and constricts venules. This leads to an elevation of capillary hydrostatic pressure (161). In the rodent (but not the human), serotonin, like histamine, increases capillary permeability to proteins. Thus, these two actions of serotonin can lead to formation of additional tissue fluid. Serotonin also can produce vasodilation by stimulating release of nitric oxide from the vascular endothelium (see below).

Autocrine regulation of VSM tone in the peripheral vasculature is classically exemplified by the family of 20 carbon, oxygenated fatty acids termed *eicosanoids* (i.e., leukotrienes, thromboxanes, and prostaglandins), that are derived from the common precursor, *arachidonic acid* (AA). As autocrine regulators (i.e., compounds that alter the activities of cells in which they are synthesized), eicosanoids are members of the class of biologically active compounds known as *autacoids.* Their arachidonic acid precursor is a 20 carbon, unsaturated (four double bond), fatty acid that is liberated from phospholipids in the plasma membrane of VSM and endothelial cells by a variety of physiologic, pharmacologic, and pathologic stimuli (122,170). Specific sources include diacylglycerol (DAG) through the action of diacylglycerol lipase, and phosphatidic acid (PA) through the action of phospholipase A_2. These two precursors of AA are, in turn, derived by a series of enzymatically controlled steps from two plasmalemmal membrane phospholipids, namely phosphatidylinositol 4,5-biphosphate (PIP_2), through the action of phospholipase C (Fig. 12) (203), and phosphatidylcholine (PC), through the action of phospholipase D.

Free AA is oxidatively metabolized along three major pathways by membrane-bound enzymes present in a wide variety of cells (including renal, VSM, and its endothelial cells) (Fig. 13) (35,125). The first is initiated by cyclooxygenase, which generates a labile endoperoxide from which prostaglandins, thromboxanes, and prostacyclin are derived. This enzyme is inhibited by indomethacin and nonsteroidal antiinflammatory drugs (e.g., aspirin). The second pathway is initiated by various lipoxygenases, which catalyze formation of leukotrienes, lipoxins, and hepoxilins. The third pathway (whose oxygenated products are currently under intense investigation for their potential control of VSM tone (83,122) is initiated by a family of cytochrome P 450 (CP 450)–dependent monooxygenases. Unlike cyclooxygenase and lipoxygenase, the CP 450 enzymes require a reductase and reduced nicotinamide adenine dinucleotide phosphate (NADPH) as cofactors for electron transfer in the oxidation-reduction steps coupled to their oxidative activity. The oxygenated metabolites derived from AA through the enzymatic action of CP 450 enzymes include a series of epoxides (e.g., four regioisomers of epoxyeicosatrienoic acids (EETs), their corresponding dihydroxyeicosatetraenoic acid (DHETEs), and 19- and 20-hydroxyeicosatetraenoic acids (HETEs) (35,83,122).

It is difficult to generalize about the actions of prostaglandins on the peripheral vasculature since closely related prostaglandins can act both as vasodilators and vasoconstrictors depending on animal species and vascular bed. It has been suggested that the overall action of prostaglandins in the peripheral circulation appears to be vasodilation in order to modulate blood pressure elevations (e.g., during stress) and to maintain organ blood flow (35,125). Prostacyclin (PGI_2) is the principal prostaglandin produced by large arteries, which have a much greater capacity for its production than veins (130). PGI_2 and prostaglandin E_2 (PGE_2) are vasodilators that can modulate vasoconstriction produced by other vasoactive neural and humoral stimuli. For example, PGE_2 can inhibit the release of NE from adrenergic nerve terminals. When administered systemically, PGI_2 and PGE_2 can reduce blood pressure by vasodilation predominantly in the renal, intestinal, and mesenteric vascular beds. Blood concentrations of circulating prostaglandins are extremely low since they are efficiently cleared by the lungs (PGE_2 and $PGF_{2\alpha}$), liver, and kidney (130).

The physiologic role of the leukotrienes in circulatory regulation is also unclear. Although some produce vasoconstriction in the coronary and mesenteric vascular beds, others relax activated blood vessels (6). They are mediators of immunologic and inflammatory reactions that affect leukocyte activity and vascular permeability (130).

The vascular actions of the lipoxygenase- and CP-450–derived HETEs and EETs are a function of the stereochemical configurations of their epoxide and hydroxyl side groups and the vascular beds in which they exert an effect (reviewed in 83,122). For example, the 12 (R)-HETE, which is

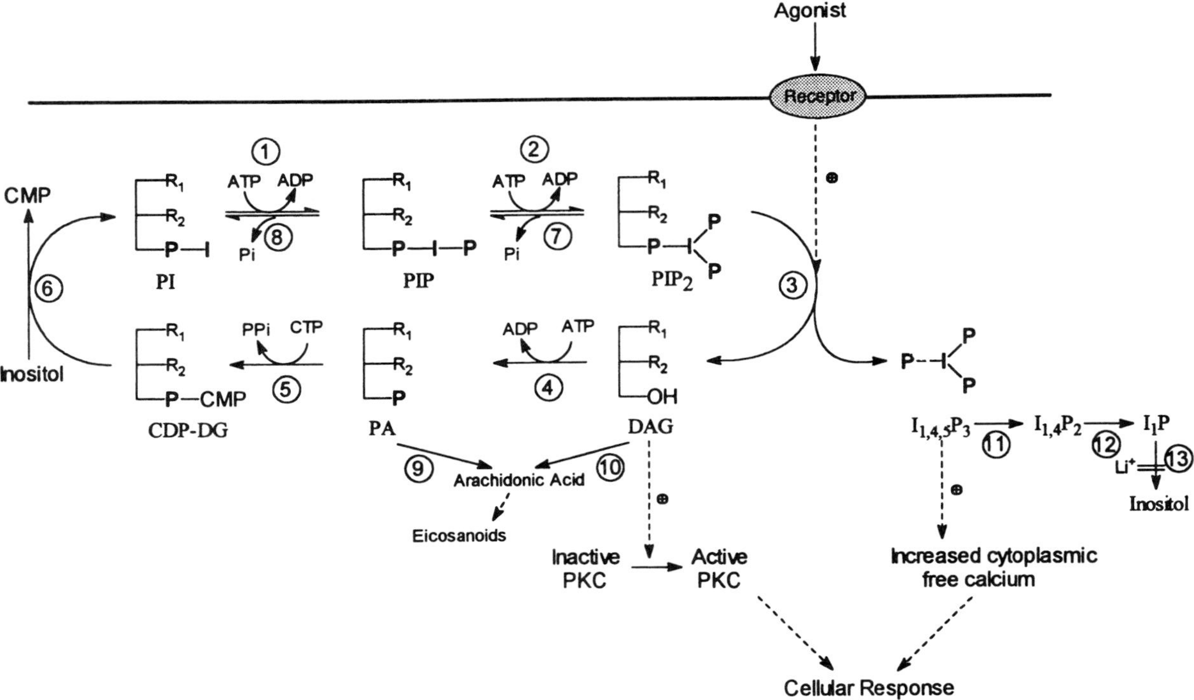

Figure 12. Biochemical steps involved in the production of vasoactive metabolites from the membrane-bound phosphatidylinositol (PI cycle). Numbered enzymes: 1, phosphatidylinositol kinase; 2, phosphatidylinositol-4-phosphate kinase; 3, phosphatidylinositol-specific phospholipase C; 4, diacylglycerol kinase; 5, phosphatidate cytidyl transferase; 6, phosphatidylserine transferase; 7, $PIP_2$5-phosphatase; 8, PIP4-phosphatase; 9, phospholipase A_2; 10, diacylglycerol lipase; 11, $I_{1,4,5}P_3$5-phosphatase; 12, $I_{1,4}P_2$-4 phosphatase; 13, I_1P phosphatase. (From ref. 203, with permission.)

formed via the CP-450 pathway, produces more potent vasoconstriction of renal arteries than 12 (S)-HETE, which is formed via the lipoxygenase pathway (115). In contrast 12 (R)-HETE has been reported to dilate arteries in the peripheral vasculature (157).

Sources of 20-HETE (via ω-hydroxylation of AA) include microvessels (but apparently not large conduit vessels) in the brain, lung, and kidney of rats and rabbits. Thus, 20-HETE may play a greater direct role in the regulation of vascular tone in the microcirculation (83). As with 12-HETE, the vas-

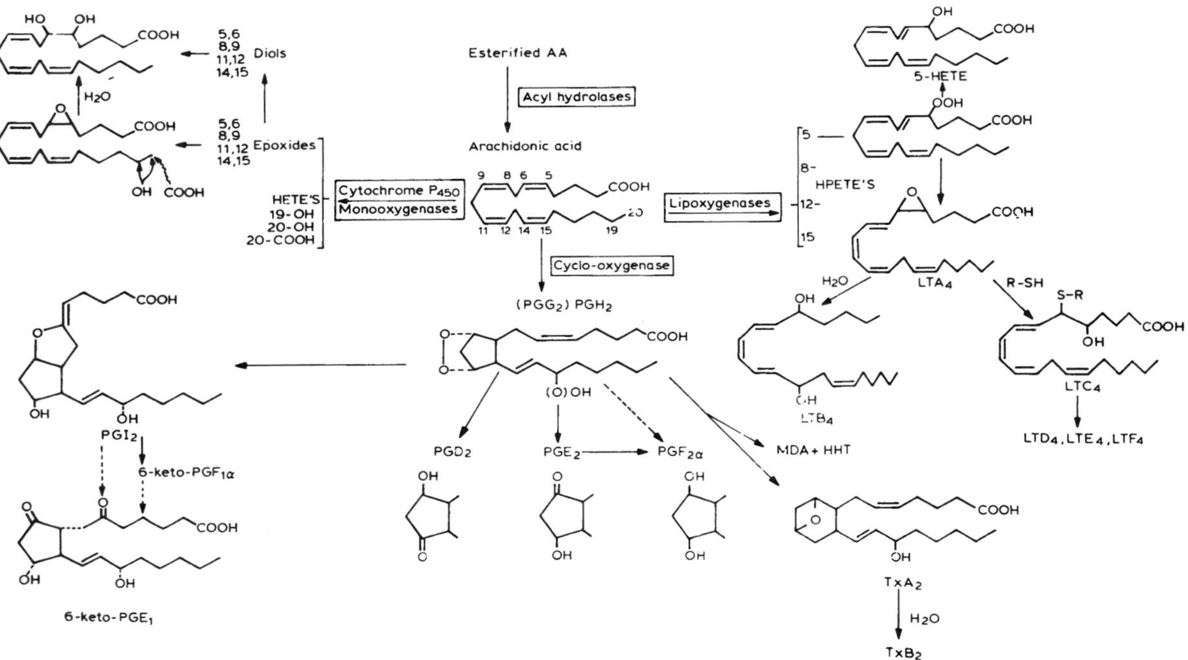

Figure 13. Three major pathways of oxygenation of arachidonic acid-forming eicosanoids: 1, cytochrome P-450 monooxygenase production of HETEs, epoxides, and diols; 2, lipoxygenase production of HETEs and leukotrienes; 3, cyclooxygenase production of prostaglandins and thromboxanes. (From ref. 125, with permission.)

cular actions of 20-HETE are also variable, again being dependent on such factors as animal species, vascular bed, and participation of the endothelium. For example, 20-HETE vasodilates the preconstricted, isolated, perfused renal and splanchnic beds in the rabbit, but is a potent vasoconstrictor of renal and cerebral microvessels. Rat aortic rings vasoconstrict in response to 20-HETE. This response is dependent on an intact endothelium and a cyclooxygenase-derived endoperoxide metabolite. On the other hand, the vasoconstrictor response to 20-HETE in the renal and cerebral microvasculature is not blocked by indomethacin (an inhibitor of cyclooxygenase), indicating that 20-HETE directly affects VSM tone in the microcirculation. [See (83,122) for references describing these studies.]

Of potential physiologic importance is the role that 20-HETE may play in the myogenic response of small vessels (i.e., the transmural pressure-induced elevation of VSM tone). The vasoconstrictor response of 20-HETE in renal and cerebral microvessels is accompanied by VSM depolarization and inhibition of the activity of Ca-activated K channels (84). Increases in the number of open K channels causes membrane hyperpolarization. Since transmural pressure mimics these actions of 20-HETE, it is possible that 20-HETE may be released in response to elevated transmural pressure and act as a second messenger to maintain depolarization when the muscle contracts as $[Ca^{2+}]_i$ rises (83).

Similar to the 12- and 20-HETEs, the action of the EETs on VSM tone in the peripheral vasculature is variable, again being dependent on such factors as animal species, vascular bed and source (i.e., VSM and endothelial cell), and steric configuration. For example, the R,S stereoisomer of 11,12 EET is the predominant form of EET in the kidney, compared to the S,R form, which predominates in the liver. The 11,12 (RS)EET is a potent vasodilator of renal preglomerular arterioles, where it enhances the activity of the large conductance Ca-activated K channel. The 11,12 (SR) EET is much less active. A detailed description of the effects of EETs and proposed mechanisms of action of the CP-450 metabolites in the peripheral vasculartlater can be found in the review by Harder and colleagues (83).

Intrinsic Regulation of Peripheral Vascular Tone

Membrane and Intracellular Biochemical Components Mediating VSM Contractile Force

The most recognized signal transduction pathway for in vivo regulation of VSM tone at the cell level by extrinsic neural and humoral agonists and by local paracrine and autocrine agonists begins with the activation of specific VSM sarcolemmal membrane receptors. When activated, these receptors trigger a cascade of biochemical steps within the VSM cell membrane and cytoplasm that ultimately lead to force generation by activated contractile proteins (108,138,206).

Central to this pathway is the regulation of the concentration of intracellular free Ca^{2+} (i.e., Ca^{2+} activity or "activator" Ca^{2+}) which, in turn, regulates the combination of the two contractile proteins, actin and myosin, to produce contractile force (108,138,183,206). The combination of specific agonists with specific membrane receptors leads to activation of specific membrane-bound guanine nucleotide (GTP)-binding proteins (G proteins) (23,90,127,143,199,222). When activated, G proteins interact with effector proteins including enzymes and ion channels, and alter activities of the latter. Such alteration may ultimately lead either to an increase or decrease in $[Ca^{2+}]_i$ depending upon the particular agonist, its specific receptor, and the specific G protein that is activated. For example, as described above, the combination of NE or Epi with α-receptors on the VSM sarcolemmal membrane leads to an elevation of VSM tone by activating a G_s protein. This, in turn, elevates $[Ca^{2+}]_i$ indirectly by the following sequential cascade: (a) activation of adenyl cyclase; (b) elevation of the second messenger cyclic adenyl monophosphate (cAMP); (c) activation of cAMP-dependent protein kinase; (d) phosphorylation of VSM membrane Ca channels, causing them to open (108).

Another sequential cascade initiated by combination of an agonist with a membrane receptor that leads to an elevation of $[Ca^{2+}]_i$ (and VSM tone) is designated as the sarcolemmal membrane phosphatidylinositol (PI) cycle. As described above, PI is one of the sources of arachidonic acid (AA) (Fig. 12) (203). In addition, two products are derived from hydrolysis of one of its phosphorylated metabolites, phosphatidylinositol 4,5-biphosphate (PIP_2), through the action of phospholipase C. These are inositoltriphosphate (IP_3) and diacylglycerol (DAG) (Fig. 12) (10,146,159,203), which also can indirectly regulate $[Ca^{2+}]_i$ by opening Ca channels in either the sarcoplasmic reticulum (SR) or sarcolemmal membrane. IP_3 elevates $[Ca^{2+}]_i$ by causing release of Ca^{2+} from the SR into the cytoplasm. DAG activates another protein kinase, protein kinase C, which also opens plasmalemmal Ca channels by phosphorylation (Fig. 12).

Contractile Force Generation in Smooth Muscle

Elevation of $[Ca^{2+}]_i$ to a concentration ranging between 10^{-7} M and 10^{-6} M causes cross-bridge attachments between actin and myosin and the generation of VSM contractile force as it does in striated muscle. However, the biochemical steps involved differ since smooth muscle does not contain troponin and Ca^{2+} regulates cross-bridge attachment indirectly. These steps are illustrated in Fig. 14 (138). Four free (activator) Ca^{2+} ions combine with a small cytoplasmic Ca-binding protein, calmodulin. A myosin-specific protein kinase (myosin light chain kinase [MLCK]) is activated upon combining with Ca-calmodulin leading to adenosine triphosphate (ATP) hydrolysis and covalent linkage of a high-energy phosphate to a serine residue on the myosin light chain that forms part of the cross-bridge (138). Figure 14 also illustrates a direct proportionality between $[Ca^{2+}]_i$ and myosin phosphorylation over the 10^{-7}–10^{-6} M concentration range (138,206). Phosphorylated myosin spontaneously forms cross-bridges with actin leading to cross-bridge flexion and consequent shortening of sarcomeres as occurs in striated muscle. Thus, phosphate bond energy is transduced into mechanical (contractile) energy. In contrast to striated muscle, the sarcomeres containing the interdigitating actin and myosin filaments in smooth muscle appear to be arranged diagonally rather than parallel to the long axis of the smooth muscle cell. Additionally, the attachment points for the thin (actin) filaments that delineate the sarcomere lengths are ellipsoidal dense bodies located both within the cytoplasm and on the sarcolemmal membrane (Fig. 15) (60,138). Upon reduction of $[Ca^{2+}]_i$ to $<10^{-7}$ M, force generation ceases as myosin is dephosphorylated by myosin phosphatase and returns to the inactive state. It is important to point out that the proportionality observed between elevations in $[Ca^{2+}]_i$ and cross-bridge cycling is observed for brief stimulations of smooth muscle resulting in phasic contractions. During generation of tonic contraction (e.g., as occurs in VSM when maintaining a constant vessel diameter under a continual transmural pressure load), the initial peak of $[Ca^{2+}]_i$ falls to a moderate steady-state level, as does cross-bridge phosphorylation. However, force generation is not necessarily reduced. Explanations for this uncoupling between $[Ca^{2+}]_i$ and force generation are controversial. One interesting hypothesis (based on plausible experimental data) is the covalent cross-bridge regulation (or latch) hypothesis (138,139). Briefly, this hypothesis postulates that contracting smooth muscle has four cross-bridge states: free, attached, phosphorylated, and dephosphorylated. These allow for two cross-bridge cycles. In the first, the phosphorylated cross-bridges cycle relatively fast and one ATP is con-

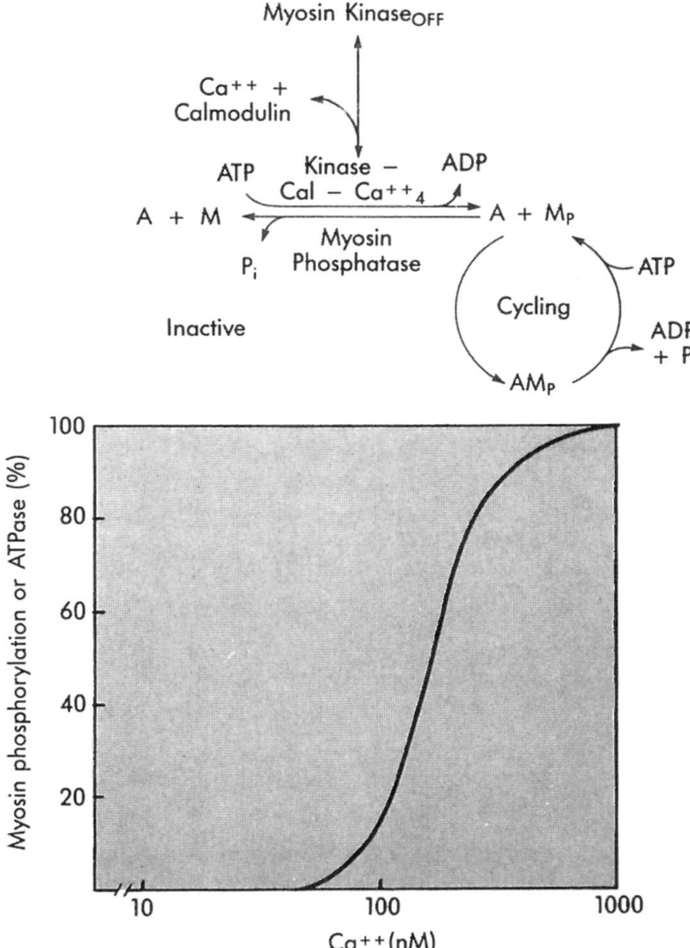

Figure 14. Regulation of smooth muscle myosin phosphorylation and ATPase activity by Ca^{2+}-calmodulin-myosin kinase complex. Note regulatory range of intracellular free Ca^{2+} concentration. (From ref. 138, with permission.)

sumed per cycle. This occurs when $[Ca^{2+}]_i$ and MLCK activity are high. Under these conditions, most of the cross-bridges will be phosphorylated, resulting in rapid force development and sarcomere shortening. If $[Ca^{2+}]_i$ falls to moderate levels (somewhat greater than 10^{-7} M), phosphorylation falls, but force is maintained by the accumulation of attached cross-bridges that are in the dephosphorylated state. This results in a slow, steady cycling rate in which contractile force is maintained with low rates of ATP consumption.

In addition to the above second messenger pathways, recent evidence indicates that agonists may also regulate VSM tone in vivo by a pathway that bypasses the membrane receptor and biochemical cascade. Thus, it has been shown in permeabilized rat mesenteric artery cells that activation of protein kinase C, either directly by a pharmacologic agent or indirectly by NE, causes an upregulation of the Ca^{2+} sensitivity of VSM contractile proteins under constant $[Ca^{2+}]_i$ (145,146). The mechanisms by which such upregulation occurs is not clear, although this process may involve a decrease in phosphatase activity and maintained phosphorylation of MLC in the absence of a marked increase in MLCK activity (206a).

Summary of Myoplasmic Ca^{2+} Balance: Sources, Sinks, and Membrane Pumps

Figure 16 (138) illustrates the principal sources and sinks involved in the regulation of $[Ca^{2+}]_i$ in both resting and activated smooth muscle. In contrast to skeletal muscle, two pools supply Ca^{2+} for regulation of contraction in VSM. Thus, as described above, sources include both extracellular Ca^{2+} that enters via Ca-specific sarcolemmal membrane channels and Ca^{2+} release from the SR. In addition to receptor-operated Ca channels (ROCs) (described above), Ca^{2+} can also enter the VSM cell through membrane voltage-dependent Ca channels (VDCC). Although much controversy had existed in the past concerning the physiologic role of VDCC in the regulation of VSM contractile force (98,206,217), it is now clear that both types of Ca channels participate in the regulation of $[Ca^{2+}]_i$. It appears that in vivo, VDCCs are opened both by the depolarization resulting from agonist-induced activation of as yet poorly defined cation and anion channels in the VSM sarcolemma and by the elevated $[Ca^{2+}]_i$ resulting from activation of ROCs. Physiologically, elevated VSM contractile force is terminated by reduction of $[Ca^{2+}]_i$ to $<10^{-7}$ M. Such reduction is achieved by three mechanisms: (a) a sarcolemmal membrane Ca^{2+}-ATPase (PMCA) that extrudes Ca^{2+} by primary active transport (i.e., direct utilization of ATP phosphate bond energy); (b) a sarcolemmal membrane Na/Ca exchange-diffusion system that utilizes the potential energy of the Na^+ gradient to extrude one Ca^{2+} ion for every three Na^+ that move into the cell (secondary active transport); (c) an ATP-dependent SR membrane Ca^{2+}-ATPase (SERCA) that returns Ca^{2+} to the SR following its release from calmodulin. It is important to note that the rate of Ca^{2+} removal by the two ATP-dependent primary active transport pumps is a first-order reaction (i.e., directly proportional to $[Ca^{2+}]_i$). Also the physiologic importance of the Na/Ca exchanger in VSM is still controversial.

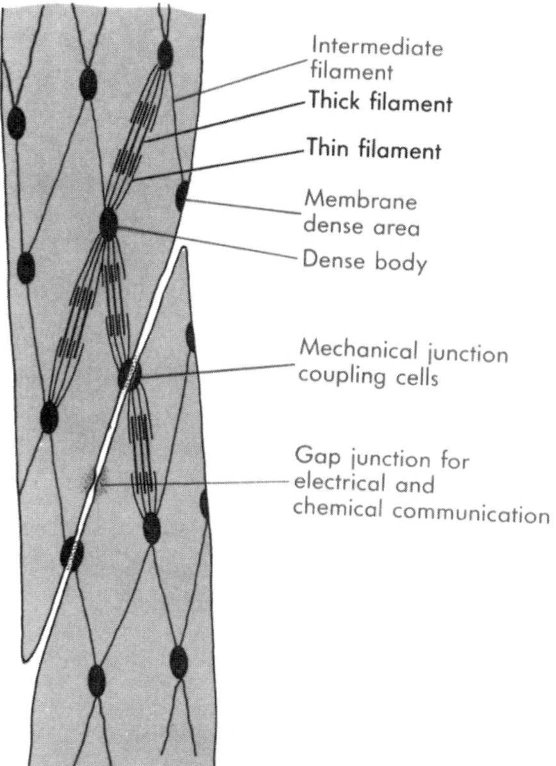

Figure 15. Diagonal orientation of muscle fibers and contractile elements (sliding filaments) in smooth muscle. Note especially the dense body attachment points for the actin and the gap junctions for electrical and chemical communication for coordinated contractions. (From ref. 138, with permission.)

Endothelial Regulation of VSM Contractile Force

In addition to neural and direct vascular smooth muscle control, the third component to be considered in the regulation of the peripheral vasculature is the endothelium. This single cell layer lining the vessels exerts significant effects on vascular function and blood flow in several distinct and yet related ways. First, these cells release vasoconstricting and relaxing factors in response to circulating hormones, local tissue factors, neurally released transmitters and modulators, as well as mechanical changes in sheer stress and pressure (66). Second, in addition to metabolizing circulating vasoactive substances and physically separating the vascular smooth muscle from these substances, the endothelial lining of the vessels is negatively charged at the surface and resists inappropriate platelet aggregation. The endothelium releases factors that in addition to having vasoactive properties also have procoagulant or anticoagulant properties. As such these cells contribute to the balance between thrombosis and thrombolysis (86). Third, endothelial cells respond to local cytokine release by expressing surface receptors that bind neutrophils and monocytes, leading to vascular infiltration by leukocytes as occurs in inflammatory processes and atherosclerosis (86). The principal focus of this discussion is on the first of these vascular endothelial functions, specifically the release of vasoactive substances that contribute to the net regulation of vascular tone. Nevertheless, it should be recognized that the endothelial effects on hemostasis, coagulation, and leukocyte aggregation also can significantly influence blood flow.

Endothelial cells have been shown to be capable of releasing a large number of vasoactive substances. Endothelium-derived NO is perhaps the most popularized of the factors and its synthesis, release, and actions have been widely studied (20,31,50,51,62,66,86,126). In endothelial cells, NO is synthesized by a membrane bound enzyme, NO synthase, which is activated by increased cytosolic Ca^{2+}. The enzyme oxidizes the amino acid substrate L–arginine utilizing NADPH and oxygen (O_2) to produce the amino acid L-citrulline and NO (99) (Fig. 17). Other related forms of NO synthase exist in other cell types such as neurons where NO acts as a neurotransmitter (as discussed previously) and in leukocytes where NO mediates cytotoxicity (50,86). Once synthesized in endothelial cells, NO diffuses into the vascular smooth muscle cells to bind the heme moiety of guanylyl cyclase, thus activating it to produce cGMP (99). As discussed previously, this increase in cGMP produces vascular smooth muscle relaxation by inhibiting Ca^{2+} influx, enhancing the plasmalemmal Ca pump as well as the sarcoplasmic uptake of Ca^{2+} and dephosphorylation of myosin light chains (16,51). This is also the mechanism of action of the nitro vasodilators such as sodium nitroprusside and nitroglycerin, which release NO when they spontaneously degrade or are metabolized. Methylene blue inhibits the vasodilating actions of these agents, as well as endothelially mediated NO-induced vasodilation (51,66). The affinity of NO for the heme moiety explains why hemoglobin will bind NO and prevent its activation of guanylyl cyclase in vascular smooth muscle cells, which produces vasodilation (66). Since O_2 is required for the synthesis of NO, hypoxia inhibits NO production and thus inhibits endothelial- (and NO-) mediated vasodilation. However, hyperoxia also inhibits NO due to the production of oxygen radicals that rapidly react with NO, which itself is a reactive molecule (51,99). The enzyme superoxide dismutase protects and prolongs the effect of NO (99). Given that NO is so susceptible to breakdown by free radicals and the fact that volatile anesthetic metabolism is associated with the formation of these reactive molecules, this represents a possible mechanism for anesthetic inhibition of endothelial (and NO) function (99).

Proposed mechanisms for the increase in intracellular endothelial Ca^{2+} leading to NO release are similar to mechanisms described previously for vascular smooth muscle. Intracellular Ca^{2+} may be increased directly by ligand binding of receptors, which activates Ca channels, or indirectly by ligand binding of receptors, which activates phospholipase C to break down membrane phospholipids to produce IP_3 and DAG (1,99). The former increases Ca^{2+} release from intracellular stores (as with vascular smooth muscle) and the latter produces protein kinase C, which in endothelial cells may produce feedback inhibition of NO synthesis (1,99). As in vascular smooth muscle, both the direct and the indirect receptor-operated mechanisms may involve G protein activation (62). Other mechanisms for regulating endothelial intracellular Ca^{2+} that have been proposed include leak-through Ca channels, alterations in Na/Ca exchange, and activation of stretch-operated K and Ca channels (1,31).

Given the above-described mechanisms of NO actions and synthesis, particularly in regard to ligand-receptor—mediated increases in intracellular Ca^{2+}, the question remains as to what physiologic stimuli actually lead to NO release and under what conditions. Endothelial cells have been shown to have receptors for and release NO in response to the binding of many humoral agents. These include acetylcholine, α_2-receptor agonists, histamine, serotonin, bradykinin ATP, ADP, thromboxane, angiotensin I and II, arginine vasopressin, and substance P (31,50,51,86,232,233). However, which of these substances actually contributes significantly to the physiologic role of endothelial-mediated vasorelaxation is a different question. The circulation would be the most likely source for humoral agents acting on the endothelium (although there is at least some evidence that neurally released norepinephrine can

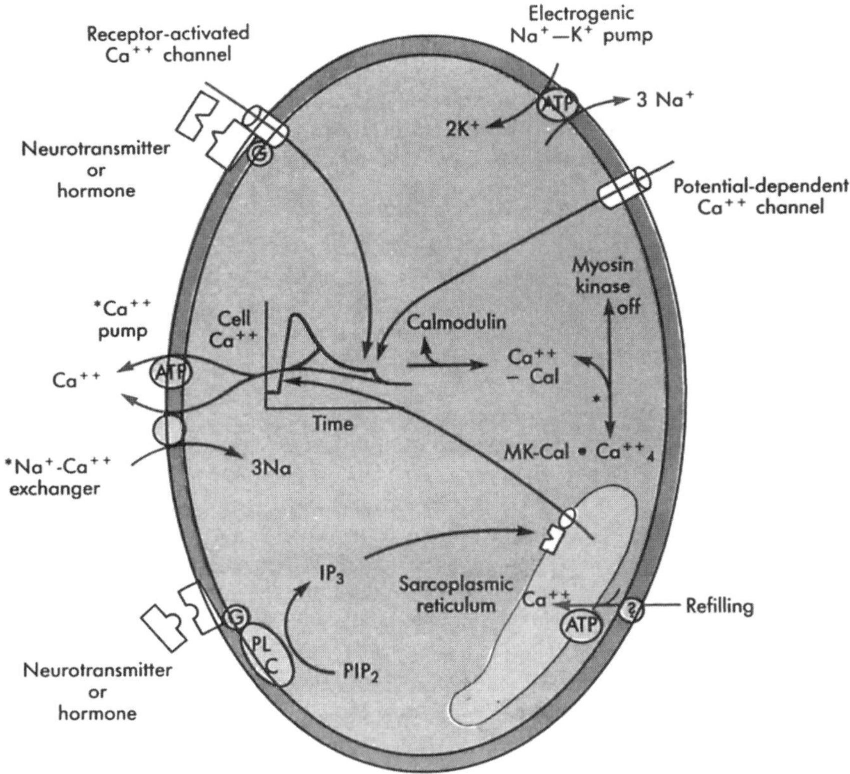

Figure 16. Diagram of principal mechanisms that regulate intracellular free Ca^{2+} concentration in a VSM cell (including extra- and intracellular sources and sinks, membrane Ca^{2+} channels, exchangers, and pumps). (From ref. 138, with permission.)

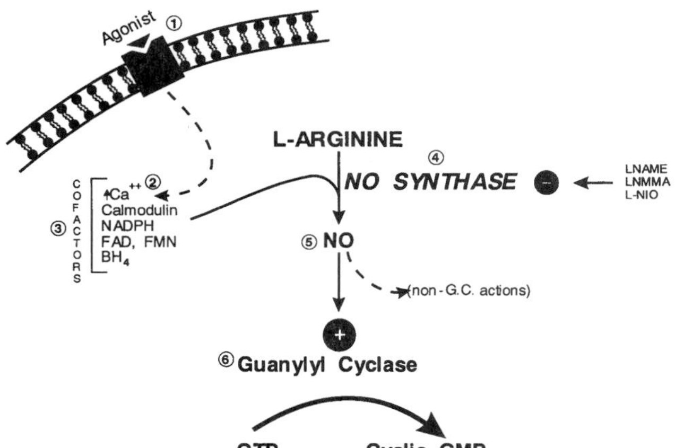

Figure 17. A schematic summarizing the synthesis of nitric oxide NO in endothelial cells. In response to an agonist-receptor interaction on the endothelial cell surface (1), cytosolic [Ca^{2+}] is increased (2). In response to increased calcium-calmodulin binding, constitutive, membrane-bound nitric oxide synthase (NOS) oxidizes L-arginine to L-citrulline producing NO in the process, which requires nicotinamide adenine denucleotide phosphate (NADP), flavin adenine dinucleotide (FAD), flavin mononucleotide (FMN), and tetrahydrobiopterin (BH4) as cofactors (3 and 4). Once synthesized, NO quickly diffuses into the vascular smooth muscle cell to bind the heme moiety of the enzyme guanylyl cyclase activating it to produce cyclic guanosine monophosphate (cGMP) from guanosine triphosphate (GTP). Nitro-L-arginine methyl ester L-NAME, N_G monomethyl-L-arginine (L-NMMA) and N-imino ornithine (L-NIO) are specific analogous of L-arginine which competitively inhibit NOS. (From ref. 99, with permission.)

affect endothelial factor release and vice versa) (126). Clearly not all of these agents are present in sufficient concentrations in the circulation to affect endothelial cells. For example, acetylcholine (31,232) and substance P (31) are metabolized too quickly to exist in the circulation. On the other hand, under certain conditions endothelial cells may be exposed to increased concentrations of catecholamines and vasopressin, which are stable in the circulation. Vascular endothelium is also exposed to circulating angiotensin I and is known (along with the lung endothelium) to contain angiotensin converting enzyme that synthesizes angiotensin II from angiotensin I (50). Histamine, bradykinin, substance P, and arachidonic acid may affect endothelial cells via their release by injured tissues and thus produce local vasodilation associated with inflammatory responses (233).

Likewise, serotonin, thromboxane, ATP, and ADP are released from locally aggregating platelets. NO released by endothelial cells in a localized area not only inhibits further platelet aggregation (86) but also may vasodilate to further limit vascular occlusion (232). Most of these mediators, which stimulate endothelial-mediated vasodilation, are known to cause constriction when vascular smooth muscle cells are directly exposed to them (31,233) in areas with damaged or denuded endothelium. Thus, in intact vasculature, platelet aggregation is inhibited and flow is maintained, but when vessels are disrupted and endothelial cells are damaged inhibitors of platelet aggregation are reduced and there is local vasoconstriction (233) (Fig. 18). In addition, endothelial cells have been shown to be capable of synthesizing and releasing many of these above-described mediators to act on themselves to release NO (31,232). Such release has been proposed to occur in response to physiologic stimuli such as

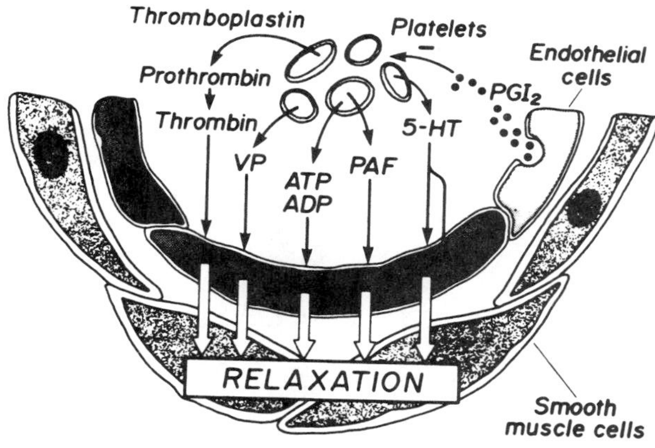

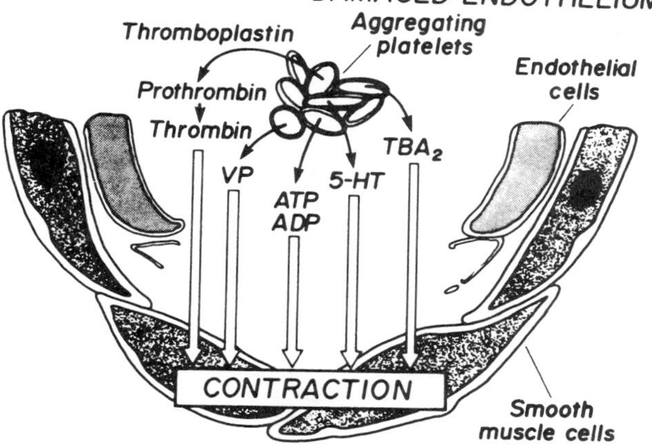

Figure 18. Aggregating platelets release adenosine triphosphate (ATP), adenosine diphosphate (ADP), serotonin (5-HT), thromboxane A_2, platelet activating factor (PAF), and vasopressin (VP). They also activate the coagulation system, leading to thrombin production. When the endothelial barrier is intact *(top)*, prostacyclin PGI_2 is released, which inhibits platelet activation, 5-HT is broken down, and agents such as VP, ATP, ADP, and thrombin stimulate endothelial-mediated vasodilation of vascular smooth muscle (VSM). Such platelet inhibition and vasodilation inhibits and flushes away developing thrombi. In contrast, when the endothelial barrier is disrupted *(bottom)*, platelet aggregation is stimulated by exposure to collagen in the vascular wall, and mediators released from aggregating platelets produce constriction of VSM. (From ref. 233, with permission.)

mechanical stimulation (31), which would represent a stretch-activated channel mechanism for NO synthesis and release in addition to the ligand-receptor mediated mechanism discussed previously. Vascular endothelial cells have been shown to be mechanosensitive in that sheer stress enhances endothelial NO release and inhibits endothelial constricting factor release, whereas cyclical strain does the opposite (166). This suggests that the vascular endothelium will act to accommodate transmission of increased flow by promoting vasodilation, and this will oppose downstream transmission of increased pressure by promoting vasoconstriction. Thus, as mechanoreceptors, endothelial cells as well as vascular smooth muscle cells themselves may participate in autoregulation.

In addition to NO, endothelial cells also produce other vasoactive substances (Fig. 19); however, the details of this synthesis and release have not been as thoroughly studied. Prostacyclin (PGI_2) is a prostaglandin with vasorelaxing properties that is synthesized in the endothelial cells by the action of the enzyme cyclooxygenase on arachidonic acid, which itself is produced from membrane phospholipid by phospholipase A_2 (50). The release of PGI_2 is stimulated by endothelial exposure to bradykinin and thrombin. Despite the potent vasorelaxing properties of PGI_2, its primary role appears to be the inhibition of platelet aggregation rather than the regulation of vascular tone (42,50,86). A third vasorelaxing substance released from endothelial cells has been termed *endothelial-derived hyperpolarizing factor* (EDHF). Although it has not been characterized, it has been shown to be chemically distinct from endothelial derived NO (126). It appears to act as a potassium channel opener on vascular smooth muscle cells to produce hyperpolarization and thus inhibit tone (86).

As indicated above, endothelial cells synthesize mediators such as histamine, substance P, acetylcholine, serotonin, ATP, and ADP, which normally cause endothelial release of NO but which cause vasoconstriction when directly exposed to vascular smooth muscle cells if endothelial cells are damaged or absent (31,233). In addition, under certain conditions, even intact undamaged endothelium may release vasoconstricting substances that act directly on smooth muscle to increase vascular tone (31,86,233). One type of endothelium-derived constricting factor is a group of prostanoids synthesized by endothelium cyclooxygenase from arachidonic acid. They include but are not exclusively thromboxane. This is illustrated by the fact that the presence of these prostanoids can still be demonstrated despite the administration of thromboxane inhibitors (50). The release of these prostaglandin endothelial-derived constricting factors appears to be caused by transmural pressure increase as well as by certain types of hypertension (86,233). A second type of endothelial constricting factor is released under conditions of hypoxia (232,233). Although this is not a prostaglandin, the substance not yet been characterized. The third and perhaps best known group of endothelial vasoconstricting substance are the endothelins, a class of polypeptides of which three distinct types have been described. Their amino acid sequence and their synthesis from precursor molecules has been described (86). Specific endothelin receptors have been identified on vascular smooth muscle cells. Binding to these receptors by endothelin results in an increase in intracellular Ca^{2+} by a G-protein–mediated phospholipase C activation, leading to production of IP_3 and DAG (50) as described previously for vascular smooth muscle. A second type of endothelin receptor has been identified on endothelial cells themselves and may be associated with increased NO and PGI_2 synthesis offsetting endothelin constriction in a type of feedback system (50). Despite being the best characterized of the endothelial constricting factors, the conditions under which endothelins are released and their precise physiologic role (126) have not been defined. Finally, as mentioned above, angiotensin II is a well-known vasoconstrictor that is produced also (from angiotensin I) and released by endothelial cells (50,51,86).

Since endothelial cells are capable of producing smooth muscle contraction and platelet aggregation as well as smooth muscle relaxation and platelet inhibition, their net effects will depend on changes in local physiologic conditions. Under normal circumstances the vasodilating and antithrombogenic effects will predominate to maintain normal blood flow. However, when the endothelium is disrupted and/or under pathologic conditions, the balance may be shifted to produce local vasoconstriction and thrombosis (50,51,86). Endothelial responses vary widely among different vessel types, and the physiologic role of these effects in conjunction with direct vascular smooth muscle responses and neurally mediated regulation of vascular tone is far from being defined in detail. The transient half-lives of endothelial factors suggest that the

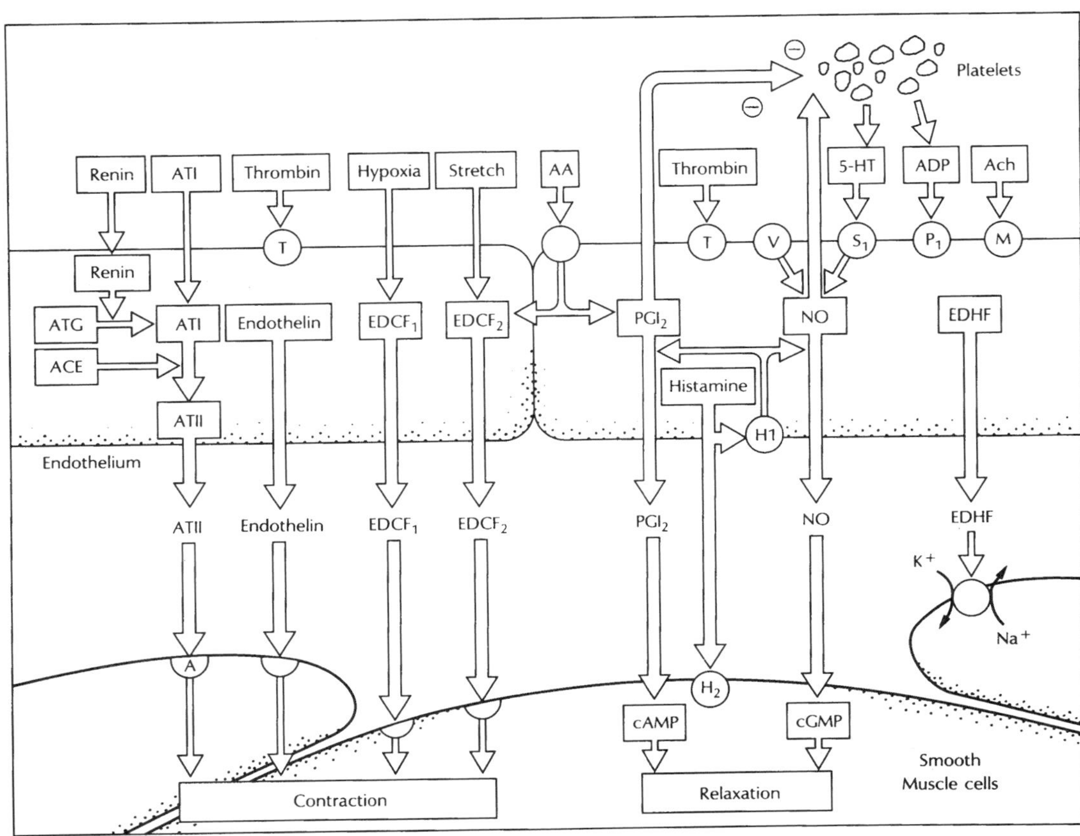

Figure 19. Summary of the vasoactive substances acting on and produced by endothelial cells to ultimately affect vascular smooth muscle cell tone. AA, arachidonic acid; ACE, angiotensin converting enzyme; Ach, acetylcholine; ADP, adenosine diphosphate; ATG, angiotensinogen; AI/II, angiotensin I and II; cAMP, cyclic adenosine monophosphate; cGMP, cyclic guanosine monophosphate; EDCF, endothelial- derived constricting factors; EDHF, endothelial-derived hyperpolarizing factor: H_1, histamine subtype 1 receptor; H_2, histamine subtype 2 receptors; m, muscarinic receptor; 5-HT, 5-hydroxytryptamine (serotonin); NO, nitric oxide; P_1, purinergic receptor; PGI_2, prostacyclin; S_1, 5-hydroxytryptamine receptor; T, thrombin receptor; V, vasopressinergic receptor. (From ref. 51, with permission.)

endothelial responses are limited to effecting changes in local control of the vascular smooth muscle (51).

FUNCTIONS OF THE PERIPHERAL CIRCULATORY COMPONENTS

Arterial Components

Large Arteries

A simplistic view of the function of the large arterial vessels (e.g., carotid, coronary, mesenteric, hepatic, renal, femoral, etc.) is that they serve as passive conduits designed primarily to distribute cardiac output to various tissues and organ systems throughout the body. However, continuing studies of the cause-effect relationship between changes in the structural and functional properties of large arterial vessels and the development of cardiovascular disease states (e.g., hypertension, arteriosclerosis, and congestive heart failure) (48,89,136,148,198) have established that in addition to acting as conduits, these vessels participate in the maintenance of cardiovascular structure and function. For example, by virtue of the effect of their viscoelastic properties and their distensibility on impedance to ventricular ejection, these vessels act as important buffers of phasic changes in pressure. In particular, such buffering of systolic blood pressure directly modulates end-systolic ventricular wall stress, which, if excessive, can lead to cardiac hypertrophy and failure (48,64,89,129,136,148,180). Reduction of such buffering function can result directly from reduction of arterial distensibility and/or compliance. Arterial compliance, formally defined as a change in volume per unit change in transmural pressure, is also equal to the product of arterial distensibility and arterial volume. Reduction of both compliance and distensibility of large conduit arteries has been reported to occur with age, systolic hypertension, and related arteriosclerotic vascular disease (48,64,136,148,180). In turn, such disease has been attributed primarily to the vascular wall injury resulting from increased flow-induced shear stress and continued exposure to elevated pulsatile pressure cycles. The latter elevation results from an increased stiffness of the arterial wall and reflected pressure pulse waves (48,148,180).

The occurrence of a reduction in compliance and distensibility of large conduit vessels in hypertension is currently a subject of debate. Thus, on the basis of their noninvasive measurement of forearm arterial cross-sectional compliance and distensibility-pressure curves in the hypertensive human as well as the direct in situ measurement of this relationship in the anesthetized spontaneously hypertensive rat, Hayoz and colleagues (89) have concluded that the elastic behavior of medium-size muscular artery (radial) in humans and of an elastic artery (carotid) in rats is not necessarily altered in the hypertensive state. This suggested conclusion has been questioned by Mulvany (136) on the basis of a lack of identification of the contribution made by the passive (structural) versus the active (smooth muscle contractile) components of the vascular wall to measured compliance or distensibility in the hypertensive subjects and animals. In his own in vitro studies Mulvany (135) has observed an increase in wall thickness and a decrease in passive wall stress per unit fractional increase in vessel diameter (defined as the elastic modulus) in small arteries from spontaneously hypertensive rats. Thus, he has concluded that despite the possible lack of a demonstrable change in compliance or distensibility in these vessels, an alteration does occur in either the characteristics or relative proportions of their individual passive wall components.

In addition to regulation by intrinsic passive structural components within the blood vessel wall, large artery diameter and compliance are also regulated by various vasoactive mechanisms. Of particular interest are the adrenergic and renin-angiotensin (RA) systems since it is well known that large arteries contain both adrenergic and AII receptors that mediate vasoconstriction in response to α_1-adrenergic agonists and AII (15,48,234). Additionally, much new knowledge has been acquired over the last decade concerning local (autocrine) cardiovascular regulatory functions of the RA system that exists in many cell types including the VSM and endothelial cell of large arteries (21,22,47,154). Thus, in addition to its role in the renal regulation of extracellular Na^+, AII produced locally within the vascular wall may also participate in the active regulation of arterial compliance by stimulating the specific AT_1 and AT_2 receptors located within the VSM cell membrane. These receptors exhibit a variable distribution in different organ systems and tissues throughout the body (21,22,54). However, all known functions mediated by AII appear to involve only the AT_1 receptor (22). One additional function of endogenous AII that may contribute to the regulation of VSM tone in large arteries (as well as in smaller vessels within the peripheral vasculature) is its ability to facilitate release of norepinephrine from postganglionic sympathetic nerve terminals via activation of prejunctional AII receptors (22,211). Such facilitated release would stimulate postjunctional vascular α_1-adrenoceptors to elevate peripheral vascular tone. Currently, evidence exists both in support of and against this possibility. Based on an observed lack of increased norepinephrine overflow in perfused skeletal muscle vascular beds during sympathetic nerve stimulation, some recent studies question whether increased circulating (exogenously administered) AII enhances norepinephrine release at the vascular neuroeffector junction under normal physiologic conditions (22,184). However, other studies provide evidence for a facilitatory action of the endogenous RA system on sympathetic neuromuscular transmission in several models of hypertension (59,165).

In summary, large arteries contribute to the regulation of cardiovascular function not only as blood conduits but also by virtue of the compliance and distensibility of their walls as buffers of phasic pressure and flow. The latter function contributes to regulation of afterload and thus to protection against deleterious cardiac hypertrophy, hypertension, peripheral vascular injury, and congestive heart failure. Large vessel compliance and distensibility are functions of both passive structural components within the vascular wall and active regulation of VSM tone. The vascular RA system contributes significantly to such regulation.

Small Arteries and Arterioles

The primary role of these smaller precapillary vessels is to regulate driving pressure and rate of blood flow to capillaries within specific vascular beds in order to maintain the requisite nutritional exchange and thus function of the tissues and organ systems that they supply. Hemodynamically such regulation is achieved by controlling the flow resistance of each vessel (Equation 1 above), which in turn is most sensitive to changes in lumen diameter (Equation 2 above). The specific size of precapillary vessel most involved in the control of flow resistance is variable, being dependent on the geometric design of the vascular bed in which it located (e.g., vessel number, length, diameter, and branching characteristics) (251).

For many years the prevailing view was that the major sites of precapillary resistance (i.e., the "true" resistance vessels) were the arterioles with diameters of <30 to 50 μm. However, as summarized by Mulvany and Aalkjaer (137), more recent measurements of intraluminal pressure as a function of vessel size and length indicate that, depending upon the particular vascular bed, up to 50% or more of the peripheral vascular resistance may lie proximal to vessels with diameters of 100 μm, e.g., rat mesentery (14), rat cerebral (85), hamster cheek pouch (44), and cat coronary (37). Of particular physiologic importance is that small arteries as well as arterioles can participate significantly in the regulation of peripheral resistance depending upon stimulus and peripheral vascular bed (137,187,218). Since elevated precapillary resistance is a hallmark of many peripheral vascular diseases, especially hypertension, much interest has been, and continues to be, focused on mechanisms underlying alteration of active (VSM tone) and passive (structural) control of the internal diameter of both of these vessel sizes (64,109,135,137,155).

Although different perfused vascular beds and in vitro isolated vessels from them vary in their sensitivity, the principal neurotransmitter mediating this control is norepinephrine (NE). Chronically, blood pressure–induced increases in the mass of passive structural components (i.e., collagen and elastin) and of active contractile components (i.e., VSM cells) within the vascular wall of small arteries as well as reduction in the numerical density of arterioles in specific vascular beds contribute to an elevation of precapillary resistance. Such structural changes have been observed not only in human essential hypertension but also in almost all animal models of hypertension (137,155).

Exchange Functions in the Microcirculation

Capillaries

Regulation of transcapillary exchange of solutes and water is of prime importance for maintenance of all body functions, including circulatory homeostasis. Both arterioles and capillaries possess highly specialized intracellular and membrane structures that are involved in the regulation of transmural exchange of solutes and water between blood and interstitial fluid. In general, such exchange is governed by passive forces. The rate of transcapillary exchange of solutes (ions and molecules) occurs by diffusion and quantitatively can be expressed by Fick's law of diffusion:

$$J = -PS(C_o - C_i) \quad (7)$$

where

J = quantity of solute moved per unit time
P = capillary permeability of the solute
S = capillary surface area
C_o = concentration of solute inside the capillary
C_i = concentration of solute outside the capillary.

Diffusion of lipid-insoluble solutes is not free but occurs along pathways (usually considered as pores) (120,197) through the capillary wall. Consequently, rate of movement is restricted as a function of size and shape of the solute molecule, attraction between solute and solvent and solute and solute molecules, pore configuration, and charge interaction between solute and endothelial wall components. All of these factors influence the numerical value of P in Equation 7. The rate of diffusion of lipid-insoluble molecules is inversely proportional to their size (and molecular weight) in nonfenestrated capillaries with finite pore sizes (e.g, skeletal muscle vascular beds). Small molecules (e.g., water, urea, NaCl, glucose) are not hindered significantly in their passage through such capillary pores; hence, their mean concentration gradient across the endothelium in these capillary beds is small and they do not contribute significantly to plasma osmotic pressure. Diffusion becomes minimal for lipid-insoluble molecules with a molecular weight above approximately 60,000 (7); hence, plasma oncotic pressure is directly proportional to their concentration difference across the endothelium. It is important to note that for lipid-insoluble solutes, the capillary surface area S in Equation 7 is that of the pores (approximately 0.02% of the capillary wall area (7). In contrast, since S is much larger for lipid-soluble solutes (e.g., respiratory gases), they move rapidly across capillary endothelium (and even across small arteries and arterioles).

The direction and magnitude of movement of solvent (i.e., water) across the capillary endothelium are determined by the algebraic sum of the hydrostatic and osmotic pressures that exist across the endothelium. This relationship can be expressed by the following equation (Starling hypothesis):

$$J_w = k[(P_c - \pi_i) - (P_i - \pi_p)] \quad (8)$$

where

J_w = volume of solvent moved per unit time
P_c = capillary hydrostatic pressure
P_i = interstitial fluid pressure
π_p = plasma protein oncotic pressure
π_i = interstitial fluid oncotic pressure
k = filtration constant for the capillary membrane.

Filtration (out of the capillary into the interstitial space) occurs when the algebraic sum is positive and absorption (into the capillary out of the interstitial space) occurs when it is negative. Each of the terms in Equation 8 can vary as a function of many factors. For example, P_c is directly proportional to arterial and venous pressure and postcapillary (venule and small vein) resistance but inversely proportional to precapillary (small artery and arteriolar) resistance. At the level of the heart, its average value is 32 mm Hg at the arterial end of the capillary and 15 mm Hg at the venous end (in human skin vessels) (7). Interestingly, changes in venous resistance affect capillary hydrostatic pressure more than do changes in arteriolar resistance. For example, approximately 80% of an increase in venous pressure is transmitted back to the capillaries (7). Thus, changes in venous tone not only can regulate venous return and cardiac output by changing vascular capacity (see above), but also by changing circulating blood volume. The value of interstitial fluid pressure (tissue pressure), P_i, which opposes P_c, is still controversial. Depending on the method of measurement, it has been reported to range from 0 to –7 mm Hg (7,77,167).

The plasma osmotic pressure, π_p, which is due primarily to the plasma proteins, is usually termed the *colloid osmotic pressure* or *oncotic pressure*. Its value is approximately 25 mm Hg. It is important to note that plasma osmotic pressure would be about 6000 mm Hg if the capillary endothelium were impermeable to all solutes in plasma (7). The amount and direction of fluid movement across the capillary endothelium by osmotic force is primarily a function of plasma protein concentration. For example, it is increased in dehydration; hence, water moves from the tissues to the vascular compartment. Under conditions where plasma protein concentration is reduced (e.g., starvation, renal loss of protein), fluid moves into the tissues and edema may result, particularly in gravity-dependent regions of the vascular system where capillary hydrostatic pressure is also elevated.

In the form that Equation 8 is written, the filtration constant, k, includes the capillary filtration coefficient (k′), the surface area of capillary available for fluid exchange (A_m), the thickness of the capillary wall Δx), and the viscosity of the filtrate (η). This relation can be expressed by the following equation:

$$k = k'A_m/\eta\Delta x \quad (9)$$

Usually, the capillary filtration coefficient, filtrate viscosity, and capillary wall thickness are relatively constant for the vascular bed within a particular tissue. Under these conditions, Equations 8 and 9 can be applied experimentally to calculate fluid exchange rate and capillary surface area available for such exchange. Of particular current interest relative to such calculations is the function and regulation of specialized protein pores termed *water channels* or *aquaporins*, which have been described in a variety of both epithelial and capillary endothelial cells (2,179). Another area of current interest is the transcapillary movement of large molecules, termed *transcytosis* (120,196,197). This movement occurs in endocytotic vesicles that shuttle across the cytoplasm through cell-spanning transient vesicle-derived channels. Such channels are considered to be the morphologic equivalent of the "large" (50 to 70 nm) pore observed in capillary endothelial cells (120).

EFFECTS OF ANESTHETIC AGENTS ON REGULATION OF PERIPHERAL VASCULAR TONE

It is now well established that peripheral vascular tone is regulated by a three-component system. (a) Vasoconstricting and relaxing factors are released from the vascular endothelium, primarily in response to local environmental changes. Simultaneously, (b) neurotransmitters released from perivascular nerve terminals in the adventitia of small arteries and arterioles can modify vascular smooth muscle tone and thus mediate regional distribution of total systemic blood flow (31). These two regulating mechanisms interact at and with the vascular smooth muscle cell membrane as well as with each other directly (126). Finally, (c) the smooth muscle cell itself incorporates a complex cell signaling system consisting of membrane bound receptors, coupled regulating proteins, ion channels, and second messenger systems that are only now being characterized at a molecular level (68). This system integrates local, humoral, and endothelial input as well as neurally mediated stimuli to produce net effects on vascular tone. Although all of these mechanisms will interact to regulate vascular smooth muscle, one or two may predominate in a particular bed depending on the needs of the tissue. Cardiac and central nervous tissue do not tolerate hypoperfusion. As such, vascular tone in these areas is particularly dependent on endothelial- and flow-dependent regulation (8). Conversely, splanchnic capacitance vessels serve as the major changeable reservoir of unstressed blood volume and, as such, are greatly affected by changes in neural activity (75). Flow to skeletal muscle is dependent on neural control at rest, but during sustained activity the effects of increased metabolic by-products and humoral agents dominate (8).

The vasodilatory properties of general anesthetic agents (particularly volatile anesthetics) have been recognized for years and are well described (38,112,113). Anticipation and management of this side effect is a standard of clinical practice. Nevertheless, the mechanisms by which these agents attenuate vascular tone is not completely understood. Early studies reported that anesthetics produced a withdrawal of sympathetic tone (156). However, direct depressive action on vascular tissue "peripheral" to the nervous system was also recognized (56,239). With recent increases in the understanding of mechanisms responsible for vascular smooth muscle contraction and its regulation, many new specific sites of anesthetic action on mechanisms of vascular control have been reported in the literature. Given the complexity of the mechanisms involved in the generation and regulation of vascular smooth muscle function and the optimal physical properties of most general anesthetic agents, which enable them to transverse membrane structures with relative ease, it is not surprising that anesthetic actions affecting vascular tone have been identified at multiple sites on and within the vascular smooth muscle cell. Nevertheless, the relative importance of many of these actions as well as some of the laboratory data that seems to contradict what is known to occur clinically, have not been clarified. In addition, the effects of volatile anesthetics on the vasculature are better understood than the effects of other general anesthetic agents (such as propofol and narcotics). Mechanisms of action of the latter have been examined in relatively few studies. This section of the chapter summarizes the data and the current understanding of the actions of general anesthetic agents on all three regulatory mechanisms of vascular smooth muscle referred to above, specifically perivascular neural control, endothelial control, and effects at the level of the vascular smooth muscle membrane signaling system itself.

Effects of Anesthetics on Neural Control of VSM Contractile Force

The inhibitory action of anesthetic agents on neural control of the vasculature is well established. The inhibitory effects of halothane (214), enflurane (209), and isoflurane (118) on baroreflex-mediated regulation of mesenteric capacitance veins have been described (Fig. 20). Similar inhibition by halothane and isoflurane (Fig. 21) of chemoreflex-mediated control of the same vessels has also been demonstrated (215,216). These studies measured vessel diameter changes in response to reflex stimuli and (in some cases resultant changes in sympathetic nerve activity) before and during the administration of inhaled anesthetics. Although they did not specifically indicate where anesthetics inhibited neural vascular control, earlier studies had indicated that (at least for baroreflex responses) halothane (186) and isoflurane (185) caused inhibition at multiple sites along the reflex pathway including afferent and efferent transmission, ganglionic transmission, and mechanisms of central integration.

Preganglionic sympathetic efferent nerve activity is attenuated during the administration of halothane (186), isoflurane (185,202), enflurane (200), and barbiturates (201). Depression of the central generation of autonomic tone is a likely explanation for this observation. Inhibition of central vasomotor centers by halothane has been recognized since the 1960s (156). Although the existence of such inhibition was somewhat controversial at that time (56,239), more recent studies have clearly established that halothane, isoflurane, etomidate, midazolam, and propofol inhibit vasomotor control at specific sites within the central nervous system (106,153,182).

In addition to these anesthetic agents, intravenous fentanyl, which is typically used clinically to offset the "stress response" associated with anesthetic induction, has been shown to attenuate reflex increases in sympathetic efferent nerve activity (93). Under at least some conditions, this occurs without any effect on baseline sympathetic tone (49). The central narcotic inhibition of the central nervous system regulatory nuclei for sympathetic tone (43) appears to predominate over peripheral actions (106).

Postganglionic sympathetic efferent nerve activity is also inhibited by halothane (186,214), isoflurane (118,185,216), enflurane (209), fentanyl, and pentobarbital (50), although it

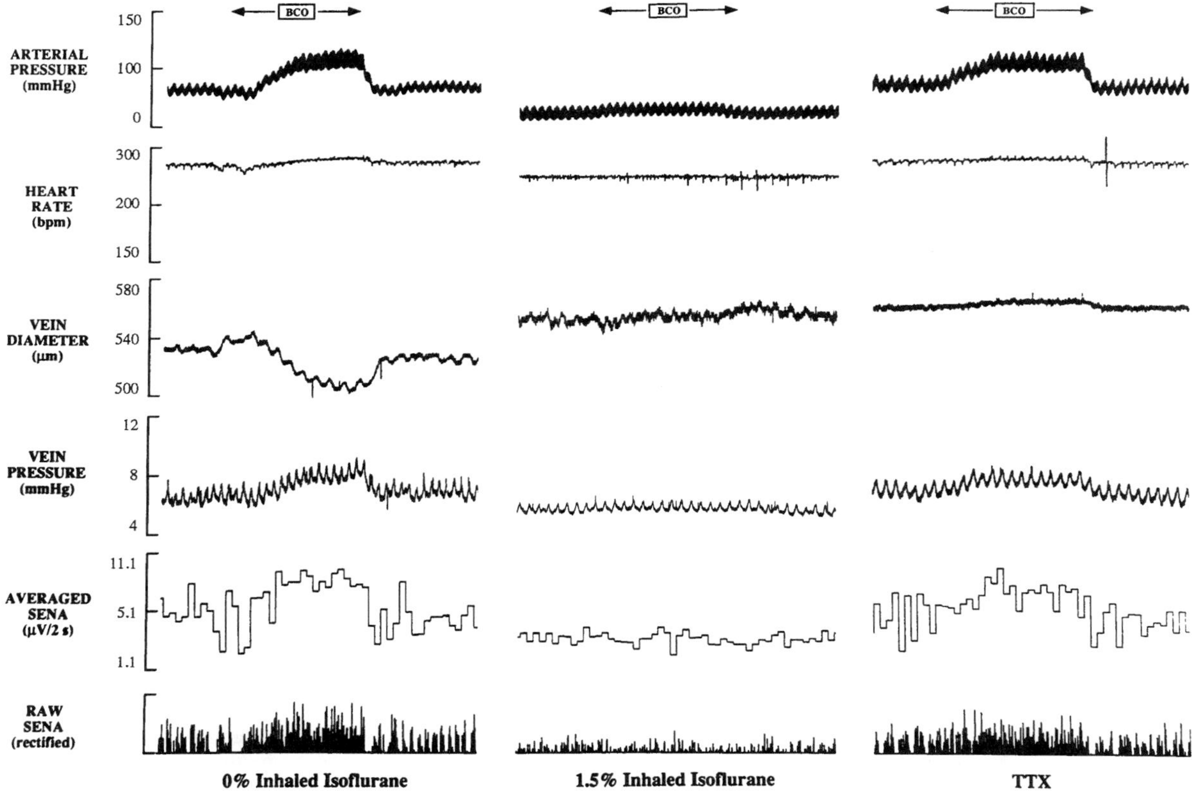

Figure 20. The response of arterial pressure, heart rate, vein diameter, intravenous pressure, and averaged and rectified sympathetic efferent nerve activity (SENA) to bilateral carotid occlusion (BCO) during 0% inhaled isoflurane, 1.5% inhaled isoflurane, and tetrodotoxin (TTX). Reduced levels of nerve activity at 0.75% (not shown) and 1.5% inhaled isoflurane were associated with an increase in vein diameter and a decrease in intravenous pressure, and reflex responses to baroreceptor stimulation were abolished by 1.5% inhaled isoflurane. However, the increase in nerve activity in response to baroreceptor stimulation was not associated with a reflex venoconstriction when the nerve traffic to the vein smooth muscle was blocked by TTX. Similar inhibition of vein diameter changes and related reflex responses was observed during enflurane (209) and halothane (214) administration. (From ref. 118, with permission.)

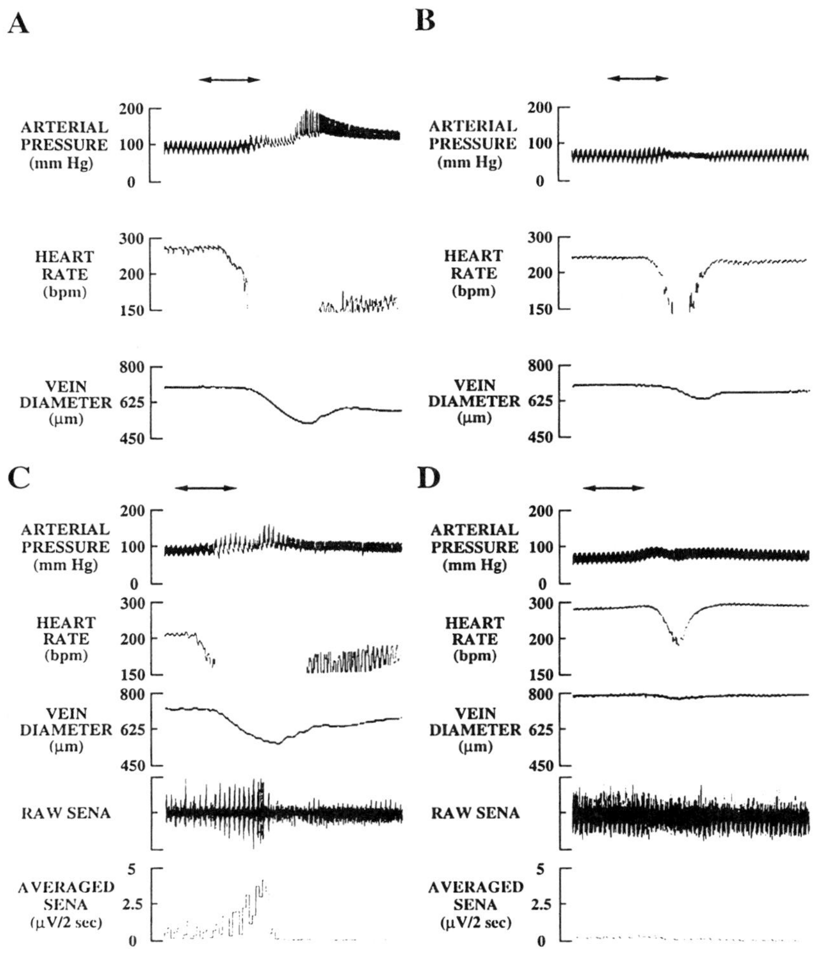

Figure 21. Representative recordings of arterial pressure, heart rate, mesenteric vein diameter, and sympathetic efferent nerve activity (SENA) responses to a 40 second period of 0% oxygen *(arrow)*. (**A** and **B**) Recordings before and during 0.75% inhaled isoflurane. (**C** and **D**) Recordings before and during 1.5% inhaled isoflurane. Similar inhibition of hypoxia-mediated reflex responses were produced by halothane (216). (From ref. 215, with permission.)

should be noted that these studies emphasized reflex rather than resting levels of nerve activity. As is the case with anesthetic attenuation of preganglionic activity, such inhibition can be the result of direct interruption of neuronal conduction and/or anesthetic depression of autonomic tone proximally. In addition to central and preganglionic attenuation, such proximal depression of measured postganglionic activity can also be the result of inhibition of ganglionic transmission. Directly measured postganglionic sympathetic efferent nerve activity is attenuated to a greater extent than preganglionic activity by the administration of both halothane (186) and isoflurane (185). Similarly, mesenteric venoconstriction in response to preganglionic but not postganglionic electrical stimulation is inhibited by isoflurane (118) supporting the concept that anesthetics inhibit ganglionic transmission. When directly measured, ganglionic transmission of compound action potentials in response to preganglionic stimulation is attenuated in the presence of clinically relevant doses of halothane (18), isoflurane (Fig. 22), and desflurane (13). Subsequently, the mechanism for this inhibition may involve attenuation of presynaptic acetylcholine release (17); however, the primary effect appears to be an altered sensitivity of the postsynaptic neuron (13).

In addition to the autonomic ganglia, anesthetics also attenuate synaptic transmission at the level of the vascular smooth

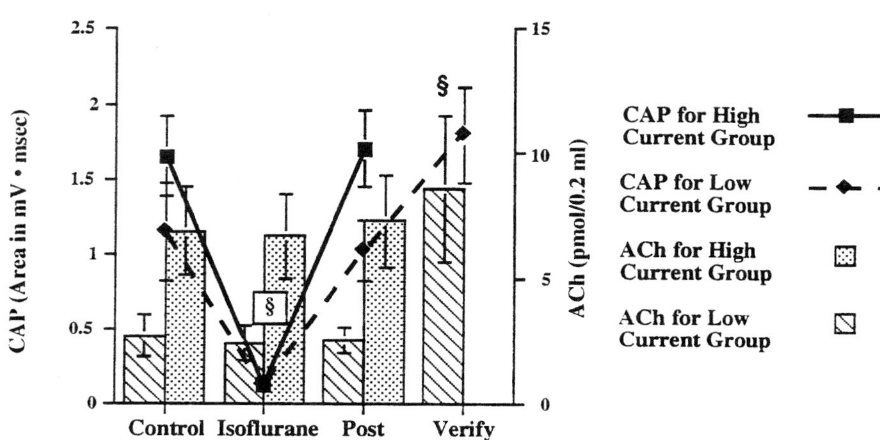

Figure 22. Isoflurane decreased the compound action potential (CAP) in response to maximum and submaximum stimulations, but acetylcholine (ACh) release was not affected by isoflurane administration during either maximum or submaximum stimulation. Increased levels of ACh release and CAP response to maximum stimulation after the study in the group with submaximum stimulations verify the current-dependent nature of synaptic transmission (high-current group, $n = 7$; low-current group, $n = 6$; §$p < .01$ versus control). Similar inhibitory effects on ganglionic transmission were observed during administration of halothane (17,18) and desflurane (13). (From ref. 13, with permission.)

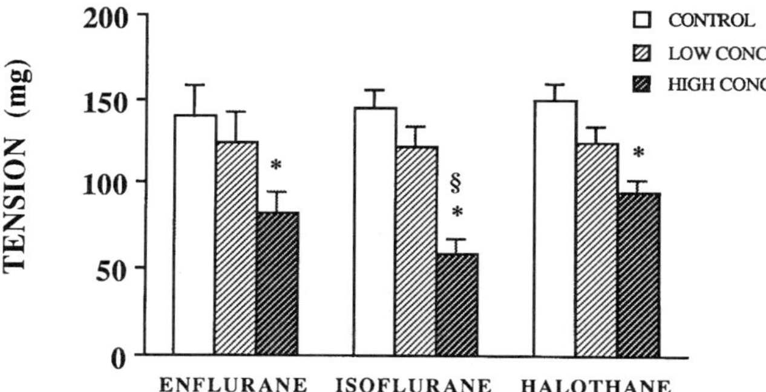

Figure 23. Effects of enflurane (31 rings, $n = 7$), halothane (16 rings, $n = 7$), and isoflurane (26 rings, $n = 7$) on contractile responses of mesenteric veins to electric field stimulation. Significant inhibition of isometric tension by high (approximately 1.0 MAC in rabbit) concentrations of volatile anesthetics. *$p \leq .01$ versus control, §$p \leq .05$ high isoflurane versus high halothane and enflurane. (From ref. 208, with permission.)

muscle neuromuscular junction. In isolated preparations of canine saphenous vein strips, halothane was shown to inhibit adrenergic neurotransmitter release in response to perivascular nerve stimulation (114,134). Subsequently, data from additional studies utilizing these preparations supported a mechanism whereby halothane modulates the prejunctional receptors that regulate neurotransmitter release from the presynaptic neuron (171). More recently, in a vessel ring preparation utilizing isolated mesenteric arteries and veins, not only halothane but also enflurane and isoflurane (Fig. 23) in clinically relevant concentrations, were shown to attenuate contractile responses to endogenous norepinephrine release during perivascular nerve stimulation (104,208).

Thus, anesthetic agents depress neural control of the peripheral vasculature by inhibition of receptor organ function and afferent transmission (when reflexes are involved), by depression of central generation of neural tone, and by attenuation of synaptic transmission both at the level of the autonomic ganglion and at the neuromuscular junction (Fig. 24). Although it is conceivable that anesthetic agents could also inhibit impulse propagation along nerve fibers, this mechanism has not been observed when studied with clinically relevant doses of halothane (18), isoflurane, or desflurane (13).

Clearly the majority of data available on the effects of anesthetic agents on the neural control of the peripheral vasculature has focused on the sympathetic nervous system, which is firmly established as a major control mechanism of vascular tone. Much less is known about anesthetic effects on other types of perivascular nerves such as parasympathetic, sensorimotor, or nitroxidergic vasodilator neurons. One recent report confirmed the presence of nitroxidergic inhibitory neurons in porcine tracheal smooth muscle. However, halothane was shown to have no effect on this mechanism of smooth muscle relaxation (111). Furthermore, the overall significance of these nonsympathetic neurons in the regulation of peripheral vascular tone remains largely speculative.

Effects of Anesthetics on Intrinsic Regulation of VSM Contractile Force

Many of the previously described vascular smooth muscle mechanisms are potential sites for inhibitory actions of anesthetic agents. Furthermore, it is clear that anesthetics can

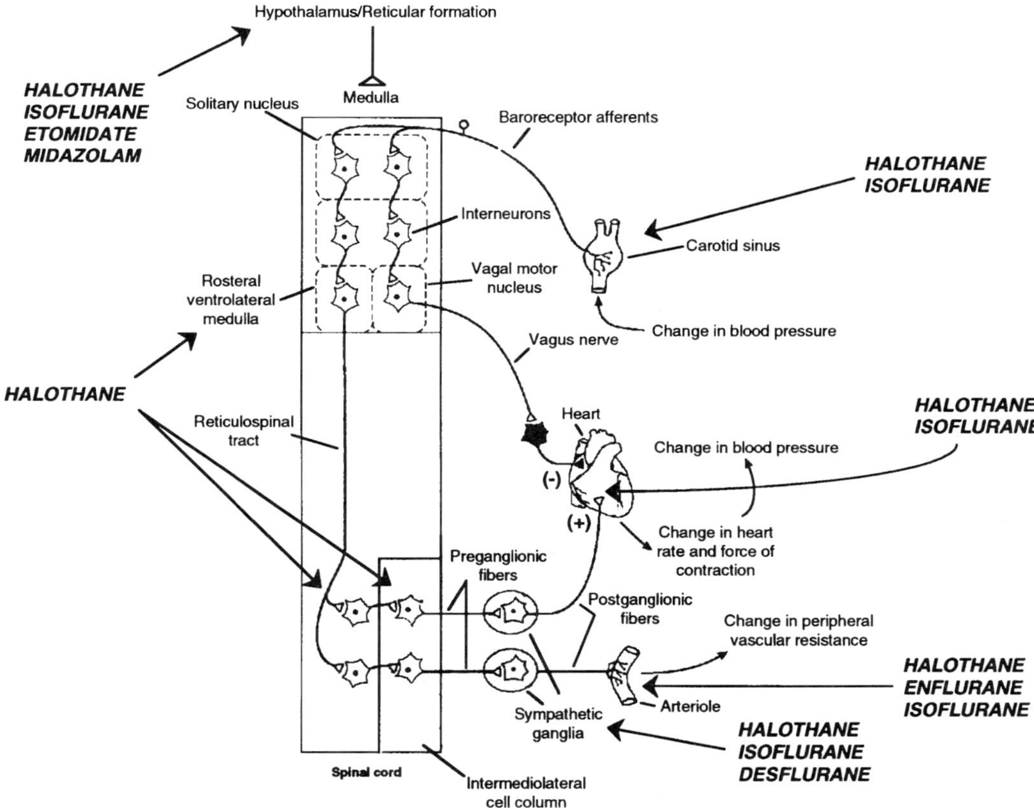

Figure 24. This schematic of the baroreflex pathway exemplifies neural mechanisms of cardiovascular control. Specific sites of anesthetic action are summarized. Other agents such as barbiturates, propofol, narcotics, and sevoflurane are also known to affect neural control of the vasculature at various levels. However, the actions of the agents at sites indicated in this figure have been specifically identified in different studies (see text). (Adapted from ref. 46, with permission.)

inhibit vascular smooth muscle directly, an action that is independent of neural or endothelial control. In the vessel ring preparation discussed previously, halothane, enflurane, and isoflurane inhibited vascular smooth muscle contraction to exogenously applied as well as endogenously released norepinephrine, suggesting direct as well as neural inhibitory effects of these agents (117,208). In other vessel ring preparations, halothane and isoflurane reduced vascular smooth muscle tone equally with endothelium intact and with endothelium removed (97). In addition to volatile anesthetics, intravenous agents also exert direct effects on vascular smooth muscle. Intravenous narcotics are used clinically as adjuncts to other anesthetics or (in higher doses) as the principal agent, particularly in patients with limited cardiovascular reserve because they tend to maintain a stable hemodynamic profile (93). Their effects on blunting the stress response associated with anesthetic induction has been mentioned above. However, fentanyl and sufentanil have also been shown to produce vasodilation by direct action on the vascular smooth muscle independent of neuronal (244) and (at least in the case of coronary arteries) endothelial integrity (246). The intravenous anesthetic propofol also directly relaxes vascular smooth muscle and attenuates the myogenic response (116).

As indicated above, vascular smooth muscle tone is proportional to intracellular calcium ion concentration ($[Ca^{2+}]_i$). The effects of anesthetic agents to produce relaxation of vascular smooth muscle appear to be mediated via a decrease in $[Ca^{2+}]_i$. However, the predominant mechanism by which this occurs seems to vary depending on which experimental preparation is used to study these effects. In cultured vascular smooth muscle–like cells halothane (194) and isoflurane (192) did not affect $[Ca^{2+}]_i$ when the cells were at rest, but they did significantly attenuate the $[Ca^{2+}]_i$ increase in response to agonist administration. Furthermore, this attenuation was associated with a decrease in inositol triphosphate (IP_3) production. Since the predominant effect of IP_3 is to stimulate Ca^{2+} release from the sarcoplasmic reticulum, Ca^{2+} release from intracellular stores may have been affected more than Ca^{2+} influx across the cell membrane. In addition, in a similar preparation using porcine coronary vascular smooth muscle cells, inhibition of agonist-induced $[Ca^{2+}]_i$ increase occurred in part at a site proximal to IP_3 production, suggesting action at the site of the membrane receptor and/or the G protein (193). In other preparations using cultured vascular smooth muscle–like cells or vascular smooth muscle cells themselves, isoflurane (96,229), halothane (96,228,229), and enflurane (221) actually enhanced Ca^{2+} release from intracellular SR stores when the cells were at rest. However, these agents inhibit the increase in $[Ca^{2+}]_i$ in response to agonist stimulation at least in part as the result of attenuation of $[Ca^{2+}]_i$ influx across the sarcolemma (96,228,229). Such a mechanism is further substantiated by recent patch clamp studies that directly demonstrated inhibitory effects of isoflurane and halothane on Ca^{2+} and K^+ current across the sarcolemma of vascular smooth muscle cells from canine coronary (Fig. 25) (25) and cerebral vessels (57). Inhibition of inward Ca^{2+} current would be expected to produce a hyperpolarization and reduced $[Ca^{2+}]_i$, thus resulting in vascular smooth muscle relaxation. Inhibition of outward K^+ current would be expected to do the opposite and therefore oppose the relaxation resulting from decreased Ca^{2+} influx. Nevertheless, the halothane- and isoflurane-mediated inhibition of Ca^{2+} current seems to be proportionally greater than that of the potassium current (16), and thus hyperpolarization and inhibition of tone would be expected to predominate. Recently, hyperpolarization of in situ single cell mesenteric arterial and venous vascular smooth muscle membrane potential measurements resulting from clinically relevant concentrations of halothane (Fig. 26), isoflurane, and sevoflurane has been demonstrated (212,213). Furthermore, hyperpolarization is directly proportional to vascular smooth muscle relaxation over the physiologic range of membrane potentials (217). In addition to the volatile anes-

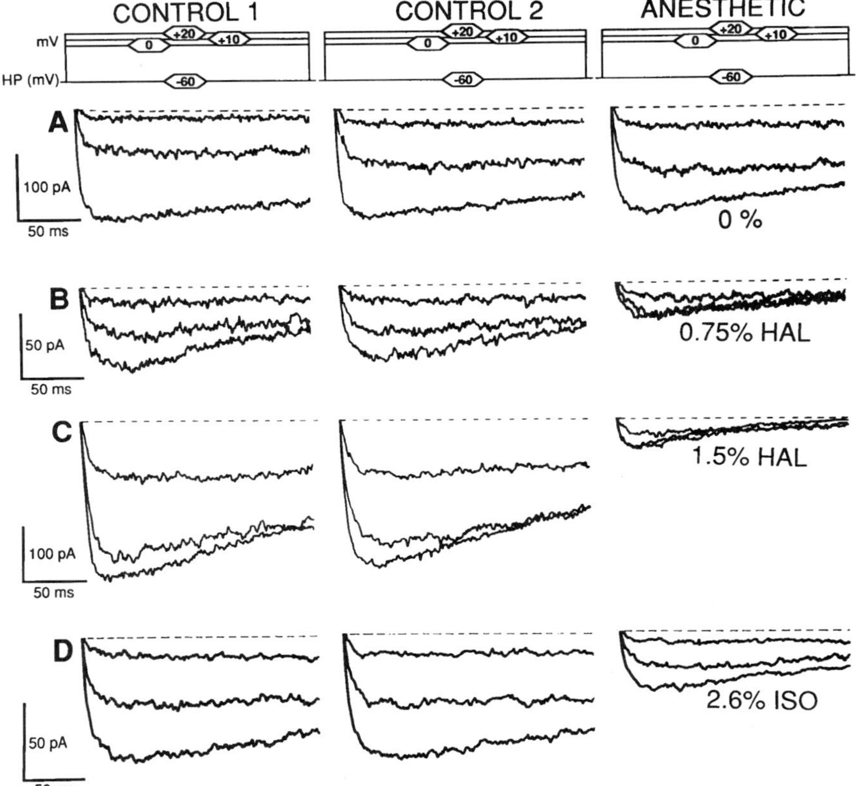

Figure 25. Recordings of Ca^{2+} current (I_{Ca}) generated by progressive depolarizing pulses from -60 mV to +40 mV (10-mV increments). Only selected episodes are shown: -60 mV *(dashed line)* and 0, +10, and +20 mV. **(A)** Three measurements (control 1, control 2, and control c) were taken 3 min apart without exposure to volatile anesthetics in order to determine time-dependent changes (decay) in I_{Ca}. **(B–D)** In other cells, recordings of I_{Ca} were obtained in control solution (control 1, control 2) and then in the presence of 0.75% halothane **(B)**, 1.5% halothane **(C)**, or 2.6% isoflurane **(D)**. Control measurements were taken 3 min apart, and measurements after anesthetic application were taken 3 min after control 2 in the same cell. (From ref. 25, with permission.)

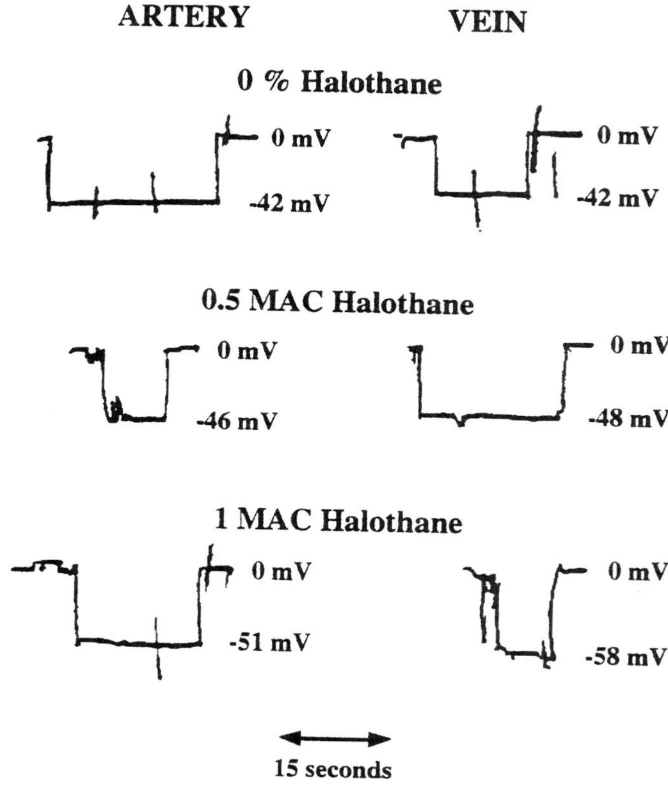

Figure 26. Recordings of single VSM cell membrane potential (E_m) from mesenteric arteries and veins illustrating the hyperpolarizing effect of inhaled halothane. Similar hyperpolarization has been observed following isoflurane (212) and sevoflurane (213) administration.

thetics, propofol has also been shown to inhibit neural and endothelium-independent influx of calcium into vascular smooth muscle (36).

Mechanisms by which anesthetics inhibit ion conductance into cells may involve direct action on the channel itself from within the membrane proper as has been proposed for the action of halothane on K channels (249). Anesthetics may also act on G proteins to uncouple the interaction between receptors, G proteins, and the channels, as has been reported for halothane in ilial smooth muscle (158) and for sevoflurane in myocytes (181). This does not appear to be a mechanism by which narcotics affect vascular smooth muscle (158). In some vascular smooth muscle preparations, halothane has been shown to increase intracellular cGMP (16,58), and both halothane and isoflurane have increased intracellular cAMP (16). In VSM cGMP as well as cAMP (in contrast to its actions in myocardial tissue) reduce muscle tone by inhibiting Ca channels (207) and by enhancing K channels, both of which lead to reduced Ca^{2+} influx (16).

In addition to producing vascular smooth muscle relaxation by inhibiting the increase of $[Ca^{2+}]_i$ via attenuation of calcium influx (and possibly by reducing its release from intracellular stores as well), anesthetic agents may also act to promote mechanisms associated with the elimination of intracellular Ca^{2+} (Fig. 27). Halothane-mediated increases in cGMP concentration and halothane and isoflurane-mediated increases in cAMP concentration (16,58) activate protein kinase, which phosphorylates and therefore activates the sodium–calcium exchanger (65), and the calcium–adenosine triphosphatase (ATPase), which drives the calcium pump, thus promoting elimination of intracellular calcium (16). At this time there does not appear to be evidence for a cGMP-mediated mechanism of vasodilation by isoflurane (20).

It is apparent from the above discussion that regulation of vascular tone at the level of vascular smooth muscle cells themselves involve many interactions between external stimuli, membrane bound and intracellular regulatory molecules, and the intracellular contractile apparatus. As one considers the direct effects of anesthetics on vascular smooth muscle, virtually every step in this series of interactions is a potential target for action by anesthetic agents. Furthermore, the understanding of these processes will undoubtedly become even more complex as new information is reported and as more exceptions are identified. This is no single universal explanation to account for all of the known effects of anesthetics at this level. Nevertheless, the most common mechanism by which most of these agents (both volatile and intravenous) ultimately act on vascular smooth muscle cells is to reduce intracellular Ca^{2+} available for excitation-contraction coupling either by inhibiting its entry, promoting its release, or both.

Effects of Anesthetics on Endothelium-Mediated Regulation of VSM Contractile Force

The general concepts of vascular endothelial cells actively contributing to the regulation of smooth muscle tone have emerged only recently. Therefore, the understanding of the effects of anesthetic agents on these mechanisms is in the early stages, and the experimental results to date that describe these effects are not entirely consistent. Initially, isoflurane was shown to facilitate endothelium-dependent dilation of canine coronary arteries (12). Subsequently enflurane (241) and halothane (240,241) were shown to offset the vasoconstricting properties of NO synthase inhibitors, suggesting that the release and/or action of endothelial-derived NO is enhanced. In addition, in a similar study using NO synthase inhibitors, the vasodilatory effect of endothelial- derived NO was greater during isoflurane than during halothane administration (74). Likewise, the intravenous anesthetic propofol has also been shown to significantly increase NO production from cultured endothelial cells and to subsequently increase cGMP in vascular smooth muscle cells in vitro (151). These observations clearly agree with the established understanding that most anesthetic agents (particularly the volatile anesthetics) clinically act as vasodilators (16,38,112,113). However, in contrast to these studies, a larger number of reports have emerged that indicate that anesthetics (particularly volatile anesthetics) do not enhance and may actually inhibit endothelial-mediated (NO regulated) vasodilation. This was initially reported for halothane (133) and later for halothane, enflurane, isoflurane, and sevoflurane (124,140,220,247).

Subsequently, studies have been conducted to identify mechanisms by which anesthetic agents inhibit endothelial derived NO-mediated vasorelaxation. One proposed mechanism is the inhibition of receptor-dependent and/or -independent increase in endothelial intracellular Ca^{2+} necessary for NO synthase activation (50,99). There is hypothetical support for this mechanism because the processes for increased cytosolic Ca^{2+} in endothelial cells are similar to those for increasing Ca^{2+} in vascular smooth muscle cells, leading to excitation-contraction coupling (99), although endothelial cells do not possess voltage-gated Ca channels. As outlined in detail above, these processes in vascular smooth muscle are known to be significantly affected by anesthetic agents. One recent study examining halothane and isoflurane concluded that these agents inhibited endothelial NO release primarily by interfering with acetylcholine receptor–mediated increase in cytosolic Ca^{2+} (225). A similar study examining halothane, isoflurane, and enflurane confirmed inhibition by these agents of receptor-mediated Ca^{2+} increases, but also demonstrated inhibition of NO release independent of alterations in endothelial cytoplasmic $[Ca^{2+}]_i$ (230). This implies anesthetic

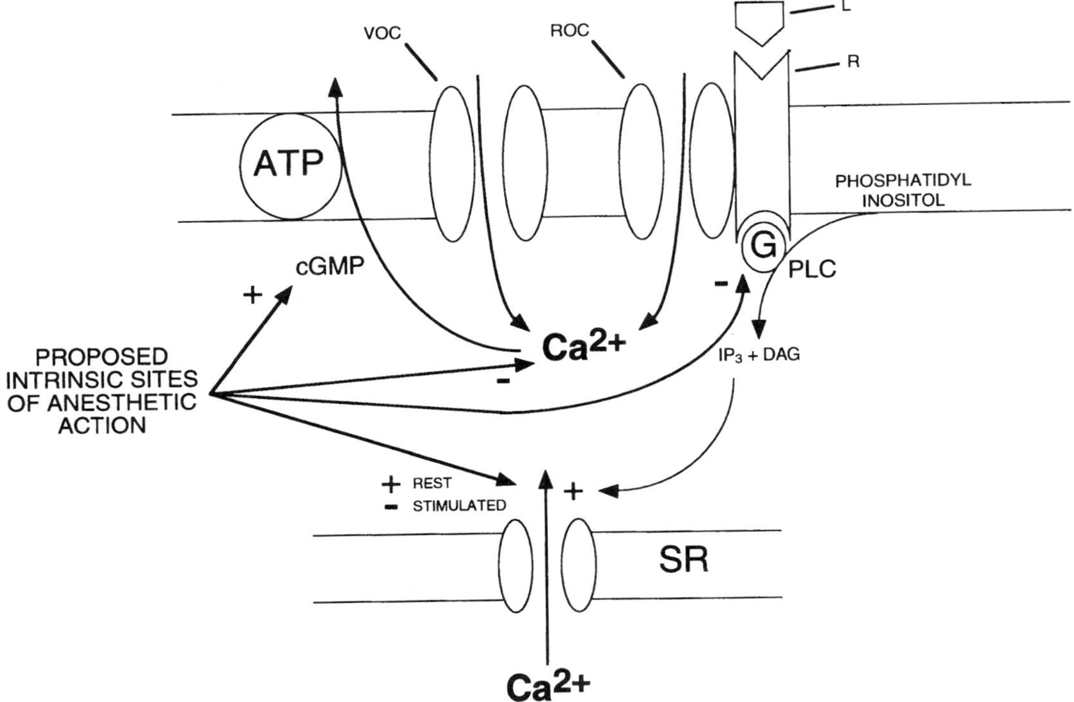

Figure 27. A schematic illustrating recognized sites of action of anesthetic agents on regulation of intracellular calcium [Ca^{2+}], which determines intrinsic (vascular smooth muscle)–mediated control of vascular tone. VOC, voltage operated calcium channel; ROC, receptor operated calcium channel; L, ligand, R, G protein–coupled receptor; G, G protein, PLC, phospholipase C; IP_3, inositol triphosphate; DAG, diacylglycerol; SR, sarcoplasmic reticulum; ATP, adenosine triphosphate–dependent calcium pump; rest, resting condition of the smooth muscle cell; stimulated, conditions when the smooth muscle cell is stimulated to contract; +, enhancement of activity; –, inhibition of activity.

inhibition of NO distal to the process of Ca^{2+}-mediated NO synthase activation. Such distal processes that could be inhibited include direct attenuation of NO synthase, interaction with the NO molecule itself, and/or interference with the cGMP-mediated vasodilation by NO within vascular smooth muscle cells (50,99).

Sevoflurane has been shown to cause free radical interaction with and inhibition of the NO molecule directly (247). More recently, some of the same authors who previously reported the isoflurane-mediated enhancement of endothelial vasodilation also reported that halothane did not inhibit endothelial-derived NO release. However, halothane did alter NO stability suggesting that halothane (like sevoflurane) may act (at least in part) by free radical inactivation of NO (12). In the studies described above in which nitroglycerine and/or nitroprusside were studied, neither halothane, enflurane, nor isoflurane affected their ability to relax vascular smooth muscle (133, 227,230). The nitro vasodilators are NO analogues that break down to release exogenous NO, which then produces vasorelaxation via cGMP production in VSM cells (50,51). A lack of anesthetic inhibition of the action of these agents suggests that anesthetics have minimal effects on NO effector targets within the vascular smooth muscle (50). This is further substantiated by the previously noted study reporting no change in soluble guanylate cyclase activity during halothane administration (58). Nevertheless, in a more recent study, authors who previously observed no inhibitory effects of halothane on VSM relaxation by nitro vasodilators now have identified these effects (87). This suggests that (at least for halothane) inhibition of endothelial NO effects not only may result from attenuation of NO synthesis and enhanced free radical inactivation of NO, but also may occur by interference with effects of endothelially released NO within the vascular smooth muscle (87). Finally, a recent study of halothane, isoflurane, and sevoflurane contributes some order to the multiplicity of results associated with inhibitory anesthetic effects on endothelially mediated NO vasodilation. The investigation concluded that isoflurane acts primarily by inhibition of endothelial NO synthesis and release, and sevoflurane inhibits NO directly via production of free radicals, while halothane inhibits NO targeted guanylyl cyclase activity within the vascular smooth muscle (140) (Fig. 28).

Only a few studies have examined the effects of anesthetics other than the volatile agents on endothelium-mediated regulation of vascular tone. As indicated previously, in one study using cultured endothelial cells, propofol enhanced endothelially released NO-mediated vasodilation (151). In a different study using a vessel ring preparation the propofol-induced vasorelaxation was found to be independent of endothelial NO (150). Likewise, in the same study, thiopental was found to have no effect on endothelial NO.

Very little information exists regarding the effects of anesthetic agents on endothelial regulation of vascular tone via mechanisms other than those involving NO. A study discussed previously with regard to inhibitory effects of halothane, enflurane, and isoflurane on endothelial NO also suggested that these anesthetics stimulated the endothelial release of a vasodilating prostaglandin substance (220). Likewise, in the study addressing the effects of propofol and thiopental (above), these agents also appeared to promote the endothelial release of prostaglandin vasodilating substances. Finally, in a different study, the inhalational agent nitrous oxide, a known (mild) sympathomimetic, was found to be associated with endothelial-dependent vasoconstriction of porcine coronary arteries. This study suggested that the mechanism involved nitrous oxide–mediated inhibition of endothelial cytosolic Ca^{2+} regulation, which led to interference with endothelial metabolism of neurotransmitter (94).

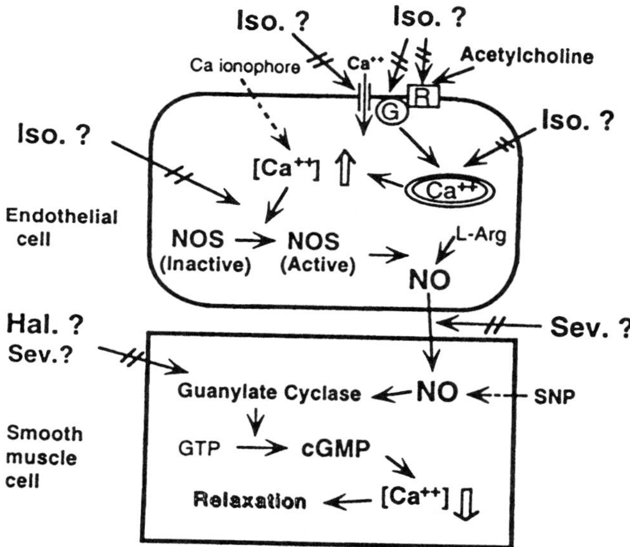

Figure 28. A schematic summarizing proposed mechanisms of inhibition by volatile anesthetics on endothelial nitric oxide–mediated vasodilation. Isoflurane (Iso) may act by interfering with the receptor-mediated (calcium dependent) synthesis of nitric oxide (NO) by constitutive membrane-bound nitric oxide synthase (NOS). Sevoflurane (sevo) may directly interfere with the stability or action of the NO molecule itself. Halothane (Hal) may inhibit NO-mediated guanylate cyclase activity within the smooth muscle cell, which normally produces cyclic guanosine monophosphate cGMP to cause vasodilation. (From ref. 140, with permission.)

It is apparent that the data describing the effects of anesthetics on the endothelial-mediated regulation of vascular smooth muscle lacks consistency as compared with the understanding of the effects of these agents on other mechanisms of vascular control. Although some evidence exists for anesthetic-induced endothelial-mediated vasodilation, the majority of studies support anesthetic inhibition of endothelial vasorelaxation. If this is true, then there is the added burden of explaining the apparent contradiction with the fact that anesthetics are recognized clinically as vasodilators. Explanations that have been advanced for these discrepancies have included differences in experimental preparations (87, 151); regional differences in responsiveness between types of vessels studied (220, 230); and difficulty in extrapolating in vitro data to explain in vivo and clinical observations (74). Although these explanations seem less than adequate in that they are only generalizations rather than specific, they merely reflect the current level of understanding of this aspect of vascular regulation.

CONCLUSIONS

Vascular tone is regulated by both extrinsic and intrinsic levels of control. The extrinsic levels consist of neural and endothelial regulation, which interact with each other as well as with intrinsic mechanisms. Intrinsic control consists of functions associated with the vascular smooth muscle itself. Specifically designed experimental conditions can and do demonstrate and emphasize particular mechanisms within each of these levels of vascular regulation. The significance of some of these mechanisms participating in overall hemodynamic control is clearly understood, such as the role of sympathetic regulation of capacitance and resistance vessels and the role of cytosolic Ca^{2+} in producing vascular smooth muscle excitation-contraction coupling. The relative importance of other mechanisms (particularly in the normal intact physiologic situation) remains to be established. For example, the predominant vasodilatory properties of intact endothelium can easily be demonstrated in preconstricted vessels in vitro (50). However, the question remains, What is the relative contribution by this endothelial mechanism in determining vascular tone when that vessel is in vivo in its natural environment with intact basal and reflex vasoconstricting sympathetic input? Similar questions could be asked about other recently identified or postulated mechanisms such as the relative role of the putative nitroxidergic peripheral vasodilating neurons (225,226,236). For clinical anesthesiologists and researchers using anesthetized animals, the effects of the anesthetic agents are also superimposed upon these many mechanisms of vascular control. As outlined in this chapter, some type of anesthetic inhibition and/or facilitation has been identified for almost every mechanism of vascular control studied. In many cases, under particular experimental conditions, dramatic effects of clinically common anesthetic agents (in clinically relevant doses) have been demonstrated to act on the mechanisms of control of vascular tone. Nevertheless, these same agents are widely used clinically every day and are well tolerated in the vast majority of patients. Clinical anesthesiologists routinely anticipate, recognize, and treat most vascular side effects of these agents. However, clinicians also recognize that there are subpopulations of patients with pathologic conditions who are at much greater risk for adverse outcome resulting from even minimal anesthetic alteration of normal mechanisms of vascular control. Examples include patients with severely compromised myocardial function, patients with altered reflex control of the vasculature, and patients with critical vascular occlusions who are at risk for end organ infarction (24). This chapter has outlined current data that describe different mechanisms of vascular control as well as many postulated sites of anesthetic interaction. The improved management of these types of patients at increased risk for anesthetics will require additional research to identify those mechanisms of vascular control that are physiologically important and how to develop anesthetics and techniques to avoid or compensate for their perturbations.

ACKNOWLEDGMENTS

This work was supported by VA Medical Research Fund and Anesthesiology Research Training Grant GM 08377. The authors thank Anita Tredeau and Edith Sulzer for their assistance with the preparation of this chapter.

REFERENCES

1. Adams DJ, Barakeh J, Laskey R, Van Breemen C. Ion channels and regulation of intracellular calcium in vascular endothelial cells. *FASEB J* 1989;3:2389–2400.
2. Agre P, Preston GM, Smith BL. Aquaporin CHIP: the archetypal molecular water channel. *Am J Physiol* 1993;265:F463–F476.
3. Augustine G. Proteins of presynaptic terminal (Poster). *TINS* 1994;17:516a–517a.
4. Baez S. Microvascular terminology. In: Kaley G, Altura BM, eds. *Microcirculation,* vol 1. Baltimore: University Park Press, 1977;23–24.
5. Bennet MR. Quantal secretion at visualized sympathetic nerve varicosities. *NIPS* 1993;8:199–201.
6. Berkowitz BA, Zabko-Potapovich B, Valocik R, Gleason JR. Effects of leukotrienes on the vasculature and blood pressure. *J Pharmacol Exp Ther* 1984;229:105–112.
7. Berne RM, Levy MN. The microcirculation and lymphatics. In: Berne RM, Levy MN, eds. *Physiology,* 3rd ed. St. Louis: Mosby Yearbook, 1993;465–477.
8. Berne RM, Levy MN. The peripheral circulation and its control. In: Berne RM, Levy MN, eds. *Physiology,* 3rd ed. St. Louis: Mosby Yearbook, 1993;478–493.
9. Berne RM, Levy MN. Control of cardiac output: coupling of heart and blood vessels. In: Berne RM, Levy MN, eds. *Physiology,* 3rd ed. St. Louis: Mosby Yearbook, 1993;494–509.
10. Berridge MJ. Inositol triphosphate and diacylglycerol: two interacting second messengers. *Annu Rev Biochem* 1987;56:159–193.
11. Bevan JA, Bevan RD, Duckles SP. Adrenergic regulation of vascular

smooth muscle. In: Bohr DF, Somlyo AP, Sparks Jr, eds. *Vascular smooth muscle vol. III, The cardiovascular, Section 2, Handbook of physiology.* Bethesda: American Physiological Society, 1980;515–566.
12. Blaise G, Sill JC, Nugent M, Van Dyke RA, Vanhoutte PM. Isoflurane causes endothelium-dependent inhibition of contractile responses of canine coronary arteries. *Anesthesiology* 1987;67:513–517.
13. Boban N, McCallum JB, Schedewie HK, Boban M, Kampine JP, Bosnjak ZJ. Direct comparative effects of isoflurane and desflurane on the sympathetic ganglionic transmission. *Anesth Analg* 1995;80:127–134.
14. Bohlen HG, Gore RW. Comparison of microvascular pressures and diameters in the innervated and denervated rat intestine. *Microvasc Res* 1977;14:251–264.
15. Bolton TB. Mechanism of action of transmitters and other substances on smooth muscle. *Physiol Rev* 1979;59:606–718.
16. Bosnjak ZJ. Ion channels in vascular smooth muscle. *Anesthesiology* 1993;79:1392–1401.
17. Bosnjak ZJ, Dujic Z, Roerig DL, Kampine JP. Effects of halothane on acetylcholine release and sympathetic ganglionic transmission. *Anesthesiology* 1988;69:56–62.
18. Bosnjak ZJ, Seagard JL, Wu A, Kampine JP. The effects of halothane on sympathetic ganglionic transmission. *Anesthesiology* 1982; 57:473–479.
19. Braun-Menendez E, Fasciolo J, Leloir L, Munoz J. The substance causing renal hypertension. *J Physiol* 1940;98:283–298.
20. Brendel JK, Johns RA. Isoflurane does not vasodilate rat thoracic aortic rings by endothelium-derived relaxing factor or other cyclic GMP-mediated mechanisms. *Anesthesiology* 1992;77:126–131.
21. Brooks DP, Ruffolo RR Jr. Functions mediated by peripheral angiotensin II receptors. In: Ruffolo RR Jr, ed. *Angiotensin II receptors.* Boca Raton: CRC Press, 1994;71–119.
22. Brooks DP, Ruffolo RR Jr. Introduction: angiotensin II receptors. In: Ruffolo RR Jr, ed. *Angiotensin II receptors.* Boca Raton: CRC Press, 1994b;1–9.
23. Brown AM. Ion channels as G protein effectors. *NIPS* 1991;6: 158–161.
24. Brown DL. *Risk and outcome in anesthesia.* Philadelphia: JB Lippincott, 1992.
25. Buljubasic N, Rusch NJ, Marijic J, Kampine JP, Bosnjak ZJ. Effects of halothane and isoflurane on calcium and potassium channel currents in canine coronary artery cells. *Anesthesiology* 1992;76: 990–998.
26. Bunnemann B, Fuxe K, Ganten D. The renin-angiotensin system in the brain: an update 1993. *Regul Peptides* 1993;46:487–509.
27. Burn JH, Rand MJ. Acetylcholine in adrenergic transmission. *Annu Rev Pharmacol* 1965;5:163–182.
28. Burnstock G. Cholinergic and purinergic regulation of blood vessels. In: Bohr DF, Somlyo AP, Sparks HV Jr, eds. *Vascular smooth muscle, vol II, The cardiovascular system, Section 2, Handbook of physiology.* Bethesda: American Physiological Society, 1980;567–612.
29. Burnstock G. Do some nerve cells release more than one transmitter? *Neuroscience* 1976;1:239–248.
30. Burnstock G. Innervation of vascular smooth muscle: and electron microscopy. *Clin Exp Pharmacol Physiol* 1975;2 (Suppl 2):7–20.
31. Burnstock G. Integration of factors controlling vascular tone. *Anesthesiology* 1993;79:1368–1380.
32. Burnstock G, Iwayama T. Fine structure identification of autonomic nerves and their relation to smooth muscle. In: Eranko O, eds. *Histochemistry of nervous transmission: progress in brain research.* Amsterdam: Elsevier Science, 1971;389–404.
33. Campbell D. Circulating and tissue angiotensin systems. *J Clin Invest* 1987;79:1–6.
34. Cannon WB. Organization for physiological homeostasis. *Physiol Rev* 1929;9:399–431.
35. Captevila JH, Falck JR, Estabrook RW. Cytochrome P450 and the arachidonate cascade. *FASEB J* 1992;6:731–744.
36. Chang KSK, Davis RF. Propofol produces endothelium-independent vasodilation and may act as a Ca^{2+} channel blocker. *Anesth Analg* 1993;76:24–32.
37. Chilian WM, Eastham CL, Marcus ML. Microvascular distribution of coronary vascular resistance in beating left ventricle. *Am J Physiol* 1986;251:H779–H788.
38. Clark SC, MacCannell KL. Vascular responses to anaesthetic agents. *Can Anaesth Soc J* 1975;22:20–33.
39. Corr L, Burnstock G. Vasodilator response of coronary smooth muscle to the sympathetic cotransmitters nor-adrenaline and adenosine triphosphate. *Br J Pharmacol* 1991;104:337–342.
40. Cryer PE. Physiology and pathophysiology of the human sympathoadrenal neuroendocrine system. *N Engl J Med* 1980;303: 436–444.
41. Dale H. *Transmission of effects from nerve endings.* Oxford: Oxford University Press, 1952.
42. Daniel TO, Ives HE. Endothelial control of vascular function. *NIPS* 1989;4:139–142.
43. Daskalpoulos NTH, Laubie M, Schmitt H. Localization of the central sympatho-inhibitory effect of narcotic analgesic fentanyl in cats. *Eur J Pharmacol* 1975;33:91–97.
44. Davis MJ, Ferrer PN, Gore RW. Vascular anatomy and hydrostatic pressure profile in the hamster cheek pouch. *Am J Physiol* 1986; 250:H291–H303.
45. Denn MJ, Stone HL. Autonomic innervation of dog coronary arteries. *J Appl Physiol* 1976;41:30–35.
46. Dodd J, Role L. The autonomic nervous system. In: Kandel E, Schwartz J, Jessel T, eds. *Principles of neuroscience,* 3rd ed. New York: Elsevier Science, 1991;761–775.
47. Dzau VJ. Circulating versus local renin-angiotensin system in cardiovascular homeostasis. *Circulation* 1988;77 (Suppl 1):1–13.
48. Dzau VJ, Safar ME. Large conduit arteries in hypertension: role of the renin-angiotensin system. *Circulation* 1988;77:947–954.
49. Ebert TJ, Kanitz D, Roerig DL, Kampine JP. Midazolam and fentanyl on muscle sympathetic nerve activity and baroreflex function in humans. *Anesth Analg* 1990;70:S96.
50. Ebert TJ, Stowe DF. Neural control of the peripheral vasculature. *J Cardiothoracic and Vascular Anesthesia* 1996;10:147–158.
51. Ebert TJ, Stowe DF. Peripheral circulation: Recent insights into autonomic nervous control and endothelial factors relevant to cardiovascular disease and anesthesia. *Curr Opin Anaesth* 1991; 4:3–11.
52. Eccles JC. *The physiology of nerve cells.* Baltimore: Johns Hopkins University Press, 1957.
53. Edvinsson L, McCulloch J, Uddmann R. Substance P: immunohistochemical localization and effect upon cat pial arteries *in vitro* and *in situ. J Physiol* 1981;318:251–258.
54. Edwards RM, Ruffolo RR Jr. Angiotensin II receptor subclassification. In: Ruffolo RR Jr, ed. *Angiotensin II receptors.* Boca Raton: CRC Press, 1994;11–31.
55. Engelson ET, Schmid-Schönbein GW, Zweifach BW. The microvasculature in skeletal muscle. II. Arteriolar network anatomy in normotensive and hypertensive rats. *Microvasc Res* 1986;31:356–374.
56. Epstein RA, Wang H-H, Bartelstone HJ. The effects of halothane on circulatory reflexes of the dog. *Anesthesiology* 1968;29:867–876.
57. Eskinder H, Gebremedhin D, Lee JG, et al. Halothane and isoflurane decrease the open state probability of K+ channels in dog cerebral arterial muscle cells. *Anesthesiology* 1995;82:479–490.
58. Eskinder H, Hillard CJ, Flynn N, Bosnjak ZJ, Kampine JP. Role of guanylate cyclase-cGMP systems in halothane-induced vasodilation in canine cerebral arteries. *Anesthesiology* 1992;77:482–487.
59. Faria FAC, Salgado MCO. Facilitation of noradrenergic transmission by angiotensin in hypertensive rats. *Hypertension* 1992;19 (suppl II):II-30–II-35.
60. Fay FS, Rees DD, Warshaw DM. The contractile mechanism in smooth muscle. In: Bittar EE, ed. *Membrane structure and function.* New York: John Wiley, 1981;79–130.
61. Ferrario C, Diz D. The renin angiotensin system: an overview. *Newsletter of AHA High Blood Pressure Council* 1995;3:17–19.
62. Flavahan NA, Vanhoutte PM. G-proteins and endothelial responses. *Blood Vessels* 1990;1990:218–229.
63. Fleming BP, Gibbins IL, Morris JL, Gannon BJ. Noradrenergic and peptidergic innervation of the extrinsic and microcirculation of the rat cremaster muscle. *Microvasc Res* 1989;38:255–268.
64. Folkow B. Physiological aspects of primary hypertension. *Physiol Rev* 1092;62:347–504.
65. Furakawa K-I, Ohshima N, Tawada-Iwata Y, Shigekawa M. Cyclic GMP stimulated Na^+/Ca^{2+} exchange in vascular smooth muscle cells in primary culture. *J Biol Chem* 191;266:12337–12341.
66. Furchgott RF, Vanhoutte PM. Endothelium-derived relaxing and contracting factors. *FASEB J* 1989;3:2007–2018.
67. Furness JB. Arrangement of blood vessels and their relation with adrenergic nerves in the rat mesentery. *J Anat* 1973;115:347–364.
68. Garcia-Sainz JA. Cell responsiveness and protein kinase C: Receptors, G proteins, and membrane effectors. 6:169–172.
69. Gibbins IL, Furness JB, Costa M, et al. Co-localization of gene-related peptide-like immunoreactivity with substance P in cuta-

neous, vascular and visceral sensory neurons of guinea pigs. *Neurosci Lett* 1985;57:125–130.
70. Goerttler K. Über den Einbau der grossen Venen des Menschliken Unterschenkels. *Z Anat Entwicklungsgeschichte* 1953;116:591–609.
71. Grau H. Zur Frage des 'elastisch-muskulösen Systems' in der Venenwand. *Gegenbaurs Morphol Jahrb* 1931;67:745–750.
72. Green HD. Circulatory system physical principles. In: Glasser O, ed. *Medical physics.* Chicago: Yearbook Medical, 1950;208–232.
73. Green HD, Rapela CE, Conrad MC. Resistance (conductance) and capacitance phenomena in terminal vascular beds. In: Hamilton WF, ed. *Handbook of physiology.* Washington: American Physiological Society, 1963;935–960.
74. Greenblatt EP, Loeb AL, Longnecker DE. Endothelium-dependent circulatory control—a mechanism for the differing peripheral vascular effects of isoflurane versus halothane. *Anesthesiology* 1992;77:1178–1185.
75. Greenway CV. Role of splanchnic venous system in overall cardiovascular homeostasis. *Fed Proc* 1983;42:1678–1684.
76. Guyton AC. *Circulatory physiology III. Arterial pressure and hypertension.* Philadelphia: WB Saunders, 1980.
77. Guyton AC, Hall JE. The circulation. In: *Textbook of medical physiology,* 9th ed. Philadelphia: WB Saunders, 1995.
78. Guyton AC, Lindsey AW, Kaufmann B. Effect of mean circulatory filling pressure and other peripheral circulatory factors on cardiac output. *Am J Physiol* 1955;180:463–468.
79. Guyton AC, Polizo D, Armstrong GG. Mean circulatory filling pressure measured immediately after cessation of heart pumping. *Am J Physiol* 1954;179:261–267.
80. Hainsworth R. The importance of vascular capacitance in cardiovascular control. *NIPS* 1990;5:250–254.
81. Hainsworth R. Vascular capacitance: its control and importance. *Rev Physiol Biochem Pharmacol* 1986;105:101–173.
82. Hales S. *Statistical essays: containing haemastaticks,* vol 2. London: Innys, Manby & Woodward, 1733.
83. Harder DR, Campbell WB, Roman RJ. Role of cytochrome P450 enzymes and metabolites in the control of vascular tone. *J Vasc Res* 1995;32:79–92.
84. Harder DR, Gebremedhin D, Narayanan J, Jeffcoate C. Formation and action of a P450 metabolite of arachidonic acid in cat cerebral microvessels. *Am J Physiol* 1994;266:H2098–H2107.
85. Harper SL, Bohlen HG. Microvascular adaptation in the cerebral cortex of adult spontaneously hypertensive rats. *Hypertension* 1984;6:408–419.
86. Harrison DG. The endothelial cell. *Heart Dis Stroke* 1992;March/April:95–99.
87. Hart JL, Jing M, Bina S, et al. Effects of halothane on EDRF/cGMP-mediated vascular smooth muscle relaxations. *Anesthesiology* 1993;79:323–331.
88. Harvey W. *Exercitatio anatomica de motu cordis et sanguinibus in animalibus.* Frankfurt: Guilielmi Fitzeri, 1628 (Reproduced with an English translation by Leake CD. Springfield, IL: Charles C. Thomas, 1928.)
89. Hayoz D, Rutschmann B, Perret FEA. Conduit artery compliance and distensibility are not necessarily reduced in hypertension. *Hypertension* 1992;20:1–6.
90. Hille B. Modulation of ion channel function by G-protein-coupled receptors. *Trends Neurosci* 1994;17:531–536.
91. Hirst GDS, Edwards FR. Sympathetic neuroeffector transmission in arteries and arterioles. *Physiol Rev* 1989;69:546–604.
92. Holmes FL. *Claude Bernard and animal chemistry: the emergence of a scientist.* Cambridge, MA: Harvard University Press, 1974.
93. Hug CC Jr. Pharmacology of opioids and antagonists. In: Nunn JF, Utting JE, Brown BR Jr, eds. *Pharmacology of narcotics,* 5th ed. London: Butterworths, 1989;135–150.
94. Hughes JM, Sill JC, Pettis M, Rorie DK. Nitrous oxide constricts epicardial coronary arteries in pigs: evidence suggesting inhibitory effects on the endothelium. *Anesth Analg* 1993;77:232–240.
95. Iadecola C. Regulation of the cerebral microcirculation during neural activity: Is nitric oxide the missing link? *Trends Neurosci* 1993;16:206–214.
96. Iaizzo PA. The effects of halothane and isoflurane on intracellular Ca^{2+} regulation in cultured cells with characteristics of vascular smooth muscle. *Cell Calcium* 1992;13:513–520.
97. Jensen NF, Todd MM, Kramer DJ, et al. A comparison of the vasodilating effects of halothane and isoflurane on the isolated rabbit basilar artery with and without intact endothelium. *Anesthesiology* 1992;76:624–634.
98. Johansson B, Somlyo AP. Electrophysiology and excitation-contraction coupling. In: Bohr DF, Somlyo AP, Sparks JH, eds. *Vascular smooth muscle, vol 2, The cardiovascular system, Sect. 2, Handbook of physiology.* Bethesda: American Physiological Society, 1980;301–323.
99. Johns RA. Endothelium, anesthetics, and vascular control. *Anesthesiology* 1993;79:1381–1391.
100. Johnson PC. *Principles of peripheral circulatory control.* New York: John Wiley, 1978.
101. Kawasaki H, Takasaki K. Vasoconstrictor responses induced by 5-hydroxytryptamine released from vascular adrenergic nerves by periarterial nerve stimulation. *J Pharmacol Exp Ther* 1984;229:816–822.
102. Kelly RB. Storage and release of neurotransmitters. *Cell/Neuron* 1993;72 (10 suppl):43–53.
103. Kennedy C, Saville VL, Burnstock G. The contributions of noradrenaline and ATP to the responses of the rabbit central ear artery to sympathetic nerve stimulation depend on the parameters of stimulation. *Eur J Pharmacol* 1986;122:291–300.
104. Kobayashi Y, Yoshida K, Noguchi M, et al. Effect of enflurane on contractile reactivity in isolated canine mesenteric arteries and veins. *Anesth Analg* 1990;70:530–536.
105. Kohlstaedt K, Helmer O, Page I. Activation of renin by blood colloids. *Proc Soc Biol Med* 1938;39:214–215.
106. Krassioukov AV, Gelb AW, Weaver LC. Action of propofol on central sympathetic mechanisms controlling blood pressure. *Can J Anaesth* 1993;40:761–769.
107. Kupfermann I. Functional studies of co-transmission. *Physiol Rev* 1991;71:683–732.
108. Kutchai HC. Membrane receptors, second messengers, and signal transduction pathways. In: Berne RM, Levy MN, eds. *Physiology.* St. Louis: Mosby Yearbook, 1993;77–89.
109. Lee RMKWE. *Blood vessel changes in hypertension: structure and function.* Boca Raton: CRC Press, 1989.
110. Lincoln TM, Cornwell TL. Intracellular cyclic GMP receptor proteins. *FASEB J* 1993;7:328–338.
111. Lindeman KS, Baker SG, Hirshman CA. Interaction between halothane and the nonadrenergic, noncholinergic inhibitory system in porcine trachealis muscle. *Anesthesiology* 1994;81:641–648.
112. Longnecker DE. Effects of general anesthetics on the microcirculation. *Microcirc Endothelium Lymphatics* 1984;1:129–150.
113. Longnecker DE, Harris PD. Anesthesia. In: Kaley G, Altura B, eds. *Microcirculation.* Baltimore: University Park Press, 1980;333–369.
114. Lunn JJ, Rorie DK. Halothane-induced changes in the release and disposition of norepinephrine at adrenergic nerve endings in dog saphenous vein. *Anesthesiology* 1984;61:377–384.
115. Ma Y-H, Harder DR, Clark JE, Roman RJ. Effects of 12-HETE on isolated dog arcuate arteries. *Am J Physiol* 1991;261:H451–H456.
116. MacPherson RD, Rasiah RL, McLeod LJ. Propofol attenuates the myogenic response of vascular smooth muscle. *Anesth Analg* 1993;76:822–829.
117. Marijic J, Madden JA, Kampine JP, Bosnjak ZJ. The effect of halothane on norepinephrine responsiveness in rabbit small mesenteric veins. *Anesthesiology* 1990:479–484.
118. McCallum JB, Stekiel TA, Bosnjak ZJ, Kampine JP. Does isoflurane alter mesenteric venous capacitance in the intact rabbit? *Anesth Analg* 1993;76:1095–1105.
119. McCulloch J, Uddmann R, Kingman TA, Edvinsson L. Calcitonin gene-related peptide: functional role in cerebrovascular regulation. *Proc Natl Acad Sci USA* 1986;83:5731–5735.
120. McCuskey RS, Krasovich MA. Anatomy of the microvascular system. In: Mortillaro NA, Taylor AE, eds. *The pathology of the microcirculation.* Boca Raton: CRC Press, 1994;1–18.
121. McDaniel NL, Chen X-L, Singer HA, et al. Nitrovasodilators relax arterial smooth muscle by decreasing $[Ca^{2+}]_i$ and uncoupling stress from myosin phosphorylation. *Am J Physiol* 1992;263:C461–C467.
122. McGiff JC. Cytochrome P450 metabolites of arachidonic acid. *Annu Rev Pharmacol* 1991;31:339–369.
123. Meisheri KD, Cipkus-Dubray LA, Hosner JM, Khan SA. Nicorandil-induced vasorelaxation: Functional evidence for K^+ channel-dependent and cyclic GMP-dependent components in a single vascular preparation. *J Cardiovasc Pharmacol* 1991;17:903–912.
124. Meyer J, Lentz CW, Herndon DN, et al. Effects of halothane anesthesia on vasoconstrictor response to N^G-nitro-L-arginine methyl ester, an inhibitor of nitric oxide synthesis, in sheep. *Anesth Analg* 1993;77:1215–1221.
125. Miller M, Quilley J, McGiff JC. Eicosanoid-dependent mechanisms and the regulation of blood pressure. In: Zanchetti A, Tarazi RC,

eds. *Pathophysiology of hypertension, vol 8: Handbook of hypertension.* New York: Elsevier Science, 1986;578–602.
126. Miller VM. Interactions between neural and endothelial mechanisms in control of vascular tone. *NIPS* 1991;6:60–63.
127. Milligan G. Mechanisms of multifunctional signalling by G protein-linked receptors. *Trends Pharmacol Sci* 1993;14:239–244.
128. Milnor WR. The circulatory system. In: *Cardiovascular physiology.* New York: University Press, 1990;3–28.
129. Milnor WR. Principles of Hemodynamics. In: *Cardiovascular physiology.* New York: Oxford University, 1990;171–218.
130. Milnor WR. Chapter 8. Autonomic and peripheral control mechanisms. In: *Cardiovascular physiology.* New York: Oxford University Press, 1990;249–326.
131. Milnor WR. *Hemodynamics.* Baltimore: Williams & Wilkins, 1989.
132. Mortillaro MA, Taylor AEE. *The pathology of the microcirculation.* Boca Raton: CRC Press, 1994.
133. Muldoon SM, Hart JL, Bowen KA, Freas W. Attenuation of endothelium-mediated vasodilation by halothane. *Anesthesiology* 1988; 68:31–37.
134. Muldoon SM, Vanhoutte PM, Lorenz RR, Van Dyke RA. Venomotor changes caused by halothane acting on the sympathetic nerves. *Anesthesiology* 1975;43:41–48.
135. Mulvany MJ. Biophysical aspects of resistance vessels studied in spontaneous and renal hypertensive rats. *Acta Physiol Scand* 1988; 133:129–138.
136. Mulvany MJ. A reduced elastic modulus of vascular wall components in hypertension. *Hypertension* 1992;20:7–9.
137. Mulvany MJ, Aalkjaer C. Structure and function of small arteries. *Physiol Rev* 1990;70:921–969.
138. Murphy RA. Chapter 19. Smooth muscle. In: Berne RM, Levy MN, eds. *Physiology,* St. Louis: Mosby Yearbook, 1993;309–324.
139. Murphy RA. What is special about smooth muscle? The significance of covalent crossbridge regulation. *FASEB J* 1994;8:311–318.
140. Nakamura K, Terasako K, Toda H, et al. Mechanisms of inhibition of endothelium-dependent relaxation by halothane, isoflurane, and sevoflurane. *Can J Anaesth* 1994;41:340–346.
141. Neil E. Peripheral Circulation: historical aspects. In: Shepherd JT, Abboud FM, Geiger SR, eds. *Peripheral circulation and organ blood flow, vol 3, The cardiovascular system, Sect. 2, Handbook of physiology.* Bethesda: Am Physiol Soc, 1983;1–19.
142. Neild TO, Braydon JE. Neural control of resistance arteries. In: Bevan JA, Halpern W, Mulvany MJ, eds. *The resistance vasculature.* Totowa: Humana Press, 1991;217–240.
143. Neubig RR. Membrane organization in G-protein mechanisms. *FASEB J* 1994;8:939–946.
144. Nilsson H, Goldstein M, Nilsson O. Adrenergic innervation and neurogenic response in large and small arteries and veins from the rat. *Acta Physiol Scand* 1986;126:121–133.
145. Nishimura J, Khalil RA, Drenth JP, van Breemen C. Evidence for increased myofilament Ca^{2+} sensitivity in norepinephrine-activated vascular smooth muscle. *Am J Physiol* 1990;259:H2–H8.
146. Nishimura J, van Breeman C. Regulation of the Ca^{2+} sensitivity of vascular smooth contractile elements. In: Cox RH, ed. *Cellular and molecular mechanisms in hypertension.* New York: Plenum Press, 1991;9–24.
147. Nishimura J, van Breemen C. Direct regulation of smooth muscle contractile elements by second messengers. *Biochem Biophys Res Commun* 1989;163:939–935.
148. O'Rourke MF. Arterial stiffness, systolic blood pressure, and logical treatment of arterial hypertension. *Hypertension* 1990;15:339–347.
149. Page IH, Helmer OM. A crystalline pressor substance (angiotonin) resulting from reaction between renin and renin activator. *J Exp Med* 1940;71:29–42.
150. Park WK, Lynch C, III, Johns RA. Effects of propofol and thiopental in isolated rat aorta and pulmonary artery. *Anesthesiology* 1992;77:956–963.
151. Petros AJ, Bogle RG, Pearson JD. Propofol stimulates nitric oxide release from cultured porcine aortic endothelial cells. *Br J Pharmacol* 1993;109:6–7.
152. Poiseuille J-L-M. Recherches expérimentales sur le mouvement des liquides dans de tubes de tres petits diametres. *Mem Savant Etrangers Paris* 1846;9:433–544.
153. Poterack KA, Kampine JP, Schmeling WT. Effects of isoflurane, midazolam, and etomidate on cardiovascular responses to stimulation of central nervous system pressor sites in chronically instrumented cats. *Anesth Analg* 1991;73:64–75.
154. Pratt JE, Dzau VJ. Molecular and cellular biology of angiotensin-mediated growth of the cardiovascular system. In: Raizda MK, Phillips MI, Summers C, eds. *Cellular and molecular biology of the renin-angiotensin system.* Boca Raton: CRC Press, 1993;471–483.
155. Prewitt RL, Wang DH, Hill MA. Hypertension. In: Mortillaro NA, Taylor AE, eds. *The pathology of the microcirculation.* Boca Raton: CRC Press, 1994;61–86.
156. Price HL, Price ML, Morse HT. Effects of cyclopropane, halothane and procaine on the vasomotor "center" of the dog. *Anesthesiology* 1965;26:55–60.
157. Proctor KG, Shatkin S Jr, Kraminski PM, Falck JR, et al. Modulation of arteriolar blood flow by inhibitors of arachidonic acid oxidation after thermal injury. Possible role for a novel class of vasodilator metabolites. *Circulation* 1988;77:1185–1196.
158. Puig MM, Turndorf H, Warner W. Synergistic interaction of morphine and halothane in the guinea pig ileum: Effects of pertussis toxin. *Anesthesiology* 1990;72:699–703.
159. Putney J Jr, Takemura H, Hughes JR, et al. How do inositol phosphates regulate calcium signalling? *FASEB J* 1989;3:1899–1905.
160. Raizda M, Phillips M, Summers C. *Cellular and molecular biology of the renin-angiotensin system.* Boca Raton: CRC Press, 1993.
161. Ralevic V, Burnstock G. *Neural-endothelial interactions in the control of local vascular tone.* Austin: RG Landis, 1993.
162. Rand MJ. Nitrergic transmission: nitric oxide as a mediator of non-adrenergic non-cholinergic neuro-effector transmission. *Clin Exp Pharmacol Physiol* 1992;19:147–169.
163. Rand MJ, Majewski H, Story DF. Modulation of neuroeffector transmission. In: Antonaccio M, eds. *Cardiovascular pharmacology.* New York: Raven Press, 1990;229–290.
164. Rand VE, Garland CJ. Endothelium-dependent relaxation to acetylcholine in the rabbit basilar artery: importance of membrane hyperpolarization. *Br J Pharmacol* 1992;106:143–150.
165. Reid IA. Interactions between angiotensin, sympathetic nervous system, and baroreceptor reflexes in regulation of blood pressure. *Am J Physiol* 1992;262:E763–E768.
166. Reneman RS. Endothelial cells as mechanoreceptors. *NIPS* 1993;8:55–56.
167. Renkin EM. Control of microcirculation and blood-tissue exchange. In: Renkin EM, Michel CC, eds. *Microcirculation, vol 4, The cardiovascular system, Sect. 2, Handbook of physiology.* Bethesda: Am Physiol Soc, 1984;627–687.
168. Rhodin JAG. Architecture of the vascular wall. In: Bohr D, Somlyo AP, Sparks JH, eds. *Vascular smooth muscle, vol 2, The cardiovascular system, Sect. 2, Handbook of physiology.* Bethesda: Am Physiol Soc, 1980;1–31.
169. Robertson G. Posterior pituitary. In: Felig PF, ed. *Endocrinology and metabolism.* New York: McGraw-Hill, 1987;347.
170. Roman RJ, Harder DR. Cytochrome P450 metabolites of arachidonic acid in the control of vascular tone. In: Rubanyi GM, ed. *Mechanoreception by the vascular wall.* Mount Kisco: Futura, 1993; 986–996.
171. Rorie DK, Tyce GM, Mackenzie RA. Evidence that halothane inhibits norepinephrine release from sympathetic nerve endings in dog saphenous vein by stimulation of presynaptic inhibitory muscarinic receptors. *Anesth Analg* 1984;63:1059–1064.
172. Rothe CF. Reflex control of the veins and vascular capacitance. *Physiol Rev* 1983;63:1281–1342.
173. Rothe CF. Venous system: physiology of capacitance vessels. In: Shepherd JT, Abboud FM, eds. *Handbook of physiology, Sect. 2, vol 3.* Bethesda: Am Physiol Soc, 1983b;397–492.
174. Rowell LB. In: *Human cardiovascular control.* New York: Oxford University Press, 1993;1–117.
175. Rowell LB. Human cardiovascular adjustments to exercise and cardiovascular stress. *Physiol Rev* 1974;54:75–149.
176. Ruffolo RR Jr. Molecular biology, biochemistry, pharmacology and clinical chemistry. In: Ruffolo RR Jr, ed. *Angiotensin II receptors,* vol 1. Boca Raton: CRC Press, 1994.
177. Ruffolo RR Jr. Medicinal chemistry. In: Ruffolo RR Jr, ed. *Angiotensin II receptors,* vol 2. Boca Raton: CRC Press, 1994.
178. Saavedra J. Brain and pituitary angiotensin. *Endocr Rev* 1992;13: 329–377.
179. Sabolić I, Brown D. Water channels in renal and nonrenal tissues. *NIPS* 1995;10:12–17.
180. Safar MJ, Simon AC, Levenson JA. Structural changes of large arteries in sustained essential hypertension. *Hypertension* 1984;6 (suppl III):III-117–III-121.
181. Sanuki M, Yuge O, Kawamoto M, et al. Sevoflurane inhibited β-

adrenoceptor-G protein bindings in myocardial membrane in rats. *Anesth Analg* 1994;79:466–471.
182. Schmeling WT, Farber NE. Anesthetic actions on cardiovascular control mechanisms in the central nervous system. *Adv Pharmacol* 1994;31:617–642.
183. Schwartz JH, Kandel ER. Synaptic transmission mediated by second messengers. In: Kandel ER, Schwartz JH, Jessell TM, eds. *Principles of neuroscience,* 3rd ed. New York: Elsevier Science, 1991;173–193.
184. Schwieler JH, Kahan T, Nussberger J, Hjemdahl P. Influence of the renin-angiotensin system on sympathetic neurotransmission in canine skeletal muscle *in vivo. Naunyn Schmiedebergs Arch Pharmacol* 1991;343:166–172.
185. Seagard JL, Elegbe EO, Hopp FA, et al. Effects of isoflurane on the baroreceptor reflex. *Anesthesiology* 1983;59:511–520.
186. Seagard JL, Hopp FA, Donegan JH, et al. Halothane and the carotid sinus reflex. *Anesthesiology* 1982;57:191–202.
187. Segal SS, Duling BR. Communication between feed arteries and microvessels in hamster striated muscle: segmental vascular responses are functionally coordinated. *Circ Res* 1986;59:283–290.
188. Shepherd JT, Abboud FM. *Peripheral circulation and organ blood flow, vol 3, The cardiovascular system, Sect. 2.* Handbook of Physiology. Bethesda: Am Physiol Soc, 1983.
189. Shepherd JT, Vanhoutte PM. Components of the cardiovascular system: how structure is geared to function. In: *The human cardiovascular system.* New York: Raven Press, 1979;13–61.
190. Shepherd JT, Vanhoutte PM. Role of venous system in circulatory control. *Mayo Clin Proc* 1978;53:247–255.
191. Shepherd JT, Vanhoutte PM. *Veins and their control.* Philadelphia: WB Saunders, 1975.
192. Sill JC, Eskuri S, Nelson R, et al. The volatile anesthetic isoflurane attenuates Ca^{++} mobilization in cultured vascular smooth muscle cells. *J Pharmacol Exp Ther* 1993;265:74–80.
193. Sill JC, Ozhan M, Nelson R, Uhl C. Isoflurane-, halothane-, and agonist-evoked responses in pig coronary arteries and vascular smooth muscle cells. In: Blank TJJ, Wheeler DM, eds. *Mechanisms of anesthetic actions in skeletal, cardiac and smooth muscle.* New York: Plenum Press, 1991;257–269.
194. Sill JC, Uhl C, Eskuri S, et al. Halothane inhibits agonist-induced inositol phosphate and Ca^{2+} signaling in A7r5 cultured vascular smooth muscle cells. *Mol Pharmacol* 1991;40:1006–1013.
195. Silverberg A, Shaw S, Haymond M, Cryer P. Norepinephrine: hormone and neurotransmitter in man. *Am J Physiol* 1978;234: E252–E256.
196. Simionescu M. Receptor-mediated transcytosis of plasma molecules by vascular endothelium. In: Simionescu N, Simionescu M, eds. *Endothelial cell biology in health and disease,* New York: Plenum Press, 1988;69–104.
197. Simionescu M, Simionescu N. Ultrastructure of the microvascular wall: functional correlations. In: Renkin EM, Michel CC, eds. *Microcirculation, vol 4, The cardiovascular system, Sect. 2, Handbook of physiology.* Bethesda: Am Physiol Soc, 1984;41–101.
198. Simon AC, Safar ME, Levenson JA, et al. An evaluation of large arteries compliance in man. *Am J Physiol* 1979;237:H550–H554.
199. Simon MI, Strathmann MP, Gautam N. Diversity of G proteins in signal transduction. *Science* 1991;252:802–808.
200. Skovsted P, Price HC. The effects of ethrane on arterial pressure, preganglionic sympathetic activity and barostatic reflexes. *Anesthesiology* 1972;36:357–262.
201. Skovsted P, Price ML, Price HC. The effects of short acting barbiturates on arterial pressure, preganglionic sympathetic activity and barostatic reflexes. *Anesthesiology* 1970;33:10–18.
202. Skovsted P, Saptlaviclukul S. The effects of isoflurane on arterial pressure, pulse rate, autonomic nervous activity and barostatic reflexes. *Can Anaesth Soc J* 1977;24:304–314.
203. Sleight RG, Lieberman MA. Signal transduction. In: Sperelakis N, ed. *Cell Physiology Source Book,* New York: Academic Press, 1995; 117–127.
204. Snyder SH, Bredt DS. Nitric oxide as a neuronal messenger. *TIPS* 1991;12:125–128.
205. Söllner T, Rothman JE. Neurotransmission: harnessing fusion machinery at the synapse. *TINS* 1994;17:344–348.
206. Somlyo AP, Somlyo AV. Smooth muscle structure and function. In: Fozzard HA, Jennings RB, Haber B, et al, eds. *The heart and cardiovascular system.* New York: Raven Press, 1991;1295–1310.
206a. Somlyo AP, Somlyo AV. Signal transduction and regulation in smooth muscle. *Nature* 1994;372:231–236.
207. Sperelakis N, Ohya Y. Regulation of calcium slow channels in vascular smooth muscle cells. In: Sperelakis N, ed. *Ion channels of vascular smooth muscle cells and endothelial cells.* New York: Elsevier Science, 1991;185–198.
208. Stadnicka A, Flynn NM, Bosnjak ZJ, Kampine JP. Enflurane, halothane, and isoflurane attenuate contractile responses to exogenous and endogenous norepinephrine in isolated small mesenteric veins of the rabbit. *Anesthesiology* 1993;78:326–334.
209. Stadnicka A, Stekiel TA, Bosnjak ZJ, Kampine JP. Inhibition by enflurane of baroreflex mediated mesenteric venoconstriction in the rabbit ileum. *Anesthesiology* 1993;78:928–936.
210. Stanton B, Koeppen BM. Control of body fluid osmolality and volume. In: Berne RM, Levy ME, eds. *Physiology.* St. Louis: Mosby Yearbook, 1993;754–783.
211. Starke K. Regulation of norepinephrine release by presynaptic receptor systems. *Rev Physiol Biochem Pharmacol* 1977;77:1–124.
212. Stekiel TA, Contney SJ, Stekiel WJ, et al. The differential effects of halothane and isoflurane on the *in situ* trans-membrane potential (E_m) of vascular smooth muscle (VSM). *Anesthesiology* 1993;79:A604.
213. Stekiel TA, Contney SJ, Stekiel WJ, et al. The effect of sevoflurane on the *in situ* trans-membrane potential (E_m) of vascular smooth muscle (VSM). *Anesthesiology* 1994;81:A666.
214. Stekiel TA, Ozono K, McCallum JB, et al. The inhibitory action of halothane on reflex constriction in mesenteric capacitance veins. *Anesthesiology* 1990;73:1169–1178.
215. Stekiel TA, Stekiel WJ, Tominaga M, et al. Isoflurane-mediated inhibition of the constriction of mesenteric capacitance veins and related circulatory responses to acute graded hypoxic hypoxia. *Anesth Analg* 1995;80:994–1001.
216. Stekiel TA, Tominaga M, Bosnjak ZJ, Kampine JP. The inhibitory effect of halothane on mesenteric venoconstriction and related reflex responses during acute graded hypoxia in rabbits. *Anesthesiology* 1992;77:709–720.
217. Stekiel WJ. Electrophysiological mechanisms of force development by vascular smooth muscle membrane in hypertension. In: Lee RMKW, ed. *Blood vessel changes in hypertension: structure and function.* Boca Raton, FL: CRC Press, 1989;127–170.
218. Stekiel WJ, Contney SJ, Lombard JH. Small vessel membrane potential, sympathetic input, and electrogenic pump rate in SHR. *Am J Physiol* 1986;250:C547–C556.
219. Stjärne L. Basic mechanisms of local modulation of nerve impulse-induced secretion of neurotransmitters from individual sympathetic nerve varicosities. *Rev Physiol Biochem Pharmacol* 1989; 112:1–137.
220. Stone DJ, Johns RA. Endothelium-dependent effects of halothane, enflurane, and isoflurane on isolated rat aortic vascular rings. *Anesthesiology* 1989;71:126–132.
221. Su JY, Chang YI, Tang LJ. Mechanisms of action of enflurane on vascular smooth muscle. *Anesthesiology* 1994;81:700–709.
222. Taylor CW. The role of G proteins in transmembrane signalling. *Biochem J* 1990;272:1–13.
223. Thiel G. Recent breakthroughs in neurotransmitter release: Paradigm for regulated exocytosis? *NIPS* 1995;10:42–46.
224. Tigerstedt R, Bergman P. Niere und kreislauf. *Scand Arch Physiol* 1898;8:223–271.
225. Toda H, Nakamura K, Hatano Y, et al. Halothane and isoflurane inhibit endothelium-dependent relaxation elicited by acetylcholine. *Anesth Analg* 1992;75:198–203.
226. Toda N, Kitamura Y, Okamura T. New idea on the mechanism of hypertension: Suppression of nitroxidergic vasodilator nerve function. *J Vasc Med Biol* 1991;3:235–241.
227. Toda N, Okamura T. Regulation by nitroxidergic nerve of arterial tone. *NIPS* 1992;7:148–152.
228. Tsuchida H, Namba H, Seki S, et al. Role of intracellular Ca^{2+} pools in the effects of halothane and isoflurane on vascular smooth muscle contraction. *Anesth Analg* 1994;78:1067–1076.
229. Tsuchida H, Namba H, Yamakage M, et al. Effects of halothane and isoflurane on cytosolic calcium ion concentrations on contraction in the vascular smooth muscle of the rat aorta. *Anesthesiology* 1993;78:531–540.
230. Uggeri MJ, Proctor GJ, Johns RA. Halothane, enflurane, and isoflurane attenuate both receptor- and non-receptor-mediated EDRF production in rat thoracic aorta. *Anesthesiology* 1992;76:1012–1017.
231. van Breemen C, Cauvin C, Johns A, et al. Ca^{2+}-regulation of vascular smooth muscle. *Fed Proc* 1986;45:2746–2651.
232. Vanhoutte PM. Endothelium and control of vascular function. *Hypertension* 1989;13:658–667.

233. Vanhoutte PM. Endothelium and the control of vascular tissue. *NIPS* 1987;2:18–22.
234. Vanhoutte PM, Verbeuren TJ, Webb RC. Local modulation of adrenergic neuroeffector. Interaction in the blood vessel wall. *Physiol Rev* 1981;61:151–247.
235. Vautrin J. Vesicular or quantal and subquantal transmitter release. *NIPS* 1994;9:59–64.
236. Vincent SR, Hope BT. Neurons that say NO. *Trends Neurosci* 1992; 15:108–13.
237. von Külgelgen A. Über das Verhältnis von Ringmuskalatur und Innendruck in menschlicken grossen Venen. *Z Zellforsch Mikroscop Anat* 1955;43:168–183.
238. von Kügelgen A. Weitere Mitteilungen über den Wandbau der grossen Venen des Menschen unter besenderer Berücksichtigung iher Kollagenstrukturen. *Z Zellforsch Microskop Anat* 1956; 44:121–174.
239. Wang H-H, Epstein RA, Markee SJ, Bartelstone HJ. The effects of halothane on peripheral and central vasomotor control mechanisms of the dog. *Anesthesiology* 1968;29:877–886.
240. Wang Y-X, Abdelrahman A, Pang CCY. Selective inhibition of pressor and haemodynamic effects of N^G-nitro-L-arginine by halothane. *J Cardiovasc Pharmacol* 1993;22:571–578.
241. Wang Y-X, Zhou T, Chua TC, Pang CCY. Effects of inhalation and intravenous anaesthetic agents on pressor response to N^G-nitro-L-arginine. *Eur J Pharmacol* 1991;198:183–188.
242. Weems WA, Downey JM. Introduction to cardiovascular physiology. In: Johnson LR, ed. *Essential medical physiology*. New York: Raven Press, 1992;147–150.
243. Welches W, Brosnihan K, Ferrario C. A comparison of the properties and enzymatic activity of three angiotensin processing enzymes: angiotensin converting enzyme, prolyl endopeptidase and neutral endopeptidase. *Life Sci* 1993;52:1461–1480.
244. White DA, Reitan JA, Kien ND, Thorup SJ. Decrease in vascular resistance in the isolated canine hindlimb after graded doses of alfentanil, fentanyl, and sufentanil. *Anesth Analg* 1990;71:29–34.
245. Wiedman MP. Architecture. In: Renkin EM, Michel CC, eds. *Microcirculation, vol 4, The cardiovascular system, Sect. 2, Handbook of physiology*. Bethesda: Am Physiol Soc, 1984;11–40.
246. Yamanoue T, Brum JM, Estafanous FG, et al. Effects of opioids on vasoresponsiveness of porcine coronary artery. *Anesth Analg* 1992; 74:889–896.
247. Yoshida K, Okabe E. Selective impairment of endothelium-dependent relaxation by sevoflurane: oxygen free radicals participation. *Anesthesiology* 1992;76:440–447.
248. Yoshida K, Okamura T, Kimura H, et al. Nitric oxide synthase-immunoreactive nerve fibers in dog cerebral and peripheral arteries. *Brain Res* 1993;629:67–72.
249. Zorn L, Kulkarni R, Anantharam V, et al. Halothane acts on many potassium channels, including a minimal potassium channel. *Neurosci Lett* 1993;161:81–84.
250. Zweifach BW. Vascular resistance. Structural and functional basis. In: Bevan JA, Halpern W, Mulvany MJ, eds. *The resistance vasculature*. Totowa: Humana Press.1;1–22.
251. Zweifach BW, Lipowsky HH. Pressure-flow relations in blood and lymph microcirculation. In: Renkin EM, Michel CC, eds. *Microcirculation, vol 4, The cardiovascular system, Sect. 2, Handbook of physiology*. Bethesda: Am Physiol Soc, 1984;251–307.
252. Zygmunt PM, Hogestatt ED. Calcium channels at the neuroeffector junction in the rabbit ear artery. *Naunyn Schmiedebergs Arch Pharmacol* 1993;347:617–623.

Anesthesia: Biologic Foundations, edited by
Tony L. Yaksh et al. Lippincott–Raven Publishers,
Philadelphia © 1997.

CHAPTER 69

THE CORONARY CIRCULATION

JUDY R. KERSTEN AND DAVID C. WARLTIER

ANATOMY OF THE CORONARY CIRCULATION

The left and right coronary arteries (Fig. 1) arise from two ostia located in the sinuses of Valsalva, usually above the extent of opening of the aortic valve leaflets in the aortic root, and subdivide into epicardial branches that traverse the surface of the heart. The left main coronary artery usually extends for up to several centimeters in length, and then bifurcates into the left anterior descending (LAD) and left circumflex branches. The LAD courses from base to apex along the anterior interventricular sulcus and gives rise to multiple septal and diagonal branches supplying the anterior interventricular septum and anterolateral aspect of the left ventricle (169). The LAD continues around the apex ascending along the posterior interventricular groove to terminate on the diaphragmatic surface of the left ventricle in approximately 78% of patients. In the remaining 22% of patients, the LAD terminates before reaching the apex, and the apex is instead supplied by the posterior descending branch of the right coronary artery (RCA) (220). The left circumflex coronary artery courses circumferentially along the left atrial-ventricular groove, providing obtuse marginal branches that supply the left ventricular free wall. The left coronary artery major branches supply the left ventricle (except for the posterior base), a portion of the anterior right ventricle, the anterior two-thirds of the septum, and the left atrium. In individuals who exhibit a "left dominant circulation," the left circumflex coronary artery continues down the posterior interventricular groove to supply the diaphragmatic surface of the heart, giving rise to several posterior left ventricular branches and the posterior descending coronary artery (PDA). The PDA, however, usually arises from the RCA.

The RCA has its origin in a separate ostia in the right aortic sinus of the aortic root and traverses the right atrial-ventricular groove, supplying the right ventricular wall and right atrium and the posterior surface of the left ventricle via the PDA. The posterior third of the interventricular septum and atrioventricular node are also supplied by the RCA. Frequently, a "double ostium" for the RCA is present, one of which gives rise to the conus artery that supplies the left anterior basal portion of the right ventricle (pulmonary outflow tract). The sinoatrial node derives perfusion from the RCA via the right atrial artery in 60% and the left circumflex in 40% of individuals (160), while the atrioventricular node is supplied by the dominant artery (169). Arterial "dominance" refers to that artery which supplies the lower interventricular septum and diaphragmatic surface of the left ventricle. A right dominant circulation is present in 80 to 85% of individuals. Of the 15 to 20% of individuals without a right dominant circulation, half exhibit a left dominant circulation and half have a balanced circulation in which both the left and right coronary arteries contribute to left ventricular diaphragmatic perfusion (169).

The epicardial coronary arteries give rise to intramural penetrating arteries that extend perpendicularly from subepicardium to subendocardium, providing extensive collateral channels and capillary networks throughout the subepicardium, midmyocardium, and subendocardium. These branches, ultimately terminating as a subendocardial vascular plexus (Fig. 2) (86), are exposed to intramural tissue pressure and forces generated during contraction of the left ventricle. These forces significantly impact the regional distribution of blood flow within

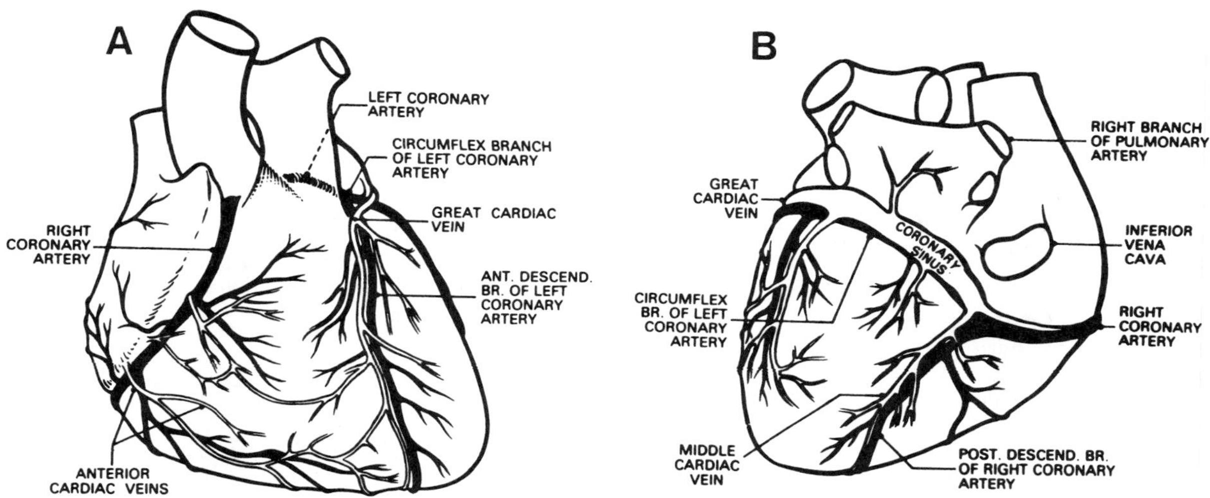

Figure 1. Coronary vessels of the human heart. Anterior view (**A**) shows the right coronary artery and anterior descending artery; posterior view (**B**) shows the left circumflex artery and the posterior descending artery. The latter may be formed by the right coronary artery in a right dominant circulation or the left circumflex in a left dominant circulation. Anterior cardiac veins drain the right ventricle, while the coronary sinus drains primarily the left ventricle, both emptying into the right atrium. (From ref. 260, with permission.)

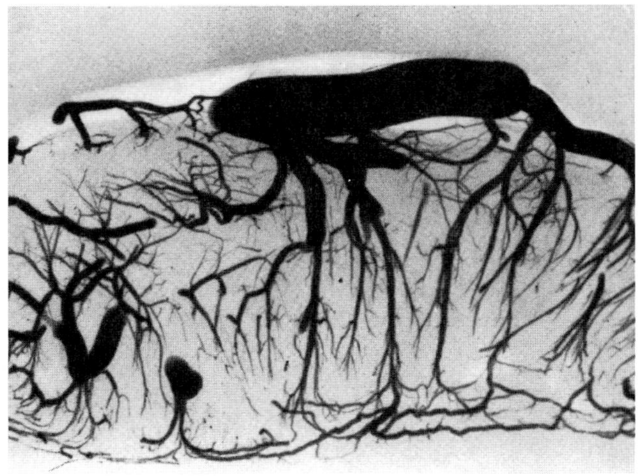

Figure 2. Injection of radiopaque dye demonstrates a large epicardial coronary artery, giving rise to transmural penetrating vessels terminating in subendocardium. Multiple interarterial anastomoses (Fulton's plexus) are visualized in subendocardium. (From ref. 86, with permission.)

the left ventricle. Visualization of large epicardial coronary arteries may be performed angiographically, but the small coronary microvessels between 15 and 500 μm in diameter are observed only by highly specialized microvascular imaging techniques.

The majority of venous return from the left ventricle (90–95%) drains into the coronary sinus located in the posterior atrial-ventricular groove, where it empties into the posterior aspect of the right atrium (Fig. 1). A small amount of venous return (2–3%) from the left ventricle and that from the right ventricle empties directly into the right atrium from the anterior cardiac veins (143). In addition, a minor portion of the venous drainage of the heart enters the right and left ventricular cavities directly via thebesian veins. The venous outflow into the left ventricle contributes a fraction of the physiologic arteriovenous shunt.

PHYSIOLOGY OF THE CORONARY CIRCULATION

Pressure-Flow Relationships

As in all vascular beds, coronary blood flow is directly proportional to driving pressure and inversely related to resistance. However, in contrast to other vascular beds, left ventricular coronary blood flow reaches its maximum during diastole and may actually reverse directions momentarily during systole (94). This phasic alteration of blood flow during the cardiac cycle occurs secondary to intramural compressive forces in the left ventricle during systole (17). In contrast, phasic blood flow to the right ventricle differs from that of the left ventricle in that the magnitude of coronary flow is nearly as high during systole as that occurring during diastole (171).

Downey and Kirk (72) and Archie (6) described coronary blood flow to be dependent on a vascular waterfall mechanism. Implicit in this concept is that the river downstream from the waterfall offers no resistance to flow. The driving pressure for coronary flow is not simply equivalent to diastolic arterial pressure less venous (coronary sinus = the downstream river) pressure. Instead, coronary perfusion pressure is equal to diastolic arterial pressure less intramural myocardial tissue pressure. Since intramural tissue pressure is greater than coronary sinus pressure, external compressive forces cause the microvasculature to collapse. Microvascular collapse secondary to compression by surrounding myocardium impedes arterial inflow, while the lower coronary sinus pressure does not (Fig. 3). The minimal driving pressure (diastolic aortic pressure) for coronary flow or that pressure at which coronary flow ceases has been studied in conscious dogs. Healthy conscious dogs have a prominent sinus arrhythmia secondary to a high parasympathetic tone. Occasional prolongation of the RR interval (equivalent to heart rates as slow as 25 to 30 bpm) provides relatively long periods of diastole during which arterial pressure slowly declines. Coronary flow is highest during early diastole and proceeds to decline, ultimately reaching zero at a pressure (critical closing pressure) preceding end-diastole. Experiments in conscious dogs have demonstrated that epicardial arterial flow may cease at perfusion pressures as high as 40 mm Hg (Fig. 4) (15) despite low coronary sinus and right atrial pressures. This finding suggests that an elevation of intramural tissue pressure may be a critical factor limiting coronary perfusion. The importance of coronary capacitance in maintaining coronary microvascular flow has recently been demonstrated. Measurement of red blood cell velocity in coronary arterioles has revealed that antegrade movement of erythrocytes continues in small coronary arterioles until coronary driving pressure is only a few mm Hg above coronary sinus pressure (138). Cessation of antegrade flow in large epicardial arteries concomitant with continuing flow in microvessels may be due to significant capacitance in the coronary circulation (177).

Coronary autoregulation refers to the ability of the coronary circulation to regulate vascular resistance such that flow remains constant despite fluctuations in perfusion pressure (134). The coronary circulation is capable of autoregulation within a range of coronary artery perfusion pressures of approximately 50 to 120 mm Hg (203). Flow is pressure dependent below or above this range because the coronary circulation becomes maximally dilated or constricted, respectively. The coronary vasculature is submaximally dilated above a perfusion pressure of 50 mm Hg, and therefore possesses a vasodilator reserve whereby flow may be further increased if metabolic demand increases (68) (Fig. 5). The capacity for autoregulatory adjustments in vascular resistance as well as the degree of vasodilator reserve decrease across the left ventricular wall from the outer subepicardial to inner subendocardial layers of myocardium (24,34,198,199). Subendocardial vessels are relatively more dilated than subepicardial vessels (126,198) at the same perfusion pressure because of the autoregulatory response to greater external compressive forces exerted on the microcirculation and a higher oxygen consumption (300) in the subendocardium. The subendocardium possesses less vasodilator reserve than the subepicardium since subendocardial vessels are relatively more dilated. It has been previously suggested that the subendocardial vessels are naturally close to being maximally vasodilated (41,95). However, other investigators have demonstrated that resting flow in the subendocardium can be increased four- to fivefold by pharmacological agents (100).

Several studies have shown that an additional pharmacologic vasodilator reserve is present at low perfusion pressures (68) (Fig. 5). Following apparent exhaustion of coronary vasodilator reserve, as produced by intense myocardial ischemia, further

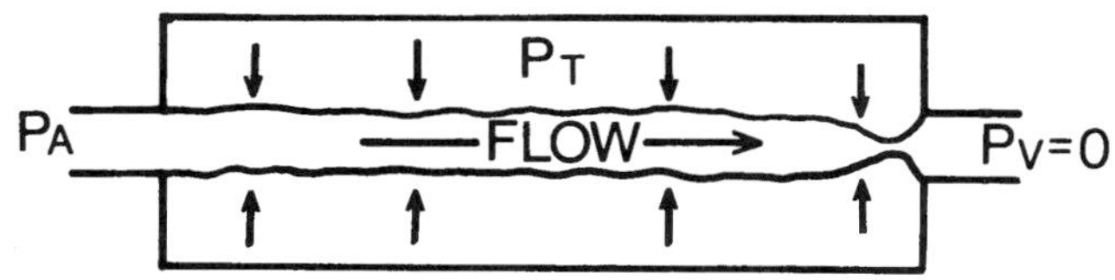

Figure 3. Vascular waterfall model. A collapsible tube is surrounded by a pressure, P_T. When P_T is less than the inflow pressure (P_A), but exceeds the outflow pressure (P_V), a region of partial collapse occurs at the outflow end. (From ref. 72, with permission.)

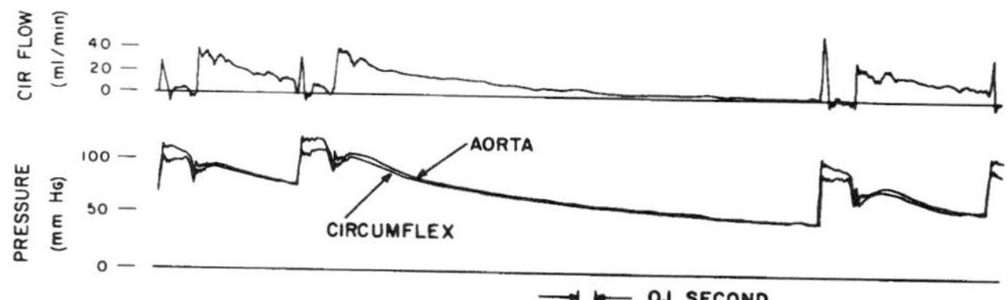

Figure 4. Phasic tracing of resting circumflex blood flow and pressure during a long diastole. Circumflex blood flow reaches zero while perfusion pressure remains 40–50 mm Hg. (From ref. 15, with permission.)

coronary dilation can nevertheless be elicited by adenosine and other vasodilator drugs (9,203,215,293). This occurs because ischemia is not homogeneous throughout the myocardium distal to a total occlusion. Subepicardial and borderline ischemic regions may contain vessels not maximally dilated by ischemia. These vessels can be dilated by pharmacologic agents (293). Pharmacologic vasodilator reserve is also exhausted more quickly in the subendocardium (95) as compared to the subepicardium. Furthermore, while subendocardial perfusion normally exceeds subepicardial perfusion as reflected by a subendocardial to subepicardial perfusion ratio (endo/epi ratio) of greater than 1 (152), the subendocardium fails to autoregulate at coronary perfusion pressures that are within the autoregulatory range of the subepicardium (24,102,236).

Theories of Autoregulation

Three theories have been advanced to explain the phenomenon of coronary autoregulation. The tissue pressure hypothesis suggests that increases in coronary perfusion pressure result in increased capillary filtration, which subsequently causes elevations in tissue pressure by Starling's forces (135). Elevated tissue pressure results in extravascular compression of intramyocardial arterioles, leading to increased resistance and decreased flow. Recent evidence demonstrates, however, that intramyocardial tissue pressure remains relatively unchanged during increases in diastolic aortic pressure (116). If tissue pressure has any importance in autoregulation it must occur over a significant period of time. Coronary pressure autoregulation, however, occurs relatively quickly. The myogenic theory of autoregulation (83) proposes that stretch of vascular smooth muscle, as produced by increases in intraluminal pressure, causes vasoconstriction. In contrast, decreases in pressure elicit vasodilation. Unfortunately, the contribution of a myogenic mechanism to coronary autoregulation has not been specifically examined experimentally (68). The most widely accepted hypothesis is the metabolic theory of autoregulation (135,239), which suggests that myocardial metabolites provide a local feedback mechanism controlling oxygen and nutrient delivery. Decreases in perfusion pressure would result in reduced substrate availability and/or increased concentrations of metabolites that would serve as stimuli for coronary vasodilation. The latter hypothesis is especially attractive because of high O_2 extraction by the myocardium under resting conditions and the strong link between coronary flow and myocardial tissue oxygen tension. During periods of increased cardiac work, coronary flow must increase to provide adequate oxygen delivery because only a small amount of additional oxygen is available through extraction.

Metabolic and Humoral Mediators of Coronary Blood Flow

The roles of several potential mediators including O_2, adenosine triphosphate (ATP), adenosine diphosphate (ADP), adenosine, nitric oxide, endothelins, and prostaglandins in regulating flow through the coronary circulation have been investigated. Dole and Nuno (69) demonstrated that coronary venous PO_2 and coronary autoregulation are closely coupled, while the association between myocardial O_2 consumption and autoregulation is relatively weak. A similar correlation between coronary venous O_2 tension and vascular resistance was demonstrated by Drake-Holland et al. (74). These findings are consistent with the hypothesis that the coronary circulation is regulated by myocardial tissue PO_2 either directly or, more likely, through the release of vasoactive mediators appearing as tissue oxygen tension is reduced. As coronary artery perfusion pressure is decreased, myocardial tissue PO_2 falls. This reduction in tissue PO_2 results in a prompt vasodilation that maintains myocardial O_2 delivery at constant levels. Increases in coronary arterial oxygen content result in a decrease in coronary blood flow.

Adenosine has been considered to be an important physiologic regulator of coronary blood flow (142,240,247). Adenosine is a potent coronary vasodilator and can be recovered from myocardial tissue demonstrating an increase in concentration during periods of hypoxia, ischemia, reactive hyperemia, and increased myocardial oxygen consumption (81). It has been suggested that during periods of increased cardiac work and energy utilization, intracellular concentrations of ATP decrease, leading to an increase in the production of adenosine. The subsequent increase in coronary blood flow maintains the balance of oxygen supply to demand. Only a portion of the adenosine found in myocardium is coupled to tissue energy state, however. Hydrolytic cleavage of interstitial adenosine monophosphate (AMP) and S-adenosylhomocysteine represents a significant source of adenosine not related to cellular energy potential (211). While adenosine may serve as a signal between myocytes and vascular smooth muscle cells to regulate coronary blood flow, a definitive role remains a subject of controversy to this day.

The role of ATP-dependent K^+ (K^+_{ATP}) channels in coronary blood flow regulation has recently been explored. Coronary vasodilation in response to hypoxia is blocked by the ATP-dependent K^+ channel antagonist glibenclamide (glyburide)

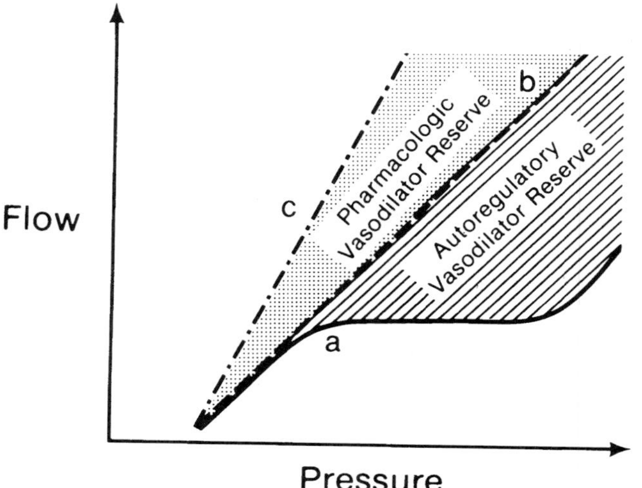

Figure 5. Autoregulation and coronary vasodilator reserve. The traditional view of autoregulation held that decreases in coronary blood flow accompanying reductions in perfusion pressure below the lower pressure limit for autoregulation indicated exhaustion of coronary vasodilator reserve. This concept may be demonstrated by examining the identity between the coronary pressure-flow relationship below the autoregulation range (line *a*) with that present in the maximally dilated bed (line *b*). Several investigations have demonstrated significant transmural flow reserve during intracoronary infusion of vasodilator agents at perfusion pressures well below the autoregulation range (line *c*). Thus, exhaustion of autoregulatory vasodilator reserve (*b* - *a*) does not necessarily imply exhaustion of pharmacologic vasodilator reserve (*c* - *a*). (From ref. 68, with permission.)

(62). This drug and other sulfonylureas such as tolbutamide are oral hypoglycemic drugs exerting their pharmacologic action to increase insulin release by blocking K^+_{ATP} channels in beta cells of the pancreas. Glibenclamide has also been shown to interfere with coronary microvascular dilation in response to reductions in perfusion pressure and coronary artery occlusion (157). ATP-dependent K^+ channel opening is thought to cause vasodilation via vascular smooth muscle cellular hyperpolarization. Hyperpolarization of the cell membrane closes voltage-gated Ca^{2+} channels, reducing intracellular Ca^{2+} concentration, and therefore causes vascular smooth muscle cell relaxation. Decreases in intracellular ATP concentration or increases in ADP concentration elicit opening of the ATP-dependent K^+ channel (75), and may represent the ultimate mechanism by which myocardial venous PO_2 is coupled to coronary arteriolar resistance. Reactive hyperemia in response to coronary occlusion is considerably reduced by ATP-dependent K^+ channel antagonists (10). Interestingly, this mechanism is inconsistent with the premise that the energy state of the myocyte is a primary determinant in regulating coronary flow, since the vascular smooth muscle cell is much less likely to become ischemic than is the myocyte (129,211,216). Adenosine may also be an important physiologic activator of ATP-dependent K^+ channels via stimulation of A_1 receptors that are linked to the channel by a G protein (101,150). In this fashion, adenosine may function as a signal between myocytes and vascular smooth muscle cells with the K^+_{ATP} channel serving a central role.

Furchgott and Zawadzki (87) demonstrated in 1980 that relaxation of blood vessels by acetylcholine is dependent on diffusion of an endothelium-derived relaxing factor (EDRF) from vascular endothelial cells. Acetylcholine produces vasoconstriction in the absence of a functional endothelium or during inhibition of the synthesis or release of EDRF. Strong evidence has shown that EDRF is equivalent to nitric oxide (NO) (214). A constitutive form of NO synthase is expressed in blood vessels that requires calcium and calmodulin for activation. Increases in intracellular Ca^{2+} concentration accompany NO release (237). NO released from endothelium activates a soluble form of guanylate cyclase in adjacent vascular smooth muscle, which causes an increase in the intracellular concentration of cGMP (228). Increases in intracellular cGMP initiate a phosphorylation cascade (223), ultimately involving many proteins and resulting in the dephosphorylation of myosin light chains. Dephosphorylation of myosin light chains, as well as activation of sarcolemmal Ca^{2+} ATPase (223) with resulting decreases in intracellular Ca^{2+} concentration, eventually causes smooth muscle cell relaxation. NO is avidly bound by hemoglobin (184) and is also deactivated by oxygen-derived free radicals (238).

NO has been shown to be released under basal conditions and by physiologic and pharmacologic stimulation. Physiologic factors eliciting NO release include increases in flow (shear stress), changes in oxygen tension, and stimulated release by platelet products, thrombin, autacoids, hormones, and neurotransmitters (285). Vasodilator drugs may or may not act by increasing local concentrations of NO at vascular smooth muscle sites. Endothelium-dependent vasodilators have been shown to preferentially increase subendocardial perfusion (219) during an increase in coronary flow. The precise role played by NO, the responses of which are variable among species and different locations in the vascular tree (211), as well as that played by other endothelial-derived hyperpolarization factors in flow regulation of the coronary circulation remains to be determined (Fig. 6).

In addition to endothelium-derived relaxant factors, a group of endothelial-derived vasoconstrictor proteins has been identified, including the endothelins (310). After binding to specific receptors endothelins activate phospholipase C, which catalyzes the hydrolysis of membrane phosphatidylinositol-4,5-bisphosphate. The cleavage product, inositol-1,4,5-trisphosphate, subsequently promotes Ca^{2+} release from intracellular stores. Additional Ca^{2+} influx through voltage-gated Ca^{2+} channels ultimately results in phosphorylation of myosin light chains, initiating contraction of smooth muscle cells (165). Endothelin-1 may be the most efficacious of all endogenous vasoconstrictors. Pathophysiologic concentrations of endothelins result in significant increases in coronary vascular resistance (166), but the role of these endogenous vasoconstrictors in the normal regulation of coronary blood flow is as yet undetermined. These agents may ultimately be responsible for vasospasm of large coronary vessels or the "no reflow phenomenon" associated with coronary artery occlusion and reperfusion injury.

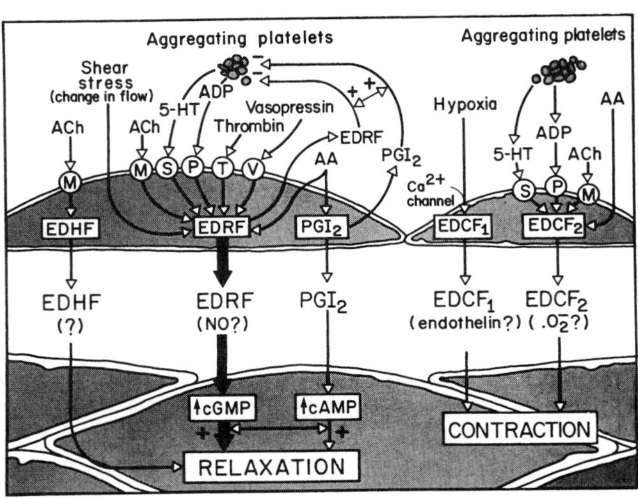

Figure 6. Current concepts of endothelium-derived factors and their modulation of vascular smooth muscle contraction. Endothelium-derived relaxing factor (EDRF), a powerful vasodilator of the underlying smooth muscle, increases cyclic GMP (cGMP) levels through activation of soluble guanylate cyclase. The chemical nature of EDRF is nitric oxide (NO). Prostacyclin (PGI_2) is another vasodilator released from the endothelium whose effects depend on elevation of cyclic AMP (cAMP) through activation of adenylate cyclase. NO and prostacyclin could act synergistically in terms of relaxing vascular smooth muscle and inhibiting platelet aggregation. The endothelial cells also secrete a hyperpolarizing factor (EDHF). The exact nature of EDHF is unknown; it most likely is a metabolite of arachidonic acid, presumably an epoxide or lipoxide. At least two endothelium-derived contracting factors exist; one is indomethacin-insensitive ($EDCF_1$), and the other is indomethacin-sensitive ($EDCF_2$). Recent data suggest that $EDCF_1$ may be endothelin, and $EDCF_2$ may be superoxide anions, although this remains to be proved. EDHF has a vasodilator effect and may contribute in part to the initial portion of endothelium-dependent relaxations. ACh, acetylcholine; 5-HT, 5-hydroxytryptamine, serotonin; ADP, adenosine diphosphate; AA, arachidonic acid; +, synergism or facilitation; –, inhibition; ?, exact nature unknown; M, muscarinic receptor; S, serotonergic receptor; P, purinergic receptor; T, thrombin receptor; V, vasopressinergic receptor. (From ref. 285, with permission.)

Coronary vascular tone is altered by a variety of vasodilating (PGI_2, PGE_2) and constricting prostanoids (thromboxane A_2) (255) and neuropeptides (211), including vasoactive intestinal peptide, substance P, calcitonin gene-related peptide, and neuropeptide Y. Present evidence suggests that eicosanoids and these peptides do not play a major role in the regulation of coronary blood flow.

Neural and Reflex Control

Autonomic control of coronary blood flow has been intensively studied over the last two decades. Large and small coronary vessels are innervated by both sympathetic and parasympathetic nerves. Stimulation of these nerves results in direct actions on the coronary vessels and also indirect effects mediated by metabolic autoregulation. The direct and indirect actions are often qualitatively opposite. Adrenergic control of the coronary circulation has been reviewed in detail by Feigl (81), Heusch (119), and Chilian et al. (50). Sympathetic nerve stimulation or intracoronary injections of norepinephrine result in metabolic coronary vasodilation secondary to increased myocardial oxygen consumption because of increases in heart rate and myocardial contractility (indirect effect) and in simultaneous α-adrenergic receptor-mediated coronary vasoconstriction (direct effect) (81). α-Adrenergic vasoconstriction during sympathetic activation limits metabolically driven canine coronary vasodilation by approximately 30% (197). Sympathetic vasoconstriction can be unmasked during β-adrenergic blockade. Antagonism of β-adrenergic receptors prevents the increases in coronary flow secondary to tachycardia and increased myocardial contractility (1,104) and allows α-receptor stimulation of the coronary vasculature to be relatively unopposed. This process may also represent a portion of the mechanism whereby coronary flow is redistributed to the subendocardium or collateral-dependent regions during nonspecific β_1- and β_2-adrenergic blockade. Blockade of these receptors in normal zones may cause localized vasoconstriction, diverting flow to relatively dilated regions.

Recently, considerable effort has been directed toward the determination of the anatomic location and physiologic role of α_1- and α_2-receptor subtypes in the coronary circulation. This is of special interest because of the current development of α_2-agonists as adjuncts for anesthesia. Canine studies suggest that α_1-receptors are uniformly present in the coronary circulation while α_2-receptors are found preferentially within the coronary microcirculation in arterioles less than 100 μm in diameter (50). While vasoconstriction can be elicited by both α_1- and α_2-receptor activation, adrenergic stimulation also causes the release of NO, which may attenuate increases in vascular tone (42,51,191). It has been shown that coronary arterioles less than 100 μm in diameter actually "escape" the effects of adrenergic activation and dilate, while coronary arteries greater than 100 μm in diameter constrict (Fig. 7) (47) in the intact autoregulating coronary circulation. These findings suggest that autoregulatory adjustments in the coronary microcirculation prevent constriction of small coronary arterioles in response to α-adrenergic activation. The physiologic significance of these findings is unknown; however, during intense sympathetic activation with increases in myocardial oxygen consumption, simultaneous functional hyperemia and vasoconstriction might prevent changes in local hydrostatic pressure that could otherwise impair water and solute exchange (48). In addition to the heterogeneous location of α_1- and α_2-receptors within the coronary microcirculation, α_2-adrenoceptors are found presynaptically on adrenergic nerves (131). Activation of presynaptic α_2-receptors decreases norepinephrine release from nerve terminals, adding further complexity to the understanding of adrenergic control of the coronary circulation.

In contrast to α-adrenergic effects, coronary vasodilation occurs in response to activation of vascular β-adrenoceptors, most likely of the β_2 subtype (81). Parasympathetic activation also produces vasodilation in canine models that can be mimicked by intracoronary administration of acetylcholine and blocked by atropine (81). Stimulation of M_1 muscarinic receptors redistributes blood flow preferentially to the subendocardium, while both M_1 and M_2 receptors are involved in increasing overall myocardial perfusion (218). In canine models, vasodilation produced by acetylcholine is endothelium dependent, secondary to release of NO via stimulation of muscarinic receptors on endothelial cells. In contrast, acetylcholine causes vasoconstriction in porcine and human coronary arteries (137). However, when isolated coronary artery rings from patients with normal endothelium free of atherosclerosis are studied in vitro, vasodilation is observed (173). These results suggest that acetylcholine has direct actions to constrict coronary vascular smooth muscle and indirect actions mediated through endothelium to cause vasodilation. Reflex control of the coronary circulation has also been investigated; however, the only well established reflex is the carotid sinus reflex (197). A decrease in perfusion pressure within the carotid sinus results in reflex α-receptor-mediated coronary vasoconstriction that is independent of changes in myocardial oxygen consumption or autoregulation (81).

Coronary blood flow is regulated at the level of the coronary microcirculation. Older theories of coronary blood flow regulation considered conductance vessels, resistance vessels, and veins to function in a homogeneous fashion. Coronary arterioles (<50 μm diameter) probably provide the greatest amount of variable resistance to flow under normal conditions, but the lengths as well as vasomotion of larger vessels may under some circumstances contribute significantly to alterations in coro-

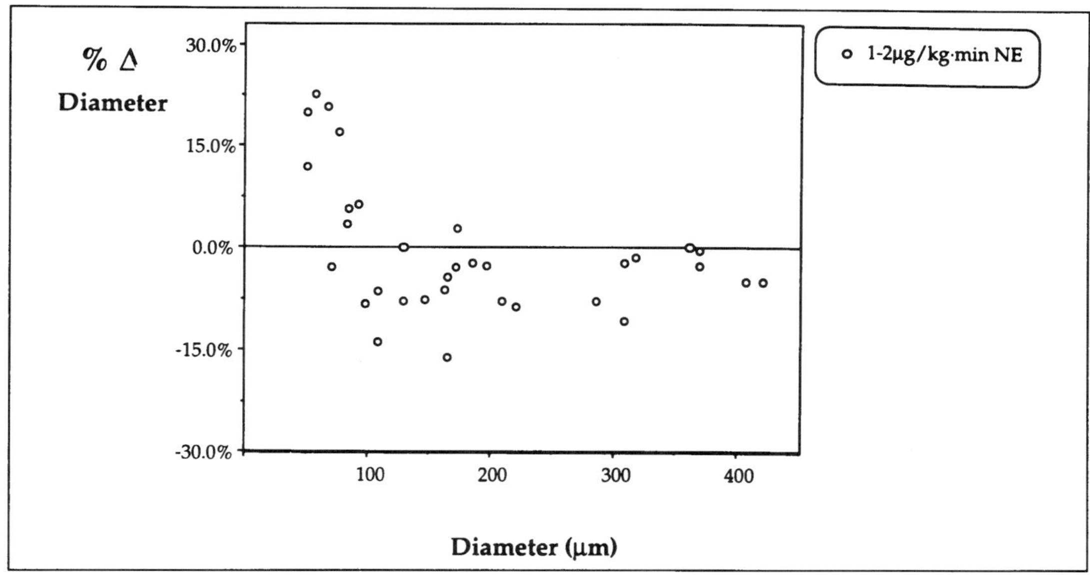

Figure 7. Coronary microvascular responses to norepinephrine infusion expressed as a percent change in diameter from the initial diameter. Small arterioles dilate during norepinephrine infusion, while larger arterioles constrict. (From ref. 47, with permission.)

nary vascular resistance. This is especially evident under conditions of maximum arteriolar vasodilation caused by drugs, exercise, or ischemia. Investigations of the coronary microcirculation have also revealed that vessels of different size respond to physiologic and pharmacologic stimuli in a heterogeneous fashion. Such heterogeneity in the response of various sizes of arterial vessels to α-receptor stimulation (50), adenosine (139), serotonin (161), vasopressin (161), and nitroglycerin (249) have all been demonstrated. In addition, NO may regulate the distribution of blood flow among arteriolar branches (97). The importance of these mechanisms has not been fully elucidated; however, it has been suggested that it is this complex ability of the coronary circulation to respond to the same stimuli in a heterogeneous fashion that enables alterations in vascular resistance to precisely regulate myocardial oxygen and nutrient delivery (177).

PATHOPHYSIOLOGY OF THE CORONARY CIRCULATION

Coronary Atherosclerosis and Thrombosis

Several risk factors have been identified that predict an increased susceptibility to coronary artery disease. These risk factors include hypertension, nicotine consumption, hypercholesterolemia, diabetes mellitus, obesity, and a family history of coronary artery disease (265). The presence of risk factors is associated with the development of atherosclerosis, but the exact pathogenesis of the atherosclerotic lesion remains unknown. The most widely held theory of atherogenesis is the "response to injury hypothesis" (235). This theory holds that some inciting injury to vascular endothelial cells occurs that triggers the release of various growth factors and results in the attraction of monocytes, macrophages, and possibly platelets to the site of injury. The interactions of these formed elements and the vessel results in smooth muscle cell proliferation and formation of a fibrous plaque (234). Platelet attachment to an uncomplicated fibrous plaque, as well as plaque rupture with exposure of thrombogenic collagen, incites thrombus formation, converting a partially occluded coronary artery into one that is severely stenosed or totally occluded (202,266). During this process, platelet aggregates can be formed, broken apart, and reformed in a cyclical process. This results in a slow reduction in flow and a sudden increase in flow, only to be followed by yet another flow reduction. This process known as coronary cyclical flow reduction occurs at a frequency of 9 to 12 times per hour in the presence of a severe stenosis in dog models of coronary artery disease. Aspirin and thromboxane A_2 antagonists inhibit this phenomenon (2,3).

Pressure-flow relationships are disturbed in myocardium supplied by atherosclerotic coronary arteries because in-flow driving pressure to the perfusion bed is no longer diastolic aortic pressure, but the pressure distal to the stenosis. With increasing severity of stenosis, resistance to flow increases and the pressure drop across the stenosis becomes greater, reducing coronary artery perfusion pressure. Furthermore, the coronary hemodynamic consequences of multiple stenoses on the same artery are additive so that stenoses of lesser severity become quite significant (291). While resting flow may be maintained early in the process of atherosclerosis, coronary vasodilator reserve is slowly exhausted. Resting coronary flow is maintained until stenosis severity reaches greater than 90% reduction in vessel cross-sectional area, but the ability of flow to increase in response to increases in oxygen demand or vasodilator agents is reduced at a stenosis severity of greater than 60% (295). Since subendocardial vasodilator reserve is normally less than that in the subepicardium, increases in myocardial oxygen demand and/or further decreases in coronary artery perfusion pressure may precipitate subendocardial ischemia and a reversal in the normal transmural perfusion gradient between

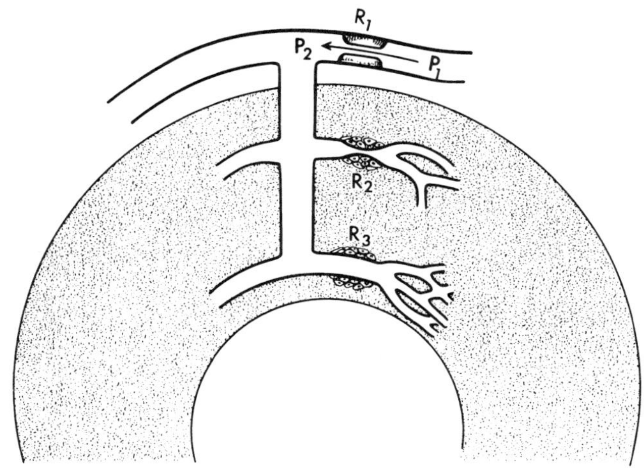

Figure 8. Effects of a stenosis on endocardial and epicardial flow. Endocardial vessels are maximally dilated, whereas epicardial vessels are not. Any vasodilator stimulus will augment transmural flow owing to dilation of subepicardial vessels. Increases in flow will cause a greater pressure drop across the stenosis. As long as the fall in resistance in subepicardial vessels is greater than the resulting fall in driving pressure, flow will increase in subepicardial region. However, because subendocardial vessels are already maximally dilated, the fall in driving pressure will not be accompanied by a fall in resistance. Hence, flow to subendocardial vessels will fall. (From ref. 76, with permission.)

subendocardium and subepicardium (76) (Fig. 8). Lower vasodilator reserve compounded with higher oxygen consumption and greater susceptibility to intramural tissue pressure predispose the subendocardium to the development of ischemia and infarction (14) (Fig. 9).

The atherosclerotic process not only alters pressure-flow relationships, but it also dramatically changes metabolic, humoral, and adrenergic control of the coronary circulation. Endothelium-dependent vascular relaxation in epicardial arteries and coronary microvessels is impaired by atherosclerosis (159) and myocardial ischemia or reperfusion (58,217,284). Impairment

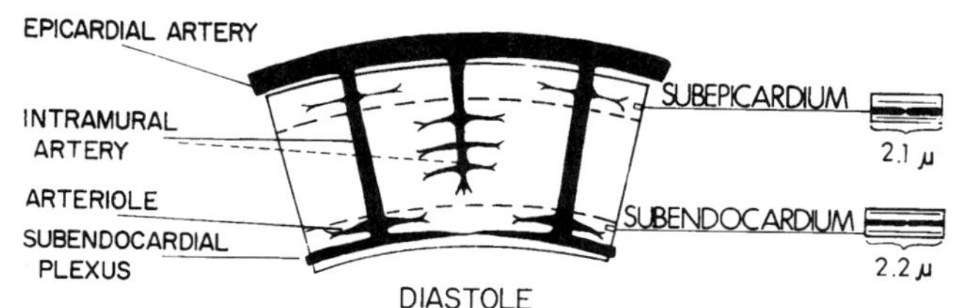

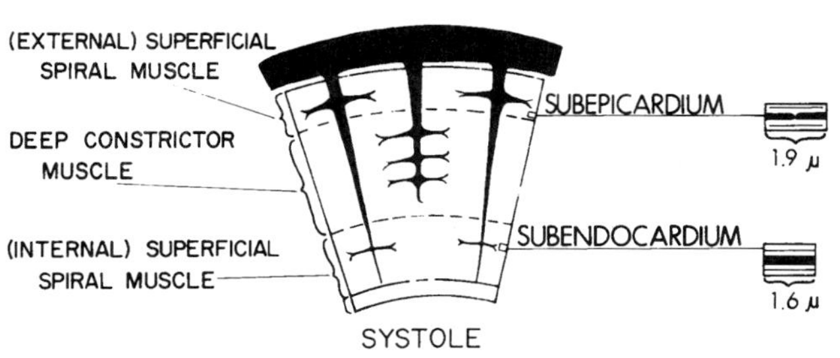

Figure 9. Cross-section of the left ventricular wall in diastole *(top)* and systole *(bottom)*. Factors involved in the susceptibility of the subendocardium to the development of ischemia include the greater dependence of this region on diastolic perfusion and the greater degree of shortening, and therefore of energy expenditure, of this region during systole. (From ref. 14, with permission.)

of endothelial function may be secondary to deficient NO production and release, or degradation of NO by oxygen-derived free radicals prior to release from endothelial cells (106). The presence of atherosclerosis and/or hypercholesterolemia also potentiates vasoconstriction to a variety of compounds including endothelin, thromboxane A_2, serotonin, acetylcholine, and histamine (159,285). NO release secondary to flow-mediated shear stress is impaired in atherosclerotic arteries and arterioles (159). Finally, the atherosclerotic process interferes with the production of prostacyclin (PGI_2), altering the balance between prostacylin produced by the vessel and thromboxane A_2 produced by circulating platelets (251). As a result, vasoconstriction caused by aggregating platelets adherent to an atherosclerotic plaque is unopposed, resulting in further platelet aggregation and vasoconstriction (Fig. 10).

Small coronary arterioles escape α_1–adrenergic vasoconstriction under normal conditions but significantly greater constrictor responses to both α_1- and α_2-adrenergic activation are exhibited during coronary hypoperfusion (48). α_2-adrenoceptor activation has been shown to increase coronary vascular resistance distal to a severe coronary stenosis in dogs (120). In contrast, α_2-adrenoceptor blockade decreases coronary blood flow in humans with a coronary artery stenosis (131). Increases in the norepinephrine concentration of coronary sinus blood concomitant with α_2-adrenergic blockade suggests that α_2-blockade reduces presynaptic inhibition of norepinephrine release. In the presence of α_2-blocking agents a greater amount of norepinephrine is released with any given level of sympathetic nerve stimulation. Thus, the beneficial versus detrimental effects of adrenergic stimulation during coronary hypoperfusion remain controversial. Feigl (80) demonstrated improved subendocardial perfusion in the presence of α-adrenergic activation compared to that observed in the presence of α-blockade during coronary hypoperfusion. In addition, α-adrenergic stimulation results in increased adenosine release and increased coronary vessel sensitivity to adenosine during myocardial ischemia (128) and hypoxia (118).

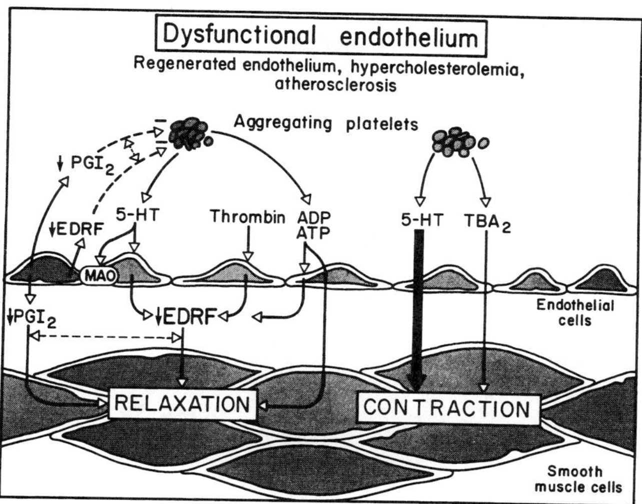

Figure 10. Illustration of endothelium-dependent responses under pathologic conditions. The endothelium is dysfunctional in a regenerated state, hypercholesterolemia and atherosclerosis, releasing less endothelium-derived relaxing factor (EDRF) or nitric oxide (NO), whereas the ability of the smooth muscle to contract is unaltered. As a result, the contractions predominate. In atherosclerosis, the production of both NO and prostacyclin (PGI_2) is reduced, and their synergistic actions against aggregating platelets may not occur. 5-HT, 5-hydroxytryptamine, serotonin; ADP, adenosine diphosphate; ATP, adenosine triphosphate; TBA_2, thromboxane A_2; MAO, monoamine oxidase; –, inhibition; +, synergism. (From ref. 285, with permission.)

Resting coronary flow eventually declines as the atherosclerotic process advances. Increases in coronary flow during exercise may decrease distending pressure across the stenosis, causing collapse of the vessel (93). Thus, a coronary stenosis should not simply be considered as a fixed resistance to flow but is dynamic in nature, with resistance changes occurring concomitant with alterations in proximal and distal vascular tone. Alterations in pre- and poststenotic vascular tone by pharmacologic agents may dramatically alter stenosis resistance (33,296). Additionally, adhesion of hyperaggregable and hyperreactive platelets to an existing atherosclerotic plaque results in intravascular thrombosis and cyclical or permanent total coronary artery occlusion. These events ultimately may lead to irreversible tissue damage. Coronary artery thrombosis is the most common cause of transmural myocardial infarction (4).

Coronary Collateral Circulation

The rapidity with which total coronary artery occlusion occurs determines the clinical consequences of the event. Some degree of perfusion may be present in the area at risk for development of infarction despite the presence of total coronary artery occlusion. The extent of myocardial injury is inversely related to the degree of collateral blood flow arising from interarterial anastomoses distal to the occluded vascular segment (297). Development of coronary collateral vessels has been examined in human, canine, and porcine hearts. While coronary collaterals are located primarily in the subepicardium in canine hearts (298), the predominant location is subendocardial in humans and porcine hearts (245). The vessels appear histologically as thin-walled arteries that subsequently acquire vascular smooth muscle over time. Coronary collaterals may be demonstrated angiographically in humans following coronary artery occlusion or high-grade stenosis (85,168). The protective role of coronary collaterals has been demonstrated in several human studies (84,136,168,248). Patients with coronary collaterals have less myocardial necrosis and better left ventricular function as compared to patients deficient in collateral development after myocardial infarction. The human coronary collateral circulation commonly supplies sufficient flow to meet only the resting needs of the myocardium (176). Increases in oxygen demand such as occur during exercise may still be associated with the onset of myocardial ischemia.

An ischemic stimulus is suspected to be necessary to induce coronary collateral development (246). In animal models of coronary collateralization, brief repetitive coronary artery occlusions are the most efficient means to induce collateral development without causing myocardial infarction (308). The mechanisms through which coronary collateral development occur are currently under investigation. Various vascular mitogens including fibroblastic growth factor, vascular endothelium growth factor, platelet-derived growth factors, and adenosine have been demonstrated to play a role in angiogenesis (11,18, 148,246).

The vascular responsiveness of coronary collateral vessels has been investigated in animal models. Endothelium-dependent vasodilation of canine coronary collaterals is intact (82), but it is attenuated in coronary microvessels perfused by the mature collateral vessels (107). Coronary collaterals have also been shown to possess β_2-adrenergic receptors, stimulation of which results in vasodilation, but α_1- and α_2-adrenoceptor mediated vasoconstriction is absent (107). Finally, both collateral vessels and microvessels present in collateral-dependent myocardium constrict dramatically in response to vasopressin at concentrations associated with physiologic stress, hemorrhage, or cardiopulmonary bypass (221). This constriction is greatly exaggerated as compared to normal coronary vessels of the same size.

Vasodilator-induced coronary artery steal has been defined as an increase in flow to nonischemic myocardium at the expense of decreasing collateral flow to an ischemic zone

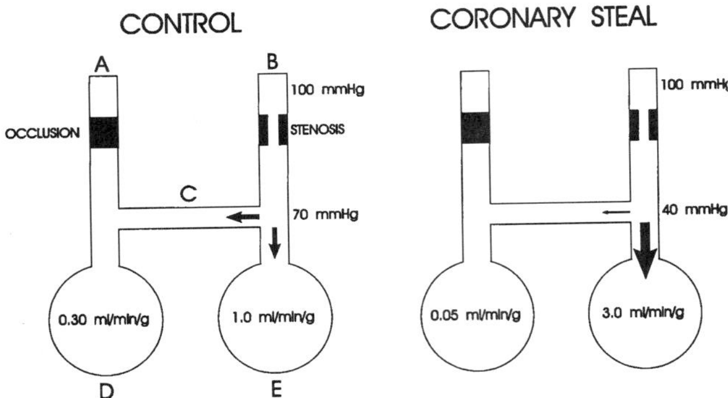

Figure 11. Schematic diagram of coronary circulation illustrating the mechanism of vasodilator-induced coronary steal. Tissue (D) supplied by coronary artery A is perfused via collaterals (C) whose artery of origin (B) possesses a proximal stenosis. Collateral vessels are maximally dilated in the control state and during coronary steal. During vasodilation perfusion pressure at the origin of the collateral vessels is reduced from 70 to 40 mm Hg, resulting in decreased perfusion of ischemic tissue (D). In contrast, vasodilation of artery B distal to the stenosis causes an increase in blood flow to tissue (E) supplied by the stenotic artery and coronary steal has occurred.

independent of change in aortic pressure and heart rate (13). Perfusion of collateral-dependent myocardium depends on the driving pressure at the origin of the collateral vessels. Arterioles in the collateral-dependent zone are relatively dilated in comparison to surrounding regions and collateral flow is considered to be pressure dependent (lack of autoregulation). As a consequence, collateral blood will decrease in direct proportion to reductions in perfusion pressure. Reduction of driving pressure at the origin of coronary collateral vessels occurs during vasodilation, especially in the presence of a stenosis. Coronary vasodilation distal to a stenosis of the artery of origin of the collaterals (e.g., as a result of exercise or administration of a potent vasodilator) reduces collateral perfusion pressure and results in coronary steal (13,100) (Fig. 11). Coronary steal can also occur in the absence of a stenosis on the artery of origin of the collateral vessels during maximum vasodilation. Under such high-flow states, even a normal proximal arterial segment may provide enough resistance such that a significant pressure drop occurs at the origin of the collateral vessels (305). Coronary steal can result in an increase in myocardial infarct size (292). In addition, transmural steal (a redistribution of flow away from the subendocardium to supepicardium) may occur distal to a single coronary artery stenosis under conditions of maximal vasodilation or high-grade coronary constriction (100,294). Transmural steal occurs because subendocardial perfusion is pressure-dependent at perfusion pressures that remain in the autoregulatory range of the subepicardium (88,102). Vasodilation causes a decrease in coronary perfusion pressure distal to the stenosis, and subendocardial flow falls while subepicardial flow increases (decrease in endo/epi ratio). The degree of stenosis and pharmacologic vasodilation needed to produce steal is interactive. The greater the degree of stenosis, the less the vasodilation required to redistribute flow.

Coronary Artery Vasospasm

Myocardial ischemia may result not only from inadequate flow through stenotic coronary arteries, but also following abrupt, focal spasm of either normal or diseased coronary arteries. The underlying mechanisms of coronary artery vasospasm have recently been under intense investigation (250). The hypothesis that increased vascular responsiveness is directly related to the atherosclerotic process is supported by postmortem evidence of atherosclerosis in "angiographically normal" coronary arteries obtained from patients sustaining acute ischemic events (170). Experimental models demonstrating augmented coronary vasoconstrictor responses in animals with early atherosclerosis but minimal luminal narrowing also support this hypothesis (89).

Augmented vascular responses may be the result of altered endothelial cell function, release of vasoconstrictors from formed elements in the blood, changes in receptor density, and neovascularization of atherosclerotic plaques (89). Endothelial-dependent vasodilation is impaired in atherosclerosis, which may result in an imbalance between vasodilator and vasoconstrictor tone in the coronary circulation (285). Platelets, macrophages, monocytes, and mast cells are attracted to the intimal surface of injured arterial walls. The release of potent vasoactive agents such as thromboxane A_2, serotonin, leukotrienes, platelet-derived growth factor, and histamine from such cells contributes to the increased vascular reactivity observed (89). Some evidence suggests that increases in serotonin (207) and histamine (H1) (174) receptor density may contribute to the augmented vasoconstriction. Platelet activation with subsequent release of tumor transforming growth factor beta and formation of thrombin stimulate release of endothelin. Endothelin-1 is a potent vasoconstrictor and has been demonstrated to potentiate human coronary artery constriction to both norepinephrine and serotonin (311). Finally, the dense microvasculature surrounding an atherosclerotic plaque may deliver higher concentrations of circulating vasoconstrictors to a focal coronary arterial segment (12), resulting in vasospasm.

A subset of individuals exists in whom angina occurs despite the presence of angiographically normal coronary arteries and the absence of large vessel coronary artery vasospasm, even during ergonovine challenge (40). This condition, referred to as "syndrome X," carries a prognosis that is considerably better than that associated with atherosclerotic coronary artery disease (186). Angina appears to occur because of abnormal vasodilator reserve present in resistance vessels, while large conductance vessels are unaffected. Increases in coronary flow and decreases in coronary vascular resistance in response to atrial pacing (40), exercise (39), and pharmacologic vasodilators (29) are impaired. Despite symptoms of ongoing chest pain and ischemia in response to exercise testing, mortality in patients with normal left ventricular function is not increased (144).

Left Ventricular Hypertrophy

Left ventricular hypertrophy (LVH) develops as an adaptive response to left ventricular pressure or volume overload. Regional hypertrophy may also occur during ventricular remodeling of normal zones following myocardial infarction. The increases in wall thickness serve to normalize left ventricular wall stress. While hypertrophy may begin as an adaptive response, abnormalities in myocardial perfusion occur. Alterations in minimal coronary vascular resistance, coronary vasodilator reserve, and coronary autoregulation have all been observed in models of LVH (66). Subendocardial autoregulation may be especially impaired (105). Findings of increased minimal coronary vascular resistance per gram of myocardium suggest that increases in left ventricular muscle mass exceed vascular growth (179,180). However, return of minimal coronary vascular resistance toward normal in the presence of prolonged LVH implies that neovascularization may occur (280). Coronary vasodilator reserve has been demonstrated to be reduced in LVH and may represent a portion of the mechanism (in conjunction with elevation of myocardial oxygen consumption) involved in the production of angina in patients with aortic stenosis and normal coronary arteries (79,178). Alterations in vascular reactivity in the presence of LVH require further investigation.

Diabetes Mellitus

Coronary artery disease is the leading cause of death among adult diabetics. The atherosclerotic process is accelerated in diabetes, resulting in more extensive and severe vascular disease (289). Not only is the risk of myocardial infarction higher in diabetes, but the morbidity and mortality resulting from myocardial infarction is also increased (303). Diabetes causes small coronary arteriolar sclerosis and microaneurysm formation (78) in addition to large vessel atherosclerosis. Diabetic cardiomyopathy may occur in the absence of significant coronary artery disease. Histologic findings in diabetic cardiomyopathic hearts are predominantly those of interstitial fibrosis unrelated to any ongoing ischemic process (274).

Metabolic and humoral control of the coronary circulation is altered in diabetes, and endothelial-dependent vasodilation is impaired in animal models of the disease (65,187,278). An increase in endothelial-dependent vasoconstrictor prostanoid production has been demonstrated in diabetic rabbit aorta (278), rat cerebral arterioles (187), and canine coronary arterial rings (156), while stimulated release of PGI_2 is reduced (155,156). Diabetes also impairs coronary microvessel dilation during a reduction in perfusion pressure (147). Hyperglycemia alone may attenuate microvascular responses to reductions in coronary flow (147) and enhance the production of endothelial-dependent vasoconstrictor eicosanoids (277).

Diabetic patients are frequently treated with sulfonylurea oral hypoglycemic drugs such as glyburide and tolbutamide, both of which are selective ATP-dependent K^+ channel antagonists. Recent evidence suggests that blockade of K^+_{ATP} channels impairs microvascular dilation during ischemia (157), delays recovery of stunned myocardium (8), increases infarct size (7), and prevents ischemic preconditioning in laboratory animals (98). Whether the findings of increased cardiovascular mortality in diabetic patients treated with tolbutamide versus insulin or placebo (188) relates specifically to K_{ATP} channel blockade is as yet unknown.

ANESTHETICS AND THE CORONARY CIRCULATION

Volatile Anesthetics

The volatile anesthetic halothane was first introduced into clinical practice in 1956, yet the mechanisms that govern its pharmacologic effects remain incompletely understood. Volatile anesthetics are known to produce relaxation of smooth muscle, but the biologic significance of any direct actions of these agents on the coronary vasculature remains controversial. The net effect of volatile anesthetic action on coronary vascular tone represents the sum of both direct and indirect effects. Volatile anesthetics cause direct coronary vasodilation; however, simultaneously occurring anesthetic-induced reductions in myocardial inotropic state, preload and afterload, and heart rate result in metabolically mediated coronary vasoconstriction. An appreciation of the directionally opposite direct and indirect effects of volatile anesthetics on coronary vascular tone may clarify what otherwise might be interpreted as conflicting experimental findings. Recent investigation of the cellular events controlling vascular smooth muscle tone will undoubtedly result in further elucidation of the mechanisms and clinical importance of the effects of anesthetics on the coronary circulation.

The direct coronary vasodilator actions of volatile anesthetics can be demonstrated in vitro, in experimental preparations in which the indirect effects of the anesthetics are minimized. The volatile anesthetics halothane, isoflurane, and enflurane cause vasodilation of isolated coronary arteries (20,26–28,114,182, 288,306). Halothane produces greater coronary artery dilation than does isoflurane at equivalent minimum alveolar concentration (MAC) (26–28,182,288) and does so in coronary arteries whose diameters are greater than 2000 μm (27,28,114,182,288). In contrast, isoflurane causes vasodilation of predominantly small (<900 μm) canine epicardial coronary arteries (114). Halothane may produce greater vasodilator effects in large coronary arteries than does isoflurane in part because halothane causes greater suppression of inward Ca^{2+} (L-type voltage dependent) currents than isoflurane (37). Inhibition of voltage-dependent Ca^{2+} channel activity by volatile anesthetics causes a decrease in vascular smooth muscle tone. Since larger diameter vessels appear to possess more intracellular Ca^{2+} stores, greater depletion of these stores by halothane versus isoflurane may also contribute.

The actions of volatile anesthetics on the coronary vasculature independent of changes in autonomic nervous system tone and systemic hemodynamics are demonstrated in isolated heart preparations. Impedance to aortic outflow and left ventricular end diastolic pressure can be independently varied, thereby controlling two important determinants of myocardial oxygen consumption. In the contracting isolated heart, anesthetic-induced negative inotropic effects cause decreases in coronary blood flow via flow-metabolism coupling. A decrease in myocardial oxygen demand is accompanied by an increase in coronary vascular resistance The direct coronary vasodilator actions of volatile anesthetics are partially discerned, however, by examining the ratio of myocardial oxygen delivery to oxygen consumption (DO_2/MVO_2) and by calculating myocardial oxygen extraction (% O_2 extraction). Examination of these variables allows detection of direct coronary vasodilation produced by anesthetic agents, concomitant with autoregulatory vasoconstriction secondary to decreases in MVO_2. If no vasodilation occurs after introduction of an anesthetic agent, DO_2/MVO_2 and % O_2 extraction remain unchanged. If, however, an anesthetic produces coronary vasodilation (even in the presence of an overall decrease in coronary blood flow secondary to reduced MVO_2), DO_2/MVO_2 increases and % O_2 extraction decreases. This occurs because "unnecessary" vasodilation results in myocardial perfusion that exceeds demand (sometimes referred to as "luxury flow") and the oxygen tension in coronary sinus blood rises. Definitive study of the "coronary vasodilator actions" of anesthetic agents in vivo requires measurement of these variables.

Interpretation of the effects of volatile anesthetics on coronary hemodynamics in vivo are often complicated by several factors, including the lack of a baseline conscious state (a basal barbiturate, chloralose-urethane, or other anesthetic is often used), the presence of anesthetic-induced alterations in systemic hemodynamics, and differing methods of measurement of coronary blood flow. Alterations of coronary vascular resistance in vivo are often interpreted as indicative of direct effects of anesthetics on coronary vascular smooth muscle tone. However, heterogeneous changes in vascular responses by vessels of differing diameter (49), pressure dependency of vascular resistance (153), and altered intramural tissue pressure may all contribute to apparent changes in coronary vascular resistance (127). Therefore, changes in the calculated value of coronary vascular resistance do not necessarily indicate active alterations in smooth muscle tone.

Halothane and isoflurane cause direct coronary vasodilation in isolated beating hearts as indicated by decreases in myocardial oxygen extraction and increases in DO_2/MVO_2 (164,242, 270,271). Halothane and isoflurane similarly reduce coronary flow reserve elicited with adenosine (163) in isolated hearts arrested with tetrodotoxin, an agent that decreases sodium channel conductance (141) and thereby blocks conduction of the cardiac action potential. Since mechanical work is not performed by the heart under these circumstances, decreases in MVO_2 produced by different anesthetics are minimized. These findings suggest that halothane and isoflurane directly cause similar degrees of coronary vasodilation.

Halothane has variable effects on coronary vascular resistance and coronary blood flow in vivo that occur concomitant with changes in MVO_2 (70,259,299,307). Decreases in MVO_2 are accompanied by metabolically coupled reductions in coronary blood flow during halothane anesthesia (5,190,286). Despite these decreases in flow, direct coronary vasodilation is evidenced by increases in the oxygen tension in coronary sinus blood and decreases in oxygen extraction (70,307). These experiments also indicate that the volatile anesthetic halothane is at best a weak coronary vasodilator because little to no change or even a decrease in total flow occurs following administration of halothane.

In a similar fashion to halothane, isoflurane variably alters coronary blood flow in vivo (32,60,121,189,190,224). Isoflurane decreases MVO_2 (189), but the simultaneous coronary vasodilator effects of isoflurane are indicated by decreases in myocardial oxygen extraction (60). Halothane and isoflurane both cause early increases in coronary blood flow during induction of anesthesia, associated with increases in MVO_2 as estimated by the pressure-work index (145). Increases in coronary blood flow are prevented by autonomic nervous system blockade (which prevents increases in heart rate and subsequently MVO_2) in halothane-, but not isoflurane-anesthetized dogs, suggesting that isoflurane causes mild coronary vasodilation independent of changes in MVO_2. Abrupt perfusion of the canine left anterior descending coronary artery at constant pressure with blood previously equilibrated with isoflurane increases coronary blood flow fourfold within minutes of exposure (61). In contrast, isoflurane caused only mild coronary vasodilator effects in similarly instrumented swine when flow was measured following a period of anesthetic equilibration (121). In addition, isoflurane increases coronary blood flow despite unchanged epicardial coronary artery cross-sectional diameter, indicating that isoflurane dilates coronary arteries of predominantly small (<900 μm) diameter (253).

Controversy exists as to the actions of enflurane on the coronary circulation (182,242,270,271). In vivo, enflurane causes a greater reduction in MVO_2 than isoflurane (55), and this reduction in MVO_2 is associated with metabolically mediated decreases in coronary blood flow (55,103). While isoflurane and enflurane both decrease myocardial oxygen extraction, isoflurane does so to a greater extent than enflurane (103). Desflurane causes similar increases in DO_2/MVO_2 and decreases in myocardial oxygen extraction in comparison to isoflurane (25). However, increases in coronary blood flow are prevented by preventing changes in heart rate by autonomic nervous system blockade during desflurane but not isoflurane anesthesia (213). Increases in coronary blood flow during isoflurane anesthesia, despite prevention of tachycardia by autonomic nervous system blockade, suggest that isoflurane produces greater direct coronary vasodilation than desflurane. In contrast to findings with isoflurane, sevoflurane has little direct coronary vasodilator action (16,56,59,163,175).

Coronary vasodilator reserve (92), expressed as the quotient of peak coronary flow following a brief coronary occlusion and baseline flow, is altered by halothane and isoflurane. Greater vasodilator reserve is present during isoflurane versus halothane anesthesia. This implies that less coronary vasodilation is produced by isoflurane versus halothane. An efficacious coronary vasodilator would reduce the ability of flow to increase further (less reserve) because flow would already be increased in its presence. This situation is more complicated when the indirect actions of the volatile anesthetics are considered. Cardiac output and stroke volume are depressed more by halothane, even during maintenance of arterial pressure at levels similar to those observed during isoflurane anesthesia. Peak flow during reactive hyperemia and percent flow debt repayment following brief coronary artery occlusion are closely related to the intensity of ischemia and the magnitude of oxygen debt accrued during the period of coronary occlusion (Fig. 12). Since halothane reduces major hemodynamic determinants of MVO_2 to a greater extent than isoflurane, oxygen debt accruing during

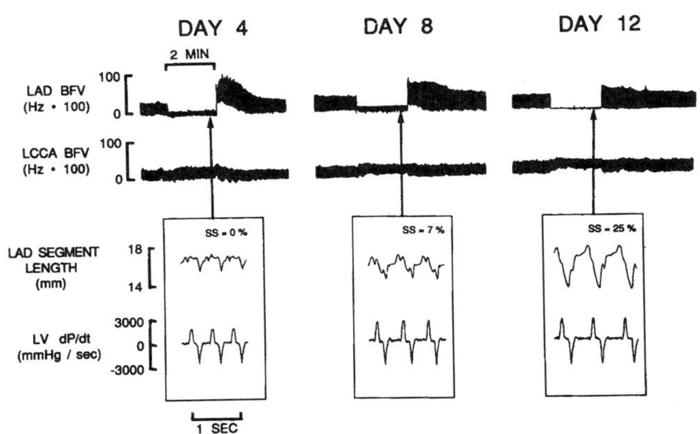

Figure 12. Left anterior descending and left circumflex coronary artery blood flow velocity (LAD and LCCA BFV, respectively) on days 4, 8, and 12 during collateral development induced by repetitive LAD occlusions in a representative dog. Coronary occlusion on day 4 causes regional akinesis [0% segment shortening (SS)] and release of LAD occlusion is followed by a dramatic increase in BFV (reactive hyperemia). As coronary collateral blood flow during coronary occlusions increases concomitantly with the progression of collateral development, the intensity of ischemia during coronary artery occlusion is reduced. As a result of decreasing ischemic intensity, reactive hyperemia is decreased. (From ref. 111, with permission.)

coronary artery occlusion in the presence of halothane is less than in the presence of isoflurane. Therefore, reductions in peak flow and percent flow debt repayment following coronary occlusion during halothane versus isoflurane anesthesia may reflect differences in the intensity of ischemia during coronary occlusion, as well as differences in vasodilator efficacy of the anesthetic agents.

The coronary microcirculation responds in a heterogeneous fashion to volatile anesthetics (53). Isoflurane causes greater dilation of small coronary microvessels (diameters less than 100 μm), than either enflurane or halothane. However, adenosine, a potent coronary vasodilator, causes greater vasodilation in microvessels less than 60 μm than does any anesthetic agent. In fact, adenosine increases coronary blood flow four- to fivefold and causes transmural flow redistribution (decreased endo/epi ratio), actions not shared by volatile anesthetic agents (53).

Dilation of arteriolar resistance vessels by volatile anesthetic agents results in alterations of autoregulation in the coronary vasculature (122). The precision of autoregulatory adjustments in coronary blood flow is determined by examining the slope of pressure-flow curves (Fig. 13) generated by variably constricting the left circumflex coronary artery. Pressure autoregulation is disrupted in anesthetized dogs as compared to the conscious state. Isoflurane interferes with autoregulation to a greater extent than does halothane or enflurane as demonstrated by greater increases in the slope of the pressure-flow relation (Fig. 14). In the presence of a volatile anesthetic, there is a greater dependence of coronary flow on coronary artery perfusion pressure. However, coronary vasodilator reserve measured with adenosine is unchanged by the volatile anesthetics. Therefore, volatile anesthetics impair coronary autoregulation, but none of these agents causes the profound degree of coronary vasodilation produced by adenosine or dipyridamole (53,103,121). The latter agents can cause maximal coronary vasodilation and inhibit pressure autoregulation such that coronary flow is directly dependent on arterial pressure.

Volatile anesthetic agents may also alter coronary blood flow through effects on ventricular relaxation. Interestingly, halothane changes the phasic pattern of coronary blood flow (Fig. 15). The overall percentage of coronary flow occurring during systole or diastole is unchanged by halothane, but peak flow during isovolumic relaxation is markedly reduced

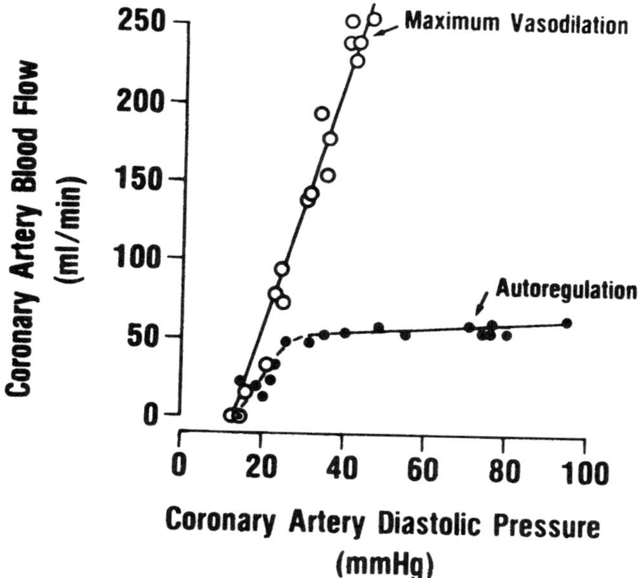

Figure 13. The coronary blood flow–pressure relationship in an awake dog. The *upper line,* labeled "Maximum Vasodilation," is obtained after the circumflex coronary artery perfusion bed is maximally dilated with adenosine. The *lower curve,* labeled "Autoregulation," has a straight horizontal portion *(solid line)* with a curved portion *(broken line)* as flow becomes pressure dependent. Note that, during maximal vasodilation, coronary artery diastolic pressure was reduced so that the maximum flow shown in this illustration was obtained at a lower pressure (50 mm Hg) than the diastolic pressure obtained in the resting state (autoregulation curve). (From ref. 122, with permission.)

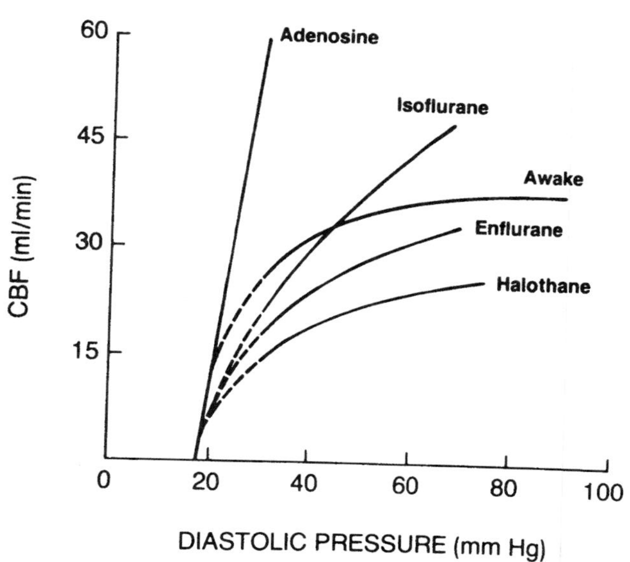

Figure 14. A qualitative description of the effects of volatile anesthetics on the coronary blood flow (CBF)-pressure relationship, and demonstrates the effect of adenosine-induced maximal coronary vasodilation in awake and anesthetized dogs. *Solid lines* are drawn from mean slopes determined by linear regression analysis. *Dashed lines* represent the nonlinear portion of the curve and are estimates. Note that, compared to values determined in awake dogs, the anesthetics affect absolute CBF variably but do tend to increase the slope of the CBF-pressure plots. During maximal coronary vasodilation by intracoronary adenosine, CBF becomes completely pressure dependent (i.e., autoregulation is lost), and CBF is greatly increased over a wide range of pressures. CBF-pressure relationships during maximal coronary vasodilation were not different in awake and anesthetized dogs, so both states are equally well represented by the single adenosine line. (From ref. 122, with permission.)

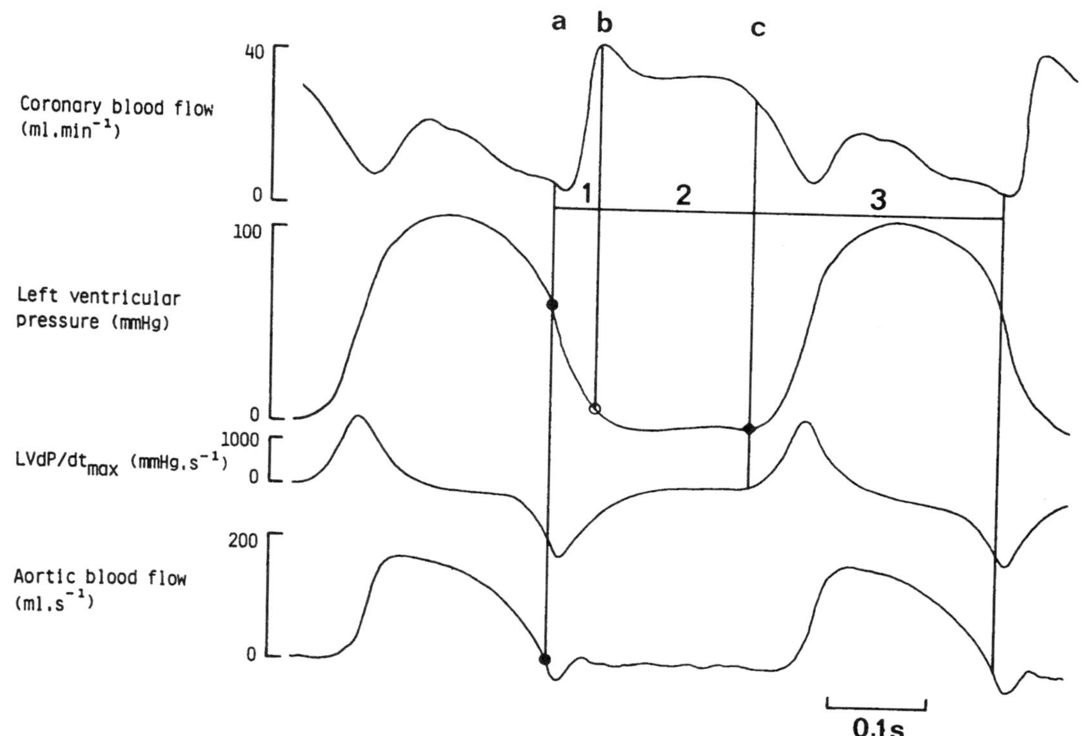

Figure 15. Coronary blood flow during three phases of the cardiac cycle. Isovolumic coronary flow *(1)* occurs after cessation of aortic flow *(a)* until completion of isovolumic relaxation *(b)* (left ventricle pressure 10 mm Hg above end-diastolic pressure). Halothane decreased that fraction of coronary blood flow occurring during isovolumic relaxation *(1)*, but had no effect on flow during diastole *(1 & 2)* or systole *(3)* (onset indicated by upslope of left ventricular dP/dt *[c]*). (From ref. 73, with permission.)

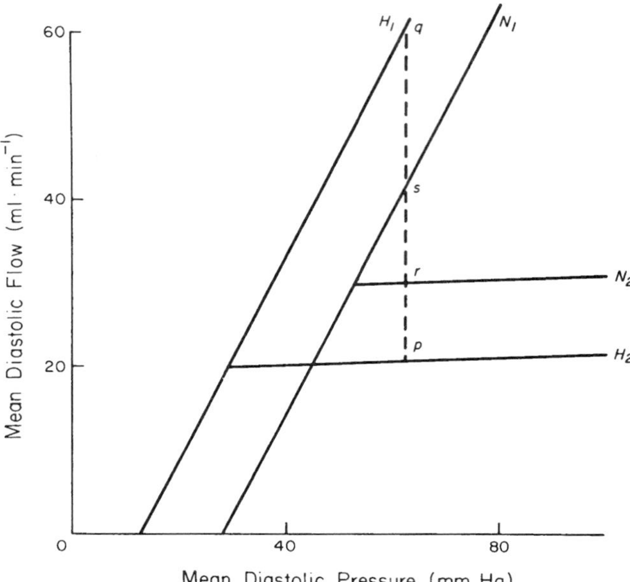

Figure 16. Composite pressure-flow relations in 11 dogs anesthetized with halothane or nitrous oxide. H_1, N_1, pressure-flow relations during maximal vasodilation; H_2, N_2, pressure-flow relations during autoregulation. The slopes of the maximal vasodilation lines are similar (H_1: 5.0 ± 0.03 SEM; N_1:5.2 ± 0.04 SEM) but the pressure-axis intercepts are significantly different (H_1:18.5 ± 1.7 SEM; N_1: 27.5 ± 1.7 SEM). At a perfusion pressure of 60 mmHg, the coronary vascular reserve during halothane anesthesia is represented by $q - p$; the coronary vascular reserve during nitrous oxide anesthesia at the same pressure is represented by $s - r$. (From ref. 287, with permission.)

(73). In addition, isovolumic coronary blood flow is inversely related to the time constant of ventricular relaxation (τ). Halothane causes a dose-dependent increase in τ, reflecting an increased time for relaxation to occur. This negative lusitropic effect of halothane may reduce early diastolic coronary flow by preventing an abrupt decrease in intramyocardial tissue pressure. Zero flow pressure (that pressure at which forward coronary flow ceases) is also decreased by halothane in comparison to nitrous oxide (Fig. 16) (287). Halothane may decrease intramural tissue pressure to a greater extent than nitrous oxide, resulting in higher levels of coronary flow for any given diastolic perfusion pressure. This also suggests that while early diastolic flow is reduced, total coronary flow will continue at lower perfusion pressures in the presence of halothane versus nitrous oxide.

Mechanisms of the Coronary Vasodilator Effects of Anesthetics

The key mechanisms that regulate smooth muscle tone in the coronary and other vascular beds ultimately depend on changes in intracellular calcium concentration (Fig. 17). Increases in intracellular calcium concentration result in phosphorylation of myosin and smooth muscle cell contraction (Fig. 18). Influx of calcium through the cell sarcolemma may be mediated via voltage- or receptor-operated channels, reversed Na^+/Ca^{2+} exchanger, and nonspecific cation channels (30). Depolarization of vascular smooth muscle membranes by high concentrations of extracellular potassium causes an influx of calcium, principally through the sarcolemma. In addition, agonist-induced release of calcium may occur by release of stored calcium from sarcoplasmic reticulum and mitochondria (205). Initiation of calcium release by sarcoplasmic reticulum occurs through activation of phospholipase C by a number of different ligands (30). Phospholipase C catalyzes the hydrolysis of phosphatidylinositol-4,5-biphosphate (261), leading to production of the second messengers inositol-1,4,5-triphosphate (IP_3) and 1,2-diacylglycerol (DAG). IP_3 causes mobilization of intracellular calcium stores from sarcoplasmic reticulum, while DAG production leads to protein kinase C activation (263), phosphorylation of sarcolemmal calcium channels, and subsequent calcium influx.

Calcium removal from the cytosol is accomplished through activation of a calcium pump and forward mode of the Na^+/Ca^{2+} exchanger in the sarcolemma. In addition, calcium is sequestered in the cell via active reuptake into mitochondria and the sarcoplasmic reticulum. Activation of adenylate- and guanylate-cyclase enzymes catalyzes the conversion of ATP and guanosine triphosphate (GTP) to adenosine 3′,5′-cyclic monophosphate (cAMP) and guanosine 3′,5′-cyclic monophosphate (cGMP), respectively (263). Inhibitory phosphorylation of protein kinase C by cAMP and cGMP results in inactivation of sarcolemmal calcium channels and activation of cellular calcium removal systems.

Volatile anesthetics potentially alter intracellular calcium regulation at any of these sites (Fig. 17). These agents may cause direct coronary vasodilation via inhibition of calcium influx through voltage- (37) and receptor-operated (20,27,182, 212,288) calcium channels, reduced calcium accumulation (via opening of ryanodine-sensitive calcium release channels) and decreased release from intracellular stores in sarcoplasmic reticulum (273), inhibition of G proteins linked to phospholipase C (212), and decreased IP_3 formation (254).

The interactions between volatile anesthetic agents and NO are incompletely understood (Figs. 17 and 19). Evidence from some investigations has suggested that the direct coronary vasodilator effects of isoflurane are endothelium dependent (20,96). Alternatively, increases in coronary blood flow during isoflurane anesthesia in vivo may cause a nonspecific flow-mediated release of NO (237), as opposed to the anesthetic agent causing a direct release of NO. Investigations of porcine coronary arteries (306) and of rabbit or rat aorta (31,204,268,273) in vitro, as well as of the canine coronary circulation in vivo (61), demonstrate that coronary vasodilation in response to volatile anesthetics is not dependent on the actions of NO. In fact, evidence in aortic preparations indicates that volatile anesthetics may inhibit either the release (by decreasing calcium entry into the endothelial cell and interfering with a calcium-dependent process), action, or stability of NO (21,31,204,268, 282), and/or may inhibit a cyclooxygenase vasodilator product (268). The findings of investigations in other vascular beds have limited applicability to the coronary circulation, but, nevertheless, such studies provide insight into potential effects of anesthetics on the coronary vasculature.

The actions of NO are mediated through activation of the soluble form of the guanylate cyclase enzyme (200), catalyzing the formation of cGMP (Fig. 17). NO-stimulated formation of cGMP in aortae is attenuated by halothane (108); however, vasodilation in response to nitroprusside or nitroglycerin (mediated by direct activation of soluble guanylate cyclase) is not affected by volatile anesthetics in aortae or mesenteric arteries (204,279,282,312). In fact, halothane increases cGMP concentration (77,206) but does so through activation of the particulate form of the guanylate cyclase enzyme (a form of guanylate cyclase not involved in NO signal transduction) (77). Halothane and isoflurane may decrease cGMP concentration (108,279) via volatile anesthetic-induced inactivation of NO released from aortic endothelial cells (Fig. 19). Pretreatment with superoxide dismutase, an oxygen-derived free radical scavenger, attenuates sevoflurane-induced impairment of endothelium-dependent vasodilation (312). These findings indicate that volatile anesthetic agents reduce the stability of NO (perhaps through anesthetic-induced generation of free radicals), while NO release and its effect on smooth muscle are unmodified (21).

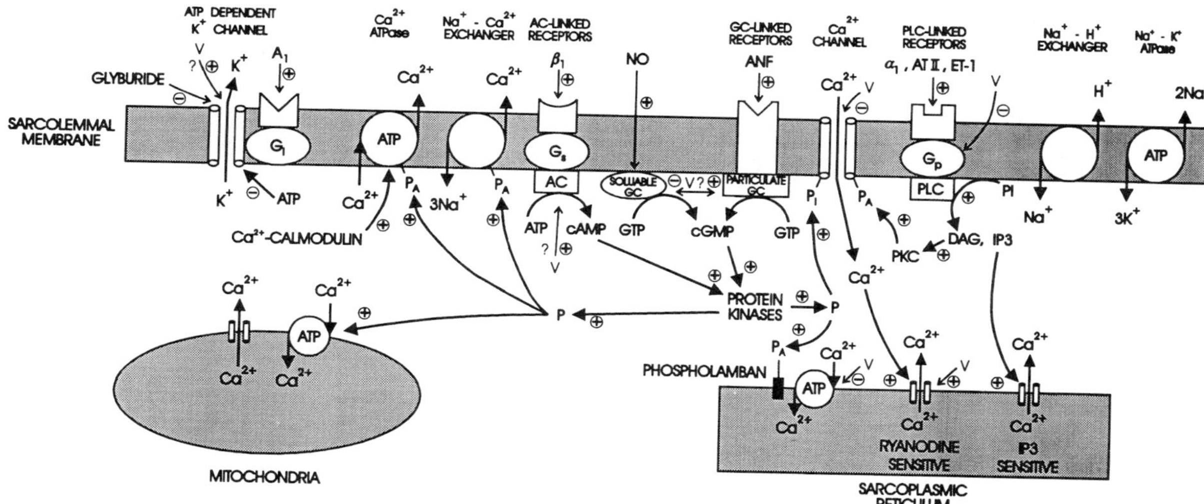

Figure 17. Regulation of calcium (Ca^{2+}) in the vascular smooth muscle cell. Sarcolemmal membrane depolarization allows influx of Ca^{2+} into cytoplasm through voltage-dependent Ca^{2+} channels, providing Ca^{2+} for contractile activation and inducing further release of Ca^{2+} from stores in sarcoplasmic reticulum (ryanodine-sensitive Ca^{2+} channels). This process is modulated by adenylate cyclase (AC), guanylate cyclase (GC), and phospholipase C (PLC)-linked receptors. Protein kinase activation by cAMP and cGMP results in inhibitory phosphorylation (P_I) of voltage-dependent Ca^{2+} channels, and in excitatory phosphorylation (P_A) of the regulatory protein of the sarcoplasmic reticular Ca^{2+} ATPase, phospholamban, mitochondrial and sarcolemmal Ca^{2+} ATPase, and sarcolemmal Na+-Ca^{2+} exchanger. These actions decrease intracellular Ca^{2+} concentration, facilitating smooth muscle cell relaxation. β-receptor activation stimulates AC via a stimulatory G protein (Gs). Soluble GC is activated by nitric oxide (NO) and particulate GC by atrial natriuretic factor (ANF). Stimulation of PLC linked receptors by α_1-agonists, angiotensin II (AT II), and endothelin-1 (ET-1) activates PLC via a G protein (GP), splitting the membrane lipid phosphatidylinositol (PI) into inositol trisphosphate (IP_3) and diacylglycerol (DAG). IP_3 directly stimulates Ca^{2+} release from the sarcoplasmic reticulum, while DAG activates protein kinase C (PKC). PKC subsequently causes excitatory phosphorylation of voltage-sensitive Ca^{2+} channels. These actions increase intracellular Ca^{2+} concentration, leading to smooth muscle cell contraction. Opening of ATP-dependent K^+ channels results in cell hyperpolarization, inhibiting Ca^{2+} influx through voltage-dependent Ca^{2+} channels. Adenosine may activate ATP-dependent K^+ channels via a G protein, while high ATP concentration and glibenclamide (glyburide) inhibit channel opening. Intracellular Ca^{2+} is also regulated by Na^+-H^+ exchangers coupled to Na^+-K^+ ATPase, and by a Ca^{2+}-ATPase (which is stimulated by Ca^{2+} bound to calmodulin) in the sarcolemmal membrane. Volatile (V) anesthetics have excitatory (+) and inhibitory (−) effects on several intracellular Ca^{2+} regulatory mechanisms. Other possible (?) sites of volatile anesthetic effects are indicated.

Volatile anesthetics may cause vascular smooth muscle relaxation via increases in cAMP concentration (264). However, halothane and isoflurane attenuate calcium mobilization in vascular smooth muscle cells independent of changes in the concentration of cAMP (212). Finally, volatile anesthetics may interact with ATP-dependent potassium channels to cause coronary vascular smooth muscle relaxation. Increases in coronary blood flow in response to halothane and isoflurane are attenuated by the ATP-dependent potassium channel antagonist glibenclamide (44,162), suggesting that volatile anesthetics cause vasodilation of coronary resistance vessels at least in part via stimulation of ATP-dependent potassium channels.

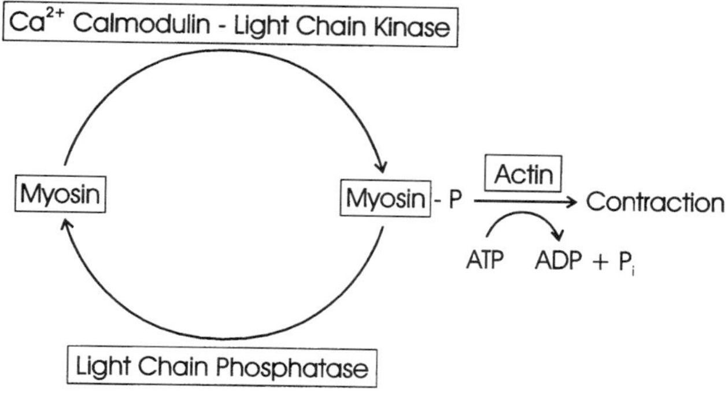

Figure 18. Cross-bridge formation between phosphorylated myosin (myosin-P) and actin filaments, an energy-dependent process, results in smooth muscle cell contraction. Myosin phosphorylation is regulated by calcium and calmodulin via activation of light chain kinase, while dephosphorylation occurs through the action of light chain phosphatase.

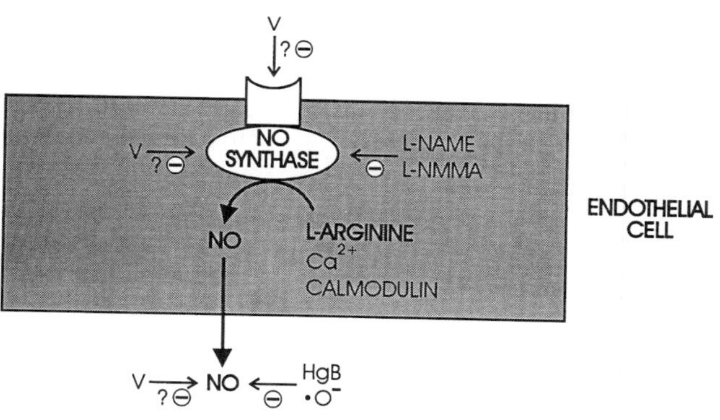

Figure 19. Nitric oxide (NO) is synthesized by NO synthase from L-arginine in the presence of Ca^{2+} and calmodulin, a process that is inhibited by L-NAME and L-NMMA. Volatile anesthetics (V) may potentially (?) act to inhibit either the production or the stability of NO, which is bound by hemoglobin (Hgb) and deactivated by oxygen-derived free radicals ($\cdot O_2^-$).

Effects of Volatile Anesthetics on Ischemic Myocardium

Volatile anesthetics produce mild direct coronary vasodilator actions in vitro by mechanisms that are as yet incompletely elucidated. The effects of these agents on myocardial perfusion in the presence of experimentally produced total coronary artery occlusion and coronary arterial stenosis have been investigated to determine whether volatile anesthetics cause a deleterious effect on myocardial perfusion. A coronary artery stenosis may be gradually produced by implanting an ameroid constrictor around an epicardial coronary artery that constricts over weeks (longer time intervals are associated with growth of collateral vessels and production of total coronary artery occlusion). Alternatively, an acute stenosis may be formed by partially constricting a coronary artery with a ligature. Models of multivessel coronary artery disease in which one coronary artery is totally occluded while an adjacent coronary artery has a severe stenosis have also been used to study the actions of volatile anesthetic agents on perfusion of collateral-dependent regions. These areas with already depleted flow reserve of different degrees may be especially sensitive to alterations in systemic and coronary hemodynamics produced by anesthetics.

Volatile anesthetics decrease subendocardial blood flow and produce regional myocardial contractile dysfunction in the presence of a coronary stenosis if coronary perfusion pressure is allowed to decrease (123,172,226). Regional ischemia in myocardium distal to a coronary artery stenosis during halothane-induced hypotension, for example, is indicated by reduced myocardial segment shortening, paradoxical systolic lengthening, and postsystolic shortening (172) (Fig. 20); decreases in subendocardial blood flow and myocardial lactate extraction; and the appearance of electrocardiographic changes (123). Isoflurane similarly reduces segment shortening and causes systolic bulging of myocardium distal to a critical coronary artery stenosis if hypotension is allowed to occur (226). During substitution of isoflurane for halothane, an increase in contractile function in the normal zone and a decrease in function in myocardium distal to the stenosis is observed, coincident with higher flows in the normal zone and lower flows in the ischemic zone (225).

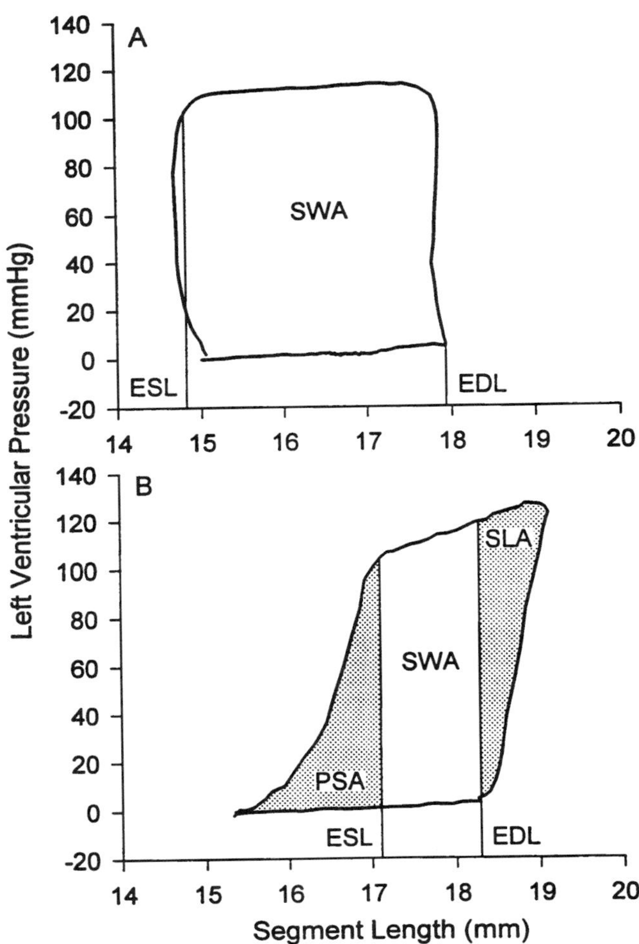

Figure 20. Left ventricular pressure-segment length loops illustrate the segmental stroke work performed during a cardiac cycle under control conditions **(A)** and during ischemia following coronary artery occlusion and reperfusion **(B)**. Stroke work is represented by the loop area (SWA) between end-diastolic (EDL) and end-systolic (ESL) segment length. During ischemia, postsystolic shortening area (PSA) and systolic lengthening area (SLA) make no contribution to ejection, and represent pure elastic recoil and work done on the ischemic segment by normal myocardium, respectively.

In contrast, adverse effects of volatile anesthetic agents on ischemic myocardium are avoided when coronary artery perfusion pressure is prevented from falling. For example, subendocardial blood flow in the perfusion territory of a critically stenosed coronary artery is reduced during hypotension produced by isoflurane, but treatment with phenylephrine to prevent a decrease in mean arterial pressure restores subendocardial blood flow to levels not different from those observed in the absence of isoflurane (276,304). The transmural distribution of coronary blood flow between subendocardium and subepicardium (endo/epi) decreases during isoflurane anesthesia with or without control of arterial pressure. However, administration of phenylephrine to raise arterial pressure increases subepicardial blood flow more than subendocardial flow. This increase in subepicardial perfusion accounts for the decreased endo/epi without the presence of transmural steal (i.e., an absolute decrease in subendocardial flow). Additionally, when mean arterial pressure is controlled at baseline levels during isoflurane anesthesia, coronary collateral blood flow increases and tissue PO_2 is normalized (54).

Buffington et al. (36) examined the effects of halothane and isoflurane on the regional distribution of coronary blood flow and contractile function in dogs 3 to 5 weeks following implantation of an ameriod constrictor to produce total left anterior descending coronary artery occlusion and enhanced collateral development. No redistribution of coronary blood flow occurred between collaterally perfused and normal myocardium, nor between subendocardium and subepicardium occurred when normal coronary blood flow was maintained during isoflurane anesthesia. When the left circumflex coronary artery was perfused at reduced flow levels to cause ischemia, both isoflurane and adenosine, but not halothane or nitrous oxide, reduced coronary collateral flow. In this model, any vasodilator reserve in the left anterior descending and left circumflex perfusion territories had already been depleted by reducing coronary flow. Thus, it is not unexpected that a further decrease in collateral perfusion pressure could produce a redistribution of collateral flow away from the totally occluded region. Other investigations conducted in dogs with a steal-prone coronary artery anatomy have repeatedly shown that isoflurane or halothane produce no change in collateral-dependent or ischemic zone myocardial blood flow (45,109–112), endo/epi flow distribution (45,109), or electrocardiogram (45) when diastolic arterial pressure is held constant by tightening an aortic snare. No change in coronary collateral perfusion is observed in dogs anesthetized with either halothane or isoflurane at a mean arterial pressure of 50 mm Hg (201). In a chronically instrumented canine model of coronary artery disease neither isoflurane (110,111), halothane (112), desflurane (113), nor sevoflurane (146) produces coronary steal. These results are independent of coronary stenosis severity (110–112)

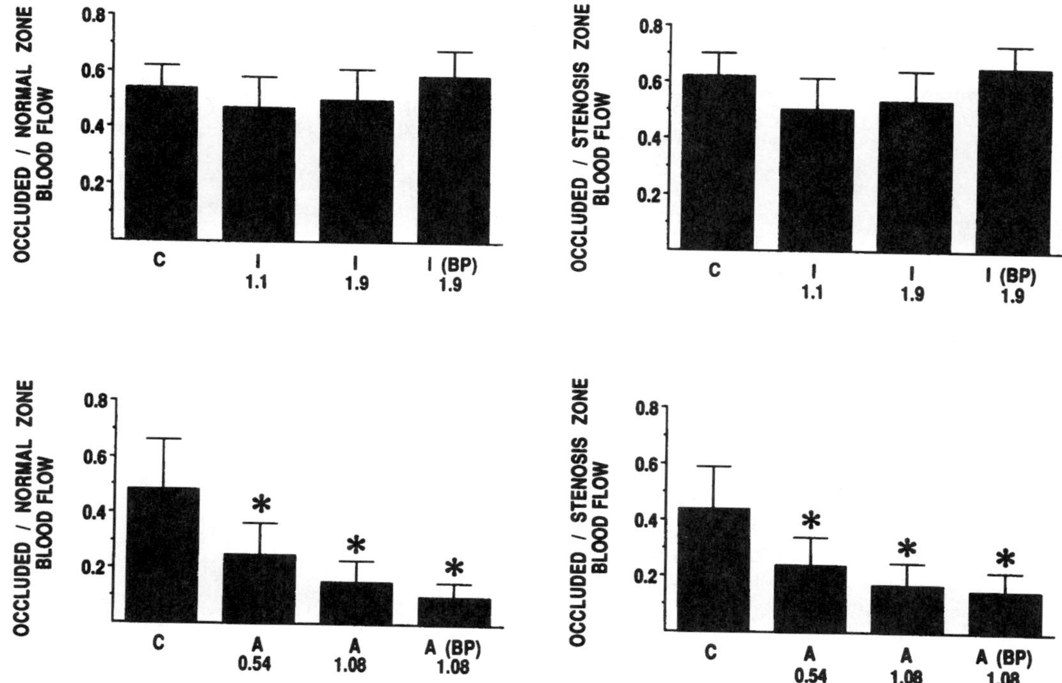

Figure 21. Occluded to normal and occluded to stenotic zone myocardial blood flow in dogs with steal-prone coronary artery anatomy during the conscious control state (C), isoflurane anesthesia (I) at 1.1% or 1.9% end-tidal concentration, or adenosine infusion (A) at 0.54 or 1.08 mg · min^{-1}, and during maintenance of blood pressure and heart rate at conscious values during the highest doses (BP). Isoflurane does not cause coronary steal, in contrast to significant (*p<.05) reductions in blood flow to collateral-dependent myocardium produced by adenosine. (From ref. 111, with permission.)

or degree of coronary collateral development (109). These findings are in stark contrast to those results obtained during an infusion of adenosine (46). Adenosine causes marked coronary steal, demonstrated by decreases in occluded to normal zone and occluded to stenotic zone blood flow when arterial pressure is maintained at control levels in a model of multivessel coronary artery disease (110,111) (Fig. 21).

The controversy about coronary vasodilation and steal overlooks an important fact. Volatile anesthetics actually have beneficial effects on ischemic myocardium. Halothane reduces ST segment elevation produced by brief coronary artery occlusion (23,91) and does so to a greater extent than does the combination of nitroprusside and propranolol, despite production of similar systemic hemodynamic changes to halothane (91). Myocardial infarct size following ligation of the left anterior descending coronary artery is reduced in dogs anesthetized with either isoflurane (64) or halothane (63), and enflurane decreases lactate production in comparison to pentobarbital in the presence of an 80% stenosis of the left descending coronary artery (283). Volatile anesthetics decrease myocardial reperfusion injury following global myocardial ischemia (38,52,85,183) and enhance functional recovery of stunned myocardium following coronary artery occlusion and reperfusion in chronically instrumented dogs (140,290). Reductions in MVO_2 produced by volatile anesthetic agents account for only a small portion of this beneficial effect.

Volatile anesthetics may produce beneficial effects on flow to ischemic myocardium. Decreases in collateral blood flow following coronary artery occlusion during halothane anesthesia are less than those decreases in flow to normal myocardium, and the ratio of myocardial oxygen delivery to oxygen consumption is increased in collateral-dependent as compared to normal myocardium (258). In a multivessel coronary artery disease model, flow to collateral-dependent myocardium is not reduced by sevoflurane but, in fact, is increased to nearly twice that observed during the conscious state, provided arterial pressure is prevented from decreasing (146) (Fig. 22). In addition, halothane may inhibit platelet thrombi formation via increases in platelet cAMP concentration and thus decrease cyclical variations in coronary flow (19). Cyclic coronary flow reductions arise in stenosed coronary arteries as occlusive platelet thrombi form, slowly decreasing flow, and break apart, suddenly increasing flow. Halothane reduces spontaneous and epinephrine-induced coronary cyclic flow reductions in dogs anesthetized with thiamylal (19).

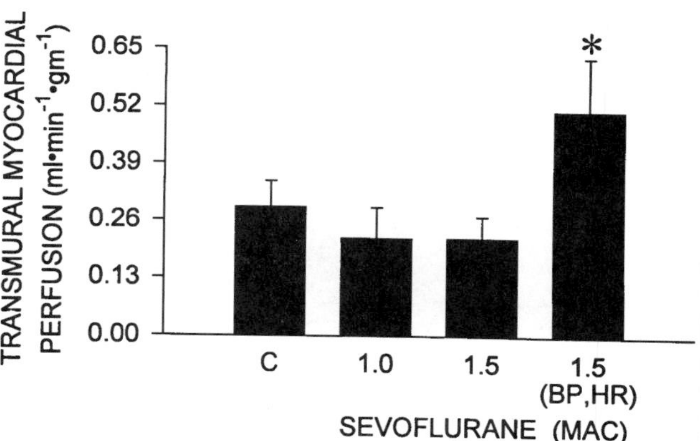

Figure 22. Transmural myocardial blood flow to collateral-dependent myocardium during conscious control (C), sevoflurane anesthesia (S) at two concentrations, and during maintenance of blood pressure and heart rate at conscious values during high-dose sevoflurane (BP). Collateral blood flow is significantly (*p<.05) increased by sevoflurane during maintenance of arterial pressure at conscious values.

The mechanisms by which volatile anesthetics exert antiischemic actions have not been elucidated but may include reductions in MVO_2, alterations in intracellular calcium metabolism, opening of ATP-dependent potassium channels, and/or enhanced collateral blood flow in relation to regional oxygen demand. The potential mechanisms by which volatile anesthetic agents may protect ischemic myocardium represent important areas for future investigation.

In summary, volatile anesthetics produce effects on the coronary circulation that are the sum of their direct and indirect actions. Potent inhalational agents are direct negative inotropes and decrease aortic blood pressure secondary to reductions in cardiac output and peripheral vascular resistance. Volatile anesthetics also depress the SA node and cardiac conduction tissue, and may cause an overall decrease in heart rate unless baroreflex-mediated tachycardia occurs simultaneously with decreases in arterial pressure. Volatile anesthetic-induced reductions in myocardial contractility, left ventricular afterload, and heart rate contribute to reductions in myocardial oxygen consumption and lead to concomitant increases in coronary vascular resistance via metabolic coronary autoregulation. Such actions in normal myocardium resulting in arteriolar vasoconstriction might actually divert flow to collateral dependent regions or areas distal to a stenosis via a "reverse steal phenomenon." Reverse coronary steal has been previously reported following administration of β-adrenergic antagonists (99). Volatile anesthetics also cause mild direct coronary vasodilation. These agents can decrease subendocardial blood flow and produce regional contractile dysfunction in the presence of a severe coronary artery stenosis if coronary perfusion pressure is allowed to decrease. Similarly, redistribution of coronary collateral blood flow away from ischemic myocardium can occur if coronary collateral perfusion pressure is reduced. Therefore, in the presence of severe coronary artery stenoses or during total coronary artery occlusion with distal collateralization, maintenance of normal arterial diastolic pressure is critical. Finally, volatile anesthetics have been shown in animals to produce favorable effects on ischemic myocardium via mechanisms that are as yet undefined. The coronary circulatory actions of volatile anesthetics in humans may be expected to result from multiple alterations in systemic hemodynamics, direct and indirect effects on coronary vascular tone, and ultimately regulation of intracellular ion concentrations.

Coronary Circulatory Effects of Volatile Anesthetics in Humans

Study of the effects of volatile anesthetics on the human coronary circulation is complicated by several methodologic barriers that pose difficulties in obtaining meaningful information. Sophisticated methods for obtaining precise measurements of myocardial perfusion in animals are available, but measurement of coronary blood flow in humans is crude by comparison. One of the more widely used techniques for measurement of coronary blood flow in clinical studies is the coronary sinus thermodilution method. This technique requires catheterization of the coronary sinus and great cardiac vein to obtain regional left ventricular flow measurements (90). Marcus et al. (181) suggest that only large changes (greater than 30%) in great cardiac vein flow are qualitatively accurate because of catheter movement in vivo, abnormal variations of venous drainage in the presence of coronary artery disease, and the lack of convincing clinical validation studies. Gas clearance methods for measuring myocardial perfusion suffer similar limitations. Coronary sinus sampling may be inaccurate in patients with coronary artery disease due to inhomogeneous left ventricular myocardial perfusion during ischemia or following myocardial infarction. Venous drainage from normally and abnormally perfused areas are mixed at the level of the coronary sinus. Sampling from specific veins draining ischemic zones is nearly impossible. Additionally, rapid changes in myocardial blood flow are undetectable. Not only are the methods used to determine coronary blood flow in humans limited, but the interpretation of clinical findings during anesthesia are complicated by concomitant changes in hemodynamics, the impact of surgery, and the use of adjuvant drugs and vasoactive agents.

Halothane decreases MVO_2 (124,231) and variably alters coronary blood flow in patients with coronary artery disease, producing no metabolic or electrocardiographic evidence of ischemia (124,149,231,244). Overall coronary blood flow may be reduced in some patients by both halothane and enflurane (194) because of decreases in oxygen demand, but concomitant decreases in myocardial oxygen extraction (194,231) reflect relative coronary vasodilation.

In 1983 Reiz et al. (232) reported the occurrence of ischemia in 10 of 21 patients anesthetized with isoflurane for major vascular surgery. Fifty percent of these patients were treated with phenylephrine and pacing to return arterial pressure and heart rate to control values. Following this intervention, 40% of patients demonstrated normalization of electrocardiographic evidence of ischemia and abnormal myocardial lactate extraction. It was proposed that isoflurane had produced coronary artery steal in these patients, despite the lack of objective evidence of blood flow redistribution between collateral-dependent and normal zones. Isoflurane causes no change in coronary blood flow in patients undergoing coronary artery bypass graft surgery; however, coronary sinus oxygen content increases (193,210,243), reflecting relative coronary vasodilation. Isoflurane produces either no electrocardiographic or metabolic evidence of ischemia (210), or if ischemia does occur during isoflurane anesthesia, it is associated with hypotension and tachycardia (149,193,233,243). Comparisons of anesthetic agents with respect to the occurrence of ischemia are also complicated by differences in patient age, operative time, and preoperative ejection fraction (67,132). Convincing evidence demonstrating redistribution of coronary blood flow away from ischemic to normal myocardium in anesthetized humans is decidedly lacking.

The reported incidence of intraoperative myocardial ischemia varies considerably among studies. It is of interest, however, that less than 50% of intraoperative ischemic events are correlated with a hemodynamic abnormality (154,227, 256,281) (Table 1). The strongest predictor of intraoperative

Table 1. INTRAOPERATIVE ISCHEMIA DURING CORONARY ARTERY BYPASS GRAFT SURGERY

	Pulley et al. (227) 1991	Slogoff and Keats (256) 1989	Tuman et al. (281) 1989	Knight et al. (154) 1988
No. of patients	40	1012	1094	50
Incidence of intraoperative ischemia (%)	37	30.6	22.1	18
Ischemia unrelated to hemodynamic abnormality (%)	44.4	33.5	—	42
Preoperative ischemia predictive of intraoperative ischemia	—	Yes (p <.0001)	—	Yes (p <.05)
Anesthetic agent predictive of intraoperative ischemia or outcome	—	No	No	—

ischemia appears to be preexisting ischemia on arrival to the operating room (154,256). The only hemodynamic event definitively related to intraoperative ischemia in a randomized trial of over 1,000 patients undergoing coronary artery bypass graft surgery is tachycardia (256). Sternotomy during morphine anesthesia causes greater increases in rate pressure product (301), hypertension requiring treatment with nitroprusside (195), and myocardial lactate production (195) than during halothane anesthesia. Induction of anesthesia with desflurane in patients undergoing coronary artery bypass graft surgery may be accompanied by tachycardia, hypertension, and a higher incidence of ischemia than that occurring during induction with sufentanil (117). Patients with a steal prone coronary anatomy do not have a greater incidence of ischemia during desflurane anesthesia as compared to other forms of coronary artery disease (117). Multivariate analysis of outcome in patients anesthetized with either volatile anesthetics, opioids, or intravenous agents for coronary artery bypass graft surgery reveals that two important predictors of poor outcome in these patients are prolonged aortic cross-clamp time and the presence of a recent myocardial infarction (281). Electrocardiographic changes, postoperative myocardial infarction, and mortality are similar in patients undergoing coronary artery bypass graft surgery, independent of volatile or opioid anesthetic agent used (115,117,167,195,227,256,257,281,301), or of the presence of a steal prone coronary artery anatomy (257), which is estimated to be present in approximately 25% of patients with coronary artery disease (35).

Interestingly, isoflurane improves the tolerance to pacing-induced ischemia in patients with coronary artery disease (275). Significantly higher heart rates are required to cause ischemia during isoflurane anesthesia than in awake patients, and the severity of ischemia (as assessed by ST segment depression and elevations in pulmonary capillary wedge pressure) is less in the presence of isoflurane. Despite findings that volatile anesthetics are mild coronary vasodilators, these agents appear to produce no deleterious redistribution of myocardial perfusion when a reduction in coronary artery perfusion pressure and tachycardia are avoided.

Nitrous Oxide

Nitrous oxide produces few if any direct effects on the coronary vasculature in vitro (130,271,272). In vivo, nitrous oxide alters coronary blood flow concomitant with directionally similar changes in MVO_2 (71,302). In the presence of experimentally produced reductions in coronary blood flow, nitrous oxide decreases myocardial segment shortening (43,209), increases postsystolic shortening (222), and redistributes transmural coronary blood flow preferentially to the subepicardium (decreased endo/epi) (209). This agent also decreases the recovery of contractile function of stunned myocardium in dogs (252). These adverse effects occur in part because of nitrous oxide–induced alterations in systemic hemodynamics (208). In patients with coronary artery disease, nitrous oxide in the presence of a volatile anesthetic agent decreases MVO_2 and myocardial oxygen extraction (196, 241), and may exacerbate myocardial ischemia if hypotension occurs (229). More recent investigations demonstrate no difference in the incidence of wall motion abnormalities as detected by transesophageal echocardiography or electrocardiographic indicators of ischemia in patients who do or do not receive nitrous oxide (158,241).

Intravenous Anesthetic Agents

The coronary circulatory effects of intravenously administered anesthetic agents are not as well characterized as those of the volatile agents. These drugs generally lack appreciable effects on the coronary vasculature. Opioids are devoid of coronary vasodilator effects in vitro (22,125) except when used in high concentrations (309). Fentanyl, in large doses, decreases MVO_2 (262) and causes relative coronary vasodilaton as indicated by increases in coronary sinus oxygen content in patients with coronary artery disease (192). Thiopental, propofol, ketamine, etomidate, and midazolam cause mild coronary vasodilation in vitro (57,269), demonstrated by decreases in oxygen extraction and increases in DO_2/MVO_2 (269). However, only very high concentrations of propofol increase coronary blood flow in vivo (133). Intravenously administered agents decrease coronary blood flow concomitant with reductions in MVO_2 in patients with coronary artery disease (185,230,267). Thallium perfusion scans performed preoperatively and following tracheal intubation in patients anesthetized with either thiopental, fentanyl, or halothane, demonstrate new perfusion defects in 45% of patients, independent of the anesthetic agent used (151).

CONCLUSIONS

Volatile anesthetics cause mild coronary vasodilation in vitro. In vivo, these agents produce effects on the coronary circulation that are the sum of their direct actions on coronary vascular smooth muscle and their indirect actions to reduce myocardial oxygen demand. The mechanisms by which volatile anesthetics alter coronary vascular smooth muscle tone are incompletely understood, but intracellular calcium regulation is likely involved. Volatile anesthetics may also alter vascular smooth muscle tone via effects on NO, cGMP, cAMP, IP_3, DAG second messenger systems, and ATP-dependent potassium channels.

In animals, volatile anesthetics impair coronary autoregulation and cause decreases in subendocardial myocardial perfusion under conditions in which coronary artery perfusion pressure is allowed to decrease. Maldistribution of perfusion between normal and collateral-dependent myocardium is avoided by maintaining arterial pressure at levels present prior to administration of anesthesia. These findings are in stark contrast to those produced by the highly efficacious coronary vasodilators adenosine, chromonar, and dipyridamole, which cause coronary steal. Volatile anesthetic agents cause only mild direct coronary artery vasodilating effects, which are counterbalanced by decreases in MVO_2 and metabolically mediated coronary vasoconstriction. In patients with coronary artery disease, no differences in outcome among anesthetic agents (volatile, intravenous, or nitrous oxide) are detected when hemodynamics are appropriately controlled. In fact, recent evidence suggests that the preoperative pattern of ischemia may be the most important predictor of intraoperative ischemia.

The potential beneficial effects of volatile anesthetics on ischemic myocardium, including actions mediated by ATP-dependent K^+ channels, represent an area for future investigation. In addition, the actions of anesthetics on the coronary vasculature in patients with altered coronary blood flow regulation secondary to ventricular dysfunction, ventricular hypertrophy, or diabetes are unknown. Investigation of the mechanisms of action of anesthetic agents and interactions with important physiologic regulators that are altered by these disease states should ultimately lead to a more complete understanding of the coronary circulatory effects of anesthetic agents.

REFERENCES

1. Adam KR, Boyles S, Scholfield PC. Cardio-selective beta-adrenoceptor blockade and the coronary circulation. *Br J Pharmacol* 1970;40:534–536.
2. Al-Wathiqui MH, Hartman JC, Brooks HL, Gross GJ, Warltier DC. Cyclical carotid artery flow reduction in conscious dogs: effect of a new thromboxane receptor antagonist. *Am Heart J* 1988;116:1482–1487.

3. Al-Wathiqui MH, Hartman JC, Brooks HL, Warltier DC. Induction of cyclic flow reduction in the coronary, carotid and femoral arteries of conscious, chronically instrumented dogs: a model for investigating the role of platelets in severely constricted arteries. *J Pharmacol Methods* 1988;20:85–92.
4. Alpert JS. Coronary vasomotion, coronary thrombosis, myocardial infarction and the camel's back. *J Am Coll Cardiol* 1985;5:617–618.
5. Amory DW, Steffenson JL, Forsyth RP. Systemic and regional blood flow changes during halothane anesthesia in the Rhesus monkey. *Anesthesiology* 1971;35:81–90.
6. Archie JP Jr. Transmural distribution of intrinsic and transmitted left ventricular diastolic intramyocardial pressure in dogs. *Cardiovasc Res* 1978;12:255–262.
7. Auchampach JA, Maruyama M, Cavero I, Gross GJ. The new K^+ channel opener Aprikalim (RP 52891) reduces experimental infarct size in dogs in the absence of hemodynamic changes. *J Pharmacol Exp Ther* 1991;259:961–967.
8. Auchampach JA, Maruyama M, Cavero I, Gross GJ. Pharmacological evidence for a role of ATP-regulated potassium channels in myocardial stunning. *Circulation* 1992;86:311–319.
9. Aversano T, Becker LC. Persistence of coronary vasodilator reserve despite functionally significant flow reduction. *Am J Physiol* 1985;248:H403–H411.
10. Aversano T, Ouyang P, Silverman H. Blockade of the ATP-sensitive potassium channel modulates reactive hyperemia in the canine coronary circulation. *Circ Res* 1991;69:618–622.
11. Banai S, Jaklitsch MT, Shou DF, et al. Angiogenic-induced enhancement of collateral blood flow to ischemic myocardium by vascular endothelial growth factor in dogs. *Circulation* 1994; 83–2189.
12. Barger AC, Beeuwkes R III, Lainey LL, Silverman KJ. Hypothesis: vasa vasorum and neovascularization of human coronary arteries. A possible role in the pathophysiology of atherosclerosis. *N Engl J Med* 1984;310:175–177.
13. Becker LC. Conditions for vasodilator-induced coronary steal in experimental myocardial ischemia. *Circulation* 57:1103–1110.
14. Bell JR, Fox AC. Pathogenesis of subendocardial ischemia. *Am J Med Sci* 1974;268:3–13.
15. Bellamy RF. Diastolic coronary pressure-flow relations in the dog. *Circ Res* 1978;43:92–101.
16. Bernard JM, Wouters PF, Doursout MF, et al. Effects of sevoflurane and isoflurane on cardiac and coronary dynamics in chronically instrumented dogs. *Anesthesiology* 1990;72:659–662.
17. Berne RM, Rubio R. Coronary circulation. In: Berne RM, Sperelakas N, Geiger SR, eds. *Handbook of physiology, Section 2:* The cardiovascular system, *vol. 1. The heart.* Bethesda: American Physiological Society, 1979;897.
18. Bernotat-Danielowski S, Sharma HS, Schott RJ, Schaper W. Generation and localisation of monoclonal antibodies against fibroblast growth factors in ischaemic collateralised porcine myocardium. *Cardiovasc Res* 1993;27:1220–1228.
19. Bertha BG, Folts JD, Nugent M, Rusy BF. Halothane, but not isoflurane or enflurane, protects against spontaneous and epinephrine-exacerbated acute thrombus formation in stenosed dog coronary arteries. *Anesthesiology* 1971;71:96–102.
20. Blaise G, Sill JC, Nugent M, Van Dyke RA, Vanhoutte PM. Isoflurane causes endothelium-dependent inhibition of contractile responses of canine coronary arteries. *Anesthesiology* 1987;67: 513–517.
21. Blaise G, To Q, Parent M, et al. Does halothane interfere with the release, action, or stability of endothelium-derived relaxing factor/nitric oxide? *Anesthesiology* 1994;80:417–426.
22. Blaise GA, Witzeling TM, Sill JC, et al. Fentanyl is devoid of major effects on coronary vasoreactivity and myocardial metabolism in experimental animals. *Anesthesiology* 1990;72:535–541.
23. Bland JHL, Chir B, Lowenstein E. Halothane-induced decrease in experimental myocardial ischemia in the non-failing canine heart. *Anesthesiology* 1976;45:287–293.
24. Boatwright RB, Downey HF, Bashour FA, Crystal GJ. Transmural variation in autoregulation of coronary blood flow in hyperperfused canine myocardium. *Circ Res* 1980;47:599–609.
25. Boban M, Stowe DF, Buljubasic N, et al. Direct comparative effects of isoflurane and desflurane in isolated guinea pig hearts. *Anesthesiology* 1992;76:775–780.
26. Bollen BA, McKlveen RE, Stevenson JA. Halothane relaxes preconstricted small and medium isolated porcine coronary artery segments more than isoflurane. *Anesth Analg* 1992;75:9–17.
27. Bollen BA, McKlveen RE, Stevenson JA. Halothane relaxes previously constricted human epicardial coronary artery segments more than isoflurane. *Anesth Analg* 1992;75:4–8.
28. Bollen BA, Tinker JH, Hermsmeyer K. Halothane relaxes previously constricted isolated porcine coronary artery segments more than isoflurane. *Anesthesiology* 1987;66:748–752.
29. Bortone AS, Hess OM, Eberli FR, et al. Abnormal coronary vasomotion during exercise in patients with normal coronary arteries and reduced coronary flow reserve. *Circulation* 1989;79:516–527.
30. Bosnjak ZJ. Ion channels in vascular smooth muscle. Physiology and pharmacology. *Anesthesiology* 1993;79:1392–1401.
31. Brendel JK, Johns RA. Isoflurane does not vasodilate rat thoracic aortic rings by endothelium-derived relaxing factor or other cyclic GMP-mediated mechanisms. *Anesthesiology* 1992;77:126–131.
32. Brett CM, Teitel DF, Heymann MA, Rudolph AM. The cardiovascular effects of isoflurane in lambs. *Anesthesiology* 1987;67:60–65.
33. Buck JD, Hardman HF, Warltier DC, Gross GJ. Changes in ischemic blood flow distribution and dynamic severity of a coronary stenosis induced by beta blockade in the canine heart. *Circulation* 1981;64:708–715.
34. Buckberg GD, Fixler DE, Archie JP, Hoffman JI. Experimental subendocardial ischemia in dogs with normal coronary arteries. *Circ Res* 1972;30:67–81.
35. Buffington CW, Davis KB, Gillispie S, Pettinger M. The prevalence of steal-prone coronary anatomy in patients with coronary artery disease: an analysis of the Coronary Artery Surgery Study Registry. *Anesthesiology* 1988;69:721–727.
36. Buffington CW, Romson JL, Levine A, et al. Isoflurane induces coronary steal in a canine model of chronic coronary occlusion. *Anesthesiology* 1987;66:280–292.
37. Buljubasic N, Rusch NJ, Marijic J, et al. Effects of halothane and isoflurane on calcium and potassium channel currents in canine coronary arterial cells. *Anesthesiology* 1992;76:990–998.
38. Buljubasic N, Stowe DF, Marijic J, et al. Halothane reduces release of adenosine, inosine, and lactate with ischemia and reperfusion in isolated hearts. *Anesth Analg* 1993;76:54–62.
39. Cannon RO, Bonow RO, Bacharach SL, et al. Left ventricular dysfunction in patients with angina pectoris, normal epicardial coronary arteries, and abnormal vasodilator reserve. *Circulation* 1985; 71:218–226.
40. Cannon RO, Schenke WH, Quyyumi A, et al. Comparison of exercise testing with studies of coronary flow reserve in patients with microvascular angina. *Circulation* 1991;83(5 suppl.):III77–81.
41. Canty JM Jr, Klocke FJ. Reduced regional myocardial perfusion in the presence of pharmacologic vasodilator reserve. *Circulation* 1985;71:370–377.
42. Carrier GO, White RE. Enhancement of alpha-1 and alpha-2 adrenergic agonist-induced vasoconstriction by removal of endothelium in rat aorta. *J Pharmacol Exp Ther* 1985;232:682–687.
43. Cason BA, Demas KA, Mazer CD, et al. Effects of nitrous oxide on coronary pressure and regional contractile function in experimental myocardial ischemia. *Anesth Analg* 1991;72:604–611.
44. Cason BA, Shubayev I, Hickey RF. Blockade of adenosine triphosphate-sensitive potassium channels eliminates isoflurane-induced coronary artery vasodilation. *Anesthesiology* 1994;81:1245–1255.
45. Cason BA, Verrier ED, London MJ, et al. Effects of isoflurane and halothane on coronary vascular resistance and collateral myocardial blood flow: their capacity to induce coronary steal. *Anesthesiology* 1987;67:665–675.
46. Cheng DCH, Moyers JR, Knutson RM, et al. Dose-response relationship of isoflurane and halothane versus coronary perfusion pressures. Effects on flow redistribution in a collateralized chronic swine model. *Anesthesiology* 1992;76:113–122.
47. Chilian WM. Adrenergic vasomotion in the coronary microcirculation. *Basic Res Cardiol* 1990;85(suppl.1):111–120.
48. Chilian WM. Functional distribution of alpha-1 and alpha-2 adrenergic receptors in the coronary microcirculation. *Circulation* 1991; 84:2108–2122.
49. Chilian WM, Eastham CL, Marcus ML. Microvascular distribution of coronary vascular resistance in beating left ventricle. *Am J Physiol* 1986;251:H779–H788.
50. Chilian WM, Layne SM, Eastham CL, Marcus ML. Heterogeneous microvascular coronary alpha-adrenergic vasoconstriction. *Circ Res* 1989;64:376–388.
51. Cocks TM, Angus JA. Endothelium-dependent relaxation of coronary arteries by noradrenaline and serotonin. *Nature* 1983;305: 627–630.

52. Coetzee A, Brits W, Genade S, Lochner A. Halothane does have protective properties in the isolated ischemic rat heart. *Anesth Analg* 1991;73:711–719.
53. Conzen PF, Habazettl H, Vollmar B, et al. Coronary microcirculation during halothane, enflurane, isoflurane, and adenosine in dogs. *Anesthesiology* 1992;76:261–270.
54. Conzen PF, Hobbhahn J, Goetz AE, et al. Regional blood flow and tissue oxygen pressures of the collateral-dependent myocardium during isoflurane anesthesia in dogs. *Anesthesiology* 1989;70: 442–452.
55. Conzen PF, Hobbhahn J, Goetz AE, et al. Myocardial contractility, blood flow, and oxygen consumption in healthy dogs during anesthesia with isoflurane or enflurane. *J Cardiothorac Anesth* 1989; 3:70–77.
56. Conzen PF, Vollmar B, Habazettl H, et al. Systemic and regional hemodynamics of isoflurane and sevoflurane in rats. *Anesth Analg* 1992;74:79–88.
57. Coughlan MG, Flynn NM, Kenny D, et al. Differential relaxant effects of high concentrations of intravenous anesthetics on endothelin-constricted proximal and distal canine coronary arteries. *Anesth Analg* 1992;74:378–383.
58. Coughlan MG, Kenny D, Kampine JP, et al. Differential sensitivity of proximal and distal coronary arteries to a nitric oxide donor following reperfusion injury or inhibition of nitric oxide synthesis. *Cardiovasc Res* 1993;27:1444–1448.
59. Crawford MW, Lerman J, Saldivia V, Carmichael FJ. Hemodynamic and organ blood flow responses to halothane and sevoflurane anesthesia during spontaneous ventilation. *Anesth Analg* 1992;75:1000–1006.
60. Crystal GJ, Kim SJ, Czinn EA, et al. Intracoronary isoflurane causes marked vasodilation in canine hearts. *Anesthesiology* 1991; 74:757–765.
61. Crystal GJ, Kim SJ, Salem MR, et al. Nitric oxide does not mediate coronary vasodilation by isoflurane. *Anesthesiology* 1994;81:209–220.
62. Daut J, Maier-Rudolph W, von Beckerath N, et al. Hypoxic dilation of coronary arteries is mediated by ATP-sensitive potassium channels. *Science* 1990;247:1341–1344.
63. Davis RF, DeBoer LWV, Rude RE, et al. The effect of halothane anesthesia on myocardial necrosis, hemodynamic performance, and regional myocardial blood flow in dogs following coronary artery occlusion. *Anesthesiology* 1983;59:402–411.
64. Davis RF, Sidi A. Effect of isoflurane on the extent of myocardial necrosis and on systemic hemodynamics, regional myocardial blood flow, and regional myocardial metabolism in dogs after coronary artery occlusion. *Anesth Analg* 1989;69:575–586.
65. Dellsperger KC, Brooks LA, Gutterman DD. Hyperglycemia attenuates coronary microvascular dilation to acetylcholine (abstr.). *FASEB J* 1992;6:A1580.
66. Dellsperger KC, Marcus ML. Effects of left ventricular hypertrophy on the coronary circulation. *Am J Cardiol* 1990;65:1504–1510.
67. Diana P, Tullock WC, Gorcsan J III, et al. Myocardial ischemia: a comparison between isoflurane and enflurane in coronary artery bypass patients. *Anesth Analg* 1993;77:221–226.
68. Dole WP. Autoregulation of the coronary circulation. *Prog Cardiovasc Dis* 1987;29:293–323.
69. Dole WP, Nuno DW. Myocardial oxygen tension determines the degree and pressure range of coronary autoregulation. *Circ Res* 1986;59:202–215.
70. Domenech RJ, Macho P, Valdes J, Penna M. Coronary vascular resistance during halothane anesthesia. *Anesthesiology* 1977;46: 236–240.
71. Dottori O, Haggendal E, Linder E, et al. The haemodynamic effects of nitrous oxide anaesthesia on myocardial blood flow in dogs. *Acta Anaesthesiol Scand* 1976;20:421–428.
72. Downey JM, Kirk ES. Inhibition of coronary blood flow by a vascular waterfall mechanism. *Circ Res* 1975;36:753–760.
73. Doyle RL, Foex P, Ryder WA, Jones LA. Effects of halothane on left ventricular relaxation and early diastolic coronary blood flow in the dog. *Anesthesiology* 1989;70:660–666.
74. Drake-Holland AJ, Laird JD, Noble MIM, et al. Oxygen and coronary vascular resistance during autoregulation and metabolic vasodilation in the dog. *J Physiol (Lond)* 1984;348:285–299.
75. Dunne MJ, West-Jordan JA, Abraham RJ, et al. The gating of nucleotide-sensitive K^+ channels in insulin-secreting cells can be modulated in changes in the ratio of ATP4-/ADP3- and by nonhydrolyzable derivatives of both ATP and ADP. *J Membr Biol* 1988; 104:165–177.
76. Epstein SE, Cannon RO III, Talbot TL. Hemodynamic principles in the control of coronary blood flow. *Am J Cardiol* 1985;56: 4E–10E.
77. Eskinder H, Hillard CJ, Flynn N, et al. Role of guanylate cyclase-cGMP systems in halothane-induced vasodilation in canine cerebral arteries. *Anesthesiology* 1992;77:482–487.
78. Factor SM, Segal BH, Van Hoeven KH. Diabetes and coronary artery disease. *Cor Art Dis* 1992;3:4–10.
79. Fallen EL, Elliott WC, Gorlin R. Mechanisms of angina in aortic stenosis. *Circulation* 1967;36:480–488.
80. Feigl EO. Adrenergic control of transmural coronary blood flow. *Basic Res Cardiol* 1990;85(suppl.1):167–176.
81. Feigl EO. Coronary physiology. *Physiol Rev* 1983;63:1–205.
82. Flynn NM, Kenny D, Pelc LR, et al. Endothelium-dependent vasodilation of canine coronary collateral vessels. *Am J Physiol* 1991;261:H1797–H1801.
83. Folkow B. Description of the myogenic hypothesis. *Circ Res* 1964; 5(suppl.1):279–287.
84. Forman MB, Collins HW, Kopelman HA, et al. Determinants of left ventricular aneurysm formation after anterior myocardial infarction: a clinical and angiographic study. *J Am Coll Cardiol* 1986;8:1256–1262.
85. Freedman BM, Hamm DP, Everson CT, et al. Enflurane enhances postischemic functional recovery in the isolated rat heart. *Anesthesiology* 1985;62:29–33.
86. Fulton WFM. *The coronary arteries; arteriography, microanatomy, and pathogenesis of obliterative coronary artery disease.* Springfield: Charles C. Thomas, 1965;95.
87. Furchgott RF, Zawadzki JV. The obligatory role of endothelial cells in the relaxation of arterial smooth muscle by acetylcholine. *Nature* 1980;288:373–376.
88. Gallagher KP. Transmural steal with isoproterenol and exercise in poststenotic myocardium. In: Heusch G, Ross J Jr, eds. *Adrenergic mechanisms in myocardial ischemia.* New York: Springer-Verlag, 1991;145–155.
89. Ganz P, Alexander RW. New insights into the cellular mechanisms of vasospasm. *Am J Cardiol* 1985;56:11E–15E.
90. Ganz W, Tamura K, Marcus HS, et al. Measurement of coronary sinus blood flow by continuous thermodilution in man. *Circulation* 1971;44:181–195.
91. Gerson JI, Hickey RF, Bainton CR. Treatment of myocardial ischemia with halothane or nitroprusside-propranolol. *Anesth Analg* 1982;61:10–14.
92. Gilbert M, Roberts SL, Mori M, et al. Comparative coronary vascular reactivity and hemodynamics during halothane and isoflurane anesthesia in swine. *Anesthesiology* 1988;68:243–253.
93. Gould KL. Dynamic coronary stenosis. *Am J Cardiol* 1980;45: 286–292.
94. Granata L, Olsson RA, Huvos A, Gregg DE. Coronary inflow and oxygen usage following cardiac sympathetic nerve stimulation in unanesthetized dogs. *Circ Res* 1965;16:114–120.
95. Grattan MT, Hanley FL, Stevens MB, Hoffman JI. Transmural coronary flow reserve patterns in dogs. *Am J Physiol* 1986;250: H276–H283.
96. Greenblatt EP, Loeb AL, Longnecker DE. Endothelium-dependent circulatory control—a mechanism for the differing peripheral vascular effects of isoflurane versus halothane. *Anesthesiology* 1992;77:1178–1185.
97. Griffith TM, Edwards DH, Davies RL, et al. EDRF coordinates the behaviour of vascular resistance vessels. *Nature* 1987;329:442–445.
98. Gross GJ, Auchampach JA. Role of ATP dependent potassium channels in myocardial ischaemia. *Cardiovasc Res* 1992;26: 1011–1016.
99. Gross GJ, Buck JD, Warltier DC, Hardman HF. Role of autoregulation in the beneficial action of propranolol on ischemic blood flow distribution and stenosis severity in the canine myocardium. *J Pharmacol Exp Ther* 1982;222:635–640.
100. Gross GJ, Warltier DC. Coronary steal in four models of single or multiple vessel obstruction in dogs. *Am J Cardiol* 1981;48:84–92.
101. Grover GJ, Sleph PG, DzwonczykS. Role of myocardial ATP-sensitive potassium channels in mediating preconditioning in the dog heart and their possible interaction with adenosine A_1-receptors. *Circulation* 1992;86:1310–1316.
102. Guyton RA, McClenathan JH, Michaelis LL. Evolution of regional ischemia distal to a proximal coronary stenosis: self-propagation of ischemia. *Am J Cardiol* 1977;40:381–392.
103. Habazettl H, Conzen PF, Hobbhahn J, et al. Left ventricular oxy-

gen tensions in dogs during coronary vasodilation by enflurane, isoflurane and dipyridamole. *Anesth Analg* 1989;68:286–294.
104. Hamilton FN, Feigl EO. Coronary vascular sympathetic beta receptor innervation. *Am J Physiol* 1976;230:1569–1576.
105. Harrison DG, Florentine MS, Brooks LA, et al. The effect of hypertension and left ventricular hypertrophy on the lower range of coronary autoregulation. *Circulation* 1988;77:1108–1115.
106. Harrison DG, Kurz MA, Quillen JE, et al. Normal and pathophysiologic considerations of endothelial regulation of vascular tone and their relevance to nitrate therapy. *Am J Cardiol* 1992;70: 11B–17B.
107. Harrison DG, Sellke FW, Quillen JE. Neurohumoral regulation of coronary collateral vasomotor tone. *Basic Res Cardiol* 1990;85 (suppl.1):121–129.
108. Hart JL, Jing M, Bina S, et al. Effects of halothane on EDRF/ cGMP-mediated vascular smooth muscle relaxations. *Anesthesiology* 1993;79:323–331.
109. Hartman JC, Kampine JP, Schmeling WT, Warltier DC. Actions of isoflurane on myocardial perfusion in chronically instrumented dogs with poor, moderate, or well-developed coronary collaterals. *J Cardiothorac Anesth* 1990;4:715–725.
110. Hartman JC, Kampine JP, Schmeling WT, Warltier DC. Alterations in collateral blood flow produced by isoflurane in a chronically instrumented canine model of multivessel coronary artery disease. *Anesthesiology* 1991;74:120–133.
111. Hartman JC, Kampine JP, Schmeling WT, Warltier DC. Steal-prone coronary circulation in chronically instrumented dogs: isoflurane versus adenosine. *Anesthesiology* 1991;74:744–756.
112. Hartman JC, Kampine JP, Schmeling WT, Warltier DC. Volatile anesthetics and regional myocardial perfusion in chronically instrumented dogs: halothane versus isoflurane in a single-vessel disease model with enhanced collateral development. *J Cardiothorac Anesth* 1990;4:588–603.
113. Hartman JC, Pagel PS, Kampine JP, et al. Influence of desflurane on regional distribution of coronary blood flow in a chronically instrumented canine model of multivessel coronary artery obstruction. *Anesth Analg* 1991;72:289–299.
114. Hatano Y, Nakamura K, Yakushiji T, et al. Comparison of the direct effects of halothane and isoflurane on large and small coronary arteries isolated from dogs. *Anesthesiology* 1990;73:513–517.
115. Heikkila H, Jalonen J, Arola M, Laaksonen V. Haemodynamics and myocardial oxygenation during anaesthesia for coronary artery surgery: comparison between enflurane and high-dose fentanyl anaesthesia. *Acta Anaesthesiol Scand* 1985;29:457–464.
116. Heineman FW, Grayson J. Transmural distribution of intramyocardial pressure measured by micropipette technique. *Am J Physiol* 1985;249:H1216–H1223.
117. Helman JD, Leung JM, Bellows WH, et al. The risk of myocardial ischemia in patients receiving desflurane versus sufentanil anesthesia for coronary artery bypass graft surgery. *Anesthesiology* 1992; 77:47–62.
118. Herrmann SC, Feigl EO. Adrenergic blockade blunts adenosine concentration and coronary vasodilation during hypoxia. *Circ Res* 1992;70:1203–1216.
119. Heusch G. Alpha-adrenergic mechanisms in myocardial ischemia. *Circulation* 1990;81:1–13.
120. Heusch G, Deussen A. The effects of cardiac sympathetic nerve stimulation on perfusion of stenotic coronary arteries in the dog. *Circ Res* 1983;53:8–15.
121. Hickey RF, Cason BA, Shubayev I. Regional vasodilating properties of isoflurane in normal swine myocardium. *Anesthesiology* 1994;80:574–581.
122. Hickey RF, Sybert PE, Verrier ED, Cason BA. Effects of halothane, enflurane, and isoflurane on coronary blood flow autoregulation and coronary vascular reserve in the canine heart. *Anesthesiology* 1988;68:21–30.
123. Hickey RF, Verrier ED, Baer RW, et al. A canine model of acute coronary stenosis: effects of deliberate hypotension. *Anesthesiology* 1983;59:226–236.
124. Hilfiker O, Larsen R, Sonntag H. Myocardial blood flow and oxygen consumption during halothane-nitrous oxide anaesthesia for coronary revascularization. *Br J Anaesth* 1983;55:927–932.
125. Hirsch LJ, Rooney MW, Mathru M, Rao TLK. Effects of fentanyl on coronary blood flow distribution and myocardial oxygen consumption in the dog. *J Cardiothorac Vasc Anesth* 1993;7:50–54.
126. Hoffman JIE. Determinants and prediction of transmural myocardial perfusion. *Circulation* 1978;58:381–391.
127. Hoffman JIE, Spaan JAE. Pressure-flow relations in coronary circulation. *Physiol Rev* 1990;70:331–390.90.
128. Hori M, Kitakaze M, Tamai J, et al. Alpha 2-adrenoceptor stimulation can augment coronary vasodilation maximally induced by adenosine in dogs. *Am J Physiol* 1989;257:H132–H140.
129. Howard RO, Richardson DW, Smith MH, Patterson JL Jr. Oxygen consumption of arterioles and venules as studied in the Cartesian diver. *Circ Res* 1965;16:187–196.
130. Hughes JM, Sill JC, Pettis M, Rorie DK. Nitrous oxide constricts epicardial coronary arteries in pigs: evidence suggesting inhibitory effects on the endothelium. *Anesth Analg* 1993;77:232–240.
131. Indolfi C, Piscione F, Villari B, et al. Role of alpha 2-adrenoceptors in normal and atherosclerotic human coronary circulation. *Circulation* 1992;86:1116–1124.
132. Inoue K, Reichelt W, El-Banayosy A, et al. Does isoflurane lead to a higher incidence of myocardial infarction and perioperative death than enflurane in coronary artery surgery? A clinical study of 1178 patients. *Anesth Analg* 1990;71:469–474.
133. Ismail EF, Kim SJ, Salem MR, Crystal GJ. Direct effects of propofol on myocardial contractility in *in situ* canine hearts. *Anesthesiology* 1992;77:964–972.
134. Johnson PC. Autoregulation of blood flow. *Circ Res* 1986;58: 483–495.
135. Johnson PC. Review of previous studies and current theories of autoregulation. *Circ Res* 1964;15(suppl.1):2–9.
136. Juilliere Y, Danchin N, Grentzinger A, et al. Role of previous angina pectoris and collateral flow to preserve left ventricular function in the presence or absence of myocardial infarction in isolated total occlusion of the left anterior descending coronary artery. *Am J Cardiol* 1990;65:277–281.
137. Kalsner S. Cholinergic mechanisms in human coronary artery preparations: implications of species differences. *J Physiol(Lond)* 1985;358:509–526.
138. Kanatsuka H, Ashikawa K, Komaru T, et al. Diameter change and pressure-red blood cell velocity relations in coronary microvessels during long diastoles in the canine left ventricle. *Circ Res* 1990;66: 503–510.
139. Kanatsuka H, Lamping KG, Eastham CL, et al. Comparison of the effects of increased myocardial oxygen consumption and adenosine on the coronary microvascular resistance. *Circ Res* 1989;65: 1296–1305.
140. Kanaya N, Fujita S. The effects of isoflurane on regional myocardial contractility and metabolism in "stunned" myocardium in acutely instrumented dogs. *Anesth Analg* 1994;79:447–454.
141. Kao CY. Pharmacology of tetrodotoxin and saxitoxin. *Fed Proc* 1972;31:1117–1123.
142. Katori M, Berne RM. Release of adenosine from anoxic hearts. Relationship to coronary flow. *Circ Res* 1966;19:420–425.
143. Katz AM. Structure of the heart and cardiac muscle. In: Katz AM, ed. *Physiology of the heart.* New York: Raven Press, 1992;15.
144. Kemp HG, Kronmal RA, Vlietstra RE, Frye RL. Seven-year survival of patients with normal or near normal coronary arteriograms: a CASS registry study. *J Am Coll Cardiol* 1986;7:479–483.
145. Kenny D, Proctor LT, Schmeling WT, et al. Isoflurane causes only minimal increases in coronary blood flow independent of oxygen demand. *Anesthesiology* 1991;75:640–649.
146. Kersten JR, Brayer AP, Pagel PS, et al. Perfusion of ischemic myocardium during anesthesia with sevoflurane. *Anesthesiology* 1994;81:995–1004.
147. Kersten JR, Brooks LA, Dellsperger KC. Impaired microvascular response to graded coronary occlusion in diabetic and hyperglycemic dogs. *Am J Physiol* 1995;268:H1667–1674.
148. Kersten JR, Pagel PS, Warltier DC. Protamine inhibits coronary collateral development in a canine model of repetitive coronary occlusion. *Am J Physiol* 1995;268:H720–728.
149. Khambatta HJ, Sonntag H, Larsen R, et al. Global and regional myocardial blood flow and metabolism during equipotent halothane and isoflurane anesthesia in patients with coronary artery disease. *Anesth Analg* 1988;67:936–942.
150. Kirsch GE, Codina J, Birnbaumer L, Brown AM. Coupling of ATP-sensitive K^+ channels to A_1 receptors by G proteins in rat ventricular myocytes. *Am J Physiol* 1990;259:H820–H826.
151. Kleinman B, Henkin RE, Glisson SN, et al. Qualitative evaluation of coronary flow during anesthetic induction using thallium-201 perfusion scans. *Anesthesiology* 1986;64:157–164.
152. Klocke FJ. Coronary blood flow in man. *Prog Cardiovasc Dis* 1976;19:117–166.

153. Klocke FJ, Mates RE, Canty JM Jr, Ellis AK. Coronary pressure-flow relationships. Controversial issues and probable implications. *Circ Res* 1985;56:310–323.
154. Knight AA, Hollenberg M, London MJ, et al. Perioperative myocardial ischemia: importance of the preoperative ischemia pattern. *Anesthesiology* 1988;68:681–688.
155. Koltai MZ, Rosen P, Hadhazy P, et al. Relationship between vascular adrenergic receptors and prostaglandin biosyntheses in canine diabetic coronary arteries. *Diabetologia* 1988;31:681–686.
156. Koltai MZ, Rosen P, Pogatsa G. Diminished vasodilation; Imbalance of synthesized cyclooxygenase products by adrenergic mediation in diabetic coronaries of the dog. *Prog Clin Biol Res* 1989; 301:449–453.
157. Komaru T, Lamping KG, Eastham CL, Dellsperger KC. Role of ATP-sensitive potassium channels in coronary microvascular autoregulatory responses. *Circ Res* 1991;69:1146–1151.
158. Kozmary SV, Lampe GH, Benefiel D, et al. No finding of increased myocardial ischemia during or after carotid endarterectomy under anesthesia with nitrous oxide. *Anesth Analg* 1990;71:591–596.
159. Kuo L, Davis MJ, Cannon MS, Chilian WM. Pathophysiological consequences of atherosclerosis extend into the coronary microcirculation. Restoration of endothelium-dependent responses by L-arginine. *Circ Res* 1992;70:465–476.
160. Kyriakidis MK, Kourouklis CB, Papaioannou JT, et al. Sinus node coronary arteries studied with angiography. *Am J Cardiol* 1983;51: 749–750.
161. Lamping KG, Kanatsuka H, Eastham CL, et al. Nonuniform vasomotor responses of the coronary microcirculation to serotonin and vasopressin. *Circ Res* 1989;65:343–351.
162. Larach DR, Schuler HG. Potassium channel blockade and halothane vasodilation in conducting and resistance coronary arteries. *J Pharmacol Exp Ther* 1993;267:72–81.
163. Larach DR, Schuler HG. Direct vasodilation by sevoflurane, isoflurane, and halothane alters coronary flow reserve in the isolated rat heart. *Anesthesiology* 1991;75:268–278.
164. Larach DR, Schuler HG, Skeehan TM, Peterson CJ. Direct effects of myocardial depressant drugs on coronary vascular tone: anesthetic vasodilation by halothane and isoflurane. *J Pharmacol Exp Ther* 1990;254:58–64.
165. Lerman A, Burnett JC Jr. Intact and altered endothelium in regulation of vasomotion. *Circulation* 1992;86:III-12–III-19.
166. Lerman A, Hildebrand FL Jr, Aarhus LL, Burnett JC Jr. Endothelin has biological actions at pathophysiological concentrations. *Circulation* 1991;83:1808–1814.
167. Leung JM, Goehner P, O'Kelly BF, et al. Isoflurane anesthesia and myocardial ischemia: comparative risk versus sufentanil anesthesia in patients undergoing coronary artery bypass graft surgery. *Anesthesiology* 1991;74:838–847.
168. Levin DC. Pathways and functional significance of the coronary collateral circulation. *Circulation* 1974;50:831–837.
169. Levin DC, Gardiner GA. Coronary arteriography. In: Braunwald E, ed. *Heart disease,* 4th ed. Philadelphia: WB Saunders, 1992; 235–275.
170. Lindsay J Jr, Dwyer S, Punja U. Angiographic demonstration of coronary occlusion during spontaneous acute myocardial infarction and subsequent angiographically normal coronary arteries. *Am J Cardiol* 1983;51:1227–1228.
171. Lowensohn HS, Khouri EM, Gregg DE, et al. Phasic right coronary artery blood flow in conscious dogs with normal and elevated right ventricular pressures. *Circ Res* 1976;39:760–766.
172. Lowenstein E, Foex P, Francis CM, et al. Regional ischemic ventricular dysfunction in myocardium supplied by a narrowed coronary artery with increasing halothane concentration in the dog. *Anesthesiology* 1981;55:349–359.
173. Ludmer PL, Selwyn AP, Shook TL, et al. Paradoxical vasoconstriction induced by acetylcholine in atherosclerotic coronary arteries. *N Engl J Med* 1986;315:1046–1051.
174. Lurie K, Bristow M, Ginsburg R, et al. Vascular H_1-receptor up-regulation in rabbits fed a high cholesterol diet (abstr). *Circulation* 1981;64:IV–272.
175. Manohar M, Parks CM. Porcine systemic and regional organ blood flow during 1.0 and 1.5 minimum alveolar concentrations of sevoflurane anesthesia without and with 50% nitrous oxide. *J Pharmacol Exp Ther* 1984;231:640–648.
176. Marcus ML. *The coronary circulation in health and disease.* New York: McGraw-Hill, 1983.
177. Marcus ML, Chilian WM, Kanatsuka H, et al. Understanding the coronary circulation through studies at the microvascular level. *Circulation* 1990;82:1–7.
178. Marcus ML, Doty DB, Hiratzka LF, et al. Decreased coronary reserve: a mechanism for angina pectoris in patients with aortic stenosis and normal coronary arteries. *N Engl J Med* 1092;307: 1362–1366.
179. Marcus ML, Mueller TM, Eastham CL. Effects of short- and long-term left ventricular hypertrophy on coronary circulation. *Am J Physiol* 1981;241:H358–H362.
180. Marcus ML, Mueller TM, Gascho JA, Kerber RE. Effects of cardiac hypertrophy secondary to hypertension on the coronary circulation. *Am J Cardiol* 1979;44:1023–1028.
181. Marcus ML, Wilson RF, White CW. Methods of measurement of myocardial blood flow in patients: a critical review. *Circulation* 1987;76:245–253.
182. Marijic J, Buljubasic N, Coughlan MG, et al. Effect of K^+ channel blockade with tetraethylammonium on anesthetic-induced relaxation in canine cerebral and coronary arteries. *Anesthesiology* 1992;77:948–955.
183. Marijic J, Stowe DF, Turner LA, et al. Differential protective effects of halothane and isoflurane against hypoxic and reoxygenation injury in the isolated guinea pig heart. *Anesthesiology* 1990;73: 976–983.
184. Martin W, Villani GM, Jothianandan D, Furchgott RF. Selective blockade of endothelium-dependent and glyceryl trinitrate-induced relaxation by hemoglobin and by methylene blue in rabbit aorta. *J Pharmacol Exp Ther* 1985;232:708–716.
185. Marty J, Nitenberg A, Blanchet F, et al. Effects of midazolam on the coronary circulation in patients with coronary artery disease. *Anesthesiology* 1986;64:206–210.
186. Maseri A, Crea F, Kaski C, Crake T. Mechanisms of angina pectoris in syndrome X. *J Am Coll Cardiol* 1991;17:499–506.
187. Mayhan WG, Simmons LK, Sharpe GM. Mechanism of impaired responses of cerebral arterioles during diabetes mellitus. *Am J Physiol* 1991;260:H319–H326.
188. Meinert CL, Knatterud GL, Prout TE, Klimt CR. A study of the effects of hypoglycemic agents on vascular complications in patients with adult-onset diabetes. II. Mortality results. *Diabetes* 1970;19:789–830.
189. Merin RG, Basch S. Are the myocardial functional and metabolic effects of isoflurane really different from those of halothane and enflurane? *Anesthesiology* 1981;55:398–408.
190. Merin RG, Kumazawa T, Luka NL. Myocardial function and metabolism in the conscious dog and during halothane anesthesia. *Anesthesiology* 1976;44:402–415.
191. Miller VM, Vanhoutte PM. Endothelial α_2 adrenoceptors in canine pulmonary and systemic blood vessels. *Eur J Pharmacol* 1985;118:123–129.
192. Moffit EA, Scovil JE, Barker RA, et al. Myocardial metabolism and haemodynamic responses during high-dose fentanyl anaesthesia for coronary patients. *Can Anaesth Soc J* 1984;31:611–618.
193. Moffitt EA, Barker RA, Glenn JJ, et al. Myocardial metabolism and hemodynamic responses with isoflurane anesthesia for coronary arterial surgery. *Anesth Analg* 1986;65:53–61.
194. Moffitt EA, Imrie DD, Scovil JE, et al. Myocardial metabolism and haemodynamic responses with enflurane anaesthesia for coronary artery surgery. *Can Anaesth Soc J* 1984;31:604–610.
195. Moffitt EA, Sethna DH, Bussell JA, et al. Myocardial metabolism and hemodynamic responses to halothane or morphine anesthesia for coronary artery surgery. *Anesth Analg* 1982;61:979–985.
196. Moffitt EA, Sethna DH, Gary RJ, et al. Nitrous oxide added to halothane reduces coronary flow and myocardial oxygen consumption in patients with coronary disease. *Can Anaesth Soc J* 1983;30:5–9.
197. Mohrman DE, Feigl EO. Competition between sympathetic vasoconstriction and metabolic vasodilation in the canine coronary circulation. *Circ Res* 1978;42:79–86.
198. Moir TW. Subendocardial distribution of coronary blood flow and the effect of antianginal drugs. *Circ Res* 1972;30:621–627.
199. Moir TW, DeBra DW. Effect of left ventricular hypertension, ischemia, and vasoactive drugs on the myocardial distribution of coronary flow. *Circ Res* 1967;21:65–74.
200. Moncada S, Palmer RM, Higgs EA. Nitric oxide: physiology, pathophysiology, and pharmacology. *Pharmacol Rev* 1991;43:109–142.
201. Moore PG, Kien ND, Reitan JA, et al. No evidence for blood flow redistribution with isoflurane or halothane during acute coronary artery occlusion in fentanyl-anesthetized dogs. *Anesthesiology* 1991; 75:854–865.

202. Moore S. Thromboatherosclerosis in normolipemic rabbits: a result of continued endothelial damage. *Lab Invest* 1973;29:478–487.
203. Mosher P, Ross J Jr, McFate PA, Shaw RF. Control of coronary blood flow by an autoregulatory mechanism. *Circ Res* 1964;14:250–259.
204. Muldoon SM, Hart JL, Bowen KA, Freas W. Attenuation of endothelium-mediated vasodilation by halothane. *Anesthesiology* 1988;68:31–37.
205. Mullett M, Gharaibeh M, Warltier DC, Gross GJ. The effect of diltiazem, a calcium channel blocking agent, on vasoconstrictor responses to norepinephrine, serotonin and potassium depolarization in canine coronary and femoral arteries. *Gen Pharmacol* 1983;14:259–264.
206. Nakamura K, Hatano Y, Toda H, et al. Halothane-induced relaxation of vascular smooth muscle: a possible contribution of increased cyclic GMP formation. *Jpn J Pharmacol* 1991;55:165–168.
207. Nanda V, Henry PD. Increased serotonergic and alpha adrenergic receptors in aortas from rabbits fed a high cholesterol diet (abstr). *Clin Res* 1982;30:209A.
208. Nathan HJ. Control of hemodynamics prevents worsening of myocardial ischemia when nitrous oxide is administered to isoflurane-anesthetized dogs. *Anesthesiology* 1989;71:686–694.
209. Nathan HJ. Nitrous oxide worsens myocardial ischemia in isoflurane-anesthetized dogs. *Anesthesiology* 1988;68:407–415.
210. O'Young J, Mastrocostopoulos G, Hilgenberg A, et al. Myocardial circulatory and metabolic effects of isoflurane and sufentanil during coronary artery surgery. *Anesthesiology* 1987;66:653–658.
211. Olsson RA, Bunger R. Coronary circulation. In: Fozzard HA, Haber E, Jennings RB, Katz AM, eds. *The heart and cardiovascular system*, vol 2, 2nd ed. New York: Raven Press, 1991;1393–1425.
212. Ozhan M, Sill JC, Atagunduz P, et al. Volatile anesthetics and agonist-induced contractions in porcine coronary artery smooth muscle and Ca^{2+} mobilization in cultured immortalized vascular smooth muscle cells. *Anesthesiology* 1994;80:1102–1113.
213. Pagel PS, Kampine JP, Schmeling WT, Warltier DC. Comparison of the systemic and coronary hemodynamic actions of desflurane, isoflurane, halothane, and enflurane in the chronically instrumented dog. *Anesthesiology* 1991;74:539–551.
214. Palmer RM, Ferrige AG, MoncadaS. Nitric oxide release accounts for the biological activity of endothelium-derived relaxing factor. *Nature* 1987;327:524–526.
215. Pantely GA, Bristow JD, Swenson LJ, et al. Incomplete coronary vasodilation during myocardial ischemia in swine. *Am J Physiol* 1985;249:H638–H647.
216. Paul RJ, Peterson JW, Caplan SR. Oxygen consumption rate in vascular smooth muscle: relation to isometric tension. *Biochem Biophys Acta* 1973;305:474–480.
217. Pelc LR, Garancis JC, Gross GJ, Warltier DC. Alteration of endothelium-dependent distribution of myocardial blood flow after coronary occlusion and reperfusion. *Circulation* 1990;81:1928–1937.
218. Pelc LR, Gross GJ, Warltier DC. Changes in regional myocardial perfusion by muscarinic receptor subtypes in dogs. *Cardiovasc Res* 1986;20:482–489.
219. Pelc LR, Gross GJ, Warltier DC. Preferential increase in subendocardial perfusion produced by endothelium-dependent vasodilators. *Circulation* 1987;76:191–200.
220. Perlmutt LM, Jay ME, Levin DC. Variations in the blood supply of the left ventricular apex. *Invest Radiol* 1983;18:138–140.
221. Peters KG, Marcus ML, Harrison DG. Vasopressin and the mature coronary collateral circulation. *Circulation* 1989;79:1324–1331.
222. Philbin DM, Foex P, Drummond G, et al. Postsystolic shortening of canine left ventricle supplied by a stenotic coronary artery when nitrous oxide is added in the presence of narcotics. *Anesthesiology* 1985;62:166–174.
223. Popescu LM, Panoiu C, Hinescu M, Nutu O. The mechanism of cGMP-induced relaxation in vascular smooth muscle. *Eur J Pharmacol* 1985;107:393–394.
224. Priebe HJ. Differential effects of isoflurane on regional right and left ventricular performances, and on coronary, systemic, and pulmonary hemodynamics in the dog. *Anesthesiology* 1987;66:262–272.
225. Priebe HJ. Isoflurane causes more severe myocardial dysfunction than halothane in dogs with a critical coronary artery stenosis. *Anesthesiology* 1988;69:72–83.
226. Priebe HJ, Foex P. Isoflurane causes regional myocardial dysfunction in dogs with critical coronary artery stenoses. *Anesthesiology* 1987;66:293–300.
227. Pulley DD, Kirvassilis GV, Kelermenos N, et al. Regional and global myocardial circulatory and metabolic effects of isoflurane and halothane in patients with steal-prone coronary anatomy. *Anesthesiology* 1991;75:756–766.
228. Rapoport RM, Murad F. Agonist-induced endothelium-dependent relaxation in rat thoracic aorta may be mediated through cGMP. *Circ Res* 1093;52:352–357.
229. Reiz S. Nitrous oxide augments the systemic and coronary haemodynamic effects of isoflurane in patients with ischaemic heart disease. *Acta Anaesthesiol Scand* 1983;27:464–469.
230. Reiz S, Balfors E, Friedman A, et al. Effects of thiopentone on cardiac performance, coronary hemodynamics and myocardial oxygen consumption in chronic ischemic heart disease. *Acta Anaesthesiol Scand* 1981;25:103–110.
231. Reiz S, Balfors E, Gustavsson B, et al. Effects of halothane on coronary haemodynamics and myocardial metabolism in patients with ischaemic heart disease and heart failure. *Acta Anaesthesiol Scand* 1982;26:133–138.
232. Reiz S, Balfors E, Sorenson MB, et al. Isoflurane—a powerful coronary vasodilator in patients with coronary artery disease. *Anesthesiology* 1983;59:91–97.
233. Reiz S, Ostman M. Regional coronary hemodynamics during isoflurane—nitrous oxide anesthesia in patients with ischemic heart disease. *Anesth Analg* 1985;64:570–576.
234. Ross R. The pathogenesis of atherosclerosis. In: Braunwald E, ed. *Heart disease*, vol 2, 4th ed. Philadelphia: WB Saunders, 1992; 1106–1124.
235. Ross R, Glomset JA. Atherosclerosis and the arterial smooth muscle cell: proliferation of smooth muscle is a key event in the genesis of the lesions of atherosclerosis. *Science* 1973;180:1332–1339.
236. Rouleau J, Boerboom LE, Surjadhana A, Hoffman JI. The role of autoregulation and tissue diastolic pressures in the transmural distribution of left ventricular blood flow in anesthetized dogs. *Circ Res* 1979;45:804–815.
237. Rubanyi GM, Romero JC, Vanhoutte PM. Flow-induced release of endothelium-derived relaxing factor. *Am J Physiol* 1986;250: H1145–H1149.
238. Rubanyi GM, Vanhoutte PM. Superoxide anions and hyperoxia inactivate endothelium-derived relaxing factor. *Am J Physiol* 1986; 250:H822–H827.
239. Rubio R, Berne RM. Regulation of coronary blood flow. *Prog Cardiovasc Dis* 1975;18:105–122.
240. Rubio R, Berne RM. Release of adenosine by the normal myocardium in dogs and its relationship to the regulation of coronary resistance. *Circ Res* 1969;25:407–415.
241. Rydvall A, Haggmark S, Nyhman H, Reiz S. Effects of enflurane on coronary haemodynamics in patients with ischaemic heart disease. *Acta Anaesthesiol Scand* 1984;28:690–695.
242. Sahlman L, Henriksson BA, Martner J, Ricksten SE. Effects of halothane, enflurane, and isoflurane on coronary vascular tone, myocardial performance, and oxygen consumption during controlled changes in aortic and left atrial pressure. Studies on isolated working rat hearts *in vitro*. *Anesthesiology* 1988;69:1–10.
243. Sahlman L, Milocco I, Appelgren L, et al. Control of intraoperative hypertension with isoflurane in patients with coronary artery disease: effects on regional myocardial blood flow and metabolism. *Anesth Analg* 1989;68:105–111.
244. Sahlman L, Milocco I, Ricksten SE. Myocardial circulatory and metabolic effects of halothane when used to control intraoperative hypertension in patients with coronary artery disease. *Acta Anaesthesiol Scand* 1992;36:283–288.
245. Schaper W, Gorge G, Winkler B, Schaper J. The collateral circulation of the heart. *Prog Cardiovasc Dis* 1988;31:57–77.
246. Schaper W, Sharma HS, Quinkler W, et al. Molecular biologic concepts of coronary anastomoses. *J Am Coll Cardiol* 1990;15:513–518.
247. Schrader J, Haddy FJ, Gerlach E. Release of adenosine, inosine and hypoxanthine from the isolated guinea pig heart during hypoxia, flow-autoregulation and reactive hyperemia. *Pflugers Arch* 1977;369:1–6.
248. Sedlis SP, Cohen KH, Sequeira JM, El-Sherif N. Preservation of left ventricular function in patients with total occlusion of the left anterior descending coronary artery and wide-caliber distal vessel filling by collateral vasculature. *Cathet Cardiovasc Diagn* 1988;15:139–142.
249. Sellke FW. Myers PR, Bates JN, Harrison DG. Influence of vessel size on the sensitivity of porcine coronary microvessels to nitroglycerin. *Am J Physiol* 1990;258:H515–H520.
250. Shepherd JT, Vanhoutte PM. Mechanisms responsible for coronary vasospasm. *J Am Coll Cardiol* 1986;8:50A–54A.

251. Shimokawa H, Vanhoutte PM. Impaired endothelium-dependent relaxation to aggregating platelets and related vasoactive substances in porcine coronary arteries in hypercholesterolemia and atherosclerosis. *Circ Res* 1989;64:900–914.
252. Siker D, Pagel PS, Pelc LR, et al. Nitrous oxide impairs functional recovery of stunned myocardium in barbiturate-anesthetized, acutely instrumented dogs. *Anesth Analg* 1992;75:539–548.
253. Sill JC, Bove AA, Nugent M, et al. Effects of isoflurane on coronary arteries and coronary arterioles in the intact dog. *Anesthesiology* 1987;66:273–279.
254. Sill JC, Eskuri S, Nelson R, et al. The volatile anesthetic isoflurane attenuates Ca^{2+} mobilization in cultured vascular smooth muscle cells. *J Pharmacol Exp Ther* 1993;265:74–80.
255. Simmet T, Peskar BA. Eicosanoids and the coronary circulation. *Rev Physiol Biochem Pharmacol* 1986;104:1–64.
256. Slogoff S, Keats AS. Randomized trial of primary anesthetic agents on outcome of coronary artery bypass operations. *Anesthesiology* 1989;70:179–188.
257. Slogoff S, Keats AS, Dear WE, et al. Steal-prone coronary anatomy and myocardial ischemia associated with four primary anesthetic agents in humans. *Anesth Analg* 1991;72:22–27.
258. Smith G, Rogers K, Thorburn J. Halothane improves the balance of oxygen supply to demand in acute experimental myocardial ischaemia. *Br J Anaesth* 1980;52:577–583.
259. Smith G, Vance JP, Brown DM, McMillan JC. Changes in canine myocardial blood flow and oxygen consumption in response to halothane. *Br J Anaesth* 1974;46:821–826.
260. Smith JJ, Kampine JP. Circulation to special regions. In: *Circulatory physiology*. Baltimore: Williams & Wilkins. 1990;193.
261. Somlyo AP, Somlyo AV. Vascular smooth muscle. II. Pharmacology of normal and hypertensive vessels. *Pharmacol Rev* 1970;22: 249–353.
262. Sonntag H, Larsen R, Hilfiker O, et al. Myocardial blood flow and oxygen consumption during high-dose fentanyl anesthesia in patients with coronary artery disease. *Anesthesiology* 1982;56:417–422.
263. Sperelakis N, Ohya Y. Regulation of calcium slow channels in vascular smooth muscle cells. In: Sperelakis N, Kuriyama H, eds. *Ion channels of vascular smooth muscle cells and endothelial cells*. New York: Elsevier Science, 1991;27–38.
264. Sprague DH, Yang JC, Ngai SH. Effects of isoflurane and halothane on contractility and the cyclic 3′,5′-adenosine monophosphate system in the rat aorta. *Anesthesiology* 1974;40:162–167.
265. Stamler J, Berkson DM, Lindberg HA. Risk factors: their role in the etiology and pathogenesis of the atherosclerotic diseases. In: Wissler RW, Geer JC, Kaufman N, eds. *The pathogenesis of atherosclerosis*. Baltimore: Williams & Wilkins, 1972;41–119.
266. Stemerman MB, Ross R. Experimental arteriosclerosis I. Fibrous plaque formation in primates, an electron microscope study. *J Exp Med* 1972;136:769–789.
267. Stephan H, Sonntag H, Schenk HD, et al. Effects of propofol on cardiovascular dynamics, myocardial blood flow and myocardial metabolism in patients with coronary artery disease. *Br J Anaesth* 1986;58:969–975.
268. Stone DJ, Johns RA. Endothelium-dependent effects of halothane, enflurane, and isoflurane on isolated rat aortic vascular rings. *Anesthesiology* 1989;71:126–132.
269. Stowe DF, Bosnjak ZJ, Kampine JP. Comparison of etomidate, ketamine, midazolam, propofol, and thiopental on function and metabolism of isolated hearts. *Anesth Analg* 1992;74:547–558.
270. Stowe DF, Marijic J, Bosnjak ZJ, Kampine JP. Direct comparative effects of halothane, enflurane, and isoflurane on oxygen supply and demand in isolated hearts. *Anesthesiology* 1991;74:1087–1095.
271. Stowe DF, Monroe SM, Marijic J, et al. Comparison of halothane, enflurane, and isoflurane with nitrous oxide on contractility and oxygen supply and demand in isolated hearts. *Anesthesiology* 1991;75:1062–1074.
272. Stowe DF, Monroe SM, Marijic J, et al. Effects of nitrous oxide on contractile function and metabolism of the isolated heart. *Anesthesiology* 1990;73:1220–1226.
273. Su JY, Zhang CC. Intracellular mechanisms of halothane's effect on isolated aortic strips of the rabbit. *Anesthesiology* 1989;71:409–417.
274. Sutherland CG, Fisher BM, Frier BM, et al. Endomyocardial biopsy pathology in insulin-dependent diabetic patients with abnormal ventricular function. *Histopathology* 1989;14:593–602.
275. Tarnow J, Markschies-Hornung A, Schulte-Sasse U. Isoflurane improves the tolerance to pacing-induced myocardial ischemia. *Anesthesiology* 1986;64:147–156.
276. Tatekawa S, Traber KB, Hantler CB, et al. Effects of isoflurane on myocardial blood flow, function, and oxygen consumption in the presence of critical coronary stenosis in dogs. *Anesth Analg* 1987; 66:1073–1082.
277. Tesfamariam B, Brown ML, Deykin D, Cohen RA. Elevated glucose promotes generation of endothelium-derived vasoconstrictor prostanoids in rabbit aorta. *J Clin Invest* 1990;85:929–932.
278. Tesfamariam B, Jakubowski JA, Cohen RA. Contraction of diabetic rabbit aorta caused by endothelium-derived PGH_2-TxA_2. *Am J Physiol* 1989;257:H1327–H1333.
279. Toda H, Nakamura K, Hatano Y, et al. Halothane and isoflurane inhibit endothelium-dependent relaxation elicited by acetylcholine. *Anesth Analg* 1992;75:198–203.
280. Tomanek RJ, Schalk KA, Marcus ML, Harrison DG. Coronary angiogenesis during long-term hypertension and left ventricular hypertrophy in dogs. *Circ Res* 1989;65:352–359.
281. Tuman KJ, McCarthy RJ, Spiess BD, et al. Does choice of anesthetic agent significantly affect outcome after coronary artery surgery? *Anesthesiology* 1989;70:189–198.
282. Uggeri MJ, Proctor GJ, Johns RA. Halothane, enflurane, and isoflurane attenuate both receptor- and non-receptor-mediated EDRF production in rat thoracic aorta. *Anesthesiology* 1992;76:1012–1017.
283. Van Ackern K, Vetter HO, Bruckner UB, et al. Effects of enflurane on myocardial ischaemia in the dog. *Br J Anaesth* 1985;57:497–504.
284. VanBenthuysen KM, McMurtry IF, Horwitz LD. Reperfusion after acute coronary occlusion in dogs impairs endothelium-dependent relaxation to acetylcholine and augments contractile reactivity *in vitro*. *J Clin Invest* 1987;79:265–274.
285. Vanhoutte PM, Shimokawa H. Endothelium-derived relaxing factor and coronary vasospasm. *Circulation* 1989;80:1–9.
286. Vatner SF, Smith NT. Effects of halothane on left ventricular function and distribution of regional blood flow in dogs and primates. *Circ Res* 1974;34:155–167.
287. Verrier ED, Edelist G, Consigny M, et al. Greater coronary vascular reserve in dogs anesthetized with halothane. *Anesthesiology* 1980;53:445–459.
288. Villeneuve E, Blaise G, Sill JC, et al. Halothane 1.5 MAC, isoflurane 1.5 MAC, and the contractile responses of coronary arteries obtained from human hearts. *Anesth Analg* 1991;72:454–461.
289. Waller BF, Palumbo JT, Lie JT, Roberts WC. Status of the coronary arteries at necropsy in diabetes mellitus with onset after age 30 years: analysis of 229 diabetic patients with and without clinical evidence of coronary heart disease and comparison to 183 control subjects. *Am J Med* 1980;69:498–506.
290. Warltier DC, Al-Wathiqui MH, Kampine JP, Schmeling WT. Recovery of contractile function of stunned myocardium in chronically instrumented dogs is enhanced by halothane or isoflurane. *Anesthesiology* 1988;69:552–565.
291. Warltier DC, Buck JD, Brooks HL, Gross GJ. Coronary hemodynamics and subendocardial perfusion distal to stenoses. *Int J Cardiol* 1983;34:173–183.
292. Warltier DC, Gross GJ, Brooks HL. Coronary steal-induced increase in myocardial infarct size after pharmacologic coronary vasodilation. *Am J Cardiol* 1980;46:83–90.
293. Warltier DC, Gross GJ, Brooks HL. Pharmacologic versus ischemia-induced coronary artery vasodilation. *Am J Physiol* 1981;240: H767–H774.
294. Warltier DC, Gross GJ, Hardman HF. Subepicardial steal and reduction of myocardial oxygen consumption by adenosine. *Eur J Pharmacol* 1980;67:101–104.
295. Warltier DC, Hardman HF, Gross GJ. Transmural perfusion gradients distal to various degrees of coronary artery stenosis during resting flow or at maximal vasodilation. *Basic Res Cardiol* 1979;74: 494–508.
296. Warltier DC, Zyvoloski M, Gross GJ, et al. Redistribution of myocardial blood flow distal to a dynamic coronary arterial stenosis by sympathomimetic amines. *Am J Cardiol* 1981;48:269–279.
297. Warltier DC, Zyvoloski MG,Gross GJ, Brooks HL. Importance of retrograde coronary flow in the prediction of experimental myocardial infarct size. *Cardiology* 1986;73:333–346.
298. Warltier DC, Zyvoloski MG, Gross GJ, Brooks HL. Subendocardial vs. transmural myocardial infarction: relationship to the collateral circulation in canine and porcine hearts. *Can J Physiol Pharmacol* 1982;60:1700–1706.
299. Weaver PC, Bailey JS, Preston TD. Coronary artery blood flow in the halothane-depressed canine heart. *Br J Anaesth* 1970;42:678–684.
300. Weiss HR, Neubauer JA, Lipp JA, Sinha AK. Quantitative determi-

nation of regional oxygen consumption in the dog heart. *Circ Res* 1978;42:394–401.

301. Wilkinson PL, Hamilton WK, Moyers JR, et al. Halothane and morphine-nitrous oxide anesthesia in patients undergoing coronary artery bypass operation. Patterns of intraoperative ischemia. *J Thorac Cardiovasc Surg* 1981;82:372–382.
302. Wilkowski DA, Sill JC, Bonta W, et al. Nitrous oxide constricts epicardial coronary arteries without effect on coronary arterioles. *Anesthesiology* 1987;66:659–665.
303. Williams GH, Braunwald E. Endocrine and nutritional disorders and heart disease. In: Braunwald E, ed. *Heart disease,* vol 2, 4th ed. Philadelphia: WB Saunders, 1992;1827–1855.
304. Wilton NCT, Knight PR, Ullrich K, et al. Transmural redistribution of myocardial blood flow during isoflurane anesthesia and its effects on regional myocardial function in a canine model of fixed coronary stenosis. *Anesthesiology* 1993;78:510–523.
305. Winbury MM, Howe BB, Hefner MA. Effect of nitrates and other coronary dilators on large and small coronary vessels. An hypothesis for the mechanism of actions of nitrates. *J Pharmacol Exp Ther* 1969;168:70–95.
306. Witzeling TM, Sill JC, Hughes JM, et al. Isoflurane and halothane attenuate coronary artery constriction evoked by serotonin in isolated porcine vessels and in intact pigs. *Anesthesiology* 1990;73: 100–108.
307. Wolff G, Claudi B, Rist M, et al. Regulation of coronary blood flow during ether and halothane anaesthesia. *Br J Anaesth* 1972;44: 1139–1149.
308. Yamamoto H, Tomoike H, Shimokawa H, et al. Development of collateral function with repetitive coronary occlusion in a canine model reduces myocardial reactive hyperemia in the absence of significant coronary stenosis. *Circ Res* 1984;55:623–632.
309. Yamanoue T, Brum JM, Estafanous FG, et al. Effects of opioids on vasoresponsiveness of porcine coronary artery. *Anesth Analg* 1992;74:889–896.
310. Yanagisawa M, Kurihara H, Kimura S, et al. A novel potent vasoconstrictor peptide produced by vascular endothelial cells. *Nature* 1988;332:411–415.
311. Yang ZH, Richard V, von Segesser J, et al. Threshold concentrations of endothelin-1 potentiate contractions to norepinephrine and serotonin in human arteries. A new mechanism of vasospasm? *Circulation* 1990;82:188–195.
312. Yoshida KI, Okabe E. Selective impairment of endothelium-dependent relaxation by sevoflurane: oxygen free radicals participation. *Anesthesiology* 1992;76:440–447.

Anesthesia: Biologic Foundations, edited by Tony L. Yaksh et al. Lippincott–Raven Publishers, Philadelphia © 1997.

CHAPTER 70

ANESTHETIC ACTION ON CEREBRAL VASCULATURE

JEFFREY R. KIRSCH AND RICHARD J. TRAYSTMAN

The main goal of this chapter is to review mechanisms of action on cerebral vasculature of anesthetics and anesthetic adjuncts. The agents that will be discussed include general anesthetics, analgesics, sedatives, and muscle relaxants. The exact mechanisms involved for alteration in cerebral blood flow (CBF) with different anesthetics appear to be different for the different classes of agents and may even be different within any particular class. However, prior to describing what is known about anesthetic actions on cerebral vasculature, we first review several basic mechanisms of control as they relate to the cerebral circulation. We then indicate, where appropriate, evidence for each of these basic control mechanisms in the vascular mechanism for anesthetic agents.

Several specific basic mechanisms of vascular control are discussed prior to a more general discussion of vascular control related to changes in physiologic variables or introduction of anesthetic agents. The basic mechanisms discussed include those involving protein kinase C, adenosine, endothelium-dependent control mechanisms (e.g., nitric oxide, endothelin), neurogenic control mechanisms (e.g., sympathetic, parasympathetic, neuropeptide Y, calcitonin gene–related peptide), cyclic adenosine monophosphate (cAMP), electrolytes (e.g., potassium, calcium), and prostaglandins.

BASIC CONTROL MECHANISMS

Protein Kinase C

Protein kinase C is an enzyme present both in cytoplasm and in association with membranes and requires calcium, phospholipids, and diacylglycerol for its full activity (129). Diacylglycerol appears to be the main regulator of protein kinase C activity. Levels of diacylglycerol in membrane are increased from membrane phosphatidylinositides by hormone or neurotransmitter activation of receptor-linked phospholipase-C. Examples of appropriate agonists include norepinephrine, angiotensin II, and arginine vasopressin. Phospholipase-C catalyzes the breakdown of phospholipids and generates inositol 1,4,5-trisphosphate and diacylglycerol. Inositol 1,4,5-triphosphate acts as an intracellular messenger to induce mobilization of calcium from sarcoplasmic reticulum (161). In the presence of diacylglycerol and a transient elevation of cytosolic calcium, protein kinase C becomes fully activated and becomes tightly associated with plasma membranes (130). Once activated, protein kinase C catalyzes phosphorylation of substrate proteins and thereby regulates ion homeostasis and neurotransmitter release by nerve cells (71). In smooth muscle cells, activation of protein kinase C causes phosphorylation of myosin light chains which results in intense contraction (148). Therefore, since this entire system appears to be very dependent on membrane function, it is likely that anesthetics may have a significant effect on this pathway.

Endothelium-Dependant Processes

Nitric Oxide

Nitric oxide (NO) or a NO-containing compound (e.g., nitrosothiol) (122,190) has been shown to be an important contributor to cerebral vascular control (81). NO is produced during conversion of L-arginine to citrulline (137) by NO synthase in vascular smooth muscle, astrocytes, and neurons (11, 121,137). Several agonists are known to cause dilation of cerebral blood vessels through a mechanism involving NO-synthase. For example, cerebral vasodilation due to acetylcholine, substance P, vasopressin, and the calcium ionophore A23187 (35,39,73), appears to be related to production of NO by endothelium. Other agents (e.g., *N*-methyl-D-aspartate) cause production of NO directly from cortical neurons (40).

Once produced, NO or related compounds activate soluble guanylyl cyclase in vascular smooth muscle. Guanylyl cyclase can also be activated by calcitonin gene–related peptide (191). Guanylyl cyclase activation results in conversion of guanosine triphosphate to 3′,5′-cyclic guanosine monophosphate (cGMP) and in vascular relaxation (65,67). The mechanism for cGMP-induced vascular relaxation appears to be related to the ability of cGMP to decrease the phosphorylation state of myosin light chains (147).

Inhibitors of NO synthase increase blood pressure and decrease CBF (51,86,87,173) without a decrease in $CMRO_2$ (51). Likewise, locally applied mono-L-arginine–containing compounds dilate piglet pial arterioles via a mechanism that can be blocked by inhibiting NO synthase (15). These data are consistent with the hypothesis that NO or a NO-containing compound is important in tonic control of CBF.

Endothelin

Although it is likely that there exist many endothelium-dependent constricting factors, endothelin is the first such compound that was identified and characterized (196). Once formed, endothelin acts at a specific receptor on vascular smooth muscle to produce contraction (62). However, the contractile response to endothelin is inhibited by L-type calcium channel blockers (50). Proposed mechanisms of action of endothelin include opening L-type calcium channels via the endothelin receptor (79) and actions to stimulate a pathway involving protein kinase C and G protein (119). Endothelin has been implicated in several disease states associated with decreased CBF; however, its production in response to pharmacologic stimulation is unclear (156).

Neurogenic Control Mechanisms

Sympathetic Nerves

Cerebral blood vessels are densely innervated with sympathetic fibers. There appears to be variability regarding the effect of stimulation of sympathetic nerves on CBF depending on the experimental conditions. For example, under control conditions sympathetic stimulation results in no change in CBF in dogs (178), whereas it is associated with a decrease in CBF during hypercapnia (22) and hypertension. There also appear to be differences in effect of stimulation between species (61).

Once norepinephrine is released from the noradrenergic nerve terminal it may affect presynaptic α_2-receptors and result in decreased release of norepinephrine from the nerve terminal and, depending on the species being studied, may affect postsynaptic α_1- or α_2-receptors and result in vasoconstriction. Because the contractile response of vascular smooth muscle in response to receptor stimulation is attenuated by calcium channel blockers, calcium is considered key in the mechanism of adrenergic mediated vasoconstriction (34). Once calcium enters the cell, it interacts with calmodulin and directly activates the smooth muscle contractile apparatus.

Parasympathetic Nerves

Parasympathetic cholinergic nerves are present in the adventitia of cerebral blood vessels (152). The origin for these cholinergic nerves appears to be the sphenopalatine, otic and internal carotid ganglia (58,168). Once acetylcholine is produced by the nerves, it diffuses through the smooth muscle to act on muscarinic receptors on endothelium to produce NO or a NO-containing compound (122,190). In addition to nerves that produce acetylcholine, the sphenopalatine ganglion also contains nerves which produce vasoactive intestinal peptide and nerves which produce NO (132). It is likely that all of these substances released from parasympathetic nerves participate in the cerebral vasodilation associated with stimulation of parasympathetic ganglia (49). Parasympathetic sensory fibers appear to originate from the trigeminal ganglion and contain substance P and calcitonin gene–related peptide (104). The potential significance of these nerves in mediating vasodilation in vivo is demonstrated by attenuation of postischemic hyperemia following trigeminal ganglionectomy (97).

Calcitonin Gene–Related Peptide

This peptide is contained within nerve fibers originating in the trigeminal ganglia and innervate cerebral arteries, pial arterioles, and cerebral veins (181). Calcitonin gene–related peptide is the most potent vasodilator contained within the trigeminal nerves. Vasodilation presumably depends on specific receptors; however, these have not yet been identified. Vasodilation does not depend on an intact endothelium (35). The mechanism for dilation appears to be due to an increase in cAMP (35). Some commonly used pharmacologic agents (e.g., nitroglycerin, nitroprusside) act to release calcitonin gene–related peptide from trigeminovascular fibers (191). However, in this paradigm, it acts by activating guanylyl cyclase and production of cGMP to produce cerebral vasodilation (191).

cAMP

Several different agonists have been found to act at specific receptors to activate adenylate cyclase to produce cAMP. Once the agonist acts on the receptor, the receptor activates a specific G protein complexing it to guanosine triphosphate (GTP) which then amplifies the extracellular hormonal signal into adenylate cyclase activity. For cerebral blood vessels agonists include calcitonin gene–related peptide, adenosine, and vasoactive intestinal polypeptide (35). Once cAMP is produced, it may block calcium-activated potassium channels (100) or inhibit the interaction of calcium with the myosin heads. On the contrary, neuropeptide Y, opiates (μ-receptor agonists), and α_2-adrenoceptor agonists are inhibitors of cAMP accumulation and produce constriction (45). Inhibitors of adenylate cyclase mediate their inhibition through a specific inhibitory G protein.

Electrolytes

Potassium

Potassium has been considered to be an important mediator of flow-metabolism coupling. This is based on the finding that in physiologic concentrations (up to 9 mM) potassium is a potent vasodilator and is released into the extracellular space during neuronal activation. However, this has been questioned because neuronal activation does not always result in appropriate changes in extracellular potassium (4). The mechanism for cerebral vasodilation from potassium presumably results from depolarization of the vascular smooth muscle. At high concentrations, potassium may also cause vasoconstriction via a mechanism which involves stimulation of voltage-sensitive calcium channels (9).

Calcium

Calcium appears to enter smooth muscle cells in one of several ways. For example, there are two types of calcium channels: voltage-activated and agonist-operated. Voltage-activated channels are opened as the potential across the cell membrane is reduced. This may occur when potassium enters the cell and depolarizes the sarcolemma. Once calcium enters the cell it interacts with calmodulin and directly activates the smooth muscle contractile apparatus.

Voltage-activated channels in smooth muscle can be further subdivided into L-type (long-lasting), T-type (transient), and N-type (neither L nor T) (131), the former being blocked by the classical (dihydropyridine) calcium antagonists they appear to have no effect on N-type calcium channels, which are present only on neurons (149). Interestingly the contractile responses of cerebral arteries to potassium, norepinephrine and neuropeptide Y are equally sensitive to calcium antagonists and, therefore, all appear to equally activate voltage-activated channels (32,34).

There also exists agonist-operated calcium channels, which allow calcium entry into cells without depolarization (9). For example, it is thought that ATP produces some of its vascular effects through activation of these receptors (7). When applied locally, excitatory amino acids stimulate agonist-operated channels and are associated with cerebral vasodilation (14). Although it is possible that these agonists directly affect vascular smooth muscle to produce vasodilation this is opposite the effect that would be anticipated from increased entry of calcium into vascular smooth muscle. A more likely explanation for the cerebral vasodilation produced by excitatory amino acids relates to their stimulatory effect on neuronal tissue which would cause an increase in CBF linked to an increase in metabolic rate (128). Recently, NO has been demonstrated to be the mediator of the vasodilation produced during local application of excitatory amino acids in cranial windows (40). This study also confirmed the hypothesis that the origin of NO is from neuronal tissue because there is no increase when the preparation is treated with tetrodotoxin. In addition, excitatory amino acids did not cause dilation of isolated middle cerebral and basilar arteries which suggests that agonist-operated calcium channels are on vascular smooth muscle and are of little physiologic significance in control of cerebral vascular tone (40).

Prostaglandins

Cerebral blood vessels are able to produce both thromboxanes, which cause platelet aggregation and vasoconstriction, and prostacyclin, which inhibits platelet aggregation and is a potent vasodilator (54). The exact cellular mechanisms for the effects on cerebrovascular tone of the cyclooxygenase metabolites have not been precisely delineated. However, prostaglandin $F_{2\alpha}$ appears to cause vasodilation through a mechanism which involves stimulation of NO-synthase in vascular endothelium (82). On the contrary, vasodilation from prostacyclin is thought to occur via a mechanism that involves cAMP (66). The vasoconstrictor thromboxane A_2 appears to effect specific vasoconstricting prostaglandin receptors which act to promote calcium uptake from low-affinity binding sites through channels activated by release of calcium from internal stores (193).

Vasodilating products of the cyclooxygenase pathway are thought to be produced tonically in the cerebral circulation since administration of cyclooxygenase inhibitors result in a decrease in resting CBF (143). In addition, products of the cyclooxygenase pathway greatly attenuate hypercapnia-induced hyperemia (143). However, this effect on hypercapnic hyperemia is specific since inhibition of the cyclooxygenase pathway has no effect on the cerebrovascular response to changes in arterial blood pressure (142), or hypoxic hyperemia (153), postischemic hyperemia (72) or hypoglycemic hyperemia (127).

As presented above there are many potential modulators of the cerebral vasculature. It is likely that anesthetics alter many of these pathways. However, only few have been tested either in vitro or in whole animal preparations. We will concentrate the remainder of the discussion on what is known mechanistically with how specific anesthetic agents alter the cerebral vasculature.

MECHANISM OF ANESTHETIC ACTION ON THE CEREBRAL VASCULATURE

Barbiturates

Barbiturates decrease both CBF and $CMRO_2$ in humans (144,188). In dogs during treatment with barbiturates $CMRO_2$ decreases progressively until the electroencephalogram becomes isoelectric. Treatment with barbiturates does not prevent CBF autoregulation (26); however, the response to hypoxia (26) and hypercapnia is attenuated in dog because of metabolic depression (47,94). The mechanism of metabolic depression by barbiturates is unknown but may be related to potentiation of chloride ion permeability due to a barbiturate effect to enhance the binding of γ-aminobutyric acid (GABA) to its receptor (135).

In addition to its effect on metabolism barbiturates may have direct effects on vascular tone. In an early study pentobarbital was noted to decrease basal vascular tone (102). However, more recently the direct vascular effects of a variety of barbiturates has been evaluated (60). In isolated cerebral arteries, thiamylal and thiopental caused a dose-related contraction, but this did not occur in arteries treated with pentobarbital. The mechanism for vasoconstriction, in these isolated vessels, appears to be due to influx of calcium from extracellular fluid into vascular smooth muscle and does not appear to be related to an effect on α-adrenergic, serotonergic or histaminergic H1-activation pathways (60). Although these isolated cerebral vessel experiments suggest that the in vivo observation of decreased CBF in response to systemic administration of barbiturates may be related to a direct vascular effect, pial vessel experiments do not support this hypothesis. For example, Levasseur and Kontos (94) have demonstrated that an anesthetic concentration of pentobarbital does not alter baseline pial vessel diameter; however, pentobarbital was associated with a decreased cerebrovascular response to hypercapnia. In this study (94), because CBF was not measured, it is unclear what effect pentobarbital had on CBF. It is possible that pentobarbital still may have been associated with a decrease in CBF because of changes in vascular diameter "upstream" (e.g., large cerebral blood vessels that are typically used in in vitro studies) or "downstream" from the site of the pial vascular measurement. Therefore, the clinical observation of a decrease in CBF with barbiturate administration appears to be a multifactorial response mediated by decreased cerebral metabolism and a direct vasoconstrictor response of some of the barbiturates (particularly thiobarbiturates).

Barbiturates also affect agonist-induced cerebral vasoconstrictor response. For example, in goat pentobarbital decreased the contraction due to norepinephrine, 5-hydroxytryptamine, and potassium chloride (102). In cat pentobarbital attenuated the vasoconstrictor response to potassium chloride, norepinephrine, and prostaglandin $F_{2\alpha}$ (36). At very high concentrations pentobarbital attenuates vasoconstriction to endothelin (169). The mechanism for decreasing the vasoconstrictor response to these agonists appears to be related to blocking influx of calcium into vascular smooth muscle cells (154). Barbiturates have inhibitory action on both calcium entry from extracellular stores as well as release from intracellular stores (102). In addition, barbiturates could also affect the vascular response to these agonists by inhibiting protein kinase C activation (113,150). The mechanism by which barbiturates interfere with protein kinase C activation probably involves an interaction with membrane components of this signal transduction pathway (113).

Volatile Anesthetics

Although a significant amount of effort has been expended there is still no consensus of opinion as to the mechanism of cerebral vasodilation with inhalational anesthetics. The goal of this section will be to present the evidence for different mechanisms that have been evaluated. Inhalational anesthetics cause an increase in CBF in vivo (21,48,95,177) and vasodilation of cerebral blood vessels in vitro (42,68). Associated with the increase in CBF is a decrease in $CMRO_2$ and consumption of glucose (56,177) with maintenance of adequate cerebral high energy phosphate content (85). The decrease in $CMRO_2$ is linked to a decrease in EEG activity and does not decrease further after the EEG becomes isoelectric (125). Desflurane also produces an increase in CBF and decrease in $CMRO_2$ that is similar in magnitude to the other potent inhalational anesthetics (96). During administration of inhalational anesthetics flow-metabolism coupling remains intact (56). Therefore, because inhalational anesthetics cause both an increase in CBF and a decrease in brain metabolism it is unlikely that vasodilation is metabolically mediated.

Although in vitro data suggest that halothane is a more potent vasodilator than is isoflurane (68), the direct vasodilator potential in vivo appears similar between isoflurane and halothane (30). It has been speculated that a finding of greater cerebral vasodilation by halothane as compared to isoflurane by some laboratories in vivo is due to greater reduction of $CMRO_2$ by isoflurane as compared to halothane (30). Still other investigators have found that isoflurane may be a more potent cerebral vasodilator than halothane (56). Interestingly, it has been speculated that some of the difference between groups for relative vascular response for the inhalational anesthetics may be due to inherent differences in tissue regions measured since these anesthetics cause different alterations in regional CBF (57). For example, halothane causes a greater increase in neocortical blood flow than does isoflurane (57).

The cerebral hyperemic response to inhalational anesthetics is only transient in subprimate mammals (13), but we have recently found it to be sustained in primates (109). Despite the transient nature of hyperemia in subprimate mammals anesthetized with isoflurane, there is no alteration in cerebral vascular response to hypercapnia over time (108). Cerebral autoregulation is preserved at 1 MAC concentration but not at higher concentrations (107,112,114).

Nitric Oxide

Many different mechanisms have been suggested for production of vasodilation which results from inhalational anesthetics. These include mechanisms involving NO, alteration in cellular calcium homeostasis, excitatory amino acids, free radicals, and prostanoids. The role of NO in the mechanism of cerebral vasodilation has been evaluated both in vivo and in vitro based predominately on the ability to block inhalational agent–induced vasodilation with agents which inhibit NO-synthase. Unfortunately, many of these experiments were done in blood vessels from outside the cerebral circulation yet the results have been generalized to the circulation in general. We have presented the data from both cerebral and extracerebral blood vessels in hopes of supplying the reader with a better understanding of the potential mechanisms of action for inhalational anesthetic–induced cerebral vasodilation. In addition, most of the data presented tend to be inferential in nature since they do not directly correlate the degree of dilation with the amount of NO being produced.

In in vitro studies in isolated precontracted ring preparations of rat thoracic aorta with intact endothelium, isoflurane and enflurane caused vasoconstriction at low concentrations and vasodilation at higher concentrations (164). In isolated thoracic rat aorta, isoflurane caused dose-dependent vasodilation that was not impaired by removal of endothelium or treatment with N-nitro-L-arginine methyl ester (L-NAME, in either endothelium-intact or endothelium-denuded vessels) or correlated with an increase in cGMP (12). In middle cerebral artery rings isoflurane produces a dose-dependent vasodilation not affected by inhibition of NO-synthase with N^G-mono-methyl-L-arginine (L-NMMA), inhibition of cyclo-oxygenase with indomethacin or removal of endothelium (42). Jensen et al (68) reported that the direct vasodilator response of halothane on basilar artery was greater than that of isoflurane in basilar artery but not in the midline ear artery. In isolated basilar artery (68), like middle cerebral artery (42), vasodilation remained intact despite removal of endothelium. However in isolated basilar artery removal of endothelium was only confirmed by "observing a *diminished* dilator response to acetylcholine," (68) not by observing an ablated response to acetylcholine.

In addition inhalational anesthetics have been demonstrated to, in fact, attenuate vasodilator mechanisms that depend on endothelium derived relaxation factor (EDRF). For example, halothane, enflurane, and isoflurane attenuate both receptor and non–receptor-mediated EDRF production in peripheral vessels (182). In canine carotid artery, although halothane decreased tension by a non–endothelium-dependent mechanism, it prevented endothelium-dependent relaxation produced by other agonists (120). Although these in vitro data would suggest that neither endothelium, NO or cGMP play an important role in vasodilation from inhalational anesthetics, halothane has recently been shown to cause an increase in diameter of canine middle cerebral arterial rings with intact endothelium, via a mechanism that involves either stimulation of particulate guanylate cyclase (but not soluble guanylate cyclase) or inhibition of cGMP phosphodiesterase (38). The mechanism for activation of particulate guanylate cyclase may involve halothane-mediated increases in membrane fluidity which is a mechanism for activation of particulate guanylate cyclase by other agonists (88). Another possible mechanism for increasing cGMP in brain may involve an interaction between inhalational agents and the α-adrenoceptor. For example, in heart, halothane causes an increase in tissue cGMP levels by a mechanism that can be blocked by both prazosin, a selective α_1-adrenergic antagonist, and yohimbine, an α_2-adrenergic antagonist (186). These investigators have also determined that the effect of halothane on the adrenergic nervous system is at the level of the receptor rather than at adrenergic nerve endings (186).

Interestingly, in endothelium-denuded rat aortae halothane causes vasodilation by a mechanism which is associated with an increase in cGMP and inhibited with methylene blue (which inhibits guanylate cyclase) (124). This finding is consistent with a mechanism for halothane-induced vasodilation, which potentially involves production of NO from a source other than endothelium (80). Other evidence for a potential role of NO in inhalational anesthetic–induced vasodilation comes from the finding that isoflurane attenuates vasoconstriction to serotonin, phenylephrine, and prostaglandin $F_{2\alpha}$ in isolated coronary artery rings in the presence, but not in the absence of endothelium (8).

In in vivo preparations inhibition of NO-synthase dose dependently and reversibly reduces the threshold for halothane anesthesia in rat (70) suggesting some interaction of NO with inhalational anesthetics. In addition, halothane causes an increase in cGMP measured in cortex but a decrease in cGMP in cerebellum (123), a region of high NO-synthase activity (11). Also consistent with a role for NO in the mechanism of vasodilation in vivo is the finding that inhibition of NO-synthase results in an increase in blood pressure, and systemic vascular resistance (52). More recently we have more directly determined the role of NO in the mechanism of vasodilation in vivo. We have found that inhibition of NO synthase prevents cerebral hyperemia to halothane, isoflurane and N_2O in dogs under baseline pentobarbital anesthesia (110). In pigs we have found that the ability of an NO-synthase inhibitor to prevent isoflurane-induced hyperemia can be reversed with L-arginine which further supports a direct role of NO in the mechanism of isoflurane-induced cerebral hyperemia (117). In rats, using a pial vessel preparation, others have also found that NO is an important mediator of halothane-induced cerebral vasodilation (84). One possible reason for the discrepancy between the finding of little or no role for NO in the mechanism for cerebral vasodilation in vitro, whereas NO appears to be very important in the mechanism of vasodilation in vivo may be because in vivo inhalation anesthetics may stimulate NO-synthase present in perivascular nerves (176), astrocytes (121), and neurons (11) that are not present in the in vitro preparation.

We conclude that NO as an important mediator of inhalational agent induced cerebral vasodilation in vivo. The source of NO production may be perivascular nerves (176), astrocytes (121), and/or parenchymal neurons (11).

Prostanoids

The role of vasodilator prostanoids in the mechanism of inhalational anesthetic–induced vasodilation has been suggested by Stone and Johns (164). In their study (164) using isolated endothelium-intact rat thoracic aortae, indomethacin was found to prevent vasodilation produced by halothane, enflurane, and isoflurane. On the contrary, other investigators (42) found that isoflurane-induced vasodilation in isolated canine middle cerebral artery rings was not dependant on endothelium and was not affected by treatment with indomethacin.

In vivo prostanoids clearly play an important role in the mechanism of isoflurane-induced vasodilation (117). This is because indomethacin markedly attenuated isoflurane-induced vasodilation and there was no further effect of inhibition of NO-synthase, whereas both agents separately also caused marked attenuation of isoflurane-induced cerebral hyperemia. These data suggest a link between a prostanoid and NO mechanism for isoflurane-induced cerebral hyperemia. Prostanoids appear to cause vasodilation by a mechanism which involves cAMP. Therefore, the finding that halothane and isoflurane increase cAMP in rat thoracic aorta strips is consistent with an effect of prostanoids in the mechanism of vasodilation in vivo (162).

NO has also been found to induce release of prostacyclin from endothelium (27). Other evidence for a link between a prostanoid and NO mechanism comes from studies by Ignarro and Kadowitz (67), which suggest that arachidonic acid may increase levels of cGMP. This effect is inhibited by methylene blue, but not by indomethacin (67). Shimokawa and Vanhoutte (157) similarly demonstrated that exogenously administered prostacyclin causes relaxation of porcine coronary arteries, an effect which is potentiated in the presence of endothelium. This potentiation is inhibited by oxyhemoglobin but not by indomethacin, suggesting that prostacyclin facilitates the release of NO. Our data (117) cannot be specific in defining the interaction between these two systems; however, it seems likely that the two are closely linked in mediating isoflurane-mediated vasodilation.

Free Radicals

As discussed above, inhalational anesthetics attenuate both receptor and non–receptor-mediated EDRF production in peripheral (182) and cerebral blood vessels (120). Oxygen radicals produced by inhalational anesthetics (197) may result in alteration of NO-mediated mechanisms by one of several mechanisms. First, oxygen radicals may cause direct injury of endothelium (189); however, we are unaware of any evidence for endothelial injury following inhalational anesthetics. Second, impairment of endothelium-dependent vasodilation may be related to direct inactivation of NO by superoxide anion (53,151). Although direct inactivation of NO by inhalational anesthetic–induced production of superoxide anion may be an explanation for altered in vitro agonist-induced endothelium-dependent vascular responses (120,182) and direct vasoconstriction of isolated vessels by inhalation anesthetics (164), we do not believe that this is clinically relevant because several NO mediated events are quite robust even in the presence of inhalational anesthetics. For example, we have found that cerebral hyperemia during administration of the cholinergic agonist oxotremorine, which causes NO-mediated vasodilation (139), is actually accentuated during isoflurane anesthesia as compared to during pentobarbital anesthesia (165). Likewise, if oxygen radicals were important in the mechanism of inhalational agent-induced cerebral hyperemia administration of oxygen radical scavengers would be expected to decrease CBF during inhalational anesthesia. Although superoxide dismutase has no effect on CBF during N_2O fentanyl anesthesia (103) its effect on CBF during anesthesia with potent inhalational anesthetics has not been reported.

Excitatory Amino Acids

Another potential mechanism for inhalational anesthetic-induced cerebral hyperemia may involve an excitatory amino acid pathway. Enflurane is an agent which produces seizure-like burst discharges from CA1 neurons in rat hippocampal slices which are completely prevented by *N*-methyl-D-aspartate receptor antagonist (98) and causes glutamate release from cortical synaptosomes (63). Halothane also caused release of glutamate but to a lessor extent than that observed with enflurane (63). Excitatory amino acids have been recently shown to cause cerebral vasodilation in a pial vessel preparation through a mechanism which involves release of NO from neurons (40). Although this excitatory amino acid–linked NO mechanism may account for some portion of in vivo hyperemia from inhalational anesthetics, it could not account for vasodilation in vitro because of the absence of neurons in in vitro preparations.

In addition, since excitatory amino acid receptors are only present in a limited number of brain regions (10,115) activation of these receptors during inhalation anesthesia would not account for the generalized increase in CBF which is observed. Although the noncompetitive NMDA receptor antagonist causes a marked reduction in CBF and $CMRO_2$ during a variety of anesthetic conditions, we have not found the competitive NMDA receptor antagonist, NPC-17742 to be associated with any reduction in CBF in cats anesthetized with halothane. Therefore, our data do not support a role for excitatory amino acids in the mechanism of vasodilation from inhalational anesthetics.

Calcium

Su and Bell (166) demonstrated that isoflurane and halothane decreased the maximal calcium-activated tension development in skeletal muscle. Su and Zhang (167) demonstrated that, in KCl-contracted isolated aortic rings, halothane produced an initial slight increase in tension followed by a decreased tension which was independent of endothelium. Halothane also caused an increase in tension in acetylcholine or nitroprusside relaxed vessels. Halothane decreased calcium accumulation in sarcoplasmic reticulum and increased release from sarcoplasmic reticulum. These investigators concluded that halothane directly caused vascular contraction or relaxation depending on the condition. In rat thoracic aorta strips (179), halothane and isoflurane increased cytosolic calcium ion concentration with a slight increase in tension in the resting state. However, these anesthetics suppressed the increases in smooth muscle tension and cytosolic calcium ion concentration in a concentration-dependent manner both during potassium- and norepinephrine-induced smooth muscle contraction. In cultured vascular smooth muscle cells (158), halothane caused impaired calcium storage in cells. In neuronal cells, halothane causes an acute increase in intracellular calcium which is associated with activation of potassium channels and depressed excitability (126). On the contrary, halothane only causes gradual depletion of calcium for internal stores (126).

In cerebral blood vessels, inhalational anesthetics cause membrane depolarization despite vascular relaxation suggesting uncoupling between membrane potential and vascular contraction (59). Volatile anesthetics also cause a depression in both calcium and potassium currents and a complex interaction for blockade of these two channels (101). The importance of these vascular mechanisms related to calcium fluxes have not yet been evaluated in vivo. The difficulty in evaluating this response in vivo is that the pharmacologic probes (e.g., ryanodine, which blocks release of calcium from sarcoplasmic reticulum) that could be used would be detrimental to other organs. Therefore, as it relates to calcium, although current data can explain how inhalational anesthetics can prevent agonist-induced vasoconstriction, these data do not fully explain why inhalational anesthetics are associated with spontaneous vasodilation.

Nitrous Oxide

In dogs and goats, nitrous oxide is associated with an increase in CBF and brain metabolism (140,174). However, in rats, nitrous oxide does not alter CBF or metabolism (16). In humans, nitrous oxide causes a small decrease in cerebral metabolism without a change in CBF (159). The difference between species on the cerebral vascular effect of nitrous oxide may be due to a difference in MAC (minimum alveolar concentration of inhaled anesthetic required to prevent 50% of subjects from responding to a painful stimulus) between species with dog having the highest MAC. At subanesthetic concentrations of nitrous oxide, cerebral excitation may occur (195). In order to minimize the excitation effects of subanesthetic concentrations of nitrous oxide, others (29) have evaluated the effect during concomitant administration of other anesthetics. In this study, it was found that the CBF response to nitrous oxide was increased with increasing concentrations of halothane but not with morphine (29). Therefore, these authors concluded that the mechanism of vasodilation following nitrous oxide administration was not likely due to a secondary effect of increased cerebral metabolism. Consistent with the conclusion that nitrous oxide does not increase CBF via a metabolic-linked mechanism, Baughman et al. (5) found that nitrous oxide increased CBF in rats without an increase in cerebral oxygen consumption or an increase in plasma catecholamines. We have found that inhibiting NO synthase prevented nitrous oxide–induced cerebral hyperemia in dogs with baseline pentobarbital anesthesia suggesting a role for NO in the mechanism of dilation (110).

We conclude that nitrous oxide causes a mild degree of cerebral vasodilation via a mechanism which involves activation of NO synthase and increasing cerebral metabolism.

Ketamine

In in vitro preparations ketamine inhibits vascular contraction by interfering with transmembrane calcium influx, and by blocking some step in release of calcium from intracellular stores. It is proposed that the main site for the direct vascular effect of ketamine is in blocking hydrolysis of phosphatydylinositol 4,5-bisphosphate (PIP_2) with impaired production of 1,4,5-triphosphate ($InsP_3$) (76). Therefore, although ketamine may interfere with synthesis of intracellular second messengers (75). This does not necessarily predict the mechanism for cerebral vasodilation during ketamine administration.

In halothane- and N_2O-anesthetized dogs ketamine results in an initial increase in CBF followed by a period of decreased

CBF in the presence of EEG activation and an increased $CMRO_2$ (25). Pretreatment with thiopental prevented the increase in CBF, $CMRO_2$, and EEG activation that occurs with ketamine suggesting that the mechanism for increased CBF is due to cerebral activation (25). In unanesthetized humans, ketamine increases CBF without an increase in cerebral metabolism (171). In unanesthetized rat, ketamine produces decreased glucose metabolism in somatosensory and auditory systems with increased metabolism in the limbic system (20) and increase in brain levels of cAMP (99). Therefore, from in vivo data ketamine-induced cerebral hyperemia may either be due to an increase in metabolism or related to some mechanism which works through increasing cAMP. Although ketamine appears to impair production of 1,4,5-triphosphate ($InsP_3$) (76) in response to specific agonists, alteration of this pathway does not appear to account for the increase in CBF which occurs with ketamine under baseline conditions.

Etomidate

Etomidate causes a reduced CBF and $CMRO_2$ while blood pressure is well maintained (46). Although the mechanism for reduction in CBF is believed to be due to a reduction in $CMRO_2$, this is not proven. Etomidate does not appear to dilate or constrict isolated blood vessels (within the cremaster muscle) (3) but may cause release of dilator prostanoids which then could result in indirect vasodilation. Because the clinical response to etomidate is a reduction in CBF, we conclude that prostanoid release must be minimal.

Opiates

In laboratory animals, systemic administration of opiates has been demonstrated to increase (64,134), decrease (170), or not change (111) CBF and either is associated with a decrease (170) or no change in $CMRO_2$ (64,111). In humans, opiates either cause no change in CBF (69,105,118) and $CMRO_2$ (69) or a decrease in $CMRO_2$ despite no change in CBF (118). We believe that the difference in response for different species relates to differences between species in indirect effects of opiates and because of differences between species in the distribution of different opiate receptors on the cerebral blood vessels.

Opiates may have indirect effects that independently affect CBF. For example, morphine causes release of histamine (175), which may cause cerebral vasodilation. Opiates may also alter CBF because they inhibit release of acetylcholine, norepinephrine, substance P, and dopamine (160) and stimulate adenylate cyclase activity (136) in the CNS (160). Therefore, some investigators have attempted to learn more about the direct effects of opiates on the cerebral vasculature by studying these drugs in vitro.

Evidence for a direct vascular effect of opiates comes from the finding of opiate receptors in association with intracerebral microvessels and Met-enkephalin–like immunoactive profiles in close proximity to cerebral arterioles (77,141). Because most of the clinically relevant opiate receptors are primarily μ-receptor agonists, dilation of isolated cerebral vessels in response to these agonists suggests the presence of μ-receptors on cerebral vessels. For example, in cat cerebral vessels opiates produce vasodilation (55,83,187) despite no change in CBF (155). In dog, however, μ and σ opiate receptors are not present on cerebral vessels, but instead these vessels appear to contain κ receptors. Although κ receptors mediate relaxation when stimulated by appropriate agonists (1) specific agonists of κ receptors are not used clinically for analgesia. In order for clinically relevant opiates (e.g., morphine) to have effects on the cerebral vasculature, very high concentrations need to be obtained (64). In piglets fentanyl, sufentanil and alfentanil constrict pial vessels (116) whereas naturally occurring opiates constrict or dilate pial vessels depending on the concentration studied and the opiate receptor which was being stimulated (2). For example, μ, δ, and κ receptor agonists vasodilated while ε receptor agonist vasoconstricted. Interestingly, in piglets blocking production of prostanoids with indomethacin also blocks vasodilation from the naturally occurring opiates (2).

We conclude that at clinically relevant doses the effect of opiates on CBF is limited. If opiates that do not cause systemic release of histamine are used, the predominant finding following systemic administration would be at most a minor reduction in CBF which would be linked to a reduction in $CMRO_2$.

Propofol

Few studies have investigated the effect of propofol on CBF. However, all studies demonstrate a decrease in CBF that is linked to a decrease in $CMRO_2$ in normal subjects (163,184, 185) and reduction in cerebral electrical activity (194). The effects of propofol on cerebral glucose metabolism are characterized by a dose-related, widespread depression which was most pronounced in forebrain (24). Reversal of metabolic suppression was consistent with the rapid duration of action of this drug (24). The cellular mechanism for propofol-induced reduction in cerebral metabolism is not known. The mechanism of reduced CBF does not appear to be due to any direct vascular effects because in vitro propofol appears to cause vasodilation (at least of systemic vessels), not vasoconstriction (138).

Propofol does not alter ability of the cerebral vasculature to autoregulate (184,194); however, it may attenuate the cerebrovascular response to alteration in CO_2 (37). In the setting of brain injury, propofol decreases both CBF and cerebral perfusion pressure without a change in cerebrovascular resistance which suggests a lack of autoregulatory ability (145). We conclude that the overall effect of propofol is to decrease CBF by a mechanism linked to a reduction in cerebral metabolism but the cellular mechanism is unknown.

α_2-Agonists

Systemic administration of the α_2-agonist dexmedetomidine results in sedation (6), a decrease in CBF and a transient decrease in ICP (199) without a change in $CMRO_2$ (78,198). Binding sites for α_2-agonists are most highly concentrated in areas of brain involved in control of cardiovascular function (183). Stimulation of α_2-adrenoceptors results in constriction of cerebral and coronary vessels, which is moderated by endogenous production of NO in the coronary circulation but not the cerebral circulation (19). Stimulation of α_2-adrenoceptors in the locus coeruleus appears to be important in the mechanism of hypnosis with dexmedetomidine (18). Cerebral arteries are enriched with postsynaptic α_2-adrenoceptors (180) which when stimulated cause vasoconstriction (19). The effector mechanism for vasoconstriction and sedation from stimulation of α_2-adrenoceptors appears to involve inhibitory G proteins (28) with inhibition of adenylate cyclase and decreased accumulation of cAMP (106). There is no evidence that the mechanism of hypnosis is linked to the mechanism for alteration in CBF since the decrease in CBF occurs without a change in $CMRO_2$. In addition, the effect on blood flow is not mediated by a change in pial vessel diameter (74). Associated with α_2-adrenoceptor activation an attenuated CBF response to hypercapnia (74).

Benzodiazepines

Benzodiazepines cause a decrease in cerebral metabolism and blood flow (41,44,133). At least a portion of their effects in brain appear to be linked to modulation of the postsynaptic response to GABA, which then acts to increase postsynaptic membrane permeability to chloride ions (135). Associated with the increase in membrane permeability is a generalized reduction in EEG and brain function (43). In addition, even though benzodiazepines decrease CBF, they result in no impairment of cerebral energy charge, brain glucose, lactate or pyruvate (133) suggesting that the decrease in CBF does not cause ischemia. The maximal reduction of CBF and $CMRO_2$ with benzodiazepines appears to be less than that observed with other anesthetics because of presumed saturation of benzodiazepine receptors. The benzodiazepine antagonist RO 15-1788 reverses the cerebral vascular and metabolic effects of midazolam in dog (41) and prevents the decrease in CBF with midazolam in humans without having any direct effects on cerebral vascular control itself (43).

Muscle Relaxants

Nondepolarizing muscle relaxants block nicotinic receptors at the neuromuscular junction. Nicotinic receptors also exist on perivascular adrenergic nerves in the cerebral circulation (33), and therefore it is possible that nondepolarizing muscle relaxants may have an indirect effect on the cerebral circulation. However, nondepolarizing muscle relaxants are typically large and charged molecules that do not readily cross the blood-brain barrier and therefore under normal circumstances nondepolarizing muscle relaxants without other systemic effects have been found to have no effect on CBF (17,91, 146,192). Agents (e.g., curare) that cause systemic histamine release may cause cerebral vasodilation (192), but this does not necessarily cause a change in CBF (17) because of other compensatory mechanisms. Likewise, even though administration of atracurium is associated with EEG activation through accumulation of its metabolite laudanosine, it is not associated with an increase in CBF (91) or alteration in ICP (31).

Interestingly some of the nondepolarizing neuromuscular antagonists (e.g., d-Tubocurarine and pancuronium) extend the lower limit of cerebral autoregulation by a mechanism which is related to their ability to cause blockade of ganglionic nicotinic receptors (17). Pancuronium has also been demonstrated to attenuate the CBF response to seizures (146). The mechanism for this has been hypothesized to be related to elimination of skeletal muscle spindle afferent input to the brain (146) but may also be due to attenuation of the blood pressure response to seizures via a mechanism which involves blockade of ganglionic nicotinic receptors (17).

Succinylcholine has been found to cause a transient increase in CBF and EEG activation without a change in $CMRO_2$ by a mechanism that involves increases in muscle afferent activity (89,92). Associated with an increase in CBF there is an increase in ICP, which is transient in nature. Although succinylcholine also causes EEG activation when applied topically on cerebral cortex (172), it is not likely that succinylcholine directly affects brain because it does not cross the blood-brain barrier (23). In addition, even when the blood-brain barrier is disrupted intravenous administration of succinylcholine is not associated with any further alteration in EEG, CBF, or $CMRO_2$ than what occurs in the presence of an intact blood-brain barrier (93). Because the increase in afferent activity does not depend on muscle movement, administration of a defasiculating dose of pancuronium does not attenuate the CBF response to succinylcholine (89). However, since the cerebral vascular response appears to depend on EEG activation administration of succinylcholine in electrically dysfunctioning brain (e.g., following cerebral ischemia (90), or presumably during deep planes of anesthesia) results in a greatly attenuated hyperemic response. We conclude that under normal clinically relevant conditions nondepolarizing and depolarizing muscle relaxants have little effect on CBF and ICP.

CONCLUSION

Despite much work published in the area, the exact mechanism of anesthetic action on cerebral blood vessels and blood flow is not known. Although important studies that evaluate anesthetic effects in vitro and at the cellular level are now emerging, in order to truly understand the mechanisms involved in humans future experiments must determine if any of these proposed pathways have relevance in vivo in animals.

REFERENCES

1. Altura BT, Altura BM, Quirion R. Identification of benzomorphan-kappa opiate receptors in cerebral arteries which subserve relaxation. *Br J Pharmacol* 1984;82:459–466.
2. Armstead WM, Mirro R, Busija DW, Leffler CW. Prostanoids modulate opioid cerebrovascular responses in newborn pigs. *J Pharmacol Exp Ther* 1990;255:1083–1089.
3. Asher EF, Alsip NL, Zhang PY, Harris PD. Prostaglandin-related microvascular dilation in pentobarbital-and etomidate-anesthetized rats. *Anesthesiology* 1992;76:271–278.
4. Astrup J, Heuser D, Lassen NA, Nilsson B, Norberg K, Siesjo BK. Evidence against H^+ and K^+ as main factors for the control of cerebral blood. 1977;110–116.
5. Baughman VL, Hoffman WE, Miletich DJ, Albrecht RF. Cerebrovascular and cerebral metabolic effects of N_2O in unrestrained rats. *Anesthesiology* 1990;73:269–272.
6. Belleville JP, Ward DS, Bloor BC, Maze M. Effects of intravenous dexmedetomidine in humans. 1. Sedation, ventilation, and metabolic rate. *Anesthesiology* 1992;77:1125–1133.
7. Benham CD, Tsien RW. A novel receptor-operated Ca^{2+}-permeable channel activated by ATP in smooth muscle. *Nature* 1987; 328:275–278.
8. Blaise G, Sill JC, Nugent M, Van Dyke RA, Vanhoutte PM. Isoflurane causes endothelium-dependent inhibition of contractile responses of canine coronary arteries. *Anesthesiology* 1987;67: 513–517.
9. Bolton TB. Mechanisms of action of transmitters and other substances on smooth muscle. *Physiol Rev* 1979;59:606–718.
10. Bowery NG, Wong EH, Hudson AL. Quantitative autoradiography of [^{3}H]-MK-801 binding sites in mammalian brain. *Br J Pharmacol* 1988;93:944–954.
11. Bredt DS, Hwang PM, Snyder SH. Localization of nitric oxide synthase indicating a neural role for nitric oxide. *Nature* 1990;347: 768–770.
12. Brendel JK, Johns RA. Isoflurane does not vasodilate rat thoracic aortic rings by endothelium-derived relaxing factor or other cyclic GMP–mediated mechanisms. *Anesthesiology* 1992;77:126–131.
13. Brian JE, Traystman RJ, McPherson RW. Changes in cerebral blood flow over time during isoflurane anesthesia in dogs. *J Neurosurg Anesth* 1990;2:122–130.
14. Busija DW, Leffler CW. Dilator effects of amino acid neurotransmitters on piglet pial arterioles. *Am J Physiol* 1989;257: H1200–H1203.
15. Busija DW, Leffler CW, Wagerle LC. Mono-L-arginine-containing compounds dilate piglet pial arterioles via an endothelium-derived relaxing factor-like substance. *Circ Res* 1990;67:1374–1380.
16. Carlsson C, Hagerdal M, Siesjo BK. The effect of nitrous oxide on oxygen consumption and blood flow in the cerebral cortex of the rat. *Acta Anaesthesiol Scand* 1976;20:91–95.
17. Chemtob S, Barna T, Beharry K, Aranda JV, Varma DR. Enhanced cerebral blood flow autoregulation in the newborn piglet by d-tubocurarine and pancuronium but not by vecuronium. *Anesthesiology* 1992;76:236–244.
18. Correa-Sales C, Rabin BC, Maze M. A hypnotic response to dexmedetomidine, an alpha-2 agonist, is mediated in the locus coeruleus in rats. *Anesthesiology* 1992;76:948–952.
19. Coughlan MG, Lee JG, Bosnjak ZJ, Schmeling WT, Kampine JP, Warltier DC. Direct coronary and cerebral vascular responses to dexmedetomidine. Significance of endogenous nitric oxide synthesis. *Anesthesiology* 1992;77:998–1006.
20. Crosby G, Crane AM, Sokoloff L. Local changes in cerebral glucose utilization during ketamine anesthesia. *Anesthesiology* 1982; 56:437–443.
21. Cucchiara RF, Theye RA, Michenfelder JD. The effects of isoflu-

rane on canine cerebral metabolism and blood flow. *Anesthesiology* 1974;40:571–574.

22. D'Alecy LG, Rose CJ, Sellers SA. Sympathetic modulation of hypercapnic cerebral vasodilation in dogs. *Circ Res* 1979;45:771–785.
23. Dal Santo G. Kinetics of distribution of radioactive labeled muscle relaxants. 3. Investigations with 14C-succinyldicholine and 14C-succinylmonocholine during controlled conditions. *Anesthesiology* 1968;29:435–443.
24. Dam M, Ori C, Pizzolato G, et al. The effects of propofol anesthesia on local cerebral glucose utilization in the rat. *Anesthesiology* 1990;73:499–505.
25. Dawson B, Michenfelder JD, Theye RA. Effects of ketamine on canine cerebral blood flow and metabolism: modification by prior administration of thiopental. *Anesth Analg* 1971;50:443–447.
26. Donegan JH, Traystman RJ, Koehler RC, Jones MD Jr, Rogers MC. Cerebrovascular hypoxic and autoregulatory responses during reduced brain metabolism. *Am J Physiol* 1985;249:H421–H429.
27. Doni MG, Whittle BJ, Palmer RM, Moncada S. Actions of nitric oxide on the release of prostacyclin from bovine endothelial cells in culture. *Eur J Pharmacol* 1988;151:19–25.
28. Doze VA, Chen B, Tinkleberg JA, Segal IS, Maze M. Pertussis toxin and 4-aminopyridine differentially affect the hypnotic-anesthetic action of dexmedetomidine and phentobarbital. *Anesthesiology* 1990;73:304–307.
29. Drummond JC, Scheller MS, Todd MM. The effect of nitrous oxide on cortical cerebral blood flow during anesthesia with halothane and isoflurane, with and without morphine, in the rabbit. *Anesth Analg* 1987;66:1083–1089.
30. Drummond JC, Todd MM, Scheller MS, Shapiro HM. A comparison of the direct cerebral vasodilating potencies of halothane and isoflurane in the New Zealand white rabbit. *Anesthesiology* 1986; 65:462–467.
31. Ducey JP, Deppe SA, Foley KT. A comparison of the effects of suxamethonium, atracurium and vecuronium on intracranial haemodynamics in swine. *Anaesth Intensive Care* 1989;17:448–455.
32. Edvinsson L. Characterization of the contractile effect of neuropeptide Y in feline cerebral arteries. *Acta Physiol Scand* 1985; 125:33–41.
33. Edvinsson L, Falck B, Owman C. Possibilities for a cholinergic action on smooth musculature and on sympathetic axons in brain vessels mediated by muscarinic and nicotinic receptors. *J Pharmacol Exp Ther* 1977;200:117–126.
34. Edvinsson L, Fallgren B, Jansen I, Horsburgh K. Mechanisms of action and interaction of perivascular peptides and nonpeptides in cerebral vasoconstriction. In: Seylaz J, MacKenzie ET, eds. *Neurotransmission and cerebrovascular function, vol. I.* Amsterdam: Elsevier Science, 1989:131–135.
35. Edvinsson L, Fredholm BB, Hamel E, Jansen I, Verrecchia C. Perivascular peptides relax cerebral arteries concomitant with stimulation of cyclic adenosine monophosphate accumulation or release of an endothelium-derived relaxing factor in the cat. *Neurosci Lett* 1985;58:213–217.
36. Edvinsson L, McCulloch J. Effects of pentobarbital on contractile responses of feline cerebral arteries. *J Cereb Blood Flow Metab* 1981; 1:437–440.
37. Eng C, Lam AM, Mayberg TS, Lee C, Mathisen T. The influence of propofol with and without nitrous oxide on cerebral blood flow velocity and CO2 reactivity in humans. *Anesthesiology* 1992;77: 872–879.
38. Eskinder H, Hillard CJ, Flynn N, Bosnjak ZJ, Kampine JP. Role of guanylate cyclase-cGMP systems in halothane-induced vasodilation in canine cerebral arteries. *Anesthesiology* 1992;77: 482–487.
39. Faraci FM. Role of nitric oxide in regulation of basilar artery tone in vivo. *Am J Physiol* 1990;259:H1216–H1221.
40. Faraci FM, Breese KR. Nitric oxide mediates vasodilatation in response to activation of N-methyl-D-aspartate receptors in brain. *Circ Res* 1993;72:476–480.
41. Fleischer JE, Milde JH, Moyer TP, Michenfelder JD. Cerebral effects of high-dose midazolam and subsequent reversal with RO15-1788 in dogs. *Anesthesiology* 1988;68:234–242.
42. Flynn NM, Buljubasic N, Bosnjak ZJ, Kampine JP. Isoflurane produces endothelium-independent relaxation in canine middle cerebral arteries. *Anesthesiology* 1992;76:461–467.
43. Forster A, Juge O, Louis M, Nahory A. Effects of a specific benzodiazepine antagonist (RO 15-1788) on cerebral blood flow. *Anesth Analg* 1987;66:309–313.
44. Forster A, Juge O, Morel D. Effects of midazolam on cerebral blood flow in human volunteers. *Anesthesiology* 1982;56:453–455.
45. Fredholm BB, Jansen I, Edvinsson L. Neuropeptide Y is a potent inhibitor of cyclic AMP accumulation in feline cerebral blood vessels. *Acta Physiol Scand* 1985;124:467–469.
46. Frizzell RT, Fichtel FM, Jordan MB, et al. Effects of etomidate and hypothermia on cerebral metabolism and blood flow in a canine model of hypoperfusion. *J Neurosurg Anesthesiol* 1993;5:104–110.
47. Fujishima M, Scheinberg P, Busto R, Reinmuth OM. The relation between cerebral oxygen consumption and cerebral vascular reactivity to carbon dioxide. *Stroke* 1971;2:251–257.
48. Gelman S, Fowler KC, Smith LR. Regional blood flow during isoflurane and halothane anesthesia. *Anesth Analg* 1984;63:557–565.
49. Goadsby PJ. Effect of stimulation of facial nerve on regional cerebral blood flow and glucose utilization in cats. *Am J Physiol* 1989; 257:R517–R521.
50. Goto K, Kasuya Y, Matsuki N, et al. Endothelin activates the dihydropyridine-sensitive, voltage-dependent Ca^{2+} channel in vascular smooth muscle. *Proc Natl Acad Sci USA* 1989;86:3915–3918.
51. Greenberg RS, Helfaer MA, Kirsch JR, Moore LE, Traystman RJ. Nitric oxide synthase inhibition with N^G-mono-methyl-L-arginine reversibly decreases cerebral blood flow in piglets. *Crit Care Med* 1994;22:384–392.
52. Greenblatt EP, Loeb AL, Longnecker DE. Endothelium-dependent circulatory control—a mechanism for the differing peripheral vascular effects of isoflurane versus halothane. *Anesthesiology* 1992;77:1178–1185.
53. Gryglewski RJ, Palmer RM, Moncada S. Superoxide anion is involved in the breakdown of endothelium-derived vascular relaxing factor. *Nature* 1986;320:454–456.
54. Hagen AA, White RP, Robertson JT. Synthesis of prostaglandins and thromboxane B2 by cerebral arteries. *Stroke* 1979;10: 306–309.
55. Hanko JH, Hardebo JE. Enkephalin-induced dilatation of pial arteries in vitro probably mediated by opiate receptors. *Eur J Pharmacol* 1978;51:295–297.
56. Hansen TD, Warner DS, Todd MM, Vust LJ. The role of cerebral metabolism in determining the local cerebral blood flow effects of volatile anesthetics: evidence for persistent flow-metabolism coupling. *J Cereb Blood Flow Metab* 1989;9:323–328.
57. Hansen TD, Warner DS, Todd MM, Vust LJ, Trawick DC. Distribution of cerebral blood flow during halothane versus isoflurane anesthesia in rats. *Anesthesiology* 1988;69:332–337.
58. Hardebo JE, Arbab M, Suzuki N, Svendgaard NA. Pathways of parasympathetic and sensory cerebrovascular nerves in monkeys. *Stroke* 1991;22:331–342.
59. Harder DR, Gradall K, Madden JA, Kampine JP. Cellular actions of halothane on cat cerebral arterial muscle. *Stroke* 1985;16: 680–683.
60. Hatano Y, Nakamura K, Moriyama S, Mori K, Toda N. The contractile responses of isolated dog cerebral and extracerebral arteries to oxybarbiturates and thiobarbiturates. *Anesthesiology* 1989;71: 80–86.
61. Heistad DD, Marcus ML, Gross PM. Effects of sympathetic nerves on cerebral vessels in dog, cat, and monkey. *Am J Physiol* 1978;235: H544–H552.
62. Hirata Y, Fukuda Y, Yoshimi H, Emori T, Shichiri M, Marumo F. Specific receptor for endothelin in cultured rat cardiocytes. *Biochem Biophys Res Commun* 1989;160:1438–1444.
63. Hirose T, Inoue M, Uchida M, Inagaki C. Enflurane-induced release of an excitatory amino acid, glutamate, from mouse brain synaptosomes. *Anesthesiology* 1992;77:109–113.
64. Hoehner PJ, Whitson JT, Kirsch JR, Traystman RJ. Effect of intracarotid and intraventricular morphine on regional cerebral blood flow and metabolism in pentobarbital-anesthetized dogs. *Anesth Analg* 1993;76:266–273.
65. Holzmann S. Endothelium-induced relaxation by acetylcholine associated with larger rises in cyclic GMP in coronary arterial strips. *J Cyclic Nucleotide Res* 1982;8:409–419.
66. Holzmann S, Kukovetz WR, Schmidt K. Mode of action of coronary arterial relaxation by prostacyclin. *J Cyclic Nucleotide Res* 1980; 6:451–460.
67. Ignarro LJ, Kadowitz PJ. The pharmacologicial and physiological role of cyclic GMP in vascular smooth muscle relaxation. *Annu Rev Pharmacol Toxicol* 1985;25:171–191.
68. Jensen NF, Todd MM, Kramer DJ, Leonard PA, Warner DS. A comparison of the vasodilating effects of halothane and isoflurane on

the isolated rabbit basilar artery with and without intact endothelium. *Anesthesiology* 1992;76:624–634.

69. Jobes DR, Kennell EM, Bush GL, et al. Cerebral blood flow and metabolism during morphine—nitrous oxide anesthesia in man. *Anesthesiology* 1977;47:16–18.
70. Johns RA, Moscicki JC, Difazio CA. Nitric oxide synthase inhibitor dose-dependently and reversibly reduces the threshold for halothane anesthesia. A role for nitric oxide in mediating consciousness? *Anesthesiology* 1992;77:779–784.
71. Kaczmarek LK. The role of protein kinase C in the regulation of ion channels and neurotransmitter release. *Trends Neurosci* 1987; 10:30–34.
72. Kagstrom E, Smith ML, Wallstedt L, Siesjo BK. Cyclo-oxygenase inhibition by indomethacin and recirculation following cerebral ischemia. *Acta Physiol Scand* 1983;118:193–201.
73. Kanamaru K, Waga S, Kojima T, Fujimoto K, Itoh H. Endothelium-dependent relaxation of canine basilar arteries. Part 1: Difference between acetylcholine- and A23187-induced relaxation and involvement of lipoxygenase metabolite(s). *Stroke* 1987;18: 932–937.
74. Kanawati IS, Yaksh TL, Anderson RE, Marsh RW. Effects of clonidine on cerebral blood flow and the response to arterial CO_2. *J Cereb Blood Flow Metab* 1986;6:358–365.
75. Kanmura Y, Kajikuri J, Itoh T, Yoshitake J. Effects of ketamine on contraction and synthesis of inositol 1,4,5-trisphosphate in smooth muscle of the rabbit mesenteric artery. *Anesthesiology* 1993; 79:571–579.
76. Kanmura Y, Yoshitake J, Casteels R. Ketamine-induced relaxation in intact and skinned smooth muscles of the rabbit ear artery. *Br J Pharmacol* 1989;97:591–597.
77. Kapadia SE, de Lanerolle NC. Immunohistochemical and electron microscopic demonstration of vascular innervation in the mammalian brainstem. *Brain Res* 1984;292:33–39.
78. Karlsson BR, Forsman M, Roald OK, Heier MS, Steen PA. Effect of dexmedetomidine, a selective and potent alpha 2-agonist, on cerebral blood flow and oxygen consumption during halothane anesthesia in dogs. *Anesth Analg* 1990;71:125–129.
79. Kasuya Y, Ishikawa T, Yanagisawa M, Kimura S, Goto K, Masaki T. Mechanism of contraction to endothelin in isolated porcine coronary artery. *Am J Physiol* 1989;257:H1828–H1835.
80. Katusic ZS. Endothelium-independent contractions to N^G-monomethyl-L-arginine in canine basilar artery. *Stroke* 1991;22: 1399–1404.
81. Katusic ZS, Marshall JJ, Kontos HA, Vanhoutte PM. Similar responsiveness of smooth muscle of the canine basilar artery to EDRF and nitric oxide. *Am J Physiol* 1989;257:H1235–H1239.
82. Kawai Y, Ohhashi T. Prostaglandin F2 alpha-induced endothelium-dependent relaxation in isolated monkey cerebral arteries. *Am J Physiol* 1991;260:H1538–H1543.
83. Kobari M, Gotoh F, Fukuuchi Y, et al. Effects of (D-Met2,Pro5)-enkephalinamide and naloxone on pial vessels in cats. *J Cereb Blood Flow Metab* 1985;5:34–39.
84. Koenig HM, Pelligrino DA, Albrecht RF. Halothane vasodilation and nitric oxide in rat pial vessels [Abstract]. *J Neurosurg Anesthesiology* 1992;4:301.
85. Kofke WA, Hawkins RA, Davis DW, Biebuyck JF. Comparison of the effects of volatile anesthetics on brain glucose metabolism in rats. *Anesthesiology* 1987;66:810–813.
86. Kovach AGB, Szabo C, Benyo Z, Csaki C, Greenberg JH, Reivich M. Effects of N^G-nitro-L-arginine and L-arginine on regional cerebral blood flow in the cat. *J Physiol (Lond)* 1992;449:183–196.
87. Kozniewska E, Oseka M, Stys T. Effects of endothelium-derived nitric oxide on cerebral circulation during normoxia and hypoxia in the rat. *J Cereb Blood Flow Metab* 1992;12:311–317.
88. Lad PJ. Activation of rat lung particulate guanylate cyclase due to filipin-induced fluidity change. *Biochem Biophys Res Commun* 1980; 96:203–210.
89. Lanier WL, Iaizzo PA, Milde JH. Cerebral function and muscle afferent activity following intravenous succinylcholine in dogs anesthetized with halothane: the effects of pretreatment with a defasciculating dose of pancuronium. *Anesthesiology* 1989;71: 87–95.
90. Lanier WL, Iaizzo PA, Milde JH. The effects of intravenous succinylcholine on cerebral function and muscle afferent activity following complete ischemia in halothane-anesthetized dogs. *Anesthesiology* 1990;73:485–490.
91. Lanier WL, Milde JH, Michenfelder JD. The cerebral effects of pancuronium and atracurium in halothane-anesthetized dogs. *Anesthesiology* 1985;63:589–597.
92. Lanier WL, Milde JH, Michenfelder JD. Cerebral stimulation following succinylcholine in dogs. *Anesthesiology* 1986;64:551–559.
93. Lanier WL, Milde JH, Sharbrough FW. Effects of suxamethonium on the cerebrum following disruption of the blood-brain barrier in dogs. *Br J Anaesth* 1990;65:708–712.
94. Levasseur JE, Kontos HA. Effects of anesthesia on cerebral arteriolar responses to hypercapnia. *Am J Physiol* 1989;257:H85–H88.
95. Lundeen G, Manohar M, Parks C. Systemic distribution of blood flow in swine while awake and during 1.0 and 1.5 MAC isoflurane anesthesia with or without 50% nitrous oxide. *Anesth Analg* 1983; 62:499–512.
96. Lutz LJ, Milde JH, Milde LN. The cerebral functional, metabolic, and hemodynamic effects of desflurane in dogs. *Anesthesiology* 1990;73:125–131.
97. Macfarlane R, Tasdemiroglu E, Moskowitz MA, Uemura Y, Wei EP, Kontos HA. Chronic trigeminal ganglionectomy or topical capsaicin application to pial vessels attenuates postocclusive cortical hyperemia but does not influence postischemic hypoperfusion. *J Cereb Blood Flow Metab* 1991;11:261–271.
98. MacIver MB, Kendig JJ. Enflurane-induced burst discharge of hippocampal CA1 neurones is blocked by the NMDA receptor antagonist APV. *Br J Anaesth* 1989;63:296–305.
99. MacMurdo SD, Nemoto EM, Nikki P, Frankenberry MJ. Brain cyclic-AMP and possible mechanisms of cerebrovascular dilation by anesthetics in rats. *Anesthesiology* 1981;55:435–438.
100. Madison DV, Nicoll RA. Cyclic adenosine 3′,5′-monophosphate mediates beta-receptor actions of noradrenaline in rat hippocampal pyramidal cells. *J Physiol* 1986;372:245–259.
101. Marijic J, Buljubasic N, Coughlan MG, Kampine JP, Bosnjak ZJ. Effect of K^+ channel blockade with tetraethylammonium on anesthetic-induced relaxation in canine cerebral and coronary arteries. *Anesthesiology* 1992;77:948–955.
102. Marin J, Rico ML, Salaices M. Interference of pentobarbitone with the contraction of vascular smooth muscle in goat middle cerebral artery. *J Pharm Pharmacol* 1981;33:357–361.
103. Matsumiya N, Koehler RC, Kirsch JR, Traystman RJ. Conjugated superoxide dismutase reduces extent of caudate injury after transient focal ischemia in cats. *Stroke* 1991;22:1193–1200.
104. Mayberg MR, Zervas NT, Moskowitz MA. Trigeminal projections to supratentorial pial and dural blood vessels in cats demonstrated by horseradish peroxidase histochemistry. *J Comp Neurol* 1984;223: 46–56.
105. Mayer N, Weinstabl C, Podreka I, Spiss CK. Sufentanil does not increase cerebral blood flow in healthy human volunteers. *Anesthesiology* 1990;73:240–243.
106. Maze M, Tranquilli W. Alpha-2 adrenoceptor agonists: defining the role in clinical anesthesia. *Anesthesiology* 1991;74:581–605.
107. McPherson RW, Briar JE, Traystman RJ. Cerebrovascular responsiveness to carbon dioxide in dogs with 1.4% and 2.8% isoflurane. *Anesthesiology* 1989;70:843–850.
108. McPherson RW, Derrer SA, Traystman RJ. Changes in cerebral CO_2 responsivity over time during isoflurane anesthesia in the dog. *J Neurosurg Anesth* 1991;3:12–19.
109. McPherson RW, Kirsch JR, Tobin JR, Ghaly RF, Traystman RJ. Cerebral blood flow in primates is increased by isoflurane over time and is decreased by nitric oxide synthase inhibition. *Anesthesiology* 1994;80:1320–1327.
110. McPherson RW, Kirsch JR, Traystman RJ. N^w-nitro-L-arginine methyl ester prevents cerebral hyperemia by inhaled anesthetics in dogs. *Anesth Analg* 1993;77:891–897.
111. McPherson RW, Traystman RJ. Fentanyl and cerebral vascular responsivity in dogs. *Anesthesiology* 1984;60:180–186.
112. McPherson RW, Traystman RJ. Effects of isoflurane on cerebral autoregulation in dogs. *Anesthesiology* 1988;69:493–499.
113. Mikawa K, Maekawa N, Hoshina H, et al. Inhibitory effect of barbiturates and local anaesthetics on protein kinase C activation. *J Int Med Res* 1990;18:153–160.
114. Miletich DJ, Ivankovich AD, Albrecht RF, Reimann CR, Rosenberg R, McKissic ED. Absence of autoregulation of cerebral blood flow during halothane and enflurane anesthesia. *Anesth Analg* 1976;55: 100–109.
115. Monaghan DT, Cotman CW. Distribution of N-methyl-D-aspartate-sensitive L-[^{3}H]glutamate-binding sites in rat brain. *J Neurosci* 1985;5:2909–2919.
116. Monitto CL, Kurth CD. The effect of fentanyl, sufentanil, and

alfentanil on cerebral arterioles in piglets. *Anesth Analg* 1993;76: 985–989.

117. Moore LE, Kirsch JR, Helfaer MA, Tobin JR, McPherson RW, Traystman RJ. Nitric oxide and prostanoids contribute to isoflurane-induced cerebral hyperemia in pigs. *Anesthesiology* 1994;80: 1328–1337.
118. Moyer JH, Pontius R, Morris G. Effect of morphine and N-allylnormorphine on cerebral hemodynamics and oxygen metabolism. *Circulation* 1957;15:379–384.
119. Muldoon LL, Rodland KD, Forsythe ML, Magun BE. Stimulation of phosphatidylinositol hydrolysis, diacylglycerol release, and gene expression in response to endothelin, a potent new agonist for fibroblasts and smooth muscle cells. *J Biol Chem* 1989;264: 8529–8536.
120. Muldoon SM, Hart JL, Bowen KA, Freas W. Attenuation of endothelium-mediated vasodilation by halothane. *Anesthesiology* 1988;68:31–37.
121. Murphy S, Minor RL Jr, Welk G, Harrison DG. Evidence for an astrocyte-derived vasorelaxing factor with properties similar to nitric oxide. *J Neurochem* 1990;55:349–351.
122. Myers PR, Minor RL Jr, Guerra R Jr, Bates JN, Harrison DG. Vasorelaxant properties of the endothelium-derived relaxing factor more closely resemble S-nitrosocysteine than nitric oxide. *Nature* 1990;345:161–163.
123. Nahrwold ML, Lust WD, Passonneau JV. Halothane-induced alterations of cyclic nucleotide concentrations in three regions of the mouse nervous system. *Anesthesiology* 1977;47:423–427.
124. Nakamura K, Hatano Y, Toda H, Nishiwada M, Baek WY, Mori K. Halothane-induced relaxation of vascular smooth muscle: a possible contribution of increased cyclic GMP formation. *Jpn J Pharmacol* 1991;55:165–168.
125. Newberg LA, Milde JH, Michenfelder JD. The cerebral metabolic effects of isoflurane at and above concentrations that suppress cortical electrical activity. *Anesthesiology* 1983;59:23–28.
126. Nicoll RA, Madison DV. General anesthetics hyperpolarize neurons in the vertebrate central nervous system. *Science* 1982;217: 1055–1057.
127. Nilsson B, Agardh CD, Ingvar M, Siesjo BK. Cerebrovascular response during and following severe insulin-induced hypoglycemia: CO_2-sensitivity, autoregulation, and influence of prostaglandin synthesis inhibition. *Acta Physiol Scand* 1981;111: 455–463.
128. Nishizaki T, Okada Y. Effects of excitatory amino acids on the oxygen consumption of hippocampal slices from the guinea pig. *Brain Res* 1988;452:11–20.
129. Nishizuka Y. The role of protein kinase C in cell surface signal transduction and tumour promotion. *Nature* 1984;308:693–698.
130. Nishizuka Y. Studies and perspectives of protein kinase C. *Science* 1986;233:305–312.
131. Nowycky MC, Fox AP, Tsien RW. Three types of neuronal calcium channel with different calcium agonist sensitivity. *Nature* 1985;316: 440–443.
132. Nozaki K, Moskowitz MA, Maynard KI, et al. Possible origins and distribution of immunoreactive nitric oxide synthase-containing nerve fibers in cerebral arteries. *J Cereb Blood Flow Metab* 1993;13: 70–79.
133. Nugent M, Artru AA, Michenfelder JD. Cerebral metabolic, vascular and protective effects of midazolam maleate: comparison to diazepam. *Anesthesiology* 1982;56:172–176.
134. Olsen GD, Hohimer AR, Mathis MD. Cerebral blood flow and metabolism during morphine-induced stimulation of breathing movements in fetal lambs. *Life Sci* 1983;33:751–754.
135. Olsen RW. GABA-benzodiazepine-barbiturate receptor interactions. *J Neurochem* 1981;37:1–13.
136. Onali P, Olianas MC. Naturally occurring opioid receptor agonists stimulate adenylate cyclase activity in rat olfactory bulb. *Mol Pharmacol* 1991;39:436–441.
137. Palmer RM, Ashton DS, Moncada S. Vascular endothelial cells synthesize nitric oxide from L-arginine. *Nature* 1988;333:664–666.
138. Park WK, Lynch C III, Johns RA. Effects of propofol and thiopental in isolated rat aorta and pulmonary artery. *Anesthesiology* 1992; 77:956–963.
139. Pelligrino DA, Miletich DJ, Albrecht RF. Diminished muscarinic receptor-mediated cerebral blood flow response in the streptozotocin-treated rat. *Am J Physiol* 1992;262:E447–E454.
140. Pelligrino DA, Miletich DJ, Hoffman WE, Albrecht RF. Nitrous oxide markedly increases cerebral cortical metabolic rate and blood flow in the goat. *Anesthesiology* 1984;60:405–412.
141. Peroutka SJ, Moskowitz MA, Reinhard JF Jr, Snyder SH. Neurotransmitter receptor binding in bovine cerebral microvessels. *Science* 1980;208:610–612.
142. Pickard JD, MacDonell LA, MacKenzie ET, Harper AM. Response of the cerebral circulation in baboons to changing perfusion pressure after indomethacin. *Circ Res* 1977;40:198–203.
143. Pickard JD, MacKenzie ET. Inhibition of prostaglandin synthesis and the response of baboon cerebral circulation to carbon dioxide. *Nature New Biol* 1973;245:187–188.
144. Pierce EC, Lambertsen JG, Deutsch S. Cerebral circulation and metabolism during thiopental anesthesia and hyperventilation in man. *J Clin Invest* 1962;41:1664–1671.
145. Pinaud M, Lelausque JN, Chetanneau A, Fauchoux N, Menegalli D, Souron R. Effects of propofol on cerebral hemodynamics and metabolism in patients with brain trauma. *Anesthesiology* 1990;73: 404–409.
146. Pourcyrous M, Leffler CW, Bada HS, Korones SB, Stidham GL, Busija DW. Effects of pancuronium bromide on cerebral blood flow changes during seizures in newborn pigs. *Pediatr Res* 1992;31: 636–639.
147. Rapoport R, Murad F. Endothelium-dependent and nitrovasodilator-induced relaxation of vascular smooth muscle: role of cyclic GMP. *J Cyclic Nucleotide Protein Phosphor Res* 1983;9:281–296.
148. Rasmussen H, Takuwa Y, Park S. Protein kinase C in the regulation of smooth muscle contraction. *FASEB J* 1987;1:177–185.
149. Reynolds IJ, Wagner JA, Snyder SH, Thayer SA, Olivera BM, Miller RJ. Brain voltage-sensitive calcium channel subtypes differentiated by omega-conotoxin fraction GVIA. *Proc Natl Acad Sci USA* 1986; 83:8804–8807.
150. Robinson White AJ, Muldoon SM, Robinson FC. Inhibition of inositol phospholipid hydrolysis in endothelial cells by pentobarbital. *Eur J Pharmacol* 1989;172:291–303.
151. Rubanyi GM, Vanhoutte PM. Superoxide anions and hyperoxia inactivate endothelium-derived relaxing factor. *Am J Physiol* 1986; 250:H822–H827.
152. Saito A, Wu JY, Lee TJ. Evidence for the presence of cholinergic nerves in cerebral arteries: an immunohistochemical demonstration of choline acetyltransferase. *J Cereb Blood Flow Metab* 1985;5: 327–334.
153. Sakabe T, Siesjo BK. The effect of indomethacin on the blood flow-metabolism couple in the brain under normal, hypercapnic and hypoxic conditions. *Acta Physiol Scand* 1979;107:283–284.
154. Sanchez Ferrer CF, Marin J, Salaices M, Rico ML, Munoz Blanco JL. Interference of pentobarbital and thiopental with the vascular contraction and noradrenaline release in human cerebral arteries. *Gen Pharmacol* 1985;16:469–473.
155. Sandor P, Gotoh F, Tomita M, Tanahashi N, Gogolak I. Effects of a stable enkephalin analogue, (D-Met2,Pro5)-enkephalinamide, and naloxone on cortical blood flow and cerebral blood volume in experimental brain ischemia in anesthetized cats. *J Cereb Blood Flow Metab* 1986;6:553–558.
156. Shigeno T, Mima T. A new vasoconstrictor peptide, endothelin: profiles as vasoconstrictor and neuropeptide. *Cerebrovasc Brain Metab Rev* 1990;2:227–239.
157. Shimokawa H, Flavahan NA, Lorenz RR, Vanhoutte PM. Prostacyclin releases endothelium-derived relaxing factor and potentiates its action in coronary arteries of the pig. *Br J Pharmacol* 1988;95: 1197–1203.
158. Sill JC, Uhl C, Eskuri S, Van Dyke R, Tarara J. Halothane inhibits agonist-induced inositol phosphate and Ca^{2+} signaling in A7r5 cultured vascular smooth muscle cells. *Mol Pharmacol* 1991;40: 1006–1013.
159. Smith AL, Wollman H. Cerebral blood flow and metabolism: effects of anesthetic drugs and techniques. *Anesthesiology* 1972;36: 378–400.
160. Snyder SH. The opiate receptor and morphine-like peptides in the brain. *Am J Psychiatry* 1978;135:645–652.
161. Somlyo AV, Bond M, Somlyo AP, Scarpa A. Inositol trisphosphate-induced calcium release and contraction in vascular smooth muscle. *Proc Natl Acad Sci USA* 1985;82:5231–5235.
162. Sprague DH, Yang JC, Ngai SH. Effects of isoflurane and halothane on contractility and the cyclic 3′,5′-adenosine monophosphate system in the rat aorta. *Anesthesiology* 1974;40: 162–167.
163. Stephan H, Sonntag H, Schenk HD, Kohlhausen S. Effect of Disoprivan (propofol) on the circulation and oxygen consumption of the brain and CO_2 reactivity of brain vessels in the human [...]. *Anaesthesist* 1987;36:60–65.

164. Stone DJ, Johns RA. Endothelium-dependent effects of halothane, enflurane, and isoflurane on isolated rat aortic vascular rings. *Anesthesiology* 1989;71:126–132.
165. Sturaitis M, Moore LE, Kirsch JR, McPherson RW. A cholinergic agonist induces cerebral hyperemia in isoflurane- but not pentobarbital-anesthetized dogs. *Anesth Analg* 1994;78:876–883.
166. Su JY, Bell JG. Intracellular mechanism of action of isoflurane and halothane on striated muscle of the rabbit. *Anesth Analg* 1986;65: 457–462.
167. Su JY, Zhang CC. Intracellular mechanisms of halothane's effect on isolated aortic strips of the rabbit. *Anesthesiology* 1989;71:409–417.
168. Suzuki N, Hardebo JE. Anatomical basis for a parasympathetic and sensory innervation of the intracranial segment of the internal carotid artery in man. Possible implication for vascular headache. *J Neurol Sci* 1991;104:19–31.
169. Taga K, Fukuda S, Nishimura N, Tsukui A, Morioka M, Shimoji K. Effects of thiopental, pentobarbital, and ketamine on endothelin-induced constriction of porcine cerebral arteries. *Anesthesiology* 1990;72:939–941.
170. Takeshita H, Michenfelder JD, Theye RA. The effects of morphine and N-allylnormorphine on canine cerebral metabolism and circulation. *Anesthesiology* 1972;37:605–612.
171. Takeshita H, Okuda Y, Sari A. The effects of ketamine on cerebral circulation and metabolism in man. *Anesthesiology* 1972;36:69–75.
172. Tan U. Electrocorticographic changes induced by topically applied succinylcholine and biperiden. *Electroencephalogr Clin Neurophysiol* 1977;42:252–258.
173. Tanaka K, Gotoh F, Gomi S, et al. Inhibition of nitric oxide synthesis induces a significant reduction in local cerebral blood flow in the rat. *Neurosci Lett* 1991;127:129–132.
174. Theye RA, Michenfelder JD. The effect of nitrous oxide on canine cerebral metabolism. *Anesthesiology* 1968;29:1119–1124.
175. Thompson WL, Walton RP. Elevation of plasma histamine levels in the dog following administration of muscle relaxants, opiates and macromolecular polymers. *J Pharmacol Exp Ther* 1964;143: 131–136.
176. Toda N, Okamura T. Role of nitric oxide in neurally induced cerebroarterial relaxation. *J Pharmacol Exp Ther* 1991;258:1027–1032.
177. Todd MM, Drummond JC. A comparison of the cerebrovascular and metabolic effects of halothane and isoflurane in the cat. *Anesthesiology* 1984;60:276–282.
178. Traystman RJ, Rapela CE. Effect of sympathetic nerve stimulation on cerebral and cephalic blood flow in dogs. *Circ Res* 1975;36: 620–630.
179. Tsuchida H, Namba H, Yamakage M, Fujita S, Notsuki E, Namiki A. Effects of halothane and isoflurane on cytosolic calcium ion concentrations and contraction in the vascular smooth muscle of the rat aorta. *Anesthesiology* 1993;78:531–540.
180. Tsukahara T, Taniguchi T, Usui H, et al. Sympathetic denervation and alpha adrenoceptors in dog cerebral arteries. *Naunyn Schmiedebergs Arch Pharmacol* 1986;334:436–443.
181. Uddman R, Edvinsson L, Ekman R, Kingman T, McCulloch J. Innervation of the feline cerebral vasculature by nerve fibers containing calcitonin gene–related peptide: trigeminal origin and coexistence with substance P. *Neurosci Lett* 1985;62:131–136.
182. Uggeri MJ, Proctor GJ, Johns RA. Halothane, enflurane, and isoflurane attenuate both receptor-and non-receptor-mediated EDRF production in rat thoracic aorta. *Anesthesiology* 1992;76: 1012–1017.
183. Unnerstall JR, Kopajtic TA, Kuhar MJ. Distribution of alpha 2 agonist binding sites in the rat and human central nervous system: analysis of some functional, anatomic correlates of the pharmacologic effects of clonidine and related adrenergic agents. *Brain Res* 1984;319:69–101.
184. Van Hemelrijck J, Fitch W, Mattheussen M, Van Aken H, Plets C, Lauwers T. Effect of propofol on cerebral circulation and autoregulation in the baboon. *Anesth Analg* 1990;71:49–54.
185. Vandesteene A, Trempont V, Engelman E, et al. Effect of propofol on cerebral blood flow and metabolism in man. *Anaesthesia* 1988; 43S:42–43.
186. Vulliemoz Y, Verosky M, Triner L. Effect of halothane on myocardial cyclic AMP and cyclic GMP content of mice. *J Pharmacol Exp Ther* 1986;236:181–186.
187. Wahl M. Effects of enkephalins, morphine, and naloxone on pial arteries during perivascular microapplication. *J Cereb Blood Flow Metab* 1985;5:451–457.
188. Wechsler RL, Dripps RD, Kety SS. Blood flow and oxygen consumption of the human brain during anesthesia produced by thiopental. *Anesthesiology* 1951;12:308–314.
189. Wei EP, Christman CW, Kontos HA, Povlishock JT. Effects of oxygen radicals on cerebral arterioles. *Am J Physiol* 1985;248:H157–H162.
190. Wei EP, Kontos HA. H_2O_2 and endothelium-dependent cerebral arteriolar dilation. Implications for the identity of endothelium-derived relaxing factor generated by acetylcholine. *Hypertension* 1990;16:162–169.
191. Wei EP, Moskowitz MA, Boccalini P, Kontos HA. Calcitonin gene–related peptide mediates nitroglycerin and sodium nitroprusside-induced vasodilation in feline cerebral arterioles. *Circ Res* 1992;70:1313–1319.
192. Weiss MH, Wertman N, Apuzzo ML, Heiden JS, Kurze T. The influence of myoneural blockers on intracranial dynamics. *Bull Los Angeles Neurol Soc* 1977;42:1–7.
193. Wendling WW, Harakal C. Effects of prostaglandin F2 alpha and thromboxane A2 analogue on bovine cerebral arterial tone and calcium fluxes. *Stroke* 1991;22:66–72.
194. Werner C, Hoffman WE, Kochs E, Schulte am Esch J, Albrecht RF. The effects of propofol on cerebral and spinal cord blood flow in rats. *Anesth Analg* 1993;76:971–975.
195. Winters WD, Ferrar Allado T, Guzman Flores C, Alcaraz M. The cataleptic state induced by ketamine: a review of the neuropharmacology of anesthesia. *Neuropharmacology* 1972;11:303–315.
196. Yanagisawa M, Kurihara H, Kimura S, et al. A novel potent vasoconstrictor peptide produced by vascular endothelial cells. *Nature* 1988;332:411–415.
197. Yoshida K, Okabe E. Selective impairment of endothelium-dependent relaxation by sevoflurane: oxygen free radicals participation. *Anesthesiology* 1992;76:440–447.
198. Zornow MH, Fleischer JE, Scheller MS, Nakakimura K, Drummond JC. Dexmedetomidine, an alpha 2-adrenergic agonist, decreases cerebral blood flow in the isoflurane-anesthetized dog. *Anesth Analg* 1990;70:624–630.
199. Zornow MH, Scheller MS, Sheehan PB, Strnat MA, Matsumoto M. Intracranial pressure effects of dexmedetomidine in rabbits. *Anesth Analg* 1992;75:232–237.

Anesthesia: Biologic Foundations, edited by Tony L. Yaksh et al. Lippincott–Raven Publishers, Philadelphia © 1997.

CHAPTER 71

CENTRAL NERVOUS SYSTEM REGULATION OF THE SYMPATHETIC AND CARDIOVAGAL VASOMOTOR OUTFLOWS

PATRICE G. GUYENET AND RUTH L. STORNETTA

The CNS exerts control over regional blood flows and arterial pressure by three distinct but interdependent means: (a) neural regulation of the vasculature, heart and kidney via sympathetic and/or cardiovagal vasomotor efferents, (b) hormonal control of kidney and vasculature, and (c) behavioral regulation of salt and water intake (thirst and salt appetite).

The best understood aspect of the autonomic nervous system (cardiovagal and sympathoadrenal) is its ability to regulate the cardiac output and regional blood flows according to behavioral demands while minimizing short-term fluctuations in arterial pressure. The relative role of the sympathetic outflow versus the kidney or the vasculature in the genesis of hypertensive states remains a hotly debated issue that will not be addressed in this chapter (58).

This chapter describes the cellular mechanisms that generate the sympathetic and vagal tones and the CNS network that underlies the most common cardiovascular reflexes. The available information derives from work done in anesthetized animals and from recordings performed in awake animals or humans (percutaneous microneurography). A brief description of the effects of opiates and centrally acting α^2-adrenergic agents on central cardiovascular regulation is also included because of their usefulness, present and potential, in anesthesiology.

GENERAL ANATOMY OF CENTRAL AUTONOMIC PATHWAYS

Major CNS Structures Involved in Autonomic Regulations

Most autonomic functions, including but not limited to hemodynamic regulations, are processed primarily within the same general set of interconnected brain stem and basal forebrain nuclei (88,119) illustrated in Fig. 1A. This network is also accessible to circulating hormones via mono- or oligosynaptic neural connections with circumventricular organs (73). Two cortical areas shown in Fig. 1B, the insular and infralimbic cortices (further described below) also appear to be specialized in autonomic regulations (23). Parts of the cerebellum and the vestibular nuclei also contribute to hemodynamic regulations, probably in connection with postural adjustments (108,153).

Autonomic Efferents: Sympathetic Preganglionic Neurons and Cardiovagal Motor Neurons

Sympathetic preganglionic neurons (SPGNs) are located primarily in the intermediolateral cell column (IML) of the thoracic and upper lumbar segments (21,30) (Fig. 2A). Within each spinal segment, a small number of these cells are also found in three additional spinal locations (lateral funicular area, intercalated cell group, and central autonomic nucleus). The axons of SPGNs project ipsilaterally through the nearest segmental ventral root and its corresponding white ramus to one or more pre- or paravertebral sympathetic ganglia. Very few SPGNs have recurrent collaterals (21) suggesting the virtual absence of Renshaw cell-style collateral feedback in this efferent motor system. A very large proportion of the dendrites of SPGNs are tightly bunched up within the confines of the IML, and they can extend over 1–2 mm in the rostrocaudal direction (21,35). Other dendrites extend toward the central canal. In combination, these dendritic projections produce a typical ladder-like arrangement.

The main transmitter of SPGNs is acetylcholine (ACh), which depolarizes postganglionic cells primarily by activation of nicotinic receptors. G-protein interactive receptors mediate muscarinic effects of ACh and that of other substances (catecholamine and peptides) directly or indirectly released by the activation of SPGNs (for a review, see ref. 76). SPGNs synthesize and presumably release neuroactive peptides (21). They also contain high levels of nitric oxide synthase (4). Nitric oxide may be potentiating ganglionic nicotinic transmission via the production of cGMP (4).

The sympathetic innervation of the heart is lateralized (120). Activation of SPGNs on the left side of the cord or stimulation of the left cardiac sympathetic nerve produces predominantly inotropic effects while the right side produces primarily chronotropic effects. This segregation suggests, but does not prove that the CNS may have the capability to fine-tune cardiac rate and myocardial contractility independently of each other.

Cardiovagal motor neurons (CVMs) are rather thinly spread out within the external formation of nucleus ambiguus, especially in its middle part (89; and for details on the subnuclear organization of nucleus ambiguus, see ref. 12). Most of these cells are, therefore, coextensive with the ventral respiratory group (VRG) (38). The remainder of CVMs are located in the dorsal motor nucleus of the vagus (DMX). The proportion of CVMs that lie in DMX varies according to the species. CVMs project to three main parasympathetic ganglia located in the fat pads surrounding the myocardium. These ganglia exert differential control over the SA and AV nodes (112) and may be controlled in turn by separate populations of CVMs. This organization suggests that the brain may have the ability to fine-tune heart rate and conduction independently of each other.

Inputs to SPGN Cells and CVMs

Powerful new tract-tracing methods based on the retrograde transsynaptic transport of neurotropic viruses—pseudorabies and herpes (132)—have revealed that monosynaptic inputs to SPGNs originate from only a few areas indicated in Fig. 2A (88,131,132): rostral ventrolateral medulla (RVL), ventromedial rostral medulla (serotonergic and other cells of the caudal raphe), A5 area (mostly noradrenergic cells) (20), and the par-

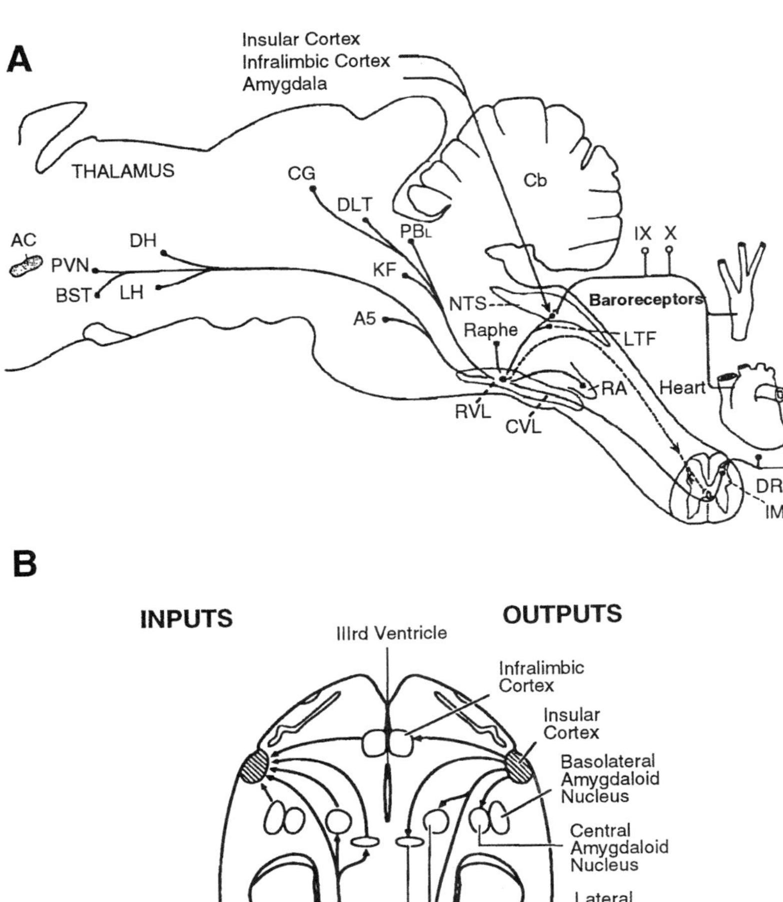

Figure 1. **(A)** Afferent inputs to rostral ventrolateral medulla (RVL) and bulbospinal efferent projections from RVL to the intermediolateral column (IML) of the spinal cord. Parasagittal view. **(B)** Horizontal section through rat brain illustrating afferent (*left,* inputs) and efferent (*right,* outputs) connections of the insular cortex and infralimbic cortex, two important cortical loci for vasomotor control. (A: Reprinted with permission from ref. 119. B: Reprinted with permission from ref 23.)

vocellular division of the paraventricular nucleus (including dopaminergic and peptidergic cells). RVL projections to SPGNs consist of a mixture of cells with and without catecholaminergic phenotype (2:1 ratio). The midbrain central gray, the lateral hypothalamus, and the Kölliker-Fuse nucleus (K-F in Fig. 3) may also project monosynaptically to the region of the intermediolateral cell column (44). The role of these last projections in vasomotor control is not fully established. Many SPGNs obviously are involved in other types of visceral control (i.e., nonvasomotor) that also require supraspinal inputs. SPGNs also receive inputs from spinal interneurons. These cells mediate spinal sympathetic reflexes (30) and probably utilize GABA and glycine as transmitters (21,66,67). The role of spinal interneurons in the supraspinal control of vasomotor SPGNs is still unclear.

Information regarding the location of brain stem neurons antecedent to CVMs is scant. Figure 2B summarizes current knowledge (127). This scheme is an interpretation of neurophysiological work done mostly in cats and, therefore, still tentative. CVMs receive monosynaptic inputs from serotonergic cells of the medullary raphe. This input is well identified anatomically, but its role remains elusive.

Organization of the Medulla Oblongata and Pons

The most basic autonomic functions (respiratory rhythmogenesis (38), generation of sympathetic and vagal tone (50), and visceral reflexes) reside in the pontomedullary regions represented in Fig. 3.

Dorsal Medulla

The nucleus of the solitary tract (NTS) is the exclusive site of termination of vagal afferents with the possible exception of peripheral chemoreceptors. The central projections of the various vagal afferents are topographically organized within the NTS in longitudinally oriented, somewhat overlapping, sheets (89). Accordingly, the NTS can be subdivided into subnuclei and regions of which only a few are thought to be specialized in the processing of cardiovascular information. For example, baroreceptor afferents project predominantly to the intermediate portion of the NTS and especially dorsally and dorsomedially to the tractus solitarius (27,32). Arterial chemoreceptor afferents project mainly to the intermediate and caudal part of the medial NTS (127).

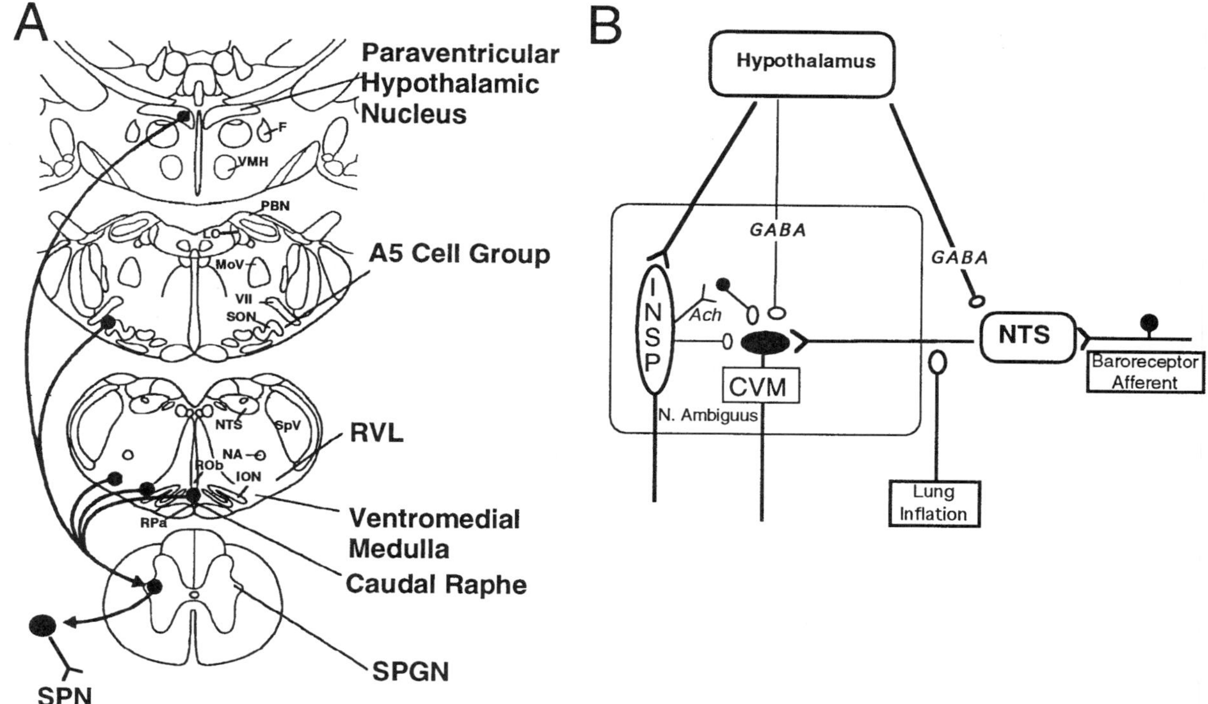

Figure 2. **(A)** Coronal sections through (bottom to top) spinal cord, rostral medulla, pons, and hypothalamus of the rat brain, illustrating the main supraspinal, presumably monosynaptic, inputs to sympathetic preganglionic neurons of spinal cord. **(B)** Some of the functionally identified inputs to CVMs: <, excitatory inputs; *open circle*, inhibitory inputs. (A: Reprinted, in adapted form, with permission from ref. 131. B: Reprinted with permission from ref. 127.)

The NTS has reciprocal connections with the area postrema (also called "chemotrigger zone"), one of several CNS circumventricular organs (73). These structures lie outside the blood-brain barrier and contain neurons with direct access to blood-borne substances via their fenestrated, peripheral-like capillaries. The area postrema contains many catecholaminergic neurons. Its major projections are to the NTS and the parabrachial nuclei. The ventrolateral medulla receives quantitatively minor direct projections from the area postrema (73), but this circumventricular organ may exert an important control on the presympathetic cells via some still unknown circuitry (136).

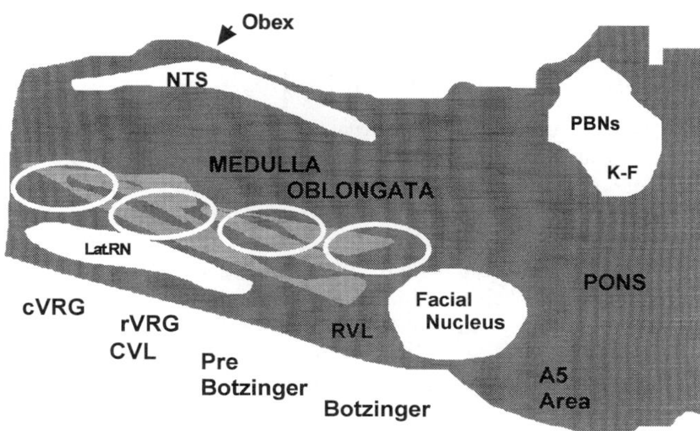

Figure 3. Parasagittal section through the lower brain stem illustrating the anatomical location of the main regions involved in cardiovascular and respiratory control. The major subdivisions of nucleus ambiguus (12) are shown (*dark stipples*). CVL, caudal ventrolateral medulla; cVRG, caudal part of ventral respiratory group; KF, Kölliker-Fuse nucleus; lat. RN, lateral reticular nucleus; NTS, nucleus of the solitary tract; PBNs, parabrachial nuclei; RVL rostral ventrolateral medulla.

Ventrolateral Medulla

The ventrolateral medulla and the dorsal motor nucleus of the vagus contain the motor or efferent side of medullary visceral reflex pathways. In addition, this area also contains the most elemental neuronal networks responsible for generation of the respiratory rhythm and the sympathetic tone.

Figure 3 illustrates the major rostrocaudal subdivisions of the ventrolateral medulla of importance to respiratory and cardiovascular control (38,50). The rostral portion, or RVL, close to the ventral surface, contains the kernel of the sympathetic tone generating mechanism to be detailed later. Various subdivisions of nucleus ambiguus (12) lie immediately dorsal and dorsolateral to this area (lightly shaded areas in Fig. 3). The compact division (dorsally) contains motoneurons innervating the striated muscle of the esophagus and the subcompact portion contains laryngeal and pharyngeal motoneurons. The subcompact portion also includes the "Botzinger nucleus" (38), a collection of neurons involved in respiratory rhythmogenesis with projections within the medulla and to the spinal cord.

Immediately caudal, within the ventrolateral medulla and nucleus ambiguus, lies the "pre-Botzinger area." This area may contain the most basic circuitry capable of generating a respiratory rhythm since its activity persists in tissue slices (125). This circuit is probably driven by neurons with bursting pacemaker activity.

Immediately caudal again, the periambigual area—the area surrounding nucleus ambiguus, called the rostral ventral respiratory group, rVRG, by respiratory physiologists (38)—is characterized by a high concentration of bulbospinal inspiratory premotor neurons that drive diaphragmatic and other relevant inspiratory muscles (Fig. 3). The very same area is commonly identified in the experimental cardiovascular field as the ventrolateral medullary "depressor area" (or "caudal" ventrolateral medulla, CVL, in contrast with the rostral portion or RVL). This nomenclature derives from the fact that increasing neuronal activity by depolarizing agents (i.e., excitatory amino acids) in this area produces hypotension whereas decreasing neuronal activity with hyperpolarizing agents (i.e., excitatory amino acid antagonists) produces increases in blood pressure (149). This effect is now attributed to the presence of inhibitory interneurons involved in the sympathetic baroreflex (83) (see Fig. 7 below).

More caudally, the ventrolateral medulla—the cVRG to respiratory physiologists (38)—contains a predominance of bulbospinal neurons involved in driving expiratory muscles. This area seems to be of lesser importance in vascular control, although some hypotension is still produced by neuronal excitation in this area (31).

Lateral Tegmental Field

The NTS and the ventrolateral medulla are heavily interconnected by a dense "transtegmental" fiber tract (119). The region outlined by this transtegmental tract seems to overlap with the portion of the "lateral tegmental field" in which cells with activity correlated with sympathetic activity have been identified—LTF (45) in Fig. 1A. Like the NTS and the ventrolateral medulla (RVL plus CVL), this region of the reticular formation is selectively targeted by inputs from most other brain regions involved in autonomic regulations, i.e., the paraventricular nucleus of hypothalamus, and the central gray area (74,88,119).

Raphe Complex and Midline Medulla

The rostral portion of the ventromedial medulla (Fig. 2A) projects heavily to the spinal cord. Projections to the IML are thought to originate from the raphe obscurus and pallidus and the outlying serotonergic areas called the lateral B3 group or parapyramidal area (65). Monosynaptic projections from serotonergic cells of the medullary raphe to SPGNs have been described (147).

Pons

The parabrachial and Kölliker-Fuse nuclei of the dorsolateral pons (identified in Figs. 1 and 3) have bilateral connections with every brain stem structure involved in cardiovascular regulation including the NTS and RVL (44). The dorsolateral pons is complex and currently subdivided in numerous subnuclei, only some of which participate in cardiorespiratory integration (44). This area also receives very heavy inputs from lamina I of the spinal cord (129) suggesting that it plays a major role in processing visceral and or nociceptive information. Also defined as the "pneumotactic area" (38), the parabrachial complex plays an essential role in respiratory pattern generation and therefore, indirectly, in controlling the sympathetic and cardiovagal outflows.

As a final remark, it should be noted that the same general areas of the medulla oblongata and pons (Fig. 3) are involved in regulating respiration and cardiovascular function (39). This proximity provides the anatomical substrate for the classic interactions between these systems.

Cortical Areas Involved in Vasomotor Regulations

This subject is covered in the anatomy section of this chapter because the bulk of our knowledge derives from the deductive reasoning of neuroanatomists (23,119). The remainder comes from a relatively modest amount of electrophysiological evidence (e.g., effects of electrical or occasionally chemical stimulation, and some unit recording, mostly in anesthetized animals).

From this body of evidence (reviewed in ref. 23), it is concluded that two cortical areas are very likely to play a predominant role in autonomic regulations (including cardiovascular function) namely, the insular and the infralimbic cortex (Fig. 1B).

The insular cortex contains an organotopic visceral sensory map. The cardiopulmonary region is primarily represented in the posterior portion of the granular insular cortex via a pathway with relays in the NTS, the parabrachial nucleus and both the ventroposterior parvocellular thalamic nucleus (VPLpc) and the lateral hypothalamic area. This portion of the insular cortex projects back to the same autonomic structures and, massively, to the infralimbic cortex. It contains units responsive to activation of baroreceptors and chemoreceptors. When stimulated, changes in respiration and arterial pressure are elicited. The insular cortex also projects to the central nucleus of the amygdala which in turn innervates most subcortical autonomic regions.

As for the infralimbic cortex, this region probably serves as the cortical autonomic motor output because it has massive descending connections with the autonomic system, including the VPLpc, parabrachial nucleus, NTS, and spinal cord lamina X, but it has few afferents from these nuclei (23). Inputs from the dorsally located prelimbic cortex provide the infralimbic cortex with information originating from the rest of the limbic system.

Finally, it is possible that the somatosensory motor cortex might also play a role in autonomic regulation. Conceivably, this area could regulate blood flow in accordance with the activity of the skeletal muscles and may serve as a central command mechanism for regional blood flow regulation (23). The evidence is controversial and the concept is only partially supported by the neuroanatomical connectivity of this cortical area.

ROSTRAL VENTROLATERAL MEDULLA: "VASOMOTOR CENTER" REVISITED

Even under anesthesia, sympathetic vasomotor efferents retain a substantial activity. The resulting vasoconstrictor and cardiomotor effects are essential to maintain arterial pressure and tissue perfusion at levels compatible with survival. This section describes the CNS circuits thought to be responsible for basal sympathetic tone generation under anesthesia.

Nucleus RVL and Sympathetic Tone

Application of the inhibitory neurotransmitter glycine on the ventral surface of the rostral ventrolateral medulla (the "glycine sensitive area") produces a fall of arterial pressure equivalent to that elicited by surgical spinalization (49). The original conclusion of this work has been that sympathetic tone requires the ongoing activity of neuronal cell bodies located close to the ventral surface of the rostral medulla oblongata. Accordingly, under anesthesia, severe hypotension is produced when intraparenchymal injections of neuronal inhibitory substances are selectively targeted to the limited region of the medulla oblongata immediately dorsal to the "glycine area" (119,149). This region of the medulla has been called by different authors rostral medullary "pressor area", nucleus reticularis rostroventrolateralis or RVL, retrofacial portion of nucleus paragigantocellularis and subretrofacial nucleus. This area (henceforth called RVL) (Fig. 3) contains the *rostral* half of the C1 cells, a group of neurons that, among other neuroactive substances, synthesize catecholamines inclusive of adrenaline and make up two thirds of the monosynaptic projection of RVL to SPGNs (119). The projection from RVL to SPGNs numbers only a few hundred neurons on each side in the rat (100). They have a very restricted localization within the reticular formation (in the rat for example, this area measures no more than 400-500 μm across and extends over less than one mm in length). The corresponding area of the human brain is identifiable by its concentration of adrenergic cells and of angiotensin AT_1 receptors (1).

RVL neurons with projections to SPGNs are tonically active "in vivo" and provide an essential excitatory input to sympathetic vasomotor preganglionic neurons (19,50,140). These RVL cells will be called "presympathetic vasomotor neurons" from this point on. Their pattern of firing is very reminiscent of that of individual sympathetic vasomotor efferents except for a generally higher discharge rate. Figure 4A illustrates some of their characteristics and the similarity between their pattern of firing and that of vasomotor sympathetic efferents (e.g., the mass discharge of a lumbar sympathetic nerve, as shown in Fig. 4B, C). Note the high level of spontaneous activity of RVL presympathetic cells at low blood pressure, their exquisite sensitivity to baroreceptor feedback (Fig. 4A1) and their pulse-related discharge pattern (Fig. 4A2, B). This cardiac-related pattern is characteristic of many of the cells directly involved in the core baroreflex circuitry, from baroreceptor afferents to vasomotor SPGNs (SND in Fig. 4C1). The major neurotransmitter of RVL presympathetic vasomotor neurons may be an excitatory amino acid (EAA), probably glutamate (36,67,103, 104). This amino acid may be released both by the C1 adrenergic and by the nonadrenergic component of the RVL-spinal pathway.

RVL presympathetic vasomotor neurons are believed to be organized in an organotopic pattern. For example some cells seem dedicated to the control of muscle vasoconstrictor sympathetic efferents while others control skin vasomotor efferents (34). The former are less barosensitive and, in keeping with the role of skin blood flow in thermoregulation, they are inhibited by increases in core temperature. The latter are very barosensitive but unaffected by temperature (93).

RVL presympathetic neurons derive their activity from (a) intrinsic pacemaker properties that are modulated by peptides and biogenic amines via G protein coupled receptors and (b) extrinsic synaptic drives.

Pacemaker Properties of Presympathetic Vasomotor Cells of RVL: Role in Basal Sympathetic Tone Generation

Many RVL bulbospinal neurons have intrinsic beating properties in tissue slices (discharge rate:2-20 Hz at 37°C). This rate of discharge is comparable to that observed under anesthesia "in vivo" in the absence of baroreceptor feedback inhibition (Fig. 5). Figure 5 also depicts the comparatively simple dendritic morphology of one such pacemaker cell and its location in the midst of the adrenergic cells of RVL (dots in "C1" area). The pacemaker theory is also supported by a large amount of congruent indirect evidence. Perhaps the most persuasive is the resistance of the sympathetic tone to blockade of receptors to GABA and excitatory amino acids (EAA) anywhere in the lower brain stem including in RVL (these transmitters are most generally involved in fast synaptic transmission). The lack of effect of EAA antagonists, for example, is in stark contrast with the powerful disruption of central respiratory rhythm generation observed when this type of agent is microinjected in widely spread out areas of the medulla oblongata. Also the pacemaker theory is supported by the fact that extensive searching within the brain stem has not uncovered any area that could be the source of a significant tonic excitatory drive to RVL presympathetic neurons.

Earlier experiments had only identified the nonadrenergic component of the RVL-IML projection as having intrinsic pacemaker properties (137). More recent evidence (Li Y. W. and P. G. Guyenet, *unpublished data*, 1995) indicates that the adrenergic component of the pathway, like many other types of catecholaminergic cells in the CNS (150), is also endowed with autoactivity.

The pharmacologic properties of C1 (adrenergic) and non-C1 cells are different (Fig. 6A). The discharge rate of the nonadrenergic RVL autoactive cells is increased by catecholamines (β-adrenergic effect) and either decreased or increased by many agonists of G protein interactive receptors: NPY, enkephalin, vasopressin, oxytocin, ATP, and adenosine (50) (summarized in Fig. 6A). Most of these substances have been detected in nerve terminals within the RVL (100), and CRF has recently been added to the list. Yet, with few exceptions (e.g., vasopressin and oxytocin that clearly originate from the parvocellular division of the hypothalamic paraventricular nucleus), the source of these inputs remains obscure at present. Via their action on the firing of RVL pacemakers, these substances could serve as long-term regulators of the vasoconstrictor output and arterial pressure. C1 adrenergic cells have a pharmacological profile that is different from the rest of the presympathetic neurons of RVL (Fig. 6A). They are predominantly inhibited by catecholamines or by drugs with α_2-adrenergic agonist activity and they are stimulated by angiotensin II via AT1, losartan-sensitive, receptors (Li Y. W. and P. G. Guyenet, *unpublished data*, 1996). Their excitation by angiotensin II may account for the sympathoexcitation caused by microinjection of this peptide into RVL (2).

Synaptic activation or inhibition of RVL presympathetic neurons via GABAergic or glutamatergic inputs underlies most vasomotor sympathetic reflexes under anesthesia. The major synaptic inputs of these cells are summarized in Fig. 6B. At the present time, it is unknown whether some of these inputs regulate C1 and other presympathetic cells in a differential manner.

Additional Bulbar Mechanisms for Sympathetic Tone Generation and Alternative Theories

The preceding section emphasized the role of RVL in AP maintenance because RVL presympathetic neurons are undoubtedly essential for sympathetic tone generation under anesthesia. However, it is probable that they represent only a fraction of all possible synaptic inputs to SPGNs. SPGNs are contacted monosynaptically by serotonergic neurons from the medullary raphe (147) that provide an additional excitatory input (95). SPGNs may also be influenced polysynaptically in complex ways by other serotinergic projections to the cord (30) and may also receive inputs (excitatory and inhibitory) from several other types of medullary raphe neurons (45,105). Intracellular recordings from SPGNs "in vivo" under anesthesia indicate that some of these cells do receive IPSPs even under anesthesia (36) and, "in vitro," IPSPs can be elicited in these cells by focal stimulation (67). Also, anatomical work indicates that SPGNs are contacted by synaptic boutons which contain the inhibitory transmitters GABA and glycine (21). Thus, although the principle of the existence of inhibitory controls of SPGN activity is well established, the origin of these inputs, the type of SPGN (vasomotor or otherwise) that receives these inhibitory contacts, and the physiological role of these inputs are not understood.

The presence of slow oscillations of the mass discharge of sympathetic nerves in anesthetized cats with resected baroreceptor afferents also indicates that some brain stem circuitry synchronizes the vasomotor output under anesthesia (9,45). These oscillations may involve an interplay between cells located in the lateral tegmental field (LTF) and putative presympathetic neurons of the raphe and RVL (45). In the

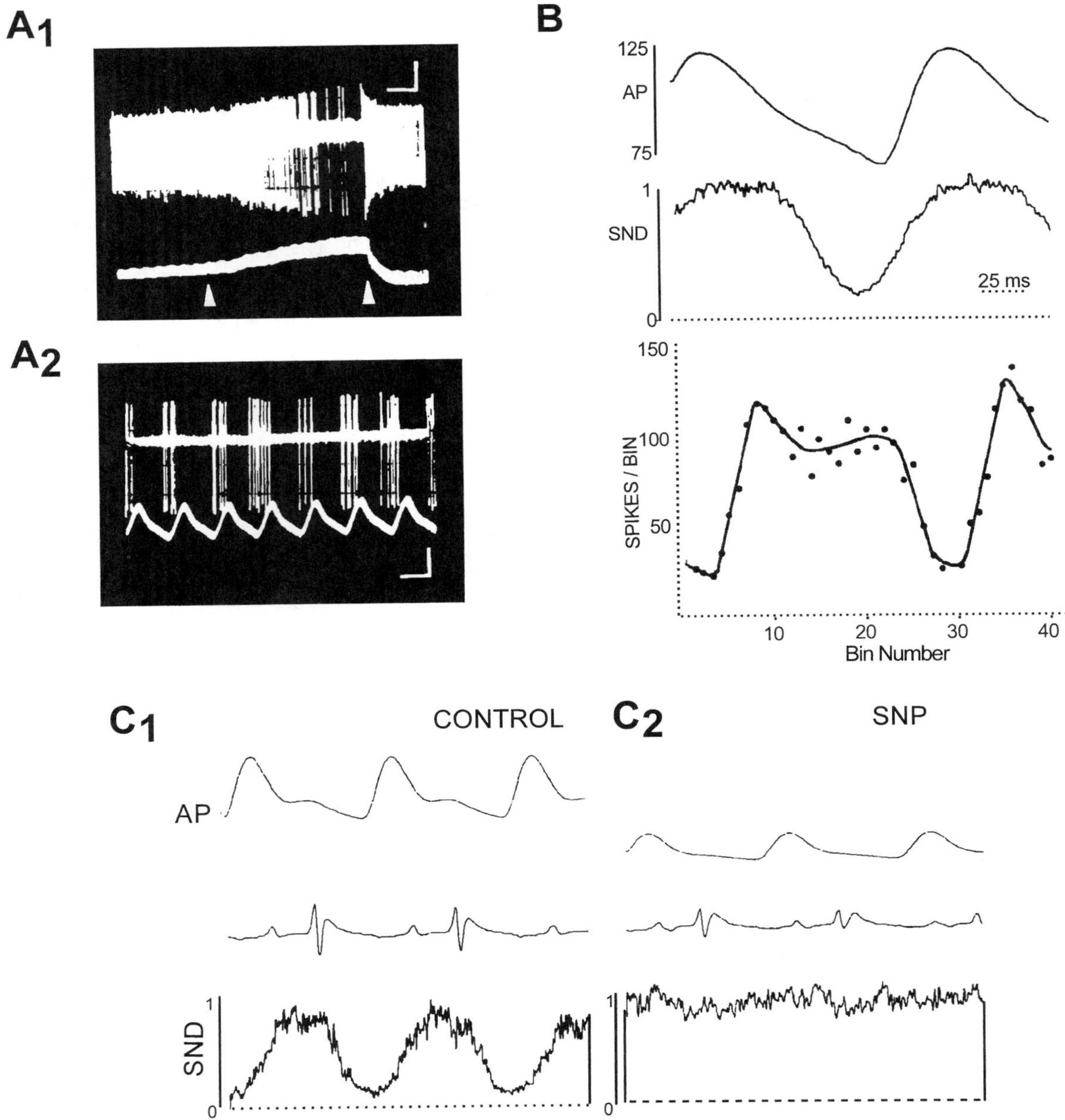

Figure 4. Electrophysiological properties of the presympathetic vasomotor cells of RVL: resemblance with discharge pattern of vasoconstrictor postganglionic cells. **(A)** Unit discharge of a single RVL presympathetic neuron in rat (*top trace,* unit; *lower trace,* AP). A_1 shows neuron's exquisite sensitivity to increases in aterial pressure (raised between *arrows* up to 150 mm Hg). A_2 shows pulse synchrony of unit discharge due to periodic inhibition of cell by polysynaptic input from baroreceptors. **(B)** Simultaneous, computer averaging of multiunit activity of vasoconstrictor nerve (SND, lumbar sympathetic chain) and unit activity of an RVL presympathetic cell (spikes/bin) triggered by pulse pressure (AP). **(C)** EKG-triggered computer averaging of AP and lumbar sympathetic nerve discharge, illustrating the fact that sympathetic vasomotor nerve activity is pulse-rhythmic at resting AP (C_2) but not synchronized to cardiac rate under conditions of lowered AP [C_2, during infusion of sodium nitroprusside (SNP)]. (A: Reprinted with permission from ref. 133. B,C: Reprinted with permission from ref. 52.)

scheme of Barman and Gebber (Fig. 7), RVLM-SE neurons (SE for sympathoexcitatory) correspond to the RVL presympathetic cells described above.

Finally, another theory considers that a common pool of neurons is responsible for generation of the sympathetic and the respiratory neural output. This particular issue is addressed below.

The vasomotor sympathetic outflow may be a pacemaker driven system, with at its "kernel" a group of autoactive neurons located in RVL that produces a glutamate-receptor mediated monosynaptic excitation of preganglionic cells. Many of these presympathetic cells of RVL also synthesize catecholamines inclusive of adrenaline and peptide hormones. The simplicity and minimal number of synapses involved in this circuit could explain why the sympathetic tone is especially resistant to general anesthesia. However, this system only represents the core of a very complex and still poorly understood network.

ARTERIAL BAROREFLEX

The core circuitry of the arterial baroreflex (circuit recruited by activation of aortic and carotid baroreceptors and leading to

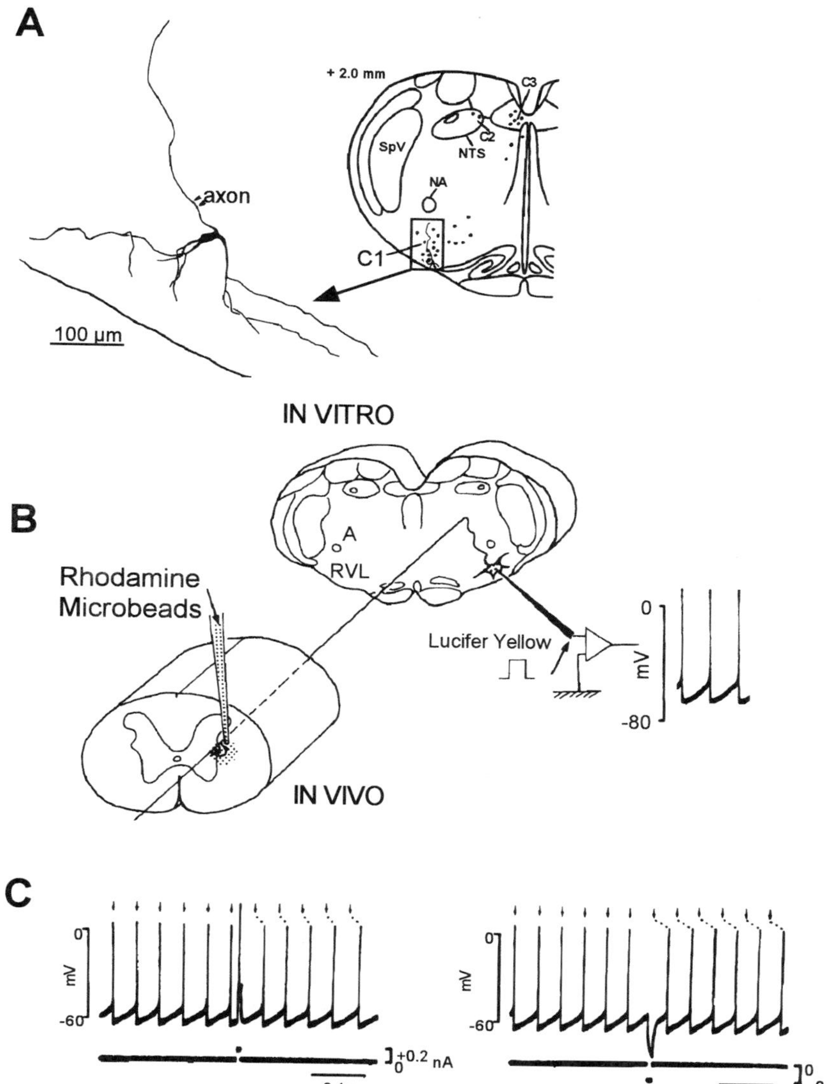

Figure 5. **(A)** Location and morphology of non-adrenergic RVL presympathetic cell with pacemaker properties shown in relation to C1 adrenergic cells (*dots* in the small-scale coronal rat brain section). **(B)** Method for anatomical identification of presympathetic vasomotor cells in "in vitro" experiments. Rhodamine microbeads are injected in spinal cord of rats "in vivo" 10 days before medullary slices are prepared for intracellular recording. Recorded cells are identified by intracellular injection of Lucifer yellow. **(C)** Intracellular current-clamp recording of RVL pacemaker neuronal activity "in vitro." Resetting of discharge rate by depolarizing and hyperpolarizing current pulses suggests cell activity is intrinsic and not a network property. (Reprinted with permission from ref. 89.)

sympathoinhibition and cardiovagal activation) is shown in Fig. 8. The salient feature of the sympathetic baroreflex under anesthesia is that the reduction in sympathetic tone produced by baroreceptor loading is primarily due to a disfacilitation of the preganglionic neurons, i.e., a reduction in the amount of excitatory drive contributed by RVL presympathetic neurons (C1 and others). Activation of bulbospinal inhibitory neurons (such as those from the raphe) may also, in theory, contribute to the reflex but definitive evidence for this option has never been clearly obtained and, therefore, will not be discussed further (for details, see ref. 30). It is very likely, although not fully documented except in the case of the NTS, that every intermediate step of the baroreceptor circuit described in Fig. 8 is synaptically regulated by inputs from the brain areas described in Fig. 1. Finally, the baroreflex circuitry is also subject to regulation by circulating hormones such as vasopressin and angiotensin II which act through the circumventricular organs (i.e., area postrema).

Arterial Baroreceptors

Arterial baroreceptors (see Chapter X and, for reviews, see refs. 25,83,85) are slowly adapting mechanoreceptors located mainly in the inner adventitia of the aortic arch and carotid bifurcation. The peripheral axons of aortic arch baroreceptor neurons travel mainly (but not exclusively) via the aortic depressor nerve and their cell bodies reside in the nodose ganglion. In many species, this nerve is physically separate from the vagal trunk and in rodents it may consist almost purely of baroreceptor fibers (83). Carotid receptors ascend via the carotid sinus nerve (a mixed nerve containing a two thirds majority of chemoreceptor afferents). Their somata reside in the petrosal ganglia. All arterial baroreceptors project selectively to a restricted number of subnuclei of the NTS and no further within the brain stem (27,83). The peripheral unmyelinated processes of the primary afferents are assumed to be directly sensitive to stretch because of the absence of specialized satellite cells. The inaccessibility of these structures has so far precluded a biophysical analysis of the mechanisms responsible for generation of the receptor potential. Most likely some form of stretch-sensitive channel is involved whose activation produces an inward current that depolarizes the nerve terminal and triggers action potentials at some preterminal site.

Aortic baroreceptors differ in their pressure threshold, adaptation to maintained stretch and conduction velocity (83,85). A fibers are in the minority, ≤ 30%, and conduct in the range of 20–55 m/s (A-β fibers) and 10–15 m/s (A-δ fibers). Their

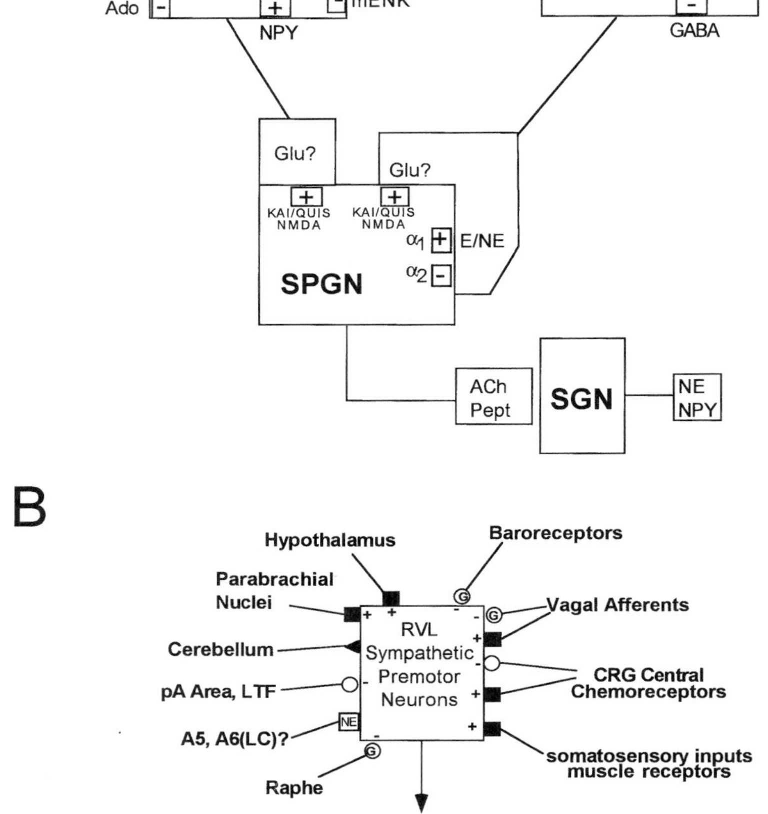

Figure 6. **(A)** Major transmitters thought to be released by C1 and non-C1 presympathetic neurons on sympathetic preganglionic neurons (SPGN). Glutamate may be the principal excitatory transmitter. C1 cells may also release neuropeptides including neuropeptide Y (not illustrated). Both C1 and non-C1 presympathetic cells have intrinsic beating properties "in vitro" that are up- or downregulated by agonists to the various receptors depicted on their respective cell bodies. The direction of the change in activity is indicated by + or - (excitation or inhibition). **(B)** Synaptic inputs (generally polysynaptic) of presympathetic cells of RVL (C1 and non-C1) based on neurophysiologic evidence "in vivo." (Reprinted with permission from ref. 55.)

threshold for activation is usually much lower than resting arterial pressure. Their discharge pattern is extremely pulse-synchronous. Although their response to mean arterial pressure suggests that their firing can encode mean arterial pressure, these cells could theoretically encode a much larger spectrum of hemodynamic variables including pulsatile pressure, heart rate, cardiac contractile force (via dP/dt) and, perhaps, blood flow. C fibers conduct in the range of 0.5–1.8 m/s and have higher pressure thresholds; only 28% of them are thought to be active at resting pressure in the rabbit (83). One of the most remarkable, if unexplained, aspects of the mechanoelectric coupling of baroreceptors is the sensitizing effect of blood flow on their response to a given level of pressure.

A single, synchronous activation of both C- and A-fiber baroreceptors is sufficient to trigger a powerful, long-lasting inhibition of the sympathetic outflow. In contrast, the selective single-shock activation of A fibers produces no effect (83). The onset latency of the sympathoinhibition evoked by single shock stimulation of C-fiber afferents is quite long (tens of milliseconds), as expected from a substantial initial delay due to the slow-conducting baroreceptor afferents and the very slow conduction velocity of the intramedullary pathway (0.2–0.5 m/s). Stimulation of A fibers produces sympathoinhibition only following train stimulation (>20 Hz), and the effect is brief (83). These results could be interpreted to mean that the C-fiber baroreceptor input is more essential for regulation of the sympathetic output than A fibers or that the effect of A-fiber activation is dramatically reduced by anesthesia.

Three forms of baroreceptor resetting are currently distinguished (25). "Instantaneous" resetting refers to the lack of baroreceptor activity during the diastolic phase although pressure may still be higher than necessary for baroreceptor activation during early systole. This form of resetting may involve mainly mechanical factors, i.e., vessel compliance.

A second form of baroreceptor resetting or "acute" resetting is typically observed within a time scale of seconds to minutes when the barosensitive areas are exposed to a sustained, nonpulsatile, elevation of intraluminal pressure (25). The hysteresis phenomenon (larger response of baroreceptors during the ascending phase of a pressure ramp than during the descending phase) is probably an avatar of the same type of resetting. This form of acute resetting is "absent or blunted" when the sustained elevation of pressure is done using a more physiological, i.e., pulsatile, pattern (26); consequently, its physiological significance remains uncertain.

Finally, both types of baroreceptors are reset to higher operating pressures by all forms of hypertension ("chronic" resetting). This resetting is essentially "complete" in the sense that the pressure threshold of baroreceptors is increased by the same amount as the degree of hypertension, with an increase in MAP (25). In addition, the slope of the pressure-activity response curve and the maximum discharge rate of

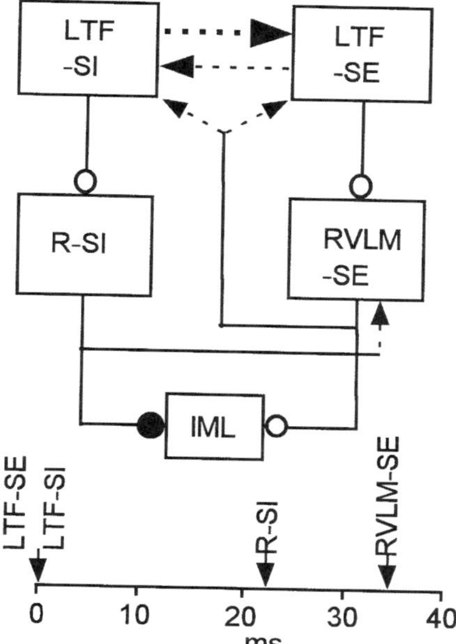

Figure 7. Generation of the slow 2–6-Hz rhythm of SND. Neuronal loops involving the lateral tegmental field, raphe, and RVL seem responsible for the existence of a slow 2–6-Hz oscillation in sympathetic nerve discharge (cats). This oscillation persists even in absence of baroreceptor input. *Open circle,* excitatory connection; *solid circle,* inhibitory connection; LTF-SE, lateral tegmental field sympathoexcitatory neuron; LTF-SI, lateral tegmental field sympathoinhibitory neuron; RVLM-SE, RVL sympathoexcitatory neuron; R-SI, medullary raphe sympathoinhibitory neuron; IML, intermediolateral spinal sympathetic nucleus. This scheme also illustrates the concept of a dual bulbospinal control of preganglionic cell activity that includes descending inhibitory inputs from the raphe nuclei. (Reprinted with permission from ref. 9.)

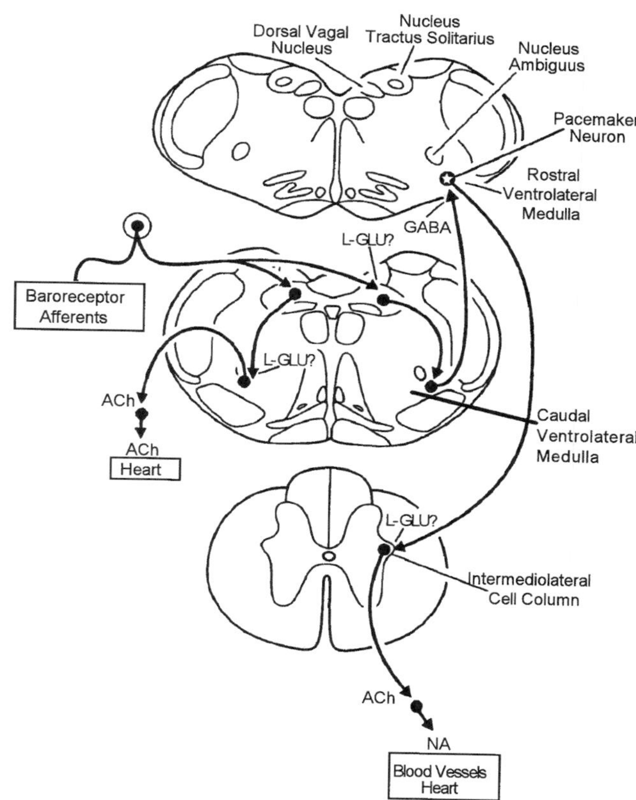

Figure 8. Model of the core circuitry involved in the baroreflex. Baroreceptor afferents (probably glutamatergic) terminate in the NTS. Second (or higher) order neurons in NTS project to CVMs by a possible glutamatergic connection (*left*) and to GABA-ergic propriobulbar neurons in the nucleus ambiguus (*right*). These GABA-ergic neurons then project to bulbospinal sympathoexcitatory neurons in RVL. The RVL neurons project to the sympathetic preganglionic neurons in the intermediolateral cell column via a mixed pathway consisting of glutamatergic neurons and adrenergic (C1) neurons. (Reprinted with permission from ref. 50.)

baroreceptor afferents is reduced in chronic hypertension. This form of resetting is probably the most important functionally as it tends to maintain rather than oppose the hypertensive process. It can occur with a $T_{1/2}$ of a few days if the hypertension is produced by an acute perturbation (aortic constriction, renal stenosis). Very importantly, some resetting may also occur before any morphological change of the arterial wall or any change in the overall distensibility of the arterial wall can be detected. The process of chronic resetting can be reversible. For example, in genetic hypertension, this reversal can be achieved by normalizing AP with a converting-enzyme inhibitor and in renal hypertension (renal arterial stenosis) by restoring flow to the kidney. Part of the resetting may be due to structural vascular changes. In addition, the mechanosensitivity of baroreceptor terminals may be altered via some unexplained neuronal plasticity phenomenon, perhaps in response to endothelial factors (25). Regardless of the mechanisms involved, this chronic resetting eliminates the ability of the baroreceptors to oppose the hypertensive process and resets the baroreflex to a higher operating range. This peculiarity suggests that the primary function of the baroreceptor feedback is to minimize short-term fluctuations of arterial pressure and not to regulate the long-term level of the sympathetic tone and arterial pressure (58).

Baroreceptor Information Processing in the Nucleus of the Solitary Tract

Baroreceptor afferents project with strong ipsilateral predominance to a narrow region dorsomedial and medial to the tractus solitarius, further restricted to the level of the obex. No projection outside the NTS has been reliably documented. The main neurotransmitter of baroreceptor afferents could be an excitatory amino acid (EAA, glutamate) because (a) the vast majority of monosynaptic EPSPs evoked in the NTS "in vitro" by stimulating tractus solitarius afferents are mediated by EAAs (5) and (b) EAA receptor antagonists injected in the NTS block the baroreflex—the cardiovagal and sympathetic (for a review, see ref. 48).

Second-Order Neurons in the Baroreflex Pathway

Two very different tactics have been used for the identification of the second-order neurons in the baroreflex pathway.

The first one has been to look specifically for NTS neurons with pulse-related firing and EPSPs locked to the cardiac cycle (32). This tactic is based on the assumption that such a pattern of firing is a necessary attribute of at least some of the second-order cells involved in the baroreflex because all other known neurons within the feedback loop also exhibit a pulse-modulated discharge, i.e., primary afferents as described above, propriomedullary interneurons of CVL, RVL presympathetic neurons, and cardiovagal and sympathetic efferents (Figs. 4, 9, and 10). In agreement with this logic, pulse-modulated cells have indeed been found in the area where arterial baroreceptor afferents arborize most (i.e., in very close proximity to the tractus solitarius at the level of the obex) and a few (n = 3) have

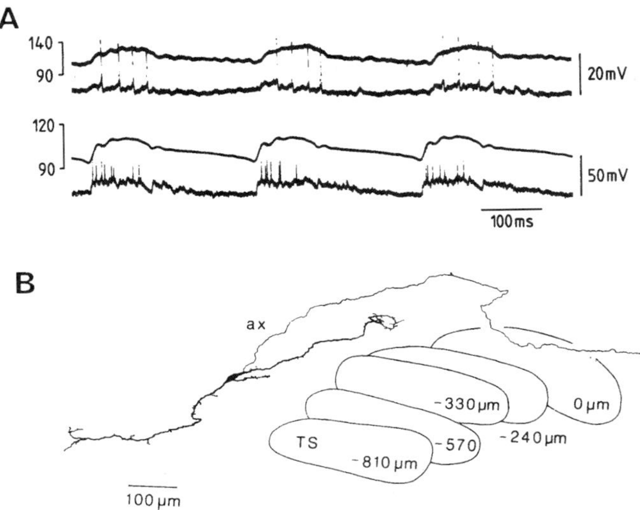

Figure 9. NTS neuron presumed to be a second-order cell in the baroreflex pathway on the basis of location and pulse-modulated pattern of firing. (Reprinted with permission from ref. 32.)

been stained following intracellular identification (32). Their structure is simple and consists of two primary dendrites extending in a rostrocaudal direction and of a laterally oriented dendrite curving medially in the dorsolateral subnucleus. The axons of these cells exit the NTS after giving off few if any local collaterals (Fig. 9). The exact destination of their axons is unfortunately unknown. The second and most common tactic to identify NTS neurons in the baroreflex pathway has been to select for neurons that appear to receive monosynaptic inputs from baroreceptor afferents. For practical purposes, the focus of the majority of these studies has been placed on NTS neurons which receive short-latency inputs of invariant latency from A-fiber baroreceptor afferents, generally activated by electrical stimulation of a buffer nerve (97,98). This approach could have overlooked the targets of the C-fiber afferents because there is no clear evidence that myelinated and C-fiber baroreceptor afferents project to the same second-order neurons. As previously indicated, the C-fiber afferents may be the major players in the baroreflex circuit (83). The vast majority of NTS neurons thus identified do not have EPSPs locked with the cardiac cycle and they respond in complex fashion to stimulation of baroreceptor afferents, i.e., by EPSPs, by EPSP-IPSP sequences, or solely by IPSPs (98,127). The absence of EPSPs linked to the cardiac pulse suggests that most of these cells may be interneurons rather than second-order baroreceptor neurons or that they are not the interneurons which are primarily involved in the cardiovagal or sympathetic baroreflex. Many other homeostatic regulations also require, or are influenced by baroreceptor afferent inputs (including vigilance, thirst, respiration, volume control, etc.). These regulations probably utilize a variety of NTS neurons in addition to those involved in the baroreflex.

Modulation of the Baroreflex Within the NTS by Other Visceral Afferents and by Inputs From the Area Postrema and Other CNS Structures

A degree of synaptic convergence between baroreceptor and selected other types of visceral afferent occurs in the case of a number of NTS cells (reviewed in ref. 102). For example, cells have been found on both sides of the NTS which seem to respond monosynaptically to baroreceptor activation or which respond monosynaptically to activation of arterial baroreceptors and vagal or superior laryngeal inputs. However, convergence between arterial baroreceptor afferent inputs and slowly adapting pulmonary stretch receptor is not observed in the NTS (102). Convergence between peripheral chemoreceptor inputs and baroreceptor inputs has been observed in some NTS neurons, but it is not certain that the cells play a role in integrating the sympathetic baroreflex and chemoreflex since the pathways of these two reflexes seem to run independent courses until the RVL level (82). As a whole, the type of synaptic interactions described above suggest the possibility that integration between arterial baroreceptor afferents and various types of cardiopulmonary afferents that are all known to produce similar tonic sympathoinhibitory effects could occur in the NTS at the very earliest steps of the baroreflex pathway (e.g., Bezold-Jarisch reflex).

In addition to this integrative function between various types of visceral afferents, baroreceptive cells of the NTS receive inputs from structures within the CNS, including the hypothalamus, (75,97); the amygdala (127); and the parabrachial nuclei (108). This is evidence that the baroreflex can be modulated or gated at the level of the NTS by the abovementioned structures. Gating (illustrated in Fig. 12B, below; a similar scheme is represented in Fig. 2B) would tend to produce temporary rises in arterial pressure and heart rate, a known effect of hypothalamic stimulation, by reducing baroreceptor feedback inhibition. This mechanism could be one of the neurophysiological substrates of the "central baroreflex resetting," which may occur in hypertension (25). The concept is illustrated in Fig. 2B. It is also supported by the observation that the baroreflex can be modulated by transmitters and other signaling molecules introduced directly into the NTS (angiotensin II, GABA agonists, catecholamines, etc.). Finally, selected receptor antagonists (notably to GABA receptors) modulate the baroreflex when they are introduced directly into the NTS suggesting that the reflex pathway may be under tonic inhibition by GABAergic neurons at this level (18,138).

α_2-Adrenergic agonists, including the clinically used antihypertensive agent clonidine, facilitate (sensitize) the baroreflex, at least in part via an action in NTS (118). Monosynaptic transmission between unknown vagal afferents and unidentified NTS second-order neurons is commonly facilitated "in vitro" by α_2-adrenergic agonists (13,63). This phenomenon may be a model of the way in which baroreceptor afferent information is modulated by these agents and consequently of how clonidine "sensitizes" the baroreflex. According to Hay and Bishop, stimulation of the area postrema also facilitates transmission between vagal afferents and NTS neurons. Because the effects of area postrema stimulation and clonidine application are both reversed by α_2-adrenoceptor antagonists, it is conceivable that clonidine might mimic an effect that may be physiologically produced by activation of the catecholaminergic neurons of the area postrema. Details of the NTS circuitry involved need to be clarified.

Hormonal Modulation of the Baroreflex: Role of the area Postrema

Within the range of concentrations that cause maximum antidiuretic effects, plasma vasopressin does not usually produce significant increases in arterial pressure. This is attributed to the fact that the direct vasoconstrictor effects of the hormone are normally offset by a reduction in heart rate, cardiac output and sympathetic outflow (14). The effectiveness of arterial baroreceptors in buffering the hypertensive effects of vasopressin thus seems unusually large when compared to other pressor hormones, especially in the dog and rabbit. In the latter species, this has been attributed to a central facilitation of the baroreflex consecutive to the activation by AVP of neuronal elements within the area postrema. Angiotensin II, via an action in the area postrema or in the subfornical organ, may also modulate the sympathetic outflow via interactions between area postrema and NTS (13,73).

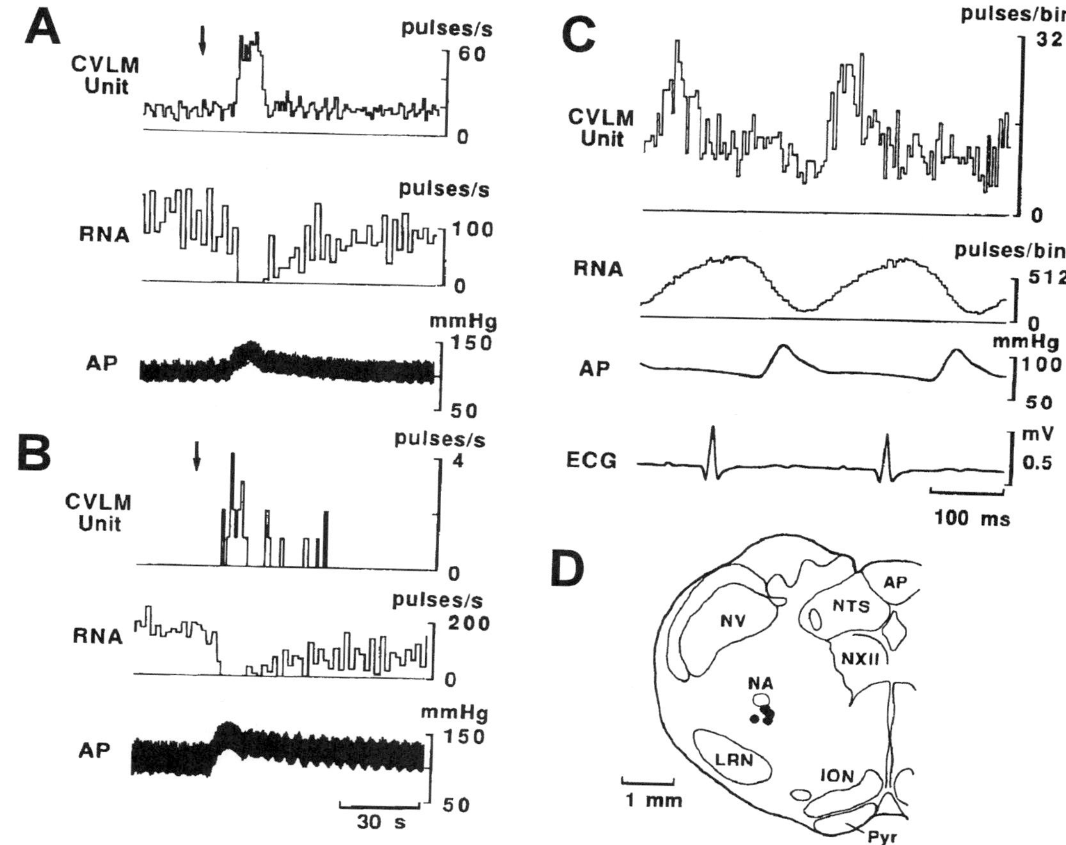

Figure 10. Properties and location of propriobulbar neurons that mediate sympathetic baroreflex by inhibition of RVL presympathetic cells. **(A,B)** Examples of two separate cells showing excitation during AP elevation and simultaneous inhibition of renal nerve activity. **(C)** Evidence that discharge pattern of these cells is synchronized with pressure pulse as is renal nerve activity (RNA). **(D)** Location of units in close proximity to nucleus ambiguus at CVL level (see location of CVL in Fig. 3). (Reprinted with permission from ref. 139.)

Second-order neurons in the baroreflex pathway may be located at obex level in the immediate proximity of the tractus solitarius. These cells are poorly characterized. It is unknown whether they project to the ventrolateral medulla directly (as illustrated in Fig. 8) or via a complex circuit within and without the NTS. The NTS also performs a complex integrative function between inputs from selected types of visceral afferents and inputs from within the CNS and the area postrema.

Caudal Ventrolateral Medulla: Third-Order Neurons of the Sympathetic Baroreflex

The activation of CVMs by baroreceptor afferents will be described later. This section is devoted to the propriomedullary cells presumed to be involved in the baroreceptor-mediated inhibition of presympathetic neurons of RVL (Figs. 8 and 10).

The first clue that the sympathetic baroreflex has a synaptic relay in the caudal ventrolateral medulla comes from experiments by Sapru and collaborators who showed that microinjection of muscimol (a GABA-mimetic agent) into the ventrolateral medulla of anesthetized rats at the level of the obex (CVL) produces AP elevation and blocks the hypotension produced by stimulation of the aortic baroreceptor nerves (149). The original interpretation that this area contains the cell bodies of propriomedullary neurons which project rostrally and inhibit the tone generating presympathetic vasomotor neurons of RVL has been validated by subsequent research whose most salient results are summarized below (50,83).

First, CVL does contain neurons projecting to RVL and which have the expected properties: they are excited by baroreceptor activation, exhibit a pressure threshold and are pulse-synchronous above this threshold (Fig. 10C). Second, stimulation of CVL produces inhibition of RVL neurons and hypotension which is reversed by administration of bicuculline (a $GABA_A$-receptor antagonist) in RVL. Third, the baroreceptor-mediated inhibition of RVL presympathetic vasomotor neurons is antagonized by iontophoretic application of bicuculline. Finally, these cells have IPSPs locked to the cardiac rate which are chloride-dependent (a characteristic of $GABA_A$-receptor mediated inhibition).

GABAergic propriomedullary interneurons with cell bodies in CVL appear to be an integral link of the sympathetic baroreflex (Fig. 8). These cells are activated by baroreceptor stimulation and are responsible for the inhibition of RVL presympathetic vasomotor neurons caused by arterial baroreceptor activation. These interneurons probably have many other inputs, unknown at the present time.

RECEPTORS AND VASOMOTOR REFLEXES FROM THE CARDIOPULMONARY REGION

The term cardiopulmonary receptors generally refers to a variety of sensory nerve endings located in the four cardiac chambers, in the great veins, the pulmonary arteries, and the lungs. Given that the vasomotor effects triggered by the activity of each individual type of afferent are not always fully understood, their central pathways are generally even more hypothetical.

Properties of Cardiopulmonary Receptors

Atrial Receptors

The right and left atria contain both myelinated and unmyelinated vagal afferents sensitive to stretch that project to the NTS. The discharge of myelinated atrial receptors (especially the predominant "B" type) is synchronous with the atrial rate and increases linearly with atrial pressure. The response of these receptors is exaggerated in volume expanded animals (59). Unmyelinated atrial receptors have a low level of activity, little or no cardiac rhythm and most can be strongly excited by various chemicals including 5-HT_3 receptor agonists, veratridine, capsaicin and prostaglandins. These sensors are also excited by increases in intraatrial pressure although their pressure threshold is somewhat higher than that of their myelinated counterparts (142). Atrial receptors, like their arterial counterparts, are reset to higher operating pressures in hypertension.

Finally, some mechanosensitive afferents have terminal fields in the atria and reach the brain via sympathetic nerves and dorsal root ganglia. These fibers ("sympathetic" afferents) generally exhibit much larger receptor fields than vagal afferents (59).

Ventricular Receptors

The ventricular wall contains mechanosensitive and chemosensitive receptors (101), which appear in this case to be largely separate. All have C-fiber axons traveling in the vagus nerve (101). Mechanosensitive receptors have a slow basal discharge rate. Their activity increases linearly with elevations of end-diastolic pressure and then becomes markedly pulse-modulated. It is also a complex function of both diastolic and systolic pressure. Chemosensitive fibers are activated by "irritant chemicals" (the same that activate atrial C fibers), and the majority are unaffected by mechanical stimuli.

Pulmonary Arterial Receptors

Pulmonary arteries have vagal myelinated mechanoreceptors with cardiac related discharges activated monotonically by the intraluminal pressure (28). The response characteristics of these receptors is quite similar to that of aortic baroreceptors except that their threshold and operating range is in line with the lower pressure prevailing in the arterial pulmonary circulation (28). The pulmonary arteries are also innervated by "chemosensitive" C-fiber afferents which respond only to extremes of arterial distention and resemble the chemosensitive fibers of the heart and lungs.

Pulmonary and Bronchial Receptors

Slowly adapting stretch receptors (SARs) with myelinated vagal afferents originate in the conducting airways. These receptors are activated by even moderate lung inflation, project to the NTS (127), and are responsible for the Hering-Breuer inspiration-inhibitory reflex (28). These mechanoreceptors are insensitive to chemical irritants.

J-receptors, located in a juxta-pulmonary capillary location, are polymodal, and their vagal axons are unmyelinated. Their threshold for lung inflation is considered to be higher than that of slowly adapting myelinated afferents but perhaps only marginally so (28,78). These receptors are also "chemosensitive"; i.e., their terminals are depolarized by 5-HT_3 receptor agonists and other agents (28).

Finally, the bronchi also contain C fibers, which are primarily chemosensitive (28).

Reflexes Elicited by Activation of Cardiopulmonary Receptors

Reflexes Elicited by Stimulation of Cardiopulmonary C Fibers

Stimulation of pulmonary C fibers by administration of chemicals into the pulmonary artery or by large lung inflation produces sympathoinhibition, reduced TPR, vagally mediated bradycardia and apnea (pulmonary chemoreflex). The bradycardia is further potentiated in spontaneously breathing animals by the withdrawal of the vagolytic feedback from activation of slowly adapting lung stretch receptors (28).

A tonic and generalized inhibitory influence on the sympathetic outflow is exerted by cardiopulmonary receptors with C-fiber vagal axons (101). Vagal cooling, for example, reversibly increases heart rate, blood pressure and vascular resistance to muscles, kidney and intestines. The use of techniques for selective blockade of unmyelinated fibers suggests that up to 80% of the tonic inhibitory influence of cardiopulmonary afferents may be due to C-fiber activity hence not to SARs (141). Receptors located in the ventricles, atria and the lungs all seem to be involved in exerting this tonic inhibitory influence but the role of ventricular receptors appear preponderant (101).

A consistent finding is that the tonic inhibitory effect of cardiopulmonary receptors on the sympathetic outflow varies according to the ongoing activity of arterial baroreceptors. For instance, denervation of the latter considerably increases the effect of the cardiopulmonary vagal receptors (101). This has led to the hypothesis that cardiopulmonary receptors may take over much of the sympathetic baroreceptor feedback control in sinoaortic denervated animals which may explain the paradoxical absence of chronic hypertension following this type of denervation. However, this theory may be incorrect since dogs previously subjected to sinoaortic denervation were not rendered chronically hypertensive by subsequent cardiac denervation (46).

In addition to their effect on the sympathetic outflow, C-fiber cardiopulmonary mechanoreceptors also exert a tonic inhibition on the release of renin. Unloading of these receptors by hemorrhage or lower body negative pressure increases renal renin release, presumably via activation of the renal sympathetic outflow. In addition, ventricular receptors, hence also probably C-fiber mechanoreceptors, appear to be primarily responsible for the release of vasopressin during hemorrhage since their selective surgical elimination severely attenuates AVP release by hemorrhage (46). Congestive heart failure also reduces cardiopulmonary reflexes which may contribute to the neurohumoral excitatory state characterizing this condition (101).

As indicated above, a significant proportion of vagal afferents with C-fiber characteristics, including those originating from the myocardial area, are "chemosensitive," i.e., their terminals have receptors which, when activated by the proper agonist, produce depolarization and propagated action potentials. The 5-HT_3 receptor (a ligand-gated nonselective cation channel activated by serotonin) is among the most notorious. Other activating substances include nicotine, prostaglandins and digitalis, the latter acting by depolarizing nerve terminals via its inhibition of Na/K ATPase. Pharmacologic activation of vagal C-fiber afferents from the myocardial and/or pulmonary region (including the pericardium) with a 5-HT_3 receptor agonist triggers a constellation of effects called the Bezold-Jarisch reflex. This consists of hypotension, sympathoinhibition, bradycardia and apnea. The central circuit responsible for the cardiovagal activation and sympathoinhibition associated with the Bezold-Jarisch reflex appears virtually identical to that of the arterial baroreflex and involves the same major transmitters (148). In humans, Bezold-Jarisch type reflexes are likely to be involved in the hemodynamic instability associated with myocardial ischemia and infarction, coronary arteriography, exertional syncope in aortic stenosis, chronic heart failure and the therapeutic effects of digitalis (for review, see ref. 92).

Vasomotor Reflexes Elicited by Activation of Myelinated Afferents From the Atria

Activation of atrial receptors by moderate atrial distention produces the following effects (46,59): increase in heart rate (sympathetically mediated) and coronary vascular resistance, no consistent change in cardiac inotropic state or peripheral vascular resistance, and an increase in urine excretion mediated by a variety of humoral agents (AVP, renin). C-fiber activation is not involved as shown by experiments utilizing differential cold block of the vagus nerve (59) hence the effects produced by moderate atrial stretch are generally attributed to activation of myelinated afferents. Denervation experiments also indicate that the activation of these receptors and not the release of atrial natriuretic peptides may be the major factor responsible for the acute effects of left atrial distention on diuresis and natriuresis (46).

Cardiovascular Reflexes From the Lungs

Activation of the myelinated slowly adapting lung stretch receptors (SAR) responsible for the Hering-Breuer inspiration-inhibitory reflex is generally credited with producing an increase in heart rate and a decrease in total peripheral resistance (33). Both effects are thought to be mediated via the central respiratory network. It is speculated that the lung SAR input reduces the central inspiratory drive to the sympathetic outflow thereby producing sympathoinhibition. Simultaneously, the SAR input would facilitate the central inspiratory inhibition of cardiovagal neurons. This second effect would result in a reduction of vagal tone, hence in cardioacceleration (28). Baroreceptor activation of the cardiovagal output is considerably attenuated during lung inflation which suggests that the myelinated slowly adapting stretch receptors (or some other cardiopulmonary receptors?) may also reduce the baroreceptor input to CVMs in some unknown fashion, perhaps independent of the central respiratory drive (127,128).

It should be noted that while lung inflation undoubtedly can produce sympathoinhibition by activation of vagal afferents, the contribution of the myelinated SAR receptors to this effect is not entirely clear or may be species dependent. The difficulty is that lung inflation not only produces the activation of myelinated SAR fibers but, as mentioned previously, it also activates numerous C-fiber mechanoreceptors within the lungs and within the cardiac chambers and intrathoracic vasculature, the latter because of changes in transmural pressure during inspiration. For example, in carefully controlled experiments in cats, only a modest sympathoexcitation (as opposed to an inhibition) occurring during central expiration could be putatively attributed to activation of low-threshold myelinated lung afferents (6), and this response seemed to parallel the activity of expiratory muscles. Sympathoinhibition was only produced when high-threshold cardiopulmonary receptors (presumably C fibers) were activated. These effects, like those produced by chemical activation of cardiopulmonary receptors, did not depend on the central respiratory drive, contrary to prior hypotheses (33). Furthermore, the effectiveness of the sympathetic baroreflex does not seem to vary with the normal lung inflation cycle in all species (16). Overall, it may be that lung SARs exert a more important control over the cardiovagal outflow than of the sympathetic system.

SOMATOSYMPATHETIC, VISCEROSYMPATHETIC, AND POSTURAL REFLEXES

Nociceptive Reflexes

The spinal cord projects to many structures involved in autonomic control, including the NTS (spinosolitary tract), the ventrolateral medulla (spinoreticular tract), the parabrachial nuclei (129), and midbrain central gray (spinomesencephalic tract), all of which are likely to contribute to nociceptive autonomic responses (24) (Fig. 11). Under anesthesia, stimulation of somatic nerves with sufficient intensity to activate cutaneous C-fiber nociceptors produces a rise in AP, activates sympathetic vasoconstrictor efferents and RVL presympathetic neurons particularly on the contralateral side since the somatic afferent pathway to the medulla is crossed (106,130) (Fig. 11). Not surprisingly, most of the activation of the sympathetic efferents

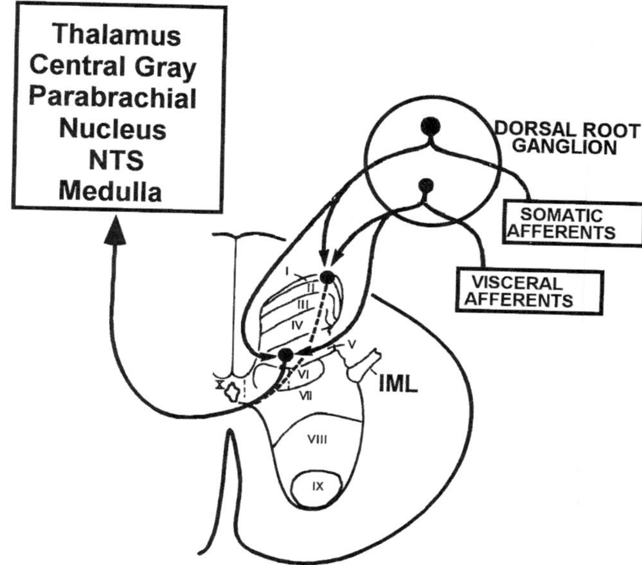

Figure 11. Inputs to laminae I and V of dorsal horn assumed to be of importance in somato- and viscerosympathetic reflexes. Convergence of visceral and somatic inputs on spinothalamic cells is also assumed to underlie the fact that pain from visceral organ is commonly referred to overlying dermatomes. (Reprinted with permission from ref. 24.)

depends primarily on the integrity of the RVL since sympathetic tone depends on this structure. Notwithstanding the existence of spinal sympathetic reflexes—best detected in spinalized preparations (30)—most of the sympathoactivation produced by nociceptive stimulation under anesthesia and in the presence of an intact neuraxis appears due to "long-loop" reflexes, which may primarily involve bulbar structures and, most notably, the activation of RVL presympathetic neurons. The circuitry is shown in Fig. 1.

Nociceptive sympathetic reflexes also originate from internal organs such as heart, peritoneum, bladder and gut (24). These nociceptive afferents travel in the sympathetic nerves, have their cell bodies in dorsal root ganglia and project mainly to laminae I and V (Fig. 11). Sympathetic and somatic nociceptors frequently activate the same pool of spinal cord polymodal cells (spinothalamic, spinoreticular, and spinomesencephalic). The viscerosomatic convergence on spinothalamic neurons is thought to underlie the fact that pain triggered by visceral nociceptors is usually referred to an overlying or nearby somatic structure, e.g., referred pain of angina pectoris (24). The autonomic effects triggered by visceral pain under anesthesia are likely to involve circuits similar to that activated by somatic pain, i.e., a medullary loop involving RVL.

Exercise Pressor Response (Muscle "Metaboreflex")

The cardiovascular adjustments to exercise probably integrate three complex processes (15): (a) a pressor reflex originating from mechano- and metaboreceptors in contracting muscles, (b) central motor command, i.e., a feedforward control of vasomotor efferents associated with the initiation and maintenance of somatomotor activity, and (c) visceral feedback from the cardiopulmonary region, baroreceptors and chemoreceptors (23,24,40). The order in which these mechanisms are recruited and their relative importance in freely behaving animals is uncertain. Clearly, chemical stimulation of skeletal muscle receptors in awake humans (e.g., by posttetanic ischemia, probably via decreases in pH) increases muscle SND—i.e., muscle metaboreflex (40). Animal experimentation indicates that skeletal muscles are innervated by slow-conducting sensory afferents (type III and IV), which respond primarily to chemical changes that would likely occur during very sustained contraction: pH reduction, lactic acid, and increases in extracellular potassium (79). Activation of group III mechanoreceptors in contracting muscles produces a generalized sympathoactivation associated with an increase in AP in animal preparations. It is speculated that, via these afferent fibers, muscle fatigue reflexively triggers an additional activation of the sympathetic system perhaps designed to increase cardiac output and blood flow in the active muscle beds. In cats the rise in AP produced by stimulation of type III mechanoreceptors during tonic muscle contraction appears to be mediated by a supraspinal neuronal loop with a relay in the rostral medulla oblongata (68).

"Central command" mechanisms are assumed to produce a feedforward control of regional blood flows during exercise. These processes are very poorly understood and very difficult to investigate. In awake humans, "central command" effects on SND, measured during hand-grip appear regionally differentiated, weak in skeletal muscle but powerful in the skin, due almost exclusively to activation of sudomotor fibers (40). It seems difficult to exclude that the modest sympathoactivation observed in vasomotor fibers is not merely due to stress. Cardiovascular adjustments to more complex forms of exercise (walking, running) are undoubtedly integrated with the activation of the respiratory centers. This issue is not addressed in this review.

Postural Autonomic Reflexes

A significant portion of vasomotor postural reflexes is undoubtedly due to venous pooling, reduction in venous return, reduction in arterial pressure, unloading of cardiopulmonary and arterial baroreceptors with consequent activation of the sympathetic outflow and withdrawal of vagal tone (127). Two additional mechanisms at least may also play a role in the hemodynamic adjustments to postural changes, namely the vestibulosympathetic reflex and the posterior vermis of the cerebellum, although the role of the latter is probably not restricted to postural changes only. Labyrinthine inputs (Fig. 12A) are capable of modulating the vasomotor outflow via the medial vestibular nucleus and its connections, direct or indirect with presympathetic cells of RVL and perhaps the raphe (153).

Recent work by Paton and Spyer (108) indicates that lobule IXb of the cerebellar vermis appears to be most effective in producing autonomic effects via two main circuits. The first involves the lateral parabrachial nuclei and RVL (Fig. 12B) and may directly modulate the medullary sympathetic tone generating circuitry (including RVL presympathetic neurons). An additional circuit operating via a loop through the NTS may gate the baroreflex.

This plot gives no part to the fastigial nucleus of the cerebellum, a structure previously thought to play a major role in autonomic control. Conceivably, these older results could be explained by the presence of fibers of passage through the fastigial nucleus.

RESPIRATORY CONTROL OF THE VASOMOTOR OUTFLOW

Precise coordination between respiration, cardiac output and regional blood flows is necessary for behaving mammals to handle the rapidly changing oxygen requirements of peripheral organs and to achieve arterial pO_2 homeostasis. Schematically, this coordination occurs via three interactive integrative processes (reviewed in refs. 39,56,115). The most fundamental level of integration is the interaction between the bulbar networks which generate the respiratory and vasomotor outputs. A second factor is the parallel processing of the multiple somatic and visceral sensory inputs which impinge on these interactive networks (e.g., baroreceptors, chemoreceptors, cardiopulmonary afferents, nociceptors, etc.). Finally, the respiratory and vasomotor networks are also both subject to central command (feedforward) mechanisms from the higher centers. The present section focuses on the basic neurophysiologic mechanisms involved in the regulation of the sympathetic vasomotor outflow by the bulbar respiratory network. The role of central and peripheral chemoreceptor activation on circulation and the related issue of hypoxia are also examined.

Control of Sympathetic Efferents by the Central Respiratory Network

Evidence for a Central Respiratory Drive of Sympathetic Vasomotor Efferents

In anesthetized, paralyzed, and ventilated preparations in which lung stretch and baroreceptor afferents are surgically removed, and in which a thoracotomy precludes the rhythmic activity of chest mechanoreceptors, the discharges of sympathetic nerves still fluctuate in synchrony with the activity of the phrenic nerve (56,99). Typically, as illustrated in Fig. 13 in the case of the rat, the amplitude of these respiratory fluctuations increases in parallel with that of the phrenic discharge. Moreover, since the mass discharge is actually slightly reduced during a portion of the respiratory cycle (inspiration in rats) and increased during another (expiration in rats) the averaged maximum increment in SND due to activation of the central respiratory drive is fairly modest (<50% in rats). Because in such a preparation peripheral feedback is interrupted and the central respiratory oscillator is free-running relative to lung ventilation, the respiratory oscillations of SND must be generated centrally. Because these oscillations are superimposed on a tonic level of sympathetic activity which persists during hyperventilation to apnea, it is concluded that a fraction of the sympathetic vasomotor outflow is generated by some element of the central respiratory network and this component is superimposed on other sources of drive which are independent of respiration. The genesis of the respiratory independent component has been examined in a previous section.

Relative Contribution of Central Respiratory and Nonrespiratory Sources of Drive to Vasoconstrictor Tone Generation

The quantitative importance of the central respiratory drive for sympathetic tone generation and arterial pressure maintenance remains undefined. It is a distinct possibility that this respiratory drive might be quantitatively significant only when peripheral or central chemoreceptors are powerfully stimulated. In deafferented and anesthetized preparations such as the one referred to above, it has been estimated that, at physiological levels of CO_2, less than a quarter of the total vasoconstrictor output to the hind quarter muscle mass might be due to the respiratory component of SND. Estimates are that this proportion could reach two thirds at levels of CO_2 assumed to have saturated central chemoreceptors (87). The actual proportion in behaving mammals is unknown. In awake humans, sympathetic vasoconstrictor activity to the muscle bed displays a very strong pulse rhythmic activity that seems dominated by an exquisitely sensitive baroreceptor feedback (126) (Fig. 14). Powerful respiratory fluctuations of this output are also usually observed but they could be largely if not exclusively accounted for by ventilation related fluctuations in AP resulting in periodic oscillations of the baroreceptor feedback (37). In addition, many published records of muscle sympathetic nerve activity in awake (and obviously breathing) humans exhibit no detectable respiratory fluctuation (see Fig. 9 of ref. 40). Thus,

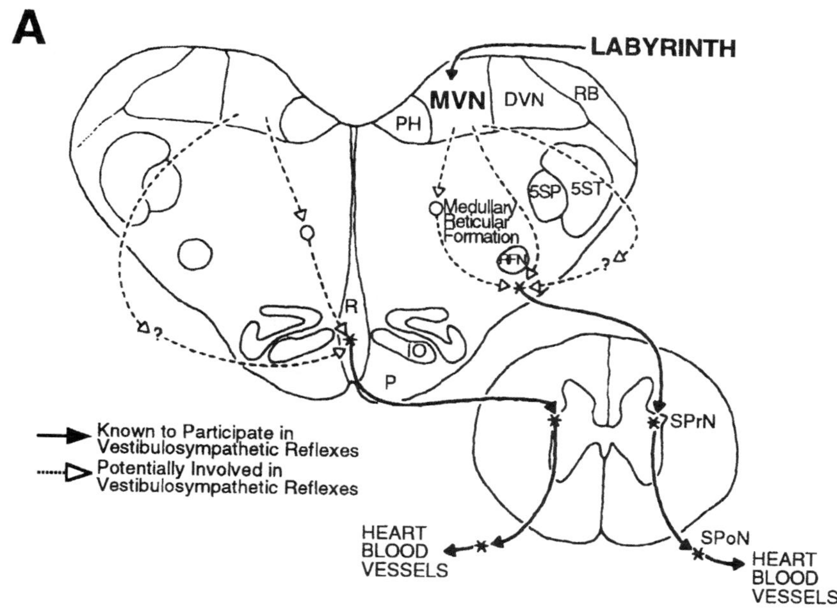

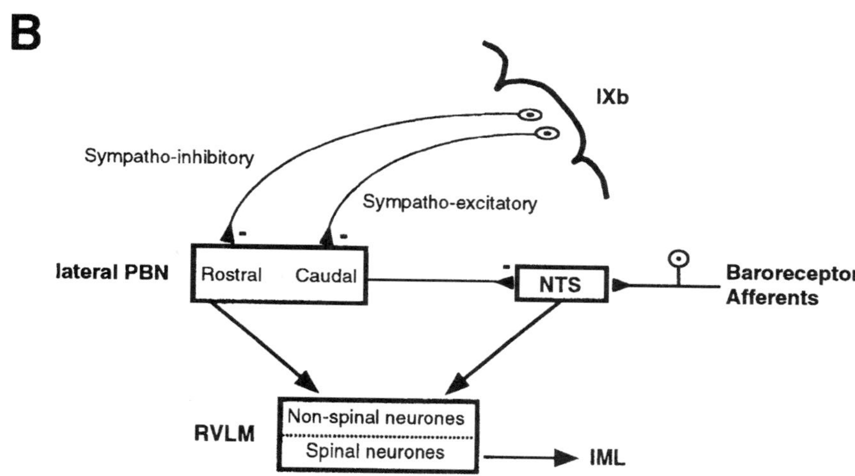

Figure 12. **(A)** Labyrinthine inputs may convey positional information needed to anticipate postural hypotension (vestibulosympathetic reflexes). **(B)** Stimulation of cerebellar lobule IXb produces hemodynamic effects via pathways represented in drawing. These circuits may be also involved in hemodynamic adjustments to change in posture. (A: Reprinted, in adapted form, with permission from ref. 153. B: Reprinted with permission from ref. 108.)

no clear evidence supports the notion that the basal human SND to muscles observed under normoxia and normocapnia might depend to a significant degree on the activity of the central respiratory network. In addition, it is clear that significant sympathetic vasomotor activity remains in humans even as respiration is virtually abolished by volatile anesthetics. Overall, these observations suggest that in humans as in lower mammals sympathetic tone generation at rest depends in large part on neural mechanisms which are independent of the central respiratory drive.

Central Respiratory Drive of Sympathetic Vasomotor Efferents: Regional Differences

Differences exist between rodents (rats and rabbits) and carnivores (cats and dogs) in terms of the phase-relationship between phrenic discharge and activity of sympathetic efferents. This specialized topic is of a comparative physiological nature and will not be covered here (for details, see ref. 56).

More importantly, when examined within a single species, the central respiratory pattern of sympathetic efferents falls into a small number of discrete categories (three in the rat) that seem to relate to the specific vascular bed targeted by the individual efferent fibers (splanchnic versus cutaneous, etc.). Their phase relationship relative to the three main components of the central respiratory cycle (inspiration, postinspiration, and expiration) are not changed by activation of central and peripheral chemoreceptors (53,82), but the amplitude of the respiratory oscillations becomes merely exaggerated by these stimuli. These regional differences in central respiratory pattern suggest that various classes of sympathetic efferents receive inputs from different sets of central respiratory neurons. In this fashion, distinct vascular beds may be differentially regulated by the central respiratory network providing the neuronal basis for the regionally differentiated effects of central and peripheral chemoreceptor stimulation (72).

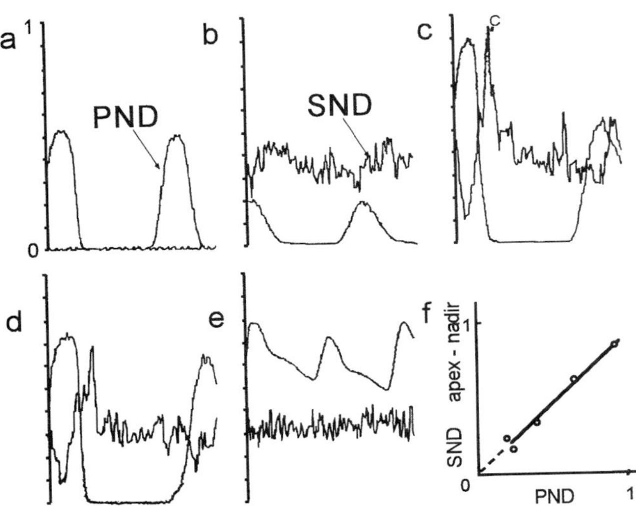

Figure 13. Relationship between activity of phrenic and sympathetic nerves in an animal in which buffer nerves and vagi have been cut. Nerve activities have been computer averaged using the phrenic burst as trigger. Increasing PND amplitude by raising CO_2 in inspired mixture increases the magnitude of the respiratory modulation of SND. The relationship between PND amplitude and respiratory modulation of SND is linear (**f**). (**e**) indicates that SND does not fluctuate with the pressure pulse in this preparation due to the fact that baroreceptors have been cut. (**a**) Control in which SND has been pharmacologically eliminated.

Putative Bulbar Circuits Responsible for the Central Respiratory Control of Sympathetic Efferents: Pathways and Transmitters

Several hypotheses have been advanced to explain the influence of the respiratory network on sympathetic vasomotor efferent activity (Fig. 15): (a) gating of baroreceptor feedback (arrows 1–3), (b) convergence at the preganglionic cell level of bulbospinal respiratory inputs and other sources of sympathetic excitatory drive (arrow 5), and (c) inputs from bulbar medullary cells involved in respiratory rhythm generation to presympathetic vasomotor neurons (such as in RVL, arrow 4). These hypotheses are not mutually exclusive, none is totally excluded at present but only the last hypothesis (i.e., respiratory input to presympathetic vasomotor neurons) is convincingly documented.

Gating Hypothesis This hypothesis has been put forward to account for the observation that, under certain experimental conditions, inhibition of the activity of vasomotor efferents by baroreceptor stimulation appears more powerful or longer lasting when the stimulation occurs during a specific phase of the central respiratory cycle (16). The gating theory derives no support from electrophysiological recordings of neurons in the nucleus of the solitary tract since few receive convergent baroreceptor and respiratory inputs. In addition, the presence of a strong respiratory rhythmicity of sympathetic efferents in debuffered animals or in intact animals below baroreceptor threshold clearly indicates that gating of the baroreceptor feedback circuit, if it exists at all, can only provide a very partial explanation of the central respiratory control of sympathetic efferents.

Respiratory Control of Sympathetic Efferents by Descending Bulbospinal Respiratory Neurons The theory that SPGNs might receive inputs (directly or via spinal interneurons) from bulbospinal "respiratory" neurons (i.e., cells distinct from those responsible for basic sympathetic tone generation—e.g., RVL inputs) rests on very tenuous evidence.

One is anatomical. Sympathetic preganglionic neurons are located dorsal to and in close proximity of ventral horn motor neurons (intercostal and abdominal), which receive inputs from respiratory cells of the caudal VRG and the pre-Botzinger complex. There is, therefore, a theoretical possibility that collaterals of these bulbospinal respiratory cells might establish direct or indirect connections with SPGNs. In addition, neurophysiological evidence indicates that, in carnivores, sympathetic activation occurs essentially in synchrony with phrenic inspiration (99,115). Since inspiratory bulbospinal cells innervate motor neurons of inspiratory muscles in thoracic spinal segments, these descending inputs are, again theoretically, poised to rhythmically activate sympathetic efferents with the proper timing. However, using selective cordotomy in cats, Connelly and Wurster (29) were able to demonstrate that the respiratory activity of intercostal nerves could be selectively eliminated without interfering with the sympathetic outflow nor with its central respiratory oscillation. Connelly and Wurster (29) concluded, therefore, that respiratory and other sources of sympathetic drive were probably integrated above the cord. In addition, sympathetic activation in rodents occurs neither during inspiration nor expiration but is "phase spanning." Therefore, it is virtually certain that SPGNs do not receive their respiratory modulation from collaterals of bulbospinal neurons which drive inspiratory or expiratory spinal motor neurons. One remaining theoretical possibility is that SPGNs are innervated by bulbar "respiratory neurons," which are distinct from the premotor neurons innervating respiratory muscles or that they receive their respiratory inputs via a complex spinal interneuronal circuit. In support of this possibility, spinal interneurons with complex phase relationships with the medullary respiratory network have occasionally been reported (11).

Respiratory Modulation of RVL Presympathetic Neurons Unit recording of presympathetic vasomotor neurons in RVL in both cats and rodents (rat and rabbit) has provided proof of convergence of respiratory and other sources of drive to the sympathetic outflow at or prior to the premotor neuronal stage (56,62).

As illustrated in Fig. 16, many RVL presympathetic neurons display a central respiratory pattern obviously similar to that of muscle sympathetic vasomotor units (cf. Fig. 13). The intensity of the central respiratory modulation of RVL presympathetic vasomotor neurons exhibits a linear relationship with phrenic nerve amplitude as is classically observed in sympathetic efferents (Figs. 13 and 16). In this species, one can recognize the same two major respiratory patterns (early inspiratory and postinspiratory, the latter being predominant) in postganglionic and RVL presympathetic vasomotor neurons (not shown). A major point, also illustrated in Fig. 16, is that RVL presympathetic neurons exhibit considerable ongoing activity below the apneic threshold. As discussed in a prior section, our laboratory has interpreted this tonic discharge as resulting essentially from the intrinsic pacemaker activity of these cells.

The ventrolateral medulla is replete with "respiratory" cells, which turn on and off at specific times of the respiratory cycle. Many of them are thought to be propriobulbar cells and some display a pattern of firing seemingly appropriate to provide the respiratory modulation of presympathetic vasomotor neurons. For example, in the rat, many cells exhibit a phasic respiratory pattern with maxima during the postinspiratory period—therefore theoretically appropriate to provide the dominant type of respiratory modulation of RVL presympathetic vasomotor neurons. Other respiratory cells with early inspiratory pattern could contribute to the early inspiratory inhibition of the presympathetic neurons (122).

In the complete absence of cardiopulmonary and baroreceptor feedback and of peripheral chemoreceptor activation, the bulbar respiratory network produces a complex phasic modulation of many sympathetic vasomotor efferents. This modulation is superimposed on a steady level of activity of these efferents generated by mechanisms independent of the central respiratory drive. The amplitude of the central respira-

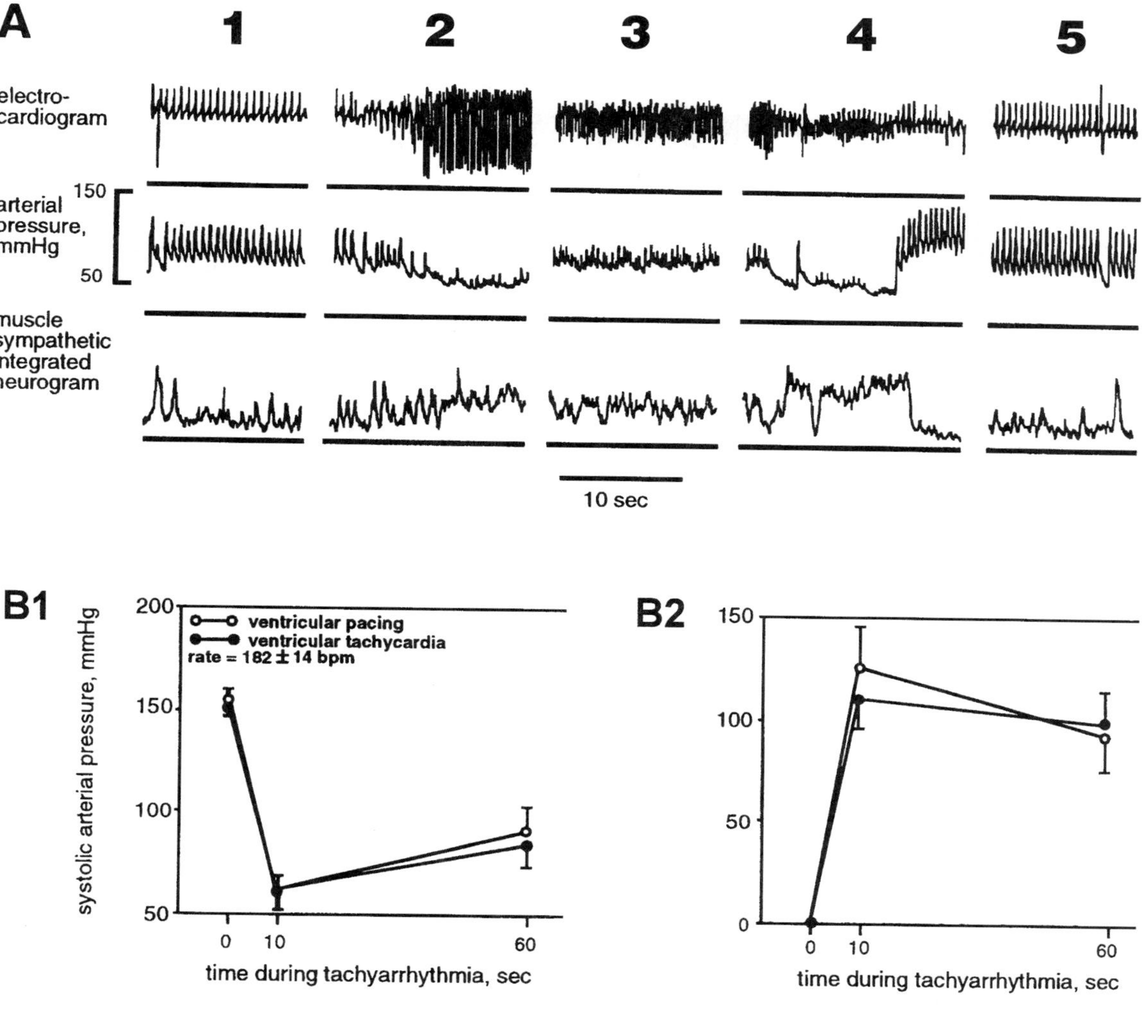

Figure 14. Muscle vasoconstrictor sympathetic nerve discharge in humans and its relation to arterial pressure (AP). SND was recorded at rest and during induced ventricular tachycardia. This example was selected from the human literature because it provides an opportunity to observe SND at very low levels of arterial pressure, presumably below baroreceptor threshold (2 and 4 in A). At rest, panel 1 in A and beginning of panel 2, muscle SND is low and characterized by a pulse synchronous pattern. As AP drops during ventricular tachycardia, SND increases and becomes tonic as in animals (cf. Fig. 4C). Note also that at low AP, SND does not display marked respiratory rhythmicity in agreement with animal SND recorded under normocapnia (cf. Fig. 13B). Both panels in B indicate existence of an inverse relationship between MAP and SND in humans, indicating the strength of the baroreceptor feedback. (Reprinted with permission from ref. 126.)

tory modulation is increased roughly in proportion with the central respiratory drive but its pattern is invariant. Under anesthesia, the largest portion of the coupling between respiratory and sympathetic networks seems to consist of a feedforward control of the discharges of the presympathetic vasomotor neurons of RVL (Fig. 15).

Central Chemosympathetic Reflex

Central chemoreceptors probably exert their action on the sympathetic outflow as a secondary consequence of their activation of the central respiratory network (53). The molecular mechanism responsible for detection by the brain of very small pH and pCO_2 fluctuations is essentially unknown and so is the nature of the cells that carry these sensors (glial cells or neurons or both). Even the location of the sensors is uncertain. Most data suggests that they reside predominantly near the ventral surface of the medulla oblongata and rostral pons (39,99), whereas other evidence points towards the NTS. It is generally considered that central chemoreceptors are not activated by hypoxia.

Peripheral Chemosympathetic Reflex

General Characteristics

Arterial chemoreflexes are thought to be significantly implicated in the maintenance of arterial pressure only during acute hypoxia, hemorrhage, and sleep. The activation of arterial chemoreceptors by hypoxia is profoundly depressed by volatile anesthetics at a fraction of 1 MAC.

Stimulation of carotid chemoreceptors by hypoxia or cyanide produces an increase in arterial pressure which is largely due to activation of sympathetic efferents (43). Some differentiation exists as to the degree of activation of various types of vasomotor efferents by carotid chemoreceptor stimula-

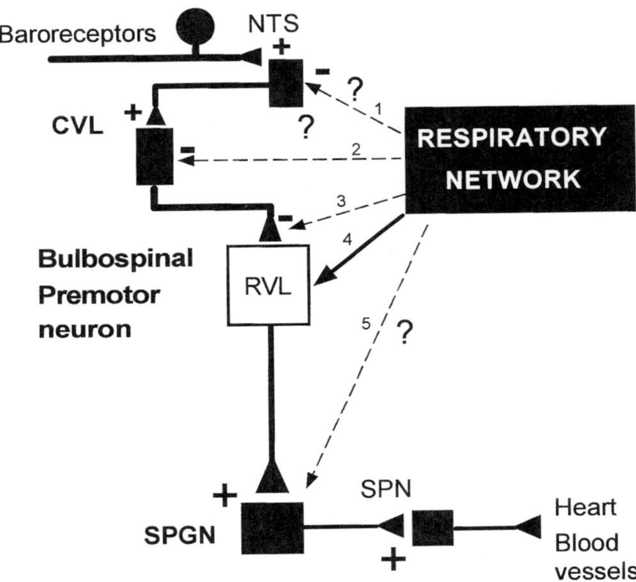

Figure 15. Control of the sympathetic vasomotor outflow by the central respiratory network. This drawing summarizes some of the schemes that have been proposed to account for the central respiratory modulation of the vasomotor outflow. *Dotted lines 1, 2, 3, and 5* represent plausible but poorly documented mechanisms. *Dark line 4* represents the best demonstrated mechanism.

tion. Those to the skeletal muscle and visceral beds are stimulated thereby increasing peripheral resistance and arterial pressure. The primary cardiac response is bradycardia due to activation of parasympathetic efferents and, possibly, reduction in sympathetic tone to the heart. If breathing is unimpeded, the pulmonary inflation reflex (vagolytic effect reflexively triggered by pulmonary stretch receptor activation) overcomes the bradycardia and tachycardia ensues (146). This section examines the central mechanisms responsible for the sympathetic activation by chemoreceptor stimulation.

Putative Pathway of the Central Chemosympathetic Reflex

Carotid chemoreceptor stimulation produces an activation of the sympathetic outflow that is synchronized with the central respiratory network and exhibits the same phase relationship to phrenic discharge observed at rest and during central chemoreceptor stimulation (56,82). An example taken from an experiment in the rat is illustrated in Fig. 17. There is also evidence that chemoreceptor inputs to sympathetic efferents may also have a tonic component which is independent of the activation of the central respiratory network (77).

The central pathway of the reflex is incompletely known (Fig. 18). Under urethan anesthesia, the sympathetic chemoreflex is preserved after midcollicular transection; therefore, its pathway is essentially contained within the pontomedullary region. Chemoreceptor primary afferents project mainly to the caudal aspects of the nucleus of the solitary tract but some projections outside the NTS have been occasionally reported (128). Some of the second-order neurons in NTS apparently do not exhibit membrane potential oscillations synchronized with the central respiratory network (128). These cells are therefore, at least theoretically, in a position to relay "pure" peripheral chemoreceptor information, i.e., not yet gated by the respiratory system. The projection pattern of these cells is unfortunately unknown.

Peripheral chemoreceptor stimulation activates RVL presympathetic neurons; therefore, these neurons constitute one of the efferent limbs of the reflex (82). Recent evidence suggests that the pontine noradrenergic A5 cells are also activated during chemoreceptor stimulation (57) (Fig. 18).

The CVL area is probably not involved in the chemoreflex because neuronal inhibition in this region (with muscimol) does not change the chemosympathetic response (82). Since this procedure blocks the baroreflex, one may conclude that these reflexes use a distinct medullary network before converging on RVL presympathetic neurons.

The pathway of the peripheral chemosympathetic reflex is roughly organized as indicated in Fig. 18. Major gaps in our understanding of this pathway remain. This is due to the fact that the chemosympathetic reflex is largely mediated via activation of the respiratory network whose organization is itself still not completely understood.

Effects of Hypoxia and Cerebral Ischemia on Sympathetic Outflow

It is essential to a comprehension of the consequences of hypoxia on the sympathetic outflow to distinguish the effects resulting from the direct depressant effects of low pO_2 in the CNS from those elicited reflexively by activation of peripheral chemoreceptors (43,116).

The initial autonomic neural effects of a severe hypoxic challenge or the sustained effects of mild hypoxia are virtually exclusively due to activation of peripheral chemoreceptors (43,82). The sympathoactivation contributes to counteract the vasodilatation consecutive to the direct effect of hypoxia on vascular smooth muscle and is part of a strategy designed to reduce oxygen consumption. This sympathoactivation disappears, as expected, after resection of the carotid sinus nerves and it is associated with a vigorous activation of the respiratory output. During this period, the sympathetic outflow is activated in bursts synchronized with the activity of the central respiratory network. As described in the preceding section, this pattern is due to the respiratory synchronous activation of RVL and perhaps other bulbospinal sympathoexcitatory neurons by elements of the medullary respiratory network (50,82).

If hypoxia is severe enough (pO_2 of <30 mm Hg), the first phase of sympathoactivation is followed by the disappearance of central respiratory activity and the appearance of a second phase of activation of the sympathetic vasomotor outflow. Sympathetic vasomotor activity during this second phase is desynchronized, a term which relates to the absence of a low (respiratory related) frequency component (by analogy with EEG terminology). This second phase is also associated with an activation of RVL presympathetic neurons (134; and for review, see ref. 135). Most likely, during this phase of the hypoxic response, the activation of RVL presympathetic neurons is due to the local hypoxic conditions prevailing in the immediate vicinity of the cells. Indeed vascular perfusion of the lower medulla with oxygen poor CSF appears to activate these cells (123) and iontophoretic application of the metabolic poison cyanide also results in their activation (134). The same maneuver usually inhibits other types of RVL neurons. Recent work suggests that the hypoxic activation of RVL presympathetic neurons is due to an increase in calcium conductance (for a review, see ref. 135).

The excitatory response of RVL presympathetic neurons to local hypoxia and cyanide underlies the concept that these cells may function as "oxygen sensors" (134). However, presently available evidence suggests that their oxygen sensing capability is limited to an extremely low range of oxygen tension that, in the adult, is inevitably associated with the disappearance of the respiratory drive and, therefore, would appear to have no survival value. However, this central hypoxic response could be conceivably of value to fetuses that are exposed to a very low pO_2.

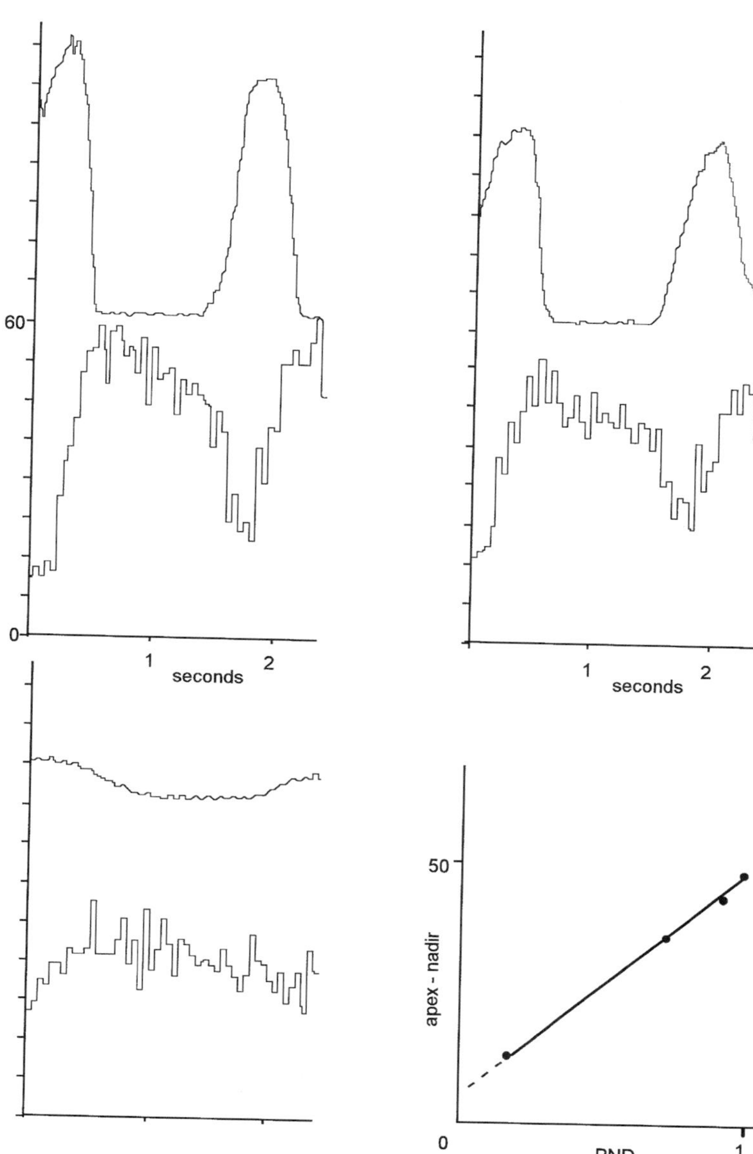

Figure 16. Respiratory input to RVL presympathetic vasomotor neuron in a vagotomized and debuffered rat. The discharge of a single cell is computer averaged using phrenic bursts as trigger (PND). The histograms represent the probability of discharge of the cell throughout the respiratory cycle. PND amplitude was adjusted to a different level by changing the concentration of CO_2 in the breathing mixture. The pattern of this cell is remarkably similar to that of vasomotor postganglionic cells (cf. Fig. 13), thus supporting the scheme illustrated in Fig. 15.

Activation of RVL presympathetic neurons also contributes to the hypertensive "cerebral ischemic response" caused by a severe restriction of blood flow to the lower brain stem (51,81). The cerebral ischemic response is triggered by an increase in intracranial pressure of a magnitude sufficient to impair brain blood flow or mimicked experimentally by purposeful reduction of arterial flow to the lower brain stem. Like the response to hypoxia, the sympathetic response to cerebral ischemia displays two phases. The first is characterized by respiratory activation (most likely due to activation of central chemoreceptors) and is accompanied by the expected increase in the respiratory modulation of the sympathetic outflow. More prolonged periods of ischemia result in a disappearance of respiratory activity and a further increase in sympathetic activity, which is aperiodic or desynchronized (81).

CARDIAC PARASYMPATHETIC EFFERENTS

Types and Location of CVMs

CVMs are few in number and, in most species examined except the rabbit, they are mainly located in the ventrolateral subdivision of the nucleus ambiguus at, and rostral to, the level of the area postrema (89). The activity of CVMs is low to absent under anesthesia, displays maxima during expiration (in cat) and is pulse-modulated when CVMs are activated by baroreceptor stimulation (89). The conduction velocity of their axons is in the B class. The direct activation of only a few CVMs within the nucleus ambiguus via iontophoresis of excitatory amino acids is sufficient to produce a detectable fall in HR suggesting that each CVM must be synaptically connected with a very large number of ganglionic cells within the myocardium (94). Right and left vagal stimulation produce different patterns of cardiac response suggesting the possibility that some CVMs may be synaptically connected with ganglionic cells regulating distinct components of the myocardial pacemaker and conduction systems. However, the presence of a topographic arrangement of projections, while suggestive, does not prove by itself that the activity of the various CVMs are ever differentially regulated. Similar unanswered questions have been raised with regard to the sympathetic innervation of the myocardium. The latter is also lateralized and left splanchnic stimulation predominantly affects rate while cardiac output is increased to a greater degree by stimulation of the right nerve.

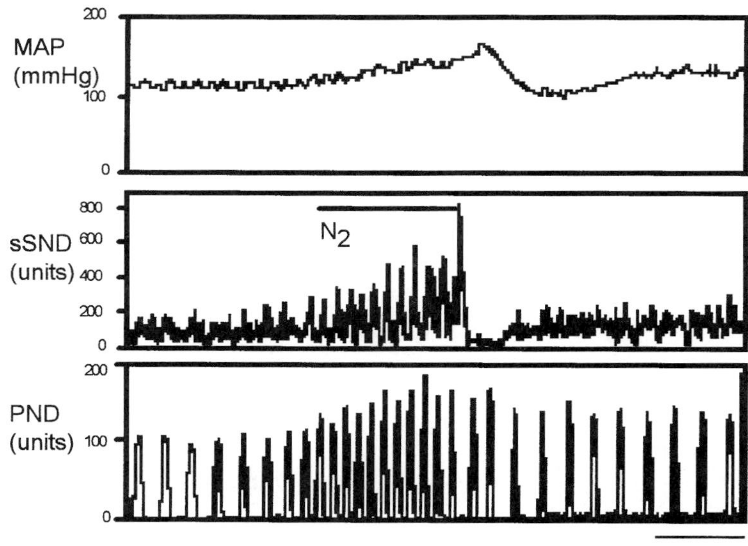

Figure 17. Sympathetic chemoreflex in rat. Mean arterial pressure, mass discharge of splanchnic nerve (sSND), and phrenic discharge (PND) were simultaneously recorded under anesthesia. Nitrogen was substituted to oxygen in the breathing mixture for 8 s (*bar*). Note the increase in MAP, PND rate and amplitude, and SND. Note that SND stimulation occurred in bursts synchronized with PND. This type of evidence supports the notion that sympathetic activation during carotid chemoreceptor activation occurs via activation of central respiratory network, which secondarily activates vasomotor cells of the medulla oblongata, as represented in Fig. 18.

Neural Control of CVMs

Vagal Tone

The neurophysiological mechanisms responsible for CVM discharges are not fully understood. Contrary to the sympathetic tone, vagal tone is dramatically reduced by general anesthesia and may be virtually nil at resting pressure. When present at rest or when triggered by arterial pressure elevation, CVM activity is synchronized with the arterial pressure pulse (89). This pattern of discharge is generally attributed to the existence of an oligosynaptic excitatory input from NTS to CVMs that is rhythmically activated by the phasic activation of arterial baroreceptors (Fig. 2B). The baroreceptor input is the only source of excitatory drive to CVMs fully identified at present. It is probably mediated by excitatory amino acids (EAAs) since the cardiovagal baroreflex is abolished by administration of an EAA receptor antagonist in the nucleus ambiguus area (54).

Under anesthesia, vagal tone may be low for two main reasons: (a) reduced excitability of CVMs and (b) depression of the polysynaptic pathway mediating the effect of arterial baroreceptor stimulation (Fig. 2B). Depression of polysynaptic pathways by anesthetics easily explains why anesthesia greatly increases the pressure threshold of the baroreflex (both sympathetic and cardiovagal) while having little impact on the pressure threshold of baroreceptor afferents.

The cardiovagal baroreflex pathway involves at least one interneuronal step. Indeed arterial baroreceptor afferents arborize exclusively within the confines of the nucleus of the solitary tract but most CVMs are located in the nucleus ambiguus. The second-order neurons involved in this reflex are believed (without the benefit of evidence) to be the same as those implicated in the sympathetic baroreflex and this issue has been addressed previously.

Like all motoneurons in the bulb and spinal cord, CVMs receive a serotonergic input from the medullary raphe (69). The activity of the medullary raphe is generally considered to be state-dependent (70). Conceivably, this serotinergic input could play a role in the increased cardiovagal tone generally thought to be associated with sleep (107).

Central Respiratory and Cardiopulmonary Reflex Control of CVM Discharges

CVM activity is influenced by the central respiratory network (127). In cats, CVM activity is actively inhibited during inspiration via chloride-mediated IPSPs, which hyperpolarize the cell and attenuate the depolarizing effect of the baroreceptor input (127). The simplest neurophysiological model that could account for these results is postsynaptic summation between an excitatory input from second-order baroreceptor neurons and postsynaptic inhibition from some unidentified GABAergic neuron of the bulbar respiratory network which fires during inspiration (Fig. 2). Note that this model provides the exact counterpoint of the way in which baroreceptor and respiratory inputs are thought to be integrated at the level of RVL presympathetic vasomotor neurons (Fig. 15).

Tachycardia and inhibition of the baroreceptor-mediated activation of the cardiovagal output occur during lung inflation (33,127). These effects are commonly attributed to the activation of slowly adapting myelinated lung-stretch receptors (SAR). It has been hypothesized that the effect of lung-stretch afferents is to potentiate the inhibitory effect of the central respiratory network on cardiovagal motoneurons; however, the

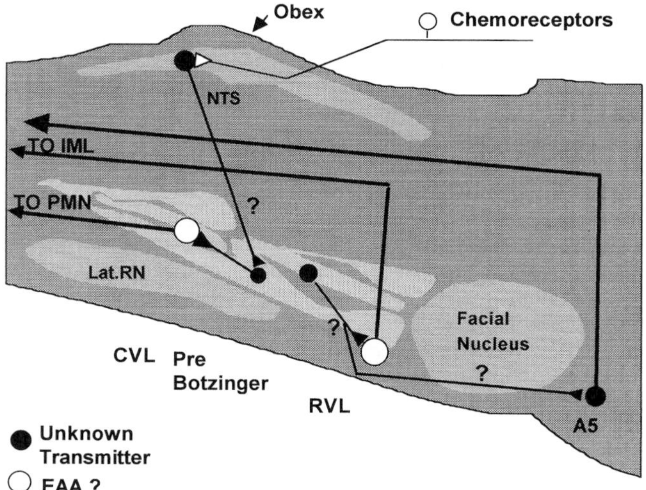

Figure 18. A working hypothesis of the central pathway of the sympathetic chemoreflex. Propriobulbar interneurons located within the RVL are assumed to act as interface between the respiratory rhythm generating network and the bulbospinal presympathetic neurons, including the pacemaker neurons of RVL and, possibly, the noradrenergic cell of the ventrolateral pons (A5 cell group).

circuit involved is not known (127). SAR afferent inputs do not appear to gate the baroreflex at the level of the NTS (127), in keeping with the fact that this gating may be relatively selective to the cardiac division of the baroreflex.

Activation of high-threshold cardiopulmonary mechanoreceptors or activation of chemosensitive cardiopulmonary afferents produces bradycardia. These effects may be due to the convergence between these and arterial baroreceptor inputs on NTS neurons as discussed in a prior section.

PERIAQUEDUCTAL GRAY MATTER (CG): ROLE IN AUTONOMIC CORRELATES OF AFFECTIVE BEHAVIORS AND NOCICEPTION

The existence of cortical and basal forebrain regions with particularly dense neuronal connections with brain stem areas involved in autonomic regulation seems the clearest evidence that the cardiovascular correlates of all behavioral states must be integrated at multiple levels of the neuraxis up to and including the cortex. However, many neuroscientists still subscribe to the notion that individual portions of this vast network can play a unique integrative role in the organization of specific forms of behavior. This notion derives from the observation that reproducible and highly complex patterns of effects (under anesthesia) or even organized behaviors (in unanesthetized animals) can be produced when the area in question is stimulated via low-level electrical pulses or, better, by microinjection of EAAs. The potential role of one such area, the midbrain central grey, is analyzed here because of its generally recognized importance in both analgesia and cardiovascular control.

Effect of CG Stimulation on Behavior

Topical stimulation of the midbrain periaqueductal gray matter (CG) of freely behaving animals with excitatory amino acids produces one of several stereotyped "defensive" or "affective" behaviors (7,74). These responses are assumed to mimic behavioral patterns that would normally occur only in response to danger (predator, social conflict, etc.). In the cat, two major types of behavior are elicited ("freezing behavior" and "forward escape behavior"). Each is accompanied by a specific array of hemodynamic changes, the presence or absence of vocalization and alterations in reactivity to somatosensory inputs. Under anesthesia, although overt behavior is of course not produced, stimulation of the CG still produces stereotyped patterns of blood flow which are reminiscent of those produced in the freely behaving animal (7,74). This has permitted an electrophysiologic analysis of some of the circuitry which underlies these patterns of autonomic activation.

A second well-studied aspect of the CG is its role in pain perception, the seminal observation being that electrical stimulation or microinjection of morphine into the area produces analgesia and, in lightly anesthetized animals, a reduction of nociceptive reflexes (152). Nociception is also normally associated with autonomic adjustments and there is reason to believe that the CG could participate in the respiratory and hemodynamic correlates of pain.

Neuroanatomical Organization of the CG

The CG has a longitudinal columnar subnuclear arrangement (22). Ventrally, the structure is occupied by the dorsal raphe, a collection of serotonergic cells with almost exclusively ascending projections (70). The dorsal raphe is considered to be of primary importance in regulating states of vigilance since its neurons have a state-dependent firing pattern, and they are relatively unaffected by sensory inputs (70). Via its projections to the cortex and the entire limbic system, the dorsal raphe influences affective behavior and, no doubt, its autonomic correlates. However, this nucleus does not appear to be primarily involved in the responses elicited by short-term stimulation of the CG, including defensive behaviors and analgesia. The most important subnuclei in this respect appear to be the ventrolateral and the lateral subnuclei (22). These elongated structures can be further divided into two main regions, a rostral pretentorial area and a caudal subtentorial portion.

This review is not the place for an exhaustive description of the input-output connections of the CG. In a nutshell, the CG has multiple, usually reciprocal, connections with diverse regions of the brain, including (a) the hypothalamus, (b) the limbic system, (c) various extrapyramidal, thalamic, and other motor pathways, and (d) most lower brain stem areas involved in autonomic regulation (10,91,96). The CG also receives heavy, topographically organized projections from most laminae of the spinal cord (80).

Descending Projections of CG Involved in Autonomic Control

Both the antinociceptive and the hemodynamic effects of CG stimulation (at least those mediated by activation of the sympathoadrenal axis) are currently accounted for by similar schemes. Both will be briefly described here to emphasize the similarities but also the anatomic separation of the pathways involved. As a caveat, consideration of the extensive connections of the CG to and from more rostral structures (10,91) should alert anyone to the distinct possibility that the emphasis placed on these descending pathways may be artificial and may simply reflect the fact that all the detailed neurophysiological work is conducted under anesthesia.

The ventrolateral CG has massive descending projections which, after sending fibers into the dorsal parabrachial nuclei of the pons (another major autonomic relay), fans out widely within the ventromedial and ventrolateral medulla, especially at rostral levels (91). The rostral half of the medulla oblongata (both ventromedial and ventrolateral divisions) is classically described as the medullary area with the heaviest projections to the spinal cord (17). Current thinking is that the antinociceptive and autonomic effects of the central gray matter are relayed through some of these descending projections.

The activation (or inhibition) of bulbospinal neurons located in the rostromedial part of the medulla oblongata (raphe magnus and juxtafacial part of nucleus paragigantocellularis) is currently assumed to result in the gating of nociceptive reflexes at the level of the spinal cord (64). This view derives from evidence that interruption of synaptic transmission at the raphe magnus/lateral paragigantocellularis nucleus level (by microinjection of morphine or excitatory amino acid receptor antagonists) negates the antinociceptive effect produced by CG stimulation (145). Several types of cells are assumed to be involved including "on cells" and "off cells"—with nomenclature referring to the timing of their firing in relation to the tail flick nociceptive paradigm (64). These cells are assumed to be involved in the gating of spinal nociceptive reflexes triggered by central gray stimulation. Raphe magnus also contains "neutral cells" now assumed to be serotinergic and which are not involved in the analgesic effect of morphine (64). These cells may produce an open-loop control of spinal nociceptive mechanisms. Interestingly, the activity of "on cells" and "off cells" has recently been shown to be pulse-rhythmic and correlated with the blood pressure changes caused by nociceptive stimuli (113). These characteristics suggest that these bulbospinal cells could also be involved in the autonomic changes elicited by CG stimulation; however, the bulk of the evidence currently available suggests that the presympathetic vasomotor neurons of RVL

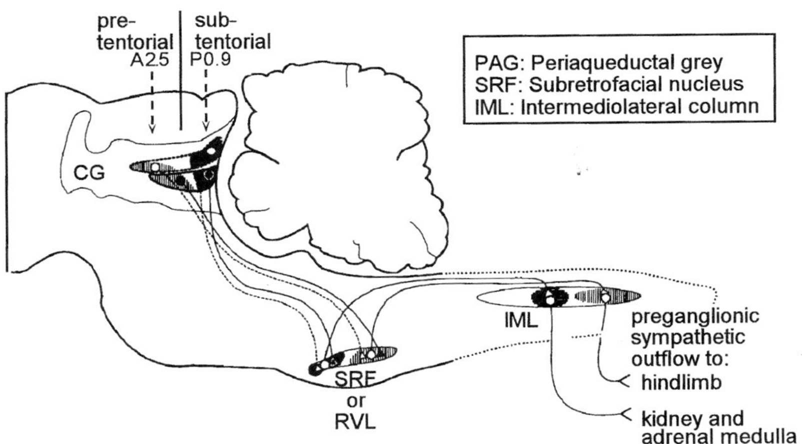

Figure 19. Topographically organized projections to RVL (called SRF by the authors of this study) underlie the hemodynamic changes produced by stimulation of the periaqueductal grey matter. This brain area is essential to the elaboration of the autonomic components of affective/defensive behaviors, which include simultaneous muscle vasodilatation and constriction of visceral areas. (Reprinted with permission from ref. 22.)

are predominantly responsible for these vasomotor effects, as summarized in Fig. 19.

This theory rests on the three following lines of evidence: (a) direct single-unit evidence that these presympathetic cells are excited or inhibited in appropriate fashion when pressor and depressor regions of the CG are stimulated (90), (b) anatomical evidence for specific topographically organized connections between regions of the CG producing muscle vasodilatation and subregions of the RVL containing a predominance of neurons controlling muscle blood flow, as well as similar evidence for visceral blood flow control (7), and (c) evidence that the antinociceptive effects of CG stimulation, in contrast to the vasomotor effects, are unaffected by selectively manipulating the activity of RVL presympathetic cells (124). Whether the projections from CG to RVL presympathetic vasomotor neurons is monosynaptic remains undetermined. The rostral paragigantocellular nucleus and the parabrachial nuclei remain viable candidates as alternate access routes between CG and RVL presympathetic vasomotor neurons.

Finally, the ventrolateral CG also sends projections to the nucleus of the solitary tract, nucleus ambiguus, retroambiguus and the periambigual area (96). These projections are likely to be involved in the cardiovagal components of the defensive behaviors, the associated vocalizations (nucleus retroambiguus) and respiratory effects (NTS, periambigual area).

Analgesia and coordinated defensive behaviors (mimicking normal motor and cardiovascular response to nociception and threat) are produced by chemical stimulation of the CG. This area probably exerts a direct control over the sympathetic and cardiovagal outflows via projections to presympathetic vasomotor neurons of RVL (and possibly CVMs). CG activation attenuates nociceptive reflexes in part by activating bulbospinal cells located in the rostral ventromedial medulla.

MECHANISM OF ACTION OF CLONIDINE AND RELATED CENTRALLY ACTING SYMPATHOLYTIC AGENTS

Molecular Mechanisms of Action

The most likely mechanism of the central hypotensive effect of clonidine and related sympatholytic drugs is an agonist activity at α_2-adrenergic receptors (for a recent review, see ref. 118).

Three subtypes of G-protein interactive α_2-adrenergic receptors (α_2-ARs) have been identified in humans and rats (61). Each exhibits a unique pharmacological profile (60) with some additional slight differences between orthologous gene products (species differences). For example, a critical amino acid difference in the structure of the α_{2A} seems responsible for the unusually low affinity of this subtype for the drug yohimbine in the rat (86). This point is of more than passing significance because the relatively low potency of yohimbine as an antagonist of clonidine in the CNS is commonly used as a critical piece of evidence for the proponents of a competing theory according to which clonidine would exert its central sympatholytic effects via interaction with "imidazoline receptors" distinct from α_2-ARs (114,143).

Cellular Mechanisms

Where investigated, activation of neuronal α_2-ARs has so far been shown to produce opening of potassium channels and/or reduction in Ca channel activation (118,150). These two effects probably underlie the postsynaptic and presynaptic inhibitory effects of these agents, respectively. α_2-AR activation also leads to a reduction in cAMP in neurons with still undefined electrophysiological consequences.

CNS Location of α_2-Adrenergic Receptors

"Generic" α_2-ARs have been mapped by radioligand autoradiography (144) and the brain stem distribution of the A subtype is available based on the use of subtype-selective antibody (117). Finally, Northern blot analysis of the mRNA content of brain parts as well as hybridization histochemistry have provided information on the sites of synthesis of the three receptor subtypes (121,154).

Within the lower brain stem, α_2 and especially α_{2A} receptors are particularly concentrated in the regions involved in autonomic control, including NTS, area postrema, RVL, ventromedial medulla, parabrachial nuclei, and intermediolateral cell column of spinal cord) (Fig. 20). The central gray, hypothalamus, and limbic system are also areas with large receptor concentrations.

Effect of α_2-Adrenergic Agonists on the Vasomotor Network

Baroreflex sensitization occurs at the level of the NTS. However, the rostral ventral medulla and the spinal cord are probably the two main sites responsible for the sympatholytic effect of clonidine under anesthesia (109,111).

Microinjection of clonidine into RVL produces hypotension and sympathoinhibition. The discharge of many RVL presympathetic vasomotor neurons is profoundly inhibited by low sympatholytic doses of clonidine given intravenously and the same cells are also inhibited by iontophoretic application of clonidine and α-methylnoradrenaline (3) (Fig. 21). The effect of both substances is blocked by iontophoretic application of

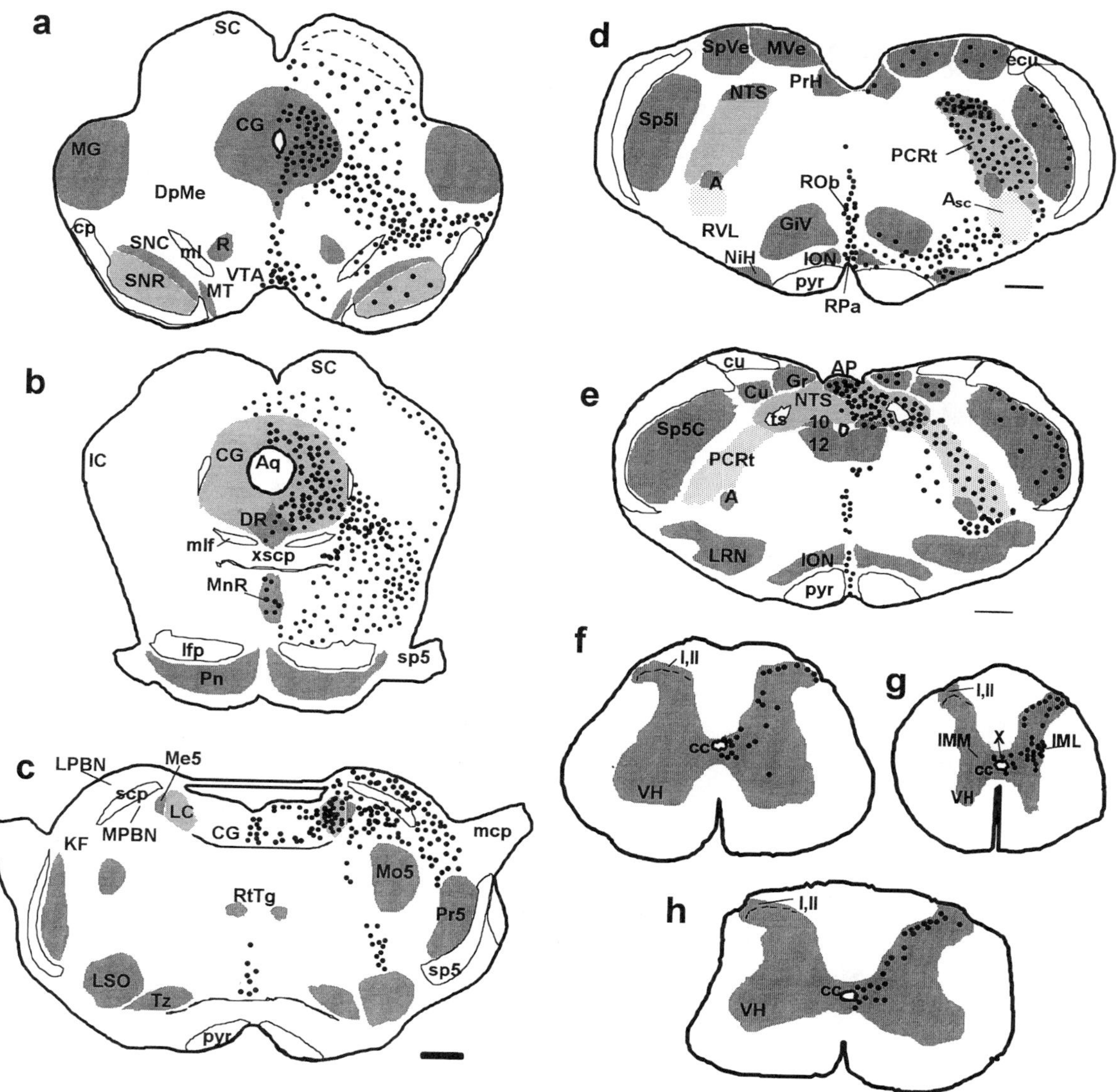

Figure 20. Distribution of α_{2A} adrenergic receptors in representative coronal sections through rat brain. Clonidine and related α_2 adrenergic receptor agonists lower arterial pressure under anaesthesia by at least three actions on the lower brain stem: inhibition of preganglionic neurons in spinal cord **(g)**, inhibition of presympathetic vasomotor neurons of RVL **(d)** and sensitization of the baroreceptor feedback via action in the nucleus of the solitary tract (NTS in **E**). (Reprinted with permission from ref. 117.)

drugs with α_2 adrenergic antagonist activity suggesting mediation of their common effect by this type of receptor (3). This result is fully congruent with anatomical evidence for the presence of α_{2A} adrenergic receptors in C1 adrenergic cells, including those with spinal projections to the intermediolateral cell column (8).

Many sympathetic preganglionic cells are also directly inhibited by α_2-AR agonists, due to somatic hyperpolarization and potassium channel opening. This and other results suggest that a significant fraction of the sympatholytic effect of clonidine may occur at a spinal level.

The three above-mentioned sites of action are likely to underlie most of the central hypotensive effect of clonidine under anesthesia but many additional sites probably also contribute in the unanesthetized state judging from the extensive distribution of α_2 receptors in more rostral brain areas with known connections with brain stem autonomic centers (118).

EFFECT OF OPIATES ON ARTERIAL PRESSURE MAINTENANCE UNDER ANESTHESIA

In humans, opiate receptor agonists are considered to produce relatively minor effects on arterial pressure unless severe hypovolemia is present. For many drugs, like morphine, it is even unclear to what degree these hypotensive effects are due to sympathoinhibition or to histamine release by mast cells (71). Fentanyl produces especially pronounced bradycardia and modest hypotension in humans and in animals. The bradycardia seems due to increased vagal tone (42). The site of these actions appears to be the caudal brain stem (42).

Opiate peptides and receptors are present in all brain stem nuclei involved in autonomic regulations including the NTS, parabrachial nuclei, the central gray and the ventrolateral medulla (41,84,100,129,151).

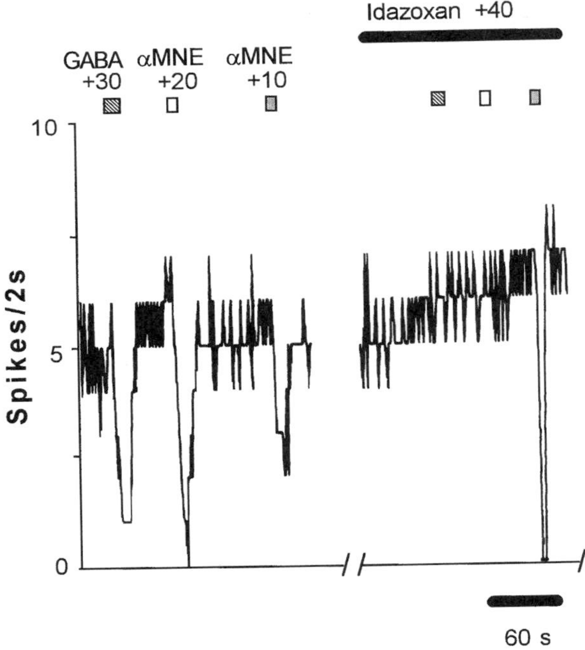

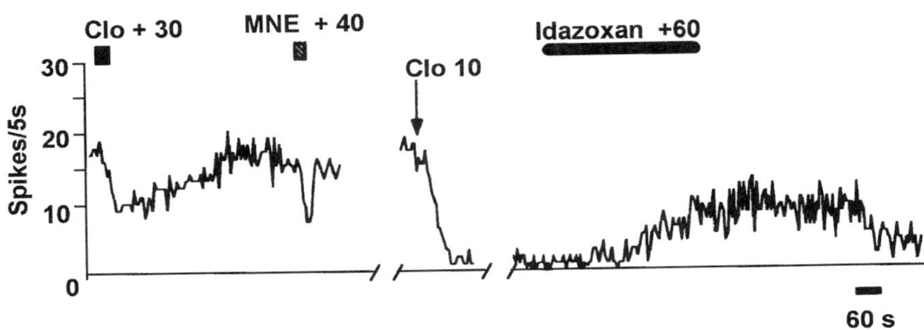

Figure 21. Inhibition of presympathetic cells in RVL by clonidine and catecholamine. *Top:* Single-unit activity of RVL presympathetic cell is inhibited in dose-dependant fashion by iontophoretic application of αmethyl-norepinephrine "in vivo" in an anesthetized rat. The effect of the catecholamine is blocked by concurrent application of idazoxan, a drug with α_2-adrenoceptor antagonist properties. *Bottom:* Different cell inhibited by low doses of clonidine i.v. and by iontophoretic application of both clonidine and αCH3-NE. The effect of i.v. clonidine is partially reversed by iontophoretic application of idazoxan suggesting that the inhibition of the cell by i.v. clonidine is due, at least in part, to an action of the drug in the immediate vicinity of the neuron. (Reprinted with permission from ref. 3.)

Experiments in animals have revealed highly complex, anesthetic dependent effects of opiates on arterial pressure, heart rate and the baroreflex (for a review, see ref. 84). In general, systemic injections of opioid agonists to anesthetized animals produce inhibition of baroreflexes, modest and regionally differentiated changes in sympathetic outflow (increases and decreases) and bradycardia (8). Most of these effects can be traced to an action in the lower brain stem. In stark contrast with the modest autonomic changes that result from systemic injections of opiate agonists, intraparenchymal microinjection of opioid agonists into the brain stem exerts large effects on cardiovascular function, even when respiration is assisted to avoid the secondary cardiovascular effects due to impairment of the central respiratory drive. Depending on the predominant role of the targeted nucleus either pressor or depressor effects are produced. For instance the microinjection of μ agonists into RVL produces a profound arterial pressure drop in anesthetized animals (110). This effect may be due in part to the direct inhibition of the presympathetic vasomotor neurons, since an inhibitory effect of metenkephalin on the discharges of RVL neurons is observed "in vitro" (50) and C1 cells receive monosynaptic contact from opioid containing terminals (100). In contrast, microinjection of similar amounts of these agents more caudally at the level of the CVL (Figs. 3, 8, and 10) produces powerful increases in pressure and a considerable attenuation of the baroreflex (110). Baroreflex impairment is also observed when these agents are given systemically or are microinjected into the NTS (47). Finally, m-receptor agonists exert powerful depressant effects on the central respiratory drive, which, indirectly, would tend to depress the sympathetic outflow (8) and could be responsible for some of the observed bradycardia.

In short, under anesthesia, the depressant effects of opiates on the central respiratory drive and on presympathetic neurons of RVL tend to reduce sympathetic outflow and lower pressure, whereas their effects in CVL and the NTS lead to attenuation of the baroreflex. These effects cancel each other functionally, leading to relatively modest overall cardiovascular effects of these drugs under normal circumstances (normovolemia in particular).

CONCLUSION

This brief survey has attempted to describe the major organizational principles of the central circuitry responsible for maintenance of arterial pressure, especially under anesthesia. Most of our knowledge of this central circuitry originates from animal work. Because significant differences between carnivores and rodents have been uncovered, it is probable that the human circuitry is also slightly different. However, comparative neuroanatomy reveals that all key brain stem structures involved in autonomic function are identifiable in humans. In addition, the sympathetic outflow to the muscle and skin of awake humans is now extensively studied and exhibits clear cut similarities with that of experimental animals. In particular, the output to the muscle is pulse-modulated at resting pressure and apparently arrhythmic at low AP (Fig. 13). This output is subject to familiar patterns of reflex control suggesting that the basic brain stem mechanisms of cardiovascular control are phylogenetically conserved.

REFERENCES

1. Allen AM, Chai SY, Clevers J, et al. Localization and characterization of angiotensin II receptor binding and angiotensin converting enzyme in the human medulla oblongata. *J Comp Neurol* 1988; 269:249–264.
2. Allen AM, Dampney RA, Mendelsohn FA. Angiotensin receptor binding and pressor effects in cat subretrofacial nucleus. *Am J Physiol* 1988; 255:H1011–H1017.
3. Allen AM, Guyenet PG. Alpha$_2$-adrenoceptor-mediated inhibition of bulbospinal barosensitive cells of rat rostral medulla. *Am J Physiol* 1993;265:R1065–R1075.
4. Anderson CR, Edwards SL, Furness JB, et al. The distribution of nitric oxide synthase-containing autonomic preganglionic terminals in the rat. *Brain Res* 1993;614:78–85.
5. Andresen MC, Young M. Non-NMDA receptors mediate sensory afferent synaptic transmission in medial nucleus tractus solitarius. *Am J Physiol* 1990;259:H1307–H1311.
6. Bachoo M, Polosa C. The pattern of sympathetic neurone activity during expiration in the cat. *J Physiol (Lond)* 1986;378:375–390.
7. Bandler R, Carrive P, Zhang SP. Integration of somatic and autonomic reactions within the midbrain periaqueductal grey: viscerotopic, somatotopic and functional organization. *Prog Brain Res* 1991;87:269–305.
8. Baraban SC, Stornetta RL, Guyenet PG. Respiratory control of sympathetic nerve activity during naloxone-precipitated morphine withdrawal in rats. *J Pharmacol Exp Ther* 1993;265:89–95.
9. Barman SM, Gebber GL. Basis for the naturally occurring activity of rostral ventrolateral medullary sympathoexcitatory neurons. *Prog Brain Res* 1989;81:117–129.
10. Beitz AJ. The organization of afferent projections to the midbrain periaquecductal gray of the rat. *Neuroscience* 1982;7:133–159.
11. Bellingham MC, Lipski J. Respiratory interneurons in the C5 segment of the spinal cord of the cat. *Brain Res* 1990;533:141–146.
12. Bieger D, Hopkins DA. Viscerotopic representation of the upper alimentary tract in the medulla oblongata in the rat: the nucleus ambiguus. *J Comp Neurol* 1987;262:546–562.
13. Bishop VS, Hay M. Involvement of the area postrema in the regulation of sympathetic outflow to the cardiovascular system. *Front Neuroendocrinol* 1993;14:57–75.
14. Bishop VS, Haywood JR. Hormonal control of cardiovascular reflexes. In: Zucker IH, Gilmore JP, eds. *Reflex control of the circulation.* Boston: CRC Press, 1991:253–271.
15. Bishop VS, Mifflin SW. Central neural mechanisms in the cardiovascular response to exercise. In: Kunos G, Ciriello J, eds. *Central neural mechanisms in cardiovascular regulation.* Boston: Birkhauser, 1992:36–51.
16. Boczek-Funcke A, Habler H-J, Janig W, et al. Rapid phasic baroreceptor inhibition of the activity in sympathetic preganglionic neurones does not change throughout the respiratory cycle. *J Autonom Nerv Syst* 1991;34:185–194.
17. Brodal A. *Neurological anatomy.* New York: Oxford University Press, 1981.
18. Brooks PA, Izzo PN, Spyer KM. Brainstem GABA pathways and the regulation of baroreflex activity. In: Kunos G, Ciriello J, eds. *Central neural mechanisms in cardiovascular regulation.* Boston: Birkhauser, 1992:321–337.
19. Brown DL, Guyenet PG. Electrophysiological study of cardiovascular neurons in the rostral ventrolateral medulla in rats. *Circ Res* 1985;56:359–369.
20. Byrum CE, Guyenet PG. Afferent and efferent connections of the A5 noradrenergic cell group in the rat. *J Comp Neurol* 1987;261: 529–542.
21. Cabot JB. Sympathetic preganglionic neurons: cytoarchitecture, ultrastructure. In: Loewy AD, Spyer KM, eds. *Central regulation of autonomic functions.* Oxford: Oxford University Press, 1990:44–67.
22. Carrive P, Bandler R. Viscerotopic organization of neurons subserving hypotensive reactions within the midbrain periaqueductal grey: a correlative functional and anatomical study. *Brain Res* 1991; 541:206–215.
23. Cechetto DF, Saper CB. Role of the cerebral cortex in autonomic function. In: Loewy AD, Spyer KM, eds. *Central regulation of autonomic functions.* New York: Oxford University Press, 1990: 208–223.
24. Cervero F, Foreman RD. Sensory innervation of the viscera. In: Loewy AD, Spyer KM, eds. *Central regulation of autonomic functions.* New York: Oxford University Press, 1990:104–125.
25. Chapleau MW, Hadjuczok G, Abboud FM. Resetting of the arterial baroreflex: peripheral and central mechanisms. In: Zucker IH, Gilmore JP, eds. *Reflex control of the circulation.* Boston: CRC Press, 1991:165–194.
26. Chapleau MW, Hajduczok G, Abboud FM. New insights into the influence of pulsatile pressure on the arterial baroreceptor reflex. *Clin Exp Hypertens* 1988;10:179–192.
27. Ciriello J. Brainstem projections of aortic baroreceptor afferent fibers in the rat. *Neurosci Lett* 1983;36:37–42.
28. Coleridge HM, Coleridge JCG. Afferent innervation of lungs, airways and pulmonary artery. In: Zucker IH, Gilmore JP, eds. *Reflex control of the circulation.* Boston: CRC Press, 1991:579–607.
29. Connelly CA, Wurster RD. Spinal pathways mediating respiratory influences on sympathetic nerves. *Am J Physiol* 1985;249:R91–R99.
30. Coote JH. The organisation of cardiovascular neurons in the spinal cord. *Rev Physiol Biochem Pharmacol* 1988;110:147–285.
31. Cravo SL, Morrison SF, Reis DJ. Differentiation of two cardiovascular regions within caudal ventrolateral medulla. *Am J Physiol* 1991;261:R985–R994.
32. Czachurski J, Dembowsky K, Seller H, et al. Morphology of electrophysiologically identified baroreceptor afferents and second order neurones in the brainstem of the cat. *Arch Ital Biol* 1988;126: 129–144.
33. Daly MD. Interactions between respiration and circulation. In: Cherniak NS, Widdicombe JG, eds. *The respiratory system, vol. 2. Control of breathing, part 2.* Bethesda: American Physiological Society, 1986:529–594.
34. Dampney RA, McAllen RM. Differential control of sympathetic fibres supplying hindlimb skin and muscle by subretrofacial neurones in the cat. *J Physiol (Lond)* 1988;395:41–56.
35. Dembowsky K, Czachurski J, Seller H. Morphology of sympathetic preganglionic neurons in the thoracic spinal cord of the cat: an intracellular horseradish peroxidase study. *J Comp Neurol* 1985; 238:453–465.
36. Dembowsky K, Czachurski J, Seller H. An intracellular study of the synaptic input to sympathetic preganglionic neurones of the third thoracic segment of the cat. *J Auton Nerv Syst*1985;13:201–244.
37. Eckberg DL, Nerhed C, Wallin BG. Respiratory modulation of muscle sympathetic and vagal cardiac outflow in man. *J Physiol (Lond)* 1985;365:181–196.
38. Feldman JL. Neurophysiology of breathing in mammals. In: Bloom FE, ed. *Handbook of physiology: the nervous system, vol. IV.* Bethesda: American Physiological Society, 1987:463–524.
39. Feldman JL, Ellenberger HH. Central coordination of respiratory and cardiovascular control in mammals. *Annu Rev Physiol* 1988;50: 593–606.
40. Ferguson DW, Mark AL. Regulation of sympathetic nerve activity in humans: new concepts regarding autonomic adjustments to exercise and neurohumoral excitation in heart failure. In: Zucker IH, Gilmore JP, eds. *Reflex control of the circulation.* Boston: CRC Press, 1991:875–906.
41. Feuerstein G, Siren AL, Vonhof S, et al. Neuropeptides: evidence for central pathways and role in cardiovascular regulation. In: Zucker IH, Gilmore JP, eds. *Reflex control of the circulation.* Boston: CRC Press, 1991:215–251.
42. Freye E, Arndt JO. Perfusion of the fourth cerebral ventricle with fentanyl induces naloxone-reversible bradycardia, hypotension, and EEG synchronization in conscious dogs. *Naunyn Scmiedebergs Arch Pharmacol* 1979;307:123–128.
43. Fukuda Y, Sato A, Suzuki A, et al. Autonomic nerve and cardiovascular responses to changing blood oxygen and carbon dioxide levels in the rat. *J Auton Nerv Syst* 1989;28:61–74.
44. Fulwiler CE, Saper CB. Subnuclear organization of the efferent connections of the parabrachial nucleus in the rat. *Brain Res* 1984; 319:229–259.
45. Gebber GL. Central determinants of sympathetic nerve discharge.

In: Loewy AD, Spyer KM, eds. *Central regulation of autonomic functions.* New York: Oxford University Press, 1990:126–144.
46. Goetz KL, Madwed JB, Leadley RJ. Atrial receptors: reflex effects in quadrupeds. In: Zucker IH, Gilmore JP, eds. *Reflex control of the circulation.* Boston: CRC Press, 1991:291–312.
47. Gordon FJ. Opioids and central baroreflex control: a site of action in the nucleus tractus solitarius. *Peptides* 1990;11:305–309.
48. Gordon FJ, Talman WT. Role of excitatory amino acids and their receptors in bulbospinal control of cardiovascular function. In: Kunos G, Ciriello J, eds. *Central neural mechanisms in cardiovascular regulation, vol. 2.* Boston: Birkhauser, 1992:209–225.
49. Guertzenstein PG, Silver A. Fall in blood pressure produced from discrete regions of the ventral surface of the medulla by glycine and lesions. *J Physiol (Lond)* 1974;242:489–503.
50. Guyenet PG. Role of the ventral medulla oblongata in blood pressure regulation. In: Loewy AD, Spyer KM, eds. *Central regulation of autonomic functions.* New York: Oxford University Press, 1990: 145–167.
51. Guyenet PG, Brown DL. Unit activity in nucleus paragigantocellularis lateralis during cerebral ischemia in the rat. *Brain Res* 1986; 364:301–314.
52. Guyenet PG, Brown DL. Nucleus paragigantocellularis lateralis and lumbar sympathetic discharge in the rat. *Am J Physiol* 1986; 250:R1081–R1094.
53. Guyenet PG, Darnall RA, Riley TA. Rostral ventrolateral medulla and sympathorespiratory integration in rats. *Am J Physiol* 1990;259: R1063–R1074.
54. Guyenet PG, Filtz TM, Donaldson SR. Role of excitatory amino acids in rat vagal and sympathetic baroreflexes. *Brain Res* 1987; 407:272–284.
55. Guyenet PG, Haselton JR, Sun MK. Sympathoexcitatory neurons of the rostroventrolateral medulla and the origin of the sympathetic vasomotor tone. *Prog Brain Res* 1989;81:105–116.
56. Guyenet PG, Koshiya N. Respiratory-Sympathetic Integration in the Medulla Oblongata. In: Kunos G, Ciriello J, eds. *Central neural mechanisms in cardiovascular regulation, vol. 2.* Boston: Birkhäuser, 1992:226–247.
57. Guyenet PG, Koshiya N, Huangfu D, et al. Central respiratory control of A5 and A6 pontine noradrenergic neurons. *Am J Physiol* 1993;264:R1035–R1044.
58. Guyton AC. Blood pressure control: special role of the kidneys and body fluids. *Science* 1991;252:1813–1816.
59. Hainsworth R. Atrial receptors. In: Zucker IH, Gilmore JP, eds. *Reflex control of the circulation.* Boston: CRC Press, 1991:273–289.
60. Harrison JK, D'Angelo DD, Zeng DW, et al. Pharmacological characterization of rat α_2-adrenergic receptors. *Mol Pharmacol* 1991;40:407–412.
61. Harrison JK, Pearson WR, Lynch KR. Molecular characterization of α_1- and α_2-adrenoceptors. *Trends Pharmacol Sci* 1991;12:62–67.
62. Haselton JR, Guyenet PG. Central respiratory modulation of medullary sympathoexcitatory neurons in rat. *Am J Physiol* 1989; 256:R739–R750.
63. Hay M, Bishop VS. Interactions of area postrema and solitary tract in the nucleus tractus solitarius. *Am J Physiol* 1991;260: H1466–H1473.
64. Heinricher MM, Morgan MM, Fields HL. Direct and indirect actions of morphine on medullary neurons that modulate nociception. *Neuroscience* 1992;48:533–543.
65. Helke CJ, Ichikawa H. Tachykinins, tachykinin receptors and the central control of the cardiovascular system. In: Kunos G, Ciriello J, eds. *Central neural mechanisms in cardiovascular regulation, vol. 2.* Boston: Birkhauser, 1992:248–265.
66. Inokuchi H, Yoshimura M, Trzebski A, et al. Fast inhibitory postsynaptic potentials and responses to inhibitory amino acids of sympathetic preganglionic neurons in the adult cat. *J Auton Nerv Syst* 1992;41:53–59.
67. Inokuchi H, Yoshimura M, Yamada S, et al. Fast excitatory postsynaptic potentials and the responses to excitant amino acids of sympathetic preganglionic neurons in the slice of the cat spinal cord. *Neuroscience* 1992;46:657–667.
68. Iwamoto GA, Kaufman MP. Caudal ventrolateral medullary cells responsive to muscular contraction. *J Appl Physiol* 1987;62: 149–157.
69. Izzo PN, Deuchars J, Spyer KM. Localization of cardiac vagal preganglionic motoneurones in the rat: immunocytochemical evidence of synaptic inputs containing 5-hydroxytryptamine. *J Comp Neurol* 1993;327:572–583.
70. Jacobs BL, Azmitia EC. Structure and function of the brain serotonin system. *Physiol Rev* 1992;72:165–229.
71. Jaffe JH, Martin WR. Opioid analgesics and antagonists. In: Gilman AG, Goodman LS, Rall TW, Murad F, eds. *The pharmacological basis of therapeutics.* New York: Macmillan, 1985:491–531.
72. Janig W. Organization of the lumbar sympathetic outflow to skeletal muscle and skin of the cat hindlimb and tail. *Rev Physiol Biochem Pharmacol* 1985;102:119–213.
73. Johnson AK, Loewy AD. Circumventricular organs and their role in visceral function. In: Loewy AD, Spyer KM, eds. *Central regulation of autonomic functions.* Oxford: Oxford University Press, 1990: 247–267.
74. Jordan D. Autonomic changes in affective behavior. In: Loewy AD, Spyer KM, eds. *Central regulation of autonomic functions.* Oxford: Oxford University Press, 1990:349–366.
75. Jordan D, Mifflin SW, Spyer KM. Hypothalamic inhibition of neurones in the nucleus tractus solitarius of the cat is GABA mediated. *J Physiol (Lond)* 1988;399:389–404.
76. Karczmar AG, Koketsu K, Nishi S. *Autonomic and enteric ganglia. Transmission and its pharmacology.* New York: Plenum, 1986.
77. Katona PG, Dembowsky K, Czachurski J, et al. Chemoreceptor stimulation on sympathetic activity: dependence on respiratory phase. *Am J Physiol* 1989;257:R1027–R1033.
78. Kaufman MP, Iwamoto GA, Ashton JH, et al. Responses to inflation of vagal afferents with endings in the lung of dogs. *Circ Res* 1982;51:525–531.
79. Kaufman MP, Longhurst JC, Rybicki KJ, et al. Effects of static muscular contraction on impulse activity of groups III and IV afferents in cats. *J Appl Physiol* 1983;55:105–112.
80. Keay KA, Bandler R. Anatomical evidence for segregated input from the upper cervical spinal cord to functionally distinct regions of the periaqueductal gray region of the cat. *Neurosci Lett* 1992;139:143–148.
81. Kocsis B, Lenkei Z. Coordination between cardiovascular and respiratory control systems during and after cerebral ischemia. *J Appl Physiol* 1992;72:1595–1603.
82. Koshiya N, Huangfu D, Guyenet PG. Ventrolateral medulla and sympathetic chemoreflex in the rat. *Brain Res* 1993;609:174–184.
83. Kumada M, Terui N, Kuwaki T. Arterial baroreceptor reflex: its central and peripheral neural mechanisms. *Prog Neurobiol* 1990;35: 331–361.
84. Kunos G, Mastrianni JA, Mosqueda-Garcia R, et al. Endorphinergic neurons in the brainstem: role in cardiovascular regulation. In: Kunos G, Ciriello J, eds. *Central neural mechanisms in cardiovascular regulation, vol. 1.* Boston: Birkhauser, 1991:122–136.
85. Kunze DL, Andresen MC. Arterial baroreceptors: excitation and modulation. In: Zucker IH, Gilmore JP, eds. *Reflex control of the circulation.* Boston: CRC Press, 1991:139–164.
86. Link R, Daunt D, Barsh G, et al. Cloning of two mouse genes encoding alpha 2–adrenergic receptor subtypes and identification of a single amino acid in the mouse alpha 2-C10 homolog responsible for an interspecies variation in antagonist binding. *Mol Pharmacol* 1992;42:16–27.
87. Lioy F, Hanna BD, Polosa C. CO_2-dependent component of the neurogenic vascular tone in the cat. *Pflugers Arch* 1937;1978: 187–191.
88. Loewy AD. Central autonomic pathways. In: Loewy AD, Spyer KM, eds. *Central regulation of autonomic functions.* New York: Oxford University Press, 1990:88–103.
89. Loewy AD, Spyer KM. Vagal preganglionic neurons. In: Loewy AD, Spyer KM, eds. *Central regulation of autonomic functions.* New York: Oxford University Press, 1990:68–87.
90. Lovick TA. Midbrain influences on ventrolateral medullo-spinal neurones in the rat. *Exp Brain Res* 1992;90:147–152.
91. Luiten PG, Ter Horst GJ, Steffens AB. The hypothalamus, intrinsic connections and outflow pathways to the endocrine system in relation to the control of feeding and metabolism. *Prog Neurobiol* 1987;28:1–54.
92. Mark AL. The Bezold-Jarisch reflex revisited: clinical implications of inhibitory reflexes originating in the heart. *J Am Coll Cardiol* 1983;1:90–102.
93. McAllen RM, May CN. Effects of preoptic warming on subretrofacial and cutaneous vasoconstrictor neurons in anesthetized cats. *J Physiol (Lond)* 1994;481:719–730.
94. McAllen RM, Spyer KM. The baroreceptor input to cardiac vagal motoneurones. *J Physiol (Lond)* 1978;282:365–374.
95. McCall RB. Central neurotransmitters involved in cardiovascular

regulation. In: Antonaccio M, ed. *Cardiovascular pharmacology.* New York: Raven Press, 1990:161–200.
96. Meller ST, Dennis BJ. Efferent projections of the periaqueductal gray in the rabbit. *Neuroscience* 1991;40:191–216.
97. Mifflin SW, Spyer KM, Withington-Wray DJ. Baroreceptor inputs to the nucleus tractus solitarius in the cat: modulation by the hypothalamus. *J Physiol (Lond)* 1988;399:369–387.
98. Mifflin SW, Spyer KM, Withington-Wray DJ. Baroreceptor inputs to the nucleus tractus solitarius in the cat: postsynaptic actions and the influence of respiration. *J Physiol (Lond)* 1988;399: 349–367.
99. Millhorn DE. Neural respiratory and circulatory interaction during chemoreceptor stimulation and cooling of ventral medulla in cats. *J Physiol (Lond)* 1986;370:217–231.
100. Milner TA, Pickel VM, Morrison SF, et al. Adrenergic neurons in the rostral ventrolateral medulla: ultrastructure and synaptic relations with other transmitter-identified neurons. In: Ciriello J, Caverson MM, Polosa C, eds. *Progress in brain research.* Amsterdam: Elsevier Science, 1989:29–47.
101. Minisi AJ, Thames MD. Reflexes from ventricular receptors with vagal afferents. In: Zucker IH, Gilmore JP, eds. *Reflex control of the circulation.* Boston: CRC Press, 1991:359–406.
102. Morris BJ, Moneta ME, ten Bruggencate G, et al. Levels of prodynorphin mRNA in rat dentate gyrus are decreased during hippocampal kindling. *Neurosci Lett* 1987;80:298–302.
103. Morrison SF, Callaway J, Milner TA, et al. Glutamate in the spinal sympathetic intermediolateral nucleus: localization by light and electron microscopy. *Brain Res* 1989;503:5–15.
104. Morrison SF, Callaway J, Milner TA, et al. Rostral ventrolateral medulla: a source of the glutamatergic innervation of the sympathetic intermediolateral nucleus. *Brain Res* 1991;562:126–135.
105. Morrison SF, Gebber GL. Raphe neurons with sympathetic-related activity: baroreceptor responses and spinal connections. *Am J Physiol* 1984;246:R338–R348.
106. Morrison SF, Reis DJ. Reticulospinal vasomotor neurons in the RVL mediate the somatosympathetic reflex. *Am J Physiol* 1989;256: R1084–R1097.
107. Parmeggiani PL, Morrison AR. Alterations in autonomic function during sleep. In: Loewy AD, Spyer KM, eds. *Central regulation of autonomic functions.* Oxford: Oxford University Press, 1990: 367–390.
108. Paton JFR, Spyer KM. Cerebellar cortical regulation of circulation. *News in Physiological Sciences* 1992;7:124–129.
109. Polosa C, Yoshimura M, Nishi S. The function of catecholamines in the control of sympathetic preganglionic neurons. In: Kunos G, Ciriello J, eds. *Central neural mechanisms in cardiovascular regulation, vol. 1.* Boston: Birkhauser, 1991:209–227.
110. Punnen S, Sapru HN. Cardiovascular responses to medullary microinjections of opiate agonists in urethane-anesthetized rats. *J Cardiovasc Pharmacol* 1986;8:950–956.
111. Punnen S, Urbanski R, Krieger AJ, et al. Ventrolateral medullary pressor area: site of hypotensive action of clonidine. *Brain Res* 1987;422:336–346.
112. Randall WC, Ardell JL. Nervous control of the heart: anatomy and pathophysiology. In: Zipes DP, Jalife J, eds. *Cardiac electrophysiology: from cell to bedside.* Philadelphia: WB Saunders, 1990:291–299.
113. Randich A. Interactions between cardiovascular and pain regulatory systems. In: Kunos G, Ciriello J, eds. *Central neural mechanisms in cardiovascular regulation, vol. 2.* Boston: Birkhauser, 1992: 297–320.
114. Reis DJ, Ernsberger PR, Meeley MP. Imidazole receptors and their endogenous ligand in the rostral ventrolateral medulla: relationship to the action of clonidine on arterial pressure. In: Kunos G, Ciriello J, eds. *Central neural mechanisms in cardiovascular regulation, vol. 1.* Boston: Birkhauser, 1991:55–68.
115. Richter DW, Spyer KM. Cardiorespiratory control. In: Loewy AD, Spyer KM, eds. *Central regulation of autonomic functions.* New York: Oxford University Press, 1990:189–207.
116. Rohlicek CV, Polosa C. Hypoxic responses of sympathetic preganglionic neurons in sinoaortic-denervated cats. *Am J Physiol* 1983; 244:H681–H686.
117. Rosin DL, Zeng D, Stornetta RL, et al. Immunohistochemical localization of α_{2A}-adrenergic receptors in catecholaminergic and other brainstem neurons in the rat. *Neuroscience* 1993;56:139–155.
118. Ruffolo RR, Nichols AJ, Stadel JM, et al. Pharmacologic and therapeutic applications of alpha 2-adrenoceptor subtypes. *Annu Rev Pharmacol Toxicol* 1993;33:243–279.
119. Ruggiero DA, Cravo SL, Arango V, et al. Central control of the circulation by the rostral ventrolateral reticular nucleus: anatomical substrates. In: Ciriello J, Caverson MM, Polosa C, eds. *Progress in brain research, vol. 81: the central neural organization of cardiovascular control.* Amsterdam: Elsevier Science, 1989:49–79.
120. Sapru HN. Spinal mechanisms in the control of cardiac function. In: Kunos G, Ciriello J, eds. *Central neural mechanisms in cardiovascular regulation, vol. 1.* Boston: Birkhauser, 1991:49–79.
121. Scheinin M, Lomasney JW, Hayden-Hixson DM, et al. Distribution of alpha 2-adrenergic receptor subtype gene expression in rat brain. *Mol Brain Res* 1994;21:133–149.
122. Schwarzacher SW, Wilhelm Z, Anders K, et al. The medullary respiratory network in the rat. *J Physiol (Lond)* 1991;435:631–644.
123. Seller H, Konig SH, Czachurski J. Chemosensitivity of sympathoexcitatory neurones in the rostroventrolateral medulla of the cat. *Pflugers Arch* 1990;416:735–741.
124. Siddall PJ, Dampney RA. Relationship between cardiovascular neurones and descending antinociceptive pathways in the rostral ventrolateral medulla of the cat. *Pain* 1989;37:347–355.
125. Smith JC, Ellenberger HH, Ballanyi K, et al. Pre-Botzinger complex: a brainstem region that may generate respiratory rhythm in mammals. *Science* 1991;254:726–729.
126. Smith ML, Ellenbogen KA, Beightol LA, et al. Sympathetic neural responses to induced ventricular tachycardia. *J Am Coll Cardiol* 1991;18:1015–1024.
127. Spyer KM. The central nervous organization of reflex circulatory control. In: Loewy AD, Spyer KM, eds. *Central regulation of autonomic functions.* New York: Oxford University Press, 1990: 168–188.
128. Spyer KM, Izzo PN, Lin RJ, et al. The central nervous organization of the carotid body chemoreceptor reflex. In: Acker H, ed. *Chemoreceptors and chemoreceptor reflexes.* New York: Plenum Press, 1990:317–321.
129. Standaert DG, Watson SJ, Houghten RA, et al. Opioid peptide immunoreactivity in spinal and trigeminal dorsal horn neurons projecting to the parabrachial nucleus in the rat. *J Neurosci* 1986; 6:1220–1226.
130. Stornetta RL, Morrison SF, Ruggiero DA, et al. Neurons of rostral ventrolateral medulla mediate somatic pressor reflex. *Am J Physiol* 1989;256:R448–R462.
131. Strack AM, Sawyer WB, Hughes JH, et al. A general pattern of CNS innervation of the sympathetic outflow demonstrated by transneuronal pseudorabies viral infections. *Brain Res* 1989;491: 156–162.
132. Strack AM, Sawyer WB, Platt KB, et al. CNS cell groups regulating the sympathetic outflow to adrenal gland as revealed by transneuronal cell body labeling with pseudorabies virus. *Brain Res* 1989; 491:274–296.
133. Sun MK, Guyenet PG. GABA-mediated baroreceptor inhibition of reticulospinal neurons. *Am J Physiol* 1985;249:R672–R680.
134. Sun MK, Jeske IT, Reis DJ. Cyanide excites medullary sympathoexcitatory neurons in rats. *Am J Physiol* 1992;262:R182–R189.
135. Sun MK, Reis DJ. Central neural mechanisms mediating excitationb of sympathetic neurons by hypoxia. *Prog Neurobiol* 1994;44: 197–219.
136. Sun MK, Spyer KM. GABA-mediated inhibition of medullary vasomotor neurones by area postrema stimulation in rats. *J Physiol (Lond)* 1991;436:669–684.
137. Sun MK, Young BS, Hackett JT, et al. Rostral ventrolateral medullary neurons with intrinsic pacemaker properties are not catecholaminergic. *Brain Res* 1988;451:345–349.
138. Sved AF, Tsukamoto K, Sved JC. GABA-B receptors in the nucleus tractus solitarius in cardiovascular regulation. In: Kunos G, Ciriello J, eds. *Central neural mechanisms in cardiovascular regulation, vol. 2.* Boston: Birkhauser, 1992:338–355.
139. Terui N, Masuda N, Saeki Y, et al. Activity of barosensitive neurons in the caudal ventrolateral medulla that send axonal projections to the rostral ventrolateral medulla in rabbits. *Neurosci Lett* 1990; 118:211–214.
140. Terui N, Saeki Y, Kumada M. Barosensory neurons in the ventrolateral medulla in rabbits and their responses to various afferent inputs from peripheral and central sources. *Jpn J Physiol* 1986;36: 1141–1164.
141. Thoren P, Shepherd JT, Donald DE. Anodal block of medullated cardiopulmonary vagal afferents in cats. *J Appl Physiol* 1977;42: 461–465.
142. Thoren PN. Atrial receptors with nonmedullated vagal afferents

in the cat. Discharge frequency and pattern in relation to atrial pressure. *Circ Res* 1976;38:357–362.
143. Tibirica E, Feldman J, Mermet C, et al. An imidazoline-specific mechanism for the hypotensive effect of clonidine: a study with yohimbine and idazoxan. *J Pharmacol Exp Ther* 1991;256: 606–613.
144. Unnerstall JR, Kopajtic TA, Kuhar MJ. Distribution of α_2 agonist binding sites in the rat and human central nervous system: analysis of some functional, anatomic correlates of the pharmacologic effects of clonidine and related adrenergic agents. *Brain Res* 1984; 319:69–101.
145. van Praag H, Frenk H. The role of glutamate in opiate descending inhibition of nociceptive spinal reflexes. *Brain Res* 1990;524: 101–105.
146. Vatner SF, Uemura N. Integrative cardiovascular control by pulmonary inflation reflexes. In: Zucker IH, Gilmore JP, eds. *Reflex control of the circulation.* Boston: CRC Press, 1991:609–626.
147. Vera PL, Holets VR, Miller KE. Ultrastructural evidence of synaptic contacts between substance P-, enkephalin-, and serotonin-immunoreactive terminals and retrogradely labeled sympathetic preganglionic neurons in the rat: a study using a double-peroxidase procedure. *Synapse* 1990;6:221–229.
148. Verberne AJM, Guyenet PG. Medullary pathway of the Bezold-Jarisch reflex in the rat. *Am J Physiol* 1992;263:R1195–R1202.
149. Willette RN, Krieger AJ, Barcas PP, et al. Medullary gamma-aminobutyric acid (GABA) receptors and the regulation of blood pressure in the rat. *J Pharmacol Exp Ther* 1983;226:893–899.
150. Williams JT, Henderson G, North RA. Characterization of α_2-adrenoceptors which increase potassium conductance in rat locus coeruleus neurones. *Neuroscience* 1985;14:95–101.
151. Xia Y, Haddad GG. Ontogeny and distribution of opioid receptors in the rat brainstem. *Brain Res* 1991;549:181–193.
152. Yaksh TL, Yeung JC, Rudy TA. Systematic examination in the rat of brain sites sensitive to the direct application of morphine: observation of differential effects within the periaqueductal gray. *Brain Res* 1976;114:83–103.
153. Yates BJ. Vestibular influences on the sympathetic nervous system. *Brain Res Rev* 1992;17:51–59.
154. Zeng DW, Lynch KR. Distribution of α_2-adrenergic receptor mRNAs in the rat CNS. *Mol Brain Res* 1991;10:219–225.

Anesthesia: Biologic Foundations, edited by Tony L. Yaksh et al. Lippincott–Raven Publishers, Philadelphia © 1997.

CHAPTER 72

AUTONOMIC NERVOUS SYSTEM: MEASUREMENT AND RESPONSE UNDER ANESTHESIA

THOMAS J. EBERT, JEANNE L. SEAGARD, AND FRANCIS A. HOPP, JR.

Anesthetics in general have been found to blunt reflex control of the cardiovascular system, reducing the ability to regulate blood pressure in both human and animal models. The sites at which anesthetics can act, leading to the reduction in blood pressure control, have been investigated in many studies, and most evidence indicates that anesthetics can affect many aspects of the reflex arc, leading ultimately to depression of reflex control. However, some anesthetics do not produce as profound a reflex depression as others. The source for this maintenance of reflex control may be due to differential effects of the reflex-sparing anesthetics on various sites in the reflex arc, although most evidence suggests that maintenance of blood pressure regulation is due to sparing effects on central nervous system control centers. Studies to examine anesthetic effects on reflex control of the cardiovascular system have evaluated the effects of anesthetics on afferent input from physiological receptors such as the baroreceptors and cardiopulmonary receptors, central integration of afferent input, and efferent responses of the autonomic nervous systems, both sympathetic and parasympathetic. In the following discussion, the effects of anesthetics on reflex control of blood pressure are described, along with techniques used by investigators to examine the anesthetic action on both afferent input and efferent sympathetic and parasympathetic nerve activity in animals and humans.

METHODS FOR ASSESSMENT OF AUTONOMIC AND REFLEX FUNCTION

Animal Studies

Methods for Recording and Analyzing Nerve Activity

To measure the effects of anesthetics on central control of autonomic outflow, sympathetic and/or parasympathetic nerve activity to many regions has been recorded before and during anesthetic exposure. Changes in afferent activity following exposure to anesthetics have been used to determine the effects of the agents on receptor firing properties. Two general types of recording techniques have been used to obtain recordings of autonomic activity—chronic and acute nerve recordings. Chronic recording techniques require implantation of electrodes prior to the day of study, while acute recordings are obtained by placement of the nerve under investigation on the electrodes at the time of the experiment. Although afferent activity has generally been analyzed using acute recording techniques, chronic recording has the advantage of being able to obtain a level of nerve activity in the conscious animal to serve as a control. Unless a chronic nerve recording technique is employed, one cannot obtain a conscious level of activity and there is usually the complicating factor of a basal or induction anesthetic. For example, if an inhalation anesthetic is the agent to be studied, and if chronic electrodes are not implanted prior to the day of study, the most common way to obtain recordings of control (preanesthetic exposure) activity is to use a different anesthetic as a basal anesthetic and then superimpose the inhalational anesthetic on a background level of the first anesthetic. A short-acting anesthetic can be used for induction, but some of the effects of this agent will still be present during at least part of the study. If sufficient time is given for the induction anesthetic to wear off, there cannot be a measurement of nerve activity without at least some of the inhalational anesthetic present. Therefore, if a fully conscious control is required, the only technique that can be utilized is chronic nerve recording. The only other method to obtain nerve activity without the presence of an anesthetic is the use of decerebration, which must initially be done under anesthesia. The animal must then be given sufficient time for the surgical anesthesia to be eliminated before study of the investigational anesthetic is initiated. However, if a low background level of anesthetic will not affect the design of the experiment, then acute recording techniques can be used. The acute recording techniques are technically easier, can employ single-fiber recordings, and have the advantage of ease in maintaining isolation of the nerve from surrounding tissue and fluids, which shunts the neuronal current and degrades signal recording. The difficulty in maintaining isolation of the nerve from fluids appears to be an important time-limiting factor for chronic recording techniques. Chronic nerve recording preparations are generally not viable for >1–2 weeks, and many last for only 3 days, especially in larger animals. Thus, the technique selected for nerve recording will depend on the intent of the study and the technical abilities of the investigator.

When sympathetic or parasympathetic efferent activity is to be recorded, care must be taken to select a nerve that contains only one or the other type of fiber. Thus, renal nerve activity is often chosen as an example of sympathetic nerve activity, since there are no parasympathetic fibers in the nerve. However, most of the close cardiac nerves, or nerves that carry efferent activity to the heart, are mixed; that is, they carry both sympathetic and parasympathetic activity. In the last case, if parasympathetic activity is desired, sympathetic input to the region must be eliminated by section of the sympathetic trunk (ansae subclavia) that carries sympathetic activity to the heart. Conversely, if sympathetic activity is desired, parasympathetic activity must be eliminated by cervical vagotomy. In both cases, as with all nerves, efferent activity must be recorded from the central end of the sectioned nerve, so that the possibility of afferent traffic in the nerve is eliminated. This process of eliminating unwanted nerve activity is much easier in acute studies, where long-term survival of the animal is not a requirement. In chronic preparations, it may not be possible to section other nerves in the region or to section the nerve under study to eliminate the afferent component, because degeneration of the nerve will begin with the section and may result in death of the efferent fibers under study. However, if afferent activity is not present, or is minimal relative to the efferent component, it may not be a major problem.

Acute Recording Techniques Acute nerve activity can be obtained by placing the nerve under study on a pair of recording electrodes after isolation of the nerve from surrounding tissue (Fig. 1). The sheaths around the nerve are carefully slit and the nerve is desheathed to better expose the fibers for recording. This technique allows recording of either pre- or postganglionic activity as long as there is sufficient length available to allow the nerve to be placed on the electrode tips. The nerve-electrode preparation must be placed under warm mineral oil or liquid paraffin to prevent the nerve from drying. This oil can be localized in a pool constructed from surrounding tissue or through the use of a recording chamber in which the nerve is drawn into a plexiglass chamber and the openings sealed with a softened material such as clay or bone wax. The electrodes are usually supported by a holder made from a nonconductive material, such as a plexiglass rod. When making comparisons of the level of nerve activity from the same nerve during different procedures, e.g., anesthetic concentrations, the nerve must not be moved, and no fluid other than the oil should be allowed to touch the nerve-electrode preparation. Because the amplitude of nerve activity recorded depends in part on the anatomical arrangement of nerve fibers that contact the electrode, any movement or disturbance that alters the nerve placement or alters contact of the nerve with the electrode can introduce changes in nerve activity levels that are "mechanical" and not reflective of true changes in nerve activity.

The types of electrodes used in acute studies are usually metal electrodes insulated with teflon, varnish, or some other nonconducting finish, except at the bared tips which contact the nerve. Bare wire electrodes, similar to those used for most chronic nerve recordings which enwrap the nerve, can also be used for acute studies (Fig. 1). With this type of electrode, a silastic embedding material is usually placed around the whole nerve-electrode wrap preparation, which replaces the mineral oil described above. This type of arrangement is useful when the animal must be moved to a different position in which the nerve cannot be maintained in a pool of oil, e.g., recording renal sympathetic nerve activity while also recording from central brainstem neurons that requires the animal be placed in a prone position. In general, multifiber activity is recorded using a pair of electrodes connected to a high input impedance differential amplifier to obtain a bipolar recording of activity. An indifferent or ground electrode is used as a reference for the recording electrodes and is placed in a fat pad or other electrically inert tissue. The amplifier measures the difference between the two recording electrodes relative to the reference electrode. Thus, any signals arriving at both the electrodes simultaneously (common mode noise signals), such as voltages produced by power line fields, generate equal and opposite voltages in the differential amplifier and are canceled (Fig. 2). However, nerve activity that is propagated along the nerve at a finite speed generates signals which arrive at each electrode at different times and therefore, depending on the interelectrode distance and conduction velocity, are minimally affected by cancellation (Fig. 3). Although noise cancellation is not perfect, amplifiers can be tuned to reduce the amplitude of 60-Hz line frequency by a factor of over a million, dramatically increasing the signal to noise ratio of nerve activity. Some investigators use a monopolar recording technique, in which the nerve is placed on one electrode of the recording pair, while the other recording electrode is placed in electrically inert tissue near the recording site. This technique also requires that a ground electrode be attached to the animal, again near the area of the recording site. This technique is often used when recording single-fiber afferent or efferent nerve activity, because it eliminates any possibility of differential cancellations of spike activity. However, because the input from the two recording electrodes are separated using this technique, the ability to reject common mode signals can be reduced or eliminated. A modification of this technique involves crushing the nerve between two recording electrodes. This method maintains high common mode rejection while generating a monopolar recording since the nerve is active at only one electrode.

Electrodes are generally connected to an amplification system that also allows filtering to eliminate some of the electronic noise which accompanies recording of low voltage nerve signals (typically $<50\ \mu V$) (Fig. 1). The amplification system used in many laboratories consists of an AC-coupled differential preamplifier which filters out some noise (bandwidth typically <1 Hz to >3 KHz) and provides a fixed gain of typically 100–1,000. This activity is then further processed by a filter amplifier, which allows additional gain and low and high frequency filtering. A high pass filter is used to set the lowest frequency that activity must exceed to pass through the amplifier. The filter cut-off frequency usually extends through the range of 0.1–400 Hz. A low pass filter is used to set the upper limit of frequency that can pass through the amplifier, with a typical range of 1–10 KHz. The amplification of the system usually extends up to a level of at least 100 times in order to amplify the microvolt signals into a range of 1–5 V. The cut-off frequencies and gain of the filter amplifier are user-selected, and choices will depend on the characteristics of the nerve activity that is being

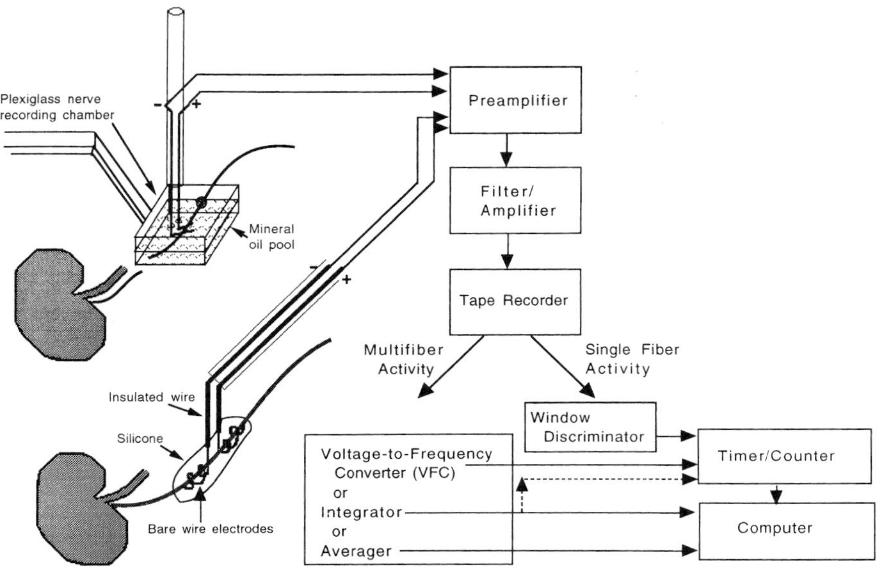

Figure 1. Two techniques for recording nerve activity and components of the recording and averaging systems. As indicated, a sectioned nerve can be placed on electrodes in a recording chamber, or the intact nerve can be circled with wire recording electrodes and encased in silicone. In both cases, the activity is recorded using a preamplifier/amplifier system and then directed toward one of the averaging systems. In general, single-fiber activity is quantitated using a discriminator/counter system to obtain spikes/time interval. Whole nerve activity is generally quantitated in terms of total voltage using voltage-to-frequency conversion, integration, or analog averaging.

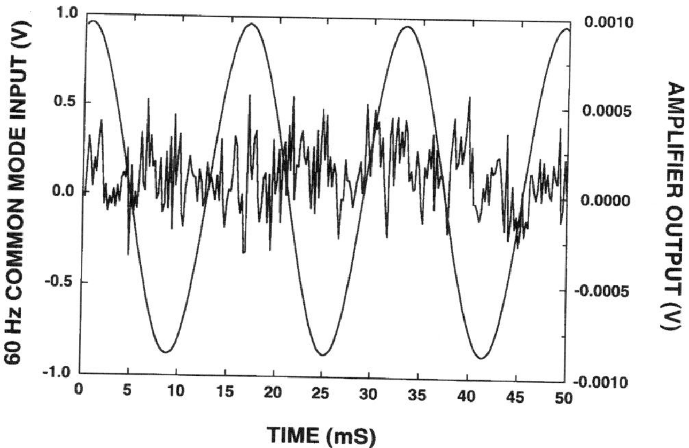

Figure 2. Demonstration of common mode rejection of noise (60-Hz common mode input) using a differential amplifier. The sine wave 60-Hz noise input is recorded simultaneously by the pair of electrodes as equal and opposite voltages. Therefore, as seen on the amplifier output tracing, the sine wave noise pattern is eliminated, and only random peaks of output are produced.

recorded. In general, the amount of filtering applied to the nerve activity signal should be kept to a minimum in order to preserve the fidelity of the signal.

Raw nerve activity is typically stored using a tape recorder for later analysis. In addition, activity can be processed on-line using a spike counter, nerve averager, or computer. The preamplifier-filter amplifier system is used to maximize the ability of the investigator to record the nerve activity signal, while minimizing noise, but there is always some relatively tonic electronic noise inherent in any recording system. The influence of tonic noise levels can be eliminated, especially in multifiber preparations, by recording the level of electronically generated noise from the nerve trunk after the active nerve fibers are destroyed by crushing or silenced by local anesthesia. Thus, after the experiment is completed, the nerve is crushed or anesthetized proximal to the recording electrodes and remaining activity is recorded for a short time. When nerve activity is analyzed, this segment of recorded activity is quantitated and then subtracted from nerve

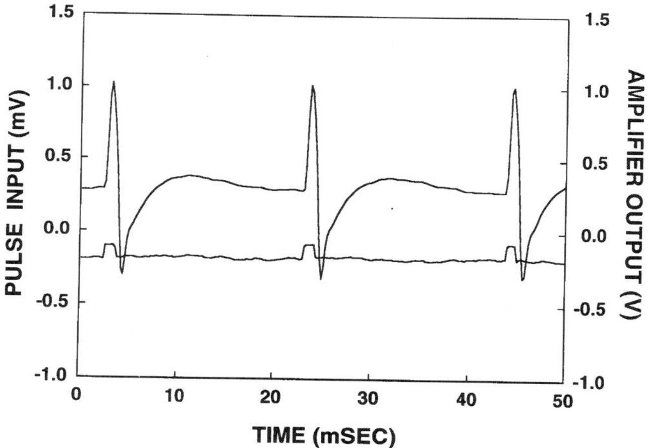

Figure 3. Demonstration of recording pulse input by the differential amplifier, simulating nerve activity, which is not eliminated by common mode rejection. Unlike noise input, which is recorded simultaneously by the electrode pair, pulse activity generated by nerve stimulation travels at a finite speed down the nerve and therefore arrives at each electrode of the pair at a different time. Thus, the pulse input from the electrodes (*lower tracing*) results in a biphasic output by the amplifier (*upper tracing*).

activity recorded during the experimental procedures, eliminating the noise component from the true nerve activity. A second method to obtain the noise level is to short the recording electrodes together by placing them in a fat pad and record the resulting level of noise, which can then be subtracted from the neural signal after quantification. Some investigators have attempted to eliminate noise by setting a voltage threshold on the recorded nerve signal such that noise lies below threshold and is not quantitated during analysis. Although this technique is adequate for few-fiber preparations where individual action potentials are discernible and actual spike counting is employed, it requires an arbitrary setting of threshold, since the actual noise level is not known (60). Thus, in multifiber nerve preparations, some low amplitude nerve activity will also be eliminated by the threshold (Fig. 4).

Chronic Recording Techniques As stated for acute recording techniques, chronic recording of autonomic activity requires that the nerve under investigation be isolated from surrounding tissue. In addition, since the animal is permitted to recover, appropriate sterile conditions must be used when implanting the electrodes. This includes sterilization of the electrodes and electrode leads that will be inserted into the animal. Chronic nerve recording has been performed in animals including the rat (61), rabbit (7,30,31), and dog (106,133), but the best success appears to be associated with use of the smaller animals. When chronic recording is to be used, one must ensure that a suitable length of nerve is isolated and exposed so that the electrode can be placed on the nerve without contacting other tissue. In addition, the electrode-nerve preparation must also be mechanically fixed to eliminate movement which can lead to leakage around the electrode preparation or death of the nerve. In general, a branch of renal nerve is the nerve most commonly recorded from to obtain a measure of sympathetic efferent nerve activity.

The preparation used by many investigators involves wrapping thin wire electrodes around an isolated segment of nerve (31) (Fig. 1). In addition, a ground wire is sutured to a nearby fat pad or area of connective tissue that does not generate any electrical activity. The electrodes wrapped around the nerve are then embedded in a silicone material which serves to isolate the electrodes from surrounding tissue. A commonly used silicone is Sil-Gel (Sil-GEl 604; Wacker, Munich, Germany), but any silicone material that cures quickly and does not contain acetic acid can be used as the insulator. The thin electrode wires are soldered to an insulated flexible wire that serves as an electrode lead which can be tunneled subcutaneously to the exterior. Again, care must be taken to ensure that the electrode connections and all portions of the lead are insulated from tissue and fluids. The recording system for these electrodes is the same as that described above for the acute studies. The implanting of the electrodes make the recording of "dead nerve noise" difficult and it is therefore difficult to determine the amount of electronic noise in the preparation. Some investigators have developed other methods to quantitate the amount of background noise and also normalize the recorded nerve activity from day to day (7,31). In the instance of sympathetic efferent activity, the maximum and minimum levels of nerve activity are obtained and equated to 100% and 0% of control, respectively. Maximum sympathetic activity in the rabbit can be obtained by exposing the animal's nostrils to smoke, which initiates an irritant response that produces peak increases in sympathetic activity (7). Minimum sympathetic activity can be obtained by infusion of a pressor agent, such as phenylephrine (123), or inflation of a vena caval cuff (30,31) to baroreflexly decrease sympathetic activity, or by administration of ganglionic blockers such as hexamethonium hydrochloride (10 mg/kg) (7). In some species, infusion of a dilator such as nitroprusside (123) has also been used to obtain maximum baroreflex increases in sympathetic activity. If these techniques are done each day prior to the actual experiment, activity

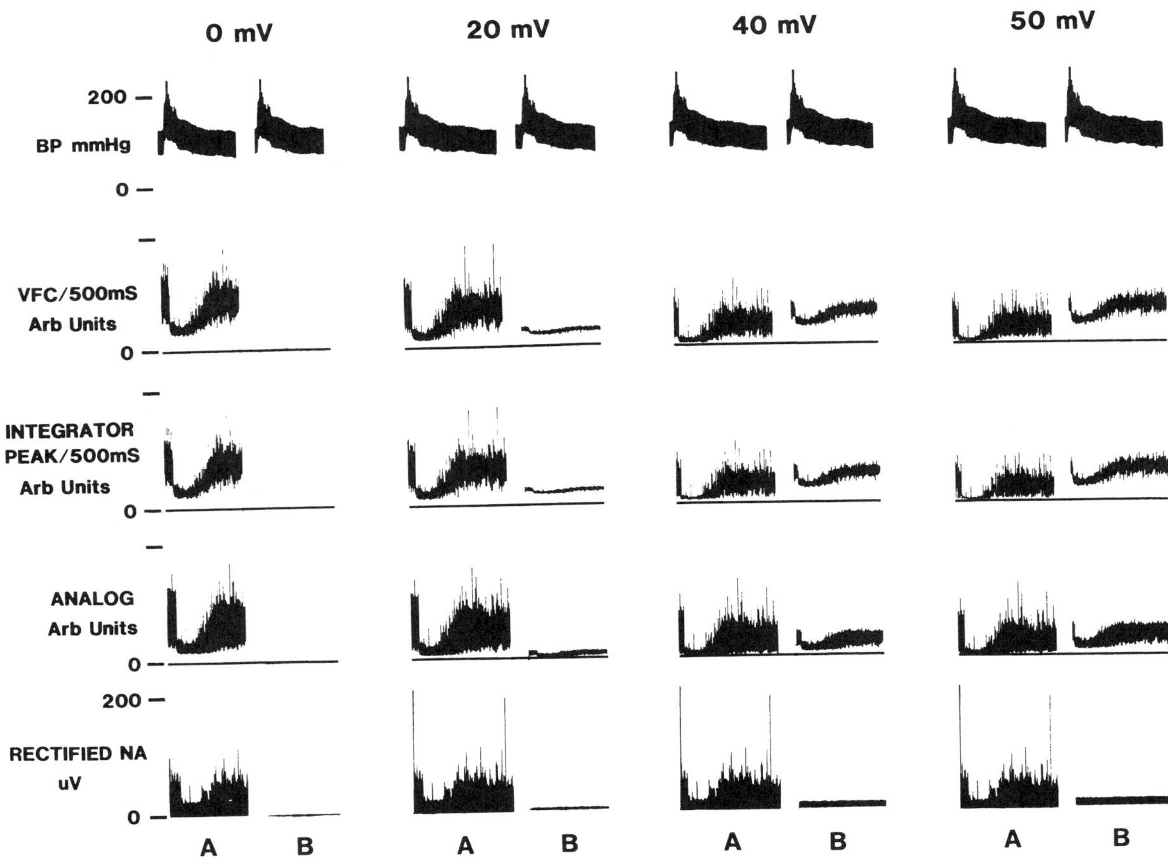

Figure 4. Effects of altering amount of noise removed by voltage threshold on average renal efferent nerve activity are shown for increasing threshold levels of 0, 20, 40, and 50 mV. **A:** Changes in average nerve activity due to increase in blood pressure. **B:** Corresponding changes in average noise level removed by threshold. As threshold is increased to remove noise, average base-line levels are shifted downward and phasic amplitude is compressed (A). Average noise levels increase, becoming more phasic as threshold increases and more signal is removed (B). (Reprinted with permission from ref. 60.)

recorded that day can be normalized as a percent of maximum control. This allows the activity recorded on different days to be compared, since the absolute level of activity recorded over time can change due to degradation of the preparation.

Single Versus Multifiber Recordings Investigators have used both single-fiber and multifiber preparations to examine the effects of many different stimuli on autonomic efferent activity and afferent input from physiological receptors. When multifiber preparations are used, the whole nerve or large bundles of fibers dissected from the desheathed nerve are placed on the recording electrodes. When single-fiber preparations are used, repeatedly smaller bundles of fibers are separated from the whole desheathed nerve until only one active spike is present in the bundle on the recording electrodes. Thus, a "single-fiber preparation" does not mean that only one fiber is present in the bundle, but that only one fiber of interest is active. In some "single-fiber preparations," more than one active fiber is present, but the action potentials of the small few-fiber preparations are of sufficiently different heights or shapes that each can be separated using a window discriminator (see below). The choice of which type of preparation to use depends on the intent of the investigation. For example, recording whole nerve sympathetic discharge to a given region, e.g., kidney or heart, will give a more global idea of how sympathetic control to that region may be modulated by given stimulus. On the other hand, to determine how baroreceptors are responding to exposure to an anesthetic, single-fiber activity from a single discharging receptor will provide the clearest picture. When using single-fiber recordings, activity from a large enough number of fibers must be recorded in order to ensure that a representative population of activity has been sampled. The same is true when examining single-fiber discharge from efferent fibers to a given region.

Methods for Analyzing Neural Signals Nerve activity has generally been analyzed by a variety of methods, as detailed by Hopp et al. (60) and summarized in the following discussion. The type of analysis depends in part on the type of nerve recording performed. When using a single-fiber recording, counting spikes/time will give an accurate picture of levels of nerve activity. However, when using multifiber preparations, some method that integrates or averages total voltage of the bursts will be more accurate than counting spikes. If counting spikes is performed and more than three active fibers are contained in the preparation, co-incidence of spikes will result in underestimating the number of spikes/time (60,117) (Fig. 5). Thus, a method that quantitates amplitude, width and number of bursts over time will provide a more accurate assessment of multifiber nerve activity. Nerve activity is often recorded and compared to other physiological parameters, including blood pressure. Thus, all methods of nerve analysis usually involve A/D conversion using a computer which allows the quantitated nerve activity to be sampled simultaneously with physiologically relevant variables. A discussion of the analysis of nerve activity versus the other physiological variables is presented in a later section.

1. *Single-Fiber Analysis:* Methods that count individual spikes can be used in preparations with only one active fiber or in

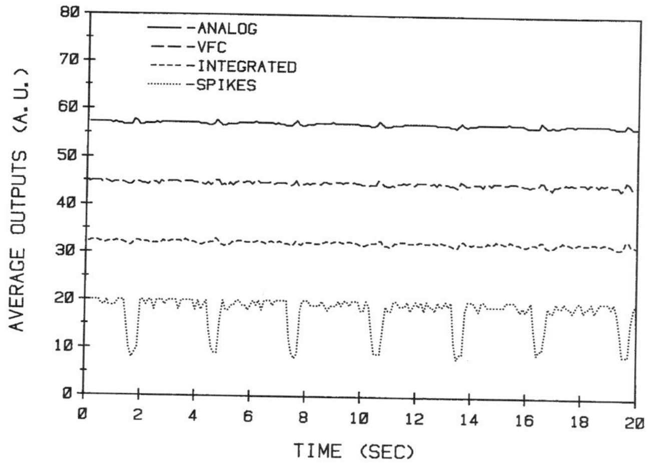

Figure 5. Response of each averaging method to summed pulse trains of ~98 and ~100 Hz. Pulse overlap can be seen in spike record as halving of frequency. Analog, VFC, and integrated maintain constant output during pulse overlap. Each method has same gain but was offset for clarity. (Reprinted with permission from ref. 60.)

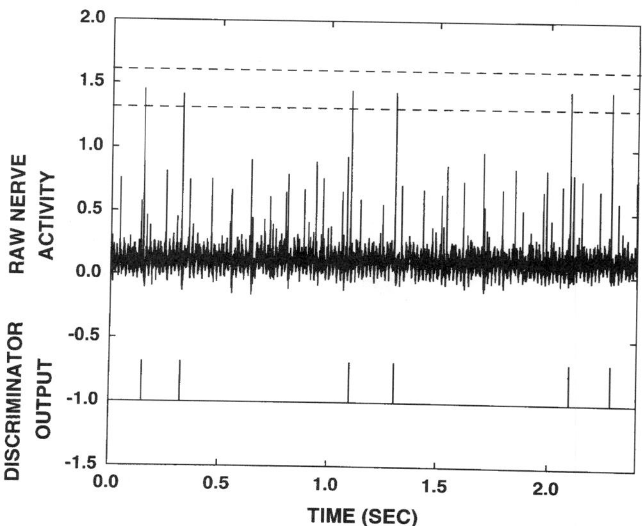

Figure 6. Demonstration of the use of a window discriminator to select a single spike from a few-fiber preparation. The adjustable voltage window set by the discriminator is shown by the *dotted lines.* Every spike which falls in the window triggers a pulse from the discriminator, which is then counted by a timer/counter. The window can be adjusted to select a spike of any height, as long as the spike of interest is from only one active fiber.

preparations in which only a few fibers are present and each action potential has an amplitude or shape different from the other spikes. In the first case, the nerve activity must be fed into a multiplexing type of circuit which allows both the neural signal and a voltage threshold to be displayed on a single oscilloscope channel. The threshold is set so that only the peak of the active spike falls above the threshold level. Each spike exceeding threshold produces a voltage pulse that can be digitally counted, integrated, or analog averaged. If more than one active fiber is present, a window discriminator can be used to separate the discharge of each spike. Several types of window discriminators are available. Amplitude discriminators generate lower and upper voltage limits which can be adjusted while viewing the spike of interest on an oscilloscope and provides a voltage "window" into which a spike must fall in order to be counted (Fig. 6). Time/amplitude discriminators allow voltage levels to be set on a particular portion of the spike, such that upper and lower voltage thresholds must be crossed in a specific time segment for a spike to be counted. This type of discriminator can sometimes differentiate spikes even if their absolute amplitudes are similar. More recently, computer-based template-matching discriminators have appeared (e.g.8701 Waveform Discriminator, Signal Processing Systems, Prospect, South Australia, Australia). These discriminators digitize the spike of interest and compare each incoming spike with the stored template. Spikes are accepted if the template is matched within a user-selected tolerance. All of these discriminators put out a voltage pulse for each windowed spike, which is then quantitated using one of the methods described below. One method to quantitate single spike discharge is to count the output of the multiplexing circuit or the window discriminator using a counter/timer, which counts voltage pulses in a user-selected predetermined interval (e.g., 500 ms, 1 s), generating a stair-step voltage proportional to averaged activity for the previous time interval (60). The width of the counting interval used will be dependent on the frequency of the spike to be analyzed, but should be fast enough to ensure that the counted average spikes/time accurately reflects the changes in spike activity induced by the stimulus. A second method uses an integrator, where voltage pulses from the discriminator are summated to produce a voltage output from the integrator that reflects total neural voltage (60). The integrator resets after a given total voltage is summated, and activity can be expressed as the time between resets or frequency of resets. In addition, the integrator can be reset using an external time base and quantified as peak voltage per unit time (60,89).

2. *Multifiber Analysis:* Multifiber activity has been analyzed using a variety of techniques, including counting spikes or bursts, integrating the neural signal, measuring a moving time average, and processing activity using a voltage-to-frequency converter (VFC) (60) (Fig. 7). As stated above, counting spikes or bursts/time may result in the underestimation of activity, although trends using this method have been found to agree with those found by integration of the same nerve activity (60). Integration, moving time averaging, and use of a VFC require that the nerve activity first be full-wave rectified before it is then processed by one of these methods to obtain a voltage output proportional to nerve activity per unit time. Each of these methods quantitates total voltage of the recorded nerve activity, which includes the numbers, amplitudes, and widths of the bursts of nerve activity. Again, the level of noise must be subtracted from the recorded activity to obtain an accurate level of nerve discharge. Use of an integrator to analyze multifiber activity is done in the same manner as when integrating single-fiber activity, with the integrator resetting at a given total voltage or triggered by an external time base. Moving time average, which is comparable to analog averaging, is performed using a low-pass filter with time constants typically ranging from 20 ms to 1 s. The longer time constants result in smoother averages, while shorter time constants are use to analyze more rapid changes in nerve activity. Different types of low-pass filters are available, and characteristics of each may make one more desirable than another, depending on the type of activity analyzed (60). However, all however provide a continuous average of activity from the previous time interval and, with the proper choice of filter (60,90), are not subjected to the delay for resetting found with true integration. A VFC can also be used to analyze rectified whole nerve activity. The VFC produces a spike output with a frequency that is proportional to the total voltage of nerve activity directed into the VFC. These spikes can be counted by a timer or integrated in a manner described for single spike analysis. Use of an integrator, moving time averager, or VFC all result in outputs that agree closely with each other

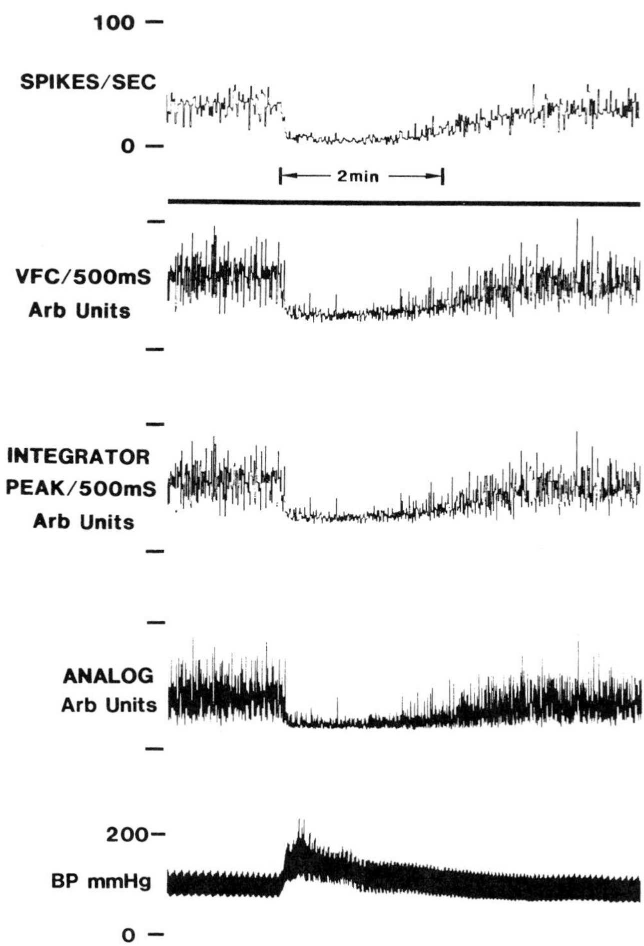

Figure 7. Typical responses in renal nerve activity due to an increase in blood pressure are shown for each averaging method. The same raw nerve activity was processed by each method for comparison. (Reprinted with permission from ref. 60.)

(60), although the integrator typically has a longer resetting delay relative to the other two methods. Moving time average is the only method that provides a continuous average of activity that is not restricted to updates every averaging interval (60).

Efferent Versus Afferent Recordings The above discussion cited many instances of recording and analyzing efferent activity. The techniques for recording afferent nerve recordings are the same as those described, with similar reservations made for the appropriateness of the analyzing technique for single- versus multifiber recordings. Most of the afferent activity recorded in investigations of cardiovascular control are from the carotid sinus baroreceptors (carotid sinus nerve), aortic baroreceptors (aortic depressor nerve), or cardiopulmonary receptors (vagi or sympathetic pathways including the ansa subclavia or white rami). The amount of efferent traffic in the carotid sinus and aortic nerves is minimal; thus, intact whole nerve recordings of these afferent pathways are possible and allow the investigator to maintain an afferent input so that reflex changes in response to afferent stimulation can be measured simultaneously with the afferent activity. Afferent activity must be recorded from the cut peripheral portions of the vagi or sympathetic nerves to eliminate the efferent activity from these recordings. When single-fiber recordings are required, the sheaths around the nerve must be slit and increasingly smaller bundles of nerve tested until a single-fiber preparation is obtained, as explained above.

An alternative technique from peripheral nerve dissection to obtain single receptor responses is to record activity from afferent neuronal cell bodies in the appropriate peripheral ganglia (carotid sinus baroreceptors/petrosal ganglion; aortic and vagal cardiopulmonary receptors/nodose ganglion) (28). This technique records extracellular activity by inserting electrodes adjacent to the cell bodies of afferent neurons in the ganglion. Verification of afferent cell type must be made to ensure that the cell studied carries information for the desired receptor type. With the petrosal ganglion, most activity with pulsatile, cardiac-related discharge is probably baroreceptor afferent activity, since carotid chemoreceptor activity does not demonstrate the same type of firing pattern. With the nodose ganglion, afferent type must be identified by stimulation of the afferent fibers of the more peripheral nerve trunks (i.e. aortic depressor nerve) or by probing of the receptor fields in the case of the cardiac receptors (e.g., left ventricle, left atrium) to directly activate the receptor. By necessity, this type of technique requires that the ganglia be accessible to electrode placement and, as with the techniques described above, movement of the ganglion must be restricted for the duration of the experiment so that artifact due to a change in electrode position is avoided.

Methods to Study Baroreflex Responses and Baroreceptor Afferent Activity

Afferent activity from arterial baroreceptors in either the carotid sinus or aortic depressor nerve has been studied using a variety of techniques, including recording activity in response to whole body changes in blood pressure produced by infusion of vasoactive agents (29,37,104,123,128) or inflation of aortic and/or vena caval cuffs (14,30,31,128); vascular isolation of the carotid sinus, to permit local controlled changes in sinus blood pressure (1,17,49,72,105,108); and in vitro perfusion of the aortic arch, which permits simultaneous measurement of arch diameter and aortic baroreceptor afferent activity (16,122). As indicated in the following discussion, two of these methods can also be used to study baroreflex control in the animal model, with or without afferent recording of baroreceptor activity. Each of the above methods can be used for both single and multifiber afferent baroreceptor recording, but there are some advantages and disadvantages specific to each technique.

When whole animal arterial blood pressure is altered via administration of vasoactive drugs or occluder cuffs, changes in afferent activity can be recorded simultaneously from both the carotid and aortic arterial baroreceptors, since both sets of baroreceptors are activated by the pressure change. This basic technique also allows reflexes from only one set of baroreceptors to be studied, if the afferent activity from the other group of baroreceptors is eliminated by section of either the aortic depressor or carotid sinus nerves. One disadvantage is that only reflex changes in heart rate or nerve activity can be used as measurements of baroreflex sensitivity, since the changes in arterial pressure per se are used to activate the baroreceptors. However, if chronic nerve recording techniques are used, reflex changes in autonomic activity and heart rate can be measured during induced changes in arterial pressure in the awake versus anesthetized animal.

With the vascularly isolated sinus technique, baroreceptor activity from the carotid sinus nerve can be measured along with reflex changes in arterial pressure, heart rate and autonomic efferent nerve activity. When this technique is used, other afferent pathways must be eliminated so the baroreceptors and cardiopulmonary receptors outside the vascularly isolated carotid sinus do not buffer the responses produced by changes in carotid sinus pressure. The vascular isolation technique permits a more controllable means to produce repeatable changes in pressure stimuli to the baroreceptors than whole body pressure changes. In addition, different patterns of pressure stimuli can be used, including pulsatile pressure changes, static pressure levels, step changes in pressure, and ramp changes in pressure. The vascular isolation of the carotid sinus can be done using a variety of techniques, depending on the species of animal under investigation. In larger animals, including dogs, cats and swine, the sinus region can be isolated by actual ligation of arterial branches in the region, and placement of cannulas in the larger ligated vessels to permit either flow-through (105,108) or blind sac preparations of the sinus (49,81). Alternatively, occlusive cuffs can be placed on the larger branches and inflated when desired to occlude flow through the vessels (75,119). This technique has been used successfully in chronic preparations examining baroreflex function when normal flow is desired, except during testing of the baroreflex (125). With smaller species, such as the rat, physical ligation of the arterial branches is more difficult. A newer technique, which utilizes vinyl plugs placed internally in the larger branches, appears to be very efficient (110). In this preparation, plugs are placed in the outflow sites of the major branches using a cannula threaded internally up the carotid artery and placed at the root of each branch. An injector system is then used to insert a plug in the branch, blocking flow.

Finally, the isolated in vitro arch preparation allows the same type of carefully controlled pressure changes to be made as in the isolated sinus preparation, while also permitting instantaneous measurement of afferent activity and arch diameter (4,84). Simultaneous measurement of baroreceptor discharge and wall dimensions allows changes in mechanical properties of the vessel wall to be equated to changes in baroreceptor activation. This may be important if one is interested in determining if changes in vessel wall mechanics such as strain or stress are involved in producing changes in baroreceptor discharge. Carotid sinus diameter has been measured to obtain similar information using sonomicrometer (8) or video (6) techniques, but the more irregular anatomy of the sinus requires some assumptions to be made using this technique. The more cylindrical nature of the arch allows a more direct measurement of diameter. However, no reflex changes in the whole animal can be made using the in vitro arch technique.

A technique which has been employed to study baroreflex function which does not permit the simultaneous recording of evoked baroreceptor afferent activity is the use of electrical stimulation of the baroreceptor afferent fibers in either the carotid sinus or aortic baroreceptor nerves (66,73,111,112, 114). This technique has the advantage of being an easily controlled, repeatable stimulus that excludes the receptors themselves from the reflex loop. This may be desired if the agent under study has been shown to directly alter baroreceptor discharge and the intent of the study is to focus on the effects of the agent at a different site in the reflex arc (104,107). However, at least for the carotid sinus nerve and for the aortic depressor nerve in dogs and cats, there are both chemoreceptor and baroreceptor afferents in the nerves that will be activated by the electrical stimulation. This simultaneous activation of the two groups of afferents can be minimized if parameters that preferentially activate larger diameter afferent A-fibers are used (low voltage or current, higher frequency, short duration), since most chemoreceptor afferents have smaller C-fiber afferents. However, there is a significant population of C-fiber baroreceptors that would be excluded from study using this technique. This problem can be avoided if the aortic nerve in rabbits or rats is used, for this nerve does not contain chemoreceptor afferent fibers.

Changes in efferent responses [e.g., heart rate (HR), blood pressure (BP), efferent nerve activity] and afferent baroreceptor activity are usually plotted versus stimulating pressure to provide a measurement of baroreflex or baroreceptor sensitivity, respectively. The slope of the stimulus (pressure)/response (HR, BP, nerve activity) curve is a measurement of the gain, or sensitivity, of the baroreflex or the baroreceptors under investigation. Determination of the slope of arterial BP versus changes in isolated carotid sinus pressure can give a measure of the sensitivity of the baroreflex as a whole, while slopes of HR or efferent nerve activity versus pressure changes can provide some insight into reflex sensitivity of components of the baroreflex. Analysis of single-fiber recordings of baroreceptor activity gives a true measure of the sensitivity of a single baroreceptor, while multifiber nerve recordings of baroreceptor afferent activity give a more global picture of baroreceptor input. Baroreflex and whole nerve baroreceptor response curves are usually sigmoidal in shape when responses are plotted versus pressure and can be analyzed using a sigmoidal logistic func-

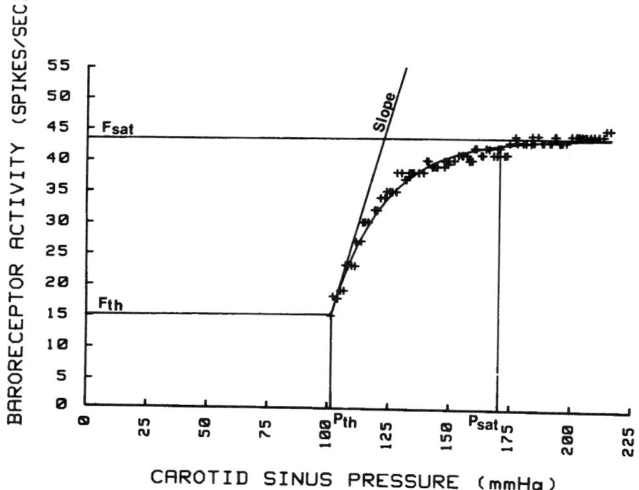

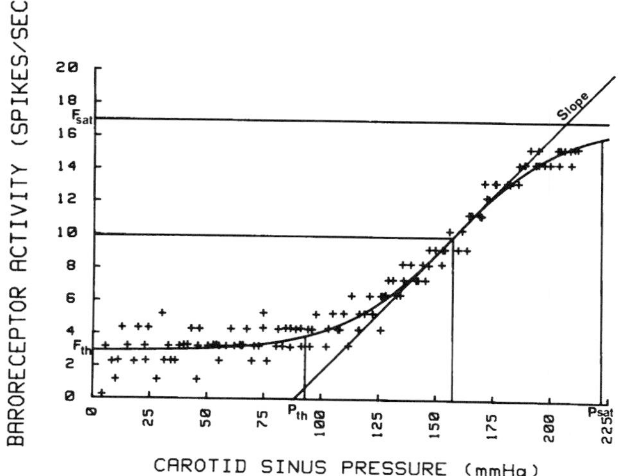

Figure 8. Stimulus-response curves for an individual type I and type II baroreceptor. The discontinuous, hyperbolic curve from the higher frequency, more sensitive type I baroreceptor is typical of curves obtained for all type I baroreceptors, although individual differences in firing characteristics could shift the curves left, right, up, or down. The continuous, sigmoidal curve from the less sensitive type II baroreceptor shows spontaneous discharge at subthreshold pressures, which is typical of this type of baroreceptor. Again, different firing characteristics for different fibers could shift the curves, but would not alter the basic shape of the response curve. Nonlinear regression techniques were used to obtain firing characteristics for each response curve, including slope, threshold (P_{th}) and saturation (P_{sat}) pressures, and threshold (F_{th}) and saturation (F_{sat}) firing rates. (Reprinted with permission from ref. 108.)

tion (31,108). Two different response curves have been obtained for single-fiber baroreceptor recordings and these curves can be analyzed with either a hyperbolic or a logistic sigmoidal curve-fit, using the analysis appropriate for the curve under study (108) (Fig. 8). In addition to slope (sensitivity), both types of curve-fitting analyses will determine other characteristics of the baroreflex or baroreceptors, including threshold (P_{th}) and saturation (P_{sat}) pressures and threshold (F_{th}) and saturation (F_{sat}) firing rates, arterial pressures, or heart rates (Fig. 8).

HUMAN STUDIES

Assessment of the Parasympathetic Nervous System in Humans

The efferent limb of the parasympathetic nervous system has multiple regulatory roles, including the control of salivation, pupil diameter, bladder function, gastrointestinal motility and cardiac function. The significance of vagal cardiac control mechanisms has been well appreciated in syndromes such as vasovagal syncope, carotid sinus syndrome and inferior wall myocardial infarction, but its importance has become emphasized in recent years because of data suggesting the parasympathetic system has a protective role in sudden death following myocardial injury (10,11,21) and a prognostic role in outcome following cardiac and neurological injury (27). Unfortunately, efferent vagal nerve activity has not been directly recorded in humans and insights have been constrained by the limitations of the various indirect techniques to assess vagal cardiac mechanisms. Resting heart rate reveals little information about vagal cardiac activity because of other simultaneous influences at the sinus node such as neurohumoral β-adrenergic receptor stimuli and intrinsic atrial pacemaker activity.

There have been three methods employed either individually or in combination to provide indirect insights into human vagal cardiac mechanisms: (a) the evaluation of heart rate responses to reflex stimuli, (b) the assessment of heart rate changes to muscarinic blocking drugs (the presumed "gold standard"), and (c) the evaluation of spontaneous heart rate fluctuations, referred to as respiratory sinus arrhythmia.

Baroreflex-Mediated Bradycardia The responsiveness of efferent vagal cardiac traffic has been inferred by quantitating the magnitude of heart rate slowing triggered by reflex stimuli. The commonly employed stimuli consist of loading the baroreceptors by various means such as the release of a Valsalva maneuver, phenylephrine injection or neck suction. The magnitude of the bradycardia in response to these stimuli in healthy young humans (96) and diabetic patients (9) has been statistically related to basal levels of vagal cardiac activity (Fig. 9). In an earlier study, we employed small intravenous doses of atropine (<3 μg/kg) to increase central vagal outflow. This increased respiratory sinus arrhythmia (an index of cardiac vagal activity) and simultaneously augmented the bradycardia triggered by neck suction. It is unknown if this association holds true in diverse patient populations, and therefore the utility of baroreceptor testing to gauge vagal cardiac activity is uncertain.

Respiratory Sinus Arrhythmia During normal respiration, the heart rate speeds during inspiration and slows during expiration. This waxing and waning of heart rate is referred to as respiratory sinus arrhythmia (RSA). The origin of RSA has been attributed to at least five factors: central vagal oscillators, stretch receptors from the lung and thorax, chemoreceptor and/or baroreceptor reflexes and the Bainbridge reflex. The efferent mechanism is well defined since either cooling of the vagi (67) or atropine (50,85,96) can virtually abolish RSA, while β-adrenergic blockade either does not consistently influence RSA (68) or slightly augments it (50). The absolute magnitude of RSA may reflect different levels of vagal cardiac traffic between individuals, while within individuals changes in RSA might reflect physiological fluctuations in vagal cardiac activity. Thus, quantification of RSA may provide the best indirect measure of vagal cardiac activity in humans. In an attempt to validate RSA as an index of vagal cardiac activity, several authors have applied the methods employed in experimental animals as described by Katona and Jih (67). RSA is calculated as the mean difference between maximum and minimum heart rates during each respiratory cycle of quiet breathing, while basal levels of efferent vagal outflow to the heart are estimated from the magnitude of heart rate acceleration produced by muscarinic receptor blockade with atropine (0.04 mg/kg) (50,59). In many cases, R-R intervals have been used instead of heart rate in these analyses. The correlation between pharmacologically determined vagal tone and RSA in humans has ranged from 0.61 to 0.91 (50,59,67,68). In addition, Eckberg has demonstrated that the mathematical calculation of the standard deviation of a consecutive series of R-R intervals during a quiet breathing period correlates closely with the average maximum to minimum R-R interval (r = 0.97), thereby simplifying RSA calculations (41).

Several limitations of RSA as an index of vagal cardiac activity have been discussed by Kollai and Mizsei (68). Variations in breathing frequency and tidal volume reduce the correlation between RSA and vagal cardiac activity (52,68). Moreover, studies that have validated RSA against the change in heart rate (HR) during muscarinic blockade may be weakened by data suggesting that the cardioacceleration produced by atropine is not merely due to blockade of cardiac vagal efferent traffic. Compared to the tachycardia produced by bilateral vagotomy, excessive or higher heart rates occur in dogs after atropine administration (98). Thus, standard measures of RSA may be constrained when attempting to define population differences in vagal cardiac activity (53), but appear to be quite useful when evaluating experimental fluctuations in vagal cardiac traffic in a given individual when respiratory parameters are controlled.

Spectral Analysis of Heart Rate One methodological problem that arises when estimating RSA from maximum to minimum R-R intervals or from standard deviation calculations has been transient surges in cardiac sympathetic outflow that trigger tachycardias that are unrelated to vagal mechanisms. These surges are not uncommon in conscious humans in which mental stress or peripheral somatic events trigger transient increases in efferent sympathetic activity despite the investigators best efforts to maintain a quiet relaxed atmosphere. Appropriately, RSA estimates of fluctuations in vagal cardiac activity have been stronger in anesthetized paralyzed animals (67) than in conscious subjects (50,59,68). One way to circumvent these estimation errors is to employ a frequency domain analysis of RSA, whereby only heart rate fluctuations that occur at the same frequency as the respiratory rate are included in analysis (52,59,76,85,91). This process is termed power spectral analysis (PSA) (2,3). This technique mathematically decodes the natural oscillations of HR into separate frequencies (Fig. 10). The relative strength of each oscillation (or power) is plotted as a function of frequency (in Hertz). To perform this analysis, a continuous segment of ECG data is converted to either R-R intervals or instantaneous HR. This signal is then either smoothed or filtered, digitized, and passed through a fast Fourier transform to discern the inherent frequencies associated within the rhythmic oscillations of HR. In this way R-R interval variations in the time domain are converted into the frequency domain. The power (or amplitude) of each contributing component is typically displayed over the frequency range of 0 Hertz (DC) to 0.5 Hertz (Hz). When displayed in this fashion, there are three primary frequencies of heart rate oscillations that contain the majority of the HR power (Fig. 10). The high-frequency peak (HFP) consists of HR oscillations due to respiration (RSA). It is typically centered ~0.25 Hz (0.15–0.4 Hz) and varies from person to person as a function of individ-

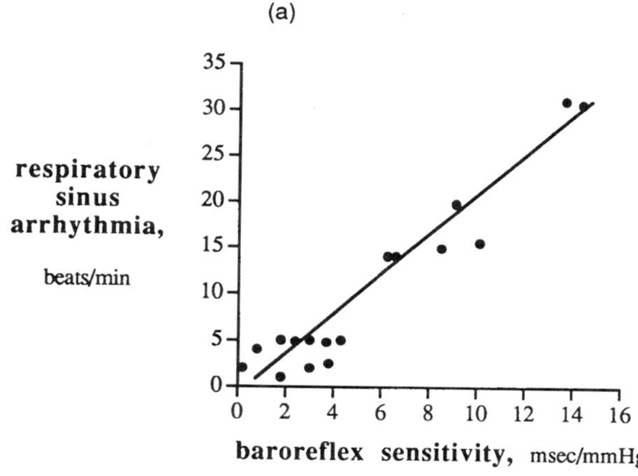

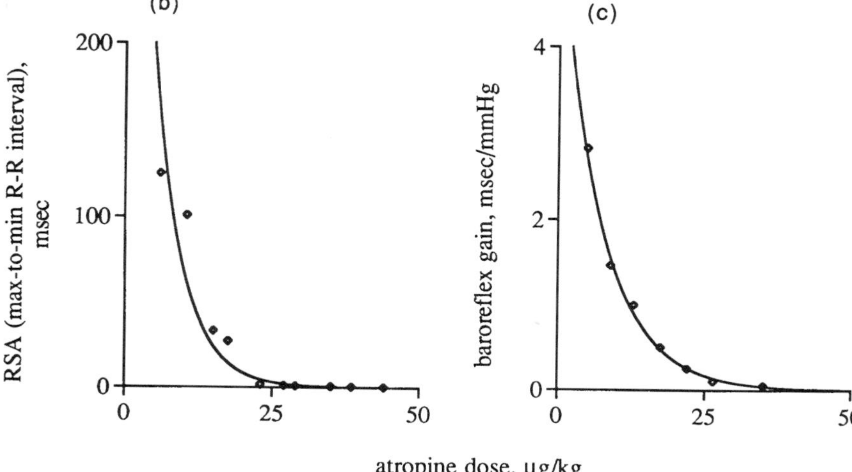

Figure 9. The close relationship between resting respiratory sinus arrhythmia (an index of cardiac vagal tone) and baroreflex gain is shown. **A**: Data from 12 diabetic patients. **B,C**: Resting vagal tone was initially augmented by low doses of atropine, then was decreased with higher doses of atropine (via cardiac muscarinic receptor blockade). (Reprinted, in adapted form, with permission from ref. 9 and ref. 96.)

ual respiratory rate (0.25 Hz is 15 breaths/min). It is quite clear that the power in this frequency is entirely due to vagal-cardiac activity (59,76,85,97). For example, we have been able to augment the power in the high frequency range by either giving low doses of atropine (which act centrally to augment vagal outflow) or by slightly raising BP with phenylephrine (which augments vagal outflow via the baroreflex) (Figs. 11 and 12). When larger doses of atropine are given, cardiac muscarinic receptors are blocked and HFP is virtually abolished (Fig. 12). Thus, derivation of the power in the HFP may provide the best estimation of fluctuations in vagal-cardiac activity in humans.

The low-frequency peak (LFP) in the HR power spectrum usually occurs at 0.05–0.15 Hz. This is the same frequency (every 10 s) as the Mayer waves first described in blood pressure recordings, and HR oscillations at this frequency therefore may be due in part to baroreceptor reflex mechanisms. It appears that both components of the autonomic nervous system contribute to the power in the LFP (59,85,97). When changing position from supine to standing, there is an increase in the LFP and a decrease in the HFP that could be attributed to sympathetic activation and simultaneous vagal withdrawal (Fig. 11). Muscarinic receptor blockade with atropine not only abolishes power in the HFP but also reduces LFP power (Fig. 12). For obvious reasons, many investigators have employed the ratio of low to high frequency power as an index of relative sympathovagal balance (76).

The very low-frequency peak (VLFP), found between DC and 0.04 Hz, represents much slower fluctuations in HR that may be related to thermoregulatory or humoral mechanisms (2,3). When continuous ECG data are displayed in the frequency domain, the powers within these three frequency ranges are reproducible from person to person and over time.

Methods for Performing Spectral Analysis of Heart Rate Initially, the raw ECG signals are digitized, R-wave peaks are detected and the inter-beat distances are determined so that a stream of R-R interval values can be derived. The ECG digitization rate determines the resolution of R-R interval measurements and should exceed 200 samples/s. The natural beat-to-beat HR variability results in unevenly spaced R wave peaks, while the Fast Fourier Transform (FFT) requires data points to be equally spaced in time. To fulfill this criteria, the R-R interval data must be resampled with evenly spaced intervals. Before resampling, the data points are interpolated by a simple sample and hold, a first-order linear interpolation from sample to sample or by some higher order spline function. If a sample and hold method is used, the resultant discontinuities in the data lead to spurious high-frequency contributions in the spectrum that may overlap the lower frequency areas of interest. This can be avoided by employing a continuous interpolation format. Once interpolated, the continuous function of R-R interval data is resampled at a rate of at least 1 Hz (typically 2 to 4 Hz or greater) and passed through the FFT. In this way, data of 0.5 Hz or less may be examined. The FFT ideally requires at least one full sinusoidal cycle to derive a power spectrum; however, more cycles improve signal-to-noise ratio in the frequency domain.

To best quantify the power within specific frequency bands one must optimize the frequency resolution while minimizing the effect of sidebands (or spectral leakage) on the various

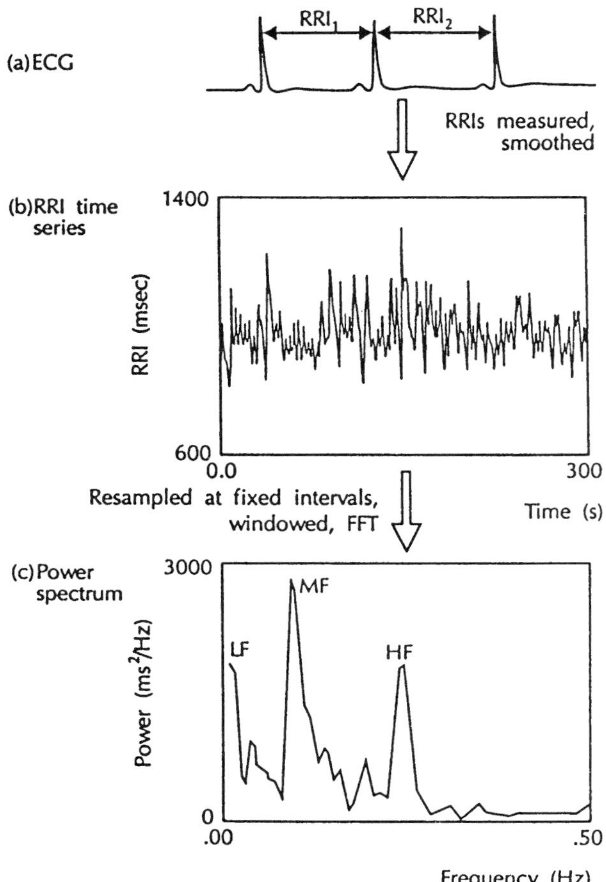

Figure 10. The technique of decomposing an epoch of R-R intervals into a time series and subsequently into its frequency components with power spectral analysis is depicted. The ECG is digitized, the R-waves are detected and the corresponding R-R intervals are measured (**a**). The resulting time series plot (**b**) is then smoothed, detrended, resampled, and windowed before being passed through the fast Fourier transformation (FFT) to derive the power spectrum (**c**). Three peaks are commonly detected in the power spectrum: the VLFP, <0.04 Hz; the LFP, 0.05–0.15 Hz; and the HFP, 0.15–0.4 Hz. (Reprinted, in adapted form, with permission from ref. 85.)

power peaks. To do this, windowing (or weighting functions) is usually performed in the time domain prior to the FFT, although it may be applied in the frequency domain after the transformation is complete for faster computation. The raised cosine function (Hamming window) lends itself to this application.

There is always nonstationarity or drift associated with the R-R interval signal. When converted to the frequency domain by the FFT method, this drift appears as a very large, low-frequency peak that approaches infinity at 0.0 Hz. Various techniques have been employed to detrend the data to reduce the magnitude of this large DC peak in order to better measure the low- and high-frequency power peaks. The simplest method is to subtract a fixed value, usually the mean R-R interval from each R-R interval value within the time series. Some have employed a first order linear approximation of the entire data set and then subtracted the value of this function from each data point. Still others have subtracted a line function formed by the first and last data points in the sample. In this way, the DC value of the frequency plot is driven to zero. The drift effect is also reduced by taking shorter samples or by windowing (which effectively shortens the sample length). The question still remains as to whether these very low frequency R-R interval fluctuations are the result of some physiologic process or from some unwanted aberrance. Much longer data sets are needed to accurately measure these low-frequency oscillations; this can typically be done with 24-hr ambulatory ECG recordings.

To improve PSA on shorter data segments, auto-regressive (AR) methods have been employed. To apply this technique, one chooses a modeling polynomial of a given size (or order). The order of the equation may be chosen automatically via an order selection algorithm. As order size increases, the original data set is more precisely modeled, but processing time lengthens. The data set is then passed through a self-modeling function that chooses the coefficients of the polynomial based on a weighted error signal (a comparison of the R-R interval signal to the polynomial). After the polynomial coefficients are "seeded" with an initial time series, smaller data segments can be passed through the self-modeling function (closed-form solution) to derive slightly new coefficients for each data segment. Once the AR coefficients are known, the spectral characteristics (i.e. power at various frequencies) can be obtained by performing an FFT on the AR parameters or poles of the equation. The closed-form solution can also be used to extrapolate the original data sequence if desired.

The advantage of the AR technique is that it can be quickly performed on shorter segments of data to yield similar results as the FFT technique. Since the analysis can be performed rapidly on smaller data segments, this method may have appli-

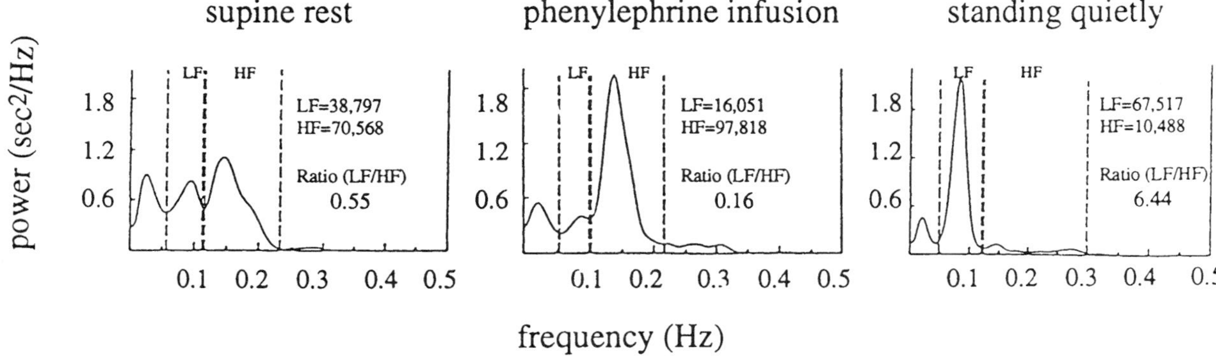

Figure 11. Changes in the power spectra in one individual in two different situations. The infusion of phenylephrine raises systemic blood pressure and slows heart rate by increasing vagal and decreasing sympathetic outflow to the heart. This is reflected by a decrease in low-frequency (LF) power and an increase in high-frequency (HF) power and a calculated reduction in the LF/HF ratio. In contrast, when standing there was a withdrawal of vagal-cardiac activity and an increase in the sympathetic outflow, as reflected by an increase in the LF power and a reduction of the HF power. The calculation of the ratio of LF to HF is substantially increased.

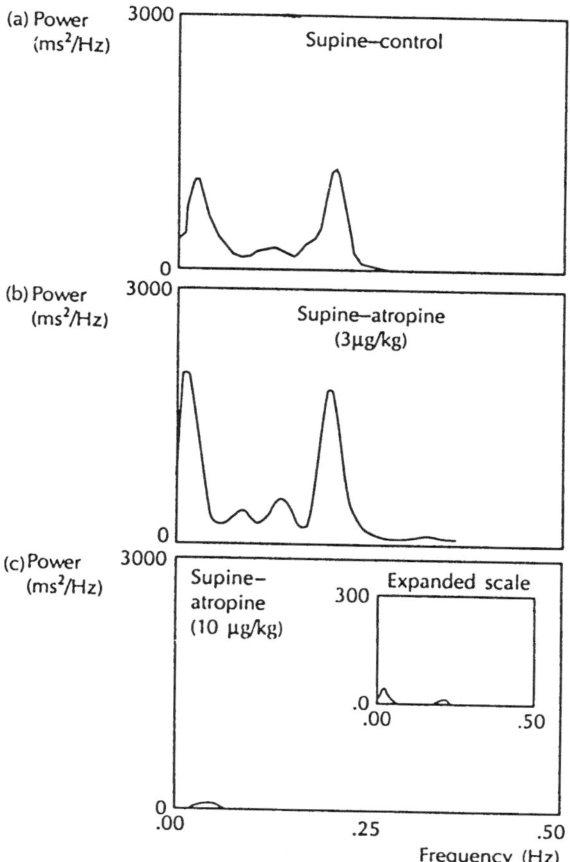

Figure 12. The effects of low and high doses of atropine sulfate on the power spectrum of a healthy volunteer. **a:** Resting power spectrum derived from 5 min of R-R interval data. **b:** Augmentation in the high-frequency peak produced by a small dose of atropine; this peak is centered between 0.15 and 0.4 Hz; this augmentation is due to enhancement of vagal outflow through atropine's central effects. **c:** Same individual after receiving a higher dose of atropine which reduces total power through cardiac muscarinic receptor blockade. Both low- and high-frequency powers are reduced substantially. (Reprinted, in adapted form, with permission from ref 85.)

cations to situations in which the conditions under study are changing rapidly. The AR technique has been shown to correlate with the FFT method in predicting the relative power in the various frequencies of interest. One caveat is that the model, no matter how precisely it defines the data, is only as good as the data itself. If the sampled data has large transients or is rapidly changing, no AR model will accurately describe the data.

One problem encountered with the application of PSA to the clinical environment is the occurrence of arrhythmias. Premature beats (typically PVCs) pose the initial problem of injecting discontinuities into the data. Some researchers fill in the void by deleting the ectopic beat and replacing it with a beat of average duration, effectively smoothing the discontinuity. Due to the effects of the PVC on the cardiovascular control mechanisms, this technique may not be valid. A PVC will reset the phase of the sinus node, activate the baroreceptors and stimulate the Bainbridge reflex, all of which may take up to 10 beats to reset to the baseline HR. It may be wise to simply avoid samples containing premature beats, although in some cases this may be impossible. Smoothing the R-R interval time series or windowing when using the FFT method should reduce the effects of transients produced by premature beats; however, this issue must be addressed with future applications.

Once the power spectrum is derived, the power within the various frequency bands can be quantified within set, predefined frequency ranges that usually encompass the three peaks of interest. These typically are the VLFP (0.0–0.05 Hz), LFP (0.05–0.15 Hz), and HFP (0.15–0.4 Hz). Because the absolute power is quite variable, the power of each peak may be normalized to the total power within the spectrum and reported as fractional percent. Total power is usually taken to be all power between ~0.03 Hz and 0.5 Hz, thus omitting the large, variable DC component. The total power can also vary considerably, however, and the normalized values may not in practice be comparable from person to person or with repeated measures within the same subject. One method to more easily compare powers of greatly changing magnitude is to use a logarithmic plot. Another relative assessment of power is made by taking the ratio of the power in the LFP to that in the HFP as a gauge of sympathovagal balance.

The quantification of power within set, predefined frequency bands may unfortunately include power elements outside of the peaks of interest. When respiratory rate varies, the HFP may override the LFP. This will occur at breathing rates <9 breaths/min (0.15 Hz). We have employed objective placement of frequency band limits based on each unique data set to delineate the peaks of interest allowing more precise power measurements. Initially, local minima about the peaks of the power spectrum are used to set these bands. For confirmation of band placement or when ambiguity exists, the coherence functions between several related spectra may assist in defining the location of the low- and high-frequency peaks (Fig. 13). This is done by applying PSA to concurrently recorded physiologic signals such as respiratory excursions, systolic blood pressure and diastolic blood pressure in a similar fashion to R-R interval data. Coherence is a measure of how closely the two spectra coincide on a scale of 0 to 1. Because the HFP of R-R interval is influenced by respiration, the coherence between these spectra should be high over the HFP and low elsewhere. Similarly, the LFP area of interest can be delineated by R-R interval versus SBP coherence peaks. Just as a linear correlation coefficient >0.5 implies a significant linear alignment of data, a coherence function of >0.5 should define a significant alignment of the two spectra. Thus, the coherence functions may allow the objective placement of frequency bands used to delineate the R-R interval power peaks for improved quantitative analysis of the spectrum.

Assessment of the Sympathetic Nervous System in Humans

The sympathetic nervous system has a central role in circulatory homeostasis in normal physiological states as well as in pathophysiological states such as hypertension, cardiac arrhythmias and autonomic insufficiency. Unfortunately, the evaluation of the sympathetic nervous system has been limited by the lack of an easily applied method for routine investigation.

There have been four primary methods which have been used for evaluating sympathetic nervous function in humans. These are (a) pharmacological methods to block prevailing levels of sympathetic activity; (b) spectral analysis of the slower components of heart rate variability (e.g., R-R interval oscillations); (c) biochemical methods to evaluate plasma norepinephrine and norepinephrine kinetics; and (d) microneurographic methods to directly record regional sympathetic nerve activity.

The pharmacological method to assess sympathetic neural tone has been infrequently employed in humans and may be the least interpretable. This consists of quantifying the magnitude of the decrease in blood pressure during ganglionic blockade. However, the measured response is imprecise because it is

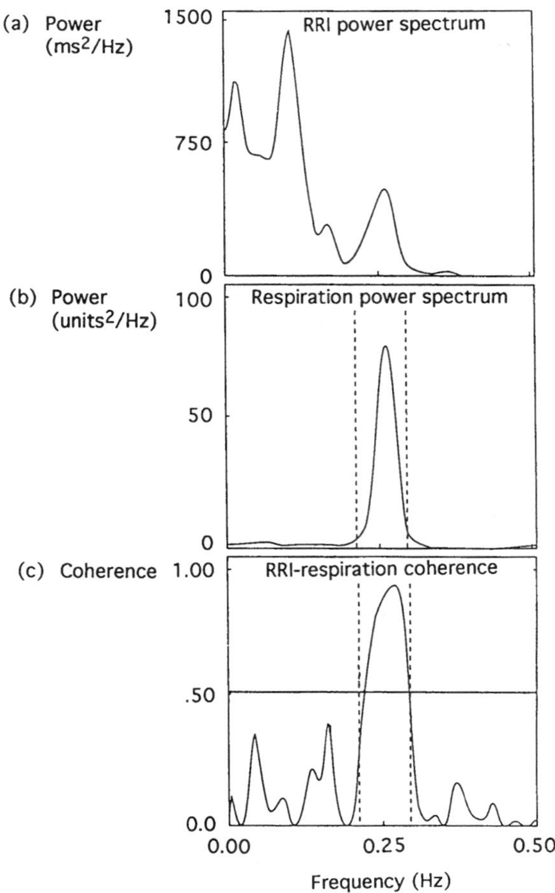

Figure 13. **a,b:** Data from simultaneously sampling both respiratory excursions and the R-R intervals during a 5-min sequence, and subsequently subjecting both signals to power spectral analysis; it is clear that the high-frequency power occurs at the same frequency as the respiration (centered at 0.25 Hz). **c:** Degree to which they coincide is the coherence. Coherence ranges from 0 to 1, and a high coherence suggests a tight correlation between these signals as they define the high frequency range. This coherence analysis can be used to more precisely define the limits of the R-R interval spectral peak in the high frequency range as indicated by the upward, dashed lines. (Reprinted, in adapted form, with permission from ref. 85.)

not only dependent upon the prevailing level of sympathetic activity, but is also influenced by autoregulation, compensatory reflex changes in cardiac output and the vascular architecture (i.e. the wall-to-lumen ratio). The use of β-adrenergic blockade to quantitate sympathetic neural drive to the heart is also limited because of compensatory responses mediated through the cardiac parasympathetic system.

Spectral Analysis of Heart Rate The noninvasive technique of PSA of heart rate variability has been employed to estimate changes in sympathetic activity in humans. The low-frequency oscillations (0.05-0.15 Hz) are influenced by changing levels of cardiac sympathetic activity (63), although contamination from parasympathetic input occurs (97). There is reasonable experimental evidence that this low-frequency component is augmented by stressors known to increase sympathetic drive, e.g., head-up tilt, mental arithmetic and hypotension (76,85). Moreover, this component is reduced in quadriplegic patients with interrupted sympathetic pathways (63) and is also reduced during syncopal episodes (76). Unfortunately, because it is likely that the power in the low frequency range is due to input from both divisions of the autonomic nervous system, the strength of this analysis is limited. A more promising use of PSA of HRV as an index to sympathetic drive has been the use of the ratio of LFP/HFP as a relative guide to the sympathovagal balance (76,85). Increases in the ratio suggest sympathetic activation and/or vagal withdrawal.

Plasma Catecholamine Analysis The simple process of sampling blood and subsequently determining the plasma concentration of norepinephrine has for years served as a "gold standard" for assessing global sympathetic outflow. It has well-known limitations (54,77,82). First, only a fraction of the norepinephrine released into the plasma actually enters the circulation. Approximately 80% is locally inactivated, primarily by reuptake of norepinephrine into the sympathetic terminals from which it was released (48). Secondly, the circulating norepinephrine concentration is determined not only by the rate of its release but by its rate of removal or clearance from the circulation (48). This may be a particularly important issue when employing plasma norepinephrine as a measure of sympathetic function during anesthesia. Clearance is a function of cardiac output, organ blood flow and neuronal and extraneuronal uptake by the vascular endothelium and other tissues, and these factors can be altered by anesthesia in unpredictable ways (22,23). Additionally, the site of blood sampling influences the measured levels of norepinephrine. For example, forearm vein sampling results in norepinephrine concentrations due primarily to sympathetic outflow to forearm skeletal muscle. This information does not reflect global sympathetic outflow because sympathetic activity can be highly differentiated and often varies remarkably in separate vascular beds at any given moment. Finally, arterial levels of norepinephrine are lower than venous concentrations because of uptake and clearance that takes place as blood traverses the pulmonary vasculature (48). Despite these many limitations, plasma catecholamine determination as an index of sympathetic nervous outflow is commonplace.

Norepinephrine Kinetics Both regional and global patterns of sympathetic nerve activation in man can be determined by evaluation of systemic or regional norepinephrine release with kinetic techniques (46-48). This process is based upon experimental data demonstrating a close relationship between experimentally manipulated sympathetic nerve firing rate to an organ and the rate of spillover of norepinephrine in the venous effluent (48). The norepinephrine that circulates is derived from sympathetic nerve terminals but represents only ~20% of the released norepinephrine which overflows into the circulation. The remainder is disposed of by reuptake back into the nerves. Kinetic techniques estimate the rate of release of norepinephrine into plasma and, assuming that the rate of reuptake is relatively fixed, provide reasonable estimates of sympathetic neural activity. A constant-rate intravenous infusion of isotope-labeled norepinephrine is employed, and the rate of norepinephrine spillover is determined by an isotope dilution method (Fig. 14). During steady state infusions, the following relationships are derived:

$$\text{NE spillover rate} = \frac{\text{Labeled NE infusion rate}}{\text{Radioactivity of plasma NE}}$$

$$\text{NE clearance} = \frac{\text{Labeled NE infusion rate}}{\text{Plasma-labeled NE concentration}}$$

The NE spillover rate is the rate at which norepinephrine enters the plasma (~20% of the release of NE from sympathetic terminals) and is directly proportional to sympathetic nerve firing rates. The calculation of clearance is important because changes in clearance uncouple the tight relationship between norepinephrine spillover and plasma NE concentrations. The reader is referred to a recent review of this method (48). This technique has been used to measure global and organ-specific

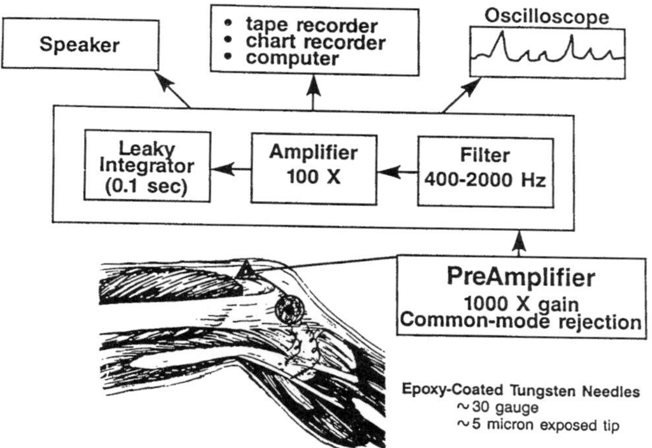

Figure 14. Depiction of the process of sympathetic microneurography as applied to recordings from the common peroneal nerve. One tungsten needle is inserted into the nerve; a second needle is placed just outside the nerve and serves as a reference electrode. A ground electrode is attached nearby. Typically, the signals are amplified 70,000–100,000 times, filtered and integrated for display and subsequent analysis.

norepinephrine release. For example, in humans, it appears that nerves to the kidneys and skeletal muscle account for about half of the total circulating norepinephrine, whereas, the heart, skin, GI tract, and liver each account for <10% of the total plasma norepinephrine concentration. Approximately 70% of the circulating norepinephrine is cleared in the lungs and splanchnic regions.

Sympathetic Microneurography Efferent sympathetic activity directed to vascular smooth muscle can be assessed from microneurographic recordings from peripheral nerves in humans (126). This technique was initially described in the 1960s (55). It consists of percutaneous placement of a needle into a peripheral nerve to record postganglionic sympathetic efferent activity (25,26). Multifiber recordings (and on occasion, single-fiber recordings) of sympathetic nerve activity directed to the vasculature of either skin or muscle have been described. Sympathetic C fibers are aggregated in discrete networks of Schwann cells interspersed within nerve fascicles, and their activity can be visually observed if recordings are filtered (200–2,000 Hz) and amplified 100,000-fold. The electronics needed to obtain recordings consists of a pair of epoxy-coated tungsten needles (32-gauge) connected to a differential preamplifier. One needle is placed into a peripheral nerve, and the second needle is located in near proximity but outside the nerve. Signals arriving at both needles simultaneously (such as 60 cycle noise and electronic glitches) are detected by the preamplifier and canceled (a process called common-mode rejection). The signal is amplified to some degree and passed to a filter amplifier that permits low and high frequency filtering using variable frequency band pass filters (Fig. 14). Additional details of the electronics are provided earlier in this chapter under "acute recording techniques" in animals.

The process of locating a sympathetic recording is a three-step process: first, identifying the course of the nerve via an external stimulator connected to a pencil-like probe; second, locating the nerve percutaneously via small pulsed electrical stimulation through the needle as it is advanced under the skin and into the peripheral nerve; and third, "tweaking" the needle until characteristic recordings are identified on an oscilloscope. The needle can enter fascicles of nerves that communicate with skin or muscle. Both afferent and efferent neural traffic run within these fascicles. If a pulsing paresthesia occurs without evidence of a muscular contraction, the needle tip is located in a fascicle of nerves supplying skin. In contrast, when a fascicle of nerves supplying muscle is entered, visible muscle contractions are observed. Additional confirmation of the location of the needle tip can be obtained when recording from the needle by observing afferent bursts of neural activity from muscle mechanoreceptors when stretching muscles or tapping tendons of muscles innervated by the nerve. In contrast, light stroking of the skin in the innervated area does not elicit afferent bursts unless the tip of the needle is located within a skin fascicle. Additional confirmation of the efferent nature of this traffic comes from studies showing that lidocaine block proximal to the recording site and/or administration of ganglionic blockers abolishes the traffic recorded from the microelectrode (25,55).

Recordings from efferent skin sympathetic fibers reveal intermittent and sporadic bursts of activity which are augmented by mental stress, startle maneuvers and body cooling, but not influenced by baroreceptor mechanisms (Fig. 15) (26,56). Recordings from skin sympathetics probably reflect both sudomotor and vasoconstrictor activity directed to skin blood vessels. Because the skin circulation represents only ~4% of the total cardiac output, bursts of skin sympathetic traffic do not necessarily initiate or correlate with subsequent blood pressure changes. In contrast, sympathetic nerve activity directed to blood vessels in skeletal muscle is tonically active and often phase-locked to the cardiac cycle (i.e. a maximum of one efferent volley of neural activity occurs each cardiac cycle) (25). This activity is under intimate control by the baroreceptor reflex (32-34,37). Reductions in arterial pressure elicit reflex augmentations in muscle sympathetic nerve activity while increases in blood pressure will inhibit sympathetic traffic (Fig. 16). This traffic can also be augmented during hypoxia, hypercarbia and exercise, and these bursts of neural activity, consistently lead to elevations in blood pressure. Thus, it appears that muscle sympathetic nerve activity plays a major role in maintaining blood pressure homeostasis in humans. This is in part due to the fact that the skeletal muscle circulation represents ~40% of the cardiac output and neurally mediated changes in muscle vascular tone importantly influence blood pressure. The microneurography technique is limited by the fact that successful recordings involve skill, sophisticated electronics and motionless subjects. A further limitation of this technique is the inaccessibility of recordings from other sympathetic nerve sites e.g., those supplying the renal, splanchnic, or cardiac beds.

Evaluation of Human Baroreflex Function

Low-Pressure Human Baroreflex Function There is strong evidence for pressure sensing receptors located within the vasculature on the low pressure side of the circulation, i.e., at the veno-atrial junction, within the pulmonary vasculature and even within the atrial and ventricular muscle (57,79,80). These receptors are tonically active and send afferent signals to the central nervous system primarily via the vagus. When central blood volume is reduced by hemorrhage or orthostatic stress, these receptors are unloaded and the reduced afferent traffic triggers increases in sympathetic outflow (80). It is thought that this reflex is activated earlier than arterial baroreflex responses and therefore exerts a rapid response that triggers vasoconstriction to maintain blood pressure in the face of mild central hypovolemia (64,80,120,132).

The evaluation of this reflex in humans has been carried out primarily with a technique called lower body negative pressure (LBNP), although other techniques have included low levels of head-up tilt (<15–20°) and venous occlusion at the upper thighs (38). Conversely, to load the low-pressure receptors, simple leg elevation or head-down tilt has been employed (101). Regardless of the technique, a sensitive measure reflecting changes in central blood volume is necessary to quantitate the stimulus.

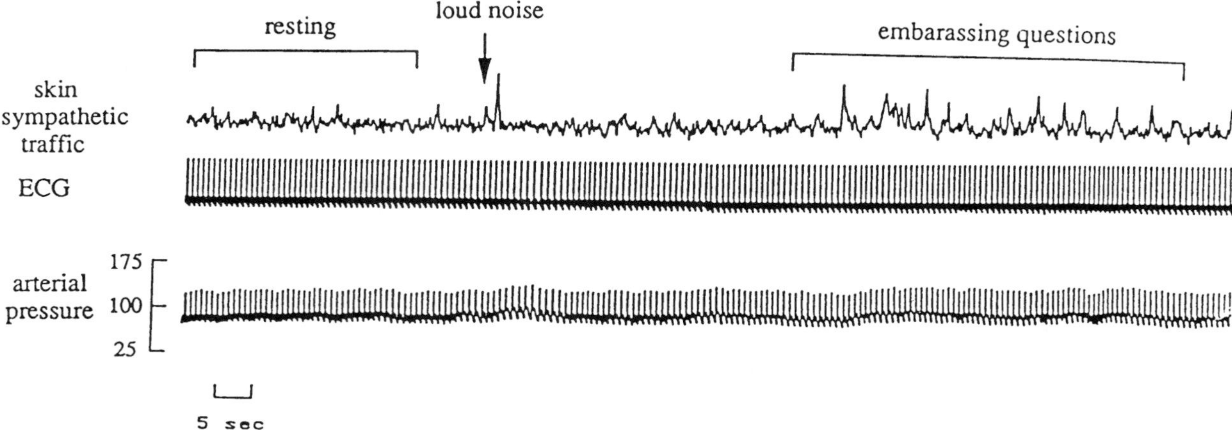

Figure 15. A recording of skin sympathetic traffic, the electrocardiogram, and arterial blood pressure from one healthy volunteer. Resting skin sympathetic traffic is highly variable and without relationship to the cardiac cycle. It is augmented by startle maneuvers such as a loud handclap and also can be increased during periods of emotional stress, such as when responding to embarrassing questions.

This measure is usually central venous pressure. The technique of LBNP is quite simple. Supine subjects are positioned in an airtight chamber that encloses the lower body caudal to the umbilicus. These chambers are often locally constructed from heavy plywood but can be cylindrical chambers constructed from metal that are commercially available (Biomedical Engineering Department, University of Iowa, Iowa City, IA). The difficult aspect of LBNP is to obtain a seal at the waist, and this has often been accomplished with a removable and adjustable template covered with a thin rubber material or a plastic bag (131). When suction is applied to the box, a seal is created against the template, which is often supplemented by heavy application of skin tape around the waist. Usually the seal is sufficient to tolerate levels of LBNP up to 60 mm Hg below atmospheric pressure. The difficulty of creating a seal to positive pressure has lead to the more common use of leg elevation or head-down tilt to increase central blood volume.

Relatively little work has been focused on the low-pressure cardiopulmonary baroreflex in humans undergoing anesthesia. We have applied sequential applications of LBNP (-5, -7.5, -10, -12.5 mm Hg) to produce incremental reductions in central blood volume in unpremedicated ASA class I patients scheduled for elective surgery (36). When these levels of LBNP were applied to patients prior to anesthesia, CVP progressively decreased and reflex increases in total peripheral resistance and forearm vascular resistance occurred. Blood pressure and heart rate remained unchanged (Fig. 17). These sympathetically mediated resistance responses in the absence of blood pressure reductions or tachycardia have been taken as strong evidence for specific unloading of the low-pressure baroreceptors without activation of the high pressure arterial baroreflex. During halothane anesthesia at 1.0 and 1.25 MAC the reflex resistance responses to LBNP were attenuated, and as a result blood pressure was not well maintained. These observations suggest that halothane may be a good choice of anesthetic agent if hypotensive anesthesia is planned, but may be a poor choice when rapid surgical blood loss is a possibility.

We also have evaluated the effects of a fentanyl/diazepam anesthetic combination on low-pressure baroreflex function (35). A similar ASA class I patient population was examined and LBNP was applied in three steps: -5, -10, and -15 mm Hg. As expected, these intensities of LBNP did not change blood pressure but decreased CVP and triggered reflex increases in vascular resistance in awake patients. During fentanyl (12.5 μg/kg)/diazepam (0.25 mg/kg) anesthesia, blood pressure and vascular resistance were decreased as is typically seen with narcotic/benzodiazepine combinations (35). Interestingly, the reflex response to LBNP was remarkably preserved and, as a

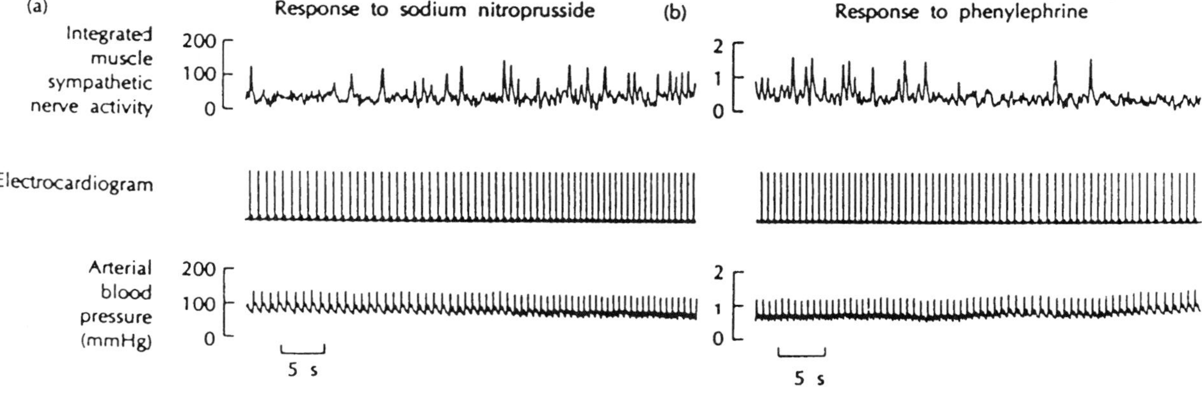

Figure 16. A recording of sympathetic traffic directed to skeletal muscle blood vessels. This traffic is pulse synchronous (only one burst of activity per cardiac cycle) and is tightly regulated through baroreceptor mechanisms. **a:** When blood pressure is lowered with nitroprusside, augmentations in the integrated neurogram are noted and increases in heart rate occur. **b:** Conversely, when blood pressure is increased subtly with phenylephrine, neural outflow decreases and heart rate slows through baroreflex mechanisms. This traffic is not altered by startle maneuvers or emotional stimuli.

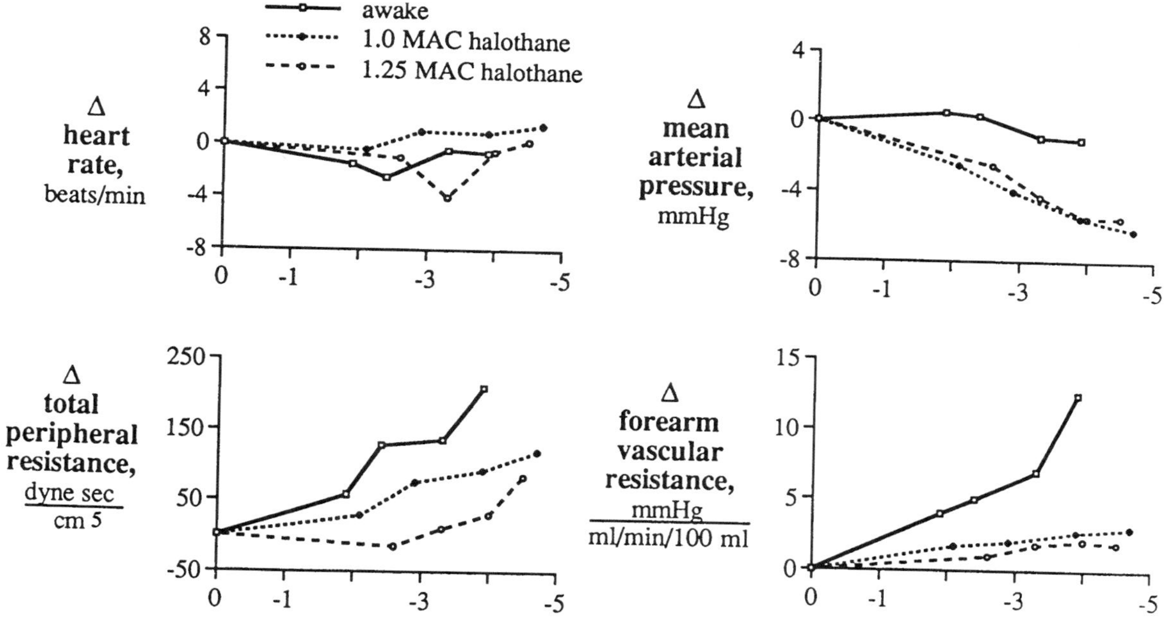

Figure 17. Cardiopulmonary baroreflex activation triggered by graded applications of lower body negative pressure (LBNP) to reduce central venous pressure. In awake volunteers, low levels of LBNP (<20 mm Hg) reduced central venous pressure without changing heart rate or blood pressure, suggesting that arterial baroreflex mechanisms were not activated. The low-pressure cardiopulmonary reflex triggered reflex increases in total and forearm vascular resistance. The same levels of LBNP applied to subjects during halothane anesthesia led to reductions in mean pressure because of impaired cardiopulmonary baroreflex-mediated increases in peripheral and forearm vascular resistance. MAC, minimum alveolar concentration. (Reprinted, in adapted form, with permission from ref. 36.)

result, blood pressure was well maintained despite significant reductions in central blood volume (Fig. 18). We conjectured that this anesthetic combination reduced central sympathetic outflow but preserved low-pressure baroreflex responses, thereby permitting blood pressure homeostasis at a new (lower) blood pressure equilibrium.

High-Pressure Baroreflex Function The baroreceptors located in the aortic arch and the carotid sinus are pressure-sensitive receptors that respond to changes in the prevailing systemic pressure and trigger reflex responses in an attempt to maintain blood pressure at equilibrium (78). One efferent limb of the baroreflex to the heart consists of vagal and, to a lesser extent, sympathetic outflow that adjust both heart rate and contractility. A second efferent limb modulates sympathetic outflow to skeletal, splanchnic and renal vascular beds. Human baroreflex research is limited by the dual location of the baroreceptive areas (carotid and aortic arch) and the inability to precisely control stimuli to these areas and by limitations of techniques to record efferent nerve activity and effector organ responses. Several techniques for provoking baroreceptor responses suffer because of the complexity of baroreceptor location and physiology (43). The heart rate and sympathetic response to standing, upright tilt or high intensity LBNP is due to the simultaneous unloading of both the low and high pressure baroreceptors. In the case of standing or tilting, the unloading of carotid baroreceptors is probably greater than aortic baroreceptors, and reflex responses may be partially mediated by somatic reflexes from the lower extremities. The Valsalva maneuver consists of increasing intrathoracic pressure for a brief time while monitoring blood pressure and recording the efferent heart rate responses. The intra- versus extra-thoracic location of the aortic and carotid baroreceptors as well as the combination of mechanical and neural factors to the integrated Valsalva response make this maneuver a relatively imprecise test of arterial baroreflex function (but perhaps an excellent test of global autonomic function) (38).

There are two accepted methods available for the study of human baroreflexes, both involving pressure changes to baroreceptor areas. One involves stretch or compression of the carotid sinus by delivering positive or negative pressure to a neck chamber. The other involves the administration of short acting vasoactive drugs to increase or decrease systemic pressure thereby loading or unloading the baroreceptor regions (often referred to as the "Oxford method")

1. *Neck Suction:* Human investigation does not permit the isolation of and application of internal and external pressure to the carotid body, as is possible with experimental animals. The neck chamber method, which specifically alters carotid baroreceptors, was originally described by Ernsting and Perry in 1957 (45) and later refined by Eckberg et al. in the late 1970s (42), then further refined in the late 1980s (118). Either the entire neck or simply the anterior portion of the neck is sealed in an airtight chamber. This has been commonly constructed of lead because it is pliable and can be molded to individual neck sizes. It is rimmed with rubber or silicone and strapped firmly in place. A commercially available model is constructed of silicone with a fiberglass backing (Engineering Development Laboratory, Newport News, VA) (Fig. 19). A pressure transducer is mounted on the collar to sense the pressure or suction delivered to the chamber. Solenoid valves are attached to or near the chamber and are in series with 0.75-in vacuum or pressure hosing that is in turn secured to commercial industrial vacuums. The vacuums are powered through

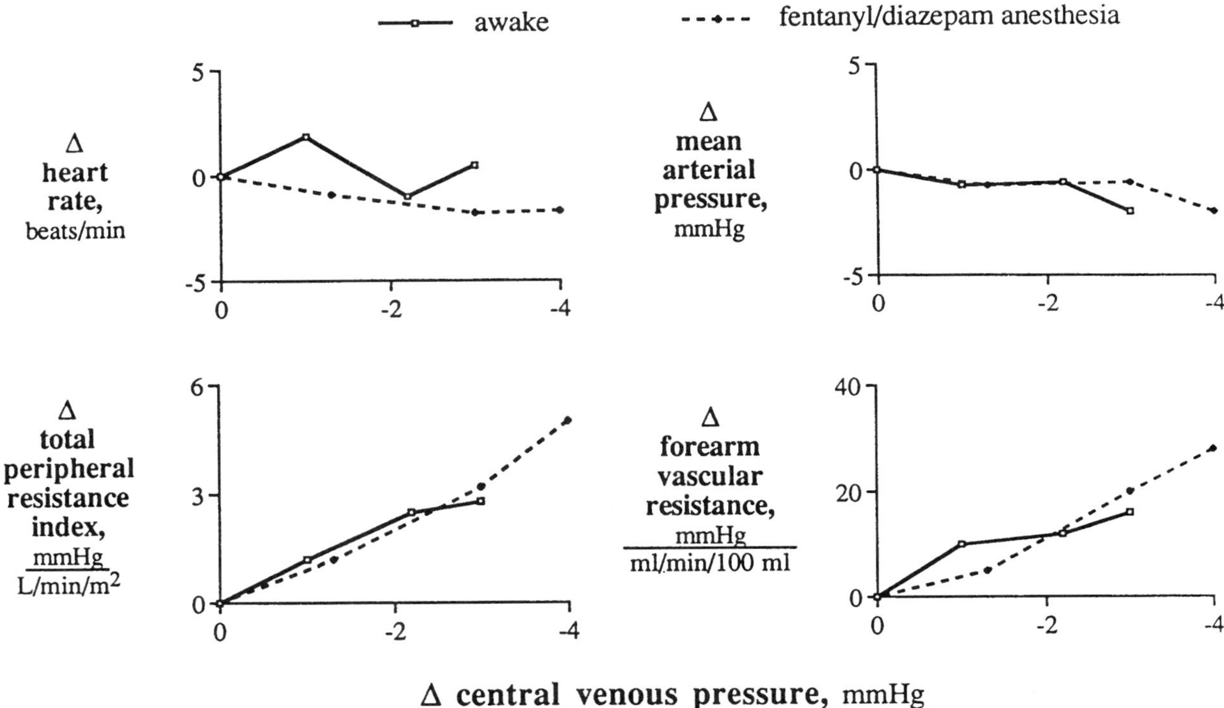

Figure 18. An example of an anesthetic combination (fentanyl and diazepam) that preserves low-pressure cardiopulmonary baroreflex function. Applications of lower body negative pressure to reduce central venous pressure triggers reflex increases in peripheral and forearm vascular resistance that prevent decreases in blood pressure. This response was preserved during anesthesia. (Reprinted, in adapted form, with permission from ref. 35.)

voltage regulators so that the level of suction or pressure loaded to the solenoids (and subsequently delivered to the neck chamber) can be regulated. Far more elaborate designs can be envisioned and have been employed (51,118). Carotid stimuli are usually given 3–4 s after beginning a relaxed breathhold at the end of expiration. The stimulus onset can either be triggered by the R-wave of the ECG or carefully timed so that it begins ~800 ms before an anticipated P wave, at a time when the sinus node is maximally responsive to the stimulus (39,40). The rate of change of pressure in the neck chamber should be at or near the physiologic systolic pressure rate of change (i.e., 300–600 mm Hg/s). The chamber pressure transmission to the carotid sinus has been measured with a fluid-filled catheter placed in the vicinity of carotid sinus in human volunteers (74). It was found that neck pressure was reduced by 14% and neck suction pressure by 36% during

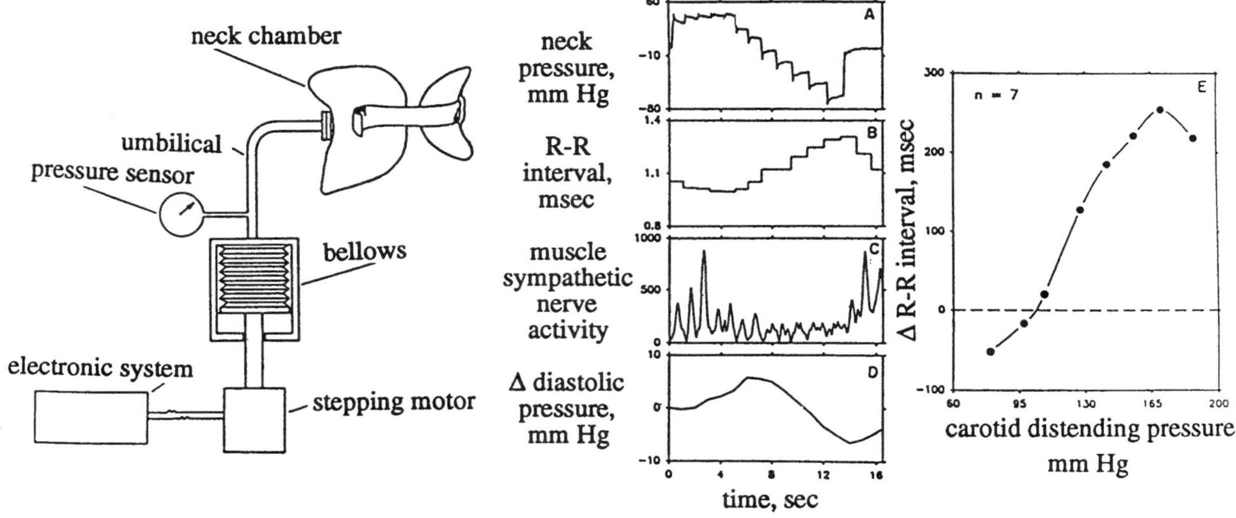

Figure 19. Commercially available, electronically controlled neck chamber device for altering carotid baroreceptor afferent traffic. The figure demonstrates an individual sequence of neck pressure changes (**A**) and the average responses to seven of these sequences (**B–E**) in one individual. (Reprinted, in adapted form, with permission from ref. 43.)

transmission through the neck tissues. Importantly, body habitus did not influence the transmission, suggesting that this technique can be applied to a diverse population without concern about individual differences in the transmitted pressure. When a stimulus is applied to the carotid baroreceptor via the neck chamber, rapid, vagal-mediated heart rate changes occur within the duration of one cardiac cycle. This results in immediate changes in heart rate and cardiac output. The peripheral sympathetic response has a longer latency than the vagal-cardiac response, in part due to sympathetic C-fiber conduction velocity of 1 m/s and in part due to neural effector response times. The combination of vagal-cardiac and sympathetic responses to neck chamber stimuli results in systemic blood pressure changing ~2–3 s after the delivery of the stimulus. Therefore, to evaluate reflex responses mediated by the carotid baroreceptors without the confounding response from aortic baroreceptors, brief (1–3 s) stimuli are usually employed. Neck stimuli have been delivered and maintained for 15–60 s periods to determine steady-state heart rate and blood pressure responses (78), however, the measured responses are due to the combined effect of carotid sinus reflexes and opposing aortic baroreflexes. Typically, different strengths of stimuli are used, ranging from +40 to -50 mm Hg, and separate stimuli are delivered during separate breathhold periods (39,40). An entire heart rate-carotid baroreflex sigmoid curve can be constructed in ~45 min of testing. A newer technique has been described in which a chamber compresses the carotid sinus with 40 mm Hg of presssure followed by 15 mm Hg neck chamber pressure reductions triggered by each subsequent cardiac cycle until a pressure of -65 mm Hg is achieved (51,118). Each pressure reduction is initiated by the ECG R-wave, and the entire sequence is delivered during one 15-sec breathhold. The authors have recommended repeating the sequence five to seven times during separate breathholds and averaging the data to derive a single stimulus-reponse relationship. The average of the last two R-R intervals immediately prior to the onset of the pressure sequences is generally taken as the control interval, and each subsequent change in R-R interval is plotted as a function of the carotid distending pressure (systolic-neck pressure) of the same interval (Fig. 19). In ~12 min, this technique can describe the sigmoid carotid baroreflex-heart period relationship which is exclusively via vagal mechanisms. It is likely that directionally opposite changes of aortic pressure oppose some of the sinus node inhibition during the later portions of the carotid baroreceptor stimulus train.

2. *Pressor and Depressor Drugs:* A second established approach to examine arterial baroreflex function is the use of vasoactive drugs to raise and lower blood pressure (32,69,116). The α-adrenergic agonist, phenylephrine, is most commonly used to raise blood pressure. It is administered intravenously as a bolus (usually 50–100 μg) and during the period of increasing blood pressure a plot of each successive R-R interval versus the preceding systolic or mean pressure yields a group of data points that are subjected to a linear regression analysis (or in some cases curvi-linear analysis). The slope of the regression

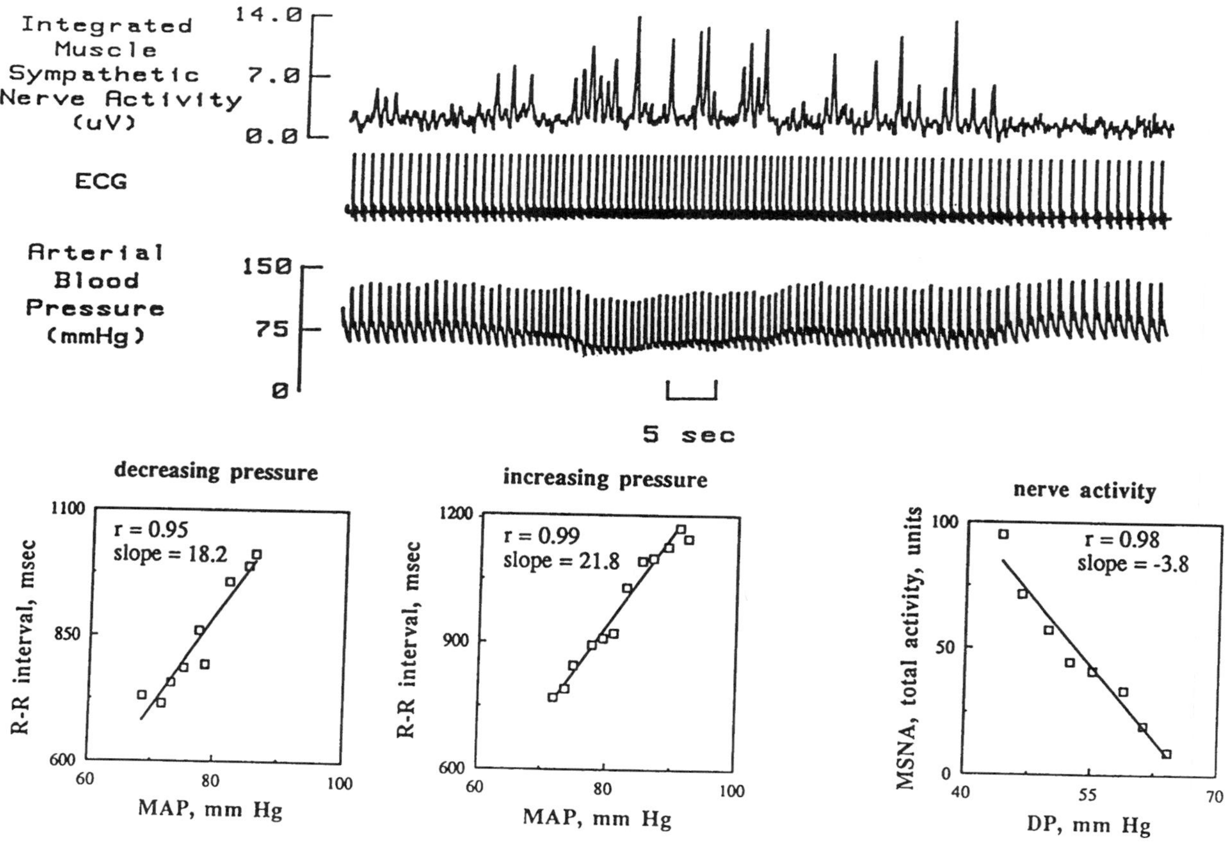

Figure 20. Process of deriving baroreflex sensitivity during sequential injections of sodium nitroprusside (100 μg) followed (1 min later) by phenylephrine (150 μg). *Top tracing:* Decrease in blood pressure and reflex increases in heart rate and sympathetic nerve activity, followed by an increase in blood pressure associated with heart rate slowing and sympathoinhibition. *Bottom tracing:* The application of linear regression analysis. The reflex R-R interval response to declining and rising pressure are separately analyzed because of hysteresis in the reflex response curve. The slope of the regression line is an index of reflex gain and can be calculated for cardiac and peripheral sympathetic baroreflex responses.

line is considered to reflect arterial baroreceptor reflex sensitivity. The same process can be carried out during intravenous injections of vasodilators such as sodium nitroprusside (1 μg/kg) or nitroglycerin (1-2 μg/kg). An alternative technique involves more gradual infusions rather than boluses of these vasoactive compounds. The primary disadvantage of this technique is that the stimulus is not confined to one set of baroreceptors, i.e. it is likely that both low- and high-pressure baroreceptors are influenced by these drugs. An important advantage of this technique is that peripheral sympathetic responses can be determined as well as heart rate responses. For example when these vasoactive compounds are given by a gradual infusion technique over several minutes, blood samples can be obtained and plasma norepinephrine levels can be determined. Plasma norepinephrine can be plotted as a function of the prevailing blood pressure at the time of blood sampling to derive a reflex gain. If sympathetic microneurography is employed, brief or bolus injections of vasoactive compound can be employed and changes in the amount of sympathetic activity can be plotted as a function of the prevailing blood pressure (Fig. 20). Although this technique is limited by the fact that all pressure sensing receptors are loaded or unloaded simultaneously, this may in fact be a highly physiological stimulus. In terms of anesthesia, consider rapid blood loss in a supine, anesthetized patient. This stress clearly unloads all baroreceptors simultaneously. A variation of the "Oxford Method" employing vasoactive drug infusions has been described by Korner and colleagues (69) in which multiple infusions of small graded doses of pressors and depressors over 20 s are given and peak or "steady-state" R-R interval and blood pressure responses are recorded. The results define a sigmoid arterial pressure to R-R interval response relationship from which the slope of the linear portion of the sigmoid curve, the threshold and saturation pressures, and a range of R-R interval responses can be determined (69). One disadvantage of this approach is that the method is time-consuming, requiring ~2–3 h to establish a complete response curve.

ANESTHETIC ALTERATIONS OF THE AUTONOMIC NERVOUS SYSTEM AND REFLEX CONTROL OF THE CARDIOVASCULAR SYSTEM

Animal Studies

Anesthetic Actions on Baroreflex Function

In general, anesthetics have been found to depress baroreflex control of blood pressure, although the extent of depression can vary from anesthetic to anesthetic. In animals, depression of the baroreflex has been reported for inhalational anesthetics, including halothane (13,19,37,44,86,103,112,124, 130), isoflurane (103,104,109,114), and enflurane (111); intravenous anesthetics, including thiopental (37,92), pentobarbital (5,19,20,88), propofol (65,100,124), ketamine (87,92,124), urethan (5), and chloralose (5,19); and induction agents, including diazepam (92,102,121), fentanyl-diazepam (121), and alfentanyl (124). However, propofol was also reported to have no effect on baroreflex sensitivity (109) or heart rate response (124) and etomidate has not been associated with a clear decrease in baroreflex function (62,124). The attenuation of the baroreflex has been attributed to depressant actions of the anesthetics at all levels of the reflex arc, including central integration of baroreceptor input and activation of autonomic activity, ganglionic transmission, and end-organ response (103,104,107). In spite of the overall depression of baroreflex function, anesthetics have actually been found to sensitize baroreceptors and similar mechanoreceptors (104, 105,107). The effects of anesthetics on mechanoreceptors and efferent autonomic activity are discussed in more detail below.

Anesthetic Actions on Afferent Activity

Afferent activity from arterial baroreceptors has been found to increase in response to exposure to some anesthetics, including halothane (12,105,107), isoflurane (104), cyclopropane (95), and ether (99) (Fig. 21). Exposure to ketamine has been reported to have no effect on baroreceptor discharge (115). Both resting discharge and sensitivity of the baroreceptors was found to increase during volatile anesthetic exposure (105). This increase in discharge appears to be a property common to many mechanoreceptors, for pulmonary stretch receptors have also been found to increase frequency when exposed to low levels of cyclopropane (129), halothane (18), and ether (18). Preliminary evidence suggests that the sensitizing effect is related to anesthetic alterations of a Ca^{2+}-dependent effect (105), but the exact mechanism is not known. The increased discharge of baroreceptors resulting from exposure to inhalational anesthetics may actually contribute to the depression of the whole baroreflex by tonically lowering the overall level of outflow of sympathetic activity, resulting in an attenuated ability of the sympathetic system to respond to produce reflex changes in blood pressure.

Anesthetic Actions on Efferent Activity

Both limbs of the autonomic nervous system have been shown to be attenuated by anesthesia. The central control of autonomic activity is measured by recording preganglionic activity, whereas all other variables are controlled. For example, if the effect of an anesthetic on resting levels of sympathetic outflow is under investigation, variables such as blood pressure, respiration, blood gases etc. must be held constant while the anesthetic is administered, so that changes in these factors do not contribute to any observed effect in preganglionic sympathetic nerve activity. Changes in postganglionic activity include any effects of the anesthetics on ganglionic transmission as well as effects on central autonomic outflow, and the difference in the magnitude of changes in pre- versus postganglionic activity can be used as an indication of attenuation of some component(s) of ganglionic transmission (104,107).

Sympathetic Efferent Activity Preganglionic sympathetic activity has been found to decrease during administration of inhalational anesthetics in both cats and dogs. Halothane did not significantly decrease activity until 2 MAC (1.5% inspired halothane) (107,112), whereas isoflurane attenuated activity at both 1.3% inspired (1 MAC) and 2.6% inspired isoflurane (2 MAC) (104,114) (Fig. 22). Enflurane depressed sympathetic activity at both 1.5% and 3.0% inspired levels in a dose-dependent manner (111). In some earlier studies, when arterial pressure was allowed to decrease in response to anesthetic administration, reflex-evoked increases in sympathetic activity prevented decreases in sympathetic nerve activity to levels comparable to those seen in animals in which arterial pressure was maintained constant (107). In these studies, little change in preganglionic nerve activity was reported for halothane (83). Decreases in preganglionic nerve activity have also been reported for thiopental (113) and etomidate (62). Postganglionic nerve activity has been found to decrease after administration of halothane (107), isoflurane (104), fentanyl (121), fentanyl-diazepam (121), and pentobarbital (58). A greater decrease in postganglionic sympathetic activity as compared to preganglionic activity in response to halothane (107) and isoflurane (104) suggested that there was also a depression of ganglionic transmission in the autonomic ganglia that contributed to the overall depression of sympathetic efferent activity. Studies that have directly examined anesthetic effects on ganglionic transmission have shown this to be true (15).

As stated earlier, many studies have examined the effects of a specific anesthetic after the use of an induction anesthetic, and therefore the attenuation in recorded sympathetic activity is the result of the combination of drugs (104,107,112,114). To

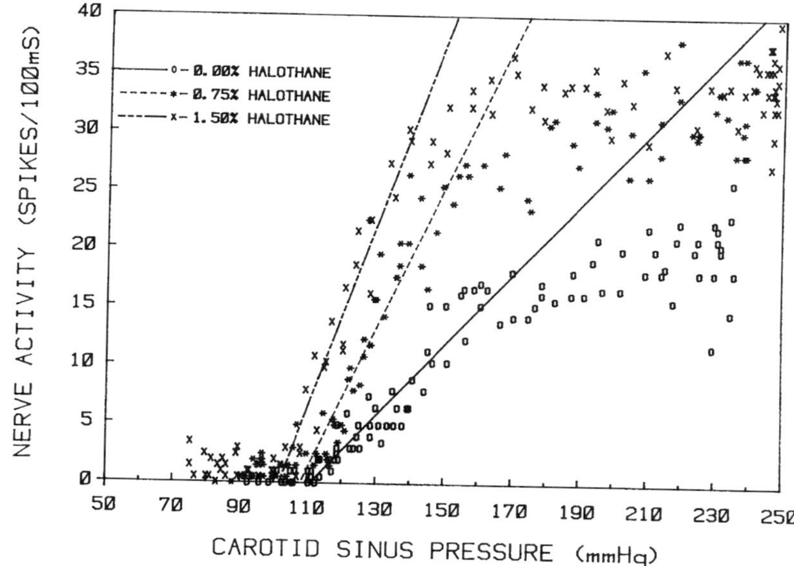

Figure 21. Graph indicating changes in carotid sinus single-fiber nerve activity (spikes/100 ms) versus increases in carotid sinus blood pressure at different levels of halothane exposure. All dogs had a basal anesthetic of sodium thiopental (25 mg/kg) and nitrous oxide. As the level of halothane increased, the sensitivity (slope) of the baroreceptor response curves increased; the curves shifted to the left, indicating a decrease in pressure threshold of the response; and the maximum firing rate of the baroreceptors increased. (Reprinted with permission from ref. 107.)

avoid this complicating factor, renal sympathetic activity was recorded in a chronic dog model in which no induction agent was used (106). At a low level of isoflurane (1.5% inspired), a baroreflex-induced increase in sympathetic activity due to the hypotension accompanying isoflurane administration was enough to prevent a significant change in sympathetic activity (Fig. 23). However, 2.5% inspired isoflurane was found to significantly depress sympathetic activity in spite of the accompanying decrease in arterial pressure. Thus, both baseline (resting) and reflex control of sympathetic outflow was altered by the higher level of anesthetic exposure.

An alternative way to examine sympathetic outflow has been the measurement of plasma levels of norepinephrine ($[NE]_p$). The assumption made when using this technique is that other factors which could alter $[NE]_p$, including uptake and metabolism of NE, are not altered by the anesthetic itself. One study (24) examining the level of $[NE]_p$ in response to administration of halothane and propofol found that $[NE]_p$ decreased in

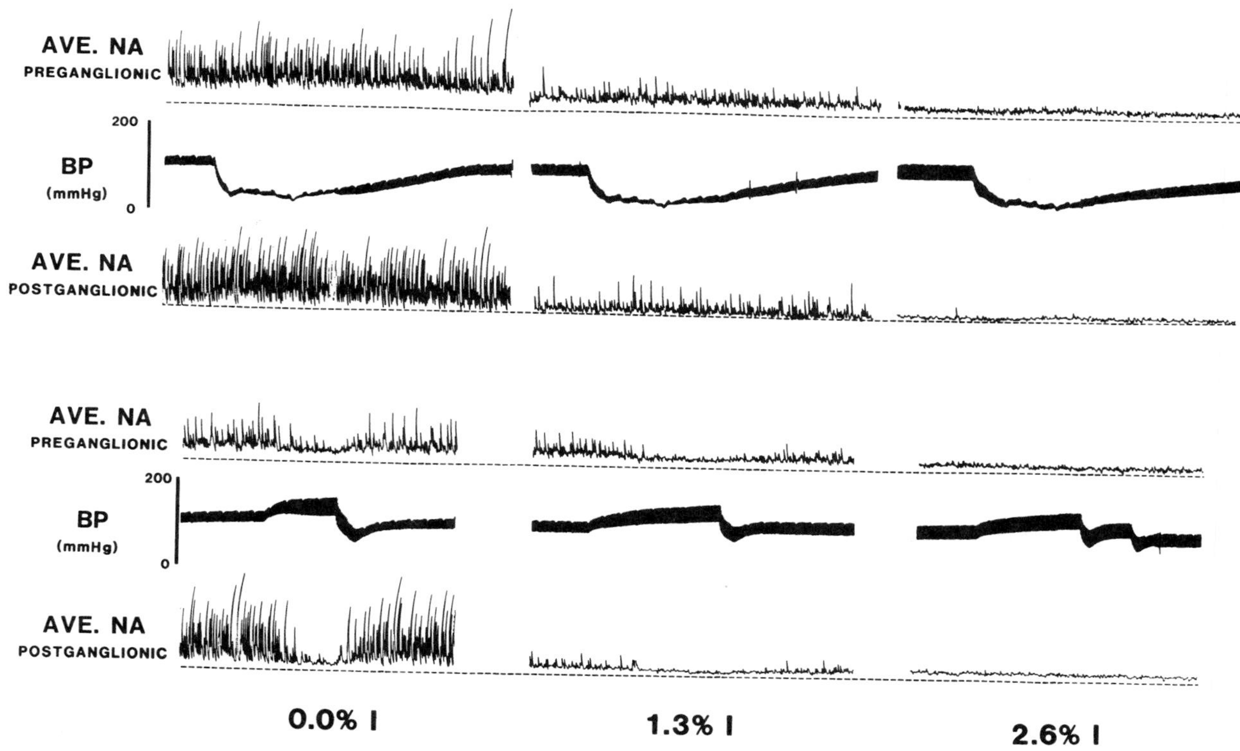

Figure 22. The baroreflex responses of sympathetic preganglionic and postganglionic nerve activities (AVE NA) to changes in pressure at 0.0%, 1.3%, and 2.6% isoflurane (I) in anesthetized dogs. All dogs were anesthetized with sodium thiopental (35 mg/kg) and had a basal level of thiopental infused at a rate of 10 mg/kg/h. Baseline levels of nerve activity were significantly less at each increasing level of isoflurane and reflex changes in nerve activity at 2.6% I were significantly attenuated compared with those at 0.0% I ($p < 0.05$). (Reprinted with permission from ref. 104.)

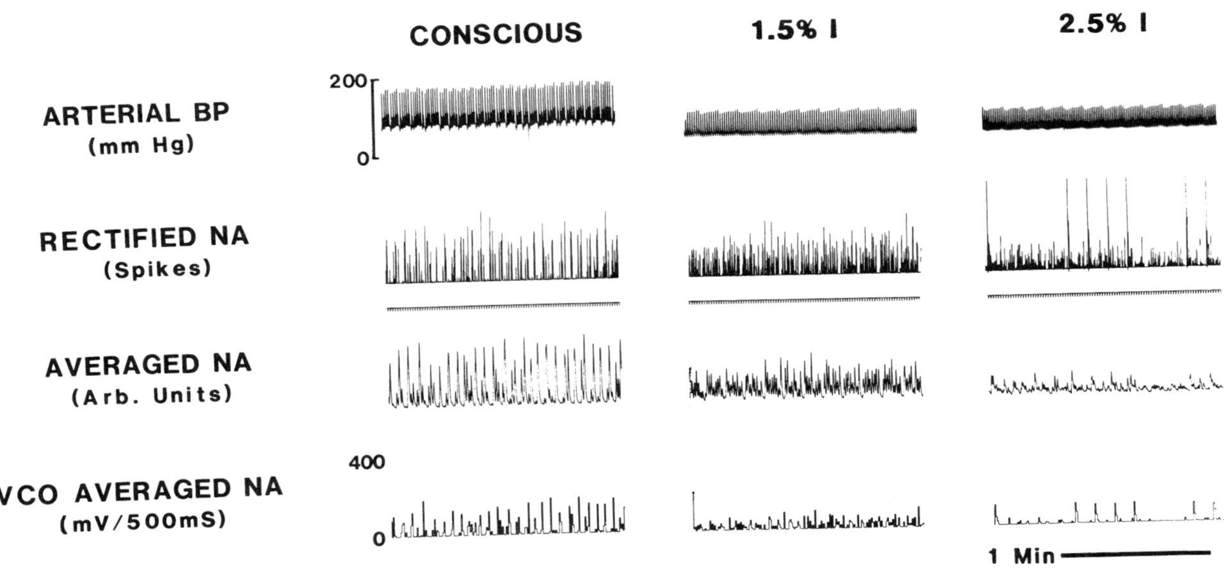

Figure 23. Baseline renal sympathetic efferent nerve activity (NA) and arterial blood pressure (BP) recorded in the conscious resting dog (*conscious*) and in the same animal anesthetized at 1.5% and 2.5% inspired isoflurane. All levels of isoflurane were maintained for 20 min prior to recording. Nerve activity was depressed at only 2.5% isoflurane, whereas blood pressure showed a dose-dependent decrease at both 1.5% and 2.5% isoflurane ($p < 0.05$). The pattern of nerve activity changed as the corresponding heart rate and pulse pressure changed during isoflurane administration. (Reprinted with permission from ref. 106.)

response to both anesthetics, with the reduction in $[NE]_P$ due to proportionally greater decreases in NE spillover than in clearance. However, halothane had a greater effect on clearance than propofol, so that decreases in $[NE]_P$ resulted from different effects of the anesthetics on NE kinetics. A similar finding was obtained in a study examining the effects of isoflurane and enflurane on NE kinetics (23). Again, both anesthetics decreased endogenous $[NE]_P$, primarily by a greater reduction in NE spillover than in clearance. Isoflurane reduced NE clearance at only the highest dose (2 MAC), while enflurane decreased clearance at both 1.0 and 1.5 MAC. Both studies demonstrated that anesthetics can vary in their mechanisms of reduction of $[NE]_P$ and therefore measurement of $[NE]_P$ alone may not give a true picture of the effects of anesthetics on sympathetic activity. Since nerve activity can be directly measured in the animal model, measurement of plasma catecholamines has not be used as much as in the human model. A thorough discussion of this technique is included in the human studies areas of this chapter.

Parasympathetic Efferent Activity Fewer studies have examined the effects of anesthetics directly on parasympathetic efferent activity. Direct recordings of parasympathetic activity have shown that halothane depresses vagal efferent activity (114). Pentobarbital was also shown to depress vagal efferent activity, in this case, to a greater extent than depression of sympathetic outflow (58). In spite of the lack of direct recordings of parasympathetic activity, many studies have indirectly examined parasympathetic activity by measuring the bradycardiac response of the heart during activation of baroreceptors by increases in arterial pressure. The attenuation of the reflex bradycardia by anesthesia found in many studies (13,92,94,100, 102,104,107,127) suggested an attenuation of parasympathetic outflow, although this response also includes the effects of the anesthetic on ganglionic transmission and the cardiac cells directly. The preferential attenuation of the tachycardic response to a decrease in blood pressure during urethane or chloralose anesthesia, without an associated decrease in the bradycardic baroreflex limb, suggested to Barringer et al. (5) that these anesthetics resulted in preferential depression of sympathetic but not parasympathetic activity. A preferential effect of diazepam was reported by Sakamoto et al. (102), who reported that diazepam attenuated the heart rate component of the baroreflex (sympathetic/parasympathetic effect) without attenuating the total peripheral resistance baroreflex response (only sympathetic limb). However, similar depression of both the depressor and pressor responses have been reported for halothane (93,94,107) and isoflurane (104), suggesting comparable depression of both autonomic outflows.

Anesthesia and Arterial Baroreflex Function in Humans

The early investigations that evaluated the effects of anesthetics on the autonomic nervous system were primarily focused on the arterial baroreceptor reflex regulation of heart rate. The studies that evaluated the effects of the inhaled anesthetics (halothane, enflurane, and isoflurane) on arterial baroreflex regulation of heart rate indicated that both halothane and enflurane had a more pronounced effect on attenuating the reflex than did isoflurane (70). In contrast, intravenous anesthesia with a combination of benzodiazepines and narcotics reduced arterial baroreflex function to a lesser degree than the inhaled agents (71).

Because of the greater difficulty in evaluating the sympathetic component of the baroreceptor reflex in humans, there is only a limited amount of information published in this area. Over the past several years, we have been employing the technique of sympathetic microneurography to directly record vasoconstrictor impulses that are directed to blood vessels within the skeletal muscles of humans. Nitrous oxide clearly increases the quantity of sympathetic traffic in human volunteers (33). Moreover, the reflex regulation of sympathetic outflow is well maintained during administration of nitrous oxide, but the reflex regulation of heart rate is significantly impaired (32). Sympathetic nerve activity has also been recorded while several of the intravenous anesthetic induction agents have been administered to patients (34,37). The administration of either thiopental or propofol leads to neural silence for a period of several minutes. Part of this sympathoinhibition may be related to the concomitant loss of consciousness. However, when etomidate is used for induction, sympathetic outflow is preserved despite a similar loss of consciousness. In addition, both thiopental and propofol appear to abolish the normal reflex sympatho-excitation associated with nitroprusside stress, whereas etomidate preserves this reflex response. Despite the remarkable sympatho-inhibition produced by thiopental and propofol, subsequent laryngoscopy and tracheal intubation elicits large increases in sympathetic traffic. This response is followed immediately by hypertension and tachycardia. Thus, the initial sympathoinhibition and hypotension produced during induction of anesthesia can be quickly reversed by proceeding to laryngoscopy and intubation in a timely manner.

REFERENCES

1. Abboud FM, Chapleau MW. Effects of pulse frequency on single-unit baroreceptor activity during sine-wave and natural pulses in dogs. *J Physiol (Lond)* 1988;401:295–308.
2. Akselrod S, Gordon D, Madwed JB, Snidman NC, Shannon DC, Cohen RJ. Hemodynamic regulation: investigation by spectral analysis. *Am J Physiol* 1985;249:H867–H875.
3. Akselrod S, Gordon D, Ubel FA, Shannon DC, Barger AC, Cohen RJ. Power spectrum analysis of heart rate fluctuation: a quantitative probe of beat-to-beat cardiovascular control. *Science* 1981;213: 220–222.
4. Andresen MC, Krauhs JM, Brown AM. Relationship of aortic wall and baroreceptor properties during development in normotensive and spontaneously hypertensive rats. *Circ Res* 1978;43:728–738.
5. Barringer DL, Bunag RD. Differential anesthetic depression of chronotropic baroreflexes in rats. *J Cardiovasc Pharmacol* 1990;15: 10–15.
6. Bell LB, Hopp FA, Seagard JL, Van Brederode JFM, Kampine JP. A continuous non-contact method for measuring in situ vascular diameter using a video camera. *J Appl Physiol* 1988;64:1279–1284.
7. Bell LB, O'Hagan KP, Clifford PS. Cardiac but not pulmonary receptors mediate depressor response to IV phenyl biguanide in conscious rabbits. *Am J Physiol* 1993;264:R1050–R1057.
8. Bell LB, Seagard JL, Zuperku EJ, Kampine JP. Mechanical effects of vasoactive drugs on carotid sinus. *Am J Physiol* 1986;250: R1074–R1080.
9. Bennett T, Farquhar IK, Hosking DJ, Hampton JR. Assessment of methods for estimating autonomic nervous control of the heart in patients with diabetes mellitus. *Diabetes* 1978;27:1167–1174.
10. Bigger JT, Hoover CA, Steinman RD, et al. Autonomic nervous system activity during myocardial ischemia in man estimated by power spectral analysis of heart period variability. *Am J Cardiol* 1990;66:497–498.
11. Bigger JT, Kleiger RE, Fleiss JL, et al. Components of heart rate variability measured during healing of acute myocardial infarction. *Am J Cardiol* 1988;61:208–215.
12. Biscoe TJ, Millar RA. The effect of halothane on carotid sinus baroreceptor activity. *J Physiol (Lond)* 1964;173:2437–2430.
13. Biscoe TJ, Millar RA. The effects of cyclopropane, halothane and ether on central baroreceptor pathways. *J Physiol (Lond)* 1966;184: 535–559.
14. Bishop VS, Hasser EM, Nair UC. Baroreflex control of renal nerve activity in conscious animals. *Circ Res* 1987;61:I76–I81.
15. Bosnjak ZJ, Seagard JL, Wu A, Kampine JP. The effects of halothane on sympathetic ganglionic transmission. *Anesthesiology* 1982;57:473–479.
16. Brown AM, Saum WR, Tuley FH. A comparison of aortic baroreceptor discharge in normotensive and spontaneously hypertensive rats. *Circ Res* 1976;39:488–496.
17. Chen HI, Chapleau MW, McDowell TS, Abboud FM. Prostaglandins contribute to activation of baroreceptors in rabbits—possible paracrine influence of endothelium. *Circ Res* 1990; 67:1394–1404.
18. Coleridge HM, Coleridge JCG, Luck JC, Norman J. The effect of four volatile anaesthetic agents on the impulse activity of two types of pulmonary receptor. *Br J Anaesth* 1968;40:484.
19. Cox RH, Bagshaw RJ. Influence of anesthesia on the response to carotid hypotension in dogs. *Am J Physiol* 1979;237:H424–H432.
20. Cox RH, Bagshaw RJ. Effects of anesthesia on carotid sinus reflex control of arterial hemodynamics in the dog. *Am J Physiol* 1980; 239:H681–H6691.
21. Craelius W, Akay M, Tangella M. Heart rate variability as an index of autonomic imbalance in patients with recent myocardial infarction. *Med Biol Eng Comput* 1992;30:385–388.
22. Deegan R, He HB, Wood AJJ, Wood M. Effects of anesthesia on norepinephrine kinetics. *Anesthesiology* 1991;75:481–488.
23. Deegan R, He HB, Wood AJJ, Wood M. Effect of enflurane and isoflurane on norepinephrine kinetics: a new approach to assessment of sympathetic function during anesthesia. *Anesth Analg* 1993;77:49–54.
24. Deegan RD, He HB, Wood AJJ, Wood M. Effects of anesthesia on norepinephrine kinetics: comparison of propofol and halothane anesthesia in dogs. *Anesthesiology* 1991;75:481–488.
25. Delius W, Hagbarth KE, Hongell A, Wallin BG. Manoeuvres affecting sympathetic outflow in human muscle nerves. *Acta Physiol Scand* 1972;84:82–94.
26. Delius W, Hagbarth KE, Hongell A, Wallin BG. Manoeuvres affecting sympathetic outflow in human skin nerves. *Acta Physiol Scand* 1972;84:177–186.
27. Donchin J, Constantini S, Szold A, Byrne EA, Porges SW. Cardiac vagal tone predicts outcome in neurosurgical patients. *Crit Care Med* 1992;20:942–949.
28. Donoghue S, Felder RB, Jordan D, Spyer KM. The central projections of carotid baroreceptors and chemoreceptors in the cat: a neurophysiological study. *J Physiol (Lond)* 1984;347:397–409.
29. Dorward PK, Andresen MC, Burke SL, Oliver JR, Korner PI. Rapid resetting of th aortic baroreceptors in the rabbit and its implications for short-term and longer term reflex control. *Circ Res* 1982;50:428–439.
30. Dorward PK, Bell LB, Rudd CD. Cardiac afferents attenuate renal sympathetic baroreceptor reflexes during acute hypertension. *Hypertension* 1990;16:131–139.
31. Dorward PK, Riedel W, Burke SL, Gipps J, Korner PI. The renal sympathetic baroreflex in the rabbit—arterial and cardiac baroreceptor influences, resetting, and effect of anesthesia. *Circ Res* 1985;57:618–633.
32. Ebert TJ. Differential effects of nitrous oxide on baroreflex control of heart rate and peripheral sympathetic nerve activity in humans. *Anesthesiology* 1990;72:16–22.
33. Ebert TJ, Kampine JP. Nitrous oxide augments sympathetic outflow: direct evidence from human peroneal nerve recordings. *Anesth Analg* 1989;69:444–449.
34. Ebert TJ, Kanitz DD, Kampine JP. Inhibition of sympathetic neural outflow during thiopental anesthesia in humans. *Anesth Analg* 1990;71:319–326.
35. Ebert TJ, Kotrly KJ, Madsen KS, Bernstein JS, Kampine JP. Fentanyl-diazepam anesthesia with or without N_2O does not attenuate cardiopulmonary baroreflex-mediated vasoconstrictor responses to controlled hypovolemia in humans. *Anesth Analg* 1988;67: 548–554.
36. Ebert TJ, Kotrly KJ, Vucins EJ, Zainer CM, Kampine JP. Effect of halothane anesthesia on cardiopulmonary baroreflex function in man. *Anesthesiology* 1985;63:668–674.
37. Ebert TJ, Muzi M, Berens R, Goff D, Kampine JP. Sympathetic responses to induction of anesthesia in humans with propofol or etomidate. *Anesthesiology* 1992;76:725–733.
38. Eckberg D. Parasympathetic cardiovascular control in human disease: a critical review of methods and results. *Am J Physiol* 1980;239:H581–H593.
39. Eckberg DL. Adaptation of the human carotid baroreceptor-cardiac reflex. *J Physiol (Lond)* 1977;269:579–589.
40. Eckberg DL. Baroreflex inhibition of the human sinus node: importance of stimulus intensity, duration, and rate of pressure change. *J Physiol (Lond)* 1977;269:561–577.
41. Eckberg DL. Human sinus arrhythmia as an index of vagal cardiac outflow. *J Appl Physiol* 1983;54:961–966.
42. Eckberg DL, Cavanaugh MS, Mark AL, Abboud FM. A simplified neck suction device for activation of carotid baroreceptors. *J Lab Clin Med* 1975;85:167–173.
43. Eckberg DL, Fritsch JM. How should human baroreflexes be tested? *NIPS* 1993;8:7–12.
44. Epstein RA, Wang H-H, Bartelstone HJ. The effects of halothane on circulatory reflexes of the dog. *Anesthesiology* 1968;29:867–876.
45. Ernsting J, Parry DJ. Some observations on the effects of stimulating the stretch receptors in the carotid artery of man. *J Physiol (Lond)* 1957;137:45P–46P.

46. Esler M, Jennings G, Korner P, Blombery P, Sacharias N, Leonard P. Measurement of total and organ-specific norepinephrine kinetics in humans. *Am J Physiol* 1984;247:E21–E28.
47. Esler M, Jennings G, Korner P, et al. Assessment of human sympathetic nervous system activity from measurements of norepinephrine turnover. *Hypertension* 1988;3:3–20.
48. Esler M, Jennings G, Lambert G, Meredith I, Horne M, Eisenhofer G. Overflow of catecholamine neurotransmitters to the circulation: source, fate, and functions. *Physiol Rev* 1990;70:963–985.
49. Felder RB, Heesch CM, Thames MD. Reflex modulation of carotid sinus baroreceptor activity in the dog. *Am J Physiol* 1983;244:H437–H447.
50. Fouad FM, Tarazi RC, Ferrario CM, Fighaly S, Alicandri C. Assessment of parasympathetic control of heart rate by a noninvasive method. *Am J Physiol* 1984;246:H838–H842.
51. Fritsch JM, Smith ML, Simmons DTF, Eckberg DL. Differential baroreflex modulation of human vagal and sympathetic activity. *Am J Physiol* 1991;260:R635–R641.
52. Grossman P, Karemaker J, Wieling W. Prediction of tonic parasympathetic cardiac control using respiratory sinus arrhythmia: the need for respiratory control. *Psychophysiology* 1991;28:201–216.
53. Grossman P, Kollai M. Respiratory sinus arrhythmia, cardiac vagal tone, and respiration: within- and between-individual relations. *Psychophysiology* 1993;30:486–495.
54. Grossman SH, Davis D, Gunnells JC, Shand DG. Plasma norepinephrine in the evaluation of baroreceptor function in humans. *Hypertension* 1982;4:566–571.
55. Hagbarth K-E, Vallbo AB. Pulse and respiratory grouping of sympathetic impulses in human muscle nerves. *Acta Physiol Scand* 1968;74:96–108.
56. Hagbarth KE, Hallin RG, Hongell A, Torebjork HE, Wallin BG. General characteristics of sympathetic activity in human skin nerves. *Acta Physiol Scand* 1972;84:164–176.
57. Hainsworth R. Reflexes from the heart. *Physiol Rev* 1991;71: 617–658.
58. Halinen MO, Hakumaki MOK, Sarajas HSS. Suppression of autonomic postganglioninc discharges by pentobarbital in dogs, with or without endotoxemia. *Acta Physiol Scand* 1978;104:167–174.
59. Hayano J, Sakakibara Y, Yamada A, et al. Accuracy of assessment of cardiac vagal tone by heart rate variability in normal subjects. *Am J Cardiol* 1991;67:199–204.
60. Hopp FA, Seagard JL, Kampine JP. Comparison of four methods of averaging nerve activity. *Am J Physiol* 1986;251:R700–R711.
61. Huang BS, Leenen HH. Dietary Na, age, and baroreflex control of heart rate and renal sympathetic nerve activity in rats. *Am J Physiol* 1992;262:H1441–H1448.
62. Hughes RL, MacKenzie JE. An investigation of the centrally and peripherally mediated cardiovascular effects of etomidate in the rabbit. *Br J Anaesth* 1978;50:101–106.
63. Inoue K, Miyake S, Kumashiro M, Ogata H, Ueta T, Akatsu T. Power spectral analysis of blood pressure variability in traumatic quadriplegic humans. *Am J Physiol* 1991;260:H842–H847.
64. Johnson JM, Rowell LB, Niederberger M, Eisman Mm. Human splanchnic and forearm vasoconstrictor responses to reductions of right atrial and aortic pressures. *Circ Res* 1974;34:515–524.
65. Kamijo Y, Goto H, Nakazawa K, Benson KT, Arakawa K. Arterial baroreflex attenuation during and after continuous propofol infusion. *Can J Anaesth* 1992;39:987–991.
66. Kardon MB, Peterson DF, Bishop VS. Reflex heart rate control via specific aortic nerve afferents in the rabbit. *Circ Res* 1975;37:41–47.
67. Katona PG, Jih F. Respiratory sinus arrhythmia: noninvasive measure of parasympathetic cardiac control. *J Appl Physiol* 1975;39: 801–805.
68. Kollai M, Mizsei G. Respiratory sinus arrhythmia is a limited measure of cardiac parasympathetic control in man. *J Physiol* 1990;424: 329–342.
69. Korner PI, West MJ, Shaw J, Uther JB. "Steady-state" properties of the baroreceptor-heart rate reflex in essential hypertension in man. *Clin Exp Pharmacol Physiol* 1974;1:65–76.
70. Kotrly KJ, Ebert TJ, Vucins EJ, Igler FO, Kampine JP. Human baroreceptor control of heart rate under isoflurane anesthesia. *Anesthesiology* 1984;60:173–179.
71. Kotrly KJ, Ebert TJ, Vucins EJ, Roerig DL, Stadnicka A, Kampine JP. Effects of fentanyl-diazepam-nitrous oxide anaesthesia on arterial baroreflex control of heart rate in man. *Br J Anaesth* 1986;58: 406–414.
72. Kunze DL. Calcium and magnesium sensitivity of the carotid baroreceptor reflex in cats. *Circ Res* 1979;45:815–821.
73. Kunze DL. Acute resetting of baroreceptor reflex in rabbits: a central component. *Am J Physiol* 1986;250:H866–H870.
74. Ludbrook J, Mancia G, Ferrari A, Zanchetti A. Factors influencing the carotid baroreceptor response to pressure changes in a neck chamber. *Clin Sci Mol Med* 1976;51:347s–349s.
75. Machado BH, Bonagamba LGH, Castania JA, Menani JV. Changes in vascular resistance during carotid occlusion in normal and baroreceptor-denervated rats. *Hypertension* 1992;19:II-149–II-153.
76. Malliani A, Pagani M, Lombardi F, Cerutti S. Cardiovascular neural regulation explored in the frequency domain. *Circulation* 1991;84:482–492.
77. Mancia G, Ferrari A, Gregorini L, et al. Plasma catecholamines do not invariably reflect sympathetically induced changes in blood pressure in man. *Clin Sci* 1983;65:227–235.
78. Mancia G, Mark AL. Arterial baroreflexes in humans. *Handbook Physiol* 1983;3:755–793.
79. Mark AL. The Bezold-Jarisch reflex revisited: clinical implications of inhibitory reflexes originating in the heart. *J Am Coll Cardiol* 1983;1:90–102.
80. Mark AL, Mancia G. Cardiopulmonary baroreflexes in humans. *Handbook Physiol* 1983;3:795–813.
81. McDowell TS, Axtelle TS, Chapleau MW, Abboud FM. Prostaglandins in carotid sinus enhance baroreflex in rabbits. *Am J Physiol* 1989;257:R445–R450.
82. Meredith IT, Eisenhofer G, Lambert GW, Jennings GL, Thompson J, Esler MD. Plasma norepinephrine responses to head-up tilt are misleading in autonomic failure. *Hypertension* 1992;19:628–633.
83. Millar RA, Biscoe TJ. Preganglionic sympathetic activity and the effects of anaesthetics. *Br J Anaesth* 1965;37:804–832.
84. Munch PA, Iwazumi T, Brown AM. Photoelectric caliper for noncontact mesurement of vascular dynamic strain in vitro. *J Appl Physiol* 1985;58:2075–2081.
85. Muzi M, Ebert TJ. Quantification of heart rate variability with power spectral analysis. *Curr Opin Anesthesiol* 1993;6:3–17.
86. Ngai SH, Bolme P. Effects of anesthetics on circulatory regulatory mechanisms in the dog. *J Pharmacol Exp Ther* 1966;153:495–504.
87. Ogawa A, Uemura M, Kataoka Y, Ol K, Inokuchi T. Effects of ketamine on cardiovascular responses mediated by *N*-methyl-D-aspartate receptor in the rat nucleus tractus solitarius. *Anesthesiology* 1993;78:163–167.
88. Peiss CN, Manning JW. Effects of sodium pentobarbital on electrical and reflex activation of the cardiovascular system. *Circ Res* 1964;14:228–235.
89. Pelletier CL, Clement DL, Sheperd JT. Comparison of afferent activity of canine aortic and sinus nerves. *Circ Res* 1972;31: 557–568.
90. Philbrick/Nexus Research. *Applications manual for operational amplifiers*. Dedham, MA: Teledyne, 1968.
91. Pomeranz B, Macaulay RJB, Caudill MA, et al. Assessment of autonomic function in humans by heart rate spectral analysis. *Am J Physiol* 1985;248:H151–H153.
92. Priano LL, Bernards C, Marrone B. Effect of anesthetic induction agents on cardiovascular neuroregulation in dogs. *Anesth Analg* 1989;68:344–349.
93. Price HL, Linde HW, Morse HT. Central nervous actions of halothane affecting the systemic circulation. *Anesthesiology* 1963; 24:770–778.
94. Price HL, Price ML, Morse HT. Effects of cyclopropane, halothane and procaine on the vasomotor "center" of the dog. *Anesthesiology* 1965;26:55–60.
95. Price HL, Widdicombe J. Actions of cyclopropane on carotid sinus baroreceptors and carotid body chemoreceptors. *J Pharmacol Exp Ther* 1962;35:233–239.
96. Raczkowska M, Ebert TJ, Eckberg DL. Muscarinic cholinergic receptors modulate vagal cardiac responses in man. *J Auton Nerv Syst* 1983;7:271–278.
97. Randall DC, Brown DR, Raisch RM, Yingling JD, Randall WC. SA nodal parasympathectomy delineates autonomic control of heart rate power spectrum. *Am J Physiol* 1991;260:H985–H988.
98. Rigel DF, Lipson D, Katona PG. Excess tachycardia: heart rate after antimuscarinic agents in conscious dogs. *Am J Physiol* 1984;246:H168–H173.
99. Robertson JD, Swan AAB, Whitteridge D. Effect of anaesthetics on systemic baroreceptors. *J Physiol (Lond)* 1956;131:463–472.

100. Rocchiccioli C, Saad MAA, Elghozi J-L. Attenuation of the baroreceptor reflex by propofol anesthesia in the rat. *J Cardiovasc Pharmacol* 1989;14:631–635.
101. Roddie IC, Shepherd JT, Whelan RF. Reflex changes in vasoconstrictor tone in human skeletal muscle in response to stimulation of receptors in a low-pressure area of the intrathoracic vascular bed. *J Physiol* 1957;139:369–376.
102. Sakamoto M, Ohsumi H, Okumura F. Effects of diazepam on the carotid sinus baroreflex control of circulation in rabbits. *Acta Physiol Scand* 1990;139:281–287.
103. Seagard JL, Bosnjak ZJ, Hopp FA, Kotrly C, Ebert T, Kampine JP. Cardiovascular effects of general anesthesia. In: Covino BG, Fozzard HA, Rehder K, Strichartz G, eds. *Effects of anesthesia.* Bethesda: American Physiological Society/Williams & Wilkins, 1985:149–178.
104. Seagard JL, Elegbe EO, Hopp FA, et al. Effects of isoflurane on the baroreceptor reflex. *Anesthesiology* 1983;59:511–520.
105. Seagard JL, Hopp FA, Bosnjak ZJ, Elegebe EO, Kampine JP. Extent and mechanism of halothane sensitization of the carotid sinus baroreceptors. *Anesthesiology* 1983;58:432–437.
106. Seagard JL, Hopp FA, Bosnjak ZJ, Osborn JL, Kampine JP. Sympathetic efferent nerve activity in conscious and isoflurane-anesthetized dogs. *Anesthesiology* 1984;61:266–270.
107. Seagard JL, Hopp FA, Donegan JH, Kalbfleisch JH, Kampine JP. Halothane and the carotid sinus reflex: evidence for multiple sites of action. *Anesthesiology* 1982;57:191–202.
108. Seagard JL, Van Brederode JFM, Dean C, Hopp FA, Gallenberg LA, Kampine JP. Firing characteristics of single-fiber carotid sinus baroreceptors. *Circ Res* 1990;66:1499–1509.
109. Sellgren J, Biber B, Henriksson B-A, Martner J, Ponten J. The effects of propofol, methohexitone and isoflurane on the baroreceptor reflex in the cat. *Acta Anaesthesiol Scand* 1992;36:784–790.
110. Shoukas AA, Callahan CA, Lash JM, Haase EB. New technique to completely isolate carotid sinus baroreceptor regions in the rat. *Am J Physiol* 1991;260:H300–H303.
111. Skovsted P, Price HL. the effects of ethrane on arterial pressure, preganglionic sympathetic activity, and barostatic reflexes. *Anesthesiology* 1972;36:257–262.
112. Skovsted P, Price ML, Price HL. The effects of halothane on arterial pressure, preganglionic sympathetic activity and barostatic reflexes. *Anesthesiology* 1969;31:507–514.
113. Skovsted P, Price ML, Price HL. The effects of short-acting barbiturates on arterial pressure, preganglionic sympathetic activity and barostatic reflexes. *Anesthesiology* 1970;33:10–18.
114. Skovsted P, Sapthavichaikul S. The effects of isoflurane on arterial pressure, pulse rate, autonomic nervous activity, and barostatic reflexes. *Can Anaesth Soc J* 1977;24:304–314.
115. Slogoff S, Allen GW. The role of baroreceptors in the cardiovascular response to ketamine. *Anesth Analg* 1974;53:704–707.
116. Smyth HS, Sleight P, Pickering GW. Reflex regulation of arterial pressure during sleep in man. *Circ Res* 1969;24:109–121.
117. Spickler J, Kezdi P. Probability of spike summations in baroreceptor electroneurogram. *J Appl Physiol* 1969;27.
118. Sprenkle JM, Eckberg DL, Goble RL, Schelhorn JJ, Halliday HC. Device for rapid quantification of human carotid baroreceptor-cardiac reflex responses. *J Appl Physiol* 1986;60:727–732.
119. Stephenson RB, Donald DE. Reversible vascular isolation of carotid sinuses in conscious dogs. *Am J Physiol* 1980;238:H809–H814.
120. Sundlof G, Wallin BG. Effect of lower body negative pressure on human muscle nerve sympathetic activity. *J Physiol* 1978;278:525–532.
121. Taneyama C, Goto H, Kohno N, Benson KT, Sasao J-I, Arakawa K. Effects of fentanyl, diazepam, and the combination of both on arterial baroreflex and sympathetic nerve activity in intact and baro-denervated dogs. *Anesth Analg* 1993;77:44–48.
122. Thoren P, Saum WR, Brown AM. Characteristics of rat aortic baroreceptors with nonmedullated afferent nerve fibers. *Circ Res* 1977;40:231–237.
123. Undresser KP, Jing-Yun P, Lynn MP, Bishop VS. Baroreflex control of sympathetic nerve activity after elevations of pressure in conscious rabbits. *Am J Physiol* 1985;248:H827–H834.
124. Van Leeuwen AF, Evans RG, Ludbrook J. Effects of halothane, ketamine, propofol and alfentanil anaesthesia on circulatory control in rabbits. *Clin Exp Pharmacol Physiol* 1990;17:781–798.
125. Walgenbach SC, Donald DE. Inhibition by carotid baroreflex of exercise-induced increase in arterial pressure. *Circ Res* 1983;52:253–262.
126. Wallin BG, Fagius J. Peripheral sympathetic neural activity in conscious humans. *Annu Rev Physiol* 1988;50:565–576.
127. Wear R, Robinson S, Gregory GA. The effect of halothane on the baroresponse of adult and baby rabbits. *Anesthesiology* 1982;56:188–191.
128. Weinstock M, Korner PI, Head GA, Dorward PK. Differentiation of cardiac baroreflex properties by cuff and drug methods in two rabbit strains. *Am J Physiol* 1988;255:R654–R664.
129. Whitteridge D. Effect of anaesthetics on mechanical receptors. *Br Med Bull* 1958;14:5–7.
130. Wilkinson PL, Stowe DF, Tyberg JV. Heart rate-systemic blood pressure relationship in dogs during halothane anesthesia. *Acta Anaesthesiol Scand* 1980;24:181–186.
131. Wolthuis R, Hoffler G, Baker J. Improved waist seal design for use with lower body negative pressure (LBNP) devices. *Aerospace Med* 1971;42:461–462.
132. Zoller RP, Mark AL, Abboud FM, Schmid PG, Heistad DD. The role of low pressure baroreceptors in reflex vasoconstrictor responses in man. *J Clin Invest* 1972;51:2967–2972.
133. Zucker IH, Chen J, Wang W. Renal sympathetic nerve and hemodynamic responses to captopril in conscious dogs: role of prostaglandins. *Am J Physiol* 1991;260:H260–H266.

D

THE RESPIRATORY SYSTEM

Anesthesia: Biologic Foundations, edited by Tony L. Yaksh et al. Lippincott–Raven Publishers, Philadelphia © 1997.

CHAPTER 73

PULMONARY SURFACTANT

JOANNA FLOROS AND DAVID S. PHELPS

HISTORICAL PERSPECTIVE

Pulmonary surfactant, a lipoprotein complex, is essential for normal lung function. It lowers the surface tension at the air-liquid interface in the alveolus and prevents alveolar collapse at low lung volumes. Deficiency of surfactant in the prematurely born infant can result in respiratory distress syndrome, a condition that can be associated with significant morbidity and mortality.

Pulmonary surfactant research can be thought of as comprising two major phases. The first phase of research includes the initial description of surfactant and the demonstration of its importance, as well as the identification of some of the hormones involved in its regulation. The second phase is centered around the success of surfactant therapy in clinical trials. Surfactants used in these trials included several preparations containing surfactant proteins in addition to lipids. The realization that the surfactant proteins are essential for function started the modern era of surfactant research with its emphasis on the study of the surfactant proteins.

Phase one began when the importance of surface tension in lung function was first reported by von Neergaard (322) in 1929. After a long period of dormancy in the field, the first observations on the nature of the alveolar lining material and its appearance late in gestation were reported in the mid-1950s (186,225). In 1957 Clements (48), by performing dynamic surface tension measurements, concluded that surfactant was an antiatelectasis factor. The clinical relevance of these observations became clear when in 1959 Avery and Mead (10) showed that extracts from lungs of infants that died from respiratory distress syndrome (RDS) or hyaline membrane disease, were less capable of reducing surface tension in vitro than lung extracts from infants who died from other causes. They suggested that the infants with RDS lacked surfactant and that this deficiency resulted in the extracts exhibiting a higher than normal surface tension. This increase in surface tension in the intact lung would increase the work of breathing by resisting inflation and causing atelectasis on expiration. In 1961 several groups of investigators further characterized surfactant by describing it as a lipoprotein (35,155,226). An association between the presence of osmiophilic bodies or surfactant-containing organelles (later known as lamellar bodies) and low surface tension in fetal mouse lung was suggested by Buchingham and Avery (36) in 1962. In 1964 the first evidence for the secretion of the osmiophilic bodies and for their potential extracellular function was presented (20).

The remainder of the first phase of surfactant research was dominated by studies of the regulation of surfactant production. The notion that fetal lung maturation might be under hormonal control was first advanced by Buckingham and coworkers (37). In the course of studying the role of hormones in parturition, Liggins (179) observed that when pregnant ewes were treated with glucocorticoids, alveolar aeration in the prematurely delivered lambs was markedly increased as compared to untreated lambs of similar gestational age. He suggested that this finding may be due to the precocious appearance of surfactant resulting from maternal glucocorticoid treatment. Liggins' suggestion was soon confirmed in fetal lamb (64) and in fetal rabbit (304), as well as in the first clinical trial showing that glucocorticoid treatment could reduce the incidence of RDS in prematurely born babies (180). Since that time, numerous studies have been carried out attempting to understand the mechanism of action of glucocorticoids in the regulation of surfactant components and to identify other hormones or agents involved in the regulation of surfactant. Today the clinical use of glucocorticoids is accepted as one form of therapy in premature labor. Its effects on surfactant production and in lung maturity in general are described elsewhere (52,267).

The second phase of surfactant research opened with the first successful clinical trial of an effective surfactant replacement preparation by Fujiwara and associates (93) in 1980. This study began the modern era of surfactant research and ended a long, frustrating period during which investigators were unable to reproduce the action of native surfactant in vivo. The presence of surfactant-associated proteins in Fujiwara's preparation suggested that these proteins were important for surfactant function and led to a flurry of research activity culminating in the characterization of these proteins and the cloning of their genes. Currently, the powerful tools of molecular biology and genetics are being used to gain insight into the regulation of gene expression of the individual surfactant proteins and other surfactant components. Some of the goals of these studies are to understand why some prematurely born infants develop RDS and others do not, and to explore the role of the surfactant proteins in pulmonary disorders other than neonatal RDS. Today surfactant replacement preparations containing surfactant proteins or other substances that mimic the actions of the proteins are widely used to treat neonatal RDS.

Since there has been enormous growth in the literature on virtually all aspects of surfactant research in recent years, and given the space constraints of this chapter, we will attempt to summarize the knowledge that has shaped the second phase of surfactant research. Areas for which recent reviews are available will not be discussed here in any detail. The reader may consult published reviews in the following areas for additional information: regulation of surfactant phospholipid synthesis and storage (17); surfactant secretion (40,190,347); surfactant clearance (351,352); and the role of surfactant in adult respiratory distress syndrome and other diseases (120,177,282).

WHAT IS SURFACTANT?

Pulmonary surfactant, produced by the type II alveolar epithelial cells, is very complex from several points of view. Biochemically, it consists of several types of lipids and proteins. Its biochemical composition has been determined by analyzing the material obtained from bronchoalveolar lavage or lung homogenates after purification by centrifugation through gradients of sucrose or sodium bromide (153,283). Surfactant prepared in this way from a number of species consists of about 90% lipid and 10% protein. The major constitutents of human surfactant are graphically depicted in Fig. 1 (283). Nearly 90% of the lipid fraction is phospholipid, 80% of which is phosphatidylcholine (PC). Most of the PC is dipalmitoylphosphatidylcholine (DPPC), a key ingredient involved in the reduction of surface tension. Phosphatidylglycerol (PG) is the second most abundant phospholipid in surfactant, constituting roughly 10% of the total phospholipid content. The percentage of PG and the nature of its constituent fatty acid

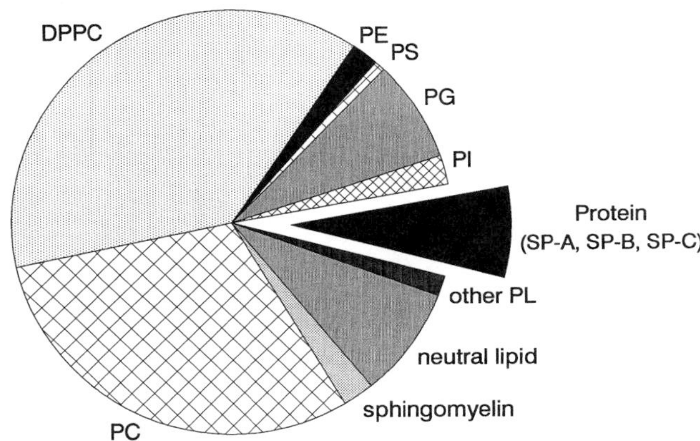

Figure 1. Composition of human pulmonary surfactant. The relative amounts of the various components in purified human pulmonary surfactant are depicted (283). DPPC, dipalmitoyl phosphatidylcholine; PC, phosphatidylcholine; PG, phosphatidylglycerol; PE, phosphatidylethanolamine; PS, phosphatidylserine; PI, phosphatidylinositol; PL, phospholipid.

subgroups vary considerably from species to species and during fetal lung development. An inverse relationship is usually observed between the levels of phosphatidylglycerol and phosphatidylinositol, another acidic phospholipid, during the course of development. The precise function of these lipids in surfactant is not known. The remainder of the phospholipid fraction consists of phosphatidylethanolamine (PE), phosphatidylserine (PS), and other phospholipids. The nonphosphorylated lipid fraction consists of neutral lipids (primarily cholesterol) and triglycerides (248). Arachidonate derivatives have been identified in surfactant during fetal development, raising the possibility that surfactant provides substrate for prostaglandin synthesis (23,204).

The protein fraction of surfactant consists of serum proteins and several other proteins that are specific to pulmonary surfactant. Of the surfactant-associated proteins (SPs), SP-A, SP-B, and SP-C are known to play important roles in the biology of surfactant. A fourth protein known as SP-D has not been shown to be involved in the surface tension-lowering function of surfactant and only a small fraction of it co-isolates with the other surfactant components. These proteins are discussed in detail below.

Structurally, surfactant is dynamic and assumes several morphologic forms during its life span in the type II alveolar cell and in the hypophase, a very thin layer of liquid that covers the alveolar surface (Fig. 2). Electron microscopic studies of the major surfactant structures associated with its anabolic pathway have identified intracellular lamellar bodies and extracellular lamellar bodies. The latter can be transformed to a lattice-like structure called tubular myelin (274). This transition is elegantly depicted in Fig. 3 and discussed in more detail elsewhere (360). Tubular myelin is thought to be the precursor of the active form of surfactant (the surface monolayer or surface film) that is found at the air/liquid interface of the alveolus (187). This structural diversity of surfactant results in considerable heterogeneity of material isolated from the alveolus. Attempts to obtain more homogeneous fractions for biochemical studies have led to the fractionation of surfactant using a variety of protocols (101,187,349,356). In each case, the heavier or more sedimentable fractions were shown to have a greater ability to reduce surface tension (i.e., more surface active) than less dense fractions. The heavier or more sedimentable fractions also have a higher protein-to-phospholipid ratio or contain higher amounts of the surfactant proteins. Morphologic analysis showed that heavier fractions were rich in tubular myelin and/or lamellar bodies (187). Lighter fractions containing disc-like material (a form of surfactant seen only in vitro) were protein poor, contained virtually no tubular myelin or lamellar bodies, and were less surface active (349).

In some cases precursor-product relationships between fractions could be demonstrated (187,356), such as the conversion of lamellar bodies to tubular myelin (91) and tubular myelin to vesicular forms. The latter change appears to require the action of a serine protease, suggesting the involvement of proteins in the transformation process (102). To study these conversions, a clever in vitro method has been devised to alternately vary the surface area of the solution to mimic surface area changes that occur during respiration. This cycling method, which simply involves rotating a surfactant-containing tube end-over-end, results in functional, biochemical, and morphologic changes in the surfactant (101,102), resembling those occurring in vivo (187,349,356).

Given the structural complexity of surfactant, one can appreciate that the typical biochemical compositional analysis of surfactant at a steady state is an averaged value derived from the multiple pools being sampled. In addition, the composition and physical and structural characteristics of surfactant differ during fetal lung development (72,248) and in disease states. The disease-related changes have been the subject of recent reviews (120,177) and will be briefly discussed in subsequent sections.

Functionally, surfactant is very complex as some of its components play multiple roles. The surfactant proteins, in particular, play important roles in the structure, function, and metabolism of surfactant as well as in the local host defense of the lung. Furthermore, genetic variation in the surfactant protein genes has also been revealed. The potential contribution of this variation to the regulation and/or function of the surfactant proteins under normal and disease states remains to be determined. The details of surfactant protein functions and of the genetic variation are presented under surfactant proteins.

METHODS AND MODELS USED TO STUDY SURFACTANT FUNCTION

Pulmonary surfactant is typically defined as the material that lines the alveolar surface of the lungs and lowers surface tension at the air/liquid interface of the alveolus. This action prevents the collapse of the alveoli at end-expiration and facilitates expansion on inspiration. Several methods and models have been employed to study the biophysical properties of surfactant, such as the reduction of surface tension, the ability to spread, the rate of adsorption, and various other respiratory measurements (reviewed in ref. 262).

In Vitro Systems

In vitro systems include surface balances, the pulsating bubble surfactometer, and others. Surface balances based on the techniques of Langmuir and Wilhelmy are used to measure the surface tension of a film as it is alternately compressed and expanded, simulating the changes of alveolar surface area during respiration (159). In dynamic surface balance measurements, a good surfactant can achieve low surface tensions of less than 10mN/m or 10–12 dynes/cm. The pulsating bubble surfactometer (76,78) mimics an alveolus. It correlates pressure and volume changes of a single bubble formed in a liquid phase and subjected to 20 oscillations per minute to simulate a normal respiratory rate. Using this instrument, a good surfactant reduces surface tension to near zero when the bubble is at minimal size (76,78). Newer versions of the surfactometer allow the solution around the bubble to be changed, enabling assessment of the effect of various proteins or other materials on the surface tension-lowering activity of

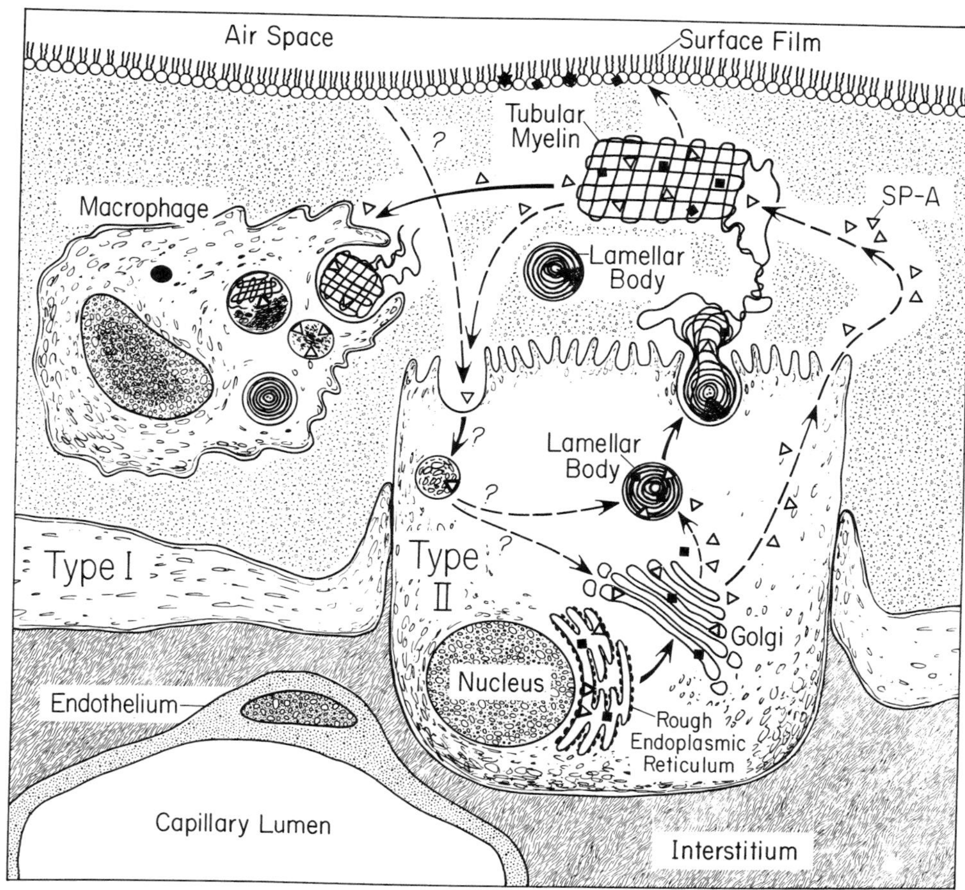

Figure 2. Life cycle of surfactant. This schematic representation depicts some of the steps in the life cycle of pulmonary surfactant. Lamellar bodies are noted both inside the type II cell and extracellularly in the hypophase. Extracellular lamellar bodies unravel to form tubular myelin, which is thought to give rise to the surface film, the active form of surfactant. An alveolar macrophage is shown in the hypophase. In addition to their involvement in the clearance of particles and pathogens, macrophages can ingest various forms of surfactant. *Triangles* in lamellar bodies, in tubular myelin, and in other locations denote SP-A. SP-A secretion is shown to follow two pathways (one via LB secretion and the other independent of LB secretion). *Squares* denote SP-B. *Stars* in the surface film denote SP-C.

surfactant (78). Both the surface balance and the bubble surfactometer allow surface tension to be tested as the area of the surface is varied, theoretically providing information about the effectiveness of a surfactant throughout the respiratory cycle (159). The adsorption characteristics or rate at which surfactant phospholipids adsorb at the surface of the air-liquid interface can also be determined with these methods.

Additional methodologies include the captive bubble method to measure adsorption, hysteresis, and surface tension (277) and methods of assessing functional surfactant levels in amniotic fluid (45,338). The excised rat lung has also been used as a model system in which surfactant function can be tested (22). These lungs assume very stable physical characteristics after multiple lavages and can be used repeatedly for instillation and testing of exogenous surfactant preparations and measurement of the resulting changes in compliance.

While these methods can provide valuable information about the physical characteristics of a surfactant preparation, in some cases they have produced results that differ from those obtained using in vivo systems, thereby necessitating the use of both types of systems.

In Vivo Systems

The most popular animal model for surfactant function studies in a surfactant deficiency state (i.e., RDS) is the fetal rabbit (59,134). Fetal rabbits taken at 27 or 28 days of gestation (term = 31 days) offer a convenient model of a surfactant deficient state (207), because they are large enough to subject to surgical procedures and physiologic monitoring, yet small enough to permit simultaneous testing of several animals. The preterm lamb (135), the rhesus monkey (247), and the rat (85,239) are also being used to study hormonal effects on surfactant components, synthesis, metabolism, and many other aspects of surfactant biology and of lung development.

Surfactant dysfunction (inhibition or inactivation) is studied in a number of models that emulate adult respiratory distress syndrome (ARDS). These models include animals lavaged extensively to deplete endogenous surfactant and animals injected with or inhaling various substances that inactivate or inhibit the function of surfactant. Antisera to the surfactant proteins, bacterial toxins, acids, oxidants, organics, and smoke are among these materials. These models and their response to surfactant treatment were recently reviewed (224).

SURFACTANT PROTEINS

As discussed above, in the 1980s a great deal of attention was focused on the surfactant proteins. During this period, it was shown that these proteins play important roles in the biology of surfactant. Since the investigation of surfactant proteins expanded rapidly in recent years and because of their importance in surfactant biology, each of the surfactant proteins will be reviewed in detail.

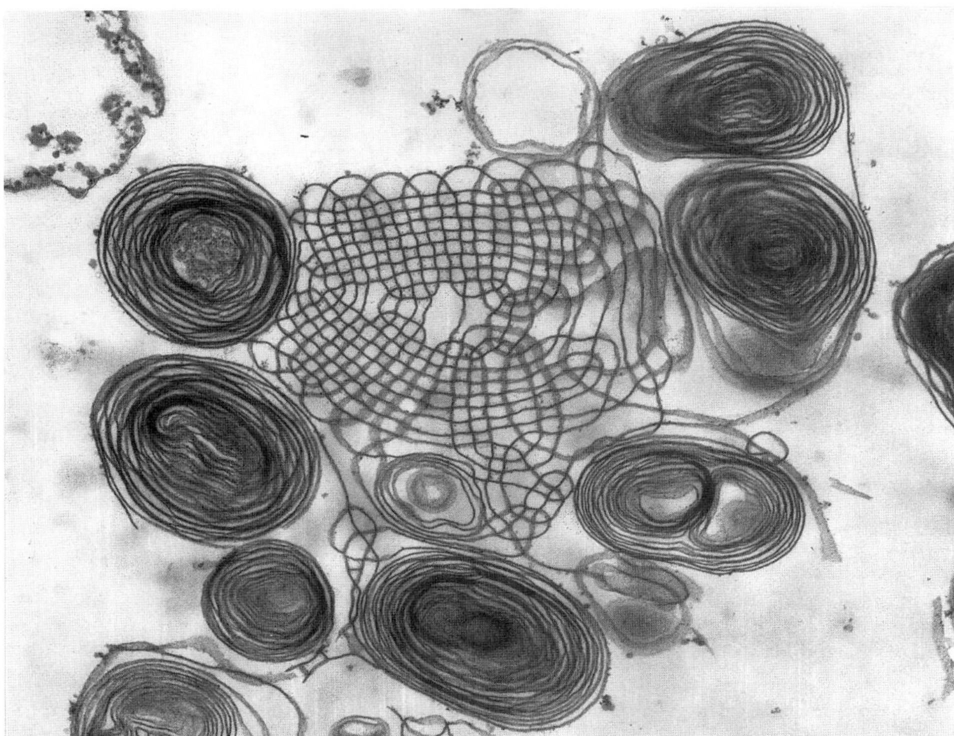

Figure 3. Micrograph showing transition of lamellar bodies to tubular myelin in rat lung tissue. This electron micrograph depicts several lamellar bodies in the process of forming tubular myelin. (For more details see ref. 360. Micrograph supplied by Dr. S. Young, Duke University Medical Center.)

SP-A

Genomic Organization

The human SP-A locus has been mapped on chromosome 10q21–24 (34,79) and consists of at least two functional genes (gene I and gene II) and one pseudogene (150,158,335). Two cDNAs, 6A and 1A, corresponding to SP-A gene I and SP-A gene II, respectively, as well as an allelic variant of 6A have been reported (86,261). These SP-A genes, although quite similar in their DNA sequences, have some diverse regions (150). Moreover, sequence analysis of the SP-A 3' untranslated region (UTR), an area that can potentially have an impact on the regulation of gene expression, revealed considerable heterogeneity and suggested the presence of many allelic variants in the population (90,261). The 3′ UTR heterogeneity was shown recently to exhibit meiotic stability over three generations (161). Within the coding region the most significant differences between SP-A gene I (6A) and gene II (1A) appear to be substitutions of leucine for proline (codon 54) and cysteine for arginine (codon 85). These changes alter the positioning of hydroxyproline residues and the formation of disulfide bonds (150). From an evolutionary point of view, it appears that all of the human SP-A genomic sequences have arisen from a single primordial primate sequence (90).

SP-A genomic and cDNA sequences for a number of animal species have been reported (21,24,42,81,160,172). Unlike the human SP-A locus with its multiple genes, in the animal species SP-A is derived from a single gene that gives rise, in most cases, to messenger RNAs of more than one size, due in part to differential polyadenylation. The genomic organization is well conserved in all species examined. In all cases there are untranslated regions at the 5′ and at the 3′ ends of the gene with four exons encoding, either in part or in their entirety, amino acids for the SP-A protein precursor (Fig. 4).

Structural Organization

Human SP-A is derived from two precursor molecules differing by only 7 amino acids (84,86) and is an extensively modified sialoglycoprotein of 30,000 to 35,000 Daltons (d) (84,232–234, 238,297). The amino acid sequence predicts a relatively hydrophilic protein using a common algorithim for hydropathicity (171). The amino-terminal part of the protein contains a signal peptide sequence and consists of a number of collagen-like Gly-X-Y triplets, with the amino acid in the Y position frequently a hydroxyproline residue (124,238). The collagen-like domains of three SP-A monomers are associated in a triple helix to form a trimer (154). Six SP-A trimers then associate to form the distinctive structure of the mature protein that has a molecular mass of about 700,000 d (154) and resembles a bouquet of flowers (326,327). The quarternary structure of SP-A is much like that of the complement component C1q (326,327).

It has been suggested that the noncollagenous carboxy-terminal portion of the protein, which has a site for N-linked glycosylation, is essential for the correct folding and assembly of the multimeric molecule. This part of the protein appears to form a nucleation center that allows a zipper-like process to occur, beginning with the interaction of the carboxy-terminal globular domains and progressing to the formation of the triple helix in the collagenous portion (293). In the human this complex requires two 6A (gene I) SP-A molecules and one IA (gene II) molecule to form each trimer (327).

SP-A exhibits some sequence similarity with the mannose binding protein and several other C-type lectins, including SP-D. Like these proteins it has the ability to bind carbohydrates in the presence of calcium and other divalent cations (70,107,271, 309). In addition to binding carbohydrates, SP-A appears to have two distinct binding sites for calcium and a lipid binding domain (109,269). Recently, SP-A was shown to bind glycolipids (46,168). Much of the glycolipid binding can be competed

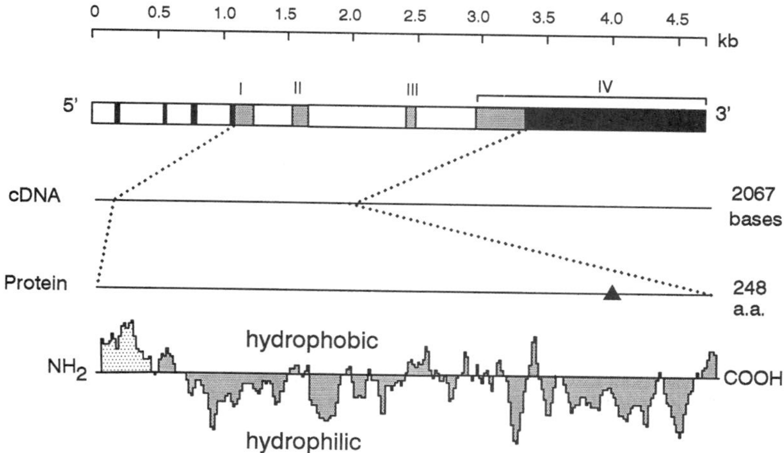

Figure 4. Genomic organization of SP-A. A schematic of the SP-A gene is shown along with a size scale. Exons with *black fill* at the 5′ and 3′ end are untranslated portions of the gene and those with *dark stipple* encode portions of the mature protein. The region with *light stipple* encodes a portion of the precursor protein that is cleaved during processing (see Figs. 5 and 6). The *dotted lines* delineate the relative positions of the translated portion of the cDNA. The lengths of the cDNA and protein are given. *Triangle* represents potential N-linked glycosylation site in the protein. The *bottom tracing* shows a hydropathicity plot of the protein based on the amino acid sequence (171). Within the hydropathicity plot, *dark stipple* represents the mature protein and *light stipple* indicates a portion of the precursor that is cleaved during processing. (From ref. 371 addendum, with permission.)

away by the addition of carbohydrates isolated from the glycolipids (168). At present it is unclear whether this interaction is mediated by a unique binding site on SP-A or whether the glycolipid binding is via the carbohydrate binding site.

SP-A aggregates phospholipids. This process is also Ca^{2+} dependent and requires the collagen region of SP-A as well as the intermolecular disulfide bond (^{9}Cys) between two SP-A monomers (110,166,270).

Rat and rabbit SP-A have been expressed in heterologous cells (3,193) and the expressed protein has physical and functional properties similar to native SP-A. The addition of the N-linked oligosaccharide to the protein appears to be required for SP-A secretion by the heterologous cells (3) and for transport of SP-A to lamellar bodies in lung organ cultures (4). When only one of the human SP-A genes was expressed in heterologous cells, several of the properties of the recombinant SP-A differed from those of the native SP-A (108), further suggesting that both SP-A gene products are required for a fully functional and stable protein.

Functional Aspects

Several diverse functions have been attributed to SP-A. Biophysically, SP-A has been shown to increase the rate of adsorption of various surfactant mixtures (47,123,125,278,362), and to reverse inhibition of surfactant by serum proteins (51). In addition, SP-A is involved in the structural organization of surfactant. It is an essential component in the formation of tubular myelin.

SP-A plays a role in the metabolism of surfactant by regulating reuptake and secretion of surfactant. The former action appears to be mediated by a specific receptor for SP-A on the type II cell membrane and is distinct from SP-A's ability to bind carbohydrates (68,164,165,310).

SP-A plays a role in local host defense. This function of SP-A was suggested following its structural characterization showing similarity to molecules involved in host defense function, such as the mannose binding protein and complement C1q (70). The details of the role of SP-A in host defense are discussed under host defense.

SP-B

Genomic Organization

Genomic and cDNA SP-B sequences for several species have been published (62,75,94,124,137,243,254,354). The gene for human SP-B (Fig. 5) is located on chromosome 2 (74) and consists of 11 exons. The first exon contains a short 5′ untranslated region and a portion of exon 10 as well as the entire exon 11 encode the 3′ untranslated region (243). The mature protein is encoded by exons 6 and 7. Structurally the SP-B gene includes a number of distinct features. Alu sequences in several introns and $(CA)_n$ repeats in human SP-B (243,311) as well as a $(CCA)_{21}$ repeat in the 3′ untranslated region of the mouse have been identified. Alterations in the CA repeats in the human SP-B gene have been identified and are implicated in pulmonary disease (our unpublished observations). Variations in the length of the 3′ untranslated region among species appear to contribute to size differences of the SP-B mRNA (62).

Structural Characteristics

Mature SP-B is derived from a larger precursor molecule of 42,000 d (137) that undergoes posttranslational cleavages of the amino- and carboxy-termini to give rise to mature SP-B, a very hydrophobic peptide isolated from bronchoalveolar lavage. The posttranslational processing of the SP-B precursor is cell specific (126), and appears to occur in an endosomal/lysosomal cellular compartment, probably in the multivesicular bodies (324). An aspartyl protease, cathespin D, or a cathespin D-like protease has been implicated in the cleavage of the amino-terminal SP-B propeptide (333). Although a number of pulmonary adenocarcinoma cell lines have been used to study SP-B processing, none of them thus far appears to have the ability to support complete processing of the SP-B precursor (212), suggesting that these cell lines may not represent useful models for this type of work.

SP-B is a cysteine-rich molecule (60), and the relative position of the cysteines is conserved among species (62). In this regard, SP-B appears to consist of four repeats with a conserved

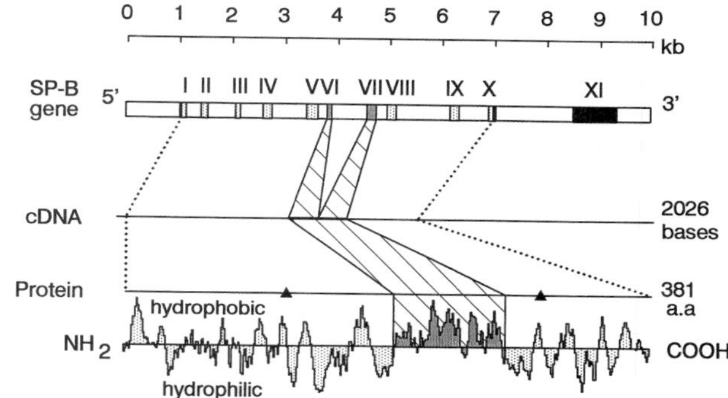

Figure 5. Genomic organization of SP-B. Details of this figure are identical to those described for Fig. 4. The *hatched areas* trace the portions of the cDNA and protein that are included in the mature protein.

periodicity of cysteine residues in each repeat. These repeats are linked by regions rich in prolines and glycines varying in length from 15 to 64 residues (126). The third repeat that contains the mature SP-B includes an additional cysteine residue that may be involved in the interchain disulfide bond formation (126). This extra cysteine is absent from the bovine SP-B (62). The remaining cysteine residues form three intrachain disulfide bridges, resulting in the formation of three loops resembling the kringle structure seen in serine proteases (141).

In human SP-B, a polymorphism in amino acid 28 has been reported (141), resulting in the presence of either an alanine residue (137), an arginine residue (94), or an isoleucine residue. In porcine SP-B, a polymorphism where either an arginine or a methionine may occur at position 64 has also been identified (141). In addition, in the porcine SP-B, some heterogeneity exists at the amino acid residue of the amino-terminus of the mature SP-B peptide (142).

Similarities of the mature SP-B with several nonsurfactant molecules have been reported. These include similarity of the mature rat SP-B with the active center of the mouse contrapsin protein inhibitor (75), with a membrane pore-forming peptide that may be involved in the cytolytic activity of the pathogen, *Entamoeba histolytica* (172), and with proteins that may bind to lipids, the prosaposin and the sulfated glycoprotein 1 (223). Among the saposins, SP-B, and the pore-forming peptide, the positions of cysteine residues are conserved (172), suggesting that this motif contributes to an important structural property common to these molecules.

Functional Aspects

As mentioned earlier and shown in Fig. 2, surfactant undergoes a number of morphologic changes. The in vivo mechanisms that promote and regulate all of these processes including the transformation from lamellar bodies to tubular myelin and from tubular myelin to the formation of the surface monolayer are currently unknown. Many in vitro studies have been carried out to enhance our understanding of these processes and the findings from these studies are summarized.

SP-B and SP-A are essential components for the in vitro formation of tubular myelin (249,303,342). Reconstitution experiments show the importance of having correct proportions of SP-A and SP-B present, to form tubular myelin with structural characteristics similar to those seen in vivo (303). The requirement of SP-A for tubular myelin formation is further suggested by the fact that tubular myelin is not detected in morphologic surveys of replacement surfactants devoid of SP-A. These surfactants include those prepared by solvent extraction (305). Furthermore, tubular myelin was not detected in lung tissue from patients with RDS, (65) subsequently shown to either lack or have reduced levels of SP-A (66).

SP-A aggregates liposomes in the presence of Ca^{2+} without disrupting their membranes, and SP-B causes lipid mixing in the presence of negatively charged phospholipids, divalent or monovalent cations, or lowered pH (219,249). The synergy of SP-A (lipid aggregation) and SP-B (lipid mixing) could lead to the formation of tubular myelin under appropriate conditions (249). In addition, the ability of SP-B to mix lipids and destabilize phospholipid bilayers may be one of the mechanisms by which lipid bilayers in tubular myelin are ultimately destabilized, adsorbed, and spread at the air/liquid interface (285).

Native SP-B and SP-C enhance adsorption of lipids to the air/liquid interface in the presence of charged lipids and Ca^{2+} (218,285) and can change the thermodynamic properties of phospholipid membranes (286). Once on the surface monolayer, SP-B has been shown by in vitro studies to carry out several functions. During monolayer compression, an experimental condition analogous to the reduction of surface area during lung deflation, SP-B appears to affect the squeeze out from the surface film of unsaturated lipids resulting in a DPPC-enriched monolayer. This DPPC monolayer in turn results in the reduction of the surface tension to near zero (192). In addition, SP-B interacts with phosphatidylglycerol at the surface (but not in the interior) of the experimental membranes bilayer in a concentration-dependent manner (11). When SP-B is present in the monolayer, the fluidity of DPPC increases (218) and the insertion of phospholipids from the hypophase into the monolayer is probably more effective (218). This phenomenon is likely to be important during the rapid increase in surface area when the lungs expand. The mechanism by which this process occurs is thought to involve binding of phospholipid vesicles, present in the hypophase, to SP-B or SP-C in the preformed monolayers via divalent ions, with the subsequent insertion of the lipids into the monolayer (217).

The hydrophobicity and the distribution of charge in the amino acid residues of SP-B peptides appear to be important factors for its structure and function as assessed by surface tension measurements (33). Based on tryptophan emission spectra, it is suggested that SP-B provides lateral stability of the phospholipid monolayer (50). This stability is achieved via interactions of electrostatic charges of the hydrophilic residues with the phospholipid polar heads and hydrophobic residues with the acyl side chains. Moreover, synthetic peptides corresponding to SP-B amphipathic sequences when mixed with lipids can also mimic several of the in vitro physicochemical and in vivo properties of the native surfactant (330).

The significance of SP-B for normal lung function has also been affirmed by in vivo studies. Treatment of neonatal rabbits with a monoclonal antibody to SP-B resulted in decreased compliance along with inflammation and lesions that included hyaline membranes (265), as well as decreased tidal volumes (156). Immunoglobulin G (IgG) treatment alone did not have any effect on lung function. Similarly, treatment of surfactant-deficient rats with surfactant preparations mixed with antibody to SP-B and SP-C did not restore normal lung function, whereas surfactant either without the antibody or mixed with control serum did restore lung function (73). Consistent with these observations on the importance of SP-B, in vivo administration of reconstituted surfactants containing SP-B to preterm rabbits could restore function to levels comparable to that of natural sheep surfactant, although the complete restoration depended on the characteristics of the accompanying mechanical ventilation (260). Perhaps the best demonstration of the pivotal role of the hydrophobic proteins for normal lung function is exemplified by surfactant replacement therapy. Surfactant preparations that include SP-B and SP-C show a significantly faster and greater improvement in lung function in animal studies than preparations that do not include these proteins (111,112).

SP-C

Genomic Organization

The gene for human SP-C (Fig. 6) is located on chromosome 8p (80) and consists of 6 exons, with exon 2 coding for the mature SP-C (95). A portion of exon 1 constitutes a short 5′ untranslated region and a portion of exon 5 as well as the entire exon 6 constitute the 3′ untranslated region (53,96). In humans, alternate splicing can result in four classes of messenger RNAs (mRNAs) of about 850 bases (95,331). Species differences have been noted in this process. Generation of heterogeneity via alternate splicing does not occur in the mouse (96). However, alternate splicing of intron 5 in the rabbit results in two types of mRNAs, with the type II mRNA (the minor type) forming a highly stable secondary (hairpin) structure (28,53). Both mRNA types appear to be regulated coordinately during fetal rabbit lung development and by hormones (28). The role of mRNA secondary structure in SP-C expression is currently unknown. Unlike SP-A (261), human SP-C is highly conserved among individuals (122) and its expression,

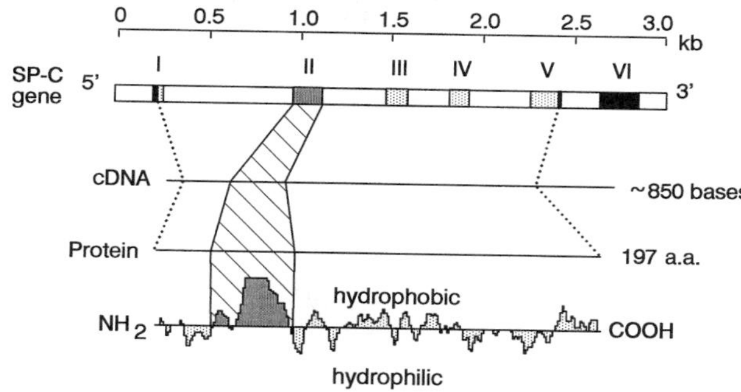

Figure 6. Genomic organization of SP-C. Details are as described in the legends of Figs. 4 and 5.

as assessed by its mRNA content, does not vary significantly among individuals (89). A high degree of similarity at the nucleotide level (77–84%) within coding sequences among species has also been reported (72) and this similarity is increased to >85% in the portion of the gene coding for the mature SP-C. Similarity in the 5′ flanking and the 3′ untranslated regions also exists among species with the similarity at the 3′ untranslated being less than that at the 5′ flanking region (53,96,122).

Structural Characteristics

Mature SP-C, the form isolated from bronchoalveolar lavage, is encoded by exon 2 and is derived from a larger precursor molecule (22,000 d) following posttranslational cleavages of the amino- and carboxy-termini (Fig. 6). Mature SP-C is a very hydrophobic protein, with its carboxy-terminus being extremely hydrophobic. It is mainly an α-helical membrane-spanning molecule and has covalently linked palmitic acids at two adjacent cysteines (except canine SP-C, which has one cysteine and therefore one palmitoyl group) near the amino-terminus (19,61,143,296). The palmitoyl group appears to increase the α-helical content of the protein and it may also stabilize the formation of the α-helix (317). The SP-C precursor has been shown in vitro to be an integral membrane protein, and the hydrophobic core of the mature SP-C appears to be important for anchoring (151) the protein in the membrane. The carboxy-terminal domain of the SP-C precursor, which is posttranslationally modified, appears to be involved in the intracellular targeting of this molecule (152). The nature of this modification is unknown, but it has been shown to be inhibited by cerulenin, an antibiotic that inhibits fatty acid synthesis (325).

Heterogeneity at the amino-terminus of the mature SP-C has been observed both within and among species (140,236,296). Although it has been reported that the relative abundance of the various SP-C forms differs in fetal and adult human lung tissue (140), the biologic significance of these differences is unknown.

Functional Aspects

A number of in vitro studies suggest that SP-C disturbs the ordering of the acyl chain region or lipid packing in DPPC bilayer models, broadens the gel-fluid phase transition temperature, and in the monolayer causes redistribution of lipids, decreases viscosity, and increases elasticity (131,222,228,288). These SP-C effects, although small, do facilitate film expansion and compression in vitro, although it is unknown how SP-C behaves under physiologic conditions.

SP-D

SP-D, although designated a surfactant-associated protein, has not been shown to contribute to the surface tension-lowering properties of surfactant and only small amounts of it are associated with purified surfactant. SP-D like SP-A is a collagenous, carbohydrate-binding glycoprotein, and its gene is located on chromosome 10q (58) as is the SP-A locus (34).

Structural Characteristics

Although SP-D and SP-A share similarities, they do differ in many respects and have been shown to be functionally dissimilar (229). These differences include the presence of irregularities in the collagenous domain in SP-A that are absent from SP-D, possibly allowing a more rigid triple helical domain in SP-D. Another difference is the absence of cysteine residues from the collagenous domain in SP-D, prohibiting interhelical disulfide cross-links. SP-D contains an intrahelical N-linked glycosylation, whereas the glycosylation site in human SP-A is near the carboxyterminus. SP-D remains primarily in the supernatant fraction of the bronchoalveolar lavage fluid following centrifugation at 33,000 × g, but SP-A and the other surfactant components are found in the pellet with only a small fraction (10%) of SP-D (229). There are charge differences between SP-A and SP-D, possibly contributed by the collagenous domain, that may result in solubility differences between the two proteins (271).

Like SP-A, SP-D is a C-type lectin exhibiting Ca^{2+} dependent carbohydrate binding activity (230). It is very similar to conglutinin, which has been shown to play a role in host defenses (182,185,287). The organizational motifs in the primary structure, the amino acid sequence in certain regions, as well as the quarternary structure, as determined by rotary shadowing and electron microscopy, are very similar between SP-D and conglutinin. These structural similarities suggest functional similarities and a role for SP-D in the local host defense of the lung.

Functional Aspects

Although SP-D by itself has not been shown to have any effect on surfactant metabolism, there is one report indicating that SP-D counteracts the inhibitory effect of SP-A on phospholipid secretion. This interaction appears to require SP-D associated lipids (167). Interestingly, SP-D binds phosphotidylinositol (PI) in a calcium concentration-dependent manner (216). Whether this SP-D:PI binding is involved in the interaction with SP-A remains to be determined. SP-D also binds to the lipopolysaccharide of *Escherichia coli* and other gram-negative bacteria, but the significance of this binding is unknown (162).

Localization and Cellular Sites of Synthesis

SP-A has been localized in the type II alveolar epithelial cells of all species that have been studied, in alveolar macrophages, and in subpopulations of bronchiolar epithelial cells of most species (49,240,329,341). In situ hybridization studies, such as those shown in Fig. 7 using rat lung tissue, indicate that both type II alveolar cells and bronchiolar cells are the sites of synthesis of SP-A (Fig. 7A,B) in all animal species examined (66, 237,240,348). Whether human SP-A is expressed in normal human bronchiolar epithelium remains controversial (8,31, 237). At the ultrastructural level, SP-A has been localized within the type II cell in the endoplasmic reticulum, the Golgi apparatus, some populations of granules and vesicles, and on the cell membrane (49,67,272,329,341). Although SP-A has been detected in lamellar bodies in many studies (49,67,147,329), in some studies SP-A was not detected in these organelles (250,272). Based on both morphologic and biochemical data, it has been suggested that, in addition to being secreted via lamellar bodies, SP-A is also secreted independently of these organelles (13,67,91,113,147). One line of evidence in support of this suggestion comes from recent studies in which the kinetics and regulation of secretion of SP-A were found to be quite different from those of phospholipids and lamellar bodies (92,136,268). Another line of evidence is the finding that the

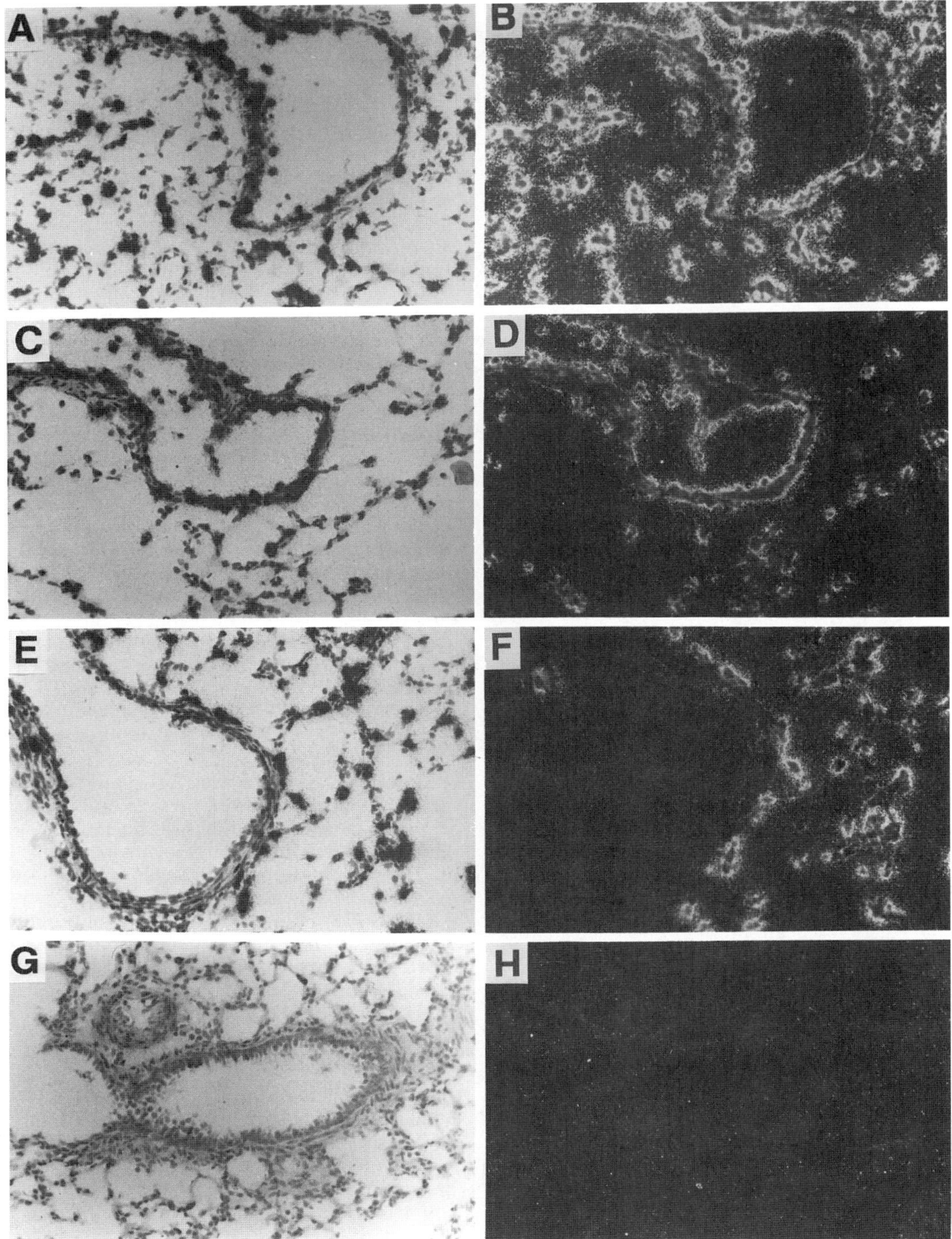

Figure 7. In situ hybridization of SP-A, SP-B, and SP-C in rat lung tissue. Frozen sections of paraformaldehyde fixed rat lung tissue were subjected to in situ hybridization (240) with cRNA antisense probes for rat SP-A **(A,B)**, SP-B **(C,D)**, and SP-C **(E,F)**. **(G,H)** The sense probe for SP-B was used as a negative control. Bright field micrographs are shown in A, C, E, G and the same areas under dark field illumination in B, D, F, H. (Original magnification: X250.)

relative concentration of SP-A is greater in tubular myelin than in lamellar bodies (67), further suggesting that some of the secreted SP-A arises from a source other than lamellar bodies (92). SP-A is present primarily in the corners of the tubular myelin lattice (323).

When SP-A is localized in alveolar macrophages, it is seen in lysosomes and other organelles associated with degradation. It is often found in conjunction with lamellar bodies and tubular myelin that have been ingested (329,341). The absence of SP-A in organelles associated with synthetic pathways and the absence of SP-A mRNA from this cell (237) indicate that the macrophage is not a site of SP-A synthesis.

Both SP-B protein and its mRNA have been identified by immunohistochemistry and tissue in situ hybridization in type II alveolar cells and in bronchiolar cells (Fig. 7C,D) in all species examined (237,240,294,348), whereas SP-C has been localized in the adult lung, exclusively in the type II cells (Fig. 7E,F) of all species examined (146,240,348). The pattern of distribution of SP-A and SP-B differs within subcellular organelles of the type II cell as suggested by immunohistochemistry (240). Recent electron microscopic studies provided further support for this observation (67).

SP-D is localized in the same cells in the rat as SP-A (type II, Clara cells, alveolar macrophages), but in different subcellular compartments, consistent with differences in function between these two proteins (57,323).

Regulation

Regulation of the expression of surfactant protein genes during lung development has been reviewed by several investigators within the last few years (14,197,332), as has the regulation of lipids (14,17). Here we will focus on the surfactant proteins by briefly summarizing earlier findings and presenting some new information.

Surfactant proteins are regulated developmentally (72,100, 181,252,275,348), hormonally (14,87,88,197,235,239,318, 332, 359), and in a tissue-specific (42,85,172) and cell-specific manner (88,132,199,239,339). Species differences in the developmental expression of surfactant proteins have been noted (72).

In Vivo Studies

Hormonal and Developmental Effects Rat SP-A mRNA is developmentally regulated (275) and is initially detected on fetal day 16 (term = 22 days) by examination of in vitro primary translation products (235) and by nuclease S1 protection assay (172). Although the level of rat SP-A mRNA increases through late gestation, it does not reach adult levels (275), whereas rabbit SP-A mRNA reaches adult levels well before term (72). The developmental profile of the surfactant protein mRNAs in the rabbit is depicted in Fig. 8. Dexamethasone treatment enhances newly synthesized SP-A and SP-A mRNA in both fetal and adult rat lung (83,87,235,276).

SP-B mRNA is detectable at 13 weeks of human gestation and increases to about 50% of adult levels by 24 weeks of gestation (181). SP-B protein appears after 18 weeks of human gestation (294). In fetal rabbit lung SP-B mRNA is detectable at 24 days (term = 31 days) (72) in the cuboidal epithelial cells and at 28 days in bronchiolar cells, whereas SP-A is detectable in type II cells at 26 days of gestation, coincident with the appearance of lamellar bodies, and at 28 days in bronchiolar cells. In neonatal and adult rabbit lungs SP-A mRNA is primarily found in type II cells and very little is seen in bronchiolar cells, whereas the SP-B mRNA level is equivalent in both type II and bronchiolar cells (348). In rat, adult levels are reached by fetal day 20 (275) and dexamethasone treatment enhances SP-B mRNA levels in both type II and bronchiolar cells (239). SP-C expression is also enhanced by in vivo glucocorticoid administration (83), as is expression of transgenes carrying the SP-C promoter (97).

Developmentally, SP-D appears in late gestation and reaches adult levels by birth (56). In vivo dexamethasone treatment enhances SP-D expression in fetal and neonatal lungs but not in the adult lung (215).

Diabetic Pregnancy (reviewed in ref. 103) In the lungs of fetuses of streptozotocin-induced diabetic rats the levels of SP-A mRNA and protein are low (104), consistent with clinical findings in amniotic fluid samples from diabetic mothers (149,291). The low levels of SP-A in the streptozotocin model (104) may in part explain why infants of diabetic mothers have a higher incidence of RDS in spite of surfactant phospholipid levels indicating lung maturity. The levels of SP-B and SP-C mRNAs are also low in the fetal lung of the streptozotocin-induced diabetic pregnancy (105). In the lungs of adult streptozotocin-induced diabetic rats the level of SP-A mRNA is found to be increased in both type II and bronchiolar cells, but the SP-A protein content in these cells was reduced (298). The reason for these differences in SP-A mRNA levels in this model during fetal and adult life is currently unknown.

Oxidants Hyperoxia, a condition that may be encountered in the treatment of RDS and other lung disorders, has differential effects on the expression of the surfactant proteins, and it also exhibits species-specific differences. In hyperoxia, SP-A and SP-B mRNAs are enhanced in rabbits in both type II and bronchiolar cells (132,319). The effect on bronchiolar cells is about ten-fold higher than that in the type II cells. Very little effect on SP-C mRNA is observed (132). In the mouse lung, however, a decrease in SP-B mRNA in type II cells and an increase in the bronchiolar cells following hyperoxia is seen (339). In a primate model hyperoxia enhances the expression of SP-B and SP-C but not that of SP-A (199).

Exposure to ozone or nitrogen dioxide can reduce the ability of SP-A to exhibit several of its properties, including self-association and lipid aggregation (203,220), as well as enhancement of phagocytosis (221). The mechanisms resulting in these effects have not yet been determined.

In Vitro Studies

SP-A Despite the consistent stimulation of SP-A expression by glucocorticoids in vivo, the effect of glucocorticoids on explant cultures appears to be complex. The data from human explant cultures suggest that glucocorticoids both stimulate and inhibit SP-A gene expression, with inhibition being the dominant effect, although there is not complete agreement on the details of these effects (26,27,133). Further complicating the interpretation of the published human studies is the fact that the experimental protocols in these studies differ in part and none of the studies distinguished between the glucocorticoid effects on each SP-A gene. Whether differential regulation of the two SP-A genes contributes to the complexity of the findings for human SP-A remains to be determined. In studies of animal lung explants, glucocorticoids exhibit a time-dependent biphasic effect on rabbit SP-A mRNA accumulation (25) and a dose-dependent increase in rat SP-A mRNA (206). A dexamethasone-induced enhancement of SP-A mRNA is observed in both type II and bronchiolar cells (206).

Other molecules and hormones that enhance SP-A protein and mRNA levels include epidermal growth factor (247,336), interferon-gamma (15), prostaglandins (1), oxygen (2), and many others (see reviews 14,197,332). Insulin reduces human SP-A protein production (63,290). Dibutyryl cAMP reduces rat SP-A mRNA levels in explant cultures, an effect that is also accomplished by sodium butyrate, but that does not occur with treatment by dibromo cAMP (206).

Transcriptional and posttranscriptional events are known to involve both *cis-* and *trans-*acting regulatory elements. The identification and characterization of such elements involved in surfactant protein gene expression are currently under intense investigation. Specific 5′ flanking conserved regions have been identified for SP-A and shown to bind lung specific nuclear proteins (160). DNAse hypersensitive sites (an indicator of transcriptionally active genes) unique to lung have also been identified for SP-A (42,172) further confirming its tissue-specific expression.

SP-B and SP-C In explant cultures, SP-B mRNA (88,211,213) and SP-C mRNA (318) levels are enhanced by glucocorticoids. Dexamethasone treatment of explant cultures results in an enhancement of SP-B mRNA levels in both rat type II and bronchiolar cells (88). Transcriptional and posttranscriptional events appear to contribute to the enhancement of human SP-B gene expression by dexamethasone (213,320). Regulatory *cis-*acting elements involved in the expression of SP-B in an adenocarcinoma cell line have been identified (29). For SP-C gene expression, transcriptional events and ongoing protein synthesis are required (97,318,320).

It is clear that developmental, hormonal, species- and cell-specific differences exist in the regulation of the surfactant protein gene expression. Similar types of regulation also exist for

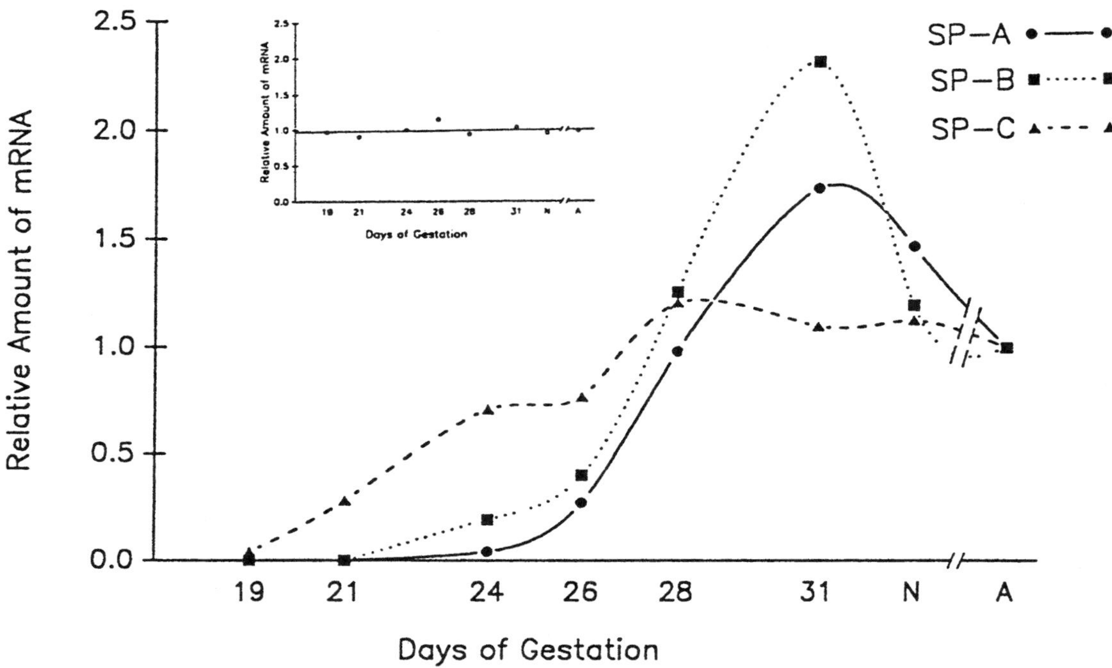

Figure 8. Ontogeny of the rabbit surfactant-associated proteins. SP-A, SP-B, SP-C mRNA levels in fetal, neonatal, and adult lung tissues were evaluated by RNA blot analysis followed by densitometry of the specific bands. Each RNA blot was also analyzed using as a control probe a rabbit cytochrome oxidase subunit II cDNA. The *insert* is a graphic representation of the densitometric values of the relative amount of cytochrome oxidase subunit II mRNA as a function of gestational age. The data for each surfactant protein mRNA are expressed as the ratio of the absorbance of the particular surfactant protein in RNA band to the absorbance of the cytochrome oxidase subunit II mRNA band in the same lane. N, neonatal; A, adult. (From ref. 72, with permission.)

some of the enzymes involved in surfactant lipid biosynthesis (reviewed in 14,17).

SURFACTANT AND HOST-DEFENSE

Surfactant is ideally suited to play a role in host-defense processes in the lung since it covers the entire alveolar surface. In this position it is the first substance encountered by pathogens reaching the alveoli in inspired air. With constant exposure to pathogens, lung host-defense processes must be efficient, while at the same time being somewhat constrained, since many substances released during a normal immune response can have a detrimental effect on lung structure and function. The literature on the effects of surfactant on lung host-defense function reflects the dichotomous nature of lung host defense, with the effects of surfactant on phagocytic cells being mainly stimulatory and its influence on other immune effector cells being inhibitory. Surfactant appears to exert its effects at multiple sites.

Alveolar Macrophages

Alveolar macrophages are considered the first line of defense for the lung. In 1973 LaForce and colleagues (174) showed that while macrophages could bind and ingest bacteria in vitro, killing of these bacteria intracellularly depended on the presence of the alveolar lining material. The lipid fraction of the alveolar lining material (145), and more specifically surfactant (210), was shown to be responsible for this effect. Other investigators, however, have reported conflicting results, describing either the lack of a surfactant effect (144) or surfactant-dependent inhibition of phagocytic potential and intracellular killing (54,127,205,284). This inhibitory influence was apparently due to interference by surfactant lipids with macrophage complement and Fc receptors (54,205).

The role surfactant proteins play in phagocytosis has been examined recently. Both SP-A and SP-D are C-type lectins with similarities to other molecules involved in host-defense function (253). It has been reported that SP-A can stimulate macrophage chemotaxis (128,353) and increase the ability of macrophages to ingest sheep erythrocytes (308) or opsonized bacteria. In addition, SP-A can enhance the production of oxygen radicals in alveolar macrophages (314). Similar enhancement of oxidative potential in alveolar macrophages can be produced by exposure to SP-D (316). However, these actions do not appear to be universal. The influence of SP-A on the interactions of various pathogens and phagocytes varies tremendously depending on the microorganism and the phagocytic cell type being studied (188,196).

Lymphocytes

Another aspect of host-defense function is the ability of lymphocytes to proliferate in response to various stimuli. Studies of lymphocytes from bronchoalveolar lavage have shown them to be less reactive than blood lymphocytes to stimulation by either mitogens or mixed lymphocyte culture (148). These differences in reactivity were subsequently shown to result from the exposure of the lymphocytes to surfactant (6,16,38,257) and its lipid constituents (344,345). The mechanism of action and impact on the in vivo immune responses of these effects are not known currently.

Natural killer cells, the lymphocyte subset responsible for cell-mediated cytotoxicity, when isolated from lung, are less active than those isolated from other sources (334). As with the differences in proliferative response, these effects on natural killer cells are caused by the lipid constituents of surfactant (38,343). The mechanism by which different types of lymphocytes exert their effects is probably different, since one process relates to cell proliferation and the other does not.

The study of the relationship between surfactant and host-defense function in the lung is still at an early stage. Much of the work cited above was completed when little was known about the surfactant proteins. Recent studies have examined the actions of isolated surfactant proteins on immune defenses and in many cases these actions are opposite to those of the surfactant lipids. It is likely that the in vivo situation, both in normal host-defense processes and in lung diseases, the relative amounts of the surfactant lipids and proteins, and the sum of their respective actions determine the status of immune defenses in the lung.

Target Cells and Organisms

Many of the effects on bacterial killing attributed to surfactant result from the interaction of surfactant with macrophages. Evidence for direct interactions between some components of surfactant and inhaled pathogens is accumulating. The ability of SP-A to bind to carbohydrates and lipids is reflected by its ability to bind to the surface of microorganisms (315) including Herpes simplex virus type I (316), the opportunistic pathogen, *Pneumocystis carinii* (363), and several types of bacteria (188,196). It is not yet known whether interaction with SP-A affects subsequent interaction between these organisms and immune cells in the lung. The recently described ability of SP-A to bind to glycolipids (46,168) raises the possibility that this interaction may be involved in host defense function by allowing SP-A to bind directly to the invading microorganisms. Furthermore, SP-D has been shown to bind to the lipopolysaccharide of some gram-negative bacteria in vitro, although the importance of this binding in vivo is unclear (162).

SURFACTANT SECRETION AND CLEARANCE

In the course of each breath, surfactant within the alveolus undergoes several physical changes to reach the air-liquid interface (Fig. 2). It has been suggested that the intracellular and extracellular reserves of surfactant are not large (reviewed in ref. 350). To meet the changing demands with each breath under a variety of conditions (e.g., exercise, birth), the various pools of surfactant must be tightly regulated by controlled processes of synthesis, secretion, and clearance. These processes and their regulation have been reviewed in detail by a number of investigators (17,40,190,347,352).

Several of the components of surfactant have been identified within lamellar bodies (secretory granules) of the type II alveolar cell. These organelles, concentric lamellated structures with a limiting membrane, move to the apical side of the cell for secretion by exocytosis (Fig. 2). Actin filaments and microtubules (32,313) have been implicated in the intracellular movement of the lamellar bodies. Exocytosis of these organelles occurs by fusion between the limiting membrane of the lamellar body and the plasma membrane. The fusion process appears to be aided by synexin (41).

Secretion can occur by both constitutive and regulated pathways. Local factors that enhance surfactant secretion include hyperventilation, stretching (346) of the surface area (e.g., deep breath), intracellular pH changes (39), and many others (reviewed in ref. 347). A variety of agonists such as tetradecanoyl phorbol acetate, adenosine triphosphate (ATP), calcium ionophores, β-adrenergic agonists, etc., enhance surfactant secretion (reviewed in ref. 190). The effects of these secretagogues, whether receptor-mediated or not, appear to involve intracellular messengers (reviewed in ref. 40). Inhibitors of surfactant secretion include lectins as well as surfactant components such as dipalmitoylphosphatidylcholine (DPPC) (301) and delipidated, purified SP-A (68,256). The inhibition by DPPC involves a novel mechanism in the type II cell. It is suggested that the physical state attained by the extracellular DPPC, when below its phase transition temperature (41°C), can serve as an inhibitor of further secretion (301). When the inhibitory effect of SP-A on surfactant secretion was tested in vivo, different results were obtained. One study suggested that SP-A inhibits secretion (55) and another suggested that it may stimulate secretion (214). The inhibitory effect of SP-A in type II cells in culture appears to be counteracted by SP-D (167).

Surfactant clearance from the alveolar space occurs via several pathways. These include uptake by type II alveolar cells, the major pathway (259,358), ingestion by the alveolar macrophage, movement up the mucociliary escalator, and others (reviewed in ref. 351). Upon reuptake, the surfactant components can follow a number of paths. They may be recycled, or degraded, or even removed from the surfactant system. A recent study has provided strong morphologic evidence that both surfactant lipids and SP-A are recycled by the type II cell (361). One study indicates that SP-B is also recycled (30). Regulators of surfactant uptake include surfactant proteins, ventilation, surfactant secretagogues, and other surfactant components (reviewed in refs. 351,352). Since surfactant uptake and secretion are regulated by some of the same molecules, questions about possible linkage of the two processes have been raised. However, the available data on this issue are discordant (82,99).

SURFACTANT REPLACEMENT

Surfactant replacement therapy is in widespread use for the treatment of neonatal RDS, and the potential usefulness of this therapy for the treatment of other lung disorders is being investigated (reviewed in ref. 138). A number of types of surfactants have been tested and several of these are currently being used clinically. These are either naturally derived surfactants that have been modified or completely synthetic surfactants. The naturally derived surfactants have been produced in several different ways.

Naturally Derived Surfactants

A preparation of human surfactant has been isolated and purified by filtration and centrifugation from human amniotic fluid obtained from full-term pregnancies. This surfactant exhibited good biophysical characteristics and proved to be effective in preventing and treating RDS in clinical trials with both prophylactic and "rescue" protocols (115,117,198). Despite the success of these studies, issues of safety and logistics preclude these preparations from widespread use.

The most extensively tested naturally derived preparations have been made by extracting native surfactant from animal lungs with organic solvents. While this approach was originally employed to separate the proteins and the lipids, it is now clear that the success of these preparations in improving lung function was due to the unexpected co-isolation of SP-B and SP-C with the surfactant lipids. Conversion of the crude extracts to reproducible preparations has been accomplished in several ways. First, organic solvent extracts of cow lung homogenate are supplemented with fixed amounts of phospholipid and fatty acid to obtain uniformity of composition and activity. This material, originally known as surfactant TA, is currently marketed in the United States as Survanta (Ross Laboratories, Columbus, Ohio). Surfactant TA was first used clinically in 1980 (93) and has been extensively characterized (305,306) and used in multiple clinical trials (130,138,157). Surfactants prepared by similar solvent extraction, using bronchoalveolar lavage as a starting material, display similar properties and do not seem to require supplementation. The best described of these surfactant preparations in the United States is known as calf lung surfactant extract (CLSE) (77,170,289).

Another well-characterized surfactant of natural origin is Curosurf (Chiesi Farmaceutici, Parma, Italy), an extract of porcine lung, which is used extensively in Europe (264,292). Rather than supplementing this preparation, its functional properties are enhanced by removing inhibitory molecules from the surfactant by chromatographic methods (59,302). Its composition is shown in Fig. 9 (263). Like the other surfactants of natural origin, Curosurf has good biophysical characteristics, is effective in the prevention and treatment of RDS, and resists inactivation by serum proteins in animal models of adult respiratory distress syndrome (ARDS).

The function of pulmonary surfactant has been shown to be inhibited under certain conditions by fibrinogen, serum protein, and other agents. An important property of the surfactant replacement preparations is their ability to resist this inhibition or inactivation. SP-B–based surfactant preparations, which include all of the naturally derived surfactants, appear to be more resistant to fibrinogen inhibition than SP-C–based surfactants (281). Surfactants containing the entire mature SP-B peptide as well as a portion of the SP-C peptide in the presence of Ca^{2+} show better resistance to inactivation by serum proteins than surfactants containing either one of these peptides alone (5).

It is important to note that although all of these naturally derived surfactants from various animal species contain proteins, the proteins (especially the hydrophobic ones) are highly conserved and not very immunogenic, particularly when only one or two doses are given intratracheally. However, immune responses to these proteins have been elicited in experimental animals by traditional immunization methods (16). The transient appearance of antibodies to these proteins in treated infants has been reported (44) but there is no evidence of any vigorous or sustained immune response against these proteins (189,337).

Synthetic Surfactants

The synthetic surfactants consist primarily of dipalmitoylphosphatidylcholine (DPPC) and contain no protein. The two best known preparations are artificial lung expanding compound (ALEC), a mixture of DPPC and phosphatidylglycerol (200,201,340), and Exosurf (Burroughs Wellcome, Research Triangle Park, North Carolina) (71,242), which uses tyloxapol and hexadecanol (Fig. 10) to enhance the spreading characteristics of the phosphatidylcholine (71,242). The absence of protein eliminates concerns over the possible immunogenicity of the preparations and simplifies their production. However, the proteins, in addition to their surface tension lowering properties, have other important functions as previously discussed. Their absence may result in synthetic surfactants having certain

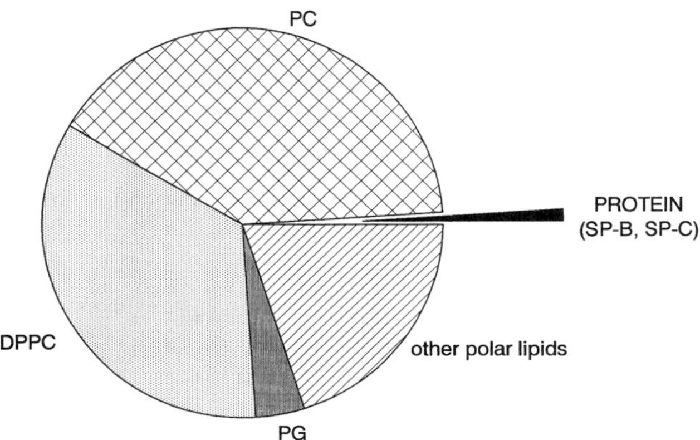

Figure 9. Composition of Curosurf (263), a surfactant replacement preparation derived from porcine lungs. Abbreviations as in Fig. 1.

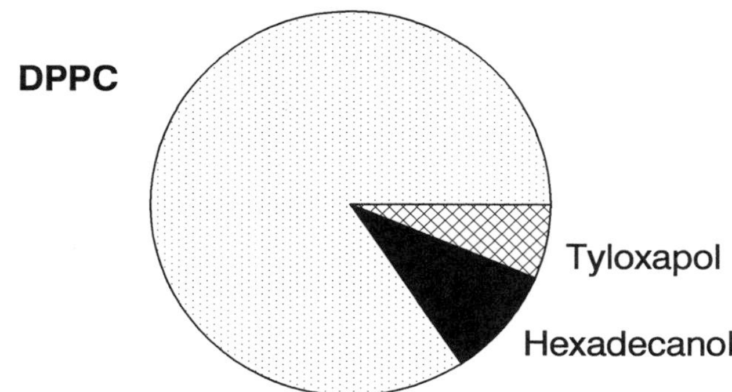

Figure 10. Composition of Exosurf, a synthetic surfactant preparation (242).

deficits as compared to naturally derived surfactants. While these protein-free surfactants reduce mortality due to RDS, the response to treatment in animals and humans differs from that seen when the natural derivatives are used (111,176). It has been suggested that the synthetic surfactants exert their beneficial effects by providing the lung with substrate for surfactant production or by combining with endogenous surfactant proteins to enhance their functional capabilities. In vitro studies support the latter possibility by showing a dramatic improvement in the biophysical characteristics of a synthetic surfactant when SP-B and SP-C are added to it (112).

"Designer" Surfactants

This class of surfactants has only been used in vitro or in animal studies. It contains synthetic lipids with either peptides or surfactant proteins that are produced by peptide synthesis or by recombinant gene technology. The surfactants containing peptides follow two main strategies. In one case peptides with sequences identical to portions of the native surfactant proteins are produced and mixed with lipids. Attention has been focused on peptides derived from the SP-B sequence due to the pivotal role of this protein in surfactant function (12,33,255). The second strategy involves designing peptides with some of the structural and charge characteristics of the surfactant proteins, but not necessarily the same amino acid residues (33,184,195,321). Although promising results have been obtained in early experiments, much testing remains to be done.

The production of surfactant proteins by recombinant gene technology is under way, with some success in expressing SP-A (3,193), mature SP-B (357), and mature SP-C (280). The major hurdle for this approach is that some of the surfactant proteins are subject to extensive posttranslational modification and that some of these modifications may not be performed by the cells employed in in vitro expression systems. Published reports of "designer" surfactant preparations with recombinant proteins, at this time, have involved only a recombinant form of human SP-C (281). While the protein performed positively in some respects, it appeared to be less resistant to inhibition or inactivation than did the native protein, perhaps due to the absence of the covalently linked palmitates in the recombinant protein.

As knowledge of surfactant biology accumulates, the potential for surfactant design will continue to increase, as will the list of conditions where surfactant replacement can be used. It is anticipated that future surfactant replacement preparations will be designed to fulfill several roles. These may include the ability to spread rapidly and reduce surface tension, to regulate endogenous surfactant production, to resist inactivation, and to modulate immune cell function.

SURFACTANT AND DISEASE

Deficiencies, dysfunctions, or alterations in the levels of the components of surfactant have been associated with several disease states (reviewed in refs. 120,178,282).

Respiratory Distress Syndrome (RDS)

Deficiency of surfactant in the prematurely born infant can result in RDS. The etiology of RDS is probably multifactorial and/or multigenic. A myriad of studies has shown an association between low levels of surfactant phospholipids and RDS (98,312). Surfactant proteins and in particular SP-A are reduced in RDS (66,67,149,291) and SP-A concentration correlates with the severity of the disease (119).

Several tests have been developed through the years to biochemically assess lung maturity at the threat of premature birth. These tests that by and large are used to predict the risk for RDS measure the concentration of the various surfactant components. Determining the ratio of lecithin or phosphatidycholine to sphingomyelin (L/S ratio) is the most widely used diagnostic test for RDS (69,98). Saturated phosphatidylcholine (312) or phosphatidyglycerol (PG) are also measured. Some studies have shown that inclusion of the surfactant protein measurements enhances the diagnostic accuracy of the L/S ratio or that of the PG levels (45,118), whereas other studies did not find improvement in the diagnostic accuracy (251). Measuring the SP-A content in samples of tracheal aspirates is a quick test for the diagnosis of RDS (43,295). Moreover, in certain cases, the concentration of SP-A in samples of amniotic fluid appears to have predictive value for RDS (149,291). These cases include the infants of diabetic mothers who often develop RDS in spite of an L/S ratio suggesting lung maturity.

Recent studies by Chida and Fujiwara (45) show that the stable microbubble test, originally described by Pattle et al. (227), appears to be a good indicator of lung maturity. The advantages of this test are its simplicity, rapidity, reliability, and low cost. In the same study, measurement of the surfactant proteins indicated that the levels of SP-B/C were good predictors for RDS and equivalent to the stable microbubble test.

Today the risk for neonatal RDS can be predicted fairly well. The morbidity and mortality from RDS can be prevented or reduced either by enhancing endogenous surfactant production in the fetus with maternal hormonal treatment (52) or by treating the newborn with surfactant replacement preparations. Experimental evidence suggests that these therapies have synergistic effects and that a combination of these therapies may provide a better outcome than either one alone (134,139,267).

Meconium Aspiration

Meconium aspiration occurs in 1% to 3% of all term and postterm births and may result in neonatal respiratory distress marked by hypoxemia and a lowering of lung compliance. In vitro studies have shown that meconium can inhibit the surface tension-lowering capabilities of surfactant (202). This inhibitory activity resides in both the water-soluble and the organic-soluble fractions of meconium, although the precise chemical nature of the inhibitory agent(s) is not known (202). However, as surfactant levels increase, much of the inhibition can be overcome, suggesting that surfactant replacement therapy might be a useful treatment for some cases of meconium aspiration. This has been confirmed in a rabbit model of meconium aspiration (300) and in limited clinical trials (9,299).

ARDS

The development of acute respiratory failure in several patients that did not respond to ordinary respiratory therapy was first described by Ashbaugh et al. (7). Because the clinical observations (reduced compliance, tachypnea, hypoxemia) and pathologic findings (hyaline membranes, atelectasis, etc.) were similar to the infant respiratory distress syndrome the term, *adult respiratory distress syndrome* was used to describe this type of respiratory failure (231).

Consequently, surfactant abnormalities have been implicated as contributing to lung dysfunction (reviewed in refs. 120, 178,282). These surfactant derangements include abnormal composition (114,116,246,279), derangements in intraalveolar metabolism (177,245), and surfactant inactivation (244,273). These and additional surfactant perturbations can lead to abnormal surfactant function with serious consequences. Although surfactant derangement may not be a primary cause of ARDS, it is likely that correction of the deranged surfactant system will improve the course of ARDS (129,178,224). Surfactant replacement therapy has been used in many animal models of lung injury (121,266) and in limited clinical situations with some encouraging results (173,209,258).

Other Diseases

Deranged levels of surfactant proteins have been associated with a variety of other disease states. In many cases these associations may not indicate a specific cause and effect relationship that would serve as a diagnostic tool for the particular disease, but they may represent derangements of a common mechanism underlying many (if not all) of the pulmonary diseases described in this regard.

In alveolar proteinosis, SP-A content is high in bronchoalveolar lavage and in sputum from these patients (191), whereas in specimens from patients with idiopathic pulmonary fibrosis SP-A content is low (194). However, in the sera from both patients with alveolar proteinosis and patients with idiopathic pulmonary fibrosis, high levels of SP-A were detected (169). In addition, some of the structural characteristics of the surfactant proteins were found to be altered in lung lavage from patients with alveolar proteinosis (328). Although both of these diseases are of unknown etiology, several years ago it was suggested that some cases of alveolar proteinosis may have a genetic component (307). Recently it was shown that a genetic defect in SP-B correlated with a case of congenital alveolar proteinosis (208). SP-B mRNA was absent in that case report, whereas SP-A and SP-C mRNA were not.

Increased SP-A was found in lavage from patients with AIDS-related pneumonia (241) and in alveolar macrophages from patients with hypersensitivity pneumonitis (106), although decreased levels have been reported in patients with bacterial pneumonia (18). In addition it has been proposed that asthma might be related to surfactant dysfunction in small airways. A study of airway morphology suggests that surface tension may be important in maintaining the patency of constricted airways (355). A technique designed to measure this property of surfactant in vitro has been described (183), and a small clinical study showed that a dose of aerosolized surfactant can improve pulmonary function in patients having asthmatic attacks (163). Although it is tempting to speculate that the production of SP-B by bronchiolar epithelial cells (240) helps maintain the patency of bronchioles, at present the possible involvement of SP-A or SP-B in these disease states is unclear.

CONCLUSIONS

The flurry of recent research on pulmonary surfactant and its protein constituents is providing some insight into the way these constituents interact to reduce surface tension in the lung. The intricacies of the genes for the surfactant proteins are being unraveled and our understanding of the molecular mechanisms regulating their expression is expanding. During this era, the use of exogenous surfactant to treat neonatal RDS has become a reality and prenatal mortality due to RDS is decreasing, although this therapy is not a panacea and some infants do not respond to treatment.

As this chapter and other recent reviews have shown, it is now becoming clear that alterations in surfactant function and metabolism may play a role in the pathogenesis of other pulmonary diseases. Exciting recent studies are beginning to forge links between some of these conditions and the structures of some of the surfactant protein genes. Furthermore, while the reduction of surface tension has always been viewed as the primary function of surfactant, rapidly accumulating evidence is linking various surfactant components to other aspects of lung function. Among these are the regulation of surfactant homeostasis and the maintenance of normal host-defense function. These and other areas will undoubtedly be the subject of numerous investigations and will be important considerations in the design of future surfactant replacement preparations. While some aspects of surfactant research are more advanced, others, such as the patients currently benefiting from it, are only in their infancy.

ADDENDUM

In the period since this chapter was written, several advances have been made with the human surfactant protein A and B loci. The human SP-B gene was localized on the short arm of chromosome 2 (2p12→2p11.2) (364). The molecular defect (121ins2) of SP-B that is implicated in the etiology of congenital alveolar proteinosis, has been identified in several unrelated infants (365,366). In patients with alveolar proteinosis, SP-B deficiency has been shown to associate with quantitative and qualitative abnormalities of the surfactant proteins A and C (366,367).

An SP-B polymorphism within intron 4, resulting from the gain or loss in the number of copies of a composite motif, has been found with significantly higher frequency in the RDS population (368). The distribution of the intron 4 SP-B alleles has also been shown to differ between Caucasians and African-Americans or Nigerians (369). This observation underscores the importance of racial composition in groups under study.

Work of the human SP-A locus has revealed extensive variability at several levels (370–372). A number of splice variants with different 5′ untranslated regions and different coding alleles have been identified and characterized for each functional SP-A gene (370,373–375). These alleles are shown to be translated in vitro and in vivo as determined by the presence of the SP-A mRNA on polysomes (373,376). Our preliminary findings indicate that the SP-A splice variants have a genetic basis and that there is a phenotype/genotype correlation between SP-A alleles and the level of SP-A mRNA (377). It would be of interest to study the regulation of expression of each SP-A allele and determine whether the impact of disease alters differentially the expression of various alleles.

It has also become clear that the influence of surfactant on the macrophage extends beyond modulating its phagocytic potential. Earlier studies on the effect of surfactant on immune cell proliferation have described the inhibition of proliferation by the major lipid components of surfactant and have also reported stimulatory effects by some of the lipid components. Recently, it has been shown that SP-A, a lectin, has the ability to stimulate immune cell proliferation in vitro, as many other lectins have been shown to do (378).

It has also been shown in a number of studies that surfactant can alter immune cell function by modulating the production and release of the proinflammatory cytokines by macrophages and monocytes. The surfactant lipids and some of the surfactant replacement preparations inhibit cytokine production by endotoxin-stimulated macrophages (379,380). SP-A, on the other hand, has been shown to be capable of stimulating the production of the proinflammatory cytokines by immune cells (381) and colony stimulating factor by epithelial cells (382). These studies raise the possibility that the inflammatory status of the lung is regulated by the relative abundance of different surfactant components and that alterations in surfactant composition may be an initiating factor in lung inflammation, rather than a consequence of it (383).

ACKNOWLEDGEMENTS

The authors thank Dr. Anne Karinch, Kevin Keough, and Mary Ellen Avery for their helpful suggestions and Beth Ditzler for typing this manuscript. This work was supported by NIH grants HL34788, HL49823, HL38288, HL48006, and GM48699.

REFERENCES

1. Acarregui MJ, Snyder JM, Mitchell MD, Mendelson CR. Prostaglandins regulate surfactant protein A (SP-A) gene expression in human fetal lung in vitro. *Endocrinology* 1990;127: 1105–1113.
2. Acarregui MJ, Snyder, JM, Mendelson, CR. Oxygen modulates the differentiation of human fetal lung in vitro and its responsiveness to cAMP. *Am J Physiol* 1993;264: (Lung Cell Mol Physiol 8) L465–L474.
3. Alcorn JL, Chen Q, Boggaram V, Mendelson CR. Expression and transport of rabbit surfactant protein A in COS-1 cells. *Am J Physiol* (Lung Cell Mol Physiol 6) 1992;262:L437–L445.
4. Alcorn JL, Mendelson CR. Trafficking of surfactant protein-A in fetal rabbit lung in organ culture. *Am J Physiol* (Lung Cell Mol Physiol 8) 1993;264:L27–L35.
5. Amirkhanian JD, Bruni R, Waring AJ, Taeusch HW. Inhibition of mixtures of surfactant lipids and synthetic sequences of surfactant proteins SP-B and SP-C. *Biochim Biophys Acta* 1991;1096:355–360.
6. Ansfield MJ, Kaltreider HB, Benson BJ, Shalaby MR. Canine surface active material and pulmonary lymphocyte function: Studies with mixed-lymphocyte culture. *Exp Lung Res* 1980;1:3–11.
7. Ashbaugh DG, Bigelow DB, Petty TL, Levine BE. Acute respiratory distress in adults. *Lancet* 1967;2:319–323.
8. Auten RL, Watkins RH, Shapiro DL, Horowitz S. Surfactant apoprotein A (SP-A) is synthesized in airway cells. *Am J Respir Cell Mol Biol* 1990;3:491–496.
9. Auten RL, Notter RH, Kendig JW, Davis JM, Shapiro DL. Surfactant treatment of full-term newborns with respiratory failure. *Pediatrics* 1991;87:101–107.
10. Avery ME, Mead J. Surface properties in relation to atelectasis and hyaline membrane disease. *Am J Dis Child* 1959;97:517–523.
11. Baatz JE, Elledge B, Whitsett JA. Surfactant protein SP-B induces ordering at the surface of model membrane bilayers. *Biochem* 1990;29:6714–6720.
12. Baatz JE, Sarin V, Absolom DR, Baxter C, Whitsett JA. Effects of surfactant-associated protein SP-B synthetic analogs on the structure and surface activity of model membrane bilayers. *Chem Phys Lipids* 1991;60:163–178.
13. Bakewell WE, Viviano CJ, Dixon D, Smith GJ, Hook GER. Confocal laser scanning immunofluorescence microscopy of lamellar bodies and pulmonary surfactant protein A in isolated alveolar type II cells. *Lab Invest* 1991;65:87–95.
14. Ballard PL. Hormonal regulation of pulmonary surfactant. *Endocr Rev* 1989;10:165–181.
15. Ballard PL, Liley HG, Gonzales LW, et al. Interferon-gamma and synthesis of surfactant components by cultured human fetal lung. *Am J Respir Cell Mol Biol* 1990;2:137–143.
16. Bartmann P, Bamberger U, Pohlandt F, Gortner L. Immunogenicity and immunomodulatory activity of bovine surfactant (SF-RI 1). *Acta Paediatr* 1992;81:383–388.
17. Batenburg JJ. Surfactant phospholipids: Synthesis and storage. *Am J Physiol* 1992;262(Lung Cell Mol Physiol 6):L367–L385.
18. Baughman RP, Sternberg RI, Hull W, Buchsbaum JA, Whitsett J. Decreased surfactant protein-A in patients with bacterial pneumonia. *Am Rev Respir Dis* 1993;147:653–657.
19. Beers MF, Fisher AB. Surfactant protein-C—A Review of its unique properties and metabolism. *Am J Physiol* (Lung Cell Mol Physiol 8) 1992;263:L151–L160.
20. Bensch K, Schaefer K, Avery ME. Granular pneumocytes: Electron microscopic evidence of their exocrinic function. *Science* 1964; 145:1318–1319.

21. Benson B, Hawgood S, Schilling J, et al. Structure of canine pulmonary surfactant apoprotein: cDNA and complete amino acid sequence. *Proc Natl Acad Sci USA* 1985;82:6379–6383.
22. Bermel MS, McBride JT, Notter RH. Lavaged excised rat lungs as a model of surfactant deficiency. *Lung* 1984;162:99–113.
23. Bernal AL, Newman GE, Phizackerley PJR, Turnbull AC. Effect of lipid and protein fractions from fetal pulmonary surfactant on prostaglandin E production by a human amnion cell line. *Eicosanoids* 1989;2:29–32.
24. Boggaram V, Mendelson CR. Transcriptional regulation of the gene encoding the major surfactant protein (SP-A) in rabbit fetal lung. *J Biol Chem* 1988;263:19060–19065.
25. Boggaram V, Qing K, Mendelson CR. The major apoprotein of rabbit pulmonary surfactant. *J Biol Chem* 1988;263:2939–2947.
26. Boggaram V, Smith ME, Mendelson CR. Regulation of expression of the gene encoding the major surfactant protein (SP-A) in human fetal lung in vitro. *J Biol Chem* 1989;264:11421–11427.
27. Boggaram V, Smith ME, Mendelson CR. Posttranscriptional regulation of surfactant protein-A messenger RNA in human fetal lung in vitro by glucocorticoids. *Mol Endocrinol* 1991;5:414–423.
28. Boggaram V, Margana RK. Rabbit surfactant protein C: cDNA cloning and regulation of alternatively spliced surfactant protein C mRNAs. *Am J Physiol* (Lung Cell Mol Physiol 7) 1992;263:L634–L644.
29. Bohinski RJ, Huffman JA, Whitsett JA, Lattier DL. Cis-active elements controlling lung cell-specific expression of human pulmonary surfactant protein B gene. *J Biol Chem* 1993;268:11160–11166.
30. Breslin JS, Weaver TE. Binding, uptake, and localization of surfactant protein-B in isolated rat alveolar Type-II cells. *Am J Physiol* (Lung Cell Mol Physiol 6) 1992;262:L699–L707.
31. Broers JLV, Jensen SM, Travis WD, et al. Expression of surfactant associated protein-A and clara cell 10 kilodalton mRNA in neoplastic and non-neoplastic human lung tissue as detected by in situ hybridization. *Lab Invest* 1992;66:337–346.
32. Brown LAS, Pasquale SM, Longmore WJ. Role of microtubules in surfactant secretion. *J Appl Physiol* 1985;58:1866–1873.
33. Bruni R, Taeusch HW, Waring AJ. Surfactant protein B: Lipid interactions of synthetic peptides representing the amino-terminal amphipathic domain. *Proc Natl Acad Sci USA* 1991;88:7451–7455.
34. Bruns G, Stroh H, Velman GM, Latt SA, Floros J. The 35kd pulmonary surfactant-associated protein is encoded on chromosome 10. *Hum Genet* 1987;76:58–62.
35. Buckingham S. Studies on the identification of an antiatelectasis factor in normal sheep lung. *Am J Dis Child* 1961;102:521–522.
36. Buckingham S, Avery ME. Time of appearance of lung surfactant in the foetal mouse. *Nature* 1962;193:688–689.
37. Buckingham S, McNary WF, Sommers SC, Rothschild J. Is lung an analog of Moog's developing intestine? I. Phosphatases and pulmonary alveolar differentiation in fetal rabbits. *Fed Proc* 1968;27:328.
38. Catanzaro A, Richman P, Batcher S, Hallman M. Immunomodulation by pulmonary surfactant. *J Lab Clin Med* 1988;112:727–734.
39. Chander A. Regulation of lung surfactant secretion by intracellular pH. *Am J Physiol* (Lung Cell Mol Physiol 1) 1989;257:L354–L360.
40. Chander A, Fisher AB. Regulation of lung surfactant secretion. *Am J Physiol* (Lung Cell Mol Physiol 2) 1990;258:L241–L253.
41. Chander A, Wu R-D. In vitro fusion of lung lamellar bodies and plasma membrane is augmented by lung synexin. *Biochim Biophys Acta* 1991;1086:157–166.
42. Chen Q, Boggaram V, Mendelson CR. Rabbit lung surfactant protein A gene: Identification of a lung-specific DNase I hypersensitive site. *Am J Physiol* (Lung Cell Mol Physiol 6) 1992;262:L662–L671.
43. Chida S, Phelps DS, Cordle C, Soll R, Floros J, Taeusch HW. Surfactant-associated proteins in tracheal aspirates of infants with respiratory distress syndrome after surfactant therapy. *Am Rev Respir Dis* 1988;137:943–947.
44. Chida S, Phelps DS, Soll RF, Taeusch HW. Surfactant proteins and anti-surfactant antibodies in sera from infants with respiratory distress syndrome with and without surfactant treatment. *Pediatrics* 1991;88(1):84–89.
45. Chida S, Fujiwara T. Stable Microbubble test for predicting the risk of respiratory distress syndrome. 1. Comparisons with other predictors of fetal lung maturity in amniotic fluid. *Eur J Pediatr* 1993;152:148–151.
46. Childs RA, Wright JR, Ross GF, et al. Specificity of lung surfactant protein SP-A for both the carbohydrate and the lipid moieties of certain neutral glycolipids. *J Biol Chem* 1992;267:9972–9979.
47. Chung J, Yu SH, Whitsett JA, Harding PGR, Possmayer F. Effect of surfactant-associated protein-A (SP-A) on the activity of lipid extract surfactant. *Biochim Biophys Acta* 1989;1002:348–358.
48. Clements JA. Surface tension of lung extracts. *Proc Soc Exp Biol Med* 1957;95:170–172.
49. Coalson JJ, Winter VT, Martin HM, King RJ. Colloidal gold immunoultrastructural localization of rat surfactant. *Am Rev Respir Dis* 1986;133:230–237.
50. Cochrane CG, Revak SD. Pulmonary surfactant protein B (SP-B): Structure-function relationships. *Science* 1991;254:566–568.
51. Cockshutt AM, Weitz J, Possmayer F. Pulmonary surfactant-associated protein A enhances the surface activity of lipid extract surfactant and reverses inhibition by blood proteins in vitro. *Biochemistry* 1990;29:8424–8429.
52. Collaborative Group on Antenatal Steroid Therapy. Effect of antenatal dexamethasone administration on the prevention of respiratory distress syndrome. *Am J Obstet Gynecol* 1981;141:276–287.
53. Connelly I, Possmayer F. cDNA sequences and alternative mRNA splicing of surfactant-associated protein C (SP-C) in rabbit lung. *Biochim Biophys Acta* 1992;1127:199–207.
54. Coonrod JD, Jarrells MC, Yoneda K. Effect of rat surfactant lipids on complement and Fc receptors of macrophages. *Infect Immun* 1986;54:371–378.
55. Corbet A, Bedi H, Owens M, Taeusch W. Surfactant protein-A inhibits lavage-induced surfactant secretion in newborn rabbits. *Am J Med Sci* 1992;304:246–251.
56. Crouch E, Rust K, Mariencheck W, Parghi D, Chang D, Persson A. Developmental expression of pulmonary surfactant protein D (SP-D). *Am J Respir Cell Mol Biol* 1991;5:13–18.
57. Crouch E, Parghi D, Kuan SF, Persson A. Surfactant protein-D - subcellular localization in nonciliated bronchiolar epithelial cells. *Am J Physiol*(Lung Cell Mol Physiol 7) 1992;263:L60–L66.
58. Crouch E, Rust K, Veile R, Doniskeller H, Grosso L. Genomic organization of human surfactant protein-D (SP-D)—SP-D is encoded on chromosome 10q22.2–23.1. *J Biol Chem* 1993;268:2976–2983.
59. Curstedt T, Jornvall H, Robertson B, Bergman T, Berggren P. Two hydrophobic low-molecular-mass protein fractions of pulmonary surfactant. Characterization and biophysical activity. *Eur J Biochem* 1987;168:255–262.
60. Curstedt T, Johansson J, Barros-Soderling J, et al. Low molecular mass surfactant protein type 1. The primary structure of a hydrophobic 8-kDa polypeptide with eight half-cystine residues. *Eur J Biochem* 1988;172:521–525.
61. Curstedt T, Johansson J, Persson P, et al. Hydrophobic surfactant-associated polypeptides: SP-C is a lipopeptide with two palmitoylated cysteine residues, whereas SP-B lacks covalently linked fatty acyl groups. *Proc Natl Acad Sci USA* 1990;87:2985–2989.
62. D'Amore-Bruno MA, Wikenheiser KA, Carter JE, Clark JC, Whitsett JA. Sequence, ontogeny, and cellular localization of murine surfactant protein B mRNA. *Am J Physiol* (Lung Cell Mol Physiol 6) 1991;262:L40–L47.
63. Dekowski SA, Snyder JM. Insulin regulation of messenger ribonucleic acid for the surfactant-associated proteins in human fetal lung in vitro. *Endocrinology* 1992;131:669–676.
64. DeLemos RA, Shermeta DW, Knelson JH, Kotas R, Avery ME. Acceleration of appearance of pulmonary surfactant in the fetal lamb by administration of corticosteroids. *Am Rev Respir Dis* 1970;102:459–461.
65. deMello DE, Chi EY, Doo E, Lagunoff D. Absence of tubular myelin in lungs of infants dying with hyaline membrane disease. *Am J Pathol* 1987;127:131–139.
66. deMello DE, Phelps DS, Patel G, Floros J, Lagunoff D. Expression of the 35kDa and low molecular weight surfactant—associated proteins in the lungs of infants dying with respiratory distress syndrome. *Am J Pathol* 1989;134:1285–1293.
67. deMello DE, Heyman S, Phelps DS, Floros J. Immunogold localization of SP-A in lungs of infants dying from respiratory distress syndrome. *Am J Pathol* 1993;142:1631–1640.
68. Dobbs LG, Wright JR, Hawgood S, Gonzalez R, Venstrom K, Nellenbogen J. Pulmonary surfactant and its components inhibit secretion of phosphatidylcholine from cultured rat alveolar type II cells. *Proc Natl Acad Sci USA* 1987;84:1010–1014.
69. Donald IR, Freeman RK, Goebelsmann U, Chan WH, Nakamura RM. Clinical experience with the amniotic fluid lecithin/sphingomyelin ratio. I. Antenatal prediction of pulmonary maturity. *Am J Obstet Gynecol* 1973;115:547–552.
70. Drickamer K, Dordal MS, Reynolds L. Mannose-binding proteins isolated from rat liver contain carbohydrate-recognition domains

linked to collagenous tails, complete primary structures and homology with pulmonary surfactant apoprotein. *J Biol Chem* 1986;261:6878–6887.

71. Durand DJ, Clyman RI, Heymann MA, et al. Effects of a protein-free, synthetic surfactant on survival and pulmonary function in preterm lambs. *J Pediatr* 1985;107:775–780.
72. Durham PL, Nanthakumar EJ, Snyder JM. Developmental regulation of surfactant-associated proteins in rabbit fetal lung in vivo. *Exp Lung Res* 1992;18:775–793.
73. Eijking EP, Strayer DS, Van Daal GJ, Lachmann B. Effects of anti-surfactant antibodies on the course of mild respiratory distress syndrome. *Pathobiology* 1991;59:96–101.
74. Emrie PA, Jones C, Hofman T, Fisher JH. The coding sequence for the human 18,000-Dalton hydrophobic pulmonary surfactant protein is located on chromosome 2 and identifies a restriction fragment length polymorphism. *Somat Cell Mol Genet* 1988;14:105–110.
75. Emrie PA, Shannon JM, Mason RJ, Fisher JH. cDNA and deduced amino acid sequence for the rat hydrophobic pulmonary surfactant- associated protein, SP-B. *Biochim Biophys Acta* 1989;994: 215–221.
76. Enhorning G. Pulsating bubble technique for evaluating pulmonary surfactant. *J Appl Physiol* 1977;43:198–203.
77. Enhorning G, Shennan A, Possmayer F, Dunn M, Chen CP, Milligan J. Prevention of neonatal respiratory distress syndrome by tracheal instillation of surfactant: a randomized clinical trial. *Pediatrics* 1985;76:145–153.
78. Enhorning G, Shennan AT. Surfactant supplementation in the neonatal period. In: Fishman AP, ed. *Update: pulmonary diseases and disorders.* New York: McGraw-Hill, 1992;213–223.
79. Fisher JH, Kao FT, Jones C, White RT, Benson BJ, Mason RJ. The coding sequence for the 32,000-dalton pulmonary surfactant-associated protein A is located on chromosome 10 and identifies two separate restriction-fragment-length polymorphisms. *Am J Hum Genet* 1987;40:503–511.
80. Fisher JH, Emrie PA, Drabkin HA, et al. The gene encoding the hydrophobic surfactant protein SP-C is located on 8p and identifies an EcoRI RFLP. *Am J Hum Genet* 1988;43:436–441.
81. Fisher JH, Emrie PA, Shannon J, Sano K, Hattler B, Mason RJ. Rat pulmonary surfactant protein A is expressed as two differently sized mRNA species which arise from differential polyadenylation of one transcript. *Biochim Biophys Acta* 1988;950:338–345.
82. Fisher AB, Dodia C, Chander A. Secretagogues for lung surfactant increase lung uptake of alveolar phospholipids. *Am J Physiol* (Lung Cell Mol Physiol 1) 1989;257:L248-L252.
83. Fisher JH, McCormack F, Park SS, Stelzner T, Shannon JM, Hofmann T. In Vivo regulation of surfactant proteins by glucocorticoids. *Am J Respir Cell Mol Biol* 1991;5:63–70.
84. Floros J, Phelps DS, Taeusch HW. Biosynthesis and in vitro translation of the major surfactant-associated protein from human lung. *J Biol Chem* 1985;260:495–500.
85. Floros J, Phelps DS, Kourembanas S, Taeusch HW. Primary translation products and tissue specificity of the major surfactant protein in rat. *J Biol Chem* 1986;261:828–831.
86. Floros J, Steinbrink R, Jacobs K, et al. Isolation and characterization of cDNA clones for the 35kDa pulmonary surfactant associated protein (PSP-A). *J Biol Chem* 1986;261:9029–9033.
87. Floros J, Phelps DS, Harding HP, Church S, Ware J. Postnatal stimulation of rat surfactant protein A synthesis by dexamethasone. *Am J Physiol*(Lung Cell Mol Physiol 1) 1989;257:137–143.
88. Floros J, Gross I, Nichols KV, et al. Hormonal effects on the surfactant protein B (SP-B) mRNA in cultured fetal rat lung. *Am J Respir Cell Mol Biol* 1991;4:449–454.
89. Floros J, Phelps DS, deMello DE, Longmate J, Harding H, Benson B, White T. The utility of post-mortem lung for RNA studies: Variability and correlation of the expression of surfactant proteins in human lung. *Exp Lung Res* 1991;17:91–104.
90. Floros J, Rishi A, Veletza SV, Rogan PK. Concerted and independent genetic events in the 3′ untranslated region of the human surfactant protein A genes. *Am J Hum Gen* 1993;53:A683.
91. Froh D, Ballard PL, Williams MC, et al. Lamellar bodies of cultured human fetal lung: content of surfactant protein A (SP-A), surface film formation and structural transformation in vitro. *Biochim Biophys Acta* 1990;1052:78–89.
92. Froh D, Gonzales LW, Ballard PL. Secretion of surfactant protein A and phosphatidylcholine from type II cells of human fetal lung. *Am J Respir Cell Mol Biol* 1993;8:556–561.
93. Fujiwara T, Maeta H, Chida S, Morita T, Watabe Y, Abe T. Artificial surfactant therapy in hyaline membrane disease. *Lancet* 1980;1: 55–59.
94. Glasser SW, Korfhagen TR, Weaver T, Pilot-Matias T, Fox JL, Whitsett JA. cDNA and deduced amino acid sequence of human pulmonary surfactant-associated proteolipid SPL (Phe). *Proc Natl Acad Sci USA* 1987;84:4007–4011.
95. Glasser SW, Korfhagen TR, Perme CM, Pilot-Matias TJ, Kister SE, Whitsett JA. Two SP-C genes encoding human pulmonary surfactant proteolipid. *J Biol Chem* 1988;263:10326–10331.
96. Glasser SW, Korfhagen TR, Bruno MD, Dey C, Whitsett JA. Structure and expression of the pulmonary surfactant protein SP-C gene in the mouse. *J Biol Chem* 1990;265:21986–21991.
97. Glasser SW, Korfhagen TR, Wert SE, Bruno MD, McWilliams KM, Vorbroker DK, Whitsett JA. Genetic element from human surfactant protein SP-C gene confers bronchiolar-alveolar cell specificty in transgenic mice. *Am J Physiol* (Lung Cell Mol Physiol 5) 1991; 261:L349–L356.
98. Gluck L, Kulovich MV, Borer RC, Brenner PH, Anderson GG, Spellacy WN. Diagnosis of the respiratory distress syndrome by amniocentesis. *Am J Obstet Gynecol* 1971;109:440–445.
99. Griese M, Gobran LI, Rooney SA. Surfactant lipid uptake and secretion in type II cells in response to lectins and secretagogues. *Am J Physiol* (Lung Cell Mol Physiol 5) 1991;261:L434–L442.
100. Gross I, Wilson CM, Floros J, Dynia DW. Initiation of fetal rat lung phospholipid and surfactant-associated protein A mRNA synthesis. *Ped Res* 1989;25:239–244.
101. Gross NJ, Narine KR. Surfactant subtypes of mice: Metabolic relationships and conversion in vitro. *J Appl Physiol* 1989;67:414–421.
102. Gross NJ, Schultz RM. Serine proteinase requirement for the extra-cellular metabolism of pulmonary surfactant. *Biochim Biophys Acta* 1990;1044:222–230.
103. Guttentag SH, Phelps DS, Floros J. Surfactant protein regulation and diabetic pregnancy. *Semin Perinatol* 1992;16:122–129.
104. Guttentag SH, Phelps DS, Stenzel W, Warshaw J, Floros J. Surfactant protein A expression is delayed in fetuses of streptozotocin-treated rats. *Am J Physiol* (Lung Cell Mol Physiol 6) 1992;262: L489–L494.
105. Guttentag SH, Phelps DS, Warshaw J, Floros J. Delayed hydrophobic surfactant protein (SP-B, SP-C) expression in fetuses of streptozotocin-treated rats. *Am J Respir Cell Mol Biol* 1992;7:190–197.
106. Guzman J, Wang Y-M, Kalaycioglu O, Schoenfeld B, Hamm H, Bartsch W, Costabel U. Increased surfactant protein A content in human alveolar macrophages in hypersensitivity pneumonitis. *Acta Cytol* 1992;36:668–673.
107. Haagsman HP, Hawgood S, Sargeant T, et al. The major lung surfactant protein, SP 28–36, is a calcium-dependent, carbohydrate-binding protein. *J Biol Chem* 1987;262:13877–13880.
108. Haagsman HP, White RT, Schilling J, et al. Studies of the structure of lung surfactant protein SP-A. *Am J Physiol* (Lung Cell Mol Physiol 1) 1989;257:L421–L429.
109. Haagsman HP, Sargeant T, Hauschka PV, Benson BJ, Hawgood S. Binding of calcium to SP-A, a surfactant-associated protein. *Biochemistry* 1990;29:8894–8990.
110. Haagsman HP, Elfring RH, van Buel BLM, Voorhout WF. The lung lectin surfactant protein A aggregates phospholipid vesicles via a novel mechanism. *Biochem J* 1991;275:273–276.
111. Häfner D, Kilian U, Bühler R, Beume R, Habel R. Comparison of a phospholipid-based protein-free surfactant and a natural bovine surfactant (SURVANTA*) during pressure and volume-controlled ventilation in an improved rabbit fetus model. *Pulmon Pharmacol* 1993;6:15–25.
112. Hall SB, Venkitaraman AR, Whitsett JA, Holm BA, Notter RH. Importance of hydrophobic apoproteins as constituents of clinical exogenous surfactants. *Am Rev Respir Dis* 1992;145:24–30.
113. Haller EM, Shelley SA, Montgomery MR, Balis JU. Immunocytochemical localization of lysozyme and surfactant protein A in rat type II cells and extracellular surfactant forms. *J Histochem Cytochem* 1992;40:1491–1500.
114. Hallman M, Spragg R, Harrell JH, Moser KM, Gluck L. Evidence of lung surfactant abnormality in respiratory failure, study of bronchoalveolar lavage phospholipids, surface activity, phospholipase activity, and plasma myoinositol. *J Clin Invest* 1982;70: 673–683.
115. Hallman M, Merritt TA, Schneider H, et al. Isolation of human surfactant from amniotic fluid and a pilot study of its efficacy in respiratory distress syndrome. *Pediatrics* 1983;71:473–482.
116. Hallman M, Arjomaa P, Tahvanainen J, Lachmann B, Spragg R.

Endobronchial surface active phospholipids in various pulmonary diseases. *Eur J Respir Res* 1985;142:37–47.
117. Hallman M, Merritt TA, Jarvenpaa AL, et al. Exogenous human surfactant for treatment of severe respiratory distress syndrome: A randomized prospective clinical trial. *J Pediatr* 1985;106: 963–969.
118. Hallman M, Arjomaa P, Mizumoto M, Akino T. Surfactant proteins in the diagnosis of fetal lung maturity: I. predictive accuracy of the 35kD protein, the lecithin/sphingomyelin ratio, and phosphatidylglycerol. *Am J Obstet Gynecol* 1988;158:531–535.
119. Hallman M, Merritt TA, Akino T, Bry K. Surfactant protein A, phosphatidycholine, and surfactant inhibitors in epithelial lining fluid. *Am Rev Resp Dis* 1991;144:1376–1384.
120. Hamm H, Fabel H, Bartsch W. The surfactant system of the adult lung: Physiology and clinical perspectives. *Clin Invest* 1992;70: 637–657.
121. Harris JD, Jackson Jr. F, Moxley MA, Longmore WJ. Effect of exogenous surfactant instillation on experimental acute lung injury. *J Appl Physiol* 1989;66:1846–1851.
122. Hatzis D, Dieter G, deMello D, Floros J. Human surfactant protein-C: Genetic homogeneity and expression in RDS; comparison with other species. *Exp Lung Res* 1993;20:57–72.
123. Hawgood S, Benson BJ, Hamilton Jr. RL. Effects of a surfactant-associated protein and calcium ions on the structure and surface activity of lung surfactant lipids. *Biochem* 1985;24:184–190.
124. Hawgood S, Efrati H, Schilling J, Benson BJ. Chemical characterization of lung surfactant apoproteins: amino acid composition, N-terminal sequence and enzymic digestion. *Biochem Society Trans* 1985;13:1092–1096.
125. Hawgood S, Benson BJ, Schilling J, Damm D, Clements JA, White RT. Nucleotide and amino acid sequences of pulmonary surfactant protein SP 18 and evidence for cooperation between SP 18 and SP 28–36 in surfactant lipid adsorption. *Proc Natl Acad Sci USA* 1987;84:66–70.
126. Hawgood S, Latham D, Borchelt J, et al. Cell-specific post-translational processing of the surfactant-associated protein SP-B. *Am J Physiol* (Lung Cell Mol Physiol 8) 1993;264:L290–L299.
127. Hayakawa H, Myrvik QN, St. Clair RW. Pulmonary surfactant inhibits priming of rabbit alveolar macrophage—Evidence that surfactant suppresses the oxidative burst of alveolar macrophage in infant rabbits. *Am Rev Respir Dis* 1989;140:1390–1397.
128. Hoffman RM, Claypool WD, Katyal SL, Singh G, Rogers RM, Dauber JH. Augmentation of rat alveolar macrophage migration by surfactant protein. *Am Rev Respir Dis* 1987;135:1358–1362.
129. Holm BA, Matalon S. Role of pulmonary surfactant in the development and treatment of adult respiratory distress syndrome. *Anesth Analg* 1989;69:805–818.
130. Horbar JD, Soll RF, Sutherland JM, et al. A multicenter randomized, placebo-controlled trial of surfactant therapy for respiratory distress syndrome. *N Eng J Med* 1989;320:959–965.
131. Horowitz AD, Elledge B, Whitsett JA, Baatz JE. Effects of lung surfactant proteolipid SP-C on the organization of model membrane lipids—a fluorescence study. *Biochim Biophys Acta* 1992;1107: 44–54.
132. Horowitz S, Watkins RH, Auten RL, Mercier CE, Cheng ERY. Differential accumulation of surfactant protein A, B, and C mRNAs in two epithelial cell types of hyperoxic lung. *Am J Respir Cell Mol Biol* 1991;5:511–515.
133. Iannuzzi DM, Ertsey R, Ballard RL. Biphasic glucocorticoid regulation of pulmonary SP-A: Characterization of inhibitory process. *Am J Physiol* (Lung Cell Mol Physiol 8) 1993;264:L236–L244.
134. Ikegami M, Jobe AH, Seidner S, Yamada T. Gestational effects of corticosteroids and surfactant in ventilated rabbits. *Pediatr Res* 1989;25:32–37.
135. Ikegami M, Polk D, Tabor B, Lewis J, Yamada T, Jobe A. Corticosteroid and thyrotropin-releasing hormone effects on preterm sheep lung function. *J Appl Physiol* 1991;70:2268–2278.
136. Ikegami M, Lewis JF, Tabor B, Rider E, Jobe AH. Surfactant protein A metabolism in preterm ventilated lambs. *Am J Physiol* 1992; 262(Lung Cell Mol Physiol 6):L765–L772.
137. Jacobs KA, Phelps DS, Steinbrink R, et al. Isolation of a cDNA clone encoding a high molecular weight precursor to a 6kDa Pulmonary surfactant-associated protein. *J Biol Chem* 1987;262: 9808–9811.
138. Jobe AH. Pulmonary surfactant therapy. *N Engl J Med* 1993;328: 861–868.
139. Jobe AH, Mitchell BR, Gunkel JH. Beneficial effects of the combined use of prenatal corticosteroids and postnatal surfactant on preterm infants. *Am J Obstet Gynecol* 1993;168:508–513.
140. Johansson J, Jornvall H, Eklund A, Christensen N, Robertson B, Curstedt T. Hydrophobic 3.7 kDa surfactant polypeptide: Structural characterization of the human and bovine forms. *FEBS Lett* 1988;232:61–64.
141. Johansson J, Curstedt T, Jornvall H. Surfactant protein B: Disulfide bridges, structural properties, and kringle similarities. *Biochemistry* 1991;30:6917–6921.
142. Johansson J, Curstedt T, Persson P, Robertson B, Lowenadler B, Jornvall H. Hydrophobic surfactant proteins SP-B and SP-C: Special analytical problems. In: Jornvall, Hoog, Gustavsson, eds. *Methods in protein sequence analysis.* Basel: Birkhauser Verlag, 1991; 197–204.
143. Johansson J, Persson P, Lowenadler B, Robertson B, Jornvall H, Curstedt T. Canine hydrophobic surfactant polypeptide SP-C; A lipopeptide with one thioester-linked palmitoyl group. *FEBS Lett* 1991;281:119–122.
144. Jonsson S, Musher DM, Goree A, Lawrence EC. Human alveolar lining material and antibacterial defenses. *Am Rev Respir Dis* 1986; 133:136–140.
145. Juers JA, Rogers RM, McCurdy JB, Cook WW. Enhancement of bactericidal capacity of alveolar macrophages by human alveolar lining material. *J Clin Invest* 1976;58:271–275.
146. Kalina M, Mason RJ, Shannon JM. Surfactant protein-C is expressed in alveolar Type-II cells but not in Clara cells of rat lung. *Am J Respir Cell Mol Biol* 1992;6:594–600.
147. Kalina M, McCormack FX, Crowley H, Voelker DR, Mason RJ. Internalization of surfactant protein A (SP-A) into lamellar bodies of rat alveolar type II cells in vitro. *J Histochem Cytochem* 1993;41: 57–70.
148. Kaltreider HB, Salmon SE. Immunology of the lower respiratory tract—functional properties of bronchoalveolar lymphocytes obtained from the normal canine lung. *J Clin Invest* 1973;52: 2211–2217.
149. Katyal SL, Amenta JS, Singh G, Silverman JA. Deficient lung surfactant apoproteins in amniotic fluid with mature phospholipid profile from diabetic pregnancies. *Am J Obstet Gynecol* 1984;148: 48–53.
150. Katyal SL, Singh G, Locker J. Characterization of a second human pulmonary surfactant-associated protein SP-A gene. *Am J Respir Cell Mol Biol* 1992;6:446–452.
151. Keller A, Eistetter HR, Voss T, Schafer KP. The pulmonary surfactant protein C (SP-C) precursor is a type II transmembrane protein. *Biochem J* 1991;277:493–499.
152. Keller A, Steinhilber W, Schafer KP, Voss T. The C-terminal domain of the pulmonary surfactant protein-C precursor contains signals for intracellular targeting. *Am J Respir Cell Mol Biol* 1992;6: 601–608.
153. King RJ, Clements JA. Surface active materials from dog lung. II. Composition and physiological correlations. *Am J Physiol* 1972; 223:715–726.
154. King RJ, Simon D, Horowitz PM. Aspects of secondary and quaternary structure of surfactant protein A from canine lung. *Biochim Biophys Acta* 1989;1001:294–301.
155. Klaus MH, Clements JA, Havel RJ. Composition of surface-active material isolated from beef lung. *Proc Natl Acad Sci USA* 1961;47: 1858–1859.
156. Kobayashi T, Nitta K, Takahashi R, Kurashima K, Robertson B, Suzuki Y. Activity of pulmonary surfactant after blocking the associated proteins SP-A and SP-B. *J Appl Physiol* 1991;71;530–536.
157. Konishi M, Fujiwara T, Naito T, et al. Surfactant replacement therapy in neonatal respiratory distress syndrome—a multi-centre, randomized clinical trial: comparison of high- versus low-dose of surfactant TA. *Eur J Pediatr* 1988;147:20–25.
158. Korfhagen TR, Glasser SW, Bruno MD, McMahan MJ, Whitsett JA. A portion of the human surfactant protein A (SP-A) gene locus consists of a pseudogene. *Am J Respir Cell Mol Biol* 1991;4:463–469.
159. Kotas RV. The physiologic assessment of lung surfactant. In: Farrell PM, ed. *Lung development: biological and clinical perspectives, vol 1: biochemistry and physiology.* New York: Academic Press, 1982;57–86.
160. Kouretas D, Karinch AM, Rishi A, Melchers K, Floros J. Cloning and sequencing of the 5′ flanking region of human and rat surfactant-associated protein A (SP-A) gene: Identification of DNA regions in rat that bind lung nuclear proteins. *Exp Lung Res* 1993; 19:485–503.

161. Krizkova K, Sakthivel R, Olowe SA, Rogan P, Floros J. Human SP-A: Genotype and single strand conformation polymorphism analysis. *Am J Physiol* 1994;266(Lung Cell. Mol. Physiol. 10):L519–L527.
162. Kuan S-F, Rust K, Crouch E. Interactions of surfactant protein D with bacterial lipopolysaccharides. Surfactant protein D is an Escherichia coli—binding protein in bronchoalveolar lavage. *J Clin Invest* 1992;90:97–106.
163. Kurashima K, Ogawa H, Ohka T, Fujimura M, Matsuda H, Kobayashi T. A pilot study of surfactant inhalation for the treatment of asthmatic attack. *Jpn J Allergol* 1991;40:160–163.
164. Kuroki Y, Mason RJ, Voelker DR. Alveolar type II cells express a high-affinity receptor for pulmonary surfactant protein A. *Proc Natl Acad Sci USA* 1988;85:5566–5570.
165. Kuroki Y, Mason RJ, Voelker DR. Chemical modification of surfactant protein A alters high affinity binding to rat alveolar type II cells and regulation of phospholipid secretion. *J Biol Chem* 1988; 263:17596–17602.
166. Kuroki Y, Akino T. Pulmonary surfactant protein A (SP-A) specifically binds dipalmitoylphosphatidylcholine. *J Biol Chem* 1991;266: 3068–3073.
167. Kuroki Y, Shiratori M, Murata Y, Akino T. Surfactant protein D (SP-D) counteracts the inhibitory effect of surfactant protein A (SP-A) on phospholipid secretion by alveolar type II cells. *Biochem J* 1991;279:115–119.
168. Kuroki Y, Gasa S, Ogasawara Y, Makita A, Akino T. Binding of pulmonary surfactant protein-A to galactosylceramide and asialo-G(M2). *Arch Biochem Biophys* 1992;299:261–267.
169. Kuroki Y, Tsutahara S, Shijubo N, et al. Elevated levels of lung surfactant protein-A in sera from patients with idiopathic pulmonary fibrosis and pulmonary alveolar proteinosis. *Am Rev Respir Dis* 1993;147:723–729.
170. Kwong MS, Egan EA, Notter RH, Shapiro DL. Double-blind clinical trial of calf lung surfactant extract for the prevention of hyaline membrane disease in extremely premature infants. *Pediatrics* 1985;76:585–592.
171. Kyte J, Doolittle RF. A simple method for displaying the hydropathic character of a protein. *J Mol Biol* 1982;157:105–132.
172. Lacaze-Masmonteil T, Fraslon C, Bourbon J, Raymondjean M, Kahn A. Characterization of the rat pulmonary surfactant protein-A promoter. *Eur J Biochem* 1992;206:613–623.
173. Lachman B. Animal models and clinical pilot studies of surfactant replacement in adult respiratory distress syndrome. *Eur Respir J* 1989;2:98s–103s.
174. LaForce FM, Kelly WJ, Huber GL. Inactivation of Staphylocooci by alveolar macrophages with preliminary observations on the importance of alveolar lining material. *Am Rev Respir Dis* 1973;108: 784–790.
175. Leippe M, Tannich E, Nickel R, et al. Primary and secondary structure of the pore-forming peptide of pathogenic Entamoeba histolytica. *EMBO J* 1992;11:3501–3506.
176. Levine D, Edwards III DK, Merritt TA. Synthetic vs. human surfactants in the treatment of respiratory distress syndrome: radiographic findings. *Am J Roentgenol* 1991;157:371–374.
177. Lewis JF, Ikegami M, Jobe AH. Altered surfactant function and metabolism in rabbits with acute lung injury. *J Appl Physiol* 1990; 69:2303–2310.
178. Lewis JF, Jobe AH. Surfactant and the adult respiratory distress syndrome. *Am Rev Respir Dis* 1993;147:218–233.
179. Liggins GC. Premature delivery of foetal lambs infused with glucocorticoids. *J Endocr* 1969;45:515–523.
180. Liggins GC, Howie RN. A controlled trial of antepartum glucocorticoid treatment for prevention of the respiratory distress syndrome in premature infants. *Pediatrics* 1972;50:515–525.
181. Liley HG, White RT, Warr RG, Benson BJ, Hawgood S, Ballard PL. Regulation of mRNAs for the hydrophobic surfactant proteins in human lung. *J Clin Invest* 1989;83:1191–1197.
182. Lim BL, Lu J, Reid KB. Structural similarity between bovine conglutinin and bovine lung surfactant protein D and demonstration of liver as a site of synthesis of conglutinin. *Immunology* 1993;78: 159–65.
183. Liu M, Wang L, Li E, Enhorning G. Pulmonary surfactant will secure free airflow through a narrow tube. *J Appl Physiol* 1991;71: 742–748.
184. Longo ML, Bisagno AM, Zasadzinski JAN, Bruni R, Waring AJ. A function of lung surfactant protein SP-B. *Science* 1993;26:453–456.
185. Lu JH, Willis AC, Reid KBM. Purification, characterization and cDNA cloning of human lung surfactant protein-D. *Biochem J* 1992;284:795–802.
186. Macklin CC. The pulmonary alveolar mucoid film and the pneumonocytes. *Lancet* 1954;1:1099–1104.
187. Magoon MW, Wright JR, Baritussio A, et al. Subfractionation of lung surfactant. Implications for metabolism and surface activity. *Biochim Biophys Acta* 1983;750:18–31.
188. Manz-Keinke H, Plattner H, Schlepper-Schafer J. Lung surfactant protein A (SP-A) enhances serum-independent phagocytosis of bacteria by alveolar macrophages. *Eur J Cell Biol* 1992;57:95–100.
189. Marraro G, Foresti B, Casiraghi G, Preti M. Follow-up on infants treated with porcine surfactant replacement for severe neonatal and infant respiratory distress syndrome: Antigenic reactivity evaluation. *Drugs Exp Clin Res* XVII 1991;(10/11):511–515.
190. Mason RJ. Surfactant secretion. In: Robertson B, van Golde LMG, Batenburg JJ, eds. *Pulmonary surfactant: from molecular biology to clinical practice.* Elsevier Science, 1992;295–312.
191. Masuda T, Shimura S, Sasaki H, Takishima T. Surfactant apoprotein-A concentration in sputum for diagnosis of pulmonary alveolar proteinosis. *Lancet* 1991;337:580–582.
192. Mathialagan N, Possmayer F. Low-molecular-weight hydrophobic proteins from bovine pulmonary surfactant. *Biochim Biophys Acta* 1990;1045:121–127.
193. McCormack FX, Fisher JH, Suwabe A, Smith DL, Shannon JM, Voelker DR. Expression and characterization of rat surfactant protein A synthesized in chinese hamster ovary cells. *Biochim Biophys Acta* 1990;1087:190–198.
194. McCormack FX, King TE, Voelker DR, Robinson PC, Mason RJ. Idiopathic pulmonary fibrosis. Abnormalities in the bronchoalveolar lavage content of surfactant protein A. *Am Rev Respir Dis* 1991; 144:160–166.
195. Mclean LR, Krstenansky JL, Jackson RL, Hagaman KA, Olsen KF, Lewis JE. Mixtures of synthetic peptides and dipalmitoyl-phosphatidylcholine as lung surfactants. *Am J Physiol* 1992;262:(Lung Cell. Mol. Physiol. 6) L292–L300.
196. McNeely TB, Coonrod JD. Comparison of the opsonic activity of human surfactant protein A for *Staphylococcus aureus* and *Streptococcus pneumoniae* with rabbit and human macrophages. *J Infect Dis* 1993;167:91–97.
197. Mendelson CR, Boggaram V. Hormonal control of the surfactant system in fetal lung. *Annu Rev Physiol* 1991;53:415–440.
198. Merritt TA, Hallman M, Holcomb K, et al. Human surfactant treatment of severe respiratory distress syndrome: Pulmonary effluent indicators of lung inflammation. *J Pediatr* 1986;108: 741–748.
199. Minoo P, Segura L, Coalson JJ, King RJ, DeLemos RA. Alterations in surfactant protein gene expression associated with premature birth and exposure to hyperoxia. *Am J Physiol* 1991;261:(Lung Cell Mol Physiol 5) L386–L392.
200. Morley CJ, Bangham AD, Miller N, Davis JA. Dry artificial lung surfactant and its effect on very premature babies. *Lancet* 1981;i: 64–68.
201. Morley CJ, Greenough A, Miller NG, et al. Randomized trial of artificial surfactant (ALEC) given at birth to babies from 23 to 34 weeks gestation. *Early Hum Dev* 1988;17:41–54.
202. Moses D, Holm BA, Spitale P, Liu M, Enhorning G. Inhibition of pulmonary surfactant function by meconium. *Am J Obstet Gynecol* 1991;164:477–481.
203. Müller B, Barth P, Von Wichert P. Structural and functional impairment of surfactant protein A after exposure to nitrogen dioxide in rats. *Am J Physiol* 1992;263(Lung Cell Mol Physiol 7) L177–L184.
204. Newman GE, Phizackerley PJR, Bernal AL. Utilization by human amniocytes for prostaglandin synthesis of [1-^{14}C]arachidonate derived from 2-[1-^{14}C]arachidonylphosphatidylcholine associated with human fetal pulmonary surfactant. *Biochim Biophys Acta* 1993; 1176:106–112.
205. Nibbering PH, van den Barselaar MT, van de Gevel JS, Leijh PCJ, van Furth R. Deficient intracellular killing of bacteria by murine alveolar macrophages. *Am J Respir Cell Mol Biol* 1989;1:417–422.
206. Nichols KV, Floros J, Dynia DW, Veletza SV, Wilson CM, Gross I. Regulation of surfactant protein A mRNA by hormones and butyrate in cultured fetal rat lung. *Am J Physiol* (Lung Cell Mol Physiol 3) 1990;259:L488–L495.
207. Nilsson R, Grossmann G, Robertson B. Lung surfactant and the pathogenesis of neonatal bronchiolar lesions induced by artificial ventilation. *Pediatr Res* 1978;12:249–255.
208. Nogee LM, DeMello DE, Dehner LP, Colten HR. Brief Report: Deficiency of pulmonary surfactant protein B in congenital alveolar proteinosis. *N Engl J Med* 1993;328:406–410.

209. Nosaka S, Sakai T, Yonekura M, Yoshikawa K. Surfactant for adults with respiratory failure. *Lancet* 1990;336:947–948.
210. O'Neill S, Lesperance E, Klass DJ. Rat lung lavage surfactant enhances bacterial phagocytosis and intracellular killing by alveolar macrophages. *Am Rev Respir Dis* 1984;130:225–230.
211. O'Reilly MA, Gazdar AF, Morris RE, Whitsett JA. Differential effects of glucocorticoid on expression of surfactant proteins in a human lung adenocarcinoma cell line. *Biochim Biophys Acta* 1988; 970:194–204.
212. O'Reilly MA, Weaver TE, Pilot-Matias TJ, Sarin VK, Gazdar AF, Whitsett JA. In vitro translation, post-translational processing and secretion of pulmonary surfactant protein B precursors. *Biochim Biophys Acta* 1989;1011:140–148.
213. O'Reilly MA, Clark JC, Whitsett JA. Glucocorticoid enhances pulmonary surfactant protein B gene transcription. *Am J Physiol* (Lung Cell Mol Biol 4) 1991;260:L37–L43.
214. Oetomo SB, Lewis J, Ikegami M, Jobe AH. Surfactant treatments alter endogenous surfactant metabolism in rabbit lungs. *J Appl Physiol* 1990;68:1590–1596.
215. Ogasawara Y, Kuroki Y, Tsuzuki A, Ueda S, Misaki H, Akino T. Pre- and postnatal stimulation of pulmonary surfactant protein D by in vivo dexamethasone treatment of rats. *Life Sci* 1992;50:1761–1767.
216. Ogasawara Y, Kuroki Y, Akino T. Pulmonary surfactant protein D specifically binds to phosphatidylinositol. *J Biol Chem* 1992;267: 21244–21249.
217. Oosterlaken-Dijksterhuis MA, Haagsman HP, van Golde LMG, Demel RA. Characterization of lipid insertion into monomolecular layers mediated by lung surfactant proteins SP-B and SP-C. *Biochemistry* 1991;30:10965–10971.
218. Oosterlaken-Dijksterhuis MA, Haagsman HP, van Golde LMG, Demel RA. Interaction of lipid vesicles with monomolecular layers containing lung surfactant proteins SP-B or SP-C. *Biochemistry* 1991;30:8276–8281.
219. Oosterlaken-Dijksterhuis MA, van Eijk M, van Golde LMG, Haagsman HP. Lipid mixing is mediated by the hydrophobic surfactant protein SP-B but not by SP-C. *Biochim Biophys Acta* 1992;1110: 45–50.
220. Oosting RS, vanGreevenbroek MJ, Verhoef J, van Golde LMG, Haagsman HP. Structural and functional changes of surfactant protein A induced by ozone. *Am J Physiol* (Lung Cell Mol Physiol 5) 1991;261:L77–L83.
221. Oosting RS, van Iwaarden JF, van Bree L, Verhoef J, van Golde LMG, Haagsman HP. Exposure of surfactant protein A to ozone in vitro and in vivo impairs its interactions with alveolar cells. *Am J Physiol* (Lung Cell Mol Physiol 6) 1992;262:L63–L68.
222. Pastrana B, Mautone AJ, Mendelsohn R. Fourier transform infrared studies of secondary structure and orientation of pulmonary surfactant SP-C and its effect on the dynamic surface properties of phospholipids. *Biochemistry* 1991;30:10058–10064.
223. Patthy L. Homology of the precursor of pulmonary surfactant-associated protein SP-B with prosaposin and sulfated glycoprotein 1. *J Biol Chem* 1991;266:6035–6037.
224. Pattishall EN, Long WA. Surfactant treatment of the adult respiratory distress syndrome. In: Fishman AP, ed. *Update: pulmonary diseases and disorders.* New York: McGraw-Hill, 1992;225–236.
225. Pattle RE. Properties, function and origin of the alveolar lining layer. *Nature* 1955;175:1125–1126.
226. Pattle RE, Thomas LC. Lipoprotein composition of the film lining the lung. *Nature* 1961;189:844.
227. Pattle RE, Kratzing CC, Parkinson CE, et al. Maturity of fetal lungs tested by production of stable microbubbles in amniotic fluid. *Br J Obstet Gynaecol* 1979;86:615–622.
228. Perez-Gil J, Nag K, Taneva S, Keough KMW. Pulmonary surfactant protein SP-C causes packing rearrangements of dipalmitoylphosphatidylcholine in spread monolayers. *Biophys J* 1992;63:197–204.
229. Persson A, Chang D, Rust K, Moxley M, Longmore W, Crouch E. Purification and biochemical characterization of CP4 (SP-D), a collagenous surfactant-associated protein. *Biochemistry* 1989;28: 6361–6367.
230. Persson, A, Chang D, Crouch E. Surfactant protein D is a divalent cation-dependent carbohydrate-binding protein. *J Biol Chem* 1990; 265:5755–5760.
231. Petty TL, Ashbaugh DG. The adult respiratory distress syndrome: Clinical features, factors influencing prognosis and principles of management. *Chest* 1971;60:233–239.
232. Phelps DS, Taeusch HW, Benson B, Hawgood S. An electrophoretic and immunochemical characterization of human surfactant-associated proteins. *Biochim Biophys Acta* 1984;791:226–238.
233. Phelps DS, Taeusch HW. A comparison of the major surfactant-associated proteins in different species. *Comp Biochem Physiol* 1985; 82B:441–446.
234. Phelps DS, Floros J, Taeusch HW. Post-translational modification of the major human surfactant-associated proteins. *Biochem J* 1986; 237:373–377.
235. Phelps DS, Church S, Kourembanas S, Taeusch HW, Floros J. Increases in the 35kDa surfactant-associated protein and its mRNA following in vivo dexamethasone treatment of fetal and neonatal rats. *Electrophoresis* 1987;8:235–238.
236. Phelps DS, Smith LM, Taeusch HW. Characterization and partial amino acid sequence of a low molecular weight surfactant protein. *Am Rev Respir Dis* 1987;135:1112–1117.
237. Phelps DS, Floros J. Localization of surfactant protein synthesis in human lung by in situ hybridization. *Am Rev Respir Dis* 1988;137: 939–942.
238. Phelps DS, Floros J. Proline hydroxylation alters the electrophoretic mobility of pulmonary surfactant-associated protein A. *Electrophoresis* 1988;9:231–233.
239. Phelps DS, Floros J. Dexamethasone in vivo raises surfactant protein B mRNA in alveolar and bronchiolar epithelium. *Am J Physiol* (Lung Cell Mol Physiol 4) 1991;4:L146–L152.
240. Phelps DS, Floros J. Localization of pulmonary surfactant proteins using immunohistochemistry and tissue *in situ* hybridization. *Exp Lung Res* 1991;17:985–995.
241. Phelps DS, Rose RM. Increased recovery of surfactant protein A in AIDS-related pneumonia. *Am Rev Respir Dis* 1991;143:1072–1075.
242. Phibbs RH, Ballard RA, Clements JA, et al. Initial clinical trial of EXOSURF, a protein-free synthetic surfactant, for the prophylaxis and early treatment of hyaline membrane disease. *Pediatrics* 1991; 88(1):1–9.
243. Pilot-Matias TJ, Kister SE, Fox JL, Kropp K, Glasser SW, Whitsett JA. Structure and organization of the gene encoding human pulmonary surfactant proteolipid SP-B. *DNA* 1989;8:75–86.
244. Pison U, Tam EK, Caughey GH, Hawgood S. Proteolytic inactivation of dog lung surfactant-associated proteins by neutrophil elastase. *Biochim Biophys Acta* 1989;992:251–257.
245. Pison U, Obertacke U, Brand M, et al. Altered pulmonary surfactant in uncomplicated and septicemia-complicated courses of acute respiratory failure. *J Trauma* 1990;30:19–26.
246. Pison U, Obertacke U, Seeger W, Hawgood S. Surfactant protein-A (SP-A) is decreased in acute parenchymal lung injury associated with polytrauma. *Eur J Clin Invest* 1992;22:712–718.
247. Plopper CG, St. George JA, Read LC, et al. Acceleration of alveolar type II cell differentiation in fetal rhesus monkey lung by administration of EGF. *Am J Physiol* (Lung Cell Mol Physiol 6) 1992;262:L313–L321.
248. Post M, van Golde LMG. Metabolic and developmental aspects of the pulmonary surfactant system. *Biochemica Biophysica Acta* 1988; 947:249–286.
249. Poulain FR, Allen L, Williams MC, Hamilton RL, Hawgood S. Effects of surfactant apolipoproteins on liposome structure: implications for tubular myelin formation. *Am J Physiol* (Lung Cell Mol Physiol 6) 1992;262:L730–L739.
250. Power JHT, Barr HA, Nicholas TE. Surfactant associated 15- and 35-kDA proteins are concentrated in different organelles in rat lung tissue. *Exp Lung Res* 1988;13:209–224.
251. Pryhuber GS, Hull WM, Fink I, McMahan MJ, Whitsett JA. Ontogeny of surfactant proteins A and B in human amniotic fluid as indices of fetal lung maturity. *Pediatr Res* 1991;30:597–605.
252. Randell SH, Silbajoris R, Young SL. Ontogeny of rat lung type II cells correlated with surfactant lipid and surfactant apoprotein expression. *Am J Physiol* (Lung Cell Mol Physiol 4) 1991;260: L562–L570.
253. Reid KBM. Structure/function relationships in the collectins (Mammalian lectins containing collagen-like regions). *Biochem Soc Trans* 1993;21:464–468.
254. Revak SD, Merritt A, Degryse E, et al. Use of human surfactant low molecular weight apoproteins in the reconstitution of surfactant biological activity. *J Clin Invest* 1988;81:826–833.
255. Revak SD, Merritt TA, Hallman M, et al. The use of synthetic peptides in the formation of biophysically and biologically active pulmonary surfactants. *Pediatr Res* 1991;29:460–465.
256. Rice WR, Ross GF, Singleton FM, Dingle S, Whitsett JA. Surfactant-associated protein inhibits phospholipid secretion from type II cells. *J Appl Physiol* 1987;63:692–698.
257. Rich EA. Pulmonary surfactant as a physiologic immunosuppressive agent. *J Lab Clin Med* 1990;116:4–5.

258. Richman PS, Spragg RG, Robertson B, Merritt TA, Curstedt T. The adult respiratory distress syndrome: First trials with surfactant replacement. *Eur Respir J* 1989;2:109s-111s.
259. Rider ED, Ikegami M, Jobe AH. Localization of alveolar surfactant clearance in rabbit lung cells. *Am J Physiol* (Lung Cell Mol Physiol 8) 1992;263:L201–L209.
260. Rider ED, Ikegami M, Whitsett JA, Hull W, Absolom D, Jobe AH. Treatment responses to surfactants containing natural surfactant proteins in preterm rabbits. *Am Rev Respir Dis* 1993;147:669–676.
261. Rishi A, Hatzis D, McAlmon K, Floros J. An allelic variant of the 6A gene for human surfactant protein A. *Am J Physiol* (Lung Cell Mol Physiol 6) 1992;262:L566–L573.
262. Robertson B, Lachmann B. Experimental evaluation of surfactants for replacement therapy. *Exp Lung Res* 1988;14:279–310.
263. Robertson B, Curstedt T, Johansson J, Jörnvall H, Kobayashi T. Structural and functional characterization of porcine surfactant isolated by liquid-gel chromatography. *Prog Respir Res,* 1990;25: 237–246.
264. Robertson B. European multicenter trials of curosurf for treatment of neonatal respiratory distress syndrome. *Lung* 1990;Suppl. 860–863.
265. Robertson B, Kobayashi T, Ganzuka M, Grossmann G, Li WZ, Suzuki Y. Experimental neonatal respiratory failure induced by a monoclonal antibody to the hydrophobic surfactant-associated protein SP-B. *Pediatr Res* 1991;30:239–243.
266. Robertson B. Surfactant inactivation and surfactant replacement in experimental models of ARDS. *Acta Anaesth Scand* 1991;35: 22–28.
267. Robertson B. Corticosteroids and surfactant for prevention of neonatal RDS. *Ann Med* 1993;25:285–288.
268. Rooney SA, Gobran LI, Umstead TM, Phelps DS. Secretion of surfactant protein-A from rat type II pneumocytes. *Am J Physiol* (Lung Cell Mol Physiol) 1993;265:L586–L590.
269. Ross GF, Notter RH, Meuth J, Whitsett JA. Phospholipid binding and biophysical activity of pulmonary surfactant—associated protein (SAP)-35 and its non-collagenous COOH-terminal domains. *J Biol Chem* 1986;261:14283–14291.
270. Ross GF, Sawyer J, O'Connor T, Whitsett JA. Intermolecular crosslinks mediate aggregation of phospholipid vesicles by pulmonary surfactant protein SP-A. *Biochemistry* 1991;30:858–865.
271. Rust K, Grosso L, Zhang V, et al. Human surfactant protein D: SP-D contains a C-type lectin carbohydrate recognition domain. *Arch Biochem Biophys* 1991;290:116–126.
272. Ryan RM, Morris RE, Rice WR, Ciraolo G, Whitsett JA. Binding and uptake of pulmonary surfactant protein (SP-A) by pulmonary type II epithelial cells. *J Histochem Cytochem* 1989;37:429–440.
273. Ryan SF, Ghassibi Y, Liau DF. Effects of activated polymorphonuclear leukocytes upon pulmonary surfactant in vitro. *Am J Respir Cell Mol Biol* 1991;4:33–41.
274. Sanderson RJ, Vatter AE. A mode of formation of tubular myelin from lamellar bodies in the lung. *J Cell Biol* 1977;74:1027–1031.
275. Schellhase DE, Emrie PA, Fisher JH, Shannon JM. Ontogeny of surfactant apoproteins in the rat. *Pediatr Res* 1989;26:167–174.
276. Schellhase DE, Shannon JM. Effects of maternal dexamethasone on expression of SP-A, SP-B, and SP-C in the fetal rat lung. *Am J Respir Cell Mol Biol* 1991;4:304–312.
277. Schurch S, Bachofen H, Goerke J, Green F. Surface properties of rat pulmonary surfactant studied with the captive bubble method—adsorption, hysteresis, stability. *Biochim Biophys Acta* 1992;1103:127–136.
278. Schurch S, Possmayer F, Cheng S, Cockshutt AM. Pulmonary SP-A enhances adsorption and appears to induce surface sorting of lipid extract surfactant. *Am J Physiol* (Lung Cell Mol Physiol 7) 1992;263:L210–L218.
279. Seeger W, Pison U, Buchhorn R, Obertacke U, Joka T. Surfactant abnormalities and adult respiratory failure. *Lung* 1990; Suppl.: 891–902.
280. Seeger W, Thede C, Gunther A, Grube C. Surface properties and sensitivity to protein-inhibition of a recombinant apoprotein C-based phospholipid mixture in vitro -comparison to natural surfactant. Biochim *Biophys Acta* 1991;1081:45–52.
281. Seeger W, Gunther A, Thede C. Differential sensitivity to fibrinogen inhibition of SP-C- based vs SP-B-based surfactants. *Am J Physiol* (Lung Cell Mol Physiol 5) 1992;261:L286–L291.
282. Seeger W, Gunther A, Walmrath HD, Grimminger F, Lasch HG. Alveolar surfactant and adult respiratory distress syndrome. *Clin Invest* 1993;71:177–190.
283. Shelley SA, Balis JU, Paciga JE, Espinoza CG, Richman AV. Biochemical composition of adult human lung surfactant. *Lung* 1982; 160:195–206.
284. Sherman MP, D'Ambola JB, Aeberhard EE, Barrett CT. Surfactant therapy of newborn rabbits impairs lung macrophage bactericidal activity. *J Appl Physiol* 1988;65(1):137–145.
285. Shiffer K, Hawgood S, Düzgünes N, Goerke J. Interactions of the low molecular weight group of surfactant associated proteins (SP 5–18) with pulmonary surfactant lipids. *Biochemistry* 1988;27: 2689–2695.
286. Shiffer K, Hawgood S, Haagsman HP, Benson B, Clements JA, Goerke J. Lung surfactant proteins, SP-B and SP-C, alter the thermodynamic properties of phospholipid membranes—A differential calorimetry study. *Biochemistry* 1993;32:590–597.
287. Shimizu H, Fisher JH, Papst P, et al. Primary structure of rat pulmonary surfactant protein D. *J Biol Chem* 1992;267:1853–1857.
288. Simatos GA, Forward KB, Morrow MR, Keough MW. Interaction between perdeuterated dimyristoylphosphatidylcholine and low molecular weight pulmonary surfactant protein SP-C. *Biochemistry* 1990;29:5807–5814.
289. Smyth JA, Metcalfe IL, Duffty P, Possmayer F, Bryan MH, Enhorning G. Hyaline membrane disease treated with bovine surfactant. *Pediatrics* 1983;71:913–917.
290. Snyder JM, Mendelson CR. Insulin inhibits the accumulation of the major lung surfactant apoprotein in human fetal lung explants maintained in vitro. *Endocrinology* 1987;120:1250–1257.
291. Snyder JM, Kwun JE, O'Brien JA, Rosenfeld CR, Odom MJ. The concentration of the 35-kDa surfactant apoprotein in amniotic fluid from normal and diabetic pregnancies. *Pediatr Res* 1988;24: 728–734.
292. Speer CP, Robertson B, Curstedt T, et al. Randomized European multicenter trial of surfactant replacement therapy for severe neonatal respiratory distress syndrome: Single versus multiple doses of curosurf. *Pediatrics* 1992;89:13–20.
293. Spissinger T, Schafer KP, Voss T. Assembly of the surfactant protein SP-A. Deletions in the globular domain interfere with the correct folding of the molecule. *Eur J Biochem* 1991;199:65–71.
294. Stahlman MT, Gray ME, Whitsett JA. The ontogeny and distribution of surfactant protein B in human fetuses and newborns. *J Histochem Cytochem* 1992;40:1471–1480.
295. Stevens PA, Schadow B, Bartholain S, Segerer H Obladen M. Surfactant protein-A in the course of respiratory distress syndrome. *Eur J Pediatr* 1992;151:596–600.
296. Stults JT, Griffin PR, Lesikar DD, Naidu A, Moffat B, Benson BJ. Lung surfactant protein SP-C from human, bovine, and canine sources contains palmityl cysteine thioester linkages. *Am J Physiol* (Lung Cell. Mol. Physiol. 5) 1991;261:L118–L125.
297. Sueishi K, Benson BJ. Isolation of a major apolipoprotein of canine and murine pulmonary surfactant biochemical and immunochemical characteristics. *Biochim Biophys Acta* 1981;665: 442–453.
298. Sugahara K, Iyama K, Sano K, Morioka T. Overexpression of pulmonary surfactant apoprotein-A messenger RNA in alveolar type-II cells and nonciliated bronchiolar (Clara) epithelial cells in streptozotocin-induced diabetic rats demonstrated by in situ hybridization. *Am J Respir Cell Mol Biol* 1992;6:307–314.
299. Sun B, Curstedt T, Robertson B. Surfactant inhibition in experimental meconium aspiration. *Acta Paediatr* 1993;82;182–189.
300. Sun B, Curstedt T, Song G-W, Robertson B. Surfactant improves lung function and morphology in newborn rabbits with meconium aspiration. *Biol Neonate* 1993;63:96–104.
301. Suwabe A, Mason RJ, Smith D, Firestone JA, Browning MD, Voelker DR. Pulmonary surfactant secretion is regulated by the physical state of extracellular phosphatidylcholine. *J Biol Chem* 1992;267:19884–19890.
302. Suzuki Y, Curstedt T, Grossmann G, et al. The role of the low-molecular weight (<15,000 daltons) apoproteins of pulmonary surfactant. *Eur J Respir Dis* 1986;69:336–345.
303. Suzuki Y, Fujita Y, Kogishi K. Reconstitution of tubular myelin from synthetic lipids and proteins associated with pig pulmonary surfactant. *Am Rev Respir Dis* 1989;140:75–81.
304. Taeusch HW, Heitner M, Avery ME. Accelerated lung maturation and increased survival in premature rabbits treated with hydrocortisone. *Am Rev Respir Dis* 1972;105:971–973.
305. Taeusch HW, Keough KMW, Williams M, et al. Characterization of an exogenous bovine surfactant for infants with respiratory distress syndrome. *Pediatrics* 1986;77:572–581.

306. Tanaka Y, Takei T, Masuda K. Lung surfactants. III. Correlations among activities in vitro, in situ and in vivo, and chemical composition. *Chem Pharm Bull* 1983;31:4110–4115.
307. Teja K, Cooper PH, Squires JE, Schnatterly PT. Pulmonary alveolar proteinosis in four siblings. *N Engl J Med* 1981;305:1390–1392.
308. Tenner AJ, Robinson SL, Borchelt J, Wright JR. Human pulmonary surfactant protein (SP-A), a protein structurally homologous to Clq, can enhance FcR- and CR1-mediated phagocytosis. *J Biol Chem* 1989;264:13923–13928.
309. Thiel S, Reid KBM. Structures and functions associated with the group of mammalian lectins containing collagen-like sequences. *FEBS Lett* 1989;250:78–84.
310. Thorkelsson T, Ciraolo GM, Ross GF, Whitsett JA, Morris RE. Lectin activity of the major surfactant protein (SP-A) may participate in, but is not required for, binding to rat type II cells. *J Histochem Cytochem* 1992;40:643–649.
311. Todd S, Naylor SL. Dinucleotide repeat polymorphism in the human surfactant-associated protein 3 gene (SFTP3). *Nucleic Acids Res* 1992;19:3756.
312. Torday J, Carson L, Lawson EE. Saturated phosphatidylcholine in amniotic fluid and prediction of the respiratory-distress syndrome. *N Engl J Med* 1979;301:1013–1018.
313. Tsilibary EC, Williams MC. Actin and secretion of surfactant. *J Histochem Cytochem* 1983;31:1298–1304.
314. van Iwaarden JF, Welmers B, Verhoef J, Haagsman HP, van Golde LMG. Pulmonary surfactant protein A enhances the host-defense mechanism of rat alveolar macrophages. *Am J Respir Cell Mol Biol* 1990;2:91–98.
315. van Iwaarden JF, van Strip JAG, Ebskamp MJM, Welmers AC, Verhoef J, van Golde LMG. Surfactant protein A is opsonin in phagocytosis of herpes simplex virus type 1 by rat alveolar macrophages. *Am J Physiol* (Lung Cell Mol Physiol 5) 1991;261:L204–L209.
316. van Iwaarden JF, Shimizu H, van Golde PHM, Voelker DR, van Golde LMG. Rat surfactant protein-D enhances the production of oxygen radicals by rat alveolar macrophages. *Biochem J* 1992;286: 5–8.
317. Vandenbussche G, Clercx A, Curstedt T, Johansson J, Jörnvall H, Ruysschaert JM. Structure and orientation of the surfactant-associated protein C in a lipid bilayer. *Eur J Biochem* 1992;203:201–209.
318. Veletza SV, Nichols KV, Gross I, Lu H, Dynia DW, Floros J. Surfactant protein C: Hormonal control of SP-C mRNA levels in vitro. *Am J Physiol* (Lung Cell Mol Physiol 6) 1992;262:L684–L687.
319. Veness-Meehan KA, Cheng ERY, Mercier CE, et al. Cell-specific alterations in expression of hyperoxia-induced mRNAs of lung. *Am J Respir Cell Mol Biol* 1991;5:516–521.
320. Venkatesh VC, Iannuzzi DM, Ertsey R, Ballard PL. Differential glucocorticoid regulation of the pulmonary hydrophobic surfactant proteins SP-B and SP-C. *Am J Respir Cell Mol Biol* 1993;8:222–228.
321. Venkitaraman AR, Hall SB, Notter RH. Hydrophobic homopolymeric peptides enhance the biophysical activity of synthetic lung phospholipids. *Chem Phys Lipids* 1990;53:157–164.
322. von Neergaard K. Neue auffassungen uber einen grundbegriff der atemmechanik. Retracktionskraft der lunge, abhangig von der oberflaschenspunnung in den alveolen. *Z Gesamte Exp Med* 1929; 66:373–394.
323. Voorhout WF, Veenendaal T, Haagsman HP, Verkleij AJ, van Golde LMG, Geuze HJ. Surfactant protein A is localized at the corners of the pulmonary tubular myelin lattice. *J Histochem Cytochem* 1991;39:1331–1336.
324. Voorhout WF, Veenendaal T, Haagsman HP, Weaver TE, Whitsett JA, van Golde LMG, Geuze HJ. Intracellular processing of pulmonary surfactant protein B in an endosomal/lysosomal compartment. *Am J Physiol* (Lung Cell Mol Physiol 7) 1992;263: L479–L486.
325. Vorbroker DK, Dey C, Weaver TE, Whitsett JA. Surfactant protein-C precursor is palmitoylated and associates with subcellular membranes. *Biochim Biophys Acta* 1992;1105:161–169.
326. Voss T, Eistetter H, Schafer KP, Engel J. Macromolecular organization of natural and recombinant lung surfactant protein SP 28–36. Structural homology with the complement factor Clq. *J Mol Biol* 1988;201:219–227.
327. Voss T, Melchers K, Scheirle G, Schafer KP. Structural comparison of recombinant pulmonary surfactant protein SP-A derived from two human coding sequences: implications for the chain composition of natural human SP-A. *Am J Respir Cell Mol Biol* 1991;4: 88–94.
328. Voss T, Schäfer KP, Nielsen PF, et al. Primary structure differences of human surfactant-associated proteins isolated from normal and proteinosis lung. *Biochim Biophys Acta* 1992;1138:261–267.
329. Walker SR, Williams MC, Benson B. Immunocytochemical localization of the major surfactant apoproteins in type II cells, clara cells, and alveolar macrophages of rat lung. *J Histochem Cytochem* 1986;34:1137–1148.
330. Waring A, Taeusch W, Bruni R, et al. Synthetic amphipathic sequences of surfactant protein-B mimic several physicochemical and in vivo properties of native pulmonary surfactant proteins. *Peptides Res* 1989;2:308–313.
331. Warr RG, Hawgood S, Buckley DI, et al. Low molecular weight human pulmonary surfactant protein (SP-5): Isolation, characterization, and cDNA and amino acid sequences. *Proc Natl Acad Sci USA* 1987;84:7915–7919.
332. Weaver TE, Whitsett JA. Function and regulation of expression of pulmonary surfactant-associated proteins. *Biochem J* 1991;273: 249–264.
333. Weaver TE, Lin S, Bogucki B, Dey C. Processing of surfactant protein-B proprotein by a cathepsin-D-like protease. *Am J Physiol* (Lung Cell Mol Physiol 7) 1992;263:L95–L103.
334. Weissler JC, Nicod LP, Lipscomb MF, Toews GB. Natural killer cell function in human lung is compartmentalized. *Am Rev Respir Dis* 1987;135:941–949.
335. White RT, Damm D, Miller J, et al. Isolation and characterization of the human pulmonary surfactant apoprotein gene. *Nature* 1985;317:361–363.
336. Whitsett JA, Weaver TE, Lieberman MA, Clark JC, Daugherty C. Differential effects of epidermal growth factor and transforming growth factor-β on synthesis of Mr|=|35,000 surfactant-associated protein in fetal lung. *J Biol Chem* 1987;262:7908–7913.
337. Whitsett JA, Hull WM, Luse S. Failure to detect surfactant protein-specific antibodies in sera of premature infants treated with survanta, a modified bovine surfactant. *Pediatrics* 1990;87:505–510.
338. Whitworth NS, Morrison JC, Whitton AC, Bowers KK. Quantified scoring of the amniotic fluid surfactant foam test and assessment of factors contributing to false negative test results. *Am J Obstet Gynecol* 1983;145:752–756.
339. Wikenheiser KA, Wert SE, Wispe JR, et al. Distinct effects of oxygen on surfactant protein B expression in bronchiolar and alveolar epithelium. *Am J Physiol* (Lung Cell Mol Physiol 6) 1992;262: L32–L39.
340. Wilkinson A, Jenkins PA, Jeffrey JA. Two controlled trials of dry artificial surfactant: Early effects and later outcome in babies with surfactant deficiency. *Lancet* 1985;2:287–291.
341. Williams MC, Benson BJ. Immunocytochemical localization and identification of the major surfactant protein in adult rat lung. *J Histochem Cytochem* 1981;29:291–305.
342. Williams MC, Hawgood S, Hamilton RL. Changes in lipid structure produced by surfactant proteins SP-A, SP-B, and SP-C. *Am J Respir Cell Mol Biol* 1991;5:41–50.
343. Wilsher ML, Hughes DA, Haslam PL. Immunomodulatory effects of pulmonary surfactant on natural killer cell and antibody-dependent cytotoxicity. *Clin Exp Immunol* 1988;74:465–470.
344. Wilsher ML, Hughes DA, Haslam PL. Immunoregulatory properties of pulmonary surfactant: effect of lung lining fluid on proliferation of human blood lymphocytes. *Thorax* 1988;43:354–359.
345. Wilsher ML, Hughes DA, Haslam PL. Immunoregulatory properties of pulmonary surfactant: influence of variations in the phospholipid profile. *Clin Exp Immunol* 1988;73:117–122.
346. Wirtz HRW, Dobbs LG. Calcium mobilization and exocytosis after one mechanical stretch of lung epithelial cells. *Science* 1990;250: 1266–1269.
347. Wirtz H, Schmidt M. Ventilation and secretion of pulmonary surfactant. *Clin Invest* 1992;70:3–13.
348. Wohlford-Lenane CL, Snyder JM. Localization of surfactant- associated proteins SP-A and SP-B messenger RNA in rabbit fetal lung tissue by in situ hybridization. *Am J Respir Cell Mol Biol* 1992;7: 335–343.
349. Wright JR, Benson BJ, Williams MC, Goerke J, Clements JA. Protein composition of rabbit alveolar surfactant subfractions. *Biochim Biophys Acta* 1984;791:320–332.
350. Wright JR, Clements JA. Metabolism and turnover of lung surfactant. *Am Rev Respir Dis* 1987;135:426–444.
351. Wright JR. Clearance and recycling of pulmonary surfactant. *Am J Physiol* (Lung Cell Mol Physiol 3) 1990;259:L1–L12.
352. Wright JR, Dobbs, LG. Regulation of pulmonary surfactant secretion and clearance. *Annu Rev Physiol* 1991;53:395–414.

353. Wright JR, Youmans DC. Pulmonary surfactant protein-A stimulates chemotaxis of alveolar macrophage. *Am J Physiol* (Lung Cell Mol Physiol 8) 1993;264:L338–L344.
354. Xu J, Richardson C, Ford C, et al. Isolation and characterization of the cDNA for pulmonary surfactant-associated protein-B (SP-B) in the rabbit. *Biochem Biophys Res Comm* 1989;160:325–332.
355. Yager D, Butler JP, Bastacky J, Israel E, Smith G, Drazen JM. Amplification of airway constriction due to liquid filling of airway interstices. *J Appl Physiol* 1989;66:2873–2884.
356. Yamada T, Ikegami M, Jobe AH. Effects of surfactant subfractions on preterm rabbit lung function. *Pediatr Res* 1990;27:592–598.
357. Yao LJ, Richardson C, Ford C, et al. Expression of mature pulmonary surfactant-associated protein B (SP-B) in *Escherichia coli* using truncated human SP-B cDNAs. *Biochem Cell Biol* 1990;68: 559–566.
358. Young, SL, Wright JR, Clements JA. Cellular uptake and processing of surfactant lipid and apoprotein SP-A by rat lung. *J Appl Physiol* 1989;66:1336–1342.
359. Young SL, Ho YS, Silbajoris RA. Surfactant apoprotein in adult rat lung compartments is increased by dexamethasone. *Am J Physiol* (Lung Cell Mol Physiol 4) 1991;260:L161–L167.
360. Young SL, Fram EK, Larson EW. Three-dimensional reconstruction of tubular myelin. *Exp Lung Res* 1992;18:497–504.
361. Young SL, Fram EK, Larson E, Wright JR. Recycling of surfactant lipid and apoprotein-A studied by electron microscopic autoradiography. *Am J Physiol* (Lung Cell Mol Physiol 9) 1993;265: L19–L26.
362. Yu S-H, Possmayer F. Adsorption, compression and stability of surface films from natural, lipid extract and reconstituted pulmonary surfactants. *Biochim Biophys Acta* 1993;1167:264–271.
363. Zimmerman PE, Voelker DR, McCormack FX, Paulsrud JR, Martin WJ II. 120-kD Surface glycoprotein of pneumocystis carinii is a ligand for surfactant protein A. *J Clin Invest* 1992;89:143–149.
364. Vamvakopoulos NC, Modi WS, Floros J. Mapping the human pulmonary surfactant-associated protein B gene (SFTP3) to chromosome 2p12→p11.2. *Cytogenet Cell Genet* 1995;68:8–10.
365. Nogee LM, Garnier G, Dietz HC, Singer L, Murphy AM, deMello DE, Colten HR. A mutation in the surfactant protein B gene responsible for fatal neonatal respiratory disease in multiple kindreds. *J Clin Invest* 1994;93:1860–1863.
366. deMello DE, Nogee LM, Heyman S, Krous HF, Hussain M, Merritt TA, Hsueh W, Haas JE, Heidelberger K, Schumacher R, Colten HR. Molecular and phenotypic variability in the congenital alveolar proteinosis syndrome associated with inherited surfactant protein B deficiency. *J Pediatr* 1994;125:43–50.
367. deMello DE, Heyman S, Phelps DS, Hamvas A, Nogee L, Cole S, Colten HR. Ultrastructure of lung in surfactant protein B deficiency. *Am J Respir Cell Mol Biol* 1994;11:230–239.
368. Floros J, Veletza SV, Kotikalapudi P, Krizkova L, Karinch AM, Friedman C, Buchter S, Marks K. Dinucleotide repeats in the human surfactant protein-B gene and respiratory-distress syndrome. *Biochem J* 1995;305:583–590.
369. Veletza SV, Rogan PK, TenHave T, Olowe SA, Floros J. Racial differences in allelic distribution at the human pulmonary surfactant protein B gene locus (SP-B). *Exp Lung Res* 1996;22:489–494.
370. Floros J, Karinch AM. Human SP-A: then and now. *Am J Physiol* (Lung Cell Mol Physiol 12) 1995;268:L162–L165.
371. Floros J, Karinch AM. Genetics of neonatal lung disease in relation to the surfactant protein genes. In: Robertson B, Taeusch HW, eds. *Surfactant therapy for lung disease* New York: Marcel Dekker, 1995;95–106.
372. Floros J, Karinch AM, Phelps DS. Sixty six years of surfactant research. *Appl Cardiopulmon Pathophysiol* 1996;6:81–88
373. Karinch AM, Floros J. 5′ Splicing and allelic variants of the human pulmonary surfactant protein A genes. *Am J Respir Cell Mol Biol* 1995;12:77–88.
374. Floros J, DiAngelo S, Koptides M, Karinch AM, Rogan P, Nielsen H, Spragg RG, Watterberg K, Deiter G. Human SP-A locus: Allele frequencies and linkage disequilibrium between the two surfactant protein A genes. *Am J Respir Cell Mol Biol* 1996;15:489–498.
375. McCormick SM, Boggaram V, Mendelson CR. Characterization of mRNA transcripts and organization of human SP-A1 and SP-A2 genes. *Am J Physiol* (Lung Cell Mol Physiol 10) 1994;266:L354–L366.
376. Karinch AM, Floros J. Translation in vivo of 58 untranslated-region splice variants of human surfactant protein-A. *Biochem J* 1995;307:327–330.
377. Karinch AM, Floros J. Effect of genotype on the levels of surfactant protein A mRNA and on SP-A2 splice variants in adult humans. *Am J Resp and Crit Care Med* 1996;153:A766.
378. Kremlev SG, Umstead TM, Phelps DS. Effects of surfactant protein A and surfactant lipids on lymphoctye proliferation in vitro. *Am J Physiol* (Lung Cell Mol Physiol 11) 1994a;11:L357–364.
379. Thomassen MJ, Antal JM, Connors MJ, Meeker DP, Wiedemann HP. Characterization of Exosurf(surfactant)-mediated suppression of stimulated human alveolar macrophage cytokine responses. *Am J Respir Cell Mol Biol* 1994;10:399–404.
380. Thomassen MJ, Meeker DP, Antal JM, Connors MJ, Wiedemann HP. Synthetic surfactant (Exosurf) inhibits endotoxin-stimulated cytokine secretion by human alveolar macrophages. *Am J Respir Cell Mol Biol* 1992;7:257–260.
381. Kremlev SG, Phelps DS. Surfactant protein A stimulation of inflammatory cytokine and immunoglobulin production. *Am J Physiol* (Lung Cell Mol Physiol 11) 1994b;11:L712–L719.
382. Blau H, Riklis S, Kravtsov V, Kalina M. Secretion of cytokines by rat alveolar epithelial cells: Possible regulatory role for SP-A. *Am J Physiol* (Lung Cell Mol Physiol 10) 1994;266:L148–L155.
383. Phelps DS. Pulmonary surfactant modulation of host-defense function. *Appl Cardiopulmon Pathophysiol* 1995;5:221–229.

Anesthesia: Biologic Foundations, edited by
Tony L. Yaksh et al. Lippincott–Raven Publishers,
Philadelphia © 1997.

CHAPTER 74

ORGANIZATION AND ROLE OF LUNG CELLS

DAVID LANGLEBEN AND ROSEMARY C. JONES

Originally thought to represent only an interface between air and blood, the lung is increasingly recognized as an exceptionally complex organ, with gas exchange, metabolic, vasoregulatory, and immunologic functions. The organization and role of the cells that form its major tissue structures are considered here, with special emphasis on ones of the alveolar region, vessels, and conducting airways. Within the constraints of this chapter, only a broad overview can be given of the cell types present. Excellent descriptions of many of the >40 cell types in the lung (29) are available elsewhere, and the reader is referred to these for detailed accounts of cell structure and function (see Chapter xx). The data now available result from the almost logarithmic growth in the number of studies of lung cell biology that has taken place since the early 1980s. These have led to major advances in our understanding of the design of the lung—both form and function.

The lung's alveolar surface and capillary bed is vast—the human adult lung has ~300,000,000 alveoli, each supplied by 1,000 capillary segments, forming an alveolar surface area of ~140 m^2 and a capillary endothelial surface area of ~126m^2 (95,340,341,342). The number of cells covering the airway surface, from the trachea to bronchioles in the human lung, is calculated as 10.5×10^9 (221), with even more (×18) covering the alveolar surface (221). Five cell types form the walls of vessels from hilum to lung periphery; three cell types line the respiratory region, and twelve cell types the conducting airways, including the surface epithelium and submucosal glands. These endothelial and epithelial surfaces are protected by resident and migratory cells, which are supported by humoral systems that maintain homeostasis. Injury, by inhaled or by circulating agents, targets surface cells as well as migratory ones, leading to their removal by apoptosis or necrosis, or to their adaptation and survival. Thus, injured lung tissue consists of surviving and new cell populations, each with their own stability and new pattern of homeostasis. Often the structural changes induced by injury become the basis for disease: An example is cell hypertrophy and hyperplasia in excess of the need for cell replacement—as of vascular cells (leading to structural restriction of the microvascular bed and rise in pulmonary artery pressure), of fibroblasts (leading to loss of alveolar architecture and efficient gas exchange), and of mucus cells (leading to plugging and blockage of small airways by mucus secretions).

Many current studies focus on the use of molecular techniques to examine gene regulation of the intracellular pathways controlling cell function and, where appropriate, correction by gene therapy (51,52,162,271,280). Typically, cells are classed by their structure and function—which is reflected by phenotype (i.e., the structural and functional properties of the cell produced by the interaction of genotype and environment). The concept that cells float restlessly between states of health and disease (126) is a useful one since it moves away from the idea of tissues being formed by "fixed" cell types to emphasize the potential diversity of cells. With only minor variation, however, in response to the modulation of steady state expression of a gene by stimuli that are part of normal homeostasis, phenotype remains stable. And in response to these stimuli or even limited forms of injury, it is likely that phenotype reflects the cell's response to an ordered sequence of events appropriate to normal tissue growth and maturation. Thus, cells swell and contract, migrate or attach, divide or differentiate, synthesize or secrete in an appropriate manner (126). Here, the phenotype acquired may resemble that of the original cell in form but not function, or both may change, as when cells that are fibroblasts synthesize organelles associated with contraction, and basement membrane, and transdifferentiate into myofibroblasts or smooth muscle cells. In response to continued injury, or disease, it is likely that gene induction or altered regulation results in a phenotype that is at the limit or even outside of the normal range for the cell population—and one that persists in response to an imbalance in local control mechanisms.

Equally important to the expression of phenotype, are the interactions between cells, and between cells and matrix, that form tissue structures, and the influence on cells of soluble molecules that mediate migration and growth, i.e., cytokines, soluble [glyco]proteins nonimmunoglobulin in nature (240). These molecules, released by lung cells to act in autocrine, juxtacrine, and paracrine regulatory loops (359), interact with matrix components to effect growth. Thus, the sythesis and release of cytokines by cells influence their synthesis of matrix and adhesion molecules which, in turn, influence cytokine synthesis (240). In response to a stimulus, it is the cell that determines the cytokine to be produced and its temporal expression: Cytokine expression then determines cytokine production by neighboring cells and regulates the expression of cell surface receptors for other cytokines (305). The basement membrane, a specialized form of extracellular matrix, plays a pivotal role in this interaction. It consists of a mesh of collagenous and noncollagenous glycoproteins—in general, type IV collagen (which is secreted as procollagen-like molecules that self-assemble into stable three-dimensional networks, and to which other components bind at specific sites), laminin (an abundant basement membrane glycoprotein that also self-assembles into polymers), entactin (a sulfated glycoprotein also known as nidogen), a specific heparan sulfate proteoglycan (perlecan), chondroitin sulfated proteoglycan and fibronectin (49,190,198,209). Anionic sites in the membrane serve as a selective charge barrier (making the membrane impermeable to proteins), and bind to integral membrane structures (i.e., type IV collagen and laminin). Synthesized to form a polarized structure to support sheets of cells, such as the endothelium or epithelium, or to surround cells, such as the smooth muscle cell (and its precursors), the membrane is multifunctional. It influences cell adhesion, spreading, polarization, movement, and proliferation, as well as phenotype (214,216). The mechanochemical forces that govern the interaction between the cytoskeleton (intracellular filaments), adhesion complexes between the cell and matrix, and components of the supporting matrix, to influence cell proliferation and differentiation in a tissue saturated with soluble mitogens has been elegantly discussed by Ingber et al. (134). How cell growth and differentiation are selectively turned on and off is an intriguing question (134). A noted feature of tissue repair (cell proliferation and tissue remodeling) in response to injury or disease is that it occurs as part of an ongoing inflammatory response, and since inflammatory cells are the source of many cytokines, it is their effect that may determine whether normal structure is restored (216).

The following account of vascular and airway cells focuses on their morphology and role in normal lung as well as in response to injury.

VASCULAR BED

The pulmonary vasculature serves first and foremost as the conduit for blood from the right ventricle, through the lung gas-exchange system, to the left atrium. A wonder of design, it operates at low-perfusion pressures, and because of the tremendous reserve of unrecruited vessels, accommodates large increases in blood flow without a significant rise in pulmonary artery pressure. Elegant vasocontrol mechanisms, influenced by shear stress, pressure and flow, oxygen tension, pH, circulating mediators, and neurohormones, constantly modify regional perfusion to match ventilation and maximize gas exchange. The pulmonary circulation also sits in a unique position as a metabolic organ through which all venous blood must pass before reaching the systemic circulation. This position, however, makes the circulation vulnerable to injury by circulating toxins, infectious agents, activated white cells and mediators. In the sections below, the structure of pulmonary vessels will be reviewed, individual cell types introduced and their major functions in health discussed, as well as their reponse to circulating mediators after injury or in disease.

For the purpose of this review, smooth muscle cells and fibroblasts will be discussed as "vascular" cells, although it must be emphasized that these cells when found in airways (or interstitium) have many common features with those described below. In addition, reference is made to similar cells from other vascular beds, which have representative common features.

Vascular Structures

Large pulmonary arteries, which share the peribronchial adventitial sheath, branch with the airways. Additional arteries branch at all levels: These supernumerary branches run a short course to supply the alveolar region. Typically, the arterial wall consists of endothelium, a layer of smooth muscle cells between an internal and external elastic lamina, and adventitial fibroblasts. In lung, however, this arrangement varies at the distal end of each vascular pathway, where a special pre- and postcapillary vessel segment is present (75,266).

The largest vessels, where several additional elastic laminae are found within the wall, are termed elastic arteries. As lumen diameter decreases the additional laminae are lost, giving rise to vessels that are termed muscular arteries. The walls of these vessels include a continuous layer of medial smooth muscle cells between an internal and external elastic lamina. Moving distally along an arterial pathway, segments are then reached in which this continuous muscle layer becomes incomplete; these are termed partially muscular arteries (75,266). Change in wall structure does not always occur in vessels of a similar size, and so is independent of the level in the vascular branching pattern; i.e., it can occur at the entrance to the acinus (at the level of the terminal or respiratory bronchiolus) or more distally (at the level of an alveolar duct or in the alveolar wall). At some point, in the distal region of the pathway, a precapillary segment is reached that is larger than a capillary but has virtually a capillary structure. These segments may or may not have a single elastic lamina in the wall. They are termed nonmuscular arteries (75,266). In this way, tissue comprising the alveolar-capillary membrane includes myriads of small muscular, partially-muscular and nonmuscular arteries entering (and draining) the capillaries. Gas exchange occurs in these vessels (and in arteries up to 200 μm in diameter) as well as across the capillary bed. The smallest muscular arteries, often found in alveolar angles, have their own adventitial coat and can be considered to lie within the interstitium. The structural arrangement of cells in the walls of these vessel segments is similar in all mammalian lungs that have been studied.

In addition to the endothelial cell, smooth muscle cell, and fibroblast, two precursor cells—the intermediate cell and pericyte—are found within the walls of themicrovessels. Internal to the single elastic lamina of nonmuscular vessels, or the nonmuscular region of partially muscular vessels, lie the cells that are termed intermediate because they have some features of the pericyte and some of the smooth muscle cell, and and lie between these two cell types in the vessel wall (230,231). In an experimental animal model (i.e., the rat) ultrastructural studies and microdissection have established the distribution of smooth muscle cells, intermediate cells and pericytes along the vessel wall in relation to the accompanying airway (55,143,144). At the level of the terminal bronchiolus the medial coat of the vessel is formed by a double layer of smooth muscle cells; at the level of the respiratory bronchiolus and first generation alveolar duct, by only a single layer. Here smooth muscle and endothelial cells are separated by their basement membranes, by an elastic lamina and by matrix. On occasion, endothelial cell processes interrupt these structures to abut the smooth muscle cell, to form a myoendothelial junction, where direct cell-cell communication is possible. At the level of the second alveolar duct, where the segment is partially muscular, and in the nonmuscular region of its wall, a thin layer of smooth muscle cells now lies directly beneath the endothelium; these cells are separated by only their basement membranes. At the level of the third alveolar duct, where the wall is nonmuscular, intermediate cells now form a thin layer beneath the endothelium, in place of smooth muscle cells, and are separated from the endothelium only by basement membrane. Gradually this intermediate cell layer becomes incomplete, until in vessel segments associated with the last alveolar duct, and in the alveolar wall, scattered pericytes are found. These cells share the endothelial basement membrane. While typical junctional processes are not evident in the distal vessel segments, the proximity here of the smooth muscle cell, intermediate cell, and pericyte, to endothelium, favors cell-cell communication, including the presence of inhibitory and stimulatory pathways.

Capillaries consist of a tube of endothelial cells lying on basement membrane. Scattered pericytes are present (340). Capillary segments connect with each other to form an open hexagonal mesh, except in the subpleural regions where blind tubes are found (124). At low lung distending pressures, the capillary mesh has a "sheet-like" appearance, while at higher pressures tubular structures are seen (298). Capillaries vary between 4 and 15 μm in diameter, and the length between their branching is sometimes <20 μm, which is much shorter than the distance from artery to vein (320). Vessels ≤300 μm in ED give rise to capillaries.

The veins run at the perphery of lung units, the most distal veins being found at the edge of acini. Venous tributaries arise from alveolar walls and the divisions of alveolar ducts, from bronchial walls (especially bifurcations), and from the pleura and connective tissue septae and sheaths. They drain to axial vessels that increase in size towards the hilum. The number of conventional veins and pulmonary arteries is similar while the number of supernumerary veins exceeds the number of supernumerary arteries (127). Conventional venous tributaries are larger than adjacent supernumerary ones (127). Nonmuscular, partially muscular and muscular venous segments are identified distally (127), and precursor cells found in nonmuscular regions (226). The adventitia around veins is usually greater than around arteries of a similar size, and distally in the lung, the vein media is typically bound by only a single (and indistinct) elastic lamina.

Bronchial arteries divide with the main bronchi, sending two divisions (one submucosal and one peribronchial) along each bronchial wall to form communicating arcades (58,59,220). The walls of bronchi and bronchioli (down to terminal and respiratory bronchioli), the perineurium of pulmonary nerves and ganglia, the lymph nodes and lymph tissue, the pleura and connective tissue septae, and the walls of arteries and veins, are each supplied by bronchial arteries. At the level of the smallest conducting airway these form a capillary network that anastomoses with the capillary network of the pulmonary arterial bed. The wall structure of the bronchial vessels is typical of systemic ones, being formed of endothelium, smooth muscle cells between well-defined internal and external elastic laminae, and fibroblasts.

Vascular Cells

Endothelial Cell

The endothelial cell, with a central flattened nucleus and cytoplasm that extends as a thin (10–20 nm) squamous sheet covering an area ~1,000–1,300 μm^2, is the most numerous cell of the alveolar region, representing >40% of all parenchymal cells (342). Once thought to represent only an inert monolayer involved in passive oxygen exchange, since the early 1980s the endothelium has been known to have high metabolic activity, and to play a major role in vascular homeostasis. Its function and response to stimuli varies with position along the arterial and venous pathway. Many functional characteristics are common, however, to endothelial cells at all sites. In addition to mediating vascular tone, the endothelium constantly interacts with cellular, plasma and hormonal components of the blood as it passes through the lung. It is also the first arbiter of passage of molecules and cells from vessels to the interstitium. Numerous microvesicles lying free in the cytoplasm, receptor mediated or nonspecific, transport or "shuttle" molecules between the cells' surfaces or link to form transport channels. Paracellular transjunctional transport also occurs. The number and complexity of junctional strands revealed by freeze fracture indicate that permeability increases from arteries to veins. This may be due to changes in endothelial pore size, but also due to electrical charge of the cell membrane and of molecules in the endothelial basement membrane. Endothelial permeability rises with increased hydrostatic pressure, in which case it is rapidly reversible, or with endothelial injury, such as is seen in the adult respiratory distress syndrome (ARDS), where the permeability is less easily reversible.

The basement membrane of the endothelial cell normally includes intrinsic components such as the fine fibrils made by the cells, collagen, a variety of sulfated proteoglycans, including heparan sulfate, and extrinsic components such as fibronectin deposited from blood. In lung, the endothelial basement membrane is highly permeable to liquids, macromolecules, and cells. The lamina densa and rara of the membrane (see below) filter selectively.

The luminal surface of pulmonary endothelium is well described as a "mosaic of domains," each with a range of chemical properties. The cell surface is expanded by microvesicles, which attach as caveolae to the luminal membrane, and are lined by enzymes that activate, inactivate, or breakdown agents circulating in the blood plasma (114,246). Angiotensin converting enzyme (ACE) converts angiotensin I to the vasoconstrictor and smooth muscle mitogen, angiotensin II. ACE also degrades bradykinin, a proinflammatory vasodilator. The enzyme 5′-nucleotidase, found predominantly in endothelial caveolae, dephosphorylates 5′-AMP to adenosine, a potent vasodilator. Carbonic anhydrase plays a part in carbon dioxide and pH homeostasis, and lipoprotein lipase mediates the conversion of triglyceride to fatty acid. The pulmonary endothelium takes up serotonin (5-hydroxytryptamine; 5-HT), propranolol and norepinephrine, but not epinephrine (103). Each of these activities may be reduced in lung injury, as in ARDS.

The endothelium releases a variety of factors, some constitutively, some inducibly, which alter vessel cross-sectional area by increasing or reducing vessel tone, by stimulating or inhibiting physical obstruction of the lumen by a thrombus, or by recruiting inflammatory cells. A fine balance is maintained between these factors, and normal function favors vessel patency while disease tips the balance in favor of lumen restriction. But, in the normal lung at rest, the ability of blood flow to reach only some areas may be beneficial in optimizing ventilation-perfusion matching. Vasodilating factors produced include prostacyclin, nitric oxide and endothelium-derived hyperpolarizing factor(s) and C-type natriuretic peptide. The former two agents also have potent platelet antiaggregatory effects. Prostacyclin acts by increasing cyclic AMP, whereas nitric oxide increases cyclic GMP in target cells. The role of nitric oxide is discussed in detail elsewhere in this volume. In normal lungs, shear-stress induced nitric oxide release may be an important short-term mechanism for pulmonary vasodilation and recruitment during high blood flow states such as exercise. Endothelium-derived hyperpolarizing factor may act via calcium-dependent potassium channels or ATP-dependent potassium channels. Endothelial-derived vasoconstrictors include thomboxane A_2, a platelet proaggregant, and endothelin-1, a potent constrictor peptide and smooth muscle mitogen. The human lung normally clears endothelin-1 from the circulation, so that pulmonary arterial blood entering the lung has higher endothelin-1 levels than pulmonary blood leaving. Reduction in the ratio of prostacyclin to thromboxane release, and reduced endothelin-1 clearance with, at times, excessive production of endothelin-1 by the endothelium, are seen in pulmonary hypertensive states, and in ARDS (43,101,184,322). Recent preliminary evidence suggests that hypoxia induces endothelin-1 synthesis by human endothelial cells in vitro and, therefore, endothelin may contribute to hypoxic pulmonary hypertension. Nitric oxide, as well as local release of prostacyclin, may moderate hypoxic vasoconstriction.

Pulmonary endothelial cells regulate local coagulation and fibrinolysis, maintaining a net balance between anticoagulant-profibrinolytic activities and procoagulant-antifibrinolytic activities. They synthesize anticoagulant-active heparan sulfate and thrombomodulin, and express protein C. The endothelial cell surface binds protein S and activated protein C, and also the thrombin-thrombomodulin complex, thereby providing a stable substrate for the interaction of these molecules in the bloodstream. Endothelial cells are the source of von-Willebrand factor. They are major producers of tissue type plasminogen activator (t-PA) and urokinase-type plasminogen activator (u-PA), which are both profibrinobrolytic, but they also produce plasminogen activator inhibitor (PAI-1) which inhibits fibrinolysis. Heparan sulfate incorporated into the subendothelial matrix may help inhibit smooth muscle proliferation in the normal vessel wall.

The pulmonary endothelial cell participates in the inflammatory response by recruiting inflammatory cells (including their attraction, adherence and migration) from the bloodstream to the interstitium and airways (9) and by binding immune complexes. It may perform these functions in response to direct injury, as in ARDS, or it may be injured indirectly as an "innocent bystander," during an inflammatory response to disease in the lung parenchyma or interstitium. Inflammatory stimuli induce leukocyte adhesion molecule expression by endothelial cells, including selectins, vascular cell adhesion molecules (VCAM), intercellular adhesion molecules (ICAM), and production of platelet activating factor (PAF; a phospholipid with a wide spectrum of proinflammatory properties affecting vascular permeability, airway hypersecretion and PMN infiltration) (286). Platelet surface glycoprotein II_bIII_a, activated during aggregation, binds to endothelial von-Willebrand factor and fibronectin, permitting platelet adhesion to endothelial cells or to the subendothelial matrix. The VCAM and ICAM glycoprotein families interact with integrin molecules on leukocyte surface membranes, and promote leukocyte adhesion and transmigration (85). PECAM-1 (also known as CD31) mediates interendothelial cell-cell interactions, and it may be important in endothelial regrowth and transendothelial leukocyte migration (6,236). Selectin receptors on the endothelial cell surface interact with complementary carbohydrate (lectin-binding) structures on inflammatory cells, and selectins on the inflammatory cells interact with carbohydrates on the endothelial surface. (Lectins bind specific sugars in the glycoconjugates that are located on the surface of all cells, and which are separate from the oligosaccharide portions of integral membrane proteins.) Endothelial E-selectin expression, induced by cytokines, including interleukin-1 (IL-1), tumor necrosis factor (TNF), and endotoxin, promotes adhesion and binding of neutrophils, monocytes, eosinophils, basophils, and some T cells to the endothelium (24). P-selectin, found in endothelial Weibel-Palade bodies, is quickly redistributed to the cell surface after cell activation by thrombin and histamine. P-selectin promotes binding of neutrophils and monocytes: L-selectin plays a role in leukocyte rolling on the vessel wall. Endothelial cells are themselves able to produce a variety of cytokines that can accentuate vascular injury and contribute to vascular remodeling and lung fibrosis, including IL-1, IL-6, and IL-8, macrophage stimulating factors, monocyte chemotaxis factor, a variety of smooth muscle and fibroblast mitogens including platelet-derived growth factor (PDGF)–like molecules, and inhibitors of smooth muscle growth including transforming growth factor–β (TGF-β) and basic fibroblast growth factor (bFGF). Endothelial cells possess complement receptors, bind immune complexes, and can phagocytose bacteria.

Endothelial cells have mechanosensitive membrane channels and generally respond to shear stress by activation of potassium and cation channels, and by altering the orientation of their microfilament network. In response to high shear stress in vitro, they increase production of prostacyclin, nitric oxide, TGF-β, and t-PA, while endothelin-1 synthesis is initially decreased (202).

Pericyte

Located immediately beneath the vascular endothelial basement membrane (306,310), and encircling distal arteries, capillaries and proximal venules in the lung, vascular pericytes are thought to represent smooth muscle-like cells of the pulmonary microvasculature. They contribute to the contol of microvascular tone. In gas exchange capillaries, pericytes cover an estimated 18% of the surface in neonatal (bovine) lungs, and in mature lungs, 26% of the surface (311).

Pericytes contain microfilaments and pinocytic vesicles along their luminal surface. They appear as elongated cells, or may be stellate. Found between endothelial cell basement membrane leaflets, their processes often penetrate through the membrane to contact or lie adjacent to the endothelial cell (37). The pericyte cytoplasmic membrane may extend into that of the endothelial cell to form a "peg and socket" contact (340). While they are uncommon, gap junctions may be present, and nucleotides can pass between the cells (188). Adhesion contacts develop at foci that are rich in fibronectin and where the cells lack plasmalemmal vesicles and basal lamina (310).

Mesodermal in origin, pericytes possess cyclic GMP (cGMP) dependent kinase (147), actin (121), tropomyosin and myosin (148,149) and they are able to contract in response to endothelin-1, and thromboxane A_2, and relax in response to prostacyclin, isoproterenol, dibutryl cAMP, and forskolin (66,158,159). But, at least in the retinal bed, pericytes of true capillaries lack the smooth muscle form of α-smooth muscle actin. Hence, it may be that microvascular blood flow is regulated by the pre- and postcapillary pericytes, with pericytes of true capillaries playing other roles (334). In the lung, it is suggested that pericytes proliferate and acquire a smooth muscle cell phenotype, thereby muscularizing previously nonmuscular microvessels, and increasing pulmonary artery pressure (227). Pericytes produce endothelin-1 (361), and produce up to ten-fold more PGF_2 and thromboxane A_2 than smooth muscle. They also release prostacyclin (78).

Pericyte phenotype and growth are affected by contact with endothelial cells, by the endothelial basement membrane and by circulating growth factors. Moreover, pericytes in contact with endothelial cells appear to inhibit endothelial cell proliferation (11), possibly by the production of TGF (293). Such an effect is likely important to the control of angiogenesis in the lung (93). Endothelial conditioned media, PDGF, and bFGF stimulate pericyte growth (122), during which time pericyte α-smooth-muscle actin levels decrease, consistent with a transition from contractile to proliferative phenotype. Inflammatory cytokines, including endotoxin and PAF, but not interleukin-1, also stimulate pericyte proliferation and might thereby contribute directly to vascular remodeling in lung injury (166,185). Endothelial-derived matrix inhibits the in vitro growth of lung pericytes, but not of smooth muscle cells (56). The matrix component (s) responsible for this effect are not yet identified, but (at low concentrations) pulmonary endothelial-derived heparan-sulfate proteoglycan, a major constituent of subendothelial matrix, inhibits (rat) lung pericyte growth in vitro (183). Exogenous heparin has similar effects, although at much higher concentrations, while other sulfated glycosaminoglycans do not alter pericyte growth (186,247). Pericytes produce an extracellular matrix, containing type I, II, and IV collagen, fibronectin, thrombospondin, laminin, and tenascin (297). In vitro, they secrete heparin sulfate and chondroitin sulfate (323). It is not known if they incorporate these glycosaminoglycans into their matrix.

Intermediate Cell

Like smooth muscle cells, and unlike pericytes, intermediate cells within the vessel wall are surrounded by their own basement membrane (231). Unlike smooth muscle cells and like pericytes, they are found only in the microvessels. Typically, they have fewer of the organelles associated with contraction than the smooth muscle cell, e.g., cytoskeletal filaments, dense bodies, attachment plaques and hemidesmosomes. Present in normal lung only as rather attenuated cells, in response to injury, intermediate cells undergo hyperplasia and acquire the phenotype of smooth muscle cells. This extends the so-called "resistance" segment of the lung's microcirculation, the vessel wall being relatively thick for external diameter, and resistance to flow increased. Relatively little is known of the function of this cell other than its role in vessel wall thickening in reponse to injury leading to pulmonary hypertension (143,144,230). This, in part, reflects an inability to grow, and so study, cells that maintain this phenotype in vitro. Studies are currently underway to identify the cytoskeletal filaments and functional properties of these cells in vivo (145).

Smooth Muscle Cell

As described above, the amount and distribution of smooth muscle cells varies along different vascular pathways of the lung. Even at a single site such as the main pulmonary artery, up to four different smooth muscle phenotypes may normally be found (91). Within these cells, organelles are distributed between extensive arrays of filaments and dense bodies. The frequency of these organelles decreases as these cells become intimal rather than medial within the wall, as do adhesion plaques on the luminal and abluminal cell membrane, and vesicles.

Although the major function of the vascular smooth muscle cell appears to be contraction, recent studies have demonstrated a variety of activities and interactions with other cells and molecules in the vessel wall. The signal transduction and growth properties of pulmonary vascular smooth muscle are discussed elsewhere in this volume. Other excellent reviews on smooth muscle also are available (115,314).

In vitro, smooth muscle cells are fusiform, form multilayers, and demonstrate great lability in phenotype by changing from differentiated cells expressing contractile organelles, to a dedifferentiated "secretory" phenotype with abundant vesicles, much rough endoplasmic reticulum, and so the ability to synthesize proteins. In differentiated cells, most of the cytoplasm is occupied by the organelles of a contractile apparatus, and cytoskeletal elements. The sarcoplasmic reticulum serves as a reservoir for calcium used in cell activation, being involved in intracellular calcium release and sequestration. Smooth muscle thin filaments include actin, tropomyosin, and filamin, and an actin-binding protein with an as yet unidentified function. Midway in size between actin microfilaments (4–6 nm diameter) and myofilaments (16 nm), desmin and vimentin are termed intermediate filaments (11 nm). These give the cell tensile strength, linking myofilaments, via the dense bodies, to the supporting structure of the cell, and these filaments, via attachment plaques, to the plasmmalemmal membrane and to elastic components of the extracellular matrix (34). Smooth muscle myosin, of at least three heavy chain isoforms in the pulmonary artery (292), forms a "thick" filament which, by forming crossbridges with actin, participates in the development of cell contraction. The dense bodies and attachment plaques contain α-actinin, vinculin, filamin, desmin, talin, and integrin (27,219) and are considered the functional equivalent of Z-bands in striated muscle.

Smooth muscle cells contract even in vitro (238). Because hypoxia induces this effect, at least part of its acute vasoconstrictive response in vivo may be due to the direct effect low oxygen, mediated via potassium channels (201,237). Hypoxia acts by increasing cytostolic calcium levels, and reducing outward potassium currents (285,355). Moreover, it reduces tropoelastin synthesis (71), increases collagen synthesis (50), and increases polyamine transport (116).

In response to stimuli, vascular smooth muscle cells, like intermediate cells, hypertrophy and undergo hyperplasia, contributing to the wall remodeling that occurs in pulmonary hypertensive states. This thickens the walls of normally muscular segments in proximal and distal lung regions. As inferred from models of atherosclerosis, endothelial injury, or at least dysfunction, is likely an important factor in initiatating smooth muscle growth (137). The neointimal plaques of smooth muscle cells typical of atherosclerosis also form in pulmonary vessels, as in the vascular sclerosis associated with interstitial lung fibrosis (117). As in systemic vessels, these arise by the migration of smooth muscle cells from the vessel media, through disrupted areas of endothelium, to the lumen surface. Increase in pulmonary artery pressure to systemic levels can also lead to wall injury and similar cell migration, as exemplified by the changes associated with high flow. The stimulation of smooth muscle proliferation by platelet-derived, endothelial-derived autocrine and class 1 and 2 heparin-binding growth factors is discussed elsewhere. 5-HT, prostaglandins, leukotrines, angiotensin II, and endothelin are also potent smooth muscle mitogens. In addition, many of these agents alter extracellular matrix synthesis by cells (154). The interactions of smooth muscle with extracellular matrix are discussed elsewhere. In general, during hypertrophy, desmin and vimentin increase (314), the relative proportions of actin isoforms, and the actin/myosin ratio are altered (203), and cells increase their synthesis and secretion of collagen and elastin precursors. The exact composition of these filaments in the smooth muscle cells of normal lung vessels, or in cells of the walls of injured vessels, is unknown. Mechanical stress, as might occur in pulmonary hypertension by increased wall tension, leads to a hypertrophic "synthetic" phenotype, with increased glycoaminoglycan synthesis (222) and decreased cell proliferation. Cell stretch also increases levels of inositol phosphate (176). The hyperplastic response to arterial injury, leading to medial thickenimg and intimal hyperplasia, involves dedifferentiation of muscle cells. In aorta, these cells then express β-actin, PDGF-B chain, cytochrome P450IA1 (CYPIA1), elastin, and osteopontin (104,169,192,301). Osteopontin may be important in directing vascular development in the embryo, and it is overexpressed in the adult in areas of smooth muscle neointimal formation (94,97,98,132). Osteopontin also acts as an adhesive and chemotactic signal for smooth muscle cells (197). The genes regulating myogenic differentiation of smooth muscle are as yet unidentified, but may resemble the MyoD, myogenin, Myf-5, and MRF-4 families of genes that regulate myogenic differentiation in striated muscle (28,57, 233,270,350).

Alteration and disruption of the internal elastic lamina is an important stage in the remodeling of vessels associated with pulmonary hypertension (258). Recently, smooth muscle cells have been shown to produce an elastase, related to the serine protease adipsin, which appears to govern this aspect of the remodellng process (358). In addition, smooth muscle cells may have to alter their pattern of integrin receptor expression in order to migrate through the vascular matrix. In vivo, they normally express α1β1 integrin receptors, but, for chemotaxis to occur, α2β2 expression is required (312).

Fibroblast and Myofibroblast

Fibroblasts are normally present in the connective tissue spaces of the lung, including the adventitial sheath of large vessels and airways, as well as septae and interstitium of the alveolar-capillary membrane. Typically, these cells have long processes that include microfilaments, lipid inclusions, and pinocytotic vesicles; high protein synthesis is marked by an extensive rough endoplasmic reticulum. They vary from the expression of a contractile phenotype, in which microfilaments increase, to one primarily involved in the synthesis of extracellular matrix components. They lack basement membrane.

Within normal lung parenchyma, fibroblasts form multicellular contractile units connected by gap-junctions and by adhering macular-junctions, which link the microfilaments bundles of adjacent cells (310). The cells express vimentin, actin isoforms, and nonmuscle myosin; they usually lack desmin, although desmin may be expressed in response to injury. Collagen fibrils and fibres form along both abluminal and adluminal margins.

In addition to the typical interstitial cell, fibroblast subsets are defined by their location or by their contractile organelles: These include the adventitial fibroblast and the myofibroblast. The adventitial cell forms part of the connective tissue sheath of a vessel or airway wall, usually lying abluminal to the external elastic lamina of the smooth muscle cell layer, and embedded in connective tissue components. Around the walls of large vessels, and around large and small airways, adventitial fibroblasts resemble interstitial ones in synthesizing and depositing collagen along both the luminal and abluminal cell margins. Around the smallest microvessels (ones <25 μm in diameter), however, fibroblasts lie abluminal to endothelium, separated from it by the endothelial basement membrane or by this membrane and an elastic lamina. Around these vessels the cells deposit collagen (mostly in a polarized manner) along their abluminal margin, to lie contiguous with the collagen mesh of the interstitium. Fibroblasts expressing contractile organelles, termed "contractile interstitial cells," are present within the interstitium of normal lung, in the thick region of the alveolar-capillary membrane and at the junctions of alveoli—around pre- and postcapillary vessels—where they exert a contractile force (151). Increased numbers of these cells occur in interstitial fibrosis (5).

The term myofibroblast is now frequently applied to interstitial fibroblasts that express many filaments. Such cells typically have several compact bundles of prominent and parallel fibrils (of actinomyosin). These resemble the fibers of the smooth muscle cell in density, are located beneath the plasma membrane and insert into the membrane to form hemidesmosome complexes (342). The fibers appear to attach (i.e., tether) the fibroblast to each side of the interstitium; they form parallel bundles that are arranged at right angles across the interstitium. The fibers do not stain for myosin and may or may not contain α-smooth muscle actin. Thus, while lung fibroblasts, and myofibroblasts, express this isoform (174,234) the "contractile interstitial cell" in normal lung does not—although it may in interstitial fibrosis (5,152). Other filaments appear in the myofibroblast in response to injury (357). In fibrosis, the distribution of intermediate and contractile filaments (desmin, vimentin, and actin) identifies phenotypic variants (291). It is proposed that fibroblasts first develop bundles of cytoplasmic actin (β- and γ-actin) filaments, followed by α-smooth muscle actin filaments, vimentin filaments and then desmin filaments (291). Certain filament combinations occur. Cells express cytoplasmic actin filaments alone, these filaments together with α-smooth muscle actin, or these filaments together with vimentin and desmin, or they may express only α-smooth actin, vimentin, and desmin filaments (291). Densities along the plasmalemmal membrane indicate attachment of the fibroblast to matrix or to adjacent cells. Contractile force when generated is transmitted to the extracellular matrix via integrins (175). In pulmonary hypertension, a subset of interstitial cells migrates to align around vessels that have no elastic lamina. Once aligned, these cells proliferate and acquire a smooth muscle phenotype (143,144).

In addition to collagen and elastin precursors, fibroblasts secrete laminin, proteoglycans (54,153), and fibronectin. The cells of both normal and fibrotic lungs secrete type I, III, and V collagens, with type I the most abundant (259). However, fibroblasts from healthy adult lungs are usually quiescent and secrete little collagen (174) while cells from fibrotic lungs secrete abundant amounts. TGF-β released by injured lung macrophages further stimulates collagen synthesis (259,163), as does TNF-α and IL-1 (64). Insulin-like growth factor (IGF) has a similar effect (108), whereas interferon-gamma (IFN-γ) reduces synthesis (44). Protein kinase C activity also modulates collagen synthesis (107). Collagenase production by fibroblasts from the lung affected by idiopathic pulmonary fibrosis is decreased, thereby favoring collagen deposition (248).

Lung fibroblast elastin is an important extracellular matrix protein which may play a role in alveolar-development (242). Elastin degradation is a hallmark of pulmonary emphysema (90), and elastolysis may be an important in the vascular wall remodeling that is associated with pulmonary hypertension (354). Elastin peptides stimulate lung fibroblast growth in vitro (96) but may decrease fibroblast elastin synthesis (90). TGF-β increases elastin synthesis (218). Whether IGF-I similarly stimulates elastin synthesis (243) or has no effect (272) remains controversial. IL-1 inhibits elastin formation (22) while heparin increases deposition of insoluble elastin into the extracellular matrix (217).

Pulmonary fibroblasts also produce and interact with other matrix components. They synthesize hyaluronic acid, and TNF-α and IFN-γ combined stimulate its synthesis. However, fibroblast can also degrade hyaluronic acid, by the release of hyaluronidase, whose function may be regulated by cytokines, and by altering fibroblast-hyaluronic acid binding (287). Fibroblasts produce syndecan (a hybrid proteoglycan), heparin sulfate, dermatan sulfate, and chrondroitin sulfate (199), and this synthesis may be altered by TGF (70). However, proliferation of normal fibroblasts is inhibited by many of these matrix glycosoaminoglycans (345) indicating a system of autologous growth control. The heparin sulfate proteoglycan binds to fibronectin (120) present in the matrix. Fibroblasts, in culture produce fibronectin (35), and fibulin, an extracellular matrix glycoprotein whose interaction with the fibronectin matrix may be important during lung development (278). Fibronectin produced by bronchial epithelial cells may also act as a lung fibroblast chemotactic factor (304).

Fibroblasts proliferate in response to a variety of growth factors released locally in the lung in disease states. They also regulate inflammatory cell function (72,276). Diseases such as idiopathic pulmonary fibrosis, silicosis and sarcoidosis all involve a mitogenic response by fibroblasts (36,196,326). Through production of IL-8 (276,277), TGF-β (160,252), fibroblast growth factor (FGF) (106), PDGF-A (84), monocytic chemotactic peptide (277), bronchial epithelial cell chemotactic factors (300), macrophage inflammatory protein 2 (69), and colony stimulating factor (356), fibroblasts can modulate the inflammatory cell response, and also the mitogenic or protein synthetic activation of neighboring lung cells. Similarly, growth factors from endothelium, alveolar macrophages or plasma (33), including PDGF (33), TGF-β (319), and endothelin (251) stimulate fibroblast growth, possibly synergistically. That TGF-β is more effective at low cell density suggests that it may be more important during early fibroblast recruitment in the process of lung injury. Exogenous TGF-β also appears to auto-induce TGF-β production by fibroblasts (161). Fibroblasts respond to IL-1, IL-2, TNF, and IFN, and increase T-lymphocyte adherence (112). IL-1β and interferon-γ inhibit fibroblast growth (32,146). However, IL-1 and TNF-α stimulate endogenous IL-1 production by the fibroblasts (73) and IL-1 stimulates IL-6 production (360). IFN and TNF-α upregulate expression of the laminin receptor integrin (86). Fibroblasts are also able to synthesize and secrete a variety of early and terminal components of the complement cascade (282).

Formation of fibrin gels in the alveoli and interstitium is an early and important event in lung injury, the gel providing a meshwork which allows ingrowth of fibroblasts. Lung fibroblasts both bind (268) and synthesize t-PA, and so regulate local fibrinolysis (89). However, in disease states, both TGF-β and TNF-α release result in increased release of PAI-1 by fibroblasts, thereby favoring persistent fibrin deposition, and contributing to alveolitis (131). Thrombin released into alveolar fluid in lung injury also stimulates fibroblast proliferation (325). Serum stimulation of quiescent fibroblasts induces the synthesis of procoagulant tissue factor (25).

In the adult human lung, attenuated fibroblasts form a thin sheath that separates the epithelial basment membrane from the connective tissue proper (81), and in asthma, subepithelial fibosis and thickening of the basement membrane are associated with the development of myofibroblast-like cells that express a-smooth muscle actin (31). Both the developing and adult lung show direct intercellular contacts between alveolar epithelial cells and fibroblasts, and after lung injury, epithelial necrosis and delayed repair both stimulate fibroblast growth (1,133). Similarly, direct contact to fibroblasts may regulate type II epithelial cell growth (1,83).

AIRWAYS AND INTERSTITIUM

Although their main purpose is gas delivery and exchange, the airway cells serve several nonrespiratory functions—protecting against the damaging effects of inhaled agents by secretion, participating in the inflammatory and immune response, and influencing the function of airway smooth muscle. This is accomplished by a complex arrangement of cell types, the function of most but not all of these being known. In the sections below, airway structure is reviewed, the individual cell types of the airway surface and submucosal gland, and alveolar surface are then introduced, and their function discussed.

Airway Structures and Interstitium

As the large airways branch, bronchi (with cartilage in their wall) give rise to bronchioli (with no cartilage) until the terminal and respiratory bronchioli are reached. The terminal bronchiolus is defined as the last bronchiolus lined by a complete layer of conducting airway epithelium. The respiratory bronchiolus is lined by conducting airway epithelium on one side and alveolar epithelium on the other. Along any one pathway the number of bronchial generations varies, being determined by the length of the segmental bronchus to the alveolar region and by an assymetrical pattern of irregular and dicotamous branching (265). The airways consist of tubes of epithelial cells, forming a polarized layer on basement membrane, surrounded by smooth muscle cells between elastic laminae, and an outer sheath of adventitial fibroblasts embedded in collagen fibers and matrix proteins.

The airway surface is hydrated and protected by secretions released into its lumen. These are removed, along with cell debris and other particles, by the ciliary escalator. This efficient system is formed by the whip-like action of the cilia that line the airways from the respiratory bronchioli to the larynx, beating in a liquid-phase (sol) layer. An incomplete solid-phase (gel) layer of viscous (sticky) mucus "rafts" floating on the surface of the sol phase assists in trapping and removing debris (221). In general, the airway surface both secretes and absorbs fluid and ions, and secretes mucus and other cell products.

The acinus, the respiratory unit of the lung, which in the adult human lung is ~1 cm in size or 1 ml in volume (265), includes all of the alveolar-capillary surface—the alveolar epithelial surface, vascular structures and interstitium. It is supplied by a terminal bronchiolus and may include several generations each of respiratory bronchioli and of alveolar ducts and, beyond, alveoli. Clusters of three to five terminal bronchioli form a lobule. In addition to gas exchange, a major function of the alveolar surface is the secretion of lipid products and glycoproteins which assist in maintaining the alveolus distended.

From the trachea to alveoli the airways are lined by cells that form a continuous surface, with regional variation in the distribution of cell types (95). The cells of the alveolar region are embedded in the interstitium—an extracellular matrix that includes fibers (e.g., elastin and collagen fibrils and microfibrils) and ground substance (343). Fibroblasts and myofibroblasts are resident cells, as are smooth muscle cells, several of these cells usually forming a cluster in the septal projections of the alveolar-capillary membrane. All the migratory cells are represented. High molecular weight amphoteric molecules in the ground substance (proteoglycans and glycoproteins) selectively bind anions and cations. Liquid and plasma proteins move through the matrix to the lymphatic plexus at the terminal bronchiolus and drain centrally through the lymphatics.

Airway Cells

Because of the variety of cell types that comprise the surface epithelium and submucosal gland the characteristic features of these cells are described first, followed by an account of features common to the cells at both sites, e.g., epithelial cell regeneration, mucus secretion, and participation in the inflammatory and immune response. A short account is then given of resident airway lymphoid and dendritic cells.

Epithelial Surface

The airways are lined by a ciliated mucus-secreting epithelium. In large airways the epithelial cells form a pseudostratified layer, and in smaller ones a single columner or cuboidal layer in which a basally placed cell occasionally intervenes. These layers consist of a variety of specialized cells (mucous, serous, Clara, ciliated, brush, indeterminate, "special," Kulchitsky, and basal). Although there are species differences, essentially similar cell types are found in mammalian lungs (138). Their distribution varies between airway generations in the same animal, and between species, and is profoundly influenced by age, sex, and estrus cycle, as well as by the environment and infection (3,267). In normal human bronchi, cell frequency is calulated as—basal cells $2{,}167 \times 10^6$, ciliated cells $2{,}295 \times 10^6$, "goblet" secretory cells 872×10^6, other secretory cells 231×10^6, and indeterminate cells $1{,}230 \times 10^6$, and in bronchioli—basal none, ciliated $1{,}552 \times 10^6$, "goblet" none, other secretory $1{,}150 \times 10^6$, and indeterminate cells 434×10^6 (221). These secretory cell groups (goblet and other secretory cell types) include the three secretory cells identified ultrastructurally, as serous, mucous, and Clara cells, the mucous cell forming the largest group within the "goblet" cell poulation; the basal cell group includes both the basal and the Kultchitsky cell.

Serous Cell The serous cell, present in large and small airways, is characterized by electron-dense cytoplasm and much rough endoplasmic reticulum. As in most secretory cells, the nucleus is located basally and lies superficial to an extensive Golgi apparatus. Characteristically, the apical region of the cell contains 1–35 discrete, spherical, secretory granules (each ~600 nm in diameter) that are limited by a membrane and electron-dense (139). In response to stimuli, the cells express, and secrete into the airway lumen, calcitonin gene-related peptide (CGRP). This neuropeptide is located in the cell's granules (18), as well as in the granules of Kultchitsky cells (see below),

Mucous Cell The distribution of organelles in the cytoplasm of the mucous cell, present mainly in the large airways, resembles that of the serous cell, although the granules are larger, electron-lucent, and confluent, with adjacent portions of the membranes incomplete (139). Prior to discharge, numerous granules distend the cell to form a chalice or goblet-shaped mass (hence the term "goblet" cell). It has long been recognized that in normal airway epithelium mucous cell differentiation is induced by vitamin A (215). These cells predominate in the injured airway characterized by hypersecretion, including proximal and distal regions.

Clara Cell Clara cells are found mainly in distal airways, where they represent almost all of the nonciliated cell population. There is considerable species variation in their location, the cells being mostly restricted to the distal conducting airways, including the last generations of bronchioli and their transition to respiratory bronchioli (253). The cells release secretory granules, process xenobiotic compounds and act as progenitor cells. Clara cells resemble serous cells in the electron density and discrete nature of their granules: They differ in the smaller size and irregular shape of their granules and low electron density of cytoplasm. The cells have extensive cytoplasmic interdigitations, and organized microfilaments. While they typically contain smooth endoplasmic reticulum (rather than the rough endoplasmic reticulum typical of the serous and mucous cell or of other protein secreting cells) its amount varies between species (253). Similarly, the content of the granules varies. These metabolically active cells, are considered important in organizing the local microenvironment. The cell produces antileukoproteases (also called secretory leukocyte proteinase inhibitor, or bronchial mucus inhibitor), protease, and elastase inhibitors, and binding proteins for toxic agents, and are a source of arachidonic acid metabolites (see below). They synthesize isozymes of cytochrome P-450, and NADPH-cytochrome P-450 reductase, as well as epoxide hydrolase, glutathiones, S-transferase isozymes, and glycuronosyl transferase (39,62,253). As a site of xenobiotic metabolism, they are susceptible to injury.

Ciliated Cell The ciliated cell, like the secretory cell, abuts the airway lumen. The nucleus is basally located and the cytoplasm contains relatively few orgenelles, with a predominance of microfilaments and microtubules. The cell is characterized by apical cilia (~200/cell), which have a specialized structure. Numerous microvilli project between the cilia. The shaft of each cilium includes a central pair of singlet tubules (composed of the protein tubulin) surrounded by nine outer doublet tubules that are bound by fine radial spokes. The tubules slide over each other to drive the cilium. The outer doublets have two arms (composed of the protein dynein). These "dynein arms" form the ratchet or base of the whip-like action of the cilium. The shaft structure condenses as it enters the cell and anchors to it via basal bodies that associate with the microfilaments and microtubules of the cell to form a dense web (342). Small claw like projections at the apex of the cilium are thought to assist in moving the mucus layer (139). Each cilium is orientated in its beat (×1,000 beats/min), and groups of ciliated cells beat in synchrony to form a metachronal wave in the direction of the larynx. The cells are grouped in fields, each being separated by areas of nonciliated cells. Ciliated cells from the trachea to the terminal bronchiolus are immmunoreactive for endopeptidase 24.15, which degrades bioactive peptides (e.g., substance P, neurotensin, bradykinin and luteinizing hormone releasing hormone) and converts dynorphin, and α- and β-neuroendorphin and other opioids to enkephalins (40). The enzyme is present in soluble cytoplasmic and membrane-bound forms. (Other noncilated cells of the airways, and gland cells, are negative.)

Brush Cell A relatively rare cell type in the lung, the brush cell is named for its characteristic brush border of blunt microvilli, which project into the airway lumen beyond the level of the microvilli on the surface of adjacent epithelial cells. A core of microfibrils extends through the center of each microvillus into the apical cytoplasm of the cell. The nucleus is basally located, and the cytoplasm contains numerous vesicles, scattered bundles of tonofilaments (specialized keratin filaments) and a Golgi apparatus (38,139). The distribution of this cell varies in different species (138): when present the cells are found mainly in the conducting airways. In some species, they appear to have a distinct spatial distribution, being present in trachea and terminal bronchiolar epithelium but rare inbetween. They are found in high numbers close to proximal alveolar ducts but then are sparse distally in the alveolar region (see below) (38). Because of the similarity of the microvilli of the airway cell to the cell in the small intestine it is believed to have an absorptive function, and to participate in maintaining the balance of fluid in the periciliary layer (228). Based on its association with afferent nerves it has been suggested that the cell acts as a chemoreceptor (200), or that it may participate in detoxification (see below) (38).

Indeterminate Cell The indeterminate or undifferentiated cell also abuts the airway lumen although it has no secretory granules or cilia. Its cytoplasm varies from electron lucent to dense. This cell, which occurs in proximal and distal airway epithelium along with secretory, ciliated and brush cells, is considered a source of these cell types.

Kultchitsky Cell The Kultchitsky cell (also called the Feyrter cell), lying against the basement membrane is found in both proximal and distal airways, either as a single cell, or as a group of cells termed a neuroepithelial body (NEB). The apices of cells forming a NEB reach (and bulge into) the airway lumen; those of single cells do not. While present in the adult lung the cells are more frequent in fetal and young lungs. Visualized by L-dopa or 5-hydroxytrytophan (which the cell converts to dopamine or serotonin) the cell forms part of the amine-precursor uptake and decarboxylation (APUD) system. The cell has electron lucent cytoplasm with numerous dense-cored, membrane-bound, vesicles. These contain a variety of bioactive agents, including serotonin, CGRP, calcitonin, and bombesin (gastrin-releasing peptide), enkephalin, somatastatin, substance P, cholecystokinin, and polypeptide YY. The distribution of these neuropeptides both in single cells and in the NEBS reveals a complex system of control (294). They have been proposed as chemo-stretch, tactile or baro-receptors (200).

Kultchitsky cells have a special relationship with airway nerves. Nerve fibers have been identified within the epithelium of the airways of several species. In the submucosal glands of the human airway, bundles of unmyelinated axons are found between acinar and single-terminal axons: they are found between serous, mucous, and duct cells, and between these cells and myoepithelial cells. In general, peptide-containing nerves extend to alveolar ducts (few are present further distally). Nerve trunks run parallel to the bronchus, outside the cartilage plates, decreasing to a single nerve fiber at the level of the terminal bronchiolus (128). In the bronchial wall, fibers form networks around and within bronchial smooth muscle, and are present within the submucosa beneath the epithelium, and in the acini of submucosal glands. In bronchi and bronchioli, single nerve fibers pass from the subepithelium between epithelial cells, decreasing in number distally. At the level of the respiratory bronchiolus single fibers are found around airway walls that consist of epithelium and muscle bundles. In this region, innervation is greater than in the accompanying pulmonary arteries, which have nerves in their adventitia (128).

The distribution of CGRP-immunoreactive (CGRP-IR) epithelial cells (and therefore possibly serous or Kulchitsky cells) has been determined in relation to nerve fibers (309). In the extrapulmonary airways, single cells are innervated by CGRP-IR nerves that form networks within the epithelium; intrapulmonary cells directly by nerve fibers from the lamina propria, indicating differences in the regulation of these cells in different airway generations. Groups of CGRP-IR cells (presumably NEBs) are found chiefly in intrapulmonary airways, about half being connected directly to nerves (309). In distal lung, the nerves are usually associated with NEBs, even in bronchiolar walls. Capsaicin causes discharge from nerves but not from single cells or cell clusters. In addition to CGRP, several other mediators have been identified in both the nerves (vasoactive intestinal peptide, histamine and leucine, substance P, neuropeptide, galanin, gastrin releasing peptide, and opioid peptides) and cells (leucine-enkephalin, bombesin, calcitonin, gastrin releasing peptide, and 5-HT) (309). CGRP interacts with these mediators to potentiate tachykinin-induced protein extravasation. Because they can activate sensory nerve fibers, it is likely that the cells transmit signals to sensory nerve terminals and so form sensory complexes (309). The epithelial nerve fibers of central airways are stimulated by irritants or by epithelial damage causing local release of CGRP which, together with tachykinins, induce neurogenic inflammation. The cells are activated by chemical and physiochemical stimuli that result in mediator release (309). The release of CGRP by cells of the epithelial surface suggests a local function, one that is supported by the expression of CGRP receptors by airway epithelial cells. It may serve to increase ciliary function or to attract inflammatory cells (18).

Basal Cell The basal cell, a moderately differentiated cell that contacts the basement membrane of the epithelium but does not reach the airway lumen, is found in the large airways, where it covers ~85% of basement membrane surface (81). It is characterized by a compact nucleus, and a small amount of electron-dense cytoplasm that usually contains tonofilaments. Basal cells attach to the epithelial basement membrane by adhesion molecules and hemidesmosomes (attachment sites between keratin filaments in the cytoplasma and basement membrane) and so form a bridge between the membrane and cells of the superficial layer (81). In turn, the basement membrane is firmly attached to the underlying connective tissue by anchoring fibrils (157). Basal cells (and cells of the superficial layer) link to adjacent cells by desmosome attachments (80,81).

Special Cell A so-called "special-cell type" within the epithelium lies basal in position; it is characterized by numerous cytoplasmic inclusions that consist of disc-shaped cyoplasmic granules (130 nm diameter) and rods (400 × 50 nm) of dense, fibrogranular material (138). Its function is not established.

Submucosal Gland

Submucosal glands extend throughout airways with cartilage in their wall. They are calculated to contribute the greatest volume (×40 volume surface cells) to mucus secretion (264). If the surface epithelial cells that line the entrance to its duct are excluded at least six cell types form the gland (duct, serous, mucous, myoepithelial, clear, and Kulchitsky). As in surface epithelial cells, the distribution of glycoproteins in mucous and serous cells of the normal airway varies (267).

Duct Cell Cells of the surface epithelium (particularly ciliated cells) line the ducts of the bronchial submucosal glands as they open to the epithelial surface. The ciliated duct is ~350 μm in length. The main gland duct, the collecting duct, is ~800 μm in length and is lined by special cells (232). The cytoplasm of these cells is eosinophilic, and filled with dense and uniformly packed mitochondria (orientated mainly parallel to the lateral cell membrane) and a well-developed discrete Gogi apparatus. Its function is largely unknown although the density of capillaries around the collecting duct indicates that fluid and ionic regulation of secretions occurs in this region of the gland.

Serous and Mucous Cell The secretory tubules of the gland (which arise from the duct) are lined by tubules consisting either of mucous or serous cells. Some of the tubules arise like buds from the lateral wall of the collecting duct; others divide randomly. The serous cells are always located at the distal ends of the mucous tubule, either as single cells or in groups (229,232). The mucous tubules are ~500 μm in length; the serous tubules 180 μm. In each gland, the lumen of the tubules and the duct is continuous: Secretions pass from the serous tubule into the mucous tubule, on into the lumen of the collecting duct, through the ciliated duct and onto the airway surface. The serous cell resembles its surface counterpart except for its wedge-shape and deep invaginations that open mainly onto its lateral surface. Typically, its granules (300—1,000 nm) are electron-dense. The mucous cell also resembles its surface counterpart morphologically. Its electron-lucent granules range in size and distribution, the smaller granules (300 nm) being found near the Golgi complex and larger ones (1,000 nm) at the cell apex, where they lose their limiting membranes and appear to fuse. Although the serous and mucous cells of the submucosal gland and airway surface appear similar in morphology and function, differences in the rate of granule synthesis and secretion, indicate that they should be considered separate cell types. In vitro, gland cells (which are mainly serous in type) appear a source of the proteoglycans in airway mucus (351).

Myoepithelial Cell Myoepithelial cells are found within the basement membrane of the gland, at the base of serous, mucous, and collecting duct cells (232). The cells contain numerous fibrils parallel to the basement membrane and it is thought that contraction of these cells may contribute to the discharge of secretory cells, including those forming the mucous and serous tubules as well as those lining the gland duct.

Clear Cell The clear cell has the features of an immunoblast, resembling those described in the human submaxillary gland (232). The cells are identifieid by their clear cytoplasm, with few organelles, numerous ribosomes and polysomes. They are found between the secretory cells and basement membrane, and between secretory cells (mucous and serous), particularly so in the collecting duct.

Kultchitsky Cell Kultchitsky cells within the submucosal gland resemble those of the airway epithelium (232). Although it is likely that the cells perform similar functions at each site, this and mechanisms of control are not established.

The integrity of airway epithelial surface is maintained by specialized junctional complexes (295): These consist of the (a) tight junction (zonula occludans); (b) intermediate junction (zonula adherens); (c) desmosomes (macular adherens); and (d) gap or communicating junction. The tight junctions prevent diffusion of fluid from the airway lumen to the basolateral surface, and segregate molecules to one of these two surfaces. The intermediate junction provides cell adhesion and recognition. Desmosomes maintain epithelial integrity, while gap junctions are cell to cell highways. The behavior of these junctinal components is critical to the permeability of the epithelium—passage into the airway lumen and absorption of material from the epithelial surface (295). Ion transport across the epithelium regulates the rate of water secretion within the airway by forming osmotic gradients in lateral intercellular spaces. Freeze-fracture techniques indicate differences in the form of the junction and the relation between junction and location along a pathway (295), and variation between species in the arrangement of the junctional complex and cell type. In human bronchi, the tight junctions between eithelial cells show little consistent pattern in relation to cell type, when assessed by junctional depth, strand number, and junctional complexity (105).

The progenitor cell of the airway epithelium—the cell dividing in response to cell loss as part of normal homeostasis or in response to injury—has long been a topic of discussion. The basal cell has been considered the airway stem cell (much as the equivalent cell in skin) although in fetal airways it has been known that basal cells develop secondarily from a columnar epithelial cell layer. Currently, it is recognized that each airway cell may give rise to daughter cells of the same type, including cells that were once considered terminally differentiated, such as the ciliated cell or secretory cell rich in granules. The basal cell, and a secretory cell-type with few granules, have a greater proliferative capacity, however, than ones that are highly specialized, and the cell(s) responsible for restoring the epithelial surface will depend on conditions.

In general, focally injured and denuded areas of the airways are covered by adjacent basal and superficial cells that become poorly differentiated, flatten and migrate. It is likely that a variety of mediators and signals from cells and matrix direct migration, including neuropeptides (273,288). Cell membrane specific markers (lectins), and monoclonal antibodies (mAbs) to cell specific epitopes, demonstrate that four days after denudation, when the epithelium is "squamoid" (one to three cell layers), it is composed of a single poorly-differentiated cell type that expresses keratin 14, and Griffonia simplicifolia I-isolectin B_4 binding sites (which recognize a α-D-galactose groups on the membrane). These cells contain glycogen and lipid and do not express ciliated or secretory cell specific-mAb epitopes. By seven days, when the epithelium is pseudostratified, cells programmed to become secretory express specific secretory-cell markers at their apex, while others, including preciliated cells (i.e., cells with apical fibrogranular bodies that are evidence of ciliogenesis) and ciliated cells, express a ciliated-cell specific epitope. Basal cells are identified by seven days, and express the same markers as the poorly-differentiated cells. While these markers are retained by the basal cell they are lost by the columnar cell as it differentiates and acquires a new set of specific epitopes (307,308). These markers also confirm that undifferentiated columnar cells are the source of all cell types in the developing airway (260). In vitro studies demonstrate that it is the secretory cell that preferentially gives rise to other secretory cells: Isolated secretory cells (seeded onto denuded tracheal grafts) give rise to an epithelium of basal, ciliated and secretory cells, while isolated basal cells give rise to an epithelium of basal and ciliated cells alone (142). In the distal airway regions, where basal cells are sparse, the de-differentiated nonciliated bronchiolar cell is the major source of new cells (30,82). Most of these cells are derived from Clara cells that are depleted of granules and of the developed Gogi and endoplasmic reticulum characteristic of the mature secretory cell (142). As cells change shape, from squamous to cuboidal to columner, and acquire secretory granules, they lose their proliferative capacity (41). Once the denuded area of the epithelium is restored, differentiation usually reestablishes the cell distribution appropriate to airway level. In response to continued injury, however, cell type and number may be inappropriate, the nature and extent of injury determining the characteristics of the epithelium re-established. For example, aberrant basal cell division will give rise to squamous epithelium, as will the transdifferentiation of secretory cells by keratinization, as in vitamin A deficiency (215). In response to an acute challenge, Clara cells of the distal airways repopulate denuded areas to reestablish an epithelium with a typical cell distribution, but the effect of long-term injury is Clara cell hyperplasia (253). In both large and small airways, persistent injury may result in an adaptative response that includes the presence of high numbers of secretory cells, especially so in response to inhaled irritants (267).

In response to injury, or in disease associated with hypersecretion, the mucus-secreting cells of the surface epithelium increase in number and appear in distal airways, and the submucosal glands increase in size (262–265). As an example, in chronic bronchitis, the surface cells increase from 5,600–8,500 mm^2 to 10,000 mm^2 (74) and increase in the size and number of gland cells shifts the gland to wall ratio (a measure of gland hypertrophy) from 0.26–0.39 to 0.45–0.85 (264,265). Typically, at both sites, such increase is accompanied by the appearance of mucous cells at the expense of serous cells. This arises from cell proliferation and the development of new mucous cells, and in the absence of cell proliferation (178,180) from transdifferentiation—as serous and Clara cells acquire a mucous cell phenotype (140,141,267,317). In vitro studies confirm that serous gland cells carry antigens to both mucous and serous cell types, indicating that, at this site, cells may readily acquire either phenotype (315).

The secretory cells of the epithelial surface and gland synthesize a variety of complex carbohydrates—sulfated or sialic acid-rich glycoconjugates (glycoproteins and glycosaminoglycans) (178,179,181,182,316). In the normal airway, these are distributed differently in the secretory cells of a single gland (mucous and serous cells) as well as in adjacent cells of a single population (179,181,182). Within mucous cells, for example, four different types of acidic glycoproteins are found alone, or in certain combinations (but not all four together) in a single cell (17). Furthermore, the distribution of glycoproteins varies between the cells of different airway generations, and between species, and also is influenced by the environment, infection, and disease (267). Mucous cell hypertrophy and increase in cell number are associated with a shift to acid glycoproteins that are sulfated. In addition to these changes, mucus-secreting cells increase their basal metabolic rate. The same range of products is identified (by histochemical techniques) inside and outside cells (267).

The visco-elastic properties of the airway mucus layer are derived from the glycoproteins—macromolecules ($>10^6$ kd) that are 60–85% carbohydrate and 40–15% protein (351). Long branching polysaccharide side chains surround the protein (apomucin) core, to which they attach by O-glycosidic linkages to produce the polydisperse structures that form airway mucus. Typically, in secretory cells, the polypeptide core of the glycoprotein is formed in the endoplasmic reticulum and the addition of some sugars (e.g., manose) occurs in this region, while most of the sugars (galactose, glucosamine, fucose, and sialic acid) are added at the Golgi membrane, as is sulfate (267,342). Recent advances have been made in understanding the primary structure of at least four mucin (core protein) genes (apomucin genes, MUC1, MUC2, MUC3, and MUC4) and possibly a fifth (MUC5), although this may derive from the same gene as MUC2 (110). MC1 is a transmembrane mucin glycoprotein found in the apical region of the epithelium: MUC2 is one of several secreted glycoproteins identified in airway secretory cells. MUC1, MUC2, and MUC5 are expressed by an SV40-transformed normal (human) bronchial epithelial cell line (335), whereas tracheobronchial tissue (including epithelium and submucosa) and isolated gland acini and cells express transcripts for MUC1 and MUC2 (88). The MUC gene cDNA gene that codes for the protein core of airway mucin and leads to the development of mucous cells, however, is not clear (10). Radiolabeled precursor studies demonstrate that tracheal gland serous cells synthesize high molecular weight-O-linked glycoproteins (both glycoprotein and proteoglycan), and the low molecular weight proteins that are specific markers for these cells—antileukoprotease, lyzozyme and lactoferrin (223). Ionic interactions between these cationic proteins and large polyanions (the glycoproteins or proteoglycans) may assist in granule packaging (223). The balance between secretion of glycoprotein and proteoglycan by these cells in vivo is still unclear, although it may be that proteoglycan is secreted preferentially by the normal airway and glycoprotein in disease (20,21). How this is linked to the transdifferentiation of serous to mucous cells that occurs in disease is as yet unclear.

Airway secretory cells discharge their granules in response to a variety of agents (205,239). Secretion from the cells of the tracheobronchial glands is regulated by multiple neural-mediated interactions (via adrenergic, cholinergic, and nonadrenergic noncholinergic [NANC] pathways): secretion from the epithelial surface secretory cells by cholinergic and NANC pathways (195). Regional differences in these control mechanisms are demonstrated by the greater sensitivity to a secretagogue of bronchial cells than tracheal or bronchiolar ones (42,67). Tracheal cells have greater amounts of (lectin-detectable) galactose, N-acetylated glactosamine, glucosamine and sialic acid than bronchial cells, with fucose similar in both, suggesting that lower levels of glycoconjugates bound to the surface of the more distal cells leaves higher numbers of binding sites for agents effecting secretion (42). Secretion is effected by nucleotides acting via 5′-nucleotide receptors, ATP being released by nerve terminals, inflammatory cells, and dead or injured airway cells (195). Extracellular ATP stimulates secretion via activation of (P2) purinoceptors located on the cell surface, via a signal transduction mechanism involving activation of GTP binding proteins and phospholipase C (167). Secretion from airway surface cells is also regulated by PAF (2,195), via a PAF receptor (2), or by a protein kinase C dependent mechanism, although this alone does not cause secretion (187). Elastase, tachykinins and purinergic compounds also stimulate secretion from airway surface cells (195). And PAF effects the release of hydroxyeicosatetraenoic acids (15-, 12-, 5-HETES), which stimulate secretion via autocrine and paracrine pathways (2). Secretion of antileukoproteases, glycoproteins and proteoglycans from the submucosal glands is stimulated by adrenergic and cholinergic agonists, secretion being potentiated by epinephrine (224). Variation in their discharge in response to stimulation reflects the distribution of receptors (α- and β-adrengeric receptors, $\alpha > \beta$ on serous cells) and different granules within cells (191,256).

Airway epithelial cells both make and respond to basement membrane components (273,328). The membrane consists, in general, of three structures—the lamina lucida (adjacent to the cell), the lamina reticularis (adjacent to the underlying basement membrane) and the lamina densa (in between). Within the airways, the organization of sulfated macromolecules in these layers demonstrates regional differences—the microdomains of the trachea, bronchi and large bronchioles being similar (where most reactive sites occur in the lamina rara and least in the lamina densa) (165), and different from ones in small bronchioles (where most reactive sites occuring in the lamina lucida). These microdomains in small bronchioles resemble those in the basement membrane of the alveolar region (165,289,330). How these anionic sites influence cell activity is not yet understood but certain growth factors show strong affinity for heparin sulfate (e.g., bFGF) and so concentrate in the membrane where (liberated by heparatinases) they regulate tissue growth and regeneration. Fibronectins, cell adhesive glycoproteins associated with the membrane, bind matrix collagens, proteoglycans, and fibrin, and fibronectin receptors link extracellular fibronectin to intracellular cytoskeletal filaments (e.g., actin). Laminin and entactin are present in the basement membrane of almost all lung regions, and there are regional differences in the distribution of chondroitin sulfate proteoglycan and heparan sulfate proteoglycan (290).

In vitro, substrata of type IV collagen, laminin or fibronectin determine the differentiation of tracheal gland serous cells; the cells responding to specific molecules by modifying their shape and synthesis of proteins (328). Collagen IV and laminin produce a profile that is similar, and one that is different from that of fibronectin. In part this sensitivity to matrix components is mediated by the expression of integrin receptors (7). The cytoplasmic domain of integrins interacts with cytoskeletal proteins via talin (130). Neutralizing antibody studies demonstrate that loss of the (β_1) integrin receptor modifies the response of these cells, shifting their normal response to substrata of collagen IV and laminin to produce the same profile as fibronectin (328). Molecules form heterodimers of α and β subunits (225) that bind major constituents of the normal basement membrane or to basement membrane proteins found during development, inflmmation and wound healing (e.g., fibronectin, fibrinogen, vitronectin, and thrombospondin) (225). Bronchial cells (in vitro) express multiple subunits that bind collagen and laminin (α_1, α_2, and α_3) and two subunits mediating adhesion to fibronectin (α_3- and α_v-containing integrins) (225). Integrin-ligand binding results in more than simple mechanical attachment, since the integrins function as signaling molecules, translating the extracellular event (i.e., ligand binding) into intracellular messages (77). And cytoplasmic signals modulate integrin activity without changing their distribution on the cell surface (perhaps via conformational changes) to alter interaction with a ligand (77).

Airway epithelial cells are both the target and source of inflammatory cell products. In addition to the presence of serum-derived protease inhibitors which are active in peripheral lung (particularly α_1 proteinase inhibitor but also α_2 macroglobulin) the airways regulate the activity of proteases released by inflammatory cells (especially neutrophils and monocytes) by the production of low molecular weight inhibitors—tissue inhibitor metalloproteinase (TIMP), antileukoprotease and an elastase specific inhibitor (elafin) (283,284). Antileukoprotease is secreted both luminally and basally by serous cells of the tracheal gland (60,173) and by Clara cells of bronchial epithelium (63). Elafin released by Clara cells is thought to minimize proteolytic damage and protect the elastic fibres of the interstitium from elastase (284). In response to injury, airway epithelial cells release and respond to a variety of cytokines (4). Detectable amounts of IL-1α and IL-1β are released (211,212), and expression of IL-1 receptors (206) amplifies the inflammatory cascade. Other amplification pathways are evident: TNF-α induces IL-8 mRNA and protein (177) and Pseudomonas infection IL-8 (135), and IL-1β and TNF induce expression of protease and elastase inhibitors (antileukoprotease and elafin). Increased production of GM-CSF by bronchial cells in response to IL-1α and IL-1β also promotes the inflammatory response, contributing to the activation and increased survival of neutrophils and eosinophils (206). Cytokine release by epithelial cells is increased by proinflammatory cytokines (45,46,156), and constitutively increased in cells derived from inflamed tissue compared with cells derived from noninflamed tissue (245,331).Irritant gases modulate IL-1β, IL-8, GM-CSF, and TNF-α synthesis by bronchial epithelial cells (61), as well as the release of PAF.

In response to challenge, bronchial epithelial cells modulate their expression of leukocytes adhesion molecules. ICAM-1 is expressed under basal conditions (but not ELAM-1, P-selectin, or VCAM-1), and ICAM-1 expression is increased in response to phorbol myristate acetate, or to the proinflammatory cytokines IFN-γ and TNF-α (26). CD44 (a family of glycoproteins that function as intercellular adhesion molecules linking the basement membrane to the cell cytoskeleton) and lymphocyte function associated antigen-3 (LFA-3) also are expressed (26). HLA-DR molecules (surface membrane glycoproteins) expressed by several lung cells that are part of the immune system (B-lymphocytes, dendritic cells, monocytes, macrophages, and activated T-cells) are also expressed by epithelial cells (281). In reponse to IFN-γ stimulation bronchial ciliated cells express HLA-DR class II antigens (281). In addition to acting as a barrier to antigenic material, epithelial cells also participate in the immune response by mediator release.

Airway cells are a source of mediators that modulate bronchoreactivity and cell growth. Cell-cell interactions lead to synthesis of nitric oxide, and so to vasodilation, and decreased cell proliferation, mediated via stimulation of guanosine 3′,5′-monophosphate (cGMP). The interaction of the free-radical NO with cells is cytotoxic. There are regional differences in airway cell expression, the inducible form of nitric oxide synthetase (iNOS) being expressed by the epithelial cells of large airways (bronchi) but not distally (bronchioli) (87,168,302), and cells may contain one or more NOS forms. In response to cytokines, bronchial cells express mRNA transcripts and protein for iNOS (274). In disease, such as asthma, the number of bronchial cells expressing iNOS increases (in vivo) and is increased further by cytokine challenge (in vitro) (111). In vitro, bronchial epithelial cells express the constitutive form of NOS (cNOS) and in response to proinflammatory cytokines (IFN-γ, IL-1β, TNF-α) and lipopolysaccharide express NOS activity similar to the iNOS form, indicating mechanisms to protect against infection and hyperreactivity (15). Airway epithelial cells produce endothelin-1 (ET-1) (213), which increases smooth muscle cell proliferation, and binds to airway cell receptors to initiate production of arachidonic acid metabolites (cyclooxygenase and lipoxygenase products), augmenting the inflammatory response and inducing bronchoconstriction (346,352). Endothelin-1 immunoreactive cells are present in airway epithelium throughout the lung, and in the submucosal glands; proendothelin-1, proendothelin-3 alone are detected in airway epithelial cells and all three isoforms in submucosal gland cells (204). While ET-1, ET-2, and ET-3 mRNA transcripts are highly expressed by cells in the developing lung (especially by neuroendocrine cells) they are, however, only minimally expressed by adult airway epithelial cells (100). In disease, as in cryptogenic fibrosing alveolitis, the number of airway cells expressing ET-1 transcripts and protein increases (99).

Airway epithelial cells express a variety of other growth mediators, and receptors that influence cell proliferation, differentiation, chemotaxis and extracellular matrix production, including PDGF (12,332), epidermal growth factor (EGF) (257), and IGF-I (113,269). Selective expression is evident, as demonstrated by expression of the three forms of TGF-β by bronchial epithelial cells, expression of transcripts and protein disappearing as terminal bronchioles become respiratory bronchioles (164,252). TGF-β can induce transcription of other growth mediators, including IL-1, PDGF, bFGF, TNF-α, and itself. Airway cells respond to growth factors secreted by other airway cells, including CGRP from serous and Kultchitsky cells; CGRP also modulates ciliary beat frequency (18,171,347,349) and airway mucus secretion (17,339).

Bronchus-Associated Lymphoid Tissue and Dendritic Cells

The airway epithelium contains two subepithelial cell populations that form an integral part of its structure and modulate the immune response—bronchus-associated lymphoid tissue (BALT) and dendritic cells (i.e., interdigitating, branched, or tree-shaped cells).

BALT BALT, nonencapsulated subepithelial aggregations of lymphoid cells, are present in the submucosa of human airways and in the airways of a variety of other species (267,329). The epithelium overlying these aggregates, which facilitates transport and processing of antigen from the airway lumen, is flattened, heavily infiltrated with lymphocytes, and does not include ciliated or secretory cells: Hence, the term lymphoepithelium has been applied. The distribution of receptor molecules (addressins) and other accessory lymphocyte adherence molecules that are likely expressed by endothelium of vessels associated with BALT is not yet clear (23). The aggregates are generally located near or at branching points of the bronchi and are quite small in human lung, although their extent varies between species. Such collections are present, however, even in gnotobiotic animals. They include distinct IgA-committed B-cell and T-cell areas, and cytokinetic studies indicate the presence of recirculating lymphocytes as well as rapidly dividing cells. It is at yet unclear how lymphocytes initially aggregate in the airway as part of normal homeostasis, although it is likely that a predetermined but latent site of exposure to antigen exists that is destined to become BALT (23). Cytokine production in response to antigen challenge in the airway may be responsible for BALT activation (23).

Dendritic Cell Dendritic cells are antigen-presenting accessory cells that play a critical role in the immune response in the lung by activating resting T cells. This effect is enhanced on exposure to cytokines such as IL-1 and GM-CSF (13). The cells, bean shaped with an eccentric nucleus and prominent cytoplasmic extensions (329), are located mainly in the subepithelium, where they may form small clusters with T cells. Fewer cells are present in the alveolar region, where they are found mainly in connective tissue forming the thick-region of the alveolar-capillary membrane and septal bifurcations (299). On occasion, several dendritic cells form a tight network, but mostly scattered cells are found along the epithelial basement membrane, and in the bronchi and bronchioli, their projections extend between epithelial cells (329). Subsets of cells have recently been isolated from lung interstium as well as from airway epithelium (13,109). Interestingly, macrophages derived from different sites in the lung exert opposing effects, interstitial macrophage releasing inflammatory cytokines that stimulate the effect of dendritic cells on T cells, and alveolar macrophage exerting an inhibitory one. Injury (tobacco smoke) increases the number of dendritic cells (313).

Alveolar Surface Cells

The alveolar surface is lined by three epithelial cell types (47, 125,210,228,296,341,342). The distended shape of the alveolus is maintained by the fibers and cells of the interstitium, as well as by a surface film of phospholipids or surfactant (189). Capillaries course through the alveolar wall, approaching closely the epithelium alternately on one side and then on the other. At their closest point, the basement membranes of the capillary endothelial cell and of the alveolar epithelial cell produce the thin region of the alveolar-capillary membrane (0.5 µm). In its thick region, these two basement membranes are separated by the interstitial space and by connective tissue, which includes matrix and both resident and migratory cells. In normal lung, solutes and liquids cross this region.

Type I Cells

The type I epithelial cell is large (40 µm diameter) but thin (0.2 µm at thinnest point) with a centrally placed nucleus, a perinuclear region containing most of the organelles, and branched cytoplasmic processes relatively poor in organelles. Its thin attenuated cytoplasm is optimal for its primary function of gas exchange. In the human lung, it has been calculated that the broad extensions of this cell cover 5,000 μm^2, although the total area covered by the cell is only 1,400 µm2 due to branching (342). It constitutes only 35% of alveolar epithelial cell number but covers 90–97% of the alveolar surface (47,342).

Type II Cells

The cuboidal type II cell, the secretory cell of the alveolar surface, is usually found in the angle of the alveolus. It constitutes 65% of alveolar epithelial cells, but covers only 3–10% of the surface area (47,342). Its tuft of surface microvilli, containing actin filaments, extends upwards from the cell apex into the surface film layer, especially so at the cell margins (342). These are thought to assist in ion transport and fluid resorption. The cell has a large number of organelles and osmophilic membrane-bound lamella bodies (150 cells) that are extruded onto the alveolar surface—a multilamellar form of surfactant in a membrane-bound structure (comprised of surfactant phospholipids and apoproteins). It is generally considered that in response to injury this cell persists, multiplies, and reconstitutes the alveolar epithelial lining by differentiation to a type I cell.

Type III Cells

A counterpart to the brush cell of the conducting airways is found in the alveolar region, although only a small part of the surface of the type III alveolar cell, the "brush" that gives the cell its name, contributes to the alveolar surface area (38,228). This consists of ~120–140 straight, blunt microvilli that protrude into the alveolus. The rest of the cell surface is covered by cytoplasmic extensions of the type I cell. The glycocalyx of this cell is rich in anionic glycoproteins. The cell resembles the more frequent brush cell of the gut, except that the fine filaments extending into the cytoplasm do not end in a terminal web. Alveolar brush cells have many vacuoles, as well as lysosomes, multivesicular bodies and glycogen granules. They are joined to neighboring cells by terminal bars. The cells are preferentially located in the central part of the acinus of proximal alveolar duct regions (distal to the terminal bronchiolus) where they may participate in maintaining fluid balance (228) or detoxification (38).

In addition to its secretory function the type II cell is considered the progenitor cell of the alveolar surface. Soluble growth factors and basement membrane components influence its proliferation (including EGF, insulin, cholera toxin, endothelial growth supplement and heparin-binding growth factors, pulmonary alveolar macrophage conditioned medium and bronchoalveolar lavage factor) (193,194,257), and matrix components modulate differentiation (261). In response to injury type II cells dedifferentiate to cover the alveolar surface and differentiate to type I or II cells (79). Proliferating cells express a type II cell phenotype (in vitro). The distribution of apical cell membrane carbohydrates (sialic acid, galactose, and N-acetylgalactosamine) then alters on differentiation—identifing differentiating type I cells from type II cells (48). These lectin-binding patterns may reflect the development of glycosylating enzymes (150), The expression of markers for differentiated type I and type II cells (mRNAs SP-A, SP-B, and SP-C), surfactant phospholipids, alkaline phosphatase, and lysozyme) indicate that the cells transdifferentiate as a function of environmental factors (348). The appearance of type I markers before type II markers, indicates that differentiation of fetal cells to an adult cell type may depend on the repression of specific genes (150). These studies suggest that the commonly accepted lineage does not apply in the fetal lung and this may equally be the case in response to injury (65).

The synthesis of components of the lamellar body of the type II cell are discussed elsewhere in this book. Briefly, the surfactant phospholipids and apoproteins, the main scretory components of the type II cell, are synthesized in the endoplasmic reticulum and packed into transport vesicles: the apoproteins undergo posttranslational modification in the endoplasmic reticulum and Golgi before fusing with the phosphlipid. SP-A is a glycoprotein, SP-B and SP-C are hydrophobic proteins with high affinity for lipids, and SP-D is a collagenous glycoprotein. It is as yet unclear if the lamellar bodies are a major source of SP-A or if any small amount of SP-A is secreted with lamellar bodies, most newly synthesized SP-A being released from vesicles by constitutive secretion (i.e., continuous secretion dependent on rate of synthesis and not stimulated by challenge), whereas secretion of the lamellar body is regulated (i.e., secretion involving intracellular packaging, concentration of secreted proteins, and increased release in response to challenge) (92). Protein 1b15 appears a major protein of the limiting membrane of the lamellar body. It may not be secreted but fuse and concentrate within the membrane (254). Gibson and Widnell (102) have discussed the endocytic pathways for surfactant in type II cells: SP-A appears located in two distinct structures involved in secretion and degradation—lamellar bodies and lysosomes. Abundant SP-A and SP-B mRNAs also are expressed by Clara cells (but not SP-C mRNAs) (16,129), and in response to injury (oxidant gas), SP-A and SP-B transcripts increase (20-fold). In type II cells, SP-A, SP-B, and SP-C each are expressed; increase in SP-A and SP-B mRNAs in response to injury (oxidant gas) is less dramatic (than in the Clara cell) and expression of SP-C transcripts does not change (129). SP-A and SP-B proteins also are found in Clara cells indicating bioactivity at this nonalveolar site (336), but it remains unclear as to whether this relates to a surfactant or nonsurfactant role.

Type II–like cells (in vitro) synthesize cytokines and cytokine receptors leading to recruitment and activation of inflammatory cells (14) and express inflammatory cell chemoattractants—interaction between the type II cell and PAMs being necessary for type II cell to express monocyte chemoattractant protein-1 (318). Type II cells respond to inflammatory cytokines by expressing iNOS, and iNOS expression is further increased by an irritant gas (ozone) (255).

In addition to the Clara cell of the epithelial surface, alveolar type II cells (as well as macrophages and capillary endothelial cells) express major components of the cytochrome P450 monooxygenase system, and so may metabolize xenobiotics and produce toxicants (39). And the alveolar lining cells (like ciliated cells) are immunoreactive for endopeptidase 24.15 (40).

EFFECT OF ANESTHETICS ON LUNG CELLS

General and Metabolic Effects

The effects of anesthetics on pulmonary vascular and bronchial tone are discussed elsewhere in this book. Despite the fact that inhaled anesthetics must diffuse through lung cells to the bloodstream, and that injected anesthetics must pass through the lung circulation, surprisingly little attention has been focused on their direct effects on lung cells or tissue.

Administration of enflurane or halothane to isolated, perfused rabbit lungs does not alter lung glucose utilization or lactate production, and thus does not influence lung carbohydrate metabolism (250). However, using varying concentrations of halothane, with or without nitrous oxide or pentobarbitone, or midazolam combined with fentanyl, Heys et al. (123) showed that lung protein synthesis was reduced by up to 30% by all these anesthetic agents. Isoflurane, ketamine or fentanyl did not affect rat lung protein synthesis (207,208).

Lung filtration is altered by anesthetics. The transpulmonary passage of venous air emboli in dogs increases with halothane anesthesia, but less than in response to fentanyl or ketamine (353). Pentobarbitone also reduces filtration of air bubbles (155). Furthermore, halothane in combination with high inspired oxygen tension increases alveolar capillary barrier permeability, as assessed by DTPA clearance in rabbits (337). Pentobarbital has no such effect. In humans, general anesthesia with N_2O in O_2 increases hyaluronic acid levels in bronchoalveolar lavage (235). These may be factors contributing to the accumulation of interstitial and alveolar fluid during general anesthesia and ARDS.

Normal pulmonary release or metabolism of vasoactive compounds is also modified by anesthetics. Nitrous oxide increases norepinephrine release at the neuroeffector junctions of dog pulmonary arteries (279). Furthermore, halothane decreases norepinephrine uptake in rat lung slices (118). The effects of anesthetics on 5-HT uptake by the lung have been examined more extensively in a variety of animal models. Halothane decreases 5-HT uptake and metabolism by the rat pulmonary circulation (119). Yet, in the rat lung, endogenous 5-HT levels are increased by halothane, possibly due to an increase in 5-HT decarboxylase activity (249). In dogs, halothane does not affect 5-HT uptake from the circulation (327). Patients undergoing coronary bypass surgery do not develop alteration of pulmonary extraction of 5-HT by anesthesia, extracorporeal circulation, or the surgery (53). Extraction of propranolol is, however, altered, suggesting that propranolol may be a more sensitive indicator of dysfunctional uptake. Ketamine reduces 5-HT uptake in perfused rat lungs, but fentanyl does not (207). Angiotensin converting enzyme activity, as assessed by hydrolysis of circulating ^{3}H-BAP substrate in perfused lungs, is not altered by ketamine, fentanyl (207), enflurane, halothane, or isoflurane (8).

Effect on Lung Cells

Endothelial cells

In addition to the effects discussed above, in studies of endothelial uptake and metabolism of circulating peptides , indicate that inhalational anesthetics have direct effects on endothelial function and resistance to injury. Halothane increases the prostacyclin, thromboxane A_2, and leukotrines C_4, D_4, E_4, and F_4 released from bovine pulmonary artery endothelial cells (19). It also increases the sensitivity of rat pulmonary artery endothelial cells to oxidant-mediated injury by activated neutrophils (303). Isoflurane also renders these cells more susceptible to injury.

Epithelial Cells

Some studies have examined the effects of anesthetics on surfactant, mucociliary clearance and tracheal contraction in animal models. Barbiturate anesthesia may reduce surfactant turnover (338). In baboons, both ketamine and pentobarbitone decrease mucociliary clearance, but the pentobarbitone has a milder inhibitory effect (68). However, in humans undergoing abdominal surgery, Konrad et al. (172) have shown that anesthesia with midazolam, fentanyl, pancuronium, and O_2/NO_2 does not alter mucociliary transport, as assessed using radiolabelled microspheres. Many inhaled anesthetics may be bronchodilators. Enflurance has been shown to reduce basal bronchomotor tone in canine isolated tracheal segments in situ (170). It also inhibits contractions induced by changes in tidal volume, and CO_2 and O_2 levels.

The halogenated hydrocarbons DDD, DBE, and trichlorethylene are recognized pneumotoxins. Their major targets of injury are Clara cells, type II pneumocytes, and alveolar macrophages (241). This injury is at least partly mediated by cytochrome P 450 oxidation and inactivation (241,244). In contrast, phenobarbital is a potent inducer of certain cytochrome P 450 enzymes. In mice, phenobarbital binding has been demonstrated in alveolar and bronchial wall cells, and in pulmonary capillary endothelial cells (136). However, in humans, first-pass lung uptake of thiopental is much lower than that of verapamil, suggesting that pulmonary uptake of circulating agents is greater with basic amine drugs that are highly lipid soluble (275).

Inflammatory Cells

Anesthetics alter the function and mobilization of inflammatory cells. Exposure to halothane as compared to ketamine reduces the intraalveolar recruitment of neutrophils, lymphocytes and macrophages following intranasal inoculation with influenza virus (324). Ketamine treated animals become "sicker," with more extensive pulmonary inflammation and consolidation. Although low-dose halothane does not appear toxic to guinea pig macrophages, a 6-h exposure to 19% halothane, or shorter exposures to 5% halothane are toxic (333). However, at clinically relevant concentrations, both enflurane and isoflurane inhibit pulmonary alveolar macrophage oxidative activity, which is reversible after 30-min exposure to air (344). Propofol, ketamine, and thiopentane induce histamine release from human lung mast cells, but do not cause release of PGD_2 or leukotrine C4, nor do they induce release from basophils (321). The hypnotics althesin and propanidid also induce histamine release from rabbit lung mast cells (76).

PERSPECTIVES

The focus of this review is the organization and role of vascular and resident airway cells in lung, including their relationship to each other and to matrix components, and their interaction with cytokines and proinflammatory mediators, to highlight the phenotype(s) acquired by these cells in response to injury. This may be an appropriate response to challenge and regulatory controls, or represent an aberrant or excessive response to injury and repair. In the past 15 years, our understanding of the complexity of the lung's structure and nonventilatory functions has greatly increased. Defining the range of normal phenotypic expression of vascular and airway cells and understanding, in response to injury, the interactions associated with a shift in phenotype, and the relationship of this to tissue remodeling, remain the challenge.

ACKNOWLEDGMENT

D.L. is a Chercheur-Boursier Clinicien, Fonds de la Recherche en Santé du Quebec, and is supported by a grant from the Heart and Stroke Foundation of Quebec. R.C.J. is supported by NIH HLB RO1 34552 and NIH HLB RO1 45737.

REFERENCES

1. Adamson IY, Hedgecock C, Bawdon DH. Epithelial cell fibroblast interactions in lung injury and repair. *Am J Pathol* 1990;137: 385–392.
2. Adler KB, Ackley NJ, Glasgow WC. Platelet-activating factor provokes release of mucin-like glycoproteins from guinea pig respiratory epithelial cells via a lipoxygenase-dependent mechanism. *Am J Respir Cell Mol Biol* 1992;6:550–556.
3. Adler KB, Cheng P-W, Kim KC. Characterization of guinea pig tracheal epithelial cells maintained in biphasic organotypic culture: cellular composition and biochemical analysis of released glycoconjugates. *Am J Respir Cell Mol Biol* 1990;2:145–154.
4. Adler KB, Fischer BM, Wright DT, Cohn LA, Becker S. Interactions between respiratory epithelial cells and cytokines: relationships to lung inflammation. *Ann NY Acad Sci* 1994;725:128–145.
5. Adler KB, Low RB, Leslie KO, Mitchell J, Evans JN. Contractile cells in normal and fibrotic lung. *Lab Invest* 1989;60:473–485.
6. Albelda SM. Endothelial and epithelial cell adhesion molecules. *Am J Respir Cell Mol Biol* 1991;4:195–203.
7. Albelda SM, Muller WA, Buck CA, Newman PJ. Molecular and cellular properties of PECAM-1. *J Cell Biol* 1991;114:1059–1068.
8. Alifimoff JK, Brandom BW, Cook DR. Enflurane, halothane and isoflurane do not inhibit angiotensin converting enzyme activity. *Can Anesth Soc J* 1985;32:351–357.
9. Allen MD, Harlan JM. The clinical role of leukocyte adhesion molecules. In: Yacoub M, Pepper J, eds. *Annual of cardiac surgery.* London: Current Science, 1993:32–40.
10. An G, Luo G, Wu R. Expression of MUC2 Gene is down-regulated *in vitro* in tracheobronchial epithelial cells. *Am J Respir Cell Mol Biol* 1994;10:546–551.
11. Antonelli-Orlidge A, Smith SR, D'Amore PA. Influence of pericytes on capillary endothelial cell growth. *Am Rev Respir Dis* 1989;140:1129–1131.
12. Antoniades HN, Bravo MA, Avila RE, et al. Platelet-derived growth factor in idiopathic pulmonary fibrosis. *J Clin Invest* 1990;86: 1055–1064.
13. Armstrong LR, Christensen PJ, Paine R III, Chen G-H. Regulation of the immunostimulatory activity of rat pulmonary interstitial dendritic cells by cell-cell interactions and cytokines. *Am J Respir Cell Mol Biol* 1994;11:682–691.
14. Arnold R, Humbert B, Werchau H, Gallati H, Konig W. Interleukin-8, interleukin-6, and soluble tumour necrosis factor receptor type I release from a human pulmonary epithelial cell line (A549) exposed to respiratory syncytial virus. *Immunology* 1994;82: 126–133.
15. Asano K. Constitutive and inducible nitric oxide synthase gene expression, regulation, and activity in human lung epithelial cells. *Proc Natl Acad Sci USA* 1994;91:10089–10093.
16. Auten RL, Watkins RH, Shapiro DL, Horowitz S. Surfactant apro-protein A (SPA) is synthesized in airway cells. *Am J Respir Cell Mol Biol* 1990;3:491–496.
17. Baker AP, Hillegass LM, Holden DA, Smith WJ. Effect of kallidin, substance P, and other basic polypeptides on the production of respiratory macromolecules. *Am Rev Respir Dis* 1977;115:811–817.
18. Baluk P, Nadel J, McDonald DM. Calcitonin gene–related peptide in secretory granules of serous cells in the rat tracheal epithelium. *Am J Respir Cell Mol Biol* 1993;8:446–453.
19. Barnes SD, Martin LD, Wetzel RC. Halothane enhances pulmonary artery eicoscenoid release. *Anesth Analg* 1992;75:1007–1013.
20. Baskhar KR, O'Sullivan DD, Seltzer J, Rossing TH, Drazen JM, Reid LM. Density gradient study of bronchial mucus aspirates from healthy volunteers (smokers and nonsmokers) and from patients with tracheostomy. *Exp Lung Res* 1985;9:289–308.
21. Baskhar KR, O'Sullivan DD, Seltzer TB, Rossing JM, Drazen JM, Reid LM. Density gradient analysis of secretions produced *in vitro* by human and canine airway mucosa: identification of lipids and protoglycans in such secretions. *Exp Lung Res* 1986;10: 401–422.
22. Berk JL, Franzblau C, Goldstein RH. Recombinant interleukin-1β inhibits elastin formation by neonatal rat lung fibroblast subtype. *J Biol Chem* 1991;266:3192–3197.
23. Berman J. Lymphocytes in the lung: should we continue to exalt only BALT? *Am J Respir Cell Mol Biol* 1990;3:101–102.
24. Bevilacqua MP. Endothelial-leukocyte adhesion molecules. *Annu Rev Immunol* 1993;11:767–804.
25. Bloem LH, Chen L, Konigsberg WH, Bach R. Serum stimulation of quiescent human fibroblasts induces the synthesis of tissue factor mRNA followed by appearance of tissue factor antigen and procoagulant activity. *J Cell Physiol* 1989;139:418–423.
26. Bloemen PGM, Van den Tweel MC, Henricks PAJ, et al. Expression and modulation of adhesion molecules on human bronchial epithelial cells. *Am J Respir Cell Mol Biol* 1993;9:586–593.
27. Bond M, Somlyo AV. Dense bodies and actin polarity in vertebrate smooth muscle. *J Cell Biol* 1982;95:403–413.
28. Braun T, Buschhausen-Denker G, Baber E, Tannich E, Arnold HH. A novel human muscle factor related to but distinct from MyoD1 induces myogenic conversion in 10T1/2 fibroblasts. *EMBO J* 1989; 8:701–709.
29. Breeze RG, Wheeldon EB. The cells of the pulmonary airways. *Am Rev Respir Dis* 1977;116:705–777.
30. Breuer R, Christensen TG, Wax Y, et al. Relationship of secretory granule content and proliferative intensity in the secretory compartment of the hamster bronchial epithelium. *Am J Respir Cell Mol Biol* 1993;8:480–485.
31. Brewster CEP, Howarth PH, Djukanovic R, Wilson J, Holgate ST, Roche WR. Myofibroblasts and subepithelial fibrosis in bronchial asthma. *Am J Respir Cell Mol Biol* 1990;3:507–511.
32. Brody AR, Bonner JC, Badgett A. Recombinant interferon-gamma reduces PDGF-induced lung fibroblasts growth but stimulates PDGF production by alveolar macrophages *in vitro. Chest* 1993; 103:121S–122S.
33. Brody AR, Bonner JC, Overby LH, et al. Interstitial pulmonary macrophages produce platelet-derived growth factor that stimulates rat lung fibroblast proliferation *in vitro. J Leukoc Biol* 1992; 51:640–648.
34. Burridge K, Fath K, Kelly T, Nuckolls G, Turner C. Focal adhesion: transmembrane junctions between the extracellular matrix and the cytoskeleton. *Annu Rev Cell Biol* 1988;4:487–525.
35. Burrows BA, Wolf G. The kinetics of fibronectin synthesis and release in normal and tumor promoter-treated lung fibroblasts. *Mol Cell Biochem* 1990;96:557–567.
36. Cantin AM, Larivee P, Begin RO. Extracellular glutathione suppresses human lung fibroblast proliferation. *Am J Respir Cell Mol Biol* 1990;3:79–85.
37. Carlson EC. Topographical specificity in isolated retinal capillary basement membrane. *Microvasc Res* 1988;35:221–235.
38. Chang L-Y, Mercer RR, Crapo JD. Differential distribution of brush cells in the rat lung. *Anat Rec* 1986;216:49–54.
39. Chichester CH, Philpot RM, Weir AJ, Buckpitt AR, Plopper CG. Characterization of the cytochrome P-450 monooxygenase system

in nonciliated bronchiolar epithelial (Clara) cells isolated from mouse lung. *Am J Respir Cell Mol Biol* 1991;4:179–186.

40. Choi HH, Lesser M, Cardozo C, Orlowski M. Immunohistochemical localization of endopeptidase 24.15 in rat trachea, lung tissue, and alveolar macrophages. *Am J Respir Cell Mol Biol* 1990;3: 619–624.
41. Christensen TG, Breuer R, Haddad CE, Niles RM. Quantitative ultrastructural analysis of the relationship between cell growth, shape change, and mucosecretory differentiation in cultured hamster tracheal epithelial cells exposed to retinoic acid. *Am J Respir Cell Mol Biol* 1993;9:287–294.
42. Christensen TG, Breuer R, Lucey EC, Hornstra LJ, Stone PJ, Snider GL. Lectin cytochemistry reveals differences between hamster trachea and bronchus in the composition of epithelial surface glycoconjugates and in the response of secretory cells to neutrophil elastase. *Am J Respir Cell Mol Biol* 1990;3:61–69.
43. Christman BW, McPherson CD, Newman JH, et al. An imbalance between the excretion of thromboxane and prostacyclin in pulmonary hypertension. *N Engl J Med* 1992;327:70–75.
44. Clark JG, Dedon TF, Wayner EA, Carter WG. Effects of interferon-gamma on expression of cell surface receptors for collagen and deposition of newly synthesized collagen by cultured human lung fibroblasts. *J Clin Invest* 1989;83:1505–1511.
45. Cox G, Gauldie J, Jordana M. Bronchial epithelial cell-derived cytokines (G-CSF and GM-CSF) promote the survival of peripheral blood neutrophils *in vitro*. *Am J Respir Cell Mol Biol* 1992;7: 507–513.
46. Cox GT. Promotion of eosinophil survival by human bronchial epithelial cells and its modulation by steroids. *Am J Respir Cell Mol Biol* 1991;4:525–531.
47. Crapo JD, Barry BE, Gehr P, Bachofen M, Weibel ER. Cell number and cell characteristics of the normal human lung. *Am Rev Respir Dis* 1982;125:332–337.
48. Crestani B, Dehoux M, Seta N, Cuer M, Aubier M. Cell surface carbohydrates of rat alveolar type II cells in primary culture. *Am J Respir Cell Mol Biol* 1993;8:145–152.
49. Crouch E, Martin G, Brodie J. Basement membranes. In: Crystal R, West G, Barnes P, Cherniak N, Weibel E, eds. *The lung: scientific foundations.* New York: Raven Press, 1991:421–437.
50. Crouch EC, Parks WC, Rosenbaum JL, et al. Regulation of collagen production by medial smooth muscle cells in hypoxic pulmonary hypertension. *Am Rev Respir Dis* 1989;140:1045–1051.
51. Crystal RG, Brantly ML, Hubbard RC, Curiel DT, States DJ, Holmes MD. The α1-antitrypsin gene and its mutations: clinical consequences and strategies for therapy. *Chest* 1989;95:196–208.
52. Curiel DT, Agarwal S, Romer MU, et al. Gene transfer to respiratory epithelial cells via the receptor–mediated endocytosis pathway. *Am J Respir Cell Mol Biol* 1992;6:247–252.
53. Dargent F, Neidhart P, Bachmann M, Suter PM, Junod AF. Simultaneous measurement of serotonin and propranolol pulmonary extraction in patients after extracorporeal circulation and surgery. *Am Rev Respir Dis* 1985;131:242–245.
54. David G, Lories V, Henemans A, Van der Schveren B, Cassiman JJ, Van den Berge H. Membrane-associated chondroitin sulfate proteoglycans of human lung fibroblasts. *J Cell Biol* 1989;108: 1165–1173.
55. Davies P, Burke G, Reid L. The structure of the wall of the rat intraacinar pulmonary artery: an electron microscopic study of microdissected preparations. *Microvasc Res* 1986;32:50–63.
56. Davies P, Smith BT, Maddalo F, et al. Characteristics of lung pericytes in culture including their growth inhibition by endothelial substrate. *Microvasc Res* 1987;33:300–314.
57. Davis RL, Weintraub H, Lassar AB. Expression of a single transfected cDNA converts fibroblasts to myoblasts. *Cell* 1987;51: 987–1000.
58. Deffebech MF, Charan NB, Lakshminarayan S, Butler J. The bronchial circulation. *Am Rev Respir Dis* 1987;135:463–481.
59. Deffebech MF, Widdicombe J. The bronchial circulation. In: Crystal R, West J, Barnes P, Cherniack N, Weibel E, eds. *The lung: scientific foundations.* New York: Raven Press, 1991:741–757.
60. Depuit F, Jacquot J, Benali R, Kinnrasky J, Puchelle E. Apical and basolateral secretion of proteins by human tracheal gland cells cultured on a permeable substra. *Eur Respir J* 1990;3:958.
61. Devalia JL, Campbell AM, Sapsford RJ, et al. Effect of nitrogen dioxide on synthesis of inflammatory cytokines expressed by human bronchial epithelial cells *in vitro*. *Am J Respir Cell Mol Biol* 1993;9:271–278.
62. Devereux TR, Serabjit-Singh CCH, Slaughter SR, Wolf CR, Philpot RM, Fouts JR. Identification of cytochrome P450 lysozymes in nonciliated bronchiolar epithelial (Clara) and alveolar type II cells isolated from rabbit lung. *Exp Lung Res* 1981;2:221–230.
63. deWater R, Willems NA, van Muijen GNP, et al. Ultrastructural localization of bronchial antileukoprotease in central and peripheral human airways by a gold-labeling technique using monoclonal antibodies. *Am Rev Respir Dis* 1986;133:882–890.
64. Diaz A, Munoz E, Johnston R, Korn JH, Jimenez SA. Regulation of human lung fibroblast aI-procollagen gene expression by tumor necrosis factor-α, interleukin-1β and prostaglandin E2. *J Biol Chem* 1993;268:10364–10371.
65. Dobbs LG, Williams MC, Brandt AE. Changes in biochemical characteristics and pattern of lectin binding of alveolar type II cells with time in culture. *Biochim Biophys Acta* 1985;846:155–166.
66. Dodge AB, Hechtman HB, Shepro D. Microvascular endothelial-derived autocoids regulate pericyte contractility. *Cell Motil Cytoskeleton* 1991;18:180–188.
67. Dodge DE, Plopper CG, Rucker RB. Regulation of Clara cell 10 kD protein secretion by pilocarpine: quantitative comparison of nonciliated cells in rat bronchi and bronchioles based on laser scanning confocal microscopy. *Am J Respir Cell Mol Biol* 1994;10: 259–270.
68. Dormehl IC, Jacobs L, Maree M, Ras G, Hugo N, Beverley G. A baboon model for *in vivo* assessment of mucociliary lung clearance. *J Med Primatol* 1991;20:235–239.
69. Driscoll KE, Hassebein DG, Carter J, et al. Macrophage inflammatory proteins 1 and 2. *Am J Respir Cell Mol Biol* 1993;8:311–318.
70. Dubaybo BA, Thet LA. Effect of transferring growth factor on synthesis of glycosaminoglycans by human lung fibroblasts. *Exp Lung Res* 1990;16:389–403.
71. Durmowicz AG, Badesch DP, Parks WC, Mechan RP, Stenmark KR. Hypoxia-induced inhibition of tropoelastin synthesis by neonatal calf pulmonary artery smooth muscle cells. *Am J Respir Cell Mol Biol* 1991;5:464–469.
72. Elias JA, Freundlich B, Kern JA, Rosenbloom J. Cytokine networks in the regulation of inflammation and fibrosis in the lung. *Chest* 1990;97:1439–1445.
73. Elias JA, Reynolds MM. Interleukin-1 and tumor necrosis factor synergistically stimulate lung fibroblast interleukin-1α production. *Am J Respir Cell Mol Biol* 1990;3:13–20.
74. Ellefsen P, Tos M. Goblet cells in human trachea: Quantitative studies of a pathological biopsy material. *Arch Otolaryngol* 1972;95: 547–555.
75. Elliott FM, Reid L. Some new facts about the pulmonary artery and its branching pattern. *Clin Radiol* 1965;16:193–198.
76. Ennis M, Lorenz W, Gerland W, Heise J. Isolation of mast cells from rabbit lung and liver. Comparison of histamine release induced by the hypnotics althesin and propanidid. *Agents Actions* 1987;20:219–222.
77. Erle DJ, Pytela R. How do integrins integrate? The role of cell adhesion receptors in differentiation and development. *Am J Respir Cell Mol Biol* 1992;6:459–460.
78. Eskenasy M, Tasca SI. Culture of pericytes isolated from rat adipose microvasculature and characterization of their prostanoid production. *Cell Biol Int Rep* 1988;12:1055–1066.
79. Evans JM, Cabral LJ, Stephens RJ, Freeman G. Transformation of alveolar type 2 cells to type I cells following exposure to NO_2. *Exp Mol Pathol* 1975;22:142–150.
80. Evans MJ, Cox RA, Shami SG, Plopper CG. Junctional adhesion mechanisms in airway basal cells. *Am J Respir Cell Mol Biol* 1990;3: 341–347.
81. Evans MJ, Guha SC, Cox RA, Moller PC. Attenuated fibroblast sheath around the basement membrane zone in the trachea. *Am J Respir Cell Mol Biol* 1993;8:188–192.
82. Evans M, Shami S, Cabral-Anderson L, Dekker N. Role of nonciliated cells in the renewal of the bronchial epithelium of rats exposed to NO_2. *Am J Pathol* 1986;123:123–126.
83. Everett MM, King RJ, Jones MB, Martin HM. Lung fibroblasts from animals breathing 100% oxygen produce growth factors for type II alveolar cells. *Am J Physiol* 1990;259:L247–L254.
84. Fabisiak JP, Absher M, Evans JN, Kelley J. Spontaneous production of PDGF-A chain homodimer by rat lung fibroblasts *in vitro*. *Am J Physiol* 1992;263:L185–L193.
85. Faruqui RM, DiCorleto PE. Mechanisms of monocyte recruitment and accumulation. *Br Heart J* 1993;69:S19–S29.
86. Felch ME, Wellis RA, Penney OP, Keng PC, Phipps R. Expression

of 6-β-1 integrin, the laminin receptor, on subsets of normal lung fibroblasts and its upregulation by the inflammatory cytokine IFN-γ and TNF-α. *Reg Immunol* 1992;4:363–370.

87. Felley-Bosco E, Ambs S, Lowenstein CJ, Keefer LK, Harris CC. Constitutive expression of inducible nitric oxide synthase in human bronchial epithelial cells induces *c-fos* and stimulates the cGMP pathway. *Am J Respir Cell Mol Biol* 1994;11:159–164.
88. Finkbeiner WE, Carrier SD, Teresi CE. Reverse transcription-polymerase chain reaction (RT-PCR) phenotypic analysis of cell cultures of human tracheal epithelium, tracheobronchial glands, and lung carcinomas. *Am J Respir Cell Mol Biol* 1993;9: 547–556.
89. Floru S, Gelvar A, Moran R, Kadouri A, Cohen AM. Modulation of tissue plasminogen activator biosynthesis by phosphatidylinositol liposomes in human fetal lung fibroblasts. *Am J Hematol* 1991;36: 100–104.
90. Foster JA, Rich CB, Miller MF. Pulmonary fibroblasts: an *in vitro* model of emphysema. *J Biol Chem* 1990;265:15544–15549.
91. Frid MG, Moiseeva EP, Stenmark K. Multiple phenotypically distinct smooth muscle cell populations exist in the adult and developing bovine pulmonary arterial media *in vivo. Circ Res* 1994; 75:669–681.
92. Froh D, Gonzales LW, Ballard PL. Secretion of surfactant protein A and phosphatidylcholine from type II cells of human fetal lung. *Am J Respir Cell Mol Biol* 1993;8:556–561.
93. Furcht LT. Critical factors controlling angiogenesis: cell products, cell matrix and growth factors. *Lab Invest* 1986;55:505–509.
94. Gadeau AP, Campan M, Millet D, Candresse T, Desranges C. Osteopontin overexpression is associated with arterial smooth muscle proliferation *in vitro. Arterioscler Thromb Vasc Biol* 1993;13: 120–125.
95. Gehr P, Bachofen M, Weibel ER. The normal lung: ultrastructure and morphometric estimation of diffusion capacity. *Respir Physiol* 1978;32:121–140.
96. Ghuysen-Itard AF, Robert L, Jacob MP. Effect of elastin peptides on cell proliferation. *Comptes Redus Acad Sci* 1992;315:473–478.
97. Giachelli CM, Bae N, Almeida M, Denhardt DT, Alpers CE, Schwartz SM. Osteopontin is elevated during neointima formation in rat arteries and is a novel component of human atherosclerotic plaques. *J Clin Invest* 1993;92:1686–1696.
98. Giachelli CM, Bae N, Lombardi D, Majesky M, Schwartz S. Molecular cloning and characterization of 2B7, a rat mRNA which distinguishes smooth muscle cell phenotypes *in vitro* and is identical to osteopontin. *Biochem Biophys Res Commun* 1991;177:867–873.
99. Giaid A, Michel RP, Stewart DJ, Sheppard M, Corrin B, Hamid Q. Expression of endothelin-1 in lungs of patients with cryptogenic fibrosing alveolitis. *Lancet* 1993;341:1550–1554.
100. Giaid A, Polak JM, Gaitonde V, et al. Distribution of endothelin-like immunoreactivity and mRNA in the developing and adult human lung. *Am J Respir Cell Mol Biol* 1991;4:50–58.
101. Giaid A, Yanagisawa M, Langleben D, et al. Expression of endothelin-1 in the lungs of patients with pulmonary hypertension. *N Engl J Med* 1993;328:1732–1739.
102. Gibson KF, Widnell CC. The relationship between lamellar bodies and lysosomes in type II pneumocytes. *Am J Respir Cell Mol Biol* 1991;4:504–513.
103. Gillis CN, Catravas JD. Altered removal of vasoactive substances in the injured lung. *Ann NY Acad Sci* 1982;384:458–474.
104. Glukhava MA, Frid MG, Koteliansky VC. Developmental changes in expression of contractile and cytoskeletal proteins in human aortic smooth muscle. *J Biol Chem* 1990;265:13042–13046.
105. Godfrey RWA, Severs NJ, Jeffery PK. Freeze-fracture morphology and quantification of human bronchial epithelial tight junctions. *Am J Respir Cell Mol Biol* 1992;6:453–458.
106. Goldsmith KT, Gammon RB, Garver Jr RI. Modulation of bFGF in lung fibroblasts by TGFβ and PDGF. *Am J Physiol* 1991;261: L378–L385.
107. Goldstein RH, Fine A, Poliks C, Polgar P. Phorbol ester-induced inhibition of collagen accumulation by human lung fibroblasts. *J Biol Chem* 1990;265:13623–13628.
108. Goldstein RH, Paliks CF, Smith BD, Fine A. Stimulation of collagen formation by insulin and insulin-like growth factor I in cultures of human lung fibroblasts. *Endocrinology* 1989;124:964–970.
109. Gong J, McCarthy J, Telford T, Tamatani T, Miyasaka M, Schneeberger E. Intraepithelial airway dendritic cells: a distinct subset of pulmonary dendritic cells obtained by microdissection. *J Exp Med* 1992;175:797–807.
110. Gum JR. Mucin genes and the proteins they encode: structure, diversity, and regulation. *Am J Respir Cell Mol Biol* 1992;7:557–564.
111. Hamid Q, Springall DR, Riveros-Moreno V, et al. Induction of nitric oxide synthase in asthma. *Lancet* 1993;1510–1513.
112. Hampson F, Manick M, Peterson MW, Hunnighake GW. Immune mediators increase adherence of T-lymphocytes to human lung fibroblasts. *Am J Physiol* 1989;256:C336–C340.
113. Han VK, Hill DJ, Strain AJ, et al. Identification of somatomedin/insulin-like growth factor immunoreactive cells in the human fetus. *Pediatr Res* 1987;22:245–249.
114. Hassoun PM, Fanberg BL, Junod AF. Endothelium: metabolic functions. In: Crystal R, West J, Barnes P, Cherniack N, Weibel E, eds. *The lung: scientific foundations.* New York: Raven Press, 1991; 313–327.
115. Hathaway DR, March KL, Cash JA, Adam LP, Wilensky RL. Vascular smooth muscle. A review of the molecular basis of contractility. *Circulation* 1991;83:382–390.
116. Haven CA, Olson JW, Arcott SS, Gillespie MN. Polyamine transport and ornithine decarboxylase activity in hypoxic pulmonary artery smooth muscle cells. *Am J Respir Cell Molec Biol* 1992;7: 286–292.
117. Hayes JA, Christensen TG, Gaensler EA. Myointimal plaques in pulmonary vascular sclerosis associated with interstitial lung fibrosis. *Lab Invest* 1979;41:268–274.
118. Hede AR. Halothane decreases uptake of noradrenaline in sliced rat lungs. *Pharmacol Toxicol* 1988;63:141–142.
119. Hede AR, Berglund BD, Post C. Trichloroethylene and halothane inhibit uptake and metabolism of 5-hydroxytryptamine in rat lung slices. *Pharmacol Toxicol* 1987;61:191–194.
120. Heremans A, De Cock B, Cassiman JJ, Vanden Berghe H, David G. The core protein of the matrix-associated heparin-sulfate proteoglycan binds to fibronectin. *J Biol Chem* 1990;265:8716–8724.
121. Herman IM, DíAmore PA. Microvascular pericytes contain muscle and non-muscle actins. *J Cell Biol* 1985;101:43–52.
122. Herman IM, Divaris N, Healy AM, Hoock TC. Regulation of pericyte growth and contractile phenotype by endothelial matrix and its associated growth factors. *J Cell Biol* 1991;115:443a.
123. Heys SD, Norton AC, Dundas CR, Erenum O, Ferguson K, Garlick PJ. Anesthetic agents and their effect on tissue protein synthesis in the rat. *Clin Sci* 1989;77:651–655.
124. Hijiya K, Okada K. Scanning electron microscope study casts of the pulmonary capillary vessels in rats. *J Electron Microsc (Tokyo)* 1978;27:49–53.
125. Hijiya K, Okada Y, Tankawa H. Ultrastructural study of the alveolar brush cell. *J Electron Microsc (Tokyo)* 1977;26:321–329.
126. Hill RB. Pathobiology and disease. In: Hill R, LaVia M, eds. *Principles of pathobiology.* New York: Oxford University Press, 1980:3–19.
127. Hislop A, Reid L. Fetal and childhood development of the intrapulmonary veins in man: branching pattern and structure. *Thorax* 1973;28:313–319.
128. Hislop AA, Wharton J, Allen KM, Polak JM, Haworth SG. Immunohistochemical localization of peptide-containing nerves in human airways: age-related changes. *Am J Respir Cell Mol Biol* 1990;3:191–198.
129. Horowitz S, Watkins RH, Auten RL, Mercier CE, Cheng ERY. Differential accumulation of surfactant protein A, B, and C mRNAs in two epithelial cell types of hyperoxic lung. *Am J Respir Cell Mol Biol* 1991;5:511–515.
130. Horwitz AF, Duggan K, Buck C, Beckerle MC, Burridge K. Interaction of plasma membrane fibronectin receptor with talinóa transmembrane linkage. *Nature* 1986;320:531–533.
131. Idell S, Zweib C, Boggaram J, Holiday D, Johnson AR, Raghu X. Mechanisms of fibrin formation and lysis by human lung fibroblasts. *Am J Physiol* 1992;263:L487–L494.
132. Ikeda T, Shirasawa T, Esaki Y, Yoshiki S, Hirokawa K. Osteopontin mRNA is expressed by smooth muscle-derived foam cells in human atherosclerotic lesions of the aorta. *J Clin Invest* 1993;92: 2814–2820.
133. Infield MD, Brennan JA, Davis PB. Human tracheobronchial epithelial cells direct migration of lung fibroblasts in three dimensional collagen gels. *Am J Physiol* 1992;262:L535–L541.
134. Ingber DE, Dike L, Hansen L, et al. Cellular tensegrity: exploring how mechanical changes in the cytoskeleton regulate cell growth, migration, and tissue pattern during morphogenesis. *Int Rev Cytol* 1994;150:173–224.
135. Inoue H, Massion PP, Ueki IF, et al. *Pseudomonas* stimulates interleukin-8 mRNA expression selectively in airway epithelium, in

gland ducts, and in recruited neutrophils. *Am J Respir Cell Mol Biol* 1994;11:651–663.

136. Ishiyana I, Mukaida M, Tanabe R, Kaiho M, Veyama M. Histochemical demonstration of phenobarbital by immunohistochemistry. *J Forensic Sci* 1987;32:1221–1234.
137. Jamal A, Bendeck M, Langille BL. Structural changes and recovery of function after arterial injury. *Arterioscler Thromb Vasc Biol* 1992;12:307–317.
138. Jeffery PK. Morphologic features of airway surface epithelial cells and glands. *Am Rev Respir Dis* 1983;128:S14–S20.
139. Jeffery PK, Reid L. New observations of rat airway epithelium: a quantitative and electron microscopy study. *J Anat* 1975;120: 295–320.
140. Jeffery PK, Reid L. The effect of tobacco smoke, with or without phenylmethyl-oxidiazole (PMO), on rat bronchial epithelium: a light and electron microscopic study. *J Pathol* 1981;133:341–359.
141. Jeffery PK, Widdicombe JG, Reid L. Anatomical and physiological features of irritation of the bronchial tree. In: Aharonson E, David A, Klinberg M, eds. *Air pollution and the lung*. New York: John Wiley, 1976:253–267.
142. Johnson NF, Hubbs AF. Epithelial progenitor cells in the rat trachea. *Am J Respir Cell Mol Biol* 1990;3:579–585.
143. Jones R. Ultrastructural analysis of contractile cell development in lung microvessels in hyperoxic pulmonary hypertension: fibroblasts and intermediate cells selectively reorganize nonmuscular segments. *Am J Pathol* 1992;141:1491–1505.
144. Jones R. Role of interstitial fibroblasts and intermediate cells in microvascular wall remodelling in pulmonary hypertension. *Eur Respir Rev* 1993;3:569–575.
145. Jones R, Rock K, Fujiwara K. Development of contractile cells in pulmonary hypertension (PH) differential expression of smooth muscle myosin by precursor cells. *Am J Respir Crit Care Med* 1994; 149:A824.
146. Jorens PG, Van Overfeld FJ, Vermeire PA, Bult H, Herman AG. Synergism between interleukin-1β and interferon gamma, an inducer of nitric oxide synthase in rat lung fibroblasts. *Eur J Pharmacol* 1992;224:7–12.
147. Joyce NC, De Camilli P, Boyles J. Pericytes, like vascular smooth muscle cells, are immunocytochemically positive for cyclic GMP dependent protein kinase. *Microvasc Res* 1984;28:206–219.
148. Joyce NC, Haire MF, Palade GE. (a) Contractile proteins in pericytes I. *J Cell Biol* 1985;100:1379–1386.
149. Joyce NC, Haire MF, Palade GE. (b) Contractile proteins in pericytes II. *J Cell Biol* 1985;100:1387–1395.
150. Joyce-Brady MF, Brody JS. Ontogeny of pulmonary alveolar epithelial makers of differentiation. *Dev Biol* 1990;137:331–348.
151. Kapanci Y, Assimocopoulos A, Zwahlen A, Gabbiani G. "Contractile interstitial cells" in pulmonary alveolar septae: a possible regulator or ventilation/perfusion ratio? *J Cell Biol* 1974;60:375–392.
152. Kapanci Y, Ribaux C, Chapponier C, Gabbiani G. Cytoskeletal features of alveolar myofibroblasts and pericytes in normal human and rat lung. *J Histochem Cytochem* 1991;40:1955–1963.
153. Karlinsky JB, Goldstein RH. Regulation of sulfated glycosaminoglycan production by prostaglandin E2 in cultured lung fibroblasts. *J Lab Clin Med* 1989;114:176–184.
154. Kato H, Suzuki H, Tajima S, et al. Angiotensin II stimulates collagen synthesis in cultured vascular smooth muscle cells. *J Hypertens* 1991;9:17–22.
155. Katz J, Leiman BC, Butler BD. Effects of inhalation anesthetics on filtration of venous gas emboli by the pulmonary vasculature. *Br J Anesth* 1988;61:200–205.
156. Kaushansky K, Lin N, Adamson JW. Interleukin-1 stimulates fibroblasts to synthesize granulocyte-macrophage and granulocyte colony-stimulating factors. *J Clin Invest* 1988;81:92–97.
157. Kawanami O, Ferrans VJ, Crystal RG. Anchoring fibrils in the normal canine respiratory system. *Am Rev Respir Dis* 1979;120:595–611.
158. Kelley C, D'Amore P, Hechtman HB, Shepro D. Vasoactive hormones and cAMP affect pericyte contraction and stress fibers *in vitro*. *J Muscle Res Cell Motil* 1988;9:184–194.
159. Kelley C, D'Amore PA, Hechtman HB, Shepro D. Microvascular pericyte contractility *in vitro*: comparison with other cells of the vascular wall. *J Cell Biol* 1987;104:483–490.
160. Kelley J, Fabisiak JP, Hawes K, Absher M. Cytokine signalling in lung. *Am J Physiol* 1991;260:L123–L128.
161. Kelley J, Shull S, Walsh JJ, Cutreno KR, Absher M. Autoinduction of transforming growth factor β in human lung fibroblasts. *Am J Respir Mol Biol* 1993;8:417–424.
162. Kerem B-T, Rommens JM, Buchanan JA. Identification of the cystic fibrosis gene: genetic analysis. *Science* 1989;245:1073–1080.
163. Khalil N, Bereznay O, Sporn M, Greenberg AH. Macrophage production of transforming growth factor and fibroblast collagen synthesis in chronic pulmonary inflammation. *J Exp Med* 1989;170: 727–737.
164. Khalil N, OíConnor RN, Unruh HW, et al. Increased production and immunohistochemical localization of transforming growth factor-β in idiopathic pulmonary fribrosis. *Am J Respir Cell Mol Biol* 1991;5:155–162.
165. Khosla J, Correa MT, Sannes PL. Heterogeneity of sulfated microdomains within basement membranes of pulmonary airway epithelium. *Am J Respir Cell Mol Biol* 1994;10:462–469.
166. Khoury J, Langleben D. Platelet-activating factor stimulates lung pericyte growth in-vitro. *FASEB J* 1994;8:A148.
167. Kim KC, Zheng Q, Van-Seuningen I. Involvement of a signal transduction mechanism in ATP-induced mucin release from cultured airway goblet cells. *Am J Respir Cell Mol Biol* 1993;8:121–125.
168. Kobzik L, Bredt S, Lowenstein CJ, et al. Nitric oxide synthase in human and rat lung: immunocytochemical and histochemical localization. *Am J Respir Cell Mol Biol* 1993;9:371–377.
169. Kocher O, Skalli O, Cerutti D, Gabbiani F, Gabbiani G. Cytoskeletal features of rat aortic cells during development. An electron microscopic, immunohistochemical and biochemical study. *Circ Res* 1985;56:829–838.
170. Kochi T, Hagiya M, Mizuguchi T. Effects of enflurane on contractile response of canine trachealis muscle. *Anesth Analg* 1989;69: 60–68.
171. Kondo MJ, Tamaoki J, Takizawa T. Neutral endopeptidase inhibitor potentiates the tachykinin-induced increase in ciliary beat frequency in rabbit trachea. *Am Rev Respir Dis* 1990;142:403–406.
172. Konrad F, Schreiber T, Grunert A, Clausen M, Ahnfeld FW. Measurement of mucociliary transport velocity in ventilated patients. Short-term effect of general anesthesia on mucociliary transport. *Chest* 1992;102:1377–1383.
173. Kramps JA, Franken C, Meijer LM, Dijkman JH. Localization of low molecular weight protease inhibitor in serous secretory cells of the respiratory tract. *J Histochem Cytochem* 1981;29:712–719.
174. Kuhn C, Boldt J, King TE, Crouch E, Vartio T, McDonald JA. An immunohistochemical study of architectural remodelling and connective tissue synthesis in pulmonary fibrosis. *Am Rev Respir Dis* 1989;40:1693–1703.
175. Kuhn C, McDonald JA. The roles of the myofibroblast in idiopathic pulmonary fibrosis. *Am J Pathol* 1991;138:1257–1265.
176. Kulik TJ, Bialecki RA, Colucci WS, Rothman A, Glennon ET, Underwood RH. Stretch increase insoitol triphosphate and inositol tetrakisphosphate in cultured pulmonary vascular smooth muscle cells. *Biochem Biophys Res Commun* 1991;180:982–987.
177. Kwon OI, Au BT, Collins PD, et al. Tumor necrosis factor-induced interleukin-8 expression in cultured human airway epithelial cells. *Am J Physiol* 1994;267:398–405.
178. Lamb D, Reid L. Mitotic rates, goblet cell increase and histochemical changes in mucus in rat bronchial epithelium during exposure to SO_2. *J Pathol Bacteriol* 1968;96:97–111.
179. Lamb D, Reid L. Histochemical types of acidic glycoprotein produced by mucous cells of the tracheobronchial glands in man. *J Pathol* 1969;98:213–229.
180. Lamb D, Reid L. Goblet cell increase in rat bronchial epithelium after exposure to cigarette and cigar tobacco smoke. *Br Med J* 1969;1:33–35.
181. Lamb D, Reid L. Histochemical and autoradiographic investigation of the serous cells of the human bronchial gland. *J Pathol* 1970;100:127–138.
182. Lamb D, Reid L. Quantitative distribution of various types of acid glycoprotein in mucous cells of human bronchi. *Histochem J* 1972;4:91–102.
183. Langleben D, Benitz W, Serban L, Spilman S. Low dose pulmonary endothelial heparan sulfate inhibits lung pericyte growth *in vitro*. *Am Rev Respir Dis* 1992;145:A479.
184. Langleben D, DeMarchie M, Laporta D, Spanier AH, Schlesinger R, Stewart DJ. Endothelin-1 in acute lung injury and the adult respiratory distress syndrome. *Am Rev Respir Dis* 1993;148:1646–1650.
185. Langleben D, Khoury J, Hirsch A. Endotoxin stimulates growth of lung pericytes *in vitro*, but IL-1β does not. *FASEB J* 1993;7:A267.
186. Langleben D, Perlin AS, DeHeuvel E. Effects of sulfated glycosaminoglycans on proliferation of rat lung pericytes *in vitro*. *FASEB J* 1989;3:A1161.

187. Larivee P, Levine SJ, Martinez A, Wu T, Logun C, Shelhamer JH. Platelet-activating factor induces airway mucin release via activation of protein kinase C: evidence for translocation of protein kinase C to membranes. *Am J Respir Cell Mol Biol* 1994;11: 199–205.
188. Larson DM, Carson MP, Haudenschild CC. Junctional transfer of small molecules in cultured bovine brain microvascular endothelial cells and pericytes. *Microvasc Res* 1987;34:184–199.
189. Laurent GJ. Lung collagen: more than scaffolding. *Thorax* 1986; 41:418–428.
190. Lauric G, Bing J, Kleinman H, Hassell J. Localization of binding sites for laminin heparan sulfate proteoglycans and fibronectin on basement membrane (type IV collagen). *J Mol Biol* 1986;189: 205–216.
191. Leikhauf GD, Ueki IF, Nadel JA. Autonomic regulation of visoelasticity of cat tracheal glands secretion. *J Appl Physiol* 1984;56: 426–430.
192. Lemire JM, Covin CW, White S, Giachelli CM, Schwartz SM. Characterization of cloned aortic smooth muscle cells from young rats. *Am J Pathol* 1994;144:1068–1081.
193. Leslie CC, McCormick-Shannon K, Mason RJ. Heparin-binding growth factors stimulate DNA synthesis in rat alveolar type II cells. *Am J Respir Cell Mol Biol* 1990;2:99–106.
194. Leslie CC, McCormick-Shannon K, Mason RJ, Shannon JM. Proliferation of rat alveolar epithelial cells in low density primary culture. *Am J Respir Cell Mol Biol* 1993;9:64–72.
195. Lethem MI, Dowell ML, Van Scott M, et al. Nucleotide regulation of goblet cells in human airway epithelial explants: normal exocytosis in cystic fibrosis. *Am J Respir Cell Mol Biol* 1993;9:315–322.
196. Li W, Kumar RK, OíGrady R, Velan GM. Role of lymphocytes in silicoses. *Int J Exp Pathol* 1992;73:793–800.
197. Liaw L, Almeida M, Hart CE, Schwartz SM, Giachelli CM. Osteopontin promotes vascular adhesion and spreading and is chemotactic for smooth muscle cells *in vitro*. *Circ Res* 1994;74:214–224.
198. Lipke D, Arcot S, Gillespie M, Olson J. Temporal alteratons in specific basement membrane components in lungs from monocrotaline-treated rats. *Am J Respir Cell Mol Biol* 1993;9:418–428.
199. Lories V, Cassiman JJ, Vanden Berghe H, David G. Differential expression of cell surface heparin sulfate proteoglycan in human mammary epithelial cells and lung fibroblasts. *J Biol Chem* 1992; 267:1116–1122.
200. Luciano L, Reale E, Rusta H. Chemoreceptive sinneszelle in der trachen der ratte. *Anat Mikrosk Anat* 1968;85:350–375.
201. Madden JA, Vadula MS, Durup VP. Effect of hypoxia and other vasoactive agents on pulmonary and cerebral artery smooth muscle cells. *Am J Physiol* 1992;263:L384–L393.
202. Malek AM, Izumo S. Molecular aspects of signal transduction of shear stress in the endothelial cell. *J Hypertens* 1994;12:989–999.
203. Malmqvist V, Arner A, Uvelius B. Contractile and cytoskeletal proteins in smooth muscle during hypertrophy and its reversal. *Am J Physiol* 1991;260:C1085–C1093.
204. Marciniak SJ, Plumpton C, Barker PJ, Huskisson NS, Davenport AP. Localization of immunoreactive endothelin and proendothelin in the human lung. *Pulm Pharmacol* 1992;5:175–182.
205. Marin MG. Pharmacology of airway secretion. *Pharmacol Rev* 1986; 38:273–289.
206. Marini M, Soloperto M, Mezzetti M, Fasoli A, Mattoli S. Interleukin-1 binds to specific receptors on human bronchial epithelial cells and upregulates granulocyte/macrophage colony-stimulating factor synthesis and release. *Am J Respir Cell Mol Biol* 1991; 4:519–524.
207. Martin DC, Carr AM, Livingston RR, Watkins CA. Effects of Kenature and Fantaryl on lung metabolism in perfused rat lungs. *Am J Physiol* 1989;257:E379–E384.
208. Martin DC, Carr AM, Watkins CA. Metabolic effects of isoflurane on rat lungs perfused *in situ*. *Gen Pharmacol* 1990;21:477–481.
209. Martin G, Temple R. Laminin and other basement membrane components. *Annu Rev Cell Biol* 1987;3:57–85.
210. Mason RJ, Williams MC. Alveolar type II cells. In: Crystal R, West J, Barnes P, Cherniack N, Weibel E, eds. *The lung: scientific foundations.* New York: Raven Press, 1991:235–246.
211. Mattioli S, Miante S, Calabro F, Mezzetti M, Allegra L. Human bronchial epithelial cells exposed to isocyanates potentiate the activation and proliferation of T cells induced by antigen receptor triggering through the release of IL1 and IL6. In: Johansson S, ed. *Cellular communication in allergic asthma. Pharmacia Allergy Foundation 1990 award book.* Uppsala: AW Grafiska, 1990:25–35.
212. Mattioli S, Miante S, Calabro F, Mezzetti M, Fasoli A, Allegra L. Bronchial epithelial cells exposed to isocyanates potentiate activation and proliferation of T cells. *Am J Physiol* 1990;259: L320–L327.
213. Mattoli S, Mezzetti M, Riva G, Allegra L, Fasoli A. Specific binding of endothelin on human bronchial smooth muscle cells in culture and secretion of endothelin-like material from bronchial epithelial cells. *Am J Respir Cell Mol Biol* 1990;3:145–151.
214. McDonald JA. Matrix regulation of cell shape and gene expression. *Curr Opin Cell Biol* 1989;1:995–999.
215. McDowell EM, Kennan KP, Huang M. Effects of vitamin A–deprivation on hamster tracheal epithelium. *Virchows Arch* 1984;45: 197–219.
216. McGowan SE. Extracellular matrix and the regulation of lung development and repair. *FASEB J* 1992;6:2895–2904.
217. McGowan SE, Liv R, Harvey CS. Effects of heparin and other glycosaminoglycans on elastin production by cultured neonatal rat lung fibroblasts. *Arch Biochem Biophys* 1993;302:322–331.
218. McGowan SE, McNamer R. Transforming growth factor-increases elastin production by neonatal rat lung fibroblasts. *Am J Respir Cell Molec Biol* 1990;3:369–376.
219. McGuiffe LJ, Mercure J, Little SA. Three dimensional structure of dense bodies in rabbit renal artery smooth muscle. *Anat Rec* 1991; 229:499–504.
220. McLaughlin RJ Jr . Bronchial artery distribution in various mammals and in humans. *Am Rev Respir Dis* 1983;S128:S57–S58.
221. Mercer RR, Russell ML, Roggli VL, Crapo JD. Cell number and distribution in human and rat airways. *Am J Respir Cell Mol Biol* 1994;10:613–624.
222. Merrilees MJ, Flint M. The effect of centrifugal force on glycosaminoglycan production by aortic smooth muscle cells in culture. *Atherosclerosis* 1977;27:259–264.
223. Merten MD, Tournier J-M, Meckler Y, Figarella C. Secretory proteins and glycoconjugates synthesized by human tracheal gland cells in culture. *Am J Respir Cell Mol Biol* 1992;7:598–605.
224. Merten MD, Tournier J-M, Meckler Y, Figarella C. Epinephrine promotes growth and differentiation of human tracheal gland cells in culture. *Am J Respir Cell Mol Biol* 1993;9:172–178.
225. Mette SA, Pilewski J, Buck CA, Albelda SM. Distribution of integrin cell adhesion receptors on normal bronchial epithelial cells and lung cancer cells *in vitro* and *in vivo*. *Am J Respir Cell Mol Biol* 1993;8:562–572.
226. Meyrick B. *Ultrastructural features of normal rat pulmonary artery and effect of a low barometric pressure.* London: University of London, 1976.
227. Meyrick B, Fujiwara K, Reid L. Smooth muscle myosin in precursor and mature smooth muscle cells in normal pulmonary arteries and the effect of hypoxia. *Exp Lung Res* 1981;1:303–313.
228. Meyrick B, Reid L. The alveolar brush cell in rat lung—a third pneumonocyte. *J Ultrastructural Res* 1968;23:71–80.
229. Meyrick B, Reid L. Ultrastructure of cells in human bronchial submucosal glands. *J Anat* 1974;107:281–299.
230. Meyrick B, Reid L. The effect of continued hypoxia on rat pulmonary arterial circulation. *Lab Invest* 1978;38:188–200.
231. Meyrick B, Reid L. Ultrastructural features of the distended pulmonary arteries of the normal rat. *Anat Rec* 1979;193:71–97.
232. Meyrick B, Sturgess J, Reid L. A reconstruction of the duct system and secretory tubules of the human bronchial submucosal gland. *Thorax* 1969;24:729–736.
233. Miner JH, Wold BJ. C-myc inhibition of MyoD and Myogenin-initiated myogenic differentiation. *Mol Cell Biol* 1991;11:2842–2851.
234. Mitchell J, Woodcock-Mitchell J, Reynolds S, et al. α-Smooth muscle actin in parenchymal cells of bleomycin-injured rat lung. *Lab Invest* 1989;60:643–650.
235. Modig J, Hallgren R. Increased hyaluronic acid production in lung. *Resuscitation* 1989;17:223–231.
236. Muller WA, Weigl SA, Deng X, Phillips DM. PECAM-1 is required for transendothelial migration of leukocytes. *J Exp Med* 1993;178: 449–460.
237. Murray TR, Chen L, Marshall BE, Macarak EJ. Hypoxic contraction of cultured pulmonary vascular smooth muscle cells. *Am J Respir Cell Mol Biol* 1990;3:457–465.
238. Murray TR, Marshall BE, Macarak EJ. Contraction of vascular smooth muscle in cell culture. *J Cell Physiol* 1990;143:26–38.
239. Nadel JA, Davis B, Phipps RJ. Control of mucus secretion and ion transport in airways. *Annu Rev Physiol* 1979;41:369–381.
240. Nathan C, Sporn N. Cytokines in context. *J Cell Biol* 1991;113: 981–986.

241. Nichols WK, Covington MO, Seiders CD, Sofiullah S, Yost GS. Bioactivation of halogeninated hydrocarbons by rabbit pulmonary cells. *Pharmacol Toxicol* 1992;71:335–339.
242. Noguchi A, Firsching K, Kursar JD, Reddy R. Developmental changes of tropoelastin synthesis by rat pulmonary fibroblasts and effects of dexamethasone. *Pediatr Res* 1990;28:379–382.
243. Noguchi A, Nelson T. IGF-1 stimulates tropoelastin synthesis in neonatal rat pulmonary fibroblasts. *Pediatr Res* 1991;30:248–251.
244. Odun J, Foster JR, Green T. A mechanism for development of Clara cell lesions in the mouse lung after exposure to tricholoroethylene. *Chem Biol Interact* 1992;83:135–153.
245. Ohtoshi T, Vancheri C, Cox G, et al. Monocyte-macrophage differentiation induced by human upper airway epithelial cells. *Am J Respir Cell Mol Biol* 1991;4:255–263.
246. Orfanos SE, Catravas JD. Metabolic functions of the pulmonary circulation. In: Yacoub M, Pepper J, eds. *Annu Rev Cardiac Surg* London: Current Science, 1993:52–59.
247. Orlidge A, D'Amore PA. Cell specific effects of glycosaminoglycans on the attachment and proliferation of vascular wall components. *Microvasc Res* 1986;31:41–53.
248. Pardo A, Silman K. Decreased collagenase production by fibroblasts derived from idiopathic pulmonary fibrosis. *Matrix* 1992;S1: 417–418.
249. Parent-Ermini A, Ben-Harari RR. Effect of volatile anesthetics on endogenous tryptophan, 5-hydroxytryptophan and 5-hydroxytryptamine in rat lung. *Lung* 1990;168:259–266.
250. Paterson JL, Sapsed-Byrne SM, Hall GM. Effects of enflurane and halothane on carbohydrate metabolism in isolated perfused rat lungs. *Br J Anesth* 1986;58:1156–1160.
251. Peacock AJ, Dawes KZE, Shock A, Gray AJ, Reeves JT, Laurent GJ. Endothelin-1 and endothelin 3 induce chemotaxis and replication of pulmonary artery fibroblasts. *Am J Respir Cell Mol Biol* 1992;7:492–499.
252. Pelton RW, Johnson MD, Perkett EA, Gold LI, Moses HL. Expression of transforming growth factor-β1, -β2, and -β3 mRNA and protein in the murine lung. *Am J Respir Cell Mol Biol* 1991;5: 522–530.
253. Plopper CG, Hyde DM, Buckpitt AR, et al., eds. *The lung: scientific foundations.* New York: Raven Press, 1991:215–228.
254. Power JHT, Barr HA, Nicholar TE. Characterization and immunohistochemical localization of the 15kd protein isolated from rat lung lamellar bodies. *Am J Respir Cell Mol Biol* 1993;8:98–105.
255. Punjabi CJ, Laskin JD, Pendino KJ, Goller NL, Durham SK, Laskin DL. Production of nitric oxide by rat type II pneumocytes: increased expression of inducible nitric oxide synthase following inhalation of a pulmonary irritant. *Am J Respir Cell Mol Biol* 1994;11: 165–172.
256. Purchelle EJ, Hinnrasky J, Tournier JM, Adnet JJ. Ultrastructural localization of bronchial inhibitor in human airways using protein A-gold technique. *Biol Cell* 1985;55:151–154.
257. Raaberg L, Poulsen SS, Nexo E. Epidermal growth factor in the rat lung. *Histochemistry* 1991;95:471–475.
258. Rabinovitch M, Bothwell T, Hayakawa BN, et al. Pulmonary artery endothelial abnormalities in patients with congenital heart defects and pulmonary hypertension. *Lab Invest* 1986;55:632–653.
259. Raghu G, Masta S, Meyers D, Narayanan AS. Collagen synthesis by normal and fibrotic human lung fibroblasts and the effect of transforming growth factor. *Am Rev Respir Dis* 1989;140:95–100.
260. Randell SH, Shimizu T, Bakerwell W, Ramaekers FCS, Nettescheim P. Phenotypic marker expression during fetal and neonatal differentiation of rat tracheal epithelial cells. *Am J Respir Cell Mol Biol* 1993;8:546–555.
261. Rannels SR, Yarnell JA, Fisher CS, Fabisiak JP, Rennels E. Role of laminin in maintenance of type II pneumocyte morphology and function. *Am J Physiol* 1987;253:C835–C845.
262. Reid L. Pathology of chronic bronchitis. *Lancet* 1954;1:275–279.
263. Reid L. Chronic bronchitis and hypersecretion of mucus. In: *Lectures on the scientific basis of medicine.* London: University Press, 1959::235–255.
264. Reid L. Measurement of the bronchial mucus gland layer: a diagnostic yardstick in chronic bronchitis. *Thorax* 1960;15:132–141.
265. Reid L. Bronchial mucus production in health and disease. In: *International Academy of Pathology monograph no. 8. The lung.* Baltimore: Williams & Wilkins, 1967:87–108.
266. Reid L. Structural and functional reappraisal of the pulmonary artery system. In: *Scientific basis of medicine, annual review.* London: Atholone Press, 1968:289–307.
267. Reid L and Jones R. Experimental chronic bronchitis. *Int Rev Exp Pathol* 1983;335–382.
268. Reilley TM, Whitfield MD, Taylor DS, Timmermans PB. Binding of tissue plasminogen activator to cultured human fibroblasts. *Thromb Haemost* 1989;61:454–458.
269. Retsch-Bogart GZ, Stiles AD, Moats-Staats BM, Van Scott MR, Boucher RC, D'Ercole AJ. Canine tracheal epithelial cells express the type 1 insulin-like growth factor receptor and proliferate in response to insulin-like growth factor I. *Am J Respir Cell Mol Biol* 1990;3:227–234.
270. Rhodes SJ, Konieczny SF. Identification of MRF4: a new member of the muscle regulatory factor gene family. *Genes Dev* 1989;3: 2050–2061.
271. Rich DP, Anderson MP, Gregory RJ, et al. Expression of cystic fibrosis transmembrane conductance regulator corrects defective chloride channel regulation in cystic fibrosis airway epithelial cells. *Nature* 1990;347:358–363.
272. Rich CB, Ewton DZ, Martin MB, et al. IGF-1 regulation of elastogenesis. *Am J Physiol* 1992;263:L276–L282.
273. Rickard KA, Taylor J, Rennard SI, Spurzem JR. Migration of bovine bronchial epithelial cells to extracellular matrix components. *Am J Respir Cell Mol Biol* 1993;8:63–68.
274. Robbins RA, Barnes PJ, Springall DR, et al. Expression of inducible nitric oxide in human lung epithelial cells. *Biochem Biophys Res Commun* 1994;209–218.
275. Roerig DL, Kotrly KJ, Dawson CA, Ahlf SB, Gualtieri JF, Kampine JD. First-pass uptake of verapamil, diltiazem and thiopental in the human lung. *Anesth Analg* 1989;69:461–466.
276. Rolfe MW, Kunkel SL, Standiford TJ, et al. Pulmonary fibroblast expression of interleukin-8. *Am J Respir Cell Mol Biol* 1991;5: 493–501.
277. Rolfe MW, Kunkel SL, Standiford TJ, et al. Expression and regulation of human pulmonary fibroblast-derived monocyte chemotactic peptide-1. *Am J Physiol* 1992;263:L536–L545.
278. Roman J, McDonald JA. Fibulinís organization into the extracellular matrix of fetal lung fibroblasts is dependent on fibronectin matrix assembly. *Am J Respir Cell Mol Biol* 1993;8:538–545.
279. Rorie DK, Tyce GM, Sill JC. Increased norepinephrine release from dog pulmonary artery caused by nitrous oxide. *Anesth Analg* 1986;65:560–564.
280. Rosenfeld MA, Siegfried W, Yoshimura K. Adenovirus-mediated transfer of a recombinant a1-antitrypsin gene to the lung epithelium *in vivo. Science* 1991;252:431–434.
281. Rossi GA, Sacco O, Balbi B, et al. Human ciliated bronchial epithelial cells: expression of the HLA-DR antigens by gamma-interferon and antigen-presenting function in the mixed leukocyte reaction. *Am J Respir Cell Mol Biol* 1990;3:431–439.
282. Rothman BL, Merrow M, Despins A, Kennedy T, Kreutzer KL. Effect of lipopolysaccharide on C3 and C5 production by human lung cells. *J Immunol* 1989;143:196–202.
283. Sallenave J, Shulmann J, Crossley J, Jordana M, Gauldie J. Regulation of secretory leukocyte proteinase inhibitor (SLPI) and elastase-specific inhibitor (ESI/elafin) in human airway epithelial cells by cytokines and neutrophilic enzymes. *Am J Respir Cell Mol Biol* 1994;11:733–741.
284. Sallenave J, Silva A, Marsden ME, Ryle AP. Secretion of mucus proteinase inhibitor and elafin by clara cell and type II pneumocyte cell lines. *Am J Respir Cell Mol Biol* 1993;8:126–133.
285. Salvaterra CG, Goldman WF. Acute hypoxia increases cytosolic calium in cultured pulmonary artery myocytes. *Am J Physiol* 1993;264: L323–L328.
286. Samet JM, Noah TL, Devlin RB, et al. Effect of ozone on platelet-activating factor production in phorbol-differentiated HL60 cells, a human bronchial epithelial cell line (BEAS S6), and primary human bronchial epithelial cells. *Am J Respir Cell Mol Biol* 1992;7: 514–522.
287. Sampson PM, Rochester CL, Freundlich B, Elias J. Cytokine regulation of human lung fibroblast hyaluronan production. *J Clin Invest* 1992;90:1492–1503.
288. Sanghavi JN, Rabe KF, Kim JS, Magnussen H, Leff AR, White SR. Migration of human and guinea pig airway epithelial cells in response to calcitonin gene-related peptide. *Am J Respir Cell Mol Biol* 1994;11:181–187.
289. Sannes PL. Differences in basement membranes associated microdomains of type I and type II pneumocytes in the rat and rabbit lung. *J Histochem Cytochem* 1984;32:827–833.
290. Sannes PL, Burch KK, Khosla J, McCarthy KJ, Couchman JR.

Immunohistochemical localization of chondroitin sulfate, chondroitin sulfate proteoglycan, heparan sulfate proteoglycan, entactin, and laminin in basement membranes of postnatal developing and adult rat lungs. *Am J Respir Cell Mol Biol* 1993;8:245–251.

291. Sappino AP, Schurch W, Gabbiani G. Differentiation of fibroblastic cells: expression of cytoskeletal proteins as a marker of phenotypic modulation. *Lab Invest* 1990;63:144–161.
292. Sartore S, DeMarzo N, Borrione AC, et al. Myosin heavy chain isoforms in human smooth muscle. *Eur J Biochem* 1989;179:79–85.
293. Sato Y, Tsuboi R, Lyons R, Moses H, Rifkin DB. Characterization of latent TGF-β by co-cultures of endothelial cells and pericytes or smooth muscle cells. *J Cell Biol* 1990;111:757–763.
294. Scheuermann DW, Adriaensen D, Timmermans JP, De Groodt-Lasseel MH. Comparative histological overview of the chemical coding of the pulmonary neuroepithelial endocrine system in health and disease. *Eur J Morphol* 1992;30:101–112.
295. Schneeberger EE. Alveolar type I cells. In: Crystal R, West J, Barnes P, Cherniack N, Weibel E, eds. *The lung: scientific foundations.* New York: Raven Press, 1991:229–234.
296. Schneeberger EE. Airway and alveolar epithelial cell junctions. In: Crystal R, West R, Barnes R, Cherniack N, Weibel E, eds. *The lung: scientific foundations.* New York: Raven Press, 1991:205–214.
297. Schor AM, Canfield AE, Sloan P, Schor SL. Differentiation of pericytes in culture is accompanied by changes in the extracellular matrix. *In Vitro* 1991;27A:651–659.
298. Schraufnagel ED, Mehta D, Harshbarger R, Traviranus K, Wang N-S. Capillary remodeling in bleomycin-induced pulmonary fibrosis. *Am J Pathol* 1986;125:97–106.
299. Sertl K, Takemura T, Tschachler E, Ferrans VJ, Kaliner MA, Shevach EM. Dendritic cells with antigen-presenting capability reside in airway epithelium, lung parenchyma and visceral pleura. *J Exp Med* 1986;163:436–451.
300. Shaji S, Rickard KA, Ertl RF, Linder J, Rennard SI. Lung fibroblasts produce chemotactic factors for bronchial epithelial cells. *Am J Physiol* 1989;257:L71–L79.
301. Shanahan CM, Weissberg PL, Metcalfe JC. Isolation of gene markers of dedifferentiated and proliferating vascular smooth muscle cells. *Circ Res* 1993;73:193–204.
302. Shaul PW, North AJ, Wu LC, et al. Endothelial nitric oxide synthase is expressed in cultured human bronchiolar epithelium. *J Clin Invest* 1994;94:2231–2236.
303. Shayevitz JR, Varani J, Ward PA, Knight PR. Halothane and isoflurane increase sensitivity to oxidant-mediated injury. *Anesthesiology* 1991;74:1067–1077.
304. Shazi S, Rickard KA, Ertl RF, Robbins RA, Linder J, Rennard SI. Bronchial epithelial cells produce lung fibroblast chemotactic factor: fibronectin. *Am J Respir Cell Mol Biol* 1989;1:13–20.
305. Shepherd V. Cytokine receptors of the lung. *Am J Respir Cell Mol Biol* 1991;5:403–410.
306. Shepro D, Morel NML. Pericyte physiology. *FASEB J* 1993;7:1031–1038.
307. Shimizu T, Nettesheim P, Ramaekers FCS, Randell SH. Expression of "cell-type-specific" markers during rat tracheal epithelial regeneration. *Am J Respir Cell Mol Biol* 1992;7:30–41.
308. Shimizu T, Nishihara M, Kawaguchi S, Sakakura Y. Expression of phenotypic markers during regeneration of rat tracheal epithelium following mechanical injury. *Am J Respir Cell Mol Biol* 1994;11:85–94.
309. Shimosegawa T, Said SI. Pulmonary calcitonin gene-related peptide immunoreactivity: nerve-endocrine cell interrelationships. *Am J Respir Cell Mol Biol* 1991;4:126–134.
310. Sims DE. Recent advances in pericyte biology. *Can J Cardiol* 1991;7:431–443.
311. Sims DE, Westfall JA. Analysis of relationships between pericytes and gas exchange capillaries in neonatal and mature bovine lungs. *Microvasc Res* 1983;25:333–342.
312. Skinner MP, Raines EW, Ross R. Dynamic expression of α1β1 and α2β1 integrin receptors by human vascular smooth muscle cells. *Am J Pathol* 1994;145:1070–1081.
313. Soler PA, Moreau A, Basset F, Hance AJ. Cigarette smoking–induced changes in the number and differentiated state of pulmonary dendritic cells/Langerhans cells. *Am Rev Respir Dis* 1989;139:1112–1117.
314. Somlyo AP, Somlyo AV. Smooth muscle structure and function. In: Fozzaard H, ed. *The heart and cardiovascular system.* New York: Raven Press, 1992:1295–1324.
315. Sommerhoff CP, Finkbeiner WE. Human tracheobronchial submucosal gland cells in culture. *Am J Respir Cell Mol Biol* 1990;2:41–50.
316. Spicer SS, Chakrin LW, Wardell Jr JR, Kendrick W. Histochemistry of mucosubstances in the canine and human respiratory tract. *Lab Invest* 1971;25:483–490.
317. Spicer SS, Schulte BA, Thomopoulos GN. Histochemical properties of the respiratory tract epithelium in different species. *Am Rev Respir Dis* 1983;128:S20–S26.
318. Standiford TJ, Kunkel SL, Phan SH, Rollins BJ, Strieter RM. Alveolar macrophage-derived cytokines induced monocyte chemoattractant protein-1 expression from human pulmonary type II–like epithelial cells. *J Biol Chem* 1991;266:9912–9918.
319. Stathakos D, Psarras S, Kletsas D. Stimulation of human embryonic lung fibroblasts by TGFβ and PDGF acting in synergism. The role of cell density. *Cell Biol Int* 1993;17:55–64.
320. Staub NC, Schultz EL. Pulmonary capillary length in dog, cat and rabbit. *Respir Physiol* 1968;5:371–378.
321. Stellato C, Cosalaro V, Ciccarelli A, Mastonardi P, Mazarella B, Marone G. General anesthetics induce only histamine release selectively from human mast cells. *J Anesth* 1991;67:751–758.
322. Stewart DJ, Levy RD, Cernacek PDL, Langleben D. Increased plasma endothelin in pulmonary hypertension: marker or mediator of disease? *Ann Intern Med* 1991;114:464–469.
323. Stramm LE, Li W, Aguirre GD, Rockey JH. Glycosaminoglycan synthesis and secretion by bovine retinal capillary pericytes in culture. *Exp Eye Res* 1987;44:17–28.
324. Tait AR, Davidson BA, Johnson KJ, Remick DG, Knight PR. Halothane inhibits the intravalvular recruitment of neutrophils, lymphocytes, and macrophages in response to influenza virus infection in mice. *Anesth Analg* 1993;76:1106–1113.
325. Tani K, Yauoka S, Ogushi F, et al. Thrombin enhances lung fibroblast proliferation in bleomycin-induced pulmonary fibrosis. *Am J Respir Cell Mol Biol* 1991;5:34–40.
326. Tani K, Yauoka S, Ogushi F, et al. Fibroblast growth-stimulating activity in bronchoalveolar lavage fluid of patients with pulmonary sarcoidosis. *Jpn J Med* 1990;29:576–582.
327. Tarkka M. Effects of mechanical ventilation and halothane on pulmonary serotonin removal in dogs. *Acta Anesthesiol Scand* 1985;69:461–466.
328. Tournier J-M, Goldstein GA, Hall DE, Damsky CH, Basbaum CB. Extracellular matrix proteins regulate morphologic and biochemical properties of tracheal gland serous cells through integrins. *Am J Respir Cell Mol Biol* 1992;6:461–471.
329. van Haarst JMW, de Wit HJ, Drexhage HA, Hoogsteden HC. Distribution and immunophenotype of mononuclear phagocytes and dendritic cells in the human lung. *Am J Respir Cell Mol Biol* 1994;10:487–492.
330. Van Kuppevelt THMSM, Cremer FPM, Domen JGN, Kuyper CMA. Staining of proteoglycans in mouse lung alveoli. 1. Ultrastructural localization of anionic sites. *Histochem J* 1984;16:657–669.
331. Vancheri C, Ohtoshi T, Cox G, et al. Neutrophilic differentiation induced by human upper airway fibroblast-derived granulocyte/macrophage colony-stimulating factor (GM-CSF). *Am J Respir Cell Mol Biol* 1991;4:11–17.
332. Vignaud J-M, Allam M, Martinet N, Pech M, Plenat F. Presence of platelet-derived growth factor in normal and fibrotic lung is specifically associated with interstitial macrophages, while both interstitial macrophages and alveolar epithelial cells express the c-*sis* proto-oncogene. *Am J Respir Cell Mol Biol* 1991;5:531–538.
333. Voisin C, Scherpereel PA, Aerts C, Lepot D. *In vitro* toxicity of halogerated anesthetics on guinea pig alveolar macrophages, surviving in gas phase. *Br J Anesth* 1984;56:415–420.
334. Volker N, Drenckhahn D. Heterogeneity of microvascular pericytes for smooth muscle type a-actin. *J Cell Biol* 1991;113:137–154.
335. Voynow JA, Rose MC. Quantitation of mucin mRNA in respiratory and intestinal epithelial cells. *Am J Respir Cell Mol Biol* 1994;11:742–750.
336. Walker SR, Williams MC, Benson B. Immunocytochemical localization of the major surfactant apoproteins in type II cells, Clara cells, and alveolar macrophages of rat lung. *J Histochem Cytochem* 1986;1137–1148.
337. Wallmer P, Schainer W, Bos JA, Bakker W, Krenning EP, Lachmann B. Pulmonary clearance on 99mTc-DTPA during halothane anesthesia. *Acta Anaesthesiol Scand* 1990;34:572–575.
338. Ward HE, Nicholas TE. Effects of artificial ventilation and anesthesia on surfactant turnover in rats. *Respir Physiol* 1992;87:115–129.
339. Webber SE, Lim JCS, Widdicombe JG. The effects of calcitonin

gene-related peptide on submucosal gland secretion and epithelial albumin transport in the ferret trachea *in vitro*. *Br J Pharmacol* 1991;102:79–84.

340. Weibel ER. On pericytes, particularly their existence in lung capillaries. *Microvasc Res* 1974;8:218–235.
341. Weibel ER. Design and structure of the human lung. In: Fishman A, ed. *Pulmonary diseases*. New York: McGraw-Hill, 1980:224–271.
342. Weibel ER. Lung cell biology. In: Fishman A, Fisher A, Geiger S, eds. *Handbook of physiology*. Bethesda: American Physiological Society, 1985:47–91.
343. Weibel ER, Crystal RG. Structural organization of the pulmonary interstitium. In: Crystal R, West J, Barnes P, Cherniack N, Weibel E, eds. *The lung: scientific foundations*. New York: Raven Press, 1991: 369–379.
344. Welch WD. Enflurane and isoflurane inhibit the oxidative activity of pulmonary alveolar macrophages. *Respiration* 1985;47:24–29.
345. Westergren-Thorsson G, Persson S, Isaksson A, et al. L-iduranate-rich glycosaminoglycans inhibit growth of normal fibroblasts independently of serum or added growth factors. *Exp Cell Res* 1993; 203:93–99.
346. White SR, Hathaway DP, Umans JG, Tallet J, Abrahams C, Leff AR. Epithelial modulation of airway smooth muscle response to endothelin-1. *Am Rev Respir Dis* 1991;144:373–378.
347. White SR, Hershenson MB, Sigrist KS, Zimmerman A, Solway J. Proliferation of guinea pig tracheal epithelial cells induced by calcitonin gene-related peptide. *Am J Respir Cell Mol Biol* 1993;8:592–596.
348. Williams MC, Dobbs LG. Expression of cell-specific markers for alveolar epithelium in fetal rat lung. *Am J Respir Cell Mol Biol* 1990; 2:533–542.
349. Wong LB, Miller IF, Yeates DB. Pathways of substance P stimulation of canine tracheal ciliary beat frequency. *J Appl Physiol* 1991; 70:267–273.
350. Wright WE, Sassoon DA, Lin VK. Myogenin, a factor regulating myogenesis, has a domain homologous to MyoD. *Cell* 1989;56: 607–617.
351. Wu R, Carlson DM. Structure and synthesis of mucins. In: Crystal R, West J, Barnes P, Chernicack N, Weibel E, eds. *The lung: scientific foundations*. New York: Raven Press, 1991:183–188.
352. Wu T, Rieves D, Larivee P, Logun C, Lawrence MG, Shelhamer JH. Production of eicosanoids in response to endothelin-1 and identification of specific endothelin-1 binding sites in airway epithelial cells. *Am J Respir Cell Mol Biol* 1993;8:282–290.
353. Yahagi N, Furuya H, Sai Y, Amakata Y. Effect of halothane, fentanyl and ketamine on the threshold for transpulmonary passage of venous air emboli in dogs. *Anesth Analg* 1992;75:720–723.
354. Ye CL, Rabinovitch M. Inhibition of elastolysis by SC-37698 reduces development and progression of monocrotaline pulmonary hypertension. *Am J Physiol* 1991;262:H1255–1267.
355. Yuan KJ, Goldman WF, Tod ML, Rubin LJ, Blaustein MP. Hypoxia reduces potassium currents in cultured rat pulmonary but not mesenteric arterial myocytes. *Am J Physiol* 1993;264:L116–L123.
356. Zambrano IR, Caceres JR, Mendoza JF, et al. Evidence that fibroblasts and epithelial cells produce a specific type of macrophage and granulocyte inducer, also known as colony stimulating factor. *Ann NY Acad Sci* 1989;554:141–155.
357. Zhang K, Rekhter MD, Gordon D, Phan SH. Myofibroblasts and their role in lung collagen gene expression during pulmonary fibrosis. *Am J Pathol* 1994;145:114–125.
358. Zhu L, Wigle D, Hinek A, et al. The endogeous vascular elastase that governs development and progression of monocrotaline-induced pulmonary hypertension in rats is a novel enzyme related to the serine proteinase adipsin. *J Clin Invest* 1994;94: 1163–1171.
359. Zimmerman GA, Lorant DE, McIntyre TM, Prescott SM. Juxtacrine intercellular signaling: another way to do it. *Am J Respir Cell Mol Biol* 1993;9:573–577.
360. Zitnik RJ, Zheng T, Elias JA. CAMP inhibition of interleukin-1 induced interleukin-6 production by human lung fibroblasts. *Am J Physiol* 1993;264:L253–L260.
361. Zoja C, Orisio S, Perico N, et al. Constitutive expression of endothelin gene in culture mesangial cells and its modulation by TGFβ thrombin and a thromboxane A_2. *Lab Invest* 1991;64:16–20.

Anesthesia: Biologic Foundations, edited by
Tony L. Yaksh et al. Lippincott–Raven Publishers,
Philadelphia © 1997.

CHAPTER 75

CELL-MATRIX RELATIONSHIPS ARE DYNAMIC AND REGULATORY

ROBERT L. TRELSTAD

Increased understanding of the roles of the extracellular matrix in the biology of anesthesia can be expected based on new information about the dynamics of cell-matrix relationships. Principal among these is the extracellular matrix as a ligand, reversibly binding biologically active agents which affect cells in an autocrine, paracrine and endocrine manner. Second is the matrix as an agonist both in solid phase, transmitting information to contiguous cells, and in soluble phase, transmitting information both through the pericellular space and the circulation. These matrix attributes of agonist add to their better known functions as adhesives, biomaterials and filters and a lesser known of the matrix as a text, recording events in the history of the organism.

In this chapter, the dynamic nature of the matrix and its multiple relationships with cells will be emphasized. Details of matrix chemistry or its macroscopic structures are available in recent reviews (25,80,105,142). The major matrix components will be described to cover matters of terminology, chemistry, intermolecular relationships, and overall organization as a three phase system: a solid phase, a fluid phase, and a cell surface phase. All three phases are comprised of components commonly known as collagens, proteoglycans, structural glycoproteins, and elastins (22,31,41,109,140,169,173).

MATRIX PHASES

Solid Phase Matrix

The solid phase extracellular matrix is well known and functions at a macroscopic level as a supporting structure. At the cellular level, the solid phase matrix serves as a substrate for cell migration; an adhesive for cell anchorage; a ligand for ions, growth factors, and other bioactive agents; signals to contacting cells; and a recording device (84,166,185). The cells that produce, store, and excrete these matrixes include nearly all cell types, ranging from circulating mast cells to neurons. The principal sources of the solid phase matrixes are fibroblasts, chondrocytes, osteoblasts, smooth muscle cells, and various epithelia (189).

Fluid Phase Matrix

Secreted matrix components are transiently in a fluid phase prior to polymerization. In addition, many of the components of the matrix may also be found in soluble forms in the extracellular fluids, lymph, or blood. The fluid phase forms may be derived from solid phase components by some form of cleavage, whereas others are unique isoforms in which the fluid form is different from the solid form (73). Hyaluronan, aggrecan, fibronectin, vitronectin, thrombospondin, cartilage matrix protein, and laminin are found intact or as fragments, in blood, lymph, synovial fluid, and bronchoalveolar lavage fluid (132, 167). Matrix components are also found in various fluid phases, from joints to the peritoneal space, following injury (10,35). Assays for tenascin in the CSF are markedly elevated in astrocytic tumors, and its measurement is useful in diagnosing and monitoring these neoplasms (187).

Cell Surface Matrix

The location of matrix components at the cell's surface is effected, in part, by membrane receptors which bind matrix components, e.g., the integrins (74); in part, as integral components of the plasma membrane, e.g., the syndecans (11); in part as covalently linked elements to membrane glycolipids, e.g., betaglycan (103); and, in part, through biosynthetic steps which result in direct transmembrane penetration of product by-passing the Golgi apparatus, e.g., hyaluronan (23). By whichever of these means, the cell surface matrix consists of polyvalent molecules which can bind other ligands and amplify and extend the surface of the cell into the pericellular space (Fig. 1). The cell-surface matrix can be indirectly or directly visualized on living cells and is several microns in thickness and in constant motion (98).

The basement membrane is an extracellular matrix which is noncovalently associated with the plasma membranes of most animal cells (Fig. 1). The term basement membrane (BM) is well engrained, even though it is neither on the "bottom" of cells nor a structure with the usual attributes of a membrane (exerts an osmotic pressure; partitions electrolytes). It coats nearly the entire surface of smooth, cardiac and skeletal muscle cells, fat cells, Schwann cells, and the basal surface of most epithelia (188). In essence, the basement membrane or basal lamina (191), is a cell surface matrix, filtering and protecting the cell surface; reversibly binding regulators and growth factors; partitioning tissues during morphogenesis and repair; and all the while traversed by components involved in nutrition, respiration and metabolic waste. The basal lamina is a heteropolymeric mixture of molecules including type IV collagen, laminin, perlecan, and entactin (6,55,123,191). These relatively constant molecular constituents undergo a variety of self-assembly reactions of both a homopolymeric and heteropolymeric nature to produce this cell surface matrix which ranges from 50 to 200 nm in thickness. The linkages to the cell surface are noncovalent, calcium dependent and mediated via a variety of its constituents acting individually and/or together (191) with receptors or through unknown means. While the filtration functions of the basement membrane are well known, particularly in the glomerulus, it plays additional important binding and storage roles for drugs, ions, enzymes and growth factors (6,135,174). Transforming growth factor–β (TGF-β), a potent regulator of cell proliferation and matrix production/degradation, is downregulated when cells are cultured on a reconstituted basement membrane. Because of their ubiquity and the polyvalency of its constituents, basement membranes play a central role in cell-matrix interactions ranging from cell anchorage to cytokine and growth factor regulation (160).

MATRIX NOMENCLATURE

The nomenclature and classification of matrix components has simultaneously blurred and come more into focus as details of their overlapping chemistries has developed. The triple helical structure of collagen, once thought to be a unique attribute, is shared with a variety of molecules including surfactant,

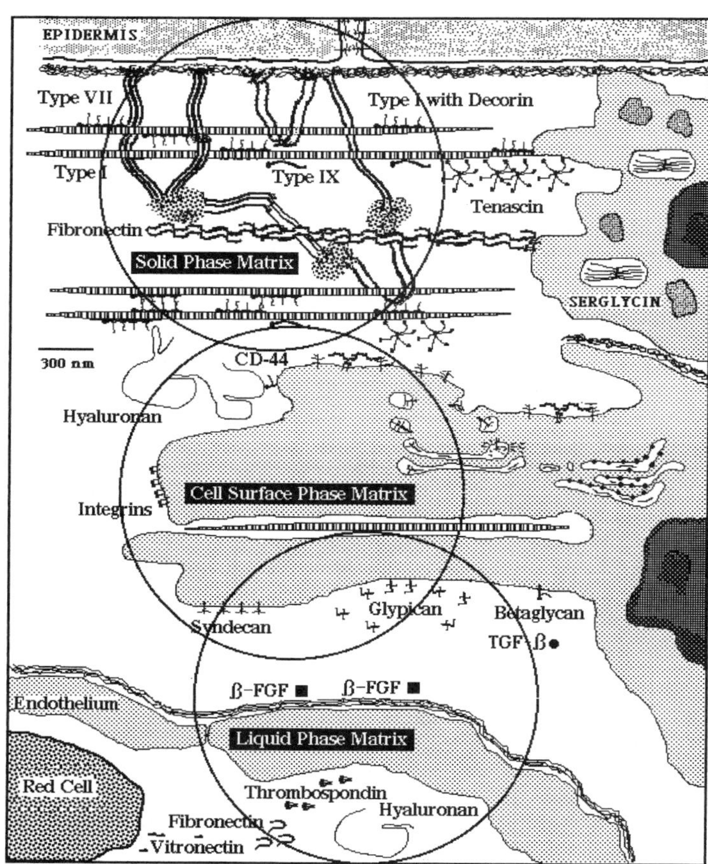

Figure 1. The three phases of the extracellular matrix are drawn to scale for both the cells and the matrix components. *Top:* Basal portion of an epidermal cell, covered on its basal surface by basement membrane. Type VII collagen aggregates are linked to the basement membrane to form anchoring fibrils, which create "loops," entrapping collagen fibrils and other matrix components. Taken together, the elements in the upper circle constitute a solid phase of the matrix. *Middle:* The fibroblast in the middle shows a convoluted topography with cell surface receptors and matrix components associated with the cell surface. Hyaluronan, bound to the cell surface by the CD44 receptor or penetrating the cell during biosynthesis, forms an extended pericellular coat. Syndecan, glypican, and betaglycan, three membrane-associated proteoglycans, are important components of the cell surface phase matrix. In that glypican is not a transmembrane protein, but rather linked by phosphoinositol, it can readily be released from the cell surface phase to enter the liquid phase matrix. *Lower left:* Capillary carrying soluble forms of fibronectin, vitronectin, hyaluronan, and thrombospondin. Fluid phase elements from the circulation and from the interstitial fluids surrounding the cells move throughout the liquid phase matrix.

macrophage scavenger receptor, C1q and acetylcholinesterase (1,38,129,144). By convention, the designation of a protein as a collagen is reserved for a structural molecule in the extracellular matrix. In that proteins are modular structures, with domains comprised of motifs often shared with unrelated molecules, the possession of a particular motif or sequence, such as that of a growth factor, does not help define a clear nosology (29,39). And since proteins often have extensive postsynthetic modifications ranging from oxidations to glycosylation, these attributes do not assist in providing clarity of definitions.

Most matrix proteins have attached one or more of four classes of carbohydrate polymers: simple hexoses; branched N-linked oligosaccharides; branched O-linked (mucinous) oligosaccharides; and unbranched O-linked glycosaminoglycans. The hexose chains on collagen are simple monosaccharides and disaccharides linked to hydroxylysine. The oligosaccharides are branched structures, often rich in mannose and sialic acid, which undergo extensive alterations during synthesis and postsynthetic modifications. Such oligosaccharides are an essential feature of a glycoprotein. The glycosaminoglycans are unbranched, long chains, which are highly sulfated and which have a disaccharide repeat motif (57). Glycosaminoglycans (GAGs) are an essential feature of a proteoglycan. The examples of types IX and XII collagens underscores the above-mentioned naming problem. Type IX collagen has covalently bound oligosaccharides and glycosaminoglycans and thus is a collagen, a glycoprotein and a proteoglycan (18). Type XII collagen presents a similar ambiguity, in that it is a chimeric molecule with reiterated fibronectin type III motifs, von Willebrand factor A motifs, a domain homologous to a noncollagenous region of type IX collagen, and short collagenous domains with an Arg-Gly-Asp (RGD) site, a classic integrin binding sequence (186).

Thus while the initial logic of earlier taxonomies of matrix components was chemistry and/or function, it is now clear that their overlapping chemistries and functions do not lend themselves to simple classifications. The current tendency is to "name" each matrix macromolecule with a new term and/or number, e.g., syndecan-1 (101) or the α1 chain of type XIX collagen (118). Although this is bound to lead to some confusion, the need to expand beyond the intellectual constraints of the prior nomenclature is clear because proteoglycans, glycoproteins and collagens are polymorphic, polyfunctional and widely distributed.

MATRIX CHEMICAL STRUCTURES

Proteins, Aggregated and/or Crosslinked, With Carbohydrates

The principal chemistry of the matrix is that of proteins with covalently attached carbohydrates. Posttranslation modifications include hydroxylation of prolyl, lysyl, and asparagine residues (50); glycosylation to form the various N- or O-linked oligosaccharides or glycosaminoglycans; acylation by the long-chained fatty acids myristate and palmitate; and tyrosine-O-sulfation (77). The proteins may also be oxidized to create covalent crosslinkages among proteins of the same group and between proteins of different groups (183). The carbohydrate polymers are covalently linked at one of four amino acids: asparagine, threonine, serine, and hydroxylysine. The linkage at the asparagine residues occurs through a nitrogen atom and is termed N-linked; those linkages through threonine, serine, and hydroxylysine are through an oxygen atom and termed O-linked.

The protein cores of matrix glycoproteins and proteoglycans vary in molecular weight from ~40 to 600 kd and in physical size from <30 to >300 nM in greatest dimension (Fig. 2). The core protein of perlecan, for example, is greater than type IV colla-

Matrix Components Solid Phase Soluble Phase Cell surface Phase	Core Protein Size (kD)	Size (nM) ——— 300 nM
Aggrecan	320	
Betaglycan	90	
Biglycan	40	
CD44	85	
Cartilage Matrix Pr.	150	
Collagen I-III & V	310	
Collagen IV	525	
Collagen VI	300	
Collagen VII	590	
Collagen IX	225	
Collagen IX	225	
Collagen X	200	
Collagen XII	590	
Decorin	40	
Entactin/Nidogen	120	
Fibrillin	350	
Fibromodulin	60	
Fibronectin	500	
Glypican	65	
Hyaluronan	0	
Integrins	220	
Laminins	840	
Link	40	
Osteocalcin	6	
Osteopontin	35	
Perlecan	600	
Serglycin	11	
SPARC/Osteonectin	40	
Syndecan	35	
Tenascin	320	
Thrombomodulin	90	
Thrombospondin	450	
Versican	250	
Vitronectin	50	

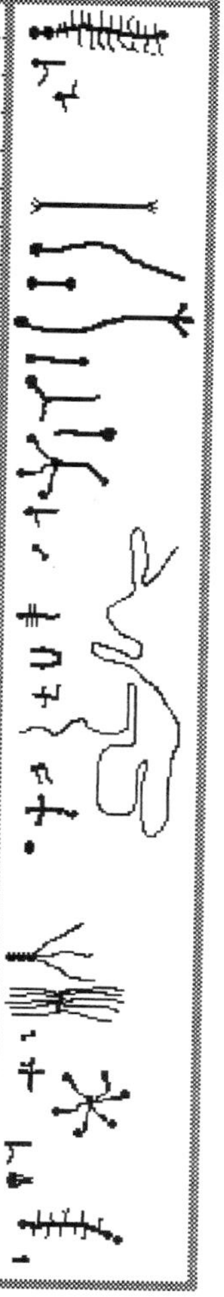

Figure 2. Major matrix components discussed in this chapter along with a listing of their core protein's molecular size in kilodaltons and their physical size in nanometers. Note that the mass of the core protein and the size of the natural configuation are not closely related.

gen in mass (450 kd versus 400 kd), but is about one fourth its size (100 nm versus 400 nm) in linear dimension. Such size/mass differences result from globular packing and indicate that the three dimension size of components cannot be predicted from simple mass. In that aggregates of matrix components establish and maintain form in most tissues in the animal kingdom, the manner of component folding, interacting and aggregating is of considerable importance (14,79,183).

Most matrix proteins are modular where the modular unit is based on sequence similarities or homologies among polypeptide stretches of 45–90 amino acids and frequently contain intramodule disulfide crosslinks. Modules presumably arise within one protein by exon duplication and among unrelated proteins by exons which have shuffled from one gene to another. Matrix proteins have an extensive modular character (51).

Carbohydrate Structures

The characters of the carbohydrate chains of both the oligosaccharides of the glycoproteins and the glycosaminoglycans of the proteoglycans are dictated by the intrinsic properties of the individual sugars, the specific sites and stereochemistry of the linkages between adjacent sugars, the order in which they are added and/or removed during biosynthesis, and postsynthetic modifications, which include epimerization and sulfation (57,69,96).

Chondroitin sulfate (CS) and dermatan sulfate (DS) glycosaminoglycan chains are similar because of the epimerization of glucuronic acid in CS to iduronic acid in DS, a conversion that occurs after the oligosaccharide is synthesized. The biologic importance of the epimerizations that occur in the iduronic acid to glucuronic acid shift should not be underestimated. A variety of agents from sulfate to Vitamin A deficiency cause reduction of GAG incorporation into the decorin class of proteoglycans and also to a decreased epimerization of D-glucuronic to L-iduronic acid (155).

MATRIX FUNCTIONS

From the preceding discussion, it is apparent that the extracellular matrix is broadly involved in functions ranging from roles as an adhesive, biomaterial, filter, ligand, signal, and text. In the following section, each of these functions is briefly presented with examples.

Adhesives

In and of themselves, matrix components are adhesives, historically as glues, binding to each other in both native and denatured forms, in homotypic and heterotypic combinations. These important practical, clinical and commercial uses of matrix continue to develop (40). However, it is the cell receptor-matrix interactions or the cell surface-matrix interactions that are new to the adhesive considerations of the matrix. Adhesion molecules and adhesive phenomena have generally excluded cell-matrix interactions. Traditional adhesion molecules dealt with homotypic cell-cell adhesions as with the calcium independent cell adhesion molecules or CAMs; the calcium dependent cadherens; the selectins; desmosomes; and a variety of receptors on lymphocytes. That cell-matrix interactions overlap with traditional adhesive interactions can be inferred from the modular chemistry of the components. In the mouse, for example, perlecan has five distinct domains: a heparan sulfate attachment domain, a LDL receptor-like domain, two different laminin-like domains and an N-CAM-like domain. This polyvalency leads to molecular interactions of considerable complexity and opens new avenues for the study of adhesion (116,185)

The most compelling argument for cell-matrix interactions as an adhesive processes is the extensive involvement of integrins in biological adhesivity (92,114,163). The regulation of integrin expression by pharmacologic means, using natural as well as synthesized agents, and the altered regulation of integrin expression in human disease suggest new avenues for study and modulation of cell-matrix adhesion (27,56,112,153, 195,196).

Microorganisms use the matrix as an adhesive substrate to establish infections. Organisms from various species express cell-surface molecules called adhesins which bind to the matrix. Typical organisms and an example of their matrix ligands include *Pneumocystis carinii* (fibronectin); *Trypanosoma cruzi* (collagen); *Aspergillus* (fibrinogen); *Staphylococcus aureus* (vitronectin); and *Plasmodium falciparum* (heparan sulfate) (127).

Biomaterials

The biomaterials properties of natural and reconstituted matrixes are well understood at macroscopic levels. The physiology of respiration is dependent on the elastic recoil of the pulmonary interstitium. Gas exchange in the lung occurs across a narrow, but stable air-blood interface comprised in great part by the opposed basement membranes of the alveolar capillary and the type I pneumocyte. These microscopic biomaterials properties of the matrix are open for exploration (122). Matrix components can be reassembled in a theoretically limitless number of combinations, in differing sizes and shapes, to form implantable devices or substrates for cells at sites of injury. It is reasonable to predict that biomaterials, comprised of extracellular matrix components will increasingly be available for clinical use (71,128,134).

Filters

All nutrients, gases, cytokines, hormones, and drugs must pass through the extracellular matrix in moving from one tissue or tissue compartment to another. In particular, most agents must traverse the basement membrane at least twice: when the agent exits the vasculature and when it enters the cell; or vice-versa. Both the matrix and/or the basement membranes bind, select, inhibit, facilitate, release and/or reversibly remove components with which they come in contact acting as a filter with physiologic consequences (120,172). In addition to these filtration functions, the glomerular basement membrane plays a major role in homeostasis and is central to a number of disease processes (95).

Ligands

Solid phase matrix components are ligands which bind, store, protect and release growth factors and other regulatory agents (9,88,119,171,181). The release of such ligands bound to the matrix may occur through matrix degradation; through specific intermediary binding factors (165); through competitive interactions with other ligands; or through some change in the ligand itself. This "storage/receptor" activity in the matrix shows considerable specificity and is a major matrix function (7).

At the same time that the solid phase matrix is a storage/receptor, cell surface matrix molecules such as the syndecans (86), CD44 (17), betaglycan (103), and glypican (26) are probably signal transducing receptors (19), although the transduction mechanisms need to be clarified.

Signals

The roles of the matrix in signaling and mediating cell-cell interactions were apparent in early studies of developing embryos and in cell culture studies in which collagen was shown to support and promote differentiation in vitro (61,70). Studies on hyaluronic acid and fibronectin opened a new view of the broad biological effects of matrix components as signals (65,84). The signaling functions of matrix macromolecules may be detected by cells when the molecules are in a complex macroaggregate and as small polypeptides or oligosaccharides, released from the parent molecule by hydrolysis (19). The solid phase signals operate in a variety of biological situations, e.g., during cell migrations in development (82), in neutrophil reactions in injury (64), in allergic reactions (168), in malignant transformations of epithelia (114) or in endometrial changes associated with menstruation or pregnancy (100). The Arg-Gly-Asp (RGD) peptide in solid phase in intact fibronectin or released from fibronectin can effectively inhibit cell binding to a number of serum and matrix components (130). Like peptides, short sequences of carbohydrates or oligosaccharides have similar regulatory effects. The replication of smooth muscle cells is significantly inhibited by oligosaccharides derived from heparin and this effect is dependent on both the size and the charge of the oligosaccharide, involves a competition between bFGF binding to cell-associated heparan sulfate proteoglycans and the released oligosaccharides and is effected by inhibition of a protein kinase C-dependent pathway (124). The matrix also has "positional information" sufficient to influence the homing and orientation of cells as shown by the effects of matrix on neural crest cell migration or the polarizing influence of the COOH-terminus of the A chain of laminin on nephrogenic mesenchyme (37,70,194).

Texts

Finally, the matrix is a text, a record of events which have taken place around a cell and within a tissue. It is a repository of information and a historical document, recording local events from the time of synthesis to later events such as cell migrations, inflammation, transformation and matrix cross-linking have occurred. These postdepositional events involve deliberate and/or accidental glycosylation (136), cross-linking (183), oxidation (89), phosphorylation, and epimerization to name but a few. Some of the history of an organism is written in this text and its epigenetic character will make it a challenge to read.

MATRIX REGULATORS

The regulatory factors which impact on matrix synthesis, degradation and function are many and include "growth factors," cytokines, hormones, vitamins, matrix metalloproteinases (MMPs), and tissue inhibitors of metalloproteinases (TIMPs). The logistics of matrix regulation is different from that for intracellular proteins in that the matrix is more distant from the genetic and biosynthetic machinery inside the cell. Nonetheless, the matrix is directly and indirectly involved in feedback on its production, polymerization, and/or degradation (60).

Vitamins

A list of matrix regulators might historically start with the recognition in the 18th century that vitamin C was an essential nutrient, required for hydroxylation of proline to hydroxyproline and consequent stability of the collagen triple helix (131) and vitamin D plays a major role in the dynamic reactions of the matrix of bone (113,145).

Hormones

The effects of hormones on matrix production, stability and degradation have been applied clinically for decades for a variety of conditions ranging from estrogens for osteoporosis to glucocorticoids for inflammatory processes which often have fibrotic sequelae. Growth factors and/or cytokines may mediate some or many of these effects while others may act directly on matrix components and/or their receptors (36).

Matrix Metalloproteinases

Matrix metalloproteinases (MMPs) are a family of enzymes that contain zinc at their active site and can degrade most of the matrix macromolecules found in connective tissues (182). The activation of some of the MMPs is linked to integrin receptors (149) and is promoted by secreted protein acidic richcysteine (SPARC) (178). MMPs are secreted by both matrix cells and infiltrating leukocytes in response to inflammatory mediators. MMPs are the major class of proteinases responsible for degradation of cartilage in rheumatoid arthritis. Zinc-binding pseudopeptide MMP inhibitors offer possible therapy for arthritis. (53).

Tissue Inhibitors of Metalloproteinases

Tissue inhibitors of metalloproteinases (TIMPs) are natural inhibitors of the matrix metalloproteinases, collagenases, stromelysins, and gelatinases, a group of zinc-binding endopeptidases involved in the degradation of the extracellular matrix.

At least three different TIMPs have been characterized, each inhibiting all known eukaryotic metalloproteinases (4). TIMPs affect activation of prometalloproteinases and modulate proteolysis of extracellular matrix components. TIMPs are particularly active in development during tissue remodeling and in pathologic disorders associated with inflammatory processes and tumor metastasis. Because of the intimate relationship between solid phase matrix components and growth regulatory agents, TIMPs play an important role in matrix cell regulation (33).

Growth Factors

TGF-β plays a major role in matrix production and degradation (5,63,106,137). It also induces leukocyte margination and accumulation both through direct chemotaxis and by inducing cell surface integrin expression on monocytes. As a consequence, TGF-β promotes monocyte adhesion to type IV collagen, laminin, and fibronectin, facilitating cellular movement through the matrix. In that TGF-β also stimulates gelatinase/type IV collagenase, it plays a major role in inflammation and repair (176). Most growth factors, directly or indirectly affect the matrix, a subject which is beyond the scope of this discussion but covered in recent articles and reviews (15,48,66,85, 138,139,147,192).

The relationships of growth factors with the matrix involves a complex set of feedback loops and ligand/storage functions (143). The growth factors which modulate matrix structure and synthesis are themselves stored in the extracellular matrix. The matrix binds these secreted bioactive agents by a number of means. For example, basic fibroblast growth factor (bFGF) has strong affinity for heparin and binds to the matrix where it is sequestered in the subendothelial matrix. Release of matrix bound bFGF occurs following exposure to proteases such as thrombin (9) or macrophage-derived urokinase-type plasminogen activator (42). Production of the macrophage plasminogen activator is enhanced by TGF-β1; thus TGF-β1 indirectly stimulates the release of bound bFGF. What makes the molecular details of this all the more interrelated is that on osteoblasts, betaglycan, a cell surface proteoglycan discussed below, binds TGF-β via its core protein and bFGF via its heparan sulfate chains (2).

MATRIX COMPONENTS

The following section is a brief overview of the various macromolecules related to the multiple phases of the matrix. The macromolecules are presented in alphabetical order and grouped by structure/function. An effort has been made to present a concise statement regarding each with references to recent literature.

Agrin, Dystroglycan

Agrin and related isoforms are secreted molecules produced by nerves and muscle that induce the aggregation of acetylcholine receptors (AChRs) (24,110). Acetylcholine receptor genes are specifically transcribed by synaptic nuclei in response to signals from the synaptic basement membrane (81). Various isoforms of agrin are generated by alternative splicing yielding molecules with differing interactive properties with proteoglycans and other components of the basement membrane (43). The C-terminus of agrin responsible for causing AChRs of muscle to aggregate contains three laminin modules separated by epidermal growth factor-like modules. Alternative splicing in the laminin modules leads to the formation of isoforms that are devoid of AChR-aggregating activity. In the N-terminus, all isoforms contain follistatin-related modules that, like those in follistatin and osteonectin, may bind the TGF-β or platelet-derived growth factor (PDGF) families (126). Structural similarities of agrin and laminin allow both to bind to the laminin receptor dystroglycan-α and dystrophin-related protein (DRP/utrophin) in a calcium-dependent manner inhibitable by heparin, and laminin, but not by fibronectin (49). α-Dystroglycan is the major agrin-binding protein in *Torpedo* and myotube membranes (161).

Aggrecan, Versican

The major proteoglycan from a variety of cartilages consists of a long core protein (350 nm) with three distinct globular domains: two near the NH_2-terminus and one at the COOH-terminus. It contains an extensive array of keratan sulfate and chondroitin sulfate glycosaminoglycan (GAG) chains giving it its classical bottle-brush appearance (Fig. 3). The amino terminal globular domain shows sequence similarity to link and the carboxy terminal globule to lectin binding proteins. The amino terminal globule binds to hyaluronan and forms a macroaggregate which contributes to the three dimensional organization of most cartilages. Aggrecan provides cartilage with osmotic properties that give articular cartilages resistance to compression (141). In the mouse, an autosomal recessive deficiency (cmd) characterized by cleft palate, short limbs, tail and snout results from a 7-bp deletion in exon 5 of aggrecan and consequent truncation of the molecule (179). The GAG chains, as well as the core protein, undergo shortening in the tissues long after synthesis and deposition possibly accounting for some of the changes that occur in cartilages with aging (20,58).

Betaglycan

Betaglycan is an integral membrane protein and part-time proteoglycan as well as soluble matrix element. Betaglycan regulates the access of TGF-β to its signaling receptors by binding TGF-β and then presenting it directly to the kinase subunit of the signaling receptor, forming a high-affinity complex (157). By itself, TGF-β binds with low affinity to this signaling receptor complex, a heteromeric serine/threonine protein kinase receptor. Betaglycan thereby enhances cell responsiveness to TGF-β and its isoforms. Soluble betaglycan binds TGF-β but does not enhance binding to membrane receptors and recombinant betaglycans act as potent inhibitors of TGF-β. Thus, in its cell surface phase, betaglycan is an enhancer of TGF-β action whereas in it soluble phase, it is a TGF-β antagonist (103)

Biglycan, Decorin, Fibromodulin, and Lumican

The small proteoglycans, biglycan, decorin, fibromodulin, and lumican, are a family of structurally similar, but distinct molecules found in a diverse array of connective tissues (47). Fibromodulin and decorin interact with collagens I and II at different sites on the respective fibrils. Fibromodulin has an average of one binding site per type I collagen molecule whereas decorin has several, some possibly mediated by the dermatan sulfate chain (177). Fibromodulin is functionally similar to decorin in that it binds to collagen types I and II during fibrillogeneis. The fibromodulin isolated from cartilage contains at least one keratan sulfate chain, suggesting that this group of molecules might show structural heterogeneities from tissue to tissue based on their GAG adducts. When decorin is present during collagen fibril assembly, fibrils of smaller diameter are formed and such fibrils will have less biomechanical strength since tensile properties of woven polymers such as collagen are dependent, in part, on the fibril diameter.

Although the "solid-phase" functions of these small proteoglycan as a structural element are important, their binding of TGF-β in a regulatory manner is likely to be of equal or greater importance. TGF-β binding presumably involves both the "solid phase" and "fluid phase" forms in vivo in that it has been demonstrated that the decorin type proteoglycans all bind to similar sites on TGF-β as betaglycan and do so in a competitive

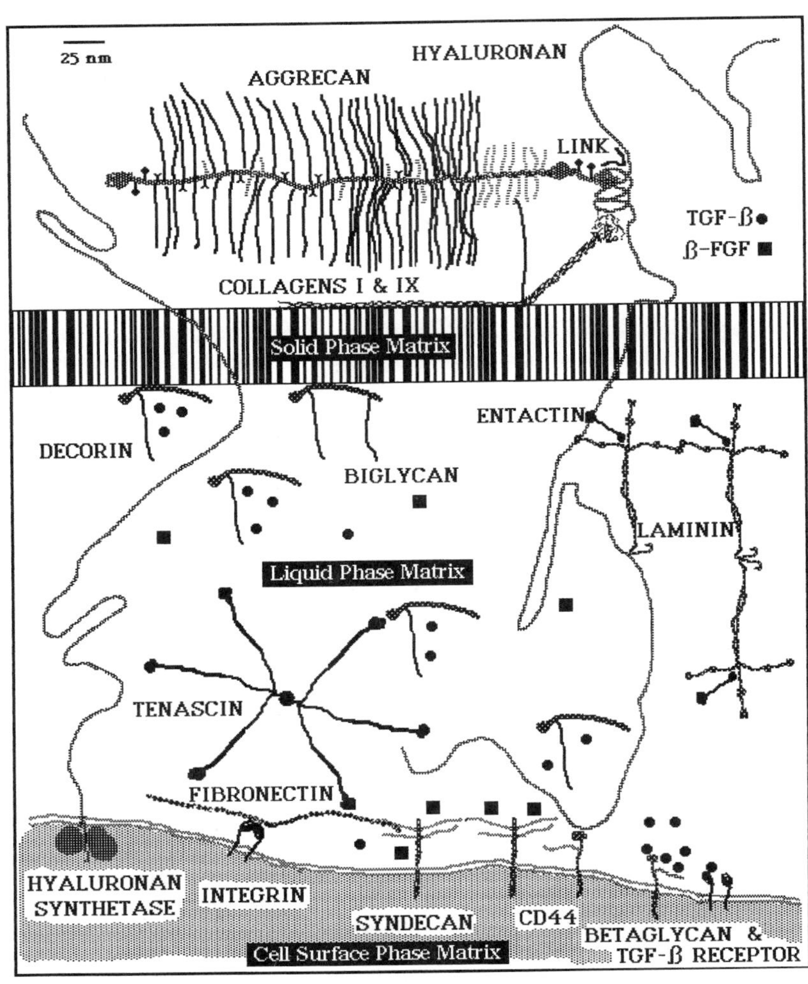

Figure 3. A detailed view of the cell surface and the pericellular matrix drawn to scale. The type I collagen fibril is present as a 67-nm striated structure with associated components, decorin, biglycan and a type IX molecule. The type IX molecule is covalently cross-linked to the type I. Decorin and biglycan both interact with the fibril and both influence fibril formation. *Upper:* Solid phase matrix. *Lower:* The external surface of the cell shows fibronectin bound to an integrin receptor with syndecan interacting with one end of the same fibronectin molecule. Syndecan is also shown interacting with β-FGF. Hyaluronan bound to the cell via CD44 as well as anchored through the membrane during synthesis leads to the formation of an extension of the cell and contributes significantly to the cell surface phase of the matrix. The binding of TGF-β to decorin, betaglycan, and its receptors occurs in all three phases of the matrix.

manner (46). In addition to their interactions with TGF-β, biglycan and decorin accelerate heparin cofactor II inhibition of thrombin an effect mediated by the GAG chains. Biglycan and decorin also bound to type V collagen in a saturable manner and in the bound state accelerated the heparin cofactor II/thrombin inhibition reaction as efficiently as the proteoglycans in solution (44,180).

Brevican, Neurocan, and Phosphacan

The extracellular matrix in the CNS is modest in its interstitial distribution, but present nonetheless. The structural roles of the matrix in the CNS are likely to be less prominent than the roles of signal, ligand and text. The following are recently described proteoglycans in the CNS which, in conjunction with hyaluronan, are serving new roles in morphogenesis and, eventually, in signaling (96).

Brevican, a part-time proteoglycan, contains chondroitin sulfate chains when glycanated, and within its short protein core (relative to aggrecan, versican or neurocan) a hyaluronan binding domain at the N-terminus, an epidermal growth factor-like repeat, a lectin-like and a complement regulatory protein-like domains in the C-terminus. Brevican is present predominantly in the brain and is expressed in primary cerebellar astrocytes but not in neurons.(184).

Neurocan is a multi-domain proteoglycan synthesized by neurons and binds to hyaluronic acid. Neurocan interacts with the adhesion molecules, Ng-CAM and N-CAM, and competes with the effects of these two adhesion molecules. In that neurocan, Ng-CAM and N-CAM colocalize in the developing cerebellum it is likely that their interactions affect neuronal adhesion and neurite growth during morphogenesis (45) Phosphacan is synthesized by glia and represents an extracellular variant of the receptor-type protein tyrosine phosphatase (107,115). Tenascin binds phosphacan and neurocan suggesting that interactions among chondroitin sulfate proteoglycans and tenascin are involved in neurogenesis, possibly by modulating signal transduction across the plasma membrane (54).

CD44, RHAMM

CD44 is a transmembrane family of proteins with various isoforms generated by alternative splicing and/or posttranslational modification which is a major hyaluronan receptor, a part-time proteoglycan and a lymphocyte homing receptor (99). The interactions of the CD44 with hyaluronan are inhibited by low concentrations of hyaluronan and high concentrations of chondroitin sulfate, suggesting that the receptor-ligand interaction may mimic the interactions of aggrecan, link and hyaluronan in the matrix, a suggestion supported by sequence homologies among the hyaluronan binding domains in aggrecan and versican with the protein core of CD44. CD44 on lymphocytes is responsible for their homing to high-endothelium during physiologic and pathologic extravasation and for the ability of macrophages to internalize hyaluronan during lung development (170). In addition to these binding and/or receptor functions, CD44 plays a role in matrix assembly where it acts to organize the immediate pericellular zone (94,98).

RMAMM is the acronym for receptor for hyaluronan-mediated motility and is a family of proteins which act the cell surface to bind hyaluronan, particularly during cell migration. RHAMM is not an integral membrane protein, but dependent on binding to the cell surface by undefined means. RHAMM contains two hyaluronan binding sites, each in a nine amino acid sequence. The RHAMM binding domains lack cysteines and are operative under reducing conditions whereas the binding domains in CD44 and link protein contain disulfides and their binding to hyaluronan is sensitive to reduction (154).

Cartilage Matrix Protein

Cartilage matrix protein is a 148 kd protein comprised of three identical units which is present in nonarticular cartilages. It can be extracted with EDTA-containing buffers indicating a divalent cation-dependent anchorage in the matrix. Its functions are not well understood, but it is released into the serum in some, but not all rheumatoid conditions. The subunits have a modular organization with one epidermal growth factor like domain and two domains which have homologies with the type A repeats of von Willebrand factor, complement factors B and C2, α chains of the integrins and a globular domain on type VI collagen. Three ellipsoid subunits, connected at the carboxy terminus by a short coiled-coil α-helical assembly domain has been observed by electron microscopy (59). In the chick limb during development, the expression of the genes for cartilage matrix protein, type II collagen, link protein, and aggrecan are all independent.

Collagens

Collagens are a family of molecules comprised of three polypeptide chains (α chains) wrapped about each other to form extended rod-shaped, triple helical regions and globular, nontriple helical regions. The globular regions are often referred to as noncollagenous, a misnomer, for the nontriple helical or globular domains. The canonical sequence of an α chain involved in triple helical formation is the triplet, (Gly-XY), with a high percentage of the Y position being *trans*-4-hydroxyproline. Each triple helical molecule belongs to a subclass whose name is denoted by a Roman numeral, i.e., type I collagen or type XIV collagen. At present there are close to 20 subclasses of collagens. Although each molecule in a subclass contains only three α chains, each collagen subclass may be comprised of as many as six different α chains. The six α chains are named α1 through α6 and their subclass is indicated by the Roman numeral assigned to that subclass. Thus α1(IV) is from type IV collagen, α2(IX) from type IX collagen and so on. The total number of biological combinations of the α chains has yet to be determined. The major collagen species in the animal kingdom, type I collagen, is comprised of $(\alpha1(I))_2\alpha2(I)$. To synthesize this molecule the cell transcribes gene products from chromosomes 7 and 17 and assembles the hetermonomer in a 2:1 stoichiometry as indicated. To date no native molecule with the chain composition of $\alpha1(I,\alpha2(I))_2$ has been isolated. Thus the combinations are probably limited. The extent to which α chains may exist in more than one subclass is not known, but present chemical data do not support much promiscuity.

The collagens are structural glycoproteins, proteoglycans and classical triple helical proteins and may contain any of the three major classes of carbohydrate additions, hydroxylysine linked neutral hexoses, N-linked high mannose or branched oligosaccharides and O-linked glycosaminoglycans. The polyvalency and multiple characters of the collagens are best described in types IX and XII. Type IX was the first collagen identified to which glycosaminoglycan chains were covalently linked. Type XII collagen has a complex modular structure with multiple homologies to other proteins. It contains a type III motif of fibronectin, followed by one homologous to the von Willebrand factor A domain, followed by more fibronectin type III modules, a second A domain from von Willebrand factor, six units of type III motif and a third A domain, 10 consecutive units of type III motif and a fourth A domain homologous type IX collagen (186).

As the chemistries and functions of the collagens have expanded, efforts to provide categories based on structures and functions have arisen. Thus fibrillar collagens are considered those forming "typical" striated fibrils such as types I, II, III, V, and XI. FACIT collagens, or *f*ibril-*a*ssociated *c*ollagens with *i*nterrupted *t*riple helix, include types IX and XII. Network forming collagens are comprised of types IV (basement membranes), type VIII (Descemet's membrane), and short-chain collagen, including types VI and X. Although such designations are transiently useful, as knowledge accrues it is likely the nosology will change.

Elastin, Elastin Binding Protein, Fibrillin

Elastin is a hydrophobic molecule that, following secretion, assembles with other elastin monomers and forms covalent crosslinks with other elastin monomers to create an extended, insoluble fabric which provides tissues with elastic properties (111). The crosslinking of the elasin monomers, also called tropoelastin, occurs primarily by oxidative deamination of lysine residues to form reactive aldehydes. This oxidized lysine crosslinking motif is similar for the collagens and is catalyzed by the copper-requiring enzyme, lysyl oxidase. Associated with the tropoelastin, both during synthesis and in the extracellular space is an elastin-binding protein that presumably prevents aggregations within the cell, mediates cell adhesion to elastin, facilitates elastin fiber assembly, and protects it from elastolytic degradation. This elastin-binding protein is very homologous to an enzymatically inactive isoform of β-galactosidase and its interactions with elastin can be dissociated by exposure to galactosugars (67).

In tissues, elastin is found in close association with another structural glycoprotein, fibrillin. The fibrillins are a family of structural glycoproteins initially identified in association with the amorphous core of elastin, but found also as isolated bundles of 10 nm diameter microfibrils in most connective tissues (193). Marfan's syndrome is associated with mutations in fibrillin-1 which are primarily located in the calcium binding domain. Fibrillin-1 contains 43 precursor epidermal growth factor-like (pEGF) domains that have a consensus sequence for calcium binding and a separate domain for an unusual β-hydroxylation of Asp/Asn (50). In the heart, fibrillin is distributed at the interface of the cardiac muscle cell surface and matrix, transferring tension from the contracting myocardial cells to the cardiac matrix. At the dermal/epidermal junction, fibrillin penetrates into the lamina densa of the basement membrane. In bone, fibrillin is found in conjunction with type III collagen and at the bone-periosteum interface is associated with linking the mineralized bone cortex to ligaments and tendons.

Entactin/Nidogen

Entactin is a major constituent of the basement membrane, and is a dumbbell-shaped molecule with a pair of NH_2-terminal globular domains linked by a relatively rigid rod to a COOH-terminal globular domain. The rodlike domain consists of EGF modules and a thyroglobulin module and with overall size of about 150 kd. Entactin is a structural element binding laminin to type IV collagen. The COOH-terminal domain of entactin has a high affinity for laminin near the intersection of the laminin arms and the NH_2-terminal domain a high affinity for calcium. Entactin contains the (RGD) Arg-Gly-Asp, sequence and potential tyrosine O-sulfation and consensus N-glycosylation sites (108).

Fibronectin

Fibronectin is an adhesive, a solid phase element, a cell surface matrix protein bound to receptors and a fluid phase element in the blood serving as an opsonin and chemoattractant. It is a polyvalent molecule with affinities for fibrin, collagen, heparin, thrombospondin, integrins, components in bacterial cell coats and itself. Fibronectin is produced early in embryogenesis and plays an important role in guiding migratory cells during early morphogenesis. In wound healing, fibronectin, as an intact molecule and as peptide fragments, is chemotactic. It also forms a substrate to which the cells involved in the repair reaction can adhere (3). Microorganisms have cell surface adhesive molecules, adhesins, which bind to fibronectin and play a role in infectivity (93). Elevated levels of fibronectin occurs in the joint fluid of patients with arthritis.

The polyfunctional binding of fibronectin is accomplished by the presence of unique domains along the axis of the two approximately 200 kd polypeptide chains. There are three types of such repeating sequences in fibronectin, types I, II, and III and over thirty of these three repeats are arranged along one fibronectin chain. The absence of a single type III repeat near the carboxy terminus determines the differences between the serum and cell-associated forms of fibronectin. The production of the plasma form of fibronectin, with the missing type III repeat, involves alternative RNA splicing. There are three exons in fibronectin which are candidates for alternative splicing making it possible to construct over 20 different proteins from one gene. The repeating domains are grouped into larger functional domains that have bindings affinities for heparin, fibrin, collagen, and cell surfaces. The binding of fibronectin to the cell is mediated by the sequence Arg-Gly-Asp (RGD). The major receptors for the fibronectins are the integrins.

The multiplicities of interactions possible because of the domain structure of monomers and/or multimers of the matrix components is well illustrated with the apparently contradictory effects fibronectin and its proteolytic fragments have on cell migration and anchorage. For example, fibroblasts interact with the integrin-binding domain and both heparin-binding domains of plasma fibronectin and this combination of interactions determines whether a cell adheres to the matrix or migrates upon it. The different fibronectin isotypes, their multiple receptors, and varying interactions of one or more domains with those receptors thus produces a spectrum of responses in different cell types. Add to this elegant complexity the competitive binding of fibronectin by other matrix components and a pattern emerges of matrix molecules as an orchestra with an unlimited repertoire (8,156).

Glypican, Cerebroglycan

Glypican is a cell surface heparan sulfate proteoglycan, with a core protein linked to the cell surface by a glycosyl-phosphatidylinositol (GPI) linkage. The core protein has both N-linked carbohydrate and four potential sites for O-linked heparan sulfate. The anchorage of the core protein to the cell surface via a phosphoinositol linkage renders it susceptible to cleavage by phospholipases and glypican is readily shed from the cell surface. Additional (GPI)-anchored heparan sulfate proteoglycans have been identified in neuronal tissues and intestinal epithelial cells, the former named cerebroglycan. Cerebroglycan appears in neurons only during their migratory phase through areas containing laminin (72) and fibronectin (152), suggesting an important role in the development of the nervous system (158).

Hyaluronan

Hyaluronan (HA) is found in all three phases of the matrix. As a solid phase matrix element it occurs in association with aggrecan and link proteins forming the compressible structure of cartilage. As a fluid phase matrix element, it circulates in the plasma and flows in the synovial space under normal and abnormal conditions. And as a cell surface matrix element, it is present on the cell surface in both a receptor bound form and as an integral membrane component (Figs. 1 and 3).

Hyaluronan is not covalently bound to protein, is the only GAG which is not sulfated and consists of a repeating disaccharide of glucuronic acid and N-acetyl-glucosamine. HA is involved in biological situations as varied as embryonic development, wound healing and tumor invasion and it is an important constituent of many tissues. Hyaluronan is present in the serum of humans and cleared by the liver. The serum levels are elevated in a variety of clinical disorders including liver disease and arthritis. Patients with rheumatoid arthritis show elevations in plasma levels, particularly early in the day in association with morning stiffness. Because of its extended conformation, it is highly hydrated and usually associated with edematous, loosely organized matrices (Figs. 1 and 3).

Hyaluronan is synthesized in the cytosol and extrudes directly through the cell membrane providing the cell with an extended "whisker" or "antenna" (94,98). After synthesis and extension into the extracellular space, non–surface bound HA is released by an unknown mechanism (23). In the matrix, HA plays a central role in tissue structure through interactions with other matrix molecules including aggrecan, link protein and type VI collagen (90).

Integrins

Integrins constitute a family of membrane-spanning, heterodimeric proteins that mediate adhesive interactions between cells and surrounding extracellular matrices (or other cells) and participate in signal transduction (74,133).

Each integrin consists of a noncovalently associated α and β subunit. The integrins are involved in both cell-cell and cell-matrix interactions. There are nearly a dozen α subunits and half as many β, which can associate in a variety of combinations leading to various binding affinities. A full review of the integrins is beyond the scope of this chapter.

Laminins

The laminins are a family of polyvalent structural glycoproteins, first isolated from the EHS sarcoma and shown to be a prominent component of most basement membranes. The monomer is comprised of three polypeptide chains, originally named A, B1, and B2, but recently renamed α, β, and γ (21). At present, three isoforms of the α and β chains and two of the γ have been described in seven different arrangements. Laminin-1 is $\alpha1,\beta1,\gamma1$; laminin-2 is $\alpha2,\beta1,\gamma1$ previously called merosin; laminin-3 is $\alpha1,\beta2,\gamma1$, previously called s-laminin; laminin-4 is $\alpha2,\beta2,\gamma1$, previously called s-merosin; laminin-5 is $\alpha3,\beta3,\gamma2$, previously called kalinin, nicein or epiligrin; laminin-6 is $\alpha x,\beta1,\gamma1$ and laminin-7 $\alpha x,\beta2,\gamma1$, called k-laminin and ks-laminin respectively(169). The three chains are entwined to form a cross-shaped structure comprised of both globular and nonglobular regions. Receptor-mediated cell attachment and heparin binding reside in the terminal region of the long arm while a separate cell attachment site, a solid phase signaling site with mitogenic capacity, binding sites for entactin and the calcium-dependent sites involved in aggregation are in the short arms (28,162,190). These various sites are principally composed of cysteine-rich regions with epidermal growth factor and perlecan homologies (188).

The list of functions of the laminins grows rapidly and range from the structural to the regulatory. As a structural element, it is a major constituent of the basement membrane; it is a major constituent of the neuromuscular junction where its structural functions are matched by its solid phase signaling; and it is a major constituent of the glomerulus where its structural functions are closely related to its being a filter and, perhaps, an incidental antigen and ligand of DNA-histone complexes. As a regulatory element, laminin is a major promoter of neurite outgrowth; it is significantly increased on the surfaces of transformed cells and may stimulate metastasis (32). Other proteolytic fragments of the laminin A chain are strongly chemotactic for mast cells which, having been attracted to a site of laminin a chain degradation, are able to produce laminin B chains, type IV collagen and heparan sulfate proteoglycan (168).

Laminin and its complex with entactin play an important modulatory role in angiogenesis, in a dose dependent manner: low concentrations stimulating, high concentrations inhibiting. These effects suggest that the basement membrane is a dynamic regulator of angiogenesis whose function varies depending on the concentration of its molecular components and on the presence of additional factors such as β-fibroblast growth factor (bFGF) (121).

Link

Link is a protein isolated from cartilage which stabilizes the interactions of the NH_2-terminus of aggrecan with hyaluronan. The structure of link shows similarities to CD44. Link is not restricted to cartilaginous structures, but has also been found in the embryonic chick mesonephros (13).

Netrins

A family of proteins from the floor plate of the neural tube during early development, called netrins (151), have been identified and they show close homologies to UNC-6, a laminin-related protein involved in the migrations of cells and axons in *Caenorhabditis elegans.* UNC-6 and the netrins, binding to the matrix and/or the surfaces of cells, within or outside the basement membrane, are likely early candidates for molecular guidance cues for cells during early development (175).

Osteocalcin

The proteins in the organic matrix of bone are many including those made by bone such as type I collagen, alkaline phosphatase, SPARC, biglycan, decorin, osteocalcin and osteopontin and others such as α2-HS-glycoprotein, TGF-β, PDGF, IGF-1, FGF-α, FGF-β, and IL-1, which are synthesized elsewhere and which bind secondarily to the bone matrix. Osteocalcin is seemingly a specific bone cell product and is one of the few matrix proteins which contains a high content of γ-carboxyglutamic acid (GLA). Osteocalcin can be detected in the circulation and is associated with an increased risk for osteoporosis and hip fracture (75,164).

Interestingly, while osteocalcin is relatively restricted to bone, its release by bone fragments does not stimulate mononuclear cells to release interleukin 1 (IL-1) and is likely not to play a role in the increased IL-1 secretion by circulating monocytes in patients with high turnover osteoporosis. Rather it appears that the collagen fragments, detected by integrin receptors on the monocytes, are responsible for IL-1 release (125).

Osteopontin

Osteopontin, originally called bone sialoprotein, is an acidic glycoprotein which is prominent in bone and teeth, but also found in other connective tissues(34). It binds to both an integrin receptor and also to the inorganic hydroxyapetite in the mineral phase of bone. Its synthesis is increased by both TGF-β and 1,25-dihydroxyvitamin D3. Osteoclast adherence to bone and its subsequent resorption stem from interactions between osteopontin and/or bone sialoprotein and an integrin receptor (87). The tartrate-resistant acid phosphatase (TRAP) of osteoclasts dephosphorylates osteopontin and bone sialoprotein reducing osteoclast binding (12). An interesting feature of osteopontin is the presence of a thrombin-cleavage site close to its integrin binding site. Cell attachment and spreading was increased on thrombin-cleaved osteopontin, possibly through exposure of the integrin binding site (150).

Perlecan

Perlecan is the major heparan sulfate proteoglycan of basement membranes and has modular structure with domains homologous to the low density lipoprotein receptor, laminin, epidermal growth factor, and neural cell adhesion molecule. At the carboxy terminus there are three GAG chains of the heparan sulfate type and sometimes of the chondroitin sulfate type (76). Perlecan plays an integral role in the structure of basement membranes (191). As a structural element, it plays a major charge-dependent sieving function in the basement membrane. It interacts with itself, both though its protein core and GAG chains and also interacts with type IV collagen, laminin, basic fibroblast growth factor and extracellular superoxide dismutase C.

The glycosaminoglycan chains of heparin and heparan sulfate can serve as potent signals if released by endoglycosidases. In addition to known effects on hemostasis, the fragments of these glycosaminoglycan chains can dampen the stimulus to replication of smooth muscle cells which have been subjected to stimulation by platelet derived growth factor. Regulation of bFGF-stimulated VSMC proliferation, by vascular cell-secreted heparin-like compounds, correlates with inhibition of bFGF binding to cell-associated heparan sulfate proteoglycans (124).

Direct relationships between perlecan production, amyloid formation and Alzheimer's disease have been demonstrated (83). Perlecan, laminin and type IV collagen are synthesized at sites of amyloid deposition, but before amyloid fibrils form. The polymerized perlecan induces serum amyloid A protein to assume a β-pleated sheet structure. Administration of low molecular weight anionic sulfate or sulphonate compounds apparently competes with the perlecan-SAA interactions with reduction of splenic AA amyloid progression in a murine model (91).

Serglycin

All types of hematopoeitic cells produce a secretory form of proteoglycans, the best know of which is serglycin, named because of the frequent sequences Ser-Gly, consensus sequences for O-linkage of GAG chains. Serglycin is produced by all types of hematopoietic cells in both a regulated and constitutive fashion including mast cells, basophils, T lymphocytes and NK cells. Serglycin is a proteinase-resistant proteoglycan whose function is to store and protect a variety of agonists with which it is copackaged. The serglycin protein core is highly glycosylated by a variety of GAG chains and this secretory, fluid phase matrix component has been implicated in the regulation of inflammation, immune responses and coagulation of blood. In circulating cells such as mast cells, platelets and NK cells, there is evidence that serglycin is complexed with cationic proteins and pharmacologic amines such as histamine, complexes that show variable sensitivities to environmental conditions such as pH and counter ions. Presumably the interactions of serglycin with these agonists, both within the cell and after discharge into the matrix represents a means for regulating the release and rates of degradation of bioactive reagents.

SPARC

SPARC, for *s*ecreted *p*rotein *a*cidic *r*ich in *c*ysteine, is also called osteonectin and BM-40 and is a solid phase, fluid phase and cell-surface phase matrix glycoprotein, found in bone, serum and in the basement membrane. It is present in platelets and released by collagen or thrombin from platelets in a dose-dependent manner; it is also present on the platelet cell surface. The platelet form of SPARC appears to be larger than that found in bone.

In vitro, SPARC induces cell rounding, as do thrombospondin and tenscin, and all three thus can act to inhibit cell spreading. Sparc interacts with collagen types III, V, and thrombospondin. The affinities of SPARC for the matrix are calcium dependent and act in concert with other regions of the molecule to inhibit cellular spreading. Endothelial cells, for example, fail to adhere to type III collagen gels which contain SPARC It has been suggested that cell shape influences might also operate in cells such as the Leydig and Sertoli cells in the testis. SPARC is released from endothelial cells when injured, leading to a rounded cell morphology and gaps between the cells. If the cells' F-actin is stabilized by with phallicidin prior to injury this effect is not seen suggesting that SPARC regulates endothelial barrier function through F-actin-dependent changes in cell shape (52).

When SPARC is added to cells in culture the effects on cell anchorage and migration are not inhibited by the RGD peptide. The biologic effects of SPARC are dependent on calcium binding at both NH_2 and COOH terminal 9E-F9 hand modules. The 90-kd protein contains a high percentage of cysteine and there is high homology among SPARC proteins obtained from various species.

Syndecan

The syndecans are a family of integral membrane cell surface proteoglycans which are found primarily on epithelial cells, but also transiently on mesenchyme at sites of epithelial-mesenchymal interactions. At present four different syndecans have been described and the nomenclature as syndecan-1, . . . syndecan-4 will presumably replace a variety of names which emerged (ryudocan, amphiglycan) for various members. The syndecans associate extracellularly with various matrix molecules and growth factors and intracellularly with the actin cytoskeleton (68).

The principal glycosaminoglycan chain linked to the syndecans is heparan sulfate. Syndecan-1 on mouse mammary epithelial cells shows preferential increase in chondroitin sulfate when treated with TGF-β and that on the vaginal epithelium of the mouse is significantly modulated by either endogenous or exogenous estrogens and progesterones (62).

Syndecans act as matrix ligands binding to most components of the interstitial matrix including collagen types I, III, and V, fibronectin, thrombospondin, and tenascin in a calcium independent manner. Syndecan is shed from the cell surface when the cells round up; conversely, epithelial cells made syndecan deficient assume a mesenchymal morphology. In the adult mouse, syndecan is predominantly distributed on the surface of epithelial cells in a variety of patterns depending on the tissue of origin; no syndecan is present on stromal cells in the adult mouse with the exception of plasma cells and Leydig cells. However in embryonic tissues, under circumstances of epithelial-mesenchymal interactions as in the tooth and limb, syndecan is transiently expressed on mesencyhme. Syndecan is expressed on the surface of plasma cells, initially when present as pre-B cells in the marrow, but not when circulating in the blood, and then again when present in tissues such as the lymph nodes and spleen (11).

Perhaps one of the major functions of the syndecans is as a coreceptor in which the syndecan presents bound ligands to adjacent receptors which possess higher ligand specificity and/or signaling capacities. This would seem to be the case with basic fibroblast growth factor, fibronectin, antithrombin III in their interactions with the syndecans and also for the interactions of TGF-β with betaglycan. A precedent for this kind of function is readily found in the multiple steps in antigen presentation and processing which occurs in the immune system and in the various binding steps and effectors of the cytokines.

Tenascin

Tenascin is a large matrix glycoprotein prominent in states of high tissue remodelling and morphogenesis. It was originally described at the myotendinous junction at which site it presumably plays an important biomechanical function. The binding of tenascin to fibronectin has been questioned, but recent studies indicate a weak affinity, which nonetheless is sufficient to block cell binding and migration on fibronectin. This effect of tenascin is probably based in its capacity to block or mask either the fibronectin and/or its receptors. Review of Fig. 3 demonstrates that the large extended configuration of tenascin could have significant, nonspecific effects not only on fibronectin/cell surface interactions, but other ligand-receptor interactions as well. In the developing chick limb, a tenascin-rich sheet has been identified which extends from the ectodermal basement membrane to the proximally located muscle anlage. This sheet lies in the position with which the tendons form and Hurle and colleagues have suggested that it represents a template which influences the spatial organization of the tendons in the limb.

Thrombomodulin

Thrombomodulin is an integral membrane protein on the endothelial cell surface and a "part-time" proteoglycan. Thrombomodulin influences coagulation by acting as a a cofactor for thrombin-induced protein C activation; altering the procoagulant activity of thrombin; andaccelerating antithrombin III inhibition of thrombin. These activities are significantly influenced by the presence or absence of solitary chondroitin sulfate chain (102). Transcriptional downregulation of thrombomodulin occurs when cultured endothelial cells are exposed to cytokines, while upregulation occurs after exposure to retinoic acid and dibutyryl cyclic AMP (30)

Thrombospondin

Thrombospondin (TSP) is a family of glycoproteins of three identical disulfide-bonded subunits, a constituent of platelet α–granules and the product of a variety of cells (16). TSP binds to cell surfaces and becomes incorporated into the extracellular matrix where it exerts a broad spectrum of activities ranging from activation of TGF-β (146) to inhibition of enzymes such as plasmin and neutrophil elastase (69). TSP forms specific complexes with active TGF-β in platelet releasate and activates endogenous latent TGF-β secreted by endothelial cells indicating that TSP is a major regulatory factor in the control of TGF-β activity (147). TSP influences platelet aggregation, fibrin formation and lysis, cell adhesion and migration, and cell proliferation (78) and promotes neutrophil adhesion and migration and monocyte recruitment at sites of injury injury site (104). TSP is also an antiadhesive in that TSP can cause a loss of focal adhesion plaques from spreading endothelial cells and fibroblasts (117).

Vitronectin

Vitronectin (VN), also known as serum spreading factor, complement S protein, or epibolin, is an adhesive glycoprotein that interacts with complement, coagulation, fibrinolytic, and immunological components as well as cells and platelets (167). The nonplasma forms of VN, abundant in platelets and subendothelium, assumes the conformation of the heparin binding form. By assuming different conformations, VN exposes unique multivalent properties and unique functions (159). Many of the interactions of VN with complement derivatives C7, C8, and C9 occur via this heparin binding domain near the COOH-terminus. Vitronectin also binds to collagens and elastins, but it does not bind to laminin and fibronectin. Vitronectin interacts with the integrin class receptors through an RGD consensus sequence and vitronectin receptor also has specificity for osteopontin (148). Cross-linked mulitmers of vitronectin can be generated by a transgluaminase and the alignment of the VN monomers during this cross-linking is facilitated by their interaction with GAG. The cross-linked forms of VN retain binding affinites to heparin, platelets and plasminogen activator inhibitor type-1 (PAI-1,97).

REFERENCES

1. Acton S, Resnick D, Freeman M, Ekkel Y, Ashkenas J, Krieger M. The collagenous domains of macrophage scavenger receptors and complement component C1q mediate their similar, but not identical, binding specificities for polyanionic ligands. *J Biol Chem* 1993;268:3530–3537.
2. Andres JL, DeFalcis D, Noda M, Massague J. Binding of two growth factor families to separate domains of the proteoglycan betaglycan. *J Biol Chem* 1992;267:5927–5930.
3. Anwar AR, Walsh GM, Cromwell O, Kay AB, Wardlaw AJ. Adhesion to fibronectin primes eosinophils via alpha 4 beta 1 (VLA-4). *Immunology* 1994;82:222–228.
4. Apte SS, Mattei MG, Olsen BR. Cloning of the cDNA encoding human tissue inhibitor of metalloproteinases-3 (TIMP-3) and mapping of the TIMP3 gene to chromosome 22. *Genomics* 1994; 19:86–90.
5. Attisano L, Wrana JL, Lopez CF, Massague J. TGF-beta receptors and actions. *Biochim Biophys Acta* 1994;1222:71–80.
6. Aumailley M, Battaglia C, Mayer U, et al. Nidogen mediates the formation of ternary complexes of basement membrane components. *Kidney Int* 1993;43:7–12.
7. Aviezer D, Levy E, Safran M, et al. Differential structural requirements of heparin and heparan sulfate proteoglycans that promote binding of basic fibroblast growth factor to its receptor. *J Biol Chem* 1994;269:114–121.
8. Barkalow FJ, Schwarzbauer JE. Interactions between fibronectin and chondroitin sulfate are modulated by molecular context. *J Biol Chem* 1994;269:3957–3962.
9. Benezra M, Vlodavsky I, Ishai MR, Neufeld G, Bar SR. Thrombin-induced release of active basic fibroblast growth factor-heparan sulfate complexes from subendothelial extracellular matrix. *Blood* 1993;81:3324–3331.
10. Berg S, Hesselvik JF, Laurent TC. Influence of surgery on serum concentrations of hyaluronan. *Crit Care Med* 1994;22:810–814.
11. Bernfield M, Kokenyesi R, Kato M, et al. Biology of the syndecans: a family of transmembrane heparan sulfate proteoglycans. *Annu Rev Cell Biol* 1992;8:365–393.
12. Binette F, Cravens J, Kahoussi B, Haudenschild DR, Goetinck PF. Dephosphorylation of osteopontin and bone sialoprotein by osteoclastic tartrate-resistant acid phosphatase. Modulation of osteoclast adhesion in vitro. *J Biol Chem* 1994;269:14853–14856.
13. Binette F, Cravens J, Kahoussi B, Haudenschild DR, Goetinck PF. Link protein is ubiquitously expressed in non-cartilaginous tissues where it enhances and stabilizes the interaction of proteoglycans with hyaluronic acid. *J Biol Chem* 1994;269:19116–19122.
14. Birk DE, Silver FH, Trelstad RL. Matrix assembly. In: Hay ED, ed. *Cell biology of extracellular matrix.* New York: Plenum Press, 1991: 221–254.
15. Bonner JC. Regulation of platelet-derived growth factor (PDGF) and alveolar macrophage-derived PDGF by alpha 2-macroglobulin. *Ann NY Acad Sci* 1994;737:324–338.
16. Bornstein P. Diversity of function is inherent in matricellular proteins: an appraisal of thrombospondin 1. *J Cell Biol* 1995;130: 503–506.
17. Bourguignon LY, Lokeshwar VB, He J, Chen X, Bourguignon GJ. A CD44-like endothelial cell transmembrane glycoprotein (GP116) interacts with extracellular matrix and ankyrin. *Mol Cell Biol* 1992; 12:4464–4471.
18. Brewton RG, Wright DW, Mayne R. Structural and functional comparison of type IX collagen-proteoglycan from chicken cartilage and vitreous humor. *J Biol Chem* 1991;266:4752–4757.
19. Brunner G, Metz CN, Nguyen H, et al. An endogenous glycosylphosphatidylinositol-specific phospholipase D releases basic fibroblast growth factor-heparan sulfate proteoglycan complexes from human bone marrow cultures. *Blood* 1994;83:2115–2125.
20. Buckwalter JA, Roughley PJ, Rosenberg LC. Age-related changes in cartilage proteoglycans: quantitative electron microscopic studies. *Microsc Res Techn* 1994;28:398–408.
21. Burgeson RE, Chiquet M, Deutzmann R, et al. A new nomenclature for laminins. *Matrix Biol* 1994;5:209–211.
22. Burgeson RE, Nimni ME. Collagen types. Molecular structure and tissue distribution. *Clin Orthop* 1992;282:250–272.
23. Calabro A, Hascall VC. Differential effects of brefeldin A on chondroitin sulfate and hyaluronan synthesis in rat chondrosarcoma cells. *J Biol Chem* 1994;269:22764–22770.
24. Campanelli JT, Roberds SL, Campbell KP, Scheller RH. A role for dystrophin-associated glycoproteins and utrophin in agrin-induced AChR clustering. *Cell* 1994;77:663–674.
25. Carey DJ. Control of growth and differentiation of vascular cells by extracellular matrix proteins. *Annu Rev Physiol* 1991;53:161–177.
26. Carey DJ, Stahl RC, Asundi VK, Tucker B. Processing and subcellular distribution of the Schwann cell lipid-anchored heparan sulfate proteoglycan and identification as glypican. *Exp Cell Res* 1993;208: 10–18.
27. Chen D, Magnuson V, Hill S, Arnaud C, Steffensen B, Klebe RJ. Regulation of integrin gene expression by substrate adherence. *J Biol Chem* 1992;267:23502–23506.
28. Colognato-Pyke H, O'Rear JJ, Yamada Y, Carbonetto S, Cheng Y, Yurchenco PD. Mapping of network-forming, heparin binding, and $\alpha 1\beta 1$ Integrin-recognition sites within the α-chain short arm of laminin-1. *J Biol Chem* (in press).
29. Colombatti A, Bonaldo P, Doliana R. Type A modules: interacting domains found in several non-fibrillar collagens and in other extracellular matrix proteins. *Matrix* 1993;13:297–306.
30. Conway EM, Liu L, Nowakowski B, Steiner MM, Jackman RW. Heat shock of vascular endothelial cells induces an up-regulatory transcriptional response of the thrombomodulin gene that is delayed in onset and does not attenuate. *J Biol Chem* 1994;269: 22804–22810.
31. David G. Integral membrane heparan sulfate proteoglycans. *FASEB J* 1993;7:1023–1030.
32. De Rosa G, Barra E, Guarino M, Staibano S, Donofrio V, Boscaino A. Fibronectin, laminin, type IV collagen distribution, and myofibroblastic stromal reaction in aggressive and nonaggressive basal cell carcinoma. *Am J Dermatopathol* 1994;16:258–267.
33. Denhardt DT, Feng B, Edwards DR, Cocuzzi ET, Malyankar UM. Tissue inhibitor of metalloproteinases (TIMP, aka EPA): structure, control of expression and biological functions. *Pharmacol Ther* 1993;59:329–341.
34. Denhardt DT, Guo X. Osteopontin: a protein with diverse functions. *FASEB J* 1993;7:1475–1482.
35. Edelstam GA, Lundkvist O, Venge P, Laurent TC. Hyaluronan and myeloperoxidase in human peritoneal fluid during genital inflammation. *Inflammation* 1994;18:141–149.
36. Eielson C, Kaplan D, Mitnick MA, Paliwal I, Insogna K. Estrogen modulates parathyroid hormone-induced fibronectin production in human and rat osteoblast-like cells. *Endocrinology* 1994;135: 1639–1644.
37. Ekblom P, Ekblom M, Fecker L, et al. Role of mesenchymal nidogen for epithelial morphogenesis in vitro. *Development* 1994;120: 2003–2014.
38. el Khoury J, Thomas CA, Loike JD, Hickman SE, Cao L, Silverstein SC. Macrophages adhere to glucose-modified basement membrane collagen IV via their scavenger receptors. *J Biol Chem* 1994; 269:10197–10200.
39. Engel J. Common structural motifs in proteins of the extracellular matrix. *Curr Opin Cell Biol* 1991;3:779–785.
40. Ennker IC, Ennker J, Schoon D, Schoon HA, Rimpler M, Hetzer R. Formaldehyde-free collagen glue in experimental lung gluing. *Ann Thorac Surg* 1994;57:1622–1627.
41. Erickson HP. Tenascin-C, tenascin-R and tenascin-X: a family of talented proteins in search of functions. *Curr Opin Cell Biol* 1993;5: 869–876.
42. Falcone DJ, McCaffrey TA, Haimovitz FA, Garcia M. Transforming growth factor-beta 1 stimulates macrophage urokinase expression and release of matrix-bound basic fibroblast growth factor. *J Cell Physiol* 1993;155:595–605.
43. Ferns M, Hoch W, Campanelli JT, Rupp F, Hall ZW, Scheller RH. RNA splicing regulates agrin-mediated acetylcholine receptor clustering activity on cultured myotubes. *Neuron* 1992;8:1079–1086.
44. Fichard A, Kleman J-P, Ruggiero F. Another look at collage V and XI molecules. *Matrix Biol* 1994;14:515–531.
45. Friedlander DR, Milev P, Karthikeyan L, Margolis RK, Margolis

RU, Grumet M. The neuronal chondroitin sulfate proteoglycan neurocan binds to the neural cell adhesion molecules Ng-CAM/L1/NILE and N-CAM, and inhibits neuronal adhesion and neurite outgrowth. *J Cell Biol* 1994;125:669–680.
46. Fukushima D, Butzow R, Hildebrand A, Ruoslahti E. Localization of transforming growth factor beta binding site in betaglycan. Comparison with small extracellular matrix proteoglycans. *J Biol Chem* 1993;268:22710–22705.
47. Funderburgh JL, Funderburgh ML, Brown SJ, et al. Sequence and structural implications of a bovine corneal keratan sulfate proteoglycan core protein. Protein 37B represents bovine lumican and proteins 37A and 25 are unique. *J Biol Chem* 1993;268: 11874–11880.
48. Gallagher JT. Heparan sulphates as membrane receptors for the fibroblast growth factors. *Eur J Clin Chem Clin Biochem* 1994;32: 239–247.
49. Gee SH, Montanaro F, Lindenbaum MH, Carbonetto S. Dystroglycan-alpha, a dystrophin-associated glycoprotein, is a functional agrin receptor. *Cell* 1994;77:675–686.
50. Glanville RW, Qian RQ, McClure DW, Maslen CL. Calcium binding, hydroxylation, and glycosylation of the precursor epidermal growth factor-like domains of fibrillin-1, the Marfan gene protein. *J Biol Chem* 1994;269:26630–26634.
51. Goetinck P, Winterbottom N. Proteoglycans: modular macromolecules of the extracellular matrix. In: Goldstein L, ed. *Biochemistry and physiology of the skin.* Oxford: Oxford University Press, 1991:558–575.
52. Goldblum SE, Ding X, Funk SE, Sage EH. SPARC (secreted protein acidic and rich in cysteine) regulates endothelial cell shape and barrier function. *Proc Natl Acad Sci USA* 1994;91:3448–3452.
53. Gordon JL, Drummond AH, Galloway WA. Metalloproteinase inhibitors as therapeutics. *Clin Exp Rheumatol* 1993;11:591–594.
54. Grumet M, Milev P, Sakurai T, et al. Interactions with tenascin and differential effects on cell adhesion of neurocan and phosphacan, two major chondroitin sulfate proteoglycans of nervous tissue. *J Biol Chem* 1994;269:12142–12146.
55. Hagen SG, Michael AF, Butkowski RJ. Immunochemical and biochemical evidence for distinct basement membrane heparan sulfate proteoglycans. *J Biol Chem* 1993;268:7261–7269.
56. Handagama P, Bainton DF, Jacques Y, Conn MT, Lazarus RA, Shuman MA. Kistrin, an integrin antagonist, blocks endocytosis of - fibrinogen into guinea pig megakaryocyte and platelet alphagranules. *J Clin Invest* 1993;91:193–200.
57. Hardingham TE, Fosang AJ. Proteoglycans: many forms and many functions. *FASEB J* 1992;6:861–870.
58. Hardingham TE, Fosang AJ, Dudhia J. The structure, function and turnover of aggrecan, the large aggregating proteoglycan from cartilage. *Eur J Clin Chem Clin Biochem* 1994;32:249–257.
59. Hauser N, Paulsson M. Native cartilage matrix protein (CMP). A compact trimer of subunits assembled via a coiled-coil alpha-helix. *J Biol Chem* 1994;269:25747–25753.
60. Hausser H, Witt O, Kresse H. Influence of membrane-associated heparan sulfate on the internalization of the small proteoglycan decorin. *Exp Cell Res* 1993;208:398–406.
61. Hay ED. Extracellular matrix alters epithelial differentiation. *Curr Opin Cell Biol* 1993;5:1029–1035.
62. Hayashi K, Hayashi M, Boutin E, Cunha GR, Bernfield M, Trelstad RL. Hormonal modification of epithelial differentiation and expression of cell surface heparan sulfate proteoglycan in the mouse vaginal epithelium. An immunohistochemical and electron microscopic study. *Lab Invest* 1988;58:68–76.
63. Heldrin C-H. Dimerization of cell surface receptors in signal transduction. *Cell* 1995;80:213–223.
64. Hermann M, Jaconi ME, Dahlgren C, Waldvogel FA, Stendahl O, Lew DP. Neutrophil bactericidal activity against *Staphylococcus aureus* adherent on biological surfaces. Surface-bound extracellular matrix proteins activate intracellular killing by oxygen-dependent and -independent mechanisms. *J Clin Invest* 1990;86:942–951.
65. Hershkoviz R, Gilat D, Miron S, et al. Extracellular matrix induces tumour necrosis factor-alpha secretion by an interaction between resting rat CD4+ T cells and macrophages. *Immunology* 1993;78: 50–57.
66. Hildebrand A, Romaris M, Rasmussen LM, et al. Interaction of the small interstitial proteoglycans biglycan, decorin and fibromodulin with transforming growth factor beta. *Biochem J* 1994;302: 527–534.
67. Hinek A, Rabinovitch M. 67-kD Elastin-binding protein is a protective "companion" of extracellular insoluble elastin and intracellular tropoelastin. *J Cell Biol* 1994;126:563–574.
68. Hinkes MT, Goldberger OA, Neumann PE, Kokenyesi R, Bernfield M. Organization and promoter activity of the mouse syndecan-1 gene. *J Biol Chem* 1993;268:11440–11448.
69. Hogg PJ, Owensby DA, Mosher DF, Misenheimer TM, Chesterman CN. Thrombospondin is a tight-binding competitive inhibitor of neutrophil elastase. *J Biol Chem* 1993;268:7139–7146.
70. Howlett AR, Bissell MJ. The influence of tissue microenvironment (stroma and extracellular matrix) on the development and function of mammary epithelium. *Epithelial Cell Biol* 1993;2:79–89.
71. Huang LL, Wu JH, Nimni ME. Effects of hyaluronan on collagen fibrillar matrix contraction by fibroblasts. *J Biomed Mater Res* 1994; 28:123–132.
72. Hunter DD, Llinas R, Ard M, Merlie JP, Sanes JR. Expression of S-laminin and laminin in developing rat central nervous system. *J Comp Neurol* 1992;323:238–251.
73. Hynes RO. *Fibronectins.* New York: Springer-Verlag, 1990.
74. Hynes RO. Integrins: versatility, modulation, and signaling in cell adhesion. *Cell* 1992;69:11–25.
75. Ingram RT, Park YK, Clarke BL, Fitzpatrick LA. Age- and gender-related changes in the distribution of osteocalcin in the extracellular matrix of normal male and female bone. Possible involvement of osteocalcin in bone remodeling. *J Clin Invest* 1994; 93:989–997.
76. Iozzo RV. Perlecan: a gem of a proteoglycan. *Matrix Biol* 1994;14: 203–208.
77. Iozzo RV, Kovalszky I, Hacobian N, Schick PK, Ellingson JS, Dodge GR. Fatty acylation of heparan sulfate proteoglycan from human colon carcinoma cells. *J Biol Chem* 1990;265:19980–19989.
78. Iruela AM, Liska DJ, Sage EH, Bornstein P. Differential expression of thrombospondin 1, 2, and 3 during murine development. *Dev Dyn* 1993;197:40–56.
79. Iwata M, Wight TN, Carlson SS. A brain extracellular matrix proteoglycan forms aggregates with hyaluronan. *J Biol Chem* 1993;268: 15061–15069.
80. Jackson RL, Busch SJ, Cardin AD. Glycosaminoglycans: molecular properties, protein interactions and role in physiological processes. *Physiol Rev* 1991;71:481–539.
81. Jennings CG, Burden SJ. Development of the neuromuscular synapse. *Curr Opin Neurobiol* 1993;3:75–81.
82. Jones PL, Schmidhauser C, Bissell MJ. Regulation of gene expression and cell function by extracellular matrix. *Crit Rev Eukaryot Gene Expr* 1993;3:137–154.
83. Jucker M, Ingram DK. Age-related fibrillar material in mouse brain. Assessing its potential as a biomarker of aging and as a model of human neurodegenerative disease. *Ann NY Acad Sci* 1994;719:238–247.
84. Juliano RL, Haskill S. Signal transduction from the extracellular matrix. *J Cell Biol* 1993;120:577–585.
85. Kagami S, Border WA, Miller DE, Noble NA. Angiotensin II stimulates extracellular matrix protein synthesis through induction of transforming growth factor-beta expression in rat glomerular mesangial cells. *J Clin Invest* 1994;93:2431–2437.
86. Kato M, Wang H, Bernfield M, Gallagher JT, Turnbull JE. Cell surface syndecan-1 on distinct cell types differs in fine structure and ligand binding of its heparan sulfate chains. *J Biol Chem* 1994;269:18881–18890.
87. Kato M, Wang H, Bernfield M, Gallagher JT, Turnbull JE. Interactions between the bone matrix proteins osteopontin and bone sialoprotein and the osteoclast integrin alpha v beta 3 potentiate bone resorption. *J Biol Chem* 1993;268:9901–9907.
88. Kato S, Ishii T, Hara H, Sugiura N, Kimata K, Akamatsu N. Hepatocyte growth factor immobilized onto culture substrates through heparin and matrigel enhances DNA synthesis in primary rat hepatocytes. *Exp Cell Res* 1994;211:53–58.
89. Kato Y, Uchida K, Kawakishi S. Oxidative fragmentation of collagen and prolyl peptide by Cu(II)/H_2O_2. Conversion of proline residue to 2-pyrrolidone. *J Biol Chem* 1992;267:23646–23651.
90. Kielty CM, Whittaker SP, Grant ME, Shuttleworth CA. Type VI collagen microfibrils: evidence for a structural association with hyaluronan. *J Cell Biol* 1992;118:979–990.
91. Kisilevsky R, Lemieux LJ, Fraser PF, Kong X, Hultin PG, Szarek WA. Arresting amyloidosis in vivo using small-molecule anionic sulphonates or sulphates: implications for Alzheimer's disease. *Nat Med* 1995;1:143–148.
92. Klein S, Giancotti FG, Presta M, Albelda SM, Buck CA, Rifkin DB.

Basic fibroblast growth factor modulates integrin expression in microvascular endothelial cells. *Mol Biol Cell* 1993;4:973–982.
93. Klotz SA, Hein RC, Smith RL, Rouse JB. The fibronectin adhesin of *Candida albicans*. *Infect Immunol* 1994;62:4679–4681.
94. Knudson W, Bartnik E, Knudson CB. Assembly of pericellular matrices by COS-7 cells transfected with CD44 lymphocyte-homing receptor genes. *Proc Natl Acad Sci USA* 1993;90:4003–4007.
95. Koide H, Hayashi T, ed. *Extracellular matrix in the kidney*. Karger, 1994.
96. Lander AD. Proteoglycans in the nervous system. *Curr Opin Neurobiol* 1993;3:716–723.
97. Lawrence DA, Berkenpas MB, Palaniappan S, Ginsburg D. Localization of vitronectin binding domain in plasminogen activator inhibitor-1. *J Biol Chem* 1994;269:15223–15228.
98. Lee GM, Johnstone B, Jacobson K, Caterson B. The dynamic structure of the pericellular matrix on living cells. *J Cell Biol* 1993;123:1899–1907.
99. Lesley J, Hyman R, Kincade PW. CD44 and its interaction with the cellular matrix. *Adv Immunol* 1993;54:271–335.
100. Lessey BA, Castelbaum AJ, Buck CA, Lei Y, Yowell CW, Sun J. Further characterization of endometrial integrins during the menstrual cycle and in pregnancy. *Fertil Steril* 1994;62:497–506.
101. Liebersbach BF, Sanderson RD. Expression of syndecan-1 inhibits cell invasion into type I collagen. *J Biol Chem* 1994;269:20013–20019.
102. Liu LW, Rezaie AR, Carson CW, Esmon NL, Esmon CT. Occupancy of anion binding exosite 2 on thrombin determines Ca^{2+} dependence of protein C activation. *J Biol Chem* 1994;269:11807–11812.
103. Lopez CF, Payne HM, Andres JL, Massague J. Betaglycan can act as a dual modulator of TGF-beta access to signaling receptors: mapping of ligand binding and GAG attachment sites. *J Cell Biol* 1994;124:557–568.
104. Mansfield PJ, Suchard SJ. Thrombospondin promotes chemotaxis and haptotaxis of human peripheral blood monocytes. *J Immunol* 1994;153:4219–29
105. Martini R. Expression and functional roles of neural cell surface molecules and extracellular matrix components during development and regeneration of peripheral nerves. *J Neurocytol* 1994;23:1–28.
106. Massague J, Attisano L, Wrana JL. The TGF-β family and its composite receptors. *Trends Cell Biol* 1994;4:172–178.
107. Maurel P, Rauch U, Flad M, Margolis RK, Margolis RU. Phosphacan, a chondroitin sulfate proteoglycan of brain that interacts with neurons and neural cell adhesion molecules, is an extracellular variant of a receptor-type protein tyrosine phosphatase. *Proc Natl Acad Sci USA* 1994;91:2512–2516.
108. Mayer U, Timpl R. Nidogen: a versatile binding protein of basement membranes. In: Yurchenco PD, Birk DE, Mecham RP, eds. *Extracellular matrix assembly and structure*. San Diego, Academic Press, 1994:389–416.
109. Mayne R, Brewton RG. New members of the collagen superfamily. *Curr Opin Cell Biol* 1993;5:883–890.
110. McMahan UJ, Horton SE, Werle MJ, et al. Agrin isoforms and their role in synaptogenesis. *Curr Opin Cell Biol* 1992;4:869–874.
111. Mecham RP, Davis EC. Elastic fibre structure and assembly. In: Yurchenco PD, Birk DE, Mecham RP, eds. *Extracellular matrix assembly and structure*. San Diego, Academic Press, 1994:281–314.
112. Medhora MM, Teitelbaum S, Chappel J, et al. 1-Alpha,25-dihydroxyvitamin D3 up-regulates expression of the osteoclast integrin alpha v beta 3. *J Biol Chem* 1993;268:1456–1461.
113. Medhora MM, Teitelbaum S, Chappel J, et al. 1-Alpha,25-dihydroxyvitamin D3 up-regulates expression of the osteoclast integrin alpha v beta 3. *J Biol Chem* 1993;268:1456–1461.
114. Mette SA, Pilewski J, Buck CA, Albelda SM. Distribution of integrin cell adhesion receptors on normal bronchial epithelial cells and lung cancer cells in vitro and in vivo. *Am J Respir Cell Mol Biol* 1993;8:562–572.
115. Milev P, Friedlander DR, Sakurai T, et al. Interactions of the chondroitin sulfate proteoglycan phosphacan, the extracellular domain of a receptor-type tyrosine phosphatase with neurons, glia and neural cell adhesion molecules. *J Cell Biol* 1994;127:1703–1715.
116. Morris JE. Proteoglycans and the modulation of cell adhesion by steric exclusion. *Dev Dyn* 1993;196:246–251.
117. Murphy UJ, Gurusiddappa S, Frazier WA, Hook M. Heparin-binding peptides from thrombospondins 1 and 2 contain focal adhesion-labilizing activity. *J Biol Chem* 1993;268:26784–26789.
118. Myers JC, Yang H, DíIppolito JA, Presente A, Miller MK, Dion AS. The triple-helical region of human type XIX collagen consists of multiple collagenous subdomains and exhibits limited sequence homology to alpha 1(XVI). *J Biol Chem* 1994;269:18549–18557.
119. Nakayama H, Ichikawa F, Andres JL, Massague J, Noda M. Dexamethasone enhancement of betaglycan (TGF-beta type III receptor) gene expression in osteoblast-like cells. *Exp Cell Res* 1994;211:301–306.
120. Nettelbladt O, Bergh J, Schenholm M, Tengblad A, Hallgren R. Accumulation of hyaluronic acid in the alveolar interstitial tissue in bleomycin-induced alveolitis. *Am Rev Respir Dis* 1989;139:759–762.
121. Nicosia RF, Bonanno E, Smith M, Yurchenco P. Modulation of angiogenesis in vitro by laminin-entactin complex. *Dev Biol* 1994;164:197–206.
122. Nishiyama T, McDonough AM, Bruns RR, Burgeson RE. Type XII and XIV collagens mediate interactions between banded collagen fibers in vitro and may modulate extracellular matrix deformability. *J Biol Chem* 1994;269:28193–28199.
123. Noonan DM, Hassell JR. Perlecan, the large low-density proteoglycan of basement membranes: structure and variant forms. *Kidney Int* 1993;43:53–60.
124. Nugent MA, Karnovsky MJ, Edelman ER. Vascular cell-derived heparan sulfate shows coupled inhibition of basic fibroblast growth factor binding and mitogenesis in vascular smooth muscle cells. *Circ Res* 1993;73:1051–1060.
125. Pacifici R, Carano A, Santoro SA, et al. Bone matrix constituents stimulate interleukin-1 release from human blood mononuclear cells. *J Clin Invest* 1991;87:221–228.
126. Patthy L, Nikolics K. Functions of agrin and agrin-related proteins. *Trends Neurosci* 1993;16:76–81.
127. Patti JM, Allen BL, McGavin M, Hook M. MSCRAMM-mediated adherence of microorganisms to host tissues. *Annu Rev Microbiol* 1994;48:585–617.
128. Petite H, Frei V, Huc A, Herbage D. Use of diphenylphosphorylazide for cross-linking collagen-based biomaterials. *J Biomed Mater Res* 1994;28:159–165.
129. Petry F, Reid KB, Loos M. Isolation, sequence analysis and characterization of cDNA clones coding for the C chain of mouse C1q. Sequence similarity of complement subcomponent C1q, collagen type VIII and type X and precerebellin. *Eur J Biochem* 1992;209:129–134.
130. Pfaff M, Aumailley M, Specks U, Knolle J, Zerwes HG, Timpl R. Integrin and Arg-Gly-Asp dependence of cell adhesion to the native and unfolded triple helix of collagen type VI. *Exp Cell Res* 1993;206:167–176.
131. Phillips CL, Combs SB, Pinnell SR. Effects of ascorbic acid on proliferation and collagen synthesis in relation to the donor age of human dermal fibroblasts. *J Invest Dermatol* 1994;103:228–232.
132. Poole AR, Ionescu M, Swan A, Dieppe PA. Changes in cartilage metabolism in arthritis are reflected by altered serum and synovial fluid levels of the cartilage proteoglycan aggrecan. Implications for pathogenesis. *J Clin Invest* 1994;94:25–33.
133. Potts JR, Campbell ID. Integrin-ligand interactions; a year in review. *Curr Opin Cell Biol* 1994;6:656–662.
134. Rao JK, Ramesh DV, Rao KP. Implantable controlled delivery systems for proteins based on collagenópHEMA hydrogels. *Biomaterials* 1994;15:383–389.
135. Reinhardt D, Mann K, Nischt R, et al. Mapping of nidogen binding sites for collagen type IV, heparan sulfate proteoglycan, and zinc. *J Biol Chem* 1993;268:10881–10887.
136. Reiser KM, Amigable MA, Last JA. Nonenzymatic glycation of type I collagen. The effects of aging on preferential glycation sites. *J Biol Chem* 1992;267:24207–24216.
137. Roberts AB, Sporn MB. Physiological actions and clinical applications of transforming growth factor-beta (TGF-beta). *Growth Factors* 1993;8:1–9.
138. Robinson CJ. Growth factors: therapeutic advances in wound healing. *Ann Med* 1993;25:535–538.
139. Roghani M, Mansukhani A, Dell'Era P, et al. Heparin increases the affinity of basic fibroblast growth factor for its receptor but is not required for binding. *J Biol Chem* 1994;269:3976–3984.
140. Rosenbloom J, Abrams WR, Mecham R. Extracellular matrix 4: the elastic fiber. *FASEB J* 1993;7:1208–1218.
141. Roughley PJ, Lee ER. Cartilage proteoglycans: structure and potential functions. *Microsc Res Techn* 1994;28:385–397.
142. Ruoslahti E. Control of cell motility and tumour invasion by extracellular matrix interactions. *Br J Cancer* 1992;66:239–242.
143. Ruoslahti E, Yamaguchi Y, Hildebrand A, Border WA. Extracellu-

lar matrix/growth factor interactions. *Cold Spring Harb Symp Quant Biol* 1992;87:309–315.
144. Sastry K, Ezekowitz RA. Collectins: pattern recognition molecules involved in first line host defense. *Curr Opin Immunol* 1993; 5:59–66.
145. Schrader M, Bendik I, Becker AM, Carlberg C. Interaction between retinoic acid and vitamin D signaling pathways. *J Biol Chem* 1993;268:17830–17836.
146. Schultz CS, Murphy UJ. Thrombospondin causes activation of latent transforming growth factor-beta secreted by endothelial cells by a novel mechanism. *J Cell Biol* 1993;122:923–932.
147. Schultz CS, Ribeiro S, Gentry L, Murphy UJ. Thrombospondin binds and activates the small and large forms of latent transforming growth factor-beta in a chemically defined system. *J Biol Chem* 1994;269:26775–26782.
148. Seiffert D, Crain K, Wagner NV, Loskutoff DJ. Vitronectin gene expression in vivo. Evidence for extrahepatic synthesis and acute phase regulation. *J Biol Chem* 1994;269:19836–19842.
149. Seltzer JL, Lee AY, Akers KT, et al. Activation of 72-kDa type IV collagenase/gelatinase by normal fibroblasts in collagen lattices is mediated by integrin receptors but is not related to lattice contraction. *Exp Cell Res* 1994;213:365–374.
150. Senger DR, Perruzzi CA, Papadopoulos SA, Van de Water L. Adhesive properties of osteopontin: regulation by a naturally occurring thrombin-cleavage in close proximity to the GRGDS cell-binding domain. *Mol Biol Cell* 1994;5:565–574.
151. Serafini T, Kennedy TE, Galko MJ, Mirzayan C, Jessell TM, Tessier LM. The netrins define a family of axon outgrowth-promoting proteins homologous to *C. elegans* UNC-6. *Cell* 1994;78:409–424.
152. Sheppard AM, Hamilton SK, Pearlman AL. Changes to the distribution of extracellular matrix components accompany early morphogeneic events of mammalian cortical development. *J Neurosci* 1991;11:3928–3942.
153. Sheppard D, Cohen DS, Wang A, Busk M. Transforming growth factor beta differentially regulates expression of integrin subunits in guinea pig airway epithelial cells. *J Biol Chem* 1992;267: 17409–17414.
154. Sherman L, Sleeman J, Herrlich P, Ponta H. Hyaluronate receptors: key players in growth, differentiation, migration and tumor progression. *Curr Opin Cell Biol* 1994;6:726–733.
155. Silbert CK, Humphries DE, Palmer ME, Silbert JE. Effects of sulfate deprivation on the production of chondroitin/dermatan sulfate by cultures of skin fibroblasts from normal and diabetic individuals. *Arch Biochem Biophys* 1991;285:137–141.
156. Sipes JM, Guo N, Negre E, Vogel T, Krutzsch HC, Roberts DD. Inhibition of fibronectin binding and fibronectin-mediated cell adhesion to collagen by a peptide from the second type I repeat of thrombospondin. *J Cell Biol* 1993;121:469–477.
157. Somers CE, Mosher DF. Localization of transforming growth factor beta binding site in betaglycan. Comparison with small extracellular matrix proteoglycans. *J Biol Chem* 1993;268: 22710–22715.
158. Stipp CS, Litwack ED, Lander AD. Cerebroglycan: An integral membrane heparan sulfate proteoglycan that is unique to the developing nervous system and expressed specifically during neuronal differentiation. *J Cell Biol* 1994;124:149–160.
159. Stockmann A, Hess S, Declerck P, Timpl R, Preissner KT. Multimeric vitronectin. Identification and characterization of conformation-dependent self-association of the adhesive protein. *J Biol Chem* 1993;268:22874–22882.
160. Streuli CH, Schmidhauser C, Kobrin M, Bissell MJ, Derynck R. Extracellular matrix regulates expression of the TGF-beta 1 gene. *J Cell Biol* 1993;120:253–260.
161. Sugiyama J, Bowen DC, Hall ZW. Dystroglycan binds nerve and muscle agrin. *Neuron* 1994;13:103–115.
162. Sung U, OíRear JJ, Yurchenco PD. Cell and heparin binding in the distal long arm of laminin: identification of active and cryptic sites with recombinant and hybrid glycoprotein. *J Cell Biol* 1993; 123:1255–1268.
163. Sutherland AE, Calarco PG, Damsky CH. Developmental regulation of integrin expression at the time of implantation in the mouse embryo. *Development* 1993;119:1175–1186.
164. Szulc P, Chapuy MC, Meunier PJ, Delmas PD. Serum undercarboxylated osteocalcin is a marker of the risk of hip fracture in elderly women. *J Clin Invest* 1993;91:1769–1774.
165. Taipale J, Miyazona K, Heldin C-H, Keski-Oja J. Latent transforming growth factor-b1 associates to fibroblast extracellular matrix via latent TGF-b binding protein. *J Cell Biol* 1994;124:171–181.
166. Tanaka Y, Adams DH, Shaw S. Proteoglycans on endothelial cells present adhesion-inducing cytokines to leukocytes. *Immunol Today* 1993;14:111–115.
167. Teschler H, Pohl WR, Thompson AB, et al. Elevated levels of bronchoalveolar lavage vitronectin in hypersensitivity pneumonitis. *Am Rev Respir Dis* 1993;147:332–337.
168. Thompson HL, Thomas L, Metcalfe DD. Murine mast cells attach to and migrate on laminin-, fibronectin-, and matrigel-coated surfaces in response to Fc epsilon RI-mediated signals. *Clin Exp Allergy* 1993;23:270–275.
169. Timpl R, Brown JC. The laminins. *Matrix Biol* 1994;14:275–281.
170. Underhill CB, Nguyen HA, Shizari M, Culty M. CD44 positive macrophages take up hyaluronan during lung development. *Dev Biol* 1993;155:324–336.
171. Upchurch HF, Conway E, Patterson MJ, Maxwell MD. Localization of cellular transglutaminase on the extracellular matrix after wounding: characteristics of the matrix bound enzyme. *J Cell Physiol* 1991;149:375–382.
172. Valeyre D, Soler P, Basset G, et al. Glucose, K^+, and albumin concentrations in the alveolar milieu of normal humans and pulmonary sarcoidosis patients. *Am Rev Respir Dis* 1991;143:1096–1101.
173. Van der Rest M, Garrone R. Collagen family of proteins. *FASEB J* 1991;5:2814–2823.
174. Vettel U, Brunner G, Bar SR, Vlodavsky I, Kramer MD. Charge-dependent binding of granzyme A (MTSP-1) to basement membranes. *Eur J Immunol* 1993;23:279–282.
175. Wadsworth WG, Hedgecock EM. Guidance of neuroblast migrations and axonal projections in *Caenorhabditis elegans*. *Curr Opin Neurobiol* 1992;2:36–41.
176. Wahl SM, Allen JB, Weeks BS, Wong HL, Klotman PE. Transforming growth factor beta enhances integrin expression and type IV collagenase secretion in human monocytes. *Proc Natl Acad Sci USA* 1993;90:4577–4581.
177. Walker A, Turnbull JE, Gallagher JT. Binding of fibromodulin and decorin to separate sites on fibrillar collagens. *J Biol Chem* 1993;268:27307–27312.
178. Wall NA, Blessing M, Wright CV, Hogan BL. SPARC, a secreted protein associated with morphogenesis and tissue remodeling, induces expression of metalloproteinases in fibroblasts through a novel extracellular matrix-dependent pathway. *J Cell Biol* 1993;121: 1433–1444.
179. Watanabe H, Kimata K, Line S, et al. Mouse cartilage matrix deficiency (cmd) caused by a 7-bp deletion in the aggrecan gene. *Nat Genet* 1994;7:154–157.
180. Whinna HC, Choi HU, Rosenberg LC, Church FC. Interaction of heparin cofactor II with biglycan and decorin. *J Biol Chem* 1993; 268:3920–3924.
181. Witt DP, Lander AD. Differential binding of chemokines to glycosaminoglcyan subpopulations. *Curr Biol* 1994;4:394–400.
182. Woessner JF. Matrix metalloproteinases and their inhibitors in connective tissue remodeling. *FASEB J* 1991;5:2145–2154.
183. Wu JJ, Woods PE, Eyre DR. Identification of cross-linking sites in bovine cartilage type IX collagen reveals an antiparallel type II–type IX molecular relationship and type IX to type IX bonding. *J Biol Chem* 1992;267:23007–23014.
184. Yamada H, Watanabe K, Shimonaka M, Yamaguchi Y. Molecular cloning of brevican, a novel brain proteoglycan of the aggrecan/versican family. *J Biol Chem* 1994;269:10119–10126.
185. Yamagata M, Saga S, Kato M, Bernfield M, Kimata K. Selective distributions of proteoglycans and their ligands in pericellular matrix of cultured fibroblasts. Implications for their roles in cell-substratum adhesion. *J Cell Sci* 1993;106:55–65.
186. Yamagata M, Yamada KM, Yamada SS, et al. The complete primary structure of type XII collagen shows a chimeric molecule with reiterated fibronectin type III motifs, von Willebrand factor A motifs, a domain homologous to a noncollagenous region of type IX collagen, and short collagenous domains with an Arg-Gly-Asp site. *J Cell Biol* 1991;115:209–221.
187. Yoshida J, Wakabayashi T, Okamoto S, et al. Tenascin in cerebrospinal fluid is a useful biomarker for the diagnosis of brain tumour. *J Neurol Neurosurg Psychiatry* 1994;57:1212–1215.
188. Yurchenco PD. Assembly of laminin and type IV collagen into basement membrane networks. In: Yurchenco PD, Birk DE, Mecham RP, eds. *Extracellular matrix assembly and structure.* San Diego: Academic Press, 1994:351–388.
189. Yurchenco PD, Birk DE, Mecham RP, ed. *Extracellular matrix assembly and structure.* San Diego: Academic Press, 1994.
190. Yurchenco PD, Cheng YS. Self-assembly and calcium binding sites

in laminin, a three-arm interaction model. *J Bioi Chem* 1993;268: 17286–17299.

191. Yurchenco PD, O'Rear JJ. Basal lamina assembly. *Curr Opin Cell Biol* 1994;5:674–681.
192. Zagzag D. Angiogenic growth factors in neural embryogenesis and neoplasia. *Am J Pathol* 1995;146:293–309.
193. Zhang H, Apfelroth SD, Hu W, et al. Structure and expression of fibrillin-2, a novel microfibrillar component preferentially located in elastic matrices. *J Cell Biol* 1994;124:855–863.
194. Zhang HY, Kluge M, Timpl R, Chu ML, Ekblom P. The extracellular matrix glycoproteins BM-90 and tenascin are expressed in the mesenchyme at sites of endothelial-mesenchymal conversion in the embryonic mouse heart. *Differentiation* 1993;52:211–220.
195. Zhang Z, Tarone G, Turner DC. Expression of integrin alpha 1 beta 1 is regulated by nerve growth factor and dexamethasone in PC12 cells. Functional consequences for adhesion and neurite outgrowth. *J Biol Chem* 1993;268:5557–5565.
196. Zhou Y, Damsky CH, Chiu K, Roberts JM, Fisher SJ. Preeclampsia is associated with abnormal expression of adhesion molecules by invasive cytotrophoblasts. *J Clin Invest* 1993;91:950–960.

Anesthesia: Biologic Foundations, edited by Tony L. Yaksh et al. Lippincott–Raven Publishers, Philadelphia © 1997.

CHAPTER 76

ANESTHETIC MODULATION OF PULMONARY VASCULAR TONE

KAREN B. DOMINO

DISTRIBUTION OF PULMONARY BLOOD FLOW

The pulmonary circulation is unique in that it is a low-pressure system through which the entire cardiac output passes. This property allows marked increases in cardiac output to occur during exercise, without severely increasing capillary pressures, which would cause fluid flux and pulmonary edema. However, the fact that the pulmonary circulation is a low-pressure system has important ramifications for the distribution of pulmonary blood flow and accounts for the interesting influences of gravity, posture, alveolar volume, edema, and vasoconstriction on its distribution.

Gravitational Distribution of Pulmonary Blood Flow

Pulmonary blood flow has been classically described as being determined by gravitational factors (192,266,267,347). The gravitational model hypothesizes that regional perfusion is determined by the relationship between local alveolar and pulmonary vascular hydrostatic pressures. The classic West model describes the vertical distribution of blood flow by three zones. It uses a Starling resistor model consisting of collapsible tubing that passes through a rigid box (Fig. 1). The tubing collapses when the pressure outside the tubing is greater than the inflow (or upstream) pressure. Blood flow cannot occur no matter what the outflow (or downstream) pressure. When the inflow pressure becomes greater than the outside pressure, blood flow begins to occur. In the gravitational model, alveolar pressure acts as a Starling resistor and thereby exerts a resistance to flow through the small collapsible vessels. In the upper zone (zone 1), the inflow or arterial pressure is less than alveolar pressure, so the vessels remain collapsed and unperfused (Fig. 2). However, in reality, a small amount of blood flow does occur in zone 1 lung through corner or extraalveolar vessels, located in junctions between alveolar septa.

In the middle zone (zone 2), the inflow pressure (arterial pressure) becomes greater than alveolar pressure and blood flow begins to occur, which has been termed by Permutt and Riley (267) as the vascular waterfall (Fig. 2). The venous pressure still does not affect flow or vascular resistance in zone 2.

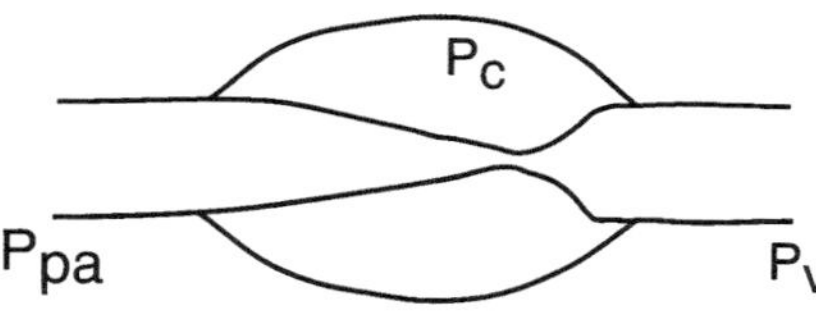

Figure 1. Starling resistor model. A thin-walled collapsible tubing is surrounded by a pressure. The tubing collapses when the pressure outside the tubing (critical pressure or Pc) is greater than the inflow pressure (pulmonary artery pressure or Ppa). Pv, venous or outflow pressure.

Blood flow increases with vertical distance because the driving pressure, the arterial/alveolar pressure difference, increases.

In the lower zone (zone 3), the venous pressure is greater than alveolar pressure (Fig. 2). The driving pressure becomes the arterial/venous pressure difference. However, as the intravascular pressures become markedly greater than alveolar pressure, the collapsible vessels become further distended and vascular resistance is progressively decreased. Flow therefore increases with vertical distance in zone 3 because of the reduced vascular resistance.

Hughes, et al. (141) added a fourth zone to explain decreases in blood flow in the most dependent regions of the lung (Fig. 2). Blood flow in vessels in zone 4 was hypothesized to be decreased because the interstitial pressure in dependent lung regions is increased and therefore the driving pressure, the arterial/interstitial pressure difference, is decreased. The area of zone 4 diminishes as overall lung volume increases (142,143). This effect suggested that the resistance of extraalveolar vessels was reduced as the increased lung held open the vessels, while the resistance of alveolar vessels was increased.

Nongravitational Distribution of Pulmonary Blood Flow

Recently the overwhelming importance of the gravitational model in determining pulmonary blood flow has been challenged by studies using new, complex technology. These studies have found that pulmonary blood flow is primarily determined by local factors, such as the three-dimensional anatomic structure and resistive properties of the pulmonary vascular tree

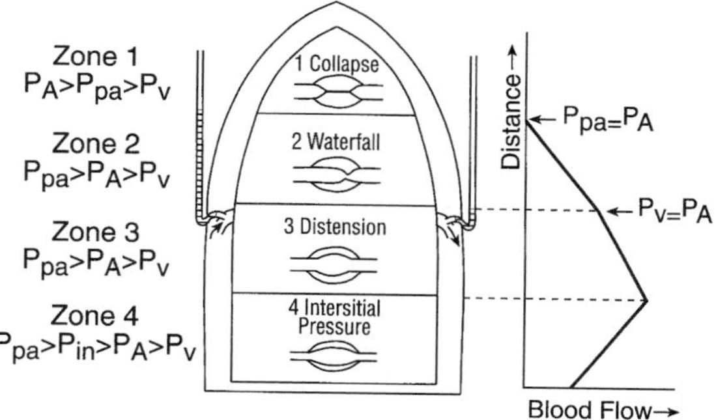

Figure 2. Four-zone model of distribution of pulmonary blood flow in a vertical distribution with respect to gravity. Blood flow in zone 1 (collapse) is absent because pulmonary artery pressure (Ppa) is less than the extravascular pressure, alveolar pressure (P_A). In zone 2 (waterfall), pulmonary blood flow is increased in a vertical distribution as the driving pressure (Ppa minus P_A) increases. In zone 3 (distention), blood flow increases with constant driving pressure (Ppa minus pulmonary venous pressure [Pv]) because the vascular resistance decreases. In zone 4 (interstitial pressure), blood flow decreases as the driving pressure (Ppa minus interstitial pressure [Pin]) decreases. (Adapted from refs. 142, 143, and 347 with permission.)

(107–110,120–123,155). Most studies supporting the gravitational model are older ones that measured blood flow in relatively large regions of the lung (38,278,347). Newer methods have far greater resolution and study blood flow to smaller areas of the lung. This methodology includes imaging techniques, such as single-photon emission computed tomography (SPECT) scanning (120–123), high-resolution computed tomography (136), and ^{99M}Technetium–labeled macroaggregates detected by planar gamma counter (108,109), and techniques that reconstruct regional blood flow by dissecting the lung into a large number of small cubic pieces and determining the perfusion of each of the cubes using radioactive-labeled (106,107,110) or fluorescent-labeled (105) microspheres. These methods permit greater accuracy, sensitivity, and resolution of regional pulmonary blood flow than was previously available.

If the distribution of blood flow is predominantly determined by gravitational factors, blood flow should increase from nondependent to dependent regions irrespective of body position. In addition, the gravitational model predicts that blood flow should be the same in all anatomic locations within the same gravitational plane. However, while pulmonary perfusion tends to follow a vertical distribution, the variability of blood flow within each isogravitational plane is greater than the change with gravity. The newer, high-resolution technology has thus suggested that regional pulmonary blood flow is *not* primarily distributed on a gravitational basis.

The anatomic properties of the pulmonary vasculature are more important than gravity in determining the distribution blood flow. For instance, perfusion is greater in the central and dorsal regions of the lung, and perfusion is reduced in the periphery of the lung (9,10,121–123,155). Using a multivariate analysis to determine the role of different factors in contributing to the variability of lung perfusion, Glenny et al. (106,107,108) found that 84% of the heterogeneity of perfusion was due to factors other than gravity. The heterogeneity of blood flow is well characterized by a fractal (or branching) model (108,109) and regional pulmonary perfusion is spatially correlated (110). It is therefore likely that the resistive properties of the pulmonary vascular tree (such as length, diameter, and branching pattern) are primarily responsible for determining regional pulmonary blood flow, with a gravitational effect as a minor determinant in the normal subject, particularly in the supine or prone position. The zones of the lung may still be present in the nongravitational model, although the anatomic distribution of zone 1 may not correspond to the classical gravitation nondependent lung regions.

Factors Affecting Regional Pulmonary Blood Flow

Central to Peripheral Gradients

Using SPECT scanning, Hakim and colleagues (120–123) have demonstrated in humans and intact dogs that pulmonary blood flow is increased in central areas and reduced in peripheral areas within each lobe (Fig. 3). Blood flow changes in the

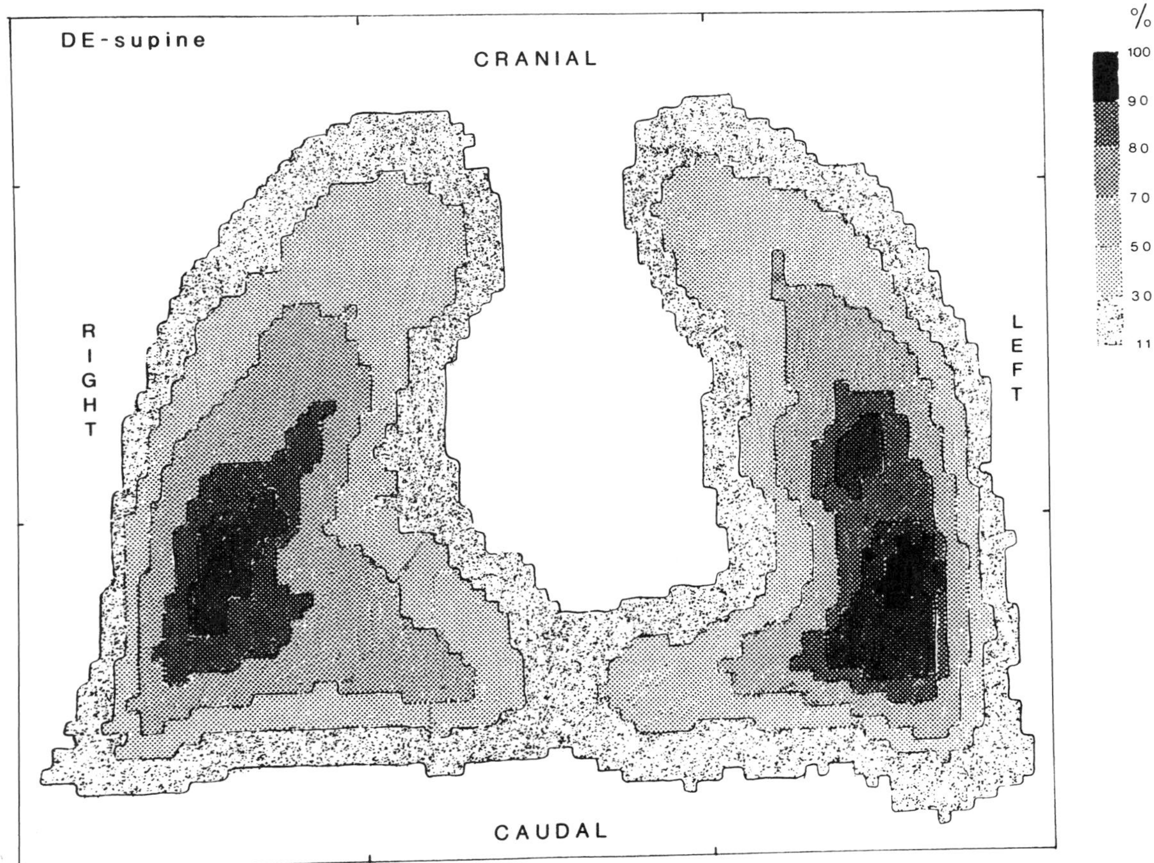

Figure 3. Midcoronal slice showing the spatial distribution of pulmonary blood flow in a supine human, determined by computerized tomography of the lung with ^{99M}TC-labeled human albumin macroaggregates. The scale on the top right shows 6 shades indicating 11–100% of maximal activity (below 10% was excluded for technical reasons). Pulmonary blood flow is greatest in central areas, with a reduction in peripheral areas in an onion skin-like effect. Zone 4 occurs in all peripheral areas and is not limited to dependent areas. (From ref. 123 with permission.)

lobe are much like an onion, with similar levels of flow in concentric spheres from the core of the lobe. The central to peripheral gradation in flow was more predominant than changes in vertical gradients due to gravity. This research suggested that the decrease in pulmonary blood flow in zone 4 may be due to the intrinsic properties of the pulmonary circulation. The decrease in perfusion from central to peripheral areas of a lobe was attributed to increases in local pulmonary vascular resistance due to the resistive properties (length, diameter, and branching pattern) of the pulmonary vascular tree (123).

Cardiac Output

Classical studies in the upright position demonstrated that exercise increased pulmonary blood flow more in the apical than in the basal lung regions, resulting in a more homogeneous distribution of blood flow (38,73,86). For instance, Bryan et al. (38) found that the ratio of apical to basal lung perfusion changed from 1:3.2 during rest to 1:1.2 with exercise. Exercise and increases in cardiac output raise pulmonary artery pressure, which would recruit vessels in zone 1 lung. In contrast, decreases in cardiac output decreased blood flow to upper lung regions, as vessels in zone 1 lung become derecruited as pulmonary artery pressure falls below alveolar pressure (134).

Using SPECT imaging, Hakim and colleagues (121) recently demonstrated that in the supine position, the distribution of pulmonary blood flow does not become more uniform with increased cardiac output. Increases in cardiac output increased blood flow in the lung in all regions in proportion to the baseline blood flow. As the vessels in the supine position are fully recruited, with no or minimal zone 1 and 2 present, increasing cardiac output in the supine or prone position does not make the perfusion distribution more uniform, in contrast to the upright position, where zone 1 would be present. Decreases in cardiac output also reduced lung blood flow in proportion to the baseline blood flow, with the exception of the appearance of zone 1 in the upper most lung regions. Thus, the distribution of perfusion, with greater blood flow to central areas (middle of the caudal lobes) and less in peripheral areas (apical and caudal areas) was not affected by changes in cardiac output. The uniform change in blood flow emphasizes the importance of the three-dimensional nature and resistive properties of the pulmonary circulation.

Lung Volume

Pulmonary blood flow is affected by lung volume as capillary resistance increases with increasing lung volume. This is balanced by decreasing resistance of extraalveolar corner vessels, located in junctions between alveolar septa, with increased lung volume. Thus, the resistance to blood flow is lowest at the lung volume at rest at the end of expiration (e.g., the functional residual capacity). When alveolar pressure and lung volume are increased by the administration of positive end-expiratory pressure, the amount of zone 1 is increased (347). Newer techniques have demonstrated a reduced perfusion in peripheral apical and ventral areas of the lung with the administration of positive end-expiratory pressure (167).

Posture

Regional pulmonary perfusion is partially dependent on posture, as would be predicted by the gravitational model. In the erect and lateral decubitus position, pulmonary blood flow increases from the top to the bottom of the lung, with an average change of 8% in regional blood flow per centimeter vertical distance (3,4,142,168,260). The reduction in pulmonary blood flow in the nondependent lung in the lateral decubitus position is in part helpful in preserving arterial oxygenation during one-lung ventilation for thoracic surgery. However, the average vertical gradient is much less pronounced in the supine and prone positions, with an average change of only 2% in regional blood flow per centimeter vertical distance (3,106, 107,120–123,168,274). Isogravitational perfusion is increased in dorsal lung regions in these positions (9,10). In these positions, nongravitational or anatomic factors have a more major role in determining regional blood flow.

The observed gradients due to gravity are also markedly influenced by lung volume. For instance, small or absent vertical gradients are observed at low lung volumes (4), while the gravitational gradients become more pronounced at high lung volumes (142,167,274). Cranial to caudal gradients (increases in blood flow to cranial compared to caudal regions) have been described in the supine position but are absent in the prone position (3,260). Using fluorescent-labeled microspheres in small cubes of lungs, Glenny et al. (106,107) found that lung blood flow was greatest in the dorsal areas of the lower lobes in both the supine and prone position. Therefore, while posture has an important role in determining the distribution of pulmonary blood flow, other anatomic factors are very important.

Pulmonary Edema/Atelectasis

The distributions of regional pulmonary blood flow during pulmonary edema and atelectasis have not been studied using the more sensitive, state-of-the-art methodology. Theoretically, alveolar edema might increase pericapillary pressure and reduce local pulmonary perfusion in much the same way as do increases in alveolar pressure. However, in contrast to changes in lung volume, pulmonary edema has small or unpredictable effects on regional pulmonary blood flow using older techniques (142,197). With atelectasis, atelectatic lung blood flow is decreased, predominantly due to the stimulation vasoconstriction (19,81,224). With total alveolar collapse, the alveolar oxygen tension (PaO_2) approaches mixed venous oxygen tension ($P\bar{v}O_2$) and hypoxic pulmonary vasoconstriction diverts blood flow away from the atelectatic lung segment. Mechanical constriction or kinking of the pulmonary vasculature is relatively unimportant in reducing blood flow (19,220,224).

DYNAMICS OF PULMONARY BLOOD FLOW

Pulmonary Vascular Resistance

Pulmonary vascular resistance (PVR), or the resistance to blood flow through the pulmonary circulation, is an important concept because it provides information about the relative tone of the pulmonary vasculature. In the usual concept of PVR that is used clinically, PVR is described by Ohm's law and is equal to the mean pulmonary arterial (Ppa) minus effective outflow pressure from the pulmonary circulation, which is usually left atrial pressure (Pla), divided by the cardiac output ($\dot{Q}_T$).

$$PVR = (Ppa - Pla)/\dot{Q}_T$$

The pulmonary capillary wedge pressure or pulmonary artery occlusion pressure (Pao) is generally used to estimate Pla in the calculation of pulmonary vascular resistance. In the usual situation, Pao is a close approximation of Pla, as the tip of the catheter measures the venous pressure at the junction of microvascular bed to veins of progressively larger sizes, which reflect left atrial pressure. In the case of high alveolar pressure, such as with use of high levels of positive end-expiratory pressure (PEEP), Pao may theoretically not accurately reflect Pla as the capillaries may be collapsed by increased alveolar pressure (133,139). However, as the catheters wedge in the regions of greatest pulmonary blood flow, in most cases Pao is a satisfactory measure of pulmonary outflow pressure for the calculation of PVR. For instance, in severe adult respiratory distress syndrome (ARDS), there is a close correspondence between Pao and left ventricular end-diastolic pressure with PEEP levels of up to 20 cm H_2O (331). This result suggests that the lung pathology of ARDS prevents transmitted alveolar pressure from collapsing adjacent pulmonary arterioles (331).

The Ohm's law calculation of PVR, although used extensively in the clinical practice of anesthesiology, is flawed (338). A major assumption of this calculation is that pulmonary blood flow follows Poiseuille's law in that flow is laminar through continuously open (rigid) vessels. In contrast, the pulmonary circulation behaves as a Starling resistor, so this calculation is meaningless. Although the effect of a therapeutic intervention on PVR can be calculated, the calculated PVR cannot distinguish between changes in pulmonary vascular tone, changes in closing pressure, or changes in vascular recruitment due to changes in cardiac output and intrathoracic volume. It is physiologically superior to interpret the changes in pulmonary artery and cardiac output together, rather than rely on a misleading single calculated variable (PVR).

Measurement by Pulmonary Pressure-Flow Curves

A superior method to determine changes in pulmonary vascular tone uses pulmonary pressure-flow curves. Pressure-flow relationships are almost universally employed in the experimental study of the action of pharmacologic agents on the pulmonary vasculature, especially in determining the effectiveness of a particular agent to lower PVR. Because several levels of pulmonary blood flow and pressure are required, they are not practical to use in the daily clinical care of patients. However, understanding pulmonary pressure-flow curves is key to understanding the pharmacology of the pulmonary vasculature and helps the clinician to pick the most logical drug to use in a particular setting. Use of pressure-flow curves helps clinicians to interpret the true effects of drugs on PVR. For instance, by analyzing pressure-flow curves, it is possible to tell whether a drug actively changes pulmonary vascular resistance or whether it only indirectly changes the calculated value, because it alters cardiac output, without directly causing a change in pulmonary vascular tone. An example of a drug that appears to reduce pulmonary vascular resistance based on a single point calculation of PVR is norepinephrine. However, pressure-flow curves showed that norepinephrine does not actually reduce pulmonary vascular tone, but only increases cardiac output (82).

Plotting pulmonary artery pressures or pulmonary arterial-venous pressure differences against pulmonary blood flow, a pressure-flow curve is obtained (Fig. 4). While pressure-flow curves are often plotted with flow as the dependent variable (on the y-axis) (as is shown in some illustrations later in the chapter), they are most logically plotted with pressure as the dependent variable (y-axis) and flow as the independent variable (x-axis), because the right ventricle acts as a flow pump rather than as a pressure source. The resulting curve shows a typical hyperbolic shape (Fig. 4) and it appears linear over the physiologic range of blood flow. The slope of the dashed line connecting with the origin at zero flow represents the calculated pulmonary vascular resistance at that $\dot{Q}_T$.

Pressure-flow curves may be interpreted by the Starling resistor model (192,267) or by the distensibility model (97,358). Although the distensibility model more accurately describes the pulmonary circulation, the Starling resistor model is the easiest for the clinician to understand and is the most useful clinically. The Starling resistor model analyzes the linear portion of the pressure-flow curve that occurs at physiologic cardiac outputs (119,227,228). It views blood flow through the pulmonary vasculature as controlled by the pulmonary artery pressure and a critical closing pressure. When Ppa approximately equals the critical closing pressure, there is no flow through a thin-walled vessel when collapsed by surrounding pressure. This pressure may be due to perivascular pressure or active tension in the muscle in vessel walls. Pulmonary blood flow occurs when Ppa is greater than the critical closing pressure (Fig. 4). At low flows, Ppa rises rapidly with increasing flow. When Ppa is high enough, all vessels are open and the slope of the pressure-flow curve becomes constant. As previously described, Starling resistors are present in human lungs under zone 2 conditions (266,347).

The resultant pressure-flow curve is illustrated in Fig. 4. The line extrapolated back to zero-flow intersects the y-axis at a pressure equal to the weighed mean of all closing pressures for the pulmonary vascular bed. Changes in critical closing pressure are said to reflect changes in Starling resistance. There are numerous variables that increase PVR by increasing Starling resistance including positive end-expiratory pressure, lung volume, and alveolar hypoxia (Fig. 5).

Drugs and experimental manipulations may also alter PVR by affecting Ohmic resistance. Ohmic resistance is the actual resistance in the pulmonary vascular bed upstream to locus of critical pressure (227,228). The Ohmic resistance is therefore independent of pulmonary blood flow, and it is measured by

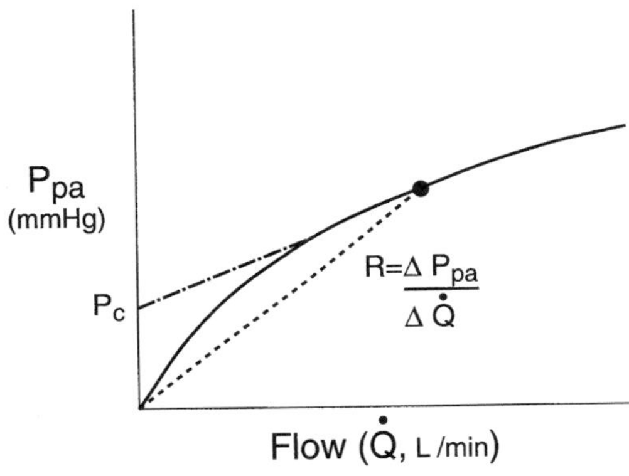

Figure 4. A typical pulmonary pressure-flow curve (solid-line) plotted with pulmonary artery pressure, Ppa, on the y-axis and blood flow, Q on the x-axis. The pressure-flow curve is hyperbolic in shape and appears linear over the middle range of blood flows, but becomes curvilinear at lower flows. The slope of the *dashed line* which connects with the origin at zero flow represents the calculated pulmonary vascular resistance (R) at that blood flow ($R = \Delta Ppa/\Delta\dot{Q}$). Extrapolation of the linear portion of the pressure-flow curve to Ppa at zero flow *(dashed-dotted line)* yields an overall critical closing pressure (Pc), as interpreted by the Starling resistor model.

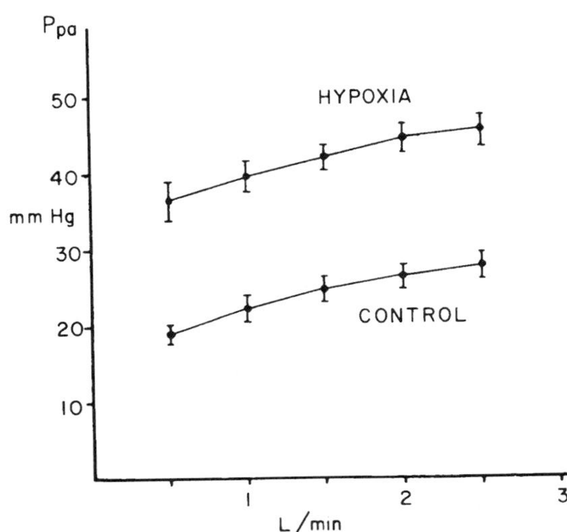

Figure 5. Example of "parallel shift" in pressure-flow curve. In this study, global alveolar hypoxia caused a parallel shift in the pressure-flow curve, which may be interpreted according to the Starling resistor model as representing an increase in critical closing pressure. (From ref. 229 with permission.)

the slope of the pressure-flow curve ($\Delta Ppa/\Delta\dot{Q}$) (Fig. 6). Direct changes in pulmonary vascular tone may therefore alter the slope of the pressure-flow curve. Increases in slope of the pressure-flow curve represent constriction or narrowing of pulmonary arteries and decreases in slope represent relaxation of pulmonary arteries (Fig. 6). In contrast, changes in Starling resistance or critical closing pressure are reflected in parallel shifts of pressure-flow curves (as in Fig. 5).

Although the concepts of Starling and Ohmic resistance are helpful in analyzing pharmacologic action, interpretation of and potential clinical significance of changes in these resistances are unclear. While the different effects suggest that there is a difference in site of action and/or type of mechanical effect, the exact relationship between site of action and type of change in pressure-flow curve is not known. What is known is that shifts in the pressure-flow curve in the absence of large changes in lung volume, pleural pressure, or left atrial pressure indicate that pulmonary vasomotor tone has changed.

In reality, the pulmonary vasculature consists of distensible and not rigid cylindrical tubes. The distensibility model of Zhuang et al. (97,358) interprets the pressure-flow curves as representing changes in the distensibility of the pulmonary vasculature. This model better describes the pulmonary circulation because the Starling resistor model is overly simplistic and relies on the incorrect assumption that the pulmonary vasculature is nondistensible. Changes in distensibility of vessels can explain the curvilinear pressure-flow curve without evoking the concept of critical closing pressure. Parallel shifts in the pressure-flow curve may occur if pulmonary vasoconstriction increases both the compliance and resistance of the constricted vessels (228). However, regardless of which model is used to interpret pressure-flow curves, changes in pressure-flow curves indicate that a drug or therapeutic manipulation actively modulates pulmonary vascular tone.

Regional Pulmonary Vascular Resistance

Calculation of PVR and pressure-flow curves, which determine resistance to blood flow of the pulmonary vasculature as a whole, are useful to assess the overall effects of drugs on pulmonary vascular tone. However, drugs may have different anatomic sites of action in the pulmonary vasculature. For instance, one drug may cause predominantly pulmonary arterial vasoconstriction, while another may be predominantly a pulmonary venous vasoconstrictor. Several experimental techniques are useful to assess the site of change in pulmonary vascular resistance. These include an indirect measurement by vascular occlusion techniques and the direct observation of vessel dimensions or blood flow. This section describes each of these techniques and illustrates their usefulness to characterize the effect of drugs on the pulmonary vasculature.

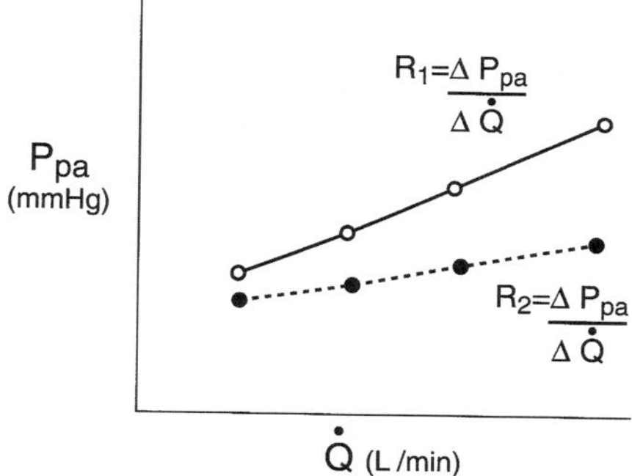

Figure 6. Schematic pressure-flow curves illustrating a change in pulmonary vascular resistance (Ohmic resistance). The slope of the pressure-flow curve ($\Delta Ppa/\Delta\dot{Q}$) represents the pulmonary vascular resistance. The resistance of the *dashed line* (R2) is less than the resistance of the *solid line* (R1). A reduction in slope indicates pulmonary vasomotor relaxation.

Indirect Measurement (Vascular Occlusion)

Vascular occlusion techniques provide information about the anatomic site of action of a drug within the pulmonary vasculature (65–69,124–126,187). By using arterial or venous occlusion, PVR can be partitioned into arterial, middle, or venous resistance. The middle segment represents pulmonary capillaries, small arterioles, and small venules. These vessels contribute relatively little to overall PVR in the normal lung (125,126). However, relatively thin-walled vessels of the middle segment tend to collapse when the extravascular pressure exceeds the intravascular pressure. This may occur under zone 1 lung conditions when alveolar pressure exceeds the intravascular pressure. Collapse of the vasculature in the middle segment also occurs because of active vasoconstriction or passively due to increases in perivascular pressure associated with edema or changes in lung volume. A critical closing pressure is thus developed upstream and downstream to the alveolar capillaries. Blood flow through the segment is determined by the arterial/venous pressure difference unless alveolar or critical closing pressure exceeds venous pressure. If so, the driving pressure is represented by the arterial/critical closing pressure difference or the arterial/alveolar pressure difference.

Arterial and venous occlusion techniques measure ongoing changes in pulmonary artery and pulmonary venous pressures after rapid occlusion of arterial inflow and venous outflow in a perfused, isolated, in situ lung or lobe. By analyzing the resultant pressure changes, the site of action of a drug may be characterized as upstream (pulmonary arteries), downstream (pulmonary veins), or middle (capillaries, small arterioles, and small venules).

The resultant pressure changes with arterial and venous occlusion are illustrated in Fig. 7. With arterial occlusion, the pulmonary arterial pressure curve exhibits a rapid fall followed by a slower exponential decrease with time (Fig. 7). Pulmonary venous outflow occlusion causes a rapid linear increase in arterial and venous pressures. The venous pressure at the instant of occlusion can be extrapolated from the linear portion of the venous pressure curve (Fig. 7). With simultaneous arterial inflow and venous outflow, the pulmonary arterial and pulmonary venous pressures rapidly converge to an equilibrium pressure, representing capillary pressure (Fig. 7).

The magnitude of the changes in pressure with occlusion are very sensitive to arterial or venous sites of action of drugs (67–69,124–126,187). Drugs may therefore be characterized as having arterial, venous, or small vessel effects on the basis of changes in the pressures obtained after vascular occlusion. For instance, using these techniques, serotonin has been characterized as having predominantly arterial vasoconstriction while histamine induces pulmonary venous vasoconstriction (67,69,125). Arterial vasoconstriction, induced by serotonin, is demonstrated by a larger initial fall in Pa (ΔPa) with arterial occlusion and an increased Pa with no change in Pv with venous occlusion compared to control (Fig. 8). In contrast, with histamine the initial fall in Pa (ΔPa) is similar to control, while the increase in Pv with venous occlusion (ΔPv) is greater than control (Fig. 8).

Direct Observation of Vessel Dimensions or Blood Flow

The site of pulmonary vasoconstriction can be determined directly by observing vessel diameters, measurement of microvascular pressures, or measurement of regional pulmonary blood flow. Vessel diameters have been observed by dimension transducers (65), microscopic techniques (174,343), and angiography (303). Regional vasoconstriction can be measured. In the microvasculature using micropuncture techniques (240), although the presence of the catheter may alter the pulmonary vascular response. Regional pulmonary perfusion has been recently measured by use of intravital fluorescence

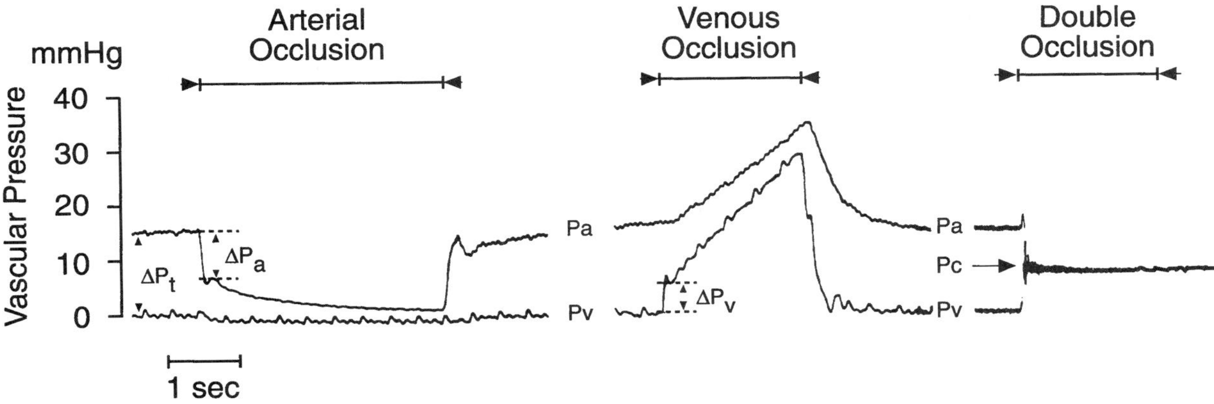

Figure 7. Typical lobar arterial (Pa) and venous (Pv) pressure curves obtained from arterial occlusion *(left),* venous occlusion *(middle),* and double occlusion *(right).* ΔPt, arterial-venous pressure difference; ΔPa, pressure drop on arterial side, ΔPv, pressure drop on venous side. Pc, pressure with double occlusion which estimates critical closing pressure. (Adapted from ref. 126 with permission.)

microscopy (115–117,174). This technique quantifies morphologic changes and regional blood flow in the pulmonary microcirculation in vivo. The technique involves creation of a window in the thoracic wall to allow the microscopic visualization of the lung. Subpleural pulmonary blood flow and microhemodynamic measurements, including arteriolar and venular diameters and red blood cell flux and velocity, are obtained by intravital microscopy of infected fluorescein-isothiocyanate–labeled red blood cells (Fig. 9). This state-of-the-art technique elegantly allows the direct visualization of the anatomic site of pulmonary vasoconstriction or vasodilation in an intact animal.

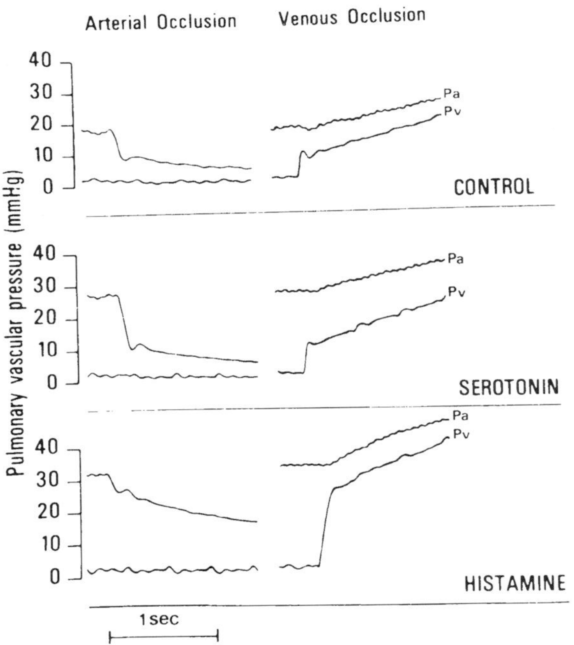

Figure 8. Effects of serotonin and histamine on pressure tracings obtained during arterial and venous occlusions. Arterial vasoconstriction, induced by serotonin *(middle),* is demonstrated by a larger initial fall in Pa with arterial occlusion and an increased Pa with no change in Pv with venous occlusion compared to control *(top).* In contrast, with histamine, a venous vasoconstrictor *(bottom),* the initial fall in Pa with arterial occlusion is similar to control, while the increase in Pv with venous occlusion (ΔPv) is greater than control. (From ref. 126 with permission.)

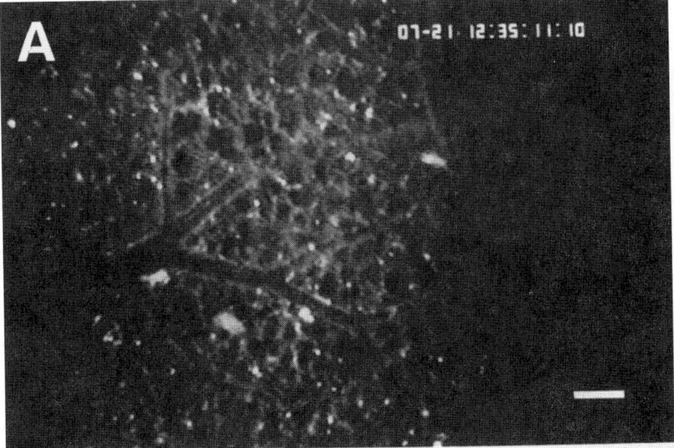

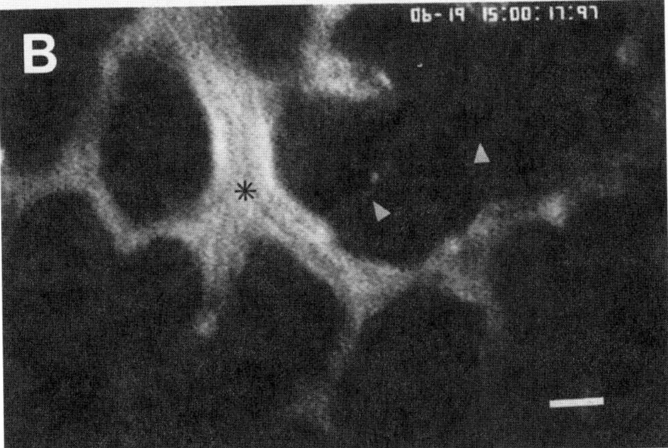

Figure 9. Intravital microscopy of the pulmonary microcirculation. **(A)** Arteriolar vessel tree at the edge of right upper lobe (x40, bar, 250pm) and **(B)** A terminal branch of venule (*), bright interalveolar sepia, and subpleural surface of alveoli with capillaries (Δ) (x225, bar 50μm): (Reproduced from ref. 174 with permission.)

REGULATION OF PULMONARY BLOOD FLOW

Hypoxic Pulmonary Vasoconstriction

General Description

The pulmonary circulation constricts in response to alveolar hypoxia, resulting in a dual response of an increase in pulmonary artery pressure and diversion of blood flow away from the hypoxic area (60,207,208). Hypoxic pulmonary vasoconstriction (HPV) is unique to the pulmonary circulation as other circulations (coronary, cerebral, and systemic) dilate in response to hypoxia (92,341). HPV is the primary adaptive mechanism of the pulmonary circulation to preserve arterial blood oxygenation by increasing pulmonary vascular resistance to hypoxic alveoli, thereby diverting pulmonary blood flow away from hypoxic alveoli. The reduction in blood flow from poorly ventilated or hypoxic alveoli to better-ventilated alveoli preserves the matching of ventilation and perfusion and arterial oxygenation (77). The success of pulmonary vasoconstriction to divert blood flow away from atelectatic or hypoxic lung regions is dependent on the size of the hypoxic region (202, 204–209,305). The smaller the hypoxic segment, the greater the blood flow reduction (e.g., flow diversion) and the smaller the rise in Ppa (Fig. 10). For instance, an 80% reduction in blood flow with a negligible increase in pulmonary artery pressure would occur when the hypoxic segment is equal to 10% of the lungs (206–208). A 50% diversion in blood flow would be expected with 60% of the lung as the hypoxic segment. When 100% of the lung is hypoxic, as is the case at high altitude, only pulmonary artery pressure increases and interregional flow diversion does not occur. However, with global alveolar hypoxia, the intraregional distribution of blood flow changes to a minor degree, as perfusion increases to the apical portions of the lung (63,64,245,342). The increase in apical perfusion is postulated to be beneficial because it increases the vascular surface area that can participate in gas exchange.

HPV increases pulmonary vascular resistance and pulmonary artery pressure according to the pressure-flow curves illustrated in Fig. 5 (global alveolar hypoxia) and Fig. 11 (one-lung hypoxia). With global hypoxia, actual experimental data show that the linear portion of the pressure-flow curves shifts in a parallel manner (189,229). On a simplistic basis, the pressure-flow curve may suggest that hypoxia increases Starling resis-

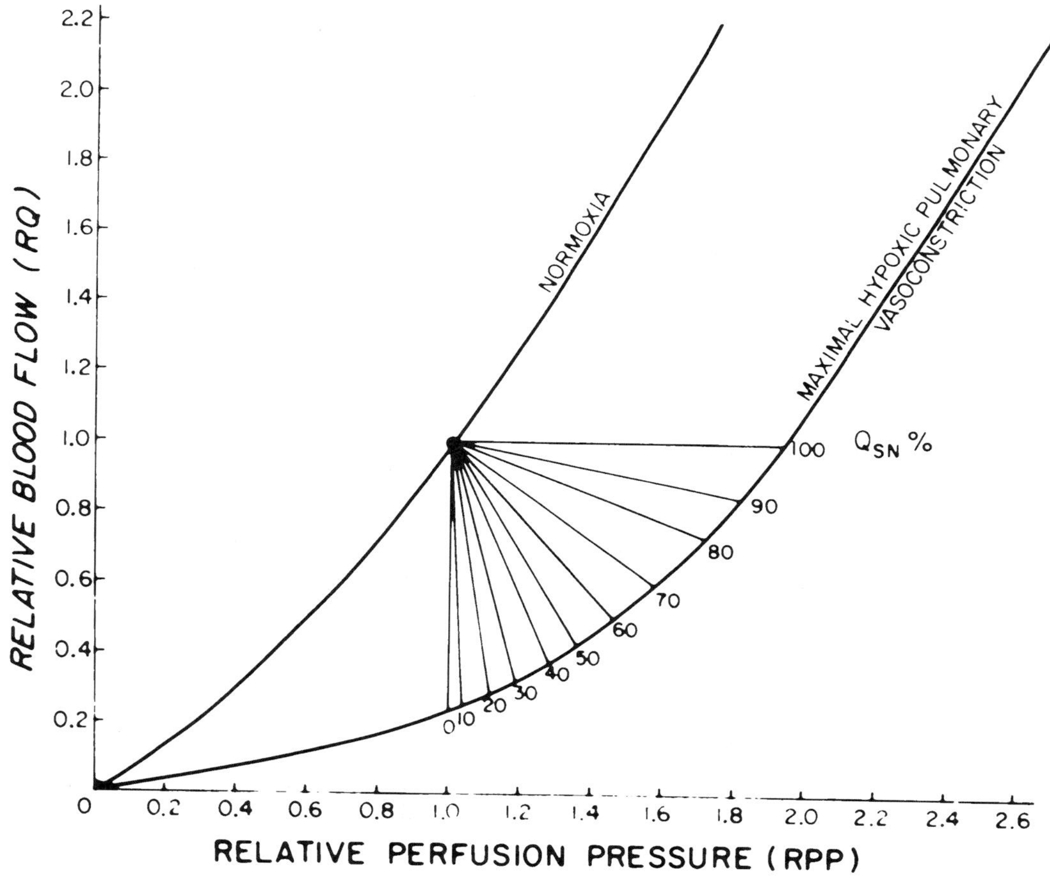

Figure 10. Influence of size of hypoxic lung segment on flow diversion and pulmonary perfusion pressure. Theoretical pressure-flow curves for normoxic and hypoxic lungs are illustrated with blood flow on the y-axis and pulmonary perfusion pressure on the x-axis, in contrast to presentations earlier in the chapter. Normal blood flow and perfusion pressure in *solid circle,* at 1.0 relative blood flow and 1.0 relative perfusion pressure. The *fans of lines* connecting the normoxic and hypoxic curves demonstrate the changes in relative blood flow and perfusion pressure with hypoxic lung segments (Q_{SN}%) of different sizes, (Q_{SN}% = 100%, [entire lung] and Q_{SN}% = 10% [small lung segment]). A large decrease in blood flow and minimal change in pulmonary perfusion pressure occurs when the hypoxic segment is small (e.g., 10%). In contrast, minimal changes in pulmonary blood flow and large increases in pulmonary perfusion pressure occur when the hypoxic segment is large (90%). (From ref. 206 with permission.)

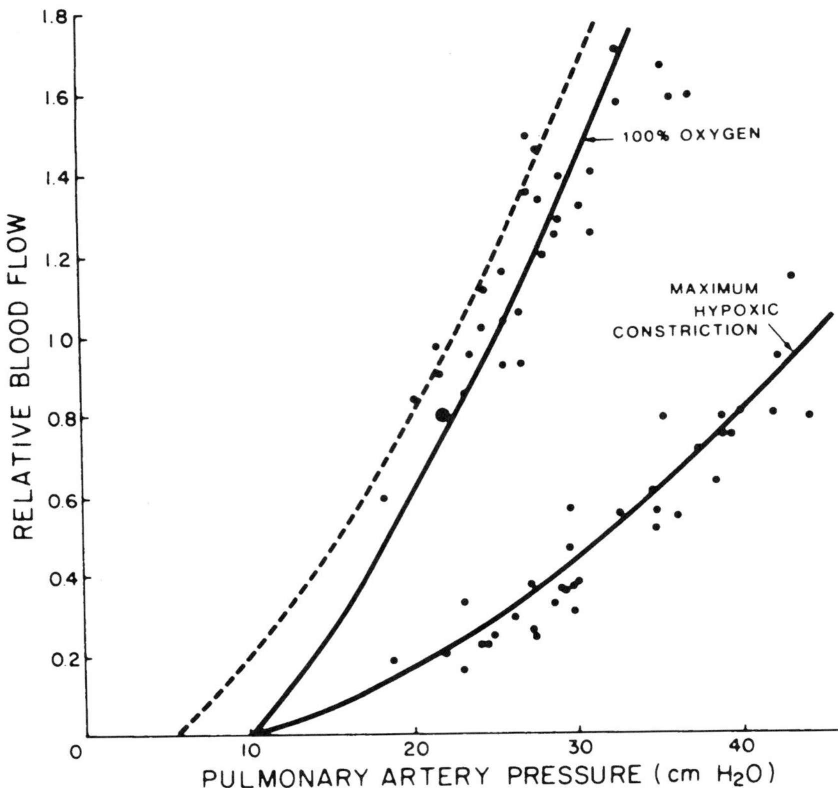

Figure 11. Pressure-flow curves for normoxic (100% oxygen ventilation) and hypoxic lungs. Each data point represents actual data from experiments. The *solid lines* represent theoretical pressure-flow curves derived from the model of Marshall and Marshall (204,205,206). The *dashed line* represents the predicted pressure-flow curve during O_2 breathing in the awake animal. The predictions are an anesthetized animal with alveolar pressure of 5cm H_2O, pleural pressure of 0 cm H_2O, left atrial pressure of 10cm H_2O, hematocrit of 35%, and resting cardiac output of 0.8 of awake value. (From ref. 204 with permission.)

tance. However, a more accurate interpretation of the curves is that hypoxia increases the distensibility of the pulmonary vasculature (97,358). Based on the Zhuang model, computer simulated pressure-flow curves with left lung hypoxia, with actual experimentally derived data points, are illustrated in Fig. 11. The pressure-flow curve of the hypoxic lung has a different curvature than in the normoxic lung.

Because HPV causes flow diversion away from hypoxic or atelectatic alveoli, it is the most important physiologic adaptation of the lung to help preserve arterial oxygen tension (PaO_2). HPV allows for the maintenance of adequate oxygenation during thoracic surgery in many patients, where the operated lung is collapsed to enhance surgical exposure. HPV is also helpful in improving oxygenation in regional lung disease, such as pneumonia or pulmonary contusion, although HPV is attenuated in most types of acute lung disease (see Modifying Factors, below). Because of the increased ability to divert blood flow away from hypoxic lung segments with smaller segments, arterial PO_2 (PaO_2) is better maintained when small rather than large areas of the lung are rendered hypoxic (202,206,208,209) (Fig. 12). For instance, if 30% of the lung is hypoxic, PaO_2 would be expected to decrease to 100 mm Hg if HPV is absent (Fig. 12). However, a PaO_2 of 400 mg Hg would be expected in the presence of HPV. With greater percentages of the lung being hypoxic, HPV is less effective in improving the observed PaO_2. HPV also appears to function as an adaptive mechanism in the normal lung, as suggested by the finding that inhibitors of HPV result in a widening of the alveolar-arterial O_2 tension difference ($P[(A\text{-}a)]O_2$) and decrease in PaO_2 (129,172).

The physiologic importance of HPV is dependent on species. HPV is strongest in cows and pigs, species that lack collateral ventilation, compared with dogs, sheep, and humans, species that have well-developed collateral ventilation (175). However, consistent and strong HPV responses are obtained in these species (12,26,37,41–43,200), and HPV is likely to be quite significant in maintaining $\dot{V}_A/\dot{Q}$ matching in lung disease (202,209).

Site/Stimulus for HPV

The primary sites for constriction of the pulmonary vasculature during acute hypoxia are the small pulmonary arterioles (30–50 µm), although constriction of capillaries and pulmonary veins contributes to a small extent (65,66,115,169,194,231,240, 289,314,342,357). Both alveolar and extraalveolar vessels constrict in response to hypoxia (328). Intravital fluorescence microscopy has demonstrated a reduction in capillary blood flow, indicated by capillary derecruitment and a reduction in red blood cell flux and velocity, in a hypoxic lung (115). Large pulmonary arterioles (>500 µm) do not participate in the usual HPV response (194) because the blood supply by the bronchial circulation increases the local vascular oxygen tension (203). However, pulmonary arteries of all sizes demonstrate HPV in vitro (195,203,235). It is likely that hypoxia acts directly on the vessel wall, as the vascular endothelium is not essential for the HPV response (214). Cultured pulmonary vascular smooth muscle cells are capable of vascular contraction (195,235). Release of endothelial-derived factors, such as nitric oxide, endothelin, and prostacyclin, while they do not mediate the HPV response, appear to modulate the intensity of the response (264,352). Autonomic innervation of the lung is not required for HPV (188), and the HPV response is present in the human transplanted lung (288,301,345). However, β-adrenergic stimulation attenuates HPV by 20% (170,312). Hypoxia may cause vasoconstriction by opening calcium channels (334) and/or closing potassium channels (290). A reduction in extracellular calcium markedly attenuates HPV in isolated ferret lungs (89).

The exact location and identity of the sensor for HPV are not known. The sensor is most likely in the vascular smooth muscle (195) and may involve the mitochondrial oxidative phosphorylation system and cytochrome P450 (225) or direct changes in the calcium or potassium channels in the vascular smooth mus-

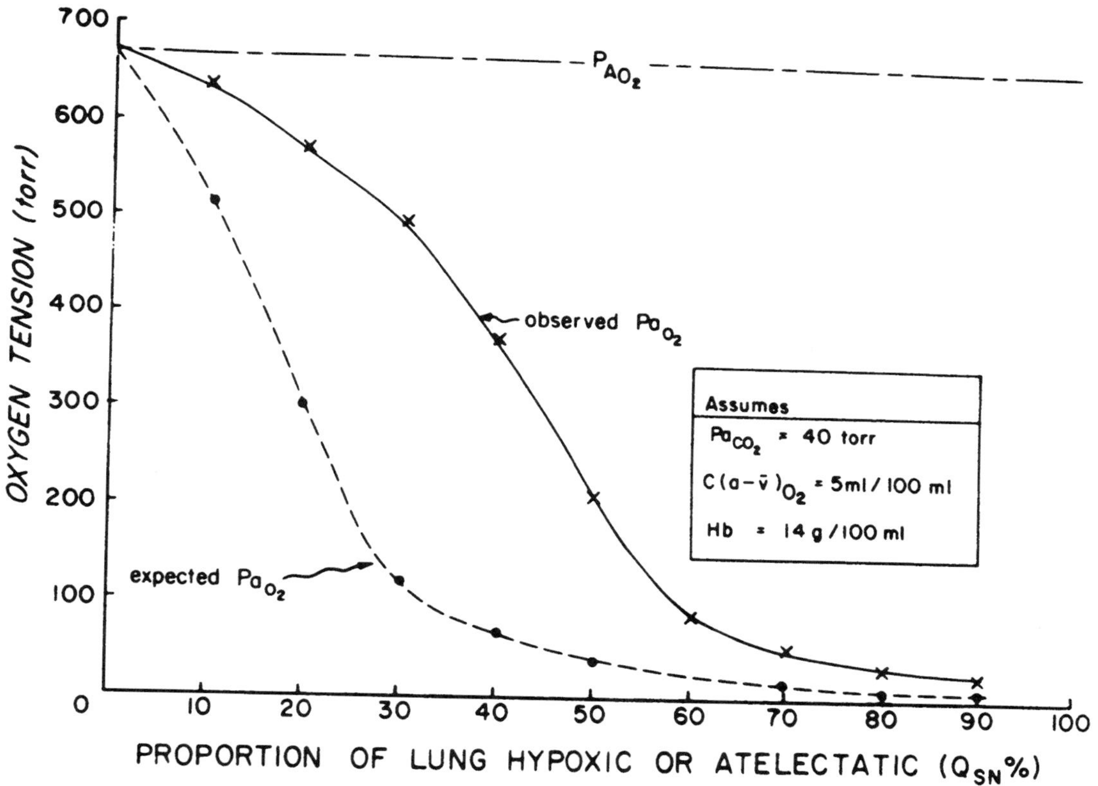

Figure 12. Arterial O_2 tension (PaO_2) predicted with hypoxic pulmonary vasoconstriction (HPV) of different-sized lung segments. In the absence of HPV, the expected PaO_2 is indicated by the *dashed line.* The observed PaO_2 with intact HPV is indicated by the *solid line.* HPV improves PaO_2, especially when 50% or less of the lung is hypoxic or atelectatic. (From ref. 206 with permission.)

cle (273,290). It is also not known whether signal transduction is necessary and if so, what is the identity of the transducer between the sensor and effector cells (221).

The stimulus for HPV response is a reduction in oxygen tension in the vicinity of the vascular smooth muscle. Although alveolar PO_2 is the predominant stimulus for HPV, $P\bar{v}O_2$ also contributes (140,151,201,212). Thus, the stimulus for HPV (PsO_2) results from the combined influence of PaO_2 and $P\bar{v}O_2$, which has been calculated by Marshall and Marshall (204,212) as:

$$PsO_2 = (P\bar{v}O_2)^{0.39} \times (PaO_2)^{0.61}$$

A similar relationship has been observed in the intact dog with one lung hypoxia (201). $P\bar{v}O_2$ becomes the predominant stimulus for HPV in atelectatic lung (81). $P\bar{v}O_2$ is also an important influence when it is unusually low (as with reduced cardiac output) and unusually high (as with severe stress or trauma) (151).

The HPV-stimulus response curve is sigmoid in shape with a maximal HPV response observed when $PsO_2 < 25$ mm Hg (Fig. 13) (6,70,130201,206,208). A 50% HPV response is observed when PsO_2 is 55 mm Hg. With a $P\bar{v}O_2$ of 40 mm Hg while breathing room air, vascular tone is increased by 15% compared to when breathing 100% O_2 and $P\bar{v}O_2$ greater than 60 mm Hg. With prolonged, severe global hypoxia ($PaO_2 = 0$ mm Hg), marked pulmonary vasodilation follows a transient pulmonary vasoconstriction (327). As vasoconstriction to known pulmonary vasoconstrictors is absent, the pulmonary vasodilation probably represents gross metabolic failure due to hypoxia (132).

In summary, HPV is critically important for the preservation of the matching of ventilation and perfusion. Clinically, HPV is most important in the presence of atelectasis, as is employed during one-lung anesthesia. The stimulus for the HPV response is a reduction in oxygen tension in the vicinity of vascular smooth muscle (reflecting both alveolar and mixed venous PO_2), with a maximal response when PsO_2 <25 mm Hg. $P\bar{v}O_2$, therefore, exerts an important influence on HPV and is the stimulus for HPV in the presence of atelectasis or flooded alveoli.

Modifying Factors

The HPV response is influenced by multiple variables including hemodynamic variables, acid-base status, and lung disease. All these factors may profoundly influence the observed effects of anesthetic drugs and inhibitors of HPV on pulmonary hemodynamics and arterial blood oxygenation. These factors are summarized in Table 1.

Hemodynamic Variables Pulmonary arterial and pulmonary venous pressures and cardiac output all affect the HPV response. Increased pulmonary arterial and venous pressure reduce the strength of HPV (14,71,118,182). In fact, the HPV response was abolished when left atrial pressure reached 25 mm Hg. Increases in Ppa attenuate the observed HPV response.

Cardiac output affects the observed HPV response because $P\bar{v}O_2$ and Ppa change with changes in cardiac output (52). Usually $P\bar{v}O_2$ increases when cardiac output increases and $P\bar{v}O_2$ decreases when cardiac output decreases. $P\bar{v}O_2$ and Ppa can act independently of each other (28,304). HPV is generally reduced with increasing cardiac output. This occurs primarily because the stimulus for HPV is reduced (e.g., PsO_2 increases) when $P\bar{v}O_2$ is increased (212). In addition, differences in pulmonary vascular recruitment and derecruitment in normoxic and hypoxic lung regions cause the curvature of the hypoxic pressure-flow curve to be increased (Fig. 11). These differences in the pressure-flow curves cause an increase in percentage blood flow to the hypoxic lung, even with the constant $P\bar{v}O_2$

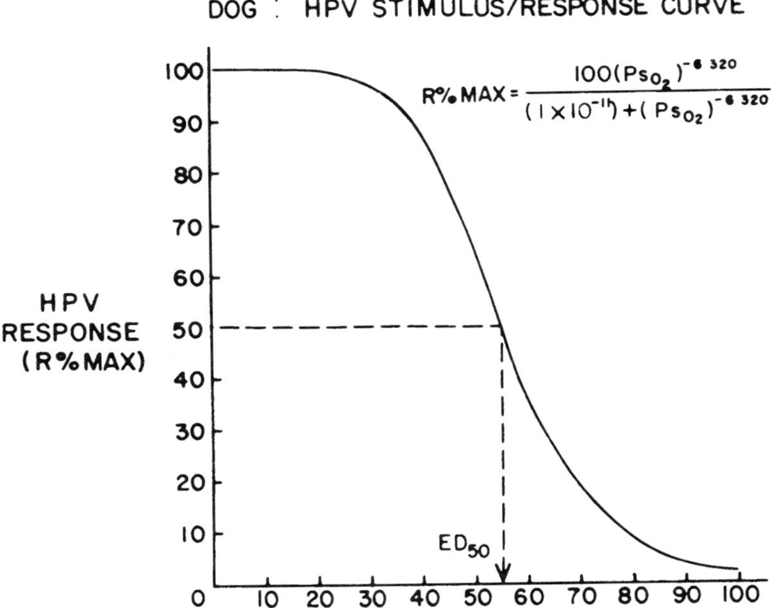

Figure 13. Stimulus-response curve for HPV in dogs. Stimulus O_2 tension (PsO_2) is derived from the contributions of alveolar PO_2 and mixed venous PO_2. HPV response is expressed as percent of maximum response (R% MAX). Equation for sigmoid function and ED_{50} at PsO_2 of 55 mm Hg are shown. (Reproduced from ref 206 with permission.)

and PsO_2 (Fig. 14). In fact, increases in pulmonary shunt (28) and ventilation-perfusion inequality (75) are observed with increases in pulmonary blood flow even in the absence of changes of $P\bar{v}O_2$. As $P\bar{v}O_2$ also increases with increasing cardiac output, the resultant attenuation of HPV is marked and hypoxic lung blood flow is markedly increased with increasing cardiac output (Fig. 14). For instance, HPV is attenuated by increased intracranial pressure, due to the resultant sympathetic activation and increase in cardiac output (76). Although HPV is reduced, PaO_2 may or may not decrease depending on whether the effect of the increase in shunt on PaO_2 is greater than the influence of $P\bar{v}O_2$ on PaO_2.

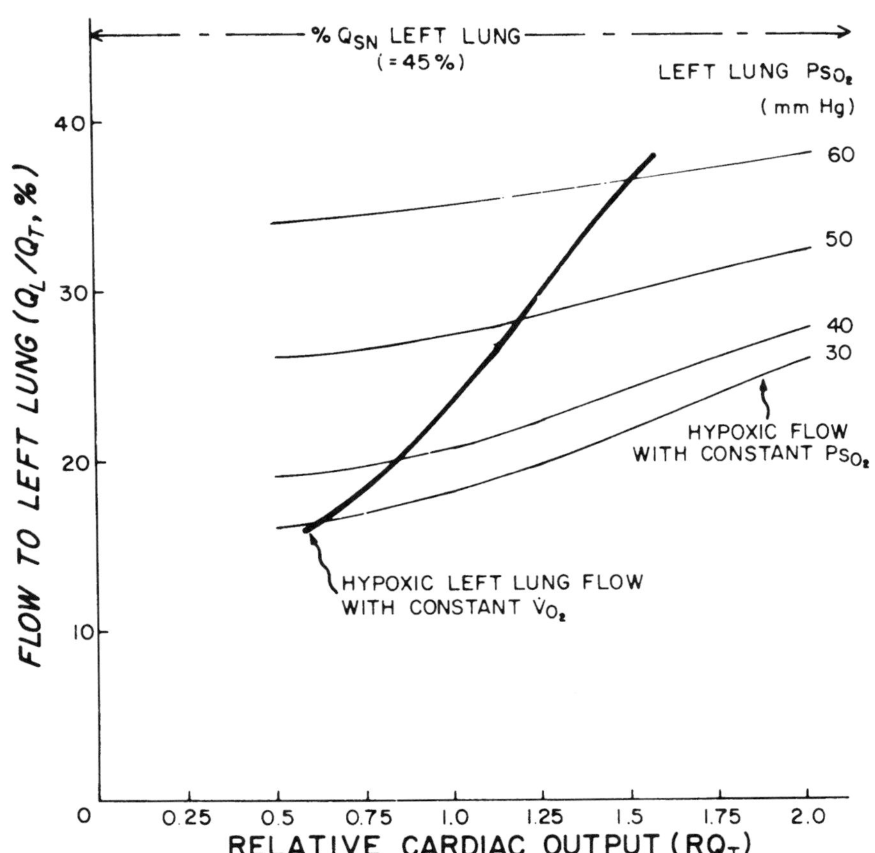

Figure 14. Change in blood flow to hypoxic left lung ($\dot{Q}L/\dot{Q}T\%$) when cardiac output is altered. The fine curves illustrate the effect of increasing cardiac output on $QL/\dot{Q}T\%$ when $P\bar{v}O_2$ (and therefore PsO_2) remain constant. The *heavy line* illustrates the effect when $P\bar{v}O_2$ s allowed to change. The *steeper slope of the line* is due to both the difference in the curvature of the normoxic and hypoxic lung pressure-flow curves and to a decreasing stimulus for HPV in the hypoxic lung. (From ref. 206 with permission.)

Table 1. FACTORS WHICH ATTENUATE HPV-INDUCED FLOW DIVERSION

1. Large hypoxic lung segment
2. Increased Ppa
3. Increased left atrial pressure
4. Increased cardiac output
5. Increased $P\bar{v}O_2$
6. Severely decreased $P\bar{v}O_2$
7. Metabolic alkalosis
8. Respiratory alkalosis
9. Acute lung injury
10. Endotoxin
11. Lung manipulation and surgery
12. Positive-end expiratory pressure (PEEP), especially normoxic lung PEEP
13. Estradiol
14. Prostacyclin (PGI_2)

Reductions in cardiac output have an even greater influence on the HPV response and arterial blood oxygenation. Ventilation-perfusion inequality is increased by reductions in pulmonary blood flow even when $P\bar{v}O_2$ is constant (75,258). A reduction in $P\bar{v}O_2$ may stimulate HPV in normal areas of the lung, resulting is less effective flow diversion away from the pathologic lung region (12,208,212,305). This is especially important in regional lung disease, where the blood flow through the hypoxic region is increased when cardiac output is low (56). As $P\bar{v}O_2$ influences PaO_2 even when pulmonary shunt is unchanged, PaO_2 may be markedly reduced with low cardiac output and regional lung disease. More modest reductions in cardiac output may not affect arterial blood oxygenation but contribute to some of the observed differences in effects of drugs on HPV in in vivo versus in vitro experiments. The impact of these changes on the influence of anesthetic agents and other drugs on HPV is discussed later in this chapter.

Acid-Base Status Acid-base status profoundly influences the HPV response (27,37,113,181,216). A metabolic acidosis enhances HPV (37,181). A metabolic alkalosis inhibits HPV, with a complete reversal noted at a pH of 7.60. HPV is blunted by a respiratory alkalosis, with an 80% inhibition observed at a pH of 7.60. However, with a chronic respiratory alkalosis, HPV is restored (114). In contrast, a respiratory acidosis does not affect HPV in dogs, due to a pH-independent vasodilating effect of CO_2 (37). The important clinical ramification is that HPV is significantly attenuated by a respiratory and metabolic alkalosis. Consequently, $\dot{V}_A/\dot{Q}$ matching and arterial blood oxygenation in normal and abnormal lungs are impaired in the presence of a metabolic alkalosis and respiratory alkalosis (78,80).

Lung Injury States HPV is attenuated by several types of acute lung injury. A diminished HPV response has been observed in lung injury in animals due to hyperoxia (246,247), endotoxin (128,146,280,345), oleic acid (178,179), *Pseudomonas* pneumonia (131,219), and platelet-activating factor (104). HPV is blunted in humans with bacterial pneumonia (176). An attenuated level of HPV was suggested by the lack of change of intrapulmonary shunt when ventilated with 100% O_2. HPV is also inhibited by tumor necrosis factor-α (TNF-α), which is released by macrophages in response to endotoxin (158). Surgical trauma and manipulation of the lungs also transiently attenuate HPV (17,200,269). Repeated intermittent exposures to hypoxia restore HPV after open-chest surgery and manipulation of pulmonary vessels (17,200,269). In contrast, repeated exposures to hypoxia do not potentiate HPV in closed-cheated animals (51) and humans (26).

In many of these lung injuries, the loss of reactivity is due to the release of vasodilator prostanoids, as treatment with cyclooxygenase inhibitors restores the HPV response and oxygenation in these diseases (128,131,178,179,247,308). In addition, variability of the baseline HPV response in dogs with alveolar hypoxia (2,127,128) and acute atelectasis (102,317) is also reduced with cyclooxygenase inhibitors. These results suggest that attenuation of HPV in lung injury is mediated by the production of vasodilating prostanoids by the endothelium. In contrast, nitric oxide probably does not mediate the loss of HPV in lung injury, such as in *Pseudomonas* pneumonia (219) and TNF-α (158).

Other Factors Lung inflation, as with PEEP, may attenuate HPV (13,79,184). PEEP especially reduces the effectiveness of HPV-induced flow diversion when it is administered to the normoxic lung regions (13,79). This is likely to be encountered clinically when PEEP is administered to the ventilated lung during one-lung anesthesia and when PEEP is used to treat regional lung disease such as a pneumonia or pulmonary contusion. In these situations, PEEP may increase blood flow through the nonventilated lung, thereby increasing pulmonary shunt and decreasing PaO_2.

HPV is also attenuated by estradiol, as the HPV response was greater in males than in females (350). The variability of the HPV response with atelectasis and alveolar hypoxia in dogs is related to the release of prostacyclin (2,102,127,128, 183,332).

In summary, HPV is attenuated by many factors that are present in the clinical care of patients, including increases in cardiac output, metabolic and respiratory alkalosis, pneumonia and endotoxin, lung inflation and surgical stress. Consequently, the effectiveness of HPV in preserving oxygenation in patients with ARDS and pneumonia is variable. However, inhibition of HPV by nonselective pulmonary vasodilators and metabolic and respiratory alkaloses will often adversely affect ventilation-perfusion matching and oxygenation.

Autonomic Control of Pulmonary Vascular Tone

In most species, the pulmonary vasculature is well innervated by sympathetic and parasympathetic nerve fibers (91,147,150, 165,285). In the dog, adrenergic nerve fibers are present in large and small pulmonary arteries (down to 25 μm) and in large intrapulmonary veins (147,165). The adrenergic terminals, which contain vesicles, are found in the adventitia of both pulmonary arteries and veins and in the outer third of the media of the arteries (165). Cholinergic nerve fibers and vesicles have also been identified in the dog within the intrapulmonary arteries, but not intrapulmonary veins (91,165).

α_1- and α_2-Adrenoreceptors, β_2-adrenoreceptors, and muscarinic cholinergic receptors are present and innervated in the pulmonary vasculature (147,148,151). The pulmonary vasculature responds to both sympathetic and parasympathetic stimulation. However, stimulation yields different responses depending on the resting level of pulmonary vascular tone (Table 2) (147,149,150,295,298). At low pulmonary vascular tone, stimulation of α_1- and α_2-adrenergic receptors and muscarinic cholinergic receptors causes vasoconstriction (147–149,295,298), whereas stimulation of β_2-adrenergic receptors causes vasodilation (147,151). However, the β_2-adrenoreceptor responses are masked at low-resting levels of pulmonary vascular tone (147). Using arterial and venous occlusion, norepinephrine and epinephrine have been found to cause predominantly venous vasoconstriction (Fig. 15) (67,69). At low pulmonary vascular tone, sympathetic stimulation causes predominantly pulmonary arterial vasoconstriction (Fig. 15), resulting in increased pulmonary vascular resistance and decreased pulmonary arterial compliance (67,69,147,148,162,164). As in the systemic circulation, sympathetic vasoconstriction is predominantly mediated by α_1-adrenergic receptors (147,148), whereas administration of norepinephrine stimulates predominantly α_2-adrenergic receptors (147,148). At low-resting tone, parasympathetic stimulation results in an inconsistent response.

At elevated pulmonary vascular tone, vasoconstrictor responses to α_2-adrenergic receptors and vasodilator responses to

Table 2. PULMONARY VASCULAR EFFECTS OF AUTONOMIC RECEPTORS AND STIMULATION

Low Pulmonary Vascular Tone	
Sympathetic	
α_1-adrenergic receptor	Vasoconstriction
α_2-adrenergic receptor	Vasoconstriction
β_2-adrenergic receptor	Vasodilation
Nerve stimulation	Vasoconstriction (α_1)
Exogenous norepinephrine	Vasoconstriction (α_2)
Parasympathetic	
Muscarinic cholinergic receptor	Vasoconstriction
Nerve stimulation	Inconsistent response
High Pulmonary Vascular Tone	
Sympathetic	
α_1-adrenergic receptor	Vasoconstriction
α_2-adrenergic receptor	Vasoconstriction (enhanced)
β_2-adrenergic receptor	Vasodilation (enhanced)
Nerve stimulation	Biphasic vasoconstriction/ vasodilation
Exogenous norepinephrine	Vasoconstriction
Parasympathetic	
Muscarinic cholinergic receptor	Vasodilation (mediated by nitric oxide)
Nerve stimulation	Vasodilation (mediated by nitric oxide)

β_2-adrenergic receptors are increased (Table 2) (147,151). Stimulation of muscarinic cholinergic receptors causes vasodilation at high pulmonary vascular tone, in contrast to its vasoconstrictor effect at low tone (147–149,295,298). At high vascular tone, parasympathetic nerve stimulation elicits vasodilation. Release of nitric oxide mediates the cholinergic response at high vascular tone, as an intact endothelium is required to elicit vasodilation with acetylcholine (53,98).

Although it is well established that autonomic innervation of the pulmonary circulation exists, the physiologic significance of and role in maintaining vascular tone and matching of ventilation and perfusion are not understood (147). The net effect of the autonomic nervous system in the conscious, intact animal is pulmonary vasodilation, predominantly mediated by β_2-adrenergic receptors (234,237). The autonomic nervous system also contributes to the regulation of pulmonary vascular tone during hemorrhage. Systemic hypotension results in pulmonary vasoconstriction mediated by α_1-adrenoreceptors (268). Activation of sympathetic β-adrenergic receptors and cholinergic muscarinic receptors does not affect the pulmonary vascular response to hypotension (268).

Autonomic stimulation may also modify the HPV response, although it does not modulate the HPV response to global hypoxia in intact dogs (188). Sympathetic nerve stimulation attenuates HPV to a mild degree (162,272) and sympathetic blockade may enhance HPV (259). In addition, widespread sympathetic activation due to stimulation of central nervous system structures and release of catecholamines plays a major role in the pathogenesis of neurogenic pulmonary edema (196). However, it is not clear what role the autonomic nervous system has in regulating pulmonary blood flow and vascular tone in most types of lung injury and in pulmonary hypertension. In addition, sympathetic blockade, as with epidural anesthesia, while it may mildly enhance HPV, has relatively little effect on ventilation-perfusion matching and oxygenation.

Humoral Regulation of Pulmonary Vascular Tone

The mechanisms responsible for the preservation of low pulmonary vascular tone in the normal state are complex and are not definitively identified. The recruitable and distensible nature of the pulmonary circulation is very important and is a passive factor that is responsible for maintenance of low vascular tone. Additionally, active pharmacologic factors are likely to maintain a low pulmonary vascular resistance. However, they probably represent a complex balance between locally and systemically produced vasoconstrictors and vasodilators. In the injured and chronically hypertensive lung, the situation becomes even more unclear as production of endothelial-cell–derived factors and membrane properties of the vascular smooth muscle cell are altered (290).

Many factors that are either circulating or are intrinsic to pulmonary vasculature may affect pulmonary vascular tone

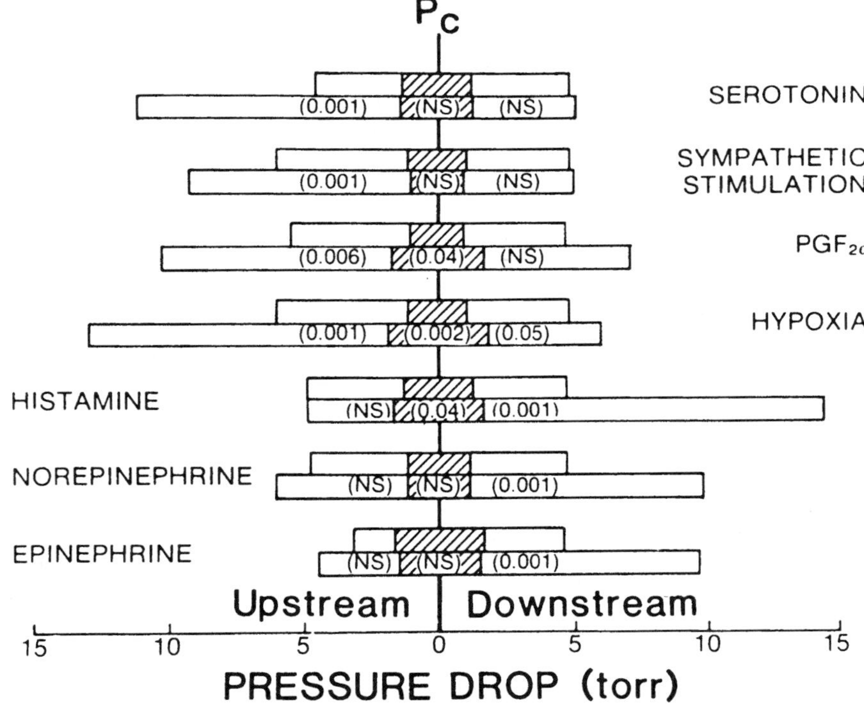

Figure 15. The effects of various vasoconstrictor substances on upstream (arterial), downstream (venous), and middle segment (small vessel and capillary) pressure drops as determined by arterial and venous occlusion techniques. The *upper bar* represents data for the control state and the *lower bar* represents data and P values after vasoconstriction with the identified substance. Pc is critical closing pressure as determined by double occlusion. (Reproduced from ref. 187 with permission.)

Table 3. **EFFECT OF VARIOUS PEPTIDES, BIOGENIC AMINES, AND LIPID MEDIATORS ON PULMONARY VASCULAR TONE**

Compound	Action
Endothelial derived	
Nitric oxide	Vasodilation
Endothelin-1	Vasoconstriction (high dose) Vasodilation (low dose)
Superoxide anion	Vasoconstriction
Peptides	
Angiotensin II	Vasoconstriction
Bradykinin	Vasodilation (mediated by nitric oxide)
Arginine vasopressin (AVP)	Vasoconstriction (exogenous) Vasodilation (endogenous release, mediated by nitric oxide)
Atrial natriuretic peptide	Vasodilation
Vasoactive intestinal peptide (VIP)	Vasodilation
Calcitonin gene-related peptide	Vasodilation
Biogenic amines	
Histamine-H_1 receptor	Vasoconstriction
Histamine-H_2 receptor	Vasodilation
Serotonin	Vasoconstriction
Lipid mediators	
Arachidonic acid	Mixed response
Platelet-activating factor (PAF)	Vasoconstriction (high dose) Vasodilation (low dose)
lyso-PAF	Inactive
Prostaglandins	
$PGF_{2\alpha}$	Vasoconstriction
PGE_2	Vasoconstriction (high dose) Vasodilation (low dose)
PGI_2 (prostacyclin)	Vasodilation
PGE_1	Vasodilation
Thromboxane	Vasoconstriction
Leukotrienes (LTC_4, LTD_4, LTE_4, LTB_4)	Vasoconstriction

(Table 3). Their effects are complex and sometimes differ among the species, with dose of the factors, and whether the factors are exogenously or endogenously released. The pulmonary endothelium produces prostanoid as well as nonprostanoid, nonpeptide mediators of vascular tone including nitric oxide, the endothelium-derived relaxing factor (EDRF) (152,261), and several endothelium-derived constricting factors—endothelin-1 and superoxide anion are two of the factors (101,291,301,353). Nitric oxide is a potent pulmonary vasodilator and inhibitor of HPV (45,94,95). Endothelin-1 is a potent vasoconstrictor (101,301,353). However, in low doses, endothelin-1 is a pulmonary vasodilator (101). Expression of endothelin-1 is increased in several pulmonary diseases, including asthma, fibrosing alveolitis, and pulmonary hypertension (8). This suggests that endothelin-1 may play a pathophysiologic role and endothelin antagonists may be useful in the treatment of various pulmonary diseases (8).

Many peptides also affect pulmonary vascular tone. Angiotensin II is a vasoconstrictor and is important for regulation of vascular tone in normal dogs (112). It is especially important during systemic hypotension, when its release causes pulmonary vasoconstriction (268). Bradykinin (153,253,254), atrial natriuretic peptide (54,138,156), vasoactive intestinal peptide (VIP) (243), and calcitonin gene-related peptide (290) are also pulmonary vasodilators. Vasodilation by bradykinin is mediated by nitric oxide (5,153). Exogenous administration of arginine vasopressin causes pulmonary vasoconstriction; however, it causes vasodilation in the presence of V1-vasopressin receptor blockade (253–255) and in the setting of acute pulmonary vasoconstriction (335). In addition, arginine vasopressin caused pulmonary vasodilation in rats (299), and endogenous release of arginine vasopressin during systemic hypotension dilates the pulmonary circulation (268). Vasodilation by arginine vasopression is mediated by release of nitric oxide (300).

Histamine is found in the perivascular structures of the lung and in the adventitia of lung vessels. The histamine type 1 (H_1) receptor mediates arterial and venous vasoconstriction (7,59, 163,244,271) and the histamine type 2 (H_2) receptor mediates pulmonary vasodilation (1). The overall effect of histamine on the pulmonary arteries may be either vasoconstriction or vasodilation, while pulmonary venous constriction is always present (313). Arterial and venous occlusion studies have revealed that histamine increases vascular resistance in the small vessel and venous circulation (Fig. 15) (67,69). In contrast, these and other studies have demonstrated that serotonin is a potent pulmonary arterial vasoconstrictor (Fig. 15) (22,59,67,69,271).

The arachidonic acid-derived metabolites also affect pulmonary vascular tone. Cell-membrane phospholipids are broken down by phospholipases into arachidonic acid and lyso-platelet-activating factor (PAF) (290). Arachidonic acid may by itself or through its metabolites alter vascular tone (Fig. 16 and Table 3). The leukotrienes (LTC_4, LTD_4, LTE_4, LTB_4) are pulmonary vasoconstrictors (290). The prostaglandin $PGF_{2\alpha}$ is a vasoconstrictor (67,302). Arterial and venous occlusion studies demonstrated that $PGF_{2\alpha}$ predominantly increases vascular resistance in arterioles and small vessels (Fig. 15) (67,69). PGE_2 is a vasoconstrictor at high doses and a vasodilator at low doses (290). PGI_2 or prostacyclin is a potent pulmonary vasodilator that acts by increasing adenosine 3',5'-cyclic monophosphate (cAMP) (302). PGE_1 causes moderate vasodilation in precontracted pulmonary arteries, an effect that is independent of the endothelium (177). Thromboxane is a vasoconstrictor, especially a venous vasoconstrictor (354). Lyso-PAF is inactive; however, its metabolite PAF causes pulmonary vasoconstriction at high doses and pulmonary vasodilation at low doses (340).

Some of the arachidonic acid-derived metabolites may have a role in modulating the HPV response. In particular, prostacyclin (PGI_2) markedly attenuates HPV and reduces flow diversion away from hypoxic alveoli, resulting in reduced PaO_2 (317). Endogenously produced PGI_2 appears to be responsible for the variability of HPV response in some animals and with acute lung injury, as the response is restored by administration of cyclooxygenase inhibitors (2,102,127,128,317).

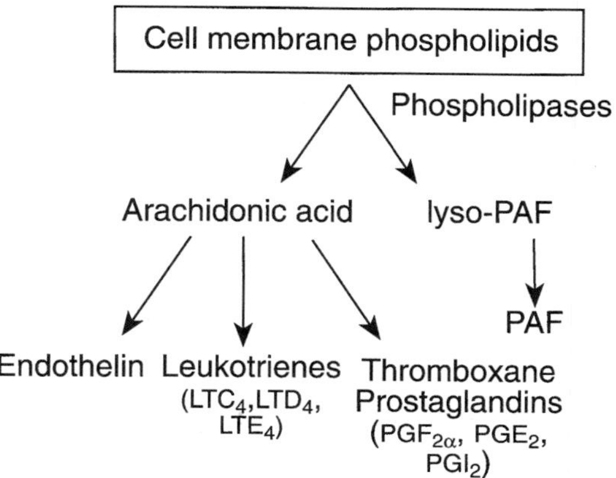

Figure 16. Vasoactive metabolites of cell membrane phospholipids. Phospholipids are broken down by phospholipases to form arachidonic acid and lyso-platelet-activating factor (lyso-PAF). Platelet-activating factor (PAF), an active metabolite of lyso-PAF, causes pulmonary vasoconstriction. Thromboxane, endothelin, and the leukotrienes (LTC_4, LTD_4, LTE_4) are also pulmonary vasoconstrictors. The prostaglandin PGI_2 causes pulmonary vasodilation and $PGF_{2\alpha}$ and PGE_2 are pulmonary vasoconstrictors.

In contrast, the leukotrienes cause pulmonary vasoconstriction and increase the pulmonary pressure response to global alveolar hypoxia (180,210). However, their effect is due to nonspecific vasoconstriction rather than a specific potentiation of HPV, as inhibitors of leukotrienes do not attenuate HPV in regional hypoxia (114,309). Pulmonary vasoconstrictor $PGF_{2\alpha}$ also is a nonspecific vasoconstrictor that does not alter HPV-induced flow diversion (50). However, infusion of $PGF_{2\alpha}$ directly into the pulmonary artery of an atelactic lung improved vasoconstriction in that lung and PaO_2 (306,307).

Regulation of pulmonary vascular tone in the basal state is dependent on two main mechanisms: cyclic-nucleotide–mediated relaxation and membrane-potential–mediated relaxation (290) (Fig. 17). There are two parallel, cyclic nucleotide-dependent systems, one dependent on cAMP, and one dependent on guanosine 3',5'-cyclic monophosphate (cGMP). Stimulation of either of these systems will reduce pulmonary vascular tone by activating regulatory enzymes that change the state of phosphorylation of the smooth muscle contractile proteins. One pathway involves stimulation of cAMP production by a receptor coupled to adenylate cyclase. Increased levels of cAMP activate cAMP-dependent protein kinase, which results in changes in the phosphorylation of myosin light chain kinase and smooth muscle relaxation. The second pathway involves stimulation of cGMP through activation of cytoplasmic guanylate cyclase by nitric oxide (EDRF). Increased levels of cGMP activate cGMP-dependent protein kinase, which causes smooth muscle relaxation by phosphorylation of myosin light chain kinase. Both cAMP and cGMP kinases affect mobilization of smooth muscle calcium from intracellular stores and alter contractile protein sensitivity to calcium (290). Pharmacologic agents that increase cGMP or cAMP also attenuate hypoxic pulmonary vasoconstriction (89).

A second mechanism for smooth muscle relaxation is mediated by changes in membrane potential (Fig. 17). Voltage-gated calcium channels open when the cell membrane depolarizes, allowing extracellular calcium to flow into the cytoplasm, which further increases calcium by activation of calcium stores. Smooth muscle relaxation occurs with closure of the voltage-gated calcium channels (290). Smooth muscle relaxation also occurs with membrane hyperpolarization by opening of potassium channels (290).

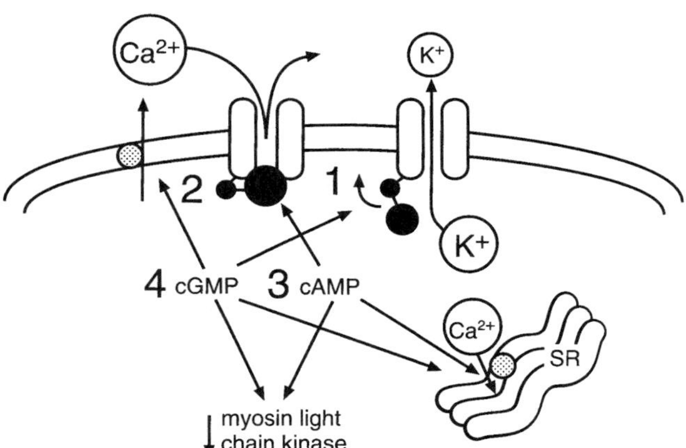

Figure 17. Regulation of pulmonary vascular tone illustrating cyclic-nucleotide and membrane-potential-mediated smooth muscle relaxation. Smooth muscle relaxation occurs with membrane hyperpolarization by opening potassium channels (1) or closure of voltage-gated calcium channels (2). Two parallel, cyclic nucleotide-dependent systems also cause smooth muscle relaxation, one dependent on cyclic 3',5'-adenosine monophosphate (cAMP, 3) and the other dependent on cyclic 3',5'-guanosine monophosphate (cGMP, 4). Increased levels of cAMP or cGMP result in vascular relaxation by the phosphorylation of myosin light chain kinase and decreased mobilization of calcium (Ca^{2+})from smooth muscle stores; the sarcoplasmic reticulum (SR). (From ref. 290 with permission.)

Many of the endogenous peptides, biogenic amines, and lipid mediators cause vasodilation by affecting the regulatory pathways (290). For instance, cAMP levels are increased by β-adrenergic receptor stimulation and PGI_2-receptor stimulation. cGMP levels are increased by nitric oxide. Membrane potential is affected by an endothelial-released hyperpolarization factor. Acetylcholine and bradykinin increase cGMP levels due to the release of nitric oxide (249). As inhibitors of each of the various factors do not cause large increases in pulmonary vascular tone (180,249), it is likely that multiple, complex systems are involved in the maintenance of normal low pulmonary tone. In diseased pulmonary vasculature, the interaction of compounds is likely to be even more complex. Release of PGI_2 and nitric oxide is stimulated by increases in pulmonary blood flow and shear force (226). Because of the complexity, the pharmacology of the pulmonary circulation in normal and diseased states are currently areas of intense active investigation.

In summary, the autonomic nervous system and humoral regulation of pulmonary vascular tone is complex. Of prime importance is the role of cAMP and cGMP systems in pulmonary vasodilation. It is through these systems that the pharmacologic effects of the cardiovascular drugs, to be discussed later in this chapter, exert their pulmonary vasodilator effects.

PHARMACOLOGY OF PULMONARY BLOOD FLOW

Anesthetic Agents

Intravenous Anesthetics

The intravenous anesthetics, including pentobarbital, opioids, droperidol, and ketamine, have been traditionally believed to have little influence on resting pulmonary vascular tone and the pulmonary vasoconstrictor response to alveolar hypoxia (15,20, 29,34,85,103,217,319). Propofol did not affect PVR in vitro when vascular tone was normal; however, propofol reduced PVR when pulmonary vascular tone was increased (337). Propofol also did not affect basal pulmonary vascular tone in intact dogs (87). The response to regional hypoxia and arterial O_2 tension is well maintained in the presence of pentobarbital (217). One-lung anesthesia with ketamine (193,279), propofol and alfentanil (318), or a mixture of diazepam, opioids, barbiturates, and/or ketamine (11,292), resulted in a more stable PaO_2 and pulmonary shunt, when compared to volatile anesthetics. Lidocaine also reversed nitrous oxide–induced depression of HPV (26,27).

However, recent studies by Murray and colleagues (48,90,233, 251,252,256,335,349) have demonstrated that pentobarbital has complex and significant effects on the regulation of pulmonary vascular tone (Table 4). When compared to the conscious state, pentobarbital did not affect (256) or had a mild vasodilatory effect on baseline pulmonary pressure-flow relationships (335). However, it alters the autonomic nervous system regulation of pulmonary vascular tone (256). In contrast to inducing pulmonary vasodilation in the conscious state, during pentobarbital anesthesia, α-adrenergic blockade caused vasoconstriction (256). β-Adrenergic blockade was associated with attenuated pulmonary vasoconstriction. Whereas cholinergic blockade resulted in vasodilation in conscious dogs, it caused pulmonary vasoconstriction in pentobarbital-anesthetized dogs (256).

Pentobarbital anesthesia augmented pulmonary vasoconstriction to cyclooxygenase inhibition (251). cGMP-mediated vasodilation by bradykinin and sodium nitroprusside were unaffected by pentobarbital anesthesia (233). Pentobarbital anesthesia resulted in an unchanged pulmonary vasoconstrictor response to angiotensin II, although it reversed pulmonary vasodilation with angiotensin-converting enzyme inhibition to pulmonary

Table 4. **COMPARISON OF PULMONARY VASCULAR EFFECTS OF PENTOBARBITAL AND HALOTHANE COMPARED TO CONSCIOUS STATE**

Effect	Pentobarbital Anesthesia	Halothane Anesthesia
Baseline pressure-flow relationship:	No change	Mild pulmonary vasoconstriction
Autonomic nervous system regulation:	Modifies	Abolishes
α-adrenergic block	Reverses vasodilation to vasoconstriction	Abolishes vasodilation
β-adrenergic block	Attenuated vasoconstriction	Abolishes vasoconstriction
cholinergic block	Reverses vasodilation to vasoconstriction	Abolishes vasodilation
Cyclooxygenase inhibition:	Augments vasoconstriction	Augments vasoconstriction
Angiotensin II:	No change	Abolishes vasoconstriction
Angiotensin converting enzyme inhibition:	Reverses vasodilation to vasoconstriction	Abolishes vasodilation
cGMP-mediated vasodilation (nitroprusside, bradykinin):	No change in vasodilation	Abolishes vasodilation
Posthypoperfusion vasoregulation:	Modifies	Modifies
Autonomic nervous system	Increased vasoconstriction (α-adrenergic stimulation)	No net change but vasoconstriction masked by vasodilation
Cyclooxygenase metabolites and angiotensin II opposing effects	Abolishes regulation	Preserves regulation
Alveolar hypoxia:	Alters	Alters
In vitro	Mild attenuation of vasoconstriction	Marked inhibition of vasoconstriction
In vivo	Mild attenuation of vasoconstriction	No change to mild attenuation of vasoconstriction
Arginine vasopressin:	Abolishes vasodilation	Reverses vasodilation to vasoconstriction

vasoconstriction (252). Arginine vasopressin-induced pulmonary vasodilation observed in the conscious state in dogs with elevated pulmonary vascular tone was abolished during pentobarbital anesthesia (335). In addition, pulmonary vasoregulation after hypoperfusion was altered in the presence of pentobarbital anesthesia (50,90). Active, flow-independent pulmonary vasoconstriction, primarily mediated by sympathetic α-vasoconstriction, occurred after hypoperfusion. The competing mechanisms of pulmonary vasoconstriction by cyclooxygenase metabolites and pulmonary vasoconstriction by angiotensin II after hypoperfusion were abolished by pentobarbital (90). In addition, the pulmonary pressor response to global hypoxia was modestly attenuated by pentobarbital when studied in vitro (349).

In summary, pentobarbital and presumably other intravenous anesthetics may affect humoral control of pulmonary vascular tone in complex ways, many of which remain to be elucidated. However, intravenous anesthetics have minimal effects on HPV, pulmonary vascular tone, and oxygenation during one-lung anesthesia. Hence, they are often used as background anesthetics in experimental studies to which the effects of the inhalational anesthetics are compared. Clinically, intravenous agents are safe and effective lung anesthesia, with minimal adverse effects on HPV and arterial blood oxygenation.

Inhalational Anesthetics

Most studies have investigated the pulmonary vascular effects of inhalational anesthetics with a background intravenous anesthetic. These studies found that the inhalational anesthetics have no or minimal vasodilating effects on normal pulmonary vascular tone, with the exception of nitrous oxide, which increases pulmonary vascular tone (326). No change in pulmonary vascular resistance was observed in isolated lungs with diethyl ether (321), trichloroethylene (321,326), enflurane (211), isoflurane (154, 211), halothane (135,191,210,211), sevoflurane (154), and desflurane (190), and modest reductions in pulmonary vascular resistance were observed with methoxylflurane (322) and halothane (135,321,326). Compared to pentobarbital anesthesia or the awake state, pulmonary vascular tone, as determined by pulmonary-pressure-flow curves, was also not affected by isoflurane in vivo (186,238). Likewise, no differences in the diameters of lung surface arterioles and venules and red blood cell flux and velocity, as measured by intravital fluorescence microscopy, were observed with isoflurane anesthesia during normoxic ventilation (117). Using arterial and venous occlusion techniques, in an isolated canine lobe, Johnson et al. (159) found that in comparison to pentobarbital, halothane reduced the percentage of resistance in the middle segment, consisting of small arterioles, venules, and capillaries. Pressure-flow curves obtained with halothane demonstrated a parallel shift with a reduction in zero-flow intercept, suggesting a critical closing pressure or Starling resistance.

However, when compared to the conscious state, halothane caused modest, active, flow-independent pulmonary vasoconstriction when prolonged changes in cardiac output were used to obtain pressure-flow relationship (46). The vasoconstriction is not mediated by reflex sympathetic α-adrenergic activation, metabolites of cyclooxygenase, or increased production or release of angiotensin II or arginine vasopressin (46). In contrast, when pressure-flow curves were generated without changes in systemic hemodynamics, halothane caused a mild reduction in pulmonary vascular tone (335). The differences are probably due to activation of sympathetic nervous system and other humoral factors with hypotension. Isoflurane had no effect on the baseline pulmonary circulation compared to the conscious state (186). Mild changes in pulmonary vascular tone are not clinically apparent when a patient is anesthetized with a volatile anesthetic, because of a concurrent decrease in cardiac output.

Halothane anesthesia alters many of the humoral mechanisms that regulate pulmonary vascular tone (Table 4). Endogenous autonomic nervous system regulation is abolished during halothane anesthesia (47). Halothane also augments oxidant-induced pulmonary vasoconstriction via alterations in arachidonic acid metabolism (311). Halothane attenuates exogenously administered angiotensin II–induced pulmonary vasoconstriction (210,252). Pulmonary vasodilation in response to angiotensin-converting enzyme inhibition is reversed to pulmonary vasoconstriction during halothane anesthesia (252). However, counteracting vasodilator effects by endogenously released cyclooxygenase metabolites, and vasoconstrictor effects by endogenously released angiotensin II, of pulmonary vasoregulation after hypoperfusion, are still active with halothane anesthesia, in contrast to pentobarbital (90). Halothane anesthesia also abolished cGMP-mediated pulmonary vasodilation with sodium nitroprusside and bradykinin, in contrast to preserved responses with pentobarbital anesthesia (233). The complex pulmonary vascular effects of other volatile agents, such as isoflurane, are under current investigation. Roughly similar effects to halothane would be expected with isoflurane. As with halothane, isoflurane anesthesia attenuated cGMP-mediated pulmonary vasodilation with bradykinin (100). Pulmonary vasodilation mediated by adenosine triphosphate (ATP)-sensitive potassium channels was also attenuated during isoflurane anesthesia (96). However, while halothane anesthesia abolished the pulmonary vascular response to neural antagonists, isoflurane potentiated cAMP-mediated vasodilation induced by isoproterenol in a canine model of elevated pulmonary vascular tone (186). These results suggest that the volatile anesthetics have complex effects on the regulation of pulmonary vascular tone.

The effect of the inhalational anesthetic agents on HPV is complex because it involves the interaction of the direct pulmonary vascular effects of the anesthetic and the secondary cardiovascular, autonomic, and humoral effects of the anesthetic. The following section reviews these effects and discusses why there are differences between what is observed in vitro in isolated lung preparations and in vivo in the intact animal or patient.

The direct pulmonary vascular effect of inhalational anesthetics is the inhibition of HPV. When studied in vitro in isolated lungs or in situ in a lobe with constant perfusion, a dose-dependent attenuation of the rise in pulmonary artery pressure with hypoxic ventilation is observed with administration of the volatile anesthetics. The marked inhibition of the response to global alveolar hypoxia has been demonstrated with ether (34,144,145,191,321), trichloroethylene (321,326), halothane (29–32,34,159,160,191,210,211,321,326), methoxyflurane (34, 322), enflurane (31,211), isoflurane (154,211), sevoflurane (154), and desflurane (190). Nitrous oxide also depresses the HPV response in the in situ perfused lung (24,25,144,145). Pulmonary vascular resistance in atelectatic lung is also reduced by the volatile anesthetics (32,161), due to an attenuation of HPV.

Using vascular occlusion techniques, Johnson et al. (160) found that halothane prevented the hypoxia-induced increase in vascular resistance in middle vascular segments. Halothane reduced the zero-flow intercept or critical closing pressure, but did not alter the slope of the pressure-flow curve during hypoxia. Halothane also reduced the resistance of the middle vascular segment in atelectatic lung (161). These data suggest that halothane and most likely other volatile agents directly inhibit HPV by reducing vascular tone in the small vessels and capillaries.

Figure 18 illustrates the typical dose-response relationship for inhibition of HPV by the volatile anesthetics in in vitro preparations with controlled perfusion. Using isolated, perfused rat lungs, Marshall et al. (211) found that halothane, enflurane, and isoflurane depressed the pulmonary presser response to global alveolar hypoxia in a dose-related manner. Fifty percent depression of HPV (ED_{50}) was observed at similar MAC units for all three agents (approximately 0.6 MAC). At 1 MAC levels, 20% or less of the baseline HPV response was observed. The slope of the dose-response curves also did not differ for the agents. Using a similar preparation in rabbits, Ishibe (154) found that the ED_{50} for inhibition of HPV by isoflurane and sevoflurane was somewhat higher (0.85 MAC for isoflurane and 1.0 MAC for sevoflurane). Therefore, based on

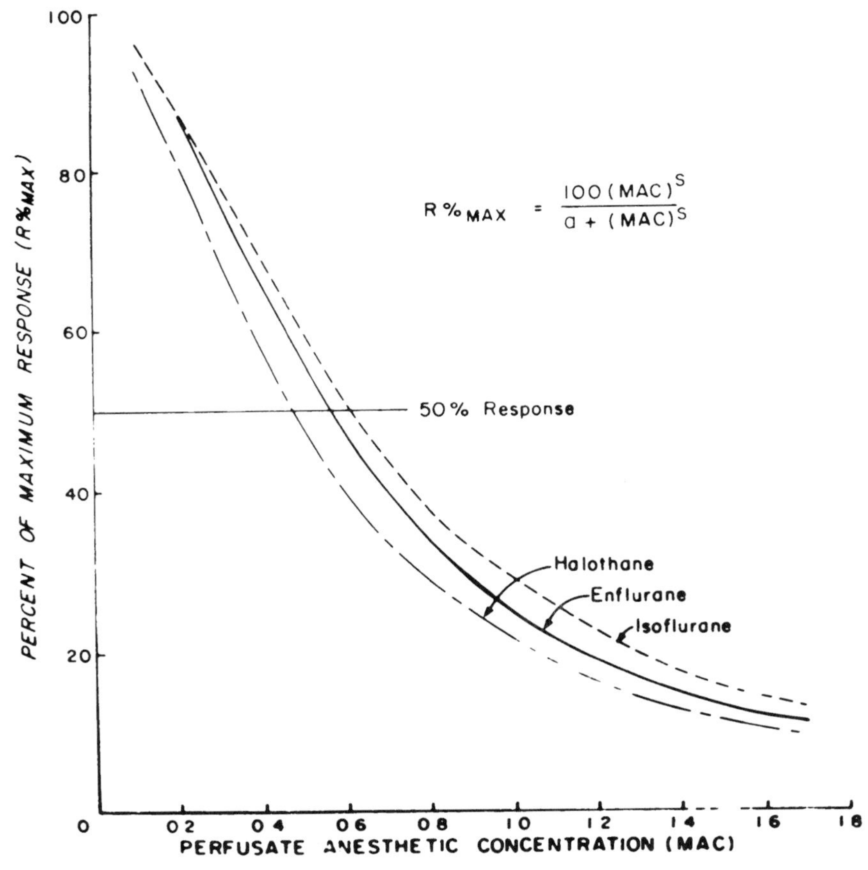

Figure 18. Effects of inhalational anesthetics in vitro in isolated rat lungs. Depression of maximal response to global alveolar hypoxia and ED_{50}s are shown. Each anesthetic curve is derived from the mean results of several animals. Anesthetic curves do not differ in slope, position, or ED_{50}. (Reproduced from ref. 211 with permission.)

studies with controlled perfused and mixed venous O_2, a significant inhibition of HPV with the volatile anesthetic agents would be expected in intact animals and human patients at clinically used concentrations.

The mechanism by which the volatile anesthetics directly inhibit HPV is unclear. Inhalational anesthetics may interact with the vascular endothelium and affect release of prostacyclin and other arachidonic metabolites from the cell membrane or endothelial-derived factors such as nitric oxide or endothelin (157,310), all factors that may modulate the intensity of the HPV response. Inhalation anesthetics interact with cell membranes and increase production of arachidonic acid mediators (311). The hypoxic pulmonary vascular effects of inhalational anesthetic agents are modulated by cyclooxygenase and lipooxygenase products of arachidonic acid metabolism. Attenuation of HPV by nitrous oxide (183), halothane (210), and isoflurane (185) was reduced or abolished by reduction in prostacyclin due to inhibition of cyclooxygenase. Reduction in leukotrienes by lipooxygenase blockade potentiated the inhibition in HPV by halothane (210).

However, inhibition of HPV by volatile anesthetics is not dependent on the endothelium. Release of nitric oxide is not essential for the reduction in HPV by inhalational anesthetics (213). The inhibition of HPV by halothane, isoflurane, and enflurane in vitro was not affected by inhibition of guanylate cyclase activity by methylene blue (213). Volatile anesthetics appear to inhibit HPV by direct effects on the vascular smooth muscle (215). Removal of endothelium from pulmonary vessels did not affect the pulmonary vasoconstrictor response to hypoxia nor the dose-dependent reduction in HPV by isoflurane and halothane (215). Because of the importance of intracellular calcium and potassium ion flux in pulmonary contraction and relaxation, alteration of these ion channels by inhalational anesthetics would affect HPV. Volatile anesthetics suppress calcium influx in other vascular beds, such as coronary artery smooth muscle cells (39), and halothane causes hyperpolarization of resting membrane potential in mesenteric arteries (35). As calcium is key to hypoxic pulmonary vasoconstriction, suppression of calcium currents by volatile anesthetics would directly attenuate HPV.

In contrast to marked inhibition of HPV in vitro, inhalational anesthetics have variable and inconclusive effects on HPV in intact animals and humans. HPV was moderately attenuated by trichloroethylene (320), diethyl ether (33,324), and nitrous oxide (14,15,183,217,325). However, mild or no inhibition of HPV was observed with methoxyflurane (198), halothane (14, 15,33,88,217,236,323), and enflurane (43,217,236). Similarly, mild inhibition (14,15,41,74,217, 236) or no inhibition (238) of HPV was observed in vivo with clinically relevant concentrations of isoflurane. Using pressure-flow curves, Naeije et al. (238) found that 1 MAC isoflurane did not affect the rise in pulmonary artery pressure with global alveolar hypoxia at each level of cardiac output (Fig. 19). On the basis of results from the in vitro studies, a 70% to 80% reduction in the HPV response would have been predicted. In human patients, 1 to 1.2 MAC levels of isoflurane did not affect HPV, as measured by lung blood flow and PaO_2, when one lung was ventilated with a hypoxia (41). Using a dog model in which isoflurane was administered only to the hypoxic lung to minimize general hemodynamic changes, Domino et al. (74) found that the ED_{50} for inhibition of regional HPV was 2.4%, or close to 2 MAC.

Recently, direct observation of the pulmonary microcirculation using intravital fluorescence microscopy has demonstrated that 1.5% isoflurane inhibits HPV in vivo (Fig. 20) (117,118). The decreases in arteriolar diameter and red blood cell flux and velocity observed with alveolar hypoxia were significantly attenuated by isoflurane.

A major reason why isolated lung and in vivo yield such disparate results is the secondary influence of cardiac output on the observed HPV response. Cardiac output profoundly influences HPV, primarily due to its effect on mixed venous O_2 tension and therefore the stimulus for HPV (Fig. 14). A linear relationship between the apparent HPV response and simultaneous change in cardiac output is observed ($r = 0.7$) (Fig. 21). The apparent HPV response with an inhalational anesthetic is unchanged when cardiac output is reduced by the anesthetics, as with halothane (217,321,323), isoflurane (217), methoxyflurane (198), or enflurane (217). In contrast, HPV appears to be attenuated in vivo when cardiac output is maintained in the presence of the anesthetic, such as nitrous oxide (325), trichlor-

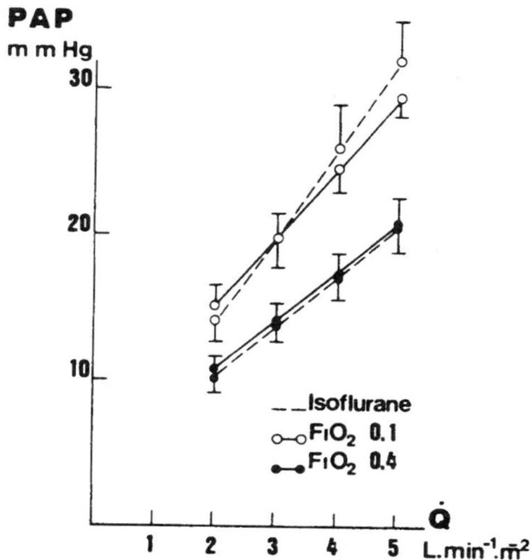

Figure 19. Pulmonary artery pressure (PAP)-flow ($\dot{Q}$) curves during hyperoxia *(solid circles)* and global alveolar hypoxia *(open circles)* before *(solid lines)* and after *(dotted lines)* isoflurane. Hypoxia increased PAP at each level of $\dot{Q}$ but this pressor response was not affected by 1 MAC isoflurane. (Reproduced from ref. 238 with permission.)

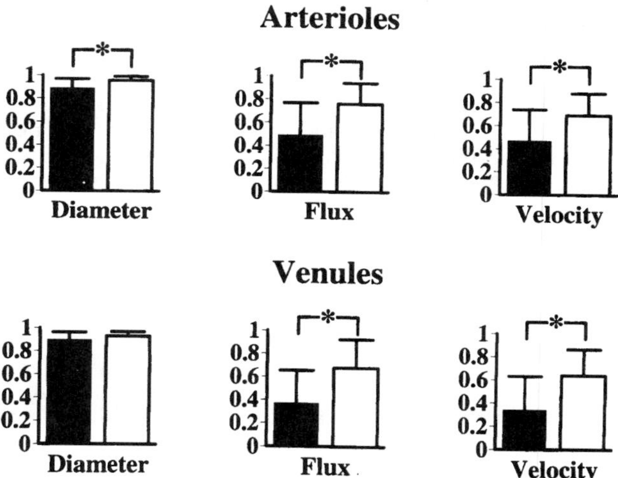

Figure 20. Effects of isoflurane on microvascular diameters and blood flow in the hypoxic lung as determined by intravital fluorescence microscopy. In comparison with baseline intravenous anesthesia *(filled columns)*, 1.5% isoflurane *(open columns)* increased the one-lung/two-lung ventilation ratio of vascular diameters in arterioles, red blood cell (RBC) flux in arterioles and venules, and RBC velocity in arterioles and venules. Therefore, direct observation of the pulmonary microcirculation demonstrated that isoflurane inhibits HPV and increases regional blood flow in the hypoxic lung. (Reproduced from ref. 118 with permission.)

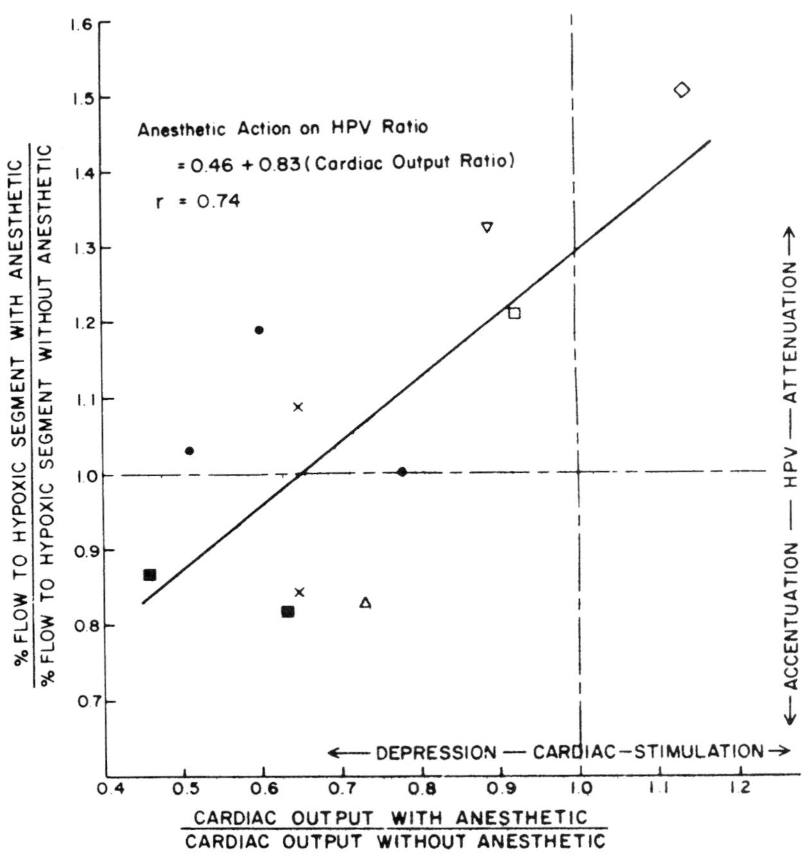

Figure 21. In vivo effects of inhalational anesthetics demonstrating the relationship between the observed changes in HPV with changes in cardiac output. Control cardiac output (x-axis) in absence of inhalational anesthetic is designated at 1.0. The effect of the anesthetic on HPV is indicated by % flow to hypoxic segment with anesthetic/without anesthetic (y-axis), with value of 1.0 indicating no effect, value >1 indicating inhibition of HPV, and value <1 indicating potentiation of HPV. There is a significant linear relationship between cardiac output and attenuation of HPV. *Solid circles,* halothane (217,323); *solid square,* isoflurane (217); *open triangle,* methoxyflurane; *open square,* nitrous oxide (325); *upside down open triangle,* trichloroethylene (320); diamond, diethyl ether (324); x, enflurane (217). (Reproduced with permission from Marshall BE and Marshall C, (206).

ethylene (320), and diethyl ether (324). Thus, during anesthesia, the effectiveness of the HPV response varies inversely with cardiac output.

Figure 22 illustrates the influence of inhalational anesthetics on the observed HPV response, depending on whether cardiac output is maintained constant or decreased by the anesthetic agent. Cardiac output inversely affects the observed HPV response both in the presence and absence of an inhalational anesthetic. However, for all cardiac outputs, the effectiveness of HPV is reduced by the inhalational anesthetic. If the hypoxic response in the presence of a volatile anesthetic that depresses cardiac output (e.g., halothane, enflurane, and isoflurane) is compared to the hypoxic response during a lightly anesthetized state, when cardiac output is high, the inhalational anesthetic would not appear to effect the HPV response. Thus, while the effectiveness of HPV is depressed by the volatile anesthetic, it is enhanced by the reduction in cardiac output. The simultaneous changes in cardiac output helps to explain some of the disparate results between studies in intact animals and people and isolated lungs or lobes with controlled perfusion.

The clinical implications are that the potent volatile anesthetics have a minimal adverse effect on HPV and oxygenation in the anesthetic care of most patients. In addition, volatile anesthetics do not exert a vasodilator influence on the pulmonary circulation in the absence of elevated pulmonary vascular tone due to hypoxia. Even in concentrations used for deliberate hypotension, isoflurane did not affect pulmonary shunt in patients free of pulmonary disease (248). The largest deterioration in arterial oxygenation would be expected during thoracotomies, as HPV is most important during one-lung ventilation. However, PaO_2 is well maintained during deliberate hypotension with isoflurane (248) and during one-lung anesthesia with isoflurane, halothane (11,20,85,292), and enflurane (316). Benumof et al. (11) found that 1 MAC halothane and isoflurane only slightly impaired arterial oxygenation compared to intravenous anesthesia during one-lung ventilation in patients undergoing thoracotomy. Their results are consistent with in vivo animal data demonstrating a 20% inhibition of HPV with 1 MAC concentrations of isoflurane (74). However, because blood flow is considerably reduced (by 50%) to the nondependent lung by the lateral decubitus position, only a 4% increase in pulmonary shunt would be expected with inhibition of HPV (18). PaO_2 is higher when isoflurane was used for one-lung anesthesia in patients undergoing thoracotomies, compared to halothane (11,20) and enflurane (316). This may be due to the higher cardiac output and P_vO_2 with isoflurane. In view of the efficacy of nondependent continuous positive airway pressure (CPAP) in improving oxygenation in one-lung ventilation, volatile anesthetics can be safely used during thoracotomy (11).

Cardiovascular Drugs

Pharmacologic agents that increase cAMP or cGMP cause pulmonary vasodilation and may attenuate hypoxic pulmonary vasoconstriction. In contrast, agents that decrease the cyclic nucleotides increase pulmonary vascular tone and may improve hypoxic pulmonary vasoconstriction, provided pulmonary artery pressures are not elevated to levels that depress HPV. The net result of a particular drug on gas exchange is complex and depends on its hemodynamic effects and whether it dilates injured as well as noninjured vessels. Some cardiovascular drugs increase cAMP by stimulating adenylate cyclase. Examples of these drugs include β_2-agonists such as isoproterenol, dobutamine, and prostacyclin. Levels of cAMP are also increased by inhibition of its breakdown by phosphodiesterases. Some phosphodiesterases also hydrolyze cGMP. Examples of phosphodiesterase inhibitors include amrinone and milrinone. Stimulation of guanylate cyclase causes pulmonary vasodilation by increasing cGMP. Nitric oxide is the pri-

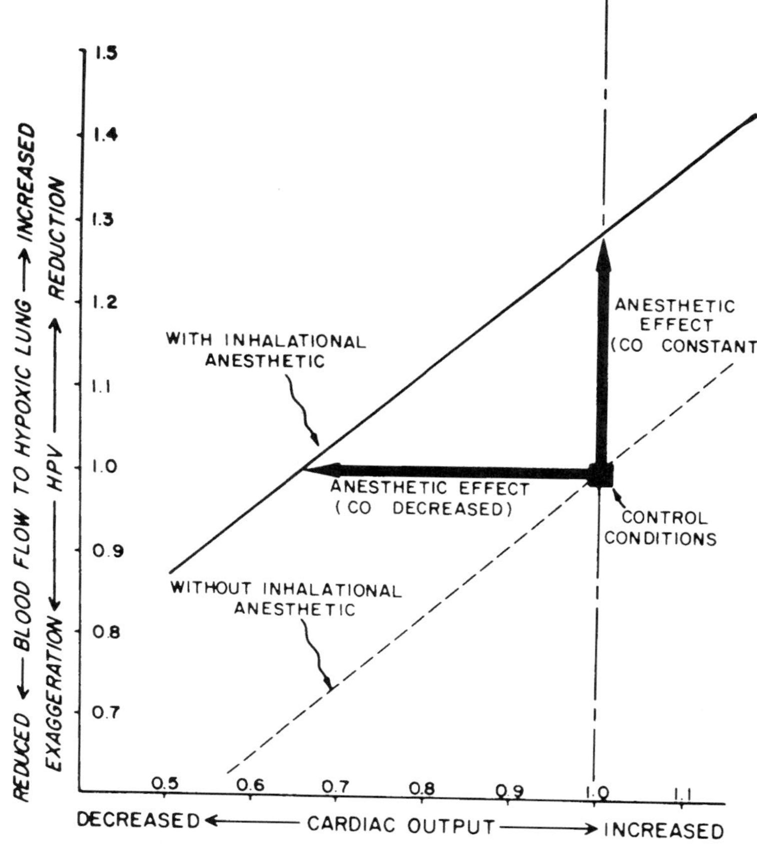

Figure 22. Schematic diagram of influence of inhalational anesthetics on the observed response to HPV. Relative cardiac output (x-axis) and apparent HPV effect (y-axis) are plotted as in Fig. 22. *Dashed line* illustrates change in blood flow to hypoxic lung as predicted by changes in cardiac output (Fig. 14). *Solid line* parallel to it shows same relationship in presence of inhalational anesthetic (from Fig. 22) *Vertical arrow* illustrates true reduction of HPV response with inhalational agent when cardiac output is not changed. *Horizontal arrows* illustrate the apparent effect when depression of cardiac output, which enhances HPV, adds to direct depression of HPV by inhalational anesthetic. This leads to an unchanged response to HPV. (Reproduced with permission from ref. 206).

mary example of a drug that stimulates cGMP. This section reviews the pulmonary vascular effects of these and other cardiovascular drugs, which are vasodilators, inotropes, and vasoconstrictors.

Vasodilators and Hypertensives

Nitric Oxide As previously described, endogenous nitric oxide is released from the pulmonary endothelium and diffuses into adjacent vascular smooth muscle, where it binds to the heme iron complex of guanylate cyclase. The activated guanylate cyclase stimulates production of cGMP, which results in smooth muscle relaxation. Exogenously administered nitric oxide has recently been advocated for the treatment of pulmonary hypertension.

Inhaled nitric oxide is a selective pulmonary vasodilator, which reduces pulmonary vascular resistance in proportion to level of initial pulmonary vascular tone (Table 5) (94,95,284, 286,294,356). Nitric oxide has little effect in reducing normal, low pulmonary vascular tone. However, inhaled nitric oxide reduces increased pulmonary vascular tone during experimental models of pulmonary hypertension, such as the infusion of a thromboxane analogue (95), oleic acid–induced pulmonary edema (294), and alveolar hypoxia (45,95,270,286,293). It also reduces elevated pulmonary vascular tone in newborns with persistent pulmonary hypertension (171,287), patients with adult respiratory distress syndrome (296), and humans breathing a hypoxic gas mixture (94). It selectively decreases pulmonary artery pressure and attenuates HPV without causing systemic vasodilation.

In contrast to many inhibitors of HPV, gas exchange is preserved during inhalation of nitric oxide (270,297). PaO_2 may be unchanged or even increased as pulmonary venous admixture is reduced following inhalation of nitric oxide. Inhaled nitric oxide increases pulmonary blood flow to ventilated but not unventilated lung regions, in contrast to other vasodilators (356). Inhaled nitric oxide also improved PaO_2 when adminis-

Table 5. EFFECTS OF SELECTED PULMONARY VASODILATORS ON PULMONARY VASCULAR TONE AND GAS EXCHANGE

Drug	PVR	HPV	Shunt	PaO_2	Mechanism of action
Nitric oxide	↓(selective)	↓	-↓	-↑	Stimulates cGMP
Prostacyclin, (PGI_2)					
Intravenous	↓	↓	↑	↓	↑ cAMP
Aerosolized	↓(selective)	↓	-↓	-↑	↑ cAMP
Sodium nitroprusside	↓	↓	↑	↓	Stimulates nitric oxide release → ↑ cGMP
Nitroglycerin	↓	↓	↑	↓	Stimulates nitric oxide release → ↑ cGMP
Nifedipine	↓	↓	↑	↓	Inhibition of voltage-dependent calcium influx
Isoproterenol	↓	↓	↑	-↓	β_2 adrenergic agonist, ↑ cAMP
Amrinone	↓	↓	↑	-↓	Phosphodiest erase-inhibitor, ↑ cAMP and ↑ cGMP

tered to the normoxic lung during unilateral hypoxia (93). This is because when nitric oxide diffuses into the intravascular space, its biologic activity is quickly terminated by binding to hemoglobin (356). Nitric oxide may also improve gas exchange by bronchodilation (84).

Prostacyclin Prostacyclin (PGI_2), when infused intravenously, is a nonspecific pulmonary vasodilator that causes vasorelaxation in both pulmonary and systemic vessels and in both ventilated and nonventilated lung regions (276,277) (Table 5). When administered intravenously, intrapulmonary shunt increased and PaO_2 decreased due to vasodilation in nonventilated lung regions (276,317). However, when administered as an aerosol, prostacyclin is a selective pulmonary vasodilator in patients with ARDS (262,344) and in newborns with congenital heart disease (359) (Table 5). PaO_2 is improved by inhaled prostacyclin because it redistributes blood flow from shunt areas to regions of normal ventilation-perfusion (262,344). Aerosolized prostacyclin selectively reduced pulmonary vascular tone when increased by alveolar hypoxia in animals, to a similar degree as inhaled nitric oxide (346). The fact that aerosolized prostacyclin has similar effects to inhaled nitric oxide compared to other drugs may be secondary to the inhaled route of administration. Because of its lack of known toxicity and convenient mode of administration, inhaled prostacyclin may become an alternative to inhaled nitric oxide in the treatment of acute pulmonary hypertension (348).

Sodium Nitroprusside/Nitroglycerin Sodium nitroprusside and nitroglycerin are pulmonary and systemic vasodilators, which act by releasing nitric oxide (356) (Table 5). As with inhaled nitric oxide, the pulmonary vasodilator responses to nitroprusside and nitroglycerin are dependent on the existing level of vasomotor tone (166). Greater pulmonary vasodilation is observed with elevated pulmonary vascular tone. These agents are nonspecific pulmonary vasodilators and affect the systemic circulation similar to intravenous prostacyclin.

Both sodium nitroprusside and nitroglycerin inhibit HPV (16,61,137,238,239,263). This is demonstrated by lack of parallel shift in the pressure-flow curve with hypoxia during infusion of nitroprusside (Fig. 23). Gas exchange is impaired because vasodilation occurs in pulmonary vessels near ventilated and nonventilated alveoli, so blood flow to abnormal lung regions is also increased. This results in an increase in venous admixture and a reduction of PaO_2 in many types of lung disease,

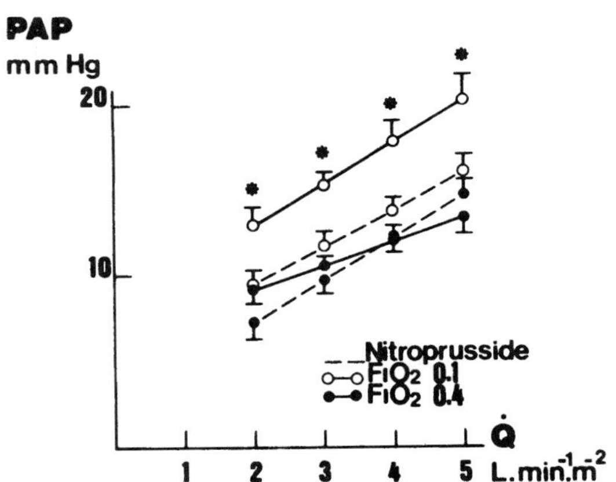

Figure 23. Pulmonary artery pressure (PAP)—flow ($\dot{Q}$) curves during hyperoxia *(solid circles)* and global alveolar hypoxia *(open circles)* before *(solid lines)* and after *(dotted lines)* administration of sodium nitroprusside. Hypoxia increased PAP at each level of $\dot{Q}$ but the pressor response was blunted by 5 μgm/kg/min of sodium nitroprusside. $*p<0.05$, nitroprusside compared with control at same fraction of inspired O_2 (FIO_2). (Reproduced from ref. 238 with permission.)

including oleic acid–induced pulmonary edema (57), one-lung atelectasis (58), pulmonary embolism (72), adult respiratory distress syndrome (276), chronic obstructive pulmonary disease (129,173,351), chronic obliterative pulmonary hypertension (62), as well as in normal lungs (129,230,239,351). In addition, sodium nitroprusside may induce changes in the pulmonary vasculature due to vascular derecruitment because of reductions in intrathoracic blood volume, as documented in patients with ARDS by increased dead space with unchanged cardiac output (275). Consequently, administration of sodium nitroprusside and nitroglycerin may cause hypoxemia during one-lung anesthesia and in the presence of lung disease such as adult respiratory distress syndrome, pneumonia, and pulmonary contusion.

Calcium-Channel Blockers Many calcium-channel blocking agents are pulmonary vasodilators (Table 5) (221,242,315,355). Nifedipine and nicardipine are more effective pulmonary vasodilators than verapamil or diltiazem, which have greater cardiac effects (242,355). The calcium-channel blockers cause vasodilation by inhibiting voltage-dependent calcium influx. These agents also inhibit HPV and may reduce PaO_2, especially in the presence of lung disease (44,221,242,315,336,355). Because diltiazem has little pulmonary vasodilating effects, HPV and oxygenation are better maintained when it is used, in contrast to nifedipine (44). The observation that the hypoxic pulmonary presser response was more susceptible to inhibition by calcium channel blockers than was pulmonary hypertension due to infusion of angiotensin II or prostaglandin $F_2\alpha$ (221) suggests that HO is especially dependent on the transmembrane flux of extracellular calcium.

Other Vasodilators and Antihypertensives

HYDRAZINE Hydralazine is a weak pulmonary vasodilator that does not impair gas exchange (83,265). While effective in reducing pulmonary vascular resistance in some settings, it is not effective in others (40). It does not directly impair HPV or PaO_2, however, increases in cardiac output and mixed venous O_2 may result in an increase in venous admixture (40).

CAPTOPRIL Angiotensin II is a potent pulmonary vasoconstrictor whose action is not dependent on the autonomic nervous system or on increased levels of arginine vasopressin (112). Converting-enzyme inhibition with captopril reduces pulmonary vascular tone in conscious dogs with normal pulmonary vascular resistance (112). These results suggest that the endogenous release of angiotensin II exerts a vasoconstrictor influence over the intact pulmonary circulation.

ADENOSINE Although adenosine is a systemic vasodilator, its effects on the pulmonary circulation are variable, being a vasoconstrictor in rats (23,333) and a vasodilator in humans (232). Adenosine receptor blockade, by the antagonist 8-phenyltheophylline, abolished the increase in pulmonary artery pressure in global hypoxia (333). When infused into a pulmonary artery, adenosine reduced pulmonary vascular tone in patients with primary pulmonary hypertension (232). Although systemic vascular resistance was mildly reduced, adenosine preferentially vasodilated the pulmonary circulation (232,281).

BETA-BLOCKERS Beta-blockade with propranolol may increase pulmonary vascular tone as pulmonary vasodilation, mediated by β_2-adrenergic receptors, is the net effect of the autonomic circulation on pulmonary vascular tone (234). Propranolol also enhances HPV (2,21,271,312), although some studies show little effect on HPV (330). Using an x-ray television system on in vitro cat lung, Shirai et al. (312) found that with propranolol pretreatment, global alveolar hypoxia reduced small pulmonary vessel diameter to a greater degree (16%) compared to global alveolar hypoxia alone (5%). They attributed the marked improvement to a reduction in β-receptor–mediated vasodilation caused by a reflex release of catecholamines during hypoxia. Beta-blockers do not adversely affect and may improve PaO_2. For instance, propranolol increased PaO_2 in acutely hypoxemic patients (339), although labetalol did not influence PaO_2 during deliberate hypotension in dogs (44). Experimentally-induced sympathectomy by total spinal block accentuated HPV to a mild degree in dogs (259). However, the small amount of improvement suggests that sympathetic blockade during subarachnoid or epidural block would probably have relatively minor effects on HPV and oxygenation during one-lung anesthesia.

In contrast, pindolol, a new nonselective beta-blocker with intrinsic sympathomimetic activity, results in pulmonary vasodilation and inhibition of HPV (330). The pulmonary vasodilation with pindolol may be due to an increased release of PGE_2 (330).

Inotropes and Vasopressors

Norepinephrine, Epinephrine, and Dopamine Norepinephrine, epinephrine, and dopamine are mixed α- and β-agonists. In high doses, these drugs may increase pulmonary vascular tone, due to stimulation of α-adrenergic receptors. However, in the presence of elevated pulmonary vascular tone, the drugs may reduce calculated pulmonary vascular resistance due to an improvement in cardiac output, without affecting pulmonary vascular tone determined by pressure-flow curves (82). These drugs usually have little adverse effect on HPV (99,111), although with high doses in which the α-adrenergic effect is marked, HPV may be impaired (199), and $\dot{V}_A/\dot{Q}$ mismatch increased (282). However, the resultant PaO_2 may or may not decrease, depending on whether the increase in $\dot{V}_A/\dot{Q}$ mismatch is offset by the improvement in $P\bar{v}O_2$ with increased cardiac output.

Isoproterenol and Dobutamine Isoproterenol, a β_1- and β_2-adrenergic agonist, and dobutamine, with predominantly β_1- and less β_2- and α-agonistic activity, are effective pulmonary vasodilators (Table 5) (82,223). Administration of isoproterenol in the presence of elevated pulmonary vascular tone directly reduces pulmonary vascular resistance, as determined by pressure-flow curves (82). However, pulmonary vasodilation induced by isoproterenol inhibits HPV (99,199), increases $\dot{V}_A/\dot{Q}$ mismatch (62), and may worsen oxygenation (172,329). Although dobutamine has similar effects on pulmonary vascular tone and HPV, PaO_2 is often well preserved when dobutamine is administered to critically ill ventilated patients because of the improvement in cardiac output (282).

Amrinone Amrinone and other phosphodiesterase inhibitors cause pulmonary vasomotor relaxation through the inhibition of hydrolysis of the cyclic nucleotides (Table 5). Amrinone and milrinone are type 3 phosphodiesterase inhibitors that inhibit the breakdown of both cAMP and cGMP. The doses required for pulmonary vasodilation are higher than those required for inotropy. Amrinone reduces pulmonary vascular resistance when pulmonary vascular tone is elevated but not normal (55,257). In the future, additional phosphodiesterase inhibitors may prove to be efficacious in selectively decreasing pulmonary vascular tone.

Potentiators of HPV

Almitrine

Almitrine bimesylate, a respiratory stimulant, increases PaO_2 in patients with chronic obstructive pulmonary disease (222) and acute respiratory failure (283). These effects occur at doses that do not stimulate peripheral chemoreceptors and increase ventilation. In the past, the improvement in PaO_2 was postulated as due to an enhancement in HPV. However, almitrine is a nonspecific pulmonary vasoconstrictor (179,241). While low doses of almitrine may potentiate HPV (241), higher doses inhibit HPV (49,179,222,241) and result in a deterioration of PaO_2 in canine oleic acid pulmonary edema (179). Therefore, almitrine is not useful in improving HPV and gas exchange in clinical situations where HPV is important, such as one-lung anesthesia for thoracic surgery.

Cyclooxygenase Inhibitors

Cyclooxygenase inhibitors, such as acetylsalicylic acid (ASA), indomethacin, and ibuprofen, enhance HPV and restore PaO_2 in many models of acute lung injury (128,131,178,179,308) and in poorly responding animals (2,102,127,128,183,205,210,236, 317). The cyclooxygenase inhibitors increase pulmonary vascular tone preferentially to the hypoxic lung segments. The increase in diversion of pulmonary blood flow away from the hypoxic or atelectatic lung regions results in an improvement in PaO_2. Cyclooxygenase inhibitors potentiate HPV when the baseline HPV response is weak and have little effect when the baseline response is strong. The diminished response in certain animals and in the presence of lung disease is due to the release of prostacyclin (PGI_2). Cyclooxygenase inhibition also reduces the attenuation of HPV by volatile anesthetics (186, 210,236). Thus, cyclooxygenase inhibitors do enhance HPV in situations and individuals in which the HPV response is weak. However, they are not used clinically to improve oxygenation, as during one-lung anesthesia for thoracic surgery, because of the lack of an intravenous preparation and their adverse effects on coagulation. It is not known whether ketorolac potentiates HPV and improves oxygenation in the doses commonly administered for the control of pain.

Other Drugs

As endogenous nitric oxide release may modulate pulmonary vasoconstriction in response to hypoxia and other vasoconstrictor substances by stimulation of cGMP, inhibitors of nitric oxide; such as, N_G-nitro-L-arginine methyl ester (L-NAME) and inhibitors of guanylate cyclase may enhance pulmonary vasoconstrictor responses to hypoxia in isolated lungs (218,250). Guanylate cyclase inhibition by methylene blue (36,213,291) or LY83583 (250) enhanced the pulmonary vasoconstrictor response to hypoxia in isolated lungs. Infusion of L-NAME enhanced HPV-induced reductions in hypoxic lobe blood flow and increased PaO_2 in pigs (93). The combination of nitric oxide inhalation to normoxic lung regions with intravenous L-NAME almost abolished perfusion of the hypoxic lobe and resulted in a restoration of PaO_2 to normoxic levels (93). Although not yet tested in humans, the marked improvement in PaO_2 with L-NAME and nitric oxide inhalation to normoxic lungs suggests that these drugs may be useful in the treatment of patients during one-lung ventilation and patients with acute respiratory failure.

CONCLUSION

The pulmonary circulation is unique in that it is a low-pressure system, in which low vascular tone is maintained by a variety of passive and active factors. The regulation of pulmonary vascular tone is complex and is under active investigation. Anesthetic agents and cardiovascular drugs commonly used in anesthetic practice modulate pulmonary flow and vascular resistance by affecting hypoxic pulmonary vasoconstriction and the autonomic and humoral regulation of the pulmonary vasculature. This chapter reviewed the current experimental findings concerning the distribution, dynamics, regulation, and pharmacology of pulmonary blood flow.

ACKNOWLEDGMENT

This work is supported in part by NHLBI grant 02507.

REFERENCES

1. Ahmed T, Mirbahar KB, Oliver W, Eyre P, Wanner A. Characterization of H_1- and H_2-receptor function in pulmonary and systemic circulations of sheep. *J Appl Physiol:* 1982;53:175–184.
2. Ahmed T, Oliver W, Wanner A. Variability of hypoxic pulmonary vasoconstriction in sheep: Role of prostaglandins. *Am Rev Respir Dis* 1983;127:59–62.

3. Amis TC, Jones HA, Hughes JMB. Effect of posture on interregional distribution of pulmonary ventilation in man. *Resp Physiol* 1984;56:145–167.
4. Anthonisen NR, Milic-Emili J. Distribution of pulmonary perfusion in erect man. *J Appl Physiol* 1966;21:760–766.
5. Archer SL, Rist K, Nelson DP, DeMaster EG, Cowan N, Weir EK. Comparison of the hemodynamic effects of nitric oxide and endothelium-dependent vasodilators in intact lungs. *J Appl Physiol* 1990; 68:735–747.
6. Barer GR, Howard P, Shaw JW. Stimulus-response curves for the pulmonary vascular bed to hypoxia and hypercapnia. *J Physiol* 1970; 211:139–155.
7. Barman SA, Taylor AE. Histamine's effect on pulmonary vascular resistance and compliance at elevated tone. *Am J Physiol* 1989;257: H618–H625.
8. Barnes PJ. Endothelins and pulmonary diseases. *J Appl Physiol* 1994;77:1051–1059.
9. Beck KC, Rehder K. Differences in regional vascular conductances in isolated dog lungs. *J Appl Physiol* 1986;61:530–538.
10. Beck KC. Regional trapping of microspheres in the lung compares well with regional blood flow. *J Appl Physiol* 1987;63: 883–889.
11. Benumof JL, Augustine SC, Gibbons JA. Halothane and isoflurane only slightly impair arterial oxygenation during one-lung ventilation in patients undergoing thoracotomy. *Anesthesiology* 1987;67: 910–915.
12. Benumof JL, Pirlo AF, Johanson I, Trousdale FR. Interaction of $P\bar{v}O_2$ with P_AO_2 on hypoxic pulmonary vasoconstriction. *J Appl Physiol* 1981;51:871–874.
13. Benumof JL, Rogers SN, Moyce PR, Berryhill RE, Wahrenbrock EA, Saidman LJ. Hypoxic pulmonary vasoconstriction and regional and whole-lung PEEP in the dog. *Anesthesiology* 1979;51: 503–507.
14. Benumof JL, Wahrenbrock EA. Blunted hypoxic pulmonary vasoconstriction by increased lung vascular pressures. *J Appl Physiol* 1975;38:846–850.
15. Benumof JL, Wahrenbrock EA. Local effects of anesthetics on regional hypoxic pulmonary vasoconstriction. *Anesthesiology* 1975; 43:525–532.
16. Benumof JL. Hypoxic pulmonary vasoconstriction and the infusion of sodium nitroprusside. *Anesthesiology* 1979;50:481–483.
17. Benumof JL. Intermittent hypoxia increases lobar hypoxic pulmonary vasoconstriction. *Anesthesiology* 1983;58:399–404.
18. Benumof JL. Isoflurane anesthesia and arterial oxygenation during one-lung ventilation. *Anesthesiology* 1986;64:419–422.
19. Benumof JL. Mechanism of decreased blood flow to atelectatic lung. *J Appl Physiol* 1979;46:1047–1048.
20. Benumof JL. One-lung ventilation and hypoxic pulmonary vasoconstriction: Implications for anesthetic management. *Anesth Analg* 1985;64:821–833.
21. Bergofsky EH. Humoral control of the pulmonary circulation. *Ann Rev Physiol* 1980;42:221–233.
22. Bhattacharya J, Nanjo S, Staub NC. Micropuncture measurement of lung microvascular pressure during 5-HT infusion. *J Appl Physiol* 1982;52:634–637.
23. Biaggioni I, King LS, Enayat N, Robertson D, Newman JH. Adenosine produces pulmonary vasoconstriction in sheep. *Circ Res* 1989; 65:1516–1525.
24. Bindlsev L, Cannon D, Sykes MK. Effect of lignocaine and nitrous oxide on hypoxic pulmonary vasoconstriction in the dog: Constant-flow perfused left lower lobe preparation. *Br J Anaesth* 1986; 53:315–320.
25. Bindslev L, Cannon D, Sykes MK. Reversal of nitrous oxide-induced depression of hypoxic pulmonary vasoconstriction by lignocaine hydrochloride during collapse and ventilation hypoxia of the left lower lobe. *Br J Anaesth* 1986;58:451–456.
26. Bindslev L, Jolin A, Hedenstierna G, Baehrendtz S, Santesson J. Hypoxic pulmonary vasoconstriction in the human lung: Effect of repeated hypoxic challenges during anesthesia. *Anesthesiology* 1985;62:621–625.
27. Bindslev L, Jolin-Carlsson A, Santesson J, Gottlieb I. Hypoxic pulmonary vasoconstriction in man: Effects of hyperventilation. *Acta Anaesthesiol Scand* 1985;29:547–551.
28. Bishop MJ, Cheney FW. Effects of pulmonary blood flow and mixed venous O_2 tension on gas exchange in dogs. *Anesthesiology* 1983;58:130–135.
29. Bjertnaes LJ, Hauge A, Kriz M. Hypoxia-induced pulmonary vasoconstriction: Effects of fentanyl following different routes of administration. *Acta Anaesthiol Scand* 1980;24:53–57.
30. Bjertnaes LJ, Hauge A, Torgrimsen T. The pulmonary vasoconstrictor response to hypoxia. The hypoxia-sensitive site studied with a volatile inhibitor. *Acta Physiol Scand* 1980;109:447–462.
31. Bjertnaes LJ, Mundal R. The pulmonary vasoconstrictor response to hypoxia during enflurane anesthesia. *Acta Anaesthesiol Scand* 1980;24:252–256.
32. Bjertnaes LJ, Mundal R., Hauge A, Nicolaysen A. Vascular resistance in atelectatic lungs: Effects of inhalation anesthetics. *Acta Anaesth Scand* 1980;24:109–118.
33. Bjertnaes LJ. Hypoxia-induced pulmonary vasoconstriction in man: Inhibition due to diethyl ether and halothane anesthesia. *Acta Anaesth Scand* 1978;22:570–588.
34. Bjertnaes LJ. Hypoxia-induced vasoconstriction in isolated perfused lungs exposed to injectable or inhalation anesthetics. *Acta Anaesthiol Scand* 1977;21:133–147.
35. Bosnjak ZJ. Ion channels in vascular smooth muscle. *Anesthesiology* 1993;79:1392–1401.
36. Brashers VL, Peach MJ, Rose CE. Augmentation of hypoxic pulmonary vasoconstriction in the isolated perfused rat lung by in vitro antagonists of endothelium-dependent relaxation. *J Clin Invest* 1988;82:1495–1502.
37. Brimioulle S, Lejeune P, Vachiery J-L, Leeman M, Mélot, Naeije R. Effect of acidosis and alkalosis on hypoxic pulmonary vasoconstriction in dogs. *Am J Physiol* 1990;258:H347–H353.
38. Bryan AC, Bentivoglio LG, Beerel F, MacLeish H, Zidulka A, Bates DV. Factors affecting regional distribution of ventilation and perfusion in the lung. *J. Appl. Physiol* 1964;19:395–402.
39. Buljubasic N, Rusch NJ, Marijic J, Kampine JP, Bosnjak ZA. Effects of halothane and isoflurane on calcium and potassium channel currents in canine coronary arterial cells. *Anesthesiology* 1992;76: 990–998.
40. Caplan RA, Bishop MJ, Cheney FW. Effect of hydralazine on cardiac output and venous admixture in experimental lung injury. *Am Rev Resp Dis* 1984;130:863–865.
41. Carlsson AJ, Bindslev L, Hedenstierna G. Hypoxia-induced pulmonary vasoconstriction in the human lung: The effect of isoflurane anesthesia. *Anesthesiology* 1987;66:312–316.
42. Carlsson AJ, Bindslev L, Santesson J, Gottlieb I, Hedenstierna G. Hypoxic pulmonary vasoconstriction in the human lung: The effect of prolonged unilateral hypoxic challenge during anaesthesia. *Acta Anaesthesiol Scand* 1985;29:346–351.
43. Carlsson AJ, Hedenstierna G, Bindslev L. Hypoxia-induced vasoconstriction in human lung exposed to enflurane anaesthesia. *Acta Anaesthesiol Scand* 1987;31:57–62.
44. Casthely PA, Villanueva R, Rabinowitz L, Gandhi P, Litwak B, Fyman PN. Intrapulmonary shunting during deliberate hypotension with nifedipine, diltiazem and labetalol in dogs. *Can Anaesth Soc J* 1985;32:119–123.
45. Channick RN, Newhart JW, Johnson FW, Moser KM. Inhaled nitric oxide reverses hypoxic pulmonary vasoconstriction in dogs. A practical nitric oxide delivery and monitoring system. *Chest* 1994;105:1842–47.
46. Chen BB, Nyhan DP, Fehr DM, Goll HM, Murray PA. Halothane anesthesia causes active flow-independent pulmonary vasoconstriction. *J Appl Physiol* 1990;259:H74–H83.
47. Chen BB, Nyhan DP, Fehr DM, Murray PA. Halothane anesthesia abolishes pulmonary vascular responses to neural antagonists. *Am J Physiol* 1992;262:H117–H122.
48. Chen BB, Nyhan DP, Goll HM, Clougherty PW, Fehr DM, Murray PA. Pentobarbital anesthesia modifies pulmonary vasoregulation after hypoperfusion. *J Appl Physiol* 1988;255:H569–H576.
49. Chen L, Miller FL, Malmkvist G, Clergue FX, Marshall C, Marshall BE. High-dose almitrine bismesylate inhibits hypoxic pulmonary vasoconstriction in closed-chest dogs. *Anesthesiology* 1987;67: 534–542.
50. Chen L, Miller FL, Malmkvist G, Cooley R, Marshall C, Marshall BE. Intravenous $PGF_{2\alpha}$ infusion does not enhance hypoxic pulmonary vasoconstriction during canine one-lung hypoxia. *Anesthesiology* 1988;68:226–233.
51. Chen L, Miller FL, Williams JJ, Alexander CM, Domino KB, Marshall C, Marshall BE. Hypoxic pulmonary vasoconstriction is not potentiated by repeated intermittent hypoxia in closed chest dogs. *Anesthesiology* 1985;63:608–610.
52. Cheney FW, Colley PS. The effect of cardiac output on arterial blood oxygenation. *Anesthesiology* 1980;52:496–503.

53. Cherry PD, Gillis CN. Evidence for the role of endothelium-derived relaxing factor in acetylcholine-induced vasodilatation in the intact lung. *J Pharmocol Exp Ther* 1987;241:516–520.
54. Cigarini I, Adnot S, Chabrier P-E, Viossat I, Braquet P, Gaujour B. Pulmonary vasodilator responses to atrial natriuretic factor and sodium nitroprusside. *J Appl Physiol* 1989;67:2269–2275.
55. Clarke WR, Morray JP, Powers K, Soltow LO'G. Amrinone reduces pulmonary vascular resistance elevated by U46619 in isolated perfused lungs. *J Cardiovasc Pharmacol* 1991;18:85–94.
56. Colley PS, Cheney FW, Butler J. Mechanism of change in pulmonary shunt flow with hemorrhage. *J Appl Physiol* 1977;42:196–201.
57. Colley PS, Cheney FW, Hlastala MP. Ventilation-perfusion and gas exchange effects of sodium nitroprusside in dogs with normal and edematous lungs. *Anesthesiology* 1979;50:489–495.
58. Colley PS, Cheney FW. Sodium nitroprusside increases $\dot{Q}s/\dot{Q}t$ in dogs with regional atelectasis. *Anesthesiology* 1977;47:338–341.
59. Cutaia M, Porcelli RJ. Pulmonary vascular reactivity after repetitive exposure to selected biogenic amines. *J Appl Physiol* 1983;55:1868–1876.
60. Cutaia M, Rounds S. Hypoxic pulmonary vasoconstriction: Physiologic significance, mechanism, and clinical relevance. *Chest* 1990;97:706–718.
61. D'Oliviera M, Sykes MK, Chakrabarti MK, Orchard C, Keslin J. Depression of hypoxic pulmonary vasoconstriction by sodium nitroprusside and nitroglycerine. *Br J Anaesth* 1981;53:11.
62. Dantzker DR, Bower JS. Pulmonary vascular tone improves $\dot{V}_A/\dot{Q}$ matching in obliterative pulmonary hypertension. *J Appl Physiol* 1981;51:607–613.
63. Dawson A, Grover RF. Regional lung function in natives and long-term residents at 3,100 m altitude. *J Appl Physiol* 1974;36:294–298.
64. Dawson A. Regional pulmonary blood flow in sitting and supine man during and after acute hypoxia. *J Clin Invest* 1969;48:301–310.
65. Dawson CA, Grimm DJ, Linehan JH. Influence of hypoxia on the longitudinal distribution of pulmonary vascular resistance. *J Appl Physiol* 1978;44:493–498.
66. Dawson CA, Grimm DJ, Linehan JH. Lung inflation and longitudinal distribution of pulmonary vascular resistance during hypoxia. *J Appl Physiol* 1979;47:532–536.
67. Dawson CA, Linehan JH, Bronikowski TA. Pressure and flow in the pulmonary vascular bed. In: Weir EK, Reeves JT, eds. *Lung Biology in Health and Disease.* Vol. 38, Lenfant series, "Pulmonary Vascular Physiology and Pathophysiology." New York, Marcel Dekker, 1989: 51–105.
68. Dawson CA, Linehan JH, Rickaby DA. Pulmonary microcirculatory hemodynamics. *Ann.N.Y.Acad.Sci.* 1982;348:90–106.
69. Dawson CA. Role of pulmonary vasomotion in physiology of the lung. *Physiol Rev* 1984;64:544–616.
70. De Cannière D, Stefanidis C, Hallemans R, Delcroix M, Brimioulle S, Naeije R. Stimulus-response curves for hypoxic pulmonary vasconstriction in piglets. *Cardiovasc Res* 1992;26:944–949.
71. De Cannière D, Stefanidis C, Hallemans R, Delcroix M, Lejeune P, Naeije R. Increased left atrial pressure inhibits hypoxic pulmonary vasoconstriction. *J Appl Physiol* 1994;76:1502–1506.
72. Delcroix M, Mélot C, Lejeune P, Leeman M, Naeije R. Effects of vasodilators on gas exchange in acute canine embolic pulmonary hypertension. *Anesthesiology* 1990;72:77–84.
73. Dollery CT, Dyson NA, Sinclair JD. Regional variations in uptake of radioactive CO in the normal lung. *J Appl Physiol* 1960;15:411–417.
74. Domino KB, Borowec L, Alexander CM, Williams JJ, Chen L, Marshall C, Marshall BE. Influence of isoflurane on hypoxic pulmonary vasoconstriction in dogs. *Anesthesiology* 1986;64:423–429.
75. Domino KB, Eisenstein BL, Cheney FW, Hlastala MP. Pulmonary blood flow and ventilation-perfusion heterogeneity. *J Appl Physiol* 1991;71:252–258.
76. Domino KB, Hlastala MP, Cheney FW. Effect of increased intracranial pressure on regional hypoxic pulmonary vasoconstriction. *Anesthesiology* 1990;72:490–495.
77. Domino KB, Hlastala MP, Eisenstein BL, Cheney FW. Effect of regional alveolar hypoxia on gas exchange in dogs. *J Appl Physiol* 1989;67:730–735.
78. Domino KB, Lu Y, Eisenstein BL, Hlastala MP. Hypocapnia worsens arterial blood oxygenation and increases $\dot{V}_A/\dot{Q}$ heterogeneity in canine pulmonary edema. *Anesthesiology* 1993;78:91–99.
79. Domino KB, Pinsky MR. Effect of positive end-expiratory pressure on hypoxic pulmonary vasoconstriction in the dog. *Am J Physiol* 1990;259:H697–H705.
80. Domino KB, Swenson ER, Polissar NL, Lu Y, Eisenstein BL, Hlastala MP. Effect of inspired CO_2 on ventilation and perfusion heterogeneity in hyperventilated dogs. *J Appl Physiol* 1993;75:1306–1314.
81. Domino KB, Wetstein L, Glasser SA, Lindgren L, Marshall C, Harken AH, Marshall BE. Influence of $P\bar{v}O_2$ on blood flow to atelectatic lung. *Anesthesiology* 1983;59:428–434.
82. Ducas J, Duval D, Dasilva H, Boiteau P, Prewitt RM. Treatment of canine pulmonary hypertension: effects of norepinephrine and isoproterenol on pulmonary vascular pressure-flow characteristics. *Circulation* 1987;75:235–242.
83. Ducas J, Girling L, Schick U, Prewitt RM. Pulmonary vascular effects of hydralazine in a canine preparation of pulmonary thromboembolism. *Circulation* 1986;73:1050–1057.
84. Dupuy PM, Shore SA, Drazen JM, Frostell C, Hill WA, Zapol WM. Bronchodilator action of inhaled nitric oxide in guinea pigs. *J Clin Invest* 1992;90:421–428.
85. Eisenkraft JB. Effects of anaesthetics on the pulmonary circulation. *Br J Anaesth* 1990;65:63–78.
86. Engel LA, Prefaut C. Cranio-caudal distribution of inspired gas and perfusion in supine man. *Resp Physiol* 1981;45:43–53.
87. Ewalenko P, Stefanidis C, Holoye A, Brimioulle S, Naeije R. Pulmonary vascular impedance vs. resistance in hypoxic and hyperoxic dogs: Effects of propofol and isoflurane. *J Appl Physiol* 1993;74:2188–2193.
88. Fargas-Babjak A, Forrest JB. Effect of halothane on the pulmonary vascular response to hypoxia in dogs. *Canad Anaesth Soc J* 1979;26:5–14.
89. Farrukh IS, Michael JR. Cellular mechanisms that control pulmonary vascular tone during hypoxia and normoxia. Possible role of Ca^{2+} ATPases. *Am Rev Respir Dis* 1992;145:1389–1397.
90. Fehr DM, Nyhan DP, Chen BB, Murray PA. Pulmonary vasoregulation by cyclooxygenase metabolites and angiotensin II after hypoperfusion in conscious, pentobarbital-anesthetized, and halothane-anesthetized dogs. *Anesthesiology* 1991;75:257–267.
91. Fillenz M. Innervation of pulmonary and bronchial blood vessels of the dog. *J Anat* 1970;106:449–461.
92. Fishman AP. Pulmonary circulation. In: Fishman AP, ed. *Handbook of Physiology.* Section 3: The respiratory system, Vol I: Circulation and nonrespiratory functions, chap 3. Baltimore: Williams & Wilkins, 1985;93–167.
93. Fredén F, Wei SZ, Berglund JE, Frostell C, Hedenstierna G. Nitric oxide modulation of pulmonary blood flow distribution in lobar hypoxia. *Anesthesiology* 1995;82:1216–1225.
94. Frostell CG, Blomqvist H, Hedenstierna G, Lundberg J, Zapol WM. Inhaled nitric oxide selectively reverses human hypoxic pulmonary vasoconstriction without causing systemic vasodilation. *Anesthesiology* 1993;78:427–435.
95. Frostell C, Fratacci M-D, Wain JC, Jones R, Zapol WM. Inhaled nitric oxide. A selective pulmonary vasodilator reversing hypoxic pulmonary vasoconstriction. *Circulation* 1991;83:2038–2047.
96. Fujiwara Y, Murray PA. Pulmonary vasodilation mediated by ATP-sensitive potassium channels is attenuated during isoflurane anesthesia (Abstract). *Anesthesiology* 1994;81:A698.
97. Fung, YC. Dynamics of blood flow and pressure-flow relationship. In: Crystal RG, West JB, Barnes PJ, Cherniack NS, Weibel ER, eds. *The Lung: Scientific Foundations.* New York: Raven Press, 1991; 1121–1134.
98. Furchgott RF, Zawadzki JV. The obligatory role of endothelial cells in the relaxation of arterial smooth muscle by acetylcholine. *Nature* 1980;288:373–376.
99. Furman WR, Summer WR, Kennedy TP, Sylvester JT. Comparison of the effects of dobutamine, dopamine, and isoproterenol on hypoxic pulmonary vasoconstriction in the pig. *Crit Care Med* 1982; 10:371–374.
100. Gambone LM, Fujiwara Y, Murray PA. Endothelium-dependent cGMP-mediated pulmonary vasodilation in conscious dogs is selectively attenuated during isoflurane anesthesia. *Am J Physiol* 1997;41:290–298.
101. Gandhi CR, Berkowitz DE, Watkins WD. Endothelins. Biochemistry and pathophysiologic actions. *Anesthesiology* 1994;80:892–905.
102. Garrett RC, Thomas HM III. Relation of prostanoids to strength of hypoxic vasoconstriction in dogs with lobar atelectasis. *J Appl Physiol* 1985;59:72–77.
103. Gibbs JM, Johnson H. Lack of effect of morphine and buprenorphine on hypoxic pulmonary vasoconstriction in the isolated perfused cat lung and the perfused lobe of the dog lung. *Br J Anaesth* 1978;50:1197–1201.

104. Gillespie MN, Bowdy BD. Impact of platelet activating factor on vascular responsiveness in isolated rat lungs. *J Pharmacol Exper Ther* 1985;23:396–402.
105. Glenny RW, Bernard S, Brinkley M. Validation of fluorescent labeled microspheres for measurement of regional organ perfusion. *J Appl Physiol* 1993;74:2585—2597.
106. Glenny RW, Lamm WJ, Albert RK, HT Robertson. Gravity is a minor determinate of pulmonary blood flow distribution. *J Appl Physiol* 1991;71:620–9.
107. Glenny RW, Polissar L, Robertson HT. Relative contribution of gravity to pulmonary perfusion heterogeneity. *J Appl Physiol* 1991; 71:2449–2452.
108. Glenny RW, Robertson HT. Fractal modeling of pulmonary blood flow heterogeneity. *J Appl Physiol* 1991;70:1024–1030.
109. Glenny RW, Robertson HT. Fractal properties of pulmonary blood flow: Characterization of spatial heterogeneity. *J Appl Physiol* 1990; 69:532–545.
110. Glenny RW. Spatial correlation of regional pulmonary perfusion. *J Appl Physiol* 1992;72:2378–2386.
111. Goldring RM, Turine GM, Cohen C, Jameson AG, Bass BG, Fishman AP. The catecholamines in the pulmonary arterial pressor response to acute hypoxia. *J Clin Invest* 1962;41:1211–1215.
112. Goll HM, Nyhan DP, Geller HS, Murray PA. Pulmonary vascular responses to angiotensin II and captopril in conscious dogs. *J Appl Physiol* 1986;61:1552–1559.
113. Gordon JB, Martinez FR, Keller PA, Tod ML, Madden JA. Differing effects of acute and prolonged alkalosis on hypoxic pulmonary vasoconstriction. *Am Rev Respir Dis* 1993;148:1651–6.
114. Gottlieb JE, McGeady M, Adkinson NF, Sylvester JT. Effects of cyclo- and lipoxygenase inhibitors on hypoxic vasoconstriction in isolated ferret lungs. *J Appl Physiol* 1988;64:936–943.
115. Groh J, Kuhnle GEH, Kuebler WM, Goetz AE. An experimental model for simultaneous quantitative analysis of pulmonary micro- and macrocirculation during unilateral hypoxia *in vivo*. *Res Exp Med* 1992;192:431–441.
116. Groh J, Kuhnle GEH, Sckell A, Ney L, Goetz AE. Effects of one-lung ventilation on pulmonary capillary perfusion (Abstract). *Anesthesiology* 1994;81:A705.
117. Groh J, Kuhnle GEH, Sckell A, Ney L, Goetz AE. Isoflurane inhibits hypoxic pulmonary vasoconstriction: An in vivo fluorescence microscopic study in rabbits. *Anesthesiology* 1994;81: 1436–1444.
118. Gu S, Ducas J, Schick U, Prewitt RM. Effects of left atrial pressure on the pulmonary vascular response to hypoxic ventilation. *J Appl Physiol* 1991;70:1991–1995.
119. Hakim TS, Chang HK, Michel RP. The rectilinear pressure-flow relationship in the pulmonary vasculature: zones 2 and 3. *Resp Physiol* 1985;61:115–123.
120. Hakim TS, Dean GW, Lisbona R. Effect of body posture on spatial distribution of pulmonary blood flow. *J Appl Physiol* 1988;64: 1160–1170.
121. Hakim TS, Lisbona R, Dean GW. Effect of cardiac output on gravity-dependent and nondependent inequality in pulmonary blood flow. *J Appl Physiol* 1989;66:1570–1578.
122. Hakim TS, Lisbona R, Dean GW. Gravity-independent inequality in pulmonary blood flow in humans. *J Appl Physiol* 1987;63:1114–1121.
123. Hakim TS, Lisbona R, Michel RP, Dean GW. Role of vasoconstriction in gravity-nondependent central-peripheral gradient in pulmonary blood flow. *J Appl Physiol* 1993;74:897–904.
124. Hakim TS, Michel RP, Chang HK. Effect of lung inflation on pulmonary vascular resistance by arterial and venous occlusion. *J Appl Physiol* 1982;53:1110–1115.
125. Hakim TS, Michel RP, Chang HK. Partitioning of pulmonary vascular resistance in dogs by arterial and venous occlusion. *J Appl Physiol* 1982;52:710–715.
126. Hakim TS, Michel RP, Minami H, Chang HK. Site of pulmonary hypoxic vasoconstriction studies with arterial and venous occlusion. *J Appl Physiol* 1983;54:1298–1302.
127. Hales CA, Rouse ET, Slate JL. Influence of aspirin and indomethacin on variability of alveolar hypoxic vasoconstriction. *J Appl Physiol* 1978;45:33–39.
128. Hales CA, Sonne L, Peterson M, Kong D, Miller M, Watkins WD. Role of thromboxane and prostacyclin in pulmonary vasomotor changes after endotoxin in dogs. *J Clin Invest* 1981;68:497–505.
129. Hales CA, Westphal D. Hypoxemia following the administration of sublingual nitroglycerin. *Am J Med* 1978b;65:911–917.
130. Hambraeus-Jonzon K, Bindsler L, Mellgard AJ, Hedenstierra G. Hypoxic pulmonary vasoconstriction in human lungs. A stimulus-response study. *Anesthesiology* 1997;86:308–315.
131. Hanly P, Sienko A, Light RB. Effect of cyclooxygenase blockade on gas exchange and hemodynamics in *Pseudomonas* pneumonia. *J Appl Physiol* 1987;63:1829–1836.
132. Harabin AL, Peake MD, Sylvester JT. Effect of severe hypoxia on the pulmonary vascular response to vasoconstrictor agents. *J Appl Physiol* 1981;50:561–565.
133. Hasan FM, Weiss WB, Braman SS, Hoppin FG. Influence of lung injury on pulmonary wedge-left atrial pressure correlation during positive end-expiratory pressure ventilation. *Am Rev Respir Dis* 1985; 131:246–250.
134. Hedenstierna G, White FC, Mazzone R, Wagner PD. Redistribution of pulmonary blood flow in the dog with PEEP ventilation. *J Appl Physiol* 1979;46:278–287.
135. Heitz DC, Jebson PJ, Boutros AR, Brody MJ. The effects of halothane on the pulmonary vascular bed of the dog. *Anesthesiology* 1971;35:61–67.
136. Herold CJ, Wetzel RC, Robotham JL, Herold SM, Zerhouni EA. Acute effects of increased intravascular volume and hypoxia on the pulmonary circulation: assessment with high-resolution CT. *Radiology* 1992;183:655–662.
137. Hill AB, Sykes MK, Reyes A. A hypoxic pulmonary vasoconstrictor response in dogs during and after infusion of sodium nitroprusside. *Anesthesiology* 1979;50:484–488.
138. Hongkui J, Yang R-H, Thornton RM, Chen Y-F, Jackson R, Oparil S. Atrial natriuretic peptide lowers pulmonary arterial pressure in hypoxia-adapted rats. *J Appl Physiol* 1988;65:1729–1735.
139. Hotchkiss RS, Katsamouris AN, Lappas DG, Mihelakos PT, Wilson RS, Long M, Coyle J, Brewster D, Greene R. Interpretation of pulmonary artery wedge pressure and pullback blood gas determinations during positive end-expiratory pressure ventilation and after exclusion of the bronchial circulation in the dog. *Am Rev Respir Dis* 1986;133:1019–1023.
140. Hughes JD, Rubin LJ. Relation between mixed venous oxygen tension and pulmonary vascular tone during normoxic, hyperoxic and hypoxic ventilation in dogs. *Am J Cardiol* 1984;54:1118–1123.
141. Hughes JMB, Glazier JB, Maloney JE, West JB. Effect of extra-alveolar vessels on distribution of blood flow in the dog lung. *J Appl Physiol* 1968;25:701–712.
142. Hughes JMB, Glazier JB, Maloney JE, West JB. Effect of lung volume on the distribution of pulmonary blood flow in man. *Resp Physiol* 1968;4:58–72.
143. Hughes JMB. Distribution of pulmonary blood flow. In: Crystal RG, West JB, Barnes PJ, Cherniack NS, Weibel ER, eds. *The Lung: Scientific Foundations.* New York:Raven Press, 1991;1135–1145.
144. Hurtig JB, Tait AR, Loh L, Sykes MK. Reduction of hypoxic pulmonary vasoconstriction by nitrous oxide administration in the isolated, perfused cat lung: The effect of acidosis and alkalosis. *Can Anaesth Soc J* 1977;24:540–549.
145. Hurtig JB, Tait AR, Sykes MK. Reduction of hypoxic pulmonary vasoconstriction by diethyl ether in the isolated, perfused cat lung: The effect of acidosis and alkalosis. *Can Anaesth Soc J* 1977; 24:433–444.
146. Hutchison AA, Ogletree ML, Snapper JR, Brigham KL. Effect of endotoxemia on hypoxic pulmonary vasoconstriction in unanesthetized sheep. *J Appl Physiol* 1985;58:1463–1468.
147. Hyman AL, Dempsey CW, Richardson DE, Lippton HL. Neural Control. In: Crystal RG, West JB, Barnes PJ, Cherniack NS, Weibel ER, eds. *The Lung: Scientific Foundations.* New York: Raven Press, 1991;1087–1102.
148. Hyman AL, Kadowitz PJ. Enhancement of a- and b-adrenoceptor responses by elevations in vascular tone in pulmonary circulation. *Am J Physiol* 1986;250:H1109–H1116.
149. Hyman AL, Kadowitz PJ. Tone-dependent responses to acetylcholine in the feline pulmonary vascular bed. *J Appl Physiol* 1988; 64:2002–2009.
150. Hyman AL, Lippton HL, Dempesy CW, Fontana CJ, Richardson DE, Rieck RW, Kadowitz PJ. Autonomic control of the pulmonary circulation. In: Weir EK, Reeves JT, eds. *Lung Biology in Health and Disease.* Vol. 38, Lenfant series, "Pulmonary Vascular Physiology and Pathophysiology." New York, Marcel Dekker, 1989:291–324.
151. Hyman AL, Nandiwada P, Knight DS, Kadowitz PJ. Pulmonary vasodilator responses to catecholamines and sympathetic nerve stimulation in the cat: Evidence that vascular β-2 adrenoreceptors are innervated. *Circ Res* 1981;48:407–415.
152. Ignarro LJ, Byrns RE, Buga GM, Wood KS. Endothelium-derived

relaxing factor from pulmonary artery and vein possesses pharmacologic and chemical properties identical to those of nitric oxide radical. *Circ Res* 1987;61:866–879.

153. Ignarro LJ, Byrns RE, Buga GM, Wood KS. Mechanisms of endothelium-dependent vascular smooth muscle relaxation elicited by bradykinin and VIP. *Am J Physiol* 1987;253:H1074–H1082.
154. Ishibe Y, Gui X, Uno H, Shiokawa Y, Umeda T, Suekane K. Effect of sevoflurane on hypoxic pulmonary vasoconstriction in the perfused rabbit lung. *Anesthesiology* 1993;79:1348–1353.
155. Jarvis KA, Steffey EP, Tyler WS, Willits N, Woliner M. Pulmonary blood flow distribution in anesthetized ponies. *J Appl Physiol* 1992; 72:1173–1178.
156. Jin H, Yang R-H, Thornton RM, Chen Y-F, Jackson R, Oparil S. Atrial natriuretic peptide lowers pulmonary arterial pressure in hypoxia-adapted rats. *J Appl Physiol* 1988;65:1729–1735.
157. Johns RA. Endothelium, Anesthetics, and Vascular Control. *Anesthesiology* 1993;79:1381–1391.
158. Johnson D, Hurst T, Wilson T, Murphy F, Saxema A, To T, Mayers I. N^G-monomethyl-L-arginine does not restore loss of hypoxic pulmonary vasconstriction induced by TNF-α. *J Appl Physiol* 1993; 75:618–625.
159. Johnson D, Mayers I, Hurst T. Halothane inhibits hypoxic pulmonary vasoconstriction in the presence of cyclooxygenase blockade. *Can Anaesth Soc J* 1990;37:287–95.
160. Johnson D, Mayers I, To T. The effects of halothane in hypoxic pulmonary vasoconstriction. *Anesthesiology* 1990;72:125–133.
161. Johnson DH, Hurst TS, Mayers I. Effects of halothane on hypoxic pulmonary vasoconstriction in canine atelectasis. *Anesth Analg* 1991;72:440–448.
162. Kadowitz PJ, Hyman AL. Effect of sympathetic nerve stimulation on pulmonary vascular resistance in the dog. *Circ Res* 1973;32: 221–227.
163. Kadowitz PJ, Hyman AL. Pulmonary vascular responses to histamine in sheep. *Am J Physiol* 1983;244:H423–H428.
164. Kadowitz PJ, Joiner PD, Hyman AL. Influence of sympathetic stimulation and vasoactive substances on the canine pulmonary veins. *J Clin Invest* 1975;56:354–365.
165. Kadowitz PJ, Knight DS, Hibbs RG, Ellison JP, Joiner PD, Brody MJ, Hyman AL. Influence of 5- and 6-hydroxydopamine on adrenergic transmission and nerve terminal morphology in the canine pulmonary vascular bed. *Circ Res* 1976;39:191–199.
166. Kadowitz PJ, Nandiwada P, Gruetter CA, Ignarro LJ, Hyman AL. Pulmonary vasodilator responses to nitroprusside and nitroglycerin in the dog. *J Clin Invest* 1981;67:893–902.
167. Kallas HJ, Domino KB, Glenny RW, Hlastala MP. Relative changes in regional pulmonary blood flow (PBF) with positive end-expiratory pressure (PEEP) are not distributed heterogenously (Abstract). *Amer J Resp Med Crit Care* 1995;151:A520.
168. Kaneko K, Milic-Emili J, Dolovich MB, Dawson A, Bates DV. Regional distribution of ventilation and perfusion as a function of body position. *J Appl Physiol* 1966;21:767–777.
169. Kato M, Staub NC. Response of small pulmonary arteries to unilobar hypoxia and hypercapnia. *Circ Res* 1966;19:426–440.
170. Kazemi H, Bruecke PE, Parsons EF. Role of the autonomic nervous system in the hypoxic response of the pulmonary vascular bed. *Respir Physiol* 1972;15:245–254.
171. Kinsella JP, Neish SR, Sheffer E, Abram SH. Low-dose inhalational nitric oxide in persistent pulmonary hypertension of the newborn. *Lancet* 1992;340:819–820.
172. Knudson RJ, Constantine HP. An effect of isoproterenol on ventilation-perfusion in asthmatic versus normal subjects. *J Appl Physiol* 1967;22:402–406.
173. Kochukoshy KN, Chick TW, Jenne JW. The effect of nitroglycerin in gas exchange on chronic obstructive pulmonary disease. *Am Rev Resp Dis* 1975;111:177–183.
174. Kuhnle GE, Leipfinger FH, Goetz AE. Measurement of microhemodynamics in the ventilated rabbit lung by intravital fluorescence microscopy. *J Appl Physiol* 1993;74:1462–1471.
175. Kuriyama T, Wagner WW. Collateral ventilation may protect against high-altitude pulmonary hypertension. *J Appl Physiol* 1981; 51:1251–1256.
176. Lampron N, Lemaire F, Teisseire B, Harf A, Palot M, Matamis D, Lorino AM. Mechanical Ventilation with 100% oxygen does not increase intrapulmonary shunt in patients with severe bacterial pneumonia. *Am Rev Respir Dis* 1985;131:409–413.
177. Lee TS, Hou X. The effect of PGE_1 on isolated rabbit pulmonary arteries (Abstract). *Anesthesiology* 1993;79:A298.
178. Leeman M, Delcroix M, Vachiéry J-L, Mélot C, Naeije R. Blunted hypoxic vasoconstriction in oleic acid lung injury: Effect of cyclooxygenase inhibitors. *J Appl Physiol* 1992;72:251–258.
179. Leeman M, Lejeune P, Hallemans R, Mélot C, Naeije R. Effects of increased pulmonary vascular tone on gas exchange in canine oleic acid pulmonary edema. *J Appl Physiol* 1988;65:662–668.
180. Leeman M, Naeije R, Lejeune P, Mélot C. Influence of cyclo-oxygenase inhibition and of leukotriene receptor blockade on pulmonary vascular pressure/cardiac index relationships in hyperoxic and in hypoxic dogs. *Clin Sci* 1987;72:717–724.
181. Lejeune P, Brimioulle S, Leeman M, Hallemans, Mélot C, Naeije R. Enhancement of hypoxic pulmonary vasoconstriction by metabolic acidosis in dogs. *Anesthesiology* 1990;73:256–264.
182. Lejeune P, De Smet J-M, De Francquen P, Leeman M, Brimioulle S, Hallemans R, Mélot C, Naeije R. Inhibition of hypoxic pulmonary vasoconstriction by increased left atrial pressure in dogs. *Am J Physiol* 1990;259:H93–H100.
183. Lejeune P, Deloof T, Leeman M, Mélot C, Naeije R. Multipoint pulmonary vascular pressure/flow relationships in hypoxic and in normoxic dogs: Effects of nitrous oxide with and without cyclooxygenase inhibition. *Anesthesiology* 1988;68:92–99.
184. Lejeune P, Vachiery J-L, De Smet J-M, Leeman M, Brimioulle S, Delcroix M, Mélot C, Naeije R. PEEP inhibits hypoxic pulmonary vasoconstriction in dogs. *J Appl Physiol* 1991;70:1867–1873.
185. Lennon PF, Murray PA. Attenuated of hypoxic pulmonary vasoconstriction during isoflurane anesthesia is abolished by cyclooxygenase inhibition in chronically instrumented dogs. *Anesthesiology* 1996;84:804–814.
186. Lennon PF, Murray PA. Isoflurane and the pulmonary vascular pressure-flow relation at baseline and during sympathetic α-and β-adrenoreceptor activation in chronically instrumented dogs. *Anesthesiology* 1995;82:723–733.
187. Linehan JH, Dawson CA. A three-component model of the pulmonary vasculature: effects of vasoconstriction. *J Appl Physiol* 1983; 55:923–928.
188. Lodato RF, Michael JR, Murray PA. Absence of neural modulation of hypoxic pulmonary vasoconstriction in conscious dogs. *J Appl Physiol* 1988;65:1481–1487.
189. Lodato RF, Michael JR, Murray PA. Multipoint pulmonary vascular pressure-cardiac output plots in conscious dogs. *Am J Physiol* 1985;249:H351–H357.
190. Loer SA, Scheeren TWL, Tarnow J. Desflurane inhibits hypoxic pulmonary vasoconstriction in isolated rabbit lungs. *Anesthesiology* 1995;83:552–556.
191. Loh L, Sykes MK, Chakrabarti MK. The effects of halothane and ether on the pulmonary circulation in the innervated perfused cat lung. *Br Anaesth* 1977;49:309–313.
192. Lopez-Muniz R, Stephens NL, Bromberger-Barnea B, Permutt S, Riley RL. Critical closure of pulmonary vessels analyzed in terms of Starling resistor model. *J Appl Physiol* 1968;24:625–635.
193. Lumb PD, Silvay G, Weinreich AI, Shiang H. A comparison of the effects of continuous ketamine infusion and halothane on oxygenation during one-lung anaesthesia in dogs. *Can Anaesth Soc J* 1979;26:394–401.
194. Madden JA, Dawson CA, Harder DR. Hypoxia-induced activation in small isolated pulmonary arteries from the cat. *J Appl Physiol* 1985;59:113–118.
195. Madden JA, Vadula MS, Kurup VP. Effects of hypoxia and other vasoactive agents on pulmonary and cerebral artery smooth muscle cells. *Am J Physiol* 1992;263:L384–L393.
196. Malik AB. Mechanisms of neurogenic pulmonary edema. *Circ Res* 1985;57:1–18.
197. Malik AB, Zee H, Neumann PH, Gertzberg NB. Effects of pulmonary edema on regional pulmonary perfusion in the intact dog lung. *J Appl Physiol* 1980;49:834–840.
198. Marin JLB, Carruthers B, Chakrabarti MK, Sykes MK. Preservation of the hypoxic pulmonary vasoconstrictor mechanism during methoxyflurane anaesthesia in the dog. *Br J Anaesth* 1979;51: 99–105.
199. Marin JLB, Orchard C, Chakrabarti MK, Sykes MK. Depression of hypoxic pulmonary vasoconstriction in the dog by dopamine and isoprenaline. *Br J Anaesth* 1979;51:303–312.
200. Marshall B. Editorial views. Another point of view on intermittent hypoxia. *Anesthesiology* 1981;55:200–202.
201. Marshall BE, Clarke WR, Costarino AT, Chen L, Miller F, Marshall C. The dose-response relationship for hypoxic pulmonary vasoconstriction. *Resp Physiol* 1994;96:231–247.

202. Marshall BE, Hanson CW, Frasch F, Marshall C. Role of hypoxic pulmonary vasoconstriction in pulmonary gas exchange and blood flow distribution. 2. Pathophysiology. *Intensive Care Med* 1994;20: 379–389.
203. Marshall BE, Marshall C, Magno M, Lilagan P, Pietra GG. Influence of bronchial arterial PO_2 on pulmonary vascular resistance. *J Appl Physiol* 1991;70:405–415.
204. Marshall BE, Marshall C. A model for hypoxic constriction of the pulmonary circulation. *J Appl Physiol* 1988;64:68–77.
205. Marshall BE, Marshall C. Active regulation of the pulmonary circulation: A model for hypoxic pulmonary vasoconstriction. In: Will JA, Dawson CA, Weir EK, Buckner CK, eds. *The Pulmonary Circulation in Health and Disease.* Orlando, FL: Academic Press, 1987: 249–275.
206. Marshall BE, Marshall C. Anesthesia and pulmonary circulation. In: Covino BG, Fozzard HA, Rehder K, Strichartz G, eds. *Effects of Anesthesia.* Bethesda, MD, American Physiological Society, 1985; 121–136.
207. Marshall BE, Marshall C. Continuity of response to hypoxic pulmonary vasoconstriction. *J Appl Physiol* 1980;49:189–196.
208. Marshall BE, Marshall C, Benumof J, Saidman LJ. Hypoxic pulmonary vasoconstriction in dogs: Effects of lung segment size and oxygen tension. *J Appl Physiol* 1981;31:1543–1551.
209. Marshall BE, Marshall C, Frasch F, Hanson CW. Role of hypoxic pulmonary vasoconstriction in pulmonary gas exchange and blood flow distribution. 1. Physiologic concepts. *Intensive Care Med* 1994;20:291–297.
210. Marshall C, Kim SD, Marshall BE. The actions of halothane, ibuprofen and BW755C on hypoxic pulmonary vasoconstriction. *Anesthesiology* 1987;66:537–542.
211. Marshall C, Lindgren L, Marshall BE. Effects of halothane, enflurane, and isoflurane on hypoxic pulmonary vasoconstriction in rat lungs *in vitro. Anesthesiology* 1984;60:304–308.
212. Marshall C, Marshall B. Site and sensitivity for stimulation of hypoxic pulmonary vasoconstriction. *J Appl Physiol* 1983;55: 711–716.
213. Marshall C, Marshall BE. Endothelium-derived relaxing factor is not responsible for inhibition of hypoxic pulmonary vasoconstriction by inhalational anesthetics. *Anesthesiology* 1990;73: 441–448.
214. Marshall C, Marshall BE. Hypoxic pulmonary vasoconstriction is not endothelium dependent. *Proc Soc Exp Biol Med* 1992;201: 267–270.
215. Marshall C, Marshall BE. Inhalational anesthetics directly inhibit hypoxic pulmonary vasoconstriction (Abstract). *Anesthesiology* 1993; 79:A1238.
216. Marshall L, Lindgren L, Marshall BE. Metabolic and respiratory hydrogen ion effects on hypoxic pulmonary vasoconstriction. *J Appl Physiol* 1984;57:545–550.
217. Mathers J, Benumof JL, Wahrenbrock EA. General anesthetics and regional hypoxic pulmonary vasoconstriction. *Anesthesiology* 1977;46:111–114.
218. Mathew R, Amar HA, Cherry PD, Gewitz MH, Wolin MS. Role of cGMP mechanism in reponse of rat pulmonary arteries to hypoxia. *Am J Physiol* 1992;263:H141–H146.
219. McCormack DG, Paterson NAM. Loss of hypoxic pulmonary vasoconstriction in chronic pneumonia is not mediated by nitric oxide. *Am J Physiol* 1993;265:H1523–H1528.
220. McFarlane PA, Gardaz J-P, Sykes MK. CO_2 and mechanical factors reduce blood flow in a collapsed lung lobe. *J Appl Physiol* 1984;57: 739–743.
221. McMurtry IF, Davidson AB, Reeves JT, Grover RF. Inhibition of hypoxic pulmonary vasoconstriction by calcium antagonists in isolated rat lungs. *Circ Res* 1976;38:99–104.
222. Mélot C, Naeije R, Rothschild T, Mertens P, Mols P, Hallemans R. Improvement in ventilation-perfusion matching by almitrine in COPD. *Chest* 1983;83:528–533.
223. Mentzer RM, Alegre CA, Nolan SP. The effects of dopamine and isoproterenol on the pulmonary circulation. *J Thorac Cardiovasc Surg* 1976;71:807–814.
224. Miller FL, Chen L, Malmkvist G, Marshall C, Marshall BE. Mechanical factors do not influence blood flow distribution in atelectasis. *Anesthesiology* 1989;70:481–488.
225. Miller MA, Hales CA. Role of cytochrome P-450 in alveolar hypoxic pulmonary vasoconstriction in dogs. *J Clin Invest* 1979; 64:666–673.
226. Miller VM, Vanhoutte PM. Enhanced release of endothelium-derived factor(s) by chronic increases in blood flow. *Am J Physiol* 1988;255:H446–H451.
227. Mitzner W. Resistance of the pulmonary circulation. *Clin Chest Med* 1983;4:127–137.
228. Mitzner W, Huang I. Interpretation of pressure-flow curves in the pulmonary vascular bed. In: Will JA, Dawson CA, Weir EK, Buckner CK, eds. *The Pulmonary Circulation in Health and Disease.* Orlando, FL: Academic Press, 1987:215–230.
229. Mitzner W, Sylvester JJ. Hypoxic vasoconstriction and fluid filtration in pig lung. *J Appl Physiol* 1981;51:1065–1071.
230. Mookherjee S, Fuleihan D, Warner RA, Vardan S, Obeid AI. Effects of sublingual nitroglycerin on resting pulmonary gas exchange and hemodynamics in man. *Circulation* 1978;57:106–110.
231. Morgan BC, Church SC, Guntheroth WG. Hypoxic constriction of pulmonary artery and vein in intact dogs. *J Appl Physiol* 1968;25: 356–361.
232. Morgan JM, McCormack DG, Griffiths MJD, Morgan CJ, Barnes PJ, Evans TW. Adenosine as a vasodilator in primary pulmonary hypertension. *Circulation* 1991;84:1145–1149.
233. Murray PA, Fehr DM, Chen BB, Rock P, Esther JW, Desai PM, Nyhan DP. Differential effects of general anesthesia on cGMP-mediated pulmonary vasodilation. *J Appl Physiol* 1992;73:721–727.
234. Murray PA, Lodato RF, Michael JR. Neural antagonists modulate pulmonary vascular pressure-flow plots in conscious dogs. *J Appl Physiol* 1986;60:1900–1907.
235. Murray TR, Chen L, Marshall BE, Macarak EJ. Hypoxic contraction of cultured pulmonary vascular smooth muscle cells. *Am J Respir Cell Mol Biol* 1990;3:457–465.
236. Naeije R, Lambert M, Lejeune P, Leeman M, Deloof T. Cardiovascular and blood gas responses to inhaled anaesthetics in normoxic and hypoxic dogs. *Acta Anaesthesiol Scand* 1987;30:538–544.
237. Naeije R, Lejeune P, Leeman M, Mélot C, Closset J. Pulmonary vascular responses to surgical chemodenervation and chemical sympathectomy in dogs. *J Appl Physiol* 1989;66:42–50.
238. Naeije R, Lejeune P, Leeman M, Mélot C, Deloof T. Pulmonary arterial pressure-flow plots in dogs: Effects of isoflurane and nitroprusside. *J Appl Physiol* 1987;63:969–977.
239. Naeije R, Mélot C, Mols P, Hallemans R. Effects of vasodilators on hypoxic pulmonary vasoconstriction in normal man. *Chest* 1982; 82:404–410.
240. Nagasaka Y, Bhattacharya J, Nanjo S, Gropper MA, Staub NC. Micropuncture measurement of lung microvascular pressure profile during hypoxia in cats. *Circ Res* 1984;54:90–95.
241. Nakanishi S, Hiramoto T, Ahmed N, Nishimoto Y. Almitrine enhances in low dose the reactivity of pulmonary vessels to hypoxia. *Resp Physiol* 1988;74:139–150.
242. Nakazawa K, Amaha K. Effect of nicardipine hydrochloride on regional hypoxic pulmonary vasoconstriction. *Br J Anaesth* 1988; 60:547–554.
243. Nandiwada PA, Kadowitz PJ, Said SI, Mojarad M, Hyman AL. Pulmonary vasodilator responses to vasoactive intestinal peptide in the cat. *J Appl Physiol* 1985;58:1723–1728.
244. Neely CF, Haile D, Nguyen J, Breit N, Matot I. Histamine (HIST) produces tone-dependent responses in the feline pulmonary vascular (PV) bed by different mechanisms (Abstract). *Anesthesiology* 1993;79:A274.
245. Neumann PH, Kivlen CM, Johnson A, Minnear FL, Malik AB. Effect of alveolar hypoxia on regional pulmonary perfusion. *J Appl Physiol* 1984;56:338–342.
246. Newman JH, Loyd JE, English DK, Ogletree ML, Fulkerson WJ, Brigham KL. Effects of 100% oxygen on lung vascular function in awake sheep. *J Appl Physiol* 1983;54:1379–1386.
247. Newman JH, McMurtry IF, Reeves JT. Blunted pulmonary pressor responses to hypoxia in blood perfused, ventilated lungs isolated from oxygen toxic rats: Possible role of prostaglandins. *Prostaglandins* 1981;22:11–20.
248. Nicholas JF, Lam AM. Isoflurane-induced hypotension does not cause impairment in pulmonary gas exchange. *Can Anaesth Soc J* 1984;31:352–358.
249. Nishiwaki K, Nyhan DP, Rock P, Desai PM, Peterson WP, Pribble CG, Murray PA. N-nitro-L-arginine and pulmonary vascular pressure-flow relationship in conscious dogs. *Am J Physiol* 1992;262: H1331–H1337.
250. Nossaman BD, Feng CJ, Kadowitz PJ. A soluble guanylate cyclase inhibitor, LY 83583, enhances the pulmonary vasoconstrictor response to intermittent hypoxia (Abstract). *Anesthesiology* 1993; 79:A1235.

251. Nyhan DP, Chen BB, Fehr DM, Goll HM, Murray PA. Pentobarbital augments pulmonary vasoconstrictor response to cyclooxygenase inhibition. *Am J Physiol* 1989;257:H1140–H1146.
252. Nyhan DP, Chen BB, Fehr DM, Rock P, Murray PA. Anesthesia alters pulmonary vasoregulation by angiotensin II and captopril. *J Appl Physiol* 1992;72:636–642.
253. Nyhan DP, Clougherty PW, Goll HM, Murray PA. Bradykinin actively modulates pulmonary vascular pressure-cardiac index relationships. *J Appl Physiol* 1987;63:145–151.
254. Nyhan DP, Clougherty PW, Murray PA. AVP-induced pulmonary vasodilation during specific V_1 receptor block in conscious dogs. *Am J Physiol* 1987;253:H493–H499.
255. Nyhan DP, Geller HS, Goll HM, Murray PA. Pulmonary vasoactive effects of exogenous and endogenous AVP in conscious dogs. *Am J Physiol* 1986;251:H1009–H1016.
256. Nyhan DP, Goll HM, Chen BB, Fehr DM, Clougherty PW, Murray PA. Pentobarbital anesthesia alters pulmonary vascular response to neural antagonists. *Am J Physiol* 1989;256:H1384–H1392.
257. Nyhan DP, Pribble CG, Peterson WP, Nishiwaki K, Trempy GA, Desai PM, Rock P, Murray PA. Amrinone and the pulmonary vascular pressure-flow relationship in conscious control dogs and following left lung autotransplantation. *Anesthesiology* 1993;78:1166–1174.
258. Ohlsson J, Middaugh M, Hlastala MP. Reduction of lung perfusion increases ($\dot{V}_A/\dot{Q}$) heterogeneity. *J Appl Physiol* 1989;66:2423–2430.
259. Ohmura A, Pace NL, Wong KC, Johansen RK. Hypoxic pulmonary vasoconstriction and the pharmacologically denervated lung. *Anaesthesia* 1982;37:152–160.
260. Orphanidou D, Hughes JMB, Myers MJ, Al-Suhali A-R, Henderson B. Tomography of regional ventilation and perfusion using krypton 81m in normal subjects and asthmatic patients *Thorax* 1986; 41:542–551.
261. Palmer RMJ, Ferrige AG, Moncada S. Nitric oxide release accounts for the biological activity of endothelium-derived relaxing factor. *Nature* 1987;327:524–526.
262. Pappert D, Busch T, Gerlach H, Lewandowski K, Radermacher P, Roissant R. Aerosolized prostacyclin versus inhaled nitric oxide in children with severe acute respiratory distress syndrome. *Anesthesiology* 1995;82:1507–1511.
263. Parsons GB, Leventhal JP, Hansen MM, Goldstein JD. Effect of sodium nitroprusside on hypoxic pulmonary vasoconstriction in the dog. *J Appl Physiol* 1981;51:288–292.
264. Peach MJ, Johns RA, Rose CE Jr. The potential role of interactions between endothelium and smooth muscle in pulmonary vascular physiology and pathophysiology. In: Weir EK, Reeves JT, eds. *Lung Biology in Health and Disease.* Vol. 38, Lenfant series, "Pulmonary Vascular Physiology and Pathophysiology." New York, Marcel Dekker, 1989:643–697.
265. Pearl RG, Siegel LC. Effects of prostaglandin E_1 and hydralazine on the longitudinal distribution of pulmonary vascular resistance during vasoconstrictor pulmonary hypertension in sheep. *Anesthesiology* 1992;76:106–112.
266. Permutt S, Howell JBL, Proctor DF, Riley RL. Effect of lung inflation on static pressure-volume characteristics of pulmonary vessels. *J Appl Physiol* 1961;16:64–70.
267. Permutt S, Riley RL. Hemodynamics of collapsible vessels with tone: The vascular waterfall. *J Appl Physiol* 1963;18:924–932.
268. Peterson WP, Trempy GA, Nishiwaki K, Nyhan DP, Murray PA. Neurohumoral regulation of the pulmonary circulation during circulatory hypotension in conscious dogs. *J Appl Physiol* 1993;75: 1675–1682.
269. Pirlo AF, Benumof JL, Trousdale FR. Potentiation of lobar hypoxic pulmonary vasoconstriction by intermittent hypoxia in dogs. *Anesthesiology* 1981;55:226–230.
270. Pison U, Lopez FA, Heidelmeyer CF, Rossaint R, Falke KJ. Inhaled nitric oxide reverses hypoxic pulmonary vasoconstriction without impairing gas exchange. *J Appl Physiol* 1993;74:1287–1292.
271. Porcelli RJ, Bergofsky EH. Adrenergic receptors in pulmonary vasoconstrictor responses to gaseous and humoral agents. *J Appl Physiol* 1973;34:483–488.
272. Porcelli RJ, Viau AT, Naftchi NE, Bergofsky EH. β-Receptor influence on lung vasoconstrictor responses to hypoxia and humoral agents. *J Appl Pysiol* 1977;43:612–616.
273. Post JM, Hume JR, Archer SL, Weir EK. Direct role for potassium channel inhibition in hypoxic pulmonary vasoconstriction. *Am J Physiol* 1992;262:C882–C890.
274. Prefaut C, Engel LA. Vertical distribution of perfusion and inspired gas in supine man. *Resp Physiol* 1981;43:209–219.
275. Radermacher P, Huet Y, Pluskwa F, Herigault R, Mal H, Teisseire B, LeMaire F. Comparison of ketanserin and sodium nitroprusside in patients with severe ARDS. *Anesthesiology* 1988;68:152–157.
276. Radermacher P, Santak B, Becker H, Falke KJ. Prostaglandin E_1 and nitroglycerin reduce pulmonary capillary pressure but worsen ventilation-perfusion distributions in patients with adult respiratory distress syndrome. *Anesthesiology* 1989;70:601–606.
277. Radermacher P, Santak B, Wüst HJ, Tarrow J, Falke KJ. Prostacyclin and right ventricular functions in patients with pulmonary hypertension associated with ARDS. *Intensive Care Med* 1990;16: 227–232.
278. Reed JH, Wood EH. Effect of body position on vertical distribution of pulmonary blood flow. *J Appl Physiol* 1970;28:303–311.
279. Rees DI, Gaines GY III. One-lung anesthesia—a comparison of pulmonary gas exchange during anesthesia with ketamine or enflurane. *Anesth Analg* 1984;63:521–525.
280. Reeves JT, Grover RF. Blockade of acute hypoxic pulmonary hypertension by endotoxin. *J Appl Physiol* 1974;36:328–332.
281. Reeves JT, Groves BM, Weir EK: Adenosine and selective reduction of pulmonary vascular resistance in primary pulmonary hypertension. *Circulation* 1991;84:1437–1439.
282. Rennotte MT, Reynaert M, Clerbaux TH, Willems E, Roeseleer J, Veriter C, Rodenstein D, Frans A. Effects of two inotropic drugs, dopamine and dobutamine, on pulmonary gas exchange in artificially ventilated patients. *Intensive Care Med* 1989;15:160–165.
283. Reyes A, López-Messa JB, Alonso P. Almitrine in acute respiratory failure: Effects on pulmonary gas exchange and circulation. *Chest* 1987;91:388–393.
284. Rich GF, Murphy GD, Roos CM, Johns RA. Inhaled nitric oxide. Selective pulmonary vasodilation in cardiac surgical patients. *Anesthesiology* 1993;78:1028–1035.
285. Richardson JB. Nerve supply to the lungs. *Am Rev Resp Dis* 1979; 119:785–802.
286. Roberts JD, Chen T-Y, Kawai N, Wain J, Dupuy P, Shimouchi A, Bloch K, Polaner D, Zapol WM. Inhaled nitric oxide reverses pulmonary vasoconstriction in the hypoxic and acidotic newborn lamb. *Circ Res* 1993;72:246–254.
287. Roberts JD, Lang P, Polaner D, Zapol WM. Inhaled nitric oxide in persistent pulmonary hypertension of the newborn. *Lancet* 1992; 340:818–819.
288. Robin ED, Theodore J, Burke CM, Oesterle SN, Fowler MB, Jamieson SW, Baldwin JC, Morris AJ, Hunt SA, Vankessel A, Stinson EB, Shumway NE. Hypoxic pulmonary vasoconstriction persists in the human transplanted lung. *Clin Sci* 1987;72:283–287.
289. Rock P, Patterson GA, Permutt S, Sylvester JT. Nature and distribution of vascular resistance in hypoxic pig lungs. *J Appl Physiol* 1985;59:1891–1901.
290. Rodman DM, Voelkel NF. Regulation of vascular tone. In: Crystal RG, West JB, Barnes PJ, Cherniack NS, Weibel ER, eds. *The Lung: Scientific Foundations.* New York: Raven Press, 1991;1105–1119.
291. Rodman DM, Yamaguchi T, O'Brien RF, McMurtry IF. Methylene blue enhances hypoxic contraction in isolated rat pulmonary arteries. *Chest* 1988;93:935–945.
292. Rogers SN, Benumof JL. Halothane and isoflurane do not decrease PaO_2 during one-lung ventilation in intravenously anesthetized patients. *Anesth Analg* 1985;64:946–954.
293. Romand JA, Pinsky MR, Firestone L, Zar HA, Lancaster JR. Inhaled nitric oxide partially reverses hypoxic pulmonary vasoconstriction in the dog. *J Appl Physiol* 1994;76:1350–1355.
294. Romand JA, Pinsky MR, Firestone L, Zar HA, Lancaster JR. Effect of inhaled nitric oxide on pulmonary hemodynamics after acute lung injury in dogs. *J Appl Physiol* 1994;76:1356–1362.
295. Rose JC. Active constriction and dilatation in pulmonary circulation in response to acetylcholine. *Proc Soc Exp Biol Med* 1957;94:734–737.
296. Rossaint R, Falke KJ, López F, Slama K, Pison U, Zapol WM. Inhaled nitric oxide for the adult respiratory distress syndrome. *N Eng J Med* 1993;328:399–405.
297. Rovira I, Chen T-Y, Winkler M, Kawai N, Bloch KD, Zapol WM. Effects of inhaled nitric oxide on pulmonary hemodynamics and gas exchange in an ovine model of ARDS. *J Appl Physiol* 1994;76: 345–355.
298. Rudolph AM, Kurland MD, Auld PAM, Paul MH. Effects of vasodilator drugs on normal and serotonin-constricted pulmonary vessels of the dog. *Am J Physiol* 1959;197:617–623.
299. Russ RD, Resta TC, Walker BR. Pulmonary vasodilatory response to neurohypophyseal peptides in the rat. *J Appl Physiol* 1992;73: 473–478.

300. Russ RD, Walker BR. Role of nitric oxide in vasopressinergic pulmonary vasodilatation. *Am J Physiol* 1992;262:H743–H747.
301. Ryan US. Receptors on pulmonary endothelial cells. *Am Rev Respir Dis* 1990;141:S132–S136.
302. Sada K, Shirai M, Ninomiya I. Effects of prostaglandin F_2 and prostacyclin on pulmonary microcirculation in the cat. *J Appl Physiol* 1987;62:1124–1132.
303. Sada K, Shirai M, Ninomiya I. X-ray TV system for measuring microcirculation in small pulmonary vessels. *J Appl Physiol* 1985; 59:1013–1018.
304. Sandoval J, Long GR, Skoog C, Wood LDH, Oppenheimer L. Independent influence of blood flow rate and mixed venous PO_2 on shunt fraction. *J Appl Physiol* 1983;55:1128–1133.
305. Scanlon TS, Benumof JL, Wahrenbrock EA, Nelson WL. Hypoxic pulmonary vasoconstriction and the ratio of hypoxic lung to perfused normoxic lung. *Anesthesiology* 1978;49:177–181.
306. Scherer R, Vigfusson G, Hultsch E, Van Aken H, Lawin P. Prostaglandin F_2 improves oxygen tension and reduces venous admixture during one-lung ventilation in anesthetized paralyzed dogs. *Anesthesiology* 1985;62:23–28.
307. Scherer R, Vigfusson G, Lawin P. Pulmonary blood flow reduction by prostaglandin F_2 and pulmonary artery balloon manipulation during one-lung ventilation in dogs. *Acta Anaesthesiol Scand* 1986; 30:2–6.
308. Schulman LL, Lennon PF, Ratner SJ, Enson Y. Meclofenamate enhances blood oxygenation in acute oleic acid lung injury. *J Appl Physiol* 1988;64:710–718.
309. Schuster DP, Dennis DR. Leukotriene inhibitors do not block hypoxic pulmonary vasoconstriction in dogs. *J Appl Physiol* 1987; 62:1808–1813.
310. Searle NR, Sahab P. Endothelial vasomotor regulation in health and disease. *Can J Anaesth* 1992;39:838–857.
311. Shayevitz JR, Traystman RJ, Adkinson F, Sciuto AM, Gurtner GH. Inhalation anesthetics augment oxidant-induced pulmonary vasoconstriction: Evidence for a membrane effect. *Anesthesiology* 1985; 63:624–632.
312. Shirai M, Shindo T, Ninomiya I. β-Adrenergic mechanisms attenuate hypoxic pulmonary vasoconstriction during systemic hypoxia in cats. *Am J Physiol* 1994;266:1777–1785.
313. Shirai M, Sada K, Ninomiya I. Nonuniform effects of histamine on small pulmonary vessels in cats. *J Appl Physiol* 1987;62:451–458.
314. Siegel LC, Pearl RG, Shafer SL, Ream AK, Prielipp RC. The longitudinal distribution of pulmonary vascular resistance during unilateral hypoxia. *Anesthesiology* 1989;70:527–532.
315. Simonneau G, Escourrou P, Duroux P, Lockhart A. Inhibition of hypoxic pulmonary vasoconstriction by nifedipine. *N Engl J Med* 1981;304:1582–1585.
316. Slinger P, Scott WAC. Arterial oxygenation during one-lung ventilation: A comparison of enflurane and isoflurane. *Anesthesiology* 1995;82:940–946.
317. Sprague RS, Stephenson AH, Lonigro AJ. Prostaglandin I_2 supports blood flow to hypoxic alveoli in anesthetized dogs. *J Appl Physiol* 1984;56:1246–1251.
318. Steegers PA, Backx PJ. Propofol and alfentanil anesthesia during one-lung ventilation. *J Cardiothoracic Anesth* 1990;4:194–199.
319. Susmano A, Passovoy M, Carleton RA. Comparison of the effects of two anesthetic agents on the production of hypoxic pulmonary hypertension in dogs. *Am Heart J* 1972;84:203–207.
320. Sykes MK, Arnot RN, Jastrzebski J, Gibbs JM, Obdrzalek J, Hurtig JB. Reduction of hypoxic pulmonary vasoconstriction during trichlorethylene anesthesia. *J Appl Physiol* 1975;39:103–108.
321. Sykes MK, Davies DM, Chakrabarti MK, Loh L. The effects of halothane, trichloroethylene and ether on the hypoxic pressor response and pulmonary vascular resistance in the isolated, perfused cat lung. *Br J Anaesth* 1973;45:655–663.
322. Sykes MK, Davies DM, Loh L, Jastrzebski J, Chakrabarti MK. The effect of methoxyflurane on pulmonary vascular resistance and hypoxic pulmonary vasoconstriction in the isolated perfused cat lung. *Br J Anaesth* 1976;48:191–194.
323. Sykes MK, Gibbs JM, Loh L, Marin JBL, Obdrzalek J, Arnot RN. Preservation of the pulmonary vasoconstrictor response to alveolar hypoxia during the administration of halothane to dogs. *Br J Anaesth* 1978;50:1185–1196.
324. Sykes MK, Hurtig JB, Tait AR, Chakrabarti MK. Reduction of hypoxic pulmonary vasoconstriction during diethyl ether anaesthesia in the dog. *Br J Anaesth* 1977;49:293–299.
325. Sykes MK, Hurtig JB, Tait AR, Chakrabarti MK. Reduction of hypoxic pulmonary vasoconstriction in the dog during administration of nitrous oxide. *Br J Anaesth* 1977;49:301–306.
326. Sykes MK, Loh L, Seed RF, Kafer ER Chakrabarti MK. The effect of inhalational anaesthetics on hypoxic pulmonary vasoconstriction and pulmonary vascular resistance in the perfused lungs of the dog and cat. *Br J Anaesth* 1972;44:776–787.
327. Sylvester JT, Harabin AL, Peake MD, Frank RS. Vasodilator and constrictor responses to hypoxia in isolated pig lungs. *J Appl Physiol* 1980;49:820–825.
328. Sylvester JT, Mitzner W, Ngeow Y, Permutt S. Hypoxic constriction of alveolar and extra-alveolar vessels in isolated pig lungs. *J Appl Physiol* 1983;54:1660–1666.
329. Tai E, Read J. Response of blood gas tensions to aminophylline and isoprenaline in patients with asthma. *Thorax* 1967;22:543–549.
330. Takashio T, Yamashita H, Onodera S. Inhibitory effect of pindolol on hypoxic pulmonary vasoconstriction. *Am J Physiol* 1992;262: H130–H135.
331. Teboul JI, Zapol WM, Brun-Buisson C, Abrouk F, Rauss A, LeMaire F. A comparison of pulmonary artery occlusion pressure and left ventricular end-diastolic pressure during mechanical ventilation with PEEP in patients with severe ARDS. *Anesthesiology* 1989;70: 261–266.
332. Thomas HM III, Garrett RC. Strength of hypoxic vasoconstriction determines shunt fraction in dogs with atelectasis. *J Appl Physiol* 1982;53:44–51.
333. Thomas T, Marshall JM. The role of adenosine in hypoxic pulmonary vasoconstriction in the anaesthetized rat. *Exper Physiol* 1993;78:541–543.
334. Tolins M, Weir EK, Chesler E, Nelson DP, From AHL. Pulmonary vascular tone is increased by a voltage-dependent calcium channel potentiator. *J Appl Physiol* 1986;60:942–948.
335. Trempy GA, Nyhan DP, Murray PA. Pulmonary vasoregulation by arginine vasopressin in conscious, halothane-anesthetized, and pentobarbital-anesthetized dogs with increased vasomotor tone. *Anesthesiology* 1994;81:632–640.
336. Tucker A, McMurtry IF, Grover RF, Reeves JT. Attenuation of hypoxic pulmonary vasoconstriction by verapamil in intact dogs. *Proc Soc Exp Biol Med* 1976;151:611–614.
337. Uezono S, Clarke WR. The effects of propofol on elevated and normal pulmonary vascular resistance (Abstract). *Anesthesiology* 1994;81:A703.
338. Versprille A. Pulmonary vascular resistance: a meaningless variable. *Intensive Care Med* 1984;10:51–53.
339. Vincent J-L, Lignian H, Gillet J-B, Berre J, Contu E. Increase in PaO_2 following intravenous administration of propranolol in acutely hypoxemic patients. *Chest* 1985;88:558–562.
340. Voelkel NF, Chang S-W, Pfeffer KD, Worthen SG, McMurtry IF, Henson PM. PAF antagonists: different effects on platelets, neutrophils, guinea pig ileum and PAF-induced vasodilation in isolated rat lung. *Prostaglandins* 1986;32:359–372.
341. Von Euler US, Liljestrand G. Observations on the pulmonary arterial blood pressure in the cat. *Acta Physiol Scand* 1946;12:301–320.
342. Wagner WW, Latham LP, Capen RL. Capillary recruitment during airway hypoxia: Role of pulmonary artery pressure. *J Appl Physiol* 1979;47:383–387.
343. Wagner WW, Latham LP. Pulmonary capillary recruitment during airway hypoxia in the dog. *J Appl Physiol* 1975;39:900–905.
344. Walmrath D, Schneider T, Pilch J, Grimminger F, Seeger W. Aerosolised prostacyclin an adult respiratory distress syndrome. *Lancet* 1993;342:961–962.
345. Weir EK, McMurtry IF, Tucker A, Reeves JT, Grover RF. Prostaglandin synthetase inhibitors do not decrease hypoxic pulmonary vasoconstriction. *J Appl Physiol* 1976;41:714–717.
346. Welte M, Zwissler B, Habazettl H, Messmer K. PGI_2 aerosol versus nitric oxide for selective pulmonary vasodilation in hypoxic pulmonary vasoconstriction. *Eur Surg Res* 1993;25:329–340.
347. West JB, Dollery CT, Naimark A. Distribution of blood flow in isolated lung: relation to vascular and alveolar pressures. *J Appl Physiol* 1964;19:713–724.
348. Wetzel RC. Aerosolized prostacyclin: in search of the ideal pulmonary vasodilator. *Anesthesiology* 1995;82:1315–1317.
349. Wetzel RC, Martin LD. Pentobarbital attenuates pulmonary vasoconstriction in isolated sheep lungs. *Am J Physiol* 1989;257: H898–H903.
350. Wetzel RC, Zacur HA, Sylvester JT. Effect of puberty and estradiol on hypoxic vasomotor response in isolated sheep lungs. *J Appl Physiol* 1984;56:1199–1203.

351. Weygandt GR, Kopman EA, Ludbrook PA. Mechanism of nitroglycerin-induced hypoxemia. *Cathet Cardiovasc Diagn* 1980;6:387–395.
352. Wong J, Vanderford PA Winters JW, Chang R, Soifer SJ, Fineman JR. Endothelin-1 does not mediate acute hypoxic pulmonary vasoconstriction in the intact newborn lamb. *J Cardiovasc Pharmacol* 1993;22:S262–S266.
353. Yanagisawa M, Kurihara H, Kimura S, Tomobe Y, Kobayashi M, Mitsui Y, Yazaki Y, Goto K, Masaki T. A novel potent vasoconstriction peptide produced by vascular endothelial cells. *Nature* 1988; 332:411–415.
354. Yoshimura K, Tod ML, Pier KG, Rubin LJ. Role of venoconstriction in thromboxane-induced pulmonary hypertension and edema in lambs. *J Appl Physiol* 1989;66:929–935.
355. Young TE, Lundquist LJ, Chesler E, Weir EK. Comparative effects of nifedipine, verapamil, and diltiazem on experimental pulmonary hypertension. *Am J Cardiol* 1983;51:195–200.
356. Zapol WM, Rimar S, Gillis N, Marletta M, Bosken CH. Nitric oxide and the lung. *Am J Respir Crit Care Med* 1994;149:1375–1380.
357. Zhao Y, Packer CS, Rhoades RA. Pulmonary vein contracts in response to hypoxia. *Am J Physiol* 1993;265:L87–L92.
358. Zhuang FY, Fung YC, Yen RT. Analysis of blood flow in cat's lung with detailed anatomical and elasticity data. *J Appl Physiol* 1983; 55:1341–1348.
359. Zwissler B, Rank N, Jaenicke U, Schurle B, Welte M, Reichart B, Netz H, Messmer K, Peter K. Selective pulmonary vasodilation by inhaled prostacyclin in a newborn with congenital heart disease and cardiopulmonary bypass. *Anesthesiology* 1995;82: 1512–1516.

Anesthesia: Biologic Foundations, edited by Tony L. Yaksh et al. Lippincott–Raven Publishers, Philadelphia © 1997.

CHAPTER 77

VENTILATION AND PERFUSION MATCHING

GÖRAN HEDENSTIERNA AND HANS ULRICH ROTHEN

This chapter reviews pertinent data on the distributions of pulmonary ventilation and blood flow under normal conditions, i.e. in the awake healthy subject and during anesthesia. The matching of alveolar ventilation (V_A), and perfusion (Q) is a major determinant of the oxygenation of arterial blood. Knowledge of the distributions of ventilation and of pulmonary blood flow may help us to understand why oxygenation of blood regularly is impaired during anesthesia and why sometimes even severe hypoxemia may develop. It may also guide in taking proper precautions to prevent hypoxemia or to choose an appropriate strategy to correct it. Furthermore, an impaired oxygenation of blood occurs in most subjects who are anesthetized (8,88,119), and it has become routine to add oxygen to the inspired gas so that the inspired O_2 fraction (F_IO_2) is kept around 0.3 to 0.4. Despite this precaution, mild to moderate hypoxemia, defined as an arterial oxygen saturation (SaO_2) between 85% and 90%, may occur in approximately half of all patients undergoing elective surgery, and the hypoxemia can last from a few seconds up to 30 minutes (83). More alarming is the fact that about 20% of the patients may suffer from severe hypoxemia, i.e., SaO_2 below 81% for up to 5 minutes (83). The cause of hypoxemia is multifactorial, including both ventilatory and circulatory dysfunctions. In this chapter causes of ventilation-perfusion ($\dot{V}_A/\dot{Q}$) mismatch, including the shunt, are discussed. Other more or less acute mechanisms of impeded gas exchange, such as upper airway obstruction, cardiac failure, and circulatory shock, are not discussed here.

VENTILATION AND PERFUSION IN THE AWAKE SUBJECT

Distribution of Ventilation

This section gives a brief summary of the major factors that determine the distributions of ventilation ($\dot{V}_A$) and perfusion ($\dot{Q}$) During quiet breathing the distribution of inspired gas is determined mainly by the pressure-volume curve of the lung and the vertical pleural pressure gradient. The nonlinear relationship between pressure and volume results in a larger volume increase for a given increment in pressure at low compared to high lung volumes. The pleural pressure increases down the pleural space by approximately 0.2 to 0.4 cm H_2O per cm distance (1,60). This results in a lower transpulmonary pressure (approximated by airway pressure minus pleural pressure) in dependent than in upper lung regions. Dependent lung regions are therefore positioned on the lower, steeper part of the pressure-volume curve (Fig. 1). During inspiration the transpulmonary pressure is increased to an equal extent all over the lung; lower and upper lung regions move along the pressure-volume curve with similar pressure increments. The change in volume (or ventilation) is therefore larger in dependent regions of the lungs.

The pleural pressure gradient is caused by the weight of the lung tissue. But in addition, differences in the shape of the thoracic cavity and the lung, and the forces exerted by the abdominal organs on the diaphragm, may also affect the distribution of ventilation (105). The influence of the latter factor may explain why ventilation apparently is more uniform from top to bottom in the prone position than supine (102). It is of interest to note that ventilation appears to be evenly distributed in the lungs if gravitational forces are absent, as evidenced by measurements in weightlessness (81).

Not only the alveolar volume but also airway caliber decreases during an expiration. This may result in closure of airways when pleural and extramural airway pressure becomes positive and higher than luminal pressure (82). Closure of airways begins in the most dependent lung regions due to the higher pleural pressure at that level, and spreads up the lung with deeper expiration. Thus, airway closure impedes ventilation mostly in dependent lung regions.

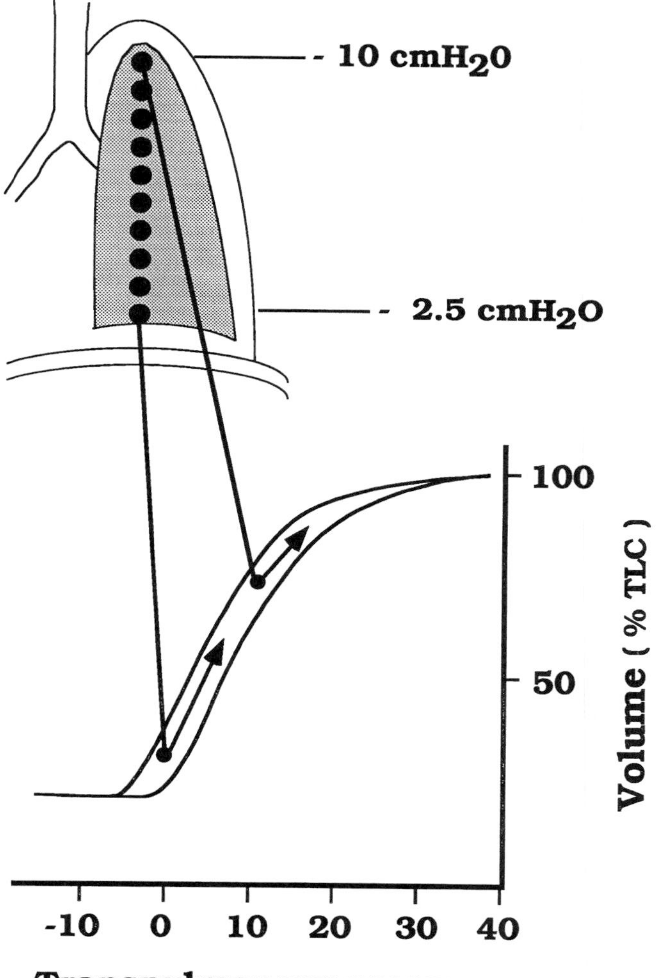

Figure 1. Static pressure-volume curve (P-V) of the total respiratory system in an upright subject. The basal lung units are on a more steep part of the P-V curve than apical units. *Arrows* show the changes during quiet tidal breathing. Note the larger volume change in dependent lung regions compared to upper ones.

The magnitude of airway closure is dependent on age. In teenagers it may be difficult to demonstrate, even after an expiration to residual volume (79). At old ages (70 years or more) airway closure may be detected at lung volumes above functional residual capacity (FRC) (72). Closure of airways appears to be independent of body position (72), but since a change from upright to supine reduces FRC by approximately 0.7 to 0.8 L (135) airway closure is seen more regularly above FRC in the supine position, and airway closure above FRC can be expected at ages 50 and older (72). Thus, ventilation of dependent lung regions decreases with age. Since blood flow goes predominantly to dependent lung regions (see below), the phenomenon of airway closure seems to be an explanation to the well-known decrease in PaO_2 with age (100).

The increase in airway closure with age is probably caused by a loss of elastic tissue in the lung. The elastic recoil of the lung decreases, making the pleural pressure less negative. This also explains why FRC slowly increases with age (corrected for changes in body size) (Fig. 2). Further causes of an increase in airway closure are, for example, a loss of elastic recoil due to lung disease (chronic bronchitis, emphysema), and an increase in airway tone (asthma) (16,78).

Inspiratory flow also affects the ventilation distribution because of an increasing influence of airway resistance. Due to the vertical pleural pressure gradient, dependent airways are less dilated than those in upper lung units. Accordingly, resistance to gas flow is higher in dependent lung regions and impedes ventilation to these regions. Thus, with increasing inspiratory flow rate, as during exercise, the distribution of ventilation within the lung becomes more uniform (6).

Distribution of Pulmonary Blood Flow

Blood flow increases down the lung, due to gravitational forces. An upper lung region may exist where alveolar pressure exceeds arterial and venous pressures, e.g., during hypotension and positive pressure ventilation. In this region the alveoli compress the alveolar capillaries and obstruct their blood flow (zone I, no blood flow zone) (93,140). Despite the fact that the alveolar capillaries are closed and blood flow has ceased through them, a persisting tiny blood flow in zone I has been demonstrated. Histologic studies on excised lung tissue have shown that this blood passes through corner vessels, i.e., vessels located in the junctions between alveolar septa (109). These vessels appear to be subject to other forces than those acting on the alveolar capillaries, and they are kept patent even when being in zone I. By using the multiple inert gas elimination technique (see below) it has also been demonstrated that this corner vessel blood flow participates in gas exchange, creating a distinct so-called high $\dot{V}_A/\dot{Q}$ mode (55).

Farther down the lung arterial pressure has increased enough to exceed alveolar pressure, the latter still being higher than venous pressure. In this region (zone II), the driving pressure equals arterial minus alveolar pressure. The effect on blood flow in this zone has variously been called the "sluice," "the waterfall phenomenon," or the "Starling resistor effect" (93,140). Because of the increasing arterial pressure down this zone, and a maintained alveolar pressure, blood flow increases down the zone. Still farther down the lung both arterial and venous pressures exceed alveolar pressure, the driving force thus being arterial pressure minus venous pressure, similar to that in the systemic circulation. Down this zone (zone III) the pressure is constant, hydrostatic pressure adding to an equal extent to both arterial and venous pressures. However, there is still a certain increase in blood flow down this zone, indicating a decrease in vascular resistance, presumably as a consequence of an increasing dilation of the alveolar capillaries. In the lowermost region of the lung, blood flow may be reduced (zone IV) (124). This may be attributed to compression of extraalveolar vessels brought about by an increasing interstitial pressure.

There appears also to be a nonhomogeneous distribution of perfusion in nongravitational planes. Studies on the perfusion-distribution in awake healthy humans using a moving gamma camera [single photon emission computed tomography (SPECT), see below] suggest a maximum blood flow in the middle of the lung (42), although different results and opinions have also been presented (86). Hakim et al. (42) have proposed that the decreasing blood flow toward the periphery of the lung is due to the increasing length of the pulmonary arterial vessels, which increases the resistance to blood flow. Glenny and Robertson (38) fitted their blood flow data, obtained in different body positions in animal experiments, to a fractal model and proposed that gravity is only a minor determinant of blood flow distribution in the lung. However, full agreement has not been reached on either the degree of nongravitational inhomogeneity of perfusion or possible mechanisms behind such inhomogeneity.

An increased intrathoracic pressure impedes the return to the right heart and therefore reduces cardiac output (124). It may also affect pulmonary vascular resistance (PVR) (93,140), although this may be a less important modifier of cardiac output. However, PVR appears to be lowest at a lung volume close to FRC and is increased whether lung volume is increased or reduced from that level. The diphasic dependence on lung volume can be explained by an increase in capillary resistance with increasing lung volume (37) and an increase in extraalveolar lung vessel resistance with decreasing lung volume (139), respectively.

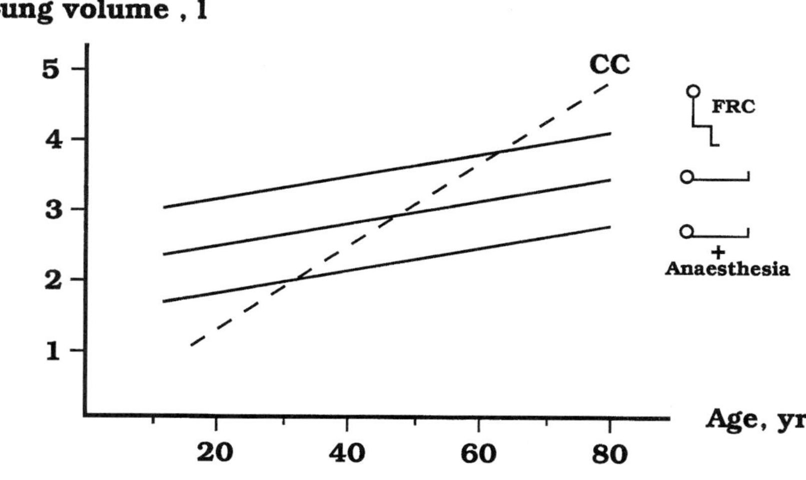

Figure 2. Schematic drawing of the age dependence of functional residual capacity (FRC) and closing capacity (CC). FRC, but not CC, is affected by body position and anesthesia, as shown by the different lines for sitting and supine positions, as well as for anesthetized subjects. For further explanations, see text. (Redrawn from ref. 49, with permission.)

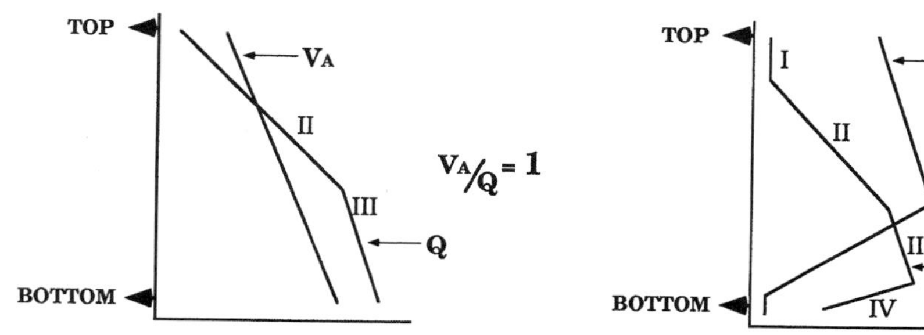

Figure 3. Schematic drawing of the vertical distribution of ventilation (V_A) and perfusion (Q) of the lung in the awake *(left)* and the anesthetized *(right)* subject. Zones I, II, III, and IV are indicated. For further details, see text. Compare with Fig 10.

Ventilation-Perfusion Relationship ($\dot{V}_A/\dot{Q}$)

Knowing the distributions of ventilation and perfusion, the ventilation-perfusion relationship ($\dot{V}_A/\dot{Q}$) can be estimated. The left panel in Fig. 3 summarizes the vertical distribution of ventilation and blood flow in an awake, healthy subject. As discussed earlier, both ventilation and blood flow increase down the lung, the fractional increase of blood flow being larger than that of ventilation. The average $\dot{V}_A/\dot{Q}$ ratio is approximately 1 with higher ratios in upper lung regions and lower ratios in lower lung regions. The $\dot{V}_A/\dot{Q}$ ratio thus varies from approximately 0.5 to 5. As will be discussed in the next section $\dot{V}_A/\dot{Q}$ can also be assessed without direct measurement of the spatial distributions of ventilation and blood flow.

TECHNIQUES FOR ASSESSING $\dot{V}_A/\dot{Q}$

The O_2/CO_2 Method (Three-Compartment Model)

An overall estimation of $\dot{V}_A/\dot{Q}$ can be obtained by simple arterial blood gas analysis, as shown in Fig. 4 (138). Three situations are shown. To the left on the diagram is a shunt, i.e., lung unit with perfusion but no ventilation. PaO_2 corresponds to the mixed venous PO_2 ($P_{\bar{V}}O_2$) and $PaCO_2$ equals $P_{\bar{V}}CO_2$. On the far right of the diagram, a lung unit that is ventilated but not perfused is shown, i.e., dead space. In this example PO_2 corresponds to the inspired O_2 tension (corrected for water vapor pressure), and PCO_2 is zero, since there is no exchange of gas across the alveolar-capillary membranes. These two situations correspond to the $\dot{V}_A/\dot{Q}$ ratios of zero and infinity, respectively. For any $\dot{V}_A/\dot{Q}$ ratio between these extremes a pair of PaO_2 and $PaCO_2$ can be deducted. This pair is located on the curve in Fig. 4. The curve is valid for air breathing and without any presence of diffusion impairment (108).

The shunt, or rather venous admixture (see below), can be calculated from the oxygenation of blood, according to the standard shunt equation (9):

$$C_aO_2 \times Q_T = C_cO_2 \times Q_c + C_vO_2 \times Q_s, \quad [1]$$

where C_aO_2, C_cO_2, and C_vO_2 are arterial, pulmonary end-capillary, and mixed venous oxygen content, respectively, and Q_T, Q_C, and Q_S are cardiac output (total lung blood flow), pulmonary capillary blood flow of ventilated lung, and shunt flow, respectively. Now we replace:

$$Q_C = Q_T - Q_S, \quad [2]$$

and rearrange:

$$\frac{Q_S}{Q_T} = \frac{C_CO_2 - C_aO_2}{C_CO_2 - C_vO_2} \quad [3]$$

The dead space ventilation can also be calculated from the CO_2 elimination according to the Bohr equation:

$$F_ECO_2 \times V_T = F_ACO_2 \times V_A + F_ICO_2 \times V_D \quad [4]$$

where F_ECO_2, F_ACO_2, and F_ICO_2 are mixed expired, alveolar, and inspired CO_2 concentrations, respectively, and V_T, V_A, and V_D are tidal volume, alveolar part of V_T that goes to perfused lung, and dead space, respectively. Rearranging, we get:

$$\frac{V_D}{V_T} = \frac{F_ACO_2 - F_ECO_2}{F_ACO_2 - F_ICO_2} \quad [5]$$

Gas fractions can be replaced by partial pressures, alveolar CO_2 tension can be approximated by arterial CO_2 tension (27), and inspired CO_2 tension can under most conditions be set to zero:

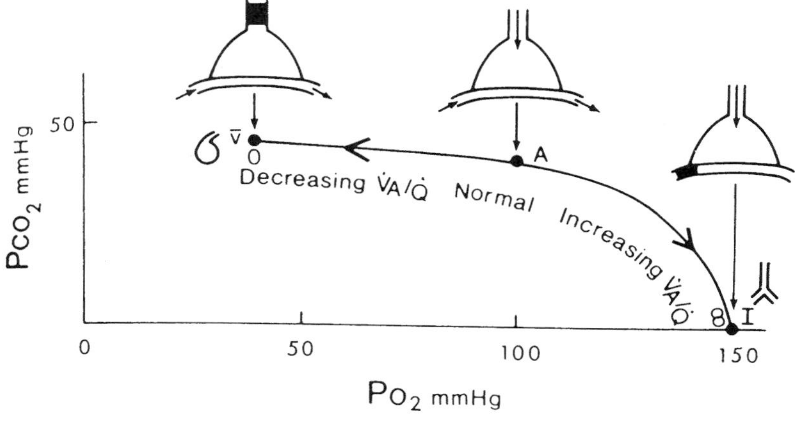

Figure 4. Oxygen-carbon dioxide diagram showing the effect of different ventilation-perfusion ratios ($\dot{V}_A/\dot{Q}$ line). Three lung units are shown: shunt (located at the mixed venous point V), normal (ideal) ventilation-perfusion ratio (A), and dead space (located at the inspired gas point I). (From ref. 138, with permission.)

$$\frac{V_D}{V_T} = \frac{PaCO_2 - P_ECO_2}{PaCO_2} \quad [6]$$

As can be seen the equations for assessing the shunt and for dead space are identical in their construction. This means a three-compartment analysis can be made, with one compartment being perfused but not ventilated ("shunt" or venous admixture), one compartment ventilated but not perfused (dead space), and an ideal compartment that is both ventilated and perfused. However, the shunt in this three-compartment model includes not only perfusion of nonventilated lung tissue (true pulmonary shunt), but also regions that are poorly ventilated, or perfused in excess of their ventilation (low $\dot{V}_A/\dot{Q}$ regions). Similarly, the dead space compartment includes not only true dead space (airways plus nonperfused alveoli) but also regions that are ventilated well in excess of their perfusion (high $\dot{V}_A/\dot{Q}$ regions).

The shunt can be better separated from regions with low $\dot{V}_A/\dot{Q}$ ratios if it is calculated during oxygen breathing, which will eliminate any contribution to the shunt value from regions with low $\dot{V}_A/\dot{Q}$ ratios. However, this analysis often yields contradictory results (96,112), and interference with the measured variable has also been noticed, such as absorption collapse (atelectasis) (20,132) and increased shunt due to inhibition of hypoxic pulmonary vasoconstriction (21).

Determination of Shunt by Infusion of a Tracer Gas with Low Solubility

Since the O_2/CO_2 method does not give a quantitative figure on true shunt but also includes regions that are perfused in excess of their ventilation, attempts have been made to find techniques that give a better description of the shunt. This can be achieved by infusing a gas of very low solubility in blood so that, when it passes through the lung capillaries it is retained only in those regions that are perfused but not at all ventilated. In gas-filled lung units, even if ventilation is poor, the low solubility of the tracer gas causes its diffusion to the alveoli and its subsequent elimination via the airways. Xenon is a gas with relatively low solubility in blood (blood:gas partition coefficient λ = 0.19). By collecting an arterial and a mixed venous blood sample, the retention (R) can be calculated as Ca/Cv, where Ca and Cv are arterial and mixed venous tracer gas concentrations. The equation

$$R = \frac{Ca}{Cv} = \frac{\lambda}{\lambda + \dot{V}_A/\dot{Q}} \quad [7]$$

gives the relation between the retention of the tracer gas, the blood gas partition coefficient and the $\dot{V}_A/\dot{Q}$ for an "inert" gas (i.e., chemically inactive in blood) (30). It can be seen that λ = 0.19 (xenon) and a normal $\dot{V}_A/\dot{Q}$ of 1.0 gives an R of 16%. For O_2 the situation is more complex since the gas is not "inert" but combines with hemoglobin according to the oxygen dissociation curve. However, if a single value for λ (O_2) of 0.9 is used, to enable a simplified comparison with the xenon retention, and a $\dot{V}_A/\dot{Q}$ of 1, the corresponding R is approximately 50%. For a lung unit with a lower $\dot{V}_A/\dot{Q}$ more of the gas is retained. Thus, there is at least a threefold difference in the degree of retention in normal $\dot{V}_A/\dot{Q}$ units for these two gases. It is obvious that xenon is the better gas for discriminating true shunt. By infusing radioactive xenon (^{133}Xe) intravenously, the shunt can be detected by external detectors, positioned over the chest (84).

Although xenon is a better gas for assessing true shunt than O_2 it is still not ideal, some gas being retained also in normal $\dot{V}_A/\dot{Q}$ units. Sulfurhexafluoride, SF_6, has extremely low solubility in blood, λ = 0.006, and is therefore almost completely eliminated from the capillary blood in lung units with normal $\dot{V}_A/\dot{Q}$ ratios, and to a major extent in lung regions with $\dot{V}_A/\dot{Q}$ ratios as low as 0.005 to 0.01, as can be calculated by entering λ SF_6 in equation (6,94). Because of its extremely low solubility, intravenous infusion of SF6 can also be used for assessing individual lung blood flow, if expired gas can be collected via a double-lumen endobronchial catheter. This is because differences in the $\dot{V}_A/\dot{Q}$ ratio and the venous/arterial tracer gas concentration ratio of each lung will have minimal impact on the elimination of SF_6 gas. By this means it compares favorably with CO_2 and xenon elimination, which have been used more frequently for such purposes (118,143). For a comparative analysis see Jolin-Carlsson et al. (64).

Despite their theoretical advantages, neither xenon nor SF_6 has been extensively used for assessing true shunt (or individual lung blood flow), mainly because of the difficulties in handling gases of low solubility and the need of sophisticated equipment for analysis (e.g., mass spectrometer or gas chromatograph).

Arterial-Alveolar Nitrogen Difference

Another approach to calculate the perfusion of low $\dot{V}_A/\dot{Q}$ regions is to measure the arterial-alveolar nitrogen difference (a-AN_2D). The method is based on the fact that in lung units where the exchange rates of O_2 and CO_2 are not equal, the N_2 fraction in blood is altered from that of the inspired gas. In alveoli with low $\dot{V}_A/\dot{Q}$ the N_2 tension rises almost in parallel with the decrease in PO_2 (the simultaneous change in PCO_2 can be no greater than the small difference in venous and arterial blood). This generates an a-AN_2D (99). Moreover, the a-AN_2D is uninfluenced by shunt blood, since that blood is not participating in any gas exchange. The technique was tested in critically ill patients and compared to multiple inert gas elimination technique (see below) by Radermacher et al. (97). They found a fair correlation between the amount of low $\dot{V}_A/\dot{Q}$ by multiple inert gas elimination technique and a-ADN_2 as well as between shunting by inert gas elimination and the difference between venous admixture (oxygen technique) and a-ADN_2. A limitation to the technique is the difficulty to measure N_2 in blood, which is based on manual gas absorption technique.

Multiple Inert Gas Elimination Technique

By using more than one or two gases with different solubilities in blood a more detailed analysis of $\dot{V}_A/\dot{Q}$ can be made. Thus, Wagner and coworkers (131,141) have developed a multiple inert gas elimination technique (MIGET) that is based on the retention and elimination of several (in practice six) "inert" gases (gases obeying Henry's law, i.e., showing a linear relationship between partial pressure and concentration in blood, e.g., SF_6 and xenon) with different solubilities in blood. The retention and excretion values for the six gases can be used in order to allocate ventilation and blood flow to a number of hypothetical compartments (e.g., 50) ranging from shunt ($\dot{V}_A/\dot{Q}$ = zero) over compartments with low, normal, and high $\dot{V}_A/\dot{Q}$ ratios to dead space ($\dot{V}_A/\dot{Q}$ = infinity). A schematic drawing of the basic principles is shown in Fig. 5. The equation is basically the same as is used above for the shunt analysis (eq. 7) for a lung containing N compartments:

$$\frac{Pa}{P_{\bar{v}}} = \frac{\left[\sum_{j=1}^{j=N} \frac{\lambda \cdot \dot{Q}_j}{\lambda + (\dot{V}A/\dot{Q})_j}\right]}{\sum_{j=1}^{j=N} \dot{Q}_j} \quad [8]$$

Note that the contribution to the overall retention value from the different compartments has to be weighted by their individual blood flows. As can be understood the equation is underdetermined, i.e., there are more unknowns than knowns.

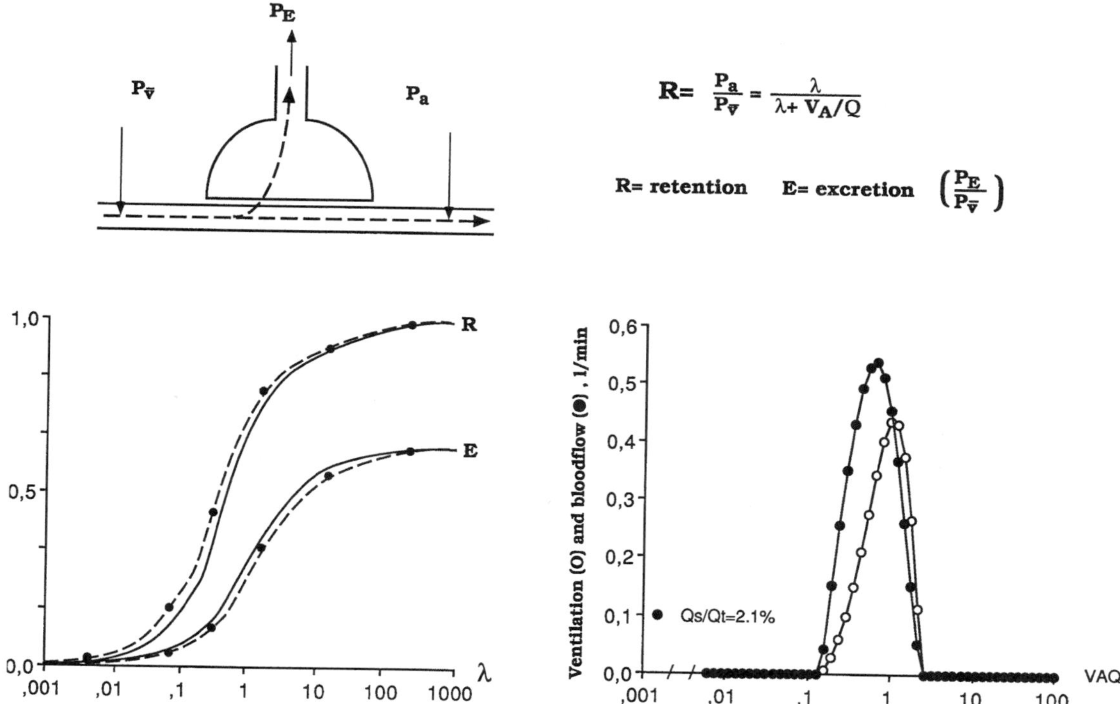

Figure 5. The basic principle of the multiple inert gas elimination technique. *Upper left:* Schematic drawing of the elimination of an inert gas during its passage through the pulmonary capillary (Pa, P_v, PE = inert gas tensions in arterial and mixed venous blood, and in expired gas). *Upper right:* The relation between retention (R), inert gas tensions, and the ventilation-perfusion relationship ($\dot{V}_A/\dot{Q}$), and the definition of excretion (E). *Lower panels:* Example of retention and excretion data *(left)* and the derived distribution of $\dot{V}_A/\dot{Q}$. *Solid curves* in the *left panel* represent measured retention-solubility and excretion-solubility curves; associated *broken curves* represent hypothetical homogeneous lungs with the same dead space as actually measured. $\dot{V}_A/\dot{Q}$ distribution *(right)*; ventilation *(open circles)*, perfusion *(filled circles)*.

A number of combinations of ventilation and perfusion values can fit the measured retention and excretion values. However, the single solution that is obtained by the mathematical analysis according to Wagner and associates (28,131,141) has been shown to give a reliable description of the $\dot{V}_A/\dot{Q}$ distribution, both in theoretical experiments (90,127) and in animal and human studies when the results have been compared with those from other techniques (52,55). Using linear programming and Monte Carlo simulation, Evans and Wagner (28) presented a technique to define the boundaries of a $\dot{V}_A/\dot{Q}$ distribution for a given set of retention and excretion data. Depending on the basic $\dot{V}_A/\dot{Q}$ pattern, the boundaries will be more or less narrow. Thus, a unimodal narrow $\dot{V}_A/\dot{Q}$ distribution has very tight boundaries, whereas a broad distribution of $\dot{V}_A/\dot{Q}$ ratios will be less precisely defined.

The MIGET requires meticulous care in preparing the gas solutions and collecting blood and gas samples, to equilibrate the blood against a gas phase and to run the samples through the gas analyzer. The latter is normally a gas chromatograph equipped with a flame ionization detector and a electron capture detector by means of a split connected to the column, or alternatively, two gas chromatographs are used. For further information on the practical aspects of the MIGET, see a comprehensive review by Wagner and Lopez (130).

The result of a run with the MIGET is shown in Fig. 5. The lower left panel shows the raw retention and excretion data (open circles). These data are entered into equation (8) (one for the retention values and another, similar one, for the excretion values). The resulting $\dot{V}_A/\dot{Q}$ distribution is shown in the lower right panel. After having derived the $\dot{V}_A/\dot{Q}$ distribution, it can be used for calculating a continuous retention-solubility curve. This curve has been entered into the left panel as the broken curve and can be compared with the curve that has been fitted to the raw data (continuous line). The difference between the two curves gives an indication of the accuracy of the data. This can be expressed as the remaining sum of squares (RSS), which is the sum of the squared differences between the values for each of the six gases on the two retention curves.

The resulting $\dot{V}_A/\dot{Q}$ distribution depends on both gravitational and nongravitational distributions of ventilation and blood flow but does not allow any spatial analysis. The $\dot{V}_A/\dot{Q}$ distribution may rather be considered as a finger print of the lungsí ability to transfer gas between alveoli and capillary blood. The $\dot{V}_A/\dot{Q}$ distribution can be described in terms of the mean $\dot{V}_A/\dot{Q}$ of ventilation and of perfusion (V_{mean}, Q_{mean}) and the scatter of the $\dot{V}_A/\dot{Q}$ ratios around V_{mean} and Q_{mean}, respectively, expressed as the logarithmic standard deviation of the ventilation and perfusion distributions (log SDV, log SDQ). Further variables that may be recovered from the measured retention and excretion of the inert gases are shunt (perfusion of regions with $\dot{V}_A/\dot{Q}$ <0.005), low $\dot{V}_A/\dot{Q}$ (perfusion of regions with 0.005 < $\dot{V}_A/\dot{Q}$ < 0.1), normal $\dot{V}_A/\dot{Q}$ (perfusion of regions with 0.1 < $\dot{V}_A/\dot{Q}$ < 10), high $\dot{V}_A/\dot{Q}$ (ventilation of regions with 10 < $\dot{V}_A/\dot{Q}$ < 100), and dead space ($\dot{V}_A/\dot{Q}$ > 100). Examples of $\dot{V}_A/\dot{Q}$ distributions in health and lung disease are shown in Fig. 6. Table 1 shows data in health and lung disease as well as during anesthesia, which will be discussed later. In samples of young healthy subjects, 95% will have a log SDQ below 0.6 and V_{mean} and Q_{mean} are approximately 1 (129). The scatter increases with age and is approximately 1.0 in 70- to 75-year-old subjects (39).

Chronic obstructive pulmonary disease (COPD) increases log SDV and log SDQ. In moderate COPD log SDQ exceeds 1.0 and in severe disease it approaches 2.0 (133). Interestingly, shunting is negligible or absent, and the often large venous admixture that has been measured by blood gas analysis is

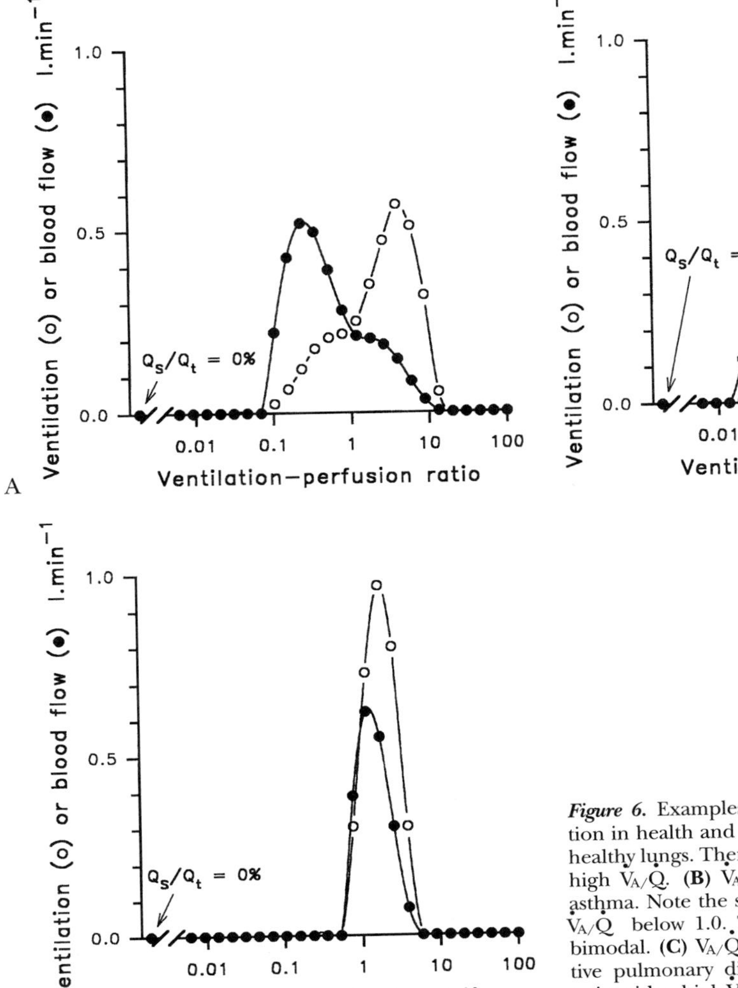

Figure 6. Examples of ventilation-perfusion distribution in health and disease. **(A)** $\dot{V}_A/\dot{Q}$ in a subject with healthy lungs. There are no units with very low or very high $\dot{V}_A/\dot{Q}$. **(B)** $\dot{V}_A/\dot{Q}$ in a patient with bronchial asthma. Note the separate population of units with a $\dot{V}_A/\dot{Q}$ below 1.0. This type of distribution is called bimodal. **(C)** $\dot{V}_A/\dot{Q}$ in a patient with chronic obstructive pulmonary disease. Note the large amount of units with a high $\dot{V}_A/\dot{Q}$. There is no shunt.

more or less due to low $\dot{V}_A/\dot{Q}$ (40,133). In patients with asthma a bimodal $\dot{V}_A/\dot{Q}$ distribution is often seen with an additional low $\dot{V}_A/\dot{Q}$ mode (128,129). This additional mode may be explained by collateral ventilation, i.e., lung units with a completely occluded airway maintain a certain gas exchange by ventilation through neighboring, better-ventilated alveoli. $\dot{V}_A/\dot{Q}$ distributions in other diseased states are not dealt with here.

Because of the assumptions and constraints that are needed for transforming the retention/excretion data to a multicompartmental $\dot{V}_A/\dot{Q}$ distribution, other approaches have been made in order to quantify the $\dot{V}_A/\dot{Q}$ mismatch. Thus, methods have been described that are based on the calculation of the area between the measured and homogeneous retention and excretion curves (59,85). However, these alternative approaches have been used to a very limited extent.

Scintigraphic Techniques

The ventilation and perfusion distributions can also be assessed by isotope techniques that give a spatial resolution. Ventilation may be assessed by the breathing of a radioactive gas or the inhalation of radiolabeled aerosols or particles. The most commonly used gas is ^{133}xenon (or ^{127}xenon, which has a higher energy level, ensuring better image quality) (18). If the gas is being rebreathed so that a steady-state condition is obtained, the activity of the gas will reflect regional lung volume. The distribution of ventilation can be assessed during the wash in or wash out of the gas, by measuring the half-time of the activity. The gas ^{81m}krypton has a very short half-life, 13 sec, and the ventilation distribution can therefore be assessed during constant ventilation of that gas (32). Breathing of krypton allows dynamic measurements, i.e., changes in the ventilation pattern can be followed. The disadvantage of ^{81m}krypton is that it must be obtained from a ^{85m}rubidium generator that can be used only over a day.

The inhalation of an aerosol or small particles results in a deposition in the airways and alveoli, that is in rough proportion to the ventilation distribution. The rather recent development of extremely small carbon particles, labeled with ^{99m}technetium, less than 1 μm in size ("technegas"), may be the most optimal ventilation agent, and comparisons have been made between the technegas and ^{133}xenon (116).

The perfusion distribution is studied by the embolization in the pulmonary vascular bed of radiolabeled particles, either macroaggregated albumin (MAA) or microspheres of polystyrene or other material (46). The particle size is approximately 15 to 40 μm and an ordinary dose contains 200,000 to 500,000 particles. This should be compared with the almost 300 million arterioles in which the particles are lodged. No measurable effect on vascular pressures should therefore be expected.

By comparing the ventilation and perfusion images the $\dot{V}_A/\dot{Q}$ can be assessed. In a gamma camera study (52) the $\dot{V}_A/\dot{Q}$ was determined for each picture element (Pixel) in a matrix (64 × 64) by dividing ventilation, assessed by aerosol technique, with perfusion, obtained by embolization with MAA. Ventilation

Table 1. VENTILATION-PERFUSION RATIOS IN AWAKE AND ANESTHETIZED ADULTS

General	n	Age (years)	Shunt (% CO)	Low $\dot{V}_A/\dot{Q}$ (% CO)	High $\dot{V}_A/\dot{Q}$ (% V_E)	Dead space (% V_E)	Log SDQ (L)	Log SDV (L)
1.	8	-/25–41	–	–	–	–	0.3 5± 0.12	0.34 ± 0.10
2. awake	10	67/55–81	1	3 ± 2	4 ± 3	–	0.62 ± 0.11	1.03 ± 0.17
EDA			1	1 ± 1	4 ± 2	–	0.55 ± 0.09	1.01 ± 0.19
3. awake	18	-/21–34	0.8 ± 0.7	–	–	–	0.43 ± 0.15	–
an.			7.8 ± 7.3	–	–	–	0.80 ± 0.32	
4. awake	45	46 ± 13	0.5 ± 1.0	1.7 ± 3.3	0.1 ± 0.3	35 ± 14	0.67 ± 0.28	0.52 ± 0.15
an.			4.8 ± 4.1	5.0 ± 4.9	1.8 ± 3.8	35 ± 10	1.04 ± 0.36	0.65 ± 0.31
5. awake	8	43 ± 3/33–55	0.5 ± 0.4	0.6 ± 0.6	0.1 ± 0.1	38 ± 1	0.50 ± 0.05	0.56 ± 0.10
an., SpB			0.9 ± 0.6	3.0 ± 2.3	1.4 ± 1.3	46 ± 3	0.58 ± 0.14	0.86 ± 0.23
an., MV			3.1 ± 0.9	3.7 ± 1.4	0.1 ± 0.1	28 ± 2	0.95 ± 0.17	0.65 ± 0.07
6. an., ZEEP	10	51 ± /37–64	8.6	1.2	15	38	1.01	0.76
an., PEEP			4.1	–	23	44	0.87	1.31
7. an., ZEEP	8	42/23–62	7.5 ± 2.3	6.6 ± 4.3	9.3 ± 2.6	26 ± 4	–	–
an., PEEP			8.3 ± 2.9	3.4 ± 2.9	13.3 ± 3.4	30 ± 4	–	–
8. awake	10	-/52–75	2.0 ± 1.8	4.5 ± 4.5	–	–	0.96 ± 0.20–	
an.			15.1 ± 9.5	20.7 ± 13.1	–	–	1.73 ± 0.36	–
9. awake	10	69 ± 8/57–77	0.6 ± 0.4	5.4 ± 5.9	2.2 ± 5.6	40 ± 8	0.99 ± 0.30	0.78 ± 0.29
an.			1.0 ± 1.1	8.5 ± 7.4	6.1 ± 7.8	35 ± 6	1.29 ± 0.31	1.00 ± 0.29
10. awake	9	69/65–75	4 ± 4	3 ± 5	2 ± 1	43 ± 11	0.86 ± 0.33	0.57 ± 0.18
an.			10 ± 9	9 ± 8	6 ± 1	26 ± 10	1.35 ± 0.44	0.58 ± 0.10
postop.			11 ± 6	1 ± 2	3 ± 1	41 ± 10	0.68 ± 0.26	0.48 ± 0.10
11 postop.	8	-/32–71	6.1	–	–	–	1.29	0.58

1. Healthy adults, supine, at rest (ref. 132).
2. Adults, supine, before and during epidural blockade (EDA), upper level 3–6 thoracic segment (74).
3. Adults, supine, awake and anesthetized (halothane, O_2/N_2 or O_2/N_2O), mechanically ventilated (95).
4. Adults with healthy lungs, among them 22 smokers, supine, awake and anesthetized (enflurane or halothane, O_2/N_2), mechanically ventilated (39).
5. Adults, supine, awake and anesthetized (ketamine), spontaneously breathing (SpB) and mechanically ventilated (MV) (123).
6. Adults, supine, anesthetized (enflurane, O_2/N_2), mechanically ventilated with zero end-expiratory pressure (ZEEP) and PEEP (13 cm H_2O) (12).
7. Adults, supine, anesthetized (halothane, O_2/N_2), mechanically ventilated with ZEEP and PEEP (10 cm H_2O) (122).
8. Adults, age > 50 years, smoking > 50 pack-years, supine, awake and anesthetized (halothane, O_2/N_2 or O_2/N_2O), mechanically ventilated (26).
9. Adults with chronic obstructive lung disease (COLD), supine, awake and anesthetized (enflurane, O_2/N_2), mechanically ventilated (40).
10. Adults, supine, coronary artery revascularization surgery, awake, anesthetized with mechanical ventilation and 20 hours postoperatively, extubated, spontaneously breathing (41).
11. Adults, supine, first day after aortic valve replacement, mechanically ventilated (35).

Data are mean ± SD except for age, where range is also given.
Shunt (% CO): $\dot{V}_A/\dot{Q} < 0.005$.
Low $\dot{V}_A/\dot{Q}$ (% CO): $0.005 < \dot{V}_A/\dot{Q} < 0.1$.
High $\dot{V}_A/\dot{Q}$ (% V_E): $10 < \dot{V}_A/\dot{Q} < 100$.
Dead space (% V_E): $100 < \dot{V}_A/\dot{Q}$.
Log SDQ: standard deviation of logarithmic perfusion distribution.
Log SDV: standard deviation of logarithmic ventilation distribution.
CO, cardiac output.
V_E, minute ventilation.
an., anesthetized.

and blood flow were plotted against $\dot{V}_A/\dot{Q}$ ratios and compared with simultaneously obtained data by MIGET. Rather good correspondence between the techniques was obtained. Other isotope studies with reference to anesthesia are referred to below (62,70).

PET

With positron emission tomography (PET) the local blood flow, ventilation, ventilation-perfusion ratios, the permeability to proteins, the density of receptors, and many other biologically relevant aspects may be estimated in vivo. Dynamic processes may be investigated with PET. The technique is based on principles developed for conventional x-ray computed tomography and measures the distribution and biologic behavior of a variety of compounds labeled with positron-emitting isotopes such as ^{15}O, ^{11}C, ^{18}F, ^{13}N (61). These positrons (positively charged antiparticles of electrons) have typically half-lifes of a few seconds up to few minutes. An interaction with a tissue electron occurs usually within a distance of 1 to 5 mm, resulting in the emission of gamma rays traveling at an 180° angle to each other. These gamma rays are registered simultaneously by two detectors operating in coincidence (61). A number of investigations with PET have been performed in awake humans (15,107).

Effect of $\dot{V}_A/\dot{Q}$ Distribution on Arterial Oxygenation and CO_2 Removal

Blood passing the lung without being oxygenated—shunting—will lower the oxygen tension when it mixes with blood from other lung regions. A mismatch of ventilation and perfusion will also cause impairment of the oxygenation of blood. In Fig. 7, left panel, the degree of gas transfer impairment is plotted against the degree of $\dot{V}_A/\dot{Q}$ mismatch, expressed as log SDQ (138). As can be seen, gas transfer is reduced to 80% of normal at a log SDQ of 1, corresponding to what can be seen in moderate obstructive lung disease (133) and during anesthesia (39) (see below). With severe $\dot{V}_A/\dot{Q}$ mismatch (log SDQ = 2), gas

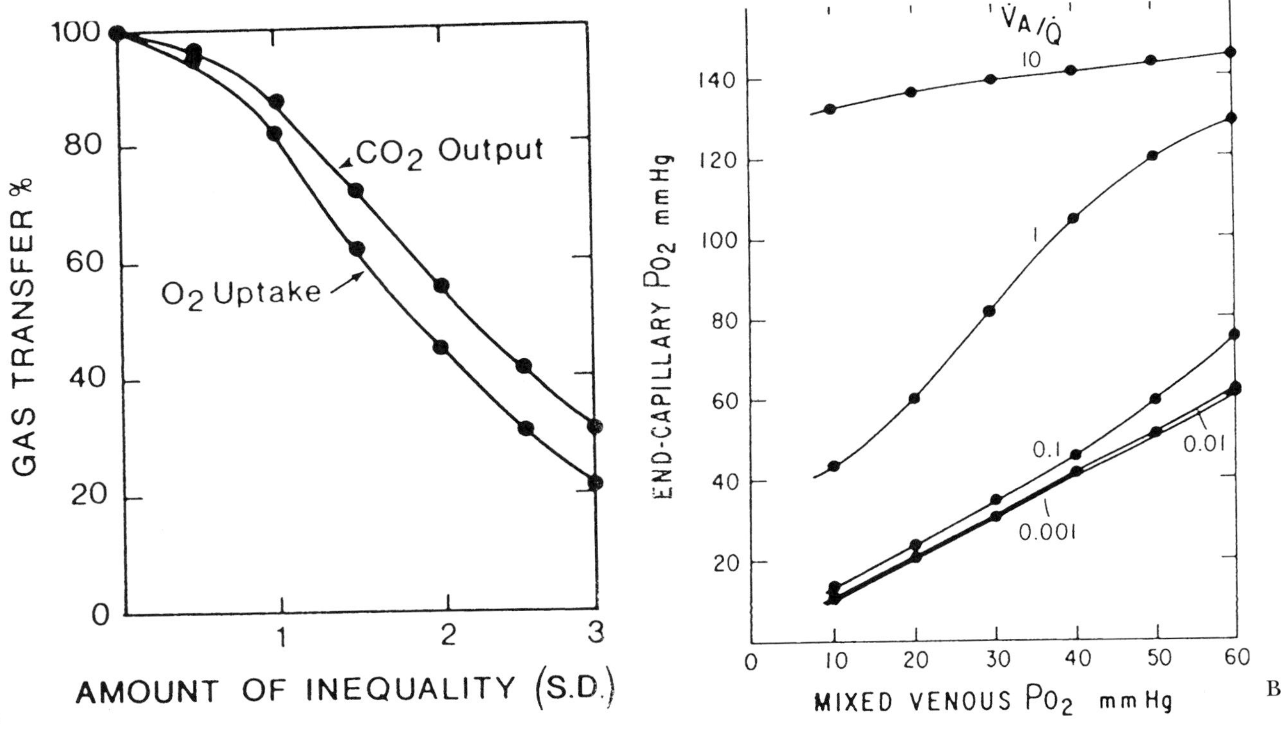

Figure 7. **(A)** The influence of ventilation-perfusion mismatch [expressed as amount of inequality of perfusion distribution (log SD)] and, **(B)**, of mixed venous PO_2 on gas transfer and end-capillary PO_2. Note that with increasing inequality of the perfusion distribution, both O_2 uptake and CO_2 output are impeded to almost the same extent *(left)*. Decreasing mixed venous PO_2 lowers the end-capillary PO_2 and thus arterial oxygenation. The effect of low mixed venous PO_2 is more marked at normal and low $\dot{V}_A/\dot{Q}$ ratios than at high *(right)*. (From ref. 138, with permission.)

transfer is only 40% of normal. Moreover, both shunt and $\dot{V}_A/\dot{Q}$ mismatch impede CO_2 removal almost to the same extent as for O_2 transfer (138). However, the latter impairment can be compensated for by an increase in ventilation. This may have contributed to the common misbelief that CO_2 elimination is not affected by a $\dot{V}_A/\dot{Q}$ disturbance.

The effect of the shunt on oxygenation can be compensated for by increasing the inspired oxygen fraction. However, with increasing shunt the supplementary oxygen causes less improvement, and with shunts above 25% almost no increase in the arterial oxygenation can be seen even with 100% oxygen (7). In the event of $\dot{V}_A/\dot{Q}$ mismatch, supplementary oxygen will always improve arterial oxygenation. This is because at high FIO_2 the alveolar oxygen tension will be much the same in lung units that are well ventilated and in units with poor ventilation. The small difference that exists is the result of differences in alveolar CO_2 tension.

Influence of Mixed Venous PO_2

It may also be obvious that if mixed venous oxygen tension is low the effect of both shunt and $\dot{V}_A/\dot{Q}$ mismatch on arterial oxygenation will be augmented. This is shown in the right panel of Fig. 7, which is taken from a review by West (138). As can be seen, the end-capillary PO_2 that for simplicity can be set equal to PaO_2, increases from 40 to 120 mm Hg for a normal lung unit with a $\dot{V}_A/\dot{Q}$ of 1 when mixed venous PO_2 increases from 10 to 60 mm Hg. The proportionate effect will be even greater for lung unit with a low $\dot{V}_A/\dot{Q}$ ratio and less marked for a unit with a high $\dot{V}_A/\dot{Q}$ ratio.

The $P_{\bar{V}}O_2$ is dependent on cardiac output, a low blood flow resulting in a larger extraction of oxygen in the systemic capillaries than at high cardiac output. This may explain why a patient with asthma but high cardiac output (due among other things to the use of sympathomimetic drugs) may have a normal PaO_2 despite certain $\dot{V}_A/\dot{Q}$ mismatch (129) and that a patient with myocardial infarction may suffer from hypoxemia despite an essentially normal $\dot{V}_A/\dot{Q}$ distribution (134).

VENTILATION AND PERFUSION IN THE ANESTHETIZED SUBJECT

General anesthesia regularly impairs the oxygenation of blood and may also interfere with the elimination of carbon dioxide from blood (for an overview, see 87).

The first studies on the regional distribution of ventilation during anesthesia were published in the early 1970s. Hulands and coworkers (62), using isotope technique in supine subjects, and Rehder and coworkers (101,102), using nitrogen washout technique in each lung in the lateral position and isotope techniques in the supine position (105), found less than expected ventilation of the dependent lung regions or the dependent lung. A difference compared to the awake state was seen both in anesthetized, spontaneously breathing subjects (102) and during muscle paralysis and mechanical ventilation (62,101,105). Hulands et al. (62) and Landmark et al. (70) also found a slight increase in the perfusion of dependent lung regions with a subsequent worsening of the ventilation-perfusion ($\dot{V}_A/\dot{Q}$).

During anesthesia pulmonary as well as systemic arterial pressure may be reduced. The fall in the former impedes perfusion of the uppermost, nondependent lung regions. Institution of mechanical ventilation increases alveolar pressure and this interferes with nondependent perfusion (56). Thus, during anesthesia and/or mechanical ventilation, dependent regions become well perfused but poorly or not at all ventilated, while nondependent regions become well ventilated but poorly or not at all perfused (Fig. 3, right panel). A $\dot{V}_A/\dot{Q}$ mismatch is established, and interferes with pulmonary gas exchange (49).

$\dot{V}_A/\dot{Q}$ During General Anesthesia: Overview

Soon after its introduction as a research tool, the multiple inert gas elimination technique was used in anesthetized subjects. Rehder and coworkers (103) studied young healthy volunteers during intravenous and inhalational anesthesia. They found that both ventilation and perfusion were distributed to wider ranges of $\dot{V}_A/\dot{Q}$ ratios after induction of anesthesia and muscle paralysis (increased log SDV and log SDQ). The shunt, on the other hand, was only little affected in this study with a mean value of approximately 1% of cardiac output. Prutow and coworkers (95) studied young subjects during anesthesia with halothane and muscle paralysis and found a much larger shunt than Rehder et al. The mean value was 8% with extremes up to 23%. Similarly to the Rehder group they found an increase in the scatter of the $\dot{V}_A/\dot{Q}$ ratios.

Middle-aged patients (mean 50 years) during halothane anesthesia and muscle paralysis prior to elective surgery were studied by Bindslev et al. (12); a significant increase in the mean shunt from approximately 1% to 9% was seen and there was also an increase in log SDQ from 0.47 awake to 1.01 during anesthesia, indicating a $\dot{V}_A/\dot{Q}$ mismatch. Finally, in elderly patients with a more marked impairment of lung function, halothane anesthesia with muscle paralysis caused considerable $\dot{V}_A/\dot{Q}$ mismatch inasmuch as log SDQ increased from 0.87 awake (i.e., already above the upper normal limit) to 1.73 during anesthesia (26). The shunt increased to a mean of 15% with a considerable variation between patients.

In conclusion, the most frequent findings during anesthesia and muscle paralysis in these studies on ventilation-perfusion relationships were an increased shunt and aggravated mismatch of ventilation and perfusion (Figs. 5 and 8, right panel). Both disturbances impede the oxygenation of blood and the elimination of CO_2. See also Table 1 for $\dot{V}_A/\dot{Q}$ data from different studies.

Causes of Ventilation-Perfusion Mismatch

Decreased Functional Residual Capacity (FRC)

Several studies have shown that the functional residual capacity (FRC) is reduced during anesthesia (for a review see 135). In the majority of these studies, gas dilution techniques (helium equilibration, nitrogen washout) have been used (e.g., 10,71). One drawback of gas distribution techniques is that the tracer gas used to assess FRC may not have been mixed with all gas in the lung because of occluded airways. This possible source of error was precluded in two studies by applying body plethysmography (43,142). This technique estimates all gas within the lung, whether located behind an occluded airway or not. Specially adapted body boxes were used to allow measurements in anesthetized, supine subjects. During anesthesia, FRC was reduced both during spontaneous breathing and after muscle paralysis without a difference between the two states (43,142). In the awake subject the change from the upright to the supine position reduces FRC by 0.7 to 0.8 L. The further

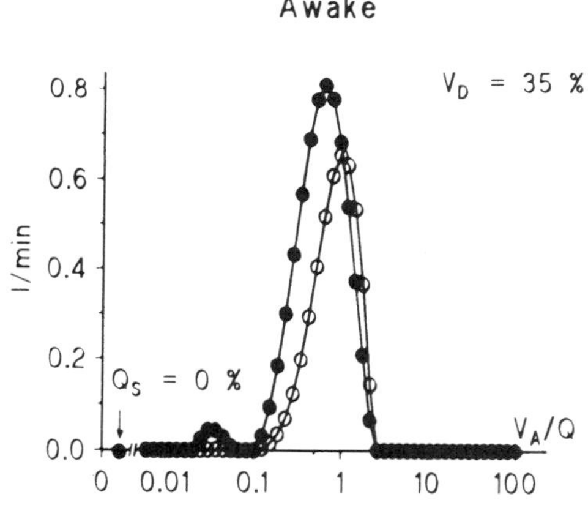

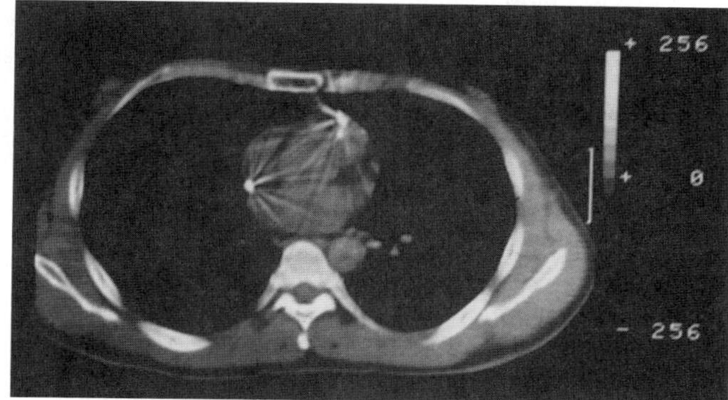

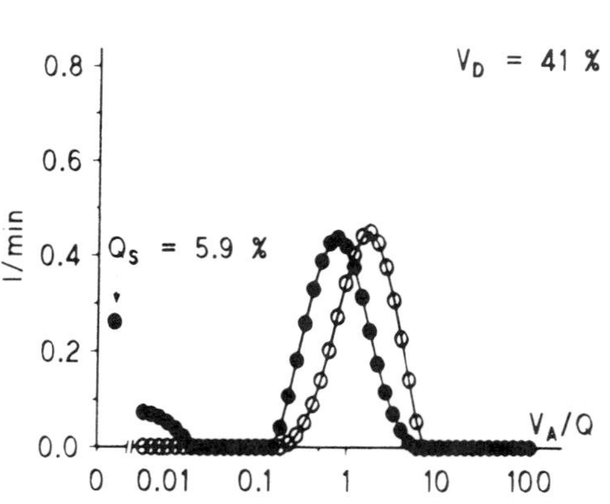

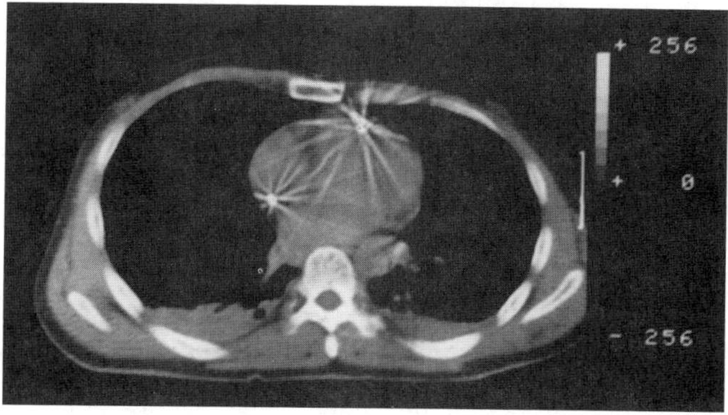

Figure 8. Example of computed x-ray tomography (CT) and of the $\dot{V}_A/\dot{Q}$ distribution. *Right:* transverse CT scans of the chest in the awake state (*upper panel*) and during anesthesia (*lower panel*). Note the appearance of densities in the dependent lung regions during anesthesia. The large white area in the right hemothorax is the diaphragm that has been moved cranially during anesthesia. *Left:* $\dot{V}_A/\dot{Q}$ distribution (*open circles* show ventilation, *filled circles* show perfusion) awake (*upper panel*) and during anesthesia (*lower panel*). Note the appearance of the shunt and an increased $\dot{V}_A/\dot{Q}$ mismatch during anesthesia. (Redrawn from ref. 39, with permission.)

decrease of FRC due to anesthesia (approximately 0.5 L or 20% of the awake value (135) results in a resting lung volume that is close to the awake residual volume.

What are the mechanisms causing a reduced FRC? Froese and Bryan (34), using cineradiography, demonstrated a cranial shift of the diaphragm during anesthesia and spontaneous breathing, without a further shift after muscle relaxation. Surprisingly, the recording of thoracoabdominal dimensions by means of external sensors such as magnetometers (126), strain gauges (65), and inductive plethysmography (44) did not show any significant change in the shape of the chest or abdomen. In a more recent study however, combining transverse exposures of the chest and abdomen (CT) with central blood volume measurement (dye dilution) and FRC recording (multiple breath nitrogen washout), a rather complex pattern of changes was noted during anesthesia with muscle paralysis and mechanical ventilation (51). Thus, the cranial shift of the diaphragm was confirmed, and in addition it was seen that the transverse area of the chest was reduced. At the same time blood was moved from the thorax and probably pooled in the abdomen, together with a small amount of blood from the extremities. The net effect on the external dimensions of the chest and abdomen was only 0.1 to 0.2 L, changes that could thus pass undetected by the recording with surface sensors.

Krayer and coworkers (69) used an advanced CT scanner that enabled several simultaneous CT exposures of the chest and abdomen. They demonstrated a reduced thoracic cross-sectional area in the anesthetized subject but had more variable results concerning shape and position of the diaphragm; some subjects showed a cranial shift of the diaphragm similarly to earlier studies, but in other subjects part of the diaphragm was unaffected or even moved caudally. Why the diaphragm may shift caudally in the anesthetized paralyzed subject at zero end-expiratory pressure remains to be shown. Nevertheless, it can be concluded that FRC is reduced in the anesthetized subject together with a possible decrease in the pulmonary blood volume, further reducing thorax volume.

Airway Closure

We now turn to the potential effect on the patency of airways and alveoli and consequently pulmonary gas exchange. In 1966 Milic-Emili and coworkers (82) suggested that airways in dependent zones of the lung will close during a deep expiration. In view of the reduced FRC, the question was raised whether airway closure develops during anesthesia. In 1972 Don et al. (22) found that gas was trapped during anesthesia, and that it could only be released by deep inflations. In the same year, Alexander et al. (2) suggested airway closure as a contributing factor to postoperative hypoxemia. Later on the occurrence of airway closure during anesthesia was confirmed by means of the single breath nitrogen washout technique as well as bolus techniques (3,23,36,47,48), although conflicting results have been presented, too (11,66). It may be concluded, hence, that there is evidence of airway closure during anesthesia but that the effect on gas exchange is less predictable. Additional factors appear to contribute to the impaired arterial oxygenation.

Atelectasis

Damgaard-Pedersen and Qvist (19) found densities in dependent lung regions in small children who had been anesthetized to enable CT studies of the spine and the abdomen, and Brismar and coworkers (14) demonstrated the prompt appearance of densities in dependent lung regions after induction of anesthesia in adults (Fig. 8, left panel). The densities appeared both during spontaneous breathing and after muscle paralysis and for inhalational or intravenous anesthesia (113). In a retrospective analysis of a larger material, 95 of 109 patients (87%) were found to develop atelectasis during anesthesia (76). The dense areas had an attenuation factor that corresponds to blood and connective tissue and indicates the absence of air. Injection of radiocontrast in the pleural space showed that the densities are located above the pleura, i.e., within the lung (115). Similar dense areas in dependent lung regions have not been seen in any of the subjects when they were awake. Interestingly, the densities in the anesthetized subject cannot be seen on a frontal or lateral conventional chest x-ray, due to difficulties in separating them from mediastinal structures or the diaphragm. This may offer an explanation as to why previous attempts to demonstrate atelectasis during anesthesia have failed. It has been over 30 years since Bendixen and coworkers (8) published their concept of a progressive alveolar collapse during general anesthesia with mechanical ventilation. It was based on the observation of a successive decrease in lung compliance and PaO_2, both of which return toward normal after deep inflations of the lungs. However, other research groups were unable to confirm the results. They rather found a prompt decrease in compliance and PaO_2 on induction of anesthesia without any further substantial changes during anesthesia and the surgical period (88,119). Moreover, atelectasis could not be demonstrated on conventional chest x-ray. Atelectasis as a mechanism of impaired gas exchange was therefore rejected at the time.

To further investigate the dense areas, different animal models have been studied. Anesthetized dogs do not show any dense areas, i.e., they are at variance with the findings in human (75). This is worth noting because dogs have been frequently used in studies on lung function changes during anesthesia. Small dense areas were found in the most dependent regions of anesthetized sheep in dorsal recumbency (supine position) (46), and large dense areas, covering more than half of the lung field, were seen in anesthetized, supine Shetland ponies (89). The morphologic analysis of excised lung tissue showed the dense regions to be atelectasis with no or only moderate interstitial edema and vascular congestion. Because the radiologic appearance is qualitatively similar to that in man, it is reasonable to conclude that the anesthetized human subject also develops atelectasis during anesthesia. Thus, *atelectasis* in this chapter refers to the dense areas seen on CT.

Good correlations between atelectasis and pulmonary shunt, assessed by the multiple inert gas elimination technique, have been demonstrated (39,54,122) (Fig. 9). Using single photon emission computed tomography (SPECT, see above) together with CT, shunt could be shown to be located within the atelectatic region (52). Thus, atelectasis is a major cause of gas exchange impairment during anesthesia.

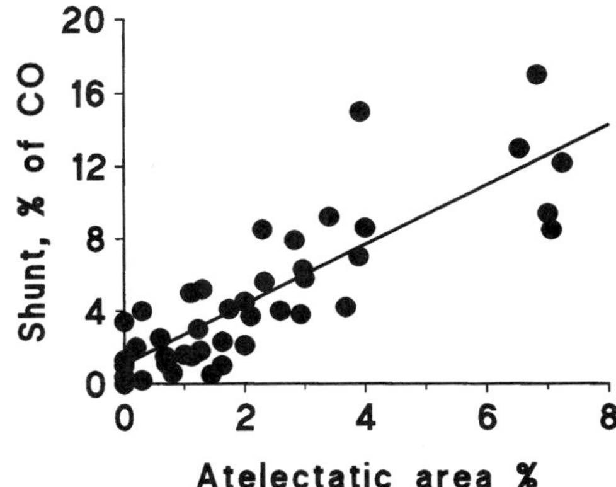

Figure 9. Shunt (in % of CO) as a function of atelectatic area (in % of intrathoracic area as recorded from CT scan) in anesthetized subjects with healthy lungs (no PEEP was applied). Regression equation: Shunt = 1.6 × atelectatic area - 1.7, $r = .81$, $p < .001$. (From ref. 39, with permission.)

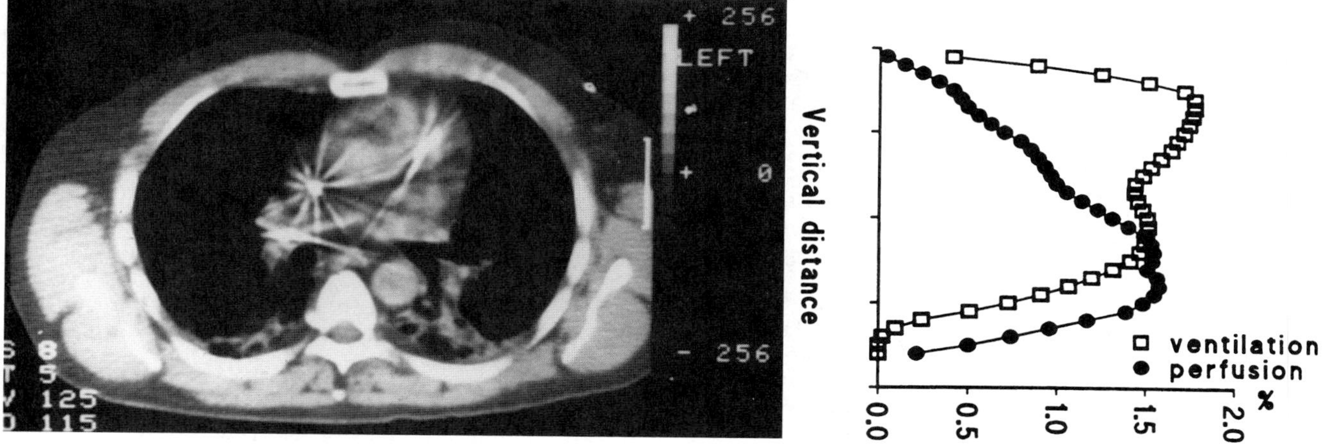

Figure 10. A transverse CT scan of the caudal lung region (*left*), and the corresponding vertical distribution of ventilation and perfusion (from the SPECT) (*right*) in an anesthetized patient (in percentage of minute ventilation and cardiac output, respectively). Note the large atelectasis in dependent lung regions, and the lack of ventilation but the abundance of blood flow corresponding to the atelectatic region. Note also the marked domination of ventilation over perfusion in nondependent lung regions. (From ref. 52, with permission). Compare also with Fig. 3, which shows the vertical distributions of ventilation and blood flow awake.

In Fig. 10, the vertical distributions of ventilation and perfusion are shown together with a CT scan of the chest in an anesthetized, paralyzed, and mechanically ventilated patient (52). The ventilation and blood flow distributions were obtained by studying the distributions of radiolabeled aerosols (ventilation) and macroaggregated albumin (perfusion), using SPECT. As can be seen ventilation was reduced in the lower half of the lung (in the vertical direction), and completely absent in the lower most, dorsal aspect of the lung. The absence of ventilation corresponding to the distribution of atelectasis as can be seen on the CT scan. The impeded ventilation above the atelectatic zone has not been fully explained yet, but may possibly be attributed to intermittent airway closure. This pattern of ventilation distribution differs from what is seen in normal subjects in the awake state (compare Fig. 3). Perfusion distribution, on the other hand, increases down the lung as has been shown in many earlier studies in awake subjects.

Mechanisms of Atelectasis Formation

Three possible mechanisms may cause atelectasis (98):

Compression
Absorption of gas behind blocked airways
Loss of surfactant.

Compression Atelectasis The diaphragm separates two spaces with different pressures as well as vertical pressure gradients. Thus, the end-expiratory intrathoracic pressure is normally lower than the abdominal pressure. The vertical pressure gradient in the pleural space of the awake subject is 0.2 to 0.4 cm H_2O per cm (see above), whereas this gradient approximates 1 cm H_2O per cm in the abdomen. If the diaphragm no longer acts as a rigid wall between these two spaces, the abdominal pressure will be transmitted into the thoracic cavity, increasing in particular the pleural pressure in dependent lung regions. This could result in compression atelectasis. Indirect evidence of this is the fact that no atelectasis developed during ketamine anesthesia (123) as this drug is known to maintain respiratory muscle function. More direct support of the role of the diaphragm is a recent study that showed that tensing the diaphragm by phrenic nerve stimulation reduced the amount of atelectasis at isovolumic conditions in anesthetized patients (53).

Gas Resorption The relationship between the reduction in FRC and atelectasis development is frequently put forward. However, chest strapping, resulting in a reduction of FRC by about 0.7 L, did not produce any atelectasis (assessed by CT) during a 20-minute period of spontaneously breathing air (121). On the other hand, already short periods of breathing 100% oxygen near the residual volume may cause atelectasis (17). Thus, an increased inspiratory fraction of oxygen may promote atelectasis formation if there is a concomitant reduction in FRC.

Surfactant The function of surfactant may be impeded by anesthesia (144). Furthermore, a lack of intermittent deep breaths (large gasps), as is usually the case during mechanical ventilation, may result in a decreased content of active forms of alveolar surfactant (91). A decreased function of surfactant results in reduced alveolar stability and may contribute to liquid bridging in the airway lumen and cause airway closure (92). However, little is known about details of these mechanisms, and an extensive discussion is beyond the scope of this chapter.

Compression may thus be an important cause of atelectasis formation during anesthesia, and resorption of gas behind occluded airways (airway closure, mucus plugging) may add to the initial lung collapse.

Attenuation of Hypoxic Pulmonary Vasoconstriction

In 1946 von Euler and Liljestrand (29) observed that hypoxia produced pulmonary vasoconstriction, a compensatory mechanism to counter hypoxemia. Attenuation of the hypoxic pulmonary vasoconstriction (HPV) is frequently considered as a mechanism of impaired gas exchange during anesthesia. Thilenius (120) showed more than 25 years ago that inhalational anesthetics attenuate HPV, and in succeeding studies Sykes and coworkers (117) showed that most inhalational anesthetics exert this effect. Intravenously given barbiturates, on the other hand, seem not to impede HPV (13). Results from human studies are inconsistent presumably because the HPV response is obscured by simultaneous changes in cardiac output, myocardial contractility, vascular tone, distribution of blood volume, blood pH, and carbon dioxide tensions and lung mechanics (80). It should also be stressed that the attenuation of HPV requires an underlying disturbance in ventilation/perfusion matching in order to produce an impaired arterial oxygenation. Unless such a disturbance exists, the release or attenuation of the HPV does not result in any impairment of gas exchange.

Since atelectasis develops during anesthesia, attenuation of HPV can be expected to increase blood flow through the atelectatic zone and thus increase the shunt. However, the commonly used inhalational anesthetics abolish only part of the HPV response at clinical concentrations of the agent. Accordingly, it can be concluded that the attenuation of HPV by the anesthetic will increase the shunt through the atelectatic zone slightly, but will not cause disturbances in an otherwise normal functioning lung.

VA/Q During Anesthesia: Specific Situations

General Anesthesia with Spontaneous Breathing or Mechanical Ventilation

Most studies on lung function have been performed in anesthetized, mechanically ventilated subjects or animals. There are relatively few data obtained during spontaneous breathing. Functional residual capacity (FRC) is reduced to the same extent during anesthesia, whether a muscle relaxant is used or not (42,142), and atelectasis occurs to almost the same extent in the anesthetized spontaneously breathing subject as during muscle paralysis (113). Furthermore, the cranial shift of the diaphragm, as reported by Froese and Bryan (34), was of the same magnitude both during general anesthesia with spontaneous breathing and with muscle paralysis, even though a difference in the movement of the diaphragm from the resting position was noted. Thus, during spontaneous breathing the lower, dependent portion of the diaphragm moved the most, whereas with muscle paralysis the upper, nondependent part showed the largest displacement. All these findings have raised the question whether regional ventilation is different between spontaneous breathing and mechanical ventilation, and whether mechanical ventilation worsens $\dot{V}_A/\dot{Q}$ as a consequence of poor ventilation of well-perfused, dependent lung regions. However, there is not much support of a worsening of gas exchange by muscle paralysis in the literature and there is also no support from the few studies on the $\dot{V}_A/\dot{Q}$ distribution that have been made. Dueck and coworkers (24) found the same increase in $\dot{V}_A/\dot{Q}$ mismatch in anesthetized sheep during anesthesia whether they were spontaneously breathing or mechanically ventilated. Log SDQ increased from 0.66 to 0.83 and 0.89 from awake to inhalational anesthesia with spontaneous breathing and mechanical ventilation, respectively. The shunt also increased with no significant difference between the two anesthesia conditions (from 1% awake to 11% and 14% during anesthesia with spontaneous breathing and mechanical ventilation). In a study on anesthetized human subjects shunt and log SDQ increased from 1% and 0.47 awake to 6% and 1.03 during anesthesia with spontaneous breathing and 8% and 1.01 during mechanical ventilation (12). Thus, most of the gas exchange effects of anesthesia can be seen already during spontaneous breathing with little or no further derangement added by muscle paralysis and mechanical ventilation.

At least one anesthetic, however, causes almost no gas exchange impairment during general anesthesia with spontaneous breathing: ketamine (123). No shunt or increase in log SDQ is found and no atelectasis could be seen with computed x-ray tomography of the lungs. As soon as the patients were paralyzed and mechanically ventilated, both atelectasis and shunt appeared, and log SDQ increased. The maintained matching of ventilation and blood flow could be due to the fact that muscle tone is maintained during anesthesia with ketamine.

Effect of Positive End-Expiratory Pressure (PEEP) or Deep Inflations of the Lungs

Positive end-expiratory pressure (PEEP) was introduced as a tool to recruit lung tissue and to improve oxygenation in severe acute respiratory failure or adult respiratory distress syndrome (ARDS) (5,31). It has been tempting to test PEEP as well in the anesthetized subject. PEEP has been shown to reduce or eliminate atelectasis (14), but on average it has no effect on pulmonary shunt (122). The lack of a uniform effect of PEEP is probably due to the fact that PEEP reduces cardiac output and forces blood flow down the lung. A remaining atelectasis may therefore receive a larger portion of lung blood flow than without PEEP. This is in line with the conclusion by Hewlett et al. (58), who proposed several years ago that the indiscriminate application of PEEP has no place in routine anesthesia.

During anesthesia and mechanical ventilation, regions with high $\dot{V}_A/\dot{Q}$ ratios may be seen that increase further during ventilation with increasing levels of PEEP (12,25). The additional high $\dot{V}_A/\dot{Q}$ mode may be explained by perfusion of corner vessels in the interalveolar septa of the lung in upper lung regions where alveolar pressure may exceed pulmonary vascular pressure (zone 1) (55) (Table 1).

To reduce the amount of atelectasis and shunt in lung healthy patients during general anesthesia, a manual hyperinflation of the lungs is often applied. However, the amount of atelectasis remains unaffected by an inflation up to an airway pressure of 10 or 20 cm H_2O (110). The latter is comparable to what is reached with a doubled tidal volume or sigh, a maneuver often proposed to be used in anesthetized subjects. At airway pressures of 30 cm H_2O, the atelectasis is reduced to approximately half the initial size and with a full inflation of the lung (airway pressure of 40 cm H_2O) the atelectasis is almost entirely eliminated (110).

Effect of an Increased Oxygen Fraction

In the studies cited so far, an inspired oxygen fraction (F_IO_2) of around 0.4 was used. Anjou-Lindskog et al. (4) induced anesthesia on air (F_IO_2 = 0.21) in middle-aged to elderly patients during intravenous anesthesia before elective lung surgery and found only small shunts of 1% to 2%, although log SDQ increased from 0.77 to 1.13. When F_IO_2 was increased to 0.5, an increase in shunt of 3% to 4% was noticed. In another study on elderly patients during halothane anesthesia (73) an increase in F_IO_2 from 0.53 to 0.85 caused an increase in shunt from 7% to 10% of cardiac output. Thus, a certain dependence on F_IO_2 appears to exist, possibly explained by the attenuation of the hypoxic pulmonary vasoconstrictor response with increasing F_IO_2 (21), or a further development of atelectasis and shunt in lung units with low $\dot{V}_A/\dot{Q}$ ratios (20).

Effects of Body Position

Because FRC is dramatically reduced by the combined effect of the supine position and anesthesia, it might be advantageous to choose a more upright position in the anesthetized subject to preserve FRC. This was tested by Heneghan et al. (57) in the healthy lungs of patients who underwent general anesthesia. However, no clear improvement in oxygenation was noticed when the patient was semirecumbent compared to a supine position. However, it can be anticipated that pulmonary blood flow is impeded by the semirecumbent position due to a possible decrease in cardiac output and enhanced inhomogeneity of blood flow distribution. The fractional perfusion of the most dependent lung regions that may still be poorly or not at all ventilated may have been increased in the semirecumbent position. In the lateral position differences in lung mechanics, resting lung volumes, and atelectasis formation between the dependent and the nondependent lung have been demonstrated (68), resulting in a further disturbance of the ventilation-perfusion match with a severe impairment of arterial oxygenation in some patients. However, there are large and unpredictable interindividual variations (67). Using isotope techniques, an increase of the $\dot{V}_A/\dot{Q}$ mismatch was also demonstrated in anesthetized, paralyzed patients in the lateral position (70).

More recent findings suggest that the vertical inhomogeneity of the perfusion distribution is less obvious in the prone position (38). This may indicate that there are regional differences in vascular configuration, promoting perfusion of dorsal lung regions, whether these are in a dependent or not dependent position. It is also worthy of note that the ventilation distribution was more uniform in anesthetized subjects who were in the prone position, in particular when the belly was not supported, i.e., hanging down through a hole in the table (104).

Effect of Age

It is well known that the arterial oxygenation is further impeded with increasing age of the patients (89). Interestingly, atelectasis formation does not increase with age in adults, and the sparse number of babies that have been studied in the CT scanner during anesthesia appear to have a greater percent of atelectasis of the transthoracic area than do older patients (39). Similarly, the shunt is independent of age in the tested range of 23 to 69 years (39). On the other hand, there appears to be an increasing $\dot{V}_A/\dot{Q}$ mismatch with age with an enhanced perfusion of low $\dot{V}_A/\dot{Q}$ regions both in awake subjects and when subsequently anesthetized (40). Figure 11 shows the relationship between the shunt, perfusion of low $\dot{V}_A/\dot{Q}$ regions, and the age of the patient. In the awake state the shunt is very small and independent of age. Perfusion of low $\dot{V}_A/\dot{Q}$ is also small, although it increases with age. During anesthesia, the shunt is much larger, but still essentially independent of age. Perfusion of low $\dot{V}_A/\dot{Q}$ regions not only is increased by anesthesia but increases also with age (39). Consequently, the major cause of gas exchange impairment during anesthesia at ages below 50 years is the shunt, whereas at higher ages mismatch (increased log SDQ) becomes increasingly important. Since the correlation between log SDQ and age during anesthesia is almost parallel with that during the awake state, it can be said that anesthesia worsens the match of ventilation and blood flow by as much as 20 years of aging. Optimally, log SDQ returns to the preanesthesia level after surgery. Why the $\dot{V}_A/\dot{Q}$ match deteriorates during anesthesia still remains to be established. A likely explanation is airway closure, which is known to increase with increasing age, at least in the awake subject (72).

Effect of Obesity

Obesity worsens the oxygenation of blood (125). A major explanation appears to be a markedly reduced FRC, promoting

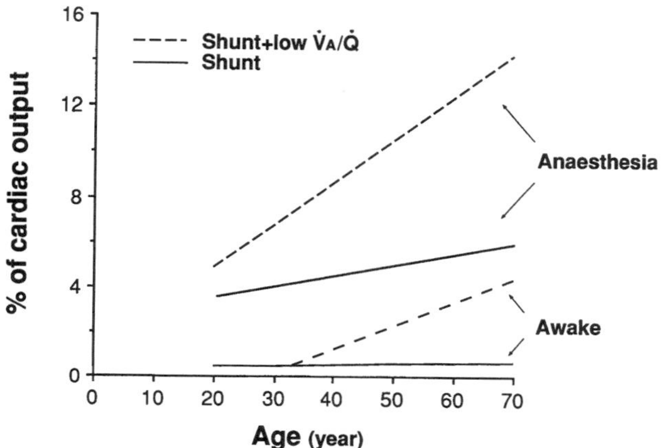

Figure 11. Schematic drawing of the shunt and the sum of shunt plus perfusion of regions with low $\dot{V}_A/\dot{Q}$ ratios by age, awake, and during anesthesia. Note the appearance or increase of the shunt during anesthesia (independent of age) and the increasing perfusion of low $\dot{V}_A/\dot{Q}$ regions with age both awake and during anesthesia. (From ref. 39, with permission.).

airway closure to a greater extent than in the normal subject (50).There is no report on atelectasis formation in the anesthetized, severely obese patient. However, correlations between Broca's index (114) or body mass index (BMI) (110) and size of atelectasis and between BMI and pulmonary shunt (95) have been presented, suggesting that an increased body weight enhances atelectasis formation and pulmonary shunt.

How can one counter hypoxemia or an increased alveolar-arterial oxygen tension difference in the anesthetized obese patient? The simplest solution is to increase the inspired oxygen fraction, but if the shunt is larger that 30%, which may well be the case in these patients, further oxygen will add little to arterial oxygenation (7). The application of PEEP has been advocated, too. As discussed earlier, this may reduce the atelectasis but will also have adverse effects such as reduced cardiac output and redistribution of blood flow toward dependent, still collapsed lung regions. A third alternative is to ventilate the lungs with a few large, near vital capacity inflations to reopen collapsed tissue (110,111,125).

Effect of Preexisting Lung Disease

Smokers and patients with lung disease show more pronounced gas exchange impairment in the awake state than healthy subjects and this difference also persists during anesthesia (26). Interestingly, smokers with moderate airflow limitation may have less shunt as measured by multiple inert gas eliminations than lung healthy subjects. Thus, in patients with mild to moderate bronchitis who were to undergo lung surgery (4) or vascular reconstructive surgery in the leg (45), only a small shunt was noticed but log SDQ was a mirror of it. More recently, patients with chronic bronchitis were studied awake and during anesthesia with both multiple inert gas elimination for assessment of $\dot{V}_A/\dot{Q}$ and CT to indicate atelectasis formation (40). Unexpectedly, these patients developed no or very little atelectasis during anesthesia and no or only minor shunting. However, a considerable $\dot{V}_A/\dot{Q}$ mismatch was seen with a large perfusion fraction to low $\dot{V}_A/\dot{Q}$ regions (Fig. 12). Consequently, the arterial oxygenation was more impaired than in lung healthy subjects, but the cause was different from that in the normal subject. A possible reason for the absence of atelectasis and shunting may be the chronic hyperinflation that changes the mechanical behavior of the lungs and the interaction with the chest wall, so that the tendency to collapse is reduced. It should be kept in mind that a patient with obstructive lung disease may have large regions with low $\dot{V}_A/\dot{Q}$ ratios that can be transferred over time to resorption atelectasis. Thus, the "protection" against atelectasis formation during anesthesia by the obstructive lung disease need not last for long. Regions with low $\dot{V}_A/\dot{Q}$ may be replaced by atelectasis, caused by slow resorption of gas behind occluded airways later during surgery and in the postoperative period.

Effect of Regional Anesthesia

Ventilatory effects of regional anesthesia depend on the type and extension of motor blockade. With extensive blocks including all thoracic and lumbar segments, inspiratory capacity is reduced by 20% and expiratory reserve volume approaches zero (33,63). The diaphragmatic function, however, is often spared even in cases of inadvertent extension of subarachnoid or epidural sensory blocking up to cervical segments (33). Skillfully handled regional anesthesia affects pulmonary gas exchange only minimally. Arterial oxygenation and carbon dioxide elimination are well maintained during spinal and epidural anesthesia (63,136,145). This is in line with the findings of unchanged relations of closing capacity to FRC (74,77) and unaltered distributions of ventilation-perfusion ratios assessed with the multiple inert gas elimination technique during epidural anesthesia (74).

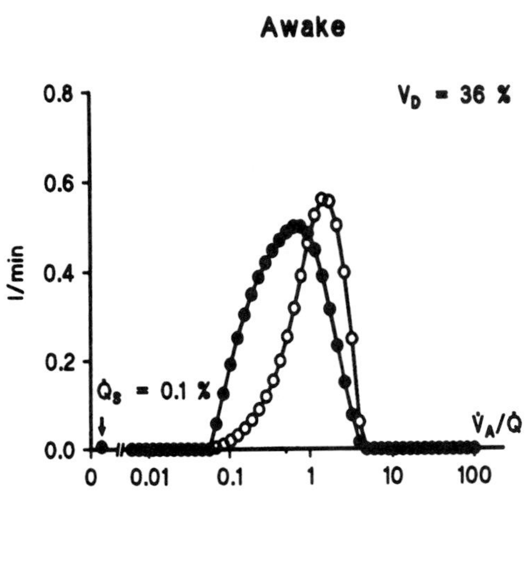

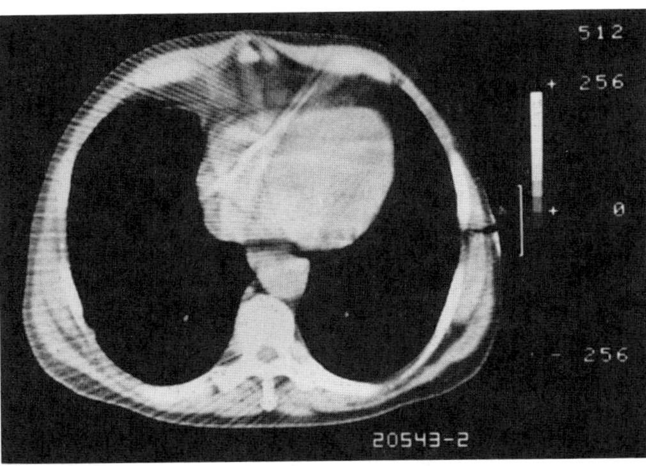

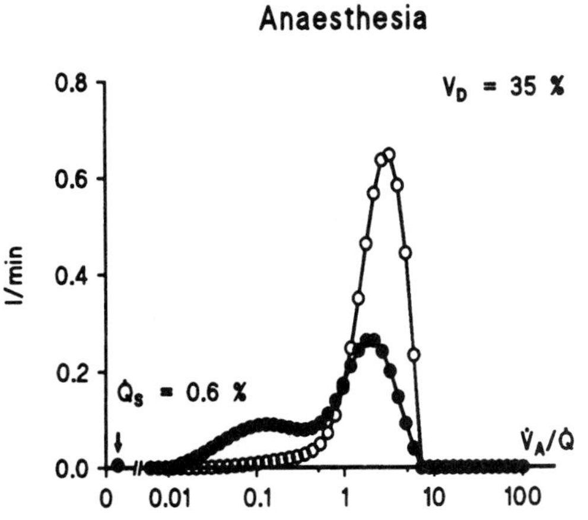

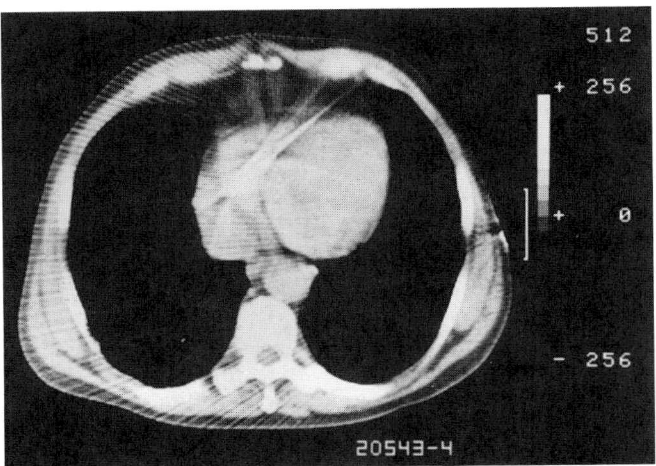

Figure 12. Computed tomography of the chest and $\dot{V}_A/\dot{Q}$ distributions (*open circle,* ventilation; *filled circle,* blood flow in L/min) in a subject with chronic obstructive pulmonary disease. Awake *(upper panel)*: note the broad $\dot{V}_A/\dot{Q}$ distribution in comparison to Fig. 8, upper panel. Anesthesia *(lower panel)*: increased perfusion of regions with low $\dot{V}_A/\dot{Q}$. Only a small shunt may be seen in this subject. For details see text. (From ref. 40, with permission.)

CONCLUSIONS

With the use of the multiple inert gas elimination technique and computed x-ray tomography, detailed insight in the impairment of gas exchange during general anesthesia has emerged. Pulmonary shunt, defined as perfusion of lung regions with $\dot{V}_A/\dot{Q}$ ratios less than 0.005, is increased in most adults and correlates with the amount of atelectasis in dependent parts of the lung. In addition, an increased dispersion of $\dot{V}_A/\dot{Q}$ ratios is usually seen. The mechanism of this phenomenon has not yet been fully established, but airway closure may be important. Dead space, defined as ventilation of lung regions with $\dot{V}_A/\dot{Q}$ ratios greater than 100, is typically unchanged, whereas regions with high $\dot{V}_A/\dot{Q}$ ratios may develop, presumably corresponding to nondependent lung regions with a poor perfusion of alveoli. Atelectasis and shunting are independent of the patient's age but tend to be larger in obese patients. $\dot{V}_A/\dot{Q}$ mismatch, on the other hand increases with age, explaining the further worsening of oxygenation that occurs in the elderly.

REFERENCES

1. Agostoni E, Miserocchi G. Vertical gradient of transpulmonary pressure with active and artificial lung expansion. *J Appl Physiol* 1970; 29(5):705–712.
2. Alexander JI, Horton PW, Millar WT, Parikh RK, Spence AA. The effect of upper abdominal surgery on the relationship of airway closing point to end tidal position. *Clin Sci* 1972;43:137–141.
3. Alexander JI, Spencer AA, Parikh RK, et al. The role of airway closure in postoperative hypoxaemia. *Br J Anaesth* 1973;45:34–40.
4. Anjou-Lindskog E, Broman L, Broman M, Holmgren A, Settergren G, Öhqvist G. Effects of intravenous anesthesia on VA/Q distribution. *Anesthesiology* 1985;62:485–492.
5. Ashbaugh DG, Bigelow DB, Petty TL, Lense BE. Acute respiratory distress in adults. *Lancet* 1967;2:319–323.
6. Bake B, Wood L, Murphy B, Macklem PI, Milic-Emili J. Effect of inspiratory flow rate on regional distribution of inspired gas. *J Appl Physiol* 1974;37:8–17.
7. Benatar SR, Hewlett AM, Nunn JF. The use of iso-shunt lines for control of oxygen therapy. *Br J Anaesth* 1973;45:711–715.
8. Bendixen HH, Hedley-Whyte J, Laver MB. Impaired oxygenation in surgical patients during general anesthesia with controlled ventilation. *N Engl J Med* 1963;269:991–996.
9. Berggren S. The oxygen deficit of arterial blood caused by nonventilating parts of the lung. *Acta Physiol Scand Suppl* 1942;1–92.
10. Bergman NA. Distribution of inspired gas during anesthesia and artificial ventilation. *J Appl Physiol* 1963;18(6):1085–1089.
11. Bergman NA, Tien YK. Contribution of the closure of pulmonary

units to impaired oxygenation during anesthesia. *Anesthesiology* 1983;59:395–401.

12. Bindslev L, Hedenstierna G, Santesson J, Gotlieb I, Carvallhas A. Ventilation-perfusion distribution during inhalation anesthesia. Effect of spontaneous breathing, mechanical ventilation and positive end-expiratory pressure. *Acta Anaesthesiol Scand* 1981;25:360–371.
13. Bjertnaes LJ. Hypoxia induced vasoconstriction in isolated perfused lungs exposed to injectable or inhalation anaesthetics. *Acta Anaesthesiol Scand* 1977;21:133–147.
14. Brismar B, Hedenstierna G, Lundquist H, Strandberg Å, Svensson L, Tokics L. Pulmonary densities during anesthesia with muscular relaxation—a proposal of atelectasis. *Anesthesiology* 1985;62:422–428.
15. Brudin LH, Rhodes CG, Valind SO, Jones T, Hughes JMB. Interrelationships between regional blood flow, blood volume and ventilation in supine man. *J Appl Physiol* 1994;76:1205–1210.
16. Buist SA, Ross BB. Quantitative analysis of the alveolar plateau in the diagnosis of early airway obstruction. *Am Rev Respir Dis* 1973;108:1078–1087.
17. Burger EJ, Macklem PT. The effect on lungs of breathing 100% O2 near residual volume. *Fed Proc* 1966;25:566.
18. Coates G, Nahmias L. Xenon-127, a comparison with xenon-133 for ventilation studies. *J Nucl Med* 1977;18:21–26.
19. Damgaard-Pedersen K, Qvist T. Pediatric pulmonary CT-scanning. *Pediatr Radiol* 1980;9:145–148.
20. Dantzker DR, Wagner PD, West JB. Instability of lung units with low VA/Q ratios during O_2 breathing. *J Appl Physiol* 1975;38(5):886–895.
21. Domino KB, Wetstein L, Glasser SA, Lindgren L, Marshall C, Harken A, Marshall BE. Influence of mixed venous oxygen tension ($P_{V}O_2$) on blood flow to atelectatic lung. *Anesthesiology* 1983;59:428–434.
22. Don HF, Wahba WM, Craig DB. Airway closure, gas trapping and the functional residual capacity during anesthesia. *Anesthesiology* 1972;36:533–539.
23. Dueck R, Prutow RJ, Davies NJH, Clausen JL, Davidson TM. The lung volume at which shunting occurs with inhalation anesthesia. *Anesthesiology* 1988;69:854–861.
24. Dueck R, Rathbun M, Greenburg AG. Lung volume and VA/Q distribution response to intravenous versus inhalation anesthesia in sheep. *Anesthesiology* 1984;61:55–65.
25. Dueck R, Wagner PD, West JB. Effects of positive end-expiratory pressure on gas exchange in dogs with normal and edematous lungs. *Anesthesiology* 1977;47:359–366.
26. Dueck R, Young I, Clausen J, Wagner PD. Altered distribution of pulmonary ventilation and blood flow following induction of inhalational anesthesia. *Anesthesiology* 1980;52:113–125.
27. Enghoff H. Volumen inefficax. Bemerkungen zur Frage des schädlichen Raumes. *Uppsala Läk För Förh* 1938;44:191.
28. Evans JW, Wagner PD. Limits on V_A/Q distributions from analysis of experimental inert gas elimination. *J Appl Physiol* 1977;42(6):889–898.
29. von Euler US, Liljestrand G. Observations on the pulmonary arterial blood pressure in cat. *Acta Physiol Scand* 1946;12:310–320.
30. Fahri LE. Elimination of inert gas by the lung. *Respir Physiol* 1967;3:1–11.
31. Falke KJ, Pontoppidan H, Kumas A, Lith DE, Geffin B, Care MB. Ventilation with an expiratory pressure in acute lung disease. *J Clin Invest* 1972;51:2315–2323.
32. Fazio F, Jones T. Assessment of regional ventilation by continuous inhalation of radioactive krypton-81m. *Br Med J* 1975;3:673–676.
33. Freund FG, Bonica JJ, Ward RJ, Akamatsu TJ, Kennedy WF. Ventilatory reserve and level of motor block during high spinal and epidural anesthesia. *Anesthesiology* 1967;28(5):834–837.
34. Froese AB, Bryan C. Effects of anesthesia and paralysis on diaphragmatic mechanics in man. *Anesthesiology* 1974;41(3):242–255.
35. Gillespie DJ, Didier EP, Rehder K. Ventilation-perfusion distribution after aortic valve replacement. *Crit Care Med* 1990;18:136–140.
36. Gilmour I, Burnham M, Craig DB. Closing capacity measurement during general anesthesia. *Anesthesiology* 1976;45(5) 477–482.
37. Glazier JB, Hughes JMB, Maloney JE, West JB, Measurements of capillary dimensions and blood volume in rapidly frozen lungs. *J Appl Physiol* 1969;26:65–76.
38. Glenny RW, Robertson TH. Fractal modeling of pulmonary blood flow heterogeneity. *J Appl Physiol* 1991;70:1024–1030.
39. Gunnarsson L, Tokics L, Gustavsson H, Hedenstierna G. Influence of age on atelectasis formation and gas exchange impairment during general anesthesia. *Br J Anaesth* 1991;66:423–432.
40. Gunnarsson L, Tokics L, Lundquist H, Brismar B, Strandberg Å, Berg B, Hedenstierna G. Chronic obstructive pulmonary disease and anesthesia: formation of atelectasis and gas exchange impairment. *Eur Respir J* 1991;4:1106–1116.
41. Hachenberg T, Tenling A Nyström SO, Tydén H, Hedenstierna G. Ventilation-perfusion inequality in patients undergoing cardiac surgery. *Anesthesiology* 1994;80:509–519.
42. Hakim TS, Dean GW, Lisbona R. Effect of body posture on spatial distribution of pulmonary blood flow. *J Appl Physiol* 1988;64:1160–1170.
43. Hedenstierna G, Järnberg P-O, Gottlieb I. Thoracic gas volume measured by body plethysmography during anesthesia and muscle paralysis. *Anesthesiology* 1981;55:439–443.
44. Hedenstierna G, Löfström B, Lundh R. Thoracic gas volume and chest-abdomen dimensions during anesthesia and muscle paralysis. *Anesthesiology* 1981;55:499–506.
45. Hedenstierna G, Lundh R, Johansson H. Alveolar stability during anesthesia for reconstructive vascular surgery in the leg. *Acta Anaesthesiol Scand* 1983;27:26–34.
46. Hedenstierna G, Lundquist H, Lundh B, Tokics L, Strandberg Å, Brismar B, et al. Pulmonary densities during anesthesia. An experimental study on lung morphology and gas exchange. *Eur Respir J* 1989;2:528–535.
47. Hedenstierna G, McCarthy G, Bergström M. Airway closure during mechanical ventilation. *Anesthesiology* 1976;44(2):114–123.
48. Hedenstierna G, Santesson J. Airway closure during anesthesia: a comparison between resident-gas and argon-bolus techniques. *J Appl Physiol* 1979;47(4):874–881.
49. Hedenstierna G, Santesson J, Bindslev L, Baehrendtz S, Klingstedt C, Norlander O. Regional differences in lung function during anesthesia and intensive care: Clinical implications. *Acta Anaesth Scand* 1982;26:429–434.
50. Hedenstierna G, Santesson J, Norlander O. Airway closure and distribution of inspired gas in the extremely obese, breathing spontaneously and during anesthesia with intermittent positive pressure ventilation. *Acta Anaesth Scand* 1976;20:334–342.
51. Hedenstierna G, Strandberg Å, Brismar B, Lundquist H, Svensson L, Tokics L. Functional residual capacity, thoracoabdominal dimensions, and central blood volume during general anesthesia with muscle paralysis and mechanical ventilation. *Anesthesiology* 1985;62:247–254.
52. Hedenstierna G, Tokics L. Determination of lung-ventilation and perfusion by isotope technique. In: Vincent JL, ed. *Update in intensive care and emergency medicine.* Heidelberg: Springer-Verlag 1990;10:138–145.
53. Hedenstierna G, Tokics L, Lundquist H, Andersson T, Strandberg Å, Brismar B. Phrenic nerve stimulation during halothane anesthesia. *Anesthesiology* 1994;80:751–760.
54. Hedenstierna G, Tokics L, Strandberg Å, Lundquist H, Brismar B. Correlation of gas exchange impairment to development of atelectasis during anesthesia and muscle paralysis. *Acta Anaesthesiol Scand* 1986;30:183–191.
55. Hedenstierna G, White FC, Mazzone R, Wagner PD. Redistribution of pulmonary blood flow in the dog with PEEP ventilation. *J Appl Physiol* 1979;46:278–287.
56. Hedenstierna G, White F, Wagner PD. Spatial distribution of pulmonary blood flow in the dog during end-expiratory pressure ventilation. *J Appl Physiol* 1979;46:278–287.
57. Heneghan CPH, Bergman NA, Jones JG. Changes in lung volume and ($PAO2-PaO_2$) during anesthesia. *Br J Anaesth* 1984;56:437–445.
58. Hewlett AM, Hulands GH, Nunn JF, Milledge JS. Functional residual capacity during anesthesia. *Br J Anaesth* 1974;46:495–503.
59. Hlastala MP, Robertson HT. Inert gas elimination characteristics of the normal and abnormal lung. *J Appl Physiol* 1978;44:258–266.
60. Hoppin FG Jr, Green ID, Mead J. Distribution of pleural surface pressure in dogs. *J Appl Physiol* 1969;27:863–871.
61. Hughes JMB, Coates G. Radionuclide imaging: positron camera. In: Potchen EJ, Grainger R, Green R, eds. *Pulmonary radiology.* Philadelphia: WB Saunders, 1993;331–339.
62. Hulands GH, Greene R, Iliff LD, Nunn JF. Influence of anesthesia on the regional distribution of perfusion and ventilation in the lung. *Clin Sci* 1970;38:451–460.
63. Ishihara Y. Respiratory functions during epidural and spinal anesthesia. *Nippon Ika Daigaku Zasshi* 1987;54(6):581–589.
64. Jolin-Carlsson Å, Hedenstierna G, Blomqvist H, Strandberg Å. Separate lung blood flow in anesthetized dogs: a comparative study

between electromagnetometry and SF6 and CO_2 elimination. *Anesthesiology* 1987;67:240–246.
65. Jones JG, Faithfull D, Jordan C, Minty B. Rib cage movement during halothane anesthesia in man. *Br J Anaesth* 1979;51:399–407.
66. Juno P, Marsh HM, Knopp TJ, Rehder K. Closing capacity in awake and anesthetized-paralyzed man. *J Appl Physiol* 1978;44(2):238–244.
67. Klingstedt C, Hedenstierna G, Baehrendtz S, Lundqvist H, Strandberg Å, Tokics L, et al. Ventilation-perfusion relationships and atelectasis formation in the supine and lateral positions during conventional mechanical and differential ventilation. *Acta Anaesthesiol Scand* 1990;34:421–429.
68. Klingstedt C, Hedenstierna G, Lundquist H, Strandberg Å, Tokics L, Brismar B. The influence of body position and differential ventilation on lung dimensions and atelectasis formation in anaesthetized man. *Acta Anaesthesiol Scand* 1990;34:315–322.
69. Krayer S, Rehder K, Beck KC, Cameron PD, Didier EP, Hoffman EA. Quantification of thoracic volumes by three-dimensional imaging. *J Appl Physiol* 1987;62(2):591–598.
70. Landmark SJ, Knopp TJ, Rehder K, Sessler AD. Regional pulmonary perfusion and V/Q in awake and anesthetized-paralyzed man. *J Appl Physiol* 1977;43(6):993–1000.
71. Laws AK. Effects of induction of anesthesia and muscle paralysis on functional residual capacity of the lungs. *Can Anaesth Soc J* 1968;15: 325–331.
72. Leblanc P, Ruff F, Milic-Emili J. Effects of age and body position on "airway closure" in man. *J Appl Physiol 1970;*28:448–451.
73. Lundh R, Hedenstierna G. Ventilation-perfusion relationships during halothane anesthesia and mechanical ventilation. Effects of varying inspired oxygen concentration. *Acta Anaesthesiol Scand* 1984;28:191–198.
74. Lundh R, Hedenstierna G, Johansson H. Ventilation-perfusion relationships during epidural analgesia. *Acta Anaesthesiol Scand* 1983;27:410–416.
75. Lundquist H, Hedenstierna G, Ringertz H. Barbiturate anesthesia does not cause pulmonary densities in dogs: a study using computerized axial tomography. *Acta Anaesthesiol Scand* 1988;32:162–165.
76. Lundquist H, Hedenstierna G, Strandberg Å, Tokics L, Brismar B. CT-assessment of dependent lung densities in man during general anesthesia. *Acta Radiol Scand* 1995;36:626–652.
77. McCarthy GS. The effect of thoracic extradural analgesia on pulmonary gas distribution, functional residual capacity and airway closure. *Br J Anaesth* 1976;48:243–248.
78. McCarthy D, Milic-Emili J. Closing volume in asymptomatic asthma. *Am Rev Respir Dis* 1973;107:559–570.
79. Mansell A, Bryan C, Levison H. Airway closure in children. *J Appl Physiol* 1972;33:711–714.
80. Marshall BE. Regulation of the pulmonary circulation. In: Stanly TH, Sperry RJ, eds. *Anesthesia and the lung,* 1st ed. London: Kluwer Academic, 1989.
81. Michels DB, West JB. Distribution of pulmonary ventilation and perfusion during short periods of weightlessness. *J Appl Physiol* 1978;45:987–998.
82. Milic-Emili J, Henderson JAM, Dolovich MB, Trop D, Kaneko K. Regional distribution of inspired gas in the lung. *J Appl Physiol* 1966;21:749–759.
83. Moller JT, Johannessen NW, Berg H, Espersen K, Larsen LE. Hypoxaemia during anesthesia—an observer study. *Br J Anaesth* 1991;66:437–444.
84. Murray JF, Davidson FF, Glazier JB. Modified technique for measuring pulmonary shunts using xenon and indocyanine green. *J Appl Physiol* 1972;32:695–700.
85. Neufeld GR, Williams JJ, Klineberg PL, Marshall BE. Inert gas a-v differences: a direct reflection of V/Q distribution. *J Appl Physiol* 1978;44:277–283.
86. Nicolaysen G, Shepard J, Onizuka M, Tanita T, Hattner RS, Staub NC. No gravity- independent gradient of blood flow distribution in dog lung. *J Appl Physiol* 1987;63:540–545.
87. Nunn JF. *Nunn's applied respiratory physiology,* 4th ed. London: Butterworth Heinemann, 1993, pp 403–413.
88. Nunn JF, Bergman NA, Coleman AJ. Factors influencing the arterial oxygen tension during anesthesia with artificial ventilation. *Br J Anaesth* 1965;37:898–914.
89. Nyman G, Funkquist B, Kvart C, Frostell C, Tokics L, Strandberg Å, et al. Atelectasis causes gas exchange impairment in the anaesthetized horse. *Equine Vet J* 1990;22(5):317–324.
90. Olszowka AJ, Waganer PD. Numerical analysis in gas exchange. In: West JB, ed. *Pulmonary gas exchange,* vol 1. New York: Academic Press, 1980;263–306.
91. Otis DR, Johnson M, Pedley TJ, Kamm RD. Role of pulmonary surfactant in airway closure: a computational study. *J Appl Physiol* 1993; 75:1323–1333.
92. Oyarzun MJ, Iturriaga R, Donso P, Dussaubat N, Santos M, Schiapacasse ME, Lathrop ME, Larrain C, Zapata P. Factors affecting distribution of alveolar surfactant during resting ventilation. *Am J Physiol* (Lung Cell Mol Physiol 5) 1991;261:L210–L217.
93. Permutt S, Bromberger-Barnea B, Bane HN. Alveolar pressure, pulmonary venous pressure and the vascular waterfall. *Med Thorac* 1962;19:239–260.
94. Pesenti A, Latini R, Riboni A, Gattinoni L. Simple estimate of the true right to left shunt (Qs/Qt) at maintenance F_IO_2 by sulphur hexafluoride retention. *Intensive Care Med* 1982;8:283–286.
95. Prutow RJ, Dueck R, Davies NJH, Clausen J. Shunt development in young adult surgical patients due to inhalation anesthesia. *Anesthesiology* 1982;57(3) A477.
96. Quan SF, Kronberg GM, Schlobohm RM, Feeley TW, Don HF, Lister G. Changes in venous admixture with alterations of inspired oxygen concentration. *Anesthesiology* 1980;52:477–482.
97. Radermacher P, Hérigault R, Teisseire B, Harf A, Lemaire F. Low V_A/Q areas: arterial-alveolar N_2 difference and multiple inert gas elimination technique. *J Appl Physiol* 1988;64(5):2224–2229.
98. Rahn H, Farhi LE. Gaseous environment and atelectasis. *Fed Proc* 1963;22:1035–1041.
99. Rahn H, Fahri LE. Ventilation, perfusion and gas exchange—the V_A/Q concept. In: *Handbook of physiology:* respiration, sect 3, vol 1. Washington, DC: Am Physiol Soc, 1964;735–766.
100. Raine RM, Bishop JM. A-a difference in O_2 tension and physiological dead space in normal man. *J Appl Physiol* 1963;18:284–288.
101. Rehder K, Hatch DJ, Sessler A, Fowler WS. The function of each lung of anesthetized and paralyzed man during mechanical ventilation. *Anesthesiology* 1972;37:16–26.
102. Rehder K, Sessler AD. Function of each lung in spontaneously breathing man anesthetized with thiopentalmeperidine. *Anesthesiology* 1973;38:320–326.
103. Rehder K, Knopp TJ, Sessler AD, Didier EP. Ventilation-perfusion relationship in young healthy awake and anesthetized-paralyzed man. *J Appl Physiol* 1979;47(4):745–753.
104. Rehder K, Knopp TJ, Sessler AD. Regional intrapulmonary gas distribution in awake and anesthetized-paralyzed prone man. *J Appl Physiol* 1978;45:528–535.
105. Rehder K, Sessler AD, Rodarte JR. Regional intrapulmonary gas distribution in awake and anesthetized-paralyzed man. *J Appl Physiol* 1977;42(3):391–402.
106. Rhodes BA, Stem HS, Buchanan JW. Lung scanning with ^{99m}Technetium microspheres. *Radiology* 1971;99:613–621.
107. Rhodes CG, Valind SO, Brudin LH, Wollmer PE, Jones T, Buckingham PD, Hughes JMB. Quantification of regional VA/Q ratios in humans by use of PET. II. Procedure and normal values. *J Appl Physiol* 1989;66:1905–1913.
108. Riley RL, Cournand A. "Ideal" alveolar air and the analysis of ventilation-perfusion relationships in the lungs. *J Appl Physiol* 1949;1: 825–847.
109. Rosenzweig DY, Hughes JMB, Glazier JB. Effects of transpulmonary and vascular pressures on pulmonary blood volume in isolated lung. *J Appl Physiol* 1970;28:553–560.
110. Rothen HU, Sporre B, Engberg G, Wegenius G, Hedenstierna G. Re-expansion of atelectasis during general anesthesia—a CT-study. *Br J Anaesth* 1993;71:788–795.
111. Rothen HU, Sporre B, Engberg G, Wegenius G, Hedenstierna G. Reexpansion of atelectasis during general anesthesia may have a prolonged effect. *Acta Anaesth Scand* 1995;39:110–125.
112. Shapiro BA, Cane RD, Harrison RA, Steiner MC. Changes in intrapulmonary shunt with administration of 100 % oxygen. *Chest* 1980;77:138–141.
113. Strandberg Å, Tokics L, Brismar B, Lundquist H, Hedenstierna G. Atelectasis during anesthesia and in the postoperative period. *Acta Anaesthesiol Scand* 1986;30:154–158.
114. Strandberg Å, Tokics L, Brismar B, Lundquist H, Hedenstierna G. Constitutional factors promoting development of atelectasis during anesthesia. *Acta Anaesthesiol Scand* 1987;31:21–24.
115. Strandberg Å, Hedenstierna G, Tokics L, Lundquist H, Brismar B. Densities in dependent lung regions during anesthesia: atelectasis or fluid accumulation? *Acta Anaesthesiol Scand* 1986;30:256–259.
116. Sullivan PJ, Burke WM, Burch WM, Lomas FE. A clinical compar-

ison of Technegas and xenon-133 in 50 patients with suspected pulmonary emboli. *Chest* 1988;94:300–304.

117. Sykes MK, Loh L, Seed RF, Kafer ER, Chakrabarti NK. The effects of inhalational anaesthetics on hypoxic pulmonary vasoconstriction and pulmonary vascular resistance in the perfused lungs of the dog and cat. *Br J Anaesth* 1972;44:776–788.
118. Sykes MK, Mill AEG, Loh L, Tait AR. Evaluation of a new method for the continuous measurement of the distribution of the blood flow between the two lungs. *Br J Anaesth* 1977;49:285–292.
119. Sykes MK, Young WE, Robinson BE. Oxygenation during anesthesia with controlled ventilation. *Br J Anaesth* 1965;37:314–325.
120. Thilenius OG. Effect of anesthesia on response of pulmonary circulation of dogs to acute hypoxia. *J Appl Physiol* 1966;21:901–904.
121. Tokics L, Hedenstierna G, Brismar B, Strandberg Å, Lundquist H. Thoracoabdominal restriction in supine men: CT and lung function measurements. *J Appl Physiol* 1988;64(2):599–604.
122. Tokics L, Hedenstierna G, Strandberg Å, Brismar B, Lundquist H. Lung collapse and gas exchange during general anesthesia: effects of spontaneous breathing, muscle paralysis, and positive end-expiratory pressure. *Anesthesiology* 1987;66:157–167.
123. Tokics L, Strandberg Å, Brismar B, Lundquist H, Hedenstierna G. Computerized tomography of the chest and gas exchange measurements during ketamine anesthesia. *Acta Anaesthesiol Scand* 1987;31:684–692.
124. Ueda H, Iio M, Kaihara S. Determination of regional pulmonary blood flow in various cardiopulmonary disorders. *Jpn Heart J* 1964; 5:431–444.
125. Vaughan RW, Wise L. Intraoperative arterial oxygenation in obese patients. *Ann Surg* 1976;184:35–42.
126. Vellody VS, Nassery M, Balasaraswathi K, Goldberg NB, Sharp JT. Compliances of human rib cage and diaphragm-abdomen pathways in relaxed versus paralyzed states. *Am Rev Respir Dis* 1978;118: 479–491.
127. Wagner PD. Calculation of the distribution of ventilation-perfusion ratios from inert gas elimination data. *Fed Proc* 1982;41: 136–139.
128. Wagner PD, Dantzker DR, Iacovoni VE, Tomlin WC, West JB. Ventilation-perfusion inequality in asymptomatic asthma. *Am Rev Respir Dis* 1978;118:511–524.
129. Wagner PD, Hedenstierna G, Bylin G. Ventilation-perfusion inequality in chronic asthma. *Am Rev Respir Dis* 1987;136:605–612.
130. Wagner PD, Lopez FA. Gas chromatography techniques in respiratory physiology. In: *Respiratory physiology.* Ireland: Elsevier Scientific, 1984;P403;1–24
131. Wagner PD, Saltzman HA, West JB. Measurement of continuous distributions of ventilation-perfusion ratios:theory. *J Appl Physiol* 1974;36(5):588–599.
132. Wagner PD, Gale GE, Moon RE, Torre-Bueno JR, Stolp BW, Saltzman HA. Pulmonary gas exchange in humans exercising at sea level and simulated altitude. *J Appl Physiol* 1986;61:260–270.
133. Wagner PD, Dantzker DR, Dueck R, Clausen JL, West JB. Ventilation-perfusion inequality in chronic obstructive pulmonary disease. *J Clin Invest* 1977;59:203–216.
134. Wagner PD, Dantzker DR, Tornabene VW, LeWinter MM, West JB. Effects of ventilation-perfusion inequality on arterial PO_2 following acute myocardial infarction (abstract). *Clin Res* 1976;24: 160A.
135. Wahba RWM. Perioperative functional residual capacity. *Can J Anaesth* 1991;38(3):384–400.
136. Ward RJ, Bonica JJ, Freund FG, Akamatsu TJ, Danziger F, Englesson S. Epidural and subarachnoid anesthesia. *JAMA* 1965;191(4): 275–278.
137. Werkö L. The influence of positive pressure breathing on the circulation in man. *Acta Med Scand* 1947;suppl 193.
138. West JB. State of the art. Ventilation-perfusion relationships. *Am Rev Respir Dis* 1977;116:919–943.
139. West JB, Dollery CT, Heard BE. Increased pulmonary vascular resistance in the dependent zone of the isolated dog lung caused by perivascular edema. *Circ Res* 1965;17:191–206.
140. West JB, Dollery CT, Naimark A. Distribution of blood flow in isolated lung: relation to vascular and alveolar pressures. *J Appl Physiol* 1964;19: 713–724.
141. West JB, Wagner PD. Ventilation-perfusion relationships. In: Crystal RG, West JB, eds. *The Lung, Scientific Foundations.* New York: Raven Press, 1991;1289–1305.
142. Westbrook PR, Stubbs SE, Sessler AD, Rehder K, Hyatt RE. Effects of anesthesia and muscle paralysis on respiratory mechanics in normal man. *J Appl Physiol* 1973;34(1):81–86.
143. Williams JJ, Chen L, Aukburg SJ, Alexander CM, Domino KB, Marshall BE. Computerized measure of CO_2 production to determine differential pulmonary blood flow (abstract). *Anesthesiology* 1983;59:A496
144. Wollmer P, Schairer W, Bos JAH, Bakker W, Krenning EP, Lachman B. Pulmonary clearance of ^{99m}Tc-DTPA during halothane anesthesia. *Acta Anaesthesiol Scand* 1990;34:572–575.
145. Yamagake M, Namiki A, Tsuchida H, Iwasaki H. Changes in ventilatory pattern and arterial oxygen saturation during spinal anesthesia in man. *Acta Anaesthesiol Scand* 1992;36:569.

Anesthesia: Biologic Foundations, edited by Tony L. Yaksh et al. Lippincott–Raven Publishers, Philadelphia © 1997.

CHAPTER 78

NEUROPHARMACOLOGY OF THE CONTROL OF VENTILATION

DENHAM S. WARD AND JOHN A. TEMP

Breathing, an amazingly complex and robust autonomic function, is normally unconscious and continuous. It continues during sleep or under light anesthesia. This autonomic function may also be interrupted abruptly, even violently, by other involuntarily acts such as coughing or sneezing. Yet, breathing also involves voluntary striated muscle. Thus, breathing may be overridden by voluntarily cortical control. During singing, for instance, the pattern of breathing accommodates the voice. And during a breath hold, breathing can be withheld even to the point of unconsciousness. Under ordinary circumstance, however, breathing regulates the chemical composition of the blood remarkably; despite a greater than tenfold change in metabolism from sleep to moderate exercise, and the accommodation of nonventilatory acts (e.g., speaking, singing, coughing, sneezing, emesis, etc.) blood pH, PCO_2, and PO_2 (see Table 1 for a list of abbreviations used in this chapter) normally fall within a very narrow range. Obviously, the neural control system needs to be complex and complete.

Elucidation of brainstem control mechanisms has proven to be formidable. Many factors can be shown to influence breathing under particular circumstances, but are clearly not of equal importance at all times. Breathing during exercise, for example, is not a simple reflex involving solely chemoreflex feedback, and thus it is qualitatively different than breathing during sleep. Many cortical stimuli add to or multiply the underlying chemical drives, and these influences greatly compound the study of the whole organism.

In animal models, a variety of techniques ranging from ablation of brainstem areas to extracellular and intracellular electrophysiologic recording have been used. These techniques, too, have often been combined with study of the chemical reflex responses to learn how the afferent information is coupled to the intrinsic generation of respiratory rhythm and coordinated ventilatory drive. New techniques have identified neurotransmitters and neuromodulators that influence breathing in very specific brainstem locations. Extensive study and progress in these fields over the last decade may lead to more exact answers to many fundamental questions in ventilatory control (e.g., the generation of the basic respiratory oscillations; identification of the central chemoreceptor cells; mechanism of CO_2 and/or H^+ signal transduction in the central chemoreceptors; mechanism of hypoxic signal transduction in the peripheral chemoreceptors; mechanism of adaptation of ventilation to prolonged hypoxia and high altitude; control of ventilation during exercise).

This chapter on the neural control of breathing presents the neural organization of the ventilatory control system with particular emphasis on the neurotransmitters and neuromodulators involved. Many drugs in anesthesia affect these transmitters or their receptors. Understanding the neuropharmacology involved in breathing may ultimately permit more rational use and design of the drugs. Much of the material in previous chapters of this book, particularly the discussion of cell-cell communication in Volume One, which relates to receptors and ligands, is fundamental to this chapter.

Figure 1 is a block diagram of the ventilatory controller. This chapter focuses on the central controller and the "closed-loop" afferent inputs to the controller (the shaded blocks in the figure). The extremely important functions of the efferent neural connections to the diaphragm, chest wall, and upper airway muscles are covered in the Chap. 79.

In the first section on the neural control of breathing, the general organization and the responses of the ventilatory controller are discussed. The difficulties and controversies surrounding drug effect studies in anesthesia are placed in the context of the physiology of the neural control of ventilation. The second section discusses the potential neuromodulators and neurotransmitters involved in the control of ventilation. In each of these sections the neuropharmacology is emphasized as a tool both to discern the roles of these neurochemicals and to provide explanations for important clinical observations.

Table 1. GLOSSARY OF SYMBOLS AND ABBREVIATIONS

ACh	Acetylcholine
CB	Carotid body
CBF	Cerebral blood flow
CNS	Central nervous system
CSF	Cerebral spinal fluid
CSN	Carotid sinus nerve
DRG	Dorsal respiratory group of neurons
ECF	Extracellular fluid
f	Breathing frequency ($1/T_B$)
GABA	γ-Aminobutyric acid
HCVR	Hypercapnic ventilatory response
HVD	Hypoxic ventilatory decline
HVR	Hypoxic ventilatory response
LC	Locus coeruleus
NA	Nucleus ambiguus
NRA	Nucleus retroambigualis
NTS	Nucleus tractus solitarius
P_aCO_2, $P_{ET}CO_2$	Arterial, end-tidal CO_2 partial pressure
P_aO_2, $P_{ET}O_2$	Arterial, end-tidal O_2 partial pressure
RRN	Respiratory-related neurons
S_aO_2, S_pO_2	Arterial O_2 hemoglobin saturation, pulse oximetry measured arterial saturation
T_I, T_E, T_P, T_B	Inspiratory, expiratory time, end expiratory pause, breath time (T_I+T_E+T_P)
$\dot{V}_A$	Alveolar ventilation
$\dot{V}_M$	Minute ventilation (breath phase unspecified but usually expiratory)
V_d	Dead space volume
V_T	Tidal volume (breath phase unspecified but usually expiratory)
V_I, V_E	Inspiratory, expiratory tidal volume
VLM	Ventrolateral medulla
VRG	Ventral respiratory group of neurons

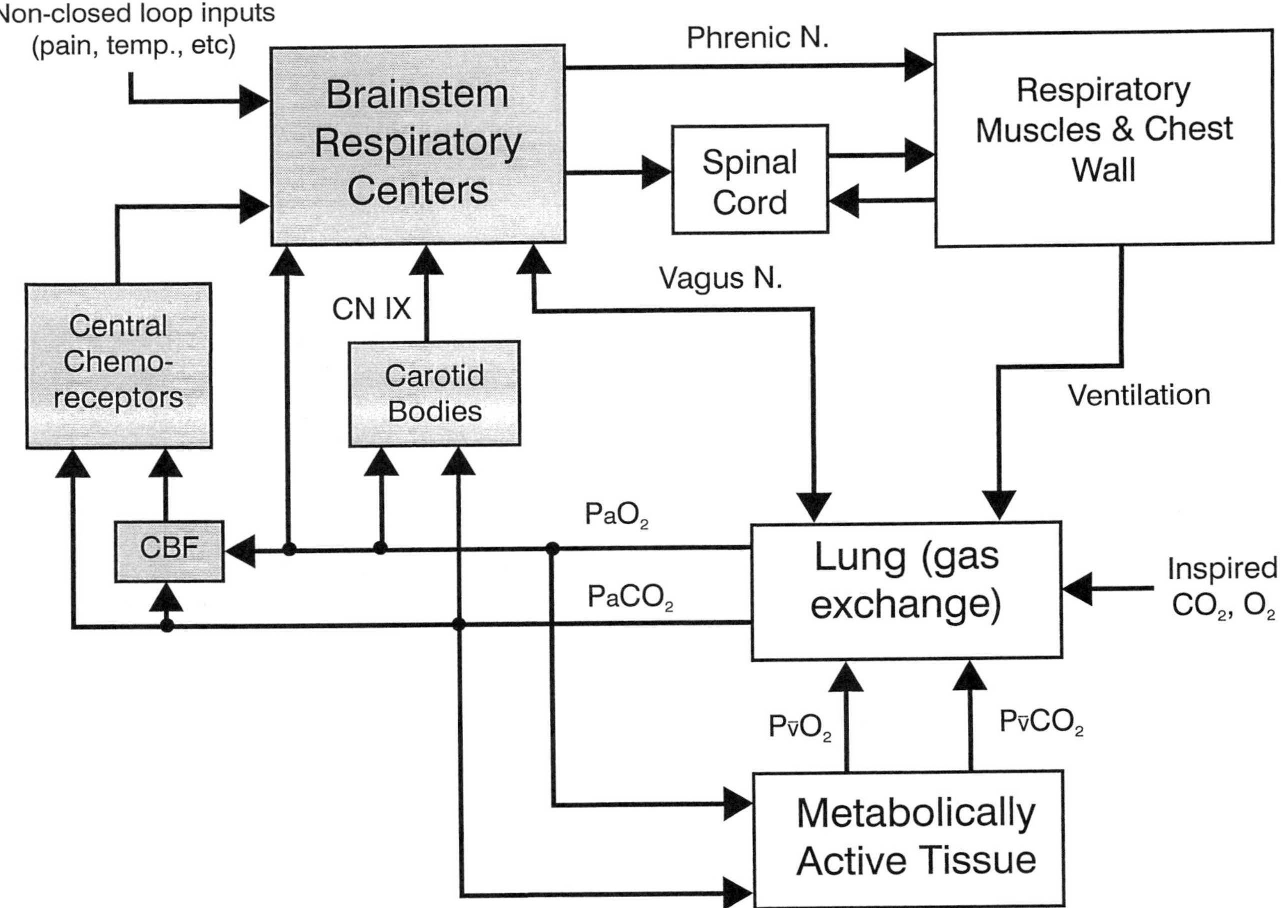

Figure 1. Block diagram of the ventilatory control system. The interconnections represent both physical quantities as well as information conducted along neural pathways. The multiple feedback connections are seen between many of the elements of the control system. The *shaded elements* are the focus of this chapter. CNIX, carotid sinus nerve, branch of the glossopharyngeal nerve.

PHYSIOLOGY OF THE NEURAL CONTROL OF BREATHING

Structure and Function

The ventilatory controller must coordinate and interact with many other voluntary and autonomic functions. Although most research on ventilation has treated the ventilatory controller in isolation from other functions, more recent work has attempted to place it within the context of a larger cardiorespiratory controller. The larger controller may integrate multiple adaptive strategies when faced with changing physiologic states (e.g., sleep, exercise) or pathophysiologic conditions (e.g., chronic lung disorder, anesthesia).

Central Neural Controller

Classical Organization Early studies of the neural control of breathing involved the section and ablation of various brainstem structures. Kellogg (129) provides a very interesting historical account of these early studies. From such structure-function experiments emerged the classical description of the ventilatory controller. In this classical organization, centers in the medulla provide the rhythmic generation of ventilatory drive, while additional areas in the pons modulate and regulate the basic rhythm. This organization, focusing on interconnected "centers," resulted because the ventilatory apparatus functions differently as central and peripheral interconnections are ablated or severed (e.g., vagus, carotid sinus nerve). The medullary centers, for instance, are capable of rhythmic respiration even when fully isolated, but the character and pattern of the ventilation is distinctly abnormal. Leaving the medulla connected to the lower and middle pons (the apneustic center) results in more regular breathing, but only if the vagi are intact. If the vagal afferents from lung stretch receptors are severed, prolonged inspirations (apneusis) with pauses at full inspiration result. If the upper third of the pons is left intact, ventilation is essentially normal, but becomes deeper and slower when the vagi are severed. The restraining influence of rostral pons resulted in the postulation of the location of the pneumotaxic center. Thus arose the concept of a pontile apneustic center as the site of inspiratory tonicity, with rhythmic inhibition of inspiration by both the pneumotaxic center and the vagi. As more knowledge of the role of neurotransmitters and neuromodulators is obtained, these concepts of respiratory centers in the brain stem is evolving. The pneumotaxic center is no longer thought to be a dominant controller of the respiratory rhythm; however, the pattern of firing of its neurons suggests a role in modulation, or fine tuning, of respiration.

Brainstem Respiratory Centers Much recent work on the organization of the respiratory centers comes from microelectrode studies. Several areas in the brain stem show neuronal firing patterns with a pronounced correlation to the respiratory cycle. While this correlation does not prove any causal relationship to the respiratory rhythm, it certainly implies some neural interconnection.

Six basic types of firing patterns have been described in respiratory related neurons (RRN). Once the general division of inspiratory (firing mainly during inspiration) and expiratory (firing mainly during expiration) neurons has been made, each can be further divided into three subtypes: those that have a constant firing rate through their respiratory phase; those with an increasing rate; and those with a decreasing rate (269). Not all of these types of neurons are common and some may not have an especially prominent role in respiratory control. Finally, some types of inspiratory neurons fire well into the expiratory phase and have been referred to as "phase-spanning" neurons.

In the medulla, two major areas of RRN have been described. The dorsal respiratory group (DRG) corresponds mainly to the nucleus of the solitary tract (NTS) and the region ventrolateral to the NTS. Primarily inspiratory neurons are found in the DRG, although a few expiratory neurons have been located. The inspiratory neurons are either of the constant or increasing firing rate types. These have been distinguished further by their response to lung inflation. So-called Iα neurons are inhibited by lung inflation and their firing can be terminated by lung inflation (as phrenic nerve activity can be), suggesting a similarity to the Hering-Breuer reflex. Iβ neurons, on the other hand, show increasing activity as the lung inflates.

The ventral respiratory group (VRG) is a much larger grouping of respiratory neurons. The VRG corresponds anatomically to the nucleus ambiguous (NA) and the nucleus retroambigualis (NRA). The most rostral end of the group has also been referred to as the Bötzinger complex. Both inspiratory and expiratory cells are found in the VRG. There appears to be some spatial organization to the group: the rostral the Bötzinger complex is primarily inspiratory while the caudal end contains more expiratory neurons. It is important to note that the NA also contains motor neurons that innervate the laryngeal muscles. Figure 2 shows the basic neuroanatomy of the respiratory centers.

In the pons, the "pneumotaxic" center (although it has been suggested that this term is useful only in a historical perspective) corresponds to the nucleus parabrachialis medialis and the Kölliker-Fuse nucleus and overlaps with the locus coeruleus and the subcoeruleus complex. Neurons of both inspiratory and expiratory type are found in these complexes but their activity is abolished during anesthesia even when respiration is otherwise still present. Thus, these areas may not be involved in the generation of respiratory rhythm, but rather may play a modulatory role. It is thought that this area integrates vagal and chemoreceptive inputs into the intrinsic oscillations of the medullary neurons.

Although the respiratory rhythm is clearly generated in the medulla, the actual mechanism or neural circuitry responsible for the rhythm has not been described. There do not seem to be pacemaker cells, which would generate a basic oscillation, as in the heart. For many years, various concepts of reciprocal inhibition and self reexcitation between pools of inspiratory and expiratory neurons have been considered. However, few anatomical correlates of such an organization have been found. Most recently, the concept of "patterning of constant excitatory input" has been the favored hypothesis. Recent reviews (80,184,269,271) as well as several older ones (20–22,183) discuss these concepts and the organization of the respiratory centers in complex detail.

Neurochemical Organization Many different neurochemicals appear to be involved in the control of breathing. Because the sites of synthesis, release, and reception may be widely separated, development of a clear picture of how these neurotransmitters function is still ongoing. The realization that some neurochemicals may act locally through classical synaptic interactions, but that others may act more remotely as longer acting modulators, has offered insight, but also added greater complexity. There seem to be different time scales of action, from direct synaptic transmission which has immediate but short-lasting effects, to more long-acting alterations that seem almost hormonal in nature (73,75). Both excitatory and inhibitory influences are present at various stages of ventilatory drive generation (45). There are many possible sites for neurotransmitter agonists and antagonists to affect ventilatory control (64,75,145,146,178,190,191). No consistent pattern of a particular neurochemical being dominant in a portion of the organization of ventilatory control has yet emerged.

Central Integration von Euler (269–271) has proposed the functional diagram of breathing shown in Fig. 3. Although studies of breathing have frequently emphasized the reflex nature of the system (i.e., the response to hypercapnia), the central integration required to produce coordinated breathing is far more complex. von Euler has emphasized three functions: (a) pattern generation, (b) pattern formation, and (c) drive integration.

Pattern generation involves the basic oscillations of the respiratory centers. A rhythmic input is not required for the oscillator, but there must be some tonic input from other neural centers. Pattern generation seems to involve primarily an inspiratory ramp generator and a central "off-switch." The off-switch represents a mechanism for termination of inspiration. It is important for determining the relative depth and duration of a tidal volume. This off-switch is not static, but rather changes depending on feedback from lung afferents and other inputs. Under quiet breathing there is little expiratory muscle activity and the expiratory ramp generator is usually "silent."

Pattern formation adapts and optimizes the basic respiratory pattern for the prevailing conditions. The influences of lung afferents and particularly nonrespiratory related feed-forward information modify the basic pattern. During much of human activity involving speech, pattern formation makes major modifications to the timing and volume determined by the basic pattern.

Drive integration pulls together the multiple, sometimes conflicting, demands on the breathing apparatus. It is at this level that the respiratory-related chemoreceptor inputs enter the scheme. These must be integrated with additional physiologic inputs (e.g., nociceptive inputs, hypothalamic inputs for temperature regulation, etc.) that will change the pattern of breathing. Drive integration can modify both the ventilatory pattern generation as well as the pattern formation. The same minute ventilation can result from different patterns of breathing and thus the drive input must modulate the ventilatory pattern generator as well as the pattern formation.

Besides integration of external inputs, there are several factors that seem to be related to previous conditions and levels of excitation of the controller. These have been extensively studied by Eldridge and Millhorn (76,180,181) and others (8,92). The most important of these phenomena seem to be short-term facilitation (also called "afterdischarge") and long-term facilitation. In many clinical and experimental situations, (76,96,255) ventilation does not immediately return to normal after a period of hyperventilation. Rather, after an initial fast decrease, it returns to the chemoreceptor-determined values with a time constant of approximately one minute. These "neural dynamics" may be caused by intrinsic neural firing patterns or may be related to transmitter/receptor changes that occur with increased stimulation. This phenomenon has been termed short-term potentiation.

In contrast, long-term potentiation refers to a longer-lasting (>30 minutes) increase in ventilation that occurs after activation of ventilation specifically by the peripheral chemoreceptors. This has been observed in anesthetized cats (180,181) and awake dogs (39). In the cat, a serotonergic mechanism (see below) has been postulated (180), but there are other possibilities (39). If the finding in dogs (39) that repetitive hypoxia can induce this

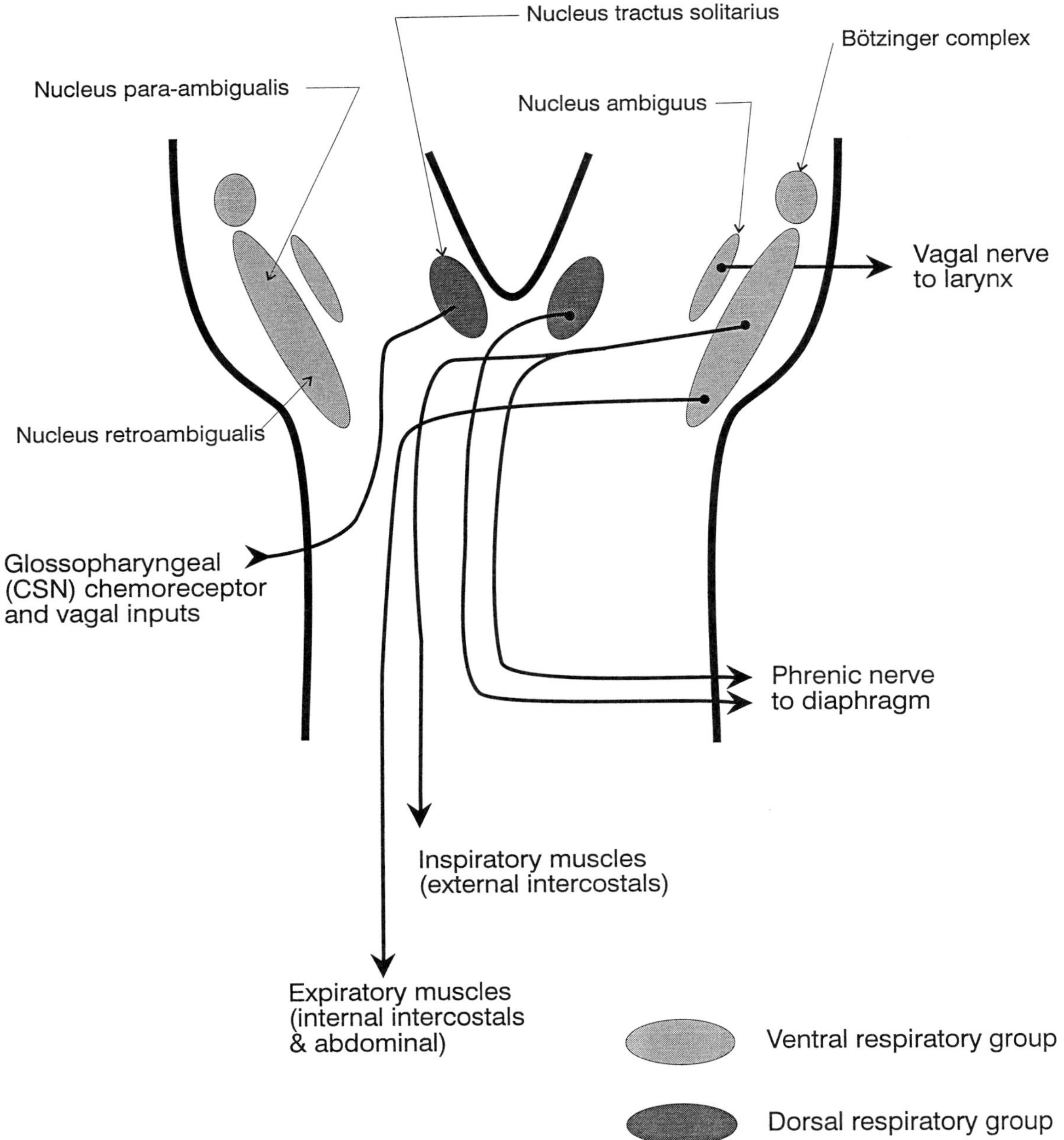

Figure 2. Schematic diagram of the anatomic medullary brain stem centers showing the connections to the respiratory muscles and the afferent connections. The interconnections between the centers are not shown. (Modified from refs. 191 and 269.)

mechanism applies to humans, then the results may have relevance to the repetitive hypoxia seen in sleep apnea (298) and during sleep in the postoperative period (42,226,288).

Afferent Information

The brain stem controller receives information from a variety of sources. Some of these involve the relatively straightforward chemoreceptor signals that provide closed-loop information on the gas exchange functions of the lung. These signals arise primarily from the central and peripheral chemoreceptors that mediate the response to hypoxia, hypercapnia, and acidemia. Because the stimuli can be relatively unambiguously defined, these reflexes have been extensively studied. However, there are many other inputs that, at various times, have pivotal roles in determining ventilatory drive. The interaction of these various stimuli are important for the short- and long-term responses of the ventilatory system. Mitchell et al. (182) have reviewed how the different sensory inputs to the ventilatory controller interact. They defined five interactions: (a) algebraic, (b) closed-loop, (c) neural, (d) mechanical, and (e) adaptive.

The states of cortical arousal and of emotion play important roles in the level of resting ventilation as well as the responses to other stimuli. This has been extensively studied in terms of sleep state (see below). The control of ventilation during exercise and during changes in metabolic rate involve afferent information from body temperature and a wide variety of joint, muscle, and nociceptive receptors. It is not known if these receptors have specific connections to ventilatory control centers or are less specifically coupled via the reticular activating network to the brain stem center (see below).

There are important receptors in the lung and the upper respiratory tract that provide afferent information to the respira-

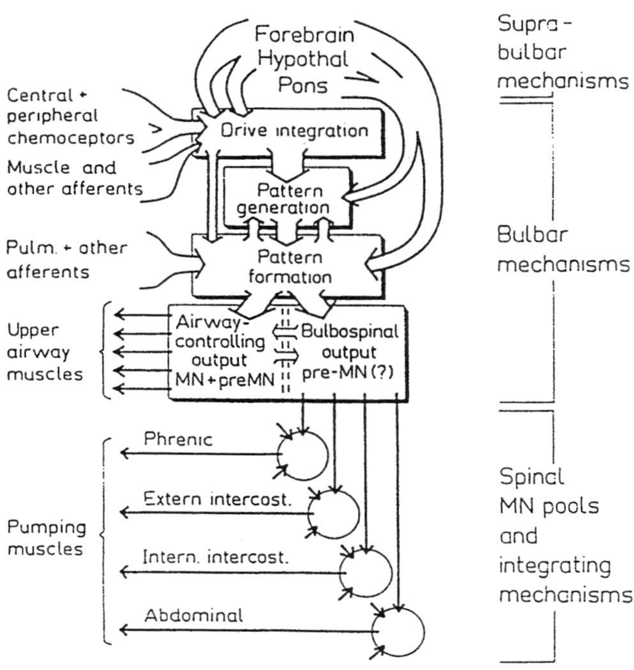

Figure 3. Functional organization of the central neural controller. The three main elements of the generation of respiratory rhythm, drive integration, pattern generation, and pattern formation, are shown. The important interconnections to the motoneuron pools for the airway and the pumping muscles are indicated. (From refs. 270 and 271, with permission.)

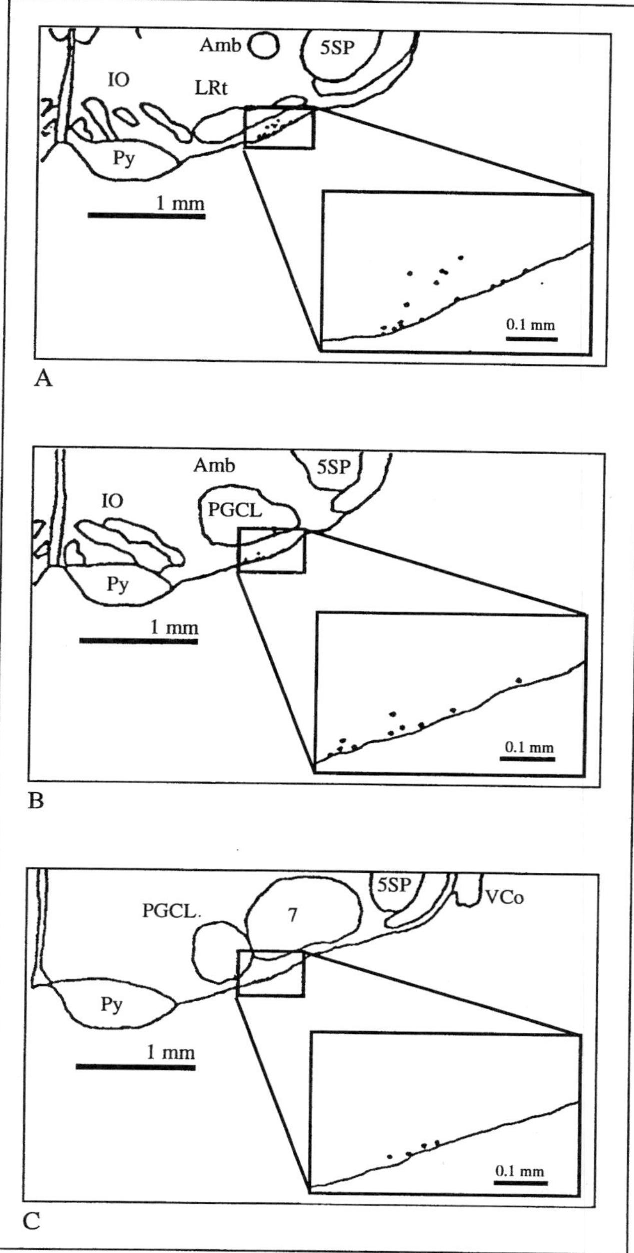

Figure 4. Distribution of *fos*-like immunoreactivity in ventral medullary surface in rats after breathing 13% CO_2 at 1.0 mm **(A)**; 1.75 mm **(B)**; and 2.25 mm **(C)** rostral to obex. 5SP, spinal trigeminal nucleus; 7, facial nucleus; Amb, nucleus ambiguus; IO, inferior olive; LRt, lateral reticular nucleus; PGCL, nucleus reticularis paragigantocellularis lateralis; Py, pyramidal tract; VCo, ventral cochlear nucleus. (From ref. 237, with permission.)

tory centers. This information is used in normal ventilation (e.g., vagal feedback of lung volume) as well as to initiate maneuvers such as sneezing and coughing that need to override the gas exchanging role of the ventilatory system. Finally, there is also important afferent information from other autonomic centers and from the cortex when nonrespiratory functions must override ventilatory functions.

Central Chemoreceptors Changes in the H^+ and/or CO_2 composition of the CSF and ECF of the brainstem make obvious changes to ventilation. Considerable work over the past 50 years has tried to answer two basic questions: (a) Where are the central chemoreceptors located in the brainstem? and (b) Is the chemoreceptor stimulus CO_2 or H^+ (or both) and how is the stimulus transduced to neural activity? There is still continuing interest and controversy concerning these questions and there are several recent reviews on the topic (28,36,43,132,179).

Following the early work of Mitchell et al. (185) the location of the chemoreceptors was felt to be in the ventral lateral medulla, close to the surface. These studies involved placing pledgets or perfusing mock CSF over specific areas of the brain and recording phrenic nerve activity. Subsequent studies using microelectrodes found that the NTS and the locus coeruleus (72) also show chemoreceptor activity but these areas have not been as directly related to changes in ventilatory drive. Although such functional studies have located possible sites for the chemoreceptors, no anatomic structures that correspond to chemoreception have been identified.

Recently Sato et al. (237) have used immunoreactivity to the *fos* protein product of the c-*fos* proto-oncogene to identify cells that increased activity in rats exposed to 13% to 15% CO_2. Cells expressing c-*fos* were located less than 150 μm from the surface of the VLM as well as in the NTS (Fig. 4). Since noxious stimuli can induce c-*fos* in many neurons, morphine 10 mg/kg was given to suppress the hyperactivity and increased ventilation induced by the hypercapnia. The morphine had no effect on the c-*fos* labeling in the VLM or the NTS, which may indicate that these cells are chemoreceptors. In contrast, however, Teppema et al. (264) subjected cats to 10% CO_2 for 1 hour. Expression of c-*fos* could be demonstrated only in one small region of the rostroventral medulla, namely the retrotrapezoid nucleus. Interestingly, the ventilatory response to hypercapnia appears to be very sensitive to local application in the retrotrapezoid nucleus of excitatory amino acid antagonists and to local lesions (195).

The retrotrapezoid nucleus has anatomic connections with both the DRG and the VRG (247), and the role of the NTS neurons as chemoreceptors in control of ventilation is uncertain, however, since local anesthetic applied to a specific area in the VLM blocks central CO_2 ventilatory response (160). The morphine data of Sato et al. would indicate that morphine causes ventilatory depression not because of a direct action on the central chemoreceptors as has been postulated.

Another recent study using microinjection of the carbonic anhydrase inhibitor acetazolamide to cause a local increase in H^+ found additional areas of chemoreception near the dorsal surface in the area of the NTS and the locus coeruleus as well as near the surface of the VLM (51). In a very reduced preparation (neonatal rat in vitro brain stem–spinal cord), Issa and Remmers (118), using a microinjection technique, identified areas in the medulla that were CO_2 responsive. They found a subsurface (100–350 μm) rostral-caudal column along the entire ventromedial medulla that contained CO_2 chemoreceptive elements.

There is an obvious difference between the large ventilatory response to hypercapnia and the much smaller response to infusion of a fixed acid. However, because of the blood-brain barrier and other local factors, this does not support a contention that the central chemoreceptors are sensitive to CO_2 rather than H^+. The Henderson-Hasselbalch equation relates CO_2, H^+, and HCO_3^- and it is obviously impossible to vary only one of these elements without at least one of the other two changing. Much of the evidence points to the extracellular pH, rather than CSF pH (132), in the brain as the final chemical signal that is converted to changes in neural activity [see Loeschcke (160) for a review]. Carbonic anhydrase may be playing an important role in the central CO_2 chemoreception (50). Other results have not supported a primary role for ECF H^+ but rather for CO_2 or carbonic acid (134). Indeed, several studies have shown that at the level of the medullary extracellular fluid, a given change in local pH due to a change PCO_2 has a much more pronounced effect on ventilation than a similar local isocapnic change in pH (74,242,263). Current thought may be turning toward a transmembrane H^+ gradient hypothesis, rather than the extracellular or intracellular H^+ concentration, as the transduction stimulus. Some of the controversies surrounding the central chemoreceptors are discussed in an editorial by Severinghaus (240).

Peripheral Chemoreceptors The peripheral chemoreceptors are found in the carotid bodies in humans (and also in the aortic bodies in some other species). The role played by the carotid bodies is more than simple reflex transduction of hypoxia and hypercapnia/acidosis; however, significant shaping of the neural signal occurs within the carotid body itself. The sensitivity of the carotid body (CB) to these stimuli is readily demonstrable, but the neuroanatomy of the organ is quite complex. Hence, controversy exists regarding the cells involved in the transduction process and the intracellular mechanism of the transduction process. Comprehensive reviews of the carotid body structure and function can be found elsewhere (82,83,106, 267). Figure 5 shows a schematic diagram of the carotid body.

Previously, the site of chemoreception was postulated to be the nerve endings themselves. Current data, however, clearly suggest the type I glomus cells are the actual sites of transduction of hypoxic and hypercapnic/acidosis stimuli. The type II cells are felt to play a vague, "supportive" role, similar to that played by glial cells. The actual mechanism of transduction is still an area of active research. Current theories of hypoxic transduction include oxygen-sensitive K^+ channels and Ca^{2+} release from intracellular stores (26,82,163). Work by Lahiri and colleagues (148,151) suggests that more than one mechanism may be involved. Finally, since interaction between hypoxia and hypercapnia occurs at the carotid body (149), the site(s) and mechanism of this interaction must also be explained.

After transduction in the type I cells, the stimulus signal needs to be coupled to the carotid sinus nerve endings. Rather than a single neurotransmitter, however, there are multiple inhibitory and excitatory neurochemicals in the carotid body that appear to function both as classical neurotransmitters and also as neuromodulators. Dopamine, for instance, appears to play an *inhibitory* role in modulating the carotid body (as opposed to its excitatory role in the CNS—see below), while tachykinin substance P plays an excitatory role in the carotid body (45). In contrast, the potential role, if any, of acetylcholine is unclear. Acetylcholine is present in the carotid body; muscarinic receptors are also present. And exogenous acetylcholine can activate the endogenous receptors. But acetylcholine antagonists have no effect on carotid body function (see below).

Finally, sympathetic and parasympathetic innervation may also modulate carotid body function. Thus, the variety of neurochemical mechanisms in the carotid body creates opportunity for extensive pharmacologic and pathophysiologic alterations in its function.

Effector Signals

The output from the respiratory centers must be highly coordinated to achieve effective ventilation. Although the phrenic nerve to the diaphragm is usually thought of as the primary efferent, the intercostal muscles, abdominal muscles (during forced expiration), other accessory muscles, bronchoconstrictor muscles, and the muscles of the larynx, pharynx, and nose are all important.

Although the purpose of ventilation is to achieve adequate gas exchange, the neural controller does not directly control alveolar ventilation. Rather, it is tidal volume (V_T) and inspiratory (T_I) and expiratory times (T_E) that are under neural control. The relationship between alveolar ventilation and these terms under direct neural control is familiar (Equation 1). Although dead space (V_d) can be altered by neural control of bronchomotor tone, usually only minute expired ventilation and tidal volume are considered to be under breath-by-breath neural control.

$$\dot{V}_A = \dot{V}_E\left(1 - \frac{V_d}{V_T}\right) \tag{1}$$

Most often minute ventilation is divided into components of tidal volume and breathing frequency (f) as shown in Equation 2. These components are readily measurable and divide ventilation into its basic components of drive amplitude and timing. It is important to note that ventilation is a multiplicative, and hence a nonlinear, function of these components. As Mitchell et al. (182) have pointed out, all three terms cannot bear a linear relationship to a stimulus (e.g., CO_2) simultaneously. However, this algebraic constraint is often overlooked.

$$\dot{V}_E = V_T \times f \tag{2}$$

Division of ventilation into tidal volume and breathing frequency, although more insightful to the neural efferent drive than just looking at ventilation, also does not reflect the true neural output. Even including the breath timing components individually and allowing for a pause in the breath time (T_P), as in Equation 3, does not directly address the issue of measuring terms reflective of the neural output.

$$\dot{V}_E = \frac{V_T}{T_I + T_E + T_P} \tag{3}$$

An alternative is to partition ventilation into average inspiratory flow and inspiratory duty cycle (fraction of the breath that is inspiration). This division (Equation 4) was proposed by Milic-Emili and Grunstein (177).

$$\dot{V}_E = \frac{V_T \wedge T_I}{T_I \times T_B} \tag{4}$$

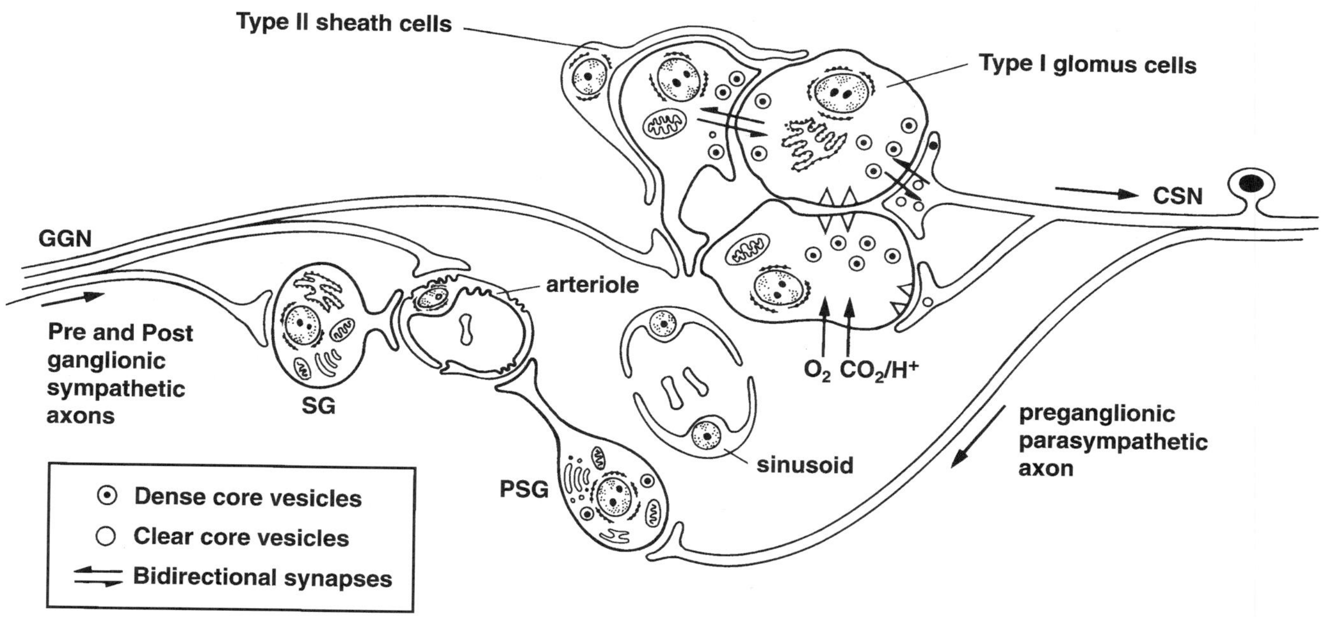

Figure 5. Carotid body structure and functional organization of neural elements. Neurochemicals found in the carotid body include substance P, acetylcholine, 5-HT, enkephalins, dopamine, norepinephrine, and atrial natriuretic peptide (see text). CSN, carotid sinus nerve; PG, petrosal ganglion; PSG, parasympathetic ganglion cell; SG, sympathetic ganglion cell; GGN, ganglio-glomerular nerve. (Modified from refs. 82 and 172.)

The purpose of this equation is to quantify the inspiratory drive. The concepts are related to the work of Clark and von Euler (49) on the relationship of inspiratory flow and the inspiratory off-switch (i.e., Hering-Breuer reflex). Clark and von Euler found that inspiration was terminated when the tidal volume reached a certain threshold. This threshold was determined by both the central pattern generator and the volume feedback from the lungs. This threshold is initially high and decreases during inspiration (i.e., a larger volume is required to terminate inspiration earlier) until a range is reached where inspiration is terminated by the central pattern generator without specific volume feedback. In awake resting humans this seemed to be the normal operating range (i.e., Hering-Breuer reflex not active in terminating inspiration). In the cat, different anesthetics affected the relative ranges differently. The slope of the inspiratory volume versus inspiratory time (V_I/T_I) appeared to be related to the central drive and was the determinate of both the inspired volume and the inspiratory time. The expiratory time was related to the inspiratory time in an approximately linear manner.

When ventilation (or even its components of tidal volume and breathing frequency) is studied, much of the detailed information that the respiratory controller must generate is lost. Control and coordination of upper airway function is an especially important role. Upper airway obstruction is a frequent and dangerous accompaniment of natural sleep as well as pharmacologically induced changes in consciousness. The specific actions that cause a preferential reduction of tone in the upper-airway muscles, more than in the main muscles of ventilation, are largely unknown.

Integrated Physiologic Responses

The respiratory controller must integrate a disparate set of inputs on a moment-by-moment basis to produce the ventilation required to provide adequate oxygen uptake and carbon dioxide elimination. Although the responses to CO_2, H^+, O_2, and exercise have been extensively studied, there are many other concurrent factors that influence ventilation. The physiology of the integrated responses has been fully reviewed in detail elsewhere (56). This section reviews important data relevant to the understanding of the neuropharmacology of ventilatory control.

Ventilatory Response to Hypercapnia and Acidosis

The increase in ventilation with increasing arterial CO_2 is probably the best studied of the ventilatory reflexes. There are many complete reviews (e.g., 56).

Both the central and peripheral chemoreceptors respond to hypercapnia. Frequently, however, the reflex is studied in hyperoxia; in humans, this markedly reduces—but does not truly eliminate—the peripheral component of the response. Under normal circumstances (i.e., normoxia at rest), the carotid body response provides only 20% to 30% of the total hypercapnic response. The carotid body response, however, is faster than the central response with a time constant of 10 to 30 seconds vs. 60 to 150 seconds for the central site (93,253). The slowness of the central response requires that hypercapnia be maintained 5 to 6 minutes in order to reach steady-state ventilation. Moreover, hypoxia increases the gain at the carotid body. Concomitant hypoxia greatly increases the carotid body response to hypercapnia. In contrast, studies in subjects who have had their carotid bodies removed show little interaction between hypoxia and hypercapnia (18,256,273). A later section discusses the relevance of these considerations to measuring the hypercapnic response.

During eucapnic ventilation, breath-to-breath variations in ventilation and P_aCO_2 do not appear to be tightly coupled. This implies that P_aCO_2 is not a particularly dominant stimulus at the resting level, and that other factors sustain ventilation in this situation. Indeed, below the eucapnic CO_2 level, the controller is only weakly responsive to changes in P_aCO_2. It is not until CO_2 rises above the eucapnic level that ventilation has an apparently linear relationship to P_aCO_2 (56).

The hypercapnic response is usually described by a slope ($l \cdot min^{-1} \cdot mm\ Hg^{-1}$) and an intercept. The intercept may be given as the intersection of the response line with either the CO_2 or the ventilation axis. However, since these intersections must be obtained by extrapolation outside the physiologic range, often an intercept within the hypercapnic range of interest is given.

At the chemoreceptor level, there has been considerable controversy over whether the stimulus is CO_2 or H^+. Hypercapnia stimulates both the central and peripheral chemoreceptors. A decrease in arterial pH also stimulates the peripheral chemoreceptors strongly, but the environment of the central chemoreceptors is less accessible to changes in blood H^+. However, decreases in ECF pH also stimulate ventilation. During metabolic acidosis this effect is not immediate and the changes in CO_2, which is more freely accessible to the CSF, must be taken into account.

The ventilatory response to hypercapnia is frequently used as a test of drug-induced ventilatory depression. However, the normal range of responses is very wide. Frequently, a quite large and statistically significant reduction in the slope results from a drug treatment, but the value is still within the normal range. How much the slope can be depressed without ventilatory failure is unknown and thus it is difficult to give a clinical interpretation to the reduced slope. A clearer indication of ventilatory depression is a concomitant increase in resting CO_2 and reduction in alveolar ventilation. Still, this also must be interpreted in light of the observation that normal sleep increases the P_aCO_2 by 3 to 7 mm Hg (211,212).

Hypoxic Ventilatory Response

The ventilatory response to hypoxia has been the subject of extensive physiologic study, particularly with regard to acclimatization to high altitude (284). This section discusses the effects of acute hypoxia, that is, hypoxia of no more than 0.5 to 1 hour. Longer periods of hypoxia have additional effects that are particularly relevant to altitude acclimatization. Since the discovery of the peripheral chemoreceptors, much work has focused on the ventilatory stimulating effects of hypoxia arising from the carotid body. However, acute hypoxia actually seems to elicit three distinct ventilatory responses: the rapid stimulation of tidal volume and respiratory rate by reflexes arising from the peripheral chemoreceptors; depression of tidal volume by action on the brainstem; and further stimulation of breathing frequency by actions on suprapontine structures. Although the initial stimulatory response is consistent under most experimental conditions, the magnitude and timing of the subsequent effects vary greatly with species, age, state of consciousness, and other experimental conditions [see Neubauer et al. (197) for a recent review]. When present, the depression of tidal volume with sustained hypoxia counteracts the initial stimulation and causes a substantial "roll-off" in ventilation. Figure 6 illustrates the ventilatory response, in human subjects, to four different levels of isocapnic hypoxia. The ventilatory response to hypoxia ultimately depends on complex interactions of several competing effects: stimulation of the carotid bodies, stimulation and/or depression of cortical and brainstem neurons, alterations in cerebral blood flow, and changes in cerebral metabolic rate. Many of these responses are mediated by neuromodulators, including monoamines, neuroactive peptides, and amino acids (45).

In intact animals and humans, the hypoxic ventilatory response is initially dominated by the acute increase in ventilation mediated by the peripheral chemoreceptors. This initial, peripheral response to acute hypoxia is a curvilinear function of the P_aO_2. There is little increase in ventilation until the P_aO_2 decreases below 70 to 80 mm Hg and then large increases occur with only small additional decreases in P_aO_2. The relationship has been described variously as an hyperbola (with and without a fixed asymptote), as exponential, or as linear with a change in hemoglobin oxygen saturation. Since there is no physiologic basis for one mathematical form over the others, and the models all fit the data equally well, the linear with saturation form is frequently chosen (144,219). However, it is important to note that the carotid bodies respond to P_aO_2 and not to arterial hemoglobin O_2 saturation or O_2 content. The increase in ventilation with decreasing P_aO_2 is very dependent on the P_aCO_2. The combination of hypoxia and hypercapnia (asphyxiation) is an extremely powerful stimulus to ventilation. The use of isolated brainstem perfusion in cats has helped clarify the central and peripheral interactions of both hypoxia and hypercapnia (24,265). The positive interaction between O_2 and CO_2 is very important and measurement of the carotid sinus nerve firing has shown that this interaction takes place at the carotid bodies.

Studies in awake animals and humans have shown that following the initial response to acute hypoxia, there is a subsequent decline in ventilation to a final steady-state ventilation that is intermediate between the peak hypoxic and the prehypoxic ventilation. This hypoxic ventilatory decline (HVD) is seen in adult humans when awake (70) or asleep (48). In human neonates, the decline can be larger with the sustained hypoxic ventilation decreasing below normoxic ventilation (55). Following bilateral neck dissection (188) or bilateral carotid endarterectomies (273), adults have lost their acute hypoxic response, but their ability to sustain ventilation during longer hypoxia was not studied. Interestingly, some studies in awake cats using a reduction in inspired oxygen have found that HVD is significant (268), but others using carbon monoxide have found a tachypneic response that was related to a suprapontine effect (94,95). Awake cats that, when intact, showed substantial HVD with hypoxia (ventilation returning to baseline with sustained hypoxia) show neither stimulation nor depression with sustained hypoxia following bilateral CSN section (161). In awake, resting humans, the actual magnitude of the HVD is quite variable, perhaps due to the additional effects of hypoxia on suprapontine structures. Perhaps as "alertness" increases, either in awake animals such as the goat (60) and dog (40) or in exercising humans (204,280), suprapontine effects predominate (primarily resulting in a progressive tachypnea) and no "roll-off" in ventilation with sustained hypoxia is seen. The reasons for these variable responses are not known but may be related to multiple effects of hypoxia with the results being dependent on how these oxygen-dependent ventilatory drives interact; it is doubtful that the interaction is solely and purely additive (130,203). Thus, for example, in some situations a peripheral input may be necessary for the central depressant effects of hypoxia to fully develop (15,161,203).

In anesthetized animals, the predominant central effect of hypoxia is a decrease in ventilation mediated primarily by a decrease in tidal volume. In cats, this has been demonstrated by the use of artificial brainstem perfusion (265,279), by peripheral denervation (5,268), and by carbon monoxide inhalation (94,198). Vizek et al. (268) found in anesthetized cats that the decrease in ventilation was accompanied by a decrease in phrenic nerve firing while carotid sinus nerve activity remained constant. This indicates a central effect of hypoxia in causing ventilatory depression without any adaptation at the peripheral chemoreceptors. However, Andronikou et al. (5), also using anesthetized cats, found no decrease in ventilation with sustained hypoxia, unless both carotid sinus nerves were sectioned. These somewhat conflicting studies are consistent in demonstrating a central depressant effect of hypoxia.

The mechanisms for the development of HVD are not fully understood. There remains considerable controversy about the relative roles of cerebral blood flow (CBF) and the Haldane effect. Both increased CBF (due to hypoxia) and a shift in CO_2 binding to hemoglobin would decrease the effective CO_2 tension at the central chemoreceptor. Most investigators, however, ascribe the major role to neuromodulators. Neubauer et al. (197) discuss these issues in detail and have classified central hypoxic depression into three types: type I, during mild hypoxia, most likely due to the increase in CBF; type II, during

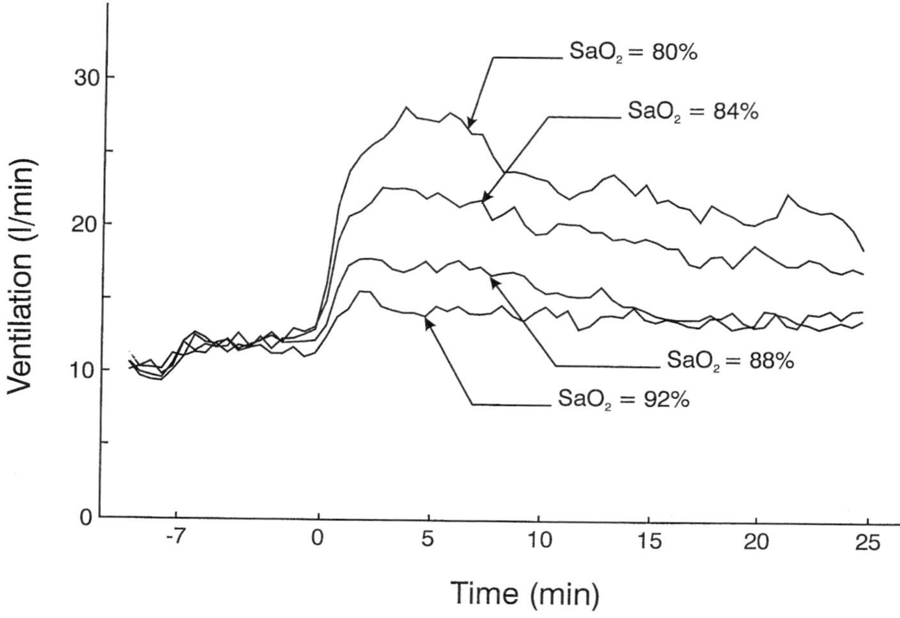

Figure 6. The biphasic ventilatory response to a 25-minute step of sustained isocapnic hypoxia starting at time zero with arterial oxygen saturations of approximately 92%, 88%, 84%, and 80%. Each curve is the ensemble average of experiments in the same eight subjects. (Modified from ref. 262a.)

moderate hypoxia, due perhaps to alterations in the balance between excitatory and inhibitory neuromodulators; and type III, during severe hypoxia, where the actual cellular metabolic process is disrupted. Endogenous opioids, adenosine, and GABA have all been studied as possible modulators of type II depression. On the other hand, Van Beek et al. (265) have shown that HVD does not reduce the slope of the CO_2 response, although the intercept is raised, suggesting that hypoxia causes a shift like that caused by an alkalosis of the CSF. This suggests the possibility of some relationship to the acid secretion in the ventrolateral medulla during hypoxia, as also suggested by Xu et al. (291,292).

Nonchemoreflex Responses

Exercise and Changes in Metabolic Rate Exercise requires more than a tenfold increase in requirements for oxygen delivery and carbon dioxide elimination. The ability to meet these requirements is one of the major, if not the most important, roles for the ventilatory controller. Since there are only small stores of oxygen in the body, without an increase in ventilation, even moderate exercise would quickly exhaust these stores and the P_aO_2 would be quickly reduced to the point of loss of consciousness. Perhaps for this very reason, the ventilatory response to exercise is very robust and determined by many highly redundant factors. Explaining the response to exercise has been one of the main problems in respiratory physiology throughout the 20th century. There is an extensive literature on this subject and many good reviews are available (e.g., 283).

The simple reflex view of ventilatory control is inadequate to explain the ventilatory response to exercise. At the onset of mild to moderate exercise, the P_aCO_2 hardly deviates; yet, ventilation increases severalfold. This remarkable coupling between ventilation and carbon dioxide production is clearly independent of any "error signal" from the chemoreceptors.

There are few studies of drug effects on the exercise response. Those that have been performed indicate that the exercise response is quite robust (235,282).

Sleep and Wakefulness Wakefulness and sleep have profound effects on ventilatory control (86,211,212), and state of consciousness interacts with other ventilatory drives. Fink (86), in 1961, postulated a separate ventilatory drive that was active during wakefulness and was absent during sleep. This results in ventilation during sleep being essentially completely dependent on chemoreflexes. The awake and sleep states also appear to modulate the chemoreceptor inputs and, during REM sleep, the output to the muscles involved in ventilation (including the muscles of the upper airway) (221). Finally, state of consciousness affects the ventilatory effects of many drugs. This has been clearly shown in the case of morphine (90), and similar principles may also explain conflicting studies of inhalational agents (223). Many drugs used in anesthesiology cause hypnosis and it may be difficult, even if desirable, to separate a specific ventilatory effect from a more indirect effect resulting from sedation.

Nociception Although it is a common observation that painful stimuli increase ventilation, it is less certain how this nociceptive input is integrated with other ventilatory drives. Bourke (34) studied the effects of relieving acute pain from upper extremity injury with a lidocaine axillary block anesthetic. Only four subjects were studied but there was a statistically significant decrease in the slope of the hypercapnic response and a shift to the right. However, the change in slope was small (a 24% decrease) and the decreased slope was within the normal range. Resting ventilation decreased and $P_{ET}CO_2$ increased slightly, but neither was statistically significant. The pattern of breathing did change significantly to a slower frequency with a larger tidal volume. The change in the hypercapnic response slope would indicate an interaction with the chemoreflexes and not just an additive input. In contrast during enflurane anesthesia, surgical stimuli shifted the hypercapnic response to the left without a change in slope (227). However, the slope was already markedly decreased by the enflurane. With 1.1 MAC enflurane, Lam et al. (155) found that surgical stimulation did not increase the anesthetically depressed hypercapnic or hypoxic responses.

Methodologic and Experimental Considerations

Considerable controversy surrounds many respiratory physiology studies because very few studies are performed under conditions similar enough to allow direct comparison. There are several reviews and book chapters that address some of these issues (44,56,162,176,218,239). Added difficulties are encountered when a drug effect is studied (125).

Three essential issues must be addressed in human studies. (a) What is the ventilatory stimulus to be studied and how are the other factors that effect ventilation to be held constant? (b) What output of the ventilatory controller is to be measured and how is this measurement to be made? (c) How is a consistent drug effect to be achieved and how is that effect to be isolated to the ventilatory controller? There is no consensus on the answers to these issues. Consistency of experimental conditions is the prevailing theme. Attention must be paid to extraneous discomforts (full bladder, cold drafts, etc.) as well as to discomforts arising from the experimental situation (anxiety, nose clips, whispering, etc.) (44,125,239). Similar circumstances also should be assured between control and test experiments (e.g., open or closed eyes, music versus quiet, light versus dark, etc.) (44,56,86). When studying women on multiple occasions, it is probably necessary to coordinate study days with the phase of the menstrual cycle.

Even with careful control of experimental conditions, however, there is considerable variability in ventilatory measurements, both between different subjects and between repeated tests on the same subject. Sahn et al. (231) repeated hypoxic and hypercapnic tests over a 2-hour period and also on different days in a group of seven subjects. The coefficient of variation over 2 hours for the hypercapnic response was 17.9% and for the hypoxic response was 19.4%. The variation between days was larger in all but one subject. Such large variability makes it difficult to detect small drug effects, particularly when comparisons are made across days. If at all possible, drug effect studies should be done with the control and the drug condition on the same day. Finally, many drugs of interest to anesthesiologists cause hypnosis. If a change in consciousness occurs, then additional changes in ventilatory drive may be found (90). There is still considerable current controversy over the proper interpretation of drug studies when hypnosis is present (223).

This section reviews some of the methodology available for human experiments. Obviously a much greater range of invasive experiments is available in animals. For clinical purposes, however, ventilatory control must be understood and measured in humans.

Resting Ventilation

Measurement of resting ventilation, with or without simultaneous blood gas measurements, is a very common way to assess a drug's effect on ventilation. However, this is not a very sensitive test. At rest, the effect of a drug is distributed across two parameters, ventilation and P_aCO_2. As a result, neither measurement may show a statistically significant change (103,136). A more sensitive method would be to compare ventilation at a set level of isocapnia, both before and after drug administration, forcing the entire effect of the drug into a change of ventilation. Although this test is practical, and perhaps one of the most clinically useful evaluations, it is not often utilized.

There are additional limitations to solely using resting ventilation as a measure of drug effect. First, little information is gained on the interaction of the drug with the various elements of the ventilatory controller. Second, the test may be a comparison between ventilation in different states. That is, when awake, the wakefulness drive may be the predominant determinate of the level of ventilation (and hence the P_aCO_2), but after a drug has induced hypnosis, the chemoreflexes (i.e., P_aCO_2 and P_aO_2) may be the principal determinates of ventilation. Thus, without appropriate precautions in interpretation, even such a simple test may give results that are difficult to interpret.

Hypercapnic Sensitivity

The ventilatory response to hypercapnia has long been used as a sensitive and useful test of the ventilatory controller. Two techniques are commonly used to assess hypercapnic sensitivity: the steady-state CO_2 response technique and variants of the Read rebreathing technique.

The stated advantages of Read's rebreathing technique include the short time required to perform it and the simplicity of the equipment involved. For these reasons, Read offered the test as a practical clinical tool (216). In reality, however, tests of hypercapnic sensitivity, including Read's, have not found a clinically useful role in practice.

Read's rebreathing test requires a small rebreathing bag (4–6 L) filled with 7% CO_2 in oxygen. The CO_2 in the bag results in a rapid equilibrium of arterial and mixed venous blood with the gas in the rebreathing bag. As a result, further increases in the $P_{ET}CO_2$ are driven by tissue CO_2 production. The oxygen (hyperoxia) effectively eliminates the effects of the peripheral chemoreceptor and the potential for hypoxic-hypercapnic interaction. As oxygen is consumed during rebreathing, the gradual increase in $P_{ET}CO_2$ on a breath-by-breath basis increasingly stimulates ventilation. Depending on the final CO_2 level, the test requires less than 5 to 10 minutes to perform. The breath-by-breath data can be fitted with a straight line by linear regression (100,101).

Steady-state CO_2 tests allow sufficient time for a constant ventilation and constant end-tidal CO_2 tension to be obtained. This must be repeated for each steady-state CO_2 level desired. To obtain the slope of the ventilatory response, at least two points must be used, and an additional point may be desirable if there is uncertainty about the factors determining resting ventilation. If a constant inspired concentration of CO_2 is used, at least 8 to 10 minutes should be allowed for steady-state conditions to be reached. If steps in end-tidal CO_2 (dynamic end-tidal forcing) are used, equilibration occurs faster, but at least 5 minutes should still be allowed (93,254).

Part of the rationale for a rebreathing test is to minimize the gradient from the point of measurement (i.e., $P_{ET}CO_2$) to the actual site of stimulation (i.e., the central chemoreceptors). End-tidal, arterial, and mixed venous CO_2 partial pressures rapidly approach equilibrium during rebreathing. This minimizes the gradient to the chemoreceptors and should also minimize effects due to other physiologic changes, such as increased cerebral blood flow (23,217). Read's original experimental study found no difference in the measured CO_2 chemosensitivity between the steady state and the rebreathing methods (216). A theoretical analysis, however, has revealed that the slope obtained by the rebreathing method could be 20% to 30% higher than that obtained by the steady-state method. This has been subsequently confirmed: both experiments and additional modeling analysis indicate that the rebreathing slope can be as much as twice the steady-state slope (23,120). This difference between rebreathing and steady-state gains many also affect the interpretation of drug studies, as can be seen in Fig. 7 (35).

Why do the two methods produce different results? The Read rebreathing method results in an initial step increase in $P_{ET}CO_2$, followed by a ramp increase, the slope of the ramp being determined by the subject's metabolic rate, lung volume, and rebreathing bag volume. Dahan et al. (57) have pointed out that the slope of the ventilatory response to the ramp is affected by the size of the initial step. They used a pseudorebreathing technique that permitted precise control of the initial step size and the rate of rise of CO_2. The measured slope was considerably sensitive to the initial size of the step. They concluded that step changes in $P_{ET}CO_2$ using the dynamic end-tidal forcing technique were the most appropriate method for drug studies. Furthermore, when a step change in $P_{ET}CO_2$ is made in normoxia, rather than hyperoxia, an appropriate mathematical model can be applied and the CO_2 gains of both the central and the peripheral chemoreflexes can be determined (18).

An additional technique, the use of a single breath of CO_2, has also been advocated occasionally. This test is subject to con-

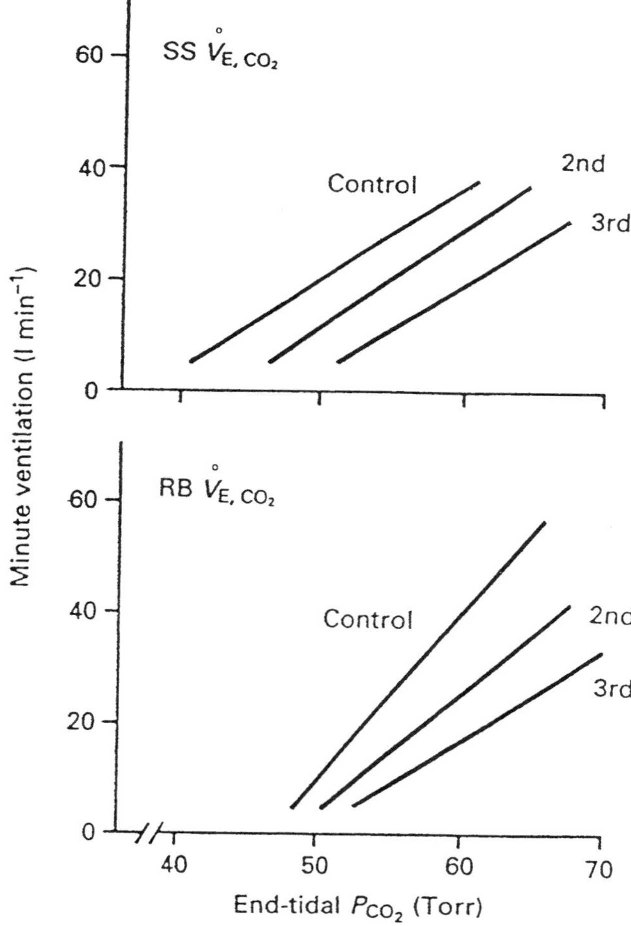

Figure 7. Comparison of hypercapnic ventilatory responses determined by the steady-state method *(top)* and the rebreathing method *(bottom)*. Control line is prior to morphine administration, 2nd line is after 0.07 mg·kg^{-1}, and 3rd line is after an additional 0.14 mg·kg^{-1} of morphine. The rebreathing method showed both a displacement and a decrease in the slope while the steady-state method showed only a shift without any change in slope. (From ref. 35, with permission.)

siderable experimental uncertainty (131), but does offer a measure of peripheral CO_2 sensitivity that may be useful in drug studies (170).

Hypoxic Sensitivity

The hypoxic response is also important clinically and various tests have been devised to measure it (44,218,219,239,241,286). There are several essential elements to an hypoxic ventilatory test. The first is the importance of maintaining isocapnia since only 1 or 2 mm Hg of change in the P_aCO_2 will greatly change the hypoxic ventilatory response (56,219). While this is particularly important during an hypoxic test as the hyperventilation induced by the hypoxia will lower the CO_2, reducing the ultimate response, it is also important when comparing hypoxic tests made under different conditions. This presents a particular problem when drug effect studies are performed since the drug may change the baseline P_aCO_2. In this situation, to have a comparison of the isolated effects on the hypoxic response, the control test would have to be the matched CO_2 level that would be anticipated to occur after the drug. An alternative would be to perform both the control and postdrug tests in hypercapnia, but this presents a problem in interpretation, since the drug may affect the hypercapnic portion of the response.

A common hypoxic test is similar to the rebreathing test for hypercapnia and uses rebreathing to lower the oxygen level while either variable CO_2 absorption or addition of CO_2 to the circuit is used to maintain isocapnia. While this test may be relatively simple to perform, there is no standardization of the rate at which the hypoxia is induced. Computer control of the composition of the fresh gas flow to an open breathing circuit has also been used to achieve breath-by-breath control of both the end-tidal CO_2 and O_2 (15,261). In either case, the length of the hypoxic test is important since central depression of ventilation begins within 5 minutes of the initiation of sustained hypoxia (70,286). In 1972 Kronenberg et al. (144) were perhaps the first to address this issue. They compared hypoxic responses as measured by (a) performing an hypercapnic response in hyperoxia and hypoxia; (b) hypoxia induced over 3 to 4 minutes at two different CO_2 levels; and (c) single vital capacity breaths of a hypoxic gas mixture. They noted that HVD occurred in some subjects in both tests a and b, and they commented that longer hypoxic ramp tests as commonly performed would presumably be more susceptible to the effects of HVD. A direct comparison of ramp and step hypoxic tests reached similar conclusions (262).

Since hypoxia is very common postoperatively, it is important to be able to assess the effects of drugs on this protective reflex. However, there is currently no consensus on the best test of the hypoxic ventilatory response that will be predictive for the clinical situation.

PHARMACOLOGY OF THE NEURAL CONTROL OF BREATHING

Amino Acid Neurotransmitters

Strictly from a quantitative standpoint, the amino acids are probably the major transmitters in the mammalian CNS, while the better-known transmitters (acetylcholine, norepinephrine, dopamine, histamine, and 5-hydroxytryptamine) probably account for transmission at only a small percentage of central sites. However, since amino acids are also involved in intermediary metabolism, it has been difficult to sift out their role solely as neurotransmitters in the mammalian CNS. Nevertheless, several amino acids are clearly major neurotransmitters. On the basis of neurophysiologic studies, these have been separated into two general classes: excitatory amino acids, which depolarize neurons in the mammalian CNS; and inhibitory amino acids, which hyperpolarize mammalian neurons. See Cooper et al. (53) for an excellent review of these neurotransmitter systems.

In general, the amino acid neurotransmitters appear to affect ventilation much as they affect basic neuronal function: excitatory amino acids stimulate ventilation, and inhibitory amino acids depress ventilation. Among the common excitatory amino acids in the mammalian CNS are aspartic acid, glutamic acid, cysteic acid, and homocysteic acid, and among the inhibitory amino acids are γ-aminobutyric acid (GABA), glycine, taurine, and alanine. While many of these have been shown to produce respiratory effects (191), recent widespread interest has focused on two, glutamate and GABA, as particularly relevant to control of breathing. Glutamate and GABA produce opposite and profound effects on respiratory and cardiovascular functions at several discrete sites on or near the surface of the medulla (128,197). They may also have indirect effects on ventilation via connections from the pons, hypothalamus, locus coeruleus, and cerebral cortex. Data on their release at the synaptic level within the medulla are lacking, however. Thus, our understanding of the precise role of amino acids in control of breathing necessarily remains somewhat speculative.

The results of the GABA and glutamate experiments reviewed here largely represent animal experiments, with a few extensions into human correlates. However, given the ubiquitous nature of these two substances in the CNS, as well as the number of anesthetics that interact with these neurotransmitter systems (particularly GABA), the role of amino acids in control of breathing deserves particular attention.

Classification of GABA and Glutamate Receptors

Both glutamate and GABA are derived from a third amino acid, glutamine, and the metabolism of the three is intricately interrelated (53). Virtually every neuron of the mammalian brain is responsive to GABA (258). However, because GABA receptors obey the principle of divergence in neurotransmitter action, GABA may have different actions depending on the nature of the postsynaptic receptors. Recent studies have demonstrated two functionally distinct GABA receptor types. A bicuculline-sensitive GABA receptor modulates chloride ion permeability and has been termed the GABA-A receptor. A second, bicuculline-*in*sensitive GABA receptor modulates potassium ion permeability and has been termed the GABA-B receptor. Activation of GABA-A receptors by synaptically released GABA is responsible for the fast inhibitory postsynaptic potential, whereas activation of GABA-B receptors underlies a much slower and longer lasting inhibition. The two receptors are not only functionally distinct, but they also belong to separate classes of receptor families and have distinct distributions within the CNS. The GABA-A receptor is a ligand-gated ion channel, whereas the GABA-B receptor is a G-protein–coupled receptor (258). In terms of breathing, most work suggests that GABA-A receptors modulate tidal volume, whereas GABA-B receptors may possibly modulate breathing pattern or frequency (210,260).

The distribution of GABA within the brain varies, with high concentrations in several brainstem nuclei, but only average concentrations within nuclei relevant to respiratory control such as the parabrachial nuclei, NTS, and LC. Animal experiments indicate that GABA mechanisms are involved in other brainstem autonomic functions as well, including thermoregulation and circulation. Mueller et al. (191) have reviewed these and other aspects of the GABA system. Of interest are several studies demonstrating an increase in GABA content, particularly in the brainstem, during moderate to severe hypoxia in adult mammals (287,289,290), neonatal mammals (119), and lower vertebrates (164). In mammals, the elevation of brain GABA is directly related to the severity of hypoxic exposure (290). Hypoxia causes an elevation of total brain GABA due to increased production, but also causes a large increase in effective extracellular concentration due to impairment of GABA reuptake systems (108). As a result, the possibility of GABA induced inhibition of brainstem functions may be greatly augmented during hypoxia (197). These observations, together with observations of the effect of GABA on breathing during normoxia, have led to the hypothesis that GABA may play a role in central hypoxic depression of ventilation (197) (see above).

Glutamate also occurs in uniquely high concentrations throughout the central nervous system and can exert powerful stimulatory effects on neuronal activity (53). Nevertheless, it has been extremely difficult to separate the role glutamate plays as a neurotransmitter from its role in intermediary metabolism. Glutamate is important in the detoxification of ammonia in the brain, as a building block in the synthesis of proteins and peptides, and also as a precursor to GABA (53). These numerous functions probably explain the lack of regional distribution of glutamate within the brain, which would otherwise argue against its role as a neurotransmitter. These various functions may also account for the highly compartmentalized and complex nature of glutamate synthesis and metabolism.

Recent efforts have defined three excitatory amino acid receptor subtypes responsive to glutamate. These receptors are termed *N*-methyl-D-aspartate (NMDA) and non-NMDA receptors, the latter subtype being further subdivided into quisqualate and kainate responsive receptors (53). Due to the availability of specific antagonists, the NMDA receptor is the most extensively characterized with respect to function and anatomic localization. The NMDA receptor is known to participate in long-term potentiation, epileptic seizure activity, and neuronal degeneration. Its function within the membrane appears to be regulated by a Mg^{2+} and voltage-dependent switch (53). Several lines of evidence demonstrate that central administration of glutamate produces excitatory effects on cardiorespiratory function by its action on or near the medullary surface (128). Additional studies also suggest glutamate may be a primary neurotransmitter released within the NTS in response to peripheral chemoreceptor stimulation (128).

Effects of GABA on Breathing in Animal Experiments

Early investigators studied the respiratory effects of GABA by intravenous administration. However, because GABA penetrates the blood-brain barrier only poorly, these experiments were difficult to interpret and often contradictory (191). In 1981 Yamada and colleagues (293) demonstrated in cats that intracisternal injections of GABA or muscimol (a GABA agonist) depressed tidal volume. Respiratory rate and timing remained unchanged until apnea ensued. Apnea produced by both agents was readily reversed by intracisternal injection of the GABA-receptor antagonist, bicuculline, whereas bicuculline injection alone caused only a small increase in ventilation. Subsequently, Yamada et al. (295) demonstrated that direct application of GABA to the ventral surface of the medulla produced the same effects, also reversed by application of bicuculline to the area. In 1986 Kneussl and colleagues (135) demonstrated reduced tidal volume in dogs utilizing ventriculocisternal perfusion of GABA. Moreover, subsequent perfusion with mock CSF readily reversed the ventilatory depression. These observations suggest that GABA plays a role in modulating tidal volume via a receptor at or near the surface of the ventral medulla (197).

The receptor that depresses tidal volume in these experiments appears to be a GABA-A receptor because other GABA-A agonists (260) and modulators (98,294) produce similar results, while baclofen (260), a GABA-B agonist, produces a quite different effect. Pentobarbital (294) and midazolam (98) administered to cats either systemically or locally produce a dose-dependent depression of tidal volume. Topical application of bicuculline (or flumazenil, in the case of midazolam) to the medullary surface promptly reverses these effects. In contrast, baclofen administered to the same animal model increases tidal volume, but decreases respiratory frequency, leading to a net depression of ventilation. Baclofen also causes an "apneustic" breathing pattern (260).

Finally, accumulation of endogenous GABA, as induced by the GABA transaminase inhibitor, aminooxoacetic acid, leads to respiratory depression in rats (109). There is relatively little work on the effects of GABA on the specific chemoreflexes. Peano et al. (208) and Waldrop (274) have shown that the posterior hypothalamus modulates the ventilatory response to hypercapnia through a GABAergic mechanism in anesthetized cats. Also, hypoxic ventilatory decline induced in cats by carbon monoxide inhalation (which avoids peripheral chemoreceptor stimulation) is fully reversed by bicuculline, suggesting the involvement of a GABA-A mechanism (175). It is worth noting, however, that carbon monoxide induces a substantial "left shift" of the hemoglobin dissociation curve (P_{50}=14 mm Hg) (299); thus, the brain tissue PO_2 levels in the study may have been very low and the results may or may not be relevant to more modest levels of hypoxia.

Effects of Glutamate on Breathing in Animal Experiments

Numerous investigators have shown that glutamate produces excitatory effects on several cardiorespiratory functions by its action on structures located near the dorsal and ventrolateral medullary surfaces (2,186; reviewed in 128). Application of glutamate to the ventral medulla results in prompt and reversible dose-dependent increases in tidal volume. Indeed, studies in cats, dogs, rhesus monkeys, and rats are all consistent with the concept that glutamate stimulates resting ventilation via an increase in tidal volume, with variable or no effect on frequency and inspiratory timing. Work by Nattie et al. (195) suggests that glutamate may play a role in the retrotrapezoid nucleus, modulating the hypercapnic response. In addition, glutamate has been shown to be released from primary afferent neurons, such as from the peripheral chemoreceptors, which terminate in the nucleus tractus solitarius in the dorsal medulla (6). During hypoxia or other peripheral chemoreceptor stimulation, these neurons may release glutamate into the NTS, causing an increase in ventilation. Hoop et al. (112) have shown that the rise in ventilation during hypoxia is correlated with some increase in central glutamate release and that chemodenervation significantly reduces normal (normoxic) glutamate turnover. Also, the increase in tidal volume that occurs during hypoxia is entirely prevented by ventriculocisternal perfusion of MK-801, a selective noncompetitive NMDA receptor antagonist (6). Although these observations are all consistent with the hypothesis that glutamate modulates tidal volume at a location near the ventrolateral surface of the medulla and/or that glutamate is a major neurotransmitter released in the NTS during activation of the peripheral chemoreceptors, it must be remembered that as with GABA, data on glutamate release at the synaptic level is lacking.

Role of Glutamate and GABA in Humans

Based on these animal findings, one may predict that GABA or its agonists should reduce tidal volume in humans. The effect of increasing GABA concentrations on human breathing, however, is unknown because GABA has not been injected intraventricularly in humans and intravenous GABA does not cross the blood-brain barrier. There are some lines of indirect evidence, however. Vigabatrin is a novel antiepileptic drug that is thought to exert its effect by preventing the breakdown of GABA. A study utilizing vigabatrin in humans found no effect on resting ventilation or the hypercapnic response (81). Interpretation of this experiment is difficult, however, because the increase in the brain GABA, if any, is unknown.

Many anesthetics interact with the GABA-A receptor. These include the barbiturates, benzodiazepines, propofol, and perhaps the inhalational agents (258). These are all positive allosteric modulators that should exaggerate GABAergic effects. Thus, if GABA tonically inhibits tidal volume, these anesthetic agents might be predicted to further reduce resting ventilation via a reduction in tidal volume as seen in the corresponding animal experiments. Such is indeed the case with thiopental, diazepam, midazolam, and propofol, as well as the potent inhalational gases. However, since these agents depress level of arousal (probably also via a GABAergic mechanism), it is unclear whether depression of ventilation is occurring through a GABAergic mechanism in the medulla or via depressed level of arousal per se.

The literature with respect to benzodiazepines and hypercapnic sensitivity is quite mixed. Gross et al. (104), Jordan et al. (126), Spaulding et al. (248), and Forster et al. (91) report decreases in the ventilatory response to hypercapnia after intravenous injection of benzodiazepines, while Bailey et al., (9) Cohen et al. (52), and Flögel et al. (89) suggest that this effect may be more variable. It seems probable that the depression seen at sedative doses is modest at most, the result depending on both the degree of sedation produced and the measurement technique. Propofol (29) and thiopental (29,105,138), are less extensively studied, but appear also to produce modest depression of hypercapnic sensitivity at sedative levels.

Extremely few studies have undertaken the complex examination of drug combinations. Interestingly, Bailey et al. (10) found no more depression of hypercapnic sensitivity (measured during hyperoxia) with midazolam and fentanyl in combination than with fentanyl alone (see Fig. 8). In this study, the combination of midazolam 0.05 mg/kg and fentanyl 2 μg/kg significantly increased the incidence (during air breathing) of hypoxemia (11 of 12 subjects) and apnea (6 of 12 subjects), compared to either drug alone. (The data suggest that central hypoxic depression may be more common with the combination, but this was not directly measured.) Clearly, chemical drives to breathe, such as the CO_2 response, are at best indirect measures of adequate respiratory function.

The interaction of the hypoxic ventilatory response with GABAergic drugs is less studied. Knill and Clement (138) found no effect of thiopental on the acute hypoxic response. Mora et al. (189), as well as Dahan and Ward (59), found variable or no effect of benzodiazepines on the acute response. Dahan and Ward found that midazolam exaggerated the hypoxic ventilatory decline when hypoxia was sustained, but Nagyova et al. (192) did not find this. Flumazenil alone did not change either the acute or sustained hypoxic ventilatory response (192) In contrast, Gross's group has reported significant depression of the acute response with both midazolam (4)

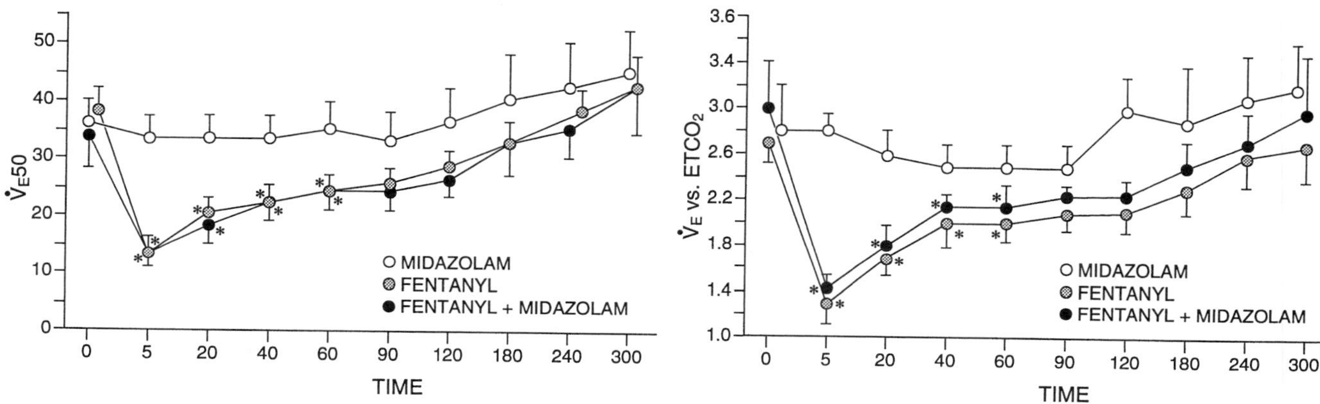

Figure 8. Effects of midazolam (0.05 mg • kg^{-1}), fentanyl (2.0 μg • kg^{-1}), and the combination of the minute ventilation at $P_{ET}CO_2$=50 mm Hg *(left)* and the slope of the HCVR *(right)*. *p<0.05 different from predrug (time zero). (From ref. 10, with permission.)

and propofol (30). Their use of an "isohypercarbic" technique, however, precludes separation of an effect on the hypoxic ventilatory response from an effect on the hypercapnic response. This is because at a constant elevated $P_{ET}CO_2$ (i.e., 46 mm Hg), the drug significantly reduces the normoxic control ventilation. The reduction must reflect a drop in hypercarbic drive. But decreased hypercarbic drive may reduce the HVR slope, just as clearly as a reduction in $P_{ET}CO_2$ would.

Finally, it should be noted that sedation induced by benzodiazepines is readily reversed by the benzodiazepine receptor antagonist flumazenil. The same, however, is not necessarily true for benzodiazepine-induced depression of chemical drive. Flumazenil only partially reverses midazolam-induced (89,104) depression of hypercapnic drive or diazepam-induced depression of hypoxic drive (189). Flumazenil does, however, "wake up" a benzodiazepine-sedated patient, and such a patient is likely to breathe more and to follow instructions.

Adenosine

Adenosine is a purine nucleoside that is found in low concentrations throughout the central and peripheral nervous systems perhaps because of its role as an intermediate in the metabolism of adenosine triphosphate. When given intravenously it is used as treatment for supraventricular tachyarrhythmias and it generally causes a reduction in blood pressure (25). However, a neuromodulator role for adenosine at presynaptic sites, postsynaptically at specific adenosine receptors, and in modulating other receptors is also likely. Since brain adenosine levels increase rapidly and dramatically during hypoxia many investigations have centered on a possible role for adenosine in the hypoxic ventilatory response particularly in neonates (145–147,190).

Maxwell et al. (168) infused adenosine at 70 to 80 $\mu g \cdot kg^{-1} \cdot min^{-1}$, which was a low enough dose not to cause symptoms or change the blood pressure. They found a small increase in resting ventilation and decrease in $P_{ET}CO_2$. They also found a significant increase in the isocapnic hypoxic ventilatory response (from a control of $-0.68 \pm 0.4\ l \cdot min^{-1} \cdot SaO_2^{-1}$ to $-2.40 \pm 1.2\ l \cdot min^{-1} \cdot SaO_2^{-1}$) without any change in the hyperoxic hypercapnic ventilatory response. This would agree with a carotid body site of action, confirming data in cats (173,228). Griffiths et al. (102) found that in patients with reduced carotid chemosensitivity following bilateral carotid endarterectomy, adenosine caused less increase in hypoxic sensitivity (as measured by a hypoxic to hyperoxic switch). Interestingly, Gleeson and Zwillich (99) found that an adenosine infusion in sleeping subjects increased ventilation slightly but caused periodic breathing that was not previously present in six of seven subjects. These periodicities were of the nonobstructive type and thus differ from the obstructive apneas seen during sleep after opioid administration. The periodicity is similar to the Cheyne-Stokes pattern of breathing of hypoxia seen in early altitude exposure in certain subjects.

Since adenosine does not readily cross the blood-brain barrier, its effects when given intravenously are predominantly from a peripheral site of action. Eldridge et al. (77) studied a long-acting analogue of adenosine in paralyzed, vagotomized, and glomectomized cats at a constant $P_{ET}CO_2$ level. They found that the analogue given either intravenously or into the third ventricle caused depression of the phrenic nerve firing (the measure of ventilation used in their preparation). The medullary extracellular fluid pH did not become alkaline as would have been expected if this was caused by vasodilation of the cerebral arterioles. Apparently, as with several other neuromodulators, adenosine has opposing peripheral and central ventilatory effects.

The ventilatory effects of antagonists may provide information on the role of endogenous adenosine. Xanthines, including theophylline, are antagonists of adenosine at therapeutic plasma levels in man. They have been used to study the role of endogenous adenosine; however, they also have inhibitory effects on cyclic nucleotide phosphodiesterase. In comparing relative adenosine antagonism and phosphodiesterase inhibition in a series of xanthines and adenosine analogues, Howell et al. (115) concluded that the respiratory effects of xanthines are more closely linked to phosphodiesterase inhibition. Nevertheless, in newborn piglets, aminophylline does reverse the ventilatory depression caused by an adenosine analogue. Another xanthine derivative, however, a weaker adenosine antagonist, does not (61). Theophylline is used clinically as a bronchodilator, and this pharmacologic effect may also be related to its adenosine antagonism. Finally, theophylline is sometimes used as a ventilatory stimulant to prevent apnea in premature infants, but this use is based primarily on empirical experience.

Dipyridamole is an intracellular uptake blocker of adenosine and thus will increase the extracellular and plasma concentrations of endogenous adenosine. It would be expected to potentiate the effects of adenosine under conditions that naturally cause its release. Although Parsons et al. (205) did not find that dipyridamole given orally had any effects on the acute hypoxic response, Yamamoto et al. (296) found that given intravenously dipyridamole increased the response. Yamamoto et al. also found that hypoxic ventilatory decline was exaggerated by dipyridamole, out of proportion to the increased acute response. This increase in HVD was attenuated by aminophylline.

Caution must be used in interpreting such results, however, as both aminophylline and dipyridamole have multiple pharmacologic effects. The result may not be due solely to the adenosine neuromodulator system. Dipyridamole is a vasodilator and also has antiplatelet activity; it is used clinically for a variety of vascular diseases.

Theophylline is often considered to be a ventilatory stimulant (233). It does increase resting ventilation, carbon dioxide production, and oxygen consumption (122). However, given orally, theophylline does not appear to augment either the hypoxic or hypercapnic ventilatory responses in several human studies (122,205,252). In contrast, intravenous aminophylline (a complex of theophylline and ethylenediamine, which increases solubility) increases the hypoxic ventilatory response but has little effect on the hypercapnic response (154,233). Since adenosine has conflicting central and peripheral effects, these differences may be related to the relative balance between these effects under specific physiologic conditions.

The effect of aminophylline on HVD has been more consistent. In cats (124), rabbit pups (229), and humans (69,97) aminophylline diminishes the ventilatory decline seen with prolonged hypoxia. This has been taken as evidence that adenosine may be a central neuromodulator of hypoxic ventilatory decline. However, it should be remembered that hypoxic ventilatory decline in humans occurs primarily via a decrease in tidal volume (rather than breathing frequency). Aminophylline attenuates the decline in ventilation by causing breathing frequency to increase during sustained hypoxia, while tidal volume remains depressed (69). This may indicate that other factors are also involved in HVD.

Opioids and Neuroactive Peptides

Although opiates (natural derivatives of extracts from the opium poppy) and opioids (synthetic compounds with activity at the same receptors that bind opiates) have dramatic effects on ventilation, there is still considerable controversy over what role, if any, natural opioid peptides play in the control of ventilation. While the endogenous opioid system has far-reaching physiologic effects, its role seems to be to provide an internal means to prevent pain from overwhelming other necessary functions (159). Perhaps it is because the endogenous opioid system is activated only in certain stressful situations that it has been difficult to delineate its role in the normal ventilatory control system. Nevertheless, the past decade has resulted in an increase in knowledge about opioid receptors and how they function in providing analgesia. Naturally occurring peptides with opioid activity include the enkephalins, β-endorphin, dynorphins, and others (191). Ligands at the endogenous opioid receptors are the most well studied and may have the greatest implication for control of breathing (41). There are several good recent reviews of opioids and ventilation (e.g., 234,243).

Various small peptides appear to function as neurotransmitters (short-acting effects at the synapse where the transmitter is released) and as neuromodulators (longer-acting effects at sites more distant from the point of release). They are frequently found colocalized with other classical neurotransmitters. Paradoxically, neuropeptides in the CNS have often been located in regions where few neuropeptide receptors exist, and vice versa. This evidence may support the hypothesis that neuropeptides exert some of their actions at sites other than local synapses. Some peptides appear to be involved especially with autonomic functions.

The discovery, in the early 1970s, of naturally occurring peptides that have opioid activity and the resulting localization and classification of receptors opened up wide avenues of research. This has led to an increased understanding of the mechanisms of action of exogenous opioids. The main opioid receptors have been classified as μ, δ, and κ, with important subtypes of the μ and κ receptors having been identified. While other receptors and subtypes have been proposed, these are the most commonly accepted. However, clinically available opioid agonists have relatively little receptor specificity. Morphine and related compounds have predominantly m activity, which is the primary receptor providing analgesia (159,206). These pain modulatory functions take place at the spinal and supraspinal levels and often act in concert with adrenergic and serotonergic systems (159). At this time, it is not known what the exact physiologic roles for the different receptors types are and how they interact.

Role of the Endogenous Opioid Peptide System in the Control of Ventilation

Opioid receptors have been found in the carotid bodies (133) as well as in the brainstem centers involved in the control of ventilation (159). In the cat, the nucleus tractus solitaris contains μ receptors; δ receptors have been found in the nucleus parabrachialis medialis (232). High densities of opioid receptors are found in other areas that have relationships to respiratory function, including the periaqueductal gray, the locus coeruleus, and the nucleus raphe magnus (7,159,206,244).

The localization of opioid receptors and opioid peptides in areas of the brain associated with ventilation suggests that endogenous opioid peptides are involved as neuromodulators in the control of breathing. Attempts to demonstrate this, however, have been surprisingly fruitless. In particular, studies using the highly specific opioid antagonist naloxone have yielded conflicting results.

Naloxone, in humans, clearly reverses the ventilatory effects of all opioids. Thus, it should reverse any tonic influence from endogenous opioid peptides. Although there is some evidence of this in the neonate (62), the evidence in adults is less than convincing. In adult humans, high doses of naloxone (50 mg) do not alter the ventilatory response to either acute hypoxia or hypercapnia (87). Similarly, during sustained hypoxia, Kagawa and colleagues (127) administered naloxone, 1.2 or 10 mg iv. As shown in Fig. 9, there is no effect on the time course of hypoxic ventilatory decline with either dose as compared to placebo. Thus, it would seem that endogenous opioids are not involved in the development of central hypoxic depression of ventilation either. On the other hand, Akiyama et al. (3) did find a significant increase in the hypercapnic hypoxic response after 3 mg of naloxone. The authors also reported a tendency for subjects with large ventilatory responses to the stimulus to have a larger augmentation of the response after naloxone. Finally, endogenous opioids do seem to blunt the ventilatory response to added external airway resistance in chronic obstructive pulmonary disease (COPD) patients, but not in normal subjects (46,236). However, recently, this too has been questioned (245).

In animal studies, relatively high doses of naloxone reverse the ventilatory depression caused by asphyxia in newborn rabbit pups (107). Lawson et al. (157) found that 0.4 mg/kg of naloxone in cats caused a small increase in phrenic nerve firing. However, experiments in which large doses of naloxone are employed in animals that have been subjected to surgery or other stressful situations must be interpreted very cautiously. Even with adequate anesthesia, surgery can induce a stress response that includes activation of the entire endogenous opioid system as well as other neuromodulator systems. The finding of an effect from an opioid antagonist, in this circumstance, may not indicate a role for endogenous opioids in the normal animal. Moreover, very large doses of naloxone may not be specific for the opioid receptor and may have effects on other transmitter systems, e.g., GABA, which could change ventilation (238).

Exogenously Administered Opioids and Opiates

If the role of endogenous opioids in ventilatory control is uncertain, it has long been known that exogenous opiates and opioids have profound effects on ventilation. Fear of ventilatory depression has resulted in many patients being undertreated for pain (1). An improved understanding of the actual ventilatory effects of systemically administered opioids can provide a better basis for their rational use.

In the normal subject, systemic opioids cause a decrease in both tidal volume and respiratory frequency. The result is a marked reduction in ventilation despite concurrent hypercapnia. Clinical "lore" holds that the respiratory rate is more depressed than is tidal volume. [This stems perhaps from the early studies of Dripps and Comroe (68) that found that intravenous morphine depressed both tidal volume and breathing frequency, but that intramuscular administration depressed predominantly breathing frequency.] Most studies in awake humans, however, have actually found the primary effect to be a reduction in tidal volume, with variable decreases in frequency (reviewed in 32,33,110). The ventilatory effects are clearly dose related, with apnea occurring at sufficiently high dosages. Once apnea occurs, the distinction between tidal volume and respiratory rate is rather academic. At high peak plasma drug concentrations, or during inhalational anesthesia, however, there seems to be more of a depressant effect on breathing frequency.

The effect of morphine on the hypercapnic ventilatory response has been repeatedly investigated with a variety of techniques (see above). A consistent displacement of the CO_2 intercept (the intersection of the extrapolated hypercapnic ventilatory response line with the CO_2 axis) to the right (toward higher CO_2 levels) has been found. This displacement corresponds to the hypercapnia seen at rest. The slope of the ventilatory response has been reported to either be reduced by 50% to 80% (110,125) or to be unaffected (35). Hypnosis may have pronounced synergistic effects (90). The measurement technique used may also change the effect of opioids on the slope. Bourke and Warley (35), after comparing rebreathing and steady-state techniques at two different morphine doses (0.07 and 0.14 mg/kg, see Fig. 7), concluded that the shift of the response was the specific opioid effect while the reduction in the slope was not.

Although the carotid body has been found to contain opioid receptors, there are relatively few studies on the effects of opioids on the hypoxic ventilatory response. The first study was by

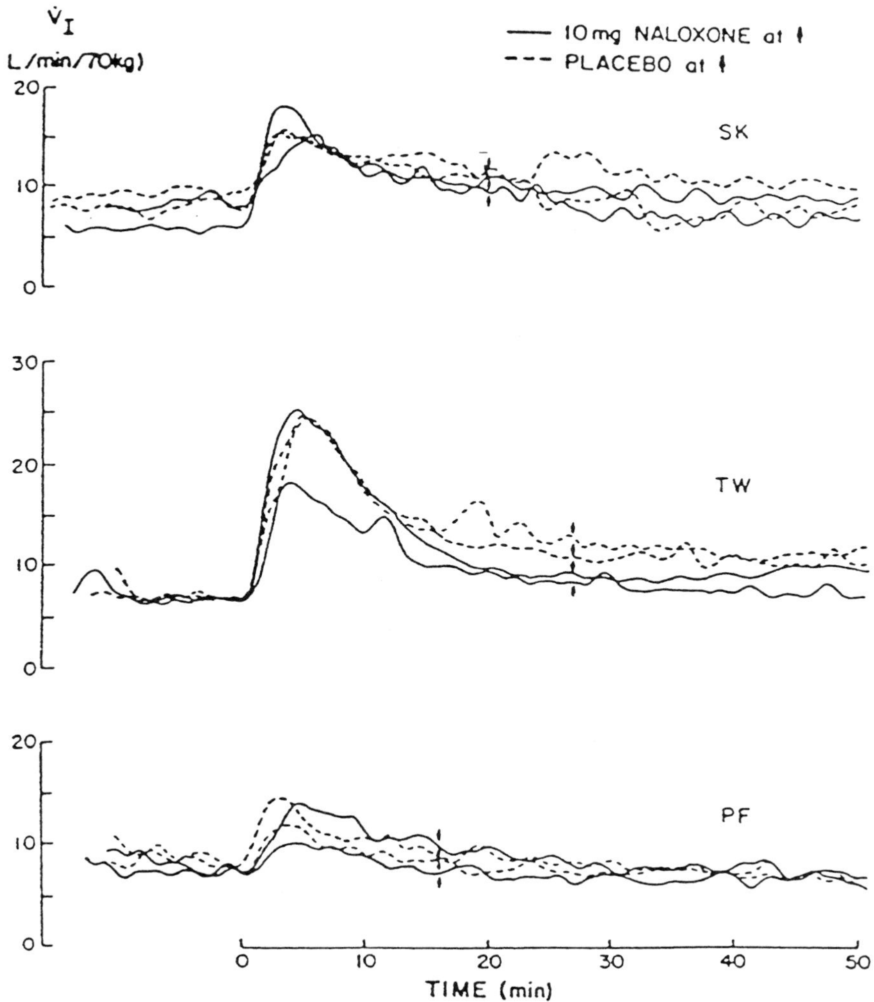

Figure 9. Time course of the ventilatory response to sustained isocapnic hypoxic in three subjects. Four experiments shown for each subject, two placebo and two 10 mg naloxone. The naloxone given after the development of hypoxic ventilatory depression did not alter the ventilation. (From ref. 127, with permission.)

Weil et al. (285), who used 7.5 mg of subcutaneous morphine in six normal subjects. The hypoxic response was measured using an isocapnic progressive hypoxia test. The resting level of CO_2 was used for both the control and the postmorphine tests and was increased by the morphine from 43 to 45 mm Hg. Despite this increase in CO_2, the hypoxic response was reduced by 60% A subsequent study by Santiago et al. (235) examined the effects of 0.2 mg/kg of intramuscular morphine on a variety of ventilatory measurements in six subjects (Table 2). In this study, at rest only, the ventilatory frequency was unaffected and both the hypoxic and hypercapnic slopes were reduced significantly. The hypoxic response was reduced even though the postmorphine $P_{ET}CO_2$ was 5 mm Hg higher. Thus, the hypoxic response seems to be depressed by morphine.

Exercise is an extremely strong stimulus to ventilation. Both morphine (235) and sufentanil (282) have been studied in normal subjects. Sufentanil causes a decrease in ventilation when given during exercise (282) and the increased P_aCO_2 caused by morphine remains elevated during exercise (235). Yet the coupling between metabolic rate with exercise and ventilation is kept relatively intact. Figure 10 shows that the relationship between ventilation and oxygen consumption was unchanged (235) in spite of a marked depression of other ventilation-related measurements (Table 2).

Table 2. EFFECTS OF 0.2 MG/KG MORPHINE INTRAMUSCULAR ON MEASUREMENTS OF THE CONTROL OF VENTILATION

	Premorphine	Postmorphine
$\dot{V}_I$ (L·min^{-1})	6.79 ± 0.78	5.06 ± 0.76*
V_T (liters)	0.68 ± 0.155	0.511 ± 0.130*
f (breaths·min^{-1})	11.5 ± 2.0	11.0 ± 1.7
P_aO_2 (mm Hg)	87.0 ± 2.0	82.7 ± 2.4*
P_aCO_2 (mm Hg)	36.8 ± 1.4	42.0 ± 1.2*
$\dot{V}O_2$ (L·min^{-1})	0.261 ± 0.021	0.226 ± 0.025*
$\dot{V}CO_2$ (L·min^{-1})	0.218 ± 0.011	0.176 ± 0.018*
$\Delta \dot{V}_I / \Delta S_aO_2$ (l·min^{-1}·%$^{-1}$)	0.500 ± 0.40	0.160 ± 0.042*
$\Delta \dot{V}_I / \Delta P_aCO_2$ (l·min^{-1}·mm Hg^{-1})	3.469 ± 1.080	1.758 ± 0.480*

Data from ref. 235, shown as mean ± standard deviation. *$p<.05$ significant from premorphine. See text.

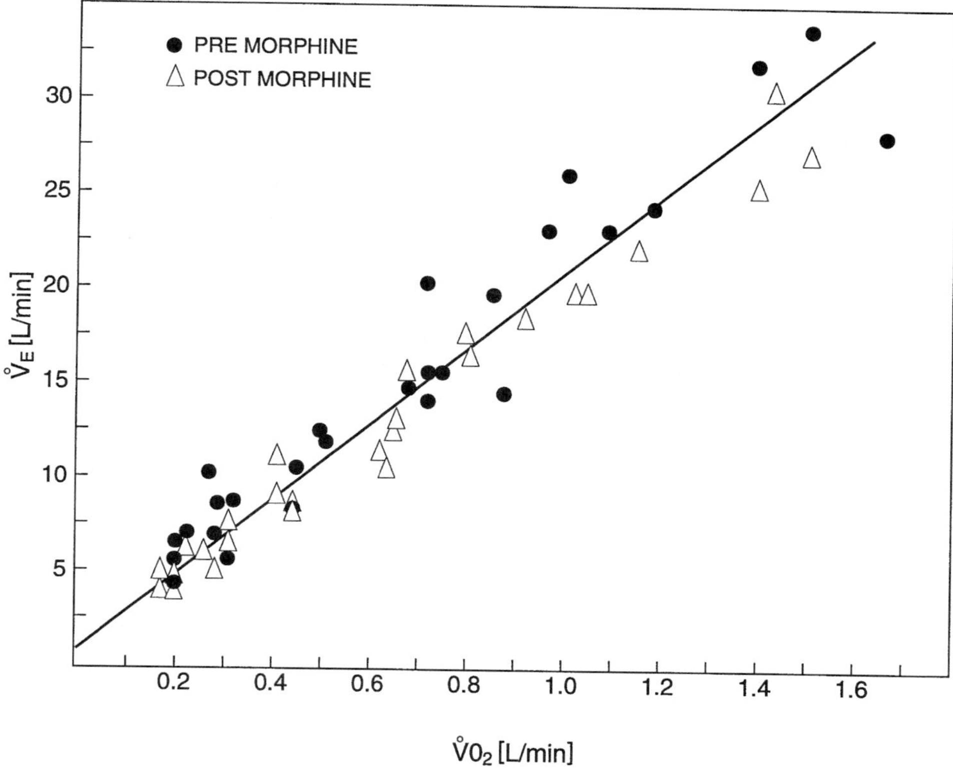

Figure 10. Ventilation versus oxygen consumption for six subjects exercising at two treadmill speeds. Data shown before and after 0.2 mg·kg^{-1} of morphine IM. Morphine did not change the relationship between oxygen consumption and ventilation. (From ref. 235, with permission.)

The interaction between sleep and opioids has important clinical implications. Forrest and Bellville (90) demonstrated that sleep and morphine have a synergistic effect on ventilatory depression. When the subjects were awake, morphine caused an increase in $P_{ET}CO_2$ of approximately 4 mm Hg, but during sleep it caused an increase of 19 mm Hg. The slope of the CO_2 response was also further depressed during sleep. These results have been confirmed by subsequent laboratory studies (142), and clinical studies have shown similar results. Catley et al. (42) found frequent central and obstructive apneic episodes only during sleep in postoperative patients receiving morphine for pain, but not in those whose pain was treated with nerve blocks. This study also found frequent partially obstructive breathing during sleep in the morphine-treated patients. Thus, morphine during sleep may decrease the hypercapnic chemoreflexes and may impair the patency of the upper airway.

Interaction with the Adrenergic Transmitter System

Many neurotransmitter systems involved in ventilatory control exhibit a high degree of interaction with one another (73,75). It would be exceedingly useful to understand these interactions since agents that affect different systems are frequently used concurrently in clinical anesthesia. There are, however, few studies of such interactions.

The adrenergic system and the opioid system appear to be especially interrelated (159,250). Interaction of these transmitter systems could take place at the presynaptic receptor, at the postsynaptic receptor, or at a second messenger level. Both opioid receptors and α_2-agonist receptors are coupled to G proteins (47). Interestingly, Vonhof and Siren (272), using a specific a_2-adrenoceptor antagonist in rats, reversed the ventilatory depression produced by a specific μ-opioid agonist, without reversing its analgesic effect. In humans, oral clonidine has been studied in conjunction with morphine (12) and alfentanil (121). Neither study found synergistic effects on ventilatory depression.

Comparison of Different Opioids Although there does seem to be some specificity of ventilatory depression and spinal analgesia to μ-1 receptors, and of supraspinal analgesia to μ-2 receptors (206), as yet there are no clinically useful opioids that are receptor subtype specific. Even with such specificity it is not yet clear that ventilatory depression can be separated from analgesia in humans. Bailey et al. (13) presented data that indicated that sufentanil produces less ventilatory depression than an equianalgesic dose of fentanyl, although the results of this study have been questioned (137). The differences in the ventilatory depression were relatively small, and of doubtful clinical significance. The opioid agonist-antagonist nalbuphine seems to cause limited ventilatory depression, even with increasing the dose, but the analgesic effects are similarly limited (224).

Epidural and Intrathecal Administration The discovery of opioid receptors in the spinal cord opened up the clinical use of neuraxial opioid administration to achieve a high concentration of the drug at an analgesia-producing site (μ-1 receptors in the dorsal horn of the spinal cord) while minimizing the concentration at the brainstem sites producing ventilatory depression. Opioids given intrathecally can still produce ventilatory depression through several mechanisms. First, nociceptive stimuli are well known to stimulate ventilation (34). By reducing the nociceptive input, neuraxial opioids may reduce the general input to the respiratory control centers. Second, systemic absorption invariably occurs, and opioids may then reach the brain stem through the circulation. Finally, the opioid may spread cephalad within the CSF itself. Incidents of delayed ventilatory depression are likely due to this latter cause. The quantity and timing of opioids reaching the brain stem via the CSF as opposed to via systemic absorption, however, is very dependent on the physicochemical properties of the particular opioid. The use of neuraxial opioids has been reviewed by Etches et al. (79).

Camporesi et al. (38) reported that 10 mg of epidural morphine causes a delayed ventilatory depression manifest as a decrease in the slope and a rightward shift of the hypercapnic response. This depression was greater than, and longer lasting than, that due to 10 mg of intravenous morphine. It started 3 hours after epidural administration, but lasted up to 22 hours. This study was in normal subjects. In postoperative patients, Doblar et al. (67) found less depression with 10 mg epidural morphine. This may again illustrate the ability of nociceptive inputs to stimulate ventilation and counter the depressive effects of opioids.

Bailey et al. (11) studied the effects of intrathecal morphine in normal subjects. After giving 0.6 mg morphine intrathecally, they found that four out of five subjects required supplemental oxygen to prevent desaturation. Maximal ventilatory depression, as measured by the increase in P_aCO_2 and the reduction in the slope of the hypercapnic ventilatory response, occurred from 6 to 10 hours after injection, and ventilatory depression remained significant for 24 hours. Much less ventilatory depression was seen with 0.2 mg.

Nociceptive input and other stimulation in the postoperative period tend to counter the depressive effects of opioids. These inputs, however, are not as effective during sleep. The combination of sleep with opioids [given systemically (42,288), into the epidural space (288), or via patient-controlled analgesia (PCA) devices (220,288)] in the postoperative period can cause dangerous levels of desaturation and may contribute to postoperative morbidity (225,226).

Other Neuroactive Peptides

Substance P Substance P was first described over 30 years ago. It is an excitatory neurotransmitter with wide distribution in the CNS. It has been especially associated with nociceptive primary afferent sensory neurons in the spinal cord. Substance P has also been found in the carotid bodies (45,215) and its concentration is known to increase in the NTS during hypoxia (158). Prabhakar (213) has recently reviewed possible roles for substance P in the carotid body. Given intracisternally, substance P stimulates ventilation (158,191).

Maxwell et al. (167) found that in humans, substance P causes an increase in the hypoxic ventilatory response, but not the hypercapnic response. However, the results of this study should be interpreted cautiously. Substance P also causes moderate hypotension, and hypotension itself may stimulate the carotid bodies. Maxwell et al. attempted to control for this hypotension by comparison with nitroprusside experiments. Unfortunately, the fact that nitroprusside stimulates the hypoxic response may not be due solely to its concomitant decrease in blood pressure. Nitroprusside also acts as a source for nitric oxide, which in turn may affect the sensitivity of the carotid bodies (214). Thus, it is very difficult to come to a firm conclusion regarding substance P in human experiments.

Somatostatin Somatostatin is a 14-amino acid peptide that was originally isolated from hypothalamic extracts. Somatostatin suppresses the release of numerous neurotransmitters, modulators, and hormones including growth hormone, insulin, glucagon, VIP, serotonin, and gastrin. A synthetic analogue of somatostatin, octreotide, has been introduced clinically and is used to treat patients with carcinoid syndrome and VIP secreting adenomas. Somatostatin and its receptors have been found throughout the CNS. The central nervous system is relatively impermeable to systemically administered somatostatin.

Maxwell et al. (166) found that somatostatin depresses the acute hypoxic response in humans, but does not change the hypercapnic response. This implies that somatostatin is an inhibitory modulator at the carotid body. Filuk et al. (85) investigated the effects of somatostatin, given intravenously to human subjects, on the prolonged ventilatory response to hypoxia. They too found a marked reduction of the initial acute hypoxic response. Moreover, after 20 minutes of hypoxia, ventilation was depressed to levels slightly (but not statistically significantly) below the prehypoxic values. Because very large doses were used in Filuk's study, a possible central effect of somatostatin should not be excluded. Neither of these studies addresses the role of endogenous somatostatin in the control of breathing. Although not explicitly studied, the clinically available somatostatin analogue octreotide would be anticipated to have similar effects when given therapeutically.

Catecholamines

The catecholamine neurotransmitters are very important and have been extensively studied in both the peripheral and central nervous systems [see Cooper et al. (53), Chaps. 9 and 10]. The principal catecholamines involved in ventilatory control are norepinephrine and dopamine. Although epinephrine has a relatively minor role in the CNS, it is very important as the principal circulating catecholamine since vascular changes can have important respiratory effects. Receptors for these transmitters are classified as alpha (with α_1 and α_2 subtypes), beta (with β_1 and β_2 subtypes), and dopaminergic (with D_1 and D_2 subtypes). Many drugs have been developed that have greater or lesser specificity to these receptors and their subtypes. This section concentrates primarily on drugs that act at the dopaminergic receptors or the a_2-adrenoceptors, as these receptors seem to have the greatest respiratory effects. Table 3 summarizes some of the ventilatory effects caused by agonists and antagonists at catecholamine receptor sites (64). Study results in intact animals may be very dose and species specific, since catecholamine agonists often have opposing effects at peripheral and control sites.

Noradrenergic System

Neuroanatomy and Neuropharmacology The central noradrenergic system has been extensively studied, in terms of its neuroanatomy and neuropharmacology (reviewed in 187). Particular attention has been focused on its role in neuroaffective disorders, and more recently on its role in the nociceptive system (159,169).

Two main areas of neuron cell bodies contain norepinephrine: a compact (in some species) group in the pons, known as the locus coeruleus, and a closely related but more diffuse group, called the subcoeruleus complex. These nuclei have extensive axonal connections both rostrally and caudally, reaching to all segments of the spinal cord. The locations of these nuclei overlap or are in close proximity to the pneumotaxic center (nucleus parabrachialis) in the pons, and extend caudally to the ventral respiratory group of the nucleus ambiguous (64). The locus coeruleus is apparently involved in arousal and sleep-waking states, with activity low in sleep (particularly REM sleep) and high during periods of arousal. Activation of the locus coeruleus increases activity in other regions of the brain, particularly in areas involved with integrating external stimuli. Suppression of locus coeruleus activity produces a behaviorally quiescent state. Some authors have ascribed a permissive or modulatory role to the locus coeruleus rather than a direct causative role in these behavioral states (251).

In many parts of the brain, the effects of the locus coeruleus seem to be coupled via β receptors (187). As discussed below, however, α_2 receptors determine the level of activity in the locus coeruleus itself (54,63). Activity is affected by a variety of external stimuli. Interestingly for ventilatory control, hypercapnia in particular causes activation, as does hypoxia to a lesser extent (72). The locus coeruleus may be the source of the arousal response seen in patients who become hypercapnic and hypoxic while asleep.

Although the noradrenergic system seems to be closely connected to the respiratory-related areas of the brain stem, many drugs affecting the noradrenergic system centrally do not have

Table 3. VENTILATORY EFFECTS OF CATECHOLAMINE AGONISTS AND ANTAGONISTS*

Receptor	Agonists	CNS effects	Peripheral effects	References
α_2	Guanabenz		↓ HVR	143
	Clonidine	± ↓ HCVR		12,121
	Dexmedetomidine	± ↓ HCVR	± ↓ HVR	17,199
β (¶)	Isoproterenol	↑ Phrenic N. firing (? β_1 receptor)	↑ CSN firing	64
D (¶)	Dopamine		↓ $\dot{V}_E$, ↓ HVR, ↓ CB HCVR, ↓ CSN firing	16,152,153, 277,278,281
	Apomorphine	↑ $\dot{V}_E$		
	Antagonists			
α_2	Atipamazole	↑ V_E		199
β	Propranolol	(?)↓ Phrenic N. firing		64
D (¶)	Haloperidol	↓ HVR		14,153
	Droperidol		↑ HVR	275
D_2	Domperidone		↑ HVR	16,123,276

*Some of the data are from animal studies, where the agonist or antagonist can be administered to either the brain stem or peripheral chemoreceptors in isolation. Since central and peripheral effects are often the opposite, the intact response depends on the relative sensitivities of central and peripheral receptors to the drug given, the particular species, and the penetration of the drug to the receptor site. ¶, receptor subtype not known or nonspecific agonist/antagonist used; $\dot{V}_E$, resting normoxic, normocapnic ventilation; HVR, hypoxic ventilatory response; HCVR, hypercapnic ventilatory response; CSN, carotid sinus nerve; CB, carotid body; ↓, decrease; ↑, increase; ±, small or variable effect.

major respiratory effects. Generally, the central noradrenergic system inhibits ventilation (75).

Norepinephrine is also found in the carotid body. The noradrenergic system seems to play a certain role in determining the carotid body response (27). This may be through direct modulation of carotid sinus nerve activity and also through vascular effects on the blood flow pattern in the carotid body.

α_2-Adrenoceptor Agonists Stimulation of central α_2-adrenoceptors causes sedation through action on the locus coeruleus (54,63). Action at other α_2 receptors, including receptors located in the spinal cord (156,257), provides analgesia. Although α_2-adrenoceptor agonists have been developed as antihypertensive agents (e.g., clonidine), their hypnotic and analgesic properties indicate a usefulness in clinical anesthesiology. Most human studies have utilized clonidine or a newer compound, dexmedetomidine. Dexmedetomidine is a full agonist at the α_2-adrenoceptor and is more specific for α_2- versus α_1-adrenoceptors than is clonidine (169).

During quiet, unstimulated breathing in humans, both clonidine (12,19,121,202) and dexmedetomidine (17) appear to cause only a small reduction in ventilation and a small increase in $P_{ET}CO_2$. The magnitude of this ventilatory depression is similar to that seen during normal sleep. This may not be surprising since the locus coeruleus is involved in the sleep/wake cycle, and the locus coeruleus may be one of the primary sites of action of these drugs.

Using the hypercapnic response as a more sensitive measurement of ventilatory depression, neither clonidine (12,121) nor dexmedetomidine (17) showed any pronounced effects. Belleville et al. (17) did not find a clear effect of dexmedetomidine on the slope, but found that the ventilation at a $P_{ET}CO_2$ of 55 mm Hg was decreased from 18.8 to 11.5 L/min after 2.0 μg/kg intravenously (see Fig 11). Bailey et al. (12) found a similar reduction after 4 to 5 μg/kg of clonidine given orally.

The effects on the hypoxic response have not been explicitly examined in humans. However, α_2-adrenoceptors have been found in the carotid body. In cats, guanabenz causes a dose-related reduction in the carotid body firing rate during hypoxia (143). However, in the dog, dexmedetomidine does not change the ventilatory response to hypoxia even in high doses (199). There may very well be a species difference in the role of α_2-adrenoceptors in the hypoxic ventilatory response.

Changes in respiratory rhythm are common during natural sleep and also during sedation with many medications. Obstructive apneic episodes are especially common in the postoperative period, and can lead to hypoxemic episodes (42,226, 288,298). Although IV dexmedetomidine is associated with brief episodes of upper airway obstruction without any hypoxemia (17), clonidine given orally (19) or epidurally (194,209) has been associated with obstructive episodes and hypoxemia, although other studies have not noted this problem (12,121). Clonidine has even been used in sleep apnea patients (117).

Dopaminergic System

Dopamine is common in the CNS as well as in many peripheral organs. Disorders of the central dopaminergic system have been implicated in the pathophysiology of Parkinson's disease and the major psychoses. Cell bodies containing dopamine are found in the substantia nigra and the hypothalamus, and they have diffuse axonal arborization throughout the brain.

Dopamine is also an important neuromodulator in the carotid body (see above). Although it was once postulated to be essential in the transduction mechanism, it now appears to function more in a modulatory role (84). Dopamine does not cross the blood-brain barrier in any appreciable amounts when given in clinical doses, and when infused intravenously, at doses that stimulate dopamine receptors but not other adrenergic receptors, dopamine reduces the chemosensitivity of the carotid body to both hypoxia and hypercapnia. Dopamine has been shown to reduce the firing of the carotid sinus nerve in cats; this effect is proportionately greater as the hypercapnic and hypoxic stimulation increases (152,153). Since dopamine is most likely contained in the glomus cells, its release is thought to reduce the firing rate of the nerve endings externally. Turnover of dopamine increases under conditions of carotid body excitation (222). Assuming that exogenous dopamine functions like

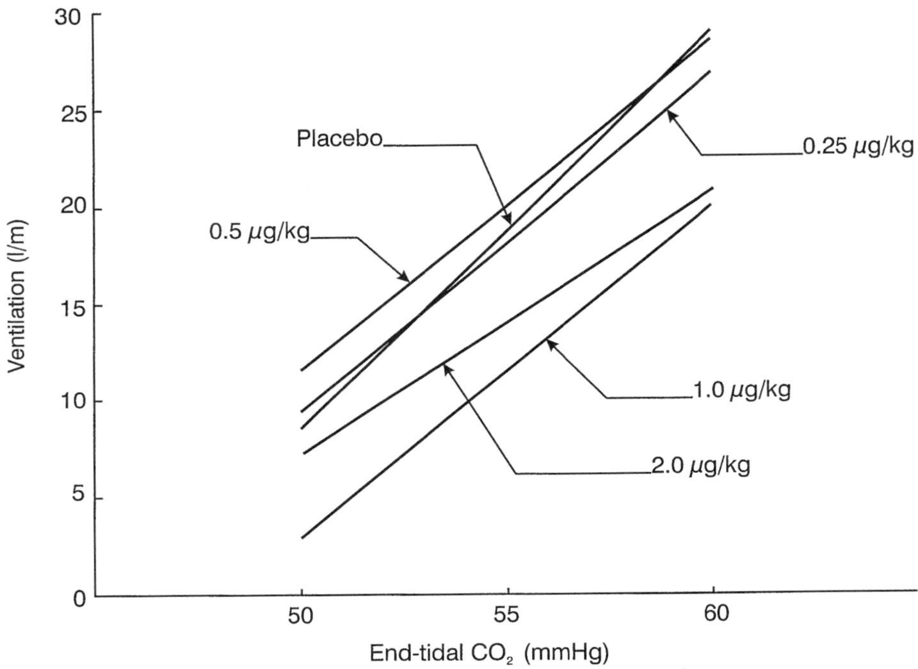

Figure 11. Ventilatory response to CO_2 at 60 minutes after placebo or four different doses of dexmedetomidine. Only the 1 and 2 μg • kg^{-1} dose groups showed a significant shift in the response. (From ref. 17, with permission.)

endogenously released dopamine, the data would indicate that dopamine plays a modulatory role; its release is stimulated by conditions that stimulate the carotid body.

The exact role for such a neuromodulator, i.e., one that decreases the sensitivity of the carotid body under conditions that arguably call for a maximum ventilatory response (e.g., asphyxia), is uncertain. It is known that increased sensitivity of the carotid bodies can cause ventilatory oscillations. Thus, a possible role for dopamine may be one of feedback compensation to prevent such oscillations. Lahiri et al. (150) found that ventilatory oscillations during hypoxia are more likely after treatment with domperidone, a peripheral dopamine antagonist.

In humans, in doses in the range of 3 to 4 μg • kg^{-1} • min^{-1}, dopamine reduces the isocapnic hypoxic sensitivity by 50% to 80% (277). Dopamine also reduces the hypercapnic sensitivity of the carotid bodies in cats (153). The carotid bodies contribute only about 20% of the hypercapnic ventilatory response (during normoxia) in humans, but this is also reduced by dopamine (278). Most, if not all, of the positive interaction between hypoxia and hypercapnia takes place at the carotid bodies; dopamine reduces this interaction as well (230).

In humans, domperidone, which does not cross the blood-brain barrier, causes an increase in the hypoxic ventilatory response (16,123), confirming a peripheral site of action for the dopamine antagonism. Since domperidone is relatively specific for D_2 dopamine receptors, this would also suggest that D_2 receptors are the predominant subtype involved. Other dopamine antagonists, including prochlorperazine (200) and droperidol (275), also increase the ventilatory response to hypoxia. Haloperidol, however, does not augment the hypoxic response (14) (but see below, and Fig. 12). Prochlorperazine also reverses the depression of the asphyxial response caused by morphine (201). Since these drugs, other than domperidone, readily cross the blood-brain barrier, the resulting effects may arise from both central and peripheral actions.

Attempts to isolate a central role for dopamine have been challenging and have often yielded contradictory results (31, 116,246). There may also be essential differences between species and/or interactions with anesthetic drugs used in the various studies. On balance, the data seem to indicate that, centrally, dopamine plays a stimulating role as opposed to its inhibitory peripheral role.

Figure 12 shows the relationship between the carotid nerve firing rate and ventilation before and after treatment with haloperidol in cats (246). Haloperidol, given after a maximal blocking dose of domperidone, paradoxically causes a decrease in the hypoxic response, although it does not affect the hypercapnic response (116). This would indicate that central dopaminergic pathways (blocked by haloperidol, but not by domperidone) normally *augment* the peripheral hypoxic response (246) (Fig. 12). Moreover, this central dopaminergic augmentation must occur *before* the peripheral pathways are integrated with the central chemoreceptor pathways since the hypercapnic response is unaffected.

Similarly, Tatsumi et al. (259) used haloperidol in cats to study the role of the dopamine in the development of hypoxia ventilatory decline (HVD; see above). After haloperidol, the initial ventilatory response to sustained hypoxia was reduced (even though the carotid sinus nerve response was augmented). HVD, however, was eliminated. In the same study, HVD did develop after domperidone administration. This experiment supports the hypothesis that central dopaminergic mechanisms are also important to the development of HVD.

In summary, in humans dopamine antagonists appear to increase the hypoxic ventilatory response. Thus, in humans as opposed to cats, the overall effects of peripheral dopamine antagonism seem to predominate over the central effects of dopaminergic antagonism. Unfortunately, this synopsis may not be true in patients without functional carotid chemoreceptors, e.g., bilateral carotid endarterectomies (188) or radical neck dissections (273). In these patients, the presumed ventilatory depressant effects of central dopamine antagonism might predominate; this has not yet been studied.

Serotonin

Cells containing serotonin, or 5-hydroxytryptamine (5-HT), have been found throughout the pons and medulla. The raphe

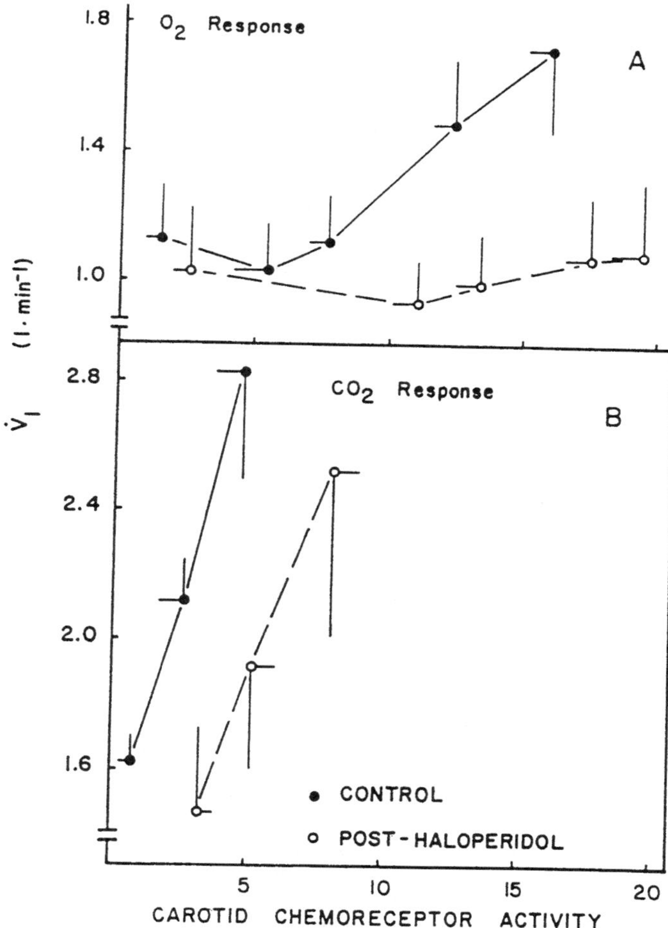

Figure 12. Effects of haloperidol (1 mg·kg^{-1} in cats) on the relationship between the steady-state ventilation and carotid chemoreceptor activity (mean ± SEM). **(A)** The relationship during normocapnic hypoxia (from *left* to *right* the points correspond to 350, 82, 67, 45, and 35 mm Hg for both curves). The posthaloperidol curve is shifted to the right (larger chemoreceptor activity for a given level of hypoxia) but paradoxically down (smaller ventilation for a given level of chemoreceptor activity). **(B)** The similar relationship for hyperoxic hypercapnia (from *left* to *right* the points are at 45, 55, and 70 mm Hg for each line). There was no significant effect of haloperidol on the slope and the ventilatory response was primarily due to the central effect of the hypercapnia. See text. (From ref. 246, with permission.)

magnus nucleus contains serotonergic neurons and has anatomical connections to the phrenic motor nucleus, the DRG, and the VRG (111). There is no particular increase in concentration of serotonin in the respiratory areas (190,191). Three types of serotonin receptors, with multiple subtypes, have been described.

Serotonin stimulates ventilation at the carotid body, but its central effects are less certain (64,191). Serotonin may be either inhibitory or excitatory in different situations. Stimulation of raphe neurons, in particular, can stimulate or depress ventilation (see ref. 114 for several references). McCrimmon and Lalley (171), using a 5-HT precursor given intravenously, found an inhibition of phrenic nerve discharge, which was overcome by hypercapnia. Hypercapnia overcame this inhibition. In different experimental models, however, 5-HT seems to have an excitatory effect on ventilation. In an extensive series of experiments Eldridge and colleagues (76) investigated the effects of brief intense carotid sinus nerve (CSN) stimulation. Immediately after cessation of electrical stimulation, the integrated phrenic nerve discharge decreased by 50% and then declined exponentially over approximately one minute. This effect has been termed "afterdischarge" or "short-term potentiation." Since it has a central origin, it is indicative of some dynamic process in the neural networks (see above). After short-term potentiation, the phrenic nerve discharge remains elevated above the prestimulation level. This residual elevation is termed "long-term potentiation." It is more pronounced after several short CSN stimulations (181). The functional role of this long-term facilitation is uncertain, but Eldridge et al. have speculated that it could be involved in the acclimatization to altitude. Subsequent investigations found that long-term facilitation was suppressed by a 5-HT receptor antagonist, by a 5-HT synthesis blocker, or by destruction of serotoninergic neurons (180).

The serotoninergic system is also closely related to the endorphin modulation of pain. The raphe magnus nucleus also contains serotonergic neurons that project descending fibers to the dorsal horn. In the dorsal horn, presynaptic release of serotonin inhibits nociceptive pathways (159). Reduction of endogenous serotonin levels antagonize morphine-induced ventilatory depression, while increased serotonin levels potentiate the depression (174). Ondansetron, a specific 5-HT type 3 receptor antagonist, does not change alfentanil-induced depression of the hypercapnic ventilation response (65).

Acetylcholine

Acetylcholine (ACh) has long been known to be the neurotransmitter at the neuromuscular junction, at preganglionic sympathetic synapses, and at all postganglionic parasympathetic fibers. Although ACh is widespread within the CNS, knowledge about many CNS pathways is still incomplete [see Cooper et al. (53), Chap. 8]. Nevertheless, ACh has been extensively studied with respect to its role in ventilatory control. In particular, ACh has been thought to play a role in the carotid body chemotransduction (82,172).

Both nicotinic and muscarinic receptors have been identified in the carotid body, but the relative density varies markedly by species (82,83). Although ACh (and nicotine) injected into the carotid artery stimulates ventilation, it is unclear whether endogenous ACh plays any particular role in the normal chemosensitivity. There does seem to be a close correlation between ACh and catecholamine release in the carotid body. Moreover, cholinergic antagonists block the effect of exogenous ACh. Still, despite considerable disparity in the literature, cholinergic antagonists do not seem to alter normal chemoreceptive responses. Of interest, though, is the observation that some neuromuscular blocking agents seem to affect the carotid body. (Neuromuscular blocking agents are active, of course, at the nicotinic receptor subtype at the neuromuscular junction, but not as active at the ganglionic or CNS subtypes.) In dogs, Bisgard et al. (27) found that d-tubocurarine, but not succinylcholine or gallamine, reduces the carotid sinus nerve chemoreceptor discharge in response to isocapnic hypoxia. Curare may have sufficient cross-reactivity to ganglionic type nicotinic receptors or the carotid body nicotinic receptors may bear a resemblance to nicotinic receptors at the neuromuscular junction. Recently, in human subjects, Eriksson et al. (78) compared the effects of partial neuromuscular blockage with vecuronium on the hypoxic and the hypercapnic ventilatory responses. The hypoxic response was much more impaired than the hypercapnic response. This implies an effect at the carotid body, and not solely at the neuromuscular junction.

The relationship between the central cholinergic system and ventilatory control is still being explored. It has long been observed that acetylcholine may play a role in central chemoreception (66,185,196). More recently, Lydic and Baghdoyan (165) presented evidence that the cholinergic system is involved in the interaction between REM sleep and ventilatory control. Important interactions also exist between the adrenergic and cholinergic systems in the ventrolateral medulla (37), an area that integrates ventilatory and cardiovascular control (179). The central ventilatory stimulating effects of salicylates may also act via a cholinergic mechanism. In dogs, atropine blocks the ventilatory stimulation induced by ventriculocisternal perfusion of sodium salicylate (88). Although anticholinergic drugs (e.g., atropine) are commonly used in the perioperative period, they do not seem to have many significant effects on ventilatory control (249).

Inhalational Anesthetics

Ventilatory effects of nitrous oxide and of the potent inhalational anesthetics are covered in recent reviews (110,207), but especially by Hornbein (113). Because of their nonspecific effect on neuronal function, it is difficult to characterize the anesthetic gases in terms of neuropharmacology or any particular neurotransmitters. Anesthetic gases also affect the neuromuscular junction and the musculature of the upper airway, rib cage, and diaphragm (see Chap. 79). Consequently, the effects of these agents on ventilation are well known, but provide little insight into the organization of the ventilatory controller, although they do reflect some common themes.

In anesthetic concentrations, all anesthetic gases depress resting ventilation. Those anesthetic gases associated with catecholamine release (ether, cyclopropane, fluroxene, and nitrous oxide) depress tidal volume and ventilation less than do other agents. They also depress the ventilatory response to CO_2, and the ventilatory response to hypoxia. The magnitude of this depression varies considerably by specific agent, but in all cases the depression is dose dependent. Anesthetic gases generally decrease resting tidal volume and increase respiratory frequency. The decrease in tidal volume is of larger magnitude than the increase in frequency, so that net minute ventilation is decreased. Since the anesthetic state leads to an increase in alveolar dead space, alveolar ventilation is reduced by a greater proportion than is minute ventilation. To a large extent, surgical stimulation counters ventilatory depression induced by all agents. Thus, a spontaneously ventilating surgical patient under 1 MAC of gaseous agent(s) may have close to a normal P_aCO_2 (71,227).

There has been recent controversy regarding the effect of subanesthetic concentrations of inhalational agents on the hypoxic response. Considerable work by Knill and colleagues (138–141) shows that many inhalational agents reduce markedly the hypoxic response at concentrations as low as 0.05 and 0.1 MAC. This is much out of proportion to their reduction of the hypercapnic response, thus implying a selective effect at the carotid body chemoreflex. Such selective reduction in hypoxic sensitivity seems relevant to the recovery period where concentrations of anesthetic agents may remain in this range for even several hours after operation, and where mild to moderate hypoxia is a frequent occurrence. Recently, however, Temp et al. (261,262) were unable to confirm Knill's results using sedative doses of isoflurane. On the other hand, Dahan et al. (58) found substantial depression of the acute response with halothane. Young et al. (297) studied the effects of 0.1% inspired halothane on HVD and found a 17% decrease in the peak hypoxic ventilation, but no difference in ventilation after 30 minutes of hypoxia. However, with 0.17% inspired enflurane, Nagyova et al. (193) found a reduction in both the acute response as well as the ventilation after 20 minutes of hypoxia. The differences in these studies appear to stem from differences in the state of arousal of the subjects during the experiments (223,266). Many of these concepts with inhalational agents illustrate again the integrative role played by the respiratory controller, and perhaps also Fink's (86) concept of the "wakefulness drive to breathe."

REFERENCES

1. *Acute pain management: operative or medical procedures and trauma.* Washington, DC: Public Health Service, 1992.
2. Abrahams TP, Hornby PJ, Walton DP, Taveira DaSilva AM. An excitatory amino acid(s) in the ventrolateral medulla is (are) required for breathing to occur in the anesthetized cat. *J Pharmacol Exp Ther* 1991;259:1388–1395.
3. Akiyama Y, Nishimura M, Suzuki A, Yamamoto M, Kishi F, Kawakami Y. Naloxone increases ventilatory response to hypercapnic hypoxia in healthy adult humans. *Am Rev Respir Dis* 1990; 142:301–305.
4. Alexander CM, Gross JB. Sedative doses of midazolam depress hypoxic ventilatory responses in humans. *Anesth Analg* 1988;67: 377–382.
5. Andronikou S, Shirahata M, Mokashi A, Lahiri S. Carotid body chemoreceptor and ventilatory responses to sustained hypoxia and hypercapnia in the cat. *Respir Physiol* 1988;72:361–374.
6. Ang RC, Hoop B, Kazemi H. Role of glutamate as the central neurotransmitter in the hypoxic ventilatory response. *J Appl Physiol* 1992;72:1480–1487.
7. Atweh SF, Kuhar MJ. Autoradiographic localization of opiate receptors in rat brain. I. spinal cord and lower medulla. *Brain Res* 1977;124:53–67.
8. Badr MS, Skatrud JB, Dempsey JA. Determinants of poststimulus potentiation in humans during NREM sleep. *J Appl Physiol* 1992; 73(5):1958–1971.
9. Bailey PL, Andriano KP, Goldman M, Stanley TH, Pace NL. Variability of the respiratory response to diazepam. *Anesthesiology* 1986; 64:460–465.
10. Bailey PL, Pace NL, Ashburn MA, Moll JWB, East KA, Stanley TH. Frequent hypoxemia and apnea after sedation with midazolam and fentanyl. *Anesthesiology* 1990;73:826–830.
11. Bailey PL, Rhondeau S, Schafer PG, et al. Dose-response pharmacology of intrathecal morphine in human volunteers. *Anesthesiology* 1993;79:49–59.
12. Bailey PL, Sperry RJ, Johnson GK, et al. Respiratory effects of clonidine alone and combined with morphine, in humans. *Anesthesiology* 1991;74:43–48.
13. Bailey PL, Streisand JB, East KA, et al. Differences in magnitude and duration of opioid-induced respiratory depression and analgesia with fentanyl and sufentanil. *Anesth Analg* 1990;70:8–15.
14. Bainbridge CW, Heistad DD. Effect of haloperidol on ventilatory responses to dopamine in man. *J Pharmacol Exp Ther* 1979;213: 13–17.
15. Bascom DA, Clement ID, Cunningham DA, Painter R, Robbins PA. Changes in peripheral chemoreflex sensitivity during sustained, isocapnic hypoxia. *Respir Physiol* 1990;82:161–176.
16. Bascom DA, Clement ID, Dorrington KL, Robbins PA. Effects of dopamine and domperidone on ventilation during isocapnic hypoxia in humans. *Respir Physiol* 1991;85:319–328.
17. Belleville JP, Ward DS, Bloor BC, Maze M. Effects of intravenous dexmedetomidine in humans I. Sedation, ventilation and metabolic rate. *Anesthesiology* 1992;77:1125–1133.
18. Bellville JW, Whipp BJ, Kaufman RD, Swanson GD, Aqleh KA, Wiberg DM. Central and peripheral chemoreflex loop gain in normal and carotid body-resected subjects. *J Appl Physiol* 1979;46: 843–853.
19. Benhamou D, Veillette Y, Narchi P, Ecoffey C. Ventilatory effects of premedication with clonidine. *Anesth Analg* 1991;73:799–803.
20. Berger AJ, Mitchell RA, Severinghaus JW. Regulation of respiration, part 1. *N Engl J Med* 1977;297:92–97.
21. Berger AJ, Mitchell RA, Severinghaus JW. Regulation of respiration, part 2. *N Engl J Med* 1977;297:138–143.
22. Berger AJ, Mitchell RA, Severinghaus JW. Regulation of respiration, part 3. *N Engl J Med* 1977;297:194–201.
23. Berkenbosch A, Bovill JG, Dahan A, DeGoede J, Olievier ICW. The ventilatory CO_2 sensitivities from Read's rebreathing method and the steady-state method are not equal in man. *J Physiol Lond* 1989;411:367–377.
24. Berkenbosch A, DeGoede J. Actions and interactions of CO_2 and O_2 on central and peripheral chemoceptive structures. In: von Euler C, Lagercrantz H, eds. *Neurobiology of the control of breathing.* New York: Raven Press, 1987;9–17.
25. Biaggioni I, Olafsson B, Robertson RM, Hollister AS, Robertson D. Cardiovascular and respiratory effects of adenosine in conscious man. *Circ Res* 1987;61:779–786.

26. Biscoe TJ, Duchen MR. Monitoring PO_2 by the carotid chemoreceptor. *NIPS* 1990;5:229–233.
27. Bisgard GE, Mitchell RA, Herbert DA. Effects of dopamine, norepinephrine and 5-hydroxytryptamine on the carotid body of the dog. *Respir Physiol* 1979;37:61–80.
28. Bledsoe SW, Hornbein TF. Central chemosensors and the regulation of their chemical environment. In: Hornbein TF, ed. *Regulation of breathing.* New York: Marcel Dekker, 1981;347–428.
29. Blouin RT, Conard PF, Gross JB. Time course of ventilatory depression following induction doses of propofol and thiopental. *Anesthesiology* 1991;75:940–944.
30. Blouin RT, Seifert HA, Babenco HD, Conrad PF, Gross JB. Propofol depresses the hypoxic ventilatory response during conscious sedation and isohypercapnia. *Anesthesiology* 1993;79:1177–1182.
31. Bonora M, Gautier H. Influence of dopamine and norepinephrine on the central ventilatory response to hypoxia in conscious cats. *Respir Physiol* 1988;71:11–24.
32. Borison HL. Central nervous respiratory depressants—narcotic analgesics. *Pharmacol Ther [B]* 1977;3:227–237.
33. Borison HL. Central nervous respiratory depressants control-systems approach to respiratory depression. *Pharmacol Ther [B]* 1977; 3:211–226.
34. Bourke DL. Respiratory effects of regional anesthesia during acute pain. *Reg Anesth* 1993;18:361–365.
35. Bourke DL, Warley A. The steady-state and rebreathing methods compared during morphine administration in humans. *J Physiol (Lond)* 1989;419:509–517.
36. Bruce EN, Cherniack NS. Central chemoreceptors. *J Appl Physiol* 1987;62:389–402.
37. Burton MD, Johnson DC, Kazemi H. Adrenergic and cholinergic interaction in central ventilatory control. *J Appl Physiol* 1990;68: 2092–2099.
38. Camporesi EM, Nielsen CH, Bromage PR, Durant PAC. Ventilatory CO_2 sensitivity after intravenous and epidural morphine in volunteers. *Anesth Analg* 1983;62:633–640.
39. Cao K, Zwillich CW, Berthon-Jones M, Sullivan CE. Increased normoxic ventilation induced by repetitive hypoxia in conscious dogs. *J Appl Physiol* 1992;73:2083–2088.
40. Cao K, Zwillich CW, Berthon-Jones M, Sullivan CE. Ventilatory response to sustained eucapnic hypoxia in the adult conscious dog. *Respir Physiol* 1992;89:65–73.
41. Carr DB. Opioids. *Int Anesth Clin* 1988;26:273–287.
42. Catley DM, Thornton M, Jordan C, et al. Pronounced, episodic oxygen desaturation in the postoperative period: its association with ventilatory pattern and analgesic regimen. *Anesthesiology* 1985;63:20–28.
43. Cherniack NS. Central chemoreceptors. In: Crystal RG, West JB, eds. *The lung: scientific foundations,* 2nd ed. New York: Raven Press, 1991;1349–1357.
44. Cherniack NS, Dempsey J, Fencl V, et al. Workshop on assessment of respiratory control in humans. I. Methods of measurement of ventilatory responses to hypoxia and hypercapnia. *Am Rev Respir Dis* 1977;115:177–181.
45. Cherniack NS, Prabhakar N, Haxhiu MA, Runold M. Excitatory and inhibitory influences on the ventilatory augmentation caused by hypoxia. In: Lahiri S, Cherniack NS, Fitzgerald RS, eds. *Response and adaptation to hypoxia.* New York: Oxford University Press, 1991;107–121.
46. Chernick V. Endorphins and ventilatory control. *N Engl J Med* 1981;304:1227–1228.
47. Childers SR. Opioid receptor-coupled second messenger systems. *Life Sci* 1991;48:1991–2003.
48. Chin K, Ohi M, Hirai M, Kuriyama T, Sagawa Y, Kuno K. Breathing during sleep with mild hypoxia. *J Appl Physiol* 1989;67: 1198–1207.
49. Clark FJ, von Euler C. On the regulation of depth and rate of breathing. *J Physiol (Lond)* 1972;222:267–295.
50. Coates EL, Li A, Nattie EE. Acetazolamide on the ventral medulla of the cat increases phrenic output and delays the ventilatory response to CO_2. *J Physiol (Lond)* 1991;441:433–451.
51. Coates EL, Li A, Nattie EE. Widespread sites of brain stem ventilatory chemoreceptors. *J Appl Physiol* 1993;75:5–14.
52. Cohen R, Finn H, Steen SN. Effect of diazepam and meperidine, alone and in combination, on respiratory response to carbon dioxide. *Anesth Analg* 1969;48:353–355.
53. Cooper JR, Bloom FE, Roth RH. *The biochemical basis of neuropharmacology,* 6th ed. New York: Oxford University Press, 1991.
54. Correa-Sales C, Rabin BC, Maze M. A hypnotic response to dexmedetomidine, an alpha 2 agonist, is mediated in the locus coeruleus in rats. *Anesthesiology* 1992;76:948–952.
55. Cotton EK, Grunstein MN. Effect of hypoxia on respiratory control in neonates at high altitude. *J Appl Physiol* 1980;48:587–595.
56. Cunningham DJC, Robbins PA, Wolff CB. Integration of respiratory responses to changes in alveolar partial pressures of CO_2 and O_2 and in arterial pH. In: Fishman AP, Cherniack NS, Widdicombe JG, Geiger SR, eds. *Handbook of physiology. The respiratory system,* vol 2. Bethesda: American Physiological Society, 1986;475–528.
57. Dahan A, Berkenbosch A, DeGoede J, Olievier ICW, Bovill JG. On a pseudo-rebreathing technique to assess the ventilatory sensitivity to carbon dioxide in man. *J Physiol (Lond)* 1990;423:615–629.
58. Dahan A, van den Elsen MJLJ, Berkenbosch A, et al. Effects of subanesthetic halothane on the ventilatory responses to hypercapnia and acute hypoxia in healthy volunteers. *Anesthesiology* 1994;80: 727–738.
59. Dahan A, Ward DS. Effect of I.V. midazolam on the ventilatory response to sustained hypoxia in man. *Br J Anaesth* 1991;66: 454–457.
60. Daristotle L, Engwall MJ, Niu W, Bisgard GE. Ventilatory effects and interactions with change in PaO2 in awake goats. *J Appl Physiol* 1991;71:1254–1260.
61. Darnall RA, Bruce RD. Effects of adenosine and xanthine derivatives on breathing during acute hypoxia in the anesthetized newborn piglet. *Pediatr Pulmonol* 1987;3:110–116.
62. De Boeck C, Van Reempts P, Rigatto H, Chernick V. Naloxone reduces decrease in ventilation induced by hypoxia in newborn infants. *J Appl Physiol* 1984;56:1507–1511.
63. De Sarro GB, Ascioti C, Froio F, Libri V, Nisticò G. Evidence that locus coeruleus is the site where clonidine and drugs acting at α_1- and a_2-adrenoceptors affect sleep and arousal mechanisms. *Br J Pharmacol* 1987;90:675–685.
64. Dempsey JA, Olson EB Jr, Skatrud JB. Hormones and neurochemicals in the regulation of breathing. In: Fishman AP, Cherniack NS, Widdicombe JG, Geiger SR, eds. *Handbook of physiology. The respiratory system,* vol 2. Bethesda: American Physiological Society, 1986;181–221.
65. Dershwitz M, Di Biase PM, Rosow CE, Wilson RS, Sanderson PE, Joslyn AF. Ondansetron does not affect alfentanil-induced ventilatory depression or sedation. *Anesthesiology* 1992;77:447–452.
66. Dev NB, Loeschcke HH. Topography of the respiratory and circulatory responses to acetylcholine and nicotine on the ventral surface of the medulla oblongata. *Pflugers Arch* 1979;379:19–27.
67. Doblar DD, Muldoon SM, Abbrecht PH, Baskoff J, Watson RL. Epidural morphine following epidural local anesthesia: effect on ventilatory and airway occlusion pressure responses to CO_2. *Anesthesiology* 1981;55:423–428.
68. Dripps RD, Comroe JH. Clinical studies on morphine. I. the immediate effect of morphine administered intravenously and intramuscularly upon the respiration of normal man. *Anesthesiology* 1945;6:462–468.
69. Easton PA, Anthonisen NR. Ventilatory response to sustained hypoxia after pretreatment with aminophylline. *J Appl Physiol* 1988; 64:1445–1450.
70. Easton PA, Slykerman LJ, Anthonisen NR. Ventilatory response to sustained hypoxia in normal adults. *J Appl Physiol* 1986;61: 906–911.
71. Eger EI, Dolan WM, Stevens WC, Miller RD, Way WL. Surgical stimulation antagonizes the respiratory depression produced by forane. *Anesthesiology* 1972;36:544–549.
72. Elam M, Yao T, Thorén P, Svensson TH. Hypercapnia and hypoxia: chemoreceptor-mediated control of locus coeruleus neurons and splanchnic, sympathetic nerves. *Brain Res* 1981;222:373–381.
73. Eldridge FL. Overview: role of neurochemicals and hormones. In: Honda Y, et al., eds. *Control of breathing and its modeling perspective.* New York: Plenum Press, 1992;187–196.
74. Eldridge FL, Kiley JP, Millhorn DE. Respiratory responses to medullary hydrogen ion changes in cats: different effects of respiratory and metabolic acidoses. *J Physiol* 1985;358:285–297.
75. Eldridge FL, Millhorn DE. Central regulation of respiration by endogenous neurotransmitters and neuromodulators. *Annu Rev Physiol* 1981;43:121–135.
76. Eldridge FL, Millhorn DE. Oscillation, gating, and memory in the respiratory control system. In: Fishman AP, Cherniack NS, Widdicombe JG, Geiger SR, eds. *Handbook of physiology. The respiratory system,* vol 2. Bethesda: American Physiological Society, 1986:93–114.

77. Eldridge FL, Millhorn DE, Kiley JP. Respiratory effects of a long-acting analog of adenosine. *Brain Res* 1984;301:273–280.
78. Eriksson LI, Sato M, Severinghaus JW. Effect of a vecuronium-induced partial neuromuscular block on hypoxic ventilatory response. *Anesthesiology* 1993;78:693–699.
79. Etches RC, Sandler AN, Daley MD. Respiratory depression and spinal opioids. *Can J Anaesth* 1989;36:165–185.
80. Ezure K. Synaptic connections between medullary respiratory neurons and considerations on the genesis of respiratory rhythm. *Prog Neurobiol* 1990;35:429–450.
81. Fennerty AG, Rimmer EM, Boulton J, Richens A. Effect of gamma-aminobutyric acid on the carbon dioxide rebreathing response of normal subjects: a study using vigabatrin. *Thorax* 1990;45:42–44.
82. Fidone SJ, Gonzalez C. Initiation and control of chemoreceptor activity in the carotid body. In: Fishman AP, Cherniack NS, Widdicombe JG, Geiger SR, eds. *Handbook of physiology. The respiratory system,* vol 2. Bethesda: American Physiological Society, 1986:247–312.
83. Fidone SJ, Gonzalez C, Dinger B, Gomez-Nino A, Obeso A, Yoshizaki K. Cellular aspects of peripheral chemoreceptor function. In: Crystal RG, West JB, eds. *The lung: scientific foundations,* 2nd ed. New York: Raven Press, 1991;1319–1332.
84. Fidone SJ, Gonzalez C, Yoshizaki K. Putative neurotransmitters in the carotid body: the case for dopamine. *Fed Proc* 1980;39: 2636–2640.
85. Filuk RB, Berezanski DJ, Anthonisen NR. Depression of hypoxic ventilatory response in humans by somatostatin. *J Appl Physiol* 1988;65:1050–1054.
86. Fink BR. Influence of cerebral activity in wakefulness on regulation of breathing. *J Appl Physiol* 1961;16:15–20.
87. Fleetham JA, Clarke H, Dhingra S, Chernick V, Anthonisen NR. Endogenous opiates and chemical control of breathing in humans. *Am Rev Respir Dis* 1980;121:1045–1049.
88. Fleming H, Burton M, Johnson DC, Kazemi H. Sodium salicylate centrally augments ventilation through cholinergic mechanisms. *J Appl Physiol* 1991;71:2299–2303.
89. Flögel CM, Ward DS, Wada DR, Ritter JW. The effects of large-dose flumazenil on midazolam-induced ventilatory depression. *Anesth Analg* 1993;77:1207–1214.
90. Forrest WH Jr, Bellville JW. The effect of sleep plus morphine on the respiratory response to carbon dioxide. *Anesthesiology* 1964; 25(2):137–141.
91. Forster A, Morel D, Bachmann M, Gemperle M. Respiratory depressant effects of different doses of midazolam and lack of reversal with naloxone-a double-blind randomized study. *Anesth Analg* 1983;62:920–924.
92. Fregosi RF. Short-term potentiation of breathing in humans. *J Appl Physiol* 1991;71(3):892–899.
93. Gardner WN. The pattern of breathing following step changes of alveolar partial pressures of carbon dioxide and oxygen in man. *J Physiol (Lond)* 1980;300:55–73.
94. Gautier H, Bonora M. Ventilatory response of intact cats to carbon monoxide hypoxia. *J Appl Physiol* 1983;55:1064–1071.
95. Gautier H, Bonora M, Zaoui D. Effects of carotid denervation and decerebration on ventilatory response to CO. *J Appl Physiol* 1990; 69:1423–1428.
96. Georgopoulos D, Bshouty Z, Younes M, Anthonisen NR. Hypoxic exposure and activation of the afterdischarge mechanism in conscious humans. *J Appl Physiol* 1990;69:1159–1164.
97. Georgopoulos D, Holtby SG, Berezanski D, Anthonisen NR. Aminophylline effects on ventilatory response to hypoxia and hyperoxia in normal adults. *J Appl Physiol* 1989;67:1150–1156.
98. Gillis RA, Namath IJ, Easington C, et al. Drug interaction with gamma aminobutyric acid/benzodiazepine receptors at the ventral surface of the medulla results in pronounced changes in cardiorespiratory activity. *J Pharmacol Exp Ther* 1988;248:863–870.
99. Gleeson K, Zwillich CW. Adenosine infusion and periodic breathing during sleep. *J Appl Physiol* 1992;72:1004–1009.
100. Goodman NW, Black AMS. Analyses of the ventilatory response to carbon dioxide. *Br J Anaesth* 1985;57:319–325.
101. Goodman NW, Curnow JSH. The ventilatory response to carbon dioxide. *Br J Anaesth* 1985;57:311–318.
102. Griffiths TL, Warren SJ, Chant ADB, Holgate ST. Ventilatory effects of hypoxia and adenosine infusion in patients after bilateral carotid endarterectomy. *Clin Sci Lond* 1990;78:25–31.
103. Gross JB. Resting ventilation measurements may be misleading. *Anesthesiology* 1984;61:110.
104. Gross JB, Weller RS, Conard P. Flumazenil antagonism of midazolam-induced ventilatory depression. *Anesthesiology* 1991;75: 179–185.
105. Gross JB, Zebrowski ME, Carel WD, Gardner S, Smith TC. Time course of ventilatory depression after thiopental and midazolam in normal subjects and in patients with chronic obstructive pulmonary disease. *Anesthesiology* 1983;58:540–544.
106. Grönblad M. Function and structure of the carotid body. *Med Biol* 1983;61:229–248.
107. Grunstein MM, Hazinski TA, Schlueter MA. Respiratory control during hypoxia in newborn rabbits: implied action of endorphins. *J Appl Physiol* 1981;51:122–130.
108. Hagberg H, Lehmann A, Sandberg M, Nystrom B, Jacobson I, Hamberger A. Ischemia-induced shift of inhibitory and excitatory amino acids from intra- to extracellular compartments. *J Cereb Blood Flow Metab* 1985;5:413–419.
109. Hedner J, Hedner T, Wessberg P, Jonason J. An analysis of the mechanism by which gamma-aminobutyric acid depresses ventilation in the rat. *J Appl Physiol* 1984;56:849–856.
110. Hickey RF, Severinghaus JW. Regulation of breathing: drug effects. In: Hornbein TF, ed. *Regulation of breathing,* 17th ed. New York: Marcel Dekker, 1981;1251–1312.
111. Holtman JR, Norman WP, Gillis RA. Projections from the raphe nuclei to the phrenic motor nucleus in the cat. *Neurosci Lett* 1984; 44:105–111.
112. Hoop B, Masjedi MR, Shih VE, Kazemi H. Brain glutamate metabolism during hypoxia and peripheral chemodenervation. *J Appl Physiol* 1990;69:147–154.
113. Hornbein TF. Anesthetics and ventilatory control. In: Covino BG, Fozzard HA, Rehder K, Stichartz G, eds. *Effects of anesthesia.* Bethesda: American Physiological Society, 1985;75–90.
114. Hosogai M, Matsuo S, Nakao S. Firing pattern and location of respiratory neurons in cat medullary raphe nuclei. *Neurosci Lett* 1993; 16:149–152.
115. Howell LL, Morse WH, Spealman RD. Respiratory effects of xanthines and adenosine analogs in rhesus monkeys. *J Pharmacol Exp Ther* 1990;254:786–791.
116. Hsiao C, Lahiri S, Mokashi A. Peripheral and central dopamine receptors in respiratory control. *Respir Physiol* 1989;76:327–336.
117. Issa FG. Effect of clonidine in obstructive sleep apnea. *Am Rev Respir Dis* 1992;145:435–439.
118. Issa FG, Remmers JE. Identification of a subsurface area in the ventral medulla sensitive to local changes in PCO_2. *J Appl Physiol* 1992;72:439–446.
119. Iversen K, Hedner T, Lundborg P. GABA concentrations and turnover in neonatal rat brain during asphyxia and recovery. *Acta Physiol Scand* 1983;118:91–94.
120. Jacobi MS, Patil CP, Saunders KB. Transient, steady-state and rebreathing responses to carbon dioxide in man, at rest and during light exercise. *J Physiol (Lond)* 1989;411:85–96.
121. Jarvis DA, Duncan SR, Segal IS, Maze M. Ventilatory effects of clonidine alone and in the presence of alfentanil, in human volunteers. *Anesthesiology* 1992;76:899–905.
122. Javaheri S, Guerra L. Lung function, hypoxic and hypercapnic ventilatory responses, and respiratory muscle strength in normal subjects taking oral theophylline. *Thorax* 1990;45:743–747.
123. Javaheri S, Guerra LF. Effects of domperidone and medroxyprogesterone acetate on ventilation in man. *Respir Physiol* 1990;81: 359–370.
124. Javaheri S, Teppema LJ, Evers JAM. Effects of aminophylline on hypoxemia-induced ventilatory depression in the cat. *J Appl Physiol* 1988;64:1837–1843.
125. Jordan C. Assessment of the effects of drugs on respiration. *Br J Anaesth* 1982;54:763–782.
126. Jordan C, Tech B, Lehane JR, Jones JG. Respiratory depression following diazepam: Reversal with high-dose naloxone. *Anesthesiology* 1980;53:293–298.
127. Kagawa S, Stafford MJ, Waggener TB, Severinghaus JW. No effect of naloxone on hypoxia-induced ventilatory depression in adults. *J Appl Physiol* 1982;52:1030–1034.
128. Kazemi H, Hoop B. Glutamic acid and gamma-aminobutyric acid neurotransmitters in central control of breathing. *J Appl Physiol* 1991;70:1–7.
129. Kellogg RH. Historical perspectives. In: Hornbein TF, ed. *Regulation of breathing.* New York: Marcel Dekker, 1993;3–66.
130. Khamnei S, Robbins PA. Hypoxic depression of ventilation in humans: alternative models for the chemoreflexes. *Respir Physiol* 1990;81:117–134.

131. Khoo MCK. A model-based evaluation of the single-breath CO[2] ventilatory response test. *J Appl Physiol* 1990;68:393–399.
132. Kiley JP, Eldridge FL, Millhorn DE. The roles of medullary extracellular and cerebrospinal fluid pH in control of respiration. *Respir Physiol* 1985;59:117–130.
133. Kirby GC, McQueen DS. Characterization of opioid receptors in the cat carotid body involved in chemosensory depression in vivo. *Br J Pharmacol* 1986;88:889–898.
134. Kiwull-Schöne H, Kiwull P. Hypoxia and the ìreaction theoryî of central respiratory chemosensitivity. In: Goldstick TK, et al., eds. *Oxygen transport to tissue XIII.* New York: Plenum Press, 1992; 347–357.
135. Kneussl MP, Pappagianopoulos P, Hoop B, Kazemi H. Reversible depression of ventilation and cardiovascular function by ventriculocisternal perfusion with gamma-aminobutyric acid in dogs. *Am Rev Respir Dis* 1986;133:1024–1028.
136. Knill RL. Wresting or resting ventilation. *Anesthesiology* 1983;59: 599–600.
137. Knill RL. Does sufentanil produce less ventilatory depression than fentanyl? *Anesth Analg* 1990;71:564–566.
138. Knill RL, Clement JL. Variable effects of anaesthetics on the ventilatory response to hypoxaemia in man. *Can Anaesth Soc J* 1982;29: 93–99.
139. Knill RL, Clement JL. Site of selective action of halothane on the peripheral chemoreflex pathway in humans. *Anesthesiology* 1984; 61:121–126.
140. Knill RL, Gelb AW. Ventilatory responses to hypoxia and hypercapnia during halothane sedation and anesthesia in man. *Anesthesiology* 1978;49:244–251.
141. Knill RL, Kieraszewicz HT, Dodgson BG, Clement JL. Chemical regulation of ventilation during isoflurane sedation and anaesthesia in humans. *Can Anaesth Soc J* 1983;30:607–614.
142. Knill RL, Moote CA, Skinner MI, Rose EA, Lok PYK. Morphine-induced ventilatory depression is potentiated by non-REM sleep. *Can J Anaesth* 1987;34:S101–S102.
143. Kou YR, Ernsberger P, Cragg PA, Cherniack NS, Prabhakar NR. Role of a_2-adrenergic receptors in the carotid body response to isocapnic hypoxia. *Respir Physiol* 1991;83:353–364.
144. Kronenberg R, Hamilton FN, Gabel R, Hickey R, Read DJC, Severinghaus J. Comparison of three methods for quantitating respiratory response to hypoxia in man. *Respir Physiol* 1972;16:109–125.
145. Lagercrantz H. Neuromodulators and respiratory control during development. *TINS* 1987;10(9):368–372.
146. Lagercrantz H. Neuromodulators and respiratory control in the infant. *Clin Perinatol* 1987;14(3):683–695.
147. Lagercrantz H, Runold M, Yamamoto Y, Fredholm B. Adenosine: A putative mediator of the hypoxic ventilatory response of the neonate. In: von Euler C, Lagercrantz H, eds. *Neurobiology of the control of breathing.* New York: Raven Press, 1987;133–139.
148. Lahiri S. Chromophores in O_2 chemoreception: the carotid body model. *NIPS* 1994;9:161–165.
149. Lahiri S, Delaney RG. Stimulus interaction in the responses of carotid body chemoreceptor single afferent fibers. *Respir Physiol* 1975;24:249–266.
150. Lahiri S, Hsiao C, Zhang R, Mokashi A, Nishino T. Peripheral chemoreceptors in respiratory oscillations. *J Appl Physiol* 1985;58: 1901–1908.
151. Lahiri S, Iturriaga R, Mokashi A, Ray DK, Chugh D. CO reveals dual mechanisms of O2 chemoreception in the cat carotid body. *Respir Physiol* 1993;94:227–240.
152. Lahiri S, Nishino T. Inhibitory and excitatory effects of dopamine on carotid chemoreceptors. *Neurosci Lett* 1980;20:313–318.
153. Lahiri S, Nishino T, Mokashi A, Mulligan E. Interaction of dopamine and haloperidol with O_2 and CO_2 chemoreception in carotid body. *J Appl Physiol* 1980;49:45–51.
154. Lakshminarayan S, Sahn SA, Weil JV. Effect of aminophylline on ventilatory responses in normal man. *Am Rev Respir Dis* 1978;117: 33–38.
155. Lam AM, Clement JL, Knill RL. Surgical stimulation does not enhance ventilatory chemoreflexes during enflurane anaesthesia in man. *Can Anaesth Soc J* 1980;27(1):22–28.
156. Lawhead RG, Blaxall HS, Bylund DB. a-2A Is the predominant a-2 adrenergic receptor subtype in human spinal cord. *Anesthesiology* 1992;77:983–991.
157. Lawson EE, Waldrop TG, Eldridge FL. Naloxone enhances respiratory output in cats. *J Appl Physiol* 1979;47:1105–1111.
158. Lindefors N, Yamamoto Y, Pantaleo T, Lagercrantz H, Brodin E, Ungerstedt U. In vivo release of substance P in the nucleus tractus solitarii increases during hypoxia. *Neurosci Lett* 1986;69: 94–97.
159. Lipp J. Possible mechanisms of morphine analgesia. *J Clin Neuropharmacol* 1991;14(2):131–147.
160. Loeschcke HH. Central chemosensitivity and the reaction theory. *J Physiol* 1982;332:1–24.
161. Long WQ, Giesbrecht GG, Anthonisen NR. Ventilatory response to moderate hypoxia in awake chemodenervated cats. *J Appl Physiol* 1993;74:805–810.
162. Lourenco RV. Clinical methods for the study of regulation of breathing. *Chest* 1976;70(Suppl):109–112.
163. López-Barneo J, Benot AR, Ureña J. Oxygen sensing and the electrophysiology of arterial chemoreceptor cells. *NIPS* 1993;8: 191–195.
164. Lutz PL, Edwards R, McMahon PM. Gamma-aminobutyric acid concentrations are maintained in anoxic turtle brain. *Am J Physiol* 1985;249:R372–R374.
165. Lydic R, Baghdoyan HA. Cholinergic pontine mechanisms causing state-dependent respiratory depression. *NIPS* 1992;7:220–224.
166. Maxwell DL, Chahal P, Nolop KB, Hughes JMB. Somatostatin inhibits the ventilatory response to hypoxia in humans. *J Appl Physiol* 1986;60:997–1002.
167. Maxwell DL, Fuller RW, Dixon CMS, Cuss FMC, Barnes PJ. Ventilatory effects of substance P, vasoactive intestinal peptide, and nitroprusside in humans. *J Appl Physiol* 1990;68:295–301.
168. Maxwell DL, Fuller RW, Nolop KB, Dixon CMS, Hughes JMB. Effects of adenosine on ventilatory responses to hypoxia and hypercapnia in humans. *J Appl Physiol* 1986;61:1762–1766.
169. Maze M, Tranquilli W. Alpha-2 adrenoceptor agonists: defining the role in clinical anesthesia. *Anesthesiology* 1991;74:581–605.
170. McClean PA, Phillipson EA, Martinez D, Zamel N. Single breath of CO_2 as a clinical test of the peripheral chemoreflex. *J Appl Physiol* 1988;64:84–89.
171. McCrimmon DR, Lalley PM. Inhibition of respiratory neural discharges by clonidine and 5-hydroxytryptophan. *J Pharmacol Exp Ther* 1982;222(3):771–777.
172. McDonald DM. Peripheral chemoreceptors. In: Hornbein TF, ed. *Regulation of breathing.* New York: Marcel Dekker, 1981;105–319.
173. McQueen DS, Ribeiro JA. Pharmacological characterization of the receptor involved in chemoexcitation induced by adenosine. *Br J Pharmacol* 1986;88:615–620.
174. Meldrum MJ, Isom GE. Role of monoaminergic systems in morphine-induced respiratory depression. *Neuropharmacology* 1981;20: 169–175.
175. Melton JE, Neubauer JA, Edelman NH. GABA antagonism reverses hypoxic respiratory depression in the cat. *J Appl Physiol* 1990; 69:1296–1301.
176. Milic-Emili J, Grassino AE, Whitelaw WA. Measurement and testing of respiratory drive. In: Hornbein TF, ed. *Regulation of breathing,* 17th ed. New York: Marcel Dekker, 1981;675–743.
177. Milic-Emili J, Grunstein MM. Drive and timing components of ventilation. *Chest* 1976;70(suppl):131–133.
178. Millhorn DE, Bayliss DA, Erickson JT, Gallman EA, Szymeczek CL, Czyzyk-Krzeska MF, Dean JB. Neurotransmission and regulation of respiration. In: Crystal RG, West JB, eds. *The lung: scientific foundations.* New York: Raven Press, 1991;1369–1382.
179. Millhorn DE, Eldridge FL. Role of ventrolateral medulla in regulation of respiratory and cardiovascular systems. *J Appl Physiol* 1986;61:1249–1263.
180. Millhorn DE, Eldridge FL, Waldrop TG. Prolonged stimulation of respiration by endogenous central serotonin. *Respir Physiol* 1980; 42:171–188.
181. Millhorn DE, Eldridge FL, Waldrop TG. Prolonged stimulation of respiration by a new central neural mechanism. *Respir Physiol* 1980;41:87–103.
182. Mitchell GS, Douse MA, Foley KT. Receptor interactions in modulating ventilatory activity. *Am J Physiol* 1990;259:R911–R920.
183. Mitchell RA, Berger AJ. Neural regulation of respiration. *Am Rev Respir Dis* 1975;3:206–224.
184. Mitchell RA, Berger AJ. Neural regulation of respiration. In: Hornbein TF, ed. *Regulation of breathing.* New York: Marcel Dekker, 1981;541–620.
185. Mitchell RA, Loeschcke HH, Severinghaus JW, Richardson BW, Massion WH. Regions of respiratory chemosensitivity on the surface of the medulla. *Ann NY Academy Sci* 1963;109(2):661–681.
186. Mitra J, Prabhakar R, Overholt JL, Cherniack NS. Respiratory and

vasomotor effects of excitatory amino acid on ventral medullary surface. *Brain Res Bull* 1987;18:681–684.

187. Moore RY, Bloom FE. Central catecholamine neuron systems: anatomy and physiology of the norepinephrine and epinephrine systems. *Annu Rev Neurosci* 1979;2:113–168.
188. Moorthy SS, Sullivan TY, Fallon JH, Dierdorf SF, Radpour S, DeAtley RE. Loss of hypoxic ventilatory response following bilateral neck dissection. *Anesth Analg* 1993;76:791–794.
189. Mora CT, Torjman M, White PF. Effects of diazepam and flumzenil on sedation and hypoxic ventilatory response. *Anesth Analg* 1989;68:473–478.
190. Moss IR, Denavit-Saubié M, Eldridge FL, Gillis RA, Herkenham M, Lahiri S. Neuromodulators and transmitters in respiratory control. *Fed Proc* 1986;45:2133–2147.
191. Mueller RA, Lundberg DBA, Breese GR, Hedner J, Hedner T, Jonason J. The neuropharmacology of respiratory control. *Pharmacol Rev* 1982;34(3):255–285.
192. Nagyova B, Dorrington KL, Robbins PA. Effects of midazolam and flumazenil on ventilation during sustained hypoxia in humans. *Respir Physiol* 1993;94:51–59.
193. Nagyova B, Dorrington KL, Robbins PA. Effect of low-dose enflurane on the ventilatory response to hypoxia in humans. *Br J Anaesth* 1994;72:509–514.
194. Narchi P, Benhamou D, Hamza J, Bouaziz H. Ventilatory effects of epidural clonidine during the first 3 hours after caesarean section. *Acta Anaesthesiol Scand* 1992;36:791–795.
195. Nattie EE, Li A, St. John WM. Lesions in retrotrapezoid nucleus decrease ventilatory output in anesthetized or decerebrate cats. *J Appl Physiol* 1991;71(4):1364–1375.
196. Nattie EE, Wood J, Mega A, Goritski W. Rostral ventrolateral medulla muscarinic receptor involvement in central ventilatory chemosensitivity. *J Appl Physiol* 1989;66:1462–1470.
197. Neubauer JA, Melton JE, Edelman NH. Modulation of respiration during brain hypoxia. *J Appl Physiol* 1990;68:441–451.
198. Neubauer JA, Santiago TV, Posner MA, Edelman NH. Ventral medullary pH and ventilatory responses to hyperperfusion and hypoxia. *J Appl Physiol* 1985;58:1659–1668.
199. Nguyen D, Abdul-Rasool I, Ward D, et al. Ventilatory effects of dexmedetomidine, atipamezole, and isoflurane in dogs. *Anesthesiology* 1992;76:573–579.
200. Olson LG, Hensley MJ, Saunders NA. Augmentation of the ventilatory response to asphyxia by prochlorperazine in human. *J Appl Physiol* 1982;53:637–643.
201. Olson LG, Hensley MJ, Saunders NA. The effects of combined morphine and prochlorperazine on ventilatory control in humans. *Am Rev Respir Dis* 1986;133:558–561.
202. Ooi R, Pattison J, Feldman SA. The effects of intravenous clonidine on ventilation. *Anaesthesia* 1991;46:632–633.
203. Painter R. Khamnei S, Robbins P. A mathematical model of the human ventilatory response to isocapnic hypoxia. *J Appl Physiol* 1993;74:2007–2015.
204. Pandit JJ, Robbins PA. The ventilatory effects of sustained isocapnic hypoxia during exercise in humans. *Respir Physiol* 1991;86:393–404.
205. Parsons ST, Griffiths TL, Christie JML, Holgate ST. Effect of theophylline and dipyridamole on the respiratory response to isocapnic hypoxia in normal human subjects. *Clin Sci Lond* 1991;80:107–112.
206. Pasternak GW. Pharmacological mechanisms of opioid analgesics. *Clin Neuropharmacol* 1993;16(1):1–18.
207. Pavlin EG, Hornbein TF. Anesthesia and the control of ventilation. In: Fishman AP, Cherniack NS, Widdicombe JG, Geiger SR, eds. *Handbook of physiology. The respiratory system,* vol II, part 2. Bethesda: American Physiological Society, 1986;793–813.
208. Peano CA, Shonis CA, Dillon GH, Waldrop TG. Hypothalamic GABAergic mechanism involved in respiratory response to hypercapnia. *Brain Res Bull* 1992;28(1):107–113.
209. Penon C, Ecoffey C, Cohen SE. Ventilatory response to carbon dioxide after epidural clonidine injection. *Anesth Analg* 1991;72:761–764.
210. Pierrefiche O, Fountz AS, Denavit-Saubié M. Effects of GABA-B receptor agonists and antagonists on the bulbar respiratory network in cat. *Brain Res* 1993;605:77–84.
211. Phillipson EA. Control of breathing during sleep. *Am Rev Respir Dis* 1978;118:909–939.
212. Phillipson EA, Bowes G. Control of breathing during sleep. In: Fishman AP, Cherniack NS, Widdicombe JG, Geiger SR, eds. *Handbook of physiology. The respiratory system,* vol II. Baltimore: Williams & Wilkins, 1986;649–689.
213. Prabhakar NR. Significance of excitatory and inhibitory neurochemicals in hypoxic chemotransmission of the carotid body. In: Honda Y, et al., eds. *Control of breathing and its modeling perspective.* New York: Plenum Press, 1992;205–212.
214. Prabhakar NR, Kumar GK, Chang CH, Agani FH, Haxhiu MA. Nitric oxide in the sensory function of the carotid body. *Brain Res* 1993;625:16–22.
215. Prabhakar NR, Runold M, Yamamoto Y, Lagercrantz H, von Euler C. Effect of substance P antagonist on the hypoxia-induced carotid chemoreceptor activity. *Acta Physiol Scand* 1984;121:301–303.
216. Read DJC. A clinical method for assessing the ventilatory response to carbon dioxide. *Australas Ann Med* 1967;16:20–32.
217. Read DJC, Leigh J. Blood-brain tissue PCO2 relationships and ventilation during rebreathing. *J Appl Physiol* 1967;23:53–70.
218. Rebuck AS, Slutsky AS. Measurement of ventilatory responses to hypercapnia and hypoxia. In: Hornbein TF, ed. *Regulation of breathing,* vol 17, part 2. New York: Marcel Dekker, 1981;745–772.
219. Rebuck AS, Woodley WE. Ventilatory effects of hypoxia and their dependence on PCO_2. *J Appl Physiol* 1975;38(1):16–19.
220. Reeder MK, Goldman MD, Loh L, et al. Postoperative hypoxaemia after major abdominal vascular surgery. *Br J Anaesth* 1992;68:23–26.
221. Remmers JE, deGroot WJ, Sauerland EK, Anch AM. Pathogenesis of upper airway occlusion during sleep. *J Appl Physiol* 1978;44:931–938.
222. Rigual R, Gonzalez E, Gonzalez C, Fidone S. Synthesis and release of catecholamines by the cat carotid body in vitro: effects of hypoxic stimulation. *Brain Res* 1986;374:101–109.
223. Robotham R. Editorial: Do low-dose inhalational anesthetic agents alter ventilatory control? *Anesthesiology* 1994;80:723–726.
224. Romagnoli A, Keats AS. Ceiling effect for respiratory depression by nalbuphine. *Clin Pharmacol Ther* 1980;27:478–485.
225. Rosenberg J, Kehlet H. Postoperative mental confusion–association with postoperative hypoxemia. *Surgery* 1993;114:76–81.
226. Rosenberg J, Rasmussen V, Von Jessen F, Ullstad T, Kehlet H. Late postoperative episodic and constant hypoxaemia and associated ECG abnormalities. *Br J Anaesth* 1990;65:684–691.
227. Rosenberg M, Tobias R, Bourke D, Kamat V. Respiratory responses to surgical stimulation during enflurane anesthesia. *Anesthesiology* 1980;52:163–165.
228. Runold M, Cherniack NS, Prabhakar NR. Effect of adenosine on isolated and superfused cat carotid body activity. *Neurosci Lett* 1990;113:111–114.
229. Runold M, Lagercrantz H, Prabhakar NR, Fredholm BB. Role of adenosine in hypoxic ventilatory depression. *J Appl Physiol* 1989;67:541–546.
230. Sabol SJ, Ward DS. Effect of dopamine on hypoxic-hypercapnic interaction in humans. *Anesth Analg* 1987;66:619–624.
231. Sahn SA, Zwillich CW, Dick N, McCullough RE, Lakshminarayan S, Weil JV. Variability of ventilatory responses to hypoxia and hypercapnia. *J Appl Physiol* 1977;43:1019–1025.
232. Sales N, Riche D, Roques BP, Denavit-Saubie M. Localization of μ- and δ-opioid receptors in cat respiratory areas: an autoradiographic study. *Brain Res* 1985;344:382–386.
233. Sanders JS, Berman TM, Bartlett MM, Kronenberg RS. Increased hypoxic ventilatory drive due to administration of aminophylline in normal men. *Chest* 1980;78(2):279–282.
234. Santiago TV, Edelman NH. Opioids and breathing. *J Appl Physiol* 1985;59:1675–1685.
235. Santiago TV, Johnson J, Riley DJ, Edelman NH. Effects of morphine on ventilatory response to exercise. *J Appl Physiol* 1979;47:112–118.
236. Santiago TV, Remolina C, Scoles V, Edelman NH. Endorphins and the control of breathing: ability of naloxone to restore flow-resistive load compensation in chronic obstructive pulmonary disease. *N Engl J Med* 1981;304:1190–1195.
237. Sato M, Severinghaus JW, Basbaum AI. Medullary CO_2 chemoreceptor neuron identification by c-fos. *J Appl Physiol* 1992;73:96–100.
238. Sawynok J, Pinsky C, LaBella FS. Minireview on the specificity of naloxone as an opiate antagonist. *Life Sci* 1979;25:1621–1631.
239. Severinghaus JW. Proposed standard determination of ventilatory responses to hypoxia and hypercapnia in man. *Chest* 1976;70:129–131.

240. Severinghaus JW. Invited editorial on ìWidespread sites of brain stem ventilatory chemoreceptors.î *J Appl Physiol* 1993;75:3–4.
241. Severinghaus J, Ozanne G, Massuda Y. Measurement of the ventilatory response to hypoxia: a step hypoxia three-minute test. *Chest* 1976;70(1)(suppl):121–123.
242. Shams H. Differential effects of CO_2 and H^+ as central stimuli of respiration in the cat. *J Appl Physiol* 1985;58(2):357–364.
243. Shook JE, Watkins WD, Camporesi EM. Differential roles of opioid receptors in respiration, respiratory disease, and opiate-induced respiratory depression. *Am Rev Respir Dis* 1990;142: 895–909.
244. Simantov R, Kuhar MJ, Uhl GR, Snyder SH. Opioid peptide enkephalin: immunohistochemical mapping in rat central nervous system. *Proc Natl Acad Sci* 1977;74(5):2167–2171.
245. Simon PM, Pope A, Lahive K, et al. Naloxone does not alter response to hypercapnia or resistive loading in chronic obstructive pulmonary disease. *Am Rev Respir Dis* 1989;139:134–138.
246. Smatresk NJ, Pokorski M, Lahiri S. Opposing effects of dopamine receptor blockade on ventilation and carotid chemoreceptor activity. *J Appl Physiol* 1983;54:1567–1573.
247. Smith JC, Morrison DE, Ellenberger HH, Otto MR, Feldman JL. Brainstem projections to the major respiratory neuron populations in the medulla of the cat. *J Comp Neurol* 1989;281:69–96.
248. Spaulding BC, Choi SD, Gross JB, Apfelbaum JL, Broderson H. The effect of physostigmine on diazepam-induced ventilatory depression: a double-blind study. *Anesthesiology* 1984;61:551–554.
249. Steinberg SS, Bellville JW, Seed JC. The effect of atropine and morphine on respiration. *J Pharmacol Exp Ther* 1957;121(1):71–77.
250. Sullivan AF, Kalso EA, McQuay HJ, Dickenson AH. Evidence for the involvement of the μ but not δ opioid receptor subtype in the synergistic interaction between opioid and alpha 2 adrenergic antinociception in the rat spinal cord. *Neurosci Lett* 1992;139:65–68.
251. Svensson TH. Brain norepinephrine neurons in the locus coeruleus and the control of arousal and respiration: implications for sudden infant death syndrome. In: von Euler C, Lagercrantz H, eds. *Neurobiology of the control of breathing.* New York: Raven Press, 1986;297–301.
252. Swaminathan S, Paton JY, Ward SLD, Sargent CW, Keens TG. Theophylline does not increase ventilatory responses to hypercapnia or hypoxia. *Am Rev Respir Dis* 1992;146:1398–1401.
253. Swanson GD, Bellville JW. Hypoxic-hypercapnic interaction in human respiratory control. *J Appl Physiol* 1974;36(4):480–487.
254. Swanson GD, Bellville JW. Step changes in end-tidal CO_2: methods and implications. *J Appl Physiol* 1975;39:377–385.
255. Swanson GD, Ward DS, Bellville JW. Post-hyperventilation isocapnic hyperpnea. *J Appl Physiol* 1976;40(4):592–596.
256. Swanson GD, Whipp BJ, Kaufman RD, Aqleh KA, Winter B, Bellville JW. Effect of hypercapnia on hypoxic ventilatory drive in carotid body-resected man. *J Appl Physiol* 1978;45:971–977.
257. Takano Y, Takano M, Yaksh TL. The effect of intrathecally administered imiloxan and WB4101: possible role of alpha 2-adrenoceptor subtypes in the spinal cord. *Eur J Pharmacol* 1992;219: 465–468.
258. Tanelian DL, Kosek P, Mody I, Maclver MB. The role of the $GABA_A$ receptor/chloride channel complex in anesthesia. *Anesthesiology* 1993;78:757–776.
259. Tatsumi K, Pickett CK, Weil JV. Effects of haloperidol and domperidone on ventilatory roll off during sustained hypoxia in cats. *J Appl Physiol* 1992;72:1945–1952.
260. Taveira Da Silva AM, Hartley B, Hamosh P, Quest JA, Gillis RA. Respiratory depressant effects of GABA a- and b-receptor agonists in the cat. *J Appl Physiol* 1987;62:2264–2272.
261. Temp JA, Henson LC, Ward DS. Does a subanesthetic concentration of isoflurane blunt the ventilatory response to hypoxia? *Anesthesiology* 1992;77:1116–1124.
262. Temp JA, Henson LC, Ward DS. Effect of a subanesthetic minimum alveolar concentration of isoflurane on two tests of the hypoxic ventilatory response. *Anesthesiology* 1994;80(4):739–750.
262a. Temp JA, Bigoni B, Ward DS. Ventilatory response at four levels of sustained hypoxia. *Anesthesiology* 1991;75:A1098.
263. Teppema LJ, Barts PWJA, Folgering HT, Evers JAM. Effects of respiratory and (isocapnic) metabolic arterial acid-base disturbances on medullary extracellular fluid pH and ventilation in cats. *Respir Physiol* 1983;53:379–395.
264. Teppema LJ, Berkenbosch A, Veening JG, Olievier CN. Hypercapnia induces c-fos expression in neurons of retrotrapezoid nucleus in cats. *Brain Res* 1994;635:353–356.
265. Van Beek JHGM, Berkenbosch A, De Goede J, Olievier CN. Effects of brain stem hypoxaemia on the regulation of breathing. *Respir Physiol* 1984;57:171–188.
266. van den Elsen MJLJ, Dahan A, Berkenbosch A, DeGoede J, van Kleef JW, Olievier ICW. Does subanesthetic isoflurane affect the ventilatory response to acute isocapnic hypoxia in healthy volunteers? *Anesthesiology* 1994;81:860–867.
267. Verna A. Ultrastructure of the carotid body in the mammals. *Int Rev Cytol* 1979;60:271–330.
268. Vizek M, Pickett CK, Weil J. Biphasic ventilatory response of adult cats to sustained hypoxia has central origin. *J Appl Physiol* 1987; 63(4):13931658–1664.
269. von Euler C. Brain stem mechanisms for generation and control of breathing pattern. In: Fishman AP, Cherniack NS, Widdicombe JG, Geiger SR, eds. *Handbook of physiology. The respiratory system,* vol II, part 1. Bethesda: American Physiological Society, 1986;1–67.
270. von Euler C. Breathing behavior. In: von Euler C, Lagercrantz H, eds. *Neurobiology of the control of breathing.* New York: Raven Press, 1987;3–8.
271. von Euler C. Neural organization and rhythm generation. In: Crystal RG, West JB, Barnes PJ, et al., eds. *The lung: scientific foundations.* New York: Raven Press, 1991;1307–1318.
272. Vonhof S, Siren AL. Reversal of μ-opioid-mediated respiratory depression by a_2-adrenoceptor antagonism. *Life Sci* 1991;49: 111–119.
273. Wade JG, Larson CP, Hickey RF, Ehrenfeld WK, Severinghaus JW. Effect of carotid endarterectomy on carotid chemoreceptor and baroreceptor function in man. *N Engl J Med* 1970;282:823–829.
274. Waldrop TG. Posterior hypothalamic modulation of the respiratory response to CO_2 in cats. *Pflugers Arch* 1991;418:7–13.
275. Ward DS. Stimulation of hypoxic ventilatory drive by droperidol. *Anesth Analg* 1984;63:106–110.
276. Ward DS. The role of the peripheral D-2 dopamine receptors in the hypoxic ventilatory response. In: Benchetrit G, Baconnier P, Demongeot J, eds. *Concepts and formalizations in the control of breathing.* Manchester, UK: Manchester University Press, 1987;157–164.
277. Ward DS, Bellville JW. Reduction of hypoxic ventilatory drive by dopamine. *Anesth Analg* 1982;61:333–337.
278. Ward DS, Bellville JW. Effect of intravenous dopamine on hypercapnic ventilatory response in human. *J Appl Physiol* 1983;55: 1418–1425.
279. Ward DS, Berkenbosch A, DeGoede J, Olievier CN. Dynamics of the ventilatory responses to central hypoxia in cats. *J Appl Physiol* 1990;68:1107–1113.
280. Ward DS, Nguyen TT. Ventilatory response to sustained hypoxia during exercise. *Med Sci Sports Exerc* 1991;23(6):719–726.
281. Ward DS, Nino M. The effects of dopamine on the ventilatory response to sustained hypoxia in humans. In: Honda Y, Miyamoto Y, Konno K, Widdicombe JG, eds. *Control of breathing and its modeling perspective.* New York: Plenum Press, 1992;291–298.
282. Ward DS, Nitti GJ. The effects of sufentanil on the hemodynamic and respiratory response to exercise. *Med Sci Sports Exerc* 1988; 20(6):579–586.
283. Wasserman K, Whipp BJ, Casaburi R. Respiratory control during exercise. In: Fishman AP, Cherniack NS, Widdicombe JG, Geiger SR, eds. *Handbook of physiology. The respiratory system,* vol II, part 2. Baltimore: American Physiological Society, 1986;595–619.
284. Weil JV. Ventilatory control at high altitude. In: Fishman AP, Cherniack NS, Widdicombe JG, Geiger SR, eds. *Handbook of physiology. The respiratory system,* vol II, part 2. Baltimore: American Physiological Society, 1986;703–727.
285. Weil JV, McCullough RE, Kline JS, Sodal IE. Diminished ventilatory response to hypoxia and hypercapnia after morphine in normal man. *N Engl J Med* 1975;292:1103–1106.
286. Weil JV, Zwillich CW. Assessment of ventilatory response to hypoxia. *Chest* 1976;70(suppl):124–128.
287. Weyne J, Van Leuven F, Leusen I. Brain amino acids in conscious rats in chronic normocapnic and hypocapnic hypoxemia. *Respir Physiol* 1977;31:231–239.
288. Wheatley RG, Somerville ID, Sapsford DJ, Jones JG. Postoperative hypoxaemia: comparison of extradural, I.M. and patient-controlled opioid analgesia. *Br J Anaesth* 1990;64:267–275.
289. Wood JD. A possible role for gamma-aminobutyric acid in the homeostatic control of brain metabolism under conditions of hypoxia. *Exp Brain Res* 1967;4:81–84.
290. Wood JD, Watson WJ, Ducker AJ. The effect of hypoxia on brain gamma-aminobutyric acid levels. *J Neurochem* 1968;15:603–608.

291. Xu FD, Sato M, Spellman MJ, Mitchell RA, Severinghaus JW. Topography of cat medullary ventral surface hypoxic acidification. *J Appl Physiol* 1992;73:2631–2637.
292. Xu FD, Spellman MJ, Sato M, Baumgartner JE, Ciricillo SF, Severinghaus JW. Anomalous hypoxic acidification of medullary ventral surface. *J Appl Physiol* 1991;71:2211–2217.
293. Yamada KA, Hamosh P, Gillis RA. Respiratory depression produced by activation of GABA receptors in hindbrain of cat. *J Appl Physiol* 1981;51:1278–1286.
294. Yamada KA, Moerschbaecher JM, Hamosh P, Gillis RA. Pentobarbital causes cardiorespiratory depression by interacting with a GABAergic system at the ventral surface of the medulla. *J Pharmacol Exp Ther* 1983;226:349–355.
295. Yamada KA, Norman WP, Hamosh P, Gillis RA. Medullary ventral surface GABA receptors affect respiratory and cardiovascular function. *Brain Res* 1982;248:71–78.
296. Yamamoto M, Nishimura M, Kobayashi S, Akiyama Y, Miyamoto K, Kawakami Y. Role of endogenous adenosine in hypoxic ventilatory response in humans: a study with dipyridamole. *J Appl Physiol* 1994;76:196–203.
297. Young CH, Drummond GB, Warren PM. Effect of a sub-anaesthetic concentration of halothane on the ventilatory response to sustained hypoxia in healthy humans. *Br J Anaesth* 1993;71:642–647.
298. Young T, Palta M, Dempsey J, Skatrud J, Weber S, Badr S. The occurrence of sleep-disordered breathing among middle-aged adults. *N Engl J Med* 1993;328:1230–1273.
299. Zwart A, Kwant G, Oeseburg B, Zijlstra WG. Human whole-blood oxygen affinity: effect of carbon monoxide. *J Appl Physiol* 1984;57:14–20.

Anesthesia: Biologic Foundations, edited by
Tony L. Yaksh et al. Lippincott–Raven Publishers,
Philadelphia © 1997.

CHAPTER 79

RESPIRATORY MUSCLE FUNCTION

DAVID O. WARNER

Anesthesiologists have long recognized that anesthetic drugs alter the neural control of the respiratory muscles. In 1858, John Snow observed that during chloroform anesthesia breathing was "sometimes performed only by the diaphragm whilst the intercostal muscles are paralyzed" (242). These alterations in chest wall motion were used for many years as a guide to the proper administration of anesthesia (102). Fortunately, the overall neural output to the respiratory muscles was relatively well preserved by early anesthetic drugs such as ether, so that anesthesia could be administered safely without assisted ventilation. However, modern drugs used during anesthesia tend to cause a more severe depression of neural output to respiratory muscles. Although anesthetic techniques have evolved to address this depression, alterations in respiratory muscle function caused by anesthesia continue to constitute a major source of morbidity and mortality in modern anesthetic practice, causing complications ranging from a mild impairment of pulmonary gas exchange (205) to the potentially catastrophic consequences of hypoventilation (30).

This chapter is concerned primarily with the distribution of motor drive to the respiratory muscles during awake and anesthetized states and the functional consequences of this activity (or its absence). Areas to be discussed include the functional anatomy and neural control of the respiratory muscles, methods used to assess their function, and their behavior before, during, and after anesthesia.

RESPIRATORY MUSCLES: FUNCTIONAL ANATOMY

The respiratory muscles supply the lungs with fresh gas. One set of muscles controls intrathoracic pressure, which drives gas in and out of the lung. These are the muscles of the chest wall, defined as those structures that participate in this manipulation of intrathoracic pressure. Another group, the upper airway muscles, maintains the patency of the extrathoracic airway proximal to the glottis. Although breathing is often considered to be a relatively simple activity involving primarily a single muscle (the diaphragm), normal breathing actually requires the complex, coordinated action of multiple chest wall and upper airway muscles. This section first considers the individual constituents of the respiratory pump.

Diaphragm

The diaphragm is a thin muscle that separates the abdominal and thoracic cavities. Anatomically, the muscle can be separated into crural and costal parts (52). The crural diaphragm arises from the first three lumbar vertebrae and arcuate ligaments attached to the posterior body wall. The costal diaphragm arises from the costal and xiphoid cartilages. Both parts insert in a broad central tendon. The two parts may have different functional actions under some circumstances (57,58), although both portions participate in most respiratory muscle behaviors.

Although the shape of the diaphragm is complex, the human diaphragm is often considered to be an elliptical cylindroid capped by an irregular dome (52) (Fig. 1). The cylindrical portion is apposed to the inner surface of the rib cage and so conforms to its shape in this "area of apposition" (164). When the diaphragm contracts, its primary motion is a descent of the dome (143,272). In recumbent postures, the axial displacement of the dorsal portion exceeds that of the ventral portion (89,143). Isolated contraction of the diaphragm also affects other chest wall structures such as the rib cage by direct mechanical actions via its insertions and by changing abdominal and thoracic pressures; the significance of these effects depends on posture, lung volume, and the activity of other chest wall muscles (41,57,58,155,178).

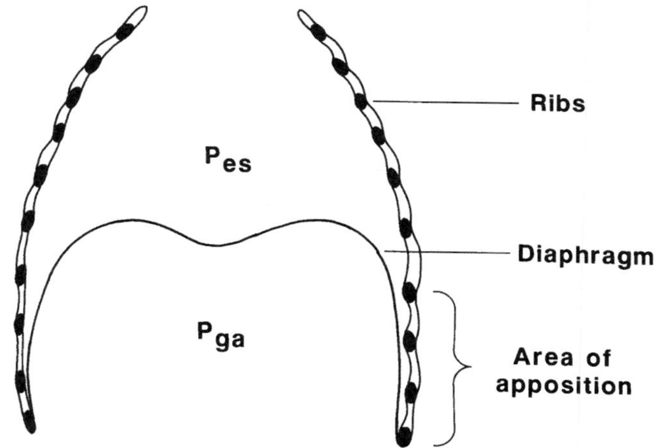

Figure 1. Coronal section of the thorax, showing the dome of the diaphragm, the area of apposition where the diaphragm is adjacent to the inner surface of the rib cage, and the regions where esophageal (P_{es}) and gastric (P_{ga}) pressures are measured to assess chest wall function.

The diaphragm is innervated by the phrenic nerves, which originate from the C_3 to C_5 roots in humans. The phrenic motoneurons are located in a narrow column in the medial part of the ventral horn of the spinal cord (172). Most motor axons are myelinated fibers in the size range of α motoneurons (7–17 μm) (8). There is also a considerable population of myelinated and unmyelinated afferent fibers, which may innervate muscle spindles (which are sparse in the diaphragm), tendon organs, and the diaphragmatic pleura and peritoneum; some may also terminate as free endings.

Rib Cage Muscles

Intercostal Muscles

There are two layers of intercostal muscle and fascia (Fig. 2). The external intercostal layer begins posteriorly at the tubercles of the ribs and runs interiorly and ventrally from the rib above to the rib below. Near the costochondral junction, it is replaced by a tendinous membrane that covers deeper layers. The internal intercostal layer runs superiorly and ventrally from the rib below to the rib above. It has two parts: a more lat-

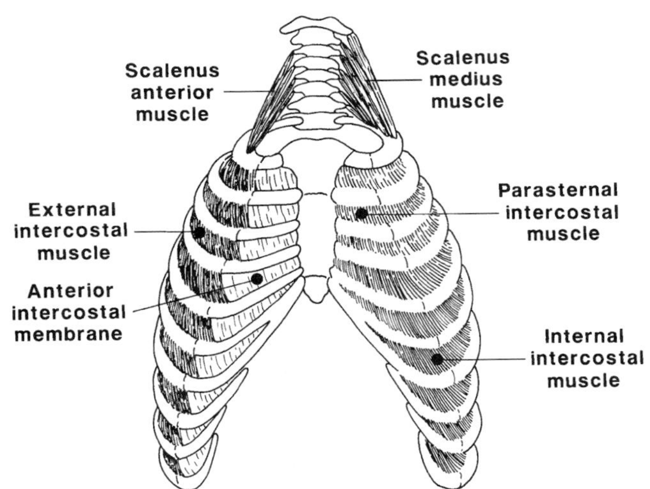

Figure 2. Anatomy of the rib cage muscles. The external intercostal muscles and anterior scalene muscles have been removed from the left side of the chest to show the internal intercostal and medial scalene muscles, respectively. (Reprinted with permission from ref. 195.)

eral intercostal portion and a more ventral interchondral portion adjacent to the sternum (often referred to as the parasternal intercostal muscle). These two portions may have different mechanical actions and patterns of electrical activation (247,273). There is an additional inner layer of muscle found deep to parasternal intercostal muscles, the triangularis sterni (transversus thoracis), which runs between the upper costal cartilages and the sternum. This layer is well developed in animals such as the dog (53) but is small in humans.

The actions of the intercostal muscles have long been debated (29). In general, the muscles of the more superficial layers are thought to promote inspiration, acting to elevate the ribs, whereas the deeper layers tend to depress the ribs and promote expiration (51,59). However, the complexity of the arrangement of these muscles is such that a single action cannot be attributed to any individual muscle. Their actions may depend on lung volume (51,60,276), activity of muscles in adjacent interspaces (51), and location (48). For example, the more ventral internal intercostal muscles (the parasternal intercostals) are inspiratory agonists (44), whereas the internal intercostal muscles in the lateral rib cage promote expiration. These muscles may also serve a stabilizing function, preventing rib cage distortion that otherwise would occur in response to the contraction of other muscles. For example, isolated diaphragmatic contraction causes a retraction of the upper rib cage secondary to decreased intrathoracic pressure (41,141, 261); normal intercostal muscle function prevents this retraction (50,178). Finally, the intercostal muscles have important nonrespiratory postural actions (274).

The intercostal muscles are innervated by segmental intercostal nerves, with motoneurons located in thoracic segments. They are richly endowed with muscle spindles and tendon organs (228).

Accessory Muscles

Other muscles attached to the rib cage may contribute to breathing. Although they have been referred to as "accessory muscles" of respiration, implying that they are used only when ventilatory demands are increased, they are often active during even quiet breathing.

The scalene muscles originate from the transverse processes of the lower five cervical vertebrae and insert on the upper surfaces of the first two ribs (Fig. 1). They are innervated by spinal segmental nerves. They elevate the ribs and sternum and, thus, have an inspiratory action.

The sternocleidomastoid muscles originate from the manubrium sterni and medial clavicle and insert on the mastoid process and occipital bone. They are innervated by the 11th cranial nerve and C2. Although their action in human subjects is unclear, they presumably also elevate the ribs and sternum.

The levator costae muscles are found posteriorly, superficial to the muscles that directly make up the thoracic wall, connecting the transverse process of each thoracic vertebra with the rib below. Innervated by segmental nerves, they have an inspiratory action on the rib cage (96).

Abdominal muscles

Four muscles compose the anterolateral abdominal wall. The fibers of the external oblique originate from the external surface of the lower ribs and run ventrally and inferiorly to the iliac crest and linea alba. The internal oblique originates from the inguinal ligament and iliac crest and run ventrally and superiorly to the lower costal cartilages and linea alba. The transversus abdominis runs circumferentially around the abdomen; attachments include the costal cartilages, the iliac crest, the lumbodorsal fascia, and the inguinal ligament. Finally, the rectus abdominis, ensheathed by the aponeuroses of the other three muscles, connects the pubic bone with the lower margins of the rib cage and xiphoid process.

Contraction of these muscles raises intraabdominal pressure, which in general tends to displace the diaphragm cephalad and to decrease lung volume (95). However, this expiratory action may be opposed by direct actions of the muscles via insertions on the rib cage (168) and by increased abdominal pressure that may inflate the lower rib cage via the area of apposition (56).

The abdominal muscles are innervated by the seventh to eleventh intercostals, subcostal, iliohypogastric, and ilioinguinal nerves.

Upper Airway Muscles

Although many muscles surround the upper airway, this section concentrates on those most likely to influence pharyngeal and laryngeal patency during anesthesia (254).

Soft Palate

The soft palate extends from the posterior border of the hard palate into the oropharynx. Its position, which directs gas flow through the mouth or nose, is regulated by five muscles, which are innervated by the pharyngeal plexus: tensor and levator veli palatini, musculus uvulae, palatoglossus, and palatopharyngeus (Fig. 3).

Pharynx

Pharyngeal caliber is narrowed by three overlapping muscles that compose the lateral and posterior walls of the pharynx: superior, middle, and inferior constrictors. The muscles originate from more anterior structures, including the tongue, hyoid bone, and thyroid and cricoid cartilages, and insert on the median fibrous raphe on the posterior pharyngeal wall (Fig. 4). These pharyngeal constrictors are all innervated by the pharyngeal plexus.

Anterior and lateral muscles dilate the pharynx. The tongue forms the anterior wall of the oropharynx, whereas the hyoid bone and associated muscles form the anterior wall of the hypopharynx.

The intrinsic muscles of the tongue (those with no attachments to external structures) primarily control shape, although they may also be involved in tongue protrusion. The position of the tongue is controlled by several extrinsic muscles that connect the tongue with surrounding structures. The genioglossus

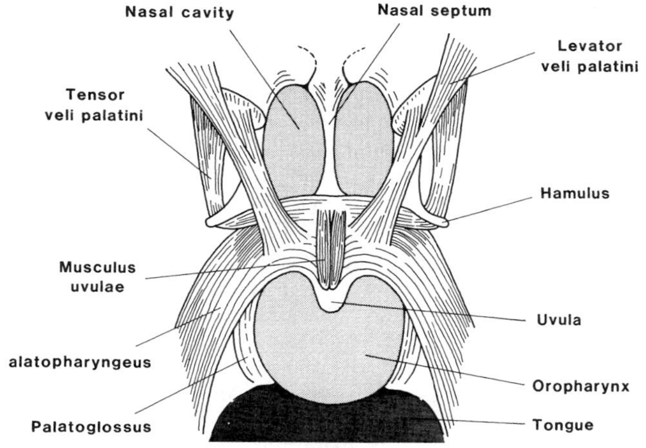

Figure 3. Anatomy of the muscles controlling the position of the soft palate, posterior view.

originates on the anterior mandible and causes tongue protrusion. It is likely that this muscle is primarily responsible for anterior motion of the posterior part of the tongue to enlarge the oropharynx (163). The genioglossus also acts with the hypoglossus, which originates on the hyoid bone, to depress the tongue. Two muscles, the styloglossus and the palatoglossus, which originate on the styloid process and palate, respectively, elevate the tongue. All tongue muscles are innervated by the hypoglossal nerve, except the palatoglossus (innervated by the pharyngeal plexus).

Several muscles attached to the hyoid bone may control pharyngeal patency. The geniohyoid, mylohyoid, stylohyoid, and digastric muscles attach to the superior hyoid and elevate it; the omohyoid, thyrohyoid, and sternohyoid muscles attach to the inferior hyoid and lower it. The coordinated activity of these muscles appears to increase upper airway size and to minimize the descent of the larynx during inspiration (2,213).

Larynx

Extrinsic laryngeal muscles control laryngeal position via attachments to outside structures such as the sternum and include many of the muscles previously described as controlling hyoid position. Intrinsic laryngeal muscles control patency of the laryngeal inlet and the position of the vocal cords (Fig. 5). The laryngeal inlet is narrowed by contraction of the transverse arytenoids, oblique arytenoids, and lateral cricothyroids. The posterior cricoarytenoids, which abduct the vocal cords, are the primary muscles that control the laryngeal aperture in adults during resting breathing (18,145). Other muscles with known respiration-related activity in humans include the cricothyroids (270), which tense the vocal cords, and the thyroarytenoids (144), which relax and adduct the vocal cords. All muscles are supplied by branches of the vagus nerve: the cricothyroid and part of the transverse arytenoid by the external branch of the superior laryngeal branch, and the remaining muscles by the recurrent laryngeal branches.

CONTROL OF RESPIRATORY MUSCLES

The focus in this chapter is on systems that regulate the neural output to specific groups of respiratory muscles.

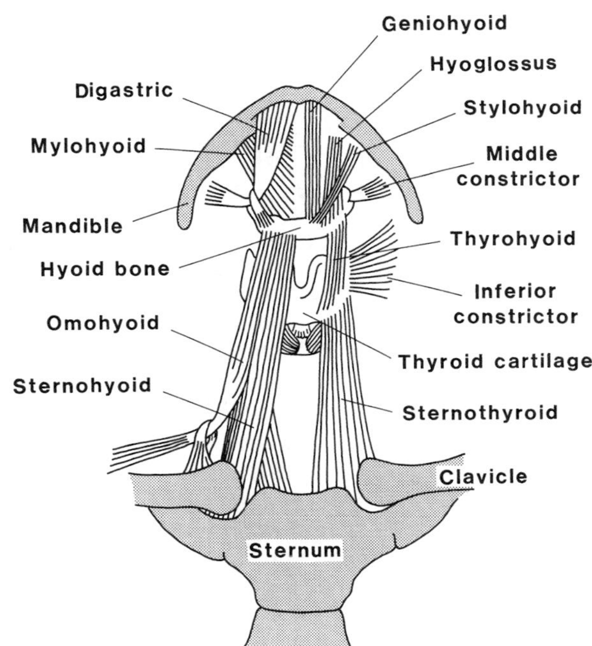

Figure 4. Anatomy of muscles attached to the hyoid bone and thyroid cartilage that may control upper airway patency. Muscles depicted on the *left* are more superficial and have been removed on the *right* for clarity.

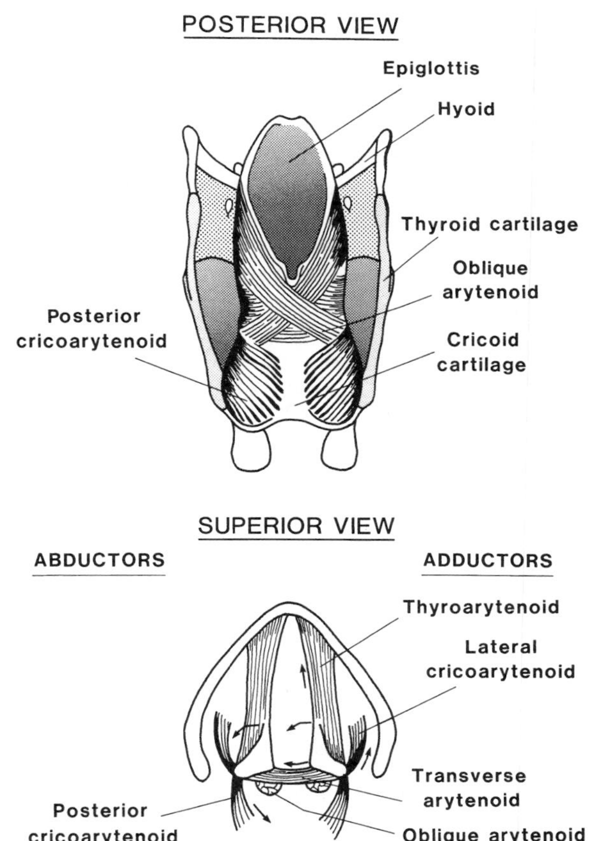

Figure 5. Anatomy of laryngeal muscles. *Upper panel:* Posterior view. *Lower panel:* Superior view of muscles controlling vocal cord position, showing actions of vocal cord abductors on the left, and the actions of adductors on the right.

Chest Wall Muscles

Output Neurons From Respiratory Centers

The respiratory muscles are innervated by motoneurons that originate in the spinal cord. These motoneurons receive input from respiratory centers in the medulla. Medullary respiratory neurons that send axons to the spinal cord are defined as bulbospinal neurons. These neurons are concentrated in two regions (172): one in the ventral nucleus of the solitary tract, referred to as the dorsal respiratory group (DRG), and the other that is an extended ventrolateral column of neurons, referred to as the ventral respiratory group (VRG) (Fig. 6). Both groups contain bulbospinal neurons that are active during inspiration; neurons active during expiration are found only in the VRG. Neurons with primarily expiratory activity are concentrated in the most rostral portion of the VRG, referred to as the Bötzinger complex, and the most caudal portion of the VRG. Thus, respiratory neurons can be classified by location (DRG or VRG) and timing of discharge (inspiratory or expiratory). Within these classifications, neurons with varying discharge patterns can be identified. Patterns of discharge may vary according to the part of the respiratory cycle when the neuron fires, the time of onset of activity, or changes in the frequency of firing during the respiratory cycle. These patterns may be influenced by collateral inputs from other respiratory neurons or afferent inputs, which may shape the output pattern transmitted to motoneurons (259).

The primary drive to phrenic motoneurons originates from inspiratory bulbospinal neurons from the DRG (34,35) and, to a lesser extent, the VRG (78,84), via monosynaptic and polysynaptic pathways (43). Amino acids and serotonin may be neurotransmitters in these pathways (179). Phrenic activity is also modulated at medullary and spinal levels by neurons with expiratory activity. Bulbospinal neurons of the Bötzinger complex inhibit inspiratory neurons of the DRG and directly inhibit phrenic motoneurons, probably via a mechanism involving γ-aminobutyric acid (82,83,166).

Inspiratory drive to intercostal motoneurons originates primarily from VRG neurons (43,114), with a lesser contribution from the DRG (212). These neurons are not inhibited during expiration (167), as are phrenic motoneurons. Pathways responsible for the control of motoneurons with expiratory activity are less well known, but appear to involve polysynaptic pathways that originate from the Bötzinger complex and caudal VRG (169). These expiratory bulbospinal neurons are strongly influenced by pulmonary stretch receptor activity via the vagus nerve (4,12).

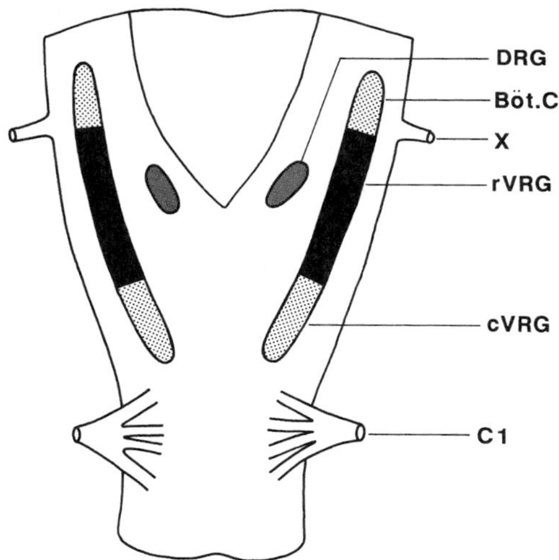

Figure 6. Location of the medullary respiratory neurons in the cat, showing a dorsal view of the medulla. Neurons primarily active during expiration in microelectrode recordings are shown in stippled areas; those in grey and black areas are primarily active during inspiration. DRG, dorsal respiratory group; rVRG and cVRG, rostral and caudal ventral respiratory group, respectively; Böt.C, Bötzinger complex; X, vagus nerve root; C1, C1 nerve root. (Reprinted with permission from ref. 172.)

Modulation of Output Neurons

As with other skeletal muscles, the final neural output to the respiratory muscles is shaped by afferent information from muscle and tendon receptors. This afferent activity is an important component of a local feedback loop at a spinal level (referred to as the motor servo) that regulates mechanical variables such as tension and stiffness that are monitored by these receptors. Afferent information is also projected to higher levels, resulting in modulation of bulbospinal neuronal activity. This complex system allows neural output to adapt to changing mechanical loads applied to the muscle, and to account for the dependence of developed force on variables such as muscle length and velocity. The system also aids in coordination between the actions of individual respiratory muscles and results in a smooth contraction that meets the needs of the respiratory system.

Compared with some other skeletal muscle systems, understanding of the exact role of afferent pathways in the respiratory muscles is limited. Although it is certain that respiratory neurons are connected by complex networks of spinal interneurons, their functional significance is unclear (172). Afferent proprioceptive information from respiratory muscles may affect respiratory activity at the spinal and medullary levels. These effects are most easily demonstrated in intercostal afferents (226,227); stimulation of some afferents can affect both inspiratory and expiratory medullary neurons (15,110,229). At a spinal level, intercostal muscle proprioceptors may modulate inspiratory muscle activity during quiet breathing, because such activity can be affected by sectioning of thoracic dorsal spinal roots (183,221); a similar role for afferent activity has been postulated for the abdominal muscles (13,217). However, it has been suggested that this proprioceptive information may be more important for the performance of nonrespiratory behaviors of the muscles such as the maintenance of posture (76). The role of afferent information from the diaphragm is more controversial (31,221,228), because there are few muscle spindles and interruption of these pathways has little effect on diaphragmatic activity.

Nonrespiratory Functions

The respiratory muscles also subserve many nonrespiratory functions such as the maintenance of posture, speech, and vomiting (172). Thus, there are significant inputs to respiratory motoneurons from nonrespiratory supramedullary centers, including the motor cortex (212) and emetic centers (170). In this way, the respiratory control of these motoneurons can be modified or superseded as necessary to perform other behaviors.

Upper Airway Muscles

Motoneurons innervating upper airway muscles are located in several nuclei; important centers include the hypoglossal nucleus (muscles of the tongue) and the retrofacial nucleus and nucleus ambiguous (laryngeal and pharyngeal muscles). Compared with the motoneurons to chest wall muscles, relatively little is known regarding the respiratory control of upper airway motoneurons (126). This lack of knowledge may reflect the fact that these muscles have important nonrespiratory functions (e.g., speech or swallowing) that make identification of specific respiratory-related inputs to these motoneurons difficult. Possible sources of such inputs include the medullary reticular formation, the pneumotaxic center in the pons, and the caudal region of the nucleus solitarius. Inputs from the reticular activating system appear to be important determinants of activity in cranial nerve nuclei (194,249). These inputs may explain the importance of the state of arousal to the function of upper airway muscle motoneurons (126).

Whatever the pathways involved, afferent information plays an important role in the control of these muscles. Even though chest wall and upper airway motoneurons must receive common inputs from the central pattern generator, their discharge patterns during lung inflation are different. Lung inflation decreases activity in upper airway motoneurons, probably via input from slowly adapting lung receptors (10,235,255), whereas phrenic nerve activity is unaffected or augmented (61,235). Other lung receptors, such as rapidly adapting receptors, can also influence upper airway muscle activity (256). There are also abundant receptors in the upper airway (275). These receptors, which respond to changes in airway pressure and a variety of mechanical and chemical stimuli (including volatile anesthetics) (187,220), can modulate the activities of upper airway and chest wall muscles. Reflex closure of the glottis, involving contraction of multiple upper airway muscles, serves an important protective function to prevent aspiration of material into the lungs (209,222).

Organization and Composition of Respiratory Motor Units

A motor unit, composed of a motoneuron and the muscle fibers that it innervates, is the final element of neural control in skeletal muscle. Motor units in respiratory muscles vary considerably in their physiologic properties, allowing for flexibility in recruitment to perform respiratory and nonrespiratory behaviors.

Different types of motor units can be classified by measuring the isometric force developed by isolated muscle preparations stimulated with electrical current (Fig. 7). Although there is a continuous distribution of twitch contraction times in such preparations, "fast" and "slow" twitch units can be distinguished by the ability of the unit to maintain force during unfused (lower frequency) tetanic stimulation (27). Units can be further classified by their resistance to fatigue. Repetitive stimulation is applied during a 2-min period, and a fatigue index is calculated as a ratio of force developed at the conclusion of this period to the initial force. On the basis of this test, "slow" twitch fibers are fatigue-resistant, whereas "fast" twitch fibers can be classified into fatigue resistant, fatigable, and intermediate types. Fibers can also be classified by staining (histochemistry) or biochemical properties (25-27).

The force generated by a muscle can be controlled by changing the number of activated muscle units, by changing the discharge frequency of recruited motor units, or by a combination of both mechanisms (233). Motor units in the diaphragm are recruited in a stereotypic order which may be related to motoneuron diameter (109), differential activation of inspiratory bulbospinal neurons (113), or other factors. It has been estimated that slow and fatigue-resistant units can provide sufficient force for quiet breathing (236,237). Intermediate and fatigable fast fibers are recruited during ventilatory stimulation and during nonrespiratory behaviors such as coughing or vomiting. Thus, the physiologic properties of individual muscle units appear to be appropriately matched to their use; fatigue-resistant units are used during sustained quiet breathing, and more fatigable units are reserved for transient behaviors requiring greater force. In a similar way, the distribution of fiber types in individual upper airway muscles may be tailored to best fulfill function (252).

In summary, respiratory motoneurons receive many inputs, including those from medullary respiratory centers via bulbospinal neurons, proprioceptive information, and nonrespiratory inputs, all of which may themselves be modulated by various neural networks. Motoneuron pools that control different muscle groups may have quite different control systems, allowing for great flexibility in the shaping of respiratory behavior to meet the demands of the organism. Heterogeneity in the physiologic properties of motor units allows for further refinement of the control of force during different muscle behaviors.

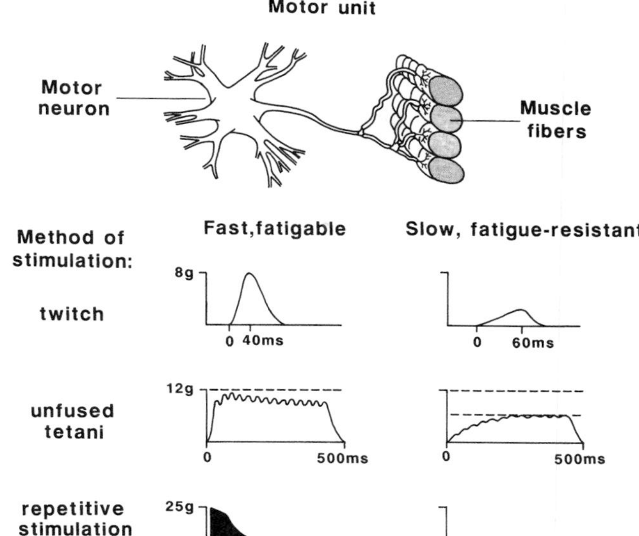

Figure 7. Individual motor unit (*upper panel*) and representative tracings of isometric force developed by two types of isolated muscles in response to different patterns of electrical stimulation (*lower panel*). Note that the fast, fatiguable muscle fiber demonstrates a rapid development of force in response to a single twitch stimulus, a "sag" in force during unfused tetanic stimulation, and considerable fatigue of response to repetitive stimulation; these characteristics are not present in slow, fatigue-resistant fibers. Fast fibers can be further classified into two additional types that are not shown. (Reprinted, in adapted form, with permission from ref. 236.)

ASSESSMENT OF RESPIRATORY MUSCLE FUNCTION

Measurement of Neural Activation

The generation and propagation of action potentials in excitable tissues creates potential differences. These differences can be measured by electrodes adjacent to nerves as the electroneurogram or by electrodes adjacent to muscles as the electromyogram (EMG). The most direct measurement of neural input to the muscle is the electroneurogram; however, such measurements are problematic in intact awake organisms. Therefore, the EMG, which represents the summation of the action potentials of individual motor units, is often used as an index of neural activation (157). However, many variables other than the neural input to the muscle can affect the EMG, including muscle length and geometry (19,133), so that the correspondence between the activity of a motor nerve and its target muscle may be imperfect. A variety of techniques are available to measure the EMG (153). Surface EMG electrodes placed on the skin are noninvasive but relatively nonselective and may detect activity from muscles other than the one of interest. Fine-wire electrodes may be placed directly in the muscle of interest but are susceptible to dislodgment and may cause discomfort.

Measurement of Mechanical Responses

Variables such as tidal volume or minute ventilation measure the overall output of the respiratory muscles but provide little insight into the function of individual muscles. Direct measurements of respiratory muscle length can be performed by ultrasonic crystals sutured directly to the surface of surgically exposed muscles (184), but these techniques have limited application in human subjects. Most current techniques suitable for human use are indirect, measuring the motion and pressures generated by the actions of the respiratory muscles on the chest wall. However, the limitations of such approaches should be clearly recognized. There is no simple, unique relationship between the motion of any chest wall structure and the activity of any single group of respiratory muscles. Also, measurements of the electrical activity generated by a muscle (i.e., the EMG) are insufficient to define the mechanical actions of that muscle; the presence of EMG activity in a muscle does not necessarily imply that the muscle has a significant mechanical action.

During inspiration, the rib cage expands and the diaphragm descends. This diaphragmatic motion requires an expansion of the abdomen, because the abdominal contents are relatively incompressible. Konno and Mead (138) demonstrated that changes in lung volume could be accurately determined from measurements of the external dimensions of the rib cage and the abdomen. These measurements can be readily obtained by using various devices that measure anteroposterior diameter, circumference, or cross-sectional area of the rib cage and abdomen. Furthermore, the tidal volume can be partitioned into a volume displaced by the rib cage and a volume displaced by the diaphragm-abdomen, providing a convenient description of the pattern of chest wall motion (Fig. 8). These volumes do not precisely correspond to volumes swept by the anatomic surfaces of the rib cage and the diaphragm, because the two structures are mechanically coupled at the area of apposition and the ventral abdominal wall (156,165). However, with newer imaging techniques, these quantities can be measured directly (see below).

Pressures in the thorax (measured in the esophagus) and the abdomen (measured in the stomach) can be used to calculate transdiaphragmatic pressure, an estimate of the effective force generated by diaphragm contraction (132,146) (Fig. 1). Various indices of diaphragm function have been calculated by using combinations of these pressures. In addition, the phrenic nerve can be electrically stimulated by surface or needle electrodes in human subjects to evaluate diaphragmatic muscle contractility (200,240). However, transdiaphragmatic pressures can also be affected by the contraction of other chest wall muscles, lung volume, and chest wall shape, so that caution must be exercised when attributing changes in these measurements solely to changes in diaphragmatic activity (115,118,197,240).

BEHAVIOR OF RESPIRATORY MUSCLES

Breathing is a complex activity, requiring the coordinated activity of several different muscle groups, even under conditions of quiet breathing (98). Like any another behavior, breathing must adapt to environmental demands. Conditions such as mechanical loads to breathing or increasing metabolic needs require a response of the respiratory muscles to maintain adequate gas exchange. Furthermore, all respiratory muscles have important nonrespiratory functions which must also be accommodated. It is important to realize that the exact mechanical consequences of activity in individual respiratory muscles are often uncertain, especially because these actions may vary according to activity in other muscles.

Chest Wall Behavior During Quiet Breathing

The pattern of breathing in awake subjects constantly changes, spontaneously (23,151) and in response to changes in behavior (such as speaking or moving). Subjects may also voluntarily alter their breathing pattern, especially when they are aware that it is being monitored. The apparatus used to monitor breathing may further affect its pattern (3,93). Thus, the state of "quiet breathing" may not be unique and reproducible.

Phasic Activity In awake human subjects, consistent phasic activity during inspiration is observed in the diaphragm, the parasternal intercostal muscles, and the scalenes (28,55,70,137, 203,247,273). This activity is seen in upright and recumbent positions. The diaphragm acts as the primary pressure generator. The relative mechanical importance of parasternal intercostal and scalene contraction to tidal breathing in human subjects is unknown, but these muscles appear to maintain normal rib cage expansion during inspiration (42,47,50,80,178), preventing rib cage retraction in response to negative intrathoracic pressure generated by the descent of the diaphragm.

Expiration during quiet breathing is primarily passive, caused by relaxation of the diaphragm and the passive recoil of the respiratory system. However, airflow during expiration is retarded by varying degrees of persistent activity in the diaphragm, parasternal intercostals, and laryngeal muscles (99, 207). The "braking" effect produced by this activity is important for the maintenance of mean lung volume in infants (36, 139,140), but not adults. The transversus thoracis and internal intercostal in the lateral rib cage show phasic activity during expiration in some individuals (54,247); the mechanical significance of this activity in generating expiratory airflow in humans is unknown.

As a result of this phasic activation of the respiratory muscles, the diaphragm descends and the rib cage expands. The relative contribution of each component to the tidal volume has recently been measured with fast computed tomographic (CT) scanning in normal subjects lying supine (266). During quiet

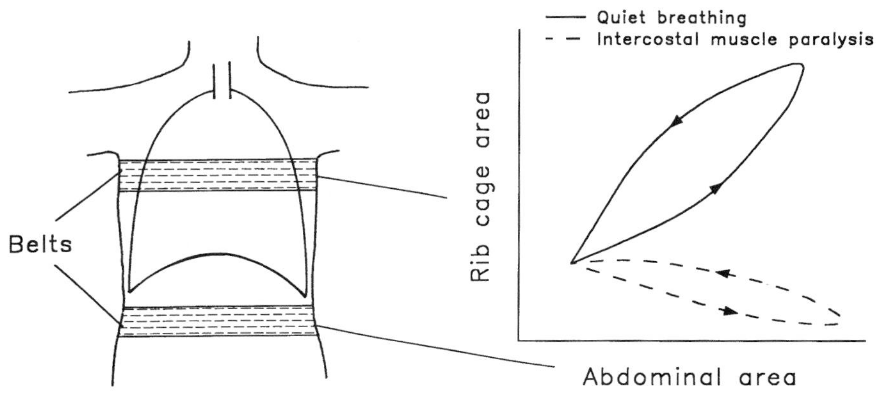

Figure 8. Schematic representation of system used to describe chest wall motion using changes in external dimensions of the rib cage and abdomen first proposed by Konno and Mead (138). *Solid line* shows typical pattern during quiet breathing; *dashed line* shows pattern during isolated diaphragmatic contraction, demonstrating paradoxic inward motion of the rib cage during inspiration.

breathing, 75% of the total change in intrathoracic volume during inspiration is produced by descent of the diaphragm, with the remaining 25% produced by expansion of the rib cage. These values agree with previous estimates from measurements of the surface dimensions of the rib cage and abdomen using Konno-Mead techniques when the mechanical linkage among abdomen, diaphragm, and rib cage is taken into account (165). In upright positions, rib cage expansion probably accounts for a greater proportion of the tidal volume (70,138,258). This difference may occur because of changes in the pattern of respiratory muscle activation (70,247), changes in the geometry of the chest wall, or a combination of these factors.

Tonic Activity

In addition to this phasic activity linked to the inspiratory and expiratory phases of the respiratory cycle, some respiratory muscles apparently exhibit tonic activity. However, the lack of association with the phases of respiration makes EMG measurements purporting to show such activity more difficult to interpret. Activity may be difficult to distinguish from noise or activity in adjacent nonrespiratory muscles, especially when surface EMG electrodes are used. In upright postures, abdominal muscles are tonically active (52,70,154,245). This activity is thought to support the abdominal contents against gravity and to prevent shortening of the diaphragm, which would impair its efficiency. Tonic abdominal muscle activity is usually not observed in supine subjects (70). Tonic activity has also been reported in the diaphragm, intercostal muscles, and scalene muscles by some, but not all, authors (46,55,67,70,180). This tonic activity may help maintain end-expiratory lung volume (the functional residual capacity; FRC). As in the abdominal muscles, this activity appears to be less in the supine compared with upright postures (70). The existence of tonic activity in the diaphragm is particularly controversial. Recent studies demonstrating that anesthesia and paralysis do not consistently change the net position of the diaphragm also argue against the presence of tonic diaphragmatic activity (142,143,263) (see below).

Upper Airway Behavior During Quiet Breathing

Several upper airway muscles demonstrate phasic activity during inspiration. The most extensively studied is the genioglossus (208,223), although other upper airway muscles such as the stylopharyngeus, styloglossus, posterior cricoarytenoid, and cricothyroid muscles may also be active (18,103,145,270). These muscles help maintain upper airway patency during the negative upper airway pressures generated by inspiratory flow. This activity is of critical importance; in its absence, even modest negative upper airway pressures can markedly narrow the upper airway of normal subjects (271) (Fig. 9). The pharyngeal constrictors may demonstrate phasic expiratory activity, although its significance is unknown (37,215).

The glottis widens during inspiration and narrows during expiration in human subjects (20), primarily due to phasic activation of the posterior cricoarytenoid muscle, a vocal cord abductor (21,250) (Fig. 10). As is true for many upper airway muscles, phasic activation of this muscle precedes activation of chest wall muscles and, consequently, inspiratory flow. This early activation may minimize airflow resistance by opening the vocal cords prior to inspiration. The activity decreases during expiration; the resulting glottic narrowing may serve to retard and control expiratory flow (21,79). Phasic expiratory activity in vocal cord adductors such as the thyroarytenoids may also serve to control expiratory flow (125,144). The cricothyroid muscle exhibits tonic activity during expiration and phasic activity during inspiration; the mechanical importance of this activity is unknown (239,270). The extrinsic laryngeal muscles can also dilate the upper airway (2,213); however, little information is available regarding the actions of these muscles in human subjects. It is likely that the coordinated activity of all these muscles is necessary to maintain normal upper airway caliber.

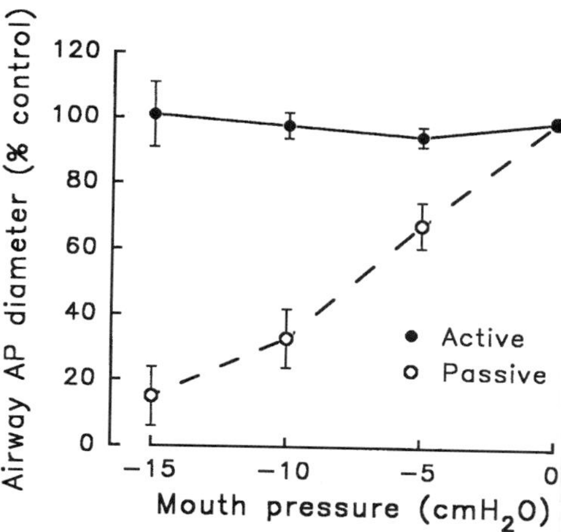

Figure 9. Relationship between anterioposterior upper airway diameter (measured by fluoroscopy) and mouth pressure in six supine subjects when mouth pressure was decreased by graded inspiratory effort against an occluded airway (*active* upper airway muscles) or negative pressure generated by an external source (*passive* upper airway muscles). Note that airway size is maintained despite negative pressures when upper airway muscles are active, and that the upper airway is markedly narrowed by relatively modest pressures in the absence of activity. (Reprinted, in adapted form, with permission from ref. 271.)

Stimulated Breathing

Ventilation may be increased by external loads to breathing (e.g., breathing through a resistance or through increased dead space) or in response to increased metabolic demands (e.g., exercise or hypoxia). There is a wide repertoire of muscle responses available to meet these demands. In general, inspiratory chest wall muscles that are normally active during quiet breathing initially increase their activities. As ventilation further increases, abdominal and rib cage expiratory muscles

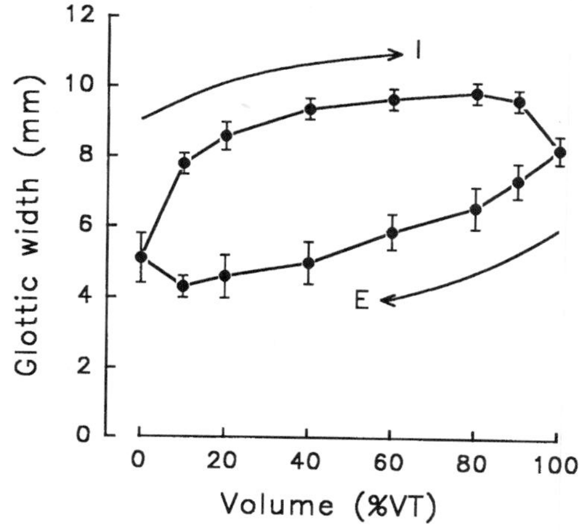

Figure 10. Relationship between glottic width (measured by fiberoptic laryngoscopy) and lung volume during quiet breathing in one subject, showing widening during inspiration. Values are mean ± SD from repeated determinations in one subject. (Reprinted with permission from ref. 20.)

develop phasic activity (101,154). This active expiration ensures that the inspired gas is fully expelled from the lung and prevents a gradual increase in end-expiratory lung volume that might otherwise occur because shortened expiratory times would not allow complete passive expiration.

The activity of laryngeal muscles can also increase in response to ventilatory stimulation, presumably to maintain airway patency in the face of more negative airway pressures generated by increased airflow (192,193,270). The opposing activity of laryngeal adductors and abductors may also play an important role in controlling airflow under such circumstances (125).

Respiratory Muscle Function in Disease

Disorders of respiratory muscle function may contribute to the pathogenesis of many diseases. Although a detailed review is beyond the scope of this chapter, respiratory muscle fatigue has attracted attention recently and may affect the perioperative management of the surgical patient.

Respiratory muscle fatigue is defined as a loss in the capacity of the respiratory muscles to develop force in response to ventilatory loads that is reversible by rest (185). Fatigue may occur at several sites, which can be classified as either central or peripheral (236). Central fatigue is characterized by a failure of motoneurons to generate action potentials, usually reflecting decreased drive from the respiratory control centers. Peripheral fatigue results from failure of motor unit function at any site from the axon to the contractile machinery of the cell. Fatigue has been postulated to be clinically significant in four groups of patients: (a) premature and newborn infants, (b) patients with chronic respiratory loads or inspiratory muscle weakness (including neuromuscular diseases), (c) patients with inadequate energy supplies (e.g., shock), and (d) patients with acute exacerbations of asthma and chronic obstructive pulmonary disease. Fatigue may exacerbate ventilatory insufficiency during acute respiratory failure and may impair weaning from mechanical ventilation (214). Neonates may be especially susceptible to fatigue because of developmental changes in the properties and distribution of motor units (87,236). Although there is no doubt that respiratory muscle fatigue can be induced experimentally, its contribution to pathophysiology remains unclear, largely because the criteria for its diagnosis are controversial (185) and because therapeutic trials of muscular "rest" for fatigue have been disappointing (230).

Species Differences

It is important to realize that respiratory muscle control may differ significantly among species. The chest wall of quadrupeds differs fundamentally from that of humans in both form and function. For example, during quiet breathing in dogs, phasic expiratory activity is prominent in the abdominal and triangularis sterni muscles, which have expiratory actions (49,53,94,186,267). Thus, expiration is an active process in the dog even while at rest, unlike humans. Consequently, the lung volume at the end of expiration is less than the lung volume when all muscles are relaxed. Dogs then initiate inspiration by relaxing their expiratory muscles and allowing lung volume to increase passively; activation of the diaphragm and other inspiratory muscles completes the inspiration. The opposite sequence occurs during expiration. This active expiratory activity may be responsible for a significant portion of the tidal volume (141,261,264). Active expiration is generally observed in normal awake human subjects only during stimulated breathing, such as occurs during exercise (108). The reason why these animals use such a markedly different strategy of breathing compared with humans is not known, but suggests that the results of animal experiments should be applied to humans only with caution.

EFFECTS OF ANESTHESIA ON RESPIRATORY MUSCLE FUNCTION

Many studies of anesthesia-induced changes in respiratory muscle function use chest wall and upper airway position and motion to infer anesthetic effects on specific muscle groups. This approach provides a convenient framework for the discussion of anesthetic effects on respiratory muscle function. However, as previously discussed, there are clear limitations to the use of chest wall motion to infer respiratory muscle activity and actions, and the neural mechanisms responsible for observed changes in chest wall motion remain largely speculative.

Functional Residual Capacity

In the majority of recumbent human subjects, the induction of general anesthesia reduces the FRC (205) (Fig. 11). This decrease occurs rapidly after anesthetic induction (9,117) and does not appear to change with time (62,112,269). During barbiturate-narcotic anesthesia, the addition of muscular paralysis does not further decrease the FRC (269). The FRC does not decrease if anesthesia is induced in the sitting position (206). Most anesthetic drugs, including thiopental, methoxyflurane, halothane, and isoflurane, decrease the FRC; however, the FRC is not affected by ketamine or, under some circumstances, methohexital anesthesia (11,161,234).

The mechanisms responsible for the decrease in FRC remain unknown. Possible mechanisms directly involving the control of respiratory muscles include a loss of tonic activity in inspiratory agonists such as the diaphragm (89,180) or a development of activity in expiratory agonists such as abdominal muscles (88,131). Other possible mechanisms, including changes in the volume of blood in the thoracoabdominal cavity and increases in lung elastic recoil, have been reviewed elsewhere (205,265).

To the extent that tonic activity in chest wall muscles is important to the maintenance of FRC (see above), abolition of such activity by anesthesia with muscular paralysis should reduce the FRC. Consistent with this idea, some studies have found that partial neuromuscular blockade decreases the FRC in seated awake subjects (45,46). However, other studies have found little change (134,225), and it is possible that changes in the volume of blood in the thorax, not changes in chest wall dimensions, are responsible for alterations in the FRC. The FRC does not change with partial paralysis in supine subjects (90).

It has been suggested that the anesthetic state itself reduces tonic muscle activity during spontaneous breathing. Such decreases in FRC could be caused by an inward motion of the rib cage, a cephalad motion of the diaphragm, or some combination of these possibilities. In the simplest case, motion of each structure suggests an effect of anesthesia on the muscles associated with that compartment.

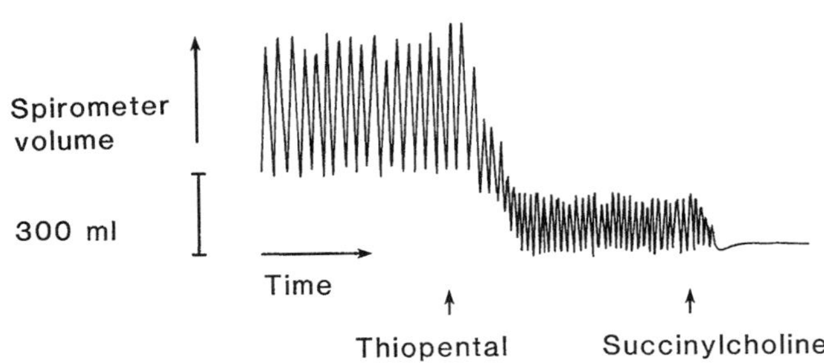

Figure 11. Spirogram during induction of anesthesia with thiopental, demonstrating an immediate decrease in functional residual capacity that is not further affected by muscular paralysis. The spirogram has been modified to account for oxygen uptake. (Reprinted, in adapted form, with permission from ref. 9.)

Inward Rib Cage Displacement

Drummond (67) found that thiopental anesthesia decreased tonic activity in intercostal, scalene, and sternocleidomastoid muscles as measured by surface electrodes. The results of this study may be questioned, because the observed pattern of awake activity in these muscles was primarily tonic, whereas all other studies have found primarily phasic activity in these muscles (46,55,70,203). Also, EMG measurements from intramuscular electrodes in supine volunteers have failed to demonstrate consistent tonic activity in parasternal intercostal or scalene muscles while the subjects were awake or during halothane anesthesia (263) (Fig. 12). However, abolition of such activity by anesthesia could explain the consistent inward motion of the rib cage observed after anesthetic induction, as measured by both surface dimensions and by three-dimensional CT images of the thorax (104,142,263). Such a change, accomplished by nonuniform changes in internal chest wall dimensions that exhibit considerable intersubject variability, is observed with anesthesia during paralysis with mechanical ventilation (104,142) and during spontaneous breathing (263).

End-expiratory rib cage dimensions could also be decreased by phasic activity in rib cage muscles with expiratory actions (lateral internal intercostals and transversus thoracis). Preliminary data suggest that the lateral internal intercostal muscles are recruited during halothane anesthesia (263) (Fig. 12). However, the mechanical consequences of such activity remain to be determined, because decreases in rib cage dimensions are observed in the absence of any muscular effort (i.e., during pharmacologic paralysis) (104,142).

Rib cage position could also be affected by other factors such as the diaphragm, acting via its insertions, and gastric pressure, acting on the lower rib cage via the area of apposition. For example, the induction of anesthesia-paralysis has been reported to reduce the end-expiratory intraabdominal pressure, which would have an expiratory action on the lower rib cage (69). The curvature of the spinal column also affects rib cage dimensions. In awake subjects, an increase in the normal thoracic kyphosis reduces rib cage dimensions without changing lung volume (241). This increase in curvature has been observed following the induction of halothane anesthesia (263) and could be due to the loss of normal tone in the muscles of the trunk (Fig. 13).

Cephalad Diaphragm Displacement

In recumbent positions, a decrease in tonic activity in the diaphragm could permit a cephalad displacement of the diaphragm by abdominal pressure during expiration and contribute to reductions in the FRC.

Froese and Bryan (89) examined the diaphragmatic silhouette with fluoroscopy in two subjects lying supine and found that the induction of anesthesia caused a cephalad shift of the end-expiratory diaphragmatic position; paralysis had no further effect. Shifts in the non-dependent regions of the diaphragm were inconsistent in these two subjects. Hedenstierna et al. (104) inferred a cephalad shift of the diaphragm from transverse CT scans of the thorax obtained before and after the induction of anesthesia with paralysis. However, both of these studies were limited by an inability to image the entire diaphragm. Three

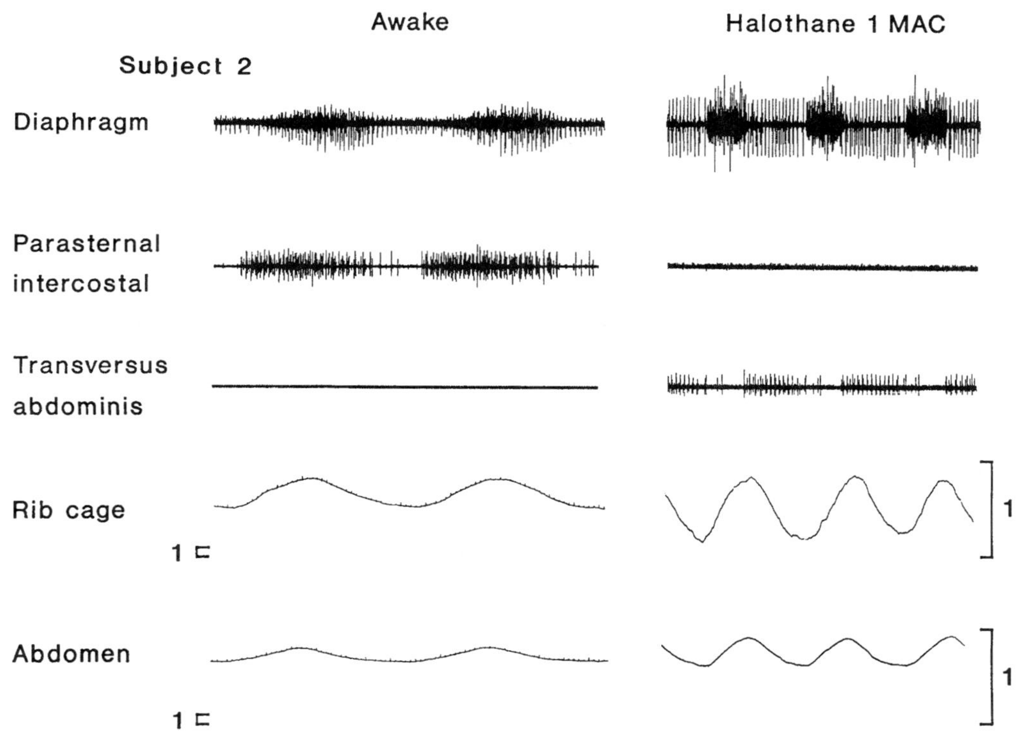

Figure 12. Pattern of breathing in one subject before (*left panel*) and after (*right panel*) the induction of halothane anesthesia, showing electromyogram activity measured with fine-wire percutaneous electrodes and the cross-sectional areas of the rib cage and abdomen during quiet breathing. The diaphragm electrode has been placed through the lateral rib cage intercostal muscles into the diaphragm at the area of apposition (Fig. 1). Halothane, 1 MAC end-tidal concentration, increases respiratory rate, abolishes activity in the parasternal intercostal muscle, and produces phasic expiratory activity in the transversus abdominis muscle. Phasic expiratory activity is also observed in the diaphragm electrode, probably representing activity in the adjacent internal intercostal muscles. Changes in rib cage and abdominal cross-sectional areas during breathing are proportionally decreased by halothane anesthesia despite the lack of parasternal intercostal activity.

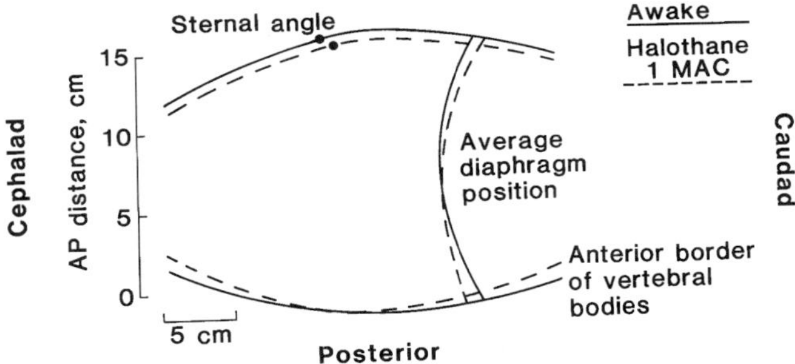

Figure 13. Diagrammatic representation of a mid-sagittal section of the chest wall of subjects lying supine, showing the position of chest wall structures at functional residual capacity during quiet breathing while awake (*solid lines*) and while anesthetized with halothane (*dashed lines*). Halothane causes an increase in spinal curvature, an inward and caudad motion of the anterior rib cage, and changes diaphragmatic shape.

studies using high-speed three-dimensional CT scans to image the entire diaphragm have found no consistent net cephalad shift in end-expiratory diaphragm position with the induction of anesthesia with or without paralysis in subjects lying supine (142,143,263); similar results have been obtained by using ultrasonography to image the diaphragm (68). However, all the later studies did note a consistent change in diaphragmatic shape; dependent diaphragmatic regions tended to shift cephalad and non-dependent regions tended to shift caudad (Fig. 13).

The results of these studies demonstrate that the diaphragm does not consistently contribute to reductions in FRC caused by anesthesia. The observed changes in shape could reflect a loss of tonic diaphragmatic activity (180). However, other factors could also change diaphragmatic shape. Phasic expiratory activity develops in abdominal muscles during thiopental-N_2O anesthesia, with or without halothane, in subjects lying supine (88,131). Such activity could increase abdominal pressure and affect diaphragmatic shape; however, the diaphragm shape changes in the absence of any muscular activity (143). Thus, the mechanical consequences of abdominal muscle activity during quiet breathing are unclear. The shape of the diaphragm could also be changed by motion of its insertions. Inward rib cage motion is associated with a caudal displacement of its inferior margin. The costal diaphragm inserts near this margin, so that this displacement could cause caudad displacement of associated regions of the diaphragm (Fig. 13). Also, the above-mentioned changes in the curvature of the spine could also change the configuration of both costal and crural attachments.

Chest Wall Motion

In addition to its effects on the end-expiratory position of the chest wall, as reflected by changes in the FRC, anesthesia can also significantly affect the pattern of chest wall motion.

When anesthesia is induced with a barbiturate and maintained with halothane in subjects lying supine, early studies found that the relative contribution of the rib cage to tidal volume during quiet breathing, as measured by changes in external thoracic dimensions, was decreased compared with the awake state in children (152,251) and adults (130). In one study, additional experiments in three adults found an abolition of the normal phasic inspiratory electrical activity of parasternal intercostal muscles during halothane anesthesia (251). However, although a recent study confirmed the loss of parasternal intercostal muscle activity with the induction of halothane anesthesia in humans, this loss had no significant effect on the relative contribution of the rib cage to tidal volume during quiet breathing, as measured directly by fast CT scanning and by measurements of external dimensions (Table 1) (Fig. 12) (266). Other recent studies have also concluded that rib cage motion is relatively well preserved during anesthesia with the volatile anesthetics in children (22) and adults (158) when airway patency is maintained during quiet breathing.

The mechanisms by which rib cage expansion is preserved in the apparent absence of parasternal intercostal muscle activity are unknown. Because isolated contraction of the diaphragm produces paradoxic (inward) motion of the rib cage during inspiration (80,178,261), some other rib cage muscles must maintain inspiratory expansion. Possibilities include other inspiratory intercostal muscles or muscles such as the scalenes that may be active during anesthesia. Rib cage muscles with expiratory actions, such as the lateral internal intercostals, may also promote expansion. If these muscles actively decrease rib cage dimensions during expiration, the rib cage may passively expand when these muscles relax at the beginning of inspiration. Also, phasic expiratory activity in the abdominal muscles may affect the pattern of chest wall expansion. However, the complex actions of these muscles make the effects of such activity difficult to predict.

Maintenance of rib cage expansion during quiet breathing does not imply normal chest wall function under all circumstances. Both halothane and isoflurane consistently affect the chest wall response to carbon dioxide rebreathing (158,251), such that there is little increase in the motion of the rib cage as minute ventilation increases. At high minute ventilation, paradoxic motion of the rib cage may occur, such that the rib cage moves inward during early inspiration, a motion that would be consistent with a loss of inspiratory intercostal muscle function. Also, the rib cage may be unable to expand normally in response to ventilatory loads, such as the partial airway obstruction produced during clinical anesthesia by anesthetic-induced depression of the muscles of the upper airway (Fig. 14). However, rib cage expansion in response to more modest loads is fairly well preserved during halothane anesthesia (174).

An impaired response to ventilatory loads may explain the abnormal rib cage motion observed clinically by early authors during administration of early volatile anesthetics such as ether or chloroform (102,242). Alternately, these older agents could have different effects on chest wall motion. Because clinical use

Table 1. VOLUME DISPLACEMENT OF CHEST WALL COMPONENTS DURING QUIET BREATHING

	Awake		Halothane 1 MAC	
	ml	Percentage of change in thoracic volume	ml	Percentage of change in thoracic volume
Total change in thoracic volume	744 ± 41	—	343 ± 29[a]	—
Rib cage displacement	185 ± 25	25 ± 4%	63 ± 11[a]	18 ± 2%
Diaphragm displacement	559 ± 49	75 ± 4%	280 ± 25[a]	82 ± 2%

[a]Significant difference from awake, $p < 0.05$. Values are M ± SE from six supine subjects, measured using fast three-dimensional CT scanning (266).

of these older agents largely predated measurements of chest wall motion, comparative studies are not available.

The effects of anesthetic drugs may be agent specific. The intravenously administered anesthetics methohexital and ketamine have no effect or actually increase the rib cage contribution to tidal volume (11,161,176). Similar effects have been noted with the benzodiazepines and with narcotics (175,211) and have been attributed to a relative sparing of intercostal muscle function, although no measurements of EMG activities are available.

Mechanisms of Anesthetic Action on Control of Chest Wall Muscles

Nothing is known regarding the mechanisms of differential anesthetic effects on the neural control of respiratory muscle groups in human subjects, and little more is known in animals.

Central Mechanisms

One possible mechanism is a differential sensitivity of motoneuron pools to anesthetic effects. Volatile anesthetics affect ventilation at least in part by a direct effect on the brain stem, and it is possible that premotor neurons or motoneurons to various groups of respiratory muscles exhibit a differential sensitivity to anesthesia-induced depression (100). In support of such a mechanism, Stuth et al. (246) found that expiratory bulbospinal neurons were more resistant to isoflurane-induced depression compared with the phrenic nerve (Fig. 15); inspiratory bulbospinal neurons were not examined. Because these dogs were vagotomized and pneumonectomized to eliminate peripheral influences, this finding suggests a differential sensitivity of inspiratory and expiratory bulbospinal neurons to this anesthetic. However, in intact animals isoflurane preferentially suppresses expiratory muscle activity (262), suggesting that peripheral influences such as that provided by the vagus nerve, which are known to be important for expiratory muscle recruitment, are important modulators of anesthetic action (202,278).

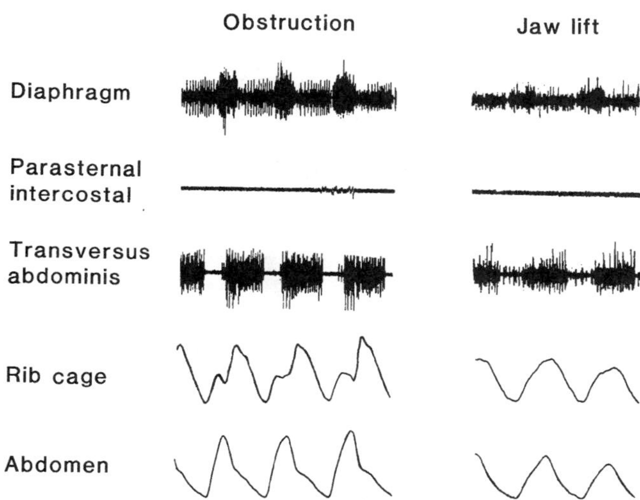

Figure 14. Patterns of breathing during and after partial airway obstruction during halothane anesthesia, showing respiratory muscle electromyograms and changes in rib cage and abdominal areas. Phasic expiratory activity is seen in the diaphragm electrode, probably representing activity in adjacent internal intercostal muscles (Fig. 9), and the transversus abdominis electrode. Note that rib cage expansion (indicated by an upward deflection) is impaired during inspiration and that rib cage motion is paradoxic during early expiration (i.e., the rib cage expands during the early part of expiration). Rib cage and abdominal expansions during inspiration become synchronous after obstruction is relieved by the insertion of an oral airway and the mandible is elevated.

Fusimotor Function

Anesthetics depress proprioceptive feedback from muscle spindles and tendon organs in skeletal muscles (40,227). It has been suggested that this depression should have a greater effect in intercostal muscles, which are richly endowed with muscle spindles, compared with the diaphragm, which has few spindles (130,251). However, the abdominal muscles also have many spindles but are recruited by volatile anesthetics in humans (88,131), so that this explanation alone is insufficient.

Neuromuscular Function

High concentrations of volatile anesthetics can depress neuromuscular transmission and contractility in skeletal muscles, so that developed muscle force is decreased for a given motoneuron activity (268). The effects of these agents on the diaphragm have been investigated by stimulating the phrenic nerve in animal preparations and measuring developed transdiaphragmatic pressure and compound muscle action potentials. Although interpretation of these studies is complicated by species and protocol differences, diaphragmatic tension in response to high-frequency stimulation (50–100 Hz) is depressed by isoflurane, enflurane, and sevoflurane (124,135,257). Little effect is seen at lower frequencies. The effects of halothane are variable, with some studies finding that halothane attenuates evoked action potentials (33) and developed diaphragmatic tension (33,75) during low-frequency phrenic nerve stimulation. However, Kochi et al. (136) found no effect of halothane on either action potentials or transdiaphragmatic pressure in dogs with either rested or fatigued diaphragms at any frequency of stimulation. Thus, it appears unlikely that depression of neuromuscular transmission or muscle contractility significantly affects muscle function during anesthesia, because such effects have not been consistently observed at the physiologic rates of phrenic nerve firing (10–30 Hz).

Comparisons With Natural Sleep

Natural sleep (i.e., not induced by anesthesia) also affects respiratory muscle function. The recognition of sleep-disordered breathing has prompted much investigation into the mechanisms responsible for these effects (97,106). It is tempting to draw parallels between drug-induced and natural sleep to explore mechanism, but the basis for such comparisons is weak. Although there are some similarities in the mechanical effects of natural sleep and anesthesia (e.g., a decrease in FRC during REM sleep and anesthesia [119]), there are also many differences, and the neurophysiologic mechanisms are probably quite different and are highly dependent on sleep stage (277). However, one important lesson is clear from studies of natural sleep that probably also applies to the anesthetized state. Many observed effects on respiratory muscle behavior are secondary to increases in upper airway resistance caused by alterations in upper airway muscle function, so much so that it has been suggested that this increase is the major effect of sleep on ventilatory control (106,107). Similar considerations may apply during anesthesia, such that anesthetic effects on chest wall motion may be critically influenced by activity in upper airway muscles.

Species Differences

Finally, recent studies suggest that there may be significant differences among species in the response of the respiratory muscles to anesthetic drugs. Parasternal intercostal activity during quiet breathing is maintained during anesthesia with the volatile agents in dogs, unlike findings in human subjects (262) (Fig. 16). More strikingly, the volatile anesthetics decrease or abolish phasic expiratory muscle activity in dogs

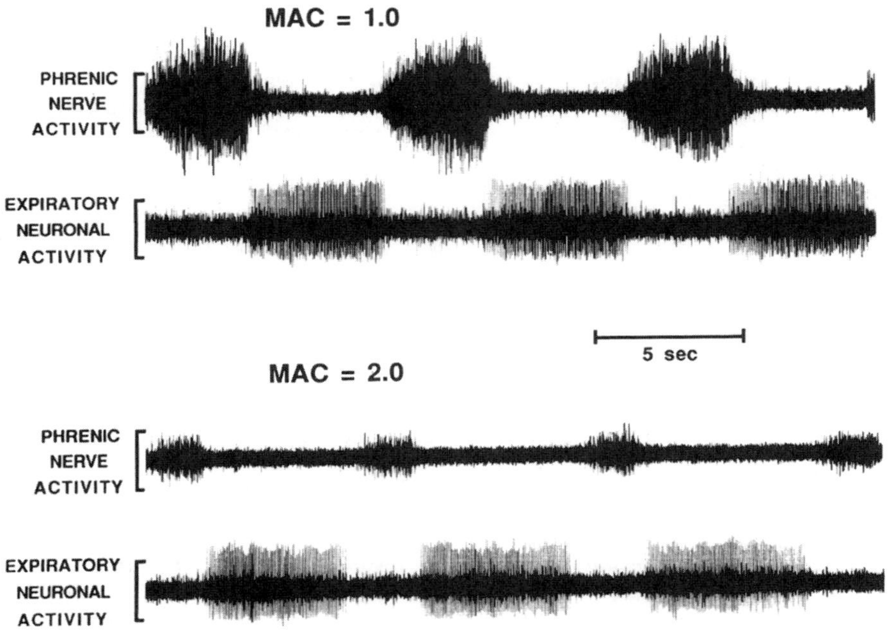

Figure 15. Recordings from the phrenic nerve and an expiratory bulbospinal neuron at 1 MAC (*upper panel*) and 2 MAC (*lower panel*) isoflurane in a vagotomized dog. Expiratory neurons discharge during phrenic nerve silence. Increasing anesthetic depth causes preferential suppression of phrenic nerve activity. (Reprinted with permission from ref. 246.)

and cats, in marked distinction to their stimulating effects on such activity in human subjects. As a result, anesthesia with the volatile agents in dogs either has no effect or may actually increase the FRC (210,262), because phasic expiratory muscle activity that reduces end-expiratory lung volume is lost with the induction of anesthesia.

Upper Airway Function

Upper Airway Dimensions

In comparison with the chest wall, relatively little is known regarding the effects of anesthesia on upper airway anatomy. Early studies in human subjects suggested that anesthesia with

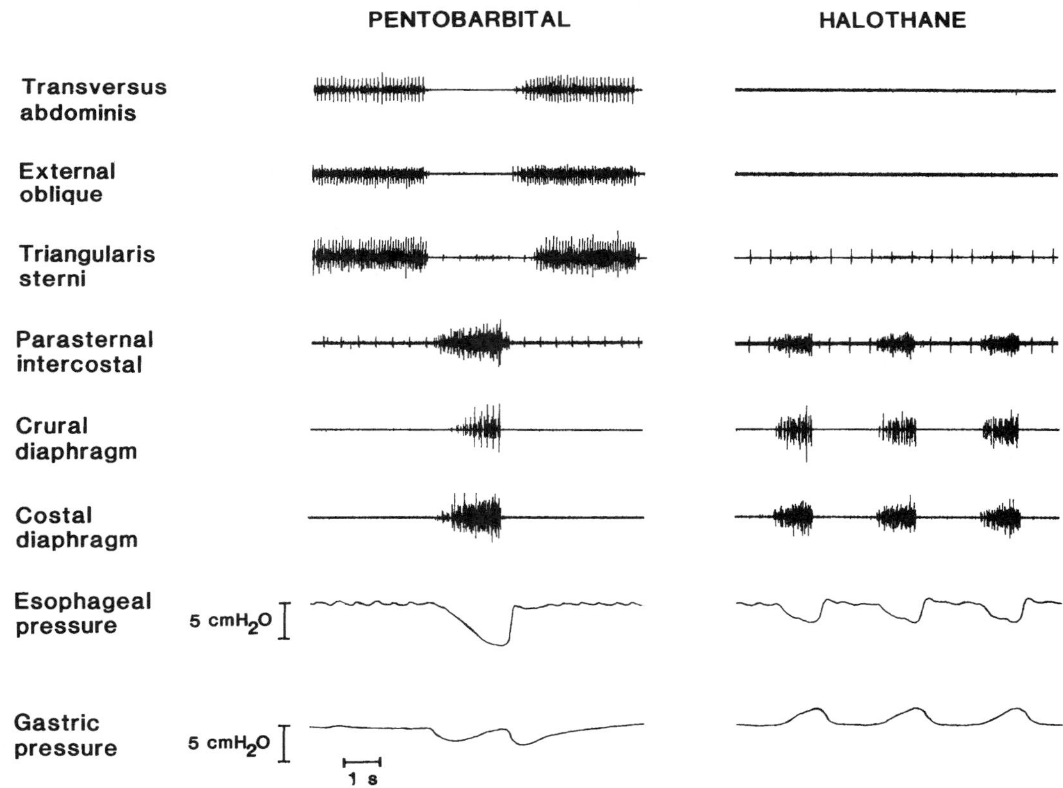

Figure 16. Pattern of respiratory muscle electromyogram activity and chest wall motion during pentobarbital (*left panel*) and halothane (*right panel*) anesthesia in one dog lying supine. The pattern of breathing during pentobarbital anesthesia resembles that present while dogs are awake, with prominent phasic activity in rib cage (triangularis sterni) and abdominal (transversus abdominis and external oblique) muscles with expiratory actions. Halothane anesthesia abolishes this activity, whereas phasic inspiratory activity in parasternal intercostal muscles is maintained. This pattern is markedly different from that observed in human subjects (compare with Fig. 9).

or without paralysis caused a posterior displacement of the tongue that produced airway obstruction at an oropharyngeal level (177,219). However, a more recent study using ultrasonography could not confirm this finding (1). Nandi et al. (182) found that, in the absence of airflow, the most consistent site of obstruction is at the nasopharyngeal level, where the soft palate becomes approximated to the posterior pharynx (Fig. 17). A similar site of obstruction has been noted in patients with obstructive sleep apnea (121,231). The epiglottis and supralaryngeal tissues may also participate in the narrowing of airway caliber (14). Inspiratory efforts decrease airway pressures and produce narrowing at multiple levels, including the base of the tongue (182).

Upper Airway Muscle Activity

In experimental animal preparations, the depth and choice of anesthetic are critical determinants of activity in the upper airway muscles (126). Normally, general anesthetics depress such activity. Laryngeal motoneurons with expiratory activities are depressed by pentobarbital (216,232). Upper airway muscles with phasic inspiratory activity are also vulnerable to depression (111,123,188–190), although one report found increases in activity when pentobarbital was given to decerebrate cats (232). Several reports have documented differential sensitivity to anesthetic depression between chest wall and upper airway muscle motoneuron activities (123,188–190). Halothane, enflurane, diazepam, and thiopental all produce a greater depression of hypoglossal nerve activity compared with phrenic nerve activity in paralyzed, ventilated, vagotomized cats (188,189). Measurements of EMG activities in intact anesthetized cats breathing spontaneously show similar results; EMG activity in the diaphragm is more resistant to depression by halothane compared with the genioglossus muscle (190) (Fig. 18). This differential suppression may be less pronounced after ketamine administration (123,189,215), suggesting that it is not a property common to all general anesthetics. Other reports also have noted an apparent preservation of upper airway motoneuron activities in animals anesthetized with ketamine (111,215). Upper airway muscles may differ in their sensitivity to anesthesia (162,188). Nishino et al. (188) found that halothane and enflurane depressed hypoglossal nerve activity more than recurrent laryngeal nerve activity.

Mechanisms of Anesthetic Action on Control of Upper Airway Muscles

Neural Mechanisms

The greater sensitivity of hypoglossal nerve activity compared with phrenic nerve activity is present in vagotomized, mechanically ventilated animals, suggesting that the effect is not caused by changes in arterial blood gases or by vagal reflexes (188,189). Differential sensitivity is also present in decerebrate animals, before and after spinal cord section at the C_1 and T_1 levels, suggesting that the action occurs at the medullary level (7). Similar results have been noted after alcohol administration (17), which also selectively depresses upper airway motoneuron activities.

Because the activity of upper airway motoneurons is highly dependent on inputs from the reticular activating system, it is possible that the sensitivity of this activity to anesthetics is related to anesthetic-induced depression of reticular activating system activity. In other words, anesthetic effects may be mediated not only by a direct effect on motoneurons, but indirectly via changes in the state of arousal. Consistent with this idea,

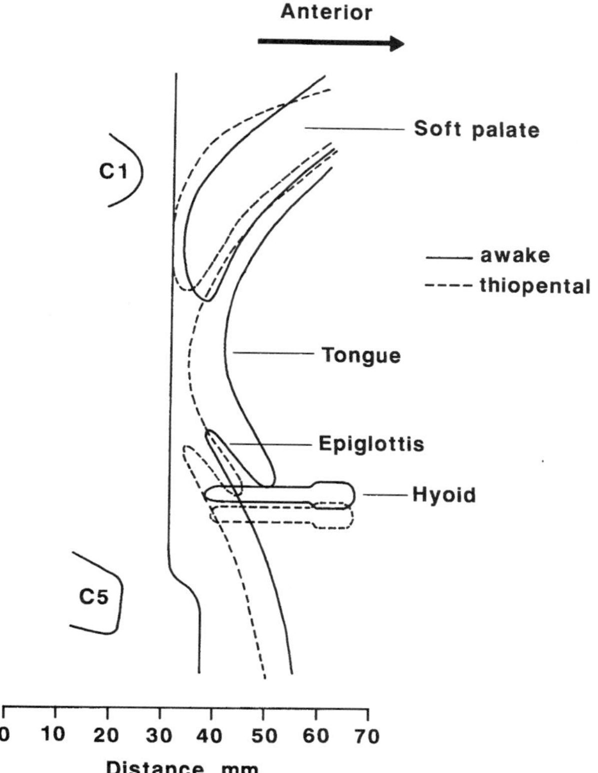

Figure 17. Mid-sagittal section through the upper airway, showing changes in upper airway anatomy during apnea following the induction of thiopental anesthesia. Note that although all dimensions are lessened, the primary site of occlusion is at the soft palate. (Reprinted, in adapted form, with permission from ref. 182.)

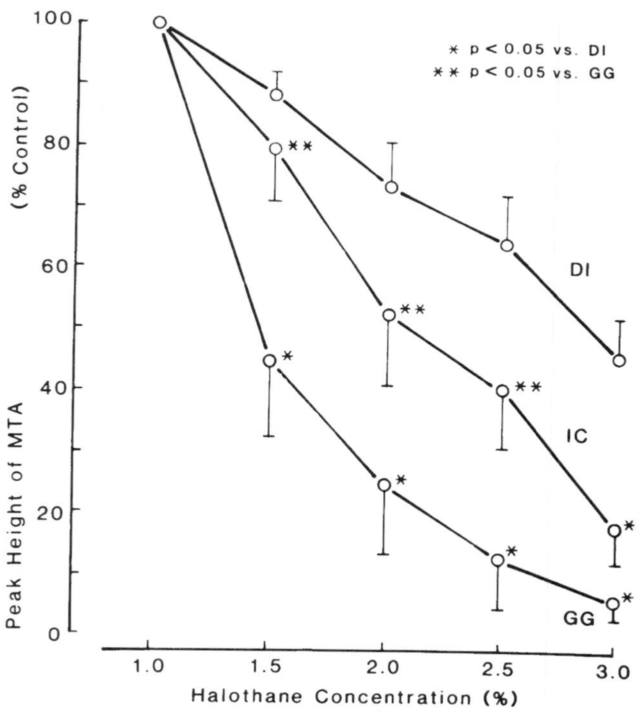

Figure 18. Phasic inspiratory muscle electromyogram activity (expressed as a percent of peak moving time average) as a function of halothane concentration for the diaphragm, intercostal, and the genioglossus muscles in spontaneously breathing cats. Note that the activity of the upper airway muscle was preferentially suppressed as anesthetic depth was increased. (Reprinted, in adapted form, with permission from ref. 190.)

some of the changes in upper airway activity caused by anesthesia mimic those seen during some stages of natural sleep, although, as with chest wall function, there are also important differences that depend on sleep state (126). Nonetheless, as a general principle, it does appear that cranial motoneurons that subserve the upper airways are more dependent on the state of arousal than motoneurons to chest wall muscles. For example, electrical stimulation of the midbrain reticular formation can partially reverse anesthetic-induced depression of upper airway activity, with a lesser effect on the diaphragm (194).

Alterations in airway reflexes that normally protect the laryngeal inlet may also affect perioperative upper airway function. These reflexes are impaired by many anesthetic drugs (181,187), and may be further impaired by techniques such as endotracheal intubation (24). The sites and mechanisms of this depression are unknown. Paradoxically, reflex irritability apparently is increased during some stages of anesthesia and may produce laryngospasm; this phenomenon, though clinically significant, is poorly understood (209,222).

Relationship of Activity to Airway Dimensions

How changes in the activity of upper airway muscles may influence upper airway caliber is uncertain. Although anesthetic effects on upper airway function may not mimic those of natural sleep, several important principles observed during natural sleep may also apply during anesthesia. Because the upper airway is a collapsible tube that is subjected to subatmospheric pressure during inspiration, upper airway muscles presumably stiffen the airway to resist collapse (149,163). However, there is not a consistent relationship between phasic EMG activity of upper airway muscles and upper airway resistance. For example, resistance changes little from non-REM to REM sleep (122), even though upper airway EMG activity is reduced (224). Similarly, Drummond found that thiopental produced alterations in the amount and pattern of activity in neck and tongue muscles measured with surface electrodes in human subjects (66). However, no reduction in activity could be related directly to the onset of airway obstruction; rather, activity was often increased, presumably in an attempt to overcome partial obstruction. Also, although benzodiazepines appear to increase upper airway resistance in human subjects (173), they decrease genioglossus activity only in older subjects (150). Thus airway obstruction may not be caused by a simple diminution of activity but by disruption of the normal coordination of activity of muscles controlling different segments of the airways (5). Disruption of the normal coordination between upper airway and chest wall muscle activities may also contribute to sleep-disordered breathing (120); this possibility has not been investigated for the anesthetic drugs.

It is possible that anesthetics could produce tonic activity in upper airway constrictors, which would explain the clinical observation that pharmacologic paralysis frequently decreases upper airway resistance following induction of anesthesia with thiopental. Factors not directly involving the upper airway muscles may also affect upper airway resistance during anesthesia. For example, the position of the head and neck may change as normal postural muscle tone decreases with the onset of anesthesia. Decreases in FRC produced by anesthesia may also increase upper airway resistance (6).

Effects of Neuromuscular Blockade

Drugs that block the neuromuscular junction are frequently used in clinical practice to inhibit respiratory muscle function, both to facilitate endotracheal intubation and to eliminate respiratory efforts during mechanical ventilation. These drugs may affect the respiratory muscles differently than other skeletal muscles, an observation that becomes clinically relevant during partial neuromuscular blockade with non-depolarizing agents.

Greater doses of pancuronium (63), vecuronium (147,148), and atracurium (147) are required to achieve a given degree of neuromuscular block in the diaphragm compared to the adductor pollicis, although the onset of block is more rapid in the diaphragm. This relative sparing of the diaphragm can allow the maintenance of respiratory effort even during complete paralysis of peripheral muscles (91,92). Other muscles amenable to monitoring by peripheral nerve stimulation such as the orbicularis oculi may better represent the degree of blockade present in the diaphragm (64). The adductor muscles of the larynx may be even more resistant to the effects of nondepolarizing drugs than the diaphragm (65). However, other upper airway muscles may not behave similarly. The susceptibility of the masseter to block appears to be equal to or greater than that of the adductor pollicis. In dogs, the geniohyoid is more susceptible to blockade than the diaphragm; this differential effect is enhanced by a low concentration of volatile anesthetic (127). The mechanisms responsible for this differential sensitivity are unknown. Nevertheless, it is apparent that upper airway patency cannot be maintained at levels of paralysis that otherwise permit maintenance of normal ventilation (199) (Fig. 19).

POSTOPERATIVE RESPIRATORY MUSCLE FUNCTION

Intraoperative alterations in respiratory mechanics can persist in the postoperative period (38,198,260). Recent attention has focused on possible postoperative respiratory muscle dysfunction and its contribution to lung-related morbidity. Although abnormalities in pulmonary mechanics and chest wall function may be observed after any type of surgery, they are most pronounced following surgery that invades the thorax

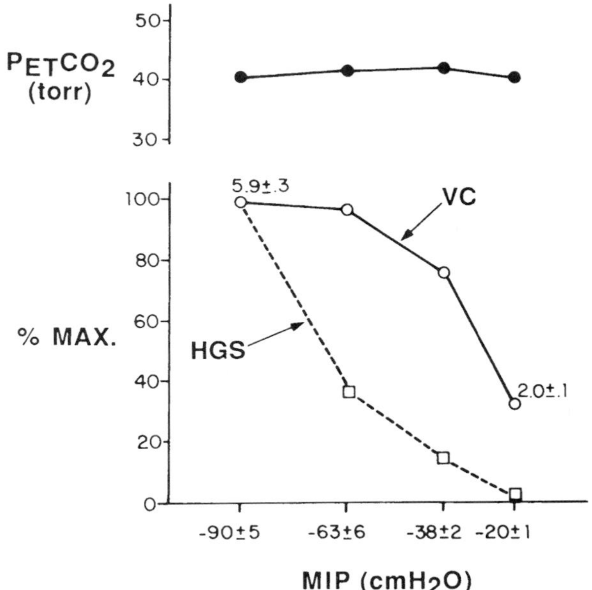

Figure 19. Handgrip strength (HGS), vital capacity (VC, with absolute values noted at the extremes of measurement), and end-tidal CO_2 ($P_{ET}CO_2$) as a function of maximum inspiratory pressure (MIP) developed at the mouth during maximum inspiration against an occluded airway at rest and during increasing degrees of paralysis with d-tubocurare. Mandibular elevation was necessary at MIP $\geq$-39 ± 5 cmH_2O to prevent upper airway obstruction. Note that ventilation can be maintained despite profound levels of peripheral muscle paralysis if airway obstruction is prevented. (Reprinted, in adapted form, with permission from ref. 199.)

or abdomen (38,260). Upper abdominal surgery causes rapid, shallow breathing, accompanied by a restrictive pattern in pulmonary function tests in human subjects. These changes have been attributed to an impairment of diaphragmatic function.

Respiratory Muscle Function

In animal models, both laparotomy and thoracotomy impair postoperative shortening of the diaphragm and alter its resting length for several days following operation (77,244,248). The presence of postoperative diaphragmatic dysfunction in human subjects is supported by several studies using indirect measurement of diaphragmatic function, such as chest wall dimensions and pressures in the esophagus and stomach (74,86,159,160,238). Upper abdominal surgery consistently decreases the contribution of abdominal motion to tidal volume. It also consistently decreases the ratio of changes in gastric pressure to changes in transdiaphragmatic pressure during inspiration. These changes can be partially reversed by aminophylline administration (73). However, interpretation of these studies is complicated by postoperative changes the pattern of respiratory muscle use. Phasic expiratory activity frequently develops in the abdominal and lower intercostal muscles (71) that significantly increases gastric pressure during expiration (72) (Fig. 20). This activity tends to decrease inspiratory changes in gastric pressure and to affect abdominal dimensions. Thus, abdominal dimension and pressures do not reflect actions of the diaphragm alone. Similar considerations would apply if rib cage muscle recruitment changes after surgery; however, no data are available. Thus, these studies suggest but do not prove the existence of postoperative diaphragmatic dysfunction.

Mechanisms of Postoperative Changes in Function

Measurements of changes in transdiaphragmatic pressure during electrical stimulation of the phrenic nerve demonstrate that the contractility of the diaphragm is not impaired after

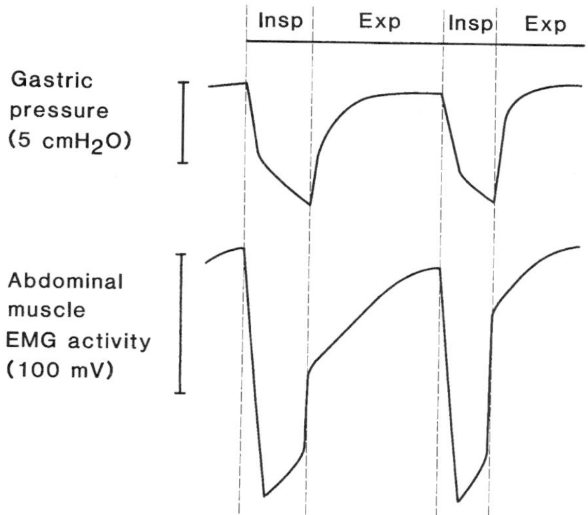

Figure 20. Diagrammatic record of gastric pressure and integrated electromyogram activity of the abdominal muscles in one subject after upper abdominal surgery. Inspiratory and expiratory phases are shown. At the onset of inspiration, abdominal EMG activity decreases and gastric pressure falls. At the onset of expiration, abdominal activity increases, increasing the gastric pressure. Thus, in this subject, gastric pressure reflects primarily abdominal muscle activity, not diaphragmatic activity. (Reprinted, in adapted form, with permission from ref. 72.)

upper abdominal surgery (74). This finding suggests that any postoperative depression of diaphragmatic activity is caused by a decrease in phrenic motoneuron output. Various reflexes from the viscera and the chest wall can influence phrenic motor output. Several studies have shown in animals that stimulation of the abdominal viscera, such as mechanical traction of the gallbladder or esophageal dilation, can markedly decrease phrenic motor output (32,85,196). These changes are only partially attenuated by vagotomy, so that the afferent pathways involved remain obscure. Such a reflex tends to minimize irritation of the abdominal peritoneum by diaphragmatic descent and could be operative after abdominal surgery. Stimulation of visceral afferents may also affect the recruitment of rib cage and abdominal muscles (81,191,196,253). Finally, patients may voluntarily change their pattern of breathing to minimize diaphragmatic descent, which may cause pain.

Effects of Analgesia

If postoperative diaphragmatic dysfunction is related to reflex inhibition or pain, it may be amenable to techniques that interrupt such pathways. Most studies have found that systemic or regional analgesia can partially, but not totally, reverse changes in chest wall motion and transdiaphragmatic pressure swings caused by upper abdominal surgery (38,260). Thoracic epidural block using local anesthetic improves these parameters after upper abdominal surgery (160,197), an improvement associated with an increase in diaphragmatic EMG (197). However, interpretation of these studies may be complicated by the abdominal expiratory muscle activity noted previously; abdominal muscle activity should also be affected by epidural block, so that results may not reflect effects only on diaphragmatic activity. These parameters are not affected by epidural opiate analgesia, despite excellent pain relief (238). Similarly, static lung volumes such as the vital capacity can be only partially normalized by analgesia. These results imply that blockade of reflex or pain pathways by these techniques is incomplete, that other unblocked pathways (e.g., vagal) are important for muscle inhibition, or that other factors such as mechanical disruption of chest wall components or changes in lung mechanics are important. For example, reflexes arising from somatic sources such as the chest wall may be susceptible to blockade by the regional application of local anesthetics or narcotics. On the other hand, inhibition arising from vagally mediated visceral reflexes may not be amenable to such techniques.

Clinically, some studies suggest that epidural analgesia significantly improves pulmonary mechanics and reduces morbidity compared with parenteral opioid analgesia (39,105,171, 204,218,243); this benefit has not been confirmed by other investigators (16,116,128,201). In perhaps the most definitive randomized study, Jayr et al. (129) compared parenteral opioid analgesia with thoracic epidural analgesia with bupivicaine and morphine. They found no differences among the groups in spirometric values or in the incidence of clinical pulmonary complications, including those patients with chronic obstructive pulmonary disease, despite excellent analgesia in the epidural group. If pain and visceral reflexes were important factors leading to pulmonary complications, their incidence should have been lessened by this excellent analgesia. Thus, there is no doubt that regional analgesic techniques can provide superb analgesia, but it appears that these techniques may not necessarily decrease pulmonary morbidity.

CONCLUSION

Breathing requires the coordinated activity of multiple respiratory muscles. The systems that control these muscles are remarkably complex, perhaps reflecting the fact that many of these muscles must simultaneously serve important nonrespiratory functions. Anesthesia and surgery can profoundly affect the activity of these muscles. Although recent studies have provided much descriptive data regarding these effects, mechanisms responsible for these changes remain poorly understood. Further advances in understanding will require better methods to assess respiratory muscle function in human subjects and better characterization of animal models to determine their applicability to human subjects. The ultimate goal of such work would be to develop drugs and techniques that could minimize perioperative alterations in respiratory muscle function and lung-related morbidity.

ACKNOWLEDGMENT

This work was supported in part by grant GM-40909 from the National Institutes of Health.

REFERENCES

1. Abernethy LJ, Allan PL, Drummond GB. Ultrasound assessment of the position of the tongue during induction of anaesthesia. *Br J Anaesth* 1990;65:744–748.
2. Andrew BL. The respiratory displacement of the larynx: a study of the innervation of accessory respiratory muscles. *J Physiol* 1955; 130:474–487.
3. Askanazi J, Silverberg PA, Foster RJ, Hyman AI, Milic-Emili J, Kinney JM. Effects of respiratory apparatus on breathing pattern. *J Appl Physiol* 1980;48:577–580.
4. Bajic J, Zuperku EJ, Tonkovi-Capin M, Hopp FA. Expiratory bulbospinal neurons of dogs: I. Control of discharge patterns by pulmonary stretch receptors. *Am J Physiol* 1992;262:R1075–R1086.
5. Bartlett D Jr, Leiter JC, Knuth SL. Control and actions of the genioglossus muscle. In: Issa FG, Suratt PM, Remmers JE, eds. *Sleep and respiration.* New York: Wiley-Liss, 1990:99–108.
6. Begle RL, Badr S, Skatrud JB, Dempsey JA. Effect of lung inflation on pulmonary resistance during NREM sleep. *Am Rev Respir Dis* 1990;141:854–860.
7. Bennett FM, St. John WM. Anesthesia selectively reduces hypoglossal nerve activity by actions upon the brain stem. *Pflugers Arch* 1984;401:421–423.
8. Berger AJ. Phrenic motoneurons in the cat: subpopulations and nature of respiratory drive potentials. *J Neurophysiol* 1979;42: 76–90.
9. Bergman NA. Reduction in resting end-expiratory position of the respiratory system with induction of anesthesia and neuromuscular paralysis. *Anesthesiology* 1982;57:14–17.
10. Bianchi AL, Barillot JC. Respiratory neurons in the region of the retrofacial nucleus: pontile, medullary, spinal and vagal projections. *Neurosci Lett* 1982;31:277–282.
11. Bickler PE, Dueck R, Prutow RJ. Effects of barbiturate anesthesia on functional residual capacity and ribcage/diaphragm contributions to ventilation. *Anesthesiology* 1987;66:147–152.
12. Bishop B. Reflex control of abdominal muscles during positive-pressure breathing. *J Appl Physiol* 1964;19:224–232.
13. Bishop B, Shaw C, Kondo T. Properties of the human abdominal monosynaptic reflexes. *Soc Neurosci Abstr* 1985;11:701.
14. Boidin MP. Airway patency in the unconscious patient. *Br J Anaesth* 1985;57:306–310.
15. Bolser DC, Lindsey BG, Shannon R. Medullary inspiratory activity: influence of intercostal tendon organs and muscle spindle endings. *J Appl Physiol* 1987;62:1046–1056.
16. Bonnet F, Blery CH, Zatan M, Simonet O, Brage D, Gaudy J. Effect of epidural morphine on post-operative pulmonary dysfunction. *Acta Anaesthesiol Scand* 1984;28:147–151.
17. Bonora M, Shields GI, Knuth SL, Bartlett D Jr, St John WM. Selective depression by ethanol of upper airway respiratory motor activity in cats. *Am Rev Respir Dis* 1984;130:156–161.
18. Brancatisano A, Dodd DS, Engel LA. Posterior cricoarytenoid activity and glottic size during hyperpnea in humans. *J Appl Physiol* 1991;71:977–982.
19. Brancatisano A, Kelly SM, Tully A, Loring SH, Engel LA. Postural changes in spontaneous and evoked regional diaphragmatic activity in dogs. *J Appl Physiol* 1989;66:1699–1705.
20. Brancatisano TP, Collett PW, Engel LA. Respiratory movements of the vocal cords. *J Appl Physiol* 1983;54:1269–1276.
21. Brancatisano TP, Dodd DS, Engel LA. Respiratory activity of posterior cricoarytenoid muscle and vocal cords in humans. *J Appl Physiol* 1984;57:1143–1149.
22. Brown KA, Bissonnette B, Holtby H, Shandling B, Ein S. Chest wall motion during halothane anaesthesia in infants and young children. *Can J Anaesth* 1992;39:21–26.
23. Brusil PJ, Waggener TB, Kronauer RE, Gulesian P Jr. Methods for identifying respiratory oscillations disclose altitude effects. *J Appl Physiol* 1980;48:545–556.
24. Burgess GE III, Cooper JR Jr, Marino RJ, Peuler MJ, Warriner RA III. Laryngeal competence after tracheal extubation. *Anesthesiology* 1979;51:73–77.
25. Burke RE. Motor units: anatomy, physiology, and functional organization. In: Brookhart JM, Mountcastle VB, eds. *Handbook of physiology, sec. 1: the nervous system.* Bethesda: American Physiological Society, 1981:345–422.
26. Burke RE, Levine DN, Tsairis P, Zajac FE III. Physiological types and histochemical profiles of motor units of the cat gastrocnemius. *J Physiol* 1973;234:723–748.
27. Burke RE, Levine DN, Zajac FE III, Tsairis P, Engel WK. Mammalian motor units: physiological-histochemical correlation in three types in cat gastrocnemius. *Science* 1971;174:709–712.
28. Campbell EJM. The role of the scalene and sternomastoid muscles in breathing in normal subjects. An electromyographic study. *J Anat* 1955;89:378–386.
29. Campbell EJM, Newsom-Davis J. The intercostal muscles and other muscles of the rib cage. In: Campbell EJM, Agostoni E, Newsom-Davis J, eds. *The respiratory muscles: mechanics and neural control.* Philadelphia: Saunders, 1970:161–174.
30. Caplan RA, Posner KL, Ward RJ, Cheney FW. Adverse respiratory events in anesthesia: a closed claims analysis. *Anesthesiology* 1990; 72:828–833.
31. Cheeseman M, Revelette WR. Phrenic afferent contribution to reflexes elicited by changes in diaphragm length. *J Appl Physiol* 1990;69:640–647.
32. Cherniack NS, Haxhiu MA, Mitra J, Strohl K, Van Lunteren E. Responses of upper airway, intercostal and diaphragm muscle activity to stimulations of oesophageal afferents in dogs. *J Physiol* 1984;349:15–25.
33. Clergue F, Viires N, Lemesle P, Aubier M, Viars P, Pariente R. Effect of halothane on diaphragmatic muscle function in pentobarbital-anesthetized dogs. *Anesthesiology* 1986;64:181–187.
34. Cohen MI, Feldman JL. Discharge properties of dorsal medullary inspiratory neurons: relation to pulmonary afferent and phrenic efferent discharges. *J Neurophysiol* 1984;51:753–776.
35. Cohen MI, Piercey MF, Gootman PM, Wolotsky P. Synaptic connections between medullary inspiratory neurons and phrenic motoneurons as revealed by cross-correlation. *Brain Res* 1974;81: 319–324.
36. Colin AA, Wohl MEB, Mead J, Ratjen FA, Glass G, Stark AR. Transition from dynamically maintained to relaxed end-expiratory volume in human infants. *J Appl Physiol* 1989;67:2107–2111.
37. Collett PW, Brancatisano AP, Engel LA. Upper airway dimensions and movements in bronchial asthma. *Am Rev Respir Dis* 1986;133: 1143–1149.
38. Craig DB. Postoperative recovery of pulmonary function. *Anesth Analg* 1981;60:46–52.
39. Cuschieri RJ, Morran CG, Howie JC, McArdle CS. Postoperative pain and pulmonary complications: comparison of three analgesic regimens. *Br J Surg* 1985;72:495–498.
40. D'Angelo E. Effects of body temperature, passive limb motion and level of anesthesia on the activity of the inspiratory muscles. *Respir Physiol* 1984;56:105–129.
41. D'Angelo E, Sant'Ambrogio G. Direct action of contracting diaphragm on the rib cage in rabbits and dogs. *J Appl Physiol* 1974; 36:715–719.
42. Danon J, Druz WS, Goldberg NB, Sharp JT. Function of the isolated paced diaphragm and the cervical accessory muscles in C1 quadriplegics. *Am Rev Respir Dis* 1979;119:909–919.
43. Davies JG, Kirkwood PA, Sears TA. The distribution of monosynaptic connexions from inspiratory bulbospinal neurones to inspiratory motoneurones in the cat. *J Physiol* 1985;368:63–87.
44. Decramer M, De Troyer A. Respiratory changes in parasternal intercostal length. *J Appl Physiol* 1984;57:1254–1260.
45. De Troyer A, Bastenier-Geens J. Effects of neuromuscular blockade on respiratory mechanics in conscious man. *J Appl Physiol* 1979;47:1162–1168.

46. De Troyer A, Bastenier J, Delhez L. Function of respiratory muscles during partial curarization in humans. *J Appl Physiol* 1980;49: 1049–1056.
47. De Troyer A, Estenne M. Coordination between rib cage muscles and diaphragm during quiet breathing in humans. *J Appl Physiol* 1984;57:899–906.
48. De Troyer A, Farkas GA. Mechanical arrangement of the parasternal intercostals in the different interspaces. *J Appl Physiol* 1989;66: 1421–1429.
49. De Troyer A, Gilmartin JJ, Ninane V. Abdominal muscle use during breathing in unanesthetized dogs. *J Appl Physiol* 1989;66: 20–27.
50. De Troyer A, Heilporn A. Respiratory mechanics in quadriplegia. The respiratory function of the intercostal muscles. *Am Rev Respir Dis* 1980;122:591–600.
51. De Troyer A, Kelly S, Macklem PT, Zin WA. Mechanics of intercostal space and actions of external and internal intercostal muscles. *J Clin Invest* 1985;75:850–857.
52. De Troyer A, Loring S. Action of the respiratory muscles. In: Fishman AP, ed. *Handbook of physiology, sec. 3: the respiratory system.* Bethesda: American Physiological Society, 1986:443–461.
53. De Troyer A, Ninane V. Triangularis sterni: a primary muscle of breathing in the dog. *J Appl Physiol* 1986;60:14–21.
54. De Troyer A, Ninane V, Gilmartin JJ, Lemerre C, Estenne M. Triangularis sterni muscle use in supine humans. *J Appl Physiol* 1987; 62:919–925.
55. De Troyer A, Sampson MG. Activation of the parasternal intercostals during breathing efforts in human subjects. *J Appl Physiol* 1982;52:524–529.
56. De Troyer A, Sampson M, Sigrist S, Kelly S. How the abdominal muscles act on the rib cage. *J Appl Physiol* 1983;54:465–469.
57. De Troyer A, Sampson M, Sigrist S, Macklem PT. The diaphragm: two muscles. *Science* 1981;213:237–238.
58. De Troyer A, Sampson M, Sigrist S, Macklem PT. Action of costal and crural parts of the diaphragm on the rib cage in dog. *J Appl Physiol* 1982;53:30–39.
59. DiMarco AF, Romaniuk JR, Supinski GS. Action of the intercostal muscles on the rib cage. *Respir Physiol* 1990;82:295–306.
60. DiMarco AF, Romaniuk JR, Supinski GS. Mechanical action of the interosseous intercostal muscles as a function of lung volume. *Am Rev Respir Dis* 1990;142:1041–1046.
61. DiMarco AF, von Euler C, Romaniuk JR, Yamamoto Y. Positive feedback facilitation of external intercostal and phrenic inspiratory activity by pulmonary stretch receptors. *Acta Physiol Scand* 1981;113:375–386.
62. Don HF, Wahba WM, Craig DB. Airway closure, gas trapping, and the functional residual capacity during anesthesia. *Anesthesiology* 1972;36:533–539.
63. Donati F, Antzaka C, Bevan DR. Potency of pancuronium at the diaphragm and the adductor pollicis muscle in humans. *Anesthesiology* 1986;65:1–5.
64. Donati F, Meistelman C, Plaud B. Vecuronium neuromuscular blockade at the diaphragm, the orbicularis oculi, and adductor pollicis muscles. *Anesthesiology* 1990;73:870–875.
65. Donati F, Meistelman C, Plaud B. Vecuronium neuromuscular blockade at the adductor muscles of the larynx and adductor pollicis. *Anesthesiology* 1991;74:833–837.
66. Drummond GB. Influence of thiopentone on upper airway muscles. *Br J Anaesth* 1989;63:12–21.
67. Drummond GB. Reduction of tonic ribcage muscle activity by anesthesia with thiopental. *Anesthesiology* 1987;67:695–700.
68. Drummond GB, Allan PL, Logan MR. Changes in diaphragmatic position in association with the induction of anaesthesia. *Br J Anaesth* 1986;58:1246–1251.
69. Drummond GB, Park GR. Changes in intragastric pressure on induction of anaesthesia. *Br J Anaesth* 1984;56:873–879.
70. Druz WS, Sharp JT. Activity of respiratory muscles in upright and recumbent humans. *J Appl Physiol* 1981;51:1552–1561.
71. Duggan J, Drummond GB. Activity of lower intercostal and abdominal muscle after upper abdominal surgery. *Anesth Analg* 1987;66:852–855.
72. Duggan JE, Drummond GB. Abdominal muscle activity and intraabdominal pressure after upper abdominal surgery. *Anesth Analg* 1989;69:598–603.
73. Dureuil B, Desmonts JM, Mankikian B, Prokocimer P. Effects of aminophylline on diaphragmatic dysfunction after upper abdominal surgery. *Anesthesiology* 1985;62:242–246.
74. Dureuil B, Viires N, Cantineau J-P, Aubier M, Desmonts J-M. Diaphragmatic contractility after upper abdominal surgery. *J Appl Physiol* 1986;61:1775–1780.
75. Dureuil B, Viires N, Nivoche Y, et al. Different effects of halothane on diaphragm and hindlimb muscle in rats. *J Appl Physiol* 1987;63: 1757–1762.
76. Duron B. Intercostal and diaphragmatic muscle endings and afferents. In: Hornbein TF, ed. *Regulation of breathing.* New York: Marcel Dekker, 1981:473–540.
77. Easton PA, Fitting J-W, Arnoux R, Guerraty A, Grassino AE. Recovery of diaphragm function after laparotomy and chronic sonomicrometer implantation. *J Appl Physiol* 1989;66:613–621.
78. Ellenberger HH, Feldman JL, Goshgarian HG. Ventral respiratory group projections to phrenic motoneurons: electron microscopic evidence for monosynaptic connections. *J Comp Neurol* 1990;302: 707–714.
79. England SJ, Bartlett D Jr. Changes in respiratory movements of the human vocal cords during hyperpnea. *J Appl Physiol* 1982;52: 780–785.
80. Estenne M, De Troyer A. Relationship between respiratory muscle electromyogram and rib cage motion in tetraplegia. *Am Rev Respir Dis* 1985;132:53–59.
81. Farkas GA, De Troyer A. Effects of midline laparotomy on expiratory muscle activation in anesthetized dogs. *J Appl Physiol* 1989;67: 599–605.
82. Fedorko L, Connelly CA, Remmers JE. Neurotransmitters mediating synaptic inhibition of phrenic motoneurons. In: Sieck GC, Gandevia SC, Cameron WE, eds. *Respiratory muscles and their neuromotor control.* New York: Alan R. Liss, 1987:167–173.
83. Fedorko L, Duffin J, England S. Inhibition of inspiratory neurons of the nucleus retroambigualis by expiratory neurons of the Bötzinger complex in the cat. *Exp Neurol* 1989;106:74–77.
84. Fedorko L, Hoskin RW, Duffin J. Projections from inspiratory neurons of the nucleus retroambigualis to phrenic motoneurons in the cat. *Exp Neurol* 1989;105:306–310.
85. Ford GT, Grant DA, Rideout KS, Davison JS, Whitelaw WA. Inhibition of breathing associated with gallbladder stimulation in dogs. *J Appl Physiol* 1988;65:72–79.
86. Ford GT, Whitelaw WA, Rosenal TW, Cruse PJ, Guenter CA. Diaphragm function after upper abdominal surgery in humans. *Am Rev Respir Dis* 1983;127:431–436.
87. Fournier M, Alula M, Sieck GC. Neuromuscular transmission failure during postnatal development. *Neurosci Lett* 1991;125:34–36.
88. Freund F, Roos A, Dodd RB. Expiratory activity of the abdominal muscles in man during general anesthesia. *J Appl Physiol* 1964;19: 693–697.
89. Froese AB, Bryan AC. Effects of anesthesia and paralysis on diaphragmatic mechanics in man. *Anesthesiology* 1974;41:242–255.
90. Gal TJ, Arora NS. Respiratory mechanics in supine subjects during progressive partial curarization. *J Appl Physiol* 1982;51:57–63.
91. Gal TJ, Goldberg SK. Diaphragmatic function in healthy subjects during partial curarization. *J Appl Physiol* 1980;48:921–926.
92. Gal TJ, Goldberg SK. Relationship between respiratory muscle strength and vital capacity during partial curarization in awake subjects. *Anesthesiology* 1981;54:141–147.
93. Gilbert R, Auchincloss JH Jr, Brodsky J, Boden W. Changes in tidal volume, frequency, and ventilation induced by their measurement. *J Appl Physiol* 1972;33:252–254.
94. Gilmartin JJ, Ninane V, De Troyer A. Abdominal muscle use during breathing in the anesthetized dog. *Respir Physiol* 1987;70:159–171.
95. Gilroy RJ Jr, Lavietes MH, Loring SH, Mangura BT, Mead J. Respiratory mechanical effects of abdominal distension. *J Appl Physiol* 1985;58:1997–2003.
96. Goldman MD, Loh L, Sears TA. The respiratory activity of human levator costae muscles and its modification by posture. *J Physiol* 1985;362:189–204.
97. Gothe B, Bruce EN, Goldman MD. Influence of sleep state on respiratory muscle function. IN: Lenfant C, ed. *Lung biology in health and disease.* New York: Marcel Dekker, 1984:241–282.
98. Grassino AE, Goldman MD. Respiratory muscle coordination. In: Fishman AP, ed. *Handbook of physiology, sec. 3: the respiratory system.* Bethesda: American Physiological Society, 1986:463–480.
99. Green JH, Howell JBL. The correlation of intercostal muscle activity with respiratory air flow in conscious human subjects. *J Physiol* 1959;149:471–476.
100. Grelot L, Bianchi AL. Differential effects of halothane anesthesia of the pattern of discharge on inspiratory and expiratory neurons

in the region of the retrofacial nucleus. *Brain Res* 1987;404: 335–338.

101. Grimby G, Goldman M, Mead J. Respiratory muscle action inferred from rib cage and abdominal V-P partitioning. *J Appl Physiol* 1976; 41:739–751.
102. Guedel AE. *Inhalation anesthesia. A fundamental guide.* New York: Macmillan, 1937.
103. Hairston LE, Sauerland EK. Electromyography of the human palate: discharge patterns of the levator and tensor veli platini. *Electromyogr Clin Neurophysiol* 1981;21:287–297.
104. Hedenstierna G, Strandberg Å, Brismar B, Lundquist H, Svensson L, Tokics L. Functional residual capacity, thoracoabdominal dimensions, and central blood volume during general anesthesia with muscle paralysis and mechanical ventilation. *Anesthesiology* 1985;62: 247–254.
105. Hendolin H, Lahtinen J, Länsimies E, Tuppurainen T, Partanen K. The effect of thoracic epidural analgesia on respiratory function after cholecystectomy. *Acta Anaesthesiol Scand* 1987;31: 645–651.
106. Henke KG, Badr MS, Skatrud JB, Dempsey JA. Load compensation and respiratory muscle function during sleep. *J Appl Physiol* 1992;72:1221–1234.
107. Henke KG, Dempsey JA, Badr MS, Kowitz JM, Skatrud JB. Effect of sleep-induced increases in upper airway resistance on respiratory muscle activity. *J Appl Physiol* 1991;70:158–168.
108. Henke KG, Sharratt M, Pegelow D, Dempsey JA. Regulation of end-expiratory lung volume during exercise. *J Appl Physiol* 1988; 64:135–146.
109. Henneman E. Relation between size of neurons and their susceptibility to discharge. *Science* 1957;126:1345–1347.
110. Hernandez YM, Lindsey BG, Shannon R. Intercostal and abdominal muscle afferent influence on caudal medullary expiratory neurons that drive abdominal muscles. *Exp Brain Res* 1989;78: 219–222.
111. Hershenson M, Brouillette RT, Olsen E, Hunt CE. The effect of chloral hydrate on genioglossus and diaphragmatic activity. *Pediatr Res* 1984;18:516–519.
112. Hewlett AM, Hulands GH, Nunn JF, Milledge JS. Functional residual capacity during anaesthesia. III: Artificial ventilation. *Br J Anaesth* 1974;46:495–503.
113. Hilaire G, Gauthier P, Monteau R. Central respiratory drive and recruitment order of phrenic and inspiratory laryngeal motoneurones. *Respir Physiol* 1983;51:341–359.
114. Hilaire G, Monteau R. Connexions entre les neurones inspiratoires bulbaires et les motoneurones phréniques et intercostaux. *J Physiol Paris* 1976;72:987–1000.
115. Hillman DR, Markos J, Finucane KE. Effect of abdominal compression on maximum transdiaphragmatic pressure. *J Appl Physiol* 1990;68:2296–2304.
116. Hjortso NC, Neumann P, Frosig F, et al. A controlled study on the effect of epidural analgesia with local anaesthetics and morphine on morbidity after abdominal surgery. *Acta Anaesthesiol Scand* 1985;29:790–796.
117. Howell JBL, Peckett BW. Studies of the elastic properties of the thorax of supine anaesthetized paralysed human subjects. *J Physiol* 1957;136:1–19.
118. Hubmayr RD, Sprung J, Nelson S. Determinants of transdiaphragmatic pressure in dogs. *J Appl Physiol* 1990;69:2050–2056.
119. Hudgel DW, Devadatta P. Decrease in functional residual capacity during sleep in normal humans. *J Appl Physiol* 1984;57: 1319–1322.
120. Hudgel DW, Harasick T. Fluctuation in timing of upper airway and chest wall inspiratory muscle activity in obstructive sleep apnea. *J Appl Physiol* 1990;69:443–450.
121. Hudgel DW, Hendricks C. Palate and hypopharnyx—sites of inspiratory narrowing of the upper airway during sleep. *Am Rev Respir Dis* 1988;138:1542–1547.
122. Hudgel DW, Martin RJ, Johnson B, Hill P. Mechanics of the respiratory system and breathing pattern during sleep in normal humans. *J Appl Physiol* 1984;56:133–137.
123. Hwang J-C, St John WM, Bartlett D Jr. Respiratory-related hypoglossal nerve activity: influence of anesthetics. *J Appl Physiol* 1983; 55:785–792.
124. Ide T, Kochi T, Isono S, Mizuguchi T. Effect of sevoflurane on diaphragmatic contractility in dogs. *Anesth Analg* 1992;74: 739–746.
125. Insalaco G, Kuna ST, Cibella F, Villeponteaux RD. Thyroarytenoid muscle activity during hypoxia, hypercapnia, and voluntary hyperventilation in humans. *J Appl Physiol* 1990;69:268–273.
126. Iscoe SD. Central control of the upper airway. In: Mathew OP, Sant'Ambrogio G, eds. *Respiratory function of the upper airway.* New York: Marcel Dekker, 1988:125–192.
127. Isono S, Kochi T, Ide T, Sugimori K, Mizuguchi T, Nishino T. Differential effects of vecuronium on diaphragm and geniohyoid muscle in anaesthetized dogs. *Br J Anaesth* 1992;68:239–243.
128. Jayr C, Mollié A, Bourgain JL, et al. Postoperative pulmonary complications: general anesthesia with postoperative parenteral morphine compared with epidural analgesia. *Surgery* 1988;104: 57–63.
129. Jayr C, Thomas H, Rey A, Farhat F, Lasser P, Bourgain J-L. Postoperative pulmonary complications: epidural analgesia using bupivicaine and opioids versus parenteral opioids. *Anesthesiology* 1993;78:666–676.
130. Jones JG, Faithfull D, Jordan C, Minty B. Rib cage movement during halothane anaesthesia in man. *Br J Anaesth* 1979;51:399–406.
131. Kaul SU, Heath JR, Nunn JF. Factors influencing the development of expiratory muscle activity during anaesthesia. *Br J Anaesth* 1973; 45:1013–1018.
132. Kim MJ, Druz WS, Danon J, Machnach W, Sharp JT. Mechanics of the canine diaphragm. *J Appl Physiol* 1976;41:369–382.
133. Kim MJ, Druz WS, Sharp JT. Effect of muscle length on electromyogram in a canine diaphragm strip preparation. *J Appl Physiol* 1985;58:1602–1607.
134. Kimball WR, Loring SH, Basta SJ, De Troyer A, Mead J. Effects of paralysis with pancuronium on chest wall statics in awake humans. *J Appl Physiol* 1985;58:1638–1645.
135. Kochi T, Ide T, Isono S, Mizuguchi T, Nishino T. Different effects of halothane and enflurane on diaphragmatic contractility in vivo. *Anesth Analg* 1990;70:362–368.
136. Kochi T, Ide T, Mizuguchi T, Nishino T. Halothane does not depress contractile function of fresh or fatigued diaphragm in pentobarbitone-anaesthetized dogs. *Br J Anaesth* 1992;68:562–566.
137. Koepke GH, Smith EM, Murphy AJ, Dickinson DG. Sequence of action of the diaphragm and intercostal muscles during respiration: I. Inspiration. *Arch Phys Med Rehabil* 1958;39:426–430.
138. Konno K, Mead J. Measurement of the separate volume changes of rib cage and abdomen during breathing. *J Appl Physiol* 1967;22: 407–422.
139. Kosch PC, Hutchison AA, Wozniak JA, Carlo WA, Stark AR. Posterior cricoarytenoid and diaphragm activities during tidal breathing in neonates. *J Appl Physiol* 1988;64:1968–1978.
140. Kosch PC, Stark AR. Dynamic maintenance of end-expiratory lung volume in full-term infants. *J Appl Physiol* 1984;57:1126–1133.
141. Krayer S, Decramer M, Vettermann J, Ritman EL, Rehder K. Volume quantification of chest wall motion in dogs. *J Appl Physiol* 1988;65:2213–2220.
142. Krayer S, Rehder K, Beck KC, Cameron PD, Didier EP, Hoffman EA. Quantification of thoracic volumes by three-dimensional imaging. *J Appl Physiol* 1987;62:591–598.
143. Krayer S, Rehder K, Vettermann J, Didier EP, Ritman EL. Position and motion of the human diaphragm during anesthesia-paralysis. *Anesthesiology* 1989;70:891–898.
144. Kuna ST, Insalaco G, Woodson GE. Thyroarytenoid muscle activity during wakefulness and sleep in normal adults. *J Appl Physiol* 1988;65:1332–1339.
145. Kuna ST, Smickley JS, Insalaco G. Posterior cricoarytenoid muscle activity during wakefulness and sleep in normal adults. *J Appl Physiol* 1990;68:1746–1754.
146. Laporta D, Grassino A. Assessment of transdiaphragmatic pressure in humans. *J Appl Physiol* 1985;58:1469–1476.
147. Laycock JRD, Donati F, Smith CE, Bevan DR. Potency of atracurium and vecuronium at the diaphragm and the adductor pollicis muscle. *Br J Anaesth* 1988;61:286–291.
148. Lebrault C, Chauvin M, Guirimand F, Duvaldestin P. Relative potency of vecuronium on the diaphragm and the adductor pollicis. *Br J Anaesth* 1989;63:389–392.
149. Leiter JC, Daubenspeck JA. Selective reflex activation of the genioglossus in humans. *J Appl Physiol* 1990;68:2581–2587.
150. Leiter JC, Knuth SL, Krol RC, Bartlett D Jr. The effect of diazepam on genioglossal muscle activity in normal human subjects. *Am Rev Respir Dis* 1985;132:216–219.
151. Lenfant C. Time-dependent variations of pulmonary gas exchange in normal man at rest. *J Appl Physiol* 1967;22:675–684.
152. Lindahl SGE, Yates AP, Hatch DJ. Respiratory depression in chil-

dren at different end tidal halothane concentrations. *Anaesthesia* 1987;42:1267–1275.
153. Loeb GE, Gans C. *Electromyography for experimentalists.* Chicago: University of Chicago Press, 1986.
154. Loring SH, Mead J. Abdominal muscle use during quiet breathing and hyperpnea in uninformed subjects. *J Appl Physiol* 1982;52: 700–704.
155. Loring SH, Mead J. Action of the diaphragm on the rib cage inferred from a force-balance analysis. *J Appl Physiol* 1982;53: 756–760.
156. Loring S, Mead J, Griscom NT. Dependence of diaphragmatic length on lung volume and thoracoabdominal configuration. *J Appl Physiol* 1985;59:1961–1970.
157. Lourenço RV, Cherniack NS, Malm JR, Fishman AP. Nervous output from the respiratory center during obstructed breathing. *J Appl Physiol* 1966;21:527–533.
158. Lumb AB, Petros AJ, Nunn JF. Rib cage contribution to resting and carbon dioxide stimulated ventilation during 1 MAC isoflurane anaesthesia. *Br J Anaesth* 1991;67:712–721.
159. Maeda H, Nakahara K, Ohno K, Kido T, Ikeda M, Kawashima Y. Diaphragm function after pulmonary resection. *Am Rev Respir Dis* 1988;137:678–681.
160. Mankikian B, Cantineau JP, Bertrand M, Kieffer E, Sartene R, Viars P. Improvement of diaphragmatic function by a thoracic extradural block after upper abdominal surgery. *Anesthesiology* 1988;68:379–386.
161. Mankikian B, Cantineau JP, Sartene R, Clergue F, Viars P. Ventilatory pattern and chest wall mechanics during ketamine anesthesia in humans. *Anesthesiology* 1986;65:492–499.
162. Masuda A, Ito Y, Haji A, Takeda R. The influence of halothane and thiopental on respiratory-related nerve activities in decerebrate cats. *Acta Anaesthesiol Scand* 1989;33:660–665.
163. Mathew OP, Abu-Osba YK, Thach BT. Influence of upper airway pressure changes on genioglossus muscle respiratory activity. *J Appl Physiol* 1982;52:438–444.
164. Mead J. Functional significance of the area of apposition of diaphragm to rib cage. *Am Rev Respir Dis* 1979;119:31–32.
165. Mead J, Loring SH. Analysis of volume displacement and length changes of the diaphragm during breathing. *J Appl Physiol* 1982; 53:750–755.
166. Merrill EG, Fedorko L. Monosynaptic inhibition of phrenic motoneurons: a long descending projection from Bötzinger neurons. *J Neurosci* 1984;4:2350–2353.
167. Merrill EG, Lipski J. Inputs to intercostal motoneurons from ventrolateral medullary respiratory neurons in the cat. *J Neurophysiol* 1987;57:1837–1853.
168. Mier A, Brophy C, Estenne M, Moxham J, Green M, De Troyer A. Action of abdominal muscles on rib cage in humans. *J Appl Physiol* 1985;58:1438–1443.
169. Miller AD, Ezure K, Suzuki I. Control of abdominal muscles by brain stem respiratory neurons in the cat. *J Neurophysiol* 1985;54: 155–167.
170. Miller AD, Tan LK, Suzuki I. Control of abdominal and expiratory intercostal muscle activity during vomiting: role of ventral respiratory group expiratory neurons. *J Neurophysiol* 1987;57: 1854–1866.
171. Miller L, Gertel M, Fox GS, MacLean LD. Comparison of effect of narcotic and epidural analgesia on postoperative respiratory function. *Am J Surg* 1976;131:291–294.
172. Monteau R, Hilaire G. Spinal respiratory motoneurons. *Prog Neurobiol* 1991;37:83–144.
173. Montravers P, Dureuil B, Desmonts JM. Effects of i.v. midazolam on upper airway resistance. *Br J Anaesth* 1992;68:27–31.
174. Moote CA, Knill RL, Clement J. Ventilatory compensation for continuous inspiratory resistive and elastic loads during halothane anesthesia in humans. *Anesthesiology* 1986;64:582–589.
175. Morel DR, Forster A, Bachmann M, Suter PM. Effect of intravenous midazolam on breathing pattern and chest wall mechanics in humans. *J Appl Physiol* 1984;57:1104–1110.
176. Morel DR, Forster A, Gemperle M. Noninvasive evaluation of breathing pattern and thoraco-abdominal motion following the infusion of ketamine or droperidol in humans. *Anesthesiology* 1986; 65:392–398.
177. Morikawa S, Safar P, DeCarlo J. Influence of the head-jaw position upon upper airway patency. *Anesthesiology* 1961;22:265–270.
178. Mortola JP, Sant'Ambrogio G. Motion of the rib cage and the abdomen in tetraplegic subjects. *Clin Sci Mol Med* 1978;54:25–32.
179. Moss IR, Denavit-Saubié M, Eldridge FL, Gillis RA, Herkenham M, Lahiri S. Neuromodulators and transmitters in respiratory control. *Fed Proc* 1986;45:2133–2147.
180. Muller N, Volgyesi G, Becker L, Bryan MH, Bryan AC. Diaphragmatic muscle tone. *J Appl Physiol* 1979;47:279–284.
181. Murphy PJ, Langton JA, Barker P, Smith G. Effect of oral diazepam on the sensitivity of upper airway reflexes. *Br J Anaesth* 1993;70:131–134.
182. Nandi PR, Charlesworth CH, Taylor SJ, Nunn JF, Doré CJ. Effect of general anaesthesia on the pharynx. *Br J Anaesth* 1991;66: 157–162.
183. Nathan PW, Sears TA. Effects of posterior root section on the activity of some muscles in man. *J Neurol Neurosurg Psychiatry* 1960; 23:10–22.
184. Newman S, Road J, Bellemare F, Clozel JP, Lavigne CM, Grassino A. Respiratory muscle length measured by sonomicrometry. *J Appl Physiol* 1984;56:753–764.
185. NHLBI Workshop Summary. Respiratory muscle fatigue. *Am Rev Respir Dis* 1990;142:474–480.
186. Ninane V, Baer RE, De Troyer A. Mechanism of triangularis sterni shortening during expiration in dogs. *J Appl Physiol* 1989;66: 2287–2292.
187. Nishino T, Hiraga K, Yokokawa N. Laryngeal and respiratory responses to tracheal irritation at different depths of enflurane anesthesia in humans. *Anesthesiology* 1990;73:46–51.
188. Nishino T, Kohchi T, Yonezawa T, Honda Y. Responses of recurrent laryngeal, hypoglossal, and phrenic nerves to increasing depths of anesthesia with halothane or enflurane in vagotomized cats. *Anesthesiology* 1985;63:404–409.
189. Nishino T, Shirahata M, Yonezawa T, Honda Y. Comparison of changes in the hypoglossal and the phrenic nerve activity in response to increasing depth of anesthesia in cats. *Anesthesiology* 1984;60:19–24.
190. Ochiai R, Guthrie RD, Motoyama EK. Effects of varying concentrations of halothane on the activity of the genioglossus, intercostals, and diaphragm in cats: an electromyographic study. *Anesthesiology* 1989;70:812–816.
191. Oliven A, Haxhiu M, Kelsen SG. Reflex effect of esophageal distension on respiratory muscle activity and pressure. *J Appl Physiol* 1989;66:536–541.
192. Önal E, Lopata M, O'Connor TD. Diaphragmatic and genioglossal electromyogram responses to isocapnic hypoxia in humans. *Am Rev Respir Dis* 1981;124:215–217.
193. Önal E, Lopata M, O'Connor TD. Diaphragmatic and genioglossal electromyogram responses to CO_2 rebreathing in humans. *J Appl Physiol* 1981;50:1052–1055.
194. Orem J, Lydic R, Norris P. Experimental control of the diaphragm and laryngeal abductor muscles by brain stem arousal systems. *Respir Physiol* 1977;38:203–221.
195. Osmond DG. Functional anatomy of the chest wall. In: Roussos C, Macklem PT, eds. *The thorax, part A.* New York: Marcel Dekker, 1985:199–233.
196. Oyer LM, Knuth SL, Ward DK, Bartlett D Jr. Reflex inhibition of crural diaphragmatic activity by esophageal distention in cats. *Respir Physiol* 1989;77:195–202.
197. Pansard J-L, Mankikian B, Bertrand M, Kieffer E, Clergue F, Viars P. Effects of thoracic extradural block on diaphragmatic electrical activity and contractility after upper abdominal surgery. *Anesthesiology* 1993;78:63–71.
198. Pasteur W. Massive collapse of the lung. *Br J Surg* 1914;1:587–601.
199. Pavlin EG, Holle RH, Schoene RB. Recovery of airway protection compared with ventilation in humans after paralysis with curare. *Anesthesiology* 1989;70:381–385.
200. Pengelly LD, Alderson AM, Milic-Emili J. Mechanics of the diaphragm. *J Appl Physiol* 1971;30:797–805.
201. Pflug AE, Murphy TM, Butler SH, Tucker GT. The effects of postoperative peridural analgesia on pulmonary therapy and pulmonary complications. *Anesthesiology* 1974;41:8–17.
202. Polacheck J, Strong R, Arens J, Davies C, Metcalf I, Younes M. Phasic vagal influence on inspiratory motor output in anesthetized human subjects. *J Appl Physiol* 1980;49:609–619.
203. Raper AJ, Thompson WT Jr, Shapiro W, Patterson JL Jr. Scalene and sternomastoid muscle function. *J Appl Physiol* 1966;21: 497–502.
204. Rawal N, Sjöstrand U, Christoffersson E, Dahlström B, Arvill A, Rydman H. Comparison of intramuscular and epidural morphine for postoperative analgesia in the grossly obese: influence on post-

operative ambulation and pulmonary function. *Anesth Analg* 1984; 63:583–592.

205. Rehder K, Marsh HM. Respiratory mechanics during anesthesia and mechanical ventilation. In: Fishman AP, ed. *Handbook of physiology, sec. 3. The respiratory system.* Bethesda: American Physiological Society, 1986:737–752.
206. Rehder K, Sittipong R, Sessler AD. The effects of thiopental-meperidine anesthesia with succinylcholine paralysis on functional residual capacity and dynamic lung compliance in normal sitting man. *Anesthesiology* 1972;37:395–398.
207. Remmers JE, Bartlett D Jr. Reflex control of expiratory airflow and duration. *J Appl Physiol* 1977;42:80–87.
208. Remmers JE, DeGroot WJ, Sauerland EK, Anch AM. Pathogenesis of upper airway occlusion during sleep. *J Appl Physiol* 1978;44: 931–938.
209. Rex MAE. A review of the structural and functional basis of laryngospasm and a discussion of the nerve pathways involved in the reflex and its clinical significance in man and animals. *Br J Anaesth* 1970;42:891–899.
210. Rich CR, Rehder K, Knopp TJ, Hyatt RE. Halothane and enflurane anesthesia and respiratory mechanics in prone dogs. *J Appl Physiol* 1979;46:646–653.
211. Rigg JRA, Rondi P. Changes in rib cage and diaphragm contribution to ventilation after morphine. *Anesthesiology* 1981;55: 507–514.
212. Rikard-Bell GC, Bystrzycka EK, Nail BS. Cells of origin of corticospinal projections to phrenic and thoracic respiratory motoneurones in the cat as shown by retrograde transport of HRP. *Brain Res Bull* 1985;14:39–47.
213. Roberts JL, Reed WR, Thach BT. Pharyngeal airway-stabilizing function of sternohyoid and sternothyroid muscles in the rabbit. *J Appl Physiol* 1984;57:1790–1795.
214. Rochester DF. Respiratory muscles and ventilatory failure: 1993 perspective. *Am J Med Sci* 1993;305:394–402.
215. Rothstein RJ, Narce SL, DeBerry-Borowiecki B, Blanks RHI. Respiratory-related activity of upper airway muscles in anesthetized rabbit. *J Appl Physiol* 1983;55:1830–1836.
216. Rudomin P. The electrical activity of the cricothyroid muscles of the cat. *Arch Int Physiol Biochem* 1966;74:135–153.
217. Russell JA, Bishop BP, Hyatt RE. Discharge of abdominal muscle α and motoneurons during expiratory loading in cats. *Exp Neurol* 1987;97:179–192.
218. Rybro L, Schurizek BA, Petersen TK, Wernberg M. Postoperative analgesia and lung function: a comparison of intramuscular with epidural morphine. *Acta Anaesthesiol Scand* 1982;26:514–518.
219. Safar P, Escarraga LA, Chang F. Upper airway obstruction in the unconscious patient. *J Appl Physiol* 1959;14:760–764.
220. Sant'Ambrogio FB, Anderson JW, Nishino T, Sant'Ambrogio G. Effects of halothane and isoflurane in the upper airway of dogs during development. *Respir Physiol* 1992;91:237–246.
221. Sant'Ambrogio G, Widdicombe JG. Respiratory reflexes acting on the diaphragm and inspiratory intercostal muscles of the rabbit. *J Physiol* 1965;180:766–779.
222. Sasaki CT, Buckwalter J. Laryngeal function. *Am J Otolaryngol* 1984; 5:281–291.
223. Sauerland EK, Harper RM. The human tongue during sleep: electromyographic activity of the genioglossus muscle. *Exp Neurol* 1976;51:160–170.
224. Sauerland EK, Orr WC, Hairston LE. EMG patterns of oropharyngeal muscles during respiration in wakefulness and sleep. *Electromyogr Clin Neurophysiol* 1981;21:307–316.
225. Saunders NA, Rigg JRA, Pengelly LD, Campbell EJM. Effect of curare on maximum static PV relationships of the respiratory system. *J Appl Physiol* 1978;44:589–595.
226. Sears TA. Activity of fusimotor fibres innervating muscle spindles in the intercostal muscles of the cat. *Nature* 1963;197:1013–1014.
227. Sears TA. Efferent discharges in alpha and fusimotor fibres of intercostal nerves of the cat. *J Physiol* 1964;174:295–315.
228. Shannon R. Reflexes from respiratory muscles and costovertebral joints. In: Fishman AP, ed. *Handbook of physiology, sec. 3: the respiratory system.* Bethesda: American Physiological Society, 1986: 431–447.
229. Shannon R, Bolser DC, Lindsey BG. Medullary expiratory activity: influence of intercostal tendon organs and muscle spindle endings. *J Appl Physiol* 1987;62:1057–1062.
230. Shapiro SH, Ernst P, Gray-Donald K, et al. Effect of negative pressure ventilation in severe chronic obstructive pulmonary disease. *Lancet* 1992;340:1425–1429.
231. Shepard JW Jr, Thawley SE. Localization of upper airway collapse during sleep in patients with obstructive sleep apnea. *Am Rev Respir Dis* 1990;141:1350–1355.
232. Sherrey JH, Megirian D. Spontaneous and reflexly evoked laryngeal abductor and adductor muscle activity of cat. *Exp Neurol* 1974; 43:487–498.
233. Sherrington CS. Ferrier lecture: Some functional problems attaching to convergence. *Proc R Soc Lond (Biol)* 1929;105:332–362.
234. Shulman D, Beardsmore CS, Aronson HB, Godfrey S. The effect of ketamine on the functional residual capacity in young children. *Anesthesiology* 1985;62:551–556.
235. Sica AL, Cohen MI, Donnelly DF, Zhang H. Responses of recurrent laryngeal motoneurons to changes of pulmonary afferent inputs. *Respir Physiol* 1985;62:153–168.
236. Sieck GC. Organization and recruitment of diaphragm motor units. In: Roussos C, ed. *The thorax.* 2nd ed. New York: Marcel Dekker (1995, in press).
237. Sieck GC, Fournier M. Diaphragm motor unit recruitment during ventilatory and nonventilatory behaviors. *J Appl Physiol* 1989;66: 2539–2545.
238. Simonneau G, Vivien A, Sartene R, et al. Diaphragm dysfunction induced by upper abdominal surgery. Role of postoperative pain. *Am Rev Respir Dis* 1983;128:899–903.
239. Sivarajan M, Fink BR. The position and the state of the larynx during general anesthesia and muscle paralysis. *Anesthesiology* 1990;72: 439–442.
240. Smith J, Bellemare F. Effect of lung volume on in vivo contraction characteristics of human diaphragm. *J Appl Physiol* 1987;62: 1893–1900.
241. Smith JC, Mead J. Three degree of freedom description of movement of the human chest wall. *J Appl Physiol* 1986;60:928–934.
242. Snow J. On chloroform and other anesthetics; their action and administration. London: John Churchill, 1858.
243. Spence AA, Smith G. Postoperative analgesia and lung function: a comparison of morphine with extradural block. *Br J Anaesth* 1971; 43:144–148.
244. Sprung J, Barnas GM, Cheng EY, Rodarte JR. Changes in functional residual capacity and regional diaphragm lengths after upper abdominal surgery in anesthetized dogs. *Anesth Analg* 1992; 977–982.
245. Strohl KP, Mead J, Banzett RB, Loring SH, Kosch PC. Regional differences in abdominal muscle activity during various maneuvers in humans. *J Appl Physiol* 1981;51:1471–1476.
246. Stuth EAE, Tonkovic-Capin M, Kampine JP, Zuperku EJ. Dose-dependent effects of isoflurane on the CO_2 responses of expiratory medullary neurons and the phrenic nerve activities in dogs. *Anesthesiology* 1992;76:763–774.
247. Taylor A. The contribution of the intercostal muscles to the effort of respiration in man. *J Physiol* 1960;151:390–402.
248. Torres A, Kimball WR, Qvist J, et al. Sonomicrometric regional diaphragmatic shortening in awake sheep after thoracic surgery. *J Appl Physiol* 1989;67:2357–2368.
249. Travers JB, Norgren R. Afferent projections to the oral motor nuclei in the rat. *J Comp Neurol* 1983;220:280–298.
250. Tully A, Brancatisano A, Loring SH, Engel LA. Influence of posterior cricoarytenoid muscle activity on pressure-flow relationship of the larynx. *J Appl Physiol* 1991;70:2252–2258.
251. Tusiewicz K, Bryan AC, Froese AB. Contributions of changing rig cage-diaphragm interactions to the ventilatory depression of halothane anesthesia. *Anesthesiology* 1977;47:327–337.
252. Van Lunteren E, Dick TE. Intrinsic properties of pharyngeal and diaphragmatic respiratory motoneurons and muscles. *J Appl Physiol* 1992;73:787–800.
253. Van Lunteren E, Haxhiu MA, Cherniack NS, Arnold JS. Rib cage and abdominal expiratory muscle responses to CO_2 and esophageal distension. *J Appl Physiol* 1988;64:846–853.
254. Van Lunteren E, Strohl KP. Striated respiratory muscles of the upper airways. In: Mathew OP, Sant'Ambrogio G, eds. *Respiratory function of the upper airway.* New York: Marcel Dekker, 1988: 87–123.
255. Van Lunteren E, Strohl KP, Parker DM, Bruce EN, Van de Graaff WB, Cherniack NS. Phasic volume-related feedback on upper airway muscle activity. *J Appl Physiol* 1984;56:730–736.
256. Van Lunteren E, Van de Graaff WB, Parker DM, et al. Activity of

upper airway muscles during augmented breaths. *Respir Physiol* 1983;53:87–98.
257. Veber B, Dureuil B, Viires N, Aubier M, Pariente R, Desmonts JM. Effects of isoflurane on contractile properties of diaphragm. *Anesthesiology* 1989;70:684–688.
258. Vellody VP, Nassery M, Druz WS, Sharp JT. Effects of body position change on thoracoabdominal motion. *J Appl Physiol* 1978;45: 581–589.
259. Von Euler C. Brain stem mechanisms for generation and control of breathing pattern. In: Fishman AP, ed. *Handbook of physiology, sec. 3: the respiratory system.* Bethesda: American Physiological Society, 1986:1–67.
260. Wahba RWM. Perioperative functional residual capacity. *Can J Anaesth* 1991;38:384–400.
261. Warner DO, Brichant J-F, Ritman EL, Rehder K. Chest wall motion during epidural anesthesia in dogs. *J Appl Physiol* 1991;70:539–547.
262. Warner DO, Joyner MJ. Halothane attenuates expiratory muscle activation in dogs. *Anesthesiology* 1992;77:A1257.
263. Warner DO, Joyner MJ, Rehder K. Electrical activation of expiratory muscles increases with time in pentobarbital-anesthetized dogs. *J Appl Physiol* 1992;72:2285–2291.
264. Warner DO, Krayer S, Rehder K, Ritman EL. Chest wall motion during spontaneous breathing and mechanical ventilation in dogs. *J Appl Physiol* 1989;66:1179–1189.
265. Warner DO, Rehder K. Influence of anesthesia on the thorax. In: Roussos C, ed. *The thorax.* 2nd ed. New York: Marcel Dekker (1995, in press).
266. Warner DO, Warner MA, Ritman EL. Chest wall configuration during halothane anesthesia with spontaneous breathing. *Anesthesiology* 1992;77:A1256.
267. Warner DO, Warner MA, Ritman EL. Inspiration during quiet breathing markedly increases intrathoracic blood volume in humans. *FASEB J* 1992;6:A1478.
268. Waud BE, Waud DR. Effects of volatile anesthetics on directly and indirectly stimulated skeletal muscle. *Anesthesiology* 1979;50: 103–110.
269. Westbrook PR, Stubbs SE, Sessler AD, Rehder K, Hyatt RE. Effects of anesthesia and muscle paralysis on respiratory mechanics in normal man. *J Appl Physiol* 1973;34:81–86.
270. Wheatley JR, Brancatisano A, Engel LA. Respiratory-related activity of cricothyroid muscle in awake normal humans. *J Appl Physiol* 1991;70:2226–2232.
271. Wheatley JR, Kelly WT, Tully A, Engel LA. Pressure-diameter relationships of the upper airway in awake supine subjects. *J Appl Physiol* 1991;70:2242–2251.
272. Whitelaw WA. Shape and size of the human diaphragm in vivo. *J Appl Physiol* 1987;62:180–186.
273. Whitelaw WA, Feroah T. Patterns of intercostal muscle activity in humans. *J Appl Physiol* 1989;67:2087–2094.
274. Whitelaw WA, Ford GT, Rimmer KP, De Troyer A. Intercostal muscles are used during rotation of the thorax in humans. *J Appl Physiol* 1992;72:1940–1944.
275. Widdicombe JG. Reflexes from the upper respiratory tract. In: Fishman AP, ed. *Handbook of physiology, sec. 3: the respiratory system.* Bethesda: American Physiological Society, 1986:363–394.
276. Wilson TA, De Troyer A. Effect of respiratory muscle tension on lung volume. *J Appl Physiol* 1992;73:2283–2288.
277. Younes M. The physiological basis of central apnea and periodic breathing. In: Simmons D, ed. *Current pulmonology.* Chicago: Yearbook, 1989:265–325.
278. Younes M, Youssef M. Effect of five human anesthetics on respiratory control in cats. *J Appl Physiol* 1978;44:596–606.

Anesthesia: Biologic Foundations, edited by
Tony L. Yaksh et al. Lippincott–Raven Publishers,
Philadelphia © 1997.

CHAPTER 80

MICROVASCULAR FLUID EXCHANGE

STEVEN J. ALLEN AND ROBERT E. DRAKE

Under normal conditions, fluid filters out of the microvasculature in all tissues. The physiologic functions of fluid filtration have not been conclusively elucidated but probably include nutrition and immunologic support. However, pathologic alterations in the factors governing fluid exchange can lead to accumulation of excess interstitial fluid/edema that frequently impairs vital organ function. In the lung, edema results in decreased compliance and hypoxemia. This chapter presents an overview of the physiologic principles governing fluid balance with particular attention to the lungs. Fluid balance refers to the transport of water and solutes, particularly large molecules such as proteins. After a description of the relevant pulmonary anatomy, the physiologic principles and the experimental techniques used in fluid balance studies along with their limitations are presented. One of the aims of this chapter is to present fluid balance concepts so that the reader can envision their application to other organs in addition to the lung.

ANATOMY OF LUNG FLUID BALANCE

Blood travels to the microcirculation by way of the pulmonary arteries which travel in proximity to the airways (Fig. 1). At the level of the alveoli, the vessels drain into capillary "sheets" surrounding the alveoli creating an enormous surface area (~70 m^2 in an adult lung) that facilitates gas exchange. The capillary blood then empties into venules and veins that drain into the left atrium. Fluid filters out of the pulmonary vessels in the vicinity of the alveoli. Filtration occurs not only in the capillaries but also in the precapillary arterioles and in the postcapillary venules. The contribution of these extracapillary filtration sites is not clear, but some investigators have estimated up to 50%. This observation has led to the term microvascular exchange vessels to refer to the anatomic location of fluid filtration. Interstitial fluid is taken up initially by the terminal lymphatics which drain into smooth muscle lined lymph vessels that carry the fluid eventually back into the veins in the neck. Although the lymph system is the conventional component used to describe interstitial fluid removal for almost all organs, there are other pathways that may also be involved. In the lung, interstitial fluid is also removed via the pleura and mediastinum (4,54). If the lymphatics cannot remove the fluid fast enough, it accumulates in the loose pier bronchial and perivascular tissue and may give rise to peribronchial cuffing seen on chest roentgengraphs. Figure 2 is a photomicrograph that demonstrates the extremely small distances that normally exists between the red cell in the capillary and the gas in the alveolus. One can easily see how edema increases diffusion distances and may impact gas exchange. However, significant pulmonary edema is often associated with alveolar flooding where edema fluid leaks out of the interstitium and into the alveolus and thereby decreases the local ventilation/perfusion ratio.

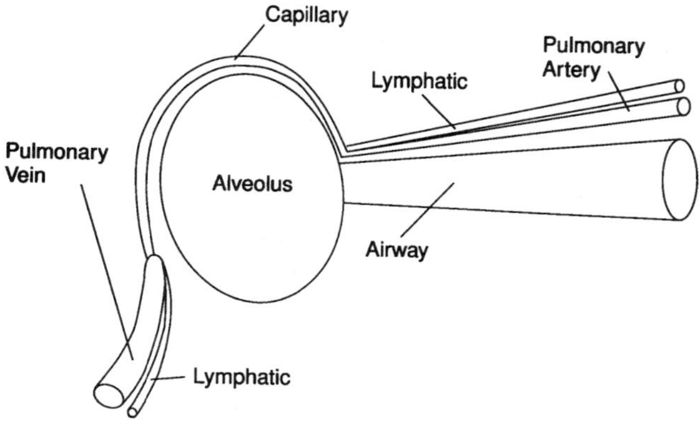

Figure 1. Lung microvascular unit. Pulmonary arteries travel with the airways down to the alveoli, and blood is drained by the venous system. Microvascular fluid filtration occurs in precapillary, capillary, and postcapillary sites. Filtered fluid is removed by the lymphatics that pass along veins and arteries. (Reprinted with permission from *Am Rev Respir Dis* 1983;127:S44–S50.)

Although thin, the pulmonary interstitium is composed of a complex structure of collagen, proteoglycans, hyaluronan, and cells. The interstitium plays an active if not well understood role in lung fluid balance as well as providing structural support. Because of its water-binding properties hyaluronan has been implicated in the regulation of interstitial water content (6). The edema in some diseases and experimental models appears to be mediated by hyaluronan accumulation (7,37).

In most tissues, including the lung, the exchange barrier is characterized by continuous endothelium (46). Fluid filters out of the vessels by way of the intercellular clefts and filtration is determined by the size and charge of the molecules that line these clefts. In contrast, hepatic microcirculation has a discontinuous endothelium and filtration occurs out of the sinusoids with little impedance of large molecule transport. In addition to intercellular cleft, there are several other proposed pathways of microvascular exchange including vascular transport and through cells (46).

HISTORY OF STARLING EQUATION

Insight into the physiologic factors governing fluid balance was long preceded by anatomic description. William Harvey's discovery of the circulation in 1628 was followed relatively shortly by the discovery of the microcirculation by the early microscopist Leeuvenhoek in 1674. However, progress in elucidating fluid exchange principles did not begin until the 19th century. Ludwig took the then recently developed concept of osmosis and applied it to the capillary in 1858. Physiologists at the end of the 19th century understood that the hydrostatic pressure within the microvascular exchange vessels was the single most important factor determining filtration. However, they still did not understand why patients with hypoproteinemia (i.e., nephrotic syndrome) but normal microvascular pressure (P_c) developed edema. Ernest Starling's central contribution to the field was his demonstration in 1896 that plasma proteins exerted an osmotic pressure that counterbalanced the hydrostatic pressure. Thus, decreased plasma protein concentration (C_p) leads to decreased plasma protein osmotic pressure (π_c), which causes increased filtration. This concept formed the first version of Starling's hypothesis of fluid filtration (eq. A in Fig. 3). Subsequently, investigators realized that the important val-

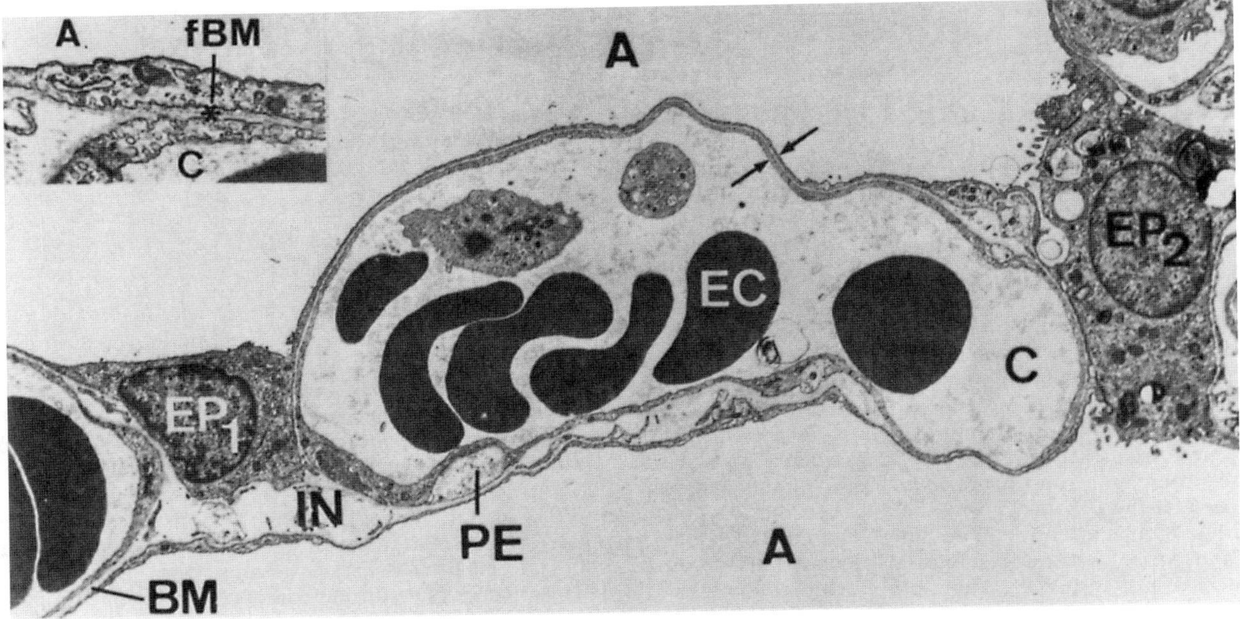

Figure 2. Photomicrograph of pulmonary microvasculature. The *arrows* highlight the thinness of the blood-gas exchange barrier. A, alveolar space; C, capillary; EC, red cell; EP_1 and EP_2, type I and II squamous epithelial cell, respectively; IN, interstitium; BM, basement membrane; fBM, fused basement membrane; PE, pericyte. (Reprinted with permission from *Am Rev Respir Dis* 1977;116:589–615.)

ues were not the absolute intravascular pressures but rather the transmembrane gradients (eq. B in Fig. 3). As will be discussed later, tissue hydrostatic (P_i) and protein osmotic pressure (π_i) measurement in most tissues is difficult and technique validity often controversial. The next step in Starling's hypothesis development was the attempt to quantitate the filtration rate by including a filtration coefficient. Landis (30) presented the third equation in Fig. 3 with F representing flow and K_f capillary filtration coefficient. This version did not take into account membrane permeability to protein. Permeability to proteins decreases the effectiveness of the transmembrane osmotic gradient to oppose hydrostatic pressures. The application of the principles of irreversible thermodynamics to membrane transport led to the incorporation of the osmotic reflection coefficient σ_d. σ_d is a unitless value that ranges from 0 to 1 and accounts for protein permeability (eq. D in Fig. 3). K_f was then defined as the product of surface area and hydraulic conductivity (L_p). This latter term is a physicochemical property that describes how fast water can cross the exchange barrier for a given pressure gradient. Thus, the contemporary Starling equation relates the filtration rate to potentially measurable pressures (P_c, P_t, π_c, and π_t) and to physical properties of the microvascular membrane (K_f and σ_d).

$$\text{A. } P = \pi$$

$$\text{B. } (P_c - P_{int}) = (\pi_p - \pi_{int})$$

$$\text{C. } F = K_f[(P_c - P_{int}) - (\pi_p - \pi_{int})]$$

$$\text{D. } J_v = L_pS[(P_c - P_{int}) - \sigma(\pi_p - \pi_{int})]$$

Figure 3. Evolution of the Starling equation. (Reprinted, in adapted form, with permission from ref. 46.)

Fluid balance in any tissue is determined by the rate at which fluid enters the tissue and the rate at which it is removed. In most cases, fluid enters the tissue spaces by filtration through the microvascular (capillary) membranes. Fluid is removed from the tissue spaces via the lymphatic vessels, and, normally, the lymphatic flow rate equals the filtration rate. Consequently, the tissue fluid volume remains constant. Under pathological circumstances, the filtration rate may exceed the lymphatic flow rate so that fluid will accumulate within the tissue.

FILTRATION COEFFICIENT: K_f

K_f is the product of two terms, hydraulic conductivity and surface area. Hydraulic conductivity is a physical property of the microvascular exchange barrier. Typically it represents how much fluid will cross a given area over a given amount of time for a given hydrostatic pressure gradient. Microvascular permeability is often modelled in terms of pores. K_f can be thought of as the sum of the hydraulic conductivity of all of the pores within an organ's microvasculature. Increases in permeability would most likely be due to increases in pore size. As changes in hydraulic conductivity are related to changes in radius to the fourth power, K_f should be a sensitive measure of hydraulic conductivity. However, K_f is also affected by changes in surface area. If capillary beds are recruited, K_f may increase without any change in permeability. Inability to account for changes in surface area during measurements of K_f is a major problem that limits its use for permeability determinations.

Measurement

Table 1 shows the variable estimates of K_f produced by experimental techniques. The best way to understand current methods for estimation of filtration coefficient is by doing series of thought experiments. Suppose you had a chamber which was divided into two parts by a membrane (Fig. 4). The membrane contains a single cylindrical pore. Both sides of the chamber contain water so that the hydrostatic pressures on side 1 and 2 are P_1 and P_2, respectively. Obviously, fluid will flow through the

Table 1. EXAMPLES OF PULMONARY K_f USING VARIOUS TECHNIQUES

Techniques	K_f, ml·min^{-1}/mm Hg^{-1}/100 g^{-1}
Weight techniques involving the production of edema	
Guyton and Lindsey (26) (anesthetized dogs)	0.07
Levine et al. (32) (anesthetized dogs)	0.03 or 0.08
Drake et al. (16) (anesthetized dogs)	0.11 ± 0.06
Ehrhart et al. (18) (isolated dog lungs)	0.07 ± 0.012
Weight-transient	
Wangensteen et al. (53) (isolated rabbit lung)	1.0
Gaar et al. (21) (isolated dog lung)	0.07 ± 0.010
Drake et al. (12) (isolated dog lungs)	0.21 ± 0.09
Lymph-flow	
Erdmann et al. (20) (unanesthetized sheep)	0.007 ± 0.011
Michel et al. (34) (anesthetized dogs)	0.006 or 0.085

membrane pore at a rate which is proportional to P_1 - P_2 times the hydraulic conductivity of the pore.

$$J_v = K_f\ (P_1 - P_2) \qquad (1)$$

There are several ways to measure K_f, but the complexity of each method depends on how much about the system we can directly measure. If we could look through a microscope and measure the dimensions of the pore (where r is radius and Δx is length), then we could calculate K_f using Poiselle's Law.

$$K_f = \frac{\pi \bullet r^4}{8 \bullet n \bullet \Delta x} \qquad (2)$$

where n is fluid viscosity.

Suppose that the membrane pore is too small to measure. In this case, we cannot calculate K_f; we would have to measure it. To do this, we could drill a hole in one side of the chamber (Fig. 5). We could then collect any water that drips from the hole, and this will allow us to measure J_v. Assume that the hole is so large that (a) J_v could never exceed the rate at which fluid can flow through the hole and (b) the side 2 water level cannot rise above the hole.

If we measure P_1, P_2, and J_v, we can calculate K_f:

$$K_f = \frac{J_V}{P_1 - P_2} \qquad (3)$$

Now let us make the problem one step more complicated. Suppose that we cannot measure P_2. This is the usual situation since it is difficult to measure tissue fluid hydrostatic pressure (P_t). Even though we do not know P_2, we can still estimate K_f if we measure J_v at several different P_1's. We could plot J_v versus P_1 and calculate K_f as $\Delta J_v/\Delta P_1$ (Fig. 6). The slope of the J_v versus P_1 relationship will equal K_f only if P_2 remains constant during the experiment. Of course, P_2 will remain constant for the system of Fig. 5 because the water level of side 2 cannot rise above the hole.

Guyton and Lindsey (26) used a modification of this technique to provide the first estimates of K_f in the lung. They raised left atrial pressure in dogs and removed the lungs after a given amount of time. They found that edema did not form unless left atrial pressure was higher than the plasma colloid osmotic pressure. From the amount of edema that formed, they calculated the rate of edema formation. They divided the change in the rates of edema formation by the change in left atrial pressure to obtain K_f. However, this method depends on two assumptions: (a) rate of edema formation differences between dogs is equal to J_v differences and (b) changes in left atrial pressure reflected changes in the actual total pressure gradient (interstitial and osmotic pressures) across the exchange barrier.

To get even closer to the real problems encountered in measuring K_f, we would have to remove the "overflow" hole in side 2 of the chamber. This creates two problems: (a) P_2 will not remain

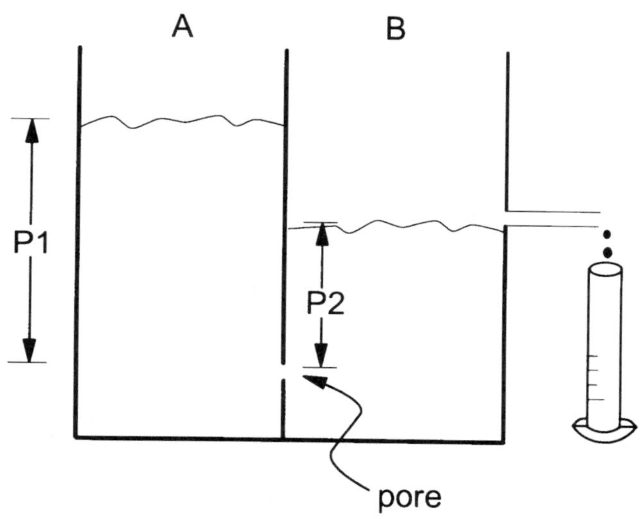

Figure 4. The filtration coefficient (K_f) of the pore can be determined by the rate of fluid (J_v) passing from **A** to **B**, divided by the pressure gradient (P_1-P_2).

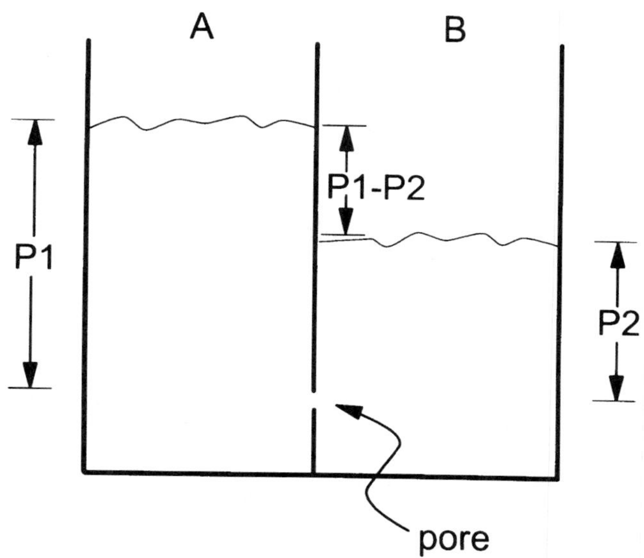

Figure 5. Rate of fluid passing through pore can be measured by amount of fluid leaving hole in side of **B**.

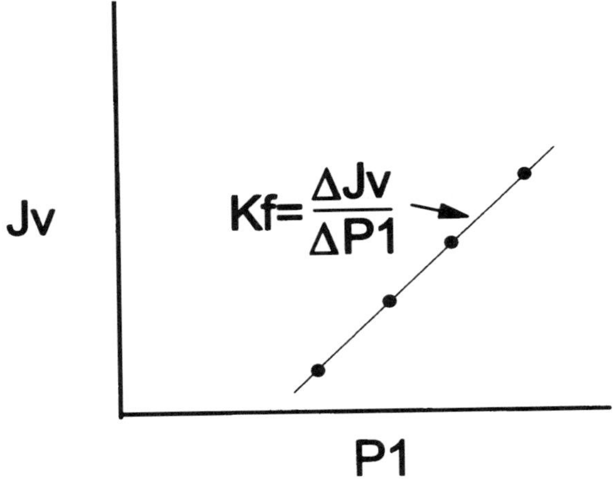

Figure 6. Without knowing P_2, we can estimate K_f as the slope of J_v versus various P_1's.

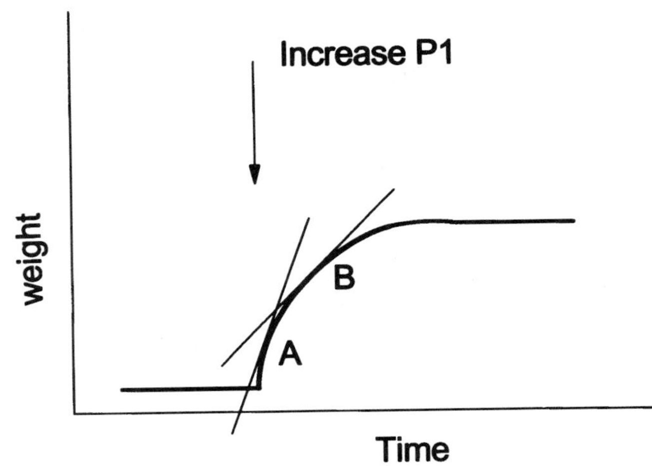

Figure 8. When microvascular pressure is increased, tissue weight increases because of both increased tissue water and increased vascular volume. K_f measurements will vary depending on how long after the pressure increase they are performed. For example, calculation at time **A** will produce a higher K_f than at time **B**.

constant, and (b) we have no direct method to measure J_v. Sometimes it is possible to remove an organ and measure weight continuously as with a lung lobe. J_v can be estimated from the rate of weight gain. This might be modeled by physically separating the two sides of the chamber and allowing the filtrate to flow from side 1 to side 2 through a flexible tube (Fig. 7). To measure K_f, we would first allow the system to come to equilibrium. In other words, we would allow fluid to filter from one side of the chamber to the other until $P_1 = P_2$. We would know that equilibrium was reached because the weight would become constant. Then we would abruptly increase P_1 by adding water to side 1. Now the filtration rate should be as follows:

$$J_v = K_f\ (\Delta P_1 + P_1' - P_2') \qquad (4)$$

where ΔP_1 is the change in P_1 and P_1' and P_2' are the values of P_1 and P_2 before we added water to side 1. The weight will begin to increase as soon as we increase P_1; however, the rate of weight gain will slowly decrease in time. The reason for the decrease in the rate of weight gain is that, as fluid accumulates in side 2, P_2 will increase. The increase in P_2 will cause J_v to gradually decrease until a new equilibrium is established (Fig. 8). At the instant that we increase P_1, $J_v = K_f \times P_1$ (eq. 4). This is

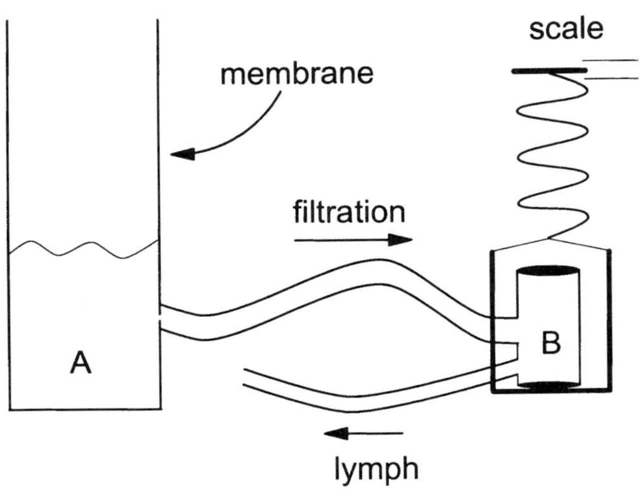

Figure 7. Changes in J_v can be estimated by tissue weight changes. The pressure in the **A** is adjusted so that the **B** is isogravimetric (not gaining or losing weight). A given pressure change is made to **B,** and the rate of rise in tissue weight is measured.

because $P_1' - P_2' = 0$ and it takes a finite amount of time for P_2 to increase above P_2'. Thus,

$$K_f = \frac{J_V\,(t = 0)}{P_1} \qquad (5)$$

According to this reasoning, it should be possible to determine the rate of weight gain immediately after increasing P_1, divide by the increase in P_1 and obtain K_f. There is a problem in applying this technique in real organs. The only way to increase microvascular pressure in an organ is to raise the vascular pressures. The increase in vascular pressures will cause blood to pool within the blood vessels. Consequently, for a brief time after we increase the vascular pressures, the organ weight will increase due to (a) fluid filtration and (b) increases in blood volume. Failing to correct for the increase in blood volume can result in overestimation of the filtration rate.

There are two ways to minimize effect of blood volume changes. Some investigators have simply waited until they felt that the blood volume shift was completed before they measured the rate of weight gain (21,51). This practice has resulted in a wide range of K_f estimates (Table 1). If an investigator measured the slope 20 s after raising P_c, then he will get a relatively high K_f estimate. If he waits 3 min, his estimate will be relatively low. The other technique to avoid the vascular volume problem is the "rate of weight gain extrapolation technique" (50). P_c is raised, and the rate of weight gain is measured every 1–2 min. The rates of weight gain are plotted versus time on semilog graph paper. The result is a curve with two slopes: one corresponding to the blood volume shift and the other corresponding to filtration. By extrapolating the second slope (filtration rate) back to zero time, the investigator may estimate the filtration rate caused by the increase in vascular pressure.

Suppose that the membrane contained two pores. Then

$$J_v = K_{f1}\ (P_1 - P_2) + K_{f2}\ (P_1 - P_2) \qquad (6)$$

where K_{f1} and K_{f2} are the filtration coefficients of the two pores. From eq. 6, it can be seen that the total membrane K_f should simply be the sum of the filtration coefficients of all the pores in the membrane. Microvascular membranes probably contain thousands of pores and each organ contains many microvascular membranes (one for each capillary). Consequently, the K_f for an organ is the sum of millions of small K_f's. If the number of perfused capillaries in an organ decreases, K_f should also decrease.

MICROVASCULAR MEMBRANE PERMEABILITY TO PROTEIN

From the Starling equation, the microvascular membrane permeability to protein is important for two reasons. First protein permeability is one of the factors determining π_t. This is because π_t depends upon the interstitial fluid protein concentration, and protein concentration depends (in part) on the rate at which protein permeates through the microvascular membrane and into the interstitium. The second way that protein permeability is important is that it determines the effectiveness of the transmembrane protein osmotic pressure gradient (π_c-π_t). This effect of permeability can be seen explicitly in the Starling equation as σ_d multiplied times (π_c-π_t). Protein osmotic pressure is discussed in a later section.

According to the pore concept of microvascular transport, there are two ways that protein moves through the microvascular membrane: (a) diffusion and (b) convection (9,15,28,40, 51). Each mechanism of transport is associated with its own permeability coefficient (PS and σ for diffusion and convection, respectively).

Diffusion

It is best to start with the basic concepts of diffusion. Suppose that you have a chamber filled with a protein solution (Fig. 9). Also suppose that there is a concentration gradient along the length of the chamber. In this case, protein will diffuse from left to right. The number of moles of protein moving past any imaginary plane within the chamber in a given amount of time will be:

$$n_D = DA\frac{dc}{dx} \tag{7}$$

where n_D is the rate of diffusion of protein, D is the diffusion coefficient of protein in water, A is the cross-sectional area of the chamber, and dc/dx is the gradient in protein concentration at the plane of interest.

The diffusion coefficient (D) can be determined from:

$$D = \frac{RT}{F_{sw}N} \tag{8}$$

where R is the universal gas constant, T is the absolute temperature, N is the number of molecules per mole (Avogadro's number), and F_{sw} is the frictional force between solute (protein) and water. The "driving force" for diffusion is derived from thermal energy and this is represented by the RT term in eq. 8. Diffusion will be slowed with larger protein molecules as the larger the protein molecule, the lower the diffusion coefficient. This is because the frictional force increases with increasing protein molecule radius (**a**) (eq. 9).

$$F_{sw} = 6\pi na \tag{9}$$

where n is the viscosity of the water.

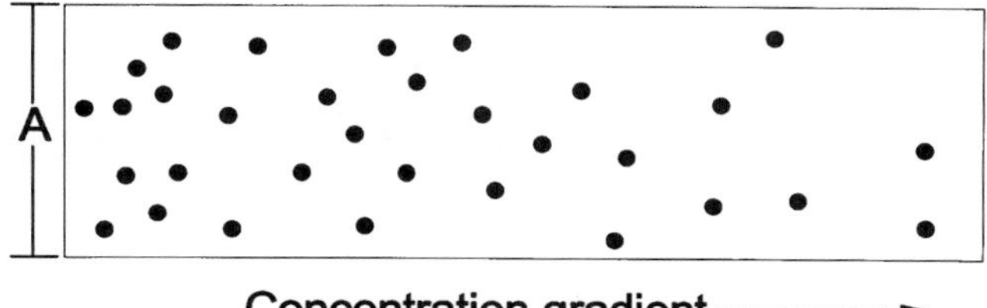

Figure 9. Diffusion gradient. The rate of solute diffusion is determined by the concentration gradient, the diffusion coefficient of the molecule, and the cross-sectional area of the chamber, **A**.

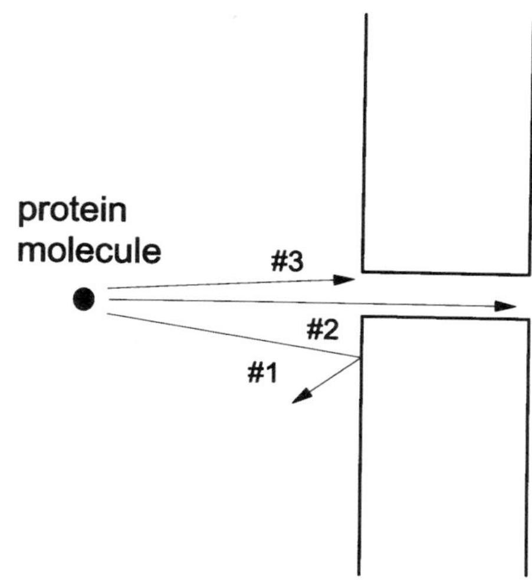

Figure 10. Possible fates of a diffusing protein molecule approaching a pore. If it travels along trajectory 1, it misses the pore and is "reflected." Along path 2, it passes through the pore. Along trajectory 3, the molecule center may be aligned with the pore, but the molecule's sides may strike the edge of the pore. The molecule's center has to be at least one molecular radius away from the pore's sides for the protein to pass through.

Now suppose that we place a membrane containing a single pore into the chamber. Obviously diffusion will be slowed considerably because only part of the chamber cross-sectional area (A) is available for diffusion. How can we calculate the rate of diffusion? If the single pore is large relative to the size of the protein molecules, we simply substitute the pore area ($A_p = \pi(r)^2$) for A in eq. 7 (where r is pore radius). The problem comes when the pore is of molecular size. In this case, several corrections must be made. First consider the probability that a protein molecule will enter the pore (Fig. 10). Diffusion depends on the random motion of the protein molecules. If a molecule approaches the membrane along trajectory 1, then it will bounce off and not diffuse through. If it goes along trajectory 2, it will go directly through the pore and thus will diffuse through the membrane. However, suppose the molecule follows trajectory 3. On this trajectory, the center of the molecule will approach the pore, but the edge of the molecule will strike the wall of the membrane and bounce away. The molecule will only go through the pore if the center of the molecule is at least one molecular radius away from the edge of the pore (Fig. 11). For this reason, the

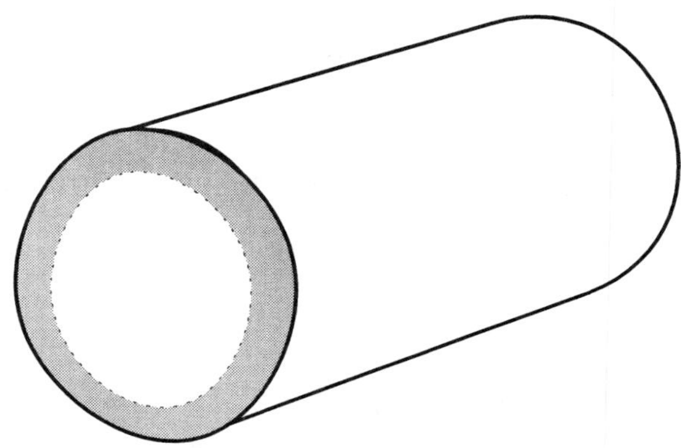

Figure 11. Effective pore area. For a given protein, the effective pore area is represented by the unshaded area and is calculated by the following: π(pore radius - protein radius)^2.

effective pore area is shown by the dashed line in Fig. 8. This effective area (A_{eff}) is:

$$A_{eff} = \pi(r - a)^2 = \pi(r)^2 (1 - a/r)^2 \qquad (10)$$

Thus, instead of substituting A_p into eq. 7, it would be necessary to substitute $A_p(1 - a/r)^2$.

The second correction that must be made to eq. 7 when a and r are similar involves the frictional forces acting on a protein molecule within the pore. According to eq. 8, the friction between the molecule and water is important in determining the free diffusion coefficient. When a protein molecule is within a pore, there is friction between the molecule and water (F_{sw}) and between the molecule and the walls of the membrane pore (F_{sm}). Thus, eq. 8 should be:

$$D = \frac{RT}{(F_{sw} + F_{sm})N} \qquad (11)$$

Considering effective pore area and friction, eq. 7 becomes:

$$n_D = A_p(1 - a/r)^2 \frac{RT}{(F_{sw} + F_{sm})N} \frac{dc}{dx} \qquad (12)$$

This can be expressed as:

$$n_D = A_p(1 - a/r)^2 D_p \frac{\Delta c}{\Delta x} \qquad (13)$$

where D_p is the diffusion coefficient within the pore, Δc is the protein concentration difference across the membrane, and Δx is the width of the membrane.

Normally, in biological membranes, there are many pores per unit surface area. Accordingly, the permeability of the membrane (P) is defined as:

$$P = \frac{N_p A_p}{S} \frac{(1 - a/r)^2 D_p}{\Delta x} \qquad (14)$$

where S is the total membrane surface area and N_p is number of pores in area S.

From eqs. 13 and 14, the total diffusion rate through a membrane containing many pores (J_{SD}) should be:

$$J_{SD} = PS\,\Delta c \qquad (15)$$

Convection

Water (the solvent), flowing through the pores, will "drag" protein molecules along. For this reason, the permeability coefficient associated with this type of transport is called the "solvent drag" reflection coefficient (σ_f).

Suppose that we have a pipe containing a protein solution. The solution flows from left to right at a velocity which is not important. Also assume that there is no diffusion. Because there is no barrier to restrict protein or water movement through the pipe, the concentration of solution going out of the pipe (C_2) is equal to the concentration of the solution entering the pipe (C_1). In this case, the amount of protein that is "reflected back" and not allowed to pass through the pipe is zero. Thus, $\sigma_f = 0.0$.

Now suppose that we put a screen into the pipe and that the holes in the screen will not allow protein to pass. In this case, the water will go through, but all the protein will be reflected or blocked by the screen. In this case, $\sigma_f = 1.0$ because 100% of the protein that is contained in the water passing through the screen is reflected and $C_2 = 0.0$.

Now suppose we put a solid plate into the pipe and thus block both water and protein. In this case, σ_f is undefined because σ_f is the fraction of protein reflected from water which passes through a barrier.

The definition is as follows: The solvent drug reflection coefficient (σ_f) is the ratio of the amount of protein reflected from a membrane to the amount of protein carried up to the membrane by water which passes through the membrane.

Although the reflection coefficient describes the fraction of protein which does not go through a barrier or membrane, it is easier to measure σ_f in terms of what does go through. For example, suppose you have a semiporous membrane in the pipe. You can measure C_1 and C_2 directly, but you would need to do some complicated measurements and calculations to figure out how much protein was reflected by the membrane and stayed on side 1. On the other hand, you know that if C_2 moles/L of protein got through, then $C_1 - C_2$ moles/L must have been reflected. Thus, the concentration of reflected protein = $C_1 - C_2$ and the fraction of protein reflected must be = $(C_1 - C_2)/C_1$. Accordingly:

$$\sigma_f = \frac{C_1 - C_2}{C_1} = 1 - C_2/C_1 \qquad (16)$$

The examples given in this discussion are based on the assumption that the reflected protein disappears. If this assumption were not made, then the reflected protein would build up on the inflow side of the pipe and increase the concentration of protein at the inflow side. As water flowed into the pipe and up to the membrane, it would carry some of the previously reflected protein with it. Thus, the concentration of protein in the water approaching the membrane would be greater than C_1. However, investigators typically assume that the reflected protein disappears rather than attempting to account for its accumulation. Fortunately, this assumption is consistent with microvascular exchange in most tissues because blood flow through the capillaries continuously washes away the reflected protein and C_1 usually remains almost constant. However, there are physiological situations, such as in the kidney, and experimental designs in which this is not the case.

Physical Factors Determining σ_f

Suppose a membrane has a single pore that has a radius (r) that is much larger than a water molecule, but is between 1 and 10 times more than the radius of a protein molecule. We need to figure out what σ_f would be in terms of the physical forces that would be acting and in terms of the geometry of the system.

The first thing to consider is the reduced area available for transport. The area available to water is just πr^2. However, the area available to the protein molecules (radius = a) is $\pi(r - a)^2$. The reason for this is that any protein molecule carried up to the membrane will strike the membrane unless the center of the pore is at least 1 molecular radius from the walls of the pore. Thus, only $\pi(r - a)^2/\pi(r)^2$ of the protein approaching the pore will get through or:

$$C_2' = C_1 (1 - a/r)^2 \qquad (17)$$

or, from eq. 16:

$$\sigma_f' = 1 - (1 - a/r)^2 \qquad (18)$$

The prime marks above C_2 and σ_f are to indicate that these are not the true estimates of C_2 and σ_f because we need to consider more factors than just the reduced area.

Another factor to be considered is that the distribution of water flow through a pore is parabolic; the water in the center of the pore moves faster than the water at the edges. Because the water in the center carries the protein, this effect will tend to raise C_2 above the level given by eq. 17. When the parabolic velocity profile is considered:

$$\sigma_f' = (1 - (1 - a/r)^2)^2 \qquad (19)$$

The derivation of eq. 19 involves integrating the product of the water velocity and protein concentration across the diameter of the pore.

The σ_f' of eq. 19 is inaccurate because it does not consider frictional forces. The derivations of equations to account for friction are quite complicated, and different authors have come up with different equations. For practical purposes, we believe that the following equation is about as good as any (11):

$$\sigma_f = \frac{16}{3}(a/r_p)^2 - \frac{20}{3}(a/r_p)^3 + \frac{7}{3}(a/r_p)^4 \qquad (20)$$

Rate of Convective Transport

We can easily calculate the rate of convective transport through a single pore (n_C) from the concentration of protein leaving the pore (C_2) and the volume flow rate through the pore (V):

$$n_C = V\,C_2 \qquad (21)$$

From eq. 16:

$$C_2 = C_1(1 - \sigma_f) \qquad (22)$$

Thus:

$$n_C = V\,C_1(1 - \sigma_f) \qquad (23)$$

We can see from eq. 14 that increasing the number of pores will increase the diffusion permeability coefficient, P. Will increasing the number of equal sized pores change σ_f? Let us take the case of two equal sized pores. The amount of protein brought up to the membrane would be $2VC_1$. The amount of protein getting through would be $2VC_2$. Thus, the amount reflected per unit time would be $2VC_1 - 2VC_2$. By definition, the membrane solvent drag reflection coefficient is the amount of protein reflected divided by the amount brought to the membrane. Thus,

$$\sigma_f = \frac{2VC_1 - 2VC_2}{2VC_1} = 1 - C_2/C_1 \qquad (24)$$

Notice that the equation for σ_f for two pores (eq. 24) is the same as the equation for σ_f for one pore (eq. 16). Thus, the membrane reflection coefficient is not dependent on the number of pores of equal size in a membrane.

Why does the number of pores in a membrane affect the diffusion permeability coefficient but not the reflection coefficient? By definition, the diffusion permeability coefficient is the rate of diffusive protein transport per unit membrane surface area(s) divided by the protein concentration gradient:

$$P = \frac{J_{SD}/S}{\Delta C} \qquad (25)$$

If the number of pores in a unit membrane area is increased, J_{SD} will increase, but S and ΔC will stay the same and P must increase.

By definition, σ_f is the amount of protein reflected divided by the amount brought up to the membrane per unit time. If the number of pores is increased, then the total volume flow rate (J_v) will increase. This will increase the amount of protein reflected per unit time ($JVC_1 - JVC_2$), but it will increase the amount of protein brought to the membrane (JVC_1) by the same proportion. Thus, σ_f will not be changed. Similarly, if there are N_p pores per unit membrane surface area (S), then an increase in S will increase the total number of pores but σ_f will not be affected. To summarize:

Increasing the number of pores in a capillary wall will (a) not change σ_f, (b) increase P proportionately, and (c) increase PS proportionately. Capillary recruitment (increasing S) will (a) not change σ_f, (b) not change P, and (c) increase PS proportionately.

Because increasing the number of pores does not affect σ_f, then the total convection transport J_{SC} should be the sum of the transports for each pore (eq. 23) so:

$$J_{SC} = J_V\,C_1(1 - \sigma_f) \qquad (26)$$

Total Protein Transport Rate

Equation 15 gives the diffusive transport for the case in which convection does not occur and eq. 26 gives the convective transport derived under conditions of no diffusion. It might seem that we could add the two to get the total transport. Unfortunately, this is not true for the following reason. In discussing convection, we assumed that protein would be brought up to the membrane (and into the pore) by convection. However, in a system involving both convection and diffusion, some protein will be brought up to the membrane by diffusion. Once a protein has entered a pore by diffusion, it will tend to be "drug" by the solvent just as if it had been carried to the membrane by convection. Similarly, molecules moving through the pore by convection will also diffuse. This means that diffusion and convection cannot actually be separated as we did in analyzing each process. Accordingly, we cannot expect the equations we arrived at in the separate analyses (eqs. 15 and 26) to be additive. The problem is currently handled by assuming that diffusion occurs as described by eq. 15, but the concentration of protein "drug" through the pores by convection is the "average" concentration within the pores (C) instead of C_1. Thus, the modified convective component of transport would be:

$$J_{SC} = J_V\,C\,(1 - \sigma_f) \qquad (27)$$

instead of eq. 26. By adding eqs. 15 and 27, we obtain the Kedem and Katchalsky equation for total protein transport (J_S) (28):

$$J_S = (1 - \sigma_f)J_V\,C + PS(C_1 - C_2) \qquad (28)$$

The problem with eq. 28 is that C is unknown. What is the "average" protein concentration in a pore?

Patlak et al. (44) derived an equation based on analysis that did not require independent consideration of diffusion or convection:

$$J_S = J_V(1 - \sigma_d)\,\frac{C_1 - C_2e^{-X}}{1 - e^{-X}} \qquad (29)$$

where X is the Peclet number [$X = (1 - \sigma_d)\,J_V/PS$].

The Patlak equation can be rearranged into another useful form:

$$\frac{C_2}{C_1} = \frac{1 - \sigma_d}{1 - \sigma_d e^{-X}} \qquad (30)$$

Note that the Patlak equations substitute the osmotic reflection coefficient (σ_d) for σ_f.

Osmotic Reflection Coefficient (σ_d)

The σ_d is the osmotic reflection coefficient and is a measure of the fraction of the total protein osmotic pressure which is effective across a semiporous membrane. Suppose that you have a solution of 5% albumin and 0.9% NaCl in water. The protein osmotic pressure (π) would be 20 mm Hg at body temperature. If you put the solution on side 1 of a semipermeable membrane and 0.9% NaCl on side 2, then water will flow through the membrane pores from side 2 to side 1. If you apply a hydrostatic pressure to side 1, the flow rate will decrease. As you apply more pressure to side 1, the net flow rate will slow more and, if enough pressure is applied, flow will reverse. If you apply just the right amount of pressure, the flow will stop.

The definition is as follows: The osmotic reflection coefficient (σ_d) is the ratio of the hydrostatic pressure required to stop the flow of fluid caused by osmotic pressure to the total protein osmotic pressure gradient across the membrane.

If it took exactly 20 mm Hg hydrostatic pressure to stop flow in the above system, then σ_d would be 20/20 = 1.0. If it took 10 mm Hg hydrostatic pressure, then σ_d would be 10/20 = 0.5. (Assume that the protein concentration on side 2 was somehow maintained at zero.) The σ_d must be between 0 and 1 for any membrane.

In a membrane with pores that are smaller than the protein molecules, $\sigma_d = 1$. However, if the pores are larger than the protein molecules, then only a fraction of the total protein osmotic pressure will be exerted across the membrane and $\sigma_d < 1.0$. Rather than discussing the physical factors which determine σ_d, suffice it to say that $\sigma_d = \sigma_f$ for a single pore.

Heteroporosity and the Two Reflection Coefficients

The purpose in this section is to deduce what σ_f and σ_d would be for a membrane containing two different sized pores. We will take σ_f first. For a given size protein, total membrane σ_f is the sum of the various pores' σ_f's to that protein, weighted by the fractional flow rate through the pore. The flow through the pore is dependent on the protein osmotic gradient difference and this gradient will not change to the same degree among pores of different σ_f's and thus of different protein osmotic gradients. As the fractional flow rate will change under diverse experimental conditions, so will the total membrane σ_f. Thus, the solvent drag reflection coefficient is not constant in a heteroporous membrane.

The total membrane σ_d for a given protein is determined by the sum of the various pore filtration coefficients which are not affected by changes in filtration flow rate. In contrast to σ_f, σ_d is constant in a heteroporous membrane and σ_f may not be equal to σ_d. However, at high filtration rates, σ_f approaches σ_d.

PROTEIN PERMEABILITY MEASUREMENT

We will review and critique the more commonly employed methods for determining the reflection coefficient. Table 2 shows the reflection coefficients determined using various techniques.

Gravimetric Technique

Similar to determining K_f, gravimetric techniques for reflection coefficient invoke a given change in π_p in an isogravimetric lung with occluded lymphatics and then measuring the resultant change in lung weight. When π_p is abruptly decreased in an isogravimetric lung, there is an initial increase in filtration rate that slows over time as compensatory changes in P_{int} and π_{int} occur. According to the Starling equation (eq. D in Fig. 3),

$$J_{vi} = \sigma_d \times K_f \times \Delta\pi_p \qquad (31)$$

where J_{vi} is the filtration rate following the change in π_p.

By using the rate of weight gain as an estimate for J_{vi} and dividing by the change in π_p and K_f, σ_d can be calculated (45,47). A major drawback of this method is the requirement of an estimation of K_f, which has its own previously noted problems.

Wash-Down Technique

Equation 30 can be written out as

$$\frac{C_L}{C_p} = \frac{1 - \sigma_d}{1 - \sigma_d \times e^{-x}} \qquad (30)$$

where C_L is the lymph protein concentration and $x = (1 - \sigma_d) \times J_v/PS$. As J_v increases the denominator on the right side of the equation approaches 1. This is because the higher the filtration rate, the less diffusion contributes to solute transport. This concept has been used experimentally to determine σ by increasing capillary pressure at successive levels until C_L/C_p decreases ("washes down") to a minimum which is independent of further increases in filtration rate (24,52). This is the most accepted method for determining σ for the following reasons. First, the high filtration rate ensures that fluid flows are distributed proportionately across various sized pores. Increased filtration rates also minimize the confounding influence of diffusion on the σ determination. The method is not dependent on surface area and any increase in C_L/C_p is due to increased permeability. The technique also does not require that lymph flow be equal or even proportional to filtration rate. This removes a significant problem from data analysis as discussed at the end of this chapter. Finally, by plotting the plasma-to-lymph solute clearance of various sized solutes against the solute radius, a technique called pore stripping can be used that allows estimates of small and large pore sizes as well as the relative distribution (41). Investigators have typically created wash-down conditions over 2–3 h in the lung and reported σ_d's of 0.06–0.75 for plasma proteins (Table 2). However, Parker et al. (42) reported that maintaining wash-down conditions for 24 h resulted in a higher σ_d of 0.89, and because of animal distress limiting the experiment, they were still not sure that C_L/C_p had reached a minimum. It may be that during 2–3 h of increased filtration interstitial protein is being washed out from a slowly equilibrating pool. If this is true, then C_L will be increased and σ_d overestimated.

Labeled Protein Technique

This method involves the intravascular injection of radiolabeled protein and monitoring radioactivity over the lung with an external probe. The rate at which radioactivity increases over time is used to estimate protein flux rate. The faster radioactivity increases, the more permeable the membrane and the lower the σ. The main advantage of this method is that it is noninvasive and can be used in humans. There are several problems with this technique. First, increases in vascular volume will contribute to an increase in the radioactivity causing an overestimation of permeability. To lessen this effect, a vascular tracer such as labeled red cells are used to account for changes in blood volume. Even in the absence of altered per-

Table 2. EXAMPLES OF PULMONARY REFLECTION COEFFICIENT ESTIMATES CATEGORIZED ACCORDING TO THE TECHNIQUE USED

Technique	Albumin	Total proteins
Gravimetric		
Rippe et al. (47) (isolated dog lungs)	$\sigma_d = 0.48$	$\sigma_d = 0.67$
Wangensteen et al. (53) (isolated rabbit lungs)	$\sigma_d = 0.40$	
Perl et al. (45) (isolated dog lungs)	$\sigma_d = 0.40$	
Washdown		
J. C. Parker et al. (39) (anesthetized dogs)	$\sigma_d = 0.50$	$\sigma_d = 0.62$
R. E. Parker et al. (43) (unanesthetized sheep)	$\sigma_d = 0.64$	$\sigma_d = 0.74$
R. E. Parker et al. (42) (24-h pressure elevation in unanesthetized sheep)	$\sigma_d = 0.840$	$\sigma_d = 0.89$

meability, increased vascular pressures will also increase surface area and filtration both of which will increase the rate of protein entering the interstitium and will also tend to result in overestimation of permeability.

PROTEIN OSMOTIC PRESSURE

The easiest way to conceptualize osmotic pressure is with gases. Suppose you have a mixture of two gases, **a** and **b**, in a box. Outside the box, the gas is 100% **a**. Assume that the molecules of gas "**a**" are small and the "**b**" molecules are large. Initially the total gas concentration inside the box equals the gas concentration outside.

Now open a cylindrical pore in one wall of the box. The pore diameter is much larger than the "**a**" molecules, but smaller than the "**b**" molecules. Because of their random motion, the "**a**" molecules will diffuse into the pore from both sides. On the other hand, the "**b**" molecules will not enter the pore at all because they are too big. Thus, even though the total concentrations of molecules inside the box equals the concentration outside, the concentrations immediately inside the two ends of the pore will be different. There will be more molecules of "**a**" within the outside end of the pore as within the inside end. Because of this concentration difference, molecules of "**a**" will diffuse through the pore to the inside of the box (osmosis). The diffusion will continue until the concentrations of "**a**" on each side are equal. Of course, the addition of "**a**" molecules to the gas in the box will cause the pressure within the box to increase. When the inside and outside "**a**" concentrations are equal, then the pressure of the "**a**" molecules inside and outside will be equal. If the gas pressure outside the box is 760 mm Hg, then the pressure of gas "**a**" will be 760 mm Hg inside the box. Thus, the pressure of gas "**b**" is "extra."The pressure of "**b**9 is the osmotic pressure, because it is the additional pressure which must be applied to the gas within the box in order to prevent osmosis of "**a**" molecules inward.

According to the universal gas law:

$$PV = nRT \tag{33}$$

where P is pressure, V is volume, n is number of moles of gas, R is universal gas constant (62.4 mm Hg L/mole°K), and T is absolute temperature. This equation can be rearranged to give the partial pressure of gas "**b**" as

$$RT(n/V) = RTC_b \tag{34}$$

where C_b is the concentration of gas "**b**." Because of the equivalence between osmotic pressure and the partial pressure of the impermeable gas (gas **b**), we can calculate the osmotic pressure (π) as:

$$\pi = RTC_b \tag{35}$$

This equation is the same as van't Hoff's eq. 31 for calculating the osmotic pressure of a solute in a solvent. For albumin solutions of concentration "C" in physiologic saline at 37°C, eq. 35 yields

$$\pi = 2.8\ C \tag{36}$$

with C expressed in g/dl and π in mm Hg.

Osmosis can be looked at from the standpoint of probability. For instance, in eq. 35 the osmotic flow of "**a**" depends on the probability that "**a**" molecules will enter the pore from the outside versus the probability that they will enter the pore from the inside. In the above example, the "**a**" concentration outside the box was initially higher than the concentration inside so there was a higher probability of molecules entering the outside end of the pore. This leads to a higher "**a**" concentration within the outside end, simply because the "**a**" concentration on the outside of the box was higher than inside. However, in the above example, we neglected the possibility that the "**a**" and "**b**" molecules might get in each other's way. Suppose, for instance, that inside the box an "**a**" molecule is on a trajectory which will take it into the pore. However, a huge "**b**" molecule hits the pore at the same time. The "**b**" molecule will block out the "**a**" molecule Because of this effect, the probability that an "**a**" molecule may strike the pore from the inside is reduced. As a result the osmotic pressure is greater than would be predicted with eq. 36.

Another factor which has to do with probability is the Donnan effect. At pH = 7.4, most plasma proteins have a negative charge so that they tend to attract positively charged ions (mostly Na^+). Suppose we have two solutions separated by a membrane. The side 1 solution contains NaCl and protein and side 2 contains only NaCl. Assume that the protein Z has negative charges. In order to have electrical neutrality for side 1:

$$[Na^+]_1 = Z[\text{Prot}] + [Cl^-]_1 \tag{37}$$

and for side 2:

$$[Na^+]_2 = [Cl^-]_2 \tag{38}$$

Now lets assume that the probability that an Na^+ or a Cl^- will enter the pore is equal to the ion concentration times the probability per unit concentration (p). We will assume that p is equal for Na and Cl and that it is equal on both sides of the membrane. Thus, the probability that an Na^+ ion will enter the pore from side 2 is $[Na^+]_{2p}$. If an Na^+ ion diffuses into the pore alone, then there will no longer be electrical neutrality and the Na^+ will be pulled back out of the pore. Thus, the only way an Na^+ ion can successfully diffuse into the pore is if a Cl^- diffuses in at the same time. The probability of the two ions entering the pore simultaneously is the product of each probability: $[Na^+]_{2p} \times [Cl^-]_{2p}$ for side 2 and $[Na^+]_{1p} \times [Cl^-]_{1p}$ for side 1.

At equilibrium, the net diffusion of Na^+ and Cl^- must be zero. Thus, the Na^+ and Cl^- pairs must enter each end of the pore with equal probability:

$$[Na^+]_{1p} \times [Cl^-]_{1p} = [Na^+]_{2p} \times [Cl^-]_{2p}$$

or

$$[Na^+]_1[Cl^-]_1 = [Na^+]_2[Cl^-]_2 \tag{39}$$

We know from eqs. 37 and 38 that $[Na^+]_2 = [Cl^-]_2$ and that $[Na^+]_1 = [Cl^-]_1$. Thus, $[Na^+]_1 + [Cl^-]_1 > [Na^+]_2 + [Cl^-]_2$. The sum of two unequal numbers will always be greater than the sum of two equal numbers which have the same product as the first two numbers. Another way to look at it is that there are two equal areas, one is a square and one is a rectangle with unequal sides. The perimeter of the rectangle will always be more than the perimeter of the square. The fact that $[Na^+]_1 + [Cl^-]_1 > [Na^+]_2 + [Cl^-]_2$ means that there is a gradient in ion concentration across the membrane. This concentration gradient would cause an osmotic pressure of

$$\pi = RT\,[Na^+_1 + Cl^-_1 - Na^+_2 - Cl^-_2] \tag{40}$$

From eqs. 37–40, and assuming the charge on an albumin molecule is -17, Landis and Pappenheimer (31) arrived at the following equation for the Donnan effect osmotic pressure:

$$\pi = 0.19C^2 \tag{41}$$

where C is albumin concentration in g/dl and the NaCl concentration is 0.15 M (physiologic).

The sum of osmotic pressure of the protein (eq. 36) and the small ions (eq. 41):

$$\pi = 2.8C + 0.19C^2 \tag{42}$$

closely resembles the equation for total osmotic pressure for albumin solutions determined from measurements of π and C:

$$\pi = 2.8C + 0.18C^2 + 0.012C^3 \tag{43}$$

The difference in eqs. 42 and 43 probably results from physical interactions between the large albumin molecules and water molecules. (As discussed above, the large albumin molecules may block the diffusion of water molecules and thus lower the probability that a water molecule may enter the pore.)

Plasma globulins have a higher molecular weight than albumin; so, for the same concentration in g/dl, they have less osmotic pressure. Landis and Pappenheimer (31) found:

$$\pi = 2.1C + 0.16C^2 + 0.009C^3 \tag{44}$$

for plasma globulins.

If you know the albumin and globulin concentrations, then you could substitute into eqs. 43 and 44 to obtain each π, then add the π's to obtain the total protein osmotic pressure. However, the Landis-Pappenheimer equations have been questioned (especially eq. 44) and there are other similar equations available. Some equations give the total π in terms of total protein concentration. However, these equations are probably less accurate than the equations which take into account the individual concentrations of albumin and globulin (36,38).

TISSUE FLUID HYDROSTATIC PRESSURE AND TISSUE COMPLIANCE

P_t is the most controversial and misunderstood of the pressures in the Starling equation. This is probably because of the complicated nature of the interstitial (tissue space) and that it is almost impossible to measure anything about the interstitium without altering it. The best approach to understanding tissue fluid pressure is to start with a simple system and then add on the complicating factors.

First consider a simple model of capillary and interstitium, where P_c is 10 mm Hg and π_c = 20 mm Hg. If the microvascular membrane is perfectly semipermeable, no protein passes so π_t = 0 and σ_d = 1. We can calculate the normal pressure within the tissue space as: $P_t = P_c - \pi_c + \pi_t$ = -10 mm Hg. On the other hand, if protein does leak through the membrane then eventually, the protein concentration in the box will equal the plasma protein concentration. Thus, at equilibrium, $\pi_t = \pi_c$ and P_t will rise to equal P_c at +10 mm Hg. This increase in P_t would be accompanied by the accumulation of a considerable amount of fluid representing edema. In order to eliminate the edema, it would be necessary to pump some of the excess fluid out of the box. Accordingly, the next step is to add a lymphatic pump to our model. Before the pump is turned on, there is no flow into or out of the interstitium because there is no pressure difference across the membrane. When the pump is turned on, P_t begins to decrease as fluid is withdrawn from the interstitium. Because P_t decreases, fluid begins to filter into the interstitium through the membrane. If we ignore protein osmotic pressure, then it should be clear that P_t will continue to decrease until $K_f(P_c - P_t)$ equals the lymphatic flow rate. However, the fluid filtered through the membrane will have a lower protein concentration than the plasma. Thus, π_t will decrease and, at equilibrium, the filtration rate J_v will equal the lymphatic flow rate, or

$$P_t = P_c - \sigma_d(\pi_c - \pi_t) - \frac{\text{Lymphatic flow rate}}{K_f} \tag{45}$$

As discussed previously, π_t depends on the tissue fluid protein concentration and thus, in turn, depends on the permeability characteristics of the membrane, the filtration rate, and the plasma protein concentration. Thus, by inspection of eq. 45 the value of P_t must depend on (a) the permeability of the membrane, (b) the plasma protein osmotic pressure, (c) the capillary hydrostatic pressure, and (d) the strength of the lymphatic pump.

The main objective in fluid exchange is not to regulate P_t, rather it is to maintain the tissue spaces in a normally hydrated condition. The amount of fluid in the interstitium will depend on (a) P_t and (b) interstitial compliance of the box. The interstitium contains a matrix of tangled collagen, proteoglycan and glycosaminoglycan molecules. The physical properties of this matrix are only partially understood, but it acts like a gel. The interstitial gel tends to imbibe fluid. Thus, if a "piece" of the interstitial gel is placed into a closed container of water, the gel will soak up some of the water. The water pressure outside the gel will decrease to a negative value until this pressure reaches the imbibition pressure of the gel. At that point the gel volume will stop increasing.

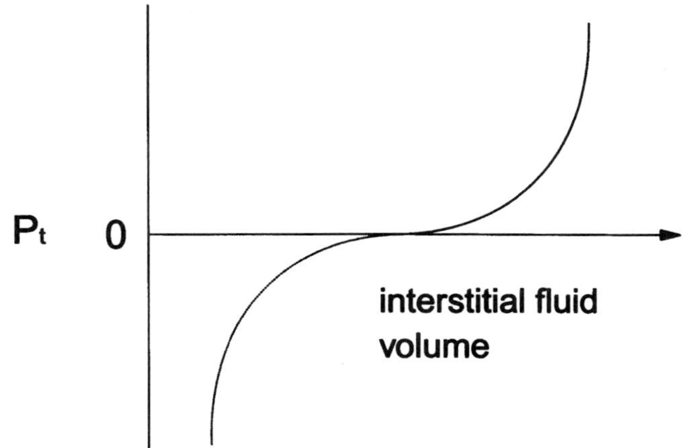

Figure 12. Interstitial compliance. This curve is characteristic of skin. P_t is interstitial hydrostatic fluid pressure. The negative pressure that results when interstitial volume is removed is referred to as the imbibition pressure and is generated by various factors including structural elements and osmotic forces. As interstitial fluid volume increases in edema, the positive curve is produced by distention of the structural elements. In contrast, pressure does not rise more than a few mm Hg in the lung as fluid leaks into the alveoli.

In many ways, water imbibition by a gel is like osmosis. In fact, many investigators believe that the imbibition pressure is a true osmotic pressure. The imbibition pressure increases (becomes less negative) as the gel becomes more hydrated, just as π decreases as a solution becomes more dilute.

In the interstitium, the gel imbibition pressure must balance P_t. If P_t is higher than the imbibition pressures, then the gel will swell until the imbibition pressure equal P_t. If P_t decreases, then fluid will be sucked from the gel until the imbibition pressure again equals P_t. Thus, much of the compliance of the interstitium is determined by the gel. Figure 12 gives a representative tissue compliance curve for skin. The increase in P_t at high interstitial volumes results from the tension exerted by the stretching of skin over the edematous tissue (25). In tissues not bounded by skin fascia or bone, this large rise in P_t probably does not occur. The lung is one example of such a tissue because, as P_t begins to rise, fluid flows into the alveoli. Thus, there is a pop-off valve effect in the lung, and P_t does not rise to high levels (>5 mm Hg).

LYMPHATIC FLOW

Lymphatic vessels serve the important role of removing excess fluid from the tissue spaces and transporting the fluid to veins within the neck. Normally, the lymphatic flow rate is low. However, if the microvascular filtration rate is increased, the lymphatic flow rate also increases. Thus, the lymphatics serve as a safety factor against edema. An organ can become edematous only if the rate at which fluid enters the tissue spaces (usually by microvascular filtration) exceeds the rate at which the fluid is removed by the lymphatics.

Lymphatic vessels contain one-way valves which allow flow only in the forward direction (from the tissue spaces to the neck veins). Furthermore, there is smooth muscle in the walls of many lymphatic vessels. This muscle actively contracts and pumps lymph fluid forward (27,33). However, in anesthetized, acutely operated animals, the lymphatic smooth muscle is often inhibited and the lymph still flows. Thus, lymph flow must be caused by a combination of active pumping and passive factors. It is easier to understand how lymphatics work if the active and passive mechanisms are considered separately.

Passive Factors That Influence Lymph Flow

Theoretically, there are several factors which probably influence lymph flow. First, the inflow end of the lymphatic vessels is in the tissue spaces. Thus, the tissue fluid pressure (P_t) should tend to push fluid into and through the lymphatics. Second, once within the lymphatic vessels, the lymph may be passively pumped forward. Passive pumping is due to compression of the lymphatic vessels by the surrounding tissue. Because of the one-way lymphatic valves, compression of a lymphatic will force fluid forward toward the neck veins. If the compression is released, the lymphatics will fill with fluid from the tissue. In a living animal, the lymphatics may be intermittently compressed by contraction of nearby muscles, by vascular pulsations, respiratory movements, etc. The third passive factor which influences lymph flow is the pressure within the neck veins (P_{NV}). P_{NV} opposes lymph flow. Finally, the resistance to flow through the lymph nodes and through the lymphatic vessels themselves must influence lymph flow. The influence of the passive factors on lymph flow may be expressed as:

$$J_L = \frac{P_t + P_{pp} - P_{NV}}{\text{Resistance}} \quad (46)$$

where P_{pp} is the pressure generated by passive lymphatic pumping (eq. 46 is accurate only if there is no active pumping).

Equation 46 implies that J_L is linearly related to the passive factors. This can be tested in anesthetized animals in which there is no active lymphatic pumping. A lymphatic vessel is cannulated so that the lymph drains through the cannula instead of into the neck veins. Then the pressure at the outflow end of the lymphatic is no longer P_{NV}. Instead, the outflow pressure (P_o) is determined by the height of the cannula and by the product of lymph flow and cannula resistance. Then eq. 46 becomes:

$$J_L = \frac{P_t + P_{pp} - P_o}{\text{Resistance}} \quad (47)$$

Although the true resistance of lymphatic vessels is difficult to measure, an effective resistance may be estimated from the relationship between lymph flow rate and lymphatic outflow pressure. The slopes of lymph flow versus outflow pressure relationships are affected by lymphatic resistance in a similar manner to the effect of vascular resistance on the slopes of venous return curves. Studies have shown that the effective lymphatic resistance decreases substantially as edema forms in most tissues. In fact, the decrease in resistance to lymph flow is the single most important factor causing the increase in lymph flow (10). Thus, increases in lymph flow are "driven" by decreased resistance rather than increased lymphatic pressure.

Active Lymphatic Vessel Pumping

There is plenty of evidence for the rhythmic contraction of lymphatic vessels in animals and humans. However, the clearest evidence that active lymphatic contractions can actually cause fluid to flow has come from studies with isolated segments of postnodal lymphatic vessel (27,33). Investigators have connected each end of the lymphatic segment to fluid-filled reservoirs, and they have shown that the lymphatic will pump fluid from the inflow reservoir to the outflow reservoir. Such studies also show that the stroke volume and frequency of lymphatic pumping vary with the transmural pressure across the vessel walls (Fig. 13). Data such as in Fig. 13 indicate that there is a stretch-induced compensation in the lymphatics similar to the heart. When the transmural pressure across the heart walls is increased, the heart pumps faster and with more force. This is similar to the Frank-Starling mechanism of the heart, and the lymphatic pump output versus pressure relationships for lymphatic vessels are similar to the "cardiac function" curves often used to analyze the blood circulation. Increased pumping allows the heart to increase its output (cardiac output) in response to an increase in venous return. Similarly, as tissue edema forms, fluid should flow into the lymphatics faster than normal. This should distend the lymphatics and stretch their walls. The increased stretch should stimulate the lymphatic vessel to pump harder and faster (Fig. 13) and thus remove the excess fluid from the tissue at a faster rate.

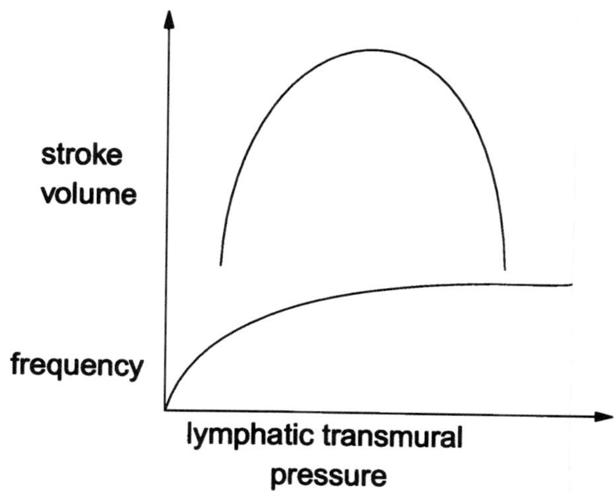

Figure 13. Lymphatic pump function. The two curves describe the impact of increasing filling (transmural) pressure on lymphatic stroke volume and frequency of contractions. Note that, although contraction increases to a plateau, stroke volume begins to decrease. As edema increases, lymphatic pumping contributes to increase lymph flow up to maximum and then further increases in lymph flow are the result of tissue driving pressure and decreased lymphatic resistance.

Combined Effect of Active and Passive Factors on Lymph Flow

The combined effects of active and passive factors are complicated and in many ways analysis of the lymphatic system is similar to analysis of the blood circulation. Recently investigators in our laboratory have methods developed for blood circulation analysis used to estimate lymphatic flow from passive lymphatic flow versus pressure as well as active lymphatic pumping versus pressure relationships (22). The results of that analysis indicate that active lymphatic pumping is particularly important in maintaining a normal rate of lymph flow. However, the lymph flow from edematous tissues seems to be determined mainly by the passive factors which influence lymph flow. These analysis results are substantiated by direct measurements of lymph flow in awake animals (13,14).

One of the most important conclusions from lymphatic analyses is that lymph flow from some tissues is driven by relatively low pressures. Because lymphatic vessels drain to veins in the neck, relatively low neck vein (or central venous) pressure may significantly slow lymphatic flow. For instance, in sheep neck vein pressures of only 10–25 cm H_2O significantly slowed lung lymph flow and causes excess edema formation in the lungs of sheep (1,29).

EDEMA

Edema can develop only if the rate at which fluid filters into the tissues exceeds the rate at which fluid is removed. Most often the edema is caused by a high filtration rate rather than a low rate of removal. There are several ways in which filtration rate (J_V) can be increased and the two most common are: an increase in microvascular pressure or an increase in microvascular permeability.

Increased Microvascular Pressure

Let us start with fluid exchange parameters for a normal, nonedematous lung: $\sigma = 0.8$; $P_c = 7$ mm Hg; $P_t = -3.6$ mm Hg; $K_f = 0.058$ ml/min/mm Hg; $\pi_c = 25.9$ mm Hg; $\pi_t = 14.8$ mm Hg; $J_V = 0.1$ ml/min; $J_L = 0.1$ ml/min.

Now suppose that P_c is elevated to 17 mm Hg. Immediately after the P_c increases, there will not have been time for any of the other Starling pressures to change. Thus, $J_V = K_f[(17 + 3.6 - \sigma(25.9 - 14.8)] = 0.679$ ml/min. Because there is a delay before lymphatic flow can increase, J_L still equals 0.1 ml/min. Thus, fluid accumulates at 0.679 - 0.100 ml/min = 0.579 ml/min. As the tissue fluid volume increases, P_t increases. Furthermore, π_t decreases because the filtrate protein concentration decreases when the filtration rate is increased. The changes in P_t and π_t both act to reduce the pressure imbalance across the microvascular membrane and bring J_V back toward control. However, P_t and π_t cannot return J_V all the way back to control because π_t is filtration rate dependent. (If J_V returned to its control level, then π_t would return to control.) Fortunately, J_L will usually increase enough so that it equals J_V and fluid no longer accumulates within the tissue. The increase in J_L is probably brought about by increases in P_t and the pressure generated by the lymphatic pump and by a decrease in the resistance to lymph flow. Because of all these adjustments, the tissue reaches a new steady-state condition with increased tissue fluid volume, increased P_t, decreased π_t, and increased lymphatic flow. In most cases, the increase in tissue fluid volume is small and the tissue is not overtly edematous. Because they helped to bring the system into a new steady state condition without the accumulation of much edema fluid, the changes in P_t, π_t, and J_L are called "safety factors against edema."

There is a maximum limit to the safety factors because P_t cannot fall to $<\sim(1 - \sigma)\pi_c$, and J_L cannot increase more than five– to ten–fold before edema occurs. Thus, at $P_c = 17$, some of each safety factor is used up. If we can continue to increase P_c, eventually we will reach a critical level at which the safety factors have been totally exhausted. If we increase P_c even slightly above the critical level, edema will form at a constant rate (Fig. 14).

Increased Microvascular Permeability

Assume that we start with the same initial conditions as in the previous example ($P_c = 7$ mm Hg, etc.). Now suppose that σ is suddenly decreased to 0.5. (For simplicity, assume that K_f remains constant even though it would usually increase as σ decreased.) J_V will abruptly increase to $K_f[(7 + 3.6 - 0.5\ (25.9 - 14.8\ ] = 0.293$ ml/min, and fluid will accumulate at 0.193 ml/min. As time progresses, the tissue fluid protein concentration will increase because σ has decreased. Consequently, the osmotic pressure gradient $[\sigma(\pi_c - \pi_t)$ will be reduced even further than it was initially. However, as fluid accumulates, P_t and J_L will both increase and they may be able to bring about a new steady state without much edema formation. However, the π_t safety factor has been injured and, in order to take up the slack, part of the P_t and J_L safety factors have been used up. Now if we increase P_c, we will find that its critical level will be lower than it was in the tissue with normal microvascular permeability.

Now let's go back to the baseline (normal) conditions. This time let us increase permeability such that only K_f is increased. Water will flow through the membrane more rapidly so that π_t will decrease. As fluid builds up in the tissue, P_t and J_L will both increase. The changes in π_t, P_t, and J_L will probably be able to return the tissue to steady state condition. However, as in the above examples, some of each safety factor will be gone. Thus, the critical level of P_c will be reduced.

Increases in permeability (increased K_f, decreased σ, or both) either injure or use up part of each safety factor against edema. Consequently, the critical level of P_c required to produce edema is reduced. If the increase in permeability is severe, then the critical level of P_c may be reduced to less than the normal P_c. In this case, edema will occur without any increase in P_c above normal. However, many toxic substances which increase increased permeability also increase P_c. Thus, edema is usually the result of both increased P_c and increased permeability.

Microvascular Hydrostatic Pressure

Microvascular hydrostatic pressure (P_c) is the most important factor determining filtration rate. When permeability is increased, P_c becomes even more important as shown in Fig. 14. However, determination of P_c is often difficult in the intact animal. The reason is that P_c lies somewhere between pulmonary artery and pulmonary venous or left atrial pressures which are normally ~18 and 5 mm Hg, respectively. The relation of P_c to these pressures is determined by the pulmonary vascular resistance distribution. Although there are many resistance sites along the pulmonary vasculature, they are typically grouped into either arterial or venous resistances and P_c can be defined as:

$$P_c = \frac{PAP * R_v + LAP * R_a}{R_a + R_v} \quad (48)$$

where PAP is pulmonary artery pressure, LAP is left atrial pressure, and R_a and R_v are arterial and venous resistance, respectively.

A key point is that resistance factors can alter P_c independently of changes in pulmonary arterial or venous pressures. Thus, a low left atrial pressure does not assure that P_c is not elevated. Allen et al. (5) induced pulmonary hypertension in

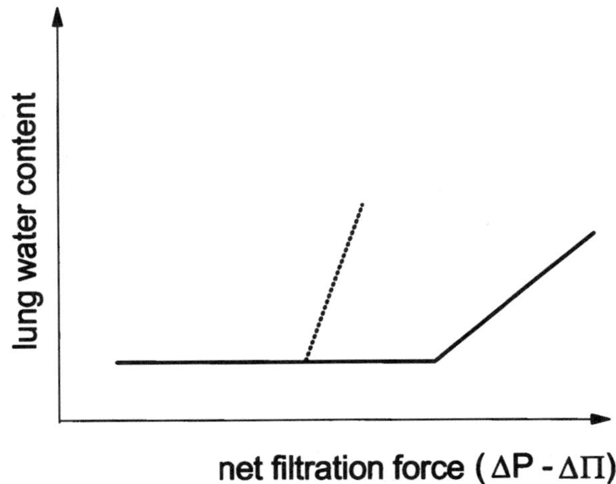

Figure 14. Increased microvascular permeability. The *solid line* represents the effect of increasing filtration pressures on pulmonary edema accumulation in a lung with normal permeability. The *dotted line* shows what happens when permeability is increased. Note that edema begins to occur at a lower filtration pressure and that fluid accumulates at a faster rate. Thus, microvascular pressures have a greater impact on filtration if permeability is increased (3).

sheep by administering endotoxin and found a significant increase in lung water after 3 h. They then gave another group of sheep endotoxin and administered sodium nitroprusside to reduce the pulmonary hypertension. In these animals, no increase in lung water was found despite an unchanged left atrial pressure (5). Some of the pulmonary hypertension was transmitted to the level of the microvascular exchange vessels but was not reflected by an increase in left atrial pressure. Because left atrial pressure does not necessarily predict P_c, attempts have been made to develop bedside techniques for estimating P_c in critically ill patients. This can be accomplished by analyzing the pressure tracing recorded from a pulmonary artery catheter as the balloon is inflated (23,55). Problems with this method include difficulty with wave analysis and the absence of a confirmatory technique.

FUTURE DIRECTIONS

From the foregoing discussion, minimizing pulmonary edema in patients will have to involve either decreasing fluid filtration or increasing lymph flow. Fluid filtration can be decreased by either decreasing P_c or preventing permeability increases. Lung injury is frequently associated with pulmonary hypertension, and as shown previously, this can contribute to increased P_c (5). Reducing pulmonary hypertension has been attempted with intravenous drugs but systemic hypotension is frequent. Intravenous pulmonary antihypertensives have the drawback of worsening ventilation/perfusion ratios. Inhaled pulmonary antihypertensives such as nitric oxide should improve gas exchange and may result in less pulmonary edema (48). Another approach to decreasing P_c is to use lung water measurements to guide fluid administration. Clinicians often infuse fluids into critically ill patients until the pulmonary artery occlusion pressure (PAOP) reaches a certain value, usually 18–20 mm Hg. PAOP is used here as an estimate for P_c, which may not be a correct assumption in pulmonary hypertension. This problem can be avoided by directly calculating extravascular lung water (EVLW) using a double dilution technique. Using EVLW to guide fluid therapy results in less pulmonary edema and there is initial evidence to suggest improved outcome in critically ill patients with ARDS (19,35). Advances in molecular biology offer the opportunity to modify the biochemical mediators that have been implicated in microvascular exchange barrier injury resulting in increased permeability. Conary et al. (8) reduced pulmonary hypertension and pulmonary edema in rabbit lungs subjected to endotoxin by transfecting them with the prostaglandin G/H gene. This gene therapy resulted in increased production of prostacyclin and PGE2 while suppressing thromboxane production.

Efforts to enhance edema fluid removal by increasing lymph flow must recognize the impact of increased venous pressure on lymphatic function. It is often impractical for hemodynamic reasons to decrease central venous pressure in patients. One alternative is to divert lymph flow. By cannulating the thoracic duct and allowing it to drain against atmospheric pressure, investigators have demonstrated improved pulmonary function in animals and patients with decreased pulmonary edema shown in the former (2,17).

REFERENCES

1. Allen SJ, Drake RE, Katz J, Gabel JC, Laine GA. Elevation of superior vena caval pressure increases extravascular lung water after endotoxemia. *J Appl Physiol* 1987;62:1006–1009.
2. Allen SJ, Drake RE, Laine GA, Gabel JC. Effect of thoracic duct drainage on hydrostatic pulmonary edema and pleural effusion in the sheep. *J Appl Physiol* 1991;71:314–316.
3. Allen SJ, Drake RE, Williams WP, Laine GA, Gabel JC. Recent advances in pulmonary edema. *Crit Care Med* 1987;15:963–970.
4. Allen S, Gabel J, Drake R. Left atrial hypertension causes pleural effusion formation in unanesthetized sheep. *Am J Physiol* 1989;257:H690–H692.
5. Allen SJ, Laine GA, Drake RE, Katz J, Gabel JC. Lowered pulmonary arterial pressure prevents edema after endotoxin in sheep. *J Appl Physiol* 1987;63:1008–1011.
6. Allen SJ, Sedin EG, Jonzon A, Wells AF, Laurent TC. Lung hyaluronan during development: a quantitative and morphological study. *Am J Physiol* 1991;260:H1449–1454.
7. Bhattacharya J, Cruz T, Bhattacharya S, Bray BA. Hyaluronan affects extravascular water in lungs of unanesthetized rabbits. *J Appl Physiol* 1989;66:2595–2599.
8. Conary JT, Parker RE, Christman BW, et al. Protection of rabbit lungs from endotoxin injury by in vivo hyperexpression of the prostaglandin G/H synthase gene. *J Clin Invest* 1994;93:1834–1840.
9. Curry FE. Mechanics and thermodynamics of transcapillary exchange. In: *Handbook of physiology. The cardiovascular system. Microcirculation.* Bethesda: American Physiological Society, 1984:309–374.
10. Drake RE, Adcock DK, Scott RL, Gabel JC. Effect of outflow pressure upon lymph flow from dog lungs. *Circ Res* 1982;50:865–869.
11. Drake RE, Davis E. A corrected equation for the calculation of reflection coefficients. *Microvasc Res* 1978;15:259.
12. Drake R, Gaar KA, Taylor AE. Estimation of the filtration coefficient of pulmonary exchange vessels. *Am J Physiol* 1978;234:H266–H274.
13. Drake RE, Gabel JC. Effect of outflow pressure on intestinal lymph flow in unanesthetized sheep. *Am J Physiol* 1991;260:R668–R671.
14. Drake R, Giesler M, Laine G, Gabel J, Hansen T. Effect of outflow pressure on lung lymph flow in unanesthetized sheep. *J Appl Physiol* 1985;58:70–76.
15. Drake RE, Laine GA. Pulmonary microvascular permeability to fluid and macromolecules. *J Appl Physiol* 1988;64:487–501.
16. Drake RE, Smith JH, Gabel JC. Estimation of the filtration coefficient in intact dog lungs. *Am J Physiol* 1980;238:H430–H438.
17. Dugernier T, Reynaert MS, Deby-Dupont G, Roeseler JJ, Carlier M. Prospective evaluation of thoracic duct drainage in the treatment of respiratory failure complicating severe acute pancreatitis. *Int Care Med* 1989;15:372–378.
18. Ehrhart IC, Granger WM, Hofman WF. Filtration coefficient obtained by stepwise pressure elevation in isolated dog lung. *J Appl Physiol* 1984;56:862–867.
19. Eisenberg PR, Hansbrough JR, Anderson D, Schaster DP. A prospective study of lung water measurements during patient management in an intensive care unit. *Am Rev Respir Dis* 1987;136:662–668.
20. Erdmann AJ III, Vaughan TR Jr, Brigham KL, Woolverton WC, Staub NC. Effect of increased vascular pressure on lung fluid balance in unanesthetized sheep. *Circ Res* 1975;37:271–284.
21. Gaar KA Jr, Taylor AE, Owens LJ, Guyton AC. Pulmonary capillary pressure and filtration coefficient in the isolated perfused lung. *Am J Physiol* 1967;213:910–914.
22. Gallagher H, Garewal D, Drake RE, Gabel JC. Estimation of lymphatic flow by equating lymphatic pump function and passive flow curves. *Lymphology* 1993;26:56–60.
23. Gilbert E, Hakim TS. Derivation of pulmonary capillary pressure from arterial occlusion in intact conditions. *Crit Care Med* 1994;22:986–993.
24. Granger DN, Taylor AE. Permeability of intestinal capillaries to endogenous macromolecules. *Am J Physiol* 1980;238:H457–H464.
25. Guyton AC, Granger HJ, Taylor AE. Interstitial fluid pressure. *Physiol Rev* 1971;51:527–563.
26. Guyton AC, Lindsey AW. Effect of elevated left atrial pressure and decreased plasma protein concentration on the development of pulmonary edema. *Circ Res* 1959;7:649–657.
27. Johnston MG, Involvement of lymphatic collecting ducts in the physiology and pathophysiology of lymph flow. In: Jonston MG, ed. *Experimental biology of the lymphatic system*, New York: Elsevier Science, 1985:81–120.
28. Kedem O, Katchalsky A. A thermodynamic analysis of the permeability of biological membranes to non-electrolytes. *Biochim Biophys Acta* 1958;27:229–246.
29. Laine GA, Allen SJ, Katz J, Gabel JC, Drake RE. Effect of systemic venous pressure elevation on lymph flow and lung edema formation. *J Appl Physiol* 1986;61:1634–1638.
30. Landis EM. Micro-injection studies of capillary permeability. II. The relation between capillary pressure and the rate at which fluid passes through the walls of single capillaries. *Am J Physiol* 1927;82:217–238.
31. Landis EM, Pappenheimer JR. Exchange of substances through the

capillary walls. In: Hamilton WF, Dow P, eds. *Handbook of physiology. Circulation.* Washington, DC: American Physiological Society, 1963: 961–1034.

32. Levine OR, Mellins RB, Senior RM, Fishman AP. The application of Starling's law of capillary exchange to the lungs. *J Clin Invest* 1967; 46:934–944.
33. McHale NG, Roddie IC. The effect of transmural pressure on pumping activity in isolated bovine lymphatic vessels. *J Physiol Lond* 1976;261:255–269.
34. Michel RP, Inoue S, Hogg JC. Pulmonary capillary permeability to HRP in dogs: a physiological and morphological study. *J Appl Physiol* 1977;42:13–21.
35. Mitchell JP, Schuller D, Calandrino FS, Schuster DP. Improved outcome based on fluid management in critically ill patients requiring pulmonary artery catherization. *Am Rev Respir Dis* 1992;145:990–998.
36. Navar PD, Navar LG. Relationship between colloid osmotic pressure and plasma protein concentration in the dog. *Am J Physiol* 1977;233:H295–H298.
37. Nettlebladt O, Tengblad A, Hällgren R. Lung accumulation of hyaluronan parallels pulmonary edema in experimental alveolitis. *Am J Physiol* 1989;257:L379–L384.
38. Nitta S, Ohnuki T, Ohkuda K, Nadada T, Staub NC. The corrected protein equation to estimate plasma colloid osmotic pressure and its development on a monogram. *Tohoku J Exp Med* 1981;135:43–49.
39. Parker JC, Parker RE, Granger DH, Taylor AE. Vascular permeability and transvascular fluid and protein transport in the dog lung. *Circ Res* 1981;48:549–561.
40. Parker JC, Perry MA, Taylor AE. Permeability of the microvascular membrane. In: Staub NC, Taylor AE, eds. *Edema.* New York: Raven Press, 1984:143–187.
41. Parker JC, Rippe B, Taylor AE. Fluid filtration and protein clearances through large and small pore populations in dog lung capillaries. *Microvasc Res* 1986;31:1–174.
42. Parker RE, Roselli RJ, Brigham KL. Effect of prolonged elevated microvascular pressure on lung fluid balance in sheep. *J Appl Physiol* 1985;58:869–874.
43. Parker RE, Roselli RJ, Harris TR, Brigham KL. Effects of raced increases in pulmonary vascular pressures on lung fluid balance in unanesthetized sheep. *Circ Res* 1981;49:1164–1172.
44. Patlak CS, Goldstein DA, Hoffman JF. The flow of solute and solvent across a two-membrane system. *J Theor Biol* 1963;5:425–442.
45. Perl W, Chowdhury P, Chinard FP. Osmotic reflection coefficient of dog lung endothelium to sodium chloride, glucose, sucrose, raffinose and albumin. *Microvasc Res* 1973;6:125–126.
46. Renkin GM. Cellular and intercellular transport pathways in exchange vessels. *Am Rev Respir Dis* 1992;146:528–531.
47. Rippe B, Townsley M, Parker JC, Taylor AE. Osmotic reflection coefficient for total plasma protein in lung microvessels. *J Appl Physiol* 1985;58:436–442.
48. Rossaint R, Falke KF, López F, Slama K, Pison U, Zapol WM. Inhaled nitric oxide for the adult respiratory distress syndrome. *N Engl J Med* 1993;328;399–405.
49. Staub NC. Pathophysiology of pulmonary edema. In: Staub NC, Taylor AE, eds. *Edema.* New York: Raven Press 1984:719–746.
50. Taylor AE, Gaar KA. Measurement of the hydraulic conductivity of the pulmonary capillary membrane in the isolated lung [Abstract]. *Int Union Physiol Sci* 1968;6:430.
51. Taylor AE, Granger DN. Exchange of macromolecules across the microcirculation. In: *Handbook of physiology. The cardiovascular system. Microcirculation.* Bethesda: American Physiological Society, 1984:467–520.
52. Taylor AE, Rippe B. Pulmonary edema. In: Andreoli TE, Fanestil DD, Hoffman JF, Schultz SG, eds. *Physiology of membrane disorders.* 2nd ed. New York: Plenum Press, 1986:1025–1039.
53. Wangensteen OD, Lysaker E, Savaryn P. Pulmonary capillary filtration and reflection coefficients in the adult rabbit. *Microvasc Res* 1977;14:81–97.
54. Wiener-Kronich JP, Broaddus VC. Interrelationship of pleural and pulmonary interstitial liquid. *Annu Rev Physiol* 1993;55:209–226.
55. Yamada Y, Komatsu K, Suzukawa M, et al. Pulmonary capillary pressure measured with a pulmonary arterial double port catheter in surgical patients. *Anesth Analg* 1993;77:1130–1134.

Anesthesia: Biologic Foundations, edited by
Tony L. Yaksh et al. Lippincott–Raven Publishers,
Philadelphia © 1997.

CHAPTER 81

INHALED NITRIC OXIDE THERAPY

WILLIAM E. HURFORD, DEAN HESS, AND WARREN M. ZAPOL

SELECTIVE PULMONARY VASODILATOR

Pulmonary hypertension and severe hypoxemia complicate the care of patients with diseases such as the adult respiratory distress syndrome, persistent pulmonary hypertension of the newborn, congenital heart disease, and following cardiopulmonary bypass. Numerous vasodilator therapies aimed at reducing pulmonary hypertension have been tested in these patients. Systemic vasodilation and hypotension occur with the use of all the currently available intravenous vasodilators infused at levels sufficient to reduce the pulmonary artery pressure. In addition, intravenous infusions of systemic vasodilators such as nitroprusside or prostacyclin (PGI_2) can markedly increase the venous admixture especially in the presence of respiratory failure (214). In 1991, inhaled NO was reported to selectively vasodilate the pulmonary circulation (62,68). The use of this novel therapy has attracted widespread interest. Research in the field has progressed rapidly along with our understanding of the many roles of endogenously produced nitric oxide.

NITRIC OXIDE: AN ENDOTHELIUM-DERIVED RELAXING FACTOR

NO-cGMP Transduction System

Nitric oxide (NO), a lipophilic, free radical, is a vasodilator which accounts for the biologic activity of endothelium-derived relaxing factor (EDRF) (109,189). Because of its short duration of action, small size, and lipophilic nature, nitric oxide is an ideal local transcellular messenger (108). The half-life of NO in tissues is a few seconds due to rapid oxidation to nitrite and nitrate (108) and its antagonism by substances containing a heme ring, such as hemoglobin, that bind NO with high affinity (78). Interestingly, the common nitroso-vasodilators, such as nitroglycerin and nitroprusside, act by releasing NO (87).

Nitric oxide activates soluble guanylate cyclase (sGC) by combining with the heme moiety of the enzyme (Fig. 1) (86,255). In perivascular smooth muscle cells, increased conversion of guanosine 5′-triphosphate (GTP) to guanosine 3′,5′-cyclic monophosphate (cGMP) is associated with reduced intracellular [Ca^{2+}] and vascular relaxation, in part through its action on cGMP-dependent protein kinase (cGDPK) (255). Cyclic GMP is inactivated by a variety of phosphodiesterase (PDE) enzymes (47,61,178).

Nitric oxide synthase (NOS) enzymes produce nitric oxide and L-citrulline from the amino acid L-arginine (200). These enzymes are divided into two classes, constitutive and inducible (174). The constitutive NO synthases are Ca^{2+} and calmodulin-dependent enzymes that release small amounts of NO (200). Constitutive NOS has been identified in endothelial cells (cNOS, eNOS, or isoform III) and neurons (nNOS, bNOS, or isoform I). Inducible NOS (iNOS or isoform II) is found in macrophages, smooth muscle cells, and many other cell types after stimulation by Gram-negative endotoxin lipopolysaccharide (LPS) and/or cytokines. Inducible NOS is Ca^{2+} and calmodulin-independent and produces large quantities of NO for long periods of time (170). The interaction of these NOS isoforms with exogenous NO is largely unstudied and controversial. While some reports suggest that increased NO concentrations may decrease NOS activity in vitro (9,31,83,125,219), other research suggests that total pulmonary iNOS activity may be unaffected by NO breathing (140). Several L-arginine analogs are competitive inhibitors of NO synthase (218).

Nitric oxide has numerous functions in addition to the relaxation of smooth muscle. The molecule is important in the central and peripheral nervous systems, where it is a neurotransmitter, and in the immune system, where it participates in macrophage cytotoxic activity (240) and tumor cell killing. Nitric oxide also inhibits proliferation of pulmonary and systemic vascular smooth muscle cells (134,227), leukocyte adhesion, and platelet aggregation (237).

Nitric oxide gas is a common environmental pollutant. It is produced in nature by lightning and the burning of fossil fuels (7). Atmospheric concentrations of NO usually range between 10 and 100 parts per billion. Present in cigarette smoke, NO is routinely inhaled for short periods in concentrations of 400–1,000 parts per million by volume (ppm) by millions of people (182). Nitric oxide is commercially manufactured from the reaction of sulfur dioxide with nitric acid (6). Alternatively, ammonia can by oxidized over a platinum catalyst at high temperatures (>500°C) (28). Following synthesis, NO is mixed with highly purified nitrogen and stored at 2,000 psi in aluminum alloy cylinders.

Nitric Oxide and the Lung

The baseline low pulmonary vascular tone of normal lungs in some species appears to be maintained in part by endogenous synthesis of nitric oxide (34,257). In normal lungs, the administration of acetylcholine (which produces vasodilation via endothelial-dependent NO production) or the addition of exogenous nitric oxide has little additional effect on pulmonary vascular resistance (66,69,97,193). In some patients with pulmonary hypertension, on the other hand, intravenous acetylcholine or inhaled nitric oxide administration can reduce pulmonary vascular resistance (66,69,193). It is possible that the production of endogenous NO is impaired in some acute and chronic pulmonary hypertensive states (3,40,49). Evidence supporting this hypothesis is indirect at this time. Giaid and Saleh (77) reported that the expression of endothelial nitric oxide synthase was decreased in patients with chronic pulmonary hypertension. In their study, the pulmonary arterial expression of endothelial NO synthase was inversely correlated with pulmonary vascular resistance in patients with plexogenic pulmonary arteriopathy (77). Studies of pulmonary vascular reactivity in response to acetylcholine infusions are consistent with the finding of decreased expression of endothelial NO synthase. Dinh Xuan et al. (48) reported that patients with cor pulmonale secondary to congenital heart disease had an impaired pulmonary vasodilatory response to intravenous acetylcholine. The same group also studied 18 patients with chronic obstructive pulmonary disease and reported that impairment of acetylcholine-induced relaxation was correlated with lower systemic arterial oxygen tensions and greater intimal thickening of pulmonary blood vessels (40). Such patients may have an intact response to inhaled NO even though their response to intravenous acetylcholine is impaired (4).

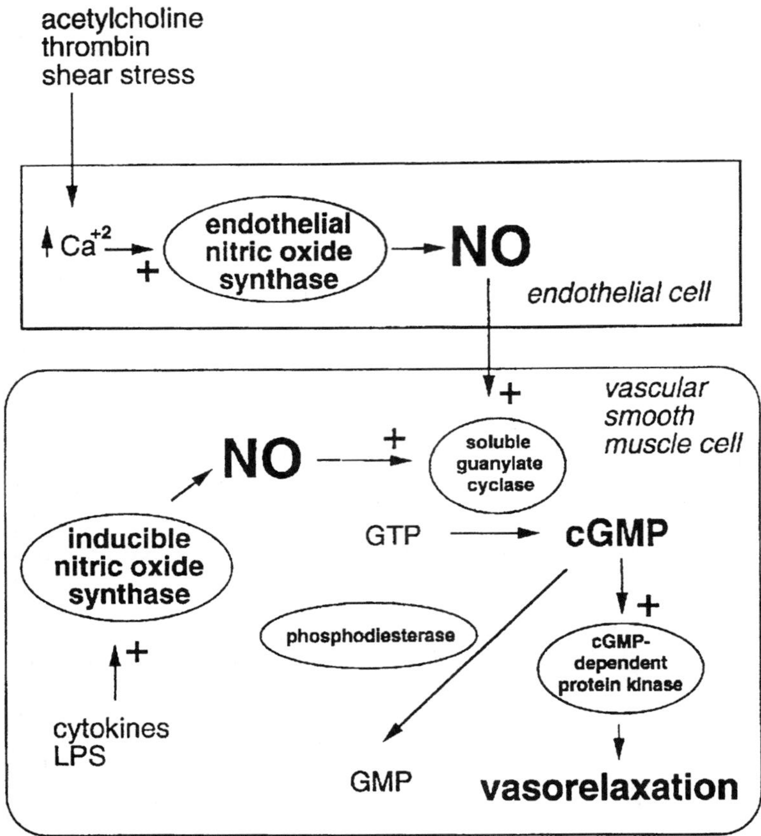

Figure 1. The nitric oxide—cGMP signal transduction system. (Reprinted with permission from ref. 107.)

Exhaled NO

Endogenous nitric oxide is present in the exhaled air of experimental animals and humans (76,89). Measurable levels of nitric oxide (0.07–0.13 ppm) are present in the human nasopharynx (76). In the paranasal sinuses, nitric oxide levels are much higher (~10 ppm). It has been suggested that the bacteriostatic effects of NO may be responsible for maintaining the sterility of the sinuses (150). Nitric oxide present in the nasopharynx is subsequently inhaled, and ~50–70% of the inhaled gas is absorbed. Gerlach et al. (76) demonstrated that when the tracheas of patients were intubated, bypassing the nasopharynx, NO levels were greatly reduced in inhaled and exhaled gas. They suggested that the inhaled endogenous NO might have a role in normal matching of perfusion to ventilation. Exhaled levels of nitric oxide are increased in inflammatory conditions such as asthma and bronchiectasis (8,76,121–123,195). The increased exhaled NO levels appears to originate in the airways (8). Increased NO levels may be due to increased inducible NOS activity of neutrophils and macrophages. Consistent with this theory, inhaled steroid therapy appears to decrease exhaled NO levels in asthmatics and patients with bronchiectasis (122,123).

Levels of exhaled NO have been reported to be decreased in smokers (96,195,239) or patients with systemic hypertension (239). In experimental animals, exhaled NO has been reported to be increased by sepsis (262), the administration of PEEP (194), and infusions of sodium nitroprusside or nitroglycerin (103).

Inhaled NO Is a Selective Pulmonary Vasodilator

Zapol et al. (62,68) hypothesized that inhaled NO should diffuse into the pulmonary vasculature of ventilated lung regions and cause relaxation of pulmonary vascular smooth muscle, thereby decreasing pulmonary hypertension. Because NO is inhaled, the gas should be distributed predominantly to well-ventilated alveoli and not to collapsed or fluid-filled areas of the lung. In the presence of increased vasomotor tone, selective vasodilation of well-ventilated lung regions should cause a "steal" or diversion of pulmonary artery blood flow towards well-ventilated alveoli and should improve the matching of ventilation to perfusion and improve arterial oxygenation. Such an effect would be in marked contrast to the effects of intravenously administered conventional vasodilators (such as nitroprusside, nitroglycerin, or prostacyclin). These intravenous agents also decrease PA pressure, but by nonselectively dilating the pulmonary vasculature, they augment blood flow to nonventilated areas, thereby increasing right-to-left shunting and reducing the PaO_2 (212–214,287). Also unlike available intravenous vasodilators, inhaled NO should not produce systemic vasodilation because it is avidly bound to hemoglobin and rapidly inactivated. This hypothesis has subsequently been proven correct in numerous animal models and clinical studies.

It is unclear whether inhaled NO has other beneficial effects in addition to its properties as a selective pulmonary vasodilator. Laboratory studies suggest that inhaled nitric oxide has important effects in reducing some forms of lung and tissue injury. These effects include the ability to scavenge oxygen free radicals (38,91,117,120,281), reduce oxygen toxicity (70,71,175), inhibit platelet and leukocyte aggregation (99,155,181,202,237), and reduce pulmonary vascular hypertrophy (227). If these effects are clinically significant, early and continued therapy with inhaled NO may be beneficial. Some of these effects may be independent of the pulmonary NO-cGMP transduction system responsible for producing selective pulmonary vasodilation.

EVALUATION OF INHALED NITRIC OXIDE IN LABORATORY MODELS

Acute Pulmonary Hypertension Models

Inhaled NO (80 ppm) had no hemodynamic effect in studies of normal awake lambs without an increased pulmonary vascular resistance (68). The pulmonary artery pressure, cardiac output, systemic arterial pressure and systemic vascular resistance were unchanged. When the pulmonary artery pressure was acutely increased, either by hypoxia, infusing the thromboxane endoperoxide analog U46619, or producing the heparin-protamine reaction, the pulmonary hypertension was reversed by inhalation of 40–80 ppm NO (62,68). Pulmonary vasodilation occurred within three minutes, lasted throughout the duration of NO inhalation, and disappeared within three minutes after the discontinuation of NO (Fig. 2). The systemic vascular resistance remained unchanged. The pulmonary vasodilator effect occurred at low levels of inhaled NO (i.e., 5 ppm). Potent vasodilation (65% of the maximal effect) occurred at 20 ppm inhaled NO. During continuous inhalation of 80 ppm NO for 1 hr, no tolerance was observed.

The anatomic sites of NO-induced vasodilation have been investigated in isolated perfused lungs (143,223,230,266). Inhaled NO dilated pulmonary arteries in these studies. The extent of pulmonary venous vasodilation appeared to depend upon the experimental model. Nitric oxide–induced dilation of pulmonary veins has been observed after extreme venous constriction (223). Perfusion of the lungs with blood prevented the dilation of large capacitance pulmonary veins by inhaled NO (223,266).

Laboratory animal models have been used to examine the effects of inhaled nitric oxide during pulmonary hypertension induced by hypoxia (17,37,63,112,176,199,228,229,231,266, 271,295), endotoxin administration (43,130,187), the infusion of vasoconstrictor substances such as NO synthase inhibitors (130,204,267), lung injury (186,204,206,228,235,245), and the heparin-protamine reaction (62). In general, these studies confirm that inhaled nitric oxide is a selective pulmonary vasodilator.

Redistribution of blood flow within the lung during NO inhalation has been demonstrated. Pison et al. (199) studied the matching of ventilation to perfusion using the multiple inert gas elimination technique in mechanically ventilated normal sheep. They reported that inhaled NO (20 ppm) redistributed blood flow to better ventilated alveoli and reversed the pulmonary hypertension caused by breathing a hypoxic gas mixture.

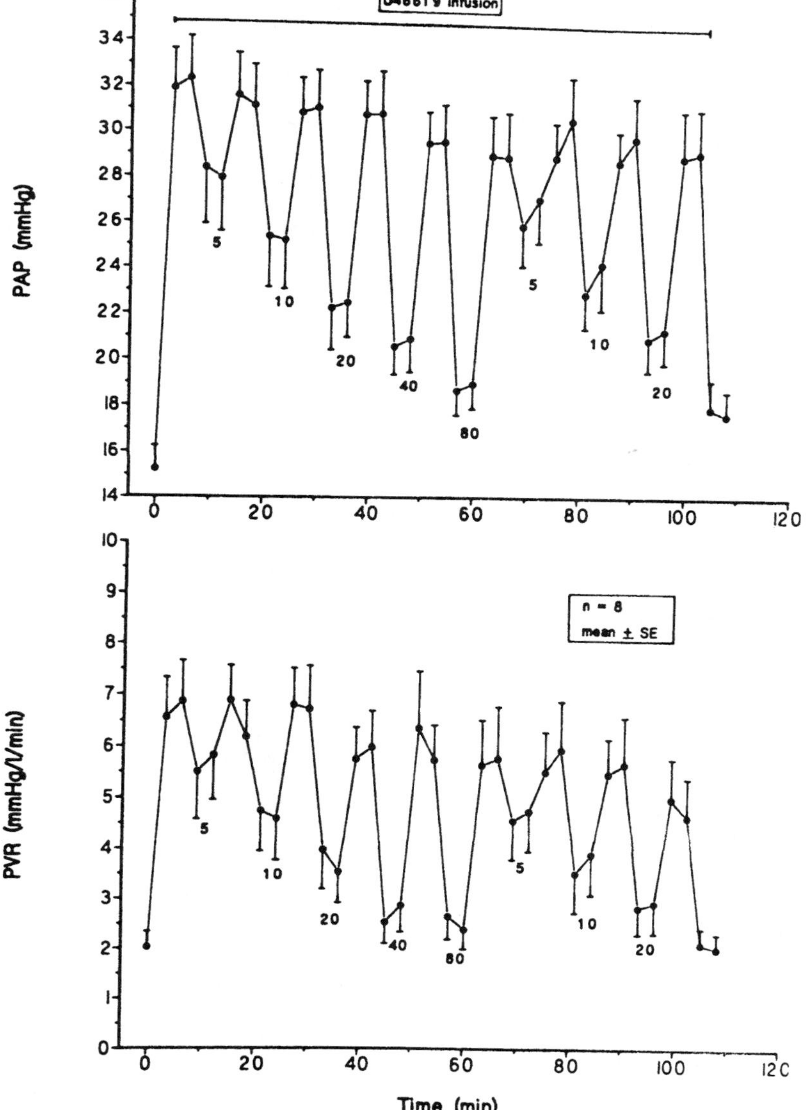

Figure 2. Plots of mean pulmonary artery pressure (PAP) and pulmonary vascular resistance (PVR) during a continuous infusion of the thromboxane analog U46619. Lambs breathed various levels of nitric oxide (5–80 ppm) at FIO_2 0.6 for 6 min, then breathed a gas mixture at FIO_2 0.6 for 6 min without nitric oxide (n = 8, mean ± SE). (Reprinted with permission from ref. 68.)

Endotoxin Administration

The effects of inhaled NO on endotoxin-induced pulmonary hypertension are complex. In a study by Weitzberg et al. (275), inhaled NO at a concentration of 10 ppm selectively decreased the acute pulmonary hypertension occurring at least 30 min after the intravenous administration of *Escherichia coli* endotoxin in anesthetized pigs. Arterial oxygenation and pH were also improved during NO inhalation. The early increase of pulmonary artery pressure (within 30 min after endotoxin administration) was unaffected by 10 ppm of inhaled nitric oxide, but was abolished by pretreatment with diclofenac (a cyclooxygenase inhibitor). No signs of tachyphylaxis were seen during 2.5 hr of NO inhalation, and the pulmonary vascular resistance increased rapidly upon cessation of NO. These results suggest that vasoconstrictor products from the cyclooxygenase pathway are involved in the initial increase in pulmonary artery pressure. This early vasoconstriction was unaffected by inhaling 10 ppm nitric oxide. Pulmonary vasoconstriction which is responsive to dilation by NO mediates the second phase of pulmonary hypertension in this pig model. The combination of intravenous L-nitroarginine (an NO synthase inhibitor) and inhaled NO reduced pulmonary artery pressure and increased the systemic vascular resistance during the second phase, but did not cause further improvement of PaO_2 or metabolic acidosis. This suggests that the additional peripheral effects of NO synthase inhibition by L-nitroarginine were not beneficial in this model.

Ogura et al. (187) reported that NO inhalation (40 ppm) decreased the late phase pulmonary hypertension following an infusion of *E. coli* endotoxin in anesthetized swine. Nitric oxide inhalation improved arterial oxygenation by redistributing blood flow from true shunt to ventilated lung regions as measured by the multiple inert gas elimination technique. The amount of pulmonary edema, as assessed by the blood-free wet-to-dry lung weight ratio, was decreased in animals breathing 40 ppm NO. Dahm et al. (43) similarly reported selective pulmonary vasodilation following nitric oxide inhalation in an anesthetized swine endotoxemia model.

Oleic Acid–Induced Lung Injury

A common animal model of acute respiratory distress syndrome (ARDS) is produced by injecting oleic acid intravenously. An injection of this 18-carbon unsaturated fatty acid produces a syndrome of acute endothelial and alveolar epithelial cell necrosis resulting in proteinaceous alveolar edema that mimics the acute phase of ARDS. In their study of a dog model of acute lung injury induced by oleic acid injections, Putensen et al. (204) examined the role of nitric oxide by giving inhaled NO and/or intravenous L-NMMA (N^G-monomethyl-L-arginine). After the induction of lung injury, inhaled NO at 40 ppm improved gas exchange by redistributing blood flow from shunting regions to lung units with a nearly ideal $\dot{V}_A/\dot{Q}_t$ ratio. The improvement of $\dot{V}_A/\dot{Q}_t$ matching and gas exchange was most pronounced when NO was inhaled in the presence of systemic L-NMMA. Systemic L-NMMA administration alone increased the pulmonary and systemic vascular resistance, but did not affect $\dot{V}_A/\dot{Q}_t$ mismatch and gas exchange. Inhaled NO reversed the pulmonary but not the systemic vasoconstriction caused by L-NMMA. This effect may be clinically important because the infusion of NO synthase inhibitors is being considered as treatment for sepsis-induced hypotension (130,204).

The effect of inhaled NO on pulmonary vascular resistance in a canine ARDS model was reported by Romand et al. (228). They found that NO inhalation (up to 145 ppm) reduced hypoxic pulmonary vasoconstriction, but not the mild pulmonary hypertension (mean pulmonary artery pressure 23 mm Hg) induced by oleic acid infusion. Gas exchange as well as dead space ventilation were not affected by inhaled NO in this study. In contrast, in a pig model of acute lung injury induced by oleic acid injection, Shah et al. (245) reported that inhaled NO (10–80 ppm) reduced mean pulmonary artery pressure and shunt fraction ($\dot{Q}_{VA}/\dot{Q}_t$) in a concentration-dependent manner, and improved oxygenation. Because a similar dose of oleic acid (0.08–0.1 ml/kg) was used to induce acute lung injury in these studies, these discrepancies in the extent of pulmonary vasodilation and improvement in oxygenation are most likely due to differences between the experimental species.

The degree of lung inflation may be an important determinant of the effects of inhaled nitric oxide. Putensen et al. (206) reported that the recruitment of lung units by the application of 10 cm H_2O continuous positive airway pressure (CPAP) augmented the improvement of oxygenation caused by inhaling 40 ppm NO in anesthetized dogs with oleic acid–induced lung injury. Application of CPAP converted extensive shunting regions [shunt = 48 ± 7% (SD) of cardiac output] to regions with a more normal $\dot{V}_A/\dot{Q}_t$ and reduced shunt to 21 ± 9%. The PaO_2 increased from 62 ± 8 mm Hg to only 64 ± 9 mm Hg in response to 40 ppm NO at ambient expiratory pressure. After adding 10 cm H_2O CPAP, however, the PaO_2 increased from 92 ± 8 to 111 ± 14 mm Hg ($p < 0.05$) with NO breathing. In this study, 40 ppm inhaled NO selectively reduced the pulmonary artery pressure from 30 ± 5 to 24 ± 6 mm Hg. The degree of pulmonary vasodilation was independent of the application of CPAP.

Inhaled NO probably mediates pulmonary vasodilation during lung injury by increasing cGMP levels within vascular smooth muscle. This increase is reflected by increased plasma cGMP concentrations. Rovira et al. (235) studied a model of acute lung injury induced by bilateral lung lavage in anesthetized lambs. When endogenous NO production was inhibited by infusing N^G-nitro-L-arginine methyl ester (L-NAME), a consistent increase of aortic, as compared with pulmonary arterial, plasma cGMP concentration could be measured within 5 min of breathing 60 ppm NO (Fig. 3). Increased aortic plasma cGMP levels were associated with selective pulmonary vasodilation, reduced venous admixture, and an increased PaO_2. However, the pulmonary vasodilatory response to inhaled NO and the salutary effects on O_2 exchange of breathing NO in this model were not enhanced by concomitant inhibition of NO synthase (NOS) by L-NAME. Levels of plasma cGMP returned to baseline within 10 minutes of discontinuing NO breathing.

Inhalation Injury

The effect of inhaled nitric oxide on lung injury caused by smoke inhalation has been studied in sheep (186). Compared with air breathing controls, pulmonary artery hypertension was reduced and oxygenation was improved in sheep breathing 20 ppm NO in air for 48 hr. However, there was no significant difference of lung wet-to-dry weight ratio, compliance, or histologic changes between the two groups. Nitric oxide inhalation neither improved nor worsened the tracheobronchial or alveolar pathologic changes occurring after inhalation injury.

Oxidant-Induced Acute Lung Injury

Oxygen-derived free radicals are important in the pathogenesis of ARDS and may contribute to pulmonary leukocyte adherence, emigration from vessels, activation and subsequent endothelial cell injury (137). Depending on the species or model used, endogenous NO appears to either enhance (101,105,156,173) or attenuate (27,104,135) the acute inflammatory response. Increased leukocyte-endothelial cell adhesion and associated albumin leakage have been demonstrated in the rat mesenteric microcirculation after NOS inhibition (138). NO donors (e.g., spermine-NO and nitroprusside) can attenuate ischemia/reperfusion injury or L-NAME-induced increase in venular albumin leakage as well as leukocyte adherence and emigration (136,139).

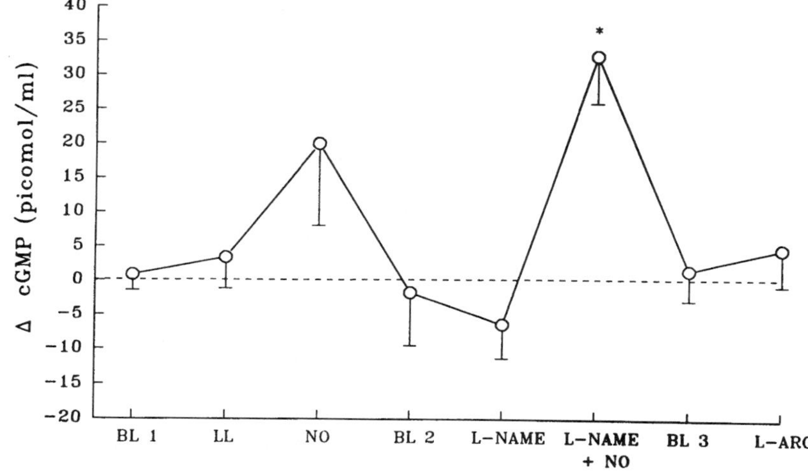

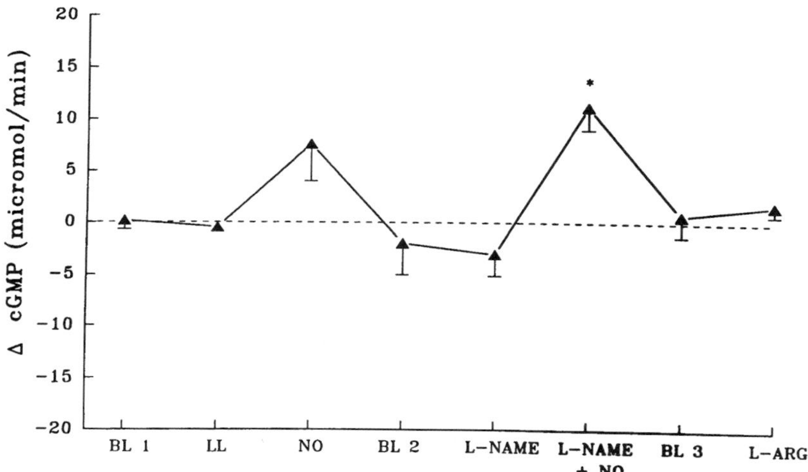

Figure 3. Aortic minus mixed venous cGMP plasma differences (*top*) and lung cGMP release (*bottom*) in six anesthetized sheep studied at baseline (BL1), after lung lavage (LL), after 10 min of 60 ppm NO inhalation (NO), 10 min after ceasing NO inhalation (BL2), after L-NAME infusion (L-NAME), again 10 min after beginning NO inhalation (L-NAME–NO), 10 min after breathing without NO (BL3), and 10 min after L-arginine infusion (L-Arg). Values are means ± SE. *$p < 0.05$ compared with period without NO. (Reprinted with permission from ref. 235.)

Nitric oxide combines with reactive oxygen species to produce intermediates such as the peroxynitrite anion which can cause cellular injury. Nozik et al. (183) reported that the administration of 1 mM L-arginine to isolated buffer-perfused rabbit lungs produced significant pulmonary hypertension and edema when the lungs were ventilated with 95% oxygen, or in the presence of a H_2O_2 generating system. This injury was attenuated by the administration of L-NAME or by pretreatment with catalase. The authors postulated that the administration of L-arginine increased the synthesis of NO within the lungs, and that NO reacted with H_2O_2 to cause lung injury via reactive intermediates.

Nitric oxide may also act as a superoxide scavenger. In the isolated buffer-perfused rabbit lung, Kavanagh et al. (120) investigated the effects of inhaled NO and endogenous NO synthase inhibition on oxidant-induced acute lung injury. Superoxide radicals were produced by the combination of purine and xanthine oxidase. Pretreatment with inhaled NO (90–120 ppm) prevented the increase of pulmonary artery pressure and capillary permeability assessed by estimating the pulmonary capillary filtration coefficient (K_{fc}). Inhibition of endogenous NOS by infusion of L-NAME increased pulmonary vascular tone without affecting capillary permeability. In addition, Guidot et al. (88) reported that inhaled NO prevented neutrophil-mediated permeability edema in isolated rat lungs, and speculated that NO may have anti-inflammatory properties. Although the mechanism by which inhaled NO protected against lung injury is unclear, it may involve alterations in cellular cGMP levels and cytoskeletal changes. These observations

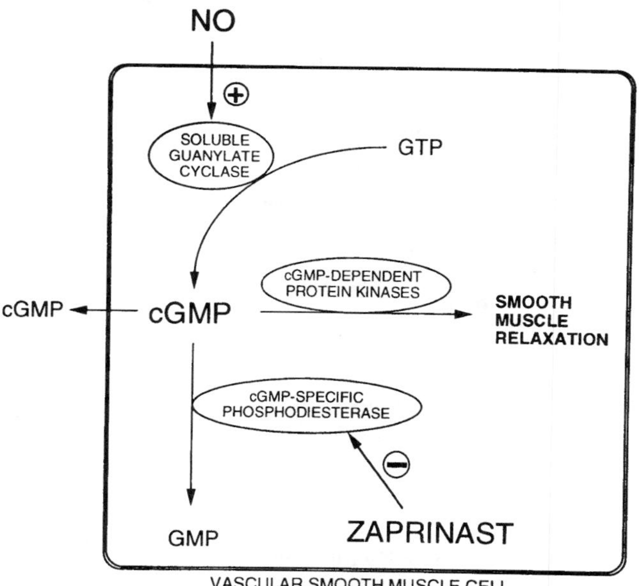

Figure 4. Putative site of action of zaprinast in vascular smooth muscle cells. NO, nitric oxide; GTP, guanosine triphosphate; GMP, guanosine monophosphate; cGMP, guanosine 3′,5′-cyclic monophosphate. (Reprinted with permission from ref. 106.)

raise the possibility that, in addition to treating the manifest abnormalities of ARDS such as pulmonary hypertension and increased intrapulmonary shunt, inhaled NO may directly attenuate neutrophil/oxidant-mediated lung injury.

Inhibition of cGMP-Specific Phosphodiesterases

The local selectivity of inhaled NO is primarily due to the inactivation of NO by its rapid combination with hemoglobin within the pulmonary circulation (222). Although this selectivity is a unique characteristic of inhaled NO, its short duration of action could be a disadvantage because many patients with chronic pulmonary hypertension or severe ARDS require continuous pulmonary vasodilator therapy. Although there is little evidence for acute pulmonary toxicity at low concentrations (<40 ppm) of inhaled NO, the toxicity of prolonged NO exposure in humans is unclear (see below) (290). Conceivably, pharmacologic agents which potentiate and/or prolong the pulmonary vasodilator effects of inhaled NO could reduce the effective dose and toxicity of NO.

Zaprinast (M&B 22948; 2-o-propoxyphenyl-8-azapurin-6-one, Rhone-Poulenc Rorer, Dagenham, Essex, U.K.) is a type V phosphodiesterase (PDE) inhibitor which selectively inhibits the hydrolysis of cGMP with minimal effects on the breakdown of adenosine 3′,5′-cyclic monophosphate (cAMP) in vascular smooth muscle cells and in isolated vascular rings (Fig. 4) (90, 149,254,269). Vasodilator responses to infusions of endothelium-dependent vasodilators and nitrosovasodilators are modified by zaprinast in newborn lambs (29) and in the isolated cat lobar artery (158). Ichinose et al. (106) investigated the effects of zaprinast on the pulmonary vasodilating effects of inhaled nitric oxide in awake spontaneously breathing lambs with pharmacologically induced pulmonary hypertension. Although the magnitude of PA pressure reduction by NO inhalation was not affected by intravenous zaprinast (Fig. 5A), the reduction of absolute values of PVR, as well as the mean percent PVR reduction (Fig. 5B) were significantly greater during the zaprinast infusion. The duration of the vasodilator response to inhaled nitric oxide ($t_{1/2}$) was markedly increased by the zaprinast infusion (Fig. 5C). Without zaprinast, the pulmonary vasodilation induced by inhaled NO persisted for only 1–2 min after NO was discontinued (Figs. 5C and 6). With zaprinast co-treatment, however, vasodilation induced by inhaled NO was maintained for 88 min with only four 4-min periods of NO (40 ppm) inhalation (Fig. 6). This reduced the time-weighted exposure to NO by 82%.

Similar results were reported in the ovine transitional circulation by Ziegler et al. (294). In this study, the effect of dipyridamole (a phosphodiesterase inhibitor which is a less specific inhibitor of cGMP PDE than zaprinast) on inhaled NO-induced pulmonary vasodilation was examined in four late-gestation

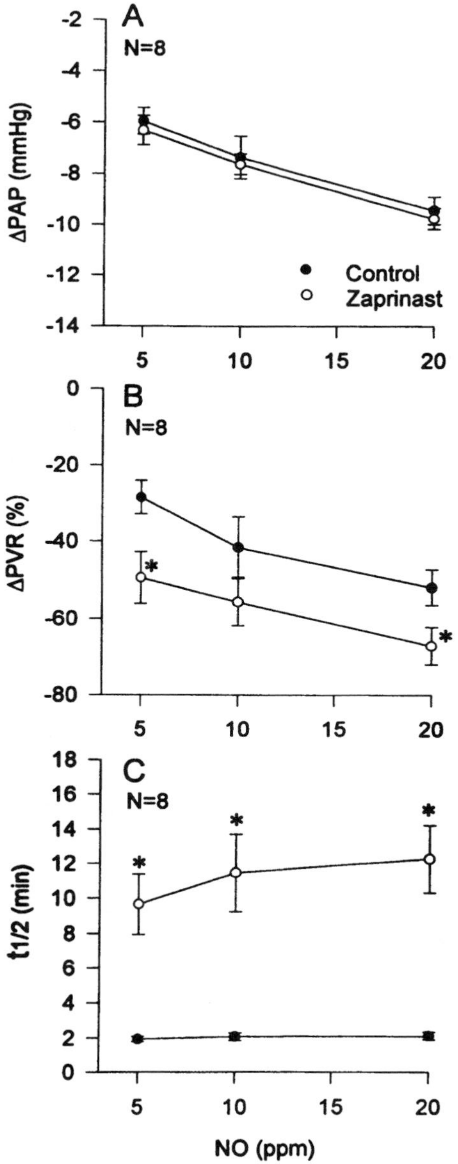

Figure 5. Influence of continuous intravenous infusion of zaprinast (0.1 mg/kg/min) on magnitude of peak decreases of mean pulmonary arterial pressures (PAP; **A**), percent change of pulmonary vascular resistance (PVR; **B**), and half times of vasodilating effect ($t_{1/2}$; **C**) in response to NO inhalation during pulmonary hypertension induced by U-46619 infusion. Values are means ± SE; N, number of lambs. *p < 0.05 compared with controls. (Reprinted with permission from ref. 106.)

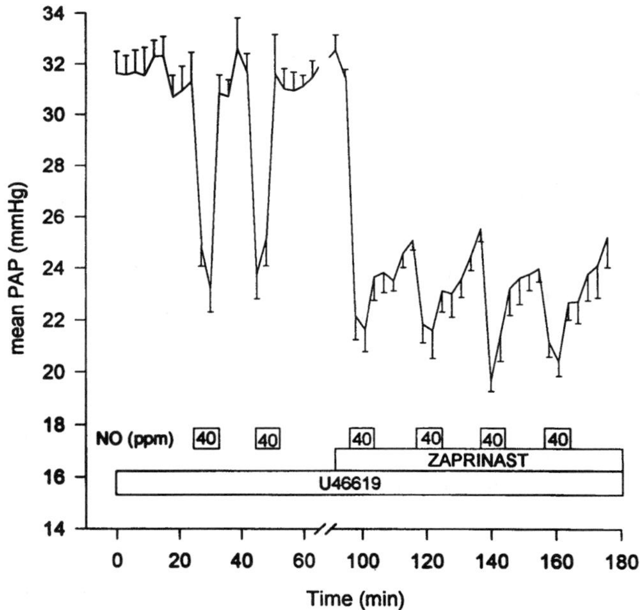

Figure 6. Demonstration of intermittent NO inhalation during pulmonary hypertension induced by U-46619 in four awake lambs. NO (40 ppm) was inhaled for 4-min periods alone and during concomitant infusion of zaprinast. During zaprinast infusion, 4-min exposures were repeated approximately every 20 min. Values are means ± SE. (Reprinted with permission from ref. 106.)

fetal lambs. Dipyridamole caused pulmonary vasodilation and augmented the pulmonary vasodilator response to inhaled NO at doses which did not alter systemic arterial pressure. Because dipyridamole can be administered to human subjects, this combination might reduce the dose of inhaled NO and improve the response to NO inhalation (152,248,294). Because high doses of zaprinast as well as dipyridamole alone may induce systemic vasodilation, further investigation is required.

NO INHALATION BY HUMANS

Short-term inhalation of NO (5–80 ppm) for diagnostic purposes was examined in patients with chronic pulmonary hypertension by Pepke-Zaba et al. (193) (Fig. 7). They reported that inhalation of 40 ppm NO decreased pulmonary vascular resistance by 5–68% without affecting systemic vascular resistance in patients with either chronic pulmonary hypertension or cardiac disease. Subsequently, Frostell et al. (69) studied the effects of breathing 40 ppm NO for 10 min in nine awake, healthy human volunteers exposed to hypoxic conditions. During air breathing, 40 ppm NO had no pulmonary or systemic vasodilatory effects. When the subjects breathed 12% oxygen to produce mild pulmonary vasoconstriction and hypertension, 40 ppm inhaled NO completely reversed the hypoxia-induced increase of pulmonary artery pressure and vascular resistance within 1–2 min (Fig. 8). Systemic blood pressure and vascular resistance were unchanged and methemoglobin levels remained below 1%.

NO breathing has since been evaluated in a wide variety of patients (Table 1), including: (a) adults with acute respiratory distress syndrome (ARDS) (16,21,45,56,141,167,208–210, 232–234,237,282,283), (b) neonatal and pediatric patients with acute respiratory failure (1,57,119,146,190,192,236,244, 264,277), (c) children with congenital heart disease and pulmonary hypertension (14,44,80,114,164,188,236,277,280), (d) adults with chronic pulmonary hypertension (249) or heart failure (23,73,145,243), (e) adults during or following cardiac surgery (142,220,253), and (f) adults with reactive airways disease (115,238).

Adult Respiratory Distress Syndrome

Acute pulmonary hypertension consistently occurs in severe ARDS. In survivors, pulmonary vascular resistance progressively decreases over time. Patients dying of acute respiratory failure tend to have a persistently increased pulmonary vascular resistance and progressive pulmonary hypertension. The increased pulmonary artery pressure is independent of changes of cardiac output and persists after the correction of systemic hypoxemia (291).

The pulmonary vascular changes in ARDS are produced by a complex combination of primary lung injury (i.e., aspiration, trauma, infection), the consequences of the pulmonary inflammatory response to injury (hypoxia, acidosis, release of cytokines and components of the complement system and the arachidonic acid pathway, as well as inhibitors of fibrinolysis), and the iatrogenic complications of intensive care therapy (oxygen toxicity and barotrauma). In severe ARDS, thromboembolic occlusion of the pulmonary vasculature is also common (289).

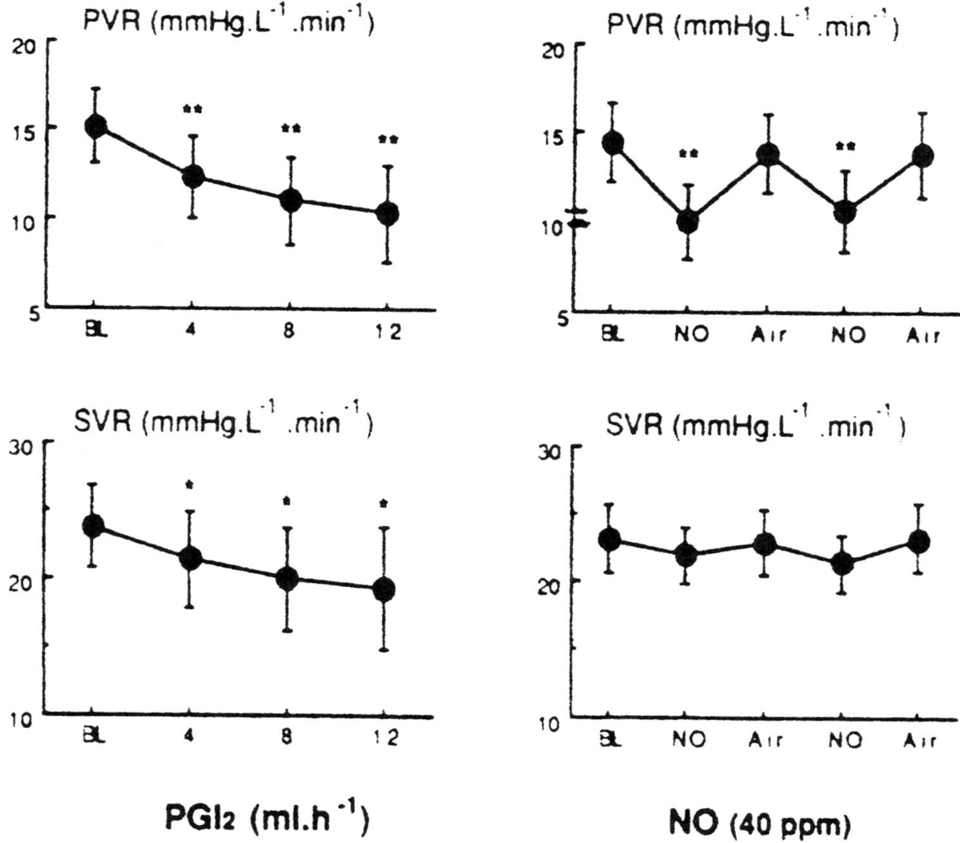

Figure 7. Pulmonary (PVR) and systemic (SVR) vascular resistance in eight patients with pulmonary hypertension receiving an intravenous infusion of prostacyclin (PGI_2) (0.5 mg in 250 ml) at rates of 4, 8, and 12 ml/hr, or inhalation of 40 ppm NO in air. Inhaled NO produced selective pulmonary vasodilation. Values are mean ± SEM. $*p < 0.05$; $**p < 0.01$. (Reprinted with permission from ref. 193.)

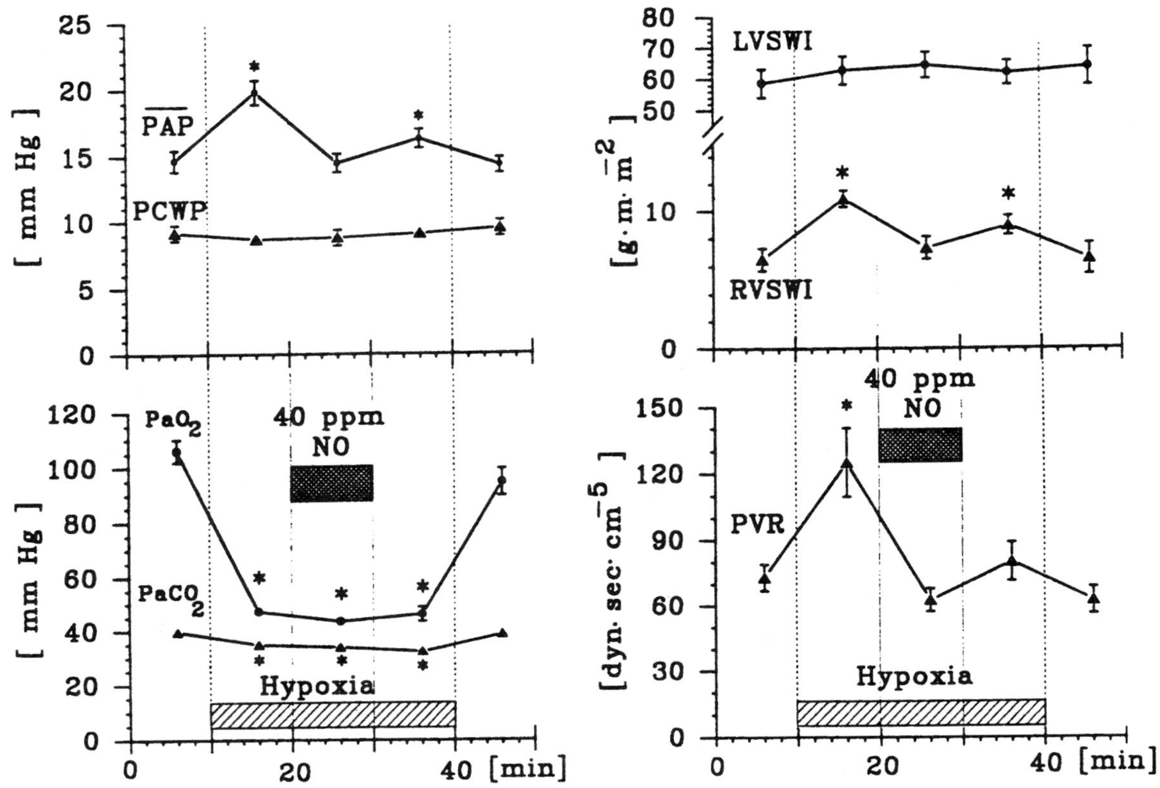

Figure 8. Nitric oxide (40 ppm) was inhaled during hypoxia by nine normal volunteers. The figure illustrates decreases of mean pulmonary artery pressure (PAP), pulmonary vascular resistance (PVR), and right ventricular stroke work index (RVSWI) during NO breathing. Pulmonary capillary wedge pressure (PCWP), PaO_2, $PaCO_2$, and left ventricular stroke work index (LVSWI) were unchanged by NO breathing. All data are mean ± SEM. *$p < 0.01$; value differs from first control breathing air. (Reprinted with permission from ref. 69.)

Rossaint et al. (232) compared the effects of NO inhalation (18 and 36 ppm) to intravenously infused prostacyclin in nine patients with ARDS. Nitric oxide selectively reduced mean pulmonary artery pressure from 37 ± 3 (SE) to 30 ± 2 mm Hg (Fig. 9). Oxygenation improved due to decreased venous admixture ($\dot{Q}_{VA}/\dot{Q}_t$). During NO breathing, the PaO_2/FIO_2 ratio increased from 152 ± 15 mm Hg to 199 ± 23 mm Hg. While the intravenous infusion of prostacyclin also reduced pulmonary artery pressure, mean arterial pressure and PaO_2 decreased.

Subsequently, numerous clinical studies have demonstrated that inhaled NO decreases pulmonary hypertension and improves hypoxemia in most patients with ARDS (Table 2). Several prospective randomized, double-blind studies of the efficacy of NO inhalation in patients with ARDS are currently underway (45). It is attractive to speculate that decreasing pulmonary capillary pressure by breathing NO may reduce the severity of lung injury in patients with ARDS. Benzing et al. (15) measured the pulmonary transvascular flux of albumin (an index of vascular fluid transfer into the pulmonary interstitium) and pulmonary capillary pressure in nine patients with acute lung injury. Pulmonary capillary pressure decreased from 24 ± 4 (SD) mm Hg to 21 ± 4 mm Hg when breathing 40 ppm NO and the pulmonary transvascular albumin flux was decreased. It is unknown if such changes are clinically significant or if they persist during long-term NO therapy.

A preliminary randomized double-blinded multicenter trial of NO inhalation in 177 patients with ARDS demonstrated that inhaled NO (1.25, 5, 20, 40, or 80 ppm) compared with placebo (nitrogen) improved PaO_2, decreased PA pressure, and decreased the intensity of mechanical ventilation over the first week of therapy (45). Overall, mortality rate and duration of mechanical ventilation were unaffected by NO breathing. Patients without extrapulmonary organ dysfunction who received 5 ppm inhaled NO, however, had an increased number of days alive and off mechanical ventilation.

It is apparent that very low concentrations of inhaled nitric oxide may effectively reduce pulmonary artery pressure and improve oxygenation in many patients with ARDS. Inhaled concentrations of <2 ppm may be effective in some patients (Fig. 10) (74,208–210,232). Right ventricular ejection fraction may increase in some patients responding to inhaled NO, suggesting that the observed decreases of pulmonary artery pressure may at times be hemodynamically important (56,234). The concomitant intravenous infusion of a novel vasoconstricting drug, almitrine, which increases the degree of hypoxic vasoconstriction in the lung, has been reported to enhance the beneficial effect of inhaled NO on PaO_2 (148,191,282). Almitrine increased mean pulmonary artery pressure and cardiac output,

Table 1. POTENTIAL CLINICAL APPLICATIONS OF INHALED NITRIC OXIDE

Adult respiratory distress syndrome (ARDS)
Neonatal and pediatric respiratory failure
Congenital heart disease
Chronic primary and secondary pulmonary hypertension
Pulmonary Hypertension following cardiopulmonary bypass
Cardiac transplantation
Lung transplantation
Bronchodilation

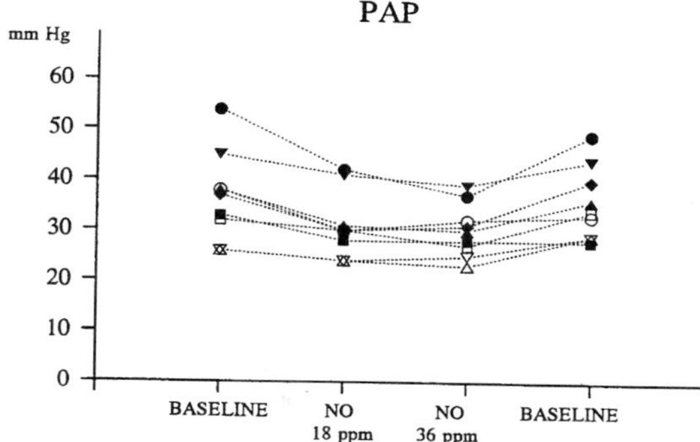

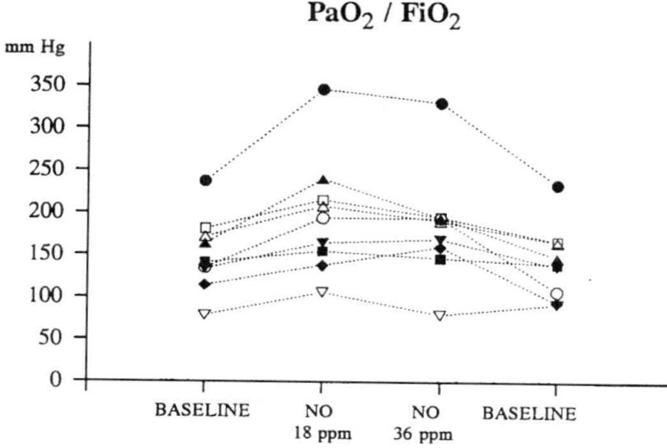

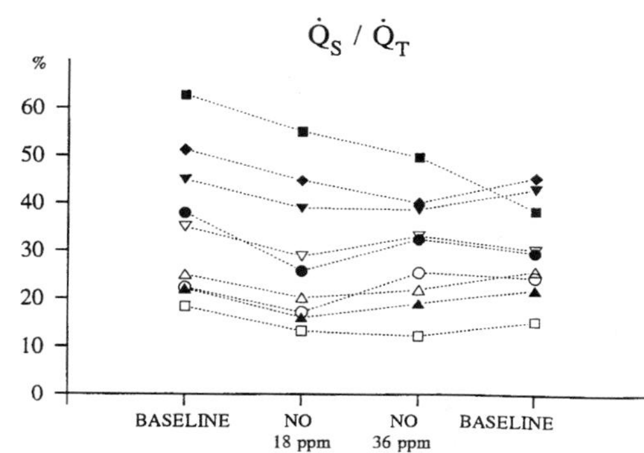

Figure 9. Mean pulmonary artery pressure (PAP), arterial oxygenation efficiency (PaO_2/FIO_2), and venous admixture ($\dot{Q}_S/\dot{Q}_T$) during inhalation of 18 and 36 ppm nitric oxide in nine patients with adult respiratory distress syndrome. *Solid symbols* represent patients treated with extracorporeal membrane oxygenation. (Reprinted with permission from ref. 232.)

but these changes were reversed by NO inhalation. Tachyphylaxis to NO inhalation has not been observed even when NO inhalation was continued for up to 53 days (232). Continuous inhalation of nitric oxide, however, is necessary. Pulmonary artery pressure increases and PaO_2 quickly falls after discontinuation of NO breathing.

Some patients do not respond to NO inhalation with pulmonary vasodilation and improved oxygenation. Sixty-five percent of patients had at least a 20% increase of PaO_2 after 4 hr of NO breathing, compared to 23% of patients receiving placebo in a prospective randomized double-blinded multicenter trial of NO inhalation in patients with ARDS (45). Varying responses to NO inhalation have been observed among different patients and during the course of acute lung injury in individual patients (21,167,233,282). In a retrospective analysis, Rossaint et al. (233) reported that 17% of patients failed to increase their PaO_2/FIO_2 by at least 10 mm Hg and 37% of patients failed to decrease their mean pulmonary artery pressure by at least 3 mm Hg. McIntyre et al. (157) reported minimal improvement of PaO_2/FIO_2 and pulmonary artery pressure in 5/16 trials (31%) and Wysocki et al. (282) reported that 10/17 (59%) patients failed to respond to inhaled NO. The precise mechanism for the variable responsiveness to inhaled NO is unknown. Clinicians are thus unable to accurately predict the responsiveness of individual patients to inhaled NO. In general, the baseline level of PVR appears to predict the degree of pulmonary vasoconstriction reversible by NO inhalation. Those with the greatest degree of pulmonary hypertension appear to respond most to NO inhalation (Fig. 11) (21,208,283). A favorable response to inhaled NO may also be related to the degree of alveolar recruitment (206,208).

If inhaled NO can improve the matching of ventilation to perfusion, it might be expected that the V_D/V_T and $PaCO_2$ might decrease during NO inhalation. While most adult studies have reported no change of $PaCO_2$ during NO inhalation, several have shown small but statistically significant decreases of V_D/V_T and $PaCO_2$ (56,209). These changes were too small to permit minute ventilation to be reduced. Interestingly, one of these studies reported a slight increase of $PaCO_2$ despite a decrease of alveolar dead space (210).

Rapid withdrawal of inhaled NO therapy has been associated with the sudden worsening of hypoxemia and pulmonary hypertension (Fig. 12) (21,74,166). This deterioration appears to be transient, but the hemodynamic consequences of this rebound may be catastrophic. The severity of the rebound may be minimized by slowly weaning the inhaled NO dose over several hours, transiently increasing the FIO_2, administering intravenous vasoactive agents as necessary, and avoiding sudden discontinuation of NO inhalation in patients with hemodynamic instability or severe hypoxemia. The mechanism for this acute pulmonary vasoconstriction is unknown and its occurrence in patients is unpredictable. It may be due to reduced NO production by endothelial NOS caused by inhaling high levels of exogenous nitric oxide, a phenomenon known as product inhibition (9,125,219). Rebound could also be due to enhanced release of vasoconstrictor substances by the pulmonary circulation or enhanced phosphodiesterase activity.

Neonatal Respiratory Failure

At birth, there is a sustained decrease of pulmonary vascular resistance and an increase of pulmonary blood flow, in part due to increasing oxygen tensions. If this does not occur, persistent pulmonary hypertension of the newborn (PPHN) may result. Persistent pulmonary hypertension of the newborn is a syndrome characterized by an increased pulmonary vascular resistance, increased right-to-left shunting across the ductus arteriosus and foramen ovale, and severe systemic hypoxemia. Extracorporeal membrane oxygenation (ECMO) is often used to support these infants, because conventional vasodilator therapy is limited by severe systemic hypotension and may reduce PaO_2 by increasing intrapulmonary right-to-left shunting. It has been hypothesized that endogenous production of NO by the pulmonary vasculature might be decreased in PPHN. If so, then inhaled NO might provide an effective therapy for these severely ill infants (129,226).

Multiple small clinical studies of NO inhalation have been performed in neonates, infants, and children with various types of acute respiratory failure (Table 3). In general, pulmonary hypertension is reduced and systemic arterial oxygenation is improved with inhalation of <20 ppm NO. In clinical studies by Roberts et al. (226), critically ill infants with PPHN rapidly increased their preductal oxygen saturation in response to NO inhalation at concentrations up to 80 ppm. In five of six infants studied, postductual oxygen saturation also increased. In one newborn, the resulting improvement in PaO_2 persisted after the discontinuation of NO, eliminating the need for ECMO.

Table 2. REPRESENTATIVE CLINICAL STUDIES OF NO INHALATION IN ARDS PATIENTS

Study	Number of patients	NO dose (ppm)	Duration of NO therapy	PA pressure	PaO_2	Remarks
Rossaint et al. (232)	10	18, 36	<1–53 days	↓	↑	$\dot{V}_A/\dot{Q}_t$ improved
Gerlach et al. (75)	12	0–100	Trial	↓	↑	Effective dose for improved of PaO_2 was less than that for pulmonary vasodilation
Gerlach et al. (74)	3	≤1	9–13 days	↓	↑	Improvement of PaO_2 occurred at <1 ppm
Benzing et al. (16)	18	40	Trial	↓	↑	Pulmonary capillary pressure decreased
Bigatello et al. (21)	13	0–40	<1 to 27 days	↓	↑	
Puybasset et al. (209)	6	0.1–5	Trial	↓	↑	
Puybasset et al. (210)	11	2	Trial	↓	↑	NO decreased PA hypertension secondary to permissive hypercapnia
Wysocki et al. (282)	17	5–10	Trial	↓	±↑	PaO_2 increased in only 7/17 patients; the effects of i.v. almitrine were additive to those of inhaled NO
Young et al. (283)	14	8–132	Trial	↓	↑	
Fierobe et al. (56)	13	5	Trial	↓	↑	RV ejection fraction increased from 32 ± 5% to 36 ± 6%
Levy et al. (141)	20	5–10	3–30 days	↓	↑	
McIntyre et al. (157)	14	0–40	<1–10 days	↓	↑	Minimal improvement in 5/16 trials
Puybasset et al. (208)	21	2	Trial	↓	↑	
Rossaint et al. (233)	30	0.01–25	2–53 days	↓	↑	PaO_2 increased in 83% of patients; PA pressure decreased in 63% of patients
Rossaint et al. (234)	10	18, 36	Trial	↓	NA	
Samama et al. (237)	6	1–100	Trial	↓	↑	Platelet aggregation was inhibited, but bleeding times were unaffected by NO inhalation
Dellinger et al. (45)	177	0, 1.25, 5, 20, 40, 80	Up to 28 days	↓	↑	Multicenter trial; 65% of pts. receiving NO had a ≥ 20% increase of PaO_2 compared with 23% of placebo patients; mortality was unaffected

NA, not applicable, results not reported; pts., patients; trial, <1-hr exposure

Kinsella et al. (129) reported the effects of inhaling 10–20 ppm NO in nine infants with severe PPHN. All nine showed a rapid improvement in oxygenation without systemic hypotension. Clinical improvement continued during treatment with 6 ppm NO for 24 hr in six of the infants. Subsequently, this group has reported that 13 of 15 patients with PPHN who were candidates for support with ECMO were successfully treated with inhaled NO. ECMO therapy was avoided in these patients (126,127). Nitric oxide inhalation in babies with PPHN currently is being studied in both open (161) and blinded and randomized multicenter trials. As in adults, the response is variable. In the neonatal lung, the degree of improvement with inhaled NO appears to depend upon the presence of a mature surfactant system (118,119).

Laboratory studies of the neonatal pulmonary circulation have also documented that inhaled nitric oxide is an effective pulmonary vasodilator (46,53,118,128,176,231,251). In hypoxic newborn lambs studied by Roberts et al. (224), NO inhalation decreased pulmonary artery pressure and increased pulmonary blood flow without reducing systemic vascular resistance. Ven-

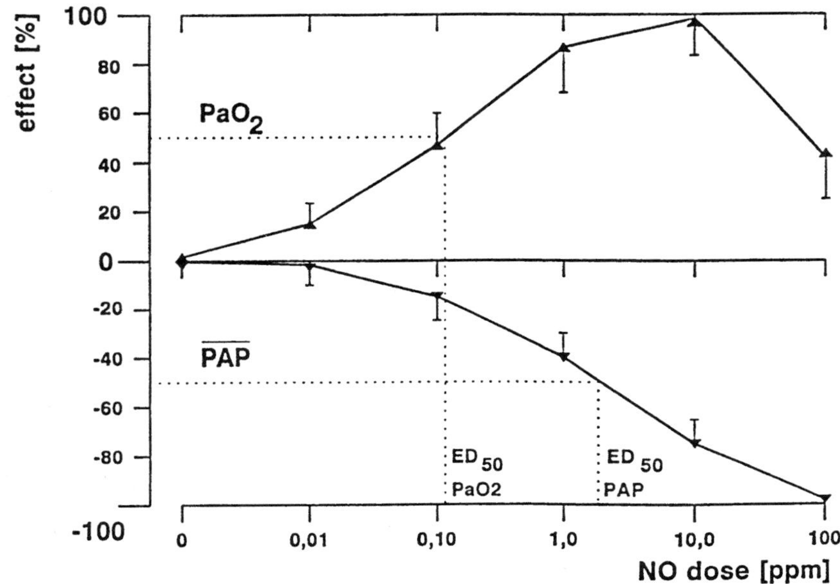

Figure 10. Dose response of inhaled NO for PaO_2 (*upper part*) and mean pulmonary artery pressure (PAP; *lower part*). Values are means ± SD (n = 12 patients with ARDS), expressed as percentage of maximal change. The estimated ED_{50} of NO for improvement of arterial oxygenation and for reduction of PAP are indicated above the *x* axis. Note the different ED_{50} for PaO_2 and PAP. (Reprinted with permission from ref. 75.)

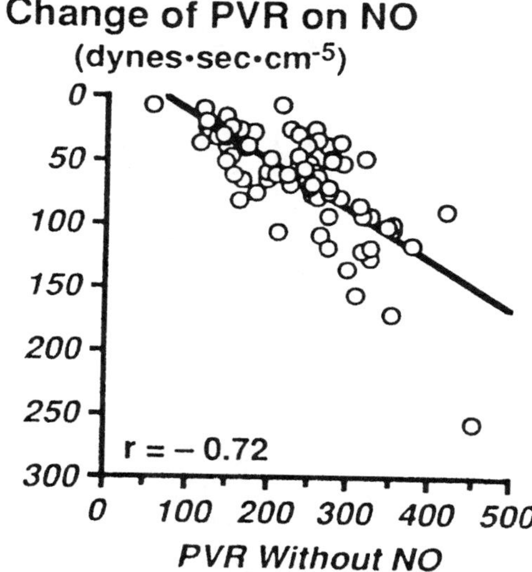

Figure 11. Change of pulmonary vascular resistance (PVR) induced by NO inhalation plotted against the baseline PVR in seven patients with severe ARDS receiving prolonged NO inhalation. The decrease of PVR during NO breathing was correlated with the patients baseline PVR. (Reprinted with permission from ref. 21.)

tilation with 80 ppm NO at an FIO_2 of 0.21 caused a threefold increase of both lung and preductal plasma cGMP concentrations. Severe respiratory acidosis did not attenuate the pulmonary vasodilation caused by inhaled NO. Zayek et al. (292) studied the effects of inhaled NO (6–100 ppm) in a model of PPHN created by prenatal ligation of the ductus arteriosus in lambs. Inhaled nitric oxide caused dose-dependent decreases of pulmonary artery pressure and pulmonary vascular resistance. Decreased right-to-left shunting of blood flow through the foramen ovale during NO inhalation resulted in an increased PaO_2 [from 43 ± 16 (SE) mm Hg to 185 ± 72 mm Hg while breathing 100 ppm NO] and arterial oxygen saturation (from 74 ± 8 to 96 ± 2%) and a decreased $PaCO_2$. Systemic blood pressure was unaffected by breathing NO (292). Using this model, Zayek et al. (293) subsequently documented an increased survival rate with NO therapy. After prenatal ligation of the ductus arteriosus and delivery 13 days later, newborn lambs were ventilated at FIO_2 0.92 and randomly allocated to breathe 80 ppm NO for 23 hr or receive no additional treatment. All seven control lambs died before the end of the study, whereas five of six lambs treated with inhaled NO survived. Arterial oxygenation was increased in the NO-breathing lambs, as compared with controls. Additionally, important experimental evidence is accumulating that the inhalation of nitric oxide attenuates hypoxic pulmonary vascular remodeling of the pulmonary circulation (134,227). Conceivably, inhaled nitric

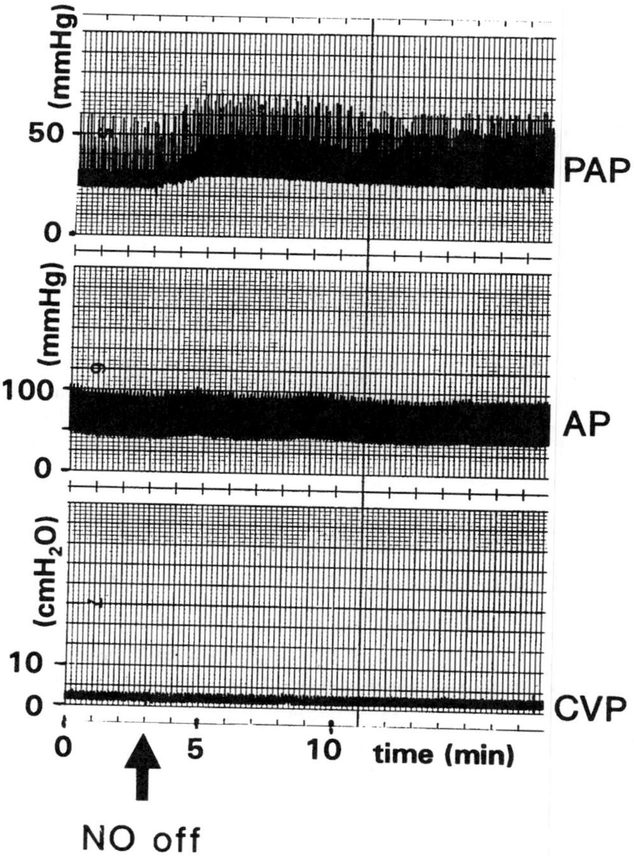

Figure 12. Continuous recording of pulmonary artery pressure (PAP), systemic artery pressure (AP), and central venous pressure (CVP) during the discontinuation of inhaled NO in a patient with ARDS. (Reprinted with permission from ref. 74.)

Table 3. REPRESENTATIVE CLINICAL STUDIES OF NO INHALATION IN NEONATAL AND PEDIATRIC ACUTE RESPIRATORY FAILURE

Study	Number of patients	NO dose (ppm)	Duration of NO therapy	PA pressure	PaO_2	Remarks
Abman et al. (1)	17	20, 3–10	30 min, then 1–24 days	↓	↑ 15/17 pts.	
Finer et al. (57)	23	5–80	1–92 hr	NA	↑ 13/23 pts.	≤20 ppm NO used for treatment after initial dose-response trial
Karamanoukian et al. (119)	9	80	20 min	NA	↑	Neonates with hypoplastic lungs improved after ECMO only
Lonnqvist et al. (146)	14	20–80	0.5–60 hr	NA	↑ 10/14 pts.	
Rozé et al. (236)	17	20 ± 32	6 hr	NA	↑	
Shah et al. (244)	4	≤20	1–6 days	NA	↑ 3/4 pts.	ECMO necessary in all 4 pts. despite use of NO
Pappert et al. (190)	3	0.1, 1, 10	30 min	↓	↑	Aerosolized prostacyclin compared with NO produced similar results
Peliowski et al. (192)	8	≤20	6–137 hr	NA	↑	Premature infants; ↓ in mean airway pressure noted with NO

NA, not applicable, results not reported; pts., patients; trial, <1-hr exposure.

oxide therapy might be used to limit the chronic pulmonary vascular remodeling which accompanies neonatal acute respiratory failure.

Chronic Pulmonary Hypertension

Clinical studies of brief periods of NO inhalation have been performed in patients with chronic pulmonary hypertension (193), patients with idiopathic or primary pulmonary hypertension (211,249), patients with COPD complicated by pulmonary hypertension (169), and patients with severe pulmonary fibrosis (36,113,133,153). Inhaled NO variably decreased pulmonary vascular resistance without affecting systemic vascular resistance in these studies. Usually, arterial oxygenation did not improve when these patients breathed NO. In some patients with severe hypoxemia due to $\dot{V}_A/\dot{Q}_t$ mismatching rather than increased venous admixture, PaO_2 has been reported to decrease slightly [from 56 ± 7 (SD) to 53 ± 7 mm Hg] when breathing 40 ppm NO (12).

Congenital and Acquired Heart Disease

Roberts et al. (225) reported that inhaled nitric oxide was an effective selective pulmonary vasodilator in children with congenital heart disease. They studied 10 children from 3 months to 6.5 years of age with chronic pulmonary hypertension due to congenital heart defects. Inhaling 20–80 ppm NO at FIO_2 0.9 for 10 min promptly decreased pulmonary artery pressure and pulmonary vascular resistance. Compared to breathing 0 ppm NO at FIO_2 0.9, NO decreased the mean pulmonary artery pressure from 48 ± 19 (SD) mm Hg to 37 ± 11 mm Hg. Under the same conditions, NO decreased the pulmonary vascular resistance from 536 ± 376 to 308 ± 260 dynes/sec^{-1}/cm^5/m^2, while systemic arterial pressure and resistance remained unchanged (Fig. 13). Inhaling 80 ppm NO at FIO_2 0.9 increased pulmonary blood flow in all of the six patients with intracardiac shunts. Subsequent studies have reported similar findings (44, 80,164,188,236,277,280).

In adult patients, Rich et al. (221) have studied the effects of inhaling 20 ppm NO in 20 patients undergoing various types of cardiac surgery requiring cardiopulmonary bypass and five patients requiring ventricular assist devices. Nitric oxide inhalation decreased the pulmonary artery pressure from 36 ± 3 (SE) to 29 ± 2 mm Hg and 32 ± 2 to 27 ± 1 mm Hg, before and after cardiopulmonary bypass, respectively, and from 68 ± 12 to 55 ± 9 mm Hg in patients requiring ventricular assist devices. The decrease of pulmonary vascular resistance during NO breathing was proportional to the patients' baseline pulmonary vascular resistance. Once again, systemic hemodynamics were unaffected. Multiple reports have documented the use of inhaled nitric oxide as short-term therapy to decrease acute pulmonary hypertension following cardiac surgery in neonates and children (Table 4) (14,18,92,114,165,242,277) and in adults (142, 220,253).

Use of Inhaled NO in Heart and/or Lung Transplantation Patients

A devastating complication after heart transplantation is right heart failure secondary to refractory pulmonary hypertension. Preoperative measurement of pulmonary vascular reactivity is believed to predict this complication. The nonselective vasodilators administered to assess the reversibility of pulmonary vasoconstriction, however, can cause severe systemic hypotension and at times lead to death. Inhaled nitric oxide could be an ideal alternative drug for this indication. The utility of inhaled nitric oxide as a selective pulmonary vasodilator patients with severe chronic heart failure has been assessed (145,243). Semigran et al. (243) compared the effects of inhaled nitric oxide with those

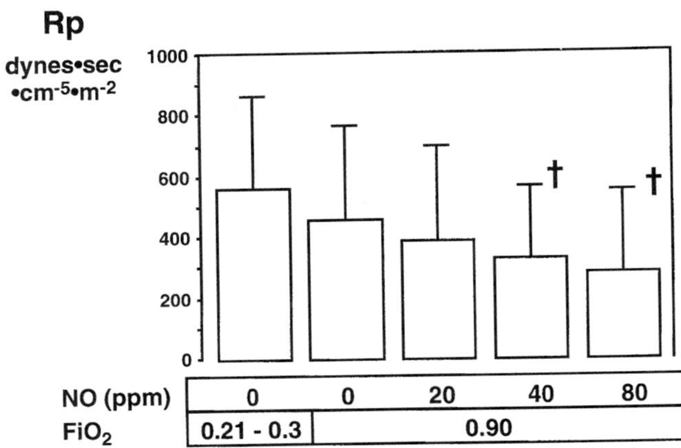

Figure 13. Pulmonary vascular resistance index (R_P) in seven pediatric patients with congenital heart disease who breathed 0, 20, 40, and 80 ppm NO at FIO_2 0.9. Nitric oxide (40 and 80 ppm) decreased R_P below levels measured both at baseline (FIO_2 0.21–0.3) and at FIO_2 0.9. (Reprinted with permission from ref. 225.)

of intravenous nitroprusside in 16 patients with New York Heart Association class III or IV heart failure referred for heart transplantation. Pulmonary vascular resistance decreased to a greater extent with 80 ppm NO than with the maximally tolerated dose of nitroprusside. Systemic arterial pressure did not change with nitric oxide but decreased with nitroprusside. Interestingly, pulmonary capillary wedge pressure increased with 80 ppm NO (26 ± 2 to 32 ± 2 mm Hg, $p < 0.05$). This finding has been reproduced by others (124,145). Pulmonary edema has occurred when inhaled nitric oxide was administered to patients with severe left ventricular failure (23). The mechanism for the increase of left ventricular filling pressure observed in these studies is unclear, but could be related to a sudden increase of left ventricular volume due to increased pulmonary venous return with NO-induced pulmonary vasodilation.

Brief clinical evaluations of NO inhalation have been performed in patients being considered for lung or heart-lung transplantation (3,249). These studies suggest that inhaled NO may be a useful alternative to drugs such as nitroprusside or prostacyclin because of the lack of systemic hypotension with inhaled NO therapy. Snell et al. (252) extended this application of inhaled NO by treating a 40-year-old woman with end-stage primary pulmonary hypertension with inhaled NO (mean dose, 50 ± 23 ppm). The nitric oxide was initially administered via a face mask and later via a transtracheal catheter. The patient received a heart-lung transplant after 68 days of inhaled NO therapy (252). Adatia et al. (2) have examined the effects of inhaled nitric oxide (80 ppm) on hemodynamics and gas exchange in six patients following lung transplantation. Oxygenation improved and PA pressure decreased in two patients treated with inhaled NO for 40 and 69 hr.

BRONCHODILATION

Since inhaled NO can diffuse through pulmonary tissue to relax upstream pulmonary artery smooth muscle cells, it seems reasonable that inhaled NO might also dilate constricted airways. However, airways have a thick epithelium and are covered by a mucus coating. Diffusion of NO, a highly lipid soluble substance with a low aqueous solubility, might be impeded by the mucus barrier (246). Dupuy et al. (51) examined the effect of inhaled NO on airway mechanics in anesthetized guinea pigs. In methacholine-bronchoconstricted animals, inhalation of 5 to 300 ppm NO produced a rapid and dose-related reduction of airway resistance and an increase of dynamic compliance. An

Table 4. REPRESENTATIVE CLINICAL STUDIES OF NO INHALATION IN NEONATAL AND PEDIATRIC CONGENITAL HEART DISEASE

Study	Number of patients	NO dose (ppm)	Duration of NO therapy	PA pressure	PaO_2	Remarks
Journois et al. (114)	17	20–80	4–250 hr	↓	↑	
Miller et al. (164)	10	2, 10, 20	7-min trials	↓	NA	Degree of PA hypertension predicted response
Winberg et al. (280)	22	40	10-min trials	↓ 13/22 pts.	NA	PA pressure ↓ only in pts. with PA hypertension
Beghetti et al. (14)	7	≤20	4–16 days	↓	↑	6/7 pts. had a favorable response to NO
Day et al. (44)	11	12, 60	<1-hr trial	↓	NA	Effects of 12 and 60 ppm were similar
Goldman et al. (80)	13	20	10-min trial	↓	↑	Inhaled nitric oxide was a more effective and selective pulmonary vasodilator than prostacyclin
Curran et al. (41)	20	5–80	<1 hr to 10 days	↓	NA	Minimal ↓ of PA pressure in infants after repair of atrioventricular canal; ↓ PA pressure in 11/15 pts. with PA hypertension and congenital heart disease

NA, not applicable, results not reported; pts., patients; trial, <1-hr exposure.

inhaled concentration of 15 ppm was able to reduce pulmonary resistance by 50%. The bronchodilating effects of NO were additive to the effects of inhaled terbutaline and were stable over 1 hr of NO breathing. Additional studies demonstrated that inhaled NO in guinea pigs could reverse bronchoconstriction due to an intravenous infusion of leukotriene D_4, histamine or neurokinin A (52).

Somewhat different results were obtained in studies of anesthetized mechanically ventilated New Zealand white rabbits (97). As in the study by Dupuy et al. (51), inhalation of 80 ppm NO blocked methacholine-induced increases of airway resistance, which primarily measures central airway tone. Pulmonary compliance, which reflects the behavior of smaller airways, and arterial oxygenation were unaffected by NO inhaled at this concentration. Apparently, peripheral airway tone in this species may be less sensitive to inhaled NO. That NO can relax constricted airways of laboratory animals has been documented in several other laboratory studies (30,100,144). In addition, the matching of perfusion to ventilation has been reported to improve following the inhalation of nitric oxide by anesthetized pigs with methacholine-induced bronchoconstriction (205).

The significance of the bronchodilator effect of nitric oxide is less clear in humans with bronchoconstriction. Sanna et al. (238) reported that the bronchodilator effect of inhaled NO in men with methacholine-induced bronchospasm was much less than that reported in animals or that regularly observed in asthmatic patients after the inhalation of beta-sympathomimetic drugs. Kacmarek et al. (115) examined 13 volunteers with mild asthma with methacholine-induced bronchospasm who breathed 100 ppm NO. Six of the patients responded to NO breathing with at least a 15% increase in FEV_1. The reason for the variable response was unclear. Similar to the study of Sanna et al. (238), the bronchodilation induced by NO was less than that induced by inhaled isoproterenol.

SAFE ADMINISTRATION OF INHALED NITRIC OXIDE

Toxicity

The interest generated by reports of the successful therapeutic use of inhaled nitric oxide is tempered by concerns over its toxicity (72). Although the U.S. Occupational Safety and Health Administration has set a time-weighted average exposure limit of 25 ppm for NO when breathed for 8 hr/day in the workplace, long-term studies of NO toxicology have not been conducted (68).

High inhaled concentrations of nitric oxide have been reported to cause acute pulmonary injury, methemoglobinemia, asphyxia and death (10,39,259). Greenbaum et al. (82) exposed anesthetized dogs to 5000 - 20,000 ppm NO. Death ensued secondary to methemoglobinemia, acidemia, and alveolar edema (82). Subsequent controlled studies demonstrated that much of the direct pulmonary toxicity of inhaled NO is due to the NO_2 contained in the gas mixtures (102,259).

Nitrogen Dioxide

Nitric oxide may form several toxic products. In oxygen mixtures, NO is oxidized to NO_2 (10,26,59,79,116,168,258). Nitrogen dioxide is cytotoxic (72) and converted in aqueous solutions to nitric and nitrous acids. Occupational safety and health standards limit the NO_2 exposure of workers to 5 ppm (35).

Because NO_2 is an atmospheric pollutant, its pulmonary toxicity has been extensively investigated. High levels (>10 ppm) of inhaled NO_2 have produced pulmonary edema, hemorrhage, changes in the surface tension of surfactant, reduced alveolar numbers, and death in studies of experimental animals (65,82,247,279). At concentrations as low as 2 ppm, alveolar cell hyperplasia, altered surfactant hysteresis, changes in the epithelium of the terminal bronchioles, and loss of epithelial cilia have been reported (55,261). In humans, exposure to 2.3 ppm NO_2 for 5 hr increased alveolar permeability (217). Airway responsiveness may also be increased at inhaled NO_2 concentrations of ≤ 2 ppm (33,60,171,261). Inhaled NO_2 may remain in the lungs for prolonged periods of time because it reacts with water to produce nitric acid and undergoes irreversible reactive absorption by pulmonary epithelial lining fluid (201). Exhaled NO_2 concentrations may not be an accurate indicator of toxic pulmonary levels. It therefore appears prudent to maintain NO_2 levels as low as possible (179).

The extent of conversion of NO to NO_2 is determined by the residence time of NO with oxygen, and is accelerated by increased NO and oxygen concentrations (5,10,26,59,79,116, 168,179,258). The conversion rate of NO to NO_2 follows second order kinetics with respect to the NO concentration and is described by the relationship (79,179):

$$-d[NO]/dt = k \cdot [NO]^2 \cdot [O_2]$$

Because the oxygen concentration is typically much greater than the NO concentration, it is assumed that the oxygen concentration remains constant. This formula also assumes that NO is exclusively converted to NO_2. Integration of the above equation yields the following:

$$1/[NO_t] - 1/[NO_o] = k \cdot [O_2] \cdot t$$

where $[NO_t]$ is the NO concentration after a residence time t, $[NO_o]$ is the initial NO concentration, $[O_2]$ is the oxygen concentration, and k is the rate constant for the conversion of NO. The difference between $[NO_t]$ and $[NO_o]$ is the nitrogen dioxide concentration. Glasson and Tuesday (79) reported the value of k as 1.57×10^{-9} $ppm^{-2}min$ at 23°C and one atmosphere. Under physical conditions similar to adult mechanical ventilation, Nishimura et al. (179) reported a rate constant of $1.46 \times 10^{-9}/ppm^2/min$ when NO was mixed with nitrogen before entering the ventilator; the rate constant increased eightfold to $1.16 \times 10^{-8}/ppm^2/min$ when NO was mixed with air prior to introduction into the ventilator. Adia et al. (5) reported that the rate constant was smaller at 37°C than 25°C, and the constant was not affected by humidity. The residence time within mechanical ventilators is dependent upon the minute ventilation and internal volume of the ventilator. Mechanical ventilators with a higher internal volume (e.g., Servo 900C) have a longer residence time and thus a greater delivered $[NO_2]$ than those with a lower internal volume (e.g., Puritan-Bennett 7200ae) (179).

A soda lime absorber can be used to remove NO_2 from the inspiratory gas (51,110,116,260). The efficacy of soda lime may vary with the preparation used and its effectiveness decreases with time (198). The soda lime also absorbs NO (5,110). Adding a soda lime canister to the inspiratory limb of a breathing circuit may introduce other problems during mechanical ventilation such as increased resistance to breathing, difficulty in triggering the ventilator, increased compression volume, and an increased risk of leaks.

Nitrosation of Metalloproteins

Nitric oxide forms complexes with transitional metal complexes, including those in metalloproteins such as hemoglobin. In tissues, nitrosation of iron-containing enzymes and iron-sulfur proteins of target cells may be responsible for the cytotoxic action of NO generated by activated macrophages (95,263).

S-nitrosothiols, mostly S-nitrosoproteins, are formed in plasma. S-nitrosothiols have been identified in human airway lining fluid and in the plasma of normal subjects (256) and patients inhaling NO mixtures. The formation of relatively stable iron-nitrosyl complexes and S-nitrosothiols may provide ways of tailoring the duration of action and transport properties of NO and a means of detoxifying NO in tissues (256,258). High levels of intracellular NO have been reported to cause DNA damage and mutations in human cell preparations (177). Damage to erythrocyte membranes may occur following long-term low-level exposures. Oda et al. (185) reported enlarged spleens and increased bilirubin levels, suggestive of increased erythrocyte turnover, in mice following 6 months of exposure to 10 ppm NO.

Methemoglobinemia

In the circulation, nitric oxide combines extremely rapidly with hemoglobin to form nitrosyl Fe(II)-hemoglobin and subsequently methemoglobin (11,50,78,111,131,151,222,268,276). Methemoglobin is produced when the heme iron of hemoglobin is oxidized from Fe^{+2} to Fe^{+3} (42). In the oxidized form, the oxygen affinity of the hemoglobin increases (i.e., shifts the oxyhemoglobin curve to the left) (32). Normal methemoglobin levels are <2%; levels <5% do not require treatment. Endogenous NO production probably accounts for the methemoglobin levels found in the blood of nonsmokers (25). Other oxidizing agents, such as nitrates, can also cause methemoglobinemia.

Methemoglobinemia may occur if its production rate is increased or its reduction rate is diminished (20). The activity of methemoglobin reductase present within erythrocytes is the predominant mechanism for metabolizing methemoglobin. The activity of methemoglobin reductase may be decreased as a result of a hereditary deficiency and is normally low in newborn infants (20). Patients with decreased methemoglobin reductase activity may develop methemoglobinemia in the face of an increased rate of hemoglobin oxidation.

Significant methemoglobinemia during NO inhalation may occur, especially in newborns, but its incidence appears low and is related to the inhaled NO dose (111,284). In a clinical study, Wessel et al. (277) reported methemoglobin concentrations of >5% in four of 123 patients who received inhaled nitric oxide. In human adults (1,21,157,232,233,283) and experimental animals (37,112,245), clinically significant methemoglobinemia is extremely rare following exposure to NO concentrations of ≤40 ppm. For example, mice exposed to 10 ppm NO for 6 months had a methemoglobin concentration of 0–0.3%, identical to unexposed animals (185). Frostell et al. (68) reported that breathing 80 ppm NO for 3 hr did not increase blood methemoglobin levels in awake spontaneously ventilating lambs. In humans, von Nieding et al. (272) found that methemoglobin levels did not rise above 0.7% in 48 normal volunteers breathing 40 ppm NO for up to 15 min. Nevertheless, it is prudent to monitor the methemoglobin levels of patients receiving inhaled NO therapy and to administer the lowest effective dose of NO. Increasing levels of methemoglobin during inhaled NO therapy can usually be controlled by decreasing the dose of NO. Methylene blue may be administered to treat severe methemoglobinemia. Because methylene blue may inhibit the activity of guanylate cyclase, methylene blue treatment could conceivably reduce the effects of inhaled NO. Young et al. (285), however, reported that methylene blue did not inhibit the action of inhaled NO in hypoxic sheep. Methylene blue may also act as a systemic vasoconstrictor in patients with septic shock and presumably increased endogenous nitric oxide production (241).

Peroxynitrite and Other Intermediates

In aqueous solutions, nitric oxide reacts rapidly with $O_2^{\cdot-}$ to form peroxynitrite ($OONO^-$) (64,72,132). This species is a strong oxidant and catalyzes membrane lipid peroxidation. In addition, nitric oxide forms complexes with iron-containing enzymes and iron-sulfur proteins. In plasma, NO is converted to nitrates and nitrites which are eliminated primarily by the kidney (112,270,278). It is unknown if the increased plasma nitrate and nitrite concentrations during NO inhalation have any deleterious effects.

Inhibition of Platelet Function

Nitric oxide inhibits platelet adhesion to endothelial cells and reverses platelet aggregation in vitro (159,216). These antiplatelet effects may be due to activation of guanylate cyclase and increased concentrations of cyclic GMP within the platelet (13,147,215,274). Minor prolongation of the bleeding time during experimental nitric oxide inhalation in rabbits (99) and human volunteers (98) has been reported. The clinical significance of this effect is uncertain. In patients with ARDS, platelet aggregation and agglutination were decreased during NO breathing at doses between 1 and 100 ppm. The effect on platelet function was not dose-dependent, however, and was not associated with any increase of the bleeding time (237).

DELIVERY AND MEASUREMENT

Technical Considerations

Several important safety considerations should be addressed in the design of clinical delivery systems for inhaled NO (67,277,288):

1. *Dependable and safe system*: Inhalation circuits should not compromise oxygenation or ventilation of the patient.

Their function should be thoroughly evaluated in the laboratory prior to their use. The design must insure the accurate delivery of nitric oxide while minimizing levels of NO_2.

2. *Precise and stable NO delivery*: Calibrated, commercially purchased stock tanks of nitric oxide in nitrogen should be used. The NO concentration of the undiluted gas should not exceed 1,000 ppm to decrease the effects of cylinder leakage or inadvertent overdosage.
3. *Administration of the lowest dose of NO which is effective*: Because the toxicity of NO remains uncertain, and NO_2 production is greater at higher NO concentrations, the smallest effective dose of inhaled NO should be sought (26,59).
4. *Continuous NO administration*: Sudden discontinuation of inhaled NO may produce severe arterial desaturation and pulmonary hypertension in some patients (21,84). Breathing circuits capable of delivering inhaled NO should therefore be available to allow manual ventilation of the patient during activities such as tracheal suctioning and transport (54,172,196). Levels of inhaled NO should be reduced slowly.
5. *Minimal NO_2 production:* Concentrations within a breathing circuit will vary with the NO and oxygen concentrations and the residence time of NO within the lungs and breathing circuit (59,179). Because conversion of NO to NO_2 is offset by minimizing the residence time of NO in the inhaled gas mixture, mixing of a stock gas of NO in nitrogen with the carrier gases (usually oxygen and air) should take place immediately before inhalation. Several studies have used large gas collection bags to store and deliver NO mixed with oxygen-containing gases. Such NO-O_2 mixtures produce steadily increasing levels of NO_2 with concomitantly decreasing levels of NO (26). This method of administration is unsuitable for clinical application because it does not allow prolonged breathing of constant levels of NO with minimal levels of NO_2. Soda lime may be useful in removing NO_2 from the breathing circuit (184).
6. *Scavenging of NO- and NO_2-containing gases:* Concerns regarding contamination of the environment with NO and NO_2 and the potential for adverse effects on health care providers working at the bedside are worthwhile. The exposure limit for NO set by the U.S. Occupational Safety and Health Administration (a time-weighted average of 25 ppm for 8 hr in the workplace) is less than the typical inhaled NO dose. In intensive care units and operating rooms which have > 6 air exchanges per hour, ambient NO and NO_2 levels should remain very low. Nevertheless, it is prudent to scavenge exhaust gases from the patient's environment. It should be appreciated that scavenging gases from the exhalation port of a breathing circuit does not eliminate ambient contamination. High-pressure leaks from valves and supply lines and the internal connections of mechanical ventilators and anesthesia machines may still occur.
7. *Monitoring of NO and NO_2*: Nomograms have been developed to estimate the administered dose of NO. Nevertheless, it is important to measure the NO and NO_2 concentrations directly because the blenders used to mix NO, nitrogen, and oxygen are imprecise and it is not possible to accurately estimate the delivered NO_2 concentration. Continuous or intermittent monitoring of NO gas concentrations can be performed easily with commercially available chemiluminescence (58) or electrochemical analyzers (54,172,196,197). Electrochemical measurements of nitrogen dioxide appear inaccurate at concentrations of $\leq$ 1 ppm (172).
8. *Monitoring of blood methemoglobin concentrations*: In addition to monitoring inhaled and ambient NO and NO_2 concentrations, blood methemoglobin concentrations should be measured regularly in each patient receiving inhaled nitric oxide.

Techniques for NO Delivery During Mechanical Ventilation

Adult Mechanical Ventilation

The most simple method to deliver NO into a breathing circuit is to continuously administer NO into the inspiratory limb (Fig. 14) (148,273,283). The average delivered NO concentration can be estimated from the flow rates of NO and the inspiratory flow rate. Most adult mechanical ventilators have gas flow within the inspiratory limb only during the inspiratory phase. With such systems, the inspiratory circuit will fill with NO during exhalation and a high concentration of NO (in a hypoxic mixture with nitrogen) will be delivered to the patient with the beginning of each breath. The delivered NO concentration will also be affected by the inspiratory flow waveform, changes of minute ventilation, and by the site at which NO is introduced into the breathing circuit.

If nitric oxide is introduced into the Y-piece of the circuit (141,207,237,282), the inspiratory limb will not fill with NO during exhalation. Instead, NO will pass out the expiratory limb of the ventilator during exhalation. With this technique, it is not possible to measure the inspired NO concentration; the NO dose can only be approximated by a mathematical calculation. Again, changes of inspiratory flow or minute ventilation will alter the NO concentration.

Nitric oxide has also been administered directly into the endotracheal tube (56). The problems associated with this technique are similar to NO administration via the Y-piece. In addition, if the patient becomes apneic, the anoxic gas mixture (NO in nitrogen) will continue to flow into the trachea and could asphyxiate the patient.

Nitric oxide may be injected into the inspiratory limb of the ventilator circuit only during the inspiratory phase of the ventilator cycle (208–210,232). This has been accomplished by a nebulizer drive mechanism which operates during inspiration. The gas supply to the nebulizer contains the NO required to achieve the desired patient dose after mixing with gas delivered from the ventilator. This method will deliver a constant NO dose only during constant flow ventilation. Because the gas flow from the nebulizer is constant during inspiration, the technique will produce varying concentrations if the inspiratory flow pattern varies (e.g., pressure control ventilation) or if tidal volume is variable (e.g., pressure support ventilation). The advantage of this system is that the residence time of NO in the oxygen-containing gas mixture is reduced and therefore oxidation of NO to NO_2 is minimized.

An alternative to the above techniques is to premix the NO with nitrogen (or air) and introduce the gas mixture proximal to the gas inlet of the ventilator or breathing circuit (21,37,157,179,207,260,265,277). The NO dose is constant throughout inspiration with this technique and is not affected by changes of minute ventilation or inspiratory flow waveform. The generation of NO_2 will be greater, however, in ventilators with large internal volumes (179). The delivered NO dose will also change when the FIO_2 setting on the ventilator is changed. This change can be easily compensated for by adjusting the concentration of NO delivered to the ventilator.

Current mechanical ventilators use microprocessors to set the FIO_2. Microprocessors coupled with precision solenoids could be designed to mix nitrogen, oxygen, and NO to achieve the desired FIO_2 and NO concentration (75). Such systems are not yet available for general use.

Pediatric Mechanical Ventilation

Nitric oxide can be titrated into the inspiratory limb of continuous flow mechanical ventilators such as those used in pedi-

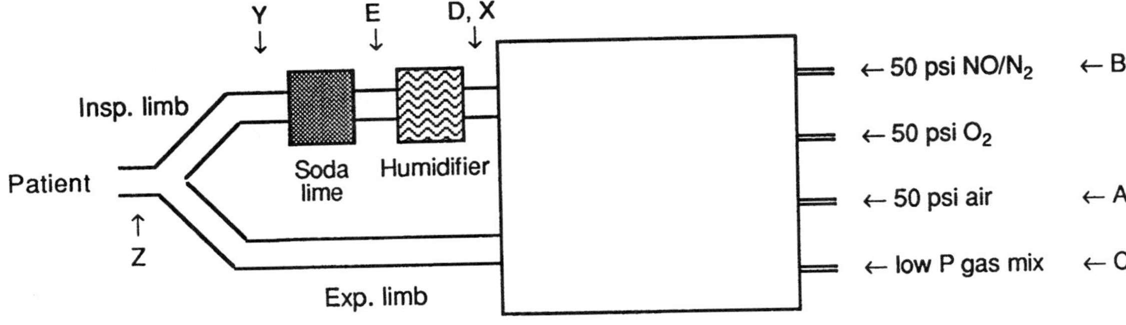

Figure 14. Diagram of systems for administration of NO via an ICU ventilator. Nitric oxide can be administered via the high-pressure air inlet, after mixing with nitrogen or air (*point A*); to the high-pressure accessory port (*point B*) present on ventilators such as the Siemens 300; to a low-pressure gas inlet (*point C*) present on the Siemens 900; or to the inspiratory limb of the ventilator circuit (*point D or E*). Suitable measurement sites are the inspiratory limb before (X) or after (Y) the soda limb canister, if used. Measurement at the Y piece will be accurate only with a very fast-response time analyzer. (Reprinted with permission from ref. 24.)

atrics (including high frequency oscillators) (19,163,250). Ideally, the nitric oxide should be administered near the outlet of the ventilator to permit adequate mixing of gases prior to inhalation by the patient. The administered NO concentration can be approximated by the formula:

$$[\text{NO}]_{\text{administered}} = (\text{NO flow} \cdot [\text{NO}]_{\text{source}}) \div (\text{NO flow} + \text{ventilator flow})$$

Once the NO concentration is established, the dose should remain constant provided that the total flow through the system is not changed. The generation of NO_2 is low because the residence time of NO within such systems is brief. The F_{IO_2} should be analyzed distal to the point at which the nitric oxide is introduced into the breathing system.

Manual Ventilators

For manual ventilators such as ambu bags, nitric oxide can be mixed with oxygen and administered into the gas inlet port of the ventilator (19). The delivered NO concentration can be approximated by the formula:

$$[\text{NO}]_{\text{administered}} = (\text{NO flow} \cdot [\text{NO}]_{\text{source}}) \div (\text{NO flow} + O_2 \text{ flow})$$

With such systems, the delivered NO concentration will change inversely with minute ventilation if the flow into the manual ventilator is less than the patient's minute ventilation. If the ventilator is not continuously flushed, the NO_2 concentration within the ventilator will increase, and high levels of NO_2 may be attained. Because such system are used only briefly, exhaled gases are usually not scavenged.

Spontaneous Ventilation

Several systems for the delivery of NO to spontaneously breathing patients have been described. A high-flow system and a tight-fitting mask have been used for brief exposures (225,243,277). Reservoir bags should be avoided with such systems because of the increased generation of NO_2 within the bag. The approximate delivered NO concentration can be estimated from the formulas described above. Exhaled gases can be easily scavenged.

Inhaled NO has also been administered by transtracheal O_2 catheters (252) or nasal cannulas (93). With such systems, however, the delivered dose varies widely with the ventilatory pattern of the patient and cannot be accurately analyzed. Scavenging of exhaled gases is difficult or impossible.

Anesthesia Machines

A standard anesthesia circuit permits gas mixing at only three sites and monitoring at two sites (Fig. 15). The possible mixing sites are at the flowmeter bank, the fresh gas flow outlet, and in the inspiratory limb of the circuit. Constant flow rates of NO into the inspiratory limb of the circuit produce very wide and unpredictable variations of NO concentration because of the varying cyclic flow and mixing within the circuit. Administration of NO at the flowmeter bank or the fresh gas outlet produces more stable concentrations (85). Because of recirculation of gas within the circle system, it is prudent to maintain high fresh gas flow rates to reduce NO_2 concentrations and to minimize errors in gas mixing. The corrosive effects of NO passing through vaporizers and other components of the anesthesia machine are unclear.

Measurement of NO and NO_2 Concentrations

Chemiluminescence Monitors

Chemiluminescence techniques for the measurement of NO and NO_2 concentrations are well described for industrial and environmental monitoring (22,58). These techniques have been adapted for biomedical use. With these methods, the sample gas reacts with O_3^- to produce activated NO_2^*:

$$NO + O_3^- \rightarrow NO_2^* + O_2$$

To ensure that the production of NO_2^* is dependent only on the concentration of NO, ozone is injected into the reaction chamber at a high constant rate to achieve concentrations which exceed the concentration of NO by several orders of magnitude. NO_2^* reverts to the ground state by emitting electromagnetic radiation:

$$NO_2^* \rightarrow NO_2 + h\nu$$

This emitted radiation has a maximum of 1200 nm and is detected by a photomultiplier tube.

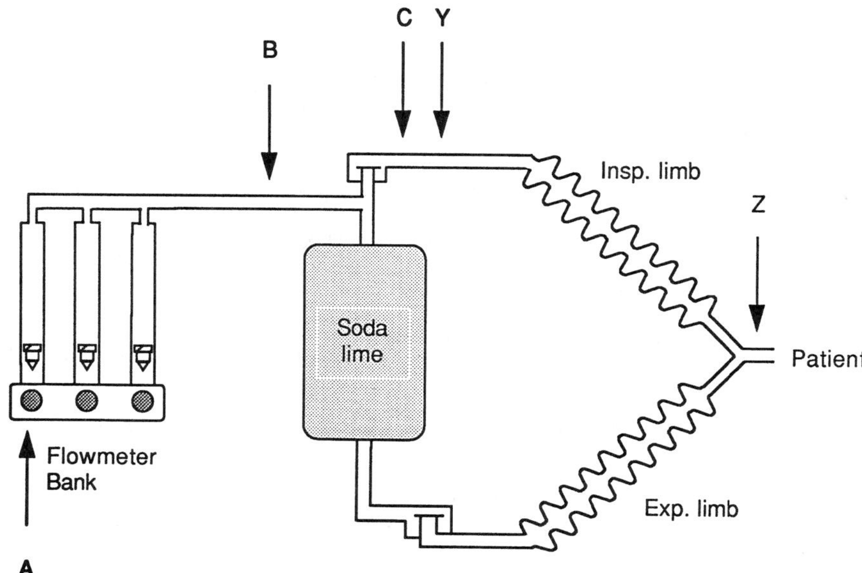

Figure 15. Diagram of systems for administration of NO via an anesthesia machine. *Points A–C* are possible points of NO delivery. *Points Y and Z* are possible points for NO and NO_2 measurement. Measurement of NO at *point Y* is constrained by the distance from the point of NO insertion (*point C* should not be used). Measurement of NO at *point Z* yields a time-weighted average of inspired and expired gas (with a slow-response analyzer) with falsely low inspired NO concentration values. (Reprinted with permission from ref. 24.)

To measure NO_2, it is first converted to NO in a thermal converter (325°C) containing molybdenum (Mo):

$$3\ NO_2 + Mo \rightarrow NO + MoO_3$$

The sum of the nitric oxide concentration measured with and without the converter is referred to as the NO_x. Most chemiluminescence analyzers measure NO and NO_x simultaneously and display [NO], [NO_2], and [NO_x]. Quenching of the emitted photons is a potential problem (81,154,162,286). Quenching occurs when some of the NO_2^* produced by ozonation of NO reverts to the ground state by reacting with other molecules (e.g., O_2, N_2, H_2O, CO_2). The greater the concentration of these molecules, the lower will be the chemiluminescence. The effects of quenching can be corrected mathematically or avoided by calibrating the analyzer with the same concentration of gases that will be present in the analyzed sample. Otherwise, the NO and NO_x values will be falsely low. Chemiluminescence analyzers, while accurate and precise, are large, expensive, and cumbersome to use.

Electrochemical Monitors

Nitric oxide and nitrogen dioxide concentrations may also be measured by electrochemical techniques. Electrochemical analyzers generate a potential difference from reactions of NO or NO_2 within an electrolyte (24). This resulting current is proportional to the NO or NO_2 concentration of the sample. Electrochemical cells have been specifically designed for biomedical use. They are small, portable, rugged, and less expensive than chemiluminescence analyzers and generally suitable for clinical use (54,160,172,196,197,203). The cells are affected by humidity and are pressure sensitive. The severity of these problems may be reduced by sampling the gas prior to humidification and by using sidestream sampling techniques. Current electrochemical analyzers for measuring NO_2 may be inaccurate at low concentrations (<1 ppm) (172).

Sampling Sites for Measurement of NO and NO_2

Most chemiluminescence and electrochemical analyzers have slow response times and provide time-weighed average measurements of NO and NO_2 concentrations (94,180). Rapid fluctuations of NO or NO_2 concentrations will not be detected by such methods. Measurement of the NO and NO_2 concentrations within the inspiratory limb of the ventilator circuit accurately reflects the NO concentration delivered to the lungs. The NO concentration has also been measured from intratracheal gas samples. The values derived from such samples are affected by changes of exhaled NO concentrations and by the ventilatory pattern (94). Chemiluminescence analyzers with faster response times are becoming available (148).

CONCLUSION

Nitric oxide inhalation has been used to successfully treat pulmonary hypertension and hypoxemia in thousands of patients worldwide since its clinical introduction in 1991. The intense interest in inhaled nitric oxide is indicative of the great need for simple and effective therapies for these critically ill patients. The clinical utility of inhaled NO therapy is being currently evaluated in prospective randomized clinical trials. As we understand why and how inhaled nitric oxide works, and why it is sometimes ineffective, we will greatly expand our knowledge of the physiology and pathophysiology of the pulmonary circulation in acute and chronic lung diseases of newborns, children, and adults.

REFERENCES

1. Abman SH, Griebel JL, Parker DK, Schmidt JM, Swanton D, Kinsella JP. Acute effects of inhaled nitric oxide in children with severe hypoxemic respiratory failure. *J Pediatr* 1994;124:881–888.
2. Adatia I, Lillehei C, Arnold JH, et al. Inhaled nitric oxide in the treatment of postoperative graft dysfunction after lung transplantation. *Ann Thorac Surg* 1994;57:1311–1318.
3. Adatia I, Perry S, Landzberg M, Moore P, Thompson JE, Wessel DL. Inhaled nitric oxide and hemodynamic evaluation of patients with pulmonary hypertension before transplantation. *J Am Coll Cardiol* 1995;25:1656–1664.
4. Adatia I, Thompson J, Landzberg M, Wessel DL. Inhaled nitric oxide in chronic obstructive lung disease. *Lancet* 1993;341:307–308.
5. Adia A, Miyamoto K, Saito S, et al. Effects of temperature and humidity on the stability of nitric oxide, and efficiency of soda lime as a selective absorber of nitrogen dioxide. *Jpn J Thorac Dis* 1995;33: 306–311.
6. Airco. *Material safety data sheet: nitric oxide in nitrogen.* Airco, 1993.
7. Alberts WM. Indoor air pollution: NO, NO_2, CO, and CO_2. *J Allergy Clin Immunol* 1994;94:524–526.
8. Alving K, Weitzberg E, Lundberg JM. Increased amount of nitric oxide in exhaled air of asthmatics. *Eur Respir J* 1993;6:1368–1370.
9. Assreuy J, Cunha FQ, Liew FY, Moncada S. Feedback inhibition of nitric oxide synthase activity by nitric oxide. *Br J Pharmacol* 1993;108: 833–837.
10. Austin AT. The chemistry of higher oxides of nitrogen as related to

the manufacture, storage and administration of nitrous oxide. *Br J Anaesth* 1967;39:345–350.

11. Azoulay E, Lachia L, Blayo MC, Pocidalo JJ. Methemoglobinemia induced by nitric oxide in whole blood. Quantitative relationship. *Toxicol Eur Res* 1978;1:7–12.
12. Barabrà JA, Roger N, Roca J, et al. Inhaled nitric oxide may worsen gas exchange in chronic obstructive pulmonary disease. *Am J Respir Crit Care Med* 1995;151:A727.
13. Bassenge E. Antiplatelet effects of endothelium-derived relaxing factor and nitric oxide donors. *Eur Heart J* 1991;12:12–15.
14. Beghetti M, Habre W, Friedli B, Berner M. Continuous low dose inhaled nitric oxide for treatment of severe pulmonary hypertension after cardiac surgery in paediatric patients. *Br Heart J* 1995;73: 65–68.
15. Benzing A, Bräutigam P, Geiger K, Loop T, Beyer U, Moser E. Inhaled nitric oxide reduces pulmonary transvascular albumin flux in patients with acute lung injury. *Anesthesiology* 1995;83:1153–1161.
16. Benzing A, Geiger K. Inhaled nitric oxide lowers pulmonary capillary pressure and changes longitudinal distribution of pulmonary vascular resistance in patients with acute lung injury. *Acta Anaesthesiol Scand* 1994;38:640–645.
17. Berger JI, Gibson RL, Redding GJ, Standaert TA, Clarke WR, Truog WE. Effect of inhaled nitric oxide during Group B Streptococcal sepsis in piglets. *Am Rev Respir Dis* 1993;147:1080–1086.
18. Berner M, Beghetti M, Ricou B, Rouge JC, Pretre R, Friedli B. Relief of severe pulmonary hypertension after closure of a large ventricular septal defect using low dose inhaled nitric oxide. *Intensive Care Med* 1993;19:75–77.
19. Betit P, Adatia I, Benjamin P, Thompson JE, Wessel DL. Inhaled nitric oxide: evaluation of a continuous titration delivery technique for infant mechanical and manual ventilation. *Respir Care* 1995;40: 706–715.
20. Beutler E. Methemoglobinemia and sulfhemoglobinemia. In: Williams WJ, Beutler E, Erslev AJ, Rundles RW, eds. *Hematology.* 2nd ed. New York: McGraw-Hill, 1977:491–494.
21. Bigatello LM, Hurford WE, Kacmarek RM, Roberts JD Jr, Zapol WM. Prolonged inhalation of low concentrations of nitric oxide in patients with severe adult respiratory distress syndrome. Effects on pulmonary hemodynamics and oxygenation. *Anesthesiology* 1994;80: 761–770.
22. Black F, Sigsby J. Chemiluminescent method for NO and NO_x (NO-NO_2) analysis. *Environ Sci Technol* 1974;8:149–152.
23. Bocchi EA, Bacal F, Auler Junior JO, Carmone MJ, Bellotti G, Pileggi F. Inhaled nitric oxide leading to pulmonary edema in stable severe heart failure. *Am J Cardiol* 1994;74:70–72.
24. Body SC, Hartigan PM, Shernan SK, Formanek V, Hurford WE. Nitric oxide: delivery, measurement, and clinical application. *J Cardiothorac Vasc Anesth* 1995;9:748–763.
25. Borland CDR, Harmes K, Cracknell N, et al. Methaemoglobin levels in smokers and non-smokers. *Arch Environ Health* 1985;40: 330–333.
26. Bouchet M, Renaudin MH, Raveau C, Mercier JC, Dehan M, Zupan V. Safety requirement for use of inhaled nitric oxide in neonates. *Lancet* 1993;341:968–969.
27. Boughton SN, Deakin AM, Whittle BJ. Actions of nitric oxide on the acute gastrointestinal damage induced by PAF in the rat. *Ann NY Acad Sci* 1992;664:126–139.
28. Braker W, Mossman A. *Matheson gas data book.* 6th ed. Lundhurst: Matheson, 1980:514–521.
29. Braner DAV, Fineman JR, Chang R, Soifer SJ. M&B 22948, a cGMP phosphodiesterase inhibitor, is a pulmonary vasodilator in lambs. *Am J Physiol* 1993;264:H252–H258.
30. Brown RH, Zerhouni EA, Hirshman CA. Reversal of bronchoconstriction by inhaled nitric oxide. Histamine versus methacholine. *Am J Respir Crit Care Med* 1994;150:233–237.
31. Buga GM, Griscavage JM, Rogers NE, Ignarro LJ. Negative feedback regulation of endothelial cell function by nitric oxide. *Circ Res* 1993;73:808–812.
32. Bunn HF. Disorders of hemoglobin. In: Wilson JD, Braunwald E, Isselbacher KJ, et al., eds. *Principles of Internal Medicine, vol. 2.* 12th ed. New York: McGraw-Hill, 1991:1543–1552.
33. Bylin G, Hedenstierna G, Lindvall T, Sundin B. Ambient nitrogen dioxide concentrations increase bronchial responsiveness in subjects with mild asthma. *Eur Respir J* 1988;1:606–612.
34. Celermajer DS, Dollery C, Burch M, Deanfield JE. Role of endothelium in the maintenance of low pulmonary vascular tone in normal children. *Circulation* 1994;89:2041–2044.
35. Centers for Disease Control. Recommendations for occupational safety and health standard. *MM WR* 1988;37 (Suppl) S–7:21.
36. Channick RN, Hoch RC, Newhart JW, Johnson FW, Smith CM. Improvement in pulmonary hypertension and hypoxemia during nitric oxide inhalation in a patient with end-stage pulmonary fibrosis. *Am J Respir Crit Care Med* 1994;149:811–814.
37. Channick RN, Newhart JW, Johnson FW, Moser KM. Inhaled nitric oxide reverses hypoxic pulmonary vasoconstriction in dogs. A practical nitric oxide delivery and monitoring system. *Chest* 1994;105:1842–1847.
38. Clancy RM, Leszynska-Piziak J, Abramson SB. Nitric oxide, an endothelial cell relaxation factor, inhibits neutrophil superoxide anion production via a direct action on the NADPH oxidase. *J Clin Invest* 1992;90:1116–1121.
39. Clutton-Brock J. Two cases of poisoning by contamination of nitrous oxide with the higher oxides of nitrogen during anaesthesia. *Br J Anaesth* 1969;39:345–350.
40. Cremona G, Dinh Xuan AT, Higenbottam TW. Endothelium-derived relaxing factor and the pulmonary circulation. *Lung* 1991;169:185–202.
41. Curran RD, Mavroudis C, Backer CL, Sautel S, Zaples VR, Wessel DL. Inhaled nitric oxide for children with congenital heart disease and pulmonary hypertension. *Ann Thorac Surg* 1995;60: 1765–1771.
42. Curry S. Methemoglobinemia. *Ann Emerg Med* 1982;11:214–221.
43. Dahm P, Blomquist S, Martensson L, Thorne J, Zoucas E. Circulatory and ventilatory effects of intermittent nitric oxide inhalation during porcine endotoxemia. *J Trauma* 1994;37:769–777.
44. Day RW, Lynch JM, Shaddy RE, Orsmond GS. Pulmonary vasodilatory effects of 12 and 60 parts per million inhaled nitric oxide in children with ventricular septal defect. *Am J Cardiol* 1995; 75:196–198.
45. Dellinger RP, Zimmerman JL, Hyers TM, et al. Inhaled nitric oxide in ARDS: preliminary results of a multicenter clinical trial. *Crit Care Med* 1996;24:A29.
46. DeMarco V, Skimming J, Ellis TM, Cassin S. Nitric oxide inhalation: effects on the ovine neonatal pulmonary and systemic circulations. *Chest* 1994;105:91S–92S.
47. Dent G, Magnussen H, Rabe KF. Cyclic nucleotide phosphodiesterases in the human lung. *Lung* 1994;172:129–146.
48. Dinh Xuan AT, Higenbottam TW, Clelland C, et al. Impairment of pulmonary endothelium-dependent relaxation in patients with Eisenmenger's syndrome. *Br J Pharmacol* 1990;99:9–10.
49. Dinh Xuan AT, Higenbottam TW, Clelland C, et al. Impairment of endothelium-dependent pulmonary artery relaxation in chronic obstructive lung disease. *N Engl J Med* 1991;324:1539–1547.
50. Doyle MP, Pickering RA, DeWeert TM, Hoekstra JW, Pater D. Kinetics and mechanism of the oxidation of human deoxyhemoglobin by nitrites. *J Biol Chem* 1981;256:12393–12398.
51. Dupuy PM, Shore SA, Drazen JM, Frostell C, Hill WA, Zapol WM. Bronchodilator action of inhaled nitric oxide in guinea pigs. *J Clin Invest* 1992;90:421–428.
52. Dupuy PM, Shore SA, Kim SA, Drazen JM, Zapol WM. Inhaled nitric oxide causes bronchodilation in histamine, leukotriene D4, or neurokinin A constricted guinea pigs. *Am J Respir Crit Care Med* (in press).
53. Etches PC, Finer NN, Barrington KJ, Graham AJ, Chan WK. Nitric oxide reverses acute hypoxic pulmonary hypertension in the newborn piglet. *Pediatr Res* 1994;35:15–19.
54. Etches PC, Harris ML, McKinley R, Finer NN. Clinical monitoring of inhaled nitric oxide: comparison of chemiluminescent and electrochemical sensors. *Biomed Instrum Technol* 1995;29: 134–140.
55. Evans MJ, Stephens RJ, Cabral LJ, Freeman G. Cell renewal in the lungs of rats exposed to low levels of NO_2. *Arch Environ Health* 1972;24:180–188.
56. Fierobe L, Brunet F, Dhainaut JF, et al. Effect of inhaled nitric oxide on right ventricular function in adult respiratory distress syndrome. *Am J Respir Crit Care Med* 1995;151:1414–1419.
57. Finer NN, Etches PC, Kamstra B, Tierney AJ, Peliowski A, Ryan CA. Inhaled nitric oxide in infants referred for extracorporeal membrane oxygenation: dose response. *J Pediatr* 1994;124: 302–308.
58. Fontijin A, Sabadell AJ, Ronco RJ. Homogeneous chemiluminescent measurement of nitric oxide and ozone. Implications for continuous selective monitoring of gaseous air pollutants. *Anal Chem* 1970;42:575–579.

59. Foubert L, Fleming B, Latimer R, et al. Safety guidelines for use of nitric oxide. *Lancet* 1992;339:1615–1616.
60. Frampton MW, Morrow PE, Cox C, Gibb R, Speers DM, Utell MJ. Effects of nitrogen dioxide exposure on pulmonary function and airway reactivity in normal humans. *Am Rev Respir Dis* 1991; 143:522–527.
61. Francis SH, Corbin JD. Purification of cGMP-binding protein phosphodiesterase from rat lung. *Methods Enzymol* 1988;159:722–729.
62. Fratacci MD, Frostell CG, Chen TY, Wain JC Jr, Robinson DR, Zapol WM. Inhaled nitric oxide. A selective pulmonary vasodilator of heparin-protamine vasoconstriction in sheep. *Anesthesiology* 1991;75:990–999.
63. Freden F, Wei SZ, Berglund JE, Frostell C, Hedenstierna G. Nitric oxide modulation of pulmonary blood flow distribution in lobar hypoxia. 1995;82:1216–1225.
64. Freeman B. Free radical chemistry of nitric oxide: looking at the dark side. *Chest* 1994;105:79S–84S.
65. Freeman G, Crane SC, Furiosi NJ, Stephens RJ, Evans MJ, Moore WD. Covert reduction in ventilatory surface in rats during prolonged exposure to subacute nitrogen dioxide. *Am Rev Respir Dis* 1972;106:563–579.
66. Fritts AW, Harris P, Clauss H, et al. The effect of acetylcholine on the human pulmonary circulation under normal and hypoxic condition. *J Clin Invest* 1958;37:99–108.
67. Frostell C. Nitric oxide inhalation—future drug or an invitation to disaster? *Paediatr Anaesth* 1994;4:147–150.
68. Frostell C, Fratacci MD, Wain JC, Jones R, Zapol WM. Inhaled nitric oxide. A selective pulmonary vasodilator reversing hypoxic pulmonary vasoconstriction. *Circulation* 1991;83:2038–2047.
69. Frostell CG, Blomqvist H, Hedenstierna G, Lundberg J, Zapol WM. Inhaled nitric oxide selectively reverses human hypoxic pulmonary vasoconstriction without causing systemic vasodilation. *Anesthesiology* 1993;78:427–435.
70. Garat C, Adnot S, Reyaiguia S, Meignan M, Jayr C. Effect of inhaled nitric oxide on 100% oxygen induced lung injury in rats. *Anesthesiology* 1994;81:A1454.
71. Garat C, Adnot S, Rezaiguia S, Kouyoumdjian C, Meignan M, Jayr C. Effect of inhaled NO or treatment with L-NAME on 100% oxygen induced lung injury in rats. *Am J Respir Crit Care Med* 1995;151:A757.
72. Gaston B, Drazen JM, Loscalzo J, Stamler JS. The biology of nitrogen oxides in the airway. *Am J Respir Crit Care Med* 1994;149: 538–551.
73. Gatecel C, Mebazaa A, Kong R, et al. Inhaled nitric oxide improves hepatic tissue oxygenation in right ventricular failure: value of hepatic venous oxygen saturation monitoring. *Anesthesiology* 1995;82:588–590.
74. Gerlach H, Pappert D, Lewandowski K, Rossaint R, Falke KJ. Long-term inhalation with evaluated low doses of nitric oxide for selective improvement of oxygenation in patients with adult respiratory distress syndrome. *Intensive Care Med* 1993;19:443–449.
75. Gerlach H, Rossaint R, Pappert D, Falke KJ. Time-course and dose-response of nitric oxide inhalation for systemic oxygenation and pulmonary hypertension in patients with adult respiratory distress syndrome. *Eur J Clin Invest* 1993;23:499–502.
76. Gerlach H, Rossaint R, Pappert D, Knorr M, Falke KJ. Autoinhalation of nitric oxide after endogenous synthesis in nasopharynx. *Lancet* 1994;343:518–519.
77. Giaid A, Saleh D. Reduced expression of endothelial nitric oxide synthase in the lungs of patients with pulmonary hypertension. *N Engl J Med* 1995;333:214–221.
78. Gibson QH, Roughton FJW. The kinetics and equilibria of the reactions of nitric oxide with sheep haemoglobin. *J Physiol (Lond)* 1957;136:507–526.
79. Glasson WA, Tuesday CS. The atmospheric thermal oxidation of nitric oxide. *J Am Chem Soc* 1963;85:2901–2904.
80. Goldman AP, Delius RE, Deanfield JE, Macrae DJ. Nitric oxide is superior to prostacyclin for pulmonary hypertension after cardiac operations. *Ann Thorac Surg* 1995;60:300–306.
81. Goldman OI, Celermajer DS, Deanfield JE, Macrae DJ. Nitrogen dioxide measurement in breathing systems. *Lancet* 1994;343:850.
82. Greenbaum R, Bay J, Hargreaves MD, et al. Effects of higher oxides of nitrogen on the anesthetized dog. *Br J Anaesth* 1967;39: 393-404.
83. Griscavage JM, Rogers NE, Sherman MP, Ignarro LJ. Inducible nitric oxide synthase from rat alveolar macrophage cell line is inhibited by nitric oxide. *J Immunol* 1993;151:6329–6337.
84. Grover R, Murdoch I, Smithies M, Mitchell I, Bihari D. Nitric oxide during hand ventilation in patient with acute respiratory failure. *Lancet* 1992;340:1038–1039.
85. Grubb W, Putensen C, Thrush D, Räsänen N. Can nitric oxide be administered accurately with a semiclosed anesthesia circuit? *Anesthesiology* 1994;81:A574.
86. Gruetter CA, Barry BK, McNamara DB, Gruetter DY, Kadowitz PJ, Ignarro LJ. Relaxation of bovine coronary artery and activiation of coronary arterial guanylate cyclase by nitric oxde, nitroprusside and a carcinogenic nitrosoamine. *J Cyclic Nucleotide Res* 1979; 5:211–224.
87. Gruetter CA, Gruetter DY, Lyon JE, Kadowitz PJ, Ignaro LJ. Relationship between cyclic 3′:58-monophosphate formation and relaxation of coronary arterial smooth muscle by glyceryl trinitrate, nitroprusside, nitrite and nitric oxide: effects of methylene bue and methemoglobin. *J Pharmacol Exp Ther* 1981;219:181–186.
88. Guidot DM, Repine MJ, Hybertson BM, Repine JE. Inhaled nitric oxide prevents neutrophil-mediated, oxygen radical-dependent leak in isolated rat lungs. *Am J Physiol* 1995;269:L2–L5.
89. Gustafsson LE, Leone AM, Persson MG, et al. Endogenous nitric oxide is present in the exhaled air of rabbits, guinea pigs and humans. *Biochem Biophys Res Commun* 1991;181:852–857.
90. Harris AL, Lemp BM, Bentley RG, Perrone MH, Hamel LT, Silver PJ. Phosphodiesterase isozyme inhibition and the potentiation by Zaprinast of endothelium-derived relaxing factor and guanylate cyclase stimulating agents in vascular smooth muscle. *J Pharmacol Exp Ther* 1989;249:394–400.
91. Hassoun PM, Yu FS, Zulueta JJ, White AC, Lanzillo JJ. Effect of nitric oxide and cell redox status on the regulation of endothelial cell xanthine dehydrogenase. *Am J Physiol* 1995;268: L809–L817.
92. Haydar A, Malhere T, Mauriat P, et al. Inhaled nitric oxide for postoperative pulmonary hypertension in patients with congenital heart defects. *Lancet* 1992;340:1545.
93. Hess D, Kacmarek R, Imanaka H, Bigatello L, Hurford W. Administration of inhaled nitric oxide by nasal cannula. *Am J Respir Crit Care Med* 1995;151:A44.
94. Hess D, Kacmarek RM, Hurford WE. Inspired versus tracheal [NO]. *Respir Care* 1995;40.
95. Hibbs JB, Taintor RR, Vavrin Z, Rachlin EM. Nitric oxide: a cytotoxic activated macrophage effector molecule. *Biochem Biophys Res Commun* 1988;157:87–94.
96. Hill G, Ruggeroli A, Pohorecki R, Alonso A, Robbins R. Cigarette smoking reduces endogenous airway nitric oxide production during cardiopulmonary bypass in humans. *Anesth Analg* 1995;81: 170–172.
97. Högman M, Frostell C, Arnberg H, Hedenstierna G. Inhalation of nitric oxide modulates methacholine-induced bronchoconstriction in the rabbit. *Eur Respir J* 1993;6:177–180.
98. Högman M, Frostell C, Arnberg H, Hedenstierna G. Bleeding time prolongation and NO inhalation. *Lancet* 1993;341:1664–1665.
99. Högman M, Frostell C, Arnberg H, Sandhagen B, Hedenstierna G. Prolonged bleeding time during nitric oxide inhalation in the rabbit. *Acta Physiol Scand* 1994;151:125–129.
100. Högman M, Wei SZ, Frostell C, Arnberg H, Hedenstierna G. Effects of inhaled nitric oxide on methacholine-induced bronchoconstriction: a concentration response study in rabbits. *Eur Respir J* 1994;7:698–702.
101. Hughes SR, Williams TJ, Brain SD. Evidence that endogenous nitric oxide modulates oedema formation induced by substance P. *Eur J Pharmacol* 1990;191:481–484.
102. Hugod C. Effect of exposure to 43 ppm nitric oxide and 3.6 ppm nitrogen dioxide on rabbit lung. *Int Arch Occup Environ Health* 1979;42:159–167.
103. Husain M, Adrie C, Ichinose F, Kavosi M, Zapol WM. Exhaled nitric oxide as a marker for organic nitrate tolerance. *Circulation* 1994;89:2498–2502.
104. Hutcheson IR, Whittle BJ, Boughton SN. Role of nitric oxide in maintaining vascular integrity in endotoxin-induced acute intestinal damage in the rat. *Eur J Pharmacol* 1990;191:485–488.
105. Ialenti A, Ianaro A, Moncada S, Di RM. Modulation of acute inflammation by endogenous nitric oxide. *Eur J Pharmacol* 1992; 211:177–182.
106. Ichinose F, Adrie C, Hurford WE, Zapol WM. Prolonged pulmonary vasodilator action of inhaled nitric oxide by Zaprinast in awake lambs. *J Appl Physiol* 1995;78:1288–1295.

107. Ichinose F, Hurford WE, Zapol WM. Evaluation of inhaled NO in experimental models of lung injury. In: Zapol WM, Bloch KD, eds. *Nitric oxide and the lung.* New York: Marcel Dekker 1997;251–270.
108. Ignarro L. Biological actions and properties of endothelium-derived nitric oxide formed and released from artery and vein. *Circ Res* 1989;65:1–21.
109. Ignarro LJ, Buga GM, Wood KS, Byrns RE, Chaudhuri G. Endothelium-derived relaxing factor produced and released from artery and vein is nitric oxide. *Proc Natl Acad Sci USA* 1987;84: 9265–9269.
110. Ishibe T, Sato T, Hayashi T, Kato N, Hata T. Absorption of nitrogen dioxide and nitric oxide by soda lime. *Br J Anaesth* 1995;75: 330–333.
111. Iwamoto J, Krasney JA, Morin FC III. Methemoglobin production by nitric oxide in fresh sheep blood. *Respir Physiol* 1994;96: 273–283.
112. Jacob TD, Nakayama DK, Seki I, et al. Hemodynamic effects and metabolic fate of inhaled nitric oxide in hypoxic piglets. *J Appl Physiol* 1994;76:1794–1801.
113. Jolliet P, Thorens JB, Chevrolet JC. Pulmonary vascular reactivity in severe pulmonary hypertension associated with mixed connective tissue disease. *Thorax* 1995;50:96–97.
114. Journois D, Pouard P, Mauriat P, Malhere T, Vouhe P, Safran D. Inhaled nitric oxide as a therapy for pulmonary hypertension after operations for congenital heart defects. *J Thorac Cardiovasc Surg* 1994;107:1129–1135.
115. Kacmarek RM, Ripple R, Cockrill BA, Bloch KJ, Zapol WM, Johnson DC. Inhaled nitric oxide: a bronchodilator in mild asthmatics with methacholine-induced bronchospasm. *Am J Respir Crit Care Med* 1996;153:128–135.
116. Kain ML. Higher oxides of nitrogen in anaesthetic gas circuits. *Br J Anaesth* 1967;39:382–387.
117. Kanner J, Harel S, Granit R. Nitric oxide as an antioxidant. *Arch Biochem Biophys* 1991;289:130–136.
118. Karamanoukian HL, Glick PL, Wilcox DT, Rossman JE, Holm BA, Morin FC III. Pathophysiology of congenital diaphragmatic hernia. VIII: inhaled nitric oxide requires exogenous surfactant therapy in the lamb model of congenital diaphragmatic hernia. *J Pediatr Surg* 1995;30:1–4.
119. Karamanoukian HL, Glick PL, Zayek M, et al. Inhaled nitric oxide in congenital hypoplasia of the lungs due to diaphragmatic hernia or oligohydramnios. *Pediatrics* 1994;94:715–718.
120. Kavanagh BP, Mouchawar A, Goldsmith J, Pearl RG. Effects of inhaled NO and inhibition of endogenous NO synthesis in oxidant-induced acute lung injury. *J Appl Physiol* 1994;76:1324–1329.
121. Kharitonov SA, O'Connor B, Evans DJ, Barnes PJ. Allergen-induced late asthmatic reactions are associated with elevation of exhaled nitric oxide. *Am J Respir Crit Care Med* 1995;151:1894–1899.
122. Kharitonov SA, Wells AU, O'Connor BJ, et al. Elevated levels of exhaled nitric oxide in bronchiectasis. *Am J Respir Crit Care Med* 1995;151:1889–1893.
123. Kharitonov SA, Yates D, Robbins RA, Logan-Sinclair R, Shinebourne EA, Barnes PJ. Increased nitric oxide in exhaled air of asthmatic patients. *Lancet* 1994;343:133–135.
124. Kieler-Jensen N, Ricksten SE, Stenqvist O, et al. Inhaled nitric oxide in the evaluation of heart transplant candidates with elevated pulmonary vascular resistance. *J Heart Lung Transplant* 1994; 13:366–375.
125. Kiff RJ, Moss DW, Moncada S. Effect of nitric oxide gas on the generation of nitric oxide by isolated blood vessels: implications for inhalation therapy. *Br J Pharmacol* 1994;113:496–498.
126. Kinsella JP, Abman SH. Inhalational nitric oxide therapy for persistent pulmonary hypertension of the newborn. *Pediatrics* 1993; 91:997–998.
127. Kinsella JP, Abman SH. Efficacy of inhalational nitric oxide therapy in the clinical management of persistent pulmonary hypertension of the newborn. *Chest* 1994;105:92S–94S.
128. Kinsella JP, Ivy DD, Abman SH. Inhaled nitric oxide improves gas exchange and lowers pulmonary vascular resistance in severe experimental hyaline membrane disease. *Pediatr Res* 1994;36: 402–408.
129. Kinsella JP, Shaffer E, Neish SR, Abman SH. Low-dose inhalational nitric oxide in persistent pulmonary hypertension of the newborn. *Lancet* 1992;340:8819–8820.
130. Klemm P, Thiemermann C, Winkmaier G, Martorana PA, Henning R. Effects of nitric oxide synthase inhibition combined with nitric oxide inhalation in a porcine model of endotoxin shock. *Br J Pharmacol* 1995;224:363–368.
131. Kon K, Maeda N, Shiga T. Effect of nitric oxide on the oxygen transport of human erythrocytes. *J Toxicol Environ Health* 1977;2: 1109–1113.
132. Kooy NW, Royall JA. Agonist-induced peroxynitrite production from endothelial cells. *Arch Biochem Biophysics* 1994;310:352–359.
133. Koppel C, von Wissmann C, Barckow D, et al. Inhaled nitric oxide in advanced paraquat intoxication. *J Toxicol Clin Toxicol* 1994;32: 205–214.
134. Kouyoumdjian C, Adnot S, Levame M, Eddahibi S, Bousbaa H, Raffestin B. Continuous inhalation of nitric oxide protects against development of pulmonary hypertension in chronically hypoxic rats. *J Clin Invest* 1994;94:578–584.
135. Kubes P. Nitric oxide modulates epithelial permeability in the feline small intestine. *Am J Physiol* 1992;262:G1138–G1142.
136. Kubes P, Granger DN. Nitric oxide modulates microvascular permeability. *Am J Physiol* 1992;262:H611–H615.
137. Kubes P, Kanwar S, Niu X-F, et al. Nitric oxide synthesis inhibition induces leukocyte adhesion via superoxide and mast cells. *FASEB J* 1993;7:1293–1299.
138. Kurose I, Kubes P, Wolf R, et al. Inhibition of nitric oxide production. Mechanisms of vascular albumin leakage. *Circ Res* 1993; 73:164–171.
139. Kurose I, Wolf R, Grisham MB, Granger DN. Modulation of ischemia/reperfusion-induced microvascular dysfunction by nitric oxide. *Circ Res* 1994;74:376–382.
140. Kurrek MM, Castillo L, Bloch KD, Tannenbaum SR, Zapol WM. Inhaled nitric oxide does not alter endotoxin-induced nitric oxide synthase activity during rat lung perfusion. *J Appl Physiol* 1995;79:1088–1092.
141. Levy B, Bollaert PE, Bauer P, Nace L, Audibert G, Larcan A. Therapeutic optimization including inhaled nitric oxide in adult respiratory distress syndrome in a polyvalent intensive care unit. *J Trauma* 1995;38:370–374.
142. Lindberg L, Larsson A, Steen S, Olsson SG, Nordstrom L. Nitric oxide gives maximal response after coronary artery bypass surgery. *J Cardiothorac Vasc Anesth* 1994;8:182–187.
143. Lindeborg DM, Kavanagh BP, Van Meurs K, Pearl RG. Inhaled nitric oxide does not alter the longitudinal distribution of pulmonary vascular resistance. *J Appl Physiol* 1995;78:341–348.
144. Lindeman KS, Aryana A, Hirshman CA. Direct effects of inhaled nitric oxide on canine peripheral airways. *J Appl Physiol* 1995;78: 1898–1903.
145. Loh E, Stamler JS, Hare JM, Loscalzo J, Colucci WS. Cardiovascular effects of inhaled nitric oxide in patients with left ventricular dysfunction. *Circulation* 1994;90:2780–2785.
146. Lonnqvist PA, Winberg P, Lundell B, Sellden H, Olsson GL. Inhaled nitric oxide in neonates and children with pulmonary hypertension. *Acta Paediatr* 1994;83:1132–1136.
147. Loscalzo J. Antiplatelet and antithrombotic effect of organic nitrates. *Am J Cardiol* 1992;70:18B–22B.
148. Lu Q, Mourgeon E, Law-Koune JD, et al. Dose-response curves of inhaled nitric oxide with and without intravenous almitrine in nitric oxide-responding patients with acute respiratory distress syndrome. *Anesthesiology* 1995;84:929–943.
149. Lugnier C, Schoeffter P, Bec AL, Strouthou E, Stoclet JC. Selective inhibition of cyclic nucleotide phosphodiesterases of human, bovine and rat aorta. *Biochem Pharmacol* 1986;35:1743–1751.
150. Lundberg JON, Farkas-Szallasi T, Weitzberg E, et al. High nitric oxide production in human paranasal sinuses. *Nat Med* 1995;1: 370–373.
151. Maeda N, Imaizumi K, Kon K, Shiga T. A kinetic study on functional impairment of nitric oxide-exposed rat erythrocytes. *Environ Health Perspect* 1987;73:171–177.
152. Martin W, Furchgott RF, Villani GM, Jothianandan D. Phosphodiesterase inhibitors induce endothelium-dependent relaxation of rat and rabbit aorta by potentiating the effects of spontaneously released endothelium-derived relaxing factor. *J Pharmacol Exp Ther* 1986;237:539–547.
153. Maruyama K, Kobayasi H, Taguchi O, Chikusa H, Muneyuki M. Higher doses of inhaled nitric oxide might be less effective in improving oxygenation in a patient with interstitial pulmonary fibrosis. *Anesth Analg* 1995;81:210–211.
154. Matthews RD, Sawyer RF, Schefer RW. Interferences in chemiluminescent measurement of NO and NO_2 emissions from combustion systems. *Environ Sci Technol* 1977;12:1092–1096.

155. May GR, Crook P, Moore PK, Page CP. The role of nitric oxide as an endogenous regulator of platelet and neutrophil activation within the pulmonary circulation of the rabbit. *Br J Pharmacol* 1991;102:759–763.
156. Mayhan WG. Role of nitric oxide in modulating permeability of hamster cheek pouch in response to adenosine 5′-diphosphate and bradykinin. *Inflammation* 1992;16:295–305.
157. McIntyre R, Moore F, Moore E, Piedalue F, Haenel J, Fullerton D. Inhaled nitric oxide variably improves oxygenation and pulmonary hypertension in patients with acute respiratory distress syndrome. *J Trauma* 1995;39:418–425.
158. McMahon TJ, Ignarro LJ, Kadowitz PJ. Influence of Zaprinast on vascular tone and vasodilator responses in the cat pulmonary vascular bed. *J Appl Physiol* 1993;74:1704–1711.
159. Mellion BT, Ignarro LJ, Ohlstein EH, Pontecorvo EG, Hyman AL, Kadowitz PJ. Evidence for the inhibitory role of guanosine 3858 monophosphate in ADP induced human platelet aggregation in the presence of nitric oxide and related vasodilators. *Blood* 1981; 57:946–955.
160. Mercier J, Zupan V, Deham M, Renaudin M, Bochet M, Raveau C. Device to monitor concentration of inhaled nitric oxide. *Lancet* 1993;342:431–432.
161. Mercier JC, Dehan M. Inhalational nitric oxide (NO) in persistent pulmonary hypertension of the newborn (PPHN). Results of the French multicenter open study. *Am J Respir Crit Care Med* 1994;149: A545.
162. Miller CC. Chemiluminescence analysis and nitrogen dioxide measurement. *Lancet* 1994;343:300–301.
163. Miller OI, Celermajer DS, Deanfield JE, Macrae DJ. Guidelines for the safe administration of inhaled nitric oxide. *Arch Dis Child* 1994;70:F47–F49.
164. Miller OI, Celermajer DS, Deanfield JE, Macrae DJ. Very-low-dose inhaled nitric oxide: a selective pulmonary vasodilator after operations for congenital heart disease. *J Thorac Cardiovasc Surg* 1994; 108:487–494.
165. Miller OI, James J, Elliott MJ. Intraoperative use of inhaled low-dose nitric oxide. *J Thorac Cardiovasc Surg* 1993;105:550–551.
166. Miller OI, Tang SF, Keech A, Celermajer DS. Rebound pulmonary hypertension on withdrawal from inhaled nitric oxide. *Lancet* 1995;346:51–52.
167. Mira JP, Monchi M, Brunet F, Fierobe L, Dhainaut JF, Dinh-Xuan AT. Lack of efficacy of inhaled nitric oxide in ARDS. *Intensive Care Med* 1994;20:532.
168. Miyamoto K, Aida A, Nishimura M, et al. Effects of humidity and temperature on nitrogen dioxide formation from nitric oxide. *Lancet* 1994;343:1099–1100.
169. Moinard J, Manier G, Pillet O, Castaing Y. Effect of inhaled nitric oxide on hemodynamics and VA/Q inequalities in patients with chronic obstructive pulmonary disease. *Am J Respir Crit Care Med* 1994;149:1482–1487.
170. Moncada S, Palmer RMJ, Higgs EA. Nitric oxide: physiology, pathophysiology, and pharmacology. *Pharmacol Rev* 1991;43: 109–142.
171. Morrow PE, Utell MJ, Bauer MA, et al. Pulmonary performance of elderly normal subjects with chronic obstructive pulmonary disease exposed to 0.3 ppm nitrogen dioxide. *Am Rev Respir Dis* 1992; 145:291–300.
172. Moutafis M, Hatahet Z, Castelain MH, Renaudin MH, Monnot A, Fischler M. Validation of a simple method assessing nitric oxide and nitrogen dioxide concentrations. *Intensive Care Med* 1995;21: 537–541.
173. Mulligan MS, Hevel JM, Marletta MA, Ward PA. Tissue injury caused by deposition of immune complexes is L-arginine dependent. *Proc Natl Acad Sci USA* 1991;88:6338–6342.
174. Nathan C, Xie Q-W. Nitric oxide synthase: roles, tolls, and controls. *Cell* 1994;78:915–918.
175. Nelin L, Dolinski S, Morrisey J, Dawson C. The effect of inhaled nitric oxide on survival of rats in oxygen. *Am J Respir Crit Care Med* 1995;151:A757.
176. Nelin LD, Moshin J, Thomas CJ, Sasidharan P, Dawson CA. The effect of inhaled nitric oxide on the pulmonary circulation of the neonatal pig. *Pediatr Res* 1994;35:20–24.
177. Nguyen T, Brunson D, Crespi CL, et al. DNA damage and mutation in human cells exposed to nitric oxide in vitro. *Proc Natl Acad Sci USA* 1992;89:3030–3034.
178. Nicholson CD, Challiss RAJ, Shadid M. Differential modulation of tissue function and therapeutic potential of selective inhibitors of cyclic nucleotide phosphodiesterase isoenzymes. *Trends Pharmacol Sci* 1991;12:19–27.
179. Nishimura M, Hess D, Kacmarek RM, Ritz R, Hurford WE. Nitrogen dioxide production during mechanical ventilation with nitric oxide in adults. Effects of ventilator internal volume, air versus nitrogen dilution, minute ventilation, and inspired oxygen fraction. *Anesthesiology* 1995;82:1246–1254.
180. Nishimura M, Tashiro C, Fujino Y, Imanaka H, Hess D, Kacmarek RM. Response of chemiluminescent analyzers on the measured value of nitric oxide (NO). *Respir Care* 1995;40:1186.
181. Niu XF, Smith W, Kubes P. Intracellular oxidative stress induced by nitric oxide synthesis inhibition increases endothelial cell adhesion to neutrophils. *Circ Res* 1994;74:1133–1140.
182. Norman V, Keith CH. Nitrogen oxides in tobacco smoke. *Nature* 1965;205:915–916.
183. Nozik ES, Huang Y-CT, Piantadosi CA. L-arginine enhances injury in the isolated rabbit lung during hyperoxia. *Respir Physiol* 1995; 100:63–74.
184. Oda H, Kusumoto S, Nakajima T. Nitrosyl-hemoglobin formation in the blood of animals exposed to nitric oxide. *Arch Environ Health* 1975;30:453–456.
185. Oda H, Nogami H, Kusumoto S, et al. Long-term exposure to nitric oxide in mice. *J Jpn Soc Air Pollut* 1976;11:150–160.
186. Ogura H, Cioffi WG Jr, Jordan BS, et al. The effect of inhaled nitric oxide on smoke inhalation injury in an ovine model. *J Trauma* 1994;37:294–302.
187. Ogura H, Cioffi WG, Offner PJ, Jordan BS, Johnson AA, Pruitt BA Jr. Effect of inhaled nitric oxide on pulmonary function after sepsis in a swine model. *Surgery* 1994;116:313–321.
188. Okamoto K, Sato T, Kurose M, Kukita I, Fujii H, Taki K. Successful use of inhaled nitric oxide for treatment of severe hypoxemia in an infant with total anomalous pulmonary venous return. *Anesthesiology* 1994;81:256–259.
189. Palmer RMJ, Ferrige AG, Moncada SA. Nitric oxide release accounts for the biological activity of endothelium-derived relaxing factor. *Nature* 1987;327:524–526.
190. Pappert D, Busch T, Gerlach H, Lewandowski K, Radermacher P, Rossaint R. Aerosolized prostacyclin versus inhaled nitric oxide in children with severe acute respiratory distress syndrome. *Anesthesiology* 1995;82:1507–1511.
191. Payen DM, Gatecel C, Plaisance P. Almitrine effect on nitric oxide inhalation in adult respiratory distress syndrome. *Lancet* 1993;341: 1164.
192. Peliowski A, Finer NN, Etches PC, Tierney AJ, Ryan CA. Inhaled nitric oxide for premature infants after prolonged rupture of the membranes. *J Pediatr* 1995;126:450–453.
193. Pepke-Zaba J, Higenbottam TW, Dinh-Xuan AT, Stone D, Wallwork J. Inhaled nitric oxide as a cause of selective pulmonary vasodilatation in pulmonary hypertension. *Lancet* 1991;338:1173–1174.
194. Persson M, Lonnqvist P, Gustafsson L. Positive end-expiratory pressure ventilation elicits increases in endogenously formed nitric oxide as detected in air exhaled from rabbits. *Anesthesiology* 1995;82:969–974.
195. Persson M, Zetterstrom O, Agrenius V, Ihre E, Gustafsson L. Single-breath nitric oxide measurements in asthmatic patients and smokers. *Lancet* 1994;343:146–147.
196. Petros AJ, Cox P, Bohn D. A simple method for monitoring the concentration of inhaled nitric oxide. *Anaesthesia* 1994;49: 317–319.
197. Petros AJ, Cox PB, Bohn D. Simple method for monitoring concentration of inhaled nitric oxide. *Lancet* 1992;340:1167.
198. Pickett JA, Moors AH, Latimer RD, Mahmood N, Ghosh S, Oduro A. The role of soda lime during administration of inhaled nitric oxide. *Br J Anaesth* 1994;72:683–685.
199. Pison U, Lopez FA, Heidelmeyer CF, Roissant R, Falke KJ. Inhaled nitric oxide reverses hypoxic pulmonary vasoconstriction without impairing gas exchange. *J Appl Physiol* 1993;74: 1287–1292.
200. Pollock JS, Forstermann U, Mitchell JA, et al. Purification and characterization of particulate endothelium-derived relaxing factor synthase from cultured and native bovine aortic endothelial cells. *Proc Natl Acad Sci USA* 1991;88:10480–10484.
201. Postlethwait EM, Langford SD, Bidani A. Kinetics of NO_2 air space absorption in isolated rat lungs. *J Appl Physiol* 1992;73: 1939–1945.
202. Provost P, Lam JYT, Lacoste L, Merhi Y, Waters D. Endothelium-derived nitric oxide attenuates neutrophil adhesion to endothe-

lium under arterial flow conditions. *Arterioscler Thromb Vasc Biol* 1994;14:331–335.
203. Purtz EP, Hess D, Kacmarek RM. Evaluation of electrochemical nitric oxide analyzers. *Respir Care* 1995;40:1186.
204. Putensen C, Rasanen J, Downs JB. Effect of endogenous and inhaled nitric oxide on the ventilation-perfusion relationships in oleic-acid lung injury. *Am J Respir Crit Care Med* 1994;150: 330–336.
205. Putensen C, Rasanen J, Lopez FA. Improvement in VA/Q distributions during inhalation of nitric oxide in pigs with methacholine-induced bronchoconstriction. *Am J Respir Crit Care Med* 1995;151:116–122.
206. Putensen C, Rasanen J, Lopez FA, Downs JB. Continuous positive airway pressure modulates effect of inhaled nitric oxide on the ventilation-perfusion distributions in canine lung injury. *Chest* 1994;106:1563–1569.
207. Putensen C, Rasanen J, Thomson MS, Braman RS. Method of delivering constant nitric oxide concentrations during full and partial ventilatory support. *J Clin Monit* 1995;11:23–31.
208. Puybasset L, Rouby JJ, Mourgeon E, et al. Factors influencing cardiopulmonary effects of inhaled nitric oxide in acute respiratory failure. *Am J Respir Crit Care Med* 1995;152:318–328.
209. Puybasset L, Rouby JJ, Mourgeon E, et al. Inhaled nitric oxide in acute respiratory failure: dose-response curves. *Intensive Care Med* 1994;20:319–327.
210. Puybasset L, Stewart T, Rouby JJ, et al. Inhaled nitric oxide reverses the increase in pulmonary vascular resistance induced by permissive hypercapnia in patients with acute respiratory distress syndrome. *Anesthesiology* 1994;80:1254–1267.
211. Radermacher P, Rammos S. Low dose inhaled nitric oxide causing selective pulmonary vasodilation in child with idiopathic pulmonary hypertension. *Eur J Pediatr* 1994;153:691–693.
212. Radermacher P, Santak B, Falke KJ. Comparison of prostaglandin E1 and nitroglycerin in patients with ARDS. *Prog Clin Biol Res* 1989;301:267–270.
213. Radermacher P, Santak B, Wust HJ, et al. Prostacyclin and right ventricular function in patients with pulmonary hypertension associated with ARDS. *Intensive Care Med* 1990;16:227–232.
214. Radermacher P, Santak B, Wust HJ, Tarnow J, Falke KJ. Prostacyclin for the treatment of pulmonary hypertension in the adult respiratory distress syndrome: Effects on pulmonary capillary pressure and ventilation-perfusion distributions. *Anesthesiology* 1990;72:238–244.
215. Radomski MW, Moncada S. Regulation of vascular homeostasis by nitric oxide. *Thromb Haemost* 1993;70:36–41.
216. Radomski MW, Palmer RMJ, Moncada S. Endogenous nitric oxide inhibits human platelet adhesion to vascular endothelium. *Lancet* 1987;2:1057–1058.
217. Rasmussen TR, Kjaergaard SK, Tapp U, Pedersen OF. Delayed effects of NO_2 exposure on alveolar permeability and glutathione peroxidase in healthy humans. *Am Rev Respir Dis* 1992; 146:654–659.
218. Rees DD, Cellek S, Palmer RMJ, Moncada S. Dexamethasone prevents the induction by endotoxin of a nitric oxide synthase and the associated effects on vascular tone: An insight into endotoxin shock. *Biochem Biophys Res Commun* 1990;173:541–547.
219. Rengasamy A, Johns RA. Regulation of nitric oxide synthase by nitric oxide. *Mol Pharmacol* 1993;44:124–128.
220. Rich GF, Lowson SM, Johns RA, Daugherty MO, Uncles DR. Inhaled nitric oxide selectively decreases pulmonary vascular resistance without impairing oxygenation during one-lung ventilation in patients undergoing cardiac surgery. *Anesthesiology* 1994;80:57–62.
221. Rich GF, Murphy GD Jr, Roos CM, Johns RA. Inhaled nitric oxide: Selective pulmonary vasodilation in cardiac surgical patients. *Anesthesiology* 1993;78:1028–1035.
222. Rimar S, Gillis CN. Selective pulmonary vasodilation by inhaled nitric oxide is due to hemoglobin inactivation. *Circulation* 1993; 88:2884–2887.
223. Rimar S, Gillis CN. Site of pulmonary vasodilation by inhaled nitric oxide in the perfused lung. *J Appl Physiol* 1995;78: 1745–1749.
224. Roberts JD Jr, Chen TY, Kawai N, et al. Inhaled nitric oxide reverses pulmonary vasoconstriction in the hypoxic and acidotic newborn lamb. *Circ Res* 1993;72:246–254.
225. Roberts JD Jr, Lang P, Bigatello LM, Vlahakes GJ, Zapol WM. Inhaled nitric oxide in congenital heart disease. *Circulation* 1993; 87:447–453.
226. Roberts JD, Polaner DM, Lang P, Zapol WM. Inhaled nitric oxide in persistent pulmonary hypertension of the newborn. *Lancet* 1992;340:818–819.
227. Roberts JD, Roberts CT, Jones RC, Zapol WM. Continuous nitric oxide inhalation reduces pulmonary arterial structural changes, right ventricular hypertrophy, and growth retardation in the hypoxic newborn rat. *Circ Res* 1995;76:215–222.
228. Romand JA, Pinsky MR, Firestone L, Zar HA, Lancaster JR Jr. Effect of inhaled nitric oxide on pulmonary hemodynamics after acute lung injury in dogs. *J Appl Physiol* 1994;76:1356–1362.
229. Romand JA, Pinsky MR, Firestone L, Zar HA, Lancaster JR Jr. Inhaled nitric oxide partially reverses hypoxic pulmonary vasoconstriction in the dog. *J Appl Physiol* 1994;76:1350–1355.
230. Roos CM, Rich GF, Uncles DR, Daugherty MO, Frank DU. Sites of vasodilation by inhaled nitric oxide vs. sodium nitroprusside in endothelin-constricted isolated rat lungs. *J Appl Physiol* 1994; 77:51–57.
231. Rosenberg AA, Kinsella JP, Abman SH. Cerebral hemodynamics and distribution of left ventricular output during inhalation of nitric oxide. *Crit Care Med* 1995;23:1391–1397.
232. Rossaint R, Falke KJ, Lopez F, Slama K, Pison U, Zapol WM. Inhaled nitric oxide for the adult respiratory distress syndrome. *N Engl J Med* 1993;328:399–405.
233. Rossaint R, Gerlach H, Schmidt-Ruhnke H, et al. Efficacy of inhaled nitric oxide in patients with severe ARDS. *Chest* 1995; 107:1107–1115.
234. Rossaint R, Slama K, Steudel W, et al. Effects of inhaled nitric oxide on right ventricular function in severe acute respiratory distress syndrome. *Intensive Care Med* 1995;21:197–203.
235. Rovira I, Chen TY, Winkler M, Kawai N, Bloch KD, Zapol WM. Effects of inhaled nitric oxide on pulmonary hemodynamics and gas exchange in an ovine model of ARDS. *J Appl Physiol* 1994;76: 345–355.
236. Rozé JC, Storme L, Zupan V, Morville P, Dinh-Xuan AT, Mercier JC. Echocardiographic investigation of inhaled nitric oxide in newborn babies with severe hypoxaemia. *Lancet* 1994;344: 303–305.
237. Samama CM, Diaby M, Fellahi JL, et al. Inhibition of platelet aggregation by inhaled nitric oxide in patients with acute respiratory distress syndrome. *Anesthesiology* 1995;83:56–65.
238. Sanna A, Kurtansky A, Veriter C, Stanescu D. Bronchodilator effect of inhaled nitric oxide in healthy men. *Am J Respir Crit Care Med* 1994;150:1702–1704.
239. Schilling J, Holzer P, Guggenbach M, Gyurech D, Marathia K, Geroulanos S. Reduced endogenous nitric oxide in the exhaled air of smokers and hypertensives. *Eur Respir J* 1994;7:467–471.
240. Schmidt HHW, Walter U. Nitric oxide at work. *Cell* 1994;78: 919–925.
241. Schneider F, Lutun P, Hasselmann M, Stoclet JC, Tempé JD. Methylene blue increases systemic vascular resistance in human septic shock. *Intensive Care Med* 1992;18:309–311.
242. Sellden H, Winberg P, Gustafsson LE, Lundell B, Book K, Frostell CG. Inhalation of nitric oxide reduced pulmonary hypertension after cardiac surgery in a 3.2-kg infant. *Anesthesiology* 1993;78: 577–580.
243. Semigran MJ, Cockrill BA, Kacmarek R, et al. Hemodynamic effects of inhaled nitric oxide in heart failure. *J Am Coll Cardiol* 1994;24:982–988.
244. Shah N, Jacob T, Exler R, et al. Inhaled nitric oxide in congenital diaphragmatic hernia. *J Pediatr Surg* 1994;29:1010–1015.
245. Shah NS, Nakayama DK, Jacob TD, et al. Efficacy of inhaled nitric oxide in a porcine model of adult respiratory distress syndrome. *Arch Surg* 1994;129:158–164.
246. Shaw AW, Vosper AJ. Solubility of nitric oxide in aqueous and nonaqueous solvents. *J Chem Soc Faraday Trans* 1977;73:1239–1244.
247. Shiel FOM. Morbid anatomical changes in the lungs of dogs after inhalation of higher oxides of nitrogen during anaesthesia. *Br J Anaesth* 1967;39:413–424.
248. Silver PJ, Hamel LJ, Perrone MH, Bentley RG, Bushover CR, Evans DB. Differential pharmacological sensitivity of cyclic nucleotide phosphodiesterase isozymes isolated from cardiac muscle, arterial and airway smooth muscle. *Eur J Pharmacol* 1988; 150:85–94.
249. Sitbon O, Brenot F, Denjean A, et al. Inhaled nitric oxide as a screening vasodilator agent in primary pulmonary hypertension. A dose-response study and comparison with prostacyclin. *Am J Respir Crit Care Med* 1995;151:384–389.

250. Skimming JW, Cassin S, Blanch PB. Nitric oxide administration using constant-flow ventilation. *Chest* 1995;108:1065–1072.
251. Skimming JW, deMarco VG, Cassin S. The effects of nitric oxide inhalation on the pulmonary circulation of preterm lambs. *Pediatr Res* 1994;37:35–40.
252. Snell GI, Salamonsen RF, Bergin P, Esmore DS, Khan S, Williams TJ. Inhaled nitric oxide used as a bridge to heart-lung transplantation in a patient with end-stage pulmonary hypertension. *Am J Respir Crit Care Med* 1995;151:1263–1266.
253. Snow DJ, Gray SJ, Ghosh S, et al. Inhaled nitric oxide in patients with normal and increased pulmonary vascular resistance after cardiac surgery. *Br J Anaesth* 1994;72:185–189.
254. Souness JE, Brazdil R, Diocee BK, Jordan R. Role of selective cyclic GMP phosphodiesterase inhibition in the myorelaxant actions of M&B 22,948, MY-54445, vinpocetine and 1-methyl-3-isobutyl-8-(methylamino) xanthine. *Br J Pharmacol* 1989;98:725–734.
255. Stamler JS. Redox signaling: nitrosylation and related target interactions of nitric oxide. *Cell* 1994;78:931–936.
256. Stamler JS, Jaraki O, Osborne J, et al. Nitric oxide circulates in mammalian plasma primarily as an S-nitroso adduct of serum albumin. *Proc Natl Acad Sci USA* 1992;89:7674–7677.
257. Stamler JS, Loh E, Roddy M-A, Currie KE, Creager MA. Nitric oxide regulates basal systemic and pulmonary vascular resistance in healthy humans. *Circulation* 1994;89:2035–2040.
258. Stamler JS, Singel DJ, Loscalzo J. Biochemistry of nitric oxide and its redox-activated forms. *Science* 1993;258:1989–1902.
259. Stavert DM, Lehnert BE. Nitric oxide and nitrogen dioxide as inducers of acute pulmonary injury when inhaled at relatively high concentrations for brief periods. *Inhal Toxicol* 1990;2:53–67.
260. Stenqvist O, Kjelltoft B, Lundin S. Evaluation of a new system for ventilatory administration of nitric oxide. *Acta Anaesthesiol Scand* 1993;37:687–691.
261. Stephens RJ, Freeman G, Evans MJ. Early response of lungs to low levels of nitrogen dioxide. *Arch Environ Health* 1972;24:160–179.
262. Stewart T, Valenza F, Ribeiro S, et al. Increased nitric oxide in exhaled gas as an early marker of lung inflammation in a model of sepsis. *Am J Respir Crit Care Med* 1995;151:713–718.
263. Stuehr DJ, Nathan CF. Nitric oxide: a macrophage product responsible for cytostasis and respiratory inhibition in tumor target cells. *J Exp Med* 1989;169:1543–1555.
264. Thompson MW, Bates JN, Klein JM. Treatment of respiratory failure in an infant with bronchopulmonary dysplasia infected with respiratory syncytial virus using inhaled nitric oxide and high frequency ventilation. *Acta Paediatr* 1995;84:100–102.
265. Tibballs J, Hochmann M, Carter B, Osborne A. An appraisal of techniques for administration of gaseous nitric oxide. *Anaesth Intensive Care* 1993;21:844–847.
266. Tod ML, DC OD, Gordon JB. Sites of inhaled NO-induced vasodilation during hypoxia and U-46619 infusion in isolated lamb lungs. *Am J Physiol* 1995;268:H1422–1427.
267. Tonz M, von Segesser LK, Schilling J, et al. Treatment of acute pulmonary hypertension with inhaled nitric oxide. *Ann Thorac Surg* 1994;58:1031–1035.
268. Toothill C. The chemistry of the in-vivo reaction between hemoglobin and various oxides of nitrogen. *Br J Anaesth* 1967;39:405–412.
269. Trapani AJ, Smits GJ, McGraw DE, McMahon EG, Blaine EH. Hemodynamic basis for the depressor activity of Zaprinast, a selective cyclic GMP phosphodiesterase Inhibitor. *J Pharmacol Exp Ther* 1991;258:269–274.
270. Valvini EM, Young JD. Serum nitrogen oxides during nitric oxide inhalation. *Br J Anaesth* 1995;74:338–339.
271. Van Camp JR, Yian C, Lupinetti FM. Regulation of pulmonary vascular resistance by endogenous and exogenous nitric oxide. *Ann Thorac Surg* 1994;58:1025–1030.
272. von Nieding G, Wagner H, Kockeler H. Investigation of the acute effects of nitrogen monoxide on lung function in man. *Staub-Reinhalt Luft* 1975;35:175–178.
273. Watkins DN, Rankin JM, Clarke GM. Inhaled nitric oxide in severe acute respiratory failure—its use in intensive care and description of a delivery system. *Anaesth Intensive Care* 1993;21:861–875.
274. Weber AA, Strobach J, Schror K. Direct inhibition of platelet function by organic nitrates via nitric oxide formation. *Eur J Pharmacol* 1993;247:29–37.
275. Weitzberg E, Rudehill A, Lundberg JM. Nitric oxide inhalation attenuates pulmonary hypertension and improves gas exchange in endotoxin shock. *Eur J Pharmacol* 1993;233:85–94.
276. Wennmalm A, Benthin G, Edlund A, et al. Metabolism and excretion of nitric oxide in humans. An experimental and clinical study. *Circ Res* 1993;73:1121–1127.
277. Wessel DL, Adatia I, Thompson JE, Hickey PR. Delivery and monitoring of inhaled nitric oxide in patients with pulmonary hypertension. *Crit Care Med* 1994;22:930–938.
278. Westfelt UN, Benthin G, Lundin S, Stenqvist O, Wennmalm A. Conversion of inhaled nitric oxide to nitrate in man. *Br J Pharmacol* 1995;114:1621–1624.
279. Williams RA, Rhoades RA, Adams WS. The response of lung tissue and surfactant to nitrogen dioxide exposure. *Arch Intern Med* 1971;128:101–108.
280. Winberg P, Lundell BP, Gustafsson LE. Effect of inhaled nitric oxide on raised pulmonary vascular resistance in children with congenital heart disease. *Br Heart J* 1994;71:282–286.
281. Wink DA, Hanbauer I, Krishna MC, DeGraff W, Gamson J, Mitchell JB. Nitric oxide protects against cellular damage and cytotoxicity from reactive oxygen species. *Proc Natl Acad Sci USA* 1993;90:9813–9817.
282. Wysocki M, Delclaux C, Roupie E, et al. Additive effect on gas exchange of inhaled nitric oxide and intravenous almitrine bismesylate in the adult respiratory distress syndrome. *Intensive Care Med* 1994;20:254–259.
283. Young JD, Brampton WJ, Knighton JD, Finfer SR. Inhaled nitric oxide in acute respiratory failure in adults. *Br J Anaesth* 1994;73:499–502.
284. Young JD, Dyar O, Xiong L, Howell S. Methaemoglobin production in normal adults inhaling low concentrations of nitric oxide. *Intensive Care Med* 1994;20:581–584.
285. Young JD, Dyar OJ, Xiong L, Zhang J, Gavaghan D. Effect of methylene blue on the vasodilator action of inhaled nitric oxide in hypoxic sheep. *Br J Anaesth* 1994;73:511–516.
286. Zableiski MF, Seery DJ, Dodge LG. Influence of mass transport and quenching on nitric oxide chemiluminescent analysis. *Environ Sci Technol* 1984;18:88–92.
287. Zapol WM. Pulmonary circulation during adult respiratory distress syndrome. In: Zapol WM, Falke KJ, eds. *Acute respiratory failure.* New York: Marcel Dekker, 1985:241–270.
288. Zapol WM, Hurford WE. Inhaled nitric oxide in the adult respiratory distress syndrome and other lung diseases. *New Horizons* 1993;1:638–650.
289. Zapol WM, Jones R. Vascular components of ARDS: clinical pulmonary hemodynamics and morphology. *Am Rev Respir Dis* 1987;136:471–474.
290. Zapol WM, Rimar S, Gillis N, Marletta M, Bosken CH. Nitric oxide and the lung. NHLBI workshop summary. *Am J Respir Crit Care Med* 1994;149:1375–1380.
291. Zapol WM, Snider MT. Pulmonary hypertension in severe acute respiratory failure. *N Engl J Med* 1977;296:476–480.
292. Zayek M, Cleveland D, Morin FC III. Treatment of persistent pulmonary hypertension in the newborn lamb by inhaled nitric oxide. *J Pediatrics* 1993;122:743–750.
293. Zayek M, Wild L, Roberts JD, Morin FC III. Effect of nitric oxide on the survival rate and incidence of lung injury in newborn lambs with persistent pulmonary hypertension. *J Pediatr* 1993;123:947–952.
294. Ziegler JW, Ivy DD, Kinsella JP, Clark WR, Abman SH. Dypyridamole, a cGMP phosphodiesterase inhibitor, augments inhaled nitric oxide induced pulmonary vasodilation in the ovine transitional circulation. *Pediatr Res* 1994;90A:527.
295. Zwissler B, Welte M, Messmer K. Effects of inhaled prostacyclin as compared with inhaled nitric oxide on right ventricular performance in hypoxic pulmonary vasoconstriction. *J Cardiothorac Vasc Anesth* 1995;9:283–289.

SUBJECT INDEX

Subject Index

P

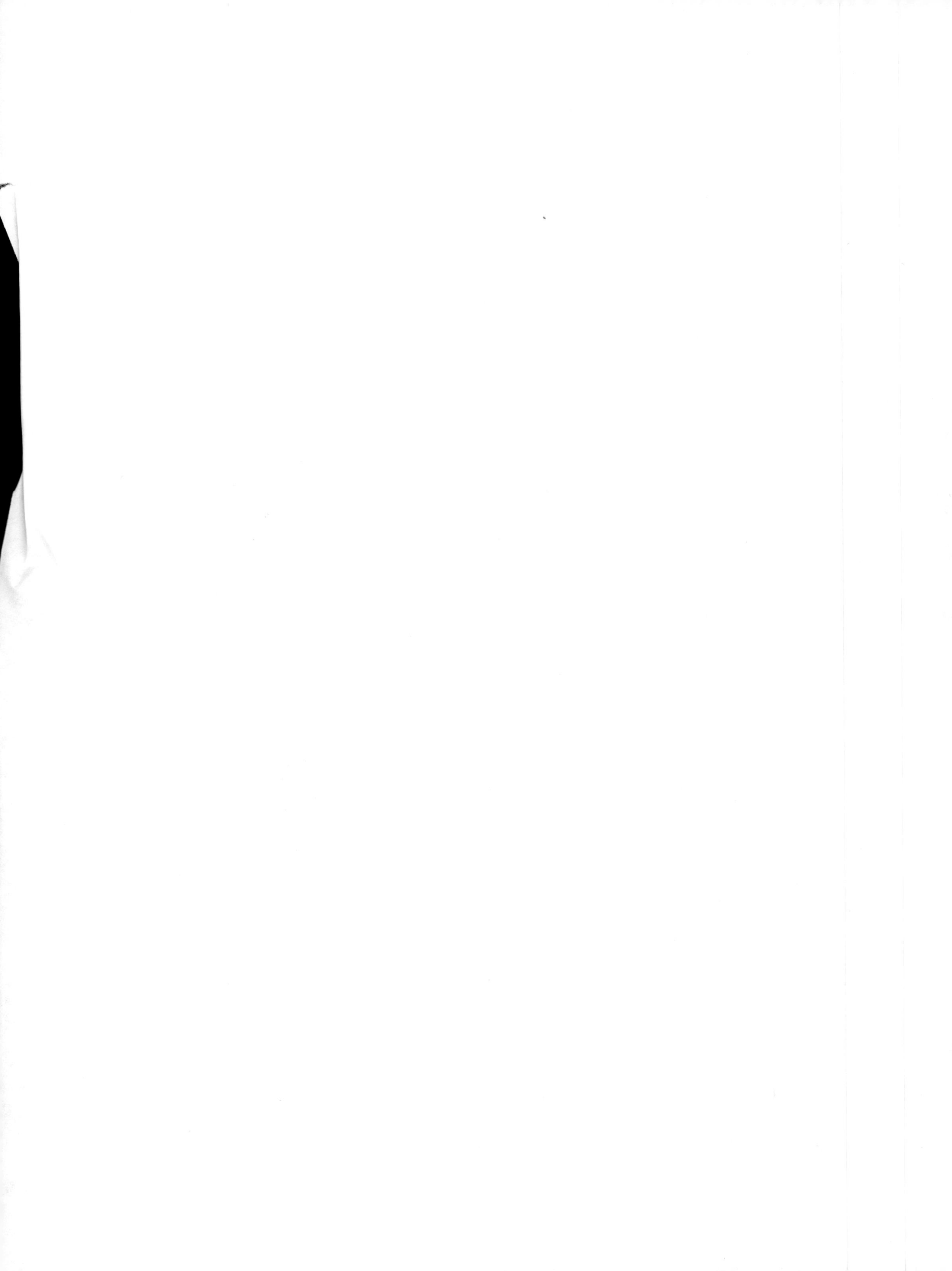